D0151229

PHARMACOTHERAPEUTICS:
A NURSING PROCESS APPROACH
2nd edition

With Special Contributions by:

Carolyn S. Brown, RN, MN, CCRN
Instructor
Louisiana State University Medical Center
School of Nursing
New Orleans, Louisiana

Marilynn E. Doenges, BSN, MA, RN, CS
Clinical Specialist
Adult Psychiatric/Mental Health Nursing
Private Practice
Colorado Springs, Colorado

Steven B. Meisel, PharmD
Assistant Director for Clinical Services
Pharmacy Department
Fairview Southdale Hospital
Minneapolis, Minnesota

Mary Frances Moorhouse, RN, CCP, CCRN, CRRN
Nurse Consultant
TNT-RN Enterprises and Fortis Corporation
Colorado Springs, Colorado

PHARMACOTHERAPEUTICS:
A NURSING PROCESS APPROACH
2nd edition

Merrily Mathewson Kuhn, PhD, RN, CCRN
President, Educational Services, Inc.
Hamburg, New York
Formerly Assistant Professor
Graduate Faculty
State University of New York at Buffalo
Buffalo, New York

 F. A. Davis Company ● **Philadelphia**

Figure 59–3 is copyright © 1989 by Beth Anne Willert and is reproduced with permission.

NOTE: As new scientific information becomes available through basic and clinical research, recommended treatments and drug therapies undergo changes. The author(s) and publisher have done everything possible to make this book accurate, up-to-date, and in accord with accepted standards at the time of publication. However, the reader is advised always to check product information (package inserts) for changes and new information regarding dose and contraindications before administering any drug. Caution is especially urged when using new or infrequently ordered drugs.

Library of Congress Cataloging-in-Publication Data

Mathewson Kuhn, Merrily, 1945–

    Pharmacotherapeutics : a nursing process approach / Merrily
Mathewson Kuhn. — 2nd ed.
      p. cm.
    Includes bibliographical references.
    ISBN 0-8036-5923-7
    1. Chemotherapy. 2. Pharmacology. 3. Nursing. I. Title.
    [DNLM: 1. Drug Therapy—nurses' instruction. 2. Nursing Process.
3. Pharmacology—nurses' instruction. WB 330 M429p]
RM262.M373 1990
615.5′8—dc20
DNLM/DLC
for Library of Congress   89-71422
                                 CIP

Dedication

To Caroline Schneggenburger
for her unending energy in typing and organizing the manuscript;

To my parents, Audrey M. and Norbert J. Kuhn
for their love and encouragement; and

To all my students.

PREFACE TO THE SECOND EDITION

The enthusiastic response of nursing instructors and, especially, their students to the first edition of PHARMACOTHERAPEUTICS: A NURSING PROCESS APPROACH has been both gratifying and challenging. Their praise has confirmed the belief that, by integrating nursing process with pharmacologic principles, the book represented something new—a nursing text on pharmacology rather than a pharmacology text with some nursing content appended to it. As nursing instructors across the country have dropped pharmacology texts that had been standards for many years in favor of PHARMACOTHERAPEUTICS, they have cited as reasons both the scope and depth of the book's nursing content, organized by the nursing process, and the quality of the book's pharmacologic coverage, made even more accessible by the extensive use of tables to summarize drug information.

The challenge, then, in preparing the second edition has been to build on the strengths of the first edition, by expanding upon and refining the book's innovative nursing-based approach while also updating and amplifying its pharmacologic content. The suggestions of instructors and students committed to the book's nursing process approach to pharmacology have been of immeasurable value in the development of this new edition, which has been improved both in its nursing and its pharmacologic content as well as in its pedagogic features.

High on the list of improvements to the nursing content is the revision of the book's nursing process tables. These tables—prepared for this edition by Marilynn Doenges and Mary Moorhouse, the authors of NURSING CARE PLANS: GUIDELINES FOR PLANNING PATIENT CARE, 2nd ed.—now include assessment parameters, nursing diagnoses (which use NANDA terminology exclusively), nursing actions with rationales, and desired outcomes/evaluation criteria. The changes to these tables have transformed them into actual care plan guidelines that can be tailored to specific patients by referring to the assessment tool and prototype care plan found at the end of Chapter 1.

Another important improvement to the nursing content is the division of the nursing implications column of the book's drug tables into assessment, intervention, and evaluation information. This change ties the nursing process firmly and directly to the book's pharmacologic information on specific drugs and aids in planning and delivering nursing care to patients receiving medications.

A third major improvement to the book's nursing content is the inclusion of NCLEX-style case study questions at the end of most chapters. With the NCLEX's increasing emphasis on pharmacologic knowledge, the inclusion of this type of question will help students prepare for this most important examination. The NCLEX-style questions are offered in addition to the multiple-choice chapter review questions that appear in Appendix A. The answers to the chapter review questions, with rationales and codes for cognitive level of the questions, appear in Appendix B. The answers to the NCLEX-style questions in the text, with rationales and codes for cognitive level and nursing process phase, are presented in Appendix C.

Improvements have also been made to the book's pharmacologic content, in both the text and the drug tables that summarize the text. Life span issues in pharmacology have been addressed in new chapters on obstetrical, neonatal/pediatric, and geriatric patients in drug therapy. New chapters have also been added for drug toxicity, blood products and blood substitutes, vaccines and immunizations, and miscellaneous and orphan drugs. Topics whose coverage has been expanded in the second edition include skeletal muscle relaxants, problems of coagulation, antihistamines, and anaphylactic reactions.

The book's drug tables have been enhanced by three changes that improve their usefulness as a quick-reference source of drug information. First, action and use statements have been added. With this change, the drug tables now offer all of the information provided by most drug handbooks. In addition, the adverse effects column of the tables has been organized by body systems, with the most frequent effects underlined and life-threatening ones in capital letters. This change makes for quicker access to this important information. Quicker access to the drug tables themselves is aided by the use of locator tabs at the edge of the pages that carry the drug tables. Also, page numbers for the drug tables (as well as for nursing process and patient teaching tables) are given inside the book's front and back covers, as well as at the opening of each chapter.

The book's pedagogic features have also been enhanced. In addition to the learning objectives that open each chapter, a list of important terms introduced in that chapter is included. These terms are italicized at their first appearance in the chapter and are defined in the new glossary at the end of the book. Once again the book provides two indices—a general index and a drug and agent index—at the end of the book.

The instructor's guide for the second edition carries all of the NCLEX-style and chapter review questions from the book, with answers, codes, and rationales. It also offers additional NCLEX-style and chapter review questions that are not found in the book. A transparency package containing the illustrations most useful for presentation in a class setting has also been prepared, and is made available free of charge to instructors adopting the textbook for their students. An annual update, which will track new and discontinued drugs and help keep the book as up to date as possible through the life of this edition, will also be made available free of charge to instructors. Photocopying of this update for distribution to students is encouraged.

The ever-expanding role of pharmacology in the practice of nursing demands that students be provided with not only reliable, current pharmacologic information, but also with an understanding of the nurse's role in applying the knowledge of drugs to patient care. The first edition of PHARMACOTHERAPEUTICS: A NURSING PROCESS APPROACH revolutionized the way nursing students learned pharmacology by integrating the nursing process with pharmacologic content. The improvements made in the second edition are intended to strengthen this integration and thus enhance the relationship between nursing and pharmacology.

PREFACE TO THE FIRST EDITION

Pharmacotherapeutics: A Nursing Process Approach has been developed in response to the need for a text that integrates nursing process with pharmacologic principles in a manner that gives precedence to the former, rather than the familiar emphasis on pharmacology as a dominant element. Thus the core and essence of nursing—nursing process—is the context used to present pharmacologic information in an easy-to-assimilate manner.

In a world of constantly increasing pharmacologic products, the nurse must acquire insights into fundamental pharmacologic principles, develop a theoretical base for the skills involved in administering medications, and have access to a ready reference for drug data. *Pharmacotherapeutics* has been designed to satisfy these needs.

The fundamentals of pharmacology include the history of drug administration as well as legal controls, how medications work in the body, and the principles of drug interactions. The text gives additional attention to the latter as appropriate throughout the book.

The nursing process approach provides a theoretical base for the skills needed to safely administer medications. Assessment skills, especially those involved in communication, are reviewed as they apply in determining drug histories, current drug information, and cues of compliance or noncompliance. Nursing diagnoses serve to define nursing practice in the pharmacologic context. Nursing intervention includes preparation and mixing techniques, and administration skills required for all age groups, together with teaching strategies. Nursing evaluation shows how the nurse may assess for effectiveness, compliance/noncompliance, sensitivity reactions, and side effects.

Twelve units present pharmacologic information utilizing a systems approach. Each unit is preceded by a brief discussion of physiology and anatomy, followed by chapters in which appropriate drugs are discussed in detail. Drug groups are presented according to action and use, and individual drugs are then delineated as to dosage, pharmacokinetics, adverse effects, contraindications, precautions, interactions, and therapeutic blood level when known. This information is also presented in accompanying tables. The dual presentation permits the use of the book both as a standard text and as a convenient drug reference source.

Each chapter presents nursing process in terms of the nursing assessment needed before administering medication; establishes appropriate nursing diagnosis; shows how short- and long-term goals are developed; discusses interventions such as mixing, administration, and patient teaching; and explains what requires evaluation when determining effectiveness, compliance, and side effects. In addition, the nursing process is featured in accompanying tables.

Patient teaching tables indicate how long the drug is to be taken, how it is to be administered, current drug-drug and drug-food interactions, what to do if a dose is omitted, how to stop medication, how—when necessary—to alter the dose, food and alcohol restrictions, common adverse effects, and proper storage.

A detailed index lists page numbers by both generic and trade names so that drug information may be located with reference to either name.

Pharmacotherapeutics: A Nursing Process Approach is thus an innovative presentation of pharmacologic information in which concepts and principles are integrated with the nursing process. I believe students, instructors, and practitioners will find the text both practical and useful, as well as an up-to-date reference for accurate drug information.

ACKNOWLEDGMENTS

Many people, over several years, have helped to make this second edition a reality.

To Caroline Schneggenburger, who typed and modified this manuscript many times. She turned handwritten material of dubious legibility into letter-perfect typed copy. Caroline also obtained permissions and kept track of artwork and table preparation and a special thank you to Caroline for the drug table preparation;

To Susan Doherty, who assisted with obtaining contracts and paying the bills during manuscript preparation;

To the contributors, who shared their expertise, generated many ideas, and rewrote their chapters many times as new concepts were incorporated into the manuscript;

To Marilynn Doenges and Mary Moorhouse, who prepared the revisions of the nursing process tables;

To Carolyn Brown, who prepared the NCLEX-style case study questions and the chapter review questions for the text and the instructor's guide;

To Steven Meisel, who prepared the extensive Glossary;

To Robert Martone, Senior Nursing Editor at F. A. Davis, who supervised the acquisition and the production of the text to this final product;

To Alan Sorkowitz, Nursing Developmental Editor, who helped design and release the final manuscript to production;

To Ruth DeGeorge, Executive Editorial Secretary, who kept track of the manuscript and reviewers;

To Herb Powell, Director of Publication, who guided the manuscript through the production process;

To Susan McCoy, Production Editor, for care and patience in finalizing galley and page proofs;

To the many reviewers who, through their constructive criticisms, helped to bring this manuscript to completion; I offer my special thanks.

M.M.K.

CONTRIBUTORS

Christine M. Bellari, MS, RN, CDE
Nursing Instructor
Erie Community College-North
Williamsville, New York

Carolyn S. Brown, RN, MN, CCRN
Instructor
Louisiana State University Medical Center
School of Nursing
New Orleans, Louisiana

Vicki L. Byers, RN, PhD, CNRN
Assistant Professor
University of Texas Health Science Center
San Antonio, Texas

Marilynn E. Doenges, BSN, MA, RN, CS
Clinical Specialist
Adult Psychiatric/Mental Health Nursing
Private Practice
Colorado Springs, Colorado

Virginia K. Drake, RN, DNSc, CS
Formerly
Assistant Administrator
and Senior Clinician
Southwest Neuropsychiatric Institute
San Antonio, Texas

Barbara L. Herlihy, RN, PhD
Professor Nursing
Incarnate Word College
San Antonio, Texas

Jeremiah T. Herlihy, Ph.D.
Associate Professor of Physiology
University of Texas Health Science Center
  at San Antonio
San Antonio, Texas

Robert W. Hirnle, MS, RRT
Director, Respiratory Care Program
Highline Community College
Des Moines, Washington

Kenneth A. Kellick, PharmD
Clinical Pharmacy Coordinator
VA Medical Center
Buffalo, New York

Carolyn Sue B. Kirsch, MSN, RN-C
Nursing Faculty
Midland College
Midland, Texas

Steven F. Kowalsky, PharmD
Associate Professor of Pharmacy
Department of Pharmacy Practice
Albany College of Pharmacy
Albany, New York

Adjunct, Associate Professor of Medicine
Department of Medicine
Division of Infectious Diseases
Albany Medical College
Albany, New York

Adjunct, Associate Professor
Department of Pharmacology/Toxicology
Albany Medical College
Albany, New York

Carol Ann Maull, RN, PhD
Nurse Coordinator
Daemon College
Buffalo, New York

Steven B. Meisel, PharmD
Assistant Director of Clinical Services
Pharmacy Department
Fairview Southdale Hospital
Minneapolis, Minnesota

Mary Frances Moorhouse, RN, CCP, CCRN, CRRN
Nurse Consultant
TNT-RN Enterprises and Fortis Corporation
Colorado Springs, Colorado

Anne Moraca-Sawicki, RN, BSN, MSN
Clinical Nurse Specialist, Surgical Coordinator for
Dr. Richard L. Sawicki
Niagara Falls, New York

On call
Staff Critical Care, Coronary Step Down Unit
Mt. St. Mary's Hospital
Lewiston, New York

Madeline A. Naegle, PhD, FAAN
Associate Professor
Division of Nursing, SEHNAP
New York University
New York, New York

Frances C. Schneider, PharmD
Clinical Associate Professor of Pharmacy
School of Pharmacy
State University of New York at Buffalo
Buffalo, New York

Nancy Keeling Shaw, MSN, RN
Faculty
Associate Degree Nursing
Midland College
Midland, Texas

Lovetta L. Smith, DNSc, RN, CS
Psychiatric Clinical Nurse Specialist
Gainesville Veteran Affairs Medical Center
Gainesville, Florida

Frances L. Stier, MSN, RNc
Clinical Nurse Educator
University Medical Center
Tucson, Arizona

Mark D. Watanabe, PharmD
Clinical Assistant Professor of Pharmacy Practice
Department of Pharmacy Practice
College of Pharmacy
University of Illinois at Chicago
Chicago, Illinois

CONSULTANTS

Paulette D. Avery, RN, MSN
Maternal Child Health Nurse
Kaiser South San Francisco
San Francisco, California

Cynthia Leahy Belcher, RN, BSN, MN
Assistant Professor of Nursing
Clemson University
Clemson, South Carolina

Katherine Camacho Carr, RN, CNM, PhD
Nurse-Midwife/Virginia Mason Medical Center
Seattle, Washington
and
Consultant, Perinatal Nursing and Midwifery
Seattle, Washington

Phyllis E. Carroll, MS, RN
Assistant Professor
St. Joseph College of Nursing
Joliet, Illinois

Meredith A. Davison, PhD
Adjunct Professor
College of Nursing and Allied Health
Tulsa University
Tulsa, Oklahoma

C. Lindsay DeVane, PharmD
Associate Professor of Pharmacy
and Associate Professor of Psychiatry
College of Pharmacy and Medicine
University of Florida
Gainesville, Florida

Marilynn E. Doenges, BSN, MA, RN, CS
Clinical Specialist
Adult Psychiatric/Mental Health Nursing
Private Practice
Colorado Springs, Colorado

Nancy Fairchild, BS, MS, RN, PhD(candidate)
Associate Professor
Boston College
School of Nursing
Chestnut Hill, Massachusetts

Alice C. Geissler, RN, CCRN
Contract Practitioner
Critical Care
Colorado Springs, Colorado

Larry Gever, PharmD
Clinical Information Coordinator
Wallace Laboratories
Cranbury, New Jersey

Barbara Given, PhD, RN, FAAN
Professor
College of Nursing
Michigan State University
East Lansing, Michigan

Edward P. Gruber, ARNP
Adult Nurse Practitioner
School of Nursing
University of Texas Health Sciences Center
San Antonio, Texas

Barbara Herlihy, PhD
Incarnate Word College
School of Nursing
San Antonio, Texas

Brenda S. Jackson, RN, PhD
Associate Professor
Incarnate Word College
School of Nursing
San Antonio, Texas

Sister Joan Klemballa, RN, PhD
Associate Professor
University of the District of Columbia
Washington, D.C.

Patricia LaMancuso, BSN, MEd, RN
Director of Nursing
Highland Pines Nursing Manor
Clearwater, Florida

Michele T. Laraia, RN, MSN
Department of Psychiatry and Behavioral Sciences
Medical University of South Carolina
Charleston, South Carolina

Susan Meeker, RN, MSN
Department of Nursing
Associate Degree Nursing Instructor
St. Clair County Community College
Port Huron, Michigan

Steven B. Meisel, PharmD
Assistant Director of Pharmacy
Fairview Southdale Hospital
Edina, Minnesota

Mary Frances Moorhouse, RN, CCP, CCRN, CRRN
Nurse Consultant
TNT-RN Enterprises and Fortis Corporation
Colorado Springs, Colorado

Gene D. Morse, PharmD
Associate Professor of Pharmacy
Erie County Medical Center
State University of New York at Buffalo
Buffalo, New York

Celeste R. Phillips, RN, EdD
President, Phillips and Fenwick
Integrated Strategies for Womens' Services
Capitola, California

Sally Phillips, RN, PhD
Assistant Professor
Undergraduate Program Director
University of Colorado
School of Nursing
Denver, Colorado

Margaret M. Priddy, RN, MSN, CCRN
Medical/Surgical Clinical Nursing Specialist
Cape Fear Valley Medical Center
Fayetteville, North Carolina

Barbara Redding, RN, EdD
Associate Professor
University of South Florida
College of Nursing
Tampa, Florida

Katy Reynolds, RN, MSN
Professor of Nursing
Long Beach City College
Long Beach, California

Kathleen Herman Scanlon, RN, MSN, MA
Elmhurst College
Elmhurst, New York

Sandra L. Schafer, MSN, ARNP
Clinical Instructor
Brevard Community College
Cocoa, Florida

Lovetta L. Smith, DNSc, RN
Veterans Administration Medical Center
Gainesville, Florida

April Hazard Vallerand, RN, MSN
Assistant Professor
University of Florida
College of Nursing
Gainesville, Florida

CONTENTS

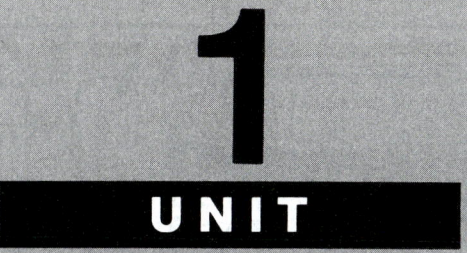

UNIT 1

THE NURSING PROCESS AND FUNDAMENTALS OF DRUG THERAPY

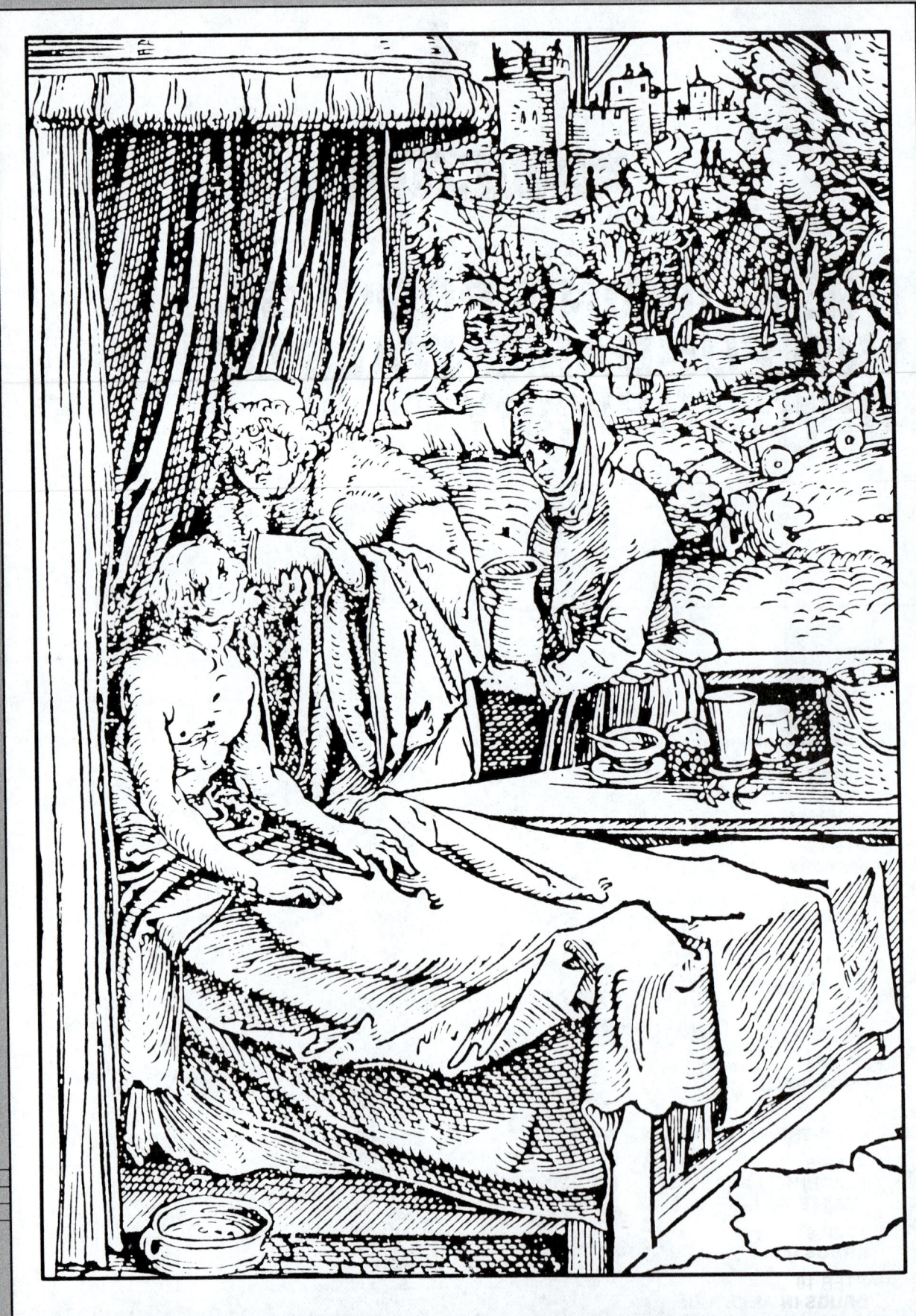

Caring for a patient, circa 1500. Free Library of Philadelphia Print Collection.

1
UNIT

THE NURSING PROCESS AND FUNDAMENTALS OF DRUG THERAPY

CHAPTER OUTLINE

PHARMACOLOGY AND NURSING
    Pharmacology
PHARMACOLOGIC APPLICATION OF THE
   NURSING PROCESS
    Assessment
    Nursing Diagnoses
    Planning
    Intervention
    Evaluation
SUMMARY
CLIENT CASE STUDY

GLOSSARY TERMS IN THIS CHAPTER

Adverse effects
Drug (medication)
Drug allergy
Idiosyncratic reaction
Nursing process
Over-the-Counter (OTC)
Pharmacology
Pharmacotherapeutics
Placebo

1
CHAPTER

THE NURSING PROCESS AND FUNDAMENTALS OF DRUG THERAPY

MERRILY MATHEWSON KUHN, R.N.C., Ph.D., CCRN

LEARNING OBJECTIVES

After reading this chapter, the student will be able to:

1. Demonstrate the importance for nurses in a modern, drug-oriented society of acquiring pharmacologic knowledge as part of their overall professional responsibility for patient care.

2. Apply the nursing process in solving problems in nursing practice related to pharmacology.

3. Articulate the components of the assessment stage of the nursing process and understand why different assessment approaches are appropriate for various types of patients.

4. Compare and contrast the elements of a nursing diagnosis and explain how they lead to the formulation of a plan for intervention involving pharmacotherapeutics.

5. Discuss the components of a plan for nursing intervention in relation to pharmacologic needs of the patient.

6. Evaluate the sources from which data are accumulated for evaluation of the nursing process and explain how criteria are determined to measure success of a treatment program.

7. Correlate the nursing process successfully to a patient case history in which drug therapy is a major component.

PHARMACOLOGY AND NURSING

Many people believe that there is a "pill" to cure every pain or symptom that can develop, and they are accustomed to consuming large numbers of drugs or medications, both prescription and *over-the-counter (OTC)*, on a daily basis. A *drug* or *medication* is a medicinal substance or agent given to produce a specific effect on the body. A drug can be derived from natural products (e.g., penicillins were first developed from molds) or from synthetics (e.g., antacids). Drugs can have various effects on the body ranging from very little effect, to therapeutic, to toxic, to fatal. By definition, a drug must have an effect.

Television and radio commercials are often responsible for the general public's medication orientation. Our society is unquestionably drug-oriented. Medications are a multimillion-dollar business that is growing each year. The drug industry spends millions of dollars annually to promote the sale of OTC drugs to consumers.

One of the major responsibilities of the nursing profession is to teach consumers of health care about the benefits and dangers of medications. Certainly, medications have a place in the field of contemporary medicine; many conditions are controlled or cured with the help of medications. Other conditions, however, are best not treated with medications but rather with alternate forms of therapy: diet, stress reduction, and exercise, for example. The health team is primarily responsible for ensuring that the patient is adequately informed about the appropriate form of therapy, and the nurse often assumes the responsibility for this patient education because of the nurse's closer contact with the patient and family.

Often, the nurse assumes primary responsibility for directing nursing care and for coordinating health care performed by other health team members in both primary and secondary health care settings. In order to direct patient care successfully, the nurse must have broad knowledge in all areas of therapy, including physiology, pathology, nutrition, psychology, and pharmacology. For example, a nurse must know which foods are high in protein when administering levodopa to a patient for control of Parkinson's disease, since a high-protein diet interferes with absorption of levodopa and thus deprives the patient of the full benefits of medication. Another example is the need to understand the pathophysiology and psychology underlying clinical depression in order to assist the patient who is receiving tranquilizers or mood elevators.

Pharmacologic comprehension is only one part of the nurse's responsibility. The nurse has an ethical and, in most states, a legal responsibility to share with patients all information needed to assist them in achieving optimal health. Every prescribed therapy has advantages and disadvantages, and the health team—including nurse, physician, pharmacist, and therapy personnel—has a responsibility to share this information with patients and their families. Often, the nurse and physician together decide what information to share, but pharmacists also are becoming more active in counseling patients about their medications.

PHARMACOLOGY

Pharmacology is a scientific study of all aspects of drugs, including their source, properties, uses, actions, and effects. *Pharmacotherapeutics* is the treatment of all aspects of disease with medication such as to diagnose, treat, or cure disease. Medication can be prescribed by a physician, dentist, osteopath, podiatrist, and in some states, by a physician's assistant, nurse practitioner, and chiropractor. Medications are prepared and dispensed in a pharmacy, usually by a licensed pharmacist. A pharmacist (druggist) is one who is licensed to prepare and sell or dispense drugs and compounds and to make up prescriptions. The pharmacist usually has a bachelor of science degree in pharmacy, but some may have more advanced degrees. Pharmacists are often a good source of information for the nurse because of the specialized education and their around-the-clock availability in most hospitals. Pharmaceutical companies also employ pharmacists to answer questions that cannot be answered by the local pharmacist. Telephone numbers for drug companies are listed in the *Physicians Desk Reference (PDR)*, which is readily available in all hospitals and nursing homes. The role of the pharmacist is discussed further in Chapter 8, "Teaching, Learning, and Evaluation Strategies for Compliance."

The pharmacist may be assisted by a pharmacologist (a specialist in pharmacology). The pharmacologist has at least a master's degree and most often a Ph.D. or M.D. degree with additional course work in pharmacology. The pharmacologist is primarily responsible for research in pharmaceutical companies, in patient populations, and in educational institutions.

PHARMACOLOGIC APPLICATION OF THE NURSING PROCESS

A process is a series of planned, logical steps that produce a definite result. The *nursing process* has 5 steps: assessment, diagnosis, planning, intervention, and evaluation. The nurse uses the nursing process each day of professional practice while caring for patients and their families in many different clinical settings: in acute-care settings, in secondary-care settings, and in the community. The nursing process is a problem-solving tool that is cyclic, dynamic, and adaptive. It is cyclic in that the nursing process is never complete; each reassessment reinitiates the process. It is dynamic in that the nursing process involves constantly changing variables and relationships, making it ongoing rather than static. It is adaptive in that the nursing process changes for each patient and for each patient condition.

Step 1 of the nursing process begins with data collection, the assessment phase. From these data, the nurse determines priorities for the care to be given. Nursing

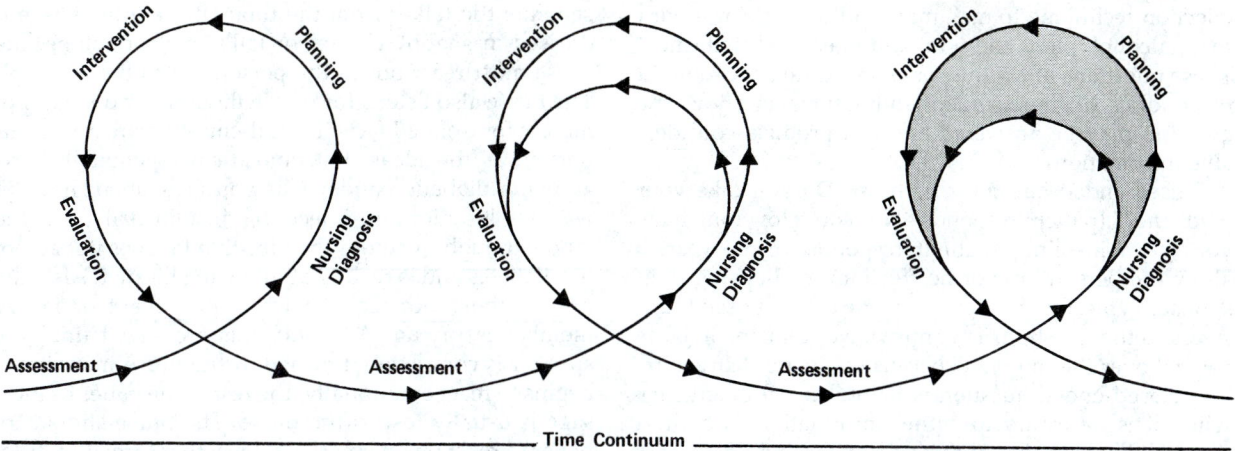

Figure 1–1. The nursing process approach to health problems. This is a five-step (assessment, diagnosis, planning, implementation, and evaluation) approach that is continuous. As the evaluation stage is entered, assessment begins again.

goals and nursing diagnoses are developed to meet the established priorities. The nurse then plans the nursing intervention necessary to implement the care. Care is given, and outcomes are subjected to evaluation. If nursing care in any phase fails to meet patient needs, or if new needs are found, the nursing process recycles to the assessment phase and begins anew. Figure 1–1 features a schematic representation of the systems approach for the nursing process. This method of operation is also the framework for theoretical approaches developed by a number of nursing theorists including Martha Rogers, Sister Callista Roy, Betty Neuman, Joanne Auger, and Dorothea Orem.

This chapter briefly reviews the five steps of the nursing process as they are implemented during medication administration. The nurse must be able to adequately assess the patient requiring medications, develop nursing diagnoses related to medication therapy, plan nursing care, implement nursing care related to medications, and then evaluate the effect of nursing interventions as well as the effects of the medication administered. The professional nurse is responsible for educating patients about their medications in order to maximize the beneficial effects and minimize adverse effects.

ASSESSMENT

Assessment, the first step of the nursing process, involves gathering information from and about each patient in order to identify the patient's disease history, current health problems, needs, problems, strengths, and weaknesses. A "need" can be for knowledge about the medication being administered. A "problem" may be the unwillingness to comply with the prescribed medication regimen. A "strength" may be a supportive family unit, whereas a "weakness" may be a lack of motivation. The nurse enters this assessment of the patient's needs, problems, strengths, and weaknesses into the data base (the body of accumulated information). The data base serves as a starting point for diagnosing,

planning, implementing, and evaluating the nursing care the patient receives. Many different tools are available for collecting the data base. A commonly used nursing assessment tool is organized by diagnostic divisions including activity/rest, circulation, ego integrity, elimination, food/fluid, hygiene, neurosensory, pain/comfort, respiration, safety, sexuality, social interaction, teaching/learning, and discharge considerations. A typical nursing assessment tool is presented later in this chapter.

The data-gathering phase has two interrelated phases: (1) verbal, or "talking and listening," phase; and (2) physical assessment, or "hands-on" phase. The verbal interchange phase occurs first, with the taking of the health history. The physical assessment, or "hands-on," phase further clarifies previously obtained information during performance of the physical examination.

The Verbal Interchange Phase

The verbal interchange phase elicits information about the total patient and the patient's significant others. The nurse uses this initial interview to learn about the patient's background, social network, feelings including fears and hopes, potential strengths and weaknesses, coping mechanisms, perception of health status, and medical history.

Both the nurse's interviewing skill and the physical environment (which should be quiet, private, and free of distractions) determine the quality of the interview. Several interviewing techniques—including open-ended questions, closed-ended questions, probing questions, hypothetical questions, and the mirror response—can be helpful in eliciting information from the patient or family. Leading and loaded questions are usually not helpful in eliciting information but are also reviewed so that the nurse understands these types of questions and can avoid them.

Open-ended questions, such as "How do you feel about your new medication?" might elicit valuable information, such as "I don't want to take it." "Explain the injection technique to me" may lead to "I clean it with soap, alcohol, pinch the skin, and inject the medicine." These questions allow the person maximum freedom in responding by imposing no limitations on how the question may be answered and can produce considerable information.

Closed-ended questions such as "Do you take your medicine?" (patient responds "No") or "How long have you taken insulin?" (patient responds "three years") allow the person little or no freedom in choosing a response. Typically, there are only one or two possible answers to the question. The interviewer remains in close control over the interview because of its rigid structure. The closed-ended question is helpful in an emergency when it is necessary to gather information in a short time. If time remains at the end of the interview, it is important to ask the patient to explain the answers to these questions in greater detail. Often, patients feel frustrated or manipulated when an interview is dominated by the closed-ended question that fails to give them an opportunity to clarify.

The probing question asks the interviewee to clarify a response for better understanding. Examples of probes are "Could you give me an example?" and "What exactly happened?" Probing questions move language from the abstract to the concrete by requiring specific and descriptive terms in the patient's answer.

The hypothetical question helps the nurse learn how the patient might handle a particular situation. Hypothetical questions include "What would you do if you felt dizzy?" and "What would you do if you noticed a rash on your body?" Hypothetical questions may be very useful in determining the extent to which the patient has learned previously presented material.

The mirror response is useful in getting at underlying meanings that might not be verbalized clearly. As an example, the patient may say, "Some days I'd like to throw this needle out the window." A mirror response might be, "Does the needle make you angry?" Now the patient is allowed to verbalize what is actually making him or her angry. The mirror response is nonevaluative and nonthreatening.

Two types of questions that should generally be avoided are leading and loaded questions. The leading question typically suggests the desired response. Examples include "The infection seems to be getting better, don't you agree?" and "This medicine really seems to be reducing the pain, doesn't it?" Leading questions reduce the range of responses, as an interviewee most commonly agrees with any leading statement.

Loaded questions, through the use of highly emotional terms, also suggest the desired response to the interviewee. Loaded questions include, "Do you ever wash your inhalator?" and "Where did you learn that injection technique?" This type of question often provokes the interviewee to "attack."

At the conclusion of the interview, the nurse summarizes the data to ensure that the patient, family, and nurse all understand the same information.

The nurse-interviewer must listen attentively to what the patient and family are saying. It is also important to separate the talker from the topic. If the interviewee is dressed in shabby clothes or talks in a monotone, the nurse must react not to the person but to the message. The nurse also listens for whole thoughts and ideas, not merely for isolated facts. Facts themselves are not as important as the ideas that bind them together. For example, a diabetic patient tells you facts about how he watches his diet and injects his insulin daily, but the whole thought includes the idea that he does not accept his diabetes and is really not following his diet. Also, the nurse should not react to what the patient or family member is saying. All comments are saved until the speaker is completely finished. If the nurse-interviewer begins to react emotionally, the rest of the patient's message is usually lost to the nurse. The nurse should try never to react on an emotional level to information from a patient.

When medications are to be administered, the nurse must ask the following questions during the assessment:

1. Does the patient have any allergies to food, animal dust, weeds, chemicals, or medications? Cross allergies are common; that is, a patient who is allergic to fish may be allergic to contrast media dyes used in diagnostic x-ray studies because the dyes contain iodine. A patient allergic to beef or pork foods may show similar allergies to insulin or heparin prepared from these animal sources. Allergic reactions (anaphylaxis) may be manifested by rash, largyngeal edema, and/or cardiovascular collapse. Some side effects such as nausea, vomiting, dizziness, and drowsiness are often inappropriately termed allergic reactions. Patients need to be questioned closely about their responses.

2. What medications does the patient currently take? The nurse asks about prescription medicines, OTC medications, vitamins, medications provided by friends, folk medicines, and drugs of abuse. Medications frequently interact with each other; therefore, it is important to know everything the patient is taking. For example, a patient taking aspirin may encounter bleeding problems when anticoagulants such as warfarin are administered. (Drug interactions are discussed further in Chapter 5.)

3. Why is the patient taking prescription and/or OTC medications? Perhaps a certain medication proved helpful to a friend or represents a new health fad, such as the use of vitamin E to improve sexual activity. Often drugs are psychosomatically effective, that is, effective because the patient desires them to be, a *placebo* effect. Patients may take a medication that interferes with the desired action of other preparations, such as a "pep" pill taken with a tranquilizer or a sleeping pill. These medications may have been obtained from friends or from physicians not involved in treating the patient's present condition.

4. What is the condition of the patient's skin, particularly if the patient has been self-administering intramuscular medication or has been taking street drugs? The nurse assesses skin for color, because a patient taking street drugs may be jaundiced from hepatitis;

for bruises, because a patient taking anticoagulants may have large hematomas on the skin; and for abscesses or infections, because a patient injecting insulin may not have good technique or may not be rotating sites properly.

5. What is the patient's current use of tobacco, marijuana, or alcohol? Daily amounts of all of these are determined. For instance, a heavy cigarette smoker (more than one pack a day) may require larger doses of theophylline, a bronchodilator, and insulin than does a nonsmoker. Conversely, if the patient stops smoking, the dose may have to be altered. The patient must notify the physician before stopping smoking so that the medication's toxic and therapeutic effects can be monitored closely.

   What is the patient's level of alcohol consumption? Alcohol interferes with or potentiates the action of many medications. It is best if the patient refrains from drinking while taking antihypertensives, tranquilizers, and all central nervous system depressants; otherwise, the patient may become overly sedated or may become dizzy or faint, resulting in a fall.

6. How much coffee, tea, cola, and other caffeine-containing beverages does the patient drink daily? Caffeine interacts with various medications. For example, the xanthine bronchodilators (theophylline) are chemically related to caffeine. The patient must limit caffeine intake to a prescribed quantity to forestall toxic effects. Coffee may also raise the blood pressure of a person with hypertension or may increase the tendency for cardiac dysrhythmias in a patient taking antidysrhythmic medication.

7. Does the patient have any current medical problems that would affect the way drugs are metabolized (broken down) in the body? Such medical problems include renal, hepatic, gastrointestinal, or cardiac diseases.

The Hands-On Phase

The next phase of the assessment process is gathering of information from the patient's physical body. This is an ongoing process that routinely continues as long as the patient is under the nurse's care. The nurse establishes privacy for the examination, readies the equipment, and explains to the patient what procedures will be performed, their rationales, and why the data they provide are valuable.

During both phases of the assessment, the nurse gathers both subjective and objective data. Subjective data consist of information told to the nurse by the patient. Objective data consist of information obtained about the patient by the nurse, who listens, observes, and physically examines the patient. Further data are obtained through laboratory and diagnostic reports, from earlier records, from other members of the health care team, and from the patient's significant others.

Once the data have been collected, the nurse proceeds to the second step of the nursing process, establishing a nursing diagnosis.

NURSING DIAGNOSES

Nursing diagnoses identify the patient's actual and potential health problems. The diagnostic statement focuses on the patient's responses to symptoms and to their underlying pathology. It is developed from the objective and subjective information obtained in the data base. Nursing diagnoses are specific to a particular patient at a particular time and lead to the development of both short- and long-term objectives during the planning stage. They are the bases upon which all nursing care is organized and delivered. The accurate diagnosis of a nursing problem can become a standard for nursing practice, understood by all who are using the plan of care and leading to improved care delivery. Once appropriate nursing diagnoses have been developed and written, the remaining steps in the nursing process proceed smoothly.

Nursing priorities are considered as the nursing diagnoses are established. Priorities are established in a hierarchical order with the most important listed first—for example, resolving threats to body integrity, either physical or psychologic, or threats that affect normal growth and development of the individual. Priorities must be re-evaluated periodically to ensure that they are being met in appropriate order and that they remain valid.

Diagnostic statements have two components: the problem and its etiology. The problem is a clear, concise statement of the condition that caused the patient to seek care. Etiology encompasses all possible factors that are related to the problem. These factors may be environmental, social, physiologic, or psychologic. The nurse writes a nursing diagnosis connecting the problem with its etiology by using the words "related to." The nursing diagnosis is further expanded in this text to include the rationale or defining characteristics for the nursing diagnosis by including "as evidenced by" after the nursing diagnosis. These statements help clarify why the nursing diagnosis was developed. The following are several examples of nursing diagnoses the nurse could develop when administering medication:

1. Knowledge deficit, related to insufficient instruction regarding new antihypertensive medication as evidenced by inability to recognize antihypertensives
2. Noncompliance, related to inability to accept diagnosis and treatment regimen as evidenced by not taking medication as ordered
3. Alterations in bowel activity, related to inappropriate administration of prescription cathartics as evidenced by diarrhea followed by constipation
4. Impairment of skin integrity, related to poor insulin injection techniques and lack of site rotation as evidenced by destruction of skin and disruption of skin surfaces
5. Anxiety, related to hair loss secondary to chemotherapy as evidenced by restlessness, facial tension, and insomnia
6. Mother's anxiety, related to administration of insulin to 6-year-old son as evidenced by increased extra-

neous body movements, hand trembling, and facial tension

Acceptable nursing diagnoses, approved by the North American Nursing Diagnosis Association (NANDA), are integrated throughout this book. Table 1–1 features the current nursing diagnoses, which are organized under various diagnostic divisions. This organization assists the nurse in choosing the specific diagnostic label to de-scribe the data accurately. By adding the etiologic fac-tors and signs and symptoms, the patient problem emerges. The nurse uses the nursing diagnosis—with its problem statement related to etiologic factors—in plan-ning nursing care. It is through the use of nursing di-agnoses that nurses are able to quantify and validate nursing care. The nurse may add more or remove nurs-ing diagnoses as the nursing process proceeds.

Table 1–1. DIAGNOSTIC DIVISONS: NURSING DIAGNOSES THROUGH THE 8th NANDA CONFERENCE

ACTIVITY/REST
Activity intolerance
Activity intolerance, potential
Disuse syndrome, potential for
Diversional activity deficit
Fatigue
Sleep pattern disturbance

CIRCULATION
Cardiac output, altered: decreased
Dysreflexia
Tissue perfusion, altered: (specify)

EGO INTEGRITY
Adjustment, impaired
*Anxiety [specify]
Coping, defensive
Coping, ineffective individual
Decisional conflict (specify)
Denial, ineffective
Fear
Grieving, anticipatory
Grieving, dysfunctional
Hopelessness
Post-trauma response
Powerlessness
Rape trauma syndrome
Self-concept, disturbance in: body image, personal identity; self-esteem
    Self-esteem, chronic low
    †Self-esteem, disturbance in
    Self-esteem, situational low
Spiritual distress (distress of the human spirit)

ELIMINATION
Bowel elimination, altered: constipation
Constipation, colonic
Constipation, perceived
Bowel elimination, altered: diarrhea
Bowel elimination, altered: incontinence
Incontinence, functional
Incontinence, reflex
Incontinence, stress
Incontinence, total
Incontinence, urge
Urinary elimination: altered patterns
*Urinary retention [acute/chronic]

FOOD/FLUID
Breastfeeding, ineffective
Fluid volume, altered: excess
*Fluid volume deficit, actual 1 [regulatory failure]
*Fluid volume deficit, actual 2 [active loss]
Fluid volume deficit, potential
Nutrition, altered: less than body requirements
Nutrition, altered: more than body requirements
Nutrition, altered: potential for more than body requirements
Oral mucous membranes, altered
Swallowing, impaired

Table 1–1. DIAGNOSTIC DIVISONS: NURSING DIAGNOSES THROUGH THE 8th NANDA CONFERENCE–*CONTINUED*

HYGIENE
Self-care deficit: feeding; bathing/hygiene; dressing/grooming; toileting

NEUROSENSORY
Neglect, unilateral
Sensory-perceptual alteration: visual; auditory; kinesthetic; gustatory; tactile; olfactory
Thought processes, altered

PAIN/COMFORT
Comfort, altered: pain, acute
Comfort, altered: pain, chronic

RESPIRATION
Airway clearance, ineffective
Aspiration, potential for
Breathing pattern, ineffective
Gas exchange, impaired

SAFETY
Body temperature, potential altered
Health maintenance, altered
Home maintenance management, impaired
Hyperthermia
†Hypothermia
Infection, potential for
Injury, potential for: poisoning; suffocation; trauma
Mobility, impaired physical
Skin integrity, impaired: actual
Skin integrity, impaired: potential
Thermoregulation, ineffective
Tissue integrity, impaired
Violence, potential for: directed at self/others

SEXUALITY (Component of Social Interaction)
Sexual dysfunction
Sexuality patterns, altered

SOCIAL INTERACTION
Communication, impaired: verbal
Coping, family: potential for growth
Coping, ineffective family: compromised
Coping, ineffective family: disabling
Family process, altered
Parental role conflict
Parenting, altered: actual or potential
Self-concept, disturbance in: role performance
Social interaction, impaired
Social isolation

TEACHING/LEARNING
Growth and development, altered
Health seeking behaviors (specify)
*Knowledge deficit [learning need] (specify)
*Noncompliance [compliance, altered] (specify)

SOURCE: Doenges, ME, et al: Nursing Care Plans: Nursing Diagnoses in Planning Patient Care, ed. 2. FA Davis, Philadelphia, 1989, with permission.

*Information that appears in brackets has been added by the authors to clarify and enhance the use of nursing diagnoses.
†Revised.

PLANNING

Planning is a systematic process in which the nurse, patient, and significant others establish short- and long-term goals and decide how they are to be implemented. These goals, in turn, become the outcomes of nursing care. During the planning phase, the design of care is developed to change or modify the patient's health status to meet new needs and/or expectations.

In an acute-care setting, such as an operating room or a critical care area, the nurse generally develops the plan of care without input from the patient. When the patient is able, as in an intermediate-care area, clinic setting, school, or physician's office, the nurse encourages the patient and significant others to participate in establishing the priorities and goals for the treatment plan. In such settings, it is important for the nurse to recognize that the locus of decision-making regarding treatment includes the patient and significant others to varying degrees and requires the patient and family to actively involve themselves in the decision-making process.

Specifically, the health-care requirements of patients are located within the following three loci of decision-making systems:

1. Centered in the nurse
2. Shared by patient and nurse
3. Centered in the patient

Planning involves establishing objectives that encompass the physical, psychologic, and sociocultural/lifestyle needs of the patient and family. All the disciplines that support nursing—arts, sciences, and humanities—are called upon as the nurse assists the patient in planning for immediate, future, and even lifelong treatment and health maintenance. For example, a patient's physical need might be to learn to live temporarily with a fractured leg or permanently with a leg amputation. A family's psychosocial need might be to respond appropriately to the impending death of the patient. Sociocultural/lifestyle needs might require changing a lifelong high-carbohydrate eating pattern because of the onset of diabetes, or changing family roles and responsibilities when the head of the household retires early because of heart disease. The patient's and the family's strengths and weaknesses are always considered when developing a plan to achieve these goals.

During the planning stage, both short- and long-term objectives are established for the medication regimen. The patient and family are actively involved with this process, and again, their strengths and weaknesses help to determine the goals. These goals actually represent the outcome criteria that will determine whether the desired patient behaviors or responses were achieved. The patient's view of the medication regimen is crucial for success. For example, if the patient is going to self-administer insulin at home, the nurse first ensures that the patient has accepted the diabetes and is willing to comply with the treatment regimen. Research has shown that the patient who is unwilling to accept the diagnosis will not comply with the treatment regimen.

During the planning stage, the nurse preparing to give medications must answer the following questions in order to proceed with medication administration:

1. What observations must be made relative to the effect of the medication? What is the action of the drug within the body? For example, is the pulse or blood pressure expected to change?
2. What route will be used to administer the medication? The patient's condition, including the ability to take medication by mouth, and level of consciousness are important considerations.
3. Are any precautions required to administer the medication, such as side rails in the upright position when narcotics are administered?
4. Are any special considerations needed because of the patient's age, physical condition, or mental state? For example, a liquid preparation should not be ordered

for a blind patient unless someone is available to ensure that the patient receives the correct dose.
5. Are specific nursing measures required to administer the medication safely? For example, the apical pulse is always taken before administering any digitalis preparation.
6. Does the patient or family have special learning needs relative to administering the medication at home, such as acquiring such specific skills as injection technique?

The long- and short-term goals or the expected outcomes developed from the nursing diagnoses become, in turn, the evaluation or outcome criteria. The nurse later evaluates the nursing intervention on the basis of these goals. The nurse, patient, and family also need to establish deadlines for meeting these goals. There are generally four major components of an outcome criterion:

1. The content
2. An action verb
3. A time frame
4. Criterion modifiers

The content describes what is to be learned or demonstrated, such as "why and how digoxin is taken" or "cheese and milk products are consumed two hours after taking tetracycline."

The action verb describes how the patient will achieve the content. Action verbs need to be easily measurable, such as describe, demonstrate, avoid, identify, or start. Verbs such as understand, believe, or know are difficult to measure.

The time frame is the period of time in which the outcome will occur, such as one day, one week, before discharge, or on the next visit. Some outcomes may need to be broken down into small steps so that they can be achieved more easily. For example, injection technique might be taught as follows:

On day 1 the patient observes nurse doing injection.
On day 3 the patient demonstrates filling of the syringe and preparation of the site for injection.
On day 5 the patient demonstrates injection technique.
On day 7 the patient states what to do if an insulin dose is missed.

Finally, the criterion modifier helps clarify what the patient is to do, such as "accurately" or "the importance of."

Several examples of patient goals or outcomes related to medication administration follow.

Before his or her discharge, the patient will describe why and how digoxin is taken.
The patient will identify the reasons for delaying the eating and drinking of cheese and milk products for at least 2 hours after taking tetracycline.
The patient will state why it is important to avoid alcohol when taking antifungal medications.

Table 1–2. TEACHING DOMAINS AND TASKS ASSOCIATED WITH LEARNING AND EVALUATION OF LEARNING

Cognitive	Affective	Psychomotor
Knowledge	Receiving	Body movements
Comprehension	Responding	Nonverbal communication
Application	Valuing	Behaviors
Analysis	Organizing	Speech
Synthesis	Characterizing	
Evaluation		

The patient will demonstrate proper injection technique.

After all feasible solutions are examined, the nursing care plan is established. The nursing care plan provides a detailed guide for patient care and generally contains nursing diagnoses, the plan of care, and the expected outcomes for each intervention.

INTERVENTION

During the intervention stage of the nursing process, the nursing care actually given is based on the nursing orders in the nursing care plan. Nursing orders developed from the nursing goals are written in behavioral terms and tell the nurse what to do. A typical nursing order would be "Explain digitalis to the patient and give him or her time to ask questions; return in one hour and offer to repeat the explanation or discuss any further questions." The nurse may implement the nursing care plan or delegate the provision of care to other health professionals. Nursing care can involve discussing diet or drugs with the patient; performing procedures, such as changing a dressing or giving an injection; or providing psychologic support to a dying patient.

The nurse is involved not only with direct care of ill people but also with health maintenance and disease prevention. Nurses usually encounter ill patients in a hospital or clinic where the immediate aim of the initial intervention is to return the patient to health. The ultimate goal, however, is to maintain the health of the entire family and to prevent future illness. Often, with good nursing care and teaching, chronic illness may be mitigated or controlled. For example, a patient with hypertension who controls weight, modifies salt intake, and takes medications as prescribed may be able to avoid a critical cerebrovascular accident.

Health teaching is an important nursing function during the intervention stage. Often, the patient and significant others must not only acquire new knowledge and skills but also radically alter behavior. Patients are unlikely to modify their behavior unless they thoroughly understand why it is necessary to do so and how they will benefit from change. Teaching, learning, and evaluation concepts are discussed in detail in Chapter 8.

Before the nurse can begin teaching, the patient and significant others must be ready to learn. The nurse presents the material in terms the patient can understand and uses teaching aids—charts, diagrams, and models—to help the patient learn. Teaching involves 3 different types of activities by the nurse, sometimes called the cognitive, affective, and psychomotor domains of learning: (1) giving factual information; (2) soliciting and evaluating feedback from the learners about their thoughts and feelings related to their new knowledge; and (3) demonstrating procedures or activities and ensuring that the learners understand the activity and can perform it (Table 1–2).

The first, or cognitive, domain emphasizes the intellectual and problem-solving tasks associated with learning. The behaviors associated with the cognitive domain range from the simple recall of facts to the synthesis of different bodies of information already learned. The major subclasses specific for the cognitive domain include knowledge, comprehension, application, analysis, synthesis, and evaluation. The nurse, for example, teaches the patient a procedure, such as injection technique, in several steps. At the conclusion of the teaching, the nurse allows the patient to perform the procedure so that the nurse can evaluate whether the patient can apply the principles. The nurse may also pose several hypothetical questions to the patient to evaluate whether the patient has learned to make valid judgments about the information. The nurse evaluates whether the patient or family member has content knowledge, comprehends it, can apply it, and is able to analyze and synthesize the new learning.

The affective domain is concerned with interests, likes, dislikes, values, attitudes, and beliefs. The major subclasses of the affective domain include receiving, responding, valuing, organizing, and characterizing by a value or value complex. An example is the nurse who uses the affective domain to determine likes and dislikes about certain foods before discussing a diet with the patient.

The psychomotor domain is concerned with gross bodily movements, finely coordinated bodily movements, nonverbal communication behaviors, and speech behaviors. In this domain, the nurse is most concerned with evaluating a patient's ability to perform a procedure such as changing a dressing or administering medications such as eye drops.

When teaching patients, keep in mind this well-known maxim: "I hear, I forget; I see, I remember; but I do, and I understand." The patient hears the nurse's explanation, sees the nurse's demonstration, and does the procedure personally while explaining it to the nurse. If the patient can "give back" what is learned, the nurse can be reasonably sure that learning has really taken place. If not, the teaching plan may have to be modified.

Health teaching may also relate to temporary side effects, such as burning at the parenteral site of injection, or to long-term needs of the patient at home. The nurse is also responsible for teaching the patient who needs special skills to continue and to comply with the medication therapy at home. In a hospital, industrial clinic, or school clinic, the nurse's essential responsibility is to provide patient teaching to ensure compliance. Teaching about the disease, its progression, and its complications is thus essential to ensure patient compliance with the medical and nursing regimens. Knowledgeable patients are more compliant because they understand why continued therapy is important. Patient compliance is discussed in detail in Chapter 8.

EVALUATION

In the first four steps in the nursing process, the patient was assessed, nursing diagnoses were developed, and care was planned and implemented. In the planning stage, the nurse determined expected outcomes, set deadlines, and developed a time frame for accumulating data to be used as criteria for evaluating the effectiveness of the plan. At the evaluation stage, the nurse ascertains whether the previously established goals have been met.

The nurse continually assesses the efficacy of nursing interventions. Ongoing evaluations are both informal (casual conversations and observations) and formal (periodic reviews of data and/or interviews). What is learned from these evaluations can be used to revise the nursing care plan as needed. Evaluation may also be delayed. In a hospital situation, evaluation may be delayed, for example, if the patient and nurse will be together for several more days. In such a case, the nurse may teach content one day and evaluate the patient's knowledge several days later. The evaluation may indicate the need for reteaching or for modifying the teaching plan.

In other situations (in an emergency room, for example), the nurse is with the patient for only a short time. The nurse must relay all information to the patient in the time available, and the patient's knowledge level must be evaluated before the patient leaves the nurse's care. Remember that patients often can repeat what they were just told (rote memorization) without being able to apply their knowledge to everyday life. Often, the nurse will have to probe and ask hypothetical questions to determine whether the patient understands what has just been taught. You might ask the patient, "Please explain this procedure to me," or "What would you do if . . . ?" Remember, knowledge that the patient cannot apply is of no use.

In situations where the patient and nurse see each other at intervals, such as in a clinic, the patient and nurse can determine what kind of evaluation will take place, when it will take place, and how it will be done. An advantage of delayed evaluation is that the patient can think about what the nurse has said, apply the information in a natural life setting, and ask questions that arise from actual experience.

Both objective and subjective data are evaluated. The nurse obtains objective data from a follow-up physical assessment or laboratory work. Subjective data, such as how the patient feels, how and whether the medication is being taken, and whether a prescribed diet is being followed, are obtained from the patient. Both subjective and objective data help the nurse evaluate the effectiveness of therapy and determine patient compliance. If the desired effects of the medication cannot be observed in the patient, the nurse helps to determine why this is so. Several plausible reasons may exist: The patient may not be taking the medication as ordered; the medication may be ineffective for this patient at this time; or the medication may not have been ordered in a correct therapeutic dose for this patient. If the patient is not complying with the treatment regimen previously established, the nurse must ascertain the reason for the lack of compliance and determine what to do to achieve compliance. Noncompliance can be due to insufficient education, poor motivation, or both. After this determination is made, the nurse, with the patient's help, rewrites the goals and objectives.

When the patient receives medications, the nurse has specific points to evaluate early in the intervention as well as later during a revisit. The nurse evaluates the following:

1. Does the patient exhibit signs or symptoms that indicate the medication is effective (or ineffective)? A reduction of blood pressure when taking antihypertensives or diminution or absence of seizure activity when taking anticonvulsants would be a sign that the medication is effective. If medications are ineffective, this is reported to the physician.
2. Is the patient experiencing any secondary effects? A secondary effect is any effect that is experienced other than the intended effect. Secondary effects include *adverse effects, drug allergies,* and *idiosyncratic reactions.* The term adverse effects describes the unwanted effects patients may experience as a result of medication therapy. Adverse effects include symptoms that are undesirable for the patient but often can be coped with, such as nausea, vomiting, fatigue, dizziness, and hypotension (Table 1–3). Toxic effects are those that can result in harm to the patient and must be treated either by stopping the drug or altering the dose. For example, leukopenia, anemia, ototoxicity, and nephrotoxicity are toxic effects that necessitate stopping a medication. The nurse reports both adverse and toxic effects to the physician.

Patients may also experience drug allergies. Drug allergies include skin reactions to systemic medications, such as rashes and urticaria, and anaphylactic

Table 1–3. COMPARISON OF ADVERSE EFFECTS AND TOXIC EFFECTS

Body System	Adverse Effects	Toxic Effects
Gastrointestinal	Nausea, vomiting, constipation, diarrhea, abdominal pain and cramps, loss of appetite (anorexia), gas distention, dry mouth	Mouth ulcers, severe change in bowel activity, hepatotoxicty
Cardiovascular	Slowing of heart rate (bradycardia), fast heart rate (tachycardia), edema, chest pain, shortness of breath, low blood pressure (hypotension), elevated blood pressure (hypertension), flushing, and palpitations	Severe change in cardiac rate, rhythm, severe change in blood pressure, pulmonary edema
Central Nervous System	Nervousness, dizziness, depression, headache, fatigue, drowsiness, lightheadedness, insomnia, and hallucinations	Seizures, ototoxicity
Dermatologic	Mild rash, itching, loss of hair (alopecia), and pigmentation of the skin	Severe rash, hives, exfoliative dermatitis, multiforme exudativum
Ophthalmic	Blurred vision, increased intraocular pressure, cataracts, and increased tearing	Retinopathy, corneal and retinal changes
Genitourinary	Urinary frequency, urinary retention, discoloration of the urine, impotence, and increased urine output	Nephrotoxicity
Other	Thirst, muscle pain, ringing in the ears (tinnitus), sweating (diaphoresis), nasal congestion, fever, and chills	Leukopenia, anemia, aplastic anemia, hemolytic anemias, thrombocytopenia, malignant hyperthermia, teratogenicity (causing changes in developing fetus)

reactions, such as respiratory embarrassment and cardiac arrest. Patients reporting drug allergies need to be evaluated carefully. Often, patients are experiencing adverse effects rather than an allergic reaction. For example, a patient may say he is allergic to Demerol (meperidine hydrochloride) because he experienced some nausea and vomiting with prior use. Nausea and vomiting are undesirable adverse effects, not signs of allergy.

Another type of reaction is an idiosyncratic reaction, which is an unexpected abnormal or peculiar reaction. An example is excitability and restlessness that barbiturates can cause in the elderly.

3. Is the patient experiencing the effects of drug interactions? Interactions may occur between two drugs (e.g., warfarin and aspirin) or between a drug and one or more foods (e.g., monoamine oxidase [MAO] inhibitors and red wine), and the result is a toxic effect (e.g., severe bleeding or a hypertensive effect) that requires investigation of the prescribed treatment and the patient's diet.
4. Does the patient comprehend all of the material previously taught about the medications?
5. Can the patient apply information when test situations are given?
6. Can the patient recognize each of his or her medications and differentiate among them?
7. Does the patient have all the knowledge or skill needed to administer the medications at home?
8. Is the patient taking the medication as ordered? The best way to elicit this information is to ask the patient, "How are you taking your medication?" The nurse should ascertain, or solicit, the following information: (1) Is the patient taking the medication as prescribed or only when he or she remembers? (2) Is the patient taking it at the correct times? and (3) Is the patient taking it in the correct way—with food or between meals—and using the correct technique, for

example, injecting it intramuscularly or subcutaneously? Is the patient rotating sites correctly?

SUMMARY

It is important for the nurse to understand (1) the expected action of the medication in the body, (2) how to teach the patient about medication to ensure compliance, and (3) how to recognize when the medication is not effective. By knowing and understanding this information, the nurse is able to use the nursing process in caring for the patient requiring medications.

A patient case study and nursing process table are included in Table 1–4 so that the student can see how the pharmacologic information can be inserted in the nursing process table and care plan.

This completes the cycle of the nursing process—assessment, diagnoses, planning, implementing, and evaluation. As the patient is assessed, goals and objectives are rewritten, and the nursing process begins again. The evaluation of goals and objectives becomes the input data for a new assessment, and the open-system nursing process begins again.

The nursing process is an effective method of planning and delivering good nursing care. The well-used nursing process promotes individual, sensitive, rational, relevant, and effective nursing care. The quality of nursing care is directly related to the sophistication of the nursing diagnoses; without complete nursing diagnoses considering all aspects of the patient, nursing care cannot be implemented. The nurse must be able to define all actual and potential health problems. It is important for the nurse to care for the "whole" patient and to consider all of the patient's physiologic, psychologic, and environmental needs.

Table 1–4. PATIENT CASE STUDY

Ken Jones, a 22-year-old male, is a 1-day postoperative appendectomy patient. His appendix had ruptured before removal and his current diagnosis is peritonitis.

His current medical orders include

IV: 2000 ml 0.45 NS and 1000 ml Ringer's lactate to infuse over 24 hours, KCl 20 mEq in IV #1 and #3.
NG to low suction: irrigate prn
Demerol 50–75 mg IM q 3–4 hr prn
Vistaril 25 mg IM q 3–4 hr prn
Tigan 200 mg IM q 4 hr prn
Mandol 1 g q 8 hr IV piggyback
Albumin 12.5 g × 2 today
Tylenol suppository T q 4 hr for T above 102° PO, 103° R
I & O
Bed rest today, OOB to chair in AM

Nursing Assessment

1. Control infection.
2. Restore/maintain circulating volume.
3. Promote comfort.
4. Maintain nutrition.
5. Provide information about disease process, possible complications and treatment needs.

Discharge Criteria

1. Infection resolved.
2. Wound healing begun.
3. Complications prevented/minimized.
4. Pain relieved/controlled.
5. Disease process, potential complications, and therapeutic regimen understood.
6. Independent in activities of daily living/appropriate support available.

Nursing Assessment

You have made the following observations on your preoperative nursing assessment:

Nursing Assessment Tool*

Name: ___Ken Jones___
Age: ___22___ DOB: ___6-16-67___ Sex: ___M___ Race: ___white___
Admission date: ___9-10___ Time: ___Midnight___ From: ___home___
Source of information: ___Ken Jones___ Reliability (1–4): ___1___
Family member/Significant other: ___none___

ACTIVITY/REST

Reports (Subjective)
Occupation: ___student___ Usual activities/Hobbies: ___swims & rides motorcycle___
Leisure time activities: ___swims daily___
Complaints of boredom: ___none___
Limitations imposed by condition: ___none when recovered___
Sleep: Hours: ___6-8 hrs___ Naps: ___none___ Aids: ___none___
Insomnia: ___none___ Related to: ___none___
Rested upon awakening: ___yes___

Exhibits (Objective)
Observed response to activity: Cardiovascular: ___normal___
Respiratory: ___normal___
Mental status (i.e., withdrawn/lethargic): ___appears tense and anxious___
Neuromuscular assessment:
Muscle mass/tone: ___normal___
Posture: ___normal___ Tremors: ___normal___
ROM: ___normal___ Strength: ___normal___
Deformity: ___none___ Other: ___

CIRCULATION

Reports (Subjective)
History of: Hypertension: ___no___ Heart trouble: ___no___
Rheumatic fever: ___no___ Ankle/leg edema: ___no___
Phlebitis: ___no___ Slow healing: ___no___
Claudication: ___no___ Other: ___
Extremities: Numbness: ___no___ Tingling: ___no___

*Source: Doenges, ME, Moorhouse, MF, and Jeffries, MF: Nursing Care Plans: Nursing Diagnoses in Planning Patient Care, ed 2. FA Davis, Philadelphia, 1989, with permission.

Table 1–4. PATIENT CASE STUDY–*CONTINUED*

Cough/hemoptysis: ___no___
Change in frequency/amount of urine: ___none___

Exhibits (Objective)
BP: R: Standing: ___0___   Sitting: ___0___   Lying: ___120/82___
    L: Standing: ___0___   Sitting: ___0___   Lying: ___120/82___
Pulse pressure: ___–___   Auscultatory gap: ___–___
Pulse (palpation): Carotid: ___normal___   Temporal: ___normal___
    Jugular: ___normal___   Radial: ___normal___
    Femoral: ___normal___   Popliteal: ___normal___
    Post Tibial: ___normal___   Dorsalis pedis: ___normal___
Cardiac (palpation): PMI: ___5 LMCS___
    Thrill: ___none___   Heaves: ___none___
Heart sounds: Rate: ___120___   Rhythm: ___regular___   Quality: ___normal___
    Friction rub: ___none___   Murmur: ___none___
Breath sounds: ___normal lung sounds, few crackles in R lower lung___
Vascular bruit: (specify): ___none___
Jugular vein distention: ___none___
Extremities: Temperature: ___normal___   Color: ___normal___
    Capillary refill: ___normal___
    Homans' sign: ___negative___   Varicosities: ___none___
    Nails (describe abnormalities): ___normal___
    Distribution/quality of hair: ___normal___
Color/cyanosis: Overall: ___pale___   Mucous membranes: ___normal___   Lips: ___normal___
    Nail beds: ___normal___   Conjunctiva: ___normal___   Sclera: ___normal___

EGO INTEGRITY

Reports (Subjective)
Report of stress factors: ___"Stress of being a senior in college trying to get good grades so I can get into graduate school"___
Ways of handling stress: ___"talking to friends"___
Financial concerns: ___paying tuition___
Relationship status: ___serious girlfriend___
Cultural factors: ___city___
Religion: ___Catholic___   Practicing: ___no___
Lifestyle: ___middle class--lives in dorms___   Recent changes: ___no___
Feelings of: Helplessness: ___no___   Hopelessness: ___no___
Powerlessness: ___no___

Exhibits (Objective)
Emotional status (check those that apply):
    Calm: ___   Anxious: ___x___   Angry: ___
    Withdrawn: ___   Fearful: ___x___   Irritable: ___
    Restive: ___   Euphoric: ___   Other (specify): ___
Observed physiologic response(s): ___occasionally sighs deeply, frowns, shrugs shoulders, anxious look on face___

ELIMINATION

Reports (Subjective)
Usual bowel pattern: ___normal___   Laxative use: ___none___
Character of stool: ___round & formed___   Last BM: ___yesterday morning___
History of bleeding: ___no___   Hemorrhoids: ___no___
Constipation: ___no___   Diarrhea: ___no___
Usual voiding pattern: ___several x daily___ Incontinence: ___no___   When: ___
    Urgency: ___no___   Frequency: ___no___   Retention: ___no___
Character of urine: ___yellow___
Pain/burning/difficulty voiding: ___no___
History of kidney/bladder disease: ___no___

Exhibits (Objective)
Abdomen: Tender: ___to palpation___   Soft/Firm: ___yes___
    Palpable mass: ___no___   Size/girth: ___appears distended___
    Bowel sounds: ___absent___
Hemorrhoids (per rectal exam): Internal: ___none___   External: ___none___
Bladder palpable: ___no___   Overflow voiding: ___no___

FOOD/FLUID

Reports (Subjective)
Usual diet (type): ___"3 squares a day"___   # meals daily: ___3___ ___"I choose food every day from the four basic food groups"___
Last meal/intake: ___lunch yesterday___   Dietary pattern: ___
Loss of appetite: ___none___   Nausea/vomiting: ___started yesterday afternoon [date]___

CONTINUED ON THE FOLLOWING PAGE

Table 1–4. PATIENT CASE STUDY–*CONTINUED*

Heartburn/indigestion: __none__ Related to: _____ Relieved by: _____
Allergy/food intolerance: __none__
Mastication/swallowing problems: __none__
    Dentures: Upper: __none__ Lower: __none__
Usual weight: __150__ Changes in weight: __none__
Use of diuretics: __none__

Exhibits (Objective)
Current weight: __150__ Height: __6'1"__ Body build: __tall & thin__
Skin turgor: __normal__ Mucous membranes moist/dry: __moist__
Hernia/masses: __no__
Edema: General: __no__ Dependent: _____
Periorbital: __no__ Ascites: __no__
Jugular vein distention: __no__
Thyroid enlarged: __no__ Halitosis: __no__
Condition of teeth/gums: __normal__
Appearance of tongue: __pink and normal__
    Mucous membranes: __pink and normal__
Bowel sounds (previously assessed): __absent__
Breath sounds (previously assessed): __lungs resonant, no adventitious sounds__
Urine S/A or Chemstix: __negative__

HYGIENE

Reports (Subjective)
Activities of daily living: Independent: __yes__
    Dependent (specify): Mobility: _____ Feeding: _____
        Hygiene: _____ Dressing: _____
        Toileting: _____ Other: _____
    Equipment/prosthetic devices required: _____
    Assistance provided by: _____
    Preferred time of bath: _____ AM _____ PM

Exhibits (Objective)
General appearance: __well-groomed__
Manner of dress: __mod__ Personal habits: __appear clean__
Body odor: __none__ Condition of scalp: __clean__
Presence of vermin: __none__

NEUROSENSORY

Reports (Subjective)
Fainting spells/dizziness: __none__
Headaches: Location: __none__ Frequency: _____
Tingling/numbness/weakness (location): __none__
Stroke (residual effects): __none__
Seizures: __none__ Aura: __none__ How controlled: _____
Eyes: Vision loss: R: __wears glasses, vision corrected to 20/20__
    Glaucoma: _____ Cataract: _____
Ears: Hearing loss: R: __none__ L: _____ none
Nose: Epistaxis: __no__ Sense of smell: __no__

Exhibits (Objective)
Mental status:
    Oriented/disoriented: Time: __yes__
        Place: __yes__
        Person: __yes__
    Alert: __x__ Drowsy: _____ Lethargic: _____
    Stuporous: _____ Comatose: _____ Other: _____
    Cooperative: _____ Combative: _____ Delusions: _____
    Hallucinations: _____ Affect (describe): _____
Memory: Recent: __normal__ Remote: _____
Speech pattern: __normal__ Content: _____
    Word choice: _____ Congruence: _____
Glasses: __yes__ Contacts: _____ Hearing Aids: _____
Pupil size/reaction: R: __PERRLA__ L: __PERRLA__
Facial droop: _____ Swallowing: _____
Handgrip/release: R: __normal__ Posturing: __no__
Deep tendon reflexes: __normal__ Paralysis: __none__

PAIN/COMFORT

Reports (Subjective)
Location: __abdomen__ Intensity (1–10): __9–10__ Frequency: __continuous__
Quality: __sharp__ Duration: __several hours__ Radiation: __to back up to shoulders__

Table 1–4. PATIENT CASE STUDY-*CONTINUED*

Precipitating factors: ___none___
How relieved: ___not relieved___

Exhibits (Objective)
Facial grimacing: ___yes___   Guarding affected area: ___yes___
Emotional response: ___anxious___   Narrowed focus: ___negative___

RESPIRATORY

Reports (Subjective)
Dyspnea (related to): ___anesthesia, splinting from abdominal pain___
Cough/sputum: ___cough nonproductive___
History of Bronchitis: ___no___   Asthma: ___no___
    Tuberculosis: ___no___   Emphysema: ___no___
    Recurrent pneumonia: ___no___   Other: ___no___
    Exposure to noxious fumes: ___no___
Smoker: ___previous___   Packs/day: ___2___   Number of years: ___4___
Use of respiratory aids: ___none___   Oxygen: ___none___

Exhibits (Objective)
                                                        chest wall moves
Respiratory: Rate: ___28/minute___   Depth: ___shallow___   Symmetry: ___symmetrically___
Use of accessory muscles: ___no___   Nasal flaring: ___no___
Fremitis: ___normal___
Breath sounds: ___normal___
Egophony: ___not present___
Cyanosis: ___not present___   Clubbing of fingers: ___negative___
Sputum characteristics: ___none___
Mentation/restlessness: ___none___
Other: _____

SAFETY

Reports (Subjective)
Allergies/Sensitivity: ___none___   Reaction: _____
Previous alteration of immune system: ___none___   Cause: _____
History of sexually transmitted disease (date/type:) ___none___
Blood transfusion: ___none___   When: _____
    Reaction (describe): _____
History of accidental injuries: ___none___
Fractures/dislocations: ___none___
Arthritis/unstable joints: ___none___
Back problems: ___none___
Changes in moles: ___none___   Enlarged nodes: ___none___
Impaired: Vision: ___none___   Hearing: ___none___
Prosthesis: ___none___   Ambulatory device: ___none___
Expressions of ideation of violence (self/others): ___none___

Exhibits (Objective)
Temperature: ___102 rectally___ Skin integrity: ___intact___
    Scars: ___none___   Rashes: ___none___
    Lacerations: ___none___   Ulcerations: ___none___
    Ecchymosis: ___none___   Blisters: ___none___
    Burns (degree/percent): ___none___
Mark location of above on diagram:

CONTINUED ON THE FOLLOWING PAGE

Table 1–4. PATIENT CASE STUDY–*CONTINUED*

General strength: __appears weak__   Muscle tone: __good__
    Gait: __unable to evaluate__   ROM: __normal__
    Paresthesia/paralysis: __negative__

SEXUALITY
Sexual concerns: __none__

Female

Reports (Subjective)
Age at menarche: _____ Length of cycle: _____ Duration: _____
Last menstrual period: _____ Menopause: _____
Vaginal discharge: _____ Bleeding between periods: _____
Practices breast self-exam: _____ Last PAP smear: _____
Method of birth control: _____

Exhibits (Objective)
Breast exam: _____
Vaginal warts/lesions: _____

Male

Reports (Subjective)
Penile discharge: __no__   Prostate disorder: __no__
Vasectomy: __no__   Use of condoms: __yes__
Practices self-exam: Breast: __no__   Testicles: __no__
Last proctoscopic exam: __never__   Last prostate exam: __yesterday__

Exhibits (Objective)
Exam: Breast __deferred__   Testicles: __deferred__

SOCIAL INTERACTION

Reports (Subjective)
Marital status: __single__   Years in relationship: __6 mo.__
    Living with: __alone in dormitory__
    Concerns/Stresses: _____
Extended family: __several close friends at school__
Other support person(s): _____
Role within family structure: __oldest of 4__
Report of problems related to illness/condition: __negative__
Coping behaviors: __seems anxious__
Do others depend on you for assistance? __no__
    How are they managing? _____
Frequency of social contacts (other than work): __daily__

Exhibits (Objective)
Speech: Clear: __yes__   Slurred: __no__
    Unintelligible: __no__   Aphasic: __no__
    Unusual speech pattern/impairment: __none__
Laryngectomy: __no__   Speech aids: __no__
Verbal/nonverbal communication with family/SO(s): __normal__

Family interaction (behavior) pattern: __not seen__

TEACHING/LEARNING

Reports (Subjective)
Dominant Language (specify): __English__
Education level: __college senior majoring in chemistry__
Learning disabilities (specify): __none__
Cognitive limitations (specify): __none__
Health beliefs/practices: __"I take care of minor problems and only see the doctor when something__
Special health care practices: __none__   __is really bothering me."__
Familial risk factors (indicate relationship):
    Diabetes: __maternal grandmother__   Tuberculosis: __no__
    Heart disease: __father__   Strokes: __no__
    High BP: __father__   Epilepsy: __no__
    Kidney disease: __none__   Cancer: __no__
    Mental illness: __none__   Other (specify): _____
Prescribed medications (circle last dose):

Drug	Dose	Times	Takes regularly	Purpose
none				

Nonprescription drugs: OTC: __aspirin on occasion for headache__
    Street drugs: __denied__

Table 1–4. PATIENT CASE STUDY–*CONTINUED*

Use of alcohol (amount/frequency): "several beers 4 or 5 times a week"
Admitting diagnosis (physician): appendicitis, possible peritonitis
Reason for hospitalization (patient): "severe pain in my belly"
History of current complaint:
Patient expectations of this hospitalization: "to get well"
Previous illnesses and/or hospitalizations/surgeries:
    none
Evidence of failure to improve: none
Last complete physical exam: 4 years ago as a preadmission to college By:

DISCHARGE CONSIDERATIONS
Date data obtained: 9-10
1. Anticipated date of discharge: 9-17
2. Resources available: Persons: home to parents
    Financial:
3. Do you anticipate changes in your living situation after discharge: yes, will go home to parents to recover
4. If Yes: Areas that may require alteration/assistance:
    Food preparation: no   Shopping: no
    Transportation: no   Ambulation: no
    Medication/IV therapy: no   Treatments: no
    Wound care: no   Supplies: no
    Self-care assistance (specify):
    Physical layout of home (specify):
    Homemaker assistance (specify):
    Living facility other than home (specify):

This care plan is individualized for Ken Jones. When designing a care plan, it must be individualized for the specific patient needs.

NURSING PROCESS TABLE: POSTOPERATIVE CARE PLAN

Assessment

Assess vital signs every hour.
Note body position.
Inspect dressing for drainage.
Assess IV site for inflammation and burning, and needle for patency.
Review laboratory results (e.g., WBC, sed rate, blood and wound cultures, Hb/Hct, electrolytes, BUN/Cr, and total protein and albumin).
Assess drug/allergy history.
Note characteristics of pain.
Evaluate level of anxiety. Observe patient for facial expression and body movement.
Evaluate vital signs, skin turgor, and mucous membranes at least every 8 hours. Calculate 24-hour fluid balance.
Assess lung sounds and respiratory rate and quality at least every 4 hours.
Assess level of knowledge about condition, self-care needs, and availability of resources.

Nursing Diagnosis	Nursing Actions	Rationale	Desired Patient Outcomes/Evaluation Criteria
Infection, potential for spread related to rupture of appendix, stasis of body fluids and invasive procedures.	Report temperature elevation and administer Tylenol suppository for oral temperature above 102/103 F rectal.	Early identification of abnormal vital signs promotes prompt treatment. Continued temperature elevation may indicate extension of infection, secondary overgrowth, inadequate treatment.	Displays vital signs within normal limits and is afebrile within 24–48 hours after surgery.
	Place in high Fowler's position as able. Monitor abdomen for abnormal amount of tenderness.	Assists in localizing peritoneal drainage to limit spread of infection.	Achieves timely healing with wound free of purulent drainage within 72 hours.

NURSING PROCESS TABLE: POSTOPERATIVE CARE PLAN–*CONTINUED*

Nursing Diagnosis	Nursing Actions	Rationale	Desired Patient Outcomes/Evaluation Criteria
	Change dressing using aseptic technique. Chart amount, character and odor of drainage. Dispose of contaminated dressings properly.	Helps to prevent spread of infection throughout the abdomen. If no drainage on dressings (along with presence of other symptoms), suspect abscess formation.	
	Monitor IV site. Discontinue IV if redness, burning, or swelling occurs at site.	IV patency is required for safe administration of antibiotics. IV site can provide an entry site for bacteria.	Free of signs of inflammation of IV site.
	Monitor lab values and report values that fail to return to normal.	Elevated lab values and positive blood cultures indicate the presence of infection and affect therapy choices.	Demonstrates return to normal/expected lab values within 48 hours of surgery.
	Note previous antibiotic therapy, presence of drug or multiple food allergies.	Reduces risk of untoward reactions.	
	Administer Mandol as ordered. Mix in 100 ml normal saline and administer over 30 minutes. Observe for side and toxic effects of Mandol such as GI effects, hypersensitivity. Monitor renal function and notify physician if output is decreased.	Antibiotics reduce the number of multiplying microorganisms. A drug reaction/decreased renal function necessitates a change in antibiotic, or possibly dosage, dependent on the situation.	
Pain related to surgical trauma, chemical irritation with inflammation (infection), anxiety evidenced by verbal complaints, muscle tension and guarding, facial grimacing, and changes in vital signs.	Administer Demerol and/or Vistaril IM q 3–4 hours as needed.	Reduces metabolic rate and intestinal irritation and aids in pain relief. The addition of Vistaril reduces nausea/vomiting which can increase level of discomfort. Vistaril also is useful in prolonging the analgesic effects of the demerol.	Reports pain is relieved/controlled within 30 minutes of drug administration. Displays a gradual resolution of abdominal pain with abdomen soft and nondistended within 72 hours.
	Notify MD if pain is not relieved with analgesics.	Changes in pain characteristics or pain which is not alleviated with analgesics may indicate an unresolved infectious process/developing complications.	
	Explore feelings with patient. Encourage verbalization of feelings.	A high anxiety level can intensify pain and may lessen analgesic effect.	Demonstrates relaxed appearance and body posture, able to sleep/rest appropriately.
	Provide calm, restful environment and comfort measures, e.g., position changes, back rub.	Promotes relaxation and may enhance patient's coping ability.	
	Maintain semi- to high-Fowler's position.	Facilitates fluid/wound drainage, reducing diaphragmatic irritation and abdominal tension.	
Fluid volume, deficit, potential related to active loss (nausea, gastric suction), increased metabolic needs (surgery, fever, healing process) and restricted intake.	Record intake and output from all sources. Measure urine specific gravity as indicated.	Decreasing output of concentrated urine with increasing specific gravity suggests dehydration/need for increased fluids. Peritonitis results in increased blood flow to perineum intensifying fluid	Maintains adequate fluid balance as evidenced by urinary output > 30 cc/hr, stable vital signs, moist mucous membranes, good skin turgor, and lab values within normal limits.

CONTINUED ON THE FOLLOWING PAGE

NURSING PROCESS TABLE: POSTOPERATIVE CARE PLAN-*CONTINUED*

Nursing Diagnosis	Nursing Actions	Rationale	Desired Patient Outcomes/Evaluation Criteria
	Provide IV fluids, 2000 ml 0.45 NS (#1–#2), 1000 ml Ringer's Lactate (#3) at 125 ml/hr.	losses through drains/ wounds. Replaces losses and maintains hydration in absence of oral intake.	
	Administer Tigan as indicated.	Reduces gastric losses related to vomiting.	
	Administer KCL IV as ordered.	Electrolytes can be lost from gastric suction/ wound drainage and coupled with lack of oral replacement can result in imbalances which may delay healing and cause further complications.	
Breathing pattern, ineffective related to muscular impairment, inflammatory process and pain evidenced by shallow respirations and crackles (R) lower lung.	Elevate head of bed at least 30 degrees. Demonstrate and encourage deep breathing and coughing exercises, use of incentive spirometry as ordered. Turn q2h. Increase activities, such as ambulation as tolerated.	Abdominal distention limits diaphragmatic excursion. Aids in inflation of all lung segments, preventing atelectasis and enhancing expectoration of secretions.	Maintains an effective respiratory pattern free of signs of cyanosis or distress. Participates in treatment regimen/breathing exercises within level of ability within 24 hours.
	Administer analgesics before activity as needed.	Abdominal pain may lead to reluctance to breath deeply. However, narcotic/analgesics must be used with caution as they can depress respiratory activity.	
	Note color of sputum, presence of adventitious breath sounds.	Indicators of developing complications.	
Nutrition, altered: potential for: less than body requirements related to inability to ingest food (NG tube), digest/absorb food (ileus) and hypermetabolic state (surgery, inflammatory process, required healing).	Administer albumin as ordered. Monitor suture line for proper healing.	There are increased nutritional needs during infection and normal wound healing. While patient is NPO there is no protein intake to maintain anabolic activity.	Maintains usual weight and positive nitrogen balance with total protein between 6–8 mg/dl and albumin between 4–4.5 gm %.
Knowledge deficit related to unfamiliarity with current health care needs and information resources evidenced by requests for information and concerns about recovery.	Provide verbal and written material about underlying disease process, drug therapy, wound care, activity restrictions/progression, nutritional needs, necessity of routine follow-up, signs and symptoms requiring medical evaluation.	Multiple methods of informational access enhances learning. Provides knowledge base on which patient can make informed choices. Promotes safe self care and aids in prevention of complications.	Participates in learning process within 24 hours. Verbalizes understanding of condition and treatment within 48 hours.
	Clarify misconceptions. Have patient explain understanding of information presented.	Includes patient as an active participant in the learning process and is useful in documenting understanding.	
	Identify post-discharge needs and personal/community resources.	Shortened length of hospital stay may require increased level of care after discharge.	Identifies available/needed resources to support individual needs.

SITUATION 1–1

Jim Case is employed as a charge nurse in a skilled nursing facility at a small rural hospital. The following questions relate to typical patient situations he encounters.

1. Jean Coyle, a 79-year-old diabetic, is being admitted to the unit for rehabilitation care following a fracture of the right hip. Which question would be *most helpful* in eliciting information for an admission nursing assessment?
   a. "You do not have problems with giving yourself insulin, do you?"
   b. "Who told you figs could be included in your diet?"
   c. "What do you do if you become shaky?"
   d. "Do you take daily laxatives?"

2. Mrs. Coyle tells Jim that she is allergic to penicillin. Which symptom indicates an allergic reaction to this drug?
   a. Rash
   b. Nausea
   c. Dizziness
   d. Drowsiness

3. Mr. Fell, an 80-year-old asthmatic, has been receiving theophylline (a bronchodilator) to decrease bronchospasm. Which statement by Mr. Fell should alert the nurse that the dosage may have to be altered to be effective?
   a. "I smoke a pack of cigarettes a day."
   b. "My bowels haven't moved in two days."
   c. "I'm not sleeping well at night."
   d. "I have a bad headache."

4. Jim is evaluating the effectiveness of barbiturates ordered for Mr. Syms, a 79-year-old patient who is very agitated. Which statement by Mr. Syms indicates that he may be having an idiosyncratic reaction to the drug?
   a. "My stomach feels upset."
   b. "I just can't sit still."
   c. "There is a rash on my neck."
   d. "It burns when I urinate."

5. Mr. Syms is started on a MAO inhibitor for depression. Jim teaches him to avoid the following food:
   a. Fish
   b. Eggs
   c. Chicken
   d. Red wine

6. Eighty-five-year-old Rose Santa has been receiving warfarin to prevent progression of neurologic deficits. Which of the following statements by Rose indicates that health teaching regarding the medication has been ineffective?
   a. "I ate a chocolate candy bar yesterday."
   b. "My legs feel heavy."
   c. "I always have a bottle of aspirin with me."
   d. "I must be catching a bad cold."

Refer to the Appendix for correct answers and additional review questions with answers.

BIBLIOGRAPHY

Carlson, C, et al: Nursing process how-to's. Ad Nurse 2(1):24–27, 1987.

Carpenito, LJ: Nursing Diagnosis: Application to Clinical Practice. JB Lippincott, Philadelphia, 1984.

Creason, NS: How do we define our diagnoses? Am J Nurs 87(2):230–231, 1987.

Doenges, ME and Moorhouse, MF: Nurse's Pocket Guide: Nursing Diagnoses with Interventions, ed 2. FA Davis, Philadelphia, 1988.

Doenges, ME, Moorhouse, MF, and Jeffries, MF: Nursing Care Plans: Nursing Diagnoses in Planning Patient Care, ed 2. FA Davis, Philadelphia, 1989.

Dougherty, C (ed): Nursing diagnosis. Nurs Clin North Am 20(4), 1985.

Gordon, M: Nursing Diagnoses: Process and Application. McGraw-Hill, New York, 1982.

Griffin, J: Writing and Using Behavioral Objectives in Nursing Education. NLN Publication 23-1670. National League for Nursing, New York, 1977.

Health & Public Policy Committee, American College of Physicians: Drug information for patients. Ann Intern Med 104(1):121, 1986.

Kim, M and Moritz, D: Classification of Nursing Diagnosis. McGraw-Hill, New York, 1982.

Physicians' Desk Reference, ed 43. Medical Economics, Oradell, NJ, 1989.

Twenty-one new diagnoses and a taxonomy. Am J Nurs 86(12):1414–1415, 1986.

2 CHAPTER

HISTORY, LEGISLATION, AND STANDARDS

2
CHAPTER

HISTORY, LEGISLATION, AND STANDARDS

ANNE MORACA-SAWICKI, R.N., M.S.N.

LEARNING OBJECTIVES

Upon the completion of this chapter, the reader will be able to:

1. List the 3 stages in the development of the science of therapeutics and define each.

2. Identify some of the early drugs utilized in the treatment of illness.

3. Identify at least one contribution to pharmacy of the Greeks—Hippocrates, Diosorides, and Galen.

4. Discuss the early pharmacopeias developed and the place of pharmacopeia in medication administration today.

5. Explain the history of the evolution of the nurse's role in the administration of medications.

6. List the five medication "rights."

7. Discuss drug laws and their impact upon how drugs are administered.

8. Explain the purpose of Drug Schedules and how drugs are classified into these categories.

9. Explain the process by which a new drug is developed and marketed.

10. Compare the similarities between the United States and Canadian controlled-drug laws.

This chapter deals with the history, legislation, and standards associated with the use of drugs in illness. Since man's awareness of disease is as old as his awareness of hunger and cold, the use of herbs and crude medications predates written history. However, through the discovery of various artifacts and drawings, it is obvious that people attempted to treat illness through medicinal intervention from earliest history. This chapter traces the history of drug development from the pre-Christian era to the modern age. In addition, the various legal and purity standards that followed the refinement of the science of pharmacology are also addressed. The role of the nurse in the preparation, administration, and recording of medicinal records is described.

The nurse's role in the administration of medications has progressed considerably since the days of Florence Nightingale, when the application of leeches and administration of enemas were the main medicinal procedures attended to by nurses. Today's nurse is responsible for the administration of oral as well as parenteral medication (parenteral refers to all routes other than oral). In addition, nurses administer intravenous doses of medications and in some states may even prescribe some medications.

PHARMACOLOGY THROUGHOUT HISTORY

ANCIENT PHARMACOLOGY

The problem of illness and disease is as old as mankind. Before there were written historical records, people left behind evidence of attempts to intervene in the disease process. Prehistoric artifacts uncovered by archaeologists attest to mankind's preoccupation with health and disease. Talismans, drawings, and other artifacts suggest some rudimentary attempts to treat or "cure" disease. Fossilized human bones give evidence of early illnesses. A thigh bone belonging to Java man (*Pithecanthropus erectus*) found in 1891 shows signs of what was almost certainly a type of cancerous bone tumor. The fact that there was evidence that the Java man so afflicted lived long enough to show disease progression suggests evidence of contemporaries who may have provided some type of support or care. Thus, 400,000 years ago man battled illness as certainly as the elements for survival. The exact details of how the most primitive cultures administered to the sick will no doubt remain a mystery. However, from their crude attempts to treat illness there developed an insatiable search for the "magic bullet" to kill off or cure disease, which persists today. Indeed, one of the oldest diseases known remains even today the number two killer in the United States, as a cancer cure still eludes us.

There is evidence that many primitive cultures nurtured or "nursed" the sick. The presence of fossilized remains with healed fractures and of children as well as adults with congenital deformities indicates cultures existed in which the sick were treated. Throughout history it seems that there have always been those who nurtured or attended to the sick and injured. The nurturing aspect of attending to the sick was the earliest form of nursing. In addition, prayers and the application of herbs, poultices, and talismans were the earliest attempts to apply medicinal intervention in illnesses. The selection of early drugs was at first fortuitous and later based upon empirical knowledge.

Stages in the Development of Therapeutic Pharmacology

There have been three distinct stages in the development of the science of therapeutics: the mystical stage, the empirical stage, and the specific stage (Table 2–1). The *mystical stage of therapeutics* is by far the oldest stage. This stage employed three major modes of therapy: prayers, surgery (crude though it may have been), and drugs. This stage was strongly influenced by religion and still persists today in remote, primitive cultures.

The use of prayer in the mystical stage demonstrated the belief that there were evil, demonic forces to contend with and that these spirits were somehow responsible for illness. The spirit of mysticism was still very much in existence as late as the 17th century in colonial Massachusetts, where 19 persons were hanged in 1692 because they were believed to be witches and capable of demonic acts. As late as the 18th century the mentally ill were believed to be possessed by evil spirits, and an important part of their care was to literally "beat the devil out of them." Thankfully, modern drug research has developed many drugs to successfully treat psychiatric patients, and such brutality remains merely an unfortunate historical fact.

The use of surgery in the mystical stage was crude and painful since the use of anesthesia was as yet unknown. Although some ancient surgeons possessed great skill, as evidenced by first century Peruvians who practiced trephining (boring of a hole into the skull), there is little evidence that the procedure was based on medical need. Possibly it was felt that the mentally ill or those suffering headaches were possessed by an evil spirit and that trephining would allow the demons to escape. Exhumed skulls of more than one person show that the "patients" so treated did survive. Some even had repeat treatments!

The use of drugs in this mystical stage of the development of therapeutics was based almost entirely upon superstition. A common belief was that through the use of plant or animal material one could transfer desired characteristics to people, such as in the drinking of tiger's blood to obtain strength. A classic form of religious mysticism still practiced in the southwestern part of the United States is the ingestion of mescal buttons (from the peyote cactus) by members of the Native American Church of North America. The use of mescal by members of the Native American Church of North America was upheld by the courts in 1962 after three Navajo members were convicted of using peyote, which is against California law. The high court decision found the Navajo's use of peyote to be a sacramental symbol

Table 2-1. STAGES IN THE DEVELOPMENT OF THERAPEUTICS

Development Stage	Explanation	Examples of Treatments/Drugs Used
Mystical stage	Oldest stage in the development of pharmacology, dates back to ancient man's earliest efforts to treat illness. This stage was steeped in religious and superstitious beliefs (magic).	Prayers, crude forms of surgery and exorcisms, unrefined medicinal herbs, and early drugs.
Empirical stage	Second stage in development of pharmacology. Based upon clinical knowledge that a drug is effective, though the mechanisms of drug action were unknown. Modern medicine still employs empirical knowledge to some extent. This stage began about the time of man's ability to leave written records. Superstition/religion still played a large role in therapeutics.	Prayers/superstitious beliefs coupled with the use of medicinal herbs, spices, ritual baths. The use of effective pharmacologic drugs appeared. Some drugs still in use first appeared then. Some examples are castor oil, opium, and colchicine.
Specific stage	Beginning of modern era of pharmacology. It began in late Middle Ages. Based upon rational principles and understanding of mechanisms of drug actions.	Refined botanical drug products as well as synthetic drugs were developed. Examples include insulins, vitamins, antineoplastics, anesthetics, antibiotics, immunizations, tranquilizers.

akin to the use of bread and wine in the Christian church, and as such, the theological heart of the religion.

The Empirical Stage of Therapeutics

The beginnings of the mystical stage of therapeutics are rooted in antiquity without recorded details. However, as man entered the empirical stage of therapeutics, written, even detailed, records were left as testament to his developing science. *Empirical therapeutics* is based upon clinical evidence that a drug is effective, although the mechanism by which it acts is unknown. An excellent example of this can be seen in the use of the drug colchicine. This drug has been employed for thousands of years in the treatment of acute attacks of gout, although the exact mechanism of its actions was a mystery until recent years. Colchicine remains in use today for acute gout attacks.

The empirical stage of therapeutics was reached at different times in different cultures and was dependent upon many factors, such as the level of scientific and religious development of the country or region. The empirical stage of therapeutics became prominent after many years of astute clinical observations. The first recorded compilations of drugs useful in the treatment of diseases is in the Egyptian medical papyri. The empirical stage persisted until the late Middle Ages when the stage of specifics emerged and the superstitious polypharmacy beliefs were attacked. An example of empirical therapeutics can be seen today in the young, who mix a variety of medicine chest products in an attempt to produce a "high."

The Specific Stage of Therapeutics

The beginning of the *specific stage of therapeutics* occurred in the late Middle Ages when rebellious individuals such as Paracelsus (1493–1541) began to question superstitious medical beliefs. This Swiss physician-scientist advocated the use of simple, specific compounds

to treat disease. This evolutionary process was the beginning of the era of modern therapeutics. Modern therapeutics is based upon rational principles and an understanding of mechanisms of drug action. Modern drug development aims at producing drugs with great specificity of action and enhanced potency with fewer undesirable side effects.

Specific details of the history of pharmacology follow. Each stage of the development of therapeutics lasted many years. Important developments in each stage are detailed in the next few pages. Keep in mind the three stages of development as each era in history is discussed.

THE PRE-CHRISTIAN ERA

During the pre-Christian era a dichotomy in the delivery of healing services developed. There were "official" healers—medicine men or priests—who were responsible for the religious and medicinal aspects of the healing arts. These male figures enjoyed status and power in their respective social groups. There were also "unofficial" healers, women who practiced the day-to-day nurturing and caring for the aged, the infirm, and the children. This nurturing or nursing of the sick by women again denotes an early form of the profession of nursing wherein specific individuals gave care and comfort to the sick. Women in these early cultures were generally responsible for the gathering of plants, herbs, and foodstuffs.

The earliest, oldest known written prescription dates back to 2100 B.C. and is contained in a tablet recorded by the ancient Sumerians. This tablet details 15 formulas for cures: spices, minerals, cereals, botanical drugs, and animal products were the main ingredients of these healing mixtures. These mixtures were used for long periods throughout history and were later replaced by pharmaceutical preparations.

One of the oldest phases in medicine is the Egyptian

period. The Egyptians made many significant discoveries in pharmacology. The Egyptian Ebers papyrus, which is more than 3000 years old (1550 B.C.), records prescriptions for the treatment of skin ulcers, sores, and other conditions. The Ebers papyrus also recommends the use of castor oil and aloe (laxatives), opium (analgesic), colchicine (antigout), and many other drugs currently employed as therapeutic agents. These writings also recommend the application of moldy bread on bruised skin, an amazing 3500 years before Alexander Fleming's discovery of penicillin from these same molds. The Egyptians were the first to employ the use of belladonna and narcotics such as mandrake and opium. The Hebrews used the same types of drugs as the Egyptians—aloe, cassia, saffron, anise, coriander, and fennel.

The history of the healing and pharmaceutical arts of the Greeks begins with legends of gods and goddesses. The Greek legends are so intertwined with the doings of real men and women that it is often difficult to determine where facts end and fiction begins. However, since the legendary tales have left their mark upon the real world, we will begin the story with them.

Greek legend begins with the centaur Chiron who supposedly began the art of pharmacology and passed this knowledge on to Asclepios, the son of Apollo. Asclepios and his daughers, Hygeia and Panacea, taught the healing arts to mortals. They taught their craft too well and incurred the wrath of the god of the underworld because of the decreased number of departed entering the underworld of Hades. Zeus destroyed Asclepios with a thunderbolt. However, through the intercession of his father, Apollo, Zeus deified Asclepios as the god of healing. The mortal followers of Asclepios formed guilds of physicians called Asclepiades. They built temples in which they practiced the healing arts. Often the temples were in mountains near mineral springs, which served as medicinal baths. The temples themselves became healing centers (hospitals). The knowledge gained in the treatment of the sick was accumulated in the temples, which served as an early form of teaching hospital. The most celebrated of these teaching/healing centers were at Cnidus and the Island of Cos.

Hippocrates was born on the Island of Cos in 460 B.C. He was a member of a long line of priest physicians and was believed to be the seventeenth in direct descent from Asclepios. He was by far the most famous of the Asclepiades. Hippocrates was scientific in his approach to healing. He denounced the then-popular superstitious beliefs and magical incantations associated with the practice of healing. Hippocrates stressed that the healing arts were a scientific skill based upon careful clinical observations. He believed that disease was the result of natural causes and could be treated through the use of medicines derived from plant and animal products. Hippocrates taught the use of the five senses in collecting data to formulate a diagnosis, as well as the use of inductive reasoning to arrive at diagnostic conclusions. By stressing principles such as observation (assessment), diagnosis, and treatment, he made a contribution to the healing arts that is still meaningful today.

Hippocrates recorded many observations and teachings in his lifetime. Hippocrates is called the Father of Medicine because his influence has lasted through the ages, and many of his teachings underlie principles of medicine in use today. He cites over 400 drugs in his writings. He had a firm belief in the recuperative nature of man and felt that the main duty of the physician was to assist nature in the healing process. His treatments always included rest, proper diet, fresh air, massage, and hydrotherapy, as well as medication. In other words, he treated the entire person as a whole and not merely the symptoms of the disease. An interesting quote from Hippocrates' writings concerns illnesses and the ways to treat or cure them. He stated, "Those diseases that medicines do not cure are cured by the knife, those the knife does not cure are cured by fire, and those not cured by fire are incurable." Obviously the term "knife" refers to surgery. Even his use of the term "fire" has modern applications todays, as seen in the fire of the laser, which is so useful in ophthalmic, gynecologic, dermatologic, and plastic surgery. The Hippocratic Physician's Oath is often recited at medical school gradua-

Table 2–2. SELECTED DRUG DISCOVERIES

Historical Era	Drugs Discovered
2700 B.C. to 1550 B.C. (Early recorded history of man)	*Ephedra vulgaris* (Cephedrine), *Cannabis indica*, vegetable laxatives, emetics, antidiarrheals
1st century A.D.	Opium, mandragora
6th century A.D.	Colchicine, iron (for anemia)
14th century A.D.	Tinctures
16th century A.D.	Ether (cough remedy)
17th century A.D.	Cinchona, crude strychnine, ipecacuanha (Ipecac), nicotine, quinine
18th century A.D.	Crude atropine, digitalis, hyoscine, nitrous oxide (analgesic), scopolamine, smallpox vaccine
19th century A.D.	Phenylbutazone, chloral hydrate/chloroform, cocaine, crude acetylsalicylic acid, ether (anesthestic use), nitroglycerin, phenacetin, potassium bromide, procaine, radiopaque dyes, refined atropine/papaverine
20th century A.D.	Antibiotics, anticonvulsants, antihypertensives, antineoplastics, oral contraceptives, immunosuppressives, insulins, measles vaccine, narcotics, polio vaccine, steroids, synthetic vitamins, tranquilizers

tions. The first line, "First do no harm . . . ," is sometimes cited in malpractice cases.

Another famous Greek physician was Dioscorides, who lived in the first century A.D. and was a contemporary of the well-known violinist Nero. Dioscorides was quite an authority on medicines and prepared a formulary arranged according to drug source (plant, animal, mineral) rather than by disease entity. He also described methods of identification of the raw materials such as plants, preparation of the drug, methods of administration, and therapeutic indications for the use of each drug so described. Dioscorides described over 700 plants, trees, spices, and wines, many of which are still in use today. His work was the main source of the pharmaceutical knowledge of antiquity. Table 2–2 lists the dates of discovery of selected pharmaceutical agents. Keep in mind while reviewing this list that the date of discovery and the use of the drugs may vary.

EARLY POST-CHRISTIAN ERA

Greek medicine migrated to Rome after the Roman conquest of Greece. The Greek physician and scientist Galen (131–201 A.D.) was the most famous physician of this era. He based his teachings and practice largely upon the work of Hippocrates. However, he did develop a system of his own. Galen's dogmatic teachings were to dominate the field of medicine for approximately 1500 years. His teachings were based upon the erroneous supposition that health was a perfect balance of four biles in the human system. His prescriptions of formulations containing dozens of ingredients (called *galenicals*) popularized the principle of polypharmacy. Galen was the first to prepare rosewater ointment (cold cream).

The decline and fall of the Roman Empire occurred over a period of approximately 4 centuries. By the end of the fifth century A.D., hordes of Germanic tribes overran Western Europe and established their own civilizations. The Dark Ages lasted about 600 years following the fall of the Roman Empire. The medicine practiced during the era consisted of little more than superstition and folklore similar to the Greeks before Hippocrates. One of the only bright spots in learning and medicine during this era was the role played by the Catholic Church. In 311 A.D. Christianity was declared the official church of Rome by Emperor Constantine. As monasteries sprang up through Europe during the Dark Ages, their role became increasingly significant to both medicine and learning as a whole. The monks collected manuscripts and painstakingly hand-copied them, preserving works of pharmacy and medicine. In addition, those in the various religious orders cared for the sick as a part of their religious duties. The religious orders, therefore, controlled much of the knowledge of healing and medicines, and their monasteries and convents became havens where the sick sought healing. Popular medicines of the time were mistletoe, primrose, henbane, clover, wormwood, belladonna, and mandragora.

The use of some modern remedies dates back to this era. Alexander of Tralles documented the use of colchi-

cine for gout, iron for anemia, and rhubarb for dysentery and liver complaints.

There was a great Arabian influence in the history of pharmacy that began in the eighth century as the Arabs spread across the Holy Land, North Africa, Spain, and Egypt. They established hospitals and medical schools and carried forward the knowledge of Greece and Rome in medicine and pharmacy. The teachings of Hippocrates and Galen furnished much of their knowledge. The Islamic world was one of the first to separate the function of pharmacy from the practice of medicine. As early as 800 A.D. the Moslems had evolved a separate profession of pharmacists who were respected members of a health care system. Pharmacists worked in their own private apothecaries or hospital dispensaries.

Moslem pharmacists contributed a great deal of knowledge to the science of pharmacy. They were the first to use ambergris, camphor, cannabis, cassia, cloves, musk, myrrh, nutmeg, sandalwood, senna, and tamarind. The Arabs originated alcohol, aromatic water, juleps, and syrups. The Arabs also introduced the use of decimal notation, which they originally acquired from India.

The Arabs compiled great *formularies*, which added significantly to the body of pharmaceutical knowledge. The pharmacologic formularies were extensive and represented the first set of drug standards produced. This served as a model for the first London *Pharmacopeia* several hundred years later. Arabian apothecaries were inspected on a regular basis, and punishment was directed upon those who were found to be selling deteriorated or spurious drugs. This idea of standards for drugs and inspecting drugs to be sure they perform as claimed, is the basis of the laws that today govern drug production and sale.

LATE MIDDLE AGES ERA

The rise of the universities began in the eighth century with the founding of the University of Salerno. Medicine was taught there, and pharmacy was a part of the training in medicine at that time. One of the most renowned pharmaceutical authorities of this era was Nicholas of Salerno, who was director of the medical school. He wrote a book entitled *The Antidotarium*, which became the standard for pharmaceutical preparations for centuries. *The Antidotarium* contained the basic units of the apothecary's system—the grain, scruple, and dram—which are still in use today. Other universities were founded during the next 200 years, including those in Paris (1110), Bologna (1113), Oxford (1167), Cambridge (1209), and Naples (1224).

The first of the Christian Crusades occurred in 1095. A profound effect on the practice of pharmacy in central and northwest Europe occurred when Crusaders brought back Arabian science and pharmacy knowledge, which was far more refined than that of the Europeans'. By the 13th century many spices, opium, and sugar were being traded from other lands to Europe. It is interesting to note that when sugar was first brought to Europe it was costly, as were most of the spices, and the use of these items was limited to their need as ingredients in medicines of the era.

During the 13th century in Europe pharmacies began to spring up as separate entities where medicines were compounded and dispensed. Thus the Europeans began to separate the function of pharmacists from that of physicians, as the Arabs had done several centuries before. By the 14th and 15th centuries there was a great awakening in the desire for knowledge in science, medicine, and pharmacy. This Renaissance appeared toward the end of the Middle Ages, and many strides in science and medicine were made. It was also during this time that epidemic disease became prevalent. Man's quest for adventure and conquest, which was spawned by the Crusades and which brought the learning of other cultures to Europe, unfortunately also helped spread disease. Diseases such as leprosy and the bubonic plague were common. During the late Middle Ages the bubonic plague, or Black Death as it was commonly called, wiped out 25% of the human race—about 60 million people. Societal stresses such as wars, natural disasters, and communicable diseases were the impetus for many of the medical and pharmacologic discoveries following the Renaissance.

During the 15th century many medical schools were established in Europe. During this century the science of alchemy became popular because of the influence of the Arabs. It was the desire of alchemists to find the *philosopher's stone* that would change base metals into gold. It was also believed that a stone of this power could restore health and youth. Although they searched for the impossible, through this work the alchemists made many important discoveries that became the foundations for the modern science of chemistry. The invention of printing in 1438 also helped the spread of knowledge, and many of the first printed books dealt with medicine and pharmacy.

THE 16TH CENTURY

Pharmacy really began to flourish during the 16th century. Drugs and prescriptions were expensive to obtain and prepare. Because of the invention of the printing press there were many formularies or books containing directions for the preparation of various medicines. It became obvious that a single authoritative standard was necessary. Valerius Cordus, the son of a professor of medicine at Marburg, produced the first *pharmacopeia* to be printed and authorized for use in a community in 1546. The pharmacopeia published by Cordus was revised five times and was in use until 1666. Editions of this publication were also in use in Venice, Paris, Lyons, and Antwerp.

Paracelsus (1493–1541), the son of a German physician and chemist, was the most outstanding figure of the 16th century. He attacked the traditional prescribing philosophies of Galen and destroyed the "humoral pathology" Galen had founded. Paracelsus taught that diseases were actual entities that should be specifically treated. He advocated the use of simple, but specific, compounds for the treatment of disease. Paracelsus in-

troduced some new remedies such as sulfur and calomel, as well as other chemical compounds. He also tried to decrease the then-popular practice of overdosing. His theories and advances had a strong influence on the medicinal science of his era and for the following centuries. The teachings of Paracelsus marked the beginning of the specific stage in the development of the science of therapeutics.

THE 17TH CENTURY

There was great interest in the sciences of pharmacy and chemistry during the 17th century. Many new drugs came into use, some of which are still available today. The first London *Pharmacopeia* was published in 1618. This volume was sponsored by the London College of Physicians, and its use was made compulsory by pharmacists throughout the British realm by King James. The London *Pharmacopeia* was extensive and contained 1028 simple drugs and 932 preparations and compounds, the most complex preparation listing 130 ingredients. Though some of the remedies listed were effective, there were many worthless preparations listed. As pharmacologic and medical science progressed, these worthless substances were dropped in favor of medicines that produced verifiable clinical results.

Some substances introduced in the 17th century are still in use today. Tincture of benzoin, senna, the alcoholic tincture of opium (laudanum), guaiacum, cinchona, and ipecac were introduced during this century. Coca was also introduced from Peru during this century, and unfortunately for modern man, abuse of this substance has become epidemic in recent years.

THE 18TH CENTURY

The 18th century saw many advances in pharmacy and medicine, although the use of many worthless compounds still abounded since there were as yet no laws requiring that safety and efficacy of medication be proven before marketing.

English hospitals in the 18th century had nursing "sisters" who cared for the ill and dispensed medications. The designation "sisters" is probably a holdover from the days when nuns were the major providers of nursing care. Unfortunately, no training or preparation in care of the sick was necessary at this time. Many nurses were social outcasts, debtors, or criminals working off jail sentences. Patient care was understandably poor and this era is often referred to as the dark ages of nursing. It persisted until the time of Florence Nightingale.

Two extremely important advances in pharmacology were introduced in the latter part of the 18th century, and these remain important to this day. The infusion of digitalis was first introduced in 1785 by William Withering of England for the treatment of heart disease. Digitalis still remains an important drug in the treatment of heart disease. A carving of the foxglove plant, from which digitalis is obtained, decorates Withering's tombstone.

Toward the end of the 18th century English physician Edward Jenner made the second major medical advance of the 18th century when he introduced immunization for smallpox in 1796. Smallpox was one of the great killers in Europe, and, unfortunately for native Americans, it was carried to the New World as well. European settlers to the United States carried the virus with them, and it killed thousands of native Americans. Jenner began public inoculations against smallpox on May 14, 1796. It did not take the physicians of that era long to accept Jenner's theory of immunization, for there were dramatic decreases in the number of smallpox cases as a result of the acquired immunity. Immunizations against many diseases are now available, and the example of Jenner's development of smallpox vaccine has served as a model for many. It is hoped by researchers in acquired immunodeficiency syndrome (AIDS) that a similar vaccine can be devised against this modern-day virus, which has now become an epidemic.

The widespread use of immunizations can even eradicate illnesses. Smallpox is an excellent case model. In 1967 the World Health Organization (WHO) instituted a global eradication program against smallpox. The last known case of this disease in the United States occurred in 1949. On October 26, 1979, two years after the last reported case occurred in Somalia, WHO officially pronounced that smallpox was eradicated. Today variola virus, the causative agent, is found only in research laboratories, and the only current indication for smallpox vaccination is for researchers working with the virus.

THE 19TH CENTURY—TOWARD A MODERN STANDARD

During the 19th century great strides were made in medicine, chemistry, and pharmacy. Chemistry became an individual, highly specialized science, and pharmaceutical chemistry became an important subdivision. The first great pharmaceutical discovery of the 19th century occurred in 1815 when Serturner isolated the alkaloid morphine from opium in his German apothecary. The discovery of morphine was the first *active principle* (that portion of a chemical substance responsible for its therapeutic effect) to be isolated, and this led to further research on other vegetable drugs as well. Initially it was believed that morphine would lack the addictive property of opium while retaining the desirable property of analgesia. This was found not to be true, although it does indeed possess excellent analgesic quality and as such, remains a useful drug.

Many other important substances were first discovered in the 19th century. Among the drugs discovered by pharmacists were quinine, strychnine, and veratrine by Pelletier and Caventou; atropine by Brandes; emetine by Pelletier and Magendie; and codeine by Robiquet. In the 19th century it also became possible to administer drugs in more palatable forms than those previously available.

Another of the important advancements of the 19th century was the attention to accuracy of dosage. Industrialization, coupled with this interest in accuracy of dosage, led to the establishment of manufacturing plants for the production of drugs. There was a great decline in the number of drugs prescribed, since drugs that were ineffective were rapidly abandoned in favor of those that were effective. The appearance of manufacturing plants decreased the amount of actual preparation work by pharmacists. However, the pharmacist continued to be much in demand for advice on prescribing drugs. The pharmacist's main function after dispensing medication became patient teaching. This patient teaching function has become more important than ever in the administration of medications.

Drs. Morton and Wells, dentists, were the first to demonstrate successful use of ether as a general anesthetic in 1846, thereby ushering in the era of painless surgery and spawning the specialty of anesthesiology. Sir J. T. Simpson used chloroform for anesthesia in 1847.

In the 1850s numerous coal tar products were discovered. The first was discovered in 1856 by Perkins, who was searching for synthetic quinine. Instead he found a coal tar dye, which became known as "Perkin's Purple," or mauve. The synthesis of salicylic and benzoic acids occurred, as well as the discovery of new agents such as acetanilid.

Along with the explosion of new drug discoveries came efforts to maintain standards of drug preparation through the publication of authoritative publications such as national pharmacopeias. The first such volume to be produced was the French *Codex* in 1818. The first *United States Pharmacopeia (USP)* was published in 1820, and the first national standard for Great Britain in 1864 replaced those of London, Dublin, and Edinburgh.

Another of the major events occurring in the 19th century was the establishment of an organized, well-trained corps of nurses by the educator practitioner Florence Nightingale. She established the first school of nursing in the 1860s to properly educate and train women for the practice of nursing. Nightingale advocated the selection of qualified, competent, well-trained nurses who could utilize a theoretical framework to practice the profession. Her extensive writings on nursing care and health stressed a general need for reform of health and sanitary conditions as a major way to promote health and wellness. The Nightingale era was the beginning of the practice of nursing as a profession, although nursing remains an evolving profession. It is obvious from Nightingale's writings that she expected and taught nurses to assume responsibility for correct technique of medication administration as well as for the preparation and application of topical treatments.

THE 20TH CENTURY AND BEYOND

Phenomenal progress has been made in both pharmacy and medicine in the 20th century. More progress has occurred in the past 50 years than in all prior years. Many of these advances can be directly tied to the increased sophistication of medicine, chemistry, and the physical sciences. The development of the germ theory and advances in the identification of diseases and their causes have spurred pharmaceutical discoveries. In addition, laws have been developed to control the manufacture and sale of drugs. Such legislation is aimed at protecting the public from ineffective, potentially hazardous drugs by requiring that safety and efficacy be demonstrated prior to marketing. The major drug legislation—the Drug Acts of 1906 and 1938 as well as the Harrison Narcotics Act of 1914 and the Controlled Substances Act of 1970—are detailed later in this chapter.

There are two pharmaceutical landmarks early in the 20th century. First was the introduction of salvarsan for the treatment of syphilis by the German physician Ehrlich in 1907. Banting's discovery of insulin for the treatment of diabetes mellitus in 1922 was a second landmark in pharmacy/medicine. Today, it is still the major mode of treatment for millions of diabetic patients.

A virtual explosion in the development of new, more effective drugs has occurred in the last 30 years. It is estimated that nearly 80% of the drugs currently prescribed were not available 30 years ago. Indeed, most of the familiar medications we now take for granted were totally unknown a scant generation ago.

In 1929 Dr. Alexander Fleming discovered penicillin while studying molds at the University of London. He observed that the mold *Penicillium notatum* secreted an antibiotic agent that inhibited the growth of certain types of gram-positive organisms although it was not toxic to animals or to white blood cells. Fleming administered penicillin-containing broths to several patients with skin infections. Although his trial cases showed excellent clinical results, little was done to develop penicillin for the next ten years. The need for a drug to combat the massive infections of war-wounded soldiers was the impetus for the commercial development of penicillin and other antibiotics in the 1940s. Dr. Howard Florey at Oxford University is credited with the isolation of the penicillin molecule, its assay and dosage, as well as definite proof of its clinical usefulness. In 1941 the first patient was treated with penicillin. Because of World War II, it was not possible for penicillin to be mass produced in England. Dr. Florey came to the Unites States in late 1941 to ask the assistance of the National Research Council, and production of penicillin was soon begun in the United States. The first patients were treated with penicillin in the United States in 1942. Since that time literally billions of doses of penicillin have been administered. During the 1940s antihistamines, antibiotics, and glucocorticoids were developed. World War II was also an important factor spurring the development of antimalarials.

The 1950s saw the development of antihypertensives and oral contraceptives. The development of oral contraceptives forever changed the definition of the term *drug*, as well as the use of drugs. Up until this time, an accurate and acceptable definition of a drug was "a chemical used in the prevention, diagnosis, treatment, or cure of a disease." However in 1955, the advent of the Pill changed that. Millions of women were soon taking daily medication in the absence of illness, trying to prevent not an illness but rather a normal biologic function. Since pregnancy is not considered a disease, the

Pill did not fit any of the previously accepted four categories of traditional drugs. Thus, a broader definition was needed. A drug may now be defined as any chemical that is capable of interacting with living organisms to produce a biologic effect.

The year 1955 also saw the development of the poliomyelitis vaccine by Dr. Jonas Salk. The mass immunization that followed helped to rid the developed world of another dreaded disease that was responsible for many deaths as well as paralysis among survivors. Small outbreaks of polio still occur, generally in nonimmunized groups such as the Amish of Pennsylvania, although the incidence in the population as a whole peaked in the 1940s and 1950s.

The 1960s saw the development of antiviral agents and levodopa as well as an oral form of polio vaccine, the Sabin vaccine. Levodopa was a breakthrough in the management of Parkinson's disease, although it is not a cure. The oral Sabin polio vaccine is available in two forms, monovalent oral polio vaccine (MOPV) and trivalent oral polio vaccine (TOPV). The trivalent Sabin vaccine is the vaccine of choice in the immunization against polio; the Salk vaccine is rarely used today.

The 1970s saw new advances in the treatment of many illnesses along with the discovery of new drugs. Introduction of the antineoplastic antibiotics adriamycin and bleomycin occurred during this decade. In the mid-1970s cimetidine, the first commercially available histamine receptor antagonist, appeared.

During the 1980s new drugs as well as new classes of drugs have been introduced. Calcium-channel blockers, also called calcium antagonists, were originally approved by the Food and Drug Administration (FDA) for use in the treatment of arrhythmias and angina pectoris. They are also useful in the treatment of hypertension.

What does the future hold in terms of pharmacologic advances? Although there is a bit of a slowdown in the introduction of new drugs, new uses for existing drugs as well as new production methods are emerging in the 1980s. The use of genetic engineering to produce quantities of insulin and other drugs has far-reaching implications for both research and treatment. Researchers in the 1980s are also working feverishly to find drugs to treat AIDS and immunize against the AIDS virus as the scientists of the 1950s did to find a vaccine for polio.

DEVELOPMENT OF THE NURSE'S ROLE IN DRUG ADMINISTRATION

As noted in the historical section of this chapter, the administration of medicinal substances in an attempt to treat illness dates back to man's earliest days. Likewise, the presence of nurturing individuals to care for or nurse the ill predates recorded history. Although there was no organized, educated corps of nurses before Florence Nightingale opened the first nursing school in the

1860s, those who practiced nursing did administer medications. When Nightingale began her school, she stressed that nurses needed to know the correct preparation, dosage, administration technique, desired effect, and side effects of the medications they administered.

By the end of the 19th century there were many hospitals with schools of nursing. By the beginning of the 20th century nurse educators were concerned with the quality of education they provided. By 1919, the National League for Nursing's Committee on Education published the earliest curriculum guidelines for nursing schools. This volume was called the *Standard Curriculum for Schools of Nursing* and included guidelines for two courses on medication administration. The introductory course, entitled "Drugs and Solutions," was meant to familiarize students with weights, measures, solutions, and symbols used in medication administration. The name of this course has had an enduring quality and has served in all or part as the title for more than one nursing text on drug doses and calculations. The second medication course advocated in this 1919 curriculum guideline was to deal with the study of drugs, their actions, administration, and reactions (adverse effects).

The National League for Nursing has updated its curriculum standards for schools of nursing throughout the 20th century. The guidelines it advocates have always included specific objectives in the area of drugs and their administration. As new and more powerful drugs are discovered and the area of drug administration becomes increasingly complex, the potential to do great harm as well as great good lies in each medication dose administered.

Nursing textbooks dealing with drug administration have been around since the turn of the century. In 1910 a drug text was written by Anna Caroline Maxwell and Amy Elizabeth Pope. It detailed drug calculations, apothecaries' weights and measures, symbols, and pediatric dosages much the same as any modern textbook does. The nurse of 1910 could administer medications in any of the following ways: oral, subcutaneous injection, dry or steam inhalation, eye drops, or enemas. At this time nurses were already using the colored cardboard medicine tickets and medications lists that are still in use today. It is only recently that the time-honored ticket system has begun to give way to medication carts with medicine log books.

A 1928 drug administration text by Bertha Harmer detailed the many aspects of medication knowledge that the nurse needed in order to safely administer drugs. Again, the principles detailed in the pages of Harmer's text could easily fit the pages of a current text. Harmer stressed the need to know the nature and action of a drug, the local and systemic effects, minimum and maximum doses, signs and symptoms of desired as well as undesired effects, and proficiency of administration technique. In 1928 intramuscular injections as well as intravenous and hypodermoclysis administrations were performed by physicians and during the 1930s drug administration responsibilities of nurses remained virtually unchanged.

During the 1940s nurses also became responsible for the administration of intramuscular injections. The growing number of drugs available to treat illnesses, the societal crisis of World War II, and various disease epidemics caused the nurses' role in the care of the sick to undergo change to meet these new demands. In 1937 the National League for Nursing's Committee on Curriculum noted the routes by which nurses could administer medication. They included all the traditional routes up to that time, as well as the administration of anesthetics in emergency situations.

During the 1950s the administration of medications constituted a great part of the professional nurse's time. Patient teaching became an important nursing task as the nurse was often responsible for teaching the patient to self-administer insulin and other medications. Nurses also began to concern themselves with the legal aspects of medication administration much more than in the past. Nursing responsibilities also began to expand into new areas of medication administration. Gradually nurses became responsible for venipuncture and for starting intravenous infusions, previously physician-only tasks.

There has been an explosive growth in health care technology since the 1960s. New drugs, new surgical techniques, life-support systems, and improved modes of therapy for chronic illnesses, as well as an aging population, have contributed to the increasingly complex needs of today's patient population. The development of critical care units and the need for specially trained nurses to staff them have also contributed to the nurse's expanded role in medication administration and all aspects of patient care.

The 1960s was an era of rights—civil rights, individual rights, patient rights. "Right" became a watchword of sorts, denoting ideas or tasks that were good, ideal, or imperative. It was during the 1960s that the idea of the *"Five Rights"* of medication came into use. These rights are ingrained into each student nurse's consciousness. The *Five Rights* (Fig. 2–1) refer to (1) the right drug, (2) the right dose, (3) by the right route, (4) at the right time, (5) to the right patient. A sixth right, the right of the patient to refuse, is also important.

Health care technology continued to grow in the 1970s and 1980s, and nursing roles expanded to fill the new niches created. Critical-care nurses, as well as nurse practitioners and clinical nurse specialists, were often the pioneers in these expanding areas. Nurses now routinely perform venipunctures and regularly administer medications through intravenous routes, central venous pressure lines, and arterial lines, depending on hospital policy.

Nurse practitioners in at least 17 states are currently allowed to prescribe medications within certain legal constraints. By 1980 a landmark new era had occurred in nursing practice. Legislation had to be passed in these states granting nurse practitioners prescriptive authority. In these states nurse practitioners who prescribe medications are limited to medications in a drug formulary or must prescribe under the supervision of a physician, or both. States allowing nurse practitioners to

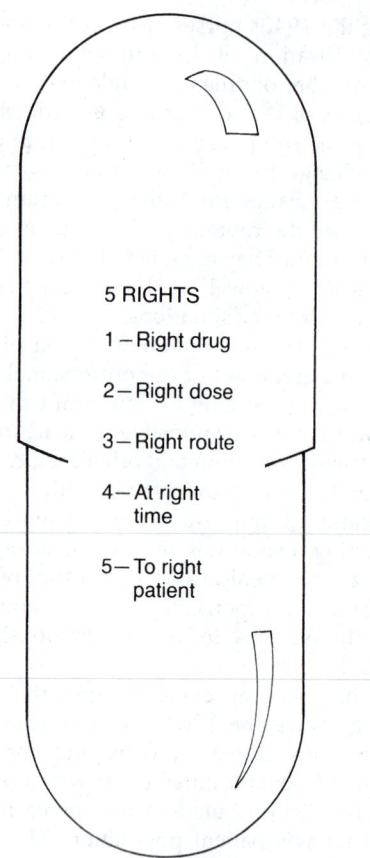

Figure 2–1. The Five Medication Rights for administering drugs.

prescribe medications include Alaska, California, Idaho, Kentucky, Maine, Maryland, Mississippi, New Hampshire, New York, New Mexico, North Carolina, Oregon, Pennsylvania, South Dakota, Tennessee, Utah, and Washington.

NEW HORIZONS IN DRUG THERAPY

The role of the professional nurse has evolved from the dependent role of "physician handmaiden" to a collaborative position in the health care team. Where once nursing practice was based upon the medical model, it is now evolving a conceptual basis of practice of its own. While no single theory of practice and unified knowledge exists, nurse theorists have proposed many useful conceptual models upon which nursing practice may be based. The nursing process, itself a theoretical tool, is a part of every nurse's daily practice. The steps of the nursing process, as detailed in Chapter 1, "The Nursing Process and Fundamentals of Drug Therapy," form a cyclic and dynamic framework upon which nurses can build to meet patient care needs relative to the administration of medications. Nursing research continues to play an integral role in medication administration as well as in other areas of nursing practice.

Administering medications to patients continues to be one of the most important—and legally most risky—aspects of nursing practice today. Nurses are responsible not only for the medications that they administer but also for the administration of medications that they direct others to give. *Liability*, a legal term denoting responsibility for a failure to act that causes harm to another (e.g., failure to administer an anticonvulsant drug, which results in patient seizures and injury), or taking an action that fails to meet minimum standards of care, thereby causing harm to another (e.g., administering a 10-fold overdose as a result of misplacing the decimal point while calculating dosage) is an important concept in the nurses' accountability for medication-related activities. Studies have shown that a frequent cause of lawsuits is related to nurse drug errors. Many drug errors can be avoided through the exercise of proper precaution and therefore are often easily preventable. Different studies in this area have reported from 9% to 30% of all malpractice claims arose from drug-related injuries (Fig. 2–2).

The preparation of drugs is another area of nursing concern. As nurses become responsible for the preparation and in some cases administration of certain drugs, notably antineoplastic agents, safety concerns have surfaced. Many antineoplastic drugs themselves are capable of producing mutagenic or carcinogenic effects, in addition to causing direct injury to eyes, skin, and mucous membranes on contact. Nurses' concerns about the safe handling of such drugs have resulted in many hospitals developing standards in this area. For detailed information on the safe handling of antineoplastic drugs refer to Chapter 48, "The Principles of Antineoplastic Chemotherapy."

Patient education and health teaching continue to grow in importance as a result of much needed concern for wellness maintenance and preventive care measures. This trend began in the 1970s as health care in general,

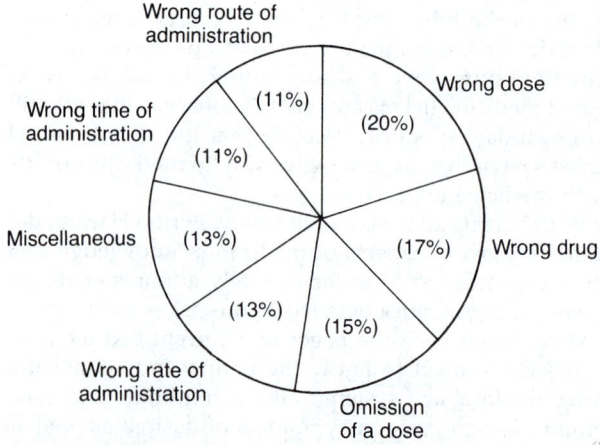

Figure 2–2. Common drug administration errors. (Adapted from Nurse's Reference Library: Practices. Nursing84 Books. Springhouse Corporation Book Division, Springhouse, PA, 1984.)

THE CLEVELAND CLINIC
9500 Euclid Avenue (At East 93rd Street)
Cleveland, Ohio 44106
Telephone No.: (216) 444-2200

NOT VALID FOR SCHEDULED DRUGS

DATE PRESCRIBED

Patient Name: History No.:

Street Address: City: State:

℞

☐ Label
☐ Do Not Refill
☐ Refill Times ______

Prescriber's Signature: ______

Prescriber's Printed Name: ______

F 37 REV. 1/83

DR. RICHARD L. SAWICKI
FELLOW AMERICAN COLLEGE OF FOOT SURGEONS
PODIATRIC MEDICINE, FOOT SURGERY AND SPORTS MEDICINE

8701 BUFFALO AVE. PHONE: 283-3338 NIAGARA FALLS, N.Y. 14304

NAME ______ AGE ______

ADDRESS ______ DATE ______

℞

THIS PRESCRIPTION WILL BE FILLED GENERICALLY UNLESS PRESCRIBER WRITES 'd a w' IN THE BOX BELOW

☐ LABEL

Dispense as Written

REFILL ______ TIMES

Figure 2–3. Samples of prescription forms currently in use. *Top* shows form used in the state of Ohio. If the prescriber wishes to allow a generic drug, then the prescriber must write out the drug to be prescribed by the generic name (furosemide rather than Lasix). *Bottom* shows form in use in New York State since July 1987. All prescriptions are filled generically unless prescriber writes DAW in box. (*Top*, Courtesy of The Cleveland Clinic, Cleveland, Ohio; *Bottom*, Courtesy of Dr. Richard L. Sawicki, Niagara Falls, New York.)

and nursing in particular, began to concentrate less on an illness model and more on health maintenance and restoration models of patient care. In the 1980s, concern over the spiraling costs of health care dramatically changed the method used by insurance companies to pay for health services. The federal government, under the Medicare program, instituted *Diagnosis Related Groups* (DRGs) to establish maximum length of hospital stays and reimbursement for various illnesses. These have quickly been adopted by private insurers. The resulting trend of discharging patients sooner has also increased the need for patient/family education on the administration of medications and observation for effectiveness and adverse effects. Nurses play an increasingly important role in patient/family teaching on medication-related matters, especially in the area of motivating patient compliance, since it is estimated that nearly half of patients do not take medications as directed.

Another big issue in the area of medications in the 1980s and beyond is generic drugs. The name-brand drug companies dominate the more than $25 billion a year market in prescription drugs. Although generic drug companies must prove that a generic version of a name-brand drug has the same amount of active ingredient and is absorbed into the bloodstream in comparable levels (called bioequivalence), the manufacturers of the original name-brand drug want physicians, pharmacists, and consumers to believe the generics are somehow inferior products. Producers of name-brand drugs spend millions of dollars promoting their products and do not wish to lose profits to generic drug companies. Name-brand drug producers cite the high cost of research and development of new drugs as a justification of higher prices. However, when a new drug is marketed, there is a period (maybe ten years or more) during which the drug enjoys patent protection; no generic versions can be produced during this time. This legal protection is designed to reward innovator drug companies and encourage them to develop new drugs, as well as to allow them to recoup research and development costs on the new drugs.

Patients are extremely concerned about the costs of medications and health care. Those with the most limited financial resources are often the patients who require the most medications. For example, although people over the age of 65 constitute approximately 12% of the population, they consume about 30% of all prescription drugs. The cost difference between a generic versus a name-brand drug can be significant. For example, a patient taking Inderal, 40 mg 3 times a day, can expect to pay almost $20.00 for a 1-month supply. The generic, propranolol hydrochloride, will cost only about $10.50 per month. The cost savings per year for such a patient would be over $125.00. In 1984, the first year of the bioequivalence law, the Federal Trade Commission (FTC) estimated that the use of generic drugs saved consumers approximately $236 million. Hospitals remain the biggest consumers of generic drugs, because their use is a significant way to cut costs without cutting services. It is thus extremely important for nurses to become familiar with the generic as well as trade names of drugs in order to avoid errors.

Generic drugs have been available since the 1970s. However, prior to the 1984 bioequivalence law it was necessary for a company to duplicate costly clinical trials rather than merely proving bioequivalence. Thus, there were not many companies producing generic drugs. Since the law went into effect, there has been an explosive increase in the production of generic drugs. Some states, such as New York, require the filling of a prescription with a generic drug if one is available. Indeed, prescription forms in New York must be filled generically unless the prescriber writes "DAW" (dispense as written) in a printed box on the form. Figure 2–3 shows samples of prescription forms.

HISTORICAL PERSPECTIVES ON DRUG STANDARDS

There was no legal control over the use or sale of any drugs until the early 1900s. This was of no particular significance because of the scarcity of effective drugs on the market. The drugs available were usually natural products prescribed and often supplied by the healer.

During the 18th and 19th centuries civilized man developed the skill to prepare and package a number of effective drugs, which the public readily embraced. The increased use of the analgesic morphine and the skyrocketing incidence of opiate addiction are testimonies to the public's awareness of drugs and their effect. The Civil War in the United States in the mid-19th century produced an incredible number of opiate addicts, partly because opium's addictive nature was not fully recognized and partly because there were no laws restricting the use or sale of drugs that we now know to be dangerous. There were likewise no laws protecting the public from bogus concoctions sold by patent medicine or "snake oil" salesmen. These mixtures generally consisted mainly of alcohol with flavorings and were touted as miracle cures for anything from cancer to bunions. Unfortunately, since the public readily believed in such quick cures, the patent medicine business was, indeed, a booming one.

The publication of the *United States Pharmacopeia (USP)* in 1820 was the first attempt to standardize drug purity. This widely recognized reference lists all approved medicines by the official name (generic); defines drugs as to source and physical and chemical properties; lists drug category, dosage, and method of storage; and provides tests for the purity and identity of an unknown compound. The *USP* is revised and updated every 5 years. Drugs are deleted when clinical use shows unacceptably high toxicity or when newer, more effective agents are developed. Originally, the *USP* restricted its coverage to single drugs. However, by the turn of the last century, it was apparent that a reference was needed for mixtures and formulas. The *National Formulary (NF)* in 1888 became such a reference and was a supplement to the *USP*. Gradually both books included both single- and multiple-drug mixtures. The *USP* was formerly the more up-to-date volume, while the *NF* continued to list drugs no longer commonly prescribed. The two books have been combined and are now called the *USP-NF*.

UNITED STATES DRUG LEGISLATION

A discussion of important United States drug legislation will be covered in this section. The important drug laws are summarized in Table 2–3, Summary of the United States Drug Laws. The Federal Food, Drug and Cos-

Table 2–3. SUMMARY OF UNITED STATES DRUG LAWS

Drug Legislation	Summary of Law
Federal Food, Drug and Cosmetic Act of 1906	First federal law designed to protect the public by restricting manufacture and sale of drugs. Set *USP* and *NF* as official standards and gave federal government authority to enforce standards. All drugs sold had to meet strength and purity standards.
Sherley Amendment of 1912	Added to FFDCA; prohibited use of fraudulent therapeutic claims by drug manufacturers.
Harrison Narcotic Act of 1914	First federal law aimed at curbing drug addiction and dependence. Established word *narcotic* as legal term.
Federal Food, Drug and Cosmetic Act of 1938	Made it mandatory for companies to perform toxicity tests on lab animals prior to seeking FDA approval to market any new drug. Labels and other literature must be included with all prescription drugs listing possible harmful effects. Requires medical devices to be safe and effective; cosmetics must be safe. FDA has power to prevent marketing or recall from market any drug it deems unsafe or not adequately tested.
Durham-Humphrey Amendment of 1952	First law to recognize class of drugs that could be sold OTC without a prescription. Two categories of drugs then existed: OTCs and prescription.
Drug Amendment of 1962 (Kefauver-Harris Act)	Required all drugs not only to be safe, but also to be proven *effective* before marketing. Also required all drugs marketed between 1938 and 1962 to be tested for effectiveness. There are five categories in addition to "effective" ("possibly effective," "probably effective," and so on). All drugs in classes other than "effective" must be so designated and upgraded to the "effective" rating or removed from the market within FDA-set time limits.
Controlled Substances Act of 1970	Strengthened existing law enforcement in area of drug abuse, provided increased research into drug abuse prevention and treatment, developed five schedules (categories) of drugs based upon abuse potential and medical effectiveness. Schedule I drugs are those with highest abuse potential and are available only for research purposes. All controlled substances have set limits on the number of times a prescription can be refilled.
Drug Regulation and Reform Act of 1978	Allows a shorter period of time for new drug investigative efforts, thus speeding up ability to get new drugs to the public.
Drug Price Competition and Patent Term Restoration Act of 1984	Allows generic drug companies to market generic drugs by proving bioequivalence rather than duplicating original companies' clinical trials. Also grants longer patent protection on new drugs.

metic Act (FFDCA) of 1906 was the first federal law designed to protect the public by restricting the manufacture and distribution of drugs. This law designated the *USP* and *NF* as the official standards and empowered the federal government to enforce those standards. All drugs sold were required to meet the strength and purity standards set down by the *USP* and *NF*. The FFDCA of 1906 was designed to protect the public from the "manufacture of adulterated or misbranded or poisonous or deleterious foods, drugs, medicines, and liquors." It also required that any drug containing an opiate must state on the label the type and amount of narcotic included. In 1912 the Sherley Amendment was added to the FFDCA. This amendment increased federal involvement in the manufacture and sale of drugs by prohibiting the use of fraudulent therapeutic claims. In recent years the Sherley Amendment was cited by the federal government in the prosecution of several aspirin producers. The government contended that the companies' advertisements contained misleading claims about the effectiveness of their products. As a result of the government lawsuit, the offending companies changed their advertisements.

The FFDCA of 1906 was a beginning step in terms of drug legislation. It helped correct some of the flagrant abuses of the era but did little to ensure the safety of drugs. Several legislative attempts to ensure drug safety for over 20 years following the FFDCA met with little success until a tragedy in 1937 made it clear that drugs must be tested to ensure safety *before* marketing is done.

In 1937 an elixir of sulfanilamide was marketed. The manufacturer used diethylene glycol as a solvent for the then-new anti-infective sulfanilamide. Because its pharmacologic effects were not tested in animals prior to marketing, its toxicity went undiscovered until reports of patient deaths came pouring in. Over 100 lives were lost in this unfortunate incident, and the public outcry to Congress in its wake resulted in new legislation to help guarantee greater safety in prescription drug products. It is difficult to believe that at one time drugs, or any product, would have been marketed without extensive prior testing.

The Federal Food, Drug and Cosmetic Act of 1938 was passed, making it mandatory for manufacturers to perform toxicity tests in laboratory animals before seeking approval from the FDA to market any new drug. This law empowered the FDA to keep a drug from being marketed and to order drug recalls if the agency decided that its safety was not adequately tested or that the drug was too dangerous for the use for which it was intended.

An important area of focus of the 1938 FFDCA was the drug label. Specific requirements for all drug labels were outlined. All drug labels must contain the following:

1. No false or misleading statements
2. The dose or frequency of use suggested. (The recommended or prescribed dose must not be toxic.)
3. The name and business address of the manufacturer, packer, or distributor
4. A list of the amount of all habit-forming drugs in a product, as well as the statement, "Warning—May Be Habit Forming"
5. The kind, quantity, and proportion of certain specified ingredients, including alcohol, atropine, digitalis, and a number of other agents that could be harmful to certain individuals
6. Adequate directions for safe use and warnings against unsafe use by children, pregnant women, and persons with pathologic conditions
7. During an experimental testing period, the statement, "Caution New Drug—Limited by Federal Law to Investigational Use"

The FFDCA was amended in 1945 and expanded to require that certain drugs such as insulin and antibiotics must be from a batch certified by the federal government before sale. The FFDCA was further amended in 1952 by the Durham-Humphrey Amendment, which was the first law to recognize over-the-counter (OTC) drugs. This allowed certain drugs such as aspirin to be sold without a prescription.

From 1938 to 1962 the approval of new drugs was based solely upon proof of safety for use in humans. Senator Estes Kefauver of Tennessee tried to initiate an investigation into the drug industry when it became known that many drug companies were raking in huge profits and some of the drug promotion was false and misleading. The Senators' efforts were largely ignored until the thalidomide tragedy. Thalidomide is a hypnotic sedative that causes toxicity in humans. When it was marketed in Europe in the early 1960s, that toxicity was unforeseen, and use of thalidomide by pregnant women in the early stages of pregnancy resulted in the birth of hundreds of deformed babies in Europe. The drug affects limb development, and many of the deformed babies were born without arms, legs, or any limbs. Some were born with stunted limbs. A tragedy of this scale was avoided in the United States because thalidomide was not yet marketed here. However, babies were born in the United States with thalidomide-associated deformities when women who traveled abroad obtained the drug outside this country.

Again, public outcry over the tragedy spurred the legislature to action. The Kefauver-Harris Amendment was passed in 1962, and this law went into effect in 1963. This law requires that both safety and efficacy of a drug be proven before it is marketed. This act also required that all drugs marketed between 1938 and 1962 be evaluated for effectiveness.

To facilitate the tremendous task of evaluating all drugs introduced between 1938 and 1962, the FDA signed a contract in 1966 with the National Academy of Sciences and its research arm, the National Research Council (NAS-NRC), to independently study all supporting data for therapeutic claims. This study was called the Drug Efficacy Study Implementation (DESI). According to the study, each drug would be rated for effectiveness and designated by one of the following categories:

Effective: There is substantial evidence of effectiveness.
Probably effective: Additional evidence is required to rate the drug effective.
Possibly effective: Effectiveness might be shown eventually, but at the present time there is little evidence of efficacy.
Ineffective: There is no substantial evidence of effectiveness.

Two other ratings were also developed, and these were as follows:

Ineffective as a fixed combination: Even though one or more components might be effective if used alone, the product is not acceptable in fixed-dosage combination for reasons of safety or because there is no evidence of contribution of each component to claimed effect.
Effective but: Although effective, there is an appropriate qualification or restriction imposed on the drug, which is still under consideration by the NAS-NRC and the FDA; the drug is effective for some recommended uses but not for all, thus requiring label changes.

Thousands of drugs and therapeutic claims were studied and the "ineffective" drugs were withdrawn from the market. Those drugs rated "possibly effective" or "probably effective" were withdrawn or reformulated. The drugs were allowed to remain on the market while claims were being modified and scientific data collected. Drugs classified "probably effective" and "possibly effective" had to be upgraded to the "effective" category within a time limit set by the FDA, or the drug would be withdrawn from the market. Drug ratings are required to be prominently displayed on the label. Substantial evidence of effectiveness must be in the form of adequate, well-controlled scientific and clinical investigations by qualified experts. Uncontrolled observations and testimonial-type endorsements are not acceptable scientific evidence.

The two most recent drug laws passed deal with the development of prescription drugs. The first deals with the development of new drugs and the second with the marketing of generic drugs. In 1978 the Drug Regulation and Reform Act was passed. This law allows for a shorter period of time for new drug investigative efforts, thereby speeding the release of new drugs to the public. The second law, The Drug Price Competition and Patent Term Restoration Act of 1984, had 2 major components: The first made it possible for generic drug companies to market generic versions of drugs by proving bioequivalence rather than duplicating costly clinical trials done when the drugs were introduced. The second provision was to grant longer patent protection to innovator drug companies for the discovery of new drugs.

CONTROLLED SUBSTANCES LAWS

The Harrison Narcotic Act passed in 1914 was the first federal law aimed at curbing drug addiction and dependence. It was also the first narcotic act passed by any nation and established the word "narcotic" as a legal term. This law regulated the importation, manufacture, sale, and use of opium, cocaine, marijuana, and all their compounds and derivatives, as well as other synthetic compounds capable of physical or psychologic dependence.

The most significant drug legislation of the modern era is the Comprehensive Drug Abuse Prevention and Control Act of 1970, which is also known as the Controlled Substances Act. This law was passed in an effort to control the rapidly increasing problem of drug abuse and misuse in the United States. The Controlled Substances Act went into effect May 1, 1971. In addition to providing increased research into drug abuse prevention and treatment of drug dependency, it also strengthened existing law enforcement and established drug schedules. In July of 1983 the Drug Enforcement Administration (DEA) in the Department of Justice became the nation's sole legal drug enforcement agency. The DEA replaced the Bureau of Narcotics and Dangerous Drugs.

In an effort to better control drug distribution and assist with the campaign against drug abuse, a classification system was developed to categorize drugs according to their abuse potential. Controlled drugs are placed into different schedules to which different regulations apply. There are five different schedules of drugs, Table 2–4 lists controlled drugs in their appropriate schedules.

SCHEDULE I

Drugs in Schedule I are available only for research (investigative) purposes. There is no other legal use for drugs in this schedule. A separate research registration and clearance from the FDA are required before any drug in Schedule I can be legally obtained. The only exception is the use of peyote by native Americans in religious rituals. Examples of drugs in Schedule I are heroin, LSD, MDA, mescaline, and psilocybin.

SCHEDULE II

Drugs in this class have accepted therapeutic uses but also have a high potential for abuse. Drugs in this class are known to be physically and/or psychologically addictive. Dependence on these drugs may readily develop if they are taken for extended periods of time or misused. Drugs in this class include amphetamines, cocaine, morphine, opium, and some barbiturates.

Prescriptions for substances in Schedule II may not be refilled; the physician must write each prescription anew. In the hospital setting an order written with a dosage schedule and an as-needed (prn) notation such as "Tuinal capsule at hs prn" is no longer valid after 72 hours. The physician must rewrite the order every three days if he wants the patient to continue to receive the medication. Hospital orders listing specific dosing schedules such as "Valium 5 mg qid" are no longer valid after 7 days and must be reordered by the physician at that time. The above reordering regulations apply to all drugs in Schedules II, III, IV, and V. In emergency situations the physician is allowed to prescribe a Schedule II substance over the telephone. The nurse obtaining such an order must record it in the patient's chart, and it must then be countersigned by the physician within 48 hours of the verbal order.

SCHEDULE III

Drugs included in Schedule III have a lower abuse potential than those in either Schedule I or II, although they may also be abused. Examples of some drugs in this class are codeine in combination with non-narcotic drugs, paregoric, butabarbital (Butisol), and some weaker stimulants such as maxindol. Telephone orders by physicians for drugs in Schedules III and IV are acceptable. Prescriptions for drugs in Schedules III and IV must be rewritten every six months or after five refills, whichever comes first.

SCHEDULE IV

Schedule IV is similar to Schedule III except for the penalties for obtaining drugs in this class illegally (illegal possession of controlled substances). Examples of some drugs included in this class are propoxyphene (Darvon), chlordiazepoxide (Librium), and diazepam (Valium). It should be noted that drugs in this class are also subject to abuse, and as a matter of fact, some drugs in this class have become quite popular among drug abusers. Oftentimes, patients become psychologically addicted or habituated to drugs of this class (especially tranquilizers and sleeping pills) without realizing they have become dependent. ("Those aren't habit-forming; I take them all the time.")

SCHEDULE V

According to federal law the drugs listed in Schedule V have a low abuse potential, do not require a prescription, and may be sold over the counter. However, most states have stricter laws than the federal statutes and therefore do require a prescription for drugs in Schedule V. Those states that do require prescriptions for drugs listed in Schedule V follow the same regulations as for drugs in Schedules III and IV. In those states where the federal law is observed (no prescription required) pharmacies are allowed to dispense only specific amounts of drugs within a specific time period. Both the drug and the time it was dispensed must be recorded in a ledger book signed by the pharmacist and the patient.

Table 2–4. SCHEDULES OF CONTROLLED DRUGS IN THE UNITED STATES

SCHEDULE I:
All nonresearch use forbidden
Narcotics heroin, cocaine
Hallucinogens
  LSD
  MDA, STP, DMT, DET, mescaline, peyote, bufoteneine, ibogaine, psilocybin, marijuana

SCHEDULE II:
No telephoned prescriptions, no refills
Narcotics
  Opium
  Opium alkaloids and derived phenanthrene alkaloids: Morphine, codeine, hydromorphone (Dilaudid), oxymorphone (Numorphan), oxycodone (14-hydroxydihydrocodeinone, a component of Percodan)
  Designated synthetic drugs: Meperidine (Demerol), alphaprodine (Nisentil), anileridine (Leritine), methadone, levorphanol (Levo-Dromoran), phenazocine (Prinadol)
Stimulants
  Coca leaves and cocaine
  Amphetamine
  Dextroamphetamine
  Methamphetamine
  Phenmetrazine (Preludin)
  Methylphenidate (Ritalin)
  Above in mixtures with other controlled or uncontrolled drugs (Dexamyl, Eskatrol)
Depressants
  Amobarbital
  Pentobarbital
  Secobarbital
  Mixtures of above (Tuinal)
  Phencyclidine (PCP)
Anti-emetic
  THC (tetrahydrocannabinol)—Nabilone

SCHEDULE III
Prescription must be rewritten after 6 months or 5 refills
Narcotics
  The following opiates in combination with one or more active non-narcotic ingredients, provided the amount does not exceed that shown:
  Codeine and dihydrocodeine: Not to exceed 1800 mg/dl or 90 mg/tablet or other dose unit
  Dihydrocodeinone (hydrocodone and in Hycodan): Not to exceed 300 mg/dl or 15 mg/tablet
  Opium: 500 mg/dl, or 25 mg/5 ml, or other dosage unit (paregoric)
Narcotic antagonist
  Nalorphine
Depressants
  Schedule II barbiturates in mixtures with uncontrolled drugs or in suppository dose form
  Butabarbital (Butisol)
  Glutethimide (Doriden)
  Methyprylon (Noludar)
Stimulants
  Benzphetamine (Didrex)
  Chlorphentermine (Pre-Sate)
  Diethylpropion (Tenuate)
  Maxindol (Sanorex)
  Phendimetrazine

SCHEDULE IV
Prescription must be rewritten after 6 months or 5 refills. Differs from Schedule III in penalties for illegal possession
Narcotics
  Pentazocine (Talwin)
  Propoxyphene (Darvon)
Stimulants
  Phentermine
  Fenfluramine (Pondimin)
Depressants
  Benzodiazepines
    Chlordiazepoxide (Librium)
    Clonazepam (Clonopin)
    Clorazepate (Tranxene)
    Diazepam (Valium)
    Flurazepam (Dalmane)
    Halazepam (Paxipam)
    Lorazepam (Ativan)
    Oxazepam (Serax)
    Prazepam (Verstran)

Table 2–4. SCHEDULES OF CONTROLLED DRUGS IN THE UNITED STATES–*CONTINUED*

> Quazepam
> Triazolam (Halcion)
> Chloral hydrate
> Ethchlorvynol (Placidyl)
> Ethinamate (Valmid)
> Meprobamate
> Mephobarbital (Mebaral)
> Paraldehyde
> Phenobarbital
>
> **SCHEDULE V**
> *As any other (non-narcotic) prescription drug; may also be dispensed without prescription unless additional state regulations apply*
> **Narcotics**
> Diphenoxylate (not more than 2.5 mg and not less than 0.025 mg of atropine per dosage unit, as in Lomotil)
> Loperamide (Imodium)
> The following drugs in combination with other active non-narcotic ingredients and provided the amount per 100 ml or 100 g does not exceed that shown:
> Codeine: 200 mg
> Dihydrocodeine: 100 mg
> Ethylmorphine: 100 mg

DRUG SCHEDULE CHANGES

It should be noted that drugs may be moved from one schedule to another. For example, propoxyphene (Darvon) was listed as a Schedule V drug several years ago. However, because of its increasing popularity for misuse and abuse, as well as its frequent involvement in overdose situations, it was moved up from Schedule V to Schedule IV. Likewise, a drug can be moved from a more restrictive class to a less restrictive one, such as from Schedule I to Schedule II. This occurred in the case of THC (tetrahydrocannabinol). This substance was listed on Schedule I for many years (investigational use only) until a legitimate clinical use for it was recently discovered: tetrahydrocannabinis (an active ingredient found in marijuana) possesses antiemetic properties especially helpful for patients undergoing cancer chemotherapy.

POSSESSION AND HANDLING OF NARCOTICS

It is unlawful for an individual to possess a controlled substance (illegal possession) unless it has been obtained by a valid prescription or order, or unless its possession is pursuant to the course of professional practice. Whenever a nurse administers controlled substances such as narcotics from stock supplies, the date, time of administration, drug name and dose, prescriber's name, patient's name, and administering nurse's name must all be recorded in the narcotics log. Stock supplies of narcotics must be kept in locked medicine cabinets or carts, and nurses are responsible for accurate accounting of all narcotics dispensed on their units. The nurse coming on duty generally double-checks the drug count with the nurse whose shift is ending.

When narcotics are ordered for patients and are not used, they must be returned to their origination point, such as the hospital pharmacy. Likewise, if a dose of narcotic is contaminated, such as when a tablet accidentally falls on the floor, it should also be returned to the pharmacy and marked as a contaminated dose. Some hospitals have narcotic return envelopes to return contaminated or refused doses of narcotics. Such doses must be signed for on the narcotics log as returned to pharmacy. The handling of controlled substances is a responsibility that should never be taken lightly. It is a crime for any individual to transfer a drug listed in Schedule II, III, or IV to anyone other than the patient for whom it was ordered. Violation of the Controlled Substances Act can result in fine, imprisonment, or both. Any nurse who violates this Act is also subject to loss of license and the right to practice nursing.

DEVELOPMENT OF NEW DRUGS

The development of a new drug begins with animal screenings to determine possible uses. New chemicals or drugs are first given to several different species of animals in an effort to determine a data base for pharmacologic use, adverse effects, and possible toxic effects. The dosage range is studied in various animals, and the minimum effective dose, effective dose, and toxic or lethal dose are determined. This type of testing can indicate possible drug actions and warn of probable dangers. Although this testing provides necessary background information, there is not yet an animal model that compares perfectly to the human model. The animal studies serve as a basis for the consideration of human studies. The FDA reviews the animal study data for safety and effectiveness before it decides whether to approve the application for Investigational New Drug (IND).

Three phases of testing occur in human subjects once IND status is granted by the FDA. These studies must provide evidence of efficacy, safety, and risk-to-benefit ratio for the new drug intended for human use. The risk-to-benefit ratio concerns itself with the risks of drug side effects or toxicity versus benefits to be obtained by taking the medication. For example, a potential antineoplastic drug or AIDS drug would be allowed more latitude of risk since the potential benefits of such drugs are worth the risk.

PHASE 1 CLINICAL STUDIES

This stage of drug development focuses on small studies of healthy volunteers under the supervision of a clinical pharmacologist. The volunteers are given the new substance and observed for absorption, distribution, metabolism, and excretion of the drug. All effects of the substance upon the volunteers are recorded and provide information useful in determining the potential of future testing.

PHASE 2 CLINICAL STUDIES

In this phase of study a small select group of volunteers determines the potential use of the substance in actual disease and determines more closely proper dosing for the achievement of therapeutic goals. Patients are again closely observed for any dangerous side effects or toxic effects. Data from long-term animal studies are also reviewed and compared to the human results. Animal studies are also observed to determine what effects, if any, the substance has upon fertility and reproduction. The refinement of dosage is generally achieved in this phase.

PHASE 3 CLINICAL TRIALS

In this phase of study large numbers of patients are treated with the substance to determine adverse effects, safety, and efficacy. Most of the risks associated with therapy are discovered at this time. Double-blind studies in which neither patient nor researcher knows if the drug or a placebo (inactive substance) was given are often used since this type of study reduces bias.

POST-MARKET SURVEILLANCE

Once all 3 phases of study are complete, the data are reviewed and evaluated by the FDA. If it finds the drug to be safe and effective, then a New Drug Application (NDA) is granted to the innovator drug company. After the NDA is approved, a post-market surveillance begins. The drug company markets the drug but keeps careful records on the results of therapy on patients, which are provided by the medical profession. The drug company must advise the FDA of any adverse effects and updates on therapy. During the years of use of a newly patented drug, the drug company is responsible for protecting the public by providing necessary updates. Sometimes a medication is discovered to be toxic in some patients, and this is only discovered in the post-market surveillance phase. Sometimes such effects are not readily observable in test populations but do become evident when a drug is marketed to large groups where rare toxic effects are noted. Such was the case several years ago when the drug Zomax was introduced. It was subsequently withdrawn from the market because of fatalities in some patients who took the drug.

CANADIAN DRUG LEGISLATION

Canadian drug laws developed in a fashion similar to that in the United States. The first Canadian drug legislation in 1875 prevented the sale of adulterated food, drink, and drugs.

The Drugs Directorate of Health Protection Branch, Department of Health and Welfare, is responsible for administering the Food and Drug Acts of Canada. The Canadian Food and Drug Acts control the research and development of new drugs, drug advertising, and product information, as well as the continuous monitoring of the safety of all drug products. The distribution of all potentially addictive drugs is also controlled by these Acts. Table 2–5 is a summary of Canadian federal and provincial laws governing prescription drug ordering, records, prescription requirements, and refills.

The most recent Canadian drug legislation is the Narcotic Control Act of 1982. This law is similar in scope to the 1970 United States Comprehensive Drug Abuse Prevention and Control Act. As in the United States, the Canadian law designates classifications of drugs with category of placement dependent upon the abuse potential of the substances involved. The classifications of the Canadian Narcotic Control Act are summarized in Table 2–5. The Canadian drug schedule lists stimulants, barbiturates, and drugs subject to potential abuse in section G of their categorization.

In Canada, as in the United States, strict accounting of all narcotic and hypnotic drugs dispensed must be kept by nurses. Hospital log records must contain the following information for each controlled drug administered: patient name, prescriber's name, medication name, date and time of administration, name of administering nurse, and the number of remaining doses in the package. These hospital records are kept by the hospital pharmacy. In Canada any nurse, physician, or pharmacist engaged in the illegal transportation or distribution of drugs may be held liable and subjected to criminal prosecution and penalties.

PATIENT PACKAGE INSERTS

Patient Package Inserts (PPIs) remain a controversial topic at this time. Although PPIs were developed for use in estrogens, estrogen products, and oral contraceptives and have been in use for some time with these products, no new PPIs have been developed since then. These information sheets with complete drug information for patient use had been proposed by the federal government for inclusion in all prescription drugs. However, their introduction was delayed because of opposition from most state regulatory agencies. The state agencies that oppose PPIs feel that the complex information obtained in them would not be wisely used or would be misunderstood by the average patient and would, therefore, be more detrimental than helpful to the patient. This system has spawned efforts to increase patient education activities in hospitals. Some drug companies have developed "commercial PPIs" for use by the health care worker in patient teaching. Patients are actively pursuing health information more than ever before. There has been explosive growth of consumer information drug books in recent years.

COMMUNITY AND INSTITUTIONAL DRUG REGULATIONS

When the laws of a community or state or the regulations of an institution differ substantially from the federal laws governing pharmaceuticals, the strictest law generally applies. The most obvious examples are Schedule V drugs in the United States, which federal law says may be dispensed without a prescription. Many states, however, have enacted requirements that these drugs must be dispensed by prescription only. Thus, in those states the strictest law, the one requiring the prescription, applies. The nurse should be familiar with all local, state, and federal laws concerning pharmaceuticals so as to practice within the regulations. Always check institutional policies when beginning a new job so that you follow procedure correctly.

INTERNATIONAL DRUG CONTROL EFFORTS

The first attempt to control drugs at the international level through legal means and treaties occurred in 1912 at the first "Opium Conference," held at the Hague. At that time international treaties were drawn up that legally obligated governments to do the following: (1) limit to medicinal and scientific needs the manufacture and trade of opium, (2) control the production and distribution of raw opium, and (3) establish a system of governmental licensing to control the manufacture and trade of drugs covered by the convention.

Government representatives in 1961 formed the Single Convention on Narcotic Drugs, which took effect in 1964. This act consolidated all existing treaties into one document for the control of all narcotic substances by the following: (1) outlawing the production, manufacture, trade, and use of narcotics for nonmedical purposes; (2) limiting the possession of all narcotic substances to authorized persons for medical and scientific purposes; (3) providing for international control of all opium transactions by the national monopolies (countries such as Turkey, which are designated to produce opium) and authorizing production only by licensed farmers in areas and on plots designated by these monopolies; and (4) requiring import certificates and export authorizations as a means of better control.

Obviously the task of enforcing such laws is monumental. An International Narcotics Control Board was established to enforce the international drug laws; however, it is not possible to stem the tide of illegal drug traffic completely. The illegal drug industry has become a multibillion-dollar-a-year industry with equipment and techniques that are state-of-the-art and often superior to the surveillance equipment of law enforcement officials. In recent years the tremendous popularity of cocaine as a drug of abuse has multiplied the problem of illegal drug traffic 100-fold. As always, the opiates remain popular drugs of abuse. Drug enforcement officials cite the following staggering statistic in relation to their job: in 1 year an estimated 1200 tons of opium are circulated in the illegal drug market in contrast to the 800 tons that are handled through proper channels and that are sufficient for world medical needs.

International drug control efforts continue. Laws in this area continue to be modified as needed and enforcement efforts are being stepped up on an international level. The United States has had several high-level meetings and has updated treaties in Central America in order to help reduce the tremendous traffic in illegal cocaine.

SUMMARY

Historical perspectives and pharmacologic developments have been traced throughout mankind's brief history on earth. Artifacts left by ancient peoples show that though there was a lack of scientific basis for their use, there were attempts at treating and curing illness. Recorded history begins with writings that show that early medicinal efforts were largely mystical—based upon magic, prayers, and in some cases, crude surgery. Some drugs were used that did provide actual relief of physical symptoms. A period of empirical therapeutics followed as man began to base therapy upon clinical evidence of medication effectiveness, even though the mechanism of drug action was as yet unknown. The specific stage of therapeutics emerged in the late Middle Ages as awareness of science developed and questions arose about the superstitious nature of medicinal beliefs. By the 19th century the science of chemistry was beginning to develop effective drugs, and toward the end of this century, a formalized educational program for nurses emerged. As medical science and chemical advances occurred the health care delivery system became more complex. Nurses have become responsible for intramuscular injections, venipuncture, intravenous drug administrations, and nurses with advanced degrees (nurse practitioners) can even prescribe medications under certain conditions in many states. The nurses' role has changed dramatically in an effort to keep pace with the evolving health care technologies of our modern era.

The task of administering medications remains one of the most time-consuming and highly risky aspects of nursing practice. There are well over a thousand prescription agents available today. It is the nurses' responsibility to know about the drugs and laws governing the

TEXT RESUMES ON PAGE 46

Table 2–5. SUMMARY OF CANADIAN FEDERAL AND PROVINCIAL LAWS GOVERNING PRESCRIPTION DRUG ORDERING, RECORDS, PRESCRIPTION REQUIREMENTS, AND REFILLS

Classification	Description	Ordering
Narcotic Drug (N) Schedule N drugs e.g., codeine, Demerol, Dilaudid, Leritine, Lomotil, morphine, Hycodan, Corutol-DH, Robidone, Tylenol #4, Percodan, Percocet, Tussionex, Novahistex-DH, Numorphan.	All straight narcotic drugs. All narcotic drugs for parenteral use. All narcotic compounds containing more than 1 narcotic drug. All narcotic compounds containing less than 2 other non-narcotic ingredients. All products containing hydrocodone and oxycodone.	Written or electronic. Written orders must be signed by the manager. The receipt for electronic orders must be signed by the pharmacist who received the drug and this receipt shall be provided to the licensed dealer within 5 working days.
Narcotic Preparations (N) (Oral prescription narcotics) Schedule N preparations e.g., AC with codeine 15, 30, or 60 mg, Cheracol, Cophylac Expectorant, Tylenol #2, #3.	All combinations containing only 1 narcotic drug and 2 or more non-narcotic medicinal ingredients in a recognized therapeutic dose not intended for parenteral use.	Verbal, written, or electronic. Written orders must be signed by the manager. The receipt for verbal or electronic orders must be signed by the pharmacist who received the drug and this receipt shall be provided to the licensed dealer within 5 working days.
Controlled Drugs (C) Schedule G Drugs e.g., Dexedrine, Mequelon, Nembutal, Seconal, Talwin, Tuinal.	All straight controlled drugs. All combinations containing more than 1 controlled drug.	Written or electronic. Written orders must be signed by the manager. The receipt for electronic orders must be signed by the pharmacist who received the drug and this receipt shall be provided to the licensed dealer within 5 working days.
Controlled Drug Preparations Schedule G preparations e.g., Carbrital, Mandrax, Talwin Compound.	All combinations containing only 1 controlled drug and 1 or more medicinal ingredients in a recognized therapeutic dose.	Verbal, written, or electronic. Written orders must be signed by the manager. The receipt for verbal or electronic orders must be signed by the pharmacist who received the drug and this receipt shall be provided to the licensed dealer within 5 working days.
Controlled drugs in Schedule to Part G of Regulation (C) e.g., Amytal, Butisol, Daybarb, Donnatal, Mebaral, Plexonal, Pre-Sate, Tenuate, Ritalin, Ionamin, Amesec, Tedral.	Barbituric acid (except secobarbital and pentobarbital), butorphanol, chlorphentermine, diethylpropion, methylphenidate, nalbuphine, phentermine, thiobarbituric acid and their salts and derivatives. All combinations containing only 1 controlled drug listed listed above and 1 or more medicinal ingredients in a therapeutic dose.	
Schedule E and F Drugs (Pr) e.g., antibiotics, antidepressants, antipsychotics, steroids, oral contraceptives.	All drugs listed in Schedule F of Food and Drug Regulations. All drugs listed in Schedule E of the Health Disciplines Act.	Verbal, written, or electronic.

NOTES: This is a summary. For complete details, reference should be made to the official information.
Prescriptions must be held in sequence as to date and number.
Prescriptions must be retained for not less than 6 years.
Drug names used are for illustrative purposes only. Not a complete listing.

Purchase Record	Sales Record	Prescription Requirements	Refills
Purchases must be recorded in Narcotic and Controlled Drug Register or other record maintained for such purposes.	Prescription on Narcotic and Controlled Drug file plus record of sales in Narcotic and Controlled Drug Register or in a computer from which a printout may be obtained on request.	A written prescription signed and dated by a physician, dentist, or veterinarian. On dispensing must show the information listed below.	Refills not permitted. All "re-orders" must be new written prescriptions. Narcotics may be prescribed to be dispensed in divided portions, subject to professional discretion.
	Prescription on Narcotic and Controlled Drug file. No record of sales in Narcotic and Controlled Drug Register required.	A written or verbal prescription by a physician, dentist, or veterinarian. Verbal prescriptions must be received by a pharmacist, intern, or registered pharmacy student under the supervision of a pharmacist. All prescriptions on dispensing must show: Name and address of patient Name, strength, quantity, and form of drug Manufacturer of drug Directions for use Name and address of prescriber Identification number Price charged Date of dispensing Signature of dispenser and when different, signature of person receiving verbal prescription.	Refills not permitted. All "re-orders" written or verbal must be new prescriptions. Narcotics may be prescribed to be dispensed in divided portions, subject to professional discretion.
	Prescription on Narcotic and Controlled Drug file plus record of sales in Narcotic and Controlled Drug Register or in a computer from which a printout may be obtained on request.		Refills not permitted, if original prescription is verbal. An original written prescription may be refilled if prescriber has indicated in writing the number of refills and dates for, or intervals between, refills.
	Prescription on Narcotic and Controlled Drug file. No record of sales in Narcotic and Controlled Drug Register required.		
Retain invoices in chronological order for auditing purposes in Narcotic and Controlled Drug Register or other record maintained for such purposes.			An original written or verbal prescription may be refilled if the prescriber has authorized in writing or verbally the number of times and dates for, or intervals between, refills.
No record required.	Prescription on regular file.		An original written or verbal prescription may be refilled if the prescriber has authorized in writing or verbally the number of times it may be refilled. For "expired" prescriptions for E, F drugs, see below. Transfer of authorized refills permitted.

Legislation can change. Keep abreast of changes in prescription requirements.

"Expired" prescriptions—When new authority is received from a prescriber for a Schedule E or F drug for which all previously authorized refills have been used up, a pharmacist may (1) transcribe this authority as a new prescription, or (2) record this authority either on the original prescription or on a manually maintained profile system.

administration of medications. It is estimated that fully 80% of the drugs currently in use were unknown just 30 years ago. In addition to administering medications and evaluating the patient for therapeutic response, the nurse is also responsible for patient teaching in relation to medications. Many patients are woefully ignorant about the medications they take. This lack of knowledge often compromises their therapy. The professional nurse can definitely make a difference for such patients by providing the information they need to obtain the maximum therapeutic benefit from their medications.

BIBLIOGRAPHY

The big lie about generic drugs. Consumer Reports :480–485, August 1987.

Brill, EL and Kilts, DF: The profession in change. In Foundations for Nursing. Appleton-Century-Crofts, New York, 1980.

Committee on Curriculum Development of the National League for Nursing (ed): A Curriculum Guide for Schools of Nursing. National League for Nursing, New York, 1937.

Committee on Education of the National League for Nursing (ed): Standard Curriculum for Schools of Nursing. National League for Nursing, New York, 1922.

Culpepper, MM and Adams, PG: Nursing in the Civil War. Am J Nurs 88(7):981–984.

Diseases. Nurse's Reference Library. Springhouse, PA, Nursing '84 Books, 1984.

Drug Enforcement Administration, New York Branch Office: Personal communication, August, 1987.

Farley, D: How FDA approves new drugs. FDA Consum 21(10):6–13, December 1987–January 1988.

Farley D: Getting outside advice for the ''close calls'' . . . Advise FDA about the safety and effectiveness of drugs and biological products. FDA Consum 21(10):14–18, December 1987–January 1988.

Fischer, RG: The meaning of FDA approval. Pediatr Nurs 13(5):360, 1987.

Gerald, MC: Drugs and Society and the Development of New Drugs in Pharmacology: An Introduction to Drugs. Englewood Cliffs, NJ, Prentice-Hall, 1974.

Gilman, G, Goodman, LS, and Gilman, A (eds): The Pharmacological Basis of Therapeutics, ed 6. Macmillan, New York, 1986.

Kozier, BB and Erb B: Fundamentals of Patient Care. WB Saunders, Philadelphia, 1980.

Nursing '88 Drug Handbook. Nursing '88 Books, Springhouse, PA, 1988.

Practices, Nurse's Reference Library. Nursing '84 Books, Springhouse, PA, 1984.

Wolfe, LV, Weitzel, MH, and Fuerst, EV: The administration of therapeutic agents. In Fundmentals of Nursing. JB Lippincott, Philadelphia, 1979.

SITUATION   2–1

Amy Forbes, a new graduate nurse, has been assigned to work on a medical-surgical unit. Many of the patients under her care are receiving controlled drugs. The following questions relate to Amy's knowledge of drug legislation and standards.

1. In administering hydromorphone (Dilaudid), a narcotic, to Jim Nesbit, who has a fractured left femur, the nurse has the responsibility to:
   a. Rewrite the prescription on the day of expiration
   b. Document and save any remaining medication
   c. Provide health teaching regarding the drug's action
   d. Obtain a telephone reorder 1 day before expiration

2. Sixty-two-year-old James Able is receiving Valium 5 mg tid for nervousness. Which of the following is true regarding Valium?
   a. It must be reordered every 7 days by the physician.
   b. As a Schedule II drug, it is reordered every 72 hours.
   c. Studies have shown Valium to have a low abuse potential.
   d. It can be dispensed without a prescription in most states.

3. Ruth Lee is being prepared for discharge following a laminectomy. The physician has ordered Talwin 50 mg PO q 6 hr prn for pain. Amy teaches that Talwin is:
   a. Nonaddictive if taken only as ordered
   b. A mild tranquilizer that is not subject to regulation
   c. Reordered by the physician every 6 months or after 5 refills

   d. A non-narcotic that can be purchased over the counter

4. Joseph Starr has been diagnosed as having AIDS. He is being considered for treatment with a new drug. Joseph asks the nurse, ''What does the term 'new drug' mean?'' All of the following statements regarding new drugs are correct *except*:
   a. The drugs are initially administered to animals to establish a data base.
   b. The FDA reviews animal study reports on safety and effectiveness.
   c. Phase I clinical studies use healthy volunteers to administer the drug.
   d. Once the FDA approves the new drug, safety is assured.

5. Amy prepares a morphine (narcotic) injection for Mr. Cane as requested. When Amy takes the medication into Mr. Cane's room, he informs her that he has changed his mind and would rather not take the shot. Amy has the legal responsibility to:
   a. Return the drug to the point of origin, such as the hospital pharmacy

SITUATION   2–1–*CONTINUED*

b. Discard the drug while another nurse observes and documents her action
c. Save the drug in the syringe in case Mr. Cane requests it later
d. Encourage Mr. Cane to take the medication since it has already been prepared

6. Bob Lockhart is receiving Demerol 50 mg IM for postoperative pain. Amy notices that the drug order has expired. She is aware that:

a. The physician must rewrite the Demerol order every 48 hours
b. A nurse cannot accept a telephone order for a drug renewal
c. The physician must countersign a verbal order within 48 hours
d. As a Schedule III drug, Demerol is only renewed one time

Refer to Appendix for correct answers and additional review questions with answers.

CHAPTER OUTLINE

MEDICATION ADMINISTRATION
    Drug Names and Preparations
    Medication Preparations—Local and Systemic
    Routes of Medication Administration
    The Medication Order
    The Medication Area
USING THE NURSING PROCESS
    Assessment
    Nursing Diagnoses
    Planning and Intervention
    Medication Administration
    Evaluation
SUMMARY

SEE APPENDIX *D*:
    Intravenous Dilution Table

GLOSSARY TERMS IN THIS CHAPTER

Aerosol
Anesthetic
Antibiotics
Anti-inflammatories
Antiseptic
Astringent
Bactericidal
Bacteriostatic
Buccal
Cleansing agent
Colloid solution
Emollients
First-pass effect
Foams
Fungicides
Gels
Generic
Intradermal
Intrathecal
Local effect
Miosis
Mydriasis
Nebulizer
Ophthalmic route
Otic route
Parenteral
Reference drug
Spray
Sublingual
Suppository
Systemic effect
Trade (brand name or proprietary name)
Transdermal
Troche

3

CHAPTER

ADMINISTERING MEDICATIONS WITH SAFETY

MERRILY MATHEWSON KUHN, R.N.C., Ph.D., CCRN

LEARNING OBJECTIVES

After reading this chapter, the student will be able to:

1. Formulate a specific plan to assess the patient who is receiving medications.

2. Plan the nursing intervention necessary to administer medications safely to any patient

3. Evaluate the nursing intervention and the patient at various stages to ensure patient safety.

MEDICATION ADMINISTRATION

All patients receiving medications have the right to have them administered safely. The nurse must assume certain responsibilities when administering medications and always follow the Five Rights of Medication Administration:

1. The Right Medication
2. The Right Patient
3. The Right Dose
4. The Right Route
5. The Right Time

In addition, the patient has the right to take or refuse the medication.

The nurse also assumes the responsibility for teaching patients all they need to know to administer the medications safely at home. Patient teaching, learning, and compliance are discussed fully in Chapter 8.

This chapter deals specifically with administering medications safely. Aspects of medication administration discussed include preparation and nursing care before, during, and after medication administration. For the actual techniques of medication administration, please refer to a fundamentals text.

DRUG NAMES AND PREPARATIONS

The majority of medications today have 4 names: chemical, *generic* (nonproprietary), *trade* (brand name or proprietary name), and official. The chemical name is primarily used by chemists and represents the chemical formulation of a drug.

The generic name can either be handed down from antiquity (colchicine), acquired from biochemistry (nitroglycerin), or assigned by the United States Adopted Name (USAN) Council. A manufacturer is given a 17-year patent on a generic drug. Once the drug is patented, the manufacturer can recover part of the investment used in research and development by licensing other companies or itself to produce or sell the drug. The trade name is created by the manufacturer and is always capitalized. If the name is registered, the trademark symbol is found at the upper right of the name e.g., Valium ®. Both generic and trade drugs are regulated by law with respect to the amount and purity of the drug. However, only a relatively small amount of a tablet or capsule is composed of active drug. The remainder is made up of nonmedicinal substances, which are not regulated. The ultimate formulation of the drug may affect the drug's action. Consumer groups claim that all chemically equivalent drug products—either generic or trade—are essentially similar. After lobbying, these consumer groups have caused legislators to enact generic drug laws in many states. These laws require pharmacists to fill prescriptions with a generic form of a prescribed drug unless the prescription is signed in a manner indicating that such substitution is not acceptable (Rodman et al, 1985). Generic drugs are often less expensive than trade drugs; therefore, the cost of medical care can be reduced by their use.

The official name, often the generic, is listed in an official compendium, *The United States Pharmacopeia-National Formulary (USP-NF)*. Canada does not designate a compendium as official.

The U.S. Food and Drug Administration (FDA) selects one formulation of a drug, usually the original of its kind, as a reference drug. The *reference drug* is the standard for all other drugs of its group. The FDA will then use this standard to test all other like drugs for potency, efficacy, bioavailability, and other criteria (concepts that are discussed fully in Chapter 4).

MEDICATION PREPARATIONS— LOCAL AND SYSTEMIC

Medications are administered to have either a local or a systemic effect. A *local effect* is one in which the effects of medications are confined to 1 area of the body; antiseptics, anti-inflammatories, and some anesthetics are used locally. A *systemic effect* is obtained when the medication is absorbed and delivered to the body tissues by way of the vascular system. Some medications, although applied locally, such as nitroglycerin ointment, nevertheless have a systemic effect due to their absorption through the skin.

Local Medications

Local medications affect only one part of the body. These medications are generally applied to the skin (topically) or to mucous membranes, or are injected into a joint cavity. When medications are applied topically, the skin usually acts as a barrier and does not allow them to be absorbed. The mucous membranes, on the other hand, line all external cavities of the body, that is, the mouth, nose, throat, rectum, vagina, and urethra, and are excellent surfaces for medication release because of the large number of capillaries directly beneath the surface. Injection of medication into a joint cavity is generally done for the purpose of reducing inflammation in the joint. Its effect is due to the presence of the large number of capillaries in the joint.

Local medications come in many forms, including aerosols, ointments, creams, pastes, powders, tinctures (medications mixed with alcohol), and lotions. Local medications can also be obtained as *gels, foams,* and *suppositories* for rectal, vaginal, and urethral application. The medication can also be administered through douche or irrigation into the vagina or through an enema or irrigation into the rectum. *Sprays, aerosols,* gases (including oxygen and carbon dioxide), and *nebulizers* are methods of introducing local or systemic medications, or both, into the respiratory system. Local medications in many different forms (gels, pastes, liquids) can be administered onto the surface of the mucous membranes and teeth to clean teeth or to freshen breath. Throat lozenges or *troches* are also used locally to produce prolonged relief for a sore mouth or throat. Many of these preparations are available over the counter (OTC).

Local medications are used for the following specific effects:

1. *Astringents* cause vasoconstriction and tissue contraction, which either decrease or arrest secretions, thereby toughening tissue.
2. *Antiseptics* and *bacteriostatic* agents inhibit the growth or multiplication of bacteria.
3. *Cleansing agents* help to remove dirt, crusts, secretions, and debris from wherever applied.
4. *Anesthetics* produce a loss of feeling or sensation in a part of the body.
5. *Emollients* soothe and soften and often reduce dryness of the skin.
6. *Antibiotics* and/or *bactericidal* agents—chemical compounds either produced by or obtained from certain living cells, especially yeasts and molds, or made from synthetic compounds—are antagonistic to other forms of life.
7. *Anti-inflammatories* reduce or counteract inflammation.
8. *Fungicides* are agents that destroy fungi.

Local medications can be water-based (aqueous) or oil-based preparations. Water-based medications are readily absorbed; oil-based medications are absorbed more slowly. Oil-based medications should not be used in the nose or respiratory tract, since the oil may be carried to the alveoli and the patient may develop a lipoid pneumonia.

Systemic Medications

Systemic medications are absorbed into the vascular system, are carried through the body, and affect 1 or more tissue groups. To give two examples, antibiotics administered orally are absorbed from the small intestine and carried in the vascular system to attack certain bacteria found in the blood stream of a patient with septicemia; digitalis, a medication for the heart, is absorbed from the small intestine and carried through the vascular system to the heart, where it effects a change on the heart muscle. How medications work and affect the body tissues is discussed fully in Chapter 4.

Systemic medications can be administered orally, topically, parenterally, or applied to mucous membranes. (*Parenteral* administration refers to a medication being introduced into the body through any route other than the gastrointestinal route, such as the intradermal; subcutaneous [SC or SQ]; intramuscular [IM]; or intravenous [IV] routes.)

ROUTES OF MEDICATION ADMINISTRATION

Oral Route

The oral route is the most common route, and is usually the safest, the most economical, and the easiest route for giving medications. Therefore, whenever possible, medications are administered orally. However, the oral route is not necessarily the best. The choice of an oral form over other methods of administration involves a consideration of both drug and patient variables. Drug vari-

ables include a prolonged absorption time, which delays the onset of action; decreased total absorption, which may cause decreased drug effect; possible gastrointestinal upset; possible interaction with food and other medications; and the possibility of a prolonged effect. The patient variables include the patient's age; how quickly the pharmacologic action is needed; the patient's mental status; neurologic state; gastrointestinal function and mobility; and ability to swallow the medication (in some cases, liquid forms of the medication may be used); and very important, the physiologic integrity of the patient, such as his or her current illness and organ function. (These variables are discussed in more detail in Chapter 4.)

Oral medications are administered with sufficient amounts of water to ensure that they enter the stomach. The administration of water with an oral medication often enhances absorption; for example, the action of expectorants such as guaifenesin and ammonium chloride may be enhanced by drinking 6–8 glasses of water daily. Exceptions include some cough medicines that are given for a local soothing effect on the throat. In addition, most cough medicines contain codeine or dextromethorphan, both of which act centrally.

The oral route of administration has some disadvantages. Patients may object to the taste of the medication or the medication may cause gastric upset, constipation, or diarrhea. Some medications may harm or stain the teeth. The medication may also be destroyed by gastrointestinal secretions and thus fail to effect its desired results. Oral medications may also be inadvertently aspirated by the seriously ill, old, or young patient.

The nurse must know the correct time to administer oral medications. Some oral medications are best administered with food to enhance absorption or to decrease their gastric irritation, whereas others are given on an empty stomach. At times, medications can upset an empty stomach. Therefore, it may be necessary to modify the time schedule so that the medication can be administered at mealtime.

Oral medications are available in two forms: solid and liquid. The solid forms currently available include tablets, capsules, caplets, and powders. (These forms are featured in Table 3–1.) Tablets, capsules, and caplets are often stamped or embossed with the pharmaceutical company's name, drug name, and/or an identifying number. Tablets, capsules, and caplets may occasionally be crushed and mixed in applesauce or other medium for patients who have difficulty swallowing, or mixed in a bowl to be administered down a feeding tube. These products may be enteric-coated, which delays the release of the medication until it reaches the small intestine. The enteric coating protects the medication and prevents its breakdown in the stomach. Enteric-coated medications are not administered concurrently with antacids, because the high pH of the antacid allows the enteric coating on the drug to break down in the stomach. Tablets and capsules may also be sustained-release or prolonged-action products. These products are designed to release over a long period of time so as to reduce the number of doses a patient must take each day. Unlike

Table 3–1. DOSAGES FORMS OF MEDICATION

Route	Form	Description	Example
Oral	Tablet	Compressed powder or granulated drugs; breaks apart quickly in the stomach	Acetylsalicylic acid (aspirin)
Oral	Tablet (coated)	Compressed powder or granulated drugs that are coated so that they dissolve slowly in the intestine	Triaminic
Oral	Capsule	Gelatin covered; dissolve in either the stomach or the intestine	Propoxyphene (Darvon)
Oral	Caplet	Compressed powder or granulated drugs with smooth outer coating resembling a capsule, which makes it easier to swallow for some patients	Acetaminophen (Tylenol)*
Oral	Syrups	Solution with sugar, water, and flavoring; may pose problems for the diabetic patient	Robitussin
Oral	Elixirs	Hydroalcoholic liquids flavored with volatile oil and slightly sweetened; may pose problems for the diabetic and alcoholic patients taking disulfiram (Antabuse)	Terpin hydrate
Oral	Emulsions	Mixtures of oils and water	Agoral Plain
Oral	Gels and magmas	Viscous suspensions of mineral precipitates in water; shake well before use	Magnesium hydroxide (Milk of Magnesia)
Oral	Aromatic water	Aqueous solution with various oils	Saturated solution potassium iodide
Oral	Tinctures	Extracts of drugs in alcohol	Camphorated tincture of opium
Oral	Fluid extracts	Concentrated liquid preparation of vegetable drugs	Fluid extract of belladonna
Oral	Extracts	Concentrated preparation made by evaporating the hydroalcoholic solvent; may be more potent than active drug	Belladonna extract
Oral	Lozenges (troches)	Flattened disk intended to be held in the mouth until dissolved; often contains sweeteners, flavors, and color	Cepacol lozenges
Oral	Effervescent tablet	Large tablets that form a bubbling solution	K-Lor
Topical	Powders	Topical products applied to dry the skin	Cornstarch
Topical	Lotion	Liquid preparation may be soothing or medicinal	Calamine
Topical	Ointment	Fatty, soft substance for external use	White petrolatum jelly (Vaseline)
Parenteral	Powders	Mixed with sterile solution for parenteral administration	Penicillin G
Parenteral	Emulsions	Mixtures of oil and water	Interlipid solutions

*Many other forms available.

tablets or capsules, enteric-coated or sustained-release products should never be crushed, because this will destroy the sustained-release property.

The liquid forms include syrups, elixirs, emulsions, gels or magmas, tinctures, aromatic waters, fluid extracts, and extracts. These forms are also featured in Table 3–1.

Parenteral Route

The parenteral route is used for medications entering the body through any route other than orally through the gastrointestinal system and commonly refers to SC, IM, intradermal, and IV routes. All medication entering the body in this manner must be sterile. Since parenteral medications usually enter the blood stream readily, great care is always taken when administering them to patients. Parenteral medications usually have a faster onset of action than do oral medications because a larger quantity of the drug is administered through systemic circulation. Parenteral medications are generally more expensive than their oral forms because of the greater cost of preparation. The administration of medications through the parenteral route often takes specialized training. Only the physician, nurse, or other specially trained persons should administer certain types of parenteral medication. The law regarding parenteral medication administration varies from state to state.

There are several parenteral routes that can be used, including the *intradermal* route, just under the surface of the skin; SC, into the subcutaneous tissue; IM, into the muscle tissue; and IV, into the vein. Parenteral medications are also given into a joint, the intra-articular route; into an artery, the intra-arterial route; into the spinal column, the intraspinal route; into the pleural space of the lung, the intrapleural route; and into the spinal or subarachnoid space, the *intrathecal* route. The drugs are

Table 3–2. INJECTION EQUIPMENT FOR PARENTERAL MEDICATION

| Type of Injection | Needle | | Syringe/Other Equipment |
	Gauge	Length (inches)	
Intradermal	26	⅜	Tuberculin
Subcutaneous	25	½	Tuberculin, insulin
Intramuscular	20–23	1–3	2–5 ml
Intravenous fluid	20, 21	1–4	Butterfly argyle, intercath connected to bottle or IV bag with tubing
Blood	16, 18	1–4	Bottle or bag with apropriate tubing
Intra-articular	18, 19	2	2–5 ml
Intraspinal	14–16	1–4	2–5 ml
Intrapleural	14–16	4	10–50 ml
Intrathecal	14–16	1–2	2–5 ml

administered from a sterile syringe through a sterile needle. The needles vary in diameter (gauge) from 14 to 26 gauge, and in length from ⅜ inch to 3 inches. The gauge and length are determined by the viscosity of the medication being administered, as well as where the medication is to be deposited. Table 3–2 features injection equipment for parenteral medication.

Many side effects can be experienced from parenteral medication administration. The medication may damage or stain the tissues; improper techniques may result in a local or systemic infection, or in nerve injury at the injection site; the skin may slough at the injection site or become abscessed; or the patient may experience prolonged pain.

SUBCUTANEOUS/INTRAMUSCULAR ROUTES. The SC and IM routes are used when medication must enter the body more quickly than by the oral route or when it would be destroyed by the gastrointestinal system if administered orally (vitamin B_{12}).

INTRADERMAL ROUTE. The intradermal route is most commonly used for testing the patient's sensitivity to an allergen, such as ragweed pollens, or for determining the presence of a disease, such as tuberculosis (the Mantoux test).

INTRAVENOUS ROUTE. The IV route administers medication directly into the vascular system, thus bypassing all barriers to drug absorption. The IV route is both the fastest and the most dangerous route. This route is usually reserved for potent drugs when a rapid onset of action is required. Many medications administered IM can also be administered IV if their action is required more quickly (digoxin, furosemide, morphine, and so on). The IV route is discussed in detail in Chapter 11.

Mucous Membrane Application

Medications are often applied to the mucous membranes of the mouth and throat, that is, the sublingual or *buccal* surfaces; the nose or other parts of the respiratory system (sprays, inhalants); the eye; the genitourinary system (vaginal douches, suppositories, creams, foams); and the gastrointestinal system (rectal suppositories or enemas). Medications applied to the mucous membranes of the nose, eye, and vagina are often given

for their local effect. On the other hand, medication may be applied to the mucous membranes for a systemic effect (e.g., an aspirin suppository given rectally for temperature control).

SUBLINGUAL ROUTE. When the *sublingual* route is used, the medication is placed under the tongue. Medications are quickly dissolved because of the dosage design, and since the tongue is a very vascular area, medications are quickly absorbed. In general, more medication is absorbed sublingually than through the oral route because the medication is not damaged by gastric secretions or metabolized by the liver through the *first-pass effect*, the combined inactivation of an orally administered medication in the liver. (This concept is explained in Chapter 4.) The patient holds the sublingual medication under the tongue until it is dissolved. The patient is instructed not to swallow the medication or drink any liquid while the medication remains under the tongue.

BUCCAL ROUTE. Several drugs (troche or lozenge) are designed to be applied to the mucous membranes of the mouth. Troches are excellent for topical application of antibiotics, antifungals, and local anesthetics in the mouth. Swallowing these products would be undesirable or impossible because they would be destroyed in the gastrointestinal tract. Drugs unsuited for troches are those whose bitter taste cannot be disguised and those not absorbed in the gastrointestinal tract. The patient is instructed to keep these products against the buccal surface of the mouth until they are completely dissolved. *Buccal absorption* takes about 5–10 minutes, but a hard-candy base can be used to delay absorption. Patients should report any irritation to the mouth that occurs.

INHALANTS. Inhalants, usually sprays, are forced through the mouth or nose by a small amount of pressure into the lower respiratory tract. These medications require a pressure device such as a hand bulb, an atomizer, or a nebulizer to deliver the medication into the lower respiratory tract. Inhalants are often used for bronchodilation, that is, dilating the lower air passages to make it easier for the patient to exchange gases. Inhalants are local-acting medications and are generally not meant to be absorbed systemically, although with some drugs systemic absorption does occur and results in occasional side effects. It is important for the nurse to teach the patient the proper technique for inhaling these products. These techniques are discussed in greater depth in Chapter 35.

VAGINAL ROUTE. Medications inserted into the vagina include foams, gels, creams, suppositories, compressed tablets, douches, troches, and irrigations. These medications, administered for their local action, are often inserted with an applicator to ensure that the medication is well positioned. Examples are contraceptives, anti-infectives, and anti-inflammatory medications. If vaginal medications are to be used by the patient at home, it is important the nurse teach the patient about proper administration.

RECTAL ROUTE. The rectum, an extremely vascular area with many small capillaries that enhance absorption, is used for administration of both local and systemic medications. Medication forms such as suppositories or enemas are administered for their local effect to treat hemorrhoids or constipation or for their systemic effect to treat respiratory conditions, to reduce temperature, and for many other effects. Suppositories are usually absorbed slowly. They are designed to melt at body temperature, so they are best stored in the refrigerator or in a cool place. Most rectal suppositories are packaged in foil wrappers. Patients are taught that the foil is removed and the suppository lubricated with water or soluble gel before insertion.

Most patients identify the rectal route with an enema. Therefore, if medications such as bronchodilators, analgesics, or antipyretics are being administered, the patient should understand that the medication is not to be expelled. Systemic rectal medications may cause irritation, burning, and itching in the rectal area. When irritation arises, the medication may need to be discontinued.

Topical Administration

Topical medication can be applied to the skin (lotions, ointments, creams, patches); the eye (drops, ointments, irrigations); and the ear (drops or irrigation). Medications administered topically are often given for their local effect. However, some medications (nitroglycerin and scopolamine) are applied topically but are absorbed and have systemic effect.

DERMAL (SKIN) MEDICATIONS. The skin can be treated topically with liquid lotions, liniments, emollients, and compresses to manage or treat local skin irritation or infections. These products are best applied to newly washed and dried skin in small amounts. Applications are made gently, by patting rather than by rubbing. When applying topical medication to large areas of a patient's body, the nurse should wear gloves to avoid skin contact with the medication.

TRANSDERMAL ROUTE. The *transdermal* route is a new form of medication administration. It uses disks of medicated dressing applied to the skin that release their medication topically for systemic absorption. Several medications, such as scopolamine, nitroglycerin, clonidine hydrochloride (Catapres), and estrogen, are available in this new long-acting form (Fig. 3–1). The adhesive-backed disks are applied to a non-hairy area.

Scopolamine applied behind the ear prevents motion sickness, nitroglycerin causes smooth muscle relaxation to protect against hypoxic coronary pain, clonidine hydrochloride disks produce smooth muscle relaxation to reduce blood pressure, and estrogen supplies female hormone. All disks can be worn safely during bathing or showering, and some of the disks remain effective even while swimming.

OPHTHALMIC ROUTE. The *ophthalmic route* is used to administer medications into the eye. Medications may be ordered to be administered to the left eye (OS), the right eye (OD), or both eyes (OU). Medications administered by this route are used to both diagnose and treat eye disorders. Eye medications can dilate the pupil *(mydriasis)*, constrict the pupil *(miosis)*, or act as a local anesthetic, anti-inflammatory, or anti-infective. Eye irrigations are performed to remove foreign substances. Patients need to receive sufficient teaching to administer these medications safely.

OTIC ROUTE. The *otic route* refers to medications that are administered into the ear canal. Many types of medications are instilled into the ear, including powders (most commonly used as antibiotics), ointments, drops, anti-inflammatories, and local anesthetics. The ear canal can also be irrigated.

THE MEDICATION ORDER

Traditionally, the nurse receives the written medication order from the physician. The order should be clearly and completely written. When the nurse receives a medication order in the hospital, it includes the name of the medication, the dose, the route, and the number of times to be given daily. The order may be written in abbreviated form (Table 3–3). As an example, the physician orders Demerol 50 mg IM q 4 hr prn (when required). This means the patient receives Demoral 50 mg intramuscularly, when the patient requires, at least 4 hours apart. Another order might read Valium 5 mg PO (by mouth) qid (4 times daily). The patient receives Valium 5 mg by mouth 4 times a day, at 10 AM, 2 PM, 6 PM, and 10 PM or at 6 AM, 12 noon, 6 PM, and 12 midnight, depending on the hospital policy. Another order might read penicillin G 400,000 units PO tid (3 times daily). This means the patient receives penicillin G 400,000 units (usually 1 tablet) by mouth, 3 times a day. Often several tid times are available to choose from: 10 AM, 2 PM, and 6 PM; 8 AM, 4 PM, and 12 midnight; 9 AM, 6 PM, and 1 AM; or 10 AM, 6 PM, and 2 AM. The nurse must know what the drug action is in order to prepare the medication card, sheet, or Kardex that dictates the proper times to administer the medication. The best time to administer penicillin G would be 8 AM, 4 PM, and 12 midnight; at 9 AM, 6 PM, and 1 AM; or 10 AM, 6 PM, and 2 AM. Any of these regimens would evenly space the dosage to maintain a constant serum level. The nurse is always able to alter the drug administration times for appropriate reasons. Antibiotics, antidysrhythmics, and bronchodilators would best be given around the clock or at regular intervals to keep the medication at a therapeutic level in the blood for the entire 24 hours.

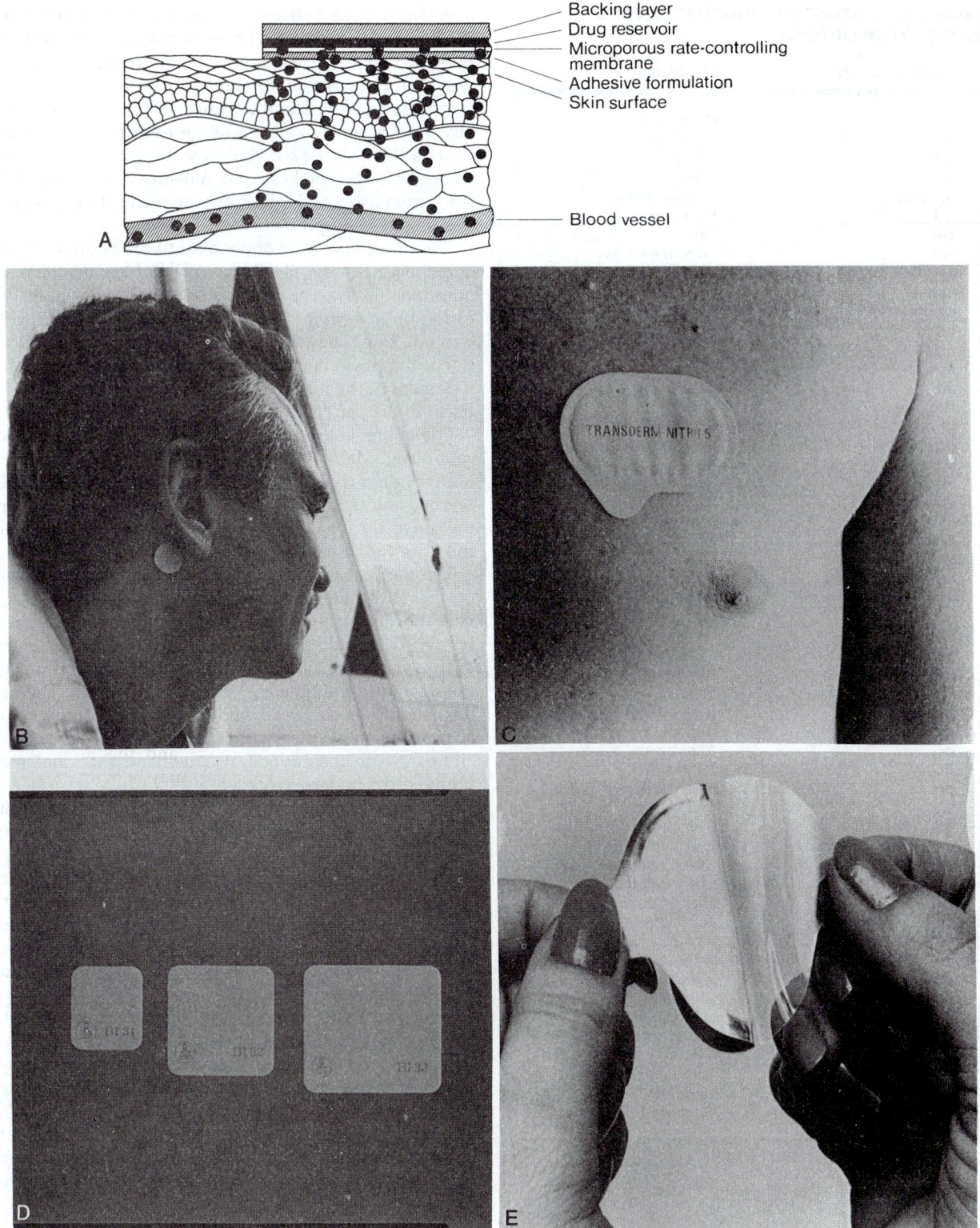

Figure 3–1. *A.* The Transderm system of transdermal medication administration has four separate layers. Applied like an adhesive bandage, the Transderm system provides a constant and controlled amount of medication through the skin and directly into the bloodstream over an extended period of time. Among the transdermal products currently available by prescription are: *B.* Transderm Scop (scopolamine) for preventing the symptoms of motion sickness; *C.* Transderm-Nitro (nitroglycerin) for treating and preventing the chest pain of angina pectoris; and *D.* Catapres-TTS (clonidine), an antihypertensive agent. *E.* The impenetrable backing of the transdermal products enables patients to undertake many activities, such as showering, bathing, or even swimming. (*A, B, C,* and *E,* courtesy of CIBA-GEIGY Corporation, Summit, NJ; *D,* courtesy of Boehringer Ingelheim Pharmaceuticals, Inc., Ridgefield, CT.)

Table 3–3. COMMON ABBREVIATIONS FOR MEDICATION ORDERS

Abbreviation	Meaning
ac	Before meals
AD	Right ear
AS	Left ear
aq	Water
aq dest	Distilled water
AU	Both ears
aur	Ear
bid	Two times a day
c̄	With
caps	Capsule
comp	Compound
dil	Dilute
dr	Dram
elix	Elixir
fld	Fluid
Gm or g	Gram
gr	Grain
gtt	A drop
h or hr	Hour
hs	Hour of sleep (bedtime)
IM	Intramuscular
IU	International unit
IV	Intravenous
L	Liter
m	A minim
mcg (μg)	Microgram
mg	Milligram
ml	Milliliter
noct	In the night
OD	Right eye
OS	Left eye
OU	Both eyes
oz	Ounce
pc	After meals
PO	By mouth
prn	When required
U	Unit
qd	Every day
qh	Every hour
q 2 h	Every 2 hours
q 3 h	Every 3 hours
q 4 h	Every 4 hours
qid	Four times a day
qs	As much as is required
s̄	Without
Sig or S	Write on label
s̄s̄	One half
stat	Immediately
supp	Suppository
tab	Tablet
tid	Three times a day
tr or tinct	Tincture
ung	Ointment

a medication card (if used) is prepared, depending on the hospital procedure. The nurse may use the medication card or sheet to administer the medication; however, the chart is the only authentic record and should be checked before administering each medication. Usually the pharmacy keeps a list of each patient's medications that is checked daily by the pharmacist, who then alerts the medical and nursing staff of possible drug interactions, duplications of medications, wrong doses, and other problems.

The nurse who is in doubt about a medication order, either because it is illegibly written or because it is of questionable dose or use, should never give the medication until verifying the order with the physician who wrote it. The nurse may also refuse to give the medication if the physician is known to be in error, or if, in the judgment of the nurse, the administration may result in harm to the patient.

The abbreviations listed in Table 3–3 should be used cautiously. Many dosing mistakes are made because of improper interpretation of abbreviations (Table 3–4). If there is any doubt in interpreting the physician's order, the nurse always verifies the order before administering the drug to the patient.

The medication order can also be verbal, often given by the physician over the phone in an emergency. All verbal orders are written in the patient's chart as they are received and are repeated back to the physician to ensure accuracy. In addition, the physician's full name, the date, and the time are written in the chart. The orders should be countersigned by the physician as soon as possible, most often within 24 hours in acute-care facilities. Some institutions also demand that the telephone order be tape-recorded.

Besides the doctor, the nurse may receive a medication order written by a nurse practitioner or physician assistant. In several states, nurse practitioners, after passing a special examination and taking at least 30 semester hours of pharmacology classes, may order more than 200 commonly used medications. In some states, the medication order may be written by physician assistants, who are licensed to practice under the direct supervision of the attending physician.

The pharmacist dispenses the correct medication to the hospital units. The nurse is then responsible for checking for the correct dose, administering the drug, and instructing the patient about the use of the drug. The nurse's responsibilities also include observing the patient for both therapeutic and nontherapeutic drug effects. Any unusual responses are reported to the physician, and the next dose of the drug is held until the physician examines the patient.

THE MEDICATION AREA

Most hospitals and other institutions keep medications in a special location that is private and quiet. Often, the medications are stored in a room or on a special medication cart, but they may also be found in the narcotic cupboard, the stock area, or the refrigerator. ("Stock" supplies are medications that are available and gener-

In general, the written medication order is written with other doctors' orders on the Doctor Order Sheet. Many hospitals use triple-copy order sheets, allowing the nurse to remove a carbon and send it to the pharmacy to be filled, rather than transcribing the medication order. This method helps to eliminate medication mistakes. If the nurse needs to transcribe the order, the medication is copied verbatim onto a pharmacy order form and sent to the pharmacy. The order is also copied into the patient Kardex or medication sheet, or both, or

Table 3–4 COMMONLY MISINTERPRETED ABBREVIATIONS

Order	Abbreviation or Problem	Intended Meaning	Misinterpretation	Correction
D/c meds: *Digoxin 0.25 mg* *Lasix 40 mg* *KCl 20 mEq*	D/C	Discharge Discontinue	Patients' medications have been prematurely discontinued when D/C, intended to mean "discharge," was misinterpreted as "discontinue," when followed by a list of drugs.	Write out "discharge" and "discontinue."
Vit B₁₂ 1 mg IM Now	μg	Microgram	When handwritten, this can easily be mistaken for "mg."	Use mcg.
Diabinese 250 mg ī/d	ī/D	Once daily	Mistaken as "t.i.d."	Write it out.
Digoxin 0.25 mg q.d.	q.d.	Every day	The period after the "q" has sometimes been mistaken for an "i," and the drug has been given qid rather than daily.	Write it out.
Lasix 200 p. today.	200	200 mg	Usual PO dose is 40–120 mg. This would have meant giving 15 tabs.	Do not write over orders.
Tylenol #3 qid prn	#3	#3 is specific dosage	Three tabs of Tylenol were administered.	Beware of ambiguous drug names.
100 ml of 5% D c̄ 100 ml HCl	HCl	KCl	KCl was misinterpreted for HCl because HCl is rarely used.	Question dose of KCl, which was too high

ally used for all patients, such as acetaminophen.) Medications are then prepared. Please refer to a nursing fundamentals text for the specific procedure. Each patient often has his or her own box or drawer that is stocked by the pharmacy.

USING THE NURSING PROCESS

ASSESSMENT

Assessment of a patient always begins with a nursing history to establish the data base. The data base is utilized later in planning and implementing patient care. It is important to include a medication history, including the use of prescription medications, over-the-counter medications, alcohol, and drugs of abuse. If the patient is taking other medications, it is important to determine why they are being taken and what information the patient understands about those medications. An allergy history is also included to prevent medication reactions. There are many cross-allergies between medications as well as between foods and medications. Current smoking history as well as intake of coffee, tea, and other caffeine beverages is also obtained.

The nurse also assesses the patient's weight, because many medications are ordered based on the patient's current weight. The nurse may need to calculate body surface area (BSA) in order to calculate proper dosage.

BSA can be calculated using a nomogram (Fig. 3–2). The nurse also assesses the patient's skin, particularly noting color, bruises, needle marks, and infection. If these are present, injections should not be performed in these areas.

During the assessment, the nurse may also be responsible for helping to select the most appropriate route for the specific medication, since the same medication often can be obtained in several different dosage forms such as a tablet, liquid, or parenteral dosage form. The patient's age and physical condition are also considered when the route is being considered. For example, a patient receiving digoxin 0.25 mg daily by mouth, who is NPO (nothing by mouth) after surgery, needs to receive digoxin by another route. The nurse has to become familiar with the medication policies within the employment setting to determine when the physician needs to be notified to rewrite the order.

If the patient will need to have the medication opened or crushed to be mixed with applesauce or with a liquid to be inserted through a nasogastric (NG) tube, the nurse must determine if this can be done safely.

During the assessment, the nurse also assesses the medication order for accuracy and completeness. If there is any doubt about the order, the physician is consulted first.

NURSING DIAGNOSES

Nursing diagnoses are established as the nurse prepares to administer medication to the patient. These nursing

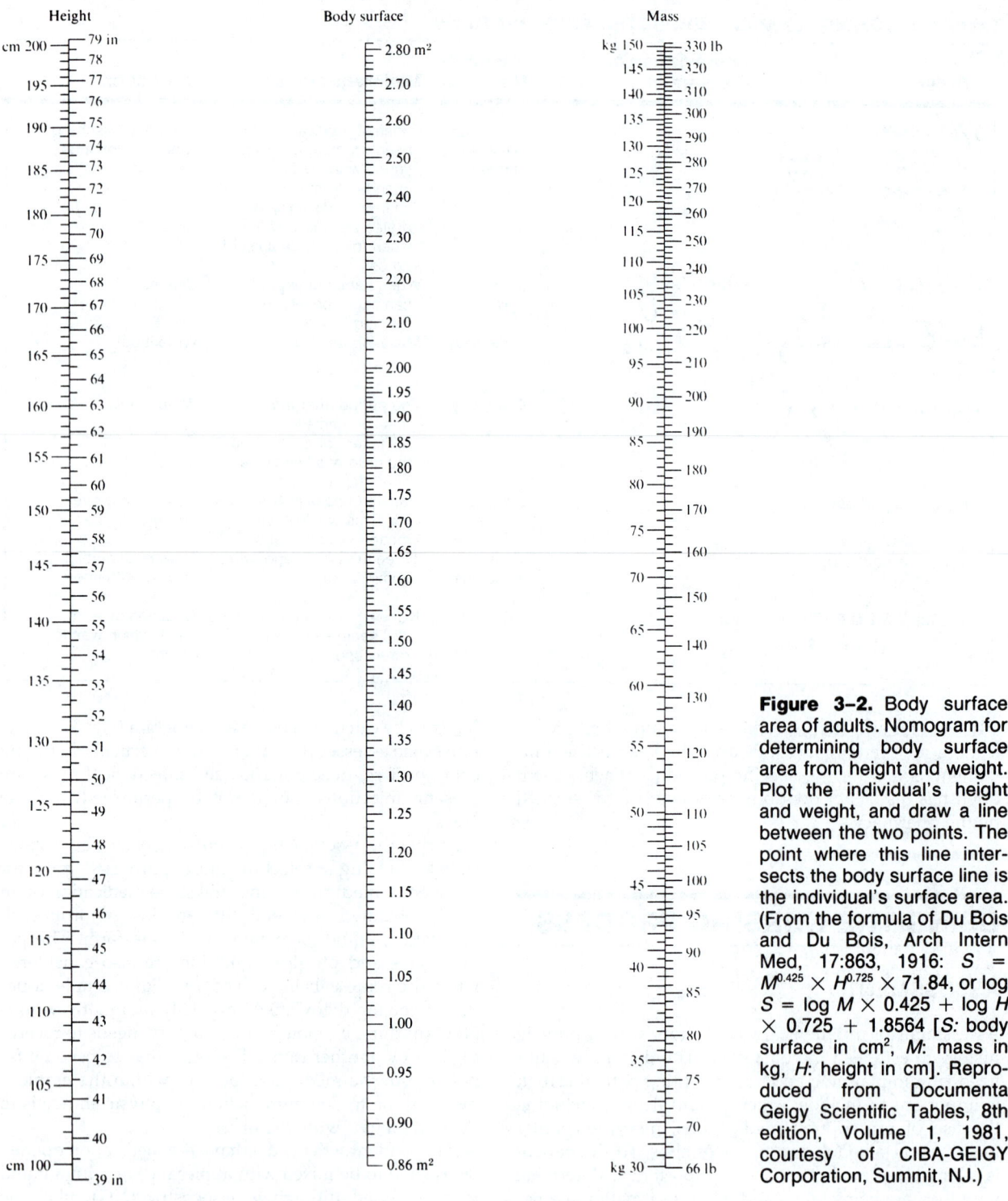

Figure 3–2. Body surface area of adults. Nomogram for determining body surface area from height and weight. Plot the individual's height and weight, and draw a line between the two points. The point where this line intersects the body surface line is the individual's surface area. (From the formula of Du Bois and Du Bois, Arch Intern Med, 17:863, 1916: $S = M^{0.425} \times H^{0.725} \times 71.84$, or log $S = \log M \times 0.425 + \log H \times 0.725 + 1.8564$ [S: body surface in cm², M: mass in kg, H: height in cm]. Reproduced from Documenta Geigy Scientific Tables, 8th edition, Volume 1, 1981, courtesy of CIBA-GEIGY Corporation, Summit, NJ.)

diagnoses may be established by the nurse when the locus of control is with the nurse, as in an acute-care situation, or by both the nurse and patient when the locus of control is shared. Typical examples of nursing diagnoses when administering medications include anxiety of patient related to IM injection; knowledge deficit related to current need for IV therapy; knowledge deficit related to the use of transdermal nitroglycerin; and potential for injury from medication administration. Additional nursing diagnoses that can be used during drug administration are reviewed throughout this text.

PLANNING AND INTERVENTION

During the planning phase, the nurse plans to administer the medication safely to the patient and to teach the patient (and/or family) information about the medication regimen. The nurse always checks the Five Rights of Medication Administration, the right medication, the right patient, the right dose, the right time, and the right route, before leaving the medication room.

Upon entering the patient's room, the nurse *always* checks the patient's identification band to compare with the name on the medication sheet, card, and/or Kardex. Special care is always taken to identify a confused or comatose patient. This habit prevents the nurse from accidentally administering the wrong medication to a patient. After identifying the correct patient, the nurse administers the medication. The right of the patient to take or refuse the medication is assessed. If the patient chooses to refuse the medication, the nurse attempts to find out why and notifies the physician of the patient's refusal. The nurse may also choose to withhold the medication at this time if any unusual or untoward adverse/toxic effect is observed.

MEDICATION ADMINISTRATION

Oral Administration

Oral preparations are taken by mouth and, with the exception of oils or cough medicines, are followed by a large glass of water. Oils and cough medicines are not meant to be diluted. They should be the last oral medication the patient takes. The nurse makes sure the patient is capable of swallowing the tablet or capsule before administering it. For the patient who has difficulty swallowing medications, there are special techniques and assistive devices that can aid in swallowing medications. (See a nursing fundamentals text for more information.)

Both small and large tablets should be followed with 100 ml water to ensure successful swallowing. Also, patients should be sitting, standing, or lying on their side—not lying supine—when oral tablets or capsules are administered. When tablets or capsules are taken when the patient is lying in a supine position, the medication often adheres to the esophageal mucosa and disintegrates, thus causing irritation of the esophageal mucosa or improper absorption. When capsules are taken, the patient should tilt the head forward so that the capsule floats to the top of the fluid in the mouth, making it easier to swallow the capsule.

The nurse may also crush tablets or open capsules when necessary. A definite rule is that if the tablet is enteric-coated, it should *not* be crushed. The enteric coating protects the medication and stomach by not allowing the tablet to disintegrate in the stomach. When enteric-coated tablets are crushed, much of the medication is destroyed by the gastric secretions and may cause gastric irritation. Not all capsules should be opened. The nurse always checks with a pharmacist before crushing tablets or opening capsules.

When the nurse has to crush a tablet, the best method is to put the tablet into a paper medicine cup, place an empty cup inside this cup, and then use a pestle or medicine crusher to crush the tablet. This method ensures that the tablet is not comtaminated with other medica-

tions as it might be if a mortar and pestle were used alone.

When the nurse gives liquid medications, it is important to measure the correct amount. Hospitals and clinics provide plastic medicine cups, so this is usually not a problem if the liquid is poured correctly. In the home, however, when a teaspoon or a tablespoon is the dosage amount ordered, the family often uses a flatware teaspoon or tablespoon. Patients are taught to use only the measuring spoons, not their flatware, as measures. Various manufacturers also supply plastic measuring devices that can be purchased at pharmacies.

Some patients, both young and old, may have difficulty taking liquids from a glass. The nurse administers the medication into the side of the patient's mouth with a syringe with a Brody tip. The fluid can then be expelled into the mouth very slowly, allowing the patient sufficient time to swallow. The nurse may also use a straw to give small quantities of medication to patients. Medication can also be inserted through a feeding tube. If the patient has an NG tube inserted, the tablets may be crushed or the capsules opened, mixed with a liquid, and, in most cases, administered through the NG tube. The NG tube is clamped for 30–60 minutes after the medication is administered to allow for it to pass into the small intestine. Again, before crushing the tablet or opening a capsule, the nurse must always make sure it can be crushed or opened. Also compatibility between the enteral feeding and the medication needs to be checked before administration.

Parenteral Administration

Parenteral medications are introduced into the body through a needle. The nurse has special education and training to administer medications by this route. Only a brief overview of parenteral medication administration is presented here. For a more detailed discussion, refer to a fundamental nursing text.

The nurse must first select the proper size syringe and needles. Syringes vary in size from 1–60 ml, and needles vary in size from a 14-gauge, which is very large in diameter, to a 27-gauge, which is very fine and small in diameter. The needle length also varies from ⅜ inch to 3 inches. The needle length and gauge depend on the route (SC, IM, IV) that is used and the condition and size of the patient. (Table 3–2 reviews injection equipment for parenteral administration.)

Medication can be found in single-dose vials, multi-dose vials, ampules, or cartridges. Occasionally, two medications may be ordered at the same time. Before mixing any medications, the nurse always checks with the pharmacist to make sure the medications are compatible; if unsure, it is always best to give the patient two injections rather than take the chance of mixing two incompatible drugs. Generally, narcotics and anticholinergics can be mixed safely, for example, meperidine (Demerol) and atropine or a similar combination. These are the usual preoperative medications. Although insulins, in general, can safely be mixed together in the same syringe, there is some current controversy about mixing of regular and long-acting insulins in the same syringe.

(More information on insulin can be found in Chapter 44.) Antibiotics may be inactivated by other medications, so compatibility always needs to be ascertained.

The medication is selected, the dose calculated, and the medication is administered to the patient.

When administering medication to the very young or old, special techniques may be useful. These techniques for pediatric and geriatric patients are reviewed in Chapters 14 and 16.

The nurse may find several strategies helpful when trying to administer a pain-free parenteral injection (IM, SC):

1. Select a site away from skin lesions, abrasions, excoriations, lipodystrophies, or lipohypertrophies.
2. Distract the patient by talking to him or her.
3. Hold the needle steady.
4. Inject the medication into or through a relaxed muscle.
5. Insert and remove the needle quickly.
6. Inject the medication slowly.
7. Hold an alcohol pad firmly against the skin as the needle is removed from the site. This provides countertraction in the skin. The needle will then not pull the tissues as it is removed and cause discomfort.
8. Rotate injection sites
9. Use a sharp needle free of burrs.
10. Select the smallest gauge needle compatible with the medication to be injected.
11. Apply an ice cube to the site before injecting the medication.
12. Apply direct pressure to the area to enhance absorption.
13. Massage the area to hasten absorption except when administering iron dextran (Imferon), heparin, or insulin.

INTRAMUSCULAR INJECTIONS. When the nurse administers an IM medication, the patient should be sitting if an injection is to be administered in the arm (deltoid), or be lying down, either on the side or prone, if an injection is to be administered in the buttocks or legs. However, it is possible to administer an IM injection while the patient is standing. The nurse asks the patient to lean forward with both hands on the table or window sill and point the toes inward toward each other. This position makes it unlikely for the patient to tighten the buttock muscles. The standing position makes it easy for a nurse to administer a medication to a patient in an office, clinic, or outpatient situation. When using the leg for IM injections, it is best to use the lateral surface. If injections are received in the anterior surface of the leg, the medication may form a hard mass that becomes painful when the patient walks. Sites for IM injection are shown in Figure 3–3.

Injections intended for the muscle may in fact not reach the muscle but are rather deposited in fat (Farley et al, 1986). This is especially true for adult women, who have a thicker gluteal fat layer than men. (Children have less gluteal fat, so injections given to them usually go into the muscle.) Injections deposited in fat may be absorbed more slowly than those deposited in muscle,

but the researchers say this has not yet been proven. The nurse must be careful to use a long enough needle to deposit the medication into the muscle.

SUBCUTANEOUS INJECTIONS. SC injections are generally administered in the outer surface of the upper arm, the anterior portion of the thigh, or the abdomen. There are fewer large blood vessels and less pain sensations felt in these locations than on the medial aspect.

When irritating medications are administered subcutaneously, a sterile abscess or tissue necrosis may result. Medications that are irritating to the subcutaneous tissue should be administered by another route.

INTRAVENOUS ROUTE. The IV route can be used for quick medication injection or for prolonged, continuous, or intermittent infusion. The medication is inserted directly into a vein and is usually given as a *bolus*, that is, a concentrated dose of medication given over a short period of time. Most bolus IV medications are given over a period of at least 1–2 minutes. Some medications need to be given over a 10- to 20-minute period. The nurse is responsible for fully understanding the medication that is being administered and knowing how it is to be administered and diluted. For more information on IV techniques, please refer to a nursing fundamentals text.

The IV route can also be used for continuous infusions. Patients can receive dextrose solutions, electrolyte solutions, proteins, fats, vitamins and minerals, plasma expanders, blood, blood components, or blood by-products through this route. The nurse must always be careful to maintain sterility when this route is used. It is the nurse's responsibility to check the site of injection and the drip rate. Infusion pumps may be used to regulate the drip rate.

Another method of administering IV medication is through intermittent therapy, often called partial-fills, piggybacks, IV series, or burettes. Medications, often antibiotics, are administered usually 1–6 times a day through this route. These are diluted and hung at a higher level (or below for a burette) than the main IV, from which they take 30–90 minutes to infuse. When this medication stops, the main IV resumes infusing at the original preset rate.

The nurse may occasionally administer medications intermittently through a heparin lock. The heparin lock is inserted into a vein and is kept patent with heparin. The heparin lock is ideal for patients who require periodic IV medications but do not require IV fluid. Often the patient is receiving IV fluids to keep the vein open (KVO) only for medication. Medication is generally preceded and followed with saline, and then heparin is inserted. The SASH method is a frequently used protocol: S—saline 1.5–2 ml before the additive; A—additive at the appropriate rate; S—saline 1.5–2 ml to flush the line; and H—heparin, usually 1 ml of 100 units/ml, to maintain line patency. The heparin lock is much more cost-effective also: $2.00 for a heparin lock compared to $12.00–$15.00/day for IV solution and tubing.

Patients with chronic disease require circulatory access for prolonged periods of time. To meet these needs, several implantable vascular access systems have been developed. The venous access port (VAP) consists of a

A   Deltoid site

B   Dorsogluteal site

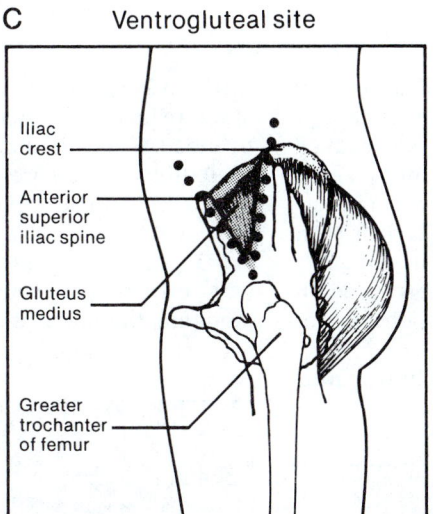

Figure 3–3. IM sites. *A)* Deltoid site: The mid-deltoid area is located by forming a rectangle, the top of which is at the level of the lower edge of the acromion, and the bottom of which is at the level of the axilla; the sides are one third and two thirds of the way around the outer aspect of the patient's arm. *B)* Dorsogluteal site: To avoid the sciatic nerve and accompanying blood vessels, an injection site is chosen above and lateral to a line drawn from the greater trochanter to the posterior superior iliac spine. *C)* Ventrogluteal site: The nurse's palm is placed on the greater trochanter and the index finger is placed on the anterior superior iliac spine; the IM injection is made into the middle of the triangle formed by the nurse's fingers and the iliac crest. *D)* Vastus lateralis site: The patient is supine or sitting for the injection. (From Deglin, JH, and Vallerand, AH: Davis's Drug Guide for Nurses. F. A. Davis, Philadelphia, 1988, p. 709, with permission.)

C   Ventrogluteal site

D   Vastus lateralis site

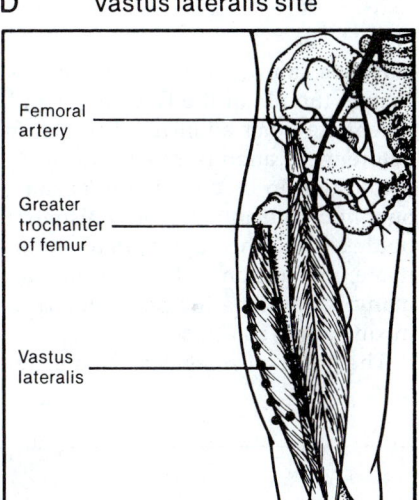

radiopaque silicone catheter and an injection port with a self-sealing silicone-rubber system. The principal differences between the VAP systems available are the size, shape, and composition (stainless steel/plastic) of the portal. Each manufacturer guarantees the septum for an indefinite number of punctures in the range of 1–2000 (Fig. 3–4). The VAPs are implanted surgically. VAPs may be used for blood sampling, bolus injection, and continuous infusions. To access the port (Fig. 3–5), it is palpated, the port is entered with special Huber needle (Fig. 3–6), and it is flushed with heparin (Fig. 3–7). For specific care of the VAP, see a fundamental nursing text.

Several long-term central venous access catheters are available (Fig. 3–8). These catheters are placed under sterile technique into the right atrium of the heart by way of a large central vein. After tip placement, the

catheter is tunneled subcutaneously for several inches to the desired exit site. A small Dacron cuff is attached to the catheter, which promotes the ingrowth of fibrous tissue. The Dacron cuff assists in securing the catheter in place and reduces the potential of infection caused by the migration of bacteria in the subcutaneous tunnel. These special catheters are available with one, two, and three inner lumens. Their main advantage is that they do not need to be heparinized after each use. (A heparin flush is used once weekly.) Only a saline flush is needed to clear the catheter. These special implantable catheters are often used in chronically ill patients who are being cared for at home. The nurse must be familiar with the type of implantable device that is being used and its care. Again, see a fundamental nursing text for detailed nursing care.

It is best not to mix medications in the same IV; many

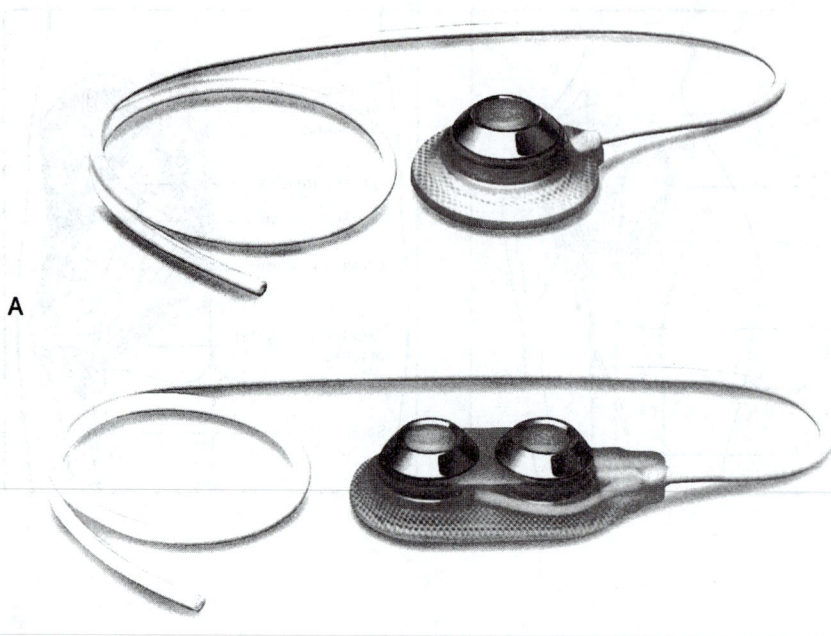

A

B

Figure 3–4. *A)* VAP/Mediport II. *B)* Mediport II DL. (Courtesy of Cormed, Inc., a subsidiary of Bard MedSystems Division, C. R. Bard, Inc., Medina, NY.)

reactions can occur. For example, one medication may change the pH of the IV solution and either destroy or potentiate other additives. The pharmacist is consulted before medication is mixed. The nurse administers each medication in its own bottle, flushing the tubing thoroughly before and after administration, and labels each bottle with the appropriate information—patient's name, medication, date, time, and the nurse's name. In many institutions the pharmacy is not responsible for mixing all IV solutions.

The nurse must regulate IV infusions carefully, partic-

ularly in very young, old, or acutely ill patients, evaluating frequently for signs of complications such as fluid overload. Signs of fluid overload include rapid pulse, elevated blood pressure, pale diaphoretic skin, and dysrhythmias. More complications are discussed in Chapter 11.

Many patients and families associate IV infusions with extremely serious illness or impending death; therefore, the nurse assesses and evaluates the feelings

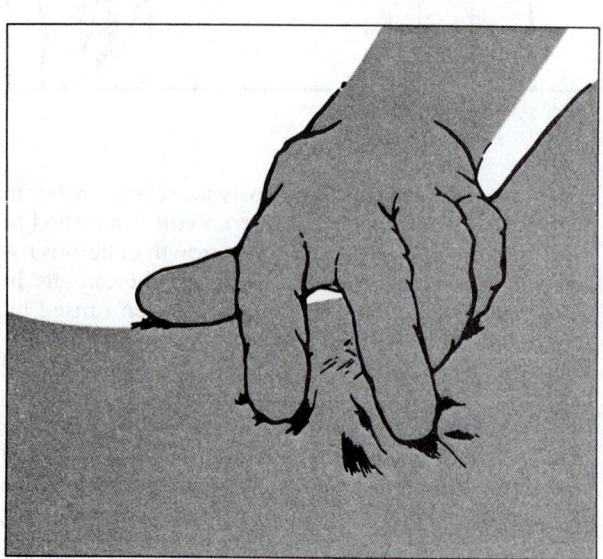

Figure 3–5. Locating the portal septum by palpation. (From Knox, LS: Implantable venous access devices. Critical Care Nurse 7(1):71, 1987, with permission.)

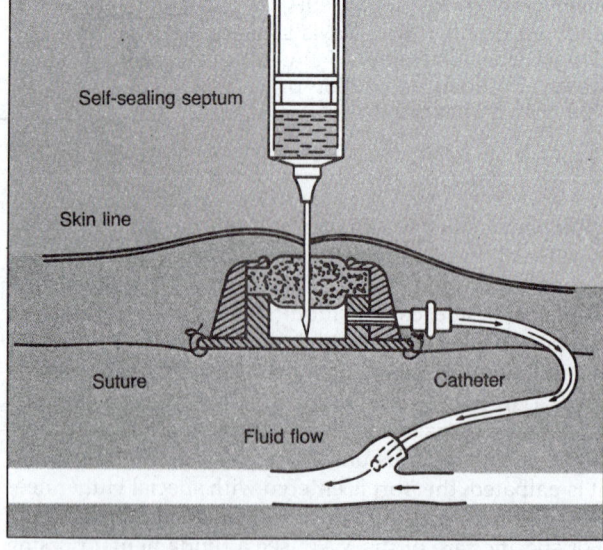

Figure 3–6. The Huber needle is pushed firmly through the skin and self-sealing septum until it hits the bottom of the portal chamber. (From Knox, LS: Implantable venous access devices. Critical Care Nurse 7(1):71, 1987, with permission.)

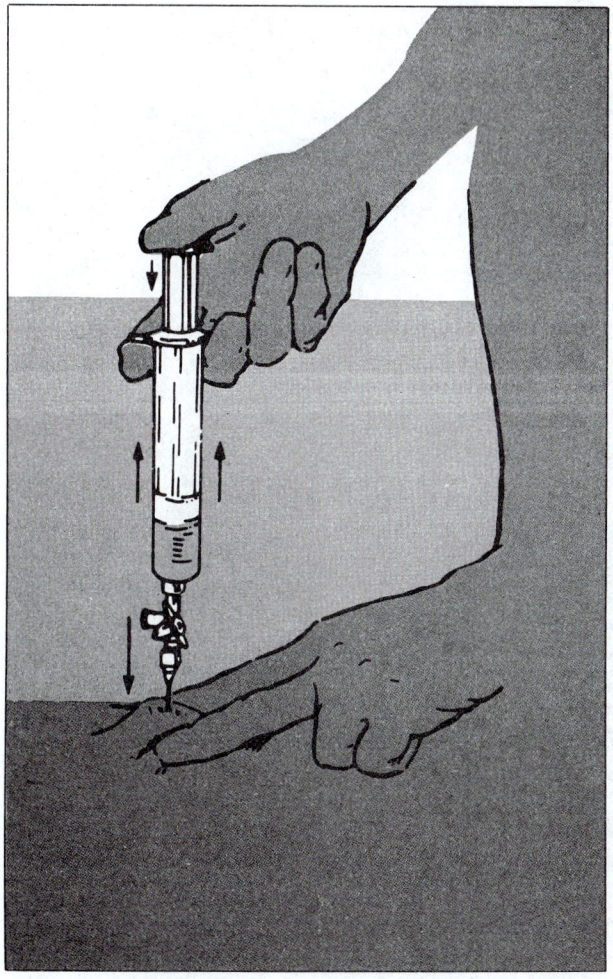

Figure 3–7. To avoid reflux, continue injecting the heparinized saline solution while simultaneously withdrawing the needle and pressing down on the portal. (From Knox, LS: Implantable venous access devices. Critical Care Nurse 7(1):72, 1987, with permission.)

of the patient and family and intervenes with appropriate health teaching when necessary.

Nursing Responsibilities of Medication Administration

Along with the Five Rights of Medication, there are some additional points the nurse must remember:

1. When preparing medications, always give full, undivided attention to this task.
2. Wash hands prior to administering any medication.
3. Never leave the medication tray or cart unattended. If the nurse must leave the patient's room, the nurse always takes the unadministered medicines.
4. Develop a habit of verifying the medicine card, sheet, or Kardex with the original doctor's orders. This helps to ensure patient safety.
5. Daily, check the patient's allergy list to ensure that the patient is not receiving a medication to which he or she is allergic.
6. Check the discontinuation date on the medication

sheet to ensure medications are given only for the ordered period.
7. Make sure that hypnotics, narcotics, and antibiotics are either discontinued or reordered on their renewal date. (See Chapter 20 for more information.)
8. Sign out narcotics and hypnotics in the appropriate location, at the time they are taken from the narcotic cabinet. Always verify the narcotic count before removing the medication.
9. Never administer medications that have been prepared by someone else. The only exception is medication prepared by the pharmacist.
10. Never administer medications from a bottle whose label is missing or illegible.
11. Never return an unused medication to a stock bottle.
12. When entering a patient's room, identify the patient by name and verify the name by checking the identification bracelet. Then compare the medication sheet with the identification bracelet.
13. The nurse always assists the patient in taking the medication. Never leave the medication for the patient on the assumption that the patient will take it.
14. Always answer all questions the patient asks about the medication.
15. If the patient expresses doubt or concern about receiving a particular medication, always recheck the medication and the original order. Often patients are very familiar with their medications and their questions help prevent a drug error.
16. Follow oral medication with sufficient amounts of water, except when administering oils and cough medications. Medications that taste particularly unpleasant may be diluted with juice or other diluents if there is no possible interaction that might occur, or they can be followed with juice or other beverage. Recent research suggests that the best fluid to follow oral medication is 3.5 ounces of cold, carbonated water (Hasselbalch et al, 1985).
17. Provide for patient privacy when administering a parenteral medication.
18. Chart the medication administration after it has been given; never chart medications before their administration.
19. Keep all equipment—carts, trays, medicine cups, and water pitchers—meticulously clean. Clean and straighten the medicine preparation area when finished. Wash hands between patients when administering parenteral medications.

The nurse is also responsible for patient education concerning both the medical and nursing regimens and all drug education. Patients have a right to know what is wrong with them, what and why products or treatments are prescribed, and what the anticipated results will be. Patient education leads to increased compliance with therapy. Patient teaching, learning, and compliance are discussed more fully in Chapter 8.

Patients need to know specific information concerning their medications. Patient teaching tables are found throughout this text. Each table includes all the information the patient should receive prior to discharge.

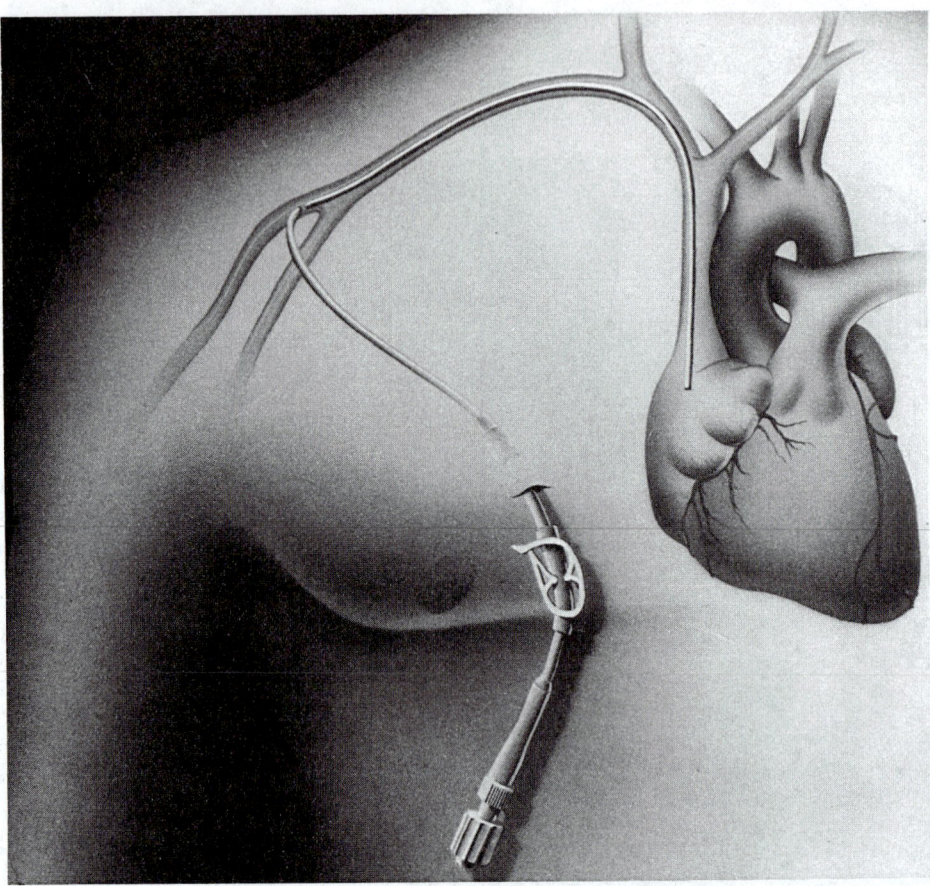

Figure 3–8. Corcath. (Courtesy of Cormed, Inc., a subsidiary of Bard MedSystems Division, C. R. Bard, Inc., Medina, NY.)

This material is discussed with the patient and family. Tables may be duplicated and given to patients for handy reference at home. The information provided in these patient teaching tables is listed in Table 3–5.

EVALUATION

During the evaluation stage, the nurse evaluates the expected outcomes and goals, the evaluation criteria. The nurse demonstrates concern for the patient's safety by asking, "Did the right patient receive the right medication, the right dose, at the right time, and by the right route?" Then the nurse evaluates the effectiveness of the medication. What was the desired action of the medication? And is that action being achieved? If not, what is the possible cause: a drug-drug or drug-food interaction, improper dosing, or lack of patient compliance? Is the patient experiencing any side effects or toxic effects?

If parenteral medications have been administered, the nurse ascertains that sites have been rotated and evaluates for complications such as abscess formation, infections, phlebitis, allergic reactions, and infiltration of IV solution.

The nurse also evaluates medications for interactions. In the 1970s, little was understood about drug interac-

tions; today, entire books feature the subject, and new information accumulates daily. Nurses must anticipate any possible drug interactions and should always check with the physician or pharmacist if they suspect a problem. Chapter 5 discusses drug interactions in detail. The nurse also evaluates the patient for toxic reactions. Toxicology has become a science of its own in recent years. Chapter 6 discusses toxicity in detail. Patient teaching is also evaluated. Does the patient understand what was taught, and can the patient apply this information in everyday life? Concepts of patient teaching, learning, and compliance are discussed in Chapter 8.

Medication errors can be made by many people: the physician, the pharmacist, the nurse, and the patient. If an error is made or found, the nurse follows the formal reporting procedure used by the institution where employed. Recent research has determined that only approximately one error out of every ten that occur is reported. It is important for the nurse to report and document medication errors as they are made. The patient's illness and recovery may be thwarted by poor reporting. Some common causes of medication error include: the wrong patient, the wrong dose, omission of a dose, the wrong time, the wrong route, and/or the wrong medication. To avoid medication errors the nurse should always

Table 3–5. INFORMATION FOUND ON PATIENT-TEACHING TABLES

1. General use
2. How long the drug will be taken
3. How the drug is to be administered, including special preparation and time of administration
4. Interactions to be aware of, including drug-food, drug-drug, drug-OTC interactions
5. Food/alcohol reactions
6. What the patient should do if he/she forgets a dose
7. How the medication will be stopped or what problems will develop if the medication is stopped abruptly
8. Information on altering the dose
9. Side effects to be aware of and those that need to be reported to the physician immediately
10. Storage instructions

1. Check ambiguous drug orders.
2. Check ambiguous drug names.
3. Beware of atypical drug names.
4. Never use the dropper of one medication to administer another medication.
5. Question the use of multiple tablets, ampules, or vials to provide a single dose.
6. Question unusually small and large doses.
7. Be suspicious of abrupt and excessive increases and decreases of medication.
8. Question the term *midnight* on an order to determine the date.
9. Refuse to interpret illegible handwriting.

The professional nurse is ultimately responsible for total patient care and safety. Only the nurse with a broad understanding of the medications being administered can confidently administer drugs with safety to patients.

SUMMARY

The nurse must assume certain responsibilities when administering medications and always follow the Five Rights of Medication Administration. The nurse must understand where a drug is to act in the body—locally, or systemically; the different routes of drug administration such as topical, oral, or parenteral, and how to read and interpret the medication order.

As the nurse prepares to administer medications, a thorough assessment is performed. This includes medication history, smoking history, current weight, and assessment of skin. The nurse then administers the medication safely to the patient and teaches the patient about the medication regimen. After the medication has been administered, the nurse evaluates the effectiveness of the medication. Was the desired action achieved? Did the patient experience any adverse or toxic effects?

BIBLIOGRAPHY

Baker, KN, et al: Effect of an automated bedside dispensing machine on medication errors. Am J Hosp Pharm 41(6):1352–1357, 1984.

Baldwin, HJ, Cosler, LE, and Schultz, RM: Opinion leadership in medication information. Communication Quarterly 35(1):84–103, 1987.

Birdsall, C, et al: How safe are generic drugs? Am J Nurs 87(4):431–432, 1987.

Clayton, M: The right way to prevent medication errors. RN 50(6):30–31, 1987.

Cobb, P, et al: Cutting down on errors and drugs. Nursing Mirror 159(12):vi–viii, 1984.

Cohen, MR: Play it safe: don't use these abbreviations. Nursing '87 87(7):46–47, 1987.

Cooke, P: Just what the doctor abbreviated. Hippocrates 9(5):22–24, 1987.

Cox, MB: Medication errors: What level of risk is acceptable? Nurse Patient Law (1):1–3, 1987.

Davis, NM, et al: Learning from mistakes: Medication errors to avoid. Nursing '87 17(5):84, 87–88, 90, 1987.

Farley, HF, et al: Will that IM needle reach the muscle? Am J Nurs 86(12):1327–1331, 1986.

Gardner, C: Risk management of medication errors, part 1. National Intravenous Therapy Association 10(3):187–196, 1987.

Gardner, C: Risk management of medication errors, part 2. National Intravenous Therapy Association 10(4):266–278, 1987.

Gilman, AG, Goodman, L, and Gilman, A (eds): Goodman and Gilman's The Pharmacological Basis of Therapeutics. Macmillan, New York, 1985.

Hasselbalch, H, et al: The best chaser for oral meds. RN 86(8):66, 1986.

Hecht, A: Know the right way to take your medicines. FDA Consum 21(4):22–24, 1987.

Howard, P: A crash course in serum drug monitoring. RN 49(4):20, 1986.

Hughes, CB: A totally implantable central venous system for chemotherapy administration. National Intravenous Therapy Association 8(6):523–527, 1985.

Knox, LS: Implantable venous access devices. Critical Care Nurse 7(1):70–73, 1987.

KVO for meds. Am J Nurs 87(1):73, 1987.

Lawrence J, et al: Helping the medicine go down. New Zealand Nursing Journal 79(3):27, 1986.

Lozenges can be lifesavers. Am J Nurs 87(9):1129–1130, 1987.

McGovern, K: 10 steps for preventing medication errors. Nursing '87 17(12):36–39, 1986.

McGovern, K: Take the first step toward reducing medication errors. Nursing '87 1(2):49, 1987.

Myths and facts of generic drugs. FDA Consum 21(7):12–14, 1987.

Rodman, M, et al: Pharmacology and Drug Therapy in Nursing. JB Lippincott, Philadelphia, 1985.

United States Pharmacopeia. Medical Economics, Oradell, NJ, 1987.

Wilkes, G, Vannicola, P, and Starck, P: Long-term venous access. Am J Nurs 85(7):793–794, 1985.

Wordell, DC: Should you crush that tablet? Nursing '88 18(1):48–49, 1988.

SITUATION 3–1

The nurse is administering medications to 28-year-old Nina Averton, who is hospitalized with bronchial pneumonia.

1. The nurse will administer several locally acting medications to Nina. All of the following types of drug preparations can produce local therapeutic effects, *except:*
   a. A troche
   b. A suppository
   c. A gel
   d. A caplet

2. Nina is ordered the expectorant guaifenesin. The nurse will administer this drug:
   a. With a glass of water
   b. On an empty stomach
   c. Through an NG tube
   d. Mixed in applesauce

3. One of Nina's respiratory medications is in the form of a sustained-release tablet. The nurse should avoid:
   a. Administering the tablet with another medication
   b. Mixing the drug with an antacid
   c. Crushing the tablet before administration
   d. Administering the tablet with water

4. The nurse is preparing to administer antibiotics to Nina. The fastest and most effective route of administration is:
   a. Oral
   b. Subcutaneous
   c. Intravenous
   d. Intramuscular

5. Nina is ordered an aspirin rectal suppository as needed for fever. The nurse is aware that the medication is:
   a. Administered with its covering intact
   b. Stored in the refrigerator
   c. Mixed with a gel before insertion
   d. Expelled within 1 minute after insertion

6. Nina is planning to take an Alaskan cruise during the next month, and her physician prescribes scopolamine disks to prevent motion sickness. The nurse instructs Nina to:
   a. Apply the disk to any hairy body surface
   b. Wear gloves when applying the disk
   c. Continue to shower while wearing the disk
   d. Rub the disk with forceful pressure after application

SITUATION 3–2

Raul Estosa is a patient in the Medical Intensive Care Unit following an automobile accident. He is on multiple drug therapy.

1. Mr. Estosa is ordered the antibiotic Wycillin 600,000 units IM tid. The *best* schedule for the nurse to follow in administering the Wycillin is:
   a. 10 AM, 2 PM, and 6 PM
   b. 7 AM, 4 PM, and 8 PM
   c. 8 AM, 1 PM, and 6 PM
   d. 9 AM, 6 PM, and 1 AM

2. When implementing drug therapy for Mr. Estosa, the nurse's responsibilities include all of the following *except:*
   a. Observing for drug effects
   b. Instructing the patient about the drug's use
   c. Checking for the correct dose of the drug
   d. Changing the dose if side effects occur

3. Each of the following is an appropriate nursing diagnosis related to administering medication to Mr. Estosa *except:*
   a. Potential for injury from medication administration
   b. Knowledge deficit related to current need for IV therapy
   c. Anxiety related to frequent intramuscular injections
   d. Impaired social interaction related to IV therapy

4. Before administering medication to Mr. Estosa, the nurse will do all of the following *except:*
   a. Withhold medication if his pulse is rapid
   b. Check his identification band
   c. Assess his mental status
   d. Honor his right to refuse medication

5. A heparin lock is placed in order to administer medications to Mr. Estosa. Nursing responsibilities associated with this device include:
   a. Preceding and following medication administration with heparin solution
   b. Mixing all multiple IV medications before injection
   c. Washing hands prior to administering medication
   d. Assessing for dehydration and decreased blood pressure following medication administration

6. The nurse administers an IV *bolus* of a bronchodilator to facilitate Mr. Estosa's breathing. A *bolus* is a:
   a. Continuous infusion given over a 24-hour period
   b. Concentrated dose given over a short time period
   c. Slow infusion given over 1 hour
   d. Diluted dose given 1–6 times a day

Refer to the Appendix for correct answers and additional review questions with answers.

4
CHAPTER

THE PHASES OF DRUG ACTION

THE PHASES OF DRUG
ACTION

CHAPTER OUTLINE

THE PHARMACEUTICAL PHASE
THE PHARMACOKINETIC PHASE
 Individual Differences
 Absorption
 Distribution
 Biotransformation
 Excretion
 Pharmacokinetic Principles
THE PHARMACODYNAMIC PHASE
 Mechanism of Drug Action
SUMMARY

GLOSSARY TERMS IN THIS CHAPTER

Absorption
Active transport
Accumulation
Agonist
Antagonist
Bioavailability
Biologic half-life
Biotransformation
Clearance
Desensitization
Diffusion
Dissolution
Distribution
Enterohepatic recirculation
Excretion
Exponential (first-order) kinetics
Facilitated diffusion
Filtration
Hepatic first-pass effect
Hyperreactivity (supersensitivity)
Ionized
Linear (zero order) kinetics
Loading dose
Maintenance dose
Michaelis-menton kinetics
Nonionized
Passive transport
Pharmaceutical phase or process
Pharmacodynamic phase
Pharmacokinetic phase
Pinocytosis
Placebo
Potency
Receptor
Selectivity
Solubility
Steady state
Volume of distribution

4
CHAPTER

THE PHASES OF DRUG ACTION

MERRILY MATHEWSON KUHN, R.N.C., Ph.D., CCRN

LEARNING OBJECTIVES

After reading this chapter, the student will be able to:

1. Differentiate among the pharmaceutical, pharmacokinetic, and pharmacodynamic phases of medication action.

2. Assess various factors that affect how the drug acts in the body.

3. Distinguish among the four pharmacokinetic phases of absorption, distribution, biotransformation, and excretion.

4. Define biologic half-life, effective concentration, peak plasma levels, therapeutic blood level, and minimum and maximum effective levels.

Medications are administered to achieve a specific result or therapeutic effect by altering body function. Medication may *treat* (e.g., aspirin for arthritic pain); *cure* (e.g., antibiotics for pneumonia); or *control* (e.g., insulin for diabetes). It is important for the nurse to understand the mechanism of action of medications in the body.

Medications may act in two ways within the body: (1) as structurally specific medications, acting on a specific cell or part of a cell; and (2) as structurally nonspecific medications, acting generally in the body but not on any specific structure.

After entering the body, most medications are dissolved, absorbed into the vascular system, distributed to the tissues to act on appropriate cells, *biotransformed* (broken down or metabolized), and excreted. As a medication passes through the body, it proceeds through three specific phases of drug activity: the *pharmaceutical phase*, the *pharmacokinetic phase*, and the *pharmacodynamic phase*.

THE PHARMACEUTICAL PHASE

The *pharmaceutical phase or process* describes that stage during which the medication enters the body in one form and changes into another form in order to be utilized. For example, a swallowed tablet or capsule is dissolved into solution by the gastrointestinal secretions. The medication is then ready for absorption into the blood stream. Liquid medications such as syrups and elixirs are already in liquid form and are generally ready for absorption faster than capsules or tablets. If the action of the drug is desired sooner, medications may be given subcutaneously, intramuscularly, or intravenously. When the medication is ready for absorption, the pharmacokinetic phase begins.

THE PHARMACOKINETIC PHASE

The pharmacokinetic phase comprises the medication's *absorption*, its *distribution* to the tissues, its *biotransformation* or metabolism, and its *excretion* from the body. Many basic principles of biochemistry and enzymology, along with principles of active and passive transport and distribution, are applied to understanding this aspect of drug administration.

INDIVIDUAL DIFFERENCES

The pharmacokinetic phase is individualized. A person can respond differently to the same medication when it is given at different times during his or her life cycle. Individual variations occur because of differences in body weight or age; because of disease states; or because of immune, psychologic, and environmental factors.

The time of day the drug is administered also influences response.

DIFFERENCES IN BODY WEIGHT. The average adult dose of aspirin is 10 grains (650 mg). Different reactions would be expected if this dose were given, for example, to a person weighing 100 lb and to one weighing 250 lb. The 100-lb person would receive a therapeutic effect, while the 250-lb person would have less-than-therapeutic effect. Therefore, many medications are ordered by body weight. Such as, an order for drug M 0.3 mg/kg body weight. If a child weighs 20 kg (2.2 lb/kg = 44 lb), the dose would be 6 mg (0.3 mg/kg × 20 kg).

The average adult dose is calculated on the premise that it will produce a specific effect in 50% of the population between ages 18 and 65 and weighing about 150 lb (70 kg). This means that very thin or obese individuals may have to receive special doses to achieve the same result. Pediatric doses are calculated on body weight expressed as milligrams per kilogram (mg/kg) or on body surface area (BSA) expressed as milligrams per square meter (mg/m²). A chart or nomogram plotting the weight in accordance with the height is used to determine the total BSA. (See Chapter 14 for more information on pediatric drug administration.)

AGE. The very young and the very old tend to react differently than the middle-aged person to medication. The immature liver or kidneys of the very young may delay drug metabolism and excretion. Delayed distribution, metabolism, and excretion are common in the elderly because of disease conditions or normal deterioration of body systems. Age may also affect the route chosen: An older person, because of poor circulation in the extremities, may not be given an intramuscular injection when acutely ill; instead, the nurse may give the medication intravenously.

PATHOLOGIC DISEASE STATES. Patients who have various pathologic diseases, such as those of the liver, kidney, or heart, react differently to medication. If a medication must be given to a patient with underlying organ disease, the patient is assessed closely for further damage to the organ and for differences in response to various medications. Therefore, the nurse must be aware of the signs and symptoms of further organ damage, such as long duration of action or toxic effects related to increased liver or kidney disease and long periods of time for absorption and circulation related to heart disease. The nurse also needs to understand the patient's current disease processes and frequently assess the patient for changes. Often a drug activates an old problem. For example, a patient taking two aspirin tablets four times a day to treat an arthritis flare-up may aggravate an ulcer condition dormant for some years, with resultant severe burning stomach pain. Using enteric-coated or buffered aspirin or taking aspirin with food may eliminate or mitigate the untoward side effect of plain aspirin.

IMMUNE FACTORS. The individual's immune system also affects how one responds to medication. Occasionally, when the patient receives a medication, the immune system is activated and produces antibodies to the foreign antigen (the medication). The next time this or a similar medication is taken, a systemic reaction may occur. As a example, a child is given penicillin for an ear infection. The ear infection is subsequently cured, and the child experiences no difficulties from the medication. Ten years later, the child develops pneumonia, and penicillin is again prescribed. This time, 30 minutes after the first penicillin tablet, the patient experiences generalized urticaria. This patient has developed antibodies against penicillin and should be told that he or she is allergic to penicillin. From now on, this patient should not receive penicillin or its related preparations and should carry a card identifying the allergy to penicillin. More is discussed on allergic drug reactions later in this chapter.

PSYCHOLOGIC FACTORS. The hopes, fears, and expectations of the individual often affect the action of the medication. If the patient is confident that the injection will relieve pain, the injection will most likely achieve that result. However, if the patient does not expect pain to lessen, it probably will not. Research indicates that the body produces natural substances called endorphins that help a person to control pain. If a person thinks the pain will be relieved, more endorphins are produced, ultimately relieving the pain. The body's release of endorphins in the brain and other body parts may be one reason why placebos are effective. (A *placebo* is an inactive substance or preparation given to satisfy the patient's perceived need for drug therapy.)

ENVIRONMENTAL FACTORS. The climate in which the patient lives may affect how he or she reacts to certain medications. This is a factor of reactivity rather than a true pharmacologic change. Temperature may affect the action/side effects of some drugs such as phenothiazines.

TIMING OF DOSAGE. Chronobiology (the study of body rhythms) has revealed countless patterns in the workings of the body. The adrenal glands of a person on a conventional schedule produce most of the day's supply of the hormone cortisol in a few hours beginning around 4:00 AM, primarily to prepare the body for stresses that are to come. Skin cells divide more rapidly at night; bone marrow make more blood cells from 6:00 PM to 10:00 PM than from 6:00 AM to 10:00 AM. The activity of the immune system is also cyclic, with the majority of natural killer cells being produced in the early morning.

Since drugs depend on enzymes and act on targets such as skin, bone, or liver, chronobiologists suggest body rhythms can have a profound effect on how drugs act. As a matter of fact, giving the same dose of the drug at a different time may be the same as giving a completely different dose. Today we know that more aspirin reaches the blood stream if it is taken at 7:00 AM than if it is taken at 11:00 PM. A single dose of antacid taken at night is more effective than two or three doses taken during the day. Alcohol, the most common of drugs, is more potent around midnight than the same amount consumed in the morning. Indomethacin (Indocin) used to treat arthritis is less likely to cause stomach pain or

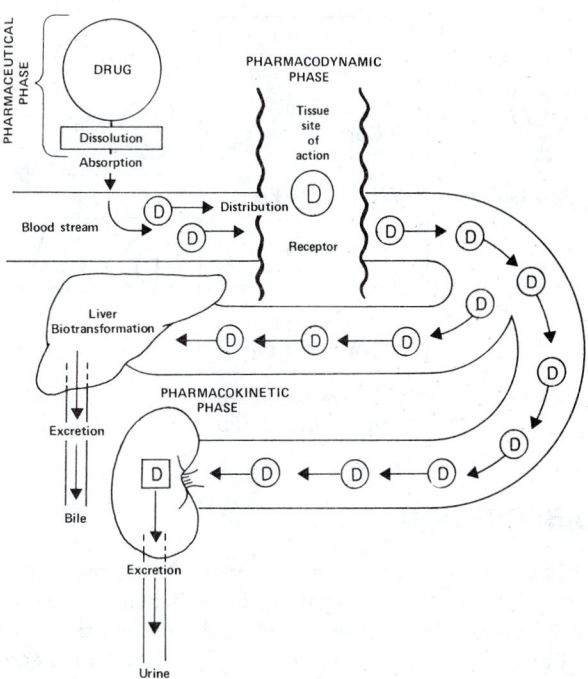

Figure 4–1. Pharmacokinetic phase of a typical medication: The medication is absorbed into the bloodstream and is distributed to its site of action. It may be biotransformed in the liver and then excreted by either the liver or the kidneys.

vertigo at bedtime. Perhaps the most dramatic effects of timing are in the treatment of cancer. Two common but extremely potent anticancer drugs are doxorubicin and cisplatin. Doxorubicin can destroy the bone marrow and elevate the heart rate, while cisplatin can cause irreversible kidney damage. It has been found that cisplatin is best administered in the evening bacause at this time the kidneys process large quantities of fluid and they may actually absorb less platinum from the cisplatin, producing less renal toxicity. Doxorubicin is best administered in the morning because the bone marrow is less vulnerable at that time when the cells are not dividing as quickly.

The question that researchers are asking today is which rhythms are the right rhythms since the body has an infinite number of rhythms that can affect each drug. Moreover, many diseases have patterns of their own, which can also affect the need for treatment. To further complicate matters, biologic cycles are easily disturbed. It would appear that in the future, chronobiology may assist patients in achieving a more therapeutic drug effect with less toxic effects.

To produce its desired effect, a medication must be present at the appropriate site in the appropriate concentration. This is usually proportional to the amount of the drug received. However, other factors, such as the extent and rate of absorption, distribution, biotransformation, and excretion, are also involved and are part of the pharmacokinetic phase (Fig.4–1).

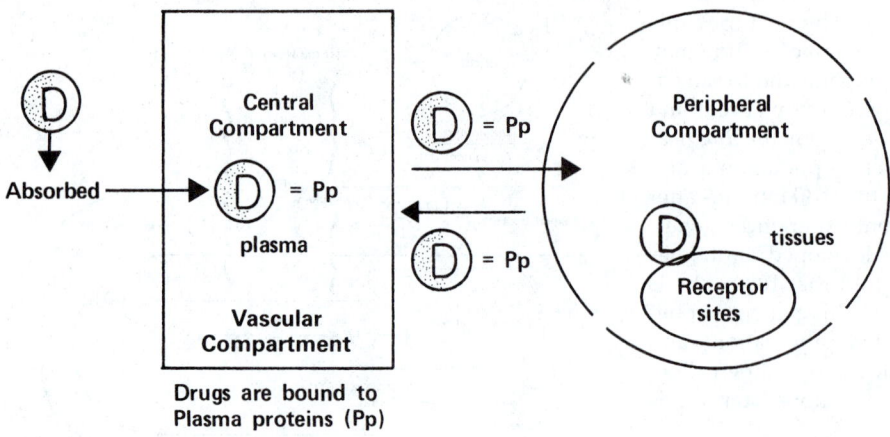

Figure 4–2. Drug distribution. Two compartments of the body hold medication, the central vascular compartment and the peripheral compartment.

ABSORPTION

Absorption is a process of movement of the medication into the central compartment, the vascular bed, which contains the blood and plasma and is where the medication travels in the body (Fig. 4–2). Medications enter the central compartment after being absorbed from the gastrointestinal tract, the rectum, any parenteral site, the skin, or the respiratory tract. Medications are also injected directly into the central compartment through the intravenous route and are therefore completely absorbed. Many factors influence the absorption of drugs and, therefore, will affect the route of administration. Factors affecting absorption include solubility, dissolution, pharmaceutical processing, concentration of the drug, circulation to the site of absorption, the absorbing surface, and the route of administration.

Factors Affecting Absorption

BIOAVAILABILITY. For a medication to be absorbed, it must be available. The bioavailability of a medication depends on the solubility of the outer covering of a tablet or capsule, pharmaceutical processing of the drug, and the pH of the medication, all of which can enhance or retard the rate of dissolution of the drug. Medication *bioavailability* can be simply stated as the percentage absorbed. Dosage forms of a drug from different manufacturers and even different lots of preparation from a single manufacturer sometimes differ in their bioavailability. Drug manufacturers and government agencies are cooperating to develop standard tests for bioavailability of pharmaceutical preparations. Bioavailability is also dependent on the presence or absence of food within the gastrointestinal tract. Drugs may have their absorption rate or extent decreased (or increased) by food. The rate is the speed at which a drug becomes available, while extent refers to the amount of drug that is absorbed and therefore available. The drug may complex with food, making less drug available for absorption, or food can actually slow the rate of drug absorption by not allowing enough drug in contact with the intestinal wall. On the other hand, the bioavailability extent can also be increased with food as a result of the increased activity within the intestinal system or the effect that food has on the pH of the intestinal system. Table 4–1 features several drugs that have their bioavailability affected by food.

DRUG SOLUBILITY. *Solubility* is the ability of a medication to dissolve and form a solution. A medication must be able to form a solution or suspension in

Table 4–1. EFFECT OF FOOD ON THE BIOAVAILABILITY OF DRUGS*

Bioavailability Rate Decreased	Bioavailability Extent Decreased	Bioavailability Extent Increased
Acetaminophen	Alcohol	Diazepam
Aspirin (effervescent tablets, tablets)	Amoxicillin	Dicumarol
Cefaclor	Ampicillin	Erythromycin ethyl succinate (coated
Cephalexin	Aspirin (enteric-coated tablets,	tablets, suspension)
Cimetidine	tablets)	Erythromycin stearate
Ciprofloxacin	Erythromycin	Griseofulvin
Digoxin (tablets)	Isoniazid	Hydralazine
Erythromycin (coated tablets, tablets)	Levodopa	Hydrochlorothiazide
Furosemide	Nafcillin	Lithium citrate
Ibuprofen	Penicillin G	Metoprolol
Nitrofurantoin	Penicillin V (suspension, tablets)	Nitrofurantoin
Phenobarbital	Rifampin	Phenytoin
	Tetracycline	Propranolol
		Spironolactone

*This is only a partial listing.

body fluids to be available for absorption into cells and tissues. The solubility of a medication affects the quantity available for absorption. Lipid-soluble products enter the vascular system more readily than other substances because most cell membranes contain a fatty acid layer. Also, only lipid-soluble substances can readily cross into the brain. Medications may react with each other (digitalis glycosides and antacids) or with substances within the body (antacids with phosphate) to form an insoluble precipitate that cannot be absorbed. The nurse must be aware of the possible reactions (discussed specifically in Chapter 5 and throughout this text) to avoid solubility problems. Medications in an aqueous solution are very quickly absorbed when given parenterally.

DISSOLUTION. *Dissolution* is the ability of a drug to move into a liquid. The ability of a drug to dissolve may be a limiting factor in absorption.

PHARMACEUTICAL PROCESSING. The pharmaceutical processing can either enhance or delay absorption. The binders or excipients used to produce and stablize the drug product, such as alcohol, dextrose, starch, oils, or other chemicals, ultimately affect the solubility of the drug. Alcohol-based products have enhanced absorption and availability, whereas oil-based products have delayed absorption and availability.

To facilitate dissolution of medication, disintegrators and chemical buffers may be added to the medication. Disintegrators, inert substances such as starch, dissolve readily, thus causing the solid drug to fragment quickly. Buffers also promote rapid dissolution through their effect on the pH of the medication at the site of absorption.

Pharmaceutical processing also includes the actual form of the product—liquids, tablets, or capsules. Liquids are available more readily becasue they are already in solution. Enteric-coated tablets are designed to be released only after they enter the relatively alkaline small

intestine. (The pH of the stomach is 1–2; the pH of the small intestine is 4–5). Time-release (sustained-release) tablets are prepared so that only a part of the medication enters solution at a time, producing a longer duration of action. Capsules, in general, are absorbed more readily than tablets. Once the capsule is destroyed, the powder or granules within have a greater surface area than a compressed tablet, thereby enhancing absorption. Time-release capsules are specially formulated capsules containing coated pellets intended to provide both immediate and sustained release of medications for as long as 8–12 hours.

Repeat-action tablets carry an initial dose in an outer shell and a second dose in an inner shell. The inner shell disintegrates later in the intestinal tract.

Osmotic pump formulations, generally tablets, have a special semipermeable membrane covering, which allows water to enter. The drug in solution can then leave the tablet, but only through a single small hole made by a laser beam during the formulation process.

pH. As medications move into solution, they become either *ionized* or *nonionized*. The ionized forms are generally lipid insoluble and nondiffusible. The nonionized forms (nonpolarized compounds) are lipid soluble and diffusible. Only nonionized forms are able to be absorbed. The availability of nonionized drugs depends on their ability to dissociate into their component parts—acids or bases. Basic drugs tend to dissociate more in acid solutions, and acid drugs tend to dissociate more in basic solutions (Fig. 4–3).

In the stomach, a very strongly acidic medium (pH 1.4), acid drugs (barbiturates, aspirin) tend to remain nonionized (nonpolarized compounds) and should be readily absorbed. However, because of the poor absorptive surface in the stomach, acidic drugs are actually better absorbed in the small intestine. By administering an antacid concurrently with an acidic drug, however, absorption can be enhanced. Basic drugs (quinidine, mor-

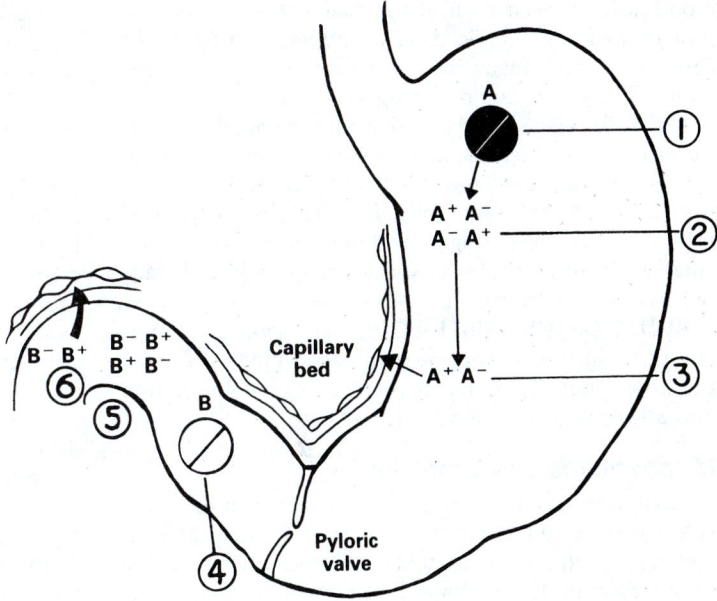

Figure 4–3. Steps in absorption of an oral tablet. (A = acid tablet, eg. aspirin; B = basic tablet, eg. quinidine). (1) acid drug reaches stomach, (2) becomes nonionized, and (3) is ready for absorption. (4) A basic drug enters duodenum where pH increases to 6.0 to 8.0, (5) becomes nonionized, and (6) is absorbed.

phine) tend to remain ionized and, therefore, are not absorbed across the stomach.

Presence or absence of food in the gastrointestinal tract will alter the rate of absorption of medications. The acidic contents of the stomach may increase the destruction of medication (e.g., penicillin G) since the food slows the emptying time of the stomach and increases the time of contact with the digestive juices. Food can also be implicated in causing absorption or adherence of the drug to the food because of chemical or physical action, resulting in decreased absorption. The calcium-containing foods, for example, greatly reduce the absorption of tetracycline, allowing less drug to be available and resulting in an inadequate systemic antibacterial action. The pH of the meal may change the amount of ionized compound formed and thus change the amount of medication absorbed since the nonpolar or nonionized molecules quickly move across membranes, while the ionized molecules do not. In general, but not always, an empty stomach enhances absorption, whereas food delays absorption.

In the intestines, pH increases to 4–5. Here, formerly ionized basic drugs (quinine, digitalis) reunite to form nonionized compounds (nonpolarized), and their absorption is enhanced. Acid drugs return to their ionized form and should have reduced absorption. However, because of the increased surface area and increased absorption of the small intestine, the majority of acidic drugs are also absorbed in the small intestine.

CONCENTRATION OF THE DRUG. The concentration of a drug influences its rate of absorption. The more concentrated a drug, the more rapidly it will be absorbed from the area of high concentration in the gastrointestinal system to a low concentration in the blood.

CIRCULATION TO THE SITE OF ABSORPTION. Blood flow in the administration and absorption site affects the amount of drug absorbed. Reduced blood flow, as occurs in peripheral vascular diseases and shock states, and with concurrent vasoconstrictor drug administration, reduces the absorption of drug. Increased blood flow, as occurs with local massage, local application of heat, metabolic disease (hyperthyroidism), or concurrent administration of vasodilator drugs, enhances the absorption of a drug.

ABSORBING SURFACE. The absorbing surface is the surface to which the drug is exposed for absorption such as the surface of the intestinal mucosa, the skin, or the pulmonary alveolar epithelium. The larger the surface area, the more drug is absorbed. Scar tissue has a small absorbing area, so medications should not be administered near scars.

ROUTE OF ADMINISTRATION. The route of administration places the drug near the absorbing surface in the appropriate form and concentration for dissolution and absorption into the vascular system.

Mechanisms of Absorption

Medications move through the body and into target cells through several mechanisms: active transport, passive transport, and pinocytosis. All mechanisms enable the medication to penetrate the cell membrane to allow the medication to act within the cell (Fig.4–4).

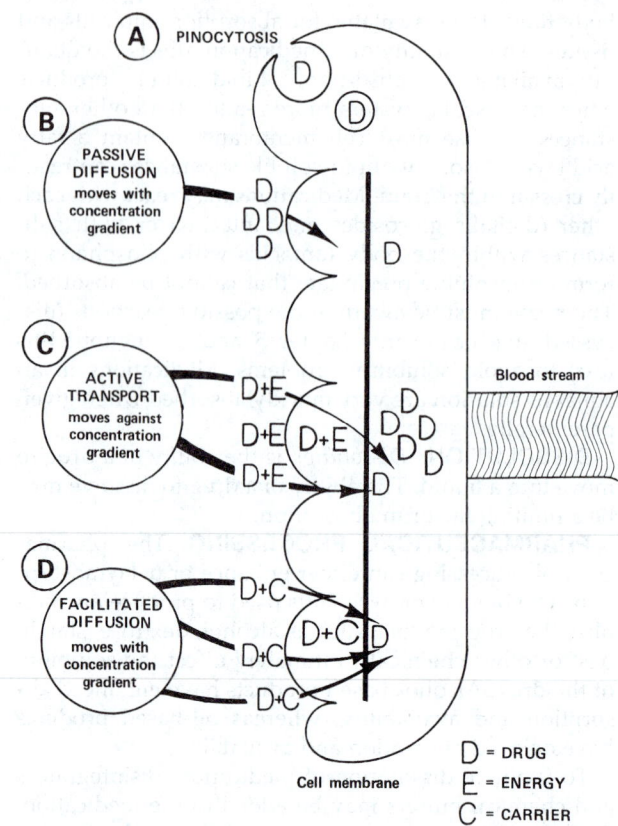

Figure 4–4. Movement of medications. Medications move across the cell membrane by passive diffusion (B)—moving with a concentration gradient; active transport (C)—moving against a concentration gradient so energy is required; facilitated diffusion (D)—moving with a concentration gradient but a carrier is needed; or pinocytosis (A), moving into the cell through an invagination into the cell wall.

Active transport requires energy and "carriers." Active transport, generally a one-way transport process, moves substances against a concentration gradient (moving from areas of low concentration to high concentration). The carriers, consisting of proteins, form complexes with the drug molecule, moving the drug across the cell membrane before dissociating from the drug, leaving the drug free to act within the cell. Energy is consumed during active transport because of the work performed by the carrier. The rate of movement against the concentration gradient is directly related to the concentration of the drug and to the amount of transport carrier available. The carrier system can reach a saturated level with drug dosing; this determines the maxium level of active transport into the cell. Also, the carrier is structurally or chemically specific and can carry only specific drugs.

Passive transport allows drug molecules to move into and out of cells without the expenditure of cellular energy. The concentration of medication is always highest in the original compartment. Therefore, absorption of the medication occurs as drugs move with the concentration gradient from high to low areas of concentration.

Passive diffusion is limited by the concentration of the drug present at the membrane site and also the area of the membrane where diffusion occurs.

Several distinct processes are involved in passive transport: filtration, diffusion, and facilitated diffusion. *Filtration* is a process of moving particles from a solution by allowing the liquid portion to pass through a membrane or other particle barrier. This barrier contains holes or spaces through which the liquid may pass but which are too small to permit the solid particles to pass. In *diffusion,* molecules move from areas of high concentration to areas of low concentration. In *facilitated diffusion,* a carrier is needed to cross the cell membrane. However, facilitated diffusion does not require energy because it does not move across a concentration gradient.

Pinocytosis is a mechanism that occurs when the cell wall invaginates, fills with the drugs, breaks off, and moves into the cell. The quantitative significance of pinocytosis in drug absorption is difficult to estimate and controversial.

Routes of Absorption

The routes of absorption of medication include skin, mucous membranes, gastrointestinal, parenteral, and inhalation.

SKIN. Medication placed on the surface of the skin may be for systemic or local action. The absorption of these drugs is proportional to their lipid solubility since the epidermis is a lipid barrier. In addition, absorption is proportional to their size: small molecules are more readily absorbed. The systemically acting medications such as nitroglycerin and scopolamine are absorbed into the vascular system and eventually reach their target tissues. Locally acting medications (anti-infectives or emollients) have their effect only in the area in which they are applied.

The skin is usually less permeable than other ports of entry, but medications enter more rapidly when the skin is abraded and covered with an occlusive dressing. Also, systemic toxicity can occur when excessive medication is absorbed. Salicylate poisoning can occur when excessive amounts of methyl salicylate (oil of wintergreen) are used to relieve arthritic pain. It is now available only with a doctor's prescription. Table 4–2 features the advantages and limitations of each route of drug administration.

MUCOUS MEMBRANES. Medication can be applied to the mucus membranes of the eye, ear, nose, vagina, urethra, and rectum. Medications may be applied for a local effect, such as a local anesthetic, antibiotic, or antiseptic, or for their systemic effect.

The rectum is at times an excellent route for medication administration. It is a vascular area, and medications quickly enter the vascular system and are not destroyed by the gastrointestinal secretions. This route is often used when the patient is not allowed anything by mouth, or when the medication can be destroyed by gastric secretions or can irritate the stomach or intestinal lining. Medications often given through the rectal route include aspirin to reduce fever and morphine to reduce severe pain. Both medications may be irritating to the upper gastrointestinal tract if given by mouth but cause fewer side effects when given rectally.

Table 4–2. ADVANTAGES AND LIMITATIONS OF VARIOUS ROUTES FOR DRUG ADMINISTRATION

Route	Advantages	Limitations	Examples of Common Medications
Skin	Easy to use	Intact epidermis generally not permeable. Inflammation or abrasion can lead to systemic absorption with toxic effects.	Local: Anesthetics, antibiotics, antiseptics, emollients, steroids Systemic: Antihistamines, vasodilators, hormones
Mucous membranes (GI tract, respiratory tract, vagina)	Easy to use	Systemic absorption can occur readily from local drugs.	Local: Anesthetics, antibiotics, miotics, mydriatics Systemic: Antipyretics, bronchodilators, vasodilators
Oral	Easy to use, most convenient, and economical	Needs cooperative patient and an intact GI system. Absorption may be sporadic and undependable.	Local: Antacids, laxatives, antidiarrheals Systemic: Steroids, antibiotics, analgesics, cardiac medications, and many others
Parenteral	Generally prompt absorption	Sterile technique is required. Possibly results in pain and necrosis at site.	Local: Steroids into joints Systemic: Antibiotics, insulin, analgesics, and many others
Inhalation	Large surface area for rapid absorption	Poor ability to regulate dose. Many drugs cause irritation.	Local: Bronchodilators, mucolytics Systemic: Oxygen, anesthetics

GASTROINTESTINAL. Most oral medications are absorbed from the small intestine. Some exceptions are alcohol, alcohol-based drugs such as elixirs, and aspirin, which are absorbed across the stomach. The convoluted lining of the duodenum contains millions of tiny capillaries that absorb medications into the central vascular compartment. The concepts previously discussed of dissolution, solubility, pharmaceutical processing, concentration of the drug, circulation to the site, and absorbing surface are all considered when administrating oral medications.

Gastric-emptying time is another important factor. The presence or absence of food and antacids will affect absorption. The patient must take some medications with food, whereas others must be taken on an empty stomach. Liquid medications are absorbed more quickly than solids. Therefore, tablets and capsules are best administered with a large glass of liquid to accelerate their dissolution and absorption. Still other medications cannot be given with certain foods; tetracycline (an antibiotic), for example, is not administered concurrently with milk, cheese, or antacids because the calcium in these substances binds with tetracycline, decreasing absorption of the drug. (More information on interactions can be found in Chapter 5 as well as throughout this text.) Antacids can prolong gastric-emptying time, thereby delaying the access of the gastric contents to the much larger absorptive area of the small intestine. Significant interactions can occur as a consequence of antacid administration.

PARENTERAL ROUTE. Parenteral medications are given through the intravenous, intramuscular, or subcutaneous route. The intravenous administration of medication provides immediate and complete absorption, while injections given intramuscularly, such as antibiotics and narcotics, or subcutaneously, such as heparin and insulin, result in penetration of tissues and eventual absorption into the vascular system. In general, parenteral medications have an onset of action earlier than oral medications do because they are more rapidly absorbed. However, patients with poor circulation or low blood pressure are given intramuscular or subcutaneous medications cautiously, because the absorption of the drugs may be delayed, thus delaying or even canceling their therapeutic effect. Patients receiving medications by this route may be unable to take the medication by mouth, or the medication itself (e.g., insulin) may be destroyed by the gastrointestinal system, leaving the parenteral route the only one available.

INHALATION. Gases, volatile medications, and aerosols may be administered into the respiratory tract, either through regular inhalation (anesthetics) or with pressure assistance (bronchodilators). These medications take the form of fine mists that easily move across the alveolar membrane into the pulmonary capillary bed to have either a local effect in the lung or a systemic effect.

DISTRIBUTION

As the medication is absorbed into the blood stream, several phases of distribution occur. The initial phase distributes medication to high blood flow areas such as the heart, liver, kidney, and brain, usually within several minutes. During the second phase, distribution occurs to areas of slower blood flow, such as the muscle, bone, middle ear, skin, and fat. Distribution to the areas may take up to several hours. Both of these phases are dependent on cardiac output and regional blood flow. When cardiac output is reduced, adequate tissue levels of medications are difficult to obtain. Superimposed on patterns of distribution of blood flow are factors that determine the rate at which drugs diffuse into tissues. Diffusion into the tissues is dependent on protein-binding of the medication as well as its solubility (lipid or aqueous solution).

Plasma Protein Binding

As the medication is absorbed into the vascular system, it is transported through protein molecules in the plasma, usually albumin, to its site of action (Fig. 4–5). The drug-protein complex is termed "bound drug," whereas the unattached drug is available to produce an effect and is termed "free drug." The plasma protein bindings range from very stable to very unstable. The plasma proteins are generally unable to exit from the vascular system because of molecular size; similarly, the units of medication that are attached to the proteins cannot exit unless they are freed from their binding sites. The stronger the binding, the slower the freeing of the medication, resulting in a longer duration of action, which may or may not be beneficial. As medication is metabolized by the body, more is usually released from the binding sites. An example of a very stable affinity between a medication and plasma protein is digitalis leaf (rarely used today because of its poor assay and better available preparations), which may have a duration of action of as long as three weeks. A patient who de-

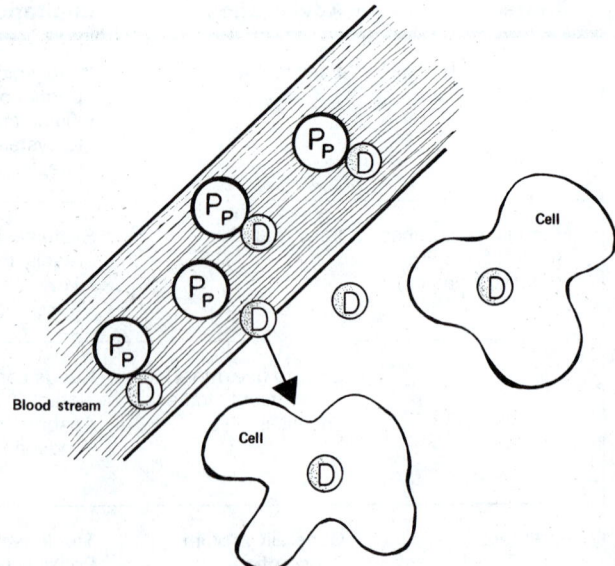

Figure 4–5. Medications (D) bind with plasma proteins (Pp) to be transported through the bloodstream. As the medication is freed from the plasma protein-binding site, it enters the tissues.

velops side effects or toxic reactions experiences them for several weeks until digitalis leaf is excreted.

Since most medications are bound in the serum to albumin, the patient has difficulty transporting medications if hypoalbuminemia exists. (Many body hormones are also carried on protein.) Because there is less protein to transport the drug molecules, excess free drug may result in an exaggerated pharmacologic effect that could prove dangerous to the patient.

Occasionally, 2 or more medications compete for the same plasma-protein-binding site. When this occurs, the drug with the strongest affinity for the binding site displaces the other drug. This is one form of drug interaction. (See Chapter 5 for more information on drug interactions.) When this interaction occurs, the drug displaced usually produces a toxic effect because a large concentration of drug is now free in the central compartment, as, for example, when aspirin, an antiarthritic medication, is given concurrently with the anticoagulant warfarin (Coumadin). Aspirin displaces warfarin from the binding site, thereby increasing the free warfarin concentration in the central compartment, causing the patient to bleed.

Solubility

Distribution is also dependent on solubility. Generally, because of the highly permeable nature of the capillary endothelial membrane, diffusion can occur rapidly. Lipid-soluble drugs readily move across the endothelial membrane, whereas lipid-insoluble drugs permeate these membranes poorly and are therefore restricted in their distribution. As an example, diazepam (Valium), a lipid-soluble drug, is distributed widely to adipose tissue and brain. Lorazepam (Ativan), a water-soluble drug, is not well distributed to the brain.

Equilibrium

Equilibrium is achieved when a stable ratio of drug is found within all body compartments including the central and the peripheral compartments. The ratio in each compartment does not have to be equal but in fact may change as the level of drug goes to a new equilibrium in the plasma or peripheral (tissue reservoir) compartment.

Drug Reservoirs

Body compartments act as reservoirs for drugs. The reservoir may fill quickly, altering distribution of the drug. Larger quantities of a drug may be required initially to provide a therapeutic level while the reservoirs are also being filled. Drugs including lipid-soluble drugs such as barbiturates, antibiotics, anesthetics, and anticoagulants are stored in fat, while other drugs such as tetracycline antibiotics, radioactive elements (e.g., ^{32}P, radium), and environmental pollutants (e.g., lead, arsenic) are stored in the bone. Both fat and bone release these stored drugs slowly over time.

Various medications have an affinity for certain body tissue. When the medication passes near that particular tissue, it will exit the blood stream to the tissue, even though it may not be the target tissue. If the blood level of drug is insufficient at the target site, increased dose or more frequent dosing intervals may be required.

Plasma Levels

The plasma concentration is the amount of both free and bound drug in plasma. Peak level or peak concentration is achieved when maximal amount of the drug is absorbed into the plasma or in the target tissue. As the peak level is reached, maximal effect usually occurs. (The term "usually" is used because peak level takes into account both bound and free drug, and all the drug may not yet be active to cause maximal effect.)

Volume of Distribution

The *volume of distribution* (V_d) of a drug refers to the volume (blood, fat, and total body water) that the drug would appear to be distributed in during its steady state if the drug existed throughout that volume at the same concentration as in the plasma. Therefore, if a drug is highly concentrated in the tissues, its apparent V_d may be many times total body water. The V_d ultimately determines the drug dosage.

A highly water-soluble drug possesses a small volume of distribution and has a high blood concentration level. A high fat-soluble drug possesses a large volume of distribution and has a low blood concentration level. Factors that tend to keep a drug in circulation (high water solubility, high serum protein binding) result in a lower volume of distribution but a high blood level. Conversely, factors that promote the movement of a drug from the blood to other compartments (high lipid solubility, high degree of tissue binding) result in a higher volume of distribution and consequently a lower blood level.

Redistribution

Drug effect is generally terminated by biotransformation and excretion but may also occur by redistribution of the drug from its site of action into other tissues. If these other tissues are fat, the drug will then be eliminated slowly from this drug reservoir. Lidocaine and diazepam (Valium) are examples of drugs that are stored in fat.

Central Nervous System and Placental Barriers

The central nervous system (brain and spinal cord) and the placenta have distribution barriers that discourage or prevent medications from entering. Usually only medications that are lipid soluble cross these barriers. Some examples are atropine, scopolamine, general anesthetics, and penicillin G. The blood–brain barrier is an important mechanism that protects the brain from chemical substances. The blood–brain barrier refers to an active transport system that pumps drug out of the brain after diffusion has allowed it to enter. If, for example, meningitis occurs, this transport system fails, and higher amounts of penicillin are allowed to remain in the brain.

Brain capillaries differ from their counterparts in most tissues by the tight junctions and absence of intercellular pores. In addition, the unique arrangement of glial cells (astrocytes) around the blood vessels contribute to slow diffusion of medications into the central nervous system.

The placenta is considered to be a lipid membrane that allows passage of substances by simple diffusion. Today, it is believed that the fetus is generally exposed to the same drug concentrations as the mother.

BIOTRANSFORMATION

Biotransformation or metabolism refers to the enzymatic alteration of a drug molecule. During biotransformation, some drugs are converted to inactive metabolites ready for excretion. However, a small number of medications become active only after this chemical reaction (e.g., 6-mercaptopurine conversion to 6-mercaptopurine ribonucleotide); still other medications are effective both before and after biotransformation (e.g., phenylbutazone conversion to oxyphenbutazone).

The majority of medications are biotransformed in the liver, but biotransformation can also occur in the renal tissue, lungs, blood plasma, and intestinal mucosa. Several factors affect biotransformation and include the extent of plasma protein binding, drug storage in reservoirs, liver function, blood flow to the liver, presence of other substances that can either induce or inhibit liver function, and age.

Biotransformation is generally classified by separating its actions into two categories—synthetic and nonsynthetic. These reactions do not refer to the origin of the medication—natural or synthetic—but only to the reaction itself. The synthetic reaction, also referred to as a conjugation reaction, occurs when the medication or its metabolite combines with an endogenous substance, usually a carbohydrate. This reaction generally produces a soluble, less active substance that is readily excreted. Additional synthetic processes include alkylation (combining the drug with an alkyl group), acetylation (combining the drug with an acetyl group), and methylation (combining the drug with a methyl group). A nonsynthetic reaction may involve the processes of oxidation, reduction, and hydrolysis, which change the activity of the drug into either a less active, equally active, or more active substance.

During either synthetic or nonsynthetic reactions, drugs may be converted through either serial or parallel transformation. In serial transformation the drug undergoes a series of steps: 1 to 2 to 3 to 4. An example would be chloral hydrate to trichloroethanol to trichloroethanol glucuronide.

In parallel transformation, the original product follows different pathways and yields various products: 1 to 2; 1 to 3; 1 to 4. An example would be salicylic acid to salicyluric acid:

salicylic phenolic glucuronide
salicylic acyl glucuronide
gentisic acid

Both synthetic and nonsynthetic biotransformations occur in the liver through an enzyme catalyst reaction. The foreign substance, the medication, is converted to a generally harmless metabolite (usually), which is then excreted by the kidney.

Some medications absorbed into the vascular system from the portal system are metabolized almost completely by the liver on their first pass. This is called the *hepatic first-pass effect*. Medications administered parenterally miss the hepatic system. Because of this metabolism, a drug such as lidocaine is not effective by the oral route and is given parenterally. Another drug, propranolol (Inderal), is also greatly metabolized by the liver on its first pass. For this reason, oral doses are much higher than parenteral doses: oral doses range from 40–160 mg, whereas parenteral (IV) doses range from 1–2 mg.

The liver has thousands of enzymes capable of catalyzing the transformation of active medication into inactive metabolites. Most medications are catalyzed by different enzymes. These enzymes usually serve to catalyze or accelerate the reaction but are not destroyed by the reaction. However, in certain instances, such as those in which the patient has hepatitis, hepatic sclerosis, or other liver degeneration, particular enzymes may exist in lowered concentration. In these cases, the medication may circulate for a longer time and trigger toxic reactions. At other times, the particular enzyme may increase in concentration (e.g., it may be triggered by another drug) and hasten the transformation of the medication into its inactive metabolite, thereby decreasing its effectiveness. For example, a person who smokes normally has an increase in several liver enzymes. If this patient also receives the bronchodilator theophylline, there will be an increase in the enzyme that helps to metabolize theophylline and thus a lower theophylline plasma level.

As mentioned previously, one drug may stimulate production of a liver enzyme that increases the biotransformation of a totally unrelated medication. For example, barbiturates stimulate the liver enzyme that biotransforms warfarin. This means that when barbiturates are given concurrently with warfarin, the dose of warfarin has to be increased to achieve optimum effects. Many other examples of drug interactions are discussed in Chapter 5.

Lipid solubility is important, but it is not the only factor for drug metabolism in the liver. Lipid solubility does favor the penetration of the drug into the endoplasmic reticulum and its binding to cytochrome P-450. Cytochrome P-450 is the primary oxidative enzyme system within the liver. The microsomal enzymes within the liver do contribute to the biotransformation of fatty acids, steroid hormones, and conjugate bilirubin.

When the nurse administers medications to the very young or old patient, the possibility of toxic drug complications must be considered. The young patient may not have a fully developed liver enzyme system, while the elderly or debilitated patient may have diminished function of the liver enzyme systems. These patients need to be assessed carefully and continually for possible toxic effects.

EXCRETION

Medications are excreted from the body unchanged or as metabolites. Medications are eliminated mostly through the renal system but also in lesser amounts through the gastrointestinal and respiratory systems, as well as through sweat, saliva, and breast milk. The rate of excretion varies with the concentration of the drug; as the drug concentration rises within the serum, excretion also rises. A *steady state* is reached when the rate of administration equals the rate of excretion. If excretion falls behind, serum levels rise, leading to a phenomenon called accumulation. *Accumulation* is the result of the gradual increase in the blood level of drugs. The increased level of the medication in the blood is likely to result in serious or toxic effects in the patient.

Clearance

Clearance is a measure of speed at which a drug leaves the body either through the kidney or the liver. A drug has a low clearance rate if it is removed from the body slowly. A drug has a high clearance rate if it is removed from the body rapidly. A drug with a high clearance often requires more frequent administration and higher doses than a drug with a low clearance. Clearance equals the V_d/Biologic half-life. Clearances are stated in milliliter per minute or liters per hour and sometimes normalized to weight. As an example, aspirin has a clearance of 9.3 ml/minute, thus, 9.3 ml is eliminated each minute per kilogram of body weight. If renal function or clearance is reduced, then the time it takes to eliminate the aspirin would be increased. Thus, it may be necessary to reduce the dose or lengthen the time between doses to prevent adverse or toxic effects.

Biologic Half-Life of Medications

The biotransformation and excretion of a medication determines the drug's *biologic half-life*. The biologic half-life of a medication is the amount of time required to reduce the original plasma concentration by 50%. The half-life of a drug ultimately determines how often the drug is to be administered. The half-life is usually not dose-dependent; therefore doubling the dose will *not* double the half-life. Half-lives do not necessarily reflect duration of action. The half-life for a given medication generally remains the same within an individual patient if all body systems are functioning normally, but a patient with renal or hepatic disease may have increased drug half-lives. For example, a 500-mg dose of a medication with a half-life of three hours is given: 250 mg remains in the body after three hours, 125 mg remains after 6 hours and 62.5 mg remains after nine hours (Fig. 4–6). It takes approximately five half-lives for a medication to be totally excreted. By understanding the concept of half-life, the nurse can appreciate why some antihypertensive medications, such as methyldopa (Aldomet) with a half-life of one hour, needs to be given two to four times daily, while others, such as guanfacine (Tenex) with a half-life of 17 hours, can be given once daily.

The difference between the daily dosage schedules of three hypoglycemic agents is based in part on their biologic half-lives. Chlorpropamide (Diabinese), with a half-life of 36 hours, is usually given once daily; tolazamide (Tolinase), with a half-life of seven to eight

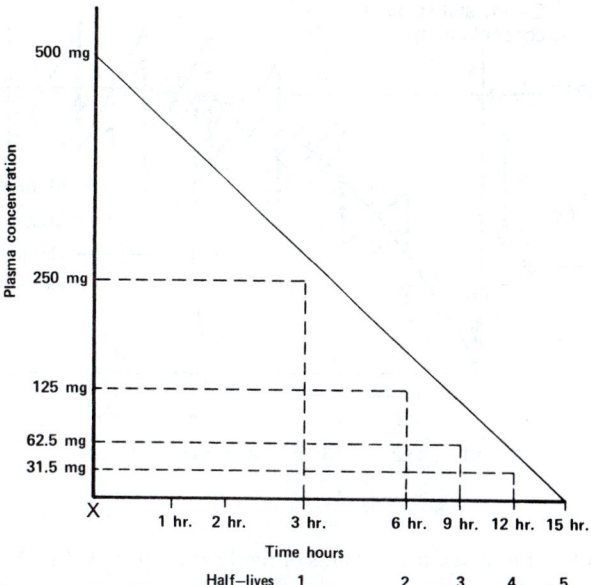

Figure 4–6. Linear medication curve shows the biologic half-life of a medication. A dose of 500 mg of the drug, which has a half-life of 3 hours, is given at point X. At 3 hours, 250 mg is excreted; at 6 hours, an additional 125 mg is excreted; at 9 hours, an additional 62.5 mg is excreted. This continues for approximately five half-lives.

hours, is given once or twice a day; and tolbutamide (Orinase), with a half-life of four to six hours, is usually given in two or three equally divided doses.

Steady State

A steady state is reached when the rate of administration equals the rate of excretion. It takes approximately five half-lives to reach a steady-state condition. Figure 4–7 examines several dosing schedules to achieve steady state. After five half-lives, all methods achieve a steady state, but the minimum/maximum plasma concentrations differ markedly.

Drug Loading Doses

The way a drug is first administered affects how quickly it reaches full therapeutic effect and steady state. When a drug is administered on a dosage schedule that is satisfactory for maintenance therapy, a partial effect occurs promptly, but full therapeutic effect will not occur for five half-lives. If the therapeutic situation is not acute, this dosage schedule may be preferred because it minimizes the risk of initial drug effects and patient dosages can be readily adjusted as the drug accumulates. However, if a full therapeutic effect is required, an initial *loading dose* may be necessary. A loading dose, however, does increase the risk of side and/or toxic effects. Sometimes, as with digitalis, an estimated loading dose is administered in divided fractions to permit at least some monitoring for efficacy and safety.

Renal Excretion

The renal system uses the processes of glomerular filtration and active tubular secretion to excrete either the ac-

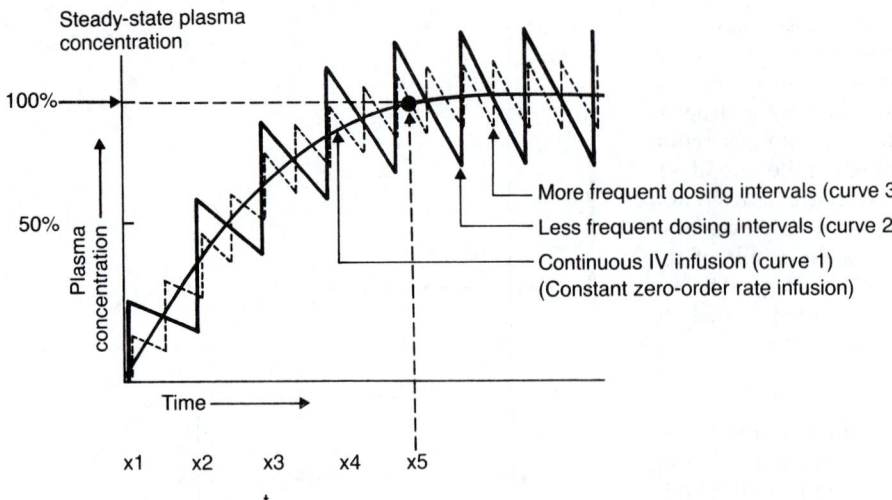

Figure 4-7. Dosing curve—relationship between dosing at a continuous IV rate with a constant zero-order rate infusion and two different rates—more frequent and less frequent—and their minimim/maximum plasma concentrations. All three methods reach steady-state at the same time—in five half-lives.

tive or inactive metabolites of medication (Fig. 4–8). The kidney usually removes the medication that is unbound and free in the plasma. Several factors directly affect the rate of excretion of medication from the kidney: the maturity of the kidney; kidney function (the absence or presence of disease); and circulatory function (the ability of the heart and blood vessels to deliver a blood supply to the kidney).

Some medications, such as penicillin, are totally excreted on the first pass through the kidney. This accounts for the medication's short duration of action. Other medications need several passes through the kidney to be totally excreted. The excretion time of some medications may depend on urinary pH. When the tubular urine is made more acidic, for example, the excretion of weak acid medications is reduced, because the formation of the nonionized (nonpolar) molecules is favored and their reabsorption into the blood is increased. In a similar fashion, the excretion of weak bases is de-

layed in an alkaline urine because of increased recovery or reabsorption in the kidney and thus reduced excretion. By altering the urinary pH, it is possible to enhance or delay excretion of certain medications. Changing the urinary pH can be effective in enhancing excretion of poisons; for example, the urinary pH can be made more alkaline in order to increase excretion of aspirin in a patient who has taken an overdose. With other treatment methods available today, however, changing the urinary pH is seldom an important part of the treatment regimen, although it may still be used.

If the kidneys are damaged, extracorporeal dialysis may be employed as a substitute. The artificial kidney is designed to perform the kidney's function to remove wastes from the body. Any medication that is normally removed by the kidney can generally be removed through dialysis. Dialysis may be particularly helpful in treating cases of accidental or deliberate poisoning or drug overdose even if the kidney is functioning. Dialysis

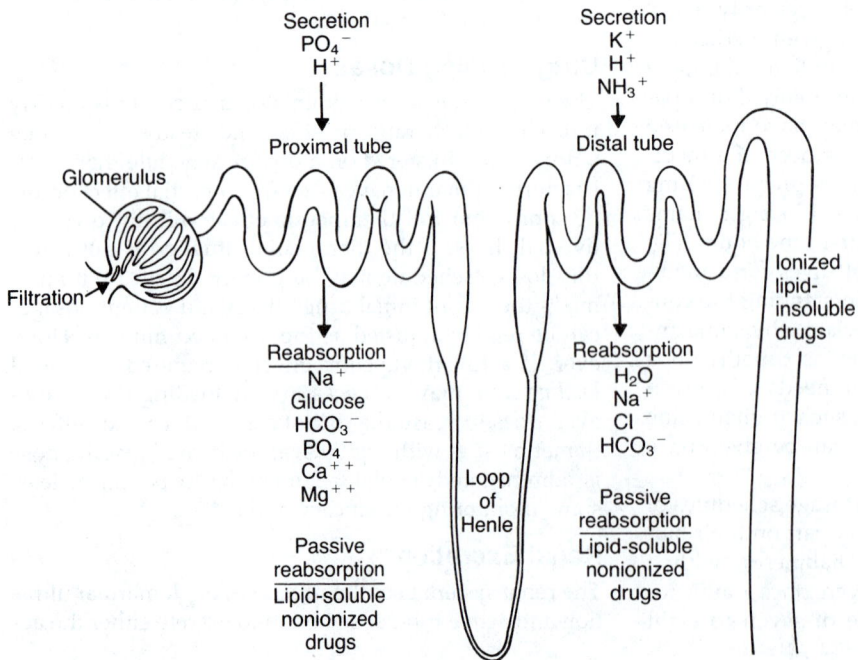

Figure 4-8. Kidney excretion. The renal system uses the processes of glomerular filtration, active tubular secretion, and passive tubular reabsorption to excrete either active or inactive metabolites of medication. Drugs are secreted in the proximal tubule and reabsorbed in both the proximal and distal tubule.

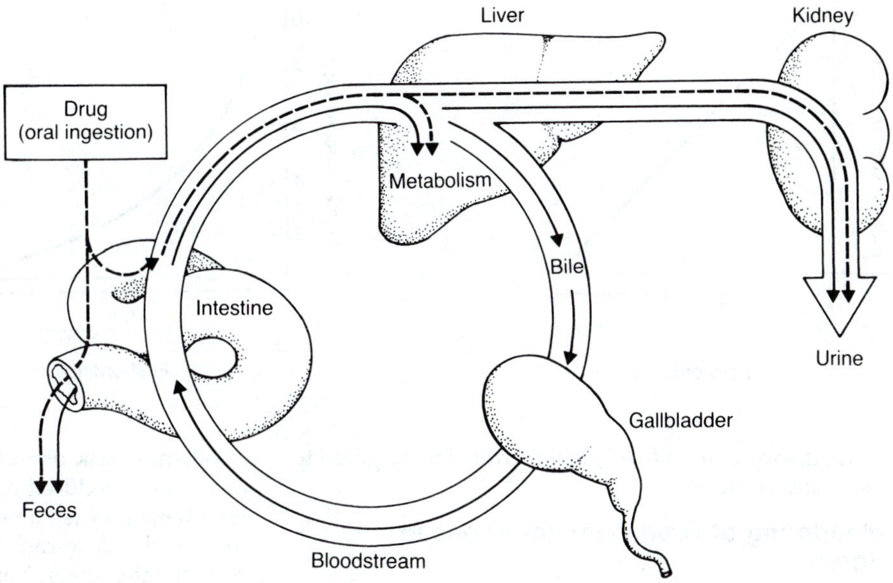

Figure 4–9. Enterohepatic recycling. A drug enters the GI system, is absorbed, and goes to the liver for metabolism. The active metabolites are secreted in bile, and bile is then excreted into the gastrointestinal system. Eighty percent of bile is reabsorbed each day so the active metabolites recirculate for a long time. Some of the active drug or metabolites may go to the kidney for excretion.

can achieve a rapid reduction of the toxic plasma level of the medication or poison.

Gastrointestinal Excretion

Medications excreted through the gastrointestinal system are mainly unabsorbed oral medications or metabolites of certain medications. Medications already absorbed can be excreted into the bile. These drugs can be reabsorbed and recirculated again *(enterohepatic recirculation)* (Fig. 4–9). The administration of laxatives or cathartics can stimulate peristalsis and thus hasten drug elimination.

Pulmonary Excretion

Pulmonary excretion occurs most commonly with gases or vapors used as anesthetic agents. (See Chapter 10 for more information.) The pulmonary system also excretes limited amounts of alcohol. Alcohol is readily absorbed through the stomach mucosa and, after entering the vascular system, is then partially excreted into the lungs and exhaled. A Breathalyzer test can be used quickly and inexpensively to calculate the percentage of alcohol consumed by an individual.

Excretion by Other Routes

The skin, although the largest organ in the body, eliminates a comparatively small amount of drugs. Several substances—arsenic, mercury, and polycyclic hydrocarbons—are all eliminated through the skin.

Excretion of drugs in sweat, saliva, and tears is relatively unimportant. Drugs excreted in saliva are usually swallowed, and their fate then follows other oral drugs. A modified epidermal structure, the hair, eliminates insignificant amounts of drug. Hair samples may be examined in forensic medicine to help determine the cause of death. Traces of mercury have been found in Mozart's hair and may have contributed to his manic behavior during the preparation of his last major work, the *Requiem.*

PHARMACOKINETIC PRINCIPLES

Pharmacokinetic principles are used to assess a patient's response to drug therapy. The primary pharmacokinetic factors affecting the patient's response and the blood concentration of the drug include the rate of drug absorption, the amount of drug absorbed, the distribution of the drug around the body, the drug's biotransformation, and the drug's rate of elimination from the body. These principles assist the physician in determining the proper dose and dosing schedule for a drug. Absorption and elimination of the drug are assumed to follow *exponential* (first-order) kinetics, that is, a constant fraction of the drug present is eliminated in a set unit of time. In first-order kinetics the half-life is independent of dose. Competitive inhibition of metabolism is absent, and metabolic characteristics are independent of dose form. If the elimination processes are saturated, *linear (zero-order) kinetics* result, where a constant amount (as opposed to percentage) of the drug is eliminated in a set unit of time. In zero-order kinetics, the drug half-life is dose-dependent. Competitive inhibition of metabolism is present, and a metabolic pattern may be influenced by dosage forms. Figure 4–10 features the difference between first-order, and zero-order dose-response relationships.

Several common drugs (phenytoin, salicylates, mezlocillin, and ethanol) exhibit nonlinear kinetics *(Michaelis-Menton kinetics)*. At typical doses these drugs saturate the enzyme systems responsible for their elimination. Special caution must be used when increasing the dose of these drugs, particularly phenytoin, because small dosing increments can result in large increases in plasma levels.

When a single dose of an intravenous drug is administered, a peak serum level is quickly achieved. Since first-order kinetics assume that a constant fraction of a drug is lost per unit of time, the half-life can be readily determined (Fig. 4–6). When repeated doses are administered, drug accumulation will occur if the dosing in-

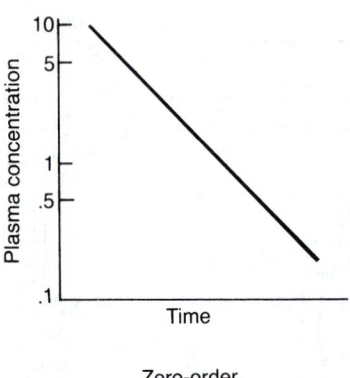

Zero-order

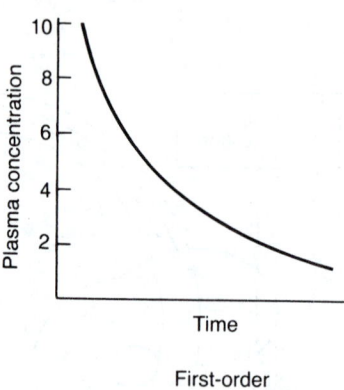

First-order

Figure 4–10. Comparison of zero-order and first-order metabolism. Zero-order metabolism has a different dose-response curve, whereas first-order metabolism follows a normal dose-response curve.

terval is shorter than five half-lives (the time required to reach steady state).

Monitoring of Drug Concentrations in Serum

In order to ensure that a therapeutic drug level is maintained, serum monitoring of the drug level may be performed. Serum drug concentrations are a guide to therapy. To monitor serum levels, two blood levels are usually obtained: the peak level, drawn ½ hour after the medication is totally administered, and the trough level, drawn ½ hour before the next dose. If levels are not drawn at these specified times, but the physician assumes they were, misinterpretation of the results will occur. Peak levels monitor possible toxic levels, whereas trough levels monitor whether or not the level remains within the therapeutic range. These blood levels are then used to determine the next dose of the medication.

Drug monitoring is of particular value in the following circumstances:

1. There is known to be considerable individual variation between the oral dose and plasma level obtained (e.g., aminophylline).
2. Therapeutic levels are close to toxic levels (e.g., lithium and gentamicin).
3. Toxicity is suspected.
4. Noncompliance is suspected.
5. Therapeutic effect must be maximized (as in sepsis).
6. Normal response to standard dosing does not occur.
7. A change in dosage or route of a drug administration is made.
8. Long-term therapy is planned. (Levels may be drawn every 4–6 months.)
9. Long-term therapy has been used, and tolerance is suspected.
10. The drug is given for an episodic syndrome such as epilepsy or cardiac dysrhythmia.

When serum levels are available, the physician and/or clinical pharmacist determine the serum level that is best suited to that patient's overall needs. For example, gentamicin (peak 4–10 μg/ml, trough 1–3 μg/ml) therapy may be prescribed for a patient in several ways:

Gentle therapy—peak 6 μg/ml, trough 1 μg/ml
Moderate therapy—peak 8 μg/ml, trough 2 μg/ml
Agressive therapy—peak 10 μg/ml, trough 3 μg/ml

When a peak or trough serum level is too high, the dose can be reduced or the time interval between doses lengthened. When a peak or trough serum level returns to low, the dose can be increased or the time interval between the doses shortened. In addition, the physician examines other causes that could elevate or reduce these levels.

THE PHARMACODYNAMIC PHASE

The pharmacodynamic phase studies the biochemical and physiologic action and effects of drugs. The pharmacodynamic phase occurs when the medication reaches the target cell and its therapeutic effect occurs. Most medications are thought to work with a receptor at their site of action.

Drugs are thought to provide their action and effects as a result of combination with enzymes, cell membranes, proteins, and cellular constituents such as nucleic acids. The combination of the cell or structure with the drug is referred to as the action, whereas the resultant occurrence is the effect of the drug. The biologic changes caused by the medications may be present for minutes, hours, or even days.

MECHANISM OF DRUG ACTION

Medications, once they have reached the desired site of action, work in various ways. They may alter the cell environment or alter cell function.

Alteration of Cell Environment

Drugs alter the environment of the cell through either physical or environmental processes. Physical processes include alteration of surface tension, as with stool softeners or mucolytics; lubrication, as with mineral oil facilitating the passage of feces; adsorption, as with activated charcoal given orally to absorb harmful chemicals in the gastrointestinal tract; osmosis, as with osmotic diuretics given intravenously to reduce cerebral edema; and ionizing radiation, as with radioactive tracers used in diagnostic testing.

Drugs also alter the chemical environment of cells through processes of inactivation, as with giving phosphate-binding antacids to bind phosphate so it can no longer be absorbed by the body; by altering pH, as with antacids to neutralize gastric acidity or vitamin C to acidify the urine; or by actually altering the body fluid chemistry, as when electrolyte solutions are administered intravenously.

Alteration of Cell Function

Drugs are also capable of interacting to change a cell function by altering cell membranes or cellular processes or by affecting specialized regions within the cell. Through these actions, cell function may be enhanced or retarded. Typically, medications alter cell function through facilitation of membrane transport, such as when insulin is injected to facilitate glucose entrance into the cells; by depression of membrane function, such as when general anesthetics are given to depress cellular reticular activity in the brain stem; by support of energy metabolism, such as when corticosteroids are administered to increase the supply of glucose so that cells may manufacture high-energy phosphate substances; and by inhibition of energy metabolism, such as when chemotherapeutic medications are given to decrease cellular function.

Drug Receptor Activity

It is thought that medications have an affinity for certain receptor sites. The term *receptor* is applied to a portion of a cell or tissue that can be occupied by a drug and result in a particular effect. Receptors are most often cellular proteins or nucleic acids, but they can also be enzymes, carbohydrate residues, and lipids. Drug concentrations in cells or organs with no receptor sites will have little effect. In many cases, similar chemical compounds can occupy the receptor and elicit either antagonist or agonist action. As an *agonist*, the drug complexes with and alters the functional properties of the receptor (e.g., terbutaline). As an *antagonist*, the drug interferes with the action of a natural agonist, either through competition for the receptor site (e.g., antihistamines) or through interaction with other components of the effector mechanism (e.g., insecticides) (Fig. 4–11). In either case, the antagonist is not capable of setting off

the sequence of biochemical events that results in a pharmacologic effect. The antagonist may act in a way that is either reversible or irreversible.

Receptors are believed to have evolved for the specific purpose of interacting with endogenous biologic compounds. If receptors are continually stimulated, their responsiveness may be decreased, which is referred to as *desensitization* or down-regulation. This decrease in responsiveness may be due to an actual decrease in number or a change in the existing receptors or both. The end state of desensitization is termed refractoriness. As an example, desensitization may occur with repeated use of beta-adrenergic bronchodilators such as isoproterenol (Isuprel) for the treatment of asthma. With repeated use, the effectiveness of the drug is reduced, thus requiring a larger dose or a change of medication.

When a receptor's activity is reduced to a chronic level, a state of *hyperreactivity* or supersensitivity to a drug may occur. The receptors must then be allowed to return to normal. Hyperreactivity can occur following long-term use of an antagonistic drug like propranolol (Inderal). If the drug is rapidly withdrawn, the patient may experience an increased number of anginal attacks or a hypertensive episode, which were previously controlled with the drug. This is due to increased sensitivity of the beta adrenergic receptors to epinephrine, which propranolol was blocking.

Some drugs are thought to produce their effects through enzymatic action. A drug may so closely resemble the enzyme that the drug may combine with the normal enzyme substrate and allow the enzyme to be freed. A group of drugs with an enzymatic action, called "antimetabolites," are discussed fully in Chapter 49.

The drug effect on nucleic acids or other cellular components can be utilized in the treatment of tumors and cancer. The ability of drugs to halve the growth of cells is the mechanism by which the medication can slow or cause regression in the spread of the disease. The ability of the antibiotics to specifically affect the production of bacterial proteins provides a safe and nonharmful treatment of infections in patients.

The influence of medications on enzymes is to produce an increase or decrease in the amount of the en-

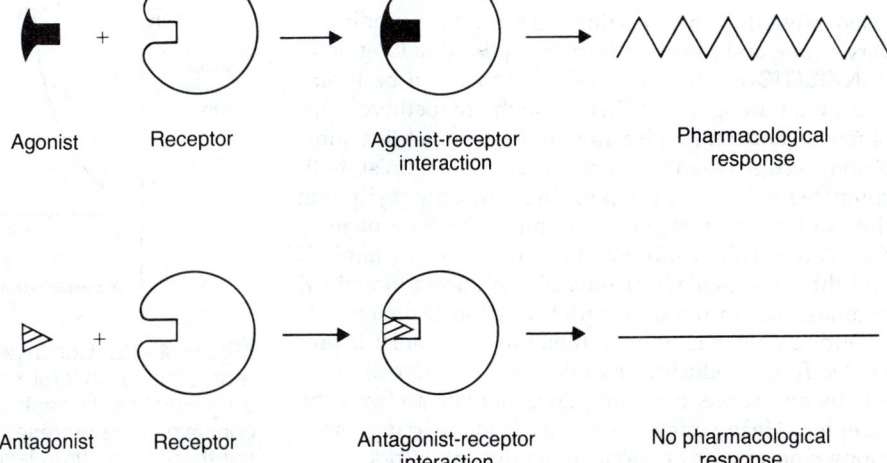

Figure 4–11. Agonist/antagonist effect. A drug acting as an agonist fits into a receptor and a drug effect occurs. A drug acting as an antagonist can combine with a receptor, but does not quite fit, so no drug response occurs.

Agonist   Receptor   Agonist-receptor   Pharmacological
                                 interaction   response

Antagonist   Receptor   Antagonist-receptor   No pharmacological
                                 interaction   response

zymes and, as a result, change cell or tissue response in the body. Since enzymes determine the rate of chemical reactions, their levels directly influence the biochemical activity of cells. The relaxation of the bronchioles in the lung is accomplished by enzyme stimulation of adenylcyclase by isoproterenol to produce more high-energy 3',5'-cyclic AMP, while aminophylline maintains the high-energy compound by inhibition of the enzyme phosphodiesterase, which breaks down 3',5'-cyclic AMP. The result of treatment with either medication is relief of bronchial constriction.

Some medications have direct action on the tissues and cells to produce effects, whereas others may have a more indirect effect on the resultant activity. The treatment of hypertension is accomplished with agents that act directly on the blood vessels (e.g., hydralazine) and indirect-acting agents that affect the brain centers for control of blood vessel tone (e.g., clonidine). The mechanism of drug action varies in its effect on the biochemical state of the cells and tissues of the body.

RECEPTOR SUBTYPES. Researchers, through the years, have identified a variety of endogenous regulators with many receptors, and now multiple receptor subtypes have also been identified. Examples include several histamine subtype receptors—H_1 and H_2—and several catecholamine subtypes—$alpha_1$, $alpha_2$, $beta_1$, and $beta_2$. Researchers have now been able to develop a number of therapeutic agents that have selectivity for specific subtype receptors. In this way, therapeutic effects can be enhanced, while unwanted effects can be minimized.

Drug Receptor Interactions

REVERSIBLE AND IRREVERSIBLE INTERACTIONS. In most cases the interaction of the drug with a receptor is reversible, that is, the drug-receptor effect is terminated by the drug leaving the receptor. If the concentration of drug remains high in the vicinity of the receptor, the drug has an effect at the receptor. As the concentration of drug goes down the receptors will no longer be filled, and drug effect is reversed.

There are drug-receptor interactions that are irreversible. With certain substances such as environmental pollutants, pesticides, and nerve gas, the drug-receptor combination alters both, so the drug receptor becomes inseparable. In other reactions, the receptor binding is very strong and remains on the receptor for a long time.

INHIBITION. The action of an agonist can be inhibited by an antagonist either through competitive inhibition or noncompetitive inhibition. Competitive inhibition occurs when the agonist and antagonist both compete for the same receptor sites. The drug occupying the most number of sites determines the type of reaction. A competitive inhibition occurs between vitamin K and the anticoagulant dicumarol and allows vitamin K to antagonize or interfere with the action of dicumarol.

During noncompetitive inhibition, the agonist is prevented from producing any effect at a receptor site usually by an irreversible acting drug that fails to leave the receptor. Heavy metals such as lead, mercury, antimony, and arsenic are noncompetitive inhibitors.

Drug Effect

The effect of the medication is dose-related (over a limited range) and is the result of its action. The dose-effect relationship is commonly derived from the drug's peak effect after a single dose of the medication. This effect can be represented by a curve that may be linear (see Fig. 4–6) or may curve upward, downward (Fig. 4–12), or sigmoidally. The sigmoid curve is the most common. Each curve has a time of onset of action when the drug is entering the central and peripheral compartments; a duration of action time, during which the therapeutic effect occurs; and the termination of action time, during which the drug is being eliminated. During this last phase, the next dose of the medication is administered to prevent the therapeutic blood level from dropping below that which is desired.

The effects of medications can be immediate or delayed; desired (beneficial or therapeutic); or undesirable (adverse or toxic). Drugs can also cause unusual effects—idiosyncratic effects—that occur in only a small percentage of individuals. Drugs can be used for their diagnostic effect (radioactive isotope, contrast medium) to diagnose the presence of disease. Drugs can be used for their ability to relieve symptoms, treat or cure a disease, or relieve pain.

Several types of dosages are administered to patients. A therapeutic dose is one that will treat the disorder effectively, while a nontherapeutic dose (too high or too low) will not produce the desired effect. A loading dose is a large dose, often given in a short period of time, in order to saturate all of the storage areas quickly. Following the loading dose, the dose is reduced to a *maintenance dose*. Digitalis products are often administered with a loading dose and then followed by maintenance dose therapy.

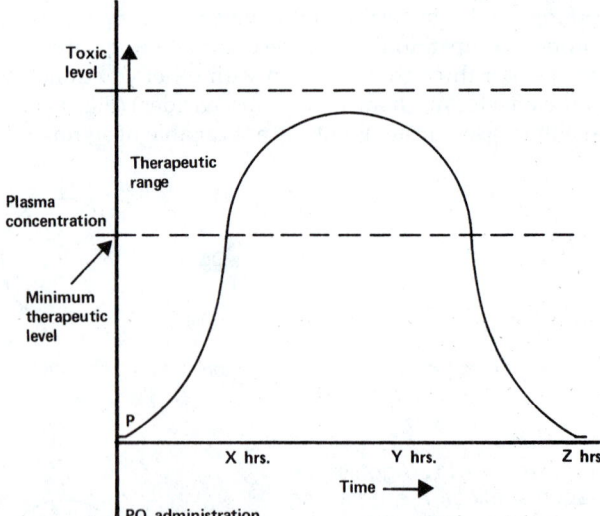

Figure 4–12. Concave time medication curve. A curve representing an oral drug administered at P time. The drug reaches its peak therapeutic level at Y hours. The concave curve represents the time arriving at and leaving the therapeutic drug level.

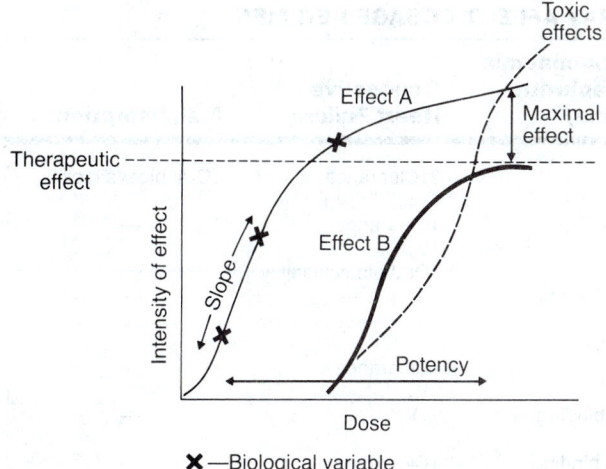

Figure 4–13. The intensity of a drug's effect is dependent on several variables: potency of the drug, the slope of the response curve, biological variables (X), and maximal effect. A drug may have several effects (A and B). However, the appearance of adverse effects may preclude using the drug to obtain effect B.

The intensity of a drug's effect is dependent on several response variables: biologic variables, potency, slope of the dose-response curve, and maximal efficacy (Fig. 4–13). When medications are given, they are all subject to known and unknown sources of biologic variation. The known factors include body weight, age, disease state, immune system function, and psychologic and environmental factors, all of which have already been discussed. Unknown variables such as individual differences account for other reasons why individuals respond differently to medications.

The *potency* of a drug is the relationship between the dose of the drug and the intensity of its effect. Potency is influenced by absorption, distribution, biotransformation, and excretion, as well as its ability to combine with receptors. Drug manufacturers take potency into consideration when drug doses are established. When switching between different drugs, such as from morphine to hydromorphone (Dilaudid), relative potency (the ratio of equieffective doses) needs to be considered by the physician. For example, 10 mg morphine equals 1 mg hydromorphone. Therefore, hydromorphone is the "most potent" drug. However, it does not matter since these doses are equally effective.

The slope of the dose-response curve (Fig. 4–13) demonstrates the ability of the drug to produce an effect. The steeper the slope, the more readily the drug will bind with receptors and the quicker the drug effect.

The efficacy of a drug refers to its maximal effect. The efficacy of a drug is indicated on Figure 4–13 by a plateau. The efficacy of a drug is clearly one of its major characteristics. Morphine is more efficacious in relieving intense pain than aspirin products.

A medication is also described in reference to its *selectivity* (or spectrum of activity), that is, with reference to the effects that the medication precipitates. Medications rarely produce a single effect. Most medications produce a spectrum of effects. The therapeutic index (margin of safety) serves as an estimate of the safety of a drug. Therapeutic index equals toxic dose/therapeutic dose. Drug selectivity is best described by summarizing the pattern and incidence of adverse and toxic effects produced by a therapeutic dose of the medication and by indicating the proportion of patients who experienced these effects and therefore had to lower the dosage or discontinue the medication. A medication reference book that lists all known adverse and toxic effects is of little use to determine selectivity. The best reference should at least indicate the most common and the least common adverse or toxic effects to assess and which effects to evaluate.

There are many pathophysiologic conditions that can alter drug effect through absorption and excretion. Table 4–3 reviews how several common drugs are affected by renal disease, hepatic disease, hypoalbuminemia, congestive heart failure, and malabsorption.

ADVERSE EFFECTS. There are several adverse effects that drugs can elicit—toxic, idiosyncratic, and allergic. Adverse effects are those that are undesirable, such as the constipation that a patient develops when codeine is administered to reduce pain. Toxic effects are those that necessitate discontinuation of a drug, such as nephrotoxicity developing secondarily to gentamicin, an antibiotic. Table 1–3 in Chapter 1 reviewed the difference between adverse and toxic effects.

Idiosyncratic reactions are those that are unexpected and may necessitate the discontinuation of the drug. For example, sedatives usually quiet the individual, but the elderly may become excitable.

DRUG ALLERGIES. Drug allergies range from very mild, with no need to discontinue the drug, to very severe, such as an anaphylactic shock reaction. Drug allergies are classified into four types: I, II, III, and IV. Drug allergies are discussed in detail in Chapter 6.

SUMMARY

For a medication to have its effect in the body, it progresses through three distinct phases—the pharmaceutic phase, the pharmacokinetic phase, and finally, the pharmacodynamic phase. Each phase is necessary and important in effecting a final positive medication effect. A patient's weight, age, general health and disease state, immune system, psychologic condition, and even the climate in which the patient lives affect the response to a particular medication at a given time, as do other drugs or medications the patient may be taking concurrently. These factors must be assessed by the nurse before medications are administered, during nursing intervention, and again when the results of intervention are evaluated. Since the nurse spends a great deal of time with the patient, the nurse is in a position to observe both the therapeutic and adverse drug effects. From these observations, the nurse can confidently suggest modification in the medication regimen, when appropriate, to ensure the patient's safety and well-being.

Table 4–3. PATHOPHYSIOLOGIC CONDITIONS THAT MAY AFFECT DOSAGE REGIMEN

Drug	Renal Failure (Uremia)	Hepatic Failure (Cirrhosis)	Hypoalbuminemia (e.g., Nephrotic Syndrome)	Congestive Heart Failure	Malabsorption
Digoxin	⇓Clearance ↓V_d	?↓Clearance	—	?↓Clearance	↓Oral bioavailability
Procainamide (Pronestyl)	↓Clearance ↑Active metabolites	↓Active metabolite	—	↓Clearance ↓V_d ↓Oral bioavailability	—
Phenytoin (Dilantin)	⇓Protein binding ↑V_d ⇑Clearance	↓Clearance	⇓Protein binding ↑V_d ⇑Clearance	—	—
Lidocaine	↑Toxic metabolites	↓Clearance	—	↓Clearance ↓V_d	—
Quinidine	↑Active metabolites	—	↓Protein binding	?↓V_d	—
Propranolol (Inderal)	—	?↓Clearance	⇓Protein binding	↓Clearance	—
Tetracycline	⇓Clearance	↓Clearance	↓Protein binding	↓Clearance	↓Oral bioavailability
Penicillin G	↓Clearance	↓Clearance	↓Protein binding	↓V_d	↓Oral bioavailability
Codeine	—	⇓Clearance	↓Protein binding	↓Clearance	↓Oral bioavailability

— no effect
↑ Moderate positive change
⇑ Major positive change
? Inconsistent effect
↓ Moderate negative change
⇓ Major negative change

BIBLIOGRAPHY

Birdsall, C, et al: How safe are generics? Am J Nurse 87(4):431–432, 1987.

Davis, L: Timing is everything. Hippocrates 2(4):22–25, 1987.

Farley, D: How FDA approves new drugs. FDA Consum 21(10):6–13, 1987.

Fischer, RG: The meaning of FDA approval. Pediatr Nurs 13(5):360, 1987.

Goodinson, SM: Fundamentals of drug action: Administration and absorption, an overview. Nursing (London) 3(10):386–390, 1986.

Goodinson, SM: Fundamentals of drug action: Drug elimination. Nursing (London) 3(12):466–467, 1986.

Hofland, S: Drug fever. Critical Care Nurse 5(4):29–35, 1985.

Howard, P: A crash course in serum drug monitoring. RN 86(4):20–25, 1986.

Jones, B: How drugs act. Nursing Mirror 158(19):17–19, 1985.

Maronde, R (ed.): Topics in Clinical Pharmacology and Therapeutics. Springer, New York, 1986.

Mason, GD and Winter ME: Appropriateness of sampling times for therapeutic drug monitoring. Am J Hosp Pharm 41:1796–1801, September 1984.

Match your meals and medicines. Changing Times 40(11):68–70, 1986.

Monitoring therapeutic levels of drugs in plasma. Laboratory Bulletin. Australian Family Physician 15(4):504–505, 1986.

Myths and facts of generic drugs. FDA Consum 21(7):12–14, 1987.

Shaikh, A: Application of pharmacokinetic principles in therapeutic drug monitoring. J Med Technol 2(9):583–587, 1985.

Smith, S: How drugs act: Elimination and cumulation. Nursing Times 80(49):44–46, 1984.

Smith, S: How drugs act: How drugs are absorbed and reach their destination. Nursing Times 80(48):24–27, 1984.

SITUATION 4–1

Ann Matlock works as a nurse in an outpatient clinic of a small community hospital. The following are situations she frequently encounters while serving in that position:

1. Mr. King has been diagnosed as having pneumonia and has been ordered penicillin 250 mg PO q 6 hr. When Ann enters the room to administer the first dose, Mr. King states that he was on penicillin 4 years ago and developed hives. Based on this information, Ann:
   a. Administers the drug as ordered and observes for a reaction
   b. Combines the drug with an antihistamine to decrease the chance of reaction
   c. Withholds the drug and informs the physician of the patient's allergy
   d. Administers the drug intramuscularly to bypass gastric absorption

2. Mr. Ames is receiving an antibiotic (erythromycin) to treat a respiratory infection. Ann informs Mr. Ames that taking erythromycin with food will:
   a. Increase the rate of absorption

SITUATION 4–1–*CONTINUED*

b. Have no effect on therapeutic action
c. Decrease gastric side effects
d. Delay the rate of absorption

3. Mr. Downs is receiving aspirin to relieve arthritic pain. Ann administers the first dose with an antacid to:
a. Increase the absorption rate in the small intestine
b. Reduce the effects of an acidic drug on absorption
c. Provide the drug in a time-release form
d. Provide a lipid base for greater absorption

4. John Foley came to the clinic complaining of headache and a stiff neck. Following a diagnosis of meningitis, the physician ordered penicillin G as part of the therapy. One reason for selection of this drug for treatment is that penicillin G is:
a. Lipid-soluble and able to cross the blood-brain barrier
b. Utilized by brain cells via an active transport system
c. Water-soluble and easily absorbed through the blood-brain barrier

d. Transported into the central nervous system via facilitated diffusion

5. Leo Cordell, a 75-year-old, comes to the clinic with a complaint of shortness of breath. During a nursing assessment, Ann learns that Mr. Cordell is an alcoholic who smokes a pack of cigarettes a day. Ann will assess Mr. Cordell for possible drug toxic effects primarily due to:
a. Increased lung capacity
b. Spasticity of the colon
c. Diminished liver function
d. Ineffective cardiac function

6. Mr. Brown, an asthmatic, complains that his bronchial inhaler (Isuprel) does not work as it used to. Ann is aware that this represents an example of:
a. Supersensitivity
b. Desensitization
c. Receptor agonist effect
d. Hypersensitivity

Refer to the Appendix for correct answers and additional review questions with answers.

GLOSSARY TERMS IN THIS CHAPTER

Additive
Antagonistic
Antidote
Complexation
Drug interaction
Incompatibility
Potentiation
Sequestration
Synergistic

5

CHAPTER

DRUG INTERACTIONS

MERRILY MATHEWSON KUHN, R.N.C., Ph.D., CCRN

LEARNING OBJECTIVES

After reading this chapter, the student will be able to:

1. Distinguish between the two concepts, drug pharmacokinetic and drug pharmacodynamic interactions.

2. Define the terms additive, synergistic, and antagonistic interactions.

3. Identify drug-food interactions.

4. Describe the different levels at which drugs may interact.

DEFINITION AND CLASSIFICATION

As drug therapy becomes more complex, medications more potent, and prescribers of drugs more specialized, the number of significant *drug interactions* will continue to grow and pose a potentially serious problem to both the patient and those who monitor patient care. A recent study at a large metropolitan teaching hospital found that over a two-month period, 5% of their admissions were attributable to adverse drug interactions and that 49% of these were preventable). Both medical and surgical patients are at risk. A recent study found that 17% of general surgical patients were at risk for drug interactions. For the ultimate benefit of the patient, nurses, pharmacists, and physicians must have a working knowledge of potential drug interactions and be able to share their experiences and knowledge with the other members of the health team (physician, nurse, and pharmacist). Communication within the health team as well as with the patient is essential. With over 700 unique pharmacologic substances available today, there is a potential for over 55 million individual, unique drug interactions.

Hayes (1981) suggests a working definition for a drug interaction: " . . . occurs whenever the diagnostic, preventive, therapeutic, or toxic action of a drug is modified in or on the body by another pharmacologically acting chemical substance, whether that be a prescription drug, an over-the-counter drug, or something in the diet or the environment." The interaction can be physical, chemical, or biologic. Unlike an incompatibility, which usually occurs in the preparation phase (of drug delivery), a drug interaction is the by-product of the administration of two or more drugs or a drug-food combination. Some drug interactions are intentional and beneficial to patient care; however, the majority are unintentional and may have a potentially deleterious effect on the patient. Drug interactions often cause patients to be hospitalized or to increase their hospital stay. The potential sites of action for drug interactions within the body are featured in Figure 5–1. The potentially harmful drug interactions are reviewed in this chapter.

INCOMPATIBILITIES

Drug *incompatibilities* are not synonymous with drug interactions. This antagonism can occur during mixing outside the body or inside the body. Drug incompatibilities are chemical or physical reactions that occur among two or more drugs.

The chemical incompatibilities between two drugs change the molecular structure of the drug, thereby rendering it different in its pharmacologic properties. Chemical incompatibilities may be beneficial, as when protamine sulfate is administered to stop the activity of heparin, an anticoagulant. These drugs form an ionic bond, which has no anticoagulant activity. Chemical incompatibilities may also be deleterious, as when multivitamins and antibiotics are mixed in the same intrave-

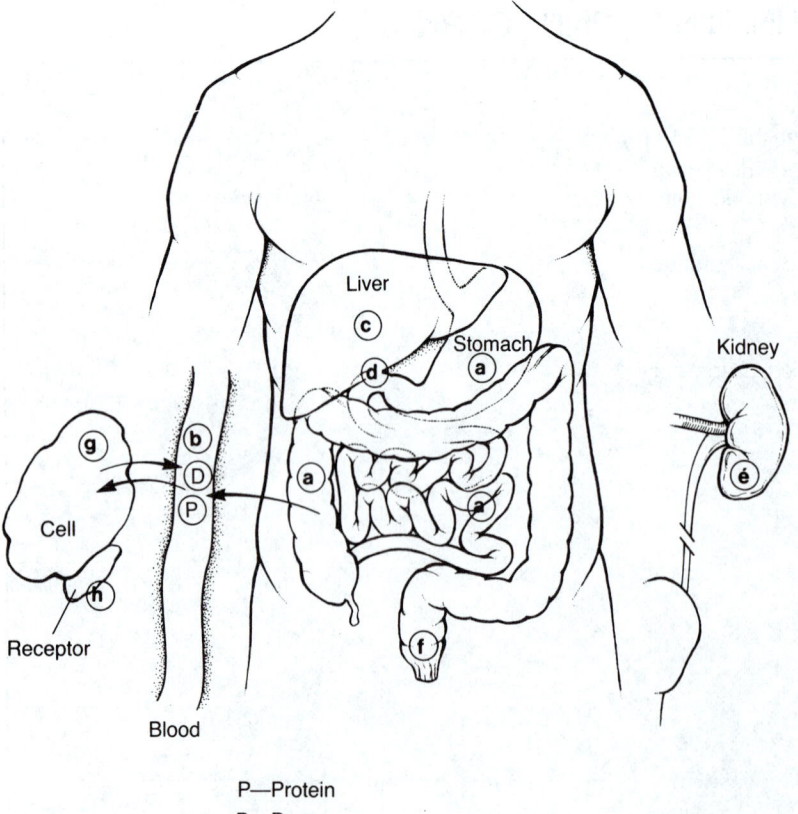

Figure 5–1. Drug interaction sites within the body. Drug interactions can occur in numerous sites within the body. Absorption can be enhanced or reduced in the gut (a); protein binding can be affected within the vasculature (b); biotransformation can be effected in the liver (c); excretion can be affected either through bile (d), the kidney (e), or in feces (f); tissue binding of one drug can be affected by another (g); and finally drugs may have an effect through action on specific receptors (h).

nous (IV) solution. Some multivitamins change the pH of the IV solution, thereby inactivating the antibiotic.

Physical incompatibilities occur when two drugs are loosely bound to each other but still retain their original pharmacologic properties. The end result of a physical incompatibility is usually a precipitate. As an example, mixing Dilantin, an anticonvulsant, with dextrose forms a precipitate in the IV bottle or IV tubing.

Incompatibilities are of prime concern in the preparation of large-volume parenterals that contain vitamin or electrolyte additives or both and in the preparation of preoperative medications where two or more drugs are to be added in the same syringe. Incompatibilities for intramuscular (IM) medications and IV medications can be found in Tables 5–1 and 5–2. Nurses can most easily obtain information on drug incompatibilities for large-volume parenterals from the reference guides available to pharmacists. Communication with the pharmacist helps the nurse avoid the potential inactivation or precipitation of two or more drugs mixed together in the same parenteral solution or syringe. When members of the health team share knowledge, they decrease the risk of causing harm or discomfort to the patient. It is essential that the nurse research incompatibility potentials before administering medication.

DRUG INTERACTION MECHANISMS

Drug interaction mechanisms can be divided into several general categories: (1) pharmacokinetic interactions, (2) pharmacodynamic interactions, and (3) combined toxicities.

Pharmacokinetic interactions comprise reactions where the absorption, distribution, biotransformation, or excretion of one drug is affected by another drug. This includes interactions in which gastrointestinal absorption of a drug is affected, plasma protein binding is modified, drug metabolism is stimulated or inhibited, or renal excretion is enhanced or inhibited.

Pharmacodynamic interactions result from the combined pharmacologic effect of drugs. They may have additive, synergistic, or antagonistic effects. Action on the same receptor may or may not be involved.

Combined toxicity results when two drugs with toxic effects on the same organ are combined for therapy. As an example, gentamicin, an aminoglycoside antibiotic, and furosemide (Lasix), a diuretic, both can cause ototoxicity. When used together, the combination could lead to permanent eighth cranial nerve damage and deafness. This combination is frequently used in intensive care units so patients need to be assessed carefully.

PHARMACOKINETIC INTERACTIONS

Through research and clinical practice, the knowledge of pharmacokinetic interactions grows daily. Constant surveillance of drug effects and continuous monitoring of drug therapy keep us abreast of new potential problems in this field of pharmacology. The primary causes of these interactions and the resulting significance of concurrent drug administration are reviewed briefly.

The major mechanisms of pharmacokinetic interactions are (1) absorption, (2) protein-binding changes, (3) changes in biotransformation, (4) changes in the excretion of drugs, and (5) other factors.

ABSORPTION

Medications given orally are absorbed through the gastrointestinal tract. Absorption depends on the function of the gastrointestinal tract itself, the physiochemical characteristics of the contents of the tract, the condition of the tract, and active and passive transport mechanisms within the tract.

Normal tract function assumes normal motility and normal bacterial flora. Absorption of most medication depends on the time it is within either the stomach or the intestine. The faster the drug passes through the intestinal tract, the less drug is absorbed. For example, patients who abuse cathartics tend to have reduced absorption of oral medications. Other drugs, such as morphine and codeine, prolong emptying time within the small intestine, which may result in increased drug absorption. Metoclopramide, which hastens gastric emptying time, may decrease drug absorption in the small intestine. Conversely, anticholinergics prolong gastric emptying time and therefore may increase drug absorption. Often, by simply giving a poorly soluble drug more time to dissolve, more may be available for absorption. Drugs affecting absorption of other drugs are featured in Table 5–3.

Modification of gastrointestinal absorption can also occur secondary to physiochemical characteristics of the contents of the gastrointestinal tract itself. By altering pH, such as with antacids or cimetidine (Tagamet), solubility and stability of medications may be affected, reducing or increasing drug absorption. When the pH is lowered, acidic drugs are absorbed more readily, whereas when the pH is elevated, basic drugs are absorbed more readily. Antacids alter the absorption of many drugs by complexing with them, thereby decreasing their absorption (e.g., digoxin and tetracycline products) or by altering the pH of the tract, thereby decreasing absorption (aspirin and barbiturates). Antacids can also increase the absorption of amphetamines, which may cause central nervous system (CNS) toxicity.

Additional problems that can occur in the bowel include *complexation* and *sequestration*. Complexation occurs when nonabsorbable complexes are formed when drug and drug or drug and food are combined (antacids and either digoxin or tetracycline products). Sequestration occurs when the drug is surrounded by a lipoid substance. For example, when the fat-soluble vitamins A, D, E, and K are combined with mineral oil, the mineral oil surrounds the vitamins and the vitamins cannot

TEXT RESUMES ON PAGE 96

Table 5–1. PHYSICAL AND CHEMICAL COMPATIBILITY FOR MIXING AND INFUSING MEDICATIONS

	Aminophylline	Ampicillin	Atropine sulfate	Bretylium	Calcium chloride	Calcium gluconate	Cefazolin	Cimetidine	Diazepam	Diazoxide	Digoxin	Dobutamine	Dopamine	Epinephrine HCl	Furosemide	Gentamicin	Heparin	Hydralazine
Aminophylline		P	N	D	N	P	S	I	N	N	P	B	P	I	B	P	P	I
Ampicillin	P		N	N	N	I	S	A	N	N	N	N	I	I	N	I	H	I
Atropine sulfate	N	N		N	N	N	N	P	N	N	N	P	N	D	N	N	P	N
Bretylium	D	N	N		C	D	N	N	N	N	D	I	C	N	N	M	N	N
Calcium chloride	N	N	N	C		N	N	N	N	N	P	I	D	I	N	N	N	N
Calcium gluconate	P	I	N	D	N		I	N	N	N	N	I	P	I	N	N	P	N
Cefazolin	S	S	N	N	N	I		P	N	N	N	N	N	N	N	I	S	N
Cimetidine	I	A	P	N	N	N	P		N	N	M	P	P	P	P	P	P	N
Diazepam	N	N	N	N	N	N	N	N		N	N	N	N	N	N	N	N	N
Diazoxide	N	N	N	N	N	N	N	N	N		N	N	N	N	N	N	N	I
Digoxin	P	N	N	D	P	N	N	M	N	N		N	N	N	N	N	N	H
Dobutamine	B	N	P	I	I	I	N	P	N	N	N		S	D	I	B	D	S
Dopamine	P	I	N	C	D	P	N	P	N	N	N	S		P	N	A	P	N
Epinephrine HCl	I	I	D	N	I	I	N	P	N	N	N	D	P		I	P	D	N
Furosemide	B	N	N	N	N	N	N	P	N	N	N	I	N	I		N	P	I
Gentamicin	P	I	N	M	N	N	I	P	N	N	N	B	A	P	N		I	N
Heparin	P	H	P	N	N	P	S	P	N	N	N	D	P	D	P	I		P
Hydralazine	I	I	N	N	N	N	N	N	N	I	H	S	N	N	I	N	P	
Insulin reg	I	N	N	P	N	N	N	A	N	N	I	I	N	N	N	N	P	P
Isoproterenol	I	P	N	I	P	P	N	P	N	N	N	P	P	N	N	P	P	P

Table 5–1. PHYSICAL AND CHEMICAL COMPATIBILITY FOR MIXING AND INFUSING MEDICATIONS—*CONTINUED*

Insulin reg	Isoproterenol	Lidocaine	Morphine sulfate	Netilmicin	Nitroglycerin	Nitroprusside	Norepinephrine	Phenytoin	Phytonadione	Potassium chloride	Procainamide	Propranolol	Quinidine	Sodium bicarbonate	Streptokinase	Tobramycin	Verapamil
I	I	P	I	N	G	N	I	N	N	P	N	N	N	B	N	N	P
N	P	P	N	N	N	N	P	N	I	P	N	N	N	N	N	N	P
N	N	N	P	P	N	N	N	N	N	P	P	N	N	I	N	N	P
P	I	C	N	N	G	N	N	N	N	P	I	N	P	C	N	N	P
N	P	P	I	N	N	N	P	N	N	P	N	N	N	I	N	I	P
N	P	D	N	N	N	N	P	N	P	P	N	N	N	I	N	I	P
N	N	I	N	P	N	N	N	N	N	S	N	N	N	N	N	N	P
A	P	D	N	N	N	N	D	N	P	D	N	N	P	P	N	N	P
N	N	N	N	N	N	N	N	N	N	N	N	N	I	N	N	N	N
N	N	N	N	N	N	N	N	N	N	N	N	I	N	N	N	N	N
I	N	P	N	N	N	N	N	N	N	Y	N	N	N	N	N	N	P
I	P	P	N	N	N	N	P	N	I	I	P	N	N	I	N	N	I
N	P	P	N	N	G	N	H	N	P	P	N	N	N	I	N	N	P
N	N	I	N	N	N	P	N	I	P	N	N	N	N	I	N	N	P
N	N	N	N	N	G	N	N	N	N	P	N	N	I	N	N	N	P
N	P	P	H	N	N	N	P	N	N	N	N	N	N	N	N	N	P
P	P	P	I	N	N	N	P	N	P	P	P	N	I	P	N	I	P
P	P	P	N	N	G	N	N	N	N	Y	N	N	N	N	N	N	S
	N	L	N	N	N	N	N	N	N	N	N	N	N	I	N	N	P
N		I	N	P	N	N	P	N	N	P	N	N	N	I	N	N	P

CONTINUED ON THE FOLLOWING PAGE

Table 5–1. PHYSICAL AND CHEMICAL COMPATIBILITY FOR MIXING AND INFUSING MEDICATIONS—*CONTINUED*

	Aminophylline	Ampicillin	Atropine sulfate	Bretylium	Calcium chloride	Calcium gluconate	Cefazolin	Cimetidine	Diazepam	Diazoxide	Digoxin	Dobutamine	Dopamine	Epinephrine HCl	Furosemide	Gentamicin	Heparin	Hydralazine
Lidocaine	P	P	N	C	P	D	I	D	N	N	P	P	P	I	N	P	P	P
Morphine sulfate	I	N	P	N	I	N	N	N	N	N	N	N	N	N	N	N	H	I	N
Netilmicin	N	N	P	N	N	N	P	N	N	N	N	N	N	N	N	N	N	N
Nitroglycerin	G	N	N	G	N	N	N	N	N	N	N	N	G	N	G	N	N	G
Nitroprusside	N	N	N	N	N	N	N	N	N	N	N	N	N	N	N	N	N	N
Norepinephrine	I	P	N	N	P	P	N	D	N	N	N	P	H	P	N	P	P	N
Phenytoin	N	N	N	N	N	N	N	N	N	N	N	N	N	N	N	N	N	N
Phytonadione	N	I	N	N	N	P	N	P	N	N	N	I	P	I	N	N	P	N
Potassium chloride	P	P	P	P	P	P	S	D	N	N	Y	I	P	P	P	N	P	Y
Procainamide	N	N	P	I	N	N	N	N	N	N	N	N	P	N	N	N	P	N
Propranolol	N	N	N	N	N	N	N	N	N	I	N	N	N	N	N	N	N	N
Quinidine	N	N	N	P	N	N	N	P	I	N	N	N	N	N	I	N	I	N
Sodium bicarbonate	B	N	I	C	I	I	N	P	N	N	N	I	I	I	N	N	P	N
Streptokinase	N	N	N	N	N	N	N	N	N	N	N	N	N	N	N	N	N	N
Tobramycin	N	N	N	N	I	I	N	N	N	N	N	N	N	N	N	N	I	N
Verapamil	P	P	P	P	P	P	P	P	N	N	P	I	P	I	P	P	P	S

C = Physically and chemically compatible
P = Physically compatible
D = Physically compatible only in D5W.
S = Physically compatible only in 0.9% NaCl.
G = Physically compatible only in a glass bottle.
H = Physically compatible for 24 hours.
A = Physically compatible for 4–8 hours.
B = Physically compatible for 4–8 hours only in D5W.
Y = Physically compatible through Y-site for at least 6 hours.
L = Regular insulin compatible with preservative free lidocaine solution.
M = Manufacturer claims medication should not be mixed with other medications but some compatibility data
    are available.
I = Incompatible.
N = Information on compatibility is not available.
  Source: Zeller, FP, et al: Compatibility of IV drugs in a coronary intensive care unit. Drug Intell Clin Pharm 20(5):352, 1986, with permission.

Table 5–1. PHYSICAL AND CHEMICAL COMPATIBILITY FOR MIXING AND INFUSING MEDICATIONS—*CONTINUED*

Insulin reg	Isoproterenol	Lidocaine	Morphine sulfate	Netilmicin	Nitroglycerin	Nitroprusside	Norepinephrine	Phenytoin	Phytonadione	Potassium chloride	Procainamide	Propranolol	Quinidine	Sodium bicarbonate	Streptokinase	Tobramycin	Verapamil
L	I		N	N	G	N	I	N	N	P	P	N	N	D	N	N	P
N	N	N		N	N	N	N	N	N	P	N	N	N	I	N	N	P
N	P	N	N		N	N	P	N	P	P	P	N	N	N	N	N	N
N	N	G	N	N		N	N	N	N	N	N	N	N	N	N	N	P
N	N	N	N	N	N		N	N	N	N	N	N	N	N	N	N	N
N	P	I	N	P	N	N		N	N	P	N	N	N	I	N	N	P
N	N	N	N	N	N	N	N		N	N	N	N	N	N	N	N	N
N	N	N	N	P	N	N	N	N		P	N	N	N	N	N	N	N
N	P	P	P	P	N	N	P	N	P		P	P	N	P	N	N	P
N	N	P	N	P	N	N	N	N	N	P		N	N	N	N	N	P
N	N	N	N	N	N	N	N	N	N	P	N		N	N	N	N	P
N	N	N	N	N	N	N	N	N	N	N	N	N		N	N	N	P
I	I	D	I	N	N	N	I	N	N	P	N	N	N		N	N	P
N	N	N	N	N	N	N	N	N	N	N	N	N	N	N		N	N
N	N	N	N	N	N	N	N	N	N	N	N	N	N	N	N		P
P	P	P	P	N	P	N	P	N	N	P	P	P	P	P	N	P	

Table 5–2. INTRAVENOUS MEDICATION COMPATIBILITY CHART

Key
★ – Compatible
☆ – Incompatible
□ – No information

	Aminophylline	Bretylium Tosylate	Cefazolin Sodium	Cimetidine	Diazepam	Dobutamine Hydrochloride	Dopamine Hydrochloride	Epinephrine Hydrochloride	Heparin Sodium	Hydrocortisone Sodium Succinate	Isoproterenol Hydrochloride	Lidocaine Hydrochloride	Methylprednisolone Sodium	Morphine Sulfate	Nitroglycerin	Phenobarbital Sodium	Phenytoin Sodium	Procainamide Hydrochloride	Propranolol Hydrochloride	Potassium Chloride	Sodium Bicarbonate	Sodium Nitroprusside
Aminophylline	★	★	★	☆	☆		☆	★	☆	☆	☆	★	★	☆	★	★	☆			★	★	☆
Ampicillin	☆		★	★			☆		★	★		☆								★		☆
Atropine Sulfate			★	☆	★			★	★				★							★	☆	☆
Bretylium Tosylate	★	★		☆	★	★		★				★			★		☆	★	★	★	☆	★
Calcium Chloride		★		★	★		★		★	★	★		☆		★				★	☆	☆	
Cefazolin Sodium	★			☆	★		★			★			☆							★		☆
Cimetidine	☆		☆	★	★	★		★	★		★	★	★	★		☆	☆		★	★	☆	
Diazepam	☆	☆	★	★	★	☆	☆	☆	☆	☆	☆	☆		☆	☆				☆	☆	☆	
Digoxin	★	★		★		★	★		★	★		★		★					★	★	☆	
Dobutamine Hydrochloride	☆	★		★	☆	★	★	★		★	★		★	★		☆	★	★	★	★	☆	☆
Dopamine Hydrochloride		★		☆	★	★		★	★	☆	★	★		★			★			★	☆	☆
Epinephrine Hydrochloride	☆		★	☆	★		★	☆	★		☆			☆			☆			★	☆	☆
Erythromycin Gluceptate	☆		☆					☆	★		☆				☆	☆				★		☆
Ethacrynate Sodium			★					★	★									☆		★		☆
Furosemide	★		★	☆	☆			★	★						★					★		☆
Gentamicin Sulfate	★		☆	☆		★		☆	☆		★											☆
Heparin Sodium	☆		★	★	☆	★	★	☆	★	☆	★	★	★	☆			☆	★	★	★	★	☆
Insulin–Regular	☆	★		★		☆			☆	★		★	☆			☆	☆			★	☆	☆
Isoproterenol Hydrochloride	☆		★	☆	★	☆		★	★	★	★									★	☆	☆
Lidocaine Hydrochloride	★	★	☆	★	☆	★	★	☆	★	★	★	★		★		☆	★	★		★	☆	☆
Magnesium Sulfate		★	★			★			★	☆	★									★	☆	☆
Meperidine Hydrochloride	☆		★	☆	★				☆						☆		☆	☆		★	☆	☆
Morphine Sulfate	☆		★	☆	★				☆	★							☆	☆		★	☆	☆
Nafcillin Sodium	☆		★	★	☆				☆			☆								★	★	☆
Nitroglycerin	★	★			☆	★	★	☆			★			★			★		☆			☆
Norepinephrine Bitartrate	☆		★	☆	★	★		★	★		☆	★					☆	☆		★	☆	☆
Penicillin G Potassium	☆		★	★			★		★	★		★	★			★	☆		★	★	★	☆
Potassium Chloride	★	★	★	★	☆	★	★	★	★	★	★	★	★	★		☆	★	★	★	★	★	☆
Sodium Bicarbonate	★	★		★	☆	☆	☆	☆	★	★	☆	☆	★	☆			☆			★	★	☆
Sodium Nitroprusside	☆	☆	☆	☆	☆	☆	☆	☆	☆	☆	☆	☆	☆	☆	☆	☆	☆	☆	☆	☆	☆	☆
Streptokinase									☆												☆	☆
Tetracycline Hydrochloride	☆		☆	★			★		☆	☆	★	★	☆			☆	☆			★	☆	☆
Ticarcillin Disodium														★								☆
Tobramycin Sulfate	☆							☆				★										☆
Trimethoprim Sulfamethoxazole	☆			☆	☆	☆		☆			☆											☆
Verapamil Hydrochloride	★	★	★	★	★	★	★	★	★	★	★	★	★	★	★	★	★	★	★	★	★	☆

SOURCE: Gorden, E: IV medication compatibility chart. Critical Care Nurse 6(4):82–83, July–August 1986, with permission.

come in contact with the bowel surface and therefore cannot be absorbed.

The initial site of potential drug interactions, the intestine, is where the heavy metals—aluminum, calcium, and magnesium—can tie up tetracycline and decrease absorption of this antibiotic. Antacids, milk, and dairy products chelate tetracycline, prevent its complete absorption, and compromise the patient's drug therapy.

How can this drug interaction be prevented in the patient using tetracycline four times a day and an antacid four times a day? The patient is instructed to take the tetracycline on an empty stomach one hour before each meal and one hour before bedtime. The antacid, which is most effective when taken after a meal, is adminis-

tered one hour after each meal and at bedtime. When drugs interfere at the point of absorption, the administration times are staggered so that the doses (of each drug) are at least 1–2 hours apart. By staggering the drugs, the patient is not denied either medication.

Drug absorption can also be affected by altering the intestinal mucosa. If the mucosa is destroyed by disease or drugs (e.g., antineoplastics), absorption within the intestinal tract may be either increased or decreased. Increased absorption may occur because destroyed mucosa leaves more vascular bed exposed, allowing more drug to be absorbed. Decreased absorption may occur because the mucosa layer of the intestine has been destroyed and no longer functions properly.

Table 5–3. EXAMPLES OF DRUG INTERACTIONS INVOLVING ABSORPTION*

Interacting Drugs	Result	Possible Mechanism
Antacid with:		
Digoxin	Decreased digoxin absorption	Adsorption
Isoniazid	Decreased isoniazid absorption	Decreased gastric emptying
Tetracycline	Decreased tetracycline absorption	Increased gastric pH and/or chelation
Ketoconazole	Decreased ketoconazole absorption	Increased gastric pH
Cimetidine	Decreased cimetidine absorption	Adsorption
Theophyllines	Decreased theophylline absorption	Adsorption
Ranitidine	Decreased ranitidine absorption	Adsorption
Ciprofloracin	Decreased ciprofloracin absorption	Adsorption
Caffeine with:		
Oral iron	Decreased iron effects	Adsorption
Cimetidine with:		
Ketoconazole	Decreased ketoconazole absorption	Increased gastric pH
Antacids	Decreased cimetidine effect	Adsorption
Oral iron	Decreased iron effect	Complexation
Cholestyramine with:		
Digitalis preparations	Decreased digitalis absorption	Complexation
Thyroid hormones	Decreased thyroid absorption	Complexation
Warfarin	Decreased warfarin effect	Complexation
Digoxin with:		
Antacids	Decreased digoxin effect	Complexation
Kaolin-pectin	Decreased digoxin effect	Adsorption
Erythromycin	Increased digoxin effect	Adsorption
Iron with:		
Tetracycline	Decreased tetracycline absorption	Chelation
Zinc	Decreased zinc effect	Chelation
Levodopa with:		
Anticholinergics	Decreased levodopa effect	Adsorption
Antidepressants	Decreased levodopa effect	Adsorption
Metoclopramide with:		
Cimetidine	Decreased cimetidine absorption	Increased gastric emptying
Tetracyclines with:		
Antacids	Decreased tetracycline effect	Complexation
Iron	Decreased tetracycline and iron effect	Complexation

*Not a complete listing.

PROTEIN AND TISSUE BINDING

Many drugs are extensively bound to plasma proteins. Drugs are pharmacologically inactive unless they are free from their binding sites on the protein. While protein-bound, the drug can neither perform its intended therapeutic action nor be eliminated from the body. (See Chapter 4 for more information on protein binding.) Table 5–4 features common drugs displacing others from their binding site.

The percentage of protein-bound drug remains constant in each individual patient and generally does not

Table 5–4. DRUGS DISPLACING OTHER DRUGS FROM BINDING SITES*

Affected Drug	Drug	Effect
Anticoagulants	Aspirin	Increased anticoagulant effect
	Chloral hydrate	Increased anticoagulant effect
	Clofibrate	Increased anticoagulant effect
	Ethacrynic acid	Increased anticoagulant effect
	Phenylbutazone	Increased anticoagulant effect
	Nalidixic acid	Increased anticoagulant effect
Hypoglycemics (sulfonylurea)	Anticoagulants	Increased anticoagulant effect
	Nonsteroidal anti-inflammatories	Hypoglycemia
Methotrexate	Probenecid	Possible increased methotrexate toxicity
	Sulfonamides	Possible increased methotrexate toxicity

*Not a complete listing.

pose any serious clinical problems. However, an increase in unbound drug in the plasma enhances not only the pharmacologic effect but also promotes the renal and/or hepatic elimination of the drug.

In general, plasma-protein-binding displacement drug interaction tends to be self-limiting, with generally only a transient increase in pharmacologic effect. It is now known that highly protein-bound drugs and their clinical effects are influenced by mechanisms other than protein-binding.

An illustration of this occurs with warfarin, an oral anticoagulant that is highly protein-bound and whose therapeutic effect is a direct result of the amount of free (or unbound) drug in the blood. Clofibrate, an antilipidemic, and phenylbutazone, an anti-inflammatory, have been shown to increase the anticoagulant effect of warfarin by displacing warfarin from its binding sites. However, of greater importance is that these agents inhibit the elimination of warfarin by the liver and prolong its anticoagulant effect. Therefore, protein displacement is not of importance alone but only when other mechanisms of interaction are involved.

Drugs are also capable of displacing other drugs from tissue-binding sites with results similar to protein-binding displacement. Quinidine (an antiarrhythmic) is known to displace digoxin from its binding sites in skeletal muscle. Therefore, if these drugs are given concurrently, the digoxin dosage needs to be reduced.

Drug interactions can also increase penetration of other drugs into tissue. Concurrent administration of acetazolamide (Diamox) and acetylsalicylic acid (aspirin) causes increased penetration of salicylic acid into the brain, although the mechanism is unknown.

BIOTRANSFORMATION

Biotransformation of many drugs is mediated largely by the liver. Biotransformation is one determinant of drug concentration at a particular site of action where a drug exerts its pharmacologic effect. Table 5–5 features drugs affecting biotransformation. Because of biotransformation, any change in the activity of drug-metabolizing enzymes in the liver can affect drug action. Metabolic changes can be divided into several categories: those medications that increase or those that inhibit enzyme activity in the liver, and those that compete for the same pathway. Enzyme induction involves the synthesis of new enzyme and takes place gradually in about 7–10 days. Enzyme inhibition usually takes place over 1–2 weeks or sometimes a longer period of time but also may occur more quickly with cimetidine (24–48 hours). It is thus important to understand the likely time course of such interaction in order to monitor the patient appropriately.

Enzyme Inducers

Phenobarbital is considered the classic stimulator (inducer) of liver drug metabolism. It stimulates the liver to produce more microsomal enzymes, which in turn increases the biotransformation of a variety of drugs and decreases their plasma concentration. The effect of phenobarbital on drug metabolism is usually seen

Table 5–5. DRUG INTERACTIONS AFFECTING BIOTRANSFORMATION*

Inducer†	Drug Affected
Phenobarbital	Warfarin
	Tricyclic antidepressants
	β-Adrenergic blockers
	Chloramphenicol
	Contraceptives, oral
	Diazepam
	Haloperidol
	Phenothiazines
	Quinidine
	Theophylline
	Phenytoin
Phenytoin	Corticosteroids
	Thyroid hormone
	Carbamazepine
	Theophylline
	Contraceptives, oral
	Haloperidol
Rifampin	Warfarin
	Tolbutamide
	Corticosteroids
	Methadone
	Quinidine
	Theophylline

Inhibitors	Drug Affected
Allopurinol	Oral anticoagulants
	Azathioprine
	Mercaptopurine
	Theophylline
Anticoagulants (oral)	Allopurinol
	Alcohol
	Amiodarone
	Disopyramide
	Erythromycin
	Isoniazid
	Metronidazole
	Phenytoin
	Ranitidine
Antidepressants (tricyclics)	Alcohol
	Cimetidine
	Contraceptives, oral
Erythromycin and ceprofloxacin	Theophylline
Cimetidine	Antidepressant, tricyclic
	Barbiturates
	Benzodiazepines
	β-Adrenergic blockers
	Digitoxin
	Lidocaine
	Nifedipine
	Phenytoin
	Quinidine
	Theophyllines

*Not a complete listing.
†The dose of the affected drug may have to be increased in order to maintain a therapeutic level.

within a few days; the maximum effect is seen after 2–3 weeks. Other well-known enzyme inducers are rifampin and phenytoin.

Alcohol is known to increase metabolism and decrease the activity of drugs such as warfarin, isoniazid, phenytoin (Dilantin), and tolbutamide. Tobacco and marijuana have been known to increase the metabolism of theophylline. Some drugs that are known to increase the metabolism of others can simultaneously increase their own metabolism as well. These include phenobarbital and carbamazepine.

Enzyme Inhibition

Enzyme inhibition is another way in which one drug can interfere with the metabolism of another drug and result in an increased pharmacologic effect. Cimetidine (Tagamet), an anti-ulcer agent, has recently been shown to interfere with the metabolism of a number of drugs. Cimetidine is known to decrease enzyme-metabolizing activity and decrease blood flow and drug delivery to the liver. Inhibition appears to occur within the first day of concurrent therapy, with maximum effect seen within one week. Other well-known interactions include inhibition of phenobarbital by valproic acid and inhibition of tolbutamide by sulfonamides and chloramphenicol.

COMPETITION FOR SAME PATHWAY. Occasionally two or more drugs given concurrently are biotransformed by the same enzyme. Their competition causes a reduced rate of biotransformation for each other and results in an increased duration of action. When phenytoin (Dilantin) and isoniazid (INH), an antituberculosis drug, are given together, there is a reduced rate of biotransformation of both drugs. Toxic levels may occur with repeated doses of these drugs.

RENAL EXCRETION

Interference with drug excretion can either delay or enhance drug effect. Excretion can be altered within the gastrointestinal tract by cathartics, food, narcotics, and stress, or through the urinary system. Any stage of urinary function can be affected, including glomerular filtration, tubular secretion, active and passive tubular reabsorption, alteration of gradients, or a change in pH. Examples of drugs that alter the urinary excretion of other drugs are listed in Table 5–6.

Some drug combinations are actively secreted by a similar process in the renal tubules, and therefore there may be interference with the elimination of one or both drugs. Examples of drugs that interact by this mechanism include penicillins, cephalosporins, probenecid, salicylates, methotrexate, and thiazide diuretics.

Diuretics (except potassium-sparing diuretics such as spironolactone, amiloride, and triamterene) decrease renal clearance of lithium and can lead to lithium intoxication. Due to lithium's narrow therapeutic index and its need for frequent monitoring of serum levels, this interaction is of serious consquence.

The use of probenecid (Benemid) to block the renal secretion of penicillin is an advantageous interaction in treating patients suspected of being noncompliant with their drug therapy. Instead of treating potentially uncooperative patients over several days with antibiotics such as penicillin, one large dose of penicillin is administered with probenecid. This two-drug combination keeps the amount of penicillin in the body at higher levels for a longer period of time than could have been achieved by giving the penicillin alone.

Drug elimination can be altered by affecting the urinary pH. Alkalization of the urine increases the amount of nonionized drug, thus promoting reabsorption of weak basic drugs and increasing their serum levels.

Table 5–6. DRUG INTERACTIONS INVOLVING RENAL EXCRETION*

Drug	Affected Drug	Adverse Effect (Probable Mechanism)
Quinidine	Digoxin	Increased digoxin effect (decreased tubular secretion)
Spironolactone	Digoxin	Increased digoxin effect (decreased tubular secretion)
Diuretics (Furosemide, ethacrynic acid, and thiazides)	Lithium	Increased lithium toxicity (increased tubular reabsorption)
Antacids	Salicylates	Decreased salicylate effect (increase in urine pH)
Sodium bicarbonate	Phenobarbital	Decreased phenobarbital effect (increase in urine pH)
	Salicylates	Decreased salicylate effect (increase in urine pH)
Probenecid	Indomethacin	Increased Indomethacin effect (decreased tubular secretion)
	Penicillins	Increased penicillin effect (decreased tubular secretion)
Cimetidine	Procainamide	Increased procainamide effect (decreased renal excretion)
Salicylates	Lithium	Possible increased lithium effect (decreased renal excretion)
	Methotrexate	Possible increased methotrexate toxicity (decreased renal excretion)
Tetracyclines	Lithium	Increased lithium toxicity (decreased renal excretion)
Allopurinol	Thiazide diuretics	Increased allopurinol toxicity (decreased renal excretion)

*Not a complete listing.

Conversely, weak acids are more ionized in alkaline urine, thus reducing tubular reabsorption and decreasing plasma levels.

Health professionals formerly relied on increasing rates of drug elimination in the treatment of acute barbiturate poisonings. Altering the pH of the urinary tract changes the chemical form of barbiturates and traps them in the urine, increasing the speed of excretion. Formerly, the response to acute barbiturate intoxication in the emergency room was rapid alkalization of the patient's urine with sodium bicarbonate to remove the drug as fast as possible from the victim's body. Today, dialysis or hemoperfusion is generally used to treat barbiturate overdose.

PHARMACODYNAMIC INTERACTIONS

Pharmacodynamic interactions can occur when drugs with similar actions or similar adverse effects are administered. The combined effect may be additive, synergistic, antagonistic, or potentiated. Table 5–7 features some examples of these interactions.

ADDITIVE

An *additive* effect occurs when two or more drugs possessing the same overt effect are combined, the result being the sum of the individual effects relative to the doses used. (For example, drug A has an effect of 1, drug B has an effect of 1, and the combination produces a 1 + 1 = 2 effect.) This additive effect may be deleterious or beneficial. The incidence of gastrointestinal bleeding is increased when alcohol is combined with a salicylate (aspirin and others). This is the result of an additive drug interaction because each agent alone can cause gastrointestinal bleeding. Combining two pain-relieving drugs such as aspirin and codeine is an example of a beneficial addition that controls pain better than either drug alone.

SYNERGISTIC

A *synergistic* effect occurs when two or more drugs, not possessing the same overt effect, are used together to yield a combined effect, the resultant outcome being greater than any single drug's active component alone. (For example, drug A has an effect of 1, drug B has an effect of 1, and the combination produces a 1 + 1 = 5 effect, rather than the 1 + 1 = 2 effect as expected.) This is exemplified by the prolonged hypnotic effect seen when alcohol is consumed with hypnotics such as chloral hydrate. Unfortunately, this interaction can potentially result in coma or death (see Chapter 24). On the positive side, the treatment of enterococcal subacute bacterial endocarditis employs the beneficial synergisitic effect of combining penicillin G with a member of the aminoglycoside family of antibiotics.

Table 5–7. PHARMACODYNAMIC INTERACTIONS*

Drug 1	+	Drug 2	Effect
ADDITIVE EFFECTS			
β-adrenergic blockers		Halothane	Hypotension
		Diltiazem and verapamil	Cardiac failure, AV conduction disturbances, and sinus bradycardia
		Diazoxide	Severe hypotension
Captopril		Most anesthetics	Hypotension
		Potassium supplements	Hyperkalemia
		Spironolactone	Hyperkalemia
Corticosteroids		Furosemide	Increased potassium loss
Furosemide		Aminoglycosides	Increased ototoxicity and nephrotoxicity
		Corticosteroids	Increased potassium loss
Smoking (marijuana)		Antidepressant (tricyclics)	Marked sinus tachycardia
Diazepam		Alcohol	Increased CNS depression
Digoxin		Methyldopa	Sinus bradycardia
Heparin		Alcohol	Increased bleeding
Nitroglycerin		Diazoxide	Severe hypotension
Nonsteroidal anti-inflammatories		Alcohol	Increased bleeding
SYNERGISM			
β-adrenergic blockers		Ergot alkaloids	Severe peripheral vasoconstriction, possible gangrene
Lithium		Carbamazepine	Increased neurotoxicity
		Phenytoin	Increased lithium toxicity
Theophylline		Halothane	Increased ventricular dysrhythmias
Amphotericin B		Aminoglycosides	Nephrotoxicity
ANTAGONISM			
β-adrenergic blockers		Sympathomimetics	Decreased antihypertensive effect, decreased bronchodilator effect

*Partial listing.
SOURCE: Adapted from the Medical Letter Handbook of Adverse Drug Interactions. The Medical Letter, New Rochelle, NY, 1989.

Another type of synergistic reaction occurs when two or more drugs produce the same type of effect but do so by exerting actions at different sites or by different mechanisms. For example, combining a diuretic, which lowers blood volume, and a β-adrenergic blocker, which dilates blood vessels to lower blood pressure, lowers blood pressure better than either drug alone.

POTENTIATION

Potentiation is best used to describe a particular type of synergistic effect, that is, a drug interaction in which only one of two drugs exerts the action that is made greater by the presence of the second drug.

ANTAGONISTIC

An *antagonistic* effect is the opposite of synergism and results in a combined effect that is less than either active component alone. In other words, adding a second drug may diminish or eliminate the effect of the first. (For example, drug A has an effect of 1, drug B has an effect of 1; when they are combined, drug A + drug B = 0 effect.) This can be seen when protamine sulfate (an anticoagulant) is administered as an *antidote* to a patient experiencing bleeding secondary to the anticoagulant action of heparin. Bleeding lessens or ceases because protamine sulfate is a strong base that neutralizes acidic heparin by binding with it to form a stable compound with no anticoagulant affect.

COMBINED TOXICITY

Combining two or more drugs with the same or similar adverse or toxic effects on the same organ may result in an additive or synergistic toxic effect. As an example, combining both furosemide (Lasix), a diuretic, and an aminoglycoside antibiotic, both of which can cause ototoxicity, may yield a combined toxicity leading to eighth cranial nerve damage and deafness.

CLINICAL SIGNIFICANCE OF COMBINING DRUGS

It is obvious from the previous discussion that many drugs are capable of interacting together. If two drugs are known to adversely interact, it does not mean that they can never be administered together. In order to prevent interactions, the dosages and/or the schedule of administration of the drugs is altered. The dosage of the drugs has to be carefully balanced and adjusted to minimize interactions. The patient needs to be taught the importance of not missing a dose of either medication. Proper scheduling of drugs can also minimize or eliminate interactions. Again, patient education is important so the patient understands why the medications are to be taken at alternate times rather than together.

Patients also have to be taught about taking over-the-counter (OTC) products. Many OTC products, when combined with prescription drugs, cause interactions. Patients are taught to always check with their pharmacist or physician before taking any OTC preparations.

DRUG-FOOD INTERACTIONS

Food is known to induce physiologic changes in the gastrointestinal tract that may decrease, increase, retard, or delay the absorption of drugs, or cause the drug to take longer to reach peak blood levels after a dose. Table 5–8 lists a number of drugs whose absorption is known to be affected when given with food.

FOODS DECREASING DRUG EFFECTIVENESS

Foods can act in various ways to decrease drug effectiveness. Foods may actually bind with drugs, allowing less to be absorbed; increase the hydrolysis of drugs in the intestine; or reduce the effect of absorbed drugs.

Several drugs are known to bind with certain foods, thus decreasing their absorption. Penicillin G and the many forms of erythromycin readily bind with any food that is present; therefore, they should be administered two hours before food ingestion. Tetracyclines bind with milk, cheese products, and all antacids; an insoluble precipitate is formed, which is excreted rather than absorbed.

Calcium binds with chocolate, oxalic acid (in spinach), and phytic acid (in nuts, legumes, and cereal grains), reducing its absorption. Patients who are taking calcium for hypocalcemia need to avoid these combinations. Calcium also inhibits the absorption of tetracycline. In addition, foods that are high in iron may also reduce the absorption of tetracycline. Tetracycline needs to be administered at least one hour before or two hours after a meal.

Table 5–8. DRUGS WHOSE ABSORPTION IS AFFECTED BY FOOD

Delayed	Reduced	Increased
Acetamino- phen	Acetaminophen	Chlorothia- zide
Aspirin	Amoxicillin	Griseofulvin
Cefaclor	Ampicillin	Hydralazine
Cephradine	Aspirin	Labetalol
Ciprofloxacin	Atenolol	Metoprolol
Digoxin	Cephalexin	Nitrofurantoin
Erythromycin	Cloxacillin	Propranolol
Furosemide	Demeclocycline	
Ibuprofen	Dicl0xacillin	
Indomethacin	Doxycycline	
Nitrofurantoin	Erythromycin	
Norfloxacin	Hydrochlorothiazide	
Metronidazole	Isoniazid	
Potassium ion	Levodopa	
Sulfisoxazole	Minocycline	
	Nafcillin	
	Oxacillin	
	Penicillin G	
	Penicillin V	
	Phenobarbital	
	Propantheline	
	Rifampin	
	Tetracycline	

Table 5–9. TYRAMINE-RICH FOODS

Aged or fermented food
Aged cheese (cheddar, Camembert, Stilton)
Chianti wine
European beer and ale
Caviar
Yeast
Pickled herring
Bananas
Beef/chicken livers
Fermented sausage (salami and pepperoni)
Yogurt
Sour cream
Avocados
Soy sauce

Bran can decrease the absorption of digoxin.

High-protein foods (eggs, meat, protein supplements) decrease the absorption of levodopa (Dopar) in the intestine. Proteins are metabolized to amino acids in the intestinal lumen. Levodopa, an amino acid derivative, competes with these amino acids for active transport across the intestinal wall. Protein intake should be spread equally in three meals a day to minimize this reaction. More than 10 mg/day of vitamin B_6 also decreases levodopa's effectiveness. Patients are cautioned to avoid B_6 supplements.

Penicillin G and erythromycin are hydrolyzed more quickly in the intestine in the presence of acid foods such as tomatoes, fruits, and vegetable and fruit juices. These foods are limited in patients taking these drugs.

Several food-drug combinations can actually reduce the effectiveness of absorbed drugs. Both natural licorice (containing glycyrrhizic acid) and tyramine-rich foods reduce the effectiveness of antihypertensives. Licorice is related to and acts like aldosterone and enhances sodium retention and potassium excretion in the distal tubule of the kidney, thus elevating blood pressure. Tyramine-rich foods (Table 5–9) enhance the release of norepinephrine from sympathetic axons, resulting in vasoconstriction and hypertension.

Patients are instructed not to eat barbecued meats while taking theophylline; the combination with charcoal-broiled meats can decrease theophylline's plasma half-life.

FOODS INCREASING DRUG EFFECTIVENESS

Food may promote the absorption of some drugs. Griseofulvin, an antifungal agent, is better absorbed when taken with meals containing fat. Patients may be encouraged to increase the fat content of their diet when taking griseofulvin. Other drugs, such as nitrofurantoin, hydrochlorothiazide (Diuril), and metoprolol (Lopressor), appear to be better absorbed after ingestion of food.

MAO inhibitors, a specific class of antidepressant medications, increase levels of norepinephrine and serotonin in the central nervous system and potentiate the cardiovascular effects of substances such as tyramine. An acute hypertensive crisis can occur, resulting in symptoms of severe occipital headache, palpitations, stiff neck, nausea, and vomiting. Tyramine-containing foods are avoided during and 2–3 weeks after MAO inhibitor therapy.

The effects of MAO inhibitors can also be enhanced by concurrent ingestion of caffeine and monosodium glutamate (MSG), a flavor enhancer. Chinese food often contains large amounts of MSG, so patients are cautioned about eating Chinese food, especially in restaurants. Consuming large amounts of MSG, even without taking any medication, can cause symptoms of throbbing in the head, lightheadedness, tightness in the jaw and shoulders, and backache. These symptoms are related to arterial vasodilatation and reflex sympathetic stimulation.

ADDITIONAL FACTORS FOR DRUG INTERACTIONS

Other patient factors that may influence the response to drug interactions are chronic disease states, diet, environment, genetic makeup, and age.

Patients affected by chronic disease states may be predisposed to the adverse effects of drug interactions. This is a consideration in patients afflicted with endocrine diseases (e.g., diabetes and thyroid conditions); alcoholism; various diseases of the gastrointestinal tract; renal failure; and hepatic dysfunction.

Dietary excesses or insufficiencies may predispose some patients to untoward effects from certain drugs. Excesses of caffeine may have an antagonistic effect with central nervous system depressants. Sucrose when taken in excess may have a tendency to suppress sexual activity, particularly in patients taking large doses of aspirin. Excessive licorice intake may cause pseudoaldosteronism (hypoaldosteronism), which causes symptoms of aldosterone suppression. Large carbohydrate intake may lower the body's resistance to toxic effects of various medications. Vitamin C may increase the secretion of weakly basic drugs such as atropine or quinidine and therefore inhibit them, or it may decrease the excretion of weak acids such as barbiturates, aspirin, and sulfonamides, thereby potentiating them. Patients taking isoniazid (INH, an antitubercular drug), should take limited amounts of Swiss cheese and tuna fish. The high histamine content of these foods may interact with this agent to cause severe headaches, redness and itching of the eyes and face, chills, palpitations, pulse rate variations, and loose stools.

Various drugs can also precipitate dietary deficiencies. Long-term use of anticonvulsants can cause folate and vitamin D deficiencies, manifested by muscle weakness, breathlessness, or bone pain. Increasing folate and vitamin D–rich foods in the diet may be helpful. Phenytoin and phenobarbital can also cause intestinal malabsorption of calcium and subsequent development of osteomalacia. Chronic aspirin ingestion can deplete folic acid, and "pseudosenility" may occur in the elderly person. Penicillamine (an antiarthritic drug) chelates zinc and copper and may precipitate these deficiencies.

Alcohol intake may also precipitate drug interactions.

In the United States, approximately 104 million people consume alcohol regularly. Alcohol can cause interactions with many types of drugs, such as antihypertensives, CNS depressants, antipsychotic agents, analgesics, anticoagulants, diuretics, cardiotonics, antiarrhythmics, and antidiabetic agents. The amount of alcohol consumed on a daily basis needs to be considered when these drugs are administered.

Environmental factors are considered in patients exposed to smoking, insecticides, and air pollution. These environmental influences are just beginning to be intensely investigated by researchers.

Another area just beginning to be actively researched is the effect a patient's genetic makeup may have on drug disposition and adverse drug interactions.

The final area of note is the effect of age on the patient's ability to handle potential drug interactions. Older patients, because of multiple chronic disease states, compromised kidney function, and possible dietary insufficiencies, must be closely monitored.

LEGAL IMPLICATIONS

As the information on drug interactions grows, the legal responsibility of nurses also increases. Current legal guidelines suggest that the nurse is responsible for only published interactions that are well known. It is the nurse's responsibility to question all orders when there is a potential for interaction that may adversely affect the patient. The nurse must always assess for symptoms of changing behavior and changing signs and symptoms, and for any unusual or unexpected modification that could indicate a drug interaction. The nurse has the legal right to withhold further doses of the medication that is suspected of causing the problem until the physician can evaluate the patient.

SUMMARY

It is becoming increasingly important for people not only to be made aware of potential adverse drug-drug interactions, but also to be properly instructed in the essential considerations of drug interactions with common foods. Many drugstore chains are currently using computer programs to assess for drug interaction before prescriptions are being filled. This is definitely an added safety feature for patients.

No list can possibly be complete and current; each day brings the chance of a new interaction that may not have been suspected previously. Health professionals must continue to stay abreast of the new data, continue to make prudent use of already documented information, and be ever aware that a new drug interaction may be as close as the next patient. It is important for the nurse to continually refer to current drug interaction texts for more complete information.

BIBLIOGRAPHY

— Match your meals and medicines. Changing Times 40(11):68–70, 72, 1986.

American Society of Hospital Pharmacists: Medication Teaching Manual. American Society of Hospital Pharmacists, Washington, DC, 1985.

Cerrato, PL: When food and drugs collide. RN 87(4):85–86, 1987.

Cerrato, PL: Drugs and food: When the dangers increase. RN 88(11):65–67, 1988.

D'Arcy, PF, et al: Drug-antacid interactions: Assessment of clinical importance. Drug Intell Clin Pharm 21(7/8), Part 1:607–617, 1987.

Durrence, C, et al: Potential drug interactions in surgical patients. Am J Hosp Pharm 42(7):1553–1556, 1985.

Gilman, AG, Goodman, LS, and Gilman, A: Goodman and Gilman's The Pharmacological Basis of Therapeutics, ed 7. Macmillan, New York, 1985.

Gordon, EL: IV medication compatibility. Critical Care Nurse 6(4):82, 1986.

Hallal, JC: Are coffee, cold tablets, and chocolate innocuous or is their caffeine hazardous to your patients' health? Am J Nurs 86(4):423–425, 1986.

Hansten, PD: Drug Interactions, ed 5. Philadelphia, Lea & Febiger, 1985.

Hansten, PD: Drug Interactions: Decision Support Tables. In Applied Therapeutics: Clinical Use of Drugs. St. Louis, Applied Therapeutics for Clinical Pharmacist Service, 1988.

Hayes, AH, Jr: How drugs affect drugs. Emergency Medicine (13):114–117, July 15, 1981.

Lakshmanan, M, et al: Hospital admissions caused by iatrogenic disease. Arch Intern Med 146(10):1931–1934, 1986.

Lerman, F and Weibert, RT: Drug Interactions Index. Medical Economics, Florence, KY, 1986.

Mathewson, Kuhn: Drug interactions. Critical Care Nurse 9(4):84–92, 1989.

Osis, M: Scheduling drug administration: Drug and food interactions. Gerontion 6(5):8–10, 1986.

Raiczyk, GB and Pinto, J: Drug-nutrient interactions, Troublesome combinations and susceptible patients. Consultant 26(7):85–105, July 1986.

Rizack, M: The Medical Letter Handbook of Adverse Drug Interactions. The Medical Letter, New Rochelle, NY, 1989.

Todd, B: Cigarettes and caffeine in drug interactions. Geriatr Nurs 8(2):97–98, 1987.

Vore, M, et al: Common adverse drug interactions. Hosp Med 22(10):94, 98, 100, 1986.

Winick, M (ed): Nutrition and Drugs. New York, John Wiley & Sons, 1983.

SITUATION 5–1

Scott Preston is a medication nurse on a medical-surgical unit in a large urban hospital. The following questions relate to situations involving drug interactions.

1. Scott checks on a patient admitted with digitalis toxicity. The patient had been taking digoxin and the antiarrhythmic agent, quinidine, for several months. Scott is aware that the presenting symptoms may be due to:
   a. Increased biotransformation of quinidine by digoxin
   b. Displacement of digoxin from its tissue-binding sites by quinidine
   c. Increased penetration of quinidine into tissue in the presence of digoxin
   d. Displacement of quinidine from its binding sites by digoxin

2. Thirty-eight-year-old Emma Smythe is receiving gentamicin, an aminoglycoside antibiotic, and furosemide (Lasix), a loop diuretic, as part of her drug therapy. Which of the following statements by Emma indicates a serious drug interaction resulting from this combination?
   a. "I've been passing my water a lot."
   b. "I didn't move my bowels today."
   c. "My mouth feels so dry."
   d. "I'm having trouble hearing you."

3. Following discharge from the hospital, which of these actions is most likely to compromise the patient's drug therapy?
   a. Taking erythromycin on an empty stomach
   b. Using antacids 2 hours after amphetamines
   c. Combining vitamin C with mineral oil
   d. Drinking a glass of milk with tetracycline

4. In administering oral medications to patients receiving cancer chemotherapy, Scott carefully considers the following patient characteristic:
   a. Blood pressure
   b. Mucosal integrity
   c. Emotional status
   d. Taste sensation

5. Which of the following patients will Scott expect to experience alterations in drug biotransformation?
   a. 52-year-old male with cirrhosis
   b. 35-year-old female with ulcerative colitis
   c. 41-year-old male with cancer of the stomach
   d. 60-year-old female with acute renal failure

6. When completing a medication history on a patient recently admitted to his unit, Scott notes the following patient statement as being significant to drug therapy while hospitalized:
   a. "I always take Tylenol when I get a headache."
   b. "I've been taking Tagamet for my ulcer."
   c. "I always take my pills with a glass of water."
   d. "I keep a list of the medications that I take."

Situation 5–2

Hillside Manor, a rural extended-care facility, has a large number of patients on multiple drug therapy. The medication nurse frequently deals with the following patient situatons.

1. Sixty-eight-year-old Mary Taggart is experiencing phantom limb pain following a recent amputation. The nurse administers aspirin and codeine together for pain relief. This is an example of which type of effect?
   a. Synergistic
   b. Antagonistic
   c. Potentiated
   d. Additive

2. Jake McBride, 72 years old, receives furosemide (Lasix), a diuretic, and propranolol (Inderal), a beta-adrenergic blocker, for control of his hypertension. The pharmacodynamic interaction responsible for the therapeutic antihypertensive effect is:
   a. Addition
   b. Antagonism
   c. Synergism
   d. Potentiation

3. Sixty-two-year-old Jane Coleman is taking calcium supplements for hypocalcemia. The nurse should avoid administering the drug with:
   a. Ginger ale
   b. Chocolate milk
   c. Orange juice
   d. Iced tea

4. Which of the following statements by a visitor to Hillside Manor reflects good insight into a serious food-drug interaction?
   a. "Mom never ate breakfast, but now she takes her digitalis pill every morning with a bowl of bran flakes."
   b. "Mom always takes her penicillin with tomato juice instead of milk in the morning."
   c. "Mom loves black licorice, but she hasn't had any since she's been taking Lasix."
   d. "Mom's been eating a lot of yogurt since she started on those blood pressure pills."

5. Seventy-year-old Mildred Rankin is on MAO inhibitor therapy for depression. After appropriate teaching by the nurse, Mildred should avoid the following menu choice:
   a. Broiled trout
   b. Tomato vegetable soup
   c. Baked stuffed flounder
   d. Chicken chow mein

6. Betty Thomas, on isoniazid (INH) for a history of tuberculosis, recently ate a large portion of tuna fish casserole for dinner. Betty would be expected to manifest this response:
   a. Severe headaches
   b. Constipation
   c. Diuresis
   d. No ill effects

Refer to the Appendix for correct answers and additional review questions with answers.

6
CHAPTER

DRUG TOXICOLOGY

GLOSSARY TERMS IN THIS CHAPTER

Anaphylactic
Anaphylactoid
Anaphylaxis
Antibody
Antigen
Antigenic
Bronchorrhea
Interstitial nephritis
Toxicology

6
CHAPTER

DRUG TOXICOLOGY

MERRILY MATHEWSON KUHN, R.N.C., Ph.D., CCRN

LEARNING OBJECTIVES

After reading this chapter, the student will be able to:

1. Differentiate among adverse, idiosyncratic, allergic, toxic, and delayed drug reactions.

2. Identify the 4 types of hypersensitivity reactions and their relationship to medication administration.

3. Understand the principles of caring for a patient who has taken a poison or drug overdose.

4. Understand drug-induced organ toxicities.

5. Identify drugs that cause toxic effects to the skin, liver, kidney, eye, ear, lung, and sexual organs.

6. Identify drugs that are removed from the body with dialysis, plasmapheresis, and hemoperfusion.

Toxicology is that aspect of pharmacology that deals with the adverse effects of drugs on living organisms. Toxicology is concerned not only with drugs used in therapy but also with many other chemicals that may be responsible for household, environmental, or industrial intoxication. Two federal agencies are responsible for the regulation of drugs and chemicals. They ensure that a low risk relative to the beneficial effect is present when the agent is used for its intended purpose in the general population. The Food and Drug Administration (FDA) regulates drugs, cosmetics, and food additives in interstate commerce (see Chapter 2), while the Environmental Protection Agency (EPA) regulates most other chemicals.

In general, when pharmacologic products are administered, the benefit should outweigh the risk. However, the use of all pharmacologic products has certain risks. This chapter briefly discusses the various types of toxic reactions to drugs and other chemicals.

The undesirable effects of drugs, or adverse reactions, fall into two classes:

1. Effects that are a predicted result of the drug's known pharmacologic effect. Toxic effects are dose-related and will occur in all persons given sufficient dosage.
2. Effects that are not related to the drug's pharmacologic effect. These effects cannot be predicted and are the result of something peculiar in that patient. Drug allergies, hypersensitivity reactions, and idiosyncratic reactions fall into this category.

Adverse drug effects may occur within a reasonably short time after a drug is started, that is, within a minute (anaphylaxis), days (gastrointestinal bleeding), or weeks (renal failure). These are generally referred to as "acute" or short-term adverse effects. On the other hand, drug toxicities may be "delayed," that is, the toxicity may become manifest only months or years after a drug is started. Assessment and evaluation of cumulative toxic effects are receiving increased attention because of chronic exposure to low concentrations of various natural and synthetic chemical substances in the environment.

ADVERSE REACTIONS

The terms "adverse" or "side effects" describe the potential unwanted effects patients experience as a result of medication therapy. Adverse effects include symptoms that are uncomfortable for the patient but may be tolerated, such as nausea, vomiting, fatigue, dizziness, and hypotension. Table 1–2 in Chapter 1 reviews typical adverse effects. Numerous studies have been done to determine the actual incidence of adverse reaction, and findings range from 10%–30% of hospitalized medical patients. In addition, 2%–3% of hospital admissions are the result of adverse reactions. Death can result from adverse reactions as well, and the incidence is approximately 0.2%–0.5% of all hospitalized medical patients.

Adverse effects are more likely to occur in females, the elderly, patients with impaired renal function, and in patients taking many medications.

PHARMACOLOGIC (PREDICTABLE) TOXICITY

Primary Reaction

It is a common occurrence when drugs are administered for a patient to experience adverse effects from overdose. These are generally effects that are merely an extension of the desired action of that drug. Several examples include excessive drowsiness and lethargy from sedatives and hypnotics, increased bleeding tendencies from anticoagulants, excessive slowing of the heart from digitalis products, and hypotension from antihypertensives. The overdose may be accidentally taken by the patient as a result of poor patient teaching or understanding; or a medication may have been ordered for the patient without regard to hepatic or renal function or age considerations, resulting in an excessive dose.

The majority of pharmacologic toxicities can be avoided by adjusting the dosage carefully to patient requirements and by vigilant monitoring on the part of the nurse.

Secondary Reaction

The majority of drugs on the market today have a wide variety of effects on the individual. Many patients can be treated effectively without the development of undesirable secondary reactions. However, there is still a group of patients who do develop these secondary reactions. Several examples include severe drowsiness and sleepiness from antihistamines used to prevent motion sickness; excessive tiredness and impotence from antihypertensives; and extreme agitation from the theophylline bronchodilators. At times, reduction of the dose may be sufficient to lessen or stop these reactions, or the drug may need to be discontinued. Nursing assessments and evaluations are important to identify these reactions and to ensure they are resolved.

Drug Allergies

Drug allergies range from very mild (e.g., urticaria or hives), with no need to discontinue the drug, to very severe, such as an anaphylactic shock reaction. Patients reporting drug allergies need to be carefully evaluated. Often, patients are merely experiencing adverse effects rather than allergic reactions (e.g., nausea or vomiting).

Drugs are relatively small molecules and have no *antigenic* activity. Therefore drugs (the *antigen*) must obtain antigenic properties and stimulate *antibody* production before they can produce an allergic reaction. This is accomplished when a drug, acting as a hapten, combines with some body protein (carrier molecule) and forms a drug-protein complex. It is this drug-protein complex that possesses antigenic activity and invokes specific antibody formation, thereby sensitizing the body to the drug (Fig. 6–1). The synthesis of antibodies usually occurs after a latent period of at least 1–2 weeks. When subsequent exposure of the individual to the

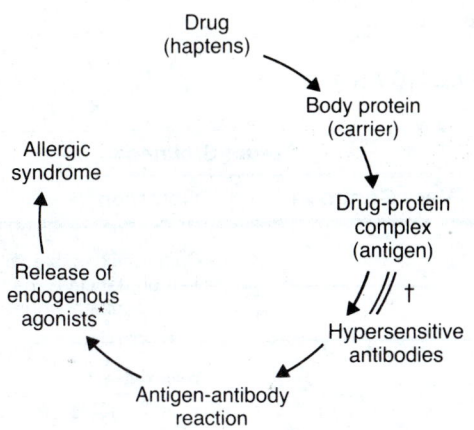

Figure 6–1. Drug allergic syndrome. (*Histamine, serotonin, bradykinins, slow-reacting substance [SRS]; †others.)

chemical occurs, an antigen-antibody interaction results in the typical allergic manifestations. Extremely small quantities of the antigen can provoke a reaction.

Drug allergies may manifest themselves over a full spectrum of immediate and delayed reaction. As an example, skin reactions may extend from mild rash to severe exfoliative dermatitis, while blood vessel reactions may extend from acute urticaria and angioedema to severe arteritis and localized degeneration.

Drug allergies are classified into four types: Types I, II, III, and IV. Each type is briefly described as to its etiology and pathology.

During an *anaphylactoid* reaction, the offending agent enters the body and works by non-immunological activating systems that cause degranulation of mast cells and basophils of the humoral system. Once the humoral system is activated the same mediators are released and the clinical symptoms are indistinguishable from anaphylaxis.

TYPE I (ANAPHYLACTIC OR ATOPIC REACTION). A type I allergic reaction is a common type of drug allergy. (This reaction can also be activated by environmental pollens, foods, insect bites, and certain household cleaning agents.) Two types of type I reactions can occur: (1) *anaphylaxis*, which refers to an acute reaction occurring in the skin and in the lung and cardiovascular systems and resulting in cardiovascular/respiratory collapse; and (2) atopy, which refers to a chronic reaction within the lung or in the skin that is dependent on the antigen, the frequency of contact, the route of contact, and the sensitivity of the organ system to the antigen. Both reactions share the same etiology and pathology. On previous exposure to the agent, such as penicillin, IgE antibodies are formed which attach to basophils, particularly mast cells. True tissue basophils are found in profusion in connective tissue, the skin, and the mucous membranes. When the drug is administered again (challenging dose), the mast cells liberate large doses of histamine and other humoral substances. These substances cause bronchoconstriction in the smooth muscles of the lung, peripheral vasodilatation, increased vascular permeability, and increased mucus production in the lung (Fig. 6–2). If this reaction remains local, erythema and local edema occur. However, if the reaction becomes systemic, many signs and symptoms occur. Table 6–1 lists common agents that can cause anaphylactic reactions.

Anaphylactic Shock. Anaphylactic shock is a systemic reaction to the antigen that consequently affects many tissues and organs in the body (Table 6–2). The release of histamine and other humoral substances results in contraction of smooth muscle and increased vascular permeability within the lung. Edema occurs

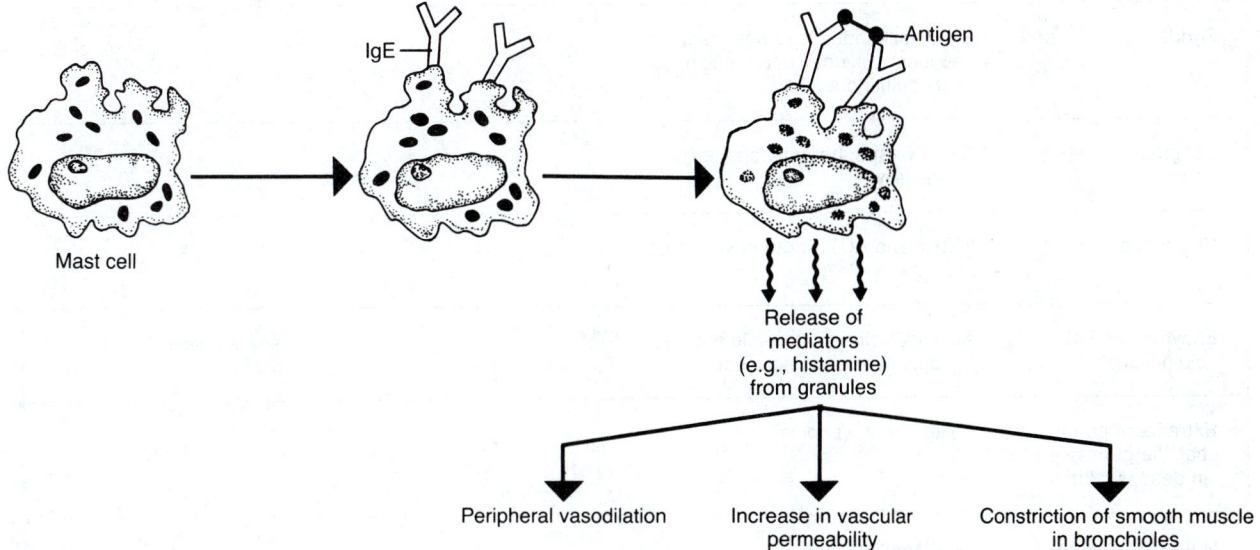

Figure 6–2. Type I hypersensitivity reaction. The mast cell in the lung and IgE antibody are attached by a specific antigen that results in the release of the vasoactive substances, histamine, and others.

Table 6–1. AGENTS COMMONLY IMPLICATED IN ANAPHYLACTIC AND ANAPHYLACTOID REACTIONS AND SERUM SICKNESS

	Anaphylactic and Anaphylactoid	Serum Sickness	
		Very Common	**Common**
Antibiotics	Penicillin and penicillin analogs, cephalosporins, tetracyclines		Sulfonamides, bleomycin, amphotericin B, penicillins, cephalosporin
Nonsteroidal anti-inflammatory agents	Salicylates		Salicylates
Narcotic analgesics	Morphine, codeine		
Other drugs	Protamine, chlorpropamide, parenteral iron, iodides, thiazide diuretics, immunotherapy	Cocaine derivatives, antihistamines, methyldopa, quinidine	Amphetamines, phenytoin, anticholinergics, procainamide
Local anesthetics	Procaine, lidocaine, cocaine		
General anesthetics	Thiopental		
Anesthetic adjuncts	Succinylcholine, tubocurarine		
Blood products and antisera	Red-cell, white-cell, and platelet transfusions, gamma globulin, rabies, tetanus, diphtheria antitoxin, snake and spider antivenom		
Diagnostic agents	Iodinated radio contrast agents		
Foods	Eggs; milk; nuts; legumes (peanuts, soybeans, kidney beans); fish; shellfish; sulfiting agents		
Venoms	Bees, wasps, hornets, snakes, spiders, jellyfish		
Hormones	Insulin and ACTH both have pituitary extract		
Enzymes and other biologicals	Acetylcysteine, pancreatic enzyme supplements, chymopapain		Asparaginase
Extracts of potential allergens used in desensitization	Pollen, food, venoms		
Nutritional agents	Lipid emulsion (rare)		

Table 6–2. CLINICAL FINDINGS—ANAPHYLAXIS

	Symptoms	Signs	Treatment
Respiratory	Nasal congestion, dysphagia, hoarseness, dyspnea	Laryngospasm, bronchospasm, rhinorrhea, oral laryngeal edema, bronchorrhea	Epinephrine, bronchodilators, oxygen, entubation and ventilation, steroids
Cardiovascular	Faintness, palpitations	Tachycardia, hypotension, shock, syncope, dysrhythmia, peripheral edema	Epinephrine, fluids, pressors, cardiotonics
Cutaneous	Pruritus, rash	Urticaria, flushing, angiodema	Antihistamines
Gastrointestinal	Bloating, nausea, cramps	Abdominal distention and pain, vomiting, diarrhea	Antihistamines
Other	Feelings of impending doom, visual changes, metallic taste		

around the eyes, on the skin, and in mucous membranes. Laryngeal edema often results in acute dyspnea. Hives or severe urticaria may appear on the skin surface. Within the vascular system the fluid shifts may result in hypotension and even cardiovascular collapse.

Anaphalaxis is an acute medical emergency that is treated with epinephrine, antihistamines, bronchodilators, vasopressors, and other emergency procedures.

Atopic Reactions. Atopic allergy from the inhalation of environmental antigens may result in bronchial asthma, with dyspnea and wheezing being early signs. Repeated exposure can result in hypertrophy of smooth muscle and can exaggerate bronchoconstriction.

Contact with irritants may cause atopic eczema resulting in urticaria, hives, and angioedema. These reactions are much more common than anaphylaxis. The urticaria involves superficial capillaries, while the angioedema affects deeper skin capillaries. Drugs can also cause dermatologic manifestations. These are discussed later in Chapter 63.

TYPE II (CYTOTOXIC REACTION). In a type II allergic reaction (cytotoxic reaction or immune complex syndromes), the foreign antigen adheres to the surface of the host's own cells (target cell). Antibodies are then formed by the host, which attach to the target cell (Fig.

6–3). Generally this reaction involves the activation of complement, a series of enzymatic proteins in normal serum that, in the presence of a specific sensitizer—often an antigen—destroy bacteria and other cells. Complement surrounds the target cells and causes destruction of the target cell, either through phagocytosis or cell lysis. The ultimate effect on the host depends on the number and type of cells destroyed.

The type II allergic reaction or serum sickness is most often seen in persons receiving penicillin and diphtheria and tetanus antitoxin. Immediately after the drug is administered, the person develops antibodies of the IgG and IgM variety. Within several days to a week the antibodies become so numerous that they begin to complex with red blood cells, platelets, and basophils. Histamine and other humoral substances are released, enter the blood stream, and are soon deposited in many tissues. The patient then presents with fever, arthralgia, rash, splenomegaly, and lymph node enlargement. In severe reactions, hemolytic reactions, glomerulonephritis, thrombocytopenia, leukopenia, and vascular purpura may be seen. Usually, the reaction is self-limiting, and recovery occurs within several days to weeks.

The exact mechanism of these drug reactions is poorly understood. Several mechanisms have been suggested:

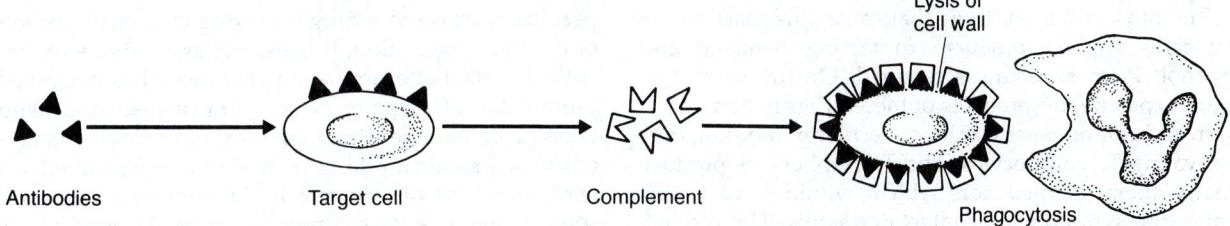

Figure 6–3. Type II hypersensitivity reaction. The target cell is covered with antibody that activates complement and sets the stage for phagocytosis.

hypersensitivity to the drug, contaminants or impurities within the drug, inflammation from the injection site, a direct pyrogenic effect, alteration of the thermoregulation center in the central nervous system, or biochemical defects within the patient.

TYPE III (AUTOIMMUNE REACTION). A type III allergic reaction, also called an autoimmune reaction or a complex-mediated hypersensitivity reaction, is associated with increased amounts of IgG. Anaphylatoxins and neutrophils release necrotizing enzymes that produce local ischemia and necrosis as a consequence of complement activation. The antigen-antibody complexes may also be present in the plasma without manifesting disease. If these complexes are not removed through phagocytosis, they may circulate through the body. They often lodge in tissue where increased vascular permeability allows them to be deposited in the extravascular space. Following deposition they initiate an inflammatory reaction leading to tissue destruction. The inflammatory process and tissue destruction are mediated through activation of complement (Fig. 6–4). The mechanism is active in autoimmune diseases such as glomerulonephritis, rheumatoid arthritis, systemic lupus erythematosus, scleroderma, and many others. Drugs capable of causing a type III reaction include penicillin, phenytoin, and streptomycin.

TYPE IV (CELL-MEDIATED HYPERSENSITIVITY). Type IV allergic reaction is mediated through T lymphocytes rather than antibodies and may be of two varieties: (1) a cell-mediated response or (2) a delayed hypersensitivity response. A cell-mediated response occurs as a result of T cell contact and destruction of the antigen. The T cell may also activate macrophages, which results in the lysis of other cells. Transplant rejection is, in part, a cell-mediated response.

Delayed hypersensitivity responses are due to the specific interaction of T cells with the antigen. The T cell/antigen reaction releases substances (macrophage migration inhibitory factor [MIF], macrophage activating factor [MAF], chemotactic factors, and others) that attract macrophages into the area. These factors also modulate the inflammatory response (Fig. 6–5). The tuberculin (TB) skin response is a good example of delayed hypersensitivity used to determine whether an individual has been sensitized to TB. If the patient was previously exposed to TB, the skin test will cause reddening and induration of the skin about 12 hours after intradermal injection. This reaction peaks within 24–72 hours. This response is only elicited when lymphocytes are present.

The most common drugs that cause this reaction are topically applied products containing benzene and phenol. Prior exposure is required. On the second or third exposure, by-products of these drugs penetrate the skin and combine with larger molecules in the skin, thus activating T lymphocytes. The T lymphocytes produce many chemical mediators which, within 6–12 hours, cause the symptoms of contact dermatitis. The product should be completely washed from the skin and not used again. Table 6–3 features a review of the four types of allergy reactions.

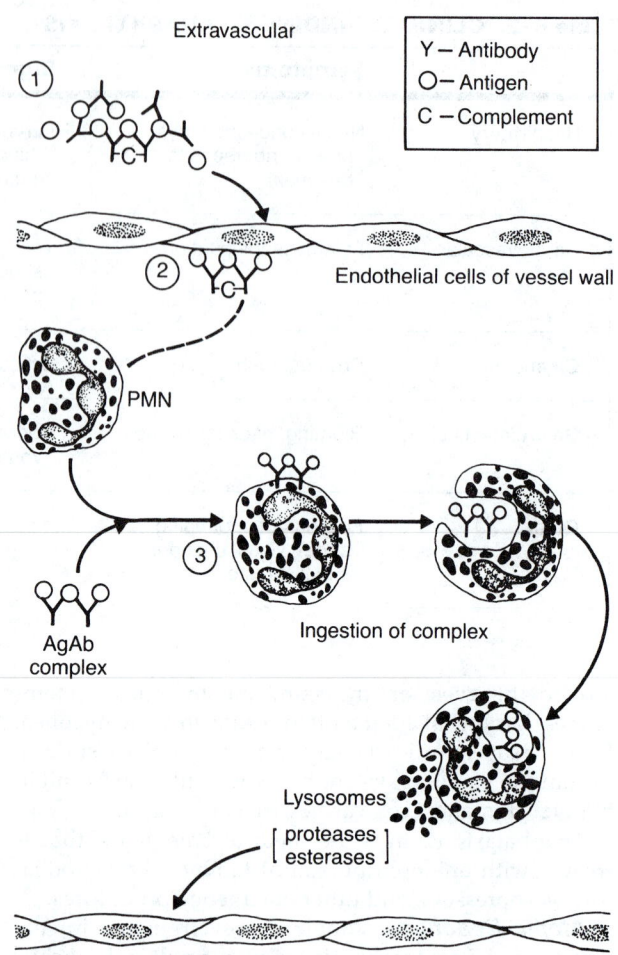

Figure 6–4. Type III hypersensitivity reaction showing the precipitation of antigen-antibody complexes in target tissues resulting in membrane destruction.

(1) In extracellular space antigen O combines with antibodies Y and complexes with complement C.

(2) The Antigen/Antibody/Complement (A/A/C) complex enters the vascular system. A polymorphyneutrophil (PMN) complexes with the A/A/C complex and injests it. The by-products of phagocytosis, lysosomes (proteases and esterases) begin to damage tissue. Here the tissue is the endothelial cells of the vessel wall.

IDIOSYNCRATIC REACTIONS

An idiosyncratic reaction is an unexpected, abnormal, or peculiar reaction to a drug occurring in a small portion of the total population. It is usually associated with genetic defects. For example, a patient who has decreased production of hepatic N-acetyltransferase and who takes procainamide (Pronestyl) will have slower metabolism of procainamide and may develop toxic effects and symptoms of systemic lupus erythematosus; persons having a decreased production of glucose-6-phosphate dehydrogenase (about 10% of black males) develop a serious hemolytic anemia when they receive primaquine (antimalarial preparation); or, persons (in

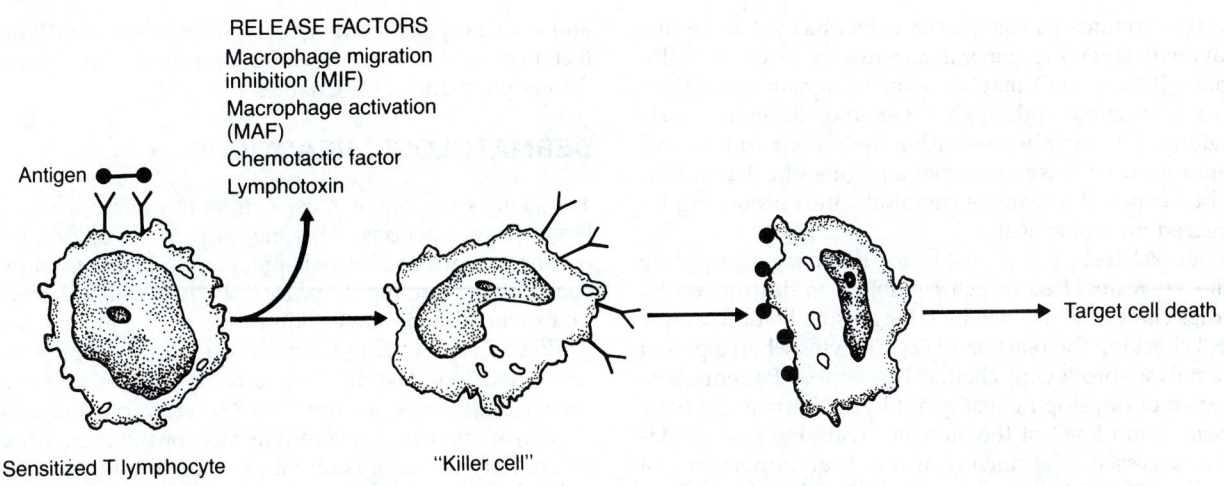

Figure 6–5. Type IV hypersensitivity reaction. The T lymphocyte contacts the foreign material and through direct intervention or the secretion of substances toxic to the foreign material causes destruction of the foreign protein.

Table 6–3. COMPARISON OF FOUR HYPERSENSITIVITY REACTIONS

Type of Reaction	Where Reaction Occurs	Drugs Causing Reaction	Time After Antigen Exposure	Observable Signs	Mechanism of Effect of Injury and Antibiody
Type I Anaphylactic reaction	Vascular system, mucous membranes, smooth muscle, skin	Antibiotics, nonsteroidal anti-inflammatories, many more (see Chapter 47)	5–20 min	Respiratory distress, bronchospasm, airway obstruction, cardiovascular shock, skin eruptions, abdominal pain, nausea, diarrhea, edema	Mast cell release of histamine, SRS-A, and other pharmacologic agents; IgE
Atopy (chronic)	Skin, mucous membranes	Iodides, sulfonamides, thiazines, and others	5–15 min and longer	Skin eruptions, bronchospasm, airway obstruction, abdominal pain, nausea, diarrhea, edema	May be related to IgA deficiency
Type II Cytotoxic (serum sickness)	Any tissue but usually vascular system or kidney	Penicillin, diphtheria and tetanus antitoxins, meprobamate	Minutes to days	Deficiency of target cell type, i.e., anemia, thrombocytopenia, leukopenia, vascular purpura, and hemolysis	Lysis of target cells due to hapten being absorbed on native cells, IgM/IgG
Type III Complex-mediated hypersensitivity (autoimmune reaction)	Systematic vascular system	Penicillin, phenytoin, streptomycin	Minutes to years	Glomerulonephritis, rheumatoid arthritis, polyarteritis nodosa, systemic lupus erythematosis, maculopapular eruptions, urticaria, vasculitis	Anaphylatoxins and neutrophil release of necrotizing lysomal enzymes, which produce local ischemic necrosis at location of antigen-antibody complement complex, IgG
Type IV Delayed hypersensitivity	In tissue	Topical benzene and phenol products, tuberculin skin testing, rabies vaccination	24–48 hr and delayed to years	Contact dermatitis, tuberculin reaction, graft rejection, allergic reactions to infection, maculopapular eruptions	Lymphokine (release and subsequent lymphocyte-mediated cytolysis), cell-mediated via lymphocytes and macrophages, antibodies, terminal inflammatory sequence

certain families whose genetic defect has yet to be discovered) receiving general anesthetics (such as halothane [Fluothane]) may develop malignant hyperthermia associated with high fever and skeletal muscle rigidity. The membranes within the muscle cells of this latter group release abnormal amounts of calcium ions when exposed to various chemicals, thus producing increased muscular heat.

Several tests are available for detecting some drug idiosyncrasies. Red cell susceptibility to destruction by drugs can be determined by taking a small blood sample and checking the reaction of erythrocytes when a potent hemolysis-producing chemical is added. Patients suspected of developing malignant hyperthermia can have their serum level of the enzyme creatinine phosphokinase assessed. The nursing history is an important tool to determine which patients, based on their family history, may be prone to this reaction. Any time the patient presents with an unusual or peculiar reaction, the suspected drug is always withheld until the physician has the opportunity to assess and evaluate the patient.

DELAYED TOXICITY

Most toxic effects occur at a predictable, usually short, time after administration. However, there are some reactions that occur several days to several years after exposure. For example, aplastic anemia caused by chloramphenicol (Chloromycetin) may appear weeks after the drug is discontinued, and hepatotoxicity after large doses of acetaminophen (Tylenol) is usually not apparent for 24–48 hours. Prolonged toxic effects, such as bronchogenic tumors, may occur many years after exposure to asbestos. Today it is speculated that women exposed to Agent Orange in Vietnam have an increased number of abortions and children born with birth defects, while men exposed to Agent Orange have an increased number of malignancies. Delayed toxicity may also occur in the offspring, such as the increased incidence of cancer of the cervix in teenage daughters born to women who received diethylstilbestrol (DES) to reduce the symptoms of morning sickness during pregnancy.

Delayed toxicities obviously cannot be assessed and/or evaluated in a short period of time. Consequently, there is an urgent need for reliable, predictive, short-term tests for such toxicities.

DRUG-INDUCED TISSUE AND ORGAN TOXICITIES

Drugs are capable of affecting tissues, structures, and organs within the body either directly or indirectly. Table 6–4 reviews the possible effects of drugs on tissues and organs. The organs most frequently affected include the skin, hematologic system, eye, kidney, liver, ear, lung,

and sexual organs. Teratogenesis (formation of birth defects) can also occur with various drugs administered during pregnancy (see Chapter 15).

DERMATOLOGIC REACTIONS

The skin is the organ most commonly affected by allergic drug reactions. The majority of "drug rashes" consist of macules (flat red spots) or papules (raised red spots), which are highly pruritic. People who are prone to, or who already have, skin problems are more prone to skin reactions. Drug reactions can also be life-threatening and long-lasting. Exfoliative dermatitis and erythema multiforme exudativum (Stevens-Johnson syndrome) are two very severe skin reactions that can occur secondarily to administration of sulfonamides and certain other drugs (see Chapter 63).

BLOOD DYSCRASIAS

Drugs are capable of affecting formed elements of the blood erythrocytes, leukocytes, and thrombocytes, resulting in hemolytic or aplastic anemia, leukopenia, and thrombocytopenia. All of these conditions are very serious and could result in death if not diagnosed early. Additional information on these conditions can be found in Chapter 32. Any complaints of generalized weakness, fatigue, infection, or easy bruising should be reported to the physician and the medication profile reviewed for potential drug-induced effects.

Hemolytic anemia can result secondarily to a type II allergic reaction. A Coombs' test of the blood can detect the presence of the abnormal immunoglobulins both in the serum and attached to the red cell. Aplastic anemia is a very serious disorder that is fatal in over half of patients despite treatment efforts. Drugs known to cause aplastic anemia include chloramphenicol, phenylbutazone, trimethadione, and certain sulfonamides. Since most patients taking these drugs do not develop aplastic anemia, this reaction is thought to be idiosyncratic. Patients need to have frequent blood counts performed to monitor for these anemias; if blood counts drop, the offending drug is discontinued.

Leukopenia, a reduction of all white cells, can occur in a more specialized form, referred to as agranulocytosis, in which only the granulocytes are affected. The white cells, the primary defense mechanism for the body, are greatly reduced. When this condition is diagnosed, the offending drug is discontinued immediately.

Thrombocytopenia, a reduction in platelets, develops occasionally. Drugs known to cause thrombocytopenia are quinidine, meprobamate (Equanil), chlorothiazide (Diuril), and some anti-infectives. Most patients recover quickly when the offending drug is discontinued.

OCULAR TOXICITY

The eye, because of its delicate structure, is particularly subject to both direct and indirect injury by drugs. Patients may complain of blurring when taking anticholinergic products and disturbances of color vision when taking digitalis products. These symptoms are gener-

Table 6-4. ORGAN/SYSTEM TOXICITIES

System or Organ	Damage	Comments
Skin	Urticaria, rashes, lesions, photo-sensitivity, alopecia	Most are minor and subside soon after drug is stopped. Careful assessment is necessary in persons having other skin lesions.
Hematologic	Blood dyscrasias; anemia (aplastic, hemolytic); thrombocytopenia; pancytopenia	Most serious of all complications. All can lead to serious illness and death.
Eye	Blurred vision to blindness	Persons taking drugs known to cause eye damage should have a thorough initial ocular examination and subsequent examinations thereafter.
Kidney	Acute/chronic renal failure, acute/chronic nephrotic syndrome, renal colic, hematuria, tubular defects, obstructive nephropathy	Patient with underlying renal disease needs thorough initial examinations. Any decreased renal function necessitates discontinuing suspected drug. Mechanisms of drug-induced renal disease are not fully understood.
Hepatic	Cholesatic, cytotoxic, mixed injuries, hepatitis	Reaction of the liver often results in hepatitis with increased enzyme levels, jaundice, and pruritus. Death rarely occurs.
Ear	Ringing in the ear (tinnitus) to total irreversible deafness	Persons taking drugs known to cause ear damage should have a thorough initial hearing examination and subsequent examinations thereafter.
Lung	Asthma, interstitial pulmonary fibrosis, pulmonary eosinophilia (infiltrates)	Uncommon complication. Exact mechanism unknown. If patient develops a respiratory condition of unknown etiology, drugs should be considered as the cause.
Sexual organs	Decreased libido to impotence	Mechanisms that cause dysfunction are poorly understood but probably involve the autonomic nervous system. These problems are probably far more common than currently reported.

ally mild and are reversible when the drugs are discontinued.

More serious complaints include changes in the cornea, lens, retina, and optic nerve. Before patients start on medications known to cause these changes, a complete eye examination should be performed and then repeated periodically thereafter during therapy. If the patient begins to note changes in vision, the drug is discontinued immediately to prevent further damage (see Chapter 60).

NEPHROTOXICITY

The kidneys are subjected to injury from drugs or chemicals that are excreted through the kidney or that are carried by blood and flow through the kidney. The kidney is at risk because it has the highest blood supply per gram of any tissue in the body. This allows circulating agents to be delivered at 50 times the "usual" rate to tissues. The kidney also has the highest oxygen consumption and glucose production per gram. *Interstitial nephritis* or toxic nephropathy can occur secondarily to various antibiotics, including the aminoglycoside class, polymyxin B, and colistin; analgesics such as salicylates; nonsteroidal anti-inflammatory drugs; anti-cancer drugs; heavy metals; and immune complex inducers such as penicillamine, captopril, or gold salts. Patients should have baseline blood urea nitrogen and creatinine levels drawn prior to therapy and then periodically during therapy. The offending drug is discontinued when these levels begin to rise. Nephrotoxicity secondary to medications is discussed more fully in Chapter 39.

LIVER INJURY

Because of the liver's anatomic location and function, it is the first organ to receive medication once it is absorbed from the intestine. This makes the liver prone to both parenchyma (the mass of functioning liver cells) and bile channel injury. Any patient with depressed liver function may be more prone to liver injury, and liver necrosis can ensue. Liver function studies are obtained prior to starting the patient on drugs known to cause liver injury and then are performed periodically during therapy (see Chapter 55).

OTOTOXICITY

Ototoxicity can result as a primary or secondary effect of medication. Toxic medications affecting the ear may affect both branches of the eighth cranial nerve—vestibular and auditory—resulting in dizziness, balance difficulties, and hearing loss. Ototoxicity often occurs in conjunction with nephrotoxicity because the medications that are not being excreted by the kidney accumulate in other tissues (see Chapter 61).

SEXUAL DYSFUNCTION

Both male and female sexual function may be affected by medication. Toxic effects may range from a decreased sexual interest to impotence (see Chapter 43).

MUTAGENIC EFFECTS

Several drugs (androgenic hormones, antineoplastic agents, caffeine, chlorpromazine, colchicine, estrogenic hormones, ether, and griseofulvin) are capable of changing the genetic composition of humans and are considered mutagenic. The largest genetic unit that can be involved in a mutation is a chromosome, while the smallest unit is a base pair present in the DNA molecule.

Today, we know that certain chemicals and drugs are capable of inducing carcinogenesis and are called carcinogens. These products (environmental pollutants) are becoming a national health problem. Chemically induced carcinogenesis usually requires long exposure periods to carcinogens.

POISONING BY DRUGS OR CHEMICALS

Poisons are described as chemical substances capable of causing harm to living substances even in small amounts. Actually, even safe therapeutic products are capable of becoming poisons if taken in large enough quantities.

Table 6–5 reviews the signs and symptoms of commonly overdosed drugs and toxic substances, and overdose management, including specific drugs used as antidotes. Typically, drugs such as aspirin and acet-

aminophen (Tylenol) are safe products. However, when taken accidentally or deliberately in large doses, death can result. Sedatives, hypnotics, and tranquilizers are all safe drugs when administered in therapeutic doses. However, these drugs can become toxic when combined with large amounts of ethanol (alcohol) or illegal drugs (cocaine, heroin, etc.). Only about 37% of poisoning is the result of a single agent. In about 25% of cases, ethanol is one of the agents named. Ethanol is the most common agent implicated in adult poisoning.

Children, left unattended, often consume drugs prescribed for parents or grandparents. Most adult medications are toxic to small children. Also toxic if consumed are household chemicals, such as cleaners and bleaches, or products found in the basement or garage, such as turpentine, petroleum distillates, gasoline, organophosphates (pesticides), and rat poisons. The signs, symptoms, and overdose management of these products can be found in Table 6–5.

Overdoses and poisonings are a common medical emergency. Poisoning is the fifth most common cause of accidental death in the United States. Recent epidemiologic data indicate that there are approximately five million cases annually with over 13,000 deaths, 1000 of them in children under five years of age. This number has been decreasing over several years. Very likely this is due to the combined effort of the American Academy of Pediatrics to prevent poisoning and the American Association of Poison Control Centers located around the country.

The toxic activity of a poison depends on a number of variables. These variables can be compared to those that affect the activity of therapeutic substances. Two variables are very important: the amount of toxic substance and its metabolic route. Generally, the more substance absorbed, the more toxic the effect. Also, poisons that are injected into the blood stream or inhaled have a more rapid onset of action. Poisons may have effects on almost all organs and tissues in the body: central nervous system, renal or hepatic systems, gastrointestinal system, and hematologic system.

USING THE NURSING PROCESS

ASSESSMENT

The diagnosis of poisoning is often difficult. Patients may arrive in the emergency department in mental states that range from alert to unconscious with seizures. The unconscious state is often difficult to differentiate from various disease states.

With an alert patient, a history is obtained as soon as possible, with therapy instituted as necessary. The history should contain

- Date and time of overdose
- Reasons for overdose
- Circumstances surrounding overdose
- Drug history

Table 6–5. COMMONLY OVERDOSED DRUGS AND TOXIC AGENTS

Agent	Signs and Symptoms	Management	Specific Drugs for Management
Acetaminophen	Anorexia, nausea, vomiting, delayed onset of symptoms of jaundice, hypoglycemia, encephalopathy, and hepatic failure.	Prevent further absorption of drug. Assess liver function for 3–5 days.	N-acetylcysteine (Mucomyst)
Alcohol	Depressed sensorium, odor on breath, hypoglycemia, dehydration, visual disturbances, slowed respiration, flushing, fast pulse, ataxia; hallucinations, tremors, and convulsions (withdrawal effects).	Assess neurologic and metabolic systems; support cardiovascular and neurologic systems. Monitor liver function.	Glucose solution IV for dehydration; diazepam (Valium) for withdrawal symptoms.
Amphetamines	Toxic (paranoid) psychosis, hyperthermia, flushing, increased blood pressure, dilated pupils, auditory and visual hallucinations, seizures, tachycardia, needle marks in intravenous users, tachypnea.	Prevent further reabsorption. Supportive treatment. Protect from further injury. Acidification of urine to increase elimination of drug.	Diazepam (Valium)
Anticholinergics (atropine, scopolamine)	Tachycardia, decreased secretions, urinary retention, dilated pupils, hallucinations, confusion, dry skin, fever, flushing.	Assess cardiac activity.	Physostigmine
Antifreeze	Metabolic acidosis, hypocalcemia, renal failure.	Prevent further reabsorption. Monitor blood alcohol and glucose levels. Include glucose in ethanol infusion.	Ethanol
Arsenic	Garlicky breath, vomiting, profuse diarrhea, abdominal colic, jaundice.	Monitor blood pressure, respiratory status. Arsenic excreted by kidneys with BAL.	Dimercaprol (BAL)
Barbiturates	Tense vesicular skin lesions, coma, nystagmus, drowsiness, ataxia, slurred speech.	Prevent further absorption. Supportive care; ventilate with oxygen if necessary. Dialyze if necessary.	Sodium bicarbonate to alkalinize the urine.
Carbon monoxide	Red skin, coal-gas odor, bullae, cyanosis.	Monitor oxyhemoglobin.	Oxygen via hyperbaric chamber.
Cocaine	Perforated nasal septum, dilated pupils, psychosis, delusions, hyperthermia, tachycardia.	See amphetamines.	See amphetamines.
Cyanide	Bitter-almond odor to breath, convulsion, coma, abnormal ECG.	Prevent further reabsorption. Administer oxygen, monitor oxygen level, ventilate if necessary.	Sodium nitrate, amyl nitrite, sodium thiosulfate.

CONTINUED ON THE FOLLOWING PAGE

Table 6–5. COMMONLY OVERDOSED DRUGS AND TOXIC AGENTS–*CONTINUED*

Agent	Signs and Symptoms	Management	Specific Drugs for Management
Diazepam (Valium)	Euphoria (sometimes), ataxia, nystagmus, progressive CNS depression.	See barbiturates.	See barbiturates.
Digitalis products	Visual disturbances, delirium, abnormal ECG, nausea, vomiting, slowed pulse.	Prevent further reabsorption. Monitor cardiac activity; treat dysrhythmias.	Potassium, phenytoin (Dilantin)
Ethchlorvynol (Placidyl)	Deep coma, pungent aromatic odor, lowered pulse and blood pressure, pink gastric aspirate.	See barbiturates.	See barbiturates.
Gasoline	Distinctive odor, choking, pulmonary infiltrates, feeling of lightness, transitory visual hallucinations.	Do not induce vomiting. Use gastric lavage to remove gasoline.	Calcium disodium edetate (EDTA) if gasoline is leaded.
Glutethimide (Doriden)	Dilated pupils, coma, prolonged respiratory depression, laryngeal spasms.	See barbiturates.	See barbiturates.
Heroin	Coma, decreased blood pressure, respiration, and pulse; miosis, needle marks.	Assess respiratory and cardiovascular systems; support as necessary.	Naloxone (Narcan)
Hydrocarbons (cleaning fluids)	Pulmonary edema, lipid pneumonia, tinnitus, convulsions, diplopia, ventricular fibrillation.	Prevent further reabsorption. Emesis or cathartics. Supportive care. Assess liver function.	Cathartics
Iron	Diarrhea, coma, bloody vomiting, radiopacity on radiograph, hypotension.	Prevent further absorption. Urine turns red as iron is being excreted. Treatment discontinued when urine returns to normal.	Desferoxamine (Desferal)
Isopropyl alcohol	Severe gastritis, acetonemia with normoglycemia, acetone odor on breath, emesis.	See alcohol.	See alcohol.
Lead	Severe abdominal pain, increased blood pressure, milky vomitus, convulsions, muscle weakness, metallic taste, anorexia, encephalopathy, ataxia, paralysis, constipation.	See arsenic.	Dimercaprol (BAL), penicillamine, calcium disodium edetate (EDTA).
LSD	Hallucinations, dilated pupils, mild tachycardia, bleeding disorder, confusion, agitation, sweating.	See amphetamines.	See amphetamines.

Table 6–5. COMMONLY OVERDOSED DRUGS AND TOXIC AGENTS–*CONTINUED*

Agent	Signs and Symptoms	Management	Specific Drugs for Management
Mercury	Stomatitis, gingivitis, colitis, nephrotic syndrome.	Monitor renal function. Prevent further reabsorption.	Penicillamine (Cuprimine)
Methadone (Dolophine)	Miosis; coma; lowered pulse, blood pressure, and respiration; transient response to narcotic antagonist naloxone.	See narcotics.	See narcotics.
Mushrooms	Nausea, vomiting, hallucinations, delayed liver failure and renal failure.	Prevent further absorption, emesis, lavage, supportive care; assess renal and hepatic systems.	Supportive therapy.
Organophosphates	Miotic pupils, cramps, bronchorrhea, salivation, lacrimation, urination, defecation, sweating, skeletal muscle weakness, and paralysis.	Prevent further reabsorption. Monitor respiratory rate; ventilate if necessary.	Atropine sulfate, pralidoxime (Protopam)
Phencyclidine (PCP)	Muscle twitching, prolonged psychosis, mild increase in blood pressure and pulse, nystagmus, altered state of consciousness.	See amphetamines; reduce sensory stimulation.	See amphetamines.
Phenothiazines	Postural hypotension, hypothermia, miosis, tremor, dystonic disorder, radiopacity on radiograph of abdomen, increased Q–T interval on ECG.	Prevent further reabsorption. Monitor vital signs; expand volume if necessary to maintain blood pressure.	Diphenhydramine (Benadryl), adsorbents (activated charcoal, kaolin, pectin).
Salicylates	Hyperventilation, vomiting, fever, bleeding, acidosis, purpura.	Prevent reabsorption by emesis or lavage. Dialysis or alkalinization of urine.	Adsorbents, sodium bicarbonate.
Strychnine	Stiff neck, status epilepticus, cyanosis, opisthotonos.	Prevent further reabsorption; supportive care. Avoid aural, visual, or tactile stimulation.	Supportive therapy.
Tricyclic antidepressants	Paralytic ileus, supraventricular dysrhythmias, convulsions, response to physostigmine, radiopacity on radiograph.	Prevent further reabsorption. Monitor cardiac activity. Antiarrhythmics may be necessary.	Physostigmine, diazepam (Valium), adsorbents.

- Drug abuse history
- Disease history
- Manifestations of overdose and prior treatment

If a friend or relative accompanies an unconscious patient, a history is obtained, including the potential of poisoning and the possible product and all information discussed above. Laboratory toxicology screening is performed from samples of blood, urine, and gastrointestinal contents to determine the causative agent. Quantitative determinations are needed for relatively few substances: acetaminophen, salicylates, Valium, barbi-

Table 6–6. ANTIDOTES

Antidote	Trade Name	Indication	Dosage	Comments
Amyl nitrite inhaler, sodium nitrite IV, sodium thiosulfate	Cyanide Antidote Kit	Cyanide poisoning	Inhale amyl nitrite for 30 seconds of each minute until sodium nitrite is administered. Children over 25 kg: Give entire ampule (300 mg) or sodium nitrite IV; follow immediately with 12.5 g sodium thiosulfate. Children under 25 kg: Adjust the doses according to hemoglobin: Hemoglobin / Initial Dose 3% Sodium nitrite (ml/kg) 8 g — 0.22 10 g — 0.27 12 g — 0.33 14 g — 0.39 Hemoglobin / Initial Dose 25% Sodium thiosulfate (ml/kg) 8 g — 1.10 10 g — 1.35 12 g — 1.65 14 g — 1.95	Follow manufacturer instructions in the kit.
Atropine		Organophosphates and carbamates poisoning	Initial dose. Children: 0.05 mg/kg IV, not to exceed 2 mg/dose	Drug should be given until excessive pulmonary secretions are effectively controlled.
Calcium disodium edetate (EDTA)	Calcium Disodium Versenate	Lead poisoning. May be used alone or in conjunction with dimercaprol; may be useful for other types of heavy metal poisoning	Children: 50–75 mg/kg/day IM in 2–3 divided doses; maximum = 500 mg/kg for each 5-day course of therapy	Usual course is 5 days; allow 2 days off and repeat course, if necessary.
Deferoxamine	Desferal	Iron poisoning	90 mg/kg IM or IV (up to 2 g q 8 hr); maximum = 6 g/day	IV use is indicated when the patient is hypotensive and blood flow to IM injection sites is poor; IV rate should not be greater than 15 mg/kg/hr.
Dimercaprol	BAL in Oil	Arsenic, gold, and mercury poisoning. For severe lead poisoning in conjunction with calcium disodium EDTA	Dosage varies according to indication; generally, 4 mg/kg IM q 4 hr	
Methylene blue		Methemoglobinemia	0.2 ml/kg IV injected over 5 min	

Table 6–6. ANTIDOTES–*CONTINUED*

Antidote	Trade Name	Indication	Dosage	Comments
N-acetyl-cysteine	Mucomyst	Acetaminophen poisoning	140 mg/kg loading dose PO followed by 70 mg/kg q 4 hr for 17 doses.	See discussion in body of chapter for specific indications.
Naloxone	Narcan	Narcotic overdose or poisoning	Children: 10 μg/kg IV bolus; repeat prn; following the bolus, an IV infusion of 0.4–0.8 mg/hr can be administered	Effect may be short-lived; repeated doses usually are necessary; patients should be monitored closely.
Penicillamine	Cuprimine	Copper, lead, mercury, and arsenic poisoning	Children: 20–40 mg/kg/day PO (maximum = 1.5 g/day)	
Physostig-mine	Antilirium	Anticholinergic poisoning Indications for physostigmine use: ● Seizures ● Severe hypertension ● Supraventricular tachy-dysrhythmias ● Severe hallucinations and delirium	Children: 0.5 mg IV slowly; repeat until a maximum dose of 2 mg is administered; repeat prn	Should be administered until desired effect is achieved or excess cholinergic symptoms develop.
Pralidoxime	Protopam	Organophosphate poisoning	Children: 25–50 mg/kg IM or IV; repeat q 8–12 hr prn (maximum 1 g/dose)	Should be used in conjunction with atropine. Of little benefit more than 36 hours after the exposure.

From Pagliaro and Pagliaro: Problems in Pediatric Drug Therapy, ed. 2. Drug Intelligence Publications, Inc., Hamilton, IL, pp. 291–295, 1987, with permission.

turates, PCP, cocaine, iron, lead, methyl alcohol, theophylline, lithium, and digitalis glycosides. For some of these, two plasma samples are obtained one or more hours apart, depending on the half-life of the drug involved, to determine if the concentration of the toxic substance is rising or falling and thus to determine what therapy is needed.

During the initial assessment, a thorough physical examination is performed to obtain the following information:

● Vital signs
● Level of consciousness
● Behavioral characteristics
● Motor signs
● Autonomic signs (diaphoresis, *bronchorrhea*, bronchospasm, urinary retention, and so on)
● Ancillary finding (pupil size, presence or absence of nystagmus, gag reflex, and status of oculocephalgyric reflex)

INTERVENTION

The primary goals of intervention are as follows:

1. Remove the toxic substance from the body, for example, wash chemicals from skin or remove from gastrointestinal system (if possible).
2. Administer antidote (if available).
3. Apply supportive measures to maintain all vital functions.

Therapy may include inducing emesis (with antiemetics discussed in detail in Chapter 53) or administration of *antidotes* (Tables 6–6 and 6–7). Figure 6–6 features an example of a chart used to treat acetaminophen toxicity. Acetaminophen is discussed in more detail in Chapter 20.

Supportive measures may include cardiopulmonary resuscitation, ventilators, control of fluid balance, chelation, diuresis, cathartics, and other supportive drugs to control blood pressure or seizures. Volume depletion

Table 6–7. PREPARATION OF MUCOMYST (N-ACETYLCYSTEINE) FOR ADMINISTRATION AS AN ANTIDOTE

Loading Dose			
BODY WEIGHT (kg)	**20% MUCOMYST (ml)**	**DILUENT (ml)**	**5% SOLUTION (TOTAL ml)**
100–110	75	225	300
90–99	70	210	280
80–89	65	195	260
70–79	55	165	220
60–69	50	150	200
50–59	45	120	160
40–49	35	105	140
30–39	30	90	120

Maintenance Dose			
BODY WEIGHT (kg)	**20% MUCOMYST (ml)**	**DILUENT (ml)**	**5% SOLUTION (TOTAL ml)**
100–110	38	113	150
90–99	35	105	140
80–89	33	98	130
70–79	28	83	110
60–69	25	75	100
50–59	20	60	80
40–49	18	53	70
30–39	15	45	60

From Gates, T: Management of Acetaminophen Overdose with N-acetylcysteine. McNeil Consumer Products Company, Fort Washington, PA, 1980, with permission.

secondary to vomiting, diarrhea, and sweating must be corrected promptly with normal saline or Ringer's solution, particularly in the young child or geriatric client. Hypotension severe enough to require correction frequently necessitates monitoring of central venous or pulmonary artery pressures to determine fluid needs.

The elimination of some drugs may be increased by altering the pH of the urine. Acid drug (aspirin, phenobarbital) excretion is promoted by alkalinizing the urine (sodium bicarbonate), whereas basic drug (amphetamines, phencyclidine) excretion is promoted by acidifying the urine (ammonium chloride).

There is a small group of severely poisoned patients, however, who may benefit from the use of artificial organs to enhance elimination of toxins from the blood. Hemodialysis, hemoperfusion, and plasmapheresis are considered state-of-the-art in invasive detoxification.

Hemodialysis exposes blood to a semipermeable membrane to remove low-molecular-weight toxins; hemoperfusion percolates blood through absorbent columns to extract lipid- or protein-bound substances. Drugs removed through dialysis are featured in Table 6–8, and drugs removed through hemoperfusion are featured in Table 6–9. Plasmapheresis is a modified phlebotomy procedure in which the cellular components of the blood are returned to the patient. The plasma and plasma proteins are replaced with fresh plasma or a suitable colloid. The use of this latest procedure in the treatment of severely intoxicated patients is growing rapidly in popularity, particularly for those strongly protein-bound toxins that are not well dialyzed or adsorbed. The ideal drug for removal by plasma exchange is one that is highly protein-bound, has a small volume of

distribution, and has a prolonged half-life. Table 6–10 features drugs that are removed through plasmapheresis.

Families need a great deal of psychological support during this period of crisis. Nurses are often in a position to teach how to avoid poisonings and the immediate steps to take if poisoning should occur. Poison control center numbers (there are over 600 in the United States) are available in most telephone books around the country. All hospital emergency rooms also have a listing of the closest centers. The Centers for Disease Control (CDC) in Atlanta, Georgia, is also a source for hard-to-find data and rare antidotes.

PREVENTION OF POISONING

Nurses are in a unique position to teach poisoning prevention, particularly school nurses and nurses who work in public health. Nurses can teach parents about storage of drugs and chemicals around the house. All chemicals should be kept in their original, labeled containers with the child-proof cap locked. Chemicals should be stored whenever possible in high, tightly shut or locked cabinets. When the container is empty, it should be discarded. Household or garden chemicals should never be mixed together. When parents are administering medications to children, they should not refer to the medications as candy.

Before taking a drug or using chemicals, always read the directions carefully. Improper use may result in ac-

TEXT RESUMES ON PAGE 126

Nomogram: Plasma or Serum Acetaminophen Concentration vs Time Post Acetaminophen Ingestion*

Estimating potential for hepatotoxicity:
The following nomogram has been developed to estimate the probability that plasma levels in relation to intervals post ingestion will result in hepatotoxicity.

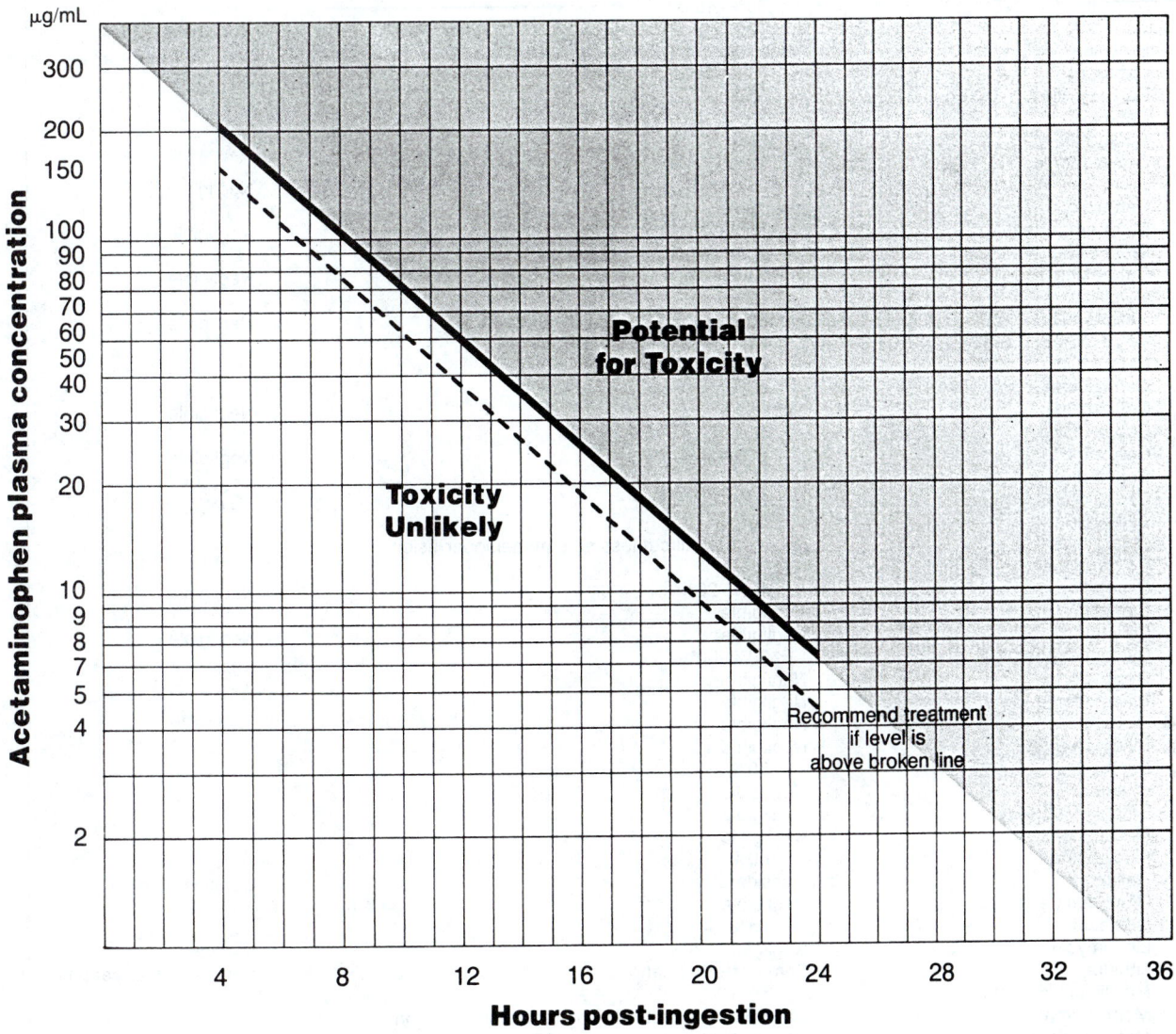

*Adapted from Rumack and Matthew, *Pediatrics* 55:871–876, 1975.

Cautions For Use of This Chart:

1. The time coordinates refer to time post ingestion.
2. The graph relates only to plasma levels following a single acute overdose ingestion.
3. The broken line, which represents a 25% allowance below the solid line, is included to allow for possible errors in acetaminophen plasma assays and estimated time from ingestion of an overdose.

For additional emergency information, call your regional poison center or the Rocky Mountain Poison Center toll-free, 1-800-525-6115.

Figure 6–6. Acetaminophen overdose nomogram. Plasma or serum acetaminophen concentration versus time after acetaminophen ingestion. The lower line defines acetaminophen plasma or serum values that are 25% below those that may be expected to cause hepatic toxicity. This line is used as a guide to treatment to allow for possible errors in assay values or errors in estimating the time that has elapsed since ingestion of the acetaminophen oversode. (Courtesy of McNeil Consumer Products Company, Fort Washington, PA.)

Table 6–8. DRUGS REMOVED WITH DIALYSIS

Drug	Hemodialysis	CAPD
Acebutolol	Negligible	
Acyclovir	60%	
Allopurinol	40%	
Amantadine	Negligible	
Aminoglycosides	50%	Negligible
Amoxicillin	30%	
Amphotericin B	Negligible	
Ampicillin	40%	
Atenolol	50%	
Azlocillin	30%–45%	
Aztreonam	40%	Negligible
Bretylium	Negligible	
Captopril	35%–40%	
Carbenicillin	50%	
Cefaclor	33%	
Cefadroxil	50%	
Cefamandole	50%	
Cefazolin	33%–50%	Negligible
Cefonicid	Negligible	
Cefoperazone	Negligible	Negligible
Ceforanide	20%	
Cefotaxime	60%	Negligible
Cefotetan	50%	
Cefoxitin	50%	Negligible
Cefroxadine	50%	
Cefsulodin	60%	
Ceftazidime	50%	
Ceftizoxime	Negligible	Negligible
Cephacetrile	50%	
Cephalexin	50%–75%	Negligible
Cephaloridine	50%	
Cephalothin	50%	
Cephapirin	20%	
Chloral hydrate	May be helpful but less so than hemoperfusion	
Chloroquine	Negligible	
Cimetidine	10%–20%	Negligible
Clonidine	Negligible	
Colistin	Negligible	Negligible
Cyclophosphamide	30%–60%	
Cyclosporine	Negligible	
Diazoxide	Negligible	
Digoxin	Negligible	
Disopyramide	Negligible	
Dyphylline	30%	
Ethambutol	Negligible	
Ethchlorvynol	Negligible	
Flecainide	Negligible	
Flucytosine	50%	
Gallamine	Considerable	Considerable
Glutethimide	Negligible	
Isoniazid	75%	
Lincomycin	Negligible	Negligible
Lithium	Same as other cations	Same as other cations
Mecillinam	50%	
Meprobamate	Can be helpful but less so than hemoperfusion	
Methaqualone	Negligible	
Methicillin	Negligible	
Methotrexate	Negligible	
Metoprolol	Negligible	
Mezlocillin	20%–25%	Negligible
Miconazole	Negligible	
Minoxidil	25%–40%	
Moxalactam	30%–50%	Negligible
N-acetylprocainamide	50%	Negligible
Nadol	50%	
Oxaprozin	Negligible	
Oxazepam	Negligible	
Para-aminosalicylic acid	75%	
Penicillin	50%	
Pethidine	Negligible	Negligible
Phenytoin	Negligible	
Piperacillin	50%	

CONTINUED ON THE FOLLOWING PAGE

Table 6–8. DRUGS REMOVED WITH DIALYSIS–*CONTINUED*

Drug	Hemodialysis	CAPD
Prednisone	Negligible	
Primidone	30%	
Procainamide	Negligible	Negligible
Propoxyphene	Negligible	Negligible
Quinine	Negligible	
Ranitidine	50%–60%	
Salicylates	Considerable at high concentrations	
Sotalol	40%	
Spectinomycin	50%	
Sulfamethoxazole	50%	Negligible
Theophylline	40%	
Ticarcillin	50%	Negligible
Tocainide	25%	
Trimethoprim	50%	Negligible
Valproic acid	Negligible	Negligible
Vancomycin	Negligible	Negligible
Warfarin	Negligible	

From Brater, DC: Handbook of Drug Use in Patients with Renal Disease, ed. 2. Dallas, 1986, with permission.

Table 6–9. DRUGS FOR WHICH RESIN HEMOPERFUSION HAS BEEN DEMONSTRATED TO REMOVE CLINICALLY IMPORTANT AMOUNTS

Barbiturates	Meprobamate
Carbamazepine	Methaqualone
Chloral hydrate (trichloroethanol)*	N-desmethylmethsuximide
Chloramphenicol	Paracetamol
Chloroquine	Phenylbutazone
Digitalis glycosides	Quinidine
Disopyramide	Salicylate
Ethchlorvynol	Theophylline
Glutethimide	Tricyclic antidepressants

*Trichloroethanol is the active metabolite; the parent, chloral hydrate, is very short-lived.
From Brater, DC: Handbook of Drug Use in Patients with Renal Disease, ed. 2. Dallas, 1986, with permission.

Table 6–10. DRUGS HIGHLY BOUND TO PLASMAPROTEINS AND REMOVED THROUGH PLASMAPHERESIS

Antimicrobials
Doxycycline
Clindamycin
Nalidixic acid
Cloxacillin
Dicloxacillin
Sulfisoxasole

Diuretics
Acetazolamide
Furosemide
Spironolactone
Bumetanide
Chlorthalidone
Metolazone

Cardiovascular Agents, Tranquilizers, Antidepressants
Large volume of distribution prevents cleaning of tissues

Anticoagulants
Warfarin
Dicumarol

Anticonvulsants
Phenytoin
Valproic acid

Hypoglycemics
Tolbutamide
Glyburide
Glibornuride
Glipizide

Anti-inflammatories
Phenylbutazone
Indomethacin
Piroxicam
Sulindac
Tolmetin
Fenoprofen
Ibuprofen
Naproxen
Mefenamid acid

Psychotropics
Tetrahydrocannabinol

Miscellaneous
Diphenhydramine
Clofibrate
Amanita (mushroom)

From Jones, JS: Current status of plasmapheresis in toxicology. Ann Emerg Med 15:474–482, 1986, with permission.

cidental poisoning. Always take or use the chemical in a well-lighted area. Taking drugs in a dimly lit room will increase the chance of error.

Teach patients to take all of their prescription medications. If for any reason medications are left over, they should be destroyed, for example, by flushing them down the toilet. Tossing a bottle of pills in the garbage or even opening the bottle and tossing loose pills in the garbage increases the likelihood of accidental poisoning. Also, patients are taught to always discard old medications. Do not save any for "a next time."

Individuals also need to know what is proper first aid after a drug overdose or poisoning. The patient with the empty container of pills or chemicals is transported to the nearest emergency room. If transportation has to be delayed, the nearest hospital should be called to determine immediate first aid. First aid may be either to induce vomiting or to give milk, depending on the substance consumed.

In summary, care of the poisoning patient includes diagnosing the toxic substance and any other underlying condition that patient may have (e.g., heat, trauma, diabetic ketosis), reducing absorption, improving elimination, and supporting the patient against the physical alterations of the poison.

SUMMARY

Toxicology is that aspect of pharmacology that deals with the adverse effects of drugs on living organisms. Undesirable effects of drugs, or adverse reactions, generally fall into two classes: (1) effects that are predicted and (2) effects that are not related to the drug's pharmacologic effect. Drug allergies, hypersensitivity reactions, and idiosyncratic reactions fall into this category. Drugs are also capable of affecting tissues, structures and organs within the body either directly or indirectly. The organs most frequently affected include the skin, hematologic system, eye, kidney, liver, ear, lung, and sexual organs.

Poisoning by drugs or chemicals can also occur. Even safe, therapeutic products are capable of becoming poisons if taken in large enough quantities.

When poisoning is expected, a thorough physical assessment and history is obtained. The primary goals during intervention are to remove the toxic substance from the body, administer an antidote (if available), and administer supportive measures to maintain all vital function.

BIBLIOGRAPHY

Anderson, M, et al: Collecting a reliable urine specimen for drug analysis. J Nurs Adm 17:25, 32, January 1987.

Ballenger, MJ: Poisoning. Emergency 17:21–49, September 1985.

Brenner, B and Rector, F: The Kidney. WB Saunders, Philadelphia, 1986.

Collins, RD: Atlas of Drug Reactions. Churchill Livingstone, New York, 1985.

Dukes, MN and Beelly, L: Side Effects of Drugs Annual, Vol 10. Elsevier, Amsterdam, 1986.

Farch, GA: Adverse drug reaction monitoring. N Engl J Med 014(24):1589–1592, June 12, 1986.

For particulars on poisons—most complete list yet of manufacturers. Emergency Medicine 17(14):142, 1985.

George, JE, et al: Drug screening in the emergency department. J Emerg Nurs 13:304–305, September–October 1987.

Gilman, AG, Goodman, LS, and Gilman, A (eds): Goodman and Gilman's The Pharmacological Basis of Therapeutics, ed. 7. Macmillan, New York, 1985.

Goldin, JM: Allergies, allergic reactions, and anaphylaxis. Emergency 18(7):18–20, 1986.

Goldstein, J: Ocular side effects of systemic drugs: A physical assessment guide for ophthalmic medical assistant. J Ophth Nurs Technol 5(3):103–106, May–June, 1986.

Gosselin, R, et al: Clinical Toxicology of Commercial Products. Williams & Wilkins, Baltimore, 1984.

Hospitalizations from adverse drug reactions. Nurses Drug Alert 11(2):15–16, February 1987.

Jones, JS: Current status of plasmapheresis in toxicology. Ann Emerg Med 15(4):474–482, 1986.

Kunkel, DB: The ills of heat: Drug and fever. Emergency Medicine 18(15):126, 1986.

Kunkel, DB: Know Your Poison Control Center . . . The Toxic Emergency. Emergency Medicine 18(17):125, October 1986.

Mackowiak, PA: Drug fever: Mechanisms, maxims and misconceptions. Am J Med Sci 294(4):275–286, 1987.

Maronde, R: Topics in Clinical Pharmacology and Therapeutics. New York, Springer-Verlag, 1986.

Miwa, LJ, et al: Adverse drug reaction program using pharm and nurse monitors. Hosp Formul 21:1140, November 1986.

Newton, M, et al: General treatment of poisoning of household products and medications. J Emerg Nurs 13:16–26, January–February 1987.

Sargent, RK: Poisoning and overdoses. Emerg Care Q 2(2):1–11, 1986.

Seldin, D and Giebisch, G: The Kidney. Raven Press, New York, 1985.

Thurkauf, GE: Acetaminophen overdose. Crit Care Nurse 7:20–29, January–February 1987.

Trombitas, ID, et al: Monitoring the world's published literature for adverse drug experiences. Drug Inf J 20(1):57–62, 1986.

Vore, M, et al: Common adverse drug interactions. Hosp Med 22(10):94, October 1986.

SITUATION   6–1

Helen Andrews is the charge nurse on nights in the emergency room at a large metropolitan hospital. She frequently encounters patients with problems related to drug toxicity.

1. A seven-year-old, Liza Steiner, has a fever (temperature 38.6C, 101.5F), rash, and enlarged lymph nodes. Helen questions Liza's mother about medications which her daughter has been taking. The mother responds, "All Liza has had is a diphtheria-tetanus shot last week." Helen is aware that this reaction represents a:
   a. type I—anaphylactic
   b. type II—serum sickness
   c. type III—auto-immune
   d. type IV—cell-mediated

2. Mike Benson arrives in the emergency room in acute respiratory distress. He also has an extensive rash and heart palpitation. A nursing assessment reveals that he recently began taking penicillin for bronchitis. Helen prepares to administer all of the following *except:*
   a. vasopressors
   b. antihistamines
   c. bronchodilators
   d. antibiotics

3. Jason Mills, a 70-year-old, complains of itching and a rash related to a topical cream containing benzene. The *first* appropriate action for Helen would be to:
   a. prepare to administer an antihistamine
   b. neutralize the benzene by applying sodium bicarbonate
   c. wash the product off of the skin
   d. prepare to administer epinephrine

4. Harry Evans, a 66-year-old with a history of a recent myocardial infarction, comes to the emergency room because of sudden symptoms related to systemic lupus erythematosus. During the assessment, Helen discovers that Mr. Evans began taking Pronestyl a week earlier. Helen is aware that this may represent the following type of reaction:
   a. idiosyncratic
   b. cell-mediated
   c. anaphylactic
   d. delayed toxicity

5. Edna Carson has been feeling very tired and presents to the emergency room after noticing a bloody stool. Lab results reveal a low platelet count and hematocrit. Helen investigates the medications that Mrs. Carson takes. Of the following list of drugs, which would most likely be related to Mrs. Carson's symptoms?
   a. digoxin
   b. quinidine
   c. theophylline
   d. captopril

6. Mr. Graham arrives in a comatose state via an ambulance from a nearby mental hospital. The patient has a history of attempted suicide by drug overdose. Helen will implement the following intervention *first:*
   a. obtain blood samples for a drug screen
   b. assess neurological function
   c. elevate the legs to increase circulation
   d. take a set of vital signs

Please refer to the Appendices for correct answers and additional review questions with answers.

GLOSSARY TERMS IN THIS CHAPTER
Antihistamine
Antipyretic
Antitussive
Expectorant
Health care provider
Neutralizing capacity
Nonpharmacologic interventions
Over-the-Counter (OTC) medications
Pharyngitis
Rhinitis
Rhinorrhea
Self-care
Self-limiting

7

CHAPTER

OVER-THE-COUNTER MEDICATIONS

FRANCES L. STIER, MSN, RNc

LEARNING OBJECTIVES

After reading this chapter, the student will be able to:

1. Recognize the role of self-treatment in providing health care.

2. Identify indications and contraindications in using over-the-counter medications.

3. Educate patients about specific uses of analgesics/ antipyretics, antacids, laxatives, and cold, cough, and allergy medications.

4. Use the nursing process when managing patient problems with over-the-counter medications.

Self-care and self-medication are major components in health care management. Nearly 60% of the health care problems treated each year are managed by the patient with *over-the-counter (OTC) medications* and other self-care measures (Covington, 1986). If this health care practice was abandoned and patients sought medical intervention for minor ailments such as colds, allergies, muscle aches, and headaches, the health care delivery system would quickly collapse. Nurses who practice in ambulatory care settings, community and public health clinics, health maintenance organizations, physicians' offices, and urgent care facilities frequently offer health care advice for minor illnesses. Knowledge of OTC drugs and self-care measures is therefore important to ensure quality health care.

OTC, nonlegend, and nonprescription are all adjectives describing drugs that an individual may purchase without a prescription. By definition, the Food and Drug Administration (FDA) has found them to be safe for use without medical supervision.

OTC drugs became a legal classification in 1951 through the passage of the Durham-Humphrey Amendment to the federal Food, Drug and Cosmetic Act, which required that each drug be classified as legend or nonlegend. Legend drugs must bear the statement, "Caution: Federal Law Prohibits Dispensing Without a Prescription," and are therefore not available for general purchase by the public. In 1962, the Kefauver-Harris Drug Amendments further required a pharmaceutical manufacturer to prove, prior to marketing, that a drug is effective for its intended indications. Before 1962, prior proof of safety was all that was necessary. This was required only for the prescription drugs; the nonprescription drugs (OTCs) had no such requirement.

In 1972, the FDA implemented a massive review of all OTC drug products to ensure that only those drugs that could be proven effective as well as safe are available for purchase. This review, which still is in progress, assesses the product ingredients for safety and effectiveness and evaluates the advertising claims and labeling. The process used in evaluating over 300,000 nonprescription products identifies the active ingredients broken down by therapeutic category and then evaluates only these ingredients. By reviewing the product labels, the FDA identified only 700 active ingredients. This finding suggests that many products may contain the same ingredients.

Although the FDA review process is not complete, changes in OTC medications have occurred. Ingredients determined to be unsafe have been removed from the market (e.g., phenacetin). Some prescription ingredients have been evaluated as safe for self-medication and changed to a nonprescription status (e.g., diphenhydramine and ibuprofen).

OTC products and drugs manufactured and marketed for self-medication are divided into groups based on the symptoms they are intended to treat. This chapter briefly reviews four of the most used and abused categories: (1) cold, cough, and allergy preparations; (2) internal analgesics; (3) antacids; and (4) laxatives. Some self-care management issues pertinent to these drugs

and the nursing process of self-medication are discussed.

THERAPEUTIC AGENTS

COLD, COUGH, AND ALLERGY PREPARATIONS

Cold Preparations

The most common illness for which an individual requests health care advice and treatment is the common cold. Symptoms associated with a cold are often temporarily disabling. The distressed individual seeks relief through home remedies, OTC cold medications, and health care consultation. Although there is no cure for the common cold, there are interventions to alleviate the discomfort.

The common cold is caused by any one of a group of viruses. Rhinoviruses and coronaviruses are the most common viral agents. The virus enters the upper respiratory tract and invades the epithelial lining of the nose, sinuses, throat, and bronchi. An inflammatory immune response occurs with subsequent degranulation of the mast cell. Histamine, released from the mast cell, is the primary substance responsible for producing "cold" symptoms: *rhinorrhea*, nasal congestion, sneezing, cough, and *pharyngitis*. Headache may occur due to impaired sinus drainage. Onset of the symptoms is abrupt, usually occurring 1–2 days after viral exposure. Prodromal symptoms, cough, scratchy throat, and body aches may occur.

Although the symptoms are self-limiting, lasting approximately 7–10 days, palliative treatment may be used. Health care management includes both pharmacologic and *nonpharmacologic interventions* (Table 7–1). Most effective drug therapy is symptom-specific. The pharmacologic interventions used most often in relieving cold symptoms include analgesics and antipyretics, antihistamines, decongestants, cough suppressants, and expectorants.

ANALGESICS AND ANTIPYRETICS. Analgesics and *antipyretics* are used to manage the symptoms of headache, malaise, fever, and sore throat often associated with a cold. Aspirin or acetaminophen is usually effective. Because it is difficult to differentiate cold from influenza symptoms, children younger than 16 years of age should receive only acetaminophen. Aspirin given during influenza is associated with the development of Reye's syndrome.

A salicylate or acetaminophen is the most common analgesic contained in OTC cold preparations. Unfortunately, the dosages of the individual drugs contained in multiagent products may be either subtherapeutic or contain the maximum strength. Managing symptoms with multiagent products is less specific than managing with single-agent medications. For example, more analgesia may be needed in the early stages of a cold than in the later stages. With combination products, the analgesic amount cannot be reduced.

Table 7–1. SELF-CARE PRACTICES FOR COMMON COLD SYMPTOMS

Symptoms	OTC Medication	Nondrug Measures
Runny nose, no nasal congestion; watery, itchy eyes	Antihistamine: chlorpheniramine, bromopheniramine	Increase rest. Fatigue diminishes the body's immune response, thus facilitating viral invasion.
Nasal congestion	Decongestant: pseudoephedrine, oral oxymetazoline	Increase hydration. Fluids help liquefy secretions by decreasing the viscosity of the mucus. Increase fluid intake to 2000 to 3000 ml per day
Nonproductive cough	Cough suppressant: dextromethorphan, diphenhydramine	Room humidification. Humidifying the inspired air relieves cough, pharyngitis, and laryngitis. Cool mist or steam vaporizers can be used. Cool mist is more effective but requires frequent disinfecting.
Productive cough without fever	Cough suppressant contraindicated	Saline gargle (½ t salt in 8 oz warm or cool water). Relieves sore throat by wetting and soothing the irritated lining.
Sore throat without fever	Unmedicated lozenges	Smoking cessation. Avoid environmental irritants, which aggravate throat symptoms.
Headache and myalgia	Analgesic: aspirin, acetaminophen if under 16 years of age, ibuprofen	Contact health care provider if fever above 101°F, sore throat with fever, productive cough, yellow or green sputum, ear pain, headache and facial tenderness, difficulty breathing, cold symptoms persist longer than 1 week.

ANTIHISTAMINES. *Antihistamines* are indicated during the initial stage of the cold when the symptoms are due to hypersecretion of the mucosal glands. Thus, rhinorrhea and rhinitis, as well as watery, itchy eyes may be alleviated. Antihistamines decrease histamine activity by blocking the receptor sites for histamine activation. Although histamine continues to be released, its effects are diminished. The anticholinergic effects of antihistamines are effective in drying secretions. There are three major chemical classes of antihistamines: alkylamines, ethanolamines, and ethylenediamines (Table 7–2). The therapeutic efficacy of all the antihistamines is the same, but the severity of side effects, duration of action, and cost differ.

Pharmacokinetics. Antihistamines begin action within 15–30 minutes, with full effect occurring within 1–2 hours. Although antihistamines may be taken every 4–6 hours, less frequent doses may be used. Antihistamines are eliminated slowly from the body, the serum half-life being approximately 30–36 hours. Time-released preparations theoretically spread out the dosage, thus decreasing the dosing interval. Unfortunately, the quantities released may be too small to be effective. Antihistamines are available in tablet, capsule, and elixir forms. There is a paucity of single-agent antihistamine products on the market. Both chlorpheniramine and brompheniramine are available as single agents. Table 7–2 contains information on some common antihistamines, related pharmacology, and nursing implications.

Adverse Effects. The most common adverse effect of antihistamines is sedation; it becomes less prominent with repeated doses. To minimize the effect of sedation on mental and physical performance, bedtime adminis-

tration is recommended. Concurrent use of other central nervous system (CNS) depressants and alcohol potentiates the sedative effect. The patient is advised to defer tasks requiring mental alertness until the effect of the antihistamine is assessed. A paradoxical excitation (insomnia, nervousness, irritability, or hyperactivity) is often observed in children. In the elderly, antihistamines may cause dizziness, sedation, confusion, and hypotension.

Adverse anticholinergic effects of antihistamines may include excessive dry mouth, tachycardia, urinary retention, constipation, and blurred vision. Patients with a history of asthma, cardiovascular disease, hypertension, hyperthyroidism, narrow-angle glaucoma, or prostate hypertrophy should use antihistamines only with physician consultation.

If the antihistamine produces untoward effects or becomes ineffective in controlling the patient's symptoms, switching to another antihistamine in the same or different chemical class may alleviate the problem. The alkylamines cause the least sedation and subsequently are the most preferred class of antihistamines. The ethylenediamines are intermediate in their effects, and the ethanolamines produce the most sedation. A prescriptive antihistamine, terfenadine (Seldane), forms a separate chemical class that does not cross the blood–brain barrier. Consequently, sedation is minimal with this agent.

DECONGESTANTS. Nasal congestion is caused by dilated blood vessels and fluid accumulation in the nasal mucosa. Nasal decongestants are classified as sympa-

TEXT RESUMES ON PAGE 146

Table 7–2. SOME COMMON OTC ANTIHISTAMINES, DECONGESTANTS, AND ANTITUSSIVES

Name	Dosage	Mode of Administration	Pharmacokinetics
ANTIHISTAMINES			

Action: Block histamine effect at the receptor site.

Use: Suppress symptoms associated with the release of histamine due to allergy.

Name	Dosage	Mode of Administration	Pharmacokinetics
Alkylamines			
Brompheniramine maleate (Dimetane, Dimetane Exten-tabs)	Adult: 4 mg q 4–6 hr prn (24 mg max/24 hr); extended-release, 8–12 mg q 8–12 hr prn Children 6 < 12 yr: 2 mg q 4–6 hr prn (12 mg max/24 hr); extended-release, 8–12 mg q 12 hr prn Children 2 < 6 yr: 1 mg q 4–6 hr prn (6 mg max/24 hr); extended-release, not recommended Children < 2 yr: consult physician	PO elixir, tablets	O:15–60 min P:3–9 hr D:4–25 hr ½ L:12–35 hr PB: UA B:liver E:renal

Key to Abbreviations in the *Pharmacokinetics* column: O-onset; P-peak; D-duration; PB-protein bound; B-biotransformed in; E-excreted in; ½L-halflife.

*Within the column listing adverse effects, underlines indicate the most common effects; CAPITALS indicate life-threatening effects.

Contraindications and Precautions	Adverse Reactions*	Interactions	Nursing Implications
FOR ALL ANTIHISTA-MINES: Contraindicated in narrow-angle glaucoma, urinary retention disorders, prostatic hypertrophy, stenosing peptic ulcer and pyloroduodendal obstruction due to anticholinergic activity. In addition, patients with asthma or COPD should use only with physician supervision because antihistamines can increase and thicken bronchial secretions. Not recommended for premature or newborn infants and contraindicated in third trimester of pregnancy. Some antihistamines have been associated with fetal malformation; therefore use is often contraindicated for entire pregnancy. Small amounts are excreted in breast milk; use not recommended in nursing mothers.	FOR ALL ANTIHISTA-MINES: Neuro: Sedation (more pronounced with ethanolamine derivatives, less with alkylamines); dizziness and confusion, especially in elderly; hyperexcitability in children. EENT: Blurred vision, diplopia, tinnitus, dry mouth, nose, throat. CV: Hypotension occasionally. RESP: Thickening of bronchial secretions. GI: Nausea, vomiting, diarrhea or constipation, anorexia. Renal: Urinary retention. Patients over age 60 are more susceptible to adverse reactions. Reduced dosing may be indicated.	FOR ALL ANTIHISTA-MINES: Drug: Concurrent use with CNS depressants or alcohol potentiates sedative effect. MAO inhibitors may prolong or potentiate the anticholinergic (drying) and CNS effects of antihistamines. Lab: Antihistamines may inhibit cutaneous histamine response in skin tests using allergen extracts producing false-negative results. Discontinue antihistamines at least 72 hours before testing.	FOR ALL ANTIHISTAMINES: ASSESSMENT: Assess patient's history for possible contraindications for antihistamine use. Obtain medication history to determine possible drug interactions. Ascertain previous effectiveness of antihistamines and adverse reactions. INTERVENTION: Recommend antihistamine use for relief of allergic rhinitis, or symptoms associated with initial stage of the common cold. Inform patient of proper administration and dose. To minimize adverse reactions have patient take a smaller initial dose and use at bedtime. Also encourage adjunctive therapy for symptoms: hydration and humidification. PATIENT TEACHING: Patient must avoid other CNS depressants while taking antihistamines, especially alcohol. Because of possible drowsiness, patient should avoid tasks requiring mental alertness: do not drive or operate heavy machinery. Drowsiness or sedation is dose-related and becomes less prominent with repeated doses. Patient should discontinue drug and notify health care provider if visual changes, weakness, fatigue, palpitations, irritability, nightmares, confusion, or urinary retention occur. EVALUATION: Antihistamines are effective in alleviating the symptoms of allergic rhinitis or common cold. If no improvement is seen, another antihistamine in the same or different chemical class can be tried. If symptoms persist beyond 5–7 days, patient should obtain health care advice.

CONTINUED ON THE FOLLOWING PAGE

Table 7–2. SOME COMMON OTC ANTIHISTAMINES, DECONGESTANTS, AND ANTITUSSIVES–CONTINUED

Name	Dosage	Mode of Administration	Pharmacokinetics
Chlorpheniramine maleate (Chlor-Trimeton, Aller-Chlor)	Adult: 4 mg q 4–6 hr prn (24 mg max/24 hr); extended-release, adult: 8 or 12 mg q 8–12 hr prn Children 6 < 12 yr: 2 mg q 4–6 hr prn (12 mg max/24 hr); extended-release, not recommended Children 2 < 6 yr: 1 mg q 4–6 hr prn (6 mg max/24 hr)	PO tablets, capsules, syrup	O:30–60 min P:2–6 hr D:4–25 hr ½ L:12–15 hr PB:72% B:liver E:renal
Triprolidine hydrochloride (Actidil)	Adult: 2.5 mg q 6–8 hr prn (10 mg max/24 hr) Children 6 < 12 yr: 1.25 mg q 6–8 hr prn (5 mg max/24 hr) Children under 6 yr: use only under direction of a physician Ages 4–6 yr: 0.9 mg q 6–8 hr prn (3.75 mg max/24 hr) Ages 2–4 yr: 0.6 mg q 6–8 hr prn (2.5 mg max/24 hr) Ages 4 months–2 yr: 0.3 mg q 6–8 hr prn (1.25 mg max/24 hr)	PO tablets, syrup	O:15–60 min P:2–3 hr D:4–25 hr ½ L:3–3.3 hr PB: UA B:liver E:renal
Ethylenediamines Tripelennamine citrate, tripelennamine HC (PBZ)	Adult: 25–50 mg q 4–6 hr prn (600 mg max/24 hr); extended-release, 100 mg q 8–12 hr prn Children: 1.25 mg/kg body weight, q 6 hr prn (300 mg max/24 hr); extended-release, not recommended	PO elixir, tablets	O:15–60 min P: 2–3 hr D:4–6 hr ½ L: UA PB: UA B:liver E:renal
Pyrilamine† maleate (Aller-stat)	Adult: 25–50 mg q 6–8 hr prn (200 mg max/24 hr) Children 6 < 12 yr: 12.5 mg–25 mg q 6–8 hr prn (100 mg max/24 hr) Children 2 < 6 yr: not recommended †Combination products only	PO tablets, capsules	O:15–60 min P: 3–6 hr D:8 hr ½ L: UA PB: UA B:liver E:renal
Ethanolamines Diphenhydramine (Benadryl)	Adult: 25–50 mg q 4–6 hr prn (300 mg max/24 hr) Children 6 < 12 yr: 12.5 mg–25 mg q 4–6 hr prn (150 mg max/24 hr)	PO capsules, elixir, syrup	O:15–60 min P:1–4 hr D:6–8 hr

Key to Abbreviations in the *Pharmacokinetics* column: O-onset; P-peak; D-duration; PB-protein bound; B-bio-transformed in; E-excreted in; ½L-halflife.
*Within the column listing adverse effects, <u>underlines</u> indicate the most common effects; CAPITALS indicate life-threatening effects.

OTC Medications

Contraindications and Precautions	Adverse Reactions*	Interactions	Nursing Implications

CONTINUED ON THE FOLLOWING PAGE

Table 7–2. SOME COMMON OTC ANTIHISTAMINES, DECONGESTANTS, AND ANTITUSSIVES–CONTINUED

Name	Dosage	Mode of Administration	Pharmacokinetics
Diphenhydramine (Benadryl)– *Continued*	Children under 6 yr: use only under direction of a physician		½ L:2.4–9.3 hr PB:80%–85%% B:liver E:renal
Carbinoxamine maleate (Clistin)	Adult: 4–8 mg q 6–8 hr prn Children over 6 yr: 4–6 mg q 6–8 hr prn Children 3–6 yr: 2–4 mg q 6–8 hr prn Children 1–3 yr: 2 mg q 6–8 hr prn	PO tablets	O:15–60 min P: 3–6 hr D:6–8 hr ½ L:10–20 hr PB: UA B:liver E:renal
Clemastine fumarate (Tavist)	Adult: 1.34 mg and 2.68 mg clemastine fumarate containing 1 mg and 2 mg clemastine, respectively, twice daily (8.04 mg max/24 hr) Children under 12 yr: safety and efficacy has not been established	PO tablets	O:15–60 min P:5–7 hr D:10–12 hr ½ L: UA PB: UA B:liver E:renal

NASAL DECONGESTANTS

Action: Stimulates the α-receptors of the adrenergic nervous system producing vasoconstriction within the nasal mucosa.

Use: Reduce nasal congestion caused by acute or chronic rhinitis.

Name	Dosage	Mode of Administration	Pharmacokinetics
Topical Ephedrine (Va-tro-nol Nose Drops)	0.5% Drops Adult: 2–3 gtt, each nostril, q 4 hr prn Children 6 < 12 yr: 1–2 gtt, each nostril, q 4 hr prn Children under 6 yr: not recommended Do not use longer than 4 consecutive days	Intranasal drops	O:1–2 min P:1 hr D:3 hr ½ L:NA PB:NA B:liver E:renal

Key to Abbreviations in the *Pharmacokinetics* column: O-onset; P-peak; D-duration; PB-protein bound; B-biotransformed in; E-excreted in; ½L-halflife.
*Within the column listing adverse effects, underlines indicate the most common effects; CAPITALS indicate life-threatening effects.

Contraindications and Precautions	Adverse Reactions*	Interactions	Nursing Implications
FOR ALL DECONGESTANTS: Contraindicated in narrow-angle glaucoma, and previous reactions manifested by sleeplessness, dizziness, lightheadedness, weakness, tremors, or cardiac arrhythmias. Patients with heart disease, high blood pressure, diabetes, or thyroid disease should use	FOR ALL DECONGESTANTS: In general, topical decongestants have less systemic reactions but are potentially addictive. Infants, children, and the elderly are more prone to systemic effects. Neuro: nervousness, headache. EENT: Rebound	FOR ALL DECONGESTANTS: Drug: Tricyclic antidepressants and MAO inhibitors can increase the sympathomimetic activity of decongestants. Concurrent use with β-adrenergic blockers may decrease the effects of both drugs. Arrhythmias may occur when digitalis	FOR ALL DECONGESTANTS: ASSESSMENT: Assess patient's history for possible contraindications for decongestant use. Obtain medication history to determine possible drug interactions. Ascertain previous effectiveness of decongestants and adverse reactions. INTERVENTION: Recommend topical decongestant

CONTINUED ON THE FOLLOWING PAGE

Table 7–2. SOME COMMON OTC ANTIHISTAMINES, DECONGESTANTS, AND ANTITUSSIVES–CONTINUED

Name	Dosage	Mode of Administration	Pharmacokinetics
Ephedrine (Va-tro-nol Nose Drops)–*Continued*			

Key to Abbreviations in the *Pharmacokinetics* column: O-onset; P-peak; D-duration; PB-protein bound; B-bio-transformed in; E-excreted in; ½L-halflife.
*Within the column listing adverse effects, underlines indicate the most common effects; CAPITALS indicate life-threatening effects.

Contraindications and Precautions	Adverse Reactions*	Interactions	Nursing Implications
only with medical supervision. For children use only decongestants designated for children. Not recommended during pregnancy or while breast-feeding.	congestion (rhinitis medicamentosa) may occur with overuse of topical decongestants. Increased intraocular pressure. **CV:** tachycardia, palpitations, irregular heart rhythm, tightness in chest, increased blood pressure. **GI:** Appetite loss, nausea, and vomiting. **Renal:** dysuria, urinary retention.	preparations and decongestants are used. Decongestants decrease effect of most antihypertensive drugs. Concurrent use with cocaine may cause dangerous cardiac stimulation. **Lab:** no known interactions.	for short-term therapy (less than 3 consecutive days) for nasal congestion due to allergy. Oral decongestants are indicated for long-term treatment, such as treatment for common cold symptoms. Inform patient of proper administration and dose. To minimize systemic absorption when administering topical decongestants apply nasal spray with the patient in an upright position, squeezing medicine into each nostril. Nasal drops are administered with head tilted back over the edge of a bed or chair. Instill the number of recommended drops into each nostril, breathe through open mouth. Keep head tilted for 3–5 minutes. Self-care measures, hydration, and humidification are also recommended. PATIENT TEACHING: Patients should understand symptoms which may be relieved with self-medication of a decongestant. Topical decongestants are used only for short-term treatment; these drugs can be habit-forming. To avoid bacterial contamination, nasal droppers and spray tips should be rinsed in hot water after use. The patient should select an oral decongestant for long-term treatment of cold symptoms. Caffeine use with decongestants may cause nervousness, tremors, or insomnia. Patient should limit caffeine intake. Patients should discontinue drug and notify health care provider if headache, nausea, vomiting, heart irregularity, extreme nervousness or restlessness, confusion, delirium, or muscle tremors occur. Decongestants should not be used longer than 5–7 days unless medical supervision is obtained. Rebound congestion may occur with prolonged or frequent use of topical decongestants.

CONTINUED ON THE FOLLOWING PAGE

Table 7–2. SOME COMMON OTC ANTIHISTAMINES, DECONGESTANTS, AND ANTITUSSIVES–CONTINUED

Name	Dosage	Mode of Administration	Pharmacokinetics
Ephedrine (Va-tro-nol Nose Drops)–*Continued*			
Oxymetazoline HCl (Afrin)	0.5% Drops or spray Adult: 2–3 gtt/spray each nostril, morning and bed-time or q 8–12 hr Children 6 < 12 yr: same as adult Children 2 < 6 yr: 2–3 gtt/ spray of 0.25% solution each nostril, morning and bedtime, q 8–10 hr	Intranasal drops or spray	O:1–2 min P:5–10 min D:up to 12 hr ½ L:NA PB:NA B:UA E:UA
Phenylephrine HCl (Neo-Synephrine)	Adult: 0.5%, 2–3 gtt/spray, q 4 hr Children 6 < 12 yr: 0.25%, 2–3 gtt/spray, q 4 hr Children 2 < 6 yr: 0.125% drops only, 2–3 gtt, q 4 hr	Intranasal drops/spray	O:1–2 min P:5–10 min D:30 min–4 hr, ½ L:UA PB:UA B:liver E:renal
Xylometazoline HCl (Neo-Synephrine II Long-Acting)	Adult: 0.1%, 2–3 gtt/spray, q 8–10 hr Children 6 < 12 yr: 0.05%, 2–3 gtt/spray, q 8–12 hr Children 2 < 6 yr: same for < 12 yr	Intranasal drops/spray	O:1–2 min P: 5–10 min D:6–12 hr ½ L:UA PB:UA B:UA E:UA
Oral Pseudoephedrine HCl (Sudafed)	Tablet Adult: 60 mg q 4–6 hr (240 mg max/24 hr)	PO tablets, capsules, liquid	O:15–30 min P:30–60 min

Key to Abbreviations in the *Pharmacokinetics* column: O-onset; P-peak; D-duration; PB-protein bound; B-bio-transformed in; E-excreted in; ½L-halflife.

*Within the column listing adverse effects, underlines indicate the most common effects; CAPITALS indicate life-threatening effects.

Contraindications and Precautions	Adverse Reactions*	Interactions	Nursing Implications
			EVALUATION: With topical decongestants patient should experience a dramatic improvement within minutes. Oral decongestants are effective within 1 hour. If patient experiences systemic adverse reactions, review proper administration and dosage of decongestant. With continued adverse reactions treatment should be discontinued and health care provider consulted.

CONTINUED ON THE FOLLOWING PAGE

OTC Medications

Table 7–2. SOME COMMON OTC ANTIHISTAMINES, DECONGESTANTS, AND ANTITUSSIVES–CONTINUED

Name	Dosage	Mode of Administration	Pharmacokinetics
Pseudoephedrine HCl (Sudafed)–*Continued*	Children 6 < 12 yr: 30 mg q 4–6 hr (120 mg max/24 hr) Children < 6 yr: not recommended		D:4–6 hr (8–12 hr for SA form) ½ L:NA
(Sudafed-SA)	Extended-release Adult: 120 mg q 12 hr Children < 12 yr: not recommended		PB:NA B:liver E:renal
(Novafed)	Liquid Adult: 60 mg q 4–6 hr Children 6 < 12 yr: 30 mg q 4–6 hr Children 2 < 6 yr: 15 mg q 4–6 hr (60 mg max/24 hr)		
Phenylpropanolamine† HCl (Triaminic, Contac)	Adult: 25 mg q 4 hr; extended-release, 75 mg q 12 hr (150 mg max/24 hr) Children 6 < 12 yr: 12.5 mg q 4 hr (75 mg max/24 hr) Children 2 < 6 yr: 6.25 mg q 4 hr	PO tablets, capsules, liquid	O:15–30 min P:1–2 hr D:3 hr: 12–16 hr extended release ½ L:3–4 hr PB:UA B:liver E:renal

†Available only in combination products

ANTITUSSIVES

Action: Suppresses cough reflex center in the brain and diminishes the sensitivity of the cough receptors in the respiratory passages.

Use: Suppress a persistent dry, nonproductive cough.

Name	Dosage	Mode of Administration	Pharmacokinetics
Codeine, codeine phosphate, codeine sulfate	Adult: 10–20 mg q 4–6 hr (120 mg max/24 hr); extended-release, 20–30 mg q 12 hr Children 6 < 12 yr: 5–10 mg q 4–6 hr (60 mg max/24 hr); extended-release, 10 mg q 12 hr Children 2 < 12 yr: 2.5–5 mg q 4–6 hr (30 mg max/24 hr); extended-release suspension not recommended	PO tablets, syrup, elixir	O:<30 min P:1–2 hr D:4 hr ½ L:2.9 hr PB:UA B:liver E:renal

　　Key to Abbreviations in the *Pharmacokinetics* column: O-onset; P-peak; D-duration; PB-protein bound; B-biotransformed in; E-excreted in; ½L-halflife.
　　*Within the column listing adverse effects, underlines indicate the most common effects; CAPITALS indicate life-threatening effects.

Contraindications and Precautions	Adverse Reactions*	Interactions	Nursing Implications
Contraindicated in patients with chronic pulmonary disease in whom use may cause respiratory insufficiency, and in patients with previous reactions to codeine or other opiates. Tolerance and physical dependence may occur following prolonged use. Not recommended for use in pregnancy or in nursing mothers.	Neuro: drowsiness, lightheadedness. CV: palpitations. Resp: bronchospasm, drying of respiratory secretions, possible respiratory depression. GI: nausea, constipation with repeated doses. Integumentary: pruritus.	Drug: Potentiates the effect of MAO inhibitors, sedatives, tranquilizers, hypnotics, tricyclic antidepressants, other opiates, and alcohol. Lab: no known interaction.	ASSESSMENT: Assess patient's history for possible contraindications for codeine use. Assess indications for codeine: presence of an exhausting, nonproductive cough. Assess patient's potential for drug abuse: history of substance abuse. Obtain medication history to determine possible drug interactions. Ascertain previous effectiveness of antitussives/ codeine and adverse reactions.

CONTINUED ON THE FOLLOWING PAGE

Table 7–2. SOME COMMON OTC ANTIHISTAMINES, DECONGESTANTS, AND ANTITUSSIVES–CONTINUED

Name	Dosage	Mode of Administration	Pharmacokinetics
Codeine, codeine phosphate, codeine sulfate–*Continued*			
Dextromethorphan (Benylin DM, Romilar CF, Robitussin DM)	Adult: 10–20 mg q 4 hr or 30 mg q 6–8 hr (120 mg max/ 24 hr); extended-release, 60 mg twice daily Children 6 < 12 yrs: 5–10 mg q 4 hr or 15 mg q 6–8 hr (60 mg max/24 hr); extended-release, 30 mg twice daily Children 2 < 6 yr: 2.5–5 mg q 4 hr or 7.5 mg q 6–8 hr (30 mg max/24 hr); extended-release, 15 mg twice daily	PO lozenges, syrup, tablets, suspension	O:15–30 min P:NA D:3–6 hr; 8–12 hr (extended release) ½ L:UA B:liver E:renal

Key to Abbreviations in the *Pharmacokinetics* column: O-onset; P-peak; D-duration; PB-protein bound; B-biotransformed in; E-excreted in; ½L-halflife.

*Within the column listing adverse effects, underlines indicate the most common effects; CAPITALS indicate life-threatening effects.

Contraindications and Precautions	Adverse Reactions*	Interactions	Nursing Implications
Use with caution in sedated or debilitated patients and in patients who have undergone thoracotomy or laparotomy.			INTERVENTION: To minimize adverse reactions and be most effective in alleviating a disruptive cough, codeine should be given at night/bedtime. Other self-care measures should be encouraged: hydration to enhance the movement of mucus, lozenges, and humidification. To prevent constipation encourage fluids, increase dietary fiber, and moderate exercise. If constipation occurs codeine is discontinued. PATIENT TEACHING: Antitussive therapy is short-term and is discontinued when the cough is diminished. Avoid alcohol and other CNS depressants that potentiate the sedative effect of antitussives. Driving or operating machinery is not recommended since drowsiness may occur. To achieve maximal soothing effect, no liquids or food are to be taken for ½ hour following ingestion of antitussives. Discontinue the drug and notify health care provider if difficulty breathing, sedation, or rash develops. EVALUATION: With proper use the cough should be alleviated without adverse reactions. If cough persists or reoccurs the patient should obtain health care consultation; the cough may be associated with a serious underlying condition.
Use with caution in patients with liver or lung disease. Not established as safe for use in pregnancy.	Rare or mild adverse reactions. Neuro: Drowsiness. GI: nausea, vomiting, diarrhea.	Drug-Drug: May potentiate the effects of MAOI.	Same as for codeine. Generally regarded as the most reliable of the non-narcotic antitussives. Available in dozens of nonprescription and prescription preparations.

thomimetic amines or α-adrenergic agonists (see Chapter 35). They reverse nasal congestion by vasoconstricting the nasal mucosal blood vessels. Swollen membranes are reduced, sinus drainage is facilitated, and air conduction is improved.

Pharmacokinetics. Decongestants (Table 7–2) are available as topical or oral agents. Topical application by a nasal spray, inhaler, or drops provides immediate effect with relatively few systemic effects. The duration of the effect, however, is short and may subsequently lead to overuse. Frequent application of topical decongestants causes a cycle of intense mucosal vasoconstriction and irritation followed by vasodilation and "rebound congestion." With prolonged use, topical nasal decongestants can become habit-forming. Topical nasal decongestants should be limited to three days and used no more than four times a day. If topical agents cannot be avoided, a nasal spray with a long duration of action—one containing oxymetazoline (Afrin and others) or xylometazoline (Sine-off Nasal Spray, Vicks Sinex Long-Acting, and others)—is recommended.

Oral decongestants are slower acting, but the beneficial effect lasts longer than most topical decongestants. Administered orally, decongestants have a higher incidence of systemic side effects affecting the general vascular bed. All decongestants stimulate α-adrenergic receptors; some others (pseudoephedrine and ephedrine) also stimulate β-adrenergic receptors.

Pseudoephedrine (Besan, NeiFed, Sudafed, Sudrin, Symptom 2, and others); phenylephrine (Allerest, Coricidin, Neo-Synephrine, Ocusol, Prefrin, Sinarest, and others); and phenylpropanolamine (Contac, Phen-lets, and others) are the only agents proven safe and effective when taken orally. Phenylephrine is available only in combination drug products at doses often less than the recommended adult dose of 10 mg. Oral preparations of ephedrine have not been proven effective in relieving nasal congestion and, therefore, are not recommended for general use.

Adverse Effects. The degree of systemic adverse effects varies with individual agents and is attributed to stimulation of the sympathetic nervous system. Most commonly, patients experience a feeling of jitteriness or wakefulness. Increases in blood pressure or blood glucose and apparent changes in thyroid function may occur. These effects are significant in patients who have borderline hypertension, glucose intolerance, or hyperthyroidism. Cardiac dysrhythmias may also occur in predisposed individuals, especially with the use of phenylpropanolamine.

Patients who have hypertension, heart disease, diabetes, hyperthyroidism, or narrow-angle glaucoma should use decongestants only with physician approval and health care supervision (Table 7–2).

Cough Preparations

One of the most irritating symptoms associated with the common cold is cough. The cough is dry and nonproductive and is usually caused by postnasal drainage into the lower respiratory tract. Initially, antihistamines and decongestants may control the cough. In the later stages of the viral respiratory infection, bronchial congestion may occur, and the cough may facilitate the removal of bronchial secretions. A nonproductive cough, the most common cough, is functionally ineffective and often causes much discomfort for the patient. Often cough can be alleviated by increasing hydration and humidification. There are two drug categories for managing cough: cough suppressants and expectorants.

SUPPRESSANTS. Cough suppressants depress the cough reflex by inhibiting the cough center in the medulla. A cough is commonly associated with the later stages of viral respiratory infections and is often the means by which bronchial congestion is cleared. Since suppression may delay this clearing, *antitussives* are used only if a persistent cough causes pain or lack of sleep or if it is nonproductive. A direct bronchial irritation and nonviral infections and carcinomas may also manifest themselves as coughs. For this reason, self-treatment with an antitussive (as well as all other OTC products) should be limited to seven days so that a serious underlying cause is not overlooked.

The only OTC antitussives recognized as safe and effective are codeine, dextromethorphan, and diphenhydramine (Table 7–2). Codeine has been the mainstay of cough suppression and the standard used to judge other agents. Although other narcotics are effective, their addiction potential is much greater, and narcotic side effects are more likely to occur. Codeine's antitussive dose (15 mg) is less than its analgesic dose, but therapeutic doses may still cause drowsiness, nausea, constipation, and some risk for addiction. Whereas in some states it can be purchased in limited quantities without a prescription, other states restrict codeine to prescription status.

Dextromethorphan (Benylin, Romilar CF, Robitussin DM, Silence Is Golden, Symptom 1) is the most commonly found cough suppressant in nonprescription products. Although it is a narcotic derivative, it does not have analgesic properties or addiction potential. Recommended doses are well tolerated, with nausea, headache, and drowsiness occurring only rarely. Larger doses may cause respiratory depression. Diphenhydramine (Benadryl) is a safe and effective antitussive, in addition to the antihistamine effect it provides. Used in the same adult dose, 25–50 mg every four hours (see Table 7–2 under antihistamines), it is effective for treating nonproductive cough associated with the common cold. Adverse effects may occur such as sedation, and it should not be given to patients with chronic lung disease who have carbon dioxide retention.

EXPECTORANTS. *Expectorants* are drugs intended to decrease the viscosity of bronchial secretions, thus facilitating their removal from the lower respiratory tract. The "productive cough" associated with the later stages of respiratory infections is the target symptom. Although expectorants have been prescribed for many years, there is much controversy concerning their usefulness. There is no convincing evidence to prove the efficacy of any marketed agent. Expectorants commonly found in OTC cough remedies include iodides, ammonium chloride, terpin hydrate, and guaifenesin. When these expectorants are used in recommended dosages, few adverse reactions occur. The most common adverse reaction is gastric upset, including nausea and vomiting. Iodinated products may interfere with thyroid function. Terpin hydrate elixir has a high alcohol content and thus may be abused. In most situations, the best approach in alleviating a tenacious cough is hydration and humidification.

Sore Throat Preparations

Sore throat associated with a common cold may be alleviated with self-care measures and local anesthetics. However, before self-treatment it is important to distinguish between viral and bacterial sore throats. A sore throat due to a streptococcal infection may lead to serious complications such as valvular heart disease or glomerulonephritis if not treated with appropriate antibiotics. Some findings suggestive of streptococcal sore throat are acute onset, high fever, tonsillar exudate, and tender and enlarged anterior cervical lymph nodes. A throat culture is needed to definitely establish whether or not the sore throat is due to group A β-hemolytic streptococci.

If the sore throat is nonbacterial in origin and no fever is present, self-care may be instituted. Salt-water gargles (½ teaspoon salt in 8 ounces warm water), unmedicated hard candies to stimulate salivation, hydration, and room humidification are the most effective measures. Systemic analgesia with aspirin or acetaminophen is also beneficial in relieving the discomfort.

The OTC products available as sore throat remedies are classified as antibacterial or anesthetic agents and are contained in sprays, lozenges, mouthwashes, gargles, and throatwashes. The topical antibacterials in mouthwashes are phenols, iodine compounds, and quaternary ammonium compounds. None of the OTC antibacterials have been proven to be effective, and there are no clinical indications for their use. Treatment of bacterial infections of the mouth or throat require systemic medication.

Local anesthetics, such as benzocaine, can relieve sore throat pain by anesthetizing pain-sensing nerve fibers. However, concentrations of 5%–20% are necessary to achieve the effect, and most OTC products have less than 5%. An allergic reaction to local anesthetics may also occur. The safest treatment for sore throat is nonpharmacologic interventions and, if indicated, smoking cessation.

Allergic Rhinitis Preparations

Rhinorrhea, lacrimation, nasal and conjunctival pruritus, nasal congestion, and spasmodic sneezing are manifestations of allergic *rhinitis*. This condition is caused when an allergen, such as pollen, enters the nasal mucosa and combines with the immunoglobulin IgE, which in turn mediates the release of histamine from the mast cell. A patient history of allergy helps to distinguish allergic rhinitis from the common cold. The most common form of allergic rhinitis is seasonal rhinitis or hay fever, with exacerbation of symptoms occurring during the pollinating seasons. Chronic rhinitis is called perennial rhinitis and is usually caused by household allergens.

The treatment for allergic rhinitis includes both preventive self-care measures and drug therapy. Antihistamines are the primary agents used to alleviate the symptoms. Preventive or prophylactic administration is ideal. Nasal congestion is best relieved with a decongestant. Because of long-term need, oral decongestants are preferred over topical. For maximal palliation, the patient may require intranasal cromolyn or nasal or systemic corticosteroids. Allergy desensitization therapy may be needed in severe cases.

INTERNAL ANALGESICS/ ANTIPYRETICS

Aspirin and Acetaminophen

Aspirin and acetaminophen remain two of the most effective analgesics for the treatment of mild-to-moderate pain of somatic origin, such as that associated with headaches, musculoskeletal disorders, and post-traumatic conditions. They also share widespread use as antipyretics for reducing the fever that is common to viral and bacterial infections. Unlike acetaminophen, aspirin is also a potent anti-inflammatory drug, making it especially useful in rheumatoid arthritis and other conditions characterized by pain and inflammation.

Although both analgesics have been available for more than 80 years, if either were newly developed today, it would represent a significant therapeutic advance. Unfortunately, the public's widespread familiarity with these drugs has led to the underestimation of their usefulness. In fact, a recommendation of aspirin or acetaminophen for a specific problem is often viewed with skepticism by the patient. (The pharmacology of these drugs and nursing process is discussed in detail in Chapter 20, Drugs That Provide Pain Relief, and Chapter 47, Anti-Inflammatory Medications.)

Aspirin and acetaminophen are each available as single-ingredient products in a variety of dosage forms (Table 7–3) and also as constituents in various combination products (Table 7–4). Together, they leave no gap in the rational treatment of fever and mild-to-moderate pain. Although acetaminophen is preferred for children because it is available as a liquid, aspirin is more useful in inflammatory conditions. If gastrointestinal (GI) side effects from aspirin are a problem, acetaminophen or enteric-coated aspirin would be the drug of choice.

Aspirin-like analgesics such as salicylamide and sodium salicylate are also available. These drugs, unlike aspirin, do not inhibit platelet aggregation, and thus their use may be advantageous in certain clinical situations. Their analgesic and antipyretic actions are not as effective as aspirin. These drugs are found in many combination products.

Enteric-coated, extended-release, and buffered aspirin preparations have been formulated to decrease GI irritation or prolong or increase absorption. Enteric-coated tablets bypass the stomach, causing less mucosal dam-

Table 7–3. ASPIRIN, ACETAMINOPHEN, AND IBUPROFEN DOSAGE RECOMMENDATION AND OTC AVAILABILITY AS SINGLE-INGREDIENT PRODUCTS

Drug and Some Common Brands	Dosage Forms	Strengths	Dosage*
Acetaminophen (Datril, Liquiprin, Phenaphen, SK-APAP, Tempra, Tylenol; generics available)	Chewable tablet Tablet Caplets Capsule Rectal suppository Drops—with calibrated dropper Liquid	80 mg, 120 mg 235 mg, 500 mg, 650 mg 500 mg 325 mg, 500 mg 120 mg, 325 mg, 650 mg 60 mg/0.6 ml 120 mg/5 ml, 165 mg/ 5 ml, 325 mg/5 ml	Adults: 325–600 mg q 4 hr, or 1000 mg q 6 hr Children: 10–15 mg/kg q 4 hr
Aspirin (A.S.A., Bayer, Ecotrin; generics available)	Tablet Enteric-coated tablet Rectal suppository	65 mg, 75 mg, 81 mg, 160 mg, 325 mg, 500 mg, 650 mg 325 mg, 650 mg 65 mg, 130 mg, 325 mg, 650 mg	Adults: 325–600 mg q 4 hr, or 100 mg q 6 hr Children: 10–15 mg/kg q 4 hr
Ibuprofen (Advil, Nuprin)	Tablet	200 mg	Adult: 200 mg q 4–6 hr (1200 mg maximum/day) Children <12 yr: not recommended without medical supervision

*Analgesic and antipyretic dosage only. Although bioavailability data for rectal suppositories are scarce and absorption appears to be significantly less than by the oral route, dosage recommendations are the same for both routes. Rectal administration should be avoided if possible.

age, and dissolve in the more alkaline pH of the small intestine. Absorption is sometimes erratic from these products and delayed, thus limiting their use if immediate effects are desired. Buffered aspirin products contain an antacid to decrease irritation. However, mucosal damage may still occur. Extended-release formulations show no therapeutic advantage when compared to plain aspirin.

ADVERSE EFFECTS. Adverse effects of these drugs may occur even with normal use. Aspirin's most common adverse effect is GI discomfort, and symptoms such as nausea, indigestion, and heartburn are frequently described. A direct gastric mucosal irritation is responsible for this discomfort. With prolonged use, occult bleeding and iron deficiency anemia may develop. For these reasons, plain aspirin is always taken with a full glass of water or food. Plain aspirin and antacid may also be taken together. However, enteric-coated aspirin should not be taken concurrently with antacids because the antacid causes the enteric-coated aspirin to break

Table 7–4. COMBINATION PRODUCTS* CONTAINING ASPIRIN AND ACETAMINOPHEN

Product	Aspirin	Sodium Bicarbonate	Caffeine	Antacid	Acetaminophen	Citric Acid	Salicylamide
Alka-Seltzer	x	x	—	—	—	x	—
Anacin	x	—	x	—	—	—	—
Anacin Arthritis Pain Formula	x	—	—	x	—	—	—
Ascriptin	x	—	—	x	—	—	—
Bufferin	x	—	—	x	—	—	—
Cope	x	—	x	x	—	—	—
ASA Compound	x	—	x	—	—	—	—
Empirin Compound	x	—	x	—	—	—	—
Excedrin	x	—	x	—	x	—	x
Bromo-Seltzer	—	x	—	—	x	—	x

*These are only a few of the possible combination drugs available.

down in the stomach. With the chronic, high doses used in inflammatory conditions, tinnitus, dizziness, headache, and mental confusion are possible, but these effects subside when the dose is reduced. Hypersensitivity reactions, such as shortness of breath, troubled breathing, tightness in chest, or wheezing may occur but are rare except in patients with chronic asthma. Aspirin is very often the cause of pediatric poisoning, resulting in hyperventilation, mental confusion, hallucinations, and convulsions. Aspirin, when given to children recovering from the flu or chickenpox, has been associated with the rare but often fatal development of Reye's syndrome.

Acetaminophen does not cause gastric irritation or bleeding as does aspirin but can cause hepatic injury at high doses. Individuals who consume alcoholic beverages regularly or have a history of liver disease should not self-medicate with acetaminophen. The increased use of acetaminophen as a household analgesic has also resulted in a greater incidence of overdoses, which cause acute hepatic necrosis. If the patient survives, recovery from the overdose is slow, over a period of weeks or months.

Ibuprofen

Ibuprofen, a nonsteroidal anti-inflammatory analgesic (NSAIA), is also available for self-medication. The OTC dose is 200 mg every 4–6 hours with a maximum daily limit of 1200 mg. This dose is less than the prescription amount, which is 300–800 mg 3–4 times a day. This low-dose ibuprofen is effective as an analgesic but ineffective as an anti-inflammatory agent. In addition, concomitant use with aspirin may further decrease the total anti-inflammatory response. Ibuprofen is available as a single-agent product (Advil, Nuprin) and in combination with other ingredients (Midol 200). This medication, like aspirin, inhibits prostaglandin synthesis, which subsequently desensitizes pain receptors. (For a detailed discussion on NSAIA, see Chapter 47, Anti-Inflammatory Medications.)

Ibuprofen is indicated for pain, fever, and dysmenorrhea. Individuals who are hypersensitive to aspirin may also be hypersensitive to ibuprofen. GI irritation and bleeding occur, but less frequently than with aspirin. Ibuprofen-induced nephrotoxicity has been reported (Moss, et al., 1986). The OTC products of ibuprofen are usually more expensive than aspirin products and in most patient situations they offer no advantage over aspirin.

In choosing an analgesic/antipyretic agent for self-medication, the patient should be familiar with the contraindications, precautions, and drug interactions. In general, patients who have bleeding disorders or take anticoagulants, or those who have peptic ulcer disease, diabetes, or asthma, should not use aspirin or ibuprofen without physician approval. Unlike aspirin, ibuprofen does not decrease the uricosuric effect of antigout agents, and therefore may be used by patients with gout.

OTC combination products for analgesia often contain caffeine additives. The use of these products with other caffeine-containing products such as coffee, tea, and soft drinks may cause caffeine overdose. Patients taking prescription medications that are derived from caffeine, aminophylline, and theophylline may also develop adverse reactions. The symptoms of caffeine overdose are manifested by jitteriness, nervousness, heart palpitations, increased gastric acid, and insomnia.

For patients with these contraindications, acetaminophen may be the drug of choice. The disadvantage of acetaminophen is its lack of anti-inflammatory activity. Contraindications for use of acetaminophen is a history of hypersensitivity or hepatic disease. Table 7–3 contains information on OTC aspirin, acetaminophen, and ibuprofen.

ANTACIDS

Antacid therapy is used in the treatment of acute GI distress or peptic ulcer disease. Only acute gastritis associated with overeating, incompatible diet selection, excessive alcohol intake, or tension should be treated by self-medication. Patients with gastric distress of unknown etiology require health care consultation. Symptoms of gastric distress may be associated with more serious illness such as coronary artery disease, perforated ulcer, gastric carcinoma, or intestinal obstruction. In addition an adverse effect of many prescription drugs, for example, antibiotics, is often indigestion. Patients should obtain health care intervention and not self-treat if any of the following situations apply:

> Any episode of severe or persistent abdominal/GI discomfort, especially if associated with sweating, weakness, breathlessness, or pleuritic chest pain
> Any episode accompanied by hematemesis
> Repeated episodes (several times a month) of gastric distress or symptoms lasting longer than two weeks
> Signs of occult bleeding

Increased fatigue, lightheadedness, dizziness, or change in color of stool should also be reported immediately to the health care provider. Even with chronic use of antacids for ulcer disease, an exacerbation of GI symptoms necessitates medical consultation.

After evaluation of the patient's history and symptoms, antacid therapy may be recommended. Antacids are sold in dosage forms ranging from chewing gums and lozenges to tablets, powders, foams, and liquids. Despite the wide selection of products, there are only four active pharmacologic agents. These agents are sodium bicarbonate, and various salts of calcium, magnesium, and aluminum.

The effectiveness of antacids is due to their ability to partially neutralize gastric acid secretions, which helps to relieve the complaints of acute gastritis such as "heartburn," "sour stomach," and "indigestion." In chronic conditions, increasing gastric pH seems to allow healing of ulcerated mucosa. (Chapter 52 contains a more complete discussion of antacids.)

Sodium Bicarbonate

Sodium bicarbonate (baking soda) is a very effective antacid. However, because it is very soluble, systemic

Table 7–5. SOME OTC ANTACID PRODUCTS THAT CONTAIN AN ALUMINUM-MAGNESIUM COMBINATION

Product	Approximate Volume Needed to Neutralize 80 mEq Acid	Volume/Day (Based on 4 Doses)	Sodium Intake/Day (Based on 4 Doses)
Aludrox	30 ml	120 ml	26 mg
A.M.T.	45 ml	180 ml	252 mg
Delcid	10 ml	40 ml	92 mg
Gelusil*	60 ml	240 ml	38 mg
Gelusil II*	30 ml	120 ml	31 mg
Gelusil M*	35 ml	140 ml	36 mg
Kolantyl	45 ml	180 ml	≤ 180 mg
Maalox	30 ml	120 ml	60 mg
Mylanta*	35 ml	140 ml	106 mg
Mylanta II*	20 ml	80 ml	129 mg
Riopan†	35 ml	140 ml	8 mg
Trisogel	50 ml	200 ml	640 mg
WinGel	35 ml	140 ml	70 mg

*Contains simethicone.
†Contains malgaldrate.

absorption is likely, and large doses may result in alkalosis. The high sodium content (476 mg per standard ½ teaspoon dose) precludes regular or frequent ingestion.

Calcium Carbonate

Calcium carbonate neutralizes gastric acid, and the systemic absorption of calcium is considered unlikely. Signs indicating hypercalcemia, however, are assessed. Calcium carbonate and other calcium-containing antacids may cause an increase in gastric secretion, referred to as acid rebound. Although the clinical significance is minimal, calcium-containing antacids are generally avoided when ulcer healing is indicated.

Magnesium

Magnesium is found as the oxide, carbonate, hydroxide, and trisilicate. An increased incidence of diarrhea in higher doses prevents its use as the sole antacid in any regimen. The possibility of hypermagnesemia exists, especially in patients with renal failure.

Aluminum

Aluminum, available as the hydroxide, carbonate, and phosphate salts, has the lowest *neutralizing capacity* of the four agents and is virtually ineffective in any form other than liquid. Antacids containing aluminum have a constipating effect. Aluminum compounds, therefore, are frequently used in combination with magnesium compounds to offset the diarrhea effect of the magnesium compounds. Chronic ingestion may cause systemic absorption of aluminum, which is a CNS toxin. Aluminum hydroxide is used alone to treat the hyperphosphatemia seen in renal failure, because it prevents absorption of phosphate from the GI tract.

The most commonly used products contain both aluminum and magnesium, a combination that maximizes antacid effect while minimizing side effects. Usually, it is a physical combination, but malgaldrate, the active ingredient, is a chemical mixture of aluminum and magnesium hydroxides. Table 7–5 lists some OTC products containing aluminum and magnesium.

Simethicone

Simethicone, an agent often found in antacids, is an antiflatulent that reduces surface tension between gas bubbles so they may be expelled more easily. Although it appears to be harmless, its inclusion in antacids is questioned because of the unlikelihood of differentiating between symptoms caused by gas or excess acid.

The first task in selecting an antacid is to choose a dosage form. To exert its effect in the stomach, an antacid must be in liquid form. Since they are relatively insoluble compounds, tablets have a big disadvantage since dissolution is a slow process. They must be chewed thoroughly and taken with plenty of water, which lessens their convenience and taste advantage. Even so, dissolution is unlikely to be complete. Undissolved fragments may coalesce to form an obstruction if numerous doses are consumed. Tablets, lozenges, and chewing gums also cannot compare to liquids with respect to effectiveness. For example, assuming complete dissolution, a 30-ml dose of Gelusil II liquid is equivalent to six Gelusil II tablets. Effervescent tablets may cause gastric distention and flatulence.

In choosing a liquid antacid product, sodium content, neutralizing capacity, volume needed per dose, cost, and palatability are considered. Sodium ingestion should be kept to a minimum, especially in patients on a low-sodium diet, such as those with cardiovascular or renal problems.

Neutralizing capacity is the amount of acid a given volume of antacid will neutralize. It is expressed as milliequivalents per milliliter and varies considerably between products. The greater the neutralizing capacity, the smaller the antacid volume needed per dose; and the smaller the volume, the more acceptable the product (see Table 7–5). In comparing costs, the volume needed per dose must be considered. Personal taste is the determining factor in selecting a palatable product.

Information on individual antacids and the nursing process for the patient requiring drugs to reduce hyperacidity is found in Chapter 52.

LAXATIVES

The most misused and abused OTC medications are laxatives, drugs that promote defecation. The misunderstanding starts primarily with the concept of normal bowel function and constipation. The proper definition of constipation is excessive hardness of stool without regard to frequency of bowel movements. Normal frequency of bowel movements can vary greatly from two to three movements daily to one every three to five days. Of importance is the change in the normal bowel function. Simple constipation, in most cases, subsides within a few days. Laxatives are rarely necessary in healthy individuals. Normal bowel function can be maintained by proper diet containing foods with high fiber content (bran), fresh fruits, vegetables, and fluids (8–10 glasses daily); regular exercise; and an established time of day for defecation. If constipation occurs, these nonpharmacologic interventions should be tried before using a laxative. Patients should see a *health care provider* and not self-medicate if abdominal pain, nausea, or vomiting is present.

Laxatives are discussed in detail in Chapter 54. The most common method used to classify laxatives is based on the mechanism of action: bulk-forming, saline (osmotic), stimulant or contact, lubricant, and stool softeners (surface-acting).

Bulk-Forming Laxatives

The mechanism of action of bulk-forming laxatives is to increase bulk volume and water content of the stool, thus promoting bowel movement. The most common active ingredients are psyllium and cellulose derivatives. Metamucil is a bulk-forming laxative containing psyllium. The onset of action with bulk-forming laxatives may occur after 24 hours but usually requires 1–3 days for maximum effect. Adverse effects include production of flatulence, obstruction, and a potential absorption of drugs concurrently administered.

Saline Laxatives

The saline laxatives, also referred to as osmotic cathartics, act by exerting an osmotic effect. Osmosis is the movement of water toward an area with high concentrations of ions, particularly sodium or magnesium. The osmotic cathartics or saline laxatives include various magnesium salts: magnesium hydroxide (Milk of Magnesia), magnesium sulfate (Epsom Salt), and magnesium citrate. Combinations of sodium and phosphate are also available, for example, Phospho-Soda, and sodium phosphate oral solution.

The use of saline laxatives is generally restricted to situations that require a prompt and complete evacuation, for example, bowel preparation prior to a diagnostic test or surgery. These laxatives act very quickly within 20–30 minutes and may cause abdominal cramping, nausea, and vomiting. Patients with cardiovascular problems such as congestive heart failure or hypertension and/or impaired renal function should not use saline laxatives.

Stimulant Laxatives

The stimulant laxatives are also referred to as contact cathartics. These agents act on the intestinal mucosa and produce effects both on motility and on net absorption of electrolytes and water. Included in this group are the

Table 7–6. SOME COMMON OTC LAXATIVES AND CATHARTICS

Class	Active Ingredient	Brand Name
Bulk-forming laxatives	Methylcellulose Psyllium preparations	Cologel Konsyl, Metamucil, Mucilose, Serutan, Syllact

Emollient laxatives
  Stool softeners
  Lubricants
	Docusate sodium
	Docusate calcium
	Mineral oil
		Colace, Doxinate
		Surfak
		Agoral Plain

Saline cathartics	Magnesium citrate Magnesium hydroxide Magnesium sulfate	— Milk of Magnesia Epsom Salt
Stimulant cathartics	Bisacodyl Castor oil Cascara sagrada Danthron Yellow phenolphthalein Senna (including sennosides A & B)	Dulcolax Alphamul Neoloid Cas-Evac Nature's Remedy Modane Dorbane Evac-U-Gen Ex-Lax Feen-A-Mint Gum Black Draught Fletcher's Castoria Senekot Swiss Kriss

diphenylmethane derivatives (phenolphthalein and bis-acodyl); the anthraquinones (senna, cascara sagrada); and castor oil. Evacuation with these agents is relatively prompt, and effects may be seen in 6–8 hours. Saline laxatives are commonly involved in OTC misuse. The major adverse effect is excessive cathartic effects with associated nausea and cramping. Laxative addiction is a potential hazard with this group.

Lubricants

Mineral oil is a petroleum derivative that is minimally absorbed. It penetrates and softens the stool and may also interfere with water absorption. The major adverse effects of mineral oil ingestion relate to its property as a fat solvent. Mineral oil may interfere with the absorption of fat-soluble drugs coadministered and may decrease the absorption of fat-soluble vitamins (A, D, E, K) in the gut.

Stool Softeners

Stool softeners are surface-acting laxatives. Dioctyl calcium sulfosuccinate (Surfax) and dioctyl sodium sulfosuccinate (Colace) are two common stool softeners. The primary mechanism of action of these laxatives is to decrease the surface tension of the stool allowing water and fats to penetrate the stool. Consequently the stool becomes soft and is easier to move.

Stool softeners are indicated for patients for whom straining at defecation is hazardous. This includes patients recovering from a myocardial infarction, stroke, or surgery. Long-term use is not recommended.

Table 7–6 lists some laxative and cathartic products commercially available and their active ingredients.

OTC DRUGS AND THE NURSING PROCESS

ASSESSMENT

The nurse, as a primary care provider in a variety of environments, interacts with patients and families, assesses presenting complaints, and intervenes with appropriate counseling and referrals. Through this process the nurse determines whether the patient's problem can be adequately treated with self-care measures and possibly OTC medications or if the patient should receive medical intervention.

Assessment begins with the collection of information. The nurse listens to the patient's description of the problem and elicits information about the symptoms (quality, location, severity, onset, duration, frequency, aggravating and alleviating factors, and associated symptoms). From this information the possible etiology and severity may be determined. If the symptoms are severe and the nurse suspects a serious underlying cause, the patient is referred to a physician for more definite assessment and intervention. In most situations the health problem is due to a minor illness and requires

Table 7–7. SYMPTOMATOLOGY REQUIRING REFERRAL

1. Symptoms indicating a serious problem
2. Persistent or recurring symptoms
3. Multiple symptoms, e.g., sore throat with fever and adenopathy
4. Failure of self-care treatment in alleviating symptoms
5. Ambiguous symptoms requiring more definite assessment
6. Any situation beyond the scope of nursing

only symptomatic treatment. High risk groups, such as the elderly, infants, children under 12 years of age, pregnant or breast-feeding women, patients with chronic disease, individuals taking prescription drugs, or those who have multiple medical problems, require a comprehensive assessment and consultation with the individual's physician before OTC medication is recommended. Table 7–7 summarizes situations when the nurse should refer the patient to a physician.

To complete the assessment, a medication history is obtained including prescription and nonprescription drugs, allergies, and adverse reactions. The patient's previous experience with OTC medication, including the successes and failures of self-medication, is assessed. Often patients do not recognize OTC products as medications or drugs. To obtain this information, the nurse asks the patient what products or agents are used when the individual has a headache, cold, upset stomach, or constipation. Chronic use or misuse of OTC medication may also cause symptoms that the nurse must evaluate. Patients are asked when and how often they use these products (Table 7–8).

NURSING DIAGNOSES

The nurse develops nursing diagnoses by synthesizing the patient's information from the assessment. Typical nursing diagnoses include alteration in comfort and knowledge deficit about self-care measures and OTC medications. More specific nursing diagnoses are developed according to the patient's individual assessment. Nursing diagnoses for a patient requiring OTC cold medications are included in Table 7–9.

Table 7–8. SOME SYMPTOMS SUGGESTIVE OF OTC MISUSE

Symptom	OTC Agent
Persistent or worsening nasal congestion (rebound congestion)	Overuse of topical nasal decongestant
Constipation, impaction in the elderly, and possibly hypophosphatemia	Chronic use or misuse of antacids
Abdominal cramping and fluid and electrolyte imbalance (especially in the elderly)	Chronic use or misuse of laxatives
Insomnia, restlessness, and nervousness	Nasal decongestants (sympathomimetics) or excessive caffeine

Table 7–9. NURSING PROCESS FOR PATIENT REQUIRING COLD PREPARATIONS

Assessment

Note abrupt onset of rhinorrhea, nasal stuffiness, sneezing, cough, and myalgia and characteristics/location of discomforts. Assess frequency and effectiveness of cough effort.

Evaluate concurrent health problems (e.g., heart disease, asthma, narrow-angle glaucoma, urinary retention, pregnancy/lactation, diabetes), and drug use (e.g., CNS depressants, tricyclic antidepressants, MAO inhibitors, β-adrenergic blockers, antihypertensives or digitalis preparations).

Ascertain previous use of antihistamines/decongestants and adverse reactions. Determine present self-medication and length of use.

Assess knowledge regarding OTC medications and self-care practices for specific cold symptoms.

Nursing Diagnosis	Nursing Actions	Rationale	Patient Outcomes/ Evaluation Criteria
Airway clearance ineffective, related to excessive secretions and inflammation of nasal membranes as evidenced by complaints of difficulty breathing, noisy respirations and cough.	Recommend an effective antihistamine and/or decongestant, e.g., chlorpheniramine, bromopheniramine; pseudoephedrine, oral oxymetazoline as appropriate. Encourage hydration with oral intake of 2–3L/day and use of cool-mist room vaporizer. Suggest use of warm fluids instead of cold. Recommend abstaining from smoking. Note complaints of persistent or worsening congestion.	Use of antihistamines can dry secretions and decongestants decrease nasal stuffiness unless contraindicated by preexisting medical conditions or concomitant drug use. Adequate hydration and use of warm fluids help counteract side effects of drug use by keeping secretions loose and facilitating expectoration. Smoking has a drying, irritating effect and decreases ciliary action impairing clearing of secretions. May indicate misuse/overuse of topical nasal decongestant.	Displays improved clearing/expectoration of secretions. Demonstrates appropriate self-care measures. Abstains from smoking.
Comfort, altered related to localized tissue inflammation, generalized immune system response, and recurrent cough as evidence by complaints of sore throat, chest tightness and malaise/myalgia.	Recommend a safe and effective analgesic, e.g., acetaminophen, aspirin, ibuprofen. Encourage use of warm salt water gargles, unmedicated lozenges, and cessation of smoking. Demonstrate chest splinting during cough. Suggest use of cough suppressant (e.g., dextromethorphan, or diphenhydramine) as appropriate.	OTC analgesics are usually effective in relieving myalgia. Stimulates salivation, wets/soothes irritated membrane lining of throat especially in presence of productive cough without fever. Provides support, helping to prevent muscle strain. Recurrent nonproductive cough increases irritation of airways and muscle fatigue, impairs rest.	Reports alleviation of localized discomfort and myalgia. Demonstrates proper use of analgesics.
Sleep pattern disturbance, related to excessive cough as evidenced by complaints of difficulty in falling asleep or maintaining sleep throughout the night.	Recommend a safe and effective cough suppressant, e.g., dextromethorphan, diphenhydramine. Provide information regarding self-care measures to decrease cough including timing of medication and adequate fluid intake.	Antitussive therapy may be used to relieve the cough by inhibiting the cough reflex. Antihistamine therapy decreases post nasal drainage and the sedative effect may also be useful in promoting sleep. Hydration facilitates expectoration, increasing effectiveness of cough effort and may help reduce frequency of cough.	Reports improvement in sleep/rest pattern and increased sense of well-being. Feels rested when awakens. Demonstrates proper use of cough suppressant and self-care measures.

CONTINUED ON THE FOLLOWING PAGE

Table 7–9. NURSING PROCESS FOR PATIENT REQUIRING COLD PREPARATIONS

Assessment

Note abrupt onset of rhinorrhea, nasal stuffiness, sneezing, cough, and myalgia and characteristics/location of discomforts. Assess frequency and effectiveness of cough effort.

Evaluate concurrent health problems (e.g., heart disease, asthma, narrow-angle glaucoma, urinary retention, pregnancy/lactation, diabetes), and drug use (e.g., CNS depressants, tricyclic antidepressants, MAO inhibitors, β-adrenergic blockers, antihypertensives or digitalis preparations).

Ascertain previous use of antihistamines/decongestants and adverse reactions. Determine present self-medication and length of use.

Assess knowledge regarding OTC medications and self-care practices for specific cold symptoms.

Nursing Diagnosis	Nursing Actions	Rationale	Patient Outcomes/ Evaluation Criteria
Knowledge deficit related to limited understanding of OTC medications and self-care measures as evidenced by inability to identify treatments to alleviate specific cold symptoms, presence of undesired side effects.	Provide information regarding OTC cold medications for specific symptoms based on individual need/circumstances. Discuss action, timing/duration of use, dosage, possible reactions, and interactions. Stress importance of reading labels of OTC products.	Knowledge of OTC cold preparations, their active ingredients, and use facilitates appropriate selection and symptom palliation and reduces potential for overmedication. OTC medications for management of common cold are generally safe and effective if used correctly.	Identifies appropriate OTC medications for specific symptom relief. Verbalizes awareness of precautions for OTC medications and possible adverse actions. Verbalizes understanding of factors that contribute to possibility of injury and takes steps to reduce risk of injury.
	Review common side effects and actions to be taken (e.g. take drug with milk/food if gastric upset occurs). Identify strategies to be used if symptoms persist, i.e., change dosage or drug instead of increasing frequency of administration.	Sedative effects are common with use of antihistamines but may also be compounded by concurrent drug use. OTC medications for management of common cold are generally safe and effective if used correctly.	
	Recommend self-care measures to alleviate discomforts associated with antihistamines, e.g., good oral hygiene, use of warm salt-water gargles, sugarless gum/lozenges.	The common cold is a self-limiting disorder, therefore, self-care is appropriate to alleviate symptoms. Dry mouth is most commonly occuring side effect.	
	Caution against driving or activities requiring alertness until individual response of drug is known.	Identifies specific safety precautions to prevent injury.	
	Recommend abstinence from alcohol or other depressant drugs. Suggest use of caffeine beverages as appropriate.	Antihistamines commonly cause drowsiness/dizziness that may abate with continued use. Stimulant effect of caffeine may help counteract drug-induced sedation but may be contraindicated in conjunction with decongestant use as nervousness, tremors or insomnia may occur.	
	Stress importance of medical follow-up if no improvement occurs or if fever, nausea/vomiting, or chest pain related to coughing or breathing develop/persist.	Allows for timely intervention and prevention of serious complications.	

Table 7–10 PATIENT GUIDELINES FOR SELF-MEDICATION

1. Do not self-medicate without advice or supervision from your health care provider if you have any of the following conditions:
   - currently taking prescription drugs
   - have history of diabetes, heart disease, asthma, emphysema, kidney disease or thyroid disease
   - pregnant or breast-feeding
2. Identify the symptoms you wish to treat
3. Select a product that is specific in treating your symptom. For example, nasal congestion is treated with a decongestant. Consult with a health care professional (pharmacist, nurse, or health care provider) if you need assistance.
4. Read instructions for use and use only as recommended. Prolonged use may lead to serious complications.
5. Use non-drug measures to help treat your symptoms. For example, drinking 1–2 quarts of water decreases nasal congestion.
6. If no relief or symptoms worsen, see your health care provider.

PLANNING AND INTERVENTION

After the assessment is made and the nursing diagnoses formulated, the health care goals for the patient are established. The primary goals when advocating self-care are as follows:

- Provide information for safe and effective use of OTC medication.
- Provide information regarding nondrug self-care measures.
- Decrease patient discomfort.
- Provide information regarding health care referral or follow-up.

Nursing interventions include health teaching, advice for a specific treatment approach, reassurance, and/or assistance in obtaining health care consultation.

Each symptom is treated separately, and both drug and nondrug treatments are considered. Typical non-drug treatments include increasing fluids to liquefy respiratory secretions, increasing rest to cure a cold, and changing dietary intake to manage chronic indigestion or bowel problems. Since coinciding symptoms do not necessarily have the same duration or severity, a "shot-gun therapy" treatment with products indicated for one symptom may possibly worsen another. Unnecessary drugs cause unnecessary side effects.

In recommending a drug, the nurse selects a product based on indications and contraindications. In addition, the beneficial effects of the drug should outweigh the risks of adverse reactions. The nurse must be very careful in performing this function and always practice within the scope of nursing.

OTC medications are chosen by selection of the specific active ingredient rather than a specific product. Single-agent products are used and are often available in generic forms, which are less expensive than the brand-name forms. To be safe and effective, the OTC medica-tion must be taken in the right amount and at the right interval and for only a specified period of time; generally seven days is the limit for OTC drug use. Patient guidelines for self-medication are listed in Table 7–10.

EVALUATION

The nurse and patient establish outcome criteria to evaluate the effectiveness of the interventions. These outcome criteria include relief of symptoms, safe use of OTC medications, absence of adverse reactions, effective application of self-care measures, and recognition of the need for follow-up or referral if symptoms worsen or fail to improve.

In most situations where self-care is being implemented, evaluation of the interventions is primarily a function the patient performs. The nurse, however, advises the patient to call or return if self-care treatment is unsuccessful or if the situation worsens. A specific time interval is given.

Self-care is an important component in health care management and is encouraged when appropriate. The nurse is in a pivotal position to ensure that patients have the knowledge and ability to safely and successfully implement self-care measures.

SUMMARY

There are many categories of OTC medications available in our health care market. The four most common categories used by patients for self-care are cold, cough, and allergy medications; internal analgesics/antipyretics; antacids; and laxatives. The indication for OTC medication is based on the presenting symptomatology.

The symptoms associated with the common cold, allergy, pain, indigestion, and constipation have been reviewed.

Self-care is an important component in health care management. The nurse needs to be knowledgeable about both nondrug measures and OTC medications which the patient can use. Knowing the indications, contraindications, precautions, and potential drug interactions of the common OTC medications is paramount in assisting patients with the selection of products.

BIBLIOGRAPHY

American Hospital Formulary Service. Drug Information 87. American Society of Hospital Pharmacists, Inc, Bethesda, 1987.

American Pharmaceutical Association. Handbook of Nonprescription Drugs, ed 8. Washington, American Pharmaceutical Association, 1986.

Covington, TR: Rational self-medication with OTC's: Whose responsibility? Drug Newsletter, 5, 1986.

Griffith, HW: Complete Guide to Prescription and Nonprescription Drugs, rev. ed. HP Books, Tucson, 1987.

Harkness, R: OTC Handbook: What to Recommend and Why, ed 2. Medical Economics Books, Oradell, NJ, 1983.

Katzung, BG: Basic and Chemical Pharmacology, ed 3. Appleton and Lange, Norwalk, CT, 1987.

Moss, A, et al: Over-the-counter ibuprofen and acute renal failure (letter). Ann Intern Med 105:303, 1986.

Olin, B (ed): Facts and Comparisons. St Louis, JB Lippincott, 1987.

Pepper, G: OTC vs. Rx for allergic rhinitis. Nurse Practitioner 12:6, 1987.

Physicians' Desk Reference for Nonprescription Drugs. Medical Economics Books, Oradell, NJ, 1988.

SITUATION 7–1

Nora Carter, RN, applies knowledge of over-the-counter medications while managing patients in the office of a physician who specializes in internal medicine.

1. Mr. Schmidt is taking an antihistamine for symptoms associated with a cold. To minimize the side effect of sedation, Nora will teach Mr. Schmidt to:
   a. take the antihistamine at bedtime
   b. ingest extra coffee during the day
   c. continue to perform his usual activities despite drowsiness
   d. combine the antihistamine with a CNS stimulant

2. When antihistamines are recommended for elderly patients, Nora will teach the patients and families to report all of the following except:
   a. dizziness
   b. confusion
   c. hypotension
   d. reduced rhinorrhea

3. An antacid is prescribed for Julia Reel, who has a duodenal ulcer. Which of the following antacids would not be indicated for treatment?
   a. sodium bicarbonate
   b. magnesium carbonate
   c. calcium carbonate
   d. aluminum hydroxide

4. Mr. Plunkett, a 67-year-old with narrow-angle glaucoma, calls to find out which medications he should take for cold and flu symptoms. Nora will tell him to avoid:
   a. antihistamines
   b. antitussives
   c. expectorants
   d. aspirin compounds

5. Mrs. Arnold has been taking Sudafed for a cold. She is also taking digoxin daily. Optimally, Mrs. Arnold should discontinue the decongestant due to
   a. decreased absorption of digoxin
   b. increased potential for arrythmias
   c. potential for digitalis toxicity
   d. decreased effects of both drugs

6. Aluminum hydroxide is the antacid recommended for Mr. Farrell, who has chronic renal failure, because it:
   a. has reduced potential for constipation
   b. prevents absorption of phosphate from the GI tract
   c. blocks absorption of calcium from the GI tract
   d. interferes with nitrogen and protein assimilation

Please refer to the Appendices for correct answers and additional review questions with answers.

8

CHAPTER

TEACHING, LEARNING, AND EVALUATION STRATEGIES FOR COMPLIANCE

TEACHING, LEARNING, AND EVALUATION STRATEGIES FOR COMPLIANCE

GLOSSARY TERMS IN THIS CHAPTER

Compliance
Comprehension
Criterion reference evaluation
Discrimination
Discovery learning
Education
Extinction
Formative evaluation
Generalization
Humanistic perspective
Learning
Meaningful/discovery learning
Meaningful/reception learning
Noncompliance
Readability
Reception learning
Reinforcement
Reinforcer
Rote/discovery learning
Rote/reception learning
Stimulus-response theory
Teaching-learning
Teaching-learning theory

8
CHAPTER

TEACHING, LEARNING, AND EVALUATION STRATEGIES FOR COMPLIANCE

CAROL ANN MAULL, R.N., Ph.D.
MERRILY MATHEWSON KUHN, R.N.C., Ph.D., CCRN

LEARNING OBJECTIVES

After reading this chapter, the student will be able to:

1. Formulate a specific plan to assess the teaching needs of a patient requiring medication.
2. Develop the nursing diagnoses relative to the teaching needs of a patient requiring medication.
3. Plan the nursing intervention necessary to teach the patient requiring medication.
4. develop teaching and evaluation tools or techniques specific to the learning needs of the patient requiring medications.
5. Compare and contrast adult learning theories and their application in a patient-nurse teaching-learning situation.
6. Employ evaluation techniques to evaluate teaching strategies.
7. Identify the components of compliant and noncompliant behaviors.
8. Identify specific areas to assess in the patient in order to predict compliant and noncompliant behaviors.
9. Formulate nursing diagnoses relevant to the patient's noncompliance with a medication regimen.
10. Formulate a plan of intervention to promote patient compliance with treatment regimen.
11. Evaluate the effectiveness of nursing intervention to promote patient compliance with the treatment regimen.

Education of patients is one of the most important functions of the professional nurse. The informed patient receives maximum benefit from medication, and education can often make the difference between patient *compliance* and *noncompliance.* Recent research has identified more than 30,000 drug-related deaths each year, and it is suspected that the number may be as high as 140,000 (Dipalma, 1979). Many of these deaths could have been avoided with adequate patient teaching. For example, a patient with inadequate understanding stops taking antihypertensive medication and has a fatal stroke two years later.

Only since the early 1970s has the importance of patient education been recognized within the medical and nursing professions. Less than two decades ago, health professionals educated patients on an intuitive basis and assumed that the patient was receptive to the message. Little effort was made to determine *comprehension* and compliance.

During the 1970s, the results of a great deal of research regarding how the adult learns became available to health professionals. Nurses began to ask questions such as:

1. When is the patient ready to learn?
2. What does the patient need to know?
3. How can the patient best learn about a particular disease and medications?
4. When is the best time to teach a patient?
5. How can the knowledge that has been imparted be best evaluated?
6. Is the patient compliant?

Sufficient research has been accomplished to answer these questions effectively.

Today, more than ever before, emphasis has been placed on the implementation and documentation of patient education within the health care system (Northrop, 1986). Policy statements by the Joint Commission on Accreditation of Hospitals (JCAH) and the American Hospital Association regarding the definition and requirements for patient education stress the significance of structuring and standardizing patient *teaching* activities within the hospital setting. To address the problem of effective patient education, this chapter is divided into three sections. Section One speaks to the need of determining the patient's readability level; Section Two focuses on adult *teaching-learning theories;* and Section Three deals with the nursing process approach to patient teaching and compliance.

DETERMINING PATIENT'S READING ABILITY

Nurse educators often utilize appropriate written materials to supplement and enhance the teaching-learning process in formal and informal educational programs in a variety of settings. Reasons for supplemental distribution of written material is to provide a review of material presented by the nurse or physician, to reinforce previous learning, or to provide additional information that is relevant to the patient's needs with the ultimate goal of compliance to a nursing and/or medical regimen.

To maximize the effectiveness of using printed materials, the nurse must be aware of the limitations inherent in their use. A major limitation of using printed materials is that they are often not appropriate for the established learning objectives. For example, if the learning objective is to learn a motor skill, both printed texts and still pictures are given a low effectiveness rating. Conversely, if the learning objective is visual identification, printed texts are rated low in effectiveness, whereas still pictures are rated high. Both printed texts and still pictures are given a medium effectiveness rating if the objective is to learn factual information, principles, concepts, and rules; and if the goal is to develop desirable attitudes, opinions, and motivations, printed texts are also given only a medium rating. Reasons for limitations of printed materials may vary but seem to focus upon concepts such as legibility, ease of reading, motivational or interest value, and particularly the ease of material comprehension.

Basically, comprehension of written information depends upon the ability to read. According to Bormuth, at least 20% of people living in the United States are functionally illiterate, that is, not able to read materials written at a fourth to fifth grade level (Bormuth, 1973–1974). Approximately 50% of health care patients have serious difficulty with reading or are unable to read instructional materials written at a fifth grade level (Doak and Doak, 1980). And more significantly, at least 20% of patients may be unable to read instructions at all (Doak and Doak, 1980). *Readability* assessments of patient materials indicate that the vast majority are written well above eighth grade level, and the standard surgical consent form used by most hospitals demands a 16th grade or college senior reading ability. At this level, a significant number of Americans may be unable to comprehend the consent form. Since few informational sources used for health teaching are available at less than an eighth grade reading level, most written materials given to patients in the course of health education simply are not comprehensible by the majority (Spadero, 1983; Table 8–1).

Nurses spend a large portion of their time in direct contact with patients in teaching-learning activities. If, as suggested by Doak and Doak, poor comprehension of written materials is a major cause of failure to achieve desired objectives and ultimately compliance to a specified regimen, a great deal of time and energy expended on the part of both nurses and patients may be unproductive, or in vain. Although the literature urges identification of a patient knowledge level and "readiness" to learn before initiation of an education program, of greater significance is the assessment of the relationship between reading level and the ability to comprehend written health care instructions before program inception. A two-prong problem exists. On one hand, the

Table 8–1. EXAMPLES OF READABILITY OF SELECTED PATIENT INFORMATION MATERIAL

Topic	Name of Pamphlet	Source	Grade Level
Contraception	Contraception? Facts on Birth Control	Patient Information Library	13
Kidney disease	Acute Glomerulonephritis	National Kidney Foundation	12
Otitis media	Understanding Otitis Media	Burroughs-Wellcome	11
Pregnancy	Drugs, Alcohol, Tobacco Abuse During Pregnancy	March of Dimes	11
Venereal disease	The Love Bugs	Patient Information Library	11

From Spadera, DC: Assessing readability of patient information materials. Pediatric Nursing, July/August 1983, pp. 276–277, with permission.

nurse must determine the degree of difficulty in printed materials and, on the other, determine if the written information presented is compatible with the patient's level of reading and comprehension ability.

A variety of formulas have been designed to predict the degree of publication complexity. The SMOG readability formula was designed in 1969 by G. H. McLaughlin and is thought to be both one of the simplest and one of the most accurate analyses of readabiity available. Unlike many others, the SMOG formula is based on 100% comprehension. For example, a reading level of grade 8 by the SMOG method means that all patients reading at the eighth grade level should comprehend the material. The SMOG formula is based on the square root of the number of polysyllabic words contained within 30 selected sentences of the reading material (McLaughlin, 1969; Table 8–2). While the SMOG method may be too involved to utilize with each teaching-learning situation, the nurse, nevertheless, must make an assessment of the patient's level of reading ability as a preliminary step to ensuring good communication between the nurse and patient whenever written materials are used for medication compliance. The following is an example of essentially the same information in a written format presented at three readability levels:

1. Coadministration of this medication with alcoholic beverages and other CNS depressing drugs (e.g.,

sedatives, tranquilizers, antihistamines) may add to the sedative effect (Patient information: Valium. Drug Consultation Guide, 1976).

Readability level: 11th grade

2. You should not take this drug while you are drinking alcoholic beverages, such as wine or beer. You should also avoid taking this drug with other medications you may be taking for sleep or tension. (Bast & Angaran, 1978).

Readability level: 5th grade

3. Don't take this drug with booze (like wine, beer, or whiskey). Don't take this drug with other drugs for tension or which help you sleep (Streiff, 1985).

Readability level: 3rd grade

Once a patient's level of reading ability has been ascertained, the nurse achieves the best results for medication compliance when both verbal and written information is presented at the appropriate readability level. Compliance may be defined as the extent to which a patient's behavior regarding the medication plan coincides with medical advice and/or health teaching. Because the nurse is the health professional most responsible for achieving patient motivation and ultimately compliance in patient procedures, therapy, and medication regimens, the nurse should also be familiar with adult learning theories as a framework for presenting both written and verbal information for teaching purposes.

Table 8–2. SMOG GRADING

1. Count 10 consecutive sentences near the beginning of the text to be assessed, 10 in the middle, and 10 near the end. Count as a sentence any string of words ending with a period, question mark, or exclamation point.
2. In the 30 selected sentences count every word of 3 or more syllables. Any string of letters or numerals beginning and ending with a space or punctuation mark should be counted if you can distinguish at least 3 syllables when you read it aloud in context. If a polysyllabic word is repeated, count each repetition.
3. Estimate the square root of the number of polysyllabic words counted. This is done by taking the square root of the nearest perfect square. For example, if the count is 95, the nearest perfect square is 100, which yields a square root of 10. If the count lies roughly between two perfect squares, choose the lower number. For instance, if the count is 110, take the square root of 100 rather than that of 121.
4. Add 3 to the approximate square root. This gives the SMOG Grade, which is the reading grade that a person must have reached if he is to understand fully the text assessed.

From McLaughlin, GH: SMOG grading—A new readability formula. Journal of Reading 12:639, 1969. Reprinted with permission of the International Reading Association.

TEACHING-LEARNING THEORIES

From the standpoint of the adult learner, three educational or teaching-learning perspectives can be directly applied to the learning experience involving the nurse, patient, and/or family. The first is B. F. Skinner's conditioning theory, focusing on reinforcement as a motivator and methodology for learning. The second is David Ausubel's cognitive theory, which assesses the learner's thinking patterns and methods of learning. Third, Carl Rogers' humanistic approach to learning stresses the value of the interpersonal relationship between teacher and learner in any given learning situation. Because of the dynamic nature of the learning experience, one or a combination of these learning theories may be used to adapt to the patient's learning needs at any point in the *teaching-learning* continuum, in a variety of settings. After these teaching-learning theories are reviewed, the nursing process section demonstrates how the nurse can implement them in daily practice.

SKINNER'S CONDITIONING-BEHAVIORISTIC PERSPECTIVE

B. F. Skinner's conditioning learning perspective is concerned with the arrangement of reinforcing (rewarding) experiences to produce the type of behavior or learning desired. When utilizing this theory, the nurse controls the learning environment by providing rewards for each correct answer so as to shape learning behavior in a step-by-step fashion that leads to a predetermined result. As expected, the conditioning perspective is also termed the S-R theory *(stimulus-response)*, wherein the nurse provides the stimulus experiences and the patient responds.

Specific principles must be considered when using the behavioristic theory in any given teaching-learning experience. The first principle is that of *reinforcement*, rewarding the desired behavior or learning to increase the probability that the behavior occurs again. Second, *extinction* is employed to eliminate unwanted behavior by abruptly withdrawing reinforcement, which results in the extinguishment of the undesired behavior. Third, a *reinforcer* can be anything that increases the probability of a desired response. Fourth, *discrimination* informs the learner that different kinds of behavior are appropriate under different conditions. Fifth, *generalization* tells the learner that behavior in a given situation continues to be valid in future learning experiences. The establishment of carefully controlled associations between stimuli and responses and the application of the principles of reinforcement, extinction, reinforcers, discrimination, and generalization result in a kind of learning that is called "conditioning." However, the cardinal principle in any given learning experience, the key to behavior control, is reinforcement.

Thus, the conditioning perspective may be useful as a teaching methodology for the nurse who subscribes to Skinner's theory that by controlling the contingencies of reinforcement, the teacher changes and guides behavior in such a way that learning occurs.

Skinner's Teaching and Learning Principles As Applied to Patient Education

The basic assumptions that underlie Skinner's conditioning perspective are, first, that learning occurs from the simple to the complex and, second, that learning continues when the behavior is reinforced at each stage in the learning process. In the application of these assumptions, all learning materials must be broken down into a very large number of very small steps, and reinforcement must be contingent on the accomplishment of each step by making each successive step as small as possible (programmed learning). Through frequent and continual reinforcement, the possibly adverse consequences of being wrong are minimized. Clearly, this learning perspective demands that the nurse be continually present in the active teaching-learning environment to provide reinforcement and observe and assess learning progress. However, this methodology does provide an impetus and motivation to learn for the insecure or anxious learner who requires an environment controlled and reinforced by the teacher and one where the learner is not threatened by failure. This perspective may be appropriate for the patient with a low readability level, as the theory provides a step-by-step process with reinforcement provided at each level.

The following is an example of the application of Skinner's principles to a specific learning situation and the role of the nurse in this learning experience. Although Skinner's principles are presented for this specific learning situation, they may be applied to any given teaching and learning experience.

As the nurse, you are confronted with teaching the procedure for insulin injections to an elderly male patient who has been newly diagnosed as having diabetes mellitus. First, as the controller of the learning environment, you select the desired behaviors to be learned. Does the patient have someone at home to assist him in insulin administration, or must he assume responsibility for the procedure himself? Once the specific behaviors or outcomes are determined, the complex learning problem is broken down into its elemental parts, and behavior objectives are listed for each learning segment. The material to be learned is presented sequentially, from simple to complex, and positive reinforcement or reinforcers are provided to increase the probability that the desired behaviors happen again. Reinforcers may be verbal ("that's good") or nonverbal (smiling). Should the patient adopt an undesirable behavior, for example, unwanted learning, a nonverbal reinforcer could be silence. Discrimination is also reinforced (rewarded) to inform the learner that certain behaviors are appropriate under different conditions. For example, one may touch the end of the syringe if it is capped.

It is important that the patient learn one step entirely before proceeding to the next, so that when all of the parts of the learning problem are assembled, they produce a unified whole. Terminal behaviors may be achieved through a variety of teaching methodologies that include, but are not limited to, charts, posters, demonstration, and discussion—whichever method is best suited to meet the unique learning needs and capabilities of each patient. In this way, learning can be individualized for each patient. Close observation of the patient's learning process, repetition of learning tasks, and continuous positive reinforcement provide a learning environment that may be appropriate for selected patients.

Summary

In summation, the behavioristic position stresses the study of overt behavior (as opposed to Ausubel's cognitive perspective), based on the assumption that learning is determined primarily by experience between teacher and learner, and the principle that learning occurs when stimuli are associated with responses that are systematically rewarded.

AUSUBEL'S COGNITIVE THEORY

David Ausubel's learning perspective is concerned with nonobservable forms of behavior (thinking) and addresses how learners solve problems and form concepts. Often, this theory is referred to as the cognitive/discovery perspective because it stresses thinking (cognition) and the ways learners discover relationships, which are basic to problem-solving and concept formation. Central to Ausubel's theory is the assumption that the most salient factors influencing learning are the stability, clarity, and organization of the learner's present knowledge. Raw perceptual information, facts, concepts, and theories constitute a learner's present knowledge and, in this perspective, are referred to as a learner's cognitive structure. This is a most significant precept when related to health teaching, because the nurse must accurately assess the make-up of the patient's cognitive structure. Simply stated, what knowledge does the patient bring to a particular teaching and learning situation? Once the patient's cognitive structure has been assessed (pretesting, questioning, open discussion), a decision must be made as to how the material should be presented for maximum learning effectiveness. According to Ausubel's theory, this can be dealt with in one of two ways. One methodology is to present the entire content of what is to be learned in final form. This is called *reception learning*. For example, the nurse may say to the patient, "It is important that you take your pulse before taking your digitalis medication." The fact is presented, and the patient is asked to internalize it so that it can be reproduced at some future time. The important point is that the learning task does not involve any independent discovery by the patient.

Using the second methodology, the principal content to be learned is not presented in final form but must be independently discovered by the patient before internalization. This is termed *discovery learning*. Using the digitalis example again, the nurse may utilize a form of

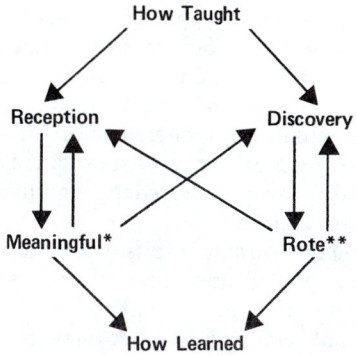

Figure 8–1. The teaching-learning theories of Ausubel.

guided discovery learning whereby, after explaining the action of digitalis, the nurse asks the patient how to determine whether to take the medication each day. The probable result would be the patient learning how to take his or her own pulse. The initial phase of discovery learning, therefore, involves a process quite different form that of reception learning. The learner must rearrange a given array of data, integrate it with existing knowledge (cognitive structure), and generate a new concept or thought. In presenting material, the nurse must choose which methodology is best suited to the learning style of the patient. Up to this point, the discussion has focused on how the material is presented to the learner.

In the second stage, the learner acts to retain the idea by relating the material to what he or she already knows and therefore to make sense of the new thought or concept. If a relationship is formed, then meaningful learning results. The new material attains meaning, and internalization of the concept follows. However, if the material is not related to what the learner already knows, then rote or meaningless learning results. In this type of learning, no relationship is formed; the patient simply memorizes the material, and the idea is not internalized or integrated with existing knowledge in a usable form. Thus, the bases of Ausubel's learning perspective are four relatively independent learning styles (Fig. 8–1):

1. Meaningful/reception
2. Meaningful/discovery
3. Rote/reception
4. Rote/discovery

The four combinations of the reception/discovery-meaningful/rote dimension learning styles can be illustrated as follows:

1. *Meaningful/reception learning* occurs when the teacher presents the generalization in its final form (reception teaching) and the learner relates it to his or her cognitive structure in some sensible way (meaningful learning).
2. *Rote/reception learning* results when the teacher pre-

sents the generalization (reception teaching) and the learner memorizes it but does not relate it to other ideas in his or her cognitive structure (rote learning).

3. *Meaningful/discovery learning* results when the learner formulates the generalization himself or herself (discovery teaching) and subsequently relates it in a sensible way to existing cognitive structure (meaningful learning).

4. *Rote/discovery learning* results when the learner discovers the generalization himself or herself (discovery teaching) and subsequently memorizes the new idea without relating it to other relevant ideas in his or her cognitive structure (rote learning).

Ausubel's Teaching and Learning Principles As Applied to Patient Education

Ausubel's theory is concerned with the formulation of significant relationships by relating meaningfully learned materials to existing concepts in the learner's cognitive structure. Most new materials that patients encounter in a health setting may not be able to be related to a previously learned background of ideas and information.

When relevant ideas are not available, Ausubel advocates the use of advance organizers. These teaching tools are presented in advance of the actual teaching and help to facilitate the learning process by providing the patient with relevant anchoring ideas. These prelearning organizers are usually in the form of introductory materials such as films, videotapes, slides, or handling of equipment (e.g., insulin syringe). In this way, the nurse educator ensures that anchoring ideas are available for the material that follows.

This is particularly true for the newly diagnosed patient—one with myocardial infarction, diabetes, cerebrovascular accident—who, until the point of incident or diagnosis, may have experienced relatively good health. Thus, it is of critical importance that the nurse completely assess the patient's existing knowledge base (cognitive structure) from which health teaching may proceed. Once this is established and when applying Ausubel's theory, the nurse must remember that logical structure, lucidity, and sequencing of the learning materials are most important because the cognitive structure is hierarchically organized. That is, as new material enters the patient's cognitive field, it interacts, relates with, and is internalized or learned under a relevant and more inclusive conceptual system. Thus, learning is structured so that it is sequential and building.

A patient is motivated to learn by being provided with potentially meaningful material that becomes meaningful as it is related to existing ideas in the cognitive structure. This provokes the beginning of further reasoning and a desire to learn. Because each patient has had different previous experiences and different ideas in the cognitive structure, it is reasonable to expect that a variety of teaching methodologies should be provided to allow for variance in learning styles.

Significantly, the relevance of the pattern formed depends on the number of items in the patient's cognitive structure to which the new material can be related.

Therefore, learning factors such as age, educational background, familiarity of subject matter, reading and comprehension ability, vocabulary, and readiness to learn (adequate background knowledge) must be evaluated in the preteaching assessment period to ensure the presentation of materials at a level appropriate to the patient's learning capabilities.

When using this teaching-learning strategy, the most appropriate evaluation tool is the pretest and posttest to measure and demonstrate evidence of learning. Because this learning perspective is most suited for the independent, motivated learner with a high level of reading ability, patient verbalization and demonstration of learned procedures (self-evaluation) may also be used as evidence of teaching effectiveness and learning. A joint evaluation by the nurse and patient may also be utilized to assess the level of individual progress. Furthermore, the ability to solve or transfer learning from original problems to other situations provides evidence of meaningful/reception, meaningful/discovery learning.

Summary

According to Ausubel's theory, learning occurs when a patient becomes aware of a new pattern of relationships. Therefore, a key variable in this perspective is the way in which material is organized for presentation to the patient, who brings prior associations to the teaching and learning experience. The role of the nurse educator takes into account the following principles:

1. Pre-assessment of the patient's learning style, readability level, and existing cognitive structure
2. Prior organization and logical sequencing of learning materials
3. Nurse's acquisition of a thorough knowledge of material to be taught
4. The utilization of meaningful/reception, meaningful/discovery strategies
5. The learner's active involvement with material over time
6. Lucidity and clarity in presentation
7. Advance organizers or anchoring ideas to facilitate relationship

ROGERS' INTERPERSONAL/ HUMANISTIC PERSPECTIVE

Carl Rogers' interpersonal learning perspective takes into consideration the way each individual modifies knowledge patterns on the basis of experience. Rogers, who began his career as a psychotherapist, came to the conclusion that the principles of client-centered or nondirective therapy (the client rather than the therapist is the central figure) could be applied just as successfully to teaching. He proposed that the teacher become learner-centered, that is, that the learner become the central figure in the teaching and learning process. In adopting this perspective, Rogers suggests that teachers try to establish the same conditions as client-centered therapists and sums up the qualities of the teacher who uses the following learner-centered approach to teaching.

In the *humanistic perspective*, the teacher assumes the role of facilitator of learning, the primary requisite of which is to develop a profound trust in the student to develop his own potentiality for learning. Once trust is established, the teacher can give the learner the opportunity to choose his or her own way of learning. Other characteristics of the facilitative teacher are sincerity, honesty, and the absence of facade. The teacher becomes a person to the learner. The facilitative teacher adopts a positive attitude toward the learner by prizing the learner's feelings and opinions and subsequently developing an empathic awareness of the ways in which the teaching-learning process appears to the learner. The teacher becomes aware of and empathizes with the anxious, the shy, the slow, or the unmotivated learner. Finally, the humanistic perspective points out that students should be helped to become aware of and clarify their values. Rogers' perspective is holistic in that not only the cognitive and psychomotor skills but also the affective domain of emotions and feelings, as well as communication skills, are considered and brought into any teaching-learning situation. Experiential or "significant" learning is a type of learning that occurs when applying the humanistic perspective to any given learning situation. Rogers has identified four elements involved in experiential learning:

1. Personal involvement. The whole person, in terms of feelings, cognition, and psychomotor aspects, is involved in the learning event.
2. Self-initiation. Even when the stimulus is external, the sense of comprehension comes from within the learner.
3. Pervasiveness. The learning makes a difference in the behavior, attitudes, or even the personality of the learner.
4. Self-evaluation. The focus of evaluation is in the learner.

For experiential learning to occur, Rogers further suggests that conventional education be replaced with a student-centered, multifaceted curriculum. The intention is to surround the learner with a multitude of learning resources, a learning environment from which the learner selects those learning experiences to meet individual needs.

Rogers' Teaching and Learning Principles As Applied to Patient Teaching

For Rogers, the goal of education is not teaching but the facilitation of change and learning. In adopting this perspective, the nurse must be cognizant of several conditions that facilitate learning, most important of which is the attitudinal quality of the interpersonal relationship between teacher and learner.

In the role of teacher, the nurse should be aware of the extent to which he or she directs and controls learning and, whenever possible, should permit and encourage patients to make choices and manage their own learning. In this way, learning can be self-paced and individualized. It is imperative that the nurse establish a

warm, positive, accepting atmosphere in which the feeling that every patient can learn is communicated. Whenever possible, the nurse functions as a facilitator, encourager, helper, and assister and assumes a supportive role. Further, the nurse helps the patient to develop a positive self-image by demonstrating sensitivity to the patient's feelings. Finally, the nurse makes himself or herself available as a resource person, remembering that self-criticism and self-evaluation are basic, whereas evaluation by the teacher is of secondary importance.

In evaluating employment of a learning environment based on Rogerian principles, the nurse may find this perspective particularly useful for the anxious, shy learner, for one who may recently have suffered a devastating blow to self-esteem (as, for example, in myocardial infarction) or for those patients with chronic diseases, such as emphysema, colitis, or rheumatoid arthritis. Initially, the nurse devotes time to establishing a warm, caring interpersonal relationship with the patient and provides an accepting atmosphere in which motivation to learn is fostered. In establishing a learning climate (regardless of the health teaching involved), a variety of teaching methodologies are available for the patient to select the approach best suited to individual needs. Allowing the learner to have control over part of the teaching and learning experience may well be the first step toward renewed self-esteem and improved attitude toward self, as the patient begins assuming responsibility for his or her own learning.

Summary

In summary, this learning perspective provides a methodology for individualized instruction, involving an interpersonal relationship where the patient learns on his or her own terms and at a rate comfortable for the individual. Also, as a result of being exposed to various curricular materials and methods, the patient develops a growing methodology that is suited to his or her own style of learning.

Perhaps the most salient aspect of this approach is the interpersonal relationship established between patient and nurse. Through personal communication, positive reinforcement, and a nonthreatening environment, the nurse may be able to change or modify the patient's ways of thinking so as to change attitudes toward health and serve as a motivation for learning. The perspective may be particularly useful for the patient who is illiterate or who has a low readability level. The nurse's sensitivity, nonjudgmental attitude, and acceptance of these factors may be the difference between patient compliance and noncompliance.

One of the major ways by which significant or experiential learning becomes responsible learning is through the evaluation of one's own learning. The patient learns to take responsibility for himself or herself and directs the learning process by setting goals to pursue and then evaluates the extent to which these goals have been achieved. For this reason, it seems critical that some degree of self-evaluation be incorporated into the attempt to promote any type of experiential learning. Although joint evaluation between teacher and learner may be used, independence and self-reliance are facilitated when self-evaluation is used and evaluation by others is of secondary importance.

The nurse, after assessing the patient's readability level, then decides which of the three theories or combination thereof, is appropriate for any given teaching and learning situation. Although a patient may have a high level of reading ability (e.g., 13), the diagnosis, prognosis, therapy, or change in life style may have increased the patient's stress and anxiety level so that learning will be more effective by incorporating Skinner's reinforcement techniques and/or Rogerian principles in addition to Ausubel's cognitive style. Combining aspects of all three theories and utilizing parts of each as the patient's teaching needs change will significantly increase the patient's knowledge level and motivation for compliance.

THE NURSING PROCESS FOR PATIENT TEACHING-LEARNING AND COMPLIANCE

ASSESSMENT

In gathering information to formulate a data base upon which a teaching and learning experience is implemented, it is to the nurse's advantage to take into consideration specific aspects of the adult learning perspective previously discussed. The nurse establishes a trusting, nonthreatening relationship with the patient, one in which the patient is made to feel worthwhile and able to learn. Since it is so important to establish initial rapport, the nurse might consider Rogers' interpersonal concept of forming a strong, caring alliance with the learner. This alliance reduces fear of failure, or perhaps lowers a high level of anxiety on the part of the learner, because the nurse conveys a sincere trust in the patient's ability to learn and succeed. In this perspective, the patient becomes the focal point in the learning process, and the nurse assumes the role of facilitator, assessing those factors such as anxiety that may inhibit learning and giving support, empathy, or encouragement in the initial development of a trusting interpersonal relationship upon which learning can proceed. The nurse performs a patient assessment in an environment totally devoid of threat to the self-esteem; and the patient assumes the role of partner in the teaching and learning process, giving freely of information and asking questions in an environment that is nonjudgmental and open.

The nurse includes in the data base an assessment of the patient's educational background; reading ability (as discussed earlier in the chapter); vocabulary level; state of readiness to learn; the level of existing knowledge of both patient and family; motivaton to learn; any cultural traditions that might affect patient and family attitudes about the disease and the treatment plan; and any ad-

ditional factors that might influence the learning environment.

Educational level and reading ability are assessed before a plan can be developed. Medical personnel who give the patient pamphlets describing various treatments or medications need to ascertain if the patient can read well enough to comprehend the material and incorporate the material into his or her existing cognitive structure.

Although Rogers' perspective is holistic in nature, Ausubel's learning theory probably is most useful in assessing the patient's readiness to learn, as well as the clarity and organization of the patient's cognitive structure, in the preteaching phase. Skinner's theory may also serve the nurse in the assessment stage. This is particularly true of the highly anxious or slow learner, who requires positive reinforcement and a teacher-controlled learning environment where the patient is rewarded for simply answering assessment questions.

Patients who have recently undergone surgery or who have just found out they have a chronic or fatal disease may not be psychologically ready to absorb and understand information. The nurse must first work to decrease the patient's level of anxiety or depression to a mild or moderate level. When a person is in a state of panic, severe anxiety, or depression, the ability to learn greatly decreases. The nurse must wait to institute the teaching plan until the patient is receptive and ready.

The nurse also needs to assess what background information the patient already has, where this knowledge came from, and what additional information must be provided. The nurse may pose questions, administer a pretest, or utilize any method deemed appropriate to establish what knowledge the patient brings to a particular teaching and learning situation. It is also important to assess the patient's motivation to understand and comply with a treatment plan. A motivated individual desires greater knowledge about practical health care than an indifferent, hostile, or detached individual.

It is important that the nurse initially approach the patient with a positive attitude and expect that the patient will comply with the treatment regimen. However, since noncompliant behaviors are prevalent, the nurse anticipates that these patterns of behavior may be demonstrated by many patients.

During the past decade, research has been undertaken to determine if it is possible to predict the patients who will not comply with their regimens. These studies have had varying results in terms of delineating specific cues that may be correlated with compliant or noncompliant behaviors. However, it is important to recognize that noncompliance has not been correlated with the potential seriousness or duration of a specific illness. Instead, noncompliance is a multifaceted problem which appears to be created by many factors. Research has identified major categories of factors appearing to promote noncompliance. These include the patient's attitudes, motivation, locus of control, level of education, and support systems. The health care regimen has also been recognized as an important factor. Table 8–3 has been developed after a review of the literature on predicting

Table 8–3. ASSESSMENT OF CUES PREDICTIVE OF NONCOMPLIANCE

Patient Factors to Be Assessed	Characteristics of Patient Factors That Correlate with Noncompliance	Method of Nursing Assessment
Feelings regarding illness	Subjectively believes illness is not as severe as perceived by health professionals	Ask "How would you describe the severity of your illness?"
Locus of control	Demonstrates cues of external locus of control, believes that powerful figures, luck, and/or fate are controlling life	Ask "What do you think caused this health problem? What do you think needs to be done to overcome this health problem? What are your goals for treatment?"
Beliefs regarding health status	Believes he or she is less susceptible to actual and potential illnesses than other people	Ask "How do you feel about the statement, 'I worry a lot about my health'?" Ask "Would you describe yourself as being healthy or unhealthy?"
Beliefs regarding the effectiveness of medical care	Believes medical care is not effective	Ask "How would you describe the effectiveness of your care?"
Feelings of satisfaction with treatment	Expresses dissatisfaction	Ask "How do you feel about your care?"
Feelings about prior care	Felt dissatisfied: "It was a waste of time and money"	Ask "How do you feel about your past care?"
Patient's perceptions of health care plan	Perceives plans to be A. Difficult to follow B. Vague and ambiguous C. Disruptive to premorbid lifestyle	Ask "How do you feel about your plan of care?" "How does this plan affect your daily routine?"
Patient's perceptions of goals of treatment	A. Does not believe goals are relevant to him or her B. Believes patient was not involved in setting the goals C. View of goals as being vague or too difficult to achieve	Ask "How do you feel about the goals of the health care plan?" "What are your goals for your treatment?" "How do you feel about this statement, 'The doctor wants me to come back even though it is not necessary'?"
Patient's perceptions of physician	A. Viewed as being unfriendly and uncaring B. Perceived as rejecting the patients concerns and feelings C. Viewed as disagreeing with the patient's goals D. Communicates in an ambiguous manner. (This feeling may be intensified with the use of medical and technical jargon) E. Experiences feelings of disruption in the continuity of care by members of the health team F. Believes the physician does not show any interest in how patient is complying with the treatment regimen	Ask "Describe your doctor." "How do you feel right after you see your doctor?"
Level of trust in physician and health care system	Believes one should not trust physicians and hospitals	Ask "Describe your doctor." "How do you feel right after you see your doctor?"

CONTINUED ON THE FOLLOWING PAGE

Table 8–3. ASSESSMENT OF CUES PREDICTIVE OF NONCOMPLIANCE–CONTINUED

Patient Factors to Be Assessed	Characteristics of Patient Factors That Correlate with Noncompliance	Method of Nursing Assessment
Intentions of compliance	Never intends to comply (Davis, 1968)	Ask "How do you intend to take your medications?" "How do you feel about this statement, 'I try to do what my doctor tells me, without question'?"
Coping mechanisms	Use of denial* and repression, which result in not recognizing need for treatment or being unable to mobilize energies to cope	Assess for cues of denial, such as "I'm not ill."
Level of self-esteem	Low	Assess for verbal cues, such as, "Don't bother with me, I'm not worth the effort," and nonverbal cues of disinterest in self.
Reactions to illness	A. Reacts with anger, aggression, and demanding behaviors B. Exhibits low level of fear and anxiety, which decreases motivation to respond to danger C. Exhibits high level of fear and panic, which immobilizes attempts to cope with danger D. Exhibits depression, which limits abilities to learn and to cope	Assess for verbal and nonverbal cues of anxiety, fear, anger, depression, hopelessness, helplessness, worthlessness. Ask "How do you feel regarding your illness?"
Methods of compliance with prior treatment regimens	Exhibited noncompliance; states, "I never take medicines"	Ask "How often did you take your medicine for a past illness?"
Methods of compliance with concurrent medication regimens	Exhibits noncompliant behaviors	Ask "How often do you take your pills for concurrent illness?"
Reactions of mothers of young children	A. Expresses feelings of being unable to get through the day with the children B. Has no situational supports to help care for the children (Becker et al, 1972)	Ask "Who helps you with your children?" "How often do you have time for yourself?"
Financial status	A. Poverty level B. Unemployed C. Lacks medical insurance D. Believes medications are not worth what they cost	Check financial data on admissions form.
Status of family	A. Family is experiencing conflict and insecurity B. Lives alone	Assess for nonverbal cues of family disharmony. As "Who do you live with?" "When you want to talk about a problem, whom do you go to?"
Level of symptoms	A. Currently asymptomatic B. Feels he or she has returned to "normal"	Ask "What are the symptoms of your illness now?"
Side effects resulting from drugs	Noncompliances increases with A. Dizziness B. Fatigue C. Gastrointestinal distress D. Impotence E. Side effects that interfere with work abilities (Daniels and Kochar, 1979)	Ask "What side effects are you experiencing now?" "How do they affect your work?" "How do they affect your daily activities?"

*The nurse must recognize that denial is considered adaptive during the initial stages of coping with a crisis. It is imperative that this mechanism be allowed unless it totally interferes with the progress of treatment.

noncompliant behaviors. It is important for the nurse to recognize that any single clue, by itself, may not be significant in predicting noncompliance. However, when a patient demonstrates a cluster of such cues, the nurse anticipates that the patient is a strong candidate to exhibit noncompliant behaviors. Table 8–3 assists the nurse in assessing whether any given patient is likely to be compliant or noncompliant.

The nurse assesses cues of noncompliant behaviors. If the patient portrays a cluster of such cues, the nurse attempts to determine whether the problem of noncompliance is actual, or merely a potential one. Furthermore, it is important to determine which factors are causing the noncompliant behaviors. This specification focuses the nurse's attention on the unique needs of the patient for a certain type of nursing intervention, rather than viewing each noncompliant patient as requiring the same approach.

For example, the attitudes of the patient and family toward health, personal health habits, chronic illness, and the health care team need to be assessed before planning and intervention can proceed. Additionally, cultural traditions and the accumulated wisdom of family members must also be assessed, especially when the nurse and family are caring for a very young or very old patient, because these factors impact upon compliance. Frequently, individuals who decided not to comply with the treatment regimen had already made this decision before leaving the health care setting. Therefore, it is important for the nurse to begin assessing the patient for cues to predict noncompliance as soon as possible. Members of the health care team must acknowledge the reality that merely telling a patient to follow a specific regimen does not guarantee compliance.

It may be useful for the nurse to select aspects from all learning theories in establishing a preteaching assessment, as principles from one or more of the perspectives may be appropriate to individualize each teaching and learning plan. Selecting the most effective principles for obtaining baseline information may well set the stage for a successful learning experience for the patient and ultimately compliance with the treatment regimen.

NURSING DIAGNOSES

In establishing nursing diagnoses relative to a teaching and learning situation, a combination of Rogerian and Skinnerian principles is useful. When a lack of knowledge or psychomotor skills is identified, the patient may become anxious, fearful, or even overwhelmed at the thought of what he or she must learn to maintain a state of health.

The whole patient—feelings, cognition, and psychomotor aspects—is considered in further developing a caring, trusting interpersonal relationship between patient and nurse. Skinner's theory suggests breaking the nursing diagnosis down into very small steps, followed by reward, to reduce anxiety and facilitate comprehension. As with nursing assessment, this stage is totally teacher-controlled. Ausubel's theory is useful in dealing with the highly motivated, confident learner, who is able to grasp new ideas and concepts because of the organized knowledge base the patient brings to the active learning environment. The nurse presents to the patient generalizations (objectives presented in final form) to be learned.

Typical diagnoses may include lack of knowledge about newly ordered antihypertensive medications, including propranolol (Inderal) and chlorothiazide (Diuril); lack of knowledge of new low-sodium diet, 1000 mg per day; fear of the technique and perceived inability to learn self-injection technique to administer insulin; anxiety concerning the health care treatment regimen; lack of correct knowledge about normal pregnancy; lack of family knowledge of health habits, including mouth care and hand washing, or noncompliance with the medication regimen related to lack of knowledge.

The patient and family should share in the development of the nursing diagnoses. When the patient feels involved in the decision-making process, the probability of patient compliance is enhanced because of shared patient interest.

The nurse, incorporating Rogers' perspective, would encourage questions in an open environment where the patient is free to express doubts, anxiety, or fear of being unable to learn.

PLANNING

Keeping in mind the patient's preteaching assessment plus the nursing diagnoses, the nurse formulates a teaching plan. In Rogers' perspective, the patient becomes an integral part of this phase, deciding which teaching and learning methodologies are most effective for him or her. Ausubel's theory suggests the planning of meaningful/reception, meaningful/discovery learning strategies, whereas Skinner's theory advocates that the nurse totally decide the learning environment and plan educational experiences accordingly.

Teaching techniques that might be used include individual lectures, closed-circuit television presentations, films, tape-slide or audio cassette presentations, videotapes, group discussions, panel presentations, and pamphlets or other reading materials to be used in a variety of ways with patients individually or in groups that may or may not include family members (Fig. 8–2). These materials may be prepared by the nurse and institution, or may be borrowed or bought from other agencies. The materials should be appropriate to the learner's previously determined visual and verbal learning ability. Most people learn best when material is presented visually, as this is the simplest way of learning. Pamphlets written to the learner's reading level can reinforce oral teachings. Group discussion or therapy groups are also effective teaching tools, particularly for patients with chronic diseases. Participating in groups sharing similar problems allows the patient and family to learn firsthand from other family groups. Patients and families have experiences to share that frequently provide solutions to problems other patients have experienced.

During the planning phase, all health team members share their individual goals with the patient. Ideally, all

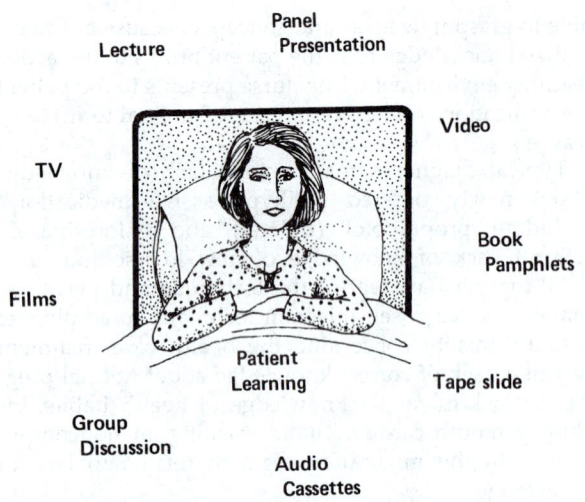

Figure 8–2. Teaching tools available today. Many vehicles are now available to assist the teaching-learning process. These include: individual or group lectures, closed-circuit television, films, audio cassettes, panel presentation, and reading materials.

health team members—physicians; pharmacists; dietitians; social workers; physical, respiratory, speech, or hearing therapists; and nurses—work together to educate the patient. Either the patient's chart or the Kardex should record the information to be taught, who taught it and when, and how comprehension was tested. Table 8–4 demonstrates the teaching file for Mr. Jones. It lists the nursing diagnosis and the material to be taught. When a health team member teaches the material, he or she records the date, initials this record of a teaching task completed, and records how the patient responded to the material. Later, during the evaluation stage, the date, teacher's initials, and the patient's response to teaching and the information are noted. The teaching file also contains several columns for evaluation to be used later.

INTERVENTION

The intervention phase is the time for teaching or presenting the new material to the learner (and family), and principles from all 3 learning perspectives may be usefully applied at this stage in the teaching and learning process. To ensure that learning can be related, according to Ausubel, meaningful/reception or meaningful/discovery learning strategies, or both are implemented. Regardless of the intervention methodology, the nurse strives to relate the new material to ideas in the patient's existing cognitive structure so that the information is comprehended and retained. Materials are presented hierarchically and are logically sequenced. To ensure that learning can be related, advance organizers, such as tapes and films, may be used before the actual teaching. Skinner's theory stresses the need to break the new learning into elemental or small steps, and then to rein-

force each step in order to facilitate the predetermined learning objective. Principles of reinforcement, extinction, discrimination, and generalization may all be employed during this phase to produce the kind of learning the nurse has decided the patient needs. Because the nurse provides the contingencies of reinforcement and determines all instructional tactics, the nurse ultimately controls the learning environment. In Roger's perspective, the patient becomes a partner in the instructional phase by selecting learning strategies believed to best fit his or her learning style. The nurse continues the role of facilitator, assisting, teaching, and advising whenever necessary, but essentialy, the instruction is patient-centered and patient-controlled.

The teaching and learning care plan is incorporated into the patient's total nursing care plan, and thus the patient's learning needs are communicated to all others involved in his or her care. The plan may be designed by the primary care nurse, team leader, or the nurse responsible for patient health teaching. Table 8–5 uses a patient situation to demonstrate a teaching and learning care plan.

The goals of teaching are achieved several days before the patient is ready for discharge. If health personnel were to give discharge instructions as the patient is going out the door of the hospital, the patient might either misunderstand or become totally disconcerted, and noncompliance would be the likely consequence (Fig. 8–3).

Teaching must occur over a span of time that allows ample periods for teaching, questions, review, and evaluation of the material. Opportunity must be provided for the patient to verbalize feelings about the material presented. Empathy at appropriate times when the patient seems to be having difficulty facilitates the learning process. The nurse's responsibility is not only to give the information to the patient but also to make sure the material is understood, retained, and accepted. During the assessment phase, the nurse began by finding out what the patient already knows about the disease and what the patient thought needed to be known. Often, if the nurse first provides the information the patient perceives to be most important, even though it is not what the nurse thinks is most important, the patient is better able to concentrate and to understand the information the nurse wants to convey.

PATIENT TEACHING

When teaching a patient about his or her pharmacology needs, the nurse must provide the following information:

1. The purpose of the medication.
2. How long the medication will be taken.
3. The correct dosage and how to measure it if it is liquid. (Liquids need to be accurately measured in measuring spoons, not in flatware.)
4. What times of day to take the medication.
5. How to take the medication, that is, whether it can be taken with (at the same time) or between meals

Table 8–4. PATIENT TEACHING GOALS

NAME _JACK JONES_   AGE _47_

DIAGNOSIS _NEW ESSENTIAL HYPERTENSION_

Nursing Diagnosis	MATERIAL TO BE TAUGHT	DATE TAUGHT & BY WHOM	PATIENT'S RESPONSE	EVALUATION OF TEACHING DATE & BY WHOM	
LACK OF KNOWLEDGE ABOUT HYPER- TENSION	ETIOLOGY OF HYPER- TENSION	4/24 MM 4/26 MM REVIEWED	ATTENTIVE RECEPTIVE	4/25 MM FAIR RECALL	4/27 MM EXCELLENT RECALL
''	DIET— 1000 mg LOW Na	4/25 KA	NOT INTERESTED	4/28 KA POOR	
		4/29 MM	RECEPTIVE	4/30 KA FAIR	
''	STRESS FACTORS	4/26 MM	INTERESTED MANY QUESTIONS		
''	EXERCISE PROGRAM	4/27 AK	ATTENTIVE INTERESTED		
''	MEDICATION DIURIL	4/26 DR.C.M.			

(one hour before or two hours after); whether it is chewed or swallowed; and whether there are any food and/or alcohol restrictions.

6. What signs are evident to indicate that the medicine is working. For example, a bronchodilator should relieve bronchospasms, and pain should be relieved after analgesics are administered.

7. What the side effects are. Without unduly alarming the patient, the nurse must encourage the patient to report any persistent or unusual symptoms, such as unplanned weight gain or loss, increasing fatigue, stomach distress, anorexia, decreasing exercise tolerance, or increasing fatigue, to name just a few.

The patient is taught the signs of toxicity of the medication, such as ototoxicity from the aminoglycoside antibiotics, congestive heart failure from β-adrenergic blockers, or severe angina from thyroid medications. Without alarming the patient, the

nurse must convey the importance of these symptoms and the need to report them immediately.

8. What the patient should do about forgetting to take a dose or an entire day's regimen of a certain medication.

9. The importance of taking the medication until it is used up and having a prescription renewed between visits to the physician. Because some medications are expensive, the patient may neglect to have a prescription refilled.

10. How to store the medication properly.

11. The patient's use of a medication profile card to keep track of all medications. Table 8–6 illustrates a profile card that lists the medication's name, time given, description, and why it is taken. On the back is the prescription number, where and how many times it was filled, and a space for additional comments. Over-the-counter medications taken by the

Table 8–5. TEACHING-LEARNING CARE PLAN

Mr. B., a 56-year old steelworker, is recovering from a myocardial infarction and has been transferred to the Intermediate Care Unit. He is married and has two grown children. The therapy regimen includes a low-sodium, low-fat, high-fiber diet and medications include digoxin 0.25 mg bid, Hydrodiuril 50 mg 8 AM daily, Procardia 20 mg qid.

Assessment	Teaching-Learning Plan	Implementation of Teaching-Learning Plan	Evaluation of Teaching-Learning Plan

1. Readability level–12th grade.
2. Reads and comprehends English.
3. Hearing and vision—wears glasses for reading.
4. Health status—no evidence of cardiac decompensation.
5. Knowledge deficit:
  a. Diet
  b. Medication
  c. Activity
  d. Pathophysiology
  e. Cardiac rehabilitation
6. Cues predictive of noncompliance—lowered self-esteem, feels worthless
	1. Adoption of Ausubel's theory. Advance organizers present material logically and sequentially.
	2. Skinner's reinforcement technique: break learning into small parts.
	3. Rogers: involve patient in teaching plan. Self-pace and individualize.
		Involve wife/family in teaching sessions. Alter plan based on patient's prognosis and needs.	Knowledge level satisfactory re
			1. Diet
			2. Medication
			3. Activity
			4. Pathophysiology
			5. Cardiac rehabilitation
			Self-esteem level satisfactory, expresses feelings of welf-worth.
			Patient compliance.

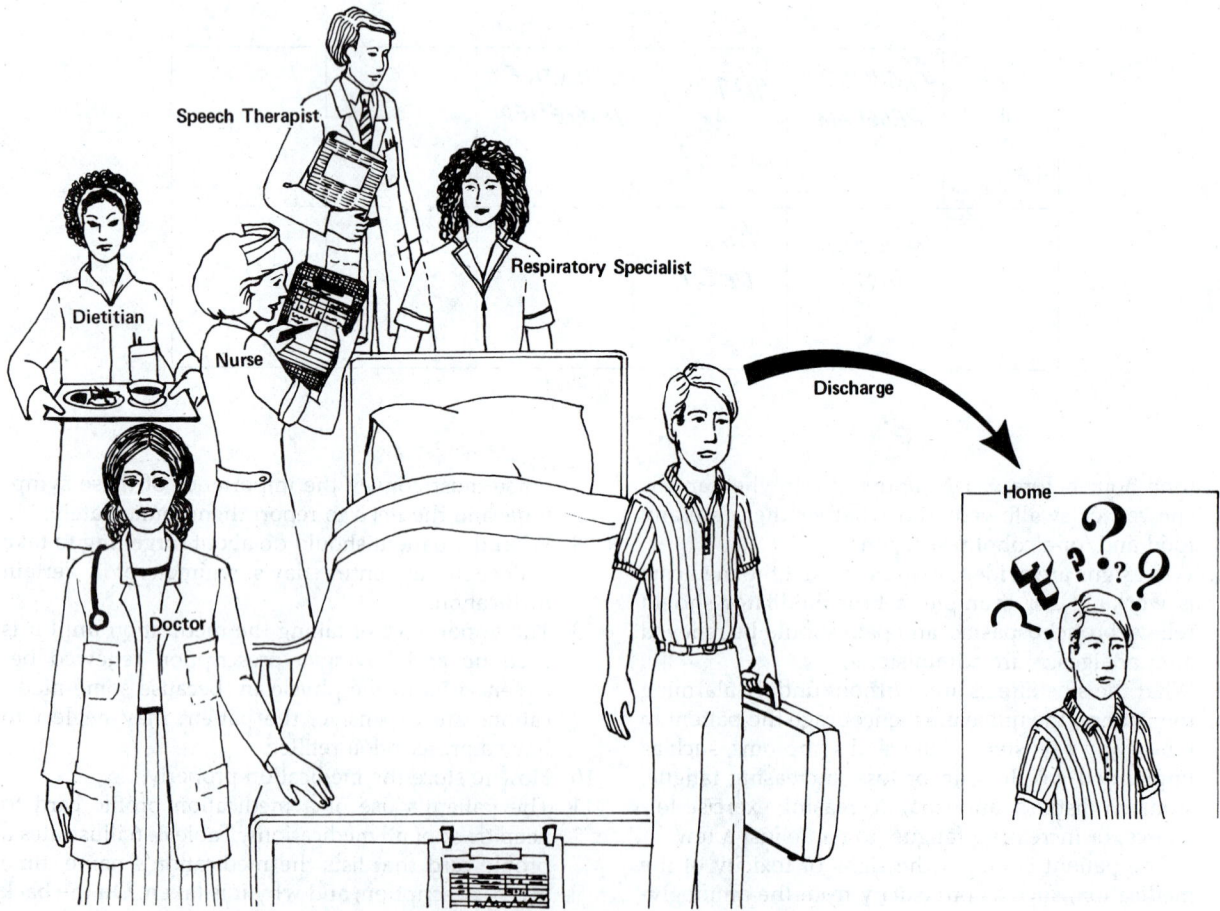

Figure 8–3. A situation to be avoided: all health professionals vying for the patient's attention before he leaves the hospital to complete their teaching. Teaching is planned and completed several days before discharge.

Table 8–6. MEDICATION PROFILE CARD

A medication profile card listing all medications, their time, description, and reason for use.

MEDICATION PROFILE FOR: Jack Jones

8A–9A Morning	12N–1P Midday	4P–5P Afternoon	8P–9P Evening	Medication	Color/ Form	Reason for Use
1	1—12N			Digoxin	White pill	Strengthen heart
				Lasix	White pill	Diuretic to reduce body water
			2	Aspirin	White pill	Thin blood and reduce clotting tendency
1 oz	1 oz—2 PM	1 oz	1 oz	Maalox	Liquid	Treat ulcer

A listing of all medications: their number, where filled, the number dispensed, and any comments.

YOU MAY WANT TO TAKE THIS PROFILE CARD WITH YOU WHEN YOU HAVE YOUR PRESCRIPTIONS FILLED BY THE PHARMACIST. PLEASE BRING THIS LIST WITH YOU WHEN YOU COME TO THE HOSPITAL OR TO YOUR DOCTOR VISITS. THIS WILL HELP YOUR DOCTORS AND PHARMACISTS TO SERVE YOU BETTER.

Rx Number	Originating Pharmacy	Medication	Number Disp.	Comments
16234	Hospital	Digoxin 0.25 mg	60	Take pulse, should be 60 or greater; do not take with Maalox.
16235	Hospital	Lasix 40 mg	60	Take early in day; drink at least 1 qt of liquid/day.

patient are also included, and this card is brought to the doctor or pharmacist at each visit.

The nurse gives the patient an information sheet on each drug. These can be made up or purchased by the institution. Figures 8–4 and 8–5, which can be obtained from ABP/Pharmex (Lea & Febiger), feature examples of patient information sheets. (The American Medical Association also produces patient information guides.) These information sheets are appropriate providing they meet the patient's readability level. The nurse can also suggest the use of a pocket personal profile, such as the one shown in Figure 8–6. When kept up-to-date by the patient and by medical personnel, the profile can help both physician and pharmacist to prevent drug interactions.

The nurse can also help the patient use a chart or graph on which to daily check off all prescribed medications as they are taken. This is particularly useful for the patient who takes multiple medications. Figure 8–7 shows one type of record that can be developed. To further facilitate the use of this chart, the medication itself can be placed to the left of its name in a glued-on pill cup. This also helps to avoid taking the wrong "little white pill" by a patient who cannot see well.

The nurse must also determine if the patient can open medication bottles. Child-proof caps can be exchanged for easy-open caps at the pharmacy if needed to prevent incidents in which patients stop taking a medication when they cannot get the bottle open. The patient and family should see and handle the medications that will

be taken at home. This helps the patient combine the teaching information with the medication to be taken.

The nurse also reviews any special precautions the patient may need to take regarding certain medications. For example, patients receiving antihypertensives are not to shower or bathe in very hot water. A patient receiving anticoagulants should shave only with an electric razor.

All special techniques the patient has to use because of a medication must also be taught, such as taking the pulse for 1 full minute before taking digitalis products or injection techniques for administering insulin.

The importance of observing proper or special diets is reviewed, such as a low-sodium diet for someone receiving diuretics or digitalis products; a low animal fat diet for someone receiving antilipemic agents; limited vitamin B_6 for someone receiving anti-Parkinson medications; or proper timing of the ingestion of cheese and milk in the diet when taking tetracycline antibiotics.

The importance of consulting with the pharmacist or physician before a patient takes any over-the-counter medications, even aspirin, is reinforced.

Any information that the nurse expects the patient to remember should be written down by the patient, checked by the nurse for accuracy, and taken home to refer to as necessary. Once the patient has received sufficient education, he or she may then make an educated decision about whether or not to comply. The ultimate choice will be the patient's.

Pharmacists are also committed to patient teaching and education. Figure 8–8 lists the guidelines for phar-

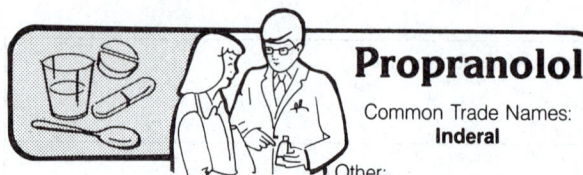

Propranolol

Common Trade Names:
Inderal

Other: _____

This medicine has many uses and the reason it was prescribed depends upon your condition. It is usually used to keep the heart beat slow and steady or to treat high blood pressure. Make sure you understand why you are taking it.

Take this medicine with a glass of water on an empty stomach at least 1 hour before (or 2 hours after) eating food unless otherwise directed. Take it at the proper time even if you skip a meal.

In some people this drug may cause drowsiness or dizziness. Do not drive a car or operate dangerous machinery or do jobs that require you to be alert until you know how you are going to react to this drug. If you become dizzy, you should be careful going up and down stairs. Sit or lie down at the first sign of dizziness.

Some non-prescription drugs, especially cough and cold remedies, may aggravate your condition. Read the label of the product you select to see if there is a warning. If there is, check with your doctor or pharmacist before using it.

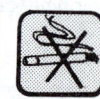

It is recommended that patients receiving this drug should stop smoking.

Call your doctor if you develop a skin rash or shortness of breath.

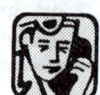

Do not stop taking this medicine suddenly without the approval of your doctor.

General Instructions for the Safe Use of Your Medicine

- Take your medicines exactly as your doctor has prescribed. Always read the prescription label carefully.
- Always tell your doctor and pharmacist if:
  — you are allergic to any drugs or other substances or have had any unpleasant reactions to drugs.
  — you have any other disease conditions.
  — you are taking any other drugs—including those products you can buy yourself without a prescription (for example: aspirin, laxatives, vitamins, cough medicines).
  — you are pregnant, plan to become pregnant or if you are breast-feeding.
  — you are planning to have dental work or surgery.
  — you are on a special diet.
  — you have been unable to take all the medicine for some reason.
- Most people experience few or no side effects from their drugs. However, if you think the medicine is bothering you and causing unusual reactions, call your doctor or pharmacist.
- Call your doctor immediately if you think you may be allergic to a medicine or if you develop a skin rash, hives, itching, swelling of the face, or difficulty in breathing.
- DO NOT take or save old medicines. Throw them away.
- STORE your drugs in a cool, dry place—NOT in the bathroom medicine cabinet. Keep all drugs out of the reach of children.
- DO NOT share your drugs with other members of your family or friends. They should see their own doctor.
- DO NOT take any other drugs (including those you can buy without a prescription) without the consent of your doctor.
- If you have any questions about your drugs, ask your pharmacist or your doctor.

◄ **Have all of your prescriptions filled at the same pharmacy** ►

These instructions may be altered by your doctor or pharmacist because of your medical condition or other drugs you may be taking.

Adapted from Smith, D.L., Medication Guide for Patient Counseling.
Exclusive permission granted by Lea & Febiger. © 1979 ABP/PHARMEX

AREA BELOW FOR DRUG MANUFACTURER'S NAME, SPECIAL INSTRUCTIONS OR YOUR STORE NAME

Figure 8–4. Propranolol drug card.

macists adopted in 1976 by the American Society of Hospital Pharmacists.

EVALUATION

The evaluation phase of the teaching-learning process may be appraised in several ways. In Ausubel's theory, the written or verbal pretest and posttest is the most appropriate tool for evaluation. In Rogers' perspective, the locus of evaluation always begins from the learner and thus mandates some form of self-evaluation. This can be accomplished through discussion, demonstration, or even a written appraisal, but the patient decides how the jointly determined educational goals are evaluated. The Skinnerian theory advocates the use of continuous feedback (formation evaluation) in the form of rewarding, or alternatively, criterion-reference evaluation,

wherein the nurse sets the standards for achievement and uses Skinnerian teaching-learning principles to guide the patient to achievement of the pre-established goals. Because the nurse is continually in the learning environment, any learner errors that are noted can be resolved immediately, preventing the interpretation of misunderstanding or confusion on the learner's part.

The evaluation process is ongoing. As material is taught and evaluated, the techniques used in the teaching are modified as necessary. Each of the goals of patient teaching is evaluated to ensure that the patient has learned the material and can use the resources given in the form of pamphlets or written materials. Any charts designed for home use should be used in the hospital for several days to avoid confusion at home. If it is possible for the patient to self-administer medications for several days prior to discharge, this also improves pa-

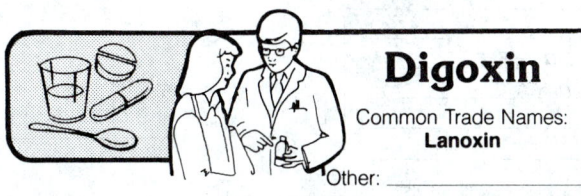

Digoxin

Common Trade Names:
Lanoxin

Other: _____

This medicine is used to help make the heart beat strong and steady.

It is very important that you take this drug as your doctor has prescribed and that you do not miss any doses. Take this medicine at the same time every day and do not go without this medicine between prescription refills.

If a dropper is used to measure the liquid dose and you do not fully understand how to use it, check with your pharmacist.

Some non-prescription drugs, especially cough and cold remedies, may aggravate your condition. Read the label of the product you select to see if there is a warning. If there is, check with your doctor or pharmacist before using it.

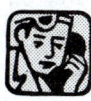

Call your doctor immediately if you develop a slow or irregular pulse, nausea, vomiting, diarrhea (loose bowel movements), loss of appetite, unusual weakness, blurred vision or changes in color vision.

General Instructions for the Safe Use of Your Medicine

- Take your medicines exactly as your doctor has prescribed. Always read the prescription label carefully.
- Always tell your doctor and pharmacist if:
  — you are allergic to any drugs or other substances or have had any unpleasant reactions to drugs.
  — you have any other disease conditions.
  — you are taking any other drugs—including those products you can buy yourself without a prescription (for example: aspirin, laxatives, vitamins, cough medicines).
  — you are pregnant, plan to become pregnant or if you are breast-feeding.
  — you are planning to have dental work or surgery.
  — you are on a special diet.
  — you have been unable to take all the medicine for some reason.
- Most people experience few or no side effects from their drugs. However, if you think the medicine is bothering you and causing unusual reactions, call your doctor or pharmacist.
- Call your doctor immediately if you think you may be allergic to a medicine or if you develop a skin rash, hives, itching, swelling of the face, or difficulty in breathing.
- DO NOT take or save old medicines. Throw them away.
- STORE your drugs in a cool, dry place—NOT in the bathroom medicine cabinet. Keep all drugs out of the reach of children.
- DO NOT share your drugs with other members of your family or friends. They should see their own doctor.
- DO NOT take any other drugs (including those you can buy without a prescription) without the consent of your doctor.
- If you have any questions about your drugs, ask your pharmacist or your doctor.

◄ Have all of your prescriptions filled at the same pharmacy ►

These instructions may be altered by your doctor or pharmacist because of your medical condition or other drugs you may be taking.

Adapted from Smith, D.L., Medication Guide for Patient Counseling.
Exclusive permission granted by Lea & Febiger. © 1979 ABP/PHARMEX

AREA BELOW FOR DRUG MANUFACTURER'S NAME, SPECIAL INSTRUCTIONS OR YOUR STORE NAME

Figure 8–5. Digoxin drug card.

tient compliance. This procedure encourages the patient to begin to take responsibility for his or her own care.

The nurse can use many techniques to evaluate the teaching effectiveness and the patient's learning. The evaluation techniques are determined jointly with the patient during the planning stage of the nursing process. The nurse gauges the effectiveness of the teaching by the amount of learning that has taken place. If minimal learning has taken place, some problem not assessed or previously predetermined prevented learning from occurring. The nurse may also use patient-completed rating scales to determine teaching effectiveness.

The evaluation process consists of three sequential steps:

1. Developing and selecting evaluation criteria
2. Collecting specific data after the nursing intervention has taken place

3. Comparing the data collected with the criteria and baseline data (when available) and then making judgments about the nature of the behavioral change

Developing and Selecting Evaluation Criteria

The first step in the evaluation process is developing and selecting the evaluation criteria. During the nursing diagnosis and planning phase, the goals of the nursing intervention were established in measurable terms. These goals now become the criteria for evaluation. For example, a goal might have been: patient will be able to demonstrate successful and correct insulin injection technique. Now the nurse needs to collect the data that substantiate the successful completion of that goal.

The conditions under which evaluation takes place are spelled out in the behavioral objectives. There are

FRONT OF CARD

MEDICATION PROFILE FOR: _JACK JONES_

PHYSICIAN: _DR. KING_   MEDICAL PROBLEM: _GASTRIC ULCER &_

DRUG ALLERGIES: _NONE_   _HEART DISEASE_

FOOD ALLERGIES: _NONE_

8A – 9A MORNING	12N – 1P MID-DAY	4P – 5P AFTER-NOON	8P – 9P EVENING	MEDICATION	COLOR/FORM	REASON FOR USE
	1^{-12}			DIGOXIN	WHITE PILL	STRENGTHEN HEART
1				LASIX	WHITE PILL	WATER PILL
		2		ASPIRIN	WHITE PILL	THIN BLOOD
1 OZ.	1 OZ. 2 PM	1 OZ.	1 OZ.	MAALOX	WHITE LIQUID	TREAT ULCER

FRONT OF CARD

BACK OF CARD

YOU MAY WANT TO TAKE THIS PROFILE CARD WITH YOU WHEN YOU HAVE YOUR PRESCRIPTIONS FILLED BY THE PHARMACIST. PLEASE BRING THIS LIST WITH YOU WHEN YOU COME TO THE HOSPITAL OR TO YOUR DOCTOR VISITS. THIS WILL HELP YOUR DOCTORS AND PHARMACISTS TO SERVE YOU BETTER.

R$_x$ NUMBER	ORIGINATING PHARMACY	MEDICATION	NUMBER DISP.	COMMENTS
16234	HOSP.	DIGOXIN 0.25 mg	60	TAKE PULSE SHOULD BE 60 OR GREATER DO NOT TAKE WITH MAALOX
16235	HOSP.	LASIX 40 mg	60	TAKE EARLY IN DAY DRINK AT LEAST 1 qt. OF LIQUID

BACK OF CARD

Figure 8–6. A pocket personal profile card that can easily be carried in a wallet. This card helps prevent drug interactions.

various forms of evaluation, but two are particularly useful in appraising the performance of the learner. The first of these, *formative evaluation,* is the process of gathering information about patient performance and providing feedback as soon as possible. This positive reinforcement by the nurse is intended to bring the patient closer to the stated objective. In the second form of evaluation, *criterion reference evaluation,* the patient's performance is compared with a relatively fixed standard that has been decided on in advance. However, criterion standards are established so that all patients can meet the conditions to demonstrate achievement. This evaluation process assumes varying time periods for achievement and provides a continuous, individualized evaluation process for the learner. Criterion reference and formative evaluation go hand in hand by providing feedback to guide and redirect the behavior being evaluated.

Methods of Evaluation

Methods of evaluation include information discussions, formal paper-and-pencil tests, oral quizzes, immediate return demonstrations, and delayed return demonstrations (several days or weeks after initial demonstration) with identified rationale for performing the procedure. The nurse and patient may have previously decided to evaluate the insulin injection technique by delayed re-

PATIENT MEDICATION RECORD (DATES)							
Medication	9/1 S	9/2 M	9/3 T	9/4 W	9/5 Th	9/6 F	9/7 S
PREDNISONE (5mg) (STEROID) SMALL PINK TABLET 3 TABLETS DAILY EVERYOTHER DAY	9		9		9		9
VALIUM (5mg) (RELAXER) SMALL BLUE TABLET 1 TABLET 4× DAILY	9 7 / 6 10	9 7 / 6 10	9 7 / 6 10	9 2 / 6 10	9 2 / 6 10	9 2 / 6 10	9 2 / 6 10
DIGOXIN (.25mg) (HEART) SMALL WHITE PILL 1 TABLET DAILY	12 PULSE—62	12 PULSE—70	12 PULSE—62	12 PULSE—	12 PULSE—	12 PULSE—	12 PULSE—
MAALOX (1 OZ.) (STOMACH) AFTER MEALS & AT BEDTIME	9 7 / 6 10	9 7 / 6 10	9 7 / 6 10	9 2 / 6 10	9 2 / 6 10	9 2 / 6 10	9 2 / 6 10
DIURIL (50 mg) (WATER) 1 TABLET DAILY	9	9	9	9	9	9	9

Figure 8–7. A patient medication record. To help a patient remember multiple medications, a chart can be developed. As the patient takes the medication, it is checked off.

turn demonstration with identified rationale for performing the procedure.

As the patient performs the return demonstration, the nurse compares the previous demonstration with that being performed by the patient. If learning is not complete, the situation is reassessed, new goals are established, and the process begins again. If the evaluation shows that the nurse/client objectives have been achieved, the nursing process is complete, and the intervention can be terminated.

Some patients may not be able to manage self-medication at home. If so, other arrangements must be made before discharge. These arrangements can include living with other family members, enlisting family or neighbors to assist the patient, suggesting visits by a visiting nurse or a home health aide, or transferring the patient to an extended care or nursing home facility.

Upon discharge from the health agency, the patient optimally returns at specified intervals to the outpatient clinic where learning retention and compliance are evaluated, using the aforementioned evaluation methodol-

ogies appropriate to each learning perspective. If the patient is unable to make follow-up visits or has never been hospitalized, a follow-up questionnaire may be a useful evaluation tool to obtain information and appraise teaching effectiveness. In other cases, a home visit or phone call may be appropriate to maintain patient contact and to evaluate compliance and learning retention.

During this evaluation phase, the nurse directly asks how the patient is following the treatment regimen. Specific questions the nurse should ask to determine compliance versus noncompliance include

● How do you take the medication?
● How often do you take the medication?
● How do you feel it is helping you?
● How often do you forget to take it?
● How often do you increase or decrease the dose?
● What is your reason for changing doses?
● What side effects are you having?
● How often do the side effects bother you?

ASHP Guidelines on Pharmacist-Conducted Patient Counseling

It is well documented that safe and effective drug therapy most frequently occurs when patients are well informed about medications and their use. Knowledgeable patients exhibit increased compliance with drug regimens, resulting in improved therapeutic outcomes. Therefore, pharmacists, as well as other health professions, have a responsibility to properly inform patients about their drug therapy.

Pharmacists' drug consultations with patients should be aimed at improving therapeutic outcomes by maximizing proper use of medications. Pharmacists, in conjunction with other health team members whenever possible, must make appropriate value judgments to determine the specific information and counseling required in each patient care situation.

Using suitable verbal, written or audiovisual communication techniques and methods, the pharmacist should inform, educate, and counsel patients (or their representative or guardian) about the following items for each medication in the patient's drug regimen.
- 1. Name--trademark, generic, common synonym or other descriptive name(s);
- 2. Intended use and expected action;
- 3. Route, dosage form, dosage and administration schedule;
- 4. Special directions for preparation;
- 5. Special directions for administration;
- 6. Precautions to be observed during administration;
- 7. Common side effects that may be encountered, including their avoidance and action required if they occur;
- 8. Techniques for self-monitoring of drug therapy;
- 9. Proper storage;
- 10. Potential drug-drug or drug-food interactions or other therapeutic contra-indications;
- 11. Prescription refill information;
- 12. Action to be taken in the event of a missed dose; and
- 13. Any other information peculiar to the specific patient or drug.

These thirteen points are applicable to nonprescription drugs as well as those ordered by a physician or other prescriber. In addition, pharmacists must counsel patients in the proper selection of nonprescription drugs as well as when and if they should be used.

Figure 8–8. ASHP Guidelines on Pharmacist-Conducted Patient Counseling. (From Medication Teaching Manual, ed 2. American Society of Hospital Pharmacists, Washington, DC, 1980, with permission.)

This kind of checking is of particular importance after the patient is well into the regimen and is once again feeling "normal." At this stage, the patient may well believe that he or she is "cured" and that it is no longer necessary to follow the plan. Thus, a follow-up call from a member of the health team is usually recommended.

Furthermore, when the nurse takes the time to focus on these issues with the patient, the patient perceives the nurse's interest in him or her as a unique human being. As noted before, giving psychosocial support tends to increase the patient's ability to comply with the treatment regimen.

After the patient has begun to comply with the plan, it is also important to follow up on issues with him or her. If the patient misses an appointment, a call emphasizes the nurse's concern and the feeling that the appointment is important.

As the nurse evaluates the effectiveness of care given, the nurse provides the patient with feedback regarding progress in complying with the treatment regimen. Ultimately, the attainment of the short-term goals leads to the achievement of the long-term goals—full understanding and compliance with the treatment regimen. This, in turn, results in the patient's illness being cured, prevented, or controlled.

SUMMARY

The nurse must be flexible in the approach to patient teaching, realizing that each stage in the nursing process may call for a different strategy, depending on the learning needs and learning style of each patient. Medication compliance may well be the ultimate outcome of a successful teaching and learning evaluation experience between nurse educator and patient.

One must suspect that a high percentage of noncompliant medication behaviors is the result of a patient's inability to read and comprehend the written instructions. Since very few educational materials are written at a level most patients can understand, the nurse must identify the patient's reading level and select all education materials appropriately before a teaching and learning plan is initiated. If poor comprehension of instruction is a major cause of failure to achieve desired goals in patient education, then it is important to distinguish between noncomprehension and noncompliance.

Table 8–7 features the principles of adult learning perspectives as they are applied to the nursing process, and Table 8–8 demonstrates application of these principles to a teaching plan.

Table 8–7. A COMPARISION OF ADULT LEARNING PRINCIPLES AS APPLIED TO THE NURSING PROCESS

Theorist	Nursing Assessment	Nursing Diagnosis	Nursing Planning	Nursing Intervention	Nursing Evaluation
Skinner	Nurse controls learning environment; determines readability level, reinforcement	Knowledge deficit(s): nurse determines.	Nurse controls simple to complex format; breaks learning into steps.	Strategies of extinction, discrimination, generalization, repetition of facts; structured environment. Reinforcement at each step.	Nurse determines: e.g., criterion reference formative evaluation.
Ausubel	Pretest to assess comprehension and readability level; nurse controls or joint determination.	Knowledge deficit(s): jointly determined.	Advance organizers such as films, written materials.	Meaningful/reception: Nurse presents in final form and patient relates to cognitive structure. Meaningful/discovery: Patient formulates generalization and relates to cognitive structure.	Post-test and/or joint evaluation.
Rogers	Patient-centered, nurse as facilitator; patient determines readability level.	Knowledge deficit(s): patient determines.	Patient is partner in planning.	Multifaceted learning environment selected by patient: e.g., open dialogue between patient and nurse.	Self-evaluation.
			Teaching begins.	Teaching–learning–evaluation continuum: open, continuous feedback system.	Learning success, compliance

Table 8–8. APPLICATION OF LEARNING PRINCIPLES TO A TEACHING PLAN FOR PROPRANOLOL (INDERAL)

Theorist	Nursing Assessment	Nursing Diagnosis	Nursing Planning	Nursing Intervention	Nursing Evaluation
Skinner	Nurse determines learning objective: e.g., patient will know when to take Inderal.	Knowledge deficit: when to take Inderal.	Break learning into steps: 1. Take on empty stomach. 2. Take 1 hr before meals. 3. Take 2 hr after meals.	Extinction—to eliminate unwanted behaviors. Discrimination—to take 1 hr before or 2 hr after meals are appropriate behaviors. Generalization—do not skip dose if at home or on vacation.	Patient is able to relate when to take Inderal.
Ausubel	Pretest, nurse or patient jointly determine learning objective: e.g., patient will know when to take Inderal.	Knowledge deficit: when to take Inderal.	Advance organizers such as drug flyer or other printed materials.	Meaningful/reception strategy: Take Inderal on an empty stomach at least 1 hr before or 2 hr after eating. Meaningful/discovery strategy: Inderal must be taken on an empty stomach. How soon before or after a meal will you take the drug?	Posttest or patient is able to relate when to take Inderal.
Rogers	Patient determines learning objective: e.g., patient will know when to take Inderal.	Knowledge deficit: when to take Inderal	Patient determines how learning will occur.	Patient selects from many options: e.g., drug flyer, self-study, A-Vs, dialogue, nurse teaching.	Patient determines learning through self-evaluation.

Research has demonstrated that patients who receive step-by-step instructions regarding medications show increased pride and confidence in their own care. They become knowledgeable about the medical regimen and can capably discuss their medications and other health responses at subsequent clinic or physician visits.

A patient and family well-educated and knowledgeable about the medication regimen can prevent unneeded hospitalizations for drug complications. Patients who have been educated are more alert to the subtle side effects some medications can cause. Early recognition can prevent possible life-threatening complications. Patient education is the key to successful medical and nursing management. The patient and the health staff share a commitment to maintaining or promoting the patient's health state.

Nursing research in the future will clearly validate approaches to patient teaching and evaluation that will prove without a doubt that patient education is, in the long run, both cost-effective and an able contributor to the improvement of medical and nursing care.

BIBLIOGRAPHY

Accreditation Manual for Hospitals. Joint Commission for Accreditation of Hospitals, Chicago, 1983.

Allensworth, DD and Luther, CR: Evaluating printed materials. Nurse Educator 11(2):18–22, 1986.

Bennett, HL: Why patients don't follow instructions. RN:45–47, March 1986.

Bormuth, JR: Reading literacy: Its definition and assessment. Reading Research Quarterly 10:7–66, 1973–1974.

Brown, CS, et al: Association between type of medication instruction and patients' knowledge, side effects, and compliance. H & CP 38:55–60, January 1987.

Brunt, B and Scott, A: Factors to consider in the development of self-instructional materials. J Contin Educ Nurs 17(3):87–93, 1986.

Doak, L and Doak, C: Patient comprehension profiles: Recent findings and strategies. Patient Counseling and Health Education 3:101–106, 1980.

Durbach, E, Goodall, R, and Wilkinson, K: Instructional objectives in patient education. Nursing Outlook 35(2):82–83, 1987.

Forman, H: Patient education and nonprescription drugs. Patient Educ Couns 8(4):415–418, December 1986.

Hill, MN: Drug compliance. Nursing '86:50–51, October 1986.

Holland, S: Teaching patients and clients. Nursing Times 82(49):34–37, 1986.

Holland, S: Teaching patients and clients. Nursing Times 83(9):56, 1987.

Johnson, MW, et al: The impact of a drug information sheet on the understanding and attitude of patients about drugs. JAMA 256(19):2721–2724, 1986.

Kasl, A and Cobb, S: Health behavior, illness behavior, and sick role behavior. Arch Environ Health 12:246, 1966.

Marchiondo, K and Kipp, C: Establishing a standardized patient education program. Critical Care Nurse 7(3):58, 1987.

Marshall, J, Penckofer, S, and Llewellyn, J: Structured postoperative teaching and knowledge and compliance of patients who had coronary artery bypass surgery. Heart Lung 15(1):76–82, 1986.

McLaughlin, HG: SMOG grading—a new readability formula. Journal of Reading 12:639, 1969.

Mooney, MA: Use of adult education principles in medication instruction—What do registered nurses know? J Contin Educ Nurs 19(3):89–92, May–June 1987.

Northrop, C: Don't overlook discharge teaching about drugs. Nursing '86 16(1):43, 1986.

A Patient's Bill of Rights. American Hospital Association, Chicago, 1975.

Quellette, F: Facilitating classroom learning: The Ausubel model. Nurse Educator 11(6):16–19, 1986.

Smith, JB: The patient who can't remember to take her meds. RN:38–41, September 1986.

Spadero, DC: Assessing readability of patient information materials. Pediatric Nursing:276–278, July/August 1983.

Streiff, LD: Can clients understand our instructions? J Nurs Scholarship 18(2):48–52, 1986.

Tullio, P, et al: Patient medication instruction and provider interactions: Effects of knowledge and attitudes. Health Education Quarterly 13:51–60, Spring 1986.

Wade, B and Bowling, A: Appropriate use of drugs by elderly people. J Adv Nurs:47–54, January 1986.

Ward, D: Why patient teaching fails, fails, fails. RN:45–57, January 1986.

SITUATION   8–1

Forty-seven-year-old Molly Black, a newly diagnosed diabetic, is prescribed teaching related to insulin administration. The nurse reviews adult teaching-learning principles before working with Ms. Black.

1. The most significant consideration for the nurse to explore prior to teaching the adult patient is:
   a. readiness to learn
   b. potential medication changes
   c. current health status
   d. age of significant others

2. The nurse plans to utilize pamphlets in teaching Ms. Black about insulin. Printed material may have limitations in patient education, due to:
   a. publication style
   b. number of illustrations used
   c. reading level of the patient
   d. number of action words used

3. The nurse plans to incorporate the concept of reinforcement during the teaching session with Ms. Black. This concept is inherent in which of the following teaching-learning theories:
   a. cognitive
   b. conditioning
   c. humanistic
   d. mechanistic

4. The nurse believes that Ms. Black should be totally involved in the teaching-learning of insulin administration. This reflects the following learning style:
   a. extinction
   b. experiential
   c. programmed
   d. rote

5. Ms. Black's ability to effectively internalize the procedure for self-administration of insulin may be *most* affected by the:
   a. type of syringe
   b. previous health care experience
   c. cultural background
   d. recent diabetic diagnosis

6. The *best* way to ensure that responsible learning about insulin administration has occurred would be through:
   a. self-evaluation
   b. standardized posttest
   c. return demonstration
   d. evaluation by the nurse

SITUATION   8–2

Ted Simmons, 56 years old, requires teaching for his cardiac medication therapy following Holter monitor evaluation.

1. In assessing Ted's readiness to learn, the nurse can *best* utilize this learning theory:
   a. Rogers'
   b. Ausubel's
   c. Skinner's
   d. McLaughlin's

2. The nurse assesses that Ted is motivated to learn about his cardiac medication because he:
   a. states that he will take his medication as ordered
   b. avoids having his wife attend the teaching session
   c. misses 50% of the questions on the medication pretest
   d. asks many questions about his health and medication

3. Ted is very anxious and overwhelmed at the thought of what he needs to learn to keep healthy. Which of the following nursing diagnoses would be *most* applicable to Ted's situation?
   a. disturbance in self-concept related to lack of understanding about cardiac medications
   b. knowledge deficit related to cardiac medications
   c. ineffective family coping related to cardiac medications

   d. alteration in compliance related to cardiac medications

4. The nurse understands that the goals of teaching should be achieved:
   a. several days before the patient is ready for discharge
   b. following instructions on day of discharge
   c. upon arriving home following discharge from the hospital
   d. immediately after presentation of material

5. The nurse would teach Ted about each of the following aspects of his cardiac medications, *except:*
   a. why he is taking the medication
   b. how to measure the correct dosage of the medication
   c. taking the medication in relation to meals
   d. how much each of the medications costs

6. In order to promote the desired learning outcomes, the nurse would use the following as a positive reinforcer for Ted:
   a. separation
   b. money
   c. smiling
   d. punishment

Please refer to the Appendices for correct answers and additional review questions with answers.

9 CHAPTER

DRUGS USED IN DIAGNOSTIC TESTING

FRANCES L. STIER, MSN, RNc

LEARNING OBJECTIVES

After reading this chapter, the student will be able to:

1. Identify the major categories of diagnostic agents.

2. Differentiate among the common diagnostic agents the indication for use, mechanism of action, mode of administration, contraindications, precautions, adverse reactions, and interactions.

3. Identify the nursing implications for the common diagnostic agents.

4. Develop a nursing teaching plan for the patient undergoing diagnostic tests.

Diagnostic testing often involves the use of chemical substances to facilitate the diagnosis of illness or to aid in the visualization of various internal structures. Although the nurse does not administer these agents, knowledge of their actions and potential adverse reactions is important in providing quality nursing care.

The diagnostic agents to be discussed are classified into the following general categories: radiopaque compounds used in diagnostic x-ray studies, agents used to stimulate glandular secretion (provocative agents), radioactive tracers used in nuclear imaging, nonradioactive dyes used in volumetric tests, and agents used in skin testing. The agents used most commonly are presented in Table 9–1.

RADIOPAQUE COMPOUNDS

Conventional x-ray studies (plain film) visualize bone and other dense structures. The x-ray beam is absorbed by the dense matter. *Radiopaque* substances inhibit the transmission of radiant energy. Thus, soft tissues (vascular structures and ductal systems, for example) have less absorption and require the presence of *radiopaque* contrast to obtain a definitive shape on x-ray films. The radiopaque contrast media used most commonly are barium sulfate and iodinated compounds.

BARIUM SULFATE

Barium sulfate is an inert, insoluble, nonabsorbable, opaque compound. It is used to visualize the gastrointestinal tract and is administered either orally or instilled rectally. The barium swallow test is used for visualizing the upper gastrointestinal tract, the pharynx, esophagus, and the stomach. The barium enema is used to examine the lower gastrointestinal tract or the colon. Barium is eliminated unchanged in the feces and may require several days for complete evacuation. Therefore, the barium enema should be performed before the barium swallow.

Contraindications and Precautions

Barium administration is contraindicated for use in individuals with fistulas, perforations of the gastrointestinal tract, or known intestinal obstructions. Because of these disorders, leakage of barium into the peritoneal cavity may result and cause peritonitis.

Adverse Effects

The most common adverse reaction following barium administration is constipation. A cathartic or cleansing enema is given after the test. Abdominal distention, cramping, or diarrhea may also occur. The patient is assessed for signs of intestinal obstruction or perforation, which include abdominal pain, distention, rigidity, vomiting, and shock. Rectal administration of barium may stimulate a vagal response resulting in bradycardia

(less than 50 beats/minute) and hypotension. This occurs more frequently in the older patient.

Nursing Implications

In preparing the patient for gastrointestinal radiographic studies using barium, the nurse assesses the patient's history for past reactions to barium and present symptoms of gastrointestinal tract obstruction or perforation. If a barium swallow is ordered, assess the patient's potential for aspiration. The patient's ability to follow directions and tolerate the procedure is also important to evaluate.

Patient Preparation

For the barium swallow the patient is allowed nothing by mouth (NPO) for 8–12 hours before the test. During the procedure the patient is required to ingest 350–425 ml of barium, which has a milkshake consistency with a chalk taste. As the patient swallows the barium, fluoroscopic image is observed and films are obtained. After the barium swallow, a cathartic is usually prescribed. The patient is informed that stools will be chalky and light-colored for 24–72 hours. Retained barium may cause fecal impaction or obstruction; therefore, the nurse must note the passage of stool. The barium should be expelled in 48–72 hours. Mouth care to remove the barium taste is also important.

The barium enema is performed before the barium swallow. Patient preparation is rigorous, and acutely ill, debilitated, or geriatric patients may not tolerate the preparation. In addition, many patients fear this test and find it painful and embarrassing.

Preparation for the barim enema varies among hospitals. The nurse should consult the policy and procedure manual for instructions. In general, the patient is put on a low-residue diet for 1–3 days or a clear liquid diet for 18–24 hours prior to the test. Laxatives are given the afternoon or evening before the test. A suppository and/or enema are administered in the evening or early morning of the test. After the test, the patient is encouraged to defecate. A cathartic or cleansing enema may be indicated. The patient's stool will be light-colored for 24–72 hours. The nurse records the passage of stool and/or the results of the enema. To avoid dehydration, the patient is encouraged to increase fluid intake. Table 9–2 is a sample of the preparation for a barium enema test.

IODINATED COMPOUNDS

The iodinated compounds are radiopaque agents that opacify structures and vessels upon contact. Visualization is maintained until significant hemodilution occurs. These agents are water-soluble. Iodinated compounds are used extensively as contrast media for a variety of diagnostic procedures including *angiography, venography, lymphography, aortography, urography, arthrography, cholecystangiography,* and *hysterosalpingography,* and in gastrointestinal radiography when barium is contraindicated. In computed tomography (CT) scans, contrast media are used to delineate soft tissue or vasculature. Iodine preparations can be administered orally or intravenously, the route depending on the area to be visualized and the method used. Oral iodinated preparations are used to assess biliary and urinary function because after absorption they are concentrated by the biliary system and excreted via the kidneys.

Nursing Implications

Prior to any test using iodinated compounds, the patient's history is obtained and any previous exposure or reaction to iodinated compounds is assessed. Allergy to foods containing iodine, for example, shellfish, is also documented and reported to the physician.

The most common reactions following intravenous iodinated compounds are pain and irritation at the injection site followed by a warm or burning sensation. Nausea and vomiting can also occur. Serious adverse reactions can occur in some individuals following the use of iodine contrast preparations. The most serious is anaphylaxis, which may result in cardiovascular collapse, CNS depression, and, if untreated, death. (See Chapter 6 for discussion on drug-induced anaphylaxis and treatment.)

AGENTS TO STIMULATE GLAND SECRETION

Agents used to stimulate glandular secretion are referred to as provocative agents because of a measurable physiologic response that is produced following their administration. There are two categories of these agents: secretagogues, which stimulate secretion of enzymes, and tropic hormones, which stimulate endocrine glands to release their hormones.

TROPIC HORMONES

Adrenocorticotropic hormone stimulates the adrenal gland to release glucocorticoids. This tropic hormone is used to diagnose adrenal insufficiency. The tropic hormone thyrotropin stimulates the thyroid gland to release thyroxine and thus aids in the differential diagnosis of primary thyroid disease versus pituitary dysfunction. Tropic hormones are reviewed in the endocrine unit.

SECRETAGOGUES

The secretagogous agents include histamine phosphate, betazole hydrochloride (Histalog), and pentagastrin (Peptavlon), which stimulate the production of gastric acid secretion; secretin, which stimulates pancreatic secretion; and sincalide, which stimulates gallbladder contraction and bile release. These agents are presented in Table 9–1.

NURSING IMPLICATIONS

Most of these agents are administered systemically, after which they move to the specific target organ and induce a measurable response. The primary function of the nurse in caring for a patient who receives a provocative agent is to monitor for physiologic responses. The agent frequently exacerbates the patient's underlying illness. The responses can be very serious. For example, when gastric acid secretion is being assessed, the increased gastric acid secretion produced by the administration of pentagastrin can cause perforation of a peptic ulcer. With administration of sincalide, acute cholecystitis may develop; and after secretion, acute pancreatitis may occur. Although these are severe responses to the provocative agents, the nurse must be prepared to know what signs and symptoms to anticipate. In addition, most secretagogues are protein substances that may stimulate an allergic reaction. Continual assessment of the patient during the testing procedure is essential.

Before the test is performed, the nurse obtains the patient's history, ascertaining information regarding the patient's underlying illness, previous history of exposure to the provocative agent, and any adverse reactions. In collaboration with the physician, the test procedure and risks are reviewed with the patient and a written consent is obtained.

For each test a procedure protocol is used. Usually the patient is NPO for 12–24 hours prior to the test, an intravenous line is inserted, and with most gastrointestinal tests a nasogastric tube is also inserted. Following the administration of the provocative agent, gastric samples and/or blood samples are obtained at timed intervals. The nurse is primarily responsible for these activities.

The patient may experience fear and anxiety prior to and during the test. Liberal reassurance and support helps to comfort the patient.

RADIOACTIVE AGENTS

Radioactive compounds are referred to as *radiopharmaceuticals*. These chemical compounds are composed of two parts: a *radionuclide*, which is an unstable nucleus with orbiting radioactive electrons, and a chemical pharmaceutical with known physiologic properties. As this unstable nucleus rearranges to become more stable, energy is emitted. This energy is radiation and is either particulate or electromagnetic. Particulate radiation is the emission of alpha and beta rays. Electromagnetic radiation is the release of gamma rays or x-rays. In diagnostic radiology, the electromagnetic radiation is measured.

A radiopharmaceutical is chosen because of its selective affinity to localize in either normal or abnormal tis-

TEXT RESUMES ON PAGE 200

Table 9–1. DRUGS USED IN DIAGNOSTIC TESTING

Name	Dosage	Mode of Administration	Pharmacokinetics
RADIOPAQUE MEDIA			
Action: Radiopaque compound.			
Use: Radiographic examination of the GI tract; barium swallow used for upper GI and barium enema for lower GI.			
Barium sulfate	Based on the region of GI tract being examined, degree of contrast needed, and technique used.	Oral: tablets, suspension Rectal: suspension	O: immediate for esophagus and stomach; 15–90 min for small intestine; immediate for colon with rectal suspensions P: variable D: 24 hr after oral administration with normal GI. For rectal administration— expelled with enema but some barium may persist for several weeks. ½ L: UA PB: UA B: unchanged E: fecal

Key to Abbreviations in the *Pharmacokinetics* column: O-onset; P-peak, D-duration; PB-protein bound; B-biotransformed in; E-excreted in; ½L-halflife.

*Within the column listing adverse effects, *underlines* indicate the most common effects; CAPITALS indicate life-threatening effects.

Contraindications/ Precautions	Adverse Effects*	Interactions	Nursing Implications
Barium swallow is contraindicated in patients with intestinal obstruction or suspected GI perforation. Use with caution in patients with obstructing lesions of the small intestine, pyloric stenosis, or tracheoesophageal fistula. Barium enema is contraindicated in patients with acute ulcerative colitis, acute diverticulitis, or suspected GI perforation. Safety in pregnancy has not been established.	GI: Constipation, intestinal obstruction, cramping from distention or diarrhea may occur. Rarely, INTESTINAL PERFORATION. Rectal administration may cause cardiac changes, bradycardia, and hypotension, especially in the elderly.	Drug: UA Lab: UA	ASSESSMENT: Obtain patient history regarding GI dysfunction and previous reactions to barium. Assess potential for aspiration. Assess the patient's ability to follow directions and tolerate the procedure. Assess the patient's understanding of the pretest dietary and fluid restrictions. If performed on outpatient status, assess the patient's ability to self-administer suppositories or enemas. After the test, assess bowel sounds to detect for possible bowel obstruction and monitor bowel movements. Monitor bowel movements to document barium evacuation and assess the patient for signs of fluid volume deficit. Notify physician if abdominal pain, decreased bowel sounds, or constipation develop. INTERVENTION: For the barium swallow the patient is NPO for 8–12 hr before the test. After the test, a cathartic is usually prescribed. Inform patient that stools will be chalky and light-colored for 24–72 hours. Record description of all stools passed. Barium should be expelled in 48–72 hours. Mouth care to remove barium taste is also important. For the barium enema follow the prescribed dietary restrictions. Give laxative, suppository, and/or enema as ordered. After the test, the patient is encouraged to defecate. A cathartic or cleansing enema is given. Stool will be light-colored for 24–72 hr. Record and describe the results of enema and stools passed. Encourage increased fluid intake to avoid dehydration.

CONTINUED ON THE FOLLOWING PAGE

Table 9–1. DRUGS USED IN DIAGNOSTIC TESTING–*CONTINUED*

Name	Dosage	Mode of Administration	Pharmacokinetics
Barium Sulfate– *Continued*			

IODINATED COMPOUNDS

Action: Organic compounds that opacify internal structures.

Use: Visualize lesions and malformations.

Name	Dosage	Mode of Administration	Pharmacokinetics
Diatrizoate sodium (Hypaque Sodium)	Dosage, mode of administration, and concentration based on the body region to be examined, technique used, and the contrast needed. Adult: 90–180 ml 25%–40% solution oral, 500–1000 ml 15%–25% solution rectal. For IV administration, dosage and concentration is individualized based on size of the vascular region to be visualized and hemodilution in the region. Children: 30–75 ml 20%–40% solution oral, 100–500 ml 10%–15% solution rectal.	Oral, rectal, IV	O: depends on region to be visualized and mode: Oral: 30–40 min (stomach) Rectal: immediate (colon) IV: immediate P: as above D: NA ½ L: 30–60 min with normal renal function, 20–140 hr with severe renal impairment PB: < 5% B: unchanged E: 95%–100% renal, 1%–2% fecal; 10%–50% fecal with severe renal impairment
Diatrizoate meglumine and diatrizoate sodium injection (Renografin 60, Hypaque M 75, Hypaque M 90)	60%, 75%, 90% solutions. Dosage and concentration are individualized and based on the size of the area to be examined and the hemodilution.	IV	O: immediate–30 min P: same D: NA ½ L: 30–60 min; 20–140 hr with severe renal impairment PB: <5% B: unchanged E: 95%–100% renal, 1%–2% fecal

Key to Abbreviations in the *Pharmacokinetics* column: O-onset; P-peak, D-duration; PB-protein bound; B-biotransformed in; E-excreted in; ½L-halflife.
   *Within the column listing adverse effects, *underlines* indicate the most common effects; CAPITALS indicate life-threatening effects.

Contraindications/ Precautions	Adverse Effects*	Interactions	Nursing Implications
			EVALUATION: Shows no adverse reaction to the barium procedure. Bowel function returned to pretest condition.
FOR ALL DIATRIZOATES: Previous hypersensitivity reaction to radiopaque agents, iodine, or shellfish. Pregnancy Use with caution in the following patient situations: severe renal impairment, severe liver impairment, hyperthyroidism, sickle cell, multiple myeloma, congestive heart disease, and pheochromocytoma.	FOR ALL DIATRIZOATES: Neuro: Headache, dizziness. CV: Hypotension or hypertension, arrhythmias (e.g., ventricular fibrillation). Resp: Wheezing, dyspnea, tightness in chest. GI: Nausea, vomiting, diarrhea, thirst. Integumentary: Warmth and flushing of skin, sweating, urticaria, rash, angioedema, chills. Hematologic: Erythrocyte sludging and agglutination, normal coagulation inhibited. Children and elderly are more sensitive.	FOR ALL DIATRIZOATES: Drug: Meperidine, morphine, and vasopressors may increase the hemodynamics and neurologic effects. Oral cholecystographic agents may cause renal toxicity when followed by IV diatrizoates. Concurrent use of IV diatrizoates with general anesthetics may increase incidence of adverse reactions. Lab: Possible interactions include decrease in leukocyte and RBC counts, increase in PT and PTT, increase in serum PBI and decrease in radioactive iodine uptake for a period of 1 week to 2 years, increase in serum amylase 6–18 hr after IV diatrizoates. Urine tests (e.g., protein, specific gravity, glucose) may be affected up to 2 days after IV diatrizoates.	FOR ALL DIATRIZOATES: ASSESSMENT: Obtain history regarding any reactions to diagnostic tests using radiopaque compounds and/or allergy to foods containing iodine (shellfish). Report positive history to physician immediately. Obtain menstrual history confirming nonpregnancy status. Assess vital signs and report any abnormalities. Obtain patient's verbal or written consent. INTERVENTION: Many different techniques are used: IV, intra-arterial, or direct instillation. Patient preparation: Usually the patient is NPO at least 8 hours prior to the test to reduce aspiration risk. Clear fluids may be given, which may prevent dehydration. This is especially important in infants, young children, geriatric, or azotemic patients. A laxative at bedtime may also be ordered. Pretreatment with corticosteroids or antihistamines may be administered to patients with a history of reactions to contrast media. Blood pressure and pulse are monitored during the examination and for at least 30–60 min after the test. EVALUATION: Shows no allergic or adverse reactions to the test. Fluid status is normal. Understands test result and follow-up.

CONTINUED ON THE FOLLOWING PAGE

Table 9-1. DRUGS USED IN DIAGNOSTIC TESTING-*CONTINUED*

Name	Dosage	Mode of Administration	Pharmacokinetics
Diatrizoate meglumine (Hypaque Meglumine injection)	30%, 60%, 76%, 85% solutions. Dosage and concentration are individualized and based on the size of the area to be examined and the hemodilution.	IV	O: immediate–30 min P: same D: NA ½ L: 30–60 min; 20–140 hr with severe renal impairment PB: very low B: unchanged E: 95%–100% renal, 1%–2% fecal

Oral Cholecystographic Agents

Action: Radiopaque organic iodine compound.

Use: Visualize gallbladder and biliary and hepatic ducts.

Name	Dosage	Mode of Administration	Pharmacokinetics
Iopanoic acid (Telepaque)	Adult: 3 g (6 tablets) 10–14 hr prior to test, or 500 mg q 1 hr × 6 doses beginning 18 hr prior to test. Not to exceed 6 g in 24 hr. Children: 50–150 mg/kg	PO	O: 4 hr P: 14–19 hr; children, 4–9 hr D: NA ½ L: 24 hr PB: high, 97% B: liver E: ⅓ renal, ⅔ fecal
Ipodate calcium	Adult: 3 g (6 capsules or 1 packet) not to exceed 6 g in 24 hr Children: 450–900 mg/kg	PO	O: 30 min for hepatic and bile ducts; 5–6 hr for gallbladder P: 1–3 hr for hepatic and bile ducts; 10 hr for gallbladder

Key to Abbreviations in the *Pharmacokinetics* column: O-onset; P-peak, D-duration; PB-protein bound; B-biotransformed in; E-excreted in; ½L-halflife.
*Within the column listing adverse effects, *underlines* indicate the most common effects; CAPITALS indicate life-threatening effects.

Contraindications/ Precautions	Adverse Effects*	Interactions	Nursing Implications
Contraindicated in patients with history of previous reaction to drug, severe renal or hepatic impairment, and severe GI disorders that prevent absorption of drug. Patients allergic to other iodinated contrast media may use iopanoic acid if premedicated with antihistamines and/or corticosteroids. Use with caution in patients with hepatic, renal, or cardiovascular disease. Patients with hyperuricemia should be well hydrated to avoid uric acid nephropathy and renal failure. Safety during pregnancy has not been established.	Neuro: Headache, dizziness CV: Coronary insufficiency, hypotension, bradycardia. Resp: Hypersensitivity reaction—bronchospasm, dyspnea, tightness in chest. GI: Nausea, vomiting, cramps, diarrhea. Hematologic: Thrombocytopenia with petechiae. Renal: Dysuria, nephrotoxicity (rare). Integumentary: Rash, pruritus, urticaria, and flushing.	Drug: Concomitant use of aspirin (600 mg) and repeated 2 hr later counteracts the uricosuric effects of iopanoic acid. Labs: False-positive results for protein in the urine may occur and last for about 3 days. Thyroid function tests based on iodine measurement are affected for several months. Sulfobromophthalein retention and serum bilirubin concentrations may be increased.	ASSESSMENT: Check patient's history for iodine allergies or previous hypersensitivity reaction to contrast media. INTERVENTION: Patient preparation: A normal diet with some fat for 1 or more days prior to the test is usually prescribed to stimulate the gallbladder. The evening meal before taking iopanoic acid tablets is low-fat or fat-free. The adult dose 3 g (6 tablets) is administered with water after the meal. Tablets are taken 1 at a time in 5-min intervals. Patient is NPO except for water until after the test. A laxative may also be prescribed to be taken 4–6 hr before taking the oral cholecystographic agent. A cleansing enema may be ordered the morning of the test to eliminate fecal contents or gas. Monitor blood pressure and pulse during and after the test. Observe for allergic or adverse reactions. EVALUATION: Understands pretest diet. Able to swallow and retain tablets. Shows no signs of adverse reactions. Understands diet modifications if gallstones are noted.
Contraindicated in patients with known allergy to ipodate calcium. Use with caution in patients with history of	Same as iopanoic acid but less common and less severe.	Drug: May partially inhibit the biliary excretion of iodipamide megulamine. The incidence and severity of adverse reactions is	Same as with iopanoic acid.

CONTINUED ON THE FOLLOWING PAGE

Table 9–1. DRUGS USED IN DIAGNOSTIC TESTING–*CONTINUED*

Name	Dosage	Mode of Administration	Pharmacokinetics
Ipodate calcium– *Continued*			D: NA ½ L: UA PB: high B: liver E: renal and fecal

SECRETAGOGUES

Gastric Function

Action: Stimulates hydrochloric acid secretion from gastric mucosa.

Use: Used in detecting achlorhydria.

Name	Dosage	Mode of Administration	Pharmacokinetics
Histamine phosphate	Expressed in terms of histamine. Adult: 0.01 ml/kg, 0.0145 ml/kg for augmented test Children: no recommended dose stated	SC; *Extreme adverse effects if inadvertently given in vein or artery. Epinephrine 1:1000, 0.5–1 ml SC, should be administered immediately.	O: immediate–15 min P: very transient D: up to 10 min ½ L: UA PB: UA B: UA E: renal
Pentagastrin (Peptavlon)	Adult: 6 μg/kg Children: not recommended	SC	O: 10 min P: 20–30 min D: 60–80 min ½ L: less than 1.0 min PB: UA B: primarily liver E: renal

Key to Abbreviations in the *Pharmacokinetics* column: O-onset; P-peak, D-duration; PB-protein bound; B-biotransformed in; E-excreted in; ½L-halflife.
*Within the column listing adverse effects, *underlines* indicate the most common effects; CAPITALS indicate life-threatening effects.

Contraindications/ Precautions	Adverse Effects*	Interactions	Nursing Implications
hypersensitivity to iodine compounds, asthma, hay fever or urticaria. Other precautions same as with iopanoic acid (Telepaque).		increased when IV iodipamide megulamine is given within 24 hr after oral ipodate calcium. Lab: Same as for iopanoic acid.	
Contraindicated in patients with asthma or other severe allergies, pregnancy, cardiac abnormalities, hypotension or severe hypertension, severe pulmonary or renal disease.	Neuro: Headache, dizziness, visual disturbances, convulsions. CV: Hypotension or marked hypertension, syncope, tachycardia, palpitations, flushing. Resp: Bronchial constriction, dyspnea. GI: Diarrhea, cramps, nausea, vomiting, metallic taste. Integumentary: Local erythema, edema, urticaria.	Drug: Unknown Labs: Unknown	ASSESSMENT: Obtain patient history, note particularly any history of dyspnea, wheezing, palpitations, syncope, or blood pressure problems. Obtain menstrual history, confirm nonpregnancy status. Assess patient's ability to follow dietary and activity restrictions. After the test, assess for adverse reactions. Monitor vital signs frequently. INTERVENTION: Patient preparation: NPO including smoking 12 hr prior to test; bedrest. Hold medications that inhibit or stimulate gastric secretion, such as antacids, anticholinergics, adrengeric blockers, and H_2 antagonists. To inhibit adverse effects of histamine, a simultaneous administration of an antihistamine may be given. Epinephrine should be available to counteract a severe reaction. Monitor blood pressure and pulse during procedure and at least 30–60 min after test. A delayed response (60 min postinjection) may occur. EVALUATION: Shows no allergic or adverse reactions. Understands test results and follow-up.
Contraindicated in patients with acute, penetrating, or bleeding peptic ulcers and in patients with known hypersensitivity. Used with caution in patients with hepatic-bili-	Infrequent and mild and less than those produced by histamine phosphate. Neuro: Headache, dizziness, blurred vision, drowsiness, fatigue, paresthesia and numbness in hands or feet. CV: Tachycardia, flushing,	Drug: Antacids prior to test decrease total effects of pentagastrin. Concurrent use of antimuscarinics, cimetidine, or ranitidine may antagonize the effect. Discontinue drugs 24 hr before test.	Same as with histamine phosphate.

CONTINUED ON THE FOLLOWING PAGE

Table 9–1. DRUGS USED IN DIAGNOSTIC TESTING–*CONTINUED*

Name	Dosage	Mode of Administration	Pharmacokinetics
Pentagastrin (Peptavlon)– *Continued*			

Pancreatic Function

Action: Increase the volume and bicarbonate content of pancreatic juice.

Use: Diagnose pancreatic exocrine disease or gastrinoma (Zollinger–Ellison syndrome).

Name	Dosage	Mode of Administration	Pharmacokinetics
Secretin (Secretin-Kabi)	1 CU†/kg (pancreatic function)	IV	O: UA P: 30 min
	2 CU†/kg (gastrinoma)	IV	D: 2 hr ½ L: 18 min PB: UA B: liver E: UA

†Clinical units

Gallbladder Function

Action: Stimulates gallbladder contraction resulting in reduction of gallbladder size and evacuation of bile.

Use: Evacuate the gallbladder after it has filled with oral cholecystographic contrast media.

Name	Dosage	Mode of Administration	Pharmacokinetics
Sincalide‡ (C8-CCK, OP-CCK)	.02 µg/kg	IV injected slowly 30–60 sec	O: NA P: 5–15 min D: 1 hr ½ L: NA PB: NA B: NA E: NA

‡Pharmacokinetics for Sincalide have not been determined (Drug Information, 88).

NONRADIOACTIVE DYES

Liver Function Tests

Action/Use: Healthy liver cells remove BSP from circulation and excrete BSP in bile; elevated levels above 5% indicate liver damage.

Name	Dosage	Mode of Administration	Pharmacokinetics
Sulfobromophthalein sodium (Bromsulphalein, BSP)	Adult: 5 mg/kg body weight; 500 mg maximal dose Children: ?	IV	O: 5 min P: 45 min following injection D: UA ½ L: UA PB: UA B: liver E: bile, fecal

Key to Abbreviations in the *Pharmacokinetics* column: O-onset; P-peak, D-duration; PB-protein bound; B-biotransformed in; E-excreted in; ½L-halflife.
*Within the column listing adverse effects, *underlines* indicate the most common effects; CAPITALS indicate life-threatening effects.

Contraindications/ Precautions	Adverse Effects*	Interactions	Nursing Implications
ary or pancreatic disease: pentagastrin can stimulate secretion of pancreatic enzymes, bicarbonate and bile. Safety in pregnancy has not been established.	palpitations, hypotension, tightness in chest. Resp: Shortness of breath. GI: Nausea, vomiting, cramps, urge to defecate, flatulence (disappear within 15 min). Integumentary: Rash, urticaria (hypersensitivity reaction), sweating, chills.	Lab: May increase bicarbonate secretion, biliary flow, and pancreatic enzymes.	
Contraindicated in patients with acute pancreatitis until attack has subsided. Safety in pregnancy or in lactation has not been established. Hyporesponsive result may occur in patients receiving anticholinergic medications or who have inflammatory bowel disease. Patients with alcoholic or liver disease may be hyperresponsive to secretin.	Possibly increases symptoms of pancreatitis (pain, nausea, vomiting). Allergic reaction may occur, manifested by skin rash to anaphylaxis.		Same as with histamine phosphate.
Use with caution in patients with suspected or known gallstones. Safety in pregnancy has not been established. Safety in children has not been established.	CV: dizziness, flushing GI: Nausea, abdominal pain or discomfort, urge to defecate.	NA	Same as with histamine phosphate.
Contraindicated in patients with asthma or any other severe allergic disease and in patients in whom a previous paravascular infiltration of BSP has occurred.	Anaphylactoid reactions especially after extravasation of BSP. Integumentary: Irritation at injection site; thrombophlebitis, cellular damage with extravasation.	Drug: Androgens, some estrogens, anabolic steroids, and oral contraceptives interfere with BSP excretion. BSP given in the same arm within a few days following	ASSESSMENT: Obtain medication history. Inform physicision if patient has been taking oral contraceptives, estrogen, androgens, or steroids. INTERVENTION: Dye is

CONTINUED ON THE FOLLOWING PAGE

Table 9–1. DRUGS USED IN DIAGNOSTIC TESTING–*CONTINUED*

Name	Dosage	Mode of Administration	Pharmacokinetics
Sulfobromophthalein Sodium (Bromosulphalein, BSP)– *Continued*			

Cardiac Function

Action/Use: Determine cardiac output by the indicator-dilution method.

Indocyanine green (Cardio-Green)	Adult: 5 mg Children: 2.5 mg Infants: 1.25 mg; total dose not to exceed 2 mg/kg	Intracardiac via cardiac catheter	O: UA P: UA D: UA ½ L: 2–3 min PB: 100% B: unchanged E: bile and fecal

DIAGNOSTIC RADIOPHARMACEUTICALS

Cardiac Function

Technetium ⁹⁹ᵐTc sodium pertechnetate ⁹⁹ᵐTc-labeled RBC

Key to Abbreviations in the *Pharmacokinetics* column: O-onset; P-peak, D-duration; PB-protein bound; B-biotransformed in; E-excreted in; ½L-halflife.

*Within the column listing adverse effects, *underlines* indicate the most common effects; CAPITALS indicate life-threatening effects.

Contraindications and Precautions	Adverse Effects*	Interactions	Nursing Implications
BSP should never be injected into an artery.		the injection of radiopaque substance will cause thrombophlebitis. Radiopaque dyes reduce the clearance and excretion. BSP can be given before or 1 week after cessation of medications and dyes. Lab: NA	injected slowly into an arm vein over a period of 5 min. Watch carefully for symptoms of a reaction. Avoid extravasation. Have epinephrine 1:1000 available for injection to counteract anaphylactoid reaction. Resuscitation equipment should also be available. For extravasation, immediately terminate the administration, elevate the extremity, and immediately apply an ice pack for 1 hr. A blood sample is drawn from opposite arm 45 min after the dye is injected to determine the clearance. EVALUATION: Shows no signs of extravasation, or allergic reaction. Understands the test results and follow-up.
Use with caution in patients with a history of iodine allergy. Safety in pregnancy has not been established.	Few and usually mild. Allergic reactions are rare.	Drug: Phenobarbital may decrease the half-life of indocyanine green. Hepatic excretion of BSP is impaired with simultaneous administration of IG. Lab: Decrease in radioactive iodide uptake for at least 1 week following use of the dye. Increase in serum inorganic iodide concentrations.	ASSESSMENT: Obtain patient history, check for allergy to iodine components. Assess vital signs and note any cardiac irregularities prior to testing. Dye is also used to assess hepatic function and blood flow. INTERVENTION: The dye is injected rapidly through catheter into the heart and timed blood measurements are made. The cardiac output is calculated using the dilution of dye over time curve. After procedure, monitor blood pressure and pulse. Check the incision for bleeding, leakage of dye, or hematoma formation. EVALUATION: Shows no signs of adverse reactions. Understands the test results and follow-up.

CONTINUED ON THE FOLLOWING PAGE

Drugs for Diagnostic Testing

Table 9–1. DRUGS USED IN DIAGNOSTIC TESTING–*CONTINUED*

Name	Dosage	Mode of Administration	Pharmacokinetics
Technetium ⁹⁹ᵐTc sodium pertechnetate ⁹⁹ᵐTc-labeled RBC–*Continued*			

Action: Attaches to RBC and emits radioactivity from the labeled RBC.

Use: Cardiac blood pool imaging and as adjunct in the diagnosis of pericardial effusion and ventricular aneurysm.

Name	Dosage	Mode of Administration	Pharmacokinetics
	Adult: 10–20 mCi (cardiac imaging) Children: individualized	IV	O: immediately P: NA D: NA ½ L: 6.02 hr PB: high E: renal, about 39%/24 hr

Technetium ⁹⁹ᵐTc pyrophos-phate

Action: Concentrates in zones of necrosis, possibly related to the calcium deposits in the infarction zones. Radionuclide uptake is increased in the infarcted myocardial tissue (hot spots). Peak uptake 48–72 hours after onset of MI, diminished uptake after 1 week.

Use: Cardiac imaging agent to aid in diagnosis of acute myocardial infarction.

Name	Dosage	Mode of Administration	Pharmacokinetics
	Adult: 15–29 mCi IV over 10–20 sec Children: individualized	IV	O: 1–2 hr, rescan in 24 hr P: UA D: UA ½ L: 6.02 hr PB: UA E: renal, 40%/24 hr

Thallous chloride Tl-201 (Thallium 201)

Action: Acts as a potassium analogue; readily diffuses across the cell membrane and accumulates in myocardial cells. Radionuclide uptake is diminished in areas where blood flow is abnormal—cold spot imaging results.

Use: Assess coronary artery blood flow, myocardial perfusion. Often used in combination with stress ECG to diagnose ischemic heart disease.

Name	Dosage	Mode of Administration	Pharmacokinetics
	Adult: 1–2 mCi Children: individualized	IV	O: immediately–10 min P: UA D: UA ½ L: 73.1 hr PB: UA E: renal, 4%–8%/24 hr

Key to Abbreviations in the *Pharmacokinetics* column: O-onset; P-peak, D-duration; PB-protein bound; B-bio-transformed in; E-excreted in; ½L-halflife.
*Within the column listing adverse effects, *underlines* indicate the most common effects; CAPITALS indicate life-threatening effects.

Contraindications and Precautions	Adverse Effects*	Interactions	Nursing Implications
Contraindicated in patients with hypersensitivity to human serum albumin. Use not recommended during pregnancy because of risk of radiation exposure to the fetus. Technetium ^{99m}Tc crosses the placenta. Breast-feeding is not recommended for at least 72 hr after administration.	None known, but hypersensitivity reactions to the albumin may occur. Radiation absorbed dose (RAD): low.	Drug: NA Lab: NA	ASSESSMENT: Obtain history regarding past exposure to ionizing radiation and adverse reactions. Confirm nonpregnancy status; obtain menstrual history. A written consent is usually obtained. INTERVENTION: Patient must follow directions regarding body position and motion during scanning. Posttest hydration to avoid accumulation of radioactivity in the bladder. Stress the necessity of proper hygiene after voiding to decrease contamination. Nursing Precaution: Wear rubber or plastic gloves when handling patient's urine specimen within 1–2 days after procedure. EVALUATION: Patient shows no adverse reactions to the procedure.
Same as technetium.	Same as technetium.	Drug: Concurrent use with sodium heparin may impair blood pool images. Estrogens and other medications that induce gynecomastia may cause localization of ^{99m}Tc pyrophosphate in breast tissue. Lab: NA	Same as technetium.
Same as for technetium.	None known. Radiation risk low.	Drug: NA Lab: NA	Same as technetium.

CONTINUED ON THE FOLLOWING PAGE

Table 9–1. DRUGS USED IN DIAGNOSTIC TESTING–*CONTINUED*

Name	Dosage	Mode of Administration	Pharmacokinetics
DIAGNOSTIC SKIN TEST AGENTS			
Tuberculin			
Action: Tuberculin antigens from *Mycobacterium tuberculosis* prepared in solution and injected into the dermis cause a hypersensitivity reaction in persons who are tuberculin-sensitive.			
Use: Aid in diagnosing active TB.			
Purified protein derivative (PPD)	Initial strength: 5 TU/0.1 ml solution of PPD 1 TU/0.1 ml Second strength: 250 TU/0.1 ml	Disposable multiple-puncture devices or by intradermal injection by the Mantoux method.	O: 5–6 hr P: 48–72 hr D: 5 days ½ L: NA PB: NA
Old tuberculin (OT)	Tine test comparable to 5 TU strength Mantoux test	Disposable multiple-puncture devices	B: NA E: NA

Key to Abbreviations in the *Pharmacokinetics* column: O-onset; P-peak, D-duration; PB-protein bound; B-biotransformed in; E-excreted in; ½L-halflife.

*Within the column listing adverse effects, *underlines* indicate the most common effects; CAPITALS indicate life-threatening effects.

sue. When a radiopharmaceutical is administered, the area is scanned with either a gamma camera or a rectilinear scanner, which detects specific localization of the drug. Pathologic findings are indicated as "cold" or "hot" spots. On the scan an area with little uptake of the radioactive agent is called a cold spot, while an area with an increased uptake is a hot spot.

As a diagnostic agent, the dose of the radiopharmaceutical is lower than the therapeutic dose. Thus, there are no pharmacologic effects of the agent. The dosing unit for the radiopharmaceutical is usually the *millicurie* (mCi) or *microcurie* (μCi), which is a measure of the radioactivity associated with a specific amount of the substance. Adverse reactions rarely occur, and the radiation

Contraindications and Precautions	Adverse Effects*	Interactions	Nursing Implications
Disease of the lymphoid system, e.g., Hodgkin's disease, may have false-negative reactions. During pregnancy, the lymphocyte response may be depressed resulting in a false-negative reaction. Safety of tuberculin skin testing during pregnancy has not been fully established. Tuberculin skin tests should not be applied to patients who have had a positive tuberculin reaction in the past. A severe reaction may result in skin ulceration or necrosis. Because of a decrease in their immune response, elderly patients may exhibit a false-negative reaction.	Integumentary: Vesiculation, ulceration, necrosis, pain or pruritus. Anaphylactoid or acute hypersensitivity reaction is rare but can occur. Epinephrine should be readily available.	Drug: Live or attenuated viral vaccines, e.g., measles, mumps, rubella, influenza, given less than 6 weeks before the tuberculin test may suppress the skin test reaction. The tuberculin test may, however, be administered before or simultaneously with the live viral vaccines. Patients taking systemic corticosteroids or aminocaproic acid may develop a false-negative reaction. Lab: None known.	ASSESSMENT: Assess history for a positive skin test reaction, recent exposure to anyone with tuberculosis, or history of tuberculosis. Assess the injection site for atopic dermatitis or other skin diseases. INTERVENTION: Explain procedure to the patient, reassure patient that test is relatively painless and the injection is only into the superficial layers of the skin. Prepare injection site. Administer tuberculin by the Mantoux method or by the multiple-puncture device. Document the location of injection in the patient's chart. PATIENT TEACHING: Patient to return within 48–72 hr to have the skin reaction assessed. Inform the patient that a hard, red, raised area may appear at the injection site, that it is temporary and will resolve. If pruritus develops, the area must not be scratched. EVALUATION: Test site is examined 48–72 hr after administration. Skin induration and erythema are assessed. Induration is the most significant clinical sign: <5 mm is negative; 5–9 mm is questionable reaction; >10 mm positive. Patients with positive skin test reactions should consult their physicians.

risk to the patient is very low. Some of the radioactive agents are discussed in Table 9–1 and include technetium (Tc) 99m, technetium (Tc) 99m pyrophosphate, and thallous chloride (Tl) 201.

NURSING IMPLICATIONS

Radioactive agents are prepared and administered by knowledgeable professionals such as nuclear medicine technicians or physicians. The nurse is primarily responsible for preparing the patient for the test and minimizing radiation contamination after the test. Patient preparation depends on the specific scan and the radioactive agent used (e.g., voiding just before a bone scan to decrease concentration of the radioactive agent in the bladder or fasting before a stress thallium scan to decrease the risk of aspiration in case of cardiac arrest). Prior to the test, the nurse should confirm the nonpregnancy status of the patient and obtain written concent.

Many patients fear radiation. The purpose of the test

Table 9–2. SAMPLE PATIENT PREPARATION FOR BARIUM ENEMA

Diet on Day Prior to Test
   Lunch—Clear liquids only: clear soup, bouillon, consommé, carbonated beverages, tea or coffee, clear juice, plain jello (no cream, milk, fruit, or other additives).
   1 PM—Drink 1 full glass or more of water.
   3 PM—Drink 1 full glass or more of water.
   5 PM—Supper: Eat ONLY a clear liquid supper, same foods as allowed for lunch.
   7 PM—Drink 1 full glass or more of water.
   8 PM—Drink bottle of magnesium citrate (cold).
   10 PM—Take 3 bisacodyl pills with 1 full glass or more of water.
   Bedtime—Drink 1 full glass or more of water.
   7 AM—Drink 1½ glasses of water and insert the bisacodyl suppository into rectum.

After Care
Use laxative to evacuate remaining barium only if you are routinely constipated.

is explained, and the procedure is described. Radionuclides are administered either orally or intravenously before scanning. The scan is done immediately or several hours later. More than one scan may be performed. The patient is given written instructions regarding the specific time to return for the scan.

When a cardiac stress (exercise) test is combined with imaging, the patient is NPO for six hours before the test and the use of alcohol, tobacco, and nonprescription medication is restricted for twenty-four hours. The physician may also have the patient discontinue specific cardiac medication before the test.

After the test, the patient is instructed to increase fluid intake and void frequently to avoid accumulation of radioactivity in the bladder. Proper hygiene after voiding is important to decrease possible radioactive contamination.

Women of childbearing age who are more than ten days postmenstruation or who are pregnant should not assist in the procedure. Pregnant nurses should avoid immediate contact with the patient for twenty-four hours after the procedure. Rubber or plastic gloves are required when handling bedpans, urine specimens, or contaminated drainage bags of patients within 1–2 days after injection of the radionuclide.

NONRADIOACTIVE DYES

Nonradioactive dyes are used to measure organ function. Flow rates, diffusion, fluid volumes, and concentraion parameters are obtained as the dye passes through the system. The dyes are relatively inert compounds. The distribution, metabolism, and excretion of the dye are the properties that make the dye useful as a diagnostic agent. Two dyes used most commonly are bromosulfophthalein sodium (Bromsulphalein, BSP), which is used to assess liver function, and idocyanine green (Cardio-Green), used to measure cardiac output. These dyes are discussed in Table 9–1.

NURSING IMPLICATIONS

Prior to the administration of the dye, the patient is assessed for dehydration or volume overload, which are contraindications. Anaphylactic reactions are rare but may occur especially following extravasation of BSP. Emergency equipment should be available.

DIAGNOSTIC SKIN TESTS

Skin testing is performed to evaluate the cellular immune response of a patient upon injection of specific antigenic preparations. These tests are used to determine the presence of allergies, to diagnose infections, or to assess cell-mediated immunity.

Three methods of skin testing are used: the patch test, wherein an adhesive patch impregnated with the antigenic substance is placed on the skin; the scratch test, wherein the skin is abraded and the testing substance is applied to the area; and the intradermal test, wherein the testing substance is injected intradermally.

The nurse is involved more frequently in administering skin tests for the diagnosis of infections such as tuberculosis, coccidioidomycosis, and histoplasmosis. Skin tests with *Candida*, mumps virus, and *Trichophyton* are used to assess for the presence of cellular immunity. This chapter discusses tuberculin skin testing because it is performed more commonly.

TUBERCULIN SKIN TESTING

The most common skin test is the tuberculin test used to detect exposure to the microorganism *Mycobacterium tuberculosis*. Skin testing involves injection of a known antigen into the superficial layers of the skin. In the tuberculin test, tuberculin purified protein derivative (PPD) or old tuberculin (OT) is the antigen. A hypersensitivity reaction evidenced by inflammation at the injection site indicates an immune response and recent or past exposure to the antigen.

Tuberculin skin testing is performed in a variety of settings: hospitals, clinics, schools, and places of employment. It is used most often as a screening test to detect carriers of tuberculosis. The nurse is the primary health professional involved in this testing; therefore, knowledge of the procedure and the interpretation of the results is important. The tuberculin reagents are discussed in Table 9–1.

Procedure

A patient history is obtained to determine whether the patient has ever had a postive skin test reaction, has recently been exposed to anyone with tuberculosis, or has had tuberculosis. Patients with a history of Calmette-Guerin bacillus (BCG) vaccination usually have a postive tuberculin skin reaction. However, the immunity obtained with this vaccination may diminish after several years. These patients may be skin-tested, but a dilute concentration of tuberculin is used. The injection site is assessed for atopic dermatitis or other skin disease prior to injection. The volar surface (inner aspect) of the upper one third of the forearm is the recommended site; if this is unacceptable, the medial aspect of the thigh or the upper back may be used.

The procedure is explained to the patient; reassure the patient that the test is relatively painless and the injection is only into the superficial layers of the skin. The injection site is cleaned with alcohol and allowed to dry before administration. There are two techniques used in administering a tuberculin skin test: the Mantoux method and the multiple-puncture devices method. For the intradermal injection of PPD by the Mantoux method, a tuberculin syringe with a ½-inch, 26–27 gauge needle is used to draw 0.1 ml solution of 5 tuberculin units (TU) of PPD. The solution is injected beneath the skin by holding the syringe nearly parallel to the skin with the bevel of the needle upward. When just the bevel becomes embedded the solution is slowly injected and a wheal (raised area), 6–10 mm in diameter, is formed (Fig. 9–1). If no wheal develops, the injection was given too deeply and must be repeated at another

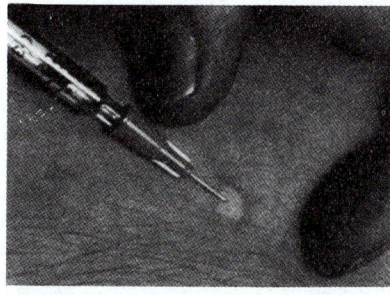

Figure 9–1. Intradermal injection on the volar surface of the forearm. Wheal forms with proper injection. (Courtesy of Parke-Davis, Division of Warner-Lambert Company, Morris Plains, NJ 07950.)

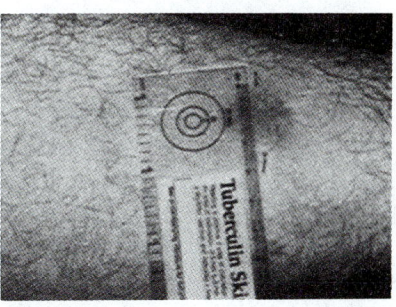

Figure 9–2. Measurement of induration. (Courtesy of Parke-Davis, Division of Warner-Lambert Company, Morris Plains, NJ 07950.)

site. The location of the injection is documented in the patient's chart.

The multiple-puncture devices contain tines that are coated with either OT or PPD. The volar surface of the forearm is prepared for injection as in the Mantoux method. The patient's forearm is held firmly and the skin is stretched taut. The tines are applied sharply and held for at least one second. If delivered accurately, the puncture sites and an imprint of the disc should be present on the skin. Slight bleeding may occur but does not require a dressing. The device is discarded properly.

Evaluation

The test site is examined 48–72 hours after the administration. Skin induration and erythema are assessed. Induration is the most significant clinical sign. To evaluate the skin reaction, the site is inspected and palpated. The induration is measured transversely to the forearm and recorded in millimeters. A felt-tipped pen is used to draw a line on each side of the reaction along the transverse axis toward the induration. The edge of induration is indicated when the pen meets resistance. The distance between the lines is measured with a ruler (Fig. 9–2). With the Mantoux method, using 0.1 ml/5 TU, an induration that measures more than 10 mm in diameter is a positive reaction and a measuremnt of less than 5 mm is negative. An induration measuring 5–9 mm is often considered a questionable reaction, and the test may be repeated. Guidelines for interpreting the skin reaction when 0.1 ml/1 TU is used have not been established.

With multiple-puncture devices, the reaction may be in the form of discrete or coalescent papules, vesicles, or erythema. Induration may also be present. A positive reaction is induration more than 2 mm and/or the presence of vesiculation. *Vesiculation* is the significant clinical response with the multiple-puncture device method. With a positive reaction, a standard Mantoux test is given to confirm the result.

In both the Mantoux and the multiple-puncture device method, erythema is a secondary sign and as a single finding is not clinically significant. The degree of erythema is graded as follows:

tr = trace discoloration
+ = pink
++ = red
+++ = purplish red
++++ = vesiculation or necrosis

Patients with positive skin test reactions require further diagnostic examinations to determine whether the reaction represents exposure to tuberculosis, or dormant infection or active infection.

USING THE NURSING PROCESS

ASSESSMENT

Before any diagnostic procedure, the nurse must assess the patient's physical and emotional status. What does the patient know about the test to be performed? How does the patient relate this to the illness? Has the patient had the test previously and thus experienced its procedures and effects? It is important for the nurse to assess the patient's level of understanding before deciding what the teaching is to include.

The patient's psychological state is also assessed to ascertain whether the individual fears the outcome of the test or the procedure itself, owing to anticipated pain, discomfort, or embarrassment; or whether the procedure is viewed as beneficial because the intent of the test is to reveal what is wrong. Assessment of the patient's feelings regarding the diagnostic procedure also helps the nurse to develop an appropriate teaching plan.

The physical status of the patient is also important to assess. How well will the patient tolerate the preparation for the procedure? The elderly patient with fluid and electrolyte problems may have difficulty tolerating the enemas and dehydration that some diagnostic tests require. Assessment of all systems just before testing is essential, as a patient's status can change suddenly. Unstable patients (medically or emotionally) may not be able to withstand the stress of the diagnostic procedure. How well will the patient tolerate the procedure itself? The elderly patient or the patient experiencing much pain will find some diagnostic procedures very difficult.

Allergies of any type are important to note before diagnostic testing. The patient is questioned regarding a history of allergies or a reaction to a dye infusion test. If a positive response is obtained, the patient is asked to describe the reaction specifically. The development of nausea, vomiting, urticaria, pruritus, dyspnea, or tachycardia following the administration of a diagnostic agent is noted in the health history and reported to the physician. The physician determines whether the reaction is significant and another diagnostic agent needs to be selected. Iodine allergies are especially significant because most dye studies are performed with an iodine-based product. Many individuals allergic to fish or other seafood may actually have an iodine allergy.

NURSING DIAGNOSES

The nursing diagnoses for a patient undergoing diagnostic tests may include knowledge deficit related to the procedure, preparation, and postprocedure care; anxiety related to the test procedure and outcome; potential alteration in comfort related to the test procedure; potential fluid volume deficit related to fluid restriction, or excessive loss of fluid (Table 9–3).

PLANNING AND INTERVENTION

The nurse plays an integral role in preparing, supporting, and assessing the patient before, during and after diagnostic tests. Nursing interventions are employed to obtain data regarding the patient's response to the test, to decrease patient anxiety, and to prevent adverse effects. A checklist containing nursing interventions in caring for a patient undergoing diagnostic tests is presented in Table 9–4.

Most patients undergoing a diagnostic procedure have questions and concerns. It is often the nurse's responsibility to explain the procedure. This is done clearly, at the patient's level of understanding, focusing on any particular concerns the patient may verbalize. Specific preparation for the procedure is stressed to ensure optimum test results. Most patients are concerned about the purpose of the test, how it is performed, the amount of discomfort associated with the procedure, and the specifics regarding scheduling.

Many patients requiring diagnostic procedures are concerned about what the tests may reveal. The patient may fear that the tests will confirm the seriousness of the illness or the need for surgery. Also, waiting for the test results often produces anxiety for the patient. Support from the nursing staff at this time is very important.

Many diagnostic procedures are performed on an outpatient basis. The time available for patient instruction prior to the procedure is limited. Preprinted instruction booklets for each procedure provide the patient with necessary information. The nurse reviews the instructions and clarifies any unclear information. The telephone number of the outpatient clinic is given to the patient if further questions arise.

The nurse is often responsible for scheduling diagnostic tests. For patient convenience, more than one test can be scheduled on a given day. The order in which procedures are scheduled is important to maintain accurate testing and avoid the need to reschedule. Thyroid studies are completed before using any iodine-based dye preparation because this alters thyroid test results. Studies using barium are usually done last because retained barium can interfere with good visualization of other organs. Barium enemas are administered before an upper gastrointestinal series or a small bowel series. Special scheduling arrangements are often necessary for the diabetic patient undergoing diagnostic tests. Insulin is not given as long as the individual is NPO. Often, the diagnostic testing department takes diabetic patients first to prevent complications.

Table 9–3. NURSING PROCESS FOR PATIENT UNDERGOING DIAGNOSTIC TESTS

Assessment

Evaluate patient's ability to follow instructions.
Evaluate the patient's reaction to previous diagnostic tests.
Identify allergies to iodine or iodine-containing foods, e.g., shellfish and type of reaction.
Assess pre-existing conditions, current drug therapy for possible interference with elimination of barium (e.g., ulcerative colitis, codeine, analgesics), or increased risk of dehydration (e.g., extremes of age; underweight patients or patients with pre-existing conditions such as diarrhea, vomiting, bleeding; or diuretic therapy).
Obtain menstrual history to confirm pregnancy status.

Nursing Diagnosis	Nursing Actions	Rationale	Patient Outcomes/ Evaluation Criteria
Knowledge, deficit related to lack of information regarding test procedures as evidenced and questions and expressions of concern.	Assess patient's knowledge or previous experience with the diagnostic test. Provide materials regarding the test procedure and preparation.	Provides starting point for individual teaching program. Use of variety of materials, e.g., written, audio/visual aids, enhances learning and retention.	Verbalizes understanding of test procedure and preparation. Demonstrates ability to follow instructions.
	Clarify the information and provide follow-up to any questions.	Facilitates patient's understanding and includes patient as an active participant in the learning process.	
	Have the patient explain the test procedure and preparation.	Return demonstration is used to document learning and patient understanding.	
Anxiety (specify level) related to threat to self from unknown procedure/sensations as evidenced by increased tension, apprehension, expressed concerns.	Ascertain the patient's expectations of the physical outcomes of test procedure and preparation.	Identifies specific concerns and degree of anxiety.	Reports anxiety level is mild and manageable.
	Provide information regarding possible physical sensations associated with the particular test (i.e., dye injections may cause a hot, flushing feeling).	Prepares patient for expected occurrences and helps reduce fear of unknown.	
	Clarify misconceptions.	Misconceptions often result in unnecessary anxiety (e.g., fear of effects of radiation from radionuclides).	
Comfort, altered potential related to test procedure and/ or preparation.	Prepare patient for possible discomfort and/or pain (i.e., bowel preparation may include enemas that cause abdominal cramping).	Patients tolerate mild discomfort and/or pain if they have been prepared for it and know it will be transient.	Verbalizes and demonstrates relief/control of pain or discomfort. Acknowledges understanding that discomfort/ pain is transient.
	Be available and provide support during uncomfortable procedures. Inform patient that any discomfort and/or pain felt will be transient not long-lasting (e.g., pain, burning sensation at injection site of iodine compounds).	Support provides reassurance, facilitating the patient's coping with discomfort.	
	Tell patient to inform the medical/nursing staff of any discomfort and/or pain.	Presence of pain may indicate need for further intervention/ medication to prevent complications.	
Fluid volume deficit, potential for, related to restricted intake, excessive fluid losses.	Monitor development of thirst, presence of nausea/vomiting, changes in skin turgor and moisture of mucous membranes.	Signs suggesting changes in hydration status.	Resumes normal fluid intake. Demonstrates no signs or symptoms of dehydration/ hypovolemia.

CONTINUED ON THE FOLLOWING PAGE

Table 9–3. NURSING PROCESS FOR PATIENT UNDERGOING DIAGNOSTIC TESTS–*CONTINUED*

Assessment

Evaluate patient's ability to follow instructions.
Evaluate the patient's reaction to previous diagnostic tests.
Identify allergies to iodine or iodine-containing foods, e.g., shellfish and type of reaction.
Assess pre-existing conditions, current drug therapy for possible interference with elimination of barium (e.g., ulcerative colitis, codeine, analgesics), or increased risk of dehydration (e.g., extremes of age; underweight patients or patients with pre-existing conditions such as diarrhea, vomiting, bleeding; or diuretic therapy).
Obtain menstrual history to confirm pregnancy status.

Nursing Diagnosis	Nursing Actions	Rationale	Patient Outcomes/ Evaluation Criteria
	Maintain accurate intake/output.	Early recognition and prompt treatment of developing deficit may prevent serious complications.	
	Follow posttest procedure in resuming fluid intake.	Excessive fluid loss may occur secondary to enemas and suppositories used for bowel studies or reaction to injected iodinated compounds requiring adequate fluid replacement to prevent complications.	
	Provide oral hygiene after barium swallow.	Relieves after taste and may help alleviate feelings of nausea.	
Constipation, potential for, related to ingestion/instillation of barium-containing solution and absence of oral intake prior to test.	Encourage increased intake of food/fluids, if able, following completion of tests and verification of presence of bowel sounds.	Stimulates gastric/intestinal motility and promotes return of usual consistency of stool.	Passes barium stool with no untoward effects. Displays usual color and consistency of stool within 48–72 hours.
	Administer laxative/enema as appropriate.	Promotes emptying of agent if not contraindicated by presence of obstructive lesions.	
	Record characteristics and frequency of stool.	Useful in determining if all of barium has been expelled.	
	Investigate changes in bowel sounds, development of abdominal distention, cramping, or diarrhea.	Signs suggestive of intestinal obstruction requiring medical evaluation and further intervention.	
	Provide nonconstipating analgesics, e.g., propacete.	Codeine based products tend to decrease gastric motility, increasing risk of constipation.	

Special consideration is necessary for elderly patients undergoing diagnostic tests. For these individuals, maintaining NPO status, waiting long periods in the diagnostic testing department, and assuming various positions during the test are uncomfortable situations and nostic tests is important. Effective bowel preparation permits better x-ray-film visualization. Hydration or dehydration orders for specific tests are followed precisely.

EVALUATION

Following the administration of any diagnostic agent, the nurse must evaluate the patient for any adverse effects. The most significant reaction is anaphylaxis. An-aphylaxis may occur during diagnostic testing, especially when iodine-based dyes are used. If evidence of allergy is present, the physician and diagnostic department are notified. During the dye infusion, the patient is watched carefully for signs of respiratory distress, sudden diaphoresis, urticaria, or instability of vital signs. Diphenhydramine (Benadryl), epinephrine, oxygen, and resuscitation equipment are available, and all personnel are prepared in management of anaphylactic shock. Prior to testing, if a hypersensitivity reaction is anticipated, antihistamine preparations may be added to the dye preparations to reduce the incidence of allergic response.

The nurse also alters the patient's care plan as needed

Table 9–4. NURSING CHECKLIST FOR THE PATIENT UNDERGOING DIAGNOSTIC TESTS

I. Patient preparation
   A. Explain purpose and procedure.
   B. Explain preparation:
      Bowel preparation
      Dietary and fluid restrictions
      Medications to be taken and action
      Time the test will be done, place, and how long it will take
   C. Explain possible adverse effects (e.g., changes in stool).
   D. Explain what specimens will be collected and how the specimens will be obtained.
II. Confirm patient's consent.
III. Check patient's allergy history:
   A. Note especially any allergy to iodine or seafood.
   B. Note any previous reaction to a diagnostic procedure.
   C. Notify physician and/or diagnostic department if an allergy is present.
IV. Administer preparatory procedures (enemas, medications, and so on).
V. Collect specimens and label.
VI. Posttest:
   A. Perform frequent physical assessment (vital signs).
   B. Observe for adverse reactions.
   C. Have emergency equipment available.
   D. Give post-test care (laxatives, increased fluids, and so on).
VII. Modify nursing care plan as appropriate and provide emotional support while patient is waiting for the test results.
VIII. Evaluate patient's understanding of the test results and follow-up care.

after the diagnostic procedure. These alterations may include increasing fluids to compensate for dehydration, giving extra laxatives to prevent constipation, and providing extra attention to the patient waiting for test results. After the test results have been discussed with the must be monitored closely. Dehydration can occur rapidly when elderly patients are NPO and undergoing numerous enemas. Following tests, it is very important to adequately replace fluids.

Physical preparation of the patient undergoing diagpatient, the nurse evaluates the patient's understanding of the results. Depending upon the outcome of the test the patient may need follow-up care and health care instructions (Table 9–5).

SUMMARY

This chapter reviewed some common diagnostic agents: radiopaque compounds, provocative agents, radioactive tracers, nonradioactive dyes, and diagnostic skin testing. Although the nurse does not usually administer these agents, except tuberculin, the nurse is responsible for reporting adverse reactions and preventing complications. As discussed, anaphylaxis can occur with these agents. The nurse must be prepared for this event. Early recognition of symptoms indicating a possible reaction and prompt treatment are vital in preventing a fatal outcome.

Table 9–5. PATIENT TEACHING INFORMATION—DIAGNOSTIC AGENTS

Before the Diagnostic Test
1. Follow the specific instructions that were given to you regarding preparation for the test.
2. Follow dietary and fluid intake restrictions as prescribed. Do not make changes without consulting your doctor.
3. Call your doctor if you have questions or are unable to follow the prescribed preparation.
4. Notify your doctor if you feel the preparation has made your condition worse.
5. Relax.

After the Diagnostic Test
1. Fluid intake is usually very important following diagnostic testing. Follow the post-test directions.
2. Drugs such as laxatives may be prescribed to remove the diagnostic agent from your body. Take according to directions.
3. Confirm whether or not you need to return for testing.
4. After some tests, such as a barium enema, you may notice changes in the color of your stool. This is normal. Ask your doctor or nurse what changes you should expect to occur after the test.
5. Ask the doctor when you will be notified regarding the results of your test.

The nurse plays an integral role in preparing the patient for diagnostic testing. Using the nursing process, the nurse obtains information to construct a plan of care. Patient preparation includes both physical and emotional preparation. Reassurance and patient education assist in relieving anxiety often associated with diagnostic testing.

BIBLIOGRAPHY

American Hospital Formulary Service: Drug Information 88. American Society of Hospital Pharmacists, Bethesda, 1988.

Diagnostic Tests Handbook. Springhouse Corporation, Springhouse, PA, 1987.

Drug Information for the Health Care Provider, Vol 1. USP DI, ed 7, 1987. Mack Printing Company, Easton, PA. Distributed by USPC, Rockville, MD.

Fischbach, F: A Manual of Laboratory Diagnostic Tests, ed 2. Lippincott, Philadelphia, 1984.

Millar, S, Sampson, L and Soukup, M: AACN Procedure Manual for Critical Care. Saunders, Philadelphia, 1985.

Nurse's Clinical Library: Gastrointestinal Disorders. Springhouse Corporation, Springhouse, PA, 1985.

Olin, B (ed): Facts & Comparisons. Lippincott, St. Louis, 1987.

Physicians' Desk Reference. Medical Economics Co., Oradell, NJ, 1987.

SITUATION 9–1

Meryl Golden is a 76-year-old female admitted to the medical-surgical unit for diagnostic testing of abdominal pain.

1. In planning the scheduling of barium studies for Mrs. Golden, the nurse is aware that:
   a. the barium swallow should be performed prior to the barium enema
   b. the barium swallow and barium enema cannot be performed during a single patient admission
   c. barium studies should be scheduled before other diagnostic tests
   d. the barium enema should be performed before the barium swallow

2. Prior to barium studies, if Mrs. Golden should complain of increasing abdominal pain with rigidity or vomiting, the nurse's *best* response would be to:
   a. administer analgesics and narcotics by intravenous route
   b. inform the physician and prepare to cancel barium studies
   c. prepare to give barium via intravenous route and keep NPO
   d. prepare to give barium sulfate via a nasogastric tube

3. All of the following would be included in planning the care for Mrs. Golden after completion of barium studies, *except:*
   a. limit oral fluid intake
   b. observe for light-colored stools
   c. provide mouth care ad lib
   d. check for bowel sounds

4. Due to Mrs. Golden's age, the nurse will be particularly concerned during rectal administration of barium, because of:
   a. hypertension
   b. tachycardia
   c. constipation
   d. vagal response

5. Mrs. Golden has been NPO since midnight and received enemas until clear the morning of the scheduled barium enema. Which of the following nursing diagnoses apply?
   a. knowledge deficit related to events of barium studies
   b. ineffective family coping related to stress of diagnostic studies
   c. potential fluid volume deficit related to NPO status and enemas
   d. disturbance in self-concept related to enema administration

6. Following the barium studies, the nurse is concerned with evaluation. Which of the following is *not* an aspect of the evaluation phase?
   a. Observe for signs of anaphylaxis.
   b. Arrange follow-up care as needed.
   c. Alter care plan to include postdiagnostic measures.
   d. Record prior experiences with diagnostic testing

Please refer to the Appendices for correct answers and additional review questions with answers.

DRUGS IN ANESTHESIA

GLOSSARY TERMS IN THIS CHAPTER

Ambulatory surgery
Anesthesia
Anesthesiologist
Anesthetist
Balanced anesthesia
Certified registered nurse anesthetist (CRNA)
Depolarizing neuromuscular blockade
General anesthesia
Induction
Inhalation anesthetic
Local anesthesia
Nondepolarizing neuromuscular blocking agents
Outpatient surgery
Same-day surgery

10

CHAPTER

DRUGS IN ANESTHESIA

ANNE MORACA-SAWICKI, M.S.N., R.N.

LEARNING OBJECTIVES

After reading this chapter, the student will be able to:

1. Identify those medications commonly used as anesthetics.

2. Differentiate among the intravenous general anesthetics as to mechanism of action, route of administration, pharmacokinetics, adverse effects, contraindications, interactions, advantages, and disadvantages.

3. Identify specific areas to assess in the patient requiring anesthetics in order to formulate appropriate nursing diagnoses relative to type of anesthesia administered.

4. Plan the nursing interventions necessary to facilitate administration of anesthetics and choose appropriate teaching strategies to facilitate patient compliance.

5. Evaluate the patient at various stages of treatment to gauge nursing interventions.

This chapter deals with anesthetic agents. Basic information on the types of anesthesia, stages of general anesthesia, and anesthetic drugs is included. Also included are various drugs used as adjuncts to the anesthetic process—certain barbiturates and opiates, for example. Discussion of these agents is limited to their use in facilitating, enhancing, or maintaining anesthesia. Nurses do not administer anesthetics unless they are specially trained and certified to do so as *Certified Registered Nurse Anesthetists (CRNA)*. However, nurses play an integral role in the administration of perioperative care. Thus, it is essential for nurses to understand the types and stages of anesthesia as well as the effects of the various drugs used to achieve this state in order to ensure the delivery of optimum patient care.

HISTORY OF ANESTHESIA

The word *anesthesia* literally means "without sensation." It is derived from the Greek words for "negative sensation." Oliver Wendell Holmes is credited with coining the term *anesthesia* and, in so doing, naming the specialty responsible for painless surgery. In order for there to be no pain, there must be no reflexes. Temporary areflexia is achieved through the use of chemical agents to produce anesthesia.

The history of modern anesthesia began in 1840 with the use of nitrous oxide for dental extractions. History does record the use of opiates by the ancient Egyptians and hashish by the Chinese to achieve varying degrees of anesthesia during surgical procedures. However, modern surgeons are indebted to the profession of dentistry and Drs. Morton and Wells for introducing anesthetics and ushering in the era of painless surgery. The first successful general anesthetic was ether. William Morton was the first to demonstrate the use of ether as an anesthetic on October 16, 1846, for a group of Boston-area physicians at the Massachusetts General Hospital. Since that time, the science of anesthesia has developed into a medical specialty, and more recently a nursing specialty, of considerable complexity.

There are three basic categories of anesthesia: local, regional, and general. Different modes of administration exist within each category. General anesthesia may be achieved through inhalation or intravenous drug administration. Local anesthesia may be achieved by topical drug application or injection, producing anesthesia of small body areas such as a finger. Regional anesthesia is used to negate sensation in large areas of the body such as in spinal anesthesia. Local anesthesia will be discussed in greater detail later in this chapter.

GENERAL ANESTHESIA

General anesthesia is the progressive, reversible stage of central nervous system depression that occurs following the administration of drugs used for this purpose. General anesthetics may be administered by the intravenous or inhalation route. Many different drugs may be used to achieve patient anesthesia, each with individual characteristics, side effects, and contraindications. The ideal agent should be nonflammable, nonexplosive if given by inhalation, and relatively nontoxic. It should achieve its desired effect without causing tissue hypoxia, laryngospasm, excessive tracheobronchial secretions, or respiratory depression. To date, no single anesthetic agent meets all of the criteria of this "ideal" drug, although isoflurane (Forane) seems to be as close to the ideal as possible. Thus, it has become common practice to combine small amounts of several intravenous drugs to achieve the most beneficial drug characteristics with a minimum of toxicity. This practice is known as *balanced anesthesia* and allows the anesthetist to select drug combinations specifically tailored to meet individual patient needs in conjunction with the type of surgery to be performed. Balanced anesthesia can also be achieved by using narcotics with inhalation gas. Balanced anesthesia is typically achieved with a combination of inhalation, narcotic, and neuromuscular blocking agents (muscle relaxants).

The anesthesia process is divided into three phases: *induction,* maintenance and recovery. The induction phase is analogous to climbing up a mountain. It requires a comparatively large amount of anesthetic to reach the height of anesthesia, just as it requires a large energy expenditure to reach the mountaintop. The maintenance dose required to remain on top, or at the desired level, is much less. In the recovery phase, anesthetic administration is stopped, or an antidote administered, so that the anesthesia is reversed as the drugs wear off.

STAGES AND CLASSIFICATION OF GENERAL ANESTHESIA

When a general anesthetic is administered, anesthesia is not achieved immediately. Induction occurs in a definite order, as the patient passes from one level of central nervous system depression to the next until an adequate stage of surgical anesthesia is achieved. Although passage from one level (stage) of anesthesia to the next occurs rapidly because of rapid onset of action of the barbiturates used, progressive signs of central nervous system depression do occur at each stage. General anesthesia is usually achieved by a combination of two types of drugs—an anesthetic and adjuncts to anesthesia such as neuromuscular blocking agents. The combination of two or more drugs is often needed to achieve and maintain the triad of anesthesia: amnesia, analgesia, and muscle relaxation.

The exact mechansim of action of general anesthetic drugs is unknown. There are several different theories of anesthetic action. One theory that has been postulated is that general anesthetics change the cell's permeability, surface tension, electrical stability, and/or cytoplasm. These agents act on the central nervous system: brain, medulla, and spinal cord. The cerebral cortex and midbrain control consciousness and are affected first.

Table 10–1. STAGES AND PLANES OF ANESTHESIA

Stage and Plane	Characteristics	Special Considerations

Stage I Analgesia
  Plane 1
  Plane 2
 	
  Plane 3
	Conscious
	Partial analgesia; total amnesia, conscious, breathing slows.
	Complete analgesia and amnesia, conscious.
		Patient may be quiet or euphoric. Since cortex is depressed in this state, it is sometimes called the cortical stage. This stage ends when consciousness is lost.

Stage II Delirium (dream)	Consciousness is lost; excitement and muscle activity may be marked or minimal; breathing is irregular. Incontinence or vomiting may occur.	Because of hyperexcitability that may occur in this transition stage, it is generally kept to a minimum. Depression of the midbrain occurs in this stage. This stage ends when automatic breathing occurs.

Stage III Surgical
  Plane 1
 	
  Plane 2
 	
  Plane 3
 	
  Plane 4
	Rhythmic breathing occurs. Hypoactivity to painful stimuli.
	Assisted respiration necessary from this point on. Somatic response to pain lost.
	Progressive intercostal paralysis occurs; visceral response to pain is lost.
	Intercostal paralysis complete; diaphragmatic breathing occurs.
		Moderate depression of subcortex occurs. Light anesthesia.
		Predominant control is by the midbrain. Moderate level of anesthesia.
		
		Moderate depression of midbrain occurs. Moderate level of anesthesia.
		
		Continued depression of midbrain; deep level of anesthesia. Approaching toxic level of anesthesia. Stage ends with apnea.

Stage IV Medullary paralysis
  Plane 1
 	
  Plane 2
	Respiratory paralysis (arrest) occurs; blood pressure falls; pupils dilate.
	
	Cardiovascular collapse (arrest) occurs; pupils fully dilated; muscles flaccid.
		Moderate depression of pons occurs; toxicity is reversible at this level; this level ends when circulatory collapse occurs.
		Irreversible level of anesthesia. Death results.

The spinal cord, involved in both sensory and motor functions, is the next site of drug action. The third site of action is the blocking of the medulla, which controls respiratory and cardiovascular function.

Guedel devised a classification (Gilman, Goodman, and Gilman, 1985) of the stages and planes of anesthesia in 1920, using ether as his model. Table 10–1 features the stages and planes of anesthesia.

Stage I is analgesia and lasts from the point of induction to the point of loss of consciousness. The patient becomes analgesic and amnesic; a minimal amount of muscular relaxation is present. Since depression of the cerebral cortex occurs during this stage, it is sometimes referred to as the cortical stage.

Stage II is the stage of delirium (also called dream stage). It begins with the patient's loss of consciousness and lasts until automatic breathing occurs. Depression of the midbrain occurs in this stage. Excitement and muscular activity may be marked or minimal; however, muscle hyperexcitability is the rule. Incontinence and vomiting with aspiration may occur. Because of the amount of exertion and excitement that can occur in this

stage, it is generally kept to a minimum so that the patient makes a smooth, rapid transition to the next stage.

Stage III, the surgical stage of anesthesia, is composed of four planes. This stage begins with the onset of automatic breathing and continues to apnea caused by intercostal and diaphragmatic paralysis. Spinal cord depression and true muscle relaxation occur in this stage. The different planes of Stage III are differentiated by changes in the quality of respiration, reflexes, and eye movements. Most general surgical procedures are performed with the patient between Planes 1 and 2. Assisted respiration is required from Plane 2 onward. Plane 4 is complete intercostal paralysis to diaphragmatic paralysis, which ends with apnea.

Stage IV is medullary paralysis, the stage of overdose. It begins with respiratory paralysis and ends with circulatory collapse. There are two planes within this stage of anesthesia: the vital centers of the medulla are depressed, leading to respiratory failure, which is reversible (Plane 1), and cardiovascular collapse, which is irreversible (Plane 2) and causes death. With proper monitoring, this type of death should never occur. Thus, patient reflexes and vital signs are constantly observed throughout the surgical procedure, and anesthetic doses are carefully adjusted to maintain the appropriate stage and plane of anesthesia. Nurses should know the effects of anesthesia so they can properly assess patient condition, especially during the immediate postoperative period.

Guedel's classification system was especially useful in the early days of anesthetic administration when induction was relatively slow because of the slow onset of the inhalation agents used. Today, almost all patients receive barbiturate induction to general anesthesia. Since these drugs have a rapid onset of action, it is not possible to observe each individual sign of the stages outlined by Guedel. However, his classification system is of historical value.

An inhalational agent to induce anesthesia is sometimes used in children. Since inhalation induction is slower than that achieved with intravenous agents, it is sometimes possible to observe the signs Guedel outlined. Inhalation induction is also used when an intravenous route is not available, such as patients who receive intravenous chemotherapy for cancer or intravenous drug abusers.

THERAPEUTIC AGENTS

INHALATION ANESTHETICS

The original anesthetics were inhalation agents, and this method of administration is still commonly used. Inhalation anesthetics are not administered in their pure form but are mixed with oxygen or nitrous oxide. Inhalation agents come in liquid form and must be vaporized by an anesthesia machine for administration to the patient by means of a mask or endotracheal tube. Once vaporized and mixed with oxygen or nitrous oxide, the anesthesia is administered and transported to the patient's lungs. These drugs may be administered by open system, closed systems, or nonrebreathing systems. The nonrebreathing valve-type delivery is used most commonly in the United States. The other methods may still be seen in less developed areas of the world. (Figure 10–1 illustrates the formation of a vapor from a liquid.) The most commonly used inhalation agents are isoflurane, halothane, and enflurane.

Inhalation agents are also referred to as volatile anesthetics, that is, a liquid or solution form that is evaporated into a vapor for administraion. Absorption, distribution, and excretion of these drugs depend on the pressure concentration gradients, moving from the area of higher concentration to the area of lower concentration. This gradient is responsible for moving oxygen from the alveoli to the arterioles and carbon dioxide from the venules back to the alveoli. Once gas exchange occurs in the patient's lungs, the heart circulates the anesthetic to the brain and other organs. Once biotransformation occurs, most of the inhalational anesthetic

agent is excreted in the form of exhaled gases. Most of the inhalational agent will be excreted by the time the patient returns to the unit, unless surgery lasts more than a few hours.

Ether

Ether was one of the first anesthetic agents used. It brought about excellent muscle relaxation and had a wide margin of safety between the anesthetic and toxic doses. Ether had a relatively long induction and recovery time as well as a distinctive odor that often made induction unpleasant for the patient. Recovery was likewise often marred by nausea and vomiting. Ether was also irritating to the mucous membranes. However, the major reason it is rarely used today is that it is highly flammable and potentially explosive and, therefore, not compatible with the electrical equipment of today's operating rooms. Although obsolete, ether may still be used in some underdeveloped countries because it is inexpensive and may be simply and effectively administered through the inexpensive open-drop system.

Cyclopropane Gas

Cyclopropane produces greater skeletal muscle relaxation than do most other anesthetic gases; hence the use of neuromuscular blocking agents is not always necessary when using this drug. There is a wide margin of safety between the anesthetic and lethal concentrations of this gas. An appropriate level of anesthesia may be achieved within 2–3 minutes of induction, and postanesthetic recovery is rapid and smooth. High concentrations of oxygen may be administered with cyclopropane, making it an excellent drug choice for persons with pulmonary or circulatory diseases. The major disadvantage of cyclopropane that has caused a decline in its use is its flammability. Special safety precautions are essential when administering this highly flammable agent, which is also explosive when mixed with oxygen.

Nitrous Oxide Gas

Nitrous oxide gas was the first modern anesthetic agent used. It is commonly referred to as "laughing gas" because inhalation of small amounts mixed with air produces an intoxicating effect: the patient feels happy and giddy and laughs. This agent was first used to produce analgesia and amnesia during dental procedures, and it remains popular for this purpose today. Because it has only relatively mild anesthetic properties, it is rarely used alone, except for dental and minor surgical procedures and during the second stage of labor. Nitrous oxide is frequently used in combination with other anesthetics for its analgesic/amnestic effects and to provide rapid induction. The major advantages of this agent are that it is not explosive and it has no clinically significant effect on the cardiovascular system as long as the patient is adequately ventilated. Nitrous oxide is relatively free from major toxicities and side effects, although chronic use may cause leukopenia. The major disadvantages of this agent are that it is too weak to produce anesthesia beyond Stage II (delirium); it rapidly diffuses out of the lungs once it is discontinued, so a "dif-

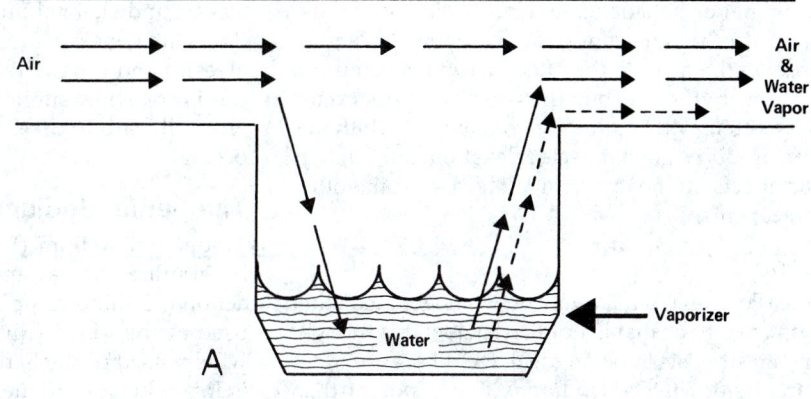

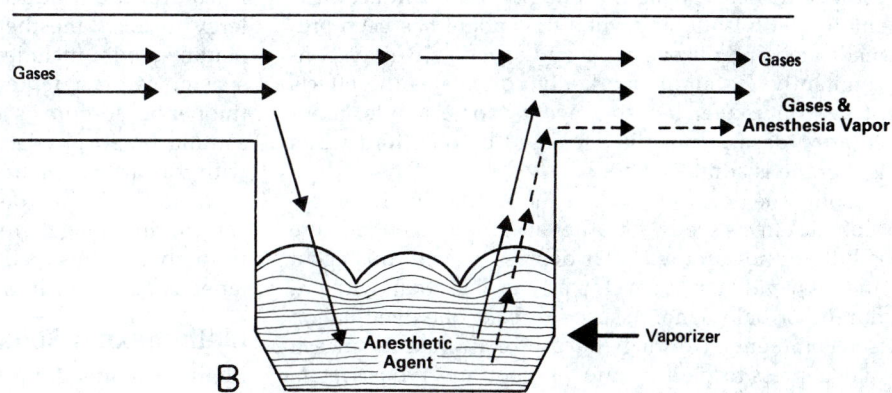

Figure 10–1. The formation of a vapor from a liquid. A) Water: As air passes through the vaporizer, some of the air passes into the water and leaves with the water vapor. An increase in temperature will increase the amount of vapor. B) Ether: Ether and other anesthetic agents are formed into vapors in the same way that water vapor is formed.

fusion hypoxia" oxygen deficiency may occur; and it tends to diffuse into open cavities, making it unacceptable for surgeries involving gastrointestinal obstruction, pneumothorax, or ear procedures.

Halothane

Halothane (Fluothane) is a halogenated hydrocarbon anesthetic that is five times more potent than ether. It is nonflammable and nonexplosive and is one of the most commonly used inhalation anesthetics. The major advantages of halothane are its pleasant, rapid induction and rapid recovery. Major disadvantages of this agent are its narrow safety range and strong circulatory, myocardial, and respiratory depressant effects. It is the only inhalation agent that can cause bradycardia. It produces poor skeletal muscle relaxation and profound uterine relaxation. Halothane sensitizes the heart to epinephrine, causing arrhythmias, and can also cause hepatotoxicity and "halothane hepatitis." It is not recommended for routine obstetric use, in cases where epinephrine may be used, or in patients with hepatic disease. Despite its narrow safety range, halothane remains a widely used inhalation anesthetic, especially for children, since they seem to have less susceptibility to "halothane hepatitis." It is the most commonly used pediatric induction agent because it is the least noxious smelling and smoothest induction agent. Specially calibrated vaporizers are available for use with halothane in order to ensure drug delivery within the safe limit range.

Methoxyflurane

Methoxyflurane (Penthrane) is the most potent of the inhalation anesthetics. It is nonflammable and nonexplosive. However, it has several important disadvantages that severely limit its use, including numerous side effects, slow induction and recovery times, narrow margin of safety, and low vapor pressure. Methoxyflurane, like halothane, sensitizes the heart to the effects of epinephrine; depresses the respiratory system (more so than halothane); and produces cardiovascular effects (less severe than halothane). It can also cause high-output renal failure. (Methoxyflurane has a high lipid and blood solubility, which slows induction and recovery times.) It is also not readily vaporized, which further delays anesthesia induction. Thus, when used, methoxyflurane is used chiefly for maintenance of anesthesia induced by other agents such as nitrous oxide, and it is supplemented with muscle relaxants. The long recovery period following use of methoxyflurane decreases the need for narcotic analgesics in the first few hours postoperatively. The long recovery following use of this drug makes it a poor agent for patients undergoing same-day surgery who will be discharged shortly after surgery.

Enflurane

Enflurane (Ethrane) is a fluorinated ether inhalation anesthetic that is nonflammable and nonexplosive. This drug and its effects are very similar to halothane. It does not cause renal or hepatic toxicity or cardiovascular depression as do the other fluorinated ethers, although it does sensitize the heart to the effects of epinephrine and may cause arrhythmias, but this cardiac effect occurs much less often with enflurane than with halothane. Enflurane produces good muscle relaxation, although its analgesic effects are not as great as those of some other anesthetic agents.

Isoflurane

Isoflurane (Forane) is a relatively new halogenated ether inhalation anesthetic that is nonflammable. It is thought by many anesthetists to be an ideal agent because it has no apparent side effects. Isoflurane is less potent than halothane. There is good patient acceptance of this anesthetic despite its slightly pungent odor. Induction is smooth with isoflurane when the patient has been premedicated and nitrous oxide and oxygen are given concomitantly. Isoflurane markedly potentiates the effects of neuromuscular blocking agents; for example, tubocurarine dosage must be decreased by one third when isoflurane is administered.

Isoflurane does not produce the renal, hepatic, or cardiotoxic effects seen with other anesthetic agents. There is little or no cardiovascular depression with this agent and less tendency to develop arrhythmias than with enflurane or halothane. Assisted or controlled ventilation is recommended during the use of isoflurane since it may depress respiratory rate. No central nervous system stimulation is evident, even when deep anesthesia is achieved with this drug. The drug has no adverse effect on intracranial or intraocular pressure as long as adequate ventilation is maintained. This agent can cause marked tachycardia at higher doses.

Postanesthesia nausea, vomiting, and excitation are rare following administration of this anesthetic. Mental alertness is generally depressed for 2–3 hrs following use of isoflurane. However, this may not be an undesirable effect because it diminishes the patient's perception of pain in the immediate postoperative period.

INTRAVENOUSLY ADMINISTERED ANESTHETIC AGENTS

The intravenous route is commonly used to induce or maintain surgical anesthesia. The drugs most commonly used for intravenous anesthesia are the ultra-short-acting barbiturates and the neuroleptics. These agents, especially the ultra-short-acting barbiturates, are excellent for inducing anesthesia before use of an inhalation agent. Intravenous agents provide pleasant, rapid induction; are easily administered; have no explosive properties; cause no respiratory tract irritation; and have rapid recovery periods. In addition to the intravenous route, barbiturates can also be administered orally (common, but not for anesthesia) and rectally (less common.) The barbiturates have a rapid onset of action (within a few seconds) and a duration of one hour or less when administered intravenously. These drugs are metabolized mainly in the liver and excreted in the urine.

Disadvantages of the barbiturates are their poor analgesic and skeletal muscle relaxation properties. These drugs are generally used in combination with potent analgesics and muscle relaxants; they produce good anesthesia for short surgical and diagnostic procedures. As with all barbiturates, the "hangover" side effect may occur.

Thiopental Sodium

Thiopental sodium (Pentothal) is an ultra-short-acting barbiturate with a rapid onset and a short duration of action (15 minutes or less). Thiopental sodium was first used at the Mayo Clinic in 1934. Today, it is the most widely used of the barbiturate anesthetics. Its major use is for induction of anesthesia, although it may be used as a sole agent for short procedures. It is sometimes used to control drug-induced convulsions resulting from allergy to local anesthetics. The adverse effects of thiopental sodium include respiratory depression, bronchospasm, cardiac depression, and hypotension. Use of thiopental sodium is contraindicated in patients with asthma or porphyria. Most of the complications seen with this drug are iatrogenic, the result of poor drug administration technique. Skin sloughing, edema, chemical arteritis, or gangrene can result if this drug is not properly administered and is delivered into the subcutaneous tissues or into an artery.

Methohexital Sodium

Methohexital sodium (Brevital) is an ultra-short-acting barbiturate that has five times the strength of thiopental sodium. It is also shorter acting than thiopental sodium and less likely to cause bronchospasm. Its disadvantages are similar to those of thiopental sodium and include respiratory depression. It also is not a good skeletal muscle relaxant or analgesic. Methohexital sodium is especially useful in examination under anesthesia procedures, oral surgery, and the setting of fractures. It is less likely to cause bronchospasm and may, therefore, be administered cautiously to patients with asthma. Intra-arterial administration of this agent can cause gangrene. Because of a shorter duration of action than thiopental, this drug is especially useful for outpatients. It is also used for patients undergoing electroconvulsive therapy (ECT).

Thiamylal Sodium

Thiamylal sodium (Surital) is the last of the ultra-short-acting barbiturates commonly used to induce anesthesia. Thiamylal sodium is also similar to thiopental in its rapid onset, short duration of effect, and recovery time. It is used as a short-duration anesthetic for diagnostic procedures. It shares the same limitations and disadvantages as the other ultra-short-acting barbiturates.

Ketamine Hydrochloride

Ketamine hydrochloride (Ketalar) is a synthetic nonbarbiturate agent and can be administered either intravenously or intramuscularly. Ketamine is metabolized by the liver and excreted primarily in the urine, with small amounts eliminated in the stool. Ketamine produces a state known as dissociative anesthesia because the patient feels dissociated or detached from the environment during induction. The exact mechansim of dissociative anesthetic action is not fully understood. It is known that ketamine selectively interrupts the higher brain centers of the cerebral cortex, causing a generalized sensory blockade that produces anesthesia. This drug has a rapid induction and produces good analgesia and amnesia but poor muscle relaxation. Ketamine does not depress the respiratory system. This drug actually increases the tone of skeletal, cardiac, and respiratory muscles and can thus raise blood pressure and heart and respiratory rates. Ketamine produces good anesthesia for 5–25 minutes with stable cardiovascular activity and good airway status. Intubation is not necessary when this drug is administered because of its negligible effect on the pharyngeal and laryngeal reflexes. This agent is often used in combination with other low-potency drugs such as nitrous oxide to produce a balanced level of anesthesia. It is a good drug of choice for short surgical or diagnostic procedures (except those involving the pharyngeal-laryngeal areas). Ketamine is often used in burn units where patients require frequent, repetitive anesthesia for procedures.

The major disadvantage of ketamine is its prolonged (up to several hours) recovery period and the occurrence of emergence reactions. Approximately 12% of persons receiving ketamine experience disturbing dreams and/or hallucinations as the drug wears off. This effect may occur more frequently in adults than in children. Diazepam (Valium) administration is recommended in conjunction with ketamine to help decrease the frequency of nightmares and hallucinations in the postoperative period. Ketamine is contraindicated in patients with hypertension or alcoholism, those who will undergo intracranial surgery, and people who have bad dreams, such as psychiatric patients. Safe use of this drug during pregnancy and delivery has not yet been established.

Droperidol/Fentanyl

Droperidol/fentanyl (Innovar) is the combination of a potent narcotic analgesic (fentanyl) with the anesthetic/antipsychotic agent droperidol. This combination is available under the trade name Innovar in a 50:1 fixed ratio. Innovar produces a state of neuroleptic analgesia: the patient is psychologically indifferent to the environment, pain free, but not necessarily asleep (depending on the dose administered). Thus, it can be useful for patients undergoing endoscopic procedures where some degree of patient cooperation may be needed. It is also an excellent agent for use as an adjunct to more potent general anesthetics for both induction and maintenance.

Droperidol/fentanyl may be administered either intramuscularly (45–60 minutes preoperatively) or intravenously. Droperidol/fentanyl can be used alone for short surgical or diagnostic procedures or in combination with other drugs. In addition to its anesthetic effects, droperidol/fentanyl produces excellent antiemetic effects, β-adrenergic blocking, and antiarrhythmic effects. The drug's major disadvantages are the slow onset of anesthesia and the degree of postoperative respira-

tory depression produced. Analgesic effects may linger several hours following surgery, so it is essential to reduce doses of all central nervous system depressant drugs, such as narcotic analgesics, by one third to one half for 8 hours after anesthesia. Droperidol/fentanyl can cause bradycardia, bronchospasm, apnea, and muscle rigidity, which is usually due to the fentanyl component in the drug. Thus, it is essential to keep atropine available (for bradycardia); keep CPR and airway intubation equipment, neuromuscular blockers, and narcotic antagonists available (for respiratory complications); and check vital signs frequently.

Alfentanil Hydrochloride

Alfentanil hydrochloride (Alfenta) is an opioid analgesic with a rapid onset of action. It is an excellent induction agent and can also be a component of balanced opioid anesthesia. Alfenta is a relatively new anesthetic agent that is useful for (1) incremental injection as an analgesic adjunct for short surgical procedures (less than one hour); (2) continuous infusion as a maintenance analgesic with nitrous oxide/oxygen for general surgical procedures; and (3) by intravenous injection for induction of general anesthesia for procedures with a minimum duration of 45 minutes. Since opioid analgesics tend to produce some muscle rigidity, use of a neuromuscular blocking agent is necessary when Alfenta is used in anesthetic doses.

The dose of Alfenta is individualized to the patient according to ideal body weight, physical status, underlying pathologic status, and the type and duration of surgical procedure and anesthesia. The dosage of Alfenta should be reduced in elderly or debilitated patients and not used in children under twelve years of age. Alfenta should be used with caution in patients with pulmonary disease, decreased respiratory reserve, potentially compromised respiration, or impaired renal or liver function. When Alfenta is administered in combination with other central nervous system depressants the magnitude and duration of central nervous system and cardiovascular effects may be enhanced, necessitating a reduction in the dose of one or both agents.

Sufentanil Citrate

Sufentanil citrate (Sufenta) is an opioid analgesic with an immediate onset of action. It is used as an analgesic adjunct in the maintenance of balanced general anesthesia, as well as a primary anesthetic agent for the induction and maintenance of anesthesia with 100% oxygen in patients undergoing major surgical procedures. Sufenta is useful in cardiovascular surgery or neurosurgical procedures and provides favorable myocardial and cerebral oxygen balance. It is also useful when extended postoperative ventilation is anticipated. Use of a neuromuscular agent is needed with Sufenta because of the muscle rigidity this opioid produces.

Sufenta dosages are based upon lean body weight and should be reduced in elderly or debilitated patients and used with caution in patients with pulmonary disease, compromised pulmonary status, or liver or renal impairment. When Sufenta is used in combination with other central nervous system depressants, the magnitude and duration of central nervous system and cardiovascular effects may be enhanced; thus the dosage of one or both agents should be reduced.

OTHER PERIOPERATIVE DRUGS

In addition to the various anesthetic agents already discussed, several other drugs may be administered in the perioperative period to facilitate and/or augment the anesthetic process. These drugs will be considered only in relation to their status as anesthetic adjuncts.

Atropine, a parasympatholytic or cholinergic blocking agent, is frequently administered as a preanesthetic medication. Atropine produces many effects including mydriasis, reduced secretion of certain glands, relaxation of smooth muscles, and vagolytic activity. (For further information on atropine, see Chapter 18). The main reasons for its preanesthesia use are its ability to decrease respiratory tract secretions and to prevent anesthesia-induced bradycardia. The usual adult dose administered is 0.4–0.6 mg intramuscularly 30–60 minutes preoperatively. Since many anesthetics currently available are relatively nonirritating to the respiratory tract, use of the anticholinergic atropine may not be as common as in the past.

Promethazine Hydrochloride

Promethazine hydrochloride (Phenergan) is a phenothiazine-derivative antihistamine. It also has anticholinergic, antiemetic, antipruritic, and sedative properties. Because promethazine is a phenothiazine, all precautions and warnings applicable to the phenothiazines apply to this drug also. (For further information, see phenothiazines in Chapter 25). Promethazine is thought to potentiate analgesia even though scientific data does not support this notion, and it is also used preoperatively for its sedative effect. Usual adult preoperative dose is 50 mg, combined with an atropine-like drug. Postoperatively, promethazine is administered to combat nausea and as an adjunct to analgesics, especially the narcotics, administered for postoperative pain. Usual adult dose is 12.5–50 mg intramuscularly.

Glycopyrrolate

Glycopyrrolate (Robinul) is a synthetic anticholinergic agent that is used for preoperative medication and to help counteract the adverse effects of anticholinergics given to reverse neuromuscular blockade. This drug decreases the volume and acidity of respiratory tract secretions and is believed not to cross the blood–brain barrier. Robinul is being more frequently used than in the past because of its low level of toxicity and better ability to reduce respiratory tract secretions. Usual adult preoperative dose is 0.002 mg/lb body weight intramuscularly 30–60 minutes preoperatively. To help reverse adverse effects of neuromuscular blockade the adult dose is 0.2 mg intravenously for each 1 mg neostigmine or equivalent dose of pyridostigmine. There are no significant interactions, but use of this drug is contraindicated in narrow-angle glaucoma, unstable cardiovascular status, myasthenia gravis, and obstructive urologic or gastrointestinal diseases.

Naloxone

Naloxone (Narcan) is a narcotic antagonist frequently used to reverse the effects of narcotics. Naloxone has no respiratory depressant or agonist activity of its own and is the most frequently used narcotic antagonist drug. Usual adult dose is 0.1–0.2 mg intravenously every 2–3 minutes as needed to reverse the effects of perioperatively administered narcotics. There are no significant interactions with Narcan. Once the effects of narcotics are reversed, the patient can experience intense pain.

There are other drugs, too numerous to mention, that may be used to facilitate anesthesia by producing some degree of preanesthesia sedation. Other drugs are also used for their effects during and following anesthetic administration. Antianxiety agents such as diazepam (Valium); hypnotic sedatives such as pentobarbital sodium (Nembutal); and narcotics such as meperidine (Demerol) and midazolam (Versed) are all commonly used perioperative agents. They may be used before surgery to facilitate anesthesia; during surgery to augment anesthesia/analgesia; and after surgery to relieve nausea, promote sedation, and/or provide analgesia. (For further information on any of these drugs, turn to their respective chapters.)

NEUROMUSCULAR BLOCKING AGENTS

Neuromuscular blocking agents are commonly used as adjuncts to other anesthesia-producing drugs. Although they are commonly referred to as muscle relaxants, this term is a misnomer. Neuromusclar blocking agents work peripherally by blocking the transmission of impulses at the neuromuscular junction. A true muscle relaxant such as carisoprodol (Soma) or chlorzoxazone (Paraflex) works centrally to reduce the transmission of impulses from the spinal cord to skeletal muscle in order to provide relief from muscle strain. Centrally acting skeletal muscle relaxants are discussed in detail in Chapter 23. Neuromuscular blocking agents are powerful drugs that produce apnea and paralysis. During surgery, it is usually desirable for the patient to be paralyzed. Many general anesthetics in use today have minimal muscle-relaxing properties; therefore, in order to produce sufficient muscle relaxation for surgery, a deep level of anesthesia must be achieved. Specific neuromuscular blocking drugs capable of producing sufficient muscle paralysis for surgery while maintaining a lighter level of anesthesia are frequently combined with anesthetics. Thus, the use of neuromuscular blockers facilitates endotracheal intubation and helps maintain anesthesia sufficient for the performance of surgery requiring deep muscle relaxation, such as abdominal procedures. Two types of neuromuscular blockers are used today, the depolarizing and nondepolarizing agents. Both types paralyze the neuromuscular junction to prevent the electrochemical transmission of information, although they accomplish this by different methods.

Neuromuscular blocking agents work by interrupting or preventing the electrochemical transfer of information at the neuromuscular synapse of nerve cells (neurons). Each neuron consists of a central cell body with threadlike projections called nerve fibers extending from each end. The axon is the nerve fiber that conducts impulses of information away from the cell body. The dendrite fibers conduct information to the cell body. Although a neuron may have many dendrite fibers, it generally has only one axon. Impulses of information are transferred through a process that involves both electrical conduction of a signal down an axon and chemical transmission of the signal from one neuron to another or from a neuron to another receiving cell such as a muscle fiber.

Impulses of information flow between nerve cells and other cells through the synapses; they do not "jump across" these synaptic gaps. The electrical conduction of a signal down the axon occurs as an action potential (a series of polarizations and depolarizations). As the action potential invades the nerve ending, a presynaptic neurotransmitting substance, in this case acetylcholine, is released. The acetylcholine allows the impulse formation to diffuse across the synapse to act on the postsynaptic membrane of the receiving cell to produce a new action potential or modulate a pre-existing action. Figure 10–2 shows where neuromuscular blocking agents act. An explanation of nondepolarizing and depolarizing neuromuscular agents follows. For more information on how the neuromuscular agents work, refer to Chapter 18.

Nondepolarizing Agents

Nondepolarizing (also called competitive) *neuromuscular blocking agents* include the drugs d-tubocurarine chloride (Tubarine), vecuronium bromide (Norcuron), pancuronium bromide (Pavulon), and atracurium (Tracrium). These drugs all work by competitive inhibition on the postsynaptic membrane. They block acetylcholine by combining with the receptors usually occupied by acetylcholine. These drugs do not change membrane muscle potential. Only skeletal muscles are affected by these agents. If more than 60% of the acetylcholine receptors are occupied by the blocker (drug), the end-plate potential cannot reach threshold level and muscle contraction cannot occur. When drug concentration of the blocker at the end-plate decreases and sufficient receptors became available to acetylcholine, muscle contraction is again possible. When the nondepolarizing block is no longer needed, it can be reversed by administering an antidote mixture of neostigmine and atropine. Neostigmine causes a build-up of acetylcholine to reverse the block, and atropine minimizes the side effects of acetylcholine build-up elsewhere in the body (bradycardia, bronchospasm, and excessive salivation) caused by neostigmine. For further information on neurotransmitters such as acetylcholine, refer to Chapter 17.

Depolarizing Agents

Depolarizing (or noncompetitive) *neuromuscular blockade* is achieved with succinylcholine (Anectine, Quelicin),

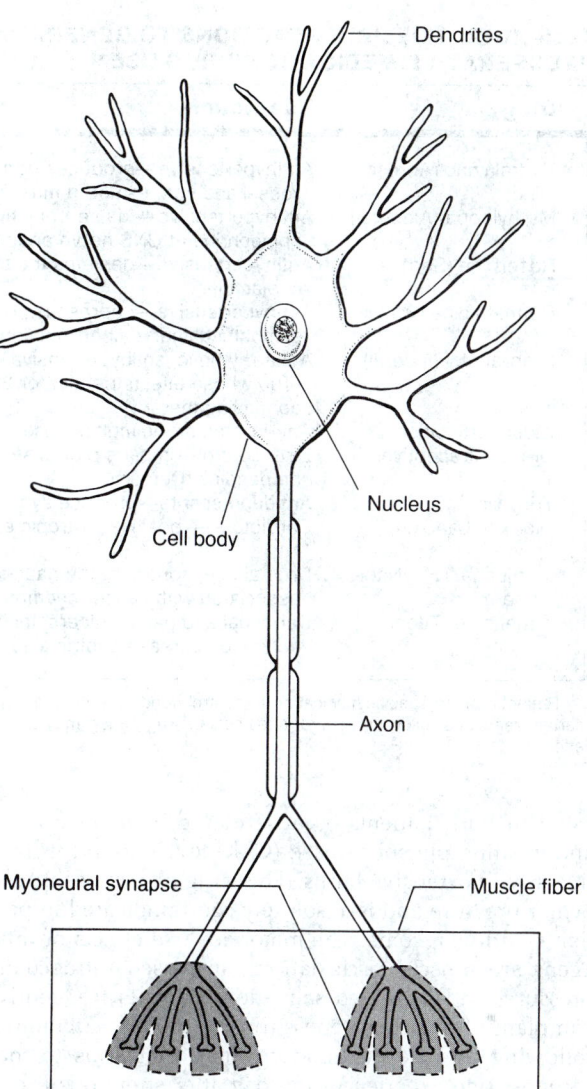

Figure 10–2. Location of neuromuscular blocking drug action in neurons. Neurons (nerve cells) receive and transmit impulses of information in a process that involves both electrical conduction of a signal down an axon and chemical transmission of this information at the synapse. The transmission of the signal at the synapse is achieved by the secretion of the neurotransmitter acetylcholine which allows the information to diffuse across the synapse to act on the receiving cell. It is in this area that neuromuscular blocking agents exert their effect and block the transmission of information (shaded area of figure).

the only drug of this type currently used. Succinylcholine is a potent skeletal muscle relaxant that achieves its effect rapidly through depolarization of the motor endplate. After the administration of this drug, muscle fasciculations occur, and potassium is forced out of the muscle cells and into the circulation. This raises potassium levels and may possibly cause digitalis toxicity. Preoperative hyperkalemia is a relative contraindication to the use of this drug. Succinylcholine is contraindi-

Table 10–2. POSSIBLE REACTIONS TO GENERAL ANESTHESIA DUE TO PREOPERATIVE MEDICATION/DRUG USE*

Drug	Use/Action	Potential Effect(s)
Hydralazine (Apresoline)	Antihypertensive—produces peripheral blood vessel and some smooth muscle relaxation.	Hypertensive crisis. Rebound hypotensive crisis may occur 48 hr following anesthesia.
Methyldopa (Aldomet)	Antihypertensive—"false transmitter" for norepinephrine at CNS nerve ending.	Hypertensive crisis.
Reserpine (Serpasil)	Antihypertensive—depletes the stores of catecholamines.	Hypertensive crisis.
Guanethidine (Ismelin)	Antihypertensive—depresses postganglionic sympathetic nerve fiber function.	Hypertensive crisis.
Propranolol (Inderal)	Antiarrhythmic; antihypertensive—β-blocking drug whose effects persist for 24 hr after discontinuing therapy.	Hypotension.
Glucocorticoids	Anti-inflammatory, multiple uses.	Hypotension.
Oral contraceptives	Birth control—impairs biotransformation of meperidine (Demerol).	Decreased effectiveness of meperidine (Demerol).
Tricyclics	Antidepressants—produce sympathetic effects.	Hypotension/hypertension, junctional rhythms.
Digoxin (Lanoxin)	Cardiotonic—positive inotropic effect.	Increased sympathetic effect of this drug on the heart.
Marijuana/THC/Nabilone	Drug abuse; control of the nausea/vomiting associated with cancer chemotherapy.	Potentiates the effects of barbiturates.
Cimetidine (Tagamet)	Duodenal and gastric ulcers. Inhibits histamine action to decrease gastric acid secretions.	Prolongs duration of action of succinylcholine.

*Patients taking specific medication to control conditions such as hypertension may be more susceptible to certain reactions following general anesthesia. Drug abuse may also precipitate certain postanesthesia side effects.

cated in burn patients because of the high potassium and creatine phosphokinase (CPK) levels found in patients with extensive burns. This drug also raises intraocular pressure and is absolutely contraindicated in patients with glaucoma. The major adverse effects of this agent are muscle fasciculations, increased intraocular pressure, and increased salivation. Patients frequently complain of muscle soreness (due to the fasciculations) following the use of this drug. It is analogous to the soreness one experiences the day after strenuous exercise following a long period of inactivity. Cimetidine (Tagamet) apparently intensifies the action of succinylcholine. Thus, the combination of these two drugs may lead to prolonged respiratory depression and extended periods of apnea (Table 10–2).

Succinylcholine is especially useful in facilitating endotracheal intubation. Its duration of effect is short (2–5 minutes), and it is rapidly broken down by the enzyme pseudocholinesterase. Approximately 1 in 2800 people has inherited atypical pseudocholinesterase, which poorly breaks down this drug. Such patients experience prolonged (3–24 hours) paralysis after a single intubation dose of succinylcholine. These patients may require prolonged ventilatory support and bear close watching until succinylcholine has sufficiently worn off. Needless to say, succinylcholine should not be administered to known pseudocholinesterase-deficient patients. There is no antidote for succinylcholine. However, the prolonged apnea caused by administration of a large dose may be reversed by neostigmine.

LOCAL ANESTHETICS

Local anesthetics stabilize the nerve cell membranes to sodium and potassium exchange, thus blocking the conduction of impulses in nerve fibers without depolarizing the cell membrane. As the anesthetic concentration increases, so too the threshold for excitation increases. These drugs can act on any part of the central nervous system and on any type of nerve cell. Onset of effect is first upon the small nonmyelinated autonomic fibers; next, ability to sense cold, warmth, pain, and touch is affected; and finally, motor function is affected. Sensation returns in reverse order.

There are several different techniques of local (sometimes called conduction) anesthesia. The types of *local anesthesia* and their sites of actions are as follows:

1. Topical (surface) anesthesia refers to the application of a readily absorbed agent to the skin or mucous membranes. Cocaine and tetracaine are topical anesthetics.
2. Infiltration anesthesia is produced by injecting the agent throughout the area to be desensitized. This is commonly done by injecting a drug along the line of an incision or the edges of a laceration to be sutured. The drug is injected into the tissue in the area and not into any specific nerves.
3. Field block anesthesia is accomplished by infiltrating the tissue around the area to be made insensitive without infiltrating the area itself. This technique is commonly used in the excision of sebaceous cysts.
4. Nerve block is the injection of the drug close to a mixed nerve so that the area innervated by that nerve will become insensitive.
5. Spinal anesthesia is achieved by injecting a local anesthetic into the subarachnoid space. Epidural anesthesia is the technique of injecting the drug between the vertebral spines and beneath the ligament into the extradural space. There are fewer complications,

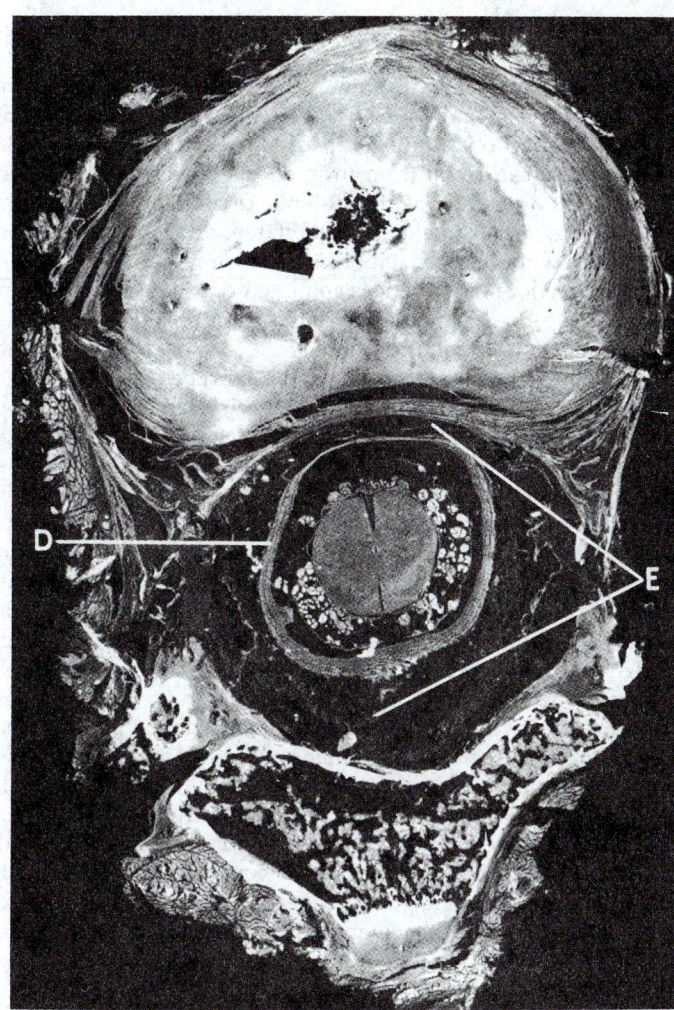

Figure 10–3. Where anesthetics are administered in the spinal canal. Traverse section of spine between 1st and 2nd lumbar vertebrae. E is the epidural space where local anesthetic agent is placed for epidural anesthesia. D is the dural and arachnoid matters separating it from the subarachnoid space. S is the subarachnoid space where anesthetic is injected to achieve spinal anesthesia. (From Norris, W. and Campbell, D.: A Nurses' Guide to Anesthetics, Resuscitation and Intensive Care, ed. 5, Williams & Wilkins, Baltimore, 1972, page 11, with permission.)

such as headache, following epidural anesthesia. Spinal and epidural anesthesia are sometimes referred to as regional anesthesia techniques (Fig. 10–3).

6. Caudal anesthesia is a technically simpler variation of spinal anesthesia technique produced by injecting the local anesthetic into the caudal or sacral canal. Caudal anesthesia is a variation of epidural anesthesia—it is just administered lower, into the caudal/sacral canal. This method of regional anesthesia is commonly used in obstetric patients.

7. Intravenous regional anesthesia is the anesthesia of the entire distal part of an extremity. This is accomplished by elevating the extremity, producing exsanguination by application of two tourniquets, and injecting the drug intravenously in the distal part of the extremity. This technique is commonly utilized in hand surgery (the Bier block) and foot surgery. Maximum length of anesthesia is 1.5 hours because of the use of the tourniquets.

Desirable characteristics of a good local anesthetic drug include complete reversibility, low systemic toxicity, action confined principally to nerve tissue, short onset time, sufficiently long duration, solubility in saline solution and water, sterilizability and storability without deterioration, compatibility with vasoconstrictor drugs, and lack of tissue irritation.

There are two types of local anesthesia, the amides and the esters. Determination of anesthetic type depends on which kind of chemical bond is present in the drug's molecular structure. Local anesthetics of the amide type include bupivacaine, dibucaine, etidocaine, lidocaine, mepivacaine, and prilocaine. Local anesthetics of the ester type are chloroprocaine, piperocaine, procaine, and tetracaine.

Epinephrine is often combined with local anesthetic drugs to slow drug absorption and thereby prolong anesthetic effect. Rapidity of drug absorption depends on drug dose, site of injection, technique of anesthesia used, and local conditions at the site of administration. The amide-type local anesthetics are metabolized almost totally by the liver and excreted in the urine. Local anesthetics of the ester group are rapidly and almost completely metabolized by blood pseudocholinesterase. The rest of the drug is metabolized in the liver. The drug metabolites are then excreted in the urine. The onset of action for all types of local anesthetics is within 15 minutes of administration. The duration of action varies according to the agent utilized, dose, technique of administration, and local tissue conditions. For example, the presence of local infection changes the pH of the tissue, causing less anesthetic to enter the cells and thereby producing less effective anesthesia.

Adverse reactions to all local anesthetic drugs may occur. These can result from toxic effects produced by an excess of drug entering the systemic circulation. Toxicity can also occur in elderly, debilitated, or acutely ill patients in whom drug metabolism is impaired. If a toxic reaction to a local anesthetic is going to occur, it usually happens within 10 minutes of administration but can occur as long as 45 minutes later.

Local anesthetics of the amide and ester types can interfere with the function of any organ or system that is dependent on the conduction or transmission of impulses, for example, the central nervous, respiratory, and cardiovascular systems. These drugs can produce arrhythmias, bradycardia, hypotension, cardiac arrest, or respiratory failure. Local anesthetics work directly on the myocardium, decreasing electrical excitability, conduction rate, and the force of contractions. This is the rationale for the clinical use of lidocaine to control an irritable heart. However, a toxic dose of lidocaine can produce cardiac arrest in a normal heart.

Hypersensitivity reactions to local anesthetics may occur but are relatively uncommon. Most reactions of this type occur with the ester rather than the amide group. Anaphylactic reactions are theoretically possible but occur extremely rarely. Early signs and symptoms of allergic reaction to a local anesthetic agent include rash, erythema, hives, itching, and edema. Treatment includes airway maintenance and administration of oxygen and diphenhydramine (Benadryl) 50 mg intravenously. Signs of severe hypersensitivity (anaphylaxis) include bronchoconstriction, asthmatic breathing, hypotension, vascular collapse, and shock. Treatment includes the above measures and intravenous fluids for hypotension and administration of appropriate bronchodilators and vasopressors. Table 10–3 features local anesthetic drugs.

USE OF THE NURSING PROCESS IN PATIENTS RECEIVING ANESTHETICS

The nursing process that follows focuses on care of the patient relative to the anesthetic drugs being administered. For other perioperative patient care details, consult a comprehensive surgical nursing text.

PREOPERATIVE ASSESSMENT

Preoperative care begins with the initial nursing assessment of the patient. For the hospitalized patient, this means the admission nursing assessment. In the ambulatory (outpatient) surgical patient, this preoperative assessment may be done just before the procedure or during the patient's preoperative visit for blood work and tests. In *ambulatory* or *outpatient surgery*, the patient arrives shortly before the procedure and leaves afterward when he or she has sufficiently recovered from the anesthetic. The short-procedure-unit approach has the patient arrive shortly before the procedure, provides a hospital bed and care for approximately eight hours postoperatively, and then discharges the patient.

Ambulatory care and short-procedure units are becoming popular for several reasons. The rising cost of all phases of health care, from insurance premiums to hospitalization, as well as the relative safety of certain routine procedures has prompted the development of this approach to surgical care. Newer anesthetic agents with rapid onset of action and rapid recovery have made it possible to discharge patients the same day of surgery following a general anesthesia, something which was unthinkable a decade ago. In addition, many insurance companies no longer will pay for the hospitalization of patients for procedures they deem to be "outpatient" or *same-day* surgical procedures. In other words, no overnight hospitalization is authorized for procedures that do not require skilled nursing care in the immediate postoperative period. An exception would be for patients with medical problems that place them at high risk for complications.

In several medical specialties, certain procedures are performed which lend themselves well to the short procedure or ambulatory care surgical approach. These include such eye surgery as cataract removal; urologic procedures such as vasectomy; gynecologic procedures such as laparoscopic tubal ligations and dilatation and curettage (D & C); podiatric procedures such as arthroplasties and bunionectomies; and other general procedures such as breast biopsies, cyst removals, and endoscopic (laparoscopy, bronchoscopy, panendoscopy) tests. Because of the shortened preoperative contact and interaction inherent in these approaches to surgery, the nursing assessment becomes more important than ever. Postoperative patient contact is likewise abbreviated at a time when patient/family teaching is essential to patient observation and care.

The initial patient assessment by the nurse includes a basic health history and psychosocial assessment. Personal health habits, eating and sleeping patterns, and drinking and smoking habits are all included in this assessment. Such information can give a more definitive focus to the nursing care regimen. Important information such as when the patient last ate or took fluids (especially for the walk-in surgical patient), allergies, and concurrent conditions or diseases are also noted prominently on the patient's chart because they can influence the choice of drugs used for the anesthesia. For example, succinylcholine is contraindicated in patients with glaucoma. Conditions such as hypertension or alcoholism (chronic or acute) contraindicate the use of ketamine. It is also important to ascertain the presence of allergies. For example, if a patient has had a hypersensitivity reaction to a drug such as procaine, the physician may avoid using other ester-type local anesthetics as a safety precaution. Patients should be asked about any previous "reactions" to anesthetic agents they may have experienced. It is also important to ask the patient if any drugs or medications (prescriptions, over-the-counter, or recreational) have been taken within the 72 hours preceding surgery, because this too may influence the choice of anesthetic or preclude the use of certain other drugs. For example, marijuana potentiates barbiturates (Table 10–2).

Patients on drugs such as cardiac medications should take them as usual, even when they are allowed nothing by mouth (NPO) before surgery. The patient should take such necessary medications with as little fluid as possible. Patients who will be discharged from the Short Procedure Unit or Ambulatory Care Center after the procedure must be accompanied by a responsible adult, even if only local anesthetization is planned.

The nurse also assesses the psychological and physiologic status of the patient, and determines the patient's understanding of the surgery in addition to noting the level of anxiety. Physiologic baseline data collected include vital signs as well as routine laboratory test results, radiographs, and electrocardiograms. Any abnormalities are reported promptly to the physician, anesthetist, or both, because they may necessitate a change in the surgical plan.

NURSING DIAGNOSES

Nursing diagnoses based on the assessment data may relate to the physical or psychological findings. For example, a nursing diagnosis of high level of anxiety might be appropriate for the excessively apprehensive patient. Other typical nursing diagnoses are included in Table 10–4. Nursing care plans will, of necessity, reflect individual patient problems or needs. The objectives (goals) of nursing care in this preoperative phase are to prepare the patient for surgery, to facilitate an uneventful operative and postoperative period, and to anticipate and plan for postoperative needs.

PREOPERATIVE NURSING INTERVENTION

Preoperative nursing interventions begin when the initial nursing assessment is completed. An explanation of preoperative procedures, anesthesia recovery, equipment likely to be in use, and the postoperative routine at this time helps answer unspoken patient questions and fosters cooperation. Ideally the patient has been well prepared for the day of surgery by both the surgeon and nurse. Most hospitals have nurse surgical coordinators who oversee outpatient testing and patient preparation before the day of surgery. Since most patients undergoing surgery have preoperative tests done on an outpatient basis several days before surgery, an initial nursing assessment often begins with this contact. Often patients are given a tour of the operating room and detailed patient teaching relative to their surgery, anesthesia, and immediate postoperative care when they report for the routine preoperative tests. Adequate explanations by the nurse in this preliminary contact can help allay patient and family fears. Table 10–5 provides general patient teaching information. The surgeon should have prepared the patient by giving specific information relative to the surgical procedure to be performed. Printed instructions from the surgeon help ensure that instructions are not misunderstood or forgotten. Figure 10–4 is an example of preoperative instructions given to patients about to undergo podiatric surgery.

When the patient is admitted and the time of surgery approaches, specific nursing care actions center around taking vital signs, administering the preanesthetic injection, and entering appropriate documentation on the patient's chart. First, preoperative laboratory reports are checked and vital signs are taken, because abrupt changes or the presence of a fever may necessitate a postponement of surgery. Any abnormalities are reported immediately. If vital signs are within normal limits and other presurgical tasks have been completed, the nurse administers the preanesthetic medication. Generally, the preclinical medication is administered 30–60 minutes before surgery. Barbiturates, analgesics, and/or cholinergic blockers are frequently given in order to dry secretions, sedate the patient, and facilitate the anesthetic induction period. Since it is common practice for more than one drug to be ordered, always check the compatibility of the drugs to be administered before mixing them. Some drugs, such as diazepam (Valium), are highly incompatible and should not be mixed with other medications. When in doubt about the compatibility of a certain combination of drugs, check with the pharmacist. Do not administer any drugs that appear cloudy or have precipitate matter present. It is essential that the preanesthetic medications be administered at the specific time ordered so the patient may derive the full benefit from the drug's effects. Once the medication is administered, have the patient lie quietly in bed with the side rails up until he or she is transported to the operating room. This promotes patient safety and facilitates drug effectiveness.

PREOPERATIVE NURSING EVALUATIONS

Preoperative nursing evaluations include many parameters. In addition to checking vital signs and preoperative medication effectiveness, the nurse also makes a final physical check of the patient to determine if he or she is indeed properly prepared for surgery. Documentation of patient status is required on a preoperative checklist in addition to the regular nurse's progress notes. It is also important at this time to give psychological and emotional reassurances to the patient. As the impending surgery draws nearer, even the best prepared patient becomes somewhat anxious. Always remember that no matter how minor or routine a procedure might be to you as a nurse, it is not routine for the patient. Studies have shown that patients having repeat procedures do not necessarily experience any less anxi-

TEXT RESUMES ON PAGE 237

Table 10–3. LOCAL ANESTHETICS

Name	Dosage	Mode of Administration	Pharmacokinetics
Action: All local anesthetics block the conduction of impulses in nerve fibers without depolarizing the cell membrane, resulting in numbness/loss of sensation in body part.			
AMIDE TYPE			
Available with or without epinephrine. All doses given for drug without epinephrine.			
Bupivacaine hydrochloride (Marcaine, Sensorcaine)			
Use: Peripheral nerve block, infiltration, caudal or epidural block, sympathetic block.			
	0.50% sol, 75–100 mg 0.50% sol, 75–100 mg 0.50% sol, 24–400 mg (max)	Epidural Caudal Peripheral nerve block	O: 4–17 min P: UA D: 3–6 hr PB: 52%–96% ½ L: 1.5–5.5 B: liver E: urine
Etidocaine hydrochloride (Duranest)			
Use: Infiltration, peripheral nerve blocks, caudal and epidural nerve blocks, vaginal.			
	0.5% sol, 4–400 mg 0.5% sol, 25–400 mg 0.5% sol, 50–150 mg 0.5% sol, 50–150 mg	Infiltration Peripheral nerve block Caudal Vaginal	O: 2–8 min P: UA D: 3–6 hr PB: 94%–96% ½ L: 1–2 hr B: liver E: urine

   Key to Abbreviations in the *Pharmacokinetics* column O-onset; P-peak; D-duration; PB-protein bound; B-bio-transformed in; E-excreted in; ½ L = halflife.
   *Within the column listing adverse effects, underlines indicate the most common effects; CAPITALS indicate life-threatening effects.

Contraindications and Precautions	Adverse Effects*	Interactions	Nursing Implications
Contraindicated for spinal anesthesia, topical anesthesia, or paracervical blocks, and in children under 12 yr. Use of 5% bupivacaine contraindicated in obstetric patients. Do not use solutions with preservatives for caudal or epidural blocks. Solutions with epinephrine used cautiously in cardiovascular disease and end arteries (fingers, toes, ears, nose).	Adverse effects related to local anesthetics are generally due to high blood levels of the drug. CV: ARRHYTHMIAS, MYOCARDIAL DEPRESSION, CARDIAC ARREST Resp: Status asthmaticus, RESPIRATORY ARREST Derm: Dermatologic reactions, edema GI: Nausea, vomiting Misc: Blurred vision, ANAPHYLAXIS	Enflurane, halothane, and related drugs: Cardiac arrhythmias can occur when used with the form of the drug containing epinephrine. Use with extreme caution. MAO inhibitors, tricyclic antidepressants: Severe and sustained hypertension can occur when used with the form of this drug containing epinephrine. Use with extreme caution.	ASSESSMENT: Assess anesthetized areas for return of sensation and motor function. INTERVENTION: Instruct patient that this drug is 4 times more potent than lidocaine. Duration of action is 3–6 hr but effects can last up to 16 hr. This drug is commonly used in ambulatory surgery for peripheral nerve blocks because of the long duration of effect, which helps postpone patient perception of pain in immediate postoperative period. Interventions following spinal anesthesia include spinal headache. Precautions: Patient should lie flat in bed for first 8–12 hr post-op. EVALUATION: Patient has pain free procedure with sensory return afterwards. Health teaching is effective and patient complies with any necessary restriction(s) of activity. If used for spinal anesthesia, spinal headache is avoided. No preventable adverse effects occur. If used for local anesthesia, trauma to anesthetized area is avoided.
Contraindicated in children under age 14; inflammation at proposed injection site; spinal deformities; spinal block; septicemia; severe hypertension; neurologic disorders. Do not use solutions with preservatives in epidural or caudal blocks. Severe	Same as bupivacaine.	Enflurane, halothane, and related drugs: Cardiac arrhythmias can occur when used with the form of this drug containing epinephrine. Use with extreme caution. MAO inhibitors, tricyclic antidepressants, phenothiazines: severe and sustained hypertension or hypoten-	ASSESSMENT: Ask females if there is any chance of pregnancy because safe use during pregnancy not established. Assess anesthetized areas for return of sensation, motor functions. Monitor patient for signs of adverse effects: allergy, respiratory distress, anaphylaxis.

CONTINUED ON THE FOLLOWING PAGE

Table 10–3. LOCAL ANESTHETICS–_CONTINUED_

Name	Dosage	Mode of Administration	Pharmacokinetics
Etidocaine hydrochloride (Duranest)–_Continued_			
Lidocaine hydrochloride (Xylocaine, Nervocaine, Ultracaine)			

Use: Topical infiltrations; nerve block; caudal; epidural; spinal; and IV regional. Also drug of choice to treat ventricular tachycardia and other arrhythmias. (Refer to Chapter 30 for cardiac use since this chapter deals with anesthetic drug use only.)

Name	Dosage	Mode of Administration	Pharmacokinetics
	Available with and without epinephrine; safe dose 7 mg/kg; maximum 200 mg without epinephrine, 500 mg with epinephrine		
	1% sol, 200–300 mg	Caudal (obstetric use) or epidural (thoracic)	O: 5–10 min P: UA
	1.5% sol, 225–300 mg	Caudal (surgery)	D: 1 hr without epinephrine; 2–3 hr with epinephrine
	5% sol, with 7.5% dextrose, 75–100 mg	Spinal surgical anesthesia	PB: 60%–80% ½ L: 100 min B: liver E: urine

Key to Abbreviations in the _Pharmacokinetics_ column O-onset; P-peak; D-duration; PB-protein bound; B-biotransformed in; E-excreted in; ½ L = halflife.
*Within the column listing adverse effects, underlines indicate the most common effects; CAPITALS indicate life-threatening effects.

Contraindications and Precautions	Adverse Effects*	Interactions	Nursing Implications
hypertension or hypotension can result if drug containing epinephrine given to patient taking MAO inhibitors, tricyclics, or phenothiazines. Solutions with epinephrine used cautiously in cardiovascular disease or in end arteries (fingers, toes, ears, nose). Safe use in pregnancy not established.		sion can occur when used with the form of this drug containing epinephrine. Use with extreme caution.	INTERVENTION: Tell patient duration of drug action can be up to 13 hr (usually 3–6 hr) so that ambulatory surgical patients know drug action lasts longer than lidocaine or typical dental anesthesia because most patients are familiar with that type of local anesthesia. Tell patient to protect area of local anesthesia from trauma since they may not be aware of injury because of numbness. EVALUATION: Same as for Bupivacaine.
Same as etidocaine.	Same as bupivacaine.	Same as bupivacaine.	ASSESSMENT: Ask patient about what other medicines/drugs they may be taking in order to determine if patient is taking MAO inhibitors or tricyclic antidepressants; severe hypertension can occur if drug containing epinephrine is given to such patients. Observe patient for signs of adverse effects: allergy, respiratory distress, anaphylaxis. INTERVENTION: Tell patient duration of drug action is 1–3 hr when used as local anesthetic. Spinal headache precautions. This drug is most popular local anesthetic and most patients are familiar with its effects, so this enhances patient teaching. Caution ambulatory patients with local anesthetic to protect area of anesthesia from trauma because injury may occur without being felt. Drug has moderate potency for surface anesthesia and is available in 4% topical form; duration of anesthesia is short when used in this form. EVALUATION: Same as Bupivacaine.

CONTINUED ON THE FOLLOWING PAGE

Local Anesthetics

Table 10–3. LOCAL ANESTHETICS–*CONTINUED*

Name	Dosage	Mode of Administration	Pharmacokinetics
Mepivacaine (Carbodaine)			
Use: Infiltration, nerve block, caudal, epidural, therapeutic blocks for pain management.			
	Doses listed are for drug without levonordefrin (a vasoconstrictor).		O: within 15 min
	1% sol, 5–200 mg	Nerve block	P: UA
	1% sol, 400 mg max	Transvaginal block	D: 3 hr
	1% sol, 150–300 mg	Caudal or epidural	PB: 60%–80%
	1% sol, 10–50 mg	Therapeutic block	½ L: 100 min
			B: liver
			E: urine
Prilocaine (Citanest)			
Use: Infiltration, peripheral nerve block, caudal or epidural block.			
	1–2% sol, 200–600 mg	Infiltration	O: 10–15 min
	1–2% sol, 30–100 mg	Peripheral nerve block (intercostal or para-cervical)	P: UA
			D: 1–3 hr
			PB: 60%–85%
	2% sol, 400–600 mg	Peripheral nerve block (surgery)	½ L: UA
			B: liver
	1% sol, 200–300 mg	Caudal nerve block (obstetrics)	E: urine, lungs (5%)
	1% sol, 200–300 mg	Epidural	

Key to Abbreviations in the *Pharmacokinetics* column O-onset; P-peak; D-duration; PB-protein bound; B-bio-transformed in; E-excreted in; ½ L = halflife.

*Within the column listing adverse effects, <u>underlines</u> indicate the most common effects; CAPITALS indicate life-threatening effects.

Contraindications and Precautions	Adverse Effects*	Interactions	Nursing Implications
Contraindicated in sensitivity to methylparaben; in heart block; or for spinal anesthesia. Use with caution in acutely ill, elderly, or debilitated patients, and for paracervical blocks. Solutions with levonordefrin should not be used in end arteries (fingers, toes, ears, nose). Use solutions without preservatives for caudal or epidural blocks.	Same as bupivacaine.	Enflurane, halothane, and related drugs: Cardiac arrhythmias can occur when used with the form of this drug containing levonordefrin (a vasoconstrictor that helps prolong the drug's anesthetic action). Use with extreme caution. MAO inhibitors, tricyclic antidepressants: Severe and sustained hypertension can occur when used with the form of this drug containing levonordefrin. Use with extreme caution.	ASSESSMENT: Observe pregnant patients closely because drug can cross placenta and cause fetal bradycardia and neonatal depression. Monitor fetal heart rate when used in delivery. Ask patient about medicines/drugs they may be taking because severe hypertension can occur if drug with levonordefrin is given to those taking MAO inhibitors or tricyclic antidepressants. Assess areas of anesthesia for return of sensation/motor function. Monitor for signs of adverse effects: allergy, respiratory distress, anaphylaxis. INTERVENTION: Tell patient that onset of drug action is rapid (within 15 min) and duration approximately 3 hr. Stress to ambulatory patients that they should protect area of local anesthesia from trauma while anesthetized. EVALUATION: Same as Bupivacaine.
Contraindicated in methemoglobinemia, severe shock, heart block, and infection at spinal injection site. Epidural and caudal use contraindicated in spinal deformities, CNS diseases, septicemia, and severe hypertension, and in children. Use with caution in acutely ill, elderly, or debilitated patients; children under 10 yr; and patients with other drug allergies.	Same as bupivacaine, but in addition, paresthesia and swelling of lips and mouth with use of 4% solutions.	None significant.	ASSESSMENT: Assess areas of anesthetization for return of sensation/motor function. Monitor for signs of adverse effects: allergy, respiratory distress, anaphylaxis. INTERVENTION: Tell patient that onset of drug action is slower than lidocaine but duration may be longer. Stress to ambulatory patients to protect area of local anesthesia from trauma while numb. Drug is about 40% less toxic than lidocaine. Drug is not used topically. EVALUATION: Same as Bupivacaine.

CONTINUED ON THE FOLLOWING PAGE

Table 10–3. LOCAL ANESTHETICS–*CONTINUED*

Name	Dosage	Mode of Administration	Pharmacokinetics
ESTER TYPE Chloroprocaine hydrochloride (Nesacine, Nesacaine-CE)			

Use: Nesacaine is used for infiltration and regional anesthesia. Nesacaine-CE is used as caudal and epidural anesthesia.

Name	Dosage	Mode of Administration	Pharmacokinetics
	Drug available without epinephrine 1% sol, 30–200 mg; 2% sol, 20–400 mg; 2–3% sol, 300–750 mg	Infiltration nerve blocks Caudal and epidural	O: within minutes P: UA D: 30–60 min PB: UA ½ L: UA B: plasma E: urine
Tetracaine hydrochloride (Pontocaine)			

Use: Low spinal (saddle block), spinal up to costal margin, topical.

Name	Dosage	Mode of Administration	Pharmacokinetics
	2–5 mg, 15 mg max.	Low spinal (for vaginal delivery)	O: 15 min P: UA
	15–20 mg, spinal doses generally do not exceed 15 mg.	Spinal up to costal margin	D: 2–3 hr PB: UA
	0.5% sol or ointment	Topical anesthesia of the eye	½ L: UA B: liver
	2% sol	Nose and throat mucous membranes	E: urine

Key to Abbreviations in the *Pharmacokinetics* column O-onset; P-peak; D-duration; PB-protein bound; B-biotransformed in; E-excreted in; ½ L = halflife.

*Within the column listing adverse effects, underlines indicate the most common effects; CAPITALS indicate life-threatening effects.

Local Anesthetics

Contraindications and Precautions	Adverse Effects*	Interactions	Nursing Implications
Contraindicated in those hypersensitive to procaine, tetracaine, or any other p-aminobenzoic acid-derived drugs. Also contraindicated for spinal or topical use. Epidural and caudal use contraindicated in presence of CNS disease. Use with caution in acutely ill, elderly, or debilitated patients, and for paracervical blocks. Use solutions without preservatives for caudal or epidural block.	Same as amide-type local anesthetics.	None significant.	ASSESSMENT: Assess areas of anesthetization for return of sensation/motor function. Monitor for signs of adverse effects: allergy, respiratory distress, anaphylaxis. INTERVENTION: Tell patient that duration of action is 30–60 min. Stress to ambulatory patients to protect area of local anesthesia from trauma. Discard any partially used vials of drug without preservatives; do not reuse. EVALUATION: Same as amide type-Bupivacaine.
Contraindicated in patients hypersensitive to chloroprocaine, procaine, or other p-aminobenzoic acid-derived drugs; in infection at injection sites; and in CNS disease. Contraindicated for obstetric use in the presence of known complications. Use with caution in patients with any of the following: shock, severe anemia, hypertension, hypotension, cardiac decompensation, increased intracranial pressure, peritonitis, and hyperexcitable states. Do not use cloudy, discolored, or crystallized solutions. Protect drug from light and store in refrigerator. When cerebrospinal fluid is used to dilute drug, the solution may become cloudy. Drug is ten times more potent and toxic than procaine.	Same as amide-type local anesthetics.	None significant.	This is the most frequently used drug for spinal anesthesia. ASSESSMENT: Assess area for signs of adverse effects: allergy, respiratory distress, anaphylaxis. INTERVENTION: Tell patient having topical anesthesia to protect area from trauma. For topical eye anesthesia, patient should not touch or rub eye and should stay indoors away from wind, drafts until numbness is gone. Use spinal headache precautions. EVALUATION: Same as Bupivacaine.

CONTINUED ON THE FOLLOWING PAGE

Table 10–3. LOCAL ANESTHETICS–_CONTINUED_

Name	Dosage	Mode of Administration	Pharmacokinetics
Piperocaine hydrochloride (Methycaine)			
Use: Caudal block in obstetrics; infiltration. Most common use is as surface anesthetic.			
	1.5% sol, 450 mg; can give additional 300 mg q 30–40 min for maintenance; 0.5% sol, 1000 mg max; 1% sol, 800 mg min 1–2% sol	Caudal Infiltration Dental infiltration	O: within minutes D: effect peaks in 20–30 min, then decreases
Procaine hydrochloride (Novocain)			
Use: Spinal anesthesia, epidural block, peripheral nerve block, infiltration.			
	Dose depends on nerves to be blocked 1.5% sol, 375 mg; 1% sol, 250 mg; 2% sol, 500 mg 0.25–0.5% sol, 250–600 mg, up to 1 g max.	Spinal Epidural Peripheral nerve block Infiltration	O: 2–5 min P: UA D: approximately 60 min but can be lengthened if solution with epinephrine is used for local nerve blocks or infiltration PB: UA ½ L: UA B: plasma E: urine

Key to Abbreviations in the _Pharmacokinetics_ column O-onset; P-peak; D-duration; PB-protein bound; B-biotransformed in; E-excreted in; ½ L = halflife.
*Within the column listing adverse effects, underlines indicate the most common effects; CAPITALS indicate life-threatening effects.

Contraindications and Precautions	Adverse Effects*	Interactions	Nursing Implications
Contraindicated in patients hypersensitive to procaine, tetracaine, or any other p-amino-benzoic acid-derived drugs and in those with CNS diseases; spinal deformities; infection at the injection site; for spinal block; and in patients with profound anemia or obesity. Use solutions without preservatives for caudal block. Do not dilute drug with sterile water; if dilution necessary, use sodium chloride or Ringer's solution. Partially used vials without preservatives should be discarded and not reused.	Same as amide-type local anesthetics.	None significant.	ASSESSMENT: Assess area of anesthesia for return of sensation/motor function. Monitor patient for adverse effects: allergy, respiratory distress, anaphylaxis. INTERVENTION: Tell patient anesthetic effect peaks at 20–30 min then begins to wear off. EVALUATION: Same as Bupivacaine.
Contraindicated in patients hypersensitive to chloroprocaine, tetracaine, or any other p-aminobenzoic acid-derived drug. Use with caution in patients with CNS disease, shock, infection at the injection site, severe anemia, sepsis, cachexia, hypertension or hypotension, GI hemorrhage, peritonitis, increased intra-abdominal pressure, cardiac decompensation, and hyperexcitable states. Reduced hydrolysis of procaine occurs in patients taking echothiophate iodine (Echodide), a miotic used to treat open-angle glaucoma; use with caution in these patients. Use for uncomplicated obstetric delivery only. Use solutions without preservatives for epidural blocks. Discard partially used vials without preservatives; do not reuse.	Same as amide-type local anesthetics.	Echothiophate iodide: reduced hydrolysis of procaine. Use together cautiously.	Procaine is the prototype local anesthetic and one of the most commonly used. Drug is not irritating to soft tissues or nerves and is widely used for dental procedures. Drug not effective as surface anesthetic. ASSESSMENT: Assess area of anesthesia for return of sensation/motor function. Monitor patient for adverse effects: allergy, respiratory distress, anaphylaxis. INTERVENTION: Tell ambulatory patients approximate duration of anesthetic effect and to protect area from trauma during that time. Use spinal headache precautions. EVALUATION: Same as Bupivacaine.

Table 10–4. NURSING PROCESS FOR THE PATIENT RECEIVING ANESTHETIC MEDICATION

Assessment (Preoperative)

Determine what patient knows/has been told about surgery and type of anesthesia planned. Assess ability to understand.
Obtain medication history, drugs patient currently taking (include alcohol or recreational drug use), noting date/time and amount of last ingestion/use.
Review history for renal, hepatic impairment; pulmonary disease; glaucoma which will affect choice of anesthetic agents.

Nursing Diagnosis	Nursing Actions	Rationale	Patient Outcomes/ Evaluation Criteria
Knowledge deficit related to unfamiliarity with drug therapy and possible/interactions as evidenced by questions and statement of concern.	Explain necessity/time of fluid restrictions and which routine drugs should be held or continued.	Patient will be more likely to comply with restrictions if he/she understands the reasons for them.	Verbalizes understanding of preoperative restrictions for general anesthesia, or restrictions and effects of any local anesthesia used. Complications minimized or prevented.
	Stress that patient should not make any major decisions or drink alcoholic beverages for 48 hours, and should avoid driving for 24 hours after procedure. Local anesthesia: Tell patient/family to protect area of local anesthetic from trauma until sensation returns.	Complications and undesired drug interactions can occur if drug/alcohol use is inappropriate. Post general anesthesia drowsiness can contribute to auto accidents. Numbness can last for several hours, increasing risk of injury.	
Anxiety related to threat to or change in health status (i.e., fear of cancer) or threat of death as evidenced by asking repetitive questions, being withdrawn and not communicating feelings or displaying anxious behavior.	Explain general anesthesia process and postanesthesia recovery room procedures. Provide appropriate information relative to outcome of the particular procedure (reinforce physician's teaching).	Many fears are founded in the unknown. If patient is properly prepared and has appropriate information, anxiety can be lessened.	Displays appropriate use of coping mechanisms. Verbalizes realistic perception of anesthesia procedures and understanding of safety of modern techniques.
	Answer questions and provide emotional support as appropriate. Discuss how patients are monitored during surgery and recovery.	Many patients fear death while under anesthesia. Appropriate teaching and emotional support can decrease fears. In addition, patients may fear cancer will be found (no matter what the surgery). Providing information can reduce unrealistic fears.	

Assessment (Postoperative)

Observe level of consciousness, ability to follow instructions (e.g., turn, cough) after general anesthesia.
Determine patient's breathing pattern, rate and depth of respirations.
Assess skin/mucous membrane color.
Assess characteristics of pain noting nonverbal cues as well.

Sensory-perceptual alterations related to chemical alteration/ pharmacologic agents,	Provide safe enviroment and close supervision as indicated. Continuously reorient patient to time, place and confirm that surgery is completed.	Some agents (e.g., Ketamine) may cause emergent reactions such as disturbing dreams/hallucinations. Provide reassurance and promote	Demonstrates uneventful recovery from anesthesia free of injury. Verbalizes understanding of limitations and seeks assistance as appropriate.

Nursing Diagnosis	Nursing Actions	Rationale	Patient Outcomes/ Evaluation Criteria
restricted environment as evidenced by decreased level of consciousness, poor verbal communication skills, altered sensorium.		patient safety during emergent stage as patient regains consciousness.	
Potential ineffective	Encourage patient cooperation with activity restrictions and provide assistance as needed.	Impaired perception, and reduced sensation increase risk of injury.	
	Monitor sensation of limbs as appropriate and protect area from trauma until sensation returns following local/regional anesthesia.	Return of function following local or spinal nerve blocks is dependent on type/amount of agent used.	
Breathing pattern, related to effects of general anesthesia or other perioperative drugs.	Monitor respiratory rate and depth. Assess for signs of air hunger, hypoxia, cyanosis.	Evaluates effectiveness of respiratory effort and identifies need for intervention.	Displays usual/effective respiratory pattern free of hypoxia, cyanosis or signs/symptoms of complications such as atelectasis and pneumonia.
	Encourage patient to cough and deep breathe.	Helps to expel anesthetic gases and prevent pooling of secretions.	
	Evaluate effectiveness of cough and expelling of secretions. Suction as needed.	Ineffective coughing and deep breathing predispose to retained secretions and complications such as atelectasis, pneumonia.	
	Demonstrate use of spirometry device if ordered.	Promotes maximal inspiratory effort to open collapsed airways and mobilize secretions.	
	Administer supplemental oxygen as needed.	Maximizes oxygen available for circulatory uptake, especially when respiratory effort is depressed.	
Comfort, status due to acute post-op pain altered as evidenced by complaints, muscle tension, restlessness, nonverbal cues.	Give ordered pain medications.	Some patients are reluctant to ask for medication even when needed. If patient is having severe pain, he/she will move less and may develop complications of immobility.	Reports pain is relieved/controlled. Displays relaxed manner and is able to mobilize, sleep/rest, appropriately.
	Provide routine comfort measures, e.g., position change, back rub.	Helps relieve muscle tension and facilitate rest.	
	Encourage appropriate diversionary activities (radio/TV)	Promotes relaxation, comfort by distracting attention from pain and may help reduce need for medication.	
	Elevate affected extremity if local anesthesia or regional limb anesthesia such as Bier Block was given. Apply ice packs to surgical site as indicated.	Can reduce swelling and associated pain and protect anesthetized limb from trauma.	
	Keep patient supine for 8–12 hours post-spinal anesthesia.	Helps prevent "spinal" headache.	

Table 10–5. PATIENT TEACHING INFORMATION—ANESTHETIC DRUGS

Dear Patient:

Anesthetic drugs will be administered prior to your surgery. This is what you should know about your planned anesthesia to avoid possible complications from your anesthesia.

FOR PATIENTS RECEIVING GENERAL ANESTHESIA

1. Food and fluid will be restricted preoperatively; usually no food or fluids are allowed from midnight before your operation.
2. Preanesthetic medication will be administered 30–60 minutes preoperatively. For safety reasons, do not get out of bed after this medication is given.
3. Following surgery, there may be additional food or fluid restrictions depending upon the procedure performed.
4. Following the surgery, there may be activity restrictions until full recovery from the anesthetics has occurred.
5. Following surgery, some nausea may be experienced because of medications given. This can be controlled by medication that the physician will order.
6. Pain will be controlled by the administration of ordered analgesics.

FOR PATIENTS HAVING OUTPATIENT SURGERY OR AMBULATORY SURGERY

1. There may be food or fluid restrictions prior to the procedure. Follow physician's orders.
2. Do not come alone; have a family member or friend accompany you, even if a local anesthetic is planned.
3. Bring in bottles of all medications you are currently taking so that the physician and/or anesthetist is aware of them.
4. If taking regular medications, check with physician to determine if alteration in dose or schedule will be necessary because of surgery. (For example, patients with diabetes may have to alter their insulin regimen.)
5. If a local anesthetic is used, protect the area from trauma because it will be numb for several hours, and injury may occur without being felt.
6. Have prescriptions for postoperative medications filled and follow postoperative instructions regarding rest, food/fluid restrictions, wound care, elevation of extremity (if appropriate), and return visits for postoperative physician care.

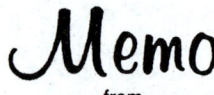

from

DR. RICHARD L. SAWICKI

DIPLOMATE AMERICAN BOARD OF PODIATRIC SURGERY

BOARD CERTIFIED FOOT SURGEON

**8701 BUFFALO AVENUE–PHONE: (716) 283 3338
NIAGARA FALLS NEW YORK 14304**

SAME DAY SURGERY PRE-OP INSTRUCTIONS

MT. ST. MARY'S HOSPITAL

You're scheduled for same day surgery (early admission the day of surgery) on _____ .

Report to the admitting office at _____ A.M. Your surgery is

_____

FOR YOUR SURGERY TO BE PERFORMED SAFELY, YOU MUST:

1. Have the necessary pre-op lab tests done. This must be done as an out-patient since most insurance companies do not pay for admission a day before surgery for testing. The hospital will call to set up your testing a few days before surgery.

2. Medical clearance is needed prior to surgery from your family doctor who will receive copies of your pre-op tests. See Dr. _____ on _____ at _____ .

3. An adult must accompany you home from the hospital.

4. You will have to remove dentures, glasses, contact lenses, make-up, jewelry, nail polish before surgery.

5. Do not drink any alcoholic beverages for 24 hours before surgery.

6. You will most likely go home later in the day you have your surgery. You will be given written instructions at that time.

You will receive a general anesthesia, therefore . . .
Do not eat or drink anything after midnight
The night before your surgery.

IF YOU HAVE ANY FURTHER QUESTIONS, CALL THE OFFICE.

_____   _____

PATIENT NAME   DATE

Figure 10–4. Same day surgery pre-op instructions. This is a copy of instructions given to patients about to undergo podiatric surgery who will be admitted to the hospital the morning before surgery and discharged the next day. The Surgical Coordinating Nurse explains the pre-operative testing and other requirements and makes the necessary appointments for the patient during this pre-op visit at the doctor's office about 10 days before surgery. The podiatrist reviews the surgery with the patient (and family) and answers questions. The post-operative routine is also explained. If necessary, arrangements are made at this time for crutch-walk training or the procurement of assistive devices such as crutches or a walker if they will be needed. The surgeon obtains informed patient consent at this time. (Courtesy of Dr. Richard L. Sawicki, Niagara Falls, NY.)

ety. Patients about to undergo surgery generally experience two major fears—fear of death and of cancer. It is common for patients receiving a general anesthesia to fear "not waking up," and even though anesthesia deaths are quite rare, patients do know it is possible, and fear this. The fear that cancer will be found during their surgery is also common. Reassure the patient without dismissing or making light of these fears. Patient care during the actual operative period and the anesthesia recovery period in the postanesthesia recovery room is generally handled by specially trained nurses and technicians. Nursing care during the period of recovery from anesthesia focuses on the facilitation of respirations and careful, frequent monitoring of vital signs. Since this care is administered only by specially trained nurses in other than patient units, we will proceed to the postoperative period.

PLANNING AND INTERVENTION

Following completion of surgery, the patient is transferred to the post-anesthesia room where frequent monitoring by specially trained nurses occurs. Respiratory status and vital signs are checked frequently. Return of the gag reflex and coughing signals that extubation is necessary. Once the anesthetist extubates the patient, respiratory status is monitored carefully to be sure it remains adequate. For the staff nurse, the postoperative nursing assessment begins as soon as the patient arrives on a cart from the postanesthesia recovery room. The nurse takes vital signs, assesses level of consciousness, and inspects the operative area. For the patient who has received a local anesthetic, take care to protect the area from injury. If an extremity is involved, make sure it is in correct alignment. Observe for color and temperature changes as well as signs of returning sensation. Once the patient is transferred to the patient care unit, complete neuromuscular function and satisfactory respiratory status should have returned. The patient should be able to lift his or her head and hold it up for 10 seconds, and should be able to grasp with a fairly firm grip, and gag/cough reflex should be present. Notify the anesthetist if these signs are absent.

Patients who have ambulatory surgery performed may have a long-acting local anesthetic such as bupivacaine (Marcaine) injected to postpone the return of sensation for 8–10 hours postoperatively. Caution these patients to rest and protect the operative area from trauma.

The postoperative nursing care plan depends on the type of anesthetic used and the procedure performed. Nursing care goals are to minimize side effects of anesthesia and surgery through use of appropriate nursing measures, to prevent complications, and to facilitate the rehabilitative process. Integral to the planning of patient care is knowledge of the type of anesthesia utilized, the symptoms of side effects associated with a particular anesthetic agent or technique, and how to prevent complications while minimizing patient discomfort. For example, following spinal anesthesia, headaches can occur that can be severe and persist for up to 36 hours. Thus,

patients are usually kept supine for 8–12 hours after spinal anesthesia to prevent a "spinal headache."

Recovery from general anesthetics is generally uneventful. However, it is not uncommon for patients to experience nausea, vomiting, or both following a general anesthetic. This usually subsides within 24 hours. From the patient's standpoint, this is probably the most troublesome postanesthesia adverse effect. Most physicians include an antiemetic in their routine postoperative orders. This can be administered if needed and appropriate comfort measures instituted. Commonly administered antiemetics include benzquinamide hydrochloride (Emete-Con), prochlorperazine maleate (Compazine), thiethylperazine maleate (Torecan), and trimethobenzamide hydrochloride (Tigan).

Pain occurs with recovery from anesthesia. This is especially true after recovery from inhalation anesthetics, because these agents leave the patient's system more rapidly and have less lingering effects than agents administered by other modes. As recovery from anesthesia progresses, the patient becomes more aware of postoperative pain and requires analgesic administration as ordered by the physician. During the initial postoperative period, the hospitalized patient may require analgesics that can be administered parenterally such as the narcotics morphine, hydromorphone hydrochloride (Dilaudid), codeine, meperidine hydrochloride (Demerol), and other analgesics such as butorphanol tartrate (Stadol), nalbuphine hydrochloride (Nubain), and pentazocine (Talwin). Patients who have ambulatory or outpatient surgery will be given a prescription for an oral analgesic such as codeine, oxycodone hydrochloride (Percodan, Percocet, Tylox), hydrocodone bitartrate (Vicodin), or propoxyphene hydrochloride (Darvon).

The frequency of assessment of vital signs as well as other patient status parameters is determined largely by the type of surgery performed, patient status, and type of anesthetic used. Progressive changes (such as gradually declining blood pressure) as well as abrupt, dramatic changes are reported to the physician. Anesthetic drugs and those drugs used to facilitate analgesia/anesthesia can remain in the patient's bloodstream for many hours. Because these drugs depress the central nervous system, observe the patient for respiratory depression and hypoventilation, which predispose to pooling of secretions. Encouraging the patient to cough and breathe deeply helps to expel anesthetic gases as well as to prevent the pooling of excretions. Since hypotension can also occur, the patient is mobilized carefully to prevent syncopal episodes.

The state of deep muscle relaxation of general anesthesia required for many surgical procedures can result in bladder atony or decreased intestinal motility. Anesthesia administration can also depress renal function temporarily. This temporary loss of bladder tone may prevent the patient from voiding for several hours following surgery. Generally, if a patient has not voided within 8 hours following return from surgery, catheterization is performed. Bladder fullness is assessed by palpation. The patient usually has a sense of fullness and may have the urge to void but be unable to do so. Following certain surgical procedures, it is routine for an indwelling catheter to be inserted postoperatively or during surgery. Instruct patients who are discharged the same day as general anesthesia administration to notify the surgeon if they are voiding only in small amounts (urinary retention with overflow) or unable to void. Patients are generally not discharged until after they void; however, a patient can still experience urinary retention, especially patients with a history of urinary or prostrate problems.

Abdominal distention can result from the decreased intestinal motility caused by anesthetic and muscle-relaxant drugs. It is not uncommon for patients to experience some discomfort from distention caused by flatus. Actions such as turning in bed and helping the patient ambulate as soon as permissible after surgery usually help relieve the discomfort caused by gas. If the patient continues to complain of discomfort, notify the physician to obtain orders for further care measures.

Early mobilization of the patient following surgery not only helps overcome such drug-related side effects as intestinal distention, but it also helps prevent other immobility-related problems. Immobility predisposes patients to hazards including urinary, circulatory, and pulmonary stasis. These hazards are the forerunners of complications such as thrombi, emboli, and pneumonia if immobility persists. Because of the lethargy or sedation produced by anesthetic/analgesic drugs, coupled with fear of incisional pain, many patients need to be coaxed into mobilization activities. This early mobilization is essential to promote an uncomplicated recovery period for the patient. Providing adequate pain relief prior to mobilization/ambulation activities can greatly enhance patient compliance and comfort. (For information on analgesic drugs see Chapter 20).

Next-day discharge following many surgical procedures as well as outpatient surgery have combined to shift the nurses' care focus from providing care to teach-

---

MOUNT ST. MARY'S HOSPITAL

Nursing Service

AMBULATORY
POST-OPERATIVE PATIENT INSTRUCTIONS

Name _____ Hospital Number _____ Procedure _____

GENERAL INSTRUCTIONS—AFTER GENERAL ANESTHESIA

1. Do not drive a motor vehicle for 24 hours.
2. Do not drink alcoholic beverages for 48 hours.
3. Do not make any major decisions regarding money for 48 hours.
4. Adults and children should be kept resting in the house all day.
5. Any signs of persistent dizziness, nausea, emesis, or bleeding—

   CALL YOUR SURGEON:

   _____   _____
              NAME   TELEPHONE

   NOTE: If you are unable to contact your surgeon, report to the Emergency Room immediately.

6. Keep incision (wound) clean and dry as per your physician's instructions.
7. Take pain medication as prescribed for control of discomfort. If pain control is not adequate or temperature is elevated, contact your surgeon.
8. After discharge, call your surgeon's office within 24 to 48 hours to schedule an appointment for suture removal.
9. You may eat a normal diet when discharged, unless otherwise advised.

Specific Instructions

_____

_____

_____

_____

_____

_____

_____

_____   _____   _____
          WITNESS   SIGNATURE OF PATIENT OR   DATE
                                               RESPONSIBLE PARTY

Figure 10–5. Sample of hospital post-operative general instruction sheet following ambulatory surgery. (Courtesy of St. Mary's Hospital of Niagara Falls, Lewiston, NY.)

DR. RICHARD L. SAWICKI

Associate American College of Foot Surgeons

**8701 BUFFALO AVENUE
NIAGARA FALLS, NEW YORK 14304**

TELEPHONE: (716) 283-3338

PODIATRY POST-OP INSTRUCTIONS

1. Call the Dr's. office for a follow-up appointment when you get home. Make appt.

   for _____ .

2. Keep operative foot clean at all times—wear protective covering—slippers, socks, etc.

3. Keep dressing or cast dry unless Dr. instructs otherwise.

4. If you are given a post-op wooden bottom shoe be sure to wear it at all times when you are walking.

5. Keep operative foot elevated when you are sitting to decrease swelling and pain.

6. Apply an ice pack to the foot while awake. Place ice pack on for 30 minutes and then leave off for 30 minutes. Do this for the first 3 days post-op.

7. Watch for and notify the Dr.'s office immediately if there is increasing redness with swelling and/or pain. Call the regular office phone # 283-3338.

8. Take any medications Dr. Sawicki has prescribed for you exactly as written.

9. If you are planning on convalescing at a place other than your home, please notify the Dr's. office of a phone number you can be reached at.

10. A local anesthesia has been used to numb the foot and its effects will last several hours. Protect the area from trauma (bumps, etc.) since you will not be able to feel any injury while the area is numb.

11. TAKE IT EASY. REST. This is important to your recovery. Adequate rest and proper diet promote healing. <u>DO NOT</u> do any yardwork or extensive housework.

_____	_____
NAME	DATE

Figure 10–6. Podiatry postoperative instructions. (Courtesy of Dr. Richard L. Sawicki, Niagara Falls, NY.)

---

ing the patient/family how to provide immediate postoperative care. For example, after outpatient surgery on an extremity (arm, hand, foot), the patient is usually advised to elevate the part in order to reduce pain and swelling and to protect the part from bumping or other trauma if a local anesthetic was given, because the numbness may mask injury. If a long-acting local anesthetic such as bupivacaine hydrochloride (Marcaine) has been given, be sure the patient is aware sensation will be absent for longer than if lidocaine (Xylocaine) had been given, because most people are well aware of the duration and effects of Xylocaine. Ice packs may be applied intermittently to reduce pain and swelling also. Patients who are discharged on the day following surgery may have to continue certain treatments at home. For example, iced compresses are often ordered following cosmetic facial surgery in order to reduce pain and swelling. The patient may have to continue this at home for a few days after surgery. Ideally, the surgeon and surgeon's staff have done preoperative teaching so that the patient/family are prepared for the postoperative instructions to patients. Routine care measures are outlined that are relative to the patient's surgery as well as the signs and symptoms that should be reported to the surgeon right away. All instructions should be verbally explained in addition to providing the printed list. The

caregiver should also repeat what is to be done so the nurse can determine if there is a clear understanding of instructions given. Refer to Figures 10–5 and 10–6 for examples of a general postoperative ambulatory surgery instruction form as well as a specific instruction sheet provided by a podiatrist for his patients following foot surgery.

POSTOPERATIVE EVALUATION

Postoperative evaluation of the success of nursing interventions to prevent or minimize the side effects of anesthetic/analgesic drugs is an ongoing part of the nursing process. Patient responses (objective as well as subjective signs) are evaluated for effectiveness of instituted nursing interventions. Once this output information is evaluated by the nurse, the pertinent information becomes new input for the problem-solving nursing process.

Many postoperative nursing interventions are preventive care measures. Those actions that aim to prevent complications such as respiratory or urinary tract problems are judged effective in the absence of corresponding problems. For example, mobilization and coughing and deep breathing activities have been done appropriately; therefore, the patient experiences no respiratory problems. In this instance, the evaluation is to continue these actions for their preventive value. Some nursing interventions are planned as problem-solving rather than preventive measures. For example, when a patient complains of pain or nausea postoperatively and an appropriate medication is administered according to the physician's standing orders to relieve the discomfort, then evaluation is based on symptom relief.

Because of the advent of ambulatory/outpatient surgery, most hospitals have a surgical coordinating nurse who calls the patient at home within 24 hours of surgery to evaluate patient status.

SUMMARY

Thorough knowledge of the drugs used to facilitate or initiate anesthesia is essential for the nurse to successfully implement the nursing care process for patients receiving these drugs. An understanding of the stages of anesthesia, drug administration techniques used to achieve anesthesia, and drug side effects is also essential to facilitiate the nursing process. The trend of short hospital stays and the increase in outpatient surgery challenge the nurse to assess and plan care to meet patient needs efficiently and effectively.

BIBLIOGRAPHY

AMA Drug Evaluations, ed 6. PSG Publishing, Littleton, MA, 1986.

Ambulatory surgery: Risk management highlighted at federated ambulatory surgery association meeting. AORN J 46(1):19–34, 1987.

Barron, S: Patient education: Preadmission made easy. Am J Nurs 87(12):1690–1691, 1987.

Burge, S, et al: Perceptions of postoperative incisional pain. Am J Nurs 86(11):1263–1265, 1986.

Chitwood, LB: Unraveling the mystery: Anesthesia. Nursing '87 17:53–55, February 1987.

Gilman, AG, Goodman, LS, and Gilman, A: Goodman and Gilman's The Pharmacological Basis of Therapeutics, ed 6. Macmillan, New York, 1985.

Ivey, DF: Local anesthesia: Implications for the perioperative nurse. AORN J 45(3):682–689, 1987.

Nurse's Drug Alert: Cimetidine-succinylcholine interaction. XI(12), December 1987.

Nursing '88 Drug Handbook. Springhouse Corporation Nursing '88 Books, Springhouse, PA, 1988.

Rogers, B: Exposure to waste anesthetic gases. AAOHN J American Association of Occupational Health Nurses Journal 34(12):574–579, 1986.

Schmidt, R and Margolin, S: Harper's Handbook of Therapeutic Pharmacology. Harper & Row, Philadelphia, 1981.

Smith, NY, Miller, RD, and Corbascio, AN: Drug Interactions in Anesthesia. Lea & Febiger, Philadelphia, 1981.

Stevens, M: Which adolescents breeze through surgery? Am J Nurs 87(12):1564–1565, 1987.

SITUATION 10–1

As a unit coordinator in a postanesthesia recovery room, Jill Henderson frequently applies knowledge of anesthetic agents.

1. Bob Wills, a 40-year-old, received halothane (Fluothane) as an induction agent. All of the following can occur with halothane administration *except:*
   a. hepatotoxicity
   b. skeletal muscle relaxation
   c. respiratory depression
   d. bradycardia and dysrhythmias

2. Amy Pallet is recovering from abdominal surgery in which isoflurane (Forane) was used as the anesthetic agent. All the following can occur after Forane administration except:
   a. nausea and vomiting
   b. postoperative excitation
   c. cardiac dysrhythmias
   d. depressed mental alertness

3. Mrs. Reeves received ketamine hydrochloride (Ketalar) for debridement of a burn. Potential effects of the drug include:
   a. frequent urination
   b. constipation
   c. disturbing dreams
   d. decreased muscle control

4. Mr. Steiner received naloxone (Narcan) 0.1 mg IV in order to reverse the effects of narcotics administered during Surgery. Jill should assess for the following after Narcan administration:
   a. respiratory difficulty
   b. dry mouth
   c. intense pain
   d. urine output

5. In order to intubate Mr. Gardner without trauma, pancuronium bromide (Pavulon) is administered by the anesthetist. Jill is aware that the antidote for this agent is a mixture of:
   a. neostigmine and atropine
   b. Narcan and neostigmine
   c. Benadryl and Robinul
   d.

6. Justine Smith, a 60-year-old, was on Inderal preoperatively. During recovery from general anesthesia, Jill will observe Ms. Smith closely for the following reaction:
   a. anxiety
   b. hypotension
   c. barbituate potentiation
   d. hypertensive crisis

Please refer to the Appendices for correct answers and additional review questions with answers.

SITUATION   10–2

Gerald Moiser is a nurse in an ambulatory surgery unit.

1. When conducting a preoperative nursing history on 18-year-old Steve Adler, Gerald discovers a history of asthma. He is aware that methohexital sodium (Brevital) is to be the anesthetic agent for oral surgery. Due to Steve's history of asthma, Gerald would anticipate:
   a. replacement of Brevital with another agent
   b. no adverse reactions
   c. administration of Brevital with caution
   d. combining Brevital with an antihistamine

2. Gerald assists with an endoscopic procedure on a patient who received droperidol/fentanyl (Innovar). In the immediate recovery period, Gerald will keep the following drug available:
   a. Atropine
   b. Demerol
   c. Lidocaine
   d. Compazine

3. The anesthesiologist administered succinylcholine to Mr. Judd in order to facilitate endotracheal intubation. Gerald is aware that the following electrolyte will be affected by this drug:
   a. sodium
   b. calcium
   c. magnesium
   d. potassium

4. Mrs. Hayes is scheduled for removal of a ganglionic cyst, using lidocaine hydrochloride (Xylocaine) with epinephrine for a field block. Gerald will review medications which Mrs. Hayes takes, because severe hypertension may result if Xylocaine with epinephrine is given to patients who are taking:
   a. beta blockers
   b. anticholinergics
   c. MAO inhibitors
   d. H_2 antagonists

5. Steve Turner is to receive an epidural using procaine hydrochloride (Novacaine). All of the following statements are correct with regard to Novacaine, *except:*
   a. Use solutions without preservatives for epidural blocks.
   b. The drug is irritating to soft tissues and nerves.
   c. Procaine should be used with caution in patients with shock.
   d. Use for uncomplicated obstetric delivery only.

6. Mr. Dominick is scheduled for surgery utilizing alfentanil hydrochloride (Alfenta) as an analgesic adjunct. Gerald will assess the following in reference to Alfenta usage:
   a. creatinine
   b. blood sugar
   c. sodium
   d. potassium

Please refer to the Appendices for correct answers and additional review questions with answers.

11
CHAPTER

INTRAVENOUS THERAPY

MERRILY MATHEWSON KUHN, R.N.C., Ph.D., CCRN

LEARNING OBJECTIVES

After reading this chapter, the student will be able to:

1. Identify those fluids commonly administered intravenously, including dextrose and electrolyte solutions.

2. Differentiate among the IV solutions as to mechanism of action, adverse effects, contraindications, and interactions.

3. Identify specific areas to assess in the patient requiring IV solutions in order to formulate appropriate nursing diagnoses.

4. Plan the nursing interventions necessary to administer IV solutions.

5. Evaluate the patient at various stages of treatment to gauge nursing interactions.

INTRAVENOUS THERAPY

Today, over half of the 40 million patients admitted to United States hospitals receive some form of intravenous (IV) therapy during their admission. Patients may require the administration of IV fluids because of (1) an inability to orally ingest adequate amounts of fluids, electrolytes, vitamins, or calories; (2) a fluid or electrolyte imbalance; or (3) a significant loss of blood volume. Fluid balance is essential to health and must be considered carefully in many diseases and disorders involving the cardiovascular, renal, and endocrine systems, as well as in burns, infections, and surgical procedures.

IV therapy involves instilling many different types of fluids directly into the circulatory system. The fluids that may be administered include dextrose solutions, electrolyte solutions, nutritional preparations, plasma expanders, and blood and blood components. (Blood and blood components are discussed in detail in Chapter 12.)

Intravenous therapy has been used in humans for more than 300 years. However, only since 1945 have major advances been made. These include the development of plastic, disposable needles and IV tubing and sterile, well-packaged fluid containers. IV therapy remained the responsibility of the physician until the mid-1960s, when state nurse practice acts began to issue policy statements pertaining to IV therapy. Today, state nurse practice acts serve as a general guide for the establishment of protocols and procedures. Each hospital or institution further clarifies this statement for its own professional staff. Hospital policies should specify the guidelines or criteria essential for nursing personnel to insert and maintain the IV line, prepare and administer admixtures, and administer IV medications.

This chapter will discuss the nurse's role in IV therapy. Specifically, IV therapy is administered to correct the following problems:

1. Water imbalance
2. Electrolyte and acid-base imbalances
3. Blood volume deficits
4. Nutritional deficiencies

This chapter will describe the administration of dextrose and electrolyte solutions. Electrolytes, as a group, are discussed in Chapter 58; blood and blood components and plasma expanders are discussed in Chapter 12; nutritional IV replacements are explained in Chapter 56; and a thorough study of vitamins and minerals is featured in Chapter 57.

WATER BALANCE

The average adult human body is approximately 60% water. (Newborns contain 70%–80% water.) Fat is mostly water-free, so the lean individual has more water

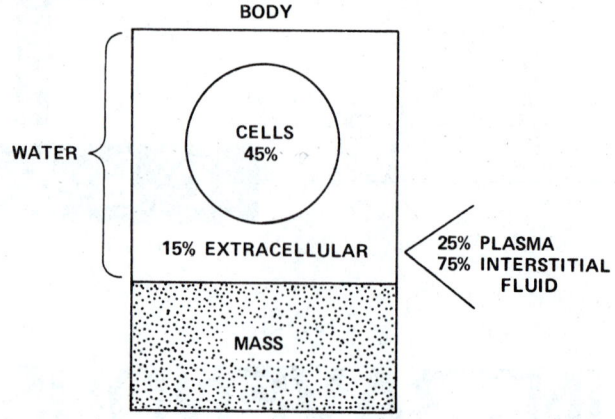

Figure 11–1. Distribution of body water. The body is composed of 60% water; 45% is found in the cells (intracellular), while 15% is outside the cells (extracellular).

per kilogram than the fat individual. The water is divided into intracellular water (approximately 45%) and extracellular water (approximately 15%) (Fig. 11–1). Intracellular fluid (ICF) is not a continuous fluid but is divided into trillions of tiny cellular compartments. ICF is not constant in its composition and varies from cell to cell in the body. Extracellular fluid (ECF) surrounds each cell in the body. The ECF moves through the circulatory and lymphatic systems and contains, in solution or suspension, plasma, electrolytes, vitamins, minerals, protein, nutrients, and waste products. The water diffuses across cell membranes into the cells, where metabolic reactions occur that are essential to life. Since these reactions occur within this water medium, water balance is crucial to healthy living.

Water balance is maintained through a dynamic balance of intake and output (Table 11–1). Water is added to the body through drinking fluids and ingesting foods, as well as from the result of metabolism. Water is lost from the body in urine, feces, perspiration, and respiration. Vomiting, diarrhea, gastric suction, or drainage of body secretions from an open wound can quickly cause water and electrolyte imbalances. Any alteration in water balance can be potentially dangerous for the individual.

The kidney is the primary regulator of water balance. The kidney regulates the amount of urine produced based on blood pressure and serum *osmolarity* (concen-

Table 11–1. NORMAL WATER BALANCE*

Intake		Output	
Water	1200 ml	Urine	1200 ml
Water in food	1000 ml	Feces	200 ml
Metabolic water	300 ml	Skin	600 ml
		Lungs	500 ml
Totals	2500 ml		2500 ml

*Normally, fluid intake equals fluid output.

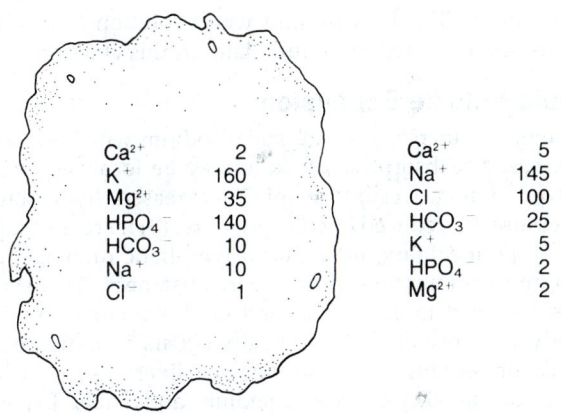

Ca²⁺	2		Ca²⁺	5
K⁺	160		Na⁺	145
Mg²⁺	35		Cl⁻	100
HPO₄	140		HCO₃	25
HCO₃⁻	10		K⁺	5
Na⁺	10		HPO₄	2
Cl⁻	1		Mg²⁺	2

Figure 11–2. Body electrolytes. Primary extracellular electrolytes include Na⁺, Cl⁻, and bicarbonate while primary intracellular electrolytes include K⁺, Mg²⁺, and phosphate. All values listed in mEq/liter.

tration of osmotically active particles in solution). Hormones secreted by the posterior pituitary—ADH (antidiuretic hormone or vasopressin)—and the adrenal cortex—aldosterone—assist in the regulation of fluid and electrolyte balance by affecting water and sodium reabsorption in the distal convoluted tubules and collecting ducts. (See Chapters 38 and 41 for further discussion.)

Water is an excellent solvent, allowing many substances to be dispersed within it. Because of its high dielectric constant (insulating ability offering a great resistance to passage of electricity by conduction), water also permits electrolytes to ionize. Electrolytes are found in both ECF and ICF and include *cations* (positively charged) and *anions* (negatively charged). The major cation in ECF is sodium (Na⁺), while the major cations in ICF are potassium (K⁺) and magnesium (Mg²⁺). The anions in ECF are chloride (Cl⁻) and bicarbonate

(HCO₃⁻) and proteins (Fig. 11–2). Small amounts of these ECF electrolytes are also found in ICF and vice versa.

FLUID VOLUME IMBALANCES

Osmolality is a term used to describe the concentration of free particles, molecules, or ions (i.e., Na⁺, K⁺, glucose) in a solution. The term osmolality is very important in classifying fluid imbalances. Terms such as dehydration and overhydration are useful but incomplete because they do not specify the composition of the fluid lost or gained. Rather, the terms *iso-osmotic*, *hypo-osmotic*, and *hyperosmotic* are more exact in defining any loss or gain in ECF volume.

Osmolarity is the concentration of osmotically active particles in solution. Electrolytes contribute the largest number of particles to osmolarity. Water moves relatively freely between intra- and extracellular compartments in order to maintain equal osmolality.

Fluid Volume Contraction

Dehydration occurs when more fluid is lost from the body than is replaced. In other words, output is greater than input. This occurs when the oral intake falls below normal, or when there is excessive loss of fluid from the body by evaporation from the skin, evaporation from the lungs, or excretion of a very dilute urine. This results in a greater concentration of particles in the extracellular compartment because of water loss and is known as a hyperosmotic contraction. Hyperosmolality is a greater concentration of particles in the extracellular space resulting from loss of water. To compensate, water shifts from the intracellular space into the extracellular space by osmosis. This results in contraction of the intracellular space as volume leaves. The overall effect is called dehydration. Cells become dehydrated and shrunken. Table 11–2 features information associated with fluid volume contractions.

Table 11–2. FLUID VOLUME CONTRACTION AND EXPANSION

Disease Causes	Pharmacologic Causes	Laboratory Findings	Therapy
FLUID VOLUME CONTRACTION Sweating, adrenal insufficiency, burns, blood loss, diarrhea	Cathartics, diuretics	Lab little help, but with severe deficit Na and Cl are reduced in urine. Urine specific gravity increased. Hemoglobin increased, Hct increased, plasma protein increased. Serum Na may be increased. BUN and creatinine may be increased.	Replace ECF with isotonic or hypotonic solutions by any route.
FLUID VOLUME EXPANSION Renal disease, liver disease, cardiac disease, Cushing's disease	Corticosteroids, excessive sodium intake, chlorpropamide	Hemodilution exists, hemoglobin decreased, Hct decreased, all electrolytes decreased, plasma protein decreased, urine specific gravity decreased.	Withhold fluids temporarily, diuretics, low Na diet, dialysis.

Additional clinical symptoms associated with hyper-osmolar contraction include thirst in mentally alert patients, poor skin turgor, dry skin and mucous membranes, soft and sunken eyeballs, apprehension, and restlessness as brain cellular dehydration occurs. A concentrated and a reduced amount of urine occurs.

Iso-osmotic contraction occurs when there is loss of fluid volume equal to solute such as NaCl and bicarbonate salts of sodium and potassium. This can be seen in patients with severe vomiting and diarrhea (i.e., cholera) or with gastric suction. The ECF compartment contracts, but there is also no shift of water in or out of the intracellular space. This is because the volume of the extracellular space decreases, but no change in the osmolality occurs. Since no change in serum osmolality occurs in the body, the cells neither shrink nor swell; consequently, there are no cerebral symptoms. Signs of an iso-osmotic contraction are assessed on physical examination by obtaining blood pressure, hematocrit, serum protein levels, and urine and sodium chloride concentrations.

A fluid volume deficit can be calculated from body weight. A liter of body fluid weighs 2.2 lb, and a kilogram also equals 2.2 lb; therefore, a loss of a liter of water equals a loss of 1 kg of weight. A mild loss is 2% of total body weight, a moderate loss is 2%–5% of body weight, and a severe loss is more than 6% of total body weight.

To demonstrate this formula, it is useful to visualize a 154-lb (70-kg) man:

- A mild loss is about 2% of total body weight. Therefore, a 2% loss of body weight in a 70-kg man is 1.4 kg (or 1.4 kg × 2.2 lb = 3 lb) or 1.4 liters.
- A moderate loss is 2%–5%. A 70-kg man losing 5% of total body weight would lose 3.5 kg (7.7 lb) or 3.5 liters of fluid.
- A severe loss is more than 6% of total body weight. A 70-kg man losing 7% of his weight has a loss of 4.9 kg (10.75 lb) or 4.9 liters (Table 11–3).

The very young and the very old are much more threatened by small changes in water balance, so they must be monitored more closely and fluids replaced as needed. Patients who become dehydrated are generally treated with an isotonic solution (0.9% sodium chloride solution or 5% dextrose and water solution). IV solutions are discussed more fully later in this chapter.

Fluid Volume Expansion

Edema, an increase in interstitial sodium with resultant increased reabsorption of fluid, may be local or generalized. Edema results from (1) increased hydrostatic pressure, (2) reduced oncotic pressure, (3) increased capillary permeability, (4) reduced lymphatic drainage, or (5) any combination of these circumstances. This state results when more sodium and fluid is retained by the body than excreted. This usually occurs in individuals with underlying heart, kidney, or liver disease who have an inability to excrete sodium and fluids. Expansion can be hyper- or hypo-osmotic. Hyperosmotic expansion can result from the excessive administration of hypertonic IV fluids (glucose 10% solutions) or excessive oral sodium chloride intake. In this situation, the extracellular space expands, the intracellular space contracts, and both have an increased osmolality. An example of a hypo-osmotic expansion is the syndrome of inappropriate secretion of ADH (SIADH), which causes the kidneys to retain water in excess. This excess water is distributed throughout the extracellular and intracellular spaces. This causes an expansion of both compartments in which solutes are diluted (i.e., electrolytes and plasma proteins), and the osmolality is lower than normal. Table 11–2 features etiologies and pharmacologic causes of these imbalances.

Clinical signs and symptoms associated with hyperosmotic expansion include headache, nausea, vomiting, muscle pain, abdominal cramps, weakness, stupor, coma, respiratory congestion, convulsions, and absence of thirst. Because of the large increase in ECF volume required to produce generalized edema, body sodium will almost always be increased, even if the serum sodium concentration is low. Clinical symptoms rarely arise until there is a greater than 10% increase in total body water.

A hypo-osmotic expansion occurs when there is either a water excess or solute deficit, such as when there has been excessive intake of water or inability to excrete water because of kidney or brain injury. In either of these states, swollen cells occur, leading primarily to neuromuscular symptoms such as twitching, hyperirri-

Table 11–3. FLUID VOLUME DEFICIT CALCULATED THROUGH WEIGHT LOSS

A liter of fluid = 2.2 lb
A kilogram = 2.2 lb, therefore
Fluid loss (L) = weight loss (kg)

154-lb (70-kg) man:

Deficit	Percentage Loss	Kilograms Loss	Pounds Loss	Fluid Loss
Mild loss	2	1.4	3	1.4 L
Moderate loss (2%–5%)	5	3.5	7.75	3.5 L
Severe loss (>6%)	7	4.9	10.75	4.9 L

tability, mental disturbances, disorientation, convulsions, and coma, all resulting from cerebral edema. In addition, there is an absence of thirst because the swollen cells inhibit the thirst osmoreceptors in the hypothalamus. If the kidneys are functioning, polyuria may occur; but if the kidneys are diseased, oliguria may be present, which further contributes to the volume excess.

Patients with a fluid volume excess are generally treated with fluid restriction and diuretics (Chapter 38). For a more detailed discussion of fluid imbalance, refer to a medical-surgical nursing text.

ELECTROLYTE AND ACID-BASE IMBALANCES

ELECTROLYTE IMBALANCES

Electrolytes are compounds that, when dissolved in water, separate into their component particles. These particles carry an electric charge—positive (cations) or negative (anions)—and are capable of conducting electricity. Electrolyte imbalances may be more dangerous than water imbalances because of their ability to change fluid distribution between body compartments and to cause other associated problems. The major cations are sodium, potassium, calcium, and magnesium ions; the anions are chloride, bicarbonate, phosphate, and sulfate ions. The electrolytes are discussed in more depth in Chapter 58. Electrolytes can be lost excessively or retained by the body. Usually, one imbalance precipitates another if it is not treated promptly.

ACID-BASE IMBALANCE

Acid-base balance is an equilibrium between the total body bases and total body acids. Acid-base balance is a reflection of hydrogen-ion (H^+) concentration in the body, and hydrogen concentration is routinely described as pH. Because pH is the negative logarithm of the concentration of hydrogen ions, the higher their concentration, the lower the pH. Balance is accomplished by maintaining the arterial pH within a narrow range in the presence of acid or alkaline loads. Any change in acid or base concentration ultimately affects the pH. As the pH shifts toward acidic, less than a pH of 7.35 units, the patient becomes acidemic. If the shift in pH is toward alkaline, greater than 7.45 units, the patient becomes alkalemic.

pH intrinsically reflects the relationship of acid to base (Fig. 11–1). Normally, the body has 1 acidic ion for 20 base ions. This relationship can be calculated by using the Henderson-Hasselbach equation: $pH = pK + \log (HCO_3^-/CO_2)$, where pK is a constant (6.1) for this buffer system. This equation is used to find the acid-base ratio that determines the blood pH rather than the absolute pH value.

Acids donate hydrogen and bases receive hydrogen.

Hydrogen ions are added to body fluids daily as metabolic by-products. To keep the pH within its normal range, the body must eliminate hydrogen ions at the same rate as they are produced. The hydrogen ion or acid produced daily in the body is either volatile or fixed. Volatile acid (carbon dioxide) is eliminated by the lung. Fixed acids, such as hydrogen sulfate and hydrochloric acid, are excreted by the kidney. Both acids are chemically buffered to protect cells from dangerous concentrations of hydrogen ion.

The maintenance of this process is the result of a number of mechanisms: body buffers (extracellular and intracellular); respiratory regulation of carbonic acid; and renal regulation of bicarbonate (HCO_3^-) and titratable acids.

Buffering Mechanisms

Body buffers are chemical substances (extracellular and intracellular) that minimize pH changes caused by acid or alkali entering the blood. Buffering operates in the ECFs and occurs in three different locations: (1) in body cells through proteins and phosphates, (2) in red cells through hemoglobin, and (3) in ECF through bicarbonate. The combination of these buffers is known as total buffer base (BB).

The bicarbonate buffering system is the most important and accounts for over half of total buffering. Dissolved carbon dioxide diffuses from the cell into the plasma and then into the red cell; there, it combines with water to form carbonic acid and quickly dissociates into hydrogen and bicarbonate ($CO_2 + H_2O \leftrightarrow H_2CO_3 \leftrightarrow H^+ + HCO_3^-$). The bicarbonate exchanges for chloride and diffuses from the red cell, combining with sodium ions to form sodium bicarbonate (combined carbon dioxide). Potassium, calcium, or both can also combine with bicarbonate.

The kidneys restore bicarbonate HCO_3^- to the blood by reclaiming or reabsorbing filtered HCO_3^- and generating new HCO_3^-. The kidneys also excrete the acids produced by the body that cannot be metabolized to carbonic acid (e.g., the fixed acids). These are known as titratable acids (H^+ buffered by HPO_4^- or by NH_3).

Respiratory System Control

The respiratory system removes carbonic acid (volatile acid) by expiration of carbon dioxide (CO_2) and water. This increases the buffering capacity of the bicarbonate/carbonic acid system. Inadequate ventilation leads to acid (P_{CO_2}) retention and respiratory acidosis; hyperventilation causes excessive acid (P_{CO_2}) loss and respiratory alkalosis.

Other Body Controls

Other buffer systems include the phosphate system (in red blood cells and kidneys); the protein system (in tissue cells and plasma); and the hemoglobin system (in red blood cells). All these systems work together to maintain normal plasma pH.

Acid-Base Disturbances

Acid-base disturbances are categorized into two major classes: metabolic and respiratory.

RESPIRATORY ACIDOSIS. Inadequate ventilation, regardless of the cause, produces an increased level of carbon dioxide, leading to respiratory acidosis. In respiratory acidosis, P_{CO_2} is always elevated, serum pH is lowered, and carbon-dioxide content combining power may be within limits or lowered. Carbon-dioxide content combining power is the amount of carbon dioxide that the blood can hold in chemical combination (normal, 50–70 volume percent; less than 50 is acidosis, above 70 is alkalosis).

The major physiologic causes of respiratory acidosis include respiratory muscle weakness (infectious polyneuritis, polio); chronic obstructive lung disease; or narcotic overdose. The primary treatment for respiratory acidosis is to improve ventilation. This improvement may be brought about through mechanical ventilation, oxygen therapy, bronchodilators, postural drainage, and breathing exercises that increase the efficiency of the respiratory system.

RESPIRATORY ALKALOSIS. Respiratory alkalosis is caused by excessive loss of carbon dioxide as a result of hyperventilation or overstimulation of the respiratory center in the brain. It is most often an aftermath of hysteria and anxiety reactions but can also be seen as a consequence of excessive ventilation with a mechanical ventilator.

Respiratory alkalosis is managed by eliminating the cause of the hyperventilation and helping the patient to breathe more slowly and deeply. The patient can use a rebreather bag or paper bag to retain carbon dioxide. On a ventilated patient, the ventilator settings may need to be adjusted (decreasing the rate or tidal volume) to reduce the amount of CO_2 being exhaled.

METABOLIC ALKALOSIS. A metabolic alkalosis is characterized by either an abnormal rise in base in the plasma that increases the alkali component of the ratio of H_2CO_3 to $NaHCO_3$, or a decrease in hydrogen concentration of the plasma with a resultant rise in blood pH. Patients prone to developing a metabolic alkalosis include those who have an excessive hydrogen loss from the body through emesis or gastrointestinal (GI) drainage (chloride is lost concurrently), or patients with peptic ulcers who often take ordinary baking soda or milk of magnesia in large concentrations, thereby increasing the alkaline concentration in the body.

To correct a metabolic alkalosis, it is necessary to diagnose and treat the underlying condition by controlling emesis or GI losses or eliminating the overuse of baking soda or milk of magnesia. To treat the alkalosis associated with GI losses, Ringer's lactate solution may be administered because it contains 10 milliequivalent (mEq) chloride and helps to correct the chloride deficiency that accompanies alkalosis. As chloride is replaced, bicarbonate is allowed to exit the red cell and is excreted rather than retained. If the alkalosis is not related to GI losses, the chloride levels are generally elevated because chloride replaces bicarbonate in ECFs.

As the pH of ECF rises, potassium moves back into the cell in exchange for hydrogen ion. Serum potassium levels need to be monitored and potassium replaced as needed, particularly if increased potassium loss through the GI tract or through the kidneys with diuretic therapy is suspected.

As the patient becomes alkalotic, the binding of ionized calcium (free or active calcium) increases and free serum calcium levels fall. Patients may experience overstimulation of the peripheral nerves, often described as a "pins and needles" feeling; muscle weakness; spasm (carpopedal spasm or spasmodic flexion of the palms of the hands); and tetany. Serum calcium levels are monitored, and calcium is administered, if necessary.

METABOLIC ACIDOSIS. A metabolic acidosis is characterized by a loss of base from the plasma. It may be related to the overproduction of metabolic acids (ketone bodies), as in diabetes mellitus, or in other clinical settings such as hyperthyroidism, starvation, or severe infection. Fatty acids are converted to ketone bodies when glucose supplies have been used and the body turns to fats for energy. Salicylate poisoning can also lead to metabolic acidosis. In addition, anaerobic metabolism increases production of lactic acid, leading to metabolic acidosis. Severe diarrhea and loss of pancreatic, biliary, or lower bowel secretions may produce acidosis as large amounts of bicarbonate are lost in those body secretions.

Whatever the underlying cause, the body instantly responds to excess acid concentration by using bicarbonate as a chemical buffer. Bicarbonate ions neutralize hydrogen ions, thus minimizing life-threatening decreases in pH. Changes in hydrogen and potassium occur concurrently. As hydrogen concentration rises in the extracellular space, potassium moves out of the cells in exchange for hydrogen. Hydrogen is excreted in the kidney tubule in exchange for sodium attached to bicarbonate. Despite the high extracellular potassium levels, a deficit of body stores of potassium may occur because intracellular levels are low.

The management of metabolic acidosis is aimed at restoring the bicarbonate level to normal and treating the underlying cause. Patients experiencing metabolic acidosis are often seriously dehydrated and need to have an adequate vascular volume restored. A frequent complication of dehydration is hyperkalemia, which may lead to cardiac arrest. Every effort is made to reduce the potassium in the plasma as well as to correct the underlying metabolic acidosis.

Decompensated/Compensated States

Acid-base disturbances can be decompensated or compensated. Decompensated states reflect an acute change affecting only one system (kidney or lung). The unaffected system remains within normal limits. A compensated state occurs when one system attempts to compensate for the other system's alterations. During compensation, the body attempts to bring the pH as close to normal as possible. In compensated states, the pH approaches normal with significant changes in both the acid and the base components. In some cases, acid-base balance can also be partially compensated. The body is attempting to compensate, but the pH has not yet returned to normal.

These conditions are the most commonly encountered acid-base disturbances and are known as simple acid-base imbalances. They also can occur in various combinations. When they do, they are more complex, occur in seriously ill patients, and are known as mixed acid-base disturbances. For a more detailed discussion of acid-base balance, the reader is referred to a medical-surgical nursing or anatomy and physiology text.

THERAPEUTIC AGENTS FOR WATER AND ELECTROLYTE IMBALANCES

Many IV solutions are available today, and a knowledge of the underlying fluid balance assists the nurse in understanding why a particular fluid is ordered. IV fluids are classified as hydrating, balanced, and gastrointestinal solutions, and each has a place in treating water, fluid, and electrolyte imbalances.

All IV solutions contain solute particles that may be either electrolytes in their ionized form (Na^+, K^+, Cl^-, HCO_3^-); particles of nonionizable urea, glucose, and others in solution or plasma. Electrolytes dissociate into more particles than do nonionizable compounds because of their existing charge.

Normally, in the healthy body, the number of cations equals the anions. When added together, they equal 310 mEq/liter in ECF. IV solutions may be equal to (isotonic), less than (hypotonic), or more than (hypertonic) 310 mEq/liter. In an *isotonic solution,* the cations and anions approximate 310 mEq/liter (some sources use 280 mEq/liter), or the same osmotic pressure as body fluids. *Hypotonic solutions* have an electrolyte content of cations and anions of less than 250 mEq/liter. *Hypertonic solutions* have an electrolyte content of greater than 375 mEq/liter.

Isotonic solutions, such as 0.9% normal saline, have concentrations of water and salt equal to those found in the ECF; they will not induce the osmotic movement of water into or out of cells.

Hypotonic solutions have a greater concentration of free water molecules than are found inside the cell. These solutions give up their water to a dehydrated cell so it can return to isotonic equilibrium. Hypotonic solutions, such as 2.5% dextrose in 0.45% sodium chloride solution or 2.5% dextrose in 0.9% sodium chloride solution, are given slowly because a sudden shift of fluid into the cells can occur.

Hypertonic solutions have a lower concentration of free water, but a higher osmotic weight, than do body fluids. These solutions, such as 10% or 50% dextrose in water, 10% fructose in water, 3% saline solutions, or 5% dextrose in lactated Ringer's solution, are given slowly (usually not greater than 150 ml/hr) because they have the ability to pull water from the cell into the circulatory system, which can cause pulmonary edema and cardiac failure. Figure 11–3 features these types of solutions and how they affect vascular volume.

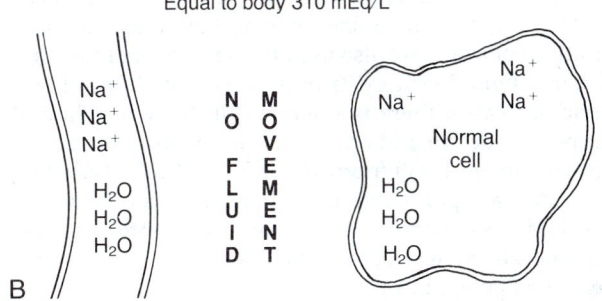

HYPOTONIC
Less than body less 250 mEq/L

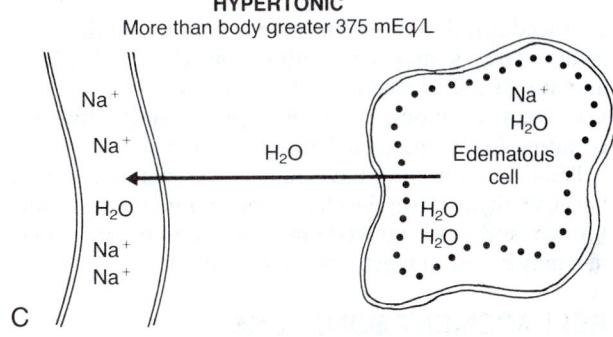

ISOTONIC
Equal to body 310 mEq/L

HYPERTONIC
More than body greater 375 mEq/L

Figure 11–3. IV solutions. A) Hypotonic solutions move from the vascular system into a dehydrated cell. B) Isotonic solutions remain within the vascular system. C) Hypertonic solutions pull free water from the edematous cell into the vascular system.

HYDRATING SOLUTIONS

Hydrating solutions are composed of water, carbohydrate, and varying amounts of sodium chloride (Table 11–4). These solutions are used primarily for simple hydration and fluid replacement and to determine the adequacy of a patient's renal function. To determine if the kidneys are still functioning, a fluid challenge is administered. A fluid challenge is a large volume (250–1000 ml) of a hydrating solution given in a short period of time (10–45 minutes). During this time, urinary output and cardiac function are monitored closely. If the kidneys are still functional, urine appears before the fluid challenge is ended. If urine does not appear, the flow

Table 11–4. HYDRATING SOLUTIONS*

Description	Cation Na (mEq/liter)	Anion Cl (mEq/liter)	Calories/liter	mOsm/liter
5% dextrose + 0.45% sodium chloride	77	77	170	405
5% dextrose + 0.33% sodium chloride	51	51	170	365
5% dextrose + 0.2% sodium chloride	34	34	170	320
2.5% dextrose + 0.45% sodium chloride	77	77	85	280

*Solutions can be obtained in 250-, 500-, and 1000-ml sizes.

rate is slowed and continued for an additional hour. If at this point there is still no urine, it may indicate serious renal disease, and renal function studies (serum creatinine, BUN, and creatinine clearance) are indicated. Hydrating solutions are also used to increase renal function when a fluid deficit exists or is suspected. As fluid volume decreases, there is a decrease in body weight and urine production and an increase in the urinary specific gravity above 1.030 (normal is 1.015–1.025). Hydrating solutions are potassium-free. (Potassium is essential to the body, but it can be toxic if the kidneys are not functioning effectively and are therefore unable to excrete the extra potassium.)

BALANCED SOLUTIONS

Balanced solutions are composed of water, carbohydrate as an energy source, and both cations (Na^+, K^+, Mg^{2+}) and anions (Cl^-, lactate, and HPO_4^-) (Table 11–5). There is a balance among the cations and anions, thus accounting for the name balanced solutions.

Balanced solutions have fallen into disfavor today, because these formulas have too many unclear, unknown, and unrecognized ingredients and because their use may result in electrolyte disturbances.

REPLACEMENT SOLUTIONS

Replacement solutions are a combination of water, carbohydrates, and electrolytes that are used to replace concurrent losses from the GI system (Table 11–6). These solutions are composed of various electrolytes that approximate losses from various GI areas through vomiting, diarrhea, fistulas, and suction. Table 11–7 describes body fluid production, composition, and probable imbalances. If more water or calories are needed, balanced solutions should be administered. Replacement solutions are available in both 5% and 10% dextrose solutions. Lactated Ringer's solution (Hartmann's solution) is a good multipurpose solution. However, it is low in potassium and, therefore, supplemental potassium may need to be added to the infusion. Replacement solutions, other than lactated Ringer's, are declining in clinical use.

CARBOHYDRATE SOLUTIONS

Carbohydrate solutions contain a carbohydrate that assists with meeting energy requirements. A liter of an IV solution of either water or normal saline with 5% dextrose has 170 calories per liter; 10% dextrose solution has 340 calories; 20% dextrose has 680 calories; 50% dextrose has 1700 calories; 5% Travert (invert sugar—a combination of levulose and dextrose formed by inversion of sucrose by enzyme invertase) solution has 190 calories; 10% Travert solution has 380 calories; and 10% fructose solution has 380 calories. Five percent solutions are approximately isotonic compared to blood. As the percent of carbohydrate increases above 5%, they become hypertonic. Hypertonic dextrose solutions are in-

Table 11–5. BALANCED IV SOLUTIONS*

Description	Cations (mEq/liter)			Anions (mEq/liter)			Calories	mOsm/liter
	Na	K	Mg	Cl	LACTATE	HPO₄		
5% or 10% Dextrose w/Electrolyte No. 48	25	20	3	24	23	3	170/340	347
5% Dextrose or Fructose w/Electrolyte No. 75	40	35	—	48	20	15	180	402
Ionosol B + 5% Dextrose	57	25	5	49	25	13	170	423
Ionosol MB + 5% Dextrose	25	20	3	22	23	3	170	350
Isolyte P + 5% Dextrose	25	19	3	23	23		175	350
Normosol M + 5% Dextrose	40	13	3	40	(Acetate) 16 (Acetate)	—	170	368
Isolyte T + 5% Dextrose	40	35	—	40	20	15	170	406

*These solutions usually can be obtained in 250-, 500-, and 1000-ml solutions.

Table 11–6. REPLACEMENT SOLUTIONS* Na$^+$ K$^+$ Ca^{2+} Mg^{2+} Cl$^-$

Description	Cations (mEq/liter)					Anions (mEq/liter)		Gluconate or Phosphate	G/I** Replacement	mOsm/liter	Calories
	Na$^+$	K$^+$	Ca^{2+}	Mg^{2+}	Cl$^-$	Lactate	Acetate				
10% Travert's (invert sugar) w/Electrolyte No. 2	56	25		6	56	25		P—12.5	G	726	384
Plasma-Lyte R + 5% Dextrose	140	10	5	3	103	8	47		I	564	170
Ionosol D-CM w/5% Dextrose	138	12	5	3	108	50			I	578	170
Normosol-R	140	5		3	98		27	G—23	I	295	—
Plasma-Lyte 148	140	5		3	98		27	G—23	I	294	—
Lactated Ringer's (Hartmann's)	130	4	3		109	28			G/I	275	—

*These solutions are mostly available in 500- and 1000-ml sizes.
**G = gastric; I = intestinal.

fused in a high-flow vein to prevent irritation to the veins. All dextrose solutions are acidic (pH 3.5–5) and may produce thrombophlebitis.

Carbohydrate solutions use natural sugars such as dextrose (glucose) and fructose (levulose). Fructose offers no advantage over dextrose injection and possesses some disadvantages. It may increase serum levels of lactate and urate if given rapidly, and it is considerably more expensive than dextrose. Travert contains both sugars. The 5% and 10% solutions cannot meet the energy needs of a severely ill patient. A patient receiving 3000 ml of a 5% dextrose in water solution receives only about 600 calories. Protein catabolism and a state of metabolic acidosis soon develop if more calories are not added. This can be achieved through total parenteral nutrition (TPN). (See Chapter 56 for more information.)

The rate of utilization of dextrose varies considerably. The average maximal rate is 300 mg/kg/hr (5 ml/kg/min of dextrose injection 5%) over periods of less than 24 hours. If more dextrose is administered than the patient can utilize, hyperglycemia, glycosuria, and excessive diuresis can result. In addition, there is increased carbon dioxide production, which may contribute to respiratory failure.

Carbohydrate in sodium chloride solution is best used when there has been an excessive loss of fluid through sweating, vomiting, or gastric suctioning. The sodium chloride solutions contain a combination of equal amounts of sodium and chloride. A 0.2% solution has 38.5 mEq of both Na and Cl; a 0.33% solution has 50 mEq of both Na and Cl; a 0.45% solution has 77 mEq of both Na and Cl; and a 0.9% solution has 154 mEq of both Na and Cl. Concentrations of 0.11%–0.45% are hypotonic, 0.9% is isotonic, and concentrations of 3%–5% are hypertonic. The 3% and 5% solutions are reserved for the treatment of severe symptomatic hyponatremia (serum Na less than 120 mEq/ml).

The simple carbohydrates in water or sodium chloride solutions are effective IV therapy solutions. However, indiscriminate use of these solutions can precipitate imbalances in patients, so they should be used with caution.

Table 11–7. BODY FLUID COMPOSITION AND LOSSES*

	Volume (ml/24hr)	pH	Composition (mEq/liter)				Probable Imbalance
			Na$^+$	K$^+$	Cl$^-$	HCO$_3^-$	
Gastric fluid	2500	1–3	10–115	1–35	90–150	0–15	Metabolic alkalosis, dec. K, dec. Na
Bile	500	7–8	130–160	3–12	90–120	40–50	Metabolic acidosis, dec. Na
Pancreatic fluid	700 (3000 total)	8	115–150	3–8	55–95	60–120	Metabolic acidosis
Intestinal fluids Jejunum	—	7.8–8	85–150	2–10	45–125	20–35	Metabolic acidosis, dec. K, dec. Na
Ileostomy (old)	—	7.8–8	40–50	3–5	20–30	—	Imbalances are unlikely

*Data are summarized from the literature for both average values and their ranges and refer to an adult in a temperate climate engaging in mild physical activity.

Table 11-8. NURSING PROCESS FOR PATIENT REQUIRING IV THERAPY

Assessment

Review present illness including routes of fluid loss (e.g., vomiting, draining wound, diuretic use), characteristics of urine. Note ability to ingest and retain fluids.
Determine current vital signs, usual/current weight.

Nursing Diagnosis	Nursing Actions	Rationale	Patient Outcomes/ Evaluation Criteria
Fluid volume deficit related to excessive loss/inadequate intake as evidenced by poor skin turgor, decreased urinary output, weight loss, decreased CVP, decreased blood pressure, confusion.	Begin/maintain intravenous fluid replacement therapy.	Replaces losses when oral route is not appropriate or rapid replacement is required.	Demonstrates improved fluid balance as evidenced by urine output of 35 cc/hour with normal specific gravity, stable vital signs, moist mucous membranes, good skin turgor and capillary refill < 3 sec.
	Observe drip rate qh.	Ensures accuracy of infusion preventing errors in intake.	
	Monitor vital signs and physical symptoms for deviation from assessed baseline. Record I/O and daily weight.	Adequate replacement of fluids should correct symptoms indicating deficit; however, continued losses and/or insufficient intake may worsen symptoms and increase imbalance between I/O and weight.	
	Note characteristics of urine and measure specific gravity.	Urine usually dark/concentrated with elevated specific gravity in presence of dehydration.	
	Review laboratory studies, e.g., Hgb/Hct, electrolytes, serum osmolality and blood cases.	Useful in identifying type and amount of fluid needed for replacement.	
	Reduce fever if present, (e.g., administer acetaminophen/ASA products), control environmental temperature, remove excessive linens.	Helps control insensible losses that contribute to fluid deficit.	
	Provide fluids for oral intake as appropriate.	Promotes patient comfort and oral route is preferred for replacement as it reduces risks associated with invasive procedures.	
Knowledge deficit related to unfamiliarity with IV therapy as evidenced by questions, statement of concern.	Provide information outlining current IV therapy to both patient and family. Allow time to ask questions and verbalize feelings/concerns.	Patient/family often have unspoken fears about what is happening and accurate information and opportunity to discuss these fears promotes understanding and may enhance cooperation with therapy.	Verbalizes understanding of condition and treatment.
Infection, potential for related to invasive procedure.	Use aseptic technique for insertion of IV device. Cover with clear dressing and observe site hourly.	Eliminates skin contaminants lowering risk of infection. Allows for early detection and prompt intervention to prevent serious complications.	Demonstrates absence of edema, erythema, or purulent drainage at insertion site, and is afebrile.
	Administer IV fluids through in-line filter.	Can prevent passage of most bacteria, yeast, and particulate matter dependent upon size of filter. (May also reduce incidence of infusion phlebitis and air emboli).	

Table 11–8. NURSING PROCESS FOR PATIENT REQUIRING IV THERAPY– CONTINUED

Name	Dosage	Mode of Administration	Pharmacokinetics
	Maintain integrity of IV system when changing bottles. Inspect bottle/bag and solution before adding to IV. Note expiration date.	Reduces risk of introduction of microbes into vascular system.	
	Change tubing and IV site at least every 72 hours or if signs of irritation/infection present.	Routine changing reduces potential for device-produced sepsis.	

USING THE NURSING PROCESS

ASSESSMENT

Assessment of the patient requiring IV therapy always begins with a thorough nursing history to develop the data base needed for preparation of a nursing care plan. The information to be obtained is featured in Table 11–8. Baseline laboratory data, particularly electrolytes, patient weights, and assessment of water balance are obtained prior to beginning IV therapy.

IV therapy is a routine part of nursing. However, it may be a traumatic event for the patient and family. Often, to the patient and family, IV therapy may erroneously indicate serious illness or impending death. The nurse should share with them the reason for and the purpose of the IV and help them to recognize and allay their fears.

The nurse must understand the reason for IV therapy in the patient, the presenting symptoms of the condition, and the type of fluid used. The nurse also assesses for symptoms of fluid and electrolyte disturbances. Table 11–9 features the major volume and electrolyte imbalances with the most common symptoms, as well as the goals of nursing care. The nurse must further assess the patient for complications that can arise from IV therapy. Complications will be discussed later in this chapter.

NURSING DIAGNOSIS

The nurse establishes the nursing diagnoses based on the information obtained during the assessment. The nursing diagnosis forms the basis for the nursing care. Typical nursing diagnoses are included in Table 11–8.

PLANNING AND INTERVENTION

The nurse develops the expected patient outcomes for the nursing intervention from the nursing diagnoses. Typical patient outcomes that are to be achieved during the nursing intervention for a patient with IV therapy are included in Table 11–8.

NURSING RESPONSIBILITIES FOR IV THERAPY

The professional nurse is often responsible for starting an IV infusion. In order to accomplish this, the nurse must

1. Explain the procedure to the patient. Patient teaching information is provided in Table 11–10.
2. Elicit the patient's cooperation. (If this is not possible because the patient is confused or unconscious, the nurse may need assistance in the actual venipuncture.)
3. Verify the IV order.
4. Gather the equipment: IV tray with alcohol or similar cleansing solution, tourniquets, adhesive bandages, tape, antiseptic ointment to apply over the site (if indicated by the hospital), a selection of needles, and an arm board. Appropriate IV tubing must also be selected as well as the correct solution.

   IV tubing comes in three basic types: regular tubing with a drip factor of 10–15 drops/ml, minidrip tubing with a drip factor of 60 drops/ml, and Y tubing used for blood administration with a drip factor of 10 drops/ml.

   In-line filters may also be used. These devices help to eliminate particulate matter that may be introduced into the IV solution by opening and adding other fluids to the IV line such as from IV additives. Recent research has demonstrated that when IV medications are drawn from single-dose glass vials, macroparticles of glass can also be drawn into the syringe and administered to the patient. The use of any size filter will trap these macroparticles. Filters come as part of the IV tubing or can be added to it (Fig. 11–4). Filters are available in three sizes: 5 μm, 0.5 μm, or 0.22 μm. The 5-μm size filters gross particulate material, whereas the 0.5-μm size prevents passage of most bacteria, yeast, and particulate matters. The 0.22-μm size filter is considered a sterilizing filter and removes nearly all bacteria, fungi, and particulate matter that find their way into IV fluids. The 0.5- and 0.22-μm filters require an infusion pump to administer fluids through them. Filters have been shown to reduce

Table 11–9. FLUID AND ELECTROLYTE IMBALANCES AND THEIR ASSESSABLE CLINICAL SYMPTOMS AND GENERAL GOALS OF INTERVENTION

Imbalance	Clinical Causes	Assessable Clinical Signs and Symptoms	Goals of Intervention
Fluid volume deficit	Hypo-osmotic: adrenal insufficiency (Addison's disease) Iso-osmotic: cholera, gastric suction, ulcerative colitis Hyperosmotic: dehydration (i.e., fever), diabetic ketoacidosis, decreased protein intake	Dry skin and mucous membranes, longitudinal wrinkling of tongue, lack of sweating, poor skin turgor, decreased urinary output, decreased systolic blood pressure, lowered body temperature, weight loss, elevated pulse, decreased central venous pressure, depressed anterior fontanelle in infants	Restore volume to normal without altering electrolyte balance by administering balanced solutions
Fluid volume excess	Hypo-osmotic: SIADH Iso-osmotic: edema Hyperosmotic: excessive administration of NaCl	Symptoms associated with congestive heart failure, edema, changes in vital signs	Restore volume to normal by correction of underlying cause, restricting fluids, diuretic therapy
Respiratory acidosis	Oversedation, COPD, pulmonary infections	Respiratory embarrassment (shallow, slow breathing); weakness; coma; disorientation	Restore pH to normal by correction of underlying pathology
Respiratory alkalosis	CNS disorders, sepsis, CNS stimulation, salicylate intoxication	Convulsions, unconsciousness, hyperventilation, possible tetany	Restore pH to normal by correcting underlying pathology
Metabolic alkalosis	Vomiting, gastric suction, primary aldosteronism	Hyperactive reflexes, depressed breathing, muscle hypertonicity, possible tetany	Restore pH to normal by replacing nonbicarbonate ions. Fluid replacement with hydrating solutions, balanced solutions, GI replacement solutions, return Ca^{++} to normal
Metabolic acidosis	Lactic acidosis, diabetic ketoacidosis, salicylate intoxication, renal failure, diarrhea	Disorientation, unconsciousness, stupor, coma, deep and rapid respirations	Restore pH to normal by correcting underlying pathology to provide bicarbonate ions and/or stop acid production. Replace fluids with hydrating solutions, balanced solutions, GI replacement solutions

the incidence of infusion phlebitis to less than 10%. The incidence of phlebitis arising from IV infusions without filters ranges between 27% and 47%. Filters can also prevent the infusion of microorganisms and air emboli. Most solutions can be filtered, except suspensions such as fats and some cytotoxins. (Blood and blood products require their own special filters.) There is disagreement on the subject of in-line filters: The Centers for Disease Control does not recommend the use of filters as a routine infection control measure, but the National Intravenous Therapy Association believes that filters should be used for all IV therapy. It must be remembered, however, that IV filters do not remove endotoxins, nor do they reduce the risk of contaminants entering the tubing below the filter. In addition, since some drugs bind to filters, using filters can reduce the drug's potency. In the final analysis, cost is a major factor in deciding whether to use IV filters. Some hospitals compromise by using them

Table 11–10. PATIENT TEACHING INFORMATION—IV THERAPY

Dear Patient:
    IV therapy has been ordered for you to _____.
Therapy is given to meet your average daily fluid, vitamin, and mineral needs. Medication can also be given IV. The most common site for the IV line is in your hand or arm. After the needle is put in, it is taped, and your hand or arm may be taped to a board to prevent movement. If you have any pain at the site of the IV line, please tell your nurse.

only for IV products that have a high concentration of particulate matter.

5. Prepare the IV solution. The solution may be a plain IV solution or an admixture. An admixture is the addition of one or more drugs and/or another solution to the main IV. Preparation of the admixture may fall under the scope of the pharmacy department or may be within the realm of nursing. When the nurse is preparing an admixture, the IV must be labeled with the drug name and dose that was added, as well as the patient's name and room number, date and time, and the nurse's name.

    Solutions come in various sizes: 100, 250, 500, and 1000 ml in either glass bottles or plastic bags. There are also 25-, 50- and 100-ml bottles available for direct administration of IV medications.

    As the nurse removes the solution from the shelf, it is inspected: the solution should be clear. The nurse checks the expiration date and sends the bottle back to the pharmacy if it is outdated. Next, the nurse checks for cracks in a glass bottle or leaks in a plastic bag. Any admixture must be prepared using sterile techniques and labeled correctly. The nurse connects the tubing to the IV container and runs fluid through the tubing to clear the air from the tubing. The solution and tubing are prepared in the medication room, where the nurse is free from distractions. (For review of medication preparation procedures see a fundamental nursing text.)

6. The nurse is now ready to enter the patient's room and perform the venipuncture. Insertion may be easier if a 2% nitroglycerin ointment is first applied to the back of the patient's hand to produce venodilatation (Roberge, et al, 1987). (See a medical-surgical textbook for procedure.) After the venipuncture, the site is labeled with the time of insertion, the date, the needle size and type used, and the nurse's name.

7. Regulate the IV. The nurse calculates the IV flow rate and regulates the rate to the proper drops per minute. If infusion pumps are being used, a nurse must understand their mechanics of operation. The drop rate is checked frequently and compared with the reading of the pump to ensure accuracy.

8. Examine the IV site for complications. At least once per hour, the nurse checks for complications at the site and on the extremity. Major complications include clotting, extravasation and infiltration, and

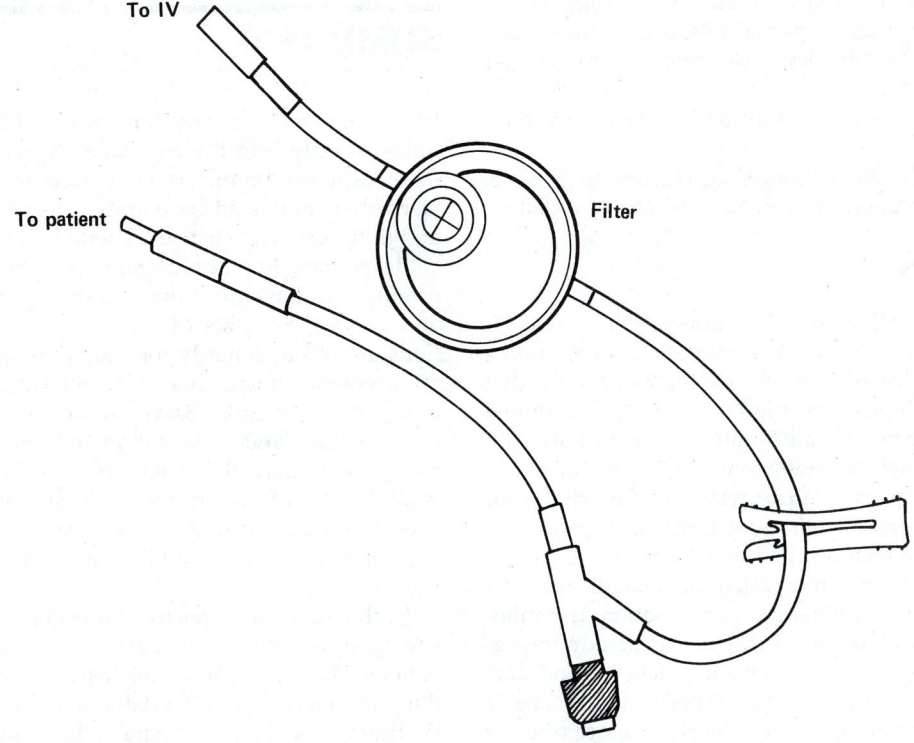

Figure 11–4. In-line IV filter.

thrombophlebitis. Complications include clotting of the cannula, which will stop the flow. Extravasation and infiltration occurs when fluid or blood enters the surrounding skin. The area will appear hard, swollen, and painful (toxic substances can even cause sloughing of the tissues). Thrombophlebitis is an inflammation at the insertion site, which may result from many possible causes including type, size, and site of the needle inserted; the fluid itself; and duration of time the IV remains in site. The site becomes red, swollen, and painful. (Refer to a medical-surgical nursing text for more detailed discussion of IV complications.)

9. Inspect the patient for generalized complications and reactions, which may include a pyrogenic reaction (when *pyrogens*, any substance that produces fever, enter through the IV line, a systemic febrile reaction follows); infection, resulting from the introduction of bacteria or fungi through the IV line; an embolism, which may occur in any central location from part of a clot breaking off near the insertion site; and fluid overload—too much fluid administered too quickly, with the heart unable to manage the extra load. Symptoms of fluid overload are those of congestive heart failure.

10. Inspect the patient for complications specific to the type of IV fluid.

11. Administer additional IV medications as ordered. Always ensure that the medications are compatible with the IV solution. (See Table 5–2 for IV drug compatibility tables.) The nurse may administer medications directly IV by push or bolus or through a device that allows a precise amount of medication to be given intermittently every four to six hours. The devices that can be used for this purpose include "piggybacks," partial fills, and volume control sets. Antibiotics are often administered intermittently.

12. Monitor intake and output and body weight on a daily basis.

13. Monitor laboratory reports for electrolyte balance. Types of solutions may need to be changed daily.

EVALUATION

During the evaluation phase, the nurse evaluates the effectiveness of IV therapy. This evaluation is based on a predetermined list of outcome evaluation criteria that have been developed in relation to the goals determined by the nurse, patient, and family. The data base, obtained in the original assessment, is used to formulate the nursing diagnoses and provide helpful criteria for measuring the treatment's effectiveness. Typical outcome criteria are included in Table 11–8.

The nurse evaluates the patient for complications of IV therapy such as infiltration, extravasation, thrombosis, cellulitis, thrombophlebitis, pain at the administration site, fluid overload, pyrogenic reactions, and bacteremia, as well as for reactions to specific fluids. The IV site and drip rate are evaluated hourly or more often, if necessary. Intravenous tubing and dressings need to be changed according to the institutional policies. Research suggests that changing tubing and dressing every 72 hours is sufficient to prevent infection.

It must be remembered that the longer the IV device remains in place, the greater the risk of infection. With appropriate infection control measures (such as aseptic initiation and maintenance of the IV system), few devices produce sepsis until they have been in place for at least 72 hours. Also, synthetic IV devices such as IV catheters have a greater risk of infection than smaller, steel "scalp vein" or "butterfly needles"—8% versus 0.1%–0.2%.

There are three exceptions to the 72-hour interval for routine IV set changes: (1) during the administration of blood products and lipid emulsion, because both these products enhance bacterial growth in parenteral solutions; (2) with arterial pressure monitoring, because of the high rate of arterial infusate contamination; (3) and in the presence of a suspected infusion-related septicemia epidemic. Because most U.S. hospitals try to replace IV cannulas every three days, researchers conclude that replacing the delivery sets along with the cannulas would be more time- and cost-effective.

The patient receiving IV fluids will also have other nursing care problems. The IV therapy may have been instituted after surgery, after trauma, or after a medical emergency. This patient is usually acutely ill and needs additional emotional support, as well as physical nursing care.

The nurse evaluates the effectiveness of treatment by a return to normal homeostasis. This is evaluated through qualitative, quantitative, and laboratory findings.

SUMMARY

IV therapy involves instilling many different types of fluids directly into the circulatory system. Specifically, IV therapy is administered to correct water imbalances, electrolyte and acid-base imbalances, blood volume, and nutritional deficiencies. Therapeutic IV solutions include isotonic, hypotonic, and hypertonic solutions. Hydrating solutions are composed of water, carbohydrate, and varying amounts of sodium chloride. These solutions are used primarily for simple hydration and fluid replacement and to determine the adequacy of a patient's renal function. Balanced are composed of water, carbohydrate, and equal cation and anion solutions are rarely used today. Balanced replacement solutions are a combination of water, carbohydrate, and electrolytes used to replace current losses from the gastrointestinal system. Replacement solutions are also declining in clinical use.

As the nurse prepares to administer IV therapy, he or she must understand the reason for IV therapy in each patient. The nurse continually assesses for symptoms of fluid and electrolyte disturbances and complications of IV therapy. Laboratory data, intake and output, and daily weights are monitored throughout therapy.

BIBLIOGRAPHY

————— Changing IV tubing. Am J Nurs 86(6):681, 1986.

————— Fluids and Electrolytes. Abbott Laboratories, North Chicago, 1980.

————— Infusion system guide. Nurse Manager 18(9):95–97, 1987.

Alexander, MR: IV infusion devices: Are they always justified? Drug Intell Clin Pharm 21(3):255–257, 1987.

Alspach, JC and Williams, SM: Core Curriculum for Critical Care Nursing, ed 3. WB Saunders, Philadelphia, 1985.

American Medical Association Drug Evaluations, ed 6. WB Saunders, Philadelphia, 1986.

Barris, D: Should you irrigate an occluded IV line? Nursing '87 17(3):63–64, 1987.

Beckwith, N: Fundamentals of fluid resuscitation. Nursinglife 7(3):49–56, 1987.

Boykoff, SL, et al: 6 ways to clear the air from an IV line. Nursing '88 18(2):46–48, 1988.

Brosnan, KM, et al: Stopcock. Am J Nurs 88(3):320–324, 1988.

Bryan, CS: CDC says . . . : The case of IV tubing replacement. Infect Control 8(6):255–256, 1987.

Cohen, MR: Improperly mixed IV additives. Nursing '87 17(5):16, 1987.

Coleman, DA: Do you need IV filters? RN 86(9):76–78, 1986.

Cyganski, JM, et al: The case for the heparin flush. Am J Nurs 87(6):796–797, 1987.

Dunn, DL, et al: The case for the saline flush. Am J Nurs 87(6):798–799, 1987.

Frey, AM: Taking the confusion out of multiple infusion: IV medications and TPN. National Intravenous Therapy Association 9(6):460–463, 1986.

Gilman, AG, Goodman, LS, and Gilman, A (eds): Goodman and Gilman's The Pharmacological Basis of Therapeutics, ed 7. Macmillan, New York, 1986.

Graham, J: How to dress an IV site. RN 87(12):10, 1987.

Hagle, ME: Implantable devices for chemotherapy: Access and delivery. Semin Oncology Nurse 3(2):95–105, 1987.

Knox, LS: Implantable venous access devices. Critical Care Nurse 7(1):70–73, 1987.

Maki, DG: Infections associated with intravascular lines. In Remington, J and Swartz, M (eds): Current Clinical Topics in Infectious Diseases. McGraw-Hill, New York, 1982.

Maki, DG: The prevention and management of device-related infection in infusion therapy. J Med 11(4):239, 1980.

Maki, DG and Botticelli, JT: Safer longer: 72-hour IV tubing changes. Am J Nurs 87(12):1539, December 1987.

Maki, DG, et al: Prospective study of replacing administration sets for IV therapy. JAMA 258(13):1777–1781, 1987.

Mathewson, M and Mathewson, R: Establishing acid-base balance. Critical Care Nurse 7(5):77–85, 1987.

Messner, RL, et al: Nursing management of peripheral intravenous sites. Focus on Critical Care 14(2):25–33, 1987.

Millam, D: Managing complications of IV therapy. Nursing '88 18(3):34–43, 1988.

Newton, GA: A better way to chart IV therapy. RN: 26–28, July 1988.

Nieweg, R, et al: A patient education program for a continuous infusion regimen on an outpatient basis. Cancer Nurs 10(4):177–182, 1987.

Northridge, JA: Calculating IV medications with confidence. Nursing '87 17(9):55–57, 1987.

Olin, B (ed): Facts and Comparisons. JB Lippincott, St Louis, 1987.

Roberge, R, et al: Facilitated intravenous access through local application of nitroglycerin ointment. JAMA 258:1237, 1987.

Shaw, N and Lyall, E: Hazards of glass ampoules. Br Med J 291:1390, 1985.

Snydman, DR, et al: Intravenous tubing containing burettes can be safely changed at 72 hour intervals. Infect Control 8(3):113–116, 1987.

Taylor, JP, et al: Vascular access devices: Uses and aftercare. J. Emergency Nursing 13(3):160–167, 1987.

Todd, B: Intravenous drug hazards: Interactions, adsorption, and inadequate mixing. Geriatr Nurs 9(1):20, 22, 1988.

Tully, JL, Friedland, GH, and Goldmann, DA: Complications of intravenous therapy with steel needles and small-bore teflon catheters (abstr). Proceedings of the 19th Interscience Conference on Antimicrobial Agents and Chemotherapy, Boston, 1979.

Wachs, T, et al: No more pokes: A review of parenteral access devices. Nutr Support Serv 7(6):12–13, 1987.

Weinstein, S: Intravenous filters. Infect Control 8(5):220–221, 1987.

SITUATION 11–1

Mr. Wells, an 86-year-old, is transferred from a nursing home to an acute care facility. The admitting diagnosis is dehydration.

1. During the admission process, the nurse will be aware of the following clinical sign of dehydration:
   a. poor skin turgor
   b. moist clammy skin
   c. pink frothy sputum
   d. abdominal cramps

2. Intravenous fluid has been ordered for Mr. Wells. It will be important for the nurse to assess the following prior to initiating therapy:
   a. ability to communicate
   b. patient height
   c. body weight
   d. cranial nerves

3. The report from the nursing home reveals that Mr. Wells has had a fever for the last three days and has not been eating or drinking adequately. The nurse is aware that the following process has probably occurred:
   a. hyperosmotic contraction
   b. hyperosmotic expansion
   c. iso-osmotic contraction
   d. hypo-osmotic expansion

4. Intravenous fluid in the form of 2.5 percent dextrose + 0.45 percent sodium chloride is started for Mr. Wells. This type of solution is:
   a. hydrating and isotonic
   b. replacement and isotonic
   c. hydrating and hypotonic
   d. replacement and isotonic

5. The rate of infusion of the intravenous fluid 2.5 percent dextrose + 0.45 percent sodium chloride should be given:
   a. rapidly in order to rehydrate as quickly as possible
   b. slowly due to rapid shift into the extracellular space
   c. rapidly in order to increase vascular volume
   d. slowly due to sudden shift of fluid into the cells

6. In evaluating Mr. Wells' intravenous therapy, all of the following outcome criteria are expected, *except:*
   a. normal electrolytes and osmolality
   b. urine output less than 30 cc per hour
   c. absence of pain at the administration site
   d. absence of infiltration, extravasation, or thrombosis

SITUATION 11–2

As an emergency room nurse, Marianne Holt encounters patients daily who require intravenous therapy and correction of acid-base imbalances.

1. Shelby Andrews presents to the emergency room, complaining of feeling "anxious" and stating that she has tingling in feet and hands. An arterial blood gas reveals respiratory alkalosis. Marianne will be prepared to treat her with:
   a. sodium bicarbonate
   b. mechanical ventilation
   c. oxygen therapy
   d. rebreather bag

2. Mr. Butler, a 72-year-old with chronic renal failure, is short of breath and restless. His wife admits that he has not been adhering to his renal diet. Marianne notes pitting edema at the ankles and crackles in the lung bases. Marianne is aware that edema results from all of the following *except:*
   a. reduced hydrostatic pressure
   b. reduced oncotic pressure
   c. increased capillary permeability
   d. reduced lymphatic drainage

3. Mr. Owens, a 62-year-old, is being treated for nausea and vomiting related to the flu syndrome. Marianne draws blood for baseline lab data. An arterial blood gas demonstrates metabolic alkalosis. Related to this, Marianne anticipates the following lab results:
   a. high potassium and low chloride levels
   b. low potassium and low chloride levels
   c. high potassium and high chloride levels
   d. low potassium and high chloride levels

4. Mr. Klein has been on oral diuretic therapy for one week after discharge from the hospital. He presents with weakness and weight loss. He currently weighs 147 lb, which represents a 7-lb decrease from his normal 154 lb. Marianne calculates this loss as:
   a. mild
   b. moderate
   c. severe
   d. extreme

5. Melinda Johnson is brought into the emergency room in diabetic ketoacidosis (DKA). An arterial blood gas reveals metabolic acidosis. Marianne is aware that intravenous therapy is ordered to:
   a. provide potassium and other necessary electrolytes
   b. administer calcium chloride to prevent teteny
   c. restore adequate vascular volume
   d. administer hyperosmotic intravenous fluid

6. Arterial blood gases on Jim Hartsman, a patient with chronic obstructive lung disease (COPD), reveal a pH of 7.39 despite elevated carbon dioxide levels. In planning nursing care for Mr. Hartsman, Marianne is aware that this represents a:
   a. decompensated state
   b. partially compensated state
   c. mixed acid-base state
   d. compensated state

Please refer to the Appendices for correct answers and additional review questions with answers.

12
CHAPTER

BLOOD PRODUCTS AND BLOOD SUBSTITUTES

GLOSSARY TERMS IN THIS CHAPTER

Acquired Immune Deficiency Syndrome (AIDS)
Antigenicity
Autologous
Centrifugation
Colloid
Colloidal osmotic pressure
Crystalloids
Human Immunodeficiency Virus
Plasma expanders
Plasmapheresis
Sensitizing lymphocytes

12
CHAPTER

BLOOD PRODUCTS AND BLOOD SUBSTITUTES

MERRILY MATHEWSON KUHN, R.N.C., Ph.D., CCRN

LEARNING OBJECTIVES

After reading this chapter, the student will be able to:

1. Identify those fluids commonly administered intravenously including plasma expanders, blood, and blood components.

2. Differentiate among the plasma expanders, blood, and blood components as to mechanism of action, adverse effects, contraindications, and interactions.

3. Identify specific areas to assess in the patient requiring plasma expanders, blood, and blood components in order to formulate appropriate nursing diagnoses.

4. Plan the nursing interventions necessary to administer plasma expanders, blood, and blood components.

5. Evaluate the patient at various stages of treatment to gauge nursing interactions.

Volume deficits develop when there is a loss of fluid volume, secondary to blood loss from hemorrhage, burns, surgery, sepsis, or other trauma. An individual can tolerate the gradual loss of up to approximately 25% (1.5 liters of a total body blood volume of 5–6 liters) of total blood volume. However, if the loss is sudden, only approximately 10% loss is tolerated before symptoms develop. In order to support vital functions, blood volume must be replaced. This can be done with plasma expanders or blood.

THERAPEUTIC AGENTS FOR VOLUME DEFICITS

BLOOD SUBSTITUTES

Blood substitutes, often referred to as *plasma expanders,* are substances obtained from sources other than blood and have the ability to expand a depleted blood volume. The substances are not artificial blood. These substances exert a *colloidal osmotic pressure* (oncotic pressure) similar to plasma proteins that balances the distribution of water between the intravascular and interstitial space. Thus, by increasing the pressure in the vascular bed, fluid is pulled from the interstitial compartment, and total blood volume is increased (Fig. 12–1). *Colloids* available today include albumin, a natural colloid discussed later in this chapter, dextran, and hetastarch.

Plasma expanders are readily available and inexpensive. They can be administered immediately, and the

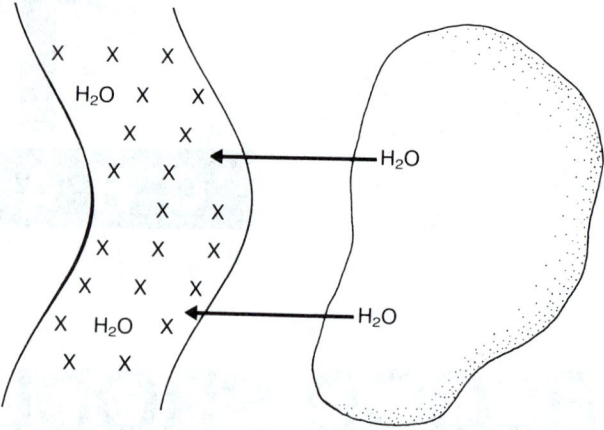

Figure 12–1. Colloid properties of plasma expanders. Plasma expanders (X) exert a high colloid oncotic pressure in the vascular system and thus pull fluid from the interstitial space into the vascular system to dilute the solute.

patient does not have to wait for a blood typing and matching of blood. These products do not transmit hepatitis virus nor *Acquired Immune Deficiency Syndrome* (AIDS) but are capable of causing an anaphylactic reaction. Therefore, patients need to be monitored carefully.

These products do not have oxygen-carrying capacity or contain plasma proteins or clotting factors. They are not meant to be a substitute for blood or plasma. Patients who have suffered a large blood loss will still need

Table 12–1. BLOOD SUBSTITUTES

Preparation/Molecular Weight	Dose and Administration of IV Solution	Pharmacokinetics
LOW-MOLECULAR-WEIGHT DEXTRAN		
Action: Synthetic polysaccharides that approximate the colloid properties of albumin and appear to disaggregate red cell sludging in the microcirculation.		
Use: Volume expansion in shock. Priming solution for extracorporeal circulation. Prophylaxis against venous thrombosis and thromboembolism.		
Dextran 40 (LMD, Rheomacrodex) 40,000	10% solution mixed with 5% dextrose (170 cal/liter) or 0.9% sodium chloride 10 ml/kg rapidly; not to exceed 20 ml/kg in first 24 hr	O: within min P: UA D: 4–6 hr ½ L:2–6 hr PB: UA B: urine E: urine

Key to Abbreviations in the *Pharmacokinetics* column O-onset; P-peak; D-duration; PB-protein bound; B-biotransformed in; E-excreted in; ½ L-halflife.
*Within the column listing adverse effects, underlines indicate the most common effects; CAPITALS indicate life-threatening effects.

the replacement of blood and blood components. Administration of large volumes of any of these products may alter coagulation and result in transient prolongation of prothrombin time (PT), partial thromboplastin time (PTT), bleeding and clotting times, and decreased hematocrit and may cause excessive dilution of plasma protein. Before administering any plasma expanders, renal function is assessed. Fluid overload may occur from lack of elimination of the newly reabsorbed fluid.

Today, there are two types of blood substitutes available: dextran and hetastarch (Table 12–1). Dextran, a polysaccharide, is prepared from sucrose. There are currently two types of dextran available: low- and high-molecular-weight dextran. Hetastarch (Hespan) is a preparation made from cornstarch and sodium chloride.

Dextran, Low-Molecular-Weight

Dextran 40, or low-molecular-weight dextran, is shorter acting and more rapidly excreted than other dextrans. It is sometimes used as a hemodiluent in the heart-lung machine because of its low viscosity and ability to keep blood cells from sludging in small blood vessels. Dextran 40 is also used to decrease the incidence of deep vein thrombosis in patients recovering from orthopedic surgery. Dextran 40 minimizes sludging of blood in the microcirculation and decreases platelet aggregation. Seventy percent of Dextran 40 is excreted within 24 hours.

Dextran 40 increases cardiac output and arterial, venous, and microcirculatory flow. It reduces mean transfer time, chiefly by expanding plasma volume and by reducing blood viscosity through hemodilution and by reducing red cell aggregation.

Antigenicity of the dextrans is related to the degree of branching in the chemical formulation. Dextran 40 has minimal branching and consequently is relatively free of antigenic effects. However, hypersensitivity reaction can occur. (See Table 12–1 for additional information.)

Dextran, High-Molecular-Weight

Dextran 70 or 75, high-molecular-weight dextran, is close in molecular weight to albumin (a part of human plasma). Because of its large molecular weight, it does not leak out of blood vessels and, therefore, has the ability to increase osmotic pressure for longer periods of time than does dextran 40. It also helps to pull fluid back into the circulatory system. It can be used when a large volume of blood has been lost; however, it does not have oxygen-carrying capacity, so red blood cells are also given as needed. Dextran 70 is primarily indicated for the management of shock or impending shock due to trauma, surgery, hemorrhage, or burns. Fifty percent of dextran 70 or 75 is excreted within 24 hours. This expansion of plasma volume improves the hemodynamic status for 24 hours or longer.

Dextran 70 has more branching in its chemical structure, and there is a greater risk of anaphylactoid reactions. These reactions generally occur early in the infusion period in patients not previously exposed to intravenous (IV) dextran. Dextran 70, when administered in large doses (15 ml/kg or over 1000 ml), can prolong bleeding time, increase bleeding tendency, and depress platelet function. Dextran 70 has also been shown to decrease factor VIII, fibrinogen, factor V, and factor

Contraindications and Precautions	Adverse Effects*	Interactions	Nursing Implications
Contraindicated in hypersensitivity, renal failure, and severe congestive heart failure. Precaution in low renal output syndromes.	All these effects are related to hypersensitivity, which usually develops within first few minutes of administration: Neuro: Headache. CV: Hypotension. Resp: Hypersensitivity. GI: Nausea and vomiting. Integ: Urticaria. Hemo: Hemodilution effect, antiplatelet effect, increased bleeding time if dose is above 15 ml/kg or over 1000 ml.	Lab: Blood glucose, bilirubin, blood typing, and cross-matching; occasionally renal and hepatic function tests.	ASSESSMENT: Obtain baseline lab data (hemoglobin, hematocrit, serum osmolality) prior to infusion. Monitor these parameters throughout course of therapy. Monitor vital signs, urine output, specific gravity, and CVP (if available) hourly throughout infusion. Notify physician promptly if urine output decreases or CVP increases >15 cm H_2O. Always do type and cross-match before administration. Assess patient for signs of congestive heart failure, and for signs and symptoms of hypersensitivity.

CONTINUED ON THE FOLLOWING PAGE

Table 12–1. BLOOD SUBSTITUTES–*CONTINUED*

Preparation/Molecular Weight	Dose and Administration of IV Solution	Pharmacokinetics**
Dextran 40–*Continued*		
HIGH-MOLECULAR-WEIGHT DEXTRAN		
Action: Synthetic polysaccharide that approximates the colloid properties of albumin which is hyperoncotic and when administered IV retains approximately 20–24 ml water/g infused. **Use:** Restore vascular volume in shock states and burns.		
Dextran 70 (Macrodex) 70,000	6% solution mixed with sodium chloride, 500 ml usual dose at 20–40 ml/min	O: within minutes P: UA D: 12 hr ½ L: 12 hr PB: UA B: urine E: urine
Dextran 75 (Gentran 75) 75,000	Children: not to exceed 20 ml/kg	
Hetastarch (Hespan) 450,000		
Action: Synthetic colloid approximating the colloid properties of albumin, which expands volume slightly more than the volume infused. **Use:** Volume expansion in shock, burns, and adjunct in leukapheresis to improve harvesting of granulocytes.		
	500–1000 ml 6% solution in 0.9% sodium chloride not to exceed 1500 ml/day or 20 mg/kg	O: immediate P: UA D: 24–36 hr ½ L: 17–48 days PB: UA B: liver E: urine

Key to Abbreviations in the *Pharmacokinetics* column O-onset; P-peak; D-duration; PB-protein bound; B-biotransformed in; E-excreted in; ½ L-halflife.
*Within the column listing adverse effects, underlines indicate the most common effects; CAPITALS indicate life-threatening effects.

IX to a greater extent than would be expected by hemodilution alone. Therefore, patients need to be assessed carefully for bleeding tendencies. When large volumes of dextran 70 are administered, plasma proteins and blood components will be decreased as hemodilution occurs. (Additional information is featured in Table 12–1.)

Hetastarch

Hetastarch (Hespan) has colloidal properties similar to those of 5% human albumin. It can be used in the treatment of shock due to hemorrhage, burns, trauma, surgery, or sepsis. It can also be used to assist with the harvesting of granulocytes through the process of leukapheresis. Hetastarch is marketed as nonantigenic;

Table 12–1. BLOOD SUBSTITUTES–*CONTINUED*

Preparation/Molecular Weight	Dose and Administration of IV Solution		Pharmacokinetics**
			INTERVENTION: Initial 500 ml may be administered over 15–30 min. Distribute remainder of daily dose over 8–24 hr depending on use. Crystallization can occur at low temperatures. Submerge in warm water and dissolve all crystals before administration and then use an IV filter. Use only clear solutions. Instruct patient to report any discomfort or dyspnea promptly throughout course of therapy. EVALUATION: Signs of shock should decrease.
Contraindicated in hypersensitivity and cardiac decompensation. Use cautiously in active hemorrhage, severe hemorrhage, severe dehydration, patients prone to congestive heart failure, and thrombocytopenia.	Same as above, but greater likelihood of allergic reactions. Hemo: Increased bleeding time, depressed platelet function. Misc: Injection site infection, phlebitis, or thrombosis.	Same as dextran 40.	Same as above. ASSESSMENT: Plasma protein levels, PT, PTT when large volumes are administered. INTERVENTION: Monitor infusion site carefully. EVALUATION: For signs of pulmonary congestion and allergic reactions.
Contraindicated in severe bleeding, severe congestive heart failure, and renal failure. Use cautiously in pregnancy and in children and persons with liver disease.	GI: Vomiting. Integ: Itching. Misc: Mild flu-like symptoms, muscle pain, chills, allergic reactions, submaxilary parotid gland enlargement.	None known at this time.	ASSESSMENT: Obtain following laboratory test results as baseline and frequently: PT, PTT, clotting time, and hematocrit. INTERVENTION: An IV filter is not needed, but if one is used, use 5-μm filter. Do not use solution if it is cloudy, deep brown, or contains crystals. EVALUATION: Same as dextrans.

however, the patient still needs to be assessed for allergic or sensitivity reactions.

The effects of hetastarch last approximately 24–36 hours. Forty percent of hetastarch is eliminated in 24 hours, 64% in 8 days, and 90% in 42 days. The elimination half-life is 17 days. The large molecules are removed and stored in the liver and spleen and are slowly degraded by amylase. Additional information is found in Table 12–1.

BLOOD PRODUCTS

Blood and its components are physiologic substances rather than pharmacologic substances (Table 12–2).

Table 12–2. BLOOD PRODUCTS

Blood or Blood Components	Volume	Shelf Life	General Indication	Nursing Implications
For all blood products				Obtain baseline vital signs before beginning any blood product. Note expiration date, blood group, and Rh factor to ensure their accuracy. Hang blood products piggyback with normal saline solution, through special blood tubing with a filter. Monitor drip rate: start at 20 gtt/min for first 10 min; if no reactions, speed to 50–70 gtt/min. Monitor vital signs and patient for reactions. At conclusion of infusion, again take vital signs and record.
Citrated whole human blood USP	500 ml	42 days	Major blood loss over 1000 ml	
Red cells	200 ml	3 yr	Blood loss, anemias	
Platelets	30 ml	3 days (cannot be cooled)	Clotting disorders	Administer within 10 min.
White cells	30 ml	6 hr	Low white cell count, depressed marrow function	Administer slowly for 45–90 min, then increase rate and finish transfusion within 4 hr. Before administering WBCs, an HLA match or a tissue match is obtained.
Normal human plasma USP (fresh/frozen)	200 ml	Fresh: 35–40 days. Frozen: 12 mo. Thawed: 2 hr	Blood loss, bleeding disorders, anticoagulant overdose, thrombotic thrombocytopenia, purpura	
Human serum albumin 5% USP (Albuminar 5%, Buminate 5%)	50 ml, 250 ml, 500 ml	3–5 yr	Low blood volume, shock, reduction of cerebral edema, burns, hypoproteinemia	Monitor blood volume and cardiac and renal function closely.
Human serum albumin 25% USP (Albuminar 25%, Buminate 25%)	50 ml, 250 ml 500 ml	3–5 yr	Low blood volume, shock, reduction of cerebral edema, burns, hypoproteinemia, exchange transfusions in erythroblastosis fetalis, cardiopulmonary bypass, renal dialysis, nephrosis, hepatic disease	Monitor blood volume and cardiac and renal function closely.
Clotting factors, fibrinogen	10 ml	Frozen: 12 mo	Clotting disorders, hemophilia A or B	

Table 12–2. BLOOD PRODUCTS–CONTINUED

Blood or Blood Components	Volume	Shelf Life	General Indication	Nursing Implications
Plasma protein fraction, human USP (Plasmanate)	Varies	3–5 yr	Similar to albumin 5%	Monitor blood volume and cardiac and renal function closely.
Immunoglobulins: gamma globulin, hepatitis B globulin	Varies	3–5 yr	Exposure to hepatitis A or B	Administer IM or IV.
Cryoprecipitate	10–20 ml	3–5 yr	Disseminated intravascular coagulation, hemophilia	Administer within 3 min.

Blood is produced by the human body and donated by an individual for one's own later use (autotransfusion) or for someone else's use. Blood is a living tissue that must be carefully preserved and stored to ensure safe and efficient use.

Blood components include red blood cells (RBC), white blood cells (WBC), platelets, and plasma. RBC, WBC, and platelets are all removed from whole blood through *centrifugation* or gravitational sedimentation. These products may be given fresh or frozen. All fresh products carry the risk of transmitting viral infections. Blood derivatives include plasma protein such as albumin and plasma protein fraction (PPF), immune-globulin G, and clotting factors such as fibrinogen. Derivatives are obtained from large pools of plasma and are sterilized and filtered. Some are heat-treated to decrease the transmission of diseases such as hepatitis A and B, and AIDS. Derivatives can be assayed and standardized.

Blood Preservation

As blood is donated by an individual, it enters a sterile plastic collection bag containing 50 ml of a preservative anticoagulant. The preservatives used today include citrate phosphate dextrose adenine solution (CPDA-1) and citrate phosphate double dextrose solution (CP2D). Both preservatives contain citric acid, which prevents clotting by combining with the free calcium in the blood. Patients who receive multiple blood transfusions may need supplemental calcium to assist clotting and to prevent tetany. Patients also need to have their acid-base balance checked for acidosis because of the accumulation of citric acid and high levels of potassium that leak out of the dying red cells.

Blood is donated in its whole form and can be used as whole blood or separated into RBC, plasma, and plasma derivatives. Preserved blood can be stored at 1°–6°C for 42 days. After 42 days, RBCs begin to die. (Lifetime for RBC in the body is 120 days.) Whole blood and its derivatives can be frozen for use at a later time. Once blood has been thawed, frozen RBC are outdated after 24 hours, and plasma is outdated after two hours.

The donated blood has the ABO group and Rh factor identified. In addition, blood is tested for hepatitis A and B, syphilis, and *human immunodeficiency virus* (HIV or

AIDS virus). Any blood found to be contaminated with any of these diseases is destroyed. Donated blood is then labeled with the following information (Circular of Information for the Use of Human Blood and Blood Components, 1985):

1. The proper name of the component, including an indication of any qualification or modification
2. The method by which the component was prepared (for example, from units of whole blood or by hemapheresis methods)
3. The temperature range in which the component should be stored
4. The preservatives and anticoagulant used in the preparation of the blood component
5. The contents or volume (standard contents, that is as prepared according to this circular, is assumed unless otherwise indicated on the label or in circular supplements)
6. The collection date (optional)
7. The collection and processing location
8. The expiration date (and time if applicable), which varies with the method of preparation (open or closed system) and the preservatives and anticoagulant used. When the expiration time is not indicated, the product expires at midnight
9. The donation (unit) number
10. The donor category (paid or volunteer)
11. Blood grouping and special handling information, as required
12. Statements regarding recipient identification, infectious diseases risk, and prescription drugs

Blood Classification Systems

Blood is classified into four major groups—A, B, AB, and O. The red blood cells are classified because of either the presence or absence of the specific A or B antigen called agglutinogens on their surface. Table 12–3 features the ABO classification system. If an RBC has antigen A on its surface, it is type A blood. If it has antigen B on its surface, it is type B blood. If both antigens are present, it is type AB blood; if neither antigen is present, it is blood type O.

Another system jointly used to classify blood is the

Table 12–3. ABO CLASSIFICATION SYSTEM

Percent	Group	Genotype	Agglutinogens (Antigens)	Agglutinins (Antibodies)
47	O	OO	None	Anti A, Anti B
41	A	OA/AA	A	Anti B
9	B	OB/BB	B	Anti A
3	AB	AB	A & B	None

Rh (for the RH(D) antigen) system. People are either Rh-negative or Rh-positive, depending on whether the Rh(D) antigen is absent or present. Rh antibodies may be produced in the blood after an immunizing event. The event may be a transfusion of Rh-positive blood to a person with Rh-negative blood. This may also occur with the absorption of blood from a Rh-positive baby to a Rh-negative mother during delivery or miscarriage. The first transfusion event merely causes immunization; only if a second event takes place will there be a problem.

When an Rh-negative mother gives birth to her first Rh-positive child, she may become sensitized to Rh antigen absorbed following placental bleeding. Any successive pregnancy with an Rh-positive baby may cause her to produce Rh antibodies, which cross the placenta and destroy fetal red blood cells, causing fetal anemia and even death. This condition, known as erythroblastosis fetalis (hemolytic disease of the newborn) is preventable. This process can be prevented by administering RhD immune globulin (RhoGAM) intramuscularly to the mother during the second or third trimester of pregnancy or within 72 hours after delivery of her first Rh-positive child. RhoGAM is a short-acting antibody preparation that coats the fetal red blood cells that may have entered the mother's circulation and prevents long-term antibody production. (More information can be found in Chapters 15 and 66.)

Type O (Rh⁻) blood, referred to as the universal donor blood, can be administered to all blood types, since it contains no antigens. Type AB (Rh⁺) is known as the universal recipient and can receive all types. Transfusion of blood containing new antigens (e.g., type A blood into a type O recipient) causes formation of antibodies to the new antigen. This is why people can receive only one type of blood unless they receive type O (Rh⁻).

In order to minimize the possibility of a transfusion reaction, particularly hemolysis, cross-matching and typing are done prior to transfusion. Typing determines whether or not the blood groups (O, A, B, AB) or donor and recipient are matched. In cross-matching, the blood of both donor and recipient are mixed together to determine whether or not an immune reaction (agglutination or clumping) takes place. If no such reaction occurs, they are considered compatible, and the patient can be transfused with this blood.

Infections Transmitted Through Blood

When blood donated by one individual is given to another, there exists the possibility of transmitting certain infections. Would-be blood donors are screened carefully with a thorough history to prevent this occurrence; however, donors may have a lack of knowledge or may deliberately falsify their answers to the questions.

Infections that can be transmitted include hepatitis non-A, non-B, malaria, syphilis, and other viral infections such as Epstein-Barr virus, herpes simplex, HIV, infectious mononucleosis, and cytomegalovirus. Hepatitis non-A, non-B is a particularly serious infection that can erupt 60 to 180 days after transfusion. The incidence of hepatitis non-A, non-B is thought to occur in about 5% of all blood transfusions.

The risk of contracting the AIDS virus through a blood transfusion is higher than previously believed, though still remote, say officials from the Centers for Disease Control (CDC). In 1984 the risk was about 1 in 2600; subsequent screening of all blood donations for antibodies to the virus was expected to reduce that threat to 1 in 200,000. But CDC statistics indicate the threat today is five times higher than expected, mostly because many donors do not develop antibodies until at least two months after infection with the virus. A CDC study of 13 people who got the virus from the blood of seven donors revealed that all but one of the donors were members of groups at high risk for AIDS, and most had ignored warnings of blood bank officials that those at high risk should not give blood.

The risk of contracting viral infections from blood has prompted many people around the country to donate their own blood for their own later use. This technique is referred to as *autologous* transfusion. Special laboratories have been developed around the United States that will process and store an individual's blood for up to three years for a fee. At the end of three years the individual is required to redonate.

Plasmapheresis

Plasmapheresis is a technique that takes only plasma, WBCs, or platelets from the donor and returns RBCs. Normally when an individual donates whole blood, he or she must wait 56 days before donating again. This is the approximate time it takes the body to replace the blood cells. When plasmapheresis is used, the donor is able to donate every 72 hours as the cells are returned to the donor. Usually, plasmapheresis donors are called to donate about once a month. The plasmapheresis technique takes about two hours. Whole blood is donated and then centrifuged; RBCs are returned to the donor, while the plasma, platelets, or WBCs are retained.

Whole Blood

Whole blood is used to restore an acute loss of blood volume, which should be greater than a 20% volume loss. Minor losses can be managed by other means. Whole fresh blood is still used in exchange transfusion treatment of newborn infants with erythroblastosis fetalis (Rh-positive infants born to an Rh-negative mother), and occasionally in Reye's syndrome and sickle-cell crisis. Stored whole blood has a low pH and calcium level and high potassium, ammonia, and low glucose and 2,3-diphosphoglycerate (2,3-DPG) levels. During storage, there is a change in RBC metabolism and hemoglobin structure and function. Ultimately, this leads to reduced survival time of transfused RBC and decreased hemoglobin function.

Blood Components

Blood components are obtained by centrifuging whole blood, which separates the cells from the plasma. The cells can then be expressed from the plastic blood pack to a smaller satellite pack. The packed cells contain RBCs, WBCs, and platelets in a volume of about 250 ml. These cells can further be separated through centrifuging into RBCs in a volume of about 200 ml and into platelets in a volume of about 30 ml. Packed cells contain less potassium, ammonia, and citrate, and a smaller volume than whole blood.

RED CELLS. RBCs are used specifically when the oxygen-carrying capacity of an individual needs to be improved. This can be due to a loss of blood or the inability to produce sufficient RBCs as in aplastic, hemolytic, and sickle-cell anemias, as well as in anemias associated with leukemias and lymphomas. Packed RBCs are often administered, along with sodium chloride solutions, to patients who have lost less than 1000 ml of their total blood volume. RBCs are available in four products: fresh, frozen, leukocyte-removed, and saline-washed. Fresh RBCs are stored like whole blood and may contain platelet and leukocyte debris and products of RBC metabolism. Packed RBCs, mixed with a glycerin and water solution to prevent cell damage from crystallization and low temperatures, can be frozen and stored for three years. This solution is removed from the cells by the laboratory before the RBCs are administered to patients. The use of frozen RBCs can reduce febrile reactions and tissue antigen sensitization because approximatley 98% of the *sensitizing lymphocytes* (WBCs, which may activate the body's immune system) are removed through this process. Frozen RBCs also contain no platelets and no plasma. Once the frozen RBCs have been prepared by the laboratory, they must be used within 24 hours.

Leukocyte-removed RBCs, also called buffy coat poor concentrate, have 70% of the leukocytes removed. RBCs, saline-washed, have 90% of the leukocytes and platelets removed through washing with saline 24 hours prior to transfusion. In the process of washing, 20% of the RBCs is also lost. All other plasma debris is present. These RBC products are used in persons who have had previous reaction to regular red cells.

PLATELETS. Platelets are administered to patients with thrombocytopenia. Platelets are less likely to be ef-
fective in conditions with increased platelet destruction such as disseminated intravascular coagulation (DIC) (because the consumptive process occurs more quickly than platelets can be replaced through transfusion); sepsis; fever; and idiopathic thrombocytopenia. Platelets share the RBC A and B antigens, but typing is often not performed prior to platelet transfusion. Platelets do not contain the Rh(D) antigen that RBCs do. A small number of RBCs may sensitize an Rh-negative female; therefore, Rh-negative females during their childbearing years should receive Rh(D) immune globulin (RhoGAM) after receiving platelets from a positive donor.

Platelets share the HLA (human leukocyte antigen) histocompatibility antigens with WBCs and other tissues. These highly immunogenic antigens are primarily responsible for isosensitization to platelets in the multiple-transfused patient. After 10–15 transfusions of random donor platelets, most patients are sensitized, and the life span of the transfused platelet is significantly reduced. Because large numbers of platelets may need to be transfused in persons with thrombocytopenia, an HLA-matched donor may be used.

Platelets are prepared from whole blood within four hours of its collection time. Platelets are stored for only seven days at 20°–24°C with gentle agitation to supply oxygen and facilitate gas exchange.

If a patient's platelet count falls below 20,000/mm³ (normal 200,000–400,000/mm³), he or she is likely to bleed spontaneously and must then be treated with platelet-rich plasma or concentrated platelets. A patient under treatment for a neoplastic disease may also have a fall in platelet count. If it falls to even 10% of normal, an average adult male may need 6–10 units of platelets to prevent further bleeding. Because of fragility of the platelets, special administration sets are used with a specially designed platelet filter. If special sets are not available, a filter with a pore size of at least 170 μm prevents excess filtration of platelets prior to circulation. Each unit should raise the platelet count by 5,000–10,000 units.

GRANULOCYTES. WBCs can also be centrifuged from whole blood and used in patients with a low leukocyte or granulocyte count. Patients with primary or secondary leukopenia may need to combat infection. WBCs are used until the marrow returns to normal function. WBCs are not appropriate therapy if marrow function is not expected to return.

WBCs are extremely fragile and must be used within 6 hours of their donation. WBCs are also matched using the ABO system because they also contain RBCs. An HLA match (tissue match) may also be performed before administering WBCs to decrease the possibility of allergic reactions.

Plasma Transfusions

Plasma is the cell-free portion of blood and constitutes 60% of the total blood volume. Plasma contains blood proteins, electrolytes, coagulation factors, and antibodies. The coagulation factors vary in stability: V is stable for ten days; VIII is stable for only two days but then

Table 12–4. SPECIFIC USES OF COLLOIDS

Uses	5% Albumin	25% Albumin	5% Plasma Protein Fraction	Dextran 40	Dextran 70	6% Hetastarch
Shock	x	x (first)	x	x	x	x
Burns	x (first)	x (after 24 hr)	—	—	x	x
Hypoproteinemia	x	x	x	—	—	—
Adult respiratory distress syndrome	—	x	—	—	—	—
Cardiopulmonary bypass	—	x	—	—	—	—
Acute liver failure	x	x	—	—	—	—
Acute nephrosis	—	x	—	—	—	—
Renal dialysis	—	x	—	—	—	—
Dialysis hyperbilirubinemia	—	x	—	—	—	—
Hemodiluent for CP bypass	—	—	—	x	—	—
Decrease incidence deep vein thrombosis	—	—	—	x	—	—

decreases by 30% over time; and VII, IX, X, XI, XII, and fibrinogen remain relatively stable. Two types of plasma are available: fresh or frozen-thawed.

Both fresh and frozen-thawed contain all clotting factors. Fresh plasma can be stored for 35–40 days. Frozen-thawed plasma is separated within four hours and frozen within six hours. Frozen plasma can be stored for one year. Both types of plasma are used for acute volume loss, to control bleeding, in thrombotic thrombocytopenic purpura, and in anticoagulant overdose.

BLOOD DERIVATIVES. Blood derivatives are obtained from pooled plasma. Several derivatives are available: plasma protein products, clotting factors, cryoprecipitate, and several immunoglobulins.

Plasma Protein Products. Plasma proteins include albumin 5% and 25% and plasma protein fraction (PPF) 5%. Plasma protein products are considered free of the danger of homologous serum hepatitis and AIDS because they are heat-treated for ten hours at 60°C. No cross-matching is required. Since these products contain no cellular elements, there is no risk of sensitization with repeated infusion. These products have many uses (Table 12–4).

Plasma protein products (PPPs) are contraindicated in patients with a history of allergic reaction to albumin because they all contain albumin, in severe anemia because plasma volume becomes even more dilute, and in cardiac failure because the increased volume can worsen failure. In chronic nephrosis, infused plasma protein products are promptly lost by the damaged nephron with consequently no relief for edema or hypoproteinemia.

During administration careful monitoring of blood pressure is performed to assess for hypertension from the returning fluid volume into the vascular space. Also, when large doses of these products are administered, blood products are given to combat the relative anemia that can result. Plasma protein products are also used cautiously in patients with hepatic or renal failure because of the added protein load that may result.

Large doses of PPPs can cause the cardiovascular system to develop fluid overload, resulting in hypertension and pulmonary edema. Hypotension can also result following rapid infusion, or in patients on cardiopulmonary bypass.

Allergic reactions can also occur resulting in fever, chills, flushing, urticaria, back pain, headache, rash, nausea, vomiting, and febrile reaction. If these symptoms occur, the infusion is discontinued and antihistamines administered.

Albumin. Albumin is separated from the plasma and administered to patients to increase or maintain their osmotic pressure, to restore albumin levels to normal, and to decrease cerebral or peripheral edema. The high-molecular-weight albumin pulls fluid into the circulatory system by osmosis and equalizes pressure on both sides of the vessel wall (Fig. 12–1). In addition, albumin is a carrier of intermediate metabolites in the transport and exchange of tissue products. Albumin comprises about 52% of the plasma proteins and provides approximately 80% of the colloid osmotic pressure. The osmotic equivalents of albumin are listed in Table 12–5. Albumin also has the ability to bind bilirubin in the circulation; for this reason, it is often used as an adjunct to exchange transfusion in an infant with erythroblastosis fetalis. It binds with the bilirubin, which helps reduce hyperbilirubinemia and decrease jaundice.

Albumin is a 96% pure product. It does not contain any blood group antibodies; therefore, there

Table 12–5. OSMOTIC EQUIVALENTS OF ALBUMIN

25% albumin = 2 U (500 ml) fresh frozen plasma
25% albumin with 100 ml normal saline = 500 ml plasma
25% albumin with 100 ml of normal saline = 2 pt whole blood
5% albumin = equal volume of citrated plasma
25% albumin = 5 times volume of citrated plasma

is no chance of incompatibility. It remains stable and can be stored for long periods of time at room temperature.

Albumin is available in 50-ml vials of both 5% and 25% solutions and has a shelf life of three to five years. Most commonly, a 5% solution is used undiluted and administered at a rate of 2–4 ml/min. In children, the rate is 0.25–0.5 the adult rate. In patients with a low cardiac reserve, give at a rate of 1 ml/min to prevent pulmonary edema. Since albumin in the 5% concentration provides additional fluid for plasma volume expansion, the rate of infusion should be slow enough to prevent too rapid expansion of the plasma volume.

A 5% albumin solution is used in patients with shock and burns to restore vascular volume and in hypoproteinemia to replace protein lost in hypoproteinemia conditions. However, if edema is present or a large amount of albumin is lost, albumin 25% is the better product because of the greater protein concentration.

The 25% albumin solution is used in persons with hypoproteinemia with or without edema to restore protein levels. The suggested rate of admission is 2 ml/min. A more rapid administration may precipitate circulatory or pulmonary problems. The 25% albumin solution is also administered to persons with hepatic cirrhosis, nephrosis, burns, and shock to restore protein levels and vascular volume. In these states the rate of admission may vary from 2–4 ml/min to very rapidly.

Plasma Protein Fraction. PPF (Plasmante) is a 5% solution of human plasma proteins (at least 83% albumin, no more than 17% globulin, and no more than 17% of total proteins as gamma globulin) in sodium chloride injection. PPF has the same indications as 5% albumin.

PPF is administered to adults at a rate of 5–8 ml/min (1000–1500 ml total volume) and to children at 33 ml/kg at a rate of 5–10 ml/min.

Clotting Factors. The clotting factors or fractions can be removed from the plasma in approximate volumes of 10 ml per pint of blood. These can be administered to individuals with hemophilia A or B to control bleeding episodes. The factors separated are X; IX (Christmas factor); and I (fibrinogen).

Cryoprecipitate. When plasma is frozen and then thawed to 4°C, the resulting cryoprecipitate contains factors I (fibrinogen) (250 mg) and VIII (100 mg) and is used specifically to treat hemophilia and von Willebrand's disease (both hereditary bleeding disorders). One unit of cryoprecipitate raises the fibrin level by 5–10 mg/dl. Cryoprecipitate has a half-life of 12–15 hours.

Cryoprecipitate is frozen for up to twelve months. After thawing, it must be used within four to six hours. Cryoprecipitate is administered totally in three minutes. Cryoprecipitate does carry the risk of hepatitis.

Immunoglobulins. The immunoglobulins (IgA, IgD, IgE, IgG, IgM) produced by the immune system to prevent certain infections can also be removed from the plasma and administered. Immunoglobulin concentrations are used to prevent hepatitis in individuals who have beem previously exposed. The immunoglobulins in use today are gamma globulin, used to prevent hepatitis A and RH(D) immune globulin (RhoGAM) used in Rh-negative females who abort, have a tubal pregnancy, deliver an Rh-positive child, or who have been given platelets, granulocytes, or Rh-positive blood.

USING THE NURSING PROCESS

ASSESSMENT

Assessment of the patient requiring plasma expanders and blood products always begins with a thorough nursing history to develop the data base needed for preparation of a nursing care plan. The information to be obtained is featured in Table 12–6.

Laboratory tests are done, such as hematocrit and hemoglobin levels. Other tests are performed based on the patient's diagnosis. When the nurse is administering plasma expanders, it is important to obtain baseline laboratory data such as hematocrit (all products lower hematocrit by increasing plasma volume) and type and cross-match for blood or blood products, before beginning the administration.

The nurse also needs to assess whether the patient has had previous blood products. Prior transfusion increases the risk of allergic reaction to certain blood products. Prior transfusions have been shown to increase the survival of persons having renal homographs, whereas prior transfusion decreases the survival of persons having bone marrow transplantation.

The patient is assessed carefully to determine his/her fluid needs. Several categories of fluid therapy are currently available for clinical use including blood products; plasma expanders, often referred to as colloids; and balanced salt solutions referred to as *crystalloids* and discussed fully in Chapter 11. The most important rule to follow in any patient is to restore vascular volume and RBC mass. Table 12–7 compares the colloid and crystalloid products.

The volume and rate of fluid administration is initially guided by arterial pressure, central venous pressure (CVP), heart rate, hematocrit, and cardiac output. The volume and rate of fluid replacement is limited by the patient's cardiac competency, especially in older patients with hypertension or ischemic heart disease. The major risk of volume expansion with any IV fluid is pulmonary edema. Therefore, a thorough and continuous respiratory assessment is performed.

The selection of the appropriate solution is determined from the patient's presenting history and current symptoms and by determining what volume (blood or

Table 12–6. NURSING PROCESS FOR PATIENT REQUIRING BLOOD PRODUCTS

Assessment

Determine precipitating factor(s) and duration of blood loss (e.g., trauma with rapid blood loss or chronic subacute gastric bleed).
Ascertain previous transfusion/reaction history.
Note current vital signs, hemodynamic pressures, and urinary output.

Nursing Diagnosis	Nursing Actions	Rationale	Patient Outcomes/ Evaluation Criteria
Fluid Volume deficit, Actual 2 related to active loss as evidenced by hypotension, tachycardia, decreased venous filling, confusion.	Begin/maintain IV therapy replacement of blood product. Observe drip rate q 15–30 minutes. Monitor vital signs/hemodynamic parameters q 30–60 minutes as indicated. Record I/O and urine specific gravity as necessary.	Replaces losses, expanding circulating volume. Ensures accuracy of infusion rate, preventing complications, e.g., too rapid infusion. As volume is replaced, parameters should stabilize/return to near normal baseline. Increasing circulating volume should improve renal perfusion and urinary output, decreasing specific gravity.	Displays improvement of hemodynamic parameters and urine output of > 1/2 cc/kg/hour.
	Monitor laboratory studies as indicated, e.g., Hgb/Hct, electrolytes, calcium, acid-base balance.	Reflects effectiveness of therapy and additional needs. Calcium may be required to promote clotting and prevent tetany in presence of multiple transfusions. Potassium level may elevate when stored blood is transfused.	
	Auscultate breath sounds for development of crackles (rales).	The major risk of volume expansion is pulmonary edema. Volume and rate of replacement is limited by the patient's cardiac competency.	
Knowledge deficit related to unfamiliarity with therapeutic interventions as evidenced by questions, statements of concern.	Inform the patient about need for and safety of blood products. Obtain consent for administration of blood as appropriate.	Patient often has unspoken fears about what is happening and accurate information and opportunity to discuss these fears promotes understanding and may enhance cooperation with therapy.	Verbalizes understanding of reasons for use of blood products.
Anxiety (specify level) related to change in health status, perceived threat of death as evidenced by increased tension, apprehension, expressed concerns.	Visit patient hourly. Encourage verbalization of fears and concerns.	Provides assurance that staff is available for help. Identifies problem areas, realities of illness and treatment.	Verbalizes awareness of feelings. Reports anxiety reduced to manageable level.
	Monitor vital signs. Provide information about physical condition and use of blood products.	Changes in vital signs suggest degree of anxiety. Knowledge can reduce anxiety and thereby enhance coping with situation.	
Injury, potential for adverse reaction to therapy related to incompatibility.	Inspect unit of blood and verify accuracy of specific unit for the patient. Start infusion at slow rate for at least the first 10 minutes.	Reduces risk of hemolytic or febrile reactions. Anaphylactic reaction most likely to occur when blood is first initiated.	Receives blood product without untoward effect/complications.

(Continued)

Table 12–6. NURSING PROCESS FOR PATIENT REQUIRING BLOOD PRODUCTS–CONTINUED

Nursing Diagnosis	Nursing Actions	Rationale	Patient Outcomes/ Evaluation Criteria
	Hang blood products pig- gyback with normal saline and administer through a Y-tubing with filters.	Provides pathway for infu- sion of fluid when starting and terminating blood product to prevent loss of IV site. Use of dextrose- containing fluids can cause agglutination/ hemolysis of red cells. Use of Y-tubing allows for blood to be shut off and line maintained if a prob- lem develops. The filter can prevent passage of agglutinated cells.	
	Monitor for fever, chills, flushing, pain in back and tightness in chest, hypotension, hemoglo- binuria.	Indicators of hemolytic or febrile reaction requiring interventions based on institutional policy, e.g., Stop transfusion, send urine specimen, blood product to laboratory and notify physician for further orders such as diuretics, steroids, or antipyretics.	

plasma) has been lost, the approximate amount of the loss, and the etiology of the loss.

When the primary circulatory problem is hypovolemia, therapy is directed toward restoration of blood volume. Because colloid solutions expand vascular volume with far less fluid infusion than crystalloid solution, hemodynamic resuscitation is likely to be accomplished more rapidly with colloids. Table 12–8 compares various IV products as to the amount of fluid returned to the vascular system. Crystalloids equilibrate across the vascular membrane such that only $\frac{1}{10}$–$\frac{1}{4}$ of the solution remains in the plasma at the end of infusion. Crystalloids also dilute plasma proteins and consequently reduce colloid osmotic pressure. Decreases in blood colloid osmotic pressure allows for filtration of fluid from the vascular space into the interstitial space, further potentiating the volume deficit. Also as colloid osmotic pressure is reduced, the patient is at increased risk for developing pulmonary edema.

When colloids are used, colloid osmotic pressure is maintained, requiring less fluid for resuscitation. The possibility of pulmonary edema is also reduced.

A single unit of whole blood yields RBCs, plasma, platelets, WBCs, clotting components, and protein. Because few patients require all these blood constituents, the transfusion of whole blood is actually an exception rather than the rule today. The goal is always to restore fluid volume and RBC mass. Blood components are then administered as needed.

Volume loading, in the form of fluid challenges, is often performed in acutely volume-depleted patients to compensate for sequestration or pooling of blood in the splanchnic organs and maldistribution of blood flow. As a fluid challenge is administered (50–200 ml of fluid during 10 minutes repeated as necessary), the nurse carefully assesses CVP and pulmonary artery obstructive or wedge pressures (PAOP/PAOP). Disproportionate increases in CVP indicate right ventricle failure, while disproportionate increases in PAWP indicate left ventricle failure.

IV therapy is a routine part of nursing. However, it may be a traumatic event for the patient and family. Often, to the patient and family, the administration of blood may erroneously indicate serious illness or impending death. The nurse shares with the patient and family the reason for and purpose of the therapy and helps them recognize and allay their fears. Table 12–9 presents some patient teaching information for the patient receiving blood products.

The nurse must understand the reason for IV therapy in the patient, the presenting symptoms of the condition, and the type of fluid used. The nurse must also assess for signs and symptoms of transfusion reactions. Table 12–10 features the various types of transfusion reactions and their causes, presenting symptoms, prevention, and treatment.

NURSING DIAGNOSIS

The nurse establishes the nursing diagnoses based on the information obtained during the assessment. The nursing diagnosis forms the basis for the nursing care. Typical nursing diagnoses are included in Table 12–6.

PLANNING AND INTERVENTION

The nurse develops the plan for the nursing intervention from the nursing diagnoses. Typical goals for a pa-

Table 12–7. COMPARISON OF COLLOIDS AND CRYSTALLOIDS

	Albumin 5%	Albumin 25%	Hetastarch 6%	Normal Saline	Dextran 40	Dextran 70
Molecular weight	69,000	UA	69,000	—	30,000–40,000	70,000
PV Expansion (per 500 ml)	100–150	200–300+	100–172		100–200	100–156
Percent volume	500–750	1700	500–850	100	500–1000	500–750
COP (mmHg)	20	100	30	−30	60	45
Tonicity	Iso-oncotic	Markedly hyper-oncotic	Hyperoncotic	Iso-tonic	Hyperoncotic	Hyperoncotic
Duration of expansion	<24 hr	<24 hr	<36 hr	Few hr	4–6 hr	12 hr
Half-life	21 days	21 days	<2 mo (17–48 days)	—	2–6 hr	12 hr
Cautions	Pulmonary edema, CHF, active bleeding, decreased platelets	See albumin 5%; give with diuretic	See albumin 5%; greater effect on coagulation	—	May cause obstructive renal failure as molecules get caught in nephron; may interfere with blood clotting	May cause obstructive renal failure as molecules get caught in nephron; may interfere with blood clotting
Allergy incidence	0.5%	0.5%	0.085%	—	>5%	>5%
Cost to the hospital per dose (approximately)	$14.50	$20.00	$40.00	$1.00	$12.79	$7.22

PV = plasma volume; CHF = congestive heart failure; COP = colloid oncotic pressure

Table 12–8. DISTRIBUTION OF COLLOIDS AND CRYSTALLOIDS

Fluid Compartment	5% Glucose	Isotonic NaCl	Hypertonic NaCl	Iso-oncotic (5%)	Hyperoncotic (25%)
Intravascular	↑10%	↑25%	↑25%	↑100%	↑200%–300%
Interstitial	↑90%	↑75%	↑75%	—	↓Reduce fluid levels
Intracellular	↑90%	—	↓Decrease cell edema	—	↓Reduce fluid levels
To increase plasma volume by 1 liter administer	10 liters	4 liters	4 liters	1 liter	0.5 liters

(Adapted from Shoemaker, W, et al.: Textbook of Critical Care Medicine. W B Saunders, Philadelphia, 1984.)

> ### Table 12-9. PATIENT TEACHING INFORMATION—BLOOD PRODUCTS
>
> Dear Patient:
>   Blood and blood products are used to replace your own blood. These products are natural products obtained from the blood of other human donors. The possible presence of certain infectious agents in blood and blood products, and of undesirable side effects in some people, cannot be avoided. The risk of transmitting hepatitis and other infectious diseases is present. Careful donor selection and available laboratory tests reduce but do not prevent the hazard.

tient recieving blood products are included in Table 12–6. The goals of nursing intervention are designed so that the patient goals or outcome criteria are achieved during the nursing intervention. Patient goals stated as outcome criteria are included in Table 12–6.

NURSING RESPONSIBILITIES FOR IV THERAPY

In most states, the professional nurse is responsible for starting an IV infusion. Please see a nursing fundamentals text for this procedure.

When administering plasma expanders, the nurse checks the bottle carefully. If crystals appear in the dextran bottle, they may be dissolved by placing the bottle in warm water for several minutes. The flow rate of the plasma expander should be ordered by the physician. The nurse monitors the patient throughout the infusion for signs of fluid overload and allergic reactions. Transient or prolonged bleeding may also occur, because platelets are rendered less sticky and decrease their ability to function. Monitoring CVP or PAOP/PAWP is recommended during administration to monitor fluid levels. Any extreme hemodynamic changes may necessitate slowing or halting the infusion.

When the nurse is administering blood and blood components, he or she must follow the guidelines established by the hospital for their administration. Nursing intervention includes obtaining baseline temperature, pulse, respirations, and blood pressure before starting the infusion. The nurse notes the expiration date on the blood and returns the blood to the blood bank if its time has expired. The nurse carefully compares the blood group and Rh factor with those of the patient to ensure accuracy. The actual starting of the blood infusion may or may not be part of the nurse's responsibility. This is determined by the employer. CDC mandates that when drawing or administering blood the nurse and/or physician wear gloves. Blood is always administered through Y-type blood tubing with a filter (170-μm filter), which has been flushed with normal saline. If a problem develops, the blood can be turned off and normal saline solution turned on, and the IV site is not lost. Dextrose solutions should not be used because they tend to cause clumping of RBCs. The tubing should be changed after each unit of blood to prevent clogging of the filter. Blood is never given or combined with drugs in an IV line.

The nurse monitors the drip rate closely. Blood is usually started at 20 gtt per minute for the first 10 minutes. If no reactions are noted, the flow can be increased to 50–70 gtt per minute. During the infusion, the vital signs are monitored every 0.5–1 hour. The nurse is alert for signs of reactions including backache, change in vital signs, urticaria, chills and fever, headache, flushing, chest pain, and suddenly developing shock. If a reaction occurs, the nurse follows institutional policy. Usually the remaining blood, a sample of blood from the patient, and a urine specimen are sent to the laboratory for examination. Reactions (hemolytic, bacterial, overload, and anaphylactic) can occur during administration and also up to 96 hours after a transfusion (Table 12–10).

Whole blood and all types of red cells are administered as previously discussed, but other components and derivatives have specific administration techniques. Platelets and cryoprecipitates are administered quickly, within ten minutes and three minutes, respectively. WBCs are run slowly over at least a two-hour period through a standard blood filter. (Micropore filters should not be used.) Patients are often premedicated with acetaminophen and antihistamines to reduce the incidence and severity of reactions. WBCs are best not administered concurrently with amphotericin B (Fungizone) because of the increased risk of pulmonary complications. It is best to separate the infusions as far apart as possible.

During an acute bleeding, therapy is aimed at maintaining

1. Blood volume at 100% normal
2. Hemoglobin at least 8 gm/dl and hematocrit 24%
3. Total serum protein at least 60% of normal
4. Plasma coagulant factors above 35% of normal (except VIII, 50% of normal)
5. Platelets over 25% (50,000) of normal.

In an acute bleed the technique for maintaining the above criteria are featured in Table 12–11. The nurse and physician work closely together in patients with acute bleeds in order to improve the patient's chance for survival.

EVALUATION

During the evaluation phase, the nurse evaluates the effectiveness of the blood or plasma expander. This evaluation is based on a predetermined list of outcome evaluation criteria that have been developed in relation to the goals determined by the nurse, patient, and family. The data base, obtained in the original assessment, is used to formulate the nursing diagnoses and provides helpful criteria for measuring the treatment's effectiveness. Typical outcome criteria are included in Table 12–6.

Fluid administration is continued until either the clinical and hemodynamic signs of hypovolemia are reversed or until the safe limit of volume expansion has been reached. Restoration of mental alertness, warm skin, urine flow greater than 0.5 ml/kg/hr, normal blood pressure, and hemodynamic stability are appropriate findings indicating effective volume expansion.

Table 12–10. TRANSFUSION REACTIONS

Type	Etiology	Prevention	Presenting Symptom	R$_x$
Hemolytic	ABO incompatible blood causing microclots due to hemolyzing of donor RBC	Check temperature and stay with patient 15–30 min	Fever, chills, flushing, pain in back and legs, decreased BP, tightness in chest, bleeding, vomiting, tachycardia, hemoglobinemia, hemoglobinuria	Stop transfusion. Send urine to lab, check for bleeding and hemorrhage, check urinary output q 1 hr, dialysis, fluids, diuretics, osmotic diuretics.
Allergic	Antibodies react with allergins in donor blood or substances in blood	Prophylactic antihistamines, washed RBC	Mild: hives, pruritus, chills, nausea, vomiting Severe: wheezing, bronchospasm, anaphylaxis	Stop transfusion. Administer antihistamines, epinephrine; if severe, steroids.
Febrile	Sensitized to WBC, platelets, or antigens—those previously transfused or multiparas	Saline-washed or frozen RBC, use of nylon filter, antipyretics	Increased temperature (1°C); headache; chills; back pain; tachycardia; generally occurs within 15 min	Stop transfusion. Give IV steroids.
Circulatory overload	Too much or too fast volume in young/elderly, or in renal or CV disease	Packed cells rather than whole blood, diuretics, careful monitoring of infusion rate	Increased CVP, increased PCWP, increased neck veins, dyspnea, cough, crackles	Stop transfusion. Place upright with feet dependent, apply tourniquets, diuretics, digitalis.
Anaphylactic reaction	Plasma protein incompatibility due to IgA deficiency and antibody development from previous transfusions and/or pregnancy	Washed RBC, or deglycerolized RBC from which IgA has been removed	Coughing, respiratory distress, decreased BP, nausea, vomiting, shock	Stop transfusion. Give epinephrine, O$_2$, fluids, steroids.

Laboratory tests are often performed to determine if the blood was effective. A unit of packed RBCs should raise the hematocrit by about 3 gm; a unit of platelets should raise the platelet count by 5000–10,000 microliters; a unit of fibrinogen should raise the fibrinogen count by 10–20 u. If the count does not go up, further investigation needs to be performed.

The nurse evaluates the patient for the regular complications of IV therapy such as infiltration, extravasation, thrombosis, thrombophlebitis, pain at the administration site, fluid overload, respiratory complications, and pyrogenic reactions, as well as for reactions to specific fluids such as plasma expanders and blood. The IV site and drip rate are evaluated hourly or more often, if necessary. IV tubing and dressings need to be changed according to the institutional policies.

The patient receiving plasma expanders and blood will also have other nursing care problems. The IV ther-

Table 12–11. ACUTE BLEED MANAGEMENT

Blood Loss	Fluids
20% or less (slowly)	Crystalloids (e.g., balanced solutions)
20%–50%	Nonprotein plasma expanders, red cells
Over 50% (slowly) or over 20% (acutely)	Whole blood or PPF and fresh or frozen plasma
80% or more	As above. For every 5 units of blood give 1–2 units fresh frozen plasma, 1–2 units platelets to prevent hemodilution of clotting factors and bleeding.

apy may have been instituted after surgery, after trauma, or after a medical emergency. This patient is usually acutely ill and needs additional emotional support, as well as physical nursing care.

The nurse evaluates the effectiveness of treatment by a return to normal homeostasis. This is evaluated through qualitative, quantitative, and laboratory findings.

SUMMARY

Plasma expanders, such as the dextrans, hetastarch, and blood products are administered to persons who have had a loss of blood volume that is severe enough to elicit symptoms. The plasma expanders do not have oxygen-carrying capacity or contain plasma proteins or clotting factors. Blood and its components are physiologic substances rather that pharmacologic substances. Blood is living tissue that must be carefully preserved and stored to ensure safe and efficient use.

As the nurse begins to administer plasma expanders and blood products, base-line laboratory tests are obtained. It is also important to assess whether the patient has had previous blood products. The nurse must follow the guidelines established by the hospital for the administration of these products. It is important for the nurse to evaluate for the effectiveness of the blood or plasma expander. When therapy is successful, there will be a return to normal homeostasis.

BIBLIOGRAPHY

American Medical Association Drug Evaluations, ed 6. WB Saunders, Philadelphia, 1986.

American Red Cross. Circular of Information for the Use of Human Blood and Blood Components. ARC #1751. July 1985.

Autologous transfusion: Increasing in popularity. Patient Care 21(15):25, 28, 149, 1987.

Backert, LB: Making home transfusions work—compatibility testing and training nurses to perform transfusions. MLO 19(12):42–46, 1987.

Birdsall, C, et al: How is autotransfusion done? Am J Nurs 88(1):108, 110, 111, 1988.

Franklin, D: The AIDS file. Hippocrates 2(3):13, 1988.

Froberg, JH: The anemias: causes and courses of action. RN:52–56, March 1989.

Gilman, AG, Goodman, LS, and Gilman, A (eds): Goodman and Gilman's The Pharmacological Basis of Therapeutics, ed 7. Macmillan, New York, 1985.

Kastrup, E, et al (eds): Facts & Comparisons. JB Lippincott, St. Louis, 1988.

Litwack, K: Practical points for transfusion therapy. J Post Anesth Nurse 2(4):257–261, 1987.

Ley, J: Fluid therapy following intracardiac operation. Critical Care Nurse 8(1):26–37, 1988.

Mathewson, M: Autotransfusion. Critical Care Update 9(2):11–14, 1982.

Olin, B (ed): Facts & Comparisons. JB Lippincott, St. Louis, 1987.

Phillips, A: Are blood transfusions really safe? Nursing 87 17(6):63–64, 1987.

Querin, JJ: How safe is the blood supply? Nursing 87 17(12):26–27, 1987.

Robenson, L: AIDS—an update. Critical Care Nurse 4(5):75–85, 1984.

Ross, A and Angaran, D: Colloids vs crystalloids—a continuing controversey. Drug Intell Clin Pharm 18:202–212, 1984.

Shoemaker, W, et al: Textbook of Critical Care Medicine. WB Saunders, Philadelphia, 1984.

Turner, J and Williamson, K: AIDS: A challenge for contemporary nursing, part I. Focus on Critical Care 13(3):53–57, 1986.

Weil, M and Rackow, E: A guide to volume repletion. Emergency Med 16:101–110, 1984.

Wyngaarden, J and Smith, L (eds): Cecil's Textbook of Medicine. WB Saunders, Philadelphia, 1988.

SITUATION 12–1

Susan Harrison, a 26-year-old with primary leukemia, is being treated for anemia and leukopenia.

1. Susan's hemoglobin and hematocrit are both decreased, and the physician orders 2 units packed red blood cells to be infused. After carefully checking the blood unit for transfusion, the nurse will:
   a. monitor the flow rate at 100 gtt per minute
   b. infuse the cells with 5% dextrose and 0.9% sodium chloride
   c. start the infusion at 20 gtt per minute for the first 10 minutes
   d. observe patient for up to one hour after infusion for signs of reaction

2. Due to Susan's low white blood cell count (WBC), orders are given to transfuse one unit of white cells. The nurse plans to:
   a. infuse the white cells slowly over at least one hour
   b. infuse the white cells through a micropore filter
   c. premedicate with acetaminophen and antihistamines
   d. administer concurrently with an antibiotic

3. During administration of packed RBCs, Susan complains of shaking chills, She has a fever of greater than 101°F.

SITUATION 12–1–*CONTINUED*

The best action by the nurse would be to:
a. stop the infusion of RBCs and infuse 0.9% sodium chloride
b. slow the drip rate down to 20 gtt per minute until symptoms subside
c. continue the infusion and administer acetaminophen and antihistamines
d. continue infusion, but observe and record vital signs every 15 minutes

4. If Susan should receive multiple transfusions, the following may be necessary:
a. potassium supplementation
b. supplemental calcium
c. ammonia compounds
d. magnesium replacement

5. Acquired infections represent potential complications as a result of blood transfusions. All of the following may be transmitted *except*:
a. malaria
b. infectious mononucleosis
c. herpes simplex
d. von Willebrand's disease

6. The nurse will check laboratory tests performed to determine if Susan's therapy is effective. The nurse would expect:
a. one unit of packed red cells should raise the hematocrit by 6 gm
b. one unit of packed red cells should increase the hemoglobin level by 10-fold
c. one unit of packed red cells should raise the platelet count by 10,000 μl
d. one unit of packed red cells should raise the hematocrit by 3 gm

SITUATION 12–2

Stephen Weber is a charge nurse on the evening shift on a medical oncology unit.

1. Mr. Sumner has a platelet count of less than 20,000 per mm^3. Stephen prepares to administer 10 units of platelets at the following rate:
a. within 10 minutes
b. over an hour
c. within 2 hours
d. over 30 minutes

2. When Janet Adams' family discovered that she was receiving a blood transfusion, they became very upset and questioned Stephen as to the reason. Stephen's best response would be:
a. "Janet is very ill right now and needs the blood transfusion. It would be best to let her rest."
b. "I will call the doctor and have her talk to you. Then I am sure that you will understand."
c. "Janet's red blood cells are low because of the chemotherapy. This will help her feel stronger."
d. "Because of the chemotherapy, she is unable to make new red cells. We hope this works."

3. Evan Mitchell is hospitalized with idiopathic thrombocytopenia. He has received multiple blood and platelet transfusions. In preparing for another platelet transfusion, Stephen will anticipate:
a. routine typing and cross-matching for A and B antigens
b. typing for human histocompatibility antigen
c. administering RhoGAM prior to starting the transfusion
d. gamma globulin administration to prevent hepatitis B

4. In collecting the equipment necessary to administer 16 units of platelets to Mr. Mitchell, Stephen discovers that Central Supply is out of platelet administration sets. An alternative set would include:
a. regular 18 gauge needle and syringe
b. a filter with a pore size of at least 170 μm
c. 60 cc Luer lock syringe without filter
d. a filter with a pore size of at least 70 μm

5. All of the following are considered outcome criteria for the patient needing fluid volume expansion *except*:
a. restoration of mental alertness
b. normal blood pressure
c. skin warm and dry
d. urine output less than ½ ml/kg/hr

6. Thomas Winfred has received six units of packed red blood cells during the past 24 hours as the result of a clotting disorder. Stephen is aware of the potential for:
a. acid-base disturbances related to the citric acid preservative
b. increased glucose related to infusion of multiple RBCs
c. decreased potassium related to diuresis and volume expansion
d. shortened bleeding times related to increased clotting factors

13

CHAPTER

UTILIZING THE NURSING PROCESS WITH PATIENTS WHO ABUSE DRUGS AND ALCOHOL

CHAPTER OUTLINE

GLOSSARY TERMS IN THIS CHAPTER

Abuse
Addiction
Antagonists
Cobehavior
Cross tolerance
Dependence
Dual addiction
Enabling
Impairment
Mixed addiction
Psychological dependence
Tolerance
Withdrawal

13
CHAPTER

UTILIZING THE NURSING PROCESS WITH PATIENTS WHO ABUSE DRUGS AND ALCOHOL

MADELINE A. NAEGLE, Ph.D., F.A.A.N.

LEARNING OBJECTIVES:

After reading this chapter, the student will be able to:

1. Define terms related to drug abuse.

2. Identify drugs of frequent abuse.

3. Describe psychological and physical dependency states.

4. List components of a nursing assessment.

5. List nursing diagnoses relevant to a patient who abuses drugs.

6. Formulate the nursing care plan for the patient with problems related to drug abuse.

7. Describe outcomes to evaluate interventions with patients who abuse drugs.

8. Formulate patient teaching on the health consequences of drug use.

INTRODUCTION

Substance abuse constitutes a major societal problem, and alcoholism now ranks as the third major cause of death in the United States after coronary heart disease and cancer. Abuse and dependence on a variety of drugs is so common that one in four individuals is estimated to have personal experience with a family member or friend who is, or was, substance-dependent. Furthermore, at any given time, 20%–35% of all persons hospitalized in nonpsychiatric settings suffer from alcohol-related illness. The prevalence of substance abuse and related medical problems ensures that students and practitioners of nursing will care for large numbers of individuals for whom alcohol and/or drug use has been an important life issue.

The nurse, therefore, must be knowledgeable about the diseases of alcoholism and substance dependence in order to provide direct nursing care and to work effectively with individuals and families and in communities. The extent of drug dependence and related problems, such as AIDS, constitutes a major public health problem in lay and professional communities throughout the United States. Like other health professionals, the nurse must be educated on the manifestations, related risk factors, appropriate interventions, and prevention strategies with substance abuse illness. Since some percentage of health professionals will develop psychiatric illness or drug dependence, the management of such problems is linked to a number of educational and organizational issues within these professions. Nurses and other health professionals should recognize situations where practice is impaired by alcohol or drug use and be capable of implementing strategies to protect the public and move the nurse into treatment. Implications for education and organizational action derive from knowledge about substance abuse illness and its effective treatment.

CONCEPTS BASIC TO THE NURSING APPROACH

Alcohol and other drug use spans a continuum of behaviors characterized by varying frequencies in use, amounts of drug used, and severity of drug-use impact on psychological, physiologic, and social function. A significant number of individuals, probably one in 10–15, will develop the disease of alcoholism or dependency on at least one psychoactive drug. The disease phenomenon is characterized by psychological dependence, including the compulsive need to use the drug, and physiologic dependence, evidence of tolerance, or withdrawal. Psychological dependence is often manifested in heavy use and/or periodic abuse of a drug. Abuse is characterized by

1. The inability to stop using the drug or cut down on the amount used
2. Repeated attempts to control use by abstinence
3. Complications of substance intoxication such as blackouts, overdose
4. The need to use in order to function normally
5. Disturbed social relations, impairment of work patterns, legal difficulties

Dependence on a drug is synonymous with the term "addiction." Key concepts in this definition are tolerance and withdrawal. *Tolerance* develops as "markedly increased amounts of a drug are necessary to achieve the same psychoactive effects formerly attained by lesser amounts of the drug." Tolerance may also exist in the heavy-using abuser. *Withdrawal* is evidenced in a substance-specific syndrome that follows the cessation of drug taking by the physiologically dependent individual. The signs and symptoms of withdrawal vary according to the class of drug on which the individual is dependent.

Other terms are also of relevance to pharmacologically based nursing interventions with these patients. These include:

Addiction: Synonymous with dependence, a condition of psychological and physiologic habituation and tolerance to a drug, including alcohol.

Mixed Addiction: Dependence on more than one substance, such as alcohol and cocaine.

Dual Addiction: Simultaneous dependence on psychoactive drugs that have similar effects, such as alcohol and the benzodiazepines.

Cross Tolerance: The cellular adaptation that creates tolerance also functions to increase the individual's tolerance for large amounts of similarly acting drugs. For example, the individual tolerant to alcohol will also be tolerant to sedative-hypnotics and will require higher doses to achieve the same pharmacologic effects.

Physiologic dependence and its concomitant changes in health status do not result from the heavy use of all drugs but are dependent on drug properties. Psychologic dependence in and of itself, however, can be incapacitating, because it results in compulsive, out-of-control use with associated impairment. In addition, psychological dependence on the euphoric, escapist, sedative, or stimulating effects of "getting high" creates a continuing need for that experience in the user. Abstinence from one drug, such as heroin, may result in abuse of another, such as alcohol or marijuana. In recent years there has been an increasing trend in all age groups toward the use of multiple drugs and addiction to a number of drugs (polydrug addiction) or drugs in combination (dual addiction). This results in a complex clinical picture requiring thorough nursing assessment.

CLASSIFICATION OF DRUGS COMMONLY ABUSED

A variety of prescription drugs are "misused," that is, used for purposes other than those for which they are intended, especially by elderly clients, who self-medicate for a variety of reasons particular to that group. Most serious problems, however, result from *abuse*, that is, drug-taking patterns that impact negatively on psychological, physiologic, and/or social functioning. Abuse may be combined with misuse or exist as a separate entity. Commercially accessible and legal drugs fall into several classes:

1. Prescription drugs (narcotics, hypnotics, minor tranquilizers)
2. Over-the-counter drugs
3. "Social" drugs (alcohol, nicotine, and caffeine)
4. Illicit drugs (cocaine, marijuana, designer drugs manufactured by "garage" chemists, Phencyclidine [PCP]); Hallucinogens (LSD, mescaline)
5. Compounds sold for other purposes but used for psychoactive effects, such as cleaning fluid and airplane glue.

They are classified according to their psychoactive effect, determined largely by their action on the central nervous system (Table 13–1). The most addicting and widely used drug in America is nicotine, usually in the form of cigarettes but also including smokeless tobaccos. Because the psychoactive effects of nicotine are minimal, it receives little attention as an addictive substance, although mortality and morbidity rates associated with its use are very high. "Coke," a solid, smokable form of cocaine, has the next highest addictive potential.

ETIOLOGIC FACTORS

The nature of this text does not support an extensive discussion of theories on drug and alcohol abuse. In many ways the scientific understanding of addiction is at a very early point of development. The prevalence of health-related problems, however, and the widespread nature of addiction require that practitioners of nursing be able to identify and intervene in common drug problems. A brief overview of the most widely acknowledged theories follows.

Why do individuals use drugs in pathologic patterns? What explains the development of addiction in one individual and the absence of negative consequences despite ongoing use by a peer with a similar drug-using history? Theoretical models have been developed in attempts to explain the origins of addiction to alcohol and other drugs, but none adequately explains this multifaceted disease process in its entirety.

Theories of drug dependence are perspectives on human-environment interaction, and the importance of causative factors varies with each approach. Three main categories of theories examine human-environment interaction with emphasis on:

1. Traits of the individual
2. Sociocultural environments
3. Multiple factors in interaction

Traits of the individual determined by constitutional factors may predispose to addiction to alcohol or drugs. One widely discussed theory suggests that a genetic predisposition may determine individuals' varying responses to alcohol, resulting in dependence among some. Patterns of familial drug use across generations indicate that alcoholism appears frequently in generations of the same family and among siblings.

The disease model, first articulated by Jellinek (1960), addresses behaviors associated with alcoholism according to the type of alcoholism that develops. He described behaviors consistent with symptoms of addiction to other drugs as well. In this model addiction is characterized by:

1. Loss of control over intake of the drug
2. The compulsive need to continue use
3. Psychologic and behavioral change

This model describes the progression from use of a drug to facilitate sociability and promote relaxation to psychological dependence on the drug for feelings of well-being and normalcy. It refers to the physiologic changes in drug metabolism as well as psychological dependence. While Jellinek's model was one of alcoholism, the continuum of increasing dependence on drugs is now viewed as applicable to drug addiction in general. A number of theories about the motives for drug use, psychodynamics, and personality traits of the individual who becomes addicted are also included in this category.

Theories on the individual and family, as well as clinical observation, suggest that certain characteristics may place the individual at risk for the development of substance-related problems. These are:

1. Family members with substance-dependence problems
2. History of multiple losses and traumatic life events
3. Unresolved psychologic conflicts
4. Extensive emotional and/or economic deprivation

A second theoretical perspective that addresses the human-environment interaction resulting in drug abuse highlights social-psychological factors and cultural environments as sources of learned and reinforced behaviors. Such theories stress the importance of social environments that includes role models, exposure to drug-taking subcultures, and both individual and social expectations about the positive and negative aspects of drug taking. "Adaptational" theories in this category regard drug taking as "functional" in response to internal or external stresses. The idea that severe distress from

Table 13–1. CLASSES OF ABUSED DRUGS AND THEIR ACTIONS

General Type of Drug	Drug Effects	Drug Name	Site of Action	Length of Effect	Potential for Addiction
Psychedelic drugs	Euphoria; altered perceptions; somatic effects (dizziness, tremors, weakness, nausea); psychotic-like symptoms; flashbacks Objective signs: Dilated pupils, emotional swings, suspiciousness, paranoia, bizarre behavior, increased BP	LSD Psilocybin Mescaline MDA (Ecstacy) DOM DMT	CNS (modify neuro-transmitters) Taken orally	Onset: 30–40 min Usual duration: 8–12 hr STP 6–9 hr Mescaline 12–14 hr LSD 10–12 hr	Psychological dependence only
Cannabinoids	Failure in judgment/memory; mild intoxication; euphoria; relaxation; sexual arousal; panic states and psychosis in high doses Objective signs: Reddened eyes; heart rate to 140/bpm; pulse, respira-tions, BP increase	Marijuana Hashish (THC, Cannabis sativa)	CNS Cardiovascular system Smoked	Admin/dose: depen-dent Usual onset: 20–30 min Usual duration: 3–7 hr	Moderate: Psychologi-cal depen-dence and long-term effects occur
Opioids (narcotics, synthetic narcot-ics)	Analgesia; euphoria; escape; reduction in sexual and aggressive drives; sedation, sleepiness Objective signs: Hypertension; respiratory depression; constipation; impaired intellectual function	Codeine Morphine Heroin Dilaudid Methadone Demerol	Bind in receptor sites, CNS, GI tract Taken orally and injected, inhaled	Usual onset: 20–30 min Usual duration: 4–8 hr	High: Toler-ance and withdrawal occur
Sedative hypnot-ics	Drowsiness/sedation/sleep; euphoria; escape/loss of inhibition; reduction of aggressive and sexual drives; emotional instability; poor judgment	Barbiturates Seconal, Nembutal, Amytal, Tuinal Barbiturate-like (Quaa-ludes) Benzodiaza-pines, minor tranquilizers (Librium, Val-ium)	CNS (ascending retic-ular activating sys-tem) Taken orally and ingested	Usual onset: 30–45 min Usual duration: 4–5 hr	High: Toler-ance and life-threat-ening with-drawal occur Cross-toler-ance to all CNS depressants occurs
Stimulants	Euphoria/grandiosity; energy; excitation; relief of fatigue; depression; wakefulness; suppression of appetite; aggressive feelings; para-noia; reproductive dysfunc-tion in women Objective signs: Sweating; dilated pupils; weight loss; vital signs ele-vated; tremors, seizures	Amphetamine (Methaphe-tamine, Dexe-drine) Cocaine Crack (free base) Caffeine	CNS (Synapses)	Usual duration: 2–6 hr Rapid onset Brief duration: up to 30 min	High: Toler-ance and withdrawal occur High: Toler-ance and withdrawal occur
Phencyclidines	Detachment from surround-ings; decreased sensory awareness; illusions of superhuman strength; acute intoxication Objective signs: Flushing; fever; sweating; coma; agitation; incoherent speech; aggression	PCP (Angel Dust) Inhaled	CNS	Rapid onset: 2–3 min up to 45 min Prolonged effects	Psychological only

(Continued)

Table 13–1. CLASSES OF ABUSED DRUGS AND THEIR ACTIONS–*CONTINUED*

General Type of Drug	Drug Effects	Drug Name	Site of Action	Length of Effect	Potential for Addiction
Inhalants	Euphoria; giddiness; headache; fatigue Objective signs: Increase in vital signs; damage to kidneys, liver; disorientation	Benzene (paint thinner, cleaning fluid, glue) Nitrites Freons Nitrous oxide	Cardiac effects CNS Inhaled	Rapid absorption	Psychological only
Alcohol	Relaxation; sedation; release of inhibition Objective signs: Incoordination; nausea; ataxia; vomiting; impaired cognitive function; slurred speech	Beverage alcohol: beer, wine, liquor Taken orally	CNS Respiratory system	Usual onset: 20 min–1 hr Dose-related	High: Tolerance and life-threatening withdrawal occur

(From Naegle, M. A.: Psychiatric Mental Health Nursing: A Client-Centered Approach. J. B. Lippincott, Philadelphia 1989)

internal psychological sources provides the motive for drug use as an escape from psychic pain is often identified as a causative link to opiate addiction (Alexander and Hadaway, 1982).

As drug and alcohol abuse have become increasingly prevalent in society, especially among youth and young addicts, the complexity of etiology is more widely acknowledged. Addiction is being viewed as a process that cannot be explained by singular or limited factors.

The "interactive" models more recently considered identify numerous variables and factors as determining the phenomena of addiction. Heredity, psychological structure, and personality, as well as sociocultural factors, must be identified and evaluated so as to gain insights into the process of substance-abuse illness as manifested in a particular person. A positive aspect of this theory, and one that should be basic to therapeutic interventions, is that the substance-abusing individual is unique in manifesting the disease. While the disease is consistent in process and symptoms among individuals, it comes about and serves a variety of functions in the life-style and psychological processes of the individual.

ATTITUDES ABOUT DRUG ABUSE AMONG HEALTH PROFESSIONALS

Studies of health professional practitioners and students, including nurses, indicate that attitudes about alcoholics and addicts are negative and that the perspectives on successful treatment outcomes are generally pessimistic (Gurel, 1976; Harlow and Goby, 1980). Attitudes and education determine the nature of interactions between practicing nurses, social workers, and physicians and the substance-abusing client. Many health practitioners in current practice were educated before recent research findings and new knowledge about substance abuse were included in professional curricula. Without a solid theoretical base and positive clinical experiences, attitudes develop from encounters with patients and family members with long-term addictive problems. The majority of alcoholics never seek treatment. Others addicted to drugs experience a chronic and repetitive disease course, and they often appear unable to create change in their lives or their drug-using behaviors. Men and women who are treated in the early stages of alcoholism or who recognize and treat drug dependencies before losing total control of such drug use are often not represented in the population served by most health practitioners, that is, hospitalized patients. Consequently, the clinical experiences of the practitioner have often been with late-stage addicts, who manifest multiple medical problems and limited prognoses for changing the disease course.

Because addiction is so widespread in the society, most nurses have "first-hand knowledge" of problematic drinking and/or drug use in their families of origin, conjugal families, or peers. Association with a substance abuser results in problems and behaviors that are rarely recognized or resolved without some type of treatment or self-help. Denial is the key symptom of substance-abuse illness, and the addict's denial of a problem is shared by those around her/him. Behavior patterns in children, other family members, and associates of drug-dependent people reflect denial and a failure to understand the nature of the addictive process. Commonly observed behaviors are "co-dependent" or "enabling" behaviors.

Enabling behaviors are those that support the patient's continuing use of the drug by failing to confront the addict with the consequences of his or her illness and shielding him or her from the realities of the economic and emotional implications of an ongoing addiction. Families often take steps to ensure that the drug of choice is in supply, so the addict does not become upset. Community members and the police avoid reporting or enforcing driving-while-intoxicated violations, particularly those involving women or individuals prominent in the community.

Cobehavior refers to behavior patterns of such long standing that the individual is unaware of them. These are patterns that develop over the years as reactions to drug-related behaviors of one family member. They include adopting roles within the family to create some sense of consistency and stability, such as assuming parenting responsibilities; modifying life plans to meet family needs; inhibition of emotional expression; and so on. These behaviors develop and are supported rather than confronting the real problem, drug-using behavior.

Health professionals engage in enabling behavior from lack of knowledge or because of unresolved personal feelings about substance abusers. The failure to include drug-using histories in comprehensive assessment, providing medical and nursing care for drug-induced medical illness without discussing the basic problem, and a failure to make appropriate referrals all support the user's denial that there is a problem. Expressions of anger and criticism about drug use serve to reinforce the addict's rationalizations about his or her own estrangement from others and to reinforce motives to continue using and not seek treatment.

Self-assessment is an important component of providing care to the substance-abusing patient. Recognizing and questioning personal attitudes highlights personal bias and helps to explore reasons why negative views remain. Studies indicate that health professional students who have clinical experience in treatment settings for substance abusers change their beliefs about the value of treatment and develop more realistic understandings of the range of severity of this illness and the heterogeneous population it afflicts. Old stereotypes of the "revolving door" addict and the skid row alcoholic can be replaced by new insights into the illnesses afflicting large numbers of adolescents and young adults, women of all ages, and persons from all socioeconomic backgrounds and ethnic groups.

USING THE NURSING PROCESS

ASSESSMENT

The individual who is abusing, or dependent upon, psychoactive chemical agents receives a comprehensive nursing assessment, utilizing both history-taking and observational and assessment skills. In a routine history and physical examination, a short-form drug history is utilized as a screening mechanism. On admission to a detoxification or rehabilitation unit, or the initiation of long-term individual treatment for substance abuse, an extensive drug-using history is completed.

Since alcohol is a drug, it is appropriate to combine drinking and drug-taking histories in a screening interview. Because the patient may know drugs only by their street names, the nurse should be conversant with these and use them along with drug descriptions to clarify ex-

actly what the patient uses. The nurse also needs to be sensitive to the placement of these questions in the interview process. Because drug-using patients are often guilty or defensive about the extent of their use, the nurse should begin the interview with less sensitive information gathering and move to topics requiring more self-disclosure after some rapport has been established.

A short-form drug screening history should include the following material.

Alcohol consumption:
1. How often do you drink alcoholic beverages? (frequency)
2. What type of alcoholic beverages do you drink? (beer, wine, liquor)
3. When you drink each beverage type, how much do you drink? Be specific about glass size. (quantity)
4. When was the last time you drank and what did you drink?
5. Are you ever concerned about your drinking? Why?
6. Have family members or friends expressed concern about your drinking? How?

The consumption of more than two drinks daily is considered heavy drinking and five or more drinks per occasion suggests problem drinking or alcohol dependence.

Medication and other drugs:
1. What other drugs do you take?
   a. Prescription drugs
   b. Over-the-counter drugs
   c. Drugs taken for "recreation" or social reasons
   d. Do you use tobacco? Which type? How much?
2. How much of each of these types of drugs do you take?
3. How often do you take these drugs?
4. How do you take these drugs (route of administration)?
5. When did you begin using drugs and/or alcohol?
6. Are you ever concerned about your drug use?
7. Have others expressed concern over how you use drugs?
8. Have you ever been treated for a drug or alcohol problem?

Longer form drug and alcohol histories include more detailed questions about drug use and a systems review with specific inquiries about symptoms related to gastrointestinal, cardiovascular, and neurologic systems.

Nursing observations of physical signs is also an important tool in detecting drug-related problems during a routine physical or admission examination. The nurse needs to know the physical signs that suggest alcohol or drug dependence and trauma associated with this behavior. A brief list of these signs includes the following:

1. Track marks or vein scarring
2. Telangectasia and spider angioma
3. Multiple bruises on extremities
4. Abscesses
5. Malnutrition, pellagra, beriberi

6. Acne rosacea
7. Alcoholic facies
8. Persistent nonintention tremor
9. Palmar erythema

Laboratory data provide additional information to support the presence of drug- or alcohol-related problems. Commonly identified signs include:

1. Alcohol or drug metabolites found upon urinalysis
2. Abnormal findings on liver function tests
3. Anemias, particularly thrombocytopenia and macrocytic anemia

The skilled nurse interviewer will note verbal and nonverbal responses that may indicate that the respondent is less than truthful about drug-using habits. Attempts to avoid direct questions and minimize the effects of drinking on other aspects of life suggest that the respondent is in denial of his or her difficulties. The presence of the described "risk factors," particularly drug dependency in family members, suggests the need for in-depth interviewing. When observational and laboratory findings frankly contradict the respondent's verbal history, family members and the respondent should be appraised of this. Alcoholism and drug dependence, when not arrested, lead to multiple medical illnesses and premature death or shortened life span because of overdose, suicide, or medical complications. Even though the alcoholic may deny dependency on the drug, the patient should be told that the health team's assessment suggests a drinking problem and be advised of the relationship between medical symptoms and alcohol use. Similarly, the intravenous drug abuser needs facts on the risk of AIDS and other life-threatening conditions despite his or her apparent unwillingness to seek treatment and rehabilitation.

NURSING DIAGNOSES

Nursing diagnoses related to substance abuse are utilized most often in relation to acute intoxication, withdrawal from drugs, and general health and nutritional status. Diagnoses are formulated on the basis of subjective and objective data obtained in the comprehensive nursing assessment, including the short- or long-form drug history. The diagnoses should reflect priorities related to actual and potential health problems of the patient and should include drug-related nursing diagnoses as well as other health-related diagnoses. They form the basis of a comprehensive nursing care plan that addresses immediate problems in short-term goals and provides for flexibility and modification as problems are resolved or new health problems emerge. Examples follow:

—Injury, potential for trauma/poisoning related to clouded sensorium, impaired judgment, poor coordination and diminished perception of pain.
—Thought processes, altered related to physiologic changes, impaired judgment with loss of memory as evidenced by inaccurate interpretation of environment, bizarre thinking, disorientation.

—Violence, potential for: Self-directed or directed at others related to toxic reactions to drugs, exogenous chemical alteration.
—Injury, potential for trauma related to muscle incoordination, reduced eye/hand coordination, decreased response to perception of pain, clouded sensorium and impaired judgment.
—Tissue perfusion altered: cardiopulmonary/cerebral related to alterations in blood flow (hypertensive crisis).
—Injury, potential for, trauma/poisoning related to CNS depression/agitation, psychologic stress, IV drug use techniques.
—Breathing pattern, ineffective, potential related to neuromuscular impairment, decreased energy, and decreased lung expansion.
—Coping, ineffective individual related to personal vulnerability, inadequate support systems as evidenced by addictive behaviors, poor self-esteem, chronic anxiety, worry and depression.
—Breathing, ineffective, potential for related to direct effect of alcohol toxicity on respiratory center, decreased energy, presence of chronic respiratory inflammatory processes, and sedative effects of drugs given to decrease alcohol withdrawal symptoms.
—Sensory-perceptual alteration (specify) related to exogenous chemical alteration (alcohol use/sudden cessation) and endogenous (electrolyte imbalance, elevated ammonia and BUN), sleep deprivation, psychologic stress as evidenced by disorientation, bizarre thinking, exaggerated responses.
—Violence, potential for (specify) related to paranoid ideation, perceptions of threats, altered perceptions.
—Cardiac output, potential for decrease related to drug effect on myocardium/electrical conduction, and pre-existing myocardiomyopathy.
—Fear, related to paranoid delusions as evidenced by suspiciousness and concerns about actions of others.
—Sensory-perceptual alteration (specify) related to exogenous chemical affecting sensory reception, transmission, and integration as evidenced by preoccupation, with hallucinatory experiences.
—Sleep pattern disturbance related to CNS sensory alterations as evidenced by constant alertness, racing thoughts, inability to sleep.
—Nutrition altered: Less than body requirements related to anorexia secondary to drug effect and insufficent/inappropriate use of financial resources as evidenced by weight loss, inadequate intake, lack of interest in food, poor muscle tone and signs/laboratory evidence of vitamin deficiencies.

Each nursing diagnosis contains a statement referring to signs or symptoms manifested by the patient and recorded in the data base. The secondary phase of the nursing diagnosis notes the etiology of the health problem. For clients with substance-related health problems, symptoms will be similar and relatively consistent as a function of the nature of addiction. Etiologic phrases will be drug-specific.

EARLY INTERVENTION

The individual who abuses drugs or alcohol comes to the attention of others far earlier than he or she develops some understanding of the problem. Denial, a key symptom of these illnesses, interferes with the user's ability to assess the feedback of others or look realistically at the negative consequences of drug-related behavior. The early stage of addictive illness is characterized by behaviors that cause disturbance in social and family relationships. The individual withdraws from community and professional activities, may behave inappropriately at gatherings of family and friends, and experiences marital problems. Often children in these families manifest behavioral or learning difficulties at school. The employee may come to the attention of the occupational health nurse or the children may be referred to the school nurse with vague symptoms and complaints. Nurses working in mental health settings or private practice may identify drug-related problems as factors in individual or marital therapy.

Because the potential patient denies that there is a problem, health professionals often do not fully assess drug use and fail to utilize opportunities for early intervention. Many people believe that the substance-dependent individual must admit to the problem and seek help on his or her own before intervention can be effective; this is not necessarily true. While it is true that the patient must acknowledge the illness and become responsible about treating it, important actions can be taken to increase motivation and move the individual toward treatment by demonstrating the severity of the problem and refusing to accept rationalizations, excuses, and continuing dysfunctional behavior. Some of these actions include referral to family treatment for other identified problems and referral to Al-Anon for concerned family members; confrontation by colleagues who have observed behavioral changes; and counseling by the primary caregiver, whether nurse or physician, about the observed signs that suggest drug-related problems. These could include laboratory data, expressions of concern by a spouse, or failure to follow usual patterns of health maintenance. Expressions of caring and concern for the individual and his or her family must be central to such action. Attempts to coerce the patient by inducing guilt or by threatening actions that cannot be implemented only lead to further estrangement and defensiveness.

NURSING INTERVENTIONS

Acute Intoxication From Depressants

The class of drugs that has the effect of producing depression of the central nervous system includes barbiturates such as Amytal, Seconal, Tuinal; barbiturate-like substances such as Doriden, Noludar, Placidyl; benzo-

diazepines such as Librium, Valium, Dalmane, Clonopin, and the minor tranquilizer, Equanil; and sedatives such as paraldehyde, Noctec, and Somnus. Individuals who become tolerant to these drugs are usually crosstolerant to alcohol, and when they are used in combination, the effects of alcohol and these drugs combine to produce a more potent effect. Individuals who use drugs, including alcohol, to relieve anxiety or to achieve sedation and a euphoric high often abuse depressants and use them in combination with alcohol. The addictive state is characterized by tolerance, so high doses of the drug are ingested and toxicity and accidental overdoses are not uncommon.

Alcohol, which has a disinhibiting effect in small doses, acts as a depressant in greater amounts. Its effects have the same qualities as those of the drugs listed above. Acute intoxication with alcohol can occur in the uninitiated drinker or in the chronic alcoholic when certain blood alcohol levels (BAC) are reached. A BAC of 100 mg/100 ml, for instance, is manifested in behavioral changes, ataxia, and dysarthria, and used as the criterion for driving-while-intoxicated charges (0.1) in many states. Blackouts (temporary amnesic states), sleep, loss of consciousness, and coma follow at BAC levels of 1.5 and above (Loomis, 1982). Acute alcohol poisoning is not an uncommon cause of death, particularly in young adults and uninitiated drinkers who consume large quantities of alcohol in a short period of time. The effect of large amounts of beverage alcohol that cannot be metabolized adequately in a short time is to overwhelm the central nervous system and induce coma and respiratory arrest (Table 13–2).

Signs of intoxication from depressant drugs include:

1. Dysarthria
2. Ataxia
3. Belligerence
4. Agitation and anxiety
5. Loss of superficial reflexes
6. Diminished respiratory volume, possible hypoxia
7. Hypotension
8. Lethargy, confused or delirious mental state

Nursing interventions in acute intoxication induced by depressants have the overriding goals of:

1. Provision of a safe, nonthreatening environment
2. Preventation of death and the development of further pathology
3. Attainment of health at the level possible for the individual
4. Use of the crisis situation to motivate the patient toward changes in drug-using patterns

To attain these goals, the nurse:

1. Attempts to obtain information on the number and kind of drugs ingested and orients the confused or delirious patient.
2. Ensures interpersonal supervision and support by nursing staff.
3. Monitors vital signs and respiratory and cardiac activity as necessary.

Table 13–2. SOME DRUG INTERACTIONS WITH ALCOHOL

Drug	Effect	Possible Mechanism
Antabuse (disulfiram)	Flushing, diaphoresis, hyperventilation, vomiting, confusion, drowsiness	Inhibits intermediary metabolism of alcohol
Anticoagulants, oral	Increased anticoagulant effect with acute intoxication Decreased anticoagulant effect after chronic alcohol abuse	Reduced metabolism
Antihistamines	Increased CNS depression	Additive
Antimicrobials		
Chloramphenicol (Chloromycetin; and others)	Minor Antabuse-like reaction	Inhibits intermediary metabolism of alcohol
Furazolidone (Furoxone)	Minor Antabuse-like reaction	Inhibits intermediary metabolism of alcohol
Griseofulvin (Fulvicin-U/F; and others)	Minor Antabuse-like reaction	Inhibits intermediary metabolism of alcohol
Isoniazid (many mfrs.)	Decreased effect after chronic alcohol abuse	Undetermined
Metronidazole (Flagyl)	Minor Antabuse-like reaction	Possible CNS effect
Quinacrine (Atabrine)	Minor Antabuse-like reaction	Inhibits intermediary metabolism of alcohol
Hypoglycemics		
Chlorpropamide (Diabinese)	Minor Antabuse-like reaction	Inhibits intermediary metabolism of alcohol
Tolbutamide (Orinase)	Decreased hypoglycemic effect after chronic alcohol abuse	Enhanced microsomal enzyme activity
	Increased hypoglycemic effect with ingestion of alcohol, particularly in fasting patients	Suppression of gluconeogenesis
	Minor Antabuse-like reaction	Inhibits intermediary of alcohol
Narcotics	Increased CNS depression with acute intoxication	Additive
Sedatives and tranquilizers		
Barbiturates	Increased CNS depression	Additive; reduced metabolism
	Decreased sedative effect after chronic alcohol abuse	Enhanced microsomal enzyme activity; decreased CNS sensitivity
Chloral hydrate (Noctec and others)	Prolonged hypnotic effect	Mutual potentiation
Chlordiazepoxide (Librium and others)	Increased CNS depression	Additive
Chlorpromazine (Thorazine; Chlor-PZ)	Increased CNS depression	Additive; inhibits oxidation of alcohol
Chlorazepate (Azene, Tranxene)	Increased CNS depression	Additive
Diazepam (Valium)	Increased CNS depression	Additive; possible increased absorption
Meprobamate (Miltown and others)	Increased CNS depression	Additive; reduced metabolism
	Decreased sedative effect after chronic alcohol abuse	Enhanced microsomal enzyme activity
Oxazepam (Serax)	Increased CNS depression	Additive
Others*		
Phentolamine (Regitine)	Minor Antabuse-like reaction	Inhibits intermediary metabolism of alcohol
Phenytoin (Dilantin and others)	Increased anticonvulsant effect with acute intoxication	Reduced metabolism
	Decreased anticonvulsant effect after chronic alcohol abuse	Enhanced microsomal activity

*Many alcoholic beverages contain tyramine, which cause reactions with MAO inhibitors (Medical Letter 19:5, 1977)
(From Medical Letter 19:48 [Issue 471], January 28, 1977, with permission.)

4. Refrains from confrontational or judgmental comments; expresses acceptance of the patient.
5. Monitors and promotes hydration and nutritional sustenance.
6. Monitors intake and output.
7. Implements nursing care for the comatose patient as indicated.
8. Implements seizure precautions as indicated.
9. Administers medications appropriate to the manifested medical complications.
10. With resolution of the physiologic crisis, suggests or initiates consultation with psychiatric or substance-abuse resource teams. May refer the patient to a drug treatment program. Gives patient objective information and feedback about the actual and potential outcomes of the immediate drug-induced crisis.

Acute Intoxication from Stimulants

Stimulant drugs such as amphetamines, amphetamine-like substances, cocaine, and crack threaten patient well-being through overactivity of the central nervous system with the potential for death.

Signs of intoxication from stimulants include:

1. Elevation of vital signs, manifested in tachycardia, hypertension, rapid respirations, elevated body temperature
2. Grand mal seizures
3. Emotional lability
4. Confused mental state, feelings of persecution and anxiety, potential for aggressive or violent behavior, hallucinations
5. Behavioral states of irritability, restlessness, rapid speech
6. Hyperthermia or hypothermia, which may progress into shock
7. Cardiac arrhythmias and shock, which may result in cardiac arrest

The nurse:

1. Provides a calm, nonstimulating environment with supervision and support by nursing staff.
2. Obtains information on drugs ingested but limits interpersonal interactions, which might increase agitation or feelings of persecution.
3. Coordinates security personnel and health team members in the provision of a safe environment for the patient and others.
4. Monitors vital signs frequently.
5. Administers medication as ordered. Diazepam is often used to control seizure activity.
6. Implements seizure precautions.
7. Promotes hydration.
8. Monitors intake and output.
9. Assists in emergency interventions as necessary.
10. Suggests or initiates consultation with the psychiatric or substance-abuse team.
11. May refer patient to a drug treatment program.
12. Gives patient objective feedback and information about the actual and potential outcomes of the immediate drug-induced crisis.

Acute Intoxication from Phencyclidines

Intoxication from phencyclidines has occurred with growing frequency in recent years and is most commonly the result of inhalation. This drug and drugs like it have varying effects, depending on the dose and the route of administration. Response to dosage also varies over time and with the composition and strength of the drug so that toxic states are often unintentionally induced. Toxic responses and overdose occur most frequently in populations of adolescents and young adults.

Signs of phencyclidine intoxication include:

1. Nausea and vomiting
2. Severe anxiety, feelings of panic, excitability, distorted perception, poor reality testing, impaired judgment
3. Vertigo, skin flushing
4. Pupillary constriction, nystagmus, and amblyopia
5. Enhanced reflexes, tremors
6. With higher doses, stupor and/or coma
7. Muscular rigidity and possible convulsions
8. Potential for aggressive or violent behavior

The nurse:

1. Provides a calm, uncrowded environment with little visual or interpersonal stimuli, windows, or furniture.
2. Reassures patient about bodily integrity and safety and orients him or her briefly to the setting.
3. Administers medication as ordered, usually antihypertensives, anticonvulsants, major tranquilizers.
4. Monitors vital signs.
5. Obtains specimens for urinalysis, blood pH, gases, electrolytes.
6. Acidifies urine with cranberry juice to facilitate excretion.
7. Monitors intake and output.
8. Implements seizure precautions.
9. Coordinates security personnel and health team members in the provision of a safe environment for the patient and others.
10. Suggests or initiates consultation with the psychiatric or substance-abuse team. May refer the patient and family to a clinic or treatment program.

Acute Intoxication from Hallucinogens

Drugs included in this category produce highly disturbed behavior and loss of contact with reality. Depending on the quantity and type of drug ingested, responses may be immediate or delayed for several hours.

Signs of intoxication from hallucinogens include:

1. Severe anxiety or panic
2. Elevated vital signs, including elevated body temperature and diaphoresis
3. Possible shock
4. Frank hallucinations, depersonalization, confusion, and paranoia
5. Potential seizures

The nurse:

1. Provides a darkened, nonstimulating, uncrowded environment.
2. Monitors vital signs.
3. Observes for signs of shock.
4. Provides reassurance and an interpersonal presence.
5. Administers medications as ordered for medical problems. The use of chlorpromazine and other antipsychotic medications should be avoided.
6. Implements seizure precautions.
7. Contacts psychiatric or substance-abuse teams for consultation and assistance with patient management and/or refers patient to mental health or substance-abuse treatment resources.

Withdrawal from Depressants and Alcohol

Untreated withdrawal from depressant drugs, including alcohol in the dependent person, can be life-threatening. Nursing interventions and management of these syndromes require that the patient be hospitalized and closely monitored. The clinical picture is further complicated when the patient has become dependent on more than one drug, typically alcohol and benzodiazepines or sedatives and alcohol. Because these drugs can be synergistic, the withdrawal responses are manifested in greater disturbances in the central nervous system. Drugs with similar effects are utilized in decreasing dosage to allay the severity of withdrawal symptoms. With the completion of withdrawal, the use of psychoactive medication is avoided.

Table 13–3 describes the behavior of patients in states of withdrawal from alcohol. These states are precipitated by a sudden drop in blood alcohol level in the alcohol-dependent person. The individual may still be drinking at the time, and individuals with coexisting conditions have an increased chance of developing severe withdrawal symptoms. These other conditions include infection, trauma, surgery, or pancreatitis; the health care team is often unaware of the patient's alcohol dependency until signs of withdrawal appear. Withdrawal requires immediate intervention because the death rate from delirium tremens can range from 5%–30% in the untreated alcoholic (Resnick and Ruben, 1975).

Seizures are not uncommon during the first three days that the BAC declines. In mixed alcohol-barbiturate withdrawal, seizures occur around days 4–6 and between days 7–14 in patients withdrawing from alcohol-benzodiazepine (Valium, Librium) dependence.

The nurse:

1. Verifies quantity and type of drugs in the drug-using pattern.
2. Establishes a nonstimulating, quiet environment and provides light at night if the patient is disoriented.
3. Assesses fluctuations in mental and physical status in conjunction with medication administration.
4. Implements seizure precautions and provides other protections from potential injury.
5. Promotes hydration and assesses nutritional intake.
6. Monitors intake and output.
7. Provides support and reassurance that the patient

Table 13–3. STATES OF WITHDRAWAL FROM ALCOHOL

Withdrawal State	Peak Time of Onset Drink	Symptoms	Duration
Tremulousness	24 hr	Tremors, slight at rest, becoming gross and irregular with activity; easily startled	1 week
		Anorexia, nausea, and vomiting	3–4 days
		Feelings of agitation and inner shakiness	2 weeks
		Insomnia, nightmares of events that seem real, increased vital signs	2 weeks or longer
Tremors and transitory hallucinosis	24 hr	Visual hallucinations of reality-type events, e.g. seeing a son drown	3 days
Auditory hallucinosis	24 hr	Vivid auditory hallucinations that are usually of a persecutory nature, agitation, fearfulness, increased suicide potential	3 days–2 weeks
Delirium tremens	24–48 hr	Generalized tonic-clonic seizures; deliriousness; disorientation to time and place; visual hallucinations of snakes, spiders, and so on; agitation; restlessness	3–5 days
Rum fits	24–48 hr	Begins with 2–6 generalized tonic-clonic seizures, ushers in symptoms of delirium tremens	3–5 days

can achieve well-being and that addiction is treatable. Orients the patient to reality as necessary.

8. Provides nursing care for associated trauma, infection, and so on.

Withdrawal from Stimulants

Withdrawal of stimulants results in disturbance in REM sleep patterns, irritability, and feelings of sadness and depression. Depression may be manifested in feelings of despair and thoughts of suicide, particularly in withdrawal from cocaine. Symptoms may occur even while the individual is taking the drug as tolerance develops. While intense symptoms subside after four or five days, others persist for weeks or months. They include moderate-to-severe depression; sleep disturbances, lethargy and fatigue; postpsychotic suspiciousness or hostility; and mild tremor of the extremities, as well as aches and pains.

The nurse:

1. Conducts ongoing assessment of mood and suicidal potential.
2. Administers sedatives for sleep that do not induce dependence.
3. Uses nonpharmacologic nursing interventions such as therapeutic touch and relaxation techniques for sleep and relaxation.
4. Interacts verbally as desired and tolerated.
5. Promotes hydration and nutrition.
6. Assists with reality testing when suspicious or paranoid ideation persists.

Withdrawal from Hallucinogens, Phencyclidines, Cannabinoids, Inhalants

Well-defined withdrawal syndromes for hallucinogens, phencyclidines, cannabinoids (marijuana, hashish) and inhalants are not clearly documented, although withdrawal states from chronic use of marijuana and phencyclidines have been reported. Flashbacks and psychological symptoms, however, may occur following withdrawal from these drugs. Flashback reactions, or the recurrence of feelings of intoxication some time after the event (Wilford, 1981), sometimes occur with hallucinogens or marijuana when it has been used in addition to hallucinogens. The patient may experience euphoria and a sense of detachment that lasts for several hours. Flashbacks induce fear, anxiety, sadness, or paranoia in the user and require that the nurse or other health care provider explain the connection with drug use and reassure the patient that these feelings will pass. The nurse employed in substance abuse treatment centers, occupational health, high school and collegiate health services, as well as in mental health clinics and private practice should be knowledgeable about these effects. Providing information and reassurance, as well as counseling the user about risk, are important aspects of treatment and prevention.

Withdrawal from Opioids

Withdrawal from opioids and opioid-like medications is rarely life-threatening but causes a range of discomfort in the user and requires nursing intervention. The dose, length of time, frequency of use, and the health of the abuser are important factors in determining the severity of withdrawal symptoms. In the heroin addict, signs of withdrawal occur 6–12 hours after the last dose and include restlessness, yawning, anxiety, diaphoresis, chills, and gastrointestinal symptoms (Table 13–1). These signs subside after 72 hours and are replaced by restlessness, hyperactivity, insomnia, and generalized anxiety. Heart rate and blood pressure may be elevated, and dehydration and electrolyte imbalance may occur. Codeine produces withdrawal symptoms similar to morphine and heroin, and methadone withdrawal is later in onset but less severe. Symptoms subside within two weeks, although the patient may experience lethargy and anorexia for an extended period.

Meperidine (Demerol), the drug upon which many nurses and other health professionals become addicted, has an earlier onset of withdrawal sysmptoms. They occur shortly after the last dose and continue for three to five days. While the "flu-like" symptoms are less pronounced, anxiety, restlessness, and muscle spasms are more prominent.

The nurse:

1. Provides reassurance and supportive verbal interaction.
2. Monitors vital signs.
3. Administers gradually decreasing amounts of opioids, usually oral methadone as indicated.
4. Provides a comfortable, nonstimulating environment.
5. Provides nursing care for related medical problems.
6. Notes changes in mental status such as clouding or euphoria, a "high" to be avoided by regulating medication dosage.
7. Supports the patient through periods of agitation and severe "craving" for the drug.

NURSING INTERVENTIONS DIRECTED TOWARD REHABILITATION

Withdrawal or detoxification are not necessarily associated with the patient's intention to address the problem of his or her addiction. Withdrawal often occurs in association with treatment of trauma or a medical or surgical problem, or can be precipitated by legal intervention or incarceration. These situations provide opportunities for the nurse to communicate with the patient about expressed fears of physical pain, anxieties aroused by the symptoms of withdrawal, and social consequences associated with drug use. Offering frank and objective (but nonjudgmental) appraisals of the patient's health status, as well as discussing feelings precipitated by psychological or emotional changes, addresses the patient's needs for support while keeping a realistic focus on the problem. Even when the patient denies the severity of the illness, the nurse can provide information about consultation services offered within the hospital or treatment facilities and self-help groups.

The individual who enters a treatment facility for purposes of withdrawal and rehabilitation is often ambivalent, frightened, and unsure about his or her ability to successfully complete the treatment process and remain "clean and sober." Most treatment programs require a commitment to 28 days of residential treatment, so that employment, domestic life, and the usual conduct of one's affairs is suspended. While the stigma of addiction to alcohol and/or drugs has decreased greatly in recent years, the responses of family members, friends, and employers to the patient's treatment are often unpredictable. While the nurse may be unable to allay the patient's many anxieties, reassurance that addiction is a treatable disease and a hopeful attitude about the patient's ability to get well is important. Medications are sometimes administered during withdrawal. They are featured in Table 13–4. When residential treatment is not required, the nurse can refer the patient to outpatient facilities or self-help groups in the community.

EVALUATION OF NURSING INTERVENTIONS

The effectivness of nursing intervention must be assessed from the perspective of long- and short-term goals. The individual addicted to alcohol and other drugs may experience many crises of acute illness in the course of the chronic, progressive illness of addiction. While the hospitalized addict is often the one most frequently encountered by the nurse, it is important that the full spectrum of nursing interventions in prevention, treatment, and rehabilitation be considered. Education on drug and alcohol use and its associated risks is central to health education at all stages of the life cycle. While experimentation with a variety of drugs is common in adolescence, increasing numbers of individuals at all ages (including the elderly) use alcohol and develop dependence and medical complications. As research on the effects of alcohol and other drugs on physical and mental function continues, nurses must interpret the health implications of such findings to the consumer.

The anticipated outcomes of short-term nurisng intervention include a stable physiologic state evidenced in vital signs within the patient's usual range, adequate hydration and nutritional intake, and a clear sensorium with the absence of marked cognitive or emotional disturbance. The patient may or may not articulate a desire to lead a drug-free life and a willingness to become involved in treatment or support systems that will enable him or her to do so. Because denial is such a central component of addictive disease, there may be many social, legal, and medical crises in the life of the user before life without the drug can be considered an attainable goal. Many individuals addicted to alcohol and other drugs never change their use patterns or seek treatment; this does not mean that intervention has failed. The nurse must be aware that the responsibility for involvement in treatment rests with the patient. Efforts by the nurse to motivate the patient toward a healthier lifestyle and a drug-free existence include assisting the client to attain whatever level of health is possible; progress must be measured in degrees.

Long-term treatment goals include recognition of a drug problem or addiction and participation in treatment and the recovery process. Recovery, or rehabilitation of substance abuse illness is a lifetime process characterized by slips from sobriety or relapses and the need for ongoing efforts to abstain from psychoactive substances. The presence of addictive disease means that individuals can use no psychoactive substances without again placing themselves at risk for addiction. In addition to treatment for addiction, individual and family therapy are helpful in changing established dysfunctional patterns in relationships and increasing self-awareness. Family members involved with the addicted individual need assistance in understanding the impact of addictive disease on their own growth and drug-using behaviors. The nurse working as a generalist (as well as the nurse employed in a substance abuse treatment center) provides counseling on general health issues and psychotherapy to the patient and family as indicated.

Pharmacologic interventions are helpful adjuncts to short- and long-term goals. Table 13–5 lists and describes medications used to deter the ingestion of alcohol and opioid narcotics. The nurse implements health teaching and counsels the client on drug action, side effects, and the result of ingesting psychoactive drugs while taking these medications. With both Antabuse and narcotic antagonists, the patient must agree to participate in this type of therapy and must be knowledgeable about the effects of combining drugs of abuse and pharmacologic deterrents. Once the patient has established a period of sobriety, antidepressants may be prescribed to raise mood and alter depressive symptoms. Lithium may be prescribed for the patient with a mixed psychiatric-addictive disorder. Education by the nurse is an important component of care, whether the nurse is the primary caregiver or is employed in a rehabilitation clinic, such as those for methadone maintenance. The long-term goal for the addicted patient remains consistent—a drug-free lifestyle and the acquisition of realistic problem-solving techniques regarding health. The nursing process table (Table 13–6) reviews the nursing care given to an addicted person by drug class.

HEALTH CONSEQUENCES ASSOCIATED WITH SUBSTANCE ABUSE

Excessive alcohol use and abuse of prescription and illicit drugs impact the total health of the individual. The extent of that impact is a function of the drug composition, the amount of drug used, and the frequency of its use. Concurrent acute or chronic illnesses or parturitional states also determine the extent and nature of cellular and system damage by drugs to the individual and offspring.

The consequences of drug use by pregnant and nursing women were first detected in infants and children of women who were heavy consumers of alcohol. In 1973 a specific pattern of neonatal defects associated with alcohol use (fetal alcohol syndrome) was described. The syndrome is characterized by pre- and postnatal growth deficiences, patterns of facial malformation, central nervous system dysfunction, and varying degrees of major organ system malformations. Children with alcohol-re-

Table 13–4. DRUGS USED IN TREATING DRUG TOXICITY AND WITHDRAWAL

Name	Dosage	Mode of Administration	Pharmacokinetics
Narcan (Naloxone)			
Action and Uses: Narcotic antagonist to decrease narcotic-induced depression, including respiratory depression. Narcotic antagonist to combat narcotic overdose or postoperative narcotic depression, including respiratory depression.			
	0.01 mg/kg body wt	IM, IV, SC IV injection	O: 1–2 min; IM, SC 2–5 min P: same as onset D: 45 min ½L: 60–90 min PB: UA B: liver E: urine
Lorfan			
Action and Uses: Acts as a narcotic antagonist to decrease respiratory depression.			
	1 mg IV with additional doses (0.5 mg) as required	IV injection	——
Diazepam (Valium)			
Action and Uses: In alcohol withdrawal: Decrease central nervous system stimulation. With stimulant toxicity: Acts as an anticonvulsant. With PCP toxicity: Acts as tranquilizer. With hallucinogen toxicity: Acts as tranquilizer. In depressant withdrawal: Decreases central nervous system stimulation.			
	10 mg PO or IV q 3–4 hr	PO, IM	O: 30 min P: 0.5–2 hr D: up to 21 days ½L: 20–50 hr PB: 96% B: liver E: urine O: 30–120 min P: 1–4 hr

Key to Abbreviations in the *Pharmacokinetics* column O-onset; P-peak; D-duration; PB-protein bound; B-biotransformed in; E-excreted in; ½ L-halflife.
  *Within the column listing adverse effects, underlines indicate the most common effects; CAPITALS indicate life-threatening effects.

lated birth defects often manifest behavior difficulties that compromise normal development. These include hyperactivity, attentional deficits, impulsivity, and poor motor function.

The prevalence of fetal alcohol syndrome is difficult to determine but ranges from one to three cases per thousand live births in the United States (Warren, 1986). While the relationship between increasing doses of alcohol and the severity of effects is established, the amount of alcohol considered harmful and the mother's drinking patterns are less clearly linked to specific effects. Effects of alcohol have been detected in children of women identified as moderate as well as heavy drinkers; therefore, alcohol consumption should be greatly reduced or totally eliminated during pregnancy.

The exposure of fetuses and infants to drugs other than alcohol is growing in prevalence. Women in all ethnic and socioeconomic groups use cocaine, marijuana, amphetamines, and heroin as evidenced in the body fluid examination and the testing of newborns in hospitals nationwide. Fetal effects of exposure to cocaine include prenatal strokes, brain damage, seizures after birth, premature birth, respiratory problems, and structural abnormalities.

Marijuana use is reported to result in the untoward effects of lower birth weight and neurologic dysfunctions. Infants born to heroin-addicted mothers experience withdrawal syndromes in the neonatal period and manifest irritability and signs similar to those of adult opiate withdrawal.

Contraindications/ Precautions	Adverse Effects*	Interactions	Nursing Implications
	Cessation of dosage may induce withdrawal in opioid-dependent individuals.		ASSESSMENT: Assess respiratory function. Observation, documentation. Patient teaching and interpretation of effects to patient and family. Monitor vital signs. Implement complementary resuscitative measures.
Mild respiratory depression. May produce withdrawal in narcotic addicts.	Same. Use with caution in individuals with cardiovascular disease. Dysphoria, miosis, lethargy, diaphoresis, vertigo, drowsiness, gastric upset.	Rendered ineffective in respiratory depression due to barbiturates, anesthetics, or nonnarcotics.	ASSESSMENT: Assess respiratory function. Interpret drug effects to family and patient. Monitor vital signs. Implement complementary resuscitative measures. Assess mental status. Monitor vital signs. Provide secure environment.
Hypersensitivity to benzodiazepines.	Drowsiness, ataxia, fatigue. Withdrawal may be induced with cessation of dosage. Potential for psychic and physical dependence.		ASSESSMENT: Observe and report behavior change, increased vital signs. Reassure patient. Avoid excessive verbal and environmental stimulation.

Drugs to Treat Toxicity/Withdrawal

The effects of drug use on development appear to vary in relation to phase of gestational growth, the amount and nature of the drug used, and other contributing factors such as maternal smoking and nutrition. Children born with irreversible effects such as structural abnormalities, mental retardation, and the potential for lifelong behavioral disturbance require comprehensive nursing, social, and educational services. In homes where parents are heavy users of alcohol and/or other drugs, the mental health of children and other family members may be compromised because of parental inconsistency, physical and psychological abuse, and economic instability.

The health consequences of extensive alcohol use and abuse are the most far-reaching of any drugs. The development and type of health problems depend on the amount and frequency of alcohol consumption in interaction with the individual's constitution, including psychological as well as physiologic traits. The ingestion of alcohol causes tissue damage and interferes with the absorption, utilization, and storage of nutrients, as well as appetite. Malnutrition results from actual histologic abnormals and decreased absorptive capacity, intestinal permeability, and motility. Of particular note is the compromised ability to absorb B vitamins. Other gastrointestinal disturbances include acute gastritis and duodenitis. With elevated doses, the probability of cancers of the head and neck also increases.

The pancreas and liver are most often affected by chronic abuse of alcohol, and alcoholic hepatitis and

Table 13–5. DRUGS USED IN TREATING SUBSTANCE DEPENDENCE

Name	Dosage	Mode of Administration	Pharmacokinetics
Disulfiram (Antabuse)			
Action and Uses: Blocks the oxidation of alcohol at the acetaldehyde stage. High concentrations of acetaldehyde then produce a highly sensitive reaction to alcohol with unpleasant reaction.			
	200–500 mg	PO	O: 0.5–3 hr P: 3–12 hr D: 1–2 weeks ½L: UA PB: UA B: liver E: urine, lungs
Methadone hydrochloride (Dolophine)			
Action and Uses: A synthetic narcotic analgesic that acts on the CNS and smooth muscle to produce analgesia or sedation. Used primarily for detoxification and maintenance in addiction to opioids.			
		PO tablet, liquid Parenteral	O: 30–60 min P: 30–120 min D: 22–48 hr ½L: 13–47 hr PB: extreme B: liver E: urine O: immediate P: immediate
Trexan			
Action and Uses: Blocks effects of heroin			
		PO	O: 15–30 min P: 1 hr D: 24–72 hr ½L: 9.7–16.8 hr PB: 21–28% B: liver E: urine

Key to Abbreviations in the *Pharmacokinetics* column O-onset; P-peak; D-duration; PB-protein bound; B-biotransformed in; E-excreted in; ½ L-halflife.
*Within the column listing adverse effects, underlines indicate the most common effects; CAPITALS indicate life-threatening effects.

pancreatitis occur. Fatty infiltration of the liver, the most conspicuous physical effect, results from the stimulation of hepatic cholesterol synthesis. The increased disposition of fat ultimately leads to cirrhosis.

Blood disorders are also common signs of excessive alcohol use and are manifested in macrocytic and other anemias and clotting disorders resulting from its direct effect on hematopoiesis. Neurologic effects include Wernicke's and Korsakoff's syndrome and peripheral neuropathy.

Accidents are a frequent health hazard to alcohol abusers and alcoholics. Not only does calcium depletion, poor diet, and decreased activity increase the risk of traumatic fractures and osteoporosis, but automobile and boating accidents are common. In the United States, 55% of all fatal motor vehicle accidents are alcohol-related. Additionally, alcoholics are at much higher risk of suicide than the nonalcoholic population, especially males.

Unintentional death from overdose and untoward effects are the most serious outcomes. They include acute alcohol intoxication and poisoning, seen most often, but not exclusively in young, uninitiated drinkers, and convulsive seizures and heart attack in cocaine users. Violent behavior and psychotic responses to PCP and LSD can also be life-threatening.

Drugs and alcohol, used singly or in combination, result in acute and long-term health problems that shorten the life span by sudden death or debilitation. Objective, nonjudgmental assessments of these potential health problems are central to health teaching by the nurse and other health care providers.

Contraindications/ Precautions	Adverse Effects*	Interactions	Nursing Implications
Never administer while patient is intoxicated or without patient's knowledge. Recent use of metronidazole paraldehyde, alcohol, or alcohol-containing preparations. Severe myocardial disease, coronary occlusion, hypersensitivity to disulfiram or other thiuram derivates.	Flushing, nausea, vomiting, headache, weakness, dizziness, skin eruptions. Impotence.	Use with barbiturates may initiate a new addiction. Produces ataxia with isoniazid. May increase prothrombin time if given with anticoagulants.	Observation, documentation. Patient teaching. Gradual administration of increasing dosage: 500 mg for 1–2 weeks. Maintenance: 250 mg/day.
Hypersensitivity to methadone.	Produces psychic and physical dependence. High abuse potential. Diaphoresis, vertigo, sedation, respiratory depression, and arrest.	Use with other narcotic analgesics, anesthetics, major tranquilizers, depressants, and antidepressants leads to respiratory depression, hypotension, and profound sedation or coma. Use with naloxone, pentazocine, and other narcotic analgesics can precipitate withdrawal symptoms in heroin addicts and patients on methadone.	Observation, documentation. Patient teaching. Methadone may impair driving or operating machinery. Gradual administration to maintenance of 40 mg/day.
Acute hepatitis or liver failure. Sensitivity to naltrexone. Absence of an opioid-free state manifested in opioid analgesics, opioid withdrawal, or opioids in urinalysis.	Opioid-dependent patients may experience withdrawal. Anxiety, insomnia, headache, rash, delayed ejaculation, and decreased potency.	Decreases the pharmacologic effect of opioid-containing preparations, including analgesics, antidiarrheal agents, cough medicines.	Observation, documentation. Patient teaching. Warn patient that attempts to overcome the blockade with large amounts of heroin may result in life-threatening circumstances.

IMPAIRMENT AMONG NURSES AND OTHER HEALTH PROFESSIONALS

Individuals predisposed to the development of addiction and those who develop drug dependencies choose careers in health as readily as they pursue other vocations. This means that a number of health workers, perhaps 5%–8%, will develop addictions and psychiatric disorders, which may go unrecognized. Among health professionals, two factors are linked to the use of and addiction to prescription drugs: attitude and accessibility. Because medication is so frequently used with positive outcomes in the practice of nursing and other health professions, an attitude about the advantages of drug use develops. The professional's knowledge of pharmacology often supports an illusion that he or she knows enough about drugs not to become addicted. Hospitals vary widely in the security of drug monitoring and control over medication records. The ease with which drugs are available, while clearly not the cause of addiction, is a factor in abuse of drugs by physicians and nurses. In recent years, medicine, nursing, dentistry, pharmacy, and other disciplines have begun programs to educate their practitioners about the prevention, signs and symptoms, and appropriate intervention strategies

TEXT RESUMES ON PAGE 304

Drugs to Treat Substance Dependence

Table 13–6. NURSING PROCESS BY DRUG CLASS BEING ABUSED

Hallucinogen Intoxication/Withdrawal (LSD, Cannabis)
Assessment

Evaluate mental status, noting degree of agitation and psychomotor activity, presence of emotional swings, suspiciousness, paranoia, bizarre behavior.
Assess baseline vital signs, noting hypertension, tachycardia, tachypnea.

Nursing Diagnosis	Nursing Actions	Rationale	Patient Outcomes/ Evaluation Criteria
Injury, potential for trauma/poisoning related to clouded sensorium, as evidenced by impaired judgment, poor coordination, and diminished perception of pain.	Have someone known to the patient accompany him and provide support, comfort, and close observation. Provide nonthreatening environment with subdued, pleasant stimuli. Avoid use of phenothiazines. Administer Valium as indicated.	Patient is disoriented, experiencing perceptual distortions and hallucinations which can increase likelihood of injury. Antipsychotic drugs may increase anticholinergic effects of ingested drug causing hypotension. Acts as a tranquilizer with calming effect to reduce risk of injury.	Maintains physiologic stability and injury does not occur.
Thought processes, altered related to physiologic changes, impaired judgment with loss of memory as evidenced by inaccurate interpretation of environment, bizarre thinking, disorientation.	Provide safe, nonthreatening environment with close observation and diversion from disturbing internal experiences. Anticipate some form of unpredictable behavior. Tell patient that current thoughts and feelings are a result of drug effect. Administer medications, e.g., Valium, as indicated.	Alteration in thinking leads to inability to process information correctly affecting patient's response to environment. Being prepared for the unexpected allows opportunity to manage situation effectively. Provides reassurance about body integrity and safety. May provide tranquilizing effect.	Demonstrates return of memory and ability to function with absence of visual/auditory disturbances.

Phencyclidine Intoxication/Withdrawal (PCP)
Assessment

Assess baseline vital signs, presence of flushing, fever, sweating. Observe for increasing anxiety, fear, irritability, and agitation. Note changes in behavior pattern and exaggerated emotional responses.
Observe signs of neurologic irritation, hyperactivity, incoherent speech, level of consciousness.
Ascertain degree of sensory awareness, presence of delusions, detachment from surroundings.

Nursing Diagnosis	Nursing Actions	Rationale	Patient Outcomes/ Evaluation Criteria
Violence, potential for: Self-directed or directed at others related to toxic reactions to drugs, exogenous chemical alteration.	Place in a darkened, quiet, nonthreatening environment with a nonintrusive observer. Speak in a soft nonthreatening voice. Avoid use of "talk-down" techniques. Observe behavior without administering drugs before a decision about use of other drugs is made. Administer valium as indicated.	Lowers stimulation decreasing the likelihood of confusion and fear and lessening the chance of violent response. May have a calming effect but "talk-downs" may crease agitation level. Allows for a clear clinical picture to develop. Provides calming effect to help control behavior.	Acknowledges reality of situation and understanding of the relationship of behavior to drug use.

Table 13–6. NURSING PROCESS BY DRUG CLASS BEING ABUSED–CONTINUED

Phencyclidine Intoxication/Withdrawal (PCP)
Assessment *(Continued)*

Injury, potential for trauma related to muscle incoordination, reduced eye/hand coordination, decreased response to perception of pain, clouded sensorium and impaired judgment.	Ascertain which drugs have been taken when possible. Anticipate some form of unpredictability, be prepared for the unexpected.	PCP often has been adulterated with other drugs. These drugs are dangerous and can lead to bizarre thinking/harmful behavior.	Demonstrates behaviors and lifestyle changes necessary to minimize and/or prevent injury.
	Remove objects that are potentially dangerous from immediate access. Place patient away from windows, tables.	Provides protection reducing risk of injury.	
	Administer IVs and ammonium chloride or ascorbic acid as indicated.	Forced diuresis and acidifying urine enhances renal clearance of PCP.	
Tissue perfusion altered: cardiopulmonary/cerebral related to alterations in blood flow (hypertensive crisis).	Elevate head of bed, keep head in midline position.	Enhances venous drainage, reducing risk of vascular congestion and increased intracranial pressure and possibility of hemorrhage.	Maintains/achieves physiologic stability evidenced by patent airway and adequate respiratory/cardiac function. Regains/maintains usual level of consciousness free of adverse neurologic symptoms/complications.
	Observe for pupillary or vital sign changes, decreased level of consciousness.	Provides for early detection and intervention to minimize increased intracranial pressure/injury.	
	Administer antihypertensive medications as indicated.	Effective in lowering blood pressure to prevent hypertensive crisis.	

Depressant Intoxication/Withdrawal (Barbiturates, Sedatives, Opioids)
Assessment:

Assess baseline vital signs, noting hypertension, respiratory depression.
Evaluate mental/emotional state (e.g., lability, belligerence, lethargy, agitation, anxiety, presence of confusion or delerium) and degree of impairment, duration of problems.
Determine concurrent alcohol and other drug use.

Nursing Diagnosis	Nursing Actions	Rationale	Patient Outcomes/Evaluation Criteria
Injury, potential for, trauma/poisoning related to depression/agitation, psychologic stress, IV drug use techniques.	Provide quiet, lighted room with close observation.	Reduces stimuli which may potentiate agitation/seizure activity and possibility of injury.	Verbalizes understanding of risk factors of taking drugs. Completes withdrawal without injury to self, development of complications.
	Restrict activity/assist as necessary.	Presence of orthostatic hypotension, hyperreflexion and muscle cramping increases risk of traumatic injury.	

CONTINUED ON THE FOLLOWING PAGE

Table 13–6. NURSING PROCESS BY DRUG CLASS BEING ABUSED–CONTINUED

Depressant Intoxication/Withdrawal (Barbiturates, Sedatives, Opioids)
Assessment *(Continued)*

	Maintain frequent contact, reorient as needed. Provide seizure precautions.	Provides resassurance/reduces anxiety. May prevent injury if seizures occur during withdrawal.	
	Evaluate changes in behavior/emotional state.	Drug intoxication can precipitate alterations in perceptions/psychotic behavior and may result in hallucinations and precipitate suicidal/homicidal behavior.	
	Administer emetics, assist with gastric lavage if indicated.	Emptying stomach may be effective when drug has been recently ingested.	
	Administer activated charcoal per protocol. Administer phenobarbital or methadone, Trexan as indicated by drug used.	Reduces intestinal absorption of ingested drugs. Phenobarbital's prolonged effect provides smoother sedation, while methadone/Trexan replace heroin or other narcotic effects.	
	Administer Valium cautiously if indicated.	Decreases CNS stimulation/agitation but may cause respiratory depression.	
	Observe for dehydration, record I/O, monitor temperature.	Hyperpyrexia may occur with withdrawal or occur with infectious process, requiring additional fluid replacement to promote clearance of drug.	
	Maintain IV line as appropriate.	Provides avenue for emergency drugs/fluid replacement.	
Breathing pattern ineffective, potential for related to neuromuscular impairment, decreased energy, and decreased lung expansion.	Establish patent airway. Elevate head of bed and position on side as indicated. Encourage cough and deep breathing.	Respiratory depression can lead to hypoxia and eventually cardiovascular collapse.	Demonstrates normal breating pattern free of symptoms of respiratory distress and cyanosis.
	Suction as needed. Monitor level of consciousness.	Treatment and medication administration is dependent on level of consciousness.	
	Review chest x-ray.	Helps to identify need for specific treatment of common complications of opiate abuse, e.g., pneumonia, aspiration pneumonitis, lung abscess, atelectasis.	
	Administer narcotic antagonists, e.g., Narcan, Lorfan.	Used to reverse respiratory depressant effects of opioid intoxication.	
Coping, ineffective, individual related to personal vulnerability, inadequate support systems as evidenced by addictive behaviors, poor self-esteem, chronic anxiety, worry and depression.	Provide safe, nonthreatening environment.	Psychological changes, cognitive distortion and physiologic discomfort increase anxiety while CNS rebound from sedative withdrawal results in apprehension impairing coping abilities.	Demonstrates improved coping skills, e.g., acknowledging powerlessness over drug and attending groups, i.e., ed., Narcotics Anonymous.
	Determine previous methods of dealing with life problems, including suicidal ideation/attempts.	Depressants are the most widely used and abused class of drugs and are often prescribed for symptoms of anxiety, depression, and sleep disturbances without adequate treatment for underlying problem.	

Table 13–6. NURSING PROCESS BY DRUG CLASS BEING ABUSED–CONTINUED

Depressant Intoxication/Withdrawal (Barbiturates, Sedatives, Opioids)
Assessment *(Continued)*

	Encourage patient to express feelings and to look at own responsibility for current situation. Express acceptance of the patient, refraining from confrontational/judgmental comments. Provide positive reinforcement when patient acknowledges own responsibility for situation and displays new behavior.	Ready availability increases use of these drugs as a means of suicide. Learning to recognize and express feelings is a beginning point for changing behavior. Helps patient to identify and accept new ways of coping with stressors.

Alcohol Intoxication/Withdrawal
Assessment:

Evaluate respiratory rate, depth, rhythm, and breath sounds.
Assess level of consciousness, behavioral responses, presence of hallucinations/impaired cognitive function, slurred speech.
Note degree of fear and reality of threat perceived by the patient.
Observe coordination, note ataxia.
Obtain information as soon as possible on drug/alcohol ingestion.

Nursing Diagnosis	Nursing Actions	Rationale	Patient Outcomes/Evaluation Criteria
Breathing, ineffective, potiential for, related to direct effect of alcohol toxicity on respiratory center, decreased energy, presence of chronic respiratory inflammatory processes and sedative effects of drugs given to decrease alcohol withdrawal symptoms.	Establish patent airway. Elevate head of bed and position on side as indicated. Encourage cough and deep breathing. Suction as needed. Monitor level of consciousness and vital signs closely. Initiate resuscitation efforts as necessary. Administer supplemental oxygen as indicated.	Respiratory depression can lead to hypoxia and eventually cardiovascular collapse. Facilitates lung expansion and clearance of secretions reducing risk of atelectasis. Treatment and medication is administered in accordance with level of consciousness. Helpful in preventing/reducing hypoxia associated with CNS/respiratory depression.	Displays normal breathing pattern free of symptoms of respiratory distress and cyanosis.
Sensory-perceptual alteration (specify) related to exogenous chemical alteration (alcohol use/sudden cessation) and endogenous (electrolyte imbalance, elevated ammonia and BUN), sleep deprivation, psychologic stress as evidenced by disorientation, bizarre thinking, exaggerated responses.	Provide safe, quiet environment and regulate lighting as indicated. Speak in calm voice. Provide supervision and interpersonal support. Refrain from judgmental comments. Administer Valium cautiously as indicated. Administer Antabuse as indicated. Refer to substance abuse treatment program upon resolution of acute intoxication.	Promotes rest and limits hyperactive responses to aid in control of hallucinations and reduce risk of personal injury. Patient is disoriented, frightened, guilty, and needs assistance to avoid additional complications. Decreases CNS stimulation but may potentiate respiratory depression. Produces a highly sensitive reaction to alcohol with unpleasant side effects, promoting abstinence. Patient is unable to respond to health-oriented referral during acute state.	Reports absence of auditory/visual hallucinations. Maintains optimal level of consciousness.

CONTINUED ON THE FOLLOWING PAGE

Table 13–6. NURSING PROCESS BY DRUG CLASS BEING ABUSED–CONTINUED

Stimulant Intoxication/Withdrawal (Amphetamines, Cocaine/Crack)
Assessment:

Obtain information on type and kind of drugs ingested.
Assess perceptions; behavioral responses; and presence of hallucinations, paranoia, aggressive feelings.
Evaluate extent of fatigue and excitation/psychomotor acceleration (e.g., sweating, dilated pupils, tremors, seizures).
Note degree of fear and reality of threat perceived by the patient.
Assess vital signs, noting presence of tachycardia, hypertension, tachypnea, hyperpyrexia.
Note suppression of appetite, weight loss.

Nursing Diagnosis	Nursing Actions	Rationale	Patient Outcomes/ Evaluation Criteria
Violence, potential for (specify), related to paranoid ideation, perceptions of threats, altered perceptions.	Decrease stimuli; provide quiet in own room or place in stimulus-reduction room with supervision.	Reduces reactivity, enhances calm feelings. Observation allows for timely intervention.	Acknowledges fearfulness and realities of situation. Demonstrates self-control.
	Remove potentially harmful objects from environment. Allow chance for verbal expression of aggressive feelings.	Reduces opportunity to carry out suicidal ideas/plan. Encouragement of new avenue of expression helps patient learn new coping behaviors.	
	Be alert to violence potential, increased pacing, verbalization of delusional persecutory content, hypervigilance regarding specific persons in the milieu, gesturing aggressively.	Recognizing potential and assisting patient to gain control can be more effective prior to violent outbreak.	
	Isolate immediately if patient becomes violent. Negotiate conditions for coming out of isolation when the patient is calm.	Patient will feel safer if others take control until internal control can be regained by the patient.	
	Administer Thorazine, Valium as indicated.	Short-term use of major tranquilizers can assist patient in gaining self-control, promotes sedation/rest when agitated, assaultive, overstimulated.	
Cardiac output, potential for decrease related to drug effect on myocardium/electrical conduction, and pre-existing myocardiomyopathy	Monitor cardiac activity, anticipate cardiac arrest and implement resuscitative measures as necessary.	Tachycardia and dysrhythmias are common and may be life-threatening.	Demonstrates adequate cardiac output and normalization of vital signs and cardiac rhythm.
	Treat body temperature of 102°F and over with cold water, sponging, hypothermic blanket.	Hyperthermia adds additional stress to the cardiovascular system increasing metabolic and cardiac output demands.	
	Administer medications, e.g., propranolol (Inderal) and lidocaine.	β-Adrenergic blockers reduce cardiac oxygen demand. Lidocaine may be used in emergency situation to control/prevent ventricular dysrhythmias.	
Fear related to paranoid delusions as evidenced by suspiciousness and concerns about actions of others.	Be concrete, clear in communication.	Promotes accurate understanding and helps to lessen fear.	Discusses reality base of persecutory fears. Demonstrates appropriate range of feelings and lessened fear.
	Acknowledge awareness of patient's feelings. Encourage verbalization of fear.	Ventilation can lessen intensity of fearfulness.	

Table 13–6. NURSING PROCESS BY DRUG CLASS BEING ABUSED–CONTINUED

Stimulant Intoxication/Withdrawal (Amphetamines, Cocaine/Crack)
Assessment (Continued)

	Assist patient in reality checking fears.	Patient can further reduce fear by understanding difference between reality and delusions.	
Sensory-perceptual alteration (specify) related to exogenous chemical affecting sensory reception, transmission, and integration as evidenced by preoccupation with hallucinatory experiences.	Place patient in quiet, nonstimulating environment with interpersonal support. Provide clear verbal direction and reorient as needed. Administer barbiturates/Valium as indicated. Implement seizure precautions.	Helps to decrease agitation, distractibility; and reduce risk for seizure activity. Provides reassurance and may reduce anxiety. Promotes understanding and reduces anxiety and agitation as suspicious/paranoid thinking as well as watchful behavior is common. Useful in controlling side-effects of cocaine overdose and reducing risk of seizures occurring secondary to CNS rebound effect.	Distinguishes reality from altered perceptions.
Sleep pattern disturbance related to CNS sensory alterations as evidenced by constant alertness, racing thoughts, inability to sleep.	Decrease environmental stimuli. Promote timely mild exercise, fresh air, abstinence from caffeine products. Provide sleep hygiene measures, e.g., warm milk, hot bath, soothing music. Assist patient to learn techniques for relaxation, e.g., visualization, deep breathing, meditation. Use nonpharmacologic nursing measures, such as Therapeutic Touch. Adminster nonaddicting medications, e.g., L-tryptophan.	Promotes drowsiness and desire for sleep. Enhances ability to rest and attain sleep. Enables patient to take charge of own self, manage stress, reduce anxiety and promotes rest. Provides chemical assistance initially to attain proper sleep cycle.	Rests/sleeps at specific intervals in a designated area. Reports feeling rested when awakens.
Nutrition altered: Less than body requirements, related to anorexia secondary to drug effect and insufficient/inappropriate use of financial resources as evidenced by weight loss, inadequate intake, lack of interest in food, poor muscle tone, and signs/laboratory evidence of vitamin deficiencies.	Compare current weight with predrug-use normals. Monitor dietary intake/calorie count. Discuss needs, likes/dislikes about food choices. Provide meals in a relaxed, nonstimulating environment. Consult with dietitian. Administer multivitamins as indicated. Review laboratory studies, e.g., CBC, UA, serum albumin.	Stimulants decrease appetite and impair judgment regarding body needs. Provides information about adequacy of intake. Will be more likely to maintain desired intake if individual preferences are considered. Stimulus reduction aids relaxation and ability to focus on eating. Useful in establishing individual nutritional needs/dietary program. Supplementation enhances correction of deficiencies. Assessment of nutritional state is necessary to treat pre-existing deficiencies and rule out anemia, dehydration, or ketosis.	Demonstrates progressive weight gain toward goal.

with these illnesses. Professional organizations at district and state levels have implemented programs to assist peers who are experiencing problems and help them to accept treatment.

Impaired nursing practice is defined as the inability to meet standards of practice because cognitive, interpersonal, and psychomotor skills are compromised by the use of drugs and/or alcohol or by psychiatric illness. Impaired practice is most readily identified by changes in job performance and the deteriorating quality of the professional's work. Typical patterns include high absenteeism, many excuses for poor job performance, problems with documentation and medication recording, interpersonal problems with patients and coworkers, decreased productivity, and withdrawal from community and professional activities.

The practitioner whose professional judgment is impaired by alcohol, drugs, or psychiatric disturbance poses a threat to the consumer, his or her own well-being, and professional standards. Impaired practice is in violation of the ethical Code for Nurses and places the nurse at risk for legal action, which can result in loss of licensure. Coworkers must compensate for poor productivity, and low morale, coupled with a high accident rate, are not infrequent on units where the impaired nurse is employed. It is important to recognize that the nurse who practices while impaired has lost control of drug and alcohol use and continues to compulsively use drugs with little rational consideration of the consequences.

Constructive intervention takes two primary forms: (1) supervisory intervention, including objective assessment of the quality of job performance and referral of the nurse to an employee assistance program, private practitioner, or health service; and (2) peer assistant intervention by trained volunteers who contact the nurse and/or the nurse's family and attempt to involve the nurse in seeking treatment. In both situations, employing institutions are encouraged to "treat before firing" and develop policies that make available sick time, employee health care benefits, and when necessary, disability insurance for the nurse. Recognition that addiction is a treatable disease is central to the management of impaired practice and the key to changing negative attitudes and providing opportunities for recovery and a return to practice.

Many experienced and talented nurses who are recovering from addiction have returned to work. When re-employment is considered, both the nurse and the employing institution identify concerns and safeguards that support the nurse's continuing recovery and assure the employer that some monitoring of the employee's recovery will be ongoing. A contract is often drawn providing for the collection and testing of randomly collected urines from the recovering nurse, and a channel for communication with a monitoring therapist or peer assistance program representative is set up. The contract may also designate employment in settings where the nurse is not required to dispense narcotics, provide for a schedule of consistent shift time, and specify a nursing service representative who oversees the re-entry process of nurses into the agency.

The American Nurses' Association and its state association members have drafted resolutions to assist the nurse experiencing the problems associated with impaired practice. Forty-eight associations now have committees and/or peer assistance programs and are providing education, supporting legislation that recognizes the need to leave practice to enter treatment, and collaborating with state boards of nursing in program development. At the district nurses' association level, services are being developed that include peer support groups, hot lines for information and referral, and organized out-reach efforts. While every profession needs to continue to care for its members who suffer such illnesses, the incidence of impaired practice can be contained. Action by professional societies is directed toward increased awareness of the risks to practice associated with drug and alcohol abuse, prevention of its occurrence through the education of students and practitioners, and the development of policies that advocate the best treatment for the addicted individual as well as the opportunity to return to practice.

SUMMARY

Alcohol and commonly abused illicit and prescription drugs, unlike other drugs discussed in this text, place the patient at risk for the development of social and health problems. Americans have a shared belief that drugs have high potential for healing, and both professional and laypersons use large numbers of medications in attempts to enhance health and feelings of well-being.

This overreliance on drugs—alcohol, prescription, and over-the-counter medications—contributes to the prevalence of alcohol and other drug abuse and dependence. Abuse and dependence, as well as combinations of abuse and dependence of several classes of drugs, afflict as many as 15 million Americans. Large numbers of individuals begin use in late childhood and develop drug dependence as late adolescents and young adults. All age groups are represented in drug-using and drug-dependent populations, but recent trends in illicit drug and alcohol use by pregnant women present complex and disturbing health problems.

Nurses practicing in all specialties need to be knowledgeable about drugs of abuse, the detection of patterns of abuse and dependence, and intervention in acute and chronic illnesses resulting from use. Pharmacokinetics of licitly prescribed medications are presented by drug class elsewhere in this text. Designer drugs manufactured and sold illicitly are less easily described in composition and effect and show wide variation in health impact. Nursing interventions are directed toward manifest physiologic and psychological problems.

Theories on the etiology of drug and alcohol abuse and dependence identify determinants of person-environment interaction from the perspective of individual traits, social and cultural factors, and the interaction of numerous variables. While recent research promises to shed some light on the individual's susceptibilities to the development of addiction, the many theoretical perspectives fall short of explaining entirely the psychological and physiologic determinants of addictive illness.

The stigma associated with excessive drinking and drug use influences the attitudes of nurses and other health care providers. As a result, assessment and health planning may be incomplete because the care provider denies evidence of a perceived "moral" or "untreatable" problem. Knowledge of signs and symptoms of substance dependence is the foundation for comprehensive history taking, examination, and the formulation of a nursing diagnosis.

Nursing diagnoses in relation to alcohol and other drug abuse include actual and potential health problems corresponding to primary, secondary, and tertiary care. Potential problems accompany drug-using patterns in individuals of all ages. Actual problems are associated with acute and chronic drug use. Nursing interventions in acute states are generally directed toward deterring the life-threatening and/or debilitating effects of intoxication or withdrawal from a drug. Nursing interventions with intoxicated individuals and nursing action in withdrawal states derive from the specific effects of drugs on physiologic and psychologic systems. Evaluative criteria correspond to indicators that the individual has returned to normal status in psychologic and physiologic spheres. Short- and long-term goals reflect a return to normal, drug-free states. Client teaching, counseling in problem-solving techniques, and short-term group and individual psychotherapy are important components of nursing care complications when the practitioner's education and experience are the bases for such intervention.

Health consequences of drug use are manifested in changes in behavioral and physiologic function. Maternal drug use results in neonatal addiction and fetal damage, as well as in dysfunctional parenting. Accidents and unintentional overdose are common causes of death from all classes of drugs and occur according to systemic drug action, such as respiratory depression from depressants and alcohol. Long-term excessive alcohol use has the greatest scope of effect on all body systems. They are most evident in cardiovascular, central nervous, and gastrointestinal systems and are responsible for high morbidity and life span reduction of ten years or more. Death from acute intoxication occurs with stimulants, depressants, and hypnotic and tranquilizing medications and is a serious threat to uninitiated users as well as to long-term dependent individuals.

Intravenous drug use is associated with several long-term and lift-threatening complications. These include superficial as well as systemic infections, damage to the cardiovascular system, and HIV infection and AIDS. All nursing intervention with sexual partners of intravenous drug users and intravenous drug users themselves should include health teaching on the prevention of HIV transmission and health maintenance.

Nurses and other health professionals develop addictive illness at rates comparable to men and women in the general population. Professional organizations have formulated policies and outreach efforts to identify and provide assistance to practitioners with drug and alcohol problems. These efforts have resulted in changes in the employement setting to assist the nurse or other health care provider in seeking treatment as well as in re-entering practice.

BIBLIOGRAPHY

Alcohol and Health: Sixth Special Report to the U.S. Congress. National Institute of Alcohol Abuse and Alcoholism, Rockville, MD, 1987.

Alcohol Consumption and Related Problems. Alcohol and Health Monograph. National Institute of Alcohol Abuse and Alcoholism, Rockville, MD, 1982.

American Nurses' Association. Addictions and Psychological Dysfunctions in Nursing. Kansas City, MO, American Nurses' Association, 1984.

American Psychiatric Association. Diagnostic and Statistical Manual III. American Psychiatric Association, Washington, 1980.

Alexander, BK and Hadaway P: Opiate addiction: The case for an adaptive orientation. Psychological Bulletin 92:367, 1982.

Coleman, J: Abnormal Psychology and Modern Life. Scott Foresman & Co, Glenview, IL, 1982.

Galant, D: Alcoholism: A Guide to Diagnosis, Intervention and Treatment. W.W. Norton & Co, New York, 1987.

Goodwin, D: The genetics of alcoholism: A state of the art review. Alcohol Health and Research World, Spring 1978.

Gurel, M: Should courses for nurses that deal solely with alcoholism be taught in universities? Nursing Research 23:166, 1974.

Harlow, PE and Goby, MJ: Changing nursing student attitudes toward alcoholic patients: Examining the effects of a clinical practicum. Nursing Research 29:59, 1980.

Heinemann, ME, and Estes, NJ: Assessing alcohol patients. In Estes, NJ and Heinemann, ME (eds): Alcoholism: Development, Consequences, and Interventions. CV Mosby, St Louis, 1982.

Jellinek, E: Disease Concept of Alcoholism. United Printing Services, New Haven, 1960.

Kneisl, CR and Wilson, HS: Handbook of Psychosocial Nursing Care. Addison Wesley, Menlo Park, CA, 1984.

Loomis, T: The Pharmacology of Alcohol. In Estes, NJ and Heinemann, ME (eds): Alcoholism: Development, Consequences and Intervention. CV Mosby, St Louis, 1982.

Naegle, M: Creative management of impaired nursing practice. Nursing Administration Quarterly 9:16, 1985.

Naegle, M: The nurse and the alcoholic: Redefining an historically ambivalent relationship. Journal of Psychosocial and Mental Health Nursing, 24, 1983.

Powell, AH and Minick, MP: Alcohol withdrawal syndrome. Am J Nurs 88(3):313–314, 1988.

Resnick, HLP and Ruben, H: Emergency Psychiatric Care: The Management of Mental Health Crises. The Charles Press, Boston, 1975.

Stanton, D: A Family Theory of Drug Abuse. In Lettieri, D, Sayers, M, and Pearson HW (eds): Theories of Drug Abuse. National Institutes of Drug Abuse, Rockville, MD, 1984.

Streissguth, A and LaDue, R: Psychological and behavioral effects in children prenatally exposed to alcohol. Alcohol Health and Research World 10:1, 1985.

Vourakis, C and Bennett, G: Angel Dust: Not heaven sent. Am J Nurs 79:649, 1979.

Warren, K: Alcohol-related birth defects. Alcohol Health and Research World, 10:1, 1985.

Wilford, B: Drug Abuse: A Guide for the Primary Care Physician. American Medical Association, Chicago, 1981.

SITUATION   13–1

Mr. Shipley is a 46-year-old cocaine addict admitted by his wife to the acute care unit of a drug rehabilitation center.

1. The nurse admitting Mr. Shipley may observe the following physical effect of acute cocaine intoxication:
   a. pinpoint pupils
   b. cardiac arrhythmias
   c. slurred speech
   d. drowsiness

2. Mr. Shipley admits to drinking a "glass or two" of vodka along with cocaine use daily. The nurse is aware that the combination of alcohol and cocaine use represents:
   a. dual addiction
   b. cross tolerance
   c. mixed addiction
   d. dual tolerance

3. During the acute phase of intoxication related to stimulant use, the nurse will provide all of the following *except:*
   a. a safe environment for patient and others
   b. medication (Diazepam) to prevent seizures
   c. referral to the substance abuse team
   d. in-depth discussion about his drug use

4. Mr. Shipley experiences sleep disturbances related to withdrawal from cocaine. The best intervention for the nurse to include in planning care would be to:
   a. direct strenuous exercises
   b. administer strong sedatives
   c. allow long periods of privacy
   d. teach relaxation techniques

5. In planning teaching concerning the psychologic and physiologic effects of alcohol and cocaine use, the nurse will:
   a. focus on education aspects as soon as Mr. Shipley recovers from acute intoxication
   b. wait until Mr. Shipley initiates the interaction by asking questions
   c. plan initial education as an outpatient in group therapy if he consents
   d. initiate teaching concerning drug use only if ordered by the attending physician

6. Which of the following responses indicates an understanding by his wife of the best approach to take with Mr. Shipley?
   a. "He really does not have a bad problem, only when his work is stressful."
   b. "I tell him all the time that taking drugs and drinking will ruin his life."
   c. "I will no longer make excuses for him; we need to face the problem together."
   d. "He gets mad when I talk about the problem, so it's best to let him quit on his own."

SITUATION   13–2

Rebecca Long is a staff nurse working in the chemical dependency unit in a psychiatric hospital.

1. Sherry Trahan, a 17-year-old with a history of substance abuse, is in acute intoxication from Valium (depressant). Ms. Long will observe for the following:
   a. increased respiratory rate
   b. loss of superficial reflexes
   c. hypertension
   d. restlessness and rapid speech

2. Jason Williamson has been admitted with intoxication of unknown substance. He demonstrates severe anxiety and panic, needing to be restrained for violent behavior. Ms. Long is aware that these symptoms probably relate to:
   a. phencyclidines
   b. opioids
   c. sedatives
   d. marijuana

3. In planning interventions for patients in withdrawal from opioids (heroin, morphine), Ms. Long will include the following:
   a. providing a stimulating environment
   b. allowing for periods of isolation
   c. administering decreasing doses of opioids
   d. producing euphoria with medications

4. Mrs. Bruster is withdrawing from alcohol-benzodiazepine dependence. Ms. Long will anticipate the possible occurrence of seizures:
   a. around days 4 to 6
   b. between days 7 to 14
   c. within 48 hours
   d. after 2 weeks

5. When Samuel Franks, a 16-year-old, is admitted for LSD intoxication, Ms. Long prepares to implement all of the following *except:*
   a. administer antipsychotic medication
   b. provide reassurance and presence
   c. implement seizure precautions
   d. promote a quiet environment

6. Ms. Long will include all of the following as appropriate nursing goals for patients in acute intoxication induced by depressants, *except:*
   a. prevention of death and the development of further pathology
   b. promotion of health at the level possible for the patient
   c. provision of a safe, nonthreatening environment
   d. evidence of patient's desire to abstain from drug use

Please refer to the Appendices for correct answers and additional review questions with answers.

14

PHARMACOTHERAPEUTICS FOR THE NEONATE AND THE PEDIATRIC PATIENT

14

PHARMACOTHERAPEUTICS FOR THE NEONATE AND THE PEDIATRIC PATIENT

GLOSSARY TERMS IN THIS CHAPTER

Bilirubin
Botulism
Cephalocaudal
Hypertonic
Hypotonic
Isotonic
Proximodistal
Sebum
Stratum corneum

14 CHAPTER

PHARMACOTHERAPEUTICS FOR THE NEONATE AND THE PEDIATRIC PATIENT

CAROLYN SUE B. KIRSCH, M.S.N., R.N.-C.

LEARNING OBJECTIVES

After reading this chapter, the student will be able to:

1. Identify physiologic differences of neonates and children affecting the pharmacokinetic phases of drug administration.

2. Assess the neonate and pediatric patient to develop a data base utilizing principles of growth and development.

3. Formulate nursing diagnoses relevant to the neonate and pediatric patient.

4. Plan nursing interventions that are appropriate for drug administration to neonate and pediatric patients.

5. Evaluate the effectiveness of medications in patients of various ages.

6. Choose appropriate teaching strategies to gain pediatric patient compliance.

The first exposure to medication for most people occurs at an early age. Within the first hour after birth, erythromycin ophthalmic ointment or drops are put in the newborn's eyes to prevent an infectious conjunctivitis, and vitamin K is given to prevent hemorrhage. Vitamin supplements are often begun in infancy, and regular injections start at the age of two months with the first immunization. The developmental status of the child places him or her at greater risk for physical and psychological trauma related to medication administration. The nurse plays a vital role in assuring that medications are given safely and that good health habits regarding medication are begun in childhood.

Children are frequently referred to as "therapeutic orphans." A large percentage of the drugs on the market are not recommended for pediatric patients because their safety and efficacy for children have not been adequately established by drug manufacturers. Drug experimentation on children to determine whether or not a drug is safe for pediatric use has been ethically unacceptable. The primary problem is compounded by the cost of this type of research.

DOSE CALCULATIONS

There are important differences in the way children of different ages absorb, distribute, metabolize, and excrete drugs. An understanding of the physiology of the child makes it apparent that a child is not a smaller version of an adult. Size alone is not sufficient to determine drug dosage. Several formulas (Table 14–1) have been developed over the years to estimate pediatric dosage based on the adult dosage in combination with the child's weight (Clark's rule), the child's age in months (Fried's rule), and the child's age in years (Young's rule). The "150" in Fried's and Clark's rules refers to the "average" adult weight. All three formulas include the "average" adult dose. Formulas based on a child's age assume, inaccurately, that all children have the same height, weight, and physiology at the same age. These assumptions make the formulas too imprecise for determining pediatric dosages, especially the minute dosages required for newborns and infants.

A more reliable dosage method uses the body surface area (BSA) of the child, as BSA correlates more closely with the physiologic functions of the child than does age or weight. BSA is determined by plotting the child's height and weight on a nomogram (Fig. 14–1). A line is drawn between the two points. The point at which this line intersects the surface area line is the child's BSA. This value then can be used with the BSA formula in Table 14–1.

Another method is the calculation of dosages as a ratio of milligram of medication per kilogram of body weight of the child. This is a simple means of dosage determination, and many medication manuals are published with dosages expressed in this way. However, this method is not perfect because it does not consider maturation. The physiology of a normal two-month old infant weighing eleven pounds is different from a six-month old infant of the same weight with failure-to-thrive. A drug dosage based only upon weight would demonstate a different therapeutic effect in each infant, as the body systems affecting drug pharmacokinetics would be more mature in the six-month old infant.

PHARMACOKINETICS

ABSORPTION

Absorption is the process by which a drug moves from the site where the drug is given to the bloodstream. The drug administration routes that are affected mainly by physiologic differences in the pediatric patient are oral, intramuscular (IM), and topical. Intravenous (IV) administration places the drug directly into the bloodstream, and it therefore bypasses the absorption process.

Oral Medications

Several physiologic differences in the pediatric patient's gastrointenstinal tract affect the absorption of oral medications. Gastric emptying time is variable in the pediatric patient. In the newborn, the stomach empties in 2.5–3 hours. This can take up to six hours in the older infant and child. When gastric emptying is slow, drugs that are absorbed primarily in the stomach (for example, penicillins) are more completely absorbed, resulting in an increased therapeutic response. However, drugs that are absorbed in the intestines are delayed in reaching the intestine, resulting in a delayed therapeutic effect. Many conditions (such as gastritis) may cause gastric motility to increase suddenly. When the stomach rapidly empties its contents into the intestine, reverse timing of the therapeutic effects noted above is seen. As the infant matures, the stomach develops a more predictable emptying rate.

Table 14–1. FORMULAS FOR PEDIATRIC DOSAGE CALCULATION

Fried's rule (for patients under 1 year of age):

$$\frac{\text{Age in Months}}{150} \times \text{Adult Dose} = \text{Pediatric Dose}$$

Clark's rule (for patients over 2 years of age):

$$\frac{\text{Weight in Pounds}}{150} \times \text{Adult Dose} = \text{Pediatric Dose}$$

Young's rule (for patients over 2 years of age):

$$\frac{\text{Age in Years}}{\text{Age in years} + 12} \times \text{Adult Dose} = \text{Pediatric Dose}$$

BSA formula:

$$\frac{\text{Surface Area of Child}}{1.7} \times \text{Adult Dose} = \text{Pediatric Dose}$$

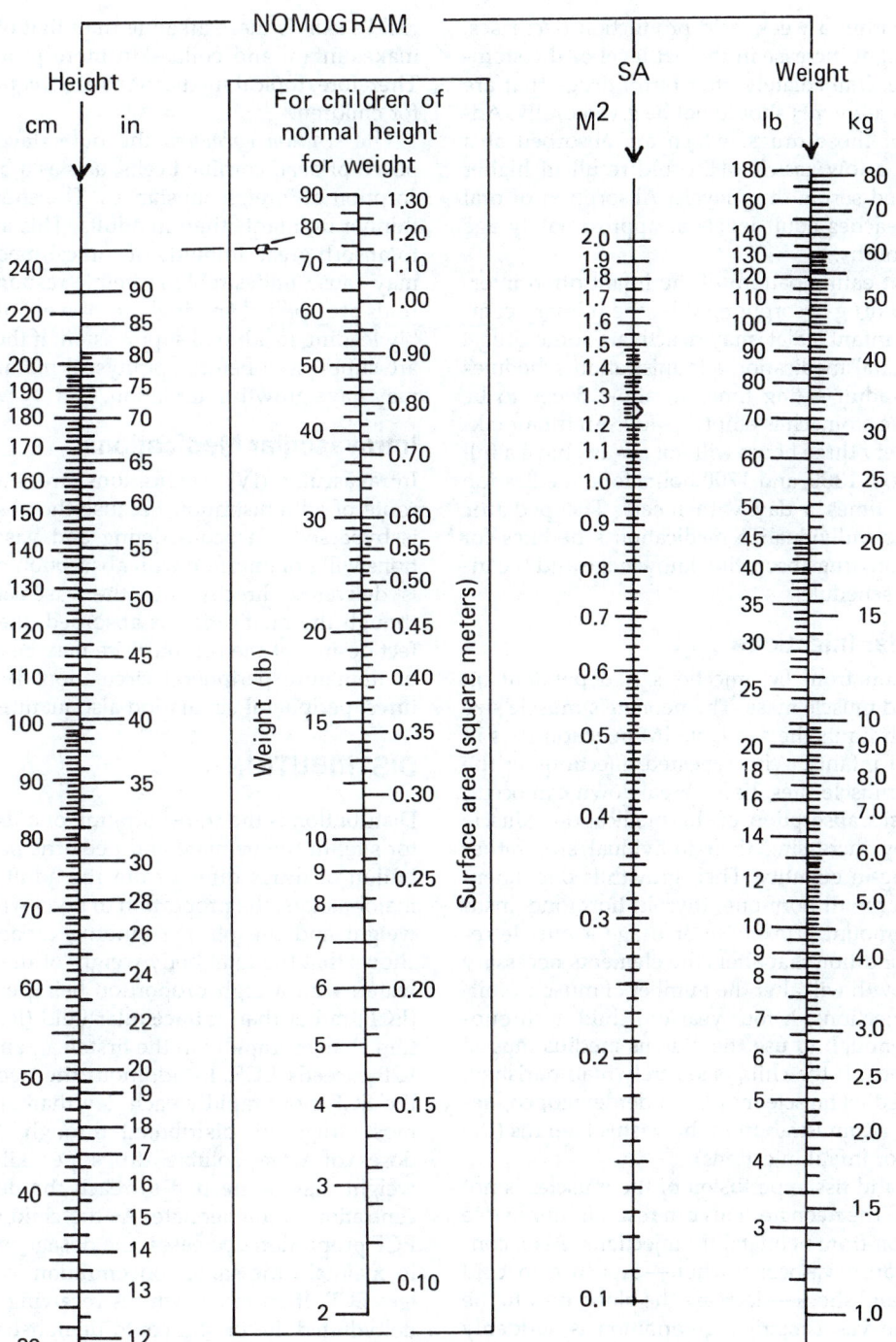

Figure 14–1. West's nomogram. Plot child's height and weight; draw a line between the two points. The point where this line intersects the surface area line is the child's surface area.

Drug absorption in the intestine is affected by the length of time the drug remains in contact with the intestinal surface. The newborn's intestine is six times his body length, and provides a proportionally greater surface area for drug absorption when compared to the adult intestine which is four to five times the adult body length. The infant's intestinal peristalsis is more rapid and unpredictable until the second year of life because of neuromuscular immaturity. When intestinal contents move rapidly through the intestines, contact time for drug absorption decreases. As a result, the medication's therapeutic effect decreases. In cases of diarrhea or the prolonged intestinal contact that results from anesthesia, an infant may be given IM or IV medications to avoid the rapid excretion of the drug that occurs when the oral route is used.

In the immediate newborn period, gastric acidity in the neonate rises, making the stomach pH similar to that of an adult. Within a week, acid production decreases, leading to a slight increase in the pH level of the stomach. Therefore, immediately after birth, drugs that are deactivated by a low pH should not be given orally. Administration of those drugs, which are absorbed at a higher rate in a low gastric pH, could result in higher than anticipated serum drug levels. Absorption of oral medications reaches adult levels at approximately age six to eight months.

The frequent eating pattern of the infant often interferes with oral drug absorption. Milk, the primary component of the infant's diet, may deactivate some drugs. Standard hospital medication administration schedules are based on adult eating times to allow drugs to be given when the stomach is empty or full. An infant taking a bottle every three hours will not always have a full stomach at 0900, 1300, and 1700 hours for a medication ordered three times a day with meals. The pediatric nurse needs to individualize medication schedules for infants based on drug absorption knowledge and the infant's feeding schedule.

Intramuscular Injections

Drug absorption from IM injections is dependent on blood flow and muscle mass. The neonate's muscle size is small, which limits the available IM injection sites in newborns and infants. With repeated injections in the few available muscle sites, tissue breakdown can occur, which decreases absorption of the medication. Muscle fibers grow by increasing their individual size rather than increasing in quantity. Their growth is dependent on nutrition, growth hormone, thyroid hormone, insulin, and the amount of exercise or usage a muscle receives. Any condition that alters the elements necessary for muscle growth will alter the number of muscles suitable for IM injections. A four-year-old child is chronologically old enough to use the gluteus medius muscle for IM injections. If the child is severely malnourished, the gluteus medius muscle may be underdeveloped, necessitating IM administration in the vastus lateralis (the muscle used for infant injections).

Blood flow and tissue perfusion of the muscles is not fully mature in the neonate. This can result in unreliable drug absorption from neonatal IM injections. Also, conditions that cause vasoconstriction—exposure to cold temperatures and shock—decrease the blood flow to the muscles. If the vasoconstricting condition is suddenly corrected, a drug previously given by IM injection would be rapidly absorbed. As the child grows, tissue perfusion increases, making the IM injection of drug administration more reliable.

Topical Medications

At birth, the sebaceous glands, which are active *in utero*, decrease their production of *sebum*. The eccrine sweat glands are immature and secrete less eccrine sweat than those of an adult. The normal acidity of the skin is due to the evaporation of sebum and eccrine sweat. The acidity of the skin acts as a bacteriocide to prevent skin infections by decreasing the multiplication of bacteria. Until the sebaceous and eccrine sweat glands mature, a slow continuous process from birth to puberty, the child's skin is more alkaline than that of the adult. This makes infant and child skin more prone to infections. Therefore, topical medications are frequently prescribed for children.

The *stratum corneum*, the outer layer of skin composed of dead cornified cells, acts as a barrier to the absorption of foreign substances. The stratum corneum is thinner in infants than in adults. This allows the infant to absorb great amounts of topical medications, which may cause undesirable systemic responses. Corticosteroids are applied sparingly to prevent absorption possibly leading to adrenal suppression. If the adrenal glands are suppressed before epiphyseal maturation, the child may have growth retardation.

Intravascular Medications

Intravascular (IV) medications are the most reliable route of administration because the absorption process is bypassed. Vasoconstricting and vasodilation conditions will not interfere with absorption because the drug is delivered directly into the vascular system. Even though the medication is absorbed, the therapeutic effect desired at the receptor site may be delayed because of immature peripheral circulation. As the child matures, peripheral circulation also matures.

DISTRIBUTION

Distribution is the transportation of a drug to the receptor site. In the neonate and pediatric patient, the distribution of drugs differs from the adult because of two major factors: the proportion of body water to total body weight and the plasma binding capacity. Table 14–2 shows that the total body weight of the neonate is 75% water, with a high proportion being extracellular fluid (ECF) rather than intracellular fluid (ICF). This proportion changes rapidly in the first year, and by adulthood, ICF exceeds ECF. In addition, the neonate exchanges the ECF more rapidly each day than an adult. Because most drugs are distributed through the ECF, higher doses of water-soluble drugs per kilogram of body weight may be needed to reach the desired drug concentration in the neonate. As the child matures and the ECF proportion decreases, the dosage may be decreased to maintain the same concentration, compensating for less ECF. If an infant who is receiving a drug becomes dehydrated, he or she could demonstrate signs of toxicity because the drug would become more concentrated until the infant can be rehydrated.

Only 15% of the neonate's body weight is fat tissue.

Table 14–2. BODY FLUIDS

Age	Total Body Fluids in Relation to Total Body Weight	Extracellular Fluid in Relation to Total Body Weight
Birth	75%	40%
One yr	60%	28%
Adult	55%	20%

Table 14–3. SERUM ALBUMIN

Neonate	3.0–4.5 g/dl
Infant	3.8–5 g/dl
Five yr to adult	4.5–6 g/dl

As the child grows, body fat increases proportionally. Therefore, a neonate needs a smaller dose of a fat-soluble drug with an increase in the dose proportional to the increase in fat tissue to maintain the same concentration for the older child.

When drugs enter the bloodstream, they bind to plasma proteins, mainly albumin. Factors influencing protein binding are the amount of albumin available for binding; the blood pH; the affinity the albumin has for a drug (binding capacity); and substances in the system competing for binding sites on the available albumin. In the neonate, there is less albumin available for binding with drugs (Table 14–3). In addition, the binding capacity of the available albumin appears to be less than in the adult (Roberts, 1984). It is the free (unbound) drug circulating in the system that causes the pharmacologic effect. Because the neonate and the infant have a larger proportion of the drug unbound, there is a greater risk for developing a toxic reaction to the drug. Most of the unbound drug is metabolized and excreted quickly. The smaller amount of the drug bound to the albumin is released slowly, resulting in a decreased pharmacologic effect. To prevent toxicity and to compensate for the shorter duration of drug action, it may be necessary to decrease the amount of the drug given and to shorten the interval between dosages. Therefore, an infant receiving 100 mg of a particular drug every four hours may receive the same therapeutic effect as an older child who is given 150 mg of the same drug every six hours.

The final consideration to be discussed in drug distribution involves the presence of other substances in the system. Hormones, drugs, and bilirubin compete for available protein binding sites. After birth, maternal hormones, which are bound to the proteins, are left in the neonate's system. Until these hormones are released

and excreted, there is a decrease in the number of available binding sites.

Bilirubin has a strong binding affinity for albumin. Immediately after birth, the serum bilirubin level rises because of the breakdown of fetal hemoglobin. This leaves few albumin binding sites available for drugs in the neonate. Normally, serum bilirubin levels begin to decrease on the fifth day. If a drug having a stronger binding power than bilirubin is given, such as a salicylate or a sulfonamide, the bilirubin could be released by the albumin. Because myelinization of the central nervous system (CNS) is incomplete at birth, the blood–brain barrier has increased permeability. This allows the free bilirubin to enter the CNS, which can cause brain damage. Conversely, if a drug with a weak binding power is given to a neonate whose available sites were saturated by bilirubin, the drug would remain unbound and a toxic effect of the drug could be seen.

METABOLISM

Metabolism or biotransformation is the breaking down of drugs into harmless substances, which are then excreted by the body. The liver is the major organ responsible for biotransformation of drugs. The neonate's liver is 4% of body weight as compared to 2% in the adult. Despite the neonate's liver size, the organ is immature at birth. This causes some of the liver enzymes to be less effective for drug biotransformation. Therefore, a drug may remain active in the neonate's body for a longer period of time (an increased half-life) and prolong the therapeutic effect of the drug. After the first two to three weeks of life, a sudden increase in metabolism occurs that can cause the half-life of a drug to decrease drastically, resulting in a shorter period of therapeutic effect.

The metabolic rate of a child peaks at about 24 months of age and then decreases as the child matures. Table 14–4 shows examples of the metabolic effect of the liver on the half-life of some commonly used drugs for children. For example, the rate of theophylline metabolism in a child can be double that of an adult. In order to maintain a therapeutically effective serum level

Table 14–4. APPROXIMATE HALF-LIVES OF VARIOUS DRUGS IN NEONATES AND ADULTS

Drug	Neonatal Age	Neonates (t − 1/2)*	Adults (t − 1/2)*
Acetaminophen		2.2–5	1.9–2.2
Diazepam		25–100	15–25
Digoxin		60–107	30–60
Phenobarbitol	0–5 days	200	64–140
	5–15 days	100	
	1–30 months	50	
Phenytoin	0–2 days	80	12–18
	3–14 days	18	
	14–50 days	6	
Salicylate		4.5–11	2–4
Theophylline	Neonate	3–10	5–6
	Child	3–4	

*Half-lives in hours.
From Cohen, MS: Principles of Drug Disposition and Therapy in Infants and Children. In Rudolph, AM (ed.): Pediatrics. Appleton-Century-Crofts, Norwalk, CT, 1982, with permission.

of the drug, it may be necessary to decrease the dosage interval.

Body temperature regulation is unstable in children. Infants and toddlers frequently develop sudden high temperatures in response to an infection, which increases their metabolic rate. For each degree centigrade rise in body temperature, the metabolic rate increases by 12%. This increased metabolism will decrease the half-life of a drug and the duration of the therapeutic effect.

EXCRETION

Drugs can be excreted by way of the skin, respiratory tract, hepatobiliary system, or kidneys. Because the majority of drugs are excreted by the kidney, it is important to note the differences between the neonate's kidney and that of the adult. The neonate has all the glomerular cells at birth, but they are functionally immature. Thus the glomerular filtration rate (GFR) of the infant is approximatley one third that of the adult. The GFR increases by 50% at three weeks of age and reaches adult levels by age six to twelve months. Digoxin is an example of a drug that is dependent on GFR. Because of the rapid increase in the GFR during the first few weeks of life, the dosage of digoxin may have to be increased to maintain the serum drug level.

Renal tubular secretory mechanisms are incompletely developed at birth, which decreases the neonate's ability to excrete drugs. This is due to a smaller number of tubular cells, a shorter tubular length, and a lower tubular blood flow. Tubular secretion reaches adult levels at about seven months of age as the tubules grow and mature. Renal blood flow increases as systemic arterial pressure increases and intrarenal vascular resistance decreases. This allows the kidneys to receive a larger proportion of the total cardiac output and the circulating medication to be excreted. Therefore, drugs that are dependent on tubular secretion, such as penicillins, have an increased half-life in the neonate and infant.

Drug excretion is also influenced by the pH of the urine, because some drugs are more rapidly excreted in acidic urine while other drugs require a more basic urine to promote excretion. An infant's kidney has a decreased ability to excrete hydrogen ions and reabsorb filtered bicarbonate ions. This makes the newborn's urine slightly less acidic than adult urine with a pH of 5–7. Drug doses may need to be adjusted to maintain an appropriate serum drug level if excretion is dependent on a more acidic urine.

USING THE NURSING PROCESS

ASSESSMENT OF THE PEDIATRIC PATIENT

The nursing assessment of the pediatric patient includes a thorough physical and developmental assessment of the child. The physical assessment relevant to medica-

tion administration includes height, weight, physical handicaps, and data concerning the current illness. The doctor uses the child's height and weight to determine the medication dose. The nurse uses this data to double-check the dose before administration. A child's physical handicap can change the nurse's approach to the child when giving a drug. For example, the nurse would let a six-year-old blind child feel the IV equipment before the infusion is started, because an explanation alone would not be as beneficial. Data relevant to the current illness is necessary for comparison with data obtained after a drug has been instituted to evaluate the therapeutic effectiveness of the medication.

A developmental assessment reveals the capabilities of the child. Growth and development have a predictable pattern which all children follow, *cephalocaudal* (head-to-toe) and *proximodistal* (near-to-far). Each child has his own individual time schedule as to when each developmental milestone is reached. One child may walk at age ten months, while another child does not walk until age fifteen months. The nurse uses knowledge of growth and development to predict his or her approach to a child and predict the child's response to the nurse. For example, the nurse knows a ten-month-old infant will probably have stranger anxiety. Therefore, it may be helpful for the parent to hold the child while the nurse administers the oral medication.

A developmental assessment reveals the capabilities of the child, such as the child's ability to take a medication and the ability to understand the situation. An alert, healthy five-year-old child can be taught to swallow pills. A five-year-old child with spastic cerebral palsy may have the intelligence to understand instructions in learning to swallow pills but may lack the coordination to do it.

A medication history would consider the following: Is the child taking any medication now? If yes, what is being taken and in what dosage? Why was it prescribed and how long has the child been taking it? Does the child or family know the side effects of the medication, and have any side effects been observed? How is the medication being administered to the child, and have there been any problems getting the child to take the medication? Does the child have any allergies?

The initial assessment also includes a family assessment, which determines how the child interacts with the parents. The nurse may identify one parent favored by the child in a stressful situation. Parental anxiety usually is increased when a child is ill, and unknowingly, the parents may transmit this anxiety to the child. A toddler sensing this anxiety may falsely believe the anxiety is due to the presence of the nurse and may react to the nurse based on this belief. All interactions during this initial encounter are beneficial to the nurse-child-parent relationship because the parents are also assessing the nurse.

NURSING DIAGNOSES AND GOALS

Data obtained during the nursing assessment is utilized by the nurse to determine nursing diagnoses and goals for the patients. Much of the data obtained from the assessment of the pediatric patient also includes information concerning the parents. This is especially evident in connection with the emotional and psychological assessment of the child-parent relationship. Therefore, many of the nursing diagnoses used for a pediatric patient will also include the parents.

All assessment data is important in developing nursing diagnoses. The pediatric patient's developmental assessment assists the nurse in determining nursing diagnoses related to medication administration. Table 14–5 demonstrates how nursing diagnoses and goals may be applied to developmental data obtained from pediatric patients of various ages.

Table 14–5. NURSING PROCESS FOR THE PEDIATRIC CLIENT

Assessment

Measure height, weight for calculation of body surface area/drug dosage.
Note developmental level.
Ascertain medication history, current drugs/dosage, length of treatment, drug form/route of administration, presence of side effects, allergies.
Evaluate family finances/ability to afford required therapy.

Nursing Diagnosis	Nursing Actions	Rationale	Patient Outcomes/ Evaluation Criteria
Aspiration, potential for related to inadequate swallowing and gag reflex.	Choose form of oral drugs appropriate to developmental level. Place small amounts of liquid medications in the side of the mouth or pocket of the cheek. Do not introduce more medication until the infant has completely swallowed.	Infant's tongue thrusts forward pushing object out of the mouth, when it is touched. (Extrusion reflex, present from birth to age four months). Toddlers resist the unknown and may struggle and scream when approached with medication.	Swallows medication without choking.
	Crush tablets, open capsules, dependent on pharmacotherapeutics of the drug. Provide drug in firm, matter-of-fact approach.	Making medication easier to take facilitates administration. Usually effective in gaining child's cooperation. Forcing drug ingestion by holding patient's nose increases danger of aspiration.	
Anxiety (specify level)/ Fear related to situational crisis, unknowns and/or previous experiences as evidenced by increased tension, apprehension, trembling, crying.	Explain procedure and the equipment in advance. Encourage child to express feelings about the procedure through play therapy and verbal expression (dependent on age/developmental level). Provide opportunity for patient input into medication administration by allowing appropriate choices.	Preparation for a procedure at appropriate developmental level promotes more effective coping and gives the child a sense of control. The adolescent is struggling to become independent from authority figures. Dependency increases feelings of inadequacy.	Displays calmer manner and cooperates with activity, receiving proper dose of medication.
	Offer medications in a nonauthoritative manner.	Children may become terrified when they are "overpowered" by a stranger who is	

CONTINUED ON THE FOLLOWING PAGE

Table 14–5. NURSING PROCESS FOR THE PEDIATRIC CLIENT–CONTINUED

Nursing Diagnosis	Nursing Actions	Rationale	Patient Outcomes/ Evaluation Criteria
		bigger and stronger making it difficult to administer drug.	
	Encourage child's participation, e.g., place pills in child's hand or in mouth. Offer liquids in cups appropriate for hand and mouth size.	Preschooler has use of many gross motor skills but is continuing to refine fine motor skills.	
	Allow parent to remain in room during procedure.	Provides emotional support.	
	Have parent hold child while nurse administers medications and continue to hold and cuddle child after medication is given.	Enhances sense of safety and promotes optimal intake of drug. Helps child to regain composure and accept situation.	
Injury, potential for poisoning/toxicity related to type of drug, dosage, route of administration, and storage method.	Calculate drug dosage correctly and double check before administering.	Prevents errors with subsequent over/under medication.	Demonstrates beneficial effects of medication with no untoward side effects. Parents identify potential hazards and formulate plan to reduce risk factors.
	Verify identity of patient via parent/identification bracelet.	Assures that medication is administered to the right patient.	
	Thoroughly shake suspensions before measuring.	Provides for uniformity in dosage.	
	Administer liquids via calibrated medication spoon/dropper.	Allows for precise measurement of dosage.	
	Administer IM injections considering blood flow and muscle mass.	Affects rate of drug absorption.	
	Apply topical medications with care.	Stratum corneum is thinner in infants allowing greater absorption of drug and increasing risk of undesirable systemic response.	
	Maintain hydration according to size and age of child.	Development of dehydration can increase risk of toxicity in infants as drug becomes more concentrated in extracellular fluid.	
	Evaluate therapeutic effectiveness of medication, monitor serum drug levels if available.	May need to alter drug dosage/choice to achieve desired effects.	
	Note development of side effects.	Side effects of medications are often difficult to evaluate but may require changes in timing (i.e., with/without food) or discontinuation dependent on type/severity of reaction.	
	Monitor body temperature.	Fluctuations alter metabolic rate affecting drug half-life and duration of therapeutic effect.	

Table 14–5. NURSING PROCESS FOR THE PEDIATRIC CLIENT–CONTINUED

Nursing Diagnosis	Nursing Actions	Rationale	Patient Outcomes/ Evaluation Criteria
	Review safety precautions with parents/care provider, e.g., proper storage and use of medications, availability of ipecac syrup, provision of emergency phone numbers.	Prevents accidental ingestion of drug. Provides for rapid action if accident occurs.	
Knowledge deficit related to lack of exposure/unfamiliarity of information resources as evidenced by questions, verbalization of concerns.	Establish individual medication schedule based on drug absorption and feeding schedule.	Increases compliance in administering drug when schedule fits particular family's routine.	Verbalizes understanding of therapeutic regimen.
	Discuss timing of food, use of milk products, acidic liquids.	May prevent side effects, inactivation of drug.	
	Suggest combining crushed pills with jelly, applesauce, pudding, not liquids.	Powder often does not dissolve and a grainy residue remains in cup reducing dosage delivered.	
	Recommend following drug with water, oral hygiene as indicated.	Clears drug and possible aftertaste, reduces potential for adverse dental effects.	
	Stress importance of continuing drug until completed or discontinued by physician.	Promotes optimal effect of medication.	
	Refer to Social Services as indicated.	May require financial assistance.	

PLANNING AND INTERVENTION

After determining that the ordered medication is appropriate and that the ordered dosage is safe, the nurse should begin the interventions by identifying an accurate, reasonable, and safe method for administration. This is especially important if the medication is to be given at home by the family. If the administration of medication becomes a complicated and time-consuming procedure, the level of compliance decreases.

If a unit dose is not available, the nurse must determine the child's dose from the available dosage form. This is a critical step in the administration of medication to pediatric patients because this is frequently where errors occur. Even the most conscientious nurse in a hectic pediatric unit can misplace a decimal point, make an addition or subtraction mistake, or accidentally read "μg" for "mg." To maintain safety, the nurse should double-check the calculation with another nurse; even a small error can be potentially lethal to a small child.

It is difficult to concentrate on calculating a child's medication dose in an emergency situation. To prevent a medication error, some hospitals require a critically ill child's crib or bed to have an emergency drug card attached stating the correct dose for resuscitation medications, based on the child's weight. The card is updated as the child's weight changes. This information will benefit all personnel, especially those who are not familiar with pediatric dosages, and protect the patient. Figure 14–2 is an example of an emergency drug card.

When administering a medication to any patient, it is vitally important to properly identify the patient. In pediatrics, this often presents more of a problem than in adult nursing. Infants are unable to identify themselves; young children may disavow their identity because they do not want the medication; and adolescents often feel it is fun to misidentify themselves to an authority figure. Therefore, the only acceptable means of identifying a pediatric patient is to read the patient's identification bracelet.

Oral Medications

Standard medicine cups and teaspoons are not totally accurate for measuring liquid medications. Household teaspoons vary in size and can cause inaccurate dose administration. Calibrated medication spoons, available at pharmacies, will allow precise measurement of one teaspoon. To measure quantities less than one teaspoon (five ml), an oral syringe, if available, is used to draw up (and possibly administer) the medication. If an oral syringe is not available, an IM syringe (tuberculin syringe for amounts of less than one ml) can be used, if care is

EMERGENCY DRUG CARD

Name _____

Doctor _____

Weight _____ Kg.   Date _____

Diagnosis _____

DRUG	NORMAL DOSE	ROUTE	CALCULATED DOSE
Atropine	0.01 to 0.02 mg/kg/dose	IV, ETT	_____
10% Calcium gluconate	1 to 2 ml/kg/dose	IV	_____
Dopamine	2 to 5 μg/kg/minute initially. 5 to 10 μg/kg/minute may be required.	IV	_____
Epinephrine 1:10,000	0.1 ml/kg	IV, ETT, IC	_____
Naloxone	0.01 mg/kg/dose	IV	_____
Na HCO$_3$	1 mEq/kg/dose every 10 minutes, × 2 doses. Dilute 1:1 with sterile water.	IV	_____

IV—Intravenous

ETT—Endotracheal tube

IC—Intracardiac

Figure 14–2. Emergency Drug Card.

taken to remove and destroy the needle immediately to prevent its being mistaken for a parenteral medication. Some liquid medications are supplied with their own calibrated droppers. These droppers should not be used for any other medication.

Children under age five years often have difficulty swallowing pills and may aspirate them. Before the nurse crushes any medication supplied only in pill form, it is important to determine if this will interfere with pharmacotherapeutics of the drug. If crushed, some enteric-coated pills are deactivated by the high gastric acidity. To crush a tablet, the nurse places it between two souffle cups or leaves it in the sealed unit package and grinds it with a pestle. The powder can then be mixed with a small amount of jelly or applesauce. Using only a small amount of jelly or fruit ensures that the child will not have a large volume to take, especially if the child is not cooperative. If the crushed tablet is mixed with a liquid, the powder often does not dissolve and a grainy residue is left in the cup, so the child does not receive a full dose. Crushed pills should not be mixed with honey for children under six months of age because some cases of infant botulism have been linked to spore-contaminated honey (Hazinski, 1984).

Liquid preparations are either suspensions or elixirs. In suspensions, the drug particles are suspended in a medium and settle out when allowed to stand. If suspensions are not shaken thoroughly, the first doses from the bottle contain less of the drug and the last doses contain more of the drug. Elixirs are alcohol-based and the

drug is evenly dissolved in the liquid, so it is not necessary to shake the container.

Many liquid medicines are bad tasting. The nurse should taste a drop of the liquid if it is not detrimental to his or her health. This helps the nurse to know which medicines should be followed by juice or formula, if these "follow-ups" do not interfere with absorption of the drug. Even though many of the liquids are artificially flavored, they may leave an unpleasant aftertaste.

Children who have a sore throat will resist a liquid medication that causes burning. Before giving the drug, allow the child to dissolve a teaspoon of crushed ice in the mouth, which has a numbing effect on the throat. This is often helpful for tonsillectomy and adenoidectomy (T and A) patients who deny pain because the acetaminophen with codeine hurts their throats.

Drug manufacturers have developed alternative oral dosage forms for children who have difficulty swallowing tablets. Some drugs are available as chewable tablets. Aspirin and vitamins are well accepted by children because they are pleasant-tasting, chewable tablets. Theo-Dur Sprinkle, a theophylline preparation, is a capsule containing small beads of medication. The capsule is opened and the beads are sprinkled over a spoonful of soft food such as ice cream or pudding. The pediatric nurse should become familiar with alternative dosage forms and become aware of new forms that may facilitate the child's ability to cooperate.

Following oral drug administration, the mouth should be rinsed and/or the teeth brushed because the sugar in the suspensions and the jelly transporting the powder can lead to dental caries. An infant or toddler not capable of rinsing can be given water to drink. This is especially important for doses given at bedtime.

Once a patient has been properly identified, the nurse proceeds in a calm manner and approaches the child as though the child is expected to take the medication. Do not give choices when the child does not have a choice. For example, the nurse should say, "Now it is time to take your medicine," rather than asking, "Do you want to take your medicine now?" Because most children, toddlers and older, want some control in a situation, offer them appropriate choices: "Do you want to wash your medicine down with water or juice?" Do not allow delaying tactics to work. Children often hope if they delay the unpleasant long enough, it will go away, but instead, this increases their anxiety. Also, do not lie, threaten, or try to bribe the child.

If the nurse assumes a matter-of-fact approach, presents the medication to the child, and offers a drink to be taken after the medication, the child usually cooperates. However, if the child refuses to cooperate, the nurse must be firm and take control of the situation. Forcing a screaming child to swallow medication by holding his or her nose is NEVER acceptable because this increases the danger of aspiration.

To administer liquid medications to an infant, small quantities of the liquid are directed toward the side of the mouth or placed in the pouch of the cheek to prevent aspiration. If the medication is being administered by oral syringe or dropper, a spoon can be used to readminister medication that is spit out. Young infants may swallow the medication more readily if a nipple is placed in the mouth after the medication is given. The use of a nipple to administer a drug is controversial because the infant may associate the nipple with medication and begin refusing the bottle at feeding time.

The nurse must be careful not to approach the child in too forceful a manner and must always explain what he or she is doing. Children, like anyone else, become terrified when they are overpowered by someone bigger and stronger. Their natural reacton is either to fight back or to become hysterical. Either reaction makes it extremely difficult to properly administer a drug. Some children do better if held by the parent. Most children, no matter how young, can accept unpleasant treatments and procedures if the explanation is at their level and is honest.

Parents' suggestions regarding medication administration may be helpful because parents are usually aware of their child's strengths and weaknesses. If, however, the nurse determines that the child is manipulating the parents and not cooperating, the nurse takes control and gives the medication.

Intramuscular Injections

Medication administered by injection can be a difficult experience for the child, the parents, and sometimes for the nurse. A child who is crying and upset because he or she is frightened and hurting is painful to observe. The nurse should keep in mind that the unpleasant and painful procedure is being done for the benefit of the child and not as a punishment. Children are very accepting if honest explanations are given.

To determine the proper injection site for a child, consult Table 14–6 and Figure 14–3. The infant's small muscle mass limits the nurse's choice of injection sites. In the infant, the gluteus is not used because it is small and the sciatic nerve is in close proximity to the muscle. The vastus lateralis is the first muscle of choice because it is well developed and does not have major nerves and blood vessels. The rectus femoris may be used as an alternative site or for rotating injection sites. It is a large muscle and promotes medication absorption. Both muscles are pinched up firmly between the thumb and forefinger of one hand and the needle is inserted at a 90° angle with the other hand. This helps the nurse instill the medication directly into the muscle without hitting the femur. When using the vastus lateralis in a neonate or infant with small muscles, the needle may be inserted at a 45° angle toward the knee to keep the needle tip within the muscle. A maximum of 1 ml is given. A very small muscle may only tolerate 0.50 ml. Even an infant needs to be restrained firmly with his knee held down as he will react to the pain of the injection by trying to move his leg. After the injection is completed, the child

Table 14–6. INTRAMUSCULAR INJECTION SITES

Age Group	Site	Needle Length	Needle Gauge	Max Sol
Infant	Vastus lateralis	⅝ in	25–27	1 ml
	Rectus femoris	⅝ in	25–27	1 ml
Toddler	Vastus lateralis	1 in	22–23	1 ml
	Rectus femoris	1 in	22–23	1 ml
	Dorsogluteal	1 in	22–23	1 ml
Preschool	Same as toddler; can also	1 in	22–23	1.5 ml
	use ventrogluteal, deltoid	1 in	22–23	1.5 ml
		1 in	22–23	1 ml
School-age and adolescent	Same as preschool-age child	1–1.5 in	22–23	2 ml

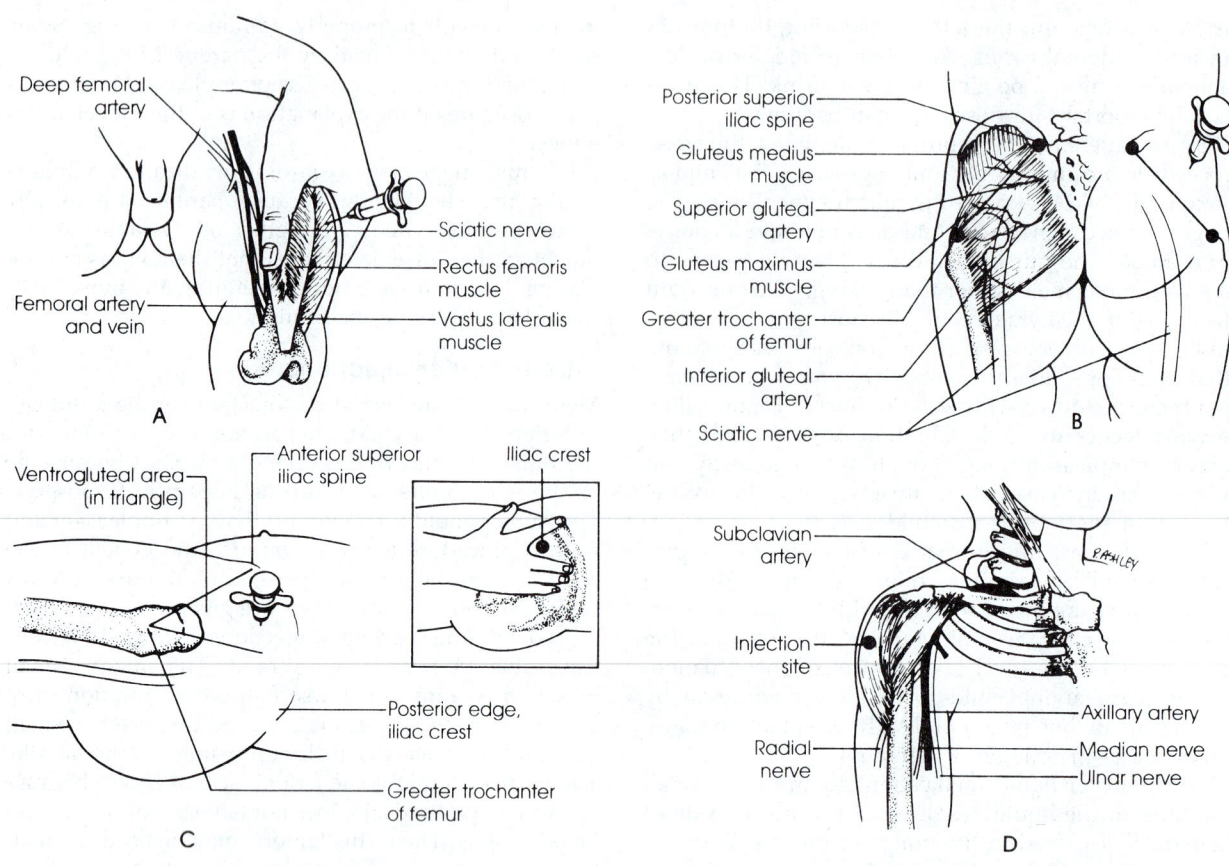

Figure 14–3. Intramuscular drug sites for the pediatric patient. A) Vastus lateralis; alternative site, rectus femoris. B) Gluteus medius muscle. C) Ventrogluteal area. D) Deltoid muscle. (From Marlow, DR: Textbook of Pediatric Nursing. WB Saunders, Philadelphia, 1988, p. 289, with permission.)

should be held and cuddled, preferably by the parents. If they are not available, the nurse should comfort the child.

The same muscles can be used for the toddler, along with the dorsogluteal muscle, after the child has been walking for one year. Because the amount of solution to be injected is determined by muscle size and walking increases the size of the muscle, up to 1.0 ml can be given with a one-inch needle. The toddler usually demonstrates resistance. Therefore, the nurse will need assistance in restraining him or her. As with the infant, the toddler should be held afterward.

In the preschooler, the ventrogluteal muscle and the deltoid muscles can be used in addition to the muscles used in the toddler. The ventrogluteal muscle is relatively free of blood vessels and nerves. The deltoid muscle is usually not used for injections prior to age three to four years because it is not well developed. In addition, the radial and ulnar nerves and the brachial artery, which lie along the humerus bone in the upper arm, can be injured. When using the deltoid muscle, the needle is angled toward the shoulder and no more than 1.0 ml is injected. The deltoid muscle is relatively small but has a rapid absorption rate. The preschooler may be very vocal and verbally lash out at the nurse in addition to physically kicking and hitting. The nurse should not take this as a personal insult. If the child was expecting

to receive an injection, he or she may be hiding, and the nurse may have to look for him or her. Adequate restraint will be needed with the preschooler.

The same muscles can be used in the school-age child and the adolescent as are used in the adult. Assessment of the muscle size determines if the nurse uses a 1- or 1.5-inch needle, with no more than 2.0 ml solution being given in one site. The school-age child may show interest in the equipment and likes to learn new words. Teaching him the word "syringe" instead of the word "needle" makes him feel important and may help to distract him during the injection. Even though many school-age children try to cooperate and be brave, the nurse will need assistance in restraining as they may forget their bravery once the needle is in the muscle. Adolescents generally react as adults.

Toddlers and preschool children are told about the injection just before the injection is given. This prevents unnecessary anxiety and fantasizing. Adolescents and school-age children are told about the injection ahead of time to allow them to prepare themselves. For example, it might be appropriate to tell a school-age child about a preoperative injection when the preoperative teaching is being done. The explanation is honest. "Yes, an injection hurts for a short time." Explain what is expected of the child. "It is okay to cry, but it is very important for you to hold still."

To help a child view the parent as a source of comfort, a parent should not be asked to help restrain a child for a painful procedure. If a child wishes the parents to be there, they should be allowed to stay but only to give emotional support to the child. Allow them to stand at the head of the bed where the child can see them and possibly hold one of their hands. It is often preferable to give children injections in the treatment room so that they have privacy and feel free to cry without fear of their peers hearing them. This also allows them to feel safe in their own hospital room and to associate painful procedures with the treatment room. An injection should never be given to a sleeping child without awakening him or her first, because the child may develop a fear of going to sleep. Telling a child to yell ''ouch'' or to squeeze someone's hand during the injection may provide enough distraction to minimize the pain. When the gluteal site is used, ask the child to turn the toes inward to help relax the gluteal muscle. Always be sure to praise the child when the procedure is done. Always finish the procedure as quickly as possible once it is started. Unnecessary delays only increase the child's anxiety. Utilizing therapeutic play also helps the child work through feelings and fears.

Intravenous Medications

The common sites for IV infusions in infants and young children can be seen in Figure 14–4. Scalp veins may be used in infants. These veins are covered with only a thin layer of subcutaneous tissue and are easily seen. A small area of the scalp is shaved to increase visualization and allow the tape to adhere to the scalp. It is preferable to insert the needle in the direction of the venous flow but it may be inserted in either direction because scalp veins do not have valves. Veins in the feet, hands, and arms may also be used for IV infusions. If the veins can be visualized in both hands, do not use the dominant extremity. Young children are in the process of developing and perfecting their fine motor skills and become frustrated when they must use the nondominant hand.

Needle size is determined by the size of the vein and the solutions to be administered. Usually 27–21 gauge needles are used for neonates and children.

All children under age twelve should have a volume control chamber in their IV line. The chambers have various names—Buratrol, Soluset, or Volutrol—depending upon the manufacturer. A volume control chamber is a safety precaution to prevent accidental fluid overload. No more than a one- or two-hour amount of solution should be put into the chamber at any time. If the IV tubing clamp becomes dislodged, the child only receives the fluid from the chamber, thus preventing fluid overload. Fluid chambers may also be used in conjunction with IV infusion pumps. If the machine malfunctions or a child plays with the dials controlling the infusion rate, the fluid chamber prevents fluid overload.

Medications may be added to the fluid chamber if they are compatible with the primary solution. If the medication is not compatible with the primary solution, it is mixed in a separate, small-volume solution bag. The primary IV tubing is flushed with 5–10 ml normal saline

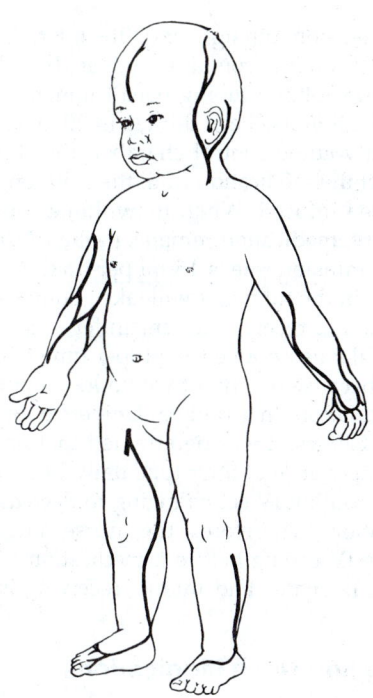

Figure 14–4. Superficial veins used most frequently for intravenous infusion. (From Kempe, CH et al.: Current Pediatric Diagnosis and Treatment, ed. 9. Appleton & Lange, E. Norwalk, CT, 1987, with permission.)

or 5% dextrose in water and the medication is piggybacked into the primary IV tubing. When the medication is finished, the primary tubing is flushed again and the primary solution is returned to the proper infusion rate. This is the same procedure used with adults receiving two incompatible medications or solutions.

Some medications will form a precipitate when mixed with the solution in the IV tubing and can clog the IV needle. This occurs when phenytoin (Dilantin) is added to 5% dextrose in water. It is important to prevent this in all patients, especially infants and small children, as it is often difficult to locate another vein for the IV infusion.

All medications must be properly diluted and should approximate an *isotonic* solution, 280–290 mOsm/liter. A *hypertonic* solution can cause a fluid shift from the ICF to the ECF in addition to being irritating to the vein. A *hypotonic* solution can cause movement in the opposite direction. Also, a large amount of diluent presents the danger of fluid overload, especially in an infant or a very small child receiving frequent IV medications. It is essential to know proper dilution amounts. These can be found in this book (see Appendix D), in manuals produced by hospital pharmacies, and in the manufacturer's insert literature packaged with the medication. If the dilution given is for an adult dose, the nurse must calculate the appropriate amount required for the child by using a proportional calculation.

The amount of solution in the IV tubing is an important consideration for the pediatric patient. This amount is different for each patient because the total amount present is dependent on the tubing size, its length (including extension tubing), and the filter. Five feet of standard IV tubing contains almost 10 ml solution, whereas low-volume tubing (small lumen) has 0.3 ml. If the medication has been diluted in 20 ml solution and placed in a volume control chamber, the child will not begin to get the medication until the solution in the tubing has been infused. When the volume control chamber is empty, medication remains in the IV tubing. If an infant's IV infusion rate is 15 ml per hour with 10 ml of medication in the tubing, it will take another 40 minutes for the infant to receive the remainder of the drug.

This would also not be the proper time to change the IV tubing because the infant would lose a portion of his or her medication. In a study at University of Iowa Hospitals and Clinics, it was determined that neonates lost approximately 36% of their total daily IV medication as a result of routine IV set changing to decrease bacterial contamination. Therefore, the nurse must plan to change the IV tubing before a medication is given, especially in neonates and infants receiving infusions at slow rates.

Eye, Ear, and Nose Medications

In administering eye, ear, or nose drops to children a major difficulty occurs with obtaining the child's cooperation, and the nurse may be required to restrain the child.

When administering eye drops, the child is placed in a supine position. The nurse rests the heel of his or her hand on the child's forehead, while holding the dropper with the forefinger and thumb. This is not only a safety precaution, but it also allows the nurse to move with the child and ensure that the medication goes into the child's eye and not onto the face. The eyelids are gently separated with the thumb and index finger of the opposite hand, and the drops or medication placed along the conjunctiva of the lower lid. The dropper or tip of the ointment tube should not touch any part of the eyelid in order to prevent contamination of the remaining medication.

To administer ear drops, the nurse must restrain the child with the head turned to the appropriate side. For children under three years of age, the pinna of the ear is pulled downward and back. For children over three years, the pinna is pulled upward and back, as for adults. The child should remain in this position for a few minutes (lying on the unaffected side) after instillation. If cotton is placed in the ear, it must be loose enough to allow discharge of any drainage.

Nose drops are instilled as for adults, with the head extending over the edge of the bed or examining table. The child should remain in this position for at least 1 minute following instillation.

Rectal Medications

Before inserting a rectal suppository, the nurse allows the child to see the suppository so the child will not think he or she is receiving an injection. The nurse tells the child that insertion will feel similar to having a rectal temperature taken. The suppository is lubricated with a water-soluble lubricant and inserted beyond the rectal sphincter with a gloved index finger. The fifth finger is used for a child under age three years. To prevent expulsion of the suppository, the nurse holds the buttocks together for several minutes.

EVALUATION

During the evaluation phase, the nurse evaluates the effectiveness of the medications. The data obtained during the initial assessment provide base criteria for measuring therapeutic medication results.

The desired therapeutic effectiveness and toxicity of a drug are evaluated in a variety of ways. Many drugs are dependent on the nurse's assessment abilities to evaluate a therapeutic response. The patient's response to furosemide (Lasix) is evaluated by an increase in urinary output. When antihypertensives are given, there should be a decrease in the blood pressure.

For some medications, the best method to evaluate therapeutic effectiveness is to obtain a blood sample to determine the serum concentration of the drug in the child's body. Many children will not demonstrate an overt positive response to a medication, yet their serum drug concentration is in the normal or above normal therapeutic range. For example, a chronic asthmatic with a serum theophylline level of 26 μg/ml (therapeutic range 10–20 μg/ml) may continue to wheeze when auscultated; a child with brain damage may continue to have seizures yet have a serum phenytoin concentration of 19 μg/ml (therapeutic range 10–20 μg/ml).

Accuracy is an important aspect of evaluation. If data obtained by the nurse are not totally accurate, the physician may increase or decrease a medication dosage based on an erroneous value. Forgetting to balance the scale when weighing a 2500-gm infant could have disastrous results. When antihypertensives are given, an accurate blood pressure reading is essential. It is sometimes difficult to obtain a blood pressure reading with a stethoscope in an infant or young child. If the nurse is unable to hear the blood pressure sounds, a Doppler ultrasound instrument is used.

Side effects of medications are often difficult to evaluate in the pediatric patient. An infant is not able to talk but uses crying and smiling as a means of communication. Young children often have trouble expressing themselves because of their lack of vocabulary and lack of experience in knowing what is normal or abnormal. The nurse listens to and asks the parents for their interpretation of the child's behavior. For example, gentamicin is an ototoxic drug that can cause auditory nerve damage. Even the astute nurse who is watching for hearing loss can miss early, subtle changes. It may be the parents who give the nurse a clue that the child is having a side effect from the gentamicin when they state that their child is not responding to them as he or she did previously.

Infants and toddlers usually do not fake pain, so the nurse should listen to the two-year-old child who complains of pain or the infant who has a change in the sound of his or her cry or is crying continuously. Preschoolers and older children may try to fool the nurse, so other assessment methods, such as vital signs, may be necessary for accurate evaluation of pain, as with an adult.

Patient Teaching

Patient teaching in pediatrics includes discovering to whom the teaching should be directed. The nurse must first determine who the primary caregiver will be. It should never be assumed that the parent who stays with the child while he or she is in the hospital or the parent who brings the child to the physician's office is the person who will be responsible for giving the medication in the home. Many children have medication administration times while they are attending day care centers, with baby-sitters, or visiting a grandparent. When the nurse is teaching the primary caregiver, it is necessary to emphasize that all persons administering the drug understand the importance of maintaining the medication schedule and know the side effects for which to observe (Table 14–7).

Many factors influence patient compliance, which affects patient teaching. Parents frequently stop a medication when the child's symptoms can no longer be seen. The importance of continuing the drug until it is gone or until the physician determines it is not necessary to continue it must be emphasized. By demonstrating concern for the child rather than just asking about the family finances, the nurse can ascertain if cost of the medication will influence compliance. A parent may not be able to afford the medication, which would indicate the need for social service assistance. A parent who is not aware of the long-term physical consequences of a disease may not feel that mild symptoms currently being exhibited are equal to the cost of the drug.

The nurse incorporates information from the original assessment into patient teaching to assist the family with compliance. For example, what is the family's home routine? What time do they eat their meals? When does the child leave for and return from school? What time does the child go to bed? A parent will increase compliance in administering the drug if a medication schedule can be individualized to fit that particular family's routine.

It is also important for the nurse to allow sufficient time in a relatively quiet atmosphere to evaluate the patient's progress. Very often, health professionals do not really listen to parents and give the impression that what they have to say is not important. If this has happened in the past, parents may be reluctant to take up the "valuable time" of the nurse unless encouraged to do so.

It has been determined that positive patient-provider interactions (i.e., a caring interaction between the nurse, child, and family) has a significant influence on compliance. The type of patient-provider relationship as determined by the family begins during the initial assessment. The relationship continues to develop with each interaction between the family and the nurse. When the family has returned home, they will increase their compliance if they feel the nurse really cared about their child.

Medication Safety

New parents have much to learn in order to allow their child to grow and develop normally. Protection of the child from potentially fatal accidents is essential. The proper storage and utilization of medications is a simple safety precaution, but one that is often not practiced. Every year many children are treated for accidental ingestion of medications.

Child-proof caps should always be replaced tightly on medicine bottles. These caps are not always an effective deterrent to a determined toddler but may slow the child's progress in opening the bottle and may give the parents time to intervene.

In a home where there is a small child, all medications should be stored in a locked container and the key hidden. Placing drugs on a high shelf beyond a child's reach is not always a safe practice. Children watch their parents and will remember where a good tasting medication is stored. After children begin walking, they quickly learn to climb. They may open drawers to use as steps and maneuver chairs into a position that allows them to reach high shelves. A child may consume an entire bottle of pills before being found by the parent.

Children also enjoy exploring women's purses that are within their reach. Many children are poisoned each year from eating birth control pills, diuretics, and antihypertensive drugs that were obtained from a purse. Parents should offer to place a visitor's purse in a safe place.

All parents of small children need the poison control

Table 14–7. PARENT TEACHING TABLE

1. A medication in suspension must be shaken well before it is given to assure all the doses in the bottle are the same strength.
2. Do not use household spoons to measure liquid medications. To assure an accurate dose, always give liquid medications using a calibrated dropper or calibrated oral spoon (available at a pharmacy).
3. If your child cannot swallow pills, ask your doctor if the medicine is available in a liquid form.
4. Do not crush pills or take the powder from a capsule until you discuss this with your child's doctor. The effectiveness of some medicines will change if they are crushed.
5. Mix crushed pills or capsule powder (if satisfactory to administer this way) with applesauce or jelly. If you mix them with a liquid, all the medicine may not dissolve and your child will not receive the correct dose.
6. Give your child the medication for the full length of time recommended by your doctor. Failure to follow the doctor's directions could result in a reoccurrence of illness symptoms or complications from the original illness.
7. All medicines should be purchased in bottles with child-proof caps. Always replace the cap on the medicine bottle to prevent your child from accidentally taking the medicine without your supervision.
8. Keep all medications in your home in cupboards outside the reach of children (or locked up).
9. Never tell your child that medicine is candy.

telephone number available for emergency use (1-800-392-8548). In addition, parents should keep ipecac syrup, an emetic, in their home for accidental medication ingestion. The emetic is given if vomiting is not contraindicated. If given immediately, the emetic will prevent much of the medication from being absorbed by the child's body. The child's doctor is notified or the child is taken to the emergency room to rule out systemic absorption. (See emetics for dosages and reactions.)

SUMMARY

Children are not little adults. The physiology of their body systems, which affects pharmacotherapeutics, is an important consideration in administering medications. Nurses giving medications to neonates and pediatric patients must be aware of the physiologic differences identified in this book. Without this knowledge, children may have therapeutic drug results different from the desired effect.

The nursing process relevant to medication administration begins at the initial encounter with both child and parents. The nurse applies principles of normal growth and development and deviations from the normal caused by the illness to develop an individualized nursing care plan for each child. This care plan will guide the nurse in medication administration and child-parent teaching. Parental education regarding medications should always be included to promote compliance with drug administration and drug safety.

BIBLIOGRAPHY

Avery, ME and Taeusch, HW: Schaffer's Diseases of the Newborn. WB Saunders, Philadelphia, 1984.

Babington, MA and Spadera, DC: Cariogenic medications. Ped Nsg 8:165, 1982.

Bavin, R: Obtaining therapeutic antibiotic blood levels in children. J Ped Nsg 1:164, 1986.

Behrman, R and Vaughan, VC: Nelson Textbook of Pediatrics. WB Saunders, Philadelphia, 1983.

Cohen, MS: Principles of Drug Disposition and Therapy in Infants and Children. In Rudolph, AM (ed.): Pediatrics. Appleton-Century-Crofts, Norwalk, CT, 1982.

Engel, J: Pocket Guide to Pediatric Assessment. CV Mosby, St Louis, 1989.

Hazinski, MF: Nursing Care of the Critically Ill Child. CV Mosby, St Louis, 1984.

Howry, LB, Binder, RM, and Tso, Y: Pediatric Medications. JB Lippincott, Philadelphia, 1981.

Kempe, CH, Silver, HK, and O'Brien, D: Current Pediatric Diagnosis and Treatment. Lange Medical Publishers, Los Altos, CA, 1984.

Marlow, DR: Textbook of Pediatric Nursing. WB Saunders, Philadelphia, 1988.

Pittitteri, A: Child Health Nursing. Little, Brown and Co, Boston, 1987.

Plumer, AL and Cosentino, F: Principles and Practices of Intravenous Therapy. Little, Brown and Co, Boston, 1987.

Reiss, BS and Melick, ME: Pharmacological Aspects of Nursing Care. Delmar Publishers, Albany, 1987.

Roberts, RJ: Drug Therapy in Infants. WB Saunders, Philadelphia, 1984.

Servonsky, J and Opas, S: Nursing Management of Children. Jones and Bartlett Publishers, Boston, 1987.

Trang, J, Kluza, RB, and Kearns, GL: Pharmacokinetics for pediatric nurses. Ped Nsg 10:267, 1984.

Whaley, LF and Wong, DL: Nursing Care of Infants and Children. CV Mosby, St Louis, 1987.

Wiener, MB and Pepper, GA: Clinical Pharmacology and Therapeutics in Nursing. McGraw-Hill, New York, 1985.

Yoos, L: Factors influencing material compliance to antibiotic regimens. Ped Nsg 2:141, 1984.

SITUATION   14-1

Darla Stevens is a 42-week-gestation newborn transferred from the operating room to the neonatal intensive care unit due to meconium aspiration.

1. Administration of intravenous fluid (5% dextrose) has been ordered for Darla at 15 cc per hour. The nurse is aware of the following in preparing to start the IV:
   a. Scalp veins may be used in the neonate, but are difficult to see.
   b. An 18 gauge needle is used for intravenous administration in neonates.
   c. The needle may be inserted in the scalp vein in either direction of blood flow.
   d. Only peripheral veins should be utilized for IV administration in neonates.

2. Darla is receiving ampicillin via intravenous piggyback. It will be best for the nurse to change the IV tubing:
   a. every 24 hours with site care
   b. immediately after medication administration
   c. per policy before a medication is given
   d. every other morning with site care

3. When giving Darla medications which are dependent on protein binding for drug distribution, the nurse is aware that it may be necessary to:
   a. decrease the amount of drug and shorten the dosage interval
   b. increase the amount of drug and give at longer intervals

SITUATION   14–1–*CONTINUED*

c. decrease the amount of drug and give at longer intervals

d. increase the amount of drug and shorten the dosage interval

4. On the fourth day, Darla's laboratory data reveal elevated bilirubin levels. At this time it will be important for the nurse to avoid administering:
   a. ampicillin
   b. aspirin
   c. acetaminophen
   d. gentamicin

5. Knowledge of the biotransformation of drugs is essential for drug administration in the neonate. During the first week of Darla's life, the nurse will observe for the following response to medication administration:
   a. reduced therapeutic effect
   b. no observable effect
   c. reduced drug half-life
   d. prolonged therapeutic effect

6. After two weeks in the neonatal unit, Darla is placed on digoxin for symptoms related to congestive failure. Repeated serum digoxin tests reveal subtherapeutic levels. The need to increase the dosage in order to reach therapeutic levels may be related to:
   a. increasing glomerular filtraton rate
   b. incomplete secretory mechanisms
   c. reduction in liver enzymes
   d. elevated bilirubin levels

SITUATION   14–2

Molly Fenderson, a two-year-old asthmatic, is recovering from pneumonia. She is a patient on a pediatric unit, and her mother stays with her. Present medications include oral penicillin and theophylline.

1. Molly develops gastritis with symptoms of gastric distress. The nurse is aware that administration of oral penicillin at this time may result in:
   a. no effect on penicillin absorption
   b. increased therapeutic response
   c. prolonged therapeutic response
   d. altered timing of the therapeutic effect

2. Oral penicillin has been discontinued, and the drug is to be given by intramuscular injection. In choosing an IM site for Molly, the nurse will avoid the deltoid muscle because of all of the following *except:*
   a. the muscle is small and not well developed
   b. it lies close to the radial and ulnar nerves
   c. the muscle has a slow rate of absorption
   d. it lies close to the brachial artery

3. Molly receives theophylline twice a day. Concerning the effect of metabolism on theophylline levels, the nurse is aware that it may be necessary to:
   a. decrease the dosage interval
   b. increase the dosage interval
   c. discontinue a dose every other day
   d. decrease the daily dosage

4. Before administering any medication to Molly, the nurse will perform all of the following actions *except:*
   a. ask her to identify herself
   b. check the armband for identification
   c. identify safe methods of administration
   d. determine if dosage is appropriate

5. The best criterion to utilize in evaluating Molly's response to theophylline therapy would be:
   a. evidence of wheezing
   b. elevated urine output
   c. therapeutic serum levels
   d. presence of shortness of breath

6. Which of the responses by Molly's mother indicates an understanding of patient teaching with regard to medication compliance?
   a. ''She stays with me during the weekdays, so I make sure she gets the medicine then.''
   b. ''We really don't have the extra money for her medicines, so I space them further apart.''
   c. ''As long as Molly feels good, I don't worry about missing a pill or two.''
   d. ''I can give Molly her medicines before breakfast and at bedtime. That way I won't forget.''

Please refer to the Appendices for correct answers and additional review questions with answers.

15
CHAPTER

PHARMACOTHERAPEUTICS FOR THE OBSTETRICAL PATIENT

NANCY K. SHAW, MSN, RN

LEARNING OBJECTIVES

After reading this chapter, the student should be able to:

1. Identify the changes in the pharmacokinetic variables related to pregnancy.

2. Identify the mechanisms that influence placental transfer of drugs.

3. Identify the drugs utilized to suppress and enhance uterine motility.

4. Differentiate among the suppression drugs and enhancement drugs as to mechanism of action, route of administration, pharmacokinetics, adverse effects, contraindications, and interactions.

5. Plan the nursing interventions necessary to administer uterine suppressant and enhancement drugs.

6. Plan the nursing interventions necessary to administer magnesium sulfate for pre-eclampsia.

7. Plan the nursing interventions necessary to administer lactation suppressants.

8. Identify the mechanisms that affect transfer of drugs into breast milk.

9. Identify the purposes of the drugs utilized in the immediate neonatal period.

Table 15–1. PATIENT TEACHING INFORMATION—DRUG USE DURING PREGNANCY

Dear Patient,

If you are attempting to become pregnant or have been told you are pregnant, there are some important considerations for you and your baby:

1. Make sure you tell your doctor ALL of your medical or obstetrical history.
2. If any medications are required for existing medical conditions, tell your doctor or nurse what the medication is, how often you take it, and how strong it is. Sometimes it is easier to take the medicine bottle with you to your doctor's office.
3. Sometimes pregnancy can require that a dosage of a medication you were using before you became pregnant be changed, but do not change your doses without checking with your doctor.
4. Do not take any medications, even over-the-counter ones, without checking with your doctor or nurse. Some drugs are safer for your baby than others.
5. Alcohol has been found to be harmful to your baby, so you should not drink alcohol during your pregnancy.

There are many physiologic changes occurring in the female during pregnancy. These changes can cause an alteration in the pharmacokinetics of drugs, which can alter their effectiveness in the pregnant female. In addition, during pregnancy there is a developing fetus, which can incur permanent damage from some drugs. This damage may not be apparent for many years. For example, the reported incidence of vaginal adenocarcinoma in young women who were exposed to diethylstilbestrol during their first trimester of gestation is well documented. Pharmacokinetic variables, effectiveness of the drug, and concern for *teratogenic* effects on the fetus all influence drug usage during pregnancy. Before any drug therapy is begun, any woman of childbearing age is always assessed for pregnancy and asked about plans for a future pregnancy.

Today, the majority of physicians limit the number of prescription medications that are given to pregnant women and counsel them to refrain from taking any over-the-counter medications. Since many women do take medications during pregnancy, education regarding their use is important (Table 15–1). When prescribed drugs are necessary for the mother, the dosage is adjusted to ensure that the drug is effective but not harmful to the fetus. Dosages may be different from those utilized for a nonpregnant female.

EFFECT OF PREGNANCY ON DRUG PHARMACOKINESIS

All the pharmacokinetic variables are affected by the physiologic changes that occur during pregnancy. These variables include absorption, distribution, biotransformation, and excretion. (For explanation of the pharmacokinetic variables, see Chapter 4.) The pharmacokinetic variables provide a rationale for the alteration of drug dosages during pregnancy. The hormones of pregnancy also alter the effectiveness of some drugs. For example, the insulin-dependent diabetic usually requires an increased insulin dosage during the second half of pregnancy because of the insulin-antagonistic effect of human placental lactogen (HPL), which is also called human chorionic somatomammotropin (HCS). HPL acts to stimulate lipolysis and exerts an antagonistic effect on insulin actions or carbohydrate metabolism. This tends to raise the plasma glucose in order to maintain the continuous flow of glucose to the fetus. Blood glucose levels and insulin dosages need to be monitored closely during pregnancy to maintain close control of the blood glucose levels. After delivery the blood glucose level is monitored to determine insulin dosage because the antagonistic hormones are not present.

ABSORPTION

The stomach emptying time is longer during pregnancy, and there is decreased gastrointestinal motility due to the influence of high levels of progesterone. While this would suggest a prolonged rate and decreased amount of drug absorption, clinical evidence does not support this conclusion, except possibly with digoxin.

DISTRIBUTION

During pregnancy there is a large increase in total body water. The greatest percentage of the increase is in the extracellular fluid. Plasma volume increases by 50%, while the concentration of plasma albumin falls. Because most drugs are bound to plasma protein, the decrease of plasma protein results in an increase of unbound drug fraction to cause pharmacologic effects. The effects can cause a difference in the volume of distribution and plasma drug concentration. The drugs affected most are those of relatively low lipid solubility, which are highly bound to plasma protein. This increased distribution volume results in a reduction in the peak plasma drug concentration after a dose. This would cause a longer half-life if not for an increase in clearance by biotransformation or excretion.

Decrease in plasma protein binding results in a larger amount of unbound drug in position to leave the blood stream, to be widely distributed, to cause pharmacologic effects, and to be biotransformed or excreted.

Elimination is increased during pregnancy; therefore there is not an increase in tissue concentration. The results during pregnancy are lower total drug concentrations in the pregnant woman's plasma. Plasma drug concentrations should be monitored closely to maintain therapeutic blood levels. For example, phenytoin levels need to be monitored during pregnancy because of the possible need to increase dosage to prevent seizure activity. After delivery, a return to the patient's prepregnant dose probably will be necessary.

BIOTRANSFORMATION

During pregnancy, it is believed that drug metabolism in the liver is stimulated, primarily by progesterone. There is also increased excretion of drug metabolizing enzymes and microscopic evidence of hyperplasia of some of the endoplasmic reticulum in the liver cells.

A small amount of drug metabolism also occurs during pregnancy in the placenta and the fetal liver. The fetoplacental unit contribution to drug metabolism is very small.

EXCRETION

If the stimulation of drug metabolism causes a measurable increase in liver clearance, elimination of drugs is accelerated, and half-life is shorter. The flow of blood through the liver is not appreciably changed during pregnancy; therefore, drugs that are dependent only on liver blood flow to be cleared from the body are cleared at the same rate as in the nonpregnant woman unless the volume of distribution is higher.

The renal plasma blood flow during pregnancy is almost twice that of the prepregnant state, and there is a substantial increase in the glomerular filtration rate and creatinine clearance. Drugs that are excreted unchanged (e.g., gentamicin and digoxin) are cleared in proportion to the creatinine clearance. Therefore, these drugs would need to be closely monitored during pregnancy to maintain an effective dosage.

It seems obvious that because of changes in the pharmacokinetic variables related to pregnancy, there may be changes needed in drug administration to the pregnant woman. However, this information is available for only a few drugs. More study is required to determine the effective dosage of all drugs for usage during pregnancy. The ethical difficulties of studies during pregnancy is a limiting factor in the progress of this research, which is evidenced by the lack of information on drug doses for the pregnant female. Before any drug is prescribed during pregnancy, the pharmacokinetic variables should be considered and researched. Table 15–2 lists drugs for which dosage information during pregnancy is available.

FETAL AND MATERNAL DRUG EFFECTS

PLACENTAL TRANSFER OF DRUGS

The effect of drugs on the fetus is dependent on whether a drug is distributed throughout the body or distributed selectively. This distribution is significant in determining whether the drug can pass through the *placental barrier*.

The placenta has the important function of allowing the transfer of substances between the mother and the fetus. The significant variables that determine the transfer of drugs across the placenta are physicochemical characteristics of the compound, physiologic properties of the placental tissue, and maternal and fetal placental blood flow. The physicochemical characteristics that determine placental transfer are molecular weight, molecular configuration, degree of ionization, lipid solubility, and tissue-binding protein properties. If the molecular weight of a substance is less than 600 (e.g., warfarin sodium), it crosses the placenta with ease. A substance with a molecular weight between 600 and 1000 crosses more slowly, while compounds with a molecular weight of greater than 1000 (e.g., heparin) meet a relatively impermeable placental barrier. The more highly ionized a drug molecule is, the lower the chance that it will cross the placenta. If a drug is highly bound to maternal plasma protein, it will not readily cross the placenta. Since only unbound drugs transfer back across the placenta, the drugs that are highly bound to fetal plasma protein concentrate in the fetus.

Maternal and fetal acid-base balance also affects the transfer of drugs across the placenta. In maternal acidosis the fetus becomes more acidotic. Maternal alkalosis, which results from hyperventilation, causes the oxyhemoglobin curve to move to the left, resulting in

Table 15–2. KNOWN EFFECTS OF PREGNANCY ON DRUGS

Drug	Dosage
Anticonvulsants	
Phenytoin	Monitor level to determine need to increase daily dose
Primidone	Monitoring levels advisable
Phenobarbital	Monitoring levels advisable
Carbamazepine	Monitoring levels advisable
Benzodiazepines	
Diazepam	No evidence of need to alter doses
Oxazepam	No evidence of need to alter doses
Lithium	Increase dose during pregnancy; dose needs to be reduced at onset of labor
Muscle relaxants	
Pancuronium	No dose alteration necessary
Analgesics and anti-inflammatories	
Salicylate	No alteration in dose
Meperidine	No alteration in dose
Digoxin	Monitor serum concentration
β-Adrenoreceptor blocking agents	
Labetalol	No alteration in dose
Furosemide	No alteration in dose
Antimicrobial agents	
Ampicillin	Dose doubled for systemic infections; for UTI, no dose change needed
Cefuroxime	Increase dosage
Sulfisoxazole	For UTI, no alteration
Metronidazole	No alteration in dose

(Adapted from Mucklow, JC: The fate of drugs in pregnancy. Clin Obstet Gynecol 13(2):161, 1986.)

fetal hypoxia and acidosis. These changes cause an accumulation of drugs that have an alkaline pH in the fetus.

The placenta also functions as an organ of metabolism. Metabolism in the placenta can result in metabolites of increased or decreased potency. The significance of the effects of this metabolic change is dependent on whether the desired effect is in the fetus or the mother. If the metabolites from placental metabolism are more potent, a toxic level may occur in the fetus.

The rate of transfer of a drug across the placenta is also dependent upon the uteroplacental blood flow. This blood flow tends to decrease near term. Blood flow will decrease because of certain conditions, such as pre-eclampsia, hypertension, and diabetes. Maternal position also affects the uteroplacental blood flow. Blood flow decreases when the female is in a supine or semi-recumbent position because of pressure from the uterus on the aorta and the vena cava. The blood flow will increase when she is in a side-lying position, particularly on her left side. The rate of transfer of drugs is decreased at times of decreased blood flow and continues to be lower in labor because of the contraction of the uterus. During uterine contraction, there is decreased blood

Table 15–3. TERATOGENIC AGENTS: EFFECTS OR ASSOCIATIONS

Agent	Reported Effects or Associations	Comments
Alcohol	Fetal alcohol syndrome: intrauterine growth retardation (IUGR), maxillary hypoplasia, reduction in width of palpebral fissures, microcephaly, mental retardation.	Direct cytotoxic effects of alcohol and indirect effects of alcoholism. Consumption of 6 oz alcohol or more per day constitutes a high risk.
Methotrexate	Hydrocephalus, cleft palate, meningomyelocele, IUGR, abnormal cranial ossification, reduction in derivatives of first branchial arch.	Folic acid antagonists that inhibit dihydrofolate reductase, resulting in cell death.
Androgens	Masculinization of female embryo: clitoromegaly with or without fusion of labia minora.	Effects are dose-dependent; stimulates growth and differentiation of receptor-containing tissue.
Warfarin	Nasal hypoplasia; stippling of secondary epiphysis; IUGR; anomalies of eyes, hands, neck; variable CNS effects	Metabolic inhibitor; bleeding is an unlikely explanation for effects. Risk from exposure 10%–25% during 8th–14th week of gestation.
Cyclophosphamide	Growth retardation, ectrodactyly, syndactyly, cardiovascular anomalies, and other minor anomalies. Magnitude of risk unknown.	Requires cytochrome P450 mono-oxidase activation; interacts with DNA, resulting in cell death.
Diethylstilbestrol	Masculinization of female: vaginal adenocarcinogenesis, anomalies of cervix and uterus. The dose that increases risk of genitourinary abnormalities in the male is controversial.	Stimulates estrogen receptor-containing tissue, may cause misplaced tissue. Vaginal adenosis from exposures before 9th week of pregnancy, 75% risk; risk of adenocarcinoma is low (1 in 10,000).
Phenytoin	Hydantoin syndrome: hypoplastic nails and distal phalanges, cleft lip/palate, microcephaly, mental retardation.	Direct effect on cell membranes, folate, and vitamin K metabolism. Wide variation in reported risk. Associations documented only with chronic exposure.
Lithium carbonate	Increased incidence of Epstein's anomaly, other heart and great vessel defects, neural tube defects.	Mechanism has not been defined. Risk is estimated at 10%.
2,4-Oxazolidine-diones (trimethadione, paramethadione)	Fetal trimethadione syndrome: V-shaped eyebrows, low-set ears with anteriorly folded helix, high-arched palate, irregular teeth, CNS anomalies, developmental delay.	Affects cell membrane permeability. Wide variation in reported risk. Associations documented only with chronic exposure.
Progestins	Masculinization of female embryo exposed to high doses.	Stimulates or interferes with growth and differentiation of receptor-containing tissue.
Tetracycline	Hypoplastic tooth enamel, tooth and bone staining.	Effects seen only if exposure is during second or third trimester.
Thalidomide	Bilateral limb reduction defects (preferential effects, phocomelia); facial hemangioma; esophageal or duodenal atresia; anomalies of external ears, kidneys, and heart.	Multiple theories have been proposed, but the primary mechanism is unknown.
Thyroid: iodine deficiency iodides, radioiodine, antithyroid drugs (propylthiouracil)	Hypothyroidism or goiter; neurologic and aural damage is variable.	Fetopathic effect of endemic iodine occurs early in development. Fetopathic effect of iodides, antithyroid drugs, and radioiodine involves metabolic block, decreases thyroid hormone synthesis and gland development. Maternal intake of 12 mg iodide per day or more increases the risk of fetal goiter.

Table 15–3. TERATOGENIC AGENTS: EFFECTS OR ASSOCIATIONS–CONTINUED

Agent	Reported Effects or Associations	Comments
Nonprescription drugs and products		
Aspirin	Heavy use may result in lowered birth weight but not an increase in malformations.	Doses toxic for the mother are likely to be fetotoxic. (May cause increased bleeding in mother and baby if taken within 5 days of delivery.)
Caffeine	Caffeine is not likely to be a human teratogen.	Excess consumption ($>$6–8 cups of coffee/day is likely to be toxic to both mother and embryo.
Smoking and nicotine	Placental lesions and IUGR but no defined malformations. Increased postnatal morbidity and mortality.	Maternal or placental complications can result in fetal death.
Vitamin A	Urogenital anomalies in humans have been associated with massive doses. ISOTRETINOIN is a human teratogen; defects include ear malformations, open neural tube, cleft palate, facial abnormalities.	Retinoic acid is cytotoxic; it may interact with DNA to delay differentiation and/or inhibit protein synthesis.
Vitamin D	Large doses given in Vitamin D prophylaxis are possibly involved in the etiology of supravalvular aortic stenosis, elfin faces, and mental retardation.	Mechanism is likely to involve a disruption of cell calcium regulation.

From Beckman, DA and Brent, RL: Mechanism of known environment teratogens: Drugs and chemicals. Clin Perinatol 13:655–658, 1986, with permission.

flow to the uterus. This decrease in blood flow may result in an accumulation of drugs in the fetus because they are unable to transfer back across the placenta into the maternal blood stream.

EFFECTS OF DRUGS ON FETUS

Whether or not a drug will cause adverse effects on the fetus depends on certain factors: the type of drug, the amount of drug, rate of elimination, distribution in the fetal tissue, gestational age, and specific receptor function in the fetus. During the first trimester of fetal development, drugs may produce major effects. The degree of *teratogenicity* is different at various times during gestation. From fertilization until after implantation, the effects range from damage that can be repaired by the developing *embryo* to demise resulting in abortion. The 18th day through approximately the 60th day or the period or organogenesis is the developmental period when the greatest damage can occur with regard to malformations. The genitourinary system and palate are the most vulnerable after the 36th day of gestation. In the *fetal period* teratogenic agents affect the cell population by causing cell death and cell growth retardation or by inhibiting cell differentiation. After the eighth week of gestation, the fetal brain is developing very rapidly and is very susceptible to damage from *teratogens*. After the first trimester, drugs do not produce gross structural abnormalities, but they can affect the growth and functional development of the fetus. They can also have toxic effects on the fetus.

The Federal Drug Administration (FDA) has developed and published a classification system for risk factors of systemic drug usage during pregnancy. The classification is based on the level of known risk the drug presents to the fetus. These classifications are A, B, C, D, and X. An A ranking indicates that studies in women have not indicated a risk to the fetus; therefore, the chance of harm to the fetus is remote. The B category indicates that human studies have not been completed to support animal studies that indicated no adverse effect. Category C drugs should be utilized by a pregnant woman ONLY if the potential benefit outweighs the risk to the fetus as indicated by studies with animals. The D category identifies a drug for which there is documented evidence of human fetal risk. These drugs may be used in life-threatening situations or pathology that is not treatable with a safer drug. Category X drugs should not be used by women any time there is the possibility of pregnancy (e.g., diethylstilbestrol and isotretinoin). It should be remembered that studies cannot rule out any possibility of harm to a fetus; therefore, drugs should not be utilized during pregnancy unless absolutely necessary and after implications for the fetus have been determined.

Because of the ethical nature of research into the effects of drugs on the fetus, most reported teratogenic effects have been based on retrospective reports. Table 15–3 lists some of the common agents known to have teratogenic effects on fetal development.

DRUGS UTILIZED IN LABOR AND DELIVERY

The progression of labor determines whether the utilization of drugs is necessary. If a labor is inefficient, *oxytocics* may be used to augment the progress. Oxytocics are also utilized to induce labor. After delivery of the placenta, ergot alkaloids and oxytocics are utilized to decrease postpartal hemorrhage by helping to maintain uterine contraction. For more information on oxytocics and ergot alkaloids, see the section of this chapter on drugs that enhance uterine motility and Table 15–7.

Relief of pain by the use of drugs during labor has the multifaceted goal of decreasing maternal discomfort with minimal effect on the fetus, minimal disruption of labor, and continued awareness in the woman. Drugs utilized during labor and delivery for the relief of pain are sedative-hypnotics, analgesics, and anesthetics.

Sedative-Hypnotics

Sedative-hypnotics are used in the latent phase of labor to induce relaxation and/or sleep in women who are exhausted or very apprehensive. The barbiturates rapidly cross the placenta and may cause adverse reactions in the fetus, such as central nervous system depression and hypotonia. Barbiturates are degraded by the placenta. Because there is no antagonist drug available, active labor with an imminent delivery is a contraindication for barbiturate administration.

The barbiturates most commonly used during labor are secobarbital sodium (Seconal), pentobarbital sodium (Nembutal), and sodium phenobarbital (Luminal). For more information regarding barbiturates see Chapter 22.

During labor, drugs are administered to decrease anxiety, apprehension, and nausea. The drugs most commonly used during labor are the phenothiazines—promazine (Sparine), promethazine (Phenergan), and hydroxyzine (Vistaril and Atarax).

Adverse maternal reactions from these drugs include maternal hypotension and drowsiness. They readily cross the placenta and therefore may cause fetal tachycardia and loss of beat-to-beat variability as seen on the electronic fetal monitor tracing. The neonate born under the influence of these drugs may demonstrate hypotonia, hypothermia, and generalized drowsiness, which causes a reluctance to feed. For more information on phenothiazines, promethazine, and hydroxyzine, see Chapter 25 in this text.

Analgesics

The most commonly used analgesics for pain during labor are meperidine hydrochloride (Demerol), nalbuphine (Nubain), butorphanol tartrate (Stadol), and, less commonly, morphine sulfate. Analgesic agents may be administered by either an intramuscular or intravenous route according to the physician's preference. The intravenous route results in a faster, more predictable means of analgesia. Intravenous analgesics are administered slowly. It is recommended by some that the analgesic be administered at the onset of a contraction and interrupted between contractions. This limits the amount of drug received by the fetus because of the decrease of uteroplacental blood flow during contractions.

Maternal vital signs and consciousness level are carefully monitored in the laboring woman receiving analgesics. Electronic monitoring is utilized to assess contraction status, fetal heart rate (FHR), and variability.

The use of meperidine may cause a decrease in baseline variability of the FHR and a decrease in *neonatal neurobehavior scores*. Safety precautions should be instituted such as bedrest with the side rails elevated and the call bell within reach. Maternal side effects to analgesics are nausea and vomiting, mild respiratory depression, transient mental impairment, postural hypotension, and urinary retention.

Analgesics may prolong the latent phase of labor, and thus they are not administered before labor is well established and cervical dilatation is progressing (at 4–5.0 cm dilatation). The analgesics readily cross the placenta and may cause deleterious effects on the fetus (e.g., respiratory depression). Neonatal depression from meperidine is less likely to occur if delivery occurs within one to two hours of administration of meperidine.

A narcotic antagonist should be available if neonatal depression is possible. The presence of unilateral or upper body hypotonia in the newborn may indicate birth trauma or asphyxia. Narcotics produce generalized motor depression. Naloxone hydrochloride (Narcan) is the preferred drug for narcotic antagonism. Naloxone will not increase depression in a neonate whose depression is not caused by narcotics. The dosage for the depressed neonate is 0.10 mg/kg, preferably into the umbilical vein, but it can be administered to the neonate intramuscularly or subcutaneously if necessary. The dose may be repeated every two to three minutes as necessary. Other resuscitative measures should be on hand and instituted (i.e., oxygen, laryngoscope, ambu bag, and so on).

Spinal opiates (morphine) have been used rarely as a means of providing labor analgesia. This analgesia lasts throughout labor and sometimes into the postpartal period. While most patients do not experience complete pain relief, the relief they do experience is prolonged without the hypotension or impaired motor function associated with spinal anesthetics because there is no sympathetic blockade. There is, however, a high incidence of nausea and itching. (See Chapter 20 for more information on analgesics and narcotic antagonists.)

Anesthetics

Anesthetics used in obstetrics are either local, regional, or general. When regional or general anesthesias are utilized, a supine position for the mother is avoided to prevent compression of the aorta and vena cava, which causes maternal hypotension and a resultant decrease in uteroplacental blood flow. A noncompressible sandbag should be placed under the patient's right hip in order to displace the uterus to the left and prevent aortic and vena caval compression. Prophylactic crystalloid solutions are administered intravenously before regular or general anesthesia.

General anesthetics are used rarely for uncomplicated vaginal deliveries because of the possible complications from the anesthesia. They are sometimes used for cesarean deliveries. The use of a general anesthetic results in an unconscious patient with an increased possibility of aspiration and respiratory depression. The pregnant patient is at a greater risk for aspiration than the nonpregnant one. The delayed gastric emptying time in pregnancy is further delayed in labor due to pain, anxiety, and analgesics and is responsible for this increased risk. Therefore, some specific precautions are utilized to minimize the risk of aspiration. Inhalation anesthesia is avoided unless absolutely necessary and is always administered by endotracheal tube. Sodium citrate (15 ml) is administered 30 minutes before induction. If the patient has had complaints of heartburn, ranitidine (150 mg orally) is administered at least 90 minutes prior to induction. These drugs decrease the acidity of stomach contents in the event of aspiration. The induction should be rapid after preoxygenation to minimize fetal depression by the anesthetic agent. Succinylcholine is utilized for tracheal intubation. It crosses the placenta but not in quantities sufficient to cause neonatal paralysis.

Since most general anesthetics reach the fetus rapidly, neonatal depression is possible with resultant respiratory distress. A time interval from anesthesia induction to delivery of the neonate of greater than eight minutes has been associated with significantly higher incidence of low one-minute Apgar scores as well as with fetal acidosis.

With a general anesthetic, delayed contact of the fetus and mother will most likely occur because a maternal recovery period is required. This lapse in immediate postpartal contact may result in delayed mother-infant bonding. Uterine relaxation is a complication following general anesthetic administration, particularly from high concentrations of halogenated hydrocarbons. This relaxation increases the postpartal woman's risk for hemorrhage. In these cases, oxytocin is used postpartally to stimulate uterine contraction.

Nitrous oxide, halothane, methoxyflurane, enflurane, and isoflurane may be used as inhalation anesthetic agents for cesarean sections and very rarely, for emergency deliveries, particularly those associated with active bleeding (i.e., placenta abruptio). Nitrous oxide, enflurane, and isoflurane are also used in analgesic concentrations during the first stage of labor. Even though these inhalation agents can rapidly cross the placenta and accumulate in the fetal brain and other tissues, there are no major fetal problems when analgesic concentrations are administered. The inhalation agent is often self-administered at the very beginning of each contraction for the analgesic effect. For more information on anesthetic agents, see Chapter 10.

Regional anesthetics are local anesthetics injected to block the nerve pathways to interrupt the transmission of pain impulses. They are utilized for labor analgesia in active labor and delivery. The woman is awake, and the absence of pain may facilitate mother-infant bonding immediately after delivery. Regional anesthetics also avoid the fetal central nervous system depression that may occur with inhalation agents. The risk of gastric content aspiration is reduced.

The regional anesthetic techniques used in obstetrics are pudendal blocks, paracervical blocks, subarachnoid blocks (spinal and saddle), and epidural blocks (lumbar and caudal). A specially trained person is needed to administer regional blocks. Labor may be prolonged if the regional block is administered too early in labor (before 4.0 cm dilation).

A pudendal block is administered by injecting a local anesthetic agent (10 ml 1% lidocaine) at the pudendal nerve on each side of the pelvis. The genitals and lower vagina are numbed to relieve pain caused by second stage labor, low forceps delivery, and repair of the episiotomy. The anesthesia lasts approximately 45 minutes. Possible maternal complications are toxic reactions to the local anesthetic, hematoma resulting from puncture of the internal pudendal artery, or abscesses at the site of the injection. Pudendal blocks are not associated with impaired neonatal neurobehavioral scores.

A paracervical block results from injecting a local anesthetic transvaginally next to the outer rim of the cervix. This provides an excellent analgesia for first stage labor and does not impair motor control required to effectively push for delivery. While systemic hypotension does not occur, paracervical blocks cause a high incidence of fetal bradycardia, which occurs within two to ten minutes after injection. Paracervical blocks are not utilized often because of the high risk of fetal bradycardia. (For more information, see an obstetrical nursing textbook.) There is also a danger of injecting the descending fetus during the transvaginal approach, which could cause a toxic reaction in the fetus. Continuous fetal monitoring is always used in conjunction with a paracervical block. If local anesthetic is injected intravenously, toxic reactions to the local anesthetic can occur.

A subarachnoid block can be either a saddle block or spinal block. A saddle block provides anesthetic for the buttocks, perineum, and inner aspects of the thighs by injecting local anesthetic *intrathecally* into the lumbar area at approximately L3–L5. A spinal block is an injection of a local anesthetic directly into the spinal fluid in the spinal canal to provide anesthetic for a vaginal delivery or cesarean section. Because the spinal anesthesia produces intense motor blockade, it is not suitable for labor analgesia. It is an excellent anesthesia for spontaneous and instrumental vaginal delivery, for manual removal of the placenta, and for a cesarean section. If patients are not prophylactically hydrated with 1500–2000 ml crystalloid solution and aortocaval compression is not avoided, any patient can develop severe systemic hypotension. Because of the possibility of rapid sympathetic blockade, spinal anesthesia must be used with great caution in patients in whom rapid sympathectomy will lead to cardiovascular compromise (i.e., patients with aortic stenosis). Other complications of spinal anesthesia are headache and nausea. Contraindications of spinal anesthesia are patient refusal, skin infection over lumbar region, and the presence of severe coagulopathy. Extreme caution is exercised when administering a subarachnoid block to the pre-eclamptic because of the sympathetic blockade that occurs from spinal anesthesia. There is little or no neurobehavior score change in the neonate following spinal anesthesia.

Epidural blocks have become the procedure of choice for labor analgesia and/or anesthesia for either vaginal delivery or cesarean section. Epidurals can be administered by either the lumbar or the caudal approach. The epidural involves the injection of a local anesthetic into the potential space between the dura mater and the ligamentum flavum, which extends from the base of the skull to the end of the sacral canal. This injection can occur either in the lumbar area (between L2, L3, or L4) or in the caudal area of the spinal canal through the sacral hiatus. The lumbar approach is preferred because larger doses of anesthetics are required for the caudal approach and the blockade necessary for labor analgesia is hard to achieve.

Epidural anesthesia is contraindicated for women who refuse, have skin infection over the injection area, or have severe coagulopathy. Epidural anesthesia is contraindicated for patients who have severe bleeding (i.e., placenta abruptio) or who require emergency cesareans.

Maternal hypotension is the most common side effect of epidural anesthesia. There is blood pooling in the lower extremities and the splanchnic bed, resulting in a decrease in venous return to the heart. This can be complicated by vena caval compression caused by the gravid uterus. Precautions that are effective in preventing maternal hypotension include (1) administration of 1000–1500 ml crystalloid solution before administering the block, and (2) placing a noncompressible sandbag under the maternal right hip to displace the uterus to the left. This will maintain vena caval blood return and maximize uteroplacental blood flow to ensure maximum possibility for fetal oxygenation. The crystalloid solution is administered in increments with assessment of maternal blood pressure following each increment. Continuous fetal monitoring with an internal lead is recommended for any woman receiving epidural anesthesia.

A test dose should be administered to check for accidental entry of the catheter into the subarachnoid space. If this occurs, the patient will complain of extensive numbness of the lower extremities and loss of motor control (occurs in three to five minutes). If the test dose is injected intravenously, the epinephrine in the test dose will promptly cause maternal and fetal tachycardia and palpitations. A properly placed catheter will not cause major sensory or motor deficit with the test dose. The remaining dosage should be administered in either one injection, repeated injections by way of epidural catheter, or by continuous infusion through a catheter and regulated by an infusion pump. Repeated injections or continuous infusion epidurals are the most commonly used in obstetrics. If repeated injections are used, blood pressure assessments should be made after each injection. During a continuous infusion, the patient should be turned from side to side at half-hour intervals. With either method of administration, continuous FHR monitoring is important, along with assessment of the maternal cardiovascular status. Occasionally, forceps may be required for delivery because the pushing reflex may be totally or partially eliminated.

There are complications that can occur following the administration of an epidural. Systemic hypotension may be treated with ephedrine 5.0–10 mg, administra-tion of oxygen, lateral positioning, and further intravenous fluid administration. Total spinal anesthesia may occur if a large volume of local anesthetic is injected into the cerebrospinal fluid. Total spinal anesthesia leads to rapid cardiovascular and respiratory collapse. This is an emergency situation. It usually results from failure to administer a test dose or from using bupivacaine for the test dose. Bupivacaine does not give a reliable test. Endotracheal intubation and ventilation, circulatory support with vasopressors, and positioning to relieve aortocaval compression are required to cope with total spinal anesthesia. The FHR must be closely monitored, and if fetal bradycardia occurs or maternal resuscitation is impossible, immediate delivery of the baby is necessary.

Intravenous injection of the anesthetic can lead to convulsions, cardiac toxicity, and respiratory arrest. Perforation of the dura mater leads to severe headache caused by cerebrospinal fluid leakage. Mild backaches and isolated nerve injuries subside with time.

Spinal opiates have been used for providing postoperative analgesia to the patient who has had a cesarean section. Morphine, fentanyl, and meperidine have been used. An epidural injection of morphine 5.0 mg will produce analgesia lasting 24 hours. The fat-soluble opiates have a shorter duration of action and will require more than one injection for relief of postoperative pain in the same time period. Therefore, the epidural catheter has to be left in place at least 24 hours.

There are advantages to the utilization of spinal opiates for postoperative analgesia. The relief of pain may enable the patient to ambulate earlier, which decreases the risk of deep vein thrombosis. The breast-feeding mother can move her baby from side to side with less discomfort. Because there are fewer parenteral injections and a smaller dose of analgesia, there is less excretion of the analgesic into the breast milk.

Respiratory depression may occur as these spinal opiates are absorbed into the vascular system. The patient is closely observed for respiratory depression for 24 hours. Pulse oximeter or apnea monitors with audible alarms are used to detect failing respirations. Other side effects can occur such as itching, nausea and vomiting, and urinary retention. If an indwelling catheter is left in the bladder, urinary retention is not a problem.

Local anesthesia is utilized in the second stage of labor for delivery and episiotomy repair. A local anesthetic agent with epinephrine is injected into the perineum just before delivery of the fetus. Epinephrine decreases the systemic absorption of the anesthetic agent and prolongs its action because of its vasoconstriction effect. Epinephrine may decrease the blood flow to the uterus and cause cardiovascular effects (i.e., tachycardia and palpitations) if absorbed in the maternal vascular system. However, the amounts of epinephrine and local anesthetic agent are small and the advantages of decreased injections because of the prolonged action that results from the addition of epinephrine make it worthwhile.

Regional anesthetic drugs are commonly 0.5%–1% solutions of lidocaine hydrochloride (Xylocaine), chloroprocaine, or tetracaine hydrochloride (Pontocaine).

For more information on these anesthetics see Chapter 10.

DRUGS THAT SUPPRESS UTERINE MOTILITY

Preterm labor is diagnosed when there are uterine contractions that lead to cervical dilation and effacement after 20 weeks gestation but before 37 weeks gestation. Preterm birth is responsible for most neonatal deaths; therefore, it is important to suppress these uterine contractions to allow the fetus the most time to mature *in utero* before birth. For suppression drugs to be effective, treatment should be begun prophylactically in high-risk patients or as soon as the diagnosis of preterm labor is made, as long as contraindications do not exist. It is not known how effective these drugs are when labor has progressed to a cervical dilatation of more than 4.0 cm and effacement of more than 50%. If the amniotic membranes are ruptured, the use of suppression drugs should be weighed against the increased risk of infection. Other contraindications to the use of these drugs include situations where the prolongation of pregnancy is deleterious to either the mother or the fetus (e.g., in cases of placenta abruptio, hypertension, cardiovascular disease, pre-eclampsia, or fetal distress).

Ethanol was used as one of the first uterine suppression drugs. It is no longer utilized for treatment of preterm labor because of the proven danger of alcohol to the fetus and because of the discomfort to the mother resulting from the intoxicating effect. Magnesium sulfate is sometimes used for preterm labor in conjunction with other suppression drugs, such as the β-sympathomimetics, or when other suppression drugs are contraindicated. For more information about magnesium sulfate see Table 15–9 and the section of this chapter regarding pre-eclampsia and eclampsia.

The β-sympathomimetics are the drugs most frequently utilized for prophylaxis and treatment of preterm labor. The most commonly used sympathomimetic is ritodrine (Yutopar), but terbutaline (Brethine, Bricanyl) and isoxsuprine (Vasodilan) have also been used to suppress uterine motility. At the present time only ritodrine is approved by the FDA for use in suppressing preterm labor.

The β-sympathomimetic drugs suppress uterine motility by stimulating the β_2 receptors found in smooth muscle, including the uterus. This leads to relaxation of the smooth muscles and thus decreases the intensity and frequency of uterine contractions. The β-sympathomimetics have a greater effect on the β_2 receptors of the uterus, bronchial, and vascular smooth muscles than on the β_1 receptors in the heart. There may be cardiovascular effects, such as an increased cardiac output, increased maternal and fetal heart rates, and widening of the maternal pulse pressure. The β_1 receptor stimulation and a reflex response to blood pressure changes caused by vascular smooth muscle relaxation are probably responsible for these changes.

The β-sympathomimetics are contraindicated in patients with a history of cardiac disease, hyperthyroidism, or hypertension. They should be used with care in patients with diabetes. β Receptor stimulation can aggravate these conditions.

The β-sympathomimetic agents, except for isoxsuprine, are administered by intravenous infusion in individually adjusted doses until contractions cease. Isoxsuprine is administered orally. Terbutaline is also administered subcutaneously. Parenteral therapy should be continued for 1–24 hours after contractions have stopped, depending on the medication used. Maintenance therapy is carried out by oral administration until the time of delivery.

RITODRINE

The most common β-sympathomimetic utilized to suppress labor is ritodrine (Yutopar). It is administered by intravenous infusion or orally. The intravenous dose of ritodrine is 50–100 μg/min with increases every 10 minutes in increments of 50 μg until an effective dose is reached. The maintenance intravenous dose of ritodrine is 150–350 μg/min. The intravenous infusion should be continued for 12–24 hours after the contractions stop. The intravenous infusion is usually followed by oral administration of ritodrine and can be reinstituted if uterine contractions resume. Oral ritodrine is administered by doses of 10 mg given 30 minutes before the intravenous infusion is discontinued, and then 10 mg every two hours for 24 hours. The oral maintenance dose is 10–20 mg every four to six hours until term or medical judgment dictates.

The onset of effect of an oral dose of ritodrine is 30–60 minutes, while the intravenous dose has an onset in five minutes when it is at the effective dosage. The peak effect is reached in the oral dose in 30–60 minutes and in the intravenous dose in 60 minutes. Ritodrine has a low protein binding. It is metabolized in the liver and excreted in the kidney. See Table 15–4 for more information on ritodrine.

TERBUTALINE

When terbutaline is administered as a preterm labor inhibitor, 2.5 mg is prescribed orally every four to six hours until term. For use as a labor suppressant, terbutaline should be infused initially at a rate of 10 μg/min. This rate should be increased by 5 μg/min every 10 minutes until contractions stop. The maximum dosage of terbutaline is 80 μg/min. After the contractions have stopped for 30 minutes–1 hour, the infusion rate should be decreased by 5 μg/min to determine the lowest effective dose. This rate should be continued for four to eight hours. A subcutaneous dosage for labor suppression is 250 mcg, which should be injected every hour until it has been effective.

Oral terbutaline has an onset of effect in one to two hours, while the parenteral onset is within 15 minutes. The peak action of the oral dose is within two to three hours, and the parenteral peak is reached in 0.50–1

Table 15–4. UTERINE SUPPRESSION DRUGS

Drug	Dosage	Mode of Administration	Pharmacokinetics
Action: All cause relaxation of smooth muscle due to stimulation of β_2 receptors.			
Use: Suppress preterm labor.			
Ritodrine (Yutopar)	PO: 10 mg 30 min before IV infusion discontinued; then increase 10 mg q 2 hr for 24 hr Maintenance (PO): 10–20 mg q 4–6 hr until term IV: 50–100 µg/min; increase q 10 min prn in increments of 50 µg to the effective dose Maintenance (IV): 150–350 µg/min	PO IV—infusion pump	O: PO—30–60 min. IV—5 min (at effective dose) P: PO: 30–60 min; IV 60 min D: NA ½ L: PO—2 phases, 1.3 and 12–20 hr. IV—3 phases, 6–9 min, 1.7–2.6 hr, 15–17 hr PB: 32% B: hepatic E: renal
Terbutaline (Brethine & Bricanyl)	2.5 mg q 4–6 hr 10 µg/min initially, increasing by 5 µg per min q 10 min until contractions cease; max. 80 µg/min 250 µg q 1 hr	PO IV SC	O: PO—1–2 hr; IV/SC—within 15 min P: PO—within 2–3 hr; IV/SC—0.5–1 hr ½ L: UA D: PO—4–8 hr; IV/SC—1.5–4 hr B: hepatic, partially E: renal
Isoxsuprine (Vasodilan, Vasoprine)	5–20 mg q 3–6 hr	PO	O: PO—1 hr D: 3 hr ½ L: approximately 1.25 hr B: partially conjugated in the blood E: primarily in urine

Key to Abbreviations in the *Pharmacokinetics* column: O-onset; P-peak; D-duration; PB-protein bound; B-biotransformed in; E-excreted in; ½ L-halflife.

*Within the column listing adverse effects, underlines indicate the most common effects; CAPITALS indicate life-threatening effects.

hour. The effects last for four to eight hours with oral administration. It is metabolized partially in the liver and excreted by the kidney. See Table 15–4 for more information on terbutaline.

ISOXSUPRINE

Isoxsuprine is administered orally to suppress uterine motility. The oral dose is 5–20 mg every three to six hours until the pregnancy is terminated. An intravenous form of this drug is also made, but it is not available commercially in the United States.

Isoxsuprine has an initial onset of one hour orally. It has a half-life of approximately 1.25 hours. Isoxsuprine

is partially conjugated in the blood and is primarily excreted in the urine. See Table 15–4 for more information on isoxsuprine.

ADVERSE REACTIONS

The use of β-sympathomimetic stimulants can result in maternal hypotension and tachycardia because of the vasodilation effect. Placing the patient on her left side, which allows adequate venous return to the heart, will minimize hypotension. Nausea, sweating, headache, and drowsiness also can occur. Hypokalemia can occur in the mother as can hypoglycemia. Pulmonary edema has been reported frequently following concurrent use

Contraindications/ Precautions	Adverse Reactions*	Interactions	Nursing Implications
Should not be used in cardiac disorders, hyperthyroidism, chorioamnionitis, hemorrhage, intrauterine fetal death or known abnormality, eclampsia and severe pre-eclampsia, pulmonary hypertension. Caution for administration in asthma, diabetes mellitus, hypertension, mild-to-moderate pre-eclampsia. Before 20 weeks gestation.	Neuro: headache, trembling, anxiety, or nervousness. CV: INCREASED MATERNAL AND FHR, PALPITATIONS; increased maternal systolic BP; decreased maternal diastolic BP; chest pain, ARRHYTHMIA; HYPOTENSION; DYSPNEA; maternal pulmonary edema. GI: nausea and vomiting, ileus, constipation. Integ: erythema. Hemo: hyperglycemia, ketoacidosis, hypokalemia. Renal: glycosuria. Neonatal effects: hypoglycemia, hyperglycemia, ileus.	Glucocorticoids: concurrent use to enhance fetal lung maturity may cause pulmonary edema. Not administered with other sympathomimetic agents due to additive effects. Concurrent administration of β-adrenergic blockers should be avoided.	ASSESSMENT: Assess medical and obstetrical hx. Assess gestational age and fetal maturity. Palpate uterine contractions. Determine FHR. Assess status of membranes. Assess vital signs, lung sounds, fluid and electrolyte status.
Same as ritodrine.	Same as ritodrine.	Same as ritodrine.	Same as ritodrine.
Not used in cardiac arrhythmic disorders, hyperthyroidism, chorioamnionitis, hemorrhage, fetal demise or known severe fetal abnormality, asthma, diabetes, hypertension, mild-to-moderate pre-eclampsia. If rash persists discontinue.	Neuro: trembling, nervousness. CV: dizziness or faintness; hypotension; unusually fast or irregular heartbeat (maternal and fetal); chest pain and shortness of breath. GI: nausea and vomiting, intestinal distention. Integ: severe rash, flushing	Same as ritodrine.	Same as above. ASSESSMENT: Assess bowel habits and bowel sounds periodically. EVALUATION: Notify MD if abdominal distention, pain, and/or decrease in bowel sounds.

with corticosteroids or in cases of multiple gestation, particularly if infused in a sodium chloride solution. Sodium chloride solutions should only be used when dextrose solutions are contraindicated (e.g., diabetic patients). In the fetus, use of these drugs often causes mild tachycardia. The neonate whose mother received β-sympathomimetics can exhibit hypoglycemia, hyperglycemia, ileus, hypocalcemia, or hypotension. For more information on β-sympathomimetic drugs see Chapter 19.

USING THE NURSING PROCESS

Assessment

Assessment of the patient requiring drugs to suppress uterine motility should begin with a thorough nursing history, which includes an obstetrical history. The presence of any contraindications for administration of β-sympathomimetics are determined and documented. Gestational age and maturity of the fetus is determined. Uterine activity with resultant cervical dilation, effacement, and status of amniotic membranes, as well as FHR, fetal heart rate, is assessed. Assessment of maternal anxiety and knowledge level regarding preterm labor is pertinent to planning nursing care. Baseline information to determine drug-induced reactions should include maternal vital signs, heart and lung sounds, and fluid electrolyte status.

Nursing Diagnoses

Based on the assessment information, nursing diagnoses are established. The nursing diagnoses form the basis for the nursing care plan. Some of the possible nursing diagnoses are featured in Table 15–5.

Table 15–5. NURSING PROCESS FOR THE PATIENT RECEIVING UTERINE SUPPRESSANTS

Assessment

Review obstetrical history including expected delivery date, education level and prenatal education, previous pregnancies and outcomes.
Assess frequency, duration and strength of uterine contractions, cervical dilation and effacement.
Evaluate concurrent medical problems, e.g., cardiac disease, hyperthyroidism, hypertension, asthma and diabetes.
Check for ruptured membranes, note signs of infection.
Determine support systems available to the patient

Nursing Diagnosis	Nursing Actions	Rationale	Patient Outcomes/ Evaluation Criteria
Activity intolerance related to muscle irritability as evidenced by uterine contractions/preterm labor.	Place on bedrest in left lateral position and explain reasons to the patient.	Activity may stimulate uterine contractions. Positioning on left side maximizes utero-placental blood flow and keeps the fetus off the cervix.	Reports/displays cessation of uterine activity.
	Provide comfort measures, e.g., backrubs, position changes, decrease lighting in room.	Decreases muscle tension and fatigue and promotes sense of well-being.	
	Offer diversional activities as appropriate.	Assists patient to refocus attention and cope with decreased activity.	
	Recheck uterine activity on a regular schedule.	Provides information about effectiveness of interventions.	
Injury, potential for poisoning related to toxic side effects of medications given to stop labor.	Obtain consent for procedures after discussion.	Indicates that information has been given and understood and patient is willing to undergo treatment.	Displays no adverse effects of therapy.
	Administer IV solutions containing tocolytics, via controlled infusion pump per protocol.	Provides for delivery of appropriate drug dosage and limits risk of inadvertent overdose.	
	Observe infusion on a periodic basis.	Verifies that drug is administered as prescribed.	
	Monitor vital signs; auscultate lung sounds, note cardiac irregularities.	Complications such as pulmonary edema, cardiac dysrhythmias, tachycardia, agitation, etc. may occur with the use of tocolytic drugs.	
	Ascertain serum glucose and potassium as indicated.	Tocolytics may interfere with potassium and glucose metabolism.	
	Administer antidote, e.g., calcium gluconate or propanolol if indicated.	May be necessary to reverse or counteract toxic effects of tocolytic drugs.	
Anxiety (specify level) related to perceived/ actual threat to self/fetus as evidenced by increased tension, tremors, restlessness, expressions of fear, distress, concern, focus on self.	Explain procedures, interventions, and treatments. Keep communication open, and discuss possible side effects and outcomes, maintaining an optimistic attitude.	Information can help to decrease fear of the unknown.	Appears relaxed, sleeps/rests appropriately. Reports anxiety is decreased to a manageable level.
	Encourage verbalization of fears.	Defines the problem, providing opportunity for resolution and a help to allay anxiety.	
	Keep patient informed of status and choices of treatment.	Assists patient to use coping skills, decreasing anxiety.	

Table 15–5. NURSING PROCESS FOR THE PATIENT RECEIVING UTERINE SUPPRESSANTS–CONTINUED

Nursing Diagnosis	Nursing Actions	Rationale	Patient Outcomes/ Evaluation Criteria
	Promote use of relaxation techniques.	Enables patient to obtain maximum benefit from rest periods; prevents muscle fatigue and improves uterine blood flow.	
	Monitor maternal/fetal vital signs.	Vital signs of patient and fetus may be altered by anxiety. Stabilization may reflect reduction of anxiety level.	
Knowledge, deficit related to lack of information/exposure, misinterpretation as evidenced by questions, request for information.	Ascertain patient's knowledge about preterm labor and possible outcomes.	Establishes data base and identifies needs.	Verbalizes awareness of implications and possible outcomes of preterm labor.
	Evaluate patient's readiness to learn.	Factors such as anxiety or lack of awareness of need for information can interfere with learning.	
	Review signs and symptoms of "early" labor.	Helps patient to recognize preterm labor so that treatment can be instituted promptly.	
	Provide information about implications of preterm labor for the fetus.	Knowledge improves possibility of patient cooperating with therapeutic regimen.	
	Include SO in explanations.	Support from SO can help allay anxiety and assist with retention of information.	
	Provide information in written form.	Provides opportunity for patient to review information frequently.	

Planning and Intervention

Nursing diagnoses are the basis for the goals of nursing intervention. Some goals that may be appropriate for a patient receiving suppression drugs are (1) the patient will experience a decrease in uterine activity so that fetal status is not jeopardized, and (2) the patient will experience minimal anxiety associated with preterm labor throughout the labor and delivery process.

An infusion pump should be utilized to assure precise control of the intravenous infusion. The nurse applies continuous external electronic fetal monitors and continuously assesses the graph to monitor fetal status and uterine activity. Manual palpation of the contractions to determine strength, duration, and frequency to adequately determine effects of suppression drugs is done periodically. Dosages of suppression drugs should be increased as necessary to reach an effective level.

Continuous monitoring of the FHR pattern is important. Mild tachycardia can occur in the fetus, but FHR should not exceed 180 beats per minute.

Since physical activity can increase uterine activity, bedrest after application of antiembolism stockings is instituted to enable the suppression drugs to be most effective. In order to maintain maximum uteroplacental blood flow, the patient is placed in a left-side-lying position.

Hydration is maintained because dehydration also stimulates uterine activity. Intake and output are kept by the nurse to determine hydration level and kidney function and to avoid fluid overload. A daily weight is also important in evaluating hydration level.

Maternal vital signs are monitored to determine if any adverse reactions to the suppression drugs are occurring (Table 15–4). The nurse is alert to the possibility of pulmonary edema. Assessments of lung sounds and hydration status as well as maternal heart rate are important. If the maternal heart rate persists at greater than 140 beats per minute, the possibility of pulmonary edema is increased. If the patient complains of chest pain or tightness, the intravenous infusion is discontinued, the physician notified, and an electrocardiogram (ECG) evaluated.

Blood glucose is monitored in the patient receiving β-sympathomimetics, particularly if she is diabetic, because of the possibility of hyperglycemia. Since ketoacidosis is also possible, acid-base status is carefully maintained.

Anxiety may be an adverse reaction to β-sympathomimetic drugs. The patient may be able to cope with this anxiety in a positive manner if she is aware of the cause and if she is kept informed of her choices, the decisions regarding her treatment, and the status of the fetus and her labor.

The patient and her significant others may be quite anxious about the onset of preterm labor as well. Anxiety can stimulate uterine activity, but knowledge can increase compliance in the patient, which will give the suppression drugs every opportunity to be effective. The nurse provides information regarding the drug being administered, the electronic fetal monitor, and any other procedure. Patients also need to be informed regarding the status of the fetus.

Since administration of β-sympathomimetics can cause a transient hypokalemia, serum potassium levels are periodically ascertained, along with continuous assessment for symptoms indicating hypokalemia such as muscle weakness, fatigue, and ECG changes. If symptoms of a toxic reaction occur (Table 15–4), the intravenous infusion is discontinued and a β-adrenergic blocking drug such as propranolol is administered.

With successful suppression of uterine contractions, the patient may be treated with oral uterine suppressants. Table 15–6 lists patient teaching information for uterine suppressants.

Evaluation

The evaluation of the effect of the suppression is based on the cessation of uterine activity until as close to term as possible or until medical judgment dictates. Material that has been previously taught to the patient is reviewed and updated if a resumption of the preterm uterine activity occurs.

DRUGS THAT ENHANCE UTERINE MOTILITY

Medications to enhance uterine motility may be prescribed to facilitate the labor process and to induce therapeutic abortion during the second trimester of pregnancy. These drugs are also used to combat uterine atony to help prevent or control postpartal hemorrhage.

Medications used to enhance uterine motility are referred to as oxytocics. Oxytocin, the ergot alkaloids, and certain prostaglandins are included in this category. The prostaglandins (PGE_2 and carboprost) function as oxytocics; however, they are not currently approved in the United States for this purpose except in experimental protocols and are used instead as *abortifacients*. Oxytocin, a posterior pituitary hormone, is the preparation used most often to induce or augment labor by enhancing uterine contractions. The ergot alkaloids—ergonovine, and methylergonovine—and oxytocin are used in the postpartal period to stimulate uterine contractions in order to control bleeding. Table 15–7 gives more information on drugs to enhance uterine motility.

OXYTOCIN

Oxytocin (Pitocin) stimulates the smooth muscle of the uterus and therefore increases both the force and frequency of contractions. High estrogen levels lower the threshold for uterine response to oxytocin. During preg-

Table 15–6. PATIENT TEACHING INFORMATION—UTERINE SUPPRESSANTS

Dear Patient,
  This drug has been prescribed for you. This is what you should know about your drug to get the most from your therapy.

1. Ritodrine (Yutopar) is taken to stop your premature labor.
2. This drug should be taken as directed by your doctor until your baby reaches term or your doctor tells you to stop taking it.
3. This drug is taken by mouth.
4. Check with your doctor or nurse before you begin taking any other drugs. Please make sure your doctor or nurse is aware of any drugs you are taking now or if you have asthma, diabetes mellitus, heart disease, high blood pressure, or an overactive thyroid.
5. If you forget a dose of this drug and remember within an hour or less of the missed dose, take it right away. If you do not remember for longer than an hour, take your next dose on the regular schedule but do not take the missed dose.
6. Contact your doctor immediately if your contractions begin again or your water breaks.
7. Since drinking alcohol can hurt your baby, you should not drink alcohol while pregnant.
8. Drugs sometimes cause some side effects along with the desired effects. Call your doctor or nurse as soon as possible if you notice any of the following: rapid irregular heartbeat, severe nausea or vomiting, severe nervousness or trembling, or shortness of breath. Some side effects occur until your body adjusts to the drug. Check with your doctor or nurse if the following symptoms do not improve or are bothering you: trembling, headache, jitteriness, nervousness, and restlessness.
9. This drug should be stored away from heat and direct light. As with all medications, keep it out of the reach of your children. The heat and moisture in your bathroom may make this medicine ineffective so do not put it in your bathroom medicine cabinet.

nancy, the uterus becomes progressively more responsive to the effects of oxytocin, becoming most sensitive at term. In fact, in early pregnancy, only large amounts of exogenous oxytocin result in contractions. Although it does not appear that oxytocin actually causes labor to begin, it is certain that oxytocin's effect on the uterus facilitates labor.

Oxytocin can be used to test uteroplacental reserve in the oxytocin challenge test (OCT). This test, administered in high-risk pregnancies, helps to determine the ability of the placenta to meet fetal oxygen needs during contractions and therefore whether or not the pregnancy can safely be continued. Small amounts of oxytocin (0.5 milliunit per minute) are infused intravenously using a double-bottle set (piggyback) and a controlled infusion device. The rate is gradually increased until the patient experiences three contractions within a ten-minute period, which generally occurs after 8–9 milliunits of oxytocin have been administered. Before, during, and after the infusion, FHR and contractions are monitored. A fetal heart pattern with late decelerations is indicative of low placental reserve and is termed a positive test, indicating the placenta may not be able to meet fetal oxygen needs during labor. Following a positive OCT, termination of the pregnancy by delivery may be indicated because of the possibility of fetal compromise. Negative tests are repeated at weekly intervals until the pregnancy is terminated. For more information, refer to an obstetrical nursing text.

Oxytocin or the ergot alkaloids may be administered during the third stage of labor to control postpartal bleeding. Pitocin is often added to an existing intravenous solution after delivery of the placenta. Methylergonovine is usually the ergot alkaloid of choice and is administered intramuscularly after the delivery of the placenta.

Oxytocin also plays a role in lactation, forcing milk into the mammary sinuses, where it is available for the suckling infant. This is usually referred to as milk ejection or milk letdown. Oxytocin is sometimes administered by nasal spray for women who experience difficulty with the letdown reflex. For more information on oxytocin nasal spray see the section in this chapter on the lactating patient.

Dosage

Oxytocin is the drug of choice for the induction and augmentation of labor. Oxytocin preparations contain 10 USP units per milliliter for intramuscular or intravenous administration. For induction of labor, continuous intravenous infusion is prepared by adding 10 units of oxytocin to 1 liter of 5% dextrose in water, 0.9% sodium chloride, or the physician's electrolyte fluid choice. The intravenous route is preferred because the dosage can be adjusted precisely and the administration discontinued quickly should problems arise. The dosage of oxytocin is individual depending on maternal (contractions) and fetal (heart rate) response. Intravenous administration of oxytocics should utilize an infusion pump with a microdrip regulator in a double-bottle setup to enable precise adjustment of the flow rate.

For induction or augmentation, the intravenous infusion should begin at a rate no greater than 1–2 milliunits per minute. The rate of the infusion should be increased every 15–30 minutes in increments of 1–2 milliunits until a relatively normal labor pattern is established. The infusion should not exceed a rate of 20 milliunits per minute and can be reduced after labor is established.

When oxytocin is utilized for a missed abortion or postpartal hemorrhage, 10 units should be diluted in a liter of solution and administered intravenously at a rate of 20–40 milliunits per minute. For control of postpartal hemorrhage, the oxytocin should be administered following the delivery of the infant(s) and preferably the placenta(s). If oxytocin is administered intramuscularly to control postpartal uterine atony, a dose of 3–10 units should be administered.

Pharmacokinetics

The onset of action of intravenous oxytocin is immediate, with the frequency and intensity of contractions increasing over a 15–60 minute period and then stabilizing. An intramuscular injection of oxytocin has an onset of action in three to five minutes. The duration of effect for an intramuscular injection is 30–60 minutes. The half-life of oxytocin is one to six minutes being at the lower level in late pregnancy and during lactation. Oxytocin has a low protein binding and is metabolized in the liver and kidney. It is excreted by the kidney with only small amounts remaining unchanged.

Contraindications and Precautions

The oxytocic dosage should be decreased with cardiovascular, hypertensive, or renal disease. It is contraindicated in cephalopelvic disproportion (CPD), placenta previa, placenta abruptio, and previous cesarean birth except under close medical supervision. If delivery is not imminent, oxytocin is contraindicated with fetal distress.

The infusion should be stopped at the first indication of uterine hyperactivity or fetal distress. It should be administered no longer than six to eight hours for *uterine inertia*, the absence or weakness of uterine contractions.

Adverse Reactions

When administering drugs that affect uterine motility, the nurse needs to be aware that these drugs can cause reactions in both the mother and the fetus. The fetal effect is usually related to the degree of uterine activity. In order to maintain effective oxygenation to the fetus, it is essential that adequate relaxation of the myometrium occurs between uterine contractions. The oxytocic drugs can lead to an increase in uterine tonus, tetanic contractions, or both, which will seriously disrupt the oxygen supply to the fetus. Fetal reactions during use of oxytocin reportedly have included bradycardia, neonatal jaundice, fetal trauma, cardiac arrhythmias, intracranial hemorrhage, and asphyxia.

In the mother, hypertension or hypotension may occur with oxytocic use. Nausea, vomiting, postpartal hemorrhage, tetanic contractions, uterine rupture, and anaphylaxis can occur. Cardiac dysrhythmias, premature ventricular contractions, and palpitations have been reported. When large amounts of oxytocins are used, water intoxication can occur. Usually a total of 40–50 units of oxytocin is required for the antidiuretic effects to occur.

Interactions

When a vasopressor or a caudal block with a vasoconstrictor is utilized concurrently with oxytocin, severe hypertension can result. When oxytocin is used in conjunction with cyclopropane, a hydrocarbon inhalation anesthetic, there can be a decrease in tachycardia caused by oxytocin and a concomitant hypotension. Enflurane, halothane, and possibly isoflurane can decrease the uterine response to oxytocin, which could lead to uterine atony and hemorrhage. Use of oxytocin with other oxytocics could cause uterine hypertonus, resulting in fetal distress, uterine rupture, or cervical laceration.

ERGOT ALKALOIDS

The ergot alkaloids were derived initially from a fungus affecting rye grain. These drugs may affect many or-

TEXT RESUMES ON PAGE 344

Table 15–7. DRUGS ENHANCING UTERINE MOTILITY (OXYTOCICS)

Drug	Dosage	Mode of Administration	Pharmacokinetics
Action: Stimulate smooth muscle of the uterus.			
Use: Induction or augmentation of labor; control of postpartal hemorrhage.			
Oxytocin (Pitocin)	Induction or stimulation: Begin no more than 1–2 milliunits per min, increasing q 15–30 min in increments of 1–2 milliunits per min until a contraction pattern similar to normal labor established; max. 20 milliunits per min Missed abortion: 10 units at rate of 20–40 milliunits per min	IV infusion pump	O: IV, immediate; IM—3–5 min D: IM, 2–3 hr; IV, 1 hr ½ L: 1–6 min PB: low B: hepatic and renal E: renal
	Control of postpartal hemorrhage: 10 units at rate of 20–40 milliunits per min 3–10 units after delivery of placenta	IM	
Ergot Alkaloids Ergonovine maleate (Ergometrine, Ergotrate)			
Action: Smooth muscle stimulation.			
Use: Control of postpartal hemorrhage.			
	0.2–0.4 mg	PO	O: PO—6–15 min; IM—2–5 min; IV—immediate
	0.2 mg	IM IV	D: PO—approximately 3 hr; IM—approximately 3 hr; IV—45 min ½ L: PO—2 hr B: hepatic E: renal
Methylergonovine maleate (Methergine, Methylergometrine)			
Action: Stimulates contraction of the uterine wall.			
Use: Contraction of uterine wall around bleeding vessels from placental site.			
	0.2–0.4 mg BID–QID	PO	P: PO—6–15 min; IM—2–5 min
		IM IV	P: IV—immediate D: PO—approximately 3 hr; IM approximately 3 hr; IV—approximately 45 min

Key to Abbreviations in the *Pharmacokinetics* column: O-onset; P-peak; D-duration; PB-protein bound; B-biotransformed in; E-excreted in; ½ L-halflife.
*Within the column listing adverse effects, underlines indicate the most common effects; CAPITALS indicate life-threatening effects.

Contraindications/ Precautions	Adverse Reactions*	Interactions	Nursing Implications
Contraindicated in OB emergencies, cephalo-pelvic disproportion, fetal distress (if delivery not imminent). Given by one route of administration only. Decrease dosage with CV, hypertensive or renal disease. Infusion should be stopped at first sign of uterine hyperactivity or fetal distress. Administered no longer than 6–8 hr for uterine inertia.	Fetal: intracranial hemor-rhage, bradycardia, cardiac arrhythmias, ASPHYXIA, neo-natal jaundice, and fetal trauma. Maternal: CV: hypertension, PVC, hypo-tension, ANAPHYLAXIS. GI: nausea and vomiting, water intoxication. Musculoskeletal: TETANIC CON-TRACTIONS, UTERINE RUPTURE, postpartal hemorrhage	Concomitant use of vaso-pressors or caudal block with vasoconstrictors can cause severe hypertension. Cyclopropane anesthesia may lessen tachycardia but worsen hypotension caused by oxytocin. Enflurane, halothane, and possibly, isoflurane may decrease uterine response to oxytocin leading to uter-ine hemorrhage. Concomitant use with other oxytocics can lead to uter-ine hypertonus and uterine rupture, cervical laceration.	ASSESSMENT: OB hx; obtain baseline data, BP, FHR, duration and fre-quency of contractions, sta-tus of membranes. Assess fluid status. INTERVENTION: Explain need for induction or aug-mentation. Utilize infusion pump piggybacked into mainline setup. Label solu-tion. Monitor I & O, position patient on left side, apply continuous fetal monitoring (internal if membranes are ruptured). Palpate fundus to evaluate contractions: intensity, frequency, dura-tion, and uterine resting tone. Document VS and T every 2 hr. EVALUATION: Relatively normal labor pattern with no fetal distress. Dilation and effacement of cervix progress. Identify adverse reactions.
Contraindicated in hyper-sensitivity, hypertension, toxemia, and prior to delivery of placenta. Hepatic or renal function impaired.	Neuro: headache, dizziness, SEIZURES, confusion. CV: sudden, severe HYPER-TENSION or HYPOTENSION, COR-ONARY VASOSPASM, DYSPNEA, CHEST PAIN. GI: nausea, vomiting, DIAR-RHEA. Musculoskeletal: uterine tetany; pain in arms, legs, or lower back. Integ: itching.	Concomitant use of vaso-pressors, ergot alkaloids, or vasoconstrictors result in severe hypertension and rupture of cerebral blood vessels.	ASSESSMENT: Same as above. Assess lochial flow and fundal height. INTERVENTION: Same as above. Monitor lochial flow and fundal height. Monitor BP. EVALUATION: Decrease in lochial flow, uterus main-tains contraction.
Same as above Protect from light.	Same as above.	Same as above.	Same as above.

CONTINUED ON THE FOLLOWING PAGE

Table 15–7. DRUGS ENHANCING UTERINE MOTILITY (OXYTOCICS)–*CONTINUED*

Drug	Dosage	Mode of Administration	Pharmacokinetics
			½ L: 0.5–2 hr B: probably hepatic with extensive 1st pass metabolism E: renal

Prostaglandins

Action: Appears to stimulate myometrium.

Use: Abortifacients

Drug	Dosage	Mode of Administration	Pharmacokinetics
Dinoprost (Prostin F2 Alpha), Dinaprost Tromethamine Injection (Prostin F2 Alpha)	40 mg 50 μg/ml in 5% dextrose at rate of 2.5 μg/min, doubled every hour prn to maximum of 20 μg/min	Intra-amniotic IV	O: 1 min P: mean abortion effect 20–24 hr ½ L: in amniotic fluid, 3–6 hr; plasma <1 min B: maternal lungs and liver E: primarily renal; 5% in feces
Dinoprostone (Prostin E2)	20 mg q 3–5 hr; max. 240 mg	Intravaginal	O: within 10 min P: mean abortion time—17 hr D: 2–3 hr B: lungs, kidneys, spleen, and other tissue E: primarily renal
Carboprost (Prostin 15M)	0.25 mg q 1.5–3.5 hr, may increase to 0.5 mg if inadequate response; max 12 mg	IM	P: 30 min B: enzymatic deactivation in tissues E: primarily renal as metabolites

Key to Abbreviations in the *Pharmacokinetics* column: O-onset; P-peak; D-duration; PB-protein bound; B-biotransformed in; E-excreted in; ½ L-halflife.
*Within the column listing adverse effects, underlines indicate the most common effects; CAPITALS indicate life-threatening effects.

gans, notably the cardiovascular system, as well as increase uterine contractility. Small doses of the ergot alkaloids increase the force and frequency of contractions. Larger doses accomplish the same but also increase the resting muscle tonus and may result in sustained contractions. This fact explains why these drugs are not used to induce or augment labor. They are used in the postpartum state to treat uterine atony and to minimize bleeding. Since the ergot derivatives cause sustained contraction of the uterus, they are not used prior to placental delivery. As with oxytocin, sensitivity of the uterus to these drugs increases with the increasing duration of pregnancy.

Ergonovine maleate (Ergotrate) and methylergonovine maleate (Methergine and Methylergometrine) are administered intramuscularly and rarely, intravenously in doses of 0.2 mg, and orally in doses of 0.2–0.4 mg two to four times daily. Intravenous administration is only utilized for emergencies such as in cases of increased uterine bleeding. Oral doses usually follow an initial parenteral dose. Intramuscular or, in cases of postpartal hemorrhage, intravenous doses may be repeated in two or four hours as necessary for up to five doses.

Onset of uterine contraction occurs two to five minutes after intramuscular administration and immediately after intravenous administration. The drug effects continue for approximately three hours after intramuscular administration and for 45 minutes after intravenous administration. The half-life of methylergonovine maleate is 0.5–2 hours.

Metabolism of ergonovine maleate occurs in the liver with excretion by the kidney. Methylergonovine maleate is probably metabolized in the liver with an extensive first-pass metabolism. Excretion of less than 5% occurs in the kidney.

Contraindications/ Precautions	Adverse Reactions*	Interactions	Nursing Implications
Contraindicated in rupture of membranes, acute peripheral vascular disorders, asthma, hypertension, glaucoma, epilepsy, diabetes, pulmonary disease, cervical stenosis, anemia, and acute PID.	Headache, hypertension, dyspnea, wheezing, nausea, vomiting, diarrhea, abdominal cramps, and fever.	May augment other prostaglandins.	Same as above.
Same as above. Handle unwrapped suppository carefully to prevent skin absorption. Store <20°C (−4°F)	Same as above.	Same as above.	Same as above. INTERVENTION: Allow suppository in foil wrapping to warm to room temperature just prior to use. Patient should remain supine for 10 min after. EVALUATION: Patient remains supine for maximum dose at cervix.
Same as above. Care should be taken not to get on skin; wash with soap and water immediately.	Same as above.	Same as above.	Same as above.

Contraindications and Precautions

Ergot alkaloids are contraindicated with a history of hypersensitivity to ergot. Since ergot alkaloids are metabolized and excreted in the liver and kidney, they are contraindicated when there is liver or kidney function impairment. Ergot alkaloids can have some serious cardiovascular side effects and therefore should not be used in patients with hypertension (pregnancy-induced or chronic); heart disease; and mitral valve stenosis.

Adverse Reactions

Headache and confusion have been reported as adverse reactions to the ergot alkaloids. The ergot alkaloids cause a vasoconstricting effect on the vascular system and are capable of causing increases in blood pressure and coronary vasospasm. The reaction indicating allergy is shortness of breath. The woman may experience nausea, vomiting, and diarrhea because of the effect on the smooth muscle of the gastrointestinal tract. Uterine tetany may result. Pain in the arms, legs, and lower back, as well as itching, has also resulted from the use of ergot alkaloids.

The concomitant use of vasopressors or vasoconstrictors, such as in local anesthetics, with ergot alkaloids may result in severe hypertension. This hypertension may result in rupture of cerebral blood vessels. The nurse must always check the blood pressure of any woman who is to receive an ergot alkaloid and not administer it if her blood pressure is elevated.

PROSTAGLANDINS

Some of the prostaglandins also stimualte uterine contractions. Their ability to do so is not confined to the end-stages of pregnancy alone. It is believed that the prostaglandins act directly on the myometrium to stimulate uterine contractions. Prostaglandins soften the cervix to assist in dilatation. Uterine contractions can be elicited early in pregnancy, thus accounting for the use of these drugs as abortifacients. Sensitivity of the uterus to the effects of prostaglandins does increase with increasing gestation, however. Three prostaglandins are currently in use as abortifacients: dinoprostone (Prostin E2), dinoprost tromethamine (Prostin F2 Alpha), and carboprost tromethamine (Prostin 15M).

Dinoprost tromethamine is administered intra-amniotically or intravenously and is used for terminating second-trimester pregnancies. Forty milligrams of the drug are injected into the amniotic sac or 50 μg/ml is mixed in 5% dextrose in water and administered intravenously at a rate of 2.5 μg/min. This administration may be doubled every hour as necessary to a maximum of 20 μg/min.

Dinoprost has an onset of effect of one minute. The mean abortion effect is 20–24 hours. The half-life of dinoprost is three to six hours in the amniotic fluid and less than 1 minute in the plasma. It is metabolized by enzymatic deactivation in the maternal lungs and liver. Excretion occurs primarily in the kidneys, but 5% of the metabolized product is found in the feces.

Dinoprostone is administered as a vaginal suppository and is used to terminate pregnancy from 12–20 weeks gestation. An initial dose of 20 mg can be repeated every three to five hours until abortion occurs. A maximum dosage of 240 mg should not be exceeded.

After the insertion of dinoprostone, contractions begin within ten minutes, with a mean abortion time of approximately 17 hours. The abortion time may range from 12–24 hours. The duration of effects is two to three hours. Metabolism occurs by enzymatic deactivation in the maternal lungs, kidneys, spleen, and other tissues, with excretion occurring mainly in the kidney as metabolites. A small amount is excreted in the feces.

The contraindications and precautions common for the prostaglandins are included at the end of this section; however, there are specific contraindications and precautions for dinoprostone. The unwrapped vaginal suppositories of dinoprostone should be handled carefully to prevent skin absorption. The suppositories are contraindicated in acute pelvic inflammatory disease.

Carboprost (Prostin 15M) is administered intramuscularly and is used between the 13th and 20th week of gestation. Deep intramuscular injection of 0.25 mg may be repeated every 1.5–3.5 hours, depending on the uterine response. The dosage may be increased to 0.5 mg if there is inadequate uterine response. Total dosage should not exceed 12 mg.

Carboprost is metabolized in maternal tissues and excreted mainly by the kidneys as metabolites. The nurse should be careful not to get the drug on the skin and should wash well with soap and water if contact does occur.

Contraindications and Precautions

Abortion may be incomplete in some cases with the use of the prostaglandins; live births may also occur, particularly when late second trimester abortions are undertaken.

The prostaglandins are contraindicated in the intra-vaginal or intra-amniotic route when the membranes are ruptured. Acute peripheral vascular disorders, hypertension, pulmonary disease, cervical stenosis, and anemia also are contraindications for use. Prostaglandins should be used cautiously in women who have histories of asthma, glaucoma, epilepsy, or diabetes mellitus. The use of more than one of the prostaglandins may augment their effect.

Adverse Reactions

Prostaglandins also affect smooth muscle of the gastrointestinal tract, leading to the occurrence of nausea, vomiting, and diarrhea. Nausea, vomiting, abdominal cramps, and diarrhea are the most common adverse reactions to prostaglandin administration and can be severe. Consequently, it is important to assess the patient's hydration status. Respiratory effects include dyspnea, bronchospasm, and hyperventilation. Headache, dizziness, and even paresthesias have been reported. Epigastric, leg, or substernal pain can occur, as can hypertension or vasovagal symptoms.

USING THE NURSING PROCESS

Assessment

A thorough nursing history is done on each patient requiring drugs to enhance uterine motility. This includes an obstetrical history, which also includes the expected delivery date. Baseline data are important for future comparison of maternal blood pressure, pulse, FHR, and duration and frequency of contractions. The nurse determines the status of the membranes and cervical dilation and effacement.

Nursing Diagnoses

Based on the assessment information nursing diagnoses are identified. The nursing diagnoses form the basis for the nursing care plan. Some of the possible nursing diagnoses are featured in Table 15–8.

Intervention

Nursing diagnoses are the basis for the goals of nursing intervention. Some goals that may be appropriate for a patient receiving drugs to enhance uterine motility are the following: the patient (and significant other) will gain knowledge about the lack of progress in labor and the need for the induction or augmentation of labor; the patient will proceed into a regular pattern of contractions; and the patient and the fetus will be able to cope with the stress of labor. For the patient requiring use of medications to enhance uterine motility, nursing interventions revolve around patient education but, most importantly, concern the safety of both the mother and the fetus. The drugs enhancing uterine motility should be used in the clinical setting under direct supervision by the physician and professional nurse.

Maternal blood pressure, FHR, and strength, duration, and frequency of contractions must be monitored. Ideally, the drug is administered by an infusion pump

Table 15–8. NURSING PROCESS FOR THE PATIENT REQUIRING OXYTOCICS

Assessment

Note obstetrical history including expected delivery date, educational level and prenatal education; prevous pregnancies and outcomes.
Assess strength, duration and frequency of contractions, cervical dilation and effacement; presentation and station of fetus.

Nursing Diagnosis	Nursing Actions	Rationale	Patient Outcomes/ Evaluation Criteria
Knowledge deficit related to unfamiliarity with procedure, lack of previous exposure as evidenced by questions, verbalization of concerns, request for information.	Provide information regarding labor induction procedures to the patient and SO. Review need for induction/ augmentation of labor. Demonstrate and explain use of equipment (external/ internal monitor, IV infusion pump), pointing out safety features and alarms. Keep patient informed of progress.	Knowing what to expect decreases anxiety, enhances coping skills, promotes involvement and sense of control. Increases understanding and control of situation, enhances coping and decreases anxiety.	Verbalizes understanding of reasons and protocol for labor induction.
Pain, related to pharmacologic intensification of muscular contractions as evidenced by verbalization, grimacing, and restlessness during contractions.	Recommend use of relaxation and deep breathing techniques. Review analgesics available and appropriate for patient, explain time factors and restrictions. Provide comfort measures, e.g., effleurage, backrubs, pillows, cool washcloths. Assist patient with periodic change of position. Provide positive feedback and keep informed of progress. Administer analgesics as indicated.	Reduces tension and fear which may intensify pain and hamper labor progress. Promotes patient participation and enhances patient sense of control. Promote relaxation, reduces tension and anxiety, enhancing coping and control. Aids circulation, helps to prevent muscle tension and fatigue. Reassures patient/couple, reduces tension and anxiety which may make pain more intense. May be used to relieve pain once dilatation and contractions are established.	Reports discomfort and pain is minimized and/or managed effectively. Able to relax between contractions.
Tissue perfusion uteroplacental, potential for decrease related to prolonged/excessive vascular constriction.	Apply continuous fetal monitoring prior to induction and throughout procedure. Note FHR immediately after membranes rupture, as well as color and amount of fluid. Position patient on left side if possible or position on back with head of bed elevated and a pillow placed under one hip, tilted to left side.	Obtain baseline of FHR and contraction activity. Bradycardia, or variable or late decelerations can indicate compromise of fetal oxygenation. Prolapse of cord can occur with membrane rupture with possibility of compromised circulation. Meconium stained fluid can indicate fetal distress. Aids in obtaining an adequate external fetal monitor stip to evaluate contraction pattern and fetal heart tones. Wedge relieves pressure of fetus on vena cava and enhances placental circulation.	Demonstrates FHR within normal limits. Displays normal Apgar scores at delivery.
Injury, potential for, maternal related to deleterious pharmacologic effects of drug administered.	Explain purpose/effects of oxytocin infusion. Administer oxytocin diluted in electrolyte solution with a two-bottle IV system, via infusion pump according to protocol.	Provides information needed for informed consent. Prevents errors or fluctuation in rate of administration which could cause inadequate contractions or uterine rupture. Oxytocin is given slowly in increasing amounts to maintain blood levels of the drug.	Produces effective labor pattern and delivery is accomplished without injury to mother or fetus.

CONTINUED ON THE FOLLOWING PAGE

Table 15–8. NURSING PROCESS FOR THE PATIENT REQUIRING OXYTOCICS–
CONTINUED

Nursing Diagnosis	Nursing Actions	Rationale	Patient Outcomes/ Evaluation Criteria
		It is rapidly metabolized and excreted by the kidneys, so constant infusion should be maintained.	
	Administer drug piggyback, close to the IV insertion site.	Can be discontinued if necessary and primary site quickly cleared and available for other drug administration as needed.	
	Check BP and pulse q 15 min after induction begins and before increasing oxytocin.	Assesses maternal well-being and detects developing hypertension or hypotension.	
	Palpate fundus to evaluate contractions. Observe for overstimulation of uterus (tetanic contraction).	External uterine monitoring indicates the frequency, intensity, of contractions. Overstimulation may cause fetal hypoxia and drug may need to be discontinued.	
	Monitor frequency, duration, intensity, and resting tone between contractions before each increase in the rate of oxytocin.	Reduces risk of uterine tetany.	
	Record intake and output. Measure urine specific gravity.	Decreased output with increased specific gravity may indicate fluid deficit or may reflect anti-diuretic effect of drug (water intoxication). May limit effectiveness of the medication.	
	Palpate bladder.	Urinary retention may impede labor and fetal descent.	
	Note presence of confusion, drowsiness, headache, edema.	Early signs of water intoxication requiring prompt intervention.	
	Discontinue oxytocin, as indicated and notify physician.	Hyperstimulation of the uterus can lead to abruptio placentae, uterine tetany, and possible rupture.	
	Administer magnesium sulfate, if necessary.	Although uterine activity from oxytocin administration should end two to three minutes after infusion is stopped, magnesium sulfate may be indicated to relieve oxytocin-induced uterine tetany.	

to allow for precise regulation of administration. The maternal contractions and FHR can best be evaluated through the use of electronic monitoring devices, either internal or external. Maternal blood pressure and pulse are monitored frequently. Use of a Y tubing or a stopcock in the infusion tubing with a double-bottle setup (piggyback setup) facilitates rapid discontinuance of the drug being administered should problems arise. The vein can be kept open with plain 5% dextrose in water.

When the ergot alkaloids are used to decrease postpartum bleeding or uterine atony, it is important also to determine the tone of the uterus. Here, relaxation is a potential problem. Routine palpation of the fundus to ascertain firmness and position is vital. Maternal pulse, blood pressure, and vaginal flow should also be observed and recorded frequently, not only to monitor the effectiveness of the drug but also to evaluate for side effects.

Evaluation

Based on the dialogue with the patient and on the list of nursing interventions, the nurse develops evaluation criteria. The patient receiving medications enhancing uterine motility should be expected to demonstrate enhanced uterine contractions culminating in the delivery of the products of conception.

The nurse should also be familiar with the common adverse effects of these drugs and continually observe the patient (mother and fetus) for them. Remember, the use of oxytocics is associated with maternal hypertension, tetanic uterine contractions, fetal bradycardia, and hypoxia. If these adverse reactions occur, the nurse discontinues the intravenous oxytocic infusion, positions the patient on her left side to maximize uteroplacental blood flow, administers oxygen, and notifies the physician.

DRUGS USED IN PRE-ECLAMPSIA AND ECLAMPSIA

Hypertension occurring during pregnancy may be a result of a chronic problem, or it may have been induced by pregnancy. Hypertension during pregnancy may be treated with antyhypertensives. Most commonly used are hydralazine (Apresoline); sodium nitroprusside (Nipride, Nitropress); and diazoxide (Hyperstat). Other hypertensives that may also be used are methyldopa and β-adrenergic blocking agents. For more information on antihypertensive agents see Chapter 29.

Pre-eclampsia (pregnancy-induced hypertension) is characterized by the triad of hypertension, edema, and proteinuria. Eclampsia represents a continuation of this condition, with the patient manifesting increased hypertension, oliguria, and convulsions. There is an increased maternal and fetal mortality associated with these disorders, especially with eclampsia. Delivery of the neonate is the only known cure for severe pre-eclampsia.

Diuretics were once utilized to decrease the retained fluid and edema of the pre-eclamptic, but they caused a decrease in the pregnant woman's blood volume and electrolyte imbalance. The blood volume decrease in turn decreased the uteroplacental blood flow, which jeopardized the fetal oxygen supply.

MAGNESIUM SULFATE

The drug most commonly utilized to treat severe pre-eclampsia and eclampsia is magnesium sulfate ($MgSO_4$). Administered parenterally, magnesium sulfate functions as a central nervous system and muscular depressant by producing peripheral neuromuscular blockade. Magnesium sulfate is used in an attempt to control seizure activity. Since it secondarily relaxes smooth muscle, there may be a decrease in blood pressure, but it is not an antihypertensive agent. It also causes a decrease in uterine contractions, so oxytocin augmentation may be indicated.

Following intramuscular injection, magnesium sulfate exerts its effects in about one hour. These effects last three to four hours. Following intravenous administration, effects begin almost immediately and last about 30 minutes. Magnesium sulfate is excreted by the kidneys at a rate proportional to the plasma concentration and the glomerular filtration rate.

Dosage regimens for treatment with magnesium sulfate vary. One dosage regimen is 8–40 mEq as a 25%–50% solution, which is administered deeply intramuscularly up to six times per day in alternating buttocks. One percent procaine may be added to decrease the pain of the injection. The intravenous dose is 8–32 mEq as a 10% to 20% solution administered at a maximum rate of 1.5 ml of a 10% solution (or its equivalent) per minute. A continuous infusion of 32 mEq in 250 ml of 5% dextrose or 0.9% sodium chloride may be administered at a rate not to exceed 4 ml/min.

Magnesium sulfate readily crosses the placenta and causes a fetal serum concentration that is similar to the maternal serum concentration. The effects on the fetus may include decreased FHR variability, hypotonia, hyporeflexia, hypotension, and respiratory depression. Adverse effects from the use of magnesium sulfate are related to the increased blood levels of magnesium (normal is 1.5–2.5 mEq per liter). The serum magnesium level should be maintained in a therapeutic range because increased levels are associated with respiratory depression. A specific clinical facility's protocol needs to be consulted regarding magnesium sulfate administration.

Earlier signs of hypermagnesemia include flushing, sweating, thirst, sedation, and hypotension. Magnesium sulfate should be used with extreme caution in patients with renal impairment and in digitalized patients. It is contraindicated for patients with heart block and myocardial damage. The use of other central nervous system depressants (barbiturates and narcotics) concurrently will cause an additive effect.

Calcium is an antidote for magnesium toxicity. An intravenous form of calcium (calcium gluconate) should be readily available during intravenous administration of magnesium sulfate. Reversal of respiratory depression or heart block caused by magnesium intoxication usually will occur with 5–10 mEq of intravenous calcium (i.e., 10–20 ml of 10% calcium gluconate).

The neonate born to a mother receiving magnesium sulfate can have low Apgar scores resulting from hypotonia and respiratory depression. Magnesium sulfate is featured in Table 15–9.

USING THE NURSING PROCESS

Assessment

Assessment of the patient with severe pre-eclampsia includes measurement of body weight changes, fluid intake and output, edema, deep tendon reflexes, clonus, and blood pressure. Urine is analyzed for protein. Indicators of impending eclampsia include restlessness, disorientation, headache, epigastric pain, hyperreflexia, and visual disturbances. FHR is also monitored and recorded frequently. A transient decrease in FHR variability can occur. Uterine contraction frequency and duration are monitored in the laboring patient to assure labor progress.

Nursing Diagnoses

Based on the assessment, the nurse develops a list of nursing diagnoses. One possible nursing diagnosis for a patient with pre-eclampsia might be alterations in comfort related to fluid retention; for the patient with eclampsia, potential for injury related to convulsive activity.

Interventions

After developing the diagnoses, the nurse plans specific interventions. Safety precautions in terms of drug administration are a major concern with magnesium sulfate administration. Since increasing blood levels of

Table 15–9. MAGNESIUM SULFATE

Drug	Dosage	Mode of Administration	Pharmacokinetics
Magnesium sulfate			
Action: Produces peripheral neuromuscular blockade causing CNS and muscular depression.			
Use: Control seizure activity occurring as a result of eclampsia.			
	8–40 mEq as a 25%–50% solution	IM—deep gluteal, 1% procaine added to decrease pain	O: IM—approximately 1 hr; IV—immediate
	8–32 mEq as a 10%–20% solution at a rate not to exceed 1.5 ml of 10% solution or equivalent per min	IV	D: IM—3–4 hr; IV—approximately 30 min
	32 mEq in 250 ml of D_5W or NS at rate not to exceed 9 ml per min	IV infusion	E: renal at rate proportional to the plasma concentration and glomerular filtration rate

Key to Abbreviations in the *Pharmacokinetics* column: O-onset; P-peak; D-duration; PB-protein bound; B-biotransformed in; E-excreted in; ½ L-halflife.
*Within the column listing adverse effects, underlines indicate the most common effects; CAPITALS indicate life-threatening effects.

magnesium are associated with severe toxic effects, it is important to accurately and frequently monitor the response of the patient to the drug.

A patient receiving parenteral magnesium sulfate is closely monitored. Respiratory paralysis and cardiac arrest can occur, necessitating the institution of resuscitation measures. An intravenous form of calcium (gluconate or gluceptate) should be readily available as an antidote should toxic effects of magnesium sulfate occur. A dose of 5–10 mEq of intravenous calcium can usually cause a reversal of respiratory depression and cardiac block caused by magnesium intoxication.

The patient who will receive repeated doses of magnesium sulfate should be evaluated carefully before these doses are given. Deep tendon reflexes (patellar are best) should be assessed; if absent, the medication should be withheld. The medication should also be withheld if respiratory rate falls below 16 per minute or if urine output is less than 100 ml in the preceding four hours.

Vital signs of the mother (pulse, blood pressure, respirations, patellar reflexes, and contractions) and fetus need to be monitored and recorded, as often as every 15 minutes if they are unstable. Fluid intake and output should be measured and recorded.

Following delivery, the neonate should be observed for any indications of respiratory or neuromuscular depression. They can occur anytime during the first 24–48 hours after birth.

Evaluation

The nurse develops evaluation criteria in observing the patient that are generally based on goals for intervention. The patient receiving medications to treat preeclampsia and eclampsia should be expected to show a decrease in blood pressure and fluid retention as evidenced by an adequate urine output. The eclamptic patient should demonstrate an absence of seizure activity as well.

In addition, the patient should be evaluated for the occurrence of side effects of magnesium sulfate, which are those of hypermagnesemia: flushing, sweating, extreme thirst, sedation, and diminished neuromuscular functioning.

POSTPARTAL DRUGS

LACTATION SUPPRESSANT

Lactation is a complex process mediated by several pituitary hormones, especially prolactin. During pregnancy, prolactin secretion and its effects on the breasts are inhibited by the high level of placental estrogen and progesterone. After delivery, prolactin levels increase because of the removal of the placenta, the primary

Contraindications/ Precautions	Adverse Reactions*	Interactions	Specific Implications for Nurse and Patient
Extreme caution if given with digitalis glycosides. Not used in patients with heart block, myocardial damage. Extreme caution in patients with severe renal function and impairment; no more than 20 g magnesium sulfate within 48-hr period. Respiratory disease.	Maternal and fetal: REDUCED RESPIRATORY RATE, CIRCULATORY COLLAPSE, hyporeflexia, flushing, transient hypotension, hypothermia, hypotonia, decreased heart rate.	Calcium neutralizes effects of parental magnesium sulfate. Concurrent use with parenteral magnesium sulfate may result in severe and unpredictable potentiation of neuromuscular blockade by neuromuscular blocking agents Digitalis glycosides: Cardiac conduction changes and heart block may occur.	ASSESSMENT: Assess weight, I&O, BP, FHR, patellar reflexes as baseline. Urine should be checked for protein. Assess neurologic status. Assess uterine activity. INTERVENTION: Monitor patient closely. Keep injectable form of calcium available at bedside. Monitor patellar reflexes: If 1 or 0 notify MD. Count respirations: If <16 notify MD. Monitor output: If urine output <30 ml q hr notify MD. Monitor VS. EVALUATION: Decrease in BP and fluid retention. Absence of seizure activity.

Magnesium Sulfate

source of estrogen and progesterone, and the stimulation of the infant suckling at the breast. Oxytocin also plays a critical role in lactation, being necessary for milk ejection (or letdown). Secretion of oxytocin, too, is stimulated by suckling. Oxytocin may be prescribed to assist in milk ejection. For more information on oxytocin prescribed to assist milk ejection, see the section in this chapter on the lactating patient.

Women who do not have the desire or the opportunity to breast-feed their babies can have lactation suppressants prescribed. Combination estrogens and androgens (i.e., testosterone and estradiol—Deladumone) were at one time utilized as lactation suppressants. They are not frequently ordered for this purpose now because of the dangers of thromboembolic disease and possible carcinogenic effects associated with large doses of estrogen.

Bromocriptine (Parlodel), an ergot alkaloid derivative, decreases serum prolactin levels by affecting dopamine-receptor sites on prolactin-secreting cells in the pituitary; it is, therefore, utilized as a lactation suppressant. It does not act on the breast itself. Bromocriptine is rapidly absorbed from the gastrointestinal tract but has a high first-pass metabolism in the liver so only a small amount reaches the bloodstream unchanged. The onset of action is two hours, with a peak effect occurring in eight hours. Bromocriptine has a very high protein binding. Excretion of bromocriptine occurs as metabolites primarily in the biliary system with some kidney excretion.

Bromocriptine is administered orally at a usual dosage of 2.5 mg twice a day with meals for 14 days. After dis-

continuance of the medication, rebound engorgement can occur and, if necessary, can be treated with an additional week of therapy.

Common side effects reported with bromocriptine include hypotension, headaches, dizziness, and nausea. Because of the possibility of hypotension, it should not be administered until postdelivery vital signs have stabilized and, in any case, no sooner than four hours after delivery. It should be used with caution when antihypertensive drugs are being used concomitantly. Bromocriptine is contraindicated during pregnancy and in children under 15 years of age. Since bromocriptine restores normal ovulatory menstrual cycles, it is necessary for the patient to use contraceptive precautions. Bromocriptine is featured in Table 15–10.

USING THE NURSING PROCESS

Assessment

Assessment of the postpartum patient using medications to suppress lactation includes palpation of the breasts for enlargement and firmness (engorgement), warmth, and tenderness.

Nursing Diagnoses

Based on assessment, nursing diagnoses are made and form a basis for the care plan. For the postpartal patients with breast engorgement, a nursing diagnosis might be (1) comfort, altered: painful breasts related to engorgement, and (2) knowledge deficit related to suppression drugs.

Table 15-10. LACTATION SUPPRESSANTS

Drug	Dosage	Mode of Administration	Pharmacokinetics
Action: Decreases serum prolactin by affecting dopamine receptor sites on prolactin-secreting cells in the pituitary.			
Use: Suppress lactation.			
Bromocriptine (Parlodel)	2.5 mg bid × 14 days	PO	O: 2 hr D: 24 hr ½ L: biphasic—alpha, 4–4.5 hr; beta, 45–50 hr P: 8 hr PB: very high B: liver E: biliary approximately 95%, renal 2.5%–5.5%

Key to Abbreviations in the *Pharmacokinetics* column: O-onset; P-peak; D-duration; PB-protein bound; B-biotransformed in; ½ L-halflife.

*Within the column listing adverse effects, <u>underlines</u> indicate the most common effects; CAPITALS indicate life-threatening effects.

Intervention

Once nursing diagnoses are established, interventions are planned. In addition to the goals related to teaching the patient about the medications she is receiving, other more specific nursing actions are planned. Nursing interventions for the patient receiving medications to suppress lactation include continuing palpation of the breasts for firmness, warmth, and tenderness, as well as familiarizing the patient with medication regimens and potential adverse effects. Patients should be informed that measures such as breast support with a well-fitting bra or binder and ice application can be used to relieve the temporary discomfort of breast engorgement. Mild analgesics can be utilized for the discomfort caused by breast engorgement.

The patient receiving bromocriptine is encouraged to take her medication with meals to lessen nausea and should be informed of the necessity for contraceptive precautions. She is also observed closely for hypotension, particularly during initial therapy. For patient teaching see Table 15–11.

Evaluation

Both the patient and the nurse determine criteria for evaluation. The evaluation of interventions for the patient receiving lactation suppressants should reveal a decrease in breast size, firmness, and tenderness or no breast engorgement.

The nurse also determines that the patient is aware of the side effects of the drugs that she is taking. Common side effects of bromocriptine therapy include hypotension, headache, dizziness, and nausea.

Rh$_O$(D) IMMUNE GLOBULIN

Rh$_O$(D) immune globulin (RhoGAM) is administered intramuscularly within 72 hours of birth when a mother who is Rh$_O$(D^u)-negative delivers an Rh$_O$(D^u)-positive baby and there is laboratory confirmation of a negative indirect Coombs test. Since sensitization of the mother can occur anytime after 8–10 weeks gestation, Rh$_O$(D) immune globulin is often administered at 28 weeks gestation to women who are Rh$_O$(Du)-negative and have a negative antibody screen (indirect Coombs test). Rh$_O$(D) immune globulin should be administered to Rh$_O$(Du)-negative women after spontaneous or induced abortions, in any pregnancy when early placental separation occurs, during amniocentesis, and to any nonpregnant women following a mismatched blood transfusion. For information on how maternal sensitization can occur, see an obstetrics textbook.

Rh$_O$(D) immune globulin promotes the lysis of fetal Rh-positive blood cells that are in the maternal circulation. This occurs before maternal antibodies are formed that would threaten pregnancies in the future. Therefore, the indirect Coombs test must be negative, indicating that the antibodies have not formed.

Dosage of Rh$_O$(D) immune globulin is 300 μg injected intramuscularly within 72 hours after delivery. This dosage of Rh immune globulin will be effective for 30 ml of fetal positive blood. A larger dose may be required

Contraindications/ Precautions	Adverse Reactions*	Interactions	Specific Implications for Nurse and Patient
Allergies to ergot derivatives. Breast-feeding. Careful use with hepatic function impairment and psychiatric disorders.	Neuro: headache, dizziness, drowsiness, fatigue, STROKE, SEIZURES. CV: HYPOTENSION, palpitation, arrhythmia, VENTRICULAR TACHYCARDIA, bradycardia. GI: dry mouth, anorexia, nausea, vomiting. Musculoskeletal: muscle cramps Integ: rash	Additive effects with concomitant use of antihypertensives. Decreased effects with amitriptyline, methyldopa, phenothiazines, reserpine.	ASSESSMENT: Palpate the breasts for enlargement and firmness, warmth, and tenderness. INTERVENTION: Monitor breasts for firmness, warmth, and tenderness. Teach patient about medication and adverse effects, using breast support and applied comfort measures such as ice. EVALAUATION: A decrease in breast size, firmness, tenderness.

Table 15–11. PATIENT TEACHING INFORMATION—LACTATION SUPPRESSANTS

Dear Patient,

This drug has been prescribed for you. This is what you should know about your drug to get the most from your therapy:

1. Bromocriptine (Parlodel) is taken to stop milk production in women who do not wish to breast feed their babies.
2. Bromocriptine is taken as directed by your doctor for 2 weeks. If you start producing milk after completing the 14 days, your doctor may prescribe it for another week.
3. Take this medication by mouth.
4. Tell your doctor if you are taking any other medication before you take bromocriptine or if you have had an allergic reaction to bromocriptine or other ergot medicines.
5. If you forget a dose and remember within 4 hours of your scheduled dose, take it when you remember it. If it has been more than 4 hours, skip the dose and take a dose at the regularly scheduled time. Do not take 2 doses.
6. Do not stop this medicine before completing the 2 weeks unless directed to do so by your doctor.
7. Do not change the amount of the medicine that you take.
8. Take this medicine with meals or milk.
9. Call your doctor immediately if you notice black tarry stools, bloody vomit, seizures, or sudden weakness. Check with your doctor if any of the following continue or are bothersome to you: dizziness or lightheadness when you get up, headache, leg cramps at night, or loss of appetite.
10. This medicine should be stored out of heat and direct light. Bathroom heat and moisture can cause the medicine to break down, so it should not be kept in the bathroom medicine cabinet. As with all medicines, keep out of reach of children.

for complications such as placenta abruptio or other third-stage abnormality where the potential exists for a large infusion of fetal Rh-positive blood into the maternal blood stream. In the case of a larger infusion of fetal blood cells, 300 μg may be injected every 12 hours until the total necessary amount is injected.

Before $Rh_O(D)$ immune globulin is administered, the patient's blood is typed and cross-matched. Since $Rh_O(D)$ immune globulin is obtained from human plasma, verification is made that lot numbers are the same as that of the cross-matched solution. The woman should be observed for symptoms of a blood transfusion reaction. There may be a mild temperature elevation, and the woman may complain of soreness at the injection site.

The nurse verifies the Rh type on each patient to be sure to identify all candidates for $Rh_O(D)$ immune globulin postpartally. If the woman is $Rh_O(Du)$-negative, the indirect Coombs test should be checked to determine whether it is negative or positive. If it is negative, there are no antiglobulins present in the red blood cells. Before administering, the nurse should provide information to the patient concerning the need for $Rh_O(D)$ immune globulin to protect future pregnancies.

THE LACTATING PATIENT

Drugs are significant to the lactating patient because they can have a variety of effects on lactation. Most drugs administered to the lactating woman are found to some extent in the breast milk. Drugs administered to the lactating woman can stimulate or inhibit lactation, change the milk composition, or pass into breast milk and affect the newborn infant.

A lactation stimulant is utilized to stimulate impaired

milk ejection. Oxytocin nasal spray (Syntocinon) stimulates the smooth muscle to facilitate ejection of milk from the breasts. It does not affect the milk production. The nasal spray is usually available in a strength of 40 units per milliliter. It is instilled intranasally in one spray or three drops into one or both nostrils. The nurse should teach women the proper use of this drug as well as the purpose for administration.

The main mechanism that enables drugs to enter breast milk are passive diffusion (either simple or facilitated) and active transport. The effect of drugs ingested by the neonate or infant through breast milk will depend on the amount of drug that is excreted in the breast milk, the oral bioavailability, the protein binding, plasma half-life, metabolism, volume of distribution and excretion of the drug, and receptor sensitivity or tolerance for the drug. Usually drugs with high bioavailability, low protein binding, small volumes of distribution, and long plasma half-lives will be excreted in breast milk. However, specific physicochemical properties of the drugs themselves are important as well. Unionized drugs are excreted in breast milk better than ionized drugs. Drugs of low molecular weight readily enter breast milk, while drugs such as insulin and heparin do not enter breast milk because of their high molecular weight. Highly lipid soluble drugs enter the breast milk easily. If the molecular weight of a water-soluble drug is less than 200, it enters the breast milk, even though drugs of high lipid solubility more readily enter the breast milk. Only drugs not bound to maternal plasma protein can enter the breast milk.

The manner in which a drug is administered to the mother also effects the drug excretion in the breast milk. The greater the dose of the drug, and the more frequently the drug is taken, the greater the chance of the drug entering the breast milk. If the mother has a dis-

Table 15–13. DRUGS TO BE USED WITH CAUTION IN BREAST-FEEDING PATIENTS

Drug	Reason
Tetracycline	Potential staining of teeth but not proven
Sulfonamides	Potential for aggravating neonatal jaundice in any infant and hemolytic anemia in G-6PD infant
Nitrofurantoin	Can cause hemolysis in G-6PD infants
Clindamycin	Potential complications such as diarrhea
Isoniazid	Monitor infants for signs of toxicity such as hepatitis, peripheral neuropathy, and vomiting
Metronidazole	Potential side effects of blood dyscrasias or neurologic disorders, although never demonstrated in nursing infant
Diazepam	Risk of accumulation in neonate
Corticosteroids (large doses)	Animal studies show problems with large doses; still under investigation
Oral contraceptive agents	Still under investigation
Acetylsalicylic acid (large doses)	Effects from ingestion of high doses over long periods have not been studied
Propylthiouracil	Still under investigation

From Kochenour, NK and Emery, MG: Drugs in lactating women. In Wynn RM (ed): Obstetrics and Gynecology Annual, Vol 10. Appleton-Century-Crofts, New York; 1981. Reprinted in Balkman, 1986.

Table 15–12. DRUGS CONTRAINDICATED IN THE NURSING MOTHER

Drug	Reason
Lithium	Significant blood levels in the infant (0.33–0.5 maternal levels)
Antimetabolites	Anti-DNA activity
Radioactive pharmaceuticals	Radioactivity in breast milk
Very lipid soluble drugs	Only elimination route through milk; measure level if any doubt of maternal body burden
Phenindione	Bleeding in 1 case report with increased PT and PTT
Chloramphenicol	Possible bone marrow depression

From Berlin, CM: Pharmacoligic considerations of drug use in the lactating mother. Obstet Gynecol (Suppl 5) 58:, 1986. Reprinted with permission from American College of Obstetricians and Gynecologists in Balkman, 1986.

ease process that decreases her ability to excrete the drug, then more of the drug can potentially enter the breast milk. (See Tables 15–12 and 15–13 for information on specific drugs and lactation.)

NEONATAL DRUGS

The neonate is not commonly given a variety of drugs. The neonatal liver and kidney are immature and therefore may be slow in metabolizing and excreting drugs that the neonate receives from the mother before birth or those given after birth.

No later than one hour after birth, the neonate receives the legally required silver nitrate, 1% solution, or erythromycin ointment in its eyes to prevent gonococcal ophthalmia neonatorum, which is caused by *Neisseria gonorrhoeae* in the maternal vaginal tract. Erythromycin ointment will also prevent neonatal chlamydial conjunctivitis contracted during delivery, while silver nitrate will not.

Silver nitrate is administered by instilling one drop of the 1% solution in each eye. It causes protein denaturation, which prevents gonorrheal ophthalmia neonatorum. The silver nitrate solution may cause periorbital edema, temporary staining of the lids and surrounding tissues, and conjunctivitis. The eyes are not irrigated following the instillation. Because of the possibility of the adverse reactions, instillation may be delayed up to one hour to enable mother-neonatal bonding. The parents are reassured regarding the reactions and told that the reactions should subside in 24–48 hours.

Because of the caustic nature of silver nitrate, erythromycin ointment (Ilotycin) is often used instead. A thin ribbon of approximately 1–1.5 cm of ointment is applied to each conjunctiva following a cesarean or vaginal delivery. Erythromycin enters the cell membrane and inhibits protein synthesis. For prophylaxis of ophthalmia neonatorum and chlamydial infections, the ointments should be instilled no later than one hour after birth.

The neonate also receives an intramuscular injection of vitamin K to prevent hemorrhagic disease of the newborn. Vitamin K promotes the formation in the liver of the clotting factors II, VII, IX, and X. The neonate does not have adequate levels of vitamin K at birth because of the small amount that crosses the placenta from the mother. In addition, the small amount of intestinal flora causes inadequate production of vitamin K in the neonate. Vitamin K (phytonadione—AquaMephyton) is injected intramuscularly or subcutaneously in a dose of 0.5–1 mg. This dosage may be repeated in six to eight hours if necessary. Higher doses may be necessary for infants whose mothers received anticoagulants or anticonvulsants during their pregnancy. See Chapter 14 for information on intramuscular injections in the neonate.

The vitamin K injection may cause pain and edema at the injection site. Allergic reactions such as rash or urticaria are possible. Hyperbilirubinemia may occur in newborns or preterm infants given more than 25 mg. This is due to the vitamin K taking the binding sites that would be utilized by the bilirubin.

The nurse assesses the newborn for bleeding as indicated by generalized ecchymoses or bleeding from the umbilical cord, circumcision site, nose, or gastrointestinal tract. The neonate, particularly a preterm neonate, is assessed for jaundice or kernicterus.

SUMMARY

The physiologic changes accompanying pregnancy affect the pharmacokinetics of drugs. During pregnancy and postpartum, drugs are prescribed as necessary for the mother, keeping in mind that many drugs cross the placenta or enter the breast milk and affect the fetus or neonate. Analgesics, sedatives and hypnotics, and anesthetics are utilized during the labor and vaginal or cesarean delivery process. The β-sympathomimetics are prescribed to suppress labor that occurs before the fetus has reached at least 38 weeks gestation. Oxytocics are prescribed to induce or augment labor or control uterine atony during the postpartal period. Some of these drugs are also used as abortifacients. Magnesium sulfate is utilized to treat pre-eclampsia, and if necessary, antihyper-

tensives are prescribed. A lactation suppressant is prescribed for the mother who is not going to breast-feed her baby. A mother who is Rh$_O$(Du)-negative is given Rh$_O$(D) immune globulin before and/or after her baby is born. The neonate receives drugs soon after birth to prevent eye infections contracted from the maternal vaginal tract and hemorrhage resulting from the normal congenital deficiency of vitamin K.

During the obstetrical period the nurse will continually be assessing the status of the fetus as well as the mother. Fetal heart tones and fetal movement patterns will assist in determining fetal well-being. Maternal vital signs, contraction pattern, and reflexes should be frequently checked to affirm maternal status and effectiveness of treatment. For the patient requiring the use of drugs during the obstetrical period, nursing interventions revolve around both patient education and, most importantly, concern for the safety of both the mother and the fetus. Nursing implications during this period are focused on the attempt to ensure that the mother and her baby will pass through pregnancy, labor, and vaginal or cesarean delivery in the healthiest manner possible with the help of drugs when necessary.

BIBLIOGRAPHY

Balkman, JAJ: Guidelines for drug therapy during lactation: J Obstet Gynecol Neonatal Nurs 65, 15: 1986.

Beall, MH: Advising the nursing mother about her medications: Contemporary Pediatrics 67, 5:2, 1988.

Beckman, DA and Brent, RL: Mechanism of known environment teratogens: Drugs and chemicals. Clin Perinatol 13(3):649, 1986.

Beeley, L: Adverse effects of drugs in later pregnancy. Clin Obstet Gynaecol 13(2):197, 1986.

Bobak, IM, Jenson, MD, and Zalar, MK: Maternity and Gynecologic Care. CV Mosby, St Louis, MO, 1989.

Brengman, SL and Burns, MK: Hypertensive crisis in L and D. Am J Nurs 88(3):325, 1987.

Briggs, GG, Freeman, RK, and Yaffee, SJ: Drugs in Pregnancy and Lactation. Williams & Wilkins, Baltimore, 1986.

Koniak-Griffin, D and Dodgson, J: Severe pregnancy-induced hypertension: Postpartum care of the critically ill patient: Heart Lung 16(6):661, 1987.

Kruse, J: Oxytocin: Pharmacology and clinical application. The Journal of Family Practice 23(5):473, 1986.

Mucklow, JC: The fate of drugs in pregnancy. Clin Obstet Gynecol 13(3):649, 1986.

Neeson, JD and May, KA: Comprehensive Maternity Nursing. JB Lippincott, Philadelphia, 1986.

Olds, SB, London, ML, and Ludewig, PA: Maternal Newborn Nursing. Addison-Wesley, Menlo Park, CA 1988.

Precup, AV (ed): Drug Information for the Health Care Provider: USP DI 1987. Mack Printing Co, Easton, PA, 1987.

Ramanathan, S: Obstetric Anesthesia. Lea & Febiger, Philadelphia, 1988.

Rivera-Calimlin, L: The significance of drugs in breast milk: Pharmacokinetic considerations. Clin Perinatol 14(1):51, 1987.

Tcheng, D: When pregnancy threatens mother and baby. RN 46:, 1986.

Yeh, TF (ed): Drug Therapy in the Neonate and Small Infant. Year Book Medical Publishers, Chicago, 1985.

Zierler, S: Maternal drugs and congenital heart disease. Obstet Gynecol 65(2):155, 1985.

SITUATION 15–1

Paula Larson, a 34-year-old G2P1, is admitted in active labor. She has been pre-eclamptic, with blood pressure controlled well with hydralazine (Apresoline).

1. The nurse will observe for one of the following characteristics of pre-eclampsia:
   a. proteinuria
   b. oliguria
   c. confusion
   d. dyspnea

2. During the first stage of labor, Paula's blood pressure increases to 170/100, and she begins to demonstrate confusion and clonic movements. The physician orders a magnesium sulfate drip. The nurse will prepare the infusion in the following manner:
   a. 100 mEq in 100 cc D_5W to run at 8 to 10 cc per hour
   b. 40 mEq in 500 cc 0.9 percent sodium chloride to run at 2 ml per minute
   c. 32 mEq in 250 cc of 5 percent dextrose to run at 1 to 4 ml per minute
   d. 8 mEq in 250 cc 0.9 percent sodium chloride to run at 1.5 ml per minute

3. In relation to the magnesium infusion, the nurse will observe for the following:
   a. dry pale skin
   b. hyporeflexia

   c. agitation
   d. increased respirations

4. In the event that Paula demonstrates symptoms related to hypermagnesemia, the nurse will be prepared to administer:
   a. oxygen
   b. epinephrine
   c. potassium phosphate
   d. calcium gluconate

5. Which of the following outcome criteria would indicate successful management of Paula's condition?
   a. decreased contractions
   b. respiratory rate <16
   c. absence of seizures
   d. absent reflexes

6. Paula safely delivers a baby boy. The infant should be monitored closely for any indications of:
   a. tachypnea
   b. hypocalcemia
   c. hyperkalemia
   d. neuromuscular depression

SITUATION 15–2

Shirley Green is a 26-year-old G1P0 presenting to the labor and delivery unit with regular contractions. During examination, the nurse confirms that Shirley is dilated 3 cm.

1. As labor progresses, Shirley requests some pain medication. Demerol 12.5 mg to 25 mg IV is ordered for the pain. The nurse is aware of the following effect with regard to the administration of meperidine hydrochloride (Demerol) during labor:
   a. reduction in signs of fetal distress
   b. promotion of fetal hyperactivity if given early
   c. prolongation of the latent stage of labor
   d. increased uterine contractions

2. After two hours of strong contractions, examination reveals complete dilation. Fetal heart rate and variability remain stable, and Mrs. Green is prepared for an epidural block. Which position will be best for Mrs. Green after epidural anesthesia?
   a. sandbag under right hip
   b. semi-Fowlers position, right side down
   c. pillow at lower back with head flat
   d. supine with head of bed elevated 30°

3. Should Mrs. Green exhibit symptoms of hypotension related to epidural anesthesia, the nurse will be prepared to administer all *except:*
   a. oxygen
   b. intravenous fluids
   c. epinephrine
   d. Trendelenburg position

4. After Mrs. Green delivers a normal infant, the nurse gives her an intramuscular injection of ergonovine maleate (Ergotrate). This drug is given to:
   a. inhibit lactation
   b. facilitate delivery of placenta
   c. treat uterine atony
   d. relax smooth muscles

5. The nurse may administer all of the following medications to Mrs. Green's baby *except:*
   a. Vitamin K
   b. silver nitrate
   c. erythromycin ointment
   d. RhoGam

6. Mrs. Green prefers to bottle feed her infant and is to receive bromocriptine (Parlodel). The nurse will include the following information during patient teaching:
   a. The drug will provide protection against pregnancy.
   b. It should be taken only if signs of breast engorgement are noted.
   c. Hypotension and dizziness are common side effects.
   d. If one dose is missed, then two doses should be taken together.

Please refer to the Appendices for correct answers and additional review questions with answers.

16
CHAPTER

PHARMACOTHERAPEUTICS FOR THE GERIATRIC PATIENT

PHARMACOTHERAPEUTICS
FOR THE GERIATRIC
PATIENT

CHAPTER OUTLINE

**AGE-INDUCED BODY CHANGES THAT AFFECT
  DRUG RESPONSE**
  The Graying of Society
  Physiologic Changes in Normal Aging
PHARMACOKINETICS AND THE AGING PROCESS
  Drug Absorption
  Drug Distribution
  Drug Metabolism
  Drug Elimination
USING THE NURSING PROCESS
  Assessment of the Older Adult
  Nursing Diagnoses for the Older Adult
  Planning and Intervention Related to the Older
    Adult and Drug Therapy
  Patient Teaching
  Evaluation of the Drug Therapy Regimen for the
    Older Adult
SUMMARY

TABLES

Nursing Process
Nursing Process for the Older Adult Taking
  Medications, 366

GLOSSARY TERMS IN THIS CHAPTER

Aged elderly
Cardiotoxicity
Drug holiday
Extravasation
Homeostasis
Lacrimation
Nephrotoxicity
Polypharmacy
Tinnitus
Vesicant

16
CHAPTER

PHARMACOTHERAPEUTICS FOR THE GERIATRIC PATIENT

ANNE MORACA-SAWICKI, R.N., M.S.N.

LEARNING OBJECTIVES

Upon completion of this chapter the reader will be able to:

1. Discuss the normal physiologic changes of aging.

2. Relate how the physiologic changes of aging affect drug disposition in the body.

3. Explain how the age-related decreases in cardiac output and function affects other metabolic processes to alter drug disposition.

4. Discuss examples of how specific drugs may cause toxicity even when normal dosages are not exceeded.

5. Summarize assessment data relative to drug regimen necessary to obtain from older patient in order to formulate nursing diagnosis and plan care.

6. List teaching strategies helpful in health care teaching of older patients.

7. List types of assistive devices and aids and approaches available to help increase patient compliance with maintaining drug dosage schedules.

Older adults, those aged 65 and older, are the fastest growing segment of the population in the United States. The average American will live to be about 74 years old and will suffer from 3 or more chronic diseases. Since cardiovascular disease is the number one cause of death in the United States, it is very likely that one of the diseases this "average" American will suffer from is a cardiovascular disorder. Other illness such as arthritis, cancer, respiratory disease, gastrointestinal disturbances, and sensory impairments are all associated with aging. Drug therapy is the primary mode of therapy in many illnesses. Those over 65 constitute about 12% of the population; however as a group, they consume about 30% of all prescription drugs. The elderly also consume the greatest number of over-the-counter drugs. Studies suggest up to 30% of older adults suffer drug adverse effects. Some studies have found that 20% of hospitalizations of adults over 65 years old are due to the effects of prescription drugs. As a person ages various anatomic and physiologic changes that are considered to be "normal" occur. These changes can alter both the therapeutic and adverse responses to drugs. Pathologic conditions can have an even greater effect upon the patient's response to drugs.

The purpose of this chapter is to review the normal changes in aging and to discuss drug therapy in the older adult. The principles of drug disposition (absorption, distribution, metabolism, and excretion) are discussed in relation to the changes caused by aging. In addition, the implementation of the nursing process is discussed relative to the needs of the elderly patient who is taking medications.

AGE-INDUCED BODY CHANGES THAT AFFECT DRUG RESPONSE

THE GRAYING OF SOCIETY

Older adults are not a homogeneous group. Many older adults are quite healthy and are not major drug consumers. About 85% of older adults reside in their homes.

The subgroups of elderly who are infirm, frail, and *aged elderly* (those 80 years and older), as well as the 15% who are residents of long-term care facilities, are the primary consumers of medications. Several recent studies of medication-prescribing practices for residents of skilled-nursing care facilities have concluded that medications are overprescribed for the elderly. Often side effects of drugs are mistaken for signs of aging or illness. For example, lethargy may be caused by various tranquilizers; forgetfulness may be caused by barbiturates; confusion may be caused by several different drugs including methyldopa, digoxin, or cimetidine; and weakness may be related to diuretic intake, which can deplete body potassium.

Drug therapy is one of the most important and often the most risky component of patient care. While it has long been understood that the very young present specific problems and needs in drug therapy, little has been done to identify the special needs of the elderly in relation to drug therapy until recently. The Surgeon General of the United States, along with the Public Health Service and Administration on Aging, is developing specific recommendations dealing with the elderly and health care, services, and medications. As an individual ages there are gradual changes in the anatomy and physiology that may alter the therapeutic and toxic effects of drugs. patients have the right to know about these and other significant aspects of drugs and their drug therapy so they can make informed choices regarding therapy. Patients do have the right to refuse a medication. To force a dose of medication upon an alert, cooperative patient constitutes battery. The nurse has a responsibility to act as patient advocate and provide appropriate health teaching to all patients. Table 16–1, Bill of Rights for the Elderly on Drug Therapy, can serve as a model for nurse advocacy for older adults.

PHYSIOLOGIC CHANGES IN NORMAL AGING

Changes in Body Composition

As a person ages there are changes in body composition. The proportions of fat, lean tissue, and water change. Total body mass and lean body mass tend to decrease

Table 16–1. BILL OF RIGHTS FOR THE ELDERLY ON DRUG THERAPY

Right to take or not take medications.
Right to keep his faculties and not be chemically restrained.
Right to know what he is being medicated with and why.
Right to know the consequences of ingesting such chemicals into his body.
Right to express his subjective response to drugs.
Right to have prescribed just enough of the drug necessary for his ailment and not be made to buy more expensive drugs than necessary.
Right to use medicines he has purchased and not be coerced into buying a new supply of the same drug just because he is hospitalized or placed in a nursing home.
Right to take his own medications as long as he is capable and competent to do so.
Right to quality medicines at the least cost.
Right to nursing and medical caregivers getting at the root of his problems before medications are given.
Right to have medications prescribed, dispensed, administered, and evaluated by persons who have an up-to-date, broad yet specific, knowledge of geriatric pharmacology.

From Alford, DM: Bill of Rights for the elderly on drug therapy. Nurs Clin North Am 17:282, June 1982, with permission.

Table 16–2. PHYSIOLOGIC CHANGES OF AGING AND PHARMACOKINETICS

Physiologic Change	Pharmacokinetic Consequence	Examples of Drugs Affected*
Decreased cardiac output→ increased circulation time.	Delayed onset of drug action. Prolonged drug effect	All cardiac drugs.
Changes in body weight and composition: Reduced total body water Reduced lean body mass per kilogram body weight and increased body fat	Changes in drug distribution and action. With some drugs peak concentrations are greater and half-lives are prolonged, increasing drug effect. This may lead to toxicity.	Water-soluble drugs such as gentamicin; fat-soluble drugs such as pentobarbital: Check pharmacology reference for specific drug effects.
Altered circulation to liver, decline in hepatic blood flow. Decreased microsomal enzymatic activity and plasma protein synthesis.	Altered drug metabolism and detoxification by the liver. Biotransformation time is lengthened and both nonmetabolized drugs and active metabolites exert their effects for extended periods of time. Drug toxicity can occur more readily.	Acetaminophen, barbituates, chlordiazepoxide, phenylbutazone, propranolol, oral anticoagulants, quinidine, tricyclic antidepressants, meperidine.
Decrease in serum albumin.	Decreased availability of protein for binding. Increased serum concentration of free drug results in increased pharmacologic effects of some drugs. For some drugs, such as phenytoin, the increased free state causes faster drug clearance and lowers therapeutic effect.	Chlorthalidone, digitoxin, furosemide, hydralazine, prazosin, propranolol, quinidine, spironolactone, warfarin.
Decreased renal function.	Impaired drug excretion, which can result in toxic build-up of drug levels in patient. Drug dose and patient response should be monitored closely. Some drug doses may need to be reduced in elderly patients.	Chlorthalidone; diazoxide; digoxin, ethambutol; furosemide; guanethidine; methyldopa; metolazone; methotrexate; phenobarbital; procainamide; tetracyclines (except doxycycline); thiazides; and all aminoglycosides.

*The aging process can affect drug disposition in all phases; therefore, one particular drug may be listed in more than one category in this chart. Also, examples are of common drugs only and are not meant to be inclusive. For more complete listings consult a pharmacology reference such as the American Hospital Formulary Service.

with age, while the proportion of body fat increases. There is a decrease in muscle mass and a loss of subcutaneous tissue. These changes in body composition vary from person to person; however, such changes definitely do affect the relationship between a drug's concentration and solubility in the body. Because the normal aging process affects every organ in the body, every phase of drug processing in the body may be affected. Table 16–2 shows some examples of how the processes of aging can affect drug action.

The decrease of lean body mass and water in the elderly can contribute to undesired toxic drug effects. For example, a water-soluble drug such as gentamicin is distributed mostly to lean body tissue and aqueous parts of the body. It is not distributed to fat. Since the elderly have less lean tissue for the drug to be distributed in, more drug remains in the bloodstream. This increased drug concentration in the bloodstream can lead to gentamicin toxicity if the dosage is not reduced. The measurement of serum drug levels plays an important role in determining adequate dosages of many drugs such as gentamicin.

Just as the changes in body composition may affect water-soluble drugs, so too may they affect fat-soluble drugs. As the elderly body increases in fat composition, fat-soluble drugs are distributed to a greater volume of tissue. This initially results in a lower drug concentration in the bloodstream. However, after body fat stores are saturated with a drug, it is then slowly released back into the circulation. This results in an increased duration of drug action. This phenomenon is a contributing factor in residual drowsiness caused by fat-soluble sleep medications the morning after drug ingestion, sometimes referred to as "hangover." Other fat-soluble drugs such as chlorpromazine (Thorazine) and phenobarbital may have prolonged duration of action because of the increased fatty tissue available for drug distribution and storage.

The loss of subcutaneous tissue seen in aging also affects the method and route of drug administration employed for the older patient. Loss of subcutaneous tissue occurs to a greater extent in the extremities than in the trunk of the body. The loss of subcutaneous tissue is especially evident on the dorsum of the hand, and this requires special caution such as avoiding excessive probing with the needle when using the blood vessels of the hand for intravenous injection. There is also a decline in the elastic fibers of the skin and vasculature, which decreases their resiliency and thereby increases the risk of drug *extravasation*. Thus, caution should be observed when administering *vesicant* drugs such as mechlorethamine (Mustargen), doxorubicin (Adriamycin), and vincristine (Oncovin).

Changes in Cardiac Function

As a person ages the myocardial contractile strength and efficiency declines. These age-associated changes are related to several factors: a decrease in cardiac muscle fiber; reduced mobilization of catecholamines; decreased amounts of adenosine triphosphate available in cardiac cells; and the inefficient utilization of oxygen. Between the third and eighth decade of life cardiac output can be reduced by as much as 50%. Coronary artery blood flow decreases with age also. By age 60 coronary artery flow is reduced by about 35%.

These age-related normal cardiac changes may sound like they would create significant functional ability impairments for older persons; however, most are not significantly limited by these age-related changes. These normal alterations in cardiac function and output do create a potential for problems, which can readily manifest themselves when illness or stresses appear or in the presence of other variables, such as the ingestion of medications. Because the older person's homeostatic adaptabilities also slow with age, any illness or stress can more easily overwhelm the body's ability to cope.

The normal aging process also affects the blood vessels. The elastic fibers in the arteries lose about 30% of their "stretch" with age. There is also increased calcium deposition and collagen proliferation within the arterial walls, which further reduce the ability of the arteries to distend. These age-related changes result in an increased peripheral vascular resistance and pulse wave velocity, which in turn cause an increase in the systolic blood pressure.

The normal cardiovascular changes associated with aging can affect all other organs of the body as well. The reduced cardiac output causes a decreased blood flow to all organs, although the brain and cardiac muscle are the least affected by the decrease. Other organs are more affected by the overall decrease in cardiac output. The renal blood flow is especially affected: Both glomerular filtration rate and renal plasma flow are significantly reduced, and this in turn can significantly alter drug distribution and excretion in the elderly.

The normal cardiovascular changes seen in aging coupled with the pathologic changes of disease states frequently seen in this population can make drug therapy problematic. Often the early signs of drug toxicity are not as clearly evident or are erroneously attributed to age-related changes when initially observed. Monitoring the elderly for drug-related side effects requires careful consideration of these age-related changes. Drugs such as propranolol, which produce a negative inotropic effect, can induce congestive heart failure sooner and more suddenly in elderly patients than in younger patients.

Some drugs are capable of producing *cardiotoxicity*. Drugs such as the antineoplastic agents cyclophosphamide (Cytoxan), methotrexate (Mexate), daunorubicin (Cerubidine), and doxurubicin (Adriamycin) are all capable of causing serious cardiotoxic effects. The elderly patient experiencing age-related decreases in cardiac function and output is especially vulnerable to the toxic effects of such drugs and must be carefully observed so cardiac effects can be recognized before serious adverse effects occur.

Changes in Gastrointestinal Function

All body systems slow in function with normal aging. The elderly show a decrease in gastric acid secretion as well as decreased gastrointestinal motility. These changes result in a slower emptying of the stomach and an overall slower movement of intestinal contents throughout the entire gastrointestinal tract. Some research has shown that the elderly may have more difficulty absorbing medications. Further research is necessary to more fully document under what circumstances this may occur and if all drugs or only specific drugs are affected. Certainly the slower movement of gastrointestinal contents has an effect upon the rate of absorption of ingested medications. A decrease in the body's ability to absorb medications can have a significant effect upon drugs that have a narrow therapeutic range. Co-administration of certain drugs with food or other drugs can also affect the amount and speed of drug absorption from the gastrintestinal tract.

Changes in Hepatic Function

The liver is responsible for the complete or partial metabolization of many drugs before they are excreted from the body. The age-related decrease in cardiac output results in a decreased blood flow to the liver. Although this decreased hepatic blood flow does not seem to result in a significant reduction in hepatic function, there is an age-related decrease in the liver's ability to metabolize certain drugs.

There are other organic changes in liver function that occur in normal aging. Vitamins C, A, B₁₂, and folic acid are often deficient in older patients. These deficiencies may result from a decreased ability to absorb the vitamins, from dietary changes, or a combination of these and other factors. Vitamin deficiencies, as well as the presence of environmental pollutants, can affect liver function adversely.

The metabolization and elimination of many drugs is highly dependent upon adequate liver function. A decrease in hepatic function may result in higher blood levels of drug, producing more intense drug effects; prolonged drug effect due to prolonged blood concentrations of drug; and increased incidence of drug toxicity. The decreased rate of hepatic metabolization is responsible in part for the hangover effect seen in older patients who take barbiturate sleeping medications. Some other drugs that are affected by these age-related hepatic changes are oral anticoagulants, propranolol (Inderal), and chlordiazepoxide (Librium).

Changes in Renal Function

Decreased cardiac output in the elderly has a significant effect upon the kidneys. Blood flow to the kidneys is especially adversely affected. The glomerular filtration rate and renal plasma flow are both significantly reduced, and the number of intact nephrons is also reduced. Although the older person's renal function is generally sufficient to eliminate excess body fluids and wastes, the older patient's ability to eliminate some drugs may be reduced by 50% or more.

The normal physiologic changes seen in the kidneys can have significant effects upon drug distribution and excretion in the elderly. Some drugs, such as digoxin and procainamide (Procan, Pronestyl), are primarily excreted by the kidneys. Since the renal changes seen in normal aging can slow excretion and prolong high blood concentrations of drug, toxicity is commonly seen. Many elderly people have cardiovascular problems and take medications such as digoxin and procainamide. The renal changes described occur with increasing age, just when the need for such medications increases. Thus drug toxicity, especially of digoxin, is a particular problem for the elderly. Careful monitoring of elderly patients is extremely important so that drug dosages can be modified to compensate for the age-related decreases in renal function.

Some drugs can cause *nephrotoxic* effects. It is especially important to observe the elderly, who already have decreased renal function, for this drug effect. The aminoglycoside antibiotics are excreted unchanged in the urine; hence renal tissue is exposed to high concentrations of these drugs. Streptomycin is the least nephrotoxic, but it is not very effective in treating gram-negative infections such as those caused by *Pseudomonas*. Amikacin (Amikin), gentamicin (Garamycin), netilmicin (Netromycin), and tobramycin (Nebcin) are the most effective aminoglycosides against such organisms. Studies have shown that of these four drugs, tobramycin is the least likely to cause nephrotoxicity. Patients receiving any of these drugs should be observed for renal effects.

Sensory and Perceptual Changes in Aging

The sensory changes associated with normal aging present special problems relative to drug safety, effectiveness, and compliance with drug therapy. Generally speaking, the sensory thresholds of response are higher in the elderly, which requires stimuli of greater intensity, while the range and speed of responses become limited by the functional and structural decline in aging.

The normal aging process affects the sensory organs of the body in several ways. In the eye, the pupil becomes smaller and less responsive to light, color discrimination decreases, the lens becomes cloudy, the ability to focus on near objects is decreased, and *lacrimation* decreases. These visual changes can impair the individual's ability to distinguish between the different medication tablets to be taken and can also impair the patient's ability to clearly read the typewriter size printing on the medicine label. The presence of cataracts or other eye conditions common in older persons can have an even greater effect upon the patient's ability to clearly see medications and read instructions.

Hearing acuity diminishes with age. There is a decrease in receptive and discriminative capacities. Often these changes occur so gradually that the patient is either not fully aware of them or develops compensatory mechanisms which mask or hide his or her handicap so that others are unaware of them. This diminished hearing acuity can interfere with patient teaching and result in misinterpretation of instructions.

All hearing loss in elder patients is not due to the changes of aging. Some drugs directly affect the ears and can result in ototoxic effects—*tinnitus*, vertigo, and hearing loss. All of the aminoglycoside antibiotics that are commonly used in hospitals to treat serious infections are capable of producing ototoxicity. Most aminoglycoside antibiotics are administered intramuscularly or intravenously; hence their use is mostly confined to hospital settings. Although the aminoglycoside antibiotics are well known for their ability to produce nephrotoxicity, it is not as well remembered that they can also produce ototoxic effects. There are other drugs that can also have ototoxic effects. For example, when furosemide (Lasix) is administered too rapidly by intravenous injection it can result in transient hearing loss. Oral drugs as routine as aspirin can affect the ears. Large doses of aspirin, taken to relieve the pain and inflammation of arthritis, can cause tinnitus.

All senses are affected by the aging process. There is diminished taste and olfactory acuity, as well as decreased sensitivity to touch (perception of pressure) and reduced manual dexterity (because of neuromuscular factors). All these factors can serve to uniquely limit the older person's ability to assume responsibility for self-administration of necessary medications. At best they impose barriers that must be recognized and surmounted whenever a nurse is administering or teaching a patient to self-administer medications. At worst, they may preclude the patient from self-administering medications. These factors are discussed in greater depth in the section of this chapter dealing with the nursing process related to older adults and medications.

PHARMACOKINETICS AND THE AGING PROCESS

The normal age-related changes that occur in major body systems and organs during the aging process have been outlined. The pharmacokinetic process can be affected by these normal, age-related changes. How these changes can affect drug absorption, distribution, metabolism, and excretion in the older adult will now be discussed.

Since even normal age-related changes in physiology can influence the pharmacokinetic process, it is obvious that pathologic changes due to disease can have even more dramatic effects upon drug therapeutics. It is therefore essential for the design of appropriate nursing intervention in older patients that the nurse understand the process of normal aging. The homeostatic mechanisms adapt less quickly in the elderly just at a time when many physiologic changes are occurring. Aging is often accompanied by many environmental and social stresses as well (death of spouse or significant others, declining ability to care for self or home, illness, or infirmity.) As previously noted, the elderly suffer from increased incidences of diseases and therefore consume about a third of all prescription drugs. When planning the care of older patients on medications it is important for the nurse to consider the following factors:

1. Changes in the size and functional capabilities of major organs and transport systems impede drug disposition processes making drug response less predictable.
2. Compensatory mechanisms become slower to respond, and as a result, side effects, toxicity, and interactions may occur which are disproportionate to actual drug dose.
3. Body tissue sensitivity and responsiveness decreases, making dosage and dose scheduling problematic.
4. The regulatory mechanisms that promote integrated activity of all body systems are less effective so that stimulation or depression of one organ may more readily affect many others.
5. The rate of readjustment to changes in the extracellular environment of the cells becomes substantially reduced so that even minor shifts in fluid-electrolyte balance can prove hazardous for the elderly.
6. Large variations in the rate of individual age-related changes make it extremely difficult to predict qualitative properties of drug response in elder patients.

Mindful of the above factors, a discussion of the normal age-related changes in physiology relative to drug disposition follows. The reader is again reminded that normal changes are being discussed, and in the presence of pathology even greater variations can occur. Every aspect of drug disposition (absorption, distribution, metabolism, and excretion) is affected by the changes that occur as a person ages.

DRUG ABSORPTION

Drug absorption is the phase of drug disposition least affected by the normal changes of aging. There are several factors that may contribute to a decrease in drug absorption in older patients: a decrease in basal and maximal gastric acid output, which raises gastric pH and can affect the solubility of some drugs such as aspirin or barbiturates; a decrease in splanchnic blood flow, which could reduce or delay absorption; slower gastric emptying; and an increase in duodenal diverticula.

Drugs that have a narrow therapeutic range, such as digoxin, would be most affected by any changes in drug absorption. Researchers are continuing to study the extent to which age-related changes affect drug absorption. Evidence thus far suggests that in most cases drug absorption is not significantly altered with increasing age. However, the age-related changes in structure and function of the gastrointestinal tract have a particular significance in effective drug administration by mouth.

Esophageal motility decreases with age so that esophageal clearance time is lengthened. This is due to weakened contractions of smooth muscle in this area and failure of the lower esophageal sphincter to relax after swallowing. These factors often combine with the elder patient's reluctance to take large capsules or tablets because of fear of difficulty swallowing them. The nurse must take the physiologic effects of aging into account when administering medications and teaching medication administration to the patient or caregiver. Simple actions such as making sure the patient is fully upright during administration so that gravity can aid the process, along with having the patient drink a full glass of water (half taken before the medicine) to assure ease of drug passage can make medication administration much easier for the patient.

Gastric motility decreases with age while gastric emptying time increases. Both of these factors contribute to a rising pH of gastric juices, which can potentiate the irritating effects of drugs such as aspirin (acidic) and phenytoin (strongly alkaline) because of the extended time during which they may be present in the stomach. Having the patient drink a full glass of water or eat a small, nonfat snack with the medication can decrease the irritation to gastric tissue. The patient can also switch to an enteric-coated aspirin tablet to reduce gastric irritation.

Drug absorption following subcutaneous or intramuscular injection occurs by rapid diffusion from the injection site into the plasma. Both these injection routes assure a more rapid onset of drug action than the oral route. The microcirculation in skeletal muscle promotes rapid drug absorption, although the age-related decrease in cardiac output can reduce blood flow to the muscles, thereby slowing drug absorption somewhat. Studies have shown that blood flow does differ in muscle groups. It is also important to select injection sites with care because the older patient does have some decrease in muscle mass, which may make a site unacceptable for the injection of some medications.

The age-related loss of subcutaneous tissues and increased fragility of the blood vessels can make intravenous drug administration more problematic for the older patient. Older patients also have an increased risk of drug infiltration and extravasation because of a decline in blood vessel wall elasticity and resiliency. While the infiltration of fluid replacing intravenous solutions to a dehydrated patient delay the receipt of necessary fluid, it generally produces no long-term effects. However, the infiltration or extravasation of antineoplastic chemotherapeutic drugs such as mechlorethamine (Mustargen), doxorubicin (Adriamycin), daunorubicin (Cerubidine), mitomycin (Mutamycin), vinblastine (Velban), and vincristine (Oncovin) can result in serious tissue damage (tissue necrosis and slough).

Topical ointments and analgesic balms are frequently used by older patients. These medications are popular remedies because of their warming effects (useful for sprains, strains, or inflamed arthritic joints) or for their numbing effects (hemorrhoid remedies). While these medications are useful, it is important to remember that, though locally applied, systemic effects can occur if large enough amounts are applied and absorbed through the skin. For example, topical anesthetics can be absorbed systemically when applied to abraded skin or over large areas of the body. Hydrocortisone-containing creams can also be absorbed systemically, especially when applied over large areas of the body.

DRUG DISTRIBUTION

Physiologic changes that occur normally in aging can produce changes in drug distribution, which may result in higher blood levels of some drugs. There is also an increased potential for more intense drug effects, toxicity, and adverse drug reactions. Among the reasons for altered patterns of drug distribution in the elderly are decreased cardiac output and changes in circulation; delayed onset of drug effect or prolongation of drug effect; changes in body weight and composition (decreases in fluid and lean body tissue, increase in fatty tissue); changes in protein binding because of decresed albumin levels; and changes in red blood cell binding.

Probably the most important factor affecting drug distribution in older patients is the change in body composition that accompanies aging. The decrease in lean body mass and increase in fatty tissue can affect the action of many drugs. Fat-soluble drugs such as chlorpromazine (Thorazine), diazepam (Valium), and phenobarbital are thus distributed more widely to the larger number of available fat cells. This increased distribution to fat cells can result in a prolonged duration of drug action, increased drug sensitivity, and/or toxic effects.

Elderly patients in general experience higher plasma levels of drugs and more erratic distribution rates. For example an equal dose of digoxin administered to a 70-year-old patient and a 40-year-old patient results in a higher blood level of drug in the older patient. This difference is due to age-related changes in body size and drug distribution. Thus, loading doses of drugs equivalent to those given to young patients can be dangerous for older patients. Careful titration of drug doses can help to reduce the number of undesirable drug reactions and toxicities seen in elderly patients.

DRUG METABOLISM

Drug metabolism as measured by prolonged drug elimination half-lives and reduced total drug clearance decreases with patient age. Other factors can also influence the rate of drug metabolism. Patient exposure to alcohol, drugs, envrionmental pollutants, as well as nutritional deficits, can significantly contribute to reduced drug metabolism in the elderly.

The aging process causes a decrease in liver mass and reduced hepatic blood flow, along with reduced protein synthesis and enzymatic activity. These changes all contribute to prolonged biotransformation, resulting in prolonged pharmacologic effects. Drugs that are quickly inactivated in the liver of a young person may therefore have a prolonged effect in elderly patients. Examples of such drugs are meperidine (Demerol), barbiturates, propranolol (Inderal), and the tricyclic antidepressants.

Many drugs bind to protein in plasma and are therefore affected by age-related decreases in serum protein levels. Hypoproteinemia causes an increase in the free, unbound fraction of circulating drug and results in a transient increase in intensity of pharmacologic action. Drugs generally highly bound to plasma protein that can be readily affected by these alterations in metabolism include diazepam (Valium); meperidine (Demerol); phenytoin (Dilantin); furosemide (Lasix); tolbutamide (Orinase); and warfarin (Coumadin).

DRUG ELIMINATION

The excretion rate of drugs is also affected by the aging process. Most drugs are excreted by the kidneys. Thus excretion is dependent upon renal blood flow, glomerular filtration rate, and urea clearance, all of which are decreased in aging. The excretion of water-soluble drugs is dependent upon glomerular filtration rate. Fat-soluble drugs are reabsorbed by the tubular epithelium and excreted following their hepatic conversion to more water-soluble compounds.

Because elderly patients have reduced rates of renal excretion of drugs, their potential for adverse drug reactions and toxicity are increased. Disease and pathologic changes in the liver or kidneys can further increase these risks in the elderly. Examples of drugs that are renally excreted which should be given in reduced doses to elderly patients include the aminoglycosides; digoxin; ethambutol (Myambutol); methotrexate (Mexate); phenobarbital; and tetracyclines (except doxycycline). Drugs such as the aminoglycosides may also be nephrotoxic; therefore elderly patients receiving such drugs need to be monitored closely for adequate renal function.

Age-related physiologic changes can affect all phases of drug disposition—absorption, distribution, metabolism, and excretion—in elder patients, thereby placing them at increased risk of side effects or toxicity. When the normal changes of aging are coupled with the multiple chronic illnesses and multiple drug regimens common to elderly patients, the implications for reduced drug effectiveness and increased potential for side effects and toxicity become greater. The key to improving drug effectiveness and reducing undesired effects lies in more accurate patient assessment and monitoring for drug effectiveness.

The following section deals with the use of the nursing process relative to the older adult and medication therapy. Careful assessment throughout the course of drug therapy assists the nurse in determining if the therapeutic goals of the drug regimen are being achieved. Understanding the processes that underlie the older patient's response to a drug results in better tailoring of nursing intervention to meet the special needs of these patients.

USING THE NURSING PROCESS

ASSESSMENT OF THE OLDER ADULT

A thorough assessment of the older patient should be done at the start of drug therapy. This assessment forms the data base upon which the nursing care plan is built. Table 16–3 lists the nursing process for the older adult taking medications.

Table 16–3. NURSING PROCESSS FOR AN OLDER ADULT TAKING MEDICATIONS

Assessment

Determine drug use: current medicines being taken (drug name, dose, what the medicine is for and side effects experienced); OTC, including vitamins, aspirin, analgesics, and laxatives; social, e.g., alcohol, nicotine and caffeine; street drugs
Note pattern of use, i.e., how often taken, what happens when taken, borrowing medication from others.
Assess current status of immunizations.
Obtain information about medical care: who patient sees, how often, and where patient fills prescriptions.
Identify dietary restrictions/needs.
Evaluate sensory acuity, cognitive skills.
Ascertain availability of support system(s), need for assistance, living conditions.

Nursing Diagnosis	Nursing Actions	Rationale	Desired Outcomes/ Evaluation Criteria
Injury, potential for under/ over dosing of medications related to emotional difficulties, inadequate drug education.	Provide information about drug, proper dosage, expected action, proper administration and possible side-effects.	Understanding of what drug can/cannot do encourages patient to cooperate with proper regimen may prevent untoward effects.	Takes drug(s) appropriately Displays no toxic reaction(s)/other complications.
	Discuss aids to maintain regimen (drug calendar, week-at-a time dispenser, etc).	Developing a system for taking medications assists with proper administration, gives patient a sense of control over therapy, decreases anxiety, and increases self-esteem.	
	Inform family/caregivers about drug regimen. Discuss symptoms which indicate need to contact physician.	SOs can monitor regimen and assist patient as needed. Prompt intervention can avoid drug related toxic effects.	
Non-compliance with medication regimen related to financial concerns, health beliefs, inadequate knowlege as evidenced by development of complications, failure to keep appointments, exacerbation of symptoms.	Review information about drug regimen, dietary intake and financial considerations.	Identifies areas of concern and provides opportunity for giving new information/reinforcing previous knowledge.	Verbalizes accurate knowledge about disease and understanding of treatment regimen.
	Discuss reasons for taking medication as ordered and checking with physician before making changes.	Accurate information can enhance cooperation, preventing complications.	
	Encourage participation in problem-solving solutions to current situation.	Enhances feelings of selfworth and promotes sense of control over own life.	
	Demonstrate ways to open drug containers, obtain easyopen containers.	Administration of medication is easier when mobility/dexterity improves.	
Grieving, dysfunctional related to death of wife/ husband as evidenced by withdrawal from activities, alterations in eating habits, alterations in concentration.	Encourage patient to verbalize feelings about loss of spouse and "getting old and helpless".	Helps to identify problems and assists patient begin resolution of grief, regaining control of life.	Verbalizes loneliness and loss. Resumes social interactions. Takes charge of own care.
	Encourage socialization and contact with family/friends.	Helps to adjust and reduce loneliness.	
	Promote activity within ability range. Suggest exercises, assistive devices as indicated.	Increased mobility enhances sense of wellbeing and control over ADLs.	
	Provide positive feedback for patient's efforts	Promotes confidence in own ability to manage self-care.	
Cardiac output decreased, potential related to alteration in rate, rhythm/electrical conduction.	Discuss how to take pulse each morning before taking Digoxin and not taking when below 60. Have patient show how she takes pulse.	Understanding of toxic effect and measures for controlling them reduces sequelae of these effects.	Maintains cardiac rate/ rhythm within prescribed limits. Verbalizes understanding of desired effects and measures for control. Displays no toxic effects of medications.
	Report presence of dysrhythmias.	May indicate need for further evaluation and treatment.	

Table 16–3. NURSING PROCESS FOR AN OLDER ADULT TAKING MEDICATIONS–*CONTINUED*

Nursing Diagnosis	Nursing Actions	Rationale	Desired Outcomes/ Evaluation Criteria
Knowledge deficit related to lack of information or misinterpretation/unfamiliarity, cognitive limitation as evidenced by questions, inaccurate follow-through of instructions/development of preventable complications.	Review dietary choices for supplemental potassium.	Understanding which foods to choose will help to maintain proper level.	Verbalizes understanding of medication regimen. Reports anxiety is decreased and is confident in own ability for self-care.
	Administer potassium replacement.	May be needed as additional supplementation.	
	Encourage verbalization of anxieties and fears.	Promotes recognition of concerns and steps which can be taken to manage own care.	
	Discuss normal aging process changes and symptoms of illness which need medical attention.	Promotes understanding of differentiation between things which can be treated.	
	Emphasize importance of not taking OTC drugs or increasing dosage of prescribed drugs without checking with physician.	Beliefs about OTC drugs not being medicine and attitudes of "if one pill is good, two must be better" can lead to untoward complications.	
	Encourage patient to wear glasses, during patient teaching sessions.	Reduces misunderstanding, speeds learning and improves self-esteem.	
	Suggest ways to mark bottles to identify different drugs, e.g., a red paper heart on the top of the digoxin bottle and a blue water drop on the furosemide.	Developing systems to help patient identify correct medication and maintain independence and safety.	
	Identify possible side-effects of ibuprofen. Instruct patient to call physician if symptoms persist or worsen.	Increasing aspirin or NSAID dosages may increase risk of GI complications such as ulcers and bleeding.	
	Provide written materials for patient to review at home.	Information is remembered better when presented in more than one format.	
	Stress importance of returning to health-care provider for regular checkups.	Monitoring physical status and medication regimen can prevent misunderstandings and complications.	

While obtaining physical information such as vital signs and health history, question the patient about any current medicines being taken. Ask the patient the drug name, dose, what the medicine is for, and the side effects associated with each drug. Many patients consume several drugs every day without knowing the drugs' names or what they are for. Be certain to specifically question the patient about ingestion of over-the-counter drugs such as vitamins, aspirin, analgesics, and laxatives. Since over-the-counter drugs can be obtained without a prescription, many people do not consider these to be "medicines." Use of social drugs such as nicotine and caffeine is also important to note. Although use of street drugs is not common in the current population of elderly (they are much more likely to be habituated or addicted legally to prescription medications), the possibility should also be considered. Keep in mind that most patients will not want to divulge this type of information. Also, many people do not recognize their frequent use of prescription (or nonprescription) drugs as out of the ordinary: "That's not habit forming—I take it all the time." Be certain that you ask not only the name of the medication but how often it is taken. When asking about alcohol consumption, a more accurate pattern of consumption may be elicited by asking "When do you drink alcoholic beverages," rather than "Do you drink?" The latter question may make the patient reluctant to answer, "yes" for fear of being labeled a heavy drinker or alcoholic. When discussing medication allergies, always ask the patient who claims an allergy, "What happens when you take this drug?" Often patients say they have an allergy when they are only experiencing a drug side effect. For example, a patient who claims penicillin allergy reveals it "upsets my stomach terribly." This is a known side effect and not an allergic reaction.

Specifically, ask if the patient ever takes medications belonging to a friend or family member. Such practices are unfortunately common and can contribute to side effects or toxic effects. Borrowing medications can also precipitate serious drug interactions.

While gathering information about the patient's medication use, it is also important to ask about their immunization history. Older adults may lack immunizations, thereby putting them at increased risk of illness. A one-time immunization with pneumococcal vaccine (Pneumovax) is recommended for all people over 65 years of age. Immunocompromised patients and those on dialysis are at increased risk for hepatitis B and should receive Heptavax-B immunization. Influenza immunization is recommended annually for patients with chronic diseases or metabolic disorders and for those over 65 years of age. Every ten years a tetanus booster, usually given as TD (tetanus-diphtheria), is needed.

Another area that is important to assess is the patient's religious and ethnic background. Orthodox Jews may object to taking pork-based insulins. Ethnic or cultural folk remedies such as herbal medicines can produce toxic effects. Sometimes older patients from a strong Catholic background may resist taking analgesics because they believe "suffering in this life will atone for sins and allow for quicker entry into heaven."

It is important to assess the patient's psychosocial status. Even in the course of a brief interview, the nurse should obtain information about marital status and significant others; living conditions (Does the patient live alone? In an apartment or house? Are there structural barriers such as stairs that present problems?); and gain insight into the patient's self-concept. Most patients, especially the elderly, are quite eager to talk about themselves and what they perceive as their problems. Be careful to listen not only to what is said but how it is said and what is not said. For example, the patient who seems adamant about not needing anyone to help look after him may be afraid that there is no one who will help.

Your nursing assessment relative to the patient's drug therapy should also include gathering information about how often the patient sees a physician, nurse practitioner, clinic, or other health care provider, as well as information about how medications are obtained. For instance, does the patient get all prescriptions filled at the same pharmacy? Some patients see more than one physician in order to obtain multiple prescriptions for pain medications or tranquilizers. Such *polypharmacy*

can lead to toxic effects. It is also important to know whether the pharmacy keeps a drug profile on each patient in order to screen for drugs that may cause untoward effects or interactions if taken together. Many pharmacies have computers to log in each patient with their medications in order to alert the pharmacist to potential problems. The patient should be told to ask about any over-the-counter drugs they want to use to see if the medication will interfere with their prescribed medications.

The nurse must be alert during the interview and gathering of physical assessment. Knowledge deficits regarding drugs and their side effects, impaired sensory acuity, noncompliant attitude, and dietary restrictions because of illness or allergy are all potential problem areas that may need to be defined in terms of establishing a nursing diagnosis, goals, and planned interventions. Patient verbalizations of misinformation, fear of drug side effects, or poor understanding of their medication regimen can all contribute to poor therapeutic response to the physician's ordered drug regimen. Almost one third of older adults fear adverse drug reactions and overmedication so much that they do not comply with their physicians' orders on the taking of medications. This lack of patient knowledge about the expected benefits of drug therapy versus the side effects of drugs does more to discourage patient compliance than the two other prime causes—advancing age and child-proof containers. Proper assessment of these factors, coupled with appropriate patient teaching, can increase patient compliance significantly.

There are three basic areas of information-gathering that are assessed. The first is the verbal and nonverbal data obtained from the patient interview or interview with family members or significant others. The second area of assessment is the physical data obtained through physical examination of vital signs and other observational skills of inspection, palpation, auscultation, and percussion. The final area of assessment is the information contained in laboratory and radiograph reports, as well as the information in the physician's history and physical examination. Coordination of information from these areas assists in the formulation of a nursing diagnosis and plan of intervention. It is important to determine goals for intervention and the outcome criteria to be evaluated in order to determine the success of planned nursing intervention.

Sample Case History

Imagine you are admitting a 73-year-old patient to your nursing unit from the Emergency Department. Sara Clingersmith was brought to the hospital by her daughter, who fears that she "has some type of severe viral infection." Mrs. Clingersmith has been anorexic for about a week, nauseated and vomiting. She has also been feeling weak, insomniac, and depressed. Her daughter states, "She has been depressed and unable to sleep—my father died three months ago after forty-five years of marriage—but her depression has gotten worse this past week." Mrs. Clingersmith has mild congestive heart failure, which has been

under control with digoxin 0.25 mg per day, furosemide (Lasix) 40 mg per day, and potassium chloride (Slo-K) tablets 3 times per day (1 with each meal) for the past 6 years. In addition, she has been experiencing generalized arthritic symptoms for the past year for which her physician has prescribed Easprin (enteric-coated 15 grain aspirin) twice a day, 1 at breakfast and 1 with dinner.

While in the Emergency Department, Mrs. Clingersmith had blood drawn for electrolytes and a digoxin level. She is transferred to your nursing unit with an intravenous infusion of 5% glucose and water at 50 ml per hour because of her

Sample Case History–*CONTINUED*

somewhat dehydrated status and to maintain an immediate intravenous access for medications if needed. She is placed on cardiac telemetry monitoring and you are to begin her assessment.

You learn that Mrs. Clingersmith has lost 25 lbs. in the last three months, often skips meals, and has not seen her physician in six months. (She is three months overdue for the appointment she canceled the week following her husband's death.) In addition, she stopped taking her potassium supplement six months ago. Concerned about the cost, she asked her physician if she could "try increasing the potassium in my diet." She was to drink a full glass of orange juice and eat a whole banana for breakfast and drink another glass of orange juice at bedtime. She was to call the doctor's office if she developed any lethargy or other signs of potassium depletion and was to be re-evaluated three months ago with electrolyte levels drawn. She never rescheduled the appointment after her husband's death.

Since the death of her husband, Mrs. Clingersmith has been depressed and has neglected her own needs. She also stopped taking the Easprin tablets after her husband's death, citing "the expense of the pills" as the main reason and fear of aspirin causing stomach problems as another. She substituted a generic acetaminophen product for the Easprin, saying that "They claim on television that it works

like aspirin and is safer." However, she has been bothered by increasing joint stiffness, inflammation, and pain in the past three months, which she has attributed to "old age."

Mrs. Clingersmith is an alert, cooperative but somewhat frail-looking woman who currently weighs 100 lbs. She is in generally stable health despite her current problems and is somewhat underweight for her 5-foot, 4-inch frame. Although she only completed the tenth grade, she is a well-read and intelligent woman. She has no medication allergies. She does not smoke and has only an occasional glass of wine on holidays. Although she lives alone in her five room ranch home, her daughter lives nearby, calls her daily, and takes her grocery shopping every Saturday. Mrs. Clingersmith has a car and knows how to drive, but she seldom drives any more.

Mrs. Clingersmith makes several statements to you about "feeling old and useless now," as well as "everyone wants me to sell my home and move into one of those apartment buildings for old folks, but that's only one step away from a nursing home and death." She likes her neighborhood because she knows everyone and is only one block from her church and a small shopping center. She used to go out daily but now seldom goes out. She even switched to a small independent pharmacy that delivers so she does not have to go out for her medicines.

Mrs. Clingersmith presents many common problems seen in older patients. As you begin to formulate a care plan based on your nursing assessment data, the laboratory phones with initial reports: an extremely low potassium level (hence her symptoms of weakness and lethargy), as well as a digoxin level in the toxic range (hence her abnormal cardiac rhythms, nausea, vomiting, insomnia, and heightened depression). Mrs. Clingersmith has a classic case of digoxin toxicity.

What assessment clues might have been attributed to causes other than drug effects? Her depression was seen by family members as caused by the loss of her spouse; however, its increased severity should have signaled a problem when coupled with the other signs. Her weight loss and subsequent loss of lean body tissue increased the amount of digoxin per kilogram, and her low potassium level compounded the body's difficulty in excreting digoxin. Hypokalemia enhances digoxin toxicity. The nausea, vomiting, and subsequent dehydration were not due to a virus but rather to digoxin toxicity. Her depression following the loss of her spouse may have caused some sleep pattern disruption. However, in this case, her insomnia was due more to digoxin toxicity. She also admitted to seeing "a vague yellow halo around objects," which she was reluctant to mention in the presence of family members for fear they would "think me crazy." This visual halo is also another classic sign of digoxin toxicity.

The discontinuation of her potassium tablets and insufficient intake of potassium in her diet compounded her cardiac problem, although she did not realize it until patient teaching was instituted. Mrs. Clingersmith, like many elderly patients, knew the purpose of the digoxin and was quite diligent about taking it every day. She perceived this "as heart medicine and essential to life."

Likewise, she was also conscientious about taking the furosemide daily "to get rid of excess water so the heart won't have to work too hard." However, she did not fully understand the need for the potassium replacement tablets, and since concern for "the high cost" of many pills made her worry about finances, she eliminated those medicines she did not think essential. Eliminating the Easprin increased her arthritic symptoms, but these problems were overshadowed by her cardiac problem.

NURSING DIAGNOSES FOR THE OLDER ADULT

What nursing diagnoses, relative to her medication therapy, would the case history of Mrs. Clingersmith suggest? Certainly she has a knowledge deficit in regard to furosemide and the need for potassium replacement. Also she has a knowledge deficit in regard to digoxin side effects and toxic signs and use of aspirin products to control the pain and inflammation of arthritis. Her dysfunctional grieving over the loss of her husband is spilling over into all aspects of her life and is contributing to her medication side effects and toxicity. Her ability to learn and her anxiety about her current health problem have increased her desire to learn more about her medicines and try to regain control over her life and health. Another nursing diagnosis for this patient is potential for decreased cardiac output related to alteration in rate, rhythm/conduction (effects of digoxin and low potassium), and alteration in nutrition status to less than body requirements as evidenced by weight loss which may be alleviated with resolution of other problems.

Nursing diagnoses for the older adult receiving drug therapy will have to be tailored to individual patient needs, such as done for Mrs. Clingersmith. Other typical nursing diagnoses for older patients could be: anxiety related to numerous medications; fear of drug side effects; potential for injury (under- or overdosing of medication), ineffective coping with life stresses resulting in noncompliance with medication regimen, inadequate drug education/proper precautions; altered compliance with medication regimen related to financial concerns, health beliefs, and inadequate knowledge. Table 16–3 Nursing Process For the Older Adult Receiving Drug Therapy can serve as a guideline for the development of individual care plans.

PLANNING AND INTERVENTION RELATED TO THE OLDER ADULT AND DRUG THERAPY

The nurse develops goals from the assessment-derived nursing diagnoses and then proceeds to plan interventions to help achieve those goals. The patient should be involved in goal setting, since this is known to foster compliance with therapy. As each patient is different, so too will the plan of care differ to reflect the needs of each individual patient. It is important to remember the physical changes that occur in aging when planning care and how these affect drug disposition and the patient's ability to understand and manage a drug regimen. Teaching a patient not to take digoxin if pulse is outside the 60–110 bpm range does no good if the patient is unable to distinguish between digoxin and furosemide tablets because of diminished visual acuity. (Both tablets are small, round, white, and approximately the same size.)

When planning nursing interventions, it is also important to include a family member or significant other in the teaching phase. This other person will have the same information about the drug regimen and can help promote compliance.

Nursing interventions for our case study patient, Mrs. Clingersmith, included (1) monitoring her closely for arrhythmias; (2) administering ordered potassium replacements; and (3) intensive patient teaching about her drug therapy. Her daughter was included in the patient teaching sessions so that she too would understand the purpose of the drug therapy and what side effects to watch for in Mrs. Clingersmith. (For a more detailed discussion of nursing care for digoxin toxicity refer to Chapter 28, Cardiac Glycosides.)

Many patients experience anxiety due to the number of medications they take. Important interventions for such patients include encouraging verbalization of anxieties so they can be recognized and overcome. Successful outcome for these patients is the ability to self-administer medicines.

Patients who experience sensory deficits due to the changes associated with aging or disease need nursing interventions that allow them as much independence as possible while maintaining their safety. For example, the patient with decreased visual acuity needs a way to distinguish between similar-looking tablets (furosemide

and digoxin). A simple solution such as cutting out a red paper heart and sticking it to the top of the digoxin bottle and cutting out a blue water drop to stick onto the top of the furosemide bottle can easily remind the patient which pill is in which bottle. Large pill bottles can be requested when prescriptions are ordered, and large type instructions or hand lettering can be requested so the patient can more easily read the label.

The potential for injury due to underdosing or overdosing of medications can be especially problematic for the elderly. In addition to normal medication dosages producing toxic effects because of slowed metabolism, there is also the problem of intentional overdosing. The philosophy of "if one pill is good, then two must be better" can create problems for the patient. The patient must be instructed always to consult the physician before making any changes in the prescribed drug regimen to avoid undesirable effects. For example, patients with increased arthritic symptoms who increase aspirin or nonsteroidal anti-inflammatory drugs such as ibuprofen (Motrin) increase their risk of gastrointestinal complications such as ulcers and bleeding. Patients should be instructed to contact the physician if they feel a medication is no longer helping or if their symptoms change because a change in drug therapy may be indicated.

Forgetting whether or not a medication was taken is a common problem for all patients. For elderly patients who take cardiac medications this can be especially problematic. Nursing interventions can be devised for such patients so that they have a way of double-checking themselves. A drug calendar can be made up so that the patient draws a line through each dose of medicine after it is taken (Fig. 16–1). Other methods include actually making up a medicine tray for the patient with each medicine poured and a label attached indicating the medicine and time of dose. This approach can include a week-long schedule for the patient, provided the drugs are individually wrapped and labeled (Fig. 16–2). If a cupcake medication tray is to be set up for the patient, it should be done on a daily basis (Fig. 16–3.).

PATIENT TEACHING

Patient teaching is a primary concern for the nurse. The nurse must assess learning needs, and then develop and implement a teaching plan. The following information deals with teaching strategies that are helpful in teaching the older adult.

People are able to learn at any age. Memory may not be as sharp in old age as in youth, the attention span may be likewise shortened, and vision and hearing less acute. These problems can be overcome if proper teaching strategies are employed. The older patient may be a much more motivated learner than the young because their health and independence are at stake—two of the most highly prized aspects of life.

Knowledge content can be categorized into three basic learning domains—the cognitive, affective, and psychomotor. For effective learning to take place, the teaching plan should address each of these specific

SUN	MON	TUES	WED	THURS	FRI	SAT
1 L 8A DIABINESE 250 10A DIGOXIN .25 10A LASIX 20 mg 10A ALDOMET 250 mg 10P ALDOMET 250 mg	**2** 8A DIABINESE 250 10A DIGOXIN .25 10A ALDOMET 250 mg 10P ALDOMET 250mg	**3** 8A DIABINESE 250 10A DIGOXIN .25 10A ALDOMET 250 mg 10A LASIX 20 mg 10P ALDOMET 250 mg	**4** 8A DIABINESE 250 mg 10A DIGOXIN .25 mg 10A ALDOMET 250 mg 10P ALDOMET 250 mg	**5** 8A DIABINESE 250 10A DIGOXIN .25 10A ALDOMET 250 mg 10P ALDOMET 250 mg	**6** 8A DIABINESE 250 mg 10A DIGOXIN .25 mg 10A ALDOMET 250mg 10P ALDOMET 250 mg	**7** L 8A DIABINESE 250 10A ALDOMET 250 mg 10A LASIX 20 mg 10P ALDOMET 250 mg
8 8A DIABINESE 250 10A DIGOXIN .25 10A ALDOMET 250 10P ALDOMET 250 mg	**9** L 8A DIABINESE 250 10A DIGOXIN .25 10A ALDOMET 250 mg 10A LASIX 20 mg 10P ALDOMET 250 mg	**10** 8A DIABINESE 250 10A DIGOXIN .25 10A ALDOMET 250 10P ALDOMET 250 mg	**11** L 8A DIABINESE 250 10A DIGOXIN .25 10A ALDOMET 250 10A LASIX 20 mg 10P ALDOMET 250 mg	**12** 8A DIABINESE 250 10A DIGOXIN .25 10A ALDOMET 250 10P ALDOMET 250 mg	**13** L 8A DIABINESE 250 10A ALDOMET 250 10A LASIX 20 mg 10P ALDOMET 250 mg	**14** 8A DIABINESE 250 10A DIGOXIN .25 10A ALDOMET 250 10P ALDOMET 250 mg
15 L 8A DIABINESE 250 10A DIGOXIN .25 10A ALDOMET 250 10A LASIX 20 mg 10P ALDOMET 250 mg	**16** 8A DIABINESE 250 10A DIGOXIN .25 10A ALDOMET 250 10P ALDOMET 250 mg	**17** L 8A DIABINESE 250 10A DIGOXIN .25 10A ALDOMET 250 10A LASIX 20 mg 10P ALDOMET 250 mg	**18** 8A DIABINESE 250 10A DIGOXIN .25 10A ALDOMET 250 10P ALDOMET 250 mg	**19** L 8A DIABINESE 250 10A DIGOXIN .25 10A ALDOMET 250 10A LASIX 20 mg 10P ALDOMET 250 mg	**20** 8A DIABINESE 250 10A DIGOXIN .25 10A ALDOMET 250 10P ALDOMET 250 mg	**21** L 8A DIABINESE 250 10A DIGOXIN .25 10A ALDOMET 250 mg 10A LASIX 20 mg 10P ALDOMET 250 mg
22 8A DIABINESE 250 10A DIGOXIN .25 10A ALDOMET 250 10P ALDOMET 250 mg	**23** L 8A DIABINESE 250 10A DIGOXIN .25 10A ALDOMET 250 10A LASIX 20 mg 10P ALDOMET 250 mg	**24** 8A DIABINESE 250 10A DIGOXIN .25 10A ALDOMET 250 10P ALDOMET 250 mg	**25** L 8A DIABINESE 250 10A DIGOXIN .25 10A ALDOMET 250 10A LASIX 20 mg 10P ALDOMET 250 mg	**26** 8A DIABINESE 250 10A DIGOXIN .25 10A ALDOMET 250 10P ALDOMET 250 mg	**27** L 8A DIABINESE 250 10A DIGOXIN .25 10A ALDOMET 250 10A LASIX 20 mg 10P ALDOMET 250 mg	**28** 8A DIABINESE 250 10A DIGOXIN .25 10A ALDOMET 250 10P ALDOMET 250 mg
29 8A DIABINESE 250 10A DIGOXIN .25 10A ALDOMET 250 10A LASIX 20 mg 10P ALDOMET 250 mg	**30** 8A DIABINESE 250 10A DIGOXIN .25 10A ALDOMET 250 10P ALDOMET 250 mg	**31** L 8A DIABINESE 250 10A DIGOXIN .25 10A ALDOMET 250 10A LASIX 20 mg 10P ALDOMET 250 mg				

Figure 16–1. Written drug calender and Sample Drug Regimen. This type of drug calendar is an aid to assist older adults in maintaining dosage regimens. To make the drug calendar, use a large piece of paper: date squares should be 4 x 4 inches. Print clearly in a legible manner. Use different colors if desired for different times, especially for nightly medications. Make certain the patient can read, and understands the calendar before discharge. Sample drug regimen for patient using drug calendar: Diabinese 250 mg qd; Digoxin 0.25 mg qd; Lasix 20 mg qod (odd days); and Aldomet 250 mg bid.

Patient instructions for use of calendar:
Check calendar every morning for medications and times.
After you take a medication, draw a line through it.

Remember every day:
Test your urine for glucose before breakfast, lunch, and dinner, and before going to bed.
Take your pulse at your wrist before taking digoxin. If your pulse is below 60, do *not* take the digoxin. Call your doctor the same day.

Every other day:
When you take Lasix, make sure you eat a banana or another fruit high in potassium.
Weigh yourself once a week.
Return to the clinic at the end of the month for a check-up and a new calendar.

areas. Goal-setting by the nurse helps to direct the health teaching process as well as motivate the patient to learn. As previously stated, independence is the goal for most aged adults. A health-teaching plan that addresses each of the learning domains and has specific goals helps the patient to more easily achieve the overall goal of independence.

In the cognitive learning domain instruction is geared towards providing information to increase knowledge and understanding. This intellectual aspect of the learning process should address the following areas.

1. What is the name and dose of each medication?
2. Why is each medication necessary?
3. How will each medication help treat my illness?
4. When and with what should the medication be taken?
5. What are the actions and side effects of each medication?
6. Under what circumstances should I not take the medication and contact my physician for immediate instructions?

Teaching strategies in the cognitive domain are best achieved by use of written materials and discussion with the patient. A one-to-one or small group setting works best with elder patients. Provide information as is necessary for the patient to understand the need for the medication and how to take it without supplying too much overly technical or background information. If too

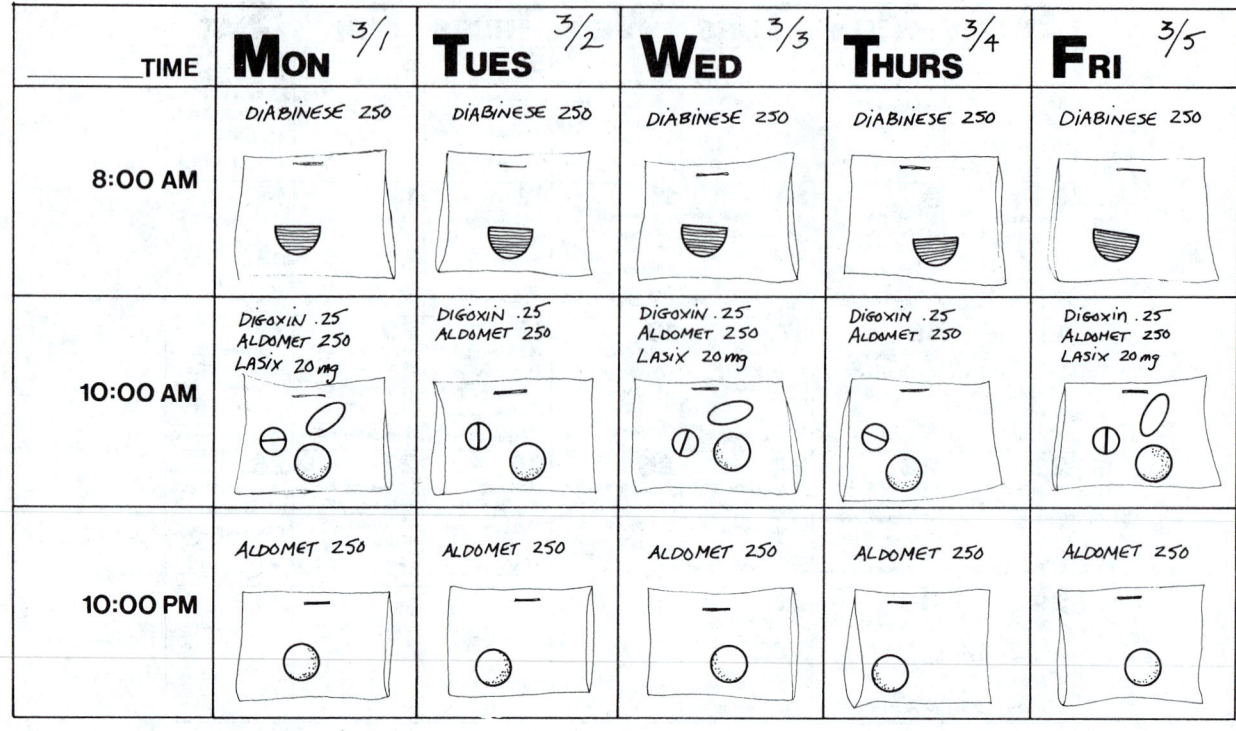

_____TIME	**M**on ³/₁	**T**ues ³/₂	**W**ed ³/₃	**T**hurs ³/₄	**F**ri ³/₅
8:00 AM	DIABINESE 250	DIABINESE 250	DIABINESE 250	DIABINESE 250	DIABINESE 250
10:00 AM	DIGOXIN .25 ALDOMET 250 LASIX 20 mg	DIGOXIN .25 ALDOMET 250	DIGOXIN .25 ALDOMET 250 LASIX 20 mg	DIGOXIN .25 ALDOMET 250	DIGOXIN .25 ALDOMET 250 LASIX 20 mg
10:00 PM	ALDOMET 250	ALDOMET 250	ALDOMET 250	ALDOMET 250	ALDOMET 250

KEY TO MEDICATIONS:

DIABINESE 250 mg

DIGOXIN .25 mg

LASIX 20 mg

ALDOMET 250 mg

Figure 16–2. Drug calendar with drugs attached. To make this calendar, use a large piece of lightweight cardboard, and write clearly. Prepare medications only up to one week in advance. Place medications in plastic wrap or plastic bags and tape or staple to appropriate time/date space. Make certain the patient can read and understands how to use the calendar fully. Make a key so that the patient can distinguish which pill is which. Sample drug regimen for patient using drug calendar with drugs attached: Diabinese 250 mg qd; Digoxin 0.25 mg qd; Lasix 20 mg qod; and Aldomet 250 mg bid.

Patient instructions for use of the calendar:
At medication time, find the right date and time, remove the pack of pills, and check them against what is written on the time/date square.
After taking the pill(s), draw a line through the drug(s).
Every day, check your urine for glucose before breakfast, lunch, and dinner, and before bedtime.
Take you pulse at your wrist before taking digoxin. If your pulse is below 60, do *not* take the digoxin. Call your doctor the same day.
When you take Lasix, make sure you eat a banana or another fruit high in potassium.
Weigh yourself once a week.
At the end of the week, call your health care provider to set up the next week's calendar.

much information is presented it can overwhelm the patient and confuse or obscure the major teaching goal—the correct self-administration of medications.

The affective domain encompasses patient attitudes toward illness, the treatment plan, and daily dependence on medications. The patient brings affective attitudes with him or her into all settings. These feelings can enhance or detract from a patient's willingness and ability to learn, as well as their compliance with the medication regimen. For example, an aged adult who is

resistant to medication instruction may be concerned about the high cost of medicines or may fear drugs and their side effects. The patient may also be preoccupied with past negative experiences with drug therapy. Patient attitudes must be recognized and problem areas overcome for information in the cognitive and psychomotor areas to be understood and utilized.

The psychomotor learning domain encompasses motor skills and performance ability. The learner must be able to translate knowledge gained in the cognitive

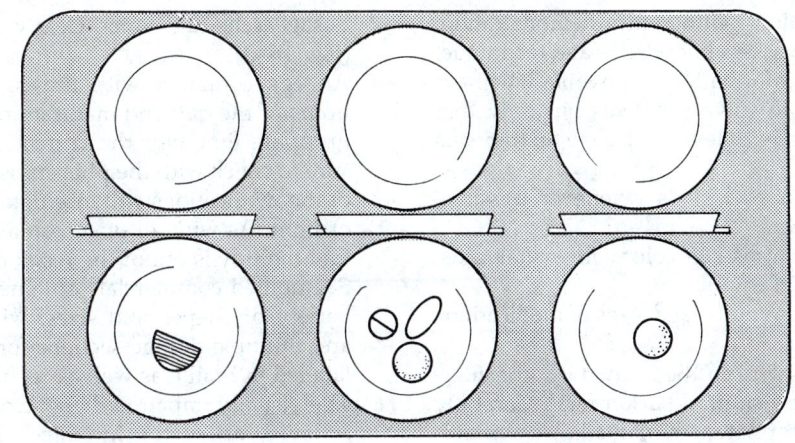

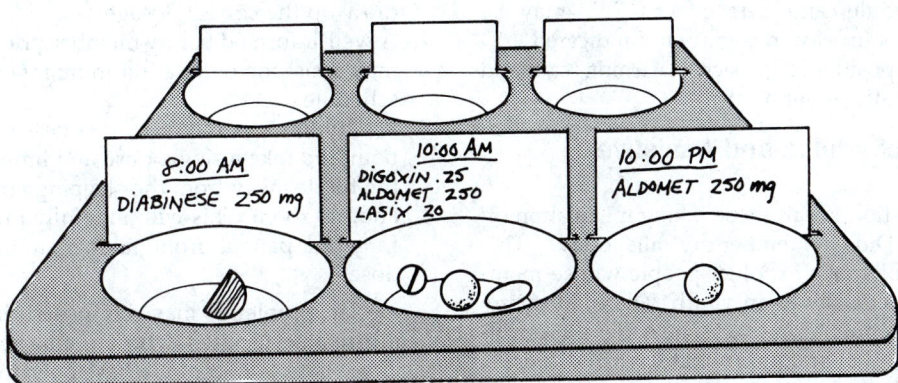

Figure 16–3. Drug tray. To set up the cupcake medication tray, use a 6- or 12-cup tray depending on the number of medication times per day. Prepare medications for only one day at a time to avoid error and contamination. (You may want two trays—one for today's medications and one for set-up.) Make a key so that the patient can distinguish which pill is which. Keep the tray well out of reach of small children. Make certain the patient can read the times and drugs and knows how to use the tray satisfactorily. Sample drug regimen for patient using cupcake medication tray: Diabinese 250 mg qd; Digoxin 0.25 mg qd; Lasix 20 mg qod; and Aldomet 250 mg bid

Patient instructions for use of the tray:

At medication time, find the right time, check the pill against what is written by the cup. Take the pill, following any special instructions.

Check your urine for glucose before breakfast, lunch, dinner, and before bedtime.

Take your pulse at your wrist before 10:00 AM. If your pulse is below 60, do *not* take the digoxin. Replace it in the tray and notify your doctor.

At lunch today and every other day, eat a banana or another fruit high in potassium.

Weigh yourself every Tuesday morning.

domain into motor skills. Classic examples here are the ability to prepare and self-administer insulin or to take a pulse accurately. Psychomotor skills are best learned through demonstration and return-demonstration.

Dall and Gresham (1982) summarized the following effective teaching strategies for the older adult:

1. Begin teaching early!
2. Assess assets and liabilities in sensory perception, central processing and integration, or motor performance before initiating a teaching plan.

3. Encourage the use of effective adaptive devices (hearing aids, glasses) whenever possible.
4. Provide only general information in a group. Avoid group learning for individuals who find groups distracting. Provide specific drug information on an individual basis. Avoid mixing the very old with the "young" old in teaching groups.
5. Keep individual teaching sessions short: 15–20 minutes at a time.
6. Seek verbalization of the steps and rationale in-

volved in skills along with return-demonstration. This allows you to assess knowledge and technique.

7. Provide as much information as possible when expecting a person to solve problems but only that which is absolutely relevant. Delete extraneous material.

8. Use concrete tasks and skills whenever possible, avoiding abstraction.

9. Choose bright contrasting colors in visual aids; avoid pale or pastel colors.

10. Use specific shapes, colors, and sizes of medications to your advantage.

11. Use words meaningful to the individual, considering educational and cultural background. Carefully consider the appropriateness of medical terminology.

12. Ensure adequate lighting, free from glare.

13. Provide medication cards to selected individuals or family members as reminders of drug purposes, dosage schedule, and side effects. Pills may be taped to cards for easy recognition if indicated.

14. Maintain a positive approach. Learning can and does occur in the older adult.

Medication Schedules and Assistive Devices

A persistent question for all those taking medication on a daily basis is "Did I remember my pills today?" This is especially problematic for older people whose memory may not be as acute as in youth. There are many ways in which the nurse can assist the patient in developing a schedule plan and appropriate assistive aids. A simple device such as turning the medicine bottle upside down once a daily medicine has been taken and then righting the bottle at bedtime serves as a definite visual confirmation that the medicine has been taken. Many patients are on multiple drugs with more than a once-daily dosage and therefore may require more elaborate assistive aids.

Because adhering to a dosage schedule is such a problem, methods of enhancing memory through various aids are extremely important. The most important factors to consider when devising a dosage schedule with a patient are (1) simplify the schedule as much as possible, and (2) schedule dosage times to coincide with routine daily activities to decrease the chances of omission (e.g., upon arising, at mealtime, at bedtime). Some patients even set wind-up alarm clocks to go off when the next dose of medicine is due. This technique is helpful when medicine dose times do not coincide with mealtime or other routine activities. Other helpful assistive aids and techniques are

1. A large calendar with room to write the drugs and times to be taken each day on which the patient crosses off each dose as taken (Fig. 16–1).

2. A guide calendar with each day's drugs wrapped in cellophane and taped to the calendar (Fig. 16–2). Such a device must be out of the way of access by visiting grandchildren.

3. A cupcake tray with the drugs to be taken and the dosage schedule times clearly labeled on the tray (Fig. 16–3).

4. An egg container with the cups labeled with the hours of the day and medications inserted in the appropriate times for the correct dosage schedule. Be sure to check with the pharmacist to determine if any of the medications will lose potency if exposed to air or light. As with all open container systems, be certain the tray is out of the reach of children.

5. Segmented commercial containers are available in a variety of shapes and sizes, with choices of single and multiple dosage sections for each day. Most are labeled in braille as well as regular alphabet letters.

6. The visually impaired diabetic on insulin can obtain a device called the Monoject Scale Magnifier that magnifies the numbers printed on an insulin syringe. Also available is the Dos-Aid Syringe Filling Device, which can be set to a precise insulin dosage on a U-100 syringe and thus allow the visually impaired to draw up the correct dosage.

7. A well-informed family member, friend, or volunteer may assist the older adult in maintaining the dosage schedule.

8. If a hypnotic is required, it is best for the patient to pour and take a single dose and immediately replace the bottle away from the sleeping area, preferably in another room. This will hopefully prevent a drowsy, forgetful patient from taking an unneeded repeat dose.

Special problems may be posed by residents of health-related facilities who are able to go outside the facility where they can purchase over-the-counter medicines. Use of a form such as represented in Figure 16–4 may help prevent such problems. It is a signed agreement between nurse and patient that spells out specific responsibilities in the self-medication plan. Basically the patient agrees to follow specific directions on prescription containers; to not share medications; to report to the pharmacy to pick up medications as directed; to discard all old, unused, or expired drugs; to not purchase or take any over-the-counter medications unless specifically ordered to do so; and to participate in medication counseling sessions. The nurse's role in this program is to interview the patient monthly to assess drug knowledge, evaluate compliance with the therapy regimen, and to observe the patient for clinical response to medications.

EVALUATION OF THE DRUG THERAPY REGIMEN FOR THE OLDER ADULT

Frequent review of patient drug profile is essential. All members of the patient's health care team should contribute towards devising a plan the patient can comply with and which meets patient needs. Evaluate the patient for inappropriate drug usage and dosage. Most pharmaceutical experts agree that the best drug regimen should be the fewest possible drugs at the minimum dosage. As previously discussed, with advancing age the margin of safety between therapeutic and toxic dose

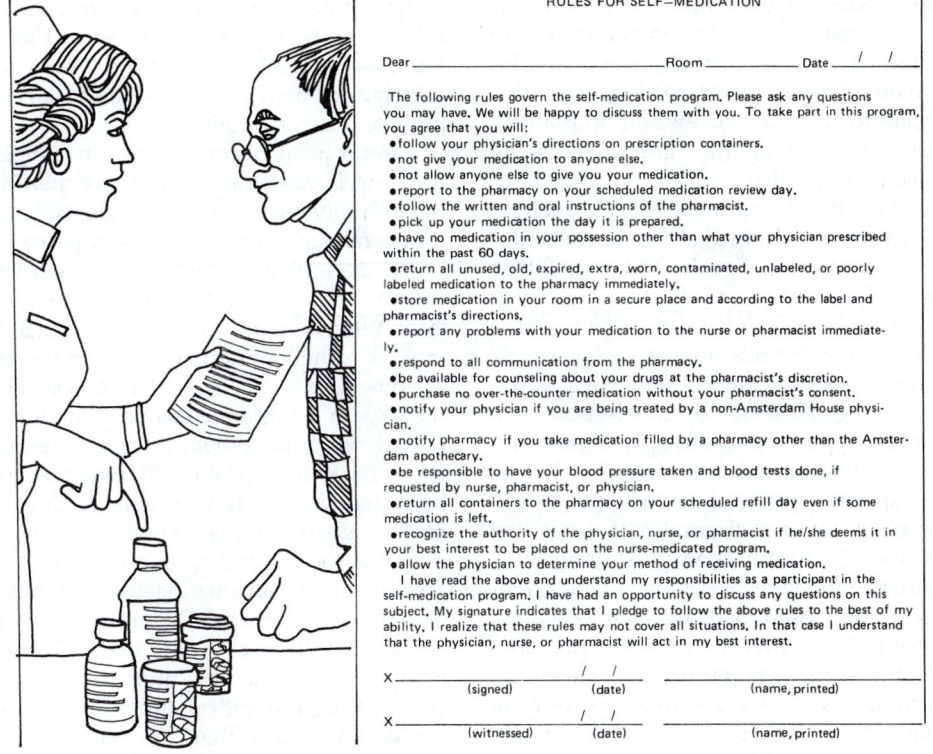

Figure 16–4. Rules for self-medication.

narrows. Therefore, the dose of a drug is often reduced. The development of geriatric dosage forms for drugs with age-dependent renal excretion would be extremely helpful for patients. The dosage for drugs metabolized by the liver may also be reduced for elderly patients without altering blood levels of the drug.

Evaluate the patient's ability to discriminate between the different drugs being taken. Many patients complain that "the medicines all look alike. " Try to consider the size, color, and shape of each drug when devising a drug regimen, so that this is not confusing for the patient.

Evaluate the patient's ability to correctly pour the proper dose. For example, liquid medications may be easier for the patient to swallow, but the patient may have great difficulty obtaining the proper dosage because of functional impairments. If tablets need to be cut in half, scored tablets should be provided. If arthritic fingers find breaking tablets too difficult, it may be necessary for someone to break the tablets for the patient. For patients who are extremely dysphagic, medication crushed and mixed with semisolid food such as applesauce is often safer to swallow than liquids. Care should be taken not to crush enteric-coated tablets, however, because gastrointestinal side effects can result and drug effectiveness may be altered.

Another important area of evaluation is patient/family ability to recognize adverse drug effects. Adverse effects is a special problem area for the older patient. Much of the current literature suggests an increased risk

of adverse drug reactions wtih increasing patient age. The presence of multiple chronic illnesses, multiple drug therapy, and the effects of aging upon drug disposition all contribute to the problem. Thus, early recognition of drug adverse effects before such effects become toxic could prevent many problems for older patients and should help to reduce hospitalizations for drug toxicity treatment.

Certain drugs pose significant risk for older patients. Those causing the greatest potential hazard for these patients include antidysrhythmics, antimicrobials, digoxin, and diuretics. These drugs are all commonly prescribed for older adults, and some have a high rate of adverse effects in this population. For example, about 20%–30% of older patients taking digoxin will experience adverse effects. Since these drugs are so essential for patients, the best way to reduce the risk of adverse effects is through patient teaching and frequent evaluation of continued patient understanding of what was taught.

Careful monitoring of patient laboratory data can give important early warning signs of such impending problems as inadequate renal function or increasing serum drug levels. Serum drug levels allow for evaluation of whether or not the drug dose administered is within the therapeutic range for the patient. Physical assessment of the patient gives clues to drug effects. Careful observations of laboratory data allows for adjustment of drug dosages before toxic effects occur. Close observation of the patient can also give important clues of beginning toxicity. Patients taking digoxin may experience anorexia, nausea, or vomiting. It is thus important not to dismiss physical signs (such as anorexia) as insignificant or attributable to moodiness. In the case of digoxin, such signs may indicate toxicity. It is likewise important to teach the patient or caregiver the signs to recognize which may indicate drug toxicity.

Drug side effects in the elderly are often mistaken for signs of aging. Among the drugs that can cause confusion are cimetidine (Tagamet); digoxin; and methyldopa (Aldomet). Depression may be an effect of digoxin or reserpine (Serpasil). Examples of drugs that can cause lethargy and drowsiness include analgesics (especially narcotics); hypnotic sedatives; and tranquilizers. Barbiturates can cause forgetfulness. Postural hypotension can result from antihypertensive therapy. Urinary incontinence may result from diuretic therapy. Furosemide (Lasix) is especially prone to cause urgency and incontinence in older patients. Examples of drugs that can cause ataxia include chlordiazepoxide (Librium); diazepam (Valium); and flurazepam (Dalmane). Gastrointestinal distress can be caused by drugs such as aspirin; ibuprofen (Motrin); indomethacin (Indocin); oral iron preparations; erythromycin; and piroxicam (Feldene).

As stated earlier, the elderly are frequent users of over-the-counter drugs. The fact that such drugs are available without a prescription lends a false sense of security. All drugs are capable of causing adverse effects and toxicity. Aspirin is frequently used by older patients for relief of arthritic symptoms. It is an especially useful drug for this purpose and much less expensive than nonsteroidal anti-inflammatory drugs. Aspirin must be taken in dosages of up to ten tablets per day to achieve adequate anti-inflammatory effects, and this can cause gastrointestinal distress, bleeding, and ulcers. Enteric-coated aspirin tablets are relatively inexpensive and decrease gastrointestinal distress. Over-the-counter antacid preparations containing magnesium hydroxide are frequently used by older persons, and these preparations can cause diarrhea. Antihistamine products, readily available over the counter, can cause drowsiness. More information on other-the-counter drugs can be found in Chapter 7. Careful evaluation of the older patient and questioning of patient/family can help to determine the cause of certain symptoms or behaviors.

Because of the prolonged blood levels seen in elderly patients, the concept of a *drug holiday* has been advocated by some. Once a steady state of a drug has been achieved, the patient skips a day of the drug. The drug holiday can reduce annual drug consumption with no loss of therapeutic effect or ill effects to patients. It can also afford patients substantial savings on the cost of medications.

Evaluation of the patient's nutritional status is also essential when trying to determine the effectiveness of a therapeutic regimen. Some drugs, such as the antineoplastic cisplatin, can have a direct effect upon the nutritional status of a patient and result in anorexia, nausea, and vomiting. Patients receiving antineoplastic chemotherapy may suffer from stomatitis and weight loss. Diarrhea, alterations in electrolytes, and interference in carbohydrate and fat metabolism can also result from other drug therapies. Patient weight loss may necessitate dose recalculation for drugs whose dose is given per kilogram of body weight. Malnutrition may prevent or impede drug absorption.

Careful evaluation of the effectiveness of health teaching is essential. Do not rely merely upon the patient/family repeating instructions to you. Rote memory is generally a short-term memory pattern. This is similar to the cramming students do before a test; material remembered for the test cannot be recalled a short time later. When you are teaching a patient a medication regimen, it is the long-term memory (necessary for self-care at home) that is most essential. An excellent way to have the patient incorporate teaching into long-term memory is by having the patient demonstrate how medications are to be poured, taken, and remembered. Have the patient demonstrate how a pulse reading is obtained before a digoxin dose is taken or how they will record or remember that a medication dose has been taken. You are not merely evaluating the patient's technique but also the effectiveness of your health teaching.

Good health teaching is the key to assuring patient compliance with a medication regimen. Also essential is patient trust and understanding of the value of the medication regimen so that compliance is motivated. Older patients are able to learn, but teaching strategies need to be modified according to the physical limitations that the aging process has imposed.

SUMMARY

Older adults are the fastest growing segment of the population. In the United States those over 65 years of age constitute 12% of the population, and this group consumes about 30% of all prescription drugs and the largest amount of over-the-counter drugs. The normal aging process affects all systems and functions of the body and results in alterations in both the therapeutic and adverse response to drugs. Pathologic conditions can have an even greater effect upon the individual's response to drugs.

The nurse's role in caring for the older adult must include appropriate health teaching to promote patient compliance with therapeutic drug regimen and help avoid adverse or toxic effects of therapy. Often the side effects or early toxic effects of drugs are erroneously attributed to aging, causing the older patient to develop more serious side effects or toxicity. The nurse, patient, and family should be aware of common side effects of patient medications and alert for early signs and symptoms of problems. The use of the nursing process in assessing individual patient areas of knowledge deficits and planning care to meet these needs is but a part of the ongoing drug therapy regimen. Follow-up evaluation of the effectiveness of health teaching, both short- and long-term, is essential for the patient to obtain the maximum therapeutic effect with the fewest adverse effects possible.

BIBLIOGRAPHY

Alford, D: Bill of rights for elderly on drug therapy. Nurs Clin North Am 17(2):282, 1982.

The big lie about generic drugs. Consumer Reports 52:480–485, 1987.

Cooper, JW: Drug-related Problems (DRPs) in the long-term care facility. Nursing Homes 35(6):13–18, 1986.

Dall, CE and Gresham, L: Promoting effective drug taking behavior in the elderly. Nurs Clin North Am 17(2):283–290, 1982.

Darnell, J, et al: Medication use by ambulatory elderly. J Am Geriatr Soc 34:1, 1986.

Doenges, ME, Jeffries, MF, and Moorhouse, MF: Nursing Care Plans. Philadelphia, FA Davis, 1984.

Elderly epileptics require less phenytoin. Nurses' Drug Alert. Am J Nurs 10:1584, 1982.

Geriatric drug-induced memory impairment. Nurse's Drug Alert 11(8):1063, 1987.

Gilman, AG, Goodman, LS, and Gilman, A (eds): The Pharmacological Basis of Therapeutics, ed 7. New York, Macmillan, 1985.

Hayes, JE: Normal changes in aging and nursing implications of drug therapy. Nurs Clin North Am 17(2):253–262, 1982.

Keenan, R: The benefits of a drug holiday. Geriatric Nursing :103–104, 1983.

Meguerdichian, D: Improving self-medication in an H.R.F. Geriatric Nursing :30–34, 1983.

NRL Drugs, ed 2: Springhouse, Nursing 84 Books, 1984.

Potempa, K and Roberts, KV: Cardiovascular drugs and the older adult. Nurs Clin North Am 17(2):263–274, 1982.

Prescribing for the elderly. FDA Drug Bulletin 18(1):9, 1988.

Shoemaker, DM: Use and abuse of OTC medications by the elderly. Journal of Gerontological Nursing 6:21–24, 1980.

Stillwell, S: Ensuring safe effective drug therapy. Nursing Life 6(6):33–39, 1986.

Treating depression in the elderly. Nurse's Drug Alert 11(7):954, 1987.

SITUATION 16–1

Marian Cantrell, an 84-year-old, is admitted to the medical-surgical floor with a diagnosis of urinary tract infection.

1. An IV is started, and the nurse administers gentamycin via an intravenous piggyback. It will be important for the nurse to assess the following in relation to gentamycin administration:
   a. magnesium level
   b. creatinine level
   c. sodium level
   d. calcium level

2. In planning nursing interventions for Mrs. Cantrell, all of the following would be included *except:*
   a. monitor serum gentamycin levels
   b. measure intake and output
   c. restrict fluids to 1000 cc per day
   d. weigh patient daily

3. The nurse will observe Mrs. Cantrell for the following sensory disturbance, indicating a toxic effect of gentamycin:
   a. visual
   b. tactile
   c. olfactory
   d. auditory

4. Mrs. Cantrell received a sleeping pill (Nembutal) for the first night in the hospital. The next day she was drowsy and wanted to sleep instead of eating her breakfast. The nurse is aware that this effect is most probably due to:
   a. reduced hepatic function
   b. reduced cardiac output
   c. gentamycin interaction
   d. delayed toxic effects

5. Mrs. Cantrell has a history of diabetes and is currently taking tolbutamide (Orinase). This drug is an example of one that is affected by:
   a. hypokalemia
   b. hyponatremia
   c. hyperlipidemia
   d. hypoproteinemia

6. On the fourth day of hospitalization, Mrs. Cantrell has an irregular heart rate and is started on oral procainamide (Pronestyl). The nurse will assess the following with regard to this medication:
   a. protein intake
   b. renal function
   c. folic acid levels
   d. subcutaneous fatty tissue

Please refer to the Appendices for correct answers and additional review questions with answers.

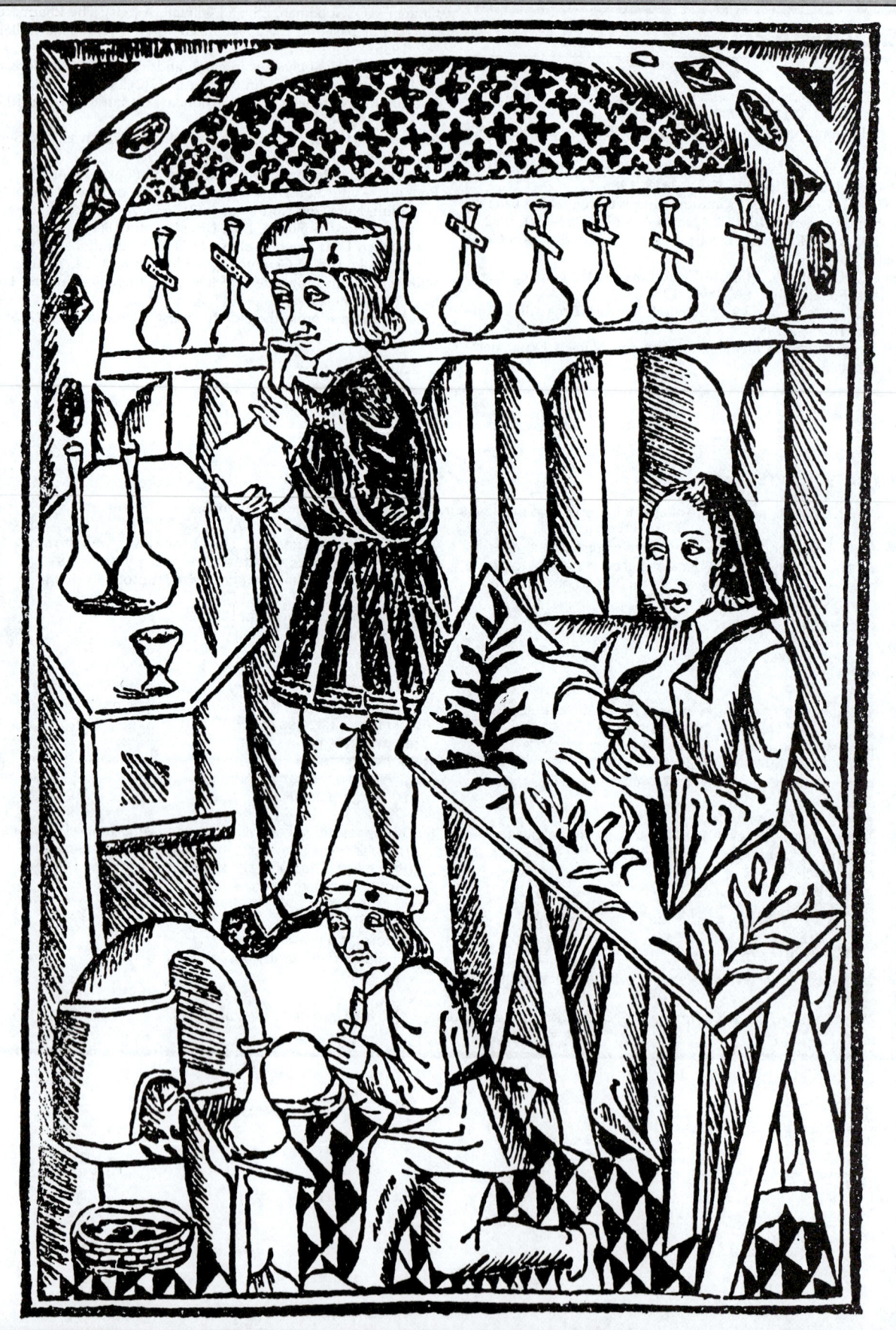

Preparing medicines, circa 1500. Free Library of Philadelphia Print Collection.

2

UNIT

DRUGS AFFECTING THE NERVOUS SYSTEM

CHAPTER OUTLINE

GLOSSARY TERMS IN THIS CHAPTER

Acetylcholine
Acetylcholinesterase
Adrenergic nerve fibers
Adrenergic receptors
Alpha receptor
Autonomic nervous system
Axon
Basal ganglia
Beta receptor
Brain stem
Catechol-O-methyl transferase (COMT)
Central nervous system
Cerebellum
Cerebral cortex
Cerebrum
Cholinergic nerve fibers
Cholinergic receptors
Cholinomimetic agent
Corpora quadrigemina
Corpus callosum
Craniosacral system
Diencephalon
Dopamine
Epinephrine (adrenaline)
Ganglia
Hypothalamus
Limbic system
Medulla oblongata
Mesencephalon
Metencephalon
Monoamine oxidase (MAO)
Motor neurons
Muscarinic receptor
Myelencephalon
Neurotransmitter
Nicotinic receptor
Norepinephrine
Parasympathetic nervous system
Paravertebral ganglia
Pons
Receptors
Reticular activating system (RAS)
Reticular formation
Somatic nervous system
Sympathetic autonomic nervous system
Sympathomimetic agent
Telencephalon
Thalamus
Thoracolumbar system

OVERVIEW OF ANATOMY AND PHYSIOLOGY OF THE CENTRAL NERVOUS SYSTEM

JEREMIAH T. HERLIHY, Ph.D.
BARBARA L. HERLIHY, R.N., Ph.D.
VICKI L. BYERS, R.N., Ph.D., CNRN

LEARNING OBJECTIVES

After reading this chapter, the student will be able to:

1. Locate and describe the functions of the major structures of the brain.

2. Identify the major sensory and motor tracts within the spinal cord.

3. Differentiate between the somatic and autonomic nervous systems.

4. Differentiate between the parasympathetic and sympathetic nervous systems.

5. Differentiate between adrenergic and cholinergic fibers.

6. Describe the adrenergic receptor subtypes (alpha and beta).

7. Describe the cholinergic receptor subtypes (muscarinic and nicotinic).

INTRODUCTION

The purpose of this chapter is to provide a brief and selective review of the nervous system, focusing primarily on those structures and functions affected by neuropharmacologic agents. In general, the nervous system serves to control and coordinate bodily functions. It receives vast amounts of information and very quickly sorts and integrates this information so as to determine the appropriate response. In addition to sensation and movement, this highly complex interconnected network of nervous tissue functions in consciousness, thought, memory, learning, emotions, and behavior. The various divisions of the nervous system are listed in Table 17–1.

CENTRAL NERVOUS SYSTEM

The *central nervous system* (CNS) is composed of the brain and the spinal cord.

Table 17–1. DIVISIONS OF THE NERVOUS SYSTEM

A. Central nervous system
  1. Brain
  2. Spinal cord
B. Peripheral nervous system
  1. Afferent system
  2. Efferent system
    a. Somatic nervous system
    b. Autonomic nervous system
      1. Sympathetic division
      2. Parasympathetic division

BRAIN

Classification systems of brain structures are numerous and often are confusing to the beginning student. Two classification systems are used: the first system is complete but sometimes cumbersome; the second system is much simpler but somewhat incomplete and admittedly oversimplified. For a number of reasons it is necessary to use terms that cut across both systems, and the student is urged to correlate both systems. Figure 17–1

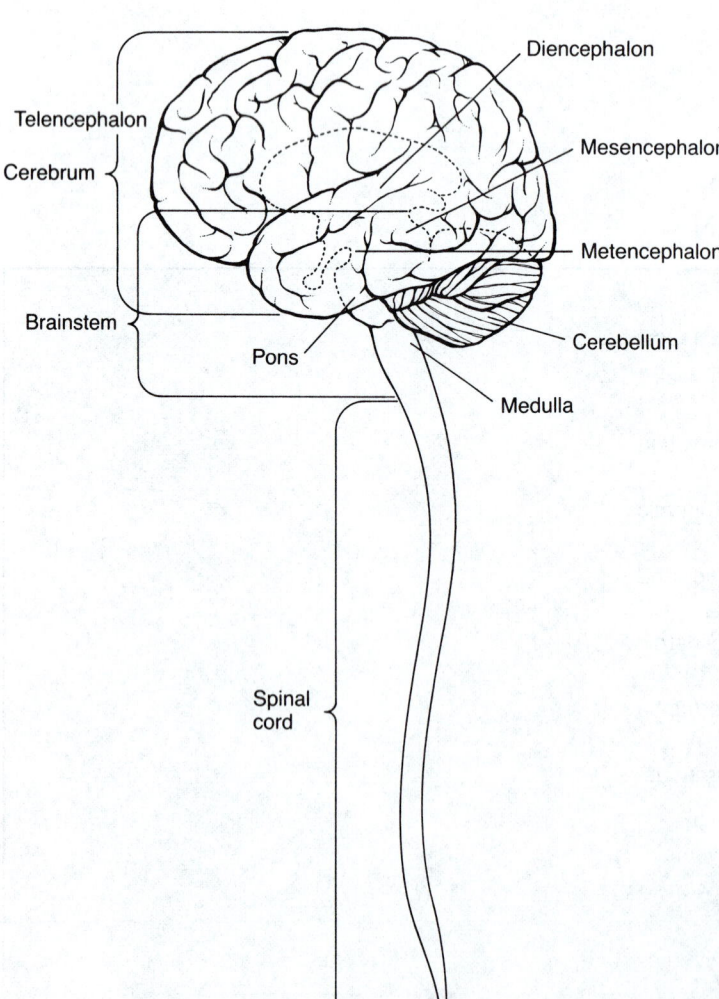

Figure 17–1. Classifications of brain structures. (Redrawn from Langley, Telford, and Christensen's: Dynamic Anatomy and Physiology, ed. 5, McGraw-Hill, New York, 1980, with permission.)

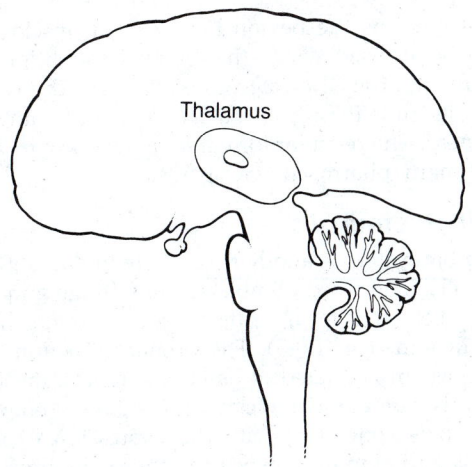

Thalamus

Figure 17–2. The reticular formation. (Redrawn from Guyton, AC: Textbook of Medical Physiology, ed. 5. WB Saunders, Philadelphia, 1986, with permission.)

graphically depicts this relationship and should be examined in light of the following discussion.

From an embryonic perspective the brain can be divided into five segments. The most rostral structure (i.e., from the top) is referred to as the (a) *telencephalon* and includes the cerebral hemispheres in which are embedded various nuclei, most notably the *basal ganglia*. Proceeding caudally (i.e., "downward") are the (b) *diencephalon*, including the *thalamus* and *hypothalamus*; (c) *mesencephalon*, including several important nuclei; (d) *metencephalon*, including the *pons* and *cerebellum*; and (e) *myelencephalon* or *medulla oblongata*. Referring to Figure 17–1, note the correlation with the more simplified system: the (a) *cerebrum*, (b) *brain stem*, and (c) cerebellum. The brain structures are described primarily in terms of the more simplified system, but it is useful to keep the more complex classification (Fig. 17–1) in mind.

In addition to these anatomic structures, there are two functional areas composed of diffuse collections of cells. These are referred to as the *reticular formation* and the *limbic system*. Both of these systems are discussed below (Fig. 17–2).

Cerebrum

The cerebrum comprises the largest part of the brain. It is divided into the right and left hemispheres, each hemisphere being joined by a band of fibers referred to as the *corpus callosum*. A thin outer layer of gray matter is referred to as the *cerebral cortex*, while the inner white matter is called the *medullary center*. Fiber tracts within the white matter connect both hemispheres and the cerebral cortex with the lower parts of the brain and spinal cord. The cerebral cortex performs the following general functions:

1. Sensory function: awareness and analysis of sensory input.

2. Motor function: initiation and control of motor activity.
3. Integrative functions: a nebulous term referring to all events that occur within the cerebral cortex in response to sensory input. In addition to the appropriate motor responses to sensory input, this term also includes consciousness, memory, learning, use of language, emotions, and mental activities of all kinds.

Embedded within the cerebral hemispheres are small gray masses called basal ganglia (see Glossary). These ganglia have numerous connections throughout the CNS and perform two general functions:

1. Control of muscle tone
2. Initiation and modulation of motor movement

The cerebrum forms connections with the diencephalon, the segment containing the thalamus and the hypothalamus. The thalamus, often referred to as the "telephone switchboard" of the brain, performs the following functions:

1. Acts as a relay center for sensory information. The thalamus produces a conscious recognition of crude sensations of pain, touch, pressure, and extremes of temperature. The cerebral cortex is required for finer discriminations of these sensations.
2. Influences emotions by associating sensory input with feelings of pleasantness and unpleasantness.
3. Plays a role in the arousal mechanism.
4. Coordinates motor movement. Complex reflexes are coordinated at this level.

The hypothalamus not only interacts extensively with other nervous tissue but also exerts widespread effects on the endocrine system. The functions of the hypothalamus include the following:

1. Coordinates autonomic activity (e.g., visceral responses).
2. Serves as a relay between the cerebral cortex and the lower autonomic centers and to spinal cord somatic centers. This "linking of the mind to the body" provides a route through which the mind can influence bodily function.
3. Participates in the regulation of water and electrolyte balance through the production of antidiuretic hormone (ADH).
4. Regulates endocrine function through the secretion of releasing hormones.
5. Participates in maintaining the waking state.
6. Participates in appetite regulation.
7. Participates in temperature regulation.

Brain Stem

The brain stem is composed of the mesencephalon, the pons, and the medulla oblongata. The brain stem performs important sensory, motor, and reflex functions and is the source of all but two of the cranial nerves (the olfactory and optic nerves originate in the diencephalon). The mesencephalon, the more rostral of these structures, contains a number of important nuclei. The *corpora quadrigemina* serve as the relay center for visual and auditory reflexes. The peduncles, red nucleus, and substantia nigra help coordinate motor activity and play an important role in postural reflexes.

The pons forms a bridge between the medulla below and the mesencephalon and cerebellum. It also forms an important structural link between the cerebral hemispheres and the cerebellum. In addition to its role of relaying sensory and motor information, the pons also contains the pneumotaxic and apneustic centers and therefore participates in the regulation of respiration.

The medulla is the part of the brain that attaches to the spinal cord. The medulla is called the "vital center" because it contains the cardiac, vasogenic, and respiratory centers, which are vital for survival. Also present in the medulla are nonvital reflex centers such as those for vomiting, coughing, sneezing, hiccupping, and swallowing. Like the other parts of the brain stem, the medulla also functions as a relay center for all ascending and descending tracts. It is at the level of the medulla that most of the major motor tracts decussate or cross over. The decussation of the fiber tracts gives the medulla its pyramid-like appearance.

Cerebellum

The cerebellum or "little brain" is a metencephalon structure that is connected to the brain stem through structures referred to as cerebellar peduncles. In general, cerebellar function is related to the control of motor activity. In concert with the cerebral cortex, the cerebellum produces skilled muscle movement, maintains equilibrium, and controls posture. It functions below the level of consciousness to smooth out jerky, awkward, and trembling movements.

In addition to the structures described above, several groups of neural tissue function as integrated systems and are often affected by pharmacologic agents. These systems include the reticular formation and the limbic system.

Reticular Formation

Groups of functionally associated neurons, collectively referred to as the reticular formation, are diffusely located throughout the entire brain stem, the diencephalon (thalamus and hypothalamus), and the lower telencephalon (Fig. 17–2). Because of its diffuse array of nuclei and fibers, the reticular formation affects and is affected by all CNS activity. The reticular formation functions to:

1. Modulate both sensory and motor activity.
2. Regulate autonomic responses.
3. Produce most of the monoamines that are distributed throughout the CNS.

Perhaps the most important role of the reticular formation is the maintenance of a state of alertness or arousal. The *reticular activating system* (RAS) consists of specific areas within the brain stem reticular formation. The RAS receives impulses from the spinal cord and relays them to the thalamus and from there to all areas of the cerebral cortex. Without such continual excitation of

cortical neurons the person becomes unconscious and cannot be aroused. Thus, the reticular formation functions as the arousal or alerting system for the cerebral cortex; its functioning is crucial for maintaining consciousness. The reticular formation is sensitive to the action of many pharmacologic agents.

Limbic System

The limbic system is another collection of diffusely scattered cells. The word "limbic" means fringe and refers to those cells that form a ring or fringe around the corpus callosum (Fig. 17–3). The primary function of the limbic system is related to emotions; hence, the limbic system is sometimes referred to as the "emotional brain." It is concerned with the expression of mood, feelings, and emotions, especially those emotions associated with sexual behavior, pleasure, fear, and rage. It also plays a role in the regulation of biologic rhythms, appetite, and learning. Like the reticular formation, the limbic system influences and is influenced by many other CNS structures.

SPINAL CORD

The second major division of the CNS is the spinal cord. The spinal cord is a slender cylinder that lies within the spinal cavity and extends from the medulla to approximately L-2. As shown in cross section in Figure 17–4, it appears as an H-shaped inner gray area surrounded by an outer area of white matter. The gray matter is composed primarily of cell bodies and interneurons. The surrounding white matter is composed primarily of nerve axons, many of which are covered by a white myelin sheath, hence the designation white matter. The white matter is arranged in pathways or tracts, each

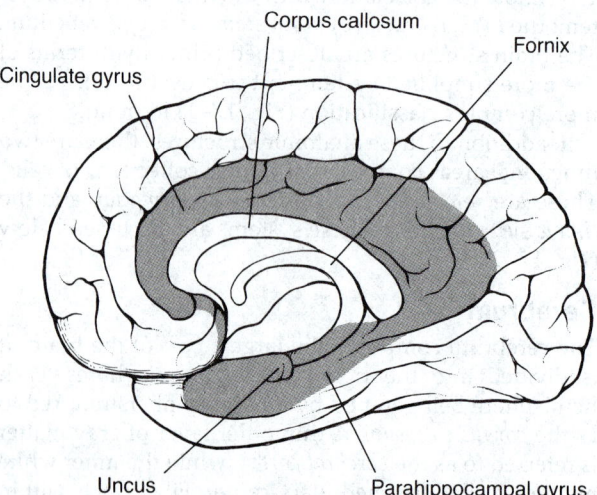

Figure 17–3. The limbic system (*shaded areas*) and other structures within it. A major function of the limbic system is the arousal of emotions. (Redrawn from Byers, VL and Guthrie, MD: The limbic system and behavior. J Neurosurg Nurs, April, Vol. 16 no. Z, 1984 p. 81, with permission.

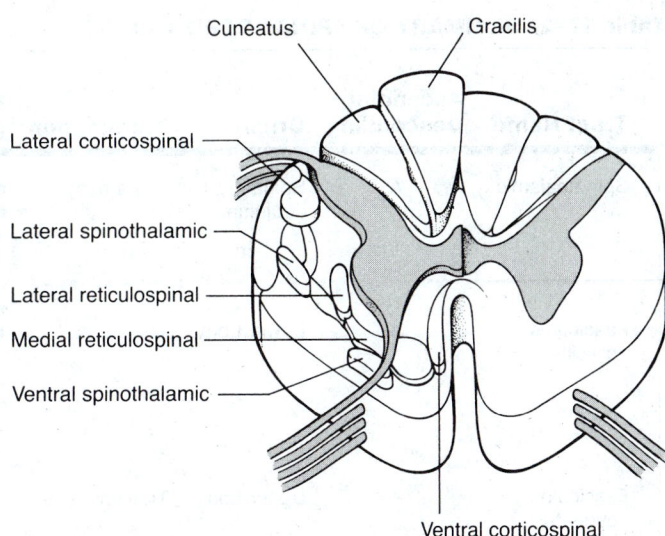

Figure 17–4. The spinal cord. This cross section indicates some of the major ascending (sensory) and descending (motor) tracts.

tract being composed of individual fibers that possess similar anatomic and functional characteristics. For instance, the fibers that comprise the spinothalamic tract have the same origin and destination and are concerned with the same general function, namely, the sensations of crude touch, pain, and temperature.

Tracts are classified as either ascending (sensory) or descending (motor). Ascending tracts conduct impulses up the cord toward the brain, while the descending tracts conduct impulses down the cord from the brain and toward the periphery. Table 17–2 contains the names of the major ascending and descending tracts.

The spinal cord performs two major functions:

1. Serves as a conducting pathway for signals going to and from the brain.
2. Serves as a center for spinal reflexes.

CENTRAL NEUROTRANSMITTERS

Information is transferred centrally and peripherally in the form of electrical messages. The process involves both electrical conduction of the signal down the axon and chemical transmission of the signal from one nerve to another or from a nerve to an effector organ across the neural synapse or across the effector cell junction, respectively. The action potential is a regenerating wave of depolarization that is conducted down the *axon*. (For a discussion of the ionic basis of the action potential refer to Chapter 27.) It does not cross (or "jump" across) directly from nerve to nerve or from nerve to muscle. Instead, the action potential, as it invades the nerve ending, releases a chemical substance presynaptically, which, in turn, diffuses across the synapse or myoneural junction and acts on the postsynaptic membrane to initiate a new action potential or modulate pre-existing activity. These chemical substances are called *neurotransmitters* and bind to specialized portions of the postsynaptic membrane called receptors. A receptor consists of chemical groups located on the cell membrane or within a cell and are capable of recognizing

specific transmitters and drugs binding to them. Only when a transmitter or agonist binds to its appropriate receptor can it effect changes in the postsynaptic cell. Agents that bind to the receptor but do not elicit the appropriate change in the effector cell are called antagonists. By occupying *receptors*, antagonists prevent agonists from binding the receptor and eliciting the appropriate cell response.

Some of the more common CNS transmitters and their characteristics are listed in Table 17–3 and include norepinephrine, serotonin, *dopamine*, and acetylcholine. Disturbances in the levels of various neurotransmitters have been implicated in certain disease states. For instance, a deficiency of dopamine within the basal ganglia has been associated with Parkinson's disease while dopamine excess within the limbic system has been implicated in schizophrenia. Alterations in neurotransmitter levels have obvious pathophysiologic and pharmacologic implications.

BLOOD–BRAIN BARRIER

The brain is perfused by two fluids, blood and cerebrospinal fluid (CSF). A rich arterial blood supply (15%–20% of the cardiac output) is provided by the circle of Willis, an intricate, interconnecting arrangement of vessels at the base of the brain.

The major sites of nutrient and end-product exchange are the cerebral capillaries. However, the exchange of substances between the blood and nervous tissue differs somewhat from the relatively unrestricted diffusion of nonprotein substances in other capillary beds. The blood–brain barrier controls both the type and rate of diffusion. This barrier to exchange is both anatomic (i.e., specialized anatomic regions) and physiologic (i.e., physiologic transport systems that handle substances in different ways). Because of the barrier, the chemical composition of the extracellular fluid within the CNS can be regulated. Moreover, the blood–brain barrier presents a formidable barrier to the diffusion of various toxins and pharmacologic agents. The ability of a drug

Table 17–2. SUMMARY OF SPINAL CORD TRACTS

Tract Name	Ascending/ Descending	Origin	Termination	Function (Transmits)	Dysfunction	Specific Names	Cross (Yes/ No)
Spinothalamic	A	Spinal column	Thalamus	• Pain • Temperature • Conscious proprioception • Light touch	Loss of pain, temperature, light touch contralaterally (opposite side) below lesion	Lateral Ventral	Yes
Fasciculus gracilis	A	Lower body	Thalamus	• Conscious proprioception • Stereognosis from lower body	Loss of conscious proprioception and stereognosis from lower body ipsilaterally (same side)	None	Yes
Fasciculus cuneatus	A	Upper body	Thalamus	• Conscious proprioception • Stereognosis from upper body	Loss of conscious proprioception and stereognosis from upper body ipsilaterally	None	Yes
Spinocerebellar	A	Spinal column	Cerebellum	• Controls equilibrium, posture, and unconscious proprioception	Ipsilateral uncoordinated postural activities	Dorsal Ventral	No Yes
Corticospinal	D	Motor cortex	Spinal cord	• Carries motor activity	Upper and lower motor neuron dysfunction produces different symptoms	Lateral Ventral	Yes Yes
Corticobulbar	D	Motor cortex	Brain stem motor nuclei	• Facial expression	Usually does not cause massive dysfunction of facial activity	None	Yes
Rubrospinal	D	Red nucleus within midbrain	Muscle groups	• Modifies muscular contractions	Loss of postural adjustments and balance	None	Yes

From Mathewson, M: Ascending and descending spinal cord tracts. Critical Care Nurse 5(5):10–14, 1985, with permission.

to cross the blood–brain barrier is an important therapeutic consideration. For instance, high plasma levels of an antibiotic may prove ineffective for the treatment of an infection within the CNS if the antibiotic is unable to cross the barrier.

The cells of the CNS are perfused by a second fluid, the cerebrospinal fluid. CSF is formed across the choroid plexus and flows through the ventricles and central canal of the spinal cord, and throughout the subarachnoid space. The CSF, thus, surrounds both the brain and spinal cord, thereby protecting these delicate structures from damage. A blood–brain barrier also exists within the choroid plexus; secretion is therefore selective and accounts for the difference in electrolyte concentrations between the CSF and plasma. The CSF eventually drains into the dural sinuses and finally into the venous drainage system.

PERIPHERAL NERVOUS SYSTEM

The peripheral nervous system consists of both afferent and efferent divisions. The efferent division includes the *somatic* and *autonomic nervous systems*, the latter of which is further subdivided into the *sympathetic* and *parasympathetic nervous systems* (see Table 17–1). The afferent division is composed of nerves that convey sensory information (pain, stretch, distention, sound, etc.) from the sensory receptors to the CNS. The cell bodies of the afferent nerves lie outside, but near, the CNS. Action potentials are initiated at the receptor end and are conducted via these afferent neurons to the CNS. The efferent division of the peripheral nervous system is more diverse, consisting of somatic and autonomic

Table 17–3. NEUROTRANSMITTERS AND NEUROHORMONES

Transmitter	Type	Characteristics
Acetylcholine	Excitatory (primarily)	Found in autonomic nervous system. Facilitates transmission over the myoneural junction. Inactivated by cholinesterase.
Norepinephrine	Excitatory	Distributed throughout brain; lower in putamen and caudate, also in the postganglionic synapse of the sympathetic division of autonomic nervous system. Inactivated by MAO.
Dopamine	Excitatory	Highest concentration in caudate and putamen. Implicated in regulation of emotional responses and complex movements. Inactivated by MAO.
Serotonin	Inhibitory	Concentrated in pons and upper brain stem, and hypothalamus. Acts as a vasoconstrictor and vasopressor and may play a role in temperature regulation, sensory perception, and the onset of sleep.
Gamma-aminobutyric acid (GABA)	Inhibitory	Present largely in gray matter of brain and cord. May regulate portions of available matter, influencing brain activity. Hyperpolarizes postsynaptic membranes.
Glutamic acid	Excitatory	Amino acid present throughout nervous system, unequally distributed in the spinal cord, and released by primary afferent nerve endings. Also implicated in neuronal metabolism.
Neuropeptides (enkephalins and endorphins)	Inhibitory	Found in some sensory neurons at their synapses with spinal cord neurons. May be involved with perception and integration of pain and emotional responses.

motor nerve fibers. The remainder of this chapter discusses the efferent system under four general headings: anatomy, physiology, neurotransmitters, and receptors.

ANATOMY

Somatic efferent nerves innervate only skeletal (voluntary) muscle. The cell bodies of these neurons are grouped within the brain and spinal cord, and synapse directly on skeletal muscle (Fig. 17–5). Action potentials initiated by local reflexes or by the activity of descending central pathways are rapidly conducted via the large-diameter, myelinated axons of these *motor neurons* to their respective skeletal muscles.

Autonomic efferent nerves differ significantly from the somatic efferent nerves. Autonomic nerves innervate cardiac and smooth muscle as well as glands and other metabolically active tissues. Unlike the somatic efferent nerves which synapse directly on their respective effector organ (skeletal muscle), preganglionic autonomic nerve fibers which originate in the spinal cord synapse on cell bodies arranged in clusters (ganglia) located outside the CNS. These postganglionic fibers in turn innervate the effector organs (heart, intestine, etc.).

Thus, an action potential is conducted peripherally to the *ganglia* via the autonomic, preganglionic nerve fibers. At the synapse, a neurotransmitter is released and diffuses across the synapse. An then action potential is then initiated in the postganglionic fiber and is conducted to the effector organ.

Several anatomic features distinguish the parasympathetic autonomic nervous system from the *sympathetic autonomic nervous system*. First, the location from which the preganglionic fibers exit from the CNS differs. Sympathetic fibers emerge from either the thoracic or lumbar sections of the spinal cord and because of this anatomic arrangement the sympathetic nervous system is referred to as the *thoracolumbar system*. In contrast, the parasympathetic preganglionic fibers originate in either the subcortical axis (cranium) while others emerge from the sacral portion of the spinal cord. The parasympathetic system is therefore referred to as the *craniosacral system*.

Another anatomic difference between the sympathetic and parasympathetic systems involves the location of their respective ganglia. The parasympathetic ganglia are situated mainly within the effector organ, while most of the sympathetic ganglia lie close to the

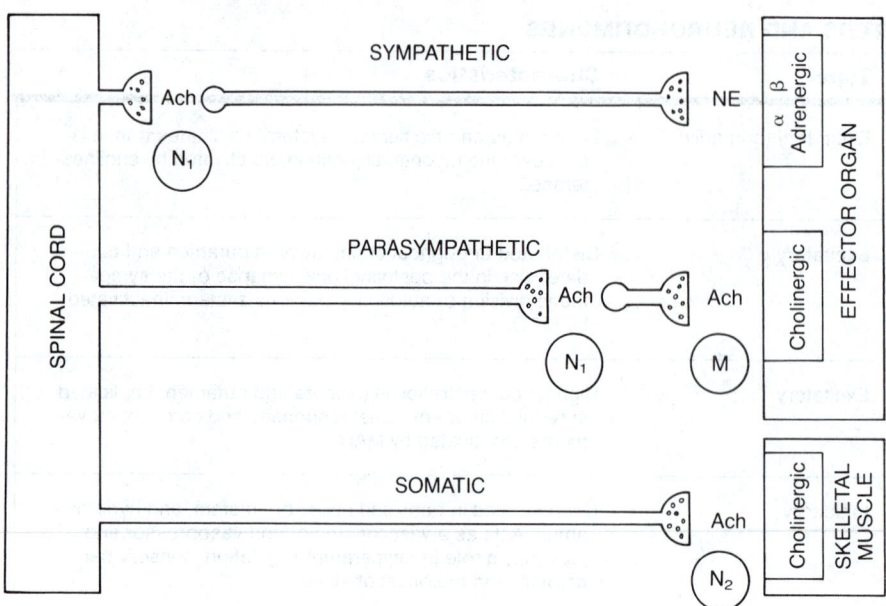

Figure 17–5. Schematic of the autonomic and somatic nervous systems. Ach = acetylcholine. NE = norepinephrine. N_1 = nicotinic type 1 receptors. N_2 = nicotinic type 2 receptors. M = muscarinic receptors. α and β = alpha and beta adrenergic receptors, respectively.

spinal cord *(paravertebral ganglia)* (see Fig. 17–5). Thus, the parasympathetic nervous system possesses long preganglionic and short postganglionic nerve fibers while the sympathetic nervous system consists of short preganglionic and long postganglionic nerve fibers.

Finally, the ratio of preganglionic to postganglionic fibers differs between the two systems. In general, in the sympathetic nervous system, one preganglionic fiber activates many postganglionic fibers, resulting in a low preganglionic-to-postganglionic fiber ratio. In the parasympathetic system, however, this ratio is quite high, and even a 1:1 correspondence is seen. The physiologic implication of this ratio difference is that sympathetic outflow tends to cause diffuse effects, whereas parasympathetic activity causes more localized effects.

PHYSIOLOGY

The function of the somatic motor system is simply to excite skeletal (voluntary) muscle to contract. Activation of this system initiates skeletal muscle contraction, and without somatic motor nerve activity this muscle remains quiescent. Since an individual neuron may innervate several skeletal muscle fibers, the functional motor unit consists of the somatic motor nerve fiber and its respective skeletal muscle fibers. Somatic motor nerves are only excitatory; that is, their activation inevitably leads to contraction or excitation of the skeletal muscle. No inhibitory somatic motor nerves have been described.

The function of the autonomic system differs in several ways from the somatic system. First, activation of the autonomic system generally does not initiate activity in the effector organs; rather, it modulates the spontaneous activity arising from the organ itself. Second, activation of the autonomic nervous system is not confined exclusively to excitation: it can enhance or inhibit the intrinsic activity of the effector organs, depending on the organ itself and which of the autonomic nerves

(sympathetic or parasympathetic) is exerting the major influence on that organ (see Table 17–4).

Much of the functional complexity of the autonomic system resides in the great diversity of effector organ responses to sympathetic and parasympathetic nerve stimulation. Table 17–4 lists the predominant effects of sympathetic and parasympathetic nerve stimulation on the function of many major organs and tissues. Note that these two systems often exert opposite effects on a given organ. In general, the sympathetic system activates those organs necessary for rapid energy expenditure, for example, the "fight-or-flight" reaction. Increase in heart rate and contractility, shunting of blood from skin and viscera to working skeletal and cardiac muscle, mobilization of glucose to supply acute demand for energy—all of these arise from enhanced sympathetic outflow. The parasympathetic system, on the other hand, is geared toward energy conservation and maintenance. Under its influence, heart rate declines, blood is shunted away from the resting muscle to the viscera and kidney, and food absorption is enhanced by activation of the gastrointestinal system. Although this generalization does not hold for all tissues, it is a useful concept for understanding the autonomic nervous system.

PERIPHERAL NEUROTRANSMITTERS

The efferent division of the peripheral nervous system utilizes many neurotransmitters but only *acetylcholine* (Ach) and *norepinephrine* (NE) are discussed here. Nerves that release Ach and receptors that bind Ach are referred to as *cholinergic nerve fibers* and *cholinergic receptors*, respectively. Nerves that release NE and receptors that bind NE are referred to as *adrenergic nerve fibers* and *adrenergic receptors*, respectively.

The somatic nervous system is completely cholinergic; that is, it utilizes only Ach as the neurotransmitter across the myoneural junction (see Fig. 17–5). Ach is synthesized in the somatic nerve terminal and stored in

Table 17–4. THE RESPONSES OF SELECTED EFFECTOR ORGANS TO AUTONOMIC NERVE STIMULATION: DIFFERENCES BETWEEN SYMPATHETIC AND PARASYMPATHETIC EFFECTS

Organ System	Receptor Subtype	Sympathetic Response	Parasympathetic Response
Cardiovascular system			
Heart rate	β_1	Increase	Decrease
Atrioventricular conduction	β_1	Increase	Decrease
Contractility	β_1	Increase	Decrease
Blood vessels*	α	Contract	Relax
	β_2	Relax	—
Pulmonary system			
Bronchial muscle	β_2	Relax	Contract
Bronchial glands	—	—	Stimulate
Gastrointestinal System			
Motility	α and β_2	Decrease	Increase
Sphincters	α	Contract	Relax
Secretion	—	—	Stimulate
Urinary bladder			
Detrusor	β_2	Relax	Contract
Trigone and sphincter	α	Contract	Relax
Miscellaneous			
Male sex organs	α	Ejaculation	Erection
Uterus (pregnant)	α	Contract	Variable
Uterus (nonpregnant)	β	Relax	Variable
Sweat glands	α	Secretion	Secretion
Liver	α	Glycogenolysis	Glycogen synthesis
	β	Gluconeogenesis	—
Fat cells	α and β	Lipolysis	—
Salivary gland secretions	α	K^+ and H_2O	K^+ and H_2O
	β	Amylase	

*The sympathetic system in skeletal muscle is cholinergic and elicits vasodilation.

synaptic vesicles (Fig. 17–6). An action potential arriving at the nerve terminal causes the vesicular and plasma membranes to fuse and break down. Ach is released from the nerve terminal, diffuses across the junction, binds to the postsynaptic receptor, and initiates a new action potential in the skeletal muscle. Contraction then ensues. The removal of Ach from the myoneural junction and postjunctional membrane terminates its action. This removal occurs by the following routes:

1. Degradation by *acetylcholinesterase*
2. Diffusion into the plasma compartment for processing by other organs of the body

The effective Ach concentration can, therefore, be altered in several ways. Any agent that decreases Ach synthesis or release, or increases its degradation compromises the action of somatic nerves on skeletal muscle. Conversely, agents that increase Ach synthesis or release, or decrease its degradation enhance the action of the somatic nervous system on skeletal muscle (see Chapter 18).

The autonomic system consists of both cholinergic and adrenergic nerve fibers and receptors, and utilizes both Ach and NE as neurotransmitters (see Fig. 17–5). It is imperative to note that all preganglionic nerve fibers (whether sympathetic or parasympathetic) are cholinergic; that is, Ach is the neurotransmitter released from preganglionic nerve terminals. Thus, agents that inter-

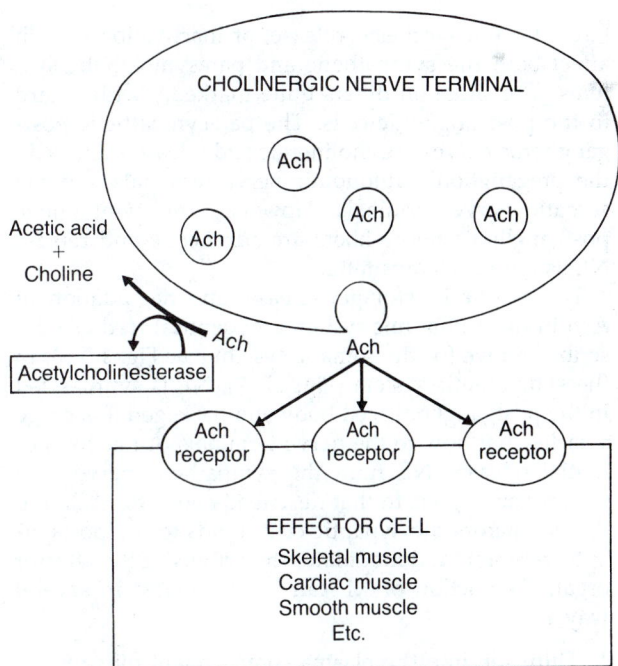

Figure 17–6. Schematic of the cholinergic nerve terminal and effector cell. Ach = acetylcholine. Acetylcholinesterase, located on the postsynaptic membrane, catalyzes the degradation of Ach to acetic acid and choline.

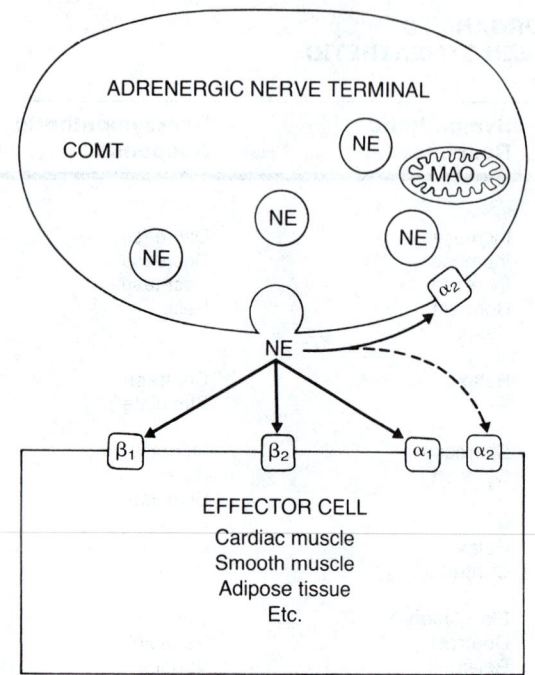

Figure 17–7. Schematic of the adrenergic nerve terminal and effector cell. NE = norepinephrine. α_1 = alpha$_1$ receptor. α_2 = alpha$_2$ receptor. β_1 = beta$_1$ receptor. β_2 = beta$_2$ receptor. COMT (cathechol-O-methyl transferase) and MAO (monoamine oxidase) are enzymes responsible for the degradation of NE. (Redrawn from Herlihy, JT, and Herlihy, BL: Adrenergic receptors. Critical Care Nurse 6(2):17, 1986, with permission.)

fere with the synthesis, release, or inactivation of Ach affect both the sympathetic and parasympathetic systems. The situation differs quite markedly with regard to the postganglionic cells. The parasympathetic postganglionic nerves are cholinergic and release Ach, as do the preganglionic autonomic nerve terminals and the somatic nerve terminals. However, the sympathetic postganglionic nerve fibers are adrenergic and release NE as the neurotransmitter.

The synthesis, storage, release, and degradation of Ach in the autonomic system are identical to those described above for the somatic system (see Fig. 17–6). In the sympathetic system (Fig. 17–7), NE is synthesized in the postganglionic cell body and packaged in storage vesicles that flow to the nerve terminals. An action potential releases NE from the sympathetic nerve in a manner analogous to that described above for Ach. NE diffuses across the synaptic cleft, binds to the postsynaptic receptor, and modulates the activity of the effector organ. The action of NE can be terminated in several ways:

1. Diffusion into the plasma compartment for processing by other organs of the body
2. Reuptake into the presynaptic terminal for repackaging or further metabolism by *monoamine oxidase* (MAO) or *catechol-O-methyl transferase* (COMT)

3. Uptake by the effector cell and degradation by COMT and MAO

As with cholinergic transmission, adrenergic transmission can be inhibited by agents that decrease synthesis or release, or enhance degradation. Transmission can be enhanced by agents that increase synthesis or release, or decrease degradation.

The sympathetic nervous system exhibits two very interesting differences with regard to transmitters. First, the adrenal medulla, which can be considered a specialized ganglion of the sympathetic nervous system, is innervated by cholinergic preganglionic fibers and releases mainly epinephrine (and some NE) directly into the blood, which in turn stimulates adrenergic receptors. Second, in skeletal muscle the postganglionic sympathetic nerves release Ach as the transmitter in contrast to NE, which is released from most other postganglionic sympathetic nerve fibers.

RECEPTORS

In addition to the cholinergic and adrenergic receptors, the efferent peripheral system contains many other types of receptors (serotoninergic, dopaminergic, purinergic, etc.). Only the cholinergic and adrenergic receptor types and their respective subtypes are discussed in this chapter, and these are shown in Figure 17–5. Cholinergic receptors specifically bind Ach whereas adrenergic receptors specifically bind NE (and epinephrine). Agents that bind to cholinergic receptors and elicit effects similar to Ach are termed *cholinomimetic agents.* Those agents which bind to adrenergic receptors and elicit effects similar to NE are called *sympathomimetic agents.* Each of these major receptor types can be divided in subtypes. A given agonist or antagonist may bind to virtually only one receptor subtype, or it may bind more broadly to more than one receptor subtype. Many of the adverse and side effects of drugs arise from the tendency of a drug to interact with more than one receptor subtype.

The cholinergic receptors are subdivided into *muscarinic* and *nicotinic* subtypes. This division is based on the observation that certain cholinergic receptors are activated by muscarine whereas other cholinergic receptors are activated by nicotine. Muscarinic receptors are located only on the effector cell membrane innervated by the parasympathetic postganglionic fibers (See Fig. 17–5). In contrast, nicotinic receptors are found in the somatic nervous system as well as in the ganglia of the autonomic (both sympathetic and parasympathetic) nervous system. The distinction between muscarinic and nicotinic receptors has important ramifications for drug therapy. Muscarinic antagonists (e.g., atropine) exert limited effects, which remain confined to the parasympathetic postganglionic nerve transmission. On the other hand, ganglionic antagonists (e.g., mecamylamine), which block nicotinic receptors, exert effects far beyond ganglionic transmission. Because ganglionic transmission is blocked, postganglionic fibers, both cholinergic (muscarinic) and adrenergic, remain quiescent (See Fig. 17–5). Thus, the total autonomic system is affected by this blockade.

Nicotinic receptors are further subdivided into nicotinic type 1 (N_1) and nicotinic type 2 (N_2), as shown in Figure 17–5. Neuromuscular blocking agents such as pancuronium, which are relatively specific for cholinergic N_2 receptors, exert very little effect on autonomic ganglionic transmission (cholinergic N_1). Other neuromuscular blocking agents such as tubocurarine also block autonomic ganglia and therefore exert broad inhibition of the autonomic system.

The adrenergic receptors are subdivided into alpha and beta subtypes (See Figs. 17–5 and 17–7). An organ's response to adrenergic stimulation is highly dependent on whether *alpha* or *beta receptors* are primarily activated (See Table 17–4). A given molecule such as NE possesses in its structure both alpha and beta receptor activity. Thus, its ability to stimulate a given organ depends on the population and density of alpha or beta receptors located in that organ. For example, the cardiac muscle possesses mainly beta receptors with few, if any, alpha receptors. Therefore, the effect of NE released from the cardiac sympathetic nerves is mediated primarily by stimulation of beta receptors. In contrast, in the peripheral vasculature the alpha receptor is the major receptor subtype and release of NE from peripheral sympathetic nerves causes vascular smooth muscle contraction via an alpha effect. NE (as well as epinephrine) is often referred to as a catecholamine because of its chemical structure. Synthetic catecholamines can activate predominantly alpha receptors (e.g., phenylephrine) or beta receptors (e.g., isoproterenol).

Both alpha and beta receptors are further subdivided into subtypes 1 and 2 (See Fig. 17–7). $Beta_1$ receptors are located in the heart, adipose tissue, and kidney, and activation of these receptors causes an increase in heart rate and contractility, adipocyte lipolysis, and release of renin from the kidney. $Beta_2$ receptors are located primarily in the peripheral vasculature as well as bronchial and intestinal smooth muscle. Activation of $beta_2$ receptors causes vasodilation, bronchodilation, and inhibition of intestinal motility. Naturally occurring compounds like epinephrine, or synthetic beta-agonists like isoproterenol, possess both $beta_1$ and $beta_2$ activity. Some synthetic compounds like albuterol possess only $beta_2$ activity. Synthetic antagonists possess similar specificities. For example, propranolol blocks both $beta_1$ and $beta_2$ receptors, respectively, while atenolol is relatively specific for $beta_1$ receptors.

The alpha-adrenergic receptors are also subdivided into $alpha_1$ and $alpha_2$ receptor subtypes (See Fig. 17–7). The $alpha_1$ receptor is located on the effector cell membrane innervated by the autonomic sympathetic nerves. In vascular smooth muscle, $alpha_1$-adrenergic stimulation leads to vasoconstriction; in bronchial and intestinal smooth muscle it causes relaxation (See Table 17–4). The newly described $alpha_2$ receptor subtype is located primarily on the presynaptic sympathetic nerve terminal, although it has been demonstrated in the post-

synaptic membrane. When activated, the presynaptic $alpha_2$ receptor inhibits the further release of NE from the nerve terminal (See Fig. 17–7).

SUMMARY

The nervous system can be divided into the central nervous system, composed of the brain and spinal cord, and the peripheral nervous system. As illustrated in Figure 17–1, the brain is composed of five subdivisions:

1. Telencephalon, which includes the cerebral hemispheres and several important nuclei including the basal ganglia
2. Diencephalon, including the thalamus and hypothalamus
3. Mesencephalon
4. Metencephalon, including the pons and cerebellum
5. Myelencephalon or medulla oblongata

Two functional areas composed of diffuse collections of cells include the reticular formation and the limbic system. The spinal cord is composed of nervous tissue appearing as white and gray matter. The arrangement allows the cord to transmit information to and from the brain and to function as a reflex center.

The peripheral efferent nerves are divided into the somatic and autonomic nervous systems. Somatic nerves innervate skeletal muscle exclusively. The transmitter is acetylcholine, which binds to nicotinic type 2 receptors on the postjunctional membrane. The autonomic system is further divided into the parasympathetic and sympathetic nervous systems and innervates most organs of the body. The nerves of the parasympathetic system exit from the cranial and sacral portions of the central nervous system (craniosacral system). Those of the sympathetic system exit from the thoracic and lumbar portions of the central nervous system (thoracolumbar system). In both systems, these nerves synapse at ganglia, which are groups of nerve bodies located outside the central nervous system. The sympathetic and parasympathetic systems tend to elicit reciprocal responses. In general, activation of the sympathetic system prepares the organism for energy-requiring activity, as in the "fight-or-flight" reaction; the parasympathetic system is geared more toward energy conservation. The preganglionic fibers of both the sympathetic and parasympathetic systems are cholinergic; that is, acetylcholine is the neurotransmitter, and postsynaptic receptors are nicotinic type 1. Parasympathetic postganglionic fibers are also cholinergic, while the postjunctional receptors are of the muscarinic type. The sympathetic postganglionic fibers are adrenergic; that is, norepinephrine is the transmitter, and the receptors are divided into alpha and beta subtypes. The distribution and density of these adrenergic receptor subtypes vary from tissue to tissue.

BIBLIOGRAPHY

Anthony, CP and Thibodeau, GA: Textbook of Anatomy and Physiology. CV Mosby, St Louis, 1983.

Guyton, AC: Textbook of Medical Physiology, ed 5. WB Saunders, Philadelphia, 1986.

Gilman, AG, Goodman, LS, and Gilman, A (eds): Goodman and Gilman's The Pharmacologic Basis of Therapeutics, ed 7. Macmillan, New York, 1985.

Herlihy, BL and Herlihy, JT: Cholinergic receptors. Critical Care Nurse, *in press.*

Herlihy, JT and Herlihy, BL: Adrenergic receptors. Critical Care Nurse 6:16–18, 1986.

Hitner, H and Nagle, BT: Basic Pharmacology for Health Occupations, ed 2. Glencoe Publishing Co, Encino, CA, 1987.

Malseed, RT: Pharmacology: Drug Therapy and Nursing Considerations. JB Lippincott, Philadelphia, 1982.

Price, SA and Wilson, LM: Pathophysiology: Clinical Concepts of Disease Processes, ed 3. McGraw-Hill, New York, 1986.

Rodman, MJ, Karch, AM, Boyd, EH, and Smith, DW: Pharamcology and Drug Therapy in Nursing, ed 3. JB Lippincott, Philadelphia, 1985.

Vander, AJ, Sherman, JH, and Luciano, DS: Human Physiology, ed 4. McGraw-Hill, New York, 1985.

18
CHAPTER

DRUGS AFFECTING THE PARASYMPATHETIC NERVOUS SYSTEM

DRUGS AFFECTING THE
PARASYMPATHETIC
NERVOUS SYSTEM

CHAPTER OUTLINE

GLOSSARY TERMS IN THIS CHAPTER

Adie's syndrome
Anticholinesterases
Antimuscarinics
Cholinesterase inhibitors
Cholinomimetic agents
Depolarizing neuromuscular blockers
Hyperhidrosis
Miosis
Muscarinic
Neuromuscular receptor
Nicotinic receptor
Nondepolarizing neuromuscular blockers
Ocusert system
Twitch monitor
Xerostomia

18
CHAPTER

DRUGS AFFECTING THE PARASYMPATHETIC NERVOUS SYSTEM

VICKI L. BYERS, R.N, Ph.D., CNRN

LEARNING OBJECTIVES

After reading this chapter, the student will be able to:

1. Compare and contrast the similarities and differences between the parasympathetic agents, anticholinesterases, anticholinergic agents, ganglionic blockers, and neuromuscular blockers.

2. Describe general drug action, therapeutic uses, pharmacokinetics, contraindications, precautions, adverse effects, and interactions of each of the classifications.

OVERVIEW OF PARASYMPATHETIC NERVOUS SYSTEM DRUGS

The parasympathetic nervous system coexists with the sympathetic nervous system to maintain homeostasis. (See Chapter 17 for a review of the parasympathetic system.) Since autonomic drugs affect multiple systems and organs of the body, the uses of these parasympathetic drugs are described in chapters corresponding to the affected body systems. This chapter does not contain a nursing process section since these drugs are used for such varied conditions; however, a short section on nursing care is included. For example, the medications used for myasthenia gravis and glaucoma are discussed in separate chapters. This chapter explores the general classifications and uses of the parasympathetic medications. Table 18–1 features the nursing process reference for the parasympathetic nervous system.

The parasympathetic agents are classified into five types: (1) cholinomimetic agents (direct-acting), (2) *anticholinesterases* (indirect-acting parasympathetic agents, *cholinesterase inhibitors*), (3) anticholinergic agents (*muscarinic* blockers, *antimuscarinics*), (4) ganglionic blockers, and (5) neuromuscular blockers. An overview of each classification of medication with its specific mechanism of action, pharmacokinetics, and adverse effects is given in this chapter.

CHOLINOMIMETICS

The drugs classified as cholinomimetics mimic the action of acetylcholine. The cholinergic receptor categories are *nicotinic, muscarinic,* and *neuromuscular.* The cholinergic receptor can be stimulated by (1) direct activation with a cholinergic agonist; (2) release of acetylcholine; and (3) by inhibiting the breakdown of acetylcholine, allowing for the build-up of endogenous acetylcholine.

In patients with urinary retention, intestinal atony, or glaucoma, drugs that stimulate muscarinic receptors are beneficial. In a patient with myasthenia gravis, drugs that stimulate the neuromuscular receptors are of therapeutic value. Other cholinomimetics are nonselective, limiting the effects of acetylcholine at the cholinergic receptors.

Direct-Acting Cholinomimetics

The direct-acting cholinomimetics mimic the actions of acetylcholine. They directly bind to and activate muscarinic or nicotinic receptors (Table 18–2). The cholinomimetics are divided into two groups: the choline esters (acetylcholine, carbachol, bethanechol) and the alkaloids (muscarine, pilocarpine, nicotine). The choline esters are similar to acetylcholine, and the natural alkaloids are derived from plant sources.

ACTION. The parasympathetic nervous system can modify organ function in two ways. First, acetylcholine can activate muscarinic receptors on the effector organ, thus altering organ function. Second, acetylcholine can interact with muscarinic receptors on sympathetic nerve

Table 18–1. NURSING PROCESS REFERENCES FOR PARASYMPATHETIC DRUGS

Drug	Classification	Indications	Nursing Process Chapter Reference
Carbachol	Parasympathomimetic	Simple glaucoma	60
		Stimulates bladder and intestine	54
Bethanechol	Parasympathomimetic	Open-angle glaucoma	60
		Prevention and treatment of postoperative bowel distention, gastric atony, and congenital megacolon	54
		Treatment of urinary retention	38
Pilocarpine	Parasympathomimetic	Decrease intraocular pressure in simple glaucoma and in treatment of detached retina	60
Neostigmine (Prostigmin)	Cholinesterase inhibitor	Myasthenia gravis	23
		Esophageal dilation and initiation of peristalsis postoperatively	54
		Treatment of postoperative dysuria	39
		Potentiation of narcotics, including morphine	20
Physostigmine (Eserine)	Cholinesterase inhibitor	Miotic to treat glaucoma	60
Atropine hydrobromide	Parasympatholytic or anticholinergic	Preoperative medication	10
Propantheline bromide (Pro-Banthine)	Anticholinergic	Reducing gastric acid secretion	52
		Decreasing spasm of the gastrointestinal tract	52
		Decreasing rigidity of Parkinson's disease	23

Table 18–2. DIRECT-ACTING CHOLINOCEPTOR STIMULANTS

Organ	Reaction
Blood vessels:	
Arteries	Dilatation
Veins	Dilatation
Heart:	
Sinoatrial node	Decrease in rate (negative chronotropy)
Atria	Decrease in contractile strength (negative inotropy). Decrease in refractory period
Atrioventricular node	Decrease in conduction velocity (negative dromotropy)
Ventricles	Small decrease in contractile strength
Lung:	
Bronchial muscle	Contraction (bronchoconstriction)
Bronchial glands	Stimulation
Gastrointestinal tract:	
Motility	Increase
Sphincters	Relaxation
Secretion	Stimulation
Urinary bladder:	
Detrusor	Contraction
Trigone and sphincter	Relaxation
Eye:	
Sphincter muscle of iris	Contraction (miosis)
Ciliary muscle	Contraction for near vision
Glands:	
Sweat, salivary, lacrimal, naropharyngeal	Secretion

terminals, thereby blocking the release of norepinephrine. This alters organ function by modifying the sympathetic nervous system.

Activation of nicotinic receptors results in depolarization of the nerve cell or neuromuscular end-plate. Activation of these receptors causes structural changes that allow sodium and potassium ions to diffuse down their concentration gradient.

USES. The major uses of cholinomimetics are for diseases of the eye (glaucoma, accommodative esotropia), gastrointestinal and urinary system (postoperative atony, neurogenic bladder), and the heart (atrial arrhythmias). Neuromuscular junction problems are discussed separately in this chapter, as are specific ocular problems (see also Chapter 60).

PHARMOCOKINETICS. The choline esters are lipid insoluble, so they are poorly absorbed and distributed in the central nervous system. They are hydrolyzed in the gastrointestinal tract. Carbachol and bethanechol are almost resistant to hydrolysis by cholinesterase.

The cholinomimetic alkaloids are absorbed from most sites of administration, including the gastrointestinal tract. Since these alkaloids are not an ester, they escape the enzymatic destruction by cholinesterases, therefore increasing the duration of action. Excretion of these agents is through the kidneys.

CONTRAINDICATIONS. Contraindications to the use of cholinomimetics include asthma, hyperthyroidism, myocardial infarction, and peptic ulcer. Any of these conditions would be aggravated by the parasympathetic effects of the drugs because of excessive muscarinic stimulation. This effect can exaggerate bronchial constriction and can increase secretion as well as have a depressant effect on the heart. The gastrointestinal tract has increased contractile activity and increased gastric secretions.

Acetylcholine

ACTION. To obtain any systemic effects from acetylcholine, the drug must be given intravenously. The effects are very short in duration because of the rapid destruction of acetylcholine by cholinesterases. After intravenous injection of acetylcholine, the muscarinic receptors are stimulated. The most pronounced effects of this drug are exerted on the cardiovascular system. Low doses of acetylcholine cause vasodilation in the vascular beds, a decrease in peripheral resistance, and decreases in systolic and diastolic blood pressures. At higher doses, acetylcholine has a depressant effect on the heart, causing a decrease in rate, atrioventricular conductivity, and force of contraction. Moderate doses of acetylcholine cause bronchial constriction and an increase in secretion; there is also urinary bladder contraction and decreased bladder capacity. When given by the intraocular route, acetylcholine causes *miosis* by eliciting contraction of the sphincter muscle of the iris.

USE. Since acetylcholine has such a short duration of action, its major clinical use is during ophthalmic surgery. It is used to obtain rapid and complete miosis during cataract removal. It is also used in anterior segment surgery and peripheral iridectomy.

PHARMACOKINETICS. Acetylcholine is lipid insoluble and therefore cannot penetrate the blood–brain barrier. It is rapidly hydrolyzed by acetylcholinesterase in the gastrointestinal tract. The half-life of acetylcholine is unknown.

DOSAGE. Acetylcholine chloride (Miochol) is instilled in the eye by a physician in 0.5–2 ml of a 1% solution. Miosis occurs immediately, and the duration of action is ten minutes.

Carbachol

ACTION. This cholinomimetic drug has greater nicotinic effects and neuromuscular activity than does acetylcholine. Therapeutic doses stimulate autonomic ganglia, the adrenal medulla, and skeletal muscle. Carbachol (Isopto, Carbachol) produces more effects on the gastrointestinal tract, the urinary bladder, and the iris than does acetylcholine.

USES. Carbachol is used to treat ocular disorders, such as glaucoma, and in ocular surgery. It is used to lower intraocular pressure. When the eyedrops are instilled, miosis occurs.

ADVERSE EFFECTS. Side effects of carbachol include headache, eye and brow pain, ciliary spasm, and hyperemia of the conjunctiva. Systemic effects include sweating, flushing, abdominal cramping with increased peristalsis, and diarrhea. A transient decrease in blood pressure with reflex tachycardia may occur. Contractions of the urinary bladder and asthma may be induced by the drug. No drug or food interactions have yet been reported.

DOSAGE. Carbachol is available in concentrations of 0.75%, 1.5%, 2.25%, and 3%. The frequency of administration is two or three times per day.

Bethanechol Chloride

ACTIONS. Bethanechol chloride (Urecholine, Duvoid) acts on postganglionic parasympathetic receptors and on muscarinic receptors of the smooth muscle of the gastrointestinal tract and bladder. The major actions of bethanechol chloride include the following: increased muscle tone and peristaltic activity in the stomach and intestines, increased esophageal sphincter pressure, increased esophageal peristalsis, increased pancreatic and gastrointestinal secretions, contraction of the detrusor muscle of the bladder, decreased bladder capacity, and an increase in the frequency of ureteral peristaltic waves. The drug can also have some cholinergic effects, such as bronchial constriction, increased bronchial secretions, and miosis. Cardiovascular responses include a decrease in blood pressure and reflex tachycardia.

USES. Bethanechol causes bladder contractions, which aid in micturition and bladder emptying. This drug is also indicated for the treatment of postoperative abdominal distention, gastric atony, or stasis. Bethanechol is used as a diagnostic agent for infantile cystic fibrosis and for neurogenic bladder. The cardiovascular effects of this drug are slight at therapeutic doses.

PHARMACOKINETICS. The onset of increased gastrointestinal motility and initiation of micturition is within 30–90 minutes after oral administration of bethanechol. Clinical effects are seen 15–30 minutes following subcutaneous doses. After oral administration of bethanechol, the duration of action is about 60 minutes. The oral absorption from the gastrointestinal tract is poor. The method of excretion of the drug is not known.

CONTRAINDICATIONS AND PRECAUTIONS. Due to the possibility of cholinergic toxicity, bethanechol should not be given intravenously or intramuscularly. Atropine sulfate should be available to counteract toxic reactions. Bethanechol is contraindicated in patients with hyperthyroidism, asthma, coronary artery disease, bradycardia, vasomotor instability, peptic ulcer, mechanical obstruction of the gastrointestinal or urinary tracts, gastrointestinal resection, inflammatory disease of the gastrointestinal tract, epilepsy, and parkinsonism; or in patients who have had recent urinary bladder surgery.

ADVERSE EFFECTS. Adverse reactions associated with bethanechol are common following subcutaneous injection but are rare following oral administration. The adverse reactions consist of flushing of the skin, sweating, lacrimation, salivation, headache, diarrhea, nausea and vomiting, bronchial constriction, belching, miosis, urinary urgency, and hypothermia.

ACUTE TOXICITY. When bethanechol is administered intravenously or intramuscularly, its effects last longer and signs of muscarinic excess can occur. The symptoms associated with this reaction include circulatory collapse, hypotension, bloody diarrhea, shock, and cardiac arrest. These symptoms have occurred rarely after subcutaneous injection.

The treatment for toxicity is administration of atropine sulfate intravenously, intramuscularly, or subcutaneously. The recommended adult dose is 0.5–1 mg; the dose for infants and children up to 12 years of age is 0.01 mg/kg, repeated every two hours until desired effect or adverse reactions occur. The maximum single dose in children should not exceed 0.5 mg.

DRUG INTERACTIONS. Bethanechol should not be used in conjunction with other cholinergic or anticholinesterase drugs, due to the additive effects and potential for toxicity. The concomitant use of bethanechol with procainamide and/or quinidine antagonizes the cholinergic effects.

LABORATORY INTERACTIONS. Bethanechol elevates serum amylase and lipase, bilirubin, aspartate aminotransferase, and sulfobromophthalein.

DOSAGE. The recommended oral dosage of bethanechol is 5–30 mg two or four times a day on an empty stomach. Dosage is adjusted on an individual basis. The recommended subcutaneous dose is 2.5–5 mg (1 ml). The drug should not be given intravenously or intramuscularly.

NURSING IMPLICATIONS. Patients will often be administering these medications at home; therefore, patient teaching is very important.

Patient teaching falls within three general areas: (1) method of administering the medication, (2) adverse reactions of the drug, and (3) storage of the medication. Due to the variability of absorption and the potential for toxicity of this drug, it is very important that the patient follow the physician's dosing instructions. The patient is informed in lay terms about the adverse reactions related to this drug. Verbal instructions are followed by written information about these side effects. It is important to stress to the patient that reporting any adverse effects to the physician is crucial. It is important to keep this medication in the original tightly closed, light-resistant container. Bethanechol should be stored in a cool place that is out of the reach of children.

Pilocarpine

ACTIONS. The mechanism of action of pilocarpine is to increase outflow of aqueous humor via the trabecular meshwork. Since the effects of the drug on outflow are shorter than effects on intraocular pressure, pilocarpine may decrease aqueous humor production. Applied locally to the eye, it causes pupillary constriction, ciliary muscle contractions, and a reduction in intraocular pressure associated with decreased resistance to the outflow of aqueous humor.

USES. Pilocarpine is effective in reducing intraocular pressure. It is the drug of choice for treating open-angle-glaucoma and for emergency treatment of acute-angle-closure glaucoma. Resistance to pilocarpine may occur and may require a brief discontinuation of the drug and substitution of another miotic agent. Pilocarpine is also used to counteract sympathomimetic mydriatic effects. Pilocarpine also serves as a diagnostic test for *Adie's syndrome*. This benign disorder is characterized by enlargement of the pupil and a delayed and slow response to light. The pupil is slow to react to accommodation. On sustained accommodation the pupil may become smaller than normal.

PHARMACOKINETICS. Miosis occurs 15–30 minutes following topical administration of pilocarpine. Maximal decrease in intraocular pressure occurs two to four hours after instillation. Miosis continues for about four to eight hours. Effective decreases in intraocular pressure have been obtained up to twelve hours after instillation. Absorption of pilocarpine is via the nasolacrimal duct.

CONTRAINDICATIONS AND PRECAUTIONS. Pilocarpine is used cautiously in patients with a history of or risk for retinal detachment. The development of conjunctival hyperemia is thought to be associated with pilocarpine allergy. Pilocarpine is contraindicated in patients who have a hypersensitivity to the drug.

ADVERSE EFFECTS. Some of the common side effects of pilocarpine include headache, nervousness, nausea, burning or itching of the eyes, blurring of vision, difficulty with night vision, decreased visual acuity, eye pain, and cholinergic side effects.

Pilocarpine produces a cortical activating response that causes headache and nervousness. This drug can increase gastric secretions that contain pepsin, which can trigger nausea. The actions of pilocarpine include constricting the pupil, stimulating the ocular muscles that move the lens, and contracting the ciliary muscle. Pilocarpine is irritating to the eye on instillation. Pupil constriction can cause pain and decreased visual acuity. Blurring of vision is a result of spasm of accommodation, secondary to sustained contraction of the ciliary muscle. Changes in ocular structures occur with long-term therapy.

DRUG INTERACTIONS. Pilocarpine's actions can be decreased when the drug is used with an adrenergic agonist. This interaction decreases stimulation of the muscarinic receptors. Pilocarpine should not be used with other cholinomimetic agents or anticholinesterases. The effects of pilocarpine are enhanced because there is stimulation of the muscarinic receptors and signs of muscarinic excess can occur.

DOSAGE. Pilocarpine is available in ophthalmic solutions of various strengths. The usual adult dose is 1–2 drops in the eyes up to six times daily.

Ocuserts are placed in the cul-de-sac of the eye at night once a week. The dosage of Ocuserts varies from 20 μg–40 μg.

NURSING IMPLICATIONS. The components of patient education are threefold: (1) method of administering eyedrops, (2) description of side effects and what to do about them, and (3) precautions connected with decreased visual acuity. Patients and family members who will be instilling eyedrops need to be instructed in how to instill the drops into the eye. A possible strategy is for the nurse to demonstrate proper administration of the drops, followed by a return demonstration by the patient or family member. As with any medication, patients are warned of side effects that can occur after drops are instilled in the eye. A burning or stinging sensation in the eye often occurs. Also following instillation of the drops, the pupil normally gets smaller, decreasing visual acuity, especially in dim light. The patient is warned to use caution when driving at night. Reducing the speed of the automobile and allowing additional response time may help with night driving. Pilocarpine may cause mild headaches, but in time this side effect should go away. If the patient uses an Ocusert, he or she needs to check the eye after waking from sleep to make sure the Ocusert is still in the eye. If the patient experiences decreased visual acuity, then he or she may wish to take precautions.

ANTICHOLINESTERASES

Anticholinesterases (cholinesterase inhibitors) are parasympathetic agents that interact with cholinesterase enzymes and block their catalytic activity. Acetylcholinesterase (AChE) normally destroys acetylcholine at the neuromuscular junctions at the various cholinergic nerve endings. The drugs that inhibit AChE are called anticholinesterase agents. Due to the blocking ability of these drugs, acetylcholine accumulates at the cholinergic receptor sites and contributes to the excessive stimulation of the cholinergic receptors in the central and peripheral nervous systems. These drugs not only serve as therapeutic agents but also are used in agricultural insecticides and in chemical warfare. Since anticholinesterases prolong the action of acetylcholine, they are also called indirect-acting cholinoceptor stimulants.

Pharmacokinetics

The cholinesterase inhibitors fall into three chemical groups: simple alcohols having a quaternary ammonium group (ambenonium chloride, edrophonium, pyridostigmine bromide), carbamic acid esters of alcohols having quaternary or tertiary ammonium groups (neostigmine), and organic derivatives of phosphoric acid (isofluorophate).

Because they are lipid insoluble, the quaternary compounds are poorly absorbed from the conjunctiva, skin, and lungs. With the exception of physostigmine, the quaternary compounds require larger doses when given by the oral route. Physostigmine, a tertiary amine, is absorbed well from the gastrointestinal tract.

Most of the organophosphate cholinesterase inhibitors are absorbed well from the skin, gut, lungs, and conjunctiva. These agents are excellent insecticides and are very dangerous to humans. The thiophosphate insecticides (parathion, malathion) are lipid soluble and are absorbed well from all sites. Some of these agents are used by the general public as insecticides. Metabolites of these agents are eliminated in the urine.

ORGAN SYSTEM EFFECTS. The pharmacologic effects of cholinesterase inhibitors involve the eye, skeletal muscle, cardiovascular, and gastrointestinal systems.

Table 18-3. EFFECTS OF ANTICHOLINESTERASE AGENTS IN HUMANS

Tissue or System	Effects
Skin	Sweating
Visual	Lacrimation, miosis, blurred vision, accommodative spasm
Digestive	Salivation; increased gastric, pancreatic, and intestinal secretions; increased tone and motility in gut (abdominal cramps, vomiting, diarrhea, and defecation)
Urinary	Urinary frequency and incontinence
Respiratory	Increased bronchial secretions, bronchoconstriction, weakness or paralysis of respiratory muscles
Skeletal muscle	Fasciculations, weakness, paralysis (depolarizing block)
Cardiovascular	Bradycardia (due to muscarinic predominance), decreased cardiac output, hypotension; effects due to ganglionic actions and activation of adrenal medulla also possible
Central nervous system	Tremor, anxiety, restlessness, disrupted concentration and memory, confusion, sleep disturbances, desynchronization of electroencephalogram, convulsions, coma, circulatory and respiratory depression

From Craig, CR and Stitzel, RE: Modern Pharmacology, ed 2. Little Brown & Co, Boston, 1986, with permission.

Table 18-3 lists the effects of anticholinesterase agents in humans.

USES. Anticholinesterase agents have a variety of clinical uses. Neostigmine, pyridostigmine, and edrophonium are used in anesthesia to reverse the neuromuscular blockade caused by nondepolarizing muscle relaxants. Anticholinesterases are used to improve muscle strength in myasthenia gravis, a disease in which neurotransmission at skeletal muscles is impaired. Anticholinesterase agents can also be used to treat glaucoma, strabismus, smooth muscle atony, and antimuscarinic toxicity. If these agents fail to lower intraocular pressure, then a long-acting anticholinesterase agent such as isoflurophate is used. Marked ciliary spasm can occur with this agent. Strong miotics can also produce iris cysts, which disappear if the agents are discontinued. Table 18-4 gives a summary of cholinesterase inhibitors and their therapeutic uses. Neostigmine, physostigmine, pyridostigmine, edrophonium, and ambenonium chloride are reviewed in depth in other chapters.

CONTRAINDICATIONS AND PRECAUTIONS. Although anticholinesterases are used in the treatment of atony of the bladder, they are contraindicated in patients with mechanical obstructions of the intestine or urinary tract. Diabetes, gangrene, coronary artery disease, heart block, ulcerative colitis, upper gastrointes-

Table 18-4. CHOLINESTERASE INHIBITORS: USES AND DURATION

	Duration of Action	Therapeutic Use
Carbamates and Related Agents		
Abenonium (Mytelase)	4-8 h	Myasthenia gravis
Demecarium (Humorsol)	4-6 h	Glaucoma
Neostigmine (Prostigmin, etc.)	0.5-2 h	Myasthenia gravis, ileus
Pyridostigmine (Mestinon, etc.)	3-6 h	Myasthenia gravis
Physostigmine	0.5-2 h	Glaucoma
Organophosphates		
Echothiophate (Phospholine, etc.)	100 h	Glaucoma
Alcohols		
Edrophonium (Tensilon)	5-15 min	Myasthenia gravis, ileus, dysrhythmias

tinal disease, hypothyroidism, myotonia congenita, and myotonia atrophica are contraindications to anticholinesterase therapy. Caution must be used if these drugs are given to patients with asthma or respiratory disorders that would further constrict the smooth muscles of the bronchioles and increase secretions. Anticholinesterases potentiate the effects of succinylcholine by inhibiting its breakdown. This becomes an important issue when patients who have been receiving anticholinesterases are given succinylcholine.

ADVERSE EFFECTS. General adverse effects of anticholinesterases involve the muscarinic, autonomic, and central nervous systems. Table 18-5 lists specific toxic effects.

ANTICHOLINERGIC AGENTS (MUSCARINIC BLOCKERS)

The third category of parasympathetic drugs are the anticholinergic agents. The agents reviewed in this section

Table 18-5. TOXIC EFFECTS OF ANTICHOLINESTERASE DRUGS ("CHOLINERGIC CRISIS")

Effects of Toxicity

Autonomic Effects
- Miosis
- Hypotension
- Vasodilation
- Bradycardia
- Salivation
- Intestinal spasm
- Nausea/vomiting
- Bronchial secretions and spasm
- Muscle fasiculations
- Blockage of neuromuscular junctions, causing paralysis of all muscles including diaphragm

CNS Effects
- Respiratory arrest

Table 18–6. EFFECTS OF MUSCARINIC BLOCKING DRUGS IN HUMANS

Tissue or System	Effects
Skin	Inhibition of sweating (hyperpyrexia may result); flushing
Visual	Cycloplegia (relaxation of ciliary muscle); mydriasis (relaxation of sphincter pupillae muscle); increase in aqueous outflow resistance (increases intraocular pressure in many cases of glaucoma)
Digestive	Decreased salivation; reduced tone and motility in the gastrointestinal tract; decrease in vagus-stimulated gastric, pancreatic, intestinal, and biliary secretions
Urinary	Urinary retention (relaxation of the detrusor muscle); relaxation of ureter
Respiratory	Bronchial dilation and decreased secretions
Cardiovascular	Bradycardia at low doses (may be a CNS effect) and tachycardia at higher doses (peripheral effect); increased cardiac output if patient is recumbent
Central nervous system	Decreased concentration and memory; drowsiness; sedation; excitation; ataxia; asynergia; decrease in alpha electroencephalogram and increase in low-voltage slow waves (as in drowsy state); hallucinations, coma

From Craig, CR and Stitzel, RE: Modern Pharmacology, ed 2. Little, Brown & Co, Boston, 1986, with permission.

include atropine, scopolamine, glycopyrrolate (Robinul), and propantheline bromide (Pro-Banthine).

The anticholinergic agents compete with acetylcholine to bind to the muscarinic receptors. These drugs have little effect on the actions of acetylcholine at nicotinic receptor sites. Table 18–6 gives the effects of anticholinergic drugs on different systems in the body.

Uses

There are various therapeutic applications for anticholinergic agents. Atropine increases heart rate and cardiac output by blocking the vagus nerve. Atropine, scopolamine, and glycopyrrolate dry up secretions and are used in anesthesiology. These anticholinergic agents inhibit gastric secretions and gastrointestinal motility and are used therapeutically for peptic ulcer disease and irritable bowel syndrome. Anticholinergic drugs such as atropine, scopolamine, homatropine, cyclopentolate, and tropicamide are used to determine the refractory state of the eye. When there is inflammation of the eye, anticholinergics may be used to relax the iris and ciliary body. Anticholinergic agents are also used in the treatment of parkinsonism (see Chapter 23) and as antidotes

for certain types of poisoning. Atropine is used as an antidote for cholinesterase-inhibitor poisoning.

Pharmacokinetics

The tertiary amines (atropine and scopolamine) are absorbed well from the gut and conjunctiva, and they cross the blood–brain barrier. The excretion of the tertiary amines occurs in the urine. The quaternary amines, in belladonna alkaloid derivatives, and the synthetic quaternary amines (glycopyrrolate) are poorly absorbed from the gut and do not cross the blood–brain barrier. Large amounts of these compounds are found in the feces.

Contraindications and Precautions

Use of anticholinergic agents is contraindicated in patients with angle-closure glaucoma. Caution is used in patients with asthma, open-angle glaucoma, hepatic and renal disease, myasthenia gravis, cardiac disease, and prostatic hypertrophy. The relaxing effects of the drug on the iris and ciliary muscles cause these structures to crowd into the angle, blocking the canals that drain the aqueous humor.

Adverse Effects

Anticholinergic agents affect many systems at the same time. Many of the adverse effects depend on the drug and dosage used. Some of the general adverse effects include dry mouth, blurred vision, constipation, difficult urination, tachycardia, dysrhythmias, contact dermatitis of the eyelids and conjunctiva, and central nervous system effects.

These agents produce an inhibitory effect on the digestive system, causing a decrease in saliva production, gastric secretion, and gastrointestinal motility because this system is under the influence of the vagus nerve. They can cause an increase or decrease in heart rate. At low doses, these agents block the parasympathetic input to the sinoatrial node, causing tachycardia. Anticholinergic agents block the excitatory effects of acetylcholine on the detrusor muscle of the bladder, resulting in urinary retention. Atropine has a mild stimulant effect on the central nervous system, causing restlessness and agitation. The cause of the contact dermatitis of the eyelids and conjunctiva is unknown.

Interactions

Additive adverse reactions from cholinergic blockade can occur when anticholinergics are administered with phenothiazines, amantadine, antiparkinsonian drugs, glutethimide, meperidine, tricyclic antidepressants, quinidine, disopyramide, and some antihistamines. Concurrent use of propantheline and slow-dissolving tablets of digoxin may result in increased digoxin absorption, placing the patient at risk for digoxin toxicity. Antacids decrease the extent of absorption of oral anticholinergics. It is important to give the anticholinergic one hour prior to use of antacids. Concurrent administration of glycopyrrolate and sustained-release potassium has been shown to increase the severity of potassium chloride-induced gastrointestinal mucosal lesions.

ATROPINE SULFATE. Atropine sulfate is a tertiary amine derived from *Atropa belladonna*.

Action. Atropine sulfate blocks acetylcholine at the cholinergic postganglionic receptor site in smooth muscle. It antagonizes histamine and serotonin. Atropine blocks the vagus nerve, thereby increasing heart rate and cardiac output. It inhibits respiratory and gastric secretions by blocking the vagus nerve.

Uses. At one time, atropine was used to treat symptoms of peptic ulcer. However, atropine does not shorten ulcer healing time and has been replaced with more efficacious drugs. Pylorospasm, spasm of intestinal and biliary tracts, ureteral spasm, and enuresis are still occasionally treated with atropine. Atropine can suppress salivation and perspiration and can be used to control respiratory tract secretions in allergies and during surgery. Atropine should be avoided in patients with respiratory infections, since it decreases the clearance of respiratory secretions, making the infection more difficult to treat. Atropine is a treatment for bradycardia and asystole, an antidote for Amanita mushroom poisoning, and a temproary measure to relieve carotid sinus hypersensitivity or heart block.

Contraindications and Precautions. Atropine sulfate is contraindicated in patients who have demonstrated previous hypersensitivity to the preparation and in patients who have accelerated cardiac rates. Atropine sulfate is also contraindicated in patients with glaucoma, because it may precipitate an attack of narrow-angle glaucoma by its dilation of the pupil and narrowing of the iridocorneal angle. It is also administered cautiously to elderly and debilitated patients, and to children under 6 years of age. The drug is also contraindicated for patients with chronic lung disease, myasthenia gravis, lactation, prostatic hypertrophy, paralytic ileus, pyloric stenosis, and severe ulcerative colitis.

Adverse Effects. Both the local and systemic adverse effects of atropine are similar to those of other anticholinergic preparations. The local effects include photophobia, loss of accommodation, contact dermatitis, edema around the eye, and conjunctivitis. Patients must be encouraged to report these symptoms as soon as they occur. Systemic symptoms include tachycardia and dryness of the mouth. If the patient is experiencing systemic adverse effects at the time of the next scheduled dose, he or she should be instructed to omit that dose. Other adverse reactions include thirst and dysphagia, bronchial plugging, headache, blurred vision, photophobia, mydriasis, cycloplegia, flushing, fever, drowsiness, vomiting, dizziness, lightheadedness, tachycardia, palpitations, urinary hesitancy, constipation, and paralytic ileus. Allergic reactions may occur. In toxic doses, the drug produces rash, hypertension, restlessness, excitement, disorientation, delirium, hallucinations, hyperthermia, respiratory depression, and death.

Interactions. Atropine may produce an additive anticholinergic effect when administered with monoamine oxidase (MAO) inhibitors, procainamide, and quinidine. Atropine antagonizes the effect of parasympathomimetic agents such as neostigmine.

Dosage. Atropine may be administered through oral, subcutaneous, intramuscular, and intravenous routes. The usual adult dosage is 0.4–0.6 mg every four to six hours. The pediatric dosage is 0.01 mg/kg every four to six hours.

Atropine sulfate is the most potent of all cycloplegic drugs. It is available in both ointment (0.25%–1% concentration) and solution (0.5%–4% concentration) and is administered one to four times daily. The dosage is adjusted to the severity of the patient's condition. Mydriasis begins 30–40 minutes after ophthalmic administration and has a duration of 5–12 days; cycloplegia is slower in onset, may require several doses over a one- to two-hour period to be effective, and may persist for five to six days.

TRIHEXYPHENIDYL HYDROCHLORIDE. Trihexyphenidyl hydrochloride (Artane, Tremin) is an anticholinergic used primarily as an antiparkinsonian agent with a relaxant effect on smooth muscle and an antispasmodic action. It is also used to prevent and control drug-induced dyskinesias and other extrapyramidal disorders.

Contraindications and Precautions. Since it is similar to atropine, precautions, contraindications, and adverse effects are common to both drugs. Trihexyphenidyl is contraindicated in patients who are hypersensitive to the drug or who have narrow-angle glaucoma. Its safety in pregnant and nursing women and in children has not been established. The drug should be used cautiously in patients with a history of hypersensitivities, arteriosclerosis, hypertension, cardiac disease, renal or hepatic disorders, or obstructed gastrointestinal or genitourinary tract, and in elderly patients with prostatic hypertrophy.

Adverse Effects. The most common adverse effects of trihexyphenidyl are dry mouth, dizziness, blurred vision, mydriasis, photophobia, nausea, nervousness, insomnia, constipation, drowsiness, and urinary hesitancy and retention. Central nervous system stimulation occurs with high dosages. Other adverse effects are similar to those of atropine.

Interactions. Trihexyphenidyl may be potentiated by MAO inhibitors. It may partially inhibit the therapeutic effect of haloperidol (Haldol) and the phenothiazines.

Dosage. The dosage is highly individualized, ranging from 6–10 mg daily in three or more divided doses, to a maximum of 12–15 mg daily.

PROPANTHELINE BROMIDE. Propantheline bromide is an anticholinergic that is similar to atropine in effect. It is used as an adjunct in treating peptic ulcer, irritable bowel syndrome, pancreatitis, ureteral and urinary bladder spasm, and excessive salivation and *hyperhidrosis*.

Contraindications, Precautions, and Adverse Effects. Contraindications, precautions, and adverse effects are similar to those of atropine.

Interactions. Propantheline exerts an additive anticholinergic effect when used with amantadine (Symmetrel) or any other drug with anticholinergic activity; it causes extrapyramidal symptoms when used with methotrimeprazine (Levoprome).

Dosage. The usual oral adult dosage is 15 mg with meals and 30 mg at bedtime or 75 mg/day. The dosage is decreased for geriatric patients and those of small stature to 7.5 mg three times per day. For children, propantheline is given as 1.5 mg/kg/24 hours in four divided doses.

SCOPOLAMINE. *Action.* Scopolamine is a naturally occurring tertiary amine antimuscarinic. The drug can be made synthetically, but it is usually obtained by extraction from members of the *Solanaceae* genus of plants. Scopolamine blocks the response of the iris sphincter muscle to cholinergic stimulation.

Uses. The major use of scopolamine is for the prevention of nausea and vomiting associated with motion. It once was used as a preoperative medication to inhibit salivation and excessive secretions from the respiratory tract; however, the use of glycopyrrolate is preferred. Scopolamine may be used to prevent cholinergic effects during surgery. The final major use of scopolamine is in obstetrics with preoperative analgesics or sedatives to provide tranquilization and amnesia.

Pharmacokinetics. Scopolamine exerts the same actions as do other anticholinergic agents. It is more potent than atropine in its action on the iris and certain secretory glands (salivary, sweat), and it has a less potent effect than atropine on the heart, bronchial muscle, and smooth muscle of the intestine. Scopolamine is very effective in the prevention of motion sickness. It is thought to correct a central imbalance of acetylcholine and norepinephrine that occurs in motion sickness.

Contraindications and Precautions. Anticholinergic agents are contraindicated in patients with known hypersensitivity to the drugs. Scopolamine is contraindicated in patients with angle-closure glaucoma. It is also contraindicated in the presence of tachycardia secondary to cardiac insufficiency or thyrotoxicosis. Scopolamine is used with caution in the geriatric patient and children since they may be more susceptible to adverse effects of the drug.

Adverse Effects. Some of the common adverse effects include the following: dry mouth, blurred vision, cycloplegia, mydriasis, photophobia, urinary hesitancy and retention, palpitation, tachycardia, constipation, drowsiness, nervousness, headache, dizziness, flushing, and rash. Anticholinergic drugs block cholinergic transmission in a number of tissues with muscarinic receptors. Since drowsiness and blurred vision are common adverse effects, patients should be warned not to engage in activities that require mental alertness and/or visual acuity (e.g., driving a car, operating machinery).

Drug Interactions. The drug interactions are the same as for anticholinergic drugs.

Dosage. Scopolamine can be given orally, intramuscularly, intravenously, subcutaneously, and percutaneously. Scopolamine must be diluted with sterile water prior to injection. For percutaneous application, the transdermal system is applied four hours prior to exposure to motion.

The adult oral dosage of scopolamine is 0.4–0.8 mg three or four times a day. For self-medication in the prevention of motion sickness, an adult oral dosage is 0.25 mg every four hours up to 1 mg daily.

The parenteral dosage of scopolamine is 0.3–0.65 mg three or four times a day. The usual pediatric intramuscular, intravenous, or subcutaneous dose is 0.006 mg/kg.

The scopolamine transdermal dosage is a system programmed to deliver 0.5 mg of scopolamine over 72 hours. Placement of the system four hours before exposure to movement is recommended. Only one patch is to be worn at any one time.

Nursing Implications. Patient teaching is aimed at three areas: (1) application of the transdermal patches, (2) possible adverse effects of this drug, and (3) drugs to avoid while taking this medication. Teaching the patient how to apply the transdermal patch is critical for its success. It is important for the nurse to see the patient apply the patch and to provide the patient with feedback. It is important for the patient to wash his or her hands after handling the patch and to avoid contact with the eyes. Since drowsiness is a common adverse effect, patients must be warned to use extreme caution if driving a car or working with machinery. It is important for the patient to notify the physician of side effects. The patient should avoid alcoholic beverages and other drugs that depress the central nervous system (over-the-counter sleep preparations, antihistamines, sedatives, tranquilizers) while taking this drug.

GLYCOPYRROLATE. *Action.* Glycopyrrolate (Robinul) is five to six times as potent as atropine in its ability to decrease pharyngeal, tracheal, and bronchial secretions. This anticholinergic drug has a longer duration of action than atropine with minimal cardiovascular, ocular, and central nervous system effects. It also lowers esophageal sphincter pressure and increases the risk of regurgitation.

Uses. Glycopyrrolate is used as a preanesthetic medication, intraoperative medication, adjunct for reversal of neuromuscular blockade, and anticholinergic agent in gastrointestinal disorders.

Pharmacokinetics. The onset of action is 10–15 minutes when administered intravenously, 20–40 minutes when given intramuscularly or subcutaneously, and 60 minutes after oral administration. The duration of action is four to six hours when administered intramuscularly or subcutaneously and six hours after an oral dose. The duration is shorter than four hours when given intravenously. When given orally, glycopyrrolate is poorly absorbed via the gastrointestinal tract. This agent does not penetrate the blood–brain barrier. It has limited access across the placenta when given in therapeutic doses.

Contraindications and Precautions. Glycopyrrolate is contraindicated in patients with hypersensitivity to anticholinergics, acute glaucoma, tachycardia, shock, obstructive gastrointestinal tract, paralytic ileus, hepatitis, obstructive uropathy, toxemia of pregnancy, and myasthenia gravis. This agent is used with caution in patients with the following disorders: autonomic neuropathy, glaucoma, hepatic disease, ulcerative colitis, hiatal hernia with reflux esophagitis, renal diseae, prostatic hypertrophy, hyperthyroidism, coronary artery disease, congestive heart failure, cardiac arrhythmias, and hypertension.

Adverse Reactions. Some of the common adverse effects of glycopyrrolate include tachycardia, risk of esophageal regurgitation, *xerostomia*, and mydriasis. These side effects are dose dependent.

Drug Interactions. When glycopyrrolate and cyclopropane are used together, ventricular dysrhythmias are produced. Concurrent use of extended-release potassium products and glycopyrrolate has been reported to increase gastrointestinal mucosal injury caused by the potassium.

Dosage. This anticholinergic agent can be administered orally, subcutaneously, intramuscularly, and intravenously. The recommended adult dosage initially is 1–2 mg three times a day, followed by maintenance dosage of 1 mg twice a day. The adult premedication dosage is 4.4 μg/kg body weight intramuscularly given 30–60 minutes prior to anesthesia. The recommended intraoperative adult dosage is 0.1 mg intravenously as a single dose repeated as needed at two- to three-minute intervals.

GANGLIONIC BLOCKING DRUGS

Action

The fourth group of parasympathetic drugs is the ganglionic blocking drugs. These agents interfere with the actions of acetylcholine and other agonists at the nicotinic receptors of both parasympathetic and sympathetic autonomic ganglia. These agents can block impulses in the autonomic ganglia by "(1) interfering with the synthesis or storage of the transmitter, (2) preventing the release of acetylcholine from the preganglionic nerve endings, (3) inactivating ganglionic cholinesterases, and (4) mimicking or preventing the actions of acetylcholine at the ganglia receptor sites" (Goodman and Gilman, 1985).

Uses

Nicotine is important because of its toxicity, its presence in tobacco, and the dependency of its users.

Mecamylamine and trimethaphan camsylate were once used for hypertension; however, since the advent of newer medications with fewer side effects, ganglionic blockers are rarely used now for hypertension. Ganglionic blockers can be used to produce controlled hypotension during surgery. Trimethaphan is used for the management of autonomic hyperreflexia.

Pharmacokinetics

Nicotine is absorbed well from the respiratory tract, buccal membranes, and skin. It is metabolized by the lungs, liver, and kidneys, and it is excreted in the urine. Mecamylamine (Inversine) and trimethaphan camsylate (Arfonad) are absorbed poorly via the gut. Both agents are excreted in the urine.

Adverse Effects

Nicotine can stimulate the sympathetic nervous system and block the parasympathetic system, or vice versa. It causes the adrenal medulla to release epinephrine, which increases both heart rate and blood pressure. Nicotine stimulates the central nervous system, causes tremors and convulsions, and increases respiration and

vomiting. The effect of nicotine on the gastrointestinal system is increased tone and motility of the bowel, causing nausea, vomiting, and diarrhea. After initial exposure to nicotine, depressant effects can occur.

Mecamylamine and trimethaphan camsylate can cause atony of the bladder and gastrointestinal tract, cycloplegia, xerostomia, decreased perspiration, abolished circulatory reflex pathways, and postural hypotension.

Dosage

Mecamylamine (Inversine) is given orally to an adult in the dose of 2.5 mg twice a day. Trimethaphan camsylate (Arfonad) is available for injection, 50 mg/ml. It has a very short duration and is administered via intravenous drip with a rate of 0.3–3 mg/minute. These drugs are discussed in detail in another chapter.

NEUROMUSCULAR BLOCKING AGENTS

The final group of drugs classified as parasympathetic drugs is the neuromuscular blocking agents. The neuromuscular blocking agents are classified as (1) nondepolarizing or competitive neuromuscular blocking agents (curare, pancuronium, vecuronium, atracurium, gallamine, tubocurarine chloride); and (2) depolarizing blocking agents or noncompetitive neuromuscular blocking agents (succinylcholine chloride).

Uses

The neuromuscular blocking agents are used to produce adequate muscle relaxation to assist with intubation and during anesthesia. The use of these agents decreases the quantity of general anesthesia required. These agents can also be used in the management of tetanus. The last use of these agents is to decrease muscular activity in electroshock therapy.

Action

Normal end-plate function can be blocked in two ways to produce paralysis. *Nondepolarizing neuromuscular blockers* (curare, pancuronium, vecuronium, atracurium) compete for sites on the acetylcholine receptor molecule with acetylcholine but do not depolarize the receptor or bind to it for long periods of time. If acetylcholine is present in adequate concentrations, neuromuscular function is not blocked by nondepolarizing blockers. The nondepolarizing neuromuscular blockade is competitive. Nondepolarizing muscle blockers can also modify the synthesis or release of acetylcholine from the presynaptic nerve terminal. Combinations of different nondepolarizing neuromuscular blockers potentiate each other's relaxant effect, suggesting that they act by different mechanisms or at different sites. Nondepolarizing blockers are reversed by anticholinesterases.

Depolarizing neuromuscular blockers (succinylcholine) bind to the acetylcholine receptor, causing the receptor to depolarize, and maintain this depolarized, inactive state for a long time. This depolarizing blockade cannot be overcome by additional acetylcholine and is, therefore, noncompetitive.

Side Effects

All of the neuromuscular blocking agents interfere with respiratory function, progressing to respiratory paralysis. Most of these agents produce residual muscle weakness. Muscle testing (5-second head lifts, hand grips, inspiring with force against a closed glottis) is performed at frequent intervals to assess recovery of neuromuscular function. The use of a *twitch monitor* also gives information about the recovery of neuromuscular function. The last side effect common to the majority of neuromuscular blockers is hypersensitivity reactions. Some of the older neuromuscular blocking agents caused hypotension, bronchospasm, and cardiac disturbances. The hypotension is due to sympathetic ganglionic blockage and histamine release. The bronchospasm is secondary to histamine release. The cardiovascular effects are due to histamine release, blocking acetylcholine at sites other than the neuromuscular junctions, and stimulation of the sympathetic nervous system.

Precautions

These very potent neuromuscular blocking agents are used only by persons familiar with their effects and under conditions where the patient can receive constant, close minitoring. Adequate equipment for endotracheal intubation, ventilation, and antidotes must be readily available.

Vecuronium

Vecuronium is a new, short-acting and nondepolarizing neuromuscular blocker similar in structure to pancuronium. The onset of action is 15 minutes, with a duration of action lasting from 34–60 minutes. Its half-life is 65–75 minutes. Vecuronium does not cause histamine release. A property of this agent is it exhibits cardiovascular stability. It is not metabolized and is excreted in the feces and urine. The rapid rate of elimination reduces the cumulative effects of this agent with repeated doses.

CONTRAINDICATIONS AND PRECAUTIONS. Vecuronium is contraindicated in patients who are hypersensitive to this agent. Vecuronium is used with caution in patients who exhibit cardiac, neuromuscular, respiratory, hepatic, and renal disease; dehydration; electrolyte imbalances; and pregnancy.

ADVERSE EFFECTS. The major central nervous system side effects are skeletal muscle weakness or paralysis. Vecuronium can cause prolonged apnea.

INTERACTIONS. An increase in neuromuscular blockade results when vecuronium is used with aminoglycosides, clindamycin, lincomycin, quinidine, local anesthetics, narcotic analgesics, thiazides, enflurane, and isoflurane. Dysrhythmias have occurred with the concurrent use of theophylline. Vecuronium is incompatible with barbiturates in the same solution or syringe.

DOSAGE. The dosage for children over nine years of age and adults is an intravenous bolus 0.08–0.1 mg/kg, then 0.01–0.015 mg/kg for procedures over 60 minutes. For prolonged procedures, vecuronium can be administered by continuous infusion.

Atracurium

Atracurium is a new, short-acting and nondepolarizing neuromuscular blocker that is similar to vecuronium in onset time, duration of action, and cardiovascular stability. The half-life is 22 minutes. Ganglionic blockade, antimuscarinic effects, and sympathetic stimulation are absent with atracurium. There is some histamine release with this agent. Atracurium undergoes an enzymatic process of degradation, and it is excreted in the feces and urine. Since there is rapid elimination of atracurium, there is no progressive or cumulative effect when given in repeated doses.

CONTRAINDICATIONS AND PRECAUTIONS. Atracurium is contraindicated in patients who are hypersensitive to this agent. Atracurium is used with caution in patients who exhibit cardiac, neuromuscular, respiratory, hepatic, and renal disease; dehydration; electrolyte imbalances; and pregnancy.

ADVERSE EFFECTS. Atracurium can cause bradycardia or tachycardia and changes in blood pressure. Atracurium can also cause prolonged apnea, bronchospasm, cyanosis, and respiratory depression. This agent can cause a rash, flushing, pruritus, and urticaria, particularly in patients sensitive to histamine release.

INTERACTIONS. An increase in the neuromuscular block results when atracurium is used with aminoglycosides, clindamycin, lincomycin, quinidine, local anesthetics, narcotic analgesics, thiazides, enflurane, and isoflurane. Dysrhythmias have occurred with the concurrent use of theophylline. Atracurium is incompatible with barbiturates in the same solution or syringe.

DOSAGE. The adult dosage by intravenous bolus is 0.4–0.5 mg/kg, then 0.08–0.1 mg/kg 20–45 minutes after the first dose for prolonged procedures. For prolonged procedures, atracurium can be administered by continuous infusion.

Succinylcholine

Succinylcholine (Anectine, Quelicin, Sucostrin), also called suxamethonium, is a depolarizing neuromuscular blocker used as an adjunct in anesthesia, to facilitate intubation and controlled respiration, and to reduce muscle contractions in pharmacologically induced convulsive disorders and electroshock convulsions.

CONTRAINDICATIONS AND PRECAUTIONS. Succinylcholine is contraindicated in patients with hypersensitivity and a family history of malignant hyperthermia. It is used with caution in patients who have renal, hepatic, pulmonary, metabolic, and cardiovascular disorders. Succinylcholine is also used cautiously in patients suffering from dehydration, electrolyte imbalance, severe burns, trauma, fractures, spinal cord injuries, neuromuscular diseases, low plasma pseudocholinesterase levels, collagen diseases, porphyria, intraocular surgery, and glaucoma, and in patients receiving digitalis therapy.

ADVERSE EFFECTS. Adverse reactions to succinylcholine are largely neuromuscular, respiratory, or cardiovascular. The patient may exhibit fasciculations, profound muscle relaxation, muscle pain, respiratory depression, bronchospasm, hypoxia, apnea, and alteration in cardiac rate and rhythm and in blood pressure. Other adverse effects include malignant hyperthermia, increased intraocular pressure, excessive salivation, enlarged salivary glands, myoglobinemia, and hyperkalemia. Hypersensitivity reactions are rare. Decreased tone and motility of the gastrointestinal tract may occur with large dosages.

INTERACTIONS. Succinylcholine may increase the possibility of cardiac irregularities in patients receiving digitalis glycosides. The action of succinylcholine may be prolonged or potentiated by acetylcholine, aminoglycoside antibiotics, benzodiazepines, cholinesterase inhibitors, polymyxins, cyclophosphamide, cyclopropane, echothiophate iodide, halothane, lidocaine, magnesium salts, phenothiazines, narcotic analgesics, organophosphate insecticides, pantothenyl alcohol, phenelzine, phenothiazines, propranolol, quinidine, quinine, and possibly thiotepa and procainamide.

Refer to Chapter 10 for information on applying the nursing process to patients receiving neuromuscular blocking agents.

DOSAGE. Succinylcholine may be administered by intravenous or intramuscular injection. The intravenous dosage is 10–30 mg over 10–30 seconds or a continuous infusion of 0.1%–2% solution at 0.5–5 mg/minute. The intramuscular dosage is 2.5 mg/kg of body weight, not to exceed 150 mg in a single dose.

SUMMARY

When administering drugs that affect the parasympathetic nervous system, it is important for the nurse to follow the nursing process (assessment, intervention, evaluation). Assessment is important prior to administration of parasympathetic agents. The direct-acting cholinomimetics can activate or aggravate peptic ulcers, so monitoring of complaints of a gnawing, aching, burning, or epigastric pain is important. Visual changes occur with the administration of direct-acting cholinomimetics, anticholinergics (antimuscarinics), and ganglionic blockers. Miosis, impaired accommodation, blurring vision, and impaired night vision occur with direct-acting cholinomimetics. Mydriasis is common with the ganglionic blockers and antimuscarinic agents. Assessment of bowel (abdominal distention, bowel sounds, constipation, diarrhea) and bladder function (urinary output, urinary retention, urinary frequency) is very important when using direct-acting cholinomimetics, indirect-acting cholinomimetics, anticholinergics, and ganglionic blockers. Monitoring of vital signs is important during administration of ganglionic and neuromuscular block-

ers. When administering the neuromuscular blockers, it is important to monitor electrolyte and neuromuscular recovery.

When administering the parasympathetic agents, it is important to know which drugs can reverse the effects of these agents. When administering indirect-acting cholinomimetics, atropine is administered to lessen the muscarinic effects. Anticholinesterase agents are given to reverse the nondepolarizing neuromuscular blockers. When administering the direct-acting cholinomimetics and anticholinergic agents, it is important to watch for cholinergic toxicity.

The nurse is also responsible for patient teaching. Patients are taught to recognize the side effects of parasympathetic agents and to know when to report them. For patients receiving ganglionic blockers, it is important to change position slowly. Monitoring of blood pressure is necessary, and the patient should be standing when blood pressures are taken. Since many of these agents affect vision, patient safety is an important consideration. The nurse should warn patients to use caution when driving.

The evaluation of parasympathetic agents is based on the therapeutic response. When administering the neuromuscular blockers, evaluate the extent of muscle weakness or paralysis. When administering the indirect-acting cholinomimetics, evaluate for an improvment in muscular function and a decrease in fatigue. When administering anticholinergic agents, evaluate for a decrease in spasms of the gastrointestinal tract. It is also important to evaluate patients for allergic reactions to these drugs and for the degree of side effects. Dry mouth is a common side effect for many of these drugs. The patient is taught to take fluids frequently, to chew gum, to suck on hard candy, or to perform frequent oral hygiene.

BIBLIOGRAPHY

American Hospital Formulary Service, Drug Information, 1988.

Craig, CR and Stitzel, RE (eds): Modern Pharmacology, ed 2. Little, Brown & Co, Boston, 1986.

Edmunds, MW: Nursing Drug Reference: A Practitioner's Guide. Prentice-Hall, Bowie, MD, 1985.

Goldberg, M and Rosenberg, H: New muscle relaxants in outpatient anesthesiology. Dent Clin North Am 31(1):117, 1987.

Jones, RM: Neuromuscular transmission and its blockade. Anesthesia 40:964, 1985.

Katzung, BG (ed): Basic and Clinical Pharmacology. Appleton & Lange, Los Altos, 1987.

Kiernan, JA: Introduction to Human Neuroscience. JB Lippincott, Philadelphia, 1987.

Weiner, N and Taylor, P: Drugs Acting at Synaptic and Neuroeffector Junctional Sites. In Goodman, AG et al (eds): Goodman and Gilman's, The Pharmacological Basis of Therapeutics, ed 7. Macmillan, New York, 1985.

SITUATION 18–1

Theresa McNeal is a 60-year-old admitted to the surgical floor and prepared for cataract removal.

1. Acetylcholine chloride (Miochol) will be given to Mrs. McNeal intraocularly during ophthalmic surgery to:
   a. relax the sphincter muscle of the iris
   b. obtain complete miosis
   c. reduce nasolacrimal secretions
   d. block the flow of aqueous humor

2. The nurse will expect the duration of effect of Miochol to be:
   a. one hour
   b. twelve hours
   c. ten minutes
   d. four hours

3. Postoperative recovery for Mrs. McNeal is uneventful; however, a recurrent problem of urinary retention is noted. Mrs. McNeal is started on bethanechol (Urecholine). The nurse is aware that this drug should be given:
   a. orally
   b. intramuscularly
   c. intravenously
   d. topically

4. Before giving bethanechol to Mrs. McNeal, the nurse will assess for the following condition, which would indicate a contraindication to its use:
   a. peptic ulcer disease
   b. abdominal distention
   c. gastric stasis
   d. neurogenic bladder

5. In planning for potential toxic effects of bethanechol, the nurse will keep the following drug available:
   a. lidocaine
   b. Prostigmin
   c. neostigmine
   d. atropine

6. Mrs. McNeal will be discharged home on an oral dose of bethanechol. Which of the following statements indicates successful patient teaching?
   a. "I should keep this drug in a warm, dry place."
   b. "It is best to take this medicine with meals."
   c. "I should not worry if I have any unusual feelings."
   d. "It is best to keep the drug away from direct light."

SITUATION 18–2

Steven Perry is a 28-year-old accountant admitted to the medical surgical floor due to upper abdominal pain and a history of tarry stools.

1. Endoscopic examination reveals peptic ulcer disease. Which of the following drug therapies would be contraindicated for Mr. Perry?
   a. anticholinergics
   b. cholinesterase inhibitors
   c. parasympatholytics
   d. muscarinic blockers

2. Mr. Perry is started on a regimen of antacids and propantheline bromide. The nurse will observe for all of the following adverse side effects of propantheline *except:*
   a. photophobia
   b. tachycardia
   c. headache
   d. urinary urgency

3. A nursing diagnosis which would be appropriate for Mr. Perry would be:
   a. alteration in bowel elimination: diarrhea related to propantheline bromide
   b. sexual dysfunction related to the side effects of antacids
   c. alteration in oral mucous membrane related to side effects of propantheline
   d. hypothermia related to the stress of peptic ulcer disease

4. The nurse will plan all of the following interventions for Mr. Perry *except:*
   a. assess bowel sounds every shift
   b. restrict oral fluid intake
   c. check temperature every four hours
   d. monitor intake and output

5. Medical treatment proves to be unsuccessful, and, after a week of hospitalization, Mr. Perry is prepared for a gastric resection. Glycopyrrolate (Robinul) is given intramuscularly as a preoperative medication. The following is an action of this drug:
   a. decreases the risk of regurgitation
   b. decreases tracheal secretions
   c. increases esophageal sphincter pressure
   d. increases neuromuscular blockade

6. When assessing Mr. Perry, the following may be observed in relation to drug therapy:
   a. dilated pupils
   b. hyperactive bowel sounds
   c. bradycardia
   d. relaxation

Refer to the Appendices for correct answers and additional review questions with answers.

GLOSSARY TERMS IN THIS CHAPTER

Adrenergic
Adrenolytic
Afterload
Dopaminergic receptors
Dromotropic effect
Ergotism
Pheochromocytoma
Vasopressors

19

CHAPTER

DRUGS AFFECTING THE SYMPATHETIC NERVOUS SYSTEM

MERRILY MATHEWSON KUHN, R.N.C., P.h.D., CCRN

LEARNING OBJECTIVES

After reading this chapter, the student will be able to:

1. Compare and contrast the sympathetic medications such as adrenergics and antiadrenergics including the beta blockers.

2. Describe general drug action, therapeutic uses, pharmacokinetics, contraindications, precautions, adverse effects, and interactions of each of the classifications.

3. Understand specific nursing implications for sympathetic medications.

OVERVIEW OF THE SYMPATHETIC NERVOUS SYSTEM

The sympathetic nervous system coexists with the parasympathetic nervous system to maintain homeostasis. A large number of peripheral autonomic fibers synthesize and release norepinephrine and are referred to as *adrenergic* fibers. Refer to Chapter 17 for a review of the synthesis and breakdown of norepinephrine.

Because of the multiple body systems and organs affected by sympathetic medications, the nursing process approach to the use of these drugs has been developed in detail in the chapter corresponding to the particular body system. (For example, beta-adrenergic blockers used for hypertension are covered in Chapter 29; their use in the management of dysrhythmias is covered in Chapter 30; the use of bronchodilators is covered in Chapter 35, which discusses drugs used to treat respiratory diseases.) Therefore, this chapter reviews the general classifications and uses of the sympathetic medications; chapter references for applying the nursing process to administration of these drugs are cited in Table 19–1.

SYMPATHETIC NERVOUS SYSTEM THERAPEUTIC AGENTS

Because adrenergic drugs mimic the effects of the sympathetic nervous system stimulation, they affect the following body systems and organs: the heart, increasing

Table 19–1. MEDICATIONS AFFECTING THE SYMPATHETIC NERVOUS SYSTEM

Classification	Drug	Indication	Chapter Reference
Adrenergic stimulant (sympathomimetic) (see above)	Epinephrine (Adrenalin)	Allergic states	35
	Isoproterenol hydrochloride (Isuprel)	Asthma, heart failure	35
	Norepinephrine (Levophed)	Hypotension, as vasoconstrictor, cardiac arrest	35
	Ephedrine	Bronchodilator, nasal decongestant, allergic states	35
	Phenylephrine hydrochloride (Neo-Synephrine)	Bronchodilator, nasal decongestant, vasoconstrictor, allergic states	35
Alpha-adrenergic blockers	Phenoxybenzamine (Dibenzyline)	Peripheral vascular disorders, Raynaud's disease, frostbite	31
	Dihydrogenated ergot alkaloids (Hydergine)	Confused elderly persons	16
Beta-adrenergic blockers	Propranolol hydrochloride (Inderal)	Hypertension, migraine headache control, dysrhythmia control	29, 30
	Metoprolol (Lopressor)	Hypertension, acute myocardial infarction	29
	Nadolol (Corgard)	Hypertension	29
	Timolol maleate (Blocadren)	Myocardial infarction: acute and prophylaxis	29, 30
	Timolol maleate ophthalmic (Timoptic)	Glaucoma	60
	Atenolol (Tenormin)	Myocardial prophylaxis, hypertension, angina, dysrhythmia control	29, 30
	Pindolol (Visken)	Hypertension	29
	Labetalol (Trandate, Normodyne)	Hypertension, angina	29
	Acebutolol (Sectral)	Hypertension, angina, arrhythmia control	29
	Esmolol (Brevibloc)	Dysrhythmia control	30
Ganglionic blockers (block both sympathetic and parasympathetic ganglia)	Mecamylamine hydrochloride (Inversine)	Hypertension	29
	Trimethaphan camsylate (Arfonad)	Hypertension	29
	Hexamethonium chloride	Hypertension	29

the rate and force of contraction; the lung and gastrointestinal tract, relaxing smooth muscle, causing bronchial dilatation and inhibition of motility; and the peripheral blood vessels (particularly in the skin), producing vasoconstriction. Adrenergic drugs work indirectly on the central nervous system to increase respiratory and cardiac rates. They also act indirectly on metabolic processes to supply more energy by releasing fatty acids from fat tissue, and increasing the breakdown of glycogen into glucose in both muscle tissue and the liver. The action of adrenergic drugs depends on the particular population of sympathetic nervous system receptors on which the drug acts. As previously discussed, adrenergic drugs may affect the receptor sites positively to enhance their effect or negatively to block their effect. Three receptor sites have been recognized: alpha-adrenergic, and beta-adrenergic, which are discussed in Chapter 17, and dopaminergic receptors.

The alpha-adrenergic receptors are found primarily in blood vessels; they are most abundant in the resistance vessels of the skin, mucosa, intestine, and kidney. Drugs with a positive effect on the alpha-adrenergic receptors, such as norepinephrine, cause greater vasoconstriction; whereas alpha-adrenergic blockers (sympatholytics), including drugs used for hypertensive crisis such as phentolamine, have a relaxant effect and produce vasodilation.

Two subtypes of beta-adrenergic receptors have been identified: beta$_1$ receptors, which are found primarily in the heart, and beta$_2$ receptors, which are found primarily in the lung and peripheral blood vessels, particularly in skeletal muscle. In general, drugs that act positively on the beta-adrenergic receptor sites increase cardiac contractility and heart rate, accelerate atrioventricular conduction in the heart, and may cause some vasodilatation in the arterioles of skeletal muscle and mesenteric vascular beds. A beta-adrenergic drug with a positive effect on beta$_1$ receptors is epinephrine (adrenalin). (Epinephrine also has an effect on the alpha receptors.) Drugs such as isoproterenol (Isuprel), which cause bronchodilatation, stimulate beta receptors in high concentrations. The beta-adrenergic blockers have a negative effect, causing profound slowing of the heart as well as inhibiting the force of contraction, and include agents to control angina or lower blood pressure such as propranolol (Inderal).

Two subtypes of dopaminergic receptors have been identified: DA-1 and DA-2. The DA-1 receptors are found primarily in the renal and mesenteric vascular beds, with a few in the coronary and cerebral circulation. Smaller arteries are more sensitive to the vasodilating actions of dopamine than are larger vessels, suggesting that greater numbers of receptors are located in smaller vessels. The DA-2 receptors are located on postganglionic sympathetic nerve terminals. When these receptors are activated, norepinephrine release is inhibited. Dopamine (Intropin) is a dopaminergic-stimulating drug that affects both DA-1 and DA-2 receptors. In small doses, it stimulates dopaminergic receptors in the renal beds and causes diuresis, and it increases cardiac output without affecting heart rate or blood pressure;

but in larger doses, alpha activity occurs and leads to more vasoconstriction, resulting in an increase in blood pressure.

The following discussion of drugs affecting the sympathetic nervous system will be divided into two sections: those drugs that mimic the sympathetic nervous system—adrenergic drugs *(sympathomimetics)*; and those that block the effects of the sympathetic nervous system—adrenergic blockers *(sympatholytics)*.

ADRENERGIC (SYMPATHOMIMETIC) AGENTS

The adrenergic drugs, which mimic the sympathetic nervous system, act in three ways. They interact directly on the adrenergic alpha or beta receptors; indirectly, they first release a catecholamine from their storage sites, which then activates the alpha and beta sites; or they act by a mixed direct and indirect effect.

DIRECT-ACTING ADRENERGIC MEDICATIONS

Action

The direct-acting adrenergic medications described in Table 19–2, the catecholamines—dopamine, norepinephrine, dobutamine, isoproterenol, and epinephrine—have many physiologic responses, including a marked inotropic effect as they increase cardiac contraction; a marked chronotropic effect as they increase cardiac rate; a positive *dromotropic effect* as they increase conduction through the heart; a stimulatory effect on the Purkinje fibers, possibly resulting in ventricular dysrhythmias; and an elevation in blood pressure due to increased peripheral resistance. Dopamine primarily affects dopaminergic receptors in low doses and then beta$_1$ and alpha$_1$ receptors. It does not combine well with beta$_2$ receptors. Epinephrine and norepinephrine act equally well on both alpha and beta receptors.

Drugs that increase sympathetic nervous system activity can produce the central nervous system effects of increased anxiety, increased alertness, and respiratory stimulation. The catecholamines also exert an effect on all nonvascular smooth muscle, in most cases leading to relaxation and less peristalsis in the gastrointestinal tract. The urinary bladder relaxes, delaying the need to void. In the eye, the radial and sphincter muscles of the iris contract, giving the patient a wide-staring appearance.

Some catecholamines, particularly isoproterenol (Isuprel) and epinephrine, have a pronounced effect on the bronchial smooth muscle, which results in bronchodi-

TEXT RESUMES ON PAGE 416

Table 19–2. DIRECT-ACTING ADRENERGIC STIMULANTS

Name	Dosage	Mode of Administration	Pharmacokinetics
Epinephrine (Adrenalin)			
Action: For All: Marked inotropic effect, marked chronotropic effect, positive dromotropic effect, increased peripheral vascular resistance.			
Use: Temporary relief of bronchospasm, restoration of cardiac activity in cardiac arrest, to treat anaphylactic shock, as mydriatic and ophthalmic decongestant.			
	1:1000 (1 mg = 1 ml), less than 0.25 mg	IV	O: 1 min P: Immediate D: 5–10 min B: liver and neuron PB: UA ½L: UA E: urine
	0.5–1.5 mg	SC/IM	O: 3–5 min P: 20 min D: 20–30 min
	1:10,000 (0.1 mg = 1 ml)	IV or trans-bronchially	O: immediate P: immediate D: 5–10 min
	Children: 0.1 ml/kg of 1:10,000 solution	IV	
Dopamine Hydro-chloride (Intropin)			
Action: Increases blood pressure and heart rate and has a positive inotropic effect on the heart; also increases mesenteric blood flow and improves renal perfusion.			
Use: Poor renal perfusion and lowered blood pressure related to shock.			
	0.5–2.0 μg/kg/min; may be increased to 20 μg/kg/min.	IV	O: 5 min D: 10 min after infusion stops P: 10–15 min ½L: 2.4 min PB: UA B: liver, neuron, kidney E: urine

Common Actions

Key for drug columns: Epinephrine: / Dopamine HCL: / Norepinephrine: / Dobutamine: / Isoproterenol:

	Epinephrine	Dopamine HCL	Norepinephrine	Dobutamine	Isoproterenol
LL	α, β_1, and β_2	dopaminergic, β_1, and α	α_1, α_2, and β_1	β_1	β_1 and β_2
KK		* CHF	—	*	†
JJ	+				+
II		+	+		
HH	+				+
GG	inc. dec.	inc. dec.			—
FF	dec. dec.	dec. dec.			—
EE	C inc.	C inc.			—
DD	D —	D —			inc. or dec.
CC	inc. 0-inc.	inc. 0-inc. inc.			systolic; dec. diastolic
BB	dec. inc./ dec./dd	inc. inc. dec.			
AA	inc. inc.	inc. inc. inc.			

*Cardiac arrest
†Heart failure

Key to Abbreviations in the *Pharmacokinetics* column O-onset; P-peak; D-duration; PB-protein bound; B-biotransformed in; E-excreted in; ½ L-halflife.

*Within the column listing adverse effects, underlines indicate the most common effects, and CAPITALS indicate life-threatening effects.

Contraindications/ Precautions	Adverse Effects*	Interactions	Nursing Implications
Contraindicated in hypersensitivity, narrow-angle glaucoma, shock, dysrhythmias, organic palpitations, and heart/brain disease. Use cautiously in debilitated persons and in those with diabetes, hyperthyroidism, and Parkinson's disease.	Neuro: anxiety, headache, fear, dizziness, sweating CV: dysrhythmias, anginal pain Resp: difficult respiration GI: nausea, vomiting	Effects potentiated with antihistamines, tricyclic antidepressants, thyroid hormones, sympathomimetic agents, and guanethidine (Ismelin). Serious ventricular dysrhythmias develop with halothane and chloroform. Increases the need for insulin and oral hypoglycemics. Antagonizes the effects of guanethidine (Ismelin) and all beta blockers.	ASSESSMENT: Assess vital signs closely. Assess the presence of bronchial obstruction through breath sounds such as wheezing or bronchiovesicular sounds, and for signs of respiratory distress. Assess subjective feelings of tightness in the chest or lung compression and signs of dyspnea. Assess cough, nature and degree and productivity. Respiratory function tests are often obtained. INTERVENTION: Massage injection site to enhance absorption. Watch for signs of extravasation at the injection site. Shake vigorously to disperse drug. Do not inject IM in buttock because gas gangrene may occur. Initial dose is usually submaximal to determine patient response. Often, second and third doses are repeated at 15- to 30-min intervals. Short duration of action is desirable in treatment of acute attacks. Many of the various preparations that are available require extra diligence in administration (e.g., not administering IM preparations IV, calculating proper dose from various concentrations that are available.) Solutions should be clear—brown color indicates oxidation has occurred; discard oxidized solutions. Do not exceed recommended doses. EVALUATION: Short duration of action makes this agent susceptible to overuse. Notify physician of failure to respond to usual dose or dizziness or the presence of chest pain. Evaluate frequently for signs of urinary retention.
Contraindicated in pheochromocytoma and tachyarrhythmias. Use cautiously in pregnancy, occlusive vascular disease, and recent use of MAO inhibitors	Neuro: headache CV: ectopic beats (greater potential for dysrhythmias than dobutamine), tachycardia, anginal pain, hypotension. GI: nausea, vomiting	Pressor effect intensified with MAO inhibitors. Enhances effect of guanethidine (Ismelin) and diuretics. Concurrent use of phenytoin may cause decreased blood pressure. Forms crystals when given concurrently with alkaline solutions.	ASSESSMENT: Check vital signs closely. INTERVENTION: Use microdrip tubing and infusion pumps. Maintain fluid volume. Discard solutions that are discolored. Use only freshly prepared solution. EVALUATION: Monitor closely for infiltration. If it occurs, 5 to 10 mg of phentolamine (Regitine) should be administered to infusion site.

CONTINUED ON THE FOLLOWING PAGE

Table 19–2. DIRECT-ACTING ADRENERGIC STIMULANTS–*CONTINUED*

Name	Dosage	Mode of Administration	Pharmacokinetics	Common Actions
Norepinephrine (Levophed)				
Action: Produces peripheral vasoconstriction and cardiac stimulation.				
Use: Hypotensive events.				
	Adults: 0.5–3 ml/min of a 0.004 mg/ml solution. (Mix 2–4 mg in 500–1000 ml.)	IV	O: 1–2 min P: NA D: 2 min after infusion stops ½L: UA PB: UA B: neuron, liver E: urine	
	Children: 2 µg/min	IV	Same as above.	
Dobutamine Hydrochloride (Dobutrex)				
Action: Increases force of cardiac contraction and improves cardiac output, increases coronary blood flow and stroke-work index, improves ejection fraction.				
Use: Poor cardiac performance with associated hypotension.				
	2.5–20 µg/kg/min *Children:* not recommended for use in children.	IV	O: within 2 min P: 8–10 min D: 5–10 min after infusion stops ½L: 2–3 min PB: UA B: liver E: urine	
Isoproterenol Hydrochloride (Isuprel)				
Action: Cardiac stimulation, bronchial dilatation, peripheral vasodilation.				
Use: Bronchodilator, cardiac stimulant.				
	5 µg/min of 1:250,000 solution (dilute 10 ml of 1:5000 solution in 500 ml diluent)	IV infusion	O: immediate P: immediate D: 2–3 min after infusion stops ½L: UA PB: UA B: liver, lung, tissues E: liver	
	0.01–0.06 mg of a 1:50,000 solution (dilute 1 ml of 1:5000 solution in 1 ml of diluent)	IV bolus	O: immediate P: immediate D: 2–3 min after infusion stops	
	Adults: 10–60 mg divided in 1–3 doses daily	SL	O: 30 min P: 1 hr D: 1–2 hr	
	Children: ½ adult dose	IV infusion	O: immediate P: immediate D: 2–3 min after infusion stops	

Common Actions (rotated column data):

	AA	BB	CC	DD	EE	FF	GG	HH	II	JJ	KK	LL
Epinephrine; Dopamine HCL:	inc. inc.	dec. inc./dec./dd	inc. 0–inc.	D –	C inc.	dec. dec.	inc. dec.	+ –	– +	+ –	* CHF	α, β₁, and β₂ dopaminergic, β₁, and α
Norepinephrine; Dobutamine; Isoproterenol:	inc. inc. inc.	inc. dec. dec.	inc. 0–inc. inc. systolic; dec. diastolic	D – inc. or dec.	C inc. –	dec. dec. –	inc. dec. –	– – +	+ – –	– – +	*Cardiac arrest †Heart failure	α₁, α₂, and β₁ β₁ β₁ and β₂ * †

Key to Abbreviations in the *Pharmacokinetics* column O-onset; P-peak; D-duration; PB-protein bound; B-biotransformed in; E-excreted in; ½ L-halflife.
*Within the column listing adverse effects, underlines indicate the most common effects, and CAPITALS indicate life-threatening effects.

Contraindications/ Precautions	Adverse Effects*	Interactions	Nursing Implications
Contraindicated in profound hypoxia, peripheral vascular thrombosis, and pregnancy. Use cautiously in hypertension, hyperthyroidism, severe cardiac disease, and with MAO inhibitors.	Neuro: headache CV: hypertension with reflex bradycardia	Potentiates pressor effects when given with ergot derivatives, guanethidine (Ismelin), methyldopa (Aldomet), tricyclics, and MAO inhibitors. Increases ventricular dysrhythmias when given with halothane and cyclopropane anesthetics.	ASSESSMENT: Assess for extravasation. Monitor vital signs closely. INTERVENTION: Dilute in dextrose solutions to protect from significant oxidation. Slowly taper infusion when stopping. Maintain fluid volume. EVALUATION: Same as for dopamine.
Contraindicated in hypersensitivity and IHSS. Use cautiously in children and pregnant women.	Neuro: headache CV: increased heart rate, increased blood pressure, increased ectopic activity, anginal pain Resp: shortness of breath GI: nausea	Incompatible with alkaline solutions; forms crystals when given concurrently with alkaline solutions. Concurrent use of halothane increases potential for dysrhythmia. MAO, tricyclic antidepressants, and oxytocics cause synergistic hypertension. Incompatible with hydrocortisone, cefazolin, cefamandole, penicillins, and heparin.	ASSESSMENT: Check vital signs closely. INTERVENTION: use microdrip tubing and infusion pumps. Maintain fluid volume. Discard solutions that are discolored. Use only freshly prepared solution. EVALUATION: If blood pressure and pulse exceed pre-established levels, notify physician.
Contraindicated in tachycardia. Use cautiously in pregnant, elderly, or debilitated patients, and in those with increased blood pressure, coronary or renal disease, or glaucoma.	Neuro: flushing of face, sweating, mild tremors, headache, dizziness CV: tachycardia, palpitations Resp: occur rarely, pulmonary edema GI: nausea and vomiting.	Effects antagonized by propranolol (Inderal). Increased dysrhythmias with cyclopropane, halogenated hydrocarbon anesthetics, epinephrine, and digitalis products.	ASSESSMENT: Assess for the presence of bronchial obstruction through breath sounds such as wheezing or bronchiovesicular sounds, and for signs of respiratory distress. Assess subjective feelings of tightness in the chest or lung compression and signs of dyspnea. Assess cough, nature and degree and productivity. Respiratory function tests are often obtained. INTERVENTION: Do not swallow; allow to dissolve on tongue. Powerful beta₁ activity may result in marked tachycar-

CONTINUED ON THE FOLLOWING PAGE

Direct-Acting Adrenergic Stimulators

Table 19–2. DIRECT-ACTING ADRENERGIC STIMULANTS–*CONTINUED*

Name	Dosage	Mode of Administration	Pharmacokinetics	Common Actions
Isoproterenol Hydrochloride–*Continued*				

Key to Abbreviations in the *Pharmacokinetics* column O-onset; P-peak; D-duration; PB-protein bound; B-biotransformed in; E-excreted in; ½ L-halflife.

*Within the column listing adverse effects, underlines indicate the most common effects, and CAPITALS indicate life-threatening effects.

AA = myocardium (heart rate)
BB = total peripheral resistance
CC = blood pressure
DD = bronchi
EE = kidneys
FF = GI tract
GG = metabolic
HH = bronchoconstriction
II = hypertension
JJ = allergic states
KK = other
LL = receptor-activated
dd = dose-dependent
inc. = increase, dec. = decrease, 0 = no effect, D = dilates, C = constricts, + = used, − = not used

lation, through beta$_2$ agonist stimulation. Epinephrine also constricts the bronchial vessels and inhibits bronchial secretions, which makes it effective in the management of bronchial asthma.

The catecholamines inhibit or stimulate metabolic activity, such as insulin secretion, depending on the sympathetic nervous system receptors stimulated. However, in a stress situation, they are responsible for making more energy available to the body; so they stimulate glycogen release from the liver and skeletal muscles, and fatty acid release as a result of lipolysis in the adipose tissue.

Pharmacokinetics

The catecholamine preparations are inactivated through uptake and metabolism at the sympathetic nerve endings. Most of these drugs are metabolized by monoamine oxidase (MAO) in the liver, kidney, and plasma, and then excreted in the urine as metabolites. All catecholamines are widely distributed in all tissues but are thought not to cross the blood–brain barrier.

Adverse Effects

The most common adverse effects of catecholamines include increased incidence of dysrhythmia, tachycardia, and anginal chest pain, which are all related to the effect on the beta$_2$ receptors. Patients also experience increased anxiety, nervousness, and possible tremors. Headache, flushing (particularly of the face), and sweating are also commonly experienced. These symptoms are all related to the increased sympathetic nervous system stimulation in the brain.

Interactions

Catecholamines commonly interact with other medications. For example, the effects of catecholamines are potentiated by antihistamines, tricyclic antidepressants, thyroid hormones, sympathomimetic agents, and guanethidine. Serious ventricular dysrhythmias may develop during surgery if catecholamines are used concurrently with halothane, chloroform, and cyclopropane anesthetics. The pressor effect of catecholamines is intensified when given concurrently with MAO inhibitors. Cat-

Contraindications/ Precautions	Adverse Effects*	Interactions	Nursing Implications
			dia and increased myocardial contractility; monitor pulse closely, especially in cardiac patients. If given IV, monitor patient closely; best administered via constant infusion pump. Short duration of action is desirable in treatment of acute attacks. Do not exceed recommended doses. Administer pressurized inhalation during the second half of inspiration because the airways are often wider and aerosol distribution is more extensive. Prepare patient for transient facial flushing. Use 72 hours or less. Stop if blood pressure increases 10–20 mm Hg systolically or if heart rate increases 5 beats/min. EVALUATION: May aggravate hypoxemia in some patients by increasing pulmonary blood flow to poorly oxygenated area; supplemental oxygen may be needed. Self-medication may lead to overuse in some patients, resulting in paradoxic bronchospasm. Notify physician of failure to respond to usual dose or of dizziness or presence of chest pain.

echolamines antagonize the effects of propranolol and guanethidine.

Nursing Actions

As the nurse administers any of the catecholamines, the vital signs are checked closely. Hemodynamic measures, including central venous pressure, pulmonary artery occlusive pressure (PAOP), and cardiac output, are monitored closely, particularly when vasopressors are administered. The *vasopressors* are those catecholamines specifically designed to elevate blood pressure, such as norepinephrine (Levophed) and dopamine hydrochloride (Intropin). When any vasopressor is administered, the nurse must continually monitor blood volume. Blood-volume depletion is continuously corrected by appropriate fluid and electrolyte replacement to maintain tissue perfusion and to avoid recurrences of hypotension when products are discontinued. The concentrations of the medications are prepared carefully. Microdrip tubing and an infusion pump are used to control the drip rate. Also, the nurse must know the exact blood pressure ranges for each patient. The medication is titrated to maintain the blood pressure within the given ranges. The nurse continually monitors mentation, skin temperature, and color of the extremities to determine the effectiveness of the therapy.

Intravenous infusion of norepinephrine in saline alone is not recommended. Dextrose solutions are used to prevent drug oxidation and thus loss of potency. Care is taken to prevent extravasation at the infusion site. If extravasation does occur, 5–10 mg of phentolamine in 10–15 ml normal saline is infiltrated throughout the affected area as soon as possible. This helps prevent tissue sloughing. If therapy is to be prolonged, it is advisable to change infusion sites at intervals to allow local va-

soconstriction effect to subside. The nurse must monitor the patient's complaints of headache, vomiting, palpitation, dysrhythmia, chest pain, photophobia, and bradycardia because these may indicate overdose. A reflex bradycardia may occur as a result of a rise in blood pressure. When therapy is to be discontinued, the infusion rate is slowed gradually. Abrupt withdrawal should be avoided.

Dopamine is generally started at a dose of 1–2 μg/kg/minute. Because of its short half-life, effects begin within minutes of starting the infusion and disappear within minutes after discontinuation of infusion.

It is important to monitor for cold extremities. If the extremities become very cold, a two-inch strip of nitroglycerin ointment is applied to the warmest areas of the chest or abdomen. This may be effective in increasing peripheral blood flow without affecting blood pressure. Signs of overdose include tachycardia, dysrhythmia, marked decrease in pulse pressure, signs of peripheral ischemia, pallor, cyanosis, and mottling. Signs and symptoms of overdose generally respond to dosage reduction or temporary discontinuation of the drug, since dopamine has a short duration of action. If these measures fail, a short-acting alpha-adrenergic blocking agent may be given.

If a patient responds to vasopressors with an increase in heart rate above 30 beats/minute or an increase in blood pressure of 50 mmHg or greater, the infusion is slowed.

When administering a catecholamine such as dobutamine, the infusion is begun at 2 μg/kg/minute and is increased as necessary. Effects are seen within seconds. The infusion is tapered slowly to avoid sudden decreases in ventricular function. If marked increases in blood pressure, heart rate, or the appearance of dysrhythmia occur, the infusion is slowed. These effects are generally reversed promptly by reduction in dosage.

Epinephrine

Epinephrine (Adrenalin), a naturally occurring catecholamine obtained from animal adrenal glands and also prepared synthetically, acts on both alpha and beta receptors and is a powerful alpha-receptor stimulator.

ACTION. Epinephrine action can be summarized as preparing the body for "flight, fright, or fight." Tachycardia and the resultant palpitation result from the stimulation of the beta$_1$ receptors. Vasoconstriction in the peripheral vessels occurs, resulting in a rise in blood pressure and cold, clammy skin as the alpha$_1$ receptors are stimulated. In contrast, vasodilatation occurs in the blood vessels of muscles where beta$_2$ receptors predominate. Gastrointestinal activity is reduced, sphincters are tightly closed, and pupil dilatation (mydriasis) occurs. Glycogen stores in the liver are released to raise the level of blood sugar.

USES. Epinephrine has many uses. It is used in the temporary relief of bronchospasm in acute asthmatic attacks, in mucosal congestion, and to restore cardiac activity in cardiac arrest. Epinephrine is the most appropriate sympathomimetic to treat anaphylactic shock (hypersensitivty reactions to animal or insect venoms, and medications) because it physiologically antagonizes the vasodilation and bronchoconstriction that occur. Epinephrine is also effective as a mydriatic and ophthalmic decongestant and is used in simple (open-angle) glaucoma.

CONTRAINDICATIONS AND PRECAUTIONS. The contraindications specific to use of epinephrine include narrow-angle glaucoma; acute shock; dysrhythmias; organic heart/brain disease, because symptoms may worsen in these conditions; and sensitivity to its ingredients. Most epinephrine products contain sulfites. Caution is used when administering epinephrine to debilitated persons because they may be more sensitive to its effects, and to diabetic persons with hyperthyroidism because symptoms may be increased, or to persons with Parkinson's disease because rigidity and tremor may be increased.

PREPARATIONS. Many forms of epinephrine are available. It may be administered parenterally, as a nasal spray, or as an ophthalmic solution.

Epinephrine Injection. Epinephrine injection is the epinephrine product most commonly administered in emergency situations. It can be administered both intravenously and subcutaneously. Solutions come as 1:1000 (1.0 mg = 1.0 ml) aqueous preparations. A milliliter of epinephrine is given: 0.5 ml is injected subcutaneously at the point of entry of the foreign substance (if known); the remaining 0.5 ml is diluted to a 1:10,000 (0.1 mg. = 1 ml) solution and is administered intravenously. The injection may be repeated intravenously every five to fifteen minutes as needed. Subcutaneously, action starts in three to five minutes and peaks in twenty minutes. Intravenously, the effect is apparent immediately. In a cardiac arrest, 1.0 ml of a 1:10,000 solution is administered either intravenously or transbronchially.

Epinephrine Inhalation. Epinephrine inhalation, available as a 1:100 (1%) solution, is administered as is, or it is diluted for nebulization directly into the lung. It is readily absorbed from the mucous membranes. Special care should be taken not to confuse the 1:100 solutions with the 1:1000 solutions. The Medihaler-Epi is a special inhaler for respiratory therapy.

Epinephrine Bitartrate. Epinephrine bitartrate (Epitrate) is a special 2% solution for ophthalmic use in treating chronic simple glaucoma.

Epinephrine (As Hydrochloride). Epinephrine (Epifrin, Glaucon) is available in various solutions (0.25%, 0.5%, 1%, and 2%) and is instilled, one to two drops, once or twice daily.

Isoproterenol Hydrochloride

Isoproterenol hydrochloride (Isuprel), a synthetic catecholamine, acts almost exclusively on beta-adrenergic receptors. Primary therapeutic effects include cardiac stimualation, bronchial dilatation, and peripheral vasodilatation. Isoproterenol hydrochloride lowers peripheral vascular resistance by vasodilating skeletal muscle and mesenteric circulation and increases venous return to the heart, which in turn slightly increases the systolic pressure and reduces the diastolic and mean pressures. A major problem with using isoproterenol hydrochloride in certain shock states is that blood pressure may be further reduced and coronary and cerebral perfusion may be compromised. Its inotropic effects may be beneficial when it is used with vasoconstricting agents.

USES. Isoproterenol hydrochloride is used primarily as a bronchodilator in both acute and chronic asthma, and as a cardiac stimulant in patients with severe bradyarrhythmias. It is discussed in greater detail in Chapter 35.

CONTRAINDICATIONS AND PRECAUTIONS. Isoproterenol hydrochloride is contraindicated in persons with tachycardia. If the pulse rate rises to between 110 and 120 beats per minute during administration, the infusion is slowed. Isoproterenol is given cautiously to persons who are pregnant, elderly, or debilitated because they are more sensitive to its effects; to those with increased blood pressure and coronary disease because it may increase blood pressure and provoke angina; to persons with diabetes and glaucoma because these conditions may worsen; and to those with renal disease because the drug is excreted through the renal system.

DOSAGE. Doses of isoproterenol hydrochloride range from 0.02–1.0 mg of a 1:50,000–1:250,000 solution given intramuscularly or intravenously. Isoproterenol is available as a 1:5000 solution. Diluting 1.0 ml of a 1:5000 solution with 10 ml of diluent results in a 1:50,000 solution. Diluting 10 ml of a 1:5000 solution in 500 ml of diluent results in a 1:250,000 solution. It is also available in oral tablets, sublingual tablets, rectal suppositories, as an inhalant, and for subcutaneous and intramuscular injection. See Chapter 35 for more information on dosage.

Norepinephrine

Norepinephrine (Levophed) is the bitartrate salt of the body's catecholamine norepinephrine. It acts primarily

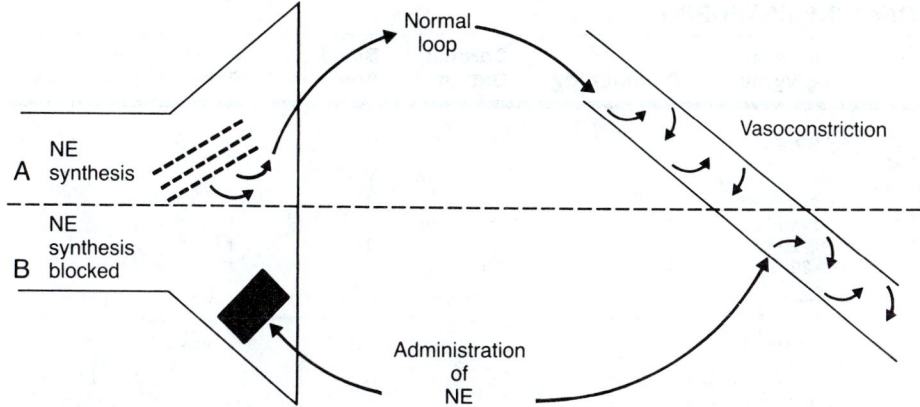

Figure 19–1. Administration of norepinephrine causes vasoconstriction in the peripheral system but also in a negative feedback loop blocking the production of new norepinephrine in the sympathetic synapse.

on alpha$_1$, alpha$_2$, and beta$_1$ receptors to cause vasoconstriction and cardiac stimulation. The blood pressure is elevated because of norepinephrine's powerful constrictor action on both resistance and capacitance blood vessels. Because of its dual action, norepinephrine increases arterial pressure more reliably than other available sympathomimetic amines. Because alpha-adrenergic receptors appear to be reduced in number in cerebral and coronary vessels, norepinephrine tends to increase blood flow to these areas. However, blood flow to the skin, skeletal muscle, and kidney is reduced and ischemia may result. For this reason, norepinephrine is used only in those patients in whom an immediate increase in arterial pressure is required to maintain life or in whom an infusion of dopamine cannot maintain perfusion pressure. Weaning patients off norepinephrine may be difficult because continued doses of norepinephrine block the synthesis of new norepinephrine in the sympathetic synapse; therefore, when the infusion is stopped, there is minimal norepinephrine in the body to effect changes in blood pressure (Fig. 19–1). Norepinephrine causes less central nervous system stimulation and has less effect on metabolism than does epinephrine.

CONTRAINDICATIONS AND PRECAUTIONS. Norepinephrine is contraindicated in profound hypoxia and peripheral vascular thrombosis because further injury may result, and in pregnancy because it crosses the placenta. Norepinephrine is also contraindicated in patients who are hypotensive from blood volume deficits; until volume is restored, severe systemic effects may occur, such as peripheral and visceral vasoconstriction, decreased renal perfusion, tissue hypoxia, and lactic acidosis. It is given cautiously to persons with hypertension, hyperthyroidism, or severe cardiac disease because these conditions may be worsened, and to patients concurrently receiving MAO inhibitors.

DOSAGE. Norepinephrine is administered intravenously through a continuous infusion. A solution is prepared by mixing 2–4.0 mg of medication in 500–1000 ml of fluid (0.004 mg/ml solution). The infusion is titrated to maintain the blood pressure within the range prescribed by the physician. During the time when the dosage is being increased or decreased, the blood pressure is recorded at least every two to three minutes. The usual dose ranges from 0.5–3 ml/minute intravenously. The action begins in one to two minutes. The dose is tapered slowly as it is being discontinued. The infusion site is watched closely to prevent extravasation of fluid, which can result in abscess, necrosis, and tissue sloughing. If infiltration does occur, the infusion is stopped immediately and phentolamine hydrochloride (Regitine), an alpha blocker, is infiltrated into the same location.

Dopamine Hydrochloride

Dopamine hydrochloride is administered to patients with poor renal perfusion and lowered blood pressure related to shock or other diseases. Dopamine hydrochloride (Intropin), the immediate precursor of norepinephrine, affects dopaminergic receptors and beta$_1$ and alpha$_1$ receptors in a dose-dependent fashion. (Table 19–3 reviews the dose-dependent effects.) Like norepinephrine, it acts as a vasopressor, and increases blood pressure, PAOP, and cardiac output. It also increases the pulse rate and has a positive inotropic effect on the heart. Dopamine may increase myocardial ischemia. However, unlike norepinephrine, it increases mesenteric blood flow, which improves renal perfusion. (In large doses, however, mesenteric blood flow is reduced.)

USES. Dopamine is used to increase cardiac output without decreasing afterload and filling pressure. It has been used successfully for cardiocirculatory support in cases of congestive heart failure with hypotension, or reduction in urinary flow, or both; for cardiogenic shock; and for other conditions that occur with critically ill patients. Low doses are also used to achieve acute diuresis in patients in whom administration of diuretic agents is not desired or is ineffective. Dopamine is the first-line sympathomimetic amine used clinically today.

CONTRAINDICATIONS AND PRECAUTIONS. Contraindications to the use of dopamine hydrochloride include pheochromocytoma tumors and tachyarrhythmias because these may be worsened. Caution is advised in pregnancy, with recent use of MAO inhibitors, and in occlusive vascular disease.

DOSAGE. At lowest infusion rates 0.5–2 µg/kg/minute, both DA-1 and DA-2 receptors are stimulated,

Table 19–3. DOPAMINE (INTROPIN)

Use	Dosage µg/kg/min	Contractility	Cardiac Output	Blood Pressure	Heart Rate	Beta Receptors	Alpha Receptors
Increased diuresis in oliguric patient, to augment diuretics	0.5–2	—	—	—	—	*	—
Shock	2–5	*	—	*	*	†	—
Shock	5–10	†	†	†	†	†	*
Shock	10–20	†	†	‡	†	‡	†
Shock	>20	†	*(*)	‡	†	‡	‡

*Mild effect
†Moderate effect
‡Great effect

which dilates mesenteric and renal beds. This rate of infusion is often used to initiate diuresis in the oliguric patient. Since the renal artery is dilated, there is increased renal blood flow, which improves urinary output and sodium excretion. Creatinine clearance also improves. Blood pressure may decrease slightly. Higher infusion rates are generally used in the treatment of shock. When infusion rates are increased to 2–5 µg/kg/minute, beta$_1$ receptors are activated, which improves cardiac contractility and cardiac output. Myocardial oxygen consumption is increased, but this does not provoke an ischemic risk. Dopamine may even increase blood flow to ischemic areas. Heart rate may increase, decrease, or remain unchanged. At infusion rates of 5–10 µg/kg/minute, contractility, cardiac output, and heart rate all improve. After about 10 minutes of this infusion rate, cardiac output may improve by 20% to 30%. At rates of 10–20 µg/kg/minute, dopamine resembles norepinephrine and alpha activity begins, which increases the blood pressure. In doses of more than 20 µg/kg/minute, only alpha receptors are activated, which increases *afterload* (force against which heart has to pump determined by the size of the *resistance vessels*). Weaning the patient from dopamine hydrochloride is often difficult. Several preliminary studies suggest that oral levodopa (used to treat Parkinson's disease), which is converted to dopamine, may be helpful during weaning. Dopamine hydrochloride, like all other catecholamines, should be given only if the total blood volume is adequate. Fluid challenges may be given concurrently to ensure adequate fluid volume.

Action begins in two minutes and lasts ten minutes after the infusion is terminated. Dopamine hydrochloride has a half-life of 1.75 minutes.

Dobutamine Hydrochloride

Dobutamine hydrochloride (Dobutrex) is a synthetic catecholamine, a form of synthetic isoproterenol, with relatively cardioselective action on beta$_1$-adrenergic receptor sites. Dobutamine exerts a relatively weak action on beta$_2$ and alpha$_1$ receptors. Unlike dopamine, it does not cause the release of endogenous norepinephrine from adrenergic nerve fibers; therefore, dobutamine is relatively selective in its ability to increase myocardial contractile force. It increases the force of cardiac contraction and cardiac output by 30%–70%, reduces the

pulmonary artery occlusive pressure, increases coronary blood flow, increases stoke-work index, and improves ejection fraction, with few vascular or cardioacceleratory effects. Dobutamine increases the blood pressure but reduces systemic vascular resistance through vasodilation. Dobutamine pulls fluid back into the vascular bed, thus increasing cardiac output. Generally, in low doses, there is little increase in heart rate; but at higher doses, these changes may become significant. These actions make dobutamine hydrochloride a particularly good drug for patients with decreased blood pressure or shock resulting from depressed myocardial function. However, if vasoconstriction is required to increase blood pressure, dobutamine hydrochloride is not appropriate. Dobutamine hydrochloride may cause cardiac ischemia, so it is important to frequently assess for ST depression. Dobutamine hydrochloride does not affect renal or mesenteric blood flow. Any effects that occur are most likely secondary to an increase in cardiac output.

USES. Dobutamine hydrochloride is useful in the short-term management of patients with myocardial infarction, cardiovascular decompensation, cardiogenic shock, or acute congestive heart failure, and for intermittent therapy for congestive heart failure. Recent research indicates that dobutamine may increase oxygen extraction by skeletal muscles and may, therefore, augment the aerobic enzyme activity of human skeletal muscles. For these reasons, dobutamine is being studied in critically ill, long-term, bed-ridden patients for its physical conditioning effect, thus decreasing the deconditioning effects of immobility and assisting in the rehabilitation of critical-care patients. Again, as with the other catecholamines, hypovolemia should be corrected before using dobutamine hydrochloride.

CONTRAINDICATIONS AND PRECAUTIONS. Dobutamine hydrochloride is specifically contraindicated in persons with any obstruction to cardiac outflow, such as idiopathic hypertrophic subaortic stenosis (IHSS), because it may be worsened. Safe use in children and pregnancy has not been established.

DOSAGE. Dobutamine hydrochloride is administered by intravenous infusion at a rate of 2.5–20 µg/kg/minute. Dosage is titrated by monitoring the effects on the pulmonary artery obstructive pressure rather than on blood pressure. In low doses, dobutamine hydrochloride has primarily an alpha$_1$ effect, causing mild va-

Table 19-4. COMBINATION DIRECT ADRENERGIC THERAPY AND OTHER DRUGS

Drug Combinations	Uses	Comments
Dobutamine: Titrate to hemodynamic response to increased CO, increased CI, decreased PAOP, increased ejection fraction. Dosage: 5–15 µg/kg/min **Dopamine:** Titrate not higher than required for renal dilation and increased renal output. Dosage: 0.5–5.0 µg/kg/min	Pump failure, pulmonary congestion, poor hemodynamic function	Superior to higher doses of either drug alone. Improves CO and arterial pressure and dilates renal arteries without increasing afterload
Dopamine: Titrate to increase CO, increase CI, decrease HR **Nitrates:** Titrate to decrease pulmonary vascular resistance, decrease PAOP to less than 17 mmHg	Congestive heart failure, hypotension, to increase peripheral vascular resistance, poor hemodynamic function	Improves CO while reducing afterload
Dobutamine: Titrate to hemodynamic response to increased CO, increased CI, decreased PAOP, increased ejection fraction. Dosage: 5–15 µg/kg/min **Nitroprusside:** Initially start at 16 µg/min	Shock, congestive heart failure	Superior to either drug alone to increase CO and reduce PAOP
Dobutamine: Titrate to hemodynamic response to increased CO, increased CI, decreased PAOP, increased ejection fraction. Dosage: 5–15 µg/kg/min **Nitrates:** Titrate to decrease pulmonary vascular resistance, decrease PAOP to less than 17 mmHg	Severe congestive heart failure	Improves CI while markedly decreasing left ventricular filling pressure and relieving congestion

CO, cardiac output; CI, cardiac index; PAOP, pulmonary artery occlusive pressure; HR, heart rate.

soconstriction. As the dosage reaches 15 µg/kg/minute, vasodilation effect occurs, which causes a reduction in afterload. The ideal dosage is 7.5 µg/kg/minute. Dobutamine has a duration of action of three to four minutes after the infusion is terminated. Infusions of up to 72 hours have demonstrated no adverse effects. Infusions for more than 72 hours may be accompanied by the development of tolerance, which may possibly be due to down-regulation of beta-adrenoreceptors.

Combination of Agents

In seriously ill patients, it is often necessary to combine several of the direct-acting adrenergics to produce a more beneficial effect. Table 19–4 describes several drug combinations that produce a beneficial effect, that is, produce the least amount of vasoconstriction while maintaining an adequate perfusion pressure.

INDIRECT- AND MIXED-ACTING ADRENERGIC MEDICATIONS

The indirect- and mixed-acting adrenergic drugs shown in Table 19–5 indirectly affect adrenergic receptors, or act either directly or indirectly on the receptors. Metaraminol bitartrate (Aramine), mephentermine sulfate (Wyamine), and methoxamine hydrochloride (Vasoxyl) are vasopressors and are similar to levarterenol bitartrate.

Adverse Effects

The adverse effects of all the indirect and mixed adrenergic stimulants include headache and nervousness from stimulation of the central nervous system, and palpitations, dysrhythmias, and tachycardia from cardiac stimulation. Patients with underlying angina pectoris may experience precordial chest pain as well.

Interactions

Many interactions exist between the adrenergic stimulants and other drugs. These are described in Table 19–5. One interaction common to all the indirect and mixed adrenergic stimulants is an increased tendency to cause severe elevations of blood pressure when given concurrently with MAO inhibitors or furazolidone (Furoxone).

Ephedrine

ACTION. Ephedrine (Ephedra, I-Sedrin plain), an indirect adrenergic stimulant that affects both alpha and beta receptors, is similar to epinephrine but is less potent, with slower onset and more prolonged action. It acts indirectly by releasing tissue stores of norepinephrine. Bronchodilation is less pronounced but more sustained than with epinephrine. Ephedrine also reduces uterine contractions. Tachyphylaxis (decreased response to repeated doses) occurs rapidly because of the depletion of norepinephrine stores.

TEXT RESUMES ON PAGE 428

Table 19–5. MIXED- AND INDIRECT-ACTING ADRENERGIC STIMULANTS

Drug	Dosage	Mode of Administration	Pharmacokinetics
Ephedrine (Ephedra)			
Action: Indirect adrenergic stimulant, reduces uterine contractions. ***Use:*** Relieves congestion, improves respiratory rate in narcotic and barbiturate poisoning, stimulant for narcolepsy.			
	Adults: 15–50 mg, q 3–4 hr prn; maximum dose in 24 hr: 150 mg	PO, SC, IM, IV (slow)	O: PO, 15–60 min; SC, IM, 5–30 min; IV, immediate P: PO, 1 hr; SC, IM, 15–60 min; IV, immediate D: PO, 4–12 hr; IM, IV, SC, 1 hr ½L: 3 hr acid urine; 6 hr alkaline urine PB: UA B: liver E: urine
Ephedrine Sulfate (Bofedrol, Ephedsol, Nasdro, Slo-fedrin)	1%–3%, 2–4 drops 4 × daily	Nasal solution	
	Children: 2–3 mg/kg/24 hr in 4–6 doses	PO, SC, IV	Same as for adults.

Common Actions

	AA	BB	CC	DD	EE	FF	GG	HH	II	JJ
Ephedrine:	inc.	D	D	inc.	C	dec.	inc.	+	+	Allergic states, myasthenia gravis
Phenylephrine HCL:	—	D	D	—	C	dec.	inc.	+	+	Mydriatic
Metaraminol Bitartrate:	inc.	—	—	—	C	dec.	—	+	+	—
Mephentermine Sulfate:	inc.	D′	D	—	C	dec	—	+	+	—
Methoxamine HCL:	—	—	—	—	dec.	dec.	—	+	+	—

Key to Abbreviations in the *Pharmacokinetics* column O-onset; P-peak; D-duration; PB-protein bound; B-biotransformed in; E-excreted in; ½ L-halflife.

*Within the column listing adverse effects, underlines indicate the most common effects, and CAPITALS indicate life-threatening effects.

Contraindications and Precautions	Adverse Effects*	Drug Interactions	Nursing Implications
Contraindicated in severe coronary artery disease or hypertension and in narrow-angle glaucoma. Use cautiously in hyperthyroidism, diabetes, bradycardia; in elderly patients.	Neuro: headache, nervousness, insomnia. CV: palpitations, tachycardia. Renal: difficult urination	Concurrent methyldopa, reserpine, and tricyclic antidepressants decrease effectiveness. Potentiated by guanethidine, MAO inhibitors, and tricyclics. Increased mydriatric activity with levodopa (L-dopa). Causes severe increase in blood pressure when used with MAO inhibitors and furazolidone (Furoxone). Increased possibility of arrhythmia when given concurrently with halothane-type anesthetics.	ASSESSMENT: Assess for the presence of bronchial obstruction through breath sounds such as wheezing or bronchiovesicular sounds, and for signs of respiratory distress. Assess subjective feelings of tightness in the chest or lung compression and signs of dyspnea. Assess cough, nature and degree and productivity. Respiratory function tests are often obtained. INTERVENTION: Generally useful only in cases of mild bronchospasm. Usually combined with barbiturate and/or theophylline compounds. If given on a daily regimen, administer in morning to avoid insomnia. Initial dose is usually submaximal to determine patient response. When patients are receiving IV solutions, monitor vital signs closely—particularly blood pressure for elevations. Blow nose before nasal administration. Rinse nasal dropper after each use to prevent contamination of medication. EVALUATION: Multiple side effects make use of this drug controversial. Rapid development of patient tolerance may lead to increased self-dosing. This can lead to habituation, or possible psychotic episodes. May cause sudden sharp rise in blood pressure as patient develops tolerance. Notify physician of failure to respond to usual dose or dizziness or of the presence of chest pain.

CONTINUED ON THE FOLLOWING PAGE

Mixed- and Indirect-Acting Adrenergic Stimulators

Table 19–5. MIXED- AND INDIRECT-ACTING ADRENERGIC STIMULANTS–*CONTINUED*

Drug	Dosage	Mode of Administration	Pharmacokinetics	Common Actions
Phenylephrine Hydrochloride (Coryban-D Nasal Decongestant, Neo-Synephrine, Prefrin)				

Action: Potent vasoconstrictor acting primarily on alpha receptors.

Use: Maintains blood pressure during anesthesia and shock, and to control tachycardia.

	Dosage	Mode of Administration	Pharmacokinetics
	Adults: 1–10 mg	SC, IM	O: 10–15 min P: 30 min D: 50 min ½L: UA PB: UA B: liver E: UA
	Children: 0.1 mg/kg	SC, IM	O: 10–15 min P: 30 min D: 50 min
	Adults: 0.1–0.5 mg	IV	O: immediate P: 10 min D: 20 min
	Adults: 0.5 mg of 1% solution	Topical	O: 1–2 min P: 30 min D: 30 min–4 hr
	Children: 0.125%–0.2% (1 drop) q 3–4 hr in infants; 0.25% q 3–4 hr in children > age 6	Topical	Same as above.
	Adults: 2.5% 10% solution	Ophthalmic	2.5% P: 15–30 min D: 1–3 hr 10% P: 10–90 min D: 3–7 hr

Drug	Dosage	Mode of Administration	Pharmacokinetics
Metaraminol Bitartrate (Aramine)			

Action: Increases venous tone, causes pulmonary vasoconstriction, and elevates pulmonary pressure.

Use: To support, restore, and maintain blood pressure during anesthesia or shock.

	Dosage	Mode of Administration	Pharmacokinetics
	Adults: 2–10 mg (at least 10 min apart)	SC, IM	O: 5–20 min P: NA D: 20–90 min ½L: UA PB: UA B: tissue uptake E: urine
	Children: 0.1 mg/kg	SC, IM	Same as above.
	Adults: 15–100 mg in 500 ml	IV infusion	O: 1–2 min P: UA D: 20 min
	Children: 0.4 mg/kg	IV infusion	Same as above.

Common Actions column (right side):

	Allergic states, myasthenia gravis	Mydriatic		
JJ			–	–
II	+		+ + + +	
HH	+		+ + +	
GG	inc.	inc.	–	–
FF	dec.	dec. dec. dec.		
EE	C	C C C	dec.	
DD	inc.		– – – –	
CC	D	D	– D	–
BB	D	D	– D'	–
AA	inc.	–	inc. inc.	–

Ephedrine:
Phenylephrine HCL:
Metaraminol Bitartrate:
Mephentermine Sulfate:
Methoxamine HCL:

Key to Abbreviations in the *Pharmacokinetics* column O-onset; P-peak; D-duration; PB-protein bound; B-biotransformed in; E-excreted in; ½ L-halflife.

*Within the column listing adverse effects, <u>underlines</u> indicate the most common effects, and CAPITALS indicate life-threatening effects.

Contraindications and Precautions	Adverse Effects*	Drug Interactions	Nursing Implications
Contraindicated in hypersensitivity, narrow-angle glaucoma, and in patients receiving MAO inhibitors, tricyclics, digitalis, and oxytocics. Use cautiously in pregnancy, hypertension, chronic heart disease, diabetes, hyperthyroidism, and prostatic hypertrophy.	Same as above; plus CV: sweating. Endo: hyperglycemia	Causes severe increase in blood pressure when used with MAO inhibitors or furazolidone (Furoxone). Causes dysrhythmias when used with halothane. Decreased effectiveness with mythyldopa (Aldomet) and reserpine (Serpasil). Blocks effect of guanethidine (Ismelin).	ASSESSMENT: Same as for ephedrine. Patients receiving IV form need constant supervision and monitoring of vital signs and intake and output. INTERVENTION: Caution patient not to overdose amount or frequency. Rinse nasal dropper after each use to prevent contamination of medication. Time doses early in the evening to prevent insomnia. EVALUATION: Rebound congestion can occur.
Contraindicated in patients receiving cyclopropane, halothane, or MAO inhibitors. Use cautiously in cardiac arrest, pulmonary edema, as sole agent in hypovolemia, in patients receiving digitalis drugs, hypertension, hyperthyroidism, diabetes, cirrhosis of liver, and in patients who have previously had malaria (may produce relapse). Not safe in pregnancy.	Same as phenylephrine, plus: necrosis and abscess formation at IV site; induration.	Enhanced pressor effect with ergot derivatives, furazolidone (Furoxone), guanethidine, MAO inhibitors, and tricyclics. Increased ventricular dysrhythmias with cyclopropane and halothane.	ASSESSMENT: When patients are receiving IV solution, monitor vital signs closely—particularly blood pressure for elevation. INTERVENTION: Correct blood volume. Carefully monitor site of IV to prevent extravasation. Gradually reduce flow rate before stopping. Monitor intake and output. Do not mix other medications in the same IV infusion.

CONTINUED ON THE FOLLOWING PAGE

Mixed- and Indirect-Acting Adrenergic Stimulators

Table 19–5. MIXED- AND INDIRECT-ACTING ADRENERGIC STIMULANTS–*CONTINUED*

Drug	Dosage	Mode of Administration	Pharmacokinetics	Common Actions
Mephentermine Sulfate (Wyamine)				
Action: Increases venous tone, causes pulmonary vasoconstriction and elevates pulmonary pressure.				
Use: To support, restore, and maintain blood pressure during anesthesia or shock.				
	15–35 mg	IM	O: 5–15 min P: UA D: 1–2 hr ½L: UA PB: UA B: liver E: urine	
	0.1% solution at 1 mg/min	IV infusion	O: immediate P: UA D: 15–30 min after infusion stops	
Methoxamine Hydrochloride (Vasoxyl)				
Action: Increases venous tone, causes pulmonary vasoconstriction, and elevates pulmonary pressure.				
Use: To support, restore, and maintain, blood pressure during anesthesia or shock.				
	3–5 mg slowly	IV	O: immediate P: 0.5–2 min D: 5–15 min ½L: UA PB: UA B: UA E: UA	
	10–15 mg, repeated if necessary, after 15 min	IM	O: 15 min P: 15–20 min D: 1½ hr B: liver E: urine	

Common Actions

Code	Ephedrine	Phenylephrine HCL	Metaraminol Bitartrate	Mephentermine Sulfate	Methoxamine HCL
JJ (Allergic states, myasthenia gravis; Mydriatic)			−	−	−
II	+	+	+	+	+
HH	+	+	+	+	+
GG	inc.	inc.	−	−	−
FF	dec.	dec.	dec.	dec.	dec.
EE	C	C	C	C	dec.
DD	inc.	−	−	−	−
CC	D	D	−	D	−
BB	D	D	D′	−	−
AA	V	−	inc.	inc.	−

Key to Abbreviations in the *Pharmacokinetics* column O-onset; P-peak; D-duration; PB-protein bound; B-biotransformed in; E-excreted in; ½ L-halflife.

*Within the column listing adverse effects, underlines indicate the most common effects, and CAPITALS indicate life-threatening effects.

AA = myocardium (heart rate)
BB = total peripheral resistance
CC = blood pressure
DD = bronchi
EE = kidneys
FF = GI tract
GG = metabolic

HH = bronchoconstriction
II = hypertension
JJ = allergic states
KK = other
LL = receptor-activated
dd = dose-dependent

inc. = increase, dec. = decrease, 0 = no effect, D = dilates, C = constricts, + = used, − = not used

Contraindications and Precautions	Adverse Effects*	Drug Interactions	Nursing Implications
Contraindicated in patients receiving cyclopropane, halothane, MAO inhibitors, and as a sole agent in hypovolemia. Not safe in pregnancy. Use cautiously in hypertension, hyperthyroidism, and diabetes.	Same as above.	Same as above, plus: decreased effectiveness with reserpine (Serpasil) and guanethidine (Ismelin).	Same as above.
Same as above.	Same as above.	Decreased effectiveness with guanethidine (Ismelin) and reserpine (Serpasil).	Same as above.

USES. Ephedrine is used to relieve congestion in allergic conditions and in the management of both mild acute asthma and chronic asthma. It is also used to improve the respiratory rate in patients with narcotic and barbiturate poisonings and to stimulate the central nervous system in patients with narcolepsy. Due to its cardiac and central nervous system toxicities, ephedrine has largely fallen into disuse.

CONTRAINDICATIONS AND PRECAUTIONS. Ephedrine is contraindicated in persons with past hypersensitivity to the drug; in persons with narrow-angle glaucoma; and in patients receiving MAO inhibitors, tricyclics, digitalis, and oxytocics. Cautious use is recommended in pregnant or hypertensive persons and in patients with chronic heart disease, diabetes, hyperthyroidism, or prostatic hypertrophy. Ephedrine causes the urinary bladder sphincter to contract, which may make the patient with prostatic hypertrophy unable to void.

INTERACTIONS. Additional interactions specific to ephedrine include an increased possibility of dysrhythmias when used concurrently with halothane or decreased action of ephedrine when the patient is receiving methyldopa and reserpine (Serpasil). Ephedrine may also block the antihypertensive effects of guanethidine (Ismelin).

DOSAGE. Ephedrine is administered by many routes. In adults, 15–50 mg is given orally or parenterally every three to four hours as needed. Orally or parenterally, the maximum dose in 24 hours is 150 mg. The action peaks in one hour and has a duration of four to twelve hours depending on the form. A 1%–3% nasal solution is administered, 2–4 drops in each nostril, four times daily. In children the dose is 2–3.0 mg/kg/24 hours by any route, administered four to six times a day.

Phenylephrine Hydrochloride

Phenylephrine hydrochloride (Neo-Synephrine) is a potent, synthetic, noncatecholamine adrenergic stimulator that is chemically related to epinephrine. Phenylephrine hydrochloride acts primarily on the alpha receptors, with little or no effect on beta receptors. Because of its alpha effect, it is a potent vasoconstrictor that elevates both the systolic and diastolic blood pressures. It has no effect on the central nervous system and little effect on the heart. It does, however, cause a reflexive bradycardia as a result of stimulation of the cardioreceptors and increased vagal activity. For this reason, it has been useful in converting paroxysmal tachycardia to a normal rate.

USES. Phenylephrine hydrochloride is used parenterally to maintain blood pressure during anesthesia and shock and to control tachycardia. Topically and orally, it is used for allergic rhinitis and sinusitis. Ophthalmically, it is used as a mydriatic in open-angle glaucoma and in eye examinations.

CONTRAINDICATIONS AND PRECAUTIONS. Phenylephrine hydrochloride is contraindicated in patients with severe coronary artery disease or hypertension and narrow-angle glaucoma. It is given cautiously to the elderly, to persons with hyperthyroidism, diabetes, or bradycardia; and to persons concurrently receiving MAO inhibitors, tricyclics, or halothane.

INTERACTIONS. Phenylephrine hydrochloride may interact with guanethidine, MAO inhibitors, and tricyclics. The action of phenylephrine hydrochloride is potentiated when these drugs are given concurrently. Concurrent use with levodopa decreases the mydriatic activity of phenylephrine.

DOSAGE. Phenylephrine hydrochloride is given parenterally, either subcutaneously or intramuscularly, in dosages of 1–10 mg in adults and 0.1 mg/kg in children every one to two hours. It has a duration of about 50 minutes. Intravenously, the dose is 0.1–0.5 mg, with a duration of 20 minutes. It should not be repeated more often than every 10–15 minutes. Topical solutions of 0.125%, 0.16%, 0.25%, 0.5%, and 1.0% are available, as are 2.5% and 10% ophthalmic solutions. The ophthalmic solution takes effect in 15–30 minutes and has a duration of one to three hours.

Other Vasopressors

Metaraminol bitartrate (Aramine), mephentermine sulfate (Wyamine), and methoxamine hydrochloride (Vasoxyl) are vasopressors. They are all used to support, restore, or maintain blood pressure during anesthesia or in shock. In most situations, these drugs have been replaced by the newer adrenergic stimulator dopamine hydrochloride.

Metaraminol increases both systolic and diastolic pressures by vasoconstriction, which is accompanied by a reflex bradycardia. It increases venous tone, causes pulmonary vasoconstriction, and elevates pulmonary pressure when cardiac output is reduced. Mephentermine sulfate acts indirectly by releasing norepinephrine. The increase in blood pressure is primarily due to an increase in cardiac output. Methoxamine hydrochloride increases peripheral resistance and has no effect on the heart.

CONTRAINDICATIONS AND PRECAUTIONS. Metaraminol, mephentermine, and methoxamine are contraindicated in patients receiving cyclopropane and halothane, because they increase the tendency for ventricular dysrhythmias, and in patients receiving MAO inhibitors, because they increase pressor effect. All three are also contraindicated for use as sole agents in treating hypovolemic shock. Their safe use in pregnancy is not established. They are given cautiously to patients with hypertension, hyperthyroidism, or diabetes. The pressor effect of these three medications is enhanced when they are given concurrently with ergot derivatives, furazolidone (Furoxone), guanethidine, tricyclics, and other antidepressants.

NURSING ACTIONS. The nursing care of patients receiving these three drugs is the same as for the vasopressors previously discussed. Care should always be taken to avoid infiltrating the intravenous infusion. No other medication is ever mixed in the same bottle or infused through the same vessel with these medications.

Metaraminol Bitartrate. Metaraminol bitartrate (Aramine) is administered to adults subcutaneously and intramusculary in doses of 2–10 mg at least ten minutes apart. The action starts in 5–20 minutes and has a duration of 90 minutes. Intravenously, 15–100 mg are

Table 19–6. EFFECTS OF ADRENERGIC BLOCKADE

Organ or System	Receptor	Effect of Adrenergic Blockade
Heart	β_1	Decreased rate of sinoatrial node discharge Decreased contractility Decreased conduction velocity in atria, AV node, and ventricles Decreased ventricular automaticity
Blood vessels	α	Vasodilatation and relaxation of arterioles and venules
	β_2	Vasoconstriction of arterioles, especially in skeletal muscle
Lungs	β_2	Constriction of bronchial smooth muscle
Gastrointestinal tract	α and β	Increase of peristalsis
Pancreas (islets of Langerhans)	α	Increased insulin release
	β	Decreased insulin release

mixed in 500 ml of solution. The infusion is titrated according to the patient's preordered blood pressure.

Mephentermine Sulfate. Mephentermine sulfate (Wyamine) can be administered in doses of 15–35 mg, as needed, intravenously or intramuscularly. The action starts in 5–15 minutes and has a duration of one to two hours. However, most commonly, a solution of 0.1% in 500 ml dextrose in water is prepared and infused. Action begins immediately and continues for 30–40 minutes after the infusion is terminated.

Methoxamine Hydrochloride. Methoxamine hydrochloride (Vasoxyl) is given slowly, intravenously, in doses of 3–5 mg as needed. Its vasopressor action begins immediately and remains for one hour after termination. Intramuscularly, 10–15 mg is given; this dose may be repeated after 15 minutes, if necessary. Action begins in 15 minutes and lasts 1.5 hours.

ADRENERGIC-BLOCKING (SYMPATHOLYTIC) AGENTS

The adrenergic blockers are a group of medications that interfere with the transmission of nerve impulses to ad-

renergic neuroeffectors. The adrenergic blockers occupy the adrenergic receptor sites (alpha or beta) without evoking any response from the effector muscle or gland. As long as the adrenergic-blocking drugs occupy these receptors sites, all normal neural or hormonal activity is blocked. The adrenergic-blocking agents include both alpha- and beta-blocking agents. Table 19–6 describes the effects of both alpha and beta blockade in the body.

ALPHA-ADRENERGIC BLOCKING MEDICATIONS

The alpha-adrenergic blocking agents inhibit the effects of alpha receptors primarily in vascular smooth muscle (Table 19–7). These agents are more effective against the action of circulating catecholamines than against catecholamines released from storage sites, and they have relatively limited usefulness. The alpha blockers are obtained from natural sources such as ergot and its derivatives, or they are synthetically prepared.

Action

The alpha blockers, since their primary site of action is in the vascular smooth muscle, have two end effects. First, the alpha blockers interfere with sympathetic stimulation in the peripheral vessels, leading to relaxation in the smooth muscle walls, and thus increase blood flow to the skin and other superficial organs. Because alpha receptors are more abundant in skin vessels than in the skeletal muscle vessels, blood flow to the skin increases. These drugs are most effective in treating Raynaud's disease. They have little effect in treating chronic occlusive peripheral vascular disease.

The second effect is a reduction in peripheral vascular resistance, which lowers blood pressure. Prazosin (Minipress) and tolazoline (Priscoline) are effective antihypertensives and are discussed in detail in Chapter 29. Unfortunately, the majority of these medications have proven disappointing in the management of hypertension. As the alpha blockers lower the blood pressure (especially in the standing position), they also cause a reflex tachycardia because they fail to block the beta receptors in the heart. The increased pulse rate can precipitate attacks of angina pectoris, coronary insufficiency, and even congestive heart failure, particularly in a person with a history of hypertensive heart disease. The alpha blocker phentolamine hydrochloride (Regitine) is used to treat infiltration of strong alpha agents like levarterenol and epinephrine.

Phenoxybenzamine Hydrochloride

Phenoxybenzamine hydrochloride (Dibenzyline) is a long-lasting alpha-adrenergic blocking agent that blocks or abolishes adrenergic activity through noncompetitive inhibition. It is particularly useful in controlling episodes of hypertension and sweating secondary to *pheochromocytoma* (tumor of the adrenal medulla). Only about 20%–30% of the oral dose is absorbed. The drug is excreted in both urine and feces and through the bile.

TEXT RESUMES ON PAGE 434

Table 19–7. ALPHA-ADRENERGIC BLOCKING DRUGS

Name	Dosage	Mode of Administration	Pharmacokinetics
Phenoxybenzamine Hydrochloride (Dibenzyline)			
Action: Blocks or abolishes adrenergic activity through noncompetitive inhibition.			
Use: To control episodes of hypertension and sweating secondary to pheochromocytoma.			
	Adults: 20–120 mg daily in single or divided doses	PO	O: 2 hr P: accumulates over 7 days D: 3–4 days ½ L: 24 hr PB: UA B: unknown E: urine, feces, bile
	Children: 0.2 mg/kg/day up to 10 mg	PO	Same as for adults.
Phentolamine Hydrochloride (Regitine)			
Action: Competitively blocks alpha-adrenergic receptors.			
Use: Secondary hypertension resulting from pheochromocytoma; to treat extravasation of vasopressors.			
	Adults: 5–10 mg in 10 ml normal saline infused into extravasation site		
	Adults: 5 mg	IV	O: immediately P: 2 min D: 10–15 min ½ L: UA PB: UA B: unknown E: urine
	Children: 1 mg	IV	Same as for adults.
	Adults: 5 mg	IM	O: immediately P: 20 min D: 3–4 hr
	Children: 1 mg	IM	Same as for adults.
Ergotamine Tartrate (Ergomar)			
Action: For all: Constrict vascular smooth muscle of uterus; reduce extracranial blood flow.			
Use for all: Acute vascular headaches.			
	Adults: 2 mg at onset of headache and repeat in 30 min (no more than 3 tablets/day or 10 tablets/wk)	SL	O: undetermined P: 2 hr D: 24 hr ½ L: 2.7 hr α phase; 21 hr β phase PB: UA B: liver E: urine

Key to Abbreviations in the *Pharmacokinetics* column O-onset; P-peak; D-duration; PB-protein bound; B-biotransformed in; E-excreted in; ½ L-halflife.
*Within the column listing adverse effects, <u>underlines</u> indicate the most common effects, and CAPITALS indicate life-threatening effects.

Contraindications/ Precautions	Adverse Effects*	Interactions	Nursing Implications
Contraindicated where a fall in blood pressure is undesirable. Use cautiously in marked cerebral or coronary ateriosclerosis, renal insufficiency, respiratory infection, reflex tachycardia, and orthostatic hypotension.	Neuro: dizziness, fainting CV: palpitations, postural hypotension, CIRCULATORY FAILURE Resp: nasal congestion GI: GI upset, vomiting GU: inhibition of ejaculation	Potentiation of hypotensive effect with concurrent antihypertensives.	ASSESSMENT: Closely observe blood pressure when dose is being started or increased. INTERVENTION: Instruct the patient to avoid cough or cold medications. Administer with milk or food to lessen GI upset. Change body position slowly to prevent orthostatic hypotension. Has cumulative effect. Protect from light.
Contraindicated in hypersensitivity, myocardial infarction, pregnancy, and lactation. Use cautiously in gastritis, peptic ulcer, coronary artery disease.	Neuro: weakness, dizziness CV: orthostatic hypotension Resp: nasal congestion GI: GI irritation	Antagonizes epinephrine and ephedrine.	ASSESSMENT: Assess patient's condition carefully during administration.
Contraindicated in hypersensitivity, pregnancy, sepsis, vascular disease, hepatic or renal disease, marked atherosclerosis, hypertension, and anemia.	Neuro: ergotism, including numbness and tingling of digits, weakness CV: gangrene GI: nausea and vomiting	Vasoconstrictors cause hypertension Nitroglycerin increases availability of ergot.	INTERVENTION: Drug therapy is begun as soon as possible after onset of headache. Patient should lie down in dark, quiet room for 2–3 hours after taking drug. Do not increase dose

CONTINUED ON THE FOLLOWING PAGE

Alpha-Adrenergic Blockers

Table 19–7. ALPHA-ADRENERGIC BLOCKING DRUGS– *CONTINUED*

Name	Dosage	Mode of Administration	Pharmacokinetics
Ergotamine Tartrate–Continued	*Older children and adolescents:* 1 mg at onset and repeat in 30 min if needed	SL	Same as for adults.
(Medihaler)	*Adults:* 1 inhalation, repeat in 5 min; maximum of 6 times in 24 hr or 15/wk	Aerosol	P: rapid

Ergotamine with Caffeine (Cafergot)

Action: Constrict vascular smooth muscle of uterus; reduce extracranial blood flow.

Use: Acute vascular headaches.

	Dosage	Mode of Administration	Pharmacokinetics
	Adults: 1–2 tablets at onset, repeated at 30 min, for a total of 6 tablets/24 hr, not to exceed 10 tablets/wk	PO	Same as ergotamine tartrate.
	Older children and adolescents: 1 tablet at onset and repeat in 30 min if needed	PO	Same as ergotamine tartrate.

Dihydroergotamine Mesylate (D.H.E. 45)

Action: Constrict vascular smooth muscle of uterus; reduce extracranial blood flow.

Use: Acute vascular headaches.

	Dosage	Mode of Administration	Pharmacokinetics
	Adults: 1 ml repeated in 1 hr if needed (total dose of 3 ml) *Children:* no dosage recommended	IM	O: 15–30 min P: 2 hr D: 3–4 hr ½ L: UA PB: UA B: liver E: urine

Methysergide (Sansert)

Action: Constrict vascular smooth muscle of uterus; reduce extracranial blood flow.

Use: Prophylaxis for vascular headaches; not used for acute attacks.

	Dosage	Mode of Administration	Pharmacokinetics
	4–8 mg daily in divided doses	PO	O: 1–days P: 2 days D: 1–2 days ½ L: 10 hr PB: UA B: liver E: urine

Key to Abbreviations in the *Pharmacokinetics* column O-onset; P-peak; D-duration; PB-protein bound; B-biotransformed in; E-excreted in; ½ L-halflife.

*Within the column listing adverse effects, underlines indicate the most common effects, and CAPITALS indicate life-threatening effects.

Contraindications/ Precautions	Adverse Effects*	Interactions	Nursing Implications
Use with caution in lactating women, the elderly, and children.			without consulting physician. Do not administer more than specifically ordered.
Same as ergotamine tartrate.	Same as ergotamine tartrate.	Same as ergotamine tartrate.	Same as ergotamine tartrate.
Same as ergotamine tartrate.	Same as ergotamine tartrate.	Same as ergotamine tartrate.	Same as ergotamine tartrate.
Contraindicated in fibrotic process, pulmonary or collagen diseases, pregnancy. Precautions are the same as with ergotamine.	Neuro: insomnia, drowsiness, mild euphoria CV: chest pain, tachycardia, edema Renal: RETROPERITONEAL FIBROSIS, including fatigue, flank pain, dysuria, increased BUN GI: nausea, vomiting, diarrhea, weight gain Hemo: neutropenia, eosinophilia Integ: facial flush, telangiectasia	None significant.	ASSESSMENT: Assess frequently for edema. INTERVENTION: Change position slowly. Instruct patient to take medication with meals and use caution when operating heavy equipment. EVALUATION: Withdraw drug slowly to prevent headache rebound. There must be a drug-free interval for 3–4 weeks every 6 months.

CONTINUED ON THE FOLLOWING PAGE

Table 19–7. ALPHA-ADRENERGIC BLOCKING DRUGS–*CONTINUED*

Name	Dosage	Mode of Administration	Pharmacokinetics
Dihydrogenated Ergot Alkaloids (Hydergine)			
Action: May increase brain metabolism.			
Use: Elderly persons who have recently had a symptomatic decline in mental capacity and self-care activities.			
	Adults: 0.5 mg 3 times daily	SL	O: SL, rapid; PO, 30–60 min P: 1 hr D: 24 hr
	1 mg 3 times daily	PO	½ L: UA PB: UA P: 0.6–3 hr (PO)
	Children: no dosage recommended		B: liver, high first pass E: urine

Key to Abbreviations in the *Pharmacokinetics* column O-onset; P-peak; D-duration; PB-protein bound; B-biotransformed in; E-excreted in; ½ L-halflife.

*Within the column listing adverse effects, underlines indicate the most common effects, and CAPITALS indicate life-threatening effects.

CONTRAINDICATIONS, PRECAUTIONS, AND ADVERSE EFFECTS. Phenoxybenzamine hydrochloride is contraindicated in patients in whom a decrease in blood pressure may be undesirable. It is given cautiously to persons with marked cerebral or coronary arteriosclerosis, renal insufficiency, and respiratory infection. The side effects include nasal congestion, palpitations, dizziness, fainting, inhibition of ejaculation, gastrointestinal irritation, and lethargy. Toxic symptoms include severe postural hypotension, vomiting, lethargy, shock, and circulatory failure.

DOSAGE. Phenoxybenzamine hydrochloride is given orally in dosages ranging from 20–120 mg daily in single or divided doses. Action begins in two hours and has a duration of 30–36 hours.

NURSING ACTION. To prevent gastrointestinal upset, phenoxybenzamine hydrochloride can be administered with milk or food. The blood pressure is observed closely during dosage increases. Patients are cautioned to change body position slowly to reduce or prevent orthostatic hypotension. Cough and cold medications that contain sympathomimetic preparations should be avoided.

Phentolamine Hydrochloride

Phentolamine hydrochloride (Regitine) competitively blocks alpha-adrenergic receptors, but its action is transient and incomplete.

USES. Phentolamine hydrochloride has several general uses. It is used to treat secondary hypertension related to increased levels of norepinephrine and epinephrine that result from a pheochromocytoma; it is used to treat extravasation of vasopressors into the subcutaneous tissue, and it is used to reduce afterload through arterial dilation. Phentolamine improves cardiac output but does not change PAOP.

CONTRAINDICATIONS, PRECAUTIONS, AND ADVERSE EFFECTS. Phentolamine hydrochloride is contraindicated in persons demonstrating acute hypersensitivity, in those who have had a myocardial infarction, and in pregnant or lactating women. It is given cautiously to persons with gastritis, peptic ulcer, or coronary artery disease. The most common side effects of phentolamine hydrochloride include weakness, dizziness, orthostatic hypotension, nasal congestion, and gastrointestinal irritation; a shock-like state occurs less commonly.

DOSAGE. The dosage used to treat extravasation is 5–10 mg in 10 ml of 0.9% sodium chloride solution injected into the infiltrated area within 12 hours. When used to reduce afterload, phentolamine is titratable due to its short half-life.

Ergot Alkaloids

The ergot alkaloids are derived from a fungus grown on rye. Besides being alpha-adrenergic blockers that reduce extracranial blood flow, the ergot derivatives constrict the vascular smooth muscle of the uterus. The gravid uterus is more sensitive to these effects.

ERGOTAMINE TARTRATE. Ergotamine tartrate (Ergomar) is a natural amino acid alkaloid of ergot that has alpha-adrenergic blocking properties. It is used primarily in the acute treatment of vascular headaches, including migraines and cluster headaches.

Contraindications and Precautions. Ergotamine tartrate and its derivatives are contraindicated in known hypersensitivity, sepsis, vascular disease, hepatic and renal disease, marked atherosclerosis, hypertension, and anemia because all of these conditions may be worsened. It is contraindicated in pregnancy because it is a powerful uterine stimulant and may cause fetal

Contraindications/ Precautions	Adverse Effects*	Interactions	Nursing Implications
Contraindicated in hypersensitivity and psychosis.	GI: buccal irritation, from SL form, nausea, GI disturbances	None significant.	ASSESSMENT: Assess for change or improvement. INTERVENTION: Instruct patient to take medication with food to decrease GI distress and to allow SL tablets to dissolve completely under tongue.

harm. It is given cautiously to lactating women, elderly persons, and children.

Adverse Effects. The most common side effects are those of nausea and vomiting, *ergotism.* Early signs of ergotism include nausea, vomiting, and complaints of abdominal cramps. Sometimes, the patient may have a headache and show signs of confusion. More serious signs are those of circulatory stasis, including itching, tingling, numbness, and coldness in the fingers and toes. This can lead to gangrene of the nose, digits, and ears. Patients may also experience seizures; rapid, weak, or irregular pulse, and confusion. Patients are encouraged to report these symptoms, and the medication should be discontinued.

Interactions. Interaction occurs between ergotamine tartrate and nitroglycerin, increasing the availability of ergot products. Concurrent vasoconstriction may cause dangerous hypertension.

Dosage. The sublingual dose of 2 mg is rapidly absorbed. The dose can be repeated in 30 minutes if relief is not obtained. Drug therapy is begun as soon as possible after onset of headache. The patient should lie down in a dark, quiet room for two to three hours after taking any ergot preparation. The patient should not take more than three tablets in a 24-hour period.

ERGOTAMINE WITH CAFFEINE. Ergotamine with caffeine (Cafergot) contains 1 mg of ergotamine tartrate and 100 mg of caffeine in each tablet. The caffeine, as a cerebral vasoconstrictor, probably increases the effectiveness of the ergotamine tartrate. The usual dose is one to two tablets at onset of headache, repeated every 30 minutes for a total of six tablets, if needed, not to exceed ten tablets per week.

DIHYDROERGOTAMINE MESYLATE. Dihydroergotamine mesylate (D.H.E. 45) is a hydrogenated ergotamine derivative that has a direct constricting effect on smooth muscle of peripheral and cranial blood vessels. It is used to prevent or relieve vascular headaches. It is available only in intramuscular form; the usual dose is

1 ml, repeated in one hour, if needed, up to a total of 3 ml. Its action starts in 15–30 minutes and lasts three to four hours. Patients should be supine when receiving parenteral doses, and the pulse rate and blood pressure are watched closely.

METHYSERGIDE. Methysergide (Sansert) is an ergot derivative, but unlike ergotamine it has weak vasoconstrictor and oxytocic actions. It exerts a potent blocking effect on serotonin activity, which may be implicated in the mechanism of vascular headaches. It is not useful in treating acute attacks, only in prophylaxis.

Contraindications, Precautions, and Adverse Effects. Contraindications include fibrotic processes, pulmonary or collagen disease, and all other precautions that apply to ergotamine tartrate. Methysergide has many severe adverse effects, including fibrosis of the retroperitoneal area (causing fatigue, flank pain, dysuria, increased blood urea nitrogen), chest pain, and tachycardia. To prevent these complications, the drug is usually stopped for four weeks every six months. When the medication is stopped, the dosage is titrated down slowly to prevent a rebound of migraine or cluster headaches. Other adverse effects include coldness and numbness in the digits, gastrointestinal complaints, flushing, and insomnia.

Dosage. The usual oral dosage is 4–8 mg daily.

DIHYDROGENATED ERGOT ALKALOIDS. Dihydrogenated ergot alkaloids (Hydergine), which contains dihydroergocornine mesylate, dihydroergocristine mesylate, and dihydroergocryptine mesylate, are indicated in elderly persons who have recently had a symptomatic decline in mental capacity and self-care activities. The efficacy of this drug is controversial. Some researchers have demonstrated that patients are more mentally alert, less confused, more cooperative, and more involved with self-care activities. Its pharmacologic action is not clearly understood but is thought to increase brain metabolism. The drug is administered either sublingually in doses of 0.5 mg three times daily, or orally in doses of 1 mg three times daily. It peaks in one hour and has a duration of 24 hours. The sublingual form is more readily absorbed and available, but it may cause buccal irritation and swelling. The oral form may cause gastrointestinal irritation. It is contraindicated in patients with known hypersensitivity and in all psychotic patients.

BETA-ADRENERGIC BLOCKING MEDICATIONS

The beta-adrenergic blockers were first introduced in the 1960s. Until 1978, the only beta blocker approved by the Food and Drug Administration in the United States was propranolol (Inderal). Since 1978, many new beta blockers have been released, including metoprolol tartrate (Lopressor), nadolol (Corgard), timolol maleate (Blocadren), atenolol (Tenormin), pindolol (Visken), acebutolol (Sectral), labetalol (Trandate, Normodyne), and esmolol (Brevibloc). The beta blockers are shown in Table 19–8. Beta blockers are classified by receptor affinity, which refers to their selectively acting on the $beta_1$ receptors in the heart or on $beta_2$ receptors found in bronchial and vascular musculature.

Action

The beta-adrenergic blockers compete with epinephrine for available beta-receptor sites. These medications inhibit the response to adrenergic stimuli in either the $beta_1$ or $beta_2$ receptors. Some beta-blocking drugs are nonspecific and block $beta_1$ and $beta_2$ receptors. $Beta_1$ receptors are found primarily in the heart whereas $beta_2$ receptors are found in peripheral circulation, pulmonary airways, and the central nervous system. Blocking the beta-adrenergic receptor sites in the heart results in a decrease in heart rate during both rest and exercise, and a decrease in myocardial contractility and ultimately in cardiac output. It is through these mechanisms that angina is most likely controlled. Conduction velocity through the atrioventricular node and the firing rate in the sinoatrial node also decrease. These effects assist in preventing exercise-induced increases in the heart rate and in effectively treating various dysrhythmias. Beta blockers do not abolish the response to catecholamines but simply require a higher concentration of catecholamine to be effective. This activity is known as competitive inhibition.

Some beta blockers have local anesthetic effects on peripheral nerves. These drugs also have a quinidine-like action on cardiac muscle, pacemakers, and conducting tissue. The general term conducting "membrane-stabilizing activity" is commonly used to characterize this property.

Uses

Over the last 25 years, beta-blockers have been used to treat cardiovascular, endocrine, neurologic, psychiatric, and gastrointestinal diseases. Beta blockers are effective in reducing the frequency and severity of anginal episodes, the consumption of nitroglycerin, and the electrocardiographic evidence of ischemia; and they are effective in increasing exercise performance in patients with chronic stable angina pectoris.

Beta-blockers are effective antihypertensive agents for managing mild, moderate, and severe hypertension. They lower systolic and diastolic supine and standing blood pressures at rest and during exercise. The entire complex and incompletely understood at this time. Possible mechanisms of action include a reduction in cardiac output, a reduction in plasma renin activity, and a central nervous system sympatholytic action. Persons more likely to respond favorably to beta blockers are young, white individuals who have a higher than normal plasma renin level, increased sympathetic activity, higher cardiac output, normal left ventricular function, and labile hypertension.

Beta-blockers are used to treat various dysrhythmias, including fast supraventricular rhythms and atrial and ventricular ectopic beats.

The newest and most promising use of beta-blockers is for cardiac protection during a myocardial infarction and secondary prevention of myocardial infarction. Several drug trials are ongoing to determine the effectiveness of beta blockers in decreasing infarct size, decreasing the incidence of ventricular dysrhythmias, and decreasing creatine phosphokinase. Preliminary findings indicate that beta blockers (metoprolol—Lopressor—is the only approved drug at this time, although the new ultra-short-acting beta blockers may prove beneficial) are best administered within 12 hours to a patient with an anterior myocardial infarction with no failure and whose heart rate is above 75 beats per minute. It is hoped that this therapy may lower post–myocardial infarction mortality.

Beta-blockers have been used for several years as a secondary prevention for a second myocardial infarction. Propranolol, 60–80 mg tid; metoprolol, 100 mg bid; and timolol, 10 mg bid are started within five to nine days of an acute myocardial infarction and are continued for six months to two years. Research has indicated that these drugs, which decrease myocardial oxygen consumption, decrease sympathetic nervous system effects on the heart, decrease overall mortality 8%–10%, and decrease the incidence of sudden death by 45%.

Beta-blockers are used in both hypertrophic and congestive cardiomyopathies to decrease contractility and to decrease heart rate, with a resultant improvement of left ventricular filling pressure.

Beta-blockers are effective in the prevention but not in the treatment of migraines. The exact mechanism of action is unknown, but it may result from the effect of beta blockers on peripheral resistance.

Beta-blockers are effective in treating the symptoms of hyperthyroidism. They may inhibit the conversion of T_4 to T_3 as well as acting as a nonspecific anti-adrenergic to inhibit sympathetic activity.

Beta-blockers are used to manage glaucoma. They decrease the production of aqueous humor, thus reducing pressure in the eye.

Lastly, beta blockers are used in a variety of neurologic and psychiatric disorders including tremor, anxiety, alcohol withdrawal syndrome, and neuroses. The mechanism of action is probably through their depressive effect on the central nervous system.

Pharmacokinetics

The beta blockers are either lipid or water soluble in the body. The solubility affects the pharmacokinetics and possibly the adverse effects of the drug. Table 19–9 identifies the lipid- and water-soluble beta blockers.

ABSORPTION. The lipid-soluble products are more readily and more completely absorbed from the gastrointestinal system than are the water-soluble products. The lipid-soluble products are best given on an empty stomach to decrease their absorption and biotransformation.

DISTRIBUTION. The lipid-soluble products are approximately 90% plasma bound and are widely distributed to tissues. They readily cross the blood–brain barrier. Propranolol (Inderal) is found in the central nervous system in concentrations 26 times higher than in the serum. This fact accounts for the adverse effects on the central nervous system, although some recent research suggests that there is no difference in central nervous system effects between lipid- and water-soluble beta blockers.

The water-soluble products are only 3% plasma bound and do not cross the blood–brain barrier and therefore have few central nervous system effects.

Both products reach maximal plasma concentrations within one to three hours.

BIOTRANSFORMATION. The lipid-soluble products are metabolized in the liver, often through presystemic elimination (first-pass effect, previously discussed in Chapter 4, Phases of Drug Action). Smoking and consumption of alcohol have an effect on the liver and therefore decrease serum levels of the lipid-soluble beta blockers. Due to their rapid metabolization in the liver, they have a short half-life, usually two to six hours.

The water-soluble products are not biotransformed in the body but are excreted unchanged in the urine. These products have a longer half-life (6–17 hours) and can often be administered once daily, improving patient compliance. Smoking and alcohol consumption do not affect plasma levels of the water-soluble beta blockers.

EXCRETION. The fat-soluble products are excreted in bile. For this reason, they are more safely administered to patients with reduced renal function. Pindolol (Visken), unlike the other fat-soluble products, has balanced excretion—half through bile and half unchanged in the urine.

The water-soluble products are excreted unchanged in the urine. For this reason, they are safely administered to patients with hepatic dysfunction.

Contraindications and Precautions

The beta blockers are contraindicated in congestive heart failure and bradycardia. In addition, many of the beta blockers are contraindicated in persons with bronchial asthma because of their beta$_2$-blocking effects. Beta blockers, especially the nonspecific drugs, are given cautiously to persons with peripheral vascular insufficiency because they decrease blood flow to the extremities through peripheral vasoconstriction; to persons with renal or hepatic impairment, because of their serum accumulation in these diseases; and to persons with hypoglycemia. The medications should not be stopped abruptly, but titrated down slowly, usually over a week, to avoid the rebound effect of an acute myocardial infarction when the patient is being treated for angina.

Adverse Effects

For most persons receiving beta blockers, the incidence of adverse effects is relatively low. Some of the adverse effects of beta blockers are due to the blockade of the beta$_2$ receptors, primarily those located in the lung. This blockade results in bronchospasm, particularly in patients with any form of chronic obstructive lung disease, including asthma. Propranolol hydrochloride, nadolol, and timolol maleate are beta$_1$ and beta$_2$ blockers. Metoprolol, atenolol, and acebutolol are administered in low doses, as highly selective beta$_1$ blockers. In larger doses, however, they also block beta$_2$ receptors and thus must be used cautiously in patients with lung disease if administered in dosages of more than 150–200 mg/day. Fatigue, a common complaint, may result from the hemodynamic effects of these agents or from peripheral metabolic effects, such as inhibition of lactic acid release from skeletal muscle. Patients with peripheral vascular impairment experience a decreasd blood flow in muscles by 30%, which may worsen existing conditions. Central nervous system complaints of vivid dreams, insomnia, depression, hallucinations, and dizziness may be more common with the lipid-soluble beta blockers. Additional adverse effects include bradycardia, drug fever, nausea, vomiting, diarrhea, transient thrombocytopenia, agranulocytosis, and sleep disorders.

The blood glucose level is usually normal at rest, but may drop during exercise. This is because the glycogenolytic and lipolytic actions of endogenous catecholamines—normally released in response to the increased energy requirements during exercise and in response to hypoglycemia—are inhibited by beta blockade. However, this does not appear to occur in practice. Therefore, beta blockers are given cautiously to patients with diabetes who are taking insulin or oral hypoglycemic drugs. Beta blockers may also mask the clinical signs of hypoglycemia: tachycardia, diaphoresis, and a slightly decreased diastolic pressure. In fact, the opposite clinical signs may appear, including increased diastolic pressure and bradycardia. Beta blockers may also precipitate hyperglycemia because they block the release of insulin.

Beta blockers, except pindolol, tend to elevate plasma levels of triglycerides and low-density lipoproteins, which may contribute to the development of atherosclerotic heart disease and lower plasma levels of high-density lipoproteins, which have a protective effect.

TEXT RESUMES ON PAGE 444

Table 19-8. BETA-ADRENERGIC BLOCKERS

Name	Dosage	Mode of Administration	Pharmacokinetics	Blocking Activity

For All Beta-Adrenergic Blockers

Action: Compete with epinephrine for available beta receptor sites. Inhibit response to adrenergic stimuli in either β_1 or β_2 receptors.

Propranolol Hydrochloride (Inderal)

Use: Dysrhythmias, myocardial infarction prophylaxis, IHSS, pheochromocytoma, hypertension, migraine prophylaxis, angina pectoris

Name	Dosage	Mode of Administration	Pharmacokinetics	Blocking Activity
	Hypertension: 80–480 mg/day in divided doses	PO (can be crushed)	O: 30 min P: 1–1.5 hr D: 6 hr ½ L: 3–5 hr PB: 90% B: liver E: urine	β_1, β_2
	80–480 mg (SR) daily *Angina:* 10–20 mg qid, 40–80 mg (SR) daily (up to 320 mg/day)	PO	P: 6 hr D: 24 hr	
	Dysrhythmias: 10–30 mg qid, up to 160–480 mg/day	PO	Same as above.	
	1–3 mg/min	IV (drug is given in separate boluses)	O: 2 min P: 15 min D: 4 hr	

Key to Abbreviations in the *Pharmacokinetics* column O-onset; P-peak; D-duration; PB-protein bound; B-biotransformed in; E-excreted in; ½ L-halflife.

*Within the column listing adverse effects, underlines indicate the most common effects, and CAPITALS indicate life-threatening effects.

Contraindications/ Precautions	Adverse Effects*	Interactions	Nursing Implications
Contraindicated in congestive heart failure, cardiogenic shock, bradycardia, greater than first-degree AV block. Use cautiously in hypersensitive patients with CHF, WPW syndrome, bronchospastic disease, pregnancy; safety in children has not been established. DO NOT STOP ABRUPTLY.	Most are mild and transient and rarely require withdrawal of therapy Neuro: dizziness, vertigo, fatigue, depression, nervousness, decreased concentration, nightmares CV: BRADYCARDIA, chest pain, worsening of angina, peripheral vascular insufficiency, DECREASED BLOOD PRESSURE, CHF Resp: bronchospasm, dyspnea, cough, crackles, wheeziness GI: gastric pain, flatulence, nausea, diarrhea Hemo: agranulocytosis, thrombocytopenia purpura Integ: rash, pruritus Allergic: pharyngitis, laryngospasm Endo: increase/decrease glucose, unstable diabetes, elevates plasma triglycerides and low-density lipoproteins GU: impotence, decreased libido, dysuria Ophth: eye irritation Muscskel: joint pain, muscle cramps	Increased potential for bradycardia and cardiac depression with cardiac glycosides—quinidine, verapamil, diltiazem Increased potential for hypoglycemia with insulin Increased hypotensive effect with diuretics, phenothiazines, and captopril Bronchodilating and cardiostimulating effects of sympathomimetics and methylzanthines are antagonized. Increased beta blockade with concurrent use of chlorpromazine, cimetidine, oral contraceptives, furosemide, and hydralazine.	ASSESSMENT: Cardiac rhythm including rate (particularly bradycardia), regularity, quality of the pulse, ECG, neurologic symptoms, urinary output, and level of anxiety should be monitored. Assess electrolytes, particularly potassium and calcium. May be discontinued prior to cardiac diagnostic tests or surgery. INTERVENTION: Caution patient not to smoke (regular cigarettes or marijuana), because this may raise the blood pressure. May produce drowsiness, dizziness, lightheadedness, blurred vision. Advise patient to observe caution in driving or performing tasks requiring alertness. May decrease libido. Teach patient to monitor own blood pressure and pulse. EVALUATION: Dosage is gradually reduced, not stopped abruptly. Evaluate for effectiveness, sensitivity, and adverse effects. Evaluate weight (report weight gain of 2 lb/week) and signs of edema and shortness of breath frequently. Monitor blood sugar in diabetics carefully. Notify physician if CHF occurs, or if a slowed pulse rate, confusion, skin rash, fever, sore throat, and unusual bleeding or bruising occur.
Contraindicated in bronchial asthma, bronchospasm, and COPD. Use cautiously in peripheral vascular insufficiency, hepatic impairment, or diabetes.	Same as above.	Decreased effectiveness with concurrent use of thyroid hormone. Lidocaine clearance is reduced. Lab: May interfere with tests for glucosuria.	INTERVENTION: Instruct patient to take with food to enhance absorption.

CONTINUED ON THE FOLLOWING PAGE

Table 19–8. BETA-ADRENERGIC BLOCKERS–*CONTINUED*

Name	Dosage	Mode of Administration	Pharmacokinetics	Blocking Activity
Propranolol Hydrochloride– *Continued*	1–2 mg *Migraine:* 160–240 mg/day in divided doses, or once daily, or SR	IV bolus PO	same as IV	

Timolol Maleate (Blocadren)

Use: Hypertension, myocardial infarction prophylaxis.

	Dosage	Mode of Administration	Pharmacokinetics	Blocking Activity
	Hypertension: 10–60 mg daily in divided doses *Myocardial prophylactic:* 10 mg bid	PO	O: 30 min P: 1–2 hr D:4–6 hr ½ L: 4 hr BP: 10%–60% B: liver E: urine	β_1, β_2

Nadolol (Corgard)

Use: Angina, hypertension.

	Dosage	Mode of Administration	Pharmacokinetics	Blocking Activity
	40–320 mg once daily	PO	O: 3–7 hr P: 7–10 hr D: 20–24 hr ½ L: 20–24 hr PB: 30% B: unchanged E: unchanged in urine	β_1, β_2

Metoprolol (Lopressor)

Use: Hypertension, myocardial infarction prophylaxis.

	Dosage	Mode of Administration	Pharmacokinetics	Blocking Activity
	Hypertension: I*: 100 mg/day in single or divided doses M*: 100–400 mg/day *MI:* As soon as patient is hemodynamically stable, 3 boluses, 5 mg each, at 2-min intervals; then after 15 min, start 50 mg q 6 hr for 48 hr; then 100 mg bid for 2 yr.	PO IV PO PO	O: 10–90 min D: up to 24 hr P: 1–3 hr Maximum effect in about 1 wk after first dose ½ L: 3–7 hr PB: 12% B: liver E: urine	β_1 (low dose only)

Atenolol (Tenormin)

Use: Angina, hypertension.

	Dosage	Mode of Administration	Pharmacokinetics	Blocking Activity
	50–100 mg once daily	PO	O: 1.0 hr P: 2–4 hr (up to 1 wk for max effect) D: 24 hr ½ L: 6–9 hr PB: 6–16%B: B: none E: unchanged in urine	β_1 (low doses)

Key to Abbreviations in the *Pharmacokinetics* column O-onset; P-peak; D-duration; PB-protein bound; B-biotransformed in; E-excreted in; ½ L-halflife.
*Within the column listing adverse effects, underlines indicate the most common effects, and CAPITALS indicate life-threatening effects.

Contraindications/ Precautions	Adverse Effects*	Interactions	Nursing Implications
Same as above.	Same as above.	Same as above.	Same as above.
Same as above. Use caution in renal disease.	Same as above.	Same as above.	Same as above. INTERVENTION: May be taken without regard to meals.
Contraindicated in treatment of myocardial infarction with heart rate less than 45 mmHg and systolic blood pressure less than 100 mmHg. Use cautiously in peripheral vascular insufficiency, hepatic impairment, diabetes, and hypoglycemia.	Same as above.	Same as above. Decreased effectiveness with concurrent thyroid hormone. Lidocaine clearance is reduced.	Same as above.
Use cautiously in hypertensive patients with CHF controlled by digitalis and diuretics, and in patients with impaired renal function or hyperthyroidism.	Same as above.	Same as above.	Same as above. INTERVENTION: Does not potentiate insulin-induced hypoglycemia or delay return of blood glucose to normal. Often administered with a diuretic. Administer 50-mg dose after renal dialysis.

CONTINUED ON THE FOLLOWING PAGE

Table 19–8. BETA-ADRENERGIC BLOCKERS–*CONTINUED*

Name	Dosage	Mode of Administration	Pharmacokinetics	Blocking Activity
Pindolol (Visken)				
Use: Hypertension.				
	15–60 mg/daily in 2–3 divided doses	PO	O: 3 hrs D: 24 hr P: 2–3 hr ½ L: 6–9 hr PB: 40%–60% B: liver E: urine	β_1 and β_2; intrinsic sympathetic
Labetalol Hydrochloride (Normodyne, Trandate)				
Use: Hypertension.				
	Initial dose: 100 mg bid; increments of 100 mg bid every 2–3 days *Maintenance:* 200–400 mg bid up to 2400 mg/day	PO	O: 1–2 hr P: 2–4 hr D: 8–24 hr ½ L: 6–8 hr PB: 50% B: liver E: urine, bile	β_1 and β_2, alpha blocker
	Initial dose: 0.25 mg/kg; then 40–80 mg given at 10-min intervals	IV	O: 2–5 min P: 5–15 min D: 16–18 hr	
	20 mg IV slowly over 2 min; additional injections of 40–80 mg every 10 min up to total of 300 mg	IV bolus		
	2 mg/min	Slow IV		
Acebutolol (Sectral)				
Use: Hypertension, ventricular dysrhythmias.				
	Hypertension: 200–1200 mg in single or divided doses *Ventricular dysrhythmias:* Initial Dose: 200 mg bid Maintenance Dose: 600–1200 mg in single or divided doses	PO	O: 1.0 hr P: 2–6 hr D: 6–10 hr ½ L: 3–4 hr (alpha); 6–12 hr (beta) PB: 11%–25% B: liver E: liver, urine	β_1 (low doses); intrinsic sympathetic activity
Esmolol Hydrochloride (Brevibloc)				
Use: Supraventricular tachycardia and noncompensatory tachycardia.				
	50–200 µg/kg/min *Loading Dose:* 500 µg/kg/min for 1 min then 50 µg/kg for 4 min continued until effect reached *Maintenance Dose:* 25–50 µg/kg/min; ideally used for 24 hr or less	IV	O: 1 min P: 5 min D: 20 min ½ L: 9 min PB: 55% B: in red blood cell E: urine	β_1

Key to Abbreviations in the *Pharmacokinetics* column O-onset; P-peak; D-duration; PB-protein bound; B-biotransformed in; E-excreted in; ½ L-halflife.
*Within the column listing adverse effects, underlines indicate the most common effects, and CAPITALS indicate life-threatening effects.

Contraindications/ Precautions	Adverse Effects*	Interactions	Nursing Implications
Same as above. Use cautiously in asthmatics and diabetics.	Same as above.	Same as above.	Same as above. INTERVENTION: May be taken without regard to meals.
Same as above.	Same as above. CNS: (parenteral) hypoesthesia (numbness), transient scalp tingling CV: (parenteral) VENTRICULAR DYSRHYTHMIAS, orthostatic hypotension GU: ejaculation failure, difficulty in micturition Ophth: visual abnormalities	Same as above. Concurrent use with tricyclic antidepressants increases tremor. Blunts reflex tachycardia produced by nitroglycerin. *Lab:* Causes falsely increased levels of urine catecholamines on laboratory tests	Same as above. INTERVENTION: Administer on an empty stomach. During IV administration, always keep patient supine. Measure blood pressure immediately before and 5– 10 min after injection. Do not administer with sodium bicarbonate.
Same as above. Cautious use in renal disease	Same as above.	Same as above.	Same as above. INTERVENTION: May be taken without regard to meals.
Contraindicated in sinus bradycardia, heart block greater than first degree, cardiogenic shock, overt heart failure. Cautious use in pregnancy and nursing mothers. *Pediatric safety not established.*	Neuro: dizziness, somnolence, confusion, headache, agitation CV: hypotension, diaphoresis, peripheral ischemia GI: nausea. Integ: at-site inflammation and induration	All catecholamine-depleting drugs may have an additive effect. May increase digoxin levels. Morphine may increase esmolol hydrochloride in steady state. Warfarin blood levels increase with concurrent esmolol hydrochloride.	Same as above. INTERVENTION: Dilute prior to administration. Not compatible with bicarbonate.

CONTINUED ON THE FOLLOWING PAGE

Table 19–8. BETA-ADRENERGIC BLOCKERS–*CONTINUED*

Name	Dosage	Mode of Administration	Pharmacokinetics	Blocking Activity
Carteolol (Cartrol)				
Use: Approved for hypertension and may be used for angina.				

	2.5–5.0 mg/day	PO	O: rapid
			P: 1–3 hr
			D: 24 hr
			½ L: 6 hr
			PB: 25–30%
			B: not
			   biotransformed
			E: unchanged
			   in urine
				β_1, β_2

Key to Abbreviations in the *Pharmacokinetics* column O-onset; P-peak; D-duration; PB-protein bound; B-biotransformed in; E-excreted in; ½ L-halflife.
  *Within the column listing adverse effects, underlines indicate the most common effects, and CAPITALS indicate life-threatening effects.

Interactions

Interactions include an increased potential for bradycardia and cardiac depression when cardiac glycosides and quinidine are given concurrently. There is also an increased hypotensive effect when diuretics and phenothiazines are given concurrently. Concurrent administration with either hydralazine or furosemide increases the plasma level of propranolol. Concurrent administration of metoprolol and hydralazine increases the plasma level of metoprolol. Coadministration of cimetidine significantly increases plasma levels of propranolol, slightly increases plasma levels of atenolol, and does not affect the plasma levels of metoprolol. Coadministration of antacids decreases the bioavailability of propranolol and atenolol. The presence of food greatly decreases the bioavailability of the lipid-soluble beta blockers. The beta blockers may falsely increase creatinine and alkaline phosphatase.

Treatment of Overdose

Clinical presentation and management of beta-blocker overdose, although rare, vary from person to person. Treatment priorities in the emergency department are directed toward reversal of life-threatening complications, including cardiovascular depression, respiratory compromise, and central nervous system disturbances. The major difficulty in treating these patients has been

Table 19–9. BETA BLOCKERS: LIPID- AND WATER-SOLUBLE PRODUCTS

Lipid-Soluble	Water Soluble
Propranolol (Inderal)	Nadolol (Corgard)
Metoprolol (Lopressor)	Atenolol (Tenormin)
Timolol (Blocadren)	Cartenolol (Cartrol)
Acebutolol (Sectral)	
Pindolol (Visken)	
Labetalol (Normodyne, Trandate)	
Esmolol (Brevibloc)	
Penbutalol (Levatol)	

their refractoriness to treatment with catecholamines and parasympatholytic agents. Glucagon, a polypeptide hormone historically used to manage hypoglycemia, has demonstrated an ability to enhance myocardial contractility in the presence of massive beta blockade. The recommended dosage of glucagon is 100–150 μg/kg (4–8 mg), IV bolus, over one minute, followed by continuous infusion at 1–5 mg/hour, titrated to the desired patient response. Effects occur in one to three minutes, with peak action being reached in five to seven minutes and lasting 15–20 minutes. The most commonly reported adverse effects are nausea and vomiting.

Propranolol Hydrochloride

Propranolol hydrochloride is the oldest and most widely used of all the beta blockers. Propranolol is often considered the standard beta blocker to which each new beta blocker is compared. Along with all the uses and actions of beta blockers already discussed, propranolol produces significant enhancement of functional capacity in the patient with coronary artery disease during exercise training.

Propranolol prolongs the sinus node cycle and slightly prolongs the atrioventricular node anterograde conduction time during sinus rhythm and during rapid atrial pacing. These electrophysiologic effects make it an ideal drug for treating both atrial and supraventricular dysrhythmias. Many reports and trials also demonstrate the efficacy of using propranolol for the treatment of ventricular dysrhythmias.

DOSAGE. Propranolol hydrochloride (Inderal) is given for hypertension in oral dosages of 80 mg bid to 240 mg/day in two to four divided doses. As an antidysrhythmic, the daily dosages of 10–30 mg po three to four times a day are used. Oral dosages may be as high as 160–480 mg/day. Intravenously, 1–3 mg can be administered for life-threatening dysrhythmias. For the treatment of angina, 40–160 mg/day, divided into three doses, is administered. For IHSS, 20–40 mg tid to qid is administered. For myocardial prophylaxis, 180–240 mg/day is administered tid or qid.

Contraindications/ Precautions	Adverse Effects*	Interactions	Nursing Implications
Same as for all plus Contraindicated in persistently severe bradycardia, patients with greater than first degree heart block, severe congestive heart failure, and COPD.	Same as for all.	Same as for all.	Same as for all.

Dosage for migraine headaches is individualized but ranges from 160–240 mg PO daily.

Propranolol starts to act in 30 minutes, peaks in 1–1.5 hours, and has a duration of six hours. Propranolol is 90%–95% bound to plasma proteins. Effects begin in two minutes, peak in 15 minutes, and have a duration of five to six hours.

Recently, a long-acting capsule, Inderal SR, was released; its therapeutic effect lasts 24 hours. However, even without the more expensive "SR" formulation, beta blockers such as metoprolol or atenolol can be given once daily to treat hypertension. SR propranolol is administered in dosages of 60, 80, 120, or 160 mg once daily.

Patients receiving propranolol are cautioned to limit smoking because of reports that smoking can elevate blood pressure in these patients.

Metoprolol

Metoprolol is a selective inhibitor of beta$_1$-adrenergic receptors. Like propranolol, metoprolol inhibits response to adrenergic stimuli by competitively blocking beta$_1$-adrenergic receptors within the myocardium. Unlike propranolol, however, metoprolol blocks beta$_2$-adrenergic receptors within bronchial and vascular smooth muscle only in high doses.

Through its myocardial beta$_1$-adrenergic blocking action, metoprolol decreases resting heart rate and reflex orthostatic tachycardia, inhibits exercise-induced increases in heart rate, decreases myocardial contractility, and decreases cardiac output at rest and during exercise without a compensatory increase in peripheral resistance. The drug increases systolic ejection time and cardiac volume; stroke volume is unchanged. Metoprolol also decreases conduction velocity through the sinoatrial and atrioventricular nodes and decreases myocardial automaticity via beta$_1$-adrenergic blockade. The drug has no intrinsic sympathomimetic activity and little or no membrane-stabilizing effect on the heart.

Metroprolol is administered to hypertensive patients and to patients who have had a myocardial infarction. For hypertension, the initial dosage is 100 mg/day in a single or divided dose, then a maintenance dosage of 100–400 mg/day. For myocardial infarction prophy-

laxis, metoprolol is started as soon as the patient is hemodynamically stable. Three IV boluses of 5 mg each are administered at two-minute intervals. After 15 minutes, 50 mg is administered orally every six hours for 48 hours. Then, 100 mg is administered twice daily for six months to two years.

Nadolol

Like propranolol, nadolol (Corgard) inhibits response to adrenergic stimuli by competitively blocking beta$_1$-adrenergic receptors within the myocardium and beta-adrenergic receptors within bronchial and vascular smooth muscle.

Through its myocardial beta$_1$-adrenergic blocking action, nadolol decreases resting heart rate, inhibits exercise-induced increases in heart rate, and decreases cardiac output at rest and during exercise. The drug decreases conduction velocity through the atrioventricular node and decreases myocardial automaticity via beta$_1$-adrenergic blockage. Nadolol apparently has little direct myocardial depressant activity and no membrane-stabilizing effect on the heart, nor does it exhibit intrinsic sympathomimetic action.

Nadolol is similar to propranolol hydrochloride; however, unlike propranolol, it is not metabolized in the liver, and it is excreted unchanged in the urine. Dosage needs to be reduced in patients with impaired renal function. The lack of hepatic metabolism gives it a relatively long plasma duration of 20–24 hours, allowing once-daily administration. The initial dose is 40 mg, with maintenance dosages ranging from 80–320 mg daily. Nadolol is used as an antihypertensive and antianginal medication.

Timolol Maleate

Timolol maleate has pharmacologic actions similar to those of other beta-adrenergic blocking agents. The principal physiologic action of timolol is to competitively block beta-adrenergic receptors within the myocardium (beta$_1$ receptors) and within bronchial and vascular smooth muscle (beta$_2$ receptors). Unlike atenolol and metoprolol, timolol is not a beta$_1$-selective adrenergic blocking agent; timolol is a nonselective beta-adrenergic blocking agent, inhibiting both beta$_1$- and beta$_2$-adrenergic receptors. Timolol also does not exhibit the intrinsic sympathomimetic activity seen with pindolol or the membrane-stabilizing activity possessed by propranol or pindolol.

By inhibiting myocardial beta$_1$-adrenergic receptors, timolol produces negative chronotropic and inotropic activity. The negative chronotropic action of timolol on the sinoatrial node results in a decrease in the rate of sinotrial node discharge and an increase in recovery time, thereby decreasing resting and exercise-stimulated heart rate and reflex orthostatic tachycardia by as much as 30%.

Timolol maleate (Blocadren) is similar to the prototype propranolol hydrochloride. It has a 50% "first-pass effect" in the liver. Dosage for control of hypertension ranges from 10–60 mg daily in divided doses; for myocardial infarction prophylaxis, the dosage is 10 mg twice daily. Therapy is started within one to four weeks following acute myocardial infarction.

Atenolol

Atenolol competitively blocks adrenergic stimulation of beta-adrenergic receptors within the myocardium and vascular smooth muscle. In low doses atenolol inhibits beta$_1$ receptors while having little effect on beta$_2$ receptors. At high doses (over 100 mg/day) this selectively diminishes and the drug competitively blocks both beta$_1$ and beta$_2$-adrenergic receptors. Atenolol does not exhibit the intrinsic sympathetic activity seen with pindolol, nor does it have the membrane-stabilizing activity of propranolol or pindolol.

Atenolol (Tenormin) is used in the treatment of hypertension and angina pectoris. Full effect requires about two to three weeks. Atenolol is administered orally in dosages of 50–100 mg once daily for hypertension. Doses need to be adjusted in patients with decreased renal function because atenolol is excreted via the kidneys.

Pindolol

Pindolol has pharmacologic actions similar to those of other beta-adrenergic blocking agents. The principal physiologic action of pindolol is to competitively block beta$_1$-adrenergic receptors within the myocardium and beta$_2$ receptors within bronchial and vascular smooth muscle. In addition to inhibiting access of physiologic or synthetic catecholamines to the beta-adrenergic receptors, pindolol causes slight activation of the beta receptors, making the drug a partial beta-agonist. This intrinsic sympathomimetic activity (ISA) of pindolol differs from the beta-agonist activity of epinephrine and isoproterenol in that the maximum beta-adrenergic stimulation that can be obtained with pindolol is less. Other beta-adrenergic blocking agents can block pindolol's ISA. Pindolol also has been shown to possess membrane-stabilizing activity or a quinidine-like effect, but this occurs only at plasma concentrations well above those obtained therapeutically. Unlike atenolol and metoprolol, pindolol is not a beta$_1$-selective adrenergic blocking agent; pindolol is a nonselective beta-adrenergic blocking agent, inhibiting both beta$_1$ and beta$_2$-adrenergic receptors.

By inhibiting myocardial beta$_1$-adrenergic receptors, pindolol produces negative chronotropic and inotropic activity. Both of these actions are reversed somewhat, but not entirely, by the drug's partial agonist activity. The negative chronotropic action of pindolol on the sinoatrial node results in a decrease in sinotrial node discharge and recovery time, thereby decreasing stress- and exercise-stimulated heart rate. Pindolol has a lesser effect on resting heart rate than do beta-adrenergic blocking agents that do not possess ISA, usually decreasing resting heart rate only by about four to eight beats/minute or not at all. The blunting of stress- and exercise-stimulated tachycardia by pindolol, however, is similar to that of the other beta blockers. Pindolol also slows conduction in the atrioventricular node but usually to a lesser extent than do the other beta-adrenergic blocking agents. Pindolol reduces exercise-stimulated cardiac output, but pindolol probably has a slightly lesser effect on cardiac output than do beta-adrenergic blocking agents without ISA. Pindolol has a lesser effect on resting cardiac output than on that stimulated by exercise. The decrease in myocardial contractility, blood pressure, and heart rate produced by pindolol during stress and exercise leads to a reduction in myocardial oxygen consumption, which accounts for the effectiveness of the drug in chronic stable angina pectoris. Pindolol is probably not effective in patients who develop angina at rest or at low exercise levels.

Pindolol (Visken) is administered in doses of 15–60 mg/day PO in two or three divided doses for the control of hypertension. Pindolol is less effective for angina but is a better choice of drug when the patient also has peripheral vascular disease because there is less vasoconstriction.

Labetalol Hydrochloride

Labetalol (Trandate) is a nonselective lipid-soluble agent with both beta- and alpha$_1$ adrenergic (postsynaptic) blocking features. The principal physiologic action of labetalol is to competitively block adrenergic stimulation of beta receptors within the myocardium (beta$_1$ receptors) and within bronchial and vascular smooth muscle (beta$_2$ receptors) and alpha$_1$ receptors within vascular smooth muscle. In addition to inhibiting access of endogenous or exogenous catecholamines to beta-adrenergic receptors, labetalol has been shown to exhibit some intrinsic beta$_2$-agonist activity in animals; however, the drug exerts little, if any, intrinsic beta$_1$-agonist activity. Labetalol does not exhibit intrinsic alpha-adrenergic agonist activity.

Labetalol produces marked vasodilation and decreased afterload with acute initiation of therapy and maintains the cardiac output despite the usual negative inotropic effects. Severe bradycardia, peripheral vascular symptoms, and congestive heart failure occur less frequently with labetalol.

Labetalol hydrochloride is used primarily for the management of hypertension either alone or with other agents. An oral dosage is started with 100 mg bid, and increments of 100 mg bid can be added every two to three days. It generally begins to lower blood pressure in one to two hours. A maintenance dosage ranges from

200–400 mg bid up to 2400 mg/day. The initial IV dosage is 0.25 mg/kg, then 40–80 mg is given at ten-minute intervals (see additional dosing in Table 19–8). The intravenous route starts to achieve a response within five minutes.

Acebutolol

Acebutolol (Sectral) is a beta$_1$-selective adrenergic blocking agent and has pharmacologic activity similar to those of other beta-adrenergic blocking agents. At low dosages, acebutolol selectively inhibits response to adrenergic stimuli by competitively blocking beta$_1$-adrenergic receptors while having little effect on the beta$_2$-adrenergic receptors of bronchial and vascular smooth muscle. At high dosages (e.g., greater than 800 mg daily), the selectivity of acebutolol for receptors usually diminishes, and the drug will competitively block both beta$_1$ and beta$_2$-adrenergic receptors. In addition to inhibiting access of physiologic or synthetic catecholamines to the beta-adrenergic receptors, acebutolol exhibits mild intrinsic sympathomimetic activity (partial beta-agonist activity). Acebutolol also has a membrane-stabilizing effect on the heart, which is similar to that of quinidine but occurs more at higher plasma concentrations and usually is not apparent at dosages used therapeutically.

Acebutolol is an oral beta blocker used for both hypertension and ventricular dysrhythmia. For hypertension the usual dosage is 200–1200 mg in a single or divided doses. Divided doses are often better at controlling high blood pressure. For ventricular dysrhythmias, the initial dosage is 200 mg bid and the maintenance dose is 600–1200 mg per day in single or divided doses. Bioavailability increases in the elderly, so dosages of more than 800 mg/day are not recommended. Reduction in dosing is required when renal function decreases.

Esmolol Hydrochloride

Esmolol hydrochloride (Brevibloc) is a rapid-onset, ultra-short-acting beta blocker. Esmolol is a short-acting beta$_1$-selective adrenergic blocking agent that has pharmacologic actions similar to those of other beta-adrenergic blocking agents. Esmolol selectiively inhibits response to adrenergic stimuli by competitively blocking cardiac beta$_1$-adrenergic receptors while having little effect on the beta$_2$-adrenergic receptors of bronchial and vascular smooth muscle. At high doses (e.g., greater than 300 μg/kg/minute), this selectivity of esmolol for beta$_1$-adrenergic receptors usually diminishes, and the drug competitively inhibits beta$_1$- and beta$_2$-adrenergic receptors.

At usual clinical doses, esmolol does not exhibit appreciable intrinsic sympathomimetic or membrane-stabilizing activity, nor does the drug exhibit alpha-adrenergic blocking activity. However, the drug may exhibit sympathomimetic and membrane-stabilizing activity at doses that substantially exceed those used clinically. It is used effectively to decrease blood pressure, ventricular heart rate in patients with acute atrial fibrillation and flutter, and the rate in noncompensatory sinus tachycardia. Esmolol has an elimination half-life of only nine minutes, which allows for a rapid, controlled titration to a desired effect and prompt reversal of beta blockade if necessary.

Esmolol is rapidly and extensively metabolized via esterases, which are principally found in erythrocytes and in highly perfused tissues that contain esterases, such as the liver and kidneys. Methanol is formed as a by-product of metabolism, but the amount of methanol does not appear to be clinically significant. Even with high dosages (150 μg/kg/minute for 24 hours), blood methanol levels remained less than 2% of those usually associated with methanol toxicity.

Esmolol is diluted just prior to administration—one 2.5-g ampule is mixed in 250 ml of solution to yield a 10 mg/ml solution. The loading dosage is 500 μg/kg/minute for one minute and then 50 μg/kg/minute for four minutes or until the desired effect is reached. A maintenance dosage of 25–50 μg/kg/minute is administered. Ideally, esmolol is used for 24 hours or less.

Penbutolol Sulfate

Penbutolol sulfate (Levatol) is used to treat mild to moderate arterial hypertension. It blocks both beta$_1$ and beta$_2$ receptors. Penbutolol sulfate has a very mild ISA. It is highly lipid soluble and close to 100% absorbed. It may be taken without regard to food.

The usual starting dose and maintenance dose is 20 mg once daily. Generally, the full antihypertensive effect is seen by the end of two weeks.

Cartenolol

Cartenolol (Cartol) is primarily used to treat hypertension. It blocks both beta$_1$ and beta$_2$ receptors. Cartenolol has a moderate ISA. Cartenolol has low lipid solubility and is about 80% absorbed. It is not biotransformed but excreted 50–70% unchanged in the urine.

The usual starting dose is 10 mg.

NURSING ACTIONS. As the nurse administers any of the beta blockers, vital signs including cardiac rate and rhythm are assessed. Baseline weight is obtained. Since beta blockers will be taken at home possibly for the rest of the patient's life, much teaching is needed. Table 19–10 describes general patient teaching for beta blockers. Patients are taught the best time to administer their beta blocker, either with or between meals. The patients are also taught information pertaining to drug interactions, typical side effects, and also the importance of always remembering to take their medication.

GANGLIONIC BLOCKERS

The ganglionic blockers prevent transmission of both sympathetic and parasympathetic nerve impulses through the ganglia. They appear to compete with acetylcholine to occupy the cholinergic synapse of the autonomic ganglia. This competition makes it impossible for the vasoconstrictive impulses to then be transmitted across the neuromuscular junction; therefore, blood vessels dilate and arterial pressure fails. Among the most potent antihypertensives available today, ganglionic blockers include mecamylamine hydrochloride (Inver-

Table 19–10. PATIENT TEACHING—BETA BLOCKERS

Dear Patient:

This drug has been prescribed for you. This is what you should know about your drug to get the most from your therapy.

1. Beta blockers work by controlling certain nerve impulses. Beta blockers are used to treat many conditions; the most common are high blood pressure, anginal pain, after a heart attack to help prevent another, irregular heart beats, migraine headaches, and many others.
2. Beta blockers will generally be taken for a long time and perhaps for the rest of your life.
3. Try to take your drug at the same time each day. You may be asked to take your heart rate or your blood pressure before you take your drug.
4. Do not take your beta blocker with antacids. There are many drugs that will interact with beta blockers so always check with your physician before taking any other drug.
5. If you forget to take your drug, take the next dose. DO NOT double dose.
6. DO NOT stop the drug on your own. If your physician does stop it, the dose will be decreased gradually over several weeks.
7. DO NOT change the dose on your own.
8. Several beta blockers are best taken in between meals. _____ is best taken (between meals) or (whenever it is convenient, food does not matter). Do not drink beer, whiskey, or wine while taking your beta blockers because these may lead to low blood pressure and dizziness. Limit your caffeinated beverages to 2/day.
9. Several side effects may occur. If any unusual symptoms occur, call your doctor. The most common side effects include dizziness and lightheadedness, unusually slow pulse, tiredness, breathing difficulties, and reduced alertness. Be careful when operating heavy equipment or driving a car.
10. Store the drug in a dry, tight, moisure-resistant container and place out of the reach of children.
11. Do not take hot baths or showers or sit in a hot tub. Limit your exposure to the sun to short periods of time. Weigh yourself weekly.

sine), trimethaphan camsylate (Arfonad), and hexamethonium chloride.

The ganglionic blockers are developed primarily from a quaternary ammonium compound—tetraethylammonium chloride. In 1950, the methonium derivatives were introduced, including hexamethonium chloride. Since 1961, other more potent, more selectively acting drugs with fewer side effects have been developed, and the ganglionic blockers are seldom used today.

When used, ganglionic blockers are most useful in the treatment of advanced stages of hypertension, including hypertensive crisis, when other medications are not effective. Ganglionic blockers are more effective than other drugs in reducing the erect blood pressure because of their sympathetic blockade of postural reflexes. The end result of this effect may be fainting because of insufficient blood flow to the brain. These drugs are discussed fully in Chapter 29.

SUMMARY

Drugs that mimic the sympathetic nervous system are adrenergic drugs. These drugs have various effects: they increase the rate and force of contraction, they relax smooth muscle in the lung and gastrointestinal system, and they produce vasoconstriction in the peripheral blood vessels. Adrenergic drugs work at alpha, beta$_1$, beta$_2$, or dopaminergic receptors to either enhance or block their effect.

Sympathomimetic drugs may act directly on the adrenergic receptors. The direct-acting adrenergic medications include dopamine, norepinephrine, dobutamine, isoproterenol, and epinephrine. Sympatholytic drugs block the transmission of nerve impulses to the adrenergic neuroeffectors. The alpha-blocking drugs include phenoxybenzamine hydrochloride, phentolamine hydrochloride, prazosin, tolazoline, and the ergot alkaloids. The beta-blocking drugs include propranolol, metoprolol tartrate, nadolol, timolol maleate, atenolol, pindolol, acebutolol, labetalol, and esmolol.

The majority of these drugs are discussed in other chapters of this book. The nursing care is discussed briefly in this chapter and in greater detail in other chapters.

BIBLIOGRAPHY

Abernethy, DR, et al: Labetalol in treatment of hypertension in elderly and young patients. J Clin Pharmacol 27(11):902–906, 1987.

AMA Drug Evaluations, ed 6. PSG Publishing, Littleton, MA, 1986.

Daley, KA and Ruksnaitis, N: Glucagon: A first-line drug for cardiotoxicity caused by beta blockade. Nurses Drug Alert 12(6):387–392.

Gilman, AG, Goodman, L, and Gilman, A (eds): Goodman and Gilman's The Pharmacological Basis of Therapeutics, ed 7. Macmillan, New York, 1985.

Jones, S, et al: L-E-A-D drugs for cardiac arrest: Lidocaine, epinephrine, atropine, and dopamine. Nursing '88 18(1):34–42, 1988.

McEvoy, G (ed): AFFS Drug Information 1988. Maryland, American Society of Hospital Pharmacists, 1988.

McGraw, JP: A graphic solution to the calculation of dopamine and other vasoactive drug dosages. J Emerg Nurs 13(3):172–174, May–June, 1987.

Miller, CL: Medications in angina. Focus Critical Care 15(4):23–29, 1988.

Miller, LG: Choice of beta blockers in hypertensive patients who smoke. Clin Pharm 6(12):924–925, 1987.

Neil-Dwyer, G, et al: Beta adrenoceptor blockers and the blood–brain barrier. Br J Clin Pharmacol 11:549, 1981.

Rude, RE, Muller, JE, and Braumwald, E: Efforts to limit the size of myocardial infarcts. Ann Intern Med 97:736, 1981.

Schactman, M, and Crawford, MV: Dobutamine rescue for intractable CHF. Am J Nurs 88:1642–1643, 1988.

Schneeweiss, A: Drug Therapy in Cardiovascular Disease. Lea & Febiger, Philadelphia, 1986.

Schulte, LK, et al: Beta-adrenocepter stimulating and blocking agents in essential hypertension: Single and combined therapy with terbutaline and metoprolol. Int J Clin Pharmacol Ther Toxicol 25(10):539–544, 1987.

Sullivan, MJ, et al: Drug-induced aerobic-enzyme activity of human skeletal muscle during bedrest deconditioning. J Cardiopulmonary Rehab 6(6):232–237, 1986.

Technical Monograph & Formulary Information—Brevibloc. Dupont Critical Care Inc, Elgin, Illinois, 1987.

Wiltse, O: For your log book—dopamine. Emerg 19(3):19–20, 1987.

SITUATION   19–1

Mr. Morris Trehan, a 52-year old, has been placed on a trial of ergotamine tartrate (Ergomar) for treatment of migraine headaches. He also has a history of diabetes and peptic ulcer disease.

1. The nurse will plan to observe Mr. Trehan for the following adverse side effect of Ergomar:
   a. hypotension
   b. constipation
   c. vomiting
   d. impaired vision

2. In teaching Mr. Trehan about Ergomar, the nurse will include all of the following information *except*:
   a. Report any itching, tingling, or numbness in fingers and toes.
   b. Take the medication with food four times a day.
   c. Lie down in a dark, quiet room after taking the drug.
   d. Have blood pressure checked on a routine basis.

3. Mr. Trehan will also be managed on a prophylactic dose of propranolol (Inderal) for prevention of migraine headaches. Which of the following conditions represents a contraindication for therapy?
   a. glaucoma
   b. hyperthyroidism
   c. alcohol withdrawal
   d. congestive heart failure

4. All of the following behaviors indicate successful patient teaching about Inderal therapy *except*:
   a. reducing or stopping cigarette smoking
   b. using antacids to decrease gastric effects
   c. taking propranolol on an empty stomach
   d. avoiding alcohol while taking the drug

5. An appropriate nursing diagnosis for Mr. Trehan would be:
   a. Noncompliance related to medication regimen for headaches
   b. Anxiety related to the side effects of beta-blocker therapy
   c. Activity intolerance: fatigue related to propranolol therapy
   d. Potential for violence related to administration of ergot derivatives

6. In planning Mr. Trehan's medication regimen, all of the following drugs would be given cautiously *except*:
   a. insulin
   b. cimetidine
   c. heparin
   d. aspirin

SITUATION   19–2

Betty Daschner is a 62-year-old with a history of renal insufficiency admitted to the intensive care unit post gastrectomy surgery. She is receiving lactated Ringer's at 100 cc per hour and has a nasogastric tube to low intermittent suction.

1. The physician orders a dopamine (Intropin) drip at 1 μg/kg/min for Mrs. Daschner. At this dosage, the nurse will expect to observe the following effect:
   a. increased blood pressure
   b. increased urine output
   c. decreased cardiac output
   d. reduced nasogastric drainage

2. In planning care for Mrs. Daschner, the nurse will include all of the following interventions with regard to dopamine infusion *except*:
   a. monitor extremities for color and temperature
   b. assess blood pressure and vital signs closely
   c. use micro drip tubing and an infusion pump
   d. discontinue intravenous infusion of lactated Ringer's

3. The nurse notes extravasation at the dopamine infusion site. After discontinuing the infusion, the nurse will:
   a. infiltrate phentolamine at the IV site
   b. wrap site in warm, moist saline dressings
   c. apply an ice pack to the area
   d. place a tourniquet above the area of infiltration

4. After four days in the intensive care unit, Mrs. Daschner demonstrates signs of septic shock. The infusion of dopamine is increased to 10 μg/kg/min. At this infusion rate, the expected outcome would be:
   a. reduced body temperature
   b. increased blood pressure
   c. reduced heart rate
   d. increased peripheral perfusion

5. Due to potential for drug interaction, all of the following agents should be used with caution *except*:
   a. MAO inhibitors
   b. thyroid hormones
   c. guanethidine
   d. nitroglycerin

6. When the dopamine infusion is no longer necessary for Mrs. Daschner, the nurse will plan to include the following measures:
   a. turn off infusion and take the blood pressure every hour
   b. restrict total fluid intake before discontinuing
   c. administer a bolus dose of dopamine and then stop infusion
   d. wean off dopamine at a slow rate, monitoring vital signs

Please refer to the Appendices for correct answers and additional review questions with answers.

GLOSSARY TERMS IN THIS CHAPTER

Acute pain
Addiction
Chronic pain
Dependence
Dynorphins
Endogenous peptides
Endorphins
Enkephalins
Epidural therapy
Intrathecal therapy
Miosis
Nociceptors
Opiate agonist
Opiate agonist-antagonist
Opiate antagonist
Opiate receptors
Opiate partial agonists
Opiates
Photophobia
Tolerance

20
CHAPTER

DRUGS THAT PROVIDE PAIN RELIEF

VICKI L. BYERS, R.N., Ph.D., CNRN

LEARNING OBJECTIVES

After reading this chapter, the student will be able to:

1. Identify medications commonly used as pain relievers.

2. Differentiate among the pain relievers' mechanisms of action, routes of administration, pharmacokinetics, adverse effects, contraindications, and interactions.

3. Identify specific areas of assessment in the patient requiring pain relievers in order to formulate appropriate nursing diagnoses.

4. Plan the nursing interventions necessary to administer pain relievers, and choose appropriate teaching strategies to gain patient compliance.

5. Evaluate the patient at various stages of treatment to measure the effectiveness of nursing interactions.

INTRODUCTION

Pain has been described as an ambiguous puzzle, man's unremitting companion and inescapable end. On the one hand, pain is beneficial because it alerts us to impending harm from the environment. It protects us from extreme temperatures, mechanical pressure, and penetrating wounds (i.e., stepping on a piece of glass). On the other hand, beyond this warning purpose, pain becomes meaningless and causes suffering. The total pain experience is defined by Bonica as "composed of the pain perception and the associated sensations, emotional reactions, affective [feeling] states, and the psychophysiological reactions consequent thereto." Nurses encounter patients in pain in a variety of clinical situations. Pain is one of the most frequent patient problems encountered, one of the most difficult to assess, and one of the most unyielding to treatment. It is very important for nurses to view the patient with pain holistically and to believe that the patient has pain.

OVERVIEW OF THE PAIN PATHWAYS

It is commonly held that pain is detected by free nerve endings in the skin, tissues, and organs. These *nociceptors* are afferent fibers. The nociceptors respond to mechanical, thermal, and chemical stimuli. These axons vary from very small-diameter myelinated (A-delta) fibers to larger unmyelinated (C) fibers. The quality of the pain evoked by A-delta fibers is a "pricking" pain while a "burning" pain is the result of stimulating C fibers. When these fibers are stimulated by noxious stimuli, the information is sent to the dorsal horn of the spinal cord. Several layers of the dorsal horn are involved with painful stimuli. The projection of these fibers in the dorsal horn are directed to higher centers in the brain. In the past, the spinothalamic pathway was considered the major pain pathway. (Fig. 20–1 traces the components of this pathway.) Although this is an important pain pathway, it is now believed that several ascending path-

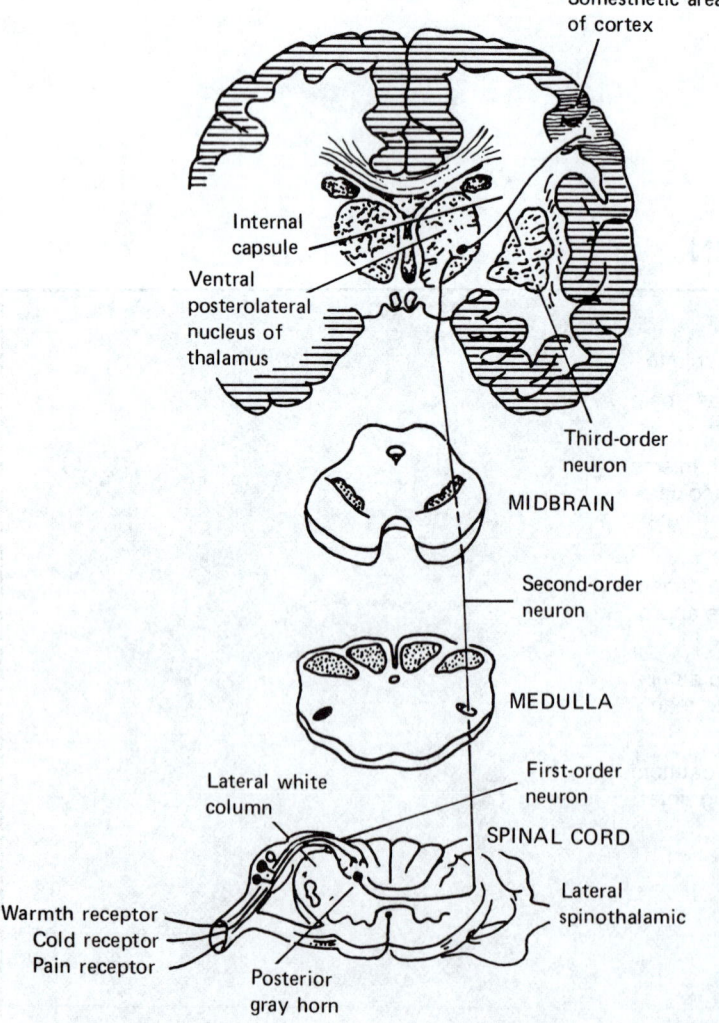

Figure 20–1. Sensory pathway for pain and temperature—the lateral spinothalmic pathway.

ways are involved in the role of pain. Willis (1985) addresses the importance of other pain pathways such as the spinoreticular and spinomesencephalic pathways. (See Table 17–2 for a description of these tracts.) In addition to these pathways, specific nuclei of the brain, such as the reticular formation, periaqueductal gray matter, and thalamus, also are components of pain pathways. Finally, the axons projecting from the thalamus to the cerebral cortex are the last component of the pain pathways. This projection system is involved in sensory-discriminative processing and motivational-affective processing, therefore refining the perception of pain.

OPIATE RECEPTORS IN THE CENTRAL NERVOUS SYSTEM

The *opiates* are of therapeutic relevance because of their calming effects and ability to change pain perceptions. A major disadvantage of the opiates is their addictive properties. This has led pharmacologists to search for nonaddicting opiates. This search has yielded information about *opiate receptors* and *endogenous peptides*.

The opiate receptors possess interesting characteristics related to the way they act, the influence of sodium, and their location in the body. These receptors act in a highly selective, stereospecific manner with opiate drugs and endogenous peptides. The highly selective receptors on neuronal membranes in the brain account for the potency of these drugs.

Table 20–1. OPIATE RECEPTORS

Receptor Type	Physiologic Effect	Opiate/Endogenous Peptide—Type of Activity
Mu	Bradycardia, bradypnea, analgesia	Morphine (agonist) Meperidine (agonist) Methadone (agonist) Codeine (agonist) Fentanyl (agonist) Levorphanol (agonist) Buprenorphine (agonist) Naloxone (antagonist) Enkephalin Endorphin
Kappa	Spinal analgesia, miosis, sedation	Morphine (agonist) Pentazocine (agonist) Naloxone (antagonist) Dynorphin
Sigma	Dysphoria, hallucinations, respiratory and vasomotor stimulation	Pentazocine (agonist)
Delta	Unknown	Enkephalin Endorphin
Epsilon	Unknown	Endorphin

Binding studies reveal that sodium influences the way opiates bind at the receptor sites. The affinity of an *opiate agonist* is reduced by sodium ions and certain guanine nucleotides. On the other hand, the affinity of *opiate antagonist* drugs is not altered by the presence of sodium.

The density of opiate receptors varies in different regions of the brain and spinal cord. This variation in opiate receptors is important to the mechanism of action of opiate drugs. The mapping of opiate receptors has revealed receptor density in the periaqueductal gray matter of the brain stem, solitary nuclei of the brain stem, medial thalamus, amygdala, and spinal cord. Binding studies have identified the following receptor types: (1) mu receptor, (2) kappa receptor, (3) sigma receptor, (4) delta receptor, and (5) epsilon receptor. (Table 20–1 summarizes the relationship between the receptors and various drugs that interact with a particular group of receptors.) The pharmacologic effects of the opiate drugs occur as the result of interactions with a particular group of receptors. Analgesia occurs with the interaction of the mu and kappa receptors, while dysphoria is associated with interaction with sigma receptors.

ENDOGENOUS PEPTIDES

The opiate receptors interact not only with opiate drugs but also with endogenous peptides. These morphine-like peptides modulate pain and serve as neurotransmitters. The three classes of endogenous peptides identified are the *enkephalins*, *endorphins*, and *dynorphins*. Each type of endogenous peptide is found in different groups of neurons. The endorphin peptides are found in the pituitary, while the enkephalin peptides are found in the brain, spinal cord, adrenal medulla, stomach, and intestines. The endogenous peptides exhibit a variety of affinities for the different types of opiate receptors.

TYPES OF PAIN

The pain experience can be either acute or chronic. Both of these experiences alter the comfort level of the patient and cause different pain reaction behaviors, thus affecting the nature of the nursing assessment.

Acute pain serves as a warning to possible or real danger. The onset of this pain is sudden and has a temporary duration. The behavioral response to this pain is based on the activation of the sympathetic nervous system with its release of epinephrine-norepinephrine. Clinically, the patient experiences increases in heart rate, respiration, blood pressure, peripheral blood flow, muscle tension, palmar sweating, and dilated pupils. The patient can also experience anxiety and restlessness.

Chronic pain, on the other hand, serves no useful pur-

Table 20–2. DIFFERENTIATING BETWEEN ACUTE AND CHRONIC PAIN

	Acute	Chronic
Time, course	Transient, lasts less than 6 months; pain subsides as healing occurs; has an ending.	Prolonged; lasts longer than 6 months; may be intractable; ending is not always in sight.
Location	Localized	Diffuse—difficult to localize
Purpose	Warns one of impending or actual tissue damage.	Serves no purpose; depletes one of energy; pain becomes the pathology.
Characteristics	Sharp, various intensity (mild to severe), can radiate; comes and goes in accordance with pathology.	Aching, burning, dull, cramping, nagging, persistent; lasts after recovery from injury/disease.
Emotional response to pain	Positive; pain is experienced on a short-term basis.	Negative; pain serves no purpose; patient is emotionally distressed and may experience alterations in life-style.
Signs/symptoms	Sympathetic activation (increased blood pressure, tachycardia, increased respirations, diaphoresis, pallor, dilated pupils, increased muscle tone, increased concentration, anxiety, weakness), facial expression.	Compensatory responses (in sympathetic response), sleep disturbances, anorexia, listlessness, apathy, personality changes (anger, withdrawal, helplessness, hostility, hopelessness, irritability, depression).

pose and has a long duration. If unrelieved, chronic pain leads to fatigue and lowers the pain threshold. The patient never becomes accustomed to having this kind of pain. The behavioral response to this type of pain is based on the long-term activation of the autonomic nervous system. The patient can exhibit sleep and appetite disturbances, irritability, decreased libido, loss of interests, and increased preoccupation with body sensations. The patient can also experience apathy, withdrawal, hopelessness, and depression. Refer to Table 20–2 for a summary of the differences between acute and chronic pain.

THERAPEUTIC AGENTS TO RELIEVE PAIN

According to Craig and Stitzel (1986) pain can be categorized as superficial or deep. Superficial pain is a quick response to a sudden onset, and deep pain lingers and aches.

Several different-sized nerve fibers conduct pain impulses. A fibers transmit fast pain, B fibers carry intermediate pain impulses, and C fibers carry impulses that are associated with slow, lingering, diffuse pain.

Drugs influence the pain experience in several ways. The first alteration to the pain experience is an interruption of the peripheral pain receptors at the free nerve endings. Nonopiate analgesics (salicylates, aniline derivatives, indene derivatives, and arylarsonic acid compounds) play a critical role in altering the pain experience at the free nerve endings. The second way drugs alter the pain experience is to modify the pain perception at the level of the central nervous system. Opiate and nonopiate agents interfere with the pain perception. Finally, drugs interfere with the pain experience by changing the pain reaction. The pain reaction is altered by an autonomic response (changes in palmar sweat index or blood pressure), skeletal muscle response (increased muscle tension, facial expressions), and the psychic component (suffering of pain). The suffering of pain is greatly modified by narcotic agents, whereas the other two types of pain reactions can be influenced by either narcotics or non-narcotics, depending on the intensity of the pain experience.

NONOPIATES

The nonopiate agents contain aspirin, acetaminophen, and nonsteroidal anti-inflammatory drugs (NSAID). These drugs are described in Table 20–3. The nonsteroidal anti-inflammatory drugs are discussed in Chapter 47.

In contrast to the opiate analgesics, which act centrally, the nonopiate analgesics have been shown to act peripherally, where they prevent the formation of prostaglandins in inflamed tissues, so that pain receptors are not stimulated. They may also affect the hypothalamus to lower body temperature and decrease capillary permeability. These drugs are generally absorbed well from the gastrointestinal tract after oral administration. They are metabolized in the liver and excreted in the urine.

Salicylates

Acetylsalicyclic acid (ASA), commonly referred to as aspirin, belongs to the family of salicylates and is one of the most effective non-narcotic pain relievers. Aspirin-like drugs (e.g., naproxen, indomethacin, ibuprofen, piroxicam, ketoprofen, sulindac, phenylbutazone, meclofenamic acid, and others) are used in the management of mild to moderate pain caused by peripheral inflammation. Although the potential of these drugs to alleviate pain is much lower than that of the narcotic analgesics, aspirin-like drugs are often preferred because they do not lead to addiction and have fewer side effects. (See Chapter 47 for specific details on these agents.)

PHARMACOKINETICS. Aspirin is absorbed well from the stomach and upper small intestine, with peak plasma salicylate level within one to two hours. The acid medium in the stomach keeps salicylate in the nonionized form, promoting absorption. If gastric pH is raised to 3.5 or higher, gastric irritation is minimized. Aspirin is metabolized in the liver by the microsomal enzymes, and it is poorly bound to the plasma proteins (40%–50%). Aspirin is cleared from the body via the kidney. When this pathway is saturated, a small increase in aspirin dose results in large increases in plasma levels of aspirin. The half-life of aspirin is two to three hours.

CONTRAINDICATIONS AND PRECAUTIONS. Aspirin is contraindicated in patients with salicylate sensitivity, in patients with gastrointestinal disease such as ulcers or bleeding, in those with glucose-6-phosphate dehydrogenase (G-6-PD) deficiency, and in newborns. Aspirin should be used with caution in hypoprothrombinemia, bleeding disorders, Hodgkin's disease, and asthma with nasal polyps, as well as in aural diseases. Caution should be used in situations in which there is risk of bleeding, because aspirin decreases platelet aggregation and prolongs bleeding time, causing the patient to bleed excessively. The use of aspirin and other salicylates in children with varicella infections or influenza-like viruses has been reported to increase the risk of developing Reye's syndrome. The mechanism for this is unknown.

ADVERSE EFFECTS. The most common adverse effect of aspirin and the other salicylates is their tendency to cause gastrointestinal upset and ulcer formation. Aspirin causes local gastric mucosal irritation by increasing the entry of acid into the mucosa. Aspirin itself has a potent antiplatelet effect in which the platelets are unable to form a clot. This may result in a dangerous prolongation of bleeding time in some persons. In toxic doses, salicylates may cause tinnitus (ringing in the ears) or a whole spectrum of adverse effects called "salicylism." These include changes in mentation and perception; changes in gastrointestinal, liver, kidney, and respiratory function; and increased uric acid production.

INTERACTIONS. Aspirin interacts with several drug types and chemical substances. Because it increases the amount of active drug in the blood by displacing other drugs from plasma proteins, aspirin increases anticoagulant effect, raises methotrexate levels, and enhances hypoglycemic response to sulfonylurea antidiabetic agents. When used with alcohol and corticosteroids, aspirin increases risk of gastrointestinal bleeding and ulceration through its irritant action. Drugs that acidify the urine such as ascorbic acid or ammonium chloride may increase the plasma concentration of the salicylates. Products that contain large amounts of alkali and sodium, such as Alka-Seltzer, are not suitable for long-term use since larger dosages of aspirin may be needed to compensate for increased excretion caused by the re-

sulting alkalosis. Aspirin decreases the uricosuric effect of probenecid and pyrazolones.

DOSAGE. The usual adult dosage of aspirin for mild pain or fever is 325–650 mg every four hours as needed. The usual pediatric dosage is 65 mg/kg of body weight over 24 hours given in divided doses every six hours. Dosages used in the treatment of rheumatoid arthritis are much higher, sometimes exceeding 5 g/day. Aspirin is available for oral administration (its most effective route) in tablets, enteric-coated tablets, and timed-release preparations. Aspirin is also available in rectal suppository form. When taken orally, aspirin should be taken with food, milk, antacid, or a very large glass of water to minimize gastrointestinal side effects. Some sources further qualify that when taken with hot water the absorption of aspirin (and hence its effectiveness) is increased. Aspirin suppositories are not suitable for long-term use because of variable rates of absorption.

Other Salicylates

Other salicylates used in analgesia include choline salicylate, sodium salicylate, and magnesium salicylate. They are generally considered to be comparable to aspirin and are used in the same manner.

Acetaminophen

Acetaminophen has analgesic and antipyretic properties roughly equivalent to those of aspirin. However, it is less likely to produce gastrointestinal and hematologic disorders and lacks anti-inflammatory properties. Acetaminophen is included in over-the-counter preparations such as Tempra, Tylenol, and Datril.

PHARMACOKINETICS. The absorption of acetaminophen is related to the rate of gastric emptying. The peak blood concentration is reached 30–60 minutes after ingestion. Acetaminophen is metabolized by the hepatic microsomal enzymes. The half-life of acetaminophen is normally two to three hours. With toxic doses or liver disease, the half-life is increased twofold or more. The highly active metabolite N-acetyl-p-benzoquinone is dangerous in high doses because of its toxicity to the liver and kidney.

CONTRAINDICATIONS AND PRECAUTIONS. The major contraindications for acetaminophen include known hypersensitivity and long-term administration in patients with anemia or cardiac, pulmonary, renal, or hepatic disease. Since the liver and kidney contain the enzymes that convert the cytotoxic metabolite in acetaminophen to a nontoxic metabolite, acetaminophen should not be given to patients with renal/liver disease nor to those with anemia and/or cardiovascular disease. Caution should be exercised when acetaminophen is administered to children under age twelve. Children tend to form methemoglobin more readily than adults, which results in cyanosis of the skin, mucosa, and fingernails and is a sign of acute p-aminophenol derivative toxicity. This is a rare complication, however, and acetaminophen is the drug of choice for children.

TEXT RESUMES ON PAGE 474

Table 20–3. DRUGS USED TO CONTROL PAIN

Name	Dosage	Mode of Administration	Pharmacokinetics
NONOPIATE ANALGESIC, ANTIINFLAMMATORY AGENTS AND ANTIPYRETIC MEDICATIONS **Aspirin** (Acetylsalicylic acid, A.S.A., Bayer, Ecotrin, Measurin)			

Action: Blocks pain impulses in the CNS that occur in response to inhibition of prostaglandin synthesis. Antipyretic action is caused by inhibition of hypothalamic neurons related to heat regulation.

Use: Mild to moderate pain or fever; used to manage arthritis, headache, thromboembolic disorders.

Name	Dosage	Mode of Administration	Pharmacokinetics
	Adult: 325–1000 mg q 4–6 hr (extended release q 8 hr) as needed (not to exceed 4 g/day) *Children (2–11 yr):* 65 mg/kg/day in 4–6 divided doses	PO	O: 5–30 min P: 1–3 hr D: 3–6 hr ½ L: 2–3 hr for low doses; for larger doses, up to 15–30 hr PB: concentration dependent 90–91% at low dose 25–60% at high dose 33% (pure aspirin) B: liver E: kidneys
	Anti-inflammatory Adults: 2.6–5.2 g in divided doses *Children:* 90–130 mg/kg/day in divided doses *Prevention of Transient Ischemic Attacks Adults:* 325 mg–1.3 g daily in 2–4 divided doses *Prevention of Myocardial Infarction Adults:* 325 mg/day	Rectal P: 4–5 hr D: 7 hr PO PO PO PO	O: 1–2 hr
Acetaminophen (Anacin-3, Datril, Panadol, Tempra, Tylenol)			

Action: Blocks pain impulses in the CNS that occur in response to inhibition of prostaglandin synthesis. Antipyretic action is inhibition of hypothalamic neurons related to heat regulation.

Use: Mild to moderate pain.

Name	Dosage	Mode of Administration	Pharmacokinetics
	Adults and Children over 12 years: 325–1000 mg q 4–6 hr not	Tablet, capsule, syrup	O: <0.5 hr P: 10–60 min D: 3–4 hr

Key to Abbreviations in the *Pharmacokinetics* column O-onset; P-peak; D-duration; PB-protein bound; B-biotransformed in; E-excreted in; ½ L-halflife.
*Within the column listing adverse effects, underlines indicate the most common effects; and CAPITALS indicate life-threatening effects.

Contraindications/ Precautions	Adverse Effects*	Interactions	Nursing Implications
Contraindicated in hypersensitivity to salicylates or other nonsteroidal anti-inflammatory agents and in patients with bleeding disorders or thrombocytopenia. Use cautiously in patients with any history of GI bleeding, ulcer disease, or severe renal or hepatic disease. Safety in pregnancy and lactation not established. Not to be used for self-medication for more than 10 days in adults or 5 days in children.	EENT: tinnitus, hearing loss GI: dyspepsia, heartburn, epigastric distress, nausea, vomiting, anorexia, abdominal pain, GI bleeding, hepatotoxicity Hema: anemia, hemolysis Misc: noncardiogenic pulmonary edema, allergic reactions including ANAPHYLAXIS, LARYNGEAL EDEMA, and Reye's syndrome	Drug–Drug: May potentiate oral anticoagulants. May enhance activity of penicillins, phenytoin, methotrexate, valproic acid, oral hypoglycemic agents, and sulfonamides. May antagonize the beneficial effects of uricosuric agents. Glucocorticoids may decrease serum salicylate levels. Urinary acidification enhances reabsorption and may increase serum salicylate levels. Alkalinization of the urine or the ingestion of large amounts of antacids promotes excretion and decreases serum salicylate levels. May blunt the therapeutic responses to diuretics. Drug–Food: Foods capable of acidifying the urine may enhance reabsorption and increase serum salicylate levels.	For all non-opiate analgesics. ASSESSMENT: Assess pain and limitation of movement; note type, location, and intensity of pain prior to and 30–60 min following administration. Assess fever and associated symptoms. INTERVENTION: Evaluate if pain is not relieved and notify MD. Pain should be relieved without a significant alteration in level of consciousness, respiratory status, or blood pressure. Food will decrease the absorption rate but will not alter the total amount absorbed. Crushing tablets increases the absorption rate. Do not crush or chew enteric-coated tablets. EVALUATION: Tablets with an acetic odor should be discarded. Patients on long-term therapy should contact physician before undergoing surgery. Drug may need to be withheld for at least a week prior to surgery. Centers for Disease Control warns against giving aspirin to children or adolescents with varicella (chickenpox) or influenza-like or viral illnesses because of a possible association with Reye's syndrome. Contact physician if tinnitus; unusual bleeding of gums; bruising; or black, tarry stools occur; or if fever returns or lasts longer than 3 days. Advise patient to avoid concurrent use of alcohol with this medication to minimize possible gastric irritation.
Contraindicated in previous hypersensitivity.	Derm: rash, urticaria GI: HEPATIC NECROSIS (overdose)	Drug–Drug: Antipyretics may cause severe hypothermia	Same as for all. ASSESSMENT: Assess

CONTINUED ON THE FOLLOWING PAGE

Table 20–3. DRUGS USED TO CONTROL PAIN-*CONTINUED*

Name	Dosage	Mode of Administration	Pharmacokinetics
Acetaminophen-*Continued*	to exceed 4 g/day, or 2.6 g/ day chronically		½ L: 1.25–3 hr PB: 25% B: liver E: urine
	Adults and Children under 12 yr: 325–650 mg q 4 hr as needed	Rectal	O: 0.5–1 hr P: 1–3 hr D: 3–4 hr
	Children 11–12 yr: 480 mg q 4–6 hr as needed	PO	
	Children 9–11 yr: 400 mg q 4–6 hr as needed	PO	
	Children 6–9 hr: 320 mg q 4–6 hr as needed	PO	
	Children 4–6 yr: 240 mg q 4–6 hr as needed	PO	
	Children 2–4 yr: 160 mg q 4–6 hr as needed	PO	
	Children 1–2 yr: 120 mg q 4–6 hr as needed	PO	
	Children 4–12 mo: 80 mg q 4–6 hr as needed	PO	
	Children under 3 mo: 40 mg q 4–6 hr as needed	PO	

OPIATE ANALGESIC–AGONIST
Morphine (Duramorph, MS Contin, RMS, Roxanol)

Action: Inhibits ascending pain pathways in the CNS and alters pain reception.

Use: Severe pain, preoperative medication.

	Adult: 10–30 mg q 4 hr (extended release tablets may be given q 8–12 hr)	PO (5 mg sublingal)	O: UA P: 60 min D: 4–5 hr ½ L: 2–3 hr PB: 33% B: liver E: urine, feces
	Adult: 5–20 mg q 4 hr	IM	O: 10–30 min P: 30–60 min D: 4–5 hr
	Same as IM.	SC	O: 20 min P: 50–90 min D: 4–5 hr
	Children: 0.1–0.2 mg/kg q 4 hr	SC	
	Adult: 2.5–15 mg q 4 hr, or IV infusion initiated at 1–10 mg/hr increased as needed (large doses of 20–150 mg/hr have been used)	IV	O: rapid P: 20 min D: 4–5 hr
	Adult: 10–20 mg q 4 hr	Rectal	O: UA P: 20–60 min D: 4–5 hr
	Adult: 5–10 mg/day	Epidural	O: 15–60 min P: UA D: >24 hr

Key to Abbreviations in the *Pharmacokinetics* column O-onset; P-peak; D-duration; PB-protein bound; B-bio-transformed in; E-excreted in; ½ L-halflife.
*Within the column listing adverse effects, underlines indicate the most common effects; and CAPITALS indi-cate life-threatening effects.

Contraindications/ Precautions	Adverse Effects*	Interactions	Nursing Implications
Use cautiously in patients with severe hepatic or renal disease. Has been used safely during pregnancy and lactation. Should not be used as self-medication for longer than 10 days in adults or 5 days in children.		when used with phenothiazine antipsychotics. Hepatotoxicity may be additive with other hepatotoxic substances including alcohol. Phenobarbital may increase liver toxicity in overdosage. Cholestyramine and colestipol decrease absorption and may decrease effectiveness of acetaminophen.	hepatic, hematologic, and renal function periodically during the course of prolonged, high-dose therapy. Assess patient's overall health status and alcohol usage before administering this medication. Patients who are malnourished or who are chronic alcohol abusers are at a higher risk of developing hepatotoxicity with chronic use of usual dose of this drug.
Contraindicated in hypersensitivity. Avoid chronic use during pregnancy or lactation. Use cautiously in patients with head trauma, increased intracranial pressure, severe renal, hepatic, or pulmonary disease, hypothryoidism, adrenal insufficiency, alcoholism, undiagnosed abdominal pain, or prostatic hypertrophy. Dosage should be reduced in elderly or debilitated patients. Has been used to relieve pain during labor; may cause respiratory depression in the newborn.	Neuro: sedation, confusion, headache, euphoria, floating feeling, unusual dreams, hallucinations, dysphoria CV: hypotension, tachycardia Resp: respiratory depression GI: nausea, vomiting, constipation GU: urinary retention EENT: dry eyes, blurred vision, lens opacities Misc: tolerance, physical and psychologic dependence, allergic reactions	Drug–Drug: Use with extreme caution in patients receiving MAO inhibitors. Additive CNS depression with alcohol, antihistamines, and sedative-hypnotics. Smoking may decrease analgesic effect. Administration of partial antagonists may precipitate narcotic withdrawal.	For all opiate analgesic-agonists. Oral doses may be administered with food or milk to minimize GI irritation. Dilute for IV administration with at least 5 ml sterile water or 0.9% NaCl. Administer slowly, 15 mg or fraction thereof, over 3–5 min. Rapid administration may lead to increased respiratory depression, hypotension, and circulatory collapse. May be added to IV solutions for continuous infusion. This method requires close titration and an infusion pump to control the rate. Dose should be titrated to ensure adequate pain relief without excessive sedation, respiratory depression, or hypotension. Medication should be discontinued gradually after long-term use to prevent withdrawal symptoms. Available in tablet, solution, suppository, and injectable forms. ASSESSMENT: Prolonged use may lead to dependence and tolerance. This

CONTINUED ON THE FOLLOWING PAGE

Table 20–3. DRUGS USED TO CONTROL PAIN-*CONTINUED*

Name	Dosage	Mode of Administration	Pharmacokinetics
Morphine-*Continued*			
Codeine			

Action: Inhibits ascending pain pathways in the CNS and alters pain reception.

Use: Moderate to severe pain, nonproductive cough.

Name	Dosage	Mode of Administration	Pharmacokinetics
	Analgesia *Adult:* 15–60 mg q 4 hr as needed *Children:* 0.5 mg/kg q 4–6 hr as needed	PO	O: 15–30 min P: 60–120 min D: 4–6 hr ½ L: 2.5–4 hr PB: 50% B: liver E: urine (5%–15% unchanged)
		IM	O: 10–30 min P: 30–60 min D: 4–6 hr
		SC	O: 10–30 min P: 30–60 min D: 4–6 hr
	Antitussive *Adult:* 10–20 mg q 4–6 hr as needed (not to exceed 120 mg/day) *Children 6–11 yr:* 5–10 mg q 4–6 hr as needed (not to exceed 60 mg/day)	PO, IM, SC	

Key to Abbreviations in the *Pharmacokinetics* column O-onset; P-peak; D-duration; PB-protein bound; B-biotransformed in; E-excreted in; ½ L-halflife.

*Within the column listing adverse effects, underlines indicate the most common effects; and CAPITALS indicate life-threatening effects.

should not prevent patient from receiving adequate analgesia. Progressively higher doses may be required to relieve pain with long-term therapy. Assess bowel function routinely. Increased intake of fluids and bulk, stool softeners, and laxatives may minimize constipating effects. Assess blood pressure, pulse, and respiratory rate before and periodically during administration. Naloxone is the antidote.

INTERVENTION: Explain therapeutic value of medication prior to administration to enhance the analgesic effect. Regularly administered doses may be more effective than prn administration. Analgesia is more effective if given before pain becomes severe. Instruct patient in how and when to ask for prn pain medication. Medication may cause drowsiness. Advise patient to call for assistance when ambulating or smoking. Advise patient to make position changes slowly to minimize orthostatic hypotension.

Contraindicated in hypersensitivity. Avoid chronic use during pregnancy and lactation.

Use cautiously in patients with head trauma; increased intracranial pressure; severe renal, hepatic, or pulmonary disease; hypothyroidism, adrenal insufficiency; alcoholism, undiagnosed abdominal pain; or prostatic hypertrophy. Reduce dosage in elderly or debilitated patients. Has been used during labor; respiratory depression may occur in the newborn.

Neuro: sedation, confusion, headache, euphoria, floating feeling, unusual dreams, hallucinations, dysphoria
CV: hypotension, bradycardia
Resp: respiratory depression
GI: nausea, vomiting, constipation
GU: urinary retention
Derm: sweating, flushing
EENT: miosis, diplopia, blurred vision
Misc: tolerance, physical and psychologic dependence

Drug–Drug: Use with extreme caution in patients receiving MAO inhibitors. Additive CNS depression with alcohol, antihistamines, and sedative-hypnotics. Smoking may decrease analgesic effect. Administration of partial antagonists may precipitate narcotic withdrawal.

Same as for all,
ASSESSMENT: Assess cough and lung sounds during antitussive use. Prolonged use may lead to dependence and tolerance. This should not prevent patient from receiving adequate analgesia. Most patients receiving codeine for medical reasons do not develop dependency. Potential for dependence is less than with morphine.
INTERVENTION: Food or milk may minimize GI irritation with oral doses. Medication should be discontinued gradually after long-term use to prevent withdrawal symptoms. Caution patient to avoid driving and activities that require alertness until effects of drug are known.

CONTINUED ON THE FOLLOWING PAGE

Table 20–3. DRUGS USED TO CONTROL PAIN-*CONTINUED*

Name	Dosage	Mode of Administration	Pharmacokinetics
Codeine-*Continued*	*Children 2–5 yr:* 2.5–5 mg q 4–6 hr (not to exceed 30 mg/day)		

Hydromorphone (Dilaudid, Dilaudid-HP)

Action: Inhibits ascending pain pathways in the CNS and alters pain perception.

Use: Moderate to severe pain.

	Analgesia *Adult:* 2–4 mg q 4–6 hr as needed	PO, IM, SC	O: 15–30 min P: UA
	1–2 mg q 4–6 hr	Slow IV	D: 4–5 hr
	Adult: 3 mg q 6–8 hr as needed	Rectal	½ L: UA
	Antitussive *Adult:* 1 mg q 3–4 hr	PO	PB: UA
	Children: 6–12 yr: 0.5 mg q 3–4 hr	PO	B: liver E: urine

Meperidine (Pethidine, Demerol)

Action: Inhibits ascending pain pathways in the CNS and alters pain perception.

Use: Moderate to severe pain, preoperative medication.

	Analgesia *Adult:* 50–150 mg q 3–4 hr	PO, IM, SC	*PO* O: 15 min P: 60 min
	Children: 1.1–1.8 mg/kg q 3–4 hr (single pediatric doses should not exceed 100 mg)	PO, IM, SC	D: 2–4 hr *IM* O: 10–15 min P: 35–50 min D: 2–4 hr
	Adult: 15–35 mg/hr as slow continuous infusion	IV	*SC* O: 10–15 min P: 40–60 min D: 2–4 hr
	Preoperative Sedation Adult: 50–100 mg, 30–90 min before anesthesia	IM, SC	*IV* O: immediate P: 5–7 min
	Children: 1–2 mg/kg, 30–90 min before anesthesia (not to exceed adult dose)	IM, SC	D: 2–4 hr ½ L: 3–8 hr PB: 60% B: liver E: urine (5% unchanged)

Key to Abbreviations in the *Pharmacokinetics* column O-onset; P-peak; D-duration; PB-protein bound; B-biotransformed in; E-excreted in; ½ L-halflife.

*Within the column listing adverse effects, underlines indicate the most common effects; and CAPITALS indicate life-threatening effects.

Contraindications/ Precautions	Adverse Effects*	Interactions	Nursing Implications
			EVALUATION: Suppression of cough determines effectiveness when used as an antitussive.
Contraindicated in hypersensitivity. Avoid chronic use during pregnancy or lactation. Use cautiously in patients with head trauma; increased intracranial pressure; severe renal, hepatic, or pulmonary disease; hypothyroidism; adrenal insufficiency; alcoholism; undiagnosed abdominal pain; or prostatic hypertrophy. Dosage should be reduced in elderly or debilitated patients.	Neuro: sedation, confusion, headache, euphoria, floating feeling, unusual dreams, hallucinations, dysphoria, dizziness CV: hypotension, bradycardia Resp: respiratory depression GI: nausea, vomiting, constipation GU: urinary retention Derm: sweating, flushing EENT: miosis, diplopia, blurred vision Misc: tolerance, physical and psychologic dependence	Drug–Drug: Use with extreme caution in patients receiving MAO inhibitors. Additive CNS depression with alcohol, antidepressants, antihistamines, and sedative-hypnotics. Smoking may decrease analgesic effect. Administration of partial antagonists may precipitate narcotic withdrawal.	Same as for all. INTERVENTION: Food or milk may minimize GI irritation with oral doses. Dilute for IV administration with at least 5 ml sterile water or 0.9% NaCl. Administer slowly at a rate not to exceed 2 mg over 3–5 min. Rapid administration may lead to increased respiratory depression, hypotension, and circulatory collapse. Do not use IV administration without having antidote available. EVALUATION: Suppression of cough demonstrates effectiveness when used as an antitussive.
Contraindicated in hypersensitivity. Avoid chronic use during pregnancy or lactation. Contraindicated in patients receiving MAO inhibitors. Use cautiously in patients with head trauma; increased intracranial pressure; severe renal, hepatic, or pulmonary disease; hypothyroidism; adrenal insufficiency; alcoholism, undiagnosed abdominal pain; or prostatic hypertrophy. Dosage should be reduced in elderly or debilitated patients. Has been used during labor; respiratory depression may occur in the newborn.	Neuro: sedation, confusion, headache, euphoria, floating feeling, unusual dreams, hallucinations, dysphoria CV: hypotension, bradycardia Resp: respiratory depression GI: nausea, vomiting, constipation GU: urinary retention Derm: sweating, flushing EENT: miosis, diplopia, blurred vision Misc: tolerance, physical and psychologic dependence	Drug–Drug: Additive CNS depression with alcohol, antihistamines, and sedative-hypnotics. Smoking may decrease analgesic effect.	Same as for all. ASSESSMENT: Oral doses may be administered with food or milk to minimize GI irritation. Syrup should be diluted in a half-glass water. Oral dose is less than 50% as effective as parenteral. When changing to oral administration, dosage may need to be increased. IM is the preferred parenteral route for repeated doses. SC administration may cause local irritation. Dilute for IV administration with at least 5 ml sterile water or 0.9% NaCl. Administer slowly, at a rate not to exceed 25 mg over 1 min. Rapid administration may lead to increased respiratory depression, hypotension, and circulatory collapse. Do not use IV administration without having antidote available.

CONTINUED ON THE FOLLOWING PAGE

Table 20–3. DRUGS USED TO CONTROL PAIN–*CONTINUED*

Name	Dosage	Mode of Administration	Pharmacokinetics
Methadone Hydrochloride (Dolophine)			
Action: Inhibits ascending pain pathways in the CNS and alters pain perception.			
Use: Severe pain, narcotic withdrawal.			
	Analgesia *Adult:* 2.5–10 mg q 3–4 hr, up to 5–20 mg q 6–8 hr *Detoxification* *Adult:* 15–40 mg/day *Maintenance* *Adult:* 20–120 mg/day	PO, IM, SC PO PO	*PO* O: 30–60 min P: 90–120 min D: 4–12 hr ½ L: 25 hr PB: 90% B: liver E: urine *IM/SC* O: 10–20 min P: 50–120 min D: 4–6 hr
Levorphanol tartrate (Levo-Dromoran)			
Action: Inhibits ascending pain pathways in the CNS and alters pain perception.			
Use: Moderate to severe pain.			
	Adult: 2–3 mg q 6–8 hr	PO, SC, slow IV	O: UA P: 20 min (IV) P: 60–90 min (SC) D: 6–8 hr ½ L: 3–4 hr PB: <50% B: liver E: urine
Oxycodone Hydrochloride (Percocet-5 [oxycodone hydrochloride, 5 mg, and acetaminophen, 325 mg]; Percodan [oxycodone hydrochloride; 4.5 mg, oxycodone terephthalate, 0.38 mg; and aspirin, 325 mg]; Percodan-Demi [oxycodone hydrochloride, 2.25 mg; oxycodone terephthalate, 0.19 mg; and aspirin 325 mg]; Tylox [oxycodone hydrochloride and Tylenol]; Oxycodone hydrochloride (5 mg]).			
Action: Inhibits ascending pain pathways in the CNS and alters pain perception.			
Use: Moderate to severe pain.			
	Adult: 1–2 tablets q 6 hr as needed	PO	O: 10–15 min P: 30–60 min D: 4–5 hr ½ L: 2–3 hr PB: <50% B: liver and kidney E: urine

Key to Abbreviations in the *Pharmacokinetics* column O-onset; P-peak; D-duration; PB-protein bound; B-biotransformed in; E-excreted in; ½ L-halflife.

*Within the column listing adverse effects, underlines indicate the most common effects; and CAPITALS indicate life-threatening effects.

Contraindications/ Precautions	Adverse Effects*	Interactions	Nursing Implications
Contraindicated in hypersensitivity. Avoid chronic use during pregnancy or lactation. Use cautiously in patients with head trauma; increased intracranial pressure; severe renal, hepatic, or pulmonary disease; hypothyroidism; adrenal insufficiency; alcoholism; undiagnosed abdominal pain; or prostatic hypertrophy. Dosage should be reduced in elderly or debilitated patients. The long half-life of methadone allows accumulation of the drug.	Neuro: sedation, confusion, headache, euphoria, floating feeling, unusual dreams, hallucinations, dysphoria. CV: hypotension, bradycardia Resp: respiratory depression GI: nausea, vomiting, constipation GU: urinary retention Derm: sweating, flushing EENT: miosis, diplopia, blurred vision Misc: tolerance, physical and psychologic dependence	Drug–Drug: Use with extreme caution in patients receiving MAO inhibitors. Additive CNS depression with alcohol, antihistamines, and sedative-hypnotics. Smoking may decrease analgesic effect. Administration of partial antagonists may precipitate narcotic withdrawal.	INTERVENTION: Food or milk may minimize GI irritation with oral doses. IM is the preferred route for repeated doses. SC administration may cause local irritation. PATIENT TEACHING: Advise patients to avoid concurrent use of alcohol or CNS depressants.
Same toxic potentials as the other opiate agonists. Safe use in pregnancy and in children has not been established.	Neuro: sedation Resp: respiratory depression GI: nausea, vomiting, constipation	Similar to those for methadone.	Same as for all. ASSESSMENT: Classified as a Schedule II drug. This drug should be given in the smallest dose possible because of its long duration. Not to be confused with levallorphan tartrate, a narcotic antagonist and antidote for levorphanol. INTERVENTION: Reduce dosage in elderly and debilitated patients.
Contraindicated in hypersensitivity, pregnancy, lactation, and in children under 6 years. Use cautiously in alcoholism, renal or hepatic disease, viral infections, Addison's disease, cardiac arrhythmias,	Neuro: lightheadedness, dizziness, sedation, euphoria, dysphoria CV: bradycardia Resp: shortness of breath GI: nausea, vomiting, anorexia, constipation Hema: unusual bleeding, bruising	Drug–Drug: Anticholinergics can cause paralytic ileus; CNS depressants increase CNS depressive effects. Lab: Evaluation of serum amylase, false decrease of blood glucose, false-positive 5-HIAA.	Same as for all. ASSESSMENT: Laboratory studies of hepatic function and hematologic status should be checked periodically in patients undergoing high-dose therapy. Re-assess patient's ongoing need for oxycodone prepa-

CONTINUED ON THE FOLLOWING PAGE

Table 20-3. DRUGS USED TO CONTROL PAIN–*CONTINUED*

Name	Dosage	Mode of Administration	Pharmacokinetics
Oxycodone Hydrochloride–*Continued*			

Oxymorphone Hydrochloride (Numorphan)

Action: Inhibits ascending pain pathways in the CNS and alters pain perception.

Use: Moderate to severe pain.

	Initial: 1–1.5 mg q 4–6 hr as needed	SC, IM	SC, IM O: 10–15 min
	Obstetric Analgesia: 0.5–1 mg, q 4–6 hr as needed	IV	IV O: 5–10 min P: 1–1.5 hr D: 3–6 hr
	Initial: 0.5–5 mg q 4–6 hr as needed		½ L: 2–3 hr PB: 33% B: liver E: urine
		Rectal suppository	O: 15–30 min (rectal)

Propoxyphene Hydrochloride (Darvocet-N, Darvon, Darvon Compound, Darvon-N, Dolene, Dolene Compound)†

Action: Inhibits ascending pain pathways in the CNS and alters pain perception.

Use: Mild to moderate pain.

	Adults: 65 mg q 4 hr (hydrochloride); 100 mg q 4 hr as needed	PO	O: 15–60 min P: 2–3 hr D: 4–6 hr ½ L: 6–12 hr

†Note Darvocet-N contains acetaminophen; Darvon Compound and Dolene Compound contain aspirin and caffeine.

Key to Abbreviations in the *Pharmacokinetics* column O-onset; P-peak; D-duration; PB-protein bound; B-biotransformed in; E-excreted in; ½ L-halflife.
*Within the column listing adverse effects, underlines indicate the most common effects; and CAPITALS indicate life-threatening effects.

Contraindications/ Precautions	Adverse Effects*	Interactions	Nursing Implications
chronic ulcerative colitis, history of drug abuse or dependency, gallbladder disease, acute abdominal conditions, head injury, intracranial lesions, hypothyroidism, prostatic hypertrophy, respiratory disease, urethral stricture, elderly or debilitated patients, peptic ulcer, or coagulation abnormalities.	GU: dysarthria, frequent urination, urinary retention Derm: rash, pruritus, jaundice		rations. Dependency and tolerance may develop with repeated use. INTERVENTION: Since many of the oxycodone preparations contain aspirin or acetaminophen, ingestion of large doses of these preparations can result in aspirin or acetaminophen poisoning. To reduce gastric irritation, administer after meals or with milk. Instruct patient to avoid hazardous activities after taking a dose of the oxycodone preparations. Inform the patient's dentist or surgeon that he or she is receiving an oxycodone preparation prior to any procedure being performed. The consumption of large amounts of alcohol while taking an oxycodone preparation can increase the risk of liver damage. Consult the patient's physician prior to recommending over-the-counter drugs for colds, upset stomachs, allergies, inability to sleep, or pain while the patient is receiving an oxycodone preparation. There is a relatively high risk for abuse of this agent.
Contraindicated in patients with pulmonary edema resulting from chemical respiratory irritants. Safe use during pregnancy (other than labor) and in children under 12 years of age has not been established.	Neuro: euphoria, dizziness GI: nausea, vomiting	Same as for morphine.	Same as for all. INTERVENTION: Protect from light. Store suppositories in refrigerator.
Contraindicated in hypersensitivity. Avoid chronic use during pregnancy and lactation. Use cautiously in patients with head trauma; increased intracranial pressure; severe renal, hepatic, or pulmonary disease; hypothyroidism; adrenal insufficiency;	Neuro: dizziness, lightheadedness, headache, weakness, sedation, drowsiness, insomnia, euphoria, dysphoria, paradoxic excitement. CV: hypotension GI: nausea, vomiting, abdominal pain, constipation Derm: rashes EENT: blurred vision	Drug–Drug: Use with extreme caution in patients receiving MAO inhibitors. Additive CNS depression with alcohol, antidepressants, antihistamines, and sedatives-hypnotics. Smoking may decrease analgesic	Same as for all. INTERVENTION: Food or milk may minimize GI irritation with oral doses. Medication should be discontinued gradually after long-term use to prevent withdrawal symptoms. Available

CONTINUED ON THE FOLLOWING PAGE

Table 20–3. DRUGS USED TO CONTROL PAIN–*CONTINUED*

Name	Dosage	Mode of Administration	Pharmacokinetics
Propoxyphrene Hydrochloride–*Continued*			PB: 50% B: liver E: urine

PARTIAL OPIATE AGONISTS
Pentazocine Hydrochloride (Talwin)

Action: Inhibits ascending pain pathways in the CNS and alters pain perception.

Use: Moderate to severe pain.

Name	Dosage	Mode of Administration	Pharmacokinetics
	Adult: 50 mg q 3–4 hr; maximum dose of 600 mg/24 hr 30 mg q 3–4 hr (excluding patients in labor). Not to exceed 60 mg IM or SC or 30 mg IV. Not to exceed 360 mg/24 hr PO. *Patients in Labor:* 20–30 mg IM; 20 mg may be repeated 1–2 times at 2–3-hr intervals as needed	PO IM, SC, IV	O: 15–30 min for PO, IM, SC O: 2–3 min (IV) P: 1–3 hr (PO) P: 15 min IV P: 15–60 min SC, IM D: 4–5 hr (PO) D: 2–3 hr (IM) ½ L: 2–3 hr PB: 60% B: liver E: urine

Action: Inhibits ascending pain pathways in the CNS and alters pain perception.

Use: Moderate to severe pain.

Name	Dosage	Mode of Administration	Pharmacokinetics
Nalbuphine Hydrochloride (Nubain)	*Adults:* 10 mg q 3–6 hr	IM, SC IV	O: <15 min P: 30–60 min D: 3–6 hr O: 2–3 min P: 30 min D: 3–6 hr ½ L: 5 hr PB: <30% B: liver E: urine, bile

Key to Abbreviations in the *Pharmacokinetics* **column** O-onset; P-peak; D-duration; PB-protein bound; B-biotransformed in; E-excreted in; ½ L-halflife.
*Within the column listing adverse effects, underlines indicate the most common effects; and CAPITALS indicate life-threatening effects.

Contraindications/ Precautions	Adverse Effects*	Interactions	Nursing Implications
alcoholism; undiagnosed abdominal pain; or prostatic hypertrophy. Dosage should be reduced in elderly or debilitated patients. Has been used safely during lactation.	Misc: tolerance, physical and psychologic dependence	effect. Administration of partial antagonists may precipitate narcotic withdrawal.	in combination with non-narcotic analgesics. PATIENT TEACHING: Caution patient to avoid concurrent use of alcohol or CNS depressants while taking this medication.
Contraindicated in patients with head injury, increased intracranial pressure, or history of drug abuse, and in emotionally unstable patients. Safe use during pregnancy or in children under 12 years of age has not been established. Use with caution in patients with impaired renal or hepatic function, respiratory depression, biliary surgery, and in those with myocardial infarction who have nausea and vomiting.	Neuro: dizziness, sedation, lightheadedness, alteration of mood, headache, weakness, insomnia, alteration of taste CV: (IV) tachycardia, hypertension GI: nausea, vomiting, constipation, dry mouth, abdominal cramps Derm: rash, diaphoresis, flushing, pruritus, injection-site reaction Eye: blurred vision, diplopia, nystagmus, miosis High Dose: respiratory depression, hypertension, palpitations, tachycardia, psychotomimetic effects, confusion, anxiety, hallucinations, disturbed dreams, bizarre thoughts, euphoria.	Drug–Drug: The effects of pentazocine are additive with those of other CNS depressants, general anesthetics, phenothiazines, sedative-hypnotics, and alcohol.	For all partial agonists. ASSESSMENT: Observe injection sites for signs of irritation or inflammation. Pentazocine may cause acute withdrawal symptoms in patients receiving opioids regularly. Observe for chills, abdominal and muscle cramps, yawning, rhinorrhea, lacrimation, itching, restlessness, anxiety, and drug-seeking behavior. INTERVENTION: Do not mix pentazocine in the same syringe with barbiturates because this causes precipitation. Pentazocine can cause withdrawal symptoms.
Contraindicated in hypersensitivity. Avoid use in opiate-dependent patients who have not been detoxified—may precipitate opiate withdrawal. Use cautiously in patients with head trauma; increased intracranial pressure; severe renal, hepatic, or pulmonary disease; hypothyroidism; adrenal insufficiency; alcoholism; undiagnosed abdominal pain; or prostatic hypertrophy. Dosage should be reduced in elderly and debilitated patients. Safe use in pregnancy, lactation,	Neuro: sedation, headache, confusion, euphoria, floating feeling, unusual dreams, hallucinations, dysphoria, dizziness, vertigo CV: hypotension, hypertension, palpitations Resp: respiratory depression GI: nausea, vomiting, constipation, ileus, dry mouth GU: urinary urgency Derm: sweating, clammy feeling EENT: miosis (high doses), blurred vision, diplopia Misc: tolerance, physical and psychologic dependence	Drug–Drug: Use with extreme caution in patients receiving MAO inhibitors. Additive CNS depression with alcohol, antihistamines, antidepressants, and sedative-hypnotics. Smoking hastens metabolism and may decrease analgesic effectiveness. May precipitate narcotic withdrawal in patients who are narcotic-dependent and have not been detoxified. Avoid concurrent use with other narcotics, which may diminish analgesic effect.	ASSESSMENT: Assess blood pressure, pulse, and respiration before and periodically during administration. Nalbuphine produces respiratory depression, but this does not markedly increase with increased doses. This drug has a low potential for dependence, but prolonged use may lead to physical and psychologic dependence and tolerance. INTERVENTION: Explain therapeutic value of medication prior to administration to enhance effectiveness. Regularly administered doses may be more effective than prn administration. Caution

CONTINUED ON THE FOLLOWING PAGE

Table 20-3. DRUGS USED TO CONTROL PAIN-*CONTINUED*

Name	Dosage	Mode of Administration	Pharmacokinetics
Nalbuphine Hydrochloride-*Continued*			

Butorphanol (Stadol)

Action: Inhibits ascending pain pathways in the limbic system, thalamus, midbrain, and hypothalamus.

Use: Moderate to severe pain.

	Adults: 1–4 mg q 3–4 hr as needed	IM	O: 10–30 min P: 30–60 min D: 3–4 hr
	Adults: 0.5–2.0 mg q 3–4 hr as needed	IV	O: 1 min P: 4–5 min D: 2–4 hr ½ L: 3–4 hr PB: 80% B: liver E: urine, feces

Buprenorphine (Buprenex)

Action: Same as butorphanol.

Use: Same as butorphanol.

	Analgesic dosage for adults and children over the age of 13 years is 0.3 mg q 6 hr. Maximum dosage is 0.6 mg q 6 hr.	IM, IV (bolus, PCA), epidural, intrathecal	O: 2–5 min (IM) P: 10 min (IM); 2 min (IV) D: 4–5 hr ½ L: 2–3 hr PB: 96% B: liver E: kidney and feces

Key to Abbreviations in the *Pharmacokinetics* column O-onset; P-peak; D-duration; PB-protein bound; B-biotransformed in; E-excreted in; ½ L-halflife.
*Within the column listing adverse effects, underlines indicate the most common effects; and CAPITALS indicate life-threatening effects.

Contraindications/ Precautions	Adverse Effects*	Interactions	Nursing Implications
and children has not been established. Has been used during labor, but may cause respiratory depression in the newborn.			ambulatory patients against operating a car or hazardous machinery after taking the drug. Administer IM injections deep into well-developed muscle. Rotate sites of injections. May give IV undiluted. Administer slowly, each 10 mg over 3–5 min. Antagonistic properties may induce withdrawal symptoms in narcotic-dependent patients.
Contraindicated in hypersensitivity. Avoid use in opiate-dependent patients who have not been detoxified; may precipitate opiate withdrawal. Use cautiously in patients with head trauma; increased intracranial pressure; severe renal, hepatic, or pulmonary disease; hypothyroidism; adrenal insufficiency; or alcoholism. Dosage should be reduced in elderly and debilitated patients. Use cautiously in patients with undiagnosed abdominal pain or prostatic hypertrophy. Safe use in pregnancy, lactation, and children has not been established. Has been used during labor, but may cause respiratory depression in the newborn.	Neuro: sedation, confusion, headache, euphoria, floating feeling, unusual dreams, hallucinations, dysphoria. CV: hypotension, hypertension, palpitations Resp: respiratory depression GI: nausea, vomiting, ileus, constipation, dry mouth GU: urinary retention Derm: sweating, clammy feeling EENT: miosis (high doses), blurred vision, diplopia Misc: sweating, tolerance, physical and psychologic dependence	Drug–Drug: Use with extreme caution in patients receiving MAO inhibitors. Additive CNS depression with alcohol, antihistamines, antidepressants, and sedative-hypnotics. Smoking hastens metabolism and may decrease analgesic effectiveness. May precipitate narcotic withdrawal in patients who are narcotic-dependent and have not been detoxified. Avoid concurrent use with other narcotics, which may diminish analgesic effect.	Same as for all. ASSESSMENT: Butorphanol, 2 mg, has approximately the same respiratory depression as 10 mg of morphine, but respiratory depression does not increase in amount, only in duration with increased dosage. Prolonged use may lead to physical and psychologic dependence and tolerance. Abrupt withdrawal following chronic administration may produce vomiting, restlessness, abdominal cramps, and increased blood pressure and temperature. INTERVENTION: Administer IM injections deep into well-developed muscle. Rotate sites of injections. May give IV undiluted. Administer over 3–5 min. Encourage patient to turn, cough, and breathe deeply every 2 hr to prevent atelectasis. Antagonistic properties may induce withdrawal symptoms in opiate-dependent patients.
Same as for the other opiate analgesics.	Neuro: sedation, headache, dizziness, vertigo, miosis CV: hypotension Resp: hypoventilation GI: nausea, vomiting, loss of appetite. GU: urinary retention Derm: sweating	CNS depressants (opiate analgesics, general anesthetics, phenothiazines, tranquilizers, sedative-hypnotics, alcohol)	Same as for the other opiate analgesics.

CONTINUED ON THE FOLLOWING PAGE

Table 20–3. DRUGS USED TO CONTROL PAIN–*CONTINUED*

Name	Dosage	Mode of Administration	Pharmacokinetics
OPIATE ANTAGONIST **Naloxone Hydrochloride** (Narcan)			
Action: Competes with opiates at opiate receptor site.			
Use: Opiate-induced respiratory depression.			
	Narcotic-Induced Respiratory Depression *Adults:* 0.4–2 mg may be repeated q 2–3 min to a total dose of 10 mg; may also be given IM, or SC if IV is not available. Can be administered as a continuous infusion.	IV IM/SC	O: 1–2 min P: dose-dependent (30–40 min) D: 45 min ½ L: 60–90 min (3 hr neonates) PB: 50% B: liver E: urine
	Children: 0.01 mg/kg; if no response, increase dose to 0.1 mg/kg; may also give IM or SC if IV is not available.	IM, SC, IV	O: 2–5 min P: UK D: >45 min.
	Neonates: 0.01 mg/kg into umbilical vein; may repeat q 2–3 min. Additional doses may be needed at 2–3-hr intervals for 3 doses; may also give IM or SC if IV is not available.	IM, SC, IV	
	Postoperative Respiratory Depression *Adult:* 0.1–0.2 mg q 2–3 min as needed, or continuous infusion of 0.25 mg/hr *Children:* 0.005–0.01 mg/kg; may repeat q 2–3 min. Additional doses may be needed at 2–3-hr intervals (up to 0.1 mg/kg may be required).		
Levallorphan Tartrate (Lorfan)			
Action: Same as naloxone.			
Use: Same as naloxone.			
	Adult: 1 mg if required. This may be followed by 1–2 additional doses of 0.5 mg at 10–15-min intervals.	IV	O: 1–2 min P: UA D: 2–5 hr ½ L: UA

Key to Abbreviations in the *Pharmacokinetics* column O-onset; P-peak; D-duration; PB-protein bound; B-biotransformed in; E-excreted in; ½ L-halflife.

*Within the column listing adverse effects, underlines indicate the most common effects; and CAPITALS indicate life-threatening effects.

Contraindications/ Precautions	Adverse Effects*	Interactions	Nursing Implications
Contraindicated in hypersensitivity. Use cautiously in patients with cardiovascular disease. May antagonize postoperative analgesia. Use cautiously in narcotic-dependent patients—may precipitate severe withdrawal. Safety in pregnancy and lactation has not been established.	CV: ventricular tachycardia, ventricular fibrillation, hypotension, hypertension. GI: nausea, vomiting	Drug–Drug: Can precipitate withdrawal in narcotic-dependent patients.	For all opiate antagonists. ASSESSMENT: Assess respiratory rate, rhythm, and depth; pulse, blood pressure, and level of consciousness frequently until effects of narcotic wear off. The effects of some narcotics may outlast the effects of antagonist and repeat doses may be necessary. Assess patient for signs and symptoms of narcotic withdrawal. Symptoms may occur within a few min to 2 hr. Severity varies. Lack of significant improvement indicates that symptoms are due to other non-narcotic CNS depressants that are not affected by antagonist or to a disease process. INTERVENTION: May be given as direct IV, undiluted, at a rate of 0.4 mg over 15 sec. Titrate to patient response. For IV infusion, dilute in 5% dextrose in water or 0.9% NaCl. The standard dilution varies according to individual hospitals. Mixture is stable for 24 hours; discard unused solution. Incompatible with preparations containing bisulfite and sulfite and solutions wth an alkaline pH. PATIENT TEACHING: As medication becomes effective, explain purpose and effects of naloxone to patient. EVALUATION: Clinical response is demonstrated by adequate ventilation and alertness without significant pain.
Contraindicated in mild narcotic-induced respiratory depression; respiratory depression due to	Neuro: drowsiness, dizziness, lethargy, dysphoria, miosis, pseudopiosis, sweating, agitation, rest-		INTERVENTION: Not to be confused with levorphanol tartrate, a narcotic analgesic. Artificial respiration with

CONTINUED ON THE FOLLOWING PAGE

Table 20–3. DRUGS USED TO CONTROL PAIN–*CONTINUED*

Name	Dosage	Mode of Administration	Pharmacokinetics
Levallorphan Tartrate– *Continued*	Total dose not to exceed 3 mg. *Neonates:* 0.05–0.1 mg diluted to 2 ml with 0.9% NaCl solution injected into umbilical cord vein immediately after delivery. If vein cannot be used, injection may be given SC or IM.		PB: 40%–50% B: liver E: urine

   Key to Abbreviations in the *Pharmacokinetics* column O-onset; P-peak; D-duration; PB-protein bound; B-bio-transformed in; E-excreted in; ½ L-halflife.
   *Within the column listing adverse effects, underlines indicate the most common effects, and CAPITALS indicate life-threatening effects.

ADVERSE EFFECTS. Adverse effects occur with hypersensitivity reactions and overdose. Rare hypersensitivity reactions may produce laryngeal edema, skin rash, fever, angioneurotic edema, and mucosal lesions. Signs of overdose include nausea, vomiting, pain, and chills, as well as blood dyscrasias, methemoglobinemia, psychologic changes, renal and hepatic damage, hypoglycemic coma, and myocardial dysfunction. Acute poisoning may be manifested by dizziness, nausea, vomiting, palpitations, and sweating. A single dose of 25 g or more can be fatal, causing fulminating hepatic failure. Acute renal failure is also possible. Both the liver and the kidney contain the enzyme systems for converting acetaminophen to the cytotoxic metabolite that causes cellular necrosis. Acetaminophen may produce a slight increase in responsiveness to oral anticoagulants. It may also cause a false increase in urinary 5-HIAA (5-hydroxyindoleacetic acid) test results. Acetaminophen combined with aspirin may be used to control severe pain. A dosage of 900–1000 mg of acetaminophen once a day on a short-term basis produces effective, long-lasting pain relief.

ANTIDOTE. If overdose of acetaminophen is suspected, syrup of ipecac is administered to the patient or gastric lavage is performed. The antidote for an overdose of acetaminophen is acetylcysteine (Mucomyst). The loading oral adult dose is 140 mg/kg body weight. The maintenance oral adult dosage is 70 mg/kg every four hours for 17 doses. Acetylcysteine is most effective when it is started within ten hours after the overdose. Acetylcysteine substitutes for a lack of glutathione and forms an inactive compound with the reactive metabolite.

DOSAGE. Acetaminophen is available in tablet, capsule, elixir, and rectal suppository forms. Acetaminophen syrup may be used to advantage even in adults since the drug is already in solution and is therefore more readily absorbed. The syrup may also be used for those who have difficulty in swallowing and who complain of nausea. The usual adult dosage is 325–650 mg three or four times daily. The pediatric dosages can be found in Table 20–3.

OPIATE ANALGESICS

Compounds similar to morphine that provide pain relief and sedation are referred to as "narcotic analgesics." The term narcotic is confusing because it implies an alteration of consciousness, and opiate analgesics work without producing a loss of consciousness. The term opiate analgesic is used in this text to refer to drugs that are the natural and semisynthetic alkaloid derivatives of opium that mimic the actions of morphine. Opiate analgesics are well known for their clinical use of pain relief. Other clinical uses include providing sedation and controlling diarrhea and cough.

Action

Many sites throughout the body produce the pharmacologic effects of opiate analgesics. The primary sites are those in the brain that are responsible for pain and psychologic reaction to pain. Sites that have a high affinity for opiate analgesics also have high concentrations of endogenous peptides (endorphins). Through the endogenous endorphin system, the body can selectively release these peptides in response to pain. The opiate analgesics mimic the action of these endorphins by binding with their receptors. Outside the brain, the dorsal horn of the spinal cord is also a binding site. The brain sites dedicated to altering the response to pain are less defined. It is thought that the pathways between the diencephalon and the frontal cortex are involved. The person is aware of pain but states that its intensity is no longer bothersome.

   Opiate analgesics inhibit neuronal firing in specific areas of the brain, thus decreasing the release of certain

Contraindications/ Precautions	Adverse Effects*	Interactions	Nursing Implications
barbiturates or other sedatives and hypnotics, anesthetics, other non-narcotic CNS depressants, or pathologic causes; and narcotic addiction (may precipitate severe and possibly fatal withdrawal symptoms).	lessness, sense of heaviness in limbs. CV: hypertension, tachycardia Resp: respiratory depression GI: nausea, vomiting High Doses: weird dreams, visual hallucinations, disorientation, feeling of unreality. Neonates: irritability, increased crying		oxygen and other resuscitative measures may accompany drug administration.

neurotransmitters. The release of transmitter substance is associated with calcium entry into the neuron. This action alters activation of postsynaptic sites.

Pharmacokinetics

The opiate analgesics are absorbed well from mucosal surfaces of the nose and gastrointestinal tract as well as from subcutaneous and intramuscular sites. The absorption from the gastrointestinal tract may be rapid, but the potency of some compounds may be lower because of the first-pass metabolism in the liver after absorption. The oral dosage of these compounds is higher than that required when parenteral administration is used. Table 20–4 details the potency of these agents.

The opiate analgesics are distributed to a variety of tissues, such as the lungs, liver, kidneys, and spleen. The skeletal muscle and fatty tissue are storage sites for these compounds, and concentrations in the brain are low compared with concentrations in other organs. The opiates are converted to metabolites and are excreted by the kidneys.

Organ-System Effects of Morphine and Other Opiates

The systemic effects described below include the opiate agonists. The effects of the antagonists and *opioid agonist-antagonists* compounds are described later in this chapter.

CENTRAL NERVOUS SYSTEM. As discussed earlier in this chapter, the opiate analgesics change the pain perception and reaction to the pain response. The opioid analgesics have an affinity for the mu receptors. The major effects are analgesia, euphoria, sedation, respiratory depression, cough suppression, miosis, truncal rigidity, and emesis. The euphoria is characterized by a floating sensation and a feeling of freedom from anxiety and distress. The sedation effect is a result of drowsiness and clouding of mentation. Patients may experience some impairment of reasoning ability. Patients, especially the elderly, may feel the need to sleep as a result of these drugs. The respiratory depression caused by the administration of opioid analgesics is a result of depres-

sion of the respiratory centers in the pons and medulla, caused by a depressed response to a carbon dioxide challenge. This is one reason why patients with increased intracranial pressure, asthma, chronic obstructive pulmonary disease, or cor pulmonale cannot tolerate opiate analgesics. Cough suppression occurs because of the depressive effects of opioid analgesics on the brain stem. Constriction of the pupil *(miosis)* is a hallmark of opiate use. Constriction of the pupil is blocked by atropine and opiate antagonists. Truncal rigidity is believed to be the result of opiate action at the level of the spinal cord. The large trunk muscles have increased tone while the drug is in the system. Emesis is a result of activation of the chemoreceptor trigger zone in the medulla. This activation is due to the opioid administration, and the result is nausea and vomiting. Prolonged use of the opiate analgesics leads to tolerance to these effects.

PERIPHERAL EFFECTS. Generally opiate analgesics do not have a direct effect on cardiac rate, rhythm, or blood pressure. If the cardiovascular system is stressed, then hypotension can result. Morphine sulfate is used as a preload reducer in myocardial infarction.

GASTROINTESTINAL TRACT. Constipation is an effect of opiate analgesics. Motility is decreased, but tone is increased. The biliary tract experiences a constriction of the biliary smooth muscle, which can cause biliary colic (occurs mainly with Demerol).

GENITOURINARY TRACT. An increase in urethral sphincter tone occurs, which contributes to urinary retention in the postoperative patient. The use of opiate analgesics in the obstetric patient can prolong labor.

OTHER SYSTEMS. The use of opiate analgesics stimulates the release of antidiuretic hormone (ADH), prolactin, and somatotropin.

Adverse Effects

The use of opiate analgesics may lead to drug *dependence, tolerance,* and *addiction.* As a whole, these drugs may interfere with ability to drive, to operate machinery, and to use accurate judgment. For the most part, the opiate analgesics have not been proven safe during

Table 20–4. COMPARISON OF OPIATE ANALGESICS WITH RESPECT TO DOSAGE, POTENCY, AND DURATION OF ACTION

Analgesic	Usual Therapeutic Dose (mg)—Adult	Potency (IM)*	Duration of Action (hr)
Morphine	5 (sublingual) 5–15 (IM, SC) 2.5–15 (IV) 10–30 (oral)	1	4–5
Codeine	15–60 (oral)	0.16–0.33	4–6
Oxymorphone (Numorphan)	10 (oral) 1–1.5 (IM)	1 (oral) 10	3–6
Hydromorphone (Dilaudid)	1–2 (IV) 2 (IM) 2–3 (oral)	1	3–4
Meperidine (Demerol)	50–150 (IM) 50–150 (oral)	0.1 0.05–0.1 (oral)	2–4
Methadone (Dolophine)	10–15 (oral) 2.5–10 (IM)	1–1.3	4–12
Levorphanol (Levo-Dromoran)	2–3 (SC, oral)	3	6–8
Fentanyl (Sublimaze)	0.05–0.1 (IM, IV)	100–200	30 min–1 hr
Pentazocine (Talwin)	30–50 (IM) 50 (oral)	0.33	3–5
Propoxyphene (Darvon)	30–60 (oral)	0.16–0.33	2–4
Oxycodone (Percodan, Percocet)	30 (oral)	1	4–5
Nalbuphine (Nubain)	10 (IM, SC, IV)	1	3–6
Butorphanol (Stadol)	0.5–2 (IV) 1–4 (IM)	1	3–4
Buprenorphine (Buprenex)	0.3 (IV, IM)	30	4–5

*Morphine = 1.
IM, intramuscular; SC, subcutaneous; IV, intravenous.

pregnancy and lactation, and they are used with caution in the very young and the very old, and in debilitated, psychotic, or hypovolemic patients, because of their central depressant effect. Common signs of opiate analgesic toxicity include pinpoint pupils, shallow respiration, and coma. Other conditions that mandate caution in administering opiate analgesics include cardiac arrhythmias, Addison's disease, and hypothyroidism, because further depression of body systems may occur; increased intracranial pressure, increased cerebrospinal fluid (CSF) pressure, seizures, and head injury, because

pressure may be increased, further worsening symptoms; acute abdominal disease, because symptoms may be masked; severe hepatitis, because these drugs are detoxified in the liver; and prostatic hypertrophy and urethral stricture, because urinary function may be further impaired. Opiate analgesics should be given in the smallest effective dose and as infrequently as possible to minimize the development of tolerance and physical dependence but not so infrequently that pain is inadequately controlled.

Another issue related to the use of opiate analgesics

is the development of tolerance. The first sign of tolerance is the patient's report that the analgesic effect is not lasting as long as it had previously. One possible solution is to switch the patient to an alternate opiate. It is also important to use nonpharmacologic approaches to pain relief, such as imagery, relaxation therapy, transcutaneous electrical nerve stimulation (TENS), biofeedback, and distraction.

The last major issue related to opioid therapy is the risk of abuse and addiction. There are very few studies that assess the degree of physical dependence, substance abuse, or psychologic dependence in patients receiving opioid analgesics. The fear of addiction does, however, limit the use of opiate analgesics.

The opioid analgesics are described in Table 20-3.

Dosage

Dosages of opiate analgesics are not interchangeable from one type of drug to another. Dosages of oral and parenteral forms of the same drug are not interchangeable. Table 20-4 lists the equianalgesic effects of selected opiate analgesics as compared with the standard, morphine. Note, for instance, that 10 mg of morphine given intramuscularly is equianalgesic to 75 mg of meperidine. Also note that 10 mg of morphine given intramuscularly is comparable in effect to 30 mg of morphine taken orally. Response to narcotics is highly individualized. Not every patient responds favorably to 75 mg of meperidine given intramuscularly every four hours as needed for pain. Some adjustment in dosage and timing may be necessary to gain optimum pain relief for each patient.

Most of the opiate analgesics are metabolized in the liver and excreted in the urine. In hepatic insufficiency, dosage reduction is recommended.

Controversies in Opiate Therapy

One of the most pressing issues in medicine today is relieving pain so patients do not suffer. Since there is a difference between acute and chronic pain, it is very difficult to find a solution to the problem of making patients free of pain. The controversies surrounding the administration of opioids include: choice of opiate analgesic, method of drug administration, route of drug administration, development of tolerance, and risk of substance abuse and addiction. The literature about choice of drug is very confusing, especially when comparisons between opiate analgesics are made. Individualization of drug and dosage seems to be the rule of thumb.

One major issue related to method of administration is the use of a fixed or an "as needed" (prn) schedule. When a fixed schedule is used, the patient experiences continuous pain relief and the pain is kept from resurfacing. There are usually minimal delays that occur in the hospital setting. This approach can be dangerous in the patient who has had no previous narcotic exposure. Repeated doses of long-acting opiate analgesics can lead to drug accumulation and side effects. In the prn approach, the drug is administered when there is recurrence of pain. This seems to work well for patients with chronic pain, although not for those with chronic acute pain. One disadvantage is that the patient may experience delays of receiving the medication. Since there are very few studies comparing these two approaches as the most appropriate means of administration, individualization of timing seems to be the current practice. If patients are not receiving relief from their pain, then the nursing assessment becomes a critical intervention.

PATIENT-CONTROLLED ANALGESIA (PCA). A method that is beneficial for the delivery of prn pain medication is patient-controlled analgesia (PCA) therapy. This system consists of an infusion pump that is electronically controlled and connected to a timing device. When a patient experiences pain, the person presses a thumb button located on the end of a cord extending from the pump. The pump then releases the preset amount of analgesia through the patient's indwelling intravenous catheter. The timer is programmed to lock out supplemental doses until the first dose has had time to reach its peak pharmacologic effect. The loading dose, lock-out interval, dose volume, and maximum volume allowed are prescribed by the physician. A wide variety of analgesic drugs (fentanyl, hydromorphone, methadone, oxymorphone, sufentanil, buprenorphine, nalbuphine, and pentazocine) are used in PCA therapy. Morphine and meperidine are the agents used most extensively (see Table 20-5 for common doses for PCA therapy). PCA allows the individual patient to overcome variations in pharmacokinetics and pharmacodynamic factors by titrating the rate of opiate administration to meet their analgesic needs (White, 1988). Patients have an opportunity to actively participate in their care and as a result exhibit decreased anxiety. The patient controls his or her care by being able to minimize the time interval between the perception of pain and the administration of the analgesic.

Table 20-5. COMMON BOLUS DOSES FOR PCA THERAPY

Drug	Bolus Dose (mg)	Lockout Interval (min)
Buprenorphine hydrochloride (A-A)*	0.03-0.2	10-20
Fentanyl citrate (A)*	0.02-0.1	3-10
Hydromorphone hydrochloride (A)	0.1-0.5	5-15
Meperidine hydrochloride (A)	5-30	5-15
Methadone hydrochloride (A)	0.5-3	10-20
Morphine sulfate (A)	0.5-3	5-20
Nalbuphine hydrochloride (A-A)	1-5	5-15
Oxymorphone hydrochloride (A)	0.2-0.8	5-15
Pentazocine hydrochloride (A-A)	5-30	5-15
Sufentanil citrate (A)	0.003-0.015	3-10

*A-A, agonist-antagonist; A, agonist

Researchers studying postoperative patients using PCA therapy reported that patients required less narcotics, experienced less sedation and pulmonary complications, experienced less postoperative fever, and increased their postoperative physical activity. When patients experience less pain and sedation, they are able to move around in bed and ambulate more easily.

Nurses need to instruct patients on the purpose and use of PCA therapy. The PCA device is used in a variety of clinical settings. Since many patients use PCA during the postoperative course, it is necessary to teach the patient in the preoperative period. Patients need time to understand PCA and to manipulate the equipment. It is important for the patient to (1) understand the PCA device; (2) realize that it does not provide complete pain relief but works to minimize distressing pain; (3) use the PCA device to avoid pain associated with transporting, ambulation, and dressing changes; and (4) attempt to minimize the size of the bolus dose during waking hours (to avoid sedation), while maximizing the dose intervals during sleeping hours. When the patient understands these important points regarding this therapy, he or she will be successful in managing pain.

Problems encountered with PCA fall into three areas: operator errors, patient errors, and mechanical errors. Operator errors consist of misprogramming the PCA device, improper loading of syringe/cartridge, failure to clamp/unclamp tubing, inability to respond to safety alarms, and misplacing the PCA pump key. Operator errors are very common in clinical practice. It is critical for the nursing staff to understand the concept of PCA therapy. In addition to understanding why this system is used for pain relief, it is also necessary to know how the system works. With this knowledge, the nurse can troubleshoot basic problems. A variety of resources are available to nurses to enhance learning in how to work PCA pumps. Some of these resources include the instruction book that accompanies the pumps, the sales representative, and other nurses. Operator errors can be overcome by becoming familiar with the particular PCA device.

Patient errors include failure to understand PCA therapy, confusion about the operation of the PCA pump, and intentional analgesia abuse. Patient errors occur for a variety of reasons, such as lack of PCA teaching, a hurried teaching/learning experience, or the patient may be a poor candidate for PCA therapy. Most patient errors can be overcome with appropriate candidate selection and a nonhurried teaching/learning experience. When nurses are not rushed during the teaching experience, the patient can ask questions and practice how to use the PCA pump. Difficulties encountered by the patient can then be resolved before actual use of the PCA pump.

Mechanical errors include failure to deliver on demand, defective one-way valves, lock malfunctions, problems with the alarms, and mechanical errors. A wide variety of PCA pumps are available today.

The side effects of administering opiates via the PCA pump are similar to the systemic effects of opiate administration. These side effects include sedation, nausea and vomiting, urinary retention, constipation, and respiratory depression. These side effects are dose-related. It is reported that sedation occurs less often in patients using PCA therapy. The risk of respiratory depression in patients receiving PCA therapy is low. Many investigators recommend the use of precautions (i.e., apnea monitors, frequent respiratory assessment, serial arterial blood gases) to minimize the risk of this life-threatening complication. When using PCA therapy, it is important to assess the dose-effect relationship at one- to three-hour intervals during the early postoperative period.

Studies that examine the cost-effectiveness of PCA therapy are needed. At present, the use of these special pumps and prefilled syringes is expensive for patients.

CONTINUOUS INTRAVENOUS INFUSION. Another method of delivering opiate analgesics is by continuous intravenous infusion. The same opiate analgesics used in PCA therapy are also used in continuous intravenous infusion therapy. An advantage of continuous intravenous infusion of opiate analgesics is better "control" of the pain because of a continuous infusion of the opiate. The disadvantages of this type of delivery system are that more nursing care is required for monitoring the patient and expensive infusion pumps are used.

The route of drug administration is an important issue in opiate therapy. The oral route has been recommended for chronic cancer pain. Continuous intravenous infusion of opioid drugs is being used increasingly for postoperative and chronic cancer pain (Portenoy, 1986).

EPIDURAL/INTRATHECAL OPIATE THERAPY. Another method of administering opiate analgesics is by the *epidural* and *intrathecal therapy* routes. Both of these routes are used in acute and chronic pain management. The use of epidural and intrathecal routes of administration is still controversial, but it seems that these routes may reduce the degree of central nervous system side effects. Properly managed, both routes offer dependable, long-acting, site-specific (some receptor binding occurs at the spinal level) pain relief with lower doses of analgesics. Many of the central depressant effects often associated with systemic opiates are avoided. The motor, sensory, and autonomic effects associated with the injection of local anesthetics are also minimized by this route of administration.

When the epidural or intrathecal approach to pain management is used, it is important to consider the pharmacologic aspects of the opiates. Important pharmacologic characteristics include lipid solubility, molecular weight and volume, specific receptor affinities (influence opiate spread), and rate of opiate clearance from the central nervous system. Knowledge of these characteristics enables the nurse to monitor the clinical effects of the opiates. It is important to predict the onset, duration of action, analgesic potency, CSF distribution, and clearance of the opiate because all of these factors determine clinical outcomes. The following examples illustrate how monitoring of the clinical effects of opiates is related to clinical outcomes. Epidural morphine is more water soluble than lipid soluble, demonstrating a slow onset of action (takes time to diffuse through the lipid neural membranes), a long duration of action, a high potency (strong receptor affinity), good distribution, and slow clearance from the CSF (due to its water solubility). Epidural fentanyl acts in the opposite way. Fentanyl is lipid soluble, entering tissues rapidly, resulting in rapid onset of effects and short duration of action. The potency of fentanyl is greater than that of morphine, and it has immediate receptor binding. The immediate receptor binding causes a limited segmental spread. Fentanyl's clearance, due to its lipid solubility, is rapid. Although many drugs are used for epidural and intrathecal administration, morphine remains the standard against which all others are measured. Drugs that contain stabilizing agents, preservatives, antioxidants, and neurolytic agents (e.g., phenol, alcohol) are not used because of damage to the spinal cord.

The common side effects associated with the administration of epidural and intrathecal opiates are urine retention, nausea and vomiting, and pruritus. All of these side effects are dose-dependent. Patients with chronic pain are less likely to experience these side effects than are patients with acute pain. Urine retention is secondary to the effect of opiates on spinal nerves innervating the bladder and influence of opiate-mediated ADH release, causing oliguria. Nausea and vomiting are the result of the stimulation of the vomiting center in the medulla and the spinal suppression of visceral inhibitory fibers that act to suppress the vomiting center. Pruritus may be related to histamine release, cephalad spread of opiates, and/or disturbances in cutaneous sensation due to opiate receptor binding. Respiratory depression is an unusual but potentially lethal complication. This problem occurs early or late following administration of the opiate. The early development of respiratory depression is related to plasma uptake, drug shunting via epidural circulation, or changes in CSF bulk flow. A late onset of respiratory depression is due to opiate penetration and distribution in the CSF and movement of the opiate via the CSF to the receptors in the medulla. These side effects can be reduced by the use of antiemetics, antipruritics, and small doses of naloxone or naloxone infusions, without reversing analgesia.

The other complications associated with epidural and intrathecal therapy are technique-related. These include catheter malposition, catheter malfunction, and infection.

Catheter malposition or migration is a complication that can occur at any time during the use of this method of opiate delivery. Catheters can migrate from the epidural space into the subarachnoid space or from the epidural space into the vascular system, or the catheter may come into contact with neural tissues (e.g., nerve roots) or compress the spinal cord. It is important for the nurse to aspirate the epidural/intrathecal catheter prior to giving the ordered opiate. Aspiration of CSF or blood from an epidural catheter may mean catheter migration. The opiate should not be administered, and the physician should be notified. As part of assessment, it is important for the nurse to recognize the signs and symptoms of dural puncture (e.g., aspiration of CSF; wet catheter dressing; patient complaining of a continuous, throbbing, occipital headache) and intravascular placement (e.g., aspiration of blood from the catheter; the patient experiences sudden nausea and vomiting, hypotension, and respiratory depression after administration of epidural opiates). Another problem that results from catheter migration is compression of nerve tissue. The nurse should be alert to signs/symptoms of paresthesias, motor weakness, paralyses, and bowel/bladder dysfunction. If these problems arise, the physician is notified.

Catheter malfunction occurs as a result of catheter kinking, knotting, compression, slippage, or shearing. Indications of catheter malfunction include patient reports of poor pain relief and difficulty administering the opiate. Medications should not be forced through the epidural/intrathecal catheter. If difficulty occurs, the patient should be repositioned with his or her spine slightly flexed. This flexion of the spine increases the intervertebral spaces and frees the catheter if it is compressed. If problems with administration remain after the patient has been repositioned, the physician is notified. When the epidural catheter is removed, the nurse should check it to make sure that it is intact and that the holes are not occluded (in many hospitals, removing an epidural catheter is a nursing function; it usually is not a nursing function to remove an intrathecal catheter). If part of the catheter is missing, the physician is notified. Surgery may be required to retrieve the missing part of the catheter.

It is necessary to use strict aseptic technique to maintain sterility of insertion site when administering solutions and starting infusion lines. Infection occurs secondary to failure to maintain aseptic conditions. Covering catheter ports maintains in-line sterility. The nurse assesses the patient for signs of infection (e.g., fever, pain/tenderness at the catheter site, red insertion site) and meningeal irritation (e.g., headache, stiff neck, pain radiating down the back, *photophobia*, mental changes).

Types of Epidural and Intrathecal Delivery Systems. The technical advancements related to catheters and pumps offer many approach options for epidural and intrathecal therapy. Examples of these approach options include intraspinal conduits, subcutaneous tunneling (i.e., Ommaya reservoir), and continuous delivery systems.

Intraspinal conduits are intended for a limited period of use (three to four days). An example of when this system is used is for postoperative pain relief. The problems with this system include accidental removal, obstruction, kinking, pain at the injection site, and local infection. Many of these problems are related to the mobility of the catheter, attachment of the catheter to the patient, and the material from which the catheter is made.

Subcutaneous tunneling is used to reduce the risk of infection of long-term placement. Several advantages of this approach include stabilization of the catheter (decreases the potential of catheter migration) and the patient's ease of access to the site. Easy access to the site allows the patient to perform self-medication and catheter care. A step beyond this approach is an implanted intrathecal or epidural catheter with an injection reservoir. This type of system is designed for long-term use. Advantages include no visual catheters hanging from the skin, the patient can perform self-medication and catheter care, and the drug dose can be changed easily. Disadvantages of this system include hemorrhagic and infectious risks associated with implanted systems, the need for bolus or periodic reservoir refills, and dependence on a bolus delivery mode.

The last approach offered is a continuous implantable infusion pump. This concept is very similar to the insulin delivery device. The continuous implantable infusion pump is approved for morphine delivery. The pump is placed in a subcutaneous pocket and anchored. The pump's catheter is then connected to a tunneled intrathecal or epidural catheter. The impact of such a delivery system is yet to be determined.

Morphine Sulfate

Morphine sulfate is one of the most widely used and potent of the opioid analgesics. Morphine sulfate reduces pain sensation by suppressing opioid receptors within the limbic system of the brain. By suppressing the limbic receptors, the unpleasant emotional responses to pain are also inhibited. Morphine also activates the production of endorphins.

Morphine may also reduce pain perception by activating certain midbrain neurons, which in turn relay inhibitory impulses down to the dorsolateral tracts to the dorsal horn neurons. These dorsal horn neurons receive pain stimuli from the periphery and thereby stop the ascent of the pain stimuli to the brain.

CONTRAINDICATIONS AND PRECAUTIONS. Morphine sulfate is contraindicated in patients with known hypersensitivity. It has a high abuse potential and is classified as a Schedule II controlled substance. It should be used cautiously in patients with head injury and increased intracranial pressure. If used in these circumstances, the patient's intracranial pressure should be monitored because morphine will depress consciousness, decrease respiration, increase carbon dioxide partial pressure, increase intracranial pressure, and alter pupil reaction to light. Morphine should also be used with caution in patients who have severe renal, hepatic, or pulmonary disease, hypothyroidism, adrenal insufficiency, alcoholism, undiagnosed abdominal pain, and in the elderly.

ADVERSE EFFECTS. The most common adverse effects of morphine sulfate administration are constipation, urinary retention, nausea, and vomiting. In the ambulatory patient, restlessness, dizziness, and lightheadedness may also occur because of central brain stimulation. In addition, the typical pupillary constriction is caused by stimulation of the oculomotor center. The patient may also experience reddened eyes as a result of cerebral vessel dilatation. This dilatation occurs secondary to respiratory depression (increased carbon dioxide and decreased oxygen), which causes cerebral

vessels to dilate. As cerebral vessels dilate, intracranial pressure increases and may result in mood changes, confusion, and flushing. Subcortical and spinal centers are also depressed, which leads to the suppression of the cough reflex. Morphine produces depression of the respiratory center in the medulla. Breathing becomes slowed and shallow, and it may even become irregular as the respiratory center fails to respond adequately to blood carbon dioxide levels.

Morphine affects the gastrointestinal system in various ways. First, there is a decreased peristaltic motility and decreased glandular secretion, which can lead to constipation. Second, there is increased spasticity of the sphincters, which can lead to biliary colic.

Morphine's effect on the cardiovascular center in the medulla is minimal. In the periphery, there is vasodilatation, which may lead to postural hypotension, dizziness, weakness, and fainting in ambulatory patients. Both this dilatory effect and its calming effect on the central nervous system contribute to morphine's effectiveness in managing the patient with acute pulmonary edema.

INTERACTIONS. Morphine sulfate interacts with certain other drugs and with some diagnostic tests. The central nervous system effects of morphine can be exaggerated or prolonged by concurrent administration of alcohol, antianxiety drugs, phenothiazines, sedative-hypnotics, barbiturates, anesthetics, and monoamine oxidase (MAO) inhibitors. Concurrent use of skeletal muscle relaxants can enhance their neuromuscular blocking action.

Diagnostic test interactions include false-positive plasma amylase and lipase determinations for 24 hours after a morphine dose. Also a false-positive urine glucose determination may occur when using Benedict's solution.

DOSAGE. The routes of administration are intramuscular (IM), subcutaneous (SC), intravenous (IV), oral (PO), rectal, and epidural. The average adult dosage is 5–15 mg SC or IM every four hours as needed. Intravenous and pediatric dosages can be found in Table 20–3.

Methylmorphine (Codeine)

The narcotic methylmorphine (codeine) provides analgesia through intramuscular, subcutaneous, intravenous, and oral routes of administration.

CONTRAINDICATIONS AND PRECAUTIONS. Codeine is contraindicated in patients with hypersensitivity to narcotics. It is also a Schedule II controlled substance (in its pure form), and tolerance and dependence may develop. Codeine is generally used with extreme caution in those conditions described under the narcotics. Codeine is the drug of choice when intracranial pressure is high. There is a ceiling effect to pain relief with codeine.

ADVERSE EFFECTS. The most common adverse effects of codeine are constipation, drowsiness, nausea and vomiting, and orthostatic hypotension. Occasionally, codeine produces itching, sweating, flushing, tolerance, dependence, respiratory depression, and suppression of the cough reflex. When combined with aspirin, codeine exerts an additive effect for pain relief.

DOSAGE. The average adult analgesic dosage is 15–60 mg four times daily. For pediatric dosages, see Table 20–3.

Hydromorphone

Hydromorphone (Dilaudid) is a Schedule II controlled substance (in pure form). It is a semisynthetic derivative of morphine and may cause tolerance, dependence, and addiction. It is ten times more potent than morphine. Newborns of mothers regularly taking opiates during pregnancy will be born dependent. Hydromorphone may exhibit an additive effect if used with other central nervous system depressant narcotics, general anesthetics, phenothiazines, tranquilizers, sedative-hypnotics, tricyclic antidepressants, or alcohol.

CONTRAINDICATIONS AND PRECAUTIONS. Hydromorphone is contraindicated in patients with the same conditions as described for morphine. This drug should also be used cautiously in patients with severe renal and hepatic disease, hypothyroidism, adrenal insufficiency, alcoholism, undiagnosed abdominal pain, or prostatic hypertrophy.

DOSAGE. Hydromorphone may be administered intramuscularly (preferred), subcutaneously (induration may occur with repeated subcutaneous injection), or intravenously. It is also available in rectal suppositories. The average adult dosage is 2 mg every four to six hours as needed. This may be increased to 4 mg every four to six hours as needed. The suppository is usually given in a 3-mg dose at bedtime. Safe use in children has not been established. The dosage of hydromorphone should be reduced in the elderly and in debilitated patients.

Meperidine

Meperidine (Demerol) is a synthetic narcotic that is used to relieve pain, as a preoperative and intraoperative medication, and during labor to ease the pain of uterine contractions.

CONTRAINDICATIONS AND PRECAUTIONS. Meperidine is contraindicated in patients with known hypersensitivity, in patients currently or recently receiving MAO inhibitors, in patients with head injury or increased intracranial or CSF pressure, and in any condition in which respiratory depression or shock is evident. Meperidine is also contraindicated in children under 12 years of age. Meperidine is a Schedule II controlled substance and may produce tolerance, dependence, and addiction. The drug is used with caution in patients with supraventricular tachycardias and convulsions.

ADVERSE EFFECTS. The adverse effects occur for the same reasons as described for morphine sulfate. The most common side effects are lightheadedness, dizziness, sedation, nausea and vomiting, and sweating. Occasionally, meperidine may cause respiratory depression and cardiovascular depression. It may produce flushing, tachycardia, bradycardia, palpitations, hypo-

tension, and syncope. Meperidine may affect the gastrointestinal system, producing dry mouth, constipation, and biliary tract spasm. Urinary retention and an antidiuretic effect may be induced. Locally, meperidine may cause pruritus, urticaria, rash, pain at the injection site, and phlebitis following intravenous injection. Tissue irritation and induration after subcutaneous injection may also occur. Meperidine may cause disturbances of mood, headache, tremor, and visual disturbances.

INTERACTIONS. Solutions of meperidine and barbiturates are chemically incompatible and should not be mixed in the same syringe. Meperidine should not be used together with, or within 14 days after therapy with, MAO inhibitors because the combination may be lethal. Meperidine, like other narcotics, potentiates the central nervous system depressant effect of general anesthetics, phenothiazines, sedatives, other narcotics, hypnotics, tricyclic antidepressants, and alcohol.

DOSAGE. Meperidine is available for intramuscular use (preferred), short-term subcutaneous use, and occasional intravenous use. It is also available in tablets and syrups for oral administration. Due to its short half-life, the usual adult dosage for pain relief is 50–150 mg every three to four hours. The usual pediatric dosage for pain relief is 0.5–0.8 mg/kg every three to four hours as needed. For other dosage information, see Table 20–3.

Methadone Hydrochloride

Methadone hydrochloride (Dolophine) is a synthetic opiate that resembles morphine and is used to relieve pain in the terminally ill, to assist an addicted person through abstinence syndrome, and to maintain the person attempting to overcome addiction. Methadone is very effective after an oral administration. It also has a long duration of action.

CONTRAINDICATIONS AND PRECAUTIONS. Methadone shares the contraindications and precautions described in the section on general opioid analgesics. In addition, methadone should not be given with, or 14 days after, therapy with MAO inhibitors.

ADVERSE EFFECTS. The most common adverse effects of methadone are lightheadedness, dizziness, nausea, vomiting, and sweating. Occasional adverse effects include cardiovascular symptoms such as bradycardia, palpitations, faintness, syncope, and flushing. Methadone hydrochloride may also produce mood disturbances, headache, and visual disturbances. Gastrointestinal effects that may develop are dry mouth, anorexia, constipation, and biliary tract spasm. Methadone may induce an antidiuretic effect, urinary retention, and decreased libido. The patient may complain of pruritus, urticaria, pain at the injection site, local tissue irritation, and induration.

DOSAGE. Methadone hydrochloride may be given intramuscularly; however, the oral form is preferred in detoxification programs. The average adult dosage for severe pain relief is 2.5–10 mg given intramuscularly every three to four hours as needed. The oral form is usually administered on a six- or eight-hour regimen. Methadone is not recommended for use in children.

Dosage schedules for detoxification and maintenance are included in Table 20–3.

Levorphanol Tartrate

Levorphanol tartrate (Levo-Dromoran) is a Schedule II controlled substance and is a derivative of morphine. This agent is three times more potent than morphine.

CONTRAINDICATIONS AND PRECAUTIONS. The drug is contraindicated in patients with known hypersensitivity, acute alcoholism, bronchial asthma, increased intracranial pressure, respiratory depression, and anoxia.

ADVERSE EFFECTS. The most common adverse effects of the drug are nausea, emesis, and dizziness. Allergic reactions, skin rash, and urticaria may also occur. Rarely, administration results in pruritus, sweating, respiratory depression, hypotension, urinary retention, and cardiac arrhythmias. Levorphanol tartrate potentiates the depressant effect of general anesthetics, other narcotics, tranquilizers, sedatives, hypnotics, tricyclic antidepressants, and MAO inhibitors.

DOSAGE. Levorphanol tartrate is usually administered orally or subcutaneously in a dosage of 2–3 mg every six to eight hours as needed. The drug is not recommended for children under 12 years of age.

Oxycodone Hydrochloride

As a Schedule II controlled substance, oxycodone hydrochloride may produce tolerance, dependence, or addiction.

CONTRAINDICATIONS AND PRECAUTIONS. Since the drug preparation may contain aspirin and caffeine, hypersensitivity to oxycodone hydrochloride or any of its major constituents is a contraindication to use. Extreme caution should be used in those conditions referred to in the section on morphine and in Table 20–3.

ADVERSE EFFECTS. The most common adverse effects of oxycodone include lightheadedness, dizziness, sedation, nausea, and vomiting. Occasionally, euphoria, dysphoria, constipation, and pruritus result. Due to the aspirin component of oxycodone preparations, an increased anticoagulant effect and a decreased uricosuric effect may be seen. Oxycodone shares the potentiating effect of other narcotics when used with medications that depress the central nervous system.

DOSAGE. Oxycodone hydrochloride is a synthetic narcotic that is administered orally in tablet form. The usual adult dosage is one tablet every six hours as needed. This drug is available as a single agent and/or combined with aspirin and caffeine (Percodan) or acetaminophen (Tylox and Percocet-5) in tablet form. A Percodan-Demi tablet is available for pediatric use; the usual dosage is one-fourth to one-half tablet every six hours as needed.

Oxymorphone Hydrochloride

Because of its potential to produce tolerance, dependence, and addiction, oxymorphone hydrochloride (Numorphan) is classified as a Schedule II controlled substance. It is similar to morphine in structure and potency. It is ten times as potent as codeine.

CONTRAINDICATIONS AND PRECAUTIONS. Oxymorphone hydrochloride shares the contraindications and precautions referred to in the section on morphine and in Table 20–3.

ADVERSE EFFECTS. The most common adverse effects of oxymorphone are nausea, vomiting, euphoria, and dizziness. Occasionally, headache, hypotension, bradycardia, miosis, red eyes, urinary retention or urgency, impotence, sweating, flushing, respiratory depression, and convulsions occur. As with the other opioid analgesics, oxymorphone also potentiates the central nervous system depressant effects of other medications and alcohol.

DOSAGE. Oxymorphone hydrochloride may be administered parenterally or by rectal suppository. The usual adult dosage is 1–1.5 mg IM or SC every four to six hours as needed. For other dosage information, refer to Table 20–3.

Propoxyphene Hydrochloride

Propoxyphene hydrochloride (Darvon) is a synthetic narcotic used alone or in combination with other drugs to relieve pain. This agent is a Schedule IV narcotic and is used for chronic pain.

PHARMACOKINETICS. Propoxyphene is absorbed well from the upper part of the small intestine. The peak serum levels occur within two to three hours. The onset of its analgesic effect is within 30 minutes after ingestion. The analgesic effect lasts up to six hours. The half-life of propoxyphene is 6–12 hours. Propoxyphene is degraded in the liver and excreted in the urine. It does cross the placenta and low concentrations have been found in breast milk.

CONTRAINDICATIONS AND PRECAUTIONS. Propoxyphene hydrochloride is not recommended for children. It is contraindicated in those with hypersensitivity to propoxyphene. Combination products (Darvon Compound-65 and Darvon A.S.A.) are contraindicated in persons with hypersensitivity to aspirin or caffeine. Propoxyphene hydrochloride is a Schedule IV drug. It may produce drug dependence when taken in higher than recommended dosages. It is also a major cause of drug-related deaths and therefore should not be prescribed for the suicidal or addiction-prone patient. Propoxyphene hydrochloride should be prescribed with caution for those taking tranquilizers or antidepressants, and for alcohol abusers. The drug may impair the patient's ability to drive or to operate machinery. Safe use in pregnancy has not been established.

ADVERSE EFFECTS. Less than 1% of patients experience side effects. The most common adverse effects include dizziness, sedation, nausea, and vomiting. Occasional adverse effects include constipation, abdominal pain, skin rash, lightheadedness, headache, weakness, euphoria, and visual disturbances. Propoxyphene hydrochloride has an additive effect when used with central nervous system depressants or alcohol. The salicylates that are used in the combination products enhance the anticoagulant effect and inhibit the uricosuric effect of this drug. Propoxyphene hydrochloride may also cause false decreases in urinary steroid-excretion tests.

DOSAGE. Propoxyphene napsylate is administered orally in capsule form. The average adult dosage is 65 mg every four hours as needed, not to exceed 390 mg in 24 hours. Propoxyphene hydrochloride, 65 mg, is equivalent to 30–45 mg of codeine or 325–600 mg of aspirin. Propoxyphene is usually not effective for single or acute dosing but may be effective with chronic dosing. Further dosage information for propoxyphene compounds is found in Table 20–3.

Phenylpiperidine Compounds

This classification of synthetic opiates, phenylpiperidine compounds, include rapid-onset, short-acting, and highly potent agents such as fentanyl, sufentanil, and alfentanil. Fentanyl is approximately 80 times more potent than morphine as an analgesic. Sufentanil is related to fentanyl and is seven times more potent than fentanyl. Alfentanil is the newest analog of fentanyl and has one fourth the potency of fentanyl.

These agents are used in the induction and maintenance of inductional anesthesia and regional and spinal anesthesia. Recently, these agents have been used to treat a variety of postoperative pain with systemic devices (i.e., PCA). These agents can be administered alone or in combination with other agents (butyrophenone droperidol, benzodiazepine).

When fentanyl is administered alone, it has a short plasma half-life (20 minutes), and an intravenous dose can be titrated to counter the patient's perception of pain. This is an advantage over morphine or meperidine.

Adverse reactions are similar to those for morphine. Fentanyl is known to cause muscle rigidity and apnea. See Chapter 10 on general anesthesia for an in-depth discussion of these agents.

OPIATE PARTIAL ANTAGONISTS

It is known that *opiate partial antagonists* have both analgesic and opiate antagonist properties. It may be that these drugs compete for opiate receptors in the brain and prevent the binding of morphine-like drugs to these sites. Because of this action, the administration of these drugs may precipitate a withdrawal syndrome in patients who have developed physical dependence on the opiates. The side effects and precautions of this class of drugs are similar to those for morphine.

Pentazocine

Pentazocine (Talwin) is a synthetic partial narcotic antagonist that does not exert an antipyretic effect.

CONTRAINDICATIONS AND PRECAUTIONS. Pentazocine is not recommended for children under 12 years of age. The use of pentazocine is contraindicated in patients with known hypersensitivity. Extreme caution should be used in patients with head injuries, respiratory depression, renal or hepatic dysfunction, myo-

cardial infarct, biliary surgery, and seizures. Pentazocine may impair the patient's ability to drive or to use machinery. Safe use in pregnancy, other than in labor, has not been established. Pentazocine may cause physical and psychological dependence in patients. Abrupt discontinuation of intramuscular injections may precipitate withdrawal. The patient receiving long-term narcotics may have developed a cross-tolerance to pentazocine. When switching from narcotics to pentazocine, care should be exercised to prevent withdrawal symptoms because pentazocine has narcotic antagonist properties.

ADVERSE EFFECTS. Adverse effects of injected pentazocine include sclerosis of skin, subcutaneous tissue, and muscle in chronic use. The most common adverse effects include tolerance, abuse, and dependency, along with nausea, dizziness, lightheadedness, vomiting, and euphoria. Occasionally, respiratory depression, hypotension, sedation, constipation, and headache occur. Rarely, pentazocine produces hallucinations, blurred vision, and allergic and toxic reactions. Injectable pentazocine interacts with soluble barbiturates when mixed in the same syringe, causing precipitation.

DOSAGE. Pentazocine is usually administered intramuscularly or orally. The tablet form for oral administration may be obtained in combination with aspirin as a pentazocine compound when an antipyretic as well as an anti-inflammatory effect is desirable. It also contains naloxone to prevent abuse. Injectable pentazocine may also be given intravenously or subcutaneously in emergency situations. The usual intramuscular adult dosage is 30 mg every three to four hours, not to exceed 360 mg over 24 hours. The usual oral adult dosage is 50 mg every three to four hours, not to exceed 600 mg in 24 hours. Further dosage recommendations may be found in Table 20–3.

Nalbuphine Hydrochloride

Nalbuphine hydrochloride (Nubain) is a synthetic opiate agonist-antagonist analgesic. It is a very potent drug that has an analgesic effect equivalent to that of morphine on a milligram-for-milligram basis.

USES. Nalbuphine is recommended for moderate to severe pain. Its onset of action occurs within two to three minutes after intravenous administration and within less than 15 minutes following subcutaneous or intramuscular injection. It can also be used for preoperative analgesia, as a supplement to surgical anesthesia, and for analgesia during labor.

PHARMACOKINETICS. Nalbuphine is metabolized in the liver and is excreted in the urine and feces. The plasma half-life of nalbuphine is five hours. Duration of action is in the range of three to six hours.

CONTRAINDICATIONS AND PRECAUTIONS. Nalbuphine should not be used in patients who are hypersensitive to it. Nalbuphine has the potential for abuse, leading to tolerance and physical dependence. Abrupt withdrawal of nalbuphine following chronic use results in opioid withdrawal symptoms.

Nalbuphine should not be used, or should be used with extreme caution, in the following situations: during pregnancy, in ambulatory patients, in children, during labor and delivery, with head injury, during the intra-operative period, with pre-existing respiratory problems, in hepatic and renal dysfunction, and in cardiac conditions.

ADVERSE REACTIONS. The most frequent adverse reaction reported is sedation. Other reactions include sweaty/clammy skin, nausea/vomiting, dizziness/vertigo, dry mouth, headache, nervousness, depression, restlessness, euphoria, floating sensation, unusual dreams, confusion, dysphoria, feeling of heaviness, hypertension, hypotension, bradycardia, tachycardia, cramps, and a bitter taste in the mouth.

DOSAGE. The recommended adult dosage is 10 mg/70 kg of body weight. The dose can be repeated every three to six hours. In nontolerant persons, the single maximum dose is 20 mg, with a maximum total daily dose of 160 mg. The route of administration is subcutaneous, intramuscular, or intravenous.

Butorphanol

Butorphanol (Stadol) is a potent synthetic opiate agonist-antagonist analgesic. The analgesic and opiate antagonistic properties reduce the liability for physical addiction. Butorphanol is more potent than morphine sulfate on a milligram-for-milligram basis.

USES. Butorphanol is recommended for moderate to severe postoperative pain. Butorphanol has also been used with excellent results for chronic pain associated with malignant diseases, neuropathy, and orthopedic pain.

PHARMACOKINETICS. Butorphanol is metabolized in the liver and is excreted via the urine, bile, and feces. The half-life of butorphanol is three to four hours. The peak plasma levels occur four to six hours after a 2-mg dose. Butorphanol is removed by dialysis.

CONTRAINDICATIONS AND PRECAUTIONS. The contraindications and precautions are the same as for nalbuphine (Nubain).

ADVERSE REACTIONS. The most common adverse reactions include sedation, nausea, drowsiness, euphoria, dizziness, agitation, and constipation.

DOSAGE. The recommended single intravenous dosage is 1 mg every three to four hours as necessary. The dosage range is 0.5–2 mg every three to four hours. The recommended single intramuscular dosage is 2 mg repeated every three to four hours. The dosage range based on severity of pain is 1–4 mg every three to four hours. Doses higher than 4 mg are not recommended. An oral form of butorphanol is currently under investigational study.

OPIATE ANTAGONISTS

The opiate antagonists compete with opiates for receptor sites, but they may also produce an agonist effect (except Narcan). They are used to reverse narcotic-induced CNS and respiratory depression. They are largely metabolized in the liver and are excreted in the urine.

Buprenorphine

ACTION. Buprenorphine (Buprenex) is a parenteral opiate analgesic that is 30 times as potent as morphine sulfate. This agent is a synthetic derivative of thebaine. It is an *opiate agonist-antagonist*. It exerts its analgesic effects by binding to the opiate receptors in the central nervous system. Buprenorphine has a low potential for abuse and is classified as a Schedule V drug.

USES. Buprenorphine is used for the treatment of moderate to severe pain. This drug relieves pain at least as well as morphine and its effects last longer in some patients.

PHARMACOKINETICS. Buprenorphine's onset of action is within 15 minutes of intramuscular administration. The peak analgesic effect occurs in one hour. It is metabolized in the liver and excreted in the urine and feces. Buprenorphine is highly bound to plasma proteins (96%). The half-life of this drug is two to three hours.

CONTRAINDICATIONS. Buprenorphine is contraindicated in persons who are hypersensitive to the drug. The other contraindications and precautions are the same as for the other opiate analgesics.

ADVERSE EFFECTS. The most frequent adverse effect of buprenorphine is sedation. Other adverse reactions are headache, dizziness, vertigo, nausea, vomiting, sweating, miosis, hypotension, hypoventilation, and urinary retention. These adverse effects are secondary to the binding of the opiate receptor sites in the central nervous system.

INTERACTIONS. The concurrent administration of buprenorphine and other central nervous system depressants (opiate analgesics, general anesthetics, phenothiazines, tranquilizers, sedative hypnotics, alcohol) can cause additive central nervous system depression. The concurrent administration of buprenorphine and MAO inhibitors is avoided.

DOSAGE. The usual dosage of buprenorphine is 0.3 mg given intramuscularly or intravenously every six hours. This is equivalent to 10 mg of morphine. The maximum recommended dose is 0.6 mg.

Naloxone Hydrochloride

USES. Naloxone hydrochloride (Narcan) may be used for neonates and for children. It is also being used in toxic shock syndrome to block endorphins that cause peripheral vasodilation and thus cardiovascular collapse.

CONTRAINDICATIONS AND PRECAUTIONS. Naloxone hydrochloride is contraindicated in patients with known hypersensitivity. It is used with caution in patients with cardiac irritability or pulmonary edema. Naloxone hydrochloride is ineffective in cases of non-narcotic respiratory depression; however, it may be used successfully to treat pentazocine- and propoxyphene-induced respiratory depression.

ADVERSE EFFECTS. Naloxone hydrochloride is essentially devoid of adverse effects, unless the patient is receiving narcotics. In those who are receiving narcotics, naloxone hydrochloride may cause reversal of analgesia and withdrawal symptoms. The latter may occur in newborns of addicted mothers as well as in addicts themselves. No other drug interactions are known at this time.

DOSAGE. Naloxone is administered intravenously to treat narcotic-induced depression. The average adult dosage is 0.4–1 mg given intravenously, followed by one or two doses of 0.5 mg at 10- to 15-minute intervals as needed, not to exceed a total dose of 3 mg.

Levallorphan Tartrate

Levallorphan tartrate (Lorfan) is another narcotic antagonist with some agonist qualities.

CONTRAINDICATIONS AND PRECAUTIONS. Levallorphan is contraindicated in patients with mild respiratory depression and in narcotic addicts, in whom it may produce withdrawal symptoms. Levallorphan tartrate is ineffective against, and may actually increase, respiratory depression produced by barbiturates, general anesthetics, and other non-narcotics. It may also increase a pre-existing mild respiratory depression. Repeated doses of levallorphan tartrate may produce tolerance to its effects.

ADVERSE EFFECTS. The most common adverse effects of levallorphan tartrate include dysphoria, miosis, pseudoptosis, lethargy, dizziness, drowsiness, gastrointestinal upset, sweating, pallor, nausea, and a sense of heaviness of the limbs. Levallorphan tartrate may produce irritability and increased crying in neonates. Rarely and only with administration of high dosage, dreams, visual hallucinations, disorientation, and feelings of unreality may occur.

INTERACTIONS. Levallorphan tartrate does not have any known drug interactions at this time.

DOSAGE. Levallorphan tartrate is given intravenously in adults and through the umbilical vein in neonates. The adult dosage schedule is 1 mg given intravenously, and followed by one or two doses of 0.5 mg at 10- or 15-minute intervals, if needed. The maximum dosage is 3 mg. See Table 20–3 for the neonatal dosage.

USING THE NURSING PROCESS

ASSESSMENT

Whether the patient is receiving narcotics or non-narcotics, the patient in pain deserves a careful, methodical assessment of his or her complaint. This assessment is performed when the patient first complains of pain and is repeated at regular intervals to determine the effectiveness or lack of effectiveness of the medication regimen. Basic information gathered is given in Table 20–6. It may be helpful to guide the patient in describing the intensity of pain by asking him or her to rate the pain on a numerical scale, on a scale of descriptive terms, or

in relation to past experience. In determining the quality of the pain or what the pain is like, it may be helpful to read off terms and allow the patient to pick those most applicable to his or her own situation. Terms that can be used to describe pain include intermittent, continuous, sharp, dull, stabbing, annoying, unbearable, and so forth. Other examples of such terms can be found in the McGill-Melzack Pain Questionnaire (Table 20–7).

The McGill-Melzack Pain Questionnaire is an excellent tool to collect information on pain and to assess pain and efficacy of treatment. Since it is a somewhat subjective tool, it is especially helpful when multiple assessments by different nurses are unavoidable. McCaffery rightfully emphasizes that the nurse's attitude in assessing the patient with pain can make a great difference between an accurate and inaccurate data base. To McCaffery, "pain is whatever the experiencing person says it is, existing when he says it does" (McCaffery, 1979). By keeping that thought in mind, the nurse focuses on the pain as perceived by the patient, rather than on the pain as perceived by the nurse. Logically then, the diagnosis, planning, and intervention are specific to the patient's pain, rather than to the nurse's prejudices or misconceptions. Such misconceptions are summarized in Table 20–8. Nurses must keep in mind that their attitudes may influence their care of the patient and should be aware that not all physical causes of pain can be identified. Psychogenic pain is as "real" to the patient as any physiologic trauma. Pain tolerance is highly individualized, and comparisons among patients in differing situations with varying conditions are not accurate. Lack of expression of pain does not mean lack of pain but is a reflection of cultural, personal, and physiologic adaptation. Health-team members are not the experts on the specific pain of an individual patient and tend, in fact, to assess the patient as experiencing less pain than the patient actually does.

The individuality of the pain experience is complemented by the individuality of responsiveness to pain therapy. For instance, it has become evident that many common beliefs regarding placebos are actually misconceptions. Researchers now feel that placebos actually enhance the endogenous curative mechanisms of the body. The patients are not tricked by the placebo but actually become physically better. Placebos provide relief in patients of all types; there is no so-called placebo personality. In addition, approximately 30%–75% of patients may respond to placebos. The nurse should not judge a patient's pain as imaginary just because the patient responds to a placebo. Any drug may have a placebo effect associated with it. The nurse should also be aware that administration of a placebo involves ethical and moral considerations regarding how much information is given to the patient and whether patient consent to placebo administration is necessary. Placebos are not administered to assess the "realness" of the patient's pain or to determine whether the patient is habituated to the current analgesic therapy. Placebos are given to produce a therapeutic response, lessening the patient's pain and improving the patient's quality of life.

Table 20–6. NURSING PROCESS FOR PATIENTS REQUIRING MEDICATION FOR PAIN

Assessment

Determine OTC analgesic use; other drugs (including alcohol, street drugs).
Note allergic reactions/hypersensitivity, previous response to drugs.
Assess pain characteristics; dull, throbbing, sharp, constant, or intermittent and review previous experiences with pain, attitudes toward pain.
Determine preexisting medical conditions, e.g., GI bleeding/ulcer, impaired renal or hepatic function, respiratory disease, cardiac dysrhythmias.
Assess current physical status/condition, including pregnancy.

Nursing Diagnosis	Nursing Actions	Rationale	Desired Patient Outcomes/Evaluation
Knowledge deficit related to unfamiliarity with prescribed medication(s), and therapeutic needs as evidenced by questions, statement of concerns.	Provide verbal and written information about pain medication, including action, use, dose, common side effects (e.g., nausea/vomiting, sedation).	Understanding promotes safe/ effective drug use and reduces risk of untoward actions/effects.	Verbalizes understanding of drug regimen.
	Discuss possible/frequent drug interactions and encourage reading of ingredient labels for OTC medications. Discuss time frame of absorption of prescribed medication.	Knowledge of potential interactions can help patient optimize drug effect/prevent adverse reactions. Allows patient to gain maximum benefit from drug and lessen undesired side-effects.	
	Stress importance of notifying physician if side-effects persist/impair activities or desired lifestyle, or adequate pain control is not achieved.	Provides for change in prescribed regimen when necessary.	
Pain, (acute/ chronic) related to injuring agents (specify) as evidenced by verbal complaints, alteration in muscle tone, guarding behavior, autonomic responses.	Provide comfort measures, e.g., backrub, change of position.	Promotes relaxation and may reduce perception of severity of pain.	Reports pain is relieved/ controlled. Follows prescribed pharmacologic regimen. Discusses/demonstrates ways in which pain can be minimized by own actions.
	Encourage use of relaxation exercises, distraction techniques, visualization.	Helps to refocus attention and enhances sense of self-control.	
	Administer pain medication through appropriate routes, e.g., oral, IM, IV/ PCA (patient controlled analgesia).	Properly administered medication enhances drug effectiveness and provides for optimal pain management.	
	Explore the way in which the patient copes with pain.	Identifies possibilities of ways in which patient may minimize own suffering and pain behavior. Promotes control over self, reducing sense of powerlessness.	
	Discuss alternate strategies. Explore ways patient does have control over situational factors, e.g., splinting of incision during cough, use of firm mattress/ proper supporting shoes for low back pain.		
	Assist patient to evaluate drug regimen; encourage decreasing dosage, alternate route, increased time span as pain lessens.	Promotes active patient participation/control in therapeutic regimen and may reduce risk of drug tolerance/dependence.	
Sleep, disturbance potential related to posi-	Provide information on creating a restful environment	Fatigue influences the way an individual responds to pain and the reduction of fatigue	Appears relaxed, able to sleep/rest appropriately. Reports increased sense

Table 20–6. NURSING PROCESS FOR PATIENTS REQUIRING MEDICATION FOR PAIN–*CONTINUED*

Nursing Diagnosis	Nursing Actions	Rationale	Desired Patient Outcomes/Evaluation
tion/proximity of pain pathways to sleep center within the brain.	Discuss nonpharmacologic pain control measures, e.g., relaxation techniques, guided imagery.	is critical for optimal functioning.	of well-being and feeling rested.
	Discuss limiting intake of caffeine and alcoholic beverages, especially prior to bedtime.	Use of these substances in excess may interfere with REM sleep.	
	Administer pain medications one hour before sleep.	Reduces transmission of pain impulses which can irritate the sleep center in the brain.	
Nutrition deficit, potential for more than body requirements related to excessive intake in relation to metabolic need.	Discuss caloric/nutritional needs reflecting current weight/activity level, disease/healing process.	Understanding that weight gain can occur as a result of changes in activity, dysfunctional eating in response to anxiety/depression enables patient to engage in preventive/corrective actions.	Maintains weight at a desirable level.
	Explore various types of activities which patient can engage in on a daily basis.	Physical activity can enhance feelings of general well-being, promote normalization of organ function, reduce risks of inactivity, e.g., weight gain.	
	Provide information regarding side effects of medication.	Increase in appetite may be noted with the use of some drugs.	
Constipation, potential for related to changes in usual pattern of activity, reduced dietary/fluid intake.	Provide information about adequate fluid intake. Identify foods high in fiber.	Adequate fluid intake and fiber in the diet normalizes consistency/amount of stool to decrease side effects of constipation.	Maintains adequate fluid/fiber intake. Establishes/returns to normal patterns of bowel functioning.
	Encourage increased activity/exercise within the limits of individual ability.	Stimulates bowel motility, enhancing transit time through the bowel reducing opportunity for excessive reabsorption of fluid from stool.	
	Discuss use of stool softeners and bulk laxatives.	Provides for normalization of stool consistency and amount to promote elimination and may decrease discomfort associated with gas decreasing the experience of pain.	
Trauma, potential for related to effects of pharmaceutical agents.	Provide information about the CNS side effects of opioid analgesics, e.g., sedation, decreased attention span, inability to concentrate, poor judgment, lightheadedness, and dizziness.	Promotes understanding of sedative effects of these drugs allowing patient to enhance own safety.	Verbalizes understanding of possible CNS side effects. Alters activities/environment to reduce risk factors.
	Caution patient not to engage in activities that require making judgments, wakefulness, and coordination (driving a car, operating power tools, heavy machinery) after taking drug.		

Table 20–7. McGILL-MELZACK PAIN QUESTIONNAIRE

McGill-Melzack PAIN QUESTIONNAIRE

Patient's name _____ Age _____

File No. _____ Date _____

Clinical category (eg. cardiac, neurological, etc.):

_____

Diagnosis : _____

_____

Analgesic (if already administered):

1. Type _____
2. Dosage _____
3. Time given in relation to this test _____

Patient's intelligence: circle number that represents best estimate

1 (low)   2   3   4   5(high)

✶✶✶✶✶✶✶✶✶✶✶✶✶✶✶

This questionnaire has been designed to tell us more about your pain. Four major questions we ask are:

1. Where is your pain?
2. What does it feel like?
3. How does it change with time?
4. How strong is it?

It is important that you tell us how your pain feels now. Please follow the instructions at the beginning of each part.

© R. Melzack, Oct. 1970

Part 1.   Where is your Pain?

Please mark, on the drawings below, the areas where you feel pain. Put E if external, or I if internal, near the areas which you mark. Put EI if both external and internal.

Part 2.   What Does Your Pain Feel Like?

Some of the words below describe your present pain. Circle ONLY those words that best describe it. Leave out any category that is not suitable. Use only a single word in each appropriate category—the one that applies best.

1	2	3	4
Flickering	Jumping	Pricking	Sharp
Quivering	Flashing	Boring	Cutting
Pulsing	Shooting	Drilling	Lacerating
Throbbing		Stabbing	
Beating		Lancinating	
Pounding			

5	6	7	8
Pinching	Tugging	Hot	Tingling
Pressing	Pulling	Burning	Itchy
Gnawing	Wrenching	Scalding	Smarting
Cramping		Searing	Stinging
Crushing			

9	10	11	12
Dull	Tender	Tiring	Sickening
Sore	Taut	Exhausting	Suffocating
Hurting	Rasping		
Aching	Splitting		
Heavy			

13	14	15	16
Fearful	Punishing	Wretched	Annoying
Frightful	Gruelling	Blinding	Troublesome
Terrifying	Cruel		Miserable
	Vicious		Intense
	Killing		Unbearable

17	18	19	20
Spreading	Tight	Cool	Nagging
Radiating	Numb	Cold	Nauseating
Penetrating	Drawing	Freezing	Agonizing
Piercing	Squeezing		Dreadful
	Tearing		Torturing

Part 3.   How Does Your Pain Change With Time?

1. Which word or words would you use to describe the pattern of your pain?

1	2	3
Continuous	Rhythmic	Brief
Steady	Periodic	Momentary
Constant	Intermittent	Transient

2. What kind of things relieve your pain?

3. What kind of things increase your pain?

Part 4.   How Strong Is Your Pain?

People agree that the following 5 words represent pain of increasing intensity. They are:

1	2	3	4	5
Mild	Discomforting	Distressing	Horrible	Excruciating

To answer each question below, write the number of the most appropriate word in the space beside the question.

1. Which word describes your pain right now?   _____
2. Which word describes it at its worst?   _____
3. Which word describes it when it is least?   _____
4. Which word describes the worst toothache you ever had?   _____
5. Which word describes the worst headache you ever had?   _____
6. Which word describes the worst stomach-ache you ever had?   _____

NURSING DIAGNOSES

When the patient assessment is complete, the nurse establishes the nursing diagnoses in order to begin the planning of interventions. Typical nursing diagnoses for a patient in pain are given in Table 20–6. The nurse individualizes the nursing diagnoses for the patient in pain, based on the nursing assessment.

PLANNING AND INTERVENTION

Goals for nursing interventions are developed from the list of nursing diagnoses. Typical goals in caring for the patient requiring analgesics are given in Table 20–6.

The nurse medicates the patient in anticipation of pain to improve pain relief. If the patient is allowd to experience severe pain, then the length of time needed for the analgesic to become effective increases and the overall analgesic effectiveness decreases. The nurse provides information to the patient and to the family regarding the nature of pain, analgesics, and common adverse effects. Information regarding acceptance of analgesia is especially important. It is not necessary for the patient to "hang in there" or "keep a stiff upper lip" or to suffer. It is necessary for the patient to achieve pain control, maintain alertness, and participate in daily activities as much as possible.

Table 20–8. MISCONCEPTIONS THAT HAMPER ASSESSMENT OF THE PATIENT WITH PAIN

Misconception	Correction
1. Health-team members are the authorities on the existence and nature of the patient's pain.	The patient is the authority on his pain. Pain is whatever the experiencing person says it is, existing whenever he says it does. The patient is believed.
2. The patient who uses his pain to obtain benefits or preferential treatment does not hurt as much as he says and may not hurt at all.	The patient who uses his pain to his own advantage may still hurt as much as he says he does.
3. The patient's pain can always be verified by the presence of certain behavioral and/or physiological expressions of pain.	Physiologic and behavioral adaptation occur, leading to periods of little or no sign of pain. Lack of pain expression does not mean lack of pain.
4. All "real" pain has an identifiable physical cause.	Not all physical causes of pain can be identified. All pain is real, regardless of its cause. Calling pain imaginary does not make it go away.
5. Psychogenic pain does not really hurt and is almost the same as malingering.	A localized sensation does exist in psychogenic pain.
6. The severity and duration of pain can be predicted accurately on the basis of the stimuli for pain.	There is no direct and invariant relationship between any stimulus and the perception of pain.
7. All patients can and should be encouraged to have a high tolerance for pain.	Pain tolerance is the person's unique response, varying between patients and in the same patient from one situation to another.
8. Health-team members tend to make accurate inferences about the severity and existence of the patient's pain.	Health-team members tend to infer less pain than the patient experiences.

From McCaffery, M: Nursing Management of the Patient With Pain, ed 2. JB Lippincott, Philadelphia, 1979, p 21, with permission.

NURSING RESPONSIBILITIES

In administering analgesics, the nurse takes advantage of the placebo effect of any drug. The placebo effect can be heightened if the nurse takes time to explain the therapeutic value of the medication and the drug action, and stresses the positive aspects of the medication. The nurse responds reassuringly to questions about the medication's effectiveness. By incorporating these ideas into the administration of medications, the nurse makes the best use of exogenous and endogenous analgesic resources.

The nurse considers which, if any, nonpharmacologic interventions for pain relief are suitable for the patient. Using nonpharmacologic interventions such as relaxation, distraction, biofeedback, or massage may increase the effectiveness of pain-relieving medications, providing the patient with optimum pain control.

If a patient requires intramuscular injections, the nurse plans to rotate sites and observes proper technique. Two weeks is the maximum time period that intramuscular injections are given on an every-4-hour basis. When using parenteral forms of narcotics, the nurse checks before mixing the narcotic with another drug (such as an anticholinergic, a tranquilizer, or a barbiturate) because the drugs often are not compatible if combined. The nurse consults with pharmacists or with a chart such as the one listed in Chapter 5 before mixing the medications.

When patients are using PCA therapy, it is necessary for the nurse to understand how the PCA device works. Many operator errors are associated with not being familiar with the equipment. Some of the problems encountered with the PCA pump are solved by the nurse. It is important to monitor the patient's respiratory status even though the risk is low for respiratory depression. The nurse monitors other side effects of opiate administration. These side effects are dose-related.

Patients receiving epidural or intrathecal opiate analgesia are monitored for nausea and vomiting, urine retention, pruritus, and respiratory depression. It is important for the nurse to anticipate cephalad spread of opiates (i.e., morphine), which may be evidenced by increasing segmental analgesia, miosis, and changes in mentation. The incidence of respiratory depression with this type of therapy is low but constant nursing surveillance is required. It is important to monitor and assess respiratory function (respiratory rate, volume, quality of effort, auscultation of lungs, for apnea, skin color changes, arterial blood gas analysis). Apnea monitors are used but not relied on solely. It is necessary for the nurse to recognize the depressant effects of other drugs in the medication regimen (e.g., hypnotics, sedatives, antianxiety agents) that may be used concurrently with opiates. Reports of respiratory depression have discouraged concurrent use of parenteral opiates and sedatives. The elderly patient is susceptible to this practice. Infusions of naloxone can reverse opiate-induced respiratory depression.

When administering a bolus or continuous drip of opiate via the epidural or intrathecal route, the nurse should make sure that the drug is a preservative-free preparation. The preparation should always be verified with another nurse before the drug is drawn up. Tubing, infusion bag, and the front of the pump should be labeled with tape reading "epidural" or "intrathecal." This alerts all care-givers to the type of infusion line to minimize confusion with similar-looking lines. Injection ports should be taped over or capped to prevent accidental injection into the epidural or intrathecal lines.

Prior to administering drugs, the nurse should aspirate the catheter to see whether there is a clear fluid or bloody return. If the catheter is in the epidural space, no fluid should be aspirated. The presence of CSF or blood signifies a migrated catheter, and the physician is notified. The drug is not given in this situation. When working with the epidural or intrathecal system, strict aseptic technique is observed. The tubing and filter of a continuous infusion should be changed in accordance with hospital policy. The nurse monitors the patient for infection (fever, excessive pain or tenderness at the catheter site, redness at the catheter site, headache, stiff neck, *photophobia,* mental changes). The patient should be instructed to notify the nurse if he or she experiences these problems.

If the patient is receiving intravenous or intramuscular medication and is switched to oral medication prior to discharge, adequate time should be allotted to "test out" the oral route for successful home therapy. In such instances, the nurse checks the equianalgesic doses and individualizes the dosage to the patient's need.

In order to provide adequate analgesia for patients in severe pain, much larger dosages of drugs than are normally considered therapeutic are in order. These larger dosages are well tolerated with few adverse effects in patients with severe pain. For such patients, medication given on a round-the-clock basis rather than every three to four hours as needed is the more effective dosage schedule.

PATIENT TEACHING

Patients require health teaching about over-the-counter analgesics (Table 20–9). The use of buffered products may cause less stomach irritation, but this has not been conclusively proven. Because many over-the-counter analgesics contain ingredients other than aspirin, the patient with medical problems (such as liver or kidney disease) and the patient who is on several medications should consult with a health-team member prior to selecting such an analgesic. Attractive packaging and flavorings of aspirin and acetaminophen may lead to ingestion by children, resulting in accidental overdosage. Special precautions should be maintained in the storage of these preparations.

Prior to PCA therapy, the nurse must teach the patient about this type of therapy. It is important for the patient to understand the concept of PCA and to know how to work the pump. For many patients, this is a new approach to pain management, and they are not aware of their role in this type of therapy. The patient must have a working knowledge of the PCA device in order to receive the analgesic, and must understand that he or she controls the frequency with which the analgesic is received. The nurse emphasizes the degree of control the patient has over the pain and what he or she can expect in relation to the activities of daily living.

Patients receiving long-term epidural or intrathecal analgesia should receive instruction prior to discharge. This teaching protocol should include self-medication regimen, signs/symptoms of infection, what to do if an infection occurs, and catheter care. Many of the subcutaneous tunneling and implanted systems are easily accessible to the patient. If the patient is unable to give his own medication and catheter care, then a significant other must be taught these concepts.

EVALUATION

During the evaluation phase of the nursing process, the nurse determines the effectiveness of the analgesic medications. This evaluation is based on goals determined by the nurse and patient. Outcome goals for the patient requiring analgesics are included in Table 20–6.

In completing the evaluation process, the nurse assesses the patient for the development of adverse effects. The most common adverse effects of the non-narcotic analgesics include gastrointestinal irritation and subsequent bleeding, prolonged bleeding time, and development of analgesic nephropathy, which may result in renal failure. Signs of gastrointestinal irritation include nausea, vomiting, tarry stools, anemia, and positive results of a test for occult blood in the stool. Irritation may be prevented or reduced by administering buffered products, or by administering the analgesics at mealtime, with food, or shortly after eating. Prolonged bleeding time is manifested by easy bruising or profuse bleeding of minor cuts and may indicate a need for a change in analgesic. Analgesic nephropathy develops after chronic long-term use or abuse of analgesics. Research suggests that the risk of analgesic nephropathy can be minimized through use of one analgesic rather than combination forms and by increasing fluid intake.

Common adverse effects of narcotic analgesic therapy include constipation, urinary retention, nausea and vomiting, orthostatic hypotension, sedation, and addiction.

Constipation may be relieved by a prophylactic bowel-management plan. This plan should provide the patient with information about fluid, food, and exercise as well as stool softeners and cathartics. Neostigmine or pyridostigmine may also be used because they enhance peristalsis, which decreases the likelihood of constipation. Urinary retention generally subsides during the first 24–48 hours of narcotic treatment. Warm baths and neostigmine may be useful in preventing and treating the spasm that causes urinary retention. Nausea and vomiting are common in patients receiving narcotics, particularly ambulatory patients. Restricting ambulation may be helpful to these patients. Two types of antiemetics are available. The antihistamine antiemetics act on vestibular sensitivity, whereas phenothiazines act on medullary trigger areas for nausea and vomiting. If initial doses of one type of antiemetic are unsuccessful, it may be more helpful to add the other type of antiemetic to the regimen than to increase the dosage of the original drug. Narcotics may be accompanied by antiemetics routinely to prevent nausea and vomiting. The possibility that nausea and vomiting are a sign of poorly controlled pain must also be considered. Orthostatic hypotension is also common in ambulatory patients. Patients should be reminded to rise slowly from the supine po-

Table 20–9. PATIENT TEACHING INFORMATION—PAIN MEDICATIONS

Non-narcotic, Nonsteroidal Anti-inflammatories

Dear Patient:
  This drug has been ordered for you. This is what you should know about your drug to get the most from your therapy. Non-narcotic, nonsteroidal anti-inflammatories are used to alleviate mild pain. Examples are aspirin, acetaminophen, ibuprofen, and indomethacin.

1. Take by mouth every 4 to 6 hours.
2. Try not to forget a dose. Do not play catch up with missed doses.
3. If the drug is relieving the pain at the ordered dose and time, then continue the pain medication. If not, then call your physician before stopping the drug.
4. Always check with your physician before changing the dose of the drug or taking over-the-counter drugs along with your ordered drugs.
5. Side effects include stomach upset and possible stomach bleeding, prolonged bleeding time, blood problems, allergic reaction, sodium and water retention, and renal and liver problems with long-term use.
6. Acetaminophen and alcohol (beer, wine, hard liquor) use (chronic or excessive) can cause liver problems. Oral anticoagulants and aspirin and/or acetaminophen can increase the bleeding effect. Birth control pills and acetaminophen cause a decrease in pain effect. Take with food to reduce stomach upset.
7. Keep medication tightly covered in light-resistant container, at room temperature. Keep out of the reach of children.

Opiate Analgesics

Dear Patient:
  This drug has been ordered for you. This is what you should know about your drug to get the most from your therapy. Opioid analgesics are used to reduce moderate pain. Several examples are codeine, codeine and aspirin, codeine and acetaminophen, propoxyphene, oxycodone, and hydrocodone.

1. Take by mouth every 4 to 6 hours.
2. Try not to forget a dose. Do not play catch up with missed doses.
3. If the drug is relieving the pain at the ordered dose and time, then continue the pain medication. If not, then notify your physician before stopping the drug.
4. Always check with your physician before changing the dose of the drug or taking over-the-counter drugs.
5. Alcohol (beer, wine, hard liquor) increases sedation, dizziness, lightheadedness, and inability to concentrate.
6. Side effects include constipation, nausea and vomiting (first 2 weeks of therapy), and drowsiness.
7. Interactions vary with each opioid analgesic.
8. Keep drug tightly covered at room temperature and out of the reach of children.

Opiate Agonists

Dear Patient:
  This drug has been ordered for you. This is what you should know about your drug to get the most from your therapy. Opioid agonists are used to reduce severe pain. Several examples are morphine, hydromorphone, methadone, and levorphanol.

1. Take by mouth every 6 to 8 hours.
2. Try not to forget a dose. Do not play catch up with missed doses.
3. If the drug is relieving the pain at the ordered dose and time, then continue to take it. If not, then notify your physician before stopping the drug.
4. Always check with your physician before changing the dose of the drug or taking over-the-counter drugs.
5. Alcohol (beer, wine, hard liquor) increases sedation, dizziness, lightheadedness, and inability to concentrate.
6. Side effects include constipation, nausea and vomiting (first 2 weeks of therapy), and drowsiness.
7. Interactions vary with each opioid agonist.
8. Keep drugs tightly covered at room temperature and out of the reach of children.

sition. Drugs such as the phenothiazines, which might potentiate this adverse effect, are used cautiously. Sedation also occurs initially. The sedation usually subsides within two or three days on a regular schedule of narcotics. Sedation may necessitate a slight reduction in analgesic dosage. Sedation should never be automatically linked with overdosage, since sedation may be the result of many factors including pain itself as well as the analgesic. Addiction, physical dependence, tolerance, and withdrawal syndrome are possible sequelae of treatment with narcotics and are reviewed in Chapter 13.

Recent advances in the body of knowledge regarding pain include the development of theories of pain, discovery of endogenous agents that mediate pain, and development of assessment tools to determine levels of pain. These advances clearly indicate a need for nurses to maintain a current working knowledge of analgesia information. They also challenge nurses to produce change and to keep pace within the sphere of nursing to perfect the process of nursing the patient with pain.

SUMMARY

This chapter has reviewed nonopiate and opiate pain medications. These agents are used in the control of pain. Various methods of administration of pain medications are discussed.

The nursing process is used to provide a framework for nursing action related to the patient in pain. Nursing implications are discussed as they relate to specific pain medications, routes of administering pain medication, and patient teaching.

BIBLIOGRAPHY

Craig, CR and Stitzel, RE: Pharmacology. Little, Brown & Co, Boston, 1986.

Deglin, JH and Vallerand, AH: Nurses Med Deck. FA Davis, Philadelphia, 1988.

Feuerstein, G and Siren, AL: The opioid system in cardiac and vascular regulation of normal and hypertensive states. Circulation 75(Suppl 1) 1:125–129, 1987.

Foley, KM: Concurrent controversies in opioid therapy. Advances in Pain Research and Therapy 8(3):124, 1986.

Katzung, BG: Basic and Clinical Pharmacology. Appleton-Lange, Los Altos, CA, 1987.

Lange, MP, Dahn, MS, and Jacobs, LA: Patient-controlled analgesia versus intermittent analgesia dosing. Heart Lung 17(5):495, 1988.

Leib, RA and Hurtig, JB: Epidural and intrathecal narcotics for pain management. Heart Lung 14(2):164, 1988.

Markowsky, C: Spinal narcotics and the implications for nursing. Canadian Critical Care Nursing Journal 5(4):15–19, 1988.

McCaffery, M: Nursing Management of Patients with Pain (2 ed). JB Lippincott, Philadelphia, PA, 1979.

Portenoy, RK: Continuous infusion of opioids. AJN 86(3):318, March, 1986.

Tartaglia, MJ: Managing chronic cancer pain effectively. Part 1. NursingLife 7(4):50, 1987.

Wall, C: The real risk of acetaminophen overdose. RN 35, August, #8 1985.

White, PF: Use of patient-controlled analgesia for management of acute pain. JAMA 259(2):243, 1988.

Willis, WD: Overview and Future Directions in the Pain System. S Karger, New York, 1985.

SITUATION 20–1

Celia Harrington has been admitted to the surgical unit with acute cholecystitis. She is being prepared for a cholecystectomy.

1. In planning for preoperative pain relief, the nurse is aware that the following medication may cause adverse effects in Ms. Harrington's case:
   a. oxycodone
   b. codeine
   c. nalbuphine
   d. meperidine

2. Butorphanol (Stadol) 2 mg IM is ordered for pain. The nurse will observe for all of the following adverse reactions with regard to this drug *except:*
   a. nausea
   b. diarrhea
   c. euphoria
   d. agitation

3. Postoperatively, Ms. Harrington will receive morphine via an epidural catheter. For management of pain control using this method, the nurse is aware that epidural morphine:
   a. demonstrates a slow onset of action
   b. provides a short duration of relief
   c. has decreased receptor affinity
   d. is quickly cleared through the CSF

4. When observing Ms. Harrington for side effects related to epidural morphine, the nurse will be aware of the following:
   a. urinary urgency
   b. polyuria
   c. pruritus
   d. tachypnea

5. Epidural catheter malposition is a complication of this type of pain therapy. The nurse will notify the physician of all of the following signs *except:*
   a. paresthesia
   b. occipital headache
   c. poor pain relief
   d. drowsiness

6. Ms. Harrington recovers from surgery without complications. For discharge, Tylenol with codeine 30 mg PO has been ordered for pain. The nurse will teach the patient to:
   a. take the drug every three to four hours with meals
   b. initiate measures to prevent constipation, such as drinking fluids
   c. observe for signs of analgesic neuropathy, which occur early
   d. continue the medication, if needed, for symptoms of arthritis

SITUATION 20–2

Mr. Van Chin is a 26-year-old who injured his back in an accident 5 years ago. He is admitted to the orthopedic floor for evaluation of recurrent back pain.

1. During the assessment phase, the nurse questions Mr. Chin about current medications. He states that he is taking Percodan, which used to help, but now the effect lasts for only an hour. The nurse is aware that this probably indicates:
   a. psychologic addiction
   b. hepatic insufficiency
   c. opiate inactivation
   d. drug tolerance

2. During the assessment, Mr. Chin describes his pain as nagging and burning. He states that it has become the "focus of [his] life." These symptoms are characteristic of which type of pain?
   a. chronic
   b. psychologic
   c. phantom
   d. acute

(cont.)

SITUATION   20-2-*CONTINUED*

3. Spinal evaluation reveals two herniated discs, and Mr. Chin undergoes a lumbar laminectomy. Postoperative orders include Dilaudid 2 mg IM every 4 hours as needed for pain. The nurse is aware of the following with regard to this drug:
   a. Dilaudid is less potent than morphine when given intramuscularly.
   b. As a partial opiate antagonist, it has less potential for abuse and addiction.
   c. Dilaudid has fewer central nervous system effects than morphine.
   d. It may have an additive effect if given with general anesthetics.

4. Mr. Chin requests medication for back pain. When administering Dilaudid to Mr. Chin, all of the following actions are appropriate *except:*
   a. maintain a positive outlook in anticipation of pain relief
   b. encourage the patient to relax and allow the drug to work
   c. wait until Mr. Chin shows signs of pain before administering
   d. take advantage of the placebo effect of the drug

5. In evaluating Mr. Chin to determine effectiveness of the pain medication regimen, the nurse is aware of the following factor:
   a. Sedation is always linked with signs of an overdose.
   b. Ambulation is encouraged for patients with nausea.
   c. Symptoms such as vomiting may indicate poorly controlled pain.
   d. Addiction is rarely a problem in patients with "real" pain.

6. If Mr. Chin has problems with urinary retention postoperatively, the following drug may be given:
   a. droperidol
   b. neostigmine
   c. levallorphan
   d. naloxone

Please refer to the Appendices for correct answers and additional review questions with answers.

GLOSSARY TERMS IN THIS CHAPTER

Anosmia
Analeptic
Asthenic
Cataplexy
Choreiform
Depolarizing postsynaptic potential
Drug holiday
Garrulous
Hyperactivity
Hyperpolarizing potential
Hyperthyroxinemia
Mydriasis
Opisthotonos
REM
Rhinorrhea

21
CHAPTER

CENTRAL NERVOUS SYSTEM STIMULANTS

VICKI L. BYERS, M.S.N., Ph.D., CNRN

LEARNING OBJECTIVES

After reading this chapter, the student will be able to:

1. Identify those medications commonly used as central nervous system stimulants.

2. Differentiate among the central nervous system stimulants as to mechanism of action, route of administration, pharmacokinetics, adverse effects, contraindications, and interactions.

3. Identify specific areas to assess in the patient requiring central nervous system stimulants in order to formulate appropriate nursing diagnoses.

4. Plan the nursing interventions necessary to administer central nervous system stimulants and choose appropriate teaching strategies to gain patient compliance.

5. Evaluate the patient at various stages of treatment to measure the effectiveness of nursing interventions.

OVERVIEW OF CENTRAL NERVOUS SYSTEM STIMULANTS

The central nervous system (CNS) stimulants are a diverse group of pharmacologic drugs whose first action is stimulation of the central nervous system. CNS stimulation is a side effect of a large number of pharmacologic drugs. CNS stimulation is demonstrated through a change in the patient's usual behavior. Some of the behavioral changes include mild elevations of alertness, increased restlessness, irritability, euphoria, nervousness, anxiety. The patient can also experience increased muscle tone and seizures. The degree of the CNS stimulation caused by a certain drug depends on both the area in the brain or spinal cord that is affected by the drug and the cellular mechanism fundamental to the increased excitability.

There is a fine balance between excitation and inhibition in the CNS. Information is transmitted along neurons by action potentials. A *depolarizing postsynaptic potential* is an excitatory postsynaptic potential (EPSP). If the degree of this action potential is of magnitude, an action potential will be produced in an all-or-nothing manner through this second neuron. The *hyperpolarizing potential*, on the other hand, is inhibitory and prevents the action potential of the second neuron. The purpose of the inhibitory postsynaptic potential (IPSP) is to decrease the number of nerve impulses generated

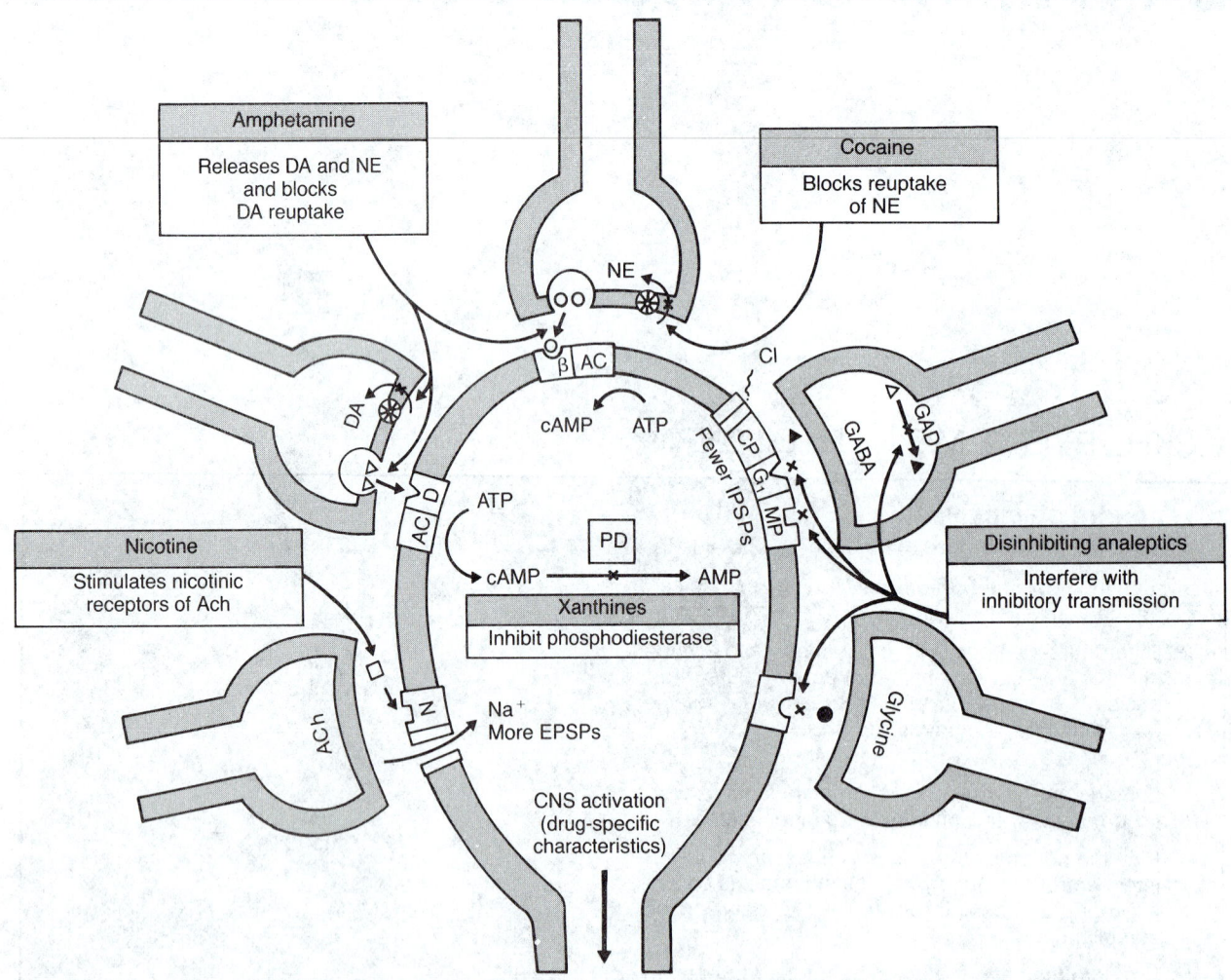

Figure 21–1. Neurochemical mechanisms of stimulants. AC, adenyl cyclase; ACh, acetylcholine; AMP, adenosine monophosphate; ATP, adenosine triphosphate; cAMP, cyclic adenosine monophosphate; *B,* Beta-adrenergic receptor; D, dopamine receptor; DA, dopamine; EPSP, excitatory postsynaptic potential; GABA, gamma-aminobutyric acid; G_1, GABA receptor, type 1; GAD, glutamic acid decarboxylase; IPSP, inhibitory postsynaptic potential; MP, modulatory protein; NE, norepinephrine; PD, phosphodiesterase. (From Alvin K. Swonger and Myrtle P. Matejski, Nursing Pharmacology: An Integrated Approach to Drug Therapy and Nursing Practice, p. 202. Copyright 1988 by Alvin K. Swonger and Myrtle P. Matejski. By permission of Scott, Foresman and Company.)

per unit of time. If this did not occur, the CNS would be in a constant state of stimulation (Fig. 21–1).

Altering the fine balance between excitatory and inhibitory influence at the level of the neuron explains how CNS stimulants produce their pharmacologic action. This action is produced by one or more of the following mechanisms: (1) to increase the effect of excitatory neurotransmission (e.g., doxapram); (2) to decrease or oppose inhibitory neurotransmission (e.g., strychnine); (3) presynaptic control of neurotransmitter release; (4) to block the uptake of catecholamines at adrenergic synapses (e.g., cocaine); or (5) to modify neurotransmitter response by altering adenosine 3':5' cyclic phosphate (cAMP) (e.g., xanthines). A review of the neurochemical mechanism of CNS stimulants is given in Figure 21–1.

The therapeutic use of stimulants has decreased over the years for a variety of reasons. The *analeptic* stimulants were used primarily as respiratory stimulants in clinical situations where there was CNS depression secondary to overdosage of CNS depressants. One factor that reduced the use of CNS stimulants was that these agents were not specific antagonists of depressant agents and, therefore, were not effective in reducing pharmacologically induced CNS depression. A second factor is that CNS stimulants have a shorter duration of action than the agents they are used to reverse. The dosage required to reverse CNS depression caused the toxic side effects of CNS stimulants, namely, seizures and cardiac dysrhythmias. The last factor leading to the reduction of the use of CNS stimulants in managing CNS depression is the development of more conservative and safer procedures such as support of a patent airway and elevation of low blood pressure.

There are three groups of CNS stimulants: analeptic stimulants, psychomotor stimulants, and methylxanthines (Table 21–1). This division of groups is based on mechanism of action or chemical composition. Descriptions of each group of stimulants and some specific agents are given in this chapter.

Table 21–1. CLASSIFICATION OF CENTRAL NERVOUS SYSTEM STIMULANTS

Analeptic Stimulants	Psychomotor Stimulants	Methylxanthines
Doxapram	Amphetamine	Caffeine
Nike-thamide	Methamphetamine	Theophylline
Pentylene-tetrazol	Methylphenidate	Theobromine
Strychnine	Pemoline	
Picrotoxin	Ephedrine	
Bicuculline	Phentermine	
	Fenfluramine	
	Phenylpropanol-amine	

From Craig, CR and Stitzel, RE: Modern Pharmacology, ed 2. Little, Brown & Co, 1986, p 492, with permission.

ANALEPTIC STIMULANTS

The agents in this group are very different in chemical composition, which makes it difficult to classify each one in reference to absorption, distribution, and metabolism. Most of these agents are absorbed orally and have short duration of action. The agents doxapram and nikethamide were historically used as CNS and respiratory stimulants. These two agents, especially doxapram, still have limited clinical use.

Mechanism of Action

Most of the agents in this group of stimulants possess the ability to interact with amino acid neurotransmitters. Recent studies have explored the gamma-amino butyric acid (GABA) receptor–chloride ionophore interaction. These experiments have postulated that the analeptic stimulants have the ability to change the way chloride ions travel across the neuronal membrane. The inhibitory action of some amino acid neurotransmitters involves an increase in chloride conductance.

Adverse Reactions

This group of agents produces adverse reactions that are exaggerations of their therapeutic effect. They produce life-threatening clonic-tonic seizures that can lead to death. Prior to these seizures, there may be an increase in respiration, tachycardia, and severe hypertension. Patients also experience extreme *opisthotonos* and increased sensitivity to sensory stimuli induced seizures (this is especially true with strychnine poisoning).

Doxapram

Doxapram is an analeptic respiratory stimulant that has a rapid onset (20–40 seconds) and a short duration of action (5–12 minutes). Doxapram produces respiratory stimulation via the peripheral carotid chemoreceptors. As the dosage level increases, the respiratory centers in the medulla are stimulated along with other parts of the CNS. This agent is used for postanesthesia respiratory depression, drug-induced CNS depression, and chronic pulmonary disease with hypercapnia (temporary measure only). The value of analeptics in the therapy of pulmonary disease is very limited. Extreme caution should be used when administering this drug. Doxapram can be given as an intravenous injection and as an intravenous infusion. Doxapram is compatible with 5% and 10% dextrose in water or normal saline. Mixing doxapram with alkaline solutions such as 2.5% thiopental sodium, bicarbonate, or aminophylline results in precipitation or gas formation. Prior to administration of doxapram, refer to the drug insert for specific instructions about the use of this drug. For dosage information, refer to Table 21–2.

CONTRAINDICATIONS AND PRECAUTIONS. Since doxapram contains benzyl alcohol, it is not used in newborns. It should not be used in any patient who is already experiencing CNS stimulation, such as epilepsy,

TEXT RESUMES ON PAGE 510

Table 21–2. CENTRAL NERVOUS SYSTEM STIMULANTS

Name	Dosage	Mode of Administration	Pharmacokinetics

Amphetamine (Benzedrine)

Action: CNS stimulant. Produces CNS stimulation by releasing norepinephrine from nerve endings. Therapeutic effects include increased motor activity, mental alertness, decreased fatigue, and brighter outlook. This agent also suppresses appetite.

Use: Used in the treatment of narcolepsy and as an adjunct in the management of attention deficit disorder (hyperkinetic syndrome of childhood, minimal brain dysfunction). Also used in the short-term management of exogenous obesity.

		Mode of Administration	Pharmacokinetics
		IV,† PO	O: rapid (PO) P: 15 min (IV) P: 30 min (PO) D: Short (IV),* 3–4 hr (PO) ½ L: 7–14 hr PB: UA B: liver E: kidneys

*Varies with the pH of the urine.
†Not legally available IV

Cocaine

Action: CNS stimulants. When applied topically, cocaine blocks nerve conduction and produces surface anesthesia with local vasoconstriction. It has an adrenergic effect by potentiating the action of endogenous epinephrine and norepinephrine.

Use: Potent CNS stimulant and local anesthetic. It is also used in the relief of cancer pain. This drug is a popular drug that is illegally abused.

	Dosage	Mode of Administration	Pharmacokinetics
	5–7.5 ml of 1%–4% solution (local anesthetic) 1–3 mg/kg, not to exceed 200 mg/70 kg over 30 min (topical)	Topical, intranasal, PO, IV	O: rapid P: 3–5 min (IV), 20–60 min (intranasal), 60–90 min (PO) D: 20–40 min (topical), 6 hr (intranasal)

Key to Abbreviations in the *Pharmacokinetics* column O-onset; P-peak; D-duration; PB-protein bound; B-biotransformed in; E-excreted in; ½ L-halflife.
*Within the column listing adverse effects, underlines indicate the most common effects, and CAPITALS indicate life-threatening effects.

Contraindications/ Precautions	Adverse Effects*	Interactions	Nursing Implications
			ASSESSMENT: Neurologic assessment establishes a baseline for mental, behavioral, and motor functioning prior to initial therapy. INTERVENTION: Monitor the patient for therapeutic response and possible adverse effects. Monitor patient's blood pressure, pulse, and respiratory status while he/she is receiving amphetamine therapy. Monitor the weight and height of children.
Contraindications: This drug should not be used in patients with advanced arteriosclerosis, symptomatic cardiovascular disease, hypertension, hyperthyroidism, glaucoma, hypersensitivity, diabetes mellitus, agitated states, drug abuse, concurrent MAO inhibitor therapy, and tics. Use cautiously in mild hypertension, children, pregnancy, patients at risk for overdose and dependency, weight loss, cigarette smoking, and heart disease.	Neuro: Euphoria, dizziness, tremor, irritability, insomnia, restlessness, dysphoria, headache, amphetamine psychosis, ataxia, choreiform movements, SEIZURES CV: Tachycardia, DYSRHYTHMIAS, hypertension, Palpitation, anginal pain Resp: PULMONARY EDEMA (overdose) GI: anorexia, abdominal pain, dry mouth, unpleasant taste, diarrhea, constipation GU: sexual dysfunction (impotence, change in libido) Endo: hyperthyroxinemia Integ: urticaria Misc: psychic dependence, addiction	Drug–Drug: Addictive adrenergic effects. Use with MAO inhibitors can result in hypertensive crisis. Alkalinization of urine (sodium bicarbonate, acetazolamide) decreases excretion and enhances effect. Acidification of urine (ammonium chloride, ascorbic acid) decreases effect. Phenothiazines may also decrease effect. Amphetamines may antagonize antihypertensives. Tricyclic antidepressants may enhance the effect of amphetamines. Drug–Food: Foods that acidify the urine (cranberry juice) can enhance the effect of amphetamines. Drug–Lab: The following lab tests have been altered with amphetamines: growth hormone, cortisol, TSH, and fecal discoloration.	Same for all, plus: EVALUATION: Side effects of amphetamines are minimized. Child's attention span is longer, concentration on tasks is greater, and hyperactivity is decreased, indicating that therapy is effective.
Contraindications: The use of cocaine is contraindicated in the following situations: hypertension, concur-	Neuro: HEADACHE, excitement, euphoria, dysphoria, psychotic reactions, tremor, HYPERREFLEXIA, insomnia, diaphoresis, mydriasis, gen-	Drug–Drug: concurrent use of anesthetics, anticholinergics, and guanethidine Drug–Lab: increases urine alkaloids	Same as for all, plus: INTERVENTION: This medication has a high dependence and abuse potential.

CONTINUED ON THE FOLLOWING PAGE

Table 21–2. CENTRAL NERVOUS SYSTEM STIMULANTS–*CONTINUED*

Name	Dosage	Mode of Administration	Pharmacokinetics
Cocaine–Continued			½ L: 75 min (topical to nasal area) PB: UA B: liver E: kidney
Methamphetamine Hydro- chloride (Desoxyn, Meth- ampex)			

Action: CNS and respiratory stimulant. It acts by releasing norepinephrine from the nerve endings and blocks the reuptake of catecholamines after their release. This agent also promotes the release of dopamine and reuptake of catecholamines after their release. Methamphetamine HCl also promotes the release of dopamine and epinephrine.

Use: Used in the treatment of attentional disorder with hyperactivity and short-term therapy of obesity. This agent is used as an adjunct for narcolepsy.

Name	Dosage	Mode of Administration	Pharmacokinetics
	Obesity 2.5–5 mg 2–3 times daily one half hour before meals; or 10–15 mg SR tablet one half hour before breakfast	PO	O: 30–45 min P: UA D: 12 hr with recommended doses; up to 24 hr with large doses ½ L: 6–12 hr but may be longer depending on urine pH PB: UA B: liver E: kidneys

Key to Abbreviations in the *Pharmacokinetics* column O-onset; P-peak; D-duration; PB-protein bound; B-bio-transformed in; E-excreted in; ½ L-halflife.
*Within the column listing adverse effects, underlines indicate the most common effects, and CAPITALS indicate life-threatening effects.

Contraindications/ Precautions	Adverse Effects*	Interactions	Nursing Implications
rent use of sympathomimetic amines, drug abuse, and hypersensitivity. Use cautiously in the following situations: concurrent therapy with cholinesterase inhibitors, succinylcholine sensitivity, and with drugs that sensitize the myocardium to catecholamines.	eralized seizures, loss of consciousness CV: CARDIOVASCULAR ARREST, tachycardia, hypertension, angina, dysrhythmias Resp: IRREGULAR RESPIRATION, RESPIRATORY ARREST, tachypnea GI: Abdominal pain, nausea, vomiting, anorexia, diarrhea GU: sexual disinterest, sexual dysfunction EENT: rhinorrhea, anosmia, clouding of the cornea, pitting, corneal ulceration		
Contraindications include hypersensitivity to sympathomimetic amines, hyperthyroidism, advanced arteriosclerosis, glaucoma, hypertension, cardiovascular disease, agitated stages, history or potential of drug abuse, pregnancy, and during or within 14 days of treatment with MAO inhibitors. Use with caution when performing activities that require mental alertness or physical coordination, with concurrent drug therapy that produces excitability, or when patient's personality is one of excitability. Use with caution in geriatric, debilitated, or asthenic patients; in psychopathic personality, in those who are allergic to the dye tartrazine, in children under 12 years of age, and in patients with diabetes mellitus.	Neuro: HYPERREFLEXIA, nervousness, insomnia, irritability, dizziness, talkativeness, headache, blurred vision, mydriasis, dysphoria, euphoria, tremor, restlessness CV: TACHYCARDIA, hypertension, hypotension, palpitation, DYSRHYTHMIAS Resp: IRREGULAR RESPIRATION, RESPIRATORY ARREST GI: ABDOMINAL PAIN, nausea, vomiting, anorexia, abdominal cramps, dry mouth, diarrhea, constipation, unpleasant taste GU: change in libido Misc: urticaria	Insulin requirements are reduced. Do not use concurrently with MAO inhibitors and some general anesthetics	Same as for all, plus: INTERVENTION: Monitor height and weight of children.

CONTINUED ON THE FOLLOWING PAGE

Table 21–2. CENTRAL NERVOUS SYSTEM STIMULANTS–*CONTINUED*

Name	Dosage	Mode of Administration	Pharmacokinetics
Doxapram Hydrochloride (Dopram)			

Action: This respiratory stimulant potentiates excitatory neurotransmission. It is thought that this mechanism is based on the ability to alter the movement of chloride ions across neuronal membranes. The central respiratory centers in the medulla are stimulated and catecholamines are released.

Use: (*A*) drug-induced postanesthesia respiratory depression or apnea; (*B*) drug-induced CNS depression; (*C*) chronic pulmonary disease with acute hypercapnia (used only for 2 hours and not in combination with mechanical ventilation).

	Dosage	Mode of Administration	Pharmacokinetics
	Postanesthetic use: *Single injection:* 0.5 mg/kg (recommended); 1.5 mg/kg (maximum dose/ single injection); 2.0 mg/kg (maximum dose/repeat injection—5-min intervals) *Infusion:*	IV	O: 20–40 sec P: 1–2 min D: 5–12 min ½L: UA PB: UA B: liver E: kidneys
	0.5–4 mg/kg (recommended); 3.0 g/kg (maximum total dose). Administer at a rate of 5 mg/min until satisfactory respiratory response is obtained. Maintenance dose of 1–3 mg/min is used to sustain the desired level of respiratory stimulation with minimal side effects.		
	For Drug-Induced CNS Depression: *Mild depression:* 1.0 mg/kg (single priming dose, repeat IV injection); 1–2 mg/kg/hr (rate of intermittent IV infusion) *Moderate depression:* 2.0 mg/kg (priming single dose, repeat IV injection); 2–3 mg/kg/hr (rate of intermittent IV infusion)	IV	

Key to Abbreviations in the *Pharmacokinetics* column: O-onset; P-peak; D-duration; PB-protein bound; B-biotransformed in; E-excreted in; ½ L-halflife.

*Within the column listing adverse effects, underlines indicate the most common effects, and CAPITALS indicate life-threatening effects.

Contraindications/ Precautions	Adverse Effects*	Interactions	Nursing Implications
Contraindicated in newborns because it contains benzyl alcohol; epilepsy/convulsive disorders; patients with mechanical disorders of ventilation such as mechanical obstruction, muscle paresis, flail chest, pneumothorax, acute bronchial asthma, pulmonary fibrosis, or other situations where there is restriction of the chest wall, muscles of respiration or alveolar expansion; head injury, cerebral vascular accident, cardiovascular impairment, or severe hypertension; or hypersensitivity to the drug. *Postanesthetic use:* Doxapram is not an antagonist to muscle relaxant drugs or narcotic antagonist. Patency or airway and oxygenation must exist prior to administration of doxapram. Administer with care in and supervise patients with hypermetabolic states such as hyperthyroidism or pheochromocytoma. *Drug-induced CNS and respiratory depression:* Use in addition to established measures and resuscitative techniques because doxapram alone may not stimulate adequate spontaneous breathing or arousal in severely depressed patients. *Chronic obstructive pulmonary disease:* Since there is an increased labor of breathing, avoid increasing the rate of infusion of doxapram in an attempt to lower Pco_2. Doxapram should not be used in combination with mechanical ventilation.	Neuro: hyperthermia, flushing, paresthesia (warmth or burning feeling especially in the area of the genitalia and perineum), apprehension, headache, disorientation, dilated pupils, dizziness, restlessness, hyperactivity, involuntary movements, increased deep tendon reflexes, CLONUS, muscle spasticity, bilateral Babinski syndrome, CONVULSIONS. Early signs of overdose include skeletal muscle hyperactivity and increased deep tendon reflexes. CV: fluctuation in heart rate, phlebitis, lowered T waves, dyshythmias, angina, tightness in chest, hypertension, hypotension. Early signs of overdose include hypertension and tachycardia. Resp: dyspnea, cough, tachypnea, LARYNGOSPASM, hiccup, BRONCHOSPASM, rebound hypoventilation GI: nausea, vomiting, diarrhea, desire to defecate GU: stimulation of urinary bladder with spontaneous voiding, urinary retention Integ: pruritus	Interactions have occurred with the following agents: sympathomimetic or MAO inhibitors, muscle relaxant drugs, and anesthetics that sensitize the myocardium to catecholamines (halothane, cyclopropane, enflurane).	Same as for all, plus: ASSESSMENT: Maintain patient airway. Monitor pulse, blood pressure, and deep tendon reflexes. Monitor arterial blood gases and respiratory status of patient. All of these assessment parameters are evaluated prior to and during infusion. INTERVENTION: Resuscitative equipment, oxygen, and short-acting barbiturates should be readily available. Place patient on seizure precautions. Discontinue doxapram if hypotension or dyspnea develops. Obtain an arterial blood gas measurement, and notify the physician. Maintain infusion at prescribed rate. It is important to remember the maximal dose for injection or infusion of doxapram. Monitor vital signs and deep tendon reflexes during infusion. Following stimulation with doxapram, narcosis may occur, so it is important to observe the patient closely for ½–1 hour after the patient is fully alert. EVALUATION: Effectiveness of therapy is evidenced by desired therapeutic effects with minimal side effects.

CONTINUED ON THE FOLLOWING PAGE

Table 21–2. CENTRAL NERVOUS SYSTEM STIMULANTS–*CONTINUED*

Name	Dosage	Mode of Administration	Pharmacokinetics
Doxapram Hydrochloride–*Continued*			

Pemoline (Cylert)

Action: CNS and respiratory stimulant; possesses weak sympathomimetic activity. CNS stimulation is mediated by brain dopamine.

Use: To treat attention deficit disorder with hyperactivity in children over 6 years of age; treatment of fatigue, mental depression, chronic schizophrenia, and as a mild stimulant for geriatric patients.

	Dosage	Mode of Administration	Pharmacokinetics
	Initial dose for children over 6 years of age is 37.5 mg administered in the morning. The daily dose is increased by 18.75 mg weekly. The usual effective range is 56.25–75.0 mg daily. Dosage for children should not exceed 112.5 mg daily.	PO	O: 30–45 min P: 2–4 hr D: 8 hr ½L: 9–14 hr in adults; nonlinear kinetics in children increase the half-life PB: 50% B: liver E: kidneys

Xanthine Derivative (Caffeine)

Action: Stimulates all levels of the CNS. Caffeine inhibits phosphodiesterase, the enzyme that degrades cAMP.

Use: Caffeine is used as a mild CNS stimulant to help fatigued persons to stay awake. It is used in combination with antihistamines to overcome sedative properties of the antihistamines; used with supportive measures to treat respiratory depression associated with overdosage of CNS depressant drugs; to treat neonatal apnea; used alone or in combination with analgesics to provide pain relief, especially for headaches; used as a diuretic for fluid retention associated with menstruation.

	Dosage	Mode of Administration	Pharmacokinetics
	Mild CNS Stimulation (Adults): 65–325 mg tid	PO	O: 30–45 min P: 50–75 min D: UA
	Neonatal Apnea: loading dose of 5–10 mg/kg, followed by 2.5–5 mg/kg daily	IV, IM, PO	½L: 3–4 hr for adults; 80 hr for neonates PB:17% B: liver
	Children Requiring CNS Stimulation: 8 mg/kg every 4 hr prn	IV, IM, PO, SC	E: kidneys

Key to Abbreviations in the *Pharmacokinetics* column: O-onset; P-peak; D-duration; PB-protein bound; B-biotransformed in; E-excreted in; ½ L-halflife.
*Within the column listing adverse effects, underlines indicate the most common effects, and CAPITALS indicate life-threatening effects.

Contraindications/ Precautions	Adverse Effects*	Interactions	Nursing Implications
This drug should be used with caution in patients with fluctuating blood pressure and/or deep tendon reflexes, lowered P_{CO_2}, and dyspnea.			
Contraindicated in children under 6 years of age, in patients with impaired hepatic function, and in those who exhibit hypersensitivity to the drug. Use with caution in patients with renal dysfunction, in those receiving pemoline over a long period of time, and in children.	Neuro: insomnia, dyskinetic movements of tongue, lips, face, and extremities; nystagmus, irritability; dizziness; headache; HALLUCINATIONS; SEIZURES; mild depression; drowsiness; malaise; spasm of eye muscle CV: TACHYCARDIA GI: anorexia, weight loss, stomach pain, nausea, diarrhea, hepatitis, jaundice Integ: rash	Drug–Drug: Unknown Drug–Lab: Elevated SGOT, SGPT, and alkaline phosphatase	Same as for all, plus: ASSESSMENT: Monitor height and weight in children. Monitor liver function tests in long-term therapy. INTERVENTION: Administer pemoline in the morning to provide maximal effectiveness during waking hours and to avoid insomnia. Insomnia and anorexia are dose-dependent. If these side effects occur, the dose may need to be reduced. Drug holidays prescribed by the physician can determine the effectiveness of therapy and the need for continuation. Monitor height and weight in children. EVALUATION: Child's attention span is longer, concentration on tasks is greater, and hyperactivity is decreased, indicating that the therapy is effective. Side effects from pemoline are minimal.
Contraindicated in acute myocardial infarction; symptomatic cardiac dysrhythmias and/or palpitations first several days post-MI; hypersensitivity to caffeine. Avoid or limit caffeine con-	Neuro: Insomnia, restlessness, excitement, flashes of light, nervousness, mild delirium CV: transient increases in heart rate, force of contraction, cardiac output, extrasystole, VENTRICULAR DYS-	Drug–Drug: interactions have been reported with the following drugs: β-adrenergic agonists, disulfiram, and phenobarbital. Drug–Lab: False-positive elevation of serum urate; increased urine levels of	Same as for all, plus: ASSESSMENT: Monitor vital signs closely. CNS effects of caffeine are more severe in children. Obtain history of caffeine intake. INTERVENTION: IM injections are painful. Explain

CONTINUED ON THE FOLLOWING PAGE

Table 21–2. CENTRAL NERVOUS SYSTEM STIMULANTS–*CONTINUED*

Name	Dosage	Mode of Administration	Pharmacokinetics
Xanthine Derivative–*Continued*			
Methylphenidate (Ritalin)			

Action: Produces CNS and respiratory stimulation with weak sympathomimetic activity. Therapeutic effects include correction of hyperactivity in hyperkinetic syndrome or increased motor activity, mental alertness, diminished sense of fatigue, and brighter outlook.

Use: Used as an adjunct in the treatment of attention deficit disorders (hyperkinetic syndrome of childhood, minimal brain dysfunction) and in the symptomatic treatment of narcolepsy.

Name	Dosage	Mode of Administration	Pharmacokinetics
	Minimal Brain Dysfunction, Children under 6 yr: 5 mg before breakfast and lunch; increase by 5–10 mg at weekly intervals (maximum 60 mg/day)	PO	O: UA P:1–3 hr D: 4–6 hr, extended release, 8 hr ½ L: 1–3 hr PB: UA
	Narcolepsy (Adults): 10 mg bid or tid (50 mg/day maximum)	PO	B: liver E: kidneys

Key to Abbreviations in the *Pharmacokinetics* column: O-onset; P-peak; D-duration; PB-protein bound; B-biotransformed in; E-excreted in; ½ L-halflife.

*Within the column listing adverse effects, underlines indicate the most common effects, and CAPITALS indicate life-threatening effects.

Contraindications/ Precautions	Adverse Effects*	Interactions	Nursing Implications
sumption during pregnancy. Use cautiously in children and in those with a history of peptic ulcer.	RHYTHMIAS, slight hypertension. Resp: TACHYPNEA GI: nausea, vomiting, GI irritation GU: diuresis Endo: increase in glycogenolysis and lipolysis Musculo: muscle tremors or twitches Misc: increase in basal metabolic rate	vanillylmandelic acid (VMA), catecholamines, and 5-hydroxyindoleacetic acid.	this to the patient prior to administration. Administer IV caffeine slowly. Overdosage can be treated with a short-acting barbiturate. EVALUATION: Patients experience minimal side effects. If given as an analgesic, ask patient whether relief is obtained.
Contraindicated in hypersensitivity, pregnancy-lactation, hyperexcitable states (hyperthyroidism, psychotic personalities, suicidal or homicidal tendencies), glaucoma, and motor tics. Use cautiously in cardiovascular disease, hypertension, diabetes mellitus, the elderly, debilitated patients, and seizure disorders. Longterm therapy may result in psychic dependence or addiction.	Neuro: HYPERREFLEXIA, CONVULSIONS, restlessness, tremor, hyperactivity, insomnia, irritability, dizziness, headache, akathisia, dyskinesia CV: TACHYCARDIA, DYSRHYTHMIA, HYPERTENSION, palpitations, hypotension GI: nausea, vomiting, anorexia, dry mouth, cramps, diarrhea, constipation, metallic taste Integ: rashes Misc: HYPERPYREXIA, hypersensitivity reactions	The following agents are reported to interact with methylphenidate: sympathomimetics, decongestants, vasoconstrictors, MAO inhibitors, guanethidine, oral anticoagulants, anticonvulsants, and tricyclic antidepressants.	Same as for all, plus: ASSESSMENT: Assess patient's behavior prior to and periodically throughout therapy. Therapy may be interrupted at intervals to determine if symptoms are sufficient to continue therapy. Monitor CBC and differential and platelet count periodically throughout therapy. Assess blood pressure and pulse periodically throughout therapy. INTERVENTION: Growth, including height and weight, are monitored in children on long-term therapy. The drug may be administered with meals if GI irritation becomes a problem. Extended-release tablets are swallowed whole; the patient should not crush, break, or chew. EVALUATION: In children with hyperkinetic syndrome, effectiveness is demonstrated by calming effect with decreased hyperactivity and prolonged attention span. In narcolepsy, effectiveness of therapy is demonstrated by increased motor activity, increased mental alertness, diminished sense of fatigue, and brighter outlook.

CONTINUED ON THE FOLLOWING PAGE

Table 21–2. CENTRAL NERVOUS SYSTEM STIMULANTS–*CONTINUED*

Name	Dosage	Mode of Administration	Pharmacokinetics

Action: Produces CNS stimulation by releasing norepinephrine from nerve endings. Pharmacologic effects include CNS and respiratory stimulation, vasoconstriction, mydriasis, and contraction of the urinary bladder sphincter. Therapeutic effects include increased motor activity, mental alertness, decreased fatigue, and brighter outlook. Suppresses appetite.

Use: Used in the treatment of narcolepsy and as an adjunct in the management of attention deficit disorders (hyperkinetic syndrome of childhood, minimal brain dysfunction). Also used as adjunctive therapy to calorie restriction in short-term management of exogenous obesity.

Name	Dosage	Mode of Administration	Pharmacokinetics
Dextroamphetamine (Dexedrine)	*Minimal Brain Dysfunction:* *Children > 6 yr:* 5–10 mg/day in 1–2 doses; increased by 5 mg at weekly intervals *Children 3–5 yr:* 2.5 mg/day, increased by 2.5 mg at weekly intervals *Narcolepsy:* *Adults:* 50–60 mg/day in divided doses *Children over 12 yr:* 10 mg/day, increased by 10 mg at weekly intervals *Children 6–12 yr:* 5 mg/day, increased by 5 mg/day at weekly intervals	PO	O: 1–2 hr P: UA D: 2–10 hr ½ L: 10.2 hr; 6.8 hr in children PB: UA B: liver E: kidneys
Metamphetamine Hydrochloride	*Attention Deficit Disorder:* 2.5–5 mg daily or bid; 20–25 mg daily is usual effective dose *Obesity (Adults):* 2.5–5 mg bid or tid, 30 min prior to meal, or 10–15-mg extended-release tablet before breakfast daily. This treatment is used for only a couple of weeks.	PO	O: 1–2 hr P: UA D: 6–12 hr ½ L: 4–5 hr (longer in alkaline urine) PB: UA B: liver E: kidneys

Key to Abbreviations in the *Pharmacokinetics* column: O-onset; P-peak; D-duration; PB-protein bound; B-biotransformed in; E-excreted in; ½ L-halflife.
*Within the column listing adverse effects, underlines indicate the most common effects, and CAPITALS indicate life-threatening effects.

Contraindications/ Precautions	Adverse Effects*	Interactions	Nursing Implications
Contraindicated in pregnancy/lactation; hyperexcitable states (hyperthyroidism, psychotic personalities, suicidal/homicidal tendencies), chemical dependence; glaucoma. Use cautiously in cardiovascular disease, hypertension, diabetes mellitus, the elderly, and debilitated patients. Long-term use of these agents may result in psychic dependence or addiction.	Neuro: restlessness, tremor, insomnia, irritability, dizziness, headache CV: TACHYCARDIA, PALPITATIONS, hypertension, hypotension Resp: PULMONARY EDEMA GI: nausea, vomiting, anorexia, dry mouth, cramps, diarrhea, constipation GU: impotence, increased libido Misc: psychic dependence, addiction	Drug–Drug: MAO inhibitors, sodium bicarbonate, acetazolamide, ammonium chloride, ascorbic acid, phenothiazines, antihypertensives, and tricyclic antidepressants Drug–Food: Foods that acidify the urine (cranberry juice, meats, fish, poultry, eggs, cheeses, grains, prunes, plums) can enhance the effect of amphetamines.	Same as for all, plus: ASSESSMENT: Monitor blood pressure, apical pulse, and respiration before administration and periodically throughout the course of therapy. These medications may produce a false sense of euphoria and well-being. Provide frequent rest periods, and observe patient for rebound depression after the effects of the medication have worn off. These medications have a high dependence and abuse potential. Tolerance to medication occurs rapidly; do not increase dose. INTERVENTION: Do not crush or chew sustained-release tablets. Capsules are swallowed whole; patient should not break, crush, or chew. EVALUATION: In children the effectiveness is demonstrated by a calming effect with decreased hyperactivity and prolonged attention span. In narcolepsy, effectiveness of therapy is demonstrated by increased motor activity, increased mental alertness, diminished sense of fatigue, and brighter outlook.
Same as above.	Same as above.	Same as above.	Same as above.

seizure disorder, agitation, head injury, or cerebral vascular accident. Due to decreased carbon dioxide induced by hyperventilation, there is cerebral vasoconstriction, which could lead to compromised cerebral circulation. Since catecholamines are released and there is a pressor effect noted with doxapram, this drug is contraindicated in patients with cardiovascular impairment and severe hypertension. Doxapram is also contraindicated in patients with mechanical disorders of ventilation (e.g., airway obstruction, muscle paresis, flail chest, pneumothorax, acute bronchial asthma, pulmonary fibrosis) and conditions where there is chest wall restriction. Doxapram's site of action is the peripheral carotid chemoreceptors and central respiratory centers in the brain, and the mechanism of action does not facilitate improvement in disorders of ventilation. Doxapram is contraindicated in persons with hypersensitivity to the drug.

Administration of doxapram is not a substitute for a patent airway. It is important to administer the minimum effective dosage to avoid side effects. In order to avoid overdosage, it is necessary to observe blood pressure and deep tendon reflexes. Intravenous short-acting barbiturates, oxygen, and resuscitative equipment should be readily available to manage overdose. Rapid infusion of doxapram can result in hemolysis. If sudden hypotension or dyspnea develops, doxapram should be discontinued.

ADVERSE REACTIONS. The major systems affected by doxapram include the central and autonomic nervous systems and the respiratory, cardiovascular, and genitourinary systems. The skin is also affected. Effects can be mild to severe. The CNS and autonomic effects include hyperthermia, flushing, paresthesia (warmth or burning feeling especially in the area of the genitalia and perineum), apprehension, headache, disorientation, dilated pupils, dizziness, restlessness, hyperactivity, involuntary movements, increased deep tendon reflexes, clonus, muscle spasticity, bilateral Babinski syndrome, and seizures. The cardiovascular effects include fluctuation in heart rate, phlebitis, lowered T waves, arrhythmias, angina, tightness in chest, hypertension, and hypotension. These are due to the combination of the release of norepinephrine from the adrenergic nerve terminals and the action on alpha and beta receptor sites. The gastrointestinal effects are nausea, vomiting, diarrhea, and the desire to defecate. These reactions are due to the release of catecholamines. The genitourinary effects of doxapram are stimulation of the urinary bladder with spontaneous voiding and urinary retention. The effects on the respiratory system include dyspnea, cough, tachypnea, laryngospasm, hiccup, bronchospasm, and rebound hypoventilation. Doxapram increases the rate of respiration by stimulating the medullary respiratory centers. There may also be activation of the carotid and aortic chemoreceptors. There have been reports of pruritus with the use of doxapram.

OVERDOSAGE. A dose of doxapram that is too large produces adverse effects and side effects that are exaggerations of the pharmacologic effects of the drug. Hypertension, tachycardia, skeletal muscle hyperactivity, and increased deep tendon reflexes are early signs of overdose. Blood pressure, pulse, and deep tendon reflexes should be monitored closely and the infusion rate adjusted on the basis of these parameters.

At the therapeutic dose, seizures are not common. The maximum recommended dosage is 3 g/24 hours. The exception to this dosage is management of chronic obstructive pulmonary disease with acute hypercapnia.

INTERACTIONS. *Drug–Drug.* When doxapram and sympathomimetics or monoamine oxidase (MAO)-inhibiting drugs are given concurrently, an additional pressor effect may occur. Doxapram can also mask the residual effects of muscle relaxant drugs. The administration of doxapram should be delayed when the patient has received general anesthetics (e.g., halothane, cyclopropane) that sensitize the myocardium to catecholamines because doxapram releases epinephrine.

PSYCHOMOTOR STIMULANTS

Many of the psychomotor agents (methamphetamine, dextroamphetamine, methylphenidate, and pemoline) have activities similar to amphetamine. Methylphenidate and pemoline have different chemical structures in comparison with amphetamine. All of these agents are absorbed following oral administration, and most are distributed in the tissues, with concentrations in the brain and cerebrospinal fluid. The psychomotor stimulants are metabolized in the liver and excreted in the urine. Alkaline urine promotes reabsorption and lengthens the duration of action of these stimulants.

Mechanism of Action

Amphetamines release catecholamines. In the peripheral system there is a release of norepinephrine from adrenergic nerve terminals and a direct stimulating action on alpha and beta receptor sites. The central mechanism of effect has not been determined. The central sites are the cerebral cortex and possibly the reticular-activating system. The inhibiting action of amine oxidase is thought to play a role in mood elevation. Amphetamines also produce an anorexigenic effect, leading to weight loss. The action of this effect is CNS stimulation. Amphetamines may cause a loss of smell and taste, which may heighten the anorexigenic effect. The overall effects of amphetamine are CNS and respiratory stimulation, *mydriasis*, bronchodilation, pressor response, anorexigenic effect, and contraction of the urinary bladder sphincter.

Uses

The therapeutic uses of the psychomotor stimulants are very limited. They are used in the management of attention deficit disorder with hyperactivity, narcolepsy, and obesity. Obesity is usually managed with amphetamine-like compounds, which will be discussed at the end of this chapter.

ATTENTION DEFICIT DISORDER. A common pediatric behavior disorder is attention deficit disorder with hyperactivity (ADDH). Evans (1987) states that the prevalence rates range from 1.2%–20%. This disorder has a male predominance of 6:1. The etiology is obscure, but there is some evidence that supports genetic transmission. There is a higher incidence of *hyperactivity* in parents of children with ADDH than in parents of children without this disorder. The diagnosis of ADDH relies on a history of inattention, impulsivity, and hyperactivity. Neurologic "soft" signs may be present, such as problems with motor coordination or perceptual difficulties. The onset is usually before six years of age. A large percentage of children with ADDH respond well to psychomotor stimulants. The stimulants used most frequently are methylphenidate, dextroamphetamine, and pemoline. The stimulant is given in the morning and at lunch. Usually, the drug is given only on school days, and *drug holidays* are used to evaluate behavioral response to the use of psychomotor stimulants. There is the possibility for reduced growth if stimulants are used over long periods of time.

NARCOLEPSY. Approximately 250,000 Americans suffer from narcolepsy. This sleep disorder occurs as a result of abnormal timing of rapid eye movement *(REM)* sleep. The symptoms associated with narcolepsy are sleep attacks, *cataplexy*, sleep paralysis, and hallucinations. The sleep attack is identified by the sudden overwhelming desire to sleep, which lasts from 5–20 minutes. The narcoleptic can be doing anything at the time the sleep attack occurs with no warning. The second symptom associated with narcolepsy is cataplexy. There is a sudden loss of muscle tone that is often associated with emotions. Many times the narcoleptic slumps in a chair or falls to the ground during the episode of cataplexy. Sleep paralysis is another symptom of narcolepsy. This muscle paralysis occurs during the interval between sleep and wakening. The sleep paralysis lasts for approximately one minute. The attack of immobility can be terminated by touch. The last symptom associated with narcolepsy is hallucinations. The hallucinations are auditory or visual and, like the sleep paralysis, occur in the interval between sleep and wakening. The narcoleptic is aware of his or her environment at the time of the hallucinations. The psychomotor stimulants used to treat this disorder include methylphenidate, amphetamine, and dextroamphetamine.

Contraindications and Precautions

Amphetamines are contraindicated in patients with hyperthyroidism, advanced arteriosclerosis, agitated states, moderate to severe hypertension, cardiovascular disease, drug abuse, glaucoma, concurrent use or use within 14 days of administration of MAO inhibitors, and hypersensitivity to amphetamines. Many of these contraindications are based on the mechanisms of action of amphetamines, such as the release of catecholamines, the pressor effect, and the direct action on alpha and beta receptor sites in the body. Amphetamines have an abuse potential and are frequently abused with alcohol or barbiturates. Amphetamines are not administered to children under 12 years of age as an anorexic agent.

Amphetamines are used with caution in situations that require the person to be mentally alert or coordinated. Performing hazardous activities (e.g., operating machinery, driving a car) should be postponed until the peak effect of the drug has occurred or the person is adjusted to a particular dose. Amphetamines are administered cautiously to persons with hyperexcitability states or who are concurrently receiving medications that produce hyperexcitability. Amphetamines are administered with caution in elderly, debilitated, or *asthenic* patients. These groups of patients may require more individualized dosages of amphetamines based on their particular situation. Caution is also used when administering amphetamines to persons with psychopathic personalities or a history of suicidal or homicidal tendencies. The psychic stimulation produced by amphetamines is followed by depression and fatigue. The psychic effects of amphetamines depend on dose, mental state, and personality of the individual. When administering amphetamines to children, there may be a temporary suppression of normal weight gain and growth. Amphetamines may also aggravate motor and vocal tics.

Adverse Reactions

The number or combination of side effects the patient may experience varies considerably among patients. The following adverse effects and side effects are reported with the use of amphetamines: nervousness, irritability, talkativeness, insomnia, dizziness, headaches, increased motor activity, mydriasis, hyperexcitability, depression, hypertension, tachycardia, palpitation, cardiac arrhythmias, nausea, anorexia, vomiting, abdominal cramping, diarrhea, constipation, dry mouth, metallic taste, and increased libido, which is related to the release of catecholamines and direct action on alpha and beta receptors.

Interactions

DRUG–DRUG. Various drug interactions occur with amphetamines. Concurrent use of an amphetamine with guanethidine, acetazolamide, tricyclic antidepressants, furazolidine, MAO inhibitors, phenothiazines, lithium carbonate, and sodium bicarbonate should be avoided. Guanethidine is displaced from its site of action, resulting in hypotension. Acetazolamide and sodium bicarbonate cause alkalinization of the urine, decreasing the renal excretion of amphetamines and resulting in an increase in the amphetamine effect. Tricyclic antidepressants release norepinephrine, increasing the effects of amphetamines. The phenothiazines and lithium carbonate cause a decreased amphetamine response. Oral dextroamphetamine-nicotine induces a dose-related increase in cigarette smoking in "normal" smokers. Evidence supports this premise because dextroamphetamine is a behavioral stimulant—it increases the rate of a variety of learned and stereotyped behaviors.

DRUG–LABORATORY. Drug–laboratory interactions also occur. These include an elevated level of growth hormone, changes in cortisol level, and fecal discoloration.

Route and Dosage

In discussing specific psychomotor stimulants, especially amphetamines, dosage requirements are the major difference between agents. The psychomotor stimulants have the same action, contraindications/precautions, and interactions.

Amphetamine Sulfate

The dosage of amphetamine sulfate (Benzedrine) for the treatment of narcolepsy is 20–60 mg/day orally. The divided doses (before breakfast and lunch) are 2.5–15 mg/day orally. The dose is age-specific and is determined by the severity of narcolepsy. Dose can be increased by 5 mg/week.

Methamphetamine Hydrochloride

The dosage of methamphetamine hydrochloride (Desoxyn, Methampex) is 2.5–5 mg once or twice daily. The usual effective dose is 20–25 mg/day orally for the treatment of attention deficit disorders.

For the treatment of obesity, methamphetamine hydrochloride is administered in a dosage of 2.5–5 mg orally, two or three times a day, 30 minutes prior to a meal, or it may be given as 10–15-mg extended-release tablets prior to breakfast. The use of amphetamines for the treatment of obesity is recommended for only a couple of weeks.

Dextroamphetamine

The dosage of dextroamphetamine (Dexedrine, d-Amphetamine) is 5–10 mg/day orally, in one or two doses, and is increased by 5 mg/week. This dosage is for children over six years of age for the treatment of attention deficit disorder. For children three to five years of age, the dosage is 2.5 mg/day orally, increasing the dosage by 2.5 mg/week. For adults with narcolepsy, the usual dose is 50–60 mg/day orally in divided doses. For children over 12 years of age with narcolepsy, the dosage is 10 mg/day orally and is increased by 10 mg/week to a maximum of 20–25 mg daily. For children ages 6–12 years with narcolepsy, the dosage is 5 mg/day orally and is increased by 5 mg/week.

Methylphenidate

Methylphenidate (Ritalin) is different from the amphetamines in chemical structure, but its action is similar. It also shares the same therapeutic uses, contraindications/precautions, adverse reactions/side effects, and interactions. It differs from amphetamines in pharmacokinetics, pharmacodynamics, and dosage.

PHARMACOKINETICS. Methylphenidate is well absorbed after oral administration, with some delay in the extended-release tablet. The exact distribution of methylphenidate is unknown. About 80% of methylphenidate is metabolized in the liver, and it is excreted in the urine. The half-life is one to three hours. The onset of methylphenidate is unknown; the peak effect occurs in one to three hours. The duration of action is four to six hours, with a longer duration of eight hours for the extended-release tablet.

DOSAGE. The adult dosage for the management of narcolepsy is 10 mg orally, two or three times daily. The maximum dose is 50 mg/day orally.

For children over six years of age, the dosage for the management of attention deficit disorder is 5 mg orally before breakfast and lunch, increased by 5–10 mg at weekly intervals. The maximum daily dose is 60 mg/day orally.

Pemoline

Pemoline (Cylert) is chemically different from amphetamines. It also differs from amphetamines in pharmacokinetics, pharmacodynamics, dosage, contraindications/precautions, and interactions.

PHARMACOKINETICS. Pemoline is well absorbed from the gastrointestinal tract. The distribution is unknown, but 50% is bound to plasma proteins. It is metabolized in the liver and excreted in the urine. The half-life is 9–14 hours in adults. Pemoline has nonlinear kinetics in children, which increases the half-life with increasing doses.

After an oral dose, the onset of this drug is 30–45 minutes. The peak effect occurs in two to four hours. The duration of action is eight hours.

CONTRAINDICATIONS AND PRECAUTIONS. Many of the contraindications and precautions are the same as those for amphetamines, but some differences do exist. Pemoline is not used in the following situations: hypersensitivity or idiosyncrasy to the drug; impaired hepatic function because the liver metabolizes this agent; and children under six years of age. Pemoline is used cautiously in children and in patients with renal dysfunction. This drug causes a temporary suppression of normal growth and weight gain in children. The drug is excreted by the kidneys, leading to the accumulation of pemoline and toxicity.

INTERACTIONS. *Drug–Laboratory.* There can be an elevated serum glutamic-oxaloacetic transaminase (SGOT), serum glutamic-pyruvic transaminase (SGPT), and alkaline phosphatase after several months of treatment. Patients should have periodic liver function tests. If these tests are abnormal, the drug is discontinued.

DOSAGE. The initial dose for children over six years of age is 37.5 mg orally, which is usually given in the morning. The dosage is increased by 18.75 mg at weekly intervals. The usual effective range is 56.25–75 mg/day orally. Doses for children should not exceed 112.5 mg/day orally.

Cocaine

Cocaine is classified as a potent CNS stimulant and a local anesthetic. As a local anesthetic, cocaine blocks initiation or conduction of nerve impulses following application. Topically, this drug also promotes vasoconstriction by indirect adrenergic effect. This adrenergic effect occurs because cocaine interferes with the uptake of norepinephrine at the adrenergic nerve terminals. The therapeutic uses of cocaine are the relief of nosebleeds and as a local anesthetic agent for the mucous membranes of the nasal, oral, and laryngeal area. Cocaine has become a popular drug that is illegally abused.

PHARMACOKINETICS. Cocaine is absorbed from all sites of application. Cocaine is well absorbed from the mucosal surfaces of the trachea, but it is not absorbed from unbroken skin. Cocaine does penetrate the CNS, but other distribution sites are unknown. This drug is metabolized in the liver by enzymatic hydrolysis and undergoes rapid biotransformation. Cocaine is excreted in the urine. The half-life of cocaine is 75 minutes (topically applied to nasal mucosa).

Cocaine has a rapid onset of action. The peak effect of this drug is three to five minutes via intravenous route, 20–60 minutes by intranasal application, and 60–90 minutes by the oral route. The duration of action is 20–40 minutes with topical application and six hours with intranasal application.

CONTRAINDICATIONS AND PRECAUTIONS. Cocaine is contraindicated in patients who have hypertension and/or cardiovascular disease. Catecholamine effects are potentiated with cocaine and can cause a variety of cardiovascular effects. For this same reason, cocaine should not be used concurrently with sympathomimetic amines.

Since cocaine is readily absorbed across the mucous membranes, caution is used when determining dosage and administration techniques. Extreme caution is used when cocaine is administered concurrently with cholinesterase inhibitors. It is hypothesized that persons receiving both types of agents would not hydrolyze cocaine as rapidly as a normal person, resulting in higher and earlier peak blood levels of cocaine. Caution is also used in situations where the person has a succinylcholine sensitivity.

ADVERSE EFFECTS. The adverse effects of cocaine are many. Cocaine represents a potential hazard to anyone with underlying fixed coronary artery disease because it causes predictable increases in heart rate, systolic blood pressure, and myocardial oxygen demand. In addition, there is a high incidence of myocardial infarction although the exact pathophysiologic features, thrombus or spasm, remain uncertain. Cocaine is also arrhythmogenic, causing sinus tachycardia, ventricular premature contractures, ventricular tachycardia, fibrillation, and asystole. Rupture of the aorta due to a large increase in systemic arterial pressure can also occur.

Central nervous system symptoms include headache, excitement, euphoria, tremor, hyperreflexia, diaphoresis, and mydriasis. Cocaine is also known to produce hyperpyrexia, which along with the effect of the drug on neurotransmitters, may contribute to the development of seizures.

Cocaine also has a deleterious influence on the outcome of pregnancy. There is a high rate of spontaneous abortion in women who use cocaine.

Sexual dysfunction is also common. In the early stages of cocaine use, cocaine may appear to be an aphrodisiac that enhances sexual performance. In men, cocaine can delay ejaculation and orgasm and cause mood elevations and heighten sensory awareness. However, with prolonged use, men have difficulty maintaining an erection and ejaculating. Women users have difficulty in achieving orgasm.

INTERACTIONS. The following drug interactions occur with cocaine: the antihypertensive effect of guanethidine is lost when used with cocaine; when cocaine is used with general anesthetics, a rise in blood pressure and pulse rate occurs; use of anticholinergic agents concurrently with cocaine results in hypertension and tachycardia.

DOSAGE. Cocaine can be administered by the oral, intranasal, and topical routes. For use as a local anesthetic, cocaine preparations are supplied as a 1%–4% solution, with a dose of 5–7.5 ml. The dose for the use of cocaine as a topical agent is 1–3 mg/kg, not to exceed 200 mg/70 kg over 30 minutes.

METHYLXANTHINES

The last group of CNS stimulants are the methylxanthines/xanthines/xanthine derivatives (caffeine, theophylline, theobromine). These alkaloids occur naturally in plants and are consumed in beverages. Coffee and cola beverages contain caffeine, while tea contains caffeine and theophylline. Most of the CNS stimulation that these beverages produce is due to caffeine. Caffeine inhibits phosphodiesterase, which degrades cAMP allowing increased levels of cAMP. Other possible mechanisms of action include blocking of the inhibitory action of adenosine and opening of the chloride channel.

All of the methylxanthines are well absorbed from the gastrointestinal tract. Intravenous administration is reserved for status asthmaticus and apnea in premature infants (theophylline). Roughly 17% of caffeine is bound to plasma proteins. These drugs are metabolized in the liver and excreted in the urine. The half-life is variable and short in adults and as long as 80 hours in neonates.

Uses

The methylxanthines have a wide variety of clinical uses. Caffeine has been used in the treatment of CNS-depressant overdosage. Many of the over-the-counter preparations of caffeine are directed toward reducing fatigue. However, these over-the-counter medications do little to overcome physical fatigue. Caffeine is also combined with some over-the-counter and prescription drugs for the treatment of headaches. Caffeine causes vasoconstriction of cerebral arteries, reducing compression of pain-sensitive structures. Theophylline has been shown to relieve paroxysmal dyspnea associated with left heart failure. Aminophylline is a bronchodilator used for the treatment of asthma, bronchospasm, and paroxysmal dyspnea. All of the methylxanthines are capable of producing some degree of diuresis. Theobromide has no clinically useful role at this time.

Adverse Reactions and Side Effects

The adverse reactions and side effects of the methylxanthines are very similar to those of CNS stimulants. The CNS and cardiovascular system are the major systems affected. Toxicity from the methylxanthines results in nervousness, insomnia, delirium, tachycardia, extrasystole, increased respiration, and diuresis (See Chapter 35).

Interactions

The methylxanthines shorten clotting time by increasing tissue prothrombin and factor V. Evidence suggests that therapeutic doses of methylxanthines alter response to oral anticoagulants.

Caffeine

Caffeine is absorbed from the gut and distributed in tissues. It is metabolized in the liver and exreted in the urine. The half-life is three to four hours in adults.

EFFECTS ON SYSTEMS. Low to moderate amounts of caffeine intake produce stimulation of the cerebral cortex. This causes an increased alertness and decreased fatigue. As one approaches 250 mg or more of caffeine (two to three cups of coffee), the chances of developing more signs of CNS stimulation increase. These include nervousness, restlessness, insomnia, and tremors.

Caffeine exerts a positive inotropic effect on the myocardium and a positive chronotropic effect at the sinoatrial node. This can cause transient increases in heart rate, force of contraction, and cardiac output. In larger amounts (more than 250 mg), the centrally mediated vagal effects of caffeine can be masked with increased sinus rates, extrasystole, or ventricular dysrhythmias. The reports of research studies are quite varied regarding the influence of caffeine on the cardiovascular system. Caffeine either lowers, raises, or does not affect heart rate and blood pressure. Caffeine may cause dysrhythmias.

Caffeine stimulates gastric acid and pepsin secretion. Persons with peptic ulcer disease are discouraged from using regular and decaffeinated coffee because both increase gastric acid secretion.

Caffeine possesses the properties of a weak diuretic. It increases renal blood flow and glomerular filtration rate and decreases proximal tubular reabsorption of sodium and water.

Caffeine has been shown to increase the basal metabolic rate. The intake of 3–9 mg/kg of body weight (225–675 mg caffeine, or two to six cups of coffee) can raise the basal metabolic rate about 10%.

CONTRAINDICATIONS AND PRECAUTIONS. Caffeine is contraindicated in persons with myocardial infarction and cardiac dysrhythmias or palpitations immediately after myocardial infarction. In patients with heart failure, venous pressure can be high and the cardiac stimulation can lead to an increase in cardiac output. Caffeine is also contraindicated in persons with a hypersensitivity to caffeine and in pregnancy. Caffeine has not been shown to be mutagenic in man; develop-mental toxicity for the fetus and neonate is unknown. Caution is used when administering caffeine to persons with peptic ulcer disease. The CNS effects are more severe in children.

STIMULANT ABUSE

Like many drugs, stimulants can be abused. Three categories of drugs are examined in this discussion of stimulant abuse: caffeine, amphetamines, and cocaine.

The use of caffeine is so customary in most cultures that it is easy not to think of it as a drug. Caffeine appears in over-the-counter medications for pain, and allergy and cold relief; and it is contained in our favorite beverages (coffee, tea, cocoa, soft drinks) and food (chocolate) (Table 21–3). There is probably no question that the use of caffeine is habituating and that certain symptoms result when intake of caffeine is reduced

Table 21-3. CAFFEINE LEVELS IN DRUGS AND BEVERAGES

Drug/Beverage	Prescription (P) or Over-the-Counter (OTC)	Amount of Caffeine (mg)
ANALGESICS		
Anacin Maximum Strength	OTC	32
Cafergot	P	100
Cope	OTC	32
Darvon	P	32.4
Excedrin	OTC	65
Fiorinal	P	40
Vanquish	OTC	33
STIMULANTS		
Cafedrine	OTC	200
Nodoz	OTC	100
Tirend	OTC	100
Vivarin	OTC	200
MENSTRUAL DRUGS		
Aqua-ban	OTC	100
Aqua-ban Plus	OTC	200
Flowaway Water Tablets	OTC	20
Midol	OTC	32.4
COLD TABLETS		
Coryban-D	OTC	30
Dristan Decongestant Tablet and Dristan-AF Tablet	OTC	16.2
Duradyne Forte	OTC	30
Triaminicin	OTC	30
CHOCOLATE AND COCOA		Average
Cocoa (150 ml/5 oz)		4
Chocolate milk (240 ml/8 oz)		5
Chocolate syrup (30 ml/1 oz)		4
Milk chocolate		6
Chocolate cake and frosting ($\frac{1}{12}$ of cake)		15.8
Dark, semi-sweet chocolate (30 ml/1 oz)		20
Baker's chocolate (30 ml/1 oz)		26

CONTINUED ON THE FOLLOWING PAGE

Table 21-3. CAFFEINE LEVELS IN DRUGS AND BEVERAGES–*CONTINUED*

Drug/Beverage	Prescription (P) or Over-the-Counter (OTC)	Amount of Caffeine (mg)
*COFFEE**		
Brewed, drip method		115
Brewed, percolator		80
Instant		65
Decaffeinated, brewed		3
Decaffeinated, instant		2
*TEA**		
US brands, brewed		40
Imported brands, brewed		60
Instant		30
Iced (360 ml/12 oz)		70
SOFT DRINKS†		
Coca-Cola		45
Dr. Pepper		40
Mello Yellow		40
Mountain Dew		53
Mr. Pibb		54
Pepsi		41
Diet Pepsi		38
Tab		47
Orange drinks		0
Other citrus soft drinks		0–54
Ginger ale, root beer		0
Tonic water		0
Soda, seltzer		0
Other soft drinks		0–43.2

*(150 ml/5 oz)
†(360 ml/12 oz)

(headache, feeling of fatigue). There is a lack of evidence to support the development of tolerance to the CNS effects of caffeine. Like other drugs used to excess, caffeine can be lethal.

Amphetamines have been produced since the 1920s. Abuse of this type of drug began in the 1940s when amphetamines were present in inhalers and nasal decongestants. One appealing effect of stimulants was anorexia. Before amphetamines were removed from over-the-counter diet pills, they were a popular method of weight control. By the 1960s, the common route of administration became intravenous injection. Giannini and colleagues (1986) report that amphetamines are the drugs most frequently abused by health-care professionals. When amphetamines were outlawed except for legitimate medical practice, more dangerous drug abuse was introduced.

Cocaine is one of the more commonly abused drugs today. In 1985 approximately one million people are addicted to cocaine. And, it is also estimated that at least 15–21 million Americans have tried cocaine once. Cocaine was once the preferred drug for the well-to-do, sophisticated social circles. Now this recreational drug is encountered in all circles of society. The half-life of cocaine is short and single dose effects persist for a couple

Table 21–4. ANOREXIANT AGENTS

Official or Generic Name	Trade Name	Usual Adult Dosage
Benzphetamine HCl	Didrex	25–50 mg 1–3 times daily
Diethylpropion HCl (USP)	Tenuate; Tepanil	25 mg tid
Fenfluramine HCl	Pondimin	20 mg tid
Mazindol	Mazanor; Sanorex	1–2 mg 1–3 times daily
Phendimetrazine tartrate	Bontril; Plegine	17.5–70 mg bid or tid
Phenmetrazine HCl (USP)	Preludin	25 mg bid or tid
Phentermine HCl	—	8 mg tid

From Rodman, MJ et al: Pharmacology and Drug Therapy in Nursing, ed 3. JB Lippincott, Philadelphia, 1985, p 1002, with permission.

of hours. Cocaine can be used many times during the day or night. The repetitive use of cocaine has been shown to have destructive effects on the individual, family, friends, and society. Addiction to cocaine involves physical and psychologic dependence. Overdoses of cocaine can be lethal.

AGENTS USED FOR WEIGHT CONTROL

In the past, dextroamphetamine or other amphetamine derivatives were used as anorexic agents. They still have very restricted use as anorexic agents; however, in the last ten years, nonamphetamine weight-reducing products have been on the market. Some of these agents include diethylpropion, fenfluramine, phenmetrazine, mazindol, and phentermine (Table 21–4). Some tolerance develops with all of these agents after a period of 6–12 weeks. These agents have some CNS effects and are also sympathomimetics. These drugs will not be reviewed in detail in this chapter.

USING THE NURSING PROCESS

ASSESSMENT

Assessment of the patient receiving CNS stimulants depends on the type of drug used and its therapeutic indication. Typical information obtained from patients and families is given in Table 21–5.

With patients receiving the amphetamines, in general, it is necessary to obtain an accurate psychologic and sociologic history, and, in particular, a history of previous drug abuse. Since the amphetamines have a high abuse potential, patients who might become abusers must be identified early and monitored carefully. See Chapter 13 for further details on assessment. In female patients, current pregnancy and future plans for childbearing should be determined, since the safety of these drugs has not been established in pregnancy. Prior to initiating amphetamine therapy in children, the nurse gathers growth and development data for comparison after therapy has begun.

If amphetamines are being used to treat the patient with narcolepsy, an additional specific assessment must be made. When taking the patient history, the nurse makes special note of seizure disorders, sleep irregularities, obesity, nervous disorders, depression, or endocrine disorders in both the patient and family. The nurse gains additional information leading up to the present illness by questioning the patient about previous head trauma, infections, and occlusive vascular disorders that may be related to the narcolepsy. A history of past medications, including stimulants and inhibitory agents, is recorded. The exact nature of the narcolepsy—including how often, how long, and the nature of the narcolepsy, as well as regular sleep and arousal patterns—is noted. The nurse also performs a baseline neurologic check, noting movement of the eyes, pupillary reaction and symmetry, and assessment of motor and sensory function. Any deviations from normal should be recorded.

In assessing the obese patient, the nurse obtains information regarding height, weight, and bone structure to determine the degree of obesity. The nurse takes a diet history and asks the patient to keep a diet diary for several weeks to record information about usual patterns of intake, exercise, and activity. The nurse assesses the patient for physical problems including high blood pressure, cardiac irregularities, or diabetes, which may restrict the available diet/drug/exercise options. A social and psychologic profile may reveal the rationale for present habits of overeating and may provide clues as to how to adjust that pattern. The patient may offer insight about why he or she overeats and what he or she feels may be the best method of weight reduction to fit his or her life-style.

When the patient receiving amphetamines is a child with attention deficit disorder with hyperactivity (ADDH), the nurse considers the health history; physical examination; family dynamics; and previous assessments of the child's behavior, activity level, and school performance. History taking includes prenatal, perinatal, and postnatal information. The nurse questions the parents about maternal infection, uterine bleeding, maternal use of drugs with teratogenic effects, and difficulties during labor and delivery with this child. Answers to these questions may offer reasons for the development of ADDH. A history of the achievement of developmental tasks may indicate the sequence of development of the symptoms of ADDH. Family history may reveal a familial pattern of the syndrome. During the physical examination, the nurse observes for external characteristics such as enlarged thyroid and exophthalmos, which may suggest hyperthyroidism. The nurse assesses the child for clumsiness, motor incoordination,

Table 21–5. NURSING PROCESS WITH PATIENTS REQUIRING STIMULANTS

Assessment

Assess mental/cognitive status, affect and general behavior.
Note support systems, family interactions, and use of coping mechanisms.
Ascertain self-image.
Note effects of illness/condition on life-style, activity/sleep.
Identify current and past drug history, including drug abuse.
Evaluate blood pressure, pulse, respiratory rate.

Nursing Diagnosis	Nursing Actions	Rationale	Desired Outcomes/ Evaluation Criteria
Thought processes, altered related to pharmacologic effects of stimulants as evidenced by short attention span, inability to concentrate, and restlessness.	Maintain a calm, supportive environment. Reduce external stimuli (TV, radio, others talking).	Stimulation of the central nervous system is the action of these drugs. Prevention of overstimulation allows patient to focus on desired activity and may enhance intake of information.	Displays usual mentation, cognitive ability, and affect with absence of adverse behaviors, e.g., restlessness, agitation, tremor, hyperactivity, insomnia, or dizziness.
	Keep instructions, conversations, and commands simple, short, and concrete.	Sensory overload alters patient's ability to process information and respond appropriately.	
	Repeat information or redirect patient as necessary. Allow the patient sufficient time to answer questions or follow directions.	May experience a short attention span or have difficulty concentrating.	

Table 21–5. NURSING PROCESS WITH PATIENTS REQUIRING STIMULANTS–
CONTINUED

Nursing Diagnosis	Nursing Actions	Rationale	Desired Outcomes/ Evaluation Criteria
Adjustment, impaired related to disability requiring change in lifestyle and impaired cognition as evidenced by emotional outbursts, poor behavioral reports from school and parents, falling asleep during the day.	Observe for therapeutic or adverse response to medication. Encourage discussion of concerns related to disability. Active-listen to feelings. Discuss expected actions of the prescribed drug.	Drug choice/dosage is dependent on effect of the drug. Promotes clarification of problems and possible solutions. Understanding reasons drug is being taken will enhance cooperation, e.g., to prevent sleepiness in narcolepsy; to decrease appetite and complement weight loss program; and to lengthen a hyperactive child's attention span.	Verbalize positive attitude toward situation. Demonstrates increased interest in self-care activities.
	Plan other activities patient can take, e.g., diet and exercise, effective parenting skills, adjunct services.	Promotes nonpharmacologic solutions to problems which can maximize the effectiveness of the drugs.	
Sleep pattern disturbance related to illness, side-effects of medications, intake of caffeine/other stimulant drugs as evidenced by verbal complaints of difficulty falling asleep, falling asleep during activities, irritability, not feeling well rested.	Provide quiet environment. Administer last dose of medication before evening.	Conditions such as narcolepsy, ADDH, and high intake of caffeine or other stimulant drugs can interfere with ability to sleep. The patient with narcolepsy can drop off to sleep but the sleep pattern is different than continual sleep at night. Also these patients may experience vivid dreams, nightmares, and hallucinations which alters the sleep pattern. The child with ADDH is constantly in motion and has great difficulty taking naps or sleeping at night. These drugs may overstimulate the CNS and may result in insomnia.	Verbalizes understanding of sleep disorder. Reports decrease in narcoleptic attacks and increased sense of well-being and feelings.
	Discuss which foods/beverages contain caffeine.	A high intake of caffeine, especially when consumed during the evening/night, may interfere with ability to sleep.	
Knowledge deficit related to unfamiliarity with resources, misunderstanding, cognitive limitations as evidenced by questions, statements of concern, development of preventable complications.	Provide information about drug purpose, action, dosage, administration/ proper timing, interactions.	Understanding promotes active participation in medication regimen and enables individual to live desired life-style. Enhances therapeutic benefit: taking pemoline in the morning provides maximal effectiveness during waking hours and avoids insomnia.	Verbalizes understanding of drug regimen and interactions of prescribed/OTC medications.
	Identify possible adverse effects, e.g., suppression of appetite/anorexia, alteration in childhood growth patterns, rebound depression.	Some effects are dose dependent and may be controlled/prevented with reduction of dosage.	
	Discuss importance/necessity of drug vacation/holiday.	Useful in determining effectiveness of therapy/need for continuation and to allow for growth spurt in children.	

difficulties with right/left discrimination, and involuntary movements or tremors. Nursing observations of difficulties in reading, writing, and speaking may be validated by school performance reports from teachers and by discussion with the family. Objective and subjective data regarding behavior patterns and activity level are recorded. Family interaction patterns are assessed to give as complete a picture as possible.

In using the analeptic agents, it is important for the nurse to develop a baseline assessment of the following parameters: blood pressure, heart rate, deep tendon reflexes, and oxygen and carbon dioxide levels of arterial blood. In addition, before using the analeptics, adequacy of airway and oxygenation must be ensured.

NURSING DIAGNOSIS

Upon completion of the patient assessment, the nurse establishes the nursing diagnoses in order to begin planning interventions. Some typical nursing diagnoses for patients receiving CNS stimulants are included in Table 21–5.

PLANNING AND INTERVENTION

Goals for nursing interventions are developed from the list of nursing diagnoses. Typical goals for the care of the patient receiving CNS stimulants are included in Table 21–5.

Because of the excitatory and euphoric effects of the amphetamines, they have a high abuse potential. In administering these medications, the lowest possible dose will be used initially and then increased gradually. Habituation, tolerance, and/or dependence may occur over a long period of time, and the nurse reassesses the patient periodically for indications of these problems. Chapter 13 describes interventions and precautions in detail. Since amphetamines may cause insomnia, the last amphetamine dose is scheduled no later than 6 hours before bedtime. The nurse instructs the patient and family to follow a similar pattern at home. If the amphetamine is not being used specifically for an anorexiant effect, then anorexia and weight loss may be undesirable side effects. The nurse monitors the patient's weight weekly and reviews intake records to make certain that adequate nutrients are being ingested. The patient and family are taught the importance of good nutrition; the elements of a basic, healthy diet; and the need to weigh the patient weekly, reporting weight loss to the health care team.

When amphetamines are administered specifically to treat narcolepsy, the nurse plans for interventions that maximize the effectiveness of these drugs. The nurse, along with other health team members, observes the patient to identify the times of the patient's peak sleepiness. Doses of the amphetamine are scheduled to coincide with these times to achieve maximum therapeutic effect. The nurse also provides a varied and interesting daily routine, using available diversions such as recreational therapy and volunteer visitors to decrease the possibility of narcoleptic attacks. The nurse teaches the patient to avoid monotony and boring routines at home and at work that are likely to precipitate narcoleptic attacks. The patient is advised to avoid shift work and frequent air travel since both can precipitate more frequent attacks. There is some indication that obesity contributes to narcolepsy. If the narcoleptic patient is obese, a sensible program of diet and exercise is initiated by the nurse and patient and is continued at home on a regular basis. Since narcolepsy may present serious social problems, compromising the patient's ability to interact as a family member or to perform at work, the nurse may refer the patient for personal counseling.

In states that allow amphetamines to be administered as anorexiants, the nurse knows that the drug is only one third of the plan, which also includes diet and exercise. This information is shared with the patient, who needs to understand that the medication alone does not produce long-lasting results. (Additional items are included in Table 21–4.) The health team helps the patient to establish a realistic weight-loss goal. Reinforcement of the weight-loss plan is important for compliance. Frequent contacts between the nurse and the patient are desirable. The nurse checks the patient's daily diet and exercise habits and observes for drug response. The nurse weighs the patient weekly and provides verbal support and encouragement during the weight-loss program. The nurse takes into account the patient's normal dietary patterns and schedules drug administration accordingly. Since amphetamines suppress appetite for a limited time (they peak in 1 hour), doses are scheduled 30 to 90 minutes before meals. If the patient skips a meal, it is senseless to take the amphetamine prior to that meal. The nurse may refer the patient for behavior modification and personal counseling in order to enhance the weight-loss plans.

When amphetamines are prescribed to treat the child with ADDH, drug therapy is usually initiated and continued on an outpatient basis. Teaching of the family assumes major importance in such circumstances. The nurse knows and informs the family that the stimulants will not be therapeutic in every case, but that a clinical trial of several weeks with dosages adjusted by the physician should clearly indicate whether the drug benefits the child. Use of the drug may enhance peer relationships, the child's self-image, and the child's ability to find satisfaction in learning. The parents are instructed that the drug is not a panacea but improves the child's ability to pay attention and to be more physically coordinated. The nurse, family, and other health team members may identify a need for adjunct services to deal with related problems. These adjunct services include family and personal counseling, psychologic testing and evaluation, and special education classes. The nurse and physician, along with the family, may plan for drug-free holidays. These holidays should fall on weekends or school vacations and should allow time to evaluate the effectiveness of and continued need for the drug. Scientific literature indicates that habituation and dependence do not occur in children when amphetamines are used for treatment of ADDH. Reasons cited for this exception include the finding that children under the age of 11 or 12 do not view medications as desirable and that therapy usually ceases before adolescence when a child might tend to experiment with excessive dosages and abuse the drug.

When analeptic drugs are administered to increase respiratory function, the nurse plans care to maximize the effects of the drugs, while maintaining a wide margin of safety. Before administering the drugs, the nurse checks for a patent airway and makes an initial assessment of respiratory status, including blood gas determinations of Po_2, Pco_2, and oxygen saturation. These blood gas levels are checked repeatedly to monitor the effectiveness of drug response. The nurse checks the readiness of emergency equipment such as additional oxygen, resuscitative equipment, and short-acting barbiturates, which are necessary to manage overdosage. The nurse institutes seizure precautions to maintain patient safety, since analeptics may precipitate a seizure. Chapter 22 discusses seizure management in detail. When analeptic therapy is initiated, the nurse maintains the intravenous flow rate prescribed by the physician. Periodic checks of the infusion site are made, since extravasation or prolonged use of a single site may cause thrombophlebitis with some analeptics. The nurse monitors the patient closely throughout the infusion. If hypotension or dyspnea develops, the nurse discontinues the infusion and notifies the physician. A mild to moderate increase in blood pressure more commonly occurs. This increase may present a problem for patients with pre-existing hypertension. If arterial blood gases show evidence of deterioration, the nurse initiates mechanical ventilation, discontinues the analeptic, and notifies the physician. Since the analeptics possess other stimulant effects, the nurse is aware that patients perceive pain more quickly. Nonpharmacologic methods for reducing pain, as discussed in Chapter 20, are instituted. If medication with an analgesic is necessary, the nurse monitors closely for signs of post-stimulation narcosis. The patient receiving analeptic drugs depends on others for care. The nurse takes time to explain the purpose of the medication to the patient and family, explaining the interventions as he or she delivers care, inviting questions, and providing support and reassurance.

Since caffeine is a substance that is ingested in large quantities through foodstuffs and over-the-counter medications in the United States, the nurse has a responsibility to educate patients about the implications of caffeine intake. In providing care for the patient with gastritis or ulcers, the nurse teaches the patient to substitute other beverages in the meal plans. The nurse cautions the patient to decrease caffeine intake slowly, because abrupt cessation of caffeine intake may result in withdrawal symptoms. Since caffeine may adversely affect the cardiovascular system of some patients with heart disese and hypertension, the nurse explores ways of modifying caffeine intake with these patients as well.

Many over-the-counter products containing caffeine are ingested to provide pep and to perk up a sleepy or tired person. If the patient's history indicates a pattern of caffeine use for this reason, then the nurse teaches the importance of adequate rest and sleep. The nurse stresses the fact that caffeine should never be used as a substitute for sleep. Although research on the effects of caffeine on growth and development are controversial, as discussed earlier in this chapter, the nurse may inform the pregnant woman of the possible teratogenic effects of caffeine ingestion. Again, modification of the dietary plan to gradually decrease caffeine is in order. The long-term effect of caffeine-containing substances in children requires further study and research. Excess ingestion of caffeine-containing products such as chocolate, colas and soft drinks, and cocoa has been implicated in hyperactivity and behavioral problems in children. Until this research is refined, the nurse may counsel parents to limit the intake of such snacks, replacing them with fruit juices and "natural" snacks and using carob as a replacement for chocolate flavor.

EVALUATION

During the evaluation phase of the nursing process, the nurse determines the effectiveness of CNS stimulants. This evaluation is based on previously determined goals. Typical outcomes for the patient receiving CNS stimulants are included in Table 21–5.

The nurse is familiar with the adverse effects of the CNS stimulants. Amphetamine therapy may cause weight loss, sleeplessness, irritability, or jitteriness. Analeptics may produce tachycardia, muscle tremors, spasticity, and hyperactive reflexes.

Patient compliance with amphetamine therapy can be increased by stressing the need for continued health care follow-up and by periodic review of health teaching and treatment goals. Overcompliance or abuse of amphetamines, as well as signs of developing tolerance, habituation, or dependence, are carefully monitored by the nurse. Patients receiving long-term amphetamine therapy may develop psychiatric syndromes, which can be evidenced by increasing irritability, paranoia, or frank psychosis. The nurse also evaluates the patient for signs of noncompliance or withdrawal. When high-dose amphetamines are prescribed, withdrawal symptoms include headache, difficult breathing, sensations of hot and cold, muscle cramps, and gastrointestinal cramps. The patient may also experience a paradoxic situation in which incredible hunger is coupled with an inability to eat, which is caused by muscular weakness. The patient may also act out aggressive impulses; may be irritable and demanding; and may experience fatigue, anxiety, nightmares, and suicidal ideation. The nurse continually stresses the need for regular follow-up and periodically reviews all previously taught material to ensure that the patient's knowledge base remains accurate. Refer to Tables 21–6 and 21–7 for the discharge teaching instructions for the patient/family on stimulants.

Table 21–6. PATIENT TEACHING INFORMATION (CHILDREN) STIMULANT THERAPY FOR ATTENTION DEFICIT DISORDER WITH HYPERACTIVITY AND NARCOLEPSY

Dear Patient:
   This drug has been prescribed for you. This is what you should know about your drug to get the most from your therapy.

1. This stimulant is taken to improve your attention span, decrease your excessive activity OR decrease your sleep attacks (narcolepsy).
2. This stimulant may be ordered by your doctor for you to take for several years. There will be days you will not take the drug. The drug may be ordered to take on school days. Over the weekend or during vacation you may not take the drug. It is very important to read the directions on the label to know when to take the medication (attention deficit disorder). If you have narcolepsy, you will be taking the drug daily.
3. Take this drug as ordered by the doctor. Take this drug 30 to 45 minutes prior to meals. Try not to take this drug after 4:00 PM because it might interfere with your sleep at night.
4. Avoid taking other drugs unless you tell your doctor.
5. Always check with your doctor or pharmacist before taking over-the-counter drugs for colds, pain, allergy, upset stomach, or obesity.
6. Do not stop your drug unless directed by your doctor.
7. If you forget a dose of your drug, eliminate that dose. Do not try and catch up by taking two doses at once.
8. If you experience any side effects from your drug, notify your doctor. Side effects can include: altered mood, dizziness, irritability, restlessness, the shakes (tremor), inability to sleep, headache, seizures, fast heart rate, high blood pressure, palpitation, loss of appetite, stomach pains, dry mouth, unpleasant taste, and itching skin. Keep a written record of the side effects that you have and time of day.
9. Loss of appetite and weight loss may be common the first three weeks of starting this drug.
10. Obtain a weekly height and weight and keep a record of this to show your doctor.
11. Limit the intake of coffee, tea, cocoa, chocolate, and caffeinated soft drinks. They can increase the side effects.
12. Good mouth care and rinsing of the mouth can decrease the dry mouth and/or bad taste in your mouth.
13. If you are a diabetic, stimulants can change the requirement of your insulin or oral hypoglycemic drug.
14. Store in a tight, light-resistant container out of the reach of other children.

Table 21-7. PATIENT TEACHING INFORMATION (ADULTS) STIMULANT THERAPY FOR NARCOLEPSY

Dear Patient:
   This drug has been prescribed for you. This is what you should know about your drug to get the most from your therapy.

1. This stimulant is taken to improve your sleep attacks.
2. This stimulant may be ordered by your doctor for you to take for several years. Please read the directions on the label for the frequency of taking the drug.
3. Take this drug as ordered usually 30-45 minutes before meals. Try taking your last dose prior to the evening hours. Stimulants can interfere with sleeping at night.
4. Avoid taking other drugs unless you tell your doctor.
5. Always check with your doctor or pharmacist before taking over-the-counter medications for colds, pain, allergy, upset stomach, or obesity.
6. Do not stop your drug unless directed by your doctor.
7. If you forget a dose of your drug, eliminate that dose. Do not try and catch up by taking two doses at one time.
8. If you have any side effects from your drug, call lyour doctor. Side effects include: altered mood, dizziness, irritability, restlessness, the shakes (tremor), inability to sleep, headache, seizures, fast heart rate, high blood pressure, palpitation, loss of appetite, stomach pain, dry mouth, unpleasant taste, and itching skin. Keep a written record of your side effects.
9. Loss of appetite and weight loss may be common the first three weeks of starting this drug.
10. Limit the intake of coffee, tea, cocoa, chocolate, and caffeinated soft drinks. They can increase the side effects.
11. This drug does not replace the body's requirement of rest and sleep.
12. Good mouth care and rinsing your mouth can decrease a dry mouth or bad taste in your mouth.
13. If you are a diabetic, stimulants can change the requirement for insulin or oral hypoglycemic drugs.
14. Store this drug in a tight, light-resistant container out of the reach of children.

SUMMARY

Stimulants exert an excitatory response in the CNS and increase systolic and diastolic blood pressure. These agents have become less important as therapeutic agents over the last few decades, but they are useful for the treatment of narcolepsy and ADDH. Stimulants have a high potential for drug abuse.

It is important for the nurse to assess patients receiving CNS stimulants prior to drug administration. It is important to observe for CNS stimulation, blood pressure, and palpitations. The height and weight of children receiving stimulant therapy should be recorded at least three times a week. To decrease insomnia, stimulants should be administered six hours prior to bedtime or if using the extended-release capsule, 12–24 hours prior to retiring.

BIBLIOGRAPHY

Chapel, JL: The hyperactive child. American Family Physician 26(4):210–215, 1982.

Craig, CR and Stitzel, RE: Modern Pharmacology, ed 2. Little, Brown & Co, Boston, 1986.

Eichlseder, W: Ten years of experience with 1000 hyperactive children in private practice. Pediatrics 76(2):176–183, 1985.

Deglin, JH and Vallerand, AH: Nurse's Med Deck. FA Davis, Philadelphia, 1988.

Evans, OB: Manual of Child Neurology. Churchill Livingstone, New York, 1984.

Franz, D: Central Nervous System Stimulants. In Goodman and Gilman's The Pharmacological Basis of Therapeutics, ed 7. Macmillan, New York, 1985.

Giannini, JA, Price, WA, and Giannini, MC: Contemporary drugs of abuse. APF 33(3):207–216, 1986.

Hallal, JC: Are coffee, cold tablets, and chocolate innocuous or is their caffeine hazardous to your patients' health? Am J Nurs: 423–425, 1986.

Miller, GW: The cocaine habit. American Family Physician: 31(2): 173–176.

SITUATION   21–1

Rodney Alterman is a 7-year-old who is exhibiting signs of attention deficit disorder (ADD). The clinic nurse is preparing teaching sessions for Rodney's parents about the disorder and its treatment.

1. Rodney will be started on methylphenidate (Ritalin) 5 mg PO. The nurse will instruct the parents to administer the drug:
   a. after each meal
   b. before breakfast and lunch
   c. after lunch and dinner
   d. before breakfast and retiring

2. The nurse will plan to include the following when teaching about psychomotor drugs:
   a. Stimulants will always demonstrate therapeutic effects.
   b. Drug holidays will be used to evaluate behavioral response.
   c. Habituation will occur in children under the age of 12.
   d. Self-image and learning ability may diminish with drug use.

3. In gathering information about Rodney's status in relationship to ADD, the nurse will include the following:
   a. the parents' sexual history
   b. usual eating patterns
   c. parents' future plans for pregnancy
   d. prenatal and perinatal information

4. Due to the adverse effects of Ritalin, the following nursing diagnostic category applies to Rodney:
   a. Altered Growth and Development
   b. Potential for Infection
   c. Impaired Swallowing
   d. Alteration in Urinary Elimination

5. In planning patient outcomes, the following goals would be included for Rodney, except:
   a. increase attention span
   b. improve physical coordination
   c. eliminate behavior problems
   d. enhance peer relationships

6. The nurse will instruct the parents to select the following snack for Rodney:
   a. soft drink
   b. carob milkshake
   c. chocolate milk
   d. iced tea

SITUATION   21–2

David Webb is a 46-year-old successful businessman complaining of a tendency to sleep at odd times during the day. A diagnosis of narcolepsy is made, and Mr. Webb is to be started on a trial of amphetamines.

1. The nurse will elicit patient information which will determine contraindications to amphetamine therapy. The following condition applies:
   a. glaucoma
   b. cataplexy
   c. hypothyroidism
   d. chronic bronchitis

2. Mr. Webb will be started on amphetamine sulfate (Benzedrine) for treatment of narcolepsy. The nurse is aware that the usual dosage of this drug is:

a. 200 to 250 mg 1/day
b. 2.5 to 10 mg once a week
c. 20 to 60 mg 1/day
d. 100 to 200 mg every other day

3. The following data are included in the assessment phase for Mr. Webb:
   a. neurologic baseline
   b. growth and development
   c. diet history
   d. reading and writing ability

CONTINUED ON THE FOLLOWING PAGE

SITUATION 21–2–*CONTINUED*

4. The nurse will instruct Mr. Webb to be alert to the following adverse effects of amphetamine, *except:*
   a. depression
   b. headaches
   c. increased motor activity
   d. rebound bradycardia

5. For Mr. Webb, the following nursing diagnostic category *best* applies in relation to the side effects of amphetamine therapy:
   a. Potential Altered Body Temperature
   b. Alteration in Cardiac Output: decreased
   c. Potential for Alteration in Nutrition
   d. Alteration in Patterns of Urinary Elimination

6. Which of the following statements indicates successful teaching with regard to therapy for narcolepsy?
   a. "It does not matter how I take my medicine, as long as I do not skip a dose."
   b. "Since I should not do any office work, I will stay at home and do simple chores."
   c. "I will plan to go for walks twice a day and vary my daily routine."
   d. "I have decided to do business travel for the company; the air travel will make me feel better."

Please refer to the Appendices for correct answers and additional review questions with answers.

22
CHAPTER

UTILIZATION OF ANTICONVULSANTS

CHAPTER OUTLINE

OVERVIEW OF ANTICONVULSANT DRUGS
  Action
  Drug Selection
  General Principles of Drug Therapy
  Monitoring Drug Concentrations
  Drug Interactions
  Withdrawal of Medication
  Use in Pregnancy
  Nonepileptic Seizures
  Status Epilepticus
ANTICONVULSANTS
  Hydantoins
  Barbiturates
  Deoxybarbiturates
  Iminostilbenes
  Branch Chain Carboxylic Acid
  Succinimides
  Oxazolidinediones
  Benzodiazepines
USING THE NURSING PROCESS
  Assessment
  Nursing Diagnosis
  Nursing Intervention
  Patient Teaching
  Evaluation
SUMMARY

TABLES

Nursing Process
Patient Teaching
Drug Tables

GLOSSARY TERMS IN THIS CHAPTER

Absence epilepsy
ADH
Aphasia
Aura
Autoinduction
EEG
Epilepsy
Hemeralopia
Heteroinduction
Ictal
Morbilliform
Postictal
Post-tetanic potentiation
Scarlatiniform
Seizure
Seizure disorder
Stevens-Johnson syndrome
Systemic lupus erythematosus

22
CHAPTER

UTILIZATION OF ANTICONVULSANTS

VICKI L. BYERS, R.N., Ph.D., CNRN

LEARNING OBJECTIVES

After reading this chapter, the student will be able to:

1. Identify those medications commonly used as anticonvulsants.

2. Differentiate among the anticonvulsants as to mechanism of action, route of administration, pharmacokinetics, adverse effects, contraindications, and interactions.

3. Identify specific areas to assess in the patient requiring anticonvulsant medication in order to formulate appropriate nursing diagnoses.

4. Plan the nursing interventions necessary to administer anticonvulsants and choose appropriate teaching strategies to gain patient compliance.

5. Evaluate the patient at various stages of treatment to measure the effect of nursing interventions on anticonvulsant therapy.

Approximately 1% of the population in the United States has epilepsy. It is the second most common neurologic disorder after cerebrovascular accident. Epilepsy can affect any age population, persons in any occupation, and at any point in time. A *seizure disorder* or epilepsy can be managed with drug therapy or surgical intervention, but the problems of the patient/family with epilepsy present a challenge to the nurse. Approximately 80% of persons with epilepsy are controlled with anticonvulsants, but there are 500,000 people in the United States with uncontrolled epilepsy.

Epilepsy is a chronic disorder that has as its hallmark recurring seizures. A *seizure* is a sudden, uncontrolled burst of neuronal firing. A century ago John Jackson, the father of the concepts of epilepsy, defined seizures as "occasional, sudden, excessive, rapid and local discharges of gray matter". A seizure is a symptom of central nervous system (CNS) dysfunction. The signs and symptoms vary with the seizure; no two seizures are alike.

A great deal of knowledge has been gained about epilepsy. Some of the various research involves studies on kindling. Kindling is the process whereby an animal receives electrical stimuli intermittently to a single area of the brain over a period of time. This results in the development of seizures that become longer and more intense with repeated stimulation. These seizures are very similar to clinical seizures. This model enables scientists to study the kindled state and epileptic propagation. The process of epileptogensis starts with synchronous high-frequency firing of a group of neurons. When this high intensity of firing continues, normal neurons can be recruited if inhibitiion does not occur. A secondary focus develops, spreading the abnormal electrical activity. This is a simplified explanation because the process is very complex and the exact mechanisms that cause seizures are not clear. One hypothesis is that the spontaneous electrical discharges result from gamma-aminobutyric acid (GABA)-neuron dysfunction. It is also unclear what anatomic pathways are involved in the progession from focal to generalized seizures.

Seizures can result from a variety of causes and can be classified in a variety of ways. A classification, based on etiology, yields idiopathic and symptomatic seizures. With idiopathic seizures, the cause is unknown. Many of these seizures start in childhood or adolescence. With symptomatic seizures, the cause has been determined. Some of these causes include congenital defects, hypoxia at birth, head injury, brain tumors, CNS infections or abscesses, vascular insufficiency, substance abuse, metabolic causes (e.g., electrolyte and glucose imbalances, hypoxia, vitamin deficiencies), and drug interactions. The Commission of Classification and Terminology of the International League Against Epilepsy classifies epilepsy into two broad groups: partial and genaralized seizures. A partial (focal) seizure is localized to one area of the brain, while generalized seizures involve both cerebral hemispheres of the brain. Each of these major categories is further subdivided. This committee classifies each seizure as a single event. Major changes have occurred in terminology, but this classification system is widely used by health professionals and lay people. See Table 22–1 for a detailed description of the subcategories.

OVERVIEW OF ANTICONVULSANT DRUGS

ACTION

Anticonvulsant drugs influence seizure activity in two ways. One way is to suppress the focus of discharge so that there is a reduction or abolishment of excessive discharge. The second way is to prevent the spread of neural excitation. This is often referred to as the "neuronal membrane stabilizing effect". These actions modify sodium, calcium, and potassium ion transport, which stabilizes the cell membrane.

The exact mechanism of drug therapy is unknown. Some of the therapeutic agents used to treat epilepsy enhance the GABA-mediated inhibitory system (clonazepam, diazepam, phenobarbital, valproic acid) by influencing chloride ion influx through chloride channels, leading to greater inhibition of the postsynaptic neuron. New agents are being developed that boost GABA-mediated inhibition (progabide, gamma-vinyl GABA).

Other neurotransmitter defects may exist in epilepsy. The enkephalinergic system may be involved in *absence epilepsy*. Therapeutic agents such as ethosuximide, valproic acid, and trimethadione block enkephalinergic-induced seizures.

DRUG SELECTION

When selecting an anticonvulsant agent, the physician must consider many factors. These include seizure type; the patient's medical history, age, sex, occupation, fatigue and stress levels; cost of medications; ingestion of large quantities of caffeine and/or alcohol; and patient acceptance of the treatment plan. Successful treatment includes consideration of the quality of the patient's life, not just a reduction in the number of seizures displayed. The goal of pharmacotherapy is to reduce or eliminate seizures with minimal side effects.

The trend is in the direction of monotherapy. The choice between drugs is debatable, and the choice should be based on the factors stated above. For the initial treatment of generalized (clonic-tonic) or partial seizures, the recommended drugs are phenytoin, phenobarbital, primidone, carbamazepine, and valproate. A growing number of neurologists are selecting carbamazepine for women and children over five years of age because it does not cause coarsening of facial features, hirsutism, or gingival hyperplasia. Phenobarbital is used initially in children under five years. The long-term use of phenobarbital in young children is being re-examined because of the evidence that phenobarbital affects cognitive ability in children and adults.

Table 22–1. EPILEPTIC SEIZURE CLASSIFICATIONS

Seizure Classification	Age	Duration	Clinical Characteristics
Generalized Seizures (Convulsive or Nonconvulsive) A. Absence seizures (petit mal seizures) 　1. Atypical absence seizure	Onset usually occurs between 4 and 8 years; rarely occurs before age 3 or after age 15	10–30 sec	An absence attack is an abrupt, brief loss of consciousness, amnesia, or unawareness characterized by staring and a 3-second spike-and-wave pattern in the EEG, which may be associated with mild clonic movements (eye-blinking, jerking movements), automatisms, or changes in postural tone. No postictal or confused state follows attack. May occur as frequently as 50–100 times a day.
B. Myoclonic seizures	Same as for Generalized Seizures.	Same as for Generalized Seizures.	Single or multiple sudden, brief, "shock-like" contractions may be generalized or confined to the face and trunk or to one or more extremities. Many cases of myoclonic jerks and action myoclonus are not classified as epileptic seizures.
C. Clonic seizures	Same as for Generalized Seizures.	Same as for Generalized Seizures.	Clonic seizures are characterized by repetitive clonic jerks that lack a tonic component. Clonic jerks may be symmetrical, asymmetrical, rhythmic, or arrhythmic; these seizures are relatively rare, occurring primarily in early childhood.
D. Tonic seizures	Same as for Generalized Seizures.	10 sec	Tonic contraction of certain muscle groups is accompanied by altered consciousness, but there is no progression to clonic phase. Ocular phenomena are common and include fixation of the eyes, eyelid retraction, superior ocular deviation, nystagmus, and mydriasis. Autonomic signs include tachycardia, hypertension, respiratory distress, and capillary restriction with cyanosis. Seizures are usually activated by sleep.
E. Tonic-clonic seizures	Same as for Generalized Seizures.	2–5 min	These types of seizures are the most commonly encountered primary and secondary generalized seizures and can occur at any age. While some patients experience a vague aura, the majority lose consciousness without premonitory signs. Seizures begin with a sudden tonic contraction of muscles (if the respiratory muscle is affected, there is stridor); the patient falls to the ground and remains rigid (10–30 sec). The tonic phase gives way to the clonic phase (30–50 sec), and muscle

CONTINUED ON THE FOLLOWING PAGE

Table 22–1. EPILEPTIC SEIZURE CLASSIFICATIONS–*CONTINUED*

Seizure Classification	Age	Duration	Clinical Characteristics
			relaxation interrupts tonic contraction. Muscle tone returns in rhythmic flexor spasms, which become less frequent as the seizure subsides. Following this, the patient remains unconscious for variable periods. Urinary and fecal incontinence may occur in the clonic phase.
F. Atonic seizures	Same as for Generalized Seizures	Same as for Generalized Seizures.	Sudden reduction of muscle tone may selectively affect muscle groups leading to head drop with slackening of the jaw, the dropping of a limb, or loss of all muscle tone, leading to a slumping to the ground. When attacks are brief, they are called drop attacks. Other conditions, such as narcolepsy cataplexy syndrome and brain-stem ischemia, also cause drop attacks.
Partial Seizures ***(Focal Seizures)*** A. Simple partial seizures 1. With motor symptoms 2. With somatosensory or special sensory symp- toms 3. With autonomic symp- toms 4. With psychic symptoms	Most commonly occur in older children and adults	1–2 min	Consciousness usually is not impaired. Paroxysmal attacks are limited to functional disturbances of sensory, motor, and/or autonomic nerves and to anatomic regions of the brain, depending on the particular cortical area of involvement. Seizures with motor (Jacksonian seizure) and special sensory symptoms (odor, taste) are most common.
B. Complex partial seizures 1. Simple partial onset fol- lowed by impairment of consciousness 2. With impairment of con- sciousness at onset	Same as for Generalized Seizures.	Same as for Generalized Seizures.	Daily episodes of impaired consciousness (e.g., amnesia, unresponsiveness), usually characterized by brief (1–2 min) loss of contact with environment. Clinical manifestations are varied; they most commonly consist of automatisms (e.g., staring, chewing movements or smacking of lips, bizarre purposeless motor or psychic performances, mumbled speech or unintelligible sounds). Confusion may persist for 1–2 min after attack subsides. The EEG is helpful for diagnosis because unusual variants of this disorder may be extremely difficult to distinguish from purely functional psychiatric disorders.
C. Partial seizures evolving to secondarily generalized sei- zures 1. Simple partial seizures evolving to generalized seizures	Same as for Generalized Seizures.	Same as for Generalized Seizures.	On occasion, partial seizures may spread and become generalized tonic-clonic seizures.

Table 22–1. EPILEPTIC SEIZURE CLASSIFICATIONS–*CONTINUED*

Seizure Classification	Age	Duration	Clinical Characteristics
2. Complex partial seizures evolving to generalized seizures 3. Simple partial seizures evolving to complex partial seizures evolving to generalized seizures			
Unclassified Epileptic Seizures	Neonate	10–30 sec	Inadequate data for classification. This category includes some neonatal seizures (e.g., rhythmic eye movements, chewing, and swimming movements).

Drugs that are effective in absence seizures include ethosuximide, valproic acid, and clonazepam. If seizures remain uncontrolled, a second agent is added to the therapy. Combination therapy is more difficult to manage because of drug interactions. See Table 22–2 for the drugs used in the treatment of seizures.

GENERAL PRINCIPLES OF DRUG THERAPY

The nurse's role in drug therapy, once it is initiated by the physician, is monitoring the patient for tolerance to the agent, side effects, and drug interactions. Another

Table 22–2. DRUG TREATMENT OF SEIZURES

Seizure Type	Commonly Used Drug Treatment	Infrequently Used Drug Treatment
Generalized Seizures Absence	Ethosuximide (Zarontin); valproic acid (Depakene, Depakote); clonazepam (Clonopin)	Acetazolamide (Diamox); clorazepate (Tranxene); diazepam (Valium); methsuximide (Celontin); phensuximide (Milontin); paramethadione (Paradione); trimethadione (Tridione)
Tonic-clonic seizures	Phenytoin (Dilantin); carbamazepine (Tegretol); phenobarbital; valproic acid (Depakene, Depakote)	Primidone (Mysoline); ethotoin (Peganone); mephenytoin (Mesantoin); mephobarbital (Mebaral)
Myoclonic seizures, infantile spasms, Lennox-Gastaut syndrome	Clonazepam (Clonopin)	Carbamazepine (Tegretol); phenytoin (Dilantin); phenobarbital; primidone (Mysoline)
Myoclonic seizures (including postanoxic myoclonus)	Valproic acid (Depakene, Depakote); clonazepam (Clonopin)	Carbamazepine (Tegretol); phenytoin (Dilantin); phenobarbital; diazepam (Valium)
Atonic seizures	Valproic acid (Depakene, Depakote); clonazepam (Clonopin)	Ethosuximide (Zarontin); trimethadione (Tridione)
Partial Seizures (Focal Seizures) Simple partial seizures Complex partial seizures Partial seizures evolving to secondarily generalized seizures	Phenytoin (Dilantin); carbamazepine (Tegretol); phenobarbital; primidone (Mysoline)	Phenacemide (Phenurone); ethotoin (Peganone); mephenytoin (Mesantoin); mephobarbital (Mebaral); valproic acid (Depakene, Depakote)

critical role of the nurse is patient teaching. Since these roles are very important, nurses need to be aware of general principles related to the selection of a therapeutic agent. When treatment is initiated with an antiepileptic agent, the goal is to control the seizures without causing intolerable adverse reactions. Drug therapy is initiated with a single drug. The initial dose is expected to fall within the therapeutic range during the plateau state. A loading dosage is used only if the benefits outweigh the risk of adverse effects. The dosage is very individualized and is based on factors discussed previously.

It is important to allow time for the drug to reach steady state prior to evaluating its effectivness. It is recommended that at least five drug half-lives pass before the steady-state serum concentrations are drawn (unless loading has occurred). Sometimes, frequent recurring seizures may require that steady state be achieved more quickly. This is accomplished by giving a loading dose. When an agent is inadequate and the patient is still having seizures with the maximal tolerated dose, then another agent is substituted or a second drug is added to the regimen. Unless serious side effects occur, the ineffective drug should be reduced gradually when being discontinued to minimize the risk of precipitating status epilepticus.

It is important to have the patient's approval of the proposed treatment plan. The patient must live with the treatment plan, and his/her support and cooperation are necessary in order for the plan to be successful. Patients need to keep a seizure diary. This diary includes a calendar in which the patient records the type(s) of seizure, number of times it occurs, the time it happens, and how long it lasted. The diary must provide space to record factors that might have precipitated the seizure. Patient education is very important to successful compliance; the role of the nurse in patient teaching is discussed later in this chapter.

Some causes of failure of anticonvulsant medication are: improper diagnosis of the type of seizure; incorrect choice of drug; inadequate or excessive dosage; too frequent changes in medication without regard to the time required for transition between plateau states; failure to fully utilize the advantages of a multiple-drug regimen; inattention to ancillary aspects of therapy; and poor compliance by the patient.

MONITORING DRUG CONCENTRATIONS

Measuring the drug concentration in plasma can help in the overall management of the patient. There is a relationship between the serum concentraion of an antiepileptic drug and its therapeutic effect. This measurement is especially helpful with initial dosage adjustment, use of multiple agents, and in providing an index of patient compliance. Since serum values vary for different institutions and laboratories, as well as among patients, the therapeutic range should serve only as a guideline. It is important to treat the patient and not just

the drug level. Some patients need a phenytoin (Dilantin) level of 10 μg/ml for seizure control.

Two pharmacokinetic factors are important when examining drug levels and drug interactions. One factor is the administration of carbamazepine. After a couple of weeks of administration, carbamazepine induces hepatic enzymes which are then responsible for its own biotransformation. Usually an increase in the dosage of the drug is required. The degree of *autoinduction* is variable. Autoinduction and *heteroinduction* contribute to drug interactions. The second factor to consider is related to the biotransformation of phenytoin, which involves dose-dependent kinetics. As the metabolism of phenytoin approaches saturation, even small dosage increases may cause unexpected toxicity as a result of disproportionately large increases in the serum concentration and half-life of the drug. Also, the biotransformation of phenytoin can be inhibited by a number of drugs causing phenytoin toxicity.

DRUG INTERACTIONS

A drug interaction occurs when one drug alters the patient's response to another drug. It can also occur when there is a change in the pharmacokinetic parameters of a drug without any change in the patient's response to the drug. Anticonvulsant agents have a high potential for drug interactions for three reasons. The first reason is that many of the anticonvulsant agents are enzyme inducers and/or inhibitors of hepatic microsomal enzymes involved in biotransformation. If they are enzyme inducers, they stimulate the synthesis of new drug-metabolizing enzymes in the liver and the new drug is metabolized at a faster rate. Enzyme inhibitors act the opposite way by causing drugs to compete with each other. Some drugs may be toxic to enzymes and inhibit their activity. Alternatively, the drug may bind to enzymes, inhibiting their actions. The second reason that anticonvulsant agents cause drug interactions is that they alter the protein binding of other anticonvulsants used in combination for mixed epilepsies. The last reason for a high potential for drug interaction is the fact that anticonvulsant agents are administered over long periods of time. The end result is that the drug interactions can cause toxicity or reduce the therapeutic effectiveness of the drug. It is critical that the patient be monitored for signs and symptoms of toxicity and that the serum concentration of the drug also be monitored.

WITHDRAWAL OF MEDICATION

Many of the seizures that start in childhood have the potential for a spontaneous remission. Other types of seizures that have an underlying pathology (head injury, brain tumor, arteriovenous malformations, etc.) may not have a remission. Guidelines for discontinuation of therapy, especially in children, are very controversial. There is agreement that the anticonvulsant agents should be tapered and never abruptly discontinued. The risk of status epilepticus is great with abrupt cessation of therapy.

There is also agreement about which factors warrant continuation of therapy. These factors include epilepsy of long duration (e.g., six years) prior to control and the presence of partial seizures, mixed seizures, and atypical febrile seizures.

USE IN PREGNANCY

Women of childbearing age who are receiving anticonvulsant drugs should be informed that there is a risk of congenital malformation in their childen. The chance of bearing a normal child is greater than 90%, but the risk for producing a child with birth defects is approximately 7%, compared with the 2%–3% for the general population. It is difficult to determine the exact cause(s), but the birth defects could be due to the effects of repeated seizures, to the teratogenic effects of anticonvulsants, and to genetic factors. The most common malformations are cleft lip and/or palate and congenital heart disease. Trimethadione is a very potent teratogen; birth defects or spontaneous abortions have occurred in 90% of fetuses exposed to this agent *in utero*. Spina bifida has been reported with the use of valproic acid. Most of the congenital malformations have occurred with the use of phenytoin or phenobarbital, either used alone or concurrently. This may be due to the fact that these two agents are used most frequently. The pattern of some of the abnormalities have been referred to as the "fetal hydantoin syndrome" or the "fetal barbiturate syndrome." These syndromes are discussed later in this chapter.

It is not recommended that anticonvulsant agents be discontinued during pregnancy. With abrupt discontinuation, the risk of status epilepticus is greater, and dangerous outcomes for mother and fetus may occur. Serum concentrations of antiepileptic drugs tend to decrease during pregnancy. It is important that drug levels be monitored frequently and the dosage adjusted when necessary. Monitoring should continue for about six weeks in the postpartum period.

Fetal monitoring should be used during labor because of the depression of clotting factors and the potential for hemorrhage. This is the greatest risk for mothers who are receiving phenobarbital, primidone, or phenytoin during pregnancy. These agents can cause a vitamin K deficiency. Bleeding can be prevented by the adminstration of vitamin K.

NONEPILEPTIC SEIZURES

Children between the ages of three months and five years of age are at risk for a febrile seizure. There is a fever but no evidence of neurologic origin. These children are at a higher risk of having another febrile seizure (30%–40%) and a slight increased risk of epilepsy. Seizure prophylaxis is not routinely instituted unless a neurologic origin is determined: febrile seizures last longer than 15 minutes with transient or persistent neurologic deficit; genetic origin of febile seizures in a sib-

ling or parent; and seizures in very young children, who have the highest risk of recurrence. Phenobarbital is the agent of choice; it is given in doses that produce a serum level of 15 μg/ml.

Seizures are also associated with drug withdrawal syndrome in persons who are physically dependent on barbiturates, alcohol, benzodiazepines, and nonbarbiturate-nonbenzodiazepine antianxiety and hypnotic drugs. Phenobarbital or benzodiazepines are used to relieve the signs and symptoms, depending on the etiology.

The use of anticonvulsant drugs in the prophylaxis of post-traumatic epilepsy is very controversial. Data is inconclusive about the effectiveness of treatment in reducing these seizures. Patients who may benefit from therapy fall into four groups: 1) penetrating head injuries, 2) closed head injuries with neurologic deficit and abnormal electroencephalogram (*EEG*), 3) closed head injury with coma lasting longer than three hours, and 4) a family history of seizures or a history of abnormal delivery or febrile seizures in childhood.

STATUS EPILEPTICUS

Status epilepticus occurs when seizures are repeated so frequently that the person does not regain his preseizure state. This situation is a neurologic emergency and must be treated immediately. There are a variety of reasons why a person experiences status epilepticus. Some of these reasons include noncompliance, abrupt withdrawal of antiepileptic medication, withdrawal of alcohol or other drugs, fever, metabolic-induced deficiencies (hypoglycemia, hypocalcemia, hyponatremia), and neurologic origin (stroke, meningitis, head injury).

If status epilepticus is not terminated, mortality is high or the patient suffers brain damage. During this state, the neurons are utilizing a large amount of energy and the metabolic demand is great. Oxygen consumption is also great during this period. Hypoxia from inadequate pulmonary ventilation compounds the problem and can cause neuronal death. If this is a major motor seizure, there is massive muscle activity, which leads to hyperthermia and neuronal cell damage or death. The excessive muscle activity can lead to fatigue and overtaxation of the cardiopulmonary system, which leads to further hypoxia, acidosis, shock, and death.

The treatment of status epilepticus is drug therapy and supportive care. The supportive care is directed at maintaining a patent airway, providing ventilatory support if needed, establishing an intravenous route for administering drugs, and ensuring patient safety. After obtaining a serum sample for glucose, a 50-ml bolus of 50% dextrose is given. Drug selection varies, but intravenous diazepam is usually the drug of choice. Lorazepam (Ativan) is being used more frequently because of its longer duration of action. A loading dose of phenytoin is usually given intravenously as well. If seizures continue despite drug therapy, general anesthesia is employed. See Table 22–3 for information about parenteral therapy for status epilepticus.

Table 22–3. PARENTERAL THERAPY FOR STATUS EPILEPTICUS

Drug	Dosage/Route
Diazepam (Valium)	*Intravenous: Adults,* 5–10 mg given at a rate of 1 ml (5 mg)/min, repeated at 5–10-minute intervals (maximum, 30 mg). This dose may be repeated in 2–4 hours if necessary. For intravenous drip, diazepam 100 mg is diluted in 500 ml of 5% dextrose in water and given at a rate of 40 ml/hr to maintain a serum concentration of 0.2–0.8 μg/ml. *Children 5 years or older,* 1 mg every 2–5 min (maximum, 10 mg), repeated in 2–4 hours if necessary. *Infants over 30 days and children under 5 years,* 0.2–0.5 mg every 2–5 min (maximum, 5 mg).
Lorazepam (Ativan)	*Intravenous: Adults,* although no dosage or rate of administration has been firmly established, 4 mg given at a rate of 1 ml (2 mg)/min has been effective (Leppik et al., 1983). This dose can be repeated at 10-min intervals if needed. *Children,* experience is limited.
Phenytoin (Dilantin)	*Intravenous: Adults and children,* a loading dose of 15 mg/kg undiluted is administered at a rate not to exceed 50 mg/min. (Pediatric loading dose also may be calculated on the basis of 250 mg/M^2 given at a rate of 1–2 mg/kg/min.) An additional 5 mg/kg is given after 12 hr. Alternatively, 20 mg/kg diluted with 0.45% or 0.9% sodium chloride solution to produce 20–30 mg/ml phenytoin is administered at a rate not to exceed 50 mg/min. This is usually the only dose required in 24 hr. With either regimen, therapeutic serum concentrations are between 10 and 25 μg/ml for 24 hr in most patients. Phenytoin should be administered in an intensive care unit so that heart rate, blood pressure, and electrocardiographic activity can be monitored.
Phenobarbital	*Intravenous, Intramuscular: Adults,* the loading dose is 5–10 mg/kg. One fifth of the total dose given intravenously undiluted at a rate of less than 50 mg/min every 5–10 min helps to prevent respiratory depression. If the patient has previously been given phenytoin without success or an unknown serum level of phenobarbital is present, 2 mg/kg of phenobarbital should be administered intravenously every 15 min until adequate response is obtained, hypotension and/or respiratory depression develops, or a cumulative dose of 1 g/24 hr has been given. Intravenous administration is preferred, but intramuscular administration may be used if necessary; the initial dose is 3–5 mg/kg. *Children,* 10–15 mg/kg. One fifth of total dose given intravenously undiluted at a rate of less than 50 mg/min every 5–10 min helps to prevent respiratory depression. Dosage is adjusted to maintain serum concentration of 15–40 μg/ml. If patient had previously been given phenytoin without success or an unknown serum level of phenobarbital is present, a dose of 2 mg/kg of phenobarbital should be administered intravenously every 15 min until an adequate response is obtained or hypotension and/or respiratory depression develops. Intravenous administration is preferred, but intramuscular administration may be used if necessary; the initial dose is 3–5 mg/kg. *Neonates,* the loading dose is 15–20 mg/kg.

ANTICONVULSANTS

HYDANTOINS

Phenytoin

ACTION. Phenytoin (Dilantin) suppresses the spread of seizures. It has a stabilizing effect on neuronal membranes, and decreases the resting fluxes of sodium ions as well as sodium currents that flow during action potentials or chemically induced depolarizations. Phenytoin also decreases the influx of calcium ion during depolarization, and the end effect is alteration of neurotransmitter release. Phenytoin is discussed in Table 22–4.

USES. Phenytoin is the primary drug used in the treatment of all types of seizures except absence seizures. The anticonvulsant activity of this drug was discovered in 1938. This agent is also used in the treatment of trigeminal and related neuralgias and digitalis-induced cardiac dysrhythmias. Phenytoin is also used for the treatment of compulsive thought disorder.

PHARMACOKINETICS. Phenytoin is absorbed slowly after oral administration, and absorption is unpredictable and incomplete. There are significant differences in bioavailability in oral pharmaceutical preparations. Once phenytoin is absorbed, it is distributed into all tissues. About 90% is bound to plasma proteins (albumin). A greater fraction of unbound phenytoin is found in the neonate, patients with hypoalbuminemia, and uremic patients. It is the unbound phenytoin that reacts with receptors to produce the pharmacologic actions. Phenytoin is metabolized by hepatic microsomal-oxidizing enzymes. The major metabolite is the p-hydroxyphenyl derivative. The parent drug brings about the anticonvulsant activity. About 5% of the dose of phenytoin is excreted unchanged in the urine. The half-life of phenytoin ranges 6–24 hours. A dose-dependent elimination is seen at higher concentrations, and the half-life increases as the concentration increases. This might be caused by saturation of the hydroxylation reaction or inhibition by metabolites.

The onset, peak, and duration of action vary with the mode of administration. This data is calculated with a loading dose. The onset of action with an oral dose is one to two hours; with an intravenous dose, one hour; and with an intramuscular dose, the onset is erratic. The peak action for an oral dose is 1.5–3 hours; for oral extended-release tablets, it is 4–12 hours; for intravenous delivery, it is rapid; and for intramuscular delivery, it is erratic. The duration of action for an oral dose is 6–12 hours; for oral extended-release tablets, 12 or 36 hours; for intravenous delivery, 12–24 hours, and for intramuscular delivery, 12–24 hours.

CONTRAINDICATIONS AND PRECAUTIONS. This agent is contraindicated in hypersensitivity, sinus bradycardia, and heart block. Phenytoin is used cautiously in patients with liver disease; dosage reduction may be required in order to prevent toxicity since this agent is metabolized in the liver. Safety in lactation has not been established. Caution should be used when administering this agent to a pregnant patient. This drug is usually discontinued if a rash appears (hypersensitivity). When given intravenously, administer slowly (50 mg/min) because it can cause hypotension and arrhythmias.

ADVERSE REACTIONS. At normal therapeutic doses, phenytoin is relatively safe with few reported side effects. The dose-related side effects are similar to those of other antiepileptic agents. The CNS, skin, gastrointestinal system, endocrine system, and hematologic system are usually involved in adverse phenytoin reactions.

Phenytoin has an excitatory effect on the cerebellar-vestibular system. The result of this action is nystagmus, ataxia, diplopia, and vertigo. Other CNS effects include blurred vision, mydriasis, hyperactive tendon reflex, hyperactivity silliness, confusion, inattention, drowsiness, dullness, headache, and coma (large doses).

Gingival hyperplasia occurs frequently with chronic therapy and is a common manifestation of toxicity in children and adolescents. This occurs only in portions of the gum that have teeth. This side effect is due to the overgrowth of tissue caused by altered collagen metabolism. This side effect can be minimized by good oral hygiene. Hirsutism and coarsening of facial features are induced by phenytoin. These effects are probably due to altered androgen levels that secondarily result from use of the drug.

Gastrointestinal problems include nausea, vomiting, anorexia, weight loss, and epigastric pain. Many of these reactions are caused by taking this agent on an empty stomach. Taking this agent with food or in more frequent divided doses reduces these reactions.

Endocrine effects such as hyperglycemia, glycosuria, and osteomalacia have been reported. The hyperglycemia and glycosuria occur secondarily to the inhibition of insulin secretion. The osteomalcia, with hypocalcemia and increased alkaline phosphatase activity, has been reported to be due to altered metabolism of vitamin D and the inhibition of intestinal absorption of calcium.

Hypersensitivity reactions include the morbilliform rash, *Stevens-Johnson syndrome, systemic lupus erythematosus,* and hepatic necrosis. Phenytoin is usually discontinued when a skin rash appears, and therefore more serious skin problems do not develop. These reactions are idiosyncratic in origin.

Hematologic reactions can also occur. These include fever, neutropenia, leukopenia, red-cell anemia, aplastic anemia, megaloblastic anemia, hypoprothrombinemia, and hemorrhage in newborns of mothers who received phenytoin. A marked phagocytosis of myeloid precursors by bone marrow histiocytes occurs in agranulocytosis. *In vitro* studies suggest that phenytoin-induced red-cell aplasia is immunologic in nature, mediated through an immunoglobulin inhibitor, requiring the presence of phenytoin to suppress erythroid colony formation. The megaloblastic anemia has been associated with altered folate absorption and metabolism. The lymphadenopathy is a secondary result of the reduction in immunoglobulin A production. The hypoprothrombinemia and hemorrhage are the secondary result of the vitamin K deficiency.

DRUG CONCENTRATIONS. Therapeutic effectiveness is obtained with concentrations over 10 μg/ml (total concentration of phenytoin), while toxic effects such as nystagmus develop at about 20 μg/ml; ataxia is present at 30 μg/ml; and lethargy at 40 μg/ml. The clinical signs of toxicity are correlated with the concentration of the unbound drug. This varies considerably among patients, so drug concentrations should serve only as a general guideline (Table 22–5). Nurses should assess the patient for signs of toxicity. Monitoring drug concentration is important for the patient on anticonvulsants because it can help in individualizing therapy to provide maximal benefit and to decrease dose-related side effects.

DRUG INTERACTIONS. Many of the drug interactions connected with phenytoin are secondary to effects on its metabolism. Some agents increase phenytoin's metabolism by inducing hepatic microsomal enzymes, while other agents decrease it by competitively inhibiting phenytoin's microsomal metabolism. Agents such as chloramphenicol, disulfiram, isoniazid, sulfonamides, and cimetidine are enzyme inhibitors, causing an increase in serum phenytoin levels and hastening signs and symptoms of toxicity. Other drugs that work by enzyme inhibition include miconazole, nifedipine, and chlorpromazine. All of these agents increase serum phenytoin levels.

Agents that displace phenytoin from its albumin-binding sites are phenylbutazone, sulfamethoxazole/trimethoprim, salicylates, and valproate. Amiodarone can also cause toxicity, but the mechanism is unclear. The chronic use of alcohol stimulates phenytoin-metabolizing enzymes, causing a decrease in anticonvulsant effect. The phenytoin–phenobarbital interaction is complex. Phenobarbital can be either an inducer (by increasing the biotransformation of phenytoin) or an inhibitor (by decreasing phenytoin activity). Rifampin causes a decrease in phenytoin level.

Phenytoin enhances the metabolism of oral contraceptives, corticosteroids, methadone, doxycycline, disopyramide, quinidine, oxazepam, and cyclosporine.

TEXT RESUMES ON PAGE 546

Table 22–4. SPECIFIC ANTICONVULSANT AGENTS

Name	Dosage	Mode of Administration	Pharmacokinetics

HYDANTOINS
Phenytoin (Dilantin Kapseals,
  Dilantin with Phenobarbital,
  Dilantin Infatabs, Dilantin
  Oral Suspension, Phenytoin
  Sodium Injection)

Action: Limits seizure propagation by altering ion transport. Antiarrhythmic properties due to improvement in AV conduction. Therapeutic effect is treatment and prevention of seizures and control of arrhythmias.

Use: Used in the treatment and prevention of tonic-clonic (generalized) seizures and complex partial seizures. Also used as an antiarrhythmic, particularly for dysrhythmias associated with digitalis glycoside toxicity. Phenytoin is also used in the treatment of compulsive thought disorders.

Name	Dosage	Mode of Administration	Pharmacokinetics
	Anticonvulsant:		O: UA; (extended release) 1–2 hr
	Adult, loading dose: 10–15 mg/kg; *maintenance dose:* 300–400 mg/day (once daily as extended-release capsules or in 3–4 divided doses). Usual maximum dose is 600 mg/day.	PO	P: 1.5–3 hr; (extended-release) 4–12 hr; D: PO: 6–12 hr; (extended-release) 12–36 hr; ½ L: 6–24 hr (average 22 hr) PB: 90% bound
	Children: initially 5 mg/kg; *maintenance dose:* 4–8 mg/kg/day in divided doses q 8–12 hr	PO	B: liver E: minimal by kidneys
	Status Epilepticus: *Adults:* 15–18 mg/kg (rate not to exceed 25–50 mg/min)	IV	O: 1–2 hr (without loading dose) P: rapid D: 12–24 hr
	Children: 250 mg/M² or up to 10–15 mg/kg (at a rate of 0.5–1.5 mg/kg/min)	IV	
	Antiarrhythmic: *Adults:* 50–100 mg q 5–15 min until dysrhythmia is abolished, 1000 mg has been given, or toxicity occurs	IV	
	Adults: 100 mg 2–4 times daily. As a last resort, dosage should be increased by 50% over previously established daily oral dose.	PO IM	O: UA P: erratic D: 12–24 hr

Key to Abbreviations in the *Pharmacokinetics* column O-onset; P-peak; D-duration; PB-protein bound; B-biotransformed in; E-excreted in; ½ L-halflife.
   *Within the column listing adverse effects, underlines indicate the most common effects, and CAPITALS indicate life-threatening effects.

Contraindications/ Precautions	Adverse Effects*	Interactions	Nursing Implications
			ASSESSMENT: Assess location, duration, and characteristics of seizure activity. CBC and platelet count, serum calcium, urinalysis, and hepatic and thyroid function tests are monitored prior to therapy and monthly for the first several months, then periodically throughout the course of therapy. Patient should have routine physical examinations, especially monitoring of skin and lymph nodes and EEG testing. EVALUATION: Effectiveness of therapy can be demonstrated by decrease or cessation of seizures without excessive sedation.
Contraindicated in hypersensitivity (including rash) and sinus bradycardia and heart block. Use with caution in severe liver disease (dosage reduction required). Safety in pregnancy has not been established; use may result in fetal hydantoin syndrome. Safety in lactation has not been established.	Neuro: nystagmus, ataxia, diplopia, drowsiness, lethargy, coma, dizziness, headache, nervousness, dyskinesia CV: hypotension (IV only) Hema: APLASTIC ANEMIA, AGRANULOCYTOSIS, leukopenia, thrombocytopenia, megaloblastic anemia Renal: hypocalcemia GI: nausea, vomiting, anorexia, weight loss, constipation, hepatitis EENT: gingival hyperplasia Integ: hypertrichosis, rashes, exfoliative dermatitis, hirsutism, coarsening facial features Muscskel: osteomalacia Misc: lymphadenopathy, fever, allergic reactions including STEVENS-JOHNSON SYNDROME	The following drugs may decrease phenytoin metabolism and increase blood levels: phenylbutazone, disulfiram, isoniazid, chloramphenicol, and cimetidine. Barbiturates, alcohol, and warfarin may stimulate phenytoin metabolism and decrease blood levels. Phenytoin may stimulate the metabolism and decrease the effectiveness of digitoxin and oral contraceptives. Tricyclic antidepressants and phenothiazines may lower seizure threshold and precipitate seizures. Additive CNS depression occurs with other CNS depressants including alcohol, antihistamines, antidepressants, narcotics, and sedative/ hypnotics. Phenytoin may alter the effect of oral anticoagulants.	Same as for all, plus: ASSESSMENT: Dental examinations, including teeth cleaning and reinforcement of plaque control for inhibition of gingival hyperplasia, should be performed at 3-month intervals. INTERVENTION: Administer with or immediately after meals to minimize GI irritation. Shake liquid preparations well before pouring. Chewable tablets must be crushed or chewed well before swallowing. Capsules may be opened and mixed with food or fluids for patients who have difficulty swallowing. To prevent direct contact of alkaline drug with mucosa, have patient swallow a fluid first, follow with mixture of medication, then follow with a full glass or water or milk,

CONTINUED ON THE FOLLOWING PAGE

Table 22–4. SPECIFIC ANTICONVULSANT AGENTS–*CONTINUED*

Name	Dosage	Mode of Administration	Pharmacokinetics
HYDANTOINS–*Continued*			

BARBITURATES—ANTICONVULSANT, BARBITURATE, SEDATIVE-HYPNOTIC
Phenobarbital (Luminal)

Action: Produces all levels of CNS depression. Depresses the sensory cortex, decreases motor activity, and alters cerebellar function. Inhibits transmission in the nervous system and raises the seizure threshold. Therapeutic effects include anticonvulsant activity and sedation. Capable of inducing enzymes in the liver that metabolize drugs, bilirubin, and other compounds.

Use: Used primarily as an anticonvulsant in tonic-clonic (generalized) seizures, partial seizures, and febrile seizures in children. Also used as a preoperative sedative and in other situations where sedation may be required and as a hypnotic. Other uses include prevention and treatment of neonatal hyperbilirubinemia and lowering of bilirubin and lipid levels in chronic cholestasis.

	Dosage	Mode of Administration	Pharmacokinetics
	Anticonvulsant: *Adults:* 100–300 mg/day, single dose or 2–3 divided doses	PO	O: PO, 30–60 min; IM and SC, 10–30 min; IV, 5 min P: IM, SC, IV, 4–6; PO, 8–12 hr (several weeks unless loading dose used)
	Children: 1–6 mg/kg/day, single or divided doses	PO	

Key to Abbreviations in the *Pharmacokinetics* column O-onset; P-peak; D-duration; PB-protein bound; B-bio-transformed in; E-excreted in; ½ L-halflife.
*Within the column listing adverse effects, underlines indicate the most common effects, and CAPITALS indicate life-threatening effects.

Contraindications/ Precautions	Adverse Effects*	Interactions	Nursing Implications
		Phenytoin may decrease absorption of folic acid and vice versa. Decreases T$_4$ levels; lowers the values for dexamethasone tests; increased liver function tests; lowered value on metapyrone tests; alters urine pregnancy tests (both false-positive and false-negative results); color changes in urine (pink, red, red-brown) in presence of an acid urinary pH.	or food. The 100-mg tablets and capsules contain 92 mg of phenytoin and are not interchangeable with two 50-mg tablets or capsules. Capsules labeled "extended" may be used for once-a-day dosage; those labeled "prompt" may result in toxic serum levels if used for once-a-day dosage. Administer direct IV at a rate not to exceed 50 mg over 1 min (25 mg/min in elderly patients). Rapid administration may result in severe hypotension or CNS depression. Administer as intermittent infusion by mixing with 0.9% NaCl in a concentration of less than 6.7 mg/ml. Administer immediately following admixture. Use tubing with a 0.22-micron in-line filter. Complete infusion within 4 hr at a rate not to exceed 50 mg/min. Monitor cardiac function and blood pressure throughout infusion. To minimize local venous irritation, follow infusion with 0.9% NaCl. Avoid extravasation; phenytoin is caustic to tissues. Do not admix with other solutions or medications, especially dextrose, because precipitation will occur. Slight yellow color will not alter solution potency. If refrigerated, may form precipitate, which dissolves after warming to room temperature. Discard solutions that are not clear. Implement seizure precautions.
Contraindicated in persons with hypersensitivity to the drug, comatose patients, or those with	Neuro: drowsiness, lethargy, vertigo, depression, hangover, excitation, delirium CV: hypotension (IV only)	Additive CNS depression with other CNS depressants, including alcohol, antidepressants, antihista-	Same as for all. ASSESSMENT: Assess sleep patterns prior to and periodically throughout the

CONTINUED ON THE FOLLOWING PAGE

Table 22–4. SPECIFIC ANTICONVULSANT AGENTS–*CONTINUED*

Name	Dosage	Mode of Administration	Pharmacokinetics
BARBITURATES–Continued	*Adults:* 100–300 mg repeated as necessary to a total of 600 mg/24-hr period	IV	D: PO, 6–24 hr; IM, SC, IV: 4–6 hr
	Children: 10–20 mg/kg as a single loading dose, followed by maintenance dose of 1–6 mg/kg/day	IV	½ L: 2–6 days PB: 20%–45% B: liver E: kidneys
	Sedation:		
	Adults: 30–120 mg/day in 2–3 divided doses	PO	
	Children: 2 mg/kg 3 times daily	PO	
	Adults: 30–120 mg/day in 2–3 divided doses	IM	
	Hypnotic:		
	Adults: 100–300 mg at bedtime	PO	
	Adults: 100–325 mg at bedtime	IV, IM, SC	
	Children: 3–5 mg/kg at bedtime	IV, IM, SC	
	Status Epilepticus:		
	Adults: 5–10 mg/kg, may be repeated at a rate of less than 50 mg/min every 5–10 min	IV	
	Children: 10–15 mg/kg at a rate of less than 50 mg/min every 5–10 min	IV	
	Hyperbilirubinemia:		
	Adults: 30–60 mg tid	PO	
	Children under 12 yr: 1–4 mg/kg tid	PO	
	Preoperative Sedation:		
	Adults: 130–200 mg 60–90 min preoperatively	IM	
	Children: 1–3 mg/kg	PO, IM, IV	

Key to Abbreviations in the *Pharmacokinetics* column O-onset; P-peak; D-duration; PB-protein bound; B-biotransformed in; E-excreted in; ½ L-halflife.
*Within the column listing adverse effects, underlines indicate the most common effects, and CAPITALS indicate life-threatening effects.

Contraindications/ Precautions	Adverse Effects*	Interactions	Nursing Implications
pre-existing CNS depression. It should not be used in patients with acute porphyria or in patients with uncontrolled severe pain. Use cautiously in hepatic dysfunction or severe renal impairment. Use with caution in patients who may be suicidal or who have been addicted to drugs. Dosage needs to be reduced in the elderly. The use of this agent as a hypnotic should be short term. Safe use in pregnancy and lactation has not been established.	Resp: respiratory depression, LARYNGOSPASM (IV only), BRONCHOSPASM (IV only) GI: nausea, vomiting, diarrhea, constipation Muscskel: myalgia, arthralgia, neuralgia Integ: rashes, urticaria, photosensitivity Misc: hypersensitivity reactions, including ANGIOEDEMA and serum sickness, phlebitis at IV site	mines, narcotics, and other sedative-hypnotics. Induces hepatic enzymes that metabolize and decrease the effectiveness of other drugs, including oral contraceptives, chloramphenicol, acebutolol, propranolol, metoprolol, timolol, doxycycline, glucocorticoids, tricyclic antidepressants, phenothiazines, phenylbutazone, and quinidine. Valproic acid inhibits phenobarbital metabolism. May enhance hepatic toxicity of acetaminophen. MAO inhibitors may block the metabolism of barbiturates. Concurrent use with primidone may lead to phenobarbital toxicity. May enhance the hematologic toxicity of cyclophosphamide.	course of therapy. Hypnotic doses of phenobarbital suppress REM sleep. Patient may experience an increase in dreaming on discontinuation of medication. Prolonged therapy may lead to psychological or physical dependence. Restrict amount of drug available to patient if patient is depressed, suicidal, or has a history of addiction. INTERVENTION: Tablets may be crushed and mixed with food or fluids (do not administer dry) for patients who have difficulty swallowing. Oral solution may be taken straight or mixed with water, milk, or fruit juice. Sterile phenobarbital sodium powder may be administered SC after reconstitution, but prediluted phenobarbital sodium injection is not recommended for SC use. IM injections should be given deep into the gluteal muscle to minimize tissue irritation. Reconstitute sterile powder for IV dose with a minimum of 10 ml of sterile water for injection. Dilute further with 10 ml of sterile water. Administer each 60 mg over at least 1 min. Titrate slowly for desired response. Rapid administration may result in respiratory depression. Solution is highly alkaline; extravasation may cause tissue damage and necrosis. If extravasation occurs, injection of 5% procaine solution into affected area and application of moist heat may be ordered. Do not use solutions that are discolored or contain particulate matter. Do not mix with other medications. Discard powder or solutions that have been exposed to air for longer than 30 min. Supervise ambulation and transfer of patients following administration. Remove cigarettes. Side rails should be raised and call bell within reach at all times.

CONTINUED ON THE FOLLOWING PAGE

Anticonvulsants

Table 22–4. SPECIFIC ANTICONVULSANT AGENTS–*CONTINUED*

Name	Dosage	Mode of Administration	Pharmacokinetics
BARBITURATES–*Continued*			

DEOXYBARBITURATES
Primidone (Mysoline)

Action: Decreases neuron excitability. Also increases the threshold of electrical stimulation of the motor cortex. Therapeutic effect is prevention of seizures.

Use: Used in the management of clonic-tonic (generalized), complex partial, and focal seizures.

Name	Dosage	Mode of Administration	Pharmacokinetics
	Adults and Children over 8 yr: Initial dose is 100–125 mg at bedtime for 3 days, then 100–125 mg bid for 3 days, then 100–125 mg tid for 3 days, then maintenance dose of 250 mg tid (not to exceed 2 g/day)	PO	O: 4–7 days P: 4 hr D: 8–24 hr after discontinue ½L: 10–21 hr; active metabolite, 24–48 hr PB: small extent B: liver (two active metabolites) E: kidneys
	Children under 8 yr: Initial dose is 50 mg at bedtime for 3 days, then 50 mg bid for 3 days, then 100 mg bid for 3 days, then maintenance dose of 125–250 mg tid (10–25 mg/kg/day). Dosage adjustment required in severe liver disease.	PO	

IMINOSTIBENES
Carbamazepine (Tegretol)

Action: Limits seizure spread by decreasing synaptic transmission. Therapeutic effect is prevention of seizures.

Use: Prophylaxis of tonic-clonic (generalized), mixed, and complex partial seizures. Also used to relieve pain in trigeminal and glossopharyngeal neuralgia.

Name	Dosage	Mode of Administration	Pharmacokinetics
	Adults: Start with 200 mg bid, increase by 200 mg/day until therapeutic levels are achieved. Usual dose is 800–1200 mg/day in divided doses given q 6–8 hr. In 12–15-year-olds, do not exceed 100 mg/day. *Children 6–12 yr:* 20 mg/kg/day in 2–4 divided doses	PO	O: 2–4 days P: 2–8 hr (Peak activity 7–14 days) D: 6–12 hr ½L: 25–65 hr initially, then 12–17 hr with multiple dosing because of autoinduction PB: 75% bound B: liver E: only 1% excreted by kidneys unchanged

Key to Abbreviations in the *Pharmacokinetics* column O-onset; P-peak; D-duration; PB-protein bound; B-biotransformed in; E-excreted in; ½ L-halflife.
*Within the column listing adverse effects, underlines indicate the most common effects, and CAPITALS indicate life-threatening effects.

Contraindications/ Precautions	Adverse Effects*	Interactions	Nursing Implications
			EVALUATION: Several weeks may be required to achieve maximum anticonvulsant effects. Effectiveness may also be demonstrated by sedation when used for this purpose.
Contraindicated in hypersensitivity or porphyria. Use cautiously in severe liver disease and pregnancy and lactation. Discontinue if rash develops.	Neuro: drowsiness, ataxia, vertigo, lethargy, excitement (children) CV: edema GI: nausea, anorexia, vomiting, hepatitis Hema: blood dyscrasias, megaloblastic anemia Integ: rashes, alopecia Misc: folic acid deficiency	Induces liver enzymes and may hasten metabolism and decrease the effectiveness of other drugs metabolized by the liver, including oral contraceptives, chloramphenicol, acebutolol, propranolol, metoprolol, timolol, doxycycline, glucocorticoids, tricyclic antidepressants, phenothiazines, phenylbutazones, and quinidine. Additive CNS depression when used with other CNS depressants, including alcohol, antihistamines, narcotics, and sedative/hypnotics. Concurrent use with phenobarbital may lead to phenobarbital toxicity. Decreases the absorption of folic acid.	Same as for all, plus: ASSESSMENT: Assess patient for allergy to phenobarbital. CBC should be monitored every 6 months throughout the course of therapy. Assess patient for signs of folic acid deficiency (mental dysfunction, unusual tiredness or weakness, psychiatric disorders, neuropathy, megaloblastic anemia). May be treated with folic acid. INTERVENTION: May be administered with food to minimize GI irritation. Tablets may be crushed and mixed with food or fluids for patients who have difficulty swallowing. Shake liquid preparations well before pouring. Implement seizure precautions. EVALUATION: May require a week or more of therapy before therapeutic response is seen.
Contraindicated in hypersensitivity. Cross-sensitivity with tricyclic antidepressants may exist. Should not be used in patients with bone marrow depression or a history of such reactions to drugs.	Neuro: vertigo, drowsiness, fatigue, ataxia, psychosis, diplopia, unsteadiness, hyperirritability, blurred vision, corneal opacities CV: congestive heart failure, syncope, hypertension, hypotension	Carbamazepine stimulates the hepatic metabolism of doxycycline, warfarin, oral contraceptives, and other anticonvulsants; may result in decreased effectiveness. Do not use with MAO inhibitors.	Same as for all, plus: ASSESSMENT: Monitor CBC, including platelet count, reticulocyte count, and serum iron, weekly during the first 3 months and monthly thereafter for evidence of potentially fatal

CONTINUED ON THE FOLLOWING PAGE

Table 22–4. SPECIFIC ANTICONVULSANT AGENTS–*CONTINUED*

Name	Dosage	Mode of Administration	Pharmacokinetics
IMINOSTIBENES*–Continued*			

BRANCH CHAIN CARBOXYLIC ACID
Valproate
Valproic Acid (Depakene
  capsules), Valproate
  Sodium (Depakene Syrup),
  Divalproex Sodium (Depak-
  ote Enteric-Coated Tablets)

Action: Increases levels of gamma-aminobutyric acid (GABA), an inhibitory neurotransmitter in the CNS. Therapeutic effect is suppression of absence seizures, partial seizures with complex symptomatology, myoclonic seizures, and tonic-clonic generalized seizures.

Use: Used in the treatment of simple and complex absence seizures, partial seizures, myoclonic seizures, and tonic-clonic generalized seizures.

Name	Dosage	Mode of Administration	Pharmacokinetics
	Adults and Children: Initial dose is 15 mg/kg/day, increased by 5–10 mg/kg/day at weekly intervals until therapeutic levels are reached (not to exceed 60 mg/kg/day). When dosage exceeds 250 mg, give in 2 divided doses.	PO	O: (liquid, capsule, enteric-coated tablet) 2–4 days (anticonvulsive effect) P: (liquid) 15–20 min; (capsule) 1–4 hr; (enteric-coated tablet) 2–5 hr (blood levels) D: 24 hr ½L: 5–20 hr (average 10.6 hr) PB: 80%–94% B: liver E: minimal by kidneys

SUCCINIMIDE
Ethosuximide (Zarontin)

Action: Elevates the seizure threshold by inhibiting central pathways.

Use: Used in the control of absence seizures. May also be useful in myoclonic or partial seizures (nonapproved use).

Key to Abbreviations in the *Pharmacokinetics* column O-onset; P-peak; D-duration; PB-protein bound; B-biotransformed in; E-excreted in; ½ L-halflife.
   *Within the column listing adverse effects, underlines indicate the most common effects, and CAPITALS indicate life-threatening effects.

Contraindications/ Precautions	Adverse Effects*	Interactions	Nursing Implications
Use cautiously in patients with cardiac or hepatic disease, elderly men with prostatic hypertrophy, and patients with increased intraocular pressure. Safe use in pregnancy and lactation has not been established.	Resp: pneumonitis GI: hepatitis, nausea, vomiting, dry mouth GU: hesitancy, urinary retention Hema: APLASTIC ANEMIA, AGRANULOCYTOSIS, THROMBOCYTOPENIA, leukopenia, leukocytosis, eosinophilia Integ: rashes, urticaria, photosensitivity, alteration in skin pigmentation Misc: fever, chills, lymphadenopathy, inappropriate secretion of ADH	Decreased values on thyroid function tests	blood dyscrasias. Liver function tests, eye examinations, urinalysis, and BUN should be routinely performed. INTERVENTION: Administer medication with food to minimize gastric irritation. Tablets may be crushed if patient has difficulty swallowing. Also available in chewable tablets. Do not discontinue this medication abruptly because this may precipitate seizures.
Contraindicated in hypersensitivity. Use cautiously in patients with hepatic impairment, bleeding disorders, and pregnancy and lactation.	Neuro: drowsiness, sedation, headache, dizziness, ataxia, confusion, incoordination, paresthesias, visual disturbances GI: nausea, vomiting, indigestion, HEPATOTOXICITY, pancreatitis, hypersalivation, anorexia, increased appetite, diarrhea, constipation, abdominal cramps Hema: prolonged bleeding time, blood dyscrasias Integ: rashes, alopecia Misc: hyperammonemia	May potentiate the effect of warfarin. Decreases the metabolism of barbiturates or benzodiazepines and increases their effect. Additive CNS depression with other CNS depressants, including alcohol, antihistamines, narcotics, and sedative-hypnotics. May increase or decrease the effects and toxicity of phenytoin. May potentiate the effect of MAO inhibitors and other antidepressants. Use with clonazepam may produce absence status. Increased alkaline phosphatase; false urinary glucose test; false-positive urine ketone test; prolongs bleeding time; increases liver function tests; alters thyroid function test	Same as for all, plus: ASSESSMENT: Therapeutic blood levels should be monitored periodically. Therapeutic levels are 50–100 μg/ml. INTERVENTION: Administer with or immediately after meals to minimize GI irritation. Single daily doses are usually administered at bedtime because of sedation. Capsules and enteric-coated tablets should be swallowed whole; patient should not break or chew, as this will cause irritation of the mouth and throat. Administering tablets with milk causes premature dissolution of the tablets. Implement seizure precautions.

CONTINUED ON THE FOLLOWING PAGE

Table 22–4. SPECIFIC ANTICONVULSANT AGENTS–*CONTINUED*

Name	Dosage	Mode of Administration	Pharmacokinetics
SUCCINIMIDE–*Continued*	*Adults and Children over 6 yr:* 250 mg bid initially; may be increased by 250 mg/day q 4–7 days up to 1.5 g/day given in 2 divided doses. *Children 3–6 yr:* 250 mg/day as a single dose or 20 mg/kg/day given in 2 divided doses.	PO	O: hours–days P: 4 hr (blood levels 4–7 days peak effect) D: 12–60 hr ½L: 60 hr for adults; 30 hr for children PB: minimal B: liver E: 20% by kidneys unchanged

BENZODIAZEPINE
Clonazepam (Clonopin)

Action: Produces anticonvulsant and sedative effects in the CNS. Mechanism is unknown, but it is known that benzodiazepines protentiate GABA-ergic neurotransmission in the CNS. Therapeutic effect is prevention of seizures.

Use: Used in the prophylaxis of absence and myoclonic seizures.

| | *Adults:* Initial daily dose not to exceed 1.5 mg given in 3 divided doses. May increase by 0.5–1 mg q 3 days until therapeutic levels are achieved. Total daily maintenance dose not to exceed 20 mg. *Children under 10 yr or 30 kg:* Initial daily dose 0.01–0.03 mg/kg (not to exceed 0.5 mg/kg) given in 2–3 divided doses. Increase by no more than 0.5 mg q 3 days until therapeutic levels are reached. Daily dose not to exceed 0.2 mg/kg. | PO | O: 20–60 min P: 1–2 hr D: 6–12 hr ½ L: 18–50 hr PB: UA B: liver E: urine and feces |

Key to Abbreviations in the *Pharmacokinetics* column O-onset; P-peak; D-duration; PB-protein bound; B-biotransformed in; E-excreted in; ½ L-halflife.
*Within the column listing adverse effects, underlines indicate the most common effects, and CAPITALS indicate life-threatening effects.

Contraindications/ Precautions	Adverse Effects*	Interactions	Nursing Implications
Contraindicated in hypersensitivity. Use cautiously in patients with hepatic and renal disease. Safe use has not been established in pregnancy and lactation.	Neuro: drowsiness, headaches, euphoria, irritability, hyperactivity, psychiatric disturbances, dizziness, blurred vision, inability to concentrate, anxiety, aggressiveness, restlessness, ataxia, increased frequency of generalized seizures. GI: anorexia, gastric upset, nausea, vomiting, cramping, weight loss, diarrhea, hiccups GU: vaginal bleeding Hema: APLASTIC ANEMIA, AGRANULOCYTOSIS, leukopenia, eosinophilia Integ: urticaria, rashes, hirsutism Misc: allergic reactions, including STEVENS-JOHNSON SYNDROME	Additive CNS depression with other CNS depressants, including alcohol, antihistamines, narcotics, and sedative-hypnotics. Valproic acid inhibits the metabolism of ethosuximide. False-positive direct Coombs' test.	Same as for all, plus: ASSESSMENT: Assess patient's mood, behavior patterns, and facial expressions. Patients with a history of psychiatric disorders have an increased risk of developing behavioral changes. These symptoms may necessitate withdrawal of the medication. INTERVENTION: Administer with food or fluids to minimize GI irritation. Available in capsules and liquid preparations. Implement seizure precautions.
Contraindicated in patients with severe hepatic disease and those who are hypersensitive to clonazepam or other benzodiazepines. Use cautiously in patients with narrow-angle glaucoma or chronic respiratory disease. Safe use in pregnancy and lactation has not been established.	Neuro: drowsiness, ataxia, hypotonia, behavioral changes, abnormal eye movement, diplopia, nystagmus CV: palpitations Resp: increased respiratory secretions GI: constipation, diarrhea, hepatitis GU: dysuria, nocturia, urinary retention Hema: blood dyscrasias Misc: fever	Additive CNS depression with other CNS depressants, including alcohol, antihistamines, narcotics, and sedative-hypnotics. May increase serum phenytoin levels. Phenytoin may decrease serum clonazepam levels.	Same as for all, plus: ASSESSMENT: Observe and record intensity, duration, and location of seizure activity. Assess patient for drowsiness, unsteadiness, and clumsiness. These symptoms are dose-related and are most severe during initial therapy; may decrease in severity or disappear with continued or long-term therapy. Prolonged high-dose therapy may lead to psychological or physical dependence. Restrict amount of drug available to patient. INTERVENTION: Administer with food to minimize gastric irritation. Tablets may be crushed if patient has difficulty swallowing. Institute seizure precautions for patients on initial therapy or undergoing dosage manipulations. EVALUATION: Dosage adjustments may be required after several months of therapy.

Table 22–5. COMMONLY USED ANTICONVULSANT DRUGS—SERUM CONCENTRATIONS AND SIGNS/SYMPTOMS OF TOXICITY

Drug	Average Daily Maintenance Dose		Signs and Symptoms Usually Associated with Elevated Serum Concentrations or Toxicity of Cited Drugs	Usual Therapeutic Serum Concentration Range (μg/ml)
	Adults (mg/kg)	Children (mg/kg)		
Carbamazepine (Tegretol)	10–20	20–30	Vertigo, lethargy, nystagmus, blurred vision, diplopia, confusion, ataxia, stupor	4–12
Clonazepam (Clonopin)	0.05–0.2	0.1–0.2	Sedation, confusion, slurred speech, somnolence, respiratory depression, coma, hypotension	0.02–0.08
Ethosuximide (Zarontin)	20–40	20–30	Nausea, vomiting, gastric distress, drowsiness, ataxia	40–100
Phenobarbital	2–3	3–5	Sedation, drowsiness, slurred speech, nystagmus, confusion, somnolence, ataxia, respiratory depression, coma, hypotension	15–40
Primidone (Mysoline)	10–25	10–25	Same as phenobarbital.	5–21
Phenytoin (Dilantin)	3–5	4–7	Vertigo, ataxia, slurred speech, nystagmus, diplopia, somnolence, coma (arrhythmias with rapid intravenous administration)	10–20
Valproic acid (Depakene, Depakote)	15–30 (monotherapy); 30–45 (combination therapy)	20–30 (monotherapy); 40–60 (combination therapy)	Sedation, gastric disturbance, diarrhea, ataxia, somnolence, coma	50–100

(American Medical Association: Drug Evaluations: Antiepileptic Drugs. 6th Ed. Chicago: American Medical Association, 1986, with permission.)

Phenytoin also increases the rate of clearance of theophylline and lidocaine. The effectiveness of these agents is diminished.

The interactions between folic acid and phenytoin are complex. Phenytoin is an inhibitor of folic acid absorption from the gut and an inducer of folic acid metabolism. See Table 22–6 for a review of anticonvulsant interactions.

Drug–Laboratory Interactions. Phenytoin inhibits thyrotropin releasing hormone-induced thyroid-stimulating hormone release. The result is a decreased serum T_4 concentration. Phenytoin also lowers the values for dexamethasone tests. It is reported that phenytoin increases liver function tests (alkaline phosphatase, alanine aminotransferase, phosphate, and prothrombin time). There may be a lowered value on metapyrone tests. There have been reports that urine pregnancy tests are altered and that false-positive and false-negative results occur. There have been some reports that phenytoin changes the color of urine (pink, red, red-brown) in the presence of an acid urinary pH; however, this has not been confirmed.

CONGENERS OF PHENYTOIN. The other three types of hydantoins are mephenytoin (Mesantoin), ethotoin (Peganone), and phenacemide (Phenurone). These agents are very similar to phenytoin, but they are not used as frequently as phenytoin. Mephenytoin and phenacemide are more toxic than phenytoin, while ethotoin has a very low efficacy.

BARBITURATES

Actions

The exact mechanism of action of the barbiturates is unknown. Phenobarbital inhibits the spread of seizure activity from a focus by increasing the threshold for neuronal firing. It might also enhance GABA-ergic inhibition. It is also thought that phenobarbital reduces the excitatory effects of glutamate.

Uses

Phenobarbital is effective in the treatment of generalized and partial seizures. It is an alternative in the treatment of status epilepticus, and it is used in the treatment

Table 22–6. SOME ANTICONVULSANT INTERACTIONS*

Interacting Drugs	Adverse Effects (Probable Mechanism)	Comments and Recommendations
***Carbamazepine,* with:** Phenytoin	Decreased carbamazepine effect (increased metabolism) Altered phenytoin effect (mechanism not established)	Monitor carbamazepine and phenytoin concentrations; both increased and decreased phenytoin concentrations have been reported.
Primidone	Decreased primidone effect and increased phenobarbital effect (increased conversion of primidone to phenobarbital)	Monitor primidone and phenobarbital concentrations.
Valproate	Decreased valproate effect (increased metabolism)	Monitor valproate concentration.
***Clonazepam,* with:** Phenobarbital	Decreased clonazepam effect (increased metabolism)	Monitor clonazepam concentration.
Phenytoin	Decreased clonazepam effect (increased metabolism) Variable effect on phenytoin concentration (mechanism not established)	Monitor clonazepam and phenytoin concentrations.
Valproate	Clonazepam may precipitate absence status (mechanism not established)	Avoid concurrent use.
***Diazepam,* with:** Valproate	Increased IV diazepam effect (displacement from binding and decreased metabolism)	Use IV diazepam with caution.
***Ethosuximide,* with:** Valproate	Possible increased ethosuximide effect (decreased metabolism)	Highly variable, clinical significance not established; monitor ethosuximide concentration.
***Phenobarbital,* with:** Clonazepam	Decreased clonazepam effect (increased metabolism)	Monitor clonazepam concentration.
Valproate	Increased phenobarbital effect (decreased metabolism)	Monitor phenobarbital concentration.
***Phenytoin,* with:** Carbamazepine	Decreased carbamazepine effect (increased metabolism) Altered phenytoin effect (mechanism not established)	Monitor carbamazepine and phenytoin concentrations; both increased and decreased phenytoin concentrations have been reported.
Clonazepam	Decreased clonazepam effect (increased metabolism) Variable effect on phenytoin concentration (mechanism not established)	Monitor clonazepam and phenytoin concentrations.
Primidone	Decreased primidone effect and increased phenobarbital effect (increased conversion of primidone to phenobarbital)	Monitor primidone and phenobarbital concentrations.

CONTINUED ON THE FOLLOWING PAGE

Table 22–6. SOME ANTICONVULSANT INTERACTIONS–*CONTINUED*

Interacting Drugs	Adverse Effects (Probable Mechanism)	Comments and Recommendations
Valproate	Increased phenytoin toxicity (displacement from binding)	Conflicting reports; monitor phenytoin concentration and clinical status.
Primidone, with: Carbamazepine	Decreased primidone effect and increased phenobarbital effect (increased conversion of primidone to phenobarbital)	Monitor primidone and phenobarbital concentrations.
Phenytoin	Decreased primidone effect and increased phenobarbital effect (increased conversion of primidone to phenobarbital)	Monitor primidone and phenobarbital concentrations.
Valproate, with: Carbamazepine	Decreased valproate effect (increased metabolism)	Monitor valproate concentration.
Clonazepam	Clonazepam may precipitate absence status (mechanism not established)	Avoid concurrent use.
Diazepam	Increased IV diazepam effect (displacement from binding and decreased metabolism)	Give IV diazepam with caution.
Ethosuximide	Possible increased ethosuximide effect (decreased metabolism)	Highly variable; clinical significance not established; monitor ethosuximide concentration.
Phenobarbital	Increased phenobarbital effect (decreased metabolism)	Monitor phenobarbital concentration.
Phenytoin	Increased phenytoin toxicity (displacement from binding)	Conflicting reports; monitor phenytoin concentration and clinical status.

*For interactions of anticonvulsants with other drugs, see the most recent edition of The Medical Letter Handbook of Adverse Drug Interactions.
From Abramowicz, M (ed.): The Medical Letter on Drugs and Therapeutics. 28:723, 1986, with permission.

of febrile seizures in infants and children. It is used in situations where sedation is necessary (preoperative sedation or hypnotic). Other uses include the prevention and treatment of neonatal hyperbilirubinemia and lowering bilirubin and lipid levels in chronic cholestasis.

Pharmacokinetics

Phenobarbital is absorbed following oral administration. Between 40% and 60% of phenobarbital is bound to plasma proteins. Phenobarbital is metabolized by microsomal enzymes. It is considered to be an enzyme-inducing drug. The primary metabolite is p-hydroxyphenobarbital. About 25% of a dose of phenobarbital is excreted by the kidneys. Phenobarbital has a long half-life of three to four days in children and five to six days in adults.

The onset of action for an oral dose of phenobarbital is 30–60 minutes. When administered by the subcutaneous and intramuscular routes, the onset of action is 10–30 minutes. When given intravenously, the onset of action is five minutes. The peak action is unknown when administered by the oral, subcutaneous, and intramuscular routes; the intravenous route achieves a peak action in 30 minutes. The duration of action varies from more than six hours when given orally, to four to six hours when given subcutaneously, intramuscularly, and intravenously.

Contraindications and Precautions

Phenobarbital is contraindicated in persons with hypersensitivity. It should not be used in comatose patients, those with pre-existing CNS depression, or in patients with acute porphyria.

Phenobarbital is used cautiously in patients who have hepatic dysfunction or severe renal impairment. These agents are metabolized in the liver and excreted to an extent by the kidneys. This could lead to poor seizure control or toxicity of barbiturates. These agents should be used cautiously in pregnant patients. The possibility of congenital malformations or coagulation defect and hemorrhage in the newborn exists. Nursing infants must be monitored for excessive sedation since phenobarbital concentrations in milk may exceed those in maternal plasma. Dosage may need to be reduced in the elderly and children due to their high susceptibility to CNS adverse effects.

Adverse Reactions

The major adverse effect of the barbiturates is neurotoxicity. This is due to the depressive effect that the barbiturates have on the brain. The side effects include cognitive and behavioral manifestations. Children and the elderly are the most susceptible to these effects. These signs and symptoms include drowsiness, depression, inattention, impaired memory, confusion, excitation, delirium, ataxia, and nystagmus. Since barbiturates depress the brain stem, respiratory depression can be seen, especially with high doses. Tolerance can develop after long-term therapy.

Another group of adverse reactions are skin rashes. These rashes are *scarlatiniform* or *morbilliform* in nature. These rashes are thought to be an allergic reaction to these agents, and discontinuation of the drug should be considered.

There are some hematologic adverse reactions reported with the use of phenobarbital. These include megaloblastic anemia, osteomalacia, and hypoprothrombinemia with hemorrhage in the newborn. The causes of these adverse reactions are the same as for phenytoin.

Drug Concentration

A precise relationship between therapeutic results and concentration of phenobarbital in plasma does not exist, but it is recommended that serum levels be monitored and serve as a guideline for treatment. For the control of seizures, plasma levels of 10–25 μg/ml are recommended. For the prophylaxis of febrile seizures, 15 μg/ml is the minimum level. Levels higher than 60 μg/ml may be associated with marked toxicity (see Table 22–5).

Drug Interactions

Additive depressive effects are seen when barbiturates are administered with other CNS depressants such as alcohol. Concurrent use of barbiturates and other CNS depressants can lead to drowsiness, lethargy, stupor, respiratory depression, coma, and death. Mental dullness, nystagmus, and staggering gait are signs of toxicity.

An increase in the phenobarbital serum level is reported with monoamine oxidase (MAO) inhibitors, propoxyphene, and valproic acid. The mechanism for this phenomenon is enzyme inhibition.

Phenobarbital has been known to decrease serum levels and to interfere with therapeutic effectiveness of certain drugs. This is due to the inducing effect phenobarbital has on drug-metabolizing enzymes. The drugs affected by phenobarbital are oral anticoagulants, tricyclic antidepressants, beta blockers, chloramphenicol, corticosteroids, estrogens in oral contraceptives, metha-

done, phenothiazine tranquilizers, quinidine, doxycycline, cimetidine, theophylline, and metronidazole. See Table 22–6 for phenobarbital's interaction with other anticonvulsants.

DEOXYBARBITURATES

Primidone

ACTION. Primidone (Mysoline) is chemically related to phenobarbital. The exact mechanism of action is unknown but may be similar to that of phenobarbital.

USES. Primidone is used for the treatment of all seizures except absence seizures. Some reports indicate that primidone is especially useful in the management of partial seizures. Primidone may be used concurrently with phenytoin or carbamazepine.

PHARMACOKINETICS. Primidone is rapidly absorbed after oral administration. It is widely distributed and crosses the placenta and enters breast milk. This agent is metabolized in the liver, where it is converted to the inactive metabolites phenobarbital and PEMA (phenylethylmalonamide). Primidone and PEMA are bound to plasma proteins to a small extent. About 40% of this agent is excreted in the urine. The half-life of primidone is 7–14 hours, and the half-life of PEMA is 16 hours.

The onset of action after oral administration is four to seven days. The peak action occurs in seven to ten days, and the duration of action is eight to twelve hours.

CONTRAINDICATIONS AND PRECAUTIONS. Primidone is contraindicated in patients with hypersensitivity or porphyria. This agent, like the barbiturates, exerts depressive effects on the brain. This drug should be used with caution in patients who have liver disease. In such patients, the dose will have to be adjusted, because the liver is the site of metabolism for this drug. Safe use in pregnancy and lactation has not been established. The use of this agent with pregnancy can result in hemorrhage in the newborn.

ADVERSE REACTIONS. The most common adverse reactions are caused by the depressive effects of primidone on the brain. Signs and symptoms of adverse reactions include sedation, vertigo, dizziness, ataxia, diplopia, nystagmus, and an acute feeling of intoxication. These adverse reactions are a result of the parent drug and its two metabolites (phenobarbital and PEMA).

Other side effects include nausea and vomiting. These gastrointestinal manifestations disappear as therapy continues or if the agent is taken with food.

As with other anticonvulsant agents, a maculopapular and morbilliform rash can occur. If this rash occurs, it is viewed as a drug allergy and the drug is discontinued.

Hematologic adverse reactions include leukopenia, thrombocytopenia, systemic lupus erythematosus, lymphadenopathy, hemorrhagic disease in the newborn, megaloblastic anemia, and osteomalacia. The mechanism of action is similar to that of phenytoin.

DRUG CONCENTRATIONS. Plasma concentrations greater than 12 μg/ml are associated with significant toxic side effects. Phenobarbital, at steady state, varies from 15–30 μg/ml. Doses of 10–20 mg/kg/day are necessary to maintain these levels. It is important to remember that the parent drug reaches its steady state in 40 hours, while the steady state of the active metabolites is reached in 4–20 days.

DRUG INTERACTIONS. Phenytoin increases the conversion of primidone to phenobarbital. Isoniazid may cause a decrease in the conversion of primidone to phenobarbital and PEMA. Other drug interactions are the same as those for phenobarbital (See Table 22–6).

IMINOSTILBENES

Carbamazepine

ACTIONS. Carbamazepine (Tegretol) acts by reducing polysynaptic responses and blocking the *post-tetanic potentiation*. The exact mechanism of action is unknown. This agent has the capacity to increase discharge of noradrenergic neurons, which may contribute to its antiepileptic actions.

USES. Carbamazepine is used for the treatment of partial, mixed, and generalized seizures. It is not used for absence seizures. This agent is also used for the management of pain associated with trigeminal and glossopharyngeal neuralgia.

PHARMACOKINETICS. Absorption is slow following oral administration. This agent is distributed to all tissues. About 75% of this agent is bound to plasma proteins. Carbamazepine is metabolized in the liver, and its metabolites are excreted in the urine. Since carbamazepine may induce its own metabolism, the half-life is variable. The average range for the half-life of this agent is 10–20 hours with repeated doses. Concurrent administration with either phenobarbital or phenytoin will reduce the half-life to nine to ten hours.

This agent is available for oral administration only. The onset of anticonvulsant activity is two to four days. Peak serum levels are achieved in two to eight hours. The duration of action is 6–12 hours.

CONTRAINDICATIONS AND PRECAUTIONS. This agent is contraindicated in persons with hypersensitivity to this agent or tricyclic compounds. This agent is structurally related to tricyclic compounds. Carbamazepine should not be used in persons with a history of bone marrow depression. Serious and sometimes fatal abnormalities of blood cells have occurred with use of carbamazepine. Concurrent use of MAO inhibitors is not recommended. Carbamazepine inhibits the uptake and release of norepinephrine from brain synapses. Patients with liver or kidney dysfunction should be monitored closely for toxic effects, because this agent is metabolized in the liver and excreted in the urine.

This drug is recommended for patients whose seizures are difficult to control or those experiencing marked side effects from other agents. Carbamazepine has some anticholinergic properties, so patients with glaucoma should be monitored closely. Carbamazepine should be used with caution in patients with mixed seizures, because an increased frequency of generalized seizures have occurred with this agent. The elderly and children are potentially at risk for developing cognitive and behavioral reactions to this drug (latent psychosis in elderly on other tricyclic agents), and dosage may need to be reduced. Carbamazepine should be used with caution in patients with cardiac disease. There may be retention of water along with decreased osmolality and concentration of sodium in plasma. This effect is due to the inappropriate secretion of antidiuretic hormone (*ADH*). Safe use in pregnancy and lactation has not been established. Carbamazepine does appear in breast milk, and there is potential for adverse reaction for nursing infants. This agent should also be used with caution by persons who have to be mentally or physically active, because drowsiness, dizziness, and unsteadiness can occur. Patients should be cautioned about the hazards of operating machinery or performing other dangerous tasks.

ADVERSE REACTIONS. Early adverse reactions are related to the depressive and anticholinergic effects of carbamazepine on the CNS. These reactions include drowsiness, fatigue, vertigo, unsteadiness, ataxia, diplopia, hyperirritability, and psychosis. Starting this agent at a low dosage can minimize these reactions.

Gastrointestinal reactions can also occur early in treatment with carbamazepine. These include nausea, vomiting, dry mouth, and hepatitis. Dry mouth is due to the anticholinergic properties of the drug, while the other reactions are idiosyncrasies of the drug.

The most severe reactions to this drug affect the skin and cardiovascular and hematologic systems. Frequent skin reactions include rashes, urticaria, photosensitivity, and alteration in skin pigmentation. More rarely, severe reactions that have been reported with the use of carbamazepine include epidermal necrosis and Stevens-Johnson syndrome. These reactions signal hypersensitivity and are difficult to predict.

The reactions of the cardiovascular system include congestive heart failure, syncope, hypertension, and hypotension. Some of these reactions are made worse by the hyponatremia and water retention that result from the inappropriate secretion of ADH.

The last group of major reactions involves the hematologic system. The mechanisms responsible for these adverse reactions are unknown and may be idiosyncratic. These reactions include aplastic anemia, agranulocytosis, thrombocytopenia, leukopenia, leukocytosis, and eosinophilia. Monitoring the complete blood count (CBC), platelet and reticulocyte counts, and serum iron level are essential, but the patient should be instructed to report early toxic signs and symptoms of hematologic dysfunction (e.g., fever, sore throat, ulcers in the mouth, easy bruising, petechial or purpuric hemorrhage).

DRUG CONCENTRATIONS. As with the other anticonvulsants, monitoring of the drug level of carbamazepine is important for management. This is particularly important when multiple drugs are being used concurrently. The usual therapeutic level of carbamazepine ranges from 4–12 μg/ml for adults. It must be remembered that these levels are variable and should serve as a guideline. CNS side effects are seen with levels above 9 μg/ml (see Table 22–5).

DRUG INTERACTIONS. Concurrent administration of carbamazepine with phenobarbital, phenytoin, or primidone or any combination of these agents causes lowering of serum levels of carbamazepine. Carbamazepine is an enzyme inducer, and the above drugs are also enzyme inducers.

Carbamazepine decreases the serum levels of warfarin, doxycycline, theophylline, and haloperidol. Since carbamazepine is an enzyme inducer, it speeds up the metabolism of these agents.

Therapeutic agents such as erythromycin, desipramine, isoniazid, cimetidine, propoxyphene, and calcium channel blockers raise serum carbamazepine levels, resulting in toxicity. Carbamazepine's metabolism is inhibited by these agents.

Dangerous interactions have occurred between tricyclic antidepressants and MAO inhibitors. Since carbamazepine is related to tricyclic agents, the potential for these interactions exists.

BRANCH CHAIN CARBOXYLIC ACID

Valproic Acid

ACTION. Valproic acid is a branch chain carboxylic acid agent that was approved for use in the United States in 1978. The exact mechanism of action is unknown. It is postulated that valproic acid has an effect on the enzymes necessary for either the production or breakdown of the inhibitory neurotransmitter GABA.

USES. Valproic acid is very effective for treatment of a variety of seizures. It is the drug of choice for absence seizures. It is also effective in treating myoclonic seizures, generalized tonic-clonic seizures, and atonic attacks. Valproic acid is less effective with partial seizures.

PHARMACOKINETICS. Valproic acid is well absorbed following an oral dose. There is a delay in absorption when the drug is taken with food. It is distributed mainly in the extracellular water. Ninety percent of valproic acid is bound to proteins, and it is highly ionized. Most of the drug is converted to the conjugate glycuronic acid, with mitochondrial metabolism (β-oxidation). Other metabolites are 2-propyl-2-pentanoic acid and 2-propyl-3-oxopentanoic acid. These metabolites also have anticonvulsant activity. About 3% of valproic acid is excreted unchanged in the urine and feces. The half-life is 15 hours, which can be reduced in patients taking other antiepileptic drugs.

Valproic acid can only be administered orally, either as a tablet or liquid. The onset of action for the liquid, capsules, and enteric-coated tablet is two to four days. The peak action for the liquid is 15–20 minutes; for the capsule, one to four hours; and for the enteric-coated tablet, two to five hours. The duration of action for the liquid is 24 hours; for the capsule, 24 hours; and for the enteric-coated tablet, 24 hours.

CONTRAINDICATIONS AND PRECAUTIONS. Valproic acid is contraindicated in hypersensitivity. This agent should be used cautiously in patients with hepatic impairment or bleeding disorders. The drug is metabolized in the liver, and liver impairment can alter metabolism of this drug. Valproic acid prolongs bleeding time by inhibiting platelet aggregation. Safe use has not been established in pregnancy and lactation. Concurrent administration with phenobarbital or clonazepam causes sedation.

ADVERSE REACTIONS. The most common side effects of the valproates are gastrointestinal disturbances. These effects include nausea, vomiting, indigestion, hepatotoxicity, pancreatitis, hypersalivation, anorexia, increased appetite, diarrhea, abdominal cramps, and constipation. These gastrointestinal effects can be minimized by administering the drug with food and by beginning therapy with a low dose. The increase in appetite is thought to be secondary to the GABA-enhancing effects. The hepatotoxicity may be an idiosyncratic reaction rather than a dose-related event. Hepatic biopsy in fatal cases reveals centrilobular necrosis and severe fatty changes in the liver. The site of injury appears to be the biosecretory apparatus, canaliculi, and ducts of Hering.

CNS depressive effects are less severe for the valproates than for other anticonvulsant agents. Side effects include drowsiness, sedation, headache, dizziness, ataxia, incoordination, confusion, and visual disturbances.

Hematologic reactions include thrombocytopenia and hemorrhage. These reactions are secondary to the inhibition of the secondary phase of platelet aggregation. Thrombocytopenia may also be due to an autoimmune mechanism. There have also been reports of hyperammonemia with administration of the valproates. The cause for this is the inhibiton of enzymes involved in intermediate cell metabolism. This reaction has appeared with hepatic dysfunction.

Other reactions that occur infrequently are rashes and alopecia. These are reversible side effects, and the cause may be idiosyncratic.

DRUG CONCENTRATION. Therapeutic values of valproic acid range from 50–100 μg/ml. Individual doses may fall anywhere within this range for seizure control. Some patients may require and tolerate levels in excess of 100 μg/ml. Again, this therapeutic range should be used as a guideline. The clearance of valproic acid is dose dependent, due to the changes in clearance and protein binding. At a low dose, valproic acid inhibits its own metabolism, decreasing the intrinsic clearance. At higher doses, there is more free valproic acid, resulting in lower serum levels. It is useful to measure the total and free drug levels (See Table 22–5).

DRUG INTERACTIONS. *Drug–Drug.* Valproic acid displaces phenytoin from its plasma proteins, interfering with its metabolism (which increases valproic acid metabolism). It also inhibits the metabolism of phenobarbital, carbamazepine, ethosuximide, and benzodiazepines, which causes excessive sedation (see Table 22–6). Use with clonazepam may cause absence status.

Drug–Laboratory. The use of valproic acid has modified several laboratory tests. These include increased alkaline phosphatase, false-positive urinary glucose test, false-positive urine ketone test, prolonged bleeding time, and elevated liver function tests.

SUCCINIMIDES

Ethosuximide (Zarontin), Methsuximide (Celontin), and Phensuximide (Milontin)

ACTIONS. The mechanism of action of succinimides is unknown, but it is related to enhancement of central inhibitory pathways.

USES. Succinimides are useful in the treatment of absence seizures. Ethosuximide is the drug of choice because methsuximide is more toxic and phensuximide is less effective in controlling seizures. Methsuximide and phensuximide are active against electroshock seizures and are also used to treat partial seizures.

PHARMACOKINETICS. The succinimides are well absorbed after oral administration. Ethosuximide is well distributed throughout tissues but does not penetrate fat. It is not protein-bound. The succinimides are metabolized by the liver through hydroxylation. About 25% of the drug is excreted unchanged in the urine. The major metabolite of methsuximide is a parahydroxyphenyl derivative. The major metabolite of phensuximide is an N-dimethyl derivative. The half-life of ethosuximide is 40–50 hours in adults and 30 hours in children. The half-life of methsuximide is less than two hours, while the half-life of phensuximide is eight hours.

Ethosuximide is available for oral administration. The onset of action is one to two hours. The peak concentration is obtained within three hours of an oral dose.

CONTRAINDICATIONS AND PRECAUTIONS. The succinimides are contraindicated in persons with a history of hypersensitivity to succinimide drugs, and another drug should be selected.

These medications should be withdrawn gradually to avoid the precipitation of absence seizure. Ethosuximide has not been proven safe for use during pregnancy and lactation. The presence of behavioral alterations is a reason to withdraw ethosuximide slowly. Since ethosuximide is metabolized in the liver and excreted from the kidneys, caution should be used when administering the drug to patients with hepatic or renal dysfunction.

ADVERSE REACTIONS. The most common side effects of the succinimides are gastrointestinal disturbances and CNS effects. The gastrointestinal reactions include anorexia, gastric upset (epigastric pain), nausea, vomiting, cramping, weight loss, diarrhea, and hiccups. The CNS effects include drowsiness, headaches, euphoria, irritability, hyperactivity, dizziness, blurred vision, inability to concentrate, aggressiveness, anxiety, and restlessness. The exact cause of complaints is unknown.

Some hematologic reactions have also been reported. These include aplastic anemia, agranulocytosis, leukopenia, and eosinophilia. These may be idiosyncratic reactions.

DRUG CONCENTRATIONS. The plateau state is reached in about 4–6 days in children and in a longer period for adults. A serum level of 40–100 μg/ml is recommended for control of absence seizures (see Table 22–5).

INTERACTIONS. Valproic acid inhibits the metabolism of ethosuximide (see Table 22–6). The concurrent use of CNS depressants causes additive CNS depression.

OXAZOLIDINEDIONES

Trimethadione (Tridione) and Paramethadione (Paradione)

ACTIONS. Trimethadione increases the after-discharge threshold in the cortex. This affects presynaptic and postsynaptic inhibition in synapses that utilize GABA as a neurotransmitter.

USES. Trimethadione was previously the agent of choice for absence seizures, but it has been replaced by newer agents such as ethosuximide and valproic acid. Trimethadione is mentioned because of its historical importance; it was the first agent to be used to treat absence seizures.

PHARMACOKINETICS. The oxazolidinediones are rapidly absorbed from the gastrointestinal tract. They are distributed to the tissues and are not bound to plasma proteins. They are metabolized by hepatic microsomal enzymes to the metabolite dimethadione. Excretion is via the kidneys. The half-life of the oxazolidinediones is 6–13 days.

CONTRAINDICATIONS AND PRECAUTIONS. These agents are contraindicated in persons who are hypersensitive to the oxazolidinediones. They should be used with caution in persons with a history of hepatic or renal dysfunction. The oxazolidinediones are metabolized in the liver and excreted by the kidney.

ADVERSE REACTIONS. The major dose-related adverse reaction of the oxazolidinediones is sedation. Another CNS side effect is *hemeralopia*. Both of these reactions are due to the CNS depression that occurs with use of these drugs.

Some idiosyncratic reactions of trimethadione are rashes, exfoliative dermatitis, blood dyscrasias, hepatitis, reversible nephrotic syndrome, and myasthenic syndrome. The causes of these reactions are not known.

DRUG CONCENTRATIONS. The exact therapeutic levels of trimethadione have not been established. It is thought that serum levels over 20 μg/ml and dimethadione levels over 700 μg/ml are acceptable.

INTERACTIONS. Very few interactions have been reported for trimethadione. Like other anticonvulsant agents, it can act as a competitive inhibitor.

BENZODIAZEPINES

Diazepam (Valium), Lorazepam (Ativan), Clonazepam (Clonopin), and Clorazepate Dipotassium (Tranxene)

ACTION. The benzodiazepines potentiate GABA-ergic neurotransmission at various levels of the brain and spinal cord. These receptor areas include the spinal cord, hypothalamus, hippocampus, substantia nigra, cerebellar cortex, and cerebral cortex. The efficiency of GABA-ergic synaptic inhibition (which leads to decreased firing rate of neurons) is enhanced with use of the benzodiazepines. There is also an increase in the chloride channel opening in the presence of benzodiazepines. These agents have broad antiepileptic properties.

USES. Clonazepam and clorazepate have been approved for the treatment of absence and myoclonic seizures. Clorazepate is used concurrently with other anticonvulsant agents for treatment of partial seizures. Diazepam is currently used for treatment of epilepticus, while lorazepam is under investigation for the treatment of status epilepticus. The other uses of the benzodiazepines are relief of anxiety, hypnosis, preoperative sedation, balanced anesthesia, control of withdrawal states, muscle relaxation, and diagnostic aids or treatment in psychiatry.

PHARMACOKINETICS. The benzodiazepines are well absorbed following oral administration. Lipid solubility plays a major role in determining the rate at which the drug enters the CNS. Diazepam is more lipid soluble than lorazepam; therefore, the CNS effect of the latter drug may be slower in onset. From the brain, the redistribution is from highly perfuse tissues to adipose tissue. The extent of protein binding correlates with lipid solubility. The benzodiazepines are metabolized in the liver. The biotransformation follows two pathways: microsomal oxidation and conjugation by glucuronyl transferases to form glucuronides. These metabolites are excreted in the urine. The major active metabolite, desmethyldiazepam, has long-lasting CNS effects. Its half-life is 40–140 hours. Desmethyldiazepam is the active metabolite of diazepam and clorazepate. The half-life of diazepam (Valium) is 20–70 hours; clonazepam (Lonopin), 18–50 hours; clorazepate (Tranxene), 48 hours; and lorazepam (Ativan), 10–20 hours.

CONTRAINDICATIONS AND PRECAUTIONS. The benzodiazepines are contraindicated in hypersensitivity. These agents should not be used in patients with severe liver disease because the liver is the site of metabolism of these agents.

The benzodiazepines should be used cautiously in patients with narrow-angle glaucoma, respiratory disease, renal insufficiency, and acute intermittent porphyria. The benzodiazepines can cause pupillary dilation and increased intraocular pressure, so caution is necessary with use in patients with narrow-angle glaucoma. It is reported that some of the benzodiazepines (clonazepam) produce an increase in salivation and respiratory depression. Since the benzodiazepines are excreted via the kidney, patients with renal insufficiency should be monitored closely while they are receiving any of these drugs. Seizure management is difficult in patients with acute intermittent porphyria. Many of the anticonvulsants induce aminolevulinic acid (ALA) synthetase and cytochrome p-450, resulting in further overproduction of heme precursors and exacerbation of the underlying disease.

Patients can develop a tolerance to the benzodiazepines with long-term therapy. As with other anticonvulsants, the abrupt withdrawal of clonazepam may precipitate status epilepticus. Safe use in pregnancy and lactation has not been established.

The benzodiazepines should be used with caution with other CNS depressants. Additive CNS depression can occur with respiratory depression. Patients on concurrent therapy need close monitoring.

ADVERSE REACTIONS. The major side effects of the benzodiazepines occur secondary to CNS depression. In ambulatory patients, low doses tend to lead to drowsiness, impaired judgment, and diminished motor skills. Signs and symptoms of CNS effects include drowsiness, somnolence, fatigue, lethargy, ataxia, dizziness, dysarthria, and behavioral disturbances (e.g., aggression, hyperactivity, irritability, difficulty in concentrating). Confusion in the elderly has been seen, which is reversible. It is important to recognize this in the elderly so that the dose can be lowered or slowly discontinued.

Cardiovascular and respiratory depression can occur after the intravenous administration of diazepam, clonazepam, or lorazepam, especially if other anticonvulsants or CNS depressants have been administered concurrently. Diazepam can be administered as an intravenous bolus or drip. If a bolus is given to adults, the dosage is 5–10 mg at a rate of 1 ml (5 mg) per minute. The dose can be repeated at five- to ten-minute intervals, but should not exceed 30 mg. The dose for children five years of age or older is 1 mg every two to five minutes, but should not exceed 10 mg. For intravenous drip, 100 mg of diazepam is added to 500 ml of 5% dextrose in water and is given at a rate of 40 ml/hour.

DRUG INTERACTIONS. The most frequent interactions involving the benzodiazepines occur with other CNS depressants, which leads to additive CNS depression. Some of these CNS depressants include alcoholic beverages, narcotic analgesics, other anticonvulsants, phenothiazines, antihistamines, and other sedative-hypnotic drugs.

Cimetidine exerts an enzyme-inhibiting action that doubles the elimination half-life of diazepam. The exact mechanism of action is poorly understood.

USING THE NURSING PROCESS

Nurses play a vital role in the care of the patient with seizures. The nurse has continuous interactions with the patient and is in a unique position to recognize abnormal behavior patterns, to witness the seizure, and to assess and monitor the postseizure behavior. The nurse has the opportunity to plan care for the patient when he/she is in the hospital and to establish a teaching plan that can assist the patient/family in planning for normal life.

ASSESSMENT

It is important to obtain a nursing history. Since alteration in consciousness often accompanies a seizure, information about patient activities prior to, during, and after the seizure may be obtained from family or friends. If the patient can remember events prior to, during, or after a seizure, then it is important to obtain the data from him or her.

It is important to establish a trend of the patient's behavior in the time prior to a seizure as well as during and after the seizure. Nursing observation plays a critical role in seizure management. Many times these observations aid the physician in diagnosing the type of seizures the patient experiences. Nursing assessment and documentation during the *ictal and postictal* periods should include the following pertinent information: data related to the precipitating event, presence of an *aura*, body area where seizure activity starts, progression of the seizure (i.e., leg jerking, lip smacking, grimacing, talking, etc.), length of time the seizure lasts, alterations in consciousness, duration of alterations in consciousness, eye movement during ictal and postictal periods, presence of tongue biting, incontinence, periods of apnea or cyanosis, head deviations, falls, behavior changes, motor weakness/paralysis, *aphasia*, and headache.

The process of diagnosis of uncontrolled seizure activity is a very difficult time for the patient and family. It is important to assess the impact of this event on the patient's psyche. It is essential to establish an effective nurse–patient relationship so that the patient feels free to discuss his/her feelings about the seizures or about his/her treatment plan. The patient's approval of and cooperation in the treatment plan are essential to successful management of the seizures. See Table 22–7 for a summary of assessment parameters for the patient receiving anticonvulsant therapy.

NURSING DIAGNOSIS

Once the nurse has compiled the data related to assessment parameters, a nursing diagnosis is formulated. Once the nursing diagnosis has been made, the nurse plans appropriate nursing interventions for the patient. See Table 22–7 for specific nursing diagnoses for the patient receiving anticonvulsant therapy.

NURSING INTERVENTION

Goals for nursing intervention are developed from a nursing diagnosis. See Table 22–7 for specific goals of intervention related to anticonvulsant therapy. The patient with seizures is managed medically with specific agents that are designed to control the seizures or with surgical intervention. It is beyond the scope of this chapter to discuss surgical interventions. Santilli and Sierzant (1987) give an excellent review of the surgical management and nursing intervention of the seizure patient.

Assessment is an ongoing part of the management of the seizure patient. Other nursing measures center on the medication regimen, seizure precautions, and the psychosocial needs of the patient. Anticonvulsant agents can be administered with food to minimize gastric distress. If the patient has difficulty swallowing pills, then other options are available. Many anticonvulsant agents are available in liquid, chewable tablet, capsule, and intravenous forms. Capsules can be opened and mixed with food. Liquids are shaken well to ensure proper mixing prior to administration. When administering an anticonvulsant agent intravenously, the nurse should check the rate to be administered over one minute to avoid unpleasant or dangerous side effects.

It is important for nurses to know the therapeutic range for particular anticonvulsant agents, potential drug interactions, and side effects of these agents. Patients need to be informed about side effects and monitored for side effects or signs and symptoms of toxicity. Drug levels should also be monitored. The timing of drawing blood is critical. Peak levels are usually measured after the drug distribution is complete to determine whether the drug level is within therapeutic range. Trough levels are measured to ensure that the serum level is above the minimum effective concentration and that the drug is being eliminated at the correct rate. Seizure precautions are implemented as needed depending on the type of seizure the patient experiences.

Nurses need to approach seizure patients in a holistic manner. It is important to address patient concerns about having a seizure disorder, the medication regimen, and other social matters. Seizures can have a significant effect on the patient's self-esteem, socialization, employment, school, and other activities. If seizures are predictable and controlled, the patient can have a flexible life-style. Seizures that are partially controlled or uncontrolled can alter one's life-style considerably.

Nursing diagnosis and interventions are highly individualized. This variability is a result of the seizure patient's unique situation based on type of seizure, degree of control, age of patient, type of therapeutic regimen, patient acceptance of the seizure state, and degree of social support the patient experiences.

PATIENT TEACHING

To involve the patient in his or her treatment plan, it is important to teach the patient and family as much as possible about the treatment plan. Teaching the patient/family about the action of the medications, its interactions with other drugs, and side effects is essential. It is important for the patient to understand the methods for taking his or her medications as well as to avoid the concurrent use of over-the-counter medications.

Women taking oral contraceptives need further teaching. Specific risks of becoming pregnant while on anticonvulsant therapy should be included in the teaching plan.

Patients need to know the importance of routine examinations to monitor progress. They also need to know to report certain signs and symptoms to the physician. These include skin rash, severe nausea or vomiting, drowsiness, slurred speech, ataxia, swollen glands, tender gums, easy bruising, mouth ulcers, nose bleeds, sore throat, chills, and fever. Since many of the anticonvulsant agents cause drowsiness, patients must be cautioned to avoid activities that require alertness (driving, using power tools, etc.). It is also important for patients

Table 22–7. NURSING PROCESS FOR PATIENTS REQUIRING ANTICONVULSANTS

Assessment

Note mentation (response to environment, orientation), noting drowsiness, confusion, restlessness; or dizziness.
Evaluate muscle strength and coordination; balance, gait and movement.
Assess respiratory rate, rhythm, and depth during seizure activity.

Nursing Diagnosis	Nursing Actions	Rationale	Desired Outcomes/ Evaluation Criteria
Trauma, potential for related to muscle weakness, balancing difficulties, loss of large or small muscle coordination, cognitive changes, altered consciousness.	Encourage patient to keep a log of activities which occur prior to a seizure. Discourage smoking in bed.	Provides information about factors which can lead to injury. Drowsiness and lack of coordination may lead to dangerous situation.	Verbalizes understanding of safety measures. Remains free from injury.
	Discuss seizure precautions, e.g., reduce the amount of sensory stimuli; leave the patient in one location; remove harmful objects from the environment or pad objects/areas as possible; take axillary temperature in patient with uncontrolled seizures.	Helping the patient/family identify ways to reduce risks promotes control of situation and prevents injury. Depending on the site of the foci, the motor system can be directly involved and during the postictal period, a motor deficit may occur.	
	Assist patient to a safe place if aura develops. Encourage the patient to rest following the seizure activity.	Prevents fall with possibility of injury. May experience extreme fatigue and exhaustion impairing function/ reflexes.	
Self-esteem, disturbance related to stigma of epilepsy, perception of loss of control, long-term need for medications as evidenced by verbalization about changed lifestyle, fear of rejection, negative feelings about body/self, withdrawal, lack of follow-through/nonparticipation in therapy.	Encourage expression of feelings. Determine patient's perception of the effect of a seizure disorder on daily life/future expectations.	Acceptance of self is important to maintenance of self esteem and to motivation and the success of therapy.	Identifies feelings and methods for coping with negative perceptions of self. Verbalizes increased sense of self-esteem in relation to current situation.
	Provide information related to developmental issues, e.g., over-protection by family, cognitive abilities, issues of dependence/ independence.	Enhances ability to manage situation more effectively and may improve cooperation with treatment regimen.	
	Give age-appropriate information.	Patient will understand information more readily when it is given on their age/developmental level.	
	Explore with patient current/ past successes and strengths.	Focusing on positive aspects can help to alleviate feelings of guilt/self-consciousness and help patient begin to accept managability of condition.	
Poisoning, potential for related to narrow therapeutic range of medications, emotional difficulties.	Discuss reasons for administering drug as prescribed.	Having information helps patient to recognize importance of following medication regimen.	Demonstrates decrease or cessation of seizures without excessive sedation, hypotension, or dysrhythmias.
	Discuss side effects, differentiating between common and life-threatening effects.	Early identification of undesired side effects allows for prompt intervention, change in drug dosage/choice.	
	Stress importance of avoiding CNS depressants such as alcohol.	Can potentiate effects of the drugs.	

CONTINUED ON THE FOLLOWING PAGE

Table 22–7. NURSING PROCESS FOR PATIENTS REQUIRING ANTICONVULSANTS–*CONTINUED*

Nursing Diagnosis	Nursing Actions	Rationale	Desired Outcomes/ Evaluation Criteria
Breathing pattern, or airway-clearance, ineffective, potential related to neuromuscular impairment, tracheobronchial obstruction, perceptual/cognitive impairment.	Implement seizure precautions, e.g., suction equipment/oral airway available. Position on side, loosen constrictive clothing. Keep airway open, suction, if necessary. Observe for labored breathing, dyspnea, apnea, tachypnea, cyanosis.	Provides for timely response to emergent situation. Maintaining airway, minimizing pooling of secretions supports ventilation/oxygenation. Indicators of airway obstruction requiring immediate intervention.	Maintains effective respiratory pattern with patent airway/ aspiration prevented.
	Administer oxygen as needed.	Maximizes oxygen delivery to support cellular activity.	
Knowledge deficit related to lack of exposure/information misinterpretation, lack of recall, cognitive limitations as evidenced by questions, failure to improve, development of preventable complications, incorrect use of medications.	Provide a supportive environment. Evaluate patient/ family for readiness to learn. Review pathology/ prognosis of condition.	When patient feels accepted and not judged, information is more apt to be heard and incorporated.	Verbalizes understanding of disorder and various stimuli that may increase/potentiate seizure activity. Initiates necessary lifestyle/behavior changes as indicated. Verbalizes understanding of drug regimen.
	Identify factors/stressors that precipitate seizures (e.g., lack of sleep, poor nutrition, illness/fever, electrolyte imbalance, emotional stress, growth spurts, hormonal changes, menstruation/pregnancy).	Promotes control over own situation, allows for adjustment of medication.	
	Identify safety factors and care during a seizure.	Helps patient/family to plan for eventualities.	
	Discuss concerns about social stigmas associated with epilepsy; explaining seizures to friends, bosses, school officials.	Patient/family can deal with these issues more effectively when they have thought/and discussed them beforehand.	
	Review purpose of medications, action, uses, dosage, adverse side effects, drug interactions.	Understanding of the medication regimen is crucial to cooperation and active participation in treatment program. Provides opportunity to minimize/prevent complications.	
	Suggest taking drug with meals if appropriate.	May reduce incidence of gastric irritation, nausea/vomiting.	
	Stress importance of following the treatment plan.	Promotes most effective control of seizure activity.	
	Encourage follow-up visits to the physician.	Monitoring of CBC, platelet count, serum calcium, urinalysis/or hepatic and thyroid function as indicated, provides opportunity to assess development of adverse/toxic reactions as well as to check on effectiveness of the treatment regimen.	
	Discuss need for good dental hygiene and routine professional examinations.	Helps to inhibit gingival hyperplasia, gum and tooth disease.	
	Recommend patient wear identification tag/bracelet stating the presence of a seizure disorder.	Expedites treatment and diagnosis in emergency setting.	
	Identify support systems, e.g., local Epilepsy groups and National Epileptic Foundation.	Provides opportunity for patient/family to interact with others with similar concerns and learn about disease and current treatment/research. Can provide positive role models.	

TABLE 22–8. PATIENT TEACHING INFORMATION—ANTICONVULSANTS

Dear Patient:

This drug has been ordered for you. This is what you should know about your drug to get the most from your drug.

1. Anticonvulsants are taken to decrease the number of or to stop your seizures.
2. Anticonvulsants are taken for a couple of years and then you are examined by your physician. You may stay on the drug, or the drug may be slowly stopped.
3. Phenytoin (Dilantin), phenobarbital (Luminal), primidone (Mysoline), carbamazepine (Tegretol), valproic acid (Depakene, Depakote), ethosuximide (Zarontin), and clonazepam (Clonopin) can be taken with meals. Do not take with milk, calcium, antacids, or milk of magnesia since these products decrease absorption of the drug.
4. Do not take your anticonvulsants with alcohol, antidepressants, phenothiazines, barbiturates, antihistamines, narcotics, sedative/hypnotics, monoamine oxidase inhibitors, and over-the-counter medications unless prescribed by your physician.
5. Always check with your physician or pharmacist before taking other drugs, as interactions may occur. Medications known to cause interactions include over-the-counter products for nasal congestion, allergy, pain, or obesity. Drugs of abuse such as marijuana may interact with your drug by increasing the side effects or lowering the seizure threshold, causing you to be at risk for seizures.
6. If you forget to take your anticonvulsant, take your forgotten dose (unless it is almost time for the next dose) to maintain your blood level. Do not try to catch up by taking two doses at the same time.
7. Do not stop your drug because this causes an increase in seizures and/or status epilepticus.
8. Do not alter the drug dosage yourself. Changes may need to be made under conditions of increasing physical stress, such as infection, or emotional stress, such as a loss of a loved one. However, the drug dosage is never changed without talking with your physician since either underdosage or overdosage can be hazardous.
9. Alcohol or alcohol withdrawal may precipitate seizures.
10. Drowsiness and unsteadiness is a frequent side effect for all patients; be cautious when operating vehicles or machinery, or when engaging in possibly hazardous activities. Often, drowsiness is an initial problem when you first begin anticonvulsant therapy; however, as therapy continues, the drowsiness lessens in severity.
11. If you have any adverse effects from your drug, talk with your physician. Side effects to anticonvulsants include drowsiness, slurred speech, dizziness, swollen glands, bleeding or tender gums, skin rash, severe nausea or vomiting, yellow skin or eyes, joint pain, fever, sore throat, unusual bleeding or bruising, and headache.
12. It is important for you to maintain good oral care and to see the dentist frequently for teeth cleaning to prevent tenderness, bleeding, and gum overgrowth.
13. Some anticonvulsants decrease the effectiveness of oral contraceptives. If you are taking oral contraceptives, consult your physician.
14. Some anticonvulsants cause sensitivity to the sun.

Use sunscreen and protective clothing when outdoors.
15. Patients receiving anticonvulsant therapy should carry identification with this information at all times.
16. It is important for you to continue your follow-up visits to your physician to monitor the effectiveness of your drug.
17. Store these products in a tight, light-resistant container to prevent deterioration.

to be advised not to use alcohol or CNS depressants concurrently with these agents.

The patient's approval of and commitment to the treatment plan are essential for obtaining and maintaining seizure control. The patient must live with this treatment plan and his or her cooperation is essential. See Table 22–8 for specific recommendations for patient teaching.

EVALUATION

An important component of the evaluation process is evaluating particular outcomes. See Table 22–7 for specific outcomes related to anticonvulsant therapy. The nurse has an important role as a member of the health team, because the nurse's observations provide needed information that enables the physician to adjust drugs and dosages. The most challenging role for the nurse is to assist the patient in assessing the results of and adjusting anticonvulsant therapy as well as in determining the impact the seizure disorder has on his or her way of life.

SUMMARY

The goal of anticonvulsant therapy is to stop the seizures that the patient experiences. Anticonvulsant agents accomplish this goal by suppressing the focus of discharge to reduce excessive discharges and to prevent the spread of neuronal excitation.

Prior to administration of anticonvulsants, the nurse must assess the patient's condition and monitor drug levels. Many of the side effects of anticonvulsant therapy are detected by nursing assessment. The nurse also has an important role in developing a patient teaching plan that helps the patient to manage the medication regimen at home.

BIBLIOGRAPHY

Abramowicz, M (ed): Drugs for epilepsy. Med Lett Drugs Ther 28(723):91, 1986.
American Medical Association: Drug Evaluations, ed 6. American Medical Association, Chicago, 1986, p 171.
Craig, CR: The pharmacological treatment of convulsive disorders. In Craig, CR and Stitzel, RE (eds): Modern Pharmacology, ed 2. Little, Brown & Co, Boston, 1986.

Deglin, JH and Vallerand, AH: Nurse's Med Deck. FA Davis, Philadelphia, 1988.

Hartshorn, JC and Hartshorn, EA: Nursing interventions for anticonvulsant drug interactions. J Neurosci Nurs 18(5):250, 1987.

Porter, RJ and Pitlick, WH: Antiepileptic Drugs. In Katzung, BG (ed): Basic and Clinical Pharmacology, ed 3. Appleton and Lange, Norwalk, CT, 1987.

Rall, TW and Schleifer, LS: Drugs effective in the therapy of the epilepsies. In Goodman and Gilman's The Pharmacological Basis of Therapeutics, ed 7. Macmillan, New York, 1985.

Santilli, N and Sierzant, TL: Advances in the treatment of epilepsy. J Neurosci Nurs 19(3):141, 1987.

Trevor, AJ and Way, WL: Sedative-hypnotics. In Katzung, BG (ed): Basic and Clinical Pharmacology, ed 3. Appleton and Lange, Norwalk, CT, 1987.

SITUATION 22–1

Randall Johnson, a 16-year-old, is admitted to the intensive care unit with clonic/tonic seizures. He has a history of a head injury due to a childhood accident. Because he had no evidence of seizures, Randall stopped taking phenytoin (Dilantin) over a year ago.

1. Randall is to receive a loading dose of phenytoin intravenously. The nurse will administer the drug at the following rate:
   a. 100 mg/minute
   b. 20 mg/minute
   c. 50 mg/minute
   d. 5 mg/minute

2. When giving the loading dose intravenously, the nurse will observe Randall closely for:
   a. allergic reaction
   b. apnea
   c. hypotension
   d. anuria

3. Two days later, the serum Dilantin level for Randall is 12 μg/ml. He is on a dosage schedule of 100 mg IV every 8 hours. The nurse will expect to:
   a. continue the dosage as ordered
   b. decrease the daily dosage
   c. hold the drug until further orders
   d. increase the daily dosage

4. In the event that Randall has continuous seizures (status epilepticus), the nurse will be prepared to administer:
   a. clonazepam (Klonopin)
   b. carbamazepine (Tegretol)
   c. phenacemide (Phenurone)
   d. diazepam (Valium)

5. Randall is to be discharged home on a maintenance dosage of Dilantin 100 mg PO tid. When performing patient teaching, the nurse will include the following information:
   a. Take the medication on an empty stomach.
   b. Discontinue the drug immediately if side effects occur.
   c. Maintain a good oral hygiene program.
   d. Use any over-the-counter medications as needed.

6. Related to the endocrine effects of phenytoin, the nurse will plan to observe for the following:
   a. hypoglycemia
   b. glycosuria
   c. hypercalcemia
   d. hyperkalemia

SITUATION 22–2

Marvel Carson is a 38-year-old who has a history of simple partial seizures. She is admitted to the medical floor for evaluation because of increased symptoms.

1. Ms. Carson has been on phenobarbital for control of partial seizures. The expected therapeutic serum concentration of phenobarbital is:
   a. 10 to 25 μg/ml
   b. 15 to 30 μg/ml
   c. 25 to 50 μg/ml
   d. 30 to 60 μg/ml

2. When giving phenobarbital, the nurse will be aware of the following major adverse effect:
   a. tachycardia
   b. diarrhea
   c. photophobia
   d. drowsiness

3. A realistic outcome for Ms. Carson would include:
   a. control of partial seizures
   b. absence of drug side effects
   c. elimination of seizure medications
   d. cure of the cause of seizures

4. In planning interventions for Ms. Carson related to phenobarbital administration, the nurse may include all of the following *except:*

   a. opening capsules and mixing with food
   b. shaking suspensions well before giving orally
   c. drawing trough levels after drug distribution
   d. implementing seizure and safety precautions

5. Ms. Carson continues to have simple partial seizures despite phenobarbital therapy, and carbamazepine (Tegretol) is to be started. The nurse will anticipate:
   a. reducing the phenobarbital gradually before discontinuing
   b. discontinuing the phenobarbital in order to prevent interactions
   c. administering diazepam prior to discontinuing phenobarbital
   d. discontinuing the phenobarbital, but observing for withdrawal

6. Concerning Tegretol administration, the nurse will monitor the following lab result:
   a. calcium
   b. sodium
   c. magnesium
   d. potassium

Please refer to the Appendices for correct answers and additional review questions with answers.

23
CHAPTER

SKELETAL MUSCLE RELAXANTS AND DRUG THERAPY FOR SPECIFIC DISEASES OF THE NERVOUS SYSTEM

23

SKELETAL MUSCLE RELAXANTS AND DRUG THERAPY FOR CHRONIC DISEASES OF THE NERVOUS SYSTEM

GLOSSARY TERMS IN THIS CHAPTER

Acetylcholinesterase inhibitors
Akinesia
Bradykinesia
Bulbar
Dyskinesia
Erythromelalgia
Fasciculation
Nuclei
Ptosis
Spasticity
Telencephalon
Tic
Tremor

23
CHAPTER

SKELETAL MUSCLE RELAXANTS AND DRUG THERAPY FOR SPECIFIC DISEASES OF THE NERVOUS SYSTEM

VICKI L. BYERS, R.N., Ph.D., CNRN
MERRILY MATHEWSON KUHN, R.N.C., Ph.D., CCRN

LEARNING OBJECTIVES

After reading this chapter, the student will be able to:

1. Describe specific disorders of the nervous system and the various medications that are commonly used to treat them.

2. Differentiate among the nervous system medications as to mechanisms of action, routes of administration, metabolism and adverse effects, contraindications, and interactions.

3. Formulate a specific plan to assess the patient with a disorder of the nervous system in order to formulate an appropriate diagnosis.

4. Plan nursing intervention necessary to administer drugs for disorders of the nervous system safely and choose appropriate teaching strategies to gain patient compliance.

5. Plan the nursing intervention necessary to counsel the families of patients who have disorders of the nervous system.

6. Evaluate the patient at various stages of treatment to gauge nursing intervention.

This chapter discusses a variety of motor disorders and the common pharmacologic agents used to treat them. Specifically, disorders associated with the basal ganglia and neuromuscular junction are examined. Anatomically, the pharmacologic agents work on the extrapyramidal system and the neuromuscular junction. The extrapyramidal system regulates muscle tone, speed of movement, and postural reflexes. This involuntary system is made up of a network of neurons located in the basal ganglia, thalamic and subthalamic nuclei, red nucleus, substantia nigra, and parts of the reticular formation, cerebellum, and cerebrum.

There are several pathways within this involuntary system. Exact functions of these pathways remain unknown. One pathway that is explored in this chapter is the nigrostriate fibers that travel from the substantia nigra to the striatum (Fig. 23–1). This pathway is rich with dopaminergic neurons. Dopamine acts as an inhibitory neurotransmitter, balancing an excitatory cholinergic system. When there is an imbalance between dopamine and acetylcholine, movement disorders become prominent.

The basal ganglia are subcortical *nuclei* of the *telencephalon.* The anatomic units that compose the basal ganglia are the caudate nucleus, putamen, globus pallidus, and the amygdaloid nuclear complex (Fig. 23–2). The caudate nucleus, putamen, and globus pallidus make up the corpus striatum.

Lesions in the involuntary system cause a variety of *dyskinesias.* The dyskinesias that are discussed in this chapter are Parkinson's disease, Huntington's chorea, dystonia musculorum deformans, spasmodic torticollis, and Gilles de la Tourette syndrome.

PARKINSON'S DISEASE

Parkinson's disease is a chronic, progressive movement disorder characterized by motor dysfunction (*bradyki-*nesia, akinesia, delayed reaction time, lack of autonomic movements, disturbance in posture), *tremor*, rigidity, and associated symptoms (autonomic nervous system dysfunction, depression, dementia). The cause of this movement disorder is neuronal degeneration of the nigrostriatal pathway. There is a loss of dopaminergic neurons in the substantia nigra and a reduction in the concentration of dopamine in the striatum and the substantia nigra. There is also a loss of the dopaminergic receptors in the striatum, which further limits the dopaminergic action. This loss of dopaminergic action causes an imbalance between dopamine (inhibitory) and acetylcholine (excitatory). This imbalance results in the enhancement of the cholinergic activity and the signs and symptoms of Parkinson's disease.

Parkinson's disease can be idiopathic or secondary. Some of the secondary causes are the "postencephalitis of 1917" (a virus-induced encephalitis causing Parkinson's disease); poisoning (carbon monoxide, manganese, other heavy metals); drug-induced (phenothiazines, butyrophenones, reserpine, MPTP [1-methyl-4-phenyl-1,2,5,6 tetrahydropyridine]); brain tumors; brain trauma; aging; and metabolic reasons (anoxic events, repeated hypoglycemic attacks). Primary Parkinson's disease usually appears in the later decades of life and slowly produces increasing disability in movement. The course of Parkinson's disease is variable. In general, parkinsonism leads to motor, posture, and tone dysfunction.

Drug therapy is directed at balancing striatal activity by reducing cholinergic activity or enhancing dopaminergic function. Very often a combination of anticholinergic and dopaminergic agents are used in the management of Parkinson's disease. Since therapy provides relief symptomatic and not curative, it is important to provide relief of symptoms and to maintain maximum independence of movement for as long as possible.

Drug therapy has been the basis of management of Parkinson's disease; however, nonpharmacologic measures are also important. Exercise, speech therapy,

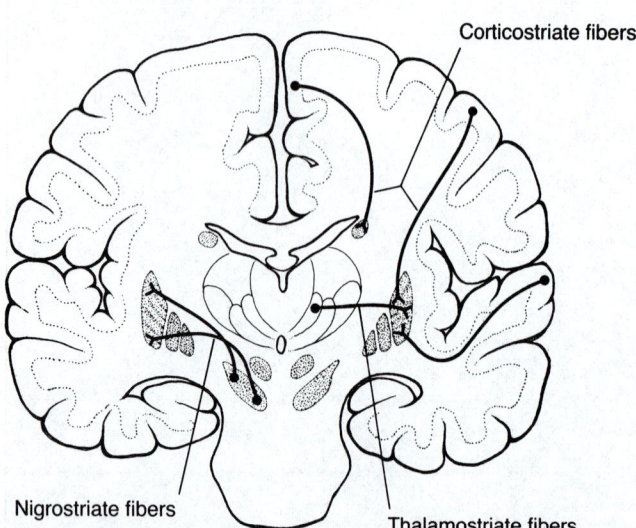

Corticostriate fibers

Nigrostriate fibers

Thalamostriate fibers

Figure 23–1. Nigrostriate pathway and other pathways of the basal ganglia. Semischematic diagram of striatal afferent fibers. Corticostriate fibers arising from broad cortical regions on the convexity of the hemisphere project to the putamen. Cortex on the medial surface projects largely to the caudate nucleus. Nigrostriatal fibers arise from cells of the pars compacta. Thalamostriate fibers arise from the centromedian-parafascicular complex. All of these striatal afferent systems are topographically organized. (From Carpenter, MB: Core Text of Neuroanatomy, ed. 2, the Williams & Wilkins Company, Baltimore, 1978, with permission.)

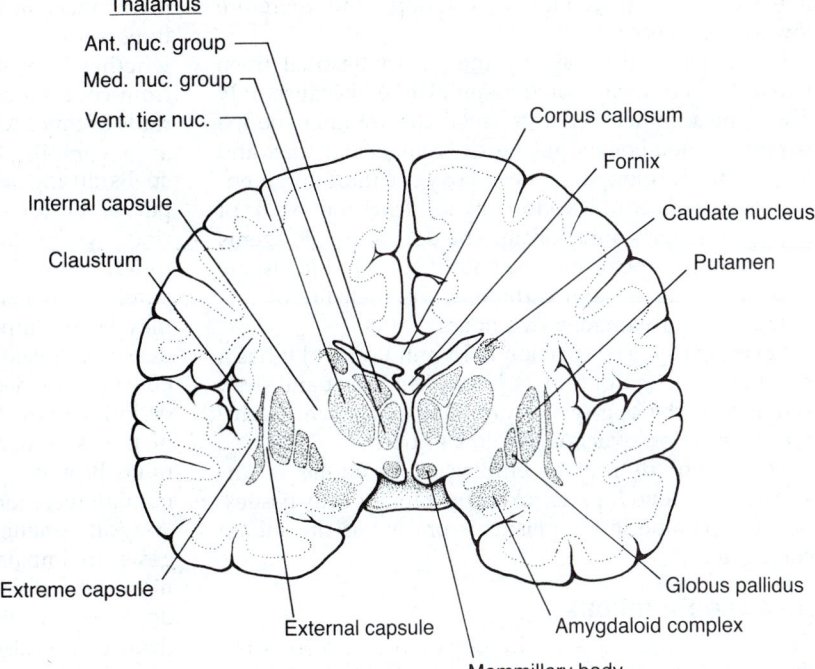

Thalamus

Ant. nuc. group

Med. nuc. group

Vent. tier nuc.

Internal capsule

Claustrum

Corpus callosum

Fornix

Caudate nucleus

Putamen

Extreme capsule

External capsule

Amygdaloid complex

Globus pallidus

Mammillary body

Figure 23–2. Structures of the basal ganglia. Photograph of a frontal section of the brain at the level of the mammillary bodies. In this section the main nuclear groups of the thalamus are identified and portions of all components of the basal ganglia are present. The amygdaloid nuclear complex lies in the temporal lobe internal to the uncus and ventral to the lentiform nucleus. (From Carpenter, MB: Core Text of Neuroanatomy, ed. 2, the Williams & Wilkins Company, Baltimore, 1978, with permission.)

physical therapy, psychotherapy, and family support are critical in the management of patients with Parkinson's disease. The recent development of cortical-adrenal autologous transplantation may offer hope for patients who are refractory to drug therapy. In this surgical procedure, the dopamine-rich cells of the adrenal cortex of the Parkinsonian patient are transplanted into his or her basal ganglia. This procedure was developed in Sweden and has been performed in Mexico and selected sites in the United States.

The choice of drug therapy depends on the severity of the disease, its progression, and the patient's ability to tolerate adverse reactions. The classifications of drugs that are reviewed in the following sections are dopaminergic agents, dopamine receptor agonists, and anticholinergic agents.

DOPAMINERGIC AGENTS (LEVODOPA, CARBIDOPA)

Action

Levodopa is a precursor to dopamine. Dopamine does not enter the brain in enough quantities to be of value for the treatment of Parkinsonism, but levodopa does. Once levodopa is converted to dopamine in the central nervous system (CNS), it serves as a neurotransmitter that facilitates movement and postural reflexes. The therapeutic effects of levodopa and side effects occur through stimulation of central and peripheral dopamine receptors.

DECARBOXYLASE INHIBITORS

Co-administration of levodopa with an inhibitor of aromatic L-amino acid decarboxylase that is unable to penetrate the CNS readily diminishes the decarboxylation of levodopa in peripheral tissues. This allows more levodopa to reach the receptor sites in the nigrostriatum. The only inhibitor that is used in the United States is carbidopa. The advantages of using a decarboxylase inhibitor with levodopa are many. These include the following: (1) the effective dose of levodopa is reduced by 75%; (2) stimulation of the receptors in the medullary emetic center is decreased, thereby decreasing nausea and vomiting; (3) antagonism of the therapeutic efficacy of levodopa by pyridoxine is avoided; (4) frequency and intensity of daily variation in control of symptoms by levodopa are reduced; (5) degree of clinical improvement is greater than with levodopa alone.

Uses

Levodopa is used to treat Parkinson's disease. This agent does not stop the progression of the pathology associated with Parkinsonism, but it does improve symptoms and prolongs life. The major symptomatic relief is associated with bradykinesia, rigidity, and to a lesser extent, tremor. Levodopa is also reported to improve the problems connected with balance, posture, gait, and handwriting. Levodopa improves the quality of life for most patients with Parkinson's disease.

Pharmacokinetics

The dopaminergic agents are well absorbed from the small bowel by an active transport system for aromatic amino acids. With the aid of L-aromatic amino acid decarboxylase, levodopa is converted to dopamine. The rate of absorption is influenced by the rate of gastric emptying, acidity of gastric juice, and competition for amino acids. Administration with food or dietary protein slows the absorption of levodopa and therefore lowers peak absorption.

Levodopa is absorbed by the gastrointestinal tract. Large doses of levodopa are administered because only 1% of the administered dose enters the brain. Levodopa is rapidly metabolized in the gastrointestinal tract and liver. Since carbidopa is a decarboxylase inhibitor, it enhances the effect of levodopa by reducing the extent of hepatic first-pass metabolism. The dopaminergic agents are excreted in the urine. The half-life of levodopa is one hour in the absence of carbidopa. The half-life of carbidopa is approximately two hours.

Levodopa's onset of action is 15 minutes, and it has a duration of action of 5 to 24 hours. The onset and peak action of carbidopa (given orally) is unknown. Carbidopa's duration of action is 5 to 24 hours.

The extent of protein binding of levodopa is unknown, but levodopa is taken up rapidly into tissues. Some dopamine in the plasma is present as the sulfate conjugate.

Adverse Reactions

The adverse reactions to the dopaminergic agents fall into two categories. The first category contains reactions that occur early in therapy and to which a tolerance may develop, such as gastrointestinal effects and cardiovascular effects. When levodopa is given without a peripheral decarboxylase inhibitor, adverse reactions such as anorexia, nausea, and vomiting occur in 80% of patients. These adverse reactions occur as a result of stimulation of the chemoreceptors in the medulla by the newly formed dopamine. These reactions are most likely to occur if the dosage of the drug is increased too rapidly. The common cardiovascular effects are orthostatic hypotension and cardiac dysrhythmias. It is thought that the mechanism for these reactions is an accumulation of dopamine innorepinephrine nerve terminals where it serves as a false transmitter. Some of the dysrhythmias reported include sinus tachycardia, atrial and ventricular extrasystoles, atrial flutter/fibrillation, and ventricular tachycardia. These dysrhythmias are caused by the beta-adrenergic action of dopamine on the heart as well as beta-adrenergic receptor stimulation by other catecholamine metabolites of the drug.

The second classification of adverse reactions occur after long-term therapy. These include abnormal involuntary movements (dyskinesias), akinetic spells, and behavioral disturbances. The abnormal involuntary movements appear several months after the introduction of dopaminergic agents. These abnormal movements usually occur at either the time of peak drug action or at the end of the period of drug action. This particular side effect is referred to as the "end-of-dose failure" because it reflects the tapering of effectiveness of the dopaminergic agents. These abnormal involuntary movements are variable in type but might include faciolingual *tic*, grimacing, head bobbing, and rocking movements of the arms, legs, or trunk. Tolerance does not develop to this side effect, and it can become worse if the amount of medication is not reduced. The pro-

posed mechanism for this side effect is the presence of hypersensitive dopamine receptors. It is not certain whether it results from denervation supersensitivity or from continuous stimulation by dopamine for long periods of time. Another group of side effects that are seen as a complication of long-term therapy are akinetic spells during which the patient is immobilized. This is part of the "on/off" phenomenon in which there are periods where the patient experiences functional ability (often with abnormal involuntary movements) alternately with periods of akinetic attacks. These attacks may be accompanied by tremor and rigidity. Tolerance does not develop to this side effect. Sometimes this side effect can be decreased by adding amantadine or bromocriptine to the therapy and adjusting the diet and times of meals. Amantadine augments the release of dopamine. Bromocriptine affects a different population of dopamine receptors than does levodopa. The cause of the "on/off" phenomenon is not fully understood but suggests an imbalance in physiologic regulatory mechanisms and usually occurs when the blood levels of levodopa are in the low therapeutic range. Behavioral disturbances also occur as side effects of long-term therapy with dopaminergic agents. This group of symptoms vary on the basis of a previous history of mental illness. The drug-induced psychosis in parkinsonism patients usually occurs after two to five years of dopaminergic therapy. These patients can experience vivid dreams or nightmares, hallucinations, confusion, delusions, insomnia, and depression. The only treatment is to reduce the amount of the dopaminergic agent, use a drug holiday, or withdraw the agent. The exact cause of the mental side effects is unknown.

Contraindications and Precautions

The dopaminergic agents are contraindicated in patients with narrow-angle glaucoma. These agents produce mydriasis, which would aggravate the glaucoma. It is also contraindicated in persons with undiagnosed skin lesions or a history of melanoma. Levodopa is the precursor of skin melanin in which exogenous levodopa induces or stimulates the growth of cutaneous melanomas. The dopaminergic agents are not used during lactation, and they are contraindicated in persons receiving monoamine oxidase (MAO) inhibitors. The concurrent use of dopaminergic agents and MAO inhibitors causes an accumulation of dopamine and other catecholamines. Hypertension and hyperpyrexia are dangerous results of this concurrent therapy. MAO inhibitors are withdrawn at least 14 days prior to the administration of a dopaminergic agent. The dopaminergic agents are also contraindicated in persons with hemolytic anemia or glucose-6-phosphate dehydrogenase deficiency. There have been reports of drug-induced hemolytic anemia. These agents should not be used in patients who exhibit hypersensitivity.

The dopaminergic agents are used with caution in patients with cardiac, psychiatric, or ulcer disease. The cardiac irregularities are due to the beta-adrenergic action of dopamine on the heart, as well as the direct beta-adrenergic receptor stimulation by other catecholamine metabolites of these agents. Persons with psychiatric disturbances, especially psychosis, should be monitored closely with dopaminergic agents because these agents can enhance hallucinations, paranoia, mania, insomnia, anxiety, nightmares, and depression, especially in the elderly. Safe use of dopaminergic agents has not been established in pregnancy, lactation, and children under 12 years of age.

There have been some reports of gastrointestinal bleeding in patients receiving dopaminergic agents. Levodopa in particular can cause gastrointestinal irritation. Patients with peptic ulcer disease are monitored closely while they are receiving dopaminergic agents.

Interactions

Certain drugs can interfere with the effectiveness of the dopaminergic agents. Pyridoxine, a cofactor in the decarboxylation of levodopa to dopamine, can reverse the effectiveness of levodopa by promoting a rapid conversion of levodopa to dopamine in the periphery, causing a decrease in the amount of levodopa transported to the brain. Patients should be aware that pyridoxine is present in multivitamin preparations in amounts greater than 5 mg. When levodopa is administered with carbidopa, this antagonistic effect of pyridoxine is lost.

Nonspecific MAO inhibitors interfere with the inactivation of dopamine, norepinephrine, and other catecholamines. They amplify the central effects of dopaminergic agents and its catecholamine metabolites, leading to hypertensive crisis and hyperpyrexia.

There is a decrease in the effectiveness of the dopaminergic agents when combined with agents such as phenothiazines, butyrophenones, thioxanthenes, rauwolfia alkaloids, phenytoin, papaverine, and metoclopramide. Many of these agents deplete stores of central dopamine (reserpine) while other agents block receptors for dopamine.

Anticholinergic agents such as trihexyphenidyl, benztropine, and procyclidine act synergistically with dopaminergic agents to improve certain symptoms associated with parkinsonism. Large doses of the anticholinergic agents can slow gastric emptying, causing a delay in the absorption of the dopaminergic agents, and can decrease the effectiveness of these agents.

Overall, the dopaminergic agents do not cause serious hematologic, renal, hepatic, or thyroid dysfunction. Large doses of levodopa can cause hypokalemia associated with increased plasma levels of aldosterone; this effect can be reduced by adding carbidopa to the therapy. Levodopa increases plasma growth hormone levels and can produce a mild carbohydrate intolerance, but not to the extent that acromegaly or diabetes mellitus develops. Dark-colored sweat and red-tinged urine have been reported but are not indications for discontinuation of these agents.

Dosage

The initial adult therapeutic dose range for levodopa is 500 to 1000 mg given orally in divided doses. This dose is increased by 100 to 750 mg every three to seven days until a maximal dosage range of 2000 to 8000 mg is given orally each day. Sinemet tablets contain 10/100, 25/100, or 25/250 mg of carbidopa and levodopa, respectively. The initial adult therapeutic dosage range for Sinemet is 75/300 to 150/1500 mg given orally in divided daily doses. Sinemet can be increased to 200/2000 mg daily. Carbidopa is available alone.

Drug Holidays

When there is a loss of the therapeutic efficacy of levodopa and the patient is experiencing the long-term side effects previously mentioned, the drug is tapered and withdrawn for up to a 14-day period. The loss of efficacy is caused by the desensitization of receptors for dopamine. The goals of drug holidays are to eliminate or reduce the adverse drug effects and to restore receptor sensitivity to dopamine. After "resensitization," lower doses of dopamine seem sufficient to alleviate symptoms of parkinsonism. During the period of the drug holidays, the patient must be monitored closely. Lannon and colleagues (1986) suggest specific guidelines for patients on drug holiday (Table 23–1).

DOPAMINE AGONISTS

The gradual loss of responsiveness to levodopa that occurs with long-term therapy has led to the investigation of specific agonists that directly act on striatal dopamine receptor sites. The two major agents available for the treatment of parkinsonism are amantadine and bromocriptine.

Amantadine

USE. Amantadine (Symmetrel) is an antiviral agent that has been found to relieve symptoms associated with parkinsonism. In the early stages of Parkinson's disease when tremor is not the major symptom, it is the drug of choice. In the advanced stages of parkinsonism, it is used concurrently with levodopa. This agent is not as effective as levodopa, but it produces a more rapid response and fewer side effects. Amantadine is also used for the prophylaxis of influenza A.

ACTION. Amantadine is thought to increase dopaminergic activity in the peripheral and central nervous systems by increasing synthesis, facilitating the release, and inhibiting cellular reuptake of dopamine. This agent may also have anticholinergic effects. The antiviral mechanism of action remains unclear. In the presence of amantadine, there is a blocking of the penetration of the virus into respiratory epithelial host cells. Amantadine also blocks uncoating of the virus and release of nucleic acid after penetration of the host cell.

PHARMACOKINETICS. Amantadine is well absorbed from the gastrointestinal tract. It is widely distributed to tissues and fluids. The onset of action after an oral dose is 15 minutes. The peak action is one to four hours, and the duration of action is 12 to 24 hours. Amantadine does cross the blood–brain barrier and is found in breast milk. Approximately 90% of amanta-

Table 23–1. GUIDELINES FOR PATIENTS ON DRUG HOLIDAY

1. Tapering medications:
   - Carbidopa/levodopa: Total dose decreased by one half every 3 days (may begin as an outpatient) to 5/50 at 7 AM; 5/50 at 11 AM before total withdrawal
   - Bromocriptine: taper and discontinue
   - Anticholinergics: taper and discontinue
   - Amantadine: discontinue
2. Duration goal of drug holiday = 14 days off carbidopa/levodopa
3. Daily assessment to include:
   - Functional abilities (out of bed, chair, roll over, etc.)
   - Ambulation
   - Tremor
   - Rigidity (cogwheeling vs. plastic; unilateral or bilateral; which extremities, trunk, etc.)
   - Mental status
   - Speech
   - Swallowing
   - Expression
   - Respiratory function
   - Circulation
   - Sleep pattern
   - Any dyskinesia/dystonia
   - Emotional response to immobility
4. If on day 7 of drug holiday, there are no major problems with swallowing, respiratory, or circulatory systems, then continue off carbidopa/levodopa until day 10.
   If still no problems at day 10, continue until day 14.
5. During drug holiday, to avoid problems of decreased mobility:
   - Change of diet to soft, mechanical soft, etc.
   - Subcutaneous heparin, 5000 units, every 12 hours
   - Water mattress
   - Elastic stockings
   - Turning assistance every 2 hours
   - Physical therapy
   - Occupational therapy
   - Recreational therapy
6. Restarting carbidopa/levodopa after a drug holiday: (Regardless of preholiday dose, *note:* doses are given 30 to 40 minutes *before* meals).
   Day 1 = 5/50 at 7 AM; 5/50 at 11 AM
   Day 3 = 5/50 at 7 AM; 5/50 at 11 AM; 5/50 at 4 PM
   Day 6 = 10/100 at 7 AM; 5/50 at 11 AM; 5/50 at 4 PM
   Day 9 = 10/100 at 7 AM; 10/100 at 11 AM; 5/50 at 4 PM
   If still in need of additional medication, the last increase would be to 10/100 three times daily before discharge. (Increments can be given after discharge according to functional requirement.) During increases, assessment should be made each day of items listed in number 3.
7. Maintenance dose is established after discharge according to targets of therapy and to avoid symptoms of excess dopaminergic stimulation.

From Lannon, MC, et al: Comprehensive care of the patient with Parkinson's disease. J Neurosci Nurs 18(3):121–131, 1986, with permission.

dine is excreted unchanged in the urine. The excretion of amantadine is increased in acidic urine. The half-life of amantadine is 24 hours.

CONTRAINDICATIONS AND PRECAUTIONS. Amantadine is contraindicated in patients who are hy-persensitive to the drug. This agent is used with caution in patients with a history of seizures, liver disease, psychiatric problems, or cardiac disease. Amantadine increases dopaminergic and catecholamine activity, thereby potentiating seizures and psychic side effects, and increasing stimulation to the heart. Safe use in pregnancy and lactation has not been established.

ADVERSE REACTIONS. Amantadine is usually well tolerated. The adverse reactions that occur are transient and reversible. The common adverse reactions are gastrointestinal disturbances (anorexia, nausea, vomiting, constipation); psychic disturbances (hallucinations, confusion, nightmares, anxiety, difficulty with concentration), which are probably related to the increased dopaminergic activity; dermatologic (mottling, peripheral edema, rash); and symptoms associated with anticholinergic agents (dry mouth, blurred vision, urinary retention, slurred speech, mood changes, dizziness, ataxia). The purplish mottling and swelling of the extremities are more common in women. They are the result of the vasoconstriction that occurs with local release of catecholamines.

INTERACTIONS. Peripheral and central adverse effects of anticholinergic drugs are increased by amantadine. Reducing high-dose anticholinergic therapy prior to amantadine administration is recommended. Concurrent use of amantadine and triamterene may reduce the plasma clearance of amantadine and increase the incidence of toxic reactions.

DOSAGE. Amantadine is administered orally. When used in the treatment of Parkinson's disease and influenza, an adult's and children's (over nine years of age) dose is 100 mg given two times a day. The pediatric dose (children one to nine years of age) is 4.4 to 8.8 mg/kg/day up to 150 mg/day given in two to three equally divided doses.

Bromocriptine Mesylate

ACTION. Bromocriptine (Parlodel) is a direct-acting dopamine receptor agonist that is used clinically for the treatment of parkinsonism. Bromocriptine is an ergot derivative. It is a potent dopaminergic agonist with preference for dopamine receptors different from those of levodopa. This agent acts on the postsynaptic dopamine receptors. The pharmacologic action of bromocriptine results from stimulation of dopamine receptors in the CNS, cardiovascular system, pituitary-hypothalamic axis, and gastrointestinal tract.

USE. Bromocriptine is used in the treatment of Parkinson's disease and hyperprolactinemia of various causes. It is used to reduce postpartum lactation and to treat abnormalities of growth hormone production. Bromocriptine is more effective than the anticholinergic drugs and amantadine in treating parkinsonism. It is an adjunct to levodopa or levodopa/carbidopa in patients experiencing significant fluctuations in therapeutic response and end-of-dose akinesia. The decrease in fluctuations may be caused by bromocriptine's longer duration of action, or it may result because the dopamine receptor sites affected by bromocriptine are different from those affected by levodopa.

PHARMACOKINETICS. Bromocriptine is partially absorbed from the gastrointestinal tract. After administration of an oral dose of bromocriptine the onset of action is 30 to 90 minutes, peak effect is one to two hours, and the duration action is 8 to 12 hours. This agent is metabolized by first-pass kinetics in the liver. The systemic bioavailability is only a small fraction of the administered dose. Ninety-eight percent of an oral dose is excreted in the feces, and the remaining 2% is excreted via the urine. The half-life of bromocriptine is biphasic. The initial phase is about 4.5 hours and the second phase is 45 to 50 hours. Bromocriptine is 90% to 96% bound to serum albumin.

CONTRAINDICATIONS AND PRECAUTIONS. This agent is contraindicated in persons who experience sensitivity to bromocriptine or ergot alkaloids. This agent is used cautiously in patients with a history of cardiac disease or psychic disturbances. This is due to the dopaminergic effect on the heart and brain. The dose of bromocriptine is reduced in patients with liver impairment since the metabolism of the drug is affected. Safety in pregnancy or children under the age of 15 has not been established.

ADVERSE REACTIONS. The response and tolerance to bromocriptine vary among patients. The drug is carefully titrated to determine the maximum benefit:risk ratio. The adverse reactions are generally related to its activity as a dopaminergic agonist. The adverse reactions are classified into two groups: effects with initial therapy and long-term effects. Initial effects include nausea, vomiting, and postural hypotension. The gastrointestinal effects can be decreased by administering bromocriptine with food or by reducing the dose. There is a "first-dose phenomenon," which is manifested by sudden cardiovascular collapse. Long-term effects include constipation, *erythromelalgia*, mental disturbances (confusion, vivid dreams, delusions, hallucinations), dyskinesia, alcohol intolerance, and digital vasospasm. All of these adverse reactions can be reversed by decreasing the dose or discontinuing bromocriptine.

INTERACTIONS. Concurrent use of bromocriptine and antihypertensive agents results in additive hypotension. The use of bromocriptine with CNS depressants (antihistamines, alcohol, sedative-hypnotics) increases sedation. Concurrent administration of phenothiazines, haloperidol, methyldopa, reserpine, and tricyclic antidepressants reduces bromocriptine's ability to decrease prolactin levels.

DOSAGE. For the treatment of parkinsonism, the adult oral dosage is 1.25 mg given two times a day, increased by 2.5 mg/day in a two- to four-week interval. The average dosage range is 30 to 90 mg/day in three divided doses.

When used for hyperprolactinemia and postpartum lactation, the adult oral dosage is 2.5 mg given two times a day.

ANTICHOLINERGIC AGENTS

The anticholinergic agents, atropine and scopolamine, were the first to be used in the treatment of parkinson-ism. These agents have been replaced by synthetic drugs that are equally as effective but have fewer adverse reactions. After dopaminergic agents were discovered, anticholinergics played a supportive role in the treatment of parkinsonism. However, these agents are still very useful for patients who have minimal symptoms, and for those unable to tolerate levodopa or levodopa/carbidopa, due to the adverse reactions or contraindications.

Actions

The anticholinergic agents inhibit the actions of endogenous acetylcholine and muscarinic agonists at the muscarinic receptors of peripheral effector tissues and in the CNS. Muscarinic receptors are distributed at sites of cholinergic transmission. The decreased amounts of dopamine in the striatum of parkinsonism patients create an intensified excitatory effect of the cholinergic system with the striatum. Anticholinergic agents (trihexyphenidyl, benztropine, biperiden, procyclidine) block the excitatory effect of the cholinergic system.

Uses

The anticholinergic agents are used in the early stages of Parkinson's disease. Many times these agents are used to treat younger patients who will require long-term therapy and for patients who are experiencing tremor. Tremor and rigidity respond well to the anticholinergic agents. There is less of a response in patients with bradykinesia and loss of the postural reflexes. Anticholinergic agents are also beneficial in the treatment of drug-induced parkinsonism. As parkinsonism progresses, the patient becomes refractory to the effects of anticholinergic agents. Responsiveness to these agents can occur by increasing the dose or by substituting another class of anticholinergic agent.

Pharmacokinetics

These agents are well absorbed from the gastrointestinal tract and can cross the blood–brain barrier. See Table 23–2 for the onset, peak, duration, and half-life of these drugs. After an oral dose of trihexyphenidyl, the onset of action is one hour, the peak of action is two to three hours, and the duration of action is 6 to 12 hours. The duration of the time-release capsule is 12 to 24 hours. After an oral dose of benztropine, the onset of action is one to two hours, the peak action is unknown, and the duration of action is 24 hours. If benztropine is administered by the parenteral route, the onset of action is a few minutes, the peak action is unknown, and the duration of action is 24 hours.

Contraindications and Precautions

Anticholinergic agents are contraindicated in patients with hypersensitivity to these drugs, narrow-angle glaucoma, and tachycardia. Anticholinergic agents can block the parasympathetic input to the sinoatrial node, producing tachycardia. The mydriatic effect of anticholinergic agents can precipitate an attack of acute glaucoma.

TEXT RESUMES ON PAGE 574

Table 23–2. ANTIPARKINSON AGENTS

Name	Dosage	Mode of Administration	Pharmacokinetics
DOPAMINERGIC AGENTS Levodopa (Dopar, L-Dopa, Larodopa); Carbidopa/Levodopa (Sinemet)			

Action: Converted to dopamine in the CNS, where it serves as a neurotransmitter. Carbidopa prevents peripheral destruction of levodopa and makes more levodopa available to the CNS.

Use: Used in the treatment of parkinsonism. Not useful for drug-induced extrapyramidal reactions.

Name	Dosage	Mode of Administration	Pharmacokinetics
	Levodopa *Adults:* Initially, 500–1000 mg given in divided doses every 6–12 hr; increase by 100–750 mg/day every 3–7 days until response occurs or dose of 8000 mg/day is reached. Usual maintenance dose is 2000–8000 mg/day.	PO	O: 10–15 min P: UA D: 5–24 hr (up to 3–5 days with prolonged therapy) ½L: 1 hr PB: UA B: GI tract and liver E: kidney
	Carbidopa/Levodopa (Tablets contain 10/100, 25/100, or 25/250 mg of carbidopa and levodopa, respectively): *Adults:* 75/300–150/1500 mg/day in 3–4 divided doses; can be increased up to 200/2000 mg/day	PO	O: UA P: UA D: 5–24 hr (up to 3–5 days with prolonged therapy) ½L: 1–2 hr carbadopa; 2 hr levodopa PB: 36%, carbadopa; UA, levodopa B: GI tract and liver E: kidney

Key to Abbreviations in the *Pharmacokinetics* column O-onset; P-peak; D-duration; PB-protein bound; B-biotransformed in; E-excreted in; ½L-halflife.
*Within the column listing adverse effects, underlines indicate the most common effects, and CAPITALS indicate life-threatening effects.

Antiparkinson Agents

Contraindications/ Precautions	Adverse Effects*	Interactions	Nursing Implications
			For all antiparkinson agents: ASSESSMENT: Assess parkinsonian symptoms prior to and throughout course of therapy. Assess blood pressure during period of dose adjustment. EVALUATION: Effectiveness of therapy can be demonstrated by a resolution of parkinsonian signs and symptoms.
Contraindicated in hypersensitivity, and in patients with narrow-angle glaucoma or those receiving MAO inhibitors. Do not use in patients with malignant melanoma or undiagnosed skin lesions. Do not use in children under 12 years of age, lactation, hemolytic anemia, and glucose-6-phosphate dehydrogenase deficiency.	Neuro: involuntary movements, memory loss, anxiety, RESTLESSNESS, psychiatric problems, nightmares, hallucinations, dizziness, PSYCHOSIS, mydriasis, blurred vision CV: hypertension, hypotension, DYSRHYTHMIA GI: nausea, vomiting, anorexia, dry mouth Hema: hemolytic anemia, leukopenia Integ: melanoma Misc: hepatotoxicity	Drug–Drug: Do not use with MAO inhibitors. Phenothiazines, haloperidol, phenytoin, and reserpine may antagonize antiparkinson agents. Large doses of pyridoxine may reverse the effect of levodopa. Additive hypotension occurs with methyldopa, guanethidine, and antidepressants. Drug–Lab: May cause false-positive urine glucose testing with copper sulfate method; use Keto-Diastix or Tes-tape. May also interfere with results of urine ketone test. Drug–Food: Diet high in pyridoxine may block the effect of levodopa.	Same as for all, plus: ASSESSMENT: In patients receiving long-term therapy, hepatic and renal functions, CBC, and serum glucose should be monitored periodically. Assess for signs of toxicity (involuntary muscle twitching, facial grimacing, spasmodic winking, exaggerated protrusion of tongue, or behavioral changes). Consult physician promptly if these symptoms occur. INTERVENTION: Administer food shortly after medication to minimize GI irritation; taking food before or concurrently may retard levodopa's effect. If patient has difficulty swallowing, confer with pharmacist. In the carbidopa/levodopa combination, the number following the drug name represents the mg of each respective drug. Wait 8 hours after last levodopa dose before switching patient to carbidopa/levodopa. Administering carbidopa shortly after a full dose of levodopa may result in toxicity. In preoperative patients who are NPO, confer with physician about continuing medication administration. EVALUATION: Therapeutic effects usually become evident after 2–3 weeks of therapy, but may require up

CONTINUED ON THE FOLLOWING PAGE

Table 23–2. ANTIPARKINSON AGENTS–*CONTINUED*

Name	Dosage	Mode of Administration	Pharmacokinetics
DOPAMINERGIC AGENTS–*Continued*			

DOPAMINE RECEPTOR AGONISTS
Amantadine (Symmetrel)

Action: Causes the release of dopamine in the CNS. Therapeutic effect is alleviation of parkinsonian symptoms. Prevents penetration of influenza A virus into host cells.

Use: Symptomatic initial and adjunct treatment of parkinsonism. Also used in prophylaxis and treatment of influenza A viral infections.

	Parkinson's Disease:		O: 10–15 min
	Adults:	PO	P: 1–4 hr
	100 mg twice daily		D: 12–24 hr
	Influenza A Viral Infection:		½L: 24 hr
	Adults and *Children over 9 yr:* 100 mg twice daily	PO	PB: UA B: minimal
	Children 1–9 yr: 4.4–8.8 mg/kg/day up to 150 mg/day in 2–3 equally divided doses	PO	E: kidneys unchanged

Bromocriptine (Parlodel)

Action: Activates dopamine receptors in the CNS. Therapeutic effect is relief of the rigidity and tremor of the parkinson syndrome. Also lowers serum prolactin levels.

Use: Treatment of parkinsonism unresponsive to levodopa therapy or in patients who cannot tolerate levodopa. Useful in conditions associated with hyperprolactinemia (amenorrhea/galactorrhea) and to suppress lactation.

Key to Abbreviations in the *Pharmacokinetics* column O-onset; P-peak; D-duration; PB-protein bound; B-biotransformed in; E-excreted in; ½L-halflife.
*Within the column listing adverse effects, underlines indicate the most common effects, and CAPITALS indicate life-threatening effects.

Contraindications/ Precautions	Adverse Effects*	Interactions	Nursing Implications
			to 6 months. Patients who receive this medication for several years may experience a decrease in its effectiveness. An increased response to the drug may occur after a drug holiday.
Contraindicated in hypersensitivity. Use cautiously in patients with a history of seizure disorders, liver disease, psychiatric problems, or cardiac disease. With renal impairment, decrease dosage. May increase susceptibility to rubella infections. Safe use in pregnancy and lactation has not been established. Taper gradually when discontinued.	Neuro: dizziness, ataxia, insomnia, depression, psychosis, anxiety, drowsiness, confusion CV: hypotension, congestive heart failure, edema GU: urinary retention Hema: leukopenia, neutropenia Integ: rashes, mottling	Additive anticholinergic effects with drugs sharing anticholinergic properties, such as antihistamines, phenothiazines, quinidine, disopyramide, and tricyclic antidepressants.	Same as for all, plus: ASSESSMENT: Monitor blood pressure periodically. Assess patient for drug-induced postural hypotension. Advise patient to make position changes slowly. INTERVENTION: Do not administer last dose of medication near bedtime, because this drug may produce insomnia in some patients. Administering drug in divided doses tends to decrease CNS side effects. The contents of capsules may be mixed with food or fluids if the patient has difficulty swallowing pills. Drug is also available as a syrup. EVALUATION: Evaluate patient for confusion, hallucinations, and mood changes. Notify physician if these occur. Assess patient for the appearance of a diffuse purple mottling of the skin. This common side effect disappears with continued therapy but may not completely resolve until several weeks after therapy has been completed. Therapeutic effects are usually apparent by the end of the first week of therapy.

CONTINUED ON THE FOLLOWING PAGE

Table 23–2. ANTIPARKINSON AGENTS–*CONTINUED*

Name	Dosage	Mode of Administration	Pharmacokinetics
Bromocriptine–*Continued*	*Parkinsonism:* *Adults:* 1.25 mg twice daily; increased by 2.5 mg/day in 2–4-week intervals (usual dosage range is 30–90 mg/day in 3 divided doses)	PO	O: 30–90 min P: 1–2 hr D: 8–12 hr ½L: Biphasic: first phase, 4–4.5 hr; terminal phase, 45–50 hr) PB: 90–96% B: liver E: feces
	Hyperprolactinemia and Postpartum Lactation: *Adults:* 2.5 mg 2–3 times daily	PO	D: 24 hr

ANTICHOLINERGIC AGENTS
Trihexyphenidyl (Aphen, Artane, Trihexane, Tri-hexy)

Action: Inhibits the action of acetylcholine, resulting in decreased sweating and salivation, mydriasis (pupillary dilation), and increased heart rate. Has a spasmolytic action on smooth muscle, inhibits cerebral motor centers, and blocks efferent impulses. Therapeutic effect is diminished signs/symptoms associated with parkinsonism syndrome.

Use: Used as an adjunct in the management of the parkinsonism syndrome, including drug-induced parkinsonism.

| | *Adults:* 1 mg/day initially; increase by 2 mg every 3–5 days. Usual maintenance dosage is 5–15 mg/day in 3–4 divided doses. Extended-release (Artane Sequels) preparations may be given every 12–24 hr once the daily dose has been determined using conventional tablets or liquids. | PO | O: 1 hr; (time-released) UA P: PO, 2–3 hr; time-released, UA D: PO, 6–12 hr; time-released, 12–24 hr ½L: UA PB: UA B: UA E: urine |

Key to Abbreviations in the *Pharmacokinetics* column O-onset; P-peak; D-duration; PB-protein bound; B-biotransformed in; E-excreted in; ½L-halflife.
*Within the column listing adverse effects, underlines indicate the most common effects, and CAPITALS indicate life-threatening effects.

Contraindications/ Precautions	Adverse Effects*	Interactions	Nursing Implications
Contraindicated in hypersensitivity to bromocriptine or ergot alkaloids. Not to be used in children under 15 years. Use cautiously in patients with a history of cardiac disease or mental disturbances. Safety in pregnancy has not been established. Suppresses lactation. Reduce dosage in severe liver impairment.	Neuro: headache, dizziness, drowsiness, insomnia, confusion, hallucinations, nightmares, burning eyes, visual disturbances, nasal stuffiness CV: hypotension, shock, leg cramps Resp: pulmonary infiltrates, effusions GI: nausea, vomiting, anorexia, abdominal pain, dry mouth, metallic taste Integ: urticaria	Additive hypotension with antihypertensives. Additive sedation with CNS depressants, including antihistamines, alcohol, and sedative-hypnotics. Additive neurologic effects with levodopa. Effectiveness in reducing prolactin levels may be antagonized by phenothiazines, haloperidol, methyldopa, tricyclic antidepressants, and reserpine.	Same as for all, plus: ASSESSMENT: Assess breasts for firmness, discomfort, and lactation (if given to suppress lactation). Assess patient for allergy to ergot derivatives. Monitor blood pressure prior to and frequently during drug therapy. Instruct patient to remain supine during and for several hours after first dose, because severe hypotension may develop. Monitor patient's mental status frequently. Psychotic symptoms have been reported with this drug. INTERVENTION: Administer with food or milk to minimize gastric distress. Tablets may be crushed if necessary. Supervise ambulation and transfer during initial dosing to prevent injury from hypotension. EVALUATION: Decreased breast engorgement, decreased galactorrhea, and a resumption of normal ovulatory menstrual cycles also demonstrate effectiveness.
Contraindicated in hypersensitivity, narrow-angle glaucoma, acute hemorrhage, tachycardia secondary to cardiac insufficiency, or thyrotoxicosis. Use cautiously in elderly and very young patients, due to increased susceptibility to adverse reactions. Use with caution in patients who may have abdominal obstruction or infection; prostatic hypertrophy; or chronic renal, hepatic, pulmonary, or cardiac disease. Safe use in pregnancy and lactation has not been established.	Neuro: dizziness, nervousness, drowsiness, weakness, headache, blurred vision, mydriasis CV: tachycardia GI: dry mouth, nausea, constipation, vomiting GU: urinary hesitancy, urinary retention Integ: decreased sweating	Additive anticholinergic effects with antihistamines, tricyclic antidepressants, and disopyramide. Additive CNS depression with alcohol, antihistamines, narcotics, and sedative-hypnotics. Anticholinergics may alter the absorption of other drugs by slowing motility of the GI tract. Antacids may decrease absorption. May increase GI mucosal lesions in patients receiving oral wax-matrix potassium chloride preparations.	Same as for all, plus: ASSESSMENT: Assess blood pressure and pulse frequently during period of dose adjustment. INTERVENTION: Usually administered after meals. May be administered before meals if patient suffers from dry mouth, or with meals if gastric distress is a problem. Sustained-release capsules should be swallowed whole; do not crush, break, or chew.

CONTINUED ON THE FOLLOWING PAGE

Table 23–2. ANTIPARKINSON AGENTS–*CONTINUED*

Name	Dosage	Mode of Administration	Pharmacokinetics
Benztropine (Cogentin)			

Action: Blocks cholinergic activity in the CNS, which is partially responsible for the symptoms of Parkinson's disease. Helps restore the natural balance of neurotransmitters in the CNS. Therapuetic effect is reduction of rigidity and tremors.

Use: Adjunctive treatment of Parkinson's disease. Also used in the treatment of drug-induced extrapyramidal effects and acute dystonic reactions.

	Dosage	Mode of Administration	Pharmacokinetics
	Parkinsonism: *Adults:* 0.5–6 mg/day in 1–2 divided doses. Start with 0.5–1.0 mg, increase by 0.5 mg every 5–6 days until response is obtained. If given as a single daily dose, administer at bedtime.	PO	O: PO, 1–2 hr P: Peak clinical effects may require 2–3 days D: 24 hr ½L: UA PB: UA B: UA E: UA
	Acute Dystonic Reactions: *Adults:* 2 mg	IM, IV	O: few minutes

Key to Abbreviations in the *Pharmacokinetics* column O-onset; P-peak; D-duration; PB-protein bound; B-biotransformed in; E-excreted in; ½L-halflife.
  *Within the column listing adverse effects, underlines indicate the most common effects, and CAPITALS indicate life-threatening effects.

These agents also increase aqueous outflow resistance, increasing intraocular pressure.

Anticholinergic agents are used with caution in patients with abdominal obstruction, prostatic hypertrophy, and in the elderly or very young due to susceptibility to adverse reactions. These agents will block the excitatory effect of acetylcholine on the detrusor muscle of the bladder, causing urinary retention. Patients with prostatic hypertrophy should be observed for urinary retention. Anticholinergic agents impair gastric secretion and gastrointestinal motility, so patients with abdominal obstruction should be observed for signs of constipation and intestinal obstruction. Safe use in pregnancy and lactation has not been established.

Adverse Reactions

The most common reactions are dry mouth, mydriasis, cycloplegia, tachycardia, constipation, urinary retention, and psychic disturbances. Anticholinergic agents inhibit salivation (which is helpful in the parkinsonism patient because excessive salivation may be a problem). Some of the frequent CNS reactions include mental confusion, hallucinations, delirium, sedation, nervousness, dizzi-

Contraindications/ Precautions	Adverse Effects*	Interactions	Nursing Implications
Contraindicated in hyper-sensitivity, children under 3 years, and patients with narrow-angle glaucoma. Used cautiously in patients who may not be able to tolerate anticho-linergic effects, particu-larly elderly patients. Safety in pregnancy and lactation has not been established.	Neuro: confusion, weakness, hallucinations, headache, sedation, depression, dizzi-ness, dry eyes, blurred vision, mydriasis (dilated pupils) CV: tachycardia, dysrhyth-mias, palpitations GI: constipation, dry mouth, nausea, ileus GU: urinary retention, hesi-tancy Misc: decreased sweating	Additive anticholinergic effects with drugs sharing anticholinergic properties, such as antihistamines, phenothiazines, quinidine, disopyramide, and tricyclic antidepressants. Counter-acts the cholinergic effects of drugs like bethanechol.	Same as for all, plus: INTERVENTION: Administer with food or immediately after meals to minimize gastric irritation. May be crushed and administered with food if patient has diffi-culty swallowing. Parenteral doses of the drug are used only in acute situations. EVALUATION: Effectiveness of therapy can be demon-strated by a decrease in drooling and rigidity and an improvement in gait and balance. Therapeutic effects are usually seen 2 to 3 days after the initiation of ther-apy. Monitor for constipa-tion, abdominal pain, dis-tention, or the absence of bowel sounds. Report abnormal findings promptly. Monitor intake:output ratios and evaluate patient for uri-nary retention (dysuria, dis-tended abdomen, infrequent voiding of small amounts, overflow incontinence). Patients with mental illness are at risk for developing exaggerated symptoms of their disorder during early therapy with this medica-tion. Withhold drug and notify physician if significant behavioral changes occur.

ness, and headache. These reactions are especially trou-blesome to the elderly patient.

Interactions

Concurrent use of anticholinergic agents with antihis-tamines, tricyclic antidepressants, phenothiazines, quin-idine, and disopyramide give additive anticholinergic ef-fects. The use of anticholinergic agents can alter the absorption of other drugs (levodopa, carbidopa) by slowing motility of the gastrointestinal tract.

All of these agents counteract the cholinergic effects of drugs such as bethanechol.

Dosage

Trihexyphenidyl is administered by the oral route. The dosage is highly individualized, based on the extent of the disease and signs and symptoms. The adult dosage is 1 mg a day initially. This is increased by 2 mg every three to five days. A maintenance dosage range is 5 to 15 mg/day in three or four divided doses. An extended-release preparation is given every 12 to 24 hours.

Benztropine is also administered by the oral route. Again, the dosage is very individualized, based on the patient's needs. The adult dosage range is 0.5 to 6.0 mg daily in divided doses. The initial dose is 0.5 to 1.0 mg, increased 0.5 mg every five to six days until the desired response is obtained. If a single daily dose is given, it should be administered at bedtime.

For a review of specific agents used in the treatment of Parkinson's disease, see Table 23–2.

OTHER AGENTS USED IN PARKINSONISM

Other drugs that are used in the treatment of parkinsonism because of their anticholinergic activity (these agents are not considered anticholinergics) include a tricyclic antidepressant, amitriptyline (Elavil); an antihistamine, diphenhydramine (Benadryl); and a phenothiazine, ethopropazine (Parsidol). These agents can be used alone or in combination with dopaminergic agents to provide mild anticholinergic activity. These agents can also be beneficial in the treatment of patients who experience adverse reactions to anticholinergic agents.

MISCELLANEOUS DISEASES

Other diseases characterized by dyskinesia are Huntington's chorea, dystonia musculorum deformans, spasmodic torticollis, and Gilles de la Tourette syndrome. Each disease has a different cause and management. Table 23–3 gives a brief description of the diseases and pharmacologic agents used to treat them. Specific therapeutic agents are discussed in other chapters of this text.

Table 23–3. MISCELLANEOUS DISEASES OF THE NERVOUS SYSTEM

AMYOTROPHIC LATERAL SCLEROSIS (ALS, LOU GEHRIG'S DISEASE)

Description
A progressive motor neuron disease in which there is anterior horn cell and pyramidal degeneration; there may be bulbar involvement. Clinical symptoms include atrophy of muscles, weakness, fasciculations in limbs, spasticity, hyperactive reflexes, and eventually paralysis of muscle groups.

Treatment
Emotional support; physical therapy; mechanical support and appliances; diazepam (Valium) and phenytoin (Dilantin) can help with spasticity and muscle cramps.

DYSTONIA MUSCULORUM DEFORMANS

Description
A degenerative cerebral cortex and basal ganglia disease characterized by twisting, turning, and writhing movements of somatic muscles. Muscular contractions are very strong and sustained. This disease can develop in childhood and progresses during a person's lifetime. Muscles may become hypertrophic, and the person can no longer perform activities of daily living.

Treatment
Levodopa; carbamazepine, diazepam, or haloperidol; ventrolateral thalamotomy and/or cerebellar electrode stimulation has variable success.

GILLES de la TOURETTE SYNDROME

Description
Syndrome often found in childhood, intermittently worsening throughout the lifetime of the person; characterized by muscle twitching (tics), use of offensive language, echolalia, incoherent grunts and gestures.

Treatment
Haloperidol (Haldol); dosage 2–10 mg/day

HUNTINGTON'S CHOREA

Description
A progressive hereditary (autosomal-dominant) disorder; appears to be a loss of GABA-ergic and cholinergic influence; characterized by involuntary twisting movements (chorea), intellectual disturbances with deterioration, incomprehensible speech with eventual aphasia.

Treatment
Haloperidol (Haldol), chlorpromazine (Thorazine); propranolol (Inderal) for the early stages of the disease. Supportive care is needed for late stage disease.

SPASMODIC TORTICOLLIS

Description
Usually intermittent spasmodic movements or distortion of the head or neck toward one side for no apparent reason; may be jerky movements of the head; the area of the lesion is the basal ganglia; usually develops between 20–40 years of age; involves the sternocleidomastoid muscle on the opposite side of the head deviation; tension and anxiety worsen the symptoms. As this chronic problem evolves, permanent head deviation to one side can occur.

Treatment
Haloperidol (Haldol), tricyclic agents; diazepam; levodopa; biofeedback; destructive surgery to cervical muscles, accessory nerves and cervical roots with reports of variable success.

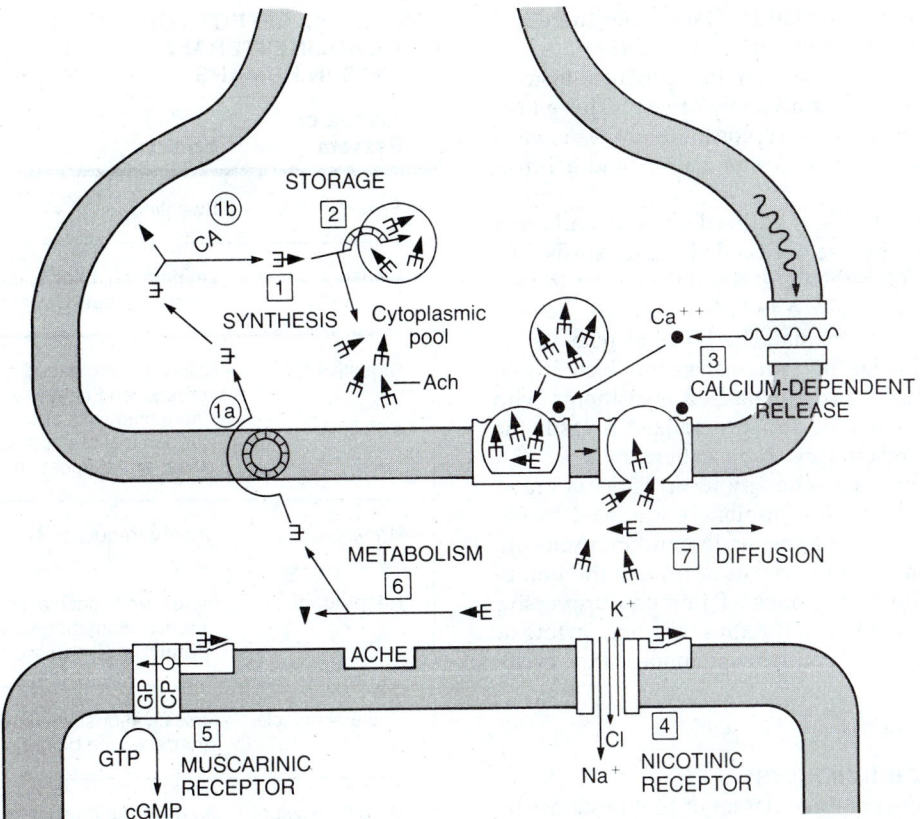

Figure 23–3. Cholinergic synapse. (1) Synthesis of acetylcholine (ACH), including (1a) choline uptake and (1b) acetylation of choline by choline acetylase (CA). (2) Storage in vesicles. (3) Calcium-dependent release. (4) Interaction with a nicotinic receptor. (5) Interaction with a muscarinic receptor linked by a coupling protein (CP) with guanadyl cyclase (GC), which catalyzes formation of cyclic-guanadyl monophosphate (cGMP) from guanadyl triphosphate (GTP). (6) Hydrolysis of ACH by acetylcholinesterase (ACHE). (From Swonger, AK, and Matejski, MP: Nursing Pharmacology, Scott, Foresman & Co., Boston, 1988, with permission.)

NEUROMUSCULAR JUNCTION DYSFUNCTION

This section focuses on the skeletal neuromuscular junction and the pharmacotherapeutic agents, *acetylcholinesterase* (AChE) *inhibitors*. It will be recalled that acetylcholine (ACh) is the neurotransmitter that is released at the skeletal neuromuscular junction (see Chapter 18).

The AChE inhibitors allow ACh to accumulate at the cholinergic receptor sites. They are capable of stimulating cholinergic receptors throughout the central and peripheral nervous systems. For a review of the cholinergic synapse, see Figure 23–3. The AChE inhibitors are used in the treatment of myasthenia gravis.

MYASTHENIA GRAVIS

Myasthenia gravis is an autoimmune neuromuscular disease that presents clinically as fluctuating weakness of one or more skeletal muscle groups. Weakness be-comes more severe with activity and improves with rest. The myasthenic can present with an acute or subacute onset precipitated by infection or emotional stress. One of the confusing aspects of myasthenia gravis is the course of the disease. It may advance irregularly, remain static for years, or spontaneously remit. Signs and symptoms are variable, fluctuating from hour to hour. They can range from mild *ptosis* to respiratory and *bulbar* failure.

The pathophysiology of myasthenia gravis involves the postjunctional receptors. There is a reduced availability of receptor sites for ACh on the postjunctional membrane caused by their blocking by antibody and the C9 component of complement to the ACh receptors. Antigenic modulation also leads to a reduction in postjunctional acetylcholine receptors. With this process, postsynaptic receptors are cross-linked, degraded, and cleared at a faster rate than normal. As a result of these pathophysiological processes, the number of interactions between the ACh release by nerve impulses and the receptors is reduced, which results in decreased muscle strength or progressive failure of contraction from repeated nerve stimulation. Many times there will also be a thymic abnormality in myasthenics.

Diagnosis is made based on the patient's history, signs and symptoms, and a variety of tests. These tests include antiacetylcholine receptor antibody tests, electromyography with repetitive stimulation, and a Tensilon test.

Drug therapy is the focus of this discussion, but other measures include thymectomy and plasmapheresis. The management of myasthenia gravis depends on the severity of the disease, the age and life-style of the patient, and the type of myasthenia. The types of myasthenia gravis include ocular myasthenia, generalized myasthenia with ocular signs, generalized myasthenia with bulbar and ocular signs, and generalized myasthenia with bulbar and respiratory complications.

The goals of pharmacotherapy in myasthenia gravis are twofold: cholinesterase inhibitors are used to enhance cholinergic nerve transmission and immunosuppressive agents are used to repair or reverse the immunologic flaw. The two groups of immunosuppressive agents are corticosteroids (prednisone) and cytotoxic agents (azathioprine, cyclophosphamide, and cyclosporine).

Cholinesterase Inhibitors

ACTION. There are three classes of cholinesterase inhibitors: quaternary ammonium compounds, carbamates, and organophosphates. This discussion addresses the ammonium compounds and carbamates. Blockage at the anionic or esteratic site of the AChE molecule prevents the hydrolysis of ACh. These two sites on the AChE molecule are chemically different. Edrophonium (quaternary ammonium amine) competes with ACh for binding at the anionic site of the active center on the AChE molecule. The carbamates (neostigmine, physostigmine, pyridostigmine) form a covalent bond to the esteratic site of the AChE molecule. The end result is inhibition of the enzyme AChE. These two classes of AChE inhibitors are reversible inhibitors. The sites of action include the neuromuscular junction, adrenal medulla, autonomic ganglia, cholinergic synapses at effector tissues of the autonomic nervous system, and cholinoceptive cells of the CNS. For a review of the effects of anticholinesterase agents on various systems in humans, see Table 23–4.

USES. The cholinesterase inhibitors have therapeutic uses in a variety of clinical situations. They are the primary agents used in the treatment of myasthenia gravis and glaucoma. They are widely used in the reversal of neuromuscular blockade and smooth muscle atony.

PHARMACOKINETICS. Most of the quaternary amines (edrophonium, ambenonium chloride) and the carbamates (pyridostigmine bromide, neostigmine) are poorly absorbed from the gastrointestinal tract, with variable absorption from the gastrointestinal tract requiring larger doses. The quaternary ammonium group does not penetrate cell membranes readily and does not

Table 23–4. EFFECTS OF ANTICHOLINESTERASE AGENTS IN HUMANS

Tissue or System	Effects
Skin	Sweating
Visual	Lacrimation, miosis, blurred vision, accommodative spasm
Digestive	Salivation; increased gastric, pancreatic, and intestinal secretions; increased tone and motility in gut (abdominal cramps, vomiting, diarrhea, and defecation)
Urinary	Urinary frequency and incontinence
Respiratory	Increased bronchial secretions, bronchoconstriction, weakness or paralysis of respiratory muscles
Skeletal muscle	Fasciculations, weakness, paralysis (depolarizing block)
Cardiovascular	Bradycardia (due to muscarinic predominance), decreased cardiac output, hypotension; effects due to ganglionic actions and activation of adrenal medulla also possible
Central nervous system	Tremor, anxiety, restlessness, disrupted concentration and memory, confusion, sleep disturbances, desynchronization of electroencephalogram, convulsions, coma, circulatory and respiratory depression

From Craig, CR and Stitzel, RE: Modern Pharmacology. Little, Brown & Co, Boston, 1986, with permission.

cross the blood–brain barrier. Physostigmine, a tertiary amine, is absorbed well from the gastrointestinal tract and is distributed throughout tissues. Edrophonium is metabolized in the liver, and some of the metabolite is excreted in bile. Carbamates undergo nonenzymatic and enzymatic hydrolysis and are excreted in the urine. Renal excretion is very important in the clearance of neostigmine, pyridostigmine, and edrophonium. The half-life of oral pyridostigmine is 3.7 hours and that of parenteral pyridostigmine is 1.9 hours. The half-life of both oral and intravenous neostigmine is 40 to 60 minutes whereas the intramuscular half-life is slightly longer, 50 to 90 minute. The onset of action for these agents varies among patients. The onset of action for ambenonium chloride is unknown; for intravenous edrophonium, the onset is 30 to 60 seconds, while the intramuscular onset is two to ten minutes. Onset for oral pyridostigmine is 30 to 45 minutes; for oral time-span pyridostigmine, 30 to 60 minutes; for intramuscular pyridostigmine, 15 minutes; for intravenous pyridostigmine, two to five minutes. The onset for oral neostigmine is 45 to 75 minutes; intramuscular, 10 to 30 minutes; and intravenous, 10 to 30 minutes. The peak effect of parenteral neostigmine is 20 to 30 minutes. The duration of action is variable. Pyridostigmine sustained-release tablets have the longest duration of action (6 to 12 hours); pyridostigmine tablets have a duration of three to six hours, and neostigmine tablets have a duration of two to four hours. Parenteral edrophonium has the shortest duration of action, 5 to 30 minutes. Pyridostigmine and neostigmine given by the parenteral route have a duration of two to four hours.

CONTRAINDICATIONS AND PRECAUTIONS. Cholinesterase inhibitors are not used in patients who are hypersensitive. These agents are contraindicated in patients with mechanical obstruction of the gastrointestinal or genitourinary tracts. These agents enhance gastric contractions and increase the secretion of gastric acid. They also increase motor activity in the small and large bowel. This effect is a combination of actions at the ganglion cells of Auerbach's plexus and at the muscle fibers, as a result of the preservation of ACh (Taylor, 1985).

Caution is used in patients with a history of asthma, ulcer disease, cardiovascular disease, epilepsy, and hyperthyroidism. The cholinesterase inhibitors cause smooth muscle constriction of the bronchioles and increase respiratory secretions. The effects of accumulated ACh on the heart and blood vessels are complex because of the involvement of both ganglionic and postganglionic fibers. The major effects are bradycardia and decreased cardiac output. The effect of ACh on the gastrointestinal tract is an increase in gastric acid secretion and contraction. The overall effect of ACh on the CNS is excitation, which can potentiate seizures. In general, the accumulation of ACh causes an increase in secretory glands that are innervated by postganglionic cholinergic fibers, as in the case of the thyroid gland. In hyperthyroidism there is already increased secretion without more ACh.

There is a fine line between the therapeutic dose and undermedication or overdose of cholinesterase inhibitors. Myasthenic weakness can occur suddenly because of the disease or undermedication or overmedication. Some of the exacerbations are due to a decrease in the responsiveness to cholinesterase inhibitors that cannot be overcome by a higher dose. Myasthenic crisis is characterized by increased weakness. The muscles affected are those associated with respiration, chewing, swallowing, and the muscles of the head and neck. The goal at this point in treatment is respiratory support, which may require patency of airway and ventilatory support.

When too many cholinesterase inhibitors are in the system, cholinergic crisis occurs. The cholinesterase inhibitors occupy the same receptors as ACh, and an excess of cholinesterase inhibitors will reduce neuromuscular transmission. The signs and symptoms of overdose are identical to those for myasthenia crisis. The goal is the same: patency of the airway and respiratory support.

ADVERSE REACTIONS. The majority of adverse reactions are caused by excessive cholinergic stimulation of the muscarinic and nicotinic receptors. The muscarinic side effects include abdominal cramps, nausea, vomiting, diarrhea, increased salivation, increased bronchial secretion, lacrimation, miosis, and diaphoresis. These side effects are uncomfortable, but usually tolerance will develop. If tolerance does not occur, the agent can be taken with food, the dose adjusted, or atropine added to the drug regimen. Atropine can alleviate these reactions, but it may also mask warning signs associated with overdosage. Masking these side effects can inadvertently lead to cholinergic crisis. The nicotinic adverse reactions are muscle cramps, *fasciculations*, and muscle weakness.

INTERACTIONS. There are many drugs that enhance or induce neuromuscular blockade (trimethaphan, neomycin sulfate, quinidine). Most of these drugs present a threat to the myasthenic because of the problems at the neuromuscular junction. Other drugs (curare, succinylcholine) induce muscle weakness in normal persons. Myasthenics are very sensitive to the normal doses of these agents. Cholinergic effects are antagonized by other drugs such as antihistamines, antidepressants, atropine, haloperidol, phenothiazines, quinidine, and disopyramide, which have anticholinergic properties.

Some drug interactions occur in the myasthenic because use of cholinesterase inhibitors with drugs such as corticosteroids, analgesics, and over-the-counter drugs that contain ephedrine can exacerbate the signs and symptoms of myasthenia gravis. Some agents, such as corticosteroids, can cause a refractoriness to cholinesterase inhibitors; other agents, such as aminoglycoside antibodies, beta blockers, and phenytoin, cause the presynaptic action of depressing ACh formation and/or release. Another problem encountered with agents such as procainamide and aminoglycoside antibodies is that they reduce the sensitivity of the postjunctional membrane to ACh. Some agents are competitive neuromuscular blockers, such as curare, succinylcholine, lidocaine, trimethaphan, quinidine (large doses), lincomycin, and chlorpromazine. Other agents potentiate hypokalemia. The diuretics are noted for this problem. As hypokalemia develops, there is muscle weakness. This clouds the picture for the myasthenic because it is difficult to determine the cause of the muscle weakness (the disease or the hypokalemia). Laxatives are problematic because they can render the patient weak after straining or diarrhea. See Table 23–5 for a summary of agents that are contraindicated or to be used with caution.

DOSAGE. The routes of administration for all cholinesterase inhibitors except edrophonium are oral, intramuscular, and intravenous. Edrophonium can be given

Table 23–5. DRUGS USED WITH CAUTION/CONTRAINDICATED IN MYASTHENIA GRAVIS

Alcohol
Analgesics (Narcotics)
Anesthetics
Antibiotics
  Aminoglycosides (neomycin, streptomycin, amikacin, tobramycin, netilmicin, gentamicin, kanamycin)
  Clindamycin
  Polymyxin B
  Sulfonamides
Anticonvulsants (Dilantin, phenobarbital, and others)
Antimalarials
Antirheumatics (D-Penicillamine, colchicine, chloroquine)
Cardiovascular
  Quinidine
  Beta blockers (Inderal and others)
  Lidocaine
Diuretics
Insecticides (Organophosphates)
Laxatives
Magnesium preparations
Over-the-counter cold preparations (antihistamines)
Psychotropics (Lithium carbonate, haloperidol, benzodiazepines, and others)
Sedative-hypnotics
Thyroid preparations

Modified from Adams, SL, Mathews, J, and Grammer, LC: Drugs that may exacerbate myasthenia gravis. Ann Emerg Med 13(7):532, 1984, with permission.

only by the parenteral route. See Table 23–6 for the dosage of specific drugs.

When discussing the dosage for cholinesterase inhibitors, it is important to consider factors related to dosage. Dosage does not lend itself to the "cookbook" approach. Myasthenia gravis can be aggravated by factors such as upper respiratory infection, general fatigue, excitement, loss of sleep, menstruation, high-carbohydrate meals, hyperthyroidism, and alcohol intake. Requirements change based on the patient's signs and symptoms. Usually, cholinesterase inhibitors are started in a low dose, with no attempt made to reach maximal muscle strength in the initial regimen. The daily doses are divided into three or four equal dosing intervals. Patients are encouraged to keep a diary of dosing times, periods of peak effect, periods of worsening, and side effects. This helps the physician to know how effective the particular cholinesterase inhibitor is for the patient. Some myasthenics become progressively refractory to these agents, and drug holidays can restore their effectiveness. Dosage is titrated against the response of the most important muscle group. It is not uncommon for the patient's response to the cholinesterase inhibitors to be an increase in muscle strength in one group of muscles and a decrease in muscle strength in other muscle groups. Oral and parenteral doses are not equal. Changing from the oral to parenteral route of administration requires reducing the dose of the agent. The most common cholinesterase inhibitors used in treatment of myasthenia gravis are pyridostigmine (Mestinon), neostigmine (Prostigmin), ambenonium chloride (Mytelase), and edrophonium (Tensilon). Edrophonium (Ten-

silon) is used for diagnostic purposes and in crisis. Pyridostigmine bromide is the drug of choice unless the patient is sensitive to bromide.

For a review of the specific cholinesterase inhibitors, see Table 23–6.

Corticosteroids

The use of corticosteroids has been beneficial in the treatment of myasthenia gravis. There are several indications for using corticosteroids: (1) inadequate control with a cholinesterase inhibitor; (2) older adults with moderate to severe disease; (3) short-term use following thymectomy, because there is a delayed response associated with the procedure; (4) patients who refuse a thymectomy or do not respond to a thymectomy; (5) maintenance therapy following a thymectomy (long-term use of corticosteroids); (6) maintenance following crisis; (7) preoperative use to prepare patients for thymectomy.

It is thought that corticosteroids act by suppressing the immune system. A proposed mechanism of action is interference in the cell cycle of activated lymphoid cells, especially lymphocytes. There are also possible lysis of the "suppresser" or helper T cells, decreased antibody response, and lowered concentration of specific antibody populations. Corticosteroids also cause vasoconstriction and decrease capillary permeability (anti-inflammatory action). These actions are very broad-based and are not aimed directly at the neuromuscular junction. Therapeutic effects of corticosteroids may not be seen for 3 to 14 months after therapy begins.

Approaches to dosage are based on low-dose or high-dose therapy. A short-acting corticosteroid (prednisone) is the drug of choice. With low-dose therapy, the agent is administered on a daily or an alternate-day basis. The dose is increased every third dose to the maximal dosage (25 mg daily or every other day, increased 12.5 mg every third dose to 100 mg). The advantage of this approach is that it minimizes the severity of "early worsening" episodes. Early worsening is a worsening of the signs and symptoms of myasthenia gravis 3 to 14 days after the initiation of corticosteroids. This response may be due to enhancing the mollification of sensitized lymphocytes. The disadvantage of this approach is that it takes weeks or months to achieve maximal dose and maximal clinical benefit. The high-dose approach also involves administration of the agent on a daily or an alternate-day basis. The dose of the agent is introduced at its high dose, which is usually 80 to 100 mg. The advantage is that initially there is rapid improvement in the patient's clinical presentation. The disadvantage is that early worsening is more common and can be more severe. The patient can also experience a period in which the myasthenia gravis is refractory to cholinesterase inhibitors.

Long-term therapy (months to years) can lead to adrenal suppression. Corticosteroids should be tapered and not abruptly discontinued. The patient should be monitored for chemically induced hyperglycemia, sodium retention with edema, hypokalemia, peptic ulcer, osteoporosis, and hidden infections. Other specific information on related corticosteroids is given in Chapter 42.

Cytotoxic Agents

When a myasthenic remains unresponsive to the conventional measures described previously, cytotoxic agents may be used. The most frequently used cytotoxic agents are azathioprine (Imuran), cyclophosphamide (Cytoxan), and cyclosporine (Sandimmune). As with corticosteroids, the benefits from this mode of therapy occur after months (4 to 15) of therapy. The major disadvantage of these agents are the serious side effects.

The proposed mechanisms of action for cytotoxic agents include interference with nucleic acid metabolism, DNA replication and RNA transcription, destruction of proliferating lymphoid cells, and alteration of antibody formation. These agents are discussed in further detail in Chapters 49 and 50.

SKELETAL MUSCLE RELAXANTS

Skeletal muscle hyperactivity is characterized by skeletal muscle *spasticity* or spasm. Spasticity of skeletal muscles occurs in a wide variety of neurologic disorders, and it varies greatly in its etiology and clinical manifestations. Spasticity results from hypertonicity of muscles. It is a form of increased muscle tone that results in increased resistance to passive movement of an extremity. As increasing force is applied to a joint or extremity, it is matched by resistance to movement. The clasp-knife phenomenon may occur. This occurs when there is sudden muscle relaxation after the initial resistance. Muscle spasticity may interfere with rehabilitation and may result in contractures, pain, and psychosocial problems. Some muscle relaxants act on the central nervous system; these include carisoprodol (Soma), chlorphene-

sin carbamate (Maolate), cyclobenzaprine hydrochloride (Flexeril), metaxalone (Skelaxin), methocarbamol (Robaxin, Robomol), orphenadrine citrate (Noradex, Marflex, etc.), baclofen (Lioresal); and diazepam (Valium). Others, such as dantrolene sodium (Dantrium), act directly on the skeletal muscle. These drugs are discussed in Table 23–7.

SKELETAL MUSCLE CONTRACTION

Skeletal muscle fibers are composed of actin and myosin filaments, which are found within the sarcoplasm. These protein molecules are responsible for muscle contraction. In order for a muscle to contract, several basic anatomic structures are involved. The skeletal muscle is stimulated by the stretch or contraction of the agonist muscle body. The impulse then travels to the spinal cord via a proprioceptor nerve (Fig. 23–4). The impulse travels through a synapse to a motor neuron and back to the muscle where it originated. This returning impulse is modified by inhibitory impulses from interneurons.

Various neurotransmitters such as ACh and norepinephrine, which excite, and glycine and gamma-aminobutyric acid (GABA), which inhibit, relay messages to the spinal motor neurons.

Acute muscle injury, severe cold, or lack of blood flow to the muscle can elicit spasm. Spasm occurs when the impulses from the muscle are transmitted to the spinal cord and back to the muscle, causing a reflex contraction. This reflex contraction stimulates the muscle even more, which increases the spinal cord stimulation, and thus increases the contraction. The central-acting muscle relaxants are believed to break the cycle by acting as CNS depressants.

TEXT RESUMES ON PAGE 593

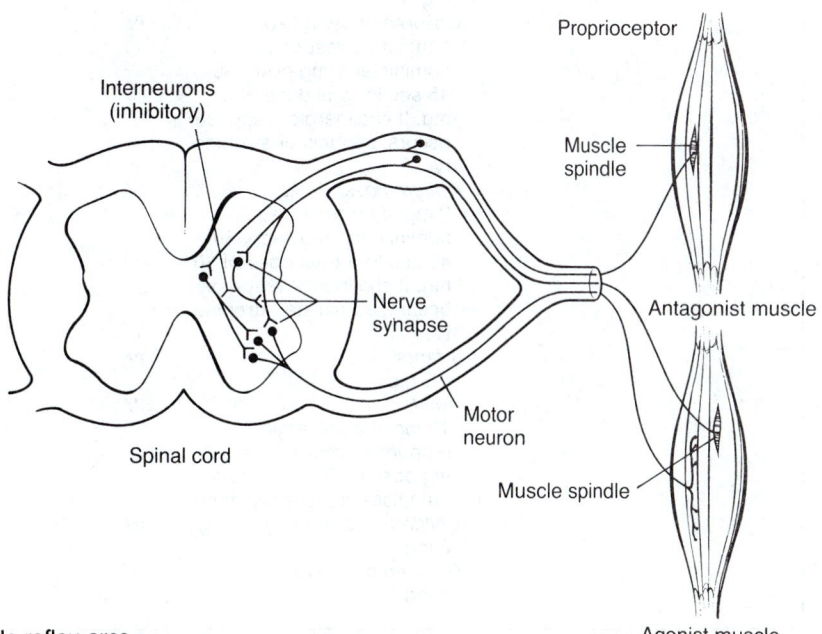

Figure 23–4. Anatomy of skeletal muscle reflex arcs.

Table 23–6. CHOLINESTERASE INHIBITORS USED IN MYASTHENIA GRAVIS

Name	Dosage	Mode of Administration	Pharmacokinetics
Edrophonium (Tensilon)			

Action: **(For all cholinesterase inhibitors)** Inhibits the breakdown of acetylcholine, prolonging its effect. Effects include miosis, increased intestinal and skeletal muscle tone, bronchial and ureteral constriction, bradycardia, increased salivation, lacrimation, and sweating. Therapeutic effects are improved muscular function in patients with myasthenia gravis, and reversal of nondepolarizing neuromuscular blockers.

Use: Used in the diagnosis of myasthenia gravis, to assess the adequacy of anticholinesterase therapy in myasthenia gravis, and to differentiate myasthenic from cholinergic crisis. Also used to reverse nondepolarizing neuromuscular blockers and to terminate paroxysmal atrial tachycardia.

Name	Dosage	Mode of Administration	Pharmacokinetics
	Diagnosis of Myasthenia Gravis: Anticholinesterase agents should be discontinued for 8 hours prior to administration.		O: IM, 2–10 min; IV, 30–60 sec P: UA D: IM, 5–30 min; IV, 5–10 min ½L: UA PB: UA B: UA E: UA
	Adults: 1 mg; if no response, administer 8 mg more. May repeat test in 30 min. If cholinergic response occurs, administer atropine, 0.4–0.5 mg IV.	IV	
	Children under 34 kg: 1 mg; if no response, administer 1 mg every 30–45 sec to total dose of 5 mg. If cholinergic response occurs, administer atropine IV.	IV	
	Children over 34 kg: 2 mg; if no response, administer 1 mg every 30–45 sec to a total dose of 10 mg. If cholinergic response occurs, administer atropine IV.	IV	
	Infants: 0.5 mg	IV	
	Adults: 10 mg; if cholinergic response occurs, repeat 2-mg dose in 30 min to rule out false-negative reaction.	IM	
	Children under 34 kg: 2 mg	IM	
	Children over 34 kg: 5 mg	IM	

Key to Abbreviations in the *Pharmacokinetics* column O-onset; P-peak; D-duration; PB-protein bound; B-biotransformed in; E-excreted in; ½L-halflife.

*Within the column listing adverse effects, underlines indicate the most common effects, and CAPITALS indicate life-threatening effects.

Contraindications/ Precautions	Adverse Effects*	Interactions	Nursing Implications
			ASSESSMENT: Assess neuromuscular status (ptosis, diplopia, vital capacity, ability to swallow, extremity strength) prior to and immediately after administration of medications. EVALUATION: Effectiveness of therapy can be demonstrated by relief of ptosis and diplopia, and improvement in chewing, swallowing, extremity strength, and breathing without the appearance of cholinergic symptoms.
Contraindicated in hypersensitivity and bromide allergies. Do not use in patients with mechanical obstruction of the GI or GU tracts. Can be used in pregnancy (may cause uterine irritability after IV administration near term; newborns may display muscle weakness) or lactation. Use cautiously in patients with a history of asthma, ulcer disease, cardiovascular disease, epilepsy, or hyperthyroidism.	Neuro: dizziness, weakness, SEIZURES, miosis, lacrimation CV: bradycardia, hypotension Resp: excess secretions, bronchospasm GI: abdominal cramps, nausea, vomiting, diarrhea, excess salivation Integ: rashes, sweating Muscskel: fasciculation	Action may be antagonized by drugs possessing anticholinergic properties, including antihistamines, antidepressants, atropine, haloperidol, phenothiazines, quinidine, and disopyramide. Prolongs action of some depolarizing muscle relaxants. Use in patients receiving digitalis glycosides may lead to excessive bradycardia.	ASSESSMENT: To differentiate myasthenic from cholinergic crisis, assess for increased weakness, diaphoresis, increased saliva and bronchial secretions, dyspnea, nausea, vomiting, diarrhea, and bradycardia. If these symptoms occur, patient is in cholinergic crisis. Monitor pulse, blood pressure, and ECG (for supraventricular tachycardia) prior to and throughout administration of this drug. INTERVENTION: Usually administered by a physician for myasthenia gravis patients. IV doses are administered undiluted with a tuberculin syringe. A dose of 2 mg is given over 15 sec; wait 45 sec while assessing neuromuscular status, and if cholinergic symptoms have not appeared, remaining dose is administered slowly. As a curare antagonist, administer 10 mg IV slowly over 30–45 sec.

CONTINUED ON THE FOLLOWING PAGE

Table 23–6. CHOLINESTERASE INHIBITORS USED IN MYASTHENIA GRAVIS– *CONTINUED*

Name	Dosage	Mode of Administration	Pharmacokinetics
Edrophonium–*Continued*	*Assessment of Anticholinesterase Therapy:* *Adults:* 1–2 mg 1 hr after oral anticholinesterase dose. *Differentiation of Cholinergic from Myasthenic Crisis:* *Adults:* 1 mg; may give additional 1 mg 1 min later. *Surgery—Reversal of Nondepolarizing Neuromuscular Blocking Agents:* *Adults:* 10 mg; may repeat every 5–10 min; not to exceed 40 mg. *Termination of Paroxysmal Atrial Tachycardia:* *Adults:* 5–10 mg *Slow Tachyarrhythmias:* *Adults:* 2-mg test dose; then 2 mg every min to a total of 10 mg. May continue therapy with infusion of 0.25–2 mg/min	IV IV IV IV IV	

Pyridostigmine (Mestinon)

Use: Used to increase muscle strength in symptomatic treatment of myasthenia gravis. Also used to reverse nondepolarizing neuromuscular blockers.

| | *Antidote for Nondepolarizing Neuromuscular Blockers:*
Adults:
10–20 mg; pretreat with 0.6–1.2 mg atropine IV
Myasthenia Gravis:
Adults:
60–180 mg 2–4 times daily (up to 1500 mg/day)
Children:
7 mg/kg/day in 5–6 divided doses
Adults:
2 mg or 1/30 of oral dose, may be repeated every 2–3 hr | IV

PO

PO

IM, IV | O: PO, 30–45 min; PO—ER, 30–60 min; IM, 15 min; IV, 2–5 min
P: UA
D: PO, 3–6 hr; PO—ER, 6–12 hr; IM, 2–4 hr; IV, 2–3 hr
½L: PO, 3.7 hr; IV, 1.9 hr
PB: UA
B: plasma cholinesterases and the liver
E: urine |

Key to Abbreviations in the *Pharmacokinetics* column O-onset; P-peak; D-duration; PB-protein bound; B-biotransformed in; E-excreted in; ½L-halflife.

*Within the column listing adverse effects, underlines indicate the most common effects, and CAPITALS indicate life-threatening effects.

Contraindications/ Precautions	Adverse Effects*	Interactions	Nursing Implications
Contraindicated in hypersensitivity. Do not use in patients with mechanical obstruction of the GI or GU tracts. Can be used in pregnancy (may cause uterine irritability after IV administration near term; newborns may display muscle weakness) or lactation. Use cautiously in patients with a history of asthma, bromide allergies, ulcer disease, cardiovascular disease, epilepsy, or hyperthyroidism.	Neuro: dizziness, weakness, SEIZURES, miosis, lacrimation CV: bradycardia, hypotension Resp: excess secretions, bronchospasm GI: abdominal cramps, nausea, vomiting, diarrhea, excess salivation Integ: rashes, sweating	Cholinergic effects may be antagonized by other drugs possessing anticholinergic properties, including antihistamines, antidepressants, atropine, haloperidol, phenothiazines, quinidine, and disopyramide. Prolongs action of depolarizing muscle-relaxing agents (succinylcholine, decamethonium).	Same as for all, plus: ASSESSMENT: Patients with myasthenia gravis may be advised to keep a daily record of their condition and the effects of this medication. Assess patient for overdose, which may induce cholinergic crisis, and underdose or resistance. Both have similar symptoms (muscle weakness, dyspnea, dysphagia). Symptoms of overdose usually occur within 1 hr after administration. Cholinergic symptoms may also include increased respiratory secretions and saliva, nausea, vomiting, cramping, diarrhea, and diaphoresis. INTERVENTION: Administer drug with food or milk to minimize side effects. Extended-release tablets should be swallowed whole; do not crush, break, or chew. Regular tablets or syrup may be administered

CONTINUED ON THE FOLLOWING PAGE

Table 23–6. CHOLINESTERASE INHIBITORS USED IN MYASTHENIA GRAVIS– *CONTINUED*

Name	Dosage	Mode of Administration	Pharmacokinetics
Pyridostigmine–*Continued*			

Neostigmine (Prostigmin)

Action: Same as for all.

Use: Used to increase muscle strength in symptomatic treatment of myasthenia gravis and to prevent and treat postoperative bladder distention and urinary retention. Also used to reverse nondepolarizing neuromuscular blockers.

	Dosage	Mode of Administration	Pharmacokinetics
	Antidote for Nondepolarizing Neuromuscular Blockers:		O: PO, 45–75 min; IM, 10–30 min; IV, 10–30 min
	Adults:	IV	P: PO, 1–2 hr (highly variable); IM, 20–30 min; IV, 20–30 min
	0.5–2 mg slowly; pretreat with 0.6–1.2 mg atropine IV		
	Bladder Atony, Abdominal Distention:		D: PO, IM, IV, 2–4 hr
	Prevention—Adults:	IM, SC	½L: 40–60 min
	0.25 mg every 4–6 hr for 2–3 days	IM, SC	PB: 15%–20%
	Treatment—Adults:	IM, SC	B: Plasma cholinesterases and liver
	0.5–1 mg; may repeat if no response after 1 hr. Repeat every 3 hr for 5 doses after bladder has been emptied.		E: urine
	Myasthenia Gravis:		
	Adults:	PO	
	Initially, 15–30 mg 3 times a day; increase at daily intervals until response is achieved. Usual maintenance dose is 150 mg/day (up to 375 mg may be needed).		
	Children:	PO	
	7.5–15 mg 3–4 times a day, up to 45 mg every 2 hr		
	Adults:	IV, IM	
	0.5–2.5 mg every 1–3 hr		

Key to Abbreviations in the *Pharmacokinetics* column O-onset; P-peak; D-duration; PB-protein bound; B-biotransformed in; E-excreted in; ½L-halflife.

*Within the column listing adverse effects, underlines indicate the most common effects, and CAPITALS indicate life-threatening effects.

Contraindications/ Precautions	Adverse Effects*	Interactions	Nursing Implications
			with extended-release tablets for optimum control of symptoms. Mottled appearance of extended-release tablets does not affect potency. To facilitate chewing, pyridostigmine may be administered 30 min before meals. Administer IV doses undiluted. Do not add to IV solutions. For myasthenia gravis, administer each 0.5 mg over 1 min. For use as muscle-relaxant antagonist, administer each 0.5 mg over 1 min. Oral dose is not interchangeable with IV dose. Parenteral form is 30 times more potent.
Same as for edrophonium.	Same as for edrophonium.	Same as for edrophonium.	Same as for pyridostigmine.

CONTINUED ON THE FOLLOWING PAGE

Cholinesterase Inhibitors

Table 23–6. CHOLINESTERASE INHIBITORS USED IN MYASTHENIA GRAVIS– *CONTINUED*

Name	Dosage	Mode of Administration	Pharmacokinetics
Ambenonium Chloride (Mytelase)			

Action: Same as for all. It is usually used only when pyridostigmine and neostigmine are unsuitable, as in patients with a history of hypersensitivity to bromides, or when a patient's weakness does not respond to pyridostigmine or neostigmine.

Use: To increase muscle strength in symptomatic treatment of myasthenia gravis. Ephedrine sulfate also may be given with ambenonium chloride. The mechanism by which ephedrine sulfate works is unknown.

Name	Dosage	Mode of Administration	Pharmacokinetics
	Adults: Initially, 5 mg 3–4 times daily; daily dosage gradually increased at 48-hr intervals; usual adult dosage ranges from 15–100 mg/day. With doses over 200 mg/day, watch for cholinergic reactions. Children: Initially, 0.3 mg/kg/day or 10 mg/M$_2$/day, 3–4 times a day. The maintenance dosage is 1.5 mg/kg/day or 50 mg/M$_2$ daily in divided doses 3–4 times a day.	PO	O: UA P: UA D: 4–8 hr. ½L: UA PB: UA B: UA E: UA

   Key to Abbreviations in the *Pharmacokinetics* column O-onset; P-peak; D-duration; PB-protein bound; B-biotransformed in; E-excreted in; ½L-halflife.
   *Within the column listing adverse effects, underlines indicate the most common effects, and CAPITALS indicate life-threatening effects.

Table 23–7. SKELETAL MUSCLE RELAXANTS

Name	Dosage	Mode of Administration	Pharmacokinetics
CENTRAL SKELETAL MUSCLE RELAXANTS			

Action: Depression of CNS in brain and spinal cord results in relaxation of striated muscles.

Use: Relief of muscle spasm of local origin caused by inflammation and trauma.

   Key to Abbreviations in the *Pharmacokinetics* column O-onset; P-peak; D-duration; PB-protein bound; B-biotransformed in; E-excreted in; ½L-halflife.
   *Within the column listing adverse effects, underlines indicate the most common effects, and CAPITALS indicate life-threatening effects.

Contraindications/ Precautions	Adverse Effects*	Interactions	Nursing Implications
Same as for edrophonium.	Same as for edrophonium.	Same as for edrophonium.	Same as for pyridostigmine.

Contraindications/ Precautions	Adverse Effects*	Interactions	Nursing Implications
For all: Contraindicated in hypersensitivity. Use with caution in persons requiring mental alertness. Safety in pregnancy, lactating women, and children has not been established.	*For all:* Neuro: drowsiness, dizziness, lightheadedness, ataxia, headache, irritability CV: palpitation, tachycardia GI: nausea, vomiting, abdominal distress, constipation, diarrhea, dry mouth	*For all:* Concurrent use of alcohol, antipsychotics, antianxiety drugs have additive effect.	*For all:* ASSESSMENT: Assess neuromuscular status before and during therapy. Assess bowel and bladder function and hepatic and renal function. INTERVENTION: Take with food to avoid GI upset. Avoid activities requiring alertness. Advise patient to avoid alcohol consumption. Drug dependence may occur; monitor the patient closely. Do not abruptly discontinue drugs. EVALUATION: Report rash, pruritus, and other evidence of hypersensitivity to physician. If symptoms are not relieved in 30 to 40 days, notify physician.

CONTINUED ON THE FOLLOWING PAGE

Table 23–7. SKELETAL MUSCLE RELAXANTS–*CONTINUED*

Name	Dosage	Mode of Administration	Pharmacokinetics
Carisoprodol (Soma, Rela, Sodol)	350 mg 3–4 times daily; last dose at bedtime	PO	O: 30 min P: 4 hr D: 4–6 hr ½L: 8 hr PB: UA B: liver E: urine
Chlorphenesin Carbamate (Maolate)	Initial: 800 mg 3 times daily Maintenance: 400 mg 4 times daily	PO	O: 1 hr P: 1–2 hr D: 4–6 hr ½L: 4 hr PB: UA B: liver E: urine
Chlorzoxazone (Paraflex, ParaFon Forte DSC)	*Adult:* 250–750 mg 3–4 times daily. *Children:* 125–500 mg 3–4 times daily	PO	O: 1 hr P: 2–4 hr D: 3–4 hr ½L: 66 min PB: UA B: liver E: urine
Cyclobenzaprine Hydrochloride (Flexeril)	10 mg 3 times daily; not to exceed 60 mg/day	PO	O: 1 hr P: 4–6 hr D: 12–24 hr ½L: 1–3 days PB: 93% B: liver E: urine
Metaxalone (Skelaxin)	800 mg 3–4 times daily	PO	O: 1 hr P: 2 hr D: 4–6 hr ½L: 2–3 hr PB: UA B: liver E: urine
Methocarbamol (Robaxin, Delaxin, Robomol, Marbaxin)	Initial: 1.5 g 4 times daily Maintenance: 1 g 4 times daily or 1.5 g 3 times daily	PO	O: 30 min P: 2 hr D: UA ½L: 1–2 hr PB: UA B: liver E: urine
	1 g undiluted, maximum rate of 3 ml/min	IV	O: immediate
Orphenadrine Citrate (Marflex, Noradex, etc.)	100 mg 2 times daily. 60 mg every 12 hours	PO IV, IM	O: 1 hr; IV, immediate P: 2 hr D: 4–6 hr ½L: 14 hr PB: UA B: liver E: urine, feces

Key to Abbreviations in the *Pharmacokinetics* column O-onset; P-peak; D-duration; PB-protein bound; B-biotransformed in; E-excreted in; ½L-halflife.
   *Within the column listing adverse effects, underlines indicate the most common effects, and CAPITALS indicate life-threatening effects.

Contraindications/ Precautions	Adverse Effects*	Interactions	Nursing Implications
Same as *for all*, plus: Contraindicated in suspected or acute intermittent porphyria. Use cautiously in patients with impaired hepatic or renal function.	Same as *for all*, plus: Neuro: ataxia, tremor CV: hypotension, tachycardia Resp: asthmatic episodes Hema: eosinophilia Integ: rash, erythema, multiforme pruritus	Same as *for all*.	Same as *for all*.
Same as *for all*, plus: Use cautiously in patients with impaired hepatic function.	Same as *for all*, plus: Neuro: headache, insomnia, confusion Resp: ANAPHYLACTIC REACTION Hema: rarely LEUKOPENIA, THROMBOCYTOPENIA, AGRANULOCYTOSIS, drug fever	Same as *for all*.	Same as *for all*, plus: INTERVENTION: Do not use for more than 8 weeks. Monitor blood studies. Administer with food or milk. EVALUATION: Evaluate for signs of blood dyscrasias.
Same as *for all*, plus: Use with caution in patients with hepatic dysfunction and known allergies.	Same as *for all*, plus: Neuro: malaise Biliary: liver damage Renal: urine discoloration Misc: allergic skin rashes, angioneurotic edema	Same as *for all*.	Same as *for all*, plus: INTERVENTION: As improvement occurs, dose is decreased. Administer with food to avoid GI upset. Monitor liver function.
Same as *for all*, plus: Contraindicated with concurrent MAO inhibitors, acute phase myocardial infarction, congestive heart failure, heart block, and hyperthyroidism. Decreases the antihypertensive effects of guanethidine.	Same as *for all*, plus: Neuro: ataxia, vertigo, dysarthria, paresthesia, disorientation CV: tachycardia, dysrhythmias GI: gastritis, dry mouth Integ: sweating, rash	Same as *for all*.	Same as *for all*, plus: INTERVENTION: Use for short-term (2–3 weeks) therapy only. EVALUATION: Evaluate for urinary output and urinary retention.
Same as *for all*, plus: Contraindicated with significantly impaired renal or liver function.	Same as *for all*, plus: Biliary: jaundice Hema: LEUKOPENIA, HEMOLYTIC ANEMIA Integ: rash	Same as *for all*.	EVALUATION: Notify physician if skin rash or yellow discoloration of skin or eyes develop. Observe for signs of blood dyscrasias.
Same as *for all*, plus: IV administration contraindicated in renal disease.	Same as *for all*, plus: Neuro: syncope CV: bradycardia GI: metallic taste Integ: urticaria, rash Ophth: blurred vision, nasal congestion, diplopia	Same as *for all*.	Same as *for all*, plus: INTERVENTION: During IV administration, patient should be recumbent. Urine may turn dark brown, black, or green when standing. EVALUATION: Notify physician if skin rash, fever, or nasal congestion occur.
Same as *for all*, plus: Contraindicated in glaucoma, pyloric and duodenal obstruction, pros-	Same as *for all*, plus: Neuro: weakness, confusion, agitation CV: tachycardia, palpitations	Concurrent use of propoxyphene results in confusion and tremors and additive effect. Cholinergic-blocking	Same as *for all*, plus: ASSESSMENT: Periodically assess blood, urine output, and liver function.

CONTINUED ON THE FOLLOWING PAGE

Table 23–7. SKELETAL MUSCLE RELAXANTS–*CONTINUED*

Name	Dosage	Mode of Administration	Pharmacokinetics
Orphenadrine Citrate–*Continued*			
Baclofen (Lioresol)	5 mg 3 times daily for 3 days. Increase 10 mg 3 times day for 3 days. Increase 15 mg 3 times day for 3 days. Increase 20 mg 3 times day for 3 days. Not to exceed 80 mg/day.	PO	O: varies from hr to weeks P: 2 hr D: 8 hr ½L: 3–4 hr PB: 30% B: liver E: urine, feces

DIRECT-ACTING SKELETAL MUSCLE RELAXANTS

Action: Interferes with intramuscular release of calcium from sarcoplasmic reticulum.

Use: To reduce spasticity of spinal cord and cerebral injuries, multiple sclerosis, cerebral palsy, and possible stroke; also used in malignant hyperthermia.

Name	Dosage	Mode of Administration	Pharmacokinetics
Dantrolene Sodium (Dantrium)	25 mg 1 time daily up to 100 mg 2–4 times daily to maximum of 400 mg	PO	O: 1 hr P: 4–6 hr D: 8 hr ½L: 9 hr PB: highly B: liver E: urine
	2.5 mg/kg over 1 hr	IV	½L: 4–8 hr

Key to Abbreviations in the *Pharmacokinetics* column O-onset; P-peak; D-duration; PB-protein bound; B-biotransformed in; E-excreted in; ½L-halflife.

*Within the column listing adverse effects, underlines indicate the most common effects, and CAPITALS indicate life-threatening effects.

Contraindications/ Precautions	Adverse Effects*	Interactions	Nursing Implications
tatic hypertrophy, and myasthenia gravis.	GI: dry mouth Hema: APLASTIC ANEMIA Renal: hesitancy, retention Ophth: blurred vision, increased intraocular pressure	agents increase anticholinergic effects.	INTERVENTION: Do not crush or chew sustained-action tablets. Give parenteral dose over 5 minutes with patient in supine position. Keep patient supine for 5–10 minutes, then help him/her to a sitting position. Educate patient about proper dosing because even mild overdoses can be toxic. EVALUATION: Notify physician of persistent skin rash, rapid heart beat, or mental confusion.
Same as *for all*, plus: Use cautiously in patients with renal dysfunction.	Same as *for all*, plus: Neuro: insomnia, weakness, fatigue, drowsiness CV: hypotension GI: nausea, vomiting, constipation, dry mouth, diarrhea, taste disorders. Renal: frequency	Same as *for all*.	Same as *for all*, plus: INTERVENTION: Do not stop abruptly. Administer with full glass of water to decrease GI irritation. EVALUATION: Notify physician of frequent urge to urinate or painful urination.
Contraindicated in hepatic disease. Use cautiously in patients with pulmonary dysfunction.	Neuro: fatigue, insomnia, depression, confusion, visual and speech disturbances, headache CV: tachycardia GI: diarrhea, GI bleeding, dysphagia Biliary: hepatitis, HEPATOTOXICITY Renal: urinary frequency, hematuria, difficult erection Integ: photosensitivity Muscskel: myalgia, backache	Increased possibility of hepatotoxicity with concurrent use of estrogen. Warfarin and clofibrate decrease plasma protein binding. Tolbutamide increases protein binding.	ASSESSMENT: Assess baseline liver function, SGPT, SGOT, and total bilirubin. INTERVENTION: Monitor liver function closely. If no benefit has been obtained within 45 days, discontinue drug. Difficulty in swallowing may occur. Patient should wear protective clothing when in sun. Reconstitute with 60 ml of sterile water, not bacteriostatic water, when administering drug IV. EVALUATION: Notify physician of persistent rash, bloody or tarry stool, or yellow discoloration of skin or eyes.

Muscle spasticity originates within the CNS. Spasticity is associated with a number of clinical conditions, such as upper motor neuron disorders, multiple sclerosis, cerebral palsy, cerebrovascular accidents, amyotrophic lateral sclerosis (Lou Gehrig's disease), and spinal cord injuries. The lesion causes an interruption of normal excitatory or inhibitory responses. The result is abnormal nerve transmission, which causes sustained contractions, relaxations, or both.

CENTRAL SKELETAL MUSCLE RELAXANTS

Action

The central skeletal muscle relaxants work by several different mechanisms. They either block the transmission of nerve impulses in the internuncial neurons in the spinal cord or have a depressant effect on the CNS (Fig. 23–5).

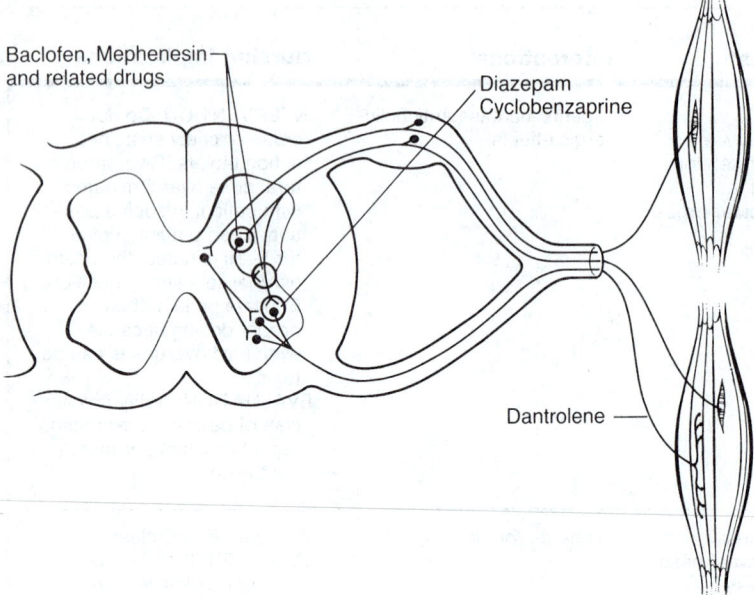

Figure 23–5. Sites of drug action for muscle relaxants.

Use

The use of central-acting muscle relaxants is controversial because of the lack of well-controlled studies to demonstrate that these drugs are safe and effective. Many of these drugs have been studied using various animal models that may or may not be an adequate reflection of responses in humans.

Central skeletal muscle relaxants are most effective in relieving muscle spasm of local origin that is caused by inflammation or trauma. They are only slightly effective in treating spasticity related to cerebrospinal trauma, cerebral palsy, or demyelinating disorders such as multiple sclerosis.

Pharmacokinetics

The pharmacokinetic properties of central skeletal muscle relaxants have not been well studied. Generally, these drugs are well absorbed after oral administration and have an onset of action of between 30 to 60 minutes. Peak effects occur between one to eight hours, with a duration of action lasting 4 to 24 hours. (For specific information, see Table 23–7.) These drugs are widely distributed to all tissues, are metabolized in the liver, and are excreted in the urine.

Contraindications and Precautions

All central skeletal muscle relaxants are contraindicated in prior hypersensitivity. Safe use in pregnancy and lactation, and in children has not been established. Because these drugs act centrally, drowsiness and dizziness frequently occur. Therefore, patients receiving central skeletal muscle relaxants should use caution when performing activities that require mental alertness. Also, caution is used when these drugs are administered with CNS depressants such as alcohol or antianxiety or antipsychotic drugs because the effects are additive. Both psychic and physical dependence may develop after

long-term use of large doses, particularly in persons with a known tendency toward drug abuse. After prolonged use, discontinuation should be gradual to prevent withdrawal symptoms, which may include seizures.

Adverse Effects

The central skeletal muscle relaxants, because they act centrally in the brain, cause drowsiness, dizziness, and lightheadedness. Elderly or debilitated patients may exhibit increased sensitization to the usual adult dosage and, therefore, should begin with lower doses and should be assessed more closely during initial therapy. Occasional gastrointestinal complaints such as nausea, vomiting, abdominal distress, constipation, and diarrhea also occur. Taking the drug with food may minimize the gastrointestinal complaints.

Carisoprodol

Carisoprodol (Soma, Rela, Sodol) is structurally similar to meprobamate, the CNS depressant. Carisoprodol reduces the transmission of impulses from the spinal cord to skeletal muscle. The mode of action of carisoprodol has not been clearly identified but may be related to its sedative properties. Carisoprodol has no peripheral or autonomic effects. It is useful as adjunctive therapy to rest and physical therapy to treat the pain of local muscle spasm. Carisoprodol is contraindicated in persons with suspected or acute intermittent porphyria because it may increase porphyrin synthesis, thereby exacerbating symptoms. Carisoprodol is administered orally in 350-mg doses three to four times daily, with the last dose administered at bedtime.

Chlorphenesin Carbamate

Chlorphenesin carbamate (Maolate) reduces the transmission of impulses from the spinal cord to skeletal muscles. It has no effect on striated muscle. Its action may be through its sedative effect. Chlorphenesin is administered in initial doses of 800 mg given three times daily until the desired effect is obtained. The dose is then reduced to 400 mg given four times daily or less for maintenance.

Chlorzoxazone

Chlorzoxazone (Paraflex, Parafon Forte DSC) is chemically distinct from other muscle relaxants. Chlorzoxazone reduces the transmission of impulses from the spinal cord to skeletal muscle through inhibition of reflex arcs. It does not directly relax tense skeletal muscles. Chlorzoxazone is administered in dosages ranging from 250 to 750 mg three to four times daily. As improvement occurs, the dose is decreased. Chlorzoxazone may be administered to children in dosages of 125 to 500 mg three to four times daily. The tablets may be crushed.

Cyclobenzaprine Hydrochloride

Cyclobenzaprine hydrochloride (Flexeril) is both structurally and pharmacologically related to the tricyclic antidepressants. Cyclobenzaprine hydrochloride acts within the brain stem to decrease tonic somatic motor activity. It relieves skeletal muscle spasm of local origin without interfering with muscle function. Cyclobenzaprine hydrochloride is used for short-term therapy (two to three weeks) only. Cyclobenzaprine hydrochloride is administered in dosages of 10 mg three times daily not to exceed 60 mg per day.

Metaxalone

Metaxalone (Skelaxin) depresses the CNS. It may block neural transmission through polysynaptic pathways in the spinal cord. Metaxalone is used to treat acute, painful musculoskeletal conditions. Metaxalone is administered to adults and children over 12 years of age in dosages of 800 mg three to four times daily.

Methocarbamol

Methocarbamol (Robaxin, Delaxin, Robomol, Marbaxin) reduces transmission of impulses from the spinal cord to skeletal muscle. The exact mechanism of action has not been established but may be due to general CNS depression. Methocarbamol does not directly relax tense skeletal muscles and has no direct action on contractile striated muscle. Methocarbamol is used to treat acute, painful musculoskeletal conditions and as an adjunct in treating tetanus. It is available orally, intravenously, and intramuscularly. The oral dosage is 1–1.5 g four times daily. Intravenously, 1 g is administered undiluted at a maximum rate of 3 ml/minute.

Orphenadrine Citrate

Orphenadrine citrate (Marflex, Noradex, etc.) is an analog of the antihistamine diphenhydramine. Orphenadrine citrate acts centrally at the brain stem. It does not directly relax tense skeletal muscles. Orphenadrine citrate is used to treat acute painful musculoskeletal conditions. It also has anticholinergic actions, which account for many of its adverse effects. These effects are generally seen with higher doses. It can be highly toxic even with mild overdosing, so the patient must be adequately educated about how to take orphenadrine citrate. Orphenadrine citrate is administered in 100-mg oral doses in the morning and at bedtime. Sustained-release tablets are available, and they must not be crushed or chewed. Doses may also be administered intramuscularly or intravenously.

Baclofen

Baclofen (Lioresol) is a chemical analog of the inhibitory neurotransmitter, gamma-aminobutyric acid (GABA). Baclofen inhibits the release of excitatory transmitters at the spinal level. It is used to relieve spinal spasticity, and it is more effective than dantrolene and diazepam in treating patients with multiple sclerosis. Baclofen is well tolerated with few adverse effects. Oral dosage is individualized until optimum effect is achieved. The daily dose should not exceed 80 mg.

DIRECT-ACTING SKELETAL MUSCLE RELAXANTS

Direct-acting skeletal muscle relaxants affect the muscle directly. There is only one currently available direct-acting skeletal muscle relaxant, dantrolene sodium.

Dantrolene Sodium

Dantrolene sodium (Dantrium) acts at the muscle and interferes with the intramuscular release of calcium ions from the sarcoplasmic reticulum, thus weakening the force of contraction. It does not interfere with nerve impulse transmission as the centrally acting muscle relaxants do. Dantrolene is effective in treating the spasticity of spinal cord and cerebral injuries, multiple sclerosis, cerebral palsy, and possibly stroke. It is particularly useful in treating patients with spasm that causes pain. Dantrolene does produce muscle weakness, so it is used with caution in patients with borderline strength. Dantrolene is also indicated in patients with a diagnosis of malignant hyperthermia.

Dantrolene has a potential for causing drug-induced hepatitis. Patients should have baseline liver function studies. Hepatitis is generally preceded by anorexia, nausea, vomiting, abdominal discomfort, and elevation of liver function studies. Patients need to be aware of these symptoms and should notify the doctor immediately if they occur. If no observable benefit is derived within 45 days, therapy is discontinued.

Dantrolene is started in low dosages of 25 mg daily and is increased to as high as 100 mg two to four times daily. Most patients respond to 400 mg per day or less.

NURSING PROCESS RELATED TO MOVEMENT DISORDERS

A major goal of therapy is to maintain or improve a patient's independent functioning. Motor system dysfunction can cause problems, some of which have been addressed in this chapter. With many of the diseases described in this chapter, chronicity, variability, and progression of the disease are common. These concepts are very important for the nurse to understand because each patient's needs are very individual and must be addressed on an individual basis. There is rarely a "classic" case, and a "cookbook" approach to these patients is not recommended.

The patient is hospitalized when there is a need for drug adjustments or drug holidays, and when he or she experiences a worsening of his or her ability to carry out activities of daily living (i.e., walking, initiating volitional movements, swallowing, bath, dressing). For a list of specific patient problems, see Table 23–8.

ASSESSMENT

Prior to the initiation of the nursing assessment, a nursing history is obtained. It is important to address specific routines or needs the patient has, such as sleep patterns, eating habits, and bowel and bladder routines.

Table 23–8. NURSING PROCESS FOR PATIENT WITH MOVEMENT DISORDERS

Assessment

Assess muscle strength, ability to initiate volitional movement, gait.
Note tremor, rigidity, bradykinesia, akinesia, dystonia, fatigue.
Assess strength of voice, ability to swallow, presence of coughing/choking following fluids/foods.
Review history for chronic diseases, use of immunosuppressive agents.
Note psychological, emotional distress and/or behavior reflective of ineffective coping skills.

Nursing Diagnosis	Nursing Actions	Rationale	Desired Outcomes Evaluation Criteria
Mobility impaired related to decreased strength/ endurance, neuromuscular impairment as evidenced by tremor, rigidity, and difficulty in movement/inability to perform desired activities.	Administer medication prior to initiating morning self-care activities or feeding. Allow time for the medication to take effect before beginning activities. Assist with activities of daily living as necessary.	Promotes independence within the individual situation. Helps to relieve symptoms so activities can be undertaken, maximizing ability to participate in activity. Provides assistance while maintaining independence.	Achieves the maximum amount of mobility possible. Reports improved level of comfort. Displays no complications associated with immobilization.
	Monitor level of fatigue or tolerance to activity and care.	Ability to perform desired activities is a good way to monitor the effectiveness of the medication. There is a fine line between therapeutic response to the medications and toxicity.	
	Promote rest periods between activities.	Prevents undue fatigue.	
	Provide range of motion on all extremities. Obtain PT/OT consult if indicated.	Maintains/improves joint flexibility and ability to participate in activities.	
	Assist with/encourage frequent change of position (at least q 2 h).	Helps prevent muscle fatigue and complications of immobility.	
Trauma, potential for related to generalized weakness of muscle groups, difficulty with volitional movements, bradykinesia, akinesia, dystonia, rigidity, gait disturbance, balance problems, fatigue, visual disturbances.	Provide a clutter free environment.	An environment free of potential hazards reduces the risk of injury.	Remains free from injury. Modifies lifestyle/environment to reduce risk factors.
	Recommend patient wear supportive shoes while walking. Suggest short walks and frequent rest periods as necessary. Allow adequate time to perform activities.	Patients with motor weakness, gait disturbances, incoordination, and poverty of movement are prone to fall.	
	Plan activity 45 minutes after taking medication.	Enhances ability to perform/participate safely in activities.	
	Suggest use of a night light.	Promotes immediate orientation if patient awakens.	

Table 23–8. NURSING PROCESS FOR PATIENT WITH MOVEMENT DISORDERS–*CONTINUED*

Nursing Diagnosis	Nursing Actions	Rationale	Desired Outcomes/ Evaluation Criteria
Aspiration, potential for related to muscle rigidity/weakness, altered cognition.	Keep head of bed slightly elevated.	Maintaining an open airway is necessary for proper oxygenation. Positioning helps reduce occurrence of gastric reflux.	Maintains patent airway free of aspiration.
	Keep a record of swallowing difficulties/related foods/fluids.	Identifies specific problems as they occur and opportunity to alter them if possible reducing risk of aspiration.	
	Provide small/frequent meals, soft foods.	Reduces muscle fatigue/rigidity (occurring with prolonged activity of chewing) which may interfere with swallowing/potentiate aspiration.	
	Promote calm/environment during meals.	Reduces distracting stimuli and enhanced concentration on eating activity.	
Communication impaired verbal/written related to decreased muscle strength/voice volume, hand tremors as evidenced by impaired articulation, inability to modulate speech, illegible handwriting, frustration.	Identify appropriate form of alternate means of communication.	Frustration can be reduced by establishing a means of letting others know needs and thoughts.	Establishes method of communication in which needs can be expressed.
	Massage neck and facial muscles. Encourage a deep breath prior to speaking. Verify meaning of patient's words/sounds. Obtain speech therapy consultation.	Relieves tension and assists patient to express words more easily. May help to relax muscles and aid in vocal expression. Promotes understanding and sense of worth. May need additional assistance to help patient be more expressive.	
Sleep pattern disturbance related to anxiety as evidenced by poor sleep history and frequent wakening.	Maintain quiet, supportive environment. Provide periodic position changes and massage muscle groups frequently. Encourage activities during the day and discourage napping for long periods.	Promotes relaxation and general comfort to decrease muscle tension/enhance sleep/ rest. Aids in expenditure of energy. Excessive napping/evening stimulation may impair ability to fall asleep.	Reports a decrease in sleep difficulty and feeling well rested upon awakening.
	Administer medication as indicated.	Sedative may be needed for brief periods to promote adequate rest.	
Adjustment, impaired potential related to presence of permanent disability requiring change in life style.	Provide information for patient/family regarding disease and management. Provide time for expression of feelings.	Helps to develop effective coping mechanisms to deal with chronic illness. Promotes identification of concerns and ways of dealing with them.	Assumes reponsibility for personal needs. Initiates lifestyle changes that permit adaptation to present life situations. Acknowledges own limitations and identifies ways to cope with them.
	Discuss ways to change lifestyle in least disruptive manner.	Helps to develop a way of living with problems without altering normal routine significantly.	

CONTINUED ON THE FOLLOWING PAGE

Table 23–8. NURSING PROCESS FOR PATIENT WITH MOVEMENT DISORDERS–*CONTINUED*

Nursing Diagnosis	Nursing Actions	Rationale	Desired Outcomes/ Evaluation Criteria
	Provide opportunity for discussion of the impact of immobility on self-concept. Active Listen to patient.	Inability to do own self-care can result in feelings of dependency and powerlessness. Communicates caring and unconditional acceptance of the patient.	
	Discuss fluctuation of the course of the disease and effectiveness of medications.	Understanding the nature of chronic disease helps with dealing with therapeutic regimen which effects all areas of life.	
Knowledge deficit related to unfamiliarity with resources, misunderstanding, cognitive limitations as evidenced by questions, statements of concern, development of preventable complications.	Review disease process.	Provides opportunity to clarify misinformation and give information as necessary.	Identifies relationship of signs/symptoms of disease process/ medication side effects and correlates with causative factors. Verbalizes understanding of drug regimen.
	Discuss dietary regimen and restrictions (limited vitamin B_6 and protein evenly spaced in three meals for the patient with Parkinson's disease).	Promotes cooperation with therapeutic regimen. Some foods contain vitamins, minerals, and other compounds that can interfere with particular medications. Other types of diets may make the symptoms of the disease worse.	
	Provide information (verbal and written) about medications, including action, use, dose, side effects, and interactions.	Understanding may enhance cooperation with the medication regimen, reducing the debilitating effects of the pathologic processes.	
	Explore with patient ways to avoid infections (e.g., avoiding crowds, or being around people with colds/ viruses).	When immunosuppressive agents are used in the medication regimen, the patient has difficulty fighting off infection.	

A basic neurologic assessment is performed and recorded. Basic screening for sight, eating, swallowing, facial expression, general movements, initiation of volitional movements, gait, and walking is performed. If deficits appear during this screening session, then a more detailed neurologic assessment is performed. In addition to this baseline data, it is important to assess the patient one hour after the administration of medications.

Another important piece of data the nurse can obtain is the patient's ability to tolerate activity. The patient's fatigue level is important to know in order to plan activities.

NURSING DIAGNOSIS

Many nursing diagnoses are possible for the patient with disorders of the nervous system. Several examples are found in Table 23–8.

PLANNING AND INTERVENTION

Once a deficit is assessed, the next step is planning the nursing action. Nurses can be very creative in problem-solving, and the patient can benefit from this creativity. If deficits related to walking are found, there are many factors to consider when planning interventions. Initially, walking is assessed on the basis of observations made by the nurse. These observations include posture, muscle tone, arm swing, rhythm, gait, coordination, and the ability to move freely in the environment. When a motor dysfunction related to walking occurs, the nurse must consider the effects this deficit has on the patient's ability to perform self-care activities. This has relevance in the planning of care as well as in the patient's plans for going home. The next concern is the influence of the deficit on the patient's self-concept. How will the patient view himself or herself? Will this deficit influence how he or she interacts with other people? Other concerns relate to the client's safety. Will the patient be able

Table 23-9 PATIENT TEACHING—ANTIPARKINSON DRUGS

Dear Patient:
    This drug has been ordered for you. This is what you should know about your drug to get the most from your therapy.
1. You will take antiparkinson drugs for the remainder of your life. Antiparkinson drugs are administered to
    _____.
2. It is best to take antiparkinson drugs during or shortly after meals to decrease upset stomach and lack of appetite. This also aids in preventing dryness of the mouth.
3. Many interactions occur. Please consult your doctor or pharmacist before taking any other medication.
4. If you forget a dose, take it, and then delay the next dose for several hours. Always take all of your drugs.
5. Do not stop taking your drug.
6. Typical side effects that may occur from your drug include: _____.
7. Protein prevents the absorption of levodopa; therefore, decrease your intake of high-protein foods (milk, meat, eggs, fish, poultry, nuts). Also, spread the protein intake over four or more small meals rather than two or three large meals. Pyridoxine (vitamin B_6) limits the amount of levodopa available to the brain. Multiple vitamins containing pyridoxine (vitamin B_6) as well as foods high in pyridoxine (yeast, whole-grain cereals, potatoes; bananas, pork, glandular meats such as liver, and oatmeal) are avoided. (Patients taking a combination drug such as Sinemet do not need to limit pyridoxine.) Alcohol (wine, beer, hard liquor) in large amounts antagonizes dopamine, and alcohol intake should be limited to one or two drinks a day.
8. It is important to maintain a normal weight. Levodopa is absorbed by fat deposits, and obese people do not receive the full effect of the dose.
9. Store in a tightly closed, dry container away from heat.

to navigate safely in the environment? If not, how much assistance is needed for this patient? It is important for the nurse to plan specific nursing interventions based on the patient's problem (see Table 23–8).

EVALUATION

The primary goal of the nursing evaluation is to maintain or enhance the patient's level of independent functioning. As humans, it is important to be as productive and independent as possible. The major concerns related to motor dysfunction are alterations in daily living, self-concept, and client safety. Nurses have a major impact in all these areas. For specific evaluation of motor problems, see Table 23–8. The evaluation of patient teaching activities is also important. See Table 23–9 for teaching of the Parkinson's patient and Table 23–10 for discharge instructions for the myasthenic patient.

Table 23-10 PATIENT TEACHING—DRUGS FOR MYASTHENIA GRAVIS

Dear Patient:
    This drug has been ordered for you. This is what you should know about your drug to get the most from your therapy.
1. The patient is an individual. Avoid evaluating your drug regimen in relation to other myasthenic patients.
2. Take your drugs on time. Avoid skipping doses. If you miss a dose of your drug, avoid doubling up on the next dose.
3. Know the action and the side effects of your drugs. If you have side effects, call your doctor. Keep a diary of the drug, time taken, your activity level, and the side effect(s).
4. Taking the drug with meals can decrease stomach discomfort.
5. Check with your doctor and/or pharmacist before taking any over-the-counter drug for colds, allergy, sleep, laxatives, or pain.
6. Take steroids during early morning hours to correspond to the natural release of cortisol.
7. If you are on alternate day steroids and you miss the morning dose and you remember it that afternoon, wait until the next morning and take it at that time. Rearrange the steroid schedule accordingly.
8. Avoid taking alcohol while on the drugs.
9. Avoid abruptly stopping your drugs without doctor's order.
10. Call the M. G. Foundation and obtain a list of drug banks in your area.
11. Tell your dentist that you have myasthenia gravis and whether or not you are taking steroids.
12. Always check the labels of your drugs to make sure you are taking the right drug at the right time.
13. Use a calendar to schedule all your drugs especially if you are on an alternate day or alternate dose schedule.
14. Keep drugs out of the reach of children.
15. Destroy leftover drugs by flushing them down the toilet.
16. If you have weakness, ask the pharmacist for a regular container instead of a childproof container.
17. Refill your drugs on time so that you will not run out.
18. When traveling, carry a supply of your drugs in your purse or carry-on luggage.
19. If you are traveling, carry a copy of your medical records and additional prescriptions.
20. Keep your drugs in a cool place. They should be stored in a dry, light-sensitive container.
21. Watch for signs of infection (fever, chills, sore throat, frequency of urination, low back pain).
22. Lab work should be checked periodically if on steroids or other immunosuppressive agents.
23. Know other prescribed drugs you are taking.
24. Obtain a medical alert bracelet.

(From Myasthenia Gravis Foundation, 53 W. Jackson Blvd. Suite 909, Chicago, IL 60604).

SUMMARY

This chapter discusses the pharmacologic agents specific to Parkinson's disease, other basal ganglia movement disorders, and myasthenia gravis. The goal of pharmacotherapy is to improve motor function and to improve the quality of the patient's life.

Nursing assessment is ongoing throughout initial drug therapy. It is important for the nurse to note the patient's response to drug therapy and any side effects that result from drug therapy. The nurse has a very active role in teaching patients about their medications.

BIBLIOGRAPHY

American Medical Association. Drug Evaluations, ed 6. AMA, Chicago, 1986.

Carpenter, MB: Core Text of Neuroanatomy, ed 2. Williams & Wilkins, Baltimore, 1978.

Deglin, JH and Vallerand, AH: Nurses Med Deck. F.A. Davis, Philadelphia, 1988.

Delgado, JM and Billo, JM: Care of the patient with Parkinson's disease: Surgical and nursing interventions. J Neurosci Nurs 20(3):142, 1988.

Hoover, DB: Muscarinic blocking drugs. In Craig, CR and Stitzel, RE: Modern Pharmacology, ed 2. Little, Brown & Co, Boston, 1986.

Jackson, L: A predictive test for Hungbon's disease: Recombinant DNA technology and implications for nursing. J Neurosci Nurs 19(5):244, 1987.

Jenson, CE: Tourette syndrome: A bizarre and frightening neurological disorder. J Neurosci Nurs 20(4):213, 1988.

Katzung, BG: Basic and Clinical Pharmacology, ed 3. Appleton & Lange, Los Altos, CA, 1987.

Lannon, MC, et al: Comprehensive care of the patient with Parkinson's disease. J Neurosci Nurs 18(3):121, 1986.

Rutledge, CO: Drug therapy in parkinsonism and other basal ganglia disorders. In Craig, CR and Stitzel, RE: Modern Pharmacology, ed 2. Little, Brown & Co, Boston, 1986.

Schelfe, RT, Hills, JR, and Munsat, TL: Myasthenia gravis: Signs, symptoms, diagnosis, immunology, and current therapy. Pharmacology 1(1):39, 1981.

Taylor, P: Cholinergic Agonists. In Goodman, LS and Gilman, AG: The Pharmacological Basis of Therapeutics, ed 7. Macmillan, New York, 1985.

SITUATION 23–1

Edmond Meyer is a 63-year-old recently diagnosed with Parkinson's disease. His condition is being managed on an outpatient basis.

1. The clinic nurse obtains a patient history and reviews Mr. Meyer's symptoms. He describes shakiness and an inability to hold items "steady." He complains that his neck and shoulders are stiff. The nurse is aware that these symptoms relate to:
   a. excitatory effect of the cholinergic system
   b. stimulation of excess dopamine at nerve junctions
   c. build-up of toxic substances in the substantia nigra
   d. lack of acetylcholine for neurotransmission

2. Mr. Meyer is to begin trihexyphenidyl (Artane) 1 mg daily PO. Prior to administration, the nurse will assess for the following condition, which contraindicates its use:
   a. diarrhea
   b. excessive salivation
   c. peptic ulcer
   d. tachycardia

3. In teaching Mr. Meyer about the drug trihexyphenidyl (Artane), the nurse will stress avoiding the concurrent use of:
   a. aspirin compounds
   b. antihistamines
   c. antacids
   d. acetaminophen

4. In addition to trihexyphenidyl, Mr. Meyer will begin taking Sinemet 25/100 PO tid. The nurse will include the following when teaching about the drug:
   a. The drug will eliminate symptoms related to Parkinson's disease.
   b. Long-term therapy with this agent may cause movement disturbances.
   c. The patient should take this drug alone with a high-protein meal.
   d. A multivitamin supplement will help in providing necessary B-vitamins.

5. The concurrent use of trihexyphenidyl and Sinemet can help to alleviate Mr. Meyer's parkinsonian symptoms. However, the nurse is aware of a potential for altered absorption of Sinemet, due to the following effect of trihexyphenidyl (Artane):
   a. reduced lipid solubility
   b. enhanced fist-pass effect
   c. rapid intestinal motility
   d. delayed gastric emptying

6. When formulating the care plan for Mr. Meyer, the nurse will observe for the following adverse reaction related to therapy with Sinemet:
   a. cardiac dysrhythmias
   b. hypertensive crisis
   c. constipation
   d. photophobia

SITUATION 23–2

Debra Paddington, a 45-year-old, is admitted to the medical intensive care unit for evaluation and treatment of myasthenia gravis.

1. During the assessment, the nurse finds which of the following to be an indication of myasthenia gravis?
   a. tremor and dyskinesia with intentional movement
   b. weakness which improves with rest
   c. complete paralysis of the lower extremities
   d. spasticity of large skeletal muscle groups

SITUATION 23-2–*CONTINUED*

2. Ms. Paddington is scheduled for a Tensilon test. Edro-phonium (Tensilon) is administered intravenously by the physician. The nurse will expect the onset of action to be:
   a. 10 minutes
   b. 30 to 60 seconds
   c. 2 to 4 minutes
   d. 5 seconds

3. Close monitoring of Ms. Paddington is important during the Tensilon test. The nurse will observe for the following:
   a. bradycardia
   b. dry cough
   c. sore throat
   c. sedation

4. The diagnosis of myasthenia is confirmed, and Ms. Pad-dington is started on pyridostigmine (Mestinon) orally. The nurse will be alert to the following adverse effect to Mestinon:

   a. constipation
   b. urinary retention
   c. diarrhea
   d. dry mouth

5. In preparing Ms. Paddington for discharge, all of the fol-lowing points will be stressed *except:*
   a. keeping a diary of the drug schedule and effects
   b. taking the medication at night to avoid adverse effects
   c. maintaining a consistent sleep schedule
   d. avoiding alcohol and high-carbohydrate meals

6. Ms. Paddington is also to be placed on Prednisone 100 mg per day. The nurse will be aware of the following ef-fect of this additional therapy:
   a. worsening of symptoms
   b. delayed therapeutic response
   c. chemically induced hypoglycemia
   d. poor skin turgor

Please refer to the Appendices for correct answers and additional review questions with answers.

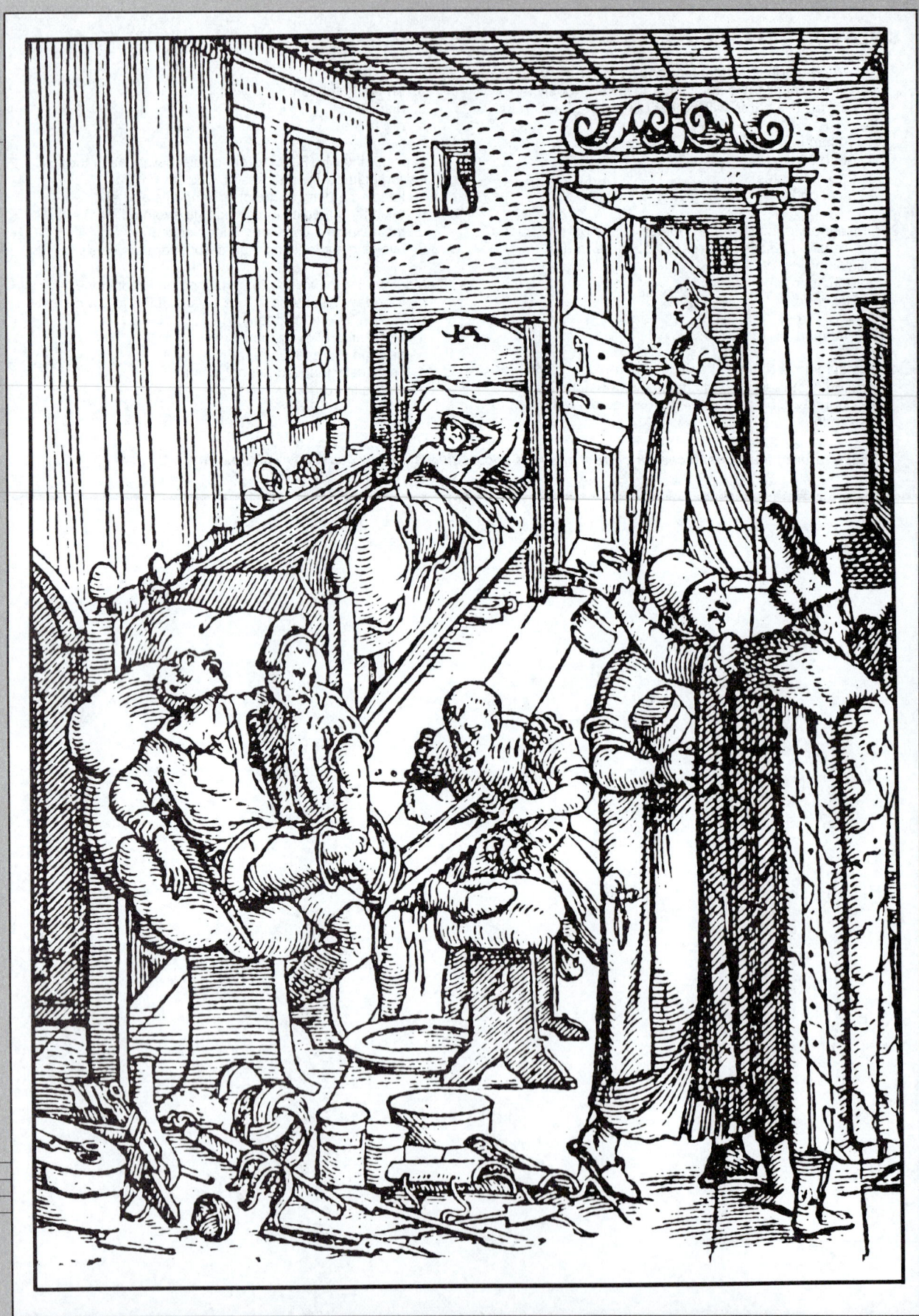

Hospital, circa 1550. Free Library of Philadelphia Print Collection.

3
UNIT

DRUGS AFFECTING MENTAL FUNCTIONING

GLOSSARY TERMS IN THIS CHAPTER

Abuse
Addiction
Anterograde amnesia
Anxiolytic
Compulsions
Cross-tolerance
Dependence
Hypnotic
Obsessions
Paradoxical reaction
Phobias
Porphyria
Rebound
Reinforcement
Relapse
REM
Sedatives
Sleep apnea
Somnambulism
Tolerance
Withdrawal

24
CHAPTER

SEDATIVES AND HYPNOTICS

FRANCES C. SCHNEIDER, Pharm.D.

LEARNING OBJECTIVES

After reading this chapter, the student will be able to:

1. Identify medications commonly used as sedative-hypnotic agents.

2. Differentiate among the sedative-hypnotic medications as to mechanism of action, route of administration, pharmacokinetics, adverse effects, contraindications, and interactions.

3. Identify specific nursing assessments in the patient requiring sedative-hypnotic medications and formulate appropriate nursing diagnoses.

4. Plan the nursing interventions necessary to administer sedative-hypnotic medications and choose appropriate teaching strategies for the patient.

5. Evaluate the patient at various stages of treatment to gauge the effectiveness of nursing interventions.

THERAPEUTIC AGENTS

The desire to reduce tension and induce sleep is an age-old phenomenon. Alcohol has been used for these purposes since ancient times. Bromide was introduced in the middle of the 19th century as a *hypnotic*. The first barbiturate, phenobarbital, was introduced in 1912; its success led to the synthesis and testing of over 2000 barbiturates, several of which are in current use. Meprobamate (Equanil), a nonbarbiturate, came into use in the early 1950s, renewing interest in more pharmacologically specific and less toxic *sedatives*. Chlordiazepoxide (Librium) was introduced in 1961 and diazepam (Valium) arrived two years later. Since then, over 3000 benzodiazepines have been synthesized and approximately 25 are currently in clinical use worldwide. Benzodiazepines were widely used in the 1960s and early 1970s. By the mid-1970s, however, there was a growing belief that they were overused and abused. Subsequently, their use declined from 87 million prescriptions in 1973 to 61 million prescriptions in 1985. The most recent significant development is the nonbenzodiazepine buspirone (BuSpar), which is touted to be effective for chronic anxiety without risks of *addiction* and psychomotor impairment.

These drugs alleviate only specific symptoms such as anxiety or sleep problems, but do not alter the factors that cause them. Therefore, these medications are used for symptomatic, noncurative treatment. The nurse and the patient must consider these drugs as aids to minimize feelings of distress so the patient may cope with the underlying causes. Table 24–1 briefly defines various anxiety disorders.

It should be noted that almost all of the sedative-hypnotic agents produce physiologic *dependence* when taken chronically. Frequently, individuals, including some nurses and other health care providers, resort to sedative-hypnotic medications to help them cope with

Table 24–1. DIAGNOSTIC CRITERIA OF ANXIETY DISORDERS

Type of Reaction	Diagnostic Criteria
Agoraphobia	Fear of being in places from which escape might be difficult or embarrassing, or in which help might not be available in the event of a panic attack. Agoraphobics restrict their travel or seek a companion when away from home.
Compulsions	Repetitive, purposeful, and intentional behaviors that are performed in response to an obsession, in some stereotypical fashion. Examples: hand washing, counting, checking, and touching.
Generalized anxiety disorder	Persistent symptoms of motor tension, automatic hyperactivity, apprehensive expectation, and/or hyperattentiveness for at least 1 month.
Obsession	Persistent ideas, thoughts, impulses, or images that are experienced as intrusive and senseless.
Obsessive-compulsive disorder	Recurrent obsessions and compulsions.
Panic disorder	Attacks of intense apprehension and feelings of impending doom in circumstances that are not correlated with life-threatening situations or physical exertion. The person is never certain when or if an attack will occur.
Post-traumatic stress disorder	Development of characteristic symptoms following a traumatic event that is outside the range of usual human experience. The symptoms include re-experiencing the event, numbing of one's reactions, withdrawal from external events, and sleep pattern disturbances.
Simple phobia	Irrational, persistent fears of an object or situation and an overwhelming desire to avoid the stimulus of the fear. Panic attacks occur immediately before or upon exposure to the phobic situation.
Social phobia	Persistent fear that the patient may do something in a social situation that will be humiliating or embarrassing. Examples: inability to speak (or stop talking) in social situations, choking on food when eating in front of others, inability to urinate in a public lavatory.

Table 24–2. CHARACTERISTICS OF THE VARIOUS STAGES OF SLEEP

Stages of Sleep	Characteristics
I	Feelings of drifting or floating off to sleep are experienced. Person experiences fleeting thoughts. Can be easily awakened. May experience suddenly occurring muscular contractions that will awaken the person. When awakened, the person may not recognize he or she was asleep.
II	Person appears relaxed. Can still be awakened easily.
III	Person appears extremely relaxed. Difficult to awaken. Decreased respirations, pulse, and blood pressure occur.
IV	Person remains in one position. Extremely difficult to awaken. If awakened, the person will appear groggy and confused. Dreams focusing on the day's activities may be experienced. Somnambulism (sleepwalking) or enuresis (bedwetting) may occur.
REM	Rapid eye movements occur. Respirations become irregular. Muscle twitching is experienced. Colorful dreams and nightmares take place.

the stresses of everyday life. The relief, or chemical escape, provided by these drugs leads to *reinforcement* of their use, without any resolution of the cause of the stress. It is easy to fall into a trap of seeking a "pill for every problem." If one drug becomes unavailable, a similar one suffices because of *cross-tolerance* and cross-dependence. This practice has led to the widespread *abuse* of these drugs. Ideally, nurses help overstressed patients develop the ability to reduce or tolerate stress while learning to cope effectively with its causes.

Some of the more potent and fast-acting sedative agents are also used to induce sleep. They appear to increase the time the person actually sleeps and may or may not promote a rested feeling. But the person may fail to achieve a rested feeling because of the increased length of time spent in sleep stages I and II, with a concurrent decrease in both the number of periods and the length of time spent in rapid-eye-movement *(REM)* sleep and deep sleep. Therefore, the person may awaken after sleeping six to eight hours without feeling rested.

The physiologic stages of sleep are described in Table 24–2. Note that patterns of sleep vary with the various stages of development, as highlighted in Table 24–3. The elderly have almost no deep sleep cycles and tend to have more nocturnal awakenings, longer times to sleep onset, and decreased total sleep times. Therefore, an older person's complaints of unrestful sleep, difficulties falling asleep, restless sleep with frequent awakenings, and inability to go back to sleep are not indications for routine hypnotic use. If a complete history does not indicate a potential cause for the complaint, appropriate interventions include environmental manipulation and patient education regarding healthy sleep habits and realistic expectations of sleep at this stage of life. Note that *sleep apnea*, which may indeed interfere with sleep, is a contraindication to the use of any hypnotic because of the danger of respiratory depression.

When REM sleep is deficient, the person feels a strong desire to make it up. When the medication is withdrawn, the person may experience a state of "REM rebound," as illustrated in Figure 24–1. REM rebound causes the individual to dream more frequently and perhaps experience nightmares that awaken him or her. The recurrence of insomnia is essentially a *relapse* caused by the medication. It is hypothesized that the problems associated with REM sleep cause people to use the *anxiolytic* agents on a chronic basis and thus become dependent on them. To date, *withdrawal* from flurazepam (Dalmane) does not appear to cause REM rebound, perhaps because of its metabolite's long half-life; this is speculative, however, since trials have often failed to follow subjects for more than a few days following discontinuation of the drug.

This chapter discusses three categories of sedative-hypnotics: benzodiazepines, barbiturates, and miscellaneous (nonbenzodiazepine, nonbarbiturate) agents. Table 24–4 lists these drugs and charts specific data. Note that some of these drugs are used as sedatives/ anxiolytics at low doses and as hypnotics at higher doses.

BENZODIAZEPINES

Uses

The major uses of benzodiazepines, once called minor tranquilizers or antianxiety agents, are to reduce anxiety and tension and to promote sleep. They are extremely effective when prescribed for individuals with anxiety disorders, but not for those with psychoses. These drugs are sometimes used to treat psychosomatic disorders,

Table 24–3. PATTERNS OF SLEEP CORRELATED WITH STAGES OF GROWTH AND DEVELOPMENT

Stages of Growth and Development	Estimated Average Daily Sleeping Hours	Percentage of REM Sleep	Characteristics
Newborn	16–20	50	Sleeps in 3–4 hour periods; minimal movement and extremely quiet respirations occur in Stage IV.
Infant	12–16	30–40	Child may fight sleep periods in later infancy.
Toddler	10–14	25	Develops ritualistic bedtime behaviors.
Preschooler	10–12	20	Frequently experiences vivid nightmares.
School-age	9–13	18–19	Fear of the dark occurs; experiences frightening dreams and nightmares.
Adolescent	8–12	20	Sleep periods may be irregular.
Young adult	7–9	22	Sleep periods may be irregular.
Middle adult	6–9	19	Insomnia may be a major concern.
Older adult	5–8	20–23	Experiences less sleep, but more rest; may demonstrate worries about the few hours he or she is sleeping.

senile agitation, and alcohol withdrawal states. Diazepam also produces relaxation of the skeletal muscles and has an anticonvulsant effect.

Action

The specific mechanisms of action of the benzodiazepines have not been completely established. Their major effects are known to stem from their effect on the limbic system and their action as central nervous system (CNS) depressants. It is believed that benzodiazepines enhance the neurotransmitter inhibitory action of gamma-aminobutyric acid (GABA), which mediates both pre- and postsynaptic inhibition in all regions of the CNS.

Pharmacokinetics

ABSORPTION. Following oral administration, benzodiazepines are well absorbed from the gastrointestinal tract, usually within one to two hours. Diazepam (Valium) and clorazepate (Tranxene) are very rapidly absorbed, whereas prazepam (Centrax) and oxazepam (Serax) are the least rapidly absorbed.

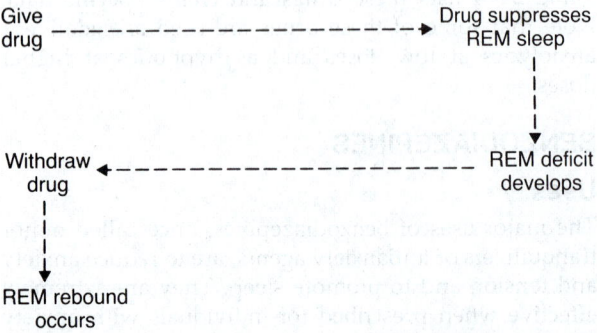

Figure 24–1. Hypnotic-induced REM suppression and REM rebound.

Following intramuscular administration of chlordiazepoxide (Librium) and diazepam, absorption may be slow and erratic, depending on the site of injection. Note: the nurse needs to recognize the effectiveness of oral benzodiazepines, rather than resorting hastily to parenteral routes.

DISTRIBUTION. Benzodiazepines and their metabolites are widely distributed into body tissues. They cross the blood–brain barrier and the placenta, and are distributed into breast milk. They are highly bound to plasma proteins. Steady-state plasma levels may be obtained after five days to two weeks.

BIOTRANSFORMATION. As illustrated in Figure 24–2, the benzodiazepines share similar pathways. Diazepam, clorazepate, and prazepam are converted to desmethyldiazepam and other active metabolites, which must be further metabolized in the liver. During chronic administration, the accumulation of desmethyldiazepam, which has a long half-life, may lead to excessive sedation. Desmethyldiazepam is eventually metabolized to oxazepam. Oxazepam, temazepam, triazolam, and lorazepam have shorter half-lives (3–20 hours); they produce no active metabolites and therefore do not produce problems resulting from metabolite build-up.

EXCRETION. Benzodiazepines with active metabolites (including desmethyldiazepam) have a cumulative effect and a half-life of up to 200 hours, which may produce problems of oversedation and ataxia. This is especially problematic for elderly clients or persons with liver problems. Small amounts of this agent are excreted in the urine.

Contraindications and Precautions

Benzodiazepines potentiate the effects of other CNS depressants (including alcohol, narcotics, and barbiturates) and should not be used in combination with these agents. The potential use of these combinations as methods for suicide attempts should therefore be kept in mind.

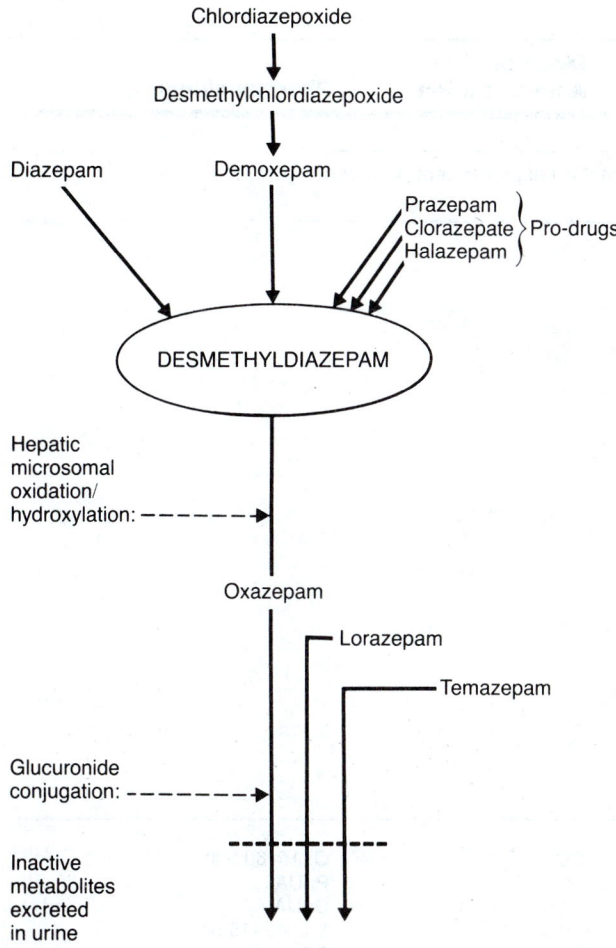

Figure 24–2. Common metabolic path of many benzodiazepine drugs.

The major risks associated with the use of benzodiazepines stem from the problems of *tolerance* and habituation. These are discussed more fully in Chapter 13. A distinct withdrawal syndrome occurs after long-term therapeutic use of benzodiazepine. Withdrawal occurs earlier in patients discontinuing short-acting agents than in those who have taken longer-acting agents. Gradual reduction of the dose is recommended.

Benzodiazepines should not be used during the first trimester of pregnancy (FDA category D and X) because the risk of congenital malformations generally outweighs potential benefit. Chronic use of benzodiazepines during pregnancy may cause physical dependence in the neonate resulting in withdrawal symptoms. Use of benzodiazepines in the last few weeks of pregnancy may cause CNS depression in the neonate.

Adverse Reactions

Drowsiness and ataxia are the most common side effects, occurring as a result of the basic pharmacologic properties of the benzodiazepines. Interestingly, patients who are taking these drugs to relieve anxiety do not typically show concern about these effects. However, those who use the drugs for other effects, for example, as an anticonvulsant, view these side effects as extremely problematic.

An infrequent but disturbing effect of hypnotics is a phenomenon known as *anterograde amnesia*. An example would be when a person takes a hypnotic with the intent of having a good night's sleep before a major presentation in another city, then cannot remember things like traveling to the airport, or making the flight, even though these were recent events. This phenomenon seems to occur most frequently with triazolam (Halcion). Table 24–5 compares the incidence of this memory impairment with various sedative-hypnotics (Allen, 1986). Anterograde amnesia is part of the intended effect when lorazepam is given preceding chemotherapy sessions that induce severe vomiting—which the patient would rather not remember! Anterograde amnesia may be a benefit when diazepam is given intravenously prior to surgery, electrical cardioversion, or labor and delivery.

Gastrointestinal discomfort, nausea, and vomiting may develop. Taking the drugs during or immediately following meals may reduce the intensity of these problems. In fact, gastric acid acts as a catalyst in the metabolism of these agents. Side effects that may occur infrequently include blurred vision, hypotension, headaches, slurred speech, insomnia, depression, shortness of breath, bradycardia, decreased libido, constipation, jaundice, urinary retention, incontinence, and rashes. Rarely, paradoxic reactions are demonstrated, with symptoms such as excitement, hostility, rage, confusion, hallucinations, and acute hyperpyrexia.

Interactions

The benzodiazepines produce fewer problematic interactions with other drugs than do most sedatives and hypnotics. The primary interaction may be seen when these drugs are combined with another CNS depressant, such as alcohol. Such combinations tend to produce oversedation and motor impairment, and may lead to impaired respiratory function and death.

Benzodiazepines metabolized by oxidation or hydroxylation (including alprazolam, chlordiazepoxide, diazepam, and others with the desmethyldiazepam metabolite) will have an increased elimination half-life when administered with cimetidine (but not with ranitidine). This enzyme-inhibition problem does not affect oxazepam and lorazepam.

The benzodiazepines alter the results of some laboratory tests, such as elevating the results of bilirubin, AST, and alkaline phosphatase tests. The nurse should not overlook this possibility.

Benzodiazepine Products
ALPRAZOLAM
Use. Alprazolam (Xanax) is a new anxiolytic agent that is especially useful in depressive and panic reactions. It may have some actions resembling the tricyclics, while maintaining the anxiolytic properties of the

TEXT RESUMES ON PAGE 622

Table 24–4. ANTIANXIETY DRUGS

Name	Dosage	Mode of Administration	Pharmacokinetics
Action: central nervous system depressant (applies to all drugs in this chapter except propranolol).			
BENZODIAZEPINES			
Alprazolam (Xanax) *Use:* anti-anxiety	0.25–5.0 mg 3 ×/day, up to 4 mg/day Pediatric: UD up to age 18 Geriatric: 0.25 mg 2–3 ×/day (increased as tolerated)	PO	O: 15–60 min P: UA D: UA ½ L: 12–15 hr PB: high B: hepatic E: rapid renal clearance after discontinuance
Chlordiazepoxide hydrochloride (Librium, Lipoxide, Mitran, Resposans-10, Sereen) *Use:* sedative and hypnotic	Sedative: 5–25 mg 3–4 ×/day Hypnotic: 50–100 mg hs Pediatric: UD under age 6; age 6 and over 5 mg 2–4 ×/day, up to 10 mg 2–3 ×/day Geriatric: 5 mg 2–4 ×/day, increase gradually, if needed Alcohol withdrawal: 50–100 mg repeated in 2–4 hr prn	PO IM, IV	O: 15–45 min (PO, IM); 1–5 min (IV) P: 0.5–2 hr (PO) D: UA ½ L: 5–30 hr PB: very high B: hepatic oxidation (active metabolites) E: renal O: 1–5 min (IV); 15–45 min (IM)
Clorazepate dipotassium (Tranxene, Tranxene SD) *Use:* antianxiety	Sedative: 7.5–15 mg 2–4 ×/day; SR 11.25–22.5 mg once daily Geriatric: 7.5–15 mg/day; increase as tolerated Anticonvulsant: 7.5 mg 3 ×/day, increased no more than 7.5 mg/week up to 90 mg/day Pediatric: age 9–12 years, 7.5 mg 2 ×/day; increased no more than 7.5 mg/week up to 60 mg/day	PO	O: 30–60 min P: 1–2 hr D: varies ½ L: 30–200 hr† PB: high B: hepatic and gastric E: renal

Key to Abbreviations in the *Pharmacokinetics* column: O-onset; P-peak; D-duration; PB-protein bound; B-biotransformed in; E-excreted in; ½ L-halflife; UA-unavailable.

*Within the column listing adverse effects, underlines indicate the most common effects; CAPITALS indicate life-threatening effects.

Contraindications/ Precautions	Adverse Effects*	Interactions	Nursing Implications
All Benzodiazepines. Contraindicated in hypersensitivity to the drug, acute alcohol intoxication, children under 6 months of age, acute narrow-angle glaucoma, shock, and coma. Use cautiously in pregnancy (first trimester risk of teratogenicity; later, dependence and withdrawal), breast feeding, patients with history of drug abuse, epilepsy, hyperkinesis, mental depression, porphyria, psychoses, hepatic and renal impairment, severe chronic obstructive lung disease.	All Benzodiazepines. Neuro: dizziness, drowsiness, CONFUSION, headache, lethargy, memory impairment, SLURRED SPEECH, SEVERE WEAKNESS. CV: palpitations, tachycardia, mild hypotension GI: constipation, dry mouth, nausea, vomiting Integ: rash	All Benzodiazepines. CNS-depressant effect potentiated when used with alcohol, barbiturates, tricyclic antidepressants, phenothiazines, antihistamines. Benzodiazepines may block therapeutic response of levodopa. May cause toxicity of phenytoin by inhibiting its breakdown. Cigarette smoking may decrease the effectiveness of the usual dose of benzodiazepines by enhancing their metabolism. Cimetidine may impede the biotransformation of certain benzodiazepines such as alprazolam, chlordiazepoxide, diazepam, and others having desmethyldiazepam as a metabolite.	All Benzodiazepines. ASSESSMENT: Is prn dose really necessary? Have nonpharmacologic approaches been tried and found to be insufficient? INTERVENTION: Give drugs orally when possible. Teach patient that drowsiness, light-headedness, or dizziness may occur. Remind patient to avoid alcoholic beverages. Note policies and legal restrictions applying to benzodiazepines. EVALUATION: Look for characteristics of tolerance to same dose (higher dose needed), physical dependence, paradoxic reactions (excitement), withdrawal reactions (REM rebound).
Same as above.	Same as above.	Same as above.	Same as above.
Same as above.	Same as above.	Same as above.	Same as above.
Same as above.	Same as above.	Same as above.	Same as above.

CONTINUED ON THE FOLLOWING PAGE

Table 24–4. ANTIANXIETY DRUGS–*CONTINUED*

Name	Dosage	Mode of Administration	Pharmacokinetics
Clorazepate dipotassium–*Continued* †desmethyldiazepam	Alcohol withdrawal: 30 mg initially, then 15 mg 2–4 × on day 1, 15 mg 3–6 × on day 2, then reduce dose on days 3, 4, and 5 to half the previous days' dose (to 3.75 mg 2–4 ×/day)		
Diazepam (Valium, Valrelease) *Use:* sedative and hypnotic	Sedative: 2–10 mg 2–4 ×/day Hypnotic: 5–10 mg repeated in 3–4 hr prn Pediatric: age 6 and over 1–2.5 mg 3–4 ×/day Geriatric: 2–2.5 mg 1–2 ×/day (increased as tolerated) Alcohol withdrawal: 10 mg 3–4 ×/day on day 1, decreased to 5 mg 3–4 ×/day as needed	PO	O: 15–45 min (PO, IM) P: 0.5–1.5 hr (PO, IM) D: varies ½ L: 20–90 hr PB: very high B: hepatic (active metabolites) E: renal
Diazepam Injection	Anticonvulsant: 2–10 mg 2–4 ×/day Skeletal muscle relaxant: 2–10 mg 3–4 ×/day Preoperative: 5–10 mg Psychoneurotic reactions: 2–5 mg repeated in 3–4 hr prn Alcohol withdrawal: 10 mg followed by 5–10 mg in 3–4 hr prn Amnestic, cardioversion: 5–15 mg 5–10 min prior to procedure Amnestic, endoscopy: up to 20 mg immediately prior to procedure; 5–10 mg about 30 min prior to procedure Status epilepticus: 5–10 mg, repeated at 10–15 min intervals up to maximum of 30 mg in 2–4 hr, repeat if necessary Skeletal muscle spasm relaxant: 5–10 mg, repeated in 3–4 hr prn	IM, IV IV IV IV IV IV, IM	O: 1–3 min (IV) P: 20 min
Flurazepam (Dalmane) *Use:* hypnotic	15–30 mg hs Pediatric: UD up to age 15 Geriatric: 15 mg hs	PO	O: 15–45 min P: 0.5–1 hr D: 7–8 hr ½L: 2–3 hr + metabolites (47–100 hr). PB: 97% B: hepatic (active metabolites) E: renal
Halazepam (Paxipam) *Use:* antianxiety	20–40 mg 3–4 Pediatric: UD up to age 18 Geriatric: 20 mg 2 ×/day	PO	O: UA (slow) P: 1–3 hr D: UA ½ L: 14 hr PB: very high B: hepatic (active metabolites) E: renal

Key to Abbreviations in the *Pharmacokinetics* column: O-onset; P-peak; D-duration; PB-protein bound; B-biotransformed in; E-excreted in; ½ L-halflife; UA-unavailable.
*Within the column listing adverse effects, underlines indicate the most common effects; CAPITALS indicate life-threatening effects.

Contraindications/ Precautions	Adverse Effects*	Interactions	Nursing Implications
Same as above.	Same as above.	Same as above.	Same as above.
Same as above.	Same as above.	Same as above.	Same as above.
Same as above.	Same as above.	Same as above.	Same as above.

CONTINUED ON THE FOLLOWING PAGE

Table 24–4. ANTIANXIETY DRUGS–*CONTINUED*

Name	Dosage	Mode of Administration	Pharmacokinetics
Lorazepam (Ativan) *Use:* sedative and hypnotic	Sedative: 1–3 mg 2–3 ×/day Preop amnestic: 0.05 mg/kg up to 4 mg total or 0.44 mg/kg up to 2 mg Hypnotic: 2–4 mg hs Pediatric: UD up to age 12 Geriatric: 1–2 mg/day, increased as tolerated	PO IM, IV PO	O: 15–40 min P: 2–5 hr O: IM 15–30 min P: 1–1.5 hr O: IV 5–15 min P: immediate D: 6–10 hr ½ L: 10–20 hr PB: 91%, high B: hepatic, no active metabolites E: renal
Oxazepam (Serax) *Use:* antianxiety	10–30 mg 3–4 ×/day Pediatric: not recommended under 6 years, UD 6–12 years Geriatric: 10 mg 3 ×/day increased as tolerated/needed to 15 mg 3–4 ×/day	PO	O: 45–90 min P: 2–4 hr D: UA ½ L: 5–15 hr PB: very high B: hepatic, no metabolites E: renal
Prazepam (Centrax) *Use:* antianxiety †desmethyldiazepam	10 mg 3 ×/day or 20–40 mg/day Pediatric: UD up to age 18 years Geriatric: 10–15 mg/day, increased as tolerated/needed	PO	O: UA, slow P: 6 hr D: varies ½ L: 30–200 hr† PB: high B: hepatic, first pass metabolism E: renal
Temazepam (Restoril) *Use:* hypnotic	15–30 mg hs Pediatric: UD up age 18 years Geriatric: 15 mg hs, increased as tolerated/needed	PO	O: 20–30 min P: 2–3 hr D: 10–17 hr ½ L: 10–20 hr PB: 98% B: hepatic, no active metabolites E: renal
Triazolam (Halcion) *Use:* hypnotic	Hypnotic: 0.125–0.5 mg hs Pediatric: UD up to age 18 years, increased as tolerated	PO	O: 15–30 min P: 1.3 hr D: 1.5–5.4 hr ½ L: 1.6–5.4 hr PB: 90% B: hepatic, no active metabolites E: renal
BARBITURATES			

Key to Abbreviations in the *Pharmacokinetics* column: O-onset; P-peak; D-duration; PB-protein bound; B-biotransformed in; E-excreted in; ½ L-halflife; UA-unavailable.
*Within the column listing adverse effects, underlines indicate the most common effects; CAPITALS indicate life-threatening effects.

Contraindications/ Precautions	Adverse Effects*	Interactions	Nursing Implications
Same as above.	Same as above.	Same as above.	Same as above.
Same as above.	Same as above.	Same as above.	Same as above.
Same as above.	Same as above.	Same as above.	Same as above.
Same as above.	Same as above.	Same as above.	Same as above.
Same as above.	Same as above.	Same as above.	Same as above.
All Barbiturates Contraindicated in sensitivity to barbiturates, severe respiratory problems, hepatic coma, porphyria, past addiction to sedative-hypnotics, uncontrolled pain, pregnancy, and lactation.	**All Barbiturates** Neuro: SEVERE CONFUSION, DECREASE IN or LOSS OF REFLEXES, FEVER or HYPOTHERMIA, NYSTAGMUS, clumsiness or unsteadiness, dizziness or lightheadedness, drowsiness, "hangover" effect. Neuro indications of possi-	**All Barbiturates** CNS depressants, including alcohol, cause increased central and respiratory depression. Valproic acid, chloramphenicol, and cimetidine cause greater effect and longer duration of barbiturates due	**All Barbiturates** ASSESSMENT: Assess the patient's suicide potential. INTERVENTION: Remember that most of these drugs are absorbed rapidly and quickly promote calmness and sleep. Remind patient to avoid alcohol. Caution

CONTINUED ON THE FOLLOWING PAGE

Table 24–4. ANTIANXIETY DRUGS–*CONTINUED*

Name	Dosage	Mode of Administration	Pharmacokinetics
BARBITURATES–*Continued*			
Short-Acting Pentobarbital (Nembutal, Nembutal Sodium) *Use:* hypnotic and anticonvulsant	Hypnotic: 100 mg hs or 120–200 mg Preop: 100–200 mg Anticonvulsant:100 mg up to 500 mg Geriatric: lower dose Pediatric preoperative: 2–6 mg/kg, up to 100 mg	PO R IV IV	O: 10–15 min (IM); 15–60 min (PO, R) P: 30–60 min D: 3–4 hr ½ L: 4 hr α phase; 35–50 hr β phase PB: 35%–45% B: hepatic E: renal
Secobarbital (Seconal, Seconal Sodium) *Use:* sedative and hypnotic	Hypnotic: 100 mg hs 200 mg 100–200 mg 50–250 mg Preop: 200–300 mg Sedative: 30–50 mg 3–4 ×/ day Geriatric: lower dose Pediatric: 50–100 mg	PO R IM IV IM PO	O: 10–15 min P: 2–4 hr (PO); 7–10 min (IM); 1–3 min (IV) D: 3–4 hr ½ L: approximately 30 hr PB: 30%–45% B: hepatic E: renal
Intermediate-Acting: Amobarbital (Amytal, Amytal Sodium) *Use:* sedative, hypnotic, and anticonvulsant	Sedative: 50–300 mg/day Hypnotic: 65–200 mg hs Anticonvulsant: 65–500 mg; pediatric up to age 6: 3–5 mg/kg Pediatric preop: 2–6 mg/kg up to 100 mg max)	PO PO IV IV	O: 45–60 min P: UA D: 6–8 hr ½ L: 16–40 hr β phase; 40 min α phase PB: 61% B: hepatic E: renal
Aprobarbital (Alurate) *Use:* hypnotic	Hypnotic: 40–160 mg hs Geriatric: lower dose Pediatric: UD	PO	O: 45–60 min P: 3 hr D: 6–8 hr ½ L: 14–34 hr PB: 35% B: hepatic E: renal (20% unchanged)
Butabarbital (Buticaps, Butisol Sodium, Butatran, Sarisol #2, Butalon) *Use:* hypnotic	Hypnotic: 50–100 mg hs or preop Geriatric: lower dose Pediatric: 2–6 mg/kg up to 100 mg	PO	O: 45–60 min P: 3–4 hr D: 6–8 hr ½ L: 66–140 hr PB: 26% B: hepatic E: renal

Key to Abbreviations in the *Pharmacokinetics* column: O-onset; P-peak; D-duration; PB-protein bound; B-biotransformed in; E-excreted in; ½ L-halflife; UA-unavailable.
*Within the column listing adverse effects, underlines indicate the most common effects; CAPITALS indicate life-threatening effects.

Contraindications/ Precautions	Adverse Effects*	Interactions	Nursing Implications
Use cautiously in hepatic function impairment, hyperkinesis (may be exaggerated), mental depression, suicidal tendencies, severe renal disease.	ble withdrawal: anxiety, restlessness, muscle twitching, trembling of hands, vision problems, increased dreaming, nightmares, insomnia CV: bradycardia Resp: wheezing, chest tightness GI: constipation, nausea or vomiting Integ: EXFOLIATIVE DERMATITIS, STEVENS-JOHNSON SYNDROME	to enzyme inhibition (delayed biotransformation). Corticosteroids have decreased effect because of barbiturate-induced enzyme induction (faster biotransformation of steroids) Estrogen-containing oral contraceptives are less effective if barbiturates are also given because enzyme induction increases the rate of estrogen metabolism. Effectiveness of coumarin derivatives is decreased because of enzyme induction (faster biotransformation of the anticoagulant).	patient regarding driving and operating machinery while taking barbiturates. Note the legal policies and restrictions regarding these drugs. EVALUATION: Remember that tolerance may develop within 7–14 days. Assess the patient routinely for signs of dependency.

CONTINUED ON THE FOLLOWING PAGE

Antianxiety Drugs

Table 24–4. ANTIANXIETY DRUGS–*CONTINUED*

Name	Dosage	Mode of Administration	Pharmacokinetics

BARBITURATES–*Continued*
Talbutal (Lotusate)
Use: sedative and hypnotic
	Hypnotic: 120 mg hs
	Sedative: 30–60 mg 2–3 ×/
	  day
	Pediatric: UD
	Geriatric: increase as toler-
	  ated
		PO	O: 45–60 min
			P: 2 hr
			D: 6–8 hr
			½ L: 15 hr
			PB: UA
			B: hepatic
			E: renal

Long-Acting:
Mephobarbital (Mebaral)
Use: anticonvulsant only
	200 mg hs to 600 mg/day in
	  divided doses
	Geriatric: lower dose
	Pediatric: up to 5 years 16–
	  32 mg 3–4 ×/day; 5 years
	  and over 32–64 mg 3–4 ×/
	  day
		PO	O: 60 min or longer
			D: 10–12 hr
			½ L: UA (converted to pheno-
			  barbital)
			PB: UA
			B: hepatic
			E: renal

Metharbital (Gemonil) *Use:* anticonvulsant only	100 mg 1–3 ×/day up to 800 mg/day Geriatric: lower dose Pediatric: UD	PO	O: 60 min or longer P: UA D: 10–12 hr ½ L: UA PB: UA B: hepatic E: renal

Phenobarbital (Luminal, Sol-
foton, Barbita, Luminal
Ovoids, Phenobarbital
Sodium)
Use: hypnotic and anticon-
vulsant
	Hypnotic: 100–320 mg hs;
	  100–300 mg hs
	Anticonvulsant: 60–250 mg/
	  day, 100–320 mg, repeated
	  prn, up to total of 600 mg/
	  day
	Pediatric: 1–6 mg/kg, 10–20
	  mg/kg as a loading dose,
	  1–6 mg/kg/day mainte-
	  nance
	Pediatric status epilepticus:
	  15–20 mg/kg over a 10–15
	  min period
		PO
		IM, IV
		PO
		
		PO
		
		IV
			O: 60 min or longer; 5 min
			  (IV)
			P: after IV admin. 15 min or
			  more; 8–12 hr (PO)
			D: 10–12 hr
			½ L: 53–118 hr (adults)
			½ L: 40–70 hr (children)
			PB: 20–45%
			B: hepatic
			E: renal

OTHER SEDATIVES AND HYPNOTICS			
Buspirone (BuSpar) *Use:* for generalized anxiety	5 mg tid up to 60 mg/day Pediatric: UD Geriatric: UD	PO	O: 1–2 wk P: 0.6–1.5 hr D: UA ½ L: 2–3 hr PB: 95% B: hepatic—> active metab- olites E: renal

Chloral hydrate (Noctec,
Somnos, Aquachloral Sup-
prettes)
Use: sedative and hypnotic
	Hypnotic: 500 mg–1 g hs
	Sedative: 250 mg 3 ×/day
	  pc, max. daily dose 2 gm
	Pediatric: 50 mg/kg hs, 8.3
	  mg/kg tid pc
	Geriatric: UD
		PO	O: <30 min
			P: UA
			D: 4–8 hr
			½ L: 7–10 hr
			PB: 35–41%
			B: hepatic
			E: renal (25% unchanged)

Key to Abbreviations in the *Pharmacokinetics* column: O-onset; P-peak; D-duration; PB-protein bound; B-bio-transformed in; E-excreted in; ½ L-halflife; UA-unavailable.
*Within the column listing adverse effects, underlines indicate the most common effects; CAPITALS indicate life-threatening effects.

Contraindications/ Precautions	Adverse Effects*	Interactions	Nursing Implications
BARBITURATES–*Continued*			
None known.	Neuro: numbness, tingling, weakness in hands or feet. Confusion or mental depression. CV: chest pain, fast or pounding heartbeat.	Concurrent use of buspirone and monoamine oxidase inhibitors may cause an elevation in blood pressure.	ASSESSMENT: Note that patients switching from another sedative need to taper it, because buspirone will not cover withdrawal symptoms.
Contraindicated in severe hepatic impairment and severe renal impairment. Use cautiously in gastritis, as condition may worsen.	Neuro: CONFUSION, CONVULSIONS GI: Nausea, vomiting, stomach pain Integ: RASH	Chloral hydrate has additive CNS depressant effects with other sedatives, alcohol, and tricyclics. Oral anticoagulants may have increased effect.	INTERVENTION: Do not break the capsule as drug has a very unpleasant taste. Give with a full glass of water to reduce gastritis. Raise siderails. Be sure call light is within reach. Caution patient against ingesting alcohol and operating machinery.

CONTINUED ON THE FOLLOWING PAGE

Table 24–4. ANTIANXIETY DRUGS–*CONTINUED*

Name	Dosage	Mode of Administration	Pharmacokinetics
Diphenhydramine (Benadryl, Nordryl, Diahist, Phen-Amin, and many others)	Hypnotic: 50–100 mg Pediatric: 1.25 mg/kg 4 ×/ day up to 30 mg	PO (IV, IM)	O: 15 min P: 1–4 hr D: 4–10 hr ½ L: 2.4–9.3 hr PB: 50%–55% B: hepatic E: renal
Action: antihistamine, CNS depressant *Use:* hypnotic, antihistamine			
Doxylamine (Unisom Night-time Sleep-Aid) *Use:* hypnotic	25 mg hs Pediatric: not recommended Geriatric: lower dose	PO	O: 30 min P: 2–3 hr D: UA ½ L: 10 hr PB: UA B: hepatic E: renal
Ethchlorvynol (Placidyl) *Use:* hypnotic	500–1000 mg Pediatric: contraindicated Geriatric: UD	PO	O: 15–60 min P: 1–2 hr D: 5 hr ½ L: 10–25 hr PB: 35% B: hepatic, kidney E: renal
Glutethimide (Doriden) *Use:* hypnotic	Hypnotic: 250–500 mg hs repeated if necessary Pediatric: UD up to age 12 Geriatric: 500 mg hs max	PO	O: 30 min P: 1–6 hr D: 4–8 hr ½ L: 10–12 hr PB: approx. 50% B: hepatic E: renal, fecal
Hydroxyzine hydrochloride (Vistaril, Atarax, and many others)	25–150 mg tid or qid Children < 6 yr: 50 mg/day Children > 6 yr: 50–100 mg/ day	PO, IM	O: 15–30 min P: UA D: 4–6 hr ½L: 3 hr PB: hepatic B: hepatic E: fecal
Hydroxyzine pamoate	25–100 mg q 4–6 hr Pediatric: 1.1 mg/kg q 4–6 hr	PO	Same as above.
Meprobamate (Equanil, Miltown, and many others) *Use:* sedative	200–1200 mg/day Pediatric: 6–12 years 25 mg/ kg/day Geriatric: UD	PO	O: 1 hr P: 1–3 hr D: 6–17 hr ½ L: approx 10 hr PB: 20% B: hepatic E: renal

Key to Abbreviations in the *Pharmacokinetics* column: O-onset; P-peak; D-duration; PB-protein bound; B-biotransformed in; E-excreted in; ½ L-halflife; UA-unavailable.

*Within the column listing adverse effects, underlines indicate the most common effects; CAPITALS indicate life-threatening effects.

Contraindications/ Precautions	Adverse Effects*	Interactions	Nursing Implications
Contraindicated in hypersensitivity and pregnancy. Use caution in asthma, prostatic hypertrophy, narrow-angle glaucoma, and GI obstruction.	Neuro: drowsiness GI: dry mouth, nausea	Concurrent use with CNS depressants results in additive CNS depression. MAO inhibitors increase and prolong antimuscarinic effects.	INTERVENTION: Administer IM injection deeply into muscle.
Same as above (antihistamine).	Same as above.	Same as above.	INTERVENTION: Caution patient against ingesting alcohol and operating machinery.
Contraindicated in patients with history of drug abuse, mental depression, porphyria, pregnancy. Use cautiously in uncontrolled pain, hepatic and renal impairment.	Same as barbiturates.	Additive CNS depressant effects. Oral anticoagulant effects may be decreased (enzyme induction by ethchlorvynol).	ASSESSMENT: Suicide potential presents especially high risk with ethchlorvynol. INTERVENTION: Giddiness and ataxia may be seen in patients who absorb it quickly. Caution patient against ingesting alcohol and operating machinery. EVALUATION: Contact physician if patient demonstrated confusion or hallucinations.
Same as above.	Same as barbiturates.	Additive effects with other CNS depressants. Oral anticoagulants may have decreased effect because of enhanced metabolism.	Same as above.
Same as diphenhydramine.	Same as diphenhydramine. (More pronounced anticholinergic effects)	Same as diphenhydramine.	Same as diphenhydramine.
Same as above.	Same as above.	Same as above.	Same as above.
Contraindicated in pregnancy, lactation, porphyria, children under 6, patients sensitive to propanediol carbamates, patients with history of drug abuse.	Neuro: "hangover effect" Integ: RASH, porphyria	Additive effects with other CNS depressants.	ASSESSMENT: suicide potential presents real risk INTERVENTION: caution patient against ingesting alcohol and operating machinery.

CONTINUED ON THE FOLLOWING PAGE

Table 24–4. ANTIANXIETY DRUGS–*CONTINUED*

Name	Dosage	Mode of Administration	Pharmacokinetics
Meprobamate–*Continued*			
Methyprylon (Noludar) *Use:* sedative-hypnotic	Sedative: 50–100 mg Pediatric: UD Geriatric: UD	PO	O: 45 min P: UA D: 5–8 hr ½ L: 3–6 hr PB: 60% B: hepatic E: renal
Paraldehyde	Sedative: 5–10 ml Pediatric: 0.15 ml/kg Hypnotic: 10–30 ml or 10 ml Pediatric: 0.3 ml/kg	R or PO R or PO R or PO IM R or PO	O: 15 min P: UA D: 8 hr ½ L: 3–9 hr PB: UA B: hepatic E: lungs

Key to Abbreviations in the *Pharmacokinetics* column: O-onset; P-peak; D-duration; PB-protein bound; B-biotransformed in; E-excreted in; ½ L-halflife; UA-unavailable.

*Within the column listing adverse effects, underlines indicate the most common effects; CAPITALS indicate life-threatening effects.

benzodiazepines. Preferably, the drug is used in conjunction with counseling.

Pharmacokinetics. When alprazolam is discontinued, it is cleared from the system very rapidly; abruptly stopping alprazolam is likely to result in seizures. It is important that patients be aware of this danger.

Table 24–5. INCIDENCE OF MEMORY IMPAIRMENT WITH VARIOUS SEDATIVE-HYPNOTICS

Generic Name	Trade Name	Incidence
Alprazolam	Xanax	+ +
Chloral Hydrate	Noctec*	+
Chlorazepate Dipotassium	Tranxene	+
Diazepam	Valium*	+ +
Diphenhydramine	Benadryl*	+ +
Flurazepam	Dalmane	+ +
Lorazepam	Ativan*	+ + +
Oxazepam	Serax	+
Secobarbital	Seconal*	+ + +
Temazepam	Restoril	+ +
Triazolam	Halcion	+ + + +

*Generics available
Key: + less frequent
+ + more frequent
+ + + quite frequent
+ + + + very frequent

CHLORAZEPATE DIPOTASSIUM

Use. Clorazepate dipotassium (Tranxene) is used in anxiety and in alcohol withdrawal. It is also indicated as an anticonvulsant.

Pharmacokinetics. Chlorazepate dipotassium is a "pro-drug." Following oral administration, it is rapidly absorbed and decarboxylated to desmethyldiazepam, its initial active form. The drug that is administered is not active until the liver converts it to another active metabolite, oxazepam.

CHLORDIAZEPOXIDE HYDROCHLORIDE

(Capsules: Librium, Lipoxide, and others; Tablets: Libritabs)

Use. Chlordiazepoxide has little usefulness as a hypnotic or for situational anxiety. With the advent of buspirone, its use in chronic anxiety will probably decrease. Chlordiazepoxide is useful in alcohol withdrawal because of its long half-life.

Pharmacokinetics. This drug is absorbed slowly, and therefore reaches its peak plasma levels two to four hours after oral administration and is excreted slowly over two to four days. Note that absorption following intramuscular injection is slower than following oral administration and is erratic. This agent is administered in the gluteus muscle when it must be given intramuscularly.

Reconstitution. For intramuscular use, prepare the ampule of powder with the special diluent provided by the manufacturer. The manufacturer cautions against in-

Contraindications/ Precautions	Adverse Effects*	Interactions	Nursing Implications
			EVALUATION: evaluate for symptoms of tolerance, dependence, and withdrawal.
Contraindicated in pregnancy, children under 12 years. Use cautiously in patients with a history of drug abuse.	Same as barbiturates	Additive effects with other CNS depressants.	INTERVENTION: Giddiness and ataxia may be seen in some patients. Caution patient against ingesting alcohol and operating machinery. EVALUATION: Contact physician if patient demonstrates confusion or hallucinations.
Contraindicated in hepatic dysfunction, lung disease, peptic ulcer.	GI: nausea, unpleasant breath odor	Disulfiram will increase blood levels of paraldehyde and acetaldehyde.	INTERVENTION: Avoid contact, paraldehyde is very irritating to skin and tissues. Use glass syringes and containers. Discard if liquid is brown or has a penetrating odor.

travenous administration of this special diluent. For intravenous use, reconstitute the powder with sterile saline.

DIAZEPAM
Use. Diazepam (Valium) is taken orally in daily doses ranging from 4–40 mg. It is appropriately used as a skeletal muscle relaxant, as a hypnotic, for situational anxiety, and for status epilepticus. Its intramuscular or intravenous dose is usually 5–10 mg every three to four hours.

Administration. If diazepam must be given intramuscularly, the preferred site is the deltoid muscle, as absorption from this site is usually rapid and complete. When administered intravenously, the rate of infusion should not exceed 5 mg/minute. Diazepam should not be mixed with other injectable solutions or drugs.

Half-Life. Its plasma half-life is age dependent, ranging from approximately 20 hours for a person who is 20 years old, to about 90 hours for an individual 90 years of age. Geriatric men may have a greater half-life extension effect than geriatric women.

FLURAZEPAM
Dosage. Flurazepam (Dalmane) is an effective hypnotic, and its usual bedtime dose is 15–30 mg orally. The elderly should be given the lower dose. It promotes drowsiness within 15–45 minutes of ingestion, and this effect lasts for seven to eight hours. Sleep cycles are minimally disrupted and total REM sleep appears to be unchanged. It is converted in the liver primarily to the active metabolite desalkylflurazepam, which has a plasma half-life of 47–100 hours. This metabolite tends

to accumulate with repeated dosages of flurazepam. Flurazepam is not maximally effective for the first few nights, but dosage is not to be increased during the initial treatment period.

HALAZEPAM
Dosage. Because halazepam (Paxipam) has the active metabolite desmethyldiazepam, geriatric and debilitated patients are given a reduced dosage of only 20 mg twice daily. The usual adult dosage is 60–160 mg daily for the relief of short-term anxiety.

LORAZEPAM
Dosage. Lorazepam (Ativan) is used for anxiety and is usually given orally in a daily dosage of 1–10 mg, with the largest dose given at bedtime. The plasma half-life of lorazepam is not age dependent or lengthened by liver disease. Dosage is reduced in geriatric patients because of their greater CNS sensitivity, not because of the drug's metabolite accumulation. Memory impairment is sometimes an intentional benefit; at other times it is an undesired effect.

OXAZEPAM *Pharmacokinetics*
Absorption. The absorption and onset of oxazepam (Serax) are too slow to make it clinically useful for inducing sleep or reducing anxiety.

Biotransformation. When oxazepam is metabolized, no active metabolites are formed. Therefore, this drug may be the anxiolytic of choice for patients who have impaired liver function. Its plasma half-life is not age dependent.

PRAZEPAM

Prazepam (Verstran, Centrax) is an antianxiety agent given orally in divided doses ranging from 20–40 mg per day. It is a "pro-drug," which must be metabolized to an active form. This activation occurs too slowly to make it useful as a hypnotic.

TEMAZEPAM

Temazepam (Restoril) is used as a hypnotic in oral dosages of 15–30 mg at bedtime. Its action is similar to that of all the other benzodiazepines.

TRIAZOLAM

Triazolam (Halcion) is a newer, fast-onset, and short-acting hypnotic, to be used only for sleep induction. Its metabolites are insignificant. Some patients may even complain that the drug interferes with sleep maintenance because its half-life is so short. Elimination may be biphasic; that is, part of the dose may be excreted later, so patients still complain about "hangover" effect. Triazolam is different from other benzodiazepines in that it does not suppress stage IV sleep, and therefore it may not be used to treat *somnambulism*.

BARBITURATES

Uses

Barbiturates (salts or derivatives of barbituric acid) have a clinical role as CNS depressants. At low dosages, they produce sedative effects; at high doses, hypnotic effects. Due to certain advantages, barbiturates have generally been replaced by benzodiazepines for daytime sedation. Some barbiturates are indicated as anticonvulsants. Some are used parenterally as anesthetics; they are also used as preoperative adjuncts to help reduce anxiety and facilitate the induction of anesthesia. Barbiturates themselves have no analgesic action and may increase the reaction to painful stimuli at subanesthetic doses.

Action

Since all barbiturates are derived from the same substance—barbituric acid—all have similar mechanisms of action and side effects. Barbiturates are capable of producing all levels of CNS depression, from mild sedation to hypnosis to death by respiratory depression. Their precise effect on neurotransmitters is unclear, but they apparently decrease the excitability of both pre- and postsynaptic membranes in the cerebral cortex and reticular formation. Relatively low doses of barbiturates depress the sensory cortex, decrease motor activity, and produce sedation and drowsiness. Judgment is often distorted and perception clouded. In some patients, however, drowsiness may be preceded by transient elation, confusion, or excitement. Barbiturates reduce REM sleep and decrease stages III and IV. Sleep disruption due to REM rebound is common following discontinuation of barbiturates. Major differences among barbiturates occur in the onset of action and duration of effect. The choice of drug is based on duration of action. Based on their half-lives, these medications are classified as being long-acting, intermediate-acting, and short-acting.

Pharmacokinetics

ABSORPTION. All of the barbiturates are absorbed rapidly when given orally. The rate of absorption slows with the presence of food in the stomach. Since the onset of effect may be rapid, the patient may initially experience feelings of dizziness and excitement. Barbiturates are also absorbed through the colon, and therefore may be administered rectally.

DISTRIBUTION. The barbiturates are distributed throughout the tissues and fluids of the body. Lipid solubility is the dominant reason that high concentrations are found in the brain. Barbiturates that are most lipid soluble, e.g., thiopental, are suitable for use as anesthetics because they penetrate the blood–brain barrier rapidly. Less lipophilic barbiturates such as phenobarbital penetrate and leave the brain more slowly and therefore have a slower onset and longer duration of action. Barbiturates cross the placental barrier and pass into the milk of nursing women. (See below for precautions during pregnancy and lactation.)

BIOTRANSFORMATION AND EXCRETION. The barbiturates are metabolized in the liver and excreted as inactive metabolites in the urine. Furthermore, these drugs stimulate microsomal enzymes in the liver; continued use may increase the rate of metabolism of certain other drugs. (See discussion under Interactions.) A tolerance develops to the effects of barbiturates, usually within 7–14 days, and use of barbiturates for a period of only one month may lead to *dependence*.

There is a wide range of half-lives for the barbiturates (see Table 24–4). The drugs tend to have a cumulative effect, creating the feeling of a hangover upon awakening.

Contraindications and Precautions

Patients with pulmonary, hepatic, or renal insufficiency and debilitated patients suffering from pulmonary insufficiency are not to be treated with barbiturates, as these patients are extremely sensitive to the respiratory depressant action of these drugs. The barbiturates must be used with extreme caution in those experiencing decreased hepatic or renal function, since these conditions alter the rate of metabolism and excretion of the drug, increasing the possibility of overdose.

Geriatric and debilitated patients are more likely to react to usual doses with excitement (*paradoxic reaction*), confusion, or mental depression. Therefore, lower doses are always advised if and when barbiturates are prescribed for geriatric patients.

PAIN. Barbiturates are contraindicated in patients with pain, because paradoxic excitement may be induced.

PREGNANCY. Barbiturates have been shown to cause an increased incidence of fetal abnormalities; risk-to-benefit ratio must be carefully considered in life-threatening situations or serious conditions for which other medications cannot be used or are ineffective (FDA Pregnancy Category D). Use of barbiturates in the third trimester of pregnancy may cause physical dependence in the newborn. Withdrawal symptoms such as seizures and hyperirritability may have a delayed onset of up to 14 days after birth.

PORPHYRIA. Barbiturate use is also contraindicated for patients with intermittent *porphyria*. Administration of a barbiturate to a person with this condition causes an increase in the level of porphyrins, leading to paralysis and death.

Adverse Reactions

The most frequently occurring adverse effects are the neurologic extensions of CNS depression. Infrequent side effects include nausea, diarrhea, headache, joint or muscle pain, vomiting, dyspnea, diarrhea, headache, joint or muscle pain, vomiting, dyspnea, hives, sore throat, fever, angioneurotic edema, bradycardia, wheezing, and jaundice. Paradoxic reactions of excitement, confusion, and hostility may be seen, mainly in the elderly and in patients with severe pain.

Drug Interactions

The barbiturates interact problematically with many other drugs. They should not be given concurrently with any other CNS depressant, since this combination creates further depressant effects, especially respiratory depression.

Barbiturates may decrease the effectiveness of estrogens, estrogen-containing contraceptives, anticoagulants (coumarin or indandione derivations), steroids, digitoxin, and quinidine. The reason is that barbiturates, and especially phenobarbital, stimulate the microsomal enzymes that are responsible for metabolizing these drugs. When these drugs are metabolized faster, lower blood levels result and their pharmacologic effects are shortened.

Barbiturates may accumulate to toxic levels when drugs such as valproic acid (Depakene) are given because the metabolism of the barbiturates is decreased. Implications of these interactions include the following:

1. Monitor asthmatics on corticosteroids to detect worsening of asthma.
2. Monitor patients on digitoxin (Purodigin) for signs of underdigitalization.
3. Check prothrombin times more frequently to see if an increase in oral anticoagulant is needed.
4. Suggest that women on estrogen-containing contraceptives discuss an alternative means of contraception.

The easier solution to these drug interactions is to use an agent other than a barbiturate.

Barbiturate Subgroups

SHORT-ACTING BARBITURATES. The short-acting barbiturates, utilized as sedative-hypnotics, include secobarbital (Seconal) and pentobarbital (Nembutal). These drugs promote sleepiness within 10–15 minutes. A single oral dose has a duration of three to four hours; however, their residual sedative effects may last as long as 48 hours. The sedative-hypnotic dosages of pentobarbital and secobarbital is 100–200 mg at bedtime, given orally, rectally, or parenterally.

INTERMEDIATE-ACTING BARBITURATES. The intermediate-acting barbiturates include butabarbital (Butisol), aprobarbital (Alurate), amobarbital (Amytal), and talbutal (Lotusate). These drugs are all used as hypnotics and as such produce sleep within 45–60 minutes. A single dose usually has a duration of six to eight hours, but the residual sedative effects may last up to two days. Amobarbital and talbutal are also used for daytime sedation in lower, divided doses.

LONG-ACTING BARBITURATES. Phenobarbital is a slow-onset, long-acting barbiturate. Its effects may begin as long as two hours following ingestion, and its residual sedative effects may last for as long as six days. Phenobarbital sodium (Luminal Sodium) is administered parenterally in doses of 100 mg but may also be administered orally as an anticonvulsant. Note that its onset is delayed even after intravenous administration; this is because it takes longer to penetrate the brain than do other intravenous barbiturates.

MISCELLANEOUS SEDATIVE-HYPNOTICS

Included in this group are buspirone, the newest agent; chloral betaine; triclofos sodium; chloral hydrate; two antihistamines, diphenhydramine and hydroxyzine; ethchlorvynol; glutethimide; meprobamate; methyprylon; paraldehyde; and propranolol.

Buspirone

Buspirone (BuSpar) is a new agent for the treatment of chronic anxiety. It appears to offer several advantages over all other sedatives. It causes less sedation and less impairment of motor skills, does not potentiate the effects of alcohol, and has no apparent abuse potential. Withdrawal symptoms are not reported, even upon abrupt discontinuation of therapy. It is not indicated for acute anxiety. It takes one to two weeks to work.

Dizziness, lightheadedness, nausea, headache, and excitement are the most commonly observed adverse reactions.

Chloral Hydrate and Derivatives

Chloral hydrate (Noctec, Somnos) is one of the oldest hypnotics and is well tolerated by elderly patients. It is absorbed rapidly when given orally and converted to trichloroethanol in the liver. This metabolite produces the hypnotic effect. This drug is an irritant and therefore produces side effects of nausea, vomiting, and flatulence. Its taste is unpleasant; therefore, it is best given with food, milk, or plenty of water. Chloral hydrate may also produce psychologic and physical dependency.

Chloral betaine (Beta-Chlor) and triclosfos sodium (Triclos) are derivatives of chloral hydrate. The hypnotic dose of chloral betaine is 870–1000 mg given orally at bedtime. The hypnotic dose of triclosfos sodium is 1500 mg given orally at bedtime. Both of these drugs promote sleep within 30 minutes, and their effects last up to ten hours.

Diphenhydramine and Hydroxyzine

Diphenhydramine (Benadryl) and hydroxyzine (Vistaril, Atarax) are not very effective in reducing anxiety, but they appear to work as mild hypnotics. Diphenhydramine is sold without a prescription as an ingredient in sleep aids. Use of this drug in treatment of individuals with anxiety associated with pruritic dermatosis may produce desired results. Doxylamine is another mild sedative available over the counter.

Ethchlorvynol

Ethchlorvynol (Placidyl) is a nonbarbiturate hypnotic. Its hypnotic dose is 500–1000 mg given orally at bedtime. Within 15–30 minutes the individual experiences its effect, which lasts about five hours. Prior to falling asleep, however, the individual may become dizzy and feel giddy. For this reason, patients are watched carefully after this drug is administered.

Glutethimide

Glutethimide (Doriden) is a nonbarbiturate hypnotic Schedule III drug used primarily on a short-term basis to treat insomnia. Its hypnotic dose is 500 mg orally. The total daily dose of glutethimide should not exceed 1000 mg. Chronic ingestion of this drug results in physical and psychologic dependence, and overdoses are highly lethal.

Meprobamate

Meprobamate (Equanil, Miltown) has been classified as a Schedule IV drug. It is addictive and has been associated with many suicides. Its daily oral dosage is 600–1200 mg.

Methyprylon

Methyprylon (Noludar) induces a hypnotic effect within 30–45 minutes of ingestion, and its action lasts five to eight hours. Its hypnotic dose is 200–400 mg given orally, whereas its sedative dose is 50–100 mg given orally three times daily.

Paraldehyde

Paraldehyde was once believed to be a safe, effective anxiolytic agent. However, it is now considered to have little value in terms of its antianxiety effect.

Other Drugs Used as Sedative/ Hypnotics

Propranolol, a beta-adrenergic blocking agent, has not yet been approved by the Food and Drug Administration for use as an antianxiety medication. The suggested anxiolytic daily dose is 30–120 mg given orally.

Tricyclic antidepressants are sometimes used for anxiety, including panic attacks, as are monoamine oxidase inhibitors. These drugs are discussed in Chapter 26. Research currently is being conducted on endorphins, which may be the next drug class to be used for anxiety disorders.

USING THE NURSING PROCESS

ASSESSMENT

Assessment of the patient's need for sedative-hypnotic medications is a difficult process because each individ-

Table 24–6. ASSESSMENT OF LEVELS OF ANXIETY

Level	Characteristics
Mild (+)	Perceptual field is broadened, perceptual abilities are intensified. Learning and problem-solving abilities are enhanced. Able to connect feelings, thoughts, and actions. Motivated to focus on the here-and-now problems. Able to make cause-and-effect relationships. Appears calm.
Moderate (+ +)	Perceptual field is narrowed. Experiences selective inattention—fails to notice what goes on in situations peripheral to the immediate focus, but can attend to the stimuli if they are pointed out. Alertness is increased, reaching its highest, most efficient level. Able to connect feelings, thoughts, and actions. Experiences feelings of tension and challenge. Utilizes ego defense mechanisms. May appear tense and restless.
Severe (+ + +)	Perceptual field is greatly decreased. Selective inattention continues but forces the person to focus on one small part of the problem or environment. Dissociation may occur. Learning and problem-solving abilities are decreased. Unable to connect feelings, thoughts, and actions. Behaviors are aimed at obtaining immediate relief from the anxiety. Appears tense and will manifest cues of physiologic response to anxiety, such as increased respirations, pulse, and blood pressure.
Panic (+ + + +)	Person experiences intense feelings of panic, awe, dread, terror, gloom and doom. Dissociation continues. Perception of reality becomes difficult: details within the environment may appear enlarged or scattered and spinning. Learning and problem-solving abilities are nonexistent. Behavior is focused on gaining or maintaining control. Symptoms of helplessness, hopelessness, rage may be observed. Symptoms of physiologic response to anxiety such as hypertension and hyperventilation syndrome may occur.

ual has a unique pattern of response to increased levels of anxiety. Persons who receive the maximum therapeutic benefit from these medications are those who demonstrate both psychological and physiologic symptoms of anxiety. An increase in a person's level of anxiety creates changes of a physiologic, cognitive, behavioral, and emotional nature. Table 24–6 reviews the response categorization to anxiety levels and highlights the physiologic, cognitive, behavioral, and emotional characteristics of each of the four levels of anxiety. The Hamilton Anxiety Rating Scale (HAM-A) is one of many scales used to evaluate anxiety (mood and somatic symptoms).

The HAM-A interview-based scale is also widely used for assessing anxiolytic efficacy.

Following an estimate of the patient's level of anxiety, assess these factors: What does the person usually do to decrease the level of anxiety? Is this coping behavior effective? Adaptive or maladaptive? What factors are pro-ducing the increase in the level of anxiety? Does the increased level of anxiety appear to be correlated with normal everyday stress or less? How does the increased level of anxiety affect the patient's ability to manage activities of daily living? Outcome evaluation criteria is found in Table 24–7.

Table 24–7. NURSING PROCESS FOR PATIENTS REQUIRING SEDATIVE-HYPNOTICS OR ANTIANXIOLYTICS

Assessment

Assess sleeping patterns during both day and night, including presleep activities/rituals, and how pattern affects patient's life.
Note history of past and current health problems.
Evaluate mental status; level of anxiety, noting presence of phobias, obsessions, compulsions.
Ascertain current/past coping behaviors.

Nursing Diagnosis	Nursing Actions	Rationale	Desired Outcomes/ Evaluation Criteria
Sleep pattern disturbance related to anxiety/ depression, inactivity, illness/pain as evidenced by difficulty falling asleep, wakening earlier or later than desired, interrupted sleep, complaints of feeling tired.	Recommend avoidance of caffeine-containing substances at least 2 hours before bedtime. Decrease environmental stimuli. Encourage use of relaxation techniques prior to bedtime. Acknowledge difficulty and frustration of insomnia. Administer medication as indicated.	Stimulation may interfere with REM sleep. Reduces muscle tension, aids in refocusing attention, promoting rest/sleep. Communicates empathy and aids in reduction of associated anxiety. Short-term use of antianxiolytics, sedatives/hypnotics may help until other problems are resolved.	Reports improvement in sleep/rest pattern with increased sense of well-being/feeling rested upon awakening.
Anxiety, moderate level related to a stressful event as evidenced by increased tension, feelings of helplessness, inability to sleep and eat, weight loss/gain.	Evaluate whether desired therapeutic effect is achieved. Encourage patient to acknowledge and express feelings. Use problem-solving techniques to help patient to make appropriate choices for individual situation. Active Listen to patient. Provide accurate information about the situation.	Promotes optimal medication response with minimal side effects. Helps to identify and deal with underlying feelings. Promotes adaptive coping behaviors which may have been impaired by high anxiety level. Promotes dealing with realities.	Appears relaxed. Vital signs are within normal limits. Reports anxiety is reduced to a manageable level. Identifies stress situations and specific actions to deal with them.
Anxiety, severe to panic level, related to perceived or actual threat to self, death, change in health status, unmet needs as evidenced by behavioral changes, apprehension, uncertainty, somatic complaints, sleeplessness, sense of impending doom, trembling, quivering voice, and focus on self.	Administer benzodiazepine medication as prescribed. Encourage use of relaxation exercises 30 min. after drug administration. Stay with patient, maintaining a calm, supportive manner. Observe patient every 15-30 min for signs of anxiety. Note cues (including vital signs) that indicate rising level of anxiety	Helps the patient to regain control and recoup ego strength. Promotes maximal effect of medication. A calm presence can help the patient to regain/maintain own composure. Allows for early intervention and treatment.	Reports anxiety reduced to a manageable level. Verbalizes awareness of feelings of anxiety and healthy ways to deal with them.

CONTINUED ON THE FOLLOWING PAGE

Table 24–7. NURSING PROCESS FOR PATIENTS REQUIRING SEDATIVE-HYPNOTICS OR ANTIANXIOLYTICS–*CONTINUED*

Nursing Diagnosis	Nursing Actions	Rationale	Desired Outcomes/ Evaluation Criteria
	and take necessary measures.		
Knowledge deficit related to unfamiliarity with medication as evidenced by questions, statements of concern.	Provide information about the medication, including action, dose, onset of effect, side effects, and interactions.	Understanding may enhance cooperation with regimen and reduce associated risks of anxiolytics and barbiturates (e.g., hangover effect, confusion, impairment of reflexes).	Verbalizes understanding of condition and treatment regimen. Initiates necessary lifestyle changes.
	Discuss problems of the condition, and resultant anxiety.	Reduction of fears enables learning to occur and enables patient to make informed decisions about treatment and medication use.	
	Review potential problems of long-term use/ habituation.	Tolerance to barbiturates may develop in 7–14 days. These medications can actually induce sleep disturbances as REM sleep cycle is suppressed. REM rebound (nightmares, poor quality of sleep, insomnia) may occur when barbiturates are withdrawn abruptly.	

The nurse also assesses for the presence of reactions such as *phobias*, *obsessions*, *compulsions*, and complaints of having symptoms of a severe physical illness (e.g., "cancer phobia"). While recognizing the person's specific reactions, the nurse continues to focus on his or her response to anxiety as the core of the illness.

Questions about the sleep-inducing techniques used by patients and whether or not a specific event or problem is causing the sleep disturbance are appropriate. When patients are treated in inpatient settings, the nurse observes them during sleep. (Refer to Tables 24–2 and 24–3 to assess the normalcy of sleep of your patients.)

Important: Listen to patients' cues regarding their ability to sleep and their preferences for medication to help them sleep. In many clinical settings, physicians routinely order medications on an as-needed (prn) basis to promote sleep when patients are admitted. These medications are then frequently administered whether or not they are required. This practice is not recommended.

A careful assessment as to whether or not the person is experiencing the desired effect from the same dosage or has developed a tolerance to the drug is essential. Since many of these drugs are addictive, the nurse should be alert to cues of physical dependency. It must be kept in mind that cues of withdrawal from certain benzodiazepines may not develop for seven to ten days after the last dose because of the relatively long halflives of some of these drugs. In addition, the potential for these drugs to cause paradoxic reactions, such as hallucinations, hostility, insomnia, and confusion, must be recognized.

Since many suicides occur because of the ingestion of alcohol with sedative-hypnotics, an assessment of the patient's suicide potential is necessary and should be done frequently.

NURSING DIAGNOSES

When the assessment has been completed, nursing diagnoses are formulated. These focus on each patient's and family's responses to anxiety disorders and/or sleep problems. Possible nursing diagnoses are featured in Table 24–7.

INTERVENTION

The goals of nursing intervention for those being treated with a sedative-hypnotic drug include reducing the target symptom, specifically anxiety or insomnia, or both; and educating patients about symptoms and treatment regimens. The data base established during the initial health history is used by the nurse and patient to develop the plan of care. Table 24–7 outlines plans of intervention related to specific nursing diagnoses.

Nursing Responsibilities

Because patients' levels of anxiety tend to fluctuate according to changes in circumstances and the environment, the nurse's primary intervention centers on monitoring these levels. The frequency of checks is correlated with the severity of patients' symptoms. The nurse recognizes the early cues that indicate a patient's level of anxiety is rising. If the physician has ordered a prn dose of benzodiazepine, the nurse administers it as the patient's anxiety level begins to rise. This tends to help the patient to avoid the intense symptoms of high anxiety levels. As noted above, the benzodiazepines are most effective when administered orally.

Patient Teaching

General information about the sedative-hypnotic medications to be included in the nurse's teaching plan for each patient is given in Table 24–8.

EVALUATION

Evaluation of the effectiveness of the nursing intervention for patients being treated with sedative-hypnotic medications is based on an appraisal of goal achievement. The overall goals of intervention are to reduce the target symptom(s), resulting from anxiety or insomnia, or both, and to educate patients about their reactions and treatment regimens.

Make a careful evaluation to ascertain whether the patient's level of anxiety has decreased. Is he or she able to focus on the current situation and to connect current feelings and thoughts with actions? (Persons who talk only of wanting to feel better may still be in the severe panic level of anxiety.) Also, evaluate whether or not the patient's pulse rate and blood pressure have decreased. Cues of a decrease in level of anxiety are usually observed within one hour of an oral dose of most of these drugs. This effect lasts from four to six hours. If the person is less anxious, symptoms of the mild to moderate level are evident. At this time, acknowledge that the patient, even though improved, may feel anxious at times. The patient's aim should be to learn adaptive methods of tolerating this feeling instead of depending on medications. The patient's levels of knowledge about the medications and anxiety are evaluated on a step-by-step basis as the material is presented.

When a patient has been receiving a sedative-hypnotic agent to induce sleep, evaluate whether or not the ability to sleep has improved. Determine whether the person wakens feeling rested or "hung over." Be alert for remarks by the patient about dreaming during the night. This is a characteristic of the REM phase of sleep. In hospitals and other settings, where there is an opportunity to make an evaluation during sleep, note whether the muscles appear to relax. Since all of the medicines, especially when combined with other CNS depressants such as alcohol, may be employed as a means of suicide, remain alert for symptoms of increased suicide potential.

EVALUATION OF INDIVIDUALS RECEIVING BENZODIAZEPINES

Along with evaluating signs of a favorable response to the anxiolytic drug, note whether there are side effects of the medications. Side effects of drowsiness and ataxia

---

Table 24–8 PATIENT TEACHING INFORMATION—SEDATIVE-HYPNOTICS

Dear Patient:
   This drug has been prescribed for you. This is what you should know about your drug to get the most from your therapy.

1. This drug will help you to relax. OR: This drug will help you to sleep.
2. This drug is usually not to be taken for more than a few months. Check with your physician to make sure if you need to continue taking it.
3. Take this medicine only as directed by your doctor. Do not take more of it. or more frequently, or for a longer period that your doctor ordered. It may become habit forming (causing mental or physical dependence) if too much is taken.
4. This medicine will add to the effects of alcohol and other medicines that slow down the nervous system, such as antihistamines, pain medications, seizure medication, tranquilizers and other sedatives. Check with your doctor before taking this with any of the above medicines.
5. If you forget to take a dose (while taking it regularly), take it immediately if you remember the missed dose within an hour or so of missing it. However, if you do not remember until later, skip the dose and go back to your regular schedule. Do not double dose.
6. Do not stop taking the medicine without first discussing this with your physician, especially if you have been taking it regularly. Your doctor may want you to gradually reduce the amount you are taking. Stopping this medicine suddenly may cause side effects.
7. The dosage should not be altered. The dose should never be altered and the time between doses should not be decreased.
   Note: For patients taking flurazepam (Dalmane): When you beging taking this medicine, your sleeping problem will improve somewhat the first night, but two or three nights may pass before you receive the full effects of this medicine.
8. Do not drink alcohol while you are taking this medicine.
9. This drug may cause you to feel drowsy, dizzy, or lightheaded. Be sure you know how the drug affects you before you drive or participate in other activities that require you to be alert, such as operating machinery.
10. Keep this medicine out of the reach of children since overdose may be especially dangerous to childern.

are most common. Recognize how frustrating these side effects can be and reassure patients that as their bodies become accustomed to the drugs, the effects tend to decrease.

Gastrointestinal discomfort, nausea, and vomiting may develop. Encourage patients to take the drugs during or immediately following meals to alleviate the intensity of these problems.

Evaluate whether clients are experiencing any of the infrequently reported side effects such as blurred vision, hypotension, depression, urinary retention, or incontinence. When these symptoms occur, the physician should be consulted.

Rarely, paradoxic reactions are demonstrated. Symptoms of these reactions include excitement, hostility, rage, confusion, hallucinations, and acute hyperpyrexia. When these symptoms appear, the nurse withholds medication and contacts the physician immediately.

EVALUATION OF INDIVIDUALS RECEIVING BARBITURATES

Observe patients who are taking barbiturates to determine whether they are experiencing side effects such as nausea, drowsiness, and slurred speech. Evaluate these patients also for any of the less frequent side effects such as mental confusion, depression, sore throat, fever, angioneurotic edema, wheezing, and paradoxic reactions of excitement or hostility. When any of these symptoms are observed, consult the physician to formulate a plan of treatment.

SUMMARY

These drugs, especially the benzodiazepines, are extremely effective in alleviating specific symptoms of anxiety and neurotic reactions. However, the potential for benzodiazepine abuse is quite high because of their widespread use, their relatively minor side effects, and the possibility for dependency. The barbiturates and other older sedative-hypnotics have even greater potential for dependency, side effects, and drug interactions. In most locations they have become less popular as

"street" drugs of abuse. Clearly, use of anxiolytic agents presents a challenge to nurses to help patients achieve the maximum therapeutic benefits from the drugs while avoiding major problems associated with their use. Whenever possible, the nurse can encourage nonpharmacologic means to relieve anxiety or induce sleep. Hypnotics are appropriate only for short-term use for situational insomnia. Nurses can help patients expect to resume normal sleep, unassisted by hypnotics, after a few weeks at most.

BIBLIOGRAPHY

Allen, RM: Tranquilizers and sedative/hypnotics: Appropriate use in the elderly. Geriatrics 41(5):75, 1986.

Brown, JT, Mulrow, CD, and Stoudemire, GA: The anxiety disorders. Ann Intern Med 100:558, 1984.

Busto, U, et al: Withdrawal reaction after long-term therapeutic use of benzodiazepines. N Engl J Med 315:854, 1986.

Csernansky, JG and Hollister, LE: Drug treatment of panic attacks. Hosp Formul 21:582, 1986.

DuPont, RL: Benzodiazepines: The social issues. Institute for Behavior and Health, Inc., Rockville, MD, 1986.

Fagan, DR and Illsley, SS: Benzodiazepine hypnotics: A comparative review of recently approved agents. Hosp Formul 20:481, 1985.

Fankhauser, MP and German, ML: Understanding the use of behavioral rating scales in studies evaluating the efficacy of antianxiety and antidepressant drugs. Am J Hosp Pharm 44:2087, 1987.

Hansten, PD: Drug Interactions, ed 5. Philadelphia, Lea & Febiger, 1985.

Harvey S: Sedatives and hypnotics. In Gilman, A and Goodman, L (eds): The Pharmacologic Basis of Therapeutics. New York, Macmillan, 1985.

McEvoy, GK: American Hospital Formulary Service Drug Information. Am Soc Hosp Pharm. Bethesda, MD, 1989.

Miller, F, et al: Unrecognized drug dependence and withdrawal in the elderly. Drug Alcohol Depend 15:177, 1985.

Sherman, JA: Identifying and treating insomnia in the elderly. The Consultant Pharmacist :71, Jan/Feb 1987.

Sussman, N: The benzodiazepines: Selection and use in treating anxiety, insomnia, and other disorders. Hosp Formul 20:298, 1985.

Taniguchi, G and Westphal, J: Long-term benzodiazepine use in anxiety states. Hosp Formul 21:179, 1986.

United States Pharmacopeial Conv, Inc: USP Drug Information 1989.

Williams, J: Diagnostic and Statistical Manual of Mental Disorders, ed 3 revised. Am Psych Assn, Washington, DC, 1987, p 235.

SITUATION 24–1

Julia Abad has been seen in the clinic frequently for difficulty sleeping after a traumatic event. She is 26 years old and is currently in counseling. In addition to insomnia, she complains of feeling "panicked" when in crowded situations.

1. Ms. Abad is to begin treatment with alprazolam (Xanax) 0.5 mg po three times a day. The clinic nurse will focus on the following during the assessment stage:
   a. response to phobic situations
   b. physiological symptoms only
   c. response to counseling
   d. psychological symptoms only

SITUATION 24–1–*CONTINUED*

2. The nurse will include the following when teaching Ms. Abad about the use of anxiolytic therapy:
   a. Discontinue if symptoms of drowsiness appear.
   b. Refrain from alcohol consumption.
   c. Increase dosage at night if unable to sleep.
   d. Take the medication as needed for anxiety.

3. Ms. Abad is concerned about the types of side effects that she may experience while taking alprazolam. The following effect applies to this agent:
   a. epilepsy
   b. slurred speech
   c. exfoliative dermatitis
   d. photophobia

4. On a follow-up visit one week later, Ms. Abad states that she is sleeping at night now, but does not feel "rested." The nurse is aware that this probably relates to reduction in:
   a. Stage I sleep
   b. Stage II sleep
   c. Stage III sleep
   d. REM sleep

5. A response by Ms. Abad that reflects adequate learning about alprazolam therapy would be:
   a. "This drug will keep me from having panic attacks in public."
   b. "I should limit my fluid intake to prevent swelling."
   c. "It would be best for me to quit smoking to receive optimal benefits."
   d. "This drug will not cause addiction, so I can take it indefinitely."

6. In planning follow-up care, the nurse will stress that Ms. Abad should not abruptly stop taking alprazolam because of the potential for:
   a. seizures
   b. headaches
   c. dermatitis
   d. rebound tachycardia

SITUATION 24–2

Karen Smith is a 70-year-old who is admitted to the surgical floor for left breast biopsy.

1. During the assessment, Ms. Smith reveals that her mother died of breast cancer. Ms. Smith is withdrawn and tense. The nurse notes that respiration, pulse, and blood pressure are elevated in comparison to admission vital signs. The nurse suspects that Ms. Smith is experiencing which of the following levels of anxiety:
   a. mild
   b. panic
   c. moderate
   d. severe

2. The nurse informs the physician regarding signs of anxiety. After an examination of Ms. Smith, the physician orders diazepam (Valium) 5 mg q 4 hours prn anxiety. As the initial dose, the nurse is to give 5 mg intramuscularly. The nurse will plan to give the drug in the following IM site:
   a. dorsogluteal
   b. deltoid
   c. ventrogluteal
   d. vastus lateralis

3. Of the following outcomes, which indicates successful therapy in Ms. Smith's situation?
   a. decreased interaction with family and friends
   b. enhanced focusing on mother's death
   c. decreased respirations, pulse, and blood pressure
   d. denial of feelings of relaxation and well-being

4. In planning nursing care for Ms. Smith, the nurse will include the following intervention:
   a. withholding the diazepam if patient appears calm
   b. providing a stimulating environment for distraction
   c. questioning the patient at length concerning feelings
   d. monitoring for unusual signs of excitement

5. A nursing responsibility associated with the care of Ms. Smith includes:
   a. encourage oral fluids
   b. limit all visitors
   c. restrict music
   d. encourage solitude and reflection

6. When evaluating Ms. Smith after several days of diazepam therapy, the nurse is aware of the possibility for the following laboratory result:
   a. reduced albumin
   b. elevated creatinine
   c. elevated bilirubin
   d. reduced platelets

Please refer to the Appendices for correct answers and additional review questions with answers.

25
CHAPTER

ANTIPSYCHOTIC MEDICATIONS

LOVETTA L. SMITH, DNSc, RN, CS

LEARNING OBJECTIVES

After reading this chapter, the student will be able to:

1. Identify commonly used antipsychotic medications.

2. Differentiate among the antipsychotic medications as to mechanism of action, route of administration, disposition in the body, adverse effects, contraindications, and interactions.

3. Identify areas of nursing assessment in the patient requiring antipsychotic medications in order to formulate appropriate nursing diagnoses.

4. Plan the nursing interventions for patients requiring antipsychotic medications.

5. Evaluate the patient at various stages of treatment to gauge the effectiveness of the nursing interventions.

ANTIPSYCHOTIC MEDICATIONS

Antipsychotic medications, also called *neuroleptics*, have been used with increasing frequency since the mid-1950s. The term "antipsychotic" is derived from the drug's ability to effectively relieve certain symptoms of acute and chronic psychoses including thought disorders, *hallucinations, delusions*, and agitation (Table 25–1). Unfortunately, another common feature of antipsychotics is their tendency to produce extrapyramidal effects that patients frequently experience as bothersome side effects and that must be managed when the drugs are used clinically. In earlier years, antipsychotics were also called "major tranquilizers." However, the term is antiquated and inaccurate since sedation and tranquilization are not the mode by which the positive actions of the drugs are realized.

There are five chemical groups of compounds that share the same pharmacologic effects. These are phenothiazines (divided into three subgroups called aliphatic, piperidine, and piperazine), thioxanthines, butyrophenones, dihydroindolones, and dibenzoxazepines. Table 25–2 lists information about the drugs in each of these classes.

The antipsychotic drugs are not curative, but they have proven effective in the control of symptoms to a degree that allows many patients a much-improved quality of life. When Thorazine (chlorpromazine, the first of the aliphatic phenothiazines) was introduced in 1954, many patients who had spent long years as patients in institutional settings were able to achieve outpatient status.

MECHANISM OF ACTION

The mechanism of action of the various antipsychotics is not definitively known. However, the link between the positive effect and the production of unwanted extrapyramidal movement disorders suggests a mechanism of dopamine blockade. Dopamine is a biogenic amine that acts as a neurotransmitter. Evidence indicates that antipsychotic agents may act to block postsynaptic dopamine receptor sites in the nigrostriatal system of the basal ganglia and therefore inhibit the transmission of the neural impulse in the brain. It has been shown that clinical potency corresponds with the level of dopamine-blocking potency. The effectiveness of the drug suggests a connection between psychotic illnesses and a biologic abnormality in dopamine release or receptor site sensitivity, a research area to which nurses may contribute in the future.

Antipsychotic medications as a class of drugs may at times be used for their antiemetic properties. The drugs have this property as a result of their ability to inhibit the chemoreceptor trigger zones in the medulla.

Antianxiety and sedative effects of the antipsychotics result from indirect reduction of stimuli to the brain stem reticular system. Additionally, an alpha-adrenergic blocking effect of the drugs results in their sedating ability.

The major neurotransmitter released at the ganglionic synapse is acetylcholine. In the parasympathetic system, the neurotransmitter between the postganglionic fiber and the effector cell is also acetylcholine. Fibers that release acetylcholine are called cholinergic fibers, and neurons in the efferent nervous system are primarily cholinergic. There are several different types of receptors for each transmitter. Experiments have demonstrated that acetylcholine receptors on the postsynaptic neurons of all autonomic ganglia respond to low doses of the drug nicotine and are therefore called nicotinic receptors. Acetylcholine receptors on smooth muscle, cardiac muscles, and gland cells are stimulated by the mushroom poison muscarine and are called muscarinic receptors. The blockade of these receptors produces a host of anticholinergic effects. The mechanism of muscarinic receptor blockade is responsible for many of the unpleasant side effects experienced by patients taking antipsychotic medications.

PHARMACOKINETICS

Absorption

Antipsychotic medications are well absorbed from the gastrointestinal tract and from parenteral sites but may be erratic, especially following oral administration. Liquid forms of drugs are most predictably absorbed, but can be reduced in the rate of absorption by the presence of food in the stomach or with concurrent administration of anticholinergic agents, antiparkinson drugs, or antacids. Administration of intramuscular preparations provides four to ten times more active drug than oral doses. Intramuscular injection is most often prescribed for initial rapid antipsychotic dosing or on a prn basis for control of potentially dangerous behavior. There is considerable variability from one individual to another in peak plasma concentrations. This variability is

Table 25–1. PSYCHOTIC DISORDERS

> *Definition*
> Group of severe mental illnesses in which the patient's abilities to perceive reality, communicate, and form stable interpersonal relationships are impaired.
>
> *Etiology*
> Unknown; many theories about physical, psychological, and social causations abound.
>
> *Symptoms*
> Three main classifications of signs and symptoms of psychotic reactions exist:
> 1. Hallucinations (visual, auditory, tactile, olfactory, gustatory).
> 2. Inappropriate affect
> 3. Delusions (somatic, religious, persecutory, grandiose)
>
> These symptoms may exist independently or in combination with each other. Frequently, patients will demonstrate symptoms of the panic level of anxiety.

thought to result from genetic differences in rates of metabolism, biodegradation of the drugs, and metabolism of the drugs. Therapeutic ranges for drug concentrations have, therefore, not been clearly established.

Distribution and Biotransformation

Antipsychotic medications are distributed into most body tissues and fluids with high concentrations into the brain, lungs, liver, kidney, and spleen. As the antipsychotics are absorbed, they bind to plasma and tissue proteins. The drugs are extensively metabolized in the liver, and many active metabolites are produced.

Elimination

The majority of the metabolites of antipsychotic medications are excreted in urine and feces; however, some may remain in the body for months beyond the time when the medication is discontinued.

The drugs are highly lipophilic, that is, they have an affinity for fatty tissue and therefore distribute widely in the body. The fatty tissues store the metabolites until a point of saturation is reached. Then, when the drug is discontinued, the material is slowly released and excreted. Most of the drugs have long elimination half-lives, in excess of 24 hours for many metabolites. Because the drugs are so extensively distributed to tissues outside the systemic circulation, hemodialysis and peritoneal dialysis methods have not proven effective in treating overdose situations.

CONTRAINDICATIONS AND PRECAUTIONS

Antipsychotic medications are generally contraindicated for patients who are also taking large amounts of barbiturates, narcotics, or alcohol. Patients who are comatose should not be given these drugs because antipsychotics further depress the CNS. Furthermore, the antipsychotics, which have a potent anticholinergic effect, are not administered to patients with prostatic hypertrophy, glaucoma, hepatic disease, and cardiac dysrhythmias. Table 25–3 features a list of medical conditions in which antipsychotic agents should be used cautiously.

ADVERSE EFFECTS

The neuroleptic agents produce many side effects. Table 25–4 identifies manifestations and mechanisms of side effects of this group of drugs. The occurrence of side effects is the major disadvantage associated with their use. Primary side-effects of neuroleptic medications are extrapyramidal reactions including *parkinsonism, dyskinesia, dystonias,* and *akathisia.* Figure 25–1 features a description of each of the extrapyramidal reactions and identifies their relative onset. Anticholinergic effects have even more serious negative potentials when ex-

TEXT RESUMES ON PAGE 640

Relative Sequence of Onset of Extrapyrimidal Side Effects

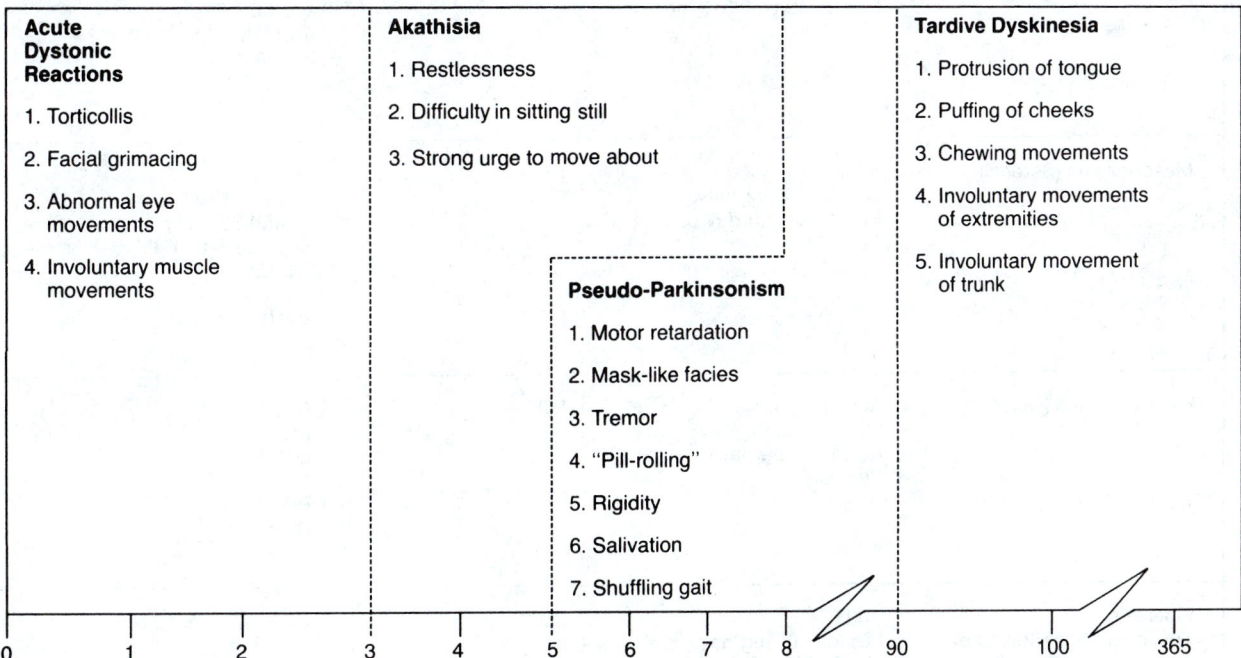

Figure 25–1. Relative sequence of onset of extrapyramidal side effects. (From Carpenter, W, and Rudo, A: Tardive dyskinesia. Behav Med 6(7):35, 1979, with permission.)

Table 25–2. ANTIPSYCHOTIC MEDICATIONS

Name	Dosage	Mode of Administration	Pharmacokinetics
Phenothiazines			
Action: For All: mechanism unknown; however, there is dopamine blockage; inhibits chemoreceptor trigger zone.			
Use: For All: control acute and chronic thought disorders, hallucinations, delusions, and agitation.			
Aliphatics: Chlorpromazine (Thorazine)	Adult: LD: 400–1500 mg/day M: 200–1000 mg/day Ped: 0.25 mg/lb, q 6–8 hr up to 40 mg/day for under 5 yr	IM, PO, Suppository, IV	O: 30 min P: 2–3 hr D: up to 12 hr ½L: UA PB: 90% B: UA E: less than 1% excreted in urine within 72 hrs.
Triflupromazine (Vesprin)	Adult: LD: 60–400 mg/day M: 20–200 mg/day Ped: 2 mg/kg, up to 150 mg/day orally or 0.2–0.25 mg/kg in div. doses	IM Rectal	O: UA P: UA D: UA ½L: UA PB: UA B: UA E: UA
Promazine (Sparine)	Adult: LD: 400–800 mg/day M: 200–800 mg/day Ped: UA	IM	See Thorazine
Piperidines: Thioridazine (Mellaril)	Adult: LD: 400–800 mg/day M: 25–800 mg/day Ped: 2–12 yr, 0.5–3 mg/kg/day	PO	O: 1 hr P: 4 hr D: 8–12 hr ½L: 26–36 hr PB: UA B: UA E: UA
Mesoridazine (Serentil)	Adult: LD: 20–600 mg/day M: 10–400 mg/day Ped: UA	IM	O: UA P: (oral) 1 hr P: (IM) 30 min D: (oral) 4–6 hr (IM) 6–8 hr ½L: UA PB: UA B: UA E: UA
Piperacetazine (Quide)	Adult: LD: 50–100 mg/day M: 15–30 mg/day Ped: UA	PO	O: UA P: 3 hr D: UA ½L: PB: UA B: UA E: UA
Piperazines: Trifluoperazine (Stelazine)	Adult: LD: 20–100 mg/day M: 10–40 mg/day Ped: UA	PO IM	O: 20–30 min; 12 hr P: 2–3 hr D: 12 hr ½L: UA PB, B, E: see Thorazine

Key to Abbreviations in the *Pharmacokinetics* column: LD-loading dose; M-maintenance; O-onset; P-peak; D-duration; PB-protein bound; B-biotransformation; E-excretion; ½L-half-life. Ped-pediatric dose; UA-unavailable
*Within the column listing adverse effects, underlines indicate the most common effects.

Contraindications and Precautions	Adverse Effects*	Interactions	Nursing Implications

For All Phenothiazines
Contraindicated in hypersensitivity to other phenothiazines; in withdrawal from alcohol and sedatives; in comatose states; bone marrow depression; pregnancy and lactation, Reye's syndrome, and myasthenia gravis.
Use cautiously in hepatic disorders, cardiovascular disorders, and previously detected breast cancer.
Pediatric precaution: Less effective than other neuroleptics in treating children.

For All Antipsychotics
Neuro: Can cause decreased seizure threshold and often act as CNS depressants.
CV: Hypotension, tachycardia, increased pulse rate and syncope have occurred, especially following the first parenteral dose, usually subsides in 30–120 min (epinephrine should not be used in combination with phenothiazines since they ameliorate epinephrine's vasopressor effect and further decrease blood pressure).
Resp: Can cause respiratory distress.
GI: Can cause anorexia, dyspepsia diarrhea; "oral syndrome" with dry mouth, redness of mucous membranes, cracking of lips and corners of mouth (may make retention of dentures difficult); nausea, adynamic ileus, atonic colon.
Hemo: Blood dyscrasias
Endocrine: Moderate engorgement of breasts with lactation, increased appetite and weight gain.
Dermatologic: pigment deposits in various tissues, photosensitivity, dermatosis.
Pediatric precautions: Should be used with caution in children with acute illnesses, e.g. chicken pox, CNS infections, measles, gastroenteritis, or dehydration since the incidence of EPS and akathisia is increased.

These agents interact with many other chemical agents. See Table 25–6.

For All Antipsychotics:
ASSESSMENT: Baseline data regarding pre-drug behavioral states (T, P, R, BP, both sitting and standing) is needed. Liver fx tests, opthalmoscopic exams, complete blood count and ECG should be completed and reviewed periodically. History of prior responses to prescribed medications.
INTERVENTIONS: Administer oral concentrate with four ounces of orange or apple juice (avoid pineapple juice). Then give 4–6 ounces of water. Care during intramuscular injections is needed to avoid irritating the subcutaneous tissues.
PATIENT TEACHING: The need for taking the drug should be emphasized to help the person avoid the merry-go-round syndrome. Teach the family and the patient that the full therapeutic response may not occur until the patient has been taking the drug for 3 weeks. Discuss that these drugs are not potentially addicting and how they differ from the anti-anxiety agents. Teach the patient precautions to follow to avoid problems resulting from orthostatic hypotension. Teach the patient to avoid the effects of exposure to sunlight. Teach the patient about extrapyramidal symptoms (EPS) and how to use prescribed medications prn as ordered. Teach the patient not to take unprescribed medications or antacids with the prescribed medications. Teach the patient about selected possible adverse effects and to contact a health care provider if such effects are experienced.
EVALUATION: Observe for decreased primary symptoms. Be cognizant and

CONTINUED ON THE FOLLOWING PAGE

Table 25–2. ANTIPSYCHOTIC MEDICATIONS–*CONTINUED*

Name	Dosage	Mode of Administration	Pharmacokinetics
Acetophenazine (Tindal)	Adult: LD: 400–600 mg/day M: 60–120 mg/day Ped: UA	PO	O: UA P: UA D: UA PB: UA B: UA E: UA
Fluphenazine hydrochloride (Permitil, Prolixin)	Adult: LD: 20–80 mg/day M: 5–40 mg/day Ped: UA	IM	O: 1 hr P: 1.5–2 hr D: 6–8 hr PB: UA B: UA E: 14.7–15.3 hr
Fluphenazine enanthate (Prolixin, Enanthate)	Adult: LD: 12.5–25 mg M: up to 100 mg/wk Ped: UA	IM	O: 24–72 hr P: 48–96 hr D: 1–3 wk PB: UA B: UA E: 3.6–3.7 days
Fluphenazine decanoate (Prolixin, Decanoate)	Adult: LD: 12.5–25 mg/2 weeks M: 25–50 mg/2 weeks	IM	O: 24–72 hr P: 48–96 hr D: 4 wk PB: UA B: UA E: 6.8–9.6 days
Perphenazine (Trilafon)	Adult: LD: 32–96 mg/day M: 6–48 mg/day Ped: UA	PO IM	O: UA P: UA D: UA PB: UA B: UA E: UA
Prochlorperazine (Compazine) Prochlorperazine edisylate (Compazine) Prochlorperazine maleate (Compazine)	Adult: LD: 50–150 mg/day M: 20–100 mg/day Ped: UA	IM Rectal PO	PO, O: 30–40 min O: (ext. release) 30–40 min O: (rectal) 60 min D: 3–4 hr PB: UA B: UA E: UA
Butaperazine (Repoise)	Adult: LD: 30–50 mg/day M: 30–100 mg/day Ped: UA	PO	O: UA P: UA D: UA PB: UA B: UA E: UA
Carphenazine (Proketazine)	Adult: LD: 400 mg/day M: 25–150 mg/day Ped: UA	PO	O: UA P: UA D: UA PB: UA B: UA E: UA
Thioxanthenes Chlorprothixene (Taractan)	Adult: M: 10–1000 mg/day	IM	O: 15–30 min P: UA

Key to Abbreviations in the *Pharmacokinetics* column: LD-loading dose; M-maintenance; O-onset; P-peak; D-duration; PB-protein bound; B-biotransformation; E-excretion; ½L-half-life. Ped-pediatric dose; UA-unavailable
*Within the column listing adverse effects, underlines indicate the most common effects.

Contraindications and Precautions	Adverse Effects*	Interactions	Nursing Implications
			observe for the possibility of secondary anxiety reactions. Evaluate for early symptoms of extrapyramidal reactions and collaborate early with physician to begin treatment as soon as possible. Patients must learn to evaluate how they react to the drug prior to driving.

CONTINUED ON THE FOLLOWING PAGE

Table 25–2. ANTIPSYCHOTIC MEDICATIONS–*CONTINUED*

Name	Dosage	Mode of Administration	Pharmacokinetics
Thioxanthenes–Continued	M: 200–100 mg/day Ped 6–12 yrs: 10–12 mg qid		PB: UA B: UA E: UA
Thiothixene (Navane)	Adult: LD: 20–100 mg/day M: 5–40 mg/day Ped: UA	IM	O: UA P: 1–3 hr D: 34 hr ½L: UA PB: UA B: UA E: UA
Butyrophenones Haloperidol (Haldol)	Adult: LD: 20–100 mg/day M: 5–40 mg/day Ped: 3–12 yr, 0.5 mg/day orally increased by 0.5 mg at intervals to a max. of 6 mg/day	IM IV PO	O: UA P: 2–6 hr D: 72 hr ½L: 12–16 hr PB: AAG 80–90% (FF 0.1–0.2) B: UA E: UA
Dihydroindolones Molindone (Moban)	Adult: LD: 50–400 mg/day M: 25–100 mg/day Ped: UA	PO IV	O: 30 min P: 30 min D: 20 hr ½L: 1.5 hr PB: UA B: UA E: UA
Dibenzoxazepines Loxapine hydrochloride (Lox-itane C) Loxapine succinate (Loxi-tane)	Adult: LD: 50–250 mg/day M: 25–100 mg/day Ped: UA	PO IV IM	O: 20–30 min P: 1½–3 hr D: 12 hr ½L: α = 5 hr, β = 19 hr PB: UA B: UA E: UA

Key to Abbreviations in the *Pharmacokinetics* column: LD-loading dose; M-maintenance; O-onset; P-peak; D-duration; PB-protein bound; B-biotransformation; E-excretion; ½L-half-life; UA-unavailable.
*Within the column listing adverse effects, underlines indicate the most common effects.

pressed through the central nervous system. Cholinergic sites blocked within the brain are likely to produce a halting or stuttering pattern of speech, impaired memory, confusion and in some cases, a toxic delirium. Approximately one third of all people who receive neuroleptic medications experience extrapyramidal symptoms. These symptoms develop as a result of the effects of the drug on the extrapyramidal tracts of the central nervous system. These tracts maintain and control involuntary movements.

Extrapyramidal symptoms can at times be mistaken for clinical psychiatric symptoms. *Hypokinesia* resembles psychomotor retardation in the depressed patient, parkinsonian rigidity resembles catatonia, and akathisia may be confused with psychotic agitation or anxiety. These symptoms are treated by reducing the amount of antipsychotic medication and through short-term use of anticholinergic antiparkinsonian agents such as benztropine or trihexyphenidyl hydrochloride.

The syndrome of *tardive dyskinesia* is not an extrapyramidal reaction per se, as it is caused by a different mechanism. The longer a patient takes antipsychotic medications the greater the possibility this syndrome will occur. It is more frequent among older patients occuring with an incidence of 10% to 20% among chronically hospitalized populations. Tardive dyskinesia is a potential risk of long-term use of antipsychotic drugs. The same mechanism thought to be responsible for the beneficial effects of the drugs, i.e., dopamine receptor site blockade, is thought to be linked to the onset of tardive dyskinesia. This may also explain why tardive dyskinesia is positively correlated with higher doses of medication rather than with lower moderate doses. It is

Contraindications and Precautions	Adverse Effects*	Interactions	Nursing Implications
Same as above.	Same as above.	Same as above.	Same as above.
Contraindicated in Parkinson's disease, seizure disorders, coma, alcoholism, CNS depression, pregnancy, lactation, and children under 3 years.	Same as above.	Same as above.	Same as above.
Same as phenothiazines.	Same as above.	Same as above.	Same as above.
Same as phenothiazines.	Same as above.	Same as above.	Same as above.

believed that none of the neuroleptics are free of the potential to be associated with this side effect.

The clinical signs of tardive dyskinesia include abnormal movements of the mouth, chewing motions, tongue thrusts and sucking, and pursing and blowing movement of the lips. The movements are involuntary and rhythmic. Often, patients with tardive dyskinesia salivate and drool excessively. These symptoms may be very embarrassing to patients and family members and may be associated with isolative behavior on the part of patients, or with the tendency to discontinue medication therapy. Patient teaching is a significant nursing intervention at this time and focuses on the relative benefits of relief from psychotic symptoms that allows the patient a more functional lifestyle versus the admittedly distressing but less impairing consequences of an abnormal movement disorder. It is also true that abrupt withdrawal of antipsychotic medications can precipitate a whole host of unpleasant side effects including withdrawal dyskinesia, which is symptomatically indistinguishable from tardive dyskinesia.

Other general classes of side effects of the neuroleptic medications include the following:

1. Sedation
2. Anticholinergic and cardiovascular effects
3. Allergic reactions
4. Skin symptoms
5. Eye symptoms
6. Endocrine symptoms
7. Psychiatric symptoms
8. Thermoregulation problems

All of the neuroleptic agents may produce any of these side effects. However, specific drugs have a greater tendency to produce specific side effects. Therefore, if a side effect develops, the physician may change the neuroleptic agent being used in order to decrease

Table 25–3. ANTIPSYCHOTICS SHOULD BE USED WITH CAUTION WHEN THE FOLLOWING MEDICAL CONDITIONS EXIST

- Bone marrow depression (could mask or exacerbate drug-induced agranulocytosis)
- Cardiovascular disease (complicated by cardiovascular effects of antipsychotics)
- Myocardial infarction
- Alcoholism
- Hepatic function impairment (could mask or exacerbate hepatic hypersensitivity to drug)
- Hypoparathyroidism (may mask endocrine effects of drugs)
- Parkinson's disease (symptoms worsened by neuroleptics)
- Glaucoma (because anticholinergic drug effects are likely to exacerbate the symptoms of this disorder)
- Gastrointestinal disturbances (as drug's antiemetic effect may mask symptoms)
- Peptic ulcer (same as glaucoma)
- Prostatic hypertrophy (same as glaucoma)
- Urinary retention (same as glaucoma)
- Respiratory problems (especially in children; some of these products contain the dye tartrazine, which may cause allergic reactions in sensitive patients)
- Reye's syndrome (because antiemetic and extrapyramidal effects may obscure the diagnosis of Reye's syndrome)

that effect. Generally speaking, aliphatics and piperidines cause fewer extrapyramidal effects and more of the above effects than do the piperazines, haloperidol, and newer agents.

Aside from the extrapyramidal reactions, other CNS side effects are caused by the neuroleptic agents. The most common one is sedation. It results especially with the use of chlorpromazine and thioridazine (Mellaril).

All neuroleptic drugs lower seizure thresholds. Patients with seizure disorders may require higher doses of prophylactic anticonvulsant medication. This side effect rarely tends to cause seizures. However, when seizures do occur, they tend to be correlated with high doses and rapid increases in dosages. The neuroleptic medications should not be used with patients being detoxified from the effects of alcohol and other medications because they tend to precipitate tonic-clonic seizures.

Anticholinergic effects, due to muscarinic receptor blockade such as blurred vision, dry mouth, constipation, and difficulty starting urination, are especially bothersome early in therapy, particularly with aliphatics and piperidines. Since some tolerance to these effects develops, it is often prescribed to start the causative drugs at a relatively low dosage and increase the dosage gradually.

Cardiovascular side effects, such as orthostatic hypotension and tachycardia, may also occur due to α-receptor blockade. A less common cardiovascular side effect includes mild changes in the electrocardiograms, which are related to altered repolarization and do not correlate with cardiac damage. ECG changes associated with therapeutic doses are increased QT duration, lowered ST segments, flattened or bimodal T waves, and infrequently U-wave production. U-wave and T-wave changes are reversible with the administration of potassium salts. Patients with cardiac problems who require

Table 25–4. UNWANTED PHARMACOLOGIC EFFECTS OF ANTIPSYCHOTIC DRUGS

Type	Manifestation	Mechanism
Adverse behavioral effects	Excitement, akinesia Supersensitivity psychosis Toxic-confusional state	Dopamine receptor blockade Denervation supersensitivity from block of dopamine receptors Block of muscarinic cholinergic receptors
Neurologic	Parkinson syndrome, akathisia, dystonias Tardive dyskinesia	Dopamine receptor blockade
Autonomic nervous system	Blurred vision, dry mouth, urinary hesitancy, constipation Orthostatic hypotension impotence, failure to ejaculate	Block of muscarinic cholinergic receptors α-adrenoreceptor blockade
Metabolic–endocrine	Amenorrhea–galactorrhea, infertility, impotence	Dopamine receptor block in tuberoinfundibular tract
Other	Heat stroke, malignant neuroleptic syndrome Cardiac toxicity	Loss of central control of body temperature Quinidine-like actions on membranes

From Hollister, LE: Clinical Pharmacology of Psychotherapeutic Drugs, ed 2. New York, Churchill Livingstone, 1983, p. 153, with permission.

neuroleptic medication should receive a drug with a low incidence of anticholinergic effect, such as haloperidol or one of the piperazine phenothiazines.

Some reactions may occur that stimulate specific allergic or toxic effects. Systemic dermatosis, usually a maculopapular rash on the face, neck, chest, arms, and legs, tends to develop two to eight weeks after the initial dose. If mild, the rash clears without any specific treatments. If the rash is severe, the specific neuroleptic agent is discontinued and another used. Two rare but extremely serious allergic syndromes are agranulocytosis and cholestatic jaundice.

Other side effects affecting the skin may also develop. Increased photosensitivity creates the most severe problems. The patient may develop a severe sunburn after only brief exposure to the sun. Because of increased photosensitivity, patient teaching about skin protection and decreased exposure is important.

A skin/eye syndrome may also occur, but rarely. The colored areas of the skin that are exposed to sunlight turn a golden brown. Eventually, the skin becomes slate gray, metallic blue, or purple. The color change is caused by the drug reacting within the body to create melanin-like granules that are deposited within the skin tissues. Melanin-like granules also build up in the conjunctiva, sclera, lens, and cornea; eyesight is not affected. If the material builds up sufficiently to be observable within the cornea and lens, it may be only slowly and partially reversed.

A more serious side effect that may cause blindness (pigmentary retinopathy) occurs with the use of thioridazine in daily doses of 800 mg or more. The patient first notices a brownish coloration to the vision. Eventually, vision becomes less and less acute. Controversy exists as to whether or not this side effect is reversible. In order to prevent the development of pigmentary retinopathy, the recommended maximum daily dose of thioridazine should not exceed 800 mg.

Endocrine system side effects may also develop.

Women may experience amenorrhea. When this occurs, the woman may believe she is pregnant. Compounding this belief is that false-positive pregnancy test results are caused by antipsychotic drugs. The woman may also develop galactorrhea related to dopamine effects on prolactin. One of the hypothalamic hormones that regulates prolactin secretion is called prolactin inhibiting factor (PIF). Some investigators believe dopamine is the PIF while others suggest that dopamine is a secondary regulator. In either case, phenothiazines induce secretion of prolactin from the anterior pituitary by inhibiting dopamine receptors in the pituitary and hypothalamus. It is therefore common to find elevated prolactin levels during long-term administration of antipsychotic drugs. Elevated prolactin levels may stimulate the development of galactorrhea. If this problem causes much discomfort, the drug is discontinued and another neuroleptic substituted.

In pregnant women the antipsychotics cross the placental barrier. The drugs do not appear to cause congenital malformations, but infants born to mothers taking the drug in their last trimester may exhibit jaundice and extrapyramidal and anticholinergic side effects at birth. It has also been shown that some drugs, such as haloperidol, are excreted in human milk and may necessitate bottle feedings versus breast feeding.

Men may experience ejaculation difficulties and *gynecomastia*. These two side effects are prominent when thioridazine is the drug of choice. Both males and females may experience a decreased libido as a result of neuroleptic use. Decreased libido may be distressing to both the client and the significant other. Patient and couple teaching is indicated to reduce the potential negative consequences of this side effect.

Manifestations of psychiatric states may also occur as side effects. To distinguish a side effect from a primary symptom requires careful assessment and documentation (Table 25–5). An atropine-like psychosis may develop. Rarely, patients using neuroleptics demonstrate

Table 25–5. POINTS TO ASSESS PRIOR TO INITIAL DOSE OF ANTIPSYCHOTIC TO DIFFERENTIATE RESPONSES RELATED TO HEALTH PROBLEMS VERSUS SIDE EFFECTS OF THE MEDICATION

Signs and Symptoms Demonstrated by the Patient	Point of Initial Observation of the Sign or Symptom	
	Prior to First Dose (Complete on Observation)	*After First Dose* (Complete on Observation)
Restlessness Dizziness Headaches Hyperactivity Dry mouth Gastrointestional distress Constipation Tremors Dermatitis Visual disturbances Hypotension Gait difficulties		

symptoms of depression. Usually, when this occurs, it is a manifestation of akinesia. Therefore, the members of the health team should consider that this may be happening and treat it accordingly.

The phenomenon of secondary anxiety reaction may also be demonstrated. This reaction is manifested by a rise in the patient's level of anxiety after a dose of a neuroleptic, instead of a decrease as anticipated. This may be a form of akathisia.

The neuroleptic agents are not addicting. However, sometimes patients may experience gastrointestinal symptoms such as nausea, vomiting, and/or diarrhea when a drug is withdrawn. Such symptoms usually occur when the person has been receiving high doses of phenothiazines that are discontinued suddenly. Controversy exists regarding the cause of this phenomenon. Withdrawal symptoms may be due to cholinergic rebound.

Phenothiazines cause thermoregulation problems (*poikilothermia*), which are of particular concern in the elderly. Hypothermia or hyperthermia may be induced by environmental temperature deviations from normal room temperature. A very rare, but potentially fatal, syndrome called *neuroleptic malignant syndrome (NMS)* can occur with the use of antipsychotics. The syndrome is characterized by muscle rigidity, hyperthermia with temperatures that may be as high as 41°C, alterations in consciousness to the point of coma, and autonomic dysfunction. Patients developing NMS exhibit tachycardia, elevated blood pressure, diaphoresis, dysphagia (difficulty swallowing), dyspnea, and incontinence. There is no definitive laboratory test to indicate the onset of NMS, but leukocytosis ranging from 15,000 to 30,000 has been reported, and CPK elevations as high as 15,000 units have been observed.

The syndrome is idiosyncratic and may appear in one patient with a first trial of an antipsychotic, whereas it may manifest in another patient only years after uneventful medication therapy. The incidence of NMS is unclear, there have been only small numbers of cases reported in the literature, and the difficulty of diagnosis makes accurate demographics difficult to obtain. One study suggests an incidence of 0.5%–1.0% with an overall mortality rate of 20%, 14% among those taking oral neuroleptics, and 38% among those receiving fluphenazine decanoate. Nursing can contribute greatly to a positive outcome in that early recognition and intervention increases the likelihood of recovery, and symptoms can occur at any time with rapid onset. Therefore, keen nursing assessment and interventions can make a critical contribution to the team effort to successfully treat the patient with NMS.

Another rare, dramatic, and potentially life-threatening extrapyramidal side effect is called *oculogyric crisis.* This side effect is demonstrated by hyperextension of the neck and rotation and fixation of the eyeballs in an upward (ceilingward) position. The experience of loss of voluntary muscle control of the eye is particularly frightening to the patient and presents a bizarre appearance to the observer. Rapid and appropriate intervention is necessary to prevent significant trauma. With counteractive medications the crisis is completely reversible without permanent damage.

It is hypothesized that the antipsychotic agents may decrease the growth rate in children by inhibiting the release of growth hormones. Therefore, the use of these drugs in children must be undertaken only with careful consideration and ongoing evaluation of growth.

Patients over 60 years of age appear to experience a greater incidence of side effects. Part of the explanation for this increase is that the half-life of antipsychotic drugs is prolonged in the elderly when compared to younger patients. Thus, the same dose administered to an elderly patient results in higher plasma concentrations, which leads to more pronounced clinical effects. In addition, the elderly may be inherently more sensitive to the anticholinergic effects of these drugs; therefore, accurate assessment and close monitoring are significant nursing contributions to the care of these patients. Elderly patients, and those with organic brain syndromes, are highly susceptible to "pseudo-psychotic" symptoms from central effects of excessive anticholinergic drug action yet, paradoxically, the more strongly anticholinergic drugs produce lower incidences of acute extrapyramidal effects. Obviously, clinical judgment will dictate the physician's pharmacologic course, and nurses must be aware, and vigilant for the potential consequences, of either option.

INTERACTIONS

The antipsychotic medications interact with a number of other drugs, potentiating the action of some and inhibiting the action of others. Peripheral symptoms and CNS symptoms are increased when antipsychotics are combined with other medications having anticholinergic activity. Some agents that may precipitate or intensify side effects when combined with antipyschotics include antimuscarinic antiparkinson agents such as benztropine mesylate (Cogentin), antihistamines such as diphenhydramine hydrochloride (Benadryl and others), atropine sulfate, narcotic analgesics such as meperidine hydrochloride (Demerol hydrochloride), and tricyclic antidepressants such as amitriptyline hydrochloride (Amitril, Elavil, and others). For interactions that can occur with these drugs, see Table 25–6.

DOSAGE REGIMEN CONSIDERATIONS

The desired outcome of pharmacotherapy is to maximize benefit and minimize risk. Since individuals respond differently to different medications, the balance point in terms of dosage, and even types of medications, may be quite different among a group of patients. Typically, a dose of medication is prescribed by the patient's physician, a therapeutic effect is realized over time, and the antipsychotic is gradually reduced until eventually the person is on a stable dosage, usually equivalent to ½–⅛ of the loading amount. If the medication does not achieve the desired effect, another in the group may be prescribed. Patients sometimes perceive this process as

**Table 25–6. DRUGS THAT
INTERACT WITH
ANTIPSYCHOTICS**

Medication	Type of Interaction
Alcohol	Potentiates and prolongs the effects of the neuroleptics and vice versa.
Amphetamines	Neuroleptics decrease the effects of the amphetamines.
Antacids or anti-diarrheal suspensions	Concurrent administration blocks the absorption of the neuroleptics.
Anticonvulsants	Neuroleptics decrease the seizure threshold; therefore, the dosage of anticonvulsants may have to be increased.
Antimuscarinics, especially atropine	Effects of these drugs are potentiated with concurrent use; these drugs may reduce the plasma levels of neuroleptics.
Antiparkinson drugs	Anticholinergic effects of these drugs may be potentiated.
Levodopa	Antiparkinsonian effects are inhibited with concurrent use.
Epinephrine	Neuroleptics may block the α-adrenergic effects of this drug, producing severe hypotension.
Guanethidine and related drugs	Neuroleptics block the antihypertensive effects of these drugs.
Central nervous system depressants	Potentiate and prolong the effects of these drugs; concurrent use with some drugs (e.g., meperidine) may produce severe respiratory depression.
Monoamine oxidase inhibitors and tricyclics	Concurrent use prolongs and potentiates the sedative effects of these drugs; potentiation of the anticholinergic effect also occurs.
Diuretics α-blocking Antihypertensives (Prazocin) and α- and β-blockers (Lubetolol)	Volume depletion produces orthostasis. α Blockade produces orthostasis.

haphazard and may express negative thoughts about medication therapy, which may predict noncompliance when the patient is in an outpatient setting. While acknowledging the inexact nature of predicting response to medication, the nurse can, with some confidence, use this opportunity to assess the patient's knowledge level. The nurse can also provide information that can reduce fears, reassure the patient of anticipated positive outcomes, and support the development of a spirit of mutual cooperation.

Divided doses are used when symptoms permit and when the patient is elderly to maximize tissue saturation and to minimize initially bothersome side effects. As soon as therapeutic response can be noted, a gradual downward dosage titration is to be prescribed to the point of lowest effective maintenance dose, which can then be prescribed once a day. Nursing observations and documentation are essential to the clinical evaluation of patient response. Liquid concentrate forms of antipsychotic drugs may be prescribed in the event that the patient experiences difficulty in swallowing or is resistant to taking medications in other forms. One may negotiate the use of a preferred route of administration with many patients, and it is important to note that coercion to take medications by threat or use of physical force in the absence of an emergency situation constitutes grounds for valid charges of battery and/or assault.

Liquid concentrate forms of the medications may be ordered for patients who have been observed "cheeking" medication in order to hoard or discard it later out of view of the nurse. Concentrate forms of the antipsychotic drugs are reported as unpleasant in taste and irritating to the gastric mucosa. For these reasons the drug is mixed with fruit juices. Orange and apple juices are frequently used, whereas pineapple juice is avoided because of its potentiation of gastric irritation. Two ounces of juice in an initial dilution, quickly followed by four or more ounces of plain juice helps to make the preparation more palatable and to dilute the drug for easier absorption. Liquid concentrates are light sensitive and should be kept in amber or opaque bottles and given immediately after diluted.

The intramuscular route of administration results in the most rapid calming effect of the antipsychotic drugs. When given in injectable form, response can be noted within as short a time as ten minutes. Thus, the intramuscular route is frequently the route of choice when antipsychotics are administered to de-escalate an emergency situation.

The injectable forms of the antipsychotics tend to irritate the subcutaneous tissues. To decrease this effect, changing the needle after filling the syringe is recommended. After selecting the appropriate site, the nurse should introduce the medicine deeply into the muscle. The injection should be administered slowly, and the site gently massaged following the injection to help promote absorption. When complete absorption has not occurred, the tissue around the site may remain hard to the touch. If such is the case when another injection is to be given, an alternate site should be selected. The in-

Table 25–7. COMPARISON OF ANTIPSYCHOTIC AGENTS' ACTIONS

| CLASSIFICATION AND GENERIC NAME | TRADE NAME | Actions | | | | | | Dosage Ranges* | |
		EPS	SEDA-TION	ANTI-CHOLIN-ERGIC	HYPO-TENSION	ANTI-EMETIC	TRADITIONAL EQUIVA-LENCE	ACUTE DOSE (MG/DAY)	MAINTENANCE DOSE (MG/DAY, PO)
Phenothiazines									
Aliphatics:									
Chlorpromazine	Thorazine	++	+++	+++	+++	Strong	100	400–1500†	200–1000
Promazine	Sparine	++	+++	+++	+++	Moderate	100	400–800	200–800
Triflupromazine	Vesprin	++	++	+++	++	Strong	NA	60–400	30–200
Piperidines:									
Thioridazine	Mellaril	+	+++	+++	+++	Weak	100	400–800	25–200–800
Mesoridazine	Serentil	+	+++	++	++	Weak	NA	20–600	10–400
Piperacetazine	Quide	++	++	+	++	Moderate	NA	50–100	15–30
Piperazines:									
Perphenazine	Trilafon	+++	+	++	+	Weak	10	32–96	6–16–48
Trifluoperazine	Stelazine	+++	+	+	+	Weak	5	20–100	10–40
Fluphenazine	Prolixin	++++	+	+	+	Weak	2	20–80	5–40
Acetophenazine	Tindal	++	++	+	+	Weak	NA	400–600	60–120
Carphenazine	Proketazine	+++	++	+	+	Weak	NA	400	25–150
Prochlorperazine	Compazine	+++	++	+	+	Strong	NA	50–150	20–100
Nonphenothiazines									
Thioxanthines									
Thiothixine	Navane						0	4	20–100†	5–40
Chlorprothixine	Taractan						0			10–100
Butyrophenones									
Haloperidol	Haldol	++++	+	+	+	0	2	20–100	5–40
Dibenzoxazepines									
Loxapine	Loxitane	+++	++	+	++	0	10	50–250†	25–100
Dihydroindolones									
Molindone	Moban, Lidone	+++	+	+	+	0		50–400	25–100

++++ = very frequent/strong
+++ = high incidence
++ = moderate incidence
+ = low incidence
* Children, adolescents, and the elderly require smaller doses. Dosages for these age groups are not established.
† = Dosage can be exceeded with caution.

jectable forms of antipsychotics are often incompatible with other injectable drugs, so if two or more medications are being given, they should be administered in separate injections, drawn up in separate syringes.

There are presently two forms of injectable antipsychotics in use, shorter-acting types (such as chlorpromazine, haloperidol, or fluphenazine hydrochloride) and long-acting types (such as fluphenazine decanoate, also known as Prolixin decanoate). The long-acting drugs use an oil-based preparation and are slowly absorbed over a two to four-week period. This means the patient receives one injection and can experience effects of the medication for a prolonged period of time with injections commonly given at intervals of every two to three weeks. Fluphenazine enanthate preceded deconoate, but is less often used because of a higher incidence of extrapyramidal side effects and a shorter drug life.

PHENOTHIAZINES

The phenothiazine class of antipsychotic medications contains the largest number of drugs. This class is further divided into three types of phenothiazines. These include the aliphatics, piperidines, and piperazines. Table 25–7 lists the specific agents in each category, compares their actions, and states dosage ranges.

Aliphatic Phenothiazines

The aliphatics often produce strong sedative effects and moderate-to-strong extrapyramidal effects. The prototype of antipsychotic medications, these drugs are particularly effective in the control of psychotic symptoms including hallucinations and delusions.

CHLORPROMAZINE. Chlorpromazine (Thorazine), classified as an aliphatic phenothiazine, was the first antipsychotic drug to be discovered, and its use is still widespread. This drug is the model for all other antipsychotic agents. It has a potent sedative effect and therefore is effectively used to calm extremely agitated patients. Depending on the patient's state, it may be administered orally or intramuscularly.

TRIFLUPROMAZINE AND PROMAZINE. Two other aliphatics are triflupromazine (Vesprin) and promazine (Sparine). Both are less frequently used antipsychotics.

Piperidine Phenothiazines

This group of medications typically has moderate to strong anticholinergic effects and strong sedative effects. The piperidines produce minimal extrapyramidal effects. The drugs in this group are sometimes used for short-term treatment of major depression, sleep disturbances, and severe behavioral problems in children.

THIORIDAZINE. Thioridazine (Mellaril) has a relatively strong sedating effect with minimal extrapyramidal and strong anticholinergic effects. Elderly patients appear to tolerate low doses of this drug well.

MESORIDAZINE. Mesoridazine (Serentil), which is a major metabolite of thioridazine, and piperacetazine (Quide) also possess sedating effects with strong anticholinergic effects and weak extrapyramidal effects. Neither is frequently used in psychosis.

Piperazine Phenothiazines

The piperazine group of phenothiazines contains the largest number of drugs in current use. These drugs have a less sedating effect on patients. They appear to be effective, especially for those experiencing depressive-type symptoms as part of their overall psychoses, and are particularly effective in treating withdrawn, apathetic patients.

Thioxanthines

The thioxanthines are another class of antipsychotics. Drugs in this group often have weak anticholinergic, hypotensive, and sedative properties. The thioxanthines are sometimes effective in treating long-term chronic schizophrenic patients who have not responded to other drugs. Chlorprothixene (Taractan), and the more frequently used thiothixene, Navane, are members of this group. None of these drugs has the advantage of being available in both oral and injectable forms.

OTHER ANTIPSYCHOTIC DRUGS

Haloperidol (Haldol), classified as a butyrophenone, has very strong extrapyramidal effects and weak anticholinergic effects. It is widely used in all age groups and is available in a variety of dosage forms. Haloperidol decanoate, a long-acting depot form for intramuscular use, requires dosing only once a month. This drug is also popularly used for its sedative effect.

Molindone (Moban) is one of the two marketed members of the dihydroindolone drug class. It has a possible advantage of causing less weight gain during long-term use, a disturbing side effect of most neuroleptics.

Loxapine is a relatively new dihydroindolone antipsychotic with effects comparable to those of haloperidol. It produces a metabolite, amoxapine, which is marketed separately as an antidepressant. Thus, loxapine is sometimes promoted as useful for patients who have both psychosis and features of depressive illness.

Clozapine, a highly anticholinergic antipsychotic was approved for widespread use in early 1990. It is used for the management of severely ill schizophrenic patients who have not responded to traditional treatment approaches. Research indicates that approximately one third of such patients have a positive response to this new drug.

Clozapine causes hyperthermia in a large proportion of patients but has an extremely low incidence of extrapyramidal side effects. Studies also show that 1–2% of patients taking clozapine may develop agranulocytosis, a potentially fatal blood disorder. For this reason the drug is only prescribed under a protocol which requires indefinite weekly blood tests. This raises the cost of treatment to approximately $10,000/year, but still may prove cost effective when compared with costs of in-patient treatment which may be avoided or reduced.

SELECTION OF ANTIPSYCHOTIC AGENTS

The differences among the various drugs within the classifications of the antipsychotic agents are difficult to determine. Therefore, the choice of which antipsychotic agent the physician uses to treat the specific patient requires a high level of medical expertise. Patient response to antipsychotics is variable, and patients who do not respond to one drug may be successfully treated with a different agent. Some of the factors the physician uses as a basis for choosing a specific drug include:

1. The patient's age
2. The type of symptoms the person is experiencing
3. Whether or not a drug with a strong sedating effect is desired
4. The patient's response to previous treatment with antipsychotics
5. The response to treatment with antipsychotic agents previously demonstrated by family members
6. The anticipated level of compliance
7. The presence of other medical conditions

USING THE NURSING PROCESS

ASSESSMENT

Assessment of the person requiring treatment with an antipsychotic medication begins with a nursing history, which establishes the data base. Frequently, the patient's high level of anxiety and behaviors limit his or her abilities to participate in this process. Therefore, the nurse contacts a significant other, obtains past records, and consults with other professionals who have worked with the patient. The nurse also assesses the patient to determine the presence of symptoms of psychotic reactions. The person may be experiencing some or all of the following symptoms: The person may demonstrate thought disorders such as delusions with ideas of reference, that is, thoughts that others are making statements about the patient. Problems such as hallucinations and other symptoms such as blunted or flat affect and mood swings are sometimes evident. The person may demonstrate sleep disturbances and a decreased fluid and food intake. Frequently, these are related to feelings of suspiciousness or paranoia that someone plans harm to the patient. Withdrawal from activities and difficulties in interpersonal relationships often occur. Unpredictable behaviors related to agitation and restlessness may lead to fear which could precede assaultive behaviors.

As the nurse gathers information related to the patient, the following factors must be considered:

1. How long has the person been experiencing these feelings and symptoms?

2. How do the symptoms and feelings affect the person's ability to manage activities of daily living?
3. Has the person previously experienced similar episodes?
4. If so, how long did they last?
5. What did the patient do then to cope with the feelings and behaviors?
6. What were the outcomes?
7. Have the person or any other family members ever been treated with antipsychotic medications? If so, which ones? What type of response to the drug did they demonstrate? What problems relevant to the drug developed?

The nurse also attempts to investigate the expectations for treatment that the patient and family members have already established. Family members may demonstrate exhaustion from trying to cope with the patient's behavior and with being frightened by threats and accusations. Therefore, their desire for treatment may be to hospitalize the person for a long time. If the patient has had repeated episodes of these behaviors or psychotic states or both, these feelings are intensified for the family members. The nurse assesses the family members' feelings of helplessness, hopelessness, and despair, and encourages them to seek counseling.

When patients are experiencing the panic level of anxiety or symptoms of a psychotic reaction, they may become very agitated. Therefore, there is the potential that the patient may lose control to the point of aggressive behavior. Usually, this results from the patient's feeling frightened, suspicious, and threatened. When such symptoms are observed in a patient, it is imperative that he or she become a focus for immediate nursing intervention.

Patients may refuse to take antipsychotics because they fear becoming addicted to the drugs. Many people base their beliefs on an assumption that "tranquilizers are addictive." Antipsychotics are not physiologically addictive. Therefore, the nurse needs to assess the patient's feelings and beliefs and correct misinformation that may form the basis of the patient's decision.

Prior to the administration of the initial dose, the patient's state of emotional and physical health must be thoroughly assessed. At this time, the nurse formulates a list of symptoms the patient is exhibiting. Then, after the patient has started on the medication regimen and begins to demonstrate a given symptom, the nurse and physician compare his or her current state with the prior list. This helps to identify whether or not the problem is specifically drug induced. Table 25–8 demonstrates the integration of the nursing process.

NURSING DIAGNOSES

When the nursing assessment is completed, the nurse formulates nursing diagnoses, which focus on identification of client-centered problems amenable to nursing intervention. Some typical nursing diagnoses are featured in Table 25–8.

PLANNING AND INTERVENTION

The goals of nursing intervention for the patient being treated with an antipsychotic medication include reducing the target symptoms, decreasing the level of anxiety and agitation, maintaining patient control of personal behavior, and educating the patient about the diagnoses and the treatment regimen and about potential adverse effects as the nurse, patient, and selected others are involved in developing the plan of care. When the patient is able to participate, his or her personal care goals should be central to the planning process.

NURSING RESPONSIBILITIES WHEN ADMINISTERING ANTIPSYCHOTICS

It is imperative for the nurse to recognize early that a patient's level of anxiety is rising. The nurse aims to intervene early in order to help return the patient to a tolerable level of comfort and thus maintain self-control. If the patient is highly agitated, an intramuscular injection or oral concentrate, as ordered by the physician, is used. The nurse remembers that the patient is extremely frightened, fearing loss of control. When the patient tells the nurse he or she feels this way, the nurse recognizes that this is a plea for immediate help. When the nurse administers the drug, a kind, firm, positive approach is used. The nurse limits phrases to as few words as possible since the patient's attention span is compromised by increased anxiety. The nurse avoids asking the patient to make decisions at this point, and postpones this until further assessment indicates that the level of anxiety is decreased. The nurse also determines whether talking with the patient increases or decreases the level of anxiety; typically, the person in this state will not want to be alone, yet does not wish to talk. The nurse empathizes with the patient regarding how frightening the situation and feelings might be. However, the nurse also avoids giving the impression of being able to read the person's mind. Thirty and 60 minutes after the injection, the nurse evaluates the need for further medication treatment and records observations.

PATIENT TEACHING

After a person has been receiving an antipsychotic drug for a period of time, two situations may arise that require anticipatory teaching on the part of the nurse. The first results from the major disadvantage of the antipsychotic medications, the wide range of side effects. Patients initially become upset with the sedation and extrapyramidal symptoms that may be experienced. These side effects frequently influence the patient to stop taking the medicine as prescribed.

The second situation develops as the person leaves the treatment facility, begins to feel well, and decides that he or she does not need the medicine or counseling sessions or both any more. This creates the "merry-go-round" syndrome, as highlighted in Figure 25–2. Most psychotic reactions recur unless the person follows a

Table 25–8. NURSING PROCESS FOR PATIENTS REQUIRING ANTIPSYCHOTIC MEDICATIONS

Assessment

Assess baseline data, e.g., TPR, BP (sitting and standing); liver function tests, opthalmoscopic exams, CBC and ECG.
Note prior responses to prescribed medications.
Determine presence of delusions, hallucinations, sleep disturbances, paranoia.
Assess affect, mood swings, unpredictable behaviors (withdrawal, aggression, agitation and restlessness) and note how these affect patient's life.
Ascertain presence of preexisting physical conditions, e.g., pregnancy/lactation, hepatic and cardiovascular disorders.

Nursing Diagnosis	Nursing Actions	Rationale	Desired Outcomes/ Evaluation Criteria
Knowledge deficit related to lack of information/ misinterpretation, cognitive limitation as evidenced by inaccurate statements, questions, refusal of medication.	Discuss reasons for taking prescribed medication, e.g., reduction of target symptoms, decreased level of anxiety/agitation, maintaining control of behavior. Review expectations of drug administration, e.g., therapeutic response may not occur for three weeks, drugs are not addicting. Caution against sudden changes in position, unprotected exposure to sunlight. Identify adverse symptoms which need to be reported to health care giver. Distinguish between significant toxic effects (e.g., onset of extrapyramidal side effects) and uncomfortable but benign side effects, (e.g., dry mouth, oral lesions). Emphasize that unprescribed medications/OTC drugs, especially antacids, should not be taken with antipsychotic drugs. Active-listen to patient feelings and concerns. Encourage continuation of antipsychotic medication as prescribed.	Understanding why medication is needed helps patient to participate with treatment. Knowing what to expect helps the patient to feel in control and may enhance participation in medication regimen. Orthostatic hypotension may occur with these drugs. Sensitivity to the sun may result in severe sunburn. Provides for timely evaluation and intervention to adjust drug regimen/prevent serious complications. Untoward interactions may interfere with absorption and desired effect of drug. Clarifies patient/ family expectations and promotes sense of control of own treatment. May be needed to control symptoms on a long-term basis.	Displays decrease in primary symptoms. Correctly explains reasons for medication/treatment regimen. Takes medications as prescribed.
Violence, potential for directed at self or others related to psychotic excitement (catatonic, manic, panic states) with indicators of	Promote quiet environment.	Decreases stimulation and allows for use of least restrictive means of assuring patient safety.	Demonstrates self-control, as evidenced by relaxed posture, absence of violent behavior.

CONTINUED ON THE FOLLOWING PAGE

Table 25–8. NURSING PROCESS FOR PATIENTS REQUIRING ANTIPYSCHOTIC MEDICATIONS—*Continued*

Nursing Diagnosis	Nursing Actions	Rationale	Desired Outcomes/ Evaluation Criteria
expressed intent/desire to harm self/others, hostile threats, overt aggressive acts, increasing anxiety/level of activity.	Use a kind, positive, firm approach. Tell the patient that the staff will protect him or her and will not allow the patient to hurt themselves or others.	Helps to reduce fear and feelings of threat to self patient is experiencing.	
	Have two or more staff members present. Use "show of force", quiet room, seclusion or restraints judiciously.	Communicates ability to maintain control over an escalating situation and reduces patient's fear of loss of control.	
	Administer medication, IM, as prescribed.	May be needed to help patient to regain/maintain control.	
Injury, potential for related to side effects of prescribed pharmaceutical agents (e.g., antipsychotic drugs).	Monitor medication regimen, observing for therapeutic effect.	Enables identification of the minimal effective dose with least adverse effects.	Reports reduction of psychotic symptoms/absence of serious side effects.
	Identify/review adverse effects of medications, hemorrhagic gingivitis, sedation, hormonal effects, reduction of seizure threshold, agranulocytosis, and extrapyramidal symptoms (tremors, akinesia/akathisia, dystonia, oculogyric crisis, and tardive dyskinesia).	Anticholinergic effects of psychotropics (and antiparkinsonian drugs which may be given concomitantly) alter automonic nervous system functioning. Most side effects occur within the first few weeks of treatment and subside with time. Signs indicative of agranulocytosis (sore throat, malaise), extrapyramidal symptoms, and tardive dyskinesia need immediate attention.	
	Emphasize importance of immediate medical attention for onset of high fever/severe muscle stiffness and to discontinue the medication until seen by the doctor.	Severe muscle stiffness and high fever are the hallmarks of neuroleptic malignant syndrome, which can usually be effectively treated before it becomes life-threatening if it is detected early.	
	Administer antiparkinsonism drugs as indicated.	Used for relief of drug-induced extrapyramidal reactions.	

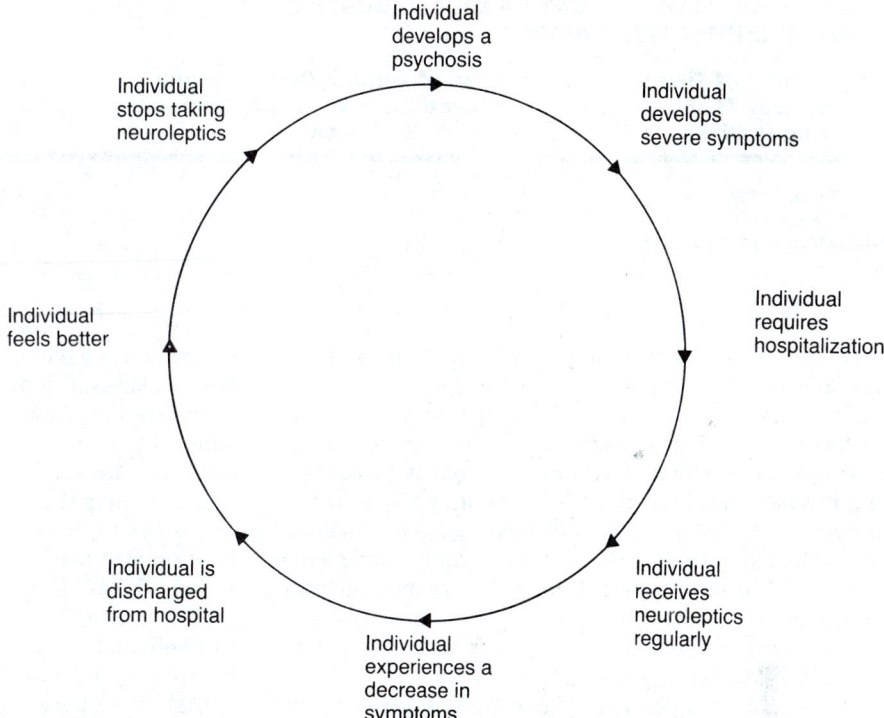

Figure 25–2. Merry-go-round syndrome associated with the utilization of neuroleptics to treat long-term psychosis.

Table 25–9. PATIENT TEACHING INFORMATION—ANTIPSYCHOTICS
Dear Patient: This drug has been prescribed for you. This is what you should know about your drug to get the most from your therapy. 1. This drug will help to relax you. As you relax, your abilities to think clearly and concentrate will improve. 2. You should never take double doses or increase the frequency of times of doses. 3. If you forget to take a pill, you should follow the regimen as outlined in Table 25–10. 4. This medicine may make you feel drowsy, dizzy, or lightheaded. You should evaluate your response to the drug before you participate in activities that require you to be alert. 5. Do not stop taking this drug without consulting with your physician. 6. Do not drink alcohol while you are taking this drug. Before you take any other drugs, discuss this with your physician. 7. This drug may increase your sensitivity to the sun. You should use a sunscreen graded R-15 and wear protective clothing when in the sun. 8. If you feel restless or excited soon after taking the medicine or develop a sore throat with no other cold symptoms or muscle stiffness, contact your physician. 9. You should not take any antacids within 1 hour of ingesting this drug. 10. This drug may be taken with food or 8 ounces of water or milk. 11. If you are using the liquid concentrate, avoid getting it on your skin or clothing. 12. This medicine may cause your urine to become pinkish red, red, or reddish brown. This effect is harmless.

long-term treatment regimen. Patient teaching focuses on highlighting positive effects to be anticipated, distinguishing significant toxic effects from uncomfortable but benign side effects, and reviewing precautions that should be exercised and dosage considerations. Some important information the nurse should teach the patient about the use of antipsychotics is highlighted in Tables 25–9 and 25–10.

EVALUATION

Evaluation of the effectiveness of the nursing intervention for patients being treated with neuroleptic medications is based on evaluating goal achievement. The overall goals of intervention include reduction of the target symptoms to decrease the patient's level of anxiety and agitation, prevention of loss of control, and education of the patient about the diagnoses and the treatment regimen and potential adverse effects. Table 25–11 identifies phases of anticipated positive response to treatment of antipsychotic agents.

The nurse carefully evaluates the patient to determine whether his or her level of anxiety has decreased. Evidence of this decrease is evaluated within one hour after an oral dose or within 30 minutes after an intramuscular dose. This effect should last four to six hours. The nurse evaluates whether or not the patient's agitated behaviors have decreased, whether the pulse rate has decreased, and whether he or she was able to sleep for at least one to two hours. If the person is less anxious, symptoms of the mild to moderate level of anxiety should be observable. A major positive response is dem-

Table 25–10. MANAGEMENT OF MISSED DOSES OF ANTIPSYCHOTIC MEDICATIONS

Number of Times Per Day That Drug Is Given	Span of Time of Remembering Missed Dose When the Dose Should Be Taken	Span of Time of Remembering a Missed Dose When It Should Not Be Taken
Once a day	12–18 hr	After 18 hr
Twice a day	6–8 hr	After 8 hr
More than twice a day	1 hr or less	After 1 hr

onstrated when the patient is able to sleep six to seven uninterrupted hours at night.

The nurse who cares for a highly anxious patient will observe a return to a premorbid level of functioning. Therefore, the patient may still have maladaptive coping mechanisms. Hopefully, as a result of experiencing a decrease in the symptoms of the psychotic reactions and establishing trust with the nurse and other members of the health care team, the patient is motivated to continue to follow the treatment regimen, including taking medications as prescribed and keeping appointments for counseling sessions.

If the patient does not demonstrate a positive response to the antipsychotic, the nurse and physician consider two possibilities. First, the patient may have stopped the medication regimen. If pills are being administered, the nurse attempts to determine whether the patient is "cheeking" them instead of swallowing them. For the client compromised in decision-making, use of an oral concentrate may be indicated. This necessitates open and honest communication and negotiation with patients who are able to be participants in their own health care.

The nurse and physician also consider whether a specific antipsychotic agent is the drug of choice for a given patient. The patient may receive a more positive effect with another neuroleptic. It is recommended that physicians administer a specific drug, in high enough doses, for at least 15 days before evaluating a course of treatment.

Evaluation of the patient's response to the medication also necessitates constant evaluation of whether or not

the person is developing side effects. Differentiating between a side effect of the medication and a consequence of the coping behaviors or illness requires keen observation by all members of the health care team, especially the nurse. The nurse is attentive to comments made by the patient and his or her situational supports, and refers to the list of symptoms exhibited by the patient prior to the initial dosage.

Since many of these side effects are potentially very problematic to the patient, the nurse is constantly alert to complaints that may indicate specific side effects. Symptoms and complaints considered indicators of potential side effects include fever, sore throat, nausea, upper right quadrant abdominal pain, pruritus, dark-colored urine, clay- or light-colored stools, sunburn, orthostatic hypotension, pulse rate over 120 bpm, brownish skin coloration, a brownish cast to vision, or symptoms of any of the extrapyramidal reactions. The earlier the appropriate intervention to decrease the severity of those side effects is initiated, the more effective and safe the overall treatment of the patient will be.

The anticholinergic actions of the antipsychotic agents create a number of side effects, which tend to be relatively mild and to decrease in severity after the first few weeks of treatment. These side effects include dry mouth, constipation, urinary retention, delayed micturition, blurred vision, diaphoresis, and atropinelike psychosis, which occurs rarely.

Table 25–12 reviews the signs and symptoms of extrapyramidal reactions and tardive dyskinesia and differentiates these side effects from the symptoms of psychoses. This differentiation is necessary to avoid

Table 25–11. PHASES OF ANTICIPATED POSITIVE RESPONSES TO TREATMENT WITH ANTIPSYCHOTIC AGENTS

Name of Phase	Time Span from Initial Dose	Cues to Assess
• Medicated cooperation	1–5 days	• Decreased motor excitement; decreased hyperactivity; sleeps 6–8 hours uninterrupted at night.
• Socialization	2 days–2 months	• Decreased withdrawal; increased socialization.
• Elimination of thought disorders	1–6 weeks	• Decreased hallucinations; decreased delusions; increased attention span.
• Maintenance phase	1 week–1 year	• Increased ability to benefit from psychotherapy; increased ability to relate with significant others; increased ability to manage activities of daily living; return to premorbid level of functioning.

**Table 25–12. SIGNS AND SYMPTOMS OF EXTRAPYRAMIDAL
REACTIONS AND TARDIVE DYSKINESIA (TD)**

Type	Symptoms	Points for Nursing Assessment
Parkinsonism	Akinesis, muscle rigidity, stooped posture, shuffling gait, tremors, masklike facies, decreased or absent swing, hypersalivation, drooling, "pill-rolling tremor," listlessness, unusual numbness or tingling sensations.	1. Cues of feeling weak, like a zombie, apathetic, being slowed down. 2. Test to see if strength in both hands has arm decreased. 3. Passive range of motion exercises will produce leadpipe or cogwheel rigidity. 4. Person will use methods other than facial gestures to express emotion. 5. Walks with forearms perpendicular to trunk of body. 6. Increasing the dose of the neuroleptic will produce catatonic-like symptoms.
Akathisia	Restlessness, agitation, compulsion to walk, facial tics, insomnia, fine hand tremor.	1. Assess for feelings of fear, anger and/or terror when patient experiences these symptoms. 2. Person will view these symptoms as being ego-alien (unlike his or her usual behavior, and outside of his or her control). 3. Symptoms will increase after a dose of a neuroleptic.
Tardive dyskinesia	Bucco-linguo-masticatory syndrome, choreiform movements of the extremities, grimacing, tongue protrusion, rocking movements.	1. Assess for earliest cues: blinking, veriform movements of the tongue. 2. Patient may view the symptoms as being "embarrassing" (Harris, 1981).
Dyskinesia and dystonias	Uncoordinated jerking or spastic movements of the neck, face, eyes, tongue, and limbs; oculogyric crisis; torticollis; respiratory distress; dysphagia; opisthotonos; carpal spasms.	1. Patient complains of having problems chewing and/or swallowing food. 2. Patient complains of "eyes rolling in head." 3. Patient will have a look of terror and fear as symptoms develop.

continuing to treat the psychotic reaction with the antipsychotic agent and thus intensifying the severity of the reactions. When recognized early, the proper intervention usually controls these side effects. Therefore, the nurse anticipates their occurrence and immediately consults with the physician. Nurses at times tend to minimize the potential seriousness of symptoms of parasympathetic blockade. Although it is true that such side effects are more annoying than dangerous, without appropriate assessment and intervention constipation may become fecal impaction, which in turn might result in peritonitis. Among elderly clients, who are more susceptible to urinary retention, there is a greater risk of urinary tract infection. Thus, ongoing application of the nursing process and competent nursing care are significant in keeping annoying symptoms from degenerating into major threats to the client's health.

Extrapyramidal reactions are treated in a number of ways. The physician attempts to minimize them by prescribing the smallest dose of the antipsychotic agent needed to achieve a therapeutic benefit. Use of antiparkinson medications also helps to decrease the extrapyramidal effects of the antipsychotic drugs. Intramuscular or intravenous doses of benztropine (Cogentin) or diphenhydramine (Benadryl) can be used to provide quick reversal of the symptoms of dyskinesias and dystonias. Antiparkinsonian medications used include benztropine, trihexyphenidyl (Artane), biperiden (Akineton), and procyclidine (Kemadrin). Refer to Chapter 23 for information on implementing the nursing process for patients receiving these drugs. Controversy exists as to whether or not these antiparkinson drugs should be given prophylactically to patients receiving neuroleptic agents. The decision of whether or not to treat a specific person in this manner is an individual one to be made jointly by the patient and the members of the health care team.

When patients do exhibit any extrapyramidal reactions, the nurse anticipates that the patients will feel frightened and upset. The nurse takes a supportive approach with honest reassurance that these symptoms are side effects of the drug. Frequently, the patient views these symptoms as proof that the condition is worsening. The nurse allows the patient to verbalize these thoughts to help him or her develop a realistic perception of the situation.

When these symptoms are observed, the nurse contacts the physician before administering another dose of the neuroleptic. Frequently at this time, the physician will decrease the dosage of the neuroleptic or change to a drug such as thioridazine (Mellaril) that has the lowest extrapyramidal effects.

During the first weeks of treatment, sedation is most severe. This tends to make the patient discouraged and frustrated because of feeling very tired. The nurse explains that the sedative effect is a side effect of the drug. Usually, after a few weeks, tolerance develops. Sedation is controlled to a limited extent by administering a single dose of the medication one to two hours before bedtime, according to the physician's order.

The potentially serious problem of agranulocytosis tends to occur within the first 8 weeks of treatment. The initial symptoms are malaise, fever, sore throat, and sores in the mouth. When any or all of these symptoms are observed, the nurse contacts the physician immediately. Medical treatment is vigorous and includes discontinuing the neuroleptic agent while using antibiotics and transfusions. Patients who have developed this reaction and survived should never receive the same neuroleptic agent again. It is imperative that nurses acknowledge the danger inherent in the patient's demonstration of malaise, fever, and sore throat, and not dismiss them as insignificant.

Early symptoms of cholestatic jaundice include malaise, fever, nausea, and right upper quadrant abdominal pain. After one week, pruritus, jaundice, dark-colored urine, and light, clay-colored stools occur. This symptom is reversible and tends to be self-limiting. Treatment includes discontinuing the neuroleptic agent, bed rest, and a high-protein, high-carbohydrate diet.

Since cardiovascular side effects may also be experienced, the nurse evaluates the person's vital signs on a regular basis. The frequency of the checks correlates with the rate and degree of stability of the vital signs. The most common cardiovascular side effect, especially among the elderly, is orthostatic hypotension. When evaluating the patient's blood pressure, the nurse checks and records the rates when the patient is sitting and standing. If the systolic rate drops more than 20–30 mm Hg from sitting to standing, the nurse withholds the medicine and notifies the physician. Orthostatic hypotension is an extremely significant problem for elderly patients. The nurse instructs such patients to change from lying to standing positions slowly. Tachycardia may also occur, and the nurse withholds the drug and notifies the physician if the pulse is over 120 bpm.

Because the possibility of the skin/eye syndrome exists, the nurse frequently evaluates the patient's skin, especially areas exposed to the sun, and contacts the physician when areas of golden brown coloration are noted. The most effective treatment occurs through prevention or detection of the problem as soon as possible.

The nurse evaluates the frequency of endocrinologic side effects and gives the patient the time and opportunity to verbalize feelings about them. Side effects, such as amenorrhea, gynecomastia, and ejaculation difficulties, may lead the patient to stop taking the medication. The nurse encourages the patient to express feelings about experiencing a decreased libido and tells the patient that as the dose of the drug is decreased, this side effect tends to be reversed.

The patient may also demonstrate weight gain. Antipsychotic agents appear to intensify a person's craving for sweet foods. Because this may occur, the nurse weighs the patient weekly. The nurse teaches the patient the components of a well-balanced, nutritional diet and emphasizes that the patient should eat fruit to satisfy this craving.

Side effects of hypothermia and, rarely, hyperthermia also may occur. Hypothermia results in the patient's experiencing changes in temperature and frequently feeling "cold." This feeling is intensified for the elderly patient receiving neuroleptic medication. The nurse offers an extra blanket at night and encourages the person to dress appropriately for the environment. Hyperthermia occurs very rarely but has caused fatalities, with temperatures of up to 108° F. Appropriate use of cool sponge baths and hypothermia blankets will safely reduce body temperature.

When it is determined that the person is experiencing an increasing level of anxiety after administration of an antipsychotic, the nurse consults with the physician about the possibility of a secondary anxiety reaction. Usually, when the patient becomes more anxious, the nursing intervention implemented is to administer another dose of the antipsychotic as needed. If this results in intense panic and possibly precipitates a violent outburst as the person tries to cope with the situation, the nurse concludes that the patient is experiencing a secondary anxiety reaction and contacts the physician. A different antipsychotic agent needs to be prescribed.

After recognizing all the problems inherent in the use of antipsychotic agents, the nurse may question the rationale for their use. The nurse needs to recognize that usually the risks of allowing the patient to function at the panic level of anxiety or in the psychotic state or both far outweighs the risks of using the drugs. The nurse, by implementing the nursing process, can help the patient receive the maximum therapeutic benefits from the drugs while attempting to decrease the risks involved.

SUMMARY

This chapter focuses on the five chemical groups that comprise the antipsychotic medications. Although these medications are not curative, they are very useful for control of psychotic symptoms such as thought disturbances, hallucinations, and delusions.

Nursing implications in the use of antipsychotics include awareness of the need for collecting baseline data to facilitate identification of possible drug-related adverse effects. Nursing care rests on the nursing process, which includes careful observation for extrapyramidal symptoms, patient teaching about such effects as increased drowsiness and photosensitivity, timely and appropriate interventions, and ongoing evaluation of patient responses to the prescribed antipsychotics.

BIBLIOGRAPHY

Carpenito, L: Handbook of Nursing Diagnosis, ed 2. JB Lippincott, Philadelphia, 1987.

Clayton, B: Mosby's Handbook of Pharmacology, ed 5. CV Mosby, St. Louis, MO, 1987.

Deglin, J and Vallerand, A: Nurse's Med Deck. FA Davis, Philadelphia, 1988.

Drug Information for the Health Care Professional, ed 8. Rockville, MD, US Pharmacopeial Convention, Inc., 1988.

Drug Information 87. Bethesda, MD, American Hospital Formulary Service, 1987.

Facts and Comparison. JB Lippincott, St. Louis, MO, 1986.

Feather, RB: The institutionalized mental health patient's right to refuse psychotropic medication. Perspect Psychiatr Care 23(2):45–68, 1985.

Gilman, AG, Goodman, L, and Gilman, A: Goodman and Gilman's The Pharmacological Basis of Therapeutics, ed 7. Macmillan, New York, 1985.

Greenblatt, D: Pharmacokinetics in Clinical Practice. WB Saunders, Philadelphia, 1985.

Grimm, P: Psychotropic medications: Nursing implications. Nurs Clin North Am 21(3):397–411, 1986.

Hollister, L: Clinical Pharmacology of Psychotherapeutic Drugs. Churchill Livingstone, New York, 1983.

Huston, LD: Do psychiatric patients really need those drugs? RN 50(2):90, 1987.

Masters, JC and Spitler, R: Neuroleptic malignant syndrome. J Psychosocial Nurs 24(9):11–15, 1986.

McGinnis, J and Foote, K: Rapid neuroleptization. J Psychosocial Nurs 24(10):17–22, 1986.

Scherer, J: Lippincott's Nurses' Drug Manual. JB Lippincott, Philadelphia, 1985.

Scrak, B and Greenstein, R: Tardive dyskinesia evaluation in a nurse managed prolixin program. J Psychosocial Nurs 24(5):10–14, 1986.

Shillcutt, S and Easterday, J: Geriatric therapeutics: Safe and effective use of antipsychotic agents. Hosp Formul 21(4):462–468, 1986.

Simpson, G, Pi, E, and Scramek, J: An update on tardive dyskinesia. Hosp Commun Psychiatr 37(4):362–369, 1986.

Taber's Cyclopedic Medical Dictionary. FA Davis, Philadelphia, 1985.

United States Pharmacopeia Dispensing Information. Easton, PA, Mack Publishing, 1984.

Vander, A, Sherman, J, and Luciano, D: Human Physiology: The Mechanisms of Body Function. McGraw-Hill, New York, 1985.

Wilson, H and Kneisl, C: Psychiatric Nursing, ed 3. Menlo Park, CA, Addison-Wesley, 1988.

SITUATION 25–1

Patty Lawson, a 22-year-old with a history of nonspecific psychiatric disorders, is admitted to the acute psychiatric unit after disrupting the peace and demonstrating delusional ideations.

1. Patty is disoriented, fearing that she is being followed and persecuted. She requires restraints and attempts to bite an orderly. It will be important for the nurse to perform the following:
   a. Question the patient about her feelings concerning drug therapy.
   b. Wait until the patient has calmed down before doing any type of assessment.
   c. Formulate a list of symptoms which the patient is exhibiting.
   d. Demonstrate aggressive, forceful behavior in order to control the patient.

2. Patty is to receive chlorpromazine (Thorazine) IM as a loading dose for acute agitation. The nurse is aware that the usual range for the loading dose is:
   a. 60 to 400 mg/day
   b. 400 to 1500 mg/day
   c. 50 to 100 mg/day
   d. 20 to 80 mg/day

3. When the nurse administers Thorazine to Patty, the following approach is appropriate:
   a. Talk with the patient in order to distract her.
   b. Demonstrate a kind but firm approach.
   c. Ask the patient at what site she would like the injection.
   d. Demonstrate an ability to read her mind.

4. The nurse will expect the onset of action of intramuscular Thorazine to be:
   a. 2 to 3 hours
   b. 5 to 10 minutes
   c. 30 minutes
   d. 1 hour

5. An expected early side effect of the antipsychotic in this case would be:
   a. secondary anxiety reaction
   b. diaphoresis
   c. sedation
   d. hypothermia

6. Which of the following behaviors would indicate an expected positive response to the antipsychotic medication after two days of therapy?
   a. return to premorbid level of functioning
   b. absence of delusions
   c. decreased attention span
   d. increased socialization

CONTINUED ON THE FOLLOWING PAGE

SITUATION 25–2

Ryan David, a 45-year-old, has a long-term history of schizophrenia and frequent readmissions to the acute psychiatric unit. He is currently admitted for a trial with new drug therapy.

1. Mr. David is scheduled to receive thiothixene (Navane). The nurse is aware that the usual route of administration of this drug is:
   a. intravenous
   b. oral
   c. subcutaneous
   d. intramuscular

2. When administering this antipsychotic medication to Mr. David, the nurse includes all of the following *except:*
   a. changing the needle after filling the syringe with medication
   b. injecting the medication deeply into the muscle tissue
   c. mixing the drug with an antiemetic to reduce side effects
   d. massaging the site following injection to promote absorption

3. The nurse will include the following when teaching Mr. David about his medication regimen:
   a. The drugs are highly addictive and require withdrawal sedation.
   b. Most psychotic reactions will recur unless he follows the treatment plan.
   c. Side effects such as sedation are rationale for stopping the drug.

   d. As he begins to feel better with the drug, he may be able to stop counseling.

4. The nurse will plan to promptly report the following symptom related to neuroleptic therapy:
   a. mild rash
   b. dry mouth
   c. sore throat
   d. photosensitivity

5. After three weeks of therapy, Mr. David complains of difficulty chewing and swallowing food. The nurse informs the physicians and is aware that these symptoms relate to:
   a. excessive anticholinergic effects of neuroleptics
   b. extrapyramidal reactions of neuroleptic agents
   c. manifestations of oculogyric crisis
   d. psychotic effects of schizophrenia

6. Should Mr. David experience right upper quadrant pain, jaundice, and clay-colored stools, the nurse will plan to:
   a. provide fresh air and exercise
   b. continue the neuroleptic at a reduced dosage
   c. encourage a high protein/carbohydrate diet
   d. place an n/g tube for enteral feedings

Please refer to the Appendices for correct answers and additional review questions with answers.

26
CHAPTER

MEDICATIONS FOR MOOD DISORDERS

CHAPTER OUTLINE

TABLES

GLOSSARY TERMS IN THIS CHAPTER

Bipolar disorder
Cyclic antidepressant
Endogenous depression
Enterohepatic recycling
Exogenous depression
Extrapyramidal syndrome
First-pass metabolism
Mania
MAOI
Monoamine oxidase inhibitor
Pheochromocytoma
Reactive depression
Reverse vegetative symptoms
"Second-messenger" systems
Tricyclic antidepressant

26
CHAPTER

MEDICATIONS FOR MOOD DISORDERS

VIRGINIA K. DRAKE, R.N., D.N.Sc., C. S.
MARK D. WATANABE, Pharm. D.

LEARNING OBJECTIVES

After reading this chapter, the student will be able to:

1. Identify medications used to treat mood disorders.

2. Differentiate among the drugs used to treat mood disorders as to mechanisms of action, routes of administration, metabolism, and adverse effects.

3. Identify nursing assessments for the patient who requires drugs to treat mood disorders in order to formulate appropriate nursing diagnoses.

4. Plan the nursing interventions necessary to administer drugs used to treat mood disorders, and to choose appropriate teaching strategies for the patient and family.

5. Evaluate the patient routinely during treatment to assess response to medication and nursing interventions.

The term "mood" is very much a part of our everyday vocabulary, and our individual conceptualization of "mood" depends in part on our stance from the perspective of philosopher, psychologist, scientist, or poet. Mood usually refers to our stable, sustained, prevailing emotional state, which colors our entire personality and psychic expression. The term "mood" also takes on personal characteristics from our experiences as we continually adapt to life with behaviors mediated in large part by our subjective emotions, both conscious and unconscious. Thus, we laugh and cry, love and hate, are happy and sad, in a variety of powerful emotional responses that set the feeling tones for our everyday lives. Our mood varies and fluctuates as part of the fabric of our perceptions and responses to our world on a continuum from normal, expected, and functional, to what we consider abnormal, overly responsive, dysfunctional, and therefore problematic.

OVERVIEW OF MOOD DISORDERS

Approaches to the understanding of mood disorders vary from the psychodynamic, the sociobehavioral, to the neurobiologic. It is commonly accepted that biologic vulnerabilities, developmental deficits, and physiologic, psychologic, social, and environmental factors are among the predisposing and precipitating stressors that affect our mood from a biochemical standpoint, resulting in behavioral changes that can be so extreme as to interrupt normal human functioning and well-being. Thus, an important component of the approach to these changes is biochemical. The last several decades have provided us with revolutionary new scientific understandings of the pathogenesis of psychiatric disorders, leading to dramatic progress in defining, classifying, and treating these disorders. Biologic research of psychiatric problems has afforded us the accessibility to powerful chemicals that affect neurochemical mechanisms, thus mediating human behavior. The first group of psychiatric disorders to be researched and treated neurochemically are the mood disorders. A description of the mood disorders as they are defined by the American Psychiatric Association in the Diagnostic and Statistical Manual III Revised (DSM III-R 1987) will provide us with the prevailing psychiatric nomenclature used in clinical settings, and with the diagnostic specificity and reliability that serve as a foundation for the selection of subjects enrolled in psychopharmacologic clinical trials, which in turn document the safety and efficacy of our psychotherapeutic agents.

DSM-III-R identifies a number of clinical conditions of mood disturbance characterized by depression and/or mania that are not due to any other physical or mental disorder. Mood disorders are divided into depressive disorders and *bipolar disorders*.

DEPRESSIVE DISORDERS

The essential feature of depressive disorders is one or more periods of depression without a history of *mania*. The essential feature of bipolar disorders is the presence of one or more manic or hypomanic episode (usually with a history of major depressive episodes).

There are two depressive disorders: major depression (one or more major depressive episode); and dysthymia, in which there is a history of a depressed mood more days than not for at least two years and in which, during the first two years, the condition does not meet the criteria for a major depressive episode. A major depression can be subclassified as mild, moderate, or severe, with or without psychotic features. A major depressive episode can also be specified as melancholic—a typically

Table 26–1. DEPRESSION

DEFINITION:
Emotional state characterized by extreme dejection, gloomy ruminations, feelings of worthlessness, hopelessness, and often of apprehension.

TYPES (SEE TABLE 26–2):
Grief reactions
Pathological grief reactions
Adjustment reaction
Major depression with melancholia
Bipolar disorder, depressed
Severe depression

ETIOLOGY:
The specific etiology of depression is unknown. There are numerous current theories relating to psychoanalytic, cognitive, psychodynamic, biologic, and sociocultural concepts. Currently, many researchers believe depression may result from a combination of many interrelated variables.

SYMPTOMS:
The major symptoms include:
a. A change in feelings toward sadness, loneliness, and apathy
b. Vegetative physical changes (anorexia, constipation, fatigue, and changes in sleeping patterns)
c. Changes in the level of activity ranging from psychomotor retardation to agitation
d. Lowered self-esteem
e. Suicidal thoughts

TREATMENT:
The goal of treatment is to have the person experience relief from the symptoms of depression. The type of treatment used will depend upon the differential diagnosis of the patient's depression. The major forms of treatments include:
1. Psychotherapy
2. Tricyclic antidepressants
3. Tetracyclic and other new types of antidepressants*
4. Monoamine oxidase inhibitors
5. Amphetamines
6. Electroconvulsive therapy
Table 26–2 correlates the various types of depression with their indicated treatments.

---

*For purposes of brevity, and because there is a minimum of information about these new drugs, in this chapter they will be considered under the information referring to tricyclics, except as noted.

severe form that is believed to be partially responsive to somatic therapy—or chronic—the current episode has lasted two consecutive years without a period of two months or longer in which there have been no depressive symptoms. In addition to a depressed mood, there can be a loss of interest or pleasure in activities; changes in appetite, weight, sleep, psychomotor activity; decreased energy, feelings of worthlessness or guilt, difficulty thinking or concentrating, and recurrent thoughts of death or suicide. The symptoms represent a change from previous functioning and are relatively persistent (Table 26–1).

BIPOLAR DISORDERS

There are two bipolar disorders: bipolar disorder, in which there is one or more manic episode (usually with one or more major depressive episode); and cyclothymia, in which there are numerous hypomanic episodes and numerous periods with depressive symptoms. Bipolar disorder is also subclassified as mild, moderate, or severe, with or without psychotic features. A manic episode is characterized by a distinct period during which the predominant mood is either elevated, expansive, or irritable, inflated self-esteem or grandiosity (which may be delusional), decreased need for sleep, pressure of speech, flight of ideas, distractability, increased involvement in goal-directed activity, psychomotor agitation, and excessive involvement in pleasurable activities, often accompanied by poor insight and poor judgment, resulting in painful consequences. The disturbance is sufficiently severe to cause marked impairment in occupational functioning or in usual social activities or relationships, or to require hospitalization (Table 26–2).

Mood disorders are further specified as having a seasonal pattern: a regular cyclic relationship between onset of the mood episodes and a particular 60-day period of the year.

NEUROTRANSMISSION AND MEDICATIONS FOR MOOD DISORDERS

As we continue to gain an understanding of the relationships between brain and behavior, we can refine the neuropsychopharmacological agents that have been successful over the past two decades in the treatment of mental illness. The action of these agents which are of interest in their role as interventions in the mood disorders takes place at the level of the neuron, the basic unit of the brain. In this chapter we will discuss antidepressants and mood-stabilizing medications as they affect the neuron, particularly at the synapse, the focal point for collecting and integrating information for the brain. The synapse, or "gap" between neurons, is the location of neurotransmission, or the chemical communication of the nervous system. These medications affect neurotransmission at the site of the synapse, as well as regulating the sites where some of these neurotransmitters are manufactured. Thus, these medications have a

direct effect on synaptic homeostasis and nervous system health. One of the direct assessments of nervous system health is the measurement of human behavior as it is influenced by "mood," and by the chemical interventions for the mood disorders.

ANTIDEPRESSANT AGENTS

Traditionally, two types of antidepressant agents have been prescribed: *tricyclics* and *monoamine oxidase inhibitors.* Currently, several types of antidepressants are being used. For purposes of brevity, and because minimal information is available about the newer agents, these agents are considered under the information referring to the tricyclics. Another group of drugs, psychomotor stimulants, is used infrequently for depression. These drugs are featured in Table 26–3.

The nurse acknowledges that antidepressants work biochemically specifically to correct an abnormal mood state, depression. Antidepressants do not influence the mood of a patient in a nondepressed state. However, these patients will experience the side effects associated with antidepressant agents.

ACTION

The modes of action of all of the antidepressants are not definitively known. Currently, the cyclic antidepressants and monoamine oxidase inhibitors are believed to achieve their therapeutic effects by regulating the biochemical processes that inactivate norepinephrine and serotonin, thereby prolonging their presence within the central nervous system synapses. Norepinephrine is a catecholamine neurotransmitter—a chemical substance within the central nervous system. Research has demonstrated that as levels of norepinephrine within the synapses are decreased, symptoms of depression can be experienced by the patient. Serotonin, an indolamine neurotransmitter, plays a similar role.

Norepinephrine is synthesized and then stored in storage granules within the presynaptic neuron. As nerve impulses pass along the presynaptic neuron, the chemical is released into the synapse. The free norepinephrine diffuses across the synapse in order to bind briefly to its postsynaptic receptor. Then, the norepinephrine migrates back into the synapse. From there, approximately 80% of the norepinephrine is reabsorbed by the presynaptic neuron and stored, once again, in the storage vesicles. This is called reuptake.

Most of the norepinephrine remaining in the synapse is metabolized by monoamine oxidase, an enzyme found in the mitochondria of the nerve cell. A by-product of norepinephrine metabolism, MHPG (3-methoxy-4-hydroxyphenylglycol), is found in blood plasma and is eventually excreted via the urinary system. The norepinephrine still remaining in the synapse may be metabolized by an extracellular enzyme, COMT (catechol-

Table 26–2. TYPES OF DEPRESSION AND INDICATED TREATMENTS

Type of Depression	Distinguishing Characteristics	Type of Treatment				
		Tricyclics	MAO Inhibitors	Amphet-amines	Electro-convulsive Therapy	Psycho-therapy
Grief reaction	Follows major loss. Shock and disbe-lief (denial) give way to sadness, crying, irritability, anger. Acceptance and some equa-nimity usually develop within 2 months.	Not indi-cated	Not indi-cated	Not indi-cated	Not indi-cated	Possible to use
Pathologic grief	Follows major loss. Prolonged grieving, excessive guilt, withdrawal from friends and activi-ties, somatic symp-toms, anniversary reactions.	Not indi-cated	Not indi-cated	Not indi-cated	Not indi-cated	Indicated
Adjustment disorder	Follows blow to self-esteem. Sadness, discontent, feelings of worthlessness, lack of initiative, hypersomnia, hyperphagia.	Not indi-cated	Not indi-cated	Possible to use	Not indi-cated	Indicated
Major depression with melan-cholia	May be related or unrelated to life events. Positive family history com-mon. Loss of inter-est, inability to respond to plea-surable stimuli, worse in a.m., early morning awakening, severe weight loss, guilt, psychomotor dis-turbance.	Indicated	Possible to use	Not indi-cated	Not indi-cated	Possible to use
Severe depression	Major depression with psychosis or severe suicidal risk.	Possible to use	Possible to use	Not indi-cated	Indicated	Indicated

From Wilson HS and Kneisl CR: Psychiatric Nursing, ed 2. Menlo Park, CA, Addison–Wesley, 1983, p 679, with permission.

O-methyltransferase). Hence, the synaptic levels of norepinephrine are carefully regulated by a delicate bal-ance of synthesis, release, reuptake, and metabolism. Levels of serotonin are handled in an analogous fashion. One of the major metabolites of serotonin is 5-HIAA (5-hydroxyindoleacetic acid).

Scientists now hypothesize that if the norepinephrine and serotonin levels at the synapse remain within a spe-cific level appropriate to the number and sensitivity of the pre- and postsynaptic receptors for those neuro-transmitters, a person experiences stable mood levels. When the levels of the neurotransmitters and the ability of the postsynaptic receptors to process them are mis-matched, the system is considered to be "dysregulated," resulting in a mood disorder. The focus of current re-search is on elucidating the complex biochemical dy-

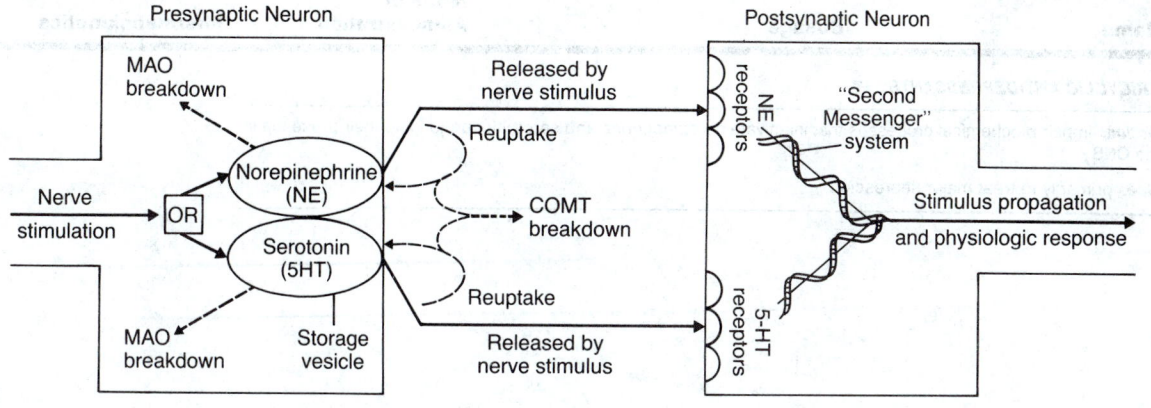

Figure 26–1. Schematic diagram showing normal release and metabolism of catecholamines at synaptic junctions.

namics of the pathophysiology involved. Figure 26–1 is a schematic diagram of the neurotransmitter systems affected by cyclic antidepressants.

TRICYCLICS AND NEWER ANTIDEPRESSANTS

Action

The primary action of the *cyclic antidepressants*, a generic term used to refer to the traditional tricyclic agents as well as the newer ones, is believed to consist of the blockage of the reuptake of norepinephrine or serotonin, or both, from the nerve synapse back into the presynaptic neuron. This process increases the level of neurotransmitter within the synapse and delays the metabolism of norepinephrine and serotonin. The associated neurotransmitter receptors will respond accordingly by altering their number and/or sensitivity. This is essentially a physiologic attempt to readjust the system so that it is more efficient and no longer "dysregulated." The time it takes for the receptors to change may account for the clinically observed delay in therapeutic effect after the initial administration of an antidepressant. Figure 26–2 illustrates a proposed scheme of how cyclic antidepressants function. The selection of a particular antidepressant is empiric. If one agent does not work after four weeks at full dosage, another agent with a different neurotransmitter blocking effect and an acceptable side effect profile could be tried. Table 26–4 shows the comparative norepinephrine and serotonin blocking of the various agents, as well as their propensity for anticholinergic and sedative side effects.

PHARMACOKINETICS

ABSORPTION. These antidepressants are highly lipid-soluble drugs that are absorbed completely from the gastrointestinal tract. The rate of absorption varies from one drug to another. Extent of absorption is reduced by significant hepatic "first-pass" metabolism. For example, average bioavailability values for amitriptyline, imipramine, and nortriptyline are 48%, 27%, and 51%, respectively. Peak plasma concentrations are usually achieved within two to four hours following a single oral dose of the tricyclic agents. Concurrent ingestion of a standardized meal has no effect on oral imipramine bioavailability, peak concentration, or the time to peak concentration.

The newer cyclic antidepressants have absorption

TEXT RESUMES ON PAGE 672

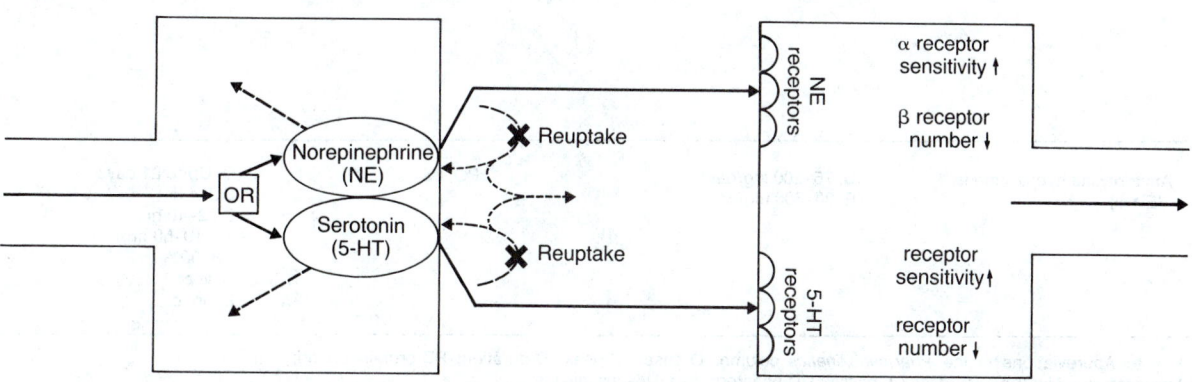

Figure 26–2. Proposed mechanism of cyclic antidepressants: blockage of catecholamine reuptake and regulation of postsynaptic receptor activity.

Table 26–3. DRUGS USED TO TREAT MOOD DISORDERS

Name	Dosage	Mode of Administration	Pharmacokinetics
TRICYCLIC ANTIDEPRESSANTS:			
Action: impair biochemical processes that inactivate norepinephrine and serotonin, prolonging their presence in the CNS			
Use: primarily to treat major depression			
Amitriptyline hydrochloride (Elavil)	U: 75–200 mg/day E: 30–300 mg/day	PO, IM	O: Up to 21 days P: 2–4 hr D: 32–40 hr ½L: 10–50 hr PB: 90% B: liver E: urine

Key to Abbreviations in the *Pharmacokinetics* column: O-onset; P-peak; D-duration; PB-protein bound; B-biotransformed in; E-excreted in; ½ L-halflife; UD-undetermined; UA-unavailable.

*Within the column listing adverse effects, underlines indicate the most common effects; CAPITALS indicate life-threatening effects.

†U-usual daily dose (mg); E-extreme daily dose (mg); LD-loading dose (mg/day); I-Initial dose; M-maintenance dose (mg/day); PO-oral; IM-intramuscular; U-undetermined

‡Although the recommended maximal dose is 100 mg, recent evidence indicates that many patients have relatively low concentrations in plasma and inferior clinical responses unless dosages exceed 100 mg. A few may have an excessive amount at doses above 150 mg/day.

Contraindications/ Precautions	Adverse Effects*	Interactions	Nursing Implications
FOR ALL TRICYCLICS AND OTHER CYCLIC AGENTS: Contraindicated in cardiovascular problems, especially left bundle branch block; in children under age 12 years, and in nursing women. Use with caution in patients with angle-closure glaucoma, thyroid disorders, history of urinary retention, seizure disorders, impaired hepatic function, or benign prostatic hypertrophy. Allergy to tartrazine (dye used in some agents). Excreted into breast milk in low concentrations.	FOR ALL TRICYCLICS AND OTHER CYCLIC AGENTS: Anticholinergic effects most frequent. CNS: dizziness, LOWERED SEIZURE THRESHOLD, sedation & drowsiness, ataxia, disturbed concentration, insomnia, nightmares. CV: DYSRHYTHMIAS, SINUS TACHYCARDIA, or orthostatic hypotension. GI: constipation, nausea & vomiting, dry mouth, paralytic ileus END: Excessive perspiration. Hemo: Petechiae, BONE MARROW DEPRESSION, AGRANULOCYTOSIS, LEUKOCYTOSIS, LEUKOPENIA Eye: blurred vision, mydriasis	FOR ALL TRICYCLICS AND OTHER CYCLIC AGENTS: Decreased effectiveness of antidepressant when given with ammonium chloride, ascorbic acid. Increased effectiveness of antidepressants with acetazolamide, methylphenidate, phenothiazines, and sodium bicarbonate. Additional interactions occur with alcohol, amphetamines, anticoagulants, antihistamines, β-blockers, diazepam, epinephrine, narcotics, phenytoin, procainamide, reserpine, thyroid drugs, and vasodilators. Diagnostic test alterations: elevate serum bilirubin, alkaline phosphatase, and blood glucose; decrease urinary 5-HIAA and VMA excretion, falsely increase excretion of urinary catecholamines.	FOR ALL TRICYCLICS AND OTHER CYCLIC AGENTS: ASSESSMENT: Assess the patient's suicidal potential frequently and routinely. Understand some patients may be at higher risk for suicide as they begin to feel better physically and emotionally. Monitor serum bilirubin, alkaline phosphatase, blood glucose, urinary catecholamines, urinary 5-HIAA, & VMA excretion levels. Assess patient's responsiveness to the medication beginning at 2–3 weeks. Understand that cyclic agents require 2–3 weeks to be effective. Assess for drug interactions. Assess patient's compliance with treatment regimen. Assess patient's nutritional intake. Assess patient's sleep patterns. Assess supine and standing BP daily. Assess patient's ability to function in activities of daily living. INTERVENTION: Teach patient and family that desired response to medication may not occur for 2–3 weeks after initial dose. Teach patient precautions to avoid problems with orthostatic hypotension. Administer drug with food or after a meal to decrease problems resulting from gastric irritation. Teach patient to consult physician before using over-the-counter medications. Do not give the drug if the patient's systolic blood pressure falls more than 20 mm Hg or if there is a sudden rise in pulse rate. Contact the physician. Teach patient the importance of oral hygiene to prevent problems from dry mucous membranes. Assist patient to maintain a balanced diet and regular bowel elimination. Provide interpersonal interaction for the patient having problems with insomnia or early morning awakening. Provide interventions that assist the patient to rest and sleep and establish normal sleep patterns. Provide a safe environment for the patient, especially during times of high suicide potential. Protect the patient from self-harm. EVALUATION: Patient reports perceived positive mood change. Sleep disturbances decrease. Patient resumes activities of daily living without assistance. Patient exhibits interest in the environment and interpersonal interactions. Patient's eating patterns return to a normal state. Patient compliant with treatment regimen. Patient learns to evaluate reaction to medication prior to driving a car, operating machinery, or engaging in other activities which require alertness.

CONTINUED ON THE FOLLOWING PAGE

Table 26-3. DRUGS USED TO TREAT MOOD DISORDERS—*Continued*

Name	Dosage	Mode of Administration	Pharmacokinetics
Desipramine hydrochloride (Norpramine, Pertofrane)	U: 100–200 mg E: 25–300 mg	PO	O: Up to 21 days P:2–4 hr D:12–54 hr ½L: 7–60 hr PB: 90% B:liver E:urine
Doxepin hydrochloride (Adapin, Sinequan)	U:75–150 mg E: 25–300 mg	PO	O: Up to 21 days P:2–4 hr D:17hr ± 6 hr ½L: 6–8 hr PB: 90% B:liver E:urine
Imipramine hydrochloride (Tofranil)	U:100–200 mg E: 25–300 mg	PO, IM	O: Up to 21 days P:2–4 hr D:6–20 hr ½L: UA PB: 90% B:liver E:urine
Nortriptyline hydrochloride (Aventyl)	U: 75–100 mg E: 20–150 mg	PO	O: Up to 21 days P:2–4 hr D:31 ± 13 hr ½L: UA PB: 90% B:liver E:urine
Protriptyline hydrochloride (Vivactyl)	U:18–40 mg E:10–60 mg	PO	O: Up to 21 days P:2–4 hr D:54–96 hr ½L: 16–90 hr PB: 90% B:liver E:urine, feces
Trimipramine maleate (Surmontil)	U:75–200 mg E:50–300 mg	PO	O: Up to 21 days P:2–4 hr D:7–30 hr ½L: 9.1 hr PB: 90% B:liver E:urine, feces
Amoxapine (Asendin)	U: 150–300 mg E: 75–600 mg	PO	O: Up to 21 days P: 90 min D: 8–30 hr ½L: 8 hr PB: 90% B: liver E: urine
Combination: Limbitrol (amitripyline & chlordiazepoxide)	U: 3–4 tabs E: 6 tabs	PO	See individual drug components
Combination: Triavil, Etrafon (amitripyline & perphenazine)	U: 3–4 tabs E: 6 tabs		See individual drug components
OTHER CYCLIC ANTIDEPRESSANTS Maprotiline hydrochloride	U: 75–150 mg E: 50–300 mg	PO	O: Up to 21 days P: 8–24 hr D: 51 hr ½L: 51 hr PB: 90 % B: liver E: urine

Key to Abbreviations in the *Pharmacokinetics* column: O-onset; P-peak; D-duration; PB-protein bound; B-biotransformed in; E-excreted in; ½ L-halflife; UD-undetermined; UA-unavailable.

*Within the column listing adverse effects, <u>underlines</u> indicate the most common effects; CAPITALS indicate life-threatening effects.

†U-usual daily dose (mg); E-extreme daily dose (mg); LD-loading dose (mg/day); I-Initial dose; M-maintenance dose (mg/day); PO-oral; IM-intramuscular; U-undetermined

‡Although the recommended maximal dose is 100 mg, recent evidence indicates that many patients have relatively low concentrations in plasma and inferior clinical responses unless dosages exceed 100 mg. A few may have an excessive amount at doses above 150 mg/day.

Contraindications/ Precautions	Adverse Effects*	Interactions	Nursing Implications
Same as for all.	Same as for all.	Same as for all.	Same as for all.
Same as for all.	Same as for all.	Same as for all.	Same as for all.
Same as for all.	Same as for all.	Same as for all.	Same as for all.
Same as for all.	Same as for all.	Same as for all.	Same as for all.
Same as for all.	Same as for all.	Same as for all.	Same as for all.
Same as for all.	Same as for all.	Same as for all.	Same as for all.
Same as for all.	Same as for all.	Same as for all.	Same as for all.
Same as for all.	Same as for all.	Same as for all.	Same as for all.
Same as for all.	Same as for all.	Same as for all.	Same as for all.
Same as for all.	Same as for all.	Same as for all.	Same as for all.

CONTINUED ON THE FOLLOWING PAGE

Table 26-3. DRUGS USED TO TREAT MOOD DISORDERS—Continued

Name	Dosage	Mode of Administration	Pharmacokinetics
Trazodone (Desyrel)	U: 150–400 mg E: 50–600 mg	PO	O: Up to 21 days P: 1–4 hr D: 4–8 hr ½L: 3–6 hr α; 5–9 hr β PB: 90% B: liver E: urine, feces
Bupropion (Wellbutrin)	U: 150–450 mg E: 150–750 mg		O: Up to 21 days P: 1–4 hr D: 10–21 hr ½L: 14 hr PB: 90% B: liver E: urine, feces
Fluoxetine (Prozac)	U: 20–20 mg E: 20–80 mg		O: P: 6–8 hr D: 2–3 days ½L: 1–30 hr PB: 90% B: liver E: urine

MONOAMINE OXIDASE INHIBITORS

Action: impairs biochemical processes that inactivate norepinephrine and serotonin, prolonging their presence in the CNS.

Use: primarily used to treat major depression.

Name	Dosage	Mode of Administration	Pharmacokinetics
Isocarboxazid (Marplan)	I: 30 mg M: 10–20 mg	PO	O: Up to 21 days P: UA

Key to Abbreviations in the *Pharmacokinetics* column: O-onset; P-peak; D-duration; PB-protein bound; B-biotransformed in; E-excreted in; ½ L-halflife; UD-undetermined; UA-unavailable.

*Within the column listing adverse effects, underlines indicate the most common effects; CAPITALS indicate life-threatening effects.

†U-usual daily dose (mg); E-extreme daily dose (mg); LD-loading dose (mg/day); I-Initial dose; M-maintenance dose (mg/day); PO-oral; IM-intramuscular; U-undetermined

‡Although the recommended maximal dose is 100 mg, recent evidence indicates that many patients have relatively low concentrations in plasma and inferior clinical responses unless dosages exceed 100 mg. A few may have an excessive amount at doses above 150 mg/day.

Contraindications/ Precautions	Adverse Effects*	Interactions	Nursing Implications
Same as for all.	Same as for all.	Same as for all.	Same as for all.
Same as for all.	Same as for all.	Same as for all.	Same as for all.
Same as for all.	Same as for all.	Same as for all.	Same as for all.

FOR ALL MONOAMINE OXIDASE INHIBITORS
Contraindicated in impaired hepatic function, pheochromocytoma, coronary artery disease, cardiac dysrhythmias, cerebrovascular accident, asthma, bronchitis, hypertension, elderly or debilitated patients, severe or frequent headaches, pregnancy, and lactation. Contraindicated within 10 days of surgery requiring general anesthesia, cocaine, or selective local anesthetics. Contraindicated in hyperactive, agitated, or schizophrenic patients.

FOR ALL MONAMINE OXIDASE INHIBITORS:
CNS: dizziness, vertigo, headache, hyperreflexia, confusion, tremors, mania, fatigue, insomnia, & memory impairment.
CV: HYPERTENSIVE CRISIS, edema, ARRHYTHMIAS, orthostatic hypotension
GI: dry mouth, anorexia, nausea, diarrhea, constipation.
GU: sexual dysfunction, urinary retention.
Metabolic system: Weight gain.
Eye: Photosensitivity.

FOR ALL MONOAMINE OXIDASE INHIBITORS
Hypertensive crisis may occur with foods containing tyramine, tryptophan, excess caffeine or chocolate, amphetamines, phenylephrine, cyclamates, reserpine, methyldopa, & tricyclic antidepressants. The MAOIs interact with many other drugs, including over-the-counter and prescription drugs, including insulin, oral antidiabetic medications, meperidine, narcotics, thiazide diuretics, guanethidine, ephedrine, phenylpropanolamine.
Use with caution and in reduced dosage when concomitant with alcohol, barbiturates, tranquilizers, dextromethorphan, and other sedatives.
Laboratory test alteration: false increase in serum bilirubin results.

FOR ALL MONOAMINE OXIDASE INHIBITORS:
ASSESSMENT: The patient's risk for suicidal behaviors must be assessed on a daily and routine basis. Be aware that some patients may be at higher risk for suicide when they begin to feel better physically and emotionally. Know that effects of MAOIs may continue for several weeks after treatment has been discontinued. Assess BP on a routine basis. Assess patient's knowledge base about dietary restrictions. Monitor laboratory values for individual taking MAOIs. Assess patient's mood response to the drug and understanding of the time lag involved from the initial dose until any benefits are observed.
INTERVENTION: Do not give this drug prior to bedtime since it can cause insomnia. Maintain patient on a low tyramine diet. Arrange a consultation with a registered dietitian for the patient and family. Instruct patient not to take any other medications, including over-the-counter medications, without consulting the physician. Teach the patient about dietary restrictions while taking MAOIs and potential for hypertensive crisis with ingestion of restricted foods. Observe for signs and symptoms of hypertension and hypotension as potential side effects. Know drug interactions with MAOIs. Maintain a safe environment for the patient at high risk for self-harm. Protect patient from self-harm. Instruct patient not to drive car, operate machinery, or engage in other activities requiring alertness until aware of drug effects.
EVALUATION: Determine patient's mood changes in response to drug therapy. Evaluate patient drug compliance.

CONTINUED ON THE FOLLOWING PAGE

Table 26–3. DRUGS USED TO TREAT MOOD DISORDERS—*Continued*

Name	Dosage	Mode of Administration	Pharmacokinetics
Phenelzine sulfate (Nardil)	I: 45–90 mg (tid) M: 15 mg (or every other day)	PO	D: Effects of drugs remain for an extended period of time, at least 2 weeks ½L: UA PB: UA B: liver E: GI tract
Tranylcypromine (Parnate)	I: 30–60 mg M: 10–30 mg	PO	P: UA D: 3–5 days B: liver E: GI tract

ANTI-MANIC AGENTS

Action: decreases catecholamine activity. Reduces release of norepinephrine from synaptic vesicles. Increases reuptake of norepinephrine and serotonin, damping effect of these neurotransmitters in the synapse.

Use: primary use is with bipolar disorder.

Name	Dosage	Mode of Administration	Pharmacokinetics
Lithium carbonate (Eskalith, Lithane, Lithonate) Lithium citrate (Lithonate-S)	M: 900–1200 mg Dosage is individualized according to plasma lithium levels and clinical condition. LD: 1800 mg; or 20–30 mg/kg in 2 or 3 divided doses	PO	O: 0.5hr P: 0.5–4 hr; 4–12 hr (SR) PB: UA D: 24 hr (adult) 18 hr (adolescent) 36 hr (elderly) E: urine

Key to Abbreviations in the *Pharmacokinetics* column: O-onset; P-peak; D-duration; PB-protein bound; B-biotransformed in; E-excreted in; ½ L-halflife; UD-undetermined; UA-unavailable.

*Within the column listing adverse effects, underlines indicate the most common effects; CAPITALS indicate life-threatening effects.

†U-usual daily dose (mg); E-extreme daily dose (mg); LD-loading dose (mg/day); I-Initial dose; M-maintenance dose (mg/day); PO-oral; IM-intramuscular; U-undetermined

‡Although the recommended maximal dose is 100 mg, recent evidence indicates that many patients have relatively low concentrations in plasma and inferior clinical responses unless dosages exceed 100 mg. A few may have an excessive amount at doses above 150 mg/day.

Contraindications/ Precautions	Adverse Effects*	Interactions	Nursing Implications
Contraindicated in cerebrovascular illnesses, renal disease, dehydration or sodium depletion, low-salt diet, schizophrenia, brain damage, diuretic therapy, children under·age 12, pregnancy, and lactation.	Correlated with serum lithium levels found in Table 26–16.	This drug interacts with many chemical agents. Do not give concurrently with theophylline, diuretics, drugs containing caffeine, chlorpromazine, iodide preparations, and norepinephrine. Laboratory test alterations: increased VMA excretion, increased serum enzymes, BUN, FBS, and magnesium levels; lower serum T_3, T_4, and PBI levels, increase ^{131}I uptake.	ASSESSMENT: Assess baseline activity level. Assess patient's involvement in inappropriate activities; for example, sexual improprieties, giving away money and possessions, excessive spending, using telephone inappropriately, Assess interactions with other people. Assess patient's ability to carry out activities of daily living. Assess patient's nutritional status and fluid intake. Assess patient's sleep patterns due to hyperactivity. Assess patient for self-destructive behaviors related to impaired judgment and grandiose ideation. INTERVENTION: Administer drug with food to decrease gastric irritation. Protect patient from self during time of hyperactivity and grandiose ideation. Protect patient from embarrassing self. Assist patient to drink 2–3 liters of fluid/day during initial treatment. Monitor patient's salt intake & report any significant changes to physician. Assist patient to comply with drug therapy treatment regimen. Monitor serum lithium levels as scheduled by the physician & noted in Table 26–13. Reduce environmental stimuli; seclude if necessary. Teach patient and family about drug actions, interactions, and continued need for probable long-term drug therapy. Observe patient for compliance with treatment regimen. Provide patient with nutritious finger foods that may be eaten during periods of hyperactivity. Provide safe environment for patient exhibiting poor judgment. Assist patient to rest whenever possible in spite of hyperactivity. EVALUATION: Patient and family understand need for drug therapy and probable long-term therapy. Patient continues to comply with treatment regimen even when feeling better and hyperactivity decreases. Evaluate for adequate food and fluid intake. Observe for effects of drug therapy after 1–2 weeks of drug administration. Serum lithium levels are in therapeutic range for patient.

Table 26–4. COMPARISON OF ANTIDEPRESSANT AGENT EFFECTS

Generic Name	Trade Name	Sedation	Anticholinergic*	Blocks Serotonin	Blocks Norepinephrine
Imipramine	Tofranil	+ +	+ +	+ +	+ +
Amitriptyline	Elavil	+ + +	+ + +	+ + +	+
Desipramine	Pertofrane, Norpramin	+	+	0	+ + +
Nortriptyline	Aventyl	+ +	+ +	+	+ +
Doxepine	Sinequan	+ + +	+ + +	0	+
Protriptyline	Vivactil	0	+ +	+ +	+ + +
Amoxapine	Asendin	+ +	+ +	+ +	+ +(+ + DA)
Trimipramine	Surmontil	+ + +	+ +	+	+
Maprotiline	Ludiomil	+ +	+ +	0	+ + +
Trazodone	Desyrel	+	+	+ +	0
Bupropion	Wellbutrin	0	+?	0? (unknown)	0? (+ DA)
Fluoxetine	Prozac	+ +	+ +	+ +	0

0 = no effect; + = little effect; + + = moderate effect; + + + = great effect; DA = dopamine blocking effect.

*Hypotensive and cardiac effects closely relate to anticholinergic effects in degree, at usual doses.

Adapted from Gilman, Goodman, and Gilman: The Pharmacological Basis of Therapeutics. Macmillan, New York, 1980, p 424; and from Katcher, B and Young, L: Applied Therapeutics: Clinical Use of Drugs, ed 3. Applied Therapeutics, Spokane, WA, 1983, p 1054.

characteristics that may differ from the tricyclics. The absorption of amoxapine, bupropion, fluoxetine, and trazodone is fairly rapid and complete, with peak concentrations achieved after one to four hours following an oral dose (six to eight hours for fluoxetine). In contrast, the absorption of maprotiline is relatively slow; peak concentrations may not be observed until 8–24 hours after administration. Lower and delayed peak concentrations of trazodone have been reported when the drug is taken with meals. The presence of food causes a slight delay in the rate but does not affect the extent of absorption of fluoxetine.

DISTRIBUTION. The tricyclic antidepressants are highly lipophilic compounds that are extensively distributed throughout body tissue. The predominant areas of concentration are found in lung, kidney, brain, small intestine, liver, skeletal muscle, and skin. Very little accumulation occurs in plasma and adipose tissue, and therefore obese patients will probably not have longer half-lives because of a larger volume of distribution. The half-life of a drug determines how long it takes to achieve a steady-state level of that drug in the body. Until a drug reaches steady state (in which the amount of drug excreted equals the amount of drug ingested), the drug level continues to fluctuate with each ingestion. Thus the optimal dose and dose schedule for each patient, a meaningful drug blood level, and a minimization of certain side effects, cannot be accomplished until steady state is reached. (Usually this takes four to six half-lives.) Tricyclics are also highly bound to plasma proteins (>90%), primarily albumin, α-1-acid glycoprotein, and lipoproteins. The distribution of the newer cyclic agents generally mimic the pattern seen for the tricyclics, with concentrations in tissue exceeding those found in plasma.

METABOLISM. All of the cyclic antidepressants undergo extensive hepatic metabolism. The extent to which this occurs varies among patients. Concurrent administration of phenobarbital or a habit of smoking may induce enzyme systems responsible for cyclic antidepressant biotransformation, resulting in an increase of metabolite formation. Many of these metabolites may also be therapeutically active as an antidepressant with potencies and half-lives that may differ from the parent drug. These active metabolites have been shown to accumulate to a significant degree. Careful studies have yet to be performed that elucidate their specific contribution to overall clinical effect. An example of this is desipramine, an active metabolite of imipramine, which can be given separately from the parent drug and generally has equal effectiveness and a lower side-effect profile.

EXCRETION. The cyclic antidepressants are primarily eliminated by a combination of hepatic metabolism (hydroxylation followed by conjugation to glucuronic acid) and renal excretion of the conjugate. Some of the parent drug and its metabolites may be excreted in the feces via the bile. There is also some evidence of *enterohepatic recycling*. The rate of elimination is relatively rapid; one-third to one-half of a single dose may be found in the urine within 24 hours. The elimination rate decreases once the plasma concentration of the drug has been stabilized. The decrease in the rate of elimination allows for detection of the drug in urine months after its ingestion has been discontinued.

Contraindications and Precautions/ Adverse Effects

Most contraindications and precautions for cyclic antidepressant administration relate to their side-effect profile. Many of these agents elicit profound anticholinergic effects, requiring caution in treating patients with angle-closure glaucoma, a history of urinary retention, or benign prostatic hypertrophy. Dry mucous membranes, blurred vision, urinary hesitancy, and constipation are common anticholinergic symptoms.

Because dysrhythmias, sinus tachycardia, and prolongation of conduction time can occur with high-dose cyclic antidepressant therapy, extreme caution should be taken in patients with cardiovascular disorders such as severe coronary heart disease with electrocardiogram abnormalities, paroxysmal tachycardia, progressive heart failure, and angina pectoris. These same concerns should be considered in patients on concomitant thyroid medication. Orthostatic hypotension is another possible cardiovascular side effect, especially in patients with decreased left ventricular performance, and those receiving α-blockers (i.e., labetalol).

Cyclic antidepressants tend to lower the seizure threshold. Seizures have been reported in patients with and without a history of seizure disorders, and an increased incidence has been associated with overdose. The sedation and drowsiness commonly seen with these agents dictate that warnings be issued regarding the impaired ability to perform tasks that are potentially hazardous or require alertness. Care should also be taken in patients with a diagnosis of schizophrenia or bipolar disorder; exacerbation of psychotic behavior or a "switch" into hypomania or mania may occur without careful titration of dosages. Lastly, as a depressed patient improves on medication, he or she may regain enough energy and motivation to act upon suicidal ideations before an actual subjective mood improvement occurs. Careful and frequent assessment of suicidal thinking is necessary, as these drugs are lethal in overdose.

Clinical experience regarding the use of these agents in pregnant women is limited, and their relative safety is undefined. Cyclic antidepressants should be used only when clearly needed and when the therapeutic benefits outweigh the potential risks to the fetus. These agents are excreted into breast milk in low concentrations.

A history of prior sensitivity to any of these agents is a contraindication. In addition, some products contain tartrazine, a dye to which some patients are allergic. Precautions against photosensitivity should be taken in predisposed patients.

Of the reported adverse effects, sedation and anticholinergic effects are the most common. Tolerance to these effects usually develops, and can often be avoided by starting therapy at lower doses with gradual increases as indicated by the clinical situation.

TOXICITY. Cases of overdosage most clearly demonstrate the dangers of cyclic antidepressant toxicity. Cardiovascular symptoms include depression of myocardial contractility, heart rate, and coronary blood flow; impaired conduction leading to atrioventricular block; intraventricular block; sinus and supraventricular tachycardias; ventricular arrhythmias or fibrillation; asystole; pulmonary edema; or hypotension. Excessive anticholinergic activity may manifest as confusion or delirium, agitation, hallucinations, hyperpyrexia, and bowel or bladder paralysis. Other central nervous system effects may include seizures, ataxia, coma, and respiratory depression, which can be monitored by ECG.

Hospitalization and supportive measures are the mainstays of treatment. The extent of toxicity may be monitored by ECG, for a prolonged QRS interval may indicate a higher risk for the development of seizures, dysrhythmias, or hypotension. Removal of the agent may be attempted in alert patients by means of emesis, gastric lavage, or administration of activated charcoal. Hemodialysis, peritoneal dialysis, exchange transfusions, and forced diuresis are generally ineffective because of the extensive tissue distribution of cyclic antidepressants. Cardiac symptoms are often difficult to manage, and therefore must be treated aggressively.

Because of their synergistic effects, quinidine, procainamide, disopyramide, and atropine are contraindicated for cyclic antidepressant overdose.

Interactions

Cyclic antidepressants may interact with a large number of concomitant medications. Some of the more important interactions are summarized in Table 26–3.

Dosage

Administration should begin at the lower end of the usual daily dosage range, and initially in divided doses. As tolerance to side effects develops, the dosage is increased to obtain maximum effectiveness. The dosage of those agents with the lesser anticholinergic and cardiovascular side effects can be increased faster than those with prominent side effects. Decreased drug metabolism in geriatric patients requires the initiation of therapy at lower doses and subsequent increases implemented more slowly. Lower dosages may also be warranted in patients with hepatic impairment and significantly reduced renal function. After effectiveness has been attained, the dosage may be decreased to the high end of the usual daily dosage. These agents should be continued for several months, depending on the patient's depressive history, and should be discontinued only gradually. Table 26–3 shows the usual daily dosage range (initial to maintenance) and the extremes in dosage, where the low dose is for adolescents and elderly persons and the high dose is for acutely depressed patients.

After the initial dosing period, these agents can be given in a single dose at bedtime. This tends to decrease the incidence of orthostatic hypotension and confusional states. Furthermore, the person who is demonstrating insomnia and agitations may actually benefit from the sedating effect of a large bedtime dose.

Table 26–3 also lists many of the properties of the cyclic antidepressants available in the United States in 1989.

Special Dosage Forms/Combination Products

Some of the cyclic antidepressants are available in dosage forms other than tablets and capsules. Doxepin (Sinequan) is available as a solution, which should be diluted with 120 ml of water, milk, or juice just before administration. It is incompatible with many carbonated beverages. Nortriptyline (Aventyl) is available as a solution that need not be diluted. Imipramine (Tofranil) and amitriptyline (Elavil) may both be given by intramuscular injection. The pamoate salt of imipramine

Table 26–5. COMBINATION DRUGS FOR ANTIDEPRESSANT ACTION

Combination Drug	Basic Products*		
	A	B	C
Etrafon 2-10 or Triavil 2-10	2	10	
Etrafon or Triavil 2-25	2	25	
Etrafon-A or Triavil 4-10	4	10	
Etrafon-Forte or Triavil 4-25	4	25	
Triavil 4-50	4	50	
Limbitrol 10-25		25	10

*Basic products: A = perphenazine, mg; B = amitriptyline hydrochloride, mg; C = chlordiazepoxide, mg.

(Tofranil PM) is marketed for once-a-day bedtime administration, but it actually has no advantage over the hydrochloride and is more expensive.

Triavil and Etrafon are brand names of combination products that contain 2–4 mg of the antipsychotic perphenazine and 10–50 mg amitriptyline. The recommended initial dose is one tablet three or four times daily. After a satisfactory response is noted, the dosage can be reduced to the smallest amount necessary to obtain relief from symptoms. However, this combination should not be used as the initial choice to treat patients with symptoms of depression and severe agitation. Individual agents should be titrated separately. Table 26–5 features a list of combination drugs that includes antidepressants.

MONOAMINE OXIDASE INHIBITORS

Action and Uses

The monoamine oxidase inhibitors interfere with the effects of monoamine oxidase (MAO). "Monoamine oxidase" refers to a number of enzymes present in cells within the brain, blood platelets, liver, spleen, and kidneys. The major function of these enzymes is to metabolize biogenic amines, such as the neurotransmitters epinephrine, norepinephrine, and serotonin. Therefore, MAO inhibitors block the action of MAO and thus increase the concentration of these amines in presynaptic neurons in the brain and elsewhere in the body. There are two types of monoamine oxidase, MAO-A and MAO-B, with different abilities to act on various substrates; the clinical significance of these differences is a topic of current research. Figure 26–3 illustrates the hypothesis of the action of monoamine oxidase inhibitors.

Currently available agents approved for the treatment of depressive disorders include isocarboxazid, phenelzine, and tranylcypromine. Whereas isocarboxazid and phenelzine bind irreversibly to MAO, tranylcypromine produces a reversible inhibition. These agents may be useful alternatives for patients who are refractory to cyclic antidepressants or intolerant to their side effects. Symptoms that appear particularly responsive to monoamine oxidase inhibitor therapy include *reverse vegetative symptoms*, nonendogenous depression, and the presence of anxiety.

PHARMACOKINETICS

ABSORPTION/DISTRIBUTION. When administered orally, the MAO inhibitors are well absorbed through the gastrointestinal tract. The actual time required for the drugs to produce inhibition of monoamine oxidase is unknown, but current estimates place the time for achievement of inhibition at about two to three days. However, when treatment of MAO inhibitors is initiated, therapeutic effects may not be observed before one to four weeks.

METABOLISM/EXCRETION. The MAO inhibitors are rapidly metabolized by means of hepatic oxidation and acetylation and the metabolites are excreted quickly through the gastrointestinal tract. Because of the irreversible nature of MAO inactivation by isocarboxazid and phenelzine, clinical effects may continue for up to two weeks after discontinuation of therapy. In contrast, when tranylcypromine is withdrawn, MAO activity may be recovered in three to five days, although the drug is excreted within 24 hours.

CONTRAINDICATIONS AND PRECAUTIONS

Most of the clinical situations in which MAO inhibitors may be contraindicated relate to the ability of these

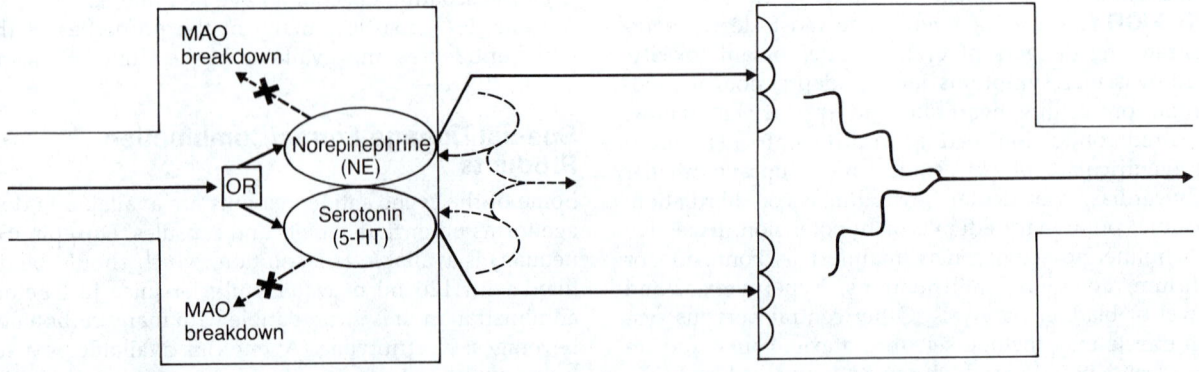

Figure 26–3. Proposed mechanism of monoamine oxidase inhibitors: decreased presynaptic metabolism of catecholamines results in increased availability in synapse.

agents to increase circulating sympathomimetic amines. Therefore, caution should be exercised when using MAO inhibitors in patients over 60 years of age, with cardiovascular disease, hypertension, history of headache, congestive heart failure, a history of liver disease or abnormal liver function tests, severe impairment of renal function, *pheochromocytoma*, or an inability to adhere to the required dietary and drug restrictions. A history of hypersensitivity to these agents is also a standard contraindication. Other precautions that must be taken are associated with potential drug and food interactions (see "interactions").

The safety of MAO inhibitors during pregnancy has not been established, nor is it known whether they are distributed into human milk.

Adverse Reactions/Toxicity

The most common adverse reactions found in MAO inhibitor therapy are orthostatic hypotension, weight gain, sexual dysfunction (i.e., retarded ejaculation, anorgasmia), and edema. These tend to diminish as the patient adjusts to the medication. Paradoxic sympatholytic effects are responsible for both the orthostatic hypotension and the sexual dysfunction. Weight gain may be related to a craving for carbohydrates or a change in metabolism, and may sometimes be indicative of a therapeutic response. Generalized edema most often occurs with isocarboxazid and phenelzine and usually subsides within a week without special intervention. Anticholinergic effects may occur, but these are less severe than those associated with the cyclic antidepressants.

Toxic symptoms of overdose include cardiovascular and neurologic manifestations. Cardiovascular symptoms reported include dizziness, flushing, tachycardia, tachypnea, hypertension or hypotension, and circulatory collapse. Neurologic symptoms reported include headache, anxiety, agitation, confusion, movement disorders, convulsions, and coma. In addition, sweating, miosis, acidosis, and hyperthermia have been seen. Treatment includes supportive measures and induction of emesis or gastric lavage. Unlike cyclic antidepressants, hemodialysis, peritoneal dialysis, and charcoal hemoperfusion have been shown to be of value in some cases of massive overdosage.

Interactions

Significant interactions involving MAO inhibitors result in either a potentiation of the normal pharmacologic action of another medication or a hypertensive crisis brought about by the supranormal release of catecholamine stores.

Potentiation of medication administered concomitantly with MAO inhibitors has been demonstrated in numerous cases. Because general anesthetics may cause additional hypotension when given with MAO inhibitors, the latter are usually discontinued at least two weeks prior to surgery. In the event of emergency surgery, intravenous hydrocortisone is preferred over pressor agents in the management of hypotension. Patients taking oral hypoglycemic agents or on insulin therapy

have been reported to develop hypoglycemia while also taking MAO inhibitors. A possibly life-threatening interaction exists between meperidine and MAO inhibitors. Because the physiologic breakdown of meperidine is impaired in this situation, there is an increased risk of hyperthermia and circulatory collapse. Of the opiates, codeine appears to offer analgesia with the lowest number of reported cases of this interaction. Addition of MAO inhibitors to a medication regimen that includes a cyclic antidepressant, levodopa, and dopamine may also increase the therapeutic and toxic effects of those agents.

Hypertensive crises are serious and can sometimes be fatal. These usually occur within several hours after ingestion of contraindicated food or medication. Severe blood pressure elevation is often preceded by nausea, vomiting, sweating, palpitations, occipital headache, and neck stiffness. Food with high tyramine content should be avoided (e.g., cheeses, meat extracts, smoked meats, soy sauce, red wines) and intake of foods and beverages containing caffeine should be limited to small amounts, since both of these agents will precipitate or exacerbate a hypertensive crisis. Table 26–6 provides a list of dietary recommendations. In addition, the use of concomitant sympathomimetics (amphetamines, phenylpropanolamine, ephedrine, pseudoephedrine, phenylephrine) and certain antihypertensive drugs (guanethidine, reserpine, methyldopa) may be contraindicated because of the risk of a hypertensive reaction. Note that other antihypertensive agents that do not release stored catecholamines may further decrease blood pressure in patients on MAO inhibitor therapy.

Dosage

Measurement of blood concentration platelet MAO activity is often recommended whenever possible before MAO inhibitor therapy is initiated (Gold et al., 1984). Most experts recommend that the patient be on a low monoamine diet for one to two weeks before drug therapy with these agents is begun (and for one week after discontinuation). The usual starting dose of phenelzine is 15 mg given three times daily, with a rapid increase to a daily dosage of 60 mg within the first two weeks. If after an additional two weeks at 60 mg/day there is no clinical response, platelet enzyme inhibition can be measured again. The dose should be adjusted to result in 85%–90% inhibition. If adequate response is not seen after two weeks at the adjusted dosage, the dose can be increased by an additional 15 mg/week up to a daily dosage of 90 mg. After maximum benefit is achieved, the dosage can gradually be decreased to a maintenance dose of 15 mg once daily or every other day. Care should be taken not to exceed 95% platelet enzyme inhibition, at which the risk of serious food and drug interactions increases.

Tranylcypromine may be given 10 mg twice daily as an initial dose. After two weeks, the dose may be increased to 30 mg daily if there is no clinical response. If there is no improvement after an additional week, an alternative agent may have to be considered, since continued administration is unlikely to show any benefit. If

Table 26–6. DIET RESTRICTIONS FOR PATIENTS RECEIVING MONOAMINE OXIDASE INHIBITORS

Foods	Restrictions
Do not eat cheese except as noted. Avoid sour cream and yogurt.	Processed cheese, cream cheese, and cottage cheese are allowed. One slice of pizza with mozzarella is believed to be safe.
Avoid stews or drinks made with meat extracts.	Meats and natural gravies are safe. See below.
Avoid foods made with yeast extracts such as marmite.	Baked goods made with yeast are allowed.
Avoid foods that have been aged without refrigeration, especially meats, poultry, or fish.	Freshly prepared frozen or tinned meats, poultry, or fish are safe.
Avoid sausages, such as bologna, salami, and pepperoni.	
Avoid pickled herring.	
Avoid chicken livers, goose livers, and paté de foie gras.	
Avoid broad bean pods, including Java beans.	These are frequently served in Chinese dishes.
Avoid avocados, raisins, figs.	Controversy exists as to whether bananas should be limited. Kline and Angst believe that the bananas are safe and that only the peel contains large quantities of tyramine.
Avoid soy sauce.	
Restrict intake of alcohol.	Limit intake of beer to 1–2 glasses per day. Limit intake of whiskey, gin, rum, etc. to 3 oz/day.
Avoid red wines (e.g., Chianti) and sherry.	Limit intake of white wine to 4–8 oz per day.
Limit intake of foods containing caffeine.	Chocolate, coffee, cola, and tea in small amounts are considered safe.
Avoid any foods or drinks that have caused problems, including allergies, in the past.	

response is achieved, slow titration to a maintenance dose of 10 or 20 mg daily may be carried out.

The usual starting dose of isocarboxazid is 30 mg daily in single or divided doses. Side effects appear to increase with daily doses greater than 30 mg. As soon as improvement is achieved, a gradual reduction to a daily dose of 10 or 20 mg is warranted. Such a therapeutic response may not be seen for three or four weeks. As with tranylcypromine, if no clinical improvement is obtained by then, continuation of therapy is unlikely to help.

PSYCHOMOTOR STIMULANTS

Psychomotor stimulants such as amphetamine, dextroamphetamine, and methylphenidate (Ritalin), have been used as adjunctive therapy to the traditional antidepressants. Their use is somewhat problematic and controversial, for there are risks of developing addic-

Table 26–7. PSYCHOMOTOR STIMULANTS

Generic Names	Trade Names
Amphetamine sulfate	
Dextroamphetamine sulfate	Dexedrine
Methamphetamine	Desoxyn
Methylphenidate	Ritalin
Pemoline	Cylert

tion, rebound depression, or a psychotic behavioral syndome. They are not primary agents in the treatment of depression; see Chapter 21 for a discussion of their properties and use. Table 26–7 lists these drugs.

USING THE NURSING PROCESS

ASSESSMENT

The nurse begins the assessment of the depressed patient with a thorough history in order to establish the data base. Particular attention is given to any previous suicide attempts or suicidal gestures by the patient as well as any positive family history of suicidal behavior. The nurse asks direct questions and identifies cues correlating etiologic factors. A suicide assessment is obtained to ascertain whether the patient has formulated a specific plan for suicide, for example, overdosing, shooting him- or herself, or staging a car accident. A specific and well-thought-out plan for suicide alerts the nurse to more imminent danger of implementation by the patient. The nurse assesses the length of time the person has been experiencing depressive symptoms. Family members may be able to provide a more accurate assessment about the length of time depressive symptoms have been present. The nurse asks specific questions about vegetative symptoms of depression (refer to a psychiatric nursing text for more specific information on obtaining a data base from depressed patients). This information helps the nurse and physician as they attempt to differentiate the specific type of depression the patient is experiencing.

The patient with depression experiences a wide range of symptoms. Table 26–8 lists these symptoms and acts as a guide for the nurse as the patient is assessed. Table 26–9 identifies information needed in the nursing data base.

Table 26–8. ASSESSMENT OF SYMPTOMS OF MOOD DISORDERS

Mode	Depression	Bipolar Reaction, Manic State
PHYSIOLOGIC:		
Rest and exercise	Extreme fatigue	Hyperactivity
	Insomnia	Restlessness
	Early morning awakening	Irritability
	Diurnal rhythm of symptoms	No time to sleep
	Decreased motivation of any activity	Constant initiation of activities, but no completion
	Psychomotor retardation	Frequent clothes changes
Oxygenation and circulation	Decreased pulse	Increased pulse
	Deep sighing	Increased blood pressure
Fluid and electrolytes	Decreased fluid intake	Frequent dehydration
Nutrition	Anorexia	No time to eat
	"Bloated" feeling	Weight loss
	Weight loss	
Elimination	Constipation	Constipation and impaction
	Decreased urine output	Bladder distention
Skin	Decreased interest in hygiene	No time for personal hygiene
		Frequent use of excessive makeup
		Frequent accidental injuries
Regulation and senses	Decreased taste (food tastes "like straw")	Hypersensitivity to environmental stimuli
	Colors all appear gray tinged	Irritability
	Decreased awareness	
	Decreased attention span	
Endocrine	Amenorrhea	Increased sexual activities
	Impotence	
	Frigidity	
Neurologic	Decreased responses to pain	Ignoring of cues to pains
	Complaints of many vague pains	Decreased attention span
	Thought retardation	
SELF-CONCEPT:		
Body image	Self-deprecation	Loves self
	Feeling of loss of control	Delusions of grandeur
	Digust with body	
	Self-mutilation	
Moral/ethical self	Extreme guilt feelings	Decreased moral and ethical standards
	Delusions of sin and guilt	Impulsive behaviors
Self-consistency	Loss of interest in all previous concerns and motivations	Unpredictability
	Self-centered preoccupations	Flight of ideas
	Delusions of poverty	Pressured speech
Self-ideal and expectancy	Hopelessness	Hopefulness
	Helplessness	Powerfulness
	Powerlessness	
	Suicidal ideation	
Self-esteem	Denial of past accomplishments	Increased delusions of grandeur
	Very low self-esteem	
	Feeling of worthlessness	
	Self-consciousness	
	High sensitivity to criticism	
Role function	Role failure	No time to fulfill responsibilities
	Decreased motivation to fulfill responsibilities	Role failure
Interdependence	Withdrawal	Independence
	Dependency	Manipulativeness
	Clinging	Seductive behavior
	Unloved feeling	Refusal of offers of help
	Views self as a burden to others	

Table 26–9. NURSING PROCESS FOR PATIENT REQUIRING ANTIDEPRESSANT MEDICATIONS

Assessment

Assess mood, coping abilities, personality styles, i.e., temperament, aggression, impulsive behavior, level of self-esteem.
Assess feelings of hopelessness, sense of being overwhelmed.
Note plan of suicide, e.g., telling people goodbye, giving away possessions, expressions of despair.
Evaluate degree of risk/suicidal potential and reevaluate periodically.

Nursing Diagnosis	Nursing Actions	Rationale	Desired Outcomes/ Evaluation Criteria
Violence, potential for directed at self related to depressed mood, self-destructive behavior with indicators of expression of intent to harm self, increased anxiety, sudden mood elevation.	Observe patient frequently, especially as mood lifts and physical/emotional state improves.	Provides for external control until patient regains internal control. As lifts, patient is more likely to have the ability to carry out suicide plan.	Verbalizes understanding of behavior and precipitating factors. Demonstrates evidence of planning for the future.
	Encourage verbalization of feelings. Active listen to patient concerns. Administer drug trial of tricyclic antidepressants (TCA) or monoamine oxidase inhibitors (MAOI).	Promotes understanding and clarification of reasons for depression. TCAs are generally considered safer and easier to manage and are given first. If a positive response is not noted in 4 to 6 wks, an MAOI may be the drug of choice.	
Coping, ineffective, individual related to personal vulnerability, multiple life changes, unmet expectations, actual/perceived loss as evidenced by perception of events and stressors in a manner that precipitates depressive episode, areas of life are seen as losses or as unfulfilled, weeping/labile affect.	Encourage verbalization of and assist in identification of feelings and relationship between feelings and event/stressor, when known. Use crisis or social skills model to teach and appropriately reinforce more effective problem-solving/coping strategies.	Talking about and labeling the feelings helps patient begin to deal with them more effectively. These models can be used effectively to increase patient's repertoire of coping techniques.	Verbalizes understanding of relationship between feelings and antecedent events. Identifies coping patterns previously used and alternative strategies to cope with this/other situations.
	Involve in activities, e.g., OT/RT, brisk walks, punching bag.	Provides safe, effective methods for releasing endorphins and discharging pentup tensions, learning to trust self, and enhancing self-esteem.	
Knowledge deficit related to unfamiliarity with resources/ misinterpretation of pathophysiology and treatment regimen, cognitive limitation as evidenced by questions, statement of misconception, development of preventable complications.	Provide information about depression and treatment regimen. Discuss drug therapy and potential side effects, e.g., anticholinergic effects of antidepressants and possibility of hypotensive crisis if foods containing tyramine are eaten while taking MAO drugs.	Promotes understanding of illness and own situation. Knowing what to expect may increase cooperation. Patient needs to be aware that improvement may not be noted for 4–6 weeks but side effects may improve/disappear within two weeks. Dietary restrictions are important to	Verbalizes understanding of condition, prognosis, and therapeutic regimen.

Table 26–9. NURSING PROCESS FOR PATIENT REQUIRING ANTIDEPRESSANT MEDICATIONS—*Continued*

Nursing Diagnosis	Nursing Actions	Rationale	Desired Outcomes/ Evaluation Criteria
		avoid precipitating crisis.	
	Encourage frequent fluids, lip salve, sugarless lozenges/gum, ice chips as indicated. Suggest taking medication at bedtime when possible.	Provides relief of dry mouth caused by anticholinergic effect of drug therapy. Sedative effect may be helpful to promote and maintain sleep.	
	Recommend slow rising from recumbent position.	Orthostatic hypotension/dizziness is a common side effect of antidepressant drugs potentiating risk of injury.	
	Reinforce importance of not stopping drug abruptly.	Sudden cessation of drugs may aggravate condition, deepening depression and withdrawal symptoms of nausea/vomiting and diarrhea.	
	Encourage use of identification bracelet/card.	Provides information if needed in emergency situation to prevent sudden termination of drug therapy.	

The nurse assesses how the patient has been seeking relief from the symptoms of depression, as well as the patient's and family members' perceptions of the depression. The nurse obtains a drug history regarding treatment with medications for depression and the patient's response to the therapeutic agent.

As part of the initial assessment, the nurse encourages the patient to verbalize feelings and thoughts about taking medications for the symptoms of depression. The nurse anticipates that the patient and family members may initially tend to exhibit one of two specific feelings regarding medication compliance. The nurse frequently observes the patient and/or the family perceiving medication as an instant, magical cure. On the other hand, because of the effects of the illness, the nurse perceives that the patient initially views all treatment efforts as being futile. The more severe the depression, the more hopeless and helpless the patient feels. These responses naturally are intensified if treatment with one or more of the antidepressant agents was previously ineffective. Such feelings frequently lead to a "why bother?" attitude, resulting in noncompliance. The nurse acknowledges the importance of the feelings expressed by the patient.

The potential for suicide is present with any person experiencing a depression. Therefore, the nurse is constantly alert to cues of the patient's position on the lethality scale. This continues to be important during the period when the patient begins to feel better physically and emotionally, but continues to believe that progress is only temporary and that the prognosis for a happy life is hopeless. At this point, the person may have the strength and concentration abilities that were lacking when too severely depressed to formulate and implement a plan of suicide. Thus, constant assessment and direct observation of the patient are necessary during this period.

NURSING DIAGNOSES

When the assessment is completed, the nursing diagnoses are formulated. These focus on the individual and family responses to the depression and the treatment regimen. Examples of nursing diagnoses related to using the antidepressants are featured in Table 26–9.

INTERVENTION

The nurse develops the goals of the nursing intervention based on the nursing diagnoses. Examples of nursing goals for the patient on medications to treat depression are included in Table 26–9. The nurse and patient use the data base established during the initial health history to develop the plan of intervention. The data base is continually updated to reflect any new or changing information.

The nurse aims to help the patient and family perceive the antidepressants as only a part of the overall treatment plan, assisting the patient to view the medication as a tool to decrease the level of depression so that the patient may participate in and benefit from other therapies. If the depression is a reactive type, one goal of therapy is to assist the patient to strengthen coping mechanisms in order to deal with future critical events more adaptively. If it has been determined that the depression is an endogenous type, one goal of therapy is to help the patient enhance abilities to identify any future recurrence of the depressive symptoms more quickly and seek treatment as soon as any symptoms are exhibited.

The nurse spends time with close family members, assisting them to understand the slow process of recovery from an altered mood state. Family members may be angry at the depressed patient "who has everything to live for" and continues to feel hopeless and helpless. Patients and family both may feel guilty for the feelings of depression and anger they are experiencing. It is important for them to understand that feelings often are not logical; feelings are "just there" and cannot be explained. Nursing staff and family will find it important to understand that mere presentation of logic does not resolve a patient's depressed or manic state. Patience with the ill person is essential; however, some family members find it difficult to tolerate the patient's behaviors.

Taking tricyclics with food decreases symptoms of gastrointestinal distress. However, it must be noted that some physicians recommend that these drugs not be taken with food because they believe doing so decreases the rate of absorption of the drug, reducing the drug's effectiveness. Therefore, the nurse and physician must discuss what instructions the patient is to be given. If the patient is taking the drug in a liquid form, it should not be diluted with grape or carbonated beverages, since these fluids decrease the effectiveness of the medication. The patient or family member is given specific written instructions about the drug therapy.

Patient Teaching

Patient teaching is an essential component of tricyclic drug therapy. The nurse teaches the patient and family the expected stages of response to tricyclic therapy and identifies any cues of improvement demonstrated by the patient. Frequently, for patients beginning treatment with one of these antidepressants, the nurse teaches the patient and the family how the tricyclic agent affects symptomatology. This assists the person in maintaining the level of motivation to continue treatment, since the drug's effects are delayed by two to three weeks or longer. The nurse teaches the necessity of continuing the medication as prescribed, even after the patient feels better. Continuation of the medication is necessary to maintain therapeutic plasma level to maintain a state of emotional equilibrium. Table 26–10 features other useful information for patient teaching.

A critical component of nursing intervention when administering MAO inhibitors is patient and family ed-

Table 26–10. PATIENT TEACHING INFORMATION—TRICYCLICS

This drug has been prescribed by your doctor. The following information will assist you to receive the most help from your total program of therapy. If you have any additional questions about the drug, please consult your doctor, nurse, or pharmacist.

1. This drug will help decrease your symptoms of depression.
2. This medicine may cause you to have feelings of dizziness and lightheadedness when you stand up. Changing positions slowly and gradually will help prevent these feelings.
3. This drug may cause you to feel drowsy. Be sure you know how the drug affects you before you drive or do other activities that require you to be alert.
4. This medicine may need to be taken for 2–3 weeks or longer before you begin to have its positive effects.
5. Do not drink alcohol (beer, wine, hard liquor) while you are taking this drug.
6. Do not change the dose or number of times when the medicine is taken. A missed dose may be taken if you remember within one hour of the scheduled time. Otherwise check with your physician as soon as possible before continuing your regular schedule.
7. Do not stop taking this medicine without first talking with your physician. It is important to continue taking the medicine even when you begin to feel better.
8. Before having any kind of surgery (including dental surgery) or emergency treatment, inform the physician or dentist that you are taking this medication.

ucation (Table 26–11). When caring for patients receiving MAO inhibitors, the nurse aims to ensure that the patient receives maximum therapeutic benefit from the drug without experiencing severe problems related to the drug. The nurse achieves this by developing a rapport with the patient, encouraging him or her to verbalize feelings about the treatment regimen, and educating the patient about the rationale underlying the drug therapy.

The nurse discusses information with the patient about the low-tyramine diet outlined in Table 26–6. The patient is encouraged to discuss feelings and thoughts about the dietary limitations and the nurse offers support as needed. Consultation with a registered dietitian is arranged to assist the patient with meal planning when returning home. A list of prohibited foods is provided for the patient to use in the hospital and take home upon discharge. The patient and family are cautioned about unusual foods that may contain tyramine. The depressed patient may need assistance with meal selection until an improved mental status is present. Until the patient experiences relief of depression from the medication and other therapies, the nurse or family member carefully monitors the dietary intake. The possibility of undermining treatment or a suicide attempt by consuming a restricted food or drink is not ruled out.

The patient is taught the importance of not taking any other prescription medications or over-the-counter preparations without first checking with the physician.

Table 26–11. PATIENT TEACHING INFORMATION—MONOAMINE OXIDASE INHIBITORS

This drug has been prescribed by your doctor. The following information will assist you to receive the most help from your total treatment program. If you have any additional questions about the drug, please consult your doctor, nurse, or pharmacist.

1. This drug will help reduce your symptoms of depression.
2. Some foods that contain tyramine, as listed in Table 26–6, may cause a rapid rise in your blood pressure. You must avoid eating the foods listed or foods not allowed by a registered dietitian.
3. Do not take any other medicine, including over-the-counter agents, without first talking to your doctor.
4. This drug may cause you to feel dizzy and lightheaded when you stand up. Changing positions slowly and gradually will help.
5. This drug needs to be taken for 1–2 weeks or longer before you begin to have its positive effects.
6. These precautions about your diet and other drugs need to be followed for 2 weeks before beginning this drug and for 2 weeks after you stop taking this drug.
7. Be certain you tell all other doctors and dentists who may treat you that you are taking this drug or have taken it in the last 2 weeks.
8. Do not change the dose or number of times the medicine is taken. If a dose is missed and you remember it within 2 hours of the scheduled time, take the dose and continue the regular schedule. If you remember after 2 hours, skip the dose and continue the regular schedule. Do not stop taking this drug without first checking with your doctor even when you begin to feel better.
9. This drug may cause some people to become drowsy or less alert than usual. Be certain you know how you react to this medicine before you drive, use machinery, or engage in other activities that require you to be alert.
10. Check with your doctor or hospital emergency room immediately if severe headache, stiff neck, chest pains, rapid heartbeat, or nausea and vomiting occur while you are taking this medicine. These may be symptoms of a serious reaction that require medical help.

Before discharge, or if the patient is being treated on an outpatient basis, the nurse teaches him or her the necessity of telling all other physicians, dentists, and health team members treating him/her for other health problems that MAO inhibitors are being taken. If the person needs to be scheduled for surgery, the physician discontinues the drug one to two weeks prior to surgery. The surgeon and anesthesiologist are informed that the patient is taking this drug. It is recommended that opium or morphine be used for pain as needed. **Meperidine is avoided since it causes severe hypertension when given with MAO inhibitors.** The precautions about diet and medications must be adhered to for two weeks before drug initiation and for two weeks following the discontinuation of the MAO inhibitors. Table 26–11 presents other information for health teaching with this group of drugs.

Consult Chapter 21 for information about use of the nursing process for the patient being treated with psychomotor stimulants.

EVALUATION

The overall goals of intervention are to reduce the severity of the symptoms of depression and to educate the patient about the illness and the treatment regimen. Therefore, the nurse evaluates the patient to ascertain whether the depression has begun to lessen. Some positive responses include: sleeping through the night, smiling, attention to personal hygiene, interacting with other people, and an increase in appetite. The nurse and the patient acknowledge that the patient, even when improved, may still feel sad, depressed, or blue on occasion, since these feelings are within the normal range of emotions. Suicidal potential of the patient is constantly assessed as the patient begins to exhibit improvement. The nurse is alert for behaviors or statements that appear to indicate improvement but in reality are signs of continued depression. The level of knowledge the patient and family exhibit about antidepressants and the illness of depression is evaluated by the nurse.

Tricyclic Antidepressants

After the patient has been on a tricyclic agent for seven to ten days, the nurse assesses how he or she is responding. At this point, the patient will not have demonstrated marked improvement. However, the patient usually has improved in terms of symptomatology though continuing to feel depressed. The patient may be sleeping and eating better, exhibiting a longer attention span, and interacting more frequently. The family members may comment that the patient appears to be improving.

The nurse is aware that the patient may continue to feel helpless, hopeless, and worthless. Although acknowledging that he/she feels better, the patient expresses concern that the improvement is only temporary. The nurse reassures and supports the patient emphasizing that treatment is in the early phase and that continuation of the medication and other treatment will assist in the patient's progress. Eventually, if the patient demonstrated initial cues of responding positively to the tricyclic agent, the patient experiences increased feelings of improvement. If the patient exhibits no progress after a trial of three to four weeks at optimum dosage, another antidepressant agent might be considered. A common reason for failure to respond to medication is underdosing.

The patient is evaluated for common anticholinergic side effects of the medication, such as dry mouth, constipation, urinary retention, delayed micturation, blurred vision, reduced sweating, and, rarely, atropine-like psychosis.

Since cardiovascular side effects may also be experienced, the nurse evaluates the patient's vital signs on a regular basis. The frequency of checks is correlated with the rate and degree of stability of the vital signs. Tachycardia may occur. The tricyclic is withheld, and the physician notified, if the patient's pulse rate exceeds 120 beats per minute.

Patients taking tricyclics commonly experience orthostatic hypotension. When assessing the patient's blood pressure, the nurse checks and records the pressure in supine and erect positions. If the systolic rate drops more than 20–30 mmHg, the nurse withholds the medication and notifies the physician. Orthostatic hypotension is recognized as an extremely significant problem, especially for elderly patients. The patient is instructed to change positions slowly.

The nurse discusses any changes in sex drive with the patient, either increased or decreased. Discussion with the male patient includes focusing on difficulties with impotency or ejaculation. The female patient may experience decreased vaginal lubrication and anorgasmia. If these side effects are present, the nurse allows the patient an opportunity to discuss his or her feelings about these side effects and how they may relate to compliance with the medication regimen. A change in medication may be required if these side effects are present.

As the depression decreases, the patient's appetite improves, permitting weight gain. The value of weight gain is dependent on the amount of weight lost during the depression and the weight of the patient prior to the weight loss. The important benefit for the patient is to return to a state of well-balanced nutrition. It is also well documented that these drugs frequently cause weight gain, apparently without an increase in food intake.

Monoamine Oxidase Inhibitors

Patients receiving MAO inhibitors must be evaluated constantly, since these drugs have potentially serious food and drug interactions. Hypertensive crisis is one of the most potentially dangerous side effects of MAO inhibitors. The patient's blood pressure is monitored on a regular basis. The nurse evaluates symptoms such as headaches, nausea, restlessness, neck stiffness, sweating, and chills, and assesses the possibility that the patient is experiencing a hypertensive crisis. Ingestion of foods high in tyramine may precipitate these symptoms; therefore, the nurse evaluates the patient's level of knowledge of low-tyramine diet and compliance with the dietary restrictions. The nurse evaluates the patient's and family's understanding of the need to go to the emergency room immediately if any of these symptoms are experienced.

The other side effects of this group of drugs tend to be less prominent than those of the tricyclics. Interestingly, considering the side effects listed above, orthostatic hypotension is the most common side effect. It tends to diminish as the patient adjusts to the medication. The patient is reminded that response to the medication takes a period of a few weeks so that the patient does not become discouraged when there is not an immediate response and stops taking the medication. The patient is also reminded not to stop the medication when there is a positive response and the depression begins to decrease.

Psychomotor Stimulants

This is the group of medications least used for the treatment of depression. However, when used, signs that the patient's depression is lifting should be observed within one week of treatment with a psychomotor stimulant. The nurse evaluates how the person is complying with the treatment regimen. The nurse acknowledges that the potential for dependence is a risk for the patient taking these drugs and therefore evaluates the patient for signs of dependence. Signs that dependence on the drug may be developing include a false sense of well-being and symptoms of withdrawal, including irritability, increased feelings of nervousness, insomnia, restlessness, tremors, hypertension, and dry mouth.

Psychomotor stimulants may be effective in treating patients with symptoms of depression; however, it is crucial that the patient's response to the drug be evaluated on a regular basis to minimize the problems inherent with the group of highly addictive medications.

TREATMENT OF BIPOLAR DISORDERS

LITHIUM SALTS

Action

The exact mechanism of action by which lithium exerts its therapeutic effect is not entirely known. However, lithium appears to decrease catecholamine activity through processes that argue for the catecholamine hypothesis of mood disorders. Lithium reduces the release of norepinephrine from synaptic vesicles, apparently by competitive inhibition with calcium ions that normally modulate this release. Lithium also increases the reuptake of norepinephrine and serotonin into synaptosomes, thereby damping the effect of these neurotransmitters in the synapse. Another proposed mechanistic contribution in the postsynaptic lithium-induced decoupling of *"second-messenger" systems* is that cyclic adenosine monophosphate [cAMP], cyclic guanosine monophosphate [cGMP], and phosphatidylinositol are responsible for eliciting the normal cellular response to neurotransmitters. The clarification of how these events correlate to the therapeutic effect of lithium in the treatment of bipolar disorder is a goal of ongoing research.

Uses

Lithium is the treatment of choice for acute manic episodes. The frequency and intensity of subsequent manic episodes are prevented or diminished by prophylactic maintenance therapy. Marked clinical improvement is seen in 70%–80% of patients after one to two weeks. Lithium may also be effective in the prophylaxis of depressive episodes in patients with known bipolar disease.

Pharmacokinetics

ABSORPTION. Lithium is generally given by the oral route. It is commercially available as both carbonate (solid dosage form) and citrate (liquid dosage form) salts. Both are well absorbed from the gastrointestinal tract without regard to food intake. Peak concentrations usually occur in one to four hours, with complete absorption in eight hours; controlled-release preparations will exhibit a slower rate. Lithium carbonate is more commonly used, having a longer shelf-life and more lithium on a percentage weight basis than the citrate salt. Lithium citrate solution may be an appropriate alternative when questions of patient compliance arise in an inpatient setting. Certain adverse effects may be related to the rate of absorption (see "Adverse Reactions").

DISTRIBUTION. Over eight to ten hours, lithium distributes throughout total body water with uneven distribution among several other tissues. Significant concentrations are found in muscle, kidney, bone, and thyroid. Distribution into brain is slow, but cerebrospinal fluid concentrations approach 40% of that found in plasma. It is not bound to plasma proteins.

METABOLISM/EXCRETION. Lithium is not metabolized, but excreted unchanged in the urine. Decreases in plasma concentrations occur in two phases. An initial steep decline occurs for a period of four to six hours, followed by a more gradual decrease continuing over 20 hours. Half of a single dose of lithium should be excreted by the kidneys within an average time of 24 hours after oral administration. These values are based on normal renal function.

Contraindications/Precautions

Extreme caution should be taken in patients with significant renal or cardiovascular disease; with severe debilitation, dehydration, or sodium depletion; or on diuretic therapy. These patients are at highest risk of developing lithium toxicity. Careful observation with hospitalization is necessary when initiating lithium therapy in these situations, at least until the clinical condition of the patient and the serum lithium concentrations have stabilized.

The decreased renal function of geriatric patients predisposes them to a higher incidence of toxicity because of the resulting decrease in the rate of lithium excretion. The use of lower doses and frequent monitoring are essential.

The use of lithium in pregnant women should be predicated on careful benefit-to-risk analysis on behalf of the mother and fetus. Lithium does cross the placenta, and fetal serum lithium concentrations will tend to equal those of the mother. The literature has suggested that lithium may cause serious cardiac abnormalities in the newborn, especially Ebstein's anomaly, if administered during the first trimester of pregnancy. If a patient becomes pregnant while taking lithium, she should be counseled regarding the potential risk to the fetus. In general, lithium should not be used in pregnant women,

particularly in their first trimester, unless the clinical benefits clearly outweigh the attendant risks.

Lithium is excreted in human breast milk, and can therefore potentially cause serious adverse reactions in nursing infants. Breast feeding should not be undertaken during lithium therapy.

Because lithium decreases renal sodium reabsorption, sodium depletion may become a problem. Sodium depletion also increases the risk of lithium toxicity. The patient should maintain a normal diet with adequate fluid and salt intake.

Lithium is contraindicated in patients with a history of leukemia, since this condition may be reactivated upon initiation of therapy.

Long-term administration of lithium may result in hypothyroidism. If this occurs, it can be treated with thyroid hormone replacement.

Lithane tablets contain tartrazine dye, which may cause allergic reactions in some individuals. An alternative preparation would have to be prescribed in the event of any hypersensitivity reaction.

Adverse Reactions/Toxicity

The adverse effect profile of lithium involves several major systems. Relationships have been suggested between lithium blood concentrations and the appearance of some adverse reactions. Toxicity is related to both the level and duration of excessive lithium concentrations. Since toxic lithium levels are close to accepted therapeutic values, careful monitoring of plasma concentrations is considered standard clinical practice.

At concentrations of less than 1.5 mEq/L, milk toxicity may manifest itself as gastrointestinal upset (nausea, vomiting, diarrhea), fine tremor, muscle weakness, and mild polyuria or polydipsia. Some of these symptoms may present as initial effects, but resolve without intervention as therapy is continued. Taking lithium with food or milk often relieves gastrointestinal symptoms.

A serum level between 1.5 and 2.5 mEq/L may cause symptoms indicative of moderate toxicity, which may include coarse tremor with twitching, a recurrence of gastrointestinal distress, slurred speech, vertigo, sedation, lethargy, and confusion.

Lithium blood concentrations that exceed 2.5 mEq/L signify a serious risk of severe toxicity. Patients can develop hyperreflexia, stupor, or seizures. Such toxic concentrations can also lead to coma, cardiovascular collapse, and death.

Some reactions that have been reported which are unrelated to dosage include hypothyroidism, leukocytosis, headache, weight gain, edema, metallic taste, and a symptomatic nephrogenic diabetes insipidus.

Early toxic symptoms can be managed by either reducing the dose or discontinuing administration of lithium. Treatment can then be restarted at a lower dose after 24 to 48 hours. Significant toxicity should be treated with gastric lavage, correction of fluid and electrolyte imbalances, and promotion of lithium excretion by use of urea, mannitol, acetazolamide, or amino-

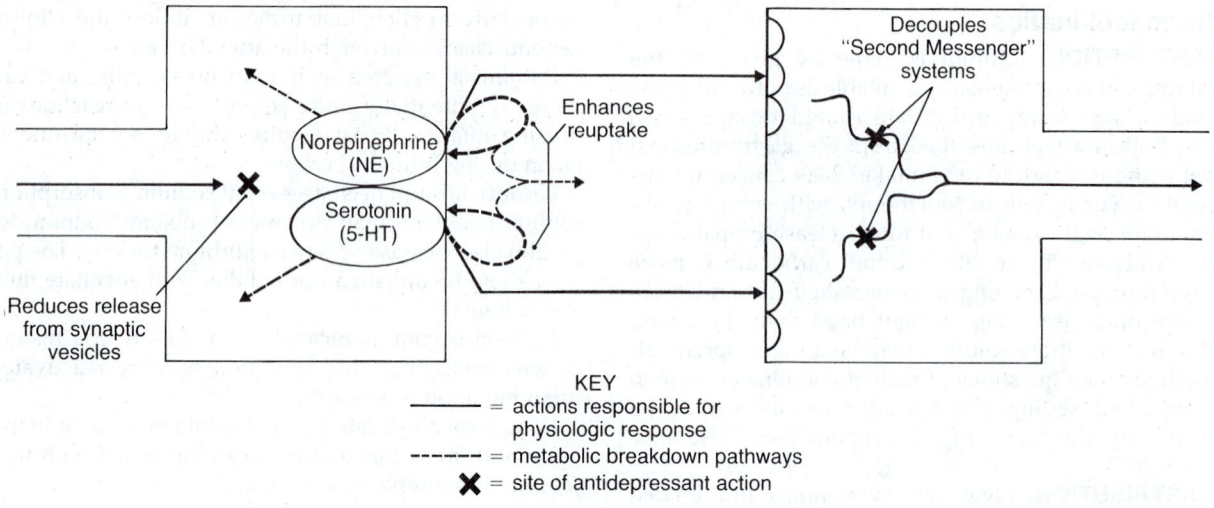

KEY

——— = actions responsible for physiologic response

- - - - - = metabolic breakdown pathways

✗ = site of antidepressant action

Figure 26–4. Hypothesized mechanism of action sites for lithium salts (compare with Fig. 26–1).

phylline. In patients with severe intoxication (e.g., serum concentrations greater than 3.0 mEq/L), impaired renal clearance, or unstable medical conditions, hemodialysis is an effective intervention.

Interactions

There are many medications that could affect lithium concentrations by altering its renal clearance. Examples of agents that reduce lithium levels by increasing renal excretion are the methylxanthines (aminophylline, caffeine, theophylline), urinary alkalinizers (acetazolamide, sodium bicarbonate), osmotic diurectics (mannitol, urea), and sodium chloride.

Conversely, agents that increase lithium concentrations by decreasing its elimination include thiazide diuretics, spironolactone, methyldopa, and several nonsteroidal anti-inflammatory drugs.

Neurotoxicity, presented as either a severe *extrapyramidal syndrome* or an organic brain syndrome with delirium, has been reported when lithium was taken concomitantly with haloperidol, the phenothiazine antipsychotics, phenytoin, and carbamazepine. The proposed mechanism of action is a synergistic effect at the receptor level.

In addition, the neuromuscular blocking effects of both depolarizing and nondepolarizing agents may be potentiated by lithium.

Dosage

If the decision is made to initiate lithium therapy, a number of laboratory tests should be performed to determine the patient's baseline status. These include complete blood count with differential, blood chemistry (including serum creatinine, blood urea nitrogen, serum calcium, and serum inorganic phosphate), serum electrolytes, urinalysis (specific gravity), thyroid function tests, electrocardiogram (if the patient is over 40 years old or has a history of cardiovascular disease), and a pregnancy test if indicated.

Determination of initial dosage is dependent on the patient's clinical presentation. For a patient with normal renal function, 900–1800 mg/day in divided doses can be given to treat acute manic episodes. Such doses generally produce serum lithium levels within a range of 1.0–1.5 mEq/L. Starting doses would be lower for hypomanic episodes or in manic patients taking concomitant antipsychotics. Although the exact therapeutic range for lithium remains controversial, current data suggest desirable serum lithium concentrations are 0.8–1.2 mEq/L for acute episodes and 0.6–1.0 mEq/L for prophylaxis. As mentioned previously, monitoring of levels should take place as often as the clinical situation dictates. Figure 26–4 is a schematic diagram of the neurotransmitter systems affected by lithium salts.

USING THE NURSING PROCESS WITH LITHIUM

ASSESSMENT

When assessing a patient experiencing an acute manic episode, the nurse observes for the criteria outlined in *DSM III-R*. The signs and symptoms include an elevated and/or irritable mood, an increase in activity and/or physical restlessness, and excessive verbalizations with high distractibility and flight of ideas. The patient exhibits increased feelings of self-esteem with grandiose ideation. This causes the person to exercise a lack of judgment regarding activities with potentially problematic consequences such as sexual indiscretions, giving money and other personal belongings away, spending money excessively, and perceived decreased need for and inability to sleep.

Since much evidence exists to formulate a theory regarding a hereditary predisposition to bipolar disorder

Table 26–12. BIPOLAR DISORDER

DEFINITION:
Group of psychotic illnesses characterized by periods of elation and overactivity and/or by periods of depression and decreased activity levels or by an alternation of the two.

TYPES:
Manic
Depressed
Mixed

SYMPTOMS:
Manic Type: increased elation and optimism; talkative, boisterous; decreased ability to concentrate; distractibility; may develop delusions of grandeur
Depressed Type: symptoms similar to ones listed in Table 21–1
Mixed Type: symptoms demonstrated will depend on whether the person is in a period of the manic type or the depressed type

TREATMENT:
Lithium carbonate or citrate is the treatment of choice. It is given to decrease symptomatology during an acute episode and prophylactically, to prevent the recurrence of the symptoms. Usually, the patient and family should have supportive psychotherapy to help them to develop insights into the illness and to cope adaptively with its long-term effects.

(Table 26–12), the nurse assesses whether any of the person's relatives have demonstrated similar patterns of mood swings. If the response is positive, the nurse determines whether the relatives were ever treated with lithium and the effectiveness of the treatment. The answers to these questions give cues about the patient's ability to be responsive to the treatment regimen.

The physician orders laboratory tests to establish baseline data on lithium levels and other serum levels prior to the start of lithium therapy. The nurse determines that the laboratory work is completed as ordered. Table 26–13 features a suggested plan of biochemical investigations for a patient on lithium therapy over the initial two-month period.

The nurse discusses both the patient's and family members' expectations from treatment. Initially, the patient may feel that no treatment is necessary because "everything is wonderful." Frequently, persons arrive for help at a treatment center just to appease the requests of significant others rather than because they believe they need help. Family members often appear overwhelmed by the patient's symptoms and fear the person's condition requires permanent institutionalization.

NURSING DIAGNOSES

When the assessment has been completed, the nurse formulates the nursing diagnosis according to the baseline data. The diagnoses focus on the patient's and family's responses to the bipolar disorder, manic state, and treatment regimen. Examples of typical nursing diagnoses for a patient being treated for bipolar disorder with lithium are highlighted in Table 26–14.

Table 26–13. PLAN OF BIOCHEMICAL INVESTIGATIONS FOR A PATIENT ON LITHIUM THERAPY OVER A 2-MONTH PERIOD

	Week					
Investigation	**0***	**1**	**2**	**4**	**6**	**8**
Urinalysis	✓		✓	✓	✓	✓
T_4 thyroxine	✓			✓		✓
T_3 resin uptake	✓			✓		✓
Free thyroxine index	✓			✓		✓
TSH	✓			✓		✓
Serum creatinine	✓			✓		✓
Serum calcium	✓					✓
Serum inorganic phosphorus	✓					✓
Serum alkaline phosphatase	✓					✓
Fasting 2-hour urinary calcium	✓					✓
Serum lithium		✓	✓	✓	✓	✓

*Week 0: the week before commencement of lithium therapy
(From Johnson, F: Handbook of Lithium Therapy. University Park Press, Baltimore, 1980, with permission.)

INTERVENTIONS

Once the physician has diagnosed the patient's specific bipolar disorder and prescribed the medications, the nurse assists the patient and family members to understand this diagnosis. The nurse encourages the patient to verbalize thoughts and feelings about the illness and the use of lithium. Frequently, the patient demonstrates a lack of information about long-term effects of this illness and the lithium treatment regimen.

The nurse develops the goals of the nursing intervention in relation to the nursing diagnoses formulated for a specific individual. When caring for the patient requiring medications to treat a bipolar disorder, the nursing goals include (1) reducing the symptoms of the illness, (2) preventing relapses of the symptoms, and (3) edu-

Table 26–14. NURSING PROCESS FOR PATIENT REQUIRING LITHIUM

Assessment
Assess level of anxiety, moderate to panic, e.g., yelling, running, withdrawn behavior, inability to concentrate. Note restlessness, inability to sleep, presence of flight of ideas, grandiose ideation and inappropriate behavior. Determine adequacy of nutritional and fluid intake, note body weight. Assess current understanding, perceptions about medications.

Nursing Diagnosis	Nursing Actions	Rationale	Desired Outcomes/ Evaluation Criteria
Trauma, potential for related to irritability and impulsive behavior, delusional thinking, angry responses.	Decrease environmental stimuli, avoid exposure to areas/situations of predictable high stimulation.	Patient may be unable to focus attention to only relevant stimuli and will be reacting/responding to all environmental stimuli.	Demonstrates self-control with decreased hyperactivity. Uses problem-solving techniques instead of violent behavior/threats or intimidation.
	Provide safe environment, removing objects and rearranging room as needed	Grandiose thinking, e.g., ''I am Superman'' and hyperactive behavior, overt/aggressive acts, can result in destructive actions/situations.	Expresses increased self-concept/esteem.
	Intervene when agitation begins to develop.	Early intervention can assist patient in regaining control, prevents escalation to violence and allow for treatment in least restrictive manner.	
	Administer medications as indicated, antimanic drugs, e.g., lithium carbonate and antipsychotic drugs, e.g., chlorpromazine, haloperidol.	Lithium is the drug of choice for mania to alleviate hyperactive symptoms. Antipsychotic drugs may decrease the level of hyperactivity and ameliorating thought disorder, if present.	
	Review consequences of own actions with patient.	Patient may have difficulty evaluating own behavior, response of others.	
Poisoning, potential for related to narrow therapeutic range of drug, lack of compliance with medication regimen, denial of need for medication or medical followup.	Provide information regarding lithium with a structured format and informational handout.	Structured education allows patient to take information in and review as necessary.	Recognizes the symptoms of lithium toxicity and appropriate actions to take.
	Stress importance of adequate sodium and fluid in diet.	Sodium and fluid are required for appropriate lithium metabolism and excretion, which is necessary to prevent toxicity.	
	Observe for/review signs of impending drug toxicity, e.g., blurred vision, ataxia, tinnitus, persistent nausea/vomiting, and severe diarrhea.	Early detection and prompt intervention may prevent serious complications.	
	Provide opportunity for patient to demonstrate learning. Clarify misconceptions, confusion about drug use/ followup.	Evaluates success of learning and helps to plan appropriate follow-up.	
	Discuss necessity of	Narrow therapeutic	

Table 26–14. NURSING PROCESS FOR PATIENT REQUIRING LITHIUM—*Continued*

Nursing Diagnosis	Nursing Actions	Rationale	Desired Outcomes/ Evaluation Criteria
	monitoring lithium levels at least twice a week upon initiation of therapy until serum levels are stable, then weekly to bi-monthly as indicated.	range increases risk of developing toxicity.	
Nutritional, altered: <u>Less than body requirements</u> related to inadequate intake in relation to metabolic expenditures as evidenced by body weight 20% or more below ideal weight.	Weigh routinely. Offer meals in a quiet, nonstimulating environment. Minimize stimuli. Offer high protein/carbohydrate diet with interval feedings. Provide finger foods. Offer foods at frequent intervals.	Provides information about therapeutic needs/effectiveness. Promotes focus on task of eating and prevents distractions from interfering with food intake. Maximizes nutritional intake and allows additional opportunity to "boost" dietary intake as patient may eat foods that are easily picked up and/or carried around.	Verbalizes importance of adequate intake. Displays increased attention to eating behaviors. Demonstrates weight gain toward goal.

cating the patient about the illness and the treatment regimen. The nurse and patient use the data base established during the initial health history to develop the plan for intervention.

During the initial stage of lithium treatment of a patient with bipolar disorder, the nurse administers the lithium according to a strict routine and monitors the results of the serum lithium level tests. The nurse schedules the blood tests early in the morning, prior to the first dose of lithium for the day and 8–12 hours after the patient's last dose of lithium. This will ensure that the lithium levels will be relatively stable. However, the nurse does not rely only on the results of the laboratory tests; instead, the patient is evaluated frequently for cues of lithium toxicity or fluid and electrolyte imbalance.

The nurse should be aware that research studies indicate that 20%–47% of patients being treated with lithium have discontinued the therapy against medical advice (Johnson, 1980). Multiple reasons have been cited for this high rate of noncompliance. These include the patient's feelings that lithium is curbing the high level of creativity and energy previously experienced during manic states. Some patients also express a strong desire to feel the high level of elation they previously felt. Another explanation for noncompliance relates to the patients' perceptions that they are being controlled by the drug instead of feeling in control of their actions. The nurse should anticipate the reality of the problem and actively encourage the patient's and family's help in preventing the complications associated with severe relapses.

General information for patient and family teaching about lithium is outlined in the nurse's teaching plan featured in Table 26–15.

Table 26–15. PATIENT TEACHING INFORMATION—LITHIUM

This drug has been ordered by your doctor. The following information will assist you to get the most help from your total treatment program. If you have any additional questions about the drug, please consult your doctor, nurse, or pharmacist.

1. This drug will help stop your mood swings.
2. You will need to take this drug for an indefinite period of time, even after your mood swings have stabilized.
3. This drug should be taken with food or milk to prevent stomach upset.
4. Drink 2–3 quarts of water per day. Avoid large amounts of food and drinks that have caffeine.
5. Do not alter salt intake without talking to your doctor.
6. You need to take this drug on a regular schedule. The dose should never be doubled. If you miss a dose, it should be taken as soon as possible unless you remember 2 hours or less before the next scheduled dose.
7. During your first weeks on this drug, you may have nausea, malaise, and very frequent urination. These problems will decrease in a few weeks.
8. Call your doctor if you have any of the following symptoms: vomiting, diarrhea, fine hand tremors, muscle weakness, or ringing in the ears.
9. You should carry with you at all times an ID card that says you are taking lithium.
10. You will need to have your lithium blood levels checked on a routine basis. *Do not fail* to get this done when ordered by your doctor.
11. This drug may make you feel drowsy, so you should check your reaction to this medicine before participating in activities that require you to be alert; for example, driving a car or operating machinery.

Table 26–16. SIDE EFFECTS AND TOXICITY OF LITHIUM

Mild (< 1.5 mEq/L)	Moderate (1.5–2.5 mEq/L)	Toxicity (2.5–7.0 mEq/L)
Metallic taste in the mouth	Severe diarrhea	Nystagmus
Fine hand tremor (resting)	Nausea and vomiting	Coarse tremor
Nausea	Mild to moderate ataxia	Dysarthria
Polyuria	Incoordination	Fasciculations
Polydipsia	Dizziness, sluggishness, giddiness, vertigo	Visual or tactile hallucinations
Diarrhea or loose stools	Slurred speech	Oliguria, anuria
Muscular weakness or fatigue	Tinnitus	Confusion
	Blurred vision	Impaired consciousness
	Increasing tremor	Dyskinesia—chorea, athetoid movements
	Muscle irritability or twitching	Tonic–clonic convulsions
	Asymmetric deep tendon reflexes	Coma
	Increased muscle tone	Death

Adapted from Harns D: Side effects and toxicity of lithium. Am J Nurs 81(7):1321, July 1981, with permission.

EVALUATION

Evaluation of the effectiveness of the nursing intervention for persons being treated with lithium is based on determining whether or not the goals were achieved. The goals of intervention were to decrease symptoms of the acute bipolar state, educate the patient and family about the illness and treatment regimen, and prevent relapses of the bipolar disorder by promoting compliance with medication recommendations.

The nurse determines if the patient is beginning to reach a level of stability by evaluating whether or not the level of anxiety has been reduced to a mild or moderate level. Also, the nurse evaluates whether the ability to sleep has improved. The nurse recognizes that as the patient stabilizes, he or she will talk and walk less. The person receiving lithium will continue to experience the emotions of joy, usual sexual desire, anger, sadness, and so forth appropriately. The effectiveness of health teaching about lithium therapy is evaluated on an ongoing basis.

The nurse also evaluates the development of side effects and toxic effects of the medication. These effects are directly correlated with serum lithium levels. Table 26–16 correlates the side effects and toxic effects of lithium with serum lithium levels.

Most patients initially experience side effects of nausea, polyuria, thirst, mild diarrhea, and a fine resting tremor of the hands. These symptoms may be felt as early as two hours after the first dose (Harris, 1981). Many patients express frustration regarding the fine hand tremor. These symptoms usually subside after the first few weeks of treatment as the patient demonstrates a positive response to the drug and the dosage is decreased.

It should be recognized by the nurse that the patient receiving lithium requires supportive, informed care in order to help him or her follow the long-term treatment regimen.

SUMMARY

Various drug therapies to treat mood disorders have been presented in this chapter. These medications have side effects that present challenging nursing care problems. Identifying the patient problems as quickly as possible and planning appropriate interventions are catalysts for assisting and increasing patient compliance with the total treatment regimen. Patient education is one of the most important interventions in any drug therapy regimen and is attended to as soon as the patient is able to comprehend the information. Drug education is repeated at various stages of the patient's illness as the level of comprehension increases.

Involvement of the family or significant others of the patient during the patient's illness assists the nurse and other members of the treatment team to achieve success with their treatment approaches. Patients experiencing mood disorders are usually unable to fully participate in their treatment plans until some improvement is experienced. The family is encouraged to assist the patient with treatment compliance and to offer support during the acute phase of the illness. The patient is consulted about his or her wishes for family involvement as soon as he or she is able to participate in the decision making process. Fortunately the length of time the patient with a mood disorder is acutely disabled has shortened significantly with the advent of antidepressant medications and lithium therapy.

BIBLIOGRAPHY

Avery, C (ed): Drug Treatment. ADIS Press, New York, 1980.
Baldessarini, RJ: Current status of antidepressants: Clinical pharmacology and therapy. J Clin Psychiatry 50(4):117–126, 1989.

Coleman, J: Abnormal Psychology and Modern Life. Scott Fores-man, Glenview, IL, 1984.

Conn, H: Current Therapy—1981. WB Saunders, Philadelphia, 1981.

DeGennaro, M, et al: Antidepressant drug therapy. Am J Nurs 81(7):1304–1309, 1981.

Deglin, JH and Vallerand, AH: Davis's Drug Guide for Nurses. FA Davis, Philadelphia, 1988.

Doenges, ME, Townsend, MC, and Moorhouse, MF: Psychiatric Care Plans: Guidelines for Client Care. FA Davis, Philadelphia, 1989.

Donlon, P and Rockwell, D: Psychiatric Disorders: Diagnosis and Treatment. Robert J. Brady, Bowie, MD, 1982.

Evans, WE, Schentag, JJ, and Jusko, WJ (eds): Clinical Pharmacokinetics—Principles of Therapeutic Drug Monitoring, ed 2. Applied Therapeutics, Spokane, WA, 1986.

Feldman, RS and Quenzer, LF: Pharmacological Treatment of Schizophrenia and the Affective Disorders: Fundamentals of Neuropharmacology. Sinauer Associates, Sunderland, MA, 1984.

Fieve, R: Moodswing—The Third Revolution in Psychiatry. William Morrow, New York, 1981.

Freedman, A, Kaplan, H, and Saddock, B: Comprehensive Textbook of Psychiatry III. Williams & Wilkins, Baltimore, 1981.

Gilman, AG, Goodman, LS, Rall, TW, and Murad, F (eds): Goodman and Gilman's The Pharmacologic Basis of Therapeutics, ed 7. Macmillan, New York, 1985.

Gold, MS, Lydiard, RB, and Carman, JD (eds): Advances in Psychopharmacology and Improving Treatment Response. CRC Press, Boca Raton, FL, 1984.

Guyton, A: Physiology of the Human Body. WB Saunders, Philadelphia, 1984.

Hanis, E: Lithium. Am J Nurs 81(7):1310–1315, 1981.

Hollister, L: Clinical Uses of Psychotherapeutic Drugs. Charles C Thomas, Springfield, IL, 1983.

Hunn, S, ET AL: Nursing care of patients on lithium. Perspect Psychiatr Care 18(5):214–220, 1980.

Iversen, L, Iversen S, and Snyder, S: Handbook of Psychopharmacology. Plenum Press, New York, 1984.

Johnson, FN: Handbook of Lithium Therapy. University Park Press, Baltimore, 1980.

Katcher, B and Young, L: Applied Therapeutics: Clinical Use of Drugs, ed 3. Applied Therapeutics, Spokane, WA, 1983.

Klein, DF, et al: Diagnosis and Drug Treatment of Psychiatric Disorders: Adults and Children. Williams & Wilkins, Baltimore, 1980.

Kline, N and Angst, J: Psychiatric Syndromes and Drug Treatment. Jason Aronson, New York, 1979.

Knoben, JE and Anderson, PO: Handbook of Clinical Drug Data, ed 6. Drug Intelligence Publications, Hamilton, IL, 1988.

McDermott, J: Ready or not here comes your patient on lithium, Nursing 83 13980: 45–48, 1983.

Perry, PJ, et al: A comparative trial of fluoxetine versus trazadone in outpatients with major depression. J Clin Psychiatry 50(8):290–294, 1989.

Stimmel, GL: Affective Disorders in Clinical Pharmacy and Therapeutics, ed 3. Williams and Wilkins, Baltimore, 1984.

Townsend, MC: Nursing Diagnoses in Psychiatric Nursing: A Pocket Guide for Care Plan Construction. FA Davis, Philadelphia, 1988.

Williams, J: Diagnostic and Statistical Manual of Mental Disorders III-R. American Psychiatric Association, Washington, DC, 1987.

Wilson, H and Kneisl, CR: Psychiatric Nursing. Addison Wesley, Menlo Park, CA, 1983.

SITUATION   26–1

Emma Ravy, a 33-year-old with recurrent depression, is an outpatient in the county mental health clinic. She is a single mother of three small children and has been unable to maintain a job for the past year.

1. Ms. Ravy is to begin psychotherapy and medication therapy with imipramine (Tofranil). During the assessment, the nurse will pay particular attention to:
   a. suicidal ideation
   b. ages of her children
   c. verbal expression
   d. occupational factors

2. The nurse is aware that the following manifestation is indicative of a major depressive episode:
   a. pressured speech
   b. feelings of omnipotence
   c. decreased energy
   d. impulsive behavior

3. Ms. Ravy is to begin taking imipramine 100 mg orally at night. Prior to administering this agent, the nurse will check for which of the following, which represents a contraindication to use?
   a. history of dysmenorrhea
   b. evidence of breastfeeding
   c. history of diabetes mellitus
   d. presence of pulmonary disease

4. The nurse will teach Ms. Ravy to avoid taking her daily dosage with:
   a. orange juice
   b. milk
   c. coffee
   d. water

5. Which of the following would be included in patient teaching regarding imipramine therapy?
   a. Take the drug as needed for depression.
   b. Expect beneficial results within 2 days.
   c. Use a strong antiseptic mouthwash.
   d. Avoid driving motor vehicles.

6. When evaluating Ms. Ravy at a return check-up, which of the following behaviors represents successful treatment?
   a. flight of ideas
   b. decreased response to pain
   c. sensitivity to criticism
   d. attention to personal hygiene

CONTINUED ON THE FOLLOWING PAGE

SITUATION 26–2

Herbert Voss is a 46-year-old with a long history of severe depression and anxiety. He is currently a patient in the chronic unit of a mental hospital. After various tricyclic antidepressant agents have proven to be ineffective alone, Mr. Voss is to begin treatment with isocarboxazid (Marplan). He is currently taking amoxapine (Asendin) 200 mg daily.

1. Before beginning therapy with isocarboxazid, the nurse will expect to:
   a. withhold all medications for at least 24 hours
   b. maintain a low monoamine diet for 1 to 2 weeks
   c. keep patient NPO for 12 hours
   d. restrict fluid intake to 1000 cc per day for 1 week

2. Mr. Voss is to begin isocarboxazid 30 mg po HS daily. The nurse will observe for the following during initial therapy:
   a. weight loss
   b. orthostatic hypotension
   c. difficulty urinating
   d. increased salivation

3. Evidence of toxic effects which would indicate altering the dosage of isocarboxazid therapy includes:
   a. headache
   b. impotence
   c. bradycardia
   d. diarrhea

4. The addition of isocarboxazid to Mr. Voss' present medication regime may result in:
   a. reduced effect of isocarboxazid
   b. increased effect of amoxapine
   c. increased effect of isocarboxazid
   d. reduced effect of amoxapine

5. With regard to food and drug interactions involving isocarboxazid, Mr. Voss is at risk for:
   a. septic shock
   b. bradycardia
   c. hypertensive crisis
   d. urticaria bullosa

6. When teaching Mr. Voss about dietary restrictions related to isocarboxazid therapy, the nurse will stress eliminating:
   a. oranges
   b. chicken
   c. eggs
   d. cheese

Please refer to the Appendices for correct answers and additional review questions with answers.

4
UNIT

DRUGS AFFECTING THE CARDIOVASCULAR SYSTEM

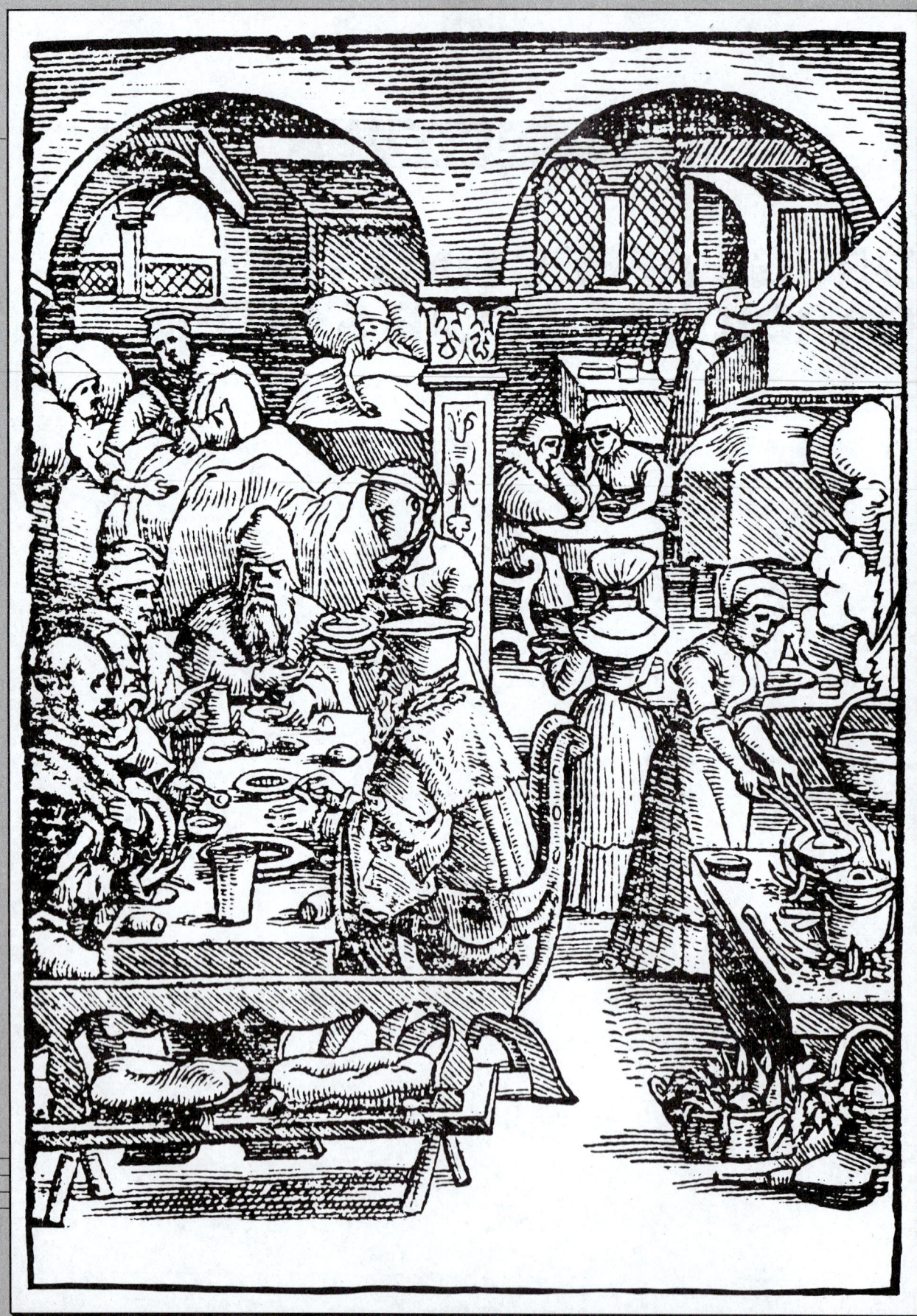

German hospital, circa 1550. Free Library of Philadelphia Print Collection.

4
U N I T

DRUGS AFFECTING THE CARDIOVASCULAR SYSTEM

GLOSSARY TERMS IN THIS CHAPTER

Afterload
Automaticity
Atrial contraction
AV block
Capillary hydrostatic pressure
Colloid osmotic pressure
Contractility
Conductivity
Diastole
Dysrhythmias
Ectopic
Elasticity
Ischemia
Mean arterial pressure
Multifocal ventricular premature beats
Mural thrombi
Peripheral resistance
Preload
Refractory period
Sarcoplasmic reticulum
Stroke volume
Systole
T-tubule

27
CHAPTER

OVERVIEW OF ANATOMY AND PHYSIOLOGY OF THE CARDIOVASCULAR SYSTEM

MERRILY MATHEWSON KUHN, R.N.C., Ph.D., CCRN

LEARNING OBJECTIVES

After reading this chapter, the student will be able to:

1. Diagram the heart, identify all four chambers, four valves, three tissue layers, and recognize the normal pressures within the heart.

2. Distinguish among the characteristics of the action potential curve and the normal electrical conduction through the heart muscle.

3. Identify characteristics of dysrhythmias including: normal sinus rhythm, sinus bradycardia and tachycardia, atrial flutter and fibrillation, sick sinus syndrome, supraventricular tachycardias, premature atrial and ventricular beats, ventricular tachycardia and fibrillation, and the conduction defects—first-, second-, and third-degree AV block.

The heart does an enormous amount of work for its size. If we take an average of 72 beats per minute, the heart will beat:

> 4,320 beats per hour
> 103,680 beats per day
> 37,843,200 beats per year
> 2,649,024,000 beats per lifetime of 70 years

This does not take into account the daily increases of heart rate caused by aerobic exercise and stress. The heart is responsible for supplying oxygenated blood to all cells of the body through about 60,000 miles of blood vessels, and for returning oxygen-poor blood to the lungs to be reoxygenated, thus beginning the cycle again.

STRUCTURE AND FUNCTION OF THE HEART

The heart, a cone-shaped hollow, muscular organ, weighing about 300 g, is located behind the sternum and is contained in the pericardial sac (Fig. 27–1). This sac is expandable and contains 5–20 ml of pericardial fluid, which lubricates the heart and prevents friction during contraction. The heart has three tissue layers: the outside tissue layer is the epicardium, a tough fibrous layer; the middle tissue layer is the myocardium, the actual muscle layer where most of the blood vessels are located; and the innermost tissue layer is the endocardium, which lines the chambers as well as the heart valves.

The heart is a four-chambered organ with two chambers on the right, the right atrium, and right ventricle, which are separated by the tricuspid valve; and two chambers on the left, the left atrium and the left ventricle, which are separated by the mitral valve. The right heart collects blood from the venous circulation and pumps it under low pressure through the pulmonic valve and pulmonary artery into the lungs. In the lungs, waste products such as carbon dioxide are removed and oxygen is absorbed. The blood then returns through the pulmonary vein to the left side of the heart into the left atrium and passes through the mitral valve into the left ventricle. The pressures generated by the left heart are much greater than those generated by the right heart. The blood exits the heart under high pressure through the aortic valve and moves into the aorta.

CORONARY CIRCULATION

Located just above the aortic valve are the two orifices of the coronary arteries (Fig. 27–2). The right coronary artery branches into the right posterior and right marginal branches, which supply blood to the right side of the heart, inferior portion of left ventricle, SA node (in 45% of the population), AV node (in 90% of the population), and posterior leaflet of the mitral valve. The left coronary artery branches into the left circumflex and the left anterior descending branches, which supply blood

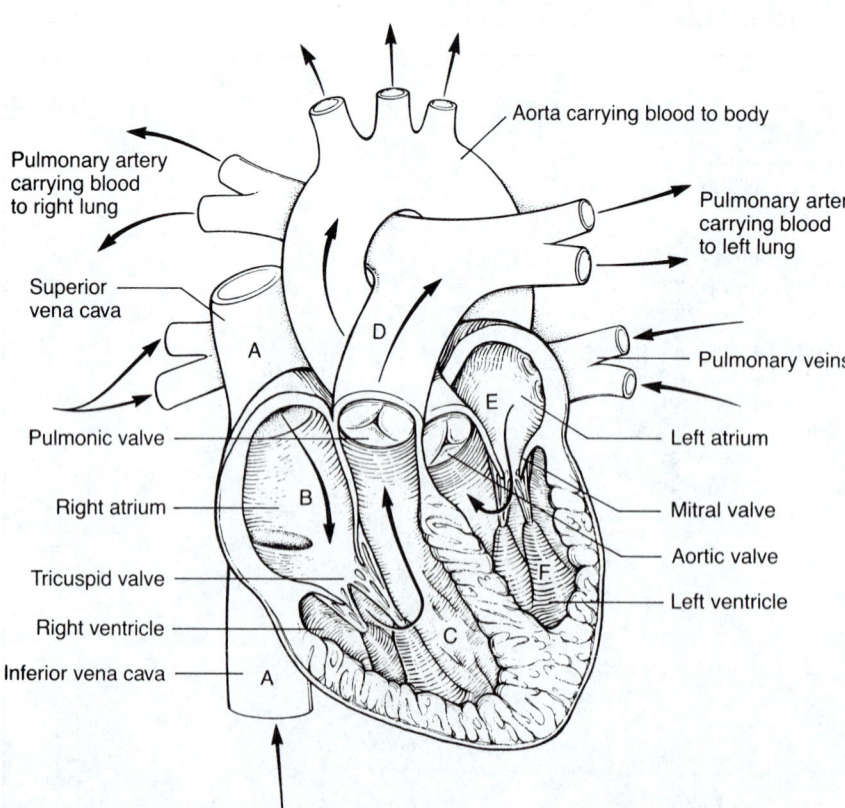

Figure 27–1. Cross section of the heart demonstrating directional flow of blood and pressures. (A) Superior/inferior vena cava 5 to 15 cm H_2O. (B) Right atrial pressure 5/0 mmHg. (C) Right ventricle 25/10 mmHg. (D) Pulmonary artery 25/10 mmHg. (E) Left atrium 10/0 mmHg. (F) Left ventricle 120/5 mmHg.

Aorta carrying blood to body

Pulmonary artery carrying blood to right lung

Pulmonary artery carrying blood to left lung

Superior vena cava

Pulmonary veins

Pulmonic valve

Left atrium

Right atrium

Mitral valve

Aortic valve

Tricuspid valve

Left ventricle

Right ventricle

Inferior vena cava

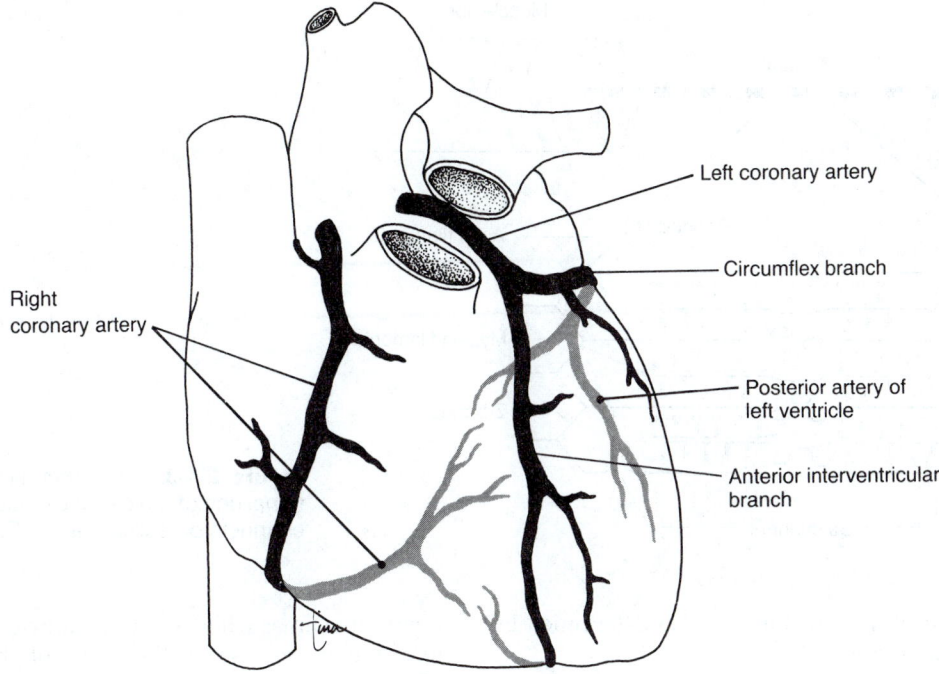

Figure 27–2. Coronary arteries.

to the left side of the heart and to the conduction system in the remaining population. Blood is returned through the coronary veins into the right atrium through the coronary sinus. When blood flows through the coronary arteries, coronary perfusion occurs, that is, the heart muscle itself receives its blood supply. Seventy to eighty percent of all coronary perfusion occurs during cardiac *diastole.*

PRESSURES WITHIN THE HEART

As blood flow returns to the right heart, pressure in the inferior and superior vena cava is low—approximately 5–15 cm water. As blood enters the right atrium, pressure rises to 5/0 mmHg. The right ventricle generates a pressure of 25/5 mmHg. As blood moves into the pulmonary artery, pressure is slightly higher at 25/10 mmHg.

Pressures in the left heart are higher, with left atrial pressure approximately 10/0 mm Hg and left ventricular pressure approximately 120/5 mmHg (see Fig. 27–1). The left heart is responsible for generating the pressure that will perfuse blood throughout the circulatory system.

CARDIAC CELL

The heart muscle comprises individual striated muscle cells called myocardial fibers. Within the *sarcoplasmic reticulum* (the inside substance of each cardiac cell), each myocardial fiber is surrounded by a cell membrane (sarcolemma) containing a nucleus and many individual strands (myofibrils). Each myofibril is composed of a

linked series of two types of contractile protein—the actin (thin) filaments and the myosin (thick) filaments. During contraction, large amounts of adenosine triphosphate (ATP) are released, allowing the actin and myosin to slide past each other and form tight cross-bridges. In order for the actin and myosin to slide, calcium must be present in the fiber. Calcium combines with a protein (troponin) found bound to actin. Normally, troponin attempts to prevent the sliding; but, when bound with calcium, it allows sliding or contraction to occur. Calcium enters the myocardial fiber through the *t-tubule* system on the surface of the cell (Fig. 27–3).

CARDIAC OUTPUT

Cardiac output (CO) is the total volume of blood ejected per unit of time. Normal CO is 5000 ml/minute. Each time the heart beats, it ejects approximately 75 ml of blood. This volume, called the *stroke volume,* is dependent on three factors: preload, contractility, and afterload.

Preload is the blood volume in the heart at the end of diastole and is measured by the degree of stretch (Frank Starling effect) of the myocardial fibers at the onset of contraction. When the heart is functioning properly, the length of heart muscle fiber is proportional to (or a function of) the amount of blood in the ventricle at the end of diastole (end-diastolic volume). In other words, stroke volume—the amount of blood ejected—is directly related to the end-diastolic volume. If stretch or preload decreases, the amount of blood in the ventricle at the end of diastole decreases (decreased end-diastolic volume), and therefore stroke volume decreases. The

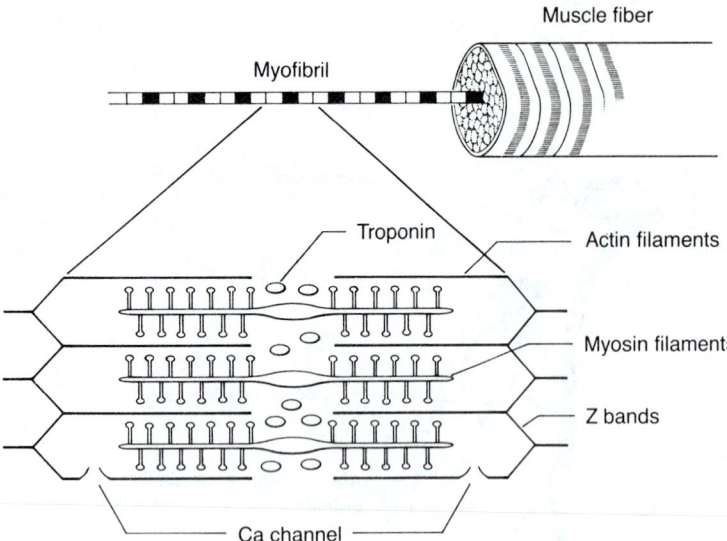

Figure 27–3. The sarcomere is the functional unit of the cardiac muscle. Calcium ion channels on surface allow Ca^{++} to enter.

amount of end-diastolic volume is also determined by three additional factors:

1. The amount of blood that has returned to the heart—venous return.
2. The strength of atrial contraction that is responsible for pushing blood into the ventricle (atrial contraction adds 20–25% to cardiac output).
3. The amount of blood that was ejected from the ventricle during the last contraction.

If any of these three factors is reduced, then stroke volume in turn is reduced.

Contractility is the ability of the ventricle to generate a force to eject the blood at particular fiber length. If the heart muscle is stretched or enlarged over its maximum because of disease, it contracts with less force and consequently is able to eject less volume. In addition, contractility is determined by the concentration of catecholamines in the heart muscle. If there is an increased level of catecholamine release (e.g., norepinephrine released through the sympathetic nervous system), there is an increase in contractility, resulting in greater stroke volume.

Afterload is the presure in the arteries leading from the ventricle that the heart must overcome for ejection to occur. It is controlled by *peripheral resistance* (pressure times the diameter of the vessel). Peripheral resistance increases in systemic hypertension, thereby forcing the heart muscle to generate a greater pressure in order to eject an adequate stroke volume.

Cardiac output (CO), the total amount of blood volume the heart ejects per minute, can be calculated by using the formula:

$$\text{cardiac output} = \text{stroke volume} \times \text{heart rate}$$

If stroke volume is 75 ml/beat and heart rate is 70 beats/min, then CO = 75 ml/beat × 70 beats/min, equaling 5250 ml, or about 5 L/min. Normal cardiac output is 5–6 L/min. Cardiac output can increase by four to five times when a healthy individual is subjected to strenuous exercise or other forms of physical or emotional stress. Cardiac output varies with the size of the individual, approximately in proportion to the surface of the body. Cardiac output is often expressed in terms of cardiac output per square meter of body area, which is called the cardiac index. The normal adult cardiac index averages 2.5–4.0 liters per square meter per minute. A cardiac index below 2.5 is abnormal.

ELECTROPHYSIOLOGY

ACTION POTENTIAL

During the past 10 to 15 years, much has been learned about the electrophysiologic events that take place inside the cardiac cells. To understand these events and how drugs work on the cardiac tissue, it is necessary to begin at the cellular level. The action potential is the electrical activity developed in a muscle or nerve during activity. Action potentials are recorded by inserting a fine electrode into any cell and observing its electrical activity, which occurs in a cardiac cell in five phases, numbered 0–4. The resting membrane potential of the cardiac muscle is approximately −80 to −90 mv (Fig. 27–4). Resting membrane potential is the potential difference across the membrane of a normal cell at rest. This resting membrane potential is a result of an unequal distribution of ions inside and outside the cell. Inside the cell there is a high concentration of potassium and a low concentration of sodium whereas outside the cell there is a reverse relationship. The difference in ion concentration on the two sides of the cell membrane results from an active transport process across the cell membrane itself. Calcium is also present in different concentrations on each side of the membrane.

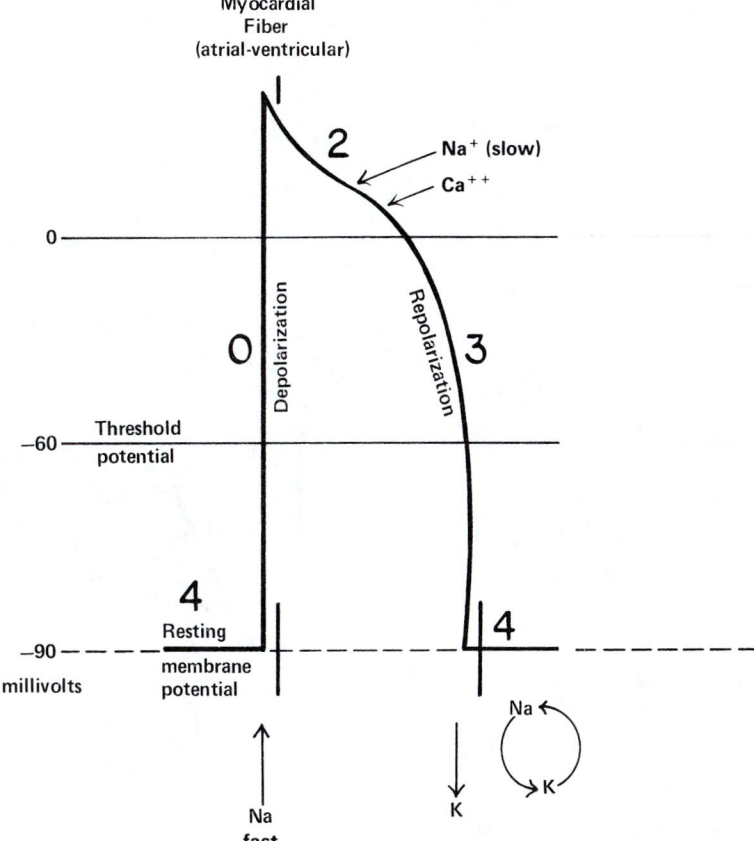

Figure 27–4. Action potential of cardiac cells. Phase 0—Sodium rapidly influxes through the fast sodium channels, and cell depolarization begins. Phase 1—The fast sodium channels close. Phase 2—The plateau phase occurs as sodium enters slowly along with Ca^{++} through the slow Ca^{++} channels. Phase 3—K^+ effluxes from the cell and late repolarization occurs. Phase 4—The cell returns to its original resting membrane potential. There is restoration of the Na^+-K^+ pump's mechanism, which actively pumps K^+ into the cell and Na^+ out of the cell.

At the beginning of rapid depolarization there is a fast influx of sodium ions through the fast sodium channels (phase 0). This is the rapid depolarization phase (See Fig. 27–3). Phases 1 and 2, often described as the plateau of the transmembrane action potential, occur when the fast sodium channels close and no longer allow sodium to enter. This is followed by a slow influx of calcium and sodium ions through the slow calcium channels. During phase 3—rapid repolarization (the return of normal negative resting membrane)—potassium effluxes from the cell. During phase 4, the cell returns to its original stable resting membrane potential, that is, with potasssium inside the cell and sodium outside the cell. Restoration of the sodium–potasssium gradient occurs through the sodium/potassium pump mechanism, which actively pumps sodium out of and potassium into the cell.

Cardiac tissue contains pacemaker and nonpacemaker cells, depending upon the function of the tissue. A nonpacemaker cardiac cell—atrial or ventricular—differs from a pacemaker cell in its action potential curve. The pacemaker cell (automatic cell) has a spontaneously depolarizing phase 4 (Fig. 27–5). This slope allows the pacemaker cell to reach threshold and fire spontaneously. The sinoatrial (SA) nodal tissue has the steepest phase 4, and the automatic cells in ventricular muscle have the shallowest phase 4. The slope allows the SA nodal tissue to reach threshold potential before other

cells; therefore, the SA node is the pacemaker of the heart. Pacemaker, or automatic, cells are found only in the conduction tissue of the heart, and all conduction tissue except the cells in the center of the atrioventricular (AV) node has automatic cells.

SYSTEMIC CIRCULATION AND BLOOD PRESSURE

Blood pressure is defined as the pressure the blood exerts on the blood vessel walls, that is, the arteries, capillaries, and veins. This pressure is generated by the left ventricle during contraction, or systole. Average blood pressure is lowest at birth and increases with age. Blood pressure increases during stress or exercise.

Blood pressure differs in the arteries, capillaries, and veins. It is greatest in the arteries and falls as blood moves into the capillaries and veins.

Arterial pressure is composed of the systolic and diastolic pressures. The systolic pressure is the maximum pressure generated by the left ventricle during its contraction (*systole*). It is usually in the range of 100–125 mmHg (torr). The diastolic pressure is the pressure exerted on the artery walls during relaxation, or the dia-

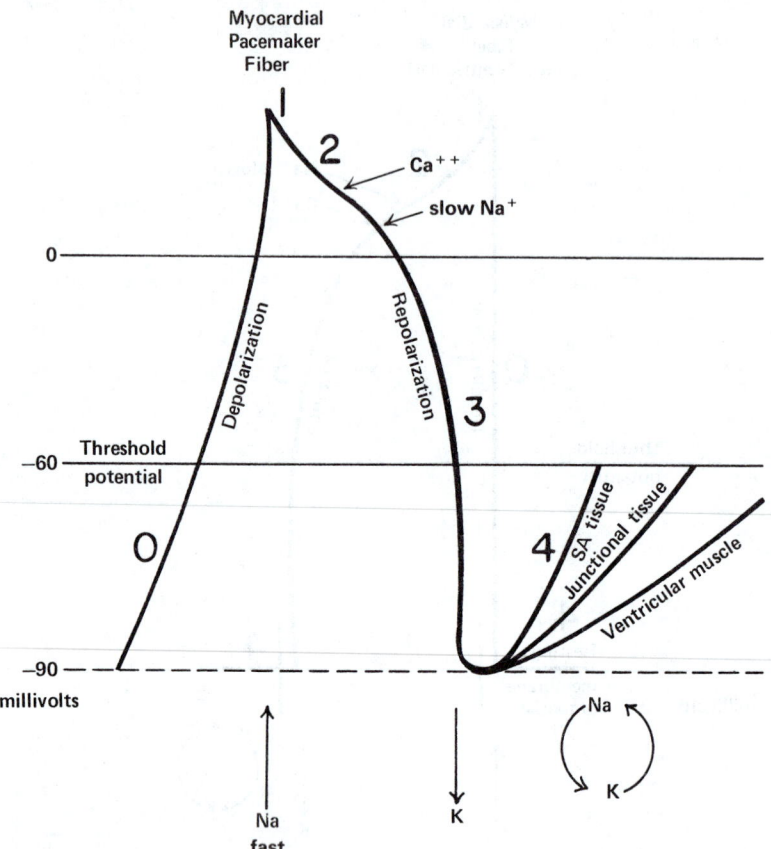

Figure 27–5. Action potential curve of pacemaker cell.

stolic phase of the cardiac cycle. It is usually 70–80 mm Hg. *Mean arterial pressure* (MAP) is a relationship between arterial and diastolic pressure:

$$MAP = CO \times \text{Total Peripheral Resistance}$$

or

$$MAP = \text{Systolic Pressure} + \frac{2(\text{Diastolic Pressure})}{3}$$

It is usually in the range of 70–90 mmHg. Blood pressure has a tendency to increase with age, as the vessels lose their *elasticity* and therefore more pressure is required to pump blood through them. The pulse pressure is the difference between the systolic and diastolic pressures and is generally about 40 mmHg.

Capillary hydrostatic pressure ranges from 30 mmHg at the arterial end to 10 mmHg at the venous end, with an overall average of 25 mmHg. Capillary hydrostatic pressure is opposed by *colloid osmotic pressure* (oncotic or protein pressure maintained primarily by albumin). The higher pressure at the arterial end is the driving force for the movement of nutrients across the capillary cell wall membrane into interstitial space (Fig. 27–6A). When the capillary hydrostatic pressure is normal and colloid osmotic pressure is low, capillary filtration increases and more fluid shifts from the vascular system to the interstitial tissues, a condition called edema (Fig. 27–6B). Conversely, if colloid osmotic pressure is high and capillary pressure is low, capillary filtration decreases, causing fluid to shift from the interstitial space to the circu-

latory system, increasing the vascular volume and producing cellular dehydration (Fig. 27–6c).

Blood pressure is maintained by the interplay of four systems: renal, endocrine, neurologic, and cardiovascular. Each of these systems is capable of elevating the blood pressure when needed.

The renal system produces and stores an enzyme called renin. It is released into the blood stream in response to a decrease in blood pressure and renal *ischemia*. In the circulatory system, renin reacts with a substrate formed in the liver, angiotensinogen, to form angiotensin I. Angiotensin I is converted to angiotensin II by a converting enzyme found, in highest quantities, in the lung. Angiotensin II is a powerful vasoconstrictor, which then constricts blood vessels in order to elevate the blood pressure. Angiotensin II also stimulates the adrenal cortex to release aldosterone. Aldosterone, a mineralocorticoid, increases the reabsorption of sodium and water in the kidney, thereby increasing blood volume and elevating blood pressure.

The anterior pituitary is also stimulated by a decrease in blood pressure. The anterior pituitary increases its release of antidiuretic hormone (ADH), or vasopressin (also a direct vasoconstrictor). Aldosterone, along with ADH, increases the reabsorption of sodium and water and causes vasoconstriction, which thereby helps to increase blood volume.

A fall in blood pressure can stimulate the sympathetic nervous system. This stimulation causes peripheral vasoconstriction, and an increased heart rate and stroke

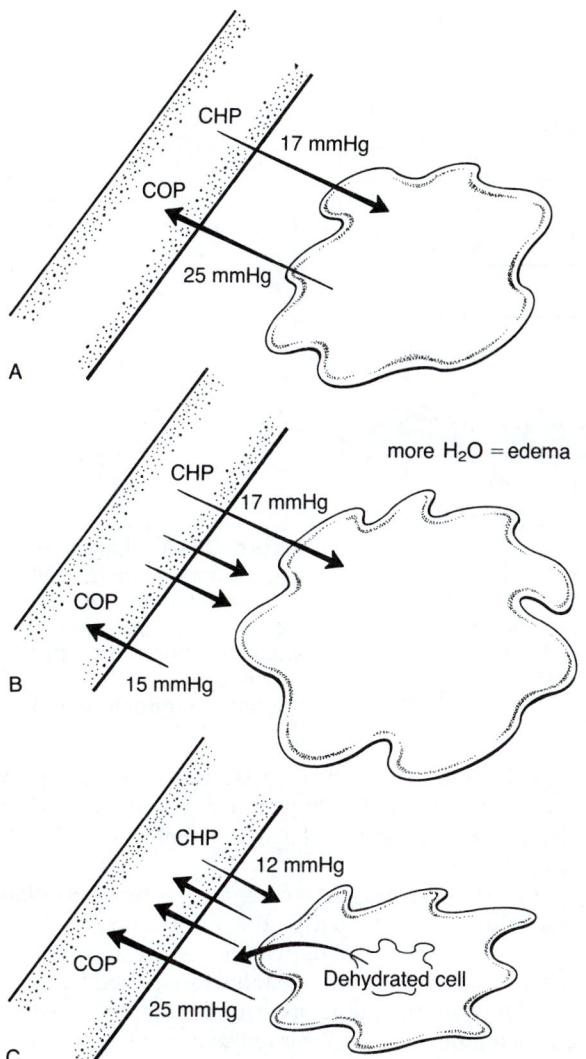

constrictor center of the medulla and excite the vagal center, resulting in peripheral vasodilation and decreased heart rate and strength of contraction, resulting in a fall in arterial pressure. Conversely, low-pressure messages from the baroreceptors elevate blood pressure.

THE CONDUCTION SYSTEM AND THE ELECTROCARDIOGRAM

The heart has its own electrical conduction system, which generally enables the heart to beat between 60 and 100 times per minute. The conduction system is composed of highly specialized cardiac cells capable of conducting electrical energy at high speeds, allowing the heart to beat rhythmically and in proper sequence. The conduction system is composed of the SA node, the AV node, bundle of His, two bundle branches (the right bundle branch [RBB] and the left bundle branch [LBB]), and the Purkinje fiber network (Fig. 27–7). The left bundle branch divides into anteroposterior, posteroinferior,

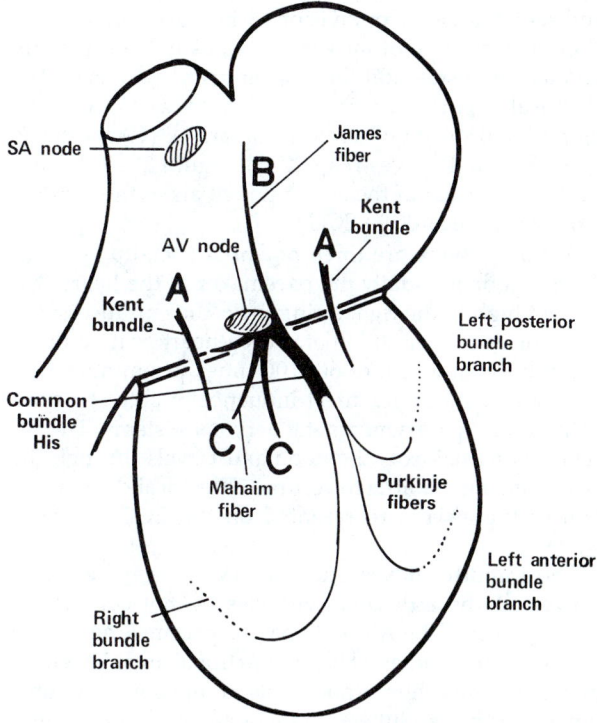

Figure 27–6. Fluid regulation. A) Normal venous capillary. Capilllary hydrostatic pressure (CHP) generated by the body in the venous system is approximately 17 mmHg. This pressure forces plasma and nutrients into the cell. Colloid osmotic pressure (COP) is pressure generated by protein that pulls plasma and waste products back into the vessel. When total protein is normal (about 7.2 mg/dl) a COP of 25 mmHg is generated in the venous system. Therefore, the net pull is always back into the vessel.

B) When capillary hydrostatic pressure is normal and colloid oncotic pressure (COP) is low, capillary filtration increases and more fluid shifts from the vascular system to the interstitial tissues. Thus, edema ensues.

C) When CHP is lower than normal, capillary filtration decreases, causing fluid to shift from the interstitial space into the circulation, increasing vascular volume and producing interstitial and ultimately cellular dehydration.

Figure 27–7. Conduction system. The normal impulse originates in the SA nodes, moves through the atrial tissue to the AV node, down the common bundle of His, and into the bundle branches (right bundle branch, left anterior bundle branch, left posterior bundle branch), and to the Purkinje fibers. Several abnormal accessory bundles can exist: (A) the Kent bundle, when activated, results in Wolf-Parkinson-White syndrome; (B) the James fiber, when activated, results in the Lawn-Ganong-Levine syndrome; and (C) the Mahaim fiber.

volume, which lead to an increase in cardiac output. The nervous system also responds to messages from the pressure-sensitive baroreceptors found between the internal and external carotids. In response to elevations in blood pressure, baroreceptor impulses inhibit the vaso-

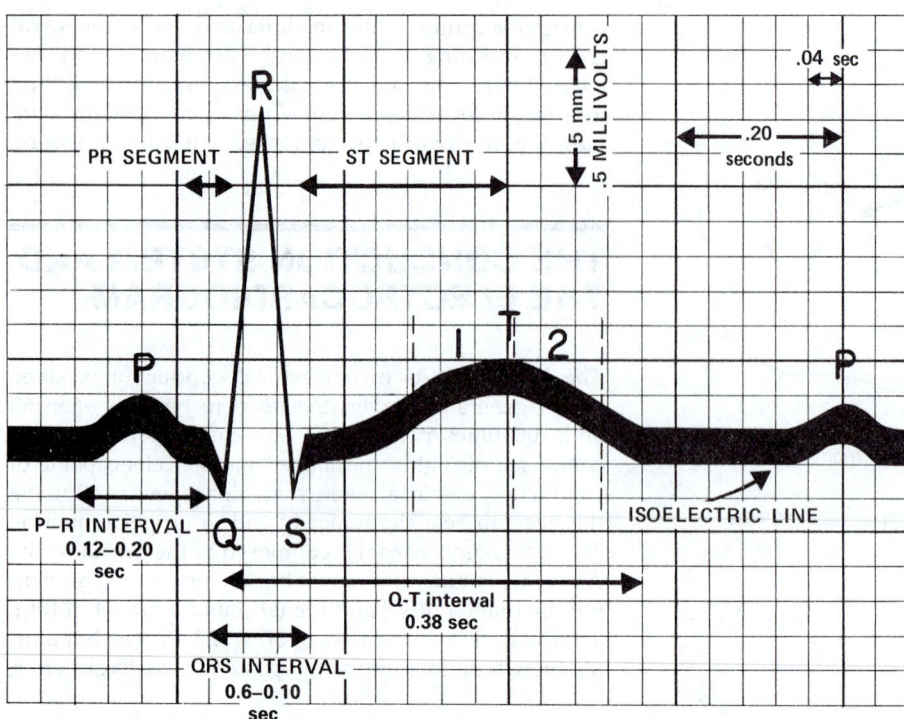

Figure 27–8. Normal electrocardiogram wave deflection and intervals. Phase 1 of the T wave represents the absolute refractory period and phase 2 of the T wave the relative refractory period.

and septal fascicles, or divisions. The Purkinje fibers are a specialized type of muscle that does not contract but acts as a transmission line for electrical impulses. The electrical events occurring in the heart are graphically represented on the electrocardiogram (ECG) by the P, Q, R, S, and T waves (Fig. 27–8). Figure 27–9 demonstrates how each of the action potentials in the conduction system record the ECG.

Although there are three potential back-up systems, the SA node is usually the pacemaker of the heart. It is located high in the right atrium near the entrance of the superior vena cava. It initiates each heart beat and normally beats at a rate of 60–100 times per minute. The SA node is under the direct influence of both the sympathetic and parasympathetic nervous systems. The SA action potential exits the node and travels through the atria, causing the atria to contract. Electrical depolarization of the atria is represented on the ECG by the P wave.

The impulse moves into the AV node, where it is slowed so the atria and ventricles do not contract simultaneously. The AV node has no pacemaking cells of its own. The bundle of His, or junctional area, generates impulses when the SA node fails to function. The junctional area has an inherent rate of 40–60 beats per minute. Atrial depolarization and the movement of the impulse through the AV node are represented by the P–R interval is 0.12–0.20 seconds in duration.

The impulse proceeds through the bundle of His into the right bundle branch to the right ventricle, and into the left anterior and left posterior bundle branch to the left ventricle. The impulse is transmitted rapidly throughout the ventricular muscle by way of the Purkinje fibers. The ventricles then depolarize or contract. The ventricular electrical depolarization is represented by the QRS wave on the ECG. The Purkinje fibers in the

ventricular muscle are also capable of generating an electrical impulse if the higher pacemakers (SA node and junction) fail to fire. Their inherent rate is 20–40 beats per minute.

The ventricular muscle now enters its repolarization phase. This is represented by the T wave on the ECG. The T wave is composed of two phases: the absolute *refractory period* and the relative refractory period (see Fig. 27–8). The absolute refractory period is the interval during which a normal cardiac impulse cannot re-excite an already excited area of cardiac muscle. The relative refractory period is the interval during which the heart can respond to an electrical stimulation if the stimulation is greater than normal. If any electrical impulse stimulates the heart during the vulnerable relative refractory period, either ventricular tachycardia or fibrillation may occur.

Between the end of the T wave and the beginning of the next QRS, the ventricles, in diastole, are filling with blood. Most of the flow into the coronary arteries occurs at this time also. Therefore, in tachycardias, there is less time for coronary perfusion. This leads to myocardial ischemia in patients with coronary obstruction. In a normal, healthy person, the decrease in coronary perfusion occurs at a pulse rate above 210 beats per minute. In an individual with heart disease, the decrease in coronary perfusion may become significant at a pulse rate over 120 beats per minute.

DYSRHYTHMIAS

Dysrhythmias are disorders of the heart rate and rhythm. Any change of rate is considered a change of rhythm.

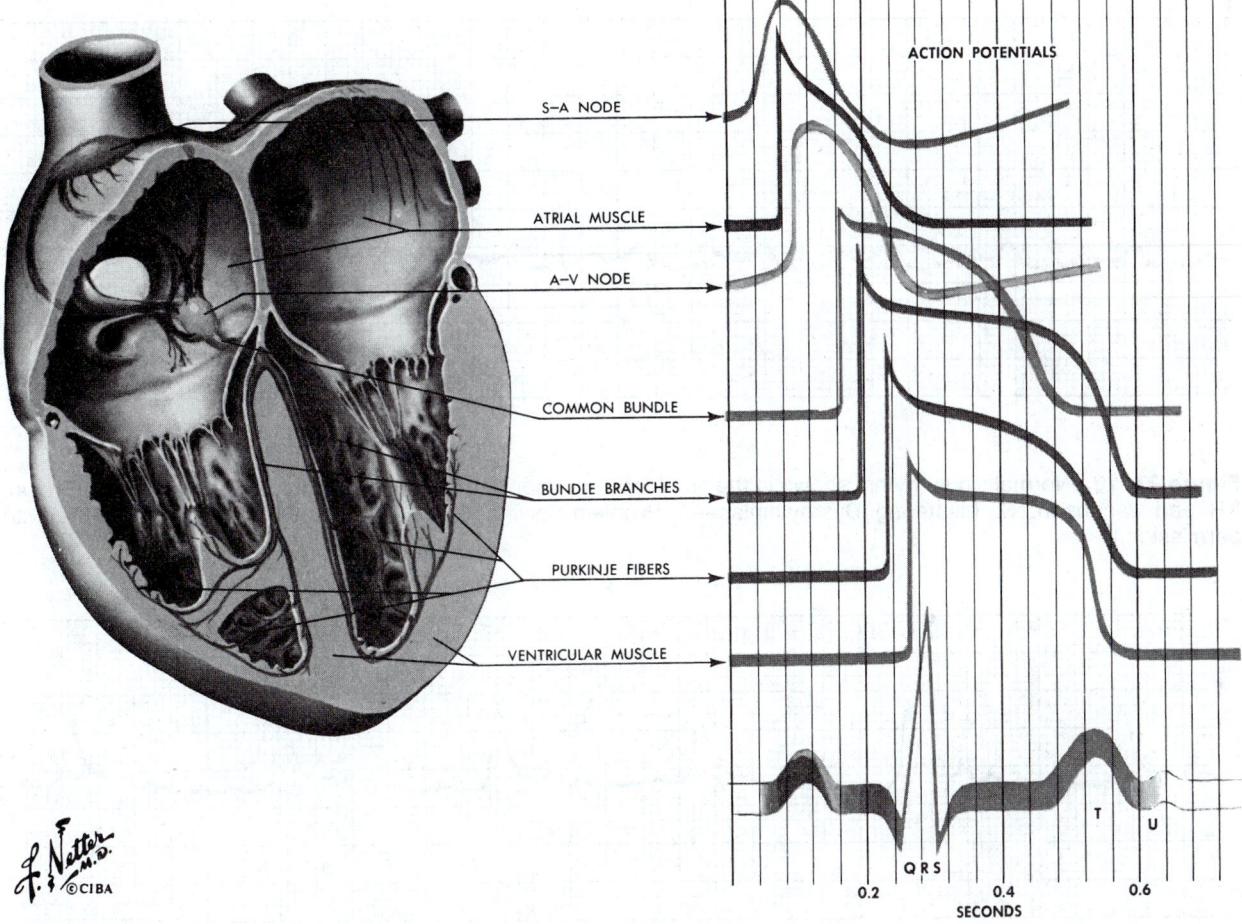

ACTION POTENTIALS

S-A NODE

ATRIAL MUSCLE

A-V NODE

COMMON BUNDLE

BUNDLE BRANCHES

PURKINJE FIBERS

VENTRICULAR MUSCLE

QRS   T   U

0.2   0.4   0.6
SECONDS

N8-65 Vol. 5/I — Heart Physiology of Conduction System II — Dr. Brian Hoffman

Figure 27–9. Composite of all the conduction system action potentials. (Redrawn from The Ciba Collection of Medical Illustrations. Vol. 5: Heart, p. 49, 1969, with permission.)

Every cell in the conduction system of the heart is capable of becoming a pacemaker, when needed, and may produce *ectopic* beats. Generally, two factors account for cardiac dysrhythmias: an increase in automaticity; and a disturbance in conduction from the SA node, or through the AV node or accessory bundles. *Automaticity* is the ability of the cells to develop an action potential spontaneously. As automaticity is increased, tachyarrhythmias or ectopic beats are produced, such as atrial or ventricular tachycardia and atrial or ventricular premature beats. When automaticity is decreased, bradyarrhythmias, such as sinus bradycardia, develop. *Conductivity* refers to the ability of the heart to conduct impulses in an orderly fashion throughout the heart muscle. Altered conductivity is associated with either a change in conduction in normal pathways or abnormal conduction through an accessory bundle. Accessory bundles are outside the normal conduction system and are known as the Kent, James, and Mahaim fibers. When these accessory bundles are activated, the patient may experience tachyarrhythmias such as the Wolff–Parkinson–White syndrome, due to activation of the Kent bundles (see Fig. 27–7A), or the Lown–Ganong–

Levine syndrome, due to the activation of the James fibers (see Fig. 27–7B).

The dysrhythmias are discussed briefly below in relation to their mechanism of action, hemodynamic results, and ECG characteristics. The rhythms discussed include normal sinus rhythm, sinus bradycardia, sinus tachycardia, and sinus arrhythmia; premature atrial beats, atrial tachycardia, atrial flutter, and atrial fibrillation; premature ventricular beats, ventricular tachycardia, and ventricular fibrillation; and the conduction defects. Please refer to other texts for additional information.

SINUS RHYTHMS

Sinus rhythms, such as normal sinus rhythm (Fig. 27–10), sinus bradycardia (Fig. 27–11), sinus tachycardia (Fig. 27–12), and sinus arrhythmia, result from variation in the rate of the SA node discharge. The SA node normally beats between 60 and 100 times per minute. Occasionally, the impulse is slower, as in sinus bradycardia (less than 60), or faster, as in sinus tachycardia with a rate usually between 100 and 150 beats per minute.

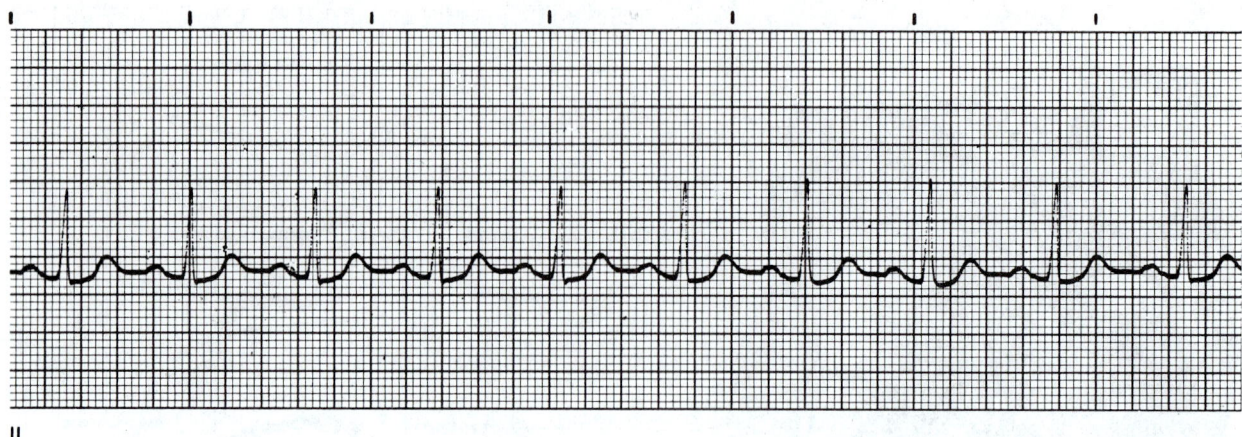

II

Figure 27–10. Normal sinus rhythm shown in the two leads commonly used for continuous monitoring. (From Brown, KR and Jacobson, S: Mastering Dysrhythmias—A Problem-Solving Guide. FA Davis, Philadelphia, 1988, with permission.)

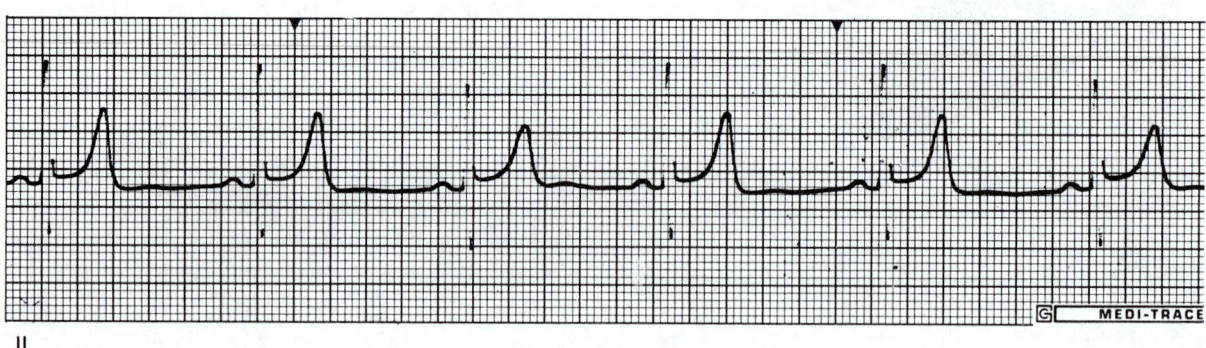

II

Figure 27–11. Sinus bradycardia (50/min). (From Brown, KR and Jacobson, S: Mastering Dysrhythmias—A Problem-Solving Guide. FA Davis, Philadelphia, 1988, with permission.)

Both of these rhythms are regular and appear normal on the ECG. There is only a change in heart rate. Both sinus bradycardia and sinus tachycardia have a similar effect on cardiac output. Although cardiac output may rise slightly in the early stages of these rhythms, eventually cardiac output falls, particularly in a patient with heart disease.

In sinus arrhythmia, the rate increases with inspiration and decreases with expiration due to an interaction or interplay of the cardiac/respiratory fibers in the medulla. This rhythm is brought about by a variation in vagal tone and occurs normally in children and young adults. This is a benign dysrhythmia that does not cause any significant hemodynamic changes.

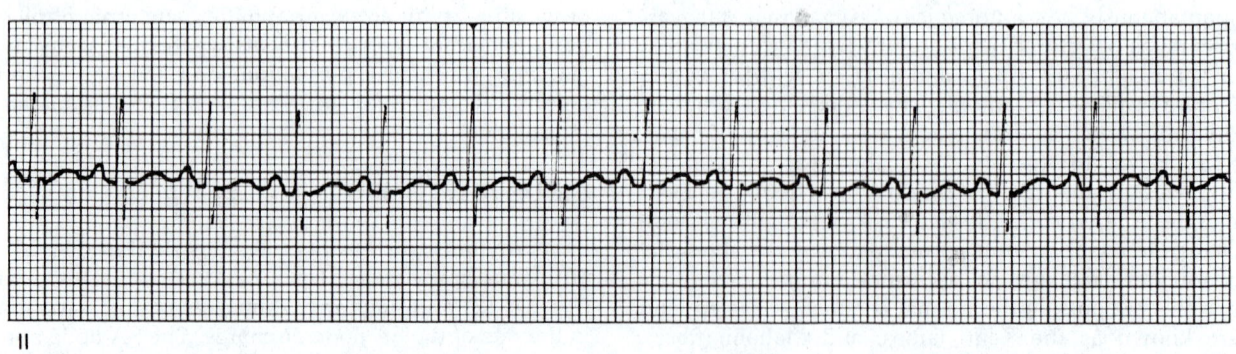

II

Figure 27–12. Sinus tachycardia (120/min). (From Brown, KR and Jacobson, S: Mastering Dysrhythmias—A Problem-Solving Guide. FA Davis, Philadelphia, 1988, with permission.)

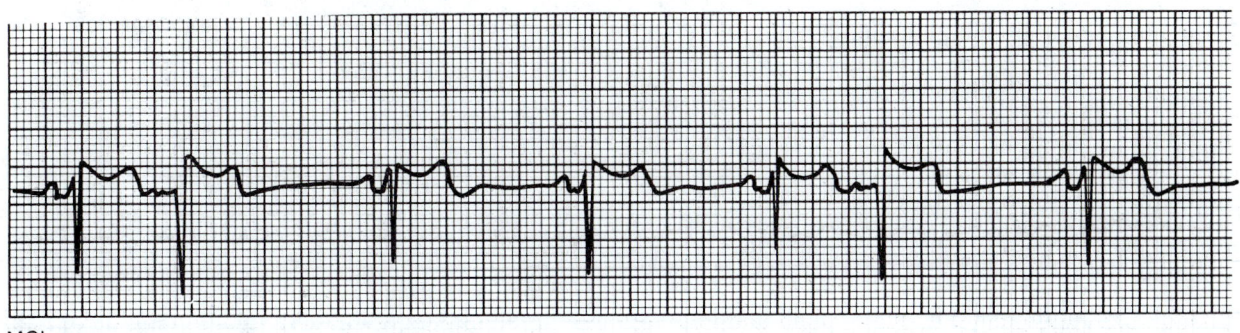

MCL₁

Figure 27–13. Premature supraventricular complexes (PACs) (beats 2 and 6). (From Brown, KR and Jacobson, S: Mastering Dysrhythmias—A Problem-Solving Guide. FA Davis, Philadelphia, 1988, with permission.)

Sick sinus syndrome is one of the most common conditions today necessitating the implantation of a pacemaker. As sick sinus syndrome occurs, the sinus node loses its ability to function as the pacemaker of the heart. A lower pacemaker, generally the junction, then takes over.

Sick sinus syndrome is generally found in the elderly and results from abnormalities of the SA node's automaticity and conduction. Sick sinus syndrome can be familial or congenital, can occur in ischemic, rheumatic, hypertensive, or infiltrative cardiac diseases, or can be idiopathic.

ATRIAL DYSRHYTHMIAS

Atrial dysrhythmias, including premature atrial contractions, atrial tachycardia, atrial flutter, and atrial fibrillation, result from a change in the pacemaker location from the SA node to the atrial tissue. The etiology of most atrial dysrhythmias is unknown. Since the direction of forces through the atria is different for every ectopic atrial focus, the P wave has a slightly different configuration on the ECG.

Premature atrial contractions (PACs) (Fig. 27–13) are premature beats that arise in the atria before the normal impulse. Because they occur early, there is a decrease in stroke volume. The P wave looks different because it arises from a site within atrial tissue rather than in the SA node, but the QRS remains the same.

Atrial tachycardia (AT) is a fast, regular atrial rhythm arising from the atrial tissue. It has a rate of 200 ($\pm$50) beats per minute. The P wave has a slightly different configuration from the normal P wave, but the QRS configuration usually remains the same. If the ventricles respond to each atrial impulse and if the ventricular rate is over 200 in a healthy heart, or at slower rates in a damaged heart, there is a resultant decrease in coronary perfusion, causing a decrease in cardiac output, myocardial ischemia, or even angina. Paroxysmal atrial tachycardia occurs when there is an abrupt beginning and end to the tachycardia.

Atrial flutter (Fig. 27–14) is usually found in patients who have heart disease. The atria beat at a rate of 300 $\pm$50 beats per minute. The AV node is incapable of transmitting impulses this fast, so there is always some degree of AV BLOCK. Therefore, a flutter-to-ventricles ratio of 2:1 or more is usual. Likewise, there is a decrease in cardiac filling because the atria are not contracting normally and do not contribute their effect. *Atrial contraction* adds 20%–25% to cardiac output.

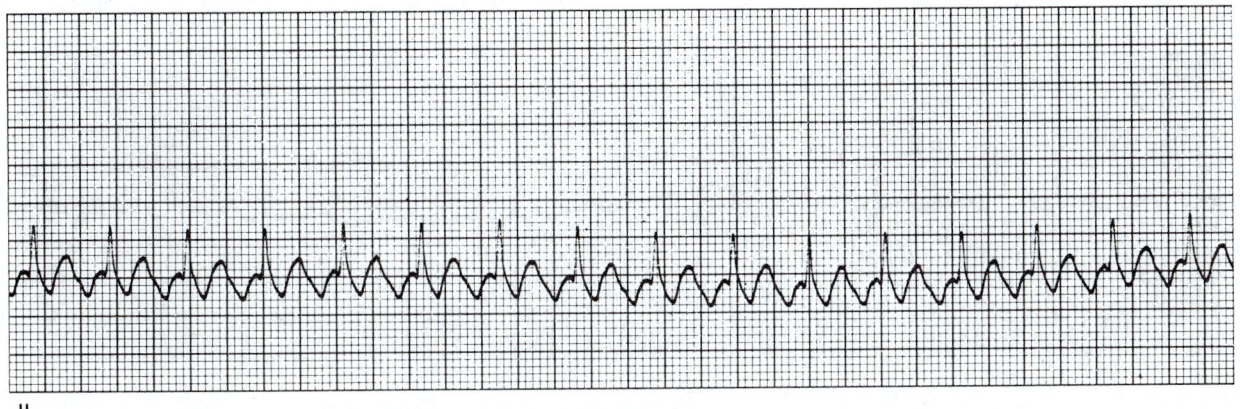

II

Figure 27–14. Atrial flutter with 2:1 AV conduction. (From Brown, KR and Jacobson, S: Mastering Dysrhythmias—A Problem-Solving Guide. FA Davis, Philadelphia, 1988, with permission.)

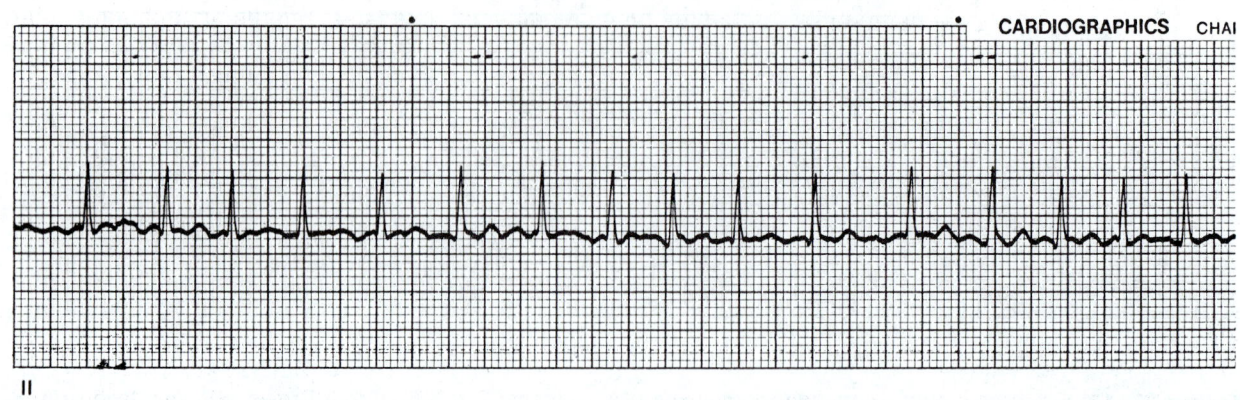

II

Figure 27–15. Atrial fibrillation with tachycardiac (120/min) ventricular response. Ventricular rate = usually 100 to 160/min; if medicated, usually less than 100/min. Ventricular rhythm = irregularly irregular R–R intervals. QRS shape = normal. QRS duration = normal unless pre-existing conduction disease exists. (From Brown, KR and Jacobson, S: Mastering Dysrhythmias—A Problem-Solving Guide. FA Davis, Philadelphia, 1988, with permission.)

Atrial contraction is often called the "booster pump" effect or atrial kick. The atrial depolarization waves resemble the teeth of a saw, often called F waves, whereas the QRS waves maintain their usual appearance.

In atrial fibrillation (Fig. 27–15), the atria no longer contract but are quivering at a rate of 400 ± 50 beats per minute. The ventricles contract sporadically, resulting in a rhythm that is totally irregular. There is a decrease in cardiac output due to the lack of atrial contraction and therefore poor ventricular filling. Since the atria are not contracting but fibrillating, there are no true P waves on the ECG, but only an irregular, chaotic baseline called f waves. The QRS waves generally maintain their usual appearance. Patients in atrial fibrillation have an increased risk of developing *mural thrombi* (thrombi involving the wall). These thrombi can break off and become emboli, often lodging in the vascular system of the brain.

Supraventricular tachycardias (SVTs) (Fig. 27–16) are tachycardias that originate in the sinus, atrial, or junctional tissue. The QRS complex is normal in shape and width, and the T waves have the same shape as the sinus beat.

None of the dysrhythmias discussed above are immediately life threatening unless the heart has already compensated for some abnormality by using all its reserve mechanisms. These dysrhythmias may, however, cause symptoms of either palpitations or heart failure of varying degrees.

VENTRICULAR DYSRHYTHMIAS

Three ventricular dysrhythmias—premature ventricular contractions (PVCs), ventricular tachycardia (VT), and ventricular fibrillation (VF)—are due to the spontaneous generation of abnormal impulses in the ventricle.

Premature ventricular contractions (Fig. 27–17A,B) arise from some ectopic focus in the ventricular muscle. Because these ectopic impulses arise prematurely, the ventricle contracts before the atrium has contracted and filled it with blood, resulting in a decreased stroke volume. Therefore, a peripheral pulse may not be palpable

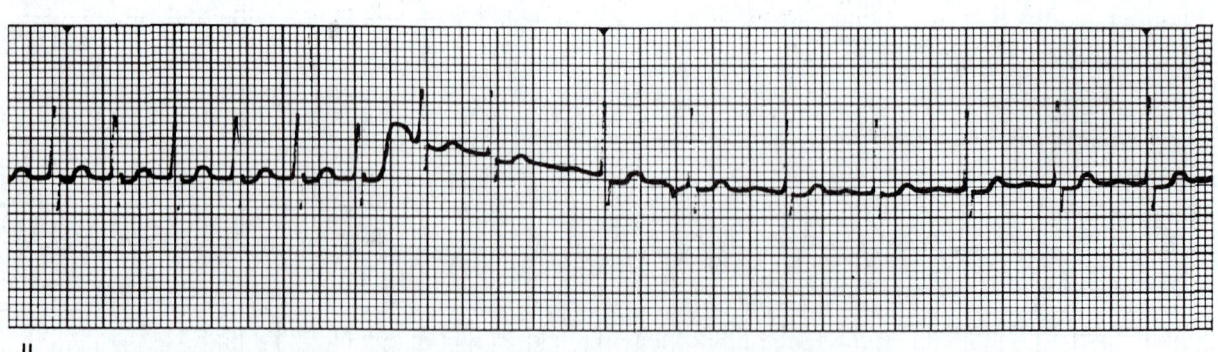

II

Figure 27–16. Supraventricular dysrhythmias. Abrupt conversion from PSVT to a sinus rhythm. (From Brown, KR and Jacobson, S: Mastering Dysrhythmias—A Problem-Solving Guide. FA Davis, Philadelphia, 1988, with permission.)

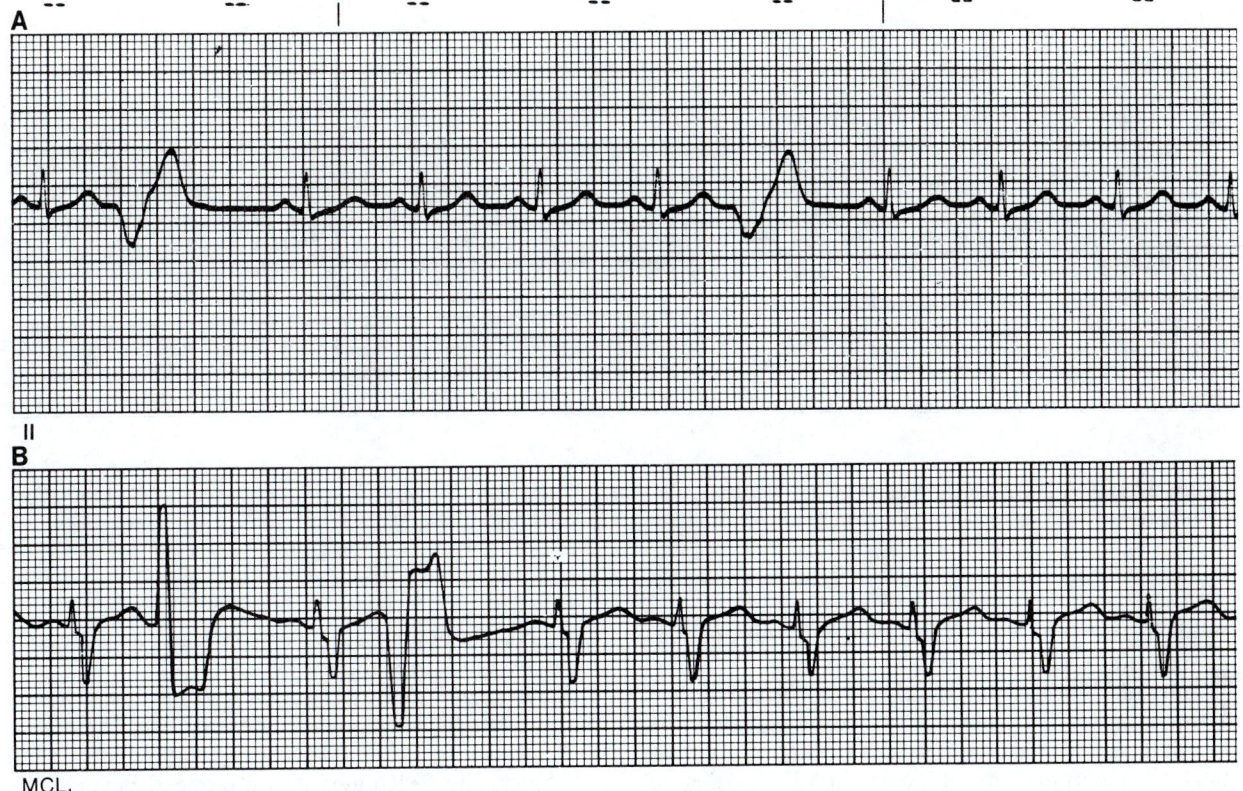

Figure 27–17. A) Premature ventricular complexes (PVCs). Two uniformed PVCs (beats 2 and 7). B) Premature ventricular complexes. Multiformed PVCs (beats 2 and 4). (From Brown, KR and Jacobson, S: Mastering Dysrhythmias—A Problem-Solving Guide. FA Davis, Philadelphia, 1988, with permission.)

during a PVC. Since PVCs originate in the ventricle, the QRS wave is wide and bizarre. PVCs are followed by a full compensatory pause. Predisposing causes for the development of PVCs include hypoxia, myocardia ischemia, and electrolyte disturbances. In a coronary care unit, PVCs must be treated if (1) there are two PVCs in a row, called paired PVCs or couplets; (2) there are *multiform* PVCs (Fig. 27–17B); (3) there are more than six PVCs per minute; or (4) the PVCs begin to move toward

or appear on the T wave (this is known as the R-on-T phenomenon). Any of these conditions can lead to lethal dysrhythmias such as VT or VF.

Ventricular tachycardia (Fig. 27–18), three or more PVCs in a row, is a result of an ectopic pacemaker in the ventricle firing faster than the higher pacemakers. There is generally very little cardiac output because of decreased filling time and poor coronary perfusion. The patient may lose consciousness in a short time. The

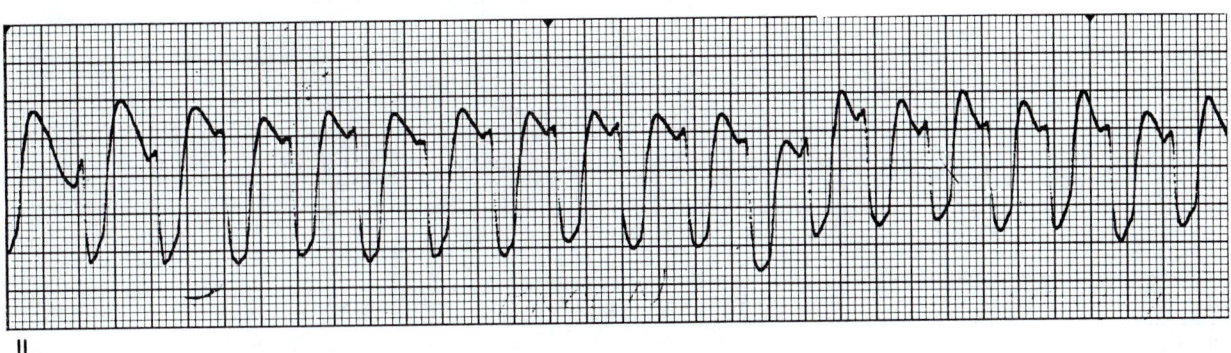

Figure 27–18. Ventricular tachycardia (160/min). (From Brown, KR and Jacobson, S: Mastering Dysrhythmias—A Problem-Solving Guide. FA Davis, Philadelphia, 1988, with permission.)

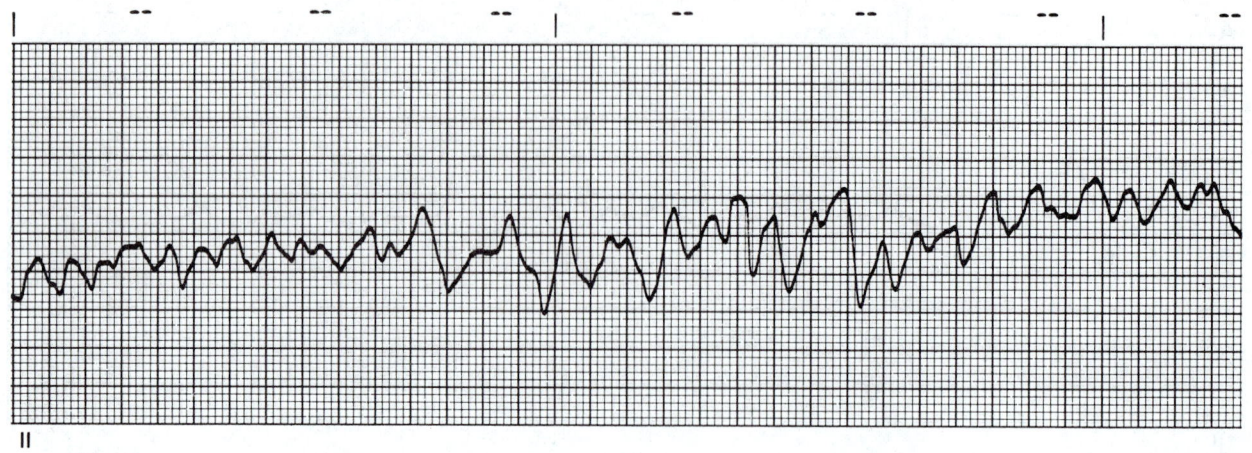

Figure 27–19. Ventricular fibrillation. Coarse ventricular fibrillation. (From Brown, KR and Jacobson, S: Mastering Dysrhythmias—A Problem-Solving Guide. FA Davis, Philadelphia, 1988, with permission.)

complexes are wide and bizarre, and P waves are usually difficult to see.

Ventricular fibrillation (Fig. 27–19) is a terminal dysrhythmia unless the patient is treated immediately. Irreversible cerebral damage begins to occur approximately four minutes after the onset of VF. There is no cardiac output or coronary perfusion because the heart is no longer contracting but is fibrillating. No peripheral pulses can be palpated, and the patient may lose consciousness within ten seconds after the onset of VF. On the ECG there is a wavy, irregular chaotic baseline with no regular P or QRS impulses.

CONDUCTION DEFECTS

Conduction defects occur because of blocks or delays in the transmission of impulses at different points among the conduction system. These can be due to the effect of ischemia, scar tissue, vagotonia, or drugs such as digitalis products on the conduction system. These blocks can be partial, as with first-degree AV block or incomplete bundle branch block, or complete, as with complete AV block or complete bundle block.

A first-degree AV block (Fig. 27–20) is due to abnormal slowing of the impulse in the AV node. The normal P–R interval is 0.12–0.20 seconds long. In first-degree AV block, the P–R interval is prolonged beyond 0.20 seconds, and only a prolonged P–R interval is seen on the ECG. In second-degree AV block (Fig. 27–21), the AV node is unable to transmit all the impulses moving through it, and therefore there are more P waves than QRS waves on the ECG. Conduction through the AV node occurs at a ratio of 2:1 or greater.

In third-degree or complete AV block (Fig. 27–22), the AV node is no longer able to transmit impulses. The atria continue to contract at their usual rate, but the impulses cannot get through the AV node. Shortly after the block occurs, a focus in the ventricle reaches threshold potential and begins to contract rhythmically at a rate of 20–40 beats per minute. There are now two pacemakers in the heart, the SA node and the ventricular pacemaker, each contracting at its own rate independent

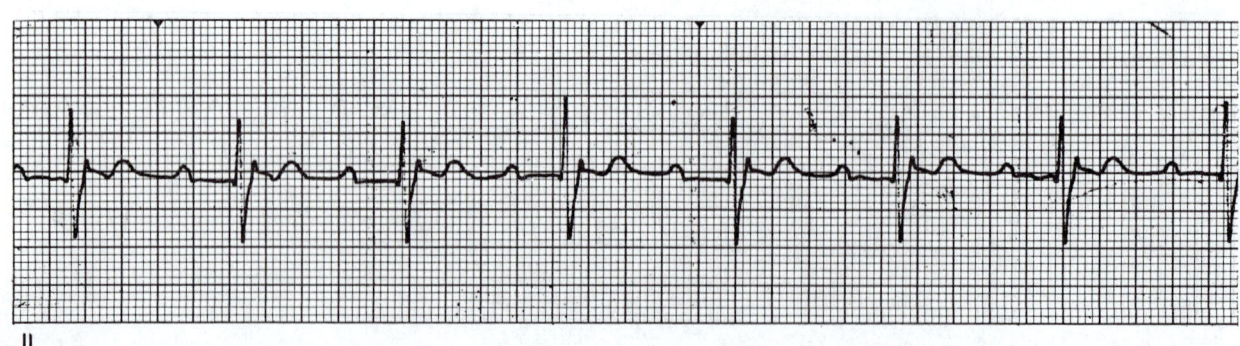

Figure 27–20. First degree AV heart block (P–R interval is 0.32 sec). (From Brown, KR and Jacobson, S: Mastering Dysrhythmias—A Problem-Solving Guide. FA Davis, Philadelphia, 1988, with permission.

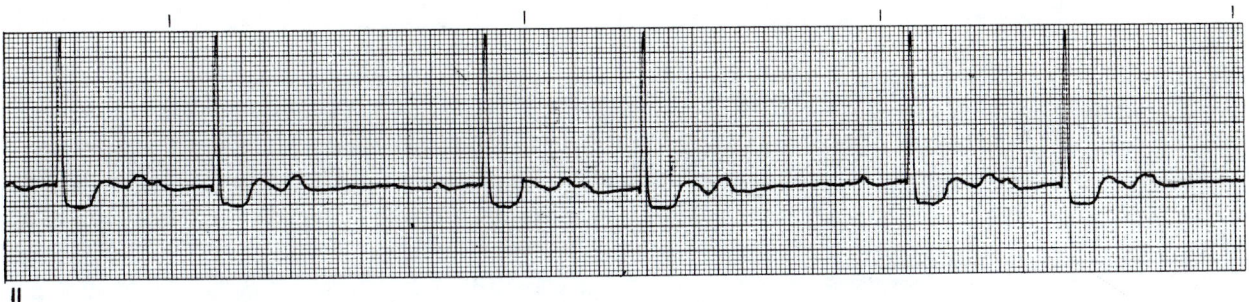

II

Figure 27-21. Second degree AV block; Mobitz type 1 (Wenckebach); 3:2 AV conduction ratio. (From Brown, KR and Jacobson, S: Mastering Dysrhythmias—A Problem-Solving Guide. FA Davis, Philadelphia, 1988, with permission.)

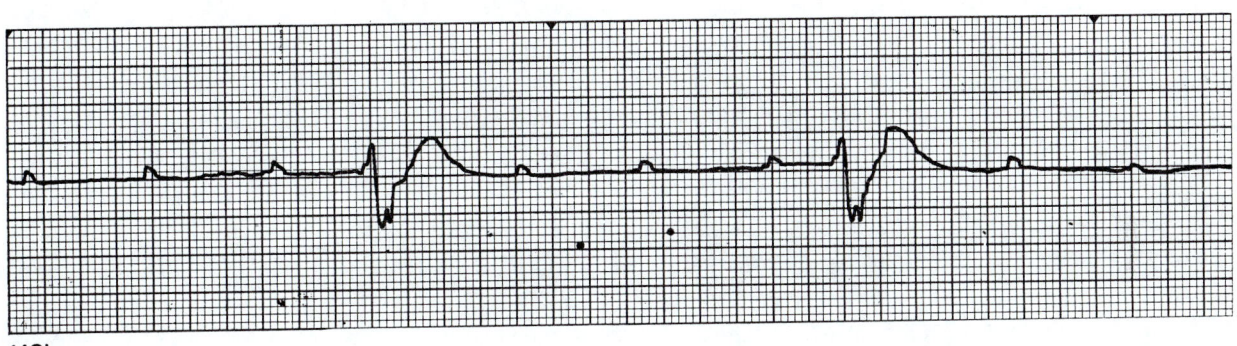

MCL₁

Figure 27-22. Third degree AV heart block (complete heart block). (From Brown, KR and Jacobson, S: Mastering Dysrhythmias—A Problem-Solving Guide. FA Davis, Philadelphia, 1988, with permission.)

of the other. Cardiac output usually falls because of the lowered heart rate. This may result in Stokes–Adams syndrome (a condition caused by heart block and characterized by sudden attacks of unconsciousness, with or without convulsions).

tem is composed of highly specialized cardiac cells capable of conducting electrical energy at high speeds, allowing the heart to beat rhythmically and in proper sequence. Dysrhythmias can occur which are disorders of either the heart rate or rhythm.

SUMMARY

The heart, a hollow cone-shaped organ located behind the sternum, is protected by the pericardial sac. The heart receives its blood supply via the coronary arteries, primarily during diastole. The heart is responsible for generating cardiac output which averages about 5 liters per minute. The stroke volume which the heart ejects per beat is dependent on preload, contractility, and afterload. Each cardiac cell is capable of generating an action potential which is the electrical activity that occurs within each cell. The heart also has its own conduction system which generally enables the heart to beat between 60 to 100 times per minute. The conduction sys-

BIBLIOGRAPHY

Brown K and Jacobson S: Mastering Dysrhythmias. FA Davis, Philadelphia, 1988.
Constant J: Learning Electrocardiography (A Complete Course). Little, Brown & Co, Boston, 1981.
Guyton A: The Textbook of Medical Physiology. WB Saunders, Philadelphia, 1986.
Hampton JR: The ECG in Practice. Churchill Livingstone, New York, 1986.
Hampton JR: The ECG Made Easy. Churchill Livingstone, New York, 1986.
Marriott H and Conover M: Advanced Concepts in Arrhythmias. CV Mosby, St. Louis, 1989.
Netter F: The CIBA Collection of Medical Illustrations—Heart, Vol 5. Ciba Pharmaceutical, New York, 1969.

28
CHAPTER

CARDIAC GLYCOSIDES

MERRILY MATHEWSON KUHN, R.N.C., Ph.D., CCRN

LEARNING OBJECTIVES

After reading this chapter, the student will be able to:

1. Identify those medications commonly used as cardiac glycosides.

2. Differentiate among the cardiac glycosides as to mechanism of action, route of administration, pharmacokinetics, adverse and toxic effects, contraindications, and interactions.

3. Identify specific areas to assess in the patient requiring cardiac glycosides in order to formulate appropriate nursing diagnoses.

4. Plan the nursing interventions necessary to administer cardiac glycosides and choose appropriate teaching strategies to gain patient compliance.

5. Evaluate the patient at various stages of treatment to gauge nursing interactions.

THERAPEUTIC AGENTS

DIGITALIS AND DIGITALIS-LIKE DRUGS

Cardiac glycosides, like other positive inotropic agents, are medications that increase the contractile force of the heart, causing the ventricles to empty more completely and thus improving cardiac output. The digitalis glycosides, including digitalis and digitalis-like drugs, are the oldest and most commonly used positive *inotropic* agents (agents increasing the force of contraction), and have been in recorded use since 1775. They were first used by William Withering of England as a "cure" for dependent edema in the lower extremities caused by heart failure, referred to as dropsy in older literature.

The term *digitalis* is sometimes used to designate the

Table 28–1. CONGESTIVE HEART FAILURE

Definition:

a group of symptoms indicating the presence of excessive amounts of blood or tissue fluid in the heart and tissue proximal to the heart resulting from failure of the heart to maintain adequate circulation of blood.

TYPES:
Chronic left-sided heart failure
Acute left-sided heart failure (acute pulmonary edema)
Chronic right-sided heart failure

ETIOLOGY: hypertension, infections, pericardial effusion, valvular insufficiency, coronary disease, congenital malformations, arteriosclerosis, constrictive pericarditis, atherosclerosis, hyperthyroidism.

Symptoms:

	Acute Left-Sided Heart Failure	Chronic Left-Sided Heart Failure	Chronic Right-Sided Heart Failure
Dyspnea	x	x	x
Cardiac asthma	x	x	–
Statis systemic and portal circulation	–	–	x
Peripheral edema	–	–	x
Cyanosis	x	x	x
Hypertrophy Heart	x	x	x
Fatigue	–	x	x
Weakness	–	x	x
Mental confusion	x	x	x
Shortness of breath	x	x	–
Pink frothy sputum	x	–	–
Paroxysmal nocturnal dyspnea	–	x	–
Hepatomegaly	–	–	x
Ascites	–	–	x
Anorexia	–	–	x
Distended neck veins	–	–	x

x = Symptoms applicable to condition

MEDICAL MANAGEMENT OF CONGESTIVE HEART FAILURE

	Acute Left-Sided Heart Failure	Chronic Left-Sided Heart Failure	Chronic Right-Sided Heart Failure
Cardiac glycosides	x	x	x
Diuretics	x	x	x
Recording I and O	x	x	x
Daily weights	x	x	x
Restriction of Na and fluids	x	x	x
Limited activities	x	x	x
Psychologic support	x	x	x
O₂ therapy	x	x	x
Morphine	x	–	–
Rotating tourniquets	x	–	–
Vasodilators	x	x	x
Angiotensin-converting enzyme inhibitors	x	x	–

x = applicable to condition

entire class of digitalis glycosides. All digitalis glycosides are potent in very low doses and their therapeutic effects on the heart are qualitatively similar. They are composed of three parts: a sugar, a steroid, and a lactone. The sugar increases the water solubility and absorption, and modifies toxicity. The steroid is similar to the sex hormones and corticosteroids. The lactone is responsible for the properties associated with the cardiac glycosides. They are all produced from a natural source, either *Digitalis purpurea*, the purple foxglove, or *Digitalis lanata*, the white foxglove, or the seed of *Strophanthus gratus* (ouabain). There is no synthetic source of cardiac glycosides at this time. Foxglove is a beautiful flowering plant native to the northern United States, Europe, and Australia. If small animals or children consume the flowers or leaves of the foxglove, they are likely to develop the signs and symptoms of digitalis overdose. Other natural sources of the digitalis glycosides include the bulb of the sea onion, the flowers of the lily of the valley and Christmas rose, and the venom of certain toads, but the expense of purifying these substances prevents their clinical use.

Approximately 10% of all hospitalized patients receive digitalis glycosides. Digoxin is reputed to be the fourth most commonly prescribed drug in the United States. Many of these patients are rehospitalized for medical problems, many of which are due to lack of patient compliance with their medical and nursing reg-imens or to the very narrow *therapeutic index* of the digitalis glycoside. Some hospitalizations could be eliminated with proper patient and family education.

Action

The digitalis glycosides have both a direct effect on cardiac muscle and on the conduction system, and an indirect action on the cardiovascular system mediated through the autonomic nervous system. These effects are dose related. Digitalis glycosides have both positive inotropic and negative *chronotropic* (reduction of heart rate) effects on the muscle cells of the myocardium. These effects are present on both the failing and non-failing heart, although a greater magnitude of effect is usually seen on the failing heart.

The positive inotropic effect causes a more complete emptying of the ventricles during systole, which is more pronounced in patients with failing hearts. The improved emptying increases the cardiac output and helps to decrease systemic venous pressure (preload reduction). At the same time, there is no overall increase in oxygen consumption. This, in turn, reduces the symptoms of congestive heart failure, that is, dyspnea, ascites, and dependent edema. A review of management of congestive heart failure is featured in Table 28–1.

The digitalis glycosides exert an inotropic effect on the heart through the inhibition of the adenosine triphosphatase (ATPase) enzyme (Fig. 28–1) required for

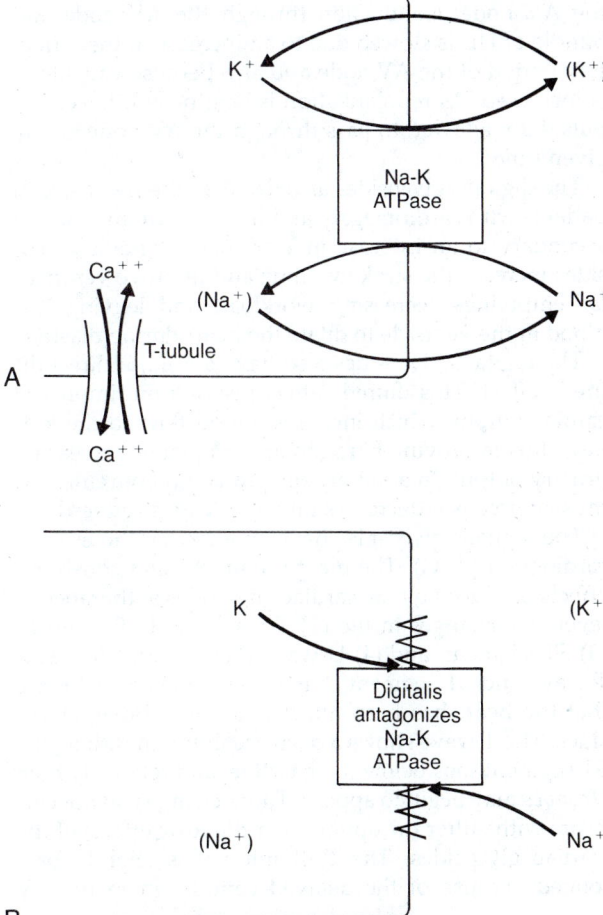

Figure 28–1. A) Adenosine triphosphatase (ATPase), the enzyme that surrounds each cardiac cell and maintained by magnesium, is responsible for active transport of sodium and calcium across the cell membrane. B) When digitalis is administered, the Na–K ATPase is depressed and Na⁺ remains in the cell and K⁺ remains outside as the Na–K pump mechanism does not work effectively.

the movement or active transport of sodium and calcium across the cell membrane into the cardiac cell, and for the movement of potassium out of the cell (often referred to as the sodium–potassium pump mechanism). By inhibiting ATPase, digitalis causes an accumulation of sodium within the cell. The intracellular sodium is exchanged for extracellular calcium through the T tubules. This calcium current moves along the T tubule, causing the cell to contract more rapidly and forcefully, thus increasing the inotropic action of the heart. The inhibition of ATPase is the reason that digitalis, at toxic levels, causes dysrhythmias. When ATPase is inhibited, more calcium is allowed to enter the cell, rendering it more irritable, and thus causing it to contract more frequently. ATPase is further inhibited if the serum potassium level is low. Often, dysrhythmias caused by digitalis can be prevented by adequate monitoring and replacement of potassium. ATPase activity is also maintained by magnesium. When magnesium levels are lower (as in acute pancreatitis, chronic alcoholism, chronic diarrhea, or chronic diuretic therapy) ATPase is inhibited further, possibly leading to dysrhythmias.

Secondary to the increase in cardiac output is a decrease in preload and end-diastolic volume. Also, a secondary concomitant reduction in the sympathetic tone with an increased sensitization of the myocardium to acetylcholine (the neurotransmitter from the vagus nerve) decrease the heart rate, thereby exerting a negative chronotropic effect.

The primary site of action of the digitalis glycosides is the AV node. Conduction through the AV node and bundle of His is slowed due to an increase in the refractory period of the AV node and also because vagal tone is increased. As repolarization is lengthened, fewer impulses are allowed to pass through the AV node at any given time.

The digitalis glycosides also decrease the heart size in patients with cardiomegaly and heart failure that occurs secondary to an increase in workload. Digitalis glycosides increase the stroke volume and improve ventricular emptying, decreasing workload and leaving less blood in the ventricle to dilate the heart during diastole.

The digitalis glycosides also have a mild, indirect diuretic effect. This diuretic effect results from improved cardiac output, which increases blood flow to the kidney, thus improving filtration and ultimately increasing urinary output. In addition, the production of renin and thus angiotensin decreases and afterload is reduced.

The digitalis glycosides have an effect on the electrocardiogram (ECG). The most prominent and consistent effects produced by the cardiac glycosides at therapeutic levels are changes in the (1) T wave, (2) P–R interval, (3) ST segment, and (4) U wave (Fig. 28–2). Clinically, T wave and ST segment changes are taken as evidence that the heart has been affected by the cardiac glycosides. The T wave shows a decrease in its amplitude, the ST segment sags below the baseline, and relatively high *U waves* may begin to appear. These changes do not correlate with either the optimum or the toxic effects of the cardiac glycosides. The P–R interval is slightly prolonged because of the delayed conduction in the AV

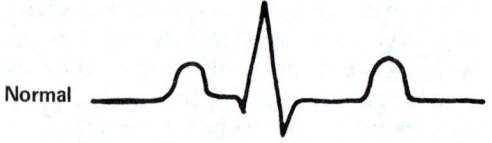

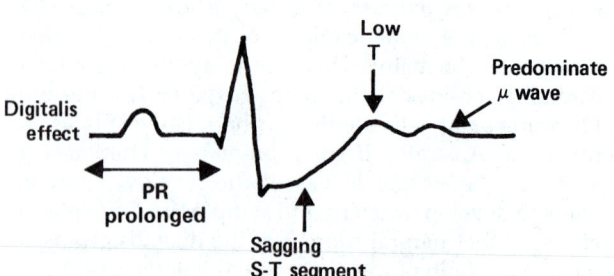

Figure 28–2. Normal ECG and effect of digitalis on the ECG.

node. The digitalis glycosides have a direct effect on the action potential curve. They shorten phase 3, which has a shortening effect on the Q–T interval (Fig. 28–3) as the ventricular cells are stimulated by digitalis.

As serum levels of the cardiac glycosides begin to rise, conduction velocity through the AV node is further delayed. As a toxic serum level is approached, the patient may develop heart block.

Digitalis glycosides cause a slight increase in blood pressure by several mechanisms: increasing cardiac output; exerting a direct vasoconstrictor effect on arteriolar smooth muscle; and sensitizing the vasoreceptors in the carotid sinus and aortic arch. The baroreceptors are stimulated even though blood pressure is not high. This is especially true following IV bolus administration.

Uses

The digitalis glycosides are currently used to treat or control congestive heart failure and certain dysrhythmias, including atrial fibrillation, atrial flutter, and supraventricular tachycardias. (See Chapter 27 for review of dysrhythmias.) If rates are not slowed with digitalis

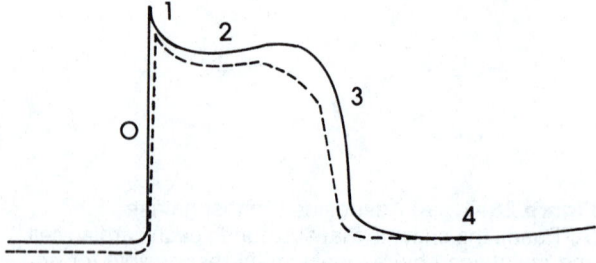

Figure 28–3. Action potential curve. A normal curve (solid line) with changes due to digitalis glycosides (dashed line).

products, magnesium levels should be assessed and corrected.

By increasing the force of contraction, which improves cardiac output, these drugs relieve the symptoms of right- and left-sided congestive heart failure. Through their effect on cardiac output, the cardiac glycosides improve both oxygen delivery to the tissues and blood flow to the kidney, which increases renal filtration and increases urinary output. Total circulating blood volume is thereby reduced. Coronary perfusion is improved by decreasing the heart rate and increasing the diastolic filling time, the period during which the coronary arteries are perfused (70%–80% of all coronary perfusion occurs during diastole).

The cardiac glycosides are most effective in low-output heart failure caused by atherosclerotic heart disease, including coronary heart disease, hypertension, and idiopathic cardiomyopathies. They are less effective in high-output failure caused by *beriberi*, thyrotoxicosis, and anemia and in mechanical disturbances such as rheumatic heart disease and other valvular lesions. Cardiac glycosides are also less effective in the treatment of right-sided heart failure. The cardiac glycosides are commonly used concomitantly with diuretics or vasodilators to treat the patient in heart failure.

The cardiac glycosides are also used to slow the heart rate by causing decreased conduction through the AV node of certain dysrhythmias such as atrial flutter, fibrillation, or atrial tachycardias such as paroxysmal atrial tachycardia (PAT).

Pharmacokinetics

The pharmacokinetics of digoxin and digitoxin are discussed fully in the following section. Information on pharmacokinetics on the remaining digitalis glycosides is found in Table 28–2.

ABSORPTION. The metabolic handling, excretion, and duration of action of the digitalis products depend on the glycoside being administered. The majority of digitalis preparations can be absorbed in part or completely from the gastrointestinal system, primarily from the jejunum. The extent of absorption (bioavailability) for the various preparations is as follows: digitoxin 100%, digoxin tablets 60%–80%, digoxin capsules 90%, digoxin elixirs 70%–85%, lanatoside C 50%, and digitalis leaf about 20%. The extent of absorption can vary from patient to patient, from manufacturer to manufacturer, and even from dose to dose in the same patient. When oral digoxin is taken with meals, the rate of absorption is slowed; however, the total amount absorbed is unchanged. The variability of absorption, particularly of digoxin, can lead to problems for patients who have been stabilized on one tablet brand and then switch to another. The digoxin content in the second tablet may be more or less bioavailable than the first. Recent regulation by the Food and Drug Administration (FDA) is designed to ensure that all marketed digoxin products have similar and uniform bioavailability.

The absorption of digoxin and digitoxin can also be reduced in malabsorption syndromes in the gastrointestinal tract and by prior radiation therapy to the gastrointestinal tract. Several drugs have the potential to reduce the absorption of these digitalis preparations (see Interactions).

DISTRIBUTION. These dugs are widely distributed throughout the body, with the highest concentrations found in the heart, kidneys, liver, intestine, stomach, and skeletal muscle. Serum levels are not significantly altered by body fat, so the distribution space best correlates with lean (ideal) body weight. The cardiac glycosides cross the placental barrier so that both fetal and maternal serum levels are equal. The cardiac glycosides are also found in breast milk. Digoxin crosses the blood–brain barrier, while digitoxin penetrates the blood–brain barrier poorly.

The difference in the duration of action of the glycosides depends on the extent that each drug is bound to plasma proteins after absorption. Digitoxin is highly bound to serum proteins, mainly albumin (90%–97%), whereas, digoxin is bound only to a small degree (20%–25%). Other medications bound to albumin such as warfarin (Coumadin) and phenylbutazone (Butazolidin) can displace digitoxin from its binding sites when they are administered concurrently. A low serum albumin level and reduced amount of digitoxin bound to albumin are also seen in renal and hepatic disease. Under these circumstances, an enhanced pharmacologic effect from the drug may occur.

Only a small amount of digoxin circulating in plasma is bound to proteins. This allows for more rapid diffusion out of the blood stream into tissues such as the myocardium. The action starts in about one hour, with maximum effects observed six to eight hours after an oral dose.

Glycoside Serum Levels. Serum levels are often evaluated to determine whether the digitalis level is within therapeutic range (Table 28–3). Serum levels may be useful to assess patient compliance, to detect underdigitalization, to monitor patients who may be at risk for becoming toxic, and to detect problems in bioavailability caused by gastrointestinal disorders, concurrent use of other drugs, or poor table dissolution.

Many factors can alter serum levels and/or the patient's response to therapy. These include electrolyte imbalance, particularly hypokalemia, renal disease, age, thyroid disease, and drug interaction. The time that the blood sample is obtained also must be taken into consideration, because serum levels are high during the absorptive and distributive phases. A delay of three to four hours after an intravenous dose of digoxin and six to eight hours after an oral dose is recommended (American Medical Association, 1986).

Serum levels often do not correlate well with actual clinical events. Serum levels are evaluated in conjunction with current symptoms, laboratory tests, and ECG findings. Even if serum levels are in the toxic range, digitalis should not be discontinued in the absence of other signs of toxicity. A serum level that is effective and safe for one patient may be excessive or inadequate for another.

TEXT RESUMES ON PAGE 720

Table 28–2. CARDIAC GLYCOSIDES AND POSITIVE INOTROPIC AGENTS

Name	Dosage	Mode of Administration	Pharmacokinetics	Therapeutic Serum Level
CARDIAC GLYCOSIDES				
Action: increases the force of myocardial contraction; prolongs refractory period of AV node; decreases conduction through SA and AV nodes; reduces heart rate; improves cardiac output; reduces preload.				
Use: treat or control congestive heart failure; slows fast rates such as atrial flutter, atrial fibrillation, and paroxysmal sypraventricular tachycardias.				
Digoxin (Lanoxin)	LD: 0.5–1 mg in divided doses over 24 hr.	PO, IV, IM (not recommended)	O: PO, 1 hr; IV, 5–30 min; IM, 30 min	0.5–2.0 ng/ml. Over 2.5 ng/ml = toxicity.
	M: O.125–0.5 mg (depending on renal function; see text).	IV slowly over 5–30 min.	P: PO, 6–8 hr; IV, 1–5 hr; IM, 4–6 hr	
		PO	D: 2–6 day	
	Children 2–5 yr: LD 25–35 μg/kg, 30–40 μg/kg, MD 8–12 μg/kg/day.	IV	½L: 30–40 hr PB: 25% B: liver (small degree)	
			E: kidney	
	Over 5 yr: LD 15–30	PO	O: ½–2 hr	
	μg/kg, 20–35 μg/kg, MD 6–10 μg/kg 1 mo–2 yr	PO	P: 2–6 hr D: 6 days	
	LD: 35–60 μg/kg in divided doses (depends on child's weight)	IV		
	M: 20%–30% of LD (elixir 0.05 mg/ml)	PO		
	Newborns (under 2 wk): 25–35 μg/kg in divided doses over 24 hr.	PO		
Digitoxin (Crystodigin, Purodigin)	LD: 1.2–1.6 mg in divided doses in 24 hr.	PO	O: 0.5–2 hr P: 4–12 hr D: 2–3 wk	14–26 ng/ml. Over 35 ng/ml = toxicity.
		IV	½L: 5–7 days PB: 97%	
	M: 0.05–0.2 mg once daily	IM (very irritating)	B: liver E: liver, urine	
		IV		
		IV		

Key to abbreviations in *Pharmacokinetics* column: M-maintenance dose; LD-loading dose; O-onset; P-peak; D-duration; PB-protein bound; B-biotransformed in; E-excreted in; ½L-halflife.

*Within the column listing adverse effects, <u>underlines</u> indicate the most common effects; CAPITALS indicate life-threatening effects.

Contraindications/ Precautions	Adverse Effects*	Interactions	Nursing Implications
For All Glycosides: Contraindicated in idiopathic hypertrophic subaortic stenosis (IHSS), constrictive pericarditis, Wolff–Parkinson–White syndrome, and heart block. Use cautiously in hypothyroidism, impaired renal or hepatic function, hypokalemia, hypomagnesia, hypercalcemia, elderly patients, pregnant or nursing women, and myocardial infarction.	For All Glycosides: Cardiovascular system: AV block, extrasystoles—all types, nonspecific ST and T changes in ECG. Virtually every type of CARDIAC DYS-RHYTHMIA has been reported (ventricular bigeminy and atrial tachycardia with atrioventricular block are particularly common). CNS: aphasia, convulsions—rare, drowsiness, fatigue, hallucinations, headache, malaise, neuralgic pain (cranial nerve v), DIZZINESS. Decreased sympathetic tone usual but perhaps increased in some situations and body systems (see GI system), increased vagal tone. Behavior: confusion, delirium, disorientation Gastrointestinal system: anorexia, abdominal pain, diarrhea, nausea (caused by a central effect on chemoreceptor zone), vomiting (caused by a central effect on chemoreceptor trigger zone), salivation Hematologic system: eosinophilia—rare, possible increased coagulability. Metabolic and Endocrine systems: gynecomastia—rare Ocular system: amblyopia, blurred vision, disturbed color vision, dyplopia, halos around dark objects, scotomas	For all Glycosides: Drugs that decrease absorption and therefore decrease effectiveness include antacids, antidiarrheals, oral aminoglycosides, and cathartics. Need to separate administration by at least 2 hr. Interact with sulfasalazine, cholestyramine, and colestipol to decrease effectiveness. Drugs that increase potential for dysrhythmias include β-blockers, edrophonium, sympathomimetic drugs, calcium salts, reserpine, thyroid preparations, and succinylcholine. Drugs that increase potential for toxicity include quinidine, thiazides and loop diuretics (potassium loss), steroids and laxatives (potassium loss), amphotericin B, anticholinergics, verapamil, and nifedipine. Barbiturates, phenytoin, rifampin, and phenylbutazone decrease effectiveness of digitoxin. May need to increase digitoxin dose. May cause increased plasma level of estrone and estrogen and decrease plasma level of luteinizing hormone and testosterone Serum I^{131} uptake may be reduced. Serum creatine kinase increases after IM injection. May alter urinary levels of 17-hydroxycorticosteroids, 17-ketosteroids, and glucose.	For All Glycosides: ASSESSMENT: Assess cardiac rate and rhythm and determine the presence of dysrhythmias. Obtain baseline serum and periodic levels of potassium, serum creatinine, BUN, and liver studies. Assess digitalis serum levels. INTERVENTION: Store in tightly closed containers and protect from excessive heat and light. Take apical pulse for 1 full minute before administering (range should be 60–110/min). Administer at the same time each day (noontime is best). Administering with food or between meals does not alter absorption. Determine pulse deficit as ordered. Administer PO or IV (IM and SC irritating to tissues). Administer IV bolus over 2–30 min. Do not discontinue medication without checking with the physician. Full loading dose is not given if other digitalis product is given within 1 week; or digitoxin, 2 weeks. EVALUATION: Weigh patient weekly to evaluate fluid retention. Notify MD if loss of appetite, lower stomach pain, nausea, vomiting, diarrhea, unusual tiredness or weakness, drowsiness, headache, blurred or yellow vision, skin rash or hives, or mental depression occurs.
Same as for all.	Same as for all.	Same as for all.	Same as for all.

CONTINUED ON THE FOLLOWING PAGE

Table 28–2. CARDIAC GLYCOSIDES AND POSITIVE INOTROPIC AGENTS–*CONTINUED*

Name	Dosage	Mode of Administration	Pharmacokinetics	Therapeutic Serum Level
Deslanoside (Cedilanid D)	LD: 0.8–1.6 mg M: 0.25–0.5 mg given in 2–3 divided doses at 3–4-hr intervals. Newborns: 0.0222 mg/kg in 2–3 divided doses at 3–4-hr intervals. Children 2 wk–3 yr 0.0225 mg/kg in 2–3 divided doses at 3–4-hr intervals Children over 3 yr: 0.0205 mg/kg in 2–3 divided doses at 3–4-hr intervals.	IV, slow IM (very irritating) no more than 0.8 mg in one site) IV, IM IV, IM IV, IM	O: 10–30 min ½L: 36 hr PB: 25% B: liver (small degree) E: kidney P: 1–3 hr D: 2–5 days	—

BIPYRIDINE DERIVATIVES (POSITIVE INOTROPIC AGENTS)

Action: improves myocardial contractility through a positive inotropic activity and a vasodilating effect. Decreases preload and afterload through a direct effect on vascular smooth muscle. Improves cardiac output.

Use: treatment of congestive heart failure.

Amrinone (Inocor)	0.75 mg/kg bolus slowly over 2–3 min, repeated in 30 min. 5–10 µg/kg/min, not to exceed 10 mg/kg/24 hr Children: dosage has not been established.	IV bolus IV drip	O: immediate P: 10 min ½L: 3.6 hr D: ½–2 hr PB: 10%–49% B: liver E: kidney	—

DIGOXIN ANTAGONIST

Action: antigen binding fragments (fab) derived from specific antidigoxin antibodies produced in sheep which binds avidly with digoxin and digitoxin and thus rapidly reduce serum levels.

Use: life-threatening digoxin and digitoxin toxicity.

Digoxin Immune Fab (Digibind)	40 mg binds 0.6 mg of digoxin, average dose 10 vials over 30 min.	IV	O: 1 min P: 15–30 min D: UA ½L: 15–20 hr B: none E: kidney	—

Key to abbreviations in *Pharmacokinetics* column: M-maintenance dose; LD-loading dose; O-onset; P-peak; D-duration; PB-protein bound; B-biotransformed in; E-excreted in; ½L-halflife.
*Within the column listing adverse effects, underlines indicate the most common effects; CAPITALS indicate life-threatening effects.

Contraindications/ Precautions	Adverse Effects*	Interactions	Nursing Implications
			Same as for all, plus INTERVENTION: Very irritating IM. Give only 0.8 mg in 1 site. Protect from light.
Contraindicated in outflow obstructions such as valvular stenosis and IHSS. Safety in children, lactation, and pregnancy not established. Not recommended in acute myocardial infarction.	Cardiovascular: dysrhythmia, hypotension, chest pain. GI: 5%–10% vomiting, dyspepsia, cramps, diarrhea, anorexia. Hemo: reversible, thrombocytopenia (10%–15%), and idiosyncratic fever.	Concurrent use with disopyramide (Norpace) causes excessive hypotension. Do not mix in glucose solutions for IV drip. Additive inotropic effect with digitalis and dobutamine.	ASSESSMENT: Assess fluid balance and electrolytes and maintain near normal so as not to precipitate reduced filling pressure and hypotension. Assess platelets weekly. INTERVENTION: Take blood pressure often. Do not mix in glucose solutions for IV drip because chemical reaction occurs slowly over a 24-hr period. Bolus administration in glucose is permissible. Protect ampuls from light. EVALUATION: Evaluate cardiac rhythm for supraventricular tachycardia and ventricular dysrhythmias.
Contraindications: none known. Precautions: cardiac function may deteriorate. Safety in children, lactation and pregnancy not established. Renal failure as the FAB-digoxin complex is very slowly	Cardiovascular: mild increase in congestive heart failure, increase in ventricular rate with atrial fibrillation, hypokalemia.	Lab: interferes with digitalis immune assay.	ASSESSMENT: Draw digoxin level and K before administration. Obtain baseline T, BP, and ECG INTERVENTION: Dissolve 1 vial in 4 ml sterile water, use immediately or refrigerate up to 4 hrs. Use 0.22 μg membrane filter.

CONTINUED ON THE FOLLOWING PAGE

Table 28-2. CARDIAC GLYCOSIDES AND POSITIVE INOTROPIC AGENTS-*CONTINUED*

Name	Dosage	Mode of Administration	Pharmacokinetics	Therapeutic Serum Level
Digoxin Immune Fab (Digibind)-*Continued*				

Key to abbreviations in *Pharmacokinetics* column: M-maintenance dose; LD-loading dose; O-onset; P-peak; D-duration; PB-protein bound; B-biotransformed in; E-excreted in; ½L-halflife.
*Within the column listing adverse effects, underlines indicate the most common effects; CAPITALS indicate life-threatening effects.

METABOLISM. As these drugs pass through the liver, digoxin is altered, but only to a minor degree, thus remaining largely unchanged. Digitoxin, however, is metabolized to other inactive and active metabolites (including digoxin), through the liver's enzyme activity. The method of biodegradation can be enhanced by concurrent administration of enzyme-inducing drugs such as phenobarbital or phenytoin. When phenobarbital is added to the drug regimen of a patient previously stabilized on a daily dose of digitoxin, increased conversion of digitoxin to its metabolites results. This may reduce the therapeutic digitoxin level.

ELIMINATION. Digitalis glycosides are eliminated from the body by different mechanisms. Digitoxin is eliminated primarily by hepatic mechanisms, whereas digoxin is eliminated primarily by renal excretion. Drug-metabolizing enzymes degrade digitoxin to several metabolites. Approximately 50%–70% are inactive with the rest active. Digitoxin is excreted into the biliary tract, and from there into the gastrointestinal tract. Once in the gastrointestinal tract, digitoxin can be reabsorbed (about 30%) into the blood stream. This process, called *enterohepatic recycling*, is in part responsible for the long serum half-life of digitoxin, six to eight days on average. Disease states that decrease hepatic enzyme activity, such as cirrhosis of the liver, can prolong digitoxin's half-life. On the other hand, several drugs known as enzyme inducers (phenobarbital, phenytoin [Dilantin], and rifampin) increase hepatic enzyme activity and can shorten the half-life of digitoxin.

Digoxin is eliminated primarily by renal excretion, with only about 14% of an administered dose metabolized first by hepatic mechanisms. Glomerular filtration and, to a lesser extent, tubular secretion processes are involved in the renal excretion of digoxin. The degree of elimination of digoxin can be correlated with measures of renal function such as serum creatinine or creati-

nine clearance. These relationships can then be used to determine the dosage of digoxin required in a patient with decreased renal function (see Preparations, Digoxin).

Digoxin is not effectively removed from the body by dialysis or exchange transfusion or during cardiopulmonary bypass, because most of the drug is in tissue rather than circulating in the blood. Digitoxin is not effectively removed by peritoneal dialysis or hemodialysis, probably because of its high degree of plasma-protein binding.

Contraindications and Precautions

The contraindications for all cardiac glycosides include idiopathic hypertrophic subaortic stenosis (IHSS), diffuse cardiomyopathies, and constrictive pericarditis, as the drugs increase the work load of the heart and worsen these conditions. Cardiac glycosides are contraindicated in Wolff–Parkinson–White (WPW) syndrome because administration may aggravate tachydysrhythmias by depressing AV nodal function and allowing accessory bundle activation. They are contraindicated in heart block because of the possibility of further slowing of AV conduction. Ventricular tachycardia and fibrillation are also contraindications to cardiac glycosides.

Precautions include hypothyroidism because such patients may suffer severe bradycardia and are more sensitive to digitalis effects; impaired renal or liver function because of delayed excretion and possible toxic effects; and hypokalemia, hypomagnesemia, and hypercalcemia because they all favor the development of digitalis toxicity. Pregnant women or nursing mothers are also given the drug cautiously because of its passage across the placenta and into breast milk. Cardiac glycosides should be given cautiously to persons with acute or toxic myocarditis since there may be an increased incidence of digitalis-induced tachydysrhythmias. The elderly are also given these products cautiously because of the increased possibility of digitalis intoxication from decreases in either liver or kidney function. Also, because the increased force of contraction raises myocardial oxygen consumption, which may increase infarct size, the cardiac glycosides are given cautiously in an acute myocardial infarction.

Table 28-3. THERAPEUTIC/TOXIC DIGITALIS SERUM LEVELS

Product	Therapeutic ng/ml	Toxic ng/ml
Digoxin	0.5–2	> 2.5
Digitoxin	14–26	> 35

Contraindications/ Precautions	Adverse Effects*	Interactions	Nursing Implications
excreted, with FAB eliminated more quickly. This may result in the release of free digoxin 1–3 weeks after therapy.			EVALUATION: ECG and K$^+$ level. Administer K as needed.

Adverse Reactions

Digitalis side-effects are the same for all preparations used and can be categorized according to noncardiac and cardiac effects. Digitalis toxicity can be life-threatening and is relatively common, occurring in 10%–20% of all people receiving digitalis products. It is, therefore, important to understand the signs and symptoms that a nurse needs to monitor to identify potential toxicity in patients.

NONCARDIAC EFFECTS. These effects include common systemic effects such as anorexia, nausea, vomiting, and diarrhea by activating the chemoreceptor trigger zone in the medulla. These gastrointestinal effects are frequently self-limiting and disappear after continued therapy. However, these symptoms can also be seen when a patient is exposed to excessive amounts of digitalis, and are digitalis toxic. Visual disturbances can manifest as blurred vision, white dots, halos, yellow or green tint to vision (*chromatopsia*), double vision, and flickering. These gastrointestinal and central nervous system (CNS) side-effects, although bothersome, are not life threatening. They may occur at lower serum concentrations than, and may precede, the more serious cardiac side-effects. It should be stressed, however, that these noncardiac signs and symptoms of digitalis may not always precede cardiac symptoms.

Gynecomastia, the enlargement of breast tissue, although rare, can be seen in both men and women. It is related to the steroid component of digitalis products and is more common with digoxin use. Other less common side-effects include mental depression, respiratory depression, and pruritis.

CARDIAC EFFECTS. Digitalis produces expected ECG changes, as previously mentioned. The effect of slowing conduction through the AV node, although beneficial and desired in the treatment of some rhythm disturbances (see Uses), can produce varying degrees of heart block. This can range from prolongation of the P–R interval to Mobitz type I heart block, where the P–R interval gets progressively longer until a beat is missed, to complete heart block. By slowing conduction through the AV node, accessory bundles can be activated, causing supraventricular tachycardias.

Dysrhythmias such as premature ventricular contractions (PVCs), premature atrial contractions (PACs), ventricular tachycardia, and supraventricular dysrhythmias can be caused by disturbances in automaticity. A com-

bination of these disturbances with delayed AV conduction can be seen. Children receiving digitalis are more likely to experience ectopic junctional or atrial beats. Since almost any dysrhythmias can present as digitalis intoxication, a good rule to use is to assume that any new rhythm disturbance observed in a patient receiving a digitalis preparation is caused by digitalis until proven otherwise.

Digitalis Toxicity

FACTORS PREDISPOSING TO DIGITALIS TOXICITY. Various factors may predispose the patient to digitalis toxicity (Table 28–4). These include electrolyte disturbances, such as hypokalemia, hypomagnesemia, and hypercalcemia, and acid–base imbalances. Patients with hypothyroidism are more susceptible to the effects of digitalis. Digitalis products are eliminated by either renal (digoxin) or hepatic (digitoxin) mechanisms; therefore, unless care is used in prescribing these products to patients with pathologic conditions that decrease renal and hepatic function, toxicity can result. This is also true when these products are used in the elderly, since both hepatic and renal functions decrease with aging. Under these circumstances, appropriate dosage adjustments and careful monitoring of serum concentrations can prevent toxicity. Rapid intravenous administration of too much digitalis can also cause toxicity.

Potassium loss may be caused by a number of conditions: vomiting; diarrhea; administration of certain diuretics, steroids, laxatives or certain antibiotics (carbenicillin, ticarcillin, piperacillin, mezlocillin, amphotericin B), which increase renal potassium excretion; poor di-

Table 28–4. DIGITALIS TOXICITY

> **PREDISPOSING FACTORS**
> Electrolyte disturbances:
>   Hypokalemia
>   Hypomagnesemia
>   Hypercalcemia
> Acid–base imbalances
> Hypothyroidism
> Renal impairment
> Hepatic impairment
> Elderly patients
> Too-rapid IV administration
>
> *CONTINUED ON THE FOLLOWING PAGE*

Table 28–4. DIGITALIS TOXICITY–*CONTINUED*

SIGNS AND SYMPTOMS
Gastrointestinal:
  *Anorexia
  *Nausea
  *Vomiting
  *Diarrhea
  Abdominal pain
Neurologic:
  Drowsiness
  Fatigue
  Dizziness
  Headache
  Restlessness
  Irritability
  Depression
  Personality change
  Lassitude
  Confusion
  Disorientation
  Insomnia
  Psychosis
  Convulsions
  Coma
Cardiac:
  Onset of bradycardia
  Onset of tachycardia
  Paroxysmal atrial/junctional rhythms†
  Atrial ectopic rhythms†
  Onset of regularity and/or irregularity
  Atrial tachycardia with varying AV block†
  Ventricular bigeminy or trigeminy*
  Ventricular tachycardia
  Second-degree AV block (Wenckebach)†
  AV dissociation
  Complete AV block†
Visual:
  Blurred or yellow vision
  Flickering lights
  White borders on dark objects
  Colored dots
  Halos
  Double vision

MANAGEMENT
Mild overdose:
  Withhold digitalis products for several days or up to 3 weeks
  Correct potassium deficit
  Reinstitute a lower maintenance dose
Severe toxicity:
  Hospitalize at once
  Support ventilation/give oxygen as necessary
  Continuously monitor ECG
  Administer potassium as needed
  Administer phenylhydantoin (Dilantin) for degenerating ventricular dysrhythmias
  Support blood pressure
  Insert a temporary demand pacemaker
  Administer digoxin antibody

*Most common early symptom in adults
†Most common early symptom in children

making the Na–K APTase enzyme system more susceptible to inhibition by digitalis.

Hypomagnesemia, as is commonly seen in alcoholics, and with use of diuretics, tends to increase sensitivity to digitalis. It can be easily corrected by administering soluble, absorbable magnesium salts.

Hypercalcemia may be seen in the immobile patient, in persons with hyperparathyroidism, and in certain malignant tumors that cause calcium to leave the bone. Hypercalcemia tends to cause increased automaticity and thus leads to tachydysrhythmias and ectopic dysrhythmias. Rapid intravenous administration of calcium may also cause digitalis toxicity.

SIGNS AND SYMPTOMS OF TOXICITY. When a patient experiences high serum concentrations of digitalis, that is, greater than 2.4 ng/ml for digoxin and greater than 35 ng/ml for digitoxin, the chemoreceptor trigger zone in the medulla is stimulated, resulting in nausea and possible emesis. In addition, anorexia, nausea, increased salivation, abdominal pain, and diarrhea can be seen.

In high doses, cardiac glycosides increase sympathetic outflow from the CNS to both cardiac and peripheral sympathetic nerves. This increase in sympathetic activity is an important factor in digitalis toxicity because most of the extracardiac manifestations are mediated by the CNS. Typical symptoms that may be associated with increased sympathetic tone include drowsiness, fatigue, dizziness, changes in vision, and, in the elderly, confusion, delirium, and even hallucinations.

Digitalis toxicity also enhances cardiac automaticity so many dysrhythmias can also occur. Unifocal or multifocal PVCs, especially in bigeminal or trigeminal patterns, are most common. In addition, paroxysmal junctional rhythms, A–V dissociation, and PAT with block may occur. Excessive slowing of the pulse, less than 50 beats per minute, is a clinical sign of overdose. ECG changes, such as ST and T wave changes, are not diagnostic of toxicity in the majority of patients.

In children, vomiting, diarrhea, and neurologic and visual disturbances are rarely seen initially. The most common and reliable signs of toxicity are cardiac dysrhythmias such as atrial dysrhythmias (atrial ectopic rhythms, PAT, and A–V block). Ventricular dysrhythmias are rarely seen.

TREATMENT OF DIGITALIS TOXICITY. When digitalis toxicity is diagnosed, the digitalis preparation is discontinued; or if the toxicity is severe, Digoxin Immune FAB (Digibind) may be administered (to be discussed later). Electrolytes (potassium, calcium, magnesium) and acid–base states are checked and returned to normal, if necessary. If the patient is receiving potassium, it is critical that the serum level of this cation be monitored closely. If this value is low, increasing the potassium can suppress many of the dysrhythmias seen. On the other hand, if the potassium level is high, administration of potassium may potentiate or intensify AV block, with the potential for the occurrence of AV block and cardiac arrest. Severe digitalis toxicity can cause an elevated serum potassium.

If the ventricular dysrhythmias (PVCs, ventricular

etary intake of potassium; and continuous use of potassium-free intravenous solutions. If any of these conditions exists and the patient is on digitalis, he or she may be more prone to developing digitalis toxicity. Low serum potassium level enhances digitalis toxicity by tachycardia) are present, they can usually be effectively suppressed by using lidocaine or phenytoin. Atrial dysrhythmias (PAT with block, atrial tachycardia) can be treated with phenytoin. The antiarrhythmics quinidine, procainamide, and propranolol may also be effective; however, they may also cause dysrhythmias. Electric shock therapy in the presence of digitalis causes dysrhythmias, and thus is not usually used to treat digitalis-induced dysrhythmias.

Bradydysrhythmias, sinoatrial arrest, and AV block can be treated with atropine. Temporary pacing may be required to maintain an adequate heart rate until digoxin levels are within the therapeutic range.

Digitalis toxicity, in addition to being a significant cause of morbidity, also adds substantially to health care costs. Patients with cardiac toxicity frequently require hospitalization and intensive monitoring until therapeutic levels have been attained and an appropriate dosage regimen achieved. Since all digitalis glycosides have long serum half-lives, this stabilization can take several days. For example, if a patient is admitted with digoxin toxicity with a serum digoxin level of 5.0 ng/ml and the drug has a half-life of three days, the serum concentration will be 2.5 ng/ml three days after admission and 1.25 ng/ml six days after admission. This, together with the seriousness of the cardiac side-effects, has led to investigations designed to enhance the removal of digitalis glycosides from the body.

Traditional methods of drug removal such as hemodialysis, charcoal hemoperfusion, and peritoneal dialysis are generally ineffective because of the wide tissue distribution of the glycosides. Removal of digitoxin, because of its high degree of enterohepatic recycling, can be enhanced by the oral administration of binding resins such as cholestyramine and colestipol. Enzyme-inducing agents (e.g., phenobarbital), although they increase the half-life of digitoxin, would be impractical to use since it takes 10–14 days for induction to occur. Administration of digoxin- or digitoxin-specific antibodies, known as Fab fragments, which bind very tightly to digoxin resulting in an inactive digoxin-antibody complex that is excreted renally, are helpful when digoxin levels are very high. This produces high serum concentrations of the complex but very low concentrations of active digoxin. Fab fragments are discussed later in this chapter.

Interactions

Cardiac glycosides adsorb to aluminum-containing antacids (Amphojel, Mylanta-II, Gelusil-II, Maalox) and kaolin-pectin (Kaopectate), forming an insoluble complex in the gut that is not absorbed. Binding resins such as cholestyramine and colestipol can reduce the absorption of cardiac glycosides by a similar mechanism. The administration of digitalis glycosides should be separated by two hours when used concurrently with any of these products. Oral aminoglycosides (neomycin, kanamycin, paromomycin, and sulfasalazine) also inhibit absorption of cardiac glycosides. Also combined chemotherapy regimens can decrease digoxin absorption 20%–50% (bleomycin, cyclophosphamide, procarbazine).

Administration of quinidine with digoxin substan-

tially increases serum digoxin concentration, producing a twofold increase on the average. This is a result of quinidine's tendency to cause both tissue displacement of digoxin with re-equilibration into serum and a reduction in the ability of the kidney to remove digoxin from serum. Along with the increase in digoxin concentration, an increase in the risk of toxicity also occurs. Frequently, the dose of digoxin needs to be reduced by 50% when quinidine is added. A similar interaction occurs with administration of the calcium antagonists verapamil (Isoptin) and nifedipine (Procardia). The magnitude of increase in digoxin level, however, is not as great as that observed with quinidine.

Several drugs can increase the elimination of digitoxin. Through interfering with the enterohepatic recycling process and increasing fecal elimination, cholestyramine and colestipol can increase the overall elimination of digitoxin. Several enzyme-inducing drugs such as rifampin, barbiturates, phenylbutazone, and phenytoin increase the hepatic metabolism of digitoxin. Because this mechanism involves an increase in synthesis of the proteins responsible for drug enzyme activity, this effect occurs over several days to weeks.

Drugs that decrease impulse formation from the sinus node, such as the beta blockers or calcium channel blockers, or increase vagal activity, such as edrophonium and succinylcholine, may increase the possibility of bradycardia. The potential for developing tachyarrhythmias and ectopic dysrhythmias may be enhanced by the administration of drugs that increase heart rate and contractility such as isoproterenol and other sympathomimetics (dopamine, dobutamine, epinephrine, ephedrine) and thyroid preparations. Intravenous administration of calcium salts, such as previously discussed, can potentiate toxicity. Drugs that can cause hypokalemia, like diuretics, thus increasing the likelihood of digoxin toxicity, have been discussed earlier.

Patients receiving cardiac glycosides also may have altered laboratory test results. Digitalis products may increase plasma levels of estrone and estrogen and decrease plasma levels of luteinizing hormone and testosterone. Cardiac glycosides may raise urine levels of ketogenic steroids and 17-hydroxycorticosteroids, as well as decreasing urine levels of 17-ketosteroids and glucose.

Foxglove Preparations

DIGOXIN. Digoxin (Lanoxin) is a hydrolytic product produced from lanatoside C. It is the most common form of digitalis used today because of its rapid onset of action and short duration.

Dosage. Digoxin can be administered as a loading dose (digitalization) if a rapid onset of action is desired. The digitalizing dose in adults is approximately 0.010–0.020 mg/kg ideal body weight (total of 0.5–1.0 mg) and is administered in three to four equally divided doses over 24 hours. The loading dose saturates the nonspecific myocardial receptor sites. Either the oral or intravenous route can be used. Intramuscular injection is not recommended because it is painful and causes muscle fasciculations and necrosis.

If the effects of digitalis are not needed quickly, a daily maintenance dose may be administered. It will take on average 11 days to reach steady state with this method of administration.

Digoxin is widely used in children. The pediatric loading dose (children one month–two years) is 35–60 μg/kg in divided doses (depending on the dose and frequency and child's age). The maintenance dose is 20%–30% of the loading dose. Digoxin is also available as an elixir of 0.05 mg/ml. For premature and newborns under two weeks, 25–35 μg/kg is given in divided doses at six to eight-hour intervals. Additional dosing information can be found in Table 28–2. Oral and intravenous doses are not equal as the bioavailability of these products must be taken into account.

The maintenance dose is based on the patient's renal function, since this is the primary route of digoxin elimination. The amount of digoxin lost per day—and hence the amount to be administered—is related to creatinine clearance (normal 85–135 ml/min) by the simple equation:

$$\text{maintenance dose} = \frac{\text{loading dose} \times 14 + C_{cr}}{5}$$

As an example, if creatinine clearance (ccr) is 10–25 ml/min, the maintenance dose is 0.125 mg/day; if creatinine clearance is 26–49 ml/min, the maintenance dose is 0.1875 mg/day; and if creatinine clearance is 50–79 ml/min, the maintenance dose is 0.25 mg/day.

Pharmacokinetics. Absorption rates vary from 40% to 90% after an oral dose. Absorption is delayed, but not reduced, by the presence of food in the gastrointestinal tract. Once absorbed, about 25% is protein bound. It is distributed to most body tissues, but is not stored in fat. Orally, the drug starts to act in one hour, peaks in six to eight hours, and has a duration of two to six days. Intravenously, it starts to act in 5–30 minutes, peaks in one to five hours, and also has a duration of two to six days. (IV boluses of digoxin can increase blood pressure in patients with limited cardiac reserve; therefore, they should be administered at least over a 5–30 minute period.) For IV use, digoxin can be mixed with 5% dextrose, normal saline, lactated Ringer's solution, and 5% dextrose in 0.45% sodium chloride and infused over 2–30 minutes. These solutions are stable for at least six hours at room temperature.

DIGITOXIN. Digitoxin (Crystodigin), available in crystalline form, is readily absorbed from the intestinal tract. Digitoxin is given orally, intramuscularly, or intravenously in a loading dose of 1.2–1.6 mg in divided doses over 24 hours. If the intramuscular route is used, the injection should be deep into the gluteal muscle, with no more than 0.4 mg at the injection site, as digitoxin is very irritating to tissues. Digitoxin may be used in patients with renal disease. Orally, action begins in one to four hours and peaks in 8–12 hours. Intravenously, it starts in 30 minutes to 2 hours and peaks in 4–12 hours. It has the longest duration of action of the digitalis products, ranging from one to three weeks. The

dosage of digitoxin needs to be reduced in patients with hepatic dysfunction.

LANATOSIDE C. Lanatoside C (Cedilanid) is a white powder that is almost insoluble in water. Lanatoside C is administered in a loading dose of 10 mg given in divided doses over three days. The maintenance dose is 0.5–1.5 mg daily. It has a duration of action of 36 hours.

DESLANOSIDE. Deslanoside (Cedilanid D), is used for rapid digitalization in emergency treatment of congestive heart failure, cardiac dysrhythmias, and cardiogenic shock. Deslanoside, derived from lanatoside C, is more soluble and stable than the original substance. It is available only in the intramuscular and intravenous injectable forms. Intramuscularly, deslanoside is very irritating to the tissues, and no more than 0.8 mg should be given in one site. Intravenous injection is made slowly. The loading dose of deslanoside is 0.8–1.6 mg. It starts its action in 10–30 minutes, peaks in two to three hours, and has a duration of 16–36 hours. The maintenance dose ranges from 0.25–0.5 mg daily.

GITALIN. Gitalin (Gitaligin) is administered in a loading dose of 6 mg given in divided doses over a 24-hour period. The maintenance dose is 0.25–1.25 mg daily. It is available orally or intravenously. It starts to act in four hours and peaks in 8–12 hours. Its duration is 7–12 days. Gitalin contains a dye that may cause an allergic reaction in patients hypersensitive to aspirin. The cardiac glycosides are featured in Table 28–2.

BIPYRIDINE DERIVATIVES

Amrinone Lactate

Use. Amrinone and milrinone are indicated for short-term management of patients with CHF who can be closely monitored and who have not responded adequately to digitalis, diuretics, dobutamine, or other vasodilators. It is important to return fluid volume and electrolytes to normal before therapy is begun if the patient has been treated vigorously with diuretics, since the patient may have insufficient cardiac filling pressures to respond adequately.

Action. Amrinone lactate (Inocor) is a positive inotropic agent with vasodilator activity. It is a bipyridine derivative that reduces afterload and preload, relaxes vascular smooth muscle, and increases cardiac output and stroke volume (Table 28–2). These drugs appear to increase myocardial contractility by inhibiting cyclic adenosine monophosphate phosphodiesterase, which increases the intracellular mediator cyclic adenosine monophosphate (cAMP). It is also possible that amrinone directly or indirectly enhances calcium ion movement into or storage within the myocardial cell. Heart rate and systemic blood pressure remain unchanged, as the increase in cardiac output compensates for the lowered vascular resistance. Pulmonary artery occlusive pressure (PAOP) and total peripheral resistance show dose-related decreases.

Pharmacokinetics. Amrinone (Inocor) is bound 10%–49% to plasma proteins. Amrinone is effective within ten minutes of administration. The duration of action is dose dependent: at a dose of 0.75 mg/kg the duration is about one-half hour, whereas at a dose of 3 mg/kg the duration is about two hours. The half-life is 3.6 hours. It is metabolized by the liver. The primary route of excretion is the urine (63%) with a small amount (18%) being excreted in the feces.

Contraindications and Precautions. Amrinone is contraindicated in patients experiencing hypersensitivity reactions to these products or bisulfites (a preservative used in amrinone solution). Amrinone and milrinone are administered cautiously in outflow obstruction such as aortic valvular disease, severe pulmonic valvular disease, and hypertrophic aortic stenosis, since they aggravate these problems. Platelet counts may be reduced because of decreased platelet survival and may precipitate thrombocytopenia. This drug is not currently recommended for use in patients with an acute myocardial infarction. Safety in children and during pregnancy and lactation has not been established. Hypersensitivity after two weeks of therapy has been reported.

Adverse Reactions. The most common adverse reactions include dysrhythmias (3%) such as supraventricular and ventricular dysrhythmias related to the increased inotropic cardiac effect; thrombocytopenia (2.4%), which is often dose dependent and probably related to decreased platelet survival time; and hypotension (1.3%) related to its vasodilation effect. Other minor side-effects include nausea (1.7%), vomiting (0.9%), abdominal pain (0.4%), anorexia (0.4%), hepatotoxicity (0.2%), chest pain (0.2%), and fever (0.9%).

Interactions. Only one interaction is known at this time. When amrinone is given concurrently with disopyramide (Norpace), there may be excessive hypotension.

Dosage. Amrinone is best diluted in a normal saline solution. A chemical reaction occurs slowly over a 24-hour period, when amrinone is mixed in glucose-containing solutions. However, amrinone can be injected into a running glucose solution through a Y-connector or directly into the tubing.

The initial dose is 0.75 mg/kg IV, given slowly over two to three minutes. An additional bolus of 0.75 mg may be administered again in 30 minutes. A maintenance dose of 5–10 µg/kg/minute is then administered. This dosing regimen creates an amrinone plasma concentration of approximately 3µg/ml. Diluted solutions should not be used after 24 hours. A daily dosage of 10 mg/kg should not be exceeded.

OTHER DRUGS USED TO TREAT CONGESTIVE HEART FAILURE

Digitalis has been a primary treatment for heart failure for over 200 years. However, other drugs such as captopril (Capoten), dobutamine (Dobutrex), and others may represent an alternative treatment.

A recent double-blind placebo-controlled study found that captopril was significantly more effective than placebo, and that it is an alternative to digoxin in patients with mild to moderate heart failure who are taking maintenance diuretic agents. More information on captopril is found in Chapter 29.

Dobutamine, a β_1-adrenergic agonist, promotes vasodilation in the peripheral vessels and reduces the heightened sympathetic drive seen in heart failure. Dobutamine also improves renal blood flow and promotes an increase in urinary output. More information on dobutamine can be found in Chapter 19.

Additional medications are also used in selected patients with congestive heart failure. They include calcium channel blockers, nitrates, sodium nitroprusside, hydralazine, and minoxidil. These drugs are all discussed in detail in other chapters.

DIGOXIN ANTAGONIST

Digoxin Immune Fab

Digoxin Immune Fab (Digibind), antigen binding fragments (fab) derived from specific antidigoxin antibodies (IgG) produced in sheep, is used in the treatment of life-threatening digoxin and digitoxin intoxications. Life-threatening episodes are indicated by shock, or impending shock, or cardiac arrest, serious ventricular dysrhythmias, bradycardia, or blocks unresponsive to atropine, and potassium levels above 6 mEq/L. Digoxin Immune Fab is administered intravenously, distributes widely to tissues, and binds avidly with digoxin and digitoxin. As a result, serum levels of digoxin and digitoxin are eventually reduced. Digoxin Immune Fab is an extremely expensive orphan drug.

PHARMACOKINETICS. Onset of action is within a minute of intravenous administration. Digoxin Immune Fab avidly binds in digoxin and digitoxin and is excreted within 15–20 hours, assuming the kidneys are normal.

CONTRAINDICATIONS AND PRECAUTIONS. No contraindications are known at this time. Caution must be used, since cardiac function may decrease rapidly and even cardiac arrest may occur. Use caution when administering Digoxin Immune Fab to pregnant or lactating women and children.

ADVERSE EFFECTS. The adverse effects of Digoxin Immune Fab include a mild increase in congestive heart failure and an increase in the ventricular rate with atrial fibrillation. There are rapid shifts of potassium in digitoxin toxicity. At first, with a high digoxin level, potassium shifts from the cell to the extracellular fluid, causing hyperkalemia. The potassium is then lost through normal renal excretion leading to hypokalemia. Digoxin Immune Fab allows potassium to move back into the cell so serum potassium levels become even lower. Potassium levels need to be monitored and potassium given cautiously.

DOSAGE. The dosage of Digoxin Immune Fab is dependent on the number of tablets of digoxin or digitoxin ingested or the serum digoxin or digitoxin concentration. One vial of Digoxin Immune Fab is mixed with 4 ml of sterile water and is administered over 30 minutes through a 0.22-µm membrane filter. Digoxin Immune Fab deteriorates rapidly once mixed, so it should be administered soon after being reconstituted.

USING THE NURSING PROCESS

ASSESSMENT

Assessment of the patient requiring cardiac glycosides always begins with a thorough nursing history to develop the data base from which to individualize drug therapy and to monitor therapeutic response, adverse reactions, and signs of toxicity. Information the nurse obtains is featured in Table 28–5. All this information is used when preparing a nursing care plan. If the patient has been or is currently taking cardiac glycosides, it is important to learn how and when the glycosides are taken, and if there are any adverse effects. A current

Table 28–5. NURSING PROCESS FOR PATIENT REQUIRING CARDIAC GLYCOSIDES

Assessment

Ascertain current/past medication history, response to drug(s) and any side effects including use of OTC drugs.
Assess concurrent health problems, e.g., impaired renal/hepatic function, electrolyte imbalances, history of hypothyroidism, pregnancy, or prior myocardial infarction/heart block.
Assess BP, skin color/temperature, peripheral pulses, mental status.
Note signs of congestion (liver/lung) and urinary output.
Obtain nutritional history (particularly use of foods high in sodium and cholesterol).
Assess current lifestyle/activities and effect of current health status on desired lifestyle.
Note the emotional and psychologic significance of illness.

Nursing Diagnosis	Nursing Actions	Rationale	Desired Outcomes/ Evaluation Criteria
Cardiac output decreased related to mechanical factors (e.g., inotropic changes in heart)/electrical changes in rate, rhythm, conduction as evidenced by fatigue, variations in hemodynamic readings, dysrhythmias, edema, dyspnea.	Administer cardiac glycoside, e.g., Lanoxin.	Increases the force of myocardial contraction; reduces preload; prolongs refractory period of AV junction, decreases conduction through SA node and AV junction reducing heart rate; improving cardiac output.	Reports decreased episodes of dyspnea, angina, and/or dysrhythmias. Displays a reduction in frequency/ duration or severity of dysrhythmias. Demonstrates an increase in activity tolerance.
	Monitor vital signs, cardiac rhythm, fluid balance and daily weight. Restrict fluid intake as indicated. Plan fluid schedule with patient.	Indicators of need for/effectiveness of therapy. Tachycardia and lower blood pressure may indicate worsening congestive heart failure. Fluid restriction (if needed) minimizes risk of fluid overload. Body weight reduction reduces myocardial workload.	
	Promote adequate rest periods, assist with self-care activities as necessary.	Prevents undue fatigue/reduces cardiac workload.	
Adjustment, impaired, potential related to anticipated change in lifestyle.	Review previous lifestyle and role changes required by current situation. Discuss coping skills already developed.	Provides information about how the patient is dealing with medical condition. Ways in which patient has dealt positively with problems in the past can be used to adjust to current situation.	Initiates lifestyle changes that will permit adaptation to present life situation.
	Develop with the patient a plan of action to meet	Provides opportunity to look at necessary changes and make	

Table 28–5. NURSING PROCESS FOR PATIENT REQUIRING CARDIAC GLYCOSIDES–*CONTINUED*

Nursing Diagnosis	Nursing Actions	Rationale	Desired Outcomes/ Evaluation Criteria
	needs. Discuss ways to implement plan.	individual choices about them.	
	Involve SOs in planning.	Facilitates cooperation with medical regimen.	
	Acknowledge feelings of frustration, focusing on the smaller factors of concern.	Promotes looking at the lifestyle changes from a less threatening perspective, one-step-at-a-time concept.	
Knowledge deficit related to lack of recall, information misinterpretation, unfamiliarity with resources, possible cognitive limitations as evidenced by questions, statement of concern, development of preventable complications.	Provide information (verbal and written formats) about cardiac glycosides including action, use, dosage, side and toxic effects (e.g., nausea/ vomiting, anorexia, weakness, headache, blurred vision or yellow halos, change in cardiac rate or rhythm) and potential interactions, especially with OTC drugs.	Understanding can facilitate adherence to prescribed regimen and prevent drug interactions/ complication.	Verbalizes understanding of disease process and measures needed to maintain/improve current health state.
	Discuss normal heart function. Include information regarding patient's variance from normal.	Helps patient to understand significance of own situation and need for continued therapy.	
	Stress importance of not discontinuing/altering drug dosage without first consulting with physician.	Prevents untoward responses that could be life-threatening.	
	Recommend storage of drug in tightly closed container, protected from excessive/heat/ light.	Maintains strength of the drug.	
	Review administration routine/ proper timing of drug, e.g., same time every day (noon often best), set pattern (with or without food).	Provides for consistent release and absorption of drug.	
	Identify foods low in sodium and cholesterol (within economic means) that can be used while maintaining a well-balanced diet.	Increased sodium expands fluid volume and further aggravates congestive heart failure. Decreased cholesterol levels may prevent further ASHD development.	

drug history is also obtained to determine if there are any possible drug interactions with digitalis products.

The nurse also assesses objective and subjective symptoms. (Refer to a medical–surgical text for review). Often, the patient being treated with cardiac glycosides has congestive heart failure or an irregular heart rhythm (atrial flutter/atrial fibrillation); therefore, signs and symptoms associated with these conditions are assessed carefully. ECG tracings and laboratory tests are obtained, including serum electrolytes such as potassium, calcium, magnesium, serum creatinine levels to evaluate kidney function, liver function studies, and serum digitalis levels if toxicity is suspected.

A serum digitalis level is a test, usually performed by radioimmunoassay, measuring the amount of digitalis in the blood. The serum level is generally checked about six to eight hours after an oral dose of digitalis, since that is when the drug equilibrates with the heart and other tissues. Therapeutic levels range from 0.5–2.0 ng/ml of serum for digoxin and 14–26 ng/ml for digitoxin. Toxic levels are above 2.5 ng/ml for digoxin and above 35 ng/ml for digitoxin.

NURSING DIAGNOSES

The nurse establishes the nursing diagnoses based on the information obtained during the assessment. The nursing diagnoses form the basis for the nursing care. Possible nursing diagnoses are featured in Table 28–5.

INTERVENTION

The goals of nursing intervention are developed based on the nursing diagnoses. The short- and long-term goals for a typical patient receiving cardiac glycosides are included in Table 28–5. The nurse-educator is responsible for teaching the patient about the disease itself including its underlying pathology, how to assess symptoms and signs of improvement or deterioration, dietary limitations (usually sodium restriction), and all requisite knowledge of the medication regimen.

NURSING RESPONSIBILITIES WHEN ADMINISTERING CARDIAC GLYCOSIDES

The nurse in the hospital situation has several nursing responsibilities when administering cardiac glycosides. (These are featured in the column marked Nursing Implications in Table 28–2). The heart rate is always taken apically for one full minute. This rate is charted along with the rhythm, regular or irregular. The nurse must know the specific pulse limitations for each patient. The physician is consulted and the limitations are written in the patient's Kardex. If the pulse rate falls below the pulse limitation set by the physician, the nurse contacts the physician to determine the recommended action. A fall in pulse rate is associated with increased digitalis levels. The physician may order an ECG or blood work to assess for signs of toxicity. If the cardiac glycoside is stopped for longer than three days, and if the glycoside

happens to be digoxin, whose duration of action averages about three days (half-life 1.5–3 days), the body would have excreted most of the digitalis and there would no longer be a therapeutic blood level. The patient may then experience an exacerbation of previous symptoms, that is, congestive heart failure. If the pulse rate goes above the limitation, the physician is also consulted. A rapid pulse may indicate the patient needs more of his or her digitalis glycoside. Weight is usually measured daily to check for fluid retention.

Determinations of pulse deficits (apical pulse minus radial pulse) may be specifically ordered for patients with atrial flutter or fibrillation. A pulse deficit occurs when a weak cardiac contraction cannot be felt in the periphery, indicating a poor cardiac output. A goal of digitalis therapy is to lower the pulse deficit to zero.

The digitalis glycosides are given at approximately the same time each day. Noon is best, since it allows the patient time to be up and active before the pulse is taken. This is of particular importance in the older adult whose resting heart rate may be low.

The oral medications may be given with or between meals, but the same routine is recommended to be followed each day. The absorption rate is slowed with food but the total amount absorbed is not affected. However, when oral medications are taken with meals high in bran fiber, the amount may be reduced.

The IM or IV route is used only when oral administration is not possible. The cardiac glycosides are irritating to both the subcutaneous and muscular tissues, and digoxin in particular may cause muscle fasciculations and necrosis. Therefore, these drugs are administered only into the gluteus maximus or ventrogluteal sites and never into the deltoid. In a patient experiencing the current signs of congestive heart failure, the absorption rate of an intramuscular injection is uncertain because of decreased perfusion to the periphery; therefore, the IV route is more certain. The IV route is best in an emergency. When administered intravenously, the cardiac glucosides are given over a 10-minute period. Slow administration helps to prevent arteriolar vasoconstriction or an increase in afterload, and thus hypertension, and allows the positive inotropic effect to keep pace with the peripheral effects. When preparing the medication, the nurse reads the label carefully to ensure that the correct product is being prepared. Many of the cardiac glycosides have similar names (digoxin and digitoxin).

DIGITALIZATION

Digitalization is the administration of enough digitalis to reach therapeutic blood level and to eliminate the signs and symptoms of heart failure or to control dysrhythmias with as few side-effects as possible. The procedure is presented earlier in this chapter.

During the period of digitalization, the serum digitalis levels may be checked to help evaluate the patient's response to therapy. Serum potassium and calcium are often checked. Hypokalemia may be caused by steroid therapy, vomiting, nasogastric suction, diarrhea, intestinal fistulas, diuretics, and insulin administration. Hy-

Table 28-6 PATIENT TEACHING INFORMATION—DIGITALIS GLYCOSIDES

Dear Patient:
  This drug has been prescribed for you. This is what you should know about your drug to get the most from your therapy.

1. Digitalis products improve the strength and efficiency of your heart and control abnormal heart rhythms.
2. Cardiac glycosides will generally be taken for the rest of your life.
3. Take your pulse before administering your drug (pulse should be between 60 and 110 beats/min). If the pulse is above or below this limit, or is different in rhythm, consult your physician before taking your medication.
4. Digitalis glycosides can be taken with or between meals. Try to take your cardiac glycoside at the same time each day. Do not alter the dose.
5. Do not take your cardiac glycosides concurrently with antacids, antidiarrheals, or laxatives. If you must take these medications, separate administration by at least 2 to 3 hours.
6. Always check with your physician or pharmacist before taking other medications, as interaction may occur. Medication known to interfere with digitalis glycosides includes barbiturates, certain antibiotics, phenytoin (Dilantin), and phenylbutazone (Butazolidin).
7. If you forget to take your digitalis glycosides for a whole day, eliminate the dose. DO NOT try to catch up by taking two doses in the same day.
8. Do not stop taking your cardiac glycosides without consulting your physician.
9. If you experience any adverse effects from your digitalis glycosides, consult your physician. Common adverse effects include loss of appetite, nausea, vomiting, weakness, fatigue, visual changes, and irregular pulse.
10. Weigh yourself weekly. A gain of 1 to 2 pounds a week may indicate fluid retention. Notify your physician if this occurs.
11. Check your lower extremities for the presence of swelling. If this occurs, notify your physician.
12. If persistent cough and shortness of breath occur, notify your physician.
13. Store these products in a tight, light-resistant, moisture-resistant container to prevent deterioration. Store out of the reach of children.

percalcemia may be associated with immobility and malignancy.

The elderly are often more sensitive to the effects of the cardiac glycosides and need lower doses and closer monitoring. Infants, however, usually need larger amounts of digoxin than expected, that is, greater than normal adult doses. This is a result of an increased elimination of water-soluble drugs in infants.

PATIENT TEACHING

General information about all cardiac glycosides that is to be included by the nurse-educator in the teaching plan for each patient is included in Table 28–6. Patients also need to be taught about signs and symptoms related to congestive heart failure that occur (pulmonary congestion, weight gain, etc.) or symptoms that indicate aggravation of their dysrhythmia.

The nurse often works with the older adult (see Chapter 16 for more information on the older adult). The nurse must work with the patient and family to establish a medication schedule that will not be forgotten. The nurse can assist the patient in developing methods to help remember the medication. Also, the nurse ensures that the patient does not confuse the cardiac glycoside, "little white pills," with other "little white pills," which may be diuretics or antiarrhythmics. The nurse also checks to see if the patient can open the child-proof caps or if the patient needs a regular cap on the medication. An older adult who has poor eyesight or arthritis may find it difficult to open child-proof caps.

Patients are also taught to store their medications in a safe place out of the reach of small children. Older adults may leave their medication on a counter when their grandchildren come to visit. Digitalis products can be toxic to small children.

EVALUATION

The evaluation of cardiac glycosides' effectiveness is based on a predetermined list of evaluation criteria. These evaluation criteria are developed on an individual basis through discussion among the nurse, patient, and family. The information in the data base, obtained in the original assessment, is used to formulate the criteria for evaluation. In most cases, the goals of intervention become the evaluation criteria. Generally, these criteria include (1) a well-informed patient and family who understand the disease and the medical and nursing regimens; (2) a reduction in the symptoms; (3) medication compliance; (4) dietary compliance; (5) understanding of and compliance with the exercise regimen; (6) minimal side-effects related to medications; and (7) the maintenance of a therapeutic blood level of digitalis.

Compliance is often a problem with patients on cardiac glycosides. (See Chapter 8 for more information on patient compliance.) This is usually because the patient does not have enough knowledge about the condition or the medication regimen. It is the nurse's responsibility to educate the patient to prevent future need for rehospitalization to control untoward effects.

When the digitalis glycosides are being administered for the first time, monitoring for hypersensitivity is important. Hypersensitivity may not be observed for five to seven days after therapy is initiated. The nurse observes for toxic reactions. Toxic reactions may result from the patient's taking too many tablets, from diminishing renal or hepatic functioning, from drug interaction, or from hypokalemia. The elderly may experience CNS symptoms early, along with anorexia. The neonate may show a slowing of the sinus rate and a prolongation of the P–R interval.

The evaluation process is ongoing. In the hospital, the

nurse continually evaluates the patient for adverse effects. The effects of the cardiac glycosides are cumulative. The most common adverse effects are anorexia, nausea, and vomiting; others are weakness, fatigue, diarrhea, and visual changes. These effects can usually be eliminated by suspension of the dose for several days. Older adults are much more likely to develop toxic side-effects of the cardiac glycosides. It is imperative that they be evaluated more closely for these signs and symptoms. If digitalis toxicity is suspected, then a serum digitalis level is measured. A blood serum creatinine level may be ordered to evaluate kidney function. Liver function may be evaluated if digitoxin is being used. The therapeutic and toxic levels vary with each digitalis preparation. The values can be found in Table 28–2. If the patient is found to have toxicity, the cardiac glycosides are withheld until the level returns to normal limits. The serum electrolytes, particularly serum potassium and calcium, are also evaluated at this time. If the potassium level is low, the patient often experiences dysrhythmias. The most common dysrhythmias caused by digitalis toxicity and low serum potassium are PVCs, either singly or in ventricular bigeminy (a continuous pattern of one normal beat followed by one PVC), and VT. When these dysrhythmias develop from digitalis toxicity, they are treated, preferably with specific antiarrhythmic medications. Ventricular tachycardia from digitalis toxicity is often best treated with IV phenytoin or lidocaine. (See Chapter 30 for more information on dysrhythmias.) In conjunction with administering these antiarrhythmic preparations, potassium chloride (KCl) is given slowly IV to increase the serum potassium level.

Digitalis rarely produces sinus bradycardia. It is much more likely to produce AV block as a manifestation of cardiotoxicity. In the presence of atrial fibrillation (AF), a junctional escape rhythm may develop because in AF digitalis may produce complete AV block. (Digitalis rarely converts AF to sinus rhythms.) If the junctional rate is over 60, then automaticity may have been increased. In patients being treated with digitalis who have a sinus rhythm, a slight first-degree AV block may occur. Again, withholding the medication for several days usually resolves these problems. The patient is usually then placed on a lower maintenance dosage.

There is also an increased potential for digitalis toxicity when patients are also receiving quinidine. (Quinidine is an antidysrhythmic often given to patients in atrial flutter and fibrillation. See Chapter 30 for more information.) Quinidine has been found to increase the serum digoxin level, possibly by displacing digoxin from tissue binding site. This interaction leads to greater potential for gastrointestinal disturbances and ventricular dysrhythmias. When starting quinidine therapy in patients already receiving digitalis, the clinical course, ECG, and serum digitalis levels are followed closely. Consequently, when quinidine is discontinued, close observation of digitalis levels is also necessary to prevent a decrease in the therapeutic blood level of digitalis.

All previously taught material is reviewed and updated with the patient and family, if necessary, to ensure that their knowledge base is still accurate. The nurse also encourages the patient to keep scheduled visits to the physician. The patient requiring cardiac glycosides may have some physical limitations. With help from the nurse, physican, and family, it is hoped that the patient will be able to live fully within these restrictions.

SUMMARY

Digitalis glycosides have a positive inotropic and negative chronotropic effect on the muscle cells of the myocardium. The primary site of action is the AV node. Digitalis glycosides are used to treat or control congestive heart failure and certain dysrhythmias. The extent of absorption depends on the product used as well as individual patient variables. Digitalis glycosides have a low therapeutic index, producing toxic reactions of increasing severity as serum concentrations rise. Common signs of digitalis toxicity include nausea, anorexia, bradycardia, and cardiac dysrhythmias.

Serum digitalis levels are evaluated often to determine proper dosing. Timing of these samples is important. A delay of three to four hours after an intravenous dose of digoxin and six to eight hours after an oral dose is recommended.

Before administering digitalis glycosides, the pulse is assessed for rate and regularity. The nurse needs to know the individual pulse limitation for each patient. The digitalis glycosides are best administered at the same time each day. When digitalis glycosides are administered IV, they are given slowly over a period of 2–30 minutes. Digitalizing doses may be administered if a rapid onset of action is required.

BIBLIOGRAPHY

Digoxin Antibody Framents for Digitalis Toxicity. Med Let 28(722):87–88, September 12, 1986.
Facts & Comparisons Drug Information. Facts & Comparisons, Inc, St Louis, MO, 1989.
When the ECG suggests digitalis toxicity. Patient Care 20(20):123, 1986.
The Captopril–Digoxin Multicenter Research Group: Comparative effects of therapy with captopril and digoxin in patients with mild to moderate heart failure. JAMA 259(4):539–544, 1988.
Daley, KA, et al: Glucagon: A first-line drug for cardiotoxicity caused by beta blockade. JEN 12(6):387–392, 1986.
Fenster, P and Bressler, R: Treating Cardiovascular Diseases in the Elderly, Part I: Digitalis glycosides and beta-blockers. Drug Therapy 14:125–132, 1984.
Few, BJ: Digoxin immune fab. MCN 12(6):431, 1987.
Gilman, AG, Goodman, LS, and Gilman, A (eds): Goodman and Gilman's The Pharmacological Basis of Therapeutics, ed 7. Macmillan, New York, 1987.

Hopkins, S: Digitalis an antidote after 200 years—digoxin-antibody product (Digibind). Nurs Times 83(28):32, 1987.

Kunkel, DB: Cardiac glycosides: Updating foxglove's toxic heritage, Part 1. Emerg Med 19(13):153+, 1987.

Mathewson, M and Curran, C: Use of cardiac glycosides in the critically ill. Critical Care Nurse 7(6):31–42, 1987.

Porterfield, L: Digoxin—Drug Interactions. Home Health Nurse 3(5):11–5, September/October 1985.

Schneeweiss, A: Drug Therapy in CV Disease. Lea & Febiger, Philadelphia, 1986.

Smith, T: Digitalis glycosides: Mechanisms and manifestations of toxicity. Prog Cardiovasc Dis 26:413–458, 1984.

Weintraub, M and Evans P: Fab: An Immunologic Treatment for Severe Digoxin Overdose. Hosp Formulary 21(12):1190+, December 1986.

SITUATION   28–1

Juliana Fortham, a 66-year-old, is admitted to the coronary care unit with symptoms of nausea, vomiting, and a heart rate of 43 beats per minute (bpm). Medications which Ms. Fortham currently takes include digoxin, Lasix, and a potassium supplement.

1. A diagnosis of digoxin toxicity is made according to serum digoxin concentrations. The nurse is aware of the following:
   a. Digoxin will be decreased slowly to prevent rebound dysrhythmias.
   b. Acid-base and electrolyte values should be checked.
   c. High doses of potassium will be necessary to restore automaticity.
   d. Cardioversion is the treatment of choice for digoxin toxicity.

2. Within a few hours, Ms. Fortham begins to have atrial dysrhythmias. Which of the following drugs would be the most appropriate in this situation?
   a. cholestyramine
   b. phenobarbital
   c. Fab fragments
   d. phenytoin

3. The nurse will check Ms. Fortham's laboratory results for the following condition which would potentiate digoxin toxicity:
   a. hyperkalemia
   b. hyperthyroidism
   c. hypocalcemia
   d. hypomagnesemia

4. After a few days of close observation, serum digoxin levels are reassessed. The nurse will check for the following therapeutic range of digoxin:
   a. 0.5 to 2.0 ng/ml
   b. 6 to 10 ng/ml
   c. 2.5 to 4.5 ng/ml
   d. 14 to 26 ng/ml

5. Ms. Fortham's serum digoxin reflects a therapeutic level, and she is to be discharged on 0.125 mg po daily. Which of the following would be included in patient teaching?
   a. taking the medication in the morning before rising
   b. monitoring pulse rate daily
   c. discontinuing the medication if pulse rate is stable
   d. eating a diet high in bran fiber

6. Ms. Fortham asks the nurse why the digoxin level was high. She states, "I thought my heart was supposed to slow down with the medicine." Which of the following represents the most appropriate nursing diagnosis for Ms. Fortham?
   a. Noncompliance related to failure to report signs and symptoms of digoxin toxicity
   b. Knowledge Deficit related to understanding of the potential toxic effects of digoxin
   c. Impaired Home Maintenance Management related to inability to take digoxin correctly
   d. Alteration in Thought Processes related to understanding the signs and symptoms of toxicity

SITUATION   28–2

Bob Norman, 49 years old, is recovering from an inferior myocardial infarction. The nurse on duty in the coronary care unit notes a change in rhythm from sinus rhythm to atrial fibrillation, heart rate of 130 bpm.

1. The physician orders a loading dose of digoxin (digitalization). The nurse is aware that the loading dosage is approximately:
   a. .0012 to .0050 mg/kg
   b. .010 to .020 mg/kg
   c. 0.5 to 1.0 mg/kg
   d. 0.25 to 1.0 mg/kg

2. Mr. Norman is complaining of difficulty breathing and weakness. The nurse will expect to administer the digoxin by the following route:
   a. subcutaneous
   b. oral
   c. intramuscular
   d. intravenous

3. When giving the digoxin, the nurse will observe for the following potential effect:
   a. hypoglycemia
   b. confusion
   c. hypertension
   d. seizures

4. After successful digitalization, serum levels of digoxin are within a therapeutic range. The maintenance dose will be determined by:
   a. creatinine clearance
   b. liver function
   c. body weight
   d. potassium levels

CONTINUED ON THE FOLLOWING PAGE

SITUATION 28–2–*Continued*

5. A nursing responsibility related to the care of Mr. Norman includes:
   a. administering digoxin in the deltoid muscle
   b. notifying the physician of a heart rate of 120 bpm
   c. relying only on patient assessment for therapeutic response
   d. drawing serum levels 10 hours after an oral dose of digoxin

6. Which of the following statements indicates successful patient teaching concerning digoxin use?

   a. "I will only have to take this drug for a month or two, until my heart heals."
   b. "If I miss a dose, I should eliminate it and not take two in one day."
   c. "If I have any nausea or vomiting, I should stop taking the medicine."
   d. "A little swelling in my feet or ankles is not uncommon with this medicine."

Please refer to the Appendices for correct answers and additional review questions with answers.

29
CHAPTER

DRUGS TO TREAT HYPERTENSION

29

DRUGS TO TREAT
HYPERTENSION

CHAPTER OUTLINE

THERAPEUTIC AGENTS
 Antiadrenergics
 Direct-Acting Vasodilators
 Calcium-Channel Blockers
 Angiotensin-Converting Enzyme Inhibitors
 Serotonin Receptor Blocking Agents
HYPERTENSIVE EMERGENCIES
USING THE NURSING PROCESS
 Assessment
 Nursing Diagnoses
 Planning and Intervention
 Patient Teaching
 Nursing Responsibilities When Administering
  Antihypertensives
 Evaluation
SUMMARY

TABLES

Nursing Process
Patient Teaching
Drug Tables

GLOSSARY TERMS IN THIS CHAPTER

Baroreceptor
Coarctation
Funduscopic exam
Hypertension
Orthostatic
Raynaud's phenomenon
Rebound hypertension
Resistance vessels

29
CHAPTER

DRUGS TO TREAT HYPERTENSION

MERRILY MATHEWSON KUHN, R.N., Ph.D., CCRN

LEARNING OBJECTIVES

After reading this chapter, the student will be able to:

1. Compare and contrast the differences and similarities among antihypertensive medications.

2. Identify medications commonly used as antihypertensives.

3. Identify mechanisms of action, routes of administration, pharmacokinetics, adverse effects, and interactions common to the antihypertensive medications.

4. Formulate a plan to assess the patient requiring antihypertensive medications in order to formulate appropriate nursing diagnoses.

5. Plan the nursing intervention necessary to administer antihypertensive medications safely, and choose appropriate teaching strategies to gain patient compliance.

6. Evaluate the patient at various stages to gauge nursing interactions.

THERAPEUTIC AGENTS

Hypertension, a disease of the circulatory system affecting about 60 million adults in North America, is characterized by persistently elevated systolic or diastolic pressure or both. In 85%–90% of patients, the specific cause of the elevated blood pressure cannot be determined. This is termed essential, or primary, hypertension. Essential hypertension is classified as mild (140/90 mmHg), moderate (160/95 mmHg), or severe (200/110 mmHg). The causes identified in the remaining 10–15% include renal artery stenosis, renal disease, primary hyperaldosteronism, pheochromocytoma—a tumor of the adrenal medulla, and *coarctation* of the aorta. Blood pressure is controlled by several systems: the renal, cardiovascular, endocrine, and neurologic systems. Blood pressure control is discussed in detail in Chapter 27. Figure 29–1 reviews blood pressure control.

Hypertensive persons often have an early increase in cardiac output followed by adaptive changes in the media of *resistance vessels*. These changes eventually cause an increase in systemic vascular resistance. Mortality associated with hypertension and hypertension-related events, including myocardial infarction, cerebrovascular accident, and renal failure, is high. In the United States, it is estimated that more than 1 million deaths occur each year from these diseases. Despite these consequences, most hypertensive patients have uncontrolled blood pressure. Factors contributing to this fact are lack of awareness and patient noncompliance with therapy. Through greater patient education and the availability of less toxic medications, the mortality and morbidity associated with hypertension have decreased. Researchers have directly confirmed that the degree of reduction of mortality obtained by treatment is related to the adequacy of blood pressure control. For a more detailed review of hypertension, see Table 29–1.

Many medications on the market today have a variety of actions that can be used in the treatment of hypertension. The antihypertensive medications do not cure hypertension; they merely lower the blood pressure, which helps to control complications. Therefore, once

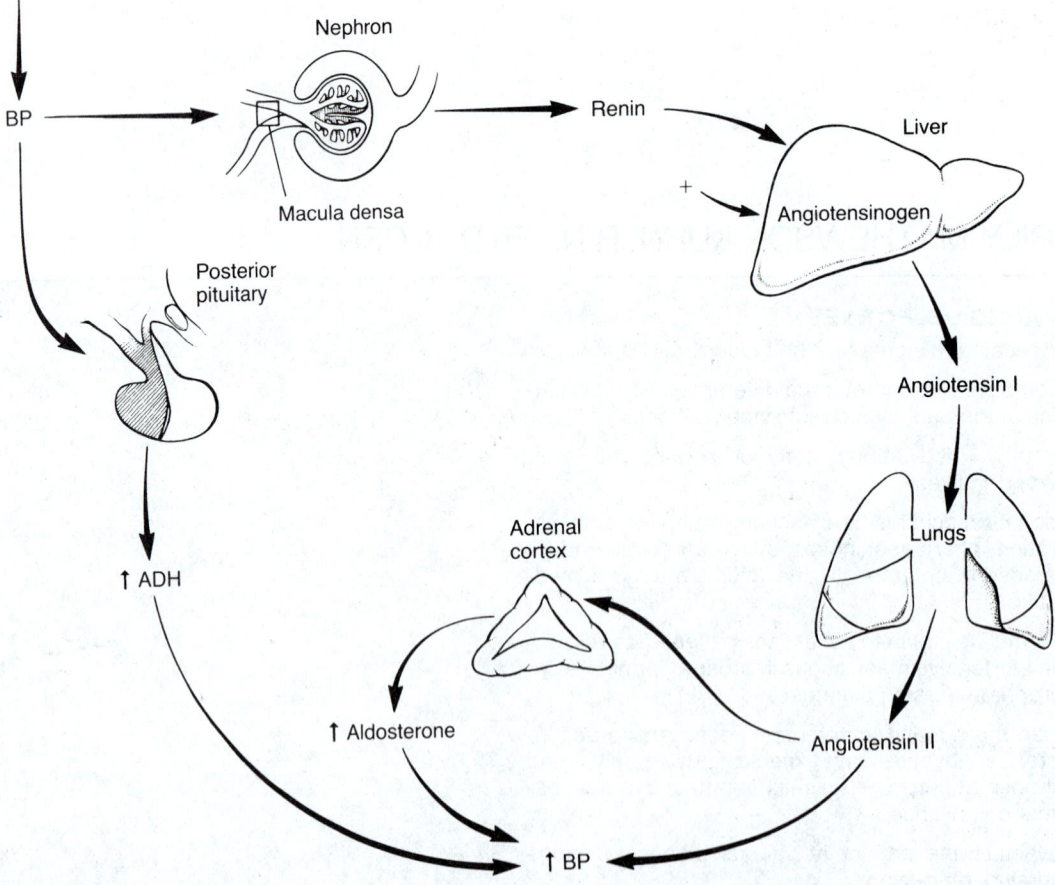

Figure 29–1. Blood pressure control. Several systems regulate blood pressure in the body. The renal system conserves volume and releases renin from the macular densa cells. Renin is eventually converted to angiotensin II, a powerful vasoconstrictor. The endocrine system releases ADH from the posterior pituitary which conserves volume and aldosterone from the adrenal cortex which conserves sodium. The nervous system, through the vasomotor center in the medulla, controls the size of the blood vessels.

Table 29–1. HYPERTENSION

DEFINITION:

Hypertension, a circulatory disease, is characterized by persistent elevated systolic or diastolic pressure, or both, over 160 mmHg (torr).

DIAGNOSIS:

Diagnosis is based on at least three consecutive daily or weekly blood pressure measurements following the criteria for high blood pressure.

	Adults
Normal	Less than 140/90
under 45	over 130/90
over 45	over 140/95

	Children
Infants	over 90/60
3–6 years	over 110/70
7–10 years	over 120/80
11–15 years	over 130/80

TYPES:

Essential, or primary, hypertension is found in 85%–90% of all persons with hypertension. The cause cannot be determined. Essential hypertension is further classified as

Range (mmHg)	**Category**
Diastolic	
<85	Normal blood pressure
85–89	High normal blood pressure
90–104	Mild hypertension
105–114	Moderate hypertension
≥115	Severe hypertension
Systolic, When Diastolic Blood Pressure Is <90	
<140	Normal blood pressure
140–159	Borderline isolated systolic hypertension
≥160	Isolated systolic hypertension

Secondary hypertension is found in the remaining 10%–15% and can be traced to a specific disease or condition. Malignant hypertension is found in any age group, and is rapidly progressive, resulting in death in two years if left untreated.

ETIOLOGY:

The cause of essential (primary) hypertension has not been elucidated, as previously mentioned. However, several contributing factors have been identified, including heredity, excessive use of sodium in the diet, smoking, hyperactive aggressive personality (type A personality), and stressful environment. There is a direct relationship between atherosclerosis and hypertension.

Secondary hypertension is secondary to renal disease, renal artery disease, pheochromocytoma, or pituitary or adrenal dysfunction.

SYMPTOMS:

Patients with hypertension are often symptom-free for many years. They experience complications of hypertension rather than symptoms, with complications occurring 10 to 20 years after the initial onset of essential hypertension.

Objective symptoms include elevated blood pressure, visual changes, coronary heart disease, renal failure, and cerebrovascular accident.

Subjective symptoms include headache, fatigue, and mental sluggishness.

MANAGEMENT (ESSENTIAL HYPERTENSION):

Stepped-care methodology of treatment:

1. Dietary restriction of sodium
2. Maintenance of normal desired weight
3. A change in lifestyle
4. Administration of diuretics
5. Administration of antihypertensive medications

Malignant hypertension is managed in a similar way but more aggressively.
Secondary hypertension is managed by determining the underlying cause and treating it.

the diagnosis of hypertension has been made, the patient is likely to be under treatment for the remainder of his or her life.

Antihypertensives are a relatively new group of drugs; the first antihypertensive was developed in the 1940s. In the 1950s, the rauwolfia preparations, such as reserpine, and several diuretics were developed. Today, there are many antihypertensive preparations, with new drugs appearing each year. The advantage of many of these new medications is their ability to control hypertension in the majority of patients with fewer adverse effects.

The actions of antihypertensives can be divided into four types: (1) centrally or peripherally acting sympathetic nervous system inhibitors, such as ganglionic blockers, neuroeffector-transmission blockers, and β-blocking agents; (2) peripheral vasodilators, such as arterial dilators or mixed arterial and venous dilators; (3) inhibitors of the renin–angiotensin system; and (4) diuretics, which are discussed fully in Chapter 38. Regardless of the method of action, the majority of antihypertensives eventually contribute to the development of peripheral vasodilation, resulting in decreased blood pressure.

The antihypertensives are used to lower blood pressure to a normal level or to the lowest level tolerated. A diastolic pressure of less than 90 mmHg usually can be achieved without producing intolerable adverse effects.

To facilitate successful management of the disease and its consequences, treatment protocols for hypertension should consider the pathophysiologic change. Hemodynamic derangements seen in hypertension have traditionally been viewed in terms of abnormalities in cardiac function (cardiac output) or as derangements of systemic resistance. Hypertension of cardiac origin is dominated by β-subtype adrenoreceptors and responds best with β antagonists, while hypertension of vascular origin is modulated by α subtype adrenoreceptors and responds best to direct α antagonists. The β adrenoreceptors are primarily found in the autonomic nervous system, where inhibitory responses occur when adrenergic agents such as norepinephrine and epinephrine are released. Beta-$_1$ receptors are found in the heart, whereas β-$_2$ receptors are found in the blood vessels and lungs. The α adrenoreceptors, found in the autonomic nervous system, release norepinephrine and epinephrine when excited. Alpha receptors are found in the blood vessels.

Because each type of antihypertensive is so different, each group of drugs is discussed individually as to its action, specific use, pharmacokinetics, contraindications, precautions, adverse effects, and interactions. Table 29–2 features all the antihypertensive medications. Nursing implications are discussed in the nursing process section of this chapter. (Fig. 29–2 reviews the general sites of action of each of these groups of medications.)

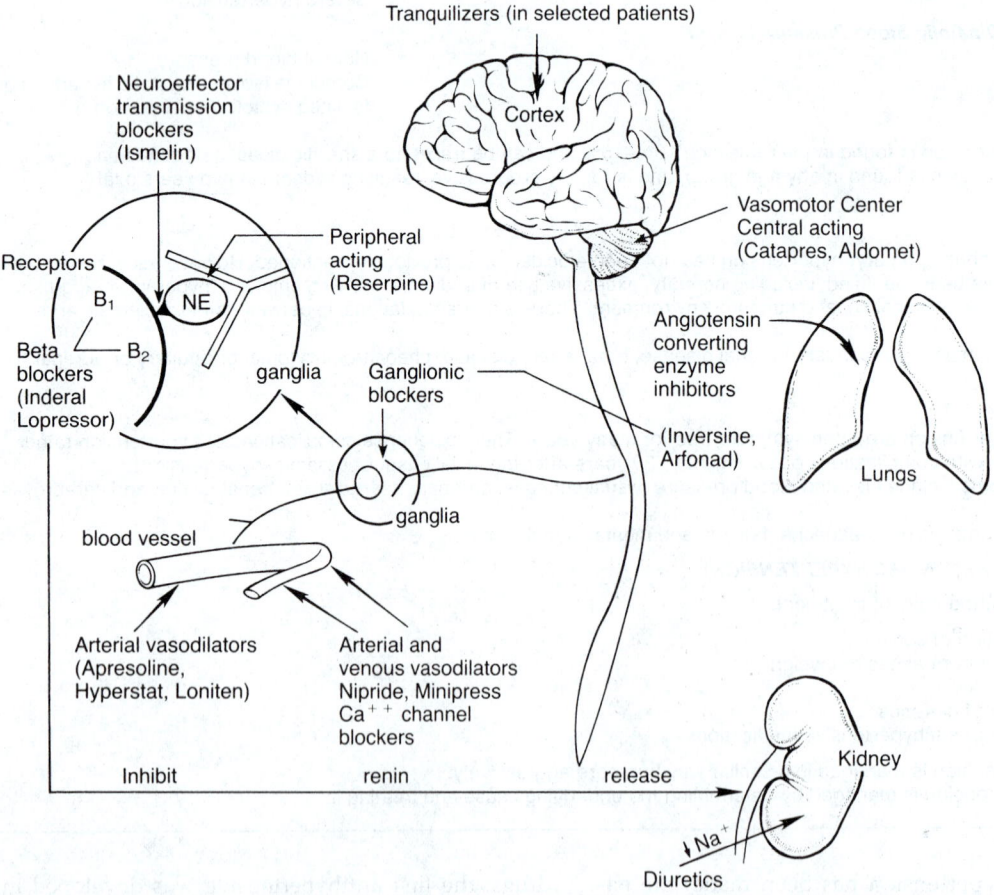

Figure 29–2. Site of action of antihypertensives.

ANTIADRENERGICS

Centrally Acting Sympathetic Nervous System Inhibitors

Sympathetic nervous system inhibitors, in addition to their use as antihypertensives, are used for a variety of other conditions. This chapter primarily reviews their actions only in relation to their ability to control hypertension. (See Chapter 19 for additional information on other uses of these drugs.) Several preparations are available as centrally-acting sympathetic nervous system inhibitors, clonidine hydrochloride (Catapres), methyldopa (Aldomet), guanabenz (Wytensin), and gaunfacine (Tenex).

ACTION. The centrally-acting α_2-adrenergic agonists stimulate receptors primarily located in the medulla oblongata. This central activity results in inhibition of peripheral sympathetic activities and vasodilatation in the peripheral blood vessels.

PRECAUTIONS. The central α_2-adrenergic agonists cause sedation or drowsiness because of their effect on the central nervous system (CNS). During beginning therapy, caution is advised in driving or operating heavy equipment to prevent injury or accident. All centrally-acting drugs are given cautiously to patients with severe coronary insufficiency and recent myocardial infarction, as the vasodilatation in the peripheral circulation may necessitate an increased heart rate and cardiac output and thus may aggravate these conditions. Patients with cerebral/vascular disease may also have their symptoms worsened due to the vasodilatation. Caution is also used in patients with renal or hepatic disease, since these drugs are metabolized and excreted by these routes.

Abrupt cessation of α_2-adrenergic agonists can result in increased plasma and urinary catecholamine levels, increases in blood pressure often to levels significantly higher than before treatment was instituted, and increased nervousness and anxiety. Dosage of these products should be slowly tapered rather than abruptly stopped.

CLONIDINE HYDROCHLORIDE. The centrally-acting agent clonidine hydrochloride (Catapres) stimulates the α_2 receptors in the CNS resulting in inhibition of peripheral sympathetic activity. Clonidine also causes an increase in vagal activity as a result of an increase in sensitivity of the *baroreceptors*. The net result is peripheral vasodilation, caused by a reduction in sympathetic activity. Bradycardia and reduction in cardiac output may also contribute to the drug's antihypertensive effects. Peripheral activity is a minor component of the overall antihypertensive effect of clonidine.

Uses. Clonidine is used in the treatment of mild to moderate hypertension. It lowers both the supine and standing blood pressures. It is often used in combination with diuretics or other antihypertensive medications to achieve a greater reduction in blood pressure.

Clonidine is currently being investigated for the prophylaxis of migraine headache and episodes of menopausal flushing, for treatment of dysmenorrhea, topi-

cally for reduction of intraocular pressure in open-angle and secondary glaucoma, and for prevention of asthma attacks by relaxing bronchial smooth muscle when it is nebulized and inhaled. It is also used for treatment of opiate withdrawal and to detoxify patients from chronic methadone administration. Sublingual clonidine may prove useful in treating hypertension in patients unable to take oral medications.

Pharmacokinetics. *Absorption and Distribution.* Clonidine is approximatley 75% absorbed from the gastrointestinal tract with peak plasma levels occurring in approximately three to five hours. Clonidine passes into cerebrospinal fluid and into the central nervous system. It is excreted in breast milk in a 1.5 milk:plasma ratio. Transdermal patches are available and achieve a peak plasma level two to three days after the initial application.

Biotransformation and Excretion. About 50% of the absorbed dose is biotransformed in the liver, and approximately 40%–60% is excreted unchanged by the kidney. The half-life in normal persons is about 12–16 hours. In persons with renal dysfunction, half-life increases to 25–40 hours.

When the transdermal patches are removed (and not replaced), plasma levels persist for about eight hours and gradually decline over several days.

Contraindications and Precautions. Clonidine is contraindicated in patients showing hypersensitivity to its oral components or to any component of the adhesive layer of the transdermal system. Clonidine should be given cautiously to patients with coronary insufficiency, recent myocardial infarction, cerebrovascular disease, chronic renal failure, or history of mental depression. Safe use in pregnancy, lactating women, and children has not been established.

Adverse Effects. The most disturbing side effects of clonidine therapy are related to the central nervous system. These include drowsiness, sedation, inability to concentrate, and vivid dreams. However, these tend to diminish as therapy continues. Because clonidine decreases salivary flow, dry mouth is a frequently observed adverse effect. Other less common adverse effects are anorexia, vomiting, impotence, rash, congestive heart failure, *orthostatic* symptoms, change in heart rate, and *Raynaud's phenomenon*. Most of these symptoms are related to the effect on the vascular system. As with other antihypertensives, sodium and fluid accumulation often occurs, necessitating administration of a diuretic.

Rebound hypertension (an overshoot in blood pressure) may occur in some patients when they are taken off long-term transdermal clonidine. Termination of the clonidine patch should be accomplished by gradual tapering. Patients who have taken clonidine for blood pressure control and who stop the medication abruptly are at risk for clonidine withdrawal symptoms, including rebound hypertension, agitation, restlessness, and tachycardia.

TEXT RESUMES ON PAGE 752

Table 29–2. ANTIHYPERTENSIVE DRUGS

Name	Dosage	Mode of Administration	Pharmacokinetics

Key to Abbreviations in the *Pharmacokinetics* column O-onset; P-peak; D-duration; PB-protein bound; B-biotransformed in; UA-Unavailable; E-excreted in; ½L-halflife.
*Within the column listing adverse effects, underlines indicate the most common effects; CAPITALS indicate life-threatening effects.

Contraindications/ Precautions	Adverse Effects*	Interactions	Nursing Implications
		FOR ALL DRUGS: Aspirin and other NSAIDs may counteract antihypertensives by inhibiting prostaglandin synthesis, causing salt and water retention.	FOR ALL DRUGS: ASSESSMENT: Thorough nursing history including history of hypertension, complete drug history including OTC, diet pills, and decongestants. Assess current smoking habits, including marijuana. Obtain baseline blood pressure, pulse, weight, and renal function studies. INTERVENTION: Check blood pressure in both the supine and standing positions. Give 1 hour before meals. For patch: wash areas with soap and water and pat dry. Apply patch to hairless site, rotate sites weekly. Apply firmly. Patient teaching: Take the medication every day near the same time. Take as directed. If forgotten, eliminate the tablet. **Do not** take two doses next time. Be cautious for at least 2 hours after taking the medication while driving or working around heavy equipment. Hot baths or showers should not be taken. Change body position slowly to prevent orthostatic hypotension. When moving from a supine position to standing, sit first. All medications are stored in a tight, light-resistant container. Avoid excessive tea, coffee, and cola (more than 4 cups per day). Caution against excessive sweating and dehydration, which may lead to excessive fall in blood pressure. Do not stop medication without physician's approval. If dry mouth occurs, use good oral hygiene. Consult pharmacist before taking OTC products. Monitor blood pressure carefully when concurrently taking aspirin and NSAIDs. EVALUATION: Notify physician of continued or severe GI pain or any change in mood or sleep habits. Evaluate weight at least twice a week to closely monitor fluid retention. Evaluate bp at intervals to determine effectiveness of drug(s).

CONTINUED ON THE FOLLOWING PAGE

Antihypertensive Drugs

Table 29–2. ANTIHYPERTENSIVE DRUGS–*CONTINUED*

Name	Dosage	Mode of Administration	Pharmacokinetics
ANTIADRENERGICS *Centrally Acting Medications*			

Action: stimulate receptors centrally in the medulla oblongata that inhibit the normal excitatory response to epinephrine and norepinephrine. This inhibition leads to dilatation in peripheral blood vessels.
Uses: treatment of hypertension, most commonly essential hypertension.

Name	Dosage	Mode of Administration	Pharmacokinetics
Clonidine hydrochloride (Catapres)	Initial: 0.1 mg bid with increments of 0.1–0.2 mg/day. Maint: 0.2–0.8 mg in 2 doses.	PO	O: 30–60 min P: 2–4 hr, may be 8 hr D: 8–30 hr ½ L: 12–16 hr PB: UA B: liver E: urine
(Catapres TTS)	0.1–0.3 mg daily Skin patch (changed every 7 days)		P: 2–3 days D: several days after removal

Use: to treat mild to moderate hypertension.

Name	Dosage	Mode of Administration	Pharmacokinetics
Methyldopa (Aldomet)	Adults: 250–500 mg 2–4 times daily Children: Initial: 10 mg/kg 2–4 times daily Max: 65 mg/kg/day	PO (can be crushed)	O: 1–2 hr P: 3–6 hr D: 24–48 hr ½ L: 1.7 hr PB: weakly B: liver/intestine E: feces/urine
	Adults: 250–500 mg q 6 hr Children: 20–40 mg/kg/day in divided doses	IV (mix dose in 100 ml of D₅W adm. over 30–60 min)	O: 2–3 hr P: 4–6 hr D: 10–16 hr

Use: to treat moderate to severe hypertension.

Name	Dosage	Mode of Administration	Pharmacokinetics
Guanfacine (Tenex)	I: 1 mg at bedtime increase q 2–3 wks to maximum of 3 mg at bedtime	PO	O: 1 hr P: 2.6–3.0 hr D: 4–5 days ½ L: 17 hr PB: 70% B: liver E: urine (50% unchanged)

Key to Abbreviations in the *Pharmacokinetics* column O-onset; P-peak; D-duration; PB-protein bound; B-biotransformed in; UA-Unavailable; E-excreted in; ½L-halflife.
*Within the column listing adverse effects, underlines indicate the most common effects; CAPITALS indicate life-threatening effects.

Contraindications/ Precautions	Adverse Effects*	Interactions	Nursing Implications
Do not discontinue abruptly. Use with caution in coronary insufficiency, recent myocardial infarction, cerebrovascular disease, chronic renal failure, and history of mental depression. Tolerance may develop. Safety in pregnant, lactating women and children not established.	Neuro: drowsiness, sedation, headache, fatigue, dreams, nightmares CV: CHF, orthostatic symptoms, change in heart rate, Raynaud's phenomenon, rebound hypertension GI: dry mouth, constipation, anorexia, malaise, nausea, vomiting, weight gain GU: impotence, loss of libido, urinary retention Integ: rash, hives (irritation from patch)	Alcohol may increase hypotensive effect. Enhances CNS depressant effects of alcohol, barbiturates, tranquilizers, and other sedatives. Increases bradycardic effect when combined with cardiac glycosides and other hypertensives.	Same as above, plus: INTERVENTION: Patients with history of mental depression require close supervision, as their depression may increase. Tolerance may develop in some patients. Withdrawal of drug should occur over 2–4 days. Abrupt withdrawal may lead to increased blood pressure. Best administered at bedtime.
Contraindicated in hypersensitivity and acute liver disease. Use with caution in history of liver disease, pregnancy, and lactating women.	Neuro: drowsiness, decreased mental alertness, headache, lightheadedness, paresthesias, depression CV: bradycardia, aggravation of angina pectoris, orthostatic hypotension, MYOCARDITIS Resp: nasal congestion GI: dry mouth, nausea, vomiting, diarrhea Biliary: abnormal liver functions, jaundice, HEPATITIS Hemo: positive Coomb's test GU: sexual dysfunction. Integ: rash	Increased hypotensive effect of other antihypertensives. Concurrent propranolol and phenothiazines may result in paradoxical hypertension. Fenfluramine & verapamil may potentiate methyldopa. Impaired tolbutamide metabolism. Amphetamines and tricyclic antidepressants may decrease antihypertensive effect of methyldopa. Alters the following laboratory test results: uric acid, creatinine, urine catecholamines, and SGOT	Same as for all antihypertensives, plus: INTERVENTION: During early drug therapy to 15 weeks, the patient should have periodic blood counts and liver function tests to assess for adverse effects. May darken the urine on standing.
Contraindicated in known hypersensitivity.	Neuro: somnolence, headache, confusion, decreased libido, asthenia CV: fatigue, bradycardia, palpitations, rebound hypertension Resp: dyspnea GI: dry mouth, constipation, abdominal pain, diarrhea, nausea Renal: incontinence GU: impotence Integ: dermatitis, pruritis, sweating	None known	Same as for all antihypertensives, plus. INTERVENTION: Used concurrently with a thiazide diuretic.

CONTINUED ON THE FOLLOWING PAGE

Antihypertensive Drugs

Table 29–2. ANTIHYPERTENSIVE DRUGS–*CONTINUED*

Name	Dosage	Mode of Administration	Pharmacokinetics
Use: to treat mild to moderate hypertension.			
Guanabenz acetate (Wytensin)	Initial: 4 mg bid increments of 4–8 mg/day every 1–2 wk to maximum 32 mg/bid	PO	O: 60 min P: 2–5 hr D: 8–12 hr ½ L: 6 hr PB: 90% B: liver E: urine

Peripherally-Acting Medications

Action: depletes the stores of catecholamines in the sympathetic nerve endings, resulting in a reduction in sympathetic output and a reduction in vasomotor tone.

Use: to treat mild to moderate hypertension.

Name	Dosage	Mode of Administration	Pharmacokinetics
Reserpine	Initial: 0.1 daily Maintenance: 0.1–0.25 mg/day	PO	O: rapid P: 2 hr D: 6–24 hr ½ L: 4.5 hr α; 11.3 day β PB: 96% B: liver E: urine/feces

Ganglionic Blockers

Action: block transmission of both sympathetic and parasympathetic nerve impulses through ganglia. Compete with acetylcholine to occupy the cholinergic receptors, thereby allowing blood vessels to dilate.

Use: severe hypertension and hypertensive crisis.

Name	Dosage	Mode of Administration	Pharmacokinetics
Mecamylamine chloride (Inversine)	Initial and Maintenance: 2.5–25 mg in divided doses 2–4 times daily	PO	O: 30 min–2 hr P: 4–6 hr D: 6–12 hr ½ L: UA PB: UA B: UA E: unchanged in urine
Trimethaphan camsylate (Arfonad)	Adult: 500 mg in 500 ml D₅W titrated to lower blood pressure, usually about 0.3–3 mg/min Children: 50–150 µg/kg/min	IV infusion	O: immediate P: immediate D: 10–30 min after infusion is stopped ½ L: UA PB: UA B: pseudocholinesterase E: kidney

Key to Abbreviations in the *Pharmacokinetics* column O-onset; P-peak; D-duration; PB-protein bound; B-biotransformed in; UA-Unavailable; E-excreted in; ½L-halflife.

*Within the column listing adverse effects, <u>underlines</u> indicate the most common effects; CAPITALS indicate life-threatening effects.

Contraindications/ Precautions	Adverse Effects*	Interactions	Nursing Implications
Contraindicated in known hypersensitivity. Precautions include severe coronary insufficiency, recent myocardial infarction, cerebral vascular disease, renal/ hepatic dysfunction, safety in pregnancy not established.	Neuro: drowsiness, sedation, dizziness, weakness, headache, depression CV: severe rebound hypertension GI: dry mouth	Concurrent CNS depressants cause increased sedation.	Same as for all antihypertensives.
Contraindicated in acute peptic ulcer and acute ulcerative colitis. Use with caution in renal insufficiency, cardiac damage and dysrhythmias, debilitated and elderly patients, and patients with depression.	Neuro: drowsiness, sleep changes, nightmares, depression, blurred vision, mental confusion CV: anginal symptoms, bradycardia Resp: nasal stuffiness GI: weight gain, abdominal cramps, diarrhea, GI bleeds GU: decreased libido, impotence Integ: rash	Increases CNS depression of barbiturates. Decreases effect of ephedrine and levodopa. May have an additive hypotensive effect with diuretics.	Same as for all antihypertensives. INTERVENTION: may cause GI upset, take with food or milk.
Contraindicated in recent myocardial infarction, severe renal insufficiency, hypovolemic shock, glaucoma, and hypersensitivity. Use cautiously in urinary retention.	Neuro: weakness, fatigue, sedation, dilated pupils, blurred vision, paresthesia CV: orthostatic dizziness GI: anorexia, dry mouth, nausea, vomiting, diarrhea/constipation GU: decreased libido, impotence	Increased hypotensive effect with other antihypertensives and diuretics.	Same as for all antihypertensives. INTERVENTION: Dosage is regulated by results of standing blood pressure. Small doses may be ordered in morning, with larger doses in afternoon to accommodate diurnal variation in blood pressure. Administer after meals for better absorption.
Contraindicated in hypovolemic shock. Use with caution in elderly, children, and debilitated since it liberates histamine.	CV: orthostatic hypotension. tachycardia GI: anorexia, nausea, vomiting, dryness of mouth GU: urinary retention EENT: mydriasis, cycloplegia	Increased hypotensive effect with anesthetics.	Same as for all. ASSESSMENT: Check intake and output carefully; assess for bladder and bowel dysfunction. INTERVENTION: Blood pressure is checked every 2 min during beginning of IV infusion, and every 5 min during maintenance. Pupillary

CONTINUED ON THE FOLLOWING PAGE

Table 29-2. ANTIHYPERTENSIVE DRUGS–*CONTINUED*

Name	Dosage	Mode of Administration	Pharmacokinetics
Trimethaphan camsylate (Arfonad)–*Continued*			

Neuroeffector Transmission Blockers

Action: produces selective blockade of efferent, peripheral sympathetic pathways. Depletes stores and release of norepinephrine from adrenergic nerve endings.

Use: Severe hypertension. Used with at least one other agent, usually a diuretic.

Name	Dosage	Mode of Administration	Pharmacokinetics
Guanethidine sulfate (Ismelin)	10–75 mg daily in single or divided doses; rarely, up to 300 mg	PO	O: 48–72 hr P: 1–3 weeks D: 7–10 days, and as long as 1–3 weeks ½ L: 5 days PB: not bound B: kidney, liver E: urine, feces
	Children: Initial: 0.2 mg/kg/24 hr Max. 3 mg/kg		
Guanadrel sulfate (Hylorel)	Initial: 5 mg bid Maintenance: 25–75 mg 1–2 times daily	PO	O: 0.5–2 hr P: 1.5–2 hr D: 10–20 hr ½ L: 10 hr PB: 20% B: liver E: urine

α-Adrenergic Blocking Drugs:

Action: selectively block α post-sympathetic adrenergic receptors dilating both arteries and veins.

Use: mild to moderate hypertension and to manage congestive heart failure.

Name	Dosage	Mode of Administration	Pharmacokinetics
Prazosin (Minipress)	Adults: I: 1 mg at bedtime M: 2–20 mg daily in divided doses Children: 0.1 mg/kg/day	PO	O: 30 min P: 1–3 hr D: 10 hr ½ L: 3 hr PB: 97% B: liver E: bile/feces 90%, urine 10%
Terazoin (Hytrin)	I: 1 mg at bedtime M: 1–5 mg up 20 mg/day	PO	O: rapid P: 1–2 hr D: 12–24 hr ½ L: 9–12 hr PB: 90%–94% B: minimally E: bile/feces 60%, urine 40%

Key to Abbreviations in the *Pharmacokinetics* column O-onset; P-peak; D-duration; PB-protein bound; B-biotransformed in; UA-Unavailable; E-excreted in; ½L-halflife.
*Within the column listing adverse effects, <u>underlines</u> indicate the most common effects; CAPITALS indicate life-threatening effects.

Contraindications/ Precautions	Adverse Effects*	Interactions	Nursing Implications
			dilatation may occur secondary to this drug. Infusions are terminated gradually. Do not mix medication with other medications in same IV bottle.
Use cautiously in coronary artery disease, recent myocardial infarction, cerebral vascular disease, concurrent digitalis, peptic ulcer, pheochromocytoma, frank CHF, concurrent MAO inhibitors.	Neuro: dizziness, weakness, syncope CV: bradycardia, fluid retention, orthostatic hypotension GI: diarrhea GU: inhibition of ejaculation. EENT: nasal stuffiness	Increased hypotensive effect with other antihypertensives, diuretics, and alcohol. Reduced antihypertensive effect with anorexiants, tricyclics, phenothiazines, haloperidol, indirect-acting sympathomimetics, and oral contraceptives.	Same as for all. INTERVENTION: Caution patient to rise slowly from bed in morning, as orthostatic hypotension is greatest in morning. Monitor intake and output for fluid retention.
Same as for guanethidine sulfate. Use with caution in CHF and peptic ulcer.	Neuro: fatigue, headache, faintness, drowsiness, visual disturbances, confusion CV: shortness of breath on exertion, palpitation, chest pain Resp: coughing GI: diarrhea, indigestion, anorexia, nausea, vomiting, excessive weight changes. Renal: nocturia, urinary frequency, impotence Musculoskeletal: aching limbs, leg cramps	Decreased antihypertensive effect—tricyclics, indirect-acting sympathomimetics, phenothiazines. Increased hypotensive effect—direct-acting sympathomimetics. Potentiation of guanadrel with adrenergic blockers.	Same as for all.
Safety in pregnant women and children has not been established.	Neuro: dizziness, headache, drowsiness, weakness CV: palpitations, edema, orthostatic hypotension GI: nausea, vomiting, change in bowel activity GU: urinary frequency, impotence, priapism Integ: rash EENT: blurred vision, tinnitis	Concurrent β-adrenergic blockers enhance postural hypotension.	Same as for all.
Same as for prazosin.	Same as for prazosin.	Same as for prazosin.	Same as for all.

CONTINUED ON THE FOLLOWING PAGE

Table 29–2. ANTIHYPERTENSIVE DRUGS–*CONTINUED*

Name	Dosage	Mode of Administration	Pharmacokinetics
DIRECT-ACTING VASODILATORS			
Hydralazine hydrochloride (Apresoline)			

Action: decrease peripheral vascular resistance in the arteries, leading to peripheral vasodilation.

Use: moderate to severe hypertension and congestive heart failure.

Name	Dosage	Mode of Administration	Pharmacokinetics
	Initial: 10 mg qid Maintenance: 50–200 mg daily in divided doses; rarely up to 400 mg/day Children: 0.75–3 mg/kg/24 hr q 6–12 hr w/max dose of 7.5 mg/kg/24 hr.	PO (can be crushed)	O: 20–30 min P: 2 hr D: 2–12 hr ½ L: 2–4 hr PB: 90% B: acetylation E: urine
	Adults: 5–20 mg repeat as necessary	IV	O: 5–20 min P: 10–80 min D: 2–6 hr
	10–40 mg Children: 0.1–0.2 mg/kg q 4–6 hr (PO, IM)	IM	O: 10–30 min D: 2–6 hr

Minoxidil (Loniten)			

Use: severe hypertension or hypertensive crisis. Often administered with diuretic and 1 or 2 other antihypertensives.

	Dosage	Mode of Administration	Pharmacokinetics
	Initial: 5 mg/day Maintenance: 2.5–20 mg/day once or bid, dose adjustments at least at 3-day intervals; maximal dose 100 mg/day. Children: Initial: 0.2 mg/kg Maintenance: 0.25–1 mg/kg/day in 1–2 divided doses. (Max. 50 mg)	PO	O: 30 min P: 2–8 hr D: 75 hr ½ L: 4.2 hr PB: not bound B: 90% by conjugation E: urine

Diazoxide (Hyperstat)			

Use: emergency treatment of malignant hypertension

	Dosage	Mode of Administration	Pharmacokinetics
	Adult: 1–3 mg/kg over 30 sec or less, may repeat in 5–15 min; do not use longer than 10 days Children: 5 mg/kg as bolus over 30 sec or less	IV bolus	O: 1–5 min P: 5 min D: 3–12 hr ½ L: 28 +/− 8 hr PB: 90% B: liver E: urine

Key to Abbreviations in the *Pharmacokinetics* column O-onset; P-peak; D-duration; PB-protein bound; B-bio-transformed in; UA-Unavailable; E-excreted in; ½L-halflife.

*Within the column listing adverse effects, underlines indicate the most common effects; CAPITALS indicate life-threatening effects.

Contraindications/ Precautions	Adverse Effects*	Interactions	Nursing Implications
Contraindicated in hypersensitivity, coronary heart disease, and valve disease.	Neuro: headache, peripheral neuritis, dizziness CV: palpitations, tachycardia, angina pectoris, sodium retention, muscle cramps GI: anorexia, nausea, vomiting, diarrhea Hemo: blood dyscrasias, lupus-like syndrome. GU: impotence Integ: rash, urticaria	Increased hypotensive effect with other antihypertensives, diuretics, quinidine, and MAO inhibitors. Positive results of laboratory tests for lupus erythematosus cells.	Same as for all. ASSESSMENT: LE prep and antinuclear antibody titer should be taken prior to and periodically during treatment. INTERVENTION: Observe mental status carefully. Monitor intake and output. Pyridoxine (vitamin B_6) may be ordered for patient experiencing peripheral neuritis due to hydralazine. Take with meals. EVALUATION: Report any prolonged tiredness, fever, muscle or joint aching, or chest pain.
Contraindicated with pheochromocytoma, myocardial infarction, dissecting aortic aneurysm. Use cautiously in recent myocardial infarction, renal disease. Safety in pregnancy, lactating women, and children not established.	CV: T-wave changes, palpitations, tachycardia, edema, pericardial effusion, CONGESTIVE HEART FAILURE Resp: pulmonary hypertension Hemo: thrombocytopenia, leukopenia Integ: hypertrichosis, rash	Concurrent guanethidine increases orthostatic hypotension. May elevate BUN, serum creatinine, and alkaline phosphatase.	Same as for all. INTERVENTION: Weigh patient daily. Suggest cosmetics to mask hypertrichosis. Auscultate lungs frequently.
Same as minoxidil. Use with caution in renal disease, ischemic heart and cerebral disease. Safety in pregnant and lactating women not established.	Neuro: dizziness, weakness, cerebral ischemia, papilledema CV: hypotension, sodium and water retention, tachycardia, angina, palpitations, chest tightness GI: nausea and vomiting, acute pancreatitis, change in bowel habits. Integ: rash Endo: hyperglycemia, hyperosmolar nonketonic coma	Potentiates warfarin, increases hepatic metabolism of hydantoins. Concurrent diuretics may potentiate hyperglycemia and hyperuricemia. Concurrent antihypertensives cause profound hypotension. May antagonize sulfonylureas. Lab test: increases renin and IgG. Decreases cortisol. Causes false-negative insulin response to glucagon.	Same as for all. INTERVENTION: Monitor IV site closely for extravasation. Monitor blood glucose level.

CONTINUED ON THE FOLLOWING PAGE

Table 29–2. ANTIHYPERTENSIVE DRUGS–*CONTINUED*

Name	Dosage	Mode of Administration	Pharmacokinetics
Mixed-Arterial/Venous Vasodilators Sodium nitroprusside (Nipride)			

Action: directly relaxes both arteries and veins reducing both afterload and preload.

Use: hypertensive crisis, reduction of preload and afterload in CHF.

Name	Dosage	Mode of Administration	Pharmacokinetics
	0.5–10 µg/kg/min only mixed in D$_5$W; if no response in 10 min to maximal dose, D/C	IV infusion	O: immediate P: 30–60 sec D: 1–10 min after infusion is stopped ½ L: 2 min PB: UA B: liver E: urine

Angiotensin-Converting Enzyme Inhibitors:

Action: compete with angiotensin II for receptor sites in vascular smooth muscle and block conversion of angiotensin I to II by inhibiting the converting enzyme.

Use: mild to severe hypertension, usually in combination with other drugs, congestive heart failure.

Name	Dosage	Mode of Administration	Pharmacokinetics
Captopril (Capoten)	For hypertension: I: 12.5 mg tid, or 25 mg bid, increase 50 mg after 1–2 wk, to maximum 100–150 mg tid, to daily maximum of 450 mg For CHF: I: 6.25 mg tid M: 50–100 mg tid	PO	O: 15 min P: 0.5–1.5 hr D: 6–12 hr ½ L: 1.7 hr PB: 25%–30% B: liver E: urine (40%–50% unchanged)

Key to Abbreviations in the *Pharmacokinetics* column O-onset; P-peak; D-duration; PB-protein bound; B-biotransformed in; UA-Unavailable; E-excreted in; ½L-halflife.

*Within the column listing adverse effects, underlines indicate the most common effects; CAPITALS indicate life-threatening effects.

Contraindications/ Precautions	Adverse Effects*	Interactions	Nursing Implications
Contraindicated with arteriovenous shunt, coarctation of aorta, pulmonary embolism. Use cautiously in hepatic and renal insufficiency and in hypothyroidism.	Neuro: headache, restlessness, agitation, muscle twitching CV: diaphoresis, chest pain, palpitations Resp: decreases arterial PO_2 GI: nausea, abdominal pain, vomiting Other: thiocyanate toxicity, cyanide toxicity	Concurrent ganglionic blockers, volatile liquid anesthetics, circulatory depressants, other antihypertensives augment hypotensive effect.	Same as for all. INTERVENTION: Solutions should be freshly prepared every 24 hours and mixed with only dextrose and water solutions. They are light sensitive and should be covered with tinfoil wrapper that comes in box. Carefully monitor the patient every 5–10 minutes when beginning or stopping the medication and 15 min during maintenance. The blood pressure range for the patient and how fast the blood pressure is to be lowered must be known. Administered IV through infusion pumps and micro-drip regulators. No other drug should be added to the IV bottle or to the IV line. Oral medication should be started as soon as possible so that IV medication can be discontinued. Monitor for thiocyanate and cyanide toxicities after 1–2 days.
		FOR ALL ACE INHIBITORS: Increased hypotensive effect with diuretics and all other antihypertensives. NSAIDS and aspirin antagonize captopril. NSAIDS increase possibility of developing renal failure. LAB: Causes false-positive laboratory test results for urine acetone, increased liver enzymes, BUN, creatinine, serum K. Concurrent allopurinol may increase possibility of hypersensitivity.	
Use cautiously in renal disease, pregnancy, and autoimmune diseases. Safety in children not yet determined.	CV: chest pain, palpitations, tachycardia, hypotension Resp: cough GI: loss of taste sensation, anorexia, nausea, vomiting, change in bowel activity. Hemo: NEUROTROPENIA, AGRANULOCYTOSIS.	Same as for all. Antacids will decrease absorption. Captopril decreases renal clearance of digoxin and may lead to digoxin toxicity. Concurrent nifedipine enhances antihypertensive response.	Same as for all. ASSESSMENT: Assess CBC frequently—every 2 weeks for 3 months, then monthly. Assess patient carefully for signs of infection such as sore throat and fever.

CONTINUED ON THE FOLLOWING PAGE

Table 29–2. ANTIHYPERTENSIVE DRUGS–*CONTINUED*

Name	Dosage	Mode of Administration	Pharmacokinetics
Captopril (Capoten)–*Continued*			
Enalapril (Vasotec)	Initial: 5 mg/day; increase dose at 1–2 wk intervals Maintenance: 10–40 mg/day; reduce dose in renal impairment and in dialysis patients	PO	O: 1 hr P: 4–8 hr D: 12–24 hr ½ L: 11 hr PB: 50%–60% B: not biotransformed E: urine (94% unchanged)
Lisinopril (Prinivil, Zestril)	Initial: 10 mg once daily Maintenance: 20–40 mg once daily; reduce dose with renal impairment	PO	O: 1 hr P: 7 hr D: 24 hr ½ L: 12 hr PB: not bound B: not biotransformed E: 100% unchanged urine

Key to Abbreviations in the *Pharmacokinetics* column O-onset; P-peak; D-duration; PB-protein bound; B-biotransformed in; UA-Unavailable; E-excreted in; ½L-halflife.

*Within the column listing adverse effects, underlines indicate the most common effects; CAPITALS indicate life-threatening effects.

Patients should be warned about the severity of this reaction and counseled to adhere strictly to their prescribed regimen. If clonidine therapy is to be discontinued, as for elective surgery or substitution of other antihypertensives, the dose should be tapered off over several days to a week.

Interactions. Tricyclic antidepressants (imipramine, desipramine, amitriptyline, nortriptyline, doxepin, and protriptyline) are α-adrenergic antagonists. At least two of these, imipramine and desipramine, have been shown to negate the hypotensive effects of clonidine. Depressed patients with hypertension should receive a different antihypertensive. CNS depression may be potentiated by other CNS-depressant drugs such as barbiturates, alcohol, and tranquilizers. Alcohol may increase clonidine's hypotensive effects secondary to its vasodilatory effects. Also, when clonidine is combined with cardiac glycosides and other antihypertensives, there may be an increased bradycardic effect.

Dosage. The initial dosage is 0.1 mg twice daily, and

Contraindications/ Precautions	Adverse Effects*	Interactions	Nursing Implications
	Renal: proteinuria, renal failure Integ: rash, pruritis		INTERVENTION: Give 1 hour before meals. Do not give with antacids. Monitor serum potassium levels. Caution against excessive sweating and dehydration, which may lead to excessive fall in blood pressure. Change body position slowly. Do not stop medication without physician's approval. Do not use K^+ supplements. Avoid cough and cold medications. EVALUATION: Notify physician if mouth sores, fever, chest pain, swelling of hands and feet, or skin rash occur.
Same as for captopril.	Neuro: dizziness, headache, fatigue, syncope, nervousness, somnolence Resp: cough CV: palpitation GI: nausea, vomiting, diarrhea Hemo: decreased hemoglobin and hematocrit Renal: hyperkalemia Reprod: impotence Integ: rash, pruritis, hyperhidrosis	Same as for all.	ASSESSMENT: Assess blood pressure carefully. Assess CBC for hemoglobin and hematocrit periodically. INTERVENTION: Avoid cough and cold medicines and K^+ supplements. Change body position slowly. EVALUATION: Notify physician of chest pains, extreme tiredness, weakness, dehydration, vomiting, diarrhea.
Same as for captopril.	Neuro: dizziness, headache, fatigue, vertigo, depression, somnolence CV: chest pain, palpitation, tachycardia, peripheral edema Resp: cough GI: diarrhea, nausea, vomiting, anorexia, constipation Hemo: decreased hemoglobin and hematocrit Renal: oliguria, hyperkalemia Reprod: impotence Integ: rash	Same as for all.	Same as for enalapril.

increments of 0.1–0.2 mg/day may be added until the desired response is achieved. Maintenance dosage is 0.2–0.8 mg daily given in two divided doses. The maximum daily dosage is 2.4 mg.

The transdermal patch (Catapres-TTS1, 2, or 3) is also started with a dosage of 0.1 mg. If after one to two weeks blood pressure is not controlled, add another 0.1 mg system or use a 0.2 mg patch. Dosage above two patches of 0.3-mg does not improve efficacy. The transdermal preparation delivers clonidine through a rate-controlling membrane.

Clonidine can also be administered sublingually in doses of 0.1–0.2 mg. Doses are given one hour apart and in most patients diastolic pressure falls. Onset of action sublingually is 30–60 minutes.

METHYLDOPA. Methyldopa (Aldomet) is structurally related to the catecholamines and their precursors. Its exact mechanism is unknown, but it may act both centrally and peripherally. Central action involves the metabolism, within central adrenergic neurons, to the active compound d-methyl norepinephrine. When the metabolite is released from these neurons, central α-adrenergic receptors are stimulated, which inhibits sympathetic outflow in a manner similar to clonidine. Methyldopa also reduces renal vascular resistance, suggesting an additional peripheral action. This effect may be useful in patients with impaired renal function and renal hypertension. The drug lowers standing and supine blood pressures and may produce orthostatic hypotension. Methyldopa has little effect on cardiac output. Sedation occurs with this drug, as it penetrates brain tissue and lowers norepinephrine levels. There is also a net reduction of tissue concentration of serotonin, dopamine, and epinephrine.

Uses. Methyldopa is used to control mild to moderate hypertension. It is commonly combined with a diuretic because it has a tendency to produce sodium and water retention. It is frequently a third-step drug (stepped-care therapy is described in the Nursing Process section of this chapter) when a thiazide alone is ineffective.

Pharmacokinetics. *Absorption and Distribution.* High first-pass metabolism results in only about 25% of unchanged methyldopa being absorbed from the gastrointestinal tract. Methyldopa is only weakly bound to plasma proteins. Approximately two days of therapy are required to establish maximal antihypertensive effects. Intravenous doses start to work in four to six hours and last for 10–16 hours.

Biotransformation/Excretion. Methyldopa is biotransformed in the gastrointestinal tract and liver. Renal excretion accounts for about 60%–70% of the drug's elimination. About 10%–20% is excreted in the feces. The elimination half-life is approximately two hours. The drug is removed by dialysis.

Contraindications and Precautions. Contraindications to methyldopa include hypersensitivity; active hepatic disease, since this is where the drug is biotransformed; and mental depression, since the drug may aggravate it. It is given cautiously to patients with a history of hepatic disease (because abnormalities of liver function can occur), renal failure (because methyldopa will accumulate), and to pregnant and lactating women. Methyldopa does cross the placenta, and has been known to reduce the blood pressure of the fetus, but no other adverse effects have been noted.

Adverse Effects. The most common adverse effects are drowsiness, decreased intellectual drive, and forgetfulness. These, together with decreased libido and impotence, limit its usefulness in young patients with hypertension. Other common adverse effects include vertigo, paresthesias, weakness, fever, and dryness of the mouth. The urine may also darken. In 25% of patients, a positive direct Coombs' test occurs. This is an incidental finding. However, in 1%–5% of patients with positive Coombs' test, hemolytic anemia will develop. Hepatic dysfunction, which can resemble either acute hepatitis or chronic active hepatitis, is sometimes seen. Although this reaction is usually reversible upon discontinuation of the drug, overt hepatic failure leading to death has been reported. Liver function tests and complete blood counts (CBCs) should be monitored on a routine basis. Lactation, associated with high prolactin concentrations, can occur in either sex.

As with other antihypertensives, sodium and water accumulation can occur, requiring treatment with diuretics. As seen with clonidine, rebound hypertension may follow abrupt discontinuation of methyldopa.

Interactions. When methyldopa is administered concurrently with amphetamines and tricyclic antidepressants, the antihypertensive effect of methyldopa is decreased. Concurrent administration of methyldopa with propranolol and phenothiazines may result in a paradoxic hypertensive effect. Fenfluramine and verapamil may potentiate the effects of methyldopa. Tolbutamide metabolism may be impaired by methyldopa, resulting in enhanced hypoglycemic effect. Several laboratory tests are also altered: uric acid, serum glutamicoxaloacetic transaminase (SGOT) and serum creatinine.

Dosage. Methyldopa can be given orally in 250–500-mg doses two to four times daily. Its maximal lowering of blood pressure occurs in three to six hours and may persist for as long as 24 hours, because of persistence of α-methylnorepinephrine in the brain. Methyldopa can usually be administered twice a day, and in some studies adequate control of blood pressure was obtained with once-a-day dosing. The maximum daily dosage should not exceed 2.5 g. Intravenous methyldopa can be given in doses of 250–500 mg every six hours. It is mixed in 100 ml of D/W and administered over a 30–60 minute period. Because of its delayed onset, four to six hours, IV methyldopa should not be used to treat hypertensive crisis.

GUANFACINE. Guanfacine (Tenex) is a centrally-acting α_2-adrenergic receptor agonist similar to clonidine and methyldopa, used to treat hypertension in patients already receiving a thiazide-type diuretic. It is not a single-control agent.

Action. Guanfacine reduces sympathetic outflow by stimulating central α_2-adrenergic receptors. Heart rate and peripheral vascular resistance are both reduced. Cardiac output is not affected or is increased slightly.

Pharmacokinetics. *Absorption and Distribution.* Guanfacine is nearly completely absorbed having a bioavailability of about 80%. Peak plasma concentrations are achieved in an average of 2.6–3.0 hours. Guanfacine is 70% bound to plasma proteins and is widely distributed. Steady-state blood levels are generally attained in four days.

Biotransformation and Excretion. Guanfacine is metabolized in the liver and excreted in the urine, probably through tubular secretion as unchanged drug (30%–75%). With normal renal function, the average elimination half-life is approximately 17 hours (10–30-hour range). Guanfacine is poorly dialyzed. Steady-state blood levels are reached in four to five days, but small increases in hypotensive effect may occur for several weeks.

Contraindications and Precautions. Guanfacine is contraindicated in patients with known hypersensitivity. Precautions are the same as for other centrally-acting products.

Adverse Effects. The adverse effects of guanfacine are usually mild and dose-related, and tend to decrease over time. The most common adverse effects are dry mouth (8%–28%), dizziness (4%), fatigue (3%–4%), and rebound hypertension if discontinued. Other, less common adverse effects include somnolence (1%–

14%), headache (2%–4%), impotence (1%–4%), and constipation (1%).

Interactions. No interactions have yet been identified, but there is a potential for increased sedation and hypotension when guanfacine is used concurrently with other CNS depressants.

Dosage. Guanfacine is available in 1-mg tablets. It should be started at 1 mg at bedtime to minimize somnolence. Dosage can be increased every two to three weeks to a total dosage of 3 mg at bedtime. Dosing once a day is possible because of its long half-life. Guanfacine is generally administered concurrently with a diuretic.

GUANABENZ ACETATE. Guanabenz acetate (Wytensin), an oral, centrally acting α_2-adrenergic agonist, causes a decreased sympathetic outflow from the brain. After chronic administration, there is a decrease in peripheral vascular resistance. Both supine and standing blood pressures are decreased, but normal postural mechanisms remain unchanged, so there is little postural hypotension. Cardiac output and left ventricular function are unchanged, but there is a slight reduction in heart rate.

Uses. Guanabenz acetate is used to treat mild to moderate hypertension and is often administered with a diuretic. Guanabenz is added to antihypertensive therapy in step 3 (discussed in the Nursing Process section).

Pharmacokinetics. Absorption and Distribution. Guanabenz is well-absorbed (75%) after an oral dose and is 90% protein bound. Onset of action begins in 60 minutes, with a peak level occurring two to five hours after a single dose.

Biotransformation and Excretion. Guanabenz is extensively biotransformed, but the exact location is unknown. Only 1% of the drug is found unchanged in the urine. The average half-life is about six hours.

Contraindications and Precautions. The only contraindication is for hypersensitivity. Guanabenz is used cautiously in patients with severe coronary insufficiency, recent myocardial infarction, or cerebrovascular disease, since these conditions may be aggravated by a decreased sympathetic outflow. Guanabenz is also given cautiously to patients with renal and/or hepatic dysfunction, since the route of biotransformation and excretion have not yet been determined.

Adverse Reactions. Guanabenz is similar to clonidine in its adverse effects. The most common adverse effects include drowsiness/sedation (20%–39%), dry mouth (28%–38%), dizziness (12%–17%), weakness (10%), and headache (5%). The CNS effects are all related to the general central action of guanabenz.

Interactions. Currently, the only interaction known is with CNS depressants. When given concurrently, increased sedation may occur.

Dosage. Initial oral dose is 4 mg twice a day with increments of 4–8 mg/day every one to two weeks. The maximum daily dose is 32 mg twice daily.

Peripherally-Acting Agents

The rauwolfia compounds are the most commonly available peripheral sympathetic vasoconstriction inhibitors. The rauwolfia compounds are natural medications extracted from Rauwolfia serpentina, a plant indigenous to India and other tropical locations. This drug was used for many years as a tranquilizer in India, and was finally introduced in the United States in the 1950s. In 1953, researchers clearly demonstrated that rauwolfia had antihypertensive qualities as well as sedative effects, and they developed reserpine, a single pure alkaloid of Rauwolfia serpentina.

RESERPINE. Reserpine (Serpasil, Sandril), considered the most potent of the rauwolfia preparations, presumably exerts its antihypertensive effects by depleting the stores of catecholamines in the sympathetic nerve ending. It may inhibit the active transport of norepinephrine to the storage site, thus further impairing its storage mechanism. The net effect is a reduction in sympathetic output, resulting in a reduced vasomotor tone. The reduction in blood pressure, however, is a combined effect of a reduction in total peripheral resistance and a decrease in cardiac output. Both the cardiovascular and the CNS effects may persist following withdrawal of these drugs.

Uses. Reserpine is used in the treatment of mild to moderate hypertension. It is often combined with diuretics or other antihypertensive agents to lower blood pressure more effectively. It is used in step three of therapy.

Pharmacokinetics. Absorption and Distribution. Following absorption, reserpine is widely distributed in the body, particularly in adipose tissue. Reserpine is extensively bound to plasma proteins (96%). Reserpine crosses the blood–brain and placenta barriers. Bioavailability of reserpine is 50%. Peak plasma levels are attained in about 3.5 hours.

Biotransformation and Excretion. Reserpine is biotransformed in the liver into inactive compounds, which are then excreted in the feces and urine. Because it is stored in adipose tissue, reserpine has a long half-life of about 33 hours.

Contraindications and Precautions. Reserpine is contraindicated in acute peptic ulcer and acute ulcerative colitis because it causes gastric and intestinal irritation. It is given cautiously to persons with renal and hepatic insufficiency, since it is biotransformed and excreted in these organs, and to patients with cardiac damage and dysrhythmias, since there is a decrease in peripheral vascular resistance and the decreased cardiac output may worsen these conditions. A Parkinsonian state may occur in debilitated or elderly patients. Reserpine is not used in depressed patients because norepinephrine levels in the brain are reduced, thus aggravating depression. Reserpine is also discontinued seven days prior to electroshock therapy to allow brain norepinephrine levels to return to normal.

Adverse Effects. The most common adverse effects include drowsiness and sleep changes owing to norepinephrine blockade, weight gain, and nasal stuffiness. Increased gastrointestinal motility, abdominal cramps, and diarrhea also are seen. Reserpine can increase gastric acid secretion and exacerbate peptic ulcer disease. In high doses, reserpine can cause gastrointestinal bleeding, and can produce nightmares and depression severe enough to cause a suicide attempt. Less common effects include angina symptoms, bradycardia, and blurred vision. Despite these adverse effects, reserpine is still used because of its low cost.

Interactions. Interactions include increasing the sedative effects of barbiturates and alcohol and decreasing the effectiveness of amphetamines and ephedrine. There may be an additive hypotensive effect when reserpine is given with diuretics, along with an increased risk of cardiac dysrhythmia when it is given concurrently with digitalis or quinidine. Concurrent theophylline can result in tachycardia.

Patients on reserpine have decreased urinary excretion of catecholamines, 17-ketosteroids, and vanillylmandelic acid because reserpine depletes the tissue stores of these substances.

Dosage. Initially, reserpine is given orally in dosages of 0.1 mg and can be increased to 0.25 mg daily. Larger doses are rarely used because of increased frequency of adverse reactions. Reserpine is not recommended for children. The effects are generally cumulative, and full antihypertensive effects may not be seen for three weeks afte therapy is initiated.

Ganglionic Blockers

The ganglionic blockers block transmission of both sympathetic and parasympathetic nerve impulses through the ganglia. They appear to compete with acetylcholine to occupy the cholinergic receptors of the autonomic ganglia. When these drugs interact with cholinergic receptors instead of acetylcholine, this makes it possible for sympathetic impulses to be transmitted from the ganglia to the neuromuscular junction; therefore, blood vessels dilate and arterial pressure falls. These drugs, some of the most potent antihypertensives available today, include mecamylamine hydrochloride (Inversine Hydrochloride) and trimethaphan camsylate (Arfonad).

The ganglionic blockers are developed primarly from a quaternary ammonium compound, tetraethyl-ammonium chloride. Since 1961, more potent and selectively acting drugs with fewer adverse effects have been developed. Thus the ganglionic blockers are seldom used.

USES. The ganglionic blockers are primarily indicated in the more advanced stages of hypertension, including hypertensive crisis, particularly acute dissecting aortic aneurysm, when other medications are not effective. These medications are most effective in reducing the erect blood pressure because of their sympathetic blockade of postural reflexes. The end result of this effect may be fainting due to insufficient blood arriving in the brain.

MECAMYLAMINE HYDROCHLORIDE. Mecamylamine hydrochloride (Inversine), a potent, long-acting secondary amine ganglionic blocker, is used in treating moderately severe to severe hypertension. It is almost completely absorbed from the gastrointestinal tract and begins acting in 30 minutes to two hours. It lasts as long as 6–12 hours. Mecamylamine is excreted slowly and is unchanged by the kidney. Mecamylamine is generally administered orally in dosages ranging from 2.5–25 mg, given in divided doses two to four times daily. For additional information, see Table 29–2.

TRIMETHAPHAN CAMSYLATE. Trimethaphan camsylate (Arfonad), a potent, short-acting ganglionic blocker, is used during hypertensive crisis associated with pulmonary edema; in patients with acute dissecting aortic aneurysm; and for short periods of time in neurosurgic or cardiovascular surgeries to prevent excessive bleeding and to allow increased visulization of the surgical field.

The usual IV dose of trimethaphan is 500 mg diluted in 500 ml of D_5W and is titrated to the desired blood pressure response. The usual dose is between 0.3 and 3 mg/min. The drug's effects are gone about five minutes after the infusion is stopped. Trimethaphan is not mixed with other medications. Because of the respiratory depression and tachycardia that can develop from its use, only those experienced in its use should administer it. Trimethaphan can stimulate the release of histamine and should be used with caution in patients with known allergies. For additional information, see Table 29–2.

Drugs That Affect Neuroeffector Transmission

GUANETHIDINE SULFATE. Guanethidine sulfate (Ismelin) acts as a neuroeffector transmission blocker. It produces a selective blockade of efferent, peripheral sympathetic pathways. This drug depletes norepinephrine from the adrenergic nerve endings and further prevents the release of norepinephrine in response to sympathetic nerve stimulation. Administration of this medication slowly reduces the catecholamine stores from the adrenergic nerve endings, producing a prolonged fall in blood pressure. It also causes a reduction in cardiac output, resulting from reduced venous return and negative chronotropic and inotropic effects and a fall in total peripheral vascular resistance. Guanethidine produces venous dilation, which results in blood pooling in the splanchnic and peripheral areas. This in turn may result in a decrease in renal, coronary, and cerebral blood flow.

Guanethidine, unlike the rauwolfia compounds, does not pentrate the CNS, so it does not have additional central actions. In addition, it does not inhibit the parasympathetic system as do the ganglionic blockers, so it does not result in anticholinergic adverse effects (dry mouth, urinary retention). Guanethidine sulfate does lower upright blood pressure more than supine and therefore can cause postural hypotensive symptoms. It also causes sexual dysfunction relatively frequently.

Uses. Guanethidine is used in the treatment of severe hypertension that does not respond to other drug regimens. It is usually used as a step five drug. As do certain other antihypertensives, it causes renal retention of sodium and water. Guanethidine is, therefore, more effective when given in conjunction with diuretics. It reduces systolic blood pressure more than diastolic, and is more effective in lowering the upright blood pressure than the supine pressure. It is not commonly used today because the dosage is difficult to regulate without causing orthostatic hypotension and diarrhea; and other effective drugs, such as captopril (Capoten), minoxidil (Loniten), are available for treating resistant hypertension. For additional information, see Table 29–2.

GUANADREL SULFATE. Guanadrel sulfate (Hylorel) is structurally and pharmacologically similar to guanethidine, but has a more rapid onset and shorter duration of action after withdrawal. Guanadrel inhibits sympathetic vasoconstriction by inhibition and depletion of norepinephrine release from neural storage sites. There is a relaxation of vascular smooth muscle with a reduction in total peripheral resistance. Guanadrel does not readily cross the blood–brain barrier, and therefore there is less sedation and fewer CNS effects than with guanethidine. Unlike the direct-acting agents, it does not inhibit parasympathetic nerve function and thus does not cause dry mouth.

Uses. Guanadrel is usually reserved for patients with severe refractory hypertension. It is used in step two and step three of therapy. It is considered as effective as guanethidine and more effective than methyldopa.

Pharmacokinetics. Absorption and Distribution. Guanadrel is readily absorbed and reaches peak plasma levels in 1.5–2 hours. It is 20% protein bound. Maximal hypotensive effect occurs in four to six hours.

Biotransformation and Excretion. The half-life is about 10 hours with wide individual variability. Forty percent of the drug is excreted unchanged in the urine, and a total of 85% is eliminated in the urine.

Contraindications and Precautions. Contraindications are similar to those associated with guanethidine—pheochromocytoma, since sensitivity to, and uptake of, circulating norepinephrine is enhanced; frank congestive heart failure, since it may be worsened by a decreased total peripheral resistance and fluid retention; and hypersensitivity.

Precautions include peptic ulcer, as symptoms may be worsened by an increase in parasympathetic tone, and asthma because the symptoms may be aggravated by catecholamine depletion. Safety of use during pregnancy and lactation and in children has not been established.

Adverse Effects. Adverse effects again are similar to guanethidine. Adverse effects are generally higher during the first eight weeks and then tend to decrease in frequency. Most common adverse effects include shortness of breath on exertion (46%) due to decreased cardiac output; fatigue (64%), headache (58%), orthostatic hypotension (47%–49%), drowsiness (45%), and aching limbs (43%) all of which are related to relaxation of vascular smooth muscle; and nocturia (48%), and peripheral edema (29%) related to increased retention of sodium and water.

Interaction. Several drugs—tricyclics, indirect-acting sympathomimetics, and possible phenothiazines— can reverse the effects of neuronal blocking agents, thus elevating blood pressure. Increased hypotensive effect can occur with concurrent direct-acting sympathomimetics. Adrenergic blocking agents can potentiate the effects of guanadrel.

Dosage. The initial dose of guanadrel is 10 mg daily, increased daily until the desired response is achieved. The usual maintenance dose is 25–75 mg once or twice daily. Tolerance may develop over time, so dosage may need to be increased.

Beta-Adrenergic Blocking Drugs

The β-adrenergic blockers propranolol hydrochloride (Inderal), acebutolol (Sectral), metoprolol (Lopressor), nadolol (Corgard), atenolol (Tenormin), pindolol (Visken), esmolol (Brevibloc), and timolol (Blocadrin) compete with epinephrine for available β-receptor sites, thereby inhibiting the response to β-adrenergic stimuli. Beta receptors are typically classified into two types, β_1 and β_2. Beta$_1$ receptors are found primarily in the heart, whereas β_2 receptors are located primarily in the lung. By blocking the β-adrenergic receptor sites in the heart, these drugs decrease heart rate, myocardial contractility, and ultimately cardiac output. Conduction velocity through the AV node and firing rate in the SA node also decrease. These effects prevent exercise-induced increases in the heart rate. The mechanism by which they lower blood pressure is much more complex and is highly controversial at this time. The most probable mechanisms of action include a reduction in cardiac output, a reduction in plasma renin activity, and a CNS sympatholytic action. Beta blockers are often administered in combination with diuretics or other antihypertensive drugs and are used in step two and step three of the antihypertensive regime. The β blockers are discussed in depth in Chapter 19 and can be found in Table 19–8.

PROPRANOLOL HYDROCHLORIDE. Propranolol hydrochloride (Inderal) is effective in treating all types of hypertension and decreases both systolic and diastolic pressures in the supine and standing positions during both rest and exercise. It is a nonselective β blocker that inhibits both β_1 and β_2 receptors. Systolic pressure decreases more than diastolic pressure, and there is a greater decrease during exercise than at rest.

Initial dose for adults begins at 40 mg bid with increments of 80 mg daily until a desired response is achieved. Maximal dose is 480 mg daily. Maximal effect may not be seen for several weeks. Children receive 1 mg/kg qid. Long-acting products (Inderal LA) are started at 80 mg daily with maintenance doses between 120 and 160 mg daily. In emergency situations, propranolol hydrochloride can be administered intravenously at a rate of 1 mg/min up to 3 mg.

ACEBUTOLOL HYDROCHLORIDE. Acebutolol hydrochloride (Sectral) acts selectively on the β_1 receptors and reduces heart rate and blood pressure at rest and during exercise. It lowers both diastolic and systolic blood pressure in the supine and standing positions. Initial dose is 400 mg singly or divided, with maintenance dosage between 200 and 800 mg daily.

METOPROLOL. Metoprolol (Lopressor) is given in an initial oral dosage of 50–250 mg twice daily. Usual maintenance dosage is 100–300 mg daily, and it can be administered as a single daily dose. If blood pressure is not controlled, metoprolol can be administered three times a day. Metoprolol acts primarily on β_1 receptors. In an emergency situation, metoprolol can be administered intravenously in three bolus injections of 5 mg at approximately two-minute intervals. Blood pressure must be carefully monitored.

NADOLOL. Nadolol (Corgard) has a longer half-life than propranolol, resulting in a longer duration of action, approximately 20–24 hours. This allows once-daily administration. Initial dosage is 20 mg with maintenance dosages ranging from 40–120 mg daily. Nadolol acts on both β_1 and β_2 receptors.

ATENOLOL. Atenolol (Tenormin), a β_1-selective β blocker, is given in once-daily doses of 50–100 mg. The maximum effect appears within three days after the initial dose. Atenolol has been used to treat essential hypertension in pregnant women and early preeclampsia.

PINDOLOL. Pindolol (Visken) is started with 10 mg bid or 5 mg tid. The dosage may be increased by 10 mg/day at two- and three-week intervals, with the maximum dosage 60 mg/day. Average dosage is usually maintained between 15 and 60 mg/day. Pindolol acts on both β_1 and β_2 receptors.

TIMOLOL. Timolol (Blocadrin) is started at 10 mg bid. Seven days should elapse before the dose is increased. Maintenance dosage is usually between 20 and 40 mg a day, with the maximum dosage being 60 mg a day in divided doses. Timolol acts on both β_1 and β_2 receptors.

Alpha- and Beta-Adrenergic Blocking Drugs

LABETALOL. Labetalol (Normodyne, Trandate) is an α/β-adrenergic blocking agent that combines both selective postsynaptic α_1-adrenergic blocking plus nonselective β-blocking actions. Because of these actions, it is used primarily to reduce hypertension. Labetalol mildly decreases cardiac output and total peripheral resistance. Plasma renin levels are reduced. Standing blood pressure is lowered more than supine, and therefore patients may experience postural hypotension. Labetalol is available in IV and PO forms. IV labetalol has a rapid onset of action (five to seven minutes) and is titratable for predictable results. Labetalol can be given in 5-mg IV bolus, every five to ten minutes, up to 100 mg, and then maintained on a 100–200-mg IV infusion over 60 minutes every four to six hours. Orally, labetalol is started at 100 mg bid with a maintenance dose of 400–800 mg. Severe hypertension may require up to 1.2 g daily in two or three divided doses. Concomitant diuretic therapy enhances the therapeutic response.

ESMOLOL HYDROCHLORIDE. Esmolol hydrochloride (Brevibloc) is a β_1 blocker with a rapid onset and short duration, and may be used to reduce the blood pressure rapidly. Esmolol is used primarily for treating supraventricular tachycardias and is discussed in detail in Chapter 19. An initial loading dose of 500 μg/kg/min for one minute is followed by a four-minute maintenance infusion of 50 μg/kg/min. This dose can be repeated in five minutes if needed. Esmolol is only for acute therapy.

Alpha-Adrenergic Blocking Drugs

A-adrenergic blockers block α-adrenergic receptors found in most blood vessels, particularly the skin, mucosa, intestine, and kidney, resulting in a lowered total peripheral resistance and a decreased blood pressure.

Prazosin (Minipress) and terazosin (Hytrin) are structurally unrelated to other antihypertensives. These drugs relax the arterial smooth muscle by blocking the α-adrenergic receptors and reducing total peripheral vascular resistance. They increase venous capacitance by dilating the venous vessels, thereby reducing preload and dilating the arterial bed, reducing afterload. Heart rate, renal blood flow, or glomerular filtration are not significantly changed; but fluid retention does occur, so often they are given concurrently with a diuretic.

USES. Prazosin and terazosin are useful in treating mild to moderate hypertension. They can increase cardiac output by reducing preload and afterload and therefore can be used in the treatment of heart failure with coexisting hypertension. Prazosin and terazosin are generally used in step two or step three. Prazosin and terazosin can be administered alone, but are much more effective when combined with a diuretic. Drug resistance frequently develops after weeks or months when prazosin and terazosin are administered alone. Prazosin is also used to treat Raynaud's syndrome.

CONTRAINDICATIONS AND PRECAUTIONS. Safety in pregnant women and in children has not been established.

ADVERSE EFFECTS. The most significant adverse effects of prazosin and terazosin are orthostatic hypotension and syncope, which occur early in therapy. They are believed to be caused by an inadequate venous return to the right side of the heart. These effects are common, therefore, in patients who are dehydrated and volume depleted. They are generally not seen in patients with an increased venous return, as in heart failure. These effects are minimized by administering the first dose, of no larger than 1 mg, at bedtime. The other adverse effects include dizziness (10% and 19%), drowsiness (8% and no report), headache (8% and 16%), palpitations (5% and 4%), and nausea (5% and 4%). Adverse effects generally disappear with continued therapy.

INTERACTIONS. Concurrent use of β adrenergic blockers may enhance postural hypotension. Since prazosin and terazosin are highly bound, they theoretically may interact with other highly bound drugs.

PRAZOSIN

Pharmacokinetics. Absorption and Distribution. Prazosin is well-absorbed from the gastrointestinal tract. Prazosin is highly bound (about 97%) to plasma proteins. Plasma concentration peaks in about one to three hours. Food does not affect the rate or extent of absorption.

Biotransformation and Excretion. Prazosin is extensively metabolized in the liver with less than 10% excreted in the urine as unchanged drug. This results in a first-pass effect, with an average bioavailability of 50%–60%. The half-life of prazosin is three hours in normal patients and is prolonged in patients with hepatic disease or congestive heart failure. The antihypertensive effects can persist for ten hours.

Dosage. The initial adult dose of prazosin is started at 1 mg at bedtime to minimize the hypotension. Dosage may then be increased gradually to 2–20 mg/day given in two to three divided doses. The maximal daily dosage is approximately 40 mg. Children receive 0.1 mg/kg/day.

TERAZOSIN

Pharmacokinetics. *Absorption and Distribution.* Terazosin has a 90% oral bioavailability, which is not affected by food. Terazosin, like prazosin, is highly bound (90% to 94%) to plasma proteins. Peak plasma level occurs within one to two hours.

Biotransformation and Excretion. Terazosin has a minimal hepatic first-pass effect, and therefore the majority of circulating drug is the parent drug. Terazosin has a half-life of 9–12 hours and is excreted 60% in bile and feces and 40% in the urine.

Dosage. Like prazosin, the first dose of terazosin is administered at bedtime. The dose is slowly increased to 1–5 mg daily until blood pressure is controlled. Some patients may receive doses as high as 20 mg/day.

DIRECT-ACTING VASODILATORS

The direct-acting vasodilators act directly on the peripheral blood vessels—either on the arteries alone or on the arteries and veins together. Both groups of drugs lower blood pressure by decreasing peripheral vascular resistance. This reduction in blood pressure can consequently stimulate the baroreceptors and, in turn, increase the heart rate, cardiac output, and force of contraction. This effect may prove dangerous for a patient with underlying ischemic cardiac disease. The peripheral vasodilators are generally given in combination with β blockers to reduce the adverse effects related to baroreceptor stimulation.

Arterial Vasodilators

The arterial vasodilators reduce blood pressure by directly relaxing the arteriolar smooth muscle. The increased caliber of the blood vessel reduces total peripheral resistance, which lowers blood pressure, decreasing afterload. Arterial vasodilators include hydralazine hydrochloride (Apresoline), diazoxide (Hyperstat), and minoxidil (Loniten). In patients without severe heart failure, all these medications increase the heart rate and cardiac output as a result of reflexes secondary to the decrease in blood pressure.

HYDRALAZINE HYDROCHLORIDE. Hydralazine (Apresoline) reduces blood pressure by directly relaxing arteriolar smooth muscle. Cardiac output is increased as afterload is reduced. Hydralazine maintains or increases renal and cerebral blood flow.

Uses. Hydralazine hydrochloride is used in the chronic management of moderate to severe hypertension. It can be used intravenously to rapidly decrease blood pressure in hypertensive emergencies. It is also used alone or in combination with nitrates to increase cardiac output (by reducing afterload) in patients with heart failure. The reflex catecholamine response can result in tachycardia and increases in heart rate. Hydralazine hydrochloride is usually a step three or four drug. Hydralazine with a diuretic is often an effective, well-tolerated treatment for the elderly hypertensive patient

because they are less likely to develop a reflex tachycardia.

Pharmacokinetics. *Absorption and Distribution.* Hydralazine is well-absorbed. Its bioavailability is relatively low (30%–50%) but can be increased by administering it with food. Peak blood levels are reached in about one hour with a duration of action of two to four hours. Hydralazine is about 90% bound to plasma proteins.

Biotransformation and Excretion. Hydralazine has an extensive first-pass hepatic metabolism. It is metabolized by several pathways; however, acetylation is most likely its major route of metabolism. Genetically determined fast "acetylators" have a lower bioavailability and lower concentrations in plasma at steady state than slow acetylators. Less than 10% of the dose is excreted unchanged in the urine. The plasma half-life is two to eight hours, but its duration of action is as long as 12 hours.

Contraindications and Precautions. Hydralazine is contraindicated in coronary artery disease because it can produce anginal attacks and in patients with mitral valvular disease because the hyperdynamic state (increased heart rate and cardiac output) may accentuate or aggravate the valvular disease. Hydralazine should be used with caution in patients with cerebral vascular accidents due to the possibility of increased cerebral ischemia, which may be precipitated. Safety in pregnant and lactating women is not yet established.

Adverse Effects. Common adverse effects include headache caused by cerebral vasodilatation, palpitation caused by reflex increase in heart rate, anorexia and nausea caused by gastrointestinal congestion, and sweating caused by increased caliber of peripheral vessels. These cardiac effects can be controlled with concurrent administration of β blockers. Less common effects are nasal congestion, flushing, lacrimation, conjunctivitis, paresthesias, edema, tremors, and muscle cramps. Tolerance to these effects can occur with continued therapy. Adverse effects that require discontinuation of therapy include rash, drug fever, polyneuritis, gastrointestinal hemorrhage, anemia, and pancytopenia (a reduction of all cellular components of blood).

A drug-induced systemic lupus erythematosus (SLE) syndrome can develop with hydralazine therapy. This syndrome usually presents with myalgias, arthralgias, and/or pleuritis. The antinuclear antigen (ANA) test is positive. Renal and CNS involvement is rare with drug-induced SLE. This syndrome is seen more commonly in slow acetylators and in patients receiving dosages greater than 400 mg/day. Upon discontinuation of the drug, the syndrome disappears.

Interactions. Interactions include an increased hypotensive effect when other antihypertensives, diuretics, quinidine, and MAO inhibitors are given concurrently.

Dosage. Hydralazine can be given both orally and parenterally. Orally, dosages range from 50 to 400 mg daily, given in divided doses. Twice-a-day administration effectively controls blood pressure. Maximal daily dosage is 300 mg. Children receive 0.75–3 mg/kg/24 hours every 6–12 hours with a maximum dose of 7.5 mg/kg/24 hours. Intravenously, 5–40 mg are given slowly to adults, and children can receive 0.1–0.2 mg/kg every four to six hours as needed. Similar doses are administered intramuscularly. Most patients can transfer to the oral form within 24–48 hours.

MINOXIDIL. Minoxidil (Loniten) is a very potent oral vasodilator with an action similar to that of hydralazine. It decreases blood pressure by reducing total peripheral resistance. Renal vascular resistance is reduced and glomerular filtration rate is not decreased. Like diazoxide and hydralazine, it can cause a reflex tachycardia, increased cardiac output, and fluid retention by increasing renin activity.

Uses. Because of serious adverse effects, the use of minoxidil is limited to patients with severe hypertension and is generally considered a step four or five drug. Minoxidil is useful for long-term therapy in patients refractory to maximum doses of standard drugs. Both a diuretic and β blocker or other sympathetic depressant drug are given concurrently to control fluid retention, prevent tachycardia, and enhance the therapeutic effectiveness. It does appear to be effective in the treatment of hypertensive patients with severe renal failure. Minoxidil, as a topical formulation, is available in Canada (Rogaine) and Europe (Regaine) for treatment of male-pattern baldness. More information can be found in Chapter 66.

Pharmacokinetics. *Absorption and Distribution.* Minoxidil is almost completely absorbed when given orally and is almost 90% bioavailable. Minoxidil is not protein-bound and concentrates in arteriolar smooth muscle. Peak plasma levels are achieved within the first hour and decline rapidly thereafter. Blood pressure starts to decline within one-half hour and reaches minimum within two to three hours.

Biotransformation and Excretion. Plasma half-life is approximately 4.2 hours. The drug is extensively metabolized (90% percent) predominantly by conjugation with glycuronic acid. Duration of effect is approximately 75 hours. Excretion is through the urine with renal clearance dependent on glomerular filtration rate.

Contraindications and Precautions. Minoxidil is contraindicated in phenochromocytoma because it may stimulate catecholamine release from the tumor, elevating blood pressure. Minoxidil is also contraindicated in myocardial infarction and dissecting aortic aneurysm because reflex cardiac stimulation may occur, aggravating these conditions.

Minoxidil is administered cautiously to patients after a myocardial infarction because the reduction in arterial pressure may further limit blood flow to the myocardium. In patients with renal disease, smaller doses may be necessary and close medical supervision is required. Safety during pregnancy, in lactating women, and in children has not been established.

Adverse Effects. The most common adverse effects are related to reflex activation of the sympathetic nervous system, resulting in palpitations, tachycardia, and increased myocardial work. These are unwanted effects in patients with ischemic heart disease that can be ef-

fectively controlled with β blockade. Changes in direction and magnitude (flattening or inversion) of T waves (60%) also occur. Fluid accumulation (7%) caused by the reduction in arterial pressure can be effectively managed with diuretics. A common adverse effect of minoxidil is hair growth (80%) most prominent in the face, arms, and back. The development of pericardial effusions (3%) is a potentially serious adverse effect. It has been recommended that patients be monitored by echocardiography for the development of this adverse effect. Pulmonary hypertension has also been described with the use of this drug and may be secondary to increased cardiac output. Minoxidil does not cause impotence and may occasionally alleviate it.

Interactions. Concurrent administration with guanethidine can result in orthostatic hypotension.

Dosage. Minoxidil is usually given twice a day in dosages ranging from 2.5 to 20 mg/day. Dosage adjustments are made at least at three-day intervals. The maximum recommended daily dose is 100 mg.

DIAZOXIDE. Diazoxide (Hyperstat) is a thiazide derivative but has no diuretic activity. It has a direct effect on the arteries. Increased heart rate and cardiac output occur as blood pressure is reduced. Renal blood flow is increased after an initial decrease.

Uses. Diazoxide is used effectively to treat patients with severe, malignant hypertension, and hypertensive crisis. The advantages of diazoxide over other antihypertensives include its rapid action time, its ability not to cause sedation or extreme hypotension, and its ability not to need a continuous infusion.

Pharmacokinetics. *Absorption and Distribution.* Diazoxide is well-absorbed orally and is useful in an oral form for treating hypertension. It is 90% bound to albumin in plasma. The extent of binding decreases in patients with renal failure, and these patients may have greater-than-expected response from the drug.

Biotransformation and Excretion. Renal excretion accounts for approximately one-third of the overall elimination of diazoxide. Plasma half-life is 28 ± 8 hours. The duration of effect is variable but generally less than 12 hours.

Contraindications and Precautions. Excessive hypotension and reflex sympathetic stimulation can produce myocardial ischemia in susceptible patients. It is also contraindicated in aortic coarctation or arteriovenous shunt and dissecting aortic aneurysm because the cardiac stimulation may aggravate these conditions. Diazoxide is used with caution in patients with ischemic heart disease. It should also be used with caution in patients with renal disease, since prologed hypotension may precipitate renal failure. Safe use in pregnancy and lactating women has not yet been established.

Adverse Effects. The most common adverse effect from diazoxide is hypotension (7%) followed by nausea and vomiting (4%), and dizziness and weakness (2%). Diazoxide also causes sodium and water retention. It is fairly common practice to administer a 20–40-mg IV dose of furosemide (Lasix) concurrently with diazoxide to overcome this adverse effect. Diazoxide can also decrease glomerular filtration rate by reducing blood pressure and renal plasma flow. Hyperglycemia can occur if it is used for several days. Under these circumstances, blood glucose levels should be monitored. If used chronically, hypertrichosis and hyperuricemia can develop.

Interactions. Diazoxide can displace warfarin from its protein-binding sites on albumin. This can potentiate the effect of warfarin. Prothrombin time should be determined in a patient stabilized on warfarin if diazoxide is adminstered. Diazoxide may increase hepatic metabolism of hydantoins. Concurrent thiazides or other diuretics may potentiate hyperglycemia and hyperuricemia. Diazoxide appears to inhibit insulin release from pancreatic islet cells and may antagonize sulfonylureas. Profound hypotension may occur when other antihypertensives are administered.

Dosage. Diazoxide is given by IV bolus over 30 seconds or less in doses of 1–3 mg/kg. Recent data suggest, however, that slower administration of diazoxide may decrease the chance of excessive hypotension. The infusion site should be watched closely, as extravasation of fluid may cause phlebitis and cellulitis. Oral therapy with other antihypertensives is usually begun as soon as the blood pressure is controlled.

Mixed Arterial and Venous Vasodilator

SODIUM NITROPRUSSIDE. The mixed arterial and venous vasodilator, sodium nitroprusside (Nipride), acts directly on both arteries and veins. By reducing afterload and preload, sodium nitroprusside improves cardiac performance and may increase cardiac output, particularly in the patient with left ventricular failure.

Use. The balanced arterial and venous vasodilator sodium nitroprusside is indicated for rapid reduction of blood pressure in patients in hypertensive crisis. It is possible to maintain blood pressure at a given level by simple titration of the dose. Nitroprusside has also been shown to be effective in treating refractory heart failure. Patients with increased pulmonary artery obstructive pressure (pulmonary capillary wedge pressure) greater than 15 mmHg and a decreased cardiac output are the most suitable candidates. Unlike the other vasodilators, nitroprusside causes minimal reflex tachycardia because of its balanced effects on preload and afterload, which result in an increase in cardiac output.

Sodium nitroprusside is a very potent agent and has to be used carefully to avoid causing inadvertent hypotension. Reflex catecholamine activity and renin–angiotensin release both interfere with the drug's action and may lead to rebound hypertension. Nitroprusside increases renal blood flow but also increases cerebral blood flow, a potential problem in the patient with intracranial hypertension.

Pharmacokinetics. *Absorption and Distribution.* Nitroprusside is used only by the IV route. It has an immediate onset of action with blood pressure reductions occurring in 30–60 seconds. Maximal effects occur within one to two minutes. The infusion flow rate is titrated until the desired results are achieved.

Biotransformation and Excretion. Nitroprusside has a very short plasma half-life (about two minutes). It is

metabolized to cyanide, which is metabolically converted in the liver to thiocyanate. The thiocyanate metabolite is excreted renally with a half-life of four days and can accumulate and cause significant adverse effects in patients receiving prolonged infusions or those with renal failure. Cyanide can also accumulate in patients receiving high doses of nitroprusside.

Contraindications and Precautions. Nitroprusside is contraindicated in arteriovenous shunt or coarctation of the aorta as the reduction inflow may worsen these conditions. Nitroprusside is also contraindicated today in persons with pulmonary embolism as it interferes with the normal intrapulmonary shunting that occurs in the lung. Nitroprusside is given with caution to patients with hepatic or renal disease. Since thiocyanate can interfere with the transport of iodine into the thyroid gland, resulting in hypothyroidism, nitroprusside should be given with care to patients with hypothyroidism. Administer to pregnant and lactating women with extreme caution and only if clearly needed.

Adverse Effects. Common adverse effects include nausea, abdominal pain, headache, diaphoresis, restlessness, agitation, chest pain, and palpitations, all related to vasodilatation and its effects within the body. These effects usually go away when the drug is discontinued. Thiocyanate toxicity, although rare, may occur if the infusion is prolonged or when renal failure is present. Symptoms include confusion, slurred speech, weakness, muscle twitching, and tinnitus. Thiocyanate levels should be monitored in patients receiving nitroprusside for more than one to two days. The thiocyanate level should be maintained under 10 mg/dl. Cyanide toxicity with subsequent methemoglobinemia can occur if infusion rates exceed 15 μg/kg/min. Cyanide toxicity, if serious enough, can also be treated by removing the compound by hemodialysis.

An important concern today is the risk of myocardial ischemia caused by diastolic hypotension and increased cardiac output. Arterial oxygen tension can decrease in patients on nitroprusside related to the increased intrapulmonary shunting. This is usually about 10 mmHg of oxygen and may be of significance in patients with compromised respiratory function or localized lung lesions.

Nitroprusside can also increase renin production; however, hypotensive effects are maintained with continuous infusion.

Interactions. Concurrent ganglionic blockers, volatile liquid anesthetics, circulatory depressants and other antihypertensives will all augment the hypotensive effects of nitroprusside.

Dosage. Nitroprusside is given in doses of 0.5–10 μg/kg/min mixed with D_5W by IV infusion. Infusion above 10 μg/kg/min should rarely be used. If blood pressure is not adequately reduced within ten minutes, administration should be stopped.

The infusion rate is usually titrated by the individual patient's response. An infusion pump is required to ensure appropriate dosage of this medication. The IV bottle and tubing are protected from light by the tinfoil wrapper included in each package. When deterioration by light occurs, the solution turns blue, green, or dark red. The solution is changed every 24 hours. The patient's blood pressure and the flow rate of the medication bottle must be monitored continually with this potent antihypertensive.

CALCIUM-CHANNEL BLOCKERS

The calcium-channel blockers, or calcium antagonists, are a group of medications used for the treatment of hypertension, dysrhythmias, and angina pectoris. They include nifedipine, nitrendipine, verapamil, verapamil SR (long-acting), and diltiazem. The calcium-channel blockers are discussed in more detail in Chapter 31.

The calcium-channel blockers have several modes of action in hypertension. In general, these agents block the slow channel in the cell membrane and prevent calcium entry into the cell. This blocking action reduces the mechanical activity of vascular smooth muscle and leads to a decrease in peripheral vascular resistance, usually without reflex tachycardia. The calcium-channel blockers also block norepinephrine-mediated vasoconstriction. This may occur because α-sympathetic vasoconstriction is produced by enhanced calcium influx into the cell. If calcium influx is decreased, then norepinephrine vasoconstriction is reduced. Another system regulated by intracellular calcium is the release of renin by the juxtaglomerular cells of the kidney. Because calcium-channel blockers inhibit renin release, the renin–angiotensin system is also suppressed.

Uses

Much research is ongoing in the use of calcium-channel blockers in hypertension. Calcium-channel blockers are used to control mild to moderate hypertension, alone or in combination with diuretics. Calcium-channel blockers are most efficacious in persons with low renin production. Calcium-channel blockers are also proving useful in hypertensive patients who also have chronic stable angina and spastic angina. The vasodilating properties of the calcium-channel blockers lead to a reduction in afterload, and their regional smooth muscle relaxant properties are useful in relieving coronary spasm. Calcium-channel blockers are also useful in treating patients who cannot take β-blocking agents.

Nifedipine

Nifedipine (Procardia, Adalat) has potent peripheral arteriolar dilating properties. It reduces blood pressure and may reflexly increase heart rate. Nifedipine is effective for long-term therapy and appears to be particularly useful in patients with severe refractory hypertension when given with a diuretic and anti-adrenergic drugs. The dosage of nifedipine ranges between 10 and 20 mg given three times a day. Doses above 100 mg are not recommended. For hypertensive emergencies, 10–20 mg is given by puncturing one or two capsules with a needle and squeezing the content under the tongue or by allowing the patient to break open the capsule and swallow the capsule and the liquid that is inside. Recent research indicates that breaking the capsule and swallowing the capsule and the liquid actually results in a faster therapeutic drug level. The oral dose is rapidly

and fully absorbed from the gastrointestinal tract. The drug is metabolized in the liver, and is highly bound to plasma proteins with a half-life of approximately two hours. (For additional information, see Chapter 31.)

Verapamil Hydrochloride

Verapamil hydrochloride (Calan, Isoptin) is given in doses of 80 mg three times a day. Sustained-release verapamil is available in 240 mg scored tablets taken once daily. Elderly or small patients may need only 120 mg/day. If blood pressure is not controlled on 240 mg, 120 mg can be added at bedtime. Dosages above 360 mg do not generally increase effectiveness. The oral dose is almost completely absorbed from the gastrointestinal tract, and there is a large first-pass hepatic effect, with only 10%–20% of the drug available after its first pass through the liver. Approximately 70% of the drug and its metabolites is excreted in the urine, and 16% in the feces within five days. (For additional information on verapamil, see Chapter 31 and the table on antiarrhythmic drugs.)

Diltiazem

The cardiovascular effects of diltiazem (Cardizem) are similar to verapamil. It dilates peripheral vessels and decreases blood pressure. Diltiazem is often administered with a diuretic to enhance its effect. The oral dosage of diltiazem for controlling hypertension is between 60 and 120 mg tid. It is well absorbed by the gastrointestinal tract, with an onset of action is less than 15 minutes, a peak effect in 30 minutes, and a half-life of approximately four hours. (For additional information, see Chapter 31.)

ANGIOTENSIN-CONVERTING ENZYME INHIBITORS

The angiotensin-converting enzyme (ACE) inhibitors block conversion of angiotensin I to angiotensin II by inhibiting ACE (see Fig. 29–1). Since angiotensin II is a powerful vasoconstrictor, interfering with its production can reduce total peripheral resistance and hence blood pressure. The ACE inhibitors also prevent degradation of the vasodilator bradykinin, and increase the urinary excretion of prostaglandins. In contrast to direct vasodilators such as hydralazine and minoxidil, ACE inhibitors do not cause reflex tachycardia, nor do they induce sodium and water retention to any substanial extent. ACE inhibitors are most effective in patients who tend to respond favorably to β blockers.

Diuretics prior to and during ACE therapy enhance the responsiveness to these drugs. In addition, ACE inhibitors blunt the hypokalemic effect of diuretics. The combination of a thiazide-type diuretic with an ACE inhibitor is generally well-tolerated and highly effective in the treatment of younger hypertensive patient who has no symptoms of coronary artery disease.

A recent study of 626 white male hypertensives suggests that the use of the ACE inhibitor captopril (Capoten) is associated with a better quality of life than treatment with the β blocker propranolol or the anti-adrenergic methyldopa. Patients taking captopril displayed the greatest improvement in standardized measures of general well-being and satisfaction with life. They also reported the most freedom from physical symptoms and the least decline in sexual function.

Captopril (Capoten), enalapril (Vasotec), and lisinopril (Prinivil) are angiotension antagonists.

Uses

The ACE inhibitors can now be recommended in initial therapy in mild to moderate hypertension. They are also effective as a vasodilator for the treatment of moderate to severe congestive heart failure. ACE inhibitors are effective alone but, in general, patients (because of their previous difficulty in controlling blood pressure) are generally placed on diuretics as well.

Contraindications and Precautions

ACE inhibitors are contraindicated in persons hypersensitive to these products. ACE inhibitors may cause a "first-dose effect"—a profound fall in blood pressure. This is more likely to occur in persons severely salt-/volume-depleted like those pretreated with diuretics. Blood pressure needs to be monitored closely. Safety in pregnancy, lactating women, and children has not been established.

ACE inhibitors are given cautiously to patients with impaired renal function because elevated BUN and serum creatinine levels have been induced after a reduction in blood pressure. Patients may also experience hyperkalemia (1%–4%), particularly if they have renal insufficiency or diabetes. Therefore, serum potassium levels need to be monitored.

Adverse Effects

ACE inhibitors have been found to cause serious adverse effects, and patients should therefore be monitored closely. Several patients have developed proteinuria, neutropenia, and agranulocytosis with captopril and decreased hemoglobin and hematocrit with enalapril and lisinopril. Rash, often with pruritus and fever (rash is usually mild and disappears within a few days with dose reduction and short-term therapy with an antihistamine), tachycardia, and chest pain may occur. Gastrointestinal symptoms may also occur such as abdominal pain, vomiting, nausea, cough, and diarrhea.

Patients receiving ACE inhibitors have also experienced elevation of liver enzymes, transient elevations of BUN and serum creatinine, and increases in serum potassium concentration. Additional adverse effects can be found in Table 29–2.

Interactions

Current ACE inhibitors enhance the hypotensive effects of diuretics and other antihypertensive medications. Potassium-sparing diuretics and potassium supplements should be given only for documented hypokalemia, as they may interact to cause a significant increase in serum potassium. All nonsteroidal anti-inflammatories (NSAIDs) and aspirin may antagonize the effectiveness of ACE inhibitors. NSAIDs also increase the possibility of renal toxicity. An interaction may occur between ACE inhibitors and diuretics causing "functional" renal failure. Renal failure is believed to develop because of a relatively greater reduction in efferent (postglomerular) than afferent (preglomerular) renal vascular resistance. As these changes occur, the pressure favoring glomerular filtration is reduced. Administer ACE inhibitors cautiously to patients receiving diuretics. Additional specific interactions are found in Table 29–2.

Captopril

Captopril is used to treat patients with hypertension and heart failure. It can also be used, in reduced dosages, in patients with renal impairment. A loop diuretic is generally administered with captopril in persons with renal impairment.

PHARMACOKINETICS. *Absorption and Distribution.* Captopril is best adminstered one hour before meals, as the presence of food in the gastrointestinal tract reduces absorption. Seventy-five percent is absorbed from the gastrointestinal system. Approximately 25%–30% of the circulating drug is bound to plasma protein. Peak serum levels are reached in 0.5–1.5 hours.

Biotransformation and Excretion. Over 95% of the absorbed drug is eliminated in the urine, with 40%–50% as unchanged drug. Captopril is dialyzable. The half-life of captopril is less than 1.7 hours.

CONTRAINDICATIONS AND PRECAUTIONS. Captopril should be given cautiously to patients with renal disease, as elevated BUN and serum cretinine levels have been induced. Captopril is administered with caution in patients who have serious autoimmune diseases, particularly SLE, or who have been exposed to drugs known to affect white cells or immune response. In patients at particular risk, white blood cell and differential counts are performed frequently during the initial stage of therapy. Patients with aortic stenosis may be at risk for decreased coronary perfusion when treated with captopril.

DOSAGE. The initial dosage of captopril to treat hypertension is 12.5 mg tid or 25 bid. If there is no satisfactory reduction of blood pressure, the dosage may be increased to 50 mg tid after one to two weeks. If blood pressure is still not controlled, a small dose of a thiazide-type diuretic is added. The usual dosage range of captopril is 25–150 mg three times a day, with a maximum daily dosage of 450 mg.

For a patient with accelerated or malignant hypertension, an initial dosage of 25 mg tid may be increased every 24 hours until a satisfactory blood pressure is obtained. However, the patient should be monitored closely.

When captopril is used to treat congestive heart failure, the initial dose is 6.25 mg tid. Most patients are controlled on 50–100 mg tid. In patients with renal dysfunction, dosage is reduced.

Enalapril

Enalapril (Vasotec) is a long-acting ACE inhibitor with pharmacologic actions similar to the other ACE inhibitors.

USES. Enalapril is useful in treating mild to severe essential hypertension and renovascular hypertension. Enalapril has also been demonstrated to decrease the mortality in patients with both acute and chronic congestive heart failure, decrease the heart size, and reduce the need for other drugs for heart failure. Enalapril is more effective in whites and younger patients than in blacks and older patients.

PHARMACOKINETICS. *Absorption and Distribution.* Enalapril is rapidly absorbed (60%) from the gastrointestinal tract, reaching peak concentrations in about one hour. Its bioavailability is not influenced by food. Onset of action is two to four hours.

Biotransformation and Excretion. The effective half-life of enalapril is 11 hours with a duration of action of 24 hours. Enalapril is excreted (94%) as unchanged drug in the urine. Enalapril is dialyzable and doses need to be decreased in patients with renal disease.

DOSAGE. The initial dose of enalapril is 5 mg/day and gradual increases at one- to two-week intervals to a maximum of 40 mg/day. A diuretic may be added to increase effectiveness.

Lisinopril

Lisinopril (Prinivil) is used to manage essential hypertension. If blood pressure is not controlled with lisinopril alone, a low dose of a thiazide diuretic may be added.

PHARMACOKINETICS. *Absorption and Distribution.* Approximately 25% of lisinopril is absorbed from the gastrointestinal tract. Its absorption is unaffected by the presence of food. Peak serum levels occur in about seven hours. Lisinopril has a duration of 24 hours.

Biotransformation and Excretion. Lisinopril is not biotransformed but is excreted 100% unchanged in the urine. Lisinopril has a half-life in persons with normal renal function of 12 hours.

DOSAGE. In patients with uncomplicated essential hypertension, the initial dose of lisinopril is 10 mg once daily. The usual maintenance dose is 20–40 mg daily as a single dose. A thiazide diuretic may be added to assist with blood pressure control. Patients with renal impairment or on dialysis will receive reduced dosage.

SEROTONIN RECEPTOR BLOCKING AGENTS

The serotonin receptor blocking agents, still investigational in the United States, block the effect of serotonin at the peripheral receptor sites, and thus prevent serotonin-induced vasoconstriction. Total peripheral resistance, and thus blood pressure, are reduced.

HYPERTENSIVE EMERGENCIES

True hypertensive emergency occurs in many clinical settings, including hypertensive encephalopathy, acute congestive heart failure, intracranial hemorrhage with hypertension, aortic dissection, acute myocardial infarction or unstable angina, acute pulmonary edema with hypertension, acute renal failure, malignant hypertension, severe hypertension after surgery, and toxemia of pregnancy. Immediate reduction in blood pressure is necessary, but an excessive decrease may be dangerous. Usually a 20% to 30% decrease of the mean arterial pressure is safe, with a minimum diastolic pressure of 100 mm Hg. Table 29–3 features drugs commonly used in hypertensive emergencies and their advantages and disadvantages.

Table 29–3. DRUGS FOR HYPERTENSIVE EMERGENCIES

Drug	Class	Route and Dose	Onset	Duration	Uses*	Advantages	Disadvantages
PARENTERAL							
Nitroprusside (Nipride, others)	Arteriolar and venous vasodilator	IV infusion pump 0.5 µg/kg/min to 10 µg/kg/min	seconds	1–10 min following cessation of infusion	1, 2, 3, 4, 5, 6, 9	Rapid onset and resolution of action; no tachyphylaxis; no sedation; decreases preload and afterload	Requires continual arterial pressure monitoring
Diazoxide (Hyperstat)	Arteriolar vasodilator	1–3 mg/kg over 30 sec or less; may repeat in 5–15 min	1–5 min	3–12 hrs	1, 2, 7, 9	No sedation	Hypotension with previously recommended dosage (300-mg bolus); hyperglycemia; increases heart rate with exacerbation of MI and aortic dissection

Table 29–3. DRUGS FOR HYPERTENSIVE EMERGENCIES–*CONTINUED*

Drug	Class	Route and Dose	Onset	Duration	Uses*	Advantages	Disadvantages
Trimethaphan (Arfonad)	Ganglionic blocker	IV infusion pump 0.3–3 mg/min	1–5 min	10–30 min	6	Rapid onset and resolution action; no reflex tachycardia; decreases preload and afterload; no sedation	Paralytic ileus; urinary retention; mydriasis; patient may need to be tilted upright for effect; requires arterial line
Labetalol (Trandate; Normodyne)	A- and β-adrenergic blocker	IV 2 mg/min or 20 mg initially, then 20–80 mg q 10 min; max cumulative dose 300 mg	5 min or less	3–6 hrs	1, 2, 3, 5, 7	No tachycardia	Contraindicated in patients with asthma, >1° heart block, severe sinus bradycardia, CHF, and pheochromocytoma
Hydralazine (Apresoline)	Arteriolar vasodilator	IV 5–20 mg	5–20 min	10–80 min	1, 2, 4, 7, 8, 9	No sedation	Less precise pressure control; increases heart rate, with exacerbation of MI and aortic dissection
Propranolol (Inderal, others)	B-adrenergic blocker	IV: 1–5 mg load then 3 mg/hr PO: 80–640 mg daily	Immediate β-adrenergic blockade	2 hr 12 hr	5, 6, 9	Useful as adjunct to prevent or treat excessive tachycardia	Will not lower blood pressure acutely
ORAL Nifedipine† (Procardia, Adalat)	Calcium-channel blocker	10–20 mg PO, sublingual, or buccal	5–15 min	3–5 hr	2, 4, 5, 9	Rapid onset (10 min), easily administered	Not yet standardized, somewhat variable response
Captopril (Capoten)	ACE inhibitor	PO 6.25–50 mg	15 min	6–12 hr	4	Easily administered	Variable, sometimes excessive response

*Uses: 1-hypertensive encephalopathy, 2-malignant hypertension, 3-subarachnoid hemorrhage, 4-acute congestive heart failure, 5-acute myocardial infarction or unstable angina, 6-aortic dissection, 7-acute renal failure, 8-pregnancy induced hypertension, 9-post-op hypertension.
†Not approved for this indication by the U.S. Food and Drug Administration.
Adapted from The Medical Letter, Drugs for Hypertensive Emergencies, Vol. 29, Issue 733 (February 13, 1987).

USING THE NURSING PROCESS

ASSESSMENT

Assessment of the patient requiring antihypertensive medications for the control of high blood pressure always begins with a thorough nursing history to develop a data base. The information obtained by the nurse is featured in Table 29–4. All of this information is used later when preparing the nursing care plan. The diagnosis of mild to moderate hypertension is made only after three consecutive tests, taken on three different days, show blood pressure to be elevated. Both standing and supine blood pressures are assessed as well as pulse pressures. Both diastolic and systolic numbers are considered. Pulse rate is also recorded, since the hyperten-

Table 29-4. NURSING PROCESS FOR PATIENT REQUIRING ANTIHYPERTENSIVE MEDICATIONS

Assessment

Measure blood pressure (standing and supine) and heart rate.
Assess smoking habits, including cigarettes, cigars, and marijuana.
Determine current weight and height.
Ascertain usual dietary pattern, including intake of sodium and use of alcohol.
Note medication history (including OTC, prescription, and any other antihypertensive medication).

Nursing Diagnosis	Nursing Actions	Rationale	Desired Outcomes/ Evaluation Criteria
Knowledge deficit related to unfamiliarity with resources, misunderstanding as evidenced by questions, statement of concern, poor control of condition, development of preventable complications.	Define and state the limits of normal blood pressure. Explain hypertension and its effects on the heart, blood vessels, kidneys, and brain.	Provides basis for understanding elevations of blood pressure and that it can be elevated without symptoms.	Verbalizes understanding of condition and therapy needs. Demonstrates behavior (e.g., monitoring of blood pressure, diet modifications designed to maintain BP at an optimal level).
	Avoid saying "normal" blood pressure, and use the term "well-controlled" when describing blood pressure within desired limits. Define and state the limits of normal blood pressure. Explain hypertension and its effects on the heart, blood vessels, kidneys, and brain.	Because treatment is lifelong, conveying the idea of "control" helps the patient to understand the need for continued treatment/medication. Provides basis for understanding elevations of blood pressure and that it can be elevated without symptoms.	
	Provide information (verbal and written) about antihypertensives including action, use, dose, adverse effects, and interactions.	Enhances knowledge base so patient is capable of making educated decisions about therapy.	
	Discuss possible drug interactions and how and when to take antihypertensive medications.	Enhances success of drug therapy. Drugs that could possibly increase blood pressure or counteract antihypertensives are eliminated.	
	Assist the patient to identify modifiable cardiovascular risk factors, e.g., obesity, diet high in saturated fats and cholesterol, sedentary lifestyle, smoking, alcohol intake, stressful lifestyle.	These risk factors have been shown to contribute to hypertension and cardiovascular/renal disease.	
	Discuss importance of eliminating smoking and assist patient in formulating a plan to quit.	Nicotine increases catecholamine discharge, resulting in increased heart rate, BP, and vasoconstriction, reducing tissue oxygenation, and increasing the myocardial workload.	
	Establish an individual exercise program incorporating aerobic exercise within patient capabilities. Stress the importance of avoiding isometric activity.	Besides helping to lower BP, aerobic activity aids in toning the cardiovascular system. Isometric exercise can increase serum catecholamine levels further elevating BP.	
	Promote use of relaxation skills, use of daily rest periods.	Identification of stress/ precipitating factors and measures to relieve them helps to maintain control.	

Table 29–4. NURSING PROCESS FOR PATIENT REQUIRING ANTIHYPERTENSIVE MEDICATIONS–*CONTINUED*

Nursing Diagnosis	Nursing Actions	Rationale	Desired Outcomes/ Evaluation Criteria
	Reinforce the importance of cooperation with treatment regimen and keeping follow-up appointments.	Lack of cooperation is a common reason for failure of antihypertensive therapy. Effective therapy reduces the incidence of stroke, heart failure, renal impairment, and possibly MI.	
	Instruct and demonstrate technique of self-monitoring of BP.	Teaching the patient/SO to monitor BP is reassuring to the patient, provides visual/positive reinforcement for patient efforts and helps in guiding therapy.	
Nutrition, altered: More than body requirements related to excessive intake in relation to metabolic need as evidenced by reported dysfunctional eating patterns, percentage of body fat greater than 18%–20% for trim women; 10%–12% for trim men.	Review individual nutritional needs and appropriate food selection within economic means. Discuss need for reduction of sodium intake, alcohol consumption, caloric intake; and importance of exercise program. Encourage weekly monitoring of weight.	Faulty eating habits contribute to weight gain, sodium retention and atherosclerosis. Exercise can assist with weight reduction, improved mental outlook, and reduction in blood pressure. Useful in evaluating therapy needs/effectiveness.	Identifies inappropriate behaviors associated with weight gain or overeating. Maintains optimal individual diet and exercise program.
Adjustment, impaired potential related to anticipated change in lifestyle, assault to self-esteem, altered locus of control.	Include patient in planning of care and encourage maximum participation in treatment plan.	Involvement provides the patient with an ongoing sense of control, improves coping skills and can enhance cooperation with therapeutic regimen.	Demonstrates increasing participation in self-care. Initiates lifestyle changes that permit adaptation to present situation.
	Encourage patient to evaluate life priorities/ goals.	Focuses patient attention on reality of present situation related to own view of what is wanted. Strong work ethic, need for "control," outward focus may have led to lack of attention to personal needs.	
	Assist patient to identify and begin planning for necessary lifestyle changes. Encourage patient to adjust, rather than abandon personal/ family goals.	Necessary changes should be realistically prioritized to prevent patient being overwhelmed with feelings of powerlessness.	
	Problem-solve with patient to identify ways in which appropriate lifestyle changes can be made to reduce the above factors.	Risk factors may accelerate the disease process or exacerbate symptoms. Changing "comfortable/usual" behavior patterns can be very stressful. Support, guidance, and empathy can enhance the patient's success in accomplishing these tasks.	
	Stress helping in developing a simple, convenient schedule for taking medications.	Individualizing medication schedule to fit the patient's personal habits/needs may facilitate	

CONTINUED ON THE FOLLOWING PAGE

Table 29–4. NURSING PROCESS FOR PATIENT REQUIRING ANTIHYPERTENSIVE MEDICATIONS–*CONTINUED*

Nursing Diagnosis	Nursing Actions	Rationale	Desired Outcomes/ Evaluation Criteria
		compliance with long-term regimen.	
	Avoid hot baths, steam rooms, and saunas and concomitant use of alcoholic beverages.	Prevents unnecessary vasodilation with dangerous side effect of syncope and hypotension.	
	Recommend monitoring own physiologic response to activity (e.g., pulse rate, shortness of breath); report a decreased tolerance to activity; and stop activity that causes chest pain, shortness of breath, dizziness, extreme fatigue, or weakness.	Involvement in monitoring own activity tolerance is vital to safely resuming and/or modifying activities of daily living.	

sive patient who is tachycardic will need different drugs than the hypertensive patient who is bradycardic.

If the patient has been or is currently taking any medication to control blood pressure, the nurse should learn what the patient is taking, for how long, and whether there are any adverse effects. Nurses also need to obtain a thorough over-the-counter (OTC) medication history. Patients can experience hypertension from combining OTC diet pills and decongestants. If such a combination is found, the medication is discontinued to determine if the blood pressure will return to normal.

The nurse also assesses the current exercise level of the patient. What are the usual type, frequency, and duration of sporting activities? How does the patient get to work? Is there job-related physical activity? How many flights of stairs does the patient climb per day? The answers to these questions help the nurse to identify persons with little exercise in their lifestyle.

Patients also are questioned about their current smoking habits, including cigarettes, cigars, and marijuana. All types of smoking should be eliminated because of the untoward side effects that can be experienced. During the intervention phase, the nurse often helps the patient devise a method to reduce or eliminate smoking.

Any misinformation the patient or family has obtained is corrected at this time. It is also important to obtain a profile of the family. Since hypertension frequently is familial, the whole family, not just the patient, is assessed to determine possible contributing factors to the development of hypertension.

Postsurgical hypertensive patients need to be assessed carefully. Occasionally naloxone, a narcotic antagonist, is administered to reverse anesthesia-induced respiratory depression, which can precipitate dramatic rises in blood pressure.

The nurse often assists with the collection of laboratory data. Typical lab tests that may be ordered include serum potassium; cholesterol and triglycerides to rule out other causes of hypertension; thyroid studies if indicated to rule out hyperthyroidism; chest radiography and ECG to determine heart size; and urine studies such as urine steroids, and vanillylmandelic acid to rule out secondary causes of hypertension.

During the physical exam, the nurse particularly notes blood pressure standing and supine and in the arms and legs using the correct-size blood-pressure cuff. Height and weight are important, and any recent changes are noted. Lungs are auscultated, and a *funduscopic exam* of the eyes is performed, to determine the presence of papilledema or retinal changes such as hemorrhages or exudates that occur as hypertension progresses.

Patients with "borderline" hypertension (diastolic blood pressure 90–94 mmHg) are generally considered at low risk. It is recommended that they be followed for four months before any form of therapy is initiated. If pharmacologic therapy is postponed, it is important to re-examine untreated patients about every six months, since their hypertension may progress or their risk profile may worsen.

NURSING DIAGNOSES

As the nursing intervention is planned, the nursing diagnoses are developed with the help of the patient and family. An involved patient and family ultimately are more compliant in the treatment and follow-up. Possible nursing diagnoses for the patient with hypertension are featured in Table 29–4.

PLANNING AND INTERVENTION

The goals of nursing intervention are developed from the nursing diagnoses. The goals of nursing intervention for a patient with hypertension are included in Table 29–4. The short-term goals include patient education and blood-pressure control, while the long-term goals include changes in lifestyle to help reduce blood pressure. It is important for the nurse to know the target blood pressure that the physician and the patient have agreed upon.

Most patients with hypertension are routinely treated at home, so it is important that both the patient and family are well-educated by the nurse. The nurse educator teaches the patient and family about the physiology of this disease; the dietary regimen (usually sodium restriction and limited alcohol) and ideal weight maintenance; the medication regimen, including adverse effects that may be experienced; and how stress and anxiety relate to the condition and how they can be controlled. Exercise counseling may be necessary based on the information obtained in the assessment phase. The nurse might suggest various relaxation techniques to the patient, including biofeedback, transcendental meditation, mind control, and yoga. All these methods have been proven effective in lowering blood pressure to some extent in selected patients. It is important that the nurse stress that these methods can be used in conjunction with medications but should not be a substitute for medical therapy.

The patient who is newly diagnosed with mild hypertension usually progresses through a stepped-care method of treatment for hypertension. (Patients with moderate to severe hypertension are started directly on antihypertensive medications.) The stepped-care method (Fig. 29–3) is supported by many clinical trials in which it has been found both effective and well tolerated over the long term in the overwhelming majority of patients.

The stepped-care method begins with non-pharmacologic approaches such as weight loss, if indicated, and dietary restriction of sodium (step one). If this treatment is not totally successful, drug therapy, or step two, is started with a single drug. (See Chapter 38 for more information on diuretics.) The physician may choose a diuretic, a β blocker, a calcium antagonist, or an ACE inhibitor. A thiazide diuretic, such as hydrochlorothiazide (Hydro-DIURIL), is usually prescribed first. Diuretics control blood pressure in a large group of patients (30%–60%) without additional therapy.

If the patient is under 50 years old or has ischemic heart disease, the physician may prescribe a β blocker initially. B blockers usually reduce blood pressure to the level achieved with diuretics.

If the first drug has some efficacy and is well tolerated but target blood pressure has not been reached, then a second drug with a different pharmacologic effect (step three) is added. Drugs may be substituted or added as necessary until the blood pressure is controlled. The use of antihypertensive drugs without diuretics is generally followed by reflex sodium and water retention and loss of antihypertensive effect. Loop diuretics are usually required in the presence of renal insufficiency or poor left ventricular function. Because of the differences in responsiveness, the regimen must be individualized. It may be necessary to try various drugs or combinations of drugs until the optimal effect is obtained. This process is often very depressing for the patient, and he or she may begin to lose confidence in the medical and nursing personnel. It is imperative that the patient have good explanations of why the drug regimen is being altered.

If the patient has not responded to a single drug reg-

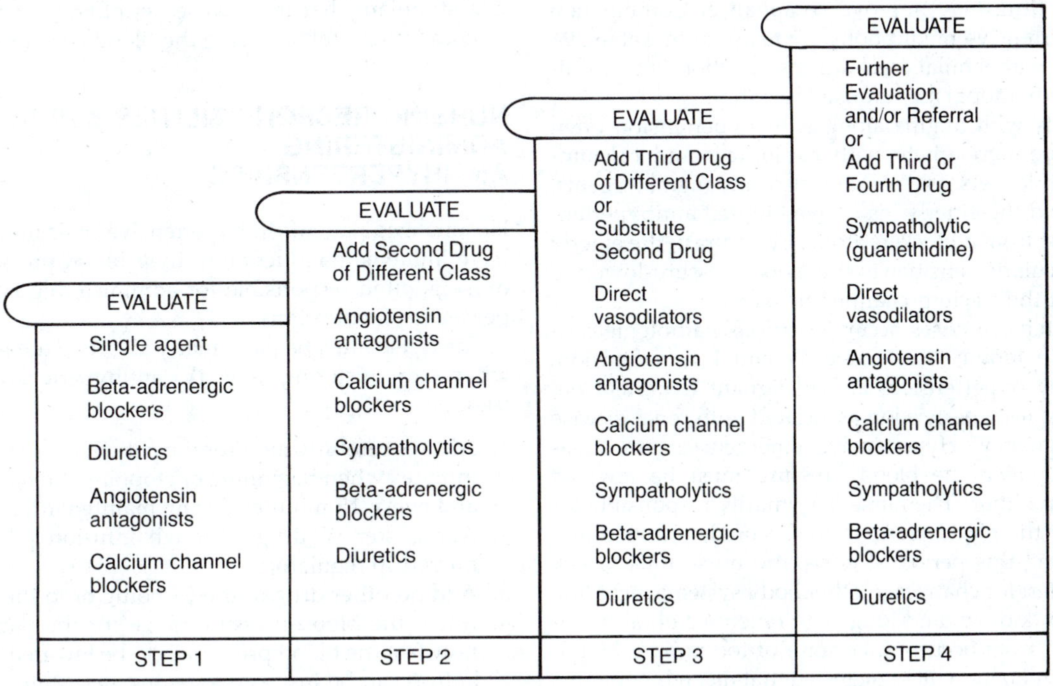

EVALUATE	EVALUATE	EVALUATE	EVALUATE
Single agent	Add Second Drug of Different Class	Add Third Drug of Different Class or Substitute Second Drug	Further Evaluation and/or Referral or Add Third or Fourth Drug
Beta-adrenergic blockers	Angiotensin antagonists	Direct vasodilators	Sympatholytic (guanethidine)
Diuretics	Calcium channel blockers	Angiotensin antagonists	Direct vasodilators
Angiotensin antagonists	Sympatholytics	Calcium channel blockers	Angiotensin antagonists
Calcium channel blockers	Beta-adrenergic blockers	Sympatholytics	Calcium channel blockers
	Diuretics	Beta-adrenergic blockers	Sympatholytics
		Diuretics	Beta-adrenergic blockers
			Diuretics
STEP 1	STEP 2	STEP 3	STEP 4

Figure 29–3. Stepped-care protocol for treating hypertension.

imen, step three begins. If the patient began therapy with a β blocker but did not respond, a diuretic is added. If this regimen does not effectively control blood pressure, a direct vasodilator, calcium-channel blocker, ACE inhibitor, α-1 blocker, or rauwolfia product is added. Smaller doses of two drugs with different mechanisms of action may prove more effective than larger doses of a single drug. This approach frequently minimizes adverse reactions without significantly reducing effectiveness.

If blood pressure is not reduced to a satisfactory level, a third drug such as hydralazine is added in step four. This drug is added to the drugs already being administered from steps one and two.

If the first four steps of therapy are ineffective and reasons other than drug failure have been ruled out, guanethidine may be added in increasing doses, as needed, or substituted for one of the step two or step three drugs. Minoxidil is held in reserve for patients who fail to respond to anything else.

The interval between drug or dosage modification is determined by the severity of the hypertension; in mild hypertension, adjustments are made at two to three month intervals, in moderate hypertension adjustments are made every two to six weeks; and in severe hypertension, adjustments may be made within hours to days depending on the blood-pressure range. When the blood-pressure goal is achieved, medication may be titrated down to avoid unnecessary overmedication of the patients.

The effective doses may vary considerably from patient to patient. Therapy usually is initiated with a single drug, and if additional agents are needed, they are added to the regimen one at a time. If the patient requires more than one drug, the use of a fixed-dose combination drug may improve compliance. Combination antihypertensive medications are featured in Table 29–5. Drugs with similar mechanisms of action (e.g., clonidine, methyldopa) are not used together.

Patients with angina along with hypertension often benefit from treatment with β blockers and calcium-channel blockers as they are also antianginal agents. Blacks and the elderly may have blunted antihypertensive effect from β blockers alone. By contrast, the elderly are particularly sensitive to the blood pressure-lowering effects of the calcium-channel blockers.

Hypertensive crises occur in various pathologic conditions including accelerated essential hypertension, secondary hypertension, and malignant hypertension, as well as in hypertension associated with renal disease and pregnancy. Hypertensive emergencies are situations in which the blood pressure must be lowered within one hour. The nurse is primarily responsible for lowering the blood pressure to the predetermined levels. During this period of crisis, the nurse must check and be alert for changes in other body systems including the brain, kidney, and lung. To prevent cerebral hypoperfusion from occurring because of too rapid a blood-pressure reduction, it is suggested that mean blood pressure be lowered no more than 20%–30% in the first 24 hours.

PATIENT TEACHING

When the patient is placed on antihypertensive medications, the nurse educator has to ensure that the patient has adequate knowledge to administer the medications safely. The information to be taught to all patients requiring antihypertensives is included in Table 29-6.

Antihypertensives are to be taken as directed, that is, once a day at a specified time; or two or more times daily at specified times and with or between meals. Medications are best taken every day near the same time. If a tablet is forgotten, that dose is eliminated. The patient should not take two tablets at the next time. Patients need to be cautious about driving or operating heavy equipment for about two hours after they take their antihypertensive medication. After several weeks, they will know how they react and this caution may no longer be necessary.

Patients are taught to change body position slowly—lying to sitting, sitting to standing—to prevent episodes of orthostatic hypotension which is common to many of the antihypertensives. Patients taking antihypertensives should not take hot baths or showers or sit in a hot tub as the excessive vasodilatation from the hot water may further lower their blood pressure. Patients also need to maintain their fluid balance and prevent dehydration, which may lead to an excessive fall in blood pressure. During hot weather or strenuous physical activities, fluids should be consumed.

Patients are taught never to discontinue their antihypertensive medication without their physician's approval. If patients experience side effects, they need to notify their physician and follow his or her guidance.

Patients should avoid excessive (more than four cups per day) intake of caffeine—coffee, tea, or cola. Caffeine is a stimulant that may cause peripheral vasoconstriction and ultimately increase the blood pressure.

NURSING RESPONSIBILITIES WHEN ADMINISTERING ANTIHYPERTENSIVES

Hospitalized patients in hypertensive crisis may need to have immediate reduction in their blood pressure. The nurse is often responsible for administering IV antihypertensive medications.

The nurse must be particularly aware of the following when administering any IV antihypertensive medication:

1. Always carefully monitor the patient every five to ten minutes when beginning or stopping the medication, and every 15 minutes during maintenance.
2. Administer IV drugs through infusion pumps and microdrip regulators.
3. Add no other drug to the IV bottle or to the IV line.
4. Know the blood-pressure range for the patient and how fast the blood pressure is to be lowered. Too fast a drop can be just as dangerous as sustained hypertension. Patients can experience angina pectoris and possibly even a myocardial infarction.

Table 29–5. COMBINATION DRUGS FOR ANTIHYPERTENSIVES

Combination Drug	Basic Products*							
	A	B	C	D	E	F	G	Other
Aldoclor-150	250	—	—					150 H
Aldoclor-250	250	—	—					250 H
Aldoril-15	250	15	—					
Aldoril-25	250	25	—					
Aldoril D30	500	30	—					
Aldoril D50	500	50	—					
Apresazide 25/25	—	25	25					
Apresazide 50/50	—	50	50					
Apresazide 100/50	—	50	100					
Apresoline-Esidrix	—	15	25					
Capozide 25/15	25/25	15 or 25	—					25 or
50/15	50/25							55AA
Combipres 0.1								15 I
								0.1 J
Combipres 0.2								15 I
								0.2 J
Corzide						5		40 or 80 X
Demi-Regroton				0.125				25 I
Diupres-250				0.125				250 H
Diupres-500				0.125				500 H
Diutensen					2.5			2 K
Diutensen-R				0.1	2.5			
Enduronyl					5			0.25 L
Enduronyl-Forte					5			0.5 L
Esimil		25						10 M
Hydromax-R				0.125				50 P
Hydropress-25		25		0.125				
Hydropress-50		50		0.125				
Hydroserp		50		0.125				
Hydrotensin-25 Tabs		25		0.125				
Hydrotensin-50 Tabs		50		0.125				
Inderide 40/25		25						40 Q
Inderide 80/25		25						80 Q
Metatensin Tablets				0.1				4 R
Minicide 1,2,5								0.5 U
								1,2,5 Z
Naquival				0.1				4 R
Oreticyl Forte		25						0.25 L
Oreticyl 25		25						0.125 L
Oreticyl 50		50						0.125 L
Rautrax							400	400 S
								50 T
Rautrax-N						4	400	50 T
Rauzide						4		50 T
Regroton				0.25				50 I
Renese-R				0.25				2 U
Salutensin				0.125				50 V
Salutensin Demi				0.125				25 V
Ser-Ap-Es		15	25	0.1				
Serpasil-Apresoline #1			25	0.1				
Serpasil-Apresoline #2			50	0.2				
Serpasil-Esidrix #1		25		0.1				
Serpasil-Esidrix #2		50		0.1				
Tenoretic 50								25 I, 50 W
Tenoretic 100								25 I, 100 W
Timolide 10/25		25						10 Y
Unipres		15	25	0.1				

*Basic Products: A-methyldopa, mg; B-hydrochlorothiazide, mg; C-hydralazine hydrochloride, mg; D-reserpine, mg; E-methyclothiazide, mg; F-bendroflumethiazide, mg; G-potassium chloride, mg; H-chlorothiazide, mg; I-chlorthalidone, mg; J-clonidine hydrochloride, mg; K-cryptenamine tannate, mg; L-deserpidine, mg; M-guanethidine monosulfate, mg; N-pargyline hydrochloride, mg; O-benzthiazide, mg; P-quinethazone, mg; Q-propranolol hydrochloride, mg; R-trichlormethiazide, mg; S-flumethiazide, mg; T-powdered rauwolfia serpentina, mg; U-polythiazide, mg; V-hydroflumethiazide, mg; W-atenolol, mg; X-nadolol, mg; Y-timolol maleate, mg; Z-prazosin, mg; AA-captopril.

Table 29–6. PATIENT TEACHING—ANTIHYPERTENSIVES*

Dear Patient:

This drug has been prescribed for you. This is what you should know about your drug to get the most from your therapy.

1. _____ is taken to lower your blood pressure. Specifically, _____ works by _____.
2. Medications are taken every day, most likely for the rest of your life.
3. Most antihypertensives can be taken with or between meals. (To nurse: If different instructions are needed, fill in.)
4. Alcohol (beer, wine, whiskey) intake is limited because of its vasodilator effect.
5. All other OTC and prescription drugs should be checked by your doctor or pharmacist before they are taken.
6. If you forget a dose, do not take it later. Never take 2 doses the next time.
7. Medication should **not** be stopped abruptly since blood pressure tends to rise higher because of increased sensitivity to substances within the body. Do not delay in refilling your prescriptions.
8. If dizziness or faintness is experienced, you should lie down or sit with your head down for a few minutes. The dizziness usually goes away.
9. If you experience any adverse effects from your medications, call your doctor. (A new drug or a change in dosage will most often stop adverse effects.)
10. Use caution for at least 2 hours after taking the medication, especially while driving or working around heavy equipment. Medications may make you drowsy, but this is usually transient and stops within a month.
11. Do not take hot baths or showers, since this may cause further vasodilation and fainting.
12. Careful exposure to sun is important, since heat increases peripheral blood flow, and some antihypertensives decrease sweating; therefore, hypotension and heat stroke may occur.
13. Change body position slowly to prevent fainting. When moving from a supine position to standing, sit first.
14. Check your weight at least twice a week and closely watch for fluid retention.
15. Avoid too much tea, coffee, and cola (more than 4 cups per day), since caffeine has been shown to raise blood pressure.
16. Blood pressures may be taken at home. Records that are kept should be reviewed periodically by the doctor or nurse.
17. Carry an ID card identifying the drug, dose, and the time taken.
18. Store all medications in a tight, light-resistant container.
19. Keep all follow-up appointments.

*In addition to these items, the specific drug's actions and side effects are discussed with the patient as well as what symptoms should be reported. Specific points about each drug can be found in Table 29–2 under "Nursing Implications." Recent studies show that 40%–70% of hypertensive patients stop taking their medication for a variety of reasons. With good health teaching, this percentage can be reduced. Through the intervention, the nurse must continually stress and reinforce the need for lifelong therapy.

5. Start oral medication as soon as possible so that IV medication can be discontinued.

Patients taking antihypertensives who are undergoing surgery should be continued on their medications until the day of surgery. Recent research has demonstrated that anesthesia is easier with fewer complications when the patient remains on drug therapy.

Secondary hypertension, often associated with pheochromocytoma (a catecholamine–producing tumor of the adrenal medulla), is often best treated with an α-adrenergic blocking agent, phentolamine (Regitine). This agent, described in Chapter 19, is only an antihypertensive agent when there are large amounts of circulating catecholamines, as produced by a pheochromocytoma or in a patient who suddenly discontinues centrally-acting antihypertensives such as clonidine.

EVALUATION

The nurse evaluates the effectiveness of antihypertensive therapy based on a predetermined list of evaluation criteria. These evaluation criteria are developed on an individual basis through discussion among the nurse, patient, and family. The data base obtained in the original assessment assists the nurse in formulating the criteria for evaluation. The evaluation criteria for patients receiving antihypertensives are included in Table 29–4.

The nurse works with the patient and family to ensure their complete assistance and support. A frequent problem with hypertensive patients is lack of compliance. The nurse can evaluate for noncompliance by direct question, pill counts, or determining whether the prescription has been refilled. Patients often never understand the importance of their medication regimen. Eighty percent of newly diagnosed hypertensive patients do not have symptoms. It is the nurse's responsibility to assist the patient in understanding that the medications will ultimately prevent complications (heart disease, cerebral vascular disease, retinal changes, and renal disease) 20–30 years later. Compliance can be enhanced with convenient medication regimens, single daily dosing, personal attention and feedback given to the patient by his or her healthcare providers, minimizing expense, education about therapy, and the avoidance of adverse effects. Patients may experience adverse effects from the medications, which, combined with their expense, increases the likelihood of noncompliance. Medical personnel have always assumed that antihypertensive medications are associated with a high rate of adverse reactions, but statistically this appears to be untrue. The most common complaints include sleepiness, fatigue, self-assessed depression, and sexual complaints (impotence and decreased sexual desire). The sexual complaints are often more age-related rather than drug-related.

If noncompliance is suspected, a program of drugs suitable for once-daily administration is developed and the patient is given a daily clinic or office appointment for five days. By week's end, pressure is nearly always lowered, and both the patient and physician can see the results that the patient will achieve with home therapy.

Patients are encouraged to keep their appointments for checkups so that their progress can be monitored. If the patient is experiencing adverse effects from one drug, alternate medications can be tried. Often, this is a trial-and-error period. It may be as long as a year before the patient's blood pressure is well controlled with a minimum of adverse effects. Since tolerance may develop from these medications, the patient must continually, for the rest of his or her life, see the physician on a regular basis.

Several antihypertensives may cause sleep disorders, including clonidine, methyldopa, and the β blockers propranolol and nadolol. Patients who experience sleep disturbances—ranging from insomnia to nightmares and sleepwalking—may be helped by taking their medication early in the day instead of at night.

Compliance may often be improved by teaching the patient to monitor and chart his or her blood pressure at home. The patient is then an active participator in the treatment.

All other evaluation criteria are assessed before the patient is discharged from hospital or clinic. All previously taught material is reviewed and updated if necessary to ensure that the patient's and family's knowledge base remains accurate.

The more the patient and family know about the treatment regimen, the more likely they are to comply with the program. Hypertension treatment is for a lifetime. Treatment is designed to lower blood pressure to an acceptable level, determined by the physician. Patients are encouraged to return to and maintain a normal weight, to reduce their intake of sodium, and to practice stress-reduction techniques. Some patients may be able to control their blood pressure using these therapies alone, but others will need to take one or more medications. Any cessation of medication allows the blood pressure to return to pretreatment levels. There is no doubt that the effective control of blood pressure and the prevention of complications enables the patient to live a longer and more satisfying life.

SUMMARY

Pharmacologic treatment of essential hypertension uses the stepped-care approach, which starts with nonpharmacologic measures and then adds drugs singly or in combination. Numerous types of antihypertensive medications are available today, including centrally-acting sympathetic nervous system inhibitors, peripherally acting agents, neuroeffector transmission blockers, β adrenergic blockers, direct-acting vasodilators, mixed arterial and venous vasodilators, calcium-channel blockers, and ACE inhibitors. These various classes of drugs have different mechanisms of actions.

Nurses need to be involved with hypertension screening and patient education. Therapy is lifelong. Patients need to understand the process of hypertension and how they can help control and treat their own condition. Patient education enhances the chances of successfully controlling blood pressure and preventing long-term complications.

BIBLIOGRAPHY

Detection, Evaluation, and Treatment of High Blood Pressure. U. S. Department of Health and Human Services Public Health Service National Institutes of Health. NIH Publication No. 88-1088, May 1988.

Drugs for hypertensive emergencies. Med Lett 29(733):20, February 13, 1987.

Guanfacine for hypertension. Med Lett 29(740):49–50, May 22, 1987.

Reactions to antihypertensives. Nurses Drug Alert 11(5):33, 1987.

Verapamil for hypertension. Med Lett 29(737):37–38, April 10, 1987.

American Medical Association: AMA Drug Evaluations. John Wiley, New York, 1987.

Borreson, RE: Drug use and misuse in hypertension therapy. Hosp Formul 21(8):851–54, August 1986.

Cherner, R: Antihypertensive agents and diabetes: Side effects that demand careful consideration. Consultant 27(2):22+, 1987.

Consensus Trial Study Group. Effects of enalapril on mortality in severe congestive heart failure. N Engl J Med 316:1429–35, 1987.

Cressman, MD, et al: Antihypertensive drugs: Practical considerations in using the newer agents, part 2. Consultant 27(5):28–31, 34, May 1987.

Croog, SH, et al: The effects of antihypertensive therapy on the quality of life. N Engl J Med 314(26):1657, June 26, 1986.

Cunningham, SG: Nonpharmacologic management of high blood pressure. Cardio-Vascular Nursing 23(4):18–22, July–August 1987.

DeMoya, D: Are women impaired by antihypertensives too? RN 34:131, 1981.

Dunn, M: Interactions of NSAIDs and antihypertensives. JAMA 260:851, August 12, 1988.

Ferguson, RK, et al: Hypertensive emergency. Pat Care 21(13):124+, 1987.

Flegel, K, et al. Adverse reaction to antihypertensive drugs. JAMA 257:1329–1330, March 13, 1987.

Gever, LN: Ace inhibitors improve compliance. Nursing 17(10):143, 1987.

Gikeson, GS, Delaney, RL: Effectiveness of sublingual clonidine in patients unable to take oral medications. Drug Intell Clin Pharm 7(21):262–263, 1987.

Gilman, AG, Goodman, LS, and Gilman, A (eds): Goodman and Gilman's The Pharmacological Basis of Therapeutics, ed 6. Macmillan, New York, 1985.

Johnson, GP and Johanson, BC: Beta Blockers. Am J Nurs 83:1034–43, July 1983.

Lindgren, BR, Andersson, RGG. The effect of inhaled clonidine in patients with asthma. Am Rev Respir Dis 134:266, August 1986.

McEntee, MA, et al: Coping with hypertension. Nurs Clin North Am 22(3):583–92, 1987.

Metz, S: Rebound hypertension after discontinuation of transdermal clonidine therapy. Am J Med 82:17–19, January 1987.

Roberts, SW: Minoxidil: A breakthrough for balding people. Health Values 11(3):14–15, 1987.

Rostand, SG: Angiotensin converting enzyme inhibitors: An overview. Hosp Form 22(3):257–58, 263, 267–269, March 1987.

Scanu, P, et al: Reversible acute renal insufficiency with combination of enalapril and diuretics. Nephron 45:321–22, 1987.

Schneeweiss, A: Drug Therapy in Cardiovascular Disease. Lea & Febiger, Philadelphia, 1986.

Vidt, DG: Beta blockers: Choosing the best one for cardiac condition and hypertension. Consultant 27(3):128–32, 24, 137–39, March 1987.

Weber, MA, et al: Transdermal continuous antihypertensive therapy. Lancet 1(9), 1984.

SITUATION 29–1

Justine Pack is a 50-year-old with essential hypertension diagnosed five years ago. She has been on a sodium-restricted diet and hydrochlorothiazide (Hydro-Diuril). Her blood pressure has been recorded consistently around 160/94. Mrs. Pack is to be started on an additional antihypertensive agent.

1. The physician prescribes prazosin (Minipress) 1 mg po daily. When teaching the patient about this drug, the nurse will stress:
   a. taking the medication early in the day
   b. limiting fluid intake to 1000 ml per day
   c. taking the drug on an empty stomach
   d. rising slowly from a supine position

2. An important area of assessment pertaining to prazosine therapy includes noting evidence of the following:
   a. hepatic disease
   b. kidney dysfunction
   c. severe depression
   d. moderate hypertension

3. When planning for follow-up care for Mrs. Pack, the nurse is aware that:
   a. a majority of patients follow the treatment plan
   b. patients with hypertension have warning symptoms
   c. most patients understand the importance of compliance
   d. patients actively involved in their care are more compliant

4. Which of the following does *not* represent an expected patient outcome for Mrs. Pack?
   a. maintenance of monthly blood pressure checkups
   b. demonstration of ability to explain drug schedule
   c. evidence of systolic blood pressure <140 and >90 mmHg
   d. documentation that prescriptions have been filled

5. Mrs. Pack will be given dietary instructions by the nurse, which will include teaching her to avoid:
   a. fresh fruits
   b. bran fiber
   c. chocolate
   d. fluid intake

6. Which of the following statements indicates an understanding of the hypertensive treatment regime?
   a. "If I miss a dose, I should take two at the next dosage time."
   b. "I should take the pills when I feel like my blood pressure is high."
   c. "For relaxation, I plan to soak in our hot tub every day."
   d. "I am not supposed to stop taking the drug if I feel dizzy."

SITUATION 29–2

Paul Mathers, a 67-year-old, is admitted to the intensive care unit in hypertensive crisis. His blood pressure on admission is 230/150.

1. Mr. Mathers is to receive nitroprusside (Nipride) intravenously. The nurse will plan to infuse the drug within the following range:
   a. .02 to .5 µg/kg/minute
   b. 10 to 20 µg/kg/minute
   c. 5 to 15 µg/kg/minute
   d. .5 to 10 µg/kg/minute

2. Pertaining to special nursing actions regarding nitroprusside administration, the following applies:
   a. The solution must be mixed in normal saline.
   b. The IV bottle should be protected from light.
   c. Nitroprusside infusions can be maintained indefinitely.
   d. When properly mixed, the solution will be dark red.

3. Should Mr. Mathers develop symptoms such as slurred speech, weakness, muscle twitching, and/or confusion, the following level should be checked:
   a. thiocyanate
   b. potassium
   c. magnesium
   d. T_3, T_4

4. Which of the following nursing interventions would be most appropriate for Mr. Mathers?

   a. lowering mean arterial blood pressure no more than 20%–30% in the first 24 hours
   b. teaching exercise and diet counseling along with stress-reduction techniques
   c. maintaining the nitroprusside infusion at a set rate regardless of the diastolic pressure
   d. checking the blood pressure hourly while on nitroprusside infusion for accelerated hypertension

5. The nurse will expect the following outcome of nitroprusside therapy:
   a. reduced cardiac output
   b. increased preload
   c. increased urine output
   d. increased afterload

6. When observing Mr. Mathers for side effects of nitroprusside therapy, which of the following apply?
   a. reflex tachycardia
   b. hyperthyroidism
   c. chest pain
   d. difficulty voiding

Please refer to the Appendices for correct answers and additional review questions with answers.

30
CHAPTER

ANTIDYSRHYTHMIC MEDICATIONS

30

CHAPTER

ANTIDYSRHYTHMIC MEDICATIONS

MERRILY MATHEWSON KUHN, R.N., Ph.D., CCRN

LEARNING OBJECTIVES

After reading this chapter, the student will be able to:

1. Identify medications commonly used as antidysrhythmics.

2. Differentiate among antidysrhythmics as to mechanism of action, route of administration, pharmacokinetics, adverse effects, contraindications, and interactions.

3. Identify specific areas to assess in the patient requiring antidysrhythmics in order to formulate appropriate nursing diagnoses.

4. Plan the nursing interventions necessary to administer antidysrhythmics and choose appropriate teaching strategies to achieve patient compliance.

5. Evaluate the patient at various stages of treatment to gauge nursing interactions.

CARDIAC DYSRHYTHMIAS

Dysrhythmias or *arrhythmias* occur in approximately 90%–95% of all patients experiencing a myocardial infarction. Complex ventricular dysrhythmias and sustained and nonsustained ventricular tachycardia in patients with ischemic heart disease cause significant mortality. Ventricular fibrillation is a major cause of sudden coronary death in patients who have experienced a previous acute myocardial infarction. During the evolution of an acute myocardial infarction, ventricular dysrhythmias are common and can lead to death if they are not identified and appropriately treated (Table 30–1 reviews acute myocardial infarction). Appropriate antidysrhythmic therapy in these patients substantially reduces mortality.

Ventricular dysrhythmias such as premature ventricular contractions (PVCs) are frequently observed in patients without ischemic heart disease and may not require treatment unless the patient is symptomatic. More complex PVCs: *coupled* (two in a row), or *R-on-T phenomenon* (QRS occurs on the T wave, which may precipitate ventricular tachycardia or fibrillation) and ventricular tachycardia are usually treated even if the patient is asymptomatic.

Atrial disturbances such as atrial fibrillation and flutter are generally not life-threatening dysrhythmias. They may, however, cause significant symptomatology, such as palpitations, dizziness and lightheadedness, decreased cardiac output secondary to the loss of atrial contraction, and embolic phenomena, and may exacerbate pre-existing congestive heart failure. These rhythm disturbances usually require treatment even if they are asymptomatic. Antidysrhythmic therapy, therefore, decreases morbidity and mortality associated with cardiac dysrhythmias.

The ideal antidysrhythmic agent should have minimal side effects, low level of toxicity, little effect on normal impulse formation, a postitive hemodynamic effect, and must be available in both oral and parenteral forms. Unfortunately, the ideal antidysrhythmic agent has not yet been developed; all the antidysrhythmics cause a variety of adverse effects and toxic reactions. Therefore, the nurse must understand how these drugs work and know what to assess and evaluate in the patient.

ANTIDYSRHYTHMIC GROUPS

Several major groups of antidysrhythmic medications have been developed—Groups I through IV. Table 30–2 summarizes the classification of antidysrhythmics. Each group works by a different mechanism to suppress dysrhythmias. The group I drugs act as local anesthetics or have a membrane-stabilizing effect that depresses phase 0 of the action potential (Fig. 30–1). There are several subgroups within group I—Ia, Ib, and Ic. The Ia group prolongs the refractoriness, slows conduction, and decreases membrane responsiveness. The Ib group shortens the duration of the refractory period but has little effect on conduction in normal tissue. The Ic group markedly slows conduction but has minimal effect on refractoriness. The group IIs are the β blockers that depress phase 4 of the depolarization. The group III drugs produce a prolongation of phase 3 depolarization. And, group IV, the calcium-channel antagonists, depress

---

Table 30–1. MYOCARDIAL INFARCTION

DEFINITION: Myocardial infarction (MI) is necrosis of the cardiac muscle caused by lack of adequate blood supply to the myocardium.

TYPES: The majority of myocardial infarctions occur in the left ventricle. They may occur at different depths of the heart muscle, such as subendocardial, or transmural; and in different areas of the left ventricle, including the anterior, posterior, lateral, inferior, apical, and septal areas.

ETIOLOGY: MIs may result from occlusion of the coronary artery due to increasing amounts of lipid deposits (atheromas) within the intima (inner lining of the artery wall) of the coronary arteries. This continued narrowing eventually causes occlusion of the blood vessel. However, sudden occlusions are thought to occur at the site of incomplete obstruction by spasm, hemorrhage into a plaque, or thrombus. Within three hours after the cessation of blood flow to the distal portion of the heart muscle, that portion of the muscle becomes necrotic.

SYMPTOMS: The chief symptom is sudden, sharp retrosternal pain often described as ''crushing,'' with radiation to the arms, throat, jaw, and back. Pallor, gastrointestinal disturbances, profuse perspiration, intense anxiety, hypotension, and cardiac rhythm disturbances may also be present. The pain is not relieved with rest or nitroglycerin, and may last for hours.

MANAGEMENT: Differentiate between Q (transmural) and non-Q (subendocardial) wave infarction. Immediate care is to stabilize the cardiac rhythm, to prevent further circulatory impairment, and to keep the hypoperfused area from evolving into a total infarct. Numerous methods are being used today to prevent or limit infarct size, including nitrates, streptokinase, tissue plasminogen activators, or similar products, coronary artery bypass surgery, intra-aortic balloon pumping, β blockers, and percutaneous transluminal angioplasty.

Metaprolol protocol for Q-wave myocardial infarction 5 mg IV q 5 min × 3, 50 mg PO q 6 hr × 48 hours, 100 mg bid maintenance.

Patients who do have an infarct are placed on bed rest, given oxygen, monitored for dysrhythmias, and given antidysrhythmics, analgesics, and antianxiety drugs as needed.

In secondary care, rehabilitation is started, which includes education about the reduction of risk factors, exercise testing, and prescription.

Table 30–2. CLASSIFICATION OF ANTIDYSRHYTHMIC AGENTS

Class	Actions*	Drugs
I	Have local anesthetic properties. Interfere with fast inward depolarizing current carried by sodium ions.	
Ia	Prolong refractoriness and slow conduction, decrease membrane responsiveness.	Quinidine, procainamide, disopyramide
Ib	Shorten duration of refractory period and have little effect on conduction in normal tissue.	Lidocaine, phenytoin, tocainide, mexiletine
Ic	Markedly slow conduction but have minimal effects on refractoriness.	Encainide, flecainide, propafenone hydrochloride
II	Have antiadrenergic properties, depress cell membrane, decrease automaticity.	B blockers
III	Prolong refractoriness, increase action potential duration.	Amiodarone, bretylium
IV	Block slow inward (calcium) current, increase refractoriness.	Verapamil

*Based on drug's predominant electrophysiologic properties in normal tissue, usually Purkinje fibers.
Adapted from Vaughan Williams, 1984; and Harrison, DC: Antidysrythmic drug classification new science and practical applications. Am J Cardiol 56:185–187, 1985.

phase 4 depolarization and lengthen phases 1 and 2 of repolarization. Table 30–3 reviews the generalized action of each type of antidysrhythmic, including several investigational drugs. Antidysrhythmic drugs are reviewed in detail in Table 30–4. Table 30–5 features the commonly observed dysrhythmias with the medications used to treat them. Table 30–6 compares the metabolism and excretion of all of the antidysrhythmics.

GROUP IA ANTIDYSRHYTHMICS

Group Ia drugs (quinidine, procainamide, disopyramide) act by depressing Na^+ conductance, slowing the action potential upstroke in phase 0, resulting in a slowing of conduction velocity. These drugs also prolong action potential duration and increase *effective refractory period* in Purkinje fibers. By decreasing automaticity and

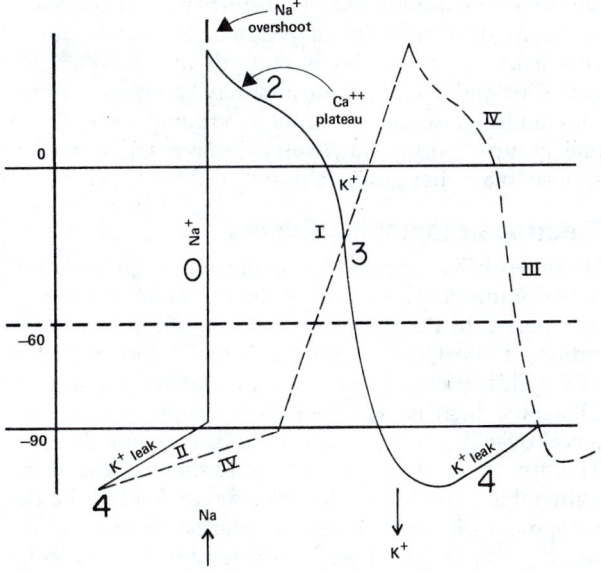

Figure 30–1. The antidysrhythmic drugs all have an effect on the action potential curve. Phase 0 is depolarization—Na^+ influx; phase I overshoot; phase II slow period that forms a plateau—K^+ efflux and Ca^{++} influx; phase III is the rapid phase of K^+ efflux; and phase IV is repolarization where Na^+ effluxes and K^+ influxes through the Na^+-K^+-ATPase pump. The group I drugs depress phase 0, group II drugs depress phase 4, group III drugs produce a prolongation of phase III, and group IV drugs depress phase 4 and lengthen phases 1 and 2 of repolarization. The effective refractory period (ERP) is also prolonged with the group I drugs.

Table 30–3. MECHANISM OF ACTION OF THE ANTIDYSRHYTHMICS

Group	Mechanism of Action	Current Medications	Investigational Preparations
Ia	Depress Na^+ conductance, increase action potential duration and effective refractory period, decrease membrane responsiveness.	Quinidine, procainamide, disopyramide	Aprindine, Pirmenol, Cifenline succinate
Ib	Increase K^+ conductance, decrease action potential duration and effective refractory period.	Lidocaine, phenytoin, mexiletine, tocainide	Ethmozine, Pirmenol, Aprindine
Ic	Cause marked depression of phase 0 through profound slowing of conduction. Just a slight effect on conduction.	Flecainide, Encainide, Propafenone	Lorcainide, Indecainide
II	Interfere with Na^+ conductance, depress cell membrane, decrease automaticity and increase effective refractory period of the AV node.	Propranolol, Nadolol, Metoprolol, Timolol, Atenolol, Pindolol	Sotalol, Practolol
III	Interfere with norepinephrine, increase action potential duration and effective refractory period.	Amiodarone, Bretylium	Sotalol, Acecainide hydrochloride
IV	Ca^{++} antagonists, increase AV nodal effective refractory period.	Verapamil	Gallopamil, Bepridil, Tiapamil

prolonging the effective refractory period, these drugs are effective in disturbances of either increased automaticity or re-entry.

Uses

Group Ia drugs are effective in suppressing dysrhythmias caused by these mechanisms of atrial or ventricular origin: atrial fibrillation; PVCs; and ventricular tachycardia. They tend to have little effect on the SA node and therefore are not used in disturbances of SA nodal function, such as sinus tachycardia. Response rate to ventricular dysrhythmias is only about 50%–70% for quinidine and disopyramide and may be higher for procainamide. A successful antidysrhythmic response to one group Ia drug, however, does not guarantee response to another group Ia drug.

Electrocardiographic Effects

Observed ECG changes are similar for all group Ia antidysrhythmics. All these drugs increase effective refractory period in Purkinje fiber cells, resulting in prolongation of the QRS complex and Q–T interval in the ECG. This effect can be used to monitor therapy. A 25%–50% increase in either QRS complex or Q–T interval over baseline is a reason to discontinue therapy. Therapy should be stopped because the increase in the vulnerable period of the ventricular can lead to the development of a ventricular tachycardia known as *Torsades de Pointes* (Fig. 30–2) (a combination of ventricular tachycardia and ventricular fibrillation, usually at a rate

of 100–300 beats/min). This effect may be related to plasma concentrations, so patients can be restarted on a lower dosage.

The lengthening Q–T interval changes more consistently as a function of drug concentration than does the widening of the QRS complex. Therefore, this is the preferable parameter to monitor.

Quinidine

Quinidine has a direct action on the cell membrane but also an indirect anticholinergic effect. The indirect anticholinergic effect of quinidine inhibits vagal action on the SA and AV nodes. The sinus node may accelerate, and often a dangerous sinus tachycardia may be provoked. If quinidine is to be administered to persons in atrial flutter or atrial fibrillation, digitalis is administered first to slow conduction at the AV node. Quinidine inhibits cation exchange (sodium influx and potassium efflux) and causes a decrease in the rate of depolarization. Through this mechanism, automaticity in ectopic sites in the atria, AV junction, and Purkinje fibers is suppressed or abolished. Ectopic tissue is more sensitive than normal pacemaker tissue, and thus the SA node is permitted to re-establish control over the cardiac impulse formation in the heart. Quinidine slows conduction velocity in all tissues and a widened QRS and prolonged P–R interval can be seen on the ECG (Fig. 30–3). A very important action of quinidine is its ability to prolong the effective refractory period of atrial and ventricular fibers. This effect probably exerts an antifibrillatory action

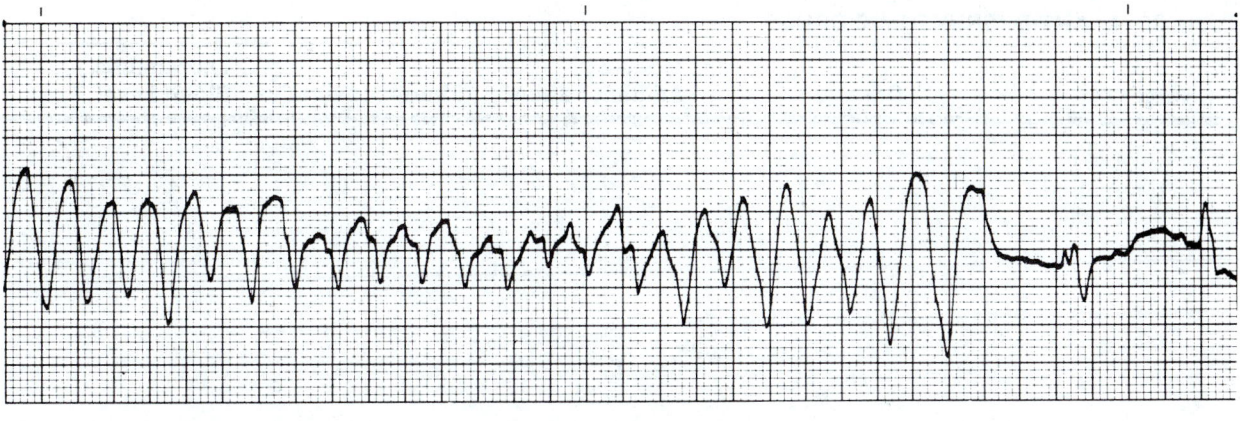

II

Figure 30-2. *Torsade de Pointes* variation of ventricular tachycardia converting spontaneously to sinus rhythm. *Torsade de Pointes* is a combination of ventricular tachycardia and ventricular fibrillation usually at a rate of 100 to 300 beats/minute. *Torsade de Pointes* is treated with beta blockers, isoproterenol, atropine, or by the insertion of a pacemaker. (From Brown, KR and Jacobson, S: Mastering Dysrhythmias—A Problem-Solving Guide. FA Davis, Philadelphia, 1986, with permission.)

by converting a unidirectional block to a bidirectional block, which thereby abolishes the re-entry type of dysrhythmias. Quinidine dilates resistance and capacitance vessels by blocking α-adrenergic receptors in the smooth muscle of peripheral tissue, which may result in hypotension.

Pharmacokinetics. Quinidine is 70%–90% absorbed when administered orally as the sulfate or gluconate salt (Quinaglute, Duraquin). The polygalacturonate preparation (Cardioquin) has a more erratic absorption profile, and its use is not recommended. Peak concentrations are seen 0.5–1.5 hours after administration of the sulfate, three to four hours after the gluconate, and 6 hours after the polygalacturonate preparation. Activity persists for 6–8 hours. Quinidine is 80%–90% bound to plasma proteins to both albumin and the acute-phase reactant protein 2, acid glycoprotein. The latter protein increases in serum when tissues become injured or inflamed, as occurs with surgery, trauma, arthritis, or acute myocardial infarction. Following an event such as an acute myocardial infarction, the free fraction of quinidine can be expected to decrease as acid glycoprotein concentrations increase twofold to threefold. Quinidine is accumulated in most tissues except the brain.

Quinidine is extensively metabolized (60%–80%) in the liver, producing several metabolites, of which at least one is active (3-hydroxyquinidine) and is present in significant amounts of serum. The half-life of quinidine in patients with normal liver function is about six to eight hours. Disease states that affect the elimination of quinidine from the body include hepatic disease and congestive heart failure. Renal disease does not influence the elimination of quinidine; however, urine acidification facilitates quinidine excretion.

Contraindications and Precautions. Specific contraindications to quinidine include hypersensitivity conduction defects, and complete AV block, as there is normal slowing through the AV node with quinidine that

can result in complete heart block and asystole. Quinidine is also contraindicated in myasthenia gravis due to its anticholinergic effects and in digitalis toxicity manifested by dysrhythmias or AV conduction disorders because they may be worsened. This drug is given cautiously to patients with impaired renal or hepatic function. The kidneys are responsible for excreting quinidine metabolites, whereas the liver is responsible for their metabolism. With hepatic disease and congestive heart failure, the dosage must be lowered.

Quinidine sulfate is also given cautiously to patients with potassium imbalance, since the effect of quinidine is enhanced by potassium or reduced if hypokalemia is present.

Adverse Effects. The most common adverse effects observed with quinidine are gastrointestinal complaints, including nausea, vomiting, and diarrhea. These symptoms can become very severe. Quinidine, as with other cinchona alkaloids (quinine), can cause cinchonism, which can manifest as tinnitus, vertigo, visual disturbances, loss of hearing, confusion, delirium, psychosis, and gastrointestinal symptoms. Quinidine exerts an α-adrenergic blocking effect that can cause vasodilation and hypotension. Less common, although still important, adverse effects include fever and thrombocytopenia. The latter reaction is a result of an antibody directed against quinidine-platelet complexes, resulting in the destruction of platelets. An asthma-like respiratory insufficiency and hepatitis reaction are other quinidine hypersensitivity reactions. Patients on long-term therapy should have periodic blood counts performed. A systemic lupus erythematosis-like syndrome can also occur.

Dysrhythmias may develop from use of quinidine and include sinus arrest, SA block, and AV block. These are most likely due to slowed conduction through the heart, and may even lead to asystole. The anticholinergic ef-

TEXT RESUMES ON PAGE 792

Table 30–4. ANTIDYSRHYTHMIC DRUGS

Name	Dosage	Mode of Administration	Pharmacokinetics	Therapeutic Blood Level

GROUP Ia

Action: Inhibits cation exchange and decreases rate of depolarization. Reduces automaticity in ectopic sites. Slows conduction velocity in all tissue. Prolongs effective refractory period of atrial and ventricular fibers. Has direct anticholinergic effect.

Use: wide variety of atrial and ventricular dysrhythmias. Maintains NSR after conversion from atrial flutter and atrial fibrillation.

Name	Dosage	Mode of Administration	Pharmacokinetics	Therapeutic Blood Level
Quinidine sulfate (Quinidex, Quinora, Cin-Quin)	200–400 mg q 4–6 hr	PO	O: 30 min P: 1–3 hr D: 6–8 hr ½L: 6–7 hr PB: 60%–80% B: liver E: urine	2–6 µg/ml (depends on assay; see text)
Sustained-release (Quinidex Extentabs)	300–600 mg q 8–12 hr	PO		
Quinidine gluconate	324 mg q 6–8 hr	PO	P: 3–4 hr D: 6–8 hr	
(Quinaglute)	324 mg q 6–8 hr	IM	O: 10 min D: 6–8 hr	
Quinidine polygalacturonate (Cardioguin)	275 mg q 8–12 hr	PO	O: UA P: 6 hr D: 8—12 hr	

Key to Abbreviations in the *Pharmacokinetics* column O-onset; P-peak; D-duration; PB-protein bound; B-biotransformed in; E-excreted in; ½ L-halflife.
*Within the column listing adverse effects, underlines indicate the most common effects, and CAPITALS indicate life-threatening effects.

Contraindications/ Precautions	Adverse Effects*	Interactions	Nursing Implications
			FOR ALL ANTIDYS-RHYTHMICS: ASSESSMENT: Monitor pulse, blood pressure, and ECG (including Q–T) frequently. INTERVENTION: Tablets may be crushed and capsules opened and mixed with food or fluids. Do not break, crush, or chew extended-release tablets. Use infusion pump to ensure accurate IV dosage. Instruct patient to take medication around the clock, as prescribed, even if feeling better. Take a missed dose as soon as possible if remembered within 2 hours (4 hours for extended-release tablets). EVALUATION: Cardiac dysrhythmias should subside without detrimental adverse effects.
Contraindicated in hypersensitivity, conduction defects, complete AV block, digitalis toxicity, and myasthenia gravis. Use cautiously in impaired renal or hepatic function, bronchial asthma, and potassium imbalance.	Neuro: headache, vertigo, confusion, restlessness, fainting CV: WIDEN ORS, PROLONG QT, cardiac asystole, HYPOTENSION, PVCS. Resp: asthmas, respiratory arrest GI: diarrhea, nausea, vomiting, anorexia, abdominal pain, hepatitis Renal: fluid and electrolyte imbalances Hemo: thrombocytopenia, purpura Integ: rash Misc: cinchonism (see text), systemic lupus erythematosus syndrome Eye: mydriasis, blurred vision	Acidifying urine increases quinidine excretion. Reserpine and othe antihypertensives increase hypotensive effects. Action of anticoagulants may be enhanced with concurrent use of quinidine. Phenobarbital, hydantoin, rifampin reduce half-life of quinidine. Nifedipine decreases serum levels of quinidine. Quinidine increases the half-life of digoxin.	Same as for all, plus: ASSESSMENT: Baseline ECG, Q–T. INTERVENTION: Take with meals to minimize GI upset. Continuously monitor apical pulse, BP, and ECG for changes. Quinidine prolongs QRS and Q–T intervals. Monitor plasma quinidine levels. Monitor intake and output—particularly for presence of diarrhea. Avoid excessive citrus fruit intake, which changes urine pH and decreases excretion of quinidine. Do not crush or chew sustained-release tablet. Whole tablet may appear in stool. EVALUATION: Same as for all. Notify physician if ringing in ears, visual disturbances, dizziness, or headache occur.

CONTINUED ON THE FOLLOWING PAGE

Table 30–4. ANTIDYSRHYTHMIC DRUGS-*CONTINUED*

Name	Dosage	Mode of Administration	Pharmacokinetics	Therapeutic Blood Level
Procainamide hydrochloride (Pronestyl)				

Action: decreases myocardial excitability, slows conduction, velocity.

Uses: wide variety of atrial and ventricular dysrhythmias; used short-term only due to adverse effects.

Name	Dosage	Mode of Administration	Pharmacokinetics	Therapeutic Blood Level
	250–500 mg q 3–4 hr	PO (may be crushed)	O: 0.5 min P: 30–90 min D: 3+ hr ½L: 2.5–4.7 hr PB: 14%–23% B: liver E: urine (40%–70%)	4–8 µg/ml (combined procainamide plus NAPA is 10–30 µg/ml) drawn 2 hr after administration
	100 mg over 5 min not to exceed 50 mg/min, then drip until 1 g has been administered, dysrhythmia disappears, or Q–T widens by 50%.	IV bolus	O: immediate D: same	
	1 g in 250 ml at 1–3 mg/min (see text)	IV drip		
(Procan SR, Pronestyl-SR)	250–1000 mg q 6 hr	PO	O: UA P: 1–2 hr D: 6 hr	

Disopyramide (Norpace)

Action: prolongs actions duration and refractory period of heart. May depress myocardial contractility. Has anticholinergic and a negative inotropic effect.

Uses: suppresses and prevents ventricular dysrhythmias.

Name	Dosage	Mode of Administration	Pharmacokinetics	Therapeutic Blood Level
	L: 300 mg followed by 150 mg q 6 hr M: 400–800 mg daily in 3–4 divided doses	PO	O: 30 min P: 0.5–3 hr D: 6–8 hr ½L: 6–8 hr	2–8 µg/ml drawn 3–4 hr after administration

Key to Abbreviations in the *Pharmacokinetics* column O-onset; P-peak; D-duration; PB-protein bound; B-biotransformed in; E-excreted in; ½ L-halflife.

*Within the column listing adverse effects, underlines indicate the most common effects, and CAPITALS indicate life-threatening effects.

Contraindications/ Precautions	Adverse Effects*	Interactions	Nursing Implications
Contraindicated in myasthenia gravis and AV block. Use cautiously in myocardial infarction, congestive heart failure, digitalis intoxication, and hepatic or renal disease. Safety in pregnancy, lactating women, and children not established.	CV: AV block, IV hypotension, bradycardia, prolonged Q–T GI: anorexia, nausea, diarrhea, vomiting, bitter taste Hemo: LUPUS ERYTHEMATOSUS, AGRANULOCYTOSIS, NEUTROPENIA, THROMBOCYTOPENIA Integ: urticaria, pruritis, rash	Antihypertensives and thiazides increase hypotensive effects. Cardiac glycosides and antidysrhythmics have additive effect. Enhances anticholinergics. Cimetidine reduces renal clearance of procainamide. Alcohol increases hepatic metabolism of procainamide.	Same as for all, plus: ASSESSMENT: Monitor ECG, pulse, and blood pressure continuously throughout IV administration and periodically during oral administration. Patient should remain supine throughout IV administration. Assess QRS and Q–T intervals during IV administration. Assess CBC and antinuclear antibody (ANA). INTERVENTION: Administer on an empty stomach with a full glass of water for faster absorption. If GI irritation occurs, may be administered with or immediately after meals. Slight yellow color of solution will not alter potency; do not use if markedly discolored or if a precipitate is present. When converting from IV to oral dose regimen, 3–4 hr should elapse between last IV dose and administration of the first oral dose. Nonabsorbable wax core may appear in stool. When administering IV procainamide, discontinue if Q–T lengthens by 50%, P–R intervals become prolonged above 0.20 seconds, or if blood pressure drops 15 mm Hg. EVALUATION: Notify physician immediately if signs of drug-induced lupus syndrome (fever, chills, joint pain or swelling, pain with breathing, skin rash), leukopenia (sore throat, mouth, or gums) or thrombocytopenia (unusual bleeding or bruising) occur.
Contraindicated in cardiogenic shock, second- or third-degree block,	Neuro: blurred vision, dizziness, headache, agitation, depression	Reduced blood levels when given with phenobarbital,	Same as for all, plus: ASSESSMENT: Monitor K$^+$

CONTINUED ON THE FOLLOWING PAGE

Antidysrhythmic Drugs

Table 30–4. ANTIDYSRHYTHMIC DRUGS–*CONTINUED*

Name	Dosage	Mode of Administration	Pharmacokinetics	Therapeutic Blood Level
Disopyramide (Norpace)– *Continued*			PB: 50%–60% B: liver E: urine, feces P: 4.9 hr (SR)	
	Time-release 200– 400 mg q 12 hr Children: 1–4 yr 10– 20 mg/kg 4–12 yr 10–15 mg/kg 12–18 yr 6–15 mg/kg	PO		

GROUP Ib

Action: depresses excessive automaticity of ectopic pacemakers in the His-Purkinje system. Has local anesthetic effect.

Uses: suppresses and prevents ventricular dysrhythmias.

Name	Dosage	Mode of Administration	Pharmacokinetics	Therapeutic Blood Level
Lidocaine hydrochloride (Xylocaine)	Adult: 1 mg/kg bolus followed by 0.5 mg/ kg in 10 min. Reduce bolus dose by 5% for patients with CHF Children: 1 mg/kg bolus followed by infusion of 10–40 µg/kg/min	IV IV	O: 10–90 sec P: minutes D: 20 min ½L: 80–108 min PB: 65%–75% B: liver E: urine	1.5–5 µg/ml
	100–500 mg	IM	O: 5–15 min P: 20–30 min D: 60–90 min	NA

Phenytoin (Dilantin)

Action: depresses spontaneous depolarization in ventricular tissue. Has mild negative inotropic effect and a peripheral vasodilator effect. Increases conduction through the AV node. Also acts as an anticonvulsant.

Uses: digitalis-induced ventricular dysrhythmias.

Name	Dosage	Mode of Administration	Pharmacokinetics	Therapeutic Blood Level
	300–500 mg/day	PO	O: slow P: 3–12 hr D: 12–24 hr ½L: 8–60 hr PB: 98% B: liver	10–20 µg/ml

Key to Abbreviations in the *Pharmacokinetics* column O-onset; P-peak; D-duration; PB-protein bound; B-bio-transformed in; E-excreted in; ½ L-halflife.
*Within the column listing adverse effects, <u>underlines</u> indicate the most common effects, and CAPITALS indicate life-threatening effects.

Contraindications/ Precautions	Adverse Effects*	Interactions	Nursing Implications
hypersensitivity, glaucoma, urinary retention, myasthenia gravis. Use cautiously in congestive heart failure. Safety in pregnant and lactating mothers has not been established.	CV: edema, fatigue, weight gain, conduction disturbances, chest pain, hypotension, congestive heart failure. Resp: shortness of breath GI: dry mouth, constipation, nausea, pain, bloating, gas, anorexia, diarrhea, vomiting Endo: hypoglycemia Renal: urinary retention, hesitancy or frequency Integ: rash, dermatoses	phenytoin, and rifampin. Concurrent antidysrhythmics may increase Q–T interval. Verapamil enhances negative inotropic effect.	levels and stabilize during therapy. INTERVENTION: Check apical pulse; if less than 60 beats/min, consult physician. Monitor vital signs, ECG (disopyramide prolongs QRS and Q–T), and intake and output closely for changes. Weigh patient daily and check extremities for edema and congestive heart failure (weight gain, dependent edema, difficulty in breathing). Sugarless gum may help dry mouth. Take on an empty stomach. Eat high-fiber diet or take bulk laxatives to treat constipation.
Contraindicated in hypersensitivity, supraventricular dysrhythmias, AV block, sinus bradycardia, Stokes–Adams syndrome, and Wolff–Parkinson–White syndrome. Use cautiously in renal or hepatic disease, congestive heart failure, respiratory depression, persons with a genetic predisposition to malignant hyperthermia, and in pregnancy and children.	Neuro: lightheadedness, dizziness, drowsiness, restlessness, confusion, blurred or double vision, sensation of heat or cold or numbness, slurred speech, unconsciousness, CONVULSIONS CV: hypotension, dysrhythmia, bradycardia, CARDIAC ARREST. Resp: RESPIRATORY ARREST, GI: vomiting Integ: phlebitis extending from the injection site	Additive neurologic depression with procainamide. Increased blood levels when given with cimetidine. Additive cardiac depression with propranolol and metoprolol. Tubocurarine and polymixin B enhance neuromuscular blockade.	Same as for all, plus: ASSESSMENT: Monitor ECG for excessive slowing or prolongation of P–R interval, blood pressure, respiratory status at onset and frequently during infusion. INTERVENTION: Read lidocaine labels carefully, so that only medications **without** epinephrine or preservatives are administered intravenously. Administer boluses over 1–2 min. Mix 1 g in 250 ml D$_5$W makes a 0.4% solution which is stable for 24 hr. Use infusion pump or microdrip system. Administer IM dosage in deltoid. EVALUATION: Serum levels periodically.
Contraindicated in history of hypersensitivity, sinus bradycardia, heart block. Use cautiously in	Neuro: nystagmus, ataxia, diplopia, drowsiness, coma, dizziness, nervousness, slurred speech, confusion	Phenytoin potentiated by oral anticoagulants, oral contraceptives, phenothiazines, salicylates, and sulfon-	INTERVENTION: Mix phenytoin with only special diluent or normal saline solution. Phenytoin, if diluted, is used

CONTINUED ON THE FOLLOWING PAGE

Table 30-4. ANTIDYSRHYTHMIC DRUGS-*CONTINUED*

Name	Dosage	Mode of Administration	Pharmacokinetics	Therapeutic Blood Level
Phenytoin (Dilantin)-*Continued*			E: urine (less than 5% unchanged) O: 3–5 min	
	50–100 mg q 5 min, up to 1 g total (mixed only in special diluent or normal saline) Not faster than 25–50 mg/min, to a max 1 g	IV		

Mexiletine hydrochloride (Mexitil)				

Action: depresses automaticity in ventricles.

Uses: suppresses and prevents ventricular tachydysrhythmias.

| | Initial: 200–400 mg q 8 hr Maintenance: 200–400 mg q 8 hr with 2–3 days in between adjustments or 300–450 mg q 12 hr | PO | O: 1–2 hr P: 2–3 hr D: 10–15 hr ½L: 8–12 hr PB: 50%–70% B: liver E: urine (10%–15% unchanged) | 0.5–2 μg/ml |

Tocainide hydrochloride (Tonocard)				

Action: decreases excitability of cardiac cells.

Uses: suppress and prevent ventricular dysrhythmias.

| | 400 mg q 8 hr Range: 1200–1800 mg/day given in divided doses | PO | O: 0.5–1 hr P: ½–3 hr D: 8–10 hr ½L: 11–15 hr PB: 10%–20% B: liver E: urine (28%–55% unchanged) | 4–10 μg/ml |

GROUP Ic:

Action: depresses sinus node automaticity and prolongs conduction throughout the heart.

Uses: suppresses and prevents all types of ventricular dysrhythmias.

Key to Abbreviations in the *Pharmacokinetics* column O-onset; P-peak; D-duration; PB-protein bound; B-biotransformed in; E-excreted in; ½ L-halflife.
*Within the column listing adverse effects, underlines indicate the most common effects, and CAPITALS indicate life-threatening effects.

Contraindications/ Precautions	Adverse Effects*	Interactions	Nursing Implications
impaired renal or hepatic function and in hypotension.	CV: hypotension GI: nausea, vomiting Integ: rashes	amides. Increased seizure activity with alcohol, barbiturates, and folic acid. Interferes with the following laboratory test results: thyroid function, urinary steroids.	immediately, as precipitation begins within 15 min after dilution. Not to exceed 50 mg/min IV (25 mg/min in elderly). Do not administer if precipitate forms. Do not mix with other solutions.
Contraindicated in cardiogenic shock, bradycardia, known hypersensitivity, or preexisting second- or third-degree block. Use cautiously in severe hepatic or renal disease. Safety in pregnancy and children has not been determined.	Neuro: tremor, dizziness/lightheadedness, nervousness, coordination difficulties, changes in sleep habits, fatigue, diplopia CV: palpitation, chest pain, increased PVCs, hypotension, bradycardia, edema Resp: dyspnea GI: GI distress, diarrhea, constipation, change in appetitie, HEPATIC NECROSIS Integ: rash Misc: fever	Morphine decreases absorption. Phenytoin, rifampin, and phenobarbital may lower serum levels. Cimetidine can increase plasma levels.	ASSESSMENT: Same as for all. INTERVENTION: Administer with food to decrease GI irritation. Do not skip or double up on doses. Use heavy equipment cautiously due to dizziness. Maintain urine pH near normal. EVALUATION: same as for all. If tiredness, yellowing of skin or eyes or sore throat persist, notify physician.
Contraindicated in hypersensitivity to amide-type local anesthetics, and in second- or third-degree AV block with no artificial pacemaker. Use cautiously in heart failure or minimal cardiac reserve, and blood dyscrasias including leukopenia, agranulocytosis, hypoplastic anemia, and thrombocytopenia, and patients with hepatic or renal impairment. Safe use in pregnancy and lactation and in children not yet established.	Neuro: dizziness, tremor, paresthesia, confusion, ataxia, anxiety, hallucination, sweating CV: VENTRICULAR FIBRILLATION, AV block, increased QRS duration, prolonged Q–T, hypotension Resp: dyspnea, pulmonary edema and embolism, PULMONARY FIBROSIS GI: nausea, anorexia, vomiting, diarrhea, epigastric pain Hemo: drug fever, BLOOD DYSCRASIAS, APLASTIC ANEMIA Integ: rash	Additive or antagonistic effects with other antidysrhythmics and β-adrenergic blockers.	ASSESSMENT: Same as for all. Monitor CBC during therapy and lungs periodically. INTERVENTION: Administer before meals. Food delays absorption. Monitor ECG (Tocainide shortens Q–T). Monitor for tremors. Observe caution while driving or performing other tasks requiring alertness or physical dexterity. EVALUATION: Notify physician immediately when dyspnea, wheezing, easy bruising or bleeding, fever, or sore throat occurs.

CONTINUED ON THE FOLLOWING PAGE

Table 30–4. ANTIDYSRHYTHMIC DRUGS–*CONTINUED*

Name	Dosage	Mode of Administration	Pharmacokinetics	Therapeutic Blood Level
Flecainide acetate (Tambocor)	I: 100 mg q 12 hr increase 50 mg every 4 days. M: 100–200 mg q 12 hr	PO	O: 0.5–1 hr P: 3 hr (1– 6 hr) D: 12–15 hr ½L: 20 hr PB: 40% B: liver E: urine (30% unchanged)	0.2–1 µg/ml

Encainide hydrochloride (Enkaid)

Action: depresses sinus node automaticity and prolongs conduction throughout the heart.

Uses: suppresses and prevents all types of ventricular dysrhythmias.

	Dosage	Mode of Administration	Pharmacokinetics	Therapeutic Blood Level
	I: 25 mg q 8 hr increase every 3–5 days. M: 50–75 mg q 8 hr	PO	O: 30–60 min P: 30–90 min D: 6–8 hr ½L: 1–2 hr (metabolites longer); 6–11 hr for certain population phenotypes PB: 75%–85% B: liver E: urine	No value secondary to ODE and MODE
Propafenone hydrochloride (Rythmol)	450–900 mg/day divided tid	PO	O: rapid P: 2–3 hr D: UA ½L: 1.8––32.3 hr PB: 77%–95% B: extensively, liver E: <1% urine	No value

CLASS III
Bretylium tosylate (Bretylol)

Action: increases action potential duration and refractory periods of Purkinje fibers. Antiadrenergic effect that prevents release of norepinephrine from sympathetic nerve terminals.

Uses: prophylaxis and treatment of life-threatening ventricular dysarhythmias.

	Dosage	Mode of Administration	Pharmacokinetics	Therapeutic Blood Level
	Loading dose: 5–10 mg/kg (to a maximum of 30 mg/kg/24 hr) mixed in 50 ml over 10–30 min; repeat in 15–30 min	IV bolus	O: 15 min P: 2–3 hr D: 6–24 hr ½L: 8–12 hr PB: 1%–10% B: not biotransformed E: urine (90% unchanged)	Not useful

Key to Abbreviations in the *Pharmacokinetics* column O-onset; P-peak; D-duration; PB-protein bound; B-biotransformed in; E-excreted in; ½ L-halflife.
*Within the column listing adverse effects, <u>underlines</u> indicate the most common effects, and CAPITALS indicate life-threatening effects.

Contraindications/ Precautions	Adverse Effects*	Interactions	Nursing Implications
Contraindicated in hypersensitivity, cardiogenic shock, heart blocks without a pacer. Use cautiously in congestive heart failure, sick sinus syndrome, potassium imbalance, liver dysfunction. Safety in pregnant and lactating women and children unknown.	Neuro: dizziness, visual disturbances, headache, temor CV: fatigue, palpitations, PROARRHYTHMIAS, decreased cardiac output, chest pain Resp: dyspnea, bronchospasm GI: nausea, vomiting, diarrhea, swollen lips, mouth, and tongue, constipation Hemo: leukopenia, thrombocytopenia Integ: rash GU: impotence, decreased libido	Increased digoxin levels increase negative inotropic effect with disopyramide and verapamil.	Same as for all, plus: ASSESSMENT: Assess blood pressure and presence of congestive heart failure during therapy. INTERVENTION: May be administered with meals to reduce GI irritation. Maintain serum K^+ levels. Monitor ECG (Flecainide can prolong P–R, Q–T, and QRS). EVALUATION: If neurologic signs occur (dizziness, visual disturbances, headache, increased fatigue), weight gain, and change in cardiac rhythm, report these to physician.
Same as for flecainide acetate.	Neuro: dizziness, blurred vision, headache CV: WORSENING OF VENTRICULAR DYSRHYTHMIAS, chest pain, palpitations GI: diarrhea, nausea, vomiting, dry mouth	Cimetidine increases plasma concentration of encainide hydrochloride.	Same as flecainide acetate.
None known	Neuro: dizziness, visual disturbances CV: proarrhythmic effect, congestive heart failure, AV block, bundle-branch block GI: nausea, vomiting, unusual metallic taste	Drug: Propafenone increases digoxin level by almost 100%. Enhances anticoagulation effects of warfarin.	Same as above.
No known contraindications. Use cautiously in renal failure and in patients with fixed cardiac output. Safety in pregnancy and children not established.	Neuro: vertigo, dizziness, lightheadedness, and syncope CV: postural hypotension, bradycardia, increased PVCs, angina, shortness of breath	Concurrent use with digitalis may increase dysrythmias; quinidine and procainamide can increase hypotension.	Same as for all. INTERVENTION: For short-term use only. Keep patient in supine position. Observe closely for hypotension. Reduce dose gradually and

CONTINUED ON THE FOLLOWING PAGE

Table 30–4. ANTIDYSRHYTHMIC DRUGS–*CONTINUED*

Name	Dosage	Mode of Administration	Pharmacokinetics	Therapeutic Blood Level
Bretylium tosylate–*Continued*	1–2 mg/min. In emergency situation, 5 mg/kg undiluted rapidly. If ventricular fibrillation continues, administer 10 mg/kg and repeat as necessary	IV drip IV bolus		

Amiodarone (Cordarone):

Action: potent smooth muscle relaxer and produces marked coronary and peripheral vasodilation. Exerts a noncompetitive blockade on both α-and β-adrenergic receptors.

Uses: Controls supraventricular and ventricular dysrhythmias in patients resistant to other antidysrhythmics.

Name	Dosage	Mode of Administration	Pharmacokinetics	Therapeutic Blood Level
	800–1600 mg daily for 1–3 weeks then 600–800 mg day for 1 month then 200–600 mg daily in single or divided doses	PO	O: 2–3 days (up to 1–3 weeks) P: 3–7 hr D: 10–150 days ½L: initial biphasic elimination 2.5–10 days, slower terminal elimination phase 26–107 days. PB: 96% B: liver E: bile	1–2.5 μg/ml

Key to Abbreviations in the *Pharmacokinetics* column O-onset; P-peak; D-duration; PB-protein bound; B-biotransformed in; E-excreted in; ½ L-halflife.
*Within the column listing adverse effects, underlines indicate the most common effects, and CAPITALS indicate life-threatening effects.

fects of quinidine on the AV node can precipitate tachycardias, particularly atrial fibrillation and atrial flutter. Ventricular dysrhythmias such as PVCs, ventrcular tachycardia, and ventrcular fibrillation may also occur. "Quinidine syncope" is due to rapid ventricular tachycardia and fibrillation (torsade de pointe). The result can be sudden death. This risk increases with higher doses and quinidine toxicity.

Interactions. The hepatic elimination of quinidine is inhibited by cimetidine (Tagamet) administration, resulting in an increase in serum levels. Concurrent quinidine and coumarin anticoagulants may reduce prothrombin levels. Quinidine may potentiate neuromuscular blocking agents. Enzyme enhancers like phenobarbital, phenytoin, or rifampin increase liver enzyme production and reduce the serum half-life of quinidine. Concurrent nifedipine decreases serum levels of quinidine, and breakthrough dysrhythmias may occur.

Quinidine can interact with other drugs such as digoxin (see Chapter 28), raising the serum levels of digoxin two to three times. Secondary to its hypotensive effects, quinidine has the potential to increase the antihypertensive effects of drugs such as nitroglycerin, reserpine, and other antihypertensives.

Dosage. Quinidine is available for oral use in a wide variety of preparations all containing different amounts of quinidine base. Quinidine sulfate contains approximately 80% quinidine base and is available in 100-, 200-, 300-mg tablets and capsules. Quinidine gluconate contains 62% quinidine base. A 324-mg tablet therefore contains a 200-mg quinidine base. Quinidine polygalacturonate contains approximately 65% quinidine base, so that 275-mg tablet contains 180 mg quinidine. Usual oral doses of quinidine sulfate range from 200–400 mg every 6 hours; quinidine gluconate, 324 mg every 8 hours; and quinidine polygalacturonate, 275 mg every 8–12 hours. A quinidine sulfate extended-release prep-

Contraindications/ Precautions	Adverse Effects*	Interactions	Nursing Implications
	GI: nausea, vomiting, diarrhea Renal: dysfunction Integ: rash		discontinue over 3–5 days if clinical status allows.
Contraindicated in bradycardia and severe sinus dysfunction, pulmonary disease or cardiomegaly. Use with caution in liver disease. Safety in pregnancy and children not established.	Neuro: neurologic problems, peripheral neuropathy, decreased libido, extrapyramidal symptoms CV: exacerbation of dysrhythmias, congestive heart failure, SA node dysfunction, PAROXYSMAL VENTRICULAR TACHYCARDIA, hypotension. Resp: PULMONARY INFILTRATES AND FIBROSIS GI: nausea, vomiting, constipation, anorexia, abdominal pain Biliary: abnormal liver function Integ: photosensitivity, blue-grey skin discoloration Eye: microdeposits, halos, photophobia, dry eyes Endo: thyroid dysfunction	Increases prothrombin time and bleeding if used with warfarin. Increased digoxin, quinidine, phenytoin and procainamide serum levels. Reduce digoxin by half when loading dose of amiodarone is given. Potentiates bradycardia and sinus arrest with concurrent β blockers and calcium antagonists. With hypokalemia, prolongs Q–T interval and may cause *Torsades de Pointes*.	Same as for all plus ASSESSMENT: Assess baseline thyroid, liver, and lung and neurologic function. Effects may not be seen for 1–3 weeks. INTERVENTION: Gradually all other antidysrhythmics are reduced. If GI symptoms develop, divide dose and give with food. Protect skin from sun exposure. Monitor K level closely. Monitor ECG (amiodarone prolongs P–R, QRS, and Q–T). EVALUATION: Chest x-ray periodically. Report increasing fatigue, dyspnea, cough, pleuritic pain to physician.

aration (Quinidex Extentabs) is also available and can be administered every 12 hours. The total daily dose of quinidine, independent of the preparation, should be approximately 10–15 mg/kg. Quinidine gluconate is available in parenteral form for both intramuscular and intravenous (IV) use, although the IV route is not recommended because it causes hypotension. Care should be used in changing from the oral sulfate to parenteral gluconate to account for the differences in quinidine base content.

Therapeutic Blood Levels. Blood levels of quinidine relate to both therapeutic efficacy and toxicity, and can be used to assess the appropriateness of a dosage regimen or significance of a drug interaction. Available assays differ substantially in their ability to measure quinidine specifically in serum. Nonspecific assays measuring quinidine metabolites as quinidine will have a higher therapeutic range (usually 2–6 μg/ml) than specific assays measuring only quinidine. A therapeutic range for these assays is 1–4 μg/ml. It is therefore important to know the specificity of the assay used before interpreting serum quinidine levels.

Procainamide Hydrochloride

Procainamide hydrochloride (Pronestyl, Procan), a group Ia antidysrhythmic, is indicated for both atrial and ventricular dysrhythmias. Its action is similar to that of quinidine.

Uses. Although the indications of quinidine and procainamide are the same, the effect achieved is not always identical. Quinidine is frequently preferred for prolonged oral therapy because of the high incidence of drug-induced lupus associated with long-term administration of procainamide.

Intravenous procainamide is preferred for terminating supraventricular or ventricular dysrhythmias. It is often the drug of choice when the dysrhythmia is resistant to lidocaine. Procainamide slows conduction in accessory pathways, and is useful for acute termination of tachyarrhythmias associated with Wolff–Parkinson–White syndrome.

Pharmacokinetics. *Absorption and Distribution.* Procainamide is well-absorbed orally as the rapid-release hydrochloride salt. Bioavailability is about 75%. Peak plasma concentrations are achieved in 30–90 min-

Table 30–5. DYSRHYTHMIAS AND THEIR USUAL MEDICATION TREATMENTS

Rhythms	Drugs of Choice	Drug Action
Bradycardias, SA block, SA arrest	Atropine, isoproterenol	Increase sinus rate and AV conduction, enhance automaticity.
Supraventricular tachycardia, paroxysmal atrial tachycardia (PAT), atrial tachycardia, sinus tachycardia	Verapamil, cardiac glycosides, propranolol, quinidine, disopyramide, procainamide, edrophonium	Depress automaticity and slow conduction velocity, and depress SA nodal automaticity and AV nodal conduction.
	Verapamil	Slows AV nodal conduction.
	Propranolol	Slows conduction velocity.
Atrial flutter, atrial fibrillation	Cardiac glycosides, verapamil, β blockers to slow rate. Quinidine, disopyramide, or procainamide for long-term suppression.	Prolongs AV nodal conduction time and refractoriness.
Premature atrial contraction (PAC)	Quinidine, procainamide, disopyramide	Depress automaticity, has local anesthetic properties.
Premature ventricular contraction (PVC)	Lidocaine for emergencies; procainamide, quinidine, tocainide, disopyramide, mexiletine, flecainide	Depress automaticity, has local anesthetic properties.
Ventricular tachycardia (VT)	Lidocaine, Ic and Ib drugs, bretylium, procainimide, amiodarone	Depress automaticity and excitability.
Ventricular fibrillation (VF)	Lidocaine, procainamide, Ic and Ib drugs, bretylium, amiodarone	Depress automaticity and excitability.
First-, second-, and third-degree AV block	Atropine, isoproterenol	Only useful temporarily to speed SA rate.

utes. Procainamide is 14%–23% protein-bound. Oral absorption of the sustained-release preparation, Procan SR, is delayed; however, the extent of absorption is similar to that of the rapid-release preparations. Procainamide is rapidly distributed to most body tissues.

Biotransformation and Excretion. Procainamide is metabolized in the liver to an equipotent metabolite, *N*-acetylprocainamide (NAPA). This metabolic process is genetically determined, with patients classified as rapid or slow acetylators. Rapid acetylators produce larger quantities of NAPA. The average half-life of procainamide is three to four hours. The active metabolite NAPA is excreted renally (50%) and has a half-life of six hours. Procainamide is used carefully, with dosage carefully titrated in patients with hepatic and renal insufficiency because of delayed elimination of procainamide and accumulation of NAPA.

Contraindications and Precautions. Procainamide is contraindicated in patients with myasthenia gravis because of its anticholinergic effects, and in persons with pre-existing disturbance of AV conduction such as AV blocks and bundle branch blocks because of its direct effects on slowing conduction through the AV node. It is used with caution in patients with digitalis intoxication because of additive effects on slowing AV conduction and precipitation of ventricular asystole or fibrilla-

tion. Procainamide is a myocardial depressant and is used with caution in patients with congestive heart failure. Procainamide is given cautiously to patients with hepatic and renal dysfunction because there is increased risk of toxicity, thus precipitating ventricular tachycardia and hypotension. Dysrhythmias can develop with procainamide, and they are similar to those seen with quinidine. Safety in pregnant and lactating women and in children is not yet established.

Adverse Effects. Gastrointestinal adverse effects occur, but less often than with quinidine. Maculopapular rashes may occur and necessitate discontinuation of the drug. A systemic lupus erythematosus (SLE) syndrome, consisting of fever, myalgias, arthralgias, and pleuritic chest pain, is seen with procainamide therapy. This reaction occurs at a higher frequency in patients who are slow acetylators of procainamide. This reaction is almost always reversible upon discontinuation of the drug. At least 50% of patients within two to eight months on procainamide develop a positive ANA (antinuclear antibody) titer and may develop a syndrome resembling SLE. This test is nonspecific for the diagnosis of procainamide-induced SLE, which therefore must be diagnosed on the basis of the time course of reaction along with symptomatology. The development of lupus in 25%–30% of patients limits the long-term usefulness

Table 30–6. COMPARISON OF THE METABOLISM AND EXCRETION OF ANTIDYSRHYTHMIC MEDICATIONS

Type	Medication	Biotransformed in Liver	Excreted by Kidneys	Other
Ia	Quinidine	90%	10%	•Active metabolite 3-hydroxyquinidine.
Ia	Procainamide hydrochloride (Pronestyle)	50%	50% unchanged	•Active metabolite NAPA half-life prolonged in renal disease.
Ia	Disopyramide phosphate (Norpace)	40%–50%	50%–60% unchanged	•Active n-dealkylated metabolite.
Ib	Lidocaine (Xylocaine)	90%	10% unchanged	•Active metabolites monoethylglycine and xylidide.
Ib	Phenytoin (Dilantin)	100%	0%	•Narrow therapeutic range.
Ib	Tocainide (Tonocard)	40%–73%	30%–50% unchanged	•No active metabolites have been identified.
Ib	Mexiletine (Mexitil)	Extensively	8% unchanged	•Several metabolites have been identified.
Ic	Encainide hydrochloride (Enkaid)	Extensively	Large amount	•Active metabolites ODE and MODE are eliminated slowly.
Ic	Flecainide (Tambocor)	Extensively	27 % unchanged	•Active metabolites have not been identified.
Ic	Propafenone (Rythmol)	Extensively	<1.0%	•Active metabolites *N*-depropylpropafenone and 5-hydroxypropafenone. 5-hydroxypropafenone has antidysrhythmic and β-blocking activity comparable to or greater than the parent drug.
II	Propranolol (Inderal)	99%	<1.0% unchanged	•Active metabolite 4-hydroxypropranolol.
III	Bretylium (Bretylol)	None	100%	•None.
III	Amiodarone (Cordarone)	Extensively	<1% unchanged	•Pharmacologic activity of active metabolite, desethylamiodarone, has not been determined.
IV	Verapamil (Isoptin, Calan)	80%–90%	<10%	•Active metabolite nor-verapamil.

of procainamide. Agranulocytosis has occurred rarely and can be fatal; it is also seen with procainamide therapy, necessitating discontinuation of therapy. Frequent complete blood counts are required during therapy to monitor for this adverse effect.

When procainamide is administered IV, hypotension, sometimes marked, may occur due to the peripheral vasodilating effect. In addition, widening of the QRS and prolongation of the P–R interval suggests toxicity. The Q–T interval is measured periodically; and if it widens by 50% above baseline, procainamide is discontinued to prevent *Torsade de Pointe*.

Interactions. The acetylation pathway for drug metabolism is generally not influenced by induction or inhibition. Therefore, these reactions are probably not significant with procainamide. Patients with hypersensitivity to procaine will have cross-sensitivity to procainamide. The addition of other antidysrhythmics can cause an additive cardiac effect or even toxic effects. Procainamide enhances anticholinergics. Concurrent thiazides and antihypertensives may potentiate hypotensive effects. Current cimetidine reduces renal clearance of procainamide. Alcohol may increase hepatic metabolism of procainamide.

Dosage. Procainamide is given most commonly orally and IV; it is rarely adminstered intramuscularly (IM). The oral dose is 250–500 mg every three to four hours (available in 250-, 375-, and 500-mg tablets or capsules). The capsules can be opened and contents administered if necessary. The short plasma half-life requires frequent dosing. This can be avoided by using the sustained-release preparation (Procan SR), a wax matrix tablet. A dosing frequency of every six hours can be used with this preparation. The tablet of this preparation remains intact as it passes through the gastrointestinal tract, and it is excreted apparently unchanged in the feces. The active contents of the capsule, however, are absorbed; what is seen in feces is the remaining inert or inactive tablet. The appearance of this tablet in the feces is of no concern. The total daily dosage, although averaging 50 mg/kg, can vary widely from patient to patient.

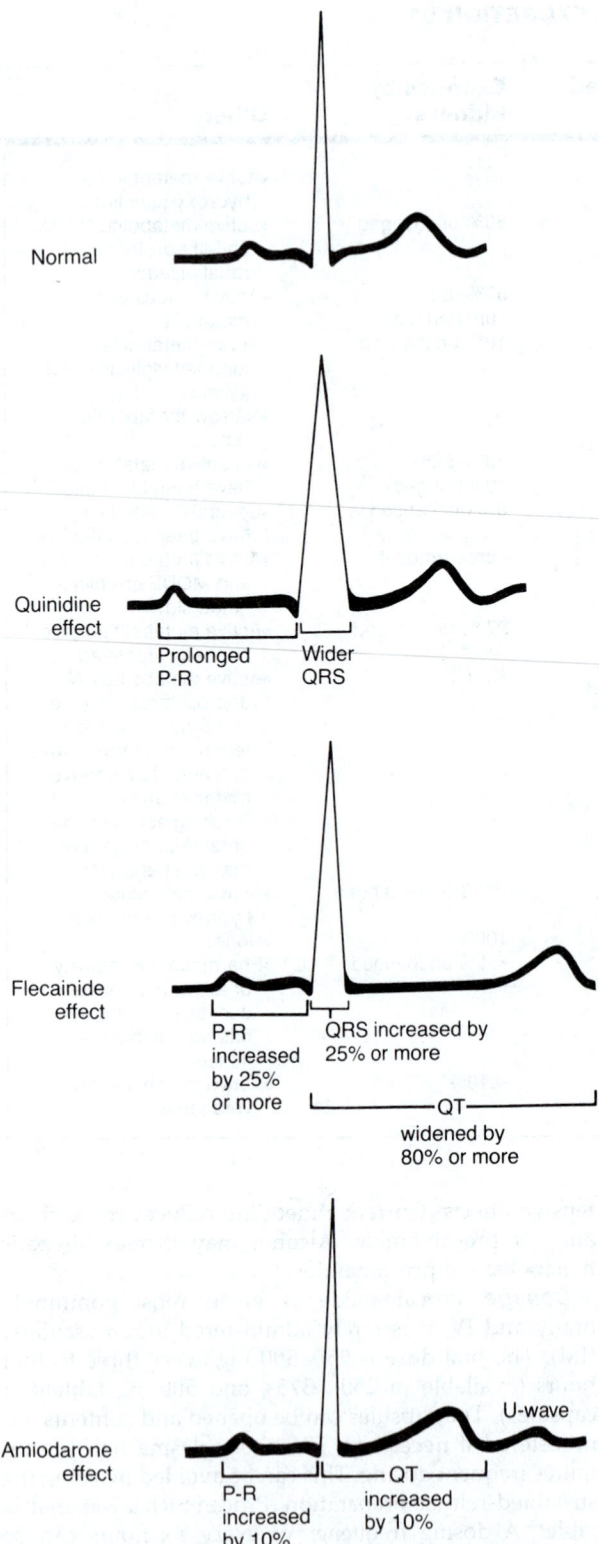

Figure 30–3. EKG effects of antidysrhythmic drugs. Quinidine widens the QRS indicating a decrease in intraventricular conduction and lengthens the P–R interval indicating a slowing of conduction through the AV node. Flecainide may increase the P–R and QRS intervals by 25% or more. The QT interval also widens by about 8%, but it is mostly due to the widened QRS. Amiodarone re-

Procainamide can be used IV, usually as a second-line drug, after lidocaine. In order to obtain therapeutic concentrations rapidly, bolus doses are administered. Since a total loading dose can cause severe hypotension, it is usually administered as a series of small injections. One safe method is to give 100 mg over five minutes, not to exceed 50 mg/min, and repeat until one of the following occurs: dysrhythmia goes away, symptomatic hypotension occurs, Q–T widens by 50% of baseline, or 1 g is administered. After a total dose of 1 g is administered, the presence of a resistant dysrhythmia is indicated.

Therapeutic Blood Levels. Therapeutic blood concentrations for procainamide would be between 4 mg and 8 μg/ml. Frequently, the active metabolite NAPA is measured as well. If this is done, a combined procainamide plus NAPA concentration of 10–30 μg/ml would be considered therapeutic.

Disopyramide Phosphate

Disopyramide phosphate (Norpace), also a group Ia drug, is similar to but chemically unrelated to procainamide and quinidine. Disopyramide affects several phases of the action potential: it prolongs the action duration and refractory period (phases 2 and 3); decreases diastolic depolarization (phase 4); and decreases the excitation velocity (phase 0). Disopyramide has an anticholinergic effect and a significant negative inotropic effect; and in contrast to quinidine and procainamide, it causes peripheral vasoconstriction.

Uses. Disopyramide is indicated for suppression and prevention of recurrence of the following cardiac dysrhythmias occurring singly or in combination: unifocal or multifocal premature ventricular contractions; paired premature ventricular contractions (couplets); and episodes of ventricular tachycardia.

Pharmacokinetics. Absorption and Distribution. Disopyramide is well-absorbed (70%–90%), with peak serum concentrations occurring 0.5–3 hours after an oral dose. As with quinidine, disopyramide is bound to plasma proteins (20%–60%) including acid glycoprotein.

Biotransformation and Excretion. Disopyramide undergoes hepatic metabolism, producing an N-dealkylated metabolite that possesses some antidysrhythmic activity. Approximately 40%–60% of an administered dose is excreted renally as unmetabolized disopyramide. The half-life of disopyramide is six to eight hours. The elimination of disopyramide is reduced in patients with hepatic or renal dysfunction or both. Patients with congestive heart failure also have a reduced elimination rate of disopyramide.

Contraindications and Precautions. Disopyramide is contraindicated in the presence of cardiogenic shock;

duces the sinus rate by 15% to 20%, and increases the P–R and QT intervals by as much as 10%. In addition, U waves may appear as well as changes in the contour of the T wave.

pre-existing second- or third-degree AV block (if no pacemaker is present); sick sinus syndrome; and Q–T prolongation, as these may worsen; and hypersensitivity.

Severe hypotension has been observed primarily in patients with primary cardiomyopathy or inadequately compensated congestive heart failure. Disopyramide should be stopped unless the hypotension is due to cardiac dysrhythmia. The drug should not be used in the presence of poorly compensated or uncompensated congestive heart failure unless the heart failure is exacerbated by or caused by a dysrhythmia, and proper treatment with cardiac glycosides and diuretics has been accomplished. Disopyramide may then suppress ectopy, and careful monitoring is necessary.

If first-degree heart block develops in a patient receiving disopyramide, the dosage is reduced. If the block persists, continuation of the drug depends on whether benefits outweigh the risk of higher degrees of block. Development of second- or third-degree AV block or *unifascicular, bifascicular,* or *trifascicular block* requires discontinuation of disopyramide unless the ventricular rate is controlled by a temporary or implanted pacemaker.

Disopyramide should not be used in patients with glaucoma, urinary retention, or myasthenia gravis because of its anticholinergic effects unless overriding measures are taken. These effects are much greater with disopyramide than with the other group Ia drugs. Urinary retention and hesitancy may occur as a consequence of disopyramide therapy; patients with benign prostatic hypertrophy are at particular risk. This drug should also be administered cautiously to patients with hypoglycemia, especially in the presence of congestive heart failure, or hepatic or renal disease.

Should significant widening of the Q–T complex occur (above 50%), disopyramide should be discontinued and dosage subsequently reduced. Patients with atrial flutter or fibrillation should be digitalized before receiving disopyramide. Disopyramide phosphate should be given with caution to patients receiving other antidysrhythmic drugs, although combination antidysrhythmic therapy may be required to control dysrhythmias.

Well-controlled studies of disopyramide have not been done in pregnant women, nor is it known whether the drug is excreted in human milk. If the drug is used in nursing mothers, an alternative method of infant feeding should be instituted. Its safe and effective use in children has not been established.

Disopyramide is given cautiously to persons with hepatic or renal dysfunction as half-life is increased. Potassium balance should be normalized before disopyramide therapy is started because disopyramide may be ineffective in hypokalemia and toxicity enhanced with hyperkalemia.

Adverse Effects. Adverse effects include anticholinergic effects such as dry mouth (32%); urinary retention (14%); urinary frequency and urgency or hesitancy (3%–4%); constipation (11%); nausea, pain, bloating, and gas (3%–9%); and blurred vision (3%–9%). Also re-

ported but less frequently are dizziness (3%–9%); general fatigue and muscle weakness (3%–9%); headache (3%–9%); edema, weight gain, cardiac conduction disturbances, shortness of breath (1%–3%); chest pain (1%–3%); hypotension (1%–3%); anorexia, diarrhea, and vomiting (1%–3%); and generalized rash (1%–3%).

Interactions. Since disopyramide is metabolized, it is highly probable that enzyme inducers such as phenobarbital, phenytoin, and rifampin increase its metabolism, thus lowering its serum concentrations. Taking other antidysrhythmics concurrently may increase the possibility of widening the QRS or Q–T interval. Verapamil may interact with disopyramide as they both have negative inotropic effects, and they should not be administered within 48 hours before or 24 hours after verapamil.

Dosage. Dosage must be individualized. Usual adult dosage is 400–800 mg/day in divided doses four times daily or as a sustained-release product 200–400 mg every 12 hours. The recommended initial loading dose is 300 mg followed by 150 mg every six hours.

For patients under 50 kg, or those with moderate renal insufficiency, hepatic insufficiency, cardiomyopathy, or possible cardiac decompensation, a loading dose of 200 mg is recommended followed by a maintenance dose of 100 mg every six hours.

Therapeutic Blood Levels. Therapeutic blood concentrations for disopyramide are between 2 μg and 8 μg/ml.

Group Ib Antidysrhythmics

Group Ib antidysrhythmic drugs include lidocaine (Xylocaine), phenytoin (Dilantin), mexiletine (Mexitil), and tocainide (Tonocard). Group Ib antidysrhythmics depress the phase 4 slope of the action potential and increase the ventricular fibrillation threshold, as shown in Figure 30–1. In Purkinje fibers, they decrease action potential duration, effective refractory period, and automaticity. They also reduce membrane responsiveness in Purkinje fibers. They have little effect on the duration of the effective refractory period in the AV node. This, however, may vary from drug to drug within this group.

Unlike group Ia, group Ib medications do not decrease conduction velocity and may, at times, actually increase the speed of propagation, which may assist in preventing re-entry dysrhythmias. Group Ib medications have no effect on speed of AV conduction, and therefore lack the potential for causing heart blocks that group Ia drugs have.

The effects of group Ib drugs on the P–R interval can vary depending on the relationship between the direct effects, which slow conduction, and the indirect vagolytic effects, which increase conduction through the AV node.

Uses. Group Ib antidysrhythmic medications are most effective when used to treat or control both acute and chronic ventricular dysrhythmias, including PVCs and ventricular tachycardia. Group Ib antidysrhythmics are generally ineffective in treating dysrhythmias of atrial origin.

LIDOCAINE. Lidocaine (Xylocaine) has been available for many years as a local and topical anesthetic agent. In the late 1960s it was approved as an antidysrhythmic drug, and today it is one of the most frequently used drugs. It is often the drug of first choice for treating ventricular dysrhythmias. Lidocaine can be administered both in and out of the hospital to control ventricular premature beats and ventricular tachycardia.

Lidocaine acts as a local anesthetic on the heart. It depresses excessive automaticity of ectopic pacemakers in the His–Purkinje system. Thus, it is very effective in suppressing the premature ventricular contractions that often arise from hypoxia or ischemic cells. Lidocaine has little or no effect on the ECG, and therefore has little potential for causing heart block, cardiac asystole, or ventricular ectopic rhythms. Unlike quinidine and procainamide, lidocaine has some effect on the effective refractory period in the AV node or purkinje fibers. This effect may prevent re-entrant types of dysrhythmias.

Pharmacokinetics. Absorption and Distribution. Lidocaine is subject to extensive first-pass hepatic metabolism, resulting in poor bioavailability when administered orally. Lidocaine is therefore always administered parenterally, either IV or IM.

Lidocaine is widely distributed in the body, readily crossing the blood–brain barrier and placenta. The fetus is therefore exposed to lidocaine if the drug is used during pregnancy or labor and delivery. Lidocaine is not highly bound to plasma proteins. The normal amount unbound in plasma is 25%–35%.

Biotransformation and Excretion. Lidocaine is extensively (90%) metabolized to several compounds, two of which, monoethylglycine and xylidide, have pharmacologic activity. The latter compound is excreted renally and can accumulate in serum of patients with renal disease. The half-life of lidocaine after a single dose is 80–108 minutes. The half-life is prolonged following continuous infusion in both healthy volunteers and patients. The average half-life in patients with ischemic heart disease after discontinuation of infusions of 24 hours' duration is four to five hours. The hepatic clearance of lidocaine is reduced in patients with congestive heart failure and hepatic disease. Urinary excretion is 10%.

Contraindications and Precautions. Lidocaine is contraindicated in patients who are sensitive to this compound or similar drugs. Lidocaine is administered with caution to persons with bradycardia and incomplete heart block. Lidocaine can cause complete block within the His–Purkinje system and is contraindicated in patients with pre-existing bundle branch block in the absence of an artificial pacemaker. Lidocaine is also contraindicated in Wolff–Parkinson–White syndrome. The elimination of lidocaine is reduced in patients with congestive heart failure and hepatic disease, and the drug is used with caution in these patients. Lidocaine is used cautiously in patients with a genetic predisposition to malignant hyperthermia, and its used in pregnancy and children has not been established.

Adverse Effects. Lidocaine distributes well into the central nervous system but serious long-term adverse effects are uncommon. Because of its anesthetic properties, it can cause significant CNS adverse effects which are usually brief and dose-related. These include mild disturbances such as paresthesias, numbness, agitation, and disorientation. Careful nursing observation is necessary to assess these symptoms. More severe adverse effects include hallucinations, decreased hearing, muscle twitching, seizures, mental confusion, and respiratory arrest. The milder adverse effects usually, but not always, precede the more serious effects and frequently disappear with a reduction in dosage. Adverse effects are also more commonly noted in patients with serum concentrations above 5.0 μg/ml. If serious adverse effects such as seizures are observed, lidocaine is discontinued. Diazepam (Valium) can be administered intravenously, but drug-induced seizures tend to be refractory to treatment. With very high serum concentrations, heart block can occur. In contrast to the group Ia drugs, lidocaine does not have anticholinergic effects and causes only negligible changes in the normal ECG. Gastrointestinal side effects may also occur, including anorexia, nausea, and vomiting.

Interactions. Drugs reducing hepatic blood flow, such as propranolol (Inderal), decrease lidocaine's elimination and increase serum concentrations. Cimetidine (Tagamet) and propranolol also reduces hepatic blood flow in addition to inhibiting lidocaine metabolism. Concurrent intravenous phenytoin may cause excessive cardiac depression. Turbocurarine or polymyxin B may enhance neuromuscular blockade by impairing transmission of impulses at the motor nerve terminal. Concurrent procainamide may produce additive neurologic effects.

Dosage. In order to achieve rapid, theapeutic serum concentrations, lidocaine therapy is initiated with a loading dose and simultaneous intravenous infusion is started to maintain therapeutic concentrations. The loading dose required, which is given at a rate of 25–50 mg/minute, is between 50 and 100 mg and depends on weight (1 mg/kg). More rapid administration increases the risk of seizures. The loading dose is reduced in congestive heart failure. Its onset of action is rapid (90 seconds); however, it is rapidly distributed from blood to tissues, resulting in a decline in plasma concentration such that subtherapeutic concentrations may be reached 15 minutes after the initial loading dose. This can cause reappearance of the dysrhythmias disturbance, which will then require treatment with a subsequent loading dose. Usually half of the initial loading dose is given at this time. No more than 200–300 mg should be given per hour.

Another method of producing and maintaining a therapeutic blood level of lidocaine is to administer an 85-mg bolus followed by an constant infusion of 2 mg/min; combined with an infusion of 175 mg mixed in a reservoir with 30 ml of fluid run with the air vent closed. (This solution has a half-life of 20 minutes.) These three approaches when used together maintain a therapeutic blood level (Fig. 30–4).

The infusion is administered using a rate-controlling pump, and the rate is titrated to 1–4 mg/min, most frequently 2 mg/min. Patients with congestive heart failure or renal or liver disease usually require lower in-

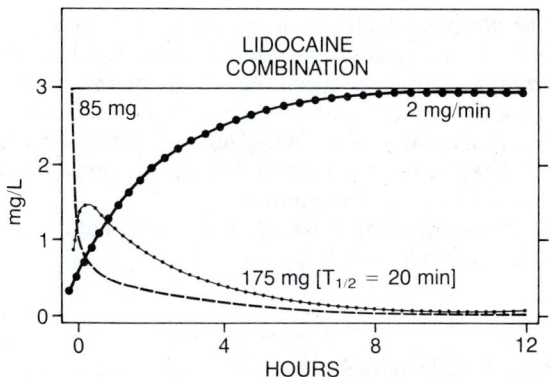

Figure 30–4. Whole-body plasma lidocaine concentrations with four dosage regimens in a healthy adult. A single injection of 85 mg and a constant infusion of 2 mg/min may be combined with an exponentially decreasing infusion of 175 mg with a half-time of 20 minutes to maintain a concentration of 3 mg/min. (Redrawn from Shoemaker, W, Thompson, W, and Holbrook, P: Textbook of Critical Care Medicine. WB Saunders, Philadelphia, 1984, p. 842, with permission.)

fusion rates, that is, 1–2 mg/min. The infusion is terminated as soon as the cardiac rhythm is stable by just turning off the IV.

Intramuscular lidocaine can be used prior to hospitalization in patients identified as having ventricular dysrhythmias at home or by paramedics. The dosage range is 100–500 mg, depending on the patient's weight. The injection is administered into the deltoid muscle.

Therapeutic Blood Levels. The usual therapeutic serum concentration range for lidocaine is 1.5–5.0 μg/ml.

PHENYTOIN. Phenytoin (Dilantin), a group Ib antidysrhythmic, depresses spontaneous depolarization in ventricular tissue. Phenytoin has a mild negative inotropic effect and a peripheral vasodilator action. Phenytoin is indicated in the management of ventricular dysrhythmias. It is effective in digitalis intoxication because it increases conduction time through the AV node, which is usually depressed in patients with digoxin intoxication. Phenytoin has few effects on the ECG. It can, however, shorten the Q–T interval. Phenytoin is discussed in more detail in Chapter 22.

Adverse Effects. Adverse effects of phenytoin include drowsiness, ataxia, blurred vision, nystagmus, and nausea. These adverse effects are usually related to serum concentrations over 20 μg/ml. If dysrhythmias do not convert with these excessive concentrations, the patient is not likely to respond to phenytoin and the drug should be discontinued. If the patient does respond and experiences these CNS adverse effects, the dosage should be reduced. This should alleviate the effects. Phenytoin has a wide range of adverse effects when administered for chronic therapy. These, as well as drug interactions, are covered in detail in Chapter 22.

Dosage. Phenytoin is generally administered intravenously in doses of 50–100 mg not to exceed 50 mg/min. It is given every five minutes until the dysrhythmia

is suppressed, up to a total of 1000 mg (12–15 mg/kg) or until toxicity develops. Care must be taken in mixing and administering phenytoin, as it forms a precipitate very easily. It is mixed only with normal saline solutions. If mixed in dextrose solution, it precipitates into white granular crystals.

Therapeutic Blood Levels. The usual accepted therapeutic blood concentration range for phenytoin is 10–20 μg/ml.

MEXILETINE HYDROCHLORIDE. Mexiletine hydrochloride (Mexitil) is structurally similar to lidocaine and is available only in oral form. Mexiletine depresses phase 0 and decreases the effective refractory period of the Purkinje fibers. Therefore, it depresses automaticity in ventricles but has little effect on atrial tissue and does not depress sinus node function.

Use. Mexiletine is used for the treatment of existing or anticipated ventricular tachydysrhythmias that are associated with myocardial infarction, ischemic heart disease, digitalis toxicity, and prosthetic heart valves. It is also used for idiopathic dysrhythmias.

Pharmacokinetics. Absorption and Distribution. Mexiletine is well-absorbed (90%) and is 88% bioavailable. However, when gastric emptying is increased or narcotics and antacids are given concurrently, absorption is decreased. Peak blood levels are reached in two to three hours. First-pass metabolism is low and mexiletine is 50%–70% plasma-bound.

Biotransformation and Excretion. Mexiletine is extensively metabolized in the liver and has a half-life of 8–12 hours in normal patients and may be as long as 18 hours in patients with acute myocardial infarction. About 10%–15% is excreted unchanged in the urine, so renal function has little effect on drug clearance. Urinary acidification accelerates excretion, whereas alkalinization retards its excretion.

Contraindications and Precautions. Mexiletine is contraindicated in patients with cardiogenic shock, bradycardia, and hypotension, and in patients with known hypersensitivity to local anesthetics of the amide type (mexiletine is chemically related to the amide anesthetics).

The drug should be used with caution in patients with hepatic disease, since this is where it is biotransformed. Safety in pregnancy and children has not been determined.

Adverse Effects. The most common adverse effects of mexiletine include gastrointestinal symptoms (41%) such as nausea, vomiting, indigestion, and unpleasant taste in the mouth; central nervous system symptoms such as confusion (2%), dizziness (18%–26%), lightheadedness (10.5%), tremor (12.6%), twitching (13%), and diplopia (5%–7%); and cardiovascular symptoms including hypotension, sinus bradycardia (0.4%), and palpitations (4%–7%). The hypotension that occurs may be reversed by atropine. Other adverse effects include rash (3%–4%), dyspnea (3%–5%), nonspecific edema (4%), and abnormal liver function tests may occur. Adverse effects can occur at doses required to treat dysrhythmias and may therefore limit the usefulness of this compound. If the dosage can be reduced, adverse effects disappear, since they are dose-related.

Interactions. Morphine, when given concurrently with mexiletine, decreases the rate of oral absorption, which may result in subtherapeutic levels being achieved at normal doses. Phenytoin, rifampin, and phenobarbital and other enzyme inducers taken concurrently may lower serum levels. Cimetidine can increase mexiletine plasma levels. Marked changes in pH effects excretion so urinary pH should be 5–8.

Dosage. The loading dose of mexiletine ranges between 200 and 400 mg, with a maintenance dose of 200–400 mg administered every eight hours. For intravenous dosage, see Table 30–4.

Therapeutic Blood Level. Therapeutic blood levels should be 0.5–2.0 µg.

TOCAINIDE. Tocainide (Tonocard) is a group Ib antidysrhythmic with electrophysiologic properties similar to lidocaine. Tocainide produces dose-dependent reductions in sodium and potassium conductance, thus decreasing excitability of cells.

Uses. Tocainide is primarily used to prevent or treat ventricular ectopy and tachycardia. Tocainide may be beneficial to patients refractory to group Ia drugs. Responsiveness to lidocaine is a fairly accurate method of selecting patients for therapy since many physicians consider tocainide the oral equivalent of lidocaine.

Pharmacokinetics. Absorption and Distribution. Tocainide is rapidly and completely absorbed (90%–100%), with peak serum levels being achieved in 0.5–3 hours. Food delays absorption, but the extent is unaffected. There is a very small first-pass liver effect, and the drug is approximately 10%–20% protein-bound.

Biotransformation and Excretion. Tocainide is eliminated by both hepatic and renal (28%–55% unchanged) mechanisms. Elevating urinary pH above 7.4 reduces urinary excretion. Elimination half-life is 11–15 hours, but is increased in severe renal failure.

Contraindications and Precautions. Tocainide is contraindicated in hypersensitivity to amide-type local anesthetics and, because of its potent negative inotropic effect, in patients with second- or third-degree heart block without a pacemaker because of its depressant effect. Tocainide also frequently causes a pro-arrhythmia effect. Tocainide is used cautiously in persons with heart failure and minimal cardiac reserves because of its potential for aggravating heart failure. Tocainide is also contraindicated in cytopenia because a fatal hematologic effect may occur.

Adverse Effects. Adverse effects usually related to the central nervous system or gastrointestinal system may require the discontinuation of tocainide in 20% of patients. The most common adverse effects are nausea, dizziness, tremor, paresthesia, and rash. Tocainide may aggravate congestive heart failure, conduction disturbances, and ventricular dysrhythmias. Leukopenia, bone marrow depression, agranulocytosis, and thrombocytopenia may all occur. If any of these disorders are identified, tocainide is discontinued and appropriate therapy instituted. CBCs are drawn periodically and patients need to report any signs of infection. Pulmonary effects such as edema, embolism, and arrest have also been reported.

Interactions. Additive or antagonistic effects occur with other antidysrhythmics and β-adrenergic blockers.

Dosage. Dosage of tocainide is individualized with a range between 1200 and 1800 mg/day in three divided doses. When patients are stabilized with administration three times a day, a twice-a-day dosing may be attempted with careful monitoring.

Therapeutic Blood Level. The therapeutic blood level of tocainide is 4–10 µg/ml.

GROUP IC DRUGS

FLECAINIDE ACETATE. Flecainide acetate (Tambocor) has local anesthetic properties like the group I antidysrhythmics and has electrophysiologic properties of the group Ic drugs. Flecainide depresses sinus node automaticity and prolongs conduction in the atria, AV node, ventricle, accessory pathways, and His–Purkinje system. Flecainide may either increase or decrease ejection fraction with usual therapeutic doses.

Uses. Flecainide is generally reserved for treatment of serious dysrhythmias that have not responded to older, better-established drugs. Flecainide may also prove useful for treating long-term prophylaxis of re-entrant tachycardias involving the AV node or accessory pathways (Fig. 30–5).

Pharmacokinetics. Absorption and Distribution. Flecainide is well-absorbed orally (90% bioavailability) with peak levels being attained in three hours (one to six hour range). Foods or antacids do not affect absorption and there is not a significant first-pass effect. Steady-state levels are reached in three to five days. Flecainide is 40% bound to plasma proteins.

Biotransformation and Excretion. Flecainide is 50% metabolized in the liver and 30% is excreted unchanged in the urine. The plasma half-life averages 20 hours (12–27 hour range) and is increased in patients with congestive heart failure.

Contraindications and Precautions. Contraindications are similar to other group I drugs: hypersensitivity, cardiogenic shock, and heart blocks without the presence of a pacemaker.

Flecainide may worsen ventricular dysrhythmia that may be life-threatening, so patients need to be monitored closely. These pro-arrhythmic effects have been reported in about 7%–10% of patients treated with flecainide and frequently necessitate stopping the drug. Patients with underlying cardiac disease and those who seem to need increasing doses to control their dysrhythmias are prone to pro-arrhythmic changes. Due to its negative inotropic effect, flecainide is given cautiously in patients with congestive heart failure. Flecainide is used with extreme caution in persons with sick sinus syndrome because of the possible slowing of the P–R interval. Hypokalemia and hyperkalemia may alter the effects of flecainide, so potassium needs to be normalized. Flecainide is given cautiously to persons with liver impairment since flecainide is extensively biotransformed in the liver. Flecainide is given cautiously in renal patients, since elimination may be impaired.

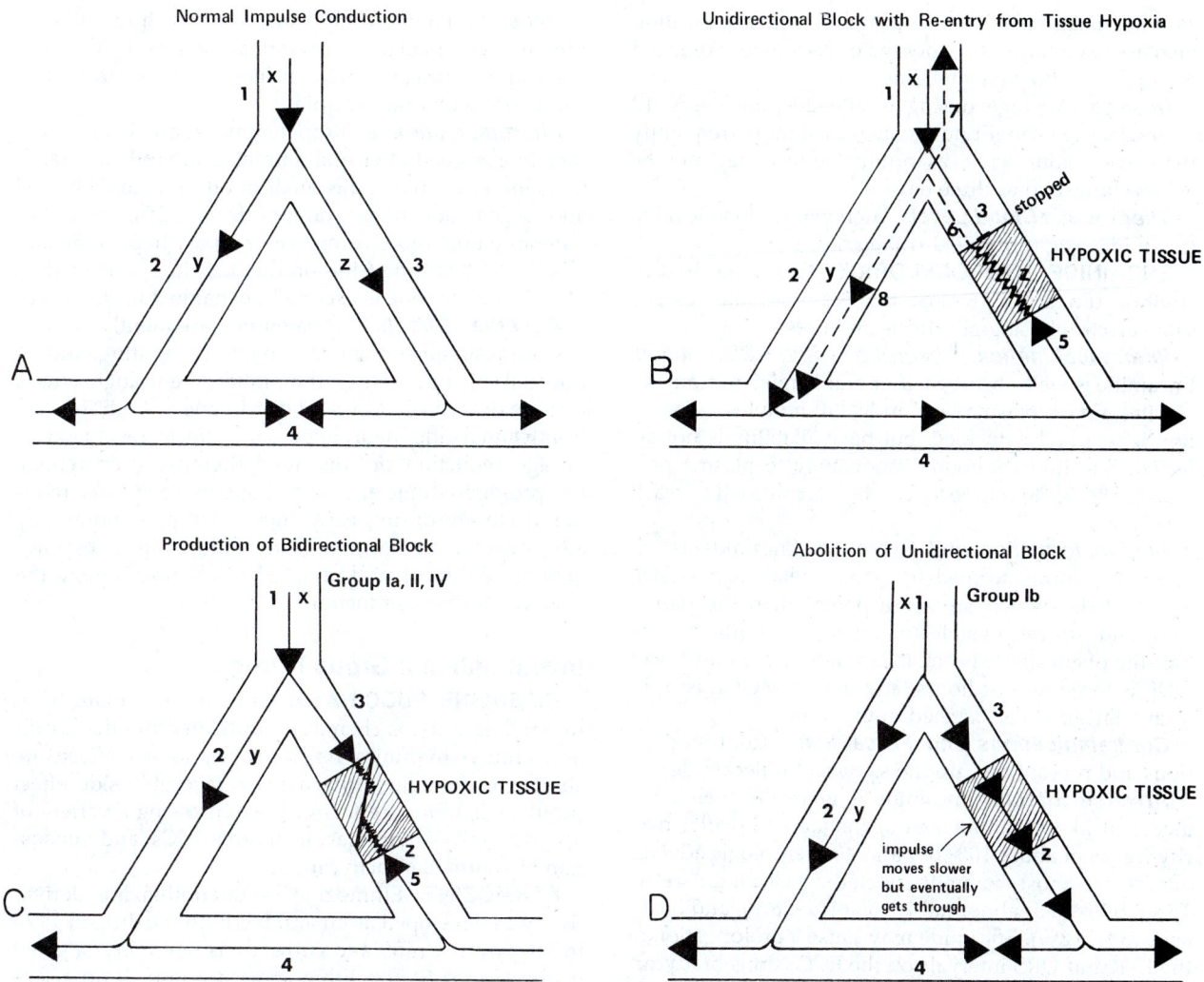

Figure 30–5. The effect of antidysrhythmic drugs on re-entry. A) represents normal conduction through the Purkinje fiber. Impulse 1, starting in x fiber, spreads through branches y and z, and with impulses 2 and 3, activates the ventricular tissue in 4. In B) an area of tissue ischemia is present in branch z. Again impulse 1 begins in fiber x; as it traverses down fiber z it is blocked. Meanwhile, impulse 2 moves quickly down fiber y and activates the ventricular muscle in area 4. Since no opposing impulse arrived in the ventricular muscles, the impulse travels through z and re-enters fibers x and y, thereby causing another beat to occur. The beat which occurs may cause a re-entry supraventricular tachycardia or may be a premature ventricular contraction. In C group Ia, II, and IV drugs increase the refractory time in the "sick" tissue so it is unable to accept either impulse 3 originally, or impulse 5 for re-entry. This produces a bidirectional block. In D) group Ib drugs enhance conduction in the "sick" tissue of fiber z, thereby allowing impulse 3 to traverse the "sick" tissue the first time, which abolishes the unidirectional block.

Safety in pregnancy, lactation, and children is unknown.

Adverse Effects. Because of the adverse effects, most physicians prefer to start flecainide in the hospital. Flecainide can aggravate existing dysrhythmias or precipitate new ones (7%–10%). Flecainide crosses the blood–brain barrier and may cause neurologic symptoms such as dizziness (19%), visual disturbances (16%), headache (9%), fatigue (8%), and tremor (5%). Additional cardiovascular adverse effects include palpitations (6%), chest pain (5%), edema (3.5%), and AV blocks and bradycardias (1%–2%). Altered taste sensation (1%) and other mild gastrointestinal symptoms

have been reported. Flecainide also has numerous effects on the ECG. The P-R, QRS, and Q-T intervals can all be prolonged from 8% to a maximum of 150% (see Fig. 30–3). If second- or third-degree AV block or right bundle branch block associated with left hemiblock occurs, flecainide is discontinued unless a ventricular pacing wire is in place.

Interactions. Flecainide may increase plasma digoxin levels (15%–25%). Concurrent propranolol increases both flecainide and propranolol serum levels. Both disopyramide and verapamil have negative inotropic effects, and administration with flecainide is not recommended at this time. Urinary pH should be 5–7, as alkalinization decreases excretion and acidification increases excretion. Also, dosage of flecainide is reduced with patients taking cimetidine.

Dosage. Average dosing is 100–200 mg every 12 hours. Dosage should not be increased more frequently than every four days, as optimal effect may not be achieved for two to three days.

Therapeutic Blood Level. Therapeutic blood level of flecainide ranges from 0.2–1.0 $\mu g/ml$.

ENCAINIDE HYDROCHLORIDE. Encainide hydrochloride (Enkaid) is related to flecainide and has the same electrophysiologic effects and uses.

Pharmacokinetics. Absorption and Distribution. Encainide is well-absorbed after oral administration and reaches a peak plasma level in 30–90 minutes. Absorption is retarded with food, but bioavailability is not affected. Encainide is bound moderately to plasma proteins (75%–85%). Three to five days are needed to reach steady state.

Biotransformation and Excretion. Encainide is extensively biotransformed to active metabolites—ODE and MODE—which are more potent than the parent drug and are responsible for much of its effects. The half-life of encainide is one to two hours, the half-life of ODE is three to four hours, and that of MODE is 6–12 hours. Encainide is excreted in the urine.

Contraindications and Precautions. Contraindications and precautions are the same as for flecainide.

Adverse Effects. Encainide is generally well-tolerated, but like flecainide can aggravate ventricular dysrhythmias in about 10% of patients. Neurologic adverse effects are most common, including dizziness (6%–18%), blurred or abnormal vision (4%–26%), and headache (3%–12%). Encainide may cause a prolongation of the P–R and QRS intervals on the ECG, sinus bradycardia, sinus pause or arrest, second- and third-degree AV block. If these dysrhythmias occur, encainide should be discontinued.

Interactions. There are no known problems with concurrent use of diuretics or cardiovascular drugs. There is no digoxin/encainide interaction. Cimetidine increases plasma concentration of encainide.

Dosage. Dosage ranges from 50–75 mg three times per day. A loading dose is not recommended. A gradual increase of dosage is recommended. Dosage begins at 25 mg. After three to five days the dose is increased to 35 mg and if a larger dose is still needed, 50 mg can be administered three to five days later.

PROPAFENONE. Propafenone (Rythmol) is also a group Ic antidysrhythmic drug that possesses weak β-blocking properties (1/40 of propranolol) and slight calcium antagonist properties (1/100 of verapamil). Propafenone depresses sinus node, intraventricular, AV nodal, and His–Purkinje functions. Propafenone also increases the refractory period and decreases conduction velocity. There is no significant effect on the Q–T interval, but there is a dose-dependent prolongation of the P–R interval and QRS duration. Propafenone increases pulmonary capillary obstructive pressure and systemic and pulmonary vascular resistance. Propafenone may also slow the heart rate and mildly depresses cardiac output.

Uses. Propafenone appears to be helpful in suppressing ventricular dysrhythmia such as PVCs, couplets, and ventricular tachycardia, as well as paroxysmal supraventricular tachycardia.

Pharmacokinetics. Propafenone is rapidly and completely absorbed after oral administration. Bioavailability is increased when this medication is given with food and is dose-dependent, ranging from 2.2%–50%. Propafenone undergoes extensive first-pass hepatic metabolism and has a half-life of 1.8–32.3 hours. Less than 1% of propafenone is excreted unchanged in the urine.

Adverse Effects. Propafenone frequently causes gastrointestinal complaints of nausea, vomiting, and an unusual metallic taste in the mouth. Neurologic effects include dizziness and visual disturbances. Both the gastrointestinal and neurologic side effects resolve with dosage reduction or continued therapy. Propafenone has pro-arrhythmic effects, so patients need to be monitored closely during early therapy. Propafenone may also develop congestive heart failure and, less frequently, AV block and bundle branch block due to the delayed cardiac conduction.

Investigational Group I Drugs

CIFENLINE SUCCINATE. Cifenline succinate (Cipralan), a Ia drug, is chemically unrelated to other available antidysrhythmics. Its electrophysiologic effects are similar to quinidine with a more favorable side effect profile. Cifenline is effective in suppressing a variety of ventricular dysrhythmias, including PVCs, and nonsustained ventricular tachycardia.

ETHMOZINE. Ethmozine, a phenothiazine derivative, was developed as an antidysrhythmic drug in 1970 in the Soviet Union and currently is being investigated in the United States. Ethmozine, a group Ib drug, appears to be quite effective in suppressing ventricular premature beats in single forms, couplets, and pairs, and ventricular tachycardia. At this time, it appears to have fewer adverse effects than do other antidysrhythmics.

LORCAINIDE. Lorcainide is a local anesthetic antidysrhythmic similar to encainide and flecainide but with minimal adverse effects. Lorcainide is used to suppress ventricular ectopic beats, ventricular tachycardia, and ventricular fibrillation when dysrhythmias are resistant to other drugs.

GROUP II ANTIDYSRHYTHMICS

Type II antidysrhythmics are drugs that exert β-blockade. Most of the antidysrhythmic effects are adequately explained by this activity. These effects include a blocking of sympathetic stimulation at the sinus node, which decreases resting heart rate only slightly, but reduces exercise-induced tachycardia substantially. Beta-blockade also reduces automaticity in Purkinje fibers. An important effect responsible for their major uses as antidysrhythmic agents is an increase in the effective refractory period of the AV node. Many β blockers are available in the United States; these include propranolol (Inderal), metoprolol (Lopressor), pindolol (Visken), atenolol (Tenormin), nadolol (Corgard), timolol (Blocadrin), and esmolol hydrochloride (Brevibloc). These drugs are discussed in detail in Chapter 19 and on Table 19–8.

Uses

Beta-blockers are used effectively to slow ventricular rate in patients with supraventricular tachydysrhythmias such as atrial fibrillation, atrial flutter, or paroxysmal supraventricular tachycardia. Digitalis and propranolol can be an effective combination when either drug fails to control ventricular rate alone. This is a result of digitalis exerting a vagal effect on the AV node while propranolol decreases sympathetic activity. B-blockers can also be used to treat and prevent recurrent tachydysrhythmias resulting from activating accessory bundles, as occurs in Wolff–Parkinson–White (WPW) syndrome.

In ventricular dysrhythmias caused by exercise or excessive catecholamines, β blockers can be used. It is also effective in treating ventricular dysrhythmias in patients with ischemic heart disease. Frequently, high doses are required to control ventricular dysrhythmias.

GROUP III ANTIDYSRHYTHMICS

The group III antidysrhythmics—bretylium tosylate and amiodarone—are relatively new antidysrhythmics whose pharmacokinetic and electrophysiologic properties are quite different.

Bretylium Tosylate

Bretylium tosylate (Bretylol), originally developed as an antihypertensive, has at least two mechanisms by which it exerts an antidysrhythmic effect. First, by a direct effect, bretylium increases action potential duration and refractory period in Purkinje fibers. It increases the threshold for developing ventricular fibrillation and in animals rapidly converts ventricular fibrillation to normal sinus rhythm through adrenergic blockade. A second effect is an antiadrenergic action as a result of its preventing the release of norepinephrine from sympathetic nerve terminals. As it is initially taken up by these terminals, however, norepinephrine is released. This can cause an initial increase in blood pressure, increased dysrhythmia, and vomiting over the first 30 minutes of therapy. These effects can be avoided by infusing the dose over eight to ten minutes if the clinical situation permits this slow infusion. Hemodynamics remain within normal ranges.

USES. Bretylium is used for the prophylaxis and treatment of life-threatening ventricular dysrhythmias unresponsive to lidocaine and procainamide.

Pharmacokinetics. Bretylium is poorly absorbed from the gastrointestinal tract and is therefore available only for use as a parenteral agent. It is absorbed from the IM injection site with an onset of action of 15 minutes; its effect peaks in two to three hours and lasts for up to ten hours. Antifibrillation effects occur within minutes of an IV injection. Protein binding is negligible.

The half-life of bretylium is 8–12 hours. In 24 hours after a single dose, up to 70%–80% of an administered dose is excreted renally as the unchanged drug. The

dosage of bretylium is therefore reduced in patients with renal failure.

Contraindications and Precautions. At this time, there are no contraindications to the administration of bretylium. Caution is used in patients with renal failure because of delayed renal excretion of bretylium. Caution is advised in administering bretylium to patients with fixed cardiac output such as aortic stenosis, pulmonary hypertension, and postural hypotension, since severe hypotension may result from a fall in peripheral resistance without a compensatory increase in cardiac output. Safety in pregnancy and in children has not been established.

Adverse Effects. Hypotension, caused by the inhibition of norepinephrine release at nerve terminals, occurs in a high percentage of patients receiving bretylium. Hypotension can be severe enough to warrant discontinuation of bretylium. In some cases, blood pressure may need to be maintained with an infusion of dopamine (Intropin). Rapid intravenous administration can cause nausea and vomiting (3%) and neurologic symptoms such as vertigo and lightheadedness (1%), as well as transient hypertension and pro-arrhythmic effects from the initial release of norepinephrine.

Interactions. Bretylium is used with caution in patients on digitalis since bretylium may aggravate digitalis-induced dysrhythmias. The hypotensive effect may be exacerbated with concurrent use of quinidine or procainamide.

Dosage. In life-threatening dysrhythmias, bretylium (5–10 mg/kg) is administered undiluted by rapid IV injection. This dose can be repeated at intervals of 15–30 minutes up to a maximum dose of 30 mg/kg. Maintenance therapy can be administered as intermittent IV bolus doses at 6-hour intervals. A continuous infusion of bretylium can also be initiated at a rate of 1–2 mg/minute. While on bretylium, patients should be kept in a supine position and observed frequently for hypotension.

Therapeutic Blood Level. Plasma levels are not useful as a guide to therapy.

Amiodarone

Amiodarone (Cordarone), an iodinated benzofuran derivative, is a unique antidysrhythmic drug that exerts a noncompetitive blockade on both α- and β-adrenergic receptors and also antagonizes the chronotropic and inotropic effects of glucagon. Amiodarone is a potent smooth muscle relaxant and produces marked coronary and peripheral vasodilation. Amiodarone increases cardiac refractory period, thus reducing automaticity. The sinus rate is reduced by 15%–20%; the P–R and Q–T intervals are increased by 10%. U waves and a change in T-wave contour may also occur (see Fig. 30–3). These changes do not require discontinuation of amiodarone. These changes may be associated with aggravation of dysrhythmias, so close monitoring of the patient is important. Amiodarone is a potent pro-arrhythmic drug and is highly toxic, so maximal efforts should be made to use alternate antidysrhythmic agents before initiating amiodarone.

Uses. Amiodarone is an effective drug in controlling

both supraventricular and ventricular dysrhythmias in patients who are resistant to most other antidysrhythmic medications. Most patients will have extensive diagnostic workups before being placed on amiodarone. Amiodarone can suppress life-threatening ventricular dysrhythmias refractory to other drugs, but its severe toxicity makes it a drug of last resort.

Pharmacokinetics. Following oral administration, amiodarone is slowly and variably absorbed with bioavailability about 50% (35%–65%). Maximal plasma concentration occurs in three to seven hours, but onset of action is approximately two to three days, and may take up to one to three weeks. Amiodarone is widely distributed and stored extensively in fat stores and highly perfused organs such as the liver, lung, and spleen. Amiodarone is highly plasma protein-bound (96%). A steady state is not achieved until 130–535 days.

Amiodarone is mainly excreted in the liver through bile. There is negligible renal excretion. After discontinuation, amiodarone has a biphasic elimination with initial half-life of 2.5–10 days. The terminal half-life is much slower, 26–107 days. Antidysrhythmic effects continue for weeks after the drug is discontinued.

Contraindications and Precautions. Amiodarone is contraindicated in patients with bradycardia and severe sinus node dysfunction. Amiodarone is administered cautiously to patients with pulmonary disease, since pulmonary toxicity (interstitial pneumonitis/alveolitis) can occur. Frequent chest radiographs and pulmonary function studies are performed.

Amiodarone is a potent pro-arrhythmic drug and can aggravate serious dysrhythmias and lead to bradycardia or sinus arrest. Amiodarone is also given cautiously to patients with liver disease because it may cause altered liver enzymes. Frequent SGOT and SGPT are obtained during therapy. Persistent elevations may necessitate reducing the dose. Use in pregnancy and children has not been established.

Adverse Effects. Amiodarone has significant adverse effects and can be highly toxic, even fatal. The most common adverse effects include corneal microdeposits, which occur in virtually all adults treated for more than six months. These deposits, however, rarely interfere with vision, and are usually dose-related. Mild gastrointestinal effects have been noticed; including nausea and vomiting (10%–33%). Amiodarone contains iodine (37% by weight) and both hypothyroidism and hyperthyroidism have been reported; therefore, thyroid studies should be done at onset of therapy and frequently during therapy. Amiodarone has also been associated with bluish-gray skin discoloration in almost *all* patients. The effect may be due to cutaneous deposits of the drug. Photosensitivity also occurs at a relatively high frequency (10%). A more serious complication is pulmonary infiltrate and fibrosis (4%–9%). This is an irreversible and often fatal adverse effect. Abnormal liver function tests (4%–9%) and nonspecific hepatic disorders including hepatitis also occur.

Interactions. Amiodarone has several significant drug interactions. It inhibits the renal excretion of digoxin, thereby increasing serum digoxin concentrations.

It also increases concentrations of quinidine and procainamide. Amiodarone potentiates the anticoagulant effect of warfarin. These effects may be caused by an inhibition of renal and hepatic clearance processes by amiodarone and its major metabolite desethylamiodarone. *Torsades de Pointes* has been reported when quinidine, mexiletine, or disopyramide has been administered in combination with amiodarone. The combination of amiodarone with β blockers or calcium antagonists can potentiate effects on the sinus or AV node, producing sinus bradycardia, sinus arrest, or AV block disturbances. During surgery, amiodarone can induce hypotension and atropine-resistant sinus bradycardia. These effects may be additive with those of the anesthetic agents used.

Dosage. Amiodarone is administered orally. The initial oral dosage is 800–1600 mg/day for several days or weeks, and is later tapered to 600–800 mg/day. Maintenance dose is usually 400 mg. Oral absorption is variable and usually very slow. In general, amiodarone needs to be administered for several days to several weeks for its full antidysrhythmic effect to be noticed. If used to treat supraventricular tachycardia, a loading dose may not be necessary.

GROUP IV ANTIDYSRHYTHMICS

Verapamil (Isoptin, Calan), and beproidil (to be released soon) are class IV antidysrhythmias, which are calcium-channel blocking agents that inhibit the transmembrane flow of calcium ions. Verapamil is the calcium-channel blocker currently used as an antidysrhythmic. These drugs are also used to treat angina and hypertension and are discussed as a group in detail in Chapter 30.

Verapamil

Verapamil (Isoptin, Calan), a synthetic derivative of papaverine, blocks the slow calcium channel and has a slight nonspecific sympathic depressant effect.

Action. Calcium plays a major role in both mechanical and electrical capabilities in the heart. Mechanically, it affects the vascular smooth muscle tone of the coronary arteries and peripheral arteries as well as the contractility of the heart muscle itself. Electrically, calcium is needed for conduction through the SA and AV nodes and "slow cells" in the conduction system. It is through the effect of slowing conduction and increasing the effective refractory period through the AV node that the calcium antagonist exerts its major antidysrhythmic effect, thus reducing the ventricular rate because of atrial flutter and atrial fibrillation. Verapamil also interferes with re-entry of impulses at the AV node, and is therefore helpful restoring normal sinus rhythms in patients with paroxysmal supraventricular tachycardia and Wolff–Parkinson–White syndrome. About 60%–80% of patients with supraventricular tachycardia convert to normal sinus rhythm within ten minutes after intravenous verapamil.

Uses. Verapamil is effective in treating supraventricular tachycardias including atrial fibrillation, atrial flutter, paroxysmal supraventricular tachycardia, and postoperative supraventricular tachycardia, including those associated with accessory bypass tracts such as Wolff–Parkinson–White and Lown–Ganong–Levine syndromes. Verapamil is often used as a first-line drug for atrial fibrillation rather than digoxin and quinidine.

Verapamil is highly effective when given intravenously in terminating an attack of AV nodal resistant tachycardia and may prevent this dysrhythmia in oral doses. Verapamil is not effective in treating ventricular dysrhythmias.

Dosage. Verapamil administered intravenously has a rapid onset of action, with peak effects occurring in three to five minutes. The duration of action corresponds well with its serum half-life. The usual intravenous bolus dose is 0.1–0.15 mg/kg (5–10 mg) administered over two to three minutes. This dose can be repeated every 30 minutes as often as necessary to regulate the heart rate. A maintenance infusion is not necessary. In addition to monitoring blood pressure, the P–R interval should be closely monitored. Oral doses range from 40–160 mg administered every six to eight hours. Onset of action and peak effects occur 30 minutes and four to five hours, respectively, after an oral verapamil dose.

CARDIAC GLYCOSIDES

The cardiac glycosides are currently used to treat or control dysrhythmias either alone or in conjunction with other antidysrhythmics. They are used to slow the ventricular rate in atrial flutter and fibrillation, and in atrial tachycardias. Digitalis acts by means of vagal stimulation on the AV node to slow conduction; therefore, fewer impulses get through to the ventricles. This effect can be obviated through sympathetic stimulation such as exercise, thus limiting the usefulness of the cardiac glycosides in therapy of chronic atrial fibrillation. The cardiac glycosides are discussed in detail in Chapter 28.

ANTIDYSRHYTHMIC DRUGS FOR BRADYARRHYTHMIAS

Atropine sulfate, a potent vagolytic, can be used acutely in IV doses of 0.4–1 mg every one to two hours as needed to treat or control bradydysrhythmias. Likewise, isoproterenol (Isuprel), a β-adrenergic agonist, can also be used for such dysrhythmias in doses of 1–2 mg of 1:5000 solution diluted in 500 ml of 5% D/W infused slowly with continual monitoring of the electrocardiogram. Dysrhythmias that are slow can result from sinus bradycardia, SA block, or AV block. Atropine and isoproterenol are used as temporary measures prior to pacing for patients with complete AV block. Atropine increases sinus rate and AV node conduction velocity and decreases the effective refractory period of the AV node by decreasing vagal tone. Isoproterenol increases myocardial oxygen demand and can aggravate ischemia and cause ventricular dysrhythmias. Isoproterenol increases the rate of the idioventricular pacemakers and therefore should not be used unless absolutely necessary in patients with acute myocardial infarctions.

USING THE NURSING PROCESS

ASSESSMENT

Assessment of the patient requiring medications for the control or treatment of dysrhythmias begins with a thorough nursing history to develop the data base needed to prepare the nursing care plans. Information the nurse obtains is included in Table 30–7.

When the patient requiring antidysrhythmic medications is acutely ill, perhaps in a critical care unit under close observation, it is necessary to perform thorough physical and psychologic nursing assessments frequently in order to evaluate possible critical changes. The nurse particularly assesses cardiac rhythm, including rate, the regularity of beats, and the quality and character of all pulses; the presence of chest pain; electrocardiogram changes such as P–R, Q–T, and QRS intervals or dysrhythmias; neurologic symptoms; urinary output; skin color, temperature, and signs of edema; abnormal respiration, including crackles; and an increased level of anxiety. The nurse then can quickly diagnose the problem and institute corrective measures before the presenting symptoms cause further deterioration in the patient's condition.

The patient and family's past history of coronary artery disease is obtained. Also, associated risk factors such as hypertension, cigarette smoking, obesity, lifestyle, diabetes, stress level, personality type, and cholesterol are examined. These factors may need to be modified during the intervention phase of the nursing process.

The nurse may be responsible for conducting frequent laboratory tests to determine acid–base balance, electrolyte levels, and blood drug levels. Blood for routine serum drug levels in drawn approximately one hour after the drug is given for a peak level and immediately before the next dose for a trough level. Any abnormalities must be corrected, as most antidysrhythmics are less effective in the presence of acid–base or electrolyte disturbances—particularly potassium.

NURSING DIAGNOSES

As the initial assessment is completed, the nurse develops the nursing diagnoses. These diagnoses become the basis for the nursing goals and later the nursing evaluation criteria. Typical nursing diagnoses for a patient requiring antidysrhythmic medications are included in Table 30–7.

PLANNING AND INTERVENTION

From the nursing diagnoses, the nurse develops the nursing/patient goals. The goals of nursing intervention for a patient requiring antidysrhythmics in the acute situation are included in Table 30–7. These goals will change as the patient progresses toward discharge from the acute care unit.

Table 30–7. NURSING PROCESS FOR PATIENT REQUIRING ANTIDYSRHYTHMICS

Assessment

Assess vital signs. Document presence of pulsus alternans, bigeminal pulse, or pulse deficit.
Determine type of dysrhythmia present, note cardiac rhythm, regularity of beats, presence of extra heart beats, dropped beats; presence of chest pain; ECG changes.
Palpate pulses noting rate, regularity, amplitude (full/thready), and symmetry.
Ascertain lifestyle, e.g., exercise, daily activities and level of stress. Note presence of risk factors, e.g., smoking, obesity, diabetes, personality type and cholesterol.
Determine sleep pattern, noting presence of long-standing problems.
Monitor laboratory findings, e.g., acid-base balance, electrolyte and serum drug levels.

Nursing Diagnosis	Nursing Actions	Rationale	Desired Outcomes/ Evaluation Criteria
Cardiac output, decreased potential related to altered electrical conduction.	Provide calm/quiet environment. Review reasons for limitations of activities during acute phase.	Reduces stimulation and release of stress-related catecholamines, which cause/aggravate dysrhythmias and vasoconstriction and increase myocardial workload.	Maintains/achieves adequate cardiac output as evidenced by absence of signs/symptoms of decompensation. Observed decrease frequency of dysrhythmia(s). Participates in activities that reduce myocardial workload.
	Demonstrate/encourage use of stress management behaviors, e.g., relaxation techniques, guided imagery, slow/ deep breathing.	Promotes patient participation, exerting some sense of control in a potentially very stressful situation.	
	Investigate complaints of chest pain documenting location, duration, intensity, relieving/aggravating factors.	Reasons for chest pain are variable, dependent on underlying cause of dysrhythmias but may indicate ischemia due to decreased myocardial perfusion or increased oxygen demand.	
	Administer antidysrhythmias according to type, e.g., atrial, ventricular, SA/AV node dysfunction.	Treatment is dependent on the kind of dysrhythmia present.	
	Administer supplemental oxygen as indicated.	Increase amount of oxygen available for myocardial uptake, which decreases irritability caused by hypoxia.	
	Be prepared for/initiate cardiopulmonary resuscitation as indicated.	Development of life-threatening dysrhythmias requires prompt intervention to prevent ischemic damage/death.	
Knowledge deficit related to lack of information/ understanding of medical condition/therapy needs as evidenced by questions, statement of concern, failure to improve and/or development of preventable complications.	Review normal cardiac function/electrical conduction.	Provides a knowledge base to understand individual variations and reasons for therapeutic interventions.	Verbalizes understanding of disease and treatment regimen, desired action and possible adverse side effects.
	Explain/reinforce specific dysrhythmia problem and therapeutic measures to patient/SO.	Ongoing/updated information can decrease anxiety associated with the unknown and prepare patient to make necessary lifestyle adaptations.	
	Identify adverse effects/ complications of specific dysrhythmias, e.g., fatigue, dependent edema, progressing changes in mentation, vertigo.	Dysrhythmias may decrease cardiac output as manifested by symptoms of developing cardiac failure/altered cerebral perfusion.	

Table 30–7. NURSING PROCESS FOR PATIENT REQUIRING ANTIDYSRHYTHMICS—*Continued*

Nursing Diagnosis	Nursing Actions	Rationale	Desired Outcomes/ Evaluation Criteria
	Provide instructions (verbal and written) regarding medications including desired action, dosage and usage particulars, expected side effects and possible adverse reactions/interactions with other prescribed/OTC drugs or substances.	Information necessary for patient to make informed choices and to manage medication regimen.	
	Encourage regular exercise routine, avoiding overexertion. Identify symptoms requiring cessation, e.g., dizziness, lightheadedness, dyspnea, chest pain.	When dysrhythmias are properly managed, normal activity should not be affected and regular exercise can enhance overall cardiovascular well being.	
	Review symptoms to be reported to the physician.	Provides for timely evaluation/intervention to prevent complications.	
	Review dietary needs/restrictions, e.g., potassium, caffeine, low cholesterol/calorie.	Depending on specific problem, may need to increase dietary potassium such as when potassium depleting diuretics are used. Limiting caffeine may prevent cardiac excitation. Reduction of weight and cholesterol levels may enhance cardiovascular functioning.	
	Stress importance of routine followup, periodic laboratory evaluations.	Evaluates therapeutic needs/effectiveness and provides for early detection of developing complications.	

NURSING RESPONSIBILITIES

In the acute situation, as the patient is being closely monitored, the nurse is responsible for administering the antidysrhythmics. The nurse must therefore know all the information featured in the column marked "Nursing Implications" in Table 30–4.

All intravenous antidysrhythmics are potentially dangerous drugs and therefore are administered through an infusion pump or volumetric pump using microdrip tubing (depending on local hospital policy and procedure). The dosage is carefully titrated in order to control dysrhythmias while minimizing the adverse effects of the drug.

No other medications are added to the IV bottle containing the antidysrhythmic or to the IV line. This prevents deterioration and precipitation of drugs. All these medications are best run piggyback on a keep-open IV line. In case there is a reaction to the medication, the keep-open IV can then be turned on.

Each medication is adequately diluted and administered according to its own special directions (see package inserts for specific directions). Most medications are normally diluted in dextrose and water to avoid the extra sodium in normal saline solutions, which may cause excessive fluid accumulation in patients with heart failure. However, when mixing phenytoin, dilute with only special diluent or normal saline and use it immediately.

The nurse must always read labels carefully, but extra care is taken when administering lidocaine. Lidocaine is available with epinephrine or preservatives or plain. Only plain lidocaine is administered intravenously. The medications with epinephrine or preservatives are meant to be used as local anesthetics; if administered intravenously, they can cause anaphylactic reactions. Lidocaine is packaged in 2-g syringes for mixing an IV drip and 100-mg syringes for IV push administration. The 2-g syringes are never to be administered IV push!

As the patient recovers from the acute illness, the focus of the nursing intervention is shifted toward health teaching. It is the primary responsibility of the nurse educator to teach the patient and family about the medical and nursing regimens. Patient education is of

Table 30–8. PATIENT TEACHING INFORMATION—ANTIDYSRHYTHMICS

Dear Patient:

This drug has been prescribed for you. This is what you should know about your drug to get the most from your therapy.

1. Antidysrhythmics are taken to regulate your heart rhythm.
2. Antidysrhythmic medications may have to be taken for the rest of your life.
3. Quinidine, procainamide hydrochloride (Pronestyl), propranolol (Inderal), and phenytoin (Dilantin) are taken with meals.
4. Do not take your antidysrhythmics concurrently with [fill in appropriate drugs].
5. Always check with your doctor or pharmacist before taking other drugs because interactions may occur. Drugs known to cause interactions include over-the-counter products for nasal congestion, allergy, pain, or obesity. Drugs of abuse such as marijuana may raise the blood pressure and stimulate heart activity and thus increase abnormal heart rhythm.
6. If you forget to take your antidysrhythmic, do not take the forgotten dose. **Do not** try to catch up by taking 2 doses at the same time.
7. Do not stop taking your drug unless directed by your doctor.
8. If you have any side effects from your drug, call your doctor. Side effects from taking antidysrhythmics include low blood pressure, lightheadedness, gastrointestinal distress, changes in rate or rhythm of the heart, and often blurred vision. Keep a written record of specific effects that are noted and the time of day that they are noted, such as in the morning upon awaking, with meals, or with activity. (Specific adverse effects are listed in Table 30–4.)
9. Weigh yourself weekly. A gain of 1–2 lb a week may be a sign of increased water. Call your doctor if this occurs.
10. Check your feet and ankles for swelling. If this occurs, notify your doctor.
11. Limit your coffee, tea, or cola drinks, since caffeine may cause an increase in abnormal heart rhythm.
12. Store these drugs in a tight, light-resistant bottle to prevent deterioration.

primary importance, since it has been demonstrated to decrease readmission to the hospital because of noncompliance. The patient and family are involved in the development of the health teaching plan. The patient and family are taught and should understand the information presented in Table 30–8.

PATIENT TEACHING

The patient going home on antidysrhythmics is taught how to administer the medications safely at home. This includes all the information in Table 30–8.

During future clinic or office visits the nurse checks the patient's blood. Patients often complain of orthostatic hypotension, dizziness, and lightheadedness. The dosage may have to be reduced to eliminate these symptoms. Also during prolonged therapy (months to years), the patient should have periodic CBC, serum electrolytes, and blood chemistry studies to determine whether any adverse effects are occurring. Renal and hepatic function are also checked. Patients need to understand the importance of taking the medication as ordered to control their dysrhythmias and the importance of diet and exercise modifications.

EVALUATION

The evaluation of the effectiveness of antidysrhythmics is based on a predetermined list of outcome evaluation criteria developed on an individual basis through discussions involving the nurse, patient, and family. The data base obtained in the original assessment is used to formulate the criteria for evaluation. Examples of these outcome evaluation criteria are included in Table 30–7.

It is extremely important to work with the patient and family to ensure their complete cooperation and support. Once patients understand the importance of their continued medical treatment, the majority usually are compliant. The fact that the patient is often recovering from a myocardial infarction, a life-threatening event, also increases compliance. Patients need to understand and recognize the adverse effects of their medication as well as the need to report these and other unusual signs to their physician.

All other evaluation criteria are assessed and evaluated before the patient is discharged. All previously taught material is reviewed and updated if necessary to ensure that the patient's understanding remains accurate. The nurse stresses the importance of continued medical care. Antidysrhythmic medications should enable the patient to live a more active life.

SUMMARY

Many groups of antidysrhythmic drugs are available today, including the medications in groups I through IV. The group I drugs act as local anesthetics or have a membrane-stabilizing effect. The group II drugs include the β blockers that depress phase 4 of depolarization. The group III drugs produce a prolongation of phase 3 depolarization. And the group IV drugs, the calcium-channel blockers, depress phase 4 depolarization and lengthen phases 1 and 2 of repolarization.

Before the nurse administers antidysrhythmics, it is important to assess the cardiac rhythm and obtain a baseline ECG. When the patient is acutely ill, the antidysrhythmics are administered intravenously through infusion or volumetric pumps. Each medication is to be diluted according to the directions on the enclosed package insert. As the patient recovers, he or she is taught how to administer these medications at home and how to monitor his or her pulse.

BIBLIOGRAPHY

AMA Drug Evaluations. PSG Publishing, Littleton, MA, 1987.

American Hospital Formulary Service 88 by the American Society of Hospital Pharmacists Inc. U.S. Library Congress Catalog Card No. 59-7620.

Amiodarone. Med Lett 28(713):49–50, May 1986.

Doom anxiety in cardiac patients: Symptom of lidocaine toxicity? Nurses Drug Alert 11(4):25–26, 1987.

Drugs for cardiac dysrythmias. Med Lett 28(727):111–116, November 1986.

Encainide for cardiac dysrythmias. Med Lett 29(740):50–52, May 1987.

Fingernail hemorrhages and procainamide lupus. Nurses Drug Alert 11(6):48, 1987.

Flecainide: A new antidysrhythmic drug. Med Lett 28(707):19–20, February 1986.

Mexiletine for dysrythmias. Med Lett 28(717):65–66, July 1986.

Tocainide agranulocytosis and anemia. Nurses Drug Alert 11(6):43–44, 1987.

Butler, JD and Harrison, BL: Keeping pace with calcium-channel blockers. Nursing 83 13:38–43, July 1983.

Catalano, JP: Antiarrhythmic medications classified by their autonomic properties. Crit Care Nurse 6(3):44–49, 1986.

Crumpley, L: An overview of antidysrhythmic drugs. Crit Care Nurse 3(4):57–64, 1983.

D'Arcy, PF, et al: Drug-antacid interactions: assessment of clinical importance. Drug Intell Clin Pharm 21(7/8):607–17, 1987.

DeAngelis, R: Amiodarone. Crit Care Nurse 6(6):12–13, 1986.

Flores, BT, et al: Amiodarone therapy: Reducing the side effects. DCCN 6(4):229–239, 1987.

Gever, LN: Flecainide: Bright prospect for better compliance. Nursing 17(5):137, 1987.

Gilman, AG, Goodman, LS, and Gilman, A (eds): Goodman and Gilman's The Pharmacological Basis of Therapeutics, ed 7. Macmillan, New York, 1986.

Harrison, DC: Antidysrhythmic drug classification new science and practical applications. Am J Cardiol 56:185–187, 1985.

Howland–Gradman, J: Flecainide Acetate. Crit Care Nurse 7(2):28–29, 1987.

Jacob, A, et al: Fatal ventricular fibrillation following verapamil in Wolff–Parkinson–White syndrome with atrial fibrillation. Ann Emerg Med 14:159–160, February 1985.

Lambrew, CT: Dysrhythmias: Evolving method of treatment. Emerg Care 2(2):65–71, August 1986.

Liem, LB, et al: A review of new antiarrhythmic drugs. Top Emerg Med 8(3):23–36, 1986.

Lute, E: Calcium blockers: The important difference. RN 84(6):36–39, 1984.

Mathewson, M: Prolapsed mitral valve. Am J Nurs 80(8):1150–1152, 1980.

Miller, K: What ever happened to bretylium? Emergency 19(1):48, 50, 1987.

Shoemaker, W, Thompson, W, and Holbrook, P: Textbook of Critical Care Medicine. WB Saunders, Philadelphia, 1984.

Singh, BN: Advances in pharmacologic control of cardiac arrhythmias: Focus on newer agents. Hosp Formul 22(7):632–636, 1987.

Venkatesh, N and Singh, BN: Interactions when new and old drugs are combined. Consultant 85(11):108–127, November 1985.

SITUATION 30–1

Five days after a myocardial infarction, Velma Tidwell, a 58-year-old, develops atrial flutter with a ventricular response of around 100 beats per minute (bpm). Ms. Tidwell is currently on digoxin 0.125 mg po daily. She is on a cardiac monitor in the telemetry unit.

1. The physician orders quinidine sulfate 200 mg IM every 6 hours times 4 doses. The nurse will obtain the following baseline data prior to starting the medication:
   a. deep tendon reflexes
   b. abdominal girth
   c. Q-T interval
   d. pupil size

2. The nurse will be aware of the following effect of combined digoxin and quinidine therapy:
   a. elevated quinidine levels
   b. reduced quinidine levels
   c. elevated digoxin levels
   d. reduced digoxin levels

3. After parenteral therapy, Ms. Tidwell is to begin quinidine 200 mg po every 6 hours. The nurse will be observant for the following common side effect associated with quinidine therapy:
   a. diarrhea
   b. hypothermia
   c. seizures
   d. dysphagia

4. Ms. Tidwell converts to sinus rhythm with a heart rate around 80 bpm. Patient teaching for Ms. Tidwell concerning quinidine therapy will include:
   a. crushing the sustained release tablets
   b. taking the medication with meals
   c. increasing the intake of citrus fruit
   d. maintaining a high bran fiber diet

5. As follow-up care, the nurse will monitor the following laboratory result, which can be altered by quinidine:
   a. lipid profile
   b. T_3, T_4
   c. potassium
   d. platelet count

6. Which of the following behaviors by Ms. Tidwell indicates successful patient teaching?
   a. neglecting to report symptoms such as nausea
   b. reporting a weight gain of over 2 pounds per week
   c. taking the pulse rate once a week
   d. maintaining yearly blood pressure check-ups

SITUATION 30–2

William Washington is a 71-year-old admitted to the emergency room with severe chest pain. He is diaphoretic and complaining of shortness of breath.

CONTINUED ON THE FOLLOWING PAGE

SITUATION 30–2–CONTINUED

1. The nurse places Mr. Washington on a cardiac monitor, which shows sinus tachycardia and frequent premature ventricular complexes (PVC's). The patient is to receive an intravenous lidocaine bolus. The nurse is prepared to deliver the following dosage:
   a. 1 mg/kg
   b. 0.5 mg/kg
   c. 2 mg/kg
   d. 4 mg/kg

2. After the loading (bolus) dose, Mr. Washington is to be placed on a lidocaine infusion. The following represents the standard range of drug dosage:
   a. 60 to 10 mg/minute
   b. .5 to 1 μg/kg/minute
   c. 5 to 10 μg/kg/minute
   d. 1 to 4 mg/minute

3. The nurse will implement the following nursing interventions for Mr. Washington:
   a. Use only lidocaine with epinephrine for intravenous use.
   b. Use an infusion pump only for low dosage lidocaine.
   c. Maintain lidocaine infusion with macrodrip tubing.
   d. Maintain lidocaine infusion separate from other drugs.

4. The nurse will plan to observe for the following side effect of lidocaine therapy:
   a. disorientation
   b. photophobia
   c. dry mouth
   d. abdominal cramps

5. Mr. Washington is cared for in the coronary care unit after a diagnosis of anterior myocardial infarction is made. The lidocaine drip is to be discontinued after several days. The nurse is aware that the half-life of lidocaine is:
   a. 30 minutes
   b. 10 hours
   c. 4 to 5 hours
   d. 1 to 2 hours

6. Mr. Washington continues to have occasional to frequent PVC's. Tocainide is to be started orally. The nurse will teach Mr. Washington to report the following with regard to Tocainide:
   a. excessive bruising
   b. difficulty voiding
   c. dry mouth
   d. photophobia

Please refer to the Appendices for correct answers and additional review questions with answers.

31
CHAPTER

VASODILATORS/ HEMORRHEOLOGIC AGENTS/SCLEROSING AGENTS

VASODILATORS/ HEMORRHEOLOGIC AGENTS/SCLEROSING AGENTS

MERRILY MATHEWSON KUHN, R.N.C., Ph.D., CCRN

LEARNING OBJECTIVES

After reading this chapter, the student will be able to:

1. Identify medications commonly used as vasodilators (coronary and peripheral) and sclerosing agents.

2. Differentiate among the vasodilators and sclerosing agents as to mechanism of action, route of administration, pharmacokinetics, adverse effects, contraindications, and interactions.

3. Identify specific areas to assess in the patient requiring vasodilators and sclerosing agents in order to formulate appropriate nursing diagnoses.

4. Plan the nursing interventions necessary to administer vasodilators and sclerosing agents and choose appropriate teaching strategies to gain patient compliance.

5. Evaluate the patient at various stages of treatment to gauge nursing interventions.

ANTIANGINAL MEDICATIONS

Angina pectoris is a disease state characterized by sudden chest pain caused by an imbalance between myocardial oxygen demand and supply (Table 31–1). The patency and diameter of the coronary arteries can be reduced by the development of *arteriosclerosis* and *atherosclerosis*. As these conditions progress, the person receives less blood to the heart muscle, and symptoms develop such as angina pectoris or, if blood flow is stopped totally to a portion of the heart, a myocardial infarction.

The heart muscle, unlike any other organ in the body, receives its blood flow during diastole. Therefore, if diastole is shortened, as with sinus tachycardia, the heart muscle experiences reduced blood flow and less coronary perfusion. As a compensatory sympathetic mechanism, the body with compromised vessels may attempt to improve coronary perfusion by increasing the heart rate. This increase in heart rate actually results in less coronary perfusion because of the shortening of diastole.

Myocardial oxygen demand is increased when heart rate rises, as with exercise; when systolic wall tension increases or left ventricular end-diastolic wall tension increases or left ventricular end-diastolic volume (LVEDV) increases; and when myocardial contractility increases. Antianginal drugs are part of a general program designed to alleviate symptoms and reduce risk factors that predispose to coronary artery disease. Drug therapy for angina is based on reducing myocardial oxygen requirements and/or increasing blood flow to ischemic myocardium.

Classic angina is managed acutely with short-acting nitroglycerin products (sublingual, transmucosal, or spray), whereas long-term prophylaxis is achieved with oral or topical nitrates, β-adrenergic blockers (discussed in detail in Chapter 19), and calcium-channel blocking agents (discussed later in this chapter). *Variant and mixed angina* are best treated with nitrates and calcium antagonists. IV nitroglycerin may alleviate symptoms of *unstable angina* or *refractory angina*, or reduce the size of myocardial infarction, and reduce symptoms in congestive heart failure (CHF). Nitrates are also used to increase exercise capacity in patients with coronary artery disease.

NITRATES

Action

Nitrates are direct-acting vasodilators. Nitrates can be conveniently classified into those that:

1. act rapidly to terminate acute anginal attacks, and
2. have a prolonged duration of action, which can prevent angina attacks.

Nitrates work by directly relaxing smooth muscle, thereby causing generalized dilatation. This dilatation is nonspecific and affects all smooth muscle in the body, including bronchial smooth muscle and smooth muscle in the biliary and gastrointestinal tracts. Nitrates act in

Table 31–1. ANGINA PECTORIS

DEFINITION
Angina pectoris is a clinical syndrome characterized by acute intermittent pain in the chest resulting from an imbalance between myocardial oxygen demand and supply.

TYPES:
Stable—angina that remains the same in nature
Unstable—angina that is changing (usually increasing) in severity and that may lead to a myocardial infarction if not treated
Nocturnal—angina whose severity is worse at night
Anginal decubitus—severe debilitating angina
Refractory—angina that cannot be treated with normal therapy
Prinzmetal's variant (vasospastic)—angina in which the attacks occur during rest and in which the S-T segment is elevated

ETIOLOGY
1. Atherosclerotic heart disease with lipid deposits (atheromas) within the intima (the inner lining of the artery wall) of the coronary blood vessels
2. Coronary spasm

PRECIPITATING FACTORS
1. Exercise
2. Stress
3. Eating a heavy meal
4. Cold
5. Drinking caffeinated beverages
6. Drugs such as hydralazine hydrochloride (Apresoline); diazoxide (Hyperstat); and isoproterenol hydrochloride (Isuprel)

7. Factors secondary to pulmonary hypertension, valvular heart disease, severe anemia
8. Smoking or even being in a smoke-filled room where there are high concentrations to carbon monoxide

SYMPTOMS
1. Retrosternal chest pain 5–10 min in duration, generally described as tightness, squeezing, or heaviness and radiating into the chin, throat, or down the left arm, usually provoked by some activity
2. ECG changes include depression of the S-T segment (the greater the depth of depression, the greater the severity of the ischemia).

MANAGEMENT
1. Educate the patient to modify or avoid activities or habits that precipitate the attacks, such as eating large meals, drinking coffee, smoking, excessive strenuous exercise, undue stress, and going out into cold, windy weather.
2. As an attack begins, the patient should cease the activity and sit down.
3. Vasodilator drugs are administered.
4. Other drugs (calcium-channel blockers, β-adrenergic blockers, and tranquilizers) may be administered.
5. Relaxation techniques such as transcendental meditation, biofeedback, and yoga may be helpful.
6. Surgical procedures to revascularize the myocardium are also effective in certain patients.

angina through their effects on coronary blood flow and myocardial oxygen demand. Nitrates relieve spasm of angiographically normal and diseased arteries.

The major systemic action is a reduction in venous tone, which leads to pooling of blood in peripheral veins, decreased venous return, and reduced venous volume, and myocardial tension (preload). This reduction in preload results in a decrease in myocardial oxygen demand. This is believed to be the most beneficial action of nitrates in patients with angina. The lowering of LVEDV through the *Frank–Starling relationship* can lower stroke volume in patients with normal and lowered cardiac reserve. Because of this effect blood pressure falls, which can cause reflex tachycardia. Blood pressure and pulse are often used to monitor therapy. At higher doses, nitrates also cause moderate decrease in peripheral vascular resistance, which reduces arterial blood pressure and ventricular outflow resistance (afterload). Venous pooling of blood, which decreases the amount of blood returning to the heart, reduces LVEDV. This can be measured as a reduction in pulmonary capillary obstructive pressure.

As other vascular beds are dilated throughout the body, the patient may notice flushing due to vasodilation of the blood vessels in the skin and a headache due to cerebral vasodilation. Cerebral vasodilation increases intracranial pressure and, in conjunction with the fall in systemic blood pressure, decreases blood flow to the brain.

Uses

Nitrates are used in the acute treatment of anginal attacks and the long-term prophylactic management of angina pectoris. Nitrates are also used in the treatment of both acute and chronic congestive heart failure. Intravenous nitroglycerin is also gaining wide acceptance in critical care units for managing severe chest pain. Intravenous nitroglycerin has been used to decrease myocardial oxygen demand which improves left ventricular function and limits myocardial ischemia. Research has demonstrated that IV nitroglycerin can potentially reduce myocardial infarction size and decrease mortality.

Pharmacokinetics

Nitroglycerin is readily absorbed from the sublingual mucosa and skin. However, gastrointestinal absorption of oral nitrates is variable. Nitroglycerin has a short half-life, estimated at one to four minutes. Plasma protein binding is approximately 60%. Therapeutic blood levels have not yet been established. Nitrates are extensively metabolized in the liver, producing nitrate derivatives and inorganic nitrites. This extensive first-pass metabolism limits the usefulness of oral therapy.

Contraindications and Precautions

Nitrates are contraindicated for patients hypersensitive to nitrates, in severe anemias (since tissue oxygenation would be reduced), and for persons with head trauma or cerebral hemorrhage (since nitrates may increase intracranial pressure). Intravenous nitroglycerin is contraindicated for patients with severe hypotension and hypovolemia because shock may ensue.

Nitrates are given cautiously in ventricular outflow obstruction such as idiopathic hypertrophic subaortic stenosis (IHSS), and with ballooned mitral valve syndrome ("floppy valve syndrome") because angina may be aggravated in these patients due to reduction in preload, or the decrease in preload may increase outflow obstruction. Nitrates are also given cautiously to persons with a history of uncontrolled hypertension, since the blood pressure may need to be maintained at a higher level to maintain organ perfusion. Nitrates are also administered cautiously to patients with carotid disease because a higher blood pressure is needed to maintain cerebral perfusion. Nitrates are also given cautiously to patients with renal and hepatic dysfunctions as these are the routes of elimination. Use with caution in patients with diuretic-induced fluid depletion or in patients with low blood pressure (< 90). In addition, give cautiously to patients with constrictive pericarditis, tamponade, and hypertropic cardiomyopathy. Safety in pregnant and lactating women and children has not been established.

Adverse Effects

In general, the adverse effects experienced from nitrates include flushing, pounding or pulsating headache in as many as 50%, nausea, and vomiting. Patients between 18 and 59 are more likely to complain of flushing than older patients, perhaps due to more sensitive autonomic nervous systems. In patients with normal cardiac function, nitrates can cause hypotension and reflex tachycardia. In patients not on β-blockers, an increase in heart rate by 10 beats/min can be used to assess adequate vasodilation. If the tachycardia is symptomatic or leads to compromises in myocardial oxygen demand, the administration of a β-blocker counteracts this adverse effect. Nitrates are usually held and dosage reduced if hypotension is symptomatic, or if systolic blood pressure decreases below 90–100 mmHg. These symptoms are all related to the generalized systemic vasodilation. Tolerance to some of these adverse effects, particularly the headache, can develop.

Interactions

Nitrates interact with alcohol, which enhances the hypotensive effects related to vasodilation. Patients are instructed to drink alcohol only in moderation (1–2 oz/day of liquor or its equivalent in beer or wine). Nitrates also interact with other drugs, such as antihypertensives, calcium-channel blockers, β-blockers, and phenothiazines. Again, the hypotensive effects are enhanced, and patients may need to have antihypertensive drug dosage reduced. Norepinephrine, acetylcholine and histamine can act as physiologic antagonists to nitrates. Nitrates also interfere with the laboratory tests, for example, falsely decreasing serum cholesterol. The coronary vasodilators are featured in Table 31–2.

Tolerance to Nitrates

Tolerance to nitrates appears to develop with sustained and chronic use. Fluctuating nitrate blood concentra-

TEXT RESUMES ON PAGE 824

Table 31–2. CORONARY VASODILATORS

Name	Dosage	Mode of Administration	Pharmacokinetics

Action: relax smooth muscle, thereby producing generalized dilatation. Relieve spasm of normal and diseased arteries. Reduce venous tone, thereby reducing preload and decreasing myocardial oxygen demand.

Uses: acute and long-term prophylactic management of angina pectoris. Also used in treatment of chronic congestive heart failure.

Name	Dosage	Mode of Administration	Pharmacokinetics
			For all nitrates: PB: 60% ½ L: NA B: liver E: liver
Nitroglycerin (Nitrostat)	0.15–0.6 mg (1/100–1/400 gr) prn (× 3 doses consecutively maximum)	SL	O: 1–3 min P: 3–5 min
	5–800 µg/min continuous 25–500 µg/ml dilute in D$_5$W or NS Low-dose therapy 5–50 µg/min = preload reduction High-dose therapy 50–100 µg/min = balanced effect on preload and afterload	IV (special IV tubing may be necessary)	O: immediate D: 3–5 min

Key to Abbreviations in the *Pharmacokinetics* **column** O-onset; P-peak; D-duration; PB-protein bound; B-biotransformed in; E-excreted in; ½L-halflife.

*Within the column listing adverse effects, underlines indicate the most common effects; CAPITALS indicate life-threatening effects.

C
o
r
o
n
a
r
y
·
V
a
s
o
d
i
l
a
t
o
r
s

Contraindication/ Precautions	Adverse Effects*	Interactions	Nursing Implications
FOR ALL NITRATES: Contraindicated in hypersensitivity, severe anemias, head trauma, cerebral hemorrhage. Use cautiously in ventricular outflow obstruction such as IHSS, prolapsed mitral valve syndrome, uncontrolled hypertension, and history of carotid disease, and in renal and hepatic dysfunction. Safety in pregnancy, lactating women, and children has not been established.	FOR ALL NITRATES: Neuro: headache, dizziness, vertigo, faintness CV: tachycardia, palpitations, hypotension, syncope, flushing GI: nausea, vomiting, involuntary passing of urine and feces, abdominal pain, burning/local irritation (sublingual, transmucosal, translingual products) Integ: rash, contact dermatitis (with transdermal products) Misc. cold sweat, perspiration, ethanol intoxication with IV doses greater than 2000 μg/min	FOR ALL NITRATES: Alcohol enhances hypotension. Antihypertensive (β-blockers, calcium-channel blockers, and all phenothiazines) enhance hypotension. May need to reduce dose of antihypertensive. Interfere with laboratory determination of serum cholesterol.	FOR ALL NITRATES: ASSESSMENT: Assess baseline cardiac function, heart rate, blood pressure. INTERVENTION: Avoid alcohol concurrently. A tolerance to nitrates may occur. Nitrates do not alter ECG patterns. See Table 31–6 for patient teaching information. All nitrates should stay in original bottle to preserve potency. EVALUATION: Report severe headache, dizziness, flushing, blurred vision, or dry mouth to physician. Symptoms should be controlled.
Same as for all nitrates.	Same as for all nitrates.	Same as for all nitrates.	Same as for all nitrates. ASSESSMENT: Assess level of consciousness, alcohol diluent may cause alcohol intoxication. Assess BP, HR often, Know BP and HR ranges. INTERVENTION: Dry mouth decreases absorption; maintain moist mouth. Tablets should cause a slight headache. Patients should sit or lie down to decrease side effects of hypotension. Patients should take no more than 3 tablets per attack, at 5-min intervals. Pain must be relieved in that time (15 min); otherwise, the patient should seek medical help. Mix in D₅W or NS only. Use proper tubing as recommended by manufacturer. Titrate dosage to desired hemodynamic function. Closely monitor heart rate, blood pressure, and obstructive pressure. Patients with low obstructive pressure are likely to be sensitive to the hypotensive effects of nitrates. Titrate infusion upward q 3–5 min following blood pressure and pulse measurement. When low-

CONTINUED ON THE FOLLOWING PAGE

Table 31–2. CORONARY VASODILATORS–*CONTINUED*

Name	Dosage	Mode of Administration	Pharmacokinetics
Nitroglycerin–*Continued*			
Nitroglycerin spray (Nitrolingual)	0.4 mg/metered dose 1–3 doses no more than 3 in 15 min	Oral spray	O: 2 min D: 3 min
Nitroglycerin sustained-release (Nitroglyn, Nitrobid, Nitrospan)	2.5–6.5 mg tablet q 8–12 hr	PO swallow whole	O: 40 min–1 hr P: 3–4 hr D: 4–8 hr
Nitroglycerin topical (Nitrobid, Nitrol)	½″ to 5″ ribbon (7.5–75 mg) q 3–4 hr	Topical, rotate sites	O: 20–60 min D: 2–12 hr, particularly useful for prevention
Nitroglycerin transdermal patches (Nitro-Dur, Transderm-Nitro, Nitro-Disc)	Release rate 2.5–15 mg/24 hr	Topical	O: 40–60 min D: 18–24 hr
Nitroglycerin transmucosal (Nitrogard)	1–3 mg q 3–5 hr while awake	Transmucosal (buccal)	O: 2–4 min D: 3–5 hr
Isosorbide dinitrate (Isordil, Sorbitrate)	2.5–5 mg prn. 40–480 mg/day in divided doses	SL, chewable PO	O: 5 min D: ½–2 hr O: 20–40 min P: 30–60 min D: 4–6 hr

Key to Abbreviations in the *Pharmacokinetcs* column O-onset; P-peak; D-duration; PB-protein bound; B-biotransformed in; E-excreted in; ½L-halflife.
*Within the column listing adverse effects, <u>underlines</u> indicate the most common effects; CAPITALS indicate life-threatening effects.

Contraindication/ Precautions	Adverse Effects*	Interactions	Nursing Implications
			dose therapy is used, titrate up by 10–20 µg; and when high-dose therapy is used, titrate up by 20–50 µg. Titration is continued until desired decline in systolic blood pressure and/or relief of chest pain is obtained.
Same as for all nitrates.	Same as for all nitrates.	Same as for all nitrates.	Same as for all nitrates. INTERVENTION: Take while seated or lying down. Highly flammable. Spray onto oral mucosa. Do not inhale spray.
Same as for all nitrates.	Same as for all nitrates.	Same as for all nitrates.	Same as for all nitrates. INTERVENTION: Take on an empty stomach. Swallow whole, do not chew. Monitor blood pressure closely.
Same as for all nitrates.	Same as for all nitrates.	Same as for all nitrates.	Same as for all nitrates. INTERVENTION: Measure correct amount of ointment on application paper. Do not touch or rub medication into your hands or into patient's skin. If medication is absorbed, it may precipitate a headache. The applicator paper may be coverd with plastic wrap for better absorption. Wash medication from hands after application. Keep tube tightly closed.
Same as for all nitrates.	Same as for all nitrates.	Same as for all nitrates.	Same as for all nitrates. INTERVENTION: Remove patch before defibrillation to avoid arcing. Rotate sites. Wash skin when patch is removed.
Same as for all nitrates.	Same as for all nitrates.	Same as for all nitrates.	Same as for all nitrates. INTERVENTION: Take tablet after meals. Remove any unused tablet at bedtime to prevent aspiration. Talking and tongue motion may dislodge tablet. Hot liquids may increase dissolution.
Same as for all nitrates. Tolerance to sustained-action vasodilator may develop.	Same as for all nitrates.	Same as for all nitrates.	Same as for all nitrates. INTERVENTION: Do not crush or chew tablets.

CONTINUED ON THE FOLLOWING PAGE

Table 31–2. CORONARY VASODILATORS–*CONTINUED*

Name	Dosage	Mode of Administration	Pharmacokinetics
Isosorbide dinitrate sustained-release (Isordil Tembids)	40 mg q 6–12 hr	PO (should not be chewed)	O: slow P: 3–4 hr D: 8–12 hr
Pentaerythritol tetranitrate (Peritrate)	1 capsule, or 10, 20, 40, 80 mg (not sustained release)	PO (take on empty stomach)	O: 20–60 min P: 3–4 hr D: 4–5 hr
Pentaerythritol tetranitrate sustained-release (Peritrate SA)	30–80 mg q 12 hr	PO	O: 30 min–1 hr D: 8–12 hr
Amyl nitrite	0.18–0.3 ml (2–5 mg)	Inhalation (small glass capsule enclosed in woven covering, which is crushed between fingers)	O: seconds P: 1–2 min D: 3–5 min E: urine (⅓)
Erythrityl tetranitrate (Cardilate)	5–30 mg tid	Chewable	O: 5 min D: 2–4 hr
		PO	O: 30 min D: 6 hr

CALCIUM-CHANNEL BLOCKERS

Action: competitively blocks the slow-channel influx of calcium into active cells. Through inhibition of calcium, coronary and systemic beds, peripheral arteries, and arterioles dilate.

Use: variant, unstable, or vasospastic angina. Antidysrhythmic effects.

Verapamil (Isoptin, Calan)

Use: as with all, controls supraventricular tachycardias.

	Angina I: 40–120 mg tid	PO	O: 30 min P: 1–2.2 hr

Key to Abbreviations in the *Pharmacokinetcs* column O-onset; P-peak; D-duration; PB-protein bound; B-biotransformed in; E-excreted in; ½L-halflife.
*Within the column listing adverse effects, underlines indicate the most common effects; CAPITALS indicate life-threatening effects.

Contraindication/ Precautions	Adverse Effects*	Interactions	Nursing Implications
Same as for all nitrates.	Same as for all nitrates.	Same as for all nitrates.	Same as for all nitrates.
Same as for all nitrates.	Same as for all nitrates.	Same as for all nitrates.	Same as for all nitrates. INTERVENTION: Take on empty stomach ½ hr before or 1 hr after meals and at bedtime.
Same as for all nitrates.	Same as for all nitrates.	Same as for all nitrates.	Same as for all nitrates. INTERVENTION: Do not crush or chew tablet.
Same as for all nitrates.	Same as for all nitrates.	Same as for all nitrates.	Same as for all nitrates. INTERVENTION: Crush the capsule and wave under patients nose. May repeat in 3–5 min. Store in a cool place.
Same as for all nitrates.	Same as for all nitrates.	Same as for all nitrates.	Same as for all nitrates. INTERVENTION: Administer on an empty stomach.
For all calcium-channel blockers.	Hemo: inhibit platelet function, may increase bleeding tendency	For all calcium-channel blockers. β-adrenergic blockers cause increased negative inotropic & chronotropic effects. Cimetidine increases bio-availability of calcium-channel blockers. Digoxins level may increase.	For all calcium-channel blockers. ASSESSMENT: Establish baseline data—vital signs, ECG, hepatic and renal function. INTERVENTION: If hypotension occurs, stay recumbent for 1 hr after taking drug. Know pulse limits: if high or irregular, notify physician. Food delays absorption and decreases plasma concentrations. EVALUATION: Notify physician of shortness of breath, swelling of feet, pronounced dizziness, constipation, nausea, and irregular heart beat. Decrease drugs gradually.
Contraindicated in hypersensitivity, sick sinus syndrome without a pacer, cardiogenic shock, and severe	Neuro: dizziness, headache CV: hypotension, CHF, bradycardia, pulmonary edema, peripheral dilitation, fatigue, edema, SINUS	Same as for all calcium-channel blockers. Verapamil and carbamazepine increase carbamazepine toxicity. Calcium salts	Same as for all calcium-channel blockers. INTERVENTION: Administer sustained-release tablet with food. Administer bolus

CONTINUED ON THE FOLLOWING PAGE

Table 31–2. CORONARY VASODILATORS–*CONTINUED*

Name	Dosage	Mode of Administration	Pharmacokinetics
Verapamil–*Continued*	dysrhythmia 240–480 mg/day in divided doses		D: 4–8 hr ½L: 3–7 hr PB: 83%–92% B: liver E: unchanged urine (3%–4%) 70% in urine
	hypertension 240–360 mg/day in divided doses, sustained-release 240 mg in a.m.		
	Adults: dysrhythmias 5–10 mg over 2 min (in older patient 3 min) repeat 10 mg in 30 min	IV	P: 3–5 min
	Children: up to 1 yr 0.1–0.2 mg/kg over 2 min; 1–15 yr 0.1–0.3 mg/kg over 2 min; repeat in 30 min		

Nifedipine (Procardia, Adalat)

Use: as with all, reduces cerebral spasm and prophylaxis of migraine headache; reduces blood pressure.

| | 30–120 mg daily increase every 7–14 days (bite and swallow capsule with water) | PO | O: 20 min
P: 0.5 hr
D: 2½–3 hr
½ L: 2–5 hr
PB: 92%–98%
B: liver
E: unchanged in urine (1%–2%) |

Diltiazem (Cardizem)

Use: as for all, improves exercise performance.

| | 30–360 mg daily in divided doses | PO | O: 30 min
P: 2–3 hr
D: 4–8 hr
½ L: 3–5 hr
PB: 70–85%
B: liver
E: unchanged in urine (2–4%) |

Nicardipine Hydrochloride (Cardene)

Use: Chronic stable effort associated angina, hypertension.

| | Angina and hypertension: 20 mg 3 times/day, increase after 3 days if needed; up to 40 mg 3 times/day | PO | O: 20 min
P: 0.5–2 hr
D: UA
½L: 2–4 hr
PB: >95%
B: liver
E: as metabolites unchanged in urine <1. |

Key to Abbreviations in the *Pharmacokinetcs* column O-onset; P-peak; D-duration; PB-protein bound; B-biotransformed in; E-excreted in; ½L-halflife.
*Within the column listing adverse effects, underlines indicate the most common effects; CAPITALS indicate life-threatening effects.

Contraindication/ Precautions	Adverse Effects*	Interactions	Nursing Implications
congestive heart failure. Use cautiously in hypotension, hepatic and renal dysfunction.	ARREST, ASYSTOLE THIRD-DEGREE HEART BLOCK GI: constipation, nausea GU: unilateral gynecomastia	and vitamin D decrease effectiveness. Lithium levels are decreased. Antihypertensives and quinidine cause acute hypotension. Warfarin and oral hypoglycemics may interact. Incompatible IV with NaCl and HCO$_3$. Incompatible IV with nafacillin.	IV doses over 2 mins. Protect IV solution from light.
Contradindicated in hypersensitivity. Use cautiously in hypotension, CHF. Safe use in pregnancy, lactating women, and children not established.	Neuro: dizziness, lightheadedness, headache, weakness, syncope, giddiness Resp: dyspnea, cough, wheezing CV: peripheral edema, myocardial infarction, weakness, CHF GI: nausea, diarrhea, constipation Hemo: thrombocytopenia, leukopenia, purpura Other: flushing, warmth, rashes	Concurrent use with quinidine decreases quinidine levels. Concurrent antihypertensive and quinidine increases hypotensive effect. Fentanyl and β-blockers cause severe hypotension. Theophylline levels increase. Lab: may increase CPK, LDH, SGOT, positive Coombs'.	Same as for all calcium-channel blockers.
Contraindicated in sinus bradycardia, second- and third-degree heart block without a pacer, and severe congestive heart failure. Use cautiously with liver problems. Safety in pregnancy, and children not determined.	Neuro: dizziness, headache, fatigue, nervousness CV: peripheral edema, hypotension, congestive heart failure, palpitation, bradycardia, dysrhythmia GI: nausea vomiting, diarrhea, constipation Integ: rash, photosensitivity	Same as for all. Cyclosporine increases serum levels. Carbamazepine increases inhibition of hepatic metabolism. Concurrent lithium causes increased neurotoxicity.	Same as for all.
Contraindicated in hypersensitivity, adverse aortic stenosis. Use with caution in patients with liver and renal disease. Discontinuing nursing when taking nicardipine.	CNS: dizziness CV: peripheral edema, palpitations, tachycardia GI: nausea, abdominal cramps Other: flushing, allergic reaction.	Increases level of cyclosporine. Concurrent cimetidine increases plasma level of nicardipine.	Same as for all.

CONTINUED ON THE FOLLOWING PAGE

Table 31–2. CORONARY VASODILATORS–*CONTINUED*

Name	Dosage	Mode of Administration	Pharmacokinetics
Nimodipine (Nimotop)			
Uses: Improve neurologic deficits due to spasm following subarachnoid hemorrhage.			
	60 mg q 4 hr for 21 days. Start within 96 hr of SAH	PO	O: NA P: 1 hr D: 3–4 hr ½L: 1–2 hr PB: 95% B: UA E: less than 1% in urine.

Key to Abbreviations in the *Pharmacokinetcs* column O-onset; P-peak; D-duration; PB-protein bound; B-bio-transformed in; E-excreted in; ½L-halflife.

*Within the column listing adverse effects, <u>underlines</u> indicate the most common effects; CAPITALS indicate life-threatening effects.

tions may be needed in order to decrease the development of tolerance. This fluctuation of blood level can be achieved by having a nitrate-free period of about eight hours per day. For most people, this is best achieved by applying patches or ointment in the morning and removing it at bedtime. A patient who has nocturnal angina may prefer to apply the medication in the late afternoon or early evening and remove it the next morning. If β-blockers or calcium channel-blockers are also prescribed, the dosing schedule can be arranged so that the peak coverage with the oral drugs occurs during the nitrate-free interval. The exact mechanism of nitrate tolerance has not as yet been elucidated.

Acute-Acting Nitrates

NITROGLYCERIN TABLETS. Nitroglycerin is used for the rapid relief of anginal pain. It is taken sublingually in doses ranging from 0.15–0.6 mg (1/100–1/400 gr) as needed for chest pain. The generally accepted maximum dosage is three consecutive doses at five-to-ten-minute intervals. If the patient continues to experience the same intensity of pain with no relief, he or she should consult the physician immediately because of the potential for myocardial infarction.

Nitroglycerin can also be used prophylactically, to prevent anginal attacks. The patient is instructed to take a nitroglycerin tablet before any activity—mild to moderate exercise or sexual activity—previously known to cause angina. This technique often prevents angina from occurring by producing adequate vasodilation and decreasing myocardial oxygen demand.

Nitroglycerin degrades when exposed to light, air, or moisture. It is stored in a tightly closed amber container away from heat. Patients are counseled to refill their supplies for periods no longer than five months. Patients are also told to keep a supply of nitroglycerin tablets on hand with them at all times.

NITROGLYCERIN IV. Nitroglycerin (Tridil, Nitro-Bid IV) is available for IV administration. It is used in the treatment of acute unstable angina, acute CHF, and often in myocardial infarction. Titration must be performed carefully according to patient's tolerance and therapeutic response. Continuous monitoring of hemodynamic parameters—arterial pressure, pulmonary artery pressures, and pulmonary capillary obstructive pressures—is extremely important and must be done throughout IV nitroglycerin administration. Often the dose of nitroglycerin is determined based on the hemodynamic trends.

In acute myocardial infarction, the greatest benefit from nitroglycerin occurs when it is administered within four hours after onset of pain. However, when given within eight hours following onset of symptoms, it can also produce positive effects. Positive effects seen include a decrease in episodes of anginal pain, ventricular ectopic beats, and left ventricular failure.

Nitroglycerin is mixed either with 5.0% dextrose or 0.9% sodium chloride solutions with dilutions ranging from 25 to 500 μg/ml. Infusion concentrations are based on the patient's fluid requirements. Dosage varies widely from 5–800 μg/min, thus requiring careful titration in a given patient.

There is currently some controversy about placing nitroglycerin in polyvinylchloride bags because the bag absorbs part of the dose. Dupont Critical Care, maker of IV Tridil, suggests that it should be mixed in glass bottles and run through special IV tubing distributed by them. On the other hand, Marion Laboratories, maker of Nitro-Bid IV, states that its product can be placed in polyvinylchloride containers. However, Marion Laboratories recommends that the preparation be mixed and allowed to stand for 15–30 minutes. At the end of this time, the polyvinylchloride bags and tubing will have absorbed all the nitroglycerin they are going to, and the infusion can then be started. Care should be taken

Contraindication/ Precautions	Adverse Effects*	Interactions	Nursing Implications
No contraindications. Use with caution in patients with liver dysfunction. Use in pregnancy only when clearly indicated and when benefits outweigh potential hazards.	CNS: headache, depression, dizziness CV: hypotension, peripheral edema, bradycardia GI: diarrhea, abdominal cramps, nausea, vomiting Integ: rash, dermatitis, urticaria Other: flushing, muscle cramps	Concurrent beta adrenergic blockers and other calcium channel blockers may enhance negative chronotropic and inotropic effects. Lab: may falsely elevate serum glucose LDH and alkaline phosphates.	Same as for all plus: INTERVENTION: If patient cannot swallow capsule, withdraw fluid from capsule and inject down nasogastric tube. Flush with 30 ml of normal saline.

to follow manufacturer's guideline when using IV nitroglycerin.

NITROGLYCERIN, TRANSLINGUAL. Nitroglycerin, translingual (Nitrolingual) is a metered spray that is available for acute relief or prophylaxis of angina due to coronary artery disease.

Dosage. The Nitrolingual is used in a fashion similar to nitroglycerin tablets. At the onset of an acute attack, one or two metered doses (0.4 mg/spray) are sprayed into the oral mucosa. Like the nitroglycerin tablets, no more than three metered doses are recommended within 15 minutes. If chest pain persists and does not change, the patient should seek medical attention. Nitrolingual can also be used prophylactically five-to-ten minutes prior to any activity known to cause angina. The spray should not be inhaled, and swallowing immediately after the spray is administered should be avoided. The canister should not be shaken.

Chronic Nitrate Therapy

NITROGLYCERIN SUSTAINED-RELEASE. Nitroglycerin sustained-release (Nitrobid) is a capsule swallowed whole and administered every 8–12 hours. Patients will most likely also use nitroglycerin sublingually for acute attacks. Nitroglycerin sustained-release is administered in 2.5–6.5-mg tablets every 8–12 hours.

NITROGLYCERIN OINTMENT. Nitroglycerin ointment (Nitro-Bid, Nitrol, Nitrong ointment) contains 2% nitroglycerin in a lanolin base. The ointment is squeezed onto special marked paper that comes with the tube (Fig. 31–1). The paper, not the fingers, is used to spread the ointment, and the paper is applied to the skin. Further discussion of administration is found in the Nursing Process section of this chapter. If the patient is able to measure his or her own dosage, the dose is more likely to be consistent. The medication can be applied anywhere on the body surface, but the skin should be clean, dry, and hairless. The tube is kept tightly closed and stored in a cool place.

Nitroglycerin ointment dosage is 7.5–75 mg (or a ½–5-inch ribbon), applied every three-to-four hours, at the same time each day. One inch of ointment contains 15 mg of nitroglycerin. The dosage is usually titrated by therapeutic response and blood pressure response. Nitroglycerin ointment is particularly beneficial in preventing noctural angina. When treatment is terminated, dosage is gradually reduced to prevent sudden withdrawal reactions.

NITROGLYCERIN TRANSDERMAL PATCHES. Nitroglycerin transdermal patches (Nitro-Dur, Transderm-Nitro, Nitrodisc) are pockets of medication containing nitroglycerin, glycerin, water, polyvinyl alcohol, and several other ingredients, surrounded by a bandage (Fig. 31–2). Once the polyester foil covering is removed from the medication, the patch resembles an ECG electrode or a round Band-Aid, and is applied to the skin. All transdermal patches can be worn during bathing, showering, and swimming.

Transdermal patches are available in several doses ranging from 20 mg to 187.5 mg of nitroglycerin and are applied only once daily. They can be applied to any non-hairy area of the body. Transdermal nitroglycerin patches rapidly become ineffective for treatment of angina pectoris if they are left in place for 24 hours and reapplied daily. They remain ineffective even if the dosage is progressively increased. Patches delivering 10 mg or more of nitroglycerin can be effective if they are removed for 10–12 hours daily.

Several manufacturers market patches, and each product contains a different amount of nitroglycerin. The release rate of nitroglycerin in milligrams per 24 hours ranges from 2.5 to 15. Patients need to be assessed carefully when alternating different manufacturers' products. The transdermal patches are compared in Table 31–3.

If a patient is changed from the nitroglycerin ointment containing 12.5 mg nitroglycerin per inch, the smallest dose size of the patch should be used, and the dose appropriately titrated.

NITROGLYCERIN, TRANSMUCOSAL. Nitroglycerin transmucosal (Nitrogard) is available for buccal application for both acute and long-term control of angina pectoris.

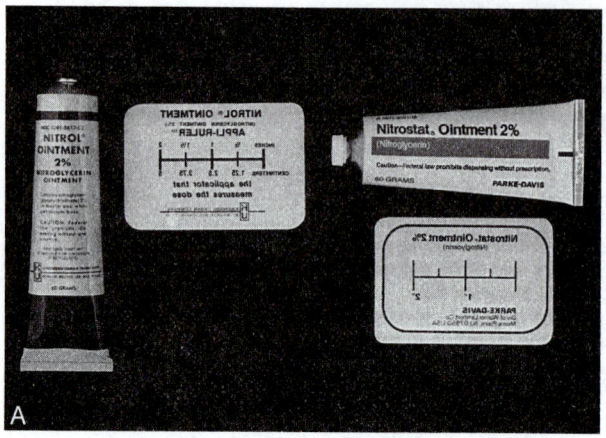

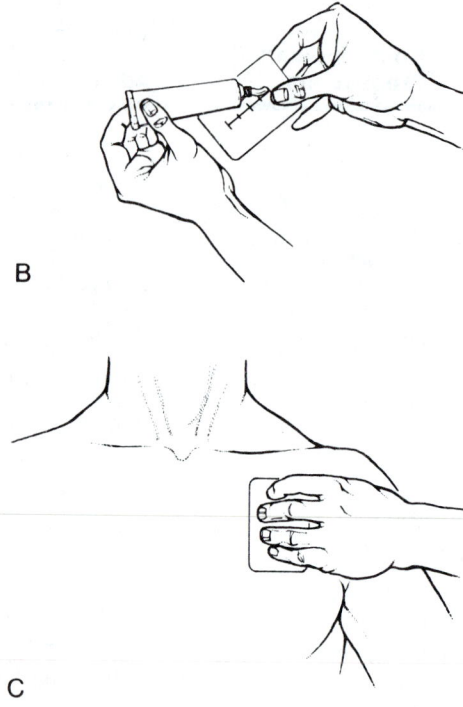

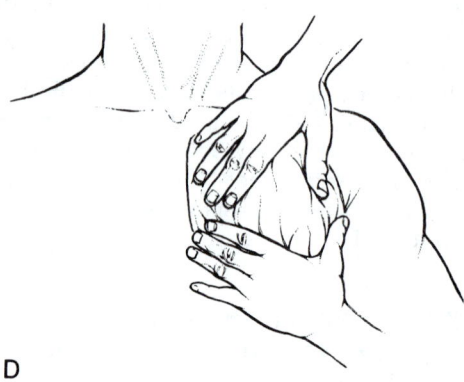

Figure 31–1. *A*) Tubes of nitroglycerin paste and the special application papers. *B*) and *C*) The correct amount of paste is squeezed onto the paper, and it is applied to the patient's skin. *D*) Clear plastic wrap is applied over the papers to enhance absorption. (Courtesy of Parke-Davis, Div. of Warner-Lambert Co., Morris Plains, NJ, and Kremers-Urban Co., Milwaukee, WI.)

Pharmacokinetics. In the transmucosal form, nitroglycerin is impregnated in an inert cellulose polymer matrix. The tablet, similar in size to sublingual nitroglycerin, is placed in the buccal cavity between the upper lip and gum, or cheek and gum. A gel forms that makes the tablet adhere to the mucosal surface, and the drug diffuses into the systemic circulation. Onset of effect occurs in two-to-four minutes. Absorption continues while the tablet remains intact (one-to-six hours). Nitroglycerin serum levels fall rapidly after the tablet is dissolved. Tolerance has not been reported with the transmucosal form of nitroglycerin, possibly because of the nitrate-free interval at night.

Adverse Effects. Irritation in the mouth such as mild erythema, mild tingling or stinging, and ulceration

can occur. The other adverse effects are similar to the group of nitroglycerin products.

Dosage. Transmucosal nitroglycerin is available in 1-, 2-, and 3-mg tablets administered every three to five hours while the patient is awake.

ISOSORBIDE DINITRATE. Isosorbide dinitrate (Isordil, Sorbitrate), like nitroglycerin, is available as sublingual and chewable tablets, oral tablets, and sustained-release tablets. Isosorbide is one of the most frequently used long-acting nitrates.

The sublingual and chewable forms are used to treat acute anginal attacks. The usual dose is 2.5–5.0 mg dissolved under the tongue or chewed, as needed.

Isosorbide dinitrate oral tablets are available in 5-, 10-, and 20-mg doses and are administered 4–6 times

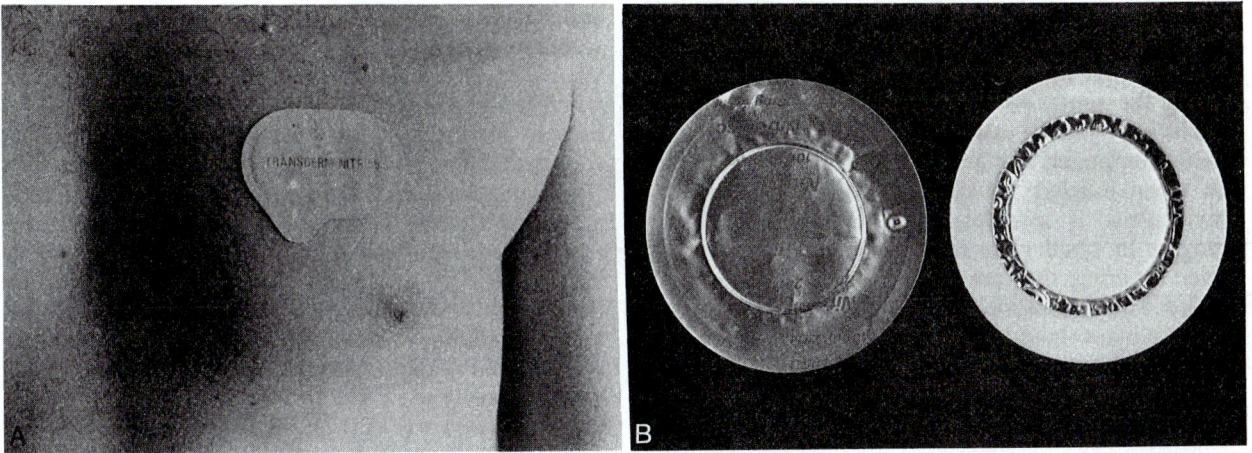

Figure 31–2. Transdermal nitroglycerin patches by CIBA (*A*) and Searle (*B*). (Courtesy of CIBA Pharmaceutical Company, Summit, NJ, and Searle Pharmaceuticals, Inc., Chicago, IL.)

daily. The daily dosage can range from 40 to 480 mg. The oral tablet would be used to prevent or decrease the number of anginal attacks. It can also be used as a part of the treatment of CHF, where it acts by reducing resistance to cardiac pumping action.

ISOSORBIDE DINITRATE SUSTAINED-RELEASE. Isosorbide dinitrate sustained-release tablets (Isordil Tembids) are given in 40-mg oral doses every 6–12 hours. The tablets should not be chewed or crushed because this eliminates the sustained-release action.

PENTAERYTHRITOL TETRANITRATE. Pentaerythritol tetranitrate (Peritrate), which is rated as ''possibly effective'' by the United States Food and Drug Administration (FDA), is available in two forms. Tablets and capsules are available in doses of 10, 20, 40, and 80 mg. Sustained-release preparations, available in doses of 30, 45, 60, and 80 mg, are slowly absorbed, which delays onset and prolongs duration to 8–12 hours. The sustained-release preparations are administered twice daily. Both tablets and sustained-release products are best administered on an empty stomach to enhance absorption.

ERYTHRITYL TETRANITRATE. Erythrityl tetranitrate (Cardilate), available in oral tablets and chewable tablets, is administered in doses of 5–30 mg three times daily.

AMYL NITRITE. Amyl nitrite is seldom used, if ever, for angina pectoris because it is expensive and incon-

Table 31–3. COMPARISON OF TRANSDERMAL NITROGLYCERIN PATCHES

Product Name	Company	Strength	Onset of Action After Initial Dose (min)	Nitroglycerin Content	Nitroglycerin Delivered Over 24 hr (mg)	Delivery System
Transderm-Nitro	Ciba	5	30–60	25	5.0	Colloid silicone and semipermeable membrane
Transderm-Nitro	Ciba	10	30–60	50	10.0	Same as above
Transderm-Nitro	Ciba	15	30–60	75	15.0	Same as above
Nitro-Dur	Key	5	30	51	5.0	Gel-like matrix
Nitro-Dur	Key	10	30	104	10.0	Same as above
Nitro-Dur II	Key	2.5	30	20	2.5	Acrylic-based polymer adhesive with a resinous cross-linking agent
Nitro-Dur II	Key	5.0	30	40	5.0	Same as above
Nitro-Dur II	Key	7.5	30	60	7.5	Same as above
Nitro-Dur II	Key	10.0	30	80	10.0	Same as above
Nitro-Dur II	Key	15.0	30	120	15.0	Same as above
Nitrodisc	Searle	5	30–60	16	5.0	Impregnated polymer
Nitrodisc	Searle	10	30–60	32	10.0	Same as above

venient, and has a high incidence of adverse effects such as headache, orthostatic symptoms, and tachycardia. In addition, amyl nitrite is sometimes abused by people seeking the sensation of lightheadedness that results from its hypotensive vasodilator effect. Amyl nitrite is a volatile compound and acts even faster than nitroglycerin when inhaled. Its effects occur within seconds. Amyl nitrite is available in 0.18–0.3-ml (2–5-mg) strengths in small glass capsule perles enclosed in a woven covering; they are crushed between fingers and inhaled. The medication has a strong, unpleasant odor, and the patient should inhale no more than two to three times to prevent overdosing.

OTHER DRUGS USED TO TREAT ANGINA PECTORIS

Other groups of drugs are used in conjunction with vasodilators, or alone, to control angina attacks. They include the β-adrenergic blockers and the calcium-channel blockers. The β-adrenergic blockers such as propranolol (Inderal), metoprolol tartrate (Lopressor), and nadolol (Corgard), all discussed in Chapter 19, cause the heart to be more resistant to the effects of catecholamines. This effect decreases the heart rate and the oxygen needs of the myocardium. B-adrenergic blockers also decrease the force of cardiac contraction, which also decreases myocardial oxygen needs. Patients usually have an increased tolerance to exercise and report a decrease in the number and the severity of their anginal attacks.

OTHER USES FOR VASODILATORS

Vasodilators are helpful in treating other diseases. Topical application, which causes cutaneous dilatation, has been used to control the symptoms of *Raynaud's disease*. (Raynaud's disease is a primary or idiopathic vasospastic disorder characterized by bilateral and symmetric pallor and cyanosis of the fingers.) Topical applications have also been used to improve healing of atrophic ulcers.

Vasodilators can also be used to treat patients with *accelerated or unstable angina*. Accelerated or unstable angina is similar to angina pectoris in its etiology and symptomatology. The pain of unstable angina, however, lasts 15–20 minutes and often must be relieved with narcotics. Vasodilators are also used to treat myocardial infarction, to reduce *vasospasm*, and possibly decrease the size of the infarct. Recent reports have shown that early use of IV nitroglycerin in acute myocardial infarction favorably affects early and long-term morbidity and mortality. Left ventricular filling pressure, volume,

and total systemic vascular resistance are reduced, resulting in a decrease in cardiac work and myocardial oxygen demand. These beneficial properties of nitrates, when combined with their coronary vasodilator effects, help to produce a favorable balance between oxygen supply and demand in the area of injury and ischemia.

Vasodilators have also proven effective in treating acute and chronic CHF. CHF is characterized by a decrease in cardiac output usually caused by an increase in peripheral vascular resistance. This is accentuated by the compensatory increase in sympathetic activity seen in heart failure. Vasodilators such as nitroglycerin decrease preload (end-diastolic volume) through venous pooling, resulting in a decrease in left ventricular end-diastolic pressure (LVEDP) and a decrease in pulmonary capillary obstructive pressure. In addition, there is a small effect on arterial tone, decreasing LVEDV and in turn helping to improve stroke volume. Nitrates are frequently combined with arterial vasodilators such as hydralazine, which decrease outflow resistance. This combination is effective in treating moderate to severe CHF. A similar effect can be seen with drugs that have major dilating effects on both venous and arterial vessels. Prazosin can be used in outpatients and nitroprusside in patients with acute heart failure treated in an intensive care setting. Angiotensin-converting enzyme inhibitors, such as captopril (Capoten), are potent vasodilators that are effective in treating patients with moderate to severe CHF. Much research is continuing in the use of vasodilators in CHF. Both nitrites and procardia are popular in treating esophageal spasm.

CALCIUM-CHANNEL BLOCKERS

Calcium-channel blockers or calcium antagonists are the newest group of cardiac drugs available to treat angina. These drugs are also used to treat hypertension and dysrhythmias and are mentioned briefly in Chapters 29 and 30. Calcium-channel blockers are a heterogeneous group of compounds with differing structures, mechanisms of actions, and therapeutic effects. Because of their inherent differences, agents are selected to meet specific needs of patients. The calcium-channel blockers are featured in Table 31–2.

All calcium-channel blockers have different pharmacologic effects while sharing the ability to competitively block the slow-channel influx of calcium into active cells. The effects of calcium-channel blockers are greatest in cells that depend on intracellular influx of calcium for activation. These are mainly vascular smooth muscle cells and cardiac tissue; however, other areas containing smooth muscle cells such as respiratory and gastrointestinal tract are also affected.

Cardiac tissue is rapidly depolarized by the rapid influx of sodium ions. This depolarization action is quickly followed by a slow inward current of calcium, which contributes to the plateau phase of the action potential and links myocardial excitation to contraction and controls energy storage and utilization. Most cardiac conducting cells depend on both fast sodium and slow calcium channels. However, the pacer cells of the SA and

Table 31–4. RELATIVE EFFECTS OF CALCIUM-CHANNEL BLOCKING AGENTS ON VARIOUS CARDIOVASCULAR FUNCTIONS

	Nifedipine	Verapamil	Diltiazem
Peripheral vascular resistance	− − −	− −	−
Coronary artery vasodilator effects	+ +	+	+ +
Myocardial contractility	+ −	− −	−
Antiarrhythmic properties	+ −	+ + +	+ +
Heart rate	+	−	−
AV node conduction	−	− − −	− −

+ − = neither positive nor negative effect; 0 = no effect; + = mild positive effect; + + = great positive effect;
− = mild negative effect; − − = moderate negative effect; − − − = great negative effect.

proximal AV nodes are depolarized primarily by the calcium current. By inhibiting calcium entry into cardiac and smooth muscle cells of the coronary and systemic beds, peripheral arteries and arterioles dilate. Specific effects of calcium-channel blockers are included in Table 31–4.

Uses

The antianginal effects of calcium antagonists are adequately explained by their ability to dilate coronary arteries, prevent vasospasm in the coronary arteries, and dilate peripheral arteries.

Nitrates and β-blockers remain standard therapy for classic angina, but calcium-channel blockers may be added to the drug regimen if nitrates are ineffective or poorly tolerated or when β-blockers produce intolerable adverse effects. Calcium-channel blockers are probably as effective as nitrates and may even be preferred to β-blockers in managing variant, unstable, or *vasospastic angina.*

In addition to their use as antidysrhythmics and antianginal drugs, calcium-channel blockers are used to treat hypertension, cerebral vascular spasm, myocardial infarction, menstrual cramps, premature labor, as prophylaxis for sudden death, and to increase the fibrillation threshold, and to improve the neurological deficits that are due to spasm following subarachnoid hemorrhage associated with ruptured congenital intracranial aneurysm.

Since the calcium-channel blockers do have different pharmacologic action, the specific uses of these drugs differ. Verapamil (Calan, Isoptin) has the most pronounced effect on AV node conduction and is the drug of choice for patients with supraventricular tachycardias with or without anginal symptoms. About 60%–80% of patients with supraventricular tachycardia convert to normal sinus rhythm within ten minutes after receiving verapamil. Also, because of its negative inotropic effect, it is an effective antihypertensive agent.

Nifedipine (Procardia, Adalat) is the most potent peripheral vasodilator but has little effect on the SA and AV nodes. It is preferred in patients with angina (all types) and coexisting sinus bradycardia, as well as cerebral spasm. It is used for prophylaxis of migraine headache. Nifedipine, although not approved, is being used to reduce blood pressure in hypertensive emergencies (sublingual dosing) in postoperative patients who are NPO with elevated blood pressure; to treat primary pulmonary hypertension and asthma; to decrease uterine contractions in premature labor; to reduce symptoms of cardiomyopathy and Raynaud's syndrome; and to relieve severe pain caused by obstruction of the bile duct or urinary tract.

Diltiazem (Cardizem) is used to manage variant angina to reduce anginal attacks and improve exercise performance. Diltiazem is also being used experimentally to treat essential hypertension.

Nicardipine (Cardene) is currently recommended for treatment of effort-associated chronic stable angina, either alone or with beta blockers and it is used for the management of essential hypertension alone or with other antihypertensives. Whether it offers any advantage over previously available calcium-channel blockers remains to be established.

Pharmacokinetics

ABSORPTION AND DISTRIBUTION. The calcium-channel blockers are all similar in that they are about 90% absorbed after oral administration. Bioavailability is different with verapamil at 10%–35% nifedipine at 45%–70%, diltiazem at 40%–67% and nicardipine at 35%. All have a rapid onset of action in 20–30 minutes and take 0.5–3 hours to reach peak serum levels. All are well-bound to plasma proteins. Specific information can be found in Table 31–2.

BIOTRANSFORMATION AND EXCRETION. All calcium-channel blockers are subject to extensive first-pass effect and converted to different metabolites (verapamil–norverapamil; nifedipine–acid or lactone; diltiazem–desacetyl diltiazem). Half-lives vary from two to seven hours. Only a small amount of drug is excreted unchanged in the urine.

Adverse Effects

Adverse effects are discussed in Table 31–2 and are summarized for each drug later in this chapter.

Interactions

The calcium-channel blocker verapamil interacts with β-adrenergic blockers, since they both have negative inotropic and chronotropic effects. This may be beneficial, but it could also be detrimental to cardiac function. Cimetidine may increase the bioavailability of calcium-channel blockers because of decreased first-pass hepatic metabolism. Digoxin levels may increase with calcium-channel blocker therapy; therefore, digoxin levels need to be monitored closely.

Verapamil

CONTRAINDICATIONS AND PRECAUTIONS. Verapamil is contraindicated in patients hypersensitive to verapamil and also in patients with sick sinus syndrome except with a functioning pacer. Verapamil is contraindicated in patients with cardiogenic shock and severe CHF because of its negative inotropic effect.

Verapamil is given cautiously in hypotensive patients because of its negative inotropic effect. It is also given cautiously in patients with hepatic and renal dysfunction, since the liver and kidney are the organs of biotransformation and excretion.

ADVERSE EFFECTS. Adverse effects of verapamil are generally not serious and rarely require discontinuation of therapy. The most common adverse effects include constipation (6%–8%), nausea (2%–3%), dizziness (4%), hypotension (3%), and possible development of CHF (1%–2%). Verapamil has also been associated with unilateral gynecomastia in men.

INTERACTION. Calcium salts and vitamin D may decrease effectiveness of verapamil because of potential antagonism. Verapamil may decrease lithium levels, thus possibly aggravating the condition that is being treated with lithium. Antihypertensive drugs used in conjunction with quinidine and verapamil may have an acute hypotensive effect. Verapamil may increase serum theophylline level, and theophylline toxicity may result. Since verapamil is highly bound, caution should be taken when coadministering other highly bound drugs like warfarin and oral hypoglycemics.

DOSAGE. Verapamil is administered orally in initial doses of 40–120 mg tid to treat angina. To manage dysrhythmias, doses range from 240 to 480 mg/day in three to four divided doses. Hypertension is treated with doses of 240 mg in divided doses up to 360 mg/day. A sustained-release tablet (240 mg) is administered with food, usually in the morning. IV verapamil is also available, and dosing is listed in Table 31–2.

Nifedipine

CONTRAINDICATIONS AND PRECAUTIONS. Nifedipine is contraindicated in hypersensitivity. It is given cautiously to patients who are hypotensive. Because nifedipine decreases peripheral vascular resistance, careful monitoring of blood pressure during initial administration and titration is suggested. Close observation is especially recommended for patients already taking medications that are known to lower blood pressure, such as β blockers and nitrates. Nifedipine is given cautiously in persons with hepatic dysfunction because of its high first-pass effect. If there is hepatic dysfunction, more drug is allowed to circulate and there may be an increased incidence of side or toxic effects. Renal dysfunction may also increase nifedipine levels.

ADVERSE EFFECTS. Adverse effects occur in a large percentage of patients and originate in either the cardiovascular system or the CNS. Rarely do these patients require discontinuation of the medication. The cardiovascular symptoms include hypotension (5%), stimulation of SA node (2%), flushing (10%–12%), peripheral edema (10%–12%), and headache (10%–12%). The CNS symptoms include dizziness and lightheadedness (10%–12%), headache (10%–12%), weakness and shakiness (8%), and nervousness (2 percent). The combination of dizziness, flushing, heat sensation, and headache is reported in 25% of patients. Nifedipine can also cause a *noncardiac dependent peripheral edema*, which is easily treated with diuretics. Nifedipine has recently been associated with unilateral gynecomastia in men.

INTERACTIONS. In addition to the general interactions of all calcium-channel blockers, nifedipine also may interact with high doses of fentanyl during coronary artery surgery, resulting in severe hypotension or increased fluid volume requirements. Concurrent administration of antihypertensives and quinidine can cause acute hypotension. Theophylline levels may increase when this drug is given concurrently with nifedipine. Use caution when mixing calcium-channel blockers with β-blockers, since there is an increased risk of hypotension, exacerbations of angina, or precipitation of CHF.

DOSAGE. Oral dosage of nifedipine is 10–30 mg administered every six to eight hours. Doses above 120 mg/day are rarely necessary. Dosage is increased every 7–14 days. Nifedipine can also be administered sublingually. In order to do this, the contents of the liquid-filled oral capsule are withdrawn into a syringe and then placed under the tongue, or the capsule can be poked with a needle or bitten and the liquid squeezed under the tongue, or cut and squeezed under the tongue. Recent research indicates that biting the capsule and then swallowing it with water causes the fastest and the highest peak plasma level, whereas the sublingual route proved the slowest and resulted in the lowest peak blood levels. There currently is not a commercially available sublingual or IV preparation for nifedipine.

Diltiazem

CONTRAINDICATIONS AND PRECAUTIONS. Diltiazem is contraindicated in patients with sick sinus syndrome, except those with functional ventricular pacemaker. It is also contraindicated in patients with second- or third-degree heart block and in patients who have hypotension with systolic pressure of less than 90 mmHg.

Diltiazem should be used cautiously in patients with congestive heart failure and hepatic dysfunction. It has not been satisfactorily evaluated in pregnancy and in children.

ADVERSE EFFECTS. Diltiazem is well-tolerated by most patients. The most common adverse effects include dizziness (4%), constipation (6%–8%), hypotension (3%), edema (2.5%), and nausea (2%–3%). CHF and bradycardia are likely to occur when diltiazem is given concurrently with β-blockers.

INTERACTIONS. Diltiazem shares the same interactions as with the other calcium-channel blockers. In addition, carbamazepine may increase inhibition of hepatic metabolism. Diltiazem and lithium act synergistically, and neurotoxicity can occur. Concurrent diltiazem and cyclosporine increases serum creatinine level and increases the danger of kidney failure.

DOSAGE. Diltiazem is administered in oral doses of 30–120 mg three times a day before meals to a maximal dose of 360 mg daily.

Nicardipine Hydrochloride

ACTION. The primary action of nicardipine hydrochloride (Cardene) is similar to the other calcium channel blockers. Specifically, nicardipine decreases his-purkinje conduction has a mixed effect on the AV node, increases the heart rate, improves cardiac output, and decreases peripheral vascular resistance.

DOSAGE. The initial dose of nicardipine to treat both angina and hypertension is 20 mg three times a day. At least three days should elapse before increasing the dose. The range is usually 20 to 40 mg three times a day. To assess blood pressure accurately, measure eight hours after dosing. When renal or hepatic impairment exists, dosage is reduced to 20 mg two times a day.

Nimodipine

USE. Nimodipine (Nimotop) improves neurological deficits that are due to spasm following sub-arachnoid hemorrhage (SAH) from rupture and congenital intracranial aneurysms in patients who are in good neurological condition post-ictus. Nimodipine has greater effect on cerebral arteries than the other calcium-channel blockers, possibly because it is highly fat soluble which allows it to cross the blood-brain barrier more readily. The exact mechanisms of action of nimodipine is unknown at this time. Nimodipine is started within 96 hours after SAH and continued for 21 days.

PHARMACOKINETICS. After oral administration, nimodipine reaches a peak serum level in about one hour and has a duration of action of three to four hours. Nimodipine is 95 percent protein bound. Nimodipine has a half-life of one to two hours. It is biotransformed in the liver and is excreted less than one percent unchanged in the urine.

CONTRAINDICATIONS AND PRECAUTIONS. Nimodipine is administered cautiously to patients with liver disease. There are no well-controlled studies in pregnant women, so it is used during pregnancy only if the benefit clearly outweighs the risks. Nimodipine does appear in breast milk so nursing should be discontinued.

ADVERSE EFFECTS. The most common side effects of nimodipine include headache and hypotension. Since it acts as a calcium-channel blocker, there is also a vasodilating effect in the periphery and some peripheral edema and flushing are experienced. Patients also ex-

perience diarrhea, nausea, vomiting, and abdominal cramps.

INTERACTIONS. Nimodipine administered concurrently with beta adrenergic and other calcium-channel blockers may enhance the negative chronotropic and inotropic effects. Nimodipine may also falsely elevate serum glucose, LDH, and alkaline phosphates.

DOSAGE. Nimodipine is started within 96 hours of SAH in patients who are neurologically intact. The usual dose is 60 mg every four hours, administered for 21 days. If the patient is unable to swallow the capsule, the liquid can be aspirated from the capsule and injected down a nasogastric tube. The tube is then flushed with 30 ml of normal saline.

USING THE NURSING PROCESS—CORONARY VASODILATORS

ASSESSMENT

Assessment of the patient requiring coronary vasodilators always begins with a thorough history to develop the data base needed for preparation of the nursing care plan. Information the nurse obtains is included in Table 31–5. A family history of coronary artery disease or any other vascular disease is obtained. If the patient has been or is currently taking coronary vasodilators, it is important to learn how and when they are taken, how many are being taken per day, how they are stored, and whether the patient experiences any side effects. The nursing history is particularly important for patients with angina because much of the nursing care is aimed at educating the patient about the condition and ways to prevent attacks.

It is important that the nurse have a thorough understanding of anginal pain in order to assist the patient in assessing the pain and in differentiating it from gastrointestinal discomfort or from more serious cardiac conditions. The pain is usually related to physical exertion or great emotion such as anger or sexual arousal. The pain may be accompanied by nausea, diaphoresis, and dyspnea. The nurse assists the patient in describing the pain, its duration, precipitating causes, and relief mechanisms to differentiate it from other diseases that produce chest pain.

The nurse also assesses the occupation and the amount of physical and psychologic stress to which the patient is exposed. Life-style, hobbies, exercise habits, and eating habits are also assessed, since they may need to be modified during the intervention phase.

The nurse also needs to assess whether the patient is physically able to measure the ointment or apply and remove the patches. Patients with physicial handicaps such as arthritis may not be able to manage their medication application.

Table 31–5. NURSING PROCESS FOR PATIENT REQUIRING CORONARY VASODILATORS

Assessment
Note history of past/present illness, including number of pain attacks per day, pain history, precipitating factors, and how patient currently seeks relief from pain. Determine drug use (OTC, prescription, street drugs, smoking, caffeine). Assess emotional and psychologic significance of illness. Note lifestyle factors, e.g., current level of activity, eating habits.

Nursing Diagnosis	Nursing Actions	Rationale	Desired Outcomes Evaluation Criteria
Pain, related to decreased myocardial blood flow, increased cardiac workload/oxygen consumption as evidenced by verbal complaints, grimacing, muscle tension, restlessness, narrowed focus.	Place patient at complete rest during anginal episodes.	Reduces myocardial oxygen demand to minimize risk of tissue injury/necrosis.	Verbalizes relief of pain. Reports anginal episodes decreased in frequency, duration and severity.
	Monitor vital signs every 5 minutes during anginal attack.	Blood pressure may rise initially due to sympathetic stimulation, then fall if cardiac output is compromised.	
	Stay with patient experiencing pain or appearing anxious.	Anxiety increases the release of catecholamines which increases the myocardial workload and can intensify/prolong ischemic attack. Presence of nurse can reduce feelings of fear and helplessness.	
	Administer anti-anginal medications promptly e.g., Nitroglycerin; Long-acting (Nitra-Dur);	Rapid vasodilator used to prevent as well as abort anginal attacks. Reduces frequency and severity of attack by producing prolonged/continuous vasodilation.	
	Beta-Blockers (Tenormin).	Reduces angina by decreasing heart rate and systolic blood pressure.	
	Provide supplemental oxygen as indicated.	May increase oxygen available for myocardial uptake/reversal of ischemia.	
Knowledge deficit related to lack of exposure, inaccurate/misinterpretation of information, as evidenced by questions, request for information, statement of concern, inaccurate followthrough of instructions.	Review pathophysiology of condition. Stress need for preventing anginal attacks and progression of atherosclerotic process.	Therapeutic management reduces likelihood of myocardial infarction.	Participates in learning process. Verbalizes understanding of condition/disease process and treatment. Participates in treatment regimen and initiates necessary lifestyle changes.
	Encourage avoidance of factors/situations that may precipitate anginal episode, e.g., emotional stress, physical exertion, ingestion of large/heavy meal, exposure to extremes in temperature.	May reduce incidence/severity of ischemic episodes.	
	Review importance of weight control, cessation of smoking, dietary changes, exercise. Encourage patient to follow prescribed reconditioning program, caution to avoid exhaustion.	Knowledge of the significance of risk factors provides patient with opportunity to make needed changes. Fear of triggering attacks may cause patient to avoid participation in activity which has been pre-	

Table 31–5. NURSING PROCESS FOR PATIENT REQUIRING CORONARY VASODILATORS-*CONTINUED*

Nursing Diagnosis	Nursing Actions	Rationale	Desired Outcomes Evaluation Criteria
		scribed to increase myocardial strength and form collateral circulation.	
	Discuss impact of illness on desired lifestyle and activities, including work, driving, sexual activity, and hobbies.	May be reluctant to resume/continue usual activities because of fear of anginal attack/death.	
	Demonstrate/encourage patient to monitor own pulse during activities.	Allows patient to identify how activities can be modified to avoid increased cardiac stress.	
	Discuss steps to take when anginal attacks occur, e.g., cessation of activity, administration of prn medication, use of relaxation techniques.	Being prepared for an event takes away the fear that patient will not know what to do if attack occurs. Promotes a sense of control.	
	Discuss proper times, doses, and medications for control/prevention of anginal attacks.	Angina is a complicated illness which often requires the use of many drugs given to decrease myocardial workload and control the occurrence of attacks.	
	Review ways to deal with possible side effects, e.g., headache, dizziness, (hypotension).	Reduces risk of injury, may enhance cooperation with therapeutic regimen.	
	Identify symptoms to be reported to physician, e.g., increase in frequency/duration of attacks, changes in reponse to medications.	Knowledge of expectations can avoid undue concern for insignificant reasons or delay in treatment of important symptoms.	
	Stress importance of not discontinuing drug without physician's knowledge.	Sudden cessation may result in rebound ischemic pain.	
Adjustment, impaired, potential related to disability requiring change in lifestyle, assault to self-esteem, altered locus of control.	Promote discussion of fears. Encourage participation of SO in discussions and planning for necessary diet, medication and lifestyle changes.	Recognizing and experiencing these feelings may help the patient to begin to deal effectively with situation. Inclusion of SO can provide support for the patient.	Initiates lifestyle changes that will assist adaptation to required treatment regimen.
	Review limitations of individual situation and importance of regular exercise program.	Modification of activities and exercise program may improve exercise tolerance. Discussion may reduce frustration and anxiety.	

The nurse may assist with the collection of blood for studies to determine the presence of myocardial damage (CPK, SGOT, LDH) and with electrocardiograms (ECGs) to determine the presence of changes indicative of angina. The nurse may also prepare patients for exercise tests to determine how much work they can perform. Patients may also have additional diagnostic studies such as echocardiograms, radioimmune assay studies, and angiograms.

NURSING DIAGNOSES

The nursing diagnoses, developed from the information obtained in the original assessment, become the basis for nursing care and later become the criteria used to evaluate the nursing intervention. Typical nursing diagnoses for a patient requiring coronary vasodilators are included in Table 31–5.

INTERVENTION

The goals of the nursing intervention are primarily to educate the patient and to reduce the number and severity of symptoms. The data base formulated during the initial health history is used to develop the teaching plan. Typical goals of intervention for a patient requiring coronary vasodilators are included in Table 31–5.

NURSING RESPONSIBILITIES

The nurse, in a hospital situation, has several responsibilities when administering coronary vasodilators. When they are administered during an acute attack, the nurse records the type of pain, its radiation, its precipitating factors, its duration, and how long before relief was obtained.

When ordered, the patient with acute angina should have a supply of nitroglycerin tablets at the bedside, to be restocked as necessary. When transferring medication from stock, make sure hands are dry, since moisture hastens deterioration of the drug. Transfer into an amber-colored bottle. The patient is told to notify the nurse whenever a tablet is taken so the nurse can assess the patient's physical condition and chart administration.

When administering IV nitroglycerin, the nurse needs to know what concentration to mix for the solution. The solution is made by mixing nitroglycerin in either D_5W or NS in a concentration of 25–500 μg/ml. After determining whether to use low-dose (5–50 μg/min) or high-dose (50–100 μg/min) therapy, the nurse is responsible for titrating the medication upward every 3–5 minutes, after assessing blood pressure and pulse. If low-dose therapy is being used, nitroglycerin is titrated by increments of 10–20 μg and if high-dose therapy is being used, nitroglycerin is titrated by 20–50 μg. Low-dose therapy is used for preload reduction, whereas high-dose therapy has a balanced effect on preload and afterload. The dose is titrated to achieve a specific end result: a reduction and/or elimination of chest pain, a change in the ECG, or a lowering of blood pressure. The nurse needs to know the hemodynamic parameter ranges that the patient is to be kept within during therapy.

If a sudden decrease in filling pressure in the left ventricle occurs following a large decline in systolic pressure (defined by a 30–40-mmHg drop in blood pressure within five minutes), temporarily stop the nitroglycerin infusion. Monitor blood pressure every two to three minutes. When the blood pressure recovers, the nitroglycerin is restarted at half the previous rate. The greatest hemodynamic changes are usually seen initially and up to one hour after relief of chest pain.

When a patient is ready to be weaned from IV nitroglycerin, the rate of titration is often left to the discretion of the nurse. The average weaning interval is 5–10 μg every 15 minutes. A blood pressure and pulse check are performed before each change. Any return of chest pain or rebound hypertension will prohibit weaning, and the physician is consulted. When weaning is complete, the effect of nitroglycerin will remain for 30–60 minutes.

PATIENT TEACHING

General information concerning coronary vasodilators needed in the teaching plan for each patient is included in Table 31–6.

Table 31–6. PATIENT TEACHING INFORMATION—CORONARY VASODILATORS

Dear Patient:
This drug has been prescribed for you. This is what you should know about your drug to get the most from your therapy.

1. Nitrates are used to prevent or treat angina pectoris (chest pain of effect).
2. Coronary vasodilators (nitrates) may be taken for the rest of your life.
3. Several forms of nitrates are available. The following instructions will include specific directions for each form of nitrate.

SHORT-ACTING PRODUCTS
Take short-acting coronary vasodilators at the first sign of pain.

Place nitroglycerin tablet under the tongue, let it dissolve, and hold saliva in the mouth for 1–2 min before swallowing. When pain is relieved, the remaining tablet is expelled from mouth.

You may take a total of 3 nitroglycerin tablets (1 tablet every 5 min) for any single attack of chest pain. If the pain is **not** relieved, you should **immediately** seek medical attention, since you may be having a heart attack.

Sit 15–20 min after taking the tablet to prevent dizziness or faintness and to help relieve the discomfort.

You may take nitroglycerin 3–5 min before beginning any activity known to trigger an attack, such as exercise or sexual intercourse. The vasodilating effects will usually be sufficient to prevent chest pain during the activity.

Medications should be kept in their original container because they lose their potency when exposed to heat, light, moisture, or other organic and inorganic materials such as cotton or paper. Note the expiration date on the bottle and refill as needed. If the medication is stored tightly closed in its original container, it is stable for approximately 5 months.

Nitroglycerin, translingual—At the onset of an attack or 10–15 min prior to an activity known to cause angina, spray 1–2 metered doses into the mouth. *Do not inhale spray.* Take no more than three metered doses in 15 min.

LONG-ACTING PRODUCTS
Take long-acting coronary vasodilators at the correct prescribed time intervals to keep a constant blood level. These products will not relieve acute anginal attacks.

Table 31–6. PATIENT TEACHING INFORMATION—CORONARY VASODILATORS-*CONTINUED*

Generally, long-acting medications can be taken with or between meals (pentaerythritol tentranitrate should be taken only between meals).

Tablets or capsules are swallowed whole and not crushed or opened.

Nitropaste—When using nitroglycerin paste, squeeze the paste onto the special application paper supplied by the manufacturer, and use the paper, not the fingers, to spread the ointment. Apply the special medicated paper to the skin, but do not rub into the skin. The medication can be applied anywhere on the body surface. Always remove the old paper and wash and dry the skin before the new dose is applied. Sites are rotated to help prevent skin irritation. Plastic wrap may also be applied over the special paper to prevent staining of the clothes and to increase absorption. If plastic wrap is used, skin irritation may occur.

The paste is kept tightly closed and stored in a cool place.

Nitro Patches—Apply patch once daily to clean, dry skin. Remove old patch and wash skin with soap and water to remove nitroglycerin.

Nitroglycerin, transmucosal—Place tablet between cheek and gum after eating. A glue forms that holds tablet in place. Tongue movement may dislodge tablet. Drinking hot fluids may increase dissolution of tablet. Remove tablet at bedtime.

Do not take coronary vasodilators with alcohol because of the possibility of lowering your blood pressure.

Always check with your physician or pharmacist before taking other medications because interaction between drugs may occur.

If a dose is forgotten, no attempt should be made to "catch up."

Do not suddenly stop coronary vasodilators without the physician's permission because of the possibility of a rebound in the number and severity of the attacks. If you are to discontinue taking coronary vasodilators, the dose will be gradually reduced over a period of time.

If you experience side effects such as dizziness, or faintness, recovery is speeded if the head is lowered and deep breathing is started. Also, a mild headache is common; but if it is severe and lasts longer than 15–20 min, the physician should be notified. The dose may have to be altered.

Nitroglycerin is not habit-forming, and you can take as many as needed during the day within reason (see above). **However,** any change in the number or severity of anginal attacks should be reported to your physician.

Carry the medication with you at all times.

Carry a medication information card to indicate that you are taking coronary vasodilators.

Inform your dentist and any other physician that you are taking coronary vasodilators.

Tell your family where the medication is kept in case you need it urgently.

It is important for the patient to be taught how to administer the nitroglycerin product correctly. The sublingual tablet, used for acute attacks of angina, are dissolved under the tongue. When the pain is relieved, the remaining tablet is removed from the mouth. Sublingual tablets are taken at the first sign of chest pain or five to ten minutes prior to an activity that is known to cause chest pain. Three tablets can be taken at five-minute intervals. If the pain is not relieved or changed, the patient should come to the hospital to be evaluated. The translingual spray is also used for acute attacks. It is sprayed onto the oral mucosa and should not be inhaled.

The sustained-release nitroglycerin tablets are swallowed whole and are not crushed or chewed. Transmucosal tablets are placed between the buccal pouch and the upper lip. The tablet creates a small glue that holds the tablet in place. The tablet is used after meals, since eating or moving the tongue vigorously may dislodge the tablet. Hot liquids may increase dissolution.

Patches are applied to clean hairless skin once a day. When the old patch is removed, the skin is washed with soap and water to remove any remaining nitroglycerin. All patches can be worn while bathing, showering, or swimming.

Ointments are placed on the correct paper, which comes with the ointment. The ointment is spread to a thin layer using an applicator, not the finger. The papers are covered with tape. Plastic wrap may be used to cover the paper, but this may increase the likelihood of skin irritation. When the paper is removed, the skin is washed with soap and water to remove all remaining nitroglycerin. If a nurse or family member is applying the ointment, care is taken not to get any ointment on their skin as this could precipitate a headache.

Nitroglycerin tablets need to be carried by the patient at all times. The bottle should not be carried close to the body to avoid body heat. The medication is best carried in a jacket pocket or handbag in the original container. Potency of the drug is indicated by a burning or stinging sensation under the tongue. However, newer, more stable preparations usually do not produce this effect. Much of the literature that supports the concept of "no burning, no efficacy" is based on a single study published in 1972. The date of publication suggests that the sublingual nitroglycerin was the conventional type without a stabilizer (Kutsop, J., 1986).

Also, the patient needs to understand the need to avoid alcoholic beverages while taking nitrates, because of a shock-like syndrome that may occur. Symptoms including flushing, weakness, pallor, hypotension, and syncope.

EVALUATION

In order to evaluate the patient's response to treatment, the nurse establishes evaluation criteria, based on the goals that both the nurse and the patient have developed previously. Successful outcome goals for the patient requiring coronary vasodilators are included in Table 31–5.

When the patient first returns home after the initial diagnosis, it is important to have him or her keep a written record of angina attacks. The list should include information such as predisposing factors, time of day, number of attacks per day, how relief was sought, and the adverse effects, if any, encountered from the coronary vasodilators. This chart is reviewed by the physician and nurse at frequent intervals to evaluate the success or failure of the prescribed treatment regimen.

The nurse discusses potential adverse effects of coronary vasodilators with the patient. The most common adverse effects include flushing, hypotension, and headache. Flushing often subsides by itself in three to five minutes. Hypotension and its resulting dizziness or faintness can be alleviated by sitting or lying down when the medication is taken and then for an additional 15–20 minutes. The headaches should subside spontaneously in three to five minutes. One common reason for noncompliance is a persistent, severe, and long-lasting headache. The intensity of these headaches can be decreased by having the physician reduce the dose.

In a recent study, the severity of headache or flushing was unrelated to any of the following factors: sex, skin color, activity level, body weight for height, drug dose, order of site rotation, previous exposure to other forms of NTG, other medications, hemodynamic parameters, medical diagnosis, or length of NTG regimen. In fact, the only predictor of a side effect was age: patients in their thirties were significantly more likely than older patients to report severe flushing.

Overcompliance, taking more than the prescribed number of tablets a day, is rarely a problem with coronary vasodilators because of the resulting headaches that are experienced. The nurse must make sure the patient understands that he or she may not take more than three short-acting nitroglycerin tablets for any angina attack. If the pain still persists at the same intensity, the patient needs to seek immediate medical attention.

Tolerance was already discussed as a problem with sustained and chronic use of coronary vasodilators. Several suggested solutions to the problem of developing nitroglycerin tolerance with the use of transdermal delivery system include higher doses of nitroglycerin delivered per 24-hour period and wearing patches intermittently for various time periods. These and other possibilities are now being tested in clinical trials.

The nurse often helps to evaluate the effectiveness of nitroglycerin paste by taking a baseline pulse and blood pressure reading and then repeating both one hour after medication administration. An effective dose decreases the blood pressure by 10 mmHg or increases the pulse rate by ten beats compared with resting values.

All general points of health teaching, which have been discussed previously, are reviewed and updated with the patient to ensure that his or her knowledge base remains accurate.

Both pharmacologic and surgical treatments are effective in controlling symptoms in patients with unstable angina pectoris. Their relative effects on survival are less clear. A recent multicenter prospective study reviewed 468 patients with unstable angina pectoris that were randomly assigned to medical or surgical intervention. No difference in the two-year survival rates or incidence of nonfatal myocardial infarction was found between patients with unstable angina pectoris treated medically

or with coronary bypass. However, patients with reduced left ventricular ejection fraction had a better outcome when treated with surgery.

PERIPHERAL VASODILATORS

Peripheral vasodilators are similar to the coronary vasodilators in that they increase the diameter of the blood

Table 31–7. PERIPHERAL VASCULAR DISEASE

DEFINITION
Disorders that diminish the supply of blood to the periphery.
CHRONIC OCCLUSIVE TYPE:
Buergers disease (thromboangiitis obliterans)
Arterial embolism/thrombosis
Cardiovascular disease
Etiology:
Reduced blood flow due to organic obstruction
Symptoms:
Objective:
  Coldness
  Trophic change (dry, scaly skin, loss of hair, hard, thickened nails)
  Decreased pulses
  Ulcers
  Gangrene
Subjective:
  Numbness
  Tingling
  Burning
  Pain
Treatment:
Supportive
Reduction of smoking
Reduction of risk factors
Surgery (sympathectomy, angioplasty, vessel grafting, endartectomy)
Vasodilators (not usually helpful)
VASOSPASTIC TYPE:
Raynaud's disease
Acrocyanosis
Primary livedo reticularis
Etiology:
Abnormally small digital blood vessels constrict with increased sympathetic stimulation. Drugs (β-adrenergic blockers).
Symptoms:
Objective:
  Coldness
  Dependent rubor
  Decreased pulses
Subjective:
  Numbness
  Tingling
  Burning
  Pain
Treatment:
Vasodilators
Reduction of risk factors
Elimination of exposure to temperature extremes
Support
Reduction of smoking
Surgery (sympathectomy)

vessel, which ultimately improves blood flow to distal tissues. These medications, however, are used to dilate blood vessels in the periphery or the cerebral circulation, or both, in arteries and veins.

Peripheral vasodilators are used to treat tissue ischemia in the specific vascular beds of the skin, skeletal muscles, and CNS. (See Chapter 23 for more information on cerebral vascular disease.) They are used primarily to reduce the vasospasm that occurs in disorders like Raynaud's disease. They may also be used, with limited value, in patients with peripheral vascular disease (Table 31–7) or cerebral vascular disease.

ACTION

Peripheral vasodilators act to dilate blood vessels in several ways. First, they act directly on and have a nonspecific relaxant effect on the vascular smooth muscle wall, resulting in dilation. This effect is independent of the sympathetic nervous system. They are not potent vasodilators when given orally, and their efficacy in peripheral vascular disease has not been established. Sec-

ond, they can stimulate β-receptors, which results in sympathetically medicated relaxation of the smooth muscle surrounding vessels. (β-adrenergic stimulation causes vasodilation.) Third, they can block α-adrenergic stimulation, which causes vasoconstriction. The relative sites of action are shown in Figure 31–3. The specific medication groups are outlined in Table 31–8 and include:

1. Direct-acting vasodilators including papaverine (Cerespan, Pavabid), ethaverine hydrochloride (Ethatab, Ethaquin), cyclandelate (Cyclospasmol), nicotinyl alcohol or tartrate (Roniacol), isoxsuprine hydrochloride (Vasodilan).
2. Sympathetic blocking agents:
   a. α-adrenergic blockers including phenoxybenzamine (Dibenzyline), reviewed in Chapter 19; and reserpine, guanethidine monosulfate (Ismelin), methyldopa (Aldomet, and prazosin hydrochloride (Minipress), reviewed in Chapter 29.

TEXT RESUMES ON PAGE 841

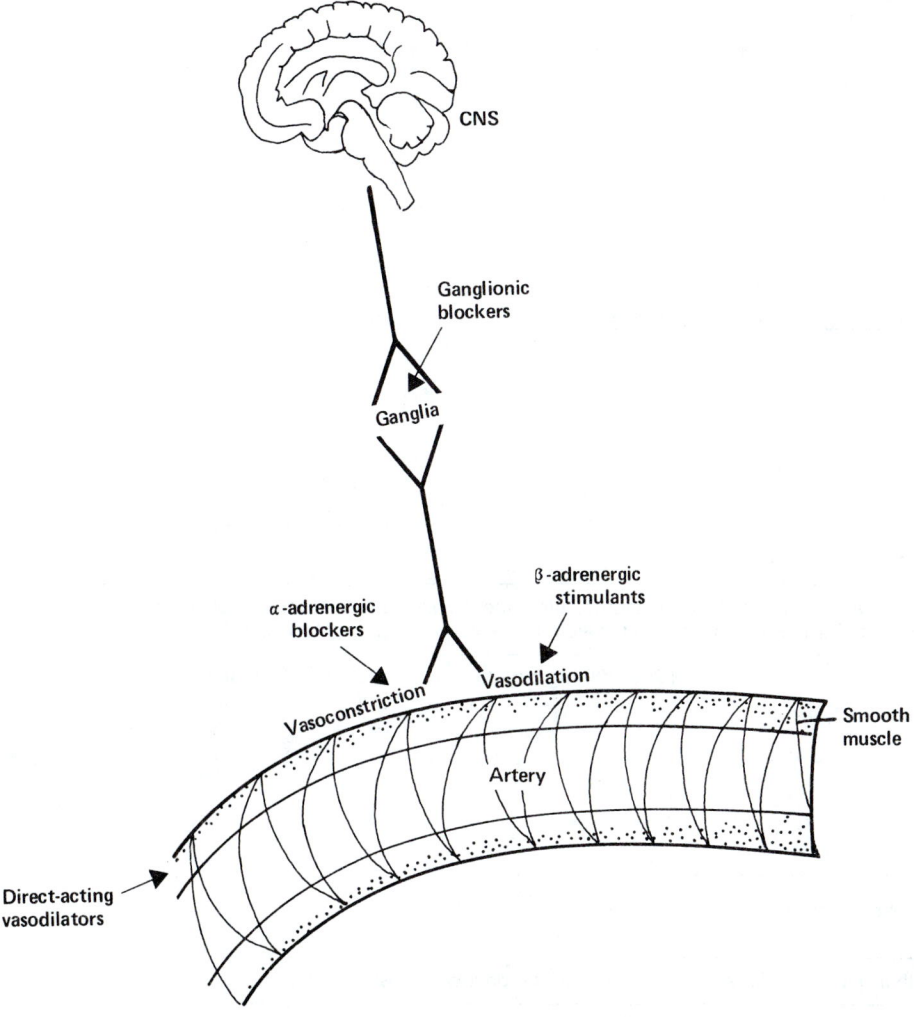

Figure 31–3. Site of action of peripheral vasodilators.

Table 31–8. PERIPHERAL VASODILATORS

Name	Dosage	Mode of Administration	Pharmacokinetics
DIRECT-ACTION VASODILATORS			
Action: act directly on the walls of the smooth muscle to cause vasodilation.			
Use: peripheral vascular disease.			
Papaverine (Pavabid)	100–300 mg 3–5 × daily	PO (cannot be crushed)	O: quickly P: 1–2 hr D: 6 hr ½L: 6 hr PB: 90% B: liver E: urine
	150–300 mg q 12 hr (timed-released) (poorly and erratically absorbed)	PO	D: 12 hr
	30–120 mg q 3 hr (IV slowly over 2 min)	IM, IV	O: immediate
Ethaverine hydrochloride (Etha-quin)	100–200 mg tid	PO	UA
Cyclandelate (Cyclospasmol)			
Use: as with all and arteriosclerosis obliterans, intermittent claudication, thrombophlebitis, nocturnal leg cramps, Raynaud's disease, and selected persons with cerebral vascular disease.			
	M 200–400 mg bid/qid	PO (can be crushed)	O: 15 min P: 1–1.5 hr D: 3–4 hr
Nicotinyl alcohol or tartrate (Roniacol)			
Use: as with all plus vascular spasm, varicose ulcers, decubitis ulcers, chilblains.			
	50–100 mg 3 × daily	PO (can be crushed)	O: 5–10 min D: 10–60 min

Key to Abbreviations in the *Pharmacokinetcs* column O-onset; P-peak; D-duration; PB-protein bound; B-bio-transformed in; E-excreted in; ½L-halflife.
*Within the column listing adverse effects, underlines indicate the most common effects; CAPITALS indicate life-threatening effects.

Contraindications/ Precautions	Adverse Effects*	Interactions	Nursing Implications
Contraindicated in AV block. Use cautiously in glaucoma, liver disease, and depressed AV function. Safety in pregnancy, lactating women, and children not established.	Neuro: malaise, vertigo, drowsiness CV: increased blood pressure, flushing of face, tachycardia Resp: increased respiratory rate GI: nausea, abdominal distress, anorexia, constipation, diarrhea, hepatic hypersensitivity Integ: rash	May decrease effectiveness of levodopa, aggravating Parkinson's disease. May decrease blood pressure with antihypertensives.	ASSESSMENT: Assess vital signs closely during therapy. Obtain baseline liver studies and monitor frequently. INTERVENTION: Change body positions slowly to reduce the possibility of orthostatic hypotension. Limit alcohol intake because of the additive vasodilation effect. Most peripheral vasodilators will be accompanied by a feeling of warmth in the extremities. Patient should be taught not to miss a dose; but if a dose is missed, patient should **not** double the dose at the next time. IV administration is incompatible with Ringer's lactate solution—this combination forms a precipitate. EVALUATION: Notify physician if flushing, headache, sweating, skin rash, abdominal pain becomes pronounced.
Contraindicated in AV dissociation. Use with caution with glaucoma. Safety in pregnancy and children not established.	Neuro: malaise, vertigo, headache, drowsiness CV: hypotension, flushing, sweating, cardiac depression Resp: respiratory depression GI: nausea, vomiting, abdominal distress, dry throat	None known	INTERVENTION: Cautious use while performing tasks requiring alertness. EVALUATION: Notify physician if flushing, sweating, nausea, or vomiting becomes severe.
Contraindicated in hypersensitivity. Caution in severe coronary or cerebral vascular disease and glaucoma. Safety in pregnancy and lactating women not established.	Neuro: headache, weakness CV: tachycardia, dizziness, mild flushing GI: heartburn, pain, and eructation, nausea	None known	INTERVENTION: Administer with food or antacid (if prescribed) to reduce GI symptoms. Improvement may occur gradually over several months.

CONTINUED ON THE FOLLOWING PAGE

Table 31–8. PERIPHERAL VASODILATORS–*CONTINUED*

Drug	Dosage	Mode of Administration	Pharmacokinetics
Nicotinyl alcohol or tartrate–*Continued*	150–300 mg 2 × daily, timed-release	PO (do not crush)	O: 30 min D: 6–12 hr
Isoxsuprine hydrochloride (Vasodilan)	10–20 mg 3–4 × daily	PO (can be crushed)	P: 1 hr D: 3 hr

β-*ADRENERGIC STIMULANT*

Action: stimulate β_2 receptors in skeletal muscle, thus dilating arterioles and increasing cardiac output.

Use: peripheral vascular disease, atherosclerotic cerebral decrease, may relieve spasm of inner ear.

Nylidrin hydrochloride (Arlidin)	3–12 mg 3–4 × daily	PO	O: 10 min P: 30 min D: 2 hr

HEMORRHEOLOGIC AGENT:

Action: increases cellular ATP thus reduces red blood cell aggregation; stimulate prostacyclin formation and release, ultimately increasing platelet cAMP and decreasing platelet aggregation; increases fibrinolytic activity, thus reducing fibrinogen concentration.

Use: chronic occlusive peripheral arterial disease and intermittent claudication.

Pentoxifylline (Trental)	400 mg 3 × day with meals	PO	O: quickly P: 2–4 hr D: UA ½L: 0.4–0.8 hr PB: UA B: liver E: urine 4% feces

Key to Abbreviations in the *Pharmacokinetcs* column O-onset; P-peak; D-duration; PB-protein bound; B-biotransformed in; E-excreted in; ½L-halflife.
*Within the column listing adverse effects, underlines indicate the most common effects; CAPITALS indicate life-threatening effects.

Contraindications/ Precautions	Adverse Effects*	Interactions	Nursing Implications
Use with caution in bleeding tendencies, angina pectoris, and pregnancy.	Neuro: flushing of face and neck, tingling GI: GI upset Integ: pruritis, rash, urticaria.	Concurrent alcohol intake may potentiate vasodilation effect.	INTERVENTION: Administer before meals. Patients frequently experience flushing and increased feeling of warmth. Tolerance may develop after prolonged use.
Contraindicated immediately postpartum and in arterial bleeding. Safety in pregnancy has not been established.	Neuro: dizziness, weakness CV: hypotension, tachycardia, chest pain GI: nausea, vomiting, abdominal distress Integ: rash (if occurs, discontinued)	Terbutaline, ritodrine, and albuterol all have additive effect.	INTERVENTION: Change position slowly. Therapeutic effect may take several weeks. EVALUATION: Notify physician if flushing, palpitation, or rash becomes bothersome.
Contraindicated in recent myocardial infarction, angina, and thyrotoxicosis. Use cautiously in uncompensated CHF, or peptic ulcer. Safety in pregnancy not established.	Neuro: tremor, nervousness, weakness, dizziness CV: postural hypotension, palpitation GI: nausea, vomiting	May enhance effects of phenothiazines.	INTERVENTION: The effects may take several weeks to occur. Avoid sudden changes in posture. Observe caution while driving or performing tasks requiring alertness. EVALUATION: Report severe palpitations, nausea, vomiting, or nervousness to physician.
Contraindicated in hypersensitivity to xanthines. Safety in pregnancy, lactating women, and children not established.	Neuro: dizziness, headache, blurred vision, earache CV: angina/chest pain, edema Resp: epistaxis, flu-like symptoms GI: dyspepsia, nausea, vomiting, flatus, bad taste Integ: brittle fingernails	Prolongs PT with warfarin. Concurrent antihypertensives may lower blood pressure.	ASSESSMENT: Assess peripheral pulses and distance walked at the onset of therapy and periodically. Assess cognitive powers as well as memory. INTERVENTION: Administer with meals to reduce nausea and vomitng. EVALUATION: If exercise pain continues or worsens, notify physician.

     b. β-adrenergic stimulants, also called musculotropic agents, including nylidrin hydrochloride (Arlidin).

3. Calcium-channel blockers nifedipine (Procardia), reviewed earlier in this chapter.

Much controversy surrounds the usefulness of these classes of drugs. There is little evidence, if any, that indicates these drugs are effective in treating chronic occlusive vascular diseases. The use of vasodilator drugs in reversing or delaying the deleterious effects of acute or chronic obstruction is questionable. Peripheral vaso-dilators, by decreasing blood pressure (since this is one of the major determinants of flow in collateral vessels), can actually reduce flow in these areas. Furthermore, studies have shown that these drugs decrease flow to ischemic areas distal to the vascular occlusions. Therefore, the use of these agents in occlusive disorders is highly questionable. There is, however, some evidence to suggest that these drugs may be of modest benefit in patients with vasospastic disease such as Raynaud's disease.

DIRECT-ACTING VASODILATORS

The direct-acting vasodilators such as papaverine, ethaverine hydrochloride, cyclandelate, nicotinyl alcohol or tartrate, and isoxsuprine hydrochloride act directly on the walls of the smooth muscle to cause vasodilation. The efficiency of these medications administered orally in treating peripheral vascular disease has not yet been established in well-controlled clinical studies.

Papaverine

Papaverine (Pavabid, Cerespan) is an alkaloid derived from opium that lacks the tolerance, habituation, and analgesic effect seen with narcotics. Although papaverine has been used for many years to relieve a number of conditions such as cerebral and peripheral ischemia associated with arterial spasm, senile dementia, cerebral ischemia, and to produce vasodilation in some radiologic procedures, there is insufficient objective evidence of any therapeutic value. Papaverine is featured in Table 31–8.

Ethaverine Hydrochloride

Ethaverine hydrochloride (Ethaquin) is closely related to papaverine and has similar actions and uses. Ethaverine hydrochloride is used in peripheral and cerebral vascular insufficiency associated with arterial spasm. It is considered "possibly effective" by the FDA for these disorders and is discussed in Table 31–8.

Cyclandelate

Cyclandelate (Cyclospasmol) exerts a papaverine-like action on the peripheral vascular smooth muscle by a direct action. It is considered "possibly effective" by the FDA in increasing peripheral circulation of the extremities and digits, and elevates the skin temperature of the extremities. It is used as adjunctive therapy in arteriosclerosis obliterans, *intermittent claudication*, thrombophlebitis, nocturnal leg cramps, Raynaud's disease, and cerebral vascular disease in some patients. Cyclandelate is featured in Table 31–8.

Nicotinyl Alcohol or Tartrate

Nicotinyl alcohol or tartrate (Roniacol) is almost identical to niacin but has a more prolonged action. It produces vasodilation through a direct action on the blood vessels and is used in patients with deficient circulation, vascular spasm, varicose ulcers, decubital ulcers, and chilblains (frostbite). Again, there are no clinical studies that support its use in these disease states.

Isoxsuprine Hydrochloride

Isoxsuprine hydrochloride (Vasodilan) is a direct-acting peripheral vasodilator that acts as an α-adrenorecep-tor antagonist with β-adrenoreceptor stimulating properties.

Isoxsuprine produces direct relaxation on vascular and uterine smooth muscle. It is "possibly effective" for relief of symptoms associated with cerebral vascular insufficiency and peripheral vascular disease, according to the FDA. In controlled studies in patients with intermittent claudication caused by arteriosclerotic disease, isoxsuprine was shown to be ineffective. Isoxsuprine should not be used in patients with obstructive arterial disease. Isoxsuprine is used in the management of dysmenorrhea, premature labor, and threatened abortion, but efficacy has not been established. Isoxsuprine is reviewed in Table 31–8.

SYMPATHETIC BLOCKING AGENTS

The medications in this group block the sympathetic vasoconstrictor impulses, either through α-adrenergic blockade or by blocking the impulse at the ganglion. This allows β stimulation to occur unopposed, producing vasodilatation (Fig. 31–4).

α-Adrenergic Blockers

The α-adrenergic blocker phenoxybenzamine (Dibenzyline) acts selectively on the α-receptor sites to block the response of the sympathetic nervous stimulation caused by circulating catecholamines. Since α-receptors are more abundant in skin vessels than in the skeletal muscle vessels, blood flow to the skin is increased. These drugs are most effective in treating Raynaud's disease. They have little effect in treating chronic occlusive peripheral vascular disease. Phenoxybenzamine is featured in Chapter 19.

β-Adrenergic Stimulants

The β-adrenergic stimulants, such as nylidrin hydrochloride (Arlidin), stimulate β_2 receptor cells in skeletal muscle, thus dilating arterioles and increasing cardiac output. Nylidrin is rated as "possibly effective" by the FDA in reducing leg cramps and pain in patients with peripheral vascular diseases because it increases the amount of blood passing through the calf muscle. Clinical studies, however, have found no effect in patients with intermittent claudication. Nylidrin is also claimed to increase cerebral blood flow in patients with atherosclerotic cerebral arteries. It is also credited with relieving the spasms of arterioles in the inner ear, and it has been used to bring relief to patients suffering from vertigo, hearing difficulties, and tinnitus (ringing in the ears). Nylidrin is reviewed in Table 31–8.

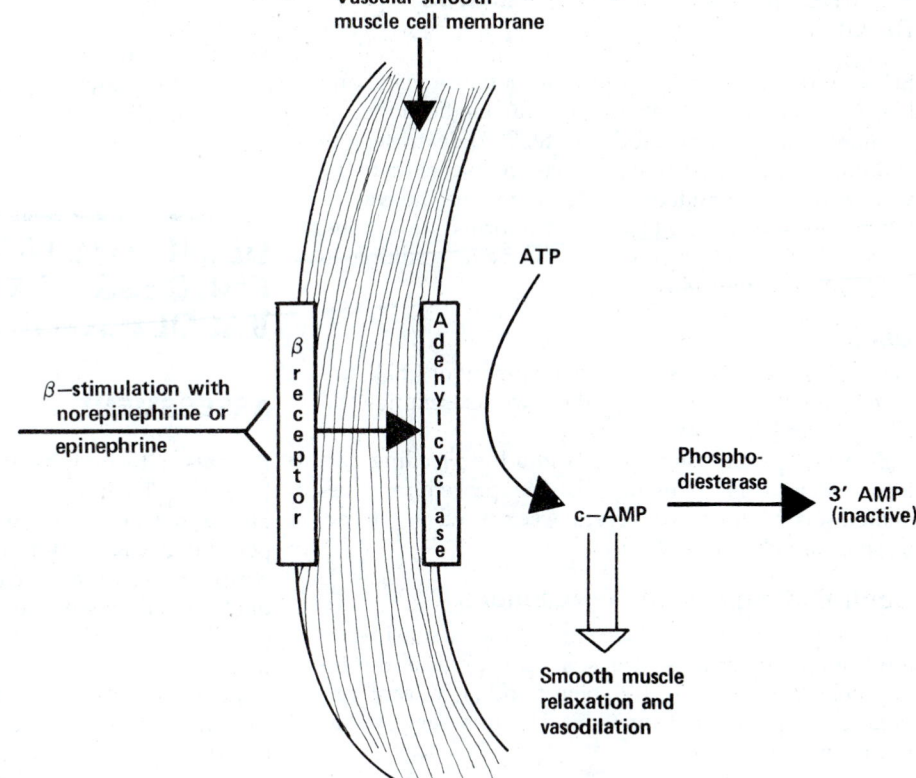

Figure 31–4. Norepineph-rine or epinephrine stimu-lates the beta receptor on the outside surface of the smooth muscle cell mem-brane. This activates adenyl cyclase, which converts ATP to cyclic adenosine mono-phosphate (cAMP), which causes the muscle to relax and produce vasodilation.

HEMORRHEOLOGIC AGENT

Pentoxifylline

Pentoxifylline (Trental) is a trisubstituted xanthine de-rivative for the treatment of intermittent claudication associated with chronic occlusive peripheral arterial dis-ease. Pentoxifylline produces dose-related hemorrheo-logic effects, lowering blood viscosity by reducing red blood cell and platelet aggregation and improving erythrocyte flexibility. The exact mechanism of action is unknown. Pentoxifylline increases cellular adenosine triphosphate (ATP) content, therefore affecting the red blood cells. It also stimulates prostacyclin formation and release, ultimately increasing platelet cAMP, thereby af-fecting the platelets. Pentoxifylline also increases blood fibrinolytic activity, thus reducing fibrinogen concentra-tion. Tissue perfusion and oxygenation is improved through a mild vasodilator effect.

PHARMACOKINETICS. Pentoxifylline is rapidly ab-sorbed after oral administration (food delays absorp-tion) and peaks in two to four hours. There is an exten-sive first-pass effect into active metabolites. The half-life is 0.4–0.8 hours for the parent drug and 1.0–1.6 hours for the metabolites. Pentoxifylline is excreted primarily in the urine.

CONTRAINDICATIONS AND PRECAUTIONS. Pentoxifylline is contraindicated in persons sensitive to other xanthine products (aminophylline, theophylline, and caffeine). It is used cautiously in chronic occlusive arterial disease, since patients with this disorder fre-quently show other manifestations of arteriosclerotic disease such as angina, hypotension, and dysrhythmias. Safety in pregnant and lactating women and in children has not been established.

ADVERSE EFFECTS. The most common adverse ef-fects are generally dose-related and include dyspepsia (2.8%), nausea (2.2%), and vomiting (1.2%). Taking the drug with meals may help prevent these symptoms. Other adverse effects involving the CNS or cardiovas-cular system are observed less frequently.

INTERACTION. Persons taking concurrent warfarin have had elevated prothrombin times, and there have been a few reports of bleeding. Patients who take con-current antihypertensives need to have periodic blood pressure monitoring as hypotension may occur.

DOSAGE. Pentoxifylline is administered in 400-mg doses with meals three times daily. Therapeutic effects may not occur for two to four weeks, and therapy should not be discontinued until at least eight weeks, unless adverse effects occur.

VENOUS DISORDERS

Several medical problems can occur in the veins, includ-ing varicose veins (incompetent valves), thrombophle-bitis (inflammation of the vein wall), and phlebothrom-bosis (a clot in the vein without inflammation).

SCLEROSING AGENTS FOR VENOUS DISORDERS

Sclerosing agents are used to treat varicose veins and bleeding esophageal varices. Several medications are available: sodium tetradecyl sulfate, 50% dextrose, and sodium morrhurate. These products are injected into the vein and cause irritation of the lining of the vessel, which tends to clot the blood, which forms a thrombus. Fibrous tissue develops within the vein, resulting in obliteration of the vein.

Uses

Sclerosing agents are used in the treatment of small, uncomplicated varicose veins of the lower extremities and to treat esophageal varices.

Sclerosing agents are injected into the bleeding varices under visual examination. The procedure is repeated several times over several weeks until all the varicosities are obliterated.

Contraindications and Precautions

The products are contraindicated in patients sensitive to any component of these drugs, acute superficial thrombophlebitis, uncontrolled diabetes, and significant valvular or deep-vein incompetence. Use in pregnancy has not been established.

Adverse Effects

When sodium morrhuate is used, local effects at the injection site may occur such as burning, cramping sensations, urticaria, tissue sloughing, and necrosis. When sodium tetradecyl sulfate is used, a permanent discoloration of the skin may occur. Postoperative sloughing may occur.

Sodium Tetradecyl Sulfate

Sodium tetradecyl sulfate (Sotradecol) is available in various solutions, 1% and 3% for IV use only. The strength of the solution is dependent on the vessel being sclerosed: 1% for very small vessels and 3% for most vessels.

Morrhuate Sodium

Morrhuate sodium (CMC) is available as a 50 mg/ml solution for IV use only. The dose depends on the size and degree of varicosity: 50–100 mg (1–2 ml) for small to medium vessels and 150–250 mg (3–5 ml) for large vessels.

OTHER DRUGS USED TO TREAT PERIPHERAL VASCULAR DISORDERS

The calcium-channel blockers diltiazem (Cardizem), nifedipine (Procardia), and synthetic compounds related to papaverine depress transmembrane calcium influx into the cell, making the blood vessel less likely to contract, and therefore acting effectively as vasodilators. Nifedipine decreases the frequency and severity of attacks in many patients with primary Raynaud's phenomenon.

USING THE NURSING PROCESS—PERIPHERAL VASODILATORS

ASSESSMENT

Patients with peripheral vascular diseases require lifelong care. Their symptoms can be relieved temporarily but cannot be cured. Assessment of patients requiring peripheral vasodilators for the control or treatment of peripheral vascular diseases always begins with a thorough nursing history to develop the data base. It is important to determine whether there has been a past history of recent injury to the extremity, hypertension, hypercholesterol levels, diabetes, renal disease, and/or cardiac disease. This underlying condition may well contribute to the development of peripheral vascular disease and need to be treated. All information is used later when preparing the nursing care plan. The information obtained is included in Table 31–9.

A history of current smoking habits (including the use of marijuana) is obtained. If the patient is still smoking, the nurse plans to work with the patient during the intervention phase to reduce the smoking habit or stop it permanently. Smoking causes further vasoconstriction in the periphery, aggravating peripheral vascular disease.

The nurse also assesses for objective and subjective symptoms of peripheral vascular disease. In addition, the patient's symptoms of pain are assessed. Intermittent claudication maybe experienced by patients with Buerger's disease (thromboangiitis obliterans). Persistent pain or rest pain is experienced if an embolism or thrombosis is present.

Occupation and leisure activities are also determined. It is important to assess whether the patient leads an active or sedentary lifestyle. Also, if the patient exercises, how often, of what type, and what difficulties are experienced during exercise?

The nurse may also assist with the collection of laboratory data such as clotting studies, hyperlipidemia studies, ECGs, doppler studies, and vascular studies.

NURSING DIAGNOSES

Nursing diagnoses are established based on the data obtained in the original assessment. The nursing diagnoses become the basis for the goals of nursing care and evaluation. Typical nursing diagnoses for a patient requiring medication to treat peripheral vascular disease are included in Table 31–9.

Table 31–9. NURSING PROCESS FOR PATIENT REQUIRING PERIPHERAL VASODILATORS

Assessment

Compare extremities/digits, noting color, temperature, sensations, pulses.
Ascertain characteristics of pain/discomfort.
Assess lifestyle, including type of work (sedentary/active) and type of leisure activities, smoking.
Note history of recent injury to the extremity, presence of hypertension, hypercholesterol levels, diabetes, renal disease, and/or cardiac disease.
Review laboratory results, e.g., clotting, hyperlipidemia studies, ECGs, doppler and vascular studies.

Nursing Diagnosis	Nursing Actions	Rationale	Desired Outcomes/ Evaluation Criteria
Tissue perfusion decreased, peripheral related to decreased blood flow as evidenced by tissue edema, diminished peripheral pulses, slow/diminished capillary refill, intermittent skin color changes, pallor/erythema, and trophic skin changes, complaints of pain.	Provide warm room free of drafts, e.g., block air conditioner vent, keep hallway door closed as indicated.	Eliminates environmental factors which may precipitate an attack.	Demonstrates improved perfusion as evidenced by peripheral pulses present/equal, skin color and temperature normal, absence of edema. Engages in behaviors/ actions to enhance tissue perfusion. Displays increasing ability to participate in desired activity.
	Promote restriction/cessation of activity or bedrest during acute phase according to individual needs.	Reduces oxygen and nutrient demands of affected extremity. Minimizes the possibility of dislodging thrombus (if present) and creating emboli.	
	Protect from injury, e.g., refrain from activities using sharp implements, requiring fine motor function, or involving heat/cold (drinking coffee) testing temperature of bath water with hand.	Sensation is often diminished during attack or chronically in advanced disease. Lack of awareness when sensation is diminished can lead to situations where the affected body parts are at increased risk for injury.	
	Administer vasodilators, e.g., Cyclospasmol, Ethequin, Roniacol; or alpha-adrenergic blockers, e.g., Dibenzyline.	Although site/mechanism of action varies, intended results are reduction of vasoconstriction, relaxation of vasospasm, a more even blood flow/narrowing of pulse pressure and elevation of skin temperature.	
	Monitor effects of medications/treatments.	Improvement may be gradual, requiring several months. Individual responses to prescribed therapies may not be adequate to control disease or may produce untoward side effects, indicating need for change in regimen.	
	Apply moist heat to extremity/immerse affected part in warm water.	Causes vasodilation which increases circulation, relaxes muscles and may stimulate release of natural endorphins.	
	Assist patient to identify precipitating factors or situations, e.g., smoking, exposure to cold, and problem-solve solutions.	Vasoconstriction is to be limited as it may lead to tissue damage and gangrene.	

CONTINUED ON THE FOLLOWING PAGE

Table 31–9. NURSING PROCESS FOR PATIENT REQUIRING PERIPHERAL VASODILATORS–*CONTINUED*

Nursing Diagnosis	Nursing Actions	Rationale	Desired Outcomes/Evaluation Criteria
	Caution patient to avoid crossing legs and hyperflexion at knee, or wearing constricting clothing (e.g., knee-high hose, girdle).	Physical restriction of circulation impairs blood flow/tissue perfusion and increases venous stasis in pelvic, popliteal and leg vessels increasing risk of thrombus formation.	
	Encourage use of stress management techniques, biofeedback, diversional activities.	Promotes relaxation/refocusing attention to help in breaking the stress/anxiety/stress cycle which can worsen vasoconstrictive response and increase pain.	
	Review importance of stopping smoking and help patient to develop program for cessation.	Cessation of smoking can improve vasodilation.	
Knowledge deficit related to lack of exposure, unfamiliarity with information resources, lack of recall as evidenced by request for information, verbalization of problem, inaccurate followthrough of instruction, development of preventable complications.	Review pathophysiology of condition and signs/symptoms of possible complications, e.g., chronic venous insufficiency, venous stasis ulcers, gangrene.	Provides a knowledge base from which patient can make informed choices and understand/identify health care needs.	Verbalizes understanding of disease process, treatment regimen and limitations. Identifies signs/symptoms requiring medical evaluation. Correctly perform therapeutic procedure(s) and explains reasons for actions.
	Discuss purpose, dosage of specific drug therapy. Emphasize importance of taking drug as prescribed.	Promotes patient safety by reducing risk of inadequate therapeutic response/deleterious side effects.	
	Identify possible drug interactions and stress need to read ingredient labels of OTC drugs.	Reduces risk of untoward reactions and possible complications.	
	Recommend avoidance of beta-blockers, e.g., Inderal.	Contraindicated as they worsen vasospasm.	
	Stress importance of continued medical follow-up.	Close supervision of therapeutic response/needs is necessary to reduce risk of complications.	
	Explain purpose of activity restrictions and need for balance between activity/rest.	Rest reduces oxygen and nutrient needs of compromised tissues. Balance of activity prevents exhaustion and further impairment of cellular perfusion.	
	Establish appropriate exercise/activity program.	May aid in developing collateral circulation, enhances venous return.	
	Instruct in meticulous skin care and routine inspection for ulcerations, lesions, gangrenous areas. Stress importance of prompt treatment of breaks in skin, reporting developing lesions/ulcers or changes in skin color.	Lesions can occur from pinpoint size to those involving the entire fingertip, etc, and may result in infection/serious tissue damage/loss.	
	Discuss importance of proper nutrition, vita-	A well-balanced diet, including adequate pro-	

Table 31–9. NURSING PROCESS FOR PATIENT REQUIRING PERIPHERAL VASODILATORS–*CONTINUED*

Nursing Diagnosis	Nursing Actions	Rationale	Desired Outcomes/ Evaluation Criteria
	mins, restriction of cholesterol.	tein and hydration, is necessary for proper healing and tissue regeneration. Lowering of cholesterol levels may reduce development/ progression of atherosclerosis which can also impair circulation.	
	Problem-solve solutions to predisposing factors that may be present, e.g., work setting that requires exposure to cold/environmental temperature below 70 degrees, drafts, or passive cigarette smoke.	Activity involves patient in identifying and intiating lifestyle/behavior changes to promote health and prevent recurrence of condition/ development of complications as possible.	

PLANNING AND INTERVENTION

As the planning phase begins, the nurse establishes the goals of nursing intervention from the nursing diagnoses. The goals of nursing intervention in caring for a patient requiring peripheral vasodilators are included in Table 31–9.

PATIENT TEACHING

In general, patients self-medicate themselves at home; therefore, the nurse needs to teach the information found in Table 31–10.

Since no specific therapy is available to cure these diseases, supportive treatment is directed at removing all the risk factors including tobacco use, trauma from chemical substances, and exposure to extremes in temperature. Surgery may be indicated to produce permanent vasodilation.

It is important that the patient and family understand that total recovery from peripheral vascular diseases as a result of medical treatment does not occur. However, medications do reduce the symptoms and may prevent further deterioration. The family must be totally involved with the treatment regimen in order to prevent further complications such as stasis ulcers and gangrene. Unfortunately, even when patients are 100% committed to their treatment, complications can and do develop. The patient should know what symptoms to report to the physician immediately such as rest pain, change in color of extremities, or ulcer formation.

EVALUTION

The nurse evaluates the effectiveness of peripheral vasodilators based on a predetermined list of outcome evaluation criteria. The outcome evaluation criteria are developed on an individual basis through discussion among the nurse, patient, and family. The information or the data base obtained in the original assessment is used to formulate the criteria for evaluation. The typical outcome evaluation criteria are included in Table 31–9.

Table 31–10. PATIENT TEACHING INFORMATION—PERIPHERAL VASODILATORS

Dear Patient:
  This drug has been prescribed for you. This is what you should know about your drug to get the most from your therapy.

1. Peripheral vasodilators are taken to reduce spasm or improve circulation to your extremities.
2. You will most likely take your vasodilator for the rest of your life.
3. Note when your medication should be taken in relationship to meals: cyclandelate (Cyclospasmol), and pentoxifylline (Trental) should be administered with food to prevent gastric irritation; nicotinyl alcohol or tartrate (Roniacol) should be taken before meals to enhance absorption.
4. If you forget your medication until your next dose, skip it; do **not** try to catch up.
5. Do not omit or stop taking your medication without your doctor's approval.
6. The side effects of your medication are (see Table 31–8 for specific information). If these occur, notify your doctor.
7. Change body positions slowly to reduce the possibility of orthostatic hypotension.
8. Limit your alcohol intake because of the additive vasodilation effect.
9. Do not expose yourself to cold, since most peripheral vasodilators are accompanied by a feeling of warmth in the extremities.
10. Avoid hot showers and hot tubs because of the additive vasodilation they cause.
11. Preserve all medications in tight, light-resistant containers.

It is extremely important to work with the patient and family to ensure their complete assistance and support. The majority of patients, once they understand the importance of their continued medical treatment, are usually compliant. Patients soon realize that it is important to prevent further deterioration and complications.

The patient is taught the side effects of the medications. Many of the medications may cause flushing of the skin and hypotension. If an unusual symptom is noted, the patient is encouraged to call the physician. The patient is encouraged to keep the extremities warm and not subject them to any unnecessary chill. The patient is also taught to change body positions slowly to prevent orthostatic hypotension.

All other evaluation criteria are also assessed and evaluated before the patient leaves the hospital. All previously taught material is reviewed and updated with the patient and family, if necessary, to ensure that the patient's knowledge base remains accurate.

The more the patient and family are involved with the planning care, the more likely they are to comply. The nurse must stress the importance of continued medical care. Peripheral vasodilators should help the patient maintain the level of functoning. Medications are not the only method of treatment, however, and the patient must comply with the other aspects of care as well.

SUMMARY

Vasodilators, including nitrates and calcium-channel blockers, are used primarily to terminate acute anginal attacks or have a prolonged effect that can prevent anginal attacks. Nitrates are primarily smooth-muscle relaxants that cause generalized dilatation. The calcium-channel blockers competitively block the slow-channel influx of calcium into active cells. By inhibiting calcium entry into cardiac and smooth muscle cells of the coronary and systemic beds, peripheral arteries and arterioles dilate.

Before the nurse begins to administer vasodilators, a thorough nursing history is obtained to determine the usual anginal pattern. It is important that the nurse have a complete understanding of anginal pain in order to assist the patient in assessing the pain and in differentiating it from gastrointestinal discomfort or from more serious cardiac conditions. It is important that the nurse know how to administer the vasodilator correctly, because many methods of administration are available. The nurse should also understand the most common adverse effects of coronary dilators, which include flushing, hypotension, and headache.

BIBLIOGRAPHY

AMA Drug Evaluations. PSG Publishing, Littleton, MA, 1986.

Bortolotti, M, et al: Nifedipine in biliary and renal colic (letter). JAMA 258:3516 December 15, 1987.

Brewer, CC, et al: Streptokinase and TPA in acute myocardial infarction. Heart Lung 15(6):552–558, 1986.

Brush, JE, et al: Combination drug therapy for chronic stable angina pectoris. Hosp Formul 22(2):146–9, February 1987.

Carlson, S: IV nitroglycerin: Reducing complications at high doses. DCCN 7(2):83, 1988.

Clinical News: Nitroglycerin headaches no easy solutions. AJN 87(1):11, 1987.

Falbe, W, Mickle, T: Avoiding medication errors with transdermal nitroglycerin products. Am J Hosp Pharm 43:2738–2740, November 1986.

Gilman, AG, Goodman, LS and Gilman, A: Goodman and Gilman's The Pharmacological Basis of Therapeutics. ed. 6. Macmillan, New York, 1986.

Herrington, D, Insley, B and Weinmann, G: Nifedine overdose. Am J Med 81:344–346, August 1986.

Hilleman, D, et al: Comment: Nifedipine in hypertensive emergencies (letter). Drug Intell Clin Pharm 21:1013–1014, December 1987.

Kutsop, J: Sublingual burning not a valid index of nitroglycerin potency (letter). Am J Hosp Pharm 43:2144, September 1986.

Luchi, RJ, Scott, SM, Deupree, RN, et al: Comparison of medical and surgical treatment for unstable angina pectoris. N Engl J Med (316):977–84, 1987.

Luke, R, et al: Transdermal nitroglycerin in angina pectoris: Efficacy of intermittent application. 10:642–646, 1987.

Mathewson, M: New uses for old drug—nitrates. Crit Care Update 9(11):7–11, 1982.

Mathewson, M: Current uses for coronary vasodilators. Focus 10(1):22–26, 1983.

Mathewson, M: Prolapsed mitral valve syndrome. Am J Nurs 80:8, 1980.

Metzer, AH, Kafka, KR, Frishman, WH: Antianginal agents part 3 calcium-entry blockers. Hosp Formul 21:299–304, March 1986.

Nitroglycerin patches: Do they work? Med Lett 31(796):65–66, July 14, 1989.

Olin, B (ed): Facts and Comparisons. St Louis, MO, JB Lippincott, 1987.

Pierce, CH: How calcium antagonists interact with cardiac glycosides. Consultant 86(9):82–89, September 1986.

Prochet, JM, Pirson, Y: Cyclosporin-diltiazem interaction (letter). Lancet 8487:979, April 26, 1986.

Reigel, B, et al: Effects of nitroglycerin ointment placement on severity of headache and flushing in patients with cardiac disease. Heart and Lung 17:462–421 July, 1988.

Riley, V, Riley, R: Nitroglycerin patches a handicap? (letter). Arch Intern Med 146:2081, October 1986.

Schakenbach, LH: Prinzmetal's angina: Current perceptions and treatments. Crit Care Nurse 7(2):90–99, 1987.

Schroeder: Calcium antagonists for CV emergencies. Top Emerg Med 8(3):37–51, October 1986.

Thadani, U: Current status of nitrates in angina pectoris. Mod Concepts Cardiovasc Dis 56(9):49–53, 1987.

Thomas, MG, Sander, GE and Giles, TD: Antianginal efficacy of nitroglycerin patches: The jury is still out. Hosp Formul 21:918–922, September 1986.

Transmucosal controlled-release nitroglycerin. Med Lett 29(737):39, April 10, 1987.

van Harten, J, et al: Negligible sublingual absorption of nifedipine. Lancet II:1363–1365, December 12, 1987.

Weinhardt, JA: Making the most of topical nitroglycerin. RN 85(12):38–40, 1985.

Wescott, BL: Tissue plasminogen activator: A new advancement in fibrinolytic therapy. Focus on Critical Care 13(6):22–25, 1986.

SITUATION 31–1

Wayne Armstrong is a 74-year-old admitted to the coronary care unit with a diagnosis of unstable angina. He has a history of mild hypertension and is current taking propranolol.

1. After 3 nitroglycerin tablets have not relieved his chest pain, Mr. Armstrong is to be started on a high-dose nitroglycerin infusion. A nursing responsibility associated with this type of medication is:
   a. checking the blood pressure and pulse every hour
   b. titrating the nitroglycerin by 20- to 50-μg increments
   c. mixing nitroglycerin in normal saline only
   d. protecting the nitroglycerin infusion from light

2. When monitoring Mr. Armstrong's EKG, the following effect may be observed related to nitroglycerin therapy:
   a. rebound bradycardia
   b. widened Q-T interval
   c. shortened P-R interval
   d. reflex tachycardia

3. Mr. Armstrong tells the nurse that he has a sudden pounding headache. The nurse is aware that this represents:
   a. an allergic reaction
   b. an adverse effect
   c. a toxic effect
   d. an impending seizure

4. After several days, the nitroglycerin infusion is discontinued. A transdermal nitroglycerin patch is to be applied in the morning and removed in the evening. The nurse is aware that this schedule of dosing reduces:
   a. nitrate dependence
   b. side effects
   c. toxic effects
   d. nitrate tolerance

5. When teaching Mr. Armstrong about administering nitroglycerin transdermal patches, the following information applies:
   a. taking off the patch when showering or swimming
   b. putting on an extra patch whenever chest pain occurs
   c. applying the patch to any non-hairy area of the body
   d. replacing the transdermal patch every six hours

6. In addition to the nitroglycerin patch, Mr. Armstrong will be advised to take sublingual nitroglycerin tablets as needed (prn) for chest pain. The nurse will teach that:
   a. if after eight consecutive doses the chest pain continues, he should notify the physician
   b. to prevent angina, he should take a tablet before exertional exercise
   c. the nitroglycerin tablets should be replaced every year to maintain freshness
   d. the bottle of nitroglycerin tablets should be kept in a warm, moist environment

SITUATION 31–2

Hazel Breaux is an 83-year-old with increasing episodes of angina with minimal exertion. She is admitted to the telemetry unit for close observation and medical management of chest pain.

1. Mrs. Breaux is to begin isosorbide dinitrate sustained-release 40 mg tablets. The nurse will instruct her to:
   a. take the dosage with milk to reduce gastric irritation
   b. allow the tablet to dissolve slowly under the tongue
   c. swallow the tablet without chewing or crushing it
   d. place the tablet between the gum and upper lip

2. In addition to the nitrate therapy, Mrs. Breaux is to begin nifedipine (Procardia) 10 mg po every 6 hours. When giving this medication along with nitrates, the nurse will observe for:
   a. hypotension
   b. tremor
   c. hyperkalemia
   d. tetany

3. When establishing baseline data for Mrs. Breaux, which of the following conditions would indicate a need to administer nifedipine with caution?
   a. kidney dysfunction
   b. migraine headaches
   c. sinus bradycardia
   d. Raynaud's syndrome

4. An important area for assessment for patients on nifedipine is to be aware of the potential for:
   a. hallucinations
   b. peripheral edema
   c. hyperglycemia
   d. photophobia

5. In order to reduce episodes of chest pain, Mrs. Breaux should be taught to avoid all of the following *except:*
   a. eating large meals
   b. smoking cigarettes
   c. performing daily exercise
   d. going out into the cold

6. Which of the following statements by Mrs. Breaux indicates adequate understanding concerning administration of coronary vasodilators?
   a. "I will only have to take these pills for a few weeks."
   b. "I can take the long-acting pill anytime during the day."
   c. "If I get a headache, I should stop taking the pills."
   d. "The nitroglycerin is not habit-forming, so I can take as needed."

Please refer to the Appendices for correct answers and additional review questions with answers.

THERAPY FOR SPECIFIC DISORDERS OF THE CARDIOVASCULAR-HEMATOLOGIC SYSTEM: HYPERLIPIDEMIA, ANEMIAS

MERRILY MATHEWSON KUHN, R.N.C., Ph.D., CCRN

LEARNING OBJECTIVES

After reading this chapter, the student will be able to:

1. Identify medications that have an effect on disorders of the cardiovascular–hematologic system, including antihyperlipemics and antianemics.

2. Differentiate among the medications as to mechanism of action, routes of administration, pharmacokinetics, adverse effects, contraindications, and interactions.

3. Identify specific areas to assess in the patient requiring various cardiovascular medications in order to formulate appropriate nursing diagnoses.

4. Plan the nursing interventions necessary to administer various cardiovascular–hematologic medications and choose appropriate teaching strategies to gain patient compliance.

5. Evaluate the patient at various stages of treatment to gauge nursing interventions.

Medications can be administered to patients with various cardiovascular–hematologic disorders. Patients may receive antihyperlipemic agents to reduce blood lipid levels and hematinic medications to treat anemias. Each group of medications is discussed separately, and is followed by a nursing process application section.

LIPIDS

High serum *cholesterol* is a known risk factor for the development of cardiovascular diseases such as hypertension, angina, acute myocardial infarction, and sudden coronary death. (See Table 32–1 for review of lipids.) Recently, it has been documented that reducing an elevated serum cholesterol level with either diet or drug therapy reduces the risk of death from cardiovascular disease (Lipid Research Clinic Program, 1984). Normal cholesterol values have traditionally been considered 200 mg/100 ml plus the patient's age. More exact values are included in Table 32–2. Recent research has indicated that patients with cholesterol values below 190 mg/100 ml have the lowest risk of developing heart disease. The Cholesterol Lowering Atherosclerosis (CLAS) Study (Blankenhorn, 1987) showed by angiography,

that lowering the serum cholesterol could arrest or even reverse atheroma formation in native coronary arteries. The most recent intervention trial, called the Helsinki Heart Study (Frick, 1987), showed data to support the hypothesis that by raising HDL levels, a corresponding decrease in CAD would follow.

It is important to understand the relationship between cholesterol concentrations and the *lipoprotein* complexes that transport cholesterol and *triglycerides*. Based on physiochemical properties, there are five major classifications of plasma lipoproteins: chylomicrons, very low-density lipoproteins (VLDLs), intermediate-density lipoproteins (IDLs), low-density lipoproteins (LDLs), and high-density lipoproteins (HDLs). Table 32–3 reviews the lipoprotein composition. The explanation for the naming of these proteins comes from the ultra-centrifugation method by which the proteins are separated according to their density. The greater the ratio of lipids to protein, the lower the density. In other words, the VLDLs carry large amounts of lipids compared with the HDLs.

Lipid compounds do not circulate freely in the blood stream, but rather are bound to plasma proteins such as albumin and globulin, which act as carriers. These complexes are called lipoproteins. In the digestive tract triglycerides are split into monoglycerides and fatty acids. These products pass through the intestinal wall and are

Table 32–1. LIPIDS

DEFINITION
Lipid, a term often used interchangeably with fat, is any organic substance that has the following properties: insolubility in water; solubility in alcohol, ether, and chloroform; utilization by living cells as a source of body fuel; and existence as part of the cell itself.

TYPES
1. Simple lipids
   a. Fatty acid
   b. Neutral fats
      1. Monoglyceride
      2. Diglyceride
      3. Triglyceride
         a. Consist of 3 molecules of fatty acid bound with 1 molecule of glycerol
         b. Most common stored fat in man
         c. Normal serum level <60 mg/100 ml
         d. Saturated—solid at room temperature and contains all hydrogen it can hold
         e. Unsaturated—liquid at room temperature and can hold more hydrogen
2. Compound lipids
   a. Phosopholipids—lipids and phosphorus
      1. Several types available; see Table 32–2
      2. Most common after triglycerides
      3. Formed in all cells of body
      4. Facilitates passage of fat in and out of cell
   b. Lipoprotein—combination of triglycerides, phospholipids, and/or cholesterol with a protein
      1. Transport insoluble lipids
      2. Formed primarily in liver
      3. Found in all body cells
      4. Four major categories; see Table 32–2
3. Derived lipids
   a. Sterols (cholesterol)
      1. Needed by body to produce corticosteroids, estrogens, androgens, progesterone, and bile salts
      2. Abnormal deposits of cholesterol (atheromas) reduce blood vessel diameter
      3. Stored and regulated by liver
      4. Normal plasma level is <220 mg/100 ml

Table 32–2. BLOOD CHOLESTEROL VALUES

Risk	Cholesterol Level
Low risk	<200 mg
Borderline	200–239 mg
High risk	>240 mg

resynthesized into molecules of triglycerides called chylomicrons. Chylomicrons, which are formed in the digestive tract, consist of 85%–95% triglyceride and 3%–5% cholesterol. Chylomicrons combine with a similar amount of protein to make them more stable. Chylomicrons are the largest and the least dense of the lipoproteins. Chylomicrons are cleared from the blood stream by the enzyme lipoprotein lipase after 12–14 hours forming chylomicron remnants. These chylomicron remnants are then transformed by the liver into VLDL, which is the precursor of IDL and eventually LDL.

Triglycerides are synthesized mainly from carbohydrates in the liver and are transported to the adipose and other peripheral tissues in the form of VLDLs. VLDLs contain triglycerides (64%–80%), and moderate concentrations of phospholipids and cholesterol (7%–14%). VLDLs are also referred to as pre-beta lipoproteins. High levels of VLDL are considered atherogenic. Patients with very high levels are also at risk of developing pancreatitis.

IDLs or broad β-lipoproteins are formed as VLDL loses its triglycerides. IDL consists of 30% cholesterol. Like VLDL, it also tends to be atherogenic. In normally healthy persons, IDL is not found in significant amounts.

LDLs are the residuals of the VLDLs after they have delivered most of their triglycerides to the tissues. LDLs contain relatively little triglyceride (7%–10%) but a very

high percentage of cholesterol (40%–50%). LDLs are also referred to as β-lipoproteins. Since LDLs contain the major portion of cholesterol in the blood, they are considered the most harmful. An evaluation of LDL suggests that a person has a high risk for developing atherosclerosis.

HDL, or α-lipoproteins, contain about 50% protein with smaller concentration of lipids: 17%–20% cholesterol and 1%–7% triglycerides. HDLs are the smallest and the most dense. HDL appears to be beneficial, since its primary function is to transport cholesterol away from peripheral tissues to the liver, where it is metabolized and then excreted. HDL, therefore, plays an important role in preventing atherosclerosis. The higher the HDL level, the lower is the potential risk for developing cardiovascular disease.

Endogenous cholesterol is metabolized in the liver to bile acids and excreted from the biliary tract into the small intestine. Cholesterol is an important substance within the body because it is used by the adrenal glands to manufacture adrenocortical hormones and the testes to form testosterone. Cholesterol is also found in the skin and makes it highly resistant to the absorption of water and to the action of many chemicals. In addition, cholesterol in the skin helps prevent water evaporation from the skin. Cholesterol as well as phospholipids are also found in the cell membrane and the membranes of internal organelles of all cells.

It is important to know the concentrations of the various lipoprotein fractions in someone with an elevated cholesterol. Lipoprotein composition is reviewed in Table 32–3. LDLs are the predominant cholesterol-transporting lipoprotein. High LDL concentrations correlate well with serum cholesterol and with risk of heart disease. On the other hand, it has been shown that patients with high HDL concentrations are at a low risk of developing heart disease because of HDL's ability to transport cholesterol away from the tissues. Disorders of

Table 32–3. LIPOPROTEIN COMPOSITION

Type	A*	B*	C*	D*	E*	Comments
Chylomicrons	1	85–95	3–5	1	8	Contain the most lipid; therefore, the least dense. Eventually stored as adipose tissue.
Very-low-density (VLDL) or pre-beta	7	64–80	7–14	6	18	Partly derived from dietary cholesterol. Stored as adipose tissue.
Low-density (LDL) or beta	21	7–10	40–50	7	23	Contains major portion of total plasma cholesterol. Thought to be responsible for atherosclerotic process.
High-density (HDL) or alpha	46	1–7	17–20	2	26	Smallest and most dense. Contains only 20% cholesterol. Least responsible for contributing to atherosclerotic process. Often referred to as the "good" cholesterol. Strenuous physical exercise increases its fraction in the serum.

This care plan is individualized for Ken Jones. When designing a care plan, it must be individualized for the specific patient needs.

Table 32–4. FREDRICKSON–LEVY LIPID PHENOTYPING

Types	I	II		III
Incidence	Rare	Common		Infrequent
Age	Child	Begins as child		Adult
Genetic	Recessive	Dominant, sporadic		Dominant, sporadic
Clinical finding	Xanthoma	Xanthoma		Xanthoma
	↑ liver	Arcus		
	Abdominal pain	↑ ASHD		↑ ASHD
CAHD Risk	Low	Very high		Very high
Electrophoresis Findings		IIa	IIb	
Cholesterol	N ↑	↑↑	↑↑	N ↑↑
Triglycerides	↑↑	N		N ↑↑
Chylomicrons	↑↑	N	N	N
VLDL	N ↑	N ↓↓	↑↑	N ↑
ILDL	N	N	N	↑↑
LDL	↓↓	↑↑	↑↑	↑↑
HDL	↓↓	N	N	N
Treatment	Diet only	Diet Diet		Diet
		IIab-cholestyramine (Questran)		Nicotinic acid
		IIab-Colestipol Hydrochloride		
		IIa-D-thyroxine (Choloxin)		
		IIab-Nicotinic acid		
		IIab-Probucol (Lorelco)		
		Lovastatin		

Types	IV	V
Incidence	Very common	Rare
Age	Adult	Adult
Genetic	Dominant, sporadic	Dominant, sporadic
Clinical finding	↑ ASHD, obesity, abdominal pain	Xanthoma, obesity
		Abdominal pain, ↑ liver
CAHD risk	High	Low
Electrophoresis Findings		
Cholesterol	N ↑	N ↑↑
Triglycerides	↑↑	↑↑↑
Chylomicrons	N	↑↑
VLDL	↑↑	↑↑
ILDL	N	N
LDL	N ↓	↓↓
HDL	N ↓	↓↓
Treatment	Diet	Gemfibrozil
	Gemfibrozil	Nicotinic acid
	Nicotinic acid	

↑ = slight increase, ↑↑ increase, ↑↑↑ large increase, ↓ slight decrease, ↓↓ decrease.

lipid metabolism have been characterized and classified as types I through V, however, the Fredrickson-Levy classifications are no longer used to guide therapy. These are outlined in Table 32–4.

ANTIHYPERLIPEMICS

Many medications on the market today interfere with normal metabolism of cholesterol, lipoproteins, or tri-glycerides. This interference ultimately reduces blood lipids. Various agents affect the lipoprotein fractions in different ways. They are not uniformly effective in reducing serum cholesterol and LDL, which would be required to decrease the risk of heart disease. Cholestyramine, colestipol, probucol, dextrothyroxine, and lovastatin are used to lower cholesterol. Clofibrate and gemfibrozil lower triglycerides more than cholesterol. If both cholesterol and triglycerides are elevated, triglycerides should be lowered first. If cholesterol is treated first, hypertriglyceridemia may occur. These medications are featured in Table 32–5.

CHOLESTEROL-LOWERING DRUGS

Bile Acid Sequestrants

The bile acid sequestrants inhibit the reabsorption of bile acids in the intestine, causing an increase in the fecal excretion of these acids. By increasing the excretion of bile acids, these compounds increase the hepatic conversion of cholesterol to bile acids, leading to lowered serum cholesterol levels. A fall in LDL is apparent in four to seven days, and the decline in cholesterol (by about 15%–20% or more) is evident by one month. Bile sequestrants may elevate triglyceride levels; therefore, they are not used in patients with triglyceride levels above 400 mg/dl. This group includes cholestyramine (Questran, and Cholybar) colestipol (Colestid).

CHOLESTYRAMINE. Cholestyramine (Questran, and Cholybar) was originally marketed as a product to reduce pruritus associated with bile stasis in patients with biliary disease, but it is now of more interest for its side effect than for its original use. Cholestyramine is a quaternary ammonium anion-exchange resin that absorbs and combines with bile salts in exchange for chloride, forming an insoluble, nonabsorbable complex that is excreted in the feces. In an attempt to compensate for the loss of bile salts, the body increases the rate of metabolism of cholesterol to bile acids. Cholestyramine is used to treat type II hyperlipidemia (Fig. 32–1).

Cholestyramine is available as a buff-colored powder. It should be mixed with any liquid or high-moisture content food to disguise the taste. It should not be given concurrently with other drugs, particularly acidic drugs, because of its ability to bind with them. Specifically, cholestyramine may interfere with absorption of oral anticoagulants, digitalis, iron preparations, thyroid products, thiazide diuretics, and phenylbutazone. Other medications are administered within 1 hour before or four to six hours after cholestyramine. The new product, Cholebar, is a 4 g/bar formula sweetened by sorbitol. It contains 50 calories/bar. Additional information is found in Table 32–5.

COLESTIPOL. Colestipol (Colestid) is very similar to cholestyramine. It is administered in 15–30 g doses, divided into two to four equal portions. For additional information see Table 32–5.

Other Agents

LOVASTATIN. Lovastatin (Mevacor) is in a new class of drugs, the 3-hydroxy-3 methylglutaryl-coenzyme A (HMG-CoA) reductase inhibitors, that inhibit cholesterol biosynthesis. Lovastatin decreases the total plasma cholesterol and LDL level by 20%–40%. In addition, the plasma concentration of the potentially atherogenic LDL or β-lipoproteins is also reduced by 20%–40%. The reduction of these lipoproteins occurs as a result of decreased synthesis and enhanced removal of LDL by the LDL receptor pathway in the liver. In addition, HDL increases in concentration during therapy. The HMG-CoA reductase inhibitors (several other products are currently undergoing research, including mevastatin, provastatin, and simvastatin) represent a new approach in the treatment of hyperlipidemia. Lovastatin is either as effective or more effective than other currently available drugs. In addition, lovastatin has few adverse effects. It is used in treating type II hyperlipidemias.

Pharmacokinetics. Lovastatin is incompletely and poorly absorbed (30%) from the gastrointestinal tract. There is extensive first-pass effect in the liver, and lovastatin is excreted primarily in bile. Peak plasma levels are achieved in two to four hours, but the peak onset of action occurs within three days of initiation of therapy. Lovastatin has a half-life of one to two hours.

Adverse Effects. Unlike the other antihyperlipidemics, lovastatin is well tolerated by most patients. A few may complain of mild transient headaches and gastrointestinal symptoms. Cataracts may occur or worsen, so baseline and periodic eye exams are performed. Also, myositis with increased CPK, *rhabdomyolysis*, and acute renal failure have been reported. Lovastatin should be used with caution if the patient is also taking gemfibrozil or Cyclosporin-A, due to an increased risk of myositis. Lovastatin does elevate the serum transaminase levels in 2%–3% of patients. No evidence of liver dysfunction has occurred, and abnormal liver function returns to normal after discontinuation of the drug. When lovastatin is discontinued, the serum cholesterol levels return to pretreatment levels.

PROBUCOL. Probucol (Lorelco) has viable efficacy and is used for the reduction of type IIa and IIb hyperlipidemia when patients are unable to tolerate bile sequestrants or nicotinic acid. It is indicated as an adjunc-

TEXT RESUMES ON PAGE 860

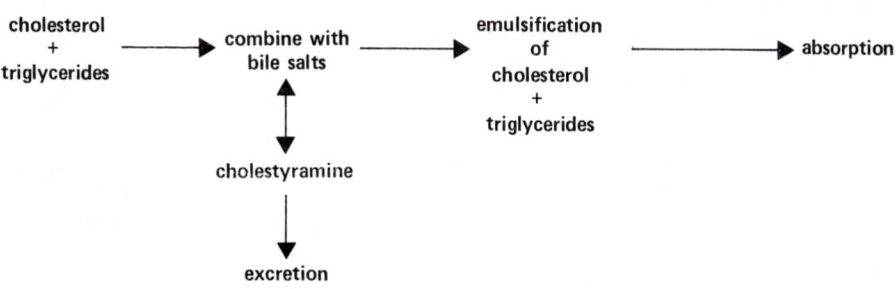

Figure 32–1. Mechanism of action of cholestyramine (Questran) and colestipol (Colestid). These drugs combine with bile salts and prevent emulsification and absorption of both cholesterol and triglycerides.

Table 32–5. ANTIHYPERLIPIDEMIC AGENTS

Name	Dosage	Mode of Administration	Pharmacokinetics
BILE ACID SEQUESTRANTS:			
Action (For all): interfere with normal metabolism of cholesterol			
Use (For all): lower blood cholesterol/triglyceride levels			
Cholestyramine (Questran) (Cholybar)			
Action: Inhibit reabsorption of bile acids in intestine, leading to increased hepatic conversion of cholesterol to bile acids, and thus increase excretion of cholesterol.			
Use: Adjunct in management of primary hypercholesterolemia. Relieves pruritis associated with elevated levels of bile acids.			
	4 g, 1–6 × daily 4g, 4–6 bars/day	PO PO	O: 4–7 days P: 1–3 wk D: 2–4 wk ½L: UA B: liver E: feces
Colestipol (Colestid)	15–30 g, 2–4 × daily	PO	O: 24–48 hr P: 1 mo D: 1 mo ½L: UA B: liver E: feces
OTHER DRUGS: Probucol (Lorelco)			
Action: Inhibit early stage of cholesterol synthesis, which increases excretion of fecal bile salts and inhibits absorption of cholesterol.			
Use: Adjunct therapy to decrease serum cholesterol but has little effect on serum triglycerides.			
	500 mg bid	PO	O: slowly P: 3–4 mo D: greater than 6 mo (stored in fat) ½L: 12–500 hr PB: UA B: liver E: bile/feces

Key to Abbreviations in the *Pharmacokinetcs* column O-onset; P-peak; D-duration; PB-protein bound; B-biotransformed in; E-excreted in; ½L-halflife.
*Within the column listing adverse effects, underlines indicate the most common effects; CAPITALS indicate life-threatening effects.

Contraindications/ Precautions	Adverse Effects*	Interactions	Nursing Implications
			For all: ASSESSMENT: serum cholesterol and triglycerides at onset and periodically during therapy. INTERVENTION: Teach patient how and when to take medications and the importance of diet therapy. EVALUATION: serum levels should decrease.
Contraindicated in complete biliary obstruction and hypersensitivity. Use cautiously in steatorrhea, preexisting constipation. Safety in pregnant and lactating women and children not established.	Neuro: headache, anxiety, vertigo, dizziness GI: constipation, abdominal pain, GI bleeding, nausea, vomiting, diarrhea, anorexia, steatorrhea, change in weight Hemo: bleeding tendency, vitamin A and D deficiency, increased prothrombin time Renal: hematuria, dysuria, burnt odor of urine, hyperchloremic acidosis Integ: rash, urticaria, dermatitis Musculoskeletal: backache, muscle and joint pain	Resins may decrease absorption of oral medications, delays or reduces absorption of oral anticoagulants, thiazide diuretics, thyroid hormones, phenylbutazone, iron preparations, phenobarbital, many antibiotics, and fat-soluble vitamins.	Same as for all. ASSESSMENT: normal bowel activity. INTERVENTION: Powder should be mixed in liquids or other high-moisture foods. Allow powder to sit on liquid and hydrate for several minutes before stirring into suspension. In solution, it has a sandy and gritty consistency. Teach patient to chew bar thoroughly and drink plenty of fluids. Supplemental vitamins A, D, E, and K may need to be taken if therapy is long-term. High-bulk diet is helpful in preventing constipation. Administer all other medications 1 hour before or 4–6 hours after. EVALUATION: If constipation occurs, contact physician.
Same as cholestyramine	Same as cholestyramine	Same as cholestyramine	Same as cholestyramine
Contraindicated in hypersensitivity and patient with current myocardial damage or indication of ventricular dysrhythmia. Use cautiously in pregnancy, and lactating women.	Neuro: headache, dizziness, syncope, blurred vision CV: prolonged Q–T interval, palpitations, chest pain GI: diarrhea, abdominal pain, nausea, vomiting Hemo: eosinophilia Integ: rash	Concurrent clofibrate may lower HDL.	As for all. ASSESSMENT: Serum cholesterol and triglycerides every 2 weeks during first several months and then monthly. Obtain baseline ECG and measure Q–T interval after 6–12 months

CONTINUED ON THE FOLLOWING PAGE

Antihyperlipidemic Agents

Table 32–5. ANTIHYPERLIPIDEMIC AGENTS–*CONTINUED*

Name	Dosage	Mode of Administration	Pharmacokinetics
Probucol–*Continued*			
Clofibrate (Atromid-S)			
Action: decreases hepatitic synthesis and accelerates breakdown of VLDL.			
	500 mg qid	PO	O: 3 hr P: 2–6 hr D: 24 hr ½L: 6–25 hr PB: 90% B: liver E: urine (40%–70% unchanged)
Gemfibrozil (Lopid)			
Action: inhibits VLDL synthesis.			
	900–1500 mg/day in 2 divided doses	PO	O: 2–5 days until VLDL is reduced P: 1–2 hr D: UA ½L: 1.5 hr PB: UA B: liver E: urine (70% unchanged)
Dextrothyroxine sodium (Choloxin)			
Action: elevates metabolic rate and metabolism of cholesterol.			
	Adult I: 1–2 mg/day M: 4–8 mg/day Children: 0.05 mg/kg/day initially. Increase 0.05 mg/kg/mo to 4 mg daily. M: 0.1 mg/kg/day	PO	O: 1–2 mo P: UA D: 6–12 wk ½L: UA PB: UA B: UA E: UA

Key to Abbreviations in the *Pharmacokinetcs* column O-onset; P-peak; D-duration; PB-protein bound; B-biotransformed in; E-excreted in; ½L-halflife.
*Within the column listing adverse effects, <u>underlines</u> indicate the most common effects; CAPITALS indicate life-threatening effects.

Contraindications/ Precautions	Adverse Effects*	Interactions	Nursing Implications
			for prolongation. Assess liver function studies at onset and during therapy. INTERVENTION: Take with meals. Should be used as adjunctive therapy and not tried alone. Therapeutic response occurs generally within 1 to 2 months. Diet therapy for reduction of cholesterol should be stressed to patients. EVALUATION: If diarrhea, abdominal pain, nausea and vomiting persist, notify physician.
Contraindicated in renal and hepatic dysfunction, pregnancy, and nursing mothers. Use cautiously in history of jaundice of hepatic disease, peptic ulcer, gout, and peripheral vascular disease.	Neuro: fatigue, weakness, drowsiness, dizziness, headache CV: increases/decreases angina, dysrhythmias Resp: pulmonary embolism GI: nausea, vomiting, diarrhea, dyspepsia, cholelithiasis, flatulence, activation of peptic ulcer, CANCER OF BILIARY TRACT Hemo: leukopenia, anemia Reprod: impotence, decreased libido Integ: rash, urticaria	Enhances oral anticoagulants, oral hypoglycemics, insulin. Rifampin decreases effectiveness. Probenecid increases therapeutic or toxic effect of Clofibrate.	As for all. INTERVENTION: Take with meals if GI upset occurs. EVALUATION: Notify physician if continued chest pain, shortness of breath, or severe stomach pain occur.
Contraindicated in hepatic or renal dysfunction, preexisting gallbladder disease. Use cautiously in pregnancy. Use in lactating women and children not established.	Neuro: headache, dizziness, blurred vision GI: abdominal pain, dry mouth, epigastric pain, diarrhea, nausea, vomiting, constipation Hemo: anemia, eosinophilia, leukopenia Misc: muscle cramps	Enhances oral anticoagulants.	As for all. ASSESSMENT: Prothrombin time and liver function studies periodically. INTERVENTION: Administer 30 min before meals.
Contraindicated in euthyroid patient with hepatic, cardiac, or renal dysfunction. Contraindicated in pregnancy and nursing mothers.	Neuro: insomnia, nervousness, headache, tinnitus, decreased sensorium, visual disturbances, insomnia	May increase insulin needs in diabetics. May potentiate anticoagulants; discontinue them 2 weeks before starting dextrothyroxine. Chole-	As for all. EVALUATION: For chest pain, sweating, diarrhea, headache. If these occur, notify physician.

CONTINUED ON THE FOLLOWING PAGE

Table 32–5. ANTIHYPERLIPIDEMIC AGENTS–*CONTINUED*

Name	Dosage	Mode of Administration	Pharmacokinetics
Dextrothyroxine sodium (Choloxin)–*Continued*			

3-HYDROXY-3 METHYLGLUTARYL-COENZYME A (HMG-COA) REDUCTASE INHIBITORS
Lovastatin (Mevacor)

Action: Decreases synthesis and enhances removal of LDL by the LDL receptor pathway in the liver. HDL is also increased.

| | 20 mg daily
Dosage can be increased at 4-wk intervals to a maximum of 80 mg daily | | O: 3 days for initial action to start
P: 2–4 hr
D: UA
½L: 1–2 hr
PB: 95%
B: liver
E: bile |

Key to Abbreviations in the *Pharmacokinetics* column O-onset; P-peak; D-duration; PB-protein bound; B-biotransformed in; E-excreted in; ½L-halflife.
*Within the column listing adverse effects, <u>underlines</u> indicate the most common effects; CAPITALS indicate life-threatening effects.

tive therapy to reduce serum cholesterol but has relatively little effect on serum triglycerides. Plasma levels of LDL are lowered 10%–15% when probucol is used in conjunction with proper diet. This, however, may be accompanied by a significant drop in HDL lipoproteins. The mechanism of action is unknown but is thought to inhibit the early stage of cholesterol synthesis, which increases the excretion of fecal bile salts and inhibits the absorption of dietary cholesterol. Probucol may exert a quinidine-like effect, with prolongation of the Q–T interval. Additional information is found in Table 32–5.

DEXTROTHYROXINE SODIUM. Dextrothyroxine sodium (Choloxin), an isomer of the thyroid hormone thyroxine, is primarily used as adjunctive therapy for reducing elevated LDL levels of type II hyperlipidemia in eythyroid patients with no known evidence of heart disease. It reduces serum cholesterol, triglycerides, and α- and β-lipoproteins. However, dextrothyroxine sodium is not consistent in reducing elevated serum levels of β lipoproteins and triglycerides. Dextrothyroxine sodium apparently stimulates the liver to increase the rate of oxidation of cholesterol and it promotes excretion of cholesterol and its by-products.

Because it is a thyroid derivative, it elevates the metabolic rate, which may be hazardous to a person with angina pectoris or hyperthyroidism. Dextrothyroxine is given cautiously to patients with diabetes, as it may elevate blood glucose levels. It is contraindicated in severe cardiac, hepatic, or renal dysfunction, as well as in pregnant and lactating women. The effects on the fetus are unknown, so women are cautioned to use strict birth control measures when taking dextrothyroxine. With the availability of newer agents, dextrothyroxine is seldom used in the treatment of hyperlipidemia. See Table 32–5 for additional information.

TRIGLYCERIDE-LOWERING AGENTS

Several triglyceride-lowering agents are currently available: clofibrate, gemfibrozil, and nicotinic acid. Clofibrate inhibits the hepatic synthesis of cholesterol and appears to enhance the intravascular conversion of VLDL to LDL. It also increases the biliary excretion of triglycerides. Gemfibrozil appears to act by inhibiting VLDL synthesis. Gemfibrozil decreases serum triglycerides, as much as 40%–55%, with a variable reduction in total serum cholesterol. In addition, gemfibrozil increases HDL levels by 17%–25%. The action of nicotinic acid includes inhibition of lipolysis in adipose tissue, hepatic de-esterification of triglycerides, and increased ac-

Contraindications/ Precautions	Adverse Effects*	Interactions	Nursing Implications
Use cautiously in cardiac disease, dysrhythmias, and patients sensitive to artrazine.	CV: angina, palpitations, dysrhythmias GI: dyspepsia, nausea, vomiting, constipation, diarrhea, decreased appetite Integ: hair loss, skin rashes	styramine and colestipol may decrease GI absorption. β-blockers decrease effectiveness of dextrothyroxine. Additive effect with digitalis.	
Use cautiously with liver dysfunction, cataracts. Safety in pregnancy, lactating women, and children not established.	Well tolerated. Neuro: mild headache, insomnia, fatigue, cataracts may develop GI: nausea, vomiting Biliary: HEPATOTOXICITY Renal: MYOSITIS WITH ACUTE RENAL FAILURE Elevated CPK, alkaline phosphates, transaminases	Unknown	As for all. ASSESSMENT: Baseline eye exam and periodically thereafter. Assess baseline lab values—CPK, renal and hepatic studies. INTERVENTION: Take with meals to increase absorption. Do not decrease unless directed by physician. EVALUATION: If prolonged muscle pain continues or visual difficulties, notify physician.

tivity of lipoprotein lipase. Triglyceride levels are reduced 20%–40% and LDLs are reduced 15%–35%. Nicotinic acid decreases the hepatic synthesis of LDL.

Clofibrate

Clofibrate (Atromid-S) has been used in the patient to reduce plasma cholesterol and triglyceride concentration. Recently, clofibrate has been associated with unexplained high death rates in clinical trials. Clofibrate is used only rarely today for the treatment of type III hyperlipoproteinemia.

PHARMACOKINETICS. Clofibrate is slowly but completely absorbed from the gastrointestinal tract and is measurable in serum 3–24 hours after administration. It is metabolized in the liver and subsequently excreted by the kidney. Clofibrate is highly bound to albumin.

CONTRAINDICATIONS. Clofibrate is contraindicated in pregnant or nursing women, and in patients with hepatic or renal dysfunction, since the drug is biotransformed and excreted in these organs.

ADVERSE EFFECTS. Adverse effects include nausea and diarrhea. Occasionally, skin rash, loss of hair, impotence, breast tenderness, and decreased libido may be seen. A high incidence of cholelithiasis and cholecystitis caused by an increased *lithogenicity* of the bile has been observed in patients treated with clofibrate. Patients taking high doses of clofibrate also appear to have a high risk of developing cancer of the biliary tract. Clofibrate is currently restricted to use as a "last resort"

drug for hyperlipidemia because of these later adverse effects and because of the unexplained high death rate.

INTERACTIONS. Clofibrate can displace warfarin from albumin, thus enhancing the pharmacologic effect of the warfarin. Hypoglycemia may occur with concurrent insulin and sulfonylurea therapy. Probenecid may increase toxicity by impairing clofibrate renal and metabolic clearance.

Gemfibrozil

Gemfibrozil (Lopid) decreases serum triglycerides by 40%–55% and VLDL by 40% with a variable reduction in total cholesterol. Gemfibrozil may increase HDL by 17%–25%, with the possible benefit of inhibiting the atherosclerotic process. Gemfibrozil may also potentiate the effect of warfarin. Gemfibrozil is used as adjunctive therapy in patients with type IV and V hyperlipidemia. The drug is generally well tolerated.

PHARMACOKINETICS. Gemfibrozil is well absorbed from the gastrointestinal tract with peak plasma levels occurring in about one to two hours. Gemfibrozil is biotransformed in the liver, has a half-life of 1.5 hours, and is excreted in the urine.

Nicotinic Acid

Nicotinic acid (Nico-Span) acts to reduce synthesis of VLDL and LDL with an average reduction of 15%–35%, in addition to increasing levels of HDL. Nicotinic acid is used as adjunctive therapy in treating the hypertriglyceride and hypercholesterol of types IIa and IIb, III, IV, and V. It is given orally in doses of 1–2 g three times daily. The usual maximal dose is 8 g/day.

The major side effect associated with nicotinic acid is intense flushing, which may be accompanied by itching, nausea, and diarrhea. These side effects are thought to be prostaglandin-mediated. Therefore, administration of one adult aspirin, a prostaglandin inhibitor, 30 minutes before the nicotinic acid dose may be helpful. Additionally, slowly increasing the doses of niacin up to the desired entry level dose is advised to ameliorate the flushing episodes.

Combined Therapy

A recent randomized, placebo-controlled angiographic trial (Blankenhorn, D. et al, 1987) tested the combination of colestipol (30 g/day) and niacin (3–12 g/day nicotinic acid). There was a significant reduction of lipids and low-density lipoproteins by 50%, which reduced the progression of coronary atherosclerotic lesion and new atheroma formation. Lovastatin has been recently shown to be effective in combination with colestipol in lowering the serum lipids of patients with familial hypercholesterolemia. Other combination therapies are currently under investigation, including gemfibrozil and niacin for resistant hypertriglyceridemia.

Fish Oils

Supermarkets, health food stores, and pharmacies are currently advertising and selling omega-3 fish oils. The omega-3 fish oils have been found in various studies to decrease serum cholesterol, low-density lipoproteins, and triglycerides; and to competitively inhibit synthesis of thromboxane A_2, a vasoconstrictor that promotes platelet aggregation. Controlled, prospective studies are currently being conducted to either prove or disprove these claims.

Several fish oil capsules are on the market (Table 32–6) with a labeled maximum dosage of 3 g or less daily (the equivalent of about 8 oz of salmon).

Table 32–6. FISH OIL PRODUCTS

Product		Omega-3 Fat Content
MaxEPA (*Scherer*)	1000-mg capsules	180 mg EPA* 120 mg DHA†
Super MaxEPA (*Twin Labs*)	1200-mg capsules	225 mg EPA 150 mg DHA
Promega (*Parke–Davis*)	1000-mg capsules	350 mg EPA 150 mg DHA
Proto-Chol (*Squibb*)	1000-mg capsules	180 mg EPA 120 mg DHA

*EPA-Eicosapentaenoic acid
†DHA-Docosahexaenoic acid

USING THE NURSING PROCESS

The positive relationship between cholesterol level and risk of coronary heart disease has led most researchers and health professionals to conclude that the cholesterol level of the U.S. population is too high. It has been proposed that ideal cholesterol levels for adults range from 130–190 mg/dl.

Nurses are often front-line educators for people in the moderate- to high-risk category. Nurses must understand the importance of cholesterol as a cardiovascular risk factor; be familiar with cholesterol-lowering approaches; and be able to teach and counsel patients and their families about lowering cholesterol. This education is multifaceted and includes diet, weight loss, exercise, and drug therapy. The approach is always individualized, based on the patient's risk factors.

ASSESSMENT

Assessment of the patient requiring antihyperlipemic medications for the control of hyperlipoproteinemia always begins with a thorough nursing history to develop the data base. This information is used later when preparing the nursing care plan. The information obtained is included in Table 32–7. The patient who requires antihyperlipemic medications may be acutely ill in a hospital or may be relatively healthy with the condition discovered on a routine medical physical examination.

During the assessment, the nurse determines both patient and family history of smoking and hyperlipidemia and related diseases such as angina, myocardial infarction, peripheral vascular disease, and hypertension. Also, dietary patterns are determined, including the amounts and types of food eaten. Current weight and percentage of body fat may be obtained. Life-style patterns, including amount and type of physical activity, leisure-time activities, and amount of stress are important to obtain.

The most important portion of the initial assessment is to rule out the underlying causes of the disease. Hyperlipidemia which is secondary to hypothyroidism, diabetes, or liver disease, does not respond well to therapies until the primary problems are addressed. Additionally, non-compliancy to treatments for the above may be exclusion criteria for the treatment of the hyperlipidemias.

Cholesterol screening facilitates the assignment to a relative risk group. Patients with borderline to high cholesterols should be further evaluated by a 12 hour fasting lipid profile. The 12 hour fast is imperative, since it takes that time for chylomicrons to clear from the circulation. Patients should also be screened for thyroid disease, liver disease, and diabetes mellitus.

Non-lipid risk factors (see Table 32–8) should be reviewed. The presence of two or more non-lipid risk factors, may change the assignment of risk from average-risk to high risk. This will affect the treatment plan.

Routine lipid screening tests should be recommended

Table 32–7. NURSING PROCESS FOR PATIENT REQUIRING ANTIHYPERLIPIDEMIC AGENTS

Assessment

Assess current dietary patterns, including amounts and types of food eaten. Note current weight and percent of body fat.
Determine lifestyle patterns, e.g., amount and type of physical/leisure activity, and amount of stress.
Note patient and family history of smoking and diseases such as angina, myocardial infarction, peripheral vascular disease, and hypertension.

Nursing Diagnosis	Nursing Actions	Rationale	Desired Outcomes/ Evaluation Criteria
Knowledge deficit related to lack of exposure/unfamiliarity with resources, information misinterpretation as evidenced by questions, statement of misconception, inaccurate follow-through of instruction, development of preventable complications.	Discuss normal pathophysiology of cardiovascular system and information about patient variance.	Becoming knowledgeable about disease process and expectations can facilitate adherance to prescribed treatment regimen.	Verbalizes understanding of condition/disease process and therapeutic regimen. Initiates necessary lifestyle changes.
	Provide information about drug action, administration and side-effects.	Understanding how the drug works can help patient to realize importance of taking it as prescribed.	
	Discuss side effects which need to be reported the physician, e.g., bleeding gums. Stress importance of followthrough care.	Promotes opportunity for patient to assume control over own treatment and seek help in a timely manner.	
	Review dietary restrictions and assist patient to plan a low-animal-fat, low-cholesterol diet including the use of oat bran. Refer for dietary consult if indicated.	Patients may believe they can continue to eat as they please as long as they take their medication. However, adherance to the diet can reduce the level of serum cholesterol significantly. In addition, reducing body weight decreases cardiac workload.	
	Encourage development of an exercise/activity program.	Supports weight loss/maintenance, improves muscle tone and feelings of general well-being.	
	Encourage supplementation of vitamins, A, D, K and E.	Antilipidemics impair absorption of fat-soluble vitamins.	
	Discuss need to stop smoking and assist with plan for cessation.	Smoking increases vasoconstriction, impairs gas exchange.	
	Identify other cardiac risk factors that may be present and problem-solve solutions, e.g. stress management.	Promotes general/cardiovascular wellness.	
Adjustment, impaired, potential related to disability requiring alterations in lifestyle.	Discuss identified changes which need to be made to achieve reduction of cholesterol/arteriosclerosis. Assist patient to develop a plan of action to meet needs.	Lack of symptoms, cost of drug therapy, presence of side-effects, e.g., nausea/constipation. Thinking about how changes can be accomplished, with as little impact on lifestyle as possible will help patient to cooperate with treatment regimen.	Initiates lifestyle changes that will permit adaptation to new life situation.
	Encourage expression of feelings and acknowledge realities of the difficulty of making required lifestyle changes.	Promotes awareness and acceptance of feelings and identifies areas of need.	

TABLE 32–8. NON-LIPID RISK FACTORS

The patient is considered to have high risk status if he or she has ONE of the following:
 Definite CHD; the characteristic picture and objective laboratory findings of either:
 Definite prior myocardial infarction, or
 Definite myocardial ischemia, such as angina pectoris
 Status post CABG or PTCA
The patient is considered to have high risk status if he or she has TWO of the following risk factors:
 Male sex
 Family history of premature CHD (definite myocardial infarction or sudden death before 55 years of age in a parent or sibling).
 Cigarette smoking (currently smokes more than ten cigarettes per day).
 Hypertension
 Low HDL-cholesterol concentration (below 35 mg/dL confirmed by repeated measurement).
 Diabetes Mellitus
 History of definite cerebrovascular or occlusive peripheral vascular disease.
 Severe obesity (≥ 30% overweight)

for relatives of those who have familial hyperlipidemia or premature atherosclerotic heart disease so that appropriate therapy can be instituted to retard atherogenesis and its consequences.

NURSING DIAGNOSES

The nurse establishes the nursing diagnoses in order to plan, implement, and evaluate nursing care. Typical nursing diagnoses for a patient receiving antihyperlipid agents are included in Table 32–7.

PLANNING AND INTERVENTION

From the nursing diagnosis, the nurse is able to plan the nursing care goals. The goals of nursing intervention for the patient who requires antihyperlipemic medications are included in Table 32–7.

Since hyperlipoproteinemia is often familial, other family members are encouraged to have regular physical examinations and blood tests. Dietary restrictions of cholesterol may be beneficial to the whole family and are encouraged by the nurse.

The hazards of smoking are also discussed. There is clear evidence in the literature that smokers have a greater incidence of coronary disease and a higher mortality. Smoking reduction is highly recommended and supported. The nurse stresses that patients who stop smoking often have a reduction in serum lipid levels that may prolong their lives and prevent further complications from coronary artery or cerebral disease or peripheral vascular disease. There is no one risk factor which emerges more important than any other. The literature is replete with experts making strong, but unfounded claims. The nurse should stress that a reasonable approach to all underlying risk factors should be

taken, with the understanding that it is still possible that despite all the "numbers" being right the patient may still have a coronary event.

PATIENT TEACHING

Most patients who require antihyperlipemic agents self-administer these medications at home. The nurse must therefore ensure that the patient has adequate knowledge about the medications and treatment program. Patient teaching information is found in Table 32–9. It is important to include dietary teaching in the education program. Many patients think they can eat whatever they like while taking their antihyperlipid agent. For information on a low–animal-fat, low-cholesterol diet, refer to a nutrition book, or consult a registered clinical dietitian.

Diet therapy is the first line treatment of hyperlipi-

TABLE 32–9. PATIENT TEACHING INFORMATION—ANTIHYPERLIPIDEMIC AGENTS

Dear Patient:
 This drug has been prescribed for you. This is what you should know about your drug to get the most from your therapy.

1. Antihyperlipidemic drugs are taken to reduce blood cholesterol and/or triglyceride levels.
2. Antihyperlipemic drugs are taken until your high lipid level is lowered, or possibly for the rest of your life.
3. When taking cholestyramine (Questran) or colestipol, mix the dry powder with fluids before taking. Any liquid—water, fruit juice, carbonated drinks—and even soft fruits like applesauce can be used. When mixing, drop the powder on top of the liquid and allow it to stand for about 2 min, then stir until it is well mixed. After taking the drug, rinse the glass with liquid and drink this as well, to ensure all the dose is received. The drug is distasteful.
4. Antihyperlipemic drugs are generally separated from other drugs by taking them 1 hour before or 4 hours after other drugs.
5. Most antihyperlipemics may be taken with meals if GI upset occurs.
6. Interactions may occur between antihyperlipemic agents and other drugs. Always check with your druggist or doctor before adding another drug or taking OTC products.
7. Do not skip a dose; however, if a dose is forgotten, do **not** double the dose to "catch up."
8. The side effects of your particular drug may include constipation. Please eat a high-bulk, high-fiber diet to avoid constipation.
9. Antihyperlipid agents may take 1–3 months before they begin to lower serum lipid levels. Your doctor will order frequent blood tests to evaluate your blood lipid level. It is also important that you continue to be on a low-cholesterol diet as ordered by your doctor.
10. Your doctor may order vitamins to prevent vitamin deficiencies. Take these as ordered.
11. Store your drugs in a tight, light-resistant container.

Table 32–10. DIETARY THERAPY

Dietary Component	Step 1	Step 2
PERCENT CALORIES		
Saturated Fat	10%	7%
Polyunsaturated fat	10%	10%
Monounsaturated fat	10–15%	10–15%
Total fat	30%	30%
Carbohydrates	50–60%	50–60%
Protein	10–20%	10–20%
Cholesterol	300 mg/Day	300 mg/Day

demia. Based on the guidelines of the American Heart Association and the NCEP, a two step diet program is implemented. As reference, the typical American diet is composed of 40%–50% caloric intake as fat, 400–600 mg/day of cholesterol, and about 40% caloric intake as carbohydrate. As noted in Table 32–10, Step I and Step II require a reduction of total fat to 30%, a reduction of cholesterol to 300 mg and 200 mg, respectively, along with an increased carbohydrate intake of 50%–60%.

Target LDL levels for diet alone are:

≤190 mg/dL in patients who are not at high risk
(2 or more non-lipid risk factors)
≤160 mg/dL in patients who are at high risk
(2 or more non-lipid risk factors)

Dietary teaching may also include the addition of oat bran to the diet. Recent research found that 1–1.5 cups (60–90 g) of dry bran a day reduced the level of serum cholesterol 13%–19%. When used with other soluble fibers, treatment with oat bran achieved total reductions in cholesterol level of 20%–25% and was maintained over two years.

This is moderated by the fact that not all patients respond to oat bran, and those who do are often so filled with gas as to be discomforting.

Patients should be taught to read food labels for fat content. Too often, those foods claiming to be cholesterol free are high in saturated fats. Moderate exercise, a low-cholesterol and low saturated fat diet are keys to the non-drug approaches to hyperlipidemia.

The use of psyllium (Metamucil) has been advocated by several researchers. Taking one teaspoonful of this OTC laxative, may have a mild to moderate effect on lowering serum cholesterol. If laxation occurs, decreasing the volume of the mixing vehicle (water or juice) will titrate the stools to the desired consistancy. Again, this product works for some patients, but is not a universally accepted therapy for hypercholesterolemia.

EVALUATION

The nurse bases the evaluation of the effectiveness of antihyperlipemic medications on a predetermined list of evaluation outcome criteria. These evaluation criteria are developed on an individual basis through discussion among the nurse, patient, and family. The information from the data base, obtained in the original assessment, is used to formulate the criteria for evaluation. Typical outcome evaluation criteria are included in Table 32–7.

It is extremely important for the nurse to work with the patient and family to ensure their complete assistance and support. The majority of patients, once they understand the importance of their continued medical treatment, usually are compliant. The fact that they may have previously had a live-threatening coronary or cerebral event may also improve their compliance. The primary reason for noncompliance is usually forgetting the medication (see Chapter 8). Noncompliance with the rest of the treatment regimen can also occur. This might include not altering or modifying diet, smoking, or lifestyle changes.

The patient should also be aware of the side effects of the medications. If the patient notes any unusual symptoms, they should be reported to the physician or nurse.

Coronary atherosclerosis is a multifactorial disease with definite evidence that certain risk factors accelerate atherogenesis. The presence of more than one risk factor is not simply additive, but synergistic. The interaction of multiple factors significantly accelerates the disease process.

The more the patient and family are involved with the planning of care, the more likely they are to comply. The nurse must stress the importance of continued medical care and continued reduction of risk factors. All other evaluation criteria are assessed and evaluated before the patient leaves the health care environment. All previously taught material is reviewed and updated with patient and family, if necessary, to ensure that the patient's knowledge base remains accurate.

THERAPEUTIC AGENTS FOR HEMATOLOGIC PROBLEMS: HEMATINICS

The anemias, in general, are a group of blood disorders of the hematopoietic system that result in a decreased number of erythrocytes (red blood cells; normally 4.2–5.7 million/mm), lowered hemoglobin concentrations (normally 12–17 g/ml), and decreased volume of packed red blood cells in the blood (hematocrit normally 42%–47%). Most anemias are not diseases in and of themselves but are manifestations of other pathologic processes such as acute and chronic diseases, dietary insufficiency, and drug toxicity.

Anemias can be characterized as those caused by a deficiency in red cell production, by excessive red cell destruction, or by a combination of the two. Production of red cells decreases when there is a deficiency of substances required for their production such as iron, vitamin B_{12}, and folic acid. Iron deficiency anemia and pernicious anemia are examples of this type of anemia.

Failure of the *stem cell* to produce red blood cell precursors in the bone marrow also causes a deficiency in the production of red blood cells, as in aplastic anemia. Irradiation and chemotherapeutic agents used in cancer may cause aplastic anemia.

Various types of pathologic states can result in increased destruction of red blood cells. These anemias are referred to as hemolytic anemias. These include conditions in which antibodies are directed at red blood cells, which results in their destruction. These can be *autoimmune disorders* or can result from drug intake (e.g., methyldopa). There can be an intrinsic metabolic disorder within the red cell that results in its destruction. These include glucose-6-phosphate dehydrogenase (G-6-PD) deficiency and paroxysmal nocturnal hemoglobinuria (PNH).

Anemias in which both decreased production and excessive destruction occur include those of chronic disease (renal, hepatic, malignancy) and hemoglobinopathies such as *sickle-cell anemia*. Acute, excessive loss of red blood cells, as occurs with hemorrhage or slow bleeding, can occur with a gastric ulcer and can also cause anemia.

Anemias can also be classified by the appearance of the red blood cell. This simple classification is *microcytic, hypochromic*, which is characteristic of iron deficiency anemia; *macrocytic*, which is characteristic of vitamin B_{12} deficiency; and *normocytic*.

Anemias are common and are produced by a wide variety of processes. It is important that the cause of an anemia be identified and the appropriate measures taken. These may include the treatment of an underlying disease state, discontinuation of an offending drug, or replacement therapy with iron, vitamin B_{12}, or folic acid. The anemias are featured in Table 32–11. The antianemic medications are featured in Table 32–12.

Iron is present in every cell in the body and is a component of hemoglobin, myoglobin, and a number of enzymes necessary for oxygen transfer. About 30% of iron is stored as hemosiderin or ferritin, primarily in hepatic cells and reticuloendothelial cells of the spleen and marrow. The remaining two-thirds of iron circulates within the red cell as hemoglobin. The total body content of iron is 50 mg/kg in men and 35 mg/kg in women.

Oral Iron Products

USES. Iron preparations correct erythropoietic abnormalities due to the deficiency of iron (see Table 32–12). Iron is of value only when the iron stores are depleted, as in hypochromic anemias. If iron supplements are given to a person with normal blood values, the hemoglobin content does not rise; there is, however, an increase in the reserve supply of iron.

When iron is administered to a person with hypochromic anemia, hematocrit and hemoglobin levels begin to increase in three days. The maximum response, however, does not occur until the second to fourth weeks. As the hemoglobin level increases, the patient notes less fatigue, improved appetite and nail condition, and improved sense of well-being.

PHARMACOKINETICS. *Absorption and Distribution.* Iron preparations are absorbed best in the duo-

Table 32–11. ANEMIAS

Etiology	Symptoms	Management	Comments
Iron deficiency: Decreased intake of iron, increased loss of iron, blood loss, frank bleeding, pregnancy	Fatigue, pallor of skin and mucous membranes, poor appetite, low vitality, severe tachycardia	Iron products, increased dietary iron, correct the underlying problem	Red blood cells can be either (a) hypochromic (low color index) or (b) microcytic (smaller in size). A 50% blood loss can be tolerated if it occurs over time. Only a 10% loss can be tolerated if it occurs quickly.
Pernicious anemia: Deficiency of vitamin B_{12} due to (a) decreased gastric intrinsic factor, (b) small bowel malabsorption, or (c) dietary deficiency	Red beefy tongue, pale colorless complexion, difficulty swallowing, digestive disturbances, fatigability, dyspnea, numbness, tingling in fingers, peripheral neuropathies, growth retardation in infants and children, mental disturbances	Parenteral vitamin B_{12}	It is a type of megaloblastic anemia—large immature cells in bone marrow and plasma.
Folic acid anemia: Poor dietary intake, malabsorption syndromes, impaired utilization, increased requirements, chemotherapeutic drugs	Similar to pernicious anemia but with no neurologic manifestations	Dietary supplements, improved diet	Red cells become macrocytic.

denum by active transport. Iron is absorbed most readily in its ferrous form, which is less ionized than the ferric form (ferrous = Fe^{++}; ferric = Fe^{+++}). Sustained-release preparations are available; however, they have been shown to be poorly absorbed and produce poor clinical responses. Iron products may be combined with ascorbic acid (vitamin C), which helps to keep the iron in its ferrous form. This is designed to enhance absorption. Studies have shown that ascorbic acid does this, but the effect is small—only about 10%. Oral preparations are best absorbed when taken between meals, but this may cause gastrointestinal irritation. If this occurs, a small snack is taken with the iron preparation.

Biotransformation and Excretion. Iron preparations have the same fate as dietary iron. Iron is removed through the loss of iron-containing cells from the bowel, skin, and genitourinary tract. Normal loss is 0.5–1 mg/day and in menstruating women the loss is 1–2 mg/day.

CONTRAINDICATIONS AND PRECAUTIONS. Oral iron is contraindicated in primary hemochromatosis, peptic ulcer, and hypersensitivity. Since it irritates the bowel, it is not given in disorders such as regional enteritis and ulcerative colitis. Iron is given cautiously to persons with renal and hepatic dysfunction. Liquid iron preparations also may stain the teeth, so they are given through a straw placed well back in the mouth.

ADVERSE EFFECTS. The local effects of orally administered iron include action as an irritant and astringent. The oral inorganic iron acts with tissue proteins to form an insoluble iron compound that can irritate the gastrointestinal tract. This local irritation can contribute to nausea, vomiting, constipation or diarrhea, and abdominal distress. This irritation can rarely cause gastrointestinal bleeding and a positive test result for fecal occult blood. If these symptoms develop, the iron products are discontinued for several days until symptoms are relieved, after which they are resumed. More commonly, dark red or black stools can occur, resulting from the insoluble iron compound in the stool.

INTERACTIONS. Iron is not given concurrently with antacids, since iron absorption is slowed due to complexation with the antacid. Coffee and tea consumed with a meal or one hour after, and eggs and milk can also inhibit iron absorption. Administration is separated by at least two to three hours. Absorption can be enhanced slightly if iron is mixed with ascorbic acid. Iron products can combine into a insoluble complex with tetracycline, decreasing its availabiltiy. They are administered two to three hours apart as well. Chloramphenicol delays iron clearance from plasma, delays iron incorporation into red blood cells, and interferes with erythropoiesis.

FERROUS SULFATE. Ferrous sulfate (Mol-Iron, Ferospace, and others), the oldest iron product, is the standard iron preparation against which all other oral preparations are usually measured. Ferrous sulfate contains 20% ferrous elemental iron. The dosage is determined according to the severity of the anemia and is included in Table 32–12.

FERROUS GLUCONATE. Ferrous gluconate (Fergon) causes less gastric irritation and is better tolerated than ferrous sulfate. This, however, is because it contains only 11.6% ferrous iron. The daily dosage range is included in Table 32–12.

FERROUS FUMARATE. Ferrous fumarate (Ircon, Femiron) is comparable to the products previously described. It contains 33% elemental iron. The usual adult dosage is included in Table 32–12.

IRON WITH VITAMIN C. Combining iron with vitamin C enhances the absorption of the iron. Several over-the-counter preparations are available in tablet, chewable tablets or time-released products. These products are featured in Table 32–13.

PARENTERAL IRON PRODUCTS

Although the preferred route of iron products is oral, it may be necessary on occasion to administer parenteral iron. The parenteral route is usually used when the patient cannot tolerate or absorb oral iron.

Iron Dextran Injection

Iron dextran injection (Imferon) is a complex ferric hydroxide with dextran in a 0.9% sodium chloride solution for injection. It contains 50 mg of elemental iron per milliliter. Reticuloendothelial cells of the liver, spleen, and bone marrow separate the iron from the dextran complex and gradually release it, which combines with transferrin for transport to the bone marrow. Iron dextran is used only after iron deficiency anemia has been confirmed and when oral therapy has failed or may further irritate gastrointestinal disease.

PHARMACOKINETICS. The majority of iron dextran is well-absorbed after IM injection within 72 hours and the remaining drug is absorbed over the next three to four weeks. The half-life of iron dextran is 5–20 hours. Iron dextran is not easily eliminated, and therefore accumulation, which may be toxic, may occur.

CONTRAINDICATIONS AND PRECAUTIONS. Iron dextran is contraindicated in persons hypersensitive to it and in all anemias other than iron deficiency anemia. It is used cautiously with impaired liver and renal function, since these organs may be further damaged. Because iron dextran has been associated with fatal anaphylactic reactions, caution is advised in administering it to patients with significant allergies or asthma. A test dose of 25 mg intramuscularly or intravenously may be administered one hour prior to determine sensitivity. If any reaction occurs, the physician is consulted. Use during pregnancy and lactation only when clearly needed. Iron dextran is not recommended in infants less than four months of age.

ADVERSE EFFECTS. The adverse effects of parenteral administration of iron include pain at the injection site, temporary or permanent discoloration of the skin at the injection site, headache, nausea and vomiting, fever, and urticaria. Parenteral iron may be deposited in the liver or pancreas and may cause hemochromatosis.

DOSAGE. Initial intramuscular dose in adults is 50 mg, with amounts as large as 250 mg administered

TEXT RESUMES ON PAGE 872

Table 32–12. ANTIANEMIC MEDICATIONS

Name	Dosage	Mode of Administration	Pharmacokinetics
IRON PREPARATIONS Ferrous sulfate (Ferospace, Mol-Iron, Fer-In-Sol, SlowFe) (20% iron)			

Action: Supplements dietary iron and is available to body for red blood cell production.

Use: To correct iron deficiency anemias.

Name	Dosage	Mode of Administration	Pharmacokinetics
	Adults: I: 300–1200 mg in divided doses daily. Children 6–12 yr: 120–600 mg/day in divided doses. Children under 6 yr: 300 mg/day in divided doses.	PO, all come as tablets, liquids, time-released capsules, elixirs, drops	O: 24–48 hr P: UA D: UA ½L: UA PB: 100% B: is not E: urine, sweat, feces
Ferrous gluconate (Fergon) (11.6% iron)	Adult: 300–640 mg 1–3 × daily Children 6–12 yr: 300 mg 1–3 × daily Children under 6 yr: 100–300 mg daily in divided doses.	PO	O: 24–48 hr P: UA D: UA ½L: UA PB: 100% B: is not E: urine, sweat, feces
Ferrous fumarate (Ircon, Femiron) (33% iron)	Adult: 200 mg 1–4 × daily. Children under 6 yr: 100–300 mg daily in divided doses.	PO	Same as ferrous gluconate
Iron dextran (Imferon) (1 ml = 50 mg elemental iron)	Given by weight. See formula in text. Approximately 250 mg iron daily for each g hemoglobin is below normal. 1 ml/min undiluted. Mix required dose in 200–250 ml, give test dose first of 25 mg over 5 min, then infuse rest in 1–2 hours.	IM IV infusion IV drip	O: slow P: 72 hr D: 3–4 wk ½L: 5–20 hr PB: 100% B: not E: not

Key to Abbreviations in the *Pharmacokinetics* column O-onset; P-peak; D-duration; PB-protein bound; B-biotransformed in; E-excreted in; ½L-halflife.

*Within the column listing adverse effects, underlines indicate the most common effects; CAPITALS indicate life-threatening effects.

Contraindications/ Precautions	Adverse Effects*	Interactions	Nursing Implications
Contraindicated in primary hemochromatosis, peptic ulcer, regional enteritis, and ulcerative colitis.	For all iron products: GI: GI irritation, anorexia, nausea, vomiting, constipation/diarrhea, stools appear dark, staining of teeth with liquid produots.	Inhibits iron absorption if given with tetracyclines, antacids, coffee, tea, milk, or eggs. Separate administration by 2–3 hr. Increases absorption of iron if administered with ascorbic acid. Chloramphenicol decreases iron clearance from serum.	ASSESSMENT: Lab blood work, dietary intake, bowel function. INTERVENTION: Medications should not be taken within 1 hr of bedtime since they are possibly corrosive to the stomach. All tablets and capsules are taken on an empty stomach between meals for best absorption. If GI distress occurs, try enteric-coated tablets or give tablets with meals. Liquid preparations are well diluted and taken through a straw placed well back in the mouth to prevent damage to enamel of the teeth. Elixir cannot be mixed with milk, fruit juice, or wine. Do not crush or chew sustained-release products. Stools may become dark green or black. EVALUATION: Iron therapy is continued 2–3 mo after hemoglobin returns to normal to assist in replenishing iron stores. If severe constipation or diarrhea, notify physician.
Same as ferrous sulfate	Same as ferrous sulfate	Same as ferrous sulfate	Same as ferrous sulfate
Same as ferrous sulfate	Same as ferrous sulfate	Same as ferrous sulfate	Same as ferrous sulfate
Contraindicated in hypersensitivity and all other anemias. Use cautiously in renal and hepatic dysfunction, and patients with significant allergies or asthma. Use in pregnant and lactating women only when clearly needed.	Neuro: convulsions, headache, weakness, fever, chills CV: chest pain, shock, hypotension, tachycardia, flushing. Resp: ANAPHYLACTIC REACTIONS, bronchospasm	Chloramphenicol delays red blood cell response. Lab: may falsely increase bilirubin, decrease calcium.	ASSESSMENT: Presence of sensitivity. A skin test should be performed before first dose to detect for the presence of allergies. 25 mg is administered IM or IV 1 hour before. If any reaction occurs, consult the doctor.

CONTINUED ON THE FOLLOWING PAGE

Antianemic Agents

Table 32–12. ANTIANEMIC MEDICATIONS–*CONTINUED*

Name	Dosage	Mode of Administration	Pharmacokinetics
Iron dextran–*Continued*			
IRON ANTIDOTE Deferoxamine (Desferal)			

Action: Chelating agent which binds iron from ferritin, hemosiderin, and transferrin and is then excreted by the kidney.

Use: Reduces serum iron level.

Name	Dosage	Mode of Administration	Pharmacokinetics
	Adult: 1 g followed by 500 mg q 4 hr $\times$ 2 doses. Additional doses 0.5 g q 4–12 hr, do not exceed 6 g daily.	IM	O: UA P: UA D: UA ½L: UA PB: UA B: plasma E: urine, bile
	Children: 50 mg/kg/dose q 6 hr up to 15 mg/kg/hr continuous IV.	IM, IV	
	Only in cerebrovascular emergencies: IV solution: not more than 15 mg/kg/hr.	IV	

VITAMINS
Cyanocobalamin (Betalin 12)

Action: Replaces dietary B_{12}, which is not being absorbed.

Use: Correct and treat pernicious anemia (B_{12} deficiency).

Name	Dosage	Mode of Administration	Pharmacokinetics
	Adults: 100–1000 μg daily for 6–7 days then 100–1000 μg monthly.	Deep IM	O: rapid P: 8 hr D: 8–12 hr ½L: UA PB: moderate amount B: is not E: urine (unchanged)
	Children: 100 μg weekly to monthly	Deep IM	

Key to Abbreviations in the *Pharmacokinetics* column O-onset; P-peak; D-duration; PB-protein bound; B-biotransformed in; E-excreted in; ½L-halflife.
*Within the column listing adverse effects, underlines indicate the most common effects; CAPITALS indicate life-threatening effects.

Contraindications/ Precautions	Adverse Effects*	Interactions	Nursing Implications
	GI: abdominal pain, nausea, vomiting, diarrhea Hemo: leukocytosis, lymph-adenopathy Renal: hematuria Musclskel: arthritis Integ: staining at IM site, pain at IM site, phlebitis at IV site.		INTERVENTION: No other medications are mixed in the syringe. Administer by Z-track technique in dorsal gluteal area of the buttock. Urine may turn dark brown or black on standing. Following IV administration, patient should remain on bed rest for 30 min. Do not administer with oral iron products. IV: give test dose first. No faster than 50 mg/min. EVALUATION: For anaphylactic reaction throughout therapy.
Use cautiously in history of pyelonephritis.	Neuro: blurred vision CV: tachycardia Renal: dysuria Integ: pain and induration at injection site, itching, rash.	None significant.	ASSESSMENT: Intake and output to assure adequate renal function. Note urine color—often reddish. Assess stool for signs of occult bleeding. Assess eyes at baseline and periodically for cataracts. INTERVENTION: Reconstituted solution should be stored for no longer than one week. Protect from light.
Contraindicated in hypersensitivity.	Neuro: optic nerve atrophy, anaphylactic shock GI: diarrhea Integ: itching, urticaria, pain at injection site.	Neomycin, colchicine, para-aminosalicylic acid, K, and alcohol may cause malabsorption of B_{12}. Cimetidine impairs absorption.	ASSESSMENT: Dietary habits for B_{12} intake. Assess patient concurrently receiving cardiotonics for hypokalemia and fluid overload. Assess for cobalt hypersensitivity. If cobalt sensitive, do an intradermal test dose first. Parenteral medications should be refrigerated and protected from light. INTERVENTION: Stress importance of monthly therapy for life for a patient with pernicious anemia. EVALUATION: Carefully for allergic reactions.

CONTINUED ON THE FOLLOWING PAGE

Table 32–12. ANTIANEMIC MEDICATIONS–*CONTINUED*

Name	Dosage	Mode of Administration	Pharmacokinetics
Hydroxocobalamin (Alphare-disol)	Adults: 1000 μg monthly Children: 100 μg monthly	Deep IM IM	O: more slowly P: 8–12 hr PB: large amount
Folic acid			
Action: Replaces dietary folic acid for use in body.			
Use: Correct and treat folic acid deficiency.			
	Adults: 0.1–2.0 mg	Deep IM IV	O: UA P: UA
	Adults: 0.4 mg/day	PO	O: rapid P: 30–60 min D: 12–24 hr ½L: UA PB: UA B: small intestine enzymes E: urine
	Children up to 4 yr: 0.3 mg/day.	PO	
	Infants: 0.1 mg/day	PO	
Levcovorin calcium (Levco-vorin, Wellcovorin)			
Action: to replace folic acid			
Use: treat methotrexate rescue, megaloblastic anemia, and counteracts effects of overdose of folic acid antagonists.			
	1 mg daily	PO	O: 20–30 min P: 2 hr D: 3–6 hr ½L: 3.5 hr PB: UA B: UA E: urine
	1 mg daily	IM	O: 10–20 min ½L: 3.7 hr

Key to Abbreviations in the *Pharmacokinetics* column O-onset; P-peak; D-duration; PB-protein bound; B-bio-transformed in; E-excreted in; ½L-halflife
*Within the column listing adverse effects, underlines indicate the most common effects; CAPITALS indicate life-threatening effects.

every other day thereafter. The dosage is calculated to reconstitute the hemoglobin mass by several formulas:

$$0.3 \times \text{wt in \#} \times$$
$$\text{or}$$
$$0.66 \times \text{wt in kg} \times$$
$$\frac{(\text{hemoglobin in g\%} \times 100)}{14.8} = \text{mg iron}$$
$$\frac{\text{mg iron}}{50} = \text{ml iron (dosage)}$$

To avoid damage to the sensitive subcutaneous tissue, iron dextran is given by Z-track technique (described in the Nursing Process section of this chapter). Dosage for children is 25–100 mg daily. The dosage for IM injection begins with 15–30 mg and may be increased by 10 mg daily to a maximum dose of 100 mg/day for a person weighing 20–110 pounds. It is given at intervals of one to two months. Iron dextran can also be administered intravenously. Only single-dose ampuls without perservatives are used. An IV infusion of 1 ml/min of undiluted iron dextran can be administered, or an IV drip can be started. The calculated dose of iron dextran is added to 200–250 ml normal saline. A test dose of 25 mg over five minutes is administered first. If no adverse effects occur, infuse the remaining solution in one to two hours.

IRON ANTIDOTE

Deferoxamine

Deferoxamine (Desferal) is a *chelating* agent with specific affinity for ferric iron and low affinity for calcium. It binds ferric ion into a stable, water-soluble chelate

Contraindications/ Precautions	Adverse Effects*	Interactions	Nursing Implications
Same as cyanocobalamin.	Same as cyanocobalamin.	Same as cyanocobalamin.	Same as cyanocobalamin.
Contraindicated in pernicious anemia, undiagnosed anemia, aplastic or normocytic anemias.	Hemo: allergic reaction	Doses above 15–20 mg daily may increase metabolism of phenobarbital and phenytoin. Oral contraceptives may impair folate metabolism. Pyrimethamine, trimethoprim, tiamterene may interfere with folate utilization.	ASSESSMENT: Lab work to diagnose folate deficiency. INTERVENTION: Do not mix with other medications for IM use. Protect from light.
Same as folic acid. Safety in pregnant and lactating women not established.	Same as folic acid.	Levcovorin decreases serum phenytoin levels.	Same as folic acid.

readily excreted by the kidneys. Its main effect is to remove iron from ferritin, hemosiderin, and transferrin.

Deferoxamine is used to treat iron overload, which may result from overtreatment with iron products or with multiple blood transfusions, iron poisoning, or abnormally high levels injected over a long time. Iron poisoning is a common occurrence in children, since iron may be readily accessible in the household. An example would be a pregnant mother taking extra iron during her pregnancy. It imparts a reddish color to the urine, which presumably means the presence of high iron level, necessitating further treatment. More information can be found in Table 32–12.

PERNICIOUS ANEMIA AGENTS

Pernicious anemia is a type of megaloblastic anemia. *Megaloblastic* is the term used to describe most anemias characterized by large *germ cells* in the bone marrow as well as large immature red cells in the plasma (see Table

32–9). Pernicious anemia is due to the lack of *intrinsic factor*, which reduces the absorption of vitamin B_{12}. Pernicious anemia occurs three months to two to five years after the onset of intrinsic factor deficiency. If not treated, pernicious anemia can result in neurologic degeneration such as degenerative spinal cord lesions.

When a vitamin B_{12} deficiency exists, the treatment is parenteral administration of vitamin B_{12}. Oral vitamin B_{12} is poorly absorbed and has no valid therapeutic role.

Vitamin B_{12}

Two preparations of vitamin B_{12} are available: hydroxocobalamin (Alpharedisol) and cyanocobalamin (Betalin 12). Hydroxocobalamin is more highly protein bound than cyanocobalamin; however, it has no advantage of cyanocobalamin. These preparations are cobalt-containing substances produced from *Streptomyces griseus* or obtained from human liver. They are absorbed into the blood stream and transported throughout the body.

Vitamin B_{12} injections, besides being used to treat per-

Table 32–13. NURSING PROCESS FOR PATIENTS REQUIRING ANTIANEMIC DRUGS

Assessment

Determine onset and type of symptoms, effect on lifestyle.
Note history of past and present illnesses including presence of allergies (food and drug), conditions/illnesses contributing to loss of blood.
Evaluate dietary patterns.
Assess medication history, including use of prescription and nonprescription vitamins and minerals.
Review laboratory results, e.g., red cell indices, blood smears, leukocyte count, and differentials, reticulocyte and platelet count.

Nursing Diagnosis	Nursing Action	Rationale	Desired Outcomes/ Evaluation Criteria
Knowledge deficit related to lack of exposure/ unfamiliarity with resources, misinterpretation of information as evidenced by questions, statement of concern, failure to improve/development of preventable complications.	Provide information (verbal and written) about anemia and therapy needs.	Understanding of condition and necessary treatments helps the patient adhere to needed dietary changes/ drug therapy.	Identifies relationship of signs/symptoms to the disease process and correlates symptoms with causative factors.
	Discuss use of antianemic medications, e.g., oral iron preparations, Vitamin B_{12}, folic acid.	Promotes correct administration and understanding of associated effects, such as dark urine, black stools.	
	Review drug history and possible interactions.	May prevent untoward response/inadequate therapeutic levels.	
	Identify dietary considerations, including sources of iron, use/avoidance of citrus juices or calcium containing foods/products.	Taking drug with food may interfere with absorption. However it may also prevent nausea/vomiting. Ascorbic acid enhances the absorption or iron but can adversely affect vitamin B_{12} stability. Calcium binds with and decreases absorption of iron products.	
	Stress need for medical follow-up.	Necessary to monitor effectiveness/need for continuation of therapy.	
Fatigue, related to decreased metabolic energy production/ reduced oxygen carrying capacity of the blood as evidenced by verbalization of lack of energy/ inability to maintain usual routines, lethargic, listless.	Develop a schedule for activity with adequate periods for rest. Monitor response to activity.	Maximizes participation while preventing undue fatigue. Tolerance varies greatly dependent on degree of anemia present.	Reports improved sense of energy. Performs ADLs and participates in desired activities at level of ability.
	Discuss signs/symptoms indicating patient needs to alter activity level.		
	Review home/work environment to identify appropriate energy conservation techniques.	Helps patient to continue necessary activities within limitations.	
Constipation, potential related to side effects of iron therapy.	Stress need for increased bulk in diet and drinking a minimum of 6 large glasses of water per day.	Promotes normalization of amount and consistency of stool.	Reports maintenance of/ return to normal patterns of bowel functioning.
	Encourage programmed exercise/activity.	Enhances intestinal motility and transit time through bowel to reduce absorption of fluid from the stool.	Demonstrates changes in lifestyle as necessitated by causative/contributing factors.
	Discuss cautious use of stool softener or mild vegetable-based laxative.	May be beneficial when other measures are unsuccessful but can decrease absorption of iron production.	

nicious anemia, are frequently used in patients with allergies, acute viral hepatitis, trigeminal neuralgia, and multiple sclerosis, and in elderly persons for the treatment of peripheral neuropathies. Usually, two to three 1000 μg injections a week are used. Some physicians still view this as controversial because these patients do not have a vitamin B_{12} deficiency; and at this point, there is no proven research data. These products are featured in Table 32–10.

FOLIC ACID ANEMIA AGENTS

Folic acid anemia (see Table 32–9) is another megaloblastic anemia resulting from a deficiency in the vitamin folic acid. Folic acid is necessary to synthesize DNA within the red cell and its lack inhibits normal hematopoiesis. Folic acid is found mostly in green leafy vegetables. In contrast to vitamin B_{12} deficiency, folic acid deficiencies are due primarily to malnutrition, the use of birth-control pills, alcoholism, and pregnancy. Folate deficiencies are more common than vitamin B_{12} deficiencies as folate stores are depleted rapidly in the presence of a dietary deficiency.

Folic Acid

Folic acid (Folvite) is most commonly administered in its oral form. Approximately 65% of oral folic acid is quickly absorbed by the body from the proximal small intestine. Folic acid is converted to an absorbable complex by enzymes in the small intestine; 75% is excreted in the urine in 24 hours. Traces of folic acid are found in breast milk. Folic acid should not be used in patients with pernicious anemia who are not receiving vitamin B_{12}. The hematologic disorder will respond; however, the neurologic sequelae will continue to progress.

Folic acid is administered in 0.04-mg tablets or injections of 0.1–2.0 mg. Doses above 15–20 mg daily may increase metabolism of phenobarbital and phenytoin (Dilantin). For more information see Table 32–12.

Leucovorin Calcium

Leucovorin calcium (Leucovorin, Wellcovorin) is a form of folic acid used to treat megaloblastic anemias due to sprue, pregnancy and infancy, nutritional deficiencies, and as a methotrexate rescue (see Chapter 49 for more information). Leucovorin is also administered to counteract the effect of overdose of folic acid antagonists. Information on leucovorin is found in Table 32–12.

USING THE NURSING PROCESS

ASSESSMENT

Assessment of the patient requiring anti-anemic medications for the control of anemias always begins with a thorough nursing history to develop the data base. All this information is used later in preparing the nursing care plan. The patient who requires anti-anemic medications may be acutely ill in a hospital, or relatively

Table 32–14. DRUGS THAT CAUSE HEMATOLOGIC TOXICITY

Drug	A*	B*	C*	D*	E*
Anitmalarials			x		
Antithyroid drugs	x				
Cephalosporins			x		
Chloramphenicol	x	x	x		x
Chlorpropamide		x			x
Diphenylhydantoin				x	
Folic acid antagonists				x	
Gold salts		x			x
Mephenytoin	x	x	x		x
Methyldopa			x		x
Nitrofurantoin			x		
Phenothiazine tranquilizers	x				
Phenylbutazone	x	x			x
Sulfonamides	x	x	x		x
Thiazides	x				x

*A = agranulocytosis, B = aplastic anemia, C = hemolytic anemia, D = megaloblastic anemia, E = thrombocytopenia.

healthy, with this condition discovered on routine physical examination. The information to be obtained from the patient is included in Table 32–13.

The nurse assesses both objective and subjective symptoms of the anemia (see Table 32–11) at the onset of treatment and periodically during treatment to determine the effectiveness of the therapy. Before therapy is undertaken, a definitive diagnosis of the anemia is essential, including its possible underlying cause. A thorough history to determine when symptoms began is important. Has the patient had a recent history of gastrointestinal tract disease, or bleeding in the lung, or epistaxis? Or, does he or she have a history of chronic disease, or drug therapy? Table 32–14 reviews drugs that are known to cause various types of hematologic toxicity. Also, it is important to determine how symptoms have changed over time.

The nurse often assists with gathering laboratory data such as red cell indices, blood smears, leukocyte count, differentials, reticulocyte count, and platelet count. Bone marrow aspiration may also be performed.

Also, dietary intake is assessed to determine whether the cause is diet related and to determine whether dietary teaching is needed later during the intervention stage (Table 32–15). Iron deficiency is the most common deficiency in the United States among children and young women. In men and postmenopausal women, the most common cause is abnormal bleeding, which may be obvious or occult. Occult gastrointestinal bleeding may be a sign of bowel cancer. Folic acid deficiencies are less common than vitamin B_{12} and other hematopoietic deficiencies are rare.

NURSING DIAGNOSES

Nursing diagnoses are established before nursing care is implemented. These diagnoses are used later to evaluate nursing care. Typical nursing diagnoses for a patient

Table 32–15. FOODS TO BE INCLUDED IN NUTRITIONAL DEFICIENCIES

	Iron Deficiency	Vitamin B₁₂ Deficiency	Folic Acid Deficiency
Normal daily recommended allowances for adults	10 mg	5 μg	1–2 mg
Rich food sources	Organ meat, shellfish, lean meat, leafy green vegetables, egg yolk, dried beans and peas, dried fruit, dark molasses, cereals	Liver, kidney, milk and dairy products, meat and eggs	Green leafy vegetables, organ meats, lean beef, wheat, eggs, fish, dry beans, lentils, cowpeas, asparagus, broccoli, yeast

who requires antianemic medication are included in Table 32–13.

PLANNING AND INTERVENTION

The goals of intervention are developed from the nursing diagnoses. The goals of nursing intervention in caring for the patient who requires antianemic medications are included in Table 32–13.

At times, it may be necessary to administer antianemic medications, such as iron products, parenterally. The nurse must remember that a skin test to detect allergies is performed before administering the first dose, since anaphylactic reactions can occur (see Table 32–10). Also, medications are administered deep IM to prevent irritation to the subcutaneous tissues.

When the nurse administers iron dextran, a special intramuscular injection technique is used. To administer this medication, first draw it up into the syringe and draw an additional 0.2–0.5 ml of air into the syringe, then change to a long needle. The best site for administration is the dorsal gluteal area of the buttock. Prepare the site, firmly displace skin laterally, insert the needle deeply, aspirate, and inject the medication slowly, including the 0.2 ml of air. Wait ten seconds and withdraw the needle and allow the skin to fall back in place at the same time. This Z-track method prevents the iron com-

pounds from leaking back into the subcutaneous tissue, causing irritation (see Fig. 32–2). Do not mix other drugs in the same syringe, and inject no more than 5 ml into one location. Monitor the patient closely for the first several hours, particularly for a fall in blood pressure. The urine may turn dark brown or black when it stands, due to its iron content.

Because the IM route is associated with several disadvantages, including pain and discoloration at the site, more physicians are ordering IV iron dextran (Imferon without perservative). The incidence of allergic reaction for both IM and IV administration is about the same. If the patient experiences vomiting, chills, fever, headache, joint pain, or urticaria, the infusion should be stopped. Phlebitis is a common side effect of IV administration, but it can be minimized by mixing the iron dextran in normal saline solution and infusing the preparation at a rate of no faster than 50 mg/min (1 ml/min). Often, the entire iron deficit can be replaced in one infusion rather than in several IM injections.

PATIENT TEACHING

The patient who requires oral antianemic medications generally administers these medications at home. The nurse must therefore ensure that the patient knows and understands the information obtained in Table 32–16.

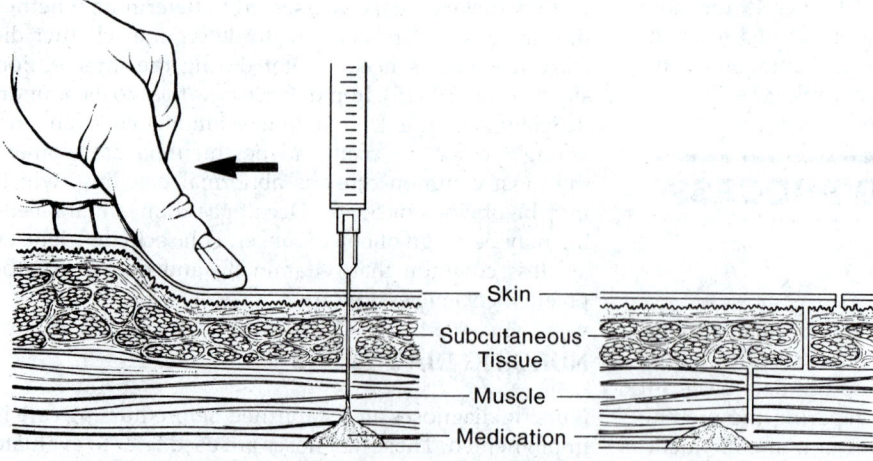

Figure 32–2. A Z-track intramuscular injection. A) The skin is pulled to one side for the injection. B) After the injection, when the skin returns to its normal position, the track is interrupted, keeping the medication from seeping back out.

Skin
Subcutaneous Tissue
Muscle
Medication

Table 32–16. PATIENT TEACHING INFORMATION—ANTIANEMICS

Dear Patient:
This drug has been ordered for you. This is what you should know about your drug to get the most from your therapy.

1. Antianemic drugs, such as _____, are taken to improve your body's ability to make healthy blood.
2. You will take antianemics until your anemia is gone. (This may be 3–5 months or a lifetime depending on the anemia.)
3. Oral iron products are absorbed best when taken between meals; however, they may be irritating to the stomach, so you may find it better to take them with or immediately following meals.
4. Liquid products are diluted in a liquid and taken through a straw to avoid staining of your teeth. Rinse your mouth immediately after taking. (Feosol elixir can be mixed with water only—**not** milk, fruit juice, or wine. Fer-In-Sol drops may be given in all liquids.)
5. Interactions between your drug and others may occur. Consult your druggist or doctor before taking other drugs.
6. If you forget a dose for more than 12 hours, skip it.
7. Do not stop taking your drugs without consulting your doctor.
8. Typical side effects of your drug are constipation, diarrhea, stomach pains, staining of the teeth, pain at the injection site, temporary or permanent skin color change at the injection site, headache, muscle ache, nausea and vomiting, fever, and mild itching.
9. Drugs may cause dark green or black stools.
10. Your dietary compliance is very important. It helps treat the present anemia and prevents further problems from occurring (Table 32–13 contains a list of foods to be included in the diet for various anemias).
11. Reversal of symptoms usually begins to occur within 2–5 days after treatment is started. You may be asked to have frequent blood testing done to evaluate progress.
12. Store drugs in tight, light-resistant containers, out of the reach of children.

EVALUATION

The evaluation of the effectiveness of antianemic medications is based on a predetermined list of outcome evaluation criteria developed on an individual basis through discussion among the nurse, patient, and family. The information in the data base obtained in the original assessment is used to formulate the criteria for evaluation. Typical outcome evaluation criteria are included in Table 32–13.

It is extremely important to work with the patient and family to ensure their complete assistance and support. The majority of patients, once they understand the importance of their continued medical treatment, usually are compliant.

Dietary knowledge is important to evaluate. Often the anemia occurred because of dietary deficiencies. Therefore, the nurse needs to evaluate daily intake of all nutrients.

The patient should know the adverse effects of his or her medications. Most side effects from hematinic medications are minimal. Since black stools can be associated with iron products and upper gastrointestinal bleeding, the patient should have periodic hemoccult tests performed on the stool. The patient should report symptoms to the physician or nurse.

The nurse must stress the importance of continued medical care. In addition, all other evaluation criteria are assessed and evaluated before the patient leaves the nurse's care. All previously taught material is reviewed and updated, if necessary to ensure that the patient's knowledge base remains accurate.

SUMMARY

Blood lipids consist of free-fatty acids, triglycerides, cholesterol, cholesterol esters, and phospholipids. These lipids form various fractions including very-low-density lipoproteins, low-density lipoproteins, intermediate-density lipoproteins, and high-density lipoproteins. Hyperlipidemia is currently associated with an increased incidence of coronary artery disease and death. Drugs are available to lower cholesterol or to lower triglycerides. Isolated hypertriglyceridemia should be treated as a separate entity. Where either the cholesterol is moderately elevated or both cholesterol and triglycerides are moderately elevated, the patient should be instructed as to dietary intervention. Once diet has been stabilized, then and only then should drug therapy be considered.

Before the nurse administers antilipidemic agents, a thorough history and laboratory data are obtained from the patient. Most patients will take antilipid agents indefinitely. Dietary teaching is important to assist with the lowering of blood lipids.

Anemias are a group of blood disorders that result in a decreased number of erythrocytes, lowered hemoglobin concentrations, and decreased volume of packed red blood cells in the blood. Anemias are either characterized as those caused by a deficiency in red cell production, those caused by excessive red blood cell destruction, or those caused by a combination of the two. Numerous products are available to treat anemia. Iron products are frequently used to treat iron deficiency anemias. Vitamin B_{12} is used to treat pernicious anemia, and folic acid is used to treat folic acid anemia.

It is important for the nurse to assess both objective and subjective symptoms of anemia. Before therapy is started, a definitive diagnosis of anemia must be made. The nurse must understand the proper administration techniques for proper administration of these products. Health and dietary teaching are also included during the intervention phase.

SITUATION 32–1

Tim Williams, a 56-year-old, has Type II hyperlipidemia uncontrolled with diet alone. He is to be managed as an outpatient through his physician's office.

1. The nurse will gather data pertinent to Mr. Williams. Which of the following items of patient information is of particular note related to hyperlipidemia?
   a. poor long-term memory
   b. high stress position in a large accounting firm
   c. rheumatic heart disease as a child
   d. history of kidney stones as an adult

2. Mr. Williams is to begin cholestyramine (Questran) 15 grams twice a day. The following represents a contraindication to the use of this drug:
   a. evidence of triglyceride levels above 400 mg/dl
   b. presence of reduced VLDL levels
   c. history of narrow angle glaucoma
   d. presence of hyperthyroidism

3. When teaching Mr. Williams about taking cholestyramine at home, the nurse includes:
   a. using over-the-counter medications as needed
   b. eating a diet low in fiber
   c. taking the drug with antacids
   d. mixing the drug with fluids before taking

4. Because of mild hypertension, Mr. Williams has been taking a thiazide diuretic for many years. When adding cholestyramine to his drug regime, the nurse will instruct him to:
   a. monitor the blood pressure daily when taking the diuretic and cholestyramine
   b. eliminate milk products which may interfere with absorption of both drugs
   c. take the diuretic 1 hour before or 6 hours after cholestyramine
   d. drink plenty of fluids after taking the diuretic and cholestyramine

5. When planning careful follow-up for Mr. Williams, the nurse will check the following laboratory result:
   a. bleeding time
   b. magnesium
   c. calcium
   d. T_3, T_4 levels

6. When Mr. Williams returns after one week for a check-up, which of the following represents successful therapy with cholestyramine?
   a. decrease in LDL levels
   b. increase in IDL levels
   c. increase in VLDL levels
   d. decrease in HDL levels

SITUATION 32–2

Martha Hampton is a 37-year-old who is admitted to the medical floor for evaluation of fatigue and anorexia.

1. Initial laboratory data indicate a diagnosis of iron deficiency anemia. When checking the results of red blood cell appearance, the following is indicative of this type of anemia:
   a. hyperchromic
   b. macrocytic
   c. hypochromic
   d. normocytic

2. Ms. Hampton is to be started on ferrous sulfate orally. Prior to administering this drug, the nurse will check for the following condition which contraindicates its use:
   a. acute glaucoma
   b. tetracycline sensitivity
   c. peptic ulcer
   d. pernicious anemia

3. When planning Ms. Hampton's care, the nurse will include monitoring for the following side effect of oral iron:
   a. clay-colored stools
   b. hypotension
   c. constipation
   d. hyperglycemia

4. The nurse will teach Ms. Hampton to avoid eating the following food within an hour of taking iron:
   a. orange juice
   b. eggs
   c. bran
   d. mustard

5. Additional patient teaching for Ms. Hampton regarding oral iron administration includes:
   a. avoid products containing ascorbic acid
   b. taking with antacids to reduce gastric irritation
   c. avoid coffee and tea with meals
   d. take with meals to enhance absorption

6. Which of the following outcomes would indicate successful treatment of anemia?
   a. elevated bleeding time
   b. increased sense of well-being
   c. reduced anxiety level
   d. elevated bilirubin levels

Rationale: As the hemoglobin level rises due to iron therapy, the patient notes less fatigue and increased feelings of well-being.

Please refer to the Appendices for correct answers and additional review questions with answers.

BIBLIOGRAPHY

AMA Drug Evaluation, WB Saunders, Philadelphia, 1986.
Becker, DM and Brown Wilder, L: Nutritional and pharmacologic approaches to hypercholesterolemia. Cardiovasc Nurs 25(3):12–16, May–June 1987.
Bell, LP et al: Cholesterol-Lowering effects of psyllium hydrophilic mucilloid. Adjunct therapy to a prudent diet for patients with mild to moderate hypercholesterolemia. JAMA 261:3419–3423, 1989.

Blair, TP, et al: Treatment of hypercholesterolemia by a clinical nurse using a stepped-care protocol in a nonvolunteer population. Arch Intern Med 148:1046–1048, 1988.

Blankenhorn, DA, Nessim, SA, Johnson, RL, et al.: Beneficial effects of combined colestipol-niacin therapy on coronary atherosclerosis and coronary venous bypass grafts. JAMA 257:3233–40, 1987.

Choice of Cholesterol-Lowering Drugs. Med Lett 30(774):81–84, September 9, 1988.

Ellison, RC: Give diet a chance in lowering cholesterol levels. Arch Intern Med 148:1017–1019, 1988.

Fish oil for the heart. Med Lett 29(731):7–9, January 16, 1987.

Fredrickson, D and Lees, R: A system for phenotyping hyperlipoproteinemia. Circulation 31:321–327, 1965.

Frick MH, et al: Helsinki heart study: Primary-prevention trial with gemfibrozil in middle-aged men with dyslipidemia. N Engl J Med 317:1237–1245, 1987.

Froberg, JH: The Anemias: Causes and courses of action. RN:24–30, January, 1989.

Gilman, AG, Goodman, LS, and Gilman, A (eds): Goodman and Gilman's The Pharmacological Basis of Therapeutics. Macmillan, New York, 1985.

Hartshorn, JC, et al: Treatment of hyperlipidemia with gemfibrozil. J Cardiovasc Nurs 1(4):76–80, August 1987.

Hoeg, J, Brewer, HB: 3-hydroxy-3-methylglutaryl-coenzyme A reductase inhibitors in treatment of hypercholesterolemia. JAMA 250 (24), December 25, 1987.

Kinosian, BP, Eisenberg, JM: Cutting into cholesterol cost-effective alternatives for treating hypercholesterolemia. JAMA 259(15):2249–2254, 1988.

Lipid Research Clinic Program. The lipid research clinics coronary primary prevent trial results. JAMA 251(3):351–64, 1984.

Lovastatin for hypercholesterolemia. Med Lett 29(752):99–101, November 6, 1987.

Lowering blood cholesterol to prevent heart disease. Consensus Conference JAMA 253:2080–2086, 1985.

Okino, K and Weibert, R: Warfarin–griseofulvin interaction. Drug intelligence and clinical pharmacy 20:291–293, April 1986.

Schucker, B, et al: Change in physician perspective on cholesterol and heart disease. JAMA 258(24):3521–3526, 1987.

Serum cholesterol determinations. Med Lett 29(738):41–42, April 24, 1987.

Sobel, B: Fibrinolysis and plasminogen, part 2. Heart Lung 16(6):775–786, November 1987.

Tranexamic acid. Med Lett 29(749):89–90, September 25, 1987.

Watson, JE: The national cholesterol education program: The role of nursing. Cardiovasc Nurs 24(3):13–18, 1988.

Witztum, JL, et al: Intensive combination drug therapy of familial hypercholesterolemia with lovastatin, probucol and colestipol hydrochloride. Circulation 79:16–28, 1989.

33
CHAPTER

PROBLEMS OF COAGULATION

MERRILY MATHEWSON KUHN, R.N.C., Ph.D., CCRN

LEARNING OBJECTIVES

After reading this chapter, the student will be able to:

1. Identify medications that affect coagulation.

2. Differentiate among the medications as to mechanism of action, routes of administration, pharmacokinetics, adverse effects, contraindications, and interactions.

3. Identify specific areas to assess in the patient who requires various medications affecting coagulation in order to formulate appropriate nursing diagnoses.

4. Plan the nursing interventions necessary to administer various medications that affect coagulation and choose appropriate teaching strategies to gain patient compliance.

5. Evaluate the patient at various stages of treatment to gauge nursing interventions.

MEDICATIONS THAT AFFECT COAGULATION

Medications that affect coagulation may act in several ways. They may prevent or retard clotting (anticoagulants), hasten clotting (hemostatics), prevent the dissolution of the clot (antifibrinolytics), or actually dissolve it (enzymes). Each drug group will be discussed individually.

HEMOSTASIS

Injury to the vascular system often results in leakage of blood from the system. To prevent or mitigate this sudden loss of fluid, the body initiates three sequential steps. First, vasoconstriction in the injured vessel occurs as a reflex response, to prevent increased blood loss. Second, a plug formed from platelets appears at the site of injury to prevent further blood loss. This platelet plug occurs because the break in the continuity of the endothelial lining of the vessel exposes collagen, a fibrous protein, to which platelets adhere. As the platelets clump together (a process known as platelet adhesion), adenosine diphosphate (ADP) is released from the injury. ADP release causes the surface of the platelets to become very sticky, thus further aiding the formation of the platelet plug. The plug is very unstable and needs the addition of fibrin to stabilize it.

The third step occurs when blood coagulates as a result of a complex series of biochemical reactions and interactions, which are not totally understood and identified. Several well-defined proteins are involved in clotting, and the remaining factors are identified by Roman numerals (Table 33–1). Several factors are identified by more than one name. Four stages of the clotting process currently have been identified: the formation of an active prothrombin-converting substance (thromboplastin) (stage I); the conversion of prothrombin to thrombin by thromboplastin (stage II); and the conversion of fibrinogen to fibrin by thrombin (stage III). Stage IV is the resolution stage in which the clot begins to break up and dissolve (Fig. 33–1).

The clotting process (hemostasis) or "cascade" can be activated by either an intrinsic or extrinsic system. The intrinsic system is activated by the introduction or presence of a surface other than the natural endothelium of the blood vessel, as when a needle is placed into a vein for the administration of IV fluids. The extrinsic system is activated as a result of injury, as when one receives a cut or scratch. Once the clotting process has been activated by either the intrinsic or extrinsic system, thromboplastin is produced. When thromboplastin formation results from the activation of the extrinsic system, factors V, VII, and X must be present. If the intrinsic system is activated, factors V, VIII, IX, X, XI, and XII are needed to form thromboplastin. In addition, calcium (factor IV) is necessary regardless of the system that is activated. When activated thromboplastin becomes available in the plasma, stage II of clotting begins. Prothrombin, synthesized in the liver only in the presence of vitamin K, is converted to thrombin in the presence of calcium and factor V. Thromboplastin is believed to act as an enzyme and catalyzes the reaction converting prothrombin to thrombin.

When thrombin becomes available in the blood, stage III of clotting begins. Thrombin acts as a catalyst that promotes the conversion of fibrinogen, also synthesized in the liver in the presence of calcium (factor IV), to fibrin, the gel-like substance which then traps other elements in the blood (calcium and platelets), forming the clot. Calcium is involved in the clotting process during all three stages. As the clot is formed, it may undergo either organization, the conversion of the clot to fibrous tissue, or resolution, the dissolution of the clot. Dysfunctions of hemostasis are summarized on Table 33–2.

The fourth stage begins with resolution. In order for resolution to begin, plasminogen and fibrinokinases must be present in the blood. Plasminogen and fibrinokinases, through an enzymatic process, are converted to fibrinolysin (plasmin). This process occurs spontaneously, and can be accelerated by the enzyme streptokinase, urokinase, or tissue plasminogen activator (tPA). The fibrin in the clot is broken down into smaller fragments, which are later dissolved.

ANTICOAGULANTS

Anticoagulants are used to retard clotting, and their use is always prophylactic. They do not dissolve the clot that is already present. Two types of anticoagulants are in current use—parenteral (heparin) and oral (coumarins and indandiones) medications. Both of these types of medications are used to treat venous conditions such as deep-vein thrombosis and pulmonary embolism. Arterial conditions such as coronary artery disease, rheumatic heart disease, atrial fibrillation alone or in com-

Table 33–1. BLOOD CLOTTING FACTORS

I	Fibrinogen
II*	Prothrombin
III	Thromboplastin
IV	Ionic calcium
V	Hereditary labile factor activator or accelerator (AC) globulin proaccelerin
VI	(No longer considered in the scheme of hemostasis)
VII*	Proconvertin—serum prothrombin conversion accelerator (SPCA)
VIII	Antihemophilic globulin factor (AHG)
IX*	Plasma thromboplastin component (PTC) or Christmas factor
X*	Stuart–Prower factor
XI	Plasma thromboplastin antecedent (PTA)
XII	Hageman factor
XIII	Fibrin-stabilizing factor
Pre-K	Prekallikrein
Ka	Kallikrein
HMW-K	High-molecular weight kininogen (Fitzgerald factor)

*Vitamin K-dependent factors

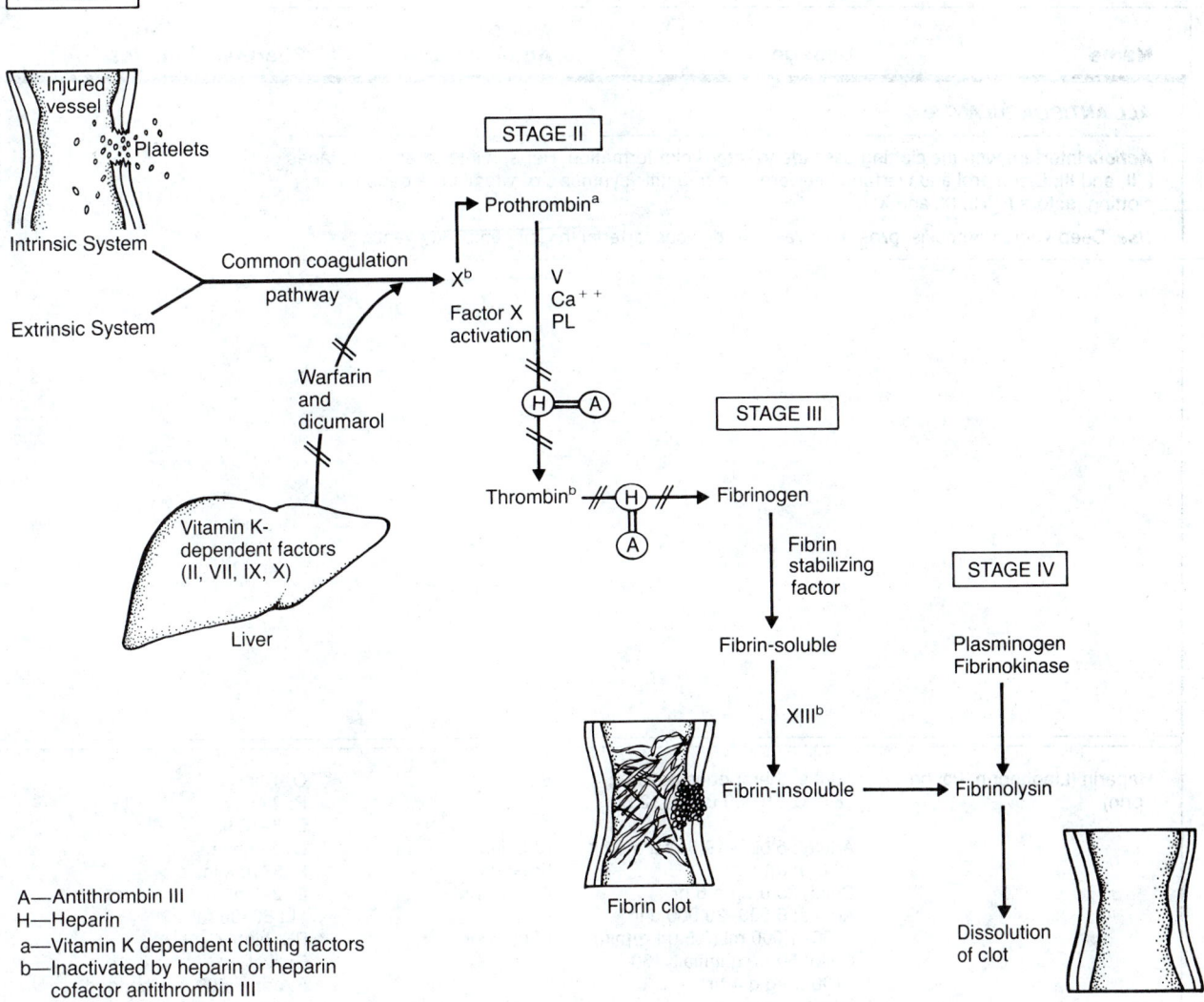

STAGE I

Injured vessel

Platelets

Intrinsic System

Extrinsic System

Common coagulation pathway

Warfarin and dicumarol

Vitamin K-dependent factors (II, VII, IX, X)

Liver

STAGE II

Prothrombin^a

X^b

Factor X activation

V
Ca^{++}
PL

(H) ═ (A)

Thrombin^b ╫ (H) ─► Fibrinogen
           (A)

STAGE III

Fibrin stabilizing factor

Fibrin-soluble

XIII^b

Fibrin-insoluble ──► Fibrinolysin

Fibrin clot

STAGE IV

Plasminogen
Fibrinokinase

Dissolution of clot

A—Antithrombin III
H—Heparin
a—Vitamin K dependent clotting factors
b—Inactivated by heparin or heparin
cofactor antithrombin III

Figure 33–1. Schematic representation of the blood coagulation mechanism.

bination with valve disease, atrial fibrillation before and after cardioversion, thromboembolic complications of prosthetic devices such as cardiac valves, and cerebral vascular disorders are also treated with anticoagulants.

Table 33–2. DYSFUNCTIONS OF HEMOSTASIS

Types	Arterial	Venous
Names	White thrombi	Red thrombi
Clotting pathway	Intrinsic	Extrinsic
Description	Large platelet head Small fibrin tail	Large fibrin head Small platelet tail
Associated with	ASHD plaques Hypertension Turbulent blood flow	Trauma to venous system Stasis

Arterial disorders, however, usually are more responsive to antiplatelet agents. Anticoagulants can also be used prophylactically to treat patients on bed rest for prolonged periods, those who have had major surgeries, or those with a history of previous clotting disorders.

Other uses for anticoagulants are being researched. Heparin lowers the level of low-density lipoproteins and also accelerates removal of fat from the blood stream. Current research indicates that heparin may therefore have some beneficial effect on patients with atherosclerosis by lowering circulating lipid levels.

Another use for anticoagulants is in the treatment of acute myocardial infarction. Several studies have demonstrated that long-term survival improves when heparin therapy is administered in the acute phase of the myocardial infarction. Anticoagulants are featured in Table 33–3.

TEXT RESUMES ON PAGE 892

Table 33–3. DRUGS THAT AFFECT COAGULATION

Name	Dosage	Mode of Administration	Pharmacokinetics
ALL ANTICOAGULANTS:			
Action: Interfere with the clotting cascade to retard clot formation. Heparin interferes with stages I, II, and III. Dicumarol and warfarin interfere with hepatitic synthesis of vitamin K—dependent clotting factors II, VII, IX, and X			
Use: Deep-vein thrombosis, prosthetic vascular devices, arterial thromboembolic events.			
Heparin (Lipoheprin, Panheprin)	Adults: therapeutic dosage: 8,000–20,000 u q 8–12 hr	SC	O: 1 hr P: 2 hr D: 8–12 hr
	Adults: 5,000–10,000 u q 6 hr (50 u/kg)	IV bolus	O: 2–3 min
		IV bolus	P: 5–10 min
	Child: 25 u/kg q 6 hr	IV infusion	D: 2–6 hr
	Adults: 5,000–20,000 u in 500–1,000 ml (0.5 u/kg/min)	IV infusion	½L: 60–90 min PB: highly
	Child: 50 u/kg initially. 50–100 u/kg q 4 hr		B: liver E: urine (50% unchanged)
	Prophylaxis:		
	Adult: 5,000 u q 8–12 hr	SC	
	Clearing heparin lock: 10–100 u/ml	IV	

Key to Abbreviations in the *Pharmacokinetics* **column** O-onset; P-peak; D-duration; PB-protein bound; B-biotransformed in; E-excreted in; ½L-halflife
*Within the column listing adverse effects, underlines indicate the most common effects; CAPITALS indicate life-threatening effects.

Contraindications/ Precautions	Adverse Effects*	Interactions	Nursing Implications
			ASSESSMENT: Frequent blood tests must be performed to assess clotting time. Carefully assess all bodily secretions and orifices for bleeding. Antagonists should be on hand. INTERVENTION: Patients should not take any medications without the physician's or nurse's approval. A flow sheet containing clotting times, the time of medication administration, and the route used should be kept on the patient's chart. EVALUATION: Evaluate mucous membranes and urine for bleeding.
Contraindicated in hypersensitivity, uncontrolled bleeding, open wounds, severe liver or kidney disease. Use cautiously in hypertension, mild liver or kidney disease, menstruation, immediately postpartum.	Neuro: fever, chills, headache CV: HEMORRHAGE, chest pain GI: nausea, vomiting, diarrhea Hemo: thrombocytopenia, BLEEDING Reprod: ovarian hemorrhage Integ: urticaria, transient alopecia, tissue necrosis Musculoskel: osteoporosis	Drugs that increase risk of bleeding include oral anticoagulants, aspirin, dextran, phenylbutazone, ibuprofen, indomethacin, penicillin. Drugs that partially counteract heparin: digitalis, tetracyclines, quinidine, antihistamines. Causes false elevations of SGOT and SGPT.	ASSESSMENT: Obtain an accurate prothrombin time (PTT or APPT); there must be at least 4–6 hr after the last IV dose and 12–24 hr after the last SC dose. INTERVENTION: Carefully administer other IM or SC medication near the time of the next heparin administration so the clotting time is almost back to normal. This will prevent prolonged bleeding at the site. Continuous IV infusions of heparin should be administered through infusion pumps and microdrip regulators. Avoid IM injection since clotting studies are always elevated with continuous drip. Follow special SC technique (in Planning and Implementation section). Older patients are started on smaller doses. Oral anticoagulants are started 3–5 days prior to discontinuing heparin. EVALUATION: Evaluate platelet counts, hemocrits, and stool for occult blood throughout therapy.

CONTINUED ON THE FOLLOWING PAGE

Drugs That Affect Coagulation

Table 33–3. DRUGS THAT AFFECT COAGULATION–*CONTINUED*

Name	Dosage	Mode of Administration	Pharmacokinetics
Heparin sodium and dihy-roergotamine mesylate (DHE) (Embolex)			
Use: Prophylaxis of deep-vein thrombosis			
	0.5 mg/DHE 5,000 u heparin 1 hr before surgery then q 12 hr after surgery for 5–7 days.	deep SC	O: 20–60 min P: 0.9–4 hr D: 8–12 hr ½L: 3–5 hr DHE, or 1–2 hr heparin PB: highly B: liver E: urine
Dicumarol (Dicoumarin)	I: 25–300 mg first day M: 25–150 mg/day Children: dosage not established.	PO	O: 1–2 days P: 3–5 days D: 2–10 days ½L: 1–2 days PB: 99% B: liver E: urine, feces
Warfarin sodium (Coumadin, Panwarfin)	I: 10 mg/day for 3–5 days M: 2–15 mg daily based on PT	PO IV IM	O: 2–12 hr P: 1.5–3 days D: 2–5 days ½L: 1.5–2.5 days PB: 99% B: liver E: urine, feces

Key to Abbreviations in the *Pharmacokinetics* column O-onset; P-peak; D-duration; PB-protein bound; B-biotransformed in; E-excreted in; ½L-halflife
*Within the column listing adverse effects, underlines indicate the most common effects; CAPITALS indicate life-threatening effects.

Contraindications/ Precautions	Adverse Effects*	Interactions	Nursing Implications
Same as heparin	Neuro: headache CV: hemorrhage, numbness and tingling of fingers and toes, precordial pain, transient tachycardia or bradycardia. GI: nausea, vomiting Integ: local irritation, mild pain, ecchymosis or hematomes at injection site.	Macrolide antibiotics and Embolex result in increased plasma levels of unchanged alkaloids. All drugs that interfere with platelet aggregation should not be used concurrently. Lab: levels of SGPT and SGOT may rise.	Same as heparin plus INTERVENTION: Use a 25- or 26-gauge needle to minimize tissue trauma. Administer deep SC into fold of anterior abdomen above iliac crest. Avoid the IM route.
Contraindicated in hypersensitivity, uncontrolled bleeding, open wounds, severe liver or kidney disease, pregnancy, threatened abortion, cerebral vascular hemorrhage, blood dyscrasias, pericardial effusion, and subacute bacterial endocarditis.	Neuro: alopecia, fever CV: HEMORRHAGE GI: nausea, vomiting, abdominal cramps, diarrhea, hepatitis, mouth ulcers Hemo: AGRANULOCYTOSIS, LEUKOPENIA, EOSINOPHILIA Renal: hematuria	Drugs that increase the chance of bleeding: salicylates, anti-inflammatory drugs, cephalosporins, antimetabolics, potassium products, plus many more too numerous to mention. Consult pharmacist. Drugs that decrease activity: barbiturates, estrogens, oral contraceptives, phenytoin, rifampin, naficillin, aluminum hydroxide, and others. Drugs enhance the anticoagulant effect: oral antibiotics, chloral hydrate, clofibrate, diazoxide, salicylates, alcohol, allopurinol, anabolic steroids, glucagon, propranolol, thyroid drugs and many more.	ASSESSMENT: Hepatic, renal function, PT. INTERVENTION: Patient should not consume high quantities of foods rich in vitamin K, such as green leafy vegetables (cabbage, spinach, kale, lettuce), cauliflower, tomatoes, fish, liver, cheese, egg yolks, and fats from red meats. Excessive alcohol intake is avoided because of its effect on the liver and an increased tendency to bleed. When traveling to a hot climate from a cold one, the dose of medication may need to be reduced. Patients are encouraged to use a soft toothbrush to prevent gum injury. Shaving is done with an electric razor to avoid scraping the skin. Patients should carry an identification card or wear a piece of jewelry that states the medication that is being taken and the physician's name and telephone number. Medications are stored in a tight, moisture-resistant container. Patient will need to take 3–5 days before PT raises. EVALUATION: PT should be kept at 1½-2½ times normal. Report abnormal bruising or bleeding to physician. Urine may turn red-orange on standing.
Same as Dicumerol, above.	Same as Dicumerol, above.	Same as Dicumerol, above.	Same as Dicumerol, above.

CONTINUED ON THE FOLLOWING PAGE

Table 33-3. DRUGS THAT AFFECT COAGULATION–*CONTINUED*

Name	Dosage	Mode of Administration	Pharmacokinetics
INDANDIONE DERIVATIVES Anisindione (Miradon)	300 mg initially; 200 mg—day 2; 100 mg—day 1; 25–50 mg maintenance	PO	O: 1–2 days P: 2–3 days D: 1–3 days ½L: 3–5 days PB: 99% B: liver E: urine, feces

ANTIPLATELET AGENTS
Dipyridamole (Persantine)

Action: Interfere with platelets' ability to adhere to each other; inhibit ADP release, thus retarding platelet aggregation.

Use: Prevention of thromboembolism in patients post-myocardial infarction with prosthetic vascular devices, history of venous/arterial thrombosis

	Dosage	Mode of Administration	Pharmacokinetics
	75–100 mg qid	PO	O: quickly P: 75 min D: 4–6 hr ½L: 40 min–10 hr PB: highly B: liver E: bile

ANTICOAGULANT ANTAGONISTS
Protamine sulfate

Action: Combines with heparin to form a stable salt that neutralizes heparin.

Use: Antagonize effects of anticoagulation and stop bleeding.

	Dosage	Mode of Administration	Pharmacokinetics
	10–50 mg, given in 1–3 min, not to exceed 20 mg/min or 50 mg in 10 min.	IV	O: 5 min P: 5–10 min D: 2 hr ½L: UA PB: UA B: UA E: UA
Vitamin K_3 (Synkayvite)	4–10 mg	PO SQ IM	O: slowly P: 6–10 hr D: UA ½L: UA PB: UA B: UA E: UA
		IV	O: 1–2 hr P: 3–6 hr D: 12–14 hr ½L: UA PB: UA B: UA E: UA

Key to Abbreviations in the *Pharmacokinetics* column O-onset; P-peak; D-duration; PB-protein bound; B-biotransformed in; E-excreted in; ½L-halflife.
*Within the column listing adverse effects, underlines indicate the most common effects; CAPITALS indicate life-threatening effects.

Contraindications/ Precautions	Adverse Effects*	Interactions	Nursing Implications
Same as Dicumerol, above.	GI: jaundice Hemo: AGRANULOCYTOSIS Renal: NEPHROPATHY Integ: dermatitis	Same as Dicumerol, above.	Same as Dicumerol, above. EVALUATION: Discolors alkaline urine orange.
No contraindications known. Use cautiously in hypotension. Use in pregnant and lactating women only if clearly needed. Safety in children not established.	Neuro: transient dizziness and headache CV: flushing, hypotension GI: abdominal distress, diarrhea, nausea, vomiting Integ: rash, pruritis	None known.	ASSESSMENT: Blood pressure prior to and during therapy. Dipyridamole may decrease blood pressure. INTERVENTION: Teach patient to change body position slowly.
Contraindicated in hemorrhage not induced by heparin. Use cautiously in cardiovascular disease and in allergy to fish. Safety in pregnancy, lactating women, and children not established.	Neuro: lassitude CV: hypotension, flushing, CV COLLAPSE, DEATH GI: nausea, vomiting Misc: allergy	None significant.	ASSESSMENT: Bleeding and clotting studies before and during therapy. Assess vital signs closely until all signs of bleeding have passed. Assess closely for allergic reactions. INTERVENTION: Dose is titrated according to clotting studies. Diluents for IV are only 0.9% sodium chloride, 5% dextrose, 5% dextrose in 0.9% sodium chloride. IV solutions are used immediately and not stored. EVALUATION: For rebleed evaluate heparin rebound, which may necessitate more protamine.
Contraindicated in hypersensitivity. Administer IV doses slowly.	Neuro: dizziness, headache CV: HYPOTENSION if administered rapid IV GI: peculiar taste sensation Integ: rash, urticaria, pain and swelling at parenteral site	Coumarins and indandiones antagonized by vitamin K.	ASSESSMENT: Baseline clotting studies. INTERVENTION: Encourage vitamin K–rich foods. EVALUATION: Bleeding should decrease.

CONTINUED ON THE FOLLOWING PAGE

Drugs That Affect Coagulation

Table 33–3. DRUGS THAT AFFECT COAGULATION–*CONTINUED*

Name	Dosage	Mode of Administration	Pharmacokinetics
Vitamin K₁ (Mephyton, Aqua-Mephyton) Konakion	2–25 mg 2.5–10 mg 2–25 mg	PO IM, IV PO, IM	Same as Vitamin K₃—Synkayvite

HEMOSTATICS (SYSTEMIC)

Action: Inhibit the resolution of the clot by inhibiting the breakdown of fibrin.

Use: Hemorrhage caused by overactivity of stage IV of clotting; as an antidote for thrombolytic agents.

Name	Dosage	Mode of Administration	Pharmacokinetics
Aminocaproic acid (Amicar)	I: 5 g M: 1–1.25 g/hr	PO, IV	O: immediate IV P: 2 hr D: 3 hr ½L: UA PB: UA B: very little E: urine (unchanged)
	I: 4–5 g in 250 ml in 1 hr followed by 1 g/50 ml/hr followed by 1–1.25 g/hr to maximum of 30 g/24 hr.	IV	
Tranexamic acid (Cyklokapron)	Before dental surgery 10 mg/kg. After surgery 25 mg/kg 3–4 × daily for 2–8 days	IV PO	O: 1–2 hr P: 3 hr D: 7–17 hr ½L: 2 hr PB: 3% to plasminogen B: very little E: urine (95% unchanged)

THROMBOLYTIC ENZYMES

Action: Dissolve clots through activation of the endogenous fibrinolytic system

Use: MI, pulmonary embolism, and to unplug central IV lines.

Name	Dosage	Mode of Administration	Pharmacokinetics
Streptokinase (Streptase, Kabikinase)	Deep vein thrombosis and pulmonary embolism: 250,000 u over 30 min loading dose; 100,000 u/hr for 24–72-hr maintenance	IV	O: immediate P: rapid D: 12–24 hr ½L: biphasic 23 min, 83 min. PB: UA
	Coronary thrombosis: 20,000 u, maintenance: 2,000 u/min for 60 min.	Intracoronary	B: antibodies and reticuloendothelial system E: UA
	1.5 million u over 1 hr	IV	
	Pulmonary embolism 250,000 u over 30 min followed by 100,000 u/hr for 24 hr	IV IV drip	

Key to Abbreviations in the *Pharmacokinetics* column O-onset; P-peak; D-duration; PB-protein bound; B-biotransformed in; E-excreted in; ½L-halflife.

*Within the column listing adverse effects, underlines indicate the most common effects; CAPITALS indicate life-threatening effects.

Contraindications/ Precautions	Adverse Effects*	Interactions	Nursing Implications
Same as above.	Same as above.	Same as above.	Same as above.
Contraindicated in active clotting process and DIC. Use with caution in renal, cardiac, hepatic dysfunction. Safe use in pregnancy has not been established.	Neuro: weakness, fatigue, dizziness, headache, auditory and visual hallucinations, nasal stuffiness CV: hypotension, malaise, bradycardia GI: nausea, vomiting, diarrhea Integ: rash	Hypercoagulability may occur with concurrent oral contraceptives and estrogen. Lab: may elevate CPK, SGOT, and serum K.	ASSESSMENT: Baseline bleeding and clotting studied. Assess routinely for clot. EVALUATION: If thrombosis occurs, aminocaproic acid may need to be discontinued.
Contraindicated in acquired defective color vision, subarrachnoid hemorrhage. Use with precaution in renal dysfunction. Use only if clearly needed in pregnancy and lactation.	Neuro: giddiness CV: hypotension (with too-rapid IV administration) GI: nausea, vomiting, diarrhea	None known.	ASSESSMENT: Bleeding and clotting studies. INTERVENTION: IV tranexamic acid can be mixed with most IV solutions. Do not mix with blood or solutions containing penicillin. Administer IV no faster than 1 ml/min.
Contraindicated in hemorrhagic disorders, recent CVA, recent intracranial or spinal surgery, recent streptokinase exposure, recent neoplasm, recent GI bleed, and infectious endocarditis. Safety in pregnancy, lactating women, and children not established.	Hemo: BLEEDING Misc: allergic reactions, febrile reactions, drug rash, ANAPHYLAXIS, urticaria	Anticoagulants increase risk of hemorrhage. Aspirin, indomethacin, phenylbutazone may alter platelet function.	ASSESSMENT: Assess laboratory values prior to and every 4 hr during therapy, including thrombin time, activated partial thromboplastin time, prothrombin time, hematocrit, fibrinogen and platelet count. Type and cross and have blood available. Assess carefully for bleeding during therapy. INTERVENTION: Handle patient as little as possible during therapy. Intramuscular injections, venipunctures, and arterial sticks should not be performed during therapy unless absolutely necessary. IV catheters that infiltrate are left in place during therapy. Follow the specific reconstitution procedures. Direct flow of diluent against side of the vial. Avoid shaking and

CONTINUED ON THE FOLLOWING PAGE

Drugs That Affect Coagulation

Table 33–3. DRUGS THAT AFFECT COAGULATION–*CONTINUED*

Name	Dosage	Mode of Administration	Pharmacokinetics
Streptokinase–*Continued*			
Urokinase (Abbokinase)	Pulmonary embolism: 4,400 u/kg over 10 min loading dose; 4,400 u/kg/hr × 12–24 hr maintenance	IV	O: immediate P: rapid D: 12–24 hr ½L: 20 min or less PB: UA B: liver E: UA
	Coronary artery occlusion: 6,000 u/min for up to 2 hr (or 500,000 units total). Occluded IV catheter 5,000 u instilled, wait 5–10 min and aspirate	IV	
Recombinant alteplase (Activase)	Acute coronary thrombosis: 100 mg over 3 hr, 6–10 mg initial bolus over 1–2 min to total 60 mg first hr, 20 mg second hr, 20 mg third hr, maximum dose 100 mg or 1.25 mg/kg	IV	O: immediate P: 5–10 min D: 3 hr ½L: biphasic: 8 min and 1.3 hr PB: UA B: liver E: urine

Key to Abbreviations in the *Pharmacokinetics* column O-onset; P-peak; D-duration; PB-protein bound; B-biotransformed in; E-excreted in; ½L-halflife.

*Within the column listing adverse effects, <u>underlines</u> indicate the most common effects; CAPITALS indicate life-threatening effects.

Heparin

Heparin, first isolated in 1916, was not used in humans until 1935. It can be extracted from many body cells, but the organs richest in heparin are the intestines and the lung, in the mast cells. Free heparin is rarely found circulating in the blood stream unless there has been massive damage to the pulmonary mast cells. However, free heparin can appear in anaphylactic shock. Nonhuman heparin is a natural product that is derived from either beef or pig lung tissue or from the mucosal linings of pig intestine. Synthetic heparin does not exist at this time.

ACTION. Heparin acts in the first three steps of the clotting cascade by combining with and activating antithrombin III–thrombin complex to prevent the ultimate formation of fibrin in stage III of the clotting cascade. In stage I of clotting, heparin has an antithromboplastin effect, reducing the amount of thromboplastin. In stage II, heparin retards the formation of thrombin from prothrombin and thereby has an antiprothrombin action. In stage III, it decreases the *agglutination* of platelets,

thereby making them less sticky and less likely to stay in the fibrin net. Also in stage III, heparin antagonizes thrombin and thereby slows conversion of fibrinogen to fibrin. (See Fig. 33–1 for sites of action of heparin.)

USES. Heparin, which is administered only parenterally, is used when rapid anticoagulant is needed and in all the conditions described above. In addition, heparin may be used during blood transfusions, hemodialysis, and extracorporeal circulation during open-heart surgery to prevent blood clotting. Heparin can also be used during pregnancy if necessary. Heparin is generally the first anticoagulant used because of its rapid action; after several days, the patient can be placed on oral anticoagulants. Heparin is also used to prevent thromboembolism in high-risk patients after myocardial infarction or surgery.

PHARMACOKINETICS. *Absorption and Distribution.* Because of its large molecular size and polarity, heparin cannot be absorbed from the gastrointestinal tract. This is also the reason for its poor penetration into

Contraindications/ Precautions	Adverse Effects*	Interactions	Nursing Implications
			agitation of solution. Use the solution within 24 hours of preparation. If it must be stored, store at 2°–4°C. Use filters during IV administration. Monitor closely and treat other problems (reperfusion angina, or dysrhythmia when given for acute MI as they occur). EVALUATION: Evaluate for allergic or febrile reactions. If they occur, decrease dose and call physician. Do not administer aspirin.
Contraindicated in hemorrhagic disorders, recent CVA, recent intracranial or spinal surgery, recent neoplasm, recent GI bleed, and infectious endocarditis. Safety in pregnancy, lactating women, and children not established.	Hemo: bleeding	Same as Streptokinase.	Same as Streptokinase.
Same as above.	CV: hemotomas at injection site GI: BLEEDING	Same as Streptokinase.	Same as Streptokinase.

the central nervous sysem (CNS) and breast milk, and its inability to cross the placental barrier. It is extensively bound to plasma proteins. Some researchers have suggested that the mast cells in the lungs may be able to absorb heparin and act as a storage depot.

Biotransformation and Excretion. Heparin is biotransformed in the liver by a heparin-inactivating enzyme called heparinase. The inactive metabolites are then excreted in the urine. The half-life of heparin is 60–90 minutes and is dose dependent. A patient with renal or hepatic disease may experience a longer anticoagulant effect.

CONTRAINDICATIONS AND PRECAUTIONS. Heparin is contraindicated in patients with hypersensitivity to it, as well as in uncontrolled bleeding, open wounds, and severe hepatic or renal disease. Heparin is given cautiously to patients with hypertension or mild hepatic or renal disease as these are the organs of elimination, to menstruating women, or to patients immediately postpartum or after surgery because bleeding may result.

ADVERSE EFFECTS. The most common adverse effect of heparin is spontaneous bleeding (10%). The most

serious and common adverse effect of heparin therapy is hemorrhage. If a patient experiences mild bleeding or excessive effects on clotting studies while receiving heparin, the drug should be discontinued and the patient monitored. The effects should dissipate in several hours. If severe bleeding occurs, the direct antagonist of its action, protamine sulfate, can be used. Protamine *in vitro* complexes with heparin to form an inactive complex. *In vitro*, this inactivates its anticoagulant effect; however, its effect of inhibiting platelet aggregation will persist. The amount of protamine required can be estimated as 1 mg of protamine for every 90–115 units of heparin remaining in the patient.

Less common adverse effects include fever, chills, burning sensation at the injection site, and rhinitis. Osteoporosis has been reported in patients taking heparin for longer than six months because heparin potentiates parathyroid hormone activity, thus producing bone resorption. Mild thrombocytopenia is frequently observed in patients receiving heparin; severe thrombocytopenia occurs less frequently.

INTERACTIONS. Several interactions occur with heparin. Drugs that increase the risk of bleeding when taken concurrently include oral anticoagulants, aspirin, dextran, and phenylbutazone, ibuprofen, indomethacin, and penicillin. This is because these drugs can prolong bleeding time or cause gastrointestinal hemorrhage. Drugs that partially counteract heparin by partially antagonizing its action when given concurrently include digitalis, aspirin, tetracyclines, and antihistamines. False elevations of serum glutamic oxaloacetic transaminase (SGOT) and serum glutamic pyruvic transaminase (SGPT) may occur.

DOSAGE. Heparin may be administered subcutaneously or by IV bolus or drip. It should not be given IM, as muscular hematomas result. The usual adult subcutaneous dose is 8,000–20,000 units administered every 8–12 hours. The best site for the subcutaneous dose is above the iliac crest or in the abdominal fat layer. After withdrawal of the needle, light pressure is applied, but no massage. This prevents damage and bleeding of the sensitive subcutaneous tissues.

When heparin is being given prophylactically to prevent thromboembolism, the usual dosage is 5000 units every 8–12 hours, usually administered subcutaneously. Bleeding rarely occurs with this protocol, and constant monitoring by laboratory tests is not required.

The adult IV bolus dosage ranges from 5,000–10,000 units (approximately 100 units/kg). A heparin lock may be used for these injections. The continuous infusion dosage is 5,000–20,000 units mixed in 500–1,000 ml of solution, administered at an initial rate of approximately 900–1,000 units/hr. These are initial guidelines, with most patients' dosage determined by regulation of clotting studies performed on each patient. (See the Nursing Process section for a discussion of the laboratory studies.)

Heparin Sodium and Dihydroergotamine Mesylate

Heparin sodium and dihydroergotamine mesylate (Embolex) is a combination of heparin (5,000 units) and dihydroergotamine (0.5 mg) (DHE). DHE is an α-adrenergic blocking agent that directly stimulates smooth muscle of peripheral blood vessels. This results in a dose-dependent constriction of capacitance vessels with variable effect on arterial resistance. Ultimately, DHE accelerates venous return, particularly from the calf, resulting in a thromboprophylactic effect.

DHE is administered two hours before surgery in a dose of 0.5 mg, then continued every 12 hours after surgery for five to seven days. DHE is administered subcutaneously using a small 25–26-gauge needle into an anterior fold of the abdomen above the iliac crest. Intramuscular injections are avoided because of the occurrence of hematomas at the injection site. With deep subcutaneous administration, patients may experience local irritation, mild pain, and ecchymosis. DHE is reviewed in Table 33–3.

Coumarin and Indandione Derivatives

The coumarin derivatives were discovered accidentally in the 1930s. Researchers investigating bleeding disorders in cattle found them to be due to ingestion of spoiled sweet clover containing a coumarin compound. Coumarin derivatives were first used in humans in 1941 and today are produced synthetically.

ACTION. Coumarin and indandione derivatives have only one main pharmacologic effect: inhibition of the blood clotting mechanism by interfering with the hepatic synthesis of vitamin K–dependent clotting factors, including factors II (prothrombin), VII, IX, and X. These derivatives compete with vitamin K, making it unavailable for synthesis of the clotting factors. (See Fig. 33–1 for site of action.) Therefore, vitamin K is an antagonist for both the coumarin and indandione derivatives. The dose of coumarin is computed on the basis of the prothrombin time. (See the Nursing Process section for an explanation of laboratory tests.)

USES. The coumarin and indandione products are used for prophylaxis and long-term anticoagulation to protect against sudden thromboembolic phenomena. Oral anticoagulants are also used to prevent recurrent transient ischemic attacks and to reduce the risk of myocardial infarction, although antiplatelet agents may be more effective. These products have several advantages: they are relatively inexpensive, are available for oral use, and need to be given only once a day to maintain their therapeutic effect.

PHARMACOKINETICS. *Absorption and Distribution.* Generally, oral anticoagulants are absorbed rapidly and completely. These drugs are highly bound to plasma proteins, and there is a potential for interaction with other highly bound drugs. Accumulations of these medications occur in the lung, liver, spleen, and kidney.

Biotransformation and Excretion. Oral anticoagulants are biotransformed by hepatic enzymes and then excreted in the urine. Unlike heparin, these products do cross the placenta and enter breast milk. Research is being conducted to determine the effect on the neonate. More information can be found in Table 33–3.

CONTRAINDICATIONS AND PRECAUTIONS. The oral anticoagulants are contraindicated in patients sensitive to its ingredients, in uncontrolled bleeding, in open wounds, and in patients with severe hepatic or renal disease. Oral anticoagulants are also contraindicated in pregnancy as they may cause fatal hemorrhage, spontaneous abortions, and other deformities. Oral anticoagulants are also contraindicated in patients with a threatened abortion, cerebral vascular hemorrhage, blood dyscrasias, precordial effusion, and subacute bacterial endocarditis, since all these conditions may result in bleeding. In patients with diseases that predispose them to bleeding, such as ulcerative diseases of the gastrointestinal tract or alcoholism, oral anticaogulants are used cautiously.

ADVERSE EFFECTS. The most significant adverse effect is hemorrhage. Consequently, oral anticoagulant therapy is closely monitored with coagulation tests and monitoring of clinical signs of bleeding, which include ecchymoses, hematuria, uterine bleeding, melena, hematoma, gingival bleeding, hemoptysis, and hematemesis. Treatment of hemorrhage involves discontinuation of the drug and administration of vitamin K. This can be administered orally in 10- and 20-mg doses.

Bleeding should stop and prothrombin time will return to normal. Severe bleeding episodes are treated with fresh frozen plasma, whole blood, or plasma concentrates of vitamin K-dependent clotting factors. If oral coagulant therapy is to be reinstituted, higher-than-normal doses may be needed until the vitamin K is eliminated from the body. This may take up to several weeks.

Other common adverse effects include anorexia, nausea, vomiting, and dermatitis. Less common adverse effects are hepatitis, jaundice, and increased menstrual flow. Tissue necrosis has also been reported with warfarin therapy.

DRUG INTERACTIONS. Many interactions occur with oral anticoagulants, which can either potentiate or inhibit their effect. Drugs can potentiate the effect of warfarin by displacing it from its protein-binding sites, inhibiting its metabolic breakdown, or decreasing the amount of vitamin K–producing bacteria in the gut. Protein-binding interactions occur when drugs such as chloral hydrate, diazoxide, ethacrynic acid, salicylates, sulfonamides, clofibrate, or phenylbutazone are administered. Almost any compound known to bind to albumin has the potential to displace oral anticoagulants. When these drugs are administered with oral anticoagulants, the patient is monitored closely for bleeding episodes for the first five to ten days of concurrent therapy. Since hepatic metabolism increases as more free drug is made available to be metabolized, often a new steady state is reached and an enhanced effect should no longer be observed.

Drugs that inhibit hepatic metabolism of coumarin and cause increased effectiveness include phenylbutazone, cimetidine, disulfiram, metronidazole, alcohol, allopurinol, amiodarone, propoxyphene, and sulfonamides. These cause an increase in plasma concentrations and an increase in response. The dosage of oral anticoagulants may need to be reduced if one of these drugs is added to a patient's therapy.

Most oral anti-infective drugs can destroy intestinal bacteria that produce vitamin K, thereby rendering the patient hypoprothrombinemic. This can result in an increased effect of oral anticoagulants.

These interactions take on an added significance if the interacting drug has an effect of its own on the hemostatic system or can cause gastrointestinal bleeding. This is particularly important when salicylates, steroids, indomethacin, phenylbutazone, antimetabolics, quinidine, potassium products, and numerous other drugs are used in someone taking oral anticoagulants.

Several drugs can decrease responsiveness to oral anticoagulants. These include enzyme inducers (barbiturates, phenytoin, rifampin), which increase the metabolism of oral anticoagulants and decrease plasma concentrations. Cholestyramine and aluminum hydroxide reduce oral anticoagulant absorption. Estrogen products and oral contraceptives can also decrease anticoagulant activity.

Warfarin Sodium. Warfarin sodium (Coumadin, Panwarfin) is almost always given once a day. A standard dosage size, however, cannot be determined since dosage is individually titrated to the amount required to increase the prothrombin time 1.5–2.5 times. The most common method to initiate warfarin therapy is to give 10 mg daily for three to five days and titrate subsequent doses based on the response to this initial regimen. Large loading doses of warfarin, that is, greater than 15–20 mg, should not be given. The usual daily maintenance dose of warfarin should be between 2–15 mg.

Dicumarol. Dicumarol (Dicoumarin) is administered orally in doses of 25–300 mg. Most physicians attempt to keep the prothrombin time the same as for warfarin. Once this level is achieved, the daily dose is generally between 25–150 mg.

Anisindione. Anisindione (Miradon) is similar in all respects to the coumarin products. However, it is potentially more dangerous, so it is reserved for patients who cannot tolerate the coumarins. Anisindione has been reported to cause dermatitis, but it may also cause agranulocytosis, jaundice, nephropathy, diarrhea, and fever. Anisindione is administered orally, 300 mg the first day, 200 mg the second day, 100 mg the third day, and the maintenance dose is 25–250 mg daily. Additional information is found in Table 33-3.

ANTIPLATELET AGENTS

Platelets are involved with the intrinsic pathway of the clotting cascade. Antiplatelet agents interfere with the platelets' ability to adhere to each other when they are exposed to *collagen*. These drugs are believed to interfere with the release of adenosine diphosphate (ADP), thus retarding platelet aggregation. Drugs in this group include salicylates (Chapter 20), dipyridamole (Persantine), sulfinpyrazone (Anturane), and Dextran 70 and 75. All these medications are currently being studied for use in preventing thromboembolism in patients with history of venous and arterial thrombosis; in patients who have recently suffered myocardial and cerebral infarction, or embolus; and in persons who have had prosthetic heart valve replacements. Prosthetic valves, particularly the ball and disk valves, increase the risk of thromboembolism. These thrombi, if they break off and migrate, may cause damage in the brain, heart, kidney, and other organs.

Salicylates have long been known to alter blood coagulability by decreasing blood clotting factor VII. Recent research has suggested that low doses of aspirin (one aspirin daily) can prevent venous thrombus by inhibiting platelet aggregation.

Dipyridamole (Persantine) is an antiplatelet agent. Researchers currently believe that dipyridamole blocks ADP-induced platelet aggregation. More information on dipyridamole can be found in Table 33-3.

Sulfinpyrazone (Anturane) is a potent uricosuric agent indicated for use in gouty arthritis that also has antithrombotic and platelet inhibitor effects. Several studies are under way to determine the effectiveness in decreasing the frequency of systemic embolization in patients with mitral valve disease and decreasing the incidence of sudden cardiac death after myocardial infarction. Sulfinpyrazone is featured in Chapter 47.

Dextran 70 and Dextran 75 are high-molecular-weight glucose polymers used as plasma expanders. These products coat the surface of erythrocytes and platelets, and the intimal surface of the blood vessel. Therefore, platelet aggregation may be decreased. These products are discussed more thoroughly in Chapter 12.

ANTICOAGULANT ANTAGONISTS

On occasion, heparin and coumarin products may cause excessive bleeding. When this occurs, each medication has its own antagonist that interferes with the anticoagulating effect. The antagonist of heparin is protamine sulfate. The basic protamine sulfate acts by combining with the acidic heparin to form a stable salt, which then neutralizes the effect of both heparin and protamine sulfate. The antagonist for coumarin derivatives is vitamin K. If bleeding is severe, blood or component therapy may also be indicated (see Table 33–3).

Protamine Sulfate

Protamine sulfate is a purified mixture of simple proteins obtained from the sperm of salmon and other fish. When used alone, it has an anticoagulant effect. Each milligram of protamine sulfate neutralizes about 90 units of heparin derived from lung tissue and 115 units of heparin derived from intestinal mucosa. The amount given should equal the amount of heparin overdose minus the heparin that was already metabolized.

PHARMACOKINETICS. Protamine sulfate has a rapid onset of action, neutralizing heparin within five minutes. The metabolic fate of the heparin–protamine complex is not known. One theory is that the protamine sulfate is partially metabolized or may be attacked by *fibrinolysis*, thus freeing the heparin.

CONTRAINDICATIONS, PRECAUTIONS, AND ADVERSE EFFECTS. Protamine sulfate is contraindicated in hemorrhage not induced by heparin and is given cautiously to patients with cardiovascular disease and to those with allergies to fish. Adverse effects include hypotension, nausea, and vomiting, and anaphylaxis has been reported.

DOSAGE. The usual dose is 10–50 mg (not to exceed 50 mg in 10 minutes or to exceed 20 mg/min) given intravenously over one to three minutes. Additional information can be found in Table 33–3.

Vitamin K

Vitamin K_3 (Synkayvite) antagonizes the effects of coumarin and indandione anticoagulants within the liver so that the normal clotting factors are again produced. Vitamin K promotes the hepatic synthesis of prothrombin and other clotting factors.

Vitamin K is routinely administered to newborns at birth to prevent hemorrhage. Prothrombin levels in the newborn are often normal at birth but begin to decline until about six days after birth, when the liver begins to form its own prothrombin.

Vitamin K is effective only in bleeding disorders that result from a low prothrombin concentration. It may be administered before surgery to persons with deficient prothrombin levels; or given to persons with hypoprothrombinemia secondary to overdoses of drugs (salicylates, quinine, sulfonamides, arsenicals, and barbiturates) or secondary to conditions limiting absorption or synthesis of vitamin K (obstructive jaundice, sprue, ulcerative colitis, celiac disease, and regional enteritis). Prothrombin levels are evaluated often.

Effects are seen 6–12 hours after oral administration, one to two hours after IM administration, and 15 minutes after IV administration. Bleeding is usually controlled within 3–8 hours. Little is known about metabolic fate. Vitamin K is contraindicated in patients with known sensitivity.

The usual dose of Synkayvite is 4–10 mg given orally, subcutaneously, intramuscularly, or intravenously. Mephyton and Konakion are given in 2–25-mg doses orally, IV, or IM. Because Konakion contains a phenol derivative, it is not administered intravenously. AquaMephyton is given in doses of 2.5–10 mg intramuscularly, and in emergency use only, it is administered intravenously. Additional information is found in Table 33–3.

TOPICAL HEMOSTATIC AGENTS

Topical hemostatic agents are preparations used to control capillary bleeding. They are designed to control oozing from minute vessels during surgery or, in an emergency situation, to combat bleeding from sources other than arteries or veins. These preparations are not directly active in the clotting process but do stop bleeding. They are either absorbable gelatin sponges (Gelfoam), sterile dry preparation (microfibrillar collagen hemostat), or specially treated surgical gauze or cotton (Oxycel, Novocell). All are placed directly on the bleeding area. These preparations either arrest bleeding by forming an artificial clot, or provide the mechanical matrix that facilitates clot formation. They are absorbed by the body after varying time periods. (See Table 33–4 for more detailed product information.)

Absorbable Gelatin Sponge

Absorbable gelatin sponge (Gelfoam) is specially prepared gelatin foam with a porous nature used to control capillary bleeding. It works by acting as a tampon at the site of injury. It is often moistened with isotonic saline solution or thrombin solution before application. However, it can be applied dry. An absorbable gelatin sponge is used to control bleeding in oral and dental surgeries and in open prostatic surgery. It is fully absorbable in four to six weeks. The presence of the foam does not cause excessive scar formation.

Oxidized Cellulose

Oxidized cellulose (Oxycel, Novocell) is a surgical gauze or cotton that causes an artificial clot to form when it is buried in the tissues. It is especially useful in controlling bleeding during dental and oral surgery and surgery of the liver, spleen, pancreas, thyroid, and prostate. It in-

Table 33–4. HEMOSTATICS

Name	Form	Completely Absorbed by Body	Comments
Absorbable gelatin sponge USP/BP (Gelfoam)	Gelatin sponge or cones	4–6 weeks	Does not produce excessive scar formation
Absorbable gelatin film (Gelfilm)	Thin film sheets	4–8 days	Used in neuro, thoracic, and ocular surgery.
Oxidized cellulose USP/BP (Oxycel, Novocell)	Surgical gauze or cotton	2–7 days	Should not be used in bone fractures or as a surface dressing on skin.
Thrombin, USP (Thrombinar)	Powder	Not available	Valuable in affixing skin transplants. Valuable as an aid in hemostasis whenever oozing capillaries are accessible.
Thromboplastin (Thrombokinase)	Powder	Not available	
Microfibrillar collagen hemostat (Avitene)	Fibrous or nonwoven web	About 84 days	Used for hemostasis in surgical procedures
Negatol (Negatan)	Colloidal product	Not available	Effective in gynecologic surgical procedures to control or stop bleeding.

terferes with the regeneration of both bone and epithelial tissue; therefore, it should not be used in either bone or surface wounds. Oxidized cellulose is completely absorbed in two to seven days; however, large blood-soaked material may take as long as six weeks.

Microfibrillar Collagen Hemostat

Microfibrillar collagen hemostat (Avitene) is an absorbable topical hemostatic agent prepared from purified bovine collagen. Two forms are available: a fibrous form applied directly to the source of bleeding or a nonwoven web form that is applied in small squares to bleeding areas. Microfibrillar collagen hemostat is used in surgical procedures as an adjunct to hemostasis when conventional procedures to halt bleeding have been ineffective.

Negatol

Negatol (Negatan) is a highly acidic colloidal product that has a coagulation effect on protein substances. It is effective as a styptic (astringent and hemostatic) in gynecology. After application, the patient should wear a perineal pad to prevent soiling of clothing by the highly acid product.

Thrombin

Thrombin is prepared from bovine plasma. Thrombin acts as a catalyst for the conversion of fibrinogen to fibrin. It is a dry powder that is mixed with sterile isotonic saline solution before use. Thrombin is marketed in powder vials containing 1,000, 5,000, or 10,000 NIH units (1 NIH unit is the amount of thrombin that will clot 1 ml of a standard solution of fibrinogen in less than one minute). Thrombin is only for topical use; it has no antigenicity and is free of serious adverse effects when used in this way. Thrombin is valuable in helping to affix skin transplants.

THROMBOLYTIC ENZYMES

Thrombolytic enzymes dissolve clots through activation of the endogenous fibrinolytic system. Several preparations are currently available as thrombolytic agents. These preparations assist the conversion of plasma proteins and plasminogen to plasmin (fibrinolysin), which, in turn, digests the fibrin threads, resulting in clot lysis. The thrombus is dissolved rather than having its extension prevented, as with anticoagulants. Several of these products alter stage IV of clotting, and consequently, bleeding is more difficult to control than the bleeding secondary to anticoagulants. These drugs are featured in Table 33–3.

Uses

Streptokinase (Kabikinase, Streptase), urokinase (Abbokinase), and recombinant alteplase (Activase) are used in various forms of thromboembolic disease such as phlebothrombosis, pulmonary embolism, thrombophlebitis, and arterial thrombosis (as in arteriovenous cannulae occlusions and acute myocardial infarction) to break up and dissolve clots and restore normal blood flow patterns. These medications are used only in controlled situations by physicians and nurses familiar with their use and are administered within several hours after embolization.

Action

These drugs are given intravenously to promote the lysis of existing fibrin clots. Streptokinase is non-selective and acts with plasminogen to produce an "activator complex" that converts plasminogen to the proteolytic enzyme plasmin. Urokinase acts directly on the fibrinolytic system to convert plasminogen into plasmin. Plasmin then degrades the fibrin clot as well as fibrinogen and other plasma proteins. This increase in fibri-

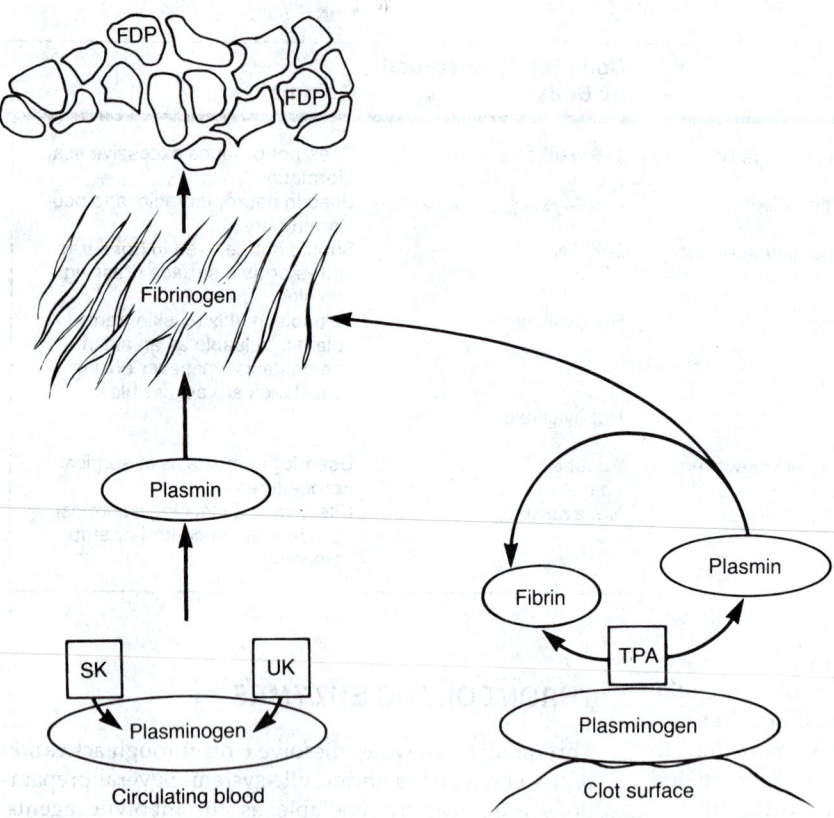

Figure 33-2. A schematic representation of the action of streptokinase (SK), urokinase (UK) which affect the exogenous circulating plasmin and tissue plasminogen activator (tPA) which affects only to fibrin-bound plasmin. Fibrin then breaks down into Fibrin Degradation Products (FDP).

nolytic activity usually disappears within a few hours after discontinuation of the medication, but may persist for up to 12–24 hours. Recombinant alteplase activates fibrin-bound plasminogen to plasmin. It is selective in that recombinant alteplase acts on new clots. It must actually act on the clot to be activated. Figure 33–2 compares the action of these products.

Contraindications and Precautions

Major relative contraindications include recent major surgery (within ten days), serious GI bleeding, organ biopsy, or obstetric delivery; severe uncontrolled arterial hypertension, that is, systolic blood pressure of 200 mmHg or more or diastolic pressure of 110 mmHg or more; cerebrovascular accident; and recent serious trauma. Minor relative contraindications include recent minor trauma, including cardiopulmonary resuscitation, high likelihood of left heart thrombus (e.g., mitral stenosis with atrial fibrillation), infectious endocarditis, pregnancy, cerebrovascular disease (within two months), diabetic hemorrhagic retinopathy, and hemostatic defects, including those associated with severe hepatic or renal disease. Safety in pregnancy, lactating women, and children is not established.

Adverse Effects

The major adverse effect of the thrombolytic enzymes is bleeding. Bleeding may occur at invaded or disturbed skin sites, or internally from many organ sites, including the brain. Should uncontrolled bleeding occur, these products are discontinued. If necessary, blood loss and reversal of bleeding tendency can be effectively managed with whole blood (fresh is preferable), packed red cells, clotting factors such as cryoprecipitate, or fresh-frozen plasma. Although the effectiveness of aminocaproic acid (Amicar) as an antidote has not been documented, it may be used in an emergency. A febrile reaction can also occur after drug administration with streptokinase (33%) as it is a foreign protein. Symptomatic treatment is usually sufficient to relieve discomfort; however, aspirin should not be used, as bleeding may occur. Allergic reaction, such as serum sickness with streptokinase, can also occur with these products.

Dysrhythmias occurring after thrombolytic therapy include ventricular tachycardia, sinus bradycardia, premature ventricular contractions, supraventricular tachycardias, and ventricular fibrillation. They are treated with appropriate antiarrhythmic medications.

Drug Interactions

Anticoagulant therapy may increase the risk of hemorrhage. Also, drugs affecting platelet function (aspirin, indomethacin, dipyridamole, phenylbutazone, and sulfinpyrazone) should be avoided.

Streptokinase

Streptokinase (Streptase, Kabikinase) is derived from bacteria protein. This causes significant antigenicity, creating the potential for allergic responses, including anaphylaxis. To open deep-vein thrombosis and pulmonary arteries, the IV loading dose is 250,000 units over 30 minutes, and the maintenance dose is 100,000 units/hr for 24–72 hours. The half-life of the initial elimination phase is 10–12 minutes, depending on the number of antibodies present. Dilution and infusion rates for IV doses are found in Table 33–3. Streptokinase is administered IV to dissolve clots in the coronary arteries that are less than three hours old, but it is best administered within 1.5 hours. The IV dosage is 1.5 million units over one hour. Because it is a foreign protein, streptokinase has the ability to cause resistance due to the development of antibodies, so therapy should not be repeated for three to six months.

Streptokinase can also be used to dissolve the thrombus in a new myocardial infarction that is less than three hours old, directly through cardiac catheterization. A catheter is inserted peripherally and passed into the affected coronary artery. A bolus of 20,000 units (u) is administered, and a maintenance dose of 2,000 u/minute for 60 minutes opens more than 75% of occlusions in less than one hour. As doses of streptokinase are given, the clot is watched on the fluoroscope. Within 30–60 minutes, the clot begins to dissolve and blood begins to flow in the blocked vessel. After streptokinase injections, the patient is heparinized for three to four days and maintained on aspirin products for six to eight months.

Streptokinase can be administered to treat pulmonary embolism. The initial dose is 250,000 u given intravenously over a period of 30 minutes followed by 100,000 u/hour given by continuous infusion for 24 hours. If concurrent deep-vein thrombosis is suspected, administer over 72 hours.

Much research is currently ongoing in order to determine the most effective way to prevent or minimize damage after a myocardial infarction. Streptokinase is best administered peripherally on admission to the hospital as soon as possible after onset of pain. If the patient experiences recurrent chest pains, the patient is then taken to the catheterization lab for a percutaneous transluminal coronary *angioplasty* to assist with opening the vessel.

Several large trials of streptokinase have recently been completed that have found that streptokinase administered within three to four hours of the onset of pain reduces muscle damage and improves the ejection fraction. The GISSI study found a reduction of mortality of 50% when streptokinase was administered within one hour. But if streptokinase is not administered until three to six hours after onset of pain, only the 30-day mortality is reduced with no increase in muscle survival. Streptokinase may also prevent recurrence of infarction.

Urokinase

Urokinase (Abbokinase) is a nonantigenic protein secreted by the human kidneys and excreted in the urine. This protein promotes *thrombolysis* through a direct action on the fibrinolytic system to convert plasminogen into the proteolytic enzyme plasmin. Urokinase is approved for use in the lysis of acute massive pulmonary emboli and for lysis of emboli accompanied by unstable hemodynamics (i.e., failure to maintain blood pressure without supportive measures) in adults. Urokinase is also used intracoronary to open occluded coronary arteries and has a recanalized rate of 62%–94% in these vessels. It is effective and can be used to restore patency to occluded IV catheters. However, because of its expense, streptokinase is more often used to restore patency to central lines. Urokinase therapy should be initiated as soon as possible. This drug is considerably more expensive than streptokinase; however, urokinase may be useful in patients who require a thrombolytic agent but have high concentrations of streptokinase antibodies.

For the treatment of pulmonary embolism, through a peripheral IV line, the usual dose is 4400 IU/kg administered over a period of 10 minutes, followed by a continuous infusion of 4400 IU/kg/hr for 12–24 hours. Thrombin time should be determined three to four hours after initiation of therapy to ensure that adequate activation (i.e., thrombin time greater than twice normal control) of the fibrinolytic system has occurred. For the treatment of coronary artery thrombosis, an infusion of 6000 IU/min for up to two hours is administered. Most studies indicate that 500,000 IU will open a coronary vessel. Continue therapy until the artery is maximally opened, usually 15–30 minutes. Adequate anticoagulation should be instituted soon after urokinase therapy is discontinued in order to minimize the risk of further clotting. (Heparin therapy should not begin until the prothrombin time has decreased to less than twice normal control value.)

For occluded IV catheters, 5000 IU is gently instilled by a tuberculin syringe in amounts equal to the internal volume of the catheter. Wait at least five to ten minutes and attempt to aspirate both the urokinase and the clot. If the catheter is not opened within 30 minutes, cap the catheter and allow the urokinase to remain for another 30–60 minutes before again attempting to aspirate. Once the clot has been aspirated, aspirate an additional 4–5 ml of blood to ensure removal of all drug and residual clot.

Recombinant Alteplase

Recombinant alteplase (Activase) is a protease enzyme purified from uterine tissue and a human melanoma cell line. Alteplase is now produced by genetic recombinant techniques (gene techology), which provides a large quantity of highly purified material. Alteplase is produced in *E. coli*. Because it is a natural protein, it is not associated with antibody formation or with allergic reaction. Alteplase is identical to the natural activator generated locally by endothelial cells of the vessel wall as part of the normal physiologic mechanism for digesting fibrin clots. The circulation half-life is three to five minutes. This is an advantage for the patient who may require immediate surgery after thrombolysis.

Alteplase currently costs about $2000 to $2500 per treatment. Alteplase given with heparin to patients with indwelling coronary catheters appears to be more effective than IV streptokinase, but is not necessarily safer for the treatment of coronary artery thrombosis.

Alteplase is administered in an IV dose of 100 mg over three hours, with 60 mg administered over the first hour (6 mg given in a bolus) followed by 40 mg over the remaining two hours. Alteplase is followed by heparin and aspirin therapy.

SYSTEMIC HEMOSTATICS

Systemic hemostatics inhibit the resolution of the clot by inhibiting the breakdown of fibrin. These products control rapid loss of blood. These drugs are featured in Table 33–3.

Aminocaproic Acid

Aminocaproic acid (Amicar), an antifibrinolytic, is administered orally or intravenously in patients with hemorrhage caused by overactivity of stage IV, clot resolution or with excessive bleeding from systemic hyperfibrinoloysis and urinary fibrinoloysis; as an antidote in patients receiving an overdose of thrombolytic agents such as streptokinase and urokinase; and in patients with hemophilia when fibrin formation is deficient. These patients often require other additional emergency measures.

PHARMACOKINETICS. Aminocaproic acid, when given orally, is rapidly absorbed from the gastrointestinal tract and reaches peak plasma levels in about two hours. Aminocaproic acid is readily distributed to tissues. It is excreted in about twelve hours unchanged in the urine.

CONTRAINDICATIONS AND PRECAUTIONS. Aminocaproic acid is contraindicated in severe renal impairment and in the presence of active intravascular clotting process. It should be used with caution in patients with renal, cardiac, and hepatic dysfunction.

ADVERSE EFFECTS. Adverse effects are generally mild and include nausea, cramping, diarrhea, dizziness, and malaise.

DOSAGE. Initial dose of 5 g orally or intravenously (mix 4–5 g in 250 ml of IV solution in one hour followed by 1 g in 50 ml/hr) followed by 1–1.25 g/hr, should achieve a satisfactory serum level. Administration of more than 30 g/24 hours is not recommended.

Tranexamic Acid

Tranexamic acid (Cyklokapion), a synthetic antifibrinolytic agent, similar to aminocaprioc acid, is designed for concurrent use with coagulation factors to prevent hemorrhage in hemophiliacs undergoing dental extractions. Tranexamic acid, a synthetic lysine analog, competitively inhibits fibrinolysis by saturating lysine binding sites where plasminogen and plasmin bind to fibrinogen and fibrin.

PHARMACOKINETICS. *Absorption and Distribution.* After an oral dose, 30%–50% of tranexamic acid is absorbed and reaches a peak in about three hours. Bioavailability is not affected by food. Tranexamic acid is widely distributed in tissues but is less concentrated

there than in blood. Tranexamic acid does not bind to albumin but is about 3% bound to plasminogen.

Biotransformation and Excretion. Only a small fraction of tranexamic acid is metabolized and the remainder (95%) is excreted unchanged in the urine. The serum half-life is about two hours but the antifibrinolytic effect remains in the serum for seven hours.

CONTRAINDICATIONS AND PRECAUTIONS. Tranexamic acid is contraindicated in *acquired defective color vision* and in subarachnoid hemorrhage because it may aggravate cerebral edema. It is used cautiously in persons with renal dysfunction, since the drug is eliminated in the kidneys.

ADVERSE EFFECTS. The most common adverse effects are nausea, vomiting, and diarrhea, all of which usually disappear as the dose is reduced. Patients may complain of visual abnormalities, including abnormalities in color vision.

DOSAGE. Tranexamic acid is available in both oral and IV forms. For dental extraction in patients with hemophilia, tranexamic acid is administered IV immediately before surgery (10 mg/kg), and orally after surgery (25 mg/kg) three to four times daily for two to eight days. The dosage needs to be reduced for patients with renal impairment.

USING THE NURSING PROCESS

ASSESSMENT

Assessment of the patient who requires medications that affect blood clotting always begins with a thorough past and recent nursing history to develop the data base. All of this information is used later when preparing the nursing care plan. The information that is obtained is included in Table 33–5. Generally, patients are hospitalized when they first require anticoagulants and then continue their therapy at home.

It is very important to assess the nutritional habits of the patient, since dietary counseling will be done when the patient is discharged on oral anticoagulants. Also, the nurse must understand that 50% of human vitamin K is synthesized by bacterial flora in the gastrointestinal tract. When a patient is allowed nothing by mouth and is taking antibiotics, the amount of vitamin K decreases because it cannot be synthesized. Therefore, people who are not eating for long periods need supplemental vitamin K. Also, to absorb vitamin K, bile must be present. If obstructive jaundice is present, bile salts cannot move into the intestine and vitamin K absorption is reduced.

A drug profile is taken to determine whether or not there are any drugs the patient is currently taking that will interfere with the drugs that affect coagulation.

Frequent blood tests are performed to assess clotting time. Table 33–6 features frequently used clotting studies. In addition, hematocrit, fibrinogen concentration,

Table 33–5. NURSING PROCESS FOR PATIENT REQUIRING AGENTS THAT AFFECT COAGULATION

Assessment

Assess color, pulses, pain and tenderness, cramping and pain.
Review lifestyle, including type of work (sedentary/active) and type of leisure activities, smoking.
Note history of recent injury to the extremity, hypertension, hypercholesterol levels, diabetes, renal disease, and/or cardiac disease.
Note respiratory rate and depth, use of accessory muscles, pursed-lip breathing.
Auscultate lungs for areas of decreased/absent breath sounds, and the presence of adventitious sounds, e.g., crackles.
Observe for generalized duskiness and cyanosis in "warm tissues" such as earlobes, lips, tongue, and buccal membranes.

Nursing Diagnosis	Nursing Actions	Rationale	Desired Outcomes/ Evaluation Criteria
Tissue perfusion decreased, peripheral related to decreased blood flow as evidenced by tissue edema, diminished peripheral pulses, slow/diminished capillary refill, skin color changes, pallor, erythema.	Promote bedrest during acute phase.	Reduces oxygen and nutrient demands on affected extremity and minimizes the possibility of dislodging thrombus and creating emboli.	Demonstrates improved perfusion as evidenced by peripheral pulses present/equal, skin color and temperature normal, absence of edema. Engages in behaviors/ actions to enhance tissue perfusion. Reports/ displays increasing tolerance to activity.
	Elevate legs when in bed or chair. Periodically elevate feet and lower legs above heart level.	Reduces tissue swelling and rapidly empties superficial and tibial veins, preventing overdistention and thereby increasing venous return.	
	Initiate/encourage active or passive exercises while in bed (e.g., flex/extend/rotate foot periodically). Assist with gradual resumption of ambulation.	These measures are designed to increase venous return from lower extremities and reduce venous stasis as well as improve general muscle tone/strength.	
	Caution patient to avoid crossing legs and hyperflexion at knee.	Physical restriction of circulation impairs blood flow and increases venous stasis in pelvic, popliteal and leg vessels.	
	Administer anticoagulation, e.g., heparin and/or coumarin derivatives.	Heparin is preferred initially because of its prompt, predictable antagonistic action on thrombin formation and its prevention of further clot formation. Coumadin, which blocks formation of prothrombin from vitamin K, may be used for long-term/post-discharge therapy.	
	Review coagulation studies, CBC as indicated.	Monitors effectiveness of anticoagulant therapy and risk factors, e.g., hemoconcentration and dehydration, which potentiate clot formation.	
Pain, related to diminished arterial circulation and oxygenation of tissues with production/ accumulation of lactic acid in tissues.	Provide foot cradle and encourage frequent position changes.	Keeps pressure of bed clothes off the affected leg, thereby reducing pressure discomfort.	Reports pain/discomfort is relieved/controlled. Verbalizes methods that provide relief. Displays relaxed manner, able to sleep/rest and engage in desired activity.
	Keep extremity elevated.	Increases venous return to minimize edema.	
	Monitor vital signs, noting elevated temperature.	Elevations in heart rate may indicate increased	

CONTINUED ON THE FOLLOWING PAGE

Table 33–5. NURSING PROCESS FOR PATIENT REQUIRING AGENTS THAT AFFECT COAGULATION–*CONTINUED*

Nursing Diagnosis	Nursing Actions	Rationale	Desired Outcomes/ Evaluation Criteria
		pain/discomfort or occur in response to fever and inflammatory process which can also increase discomfort.	
	Investigate complaints of sudden and/or sharp chest pain, accompanied by dyspnea, tachycardia, and apprehension.	Suggest presence of pulmonary emboli as a complication of DVT.	
	Administer analgesics, antipyretics as indicated.	Control of pain, muscle tension, fever and inflammation, enhances comfort and promotes healing.	
	Apply moist heat to extremity.	Causes vasodilation which increases circulation, relaxes muscles and may stimulate release of natural endorphins.	
Gas exchange, impaired, potential related to altered blood flow to alveoli, pulmonary edema/effusion, atelectasis in the presence of pulmonary emboli.	Elevate head of bed as patient requires/tolerates.	Promotes maximal chest expansion, making it easier to breathe which enhances physiologic/ psychologic comfort.	Demonstrates adequate ventilation/oxygenation by ABGs within patient's normal range. Reports/ displays resolution or absence of symptoms of respiratory distress.
	Institute measures to restore/maintain patent airways, e.g., deep breathing exercises, coughing, suctioning, etc.	Plugged/collapsed airways reduce number of functional alveoli, negatively affecting gas exchange.	
	Administer oxygen by appropriate method.	Maximizes available oxygen for gas exchange.	
	Monitor serial ABGs.	Identifies therapy needs/ effectiveness as hypoxemia is present in varying degrees, depending on the amount of airway obstruction, prior cardiopulmonary function, and presence/absence of shock.	
Knowledge deficit related to lack of exposure/ unfamiliarity with information resources, lack of recall as evidenced by request for information, verbalization of concerns, inaccurate followthrough of instructions, development of preventable complications.	Review pathophysiology of condition and signs/ symptoms of possible complications, e.g., pulmonary emboli, chronic venous insufficiency, venous stasis ulcers.	Provides a knowledge base from which patient can make informed choices and understand/ identify health care needs.	Verbalizes understanding of disease process, treatment regimen and limitations. Identifies signs/symptoms requiring medical evaluation. Correctly performs therapeutic procedure(s) and explains reasons for actions.
	Discuss purpose, dosage of anticoagulant. Emphasize importance of taking drug as prescribed.	Promotes patient safety by maintaining serum anticoagulation levels within the narrow therapeutic range reducing risk of inadequate therapeutic response/deleterious side effect.	
	Discuss possible drug interactions (e.g., salicylates, alcohol, barbiturates, Vit K). Stress need to read ingredient labels of OTC drugs and avoidance of foods high in Vit K, e.g., (green leafy vegetables).	Reduces risk of inadequate drug effect, untoward reactions and possible complications.	

Table 33–5. NURSING PROCESS FOR PATIENT REQUIRING AGENTS THAT AFFECT COAGULATION–*CONTINUED*

Nursing Diagnosis	Nursing Actions	Rationale	Desired Outcomes/ Evaluation Criteria
	Identify untoward anticoagulant effects requiring medical attention, e.g., bleeding from mucous membranes, bruising with little or no trauma, development of petechiae.	Early detection of deleterious effects of therapy allows for timely intervention/prevention of serious complications.	
	Stress importance of medical follow-up/laboratory testing.	Encourages patient participation. Close supervision of anticoagulant therapy is necessary, to maintain therapeutic effectiveness/prevent complications.	
	Recommend appropriate safety precautions, e.g., use of soft toothbrush, electric razors, avoidance of forceful blowing of nose, walking barefoot.	Reduces risk of traumatic injury/bleeding.	
	Explain purpose of activity restrictions and need for balance between activity/rest.	Rest reduces oxygen and nutrient needs of compromised tissues. Balance of activity prevents exhaustion and further impairment of cellular perfusion.	
	Establish appropriate exercise/activity program.	Aids in developing collateral circulation, enhances venous return and aids in prevention of recurrence.	
	Problem-solve solutions to predisposing factors that may be present, e.g., work setting that requires prolonged standing/sitting, wearing of restrictive clothing, use of oral contraceptives, obesity, prolonged bedrest/immobility, dehydration.	Activity involves patient in identifying and initiating lifestyle/behavior changes to promote health and prevent recurrence of condition/development of complications as possible.	
	Instruct in meticulous skin care of lower extremities, e.g., prevent/promptly treat breaks in skin, report development of lesions/ulcers or changes in skin color.	Chronic venous congestion/postphlebotic syndrome may develop potentiating risk of stasis ulcers/infection.	
	Review purpose and demonstrate correct application/removal of antiembolic hose.	May enhance cooperation with prescribed therapy and prevent improper/ineffective use.	

and platelet counts are done. The patient must understand the importance of these clotting tests because medication dosage is regulated by their results. During the first several days, laboratory tests may be needed daily. The frequency of the tests may be reduced to weekly for about a month, and then monthly, until the medication can be discontinued. Drug administration generally does not begin until after the laboratory results are received.

If the patient is being placed on thrombolytic enzymes, the thrombin time and activated partial thromboplastin time should be less than twice the normal control times before therapy is started. Also heparin and/or coumarin products need to be discontinued.

Table 33–6. TESTS OF BLOOD COAGULATION

Test	Normal Value	Therapeutic Value	Medications Monitored
Prothrombin time (PT)	11–12 sec	20–25 sec	Coumarin derivatives
Partial thromboplastin time (PTT)	60–90 sec	90–180 sec	Heparin
Lee–White clotting time (LWCT) (done on whole blood)	9–14 min	20–30 min	Heparin
Activated partial thromboplastin time (APTT)	24–36 sec	48–60 sec	Heparin
Activated clotting time (ACT)	80–135 sec	3 min	Heparin
Thrombin time (TT)	10–15 sec	20–25 sec	Heparin

NURSING DIAGNOSES

The nurse establishes the nursing diagnoses, which become the basis for nursing care and nursing evaluation. Typical nursing diagnoses for a patient with problems of coagulation are included in Table 33–5.

PLANNING AND INTERVENTION

The goals of nursing intervention are developed from the nursing diagnoses. The goals of nursing intervention in caring for the patient who requires medications that affect blood coagulation are included in Table 33–5.

NURSING RESPONSIBILITIES

Anticoagulants

When the nurse administers the anticoagulant heparin parenterally, the following procedures are followed: clotting studies are performed, usually every 6–12 hours during early therapy and once daily when stable, before the next dose of heparin is administered. (When heparin is being given prophylactically [5000 units every 12 hours], clotting studies are not necessary.) All body secretions are also examined to detect bleeding. Other IM or subcutaneous medications are best scheduled near to the time of the next heparin administration so that the clotting time is almost back to normal. This prevents prolonged bleeding at the site.

When the nurse administers heparin subcutaneously, the best location is the abdomen. The medication is administered deep using a 25- or 26-gauge, ½–⅝-inch needle. The technique is as follows: cleanse with alcohol (do not rub, however, because tissue may be traumatized), allow to dry. Bunch up fat, insert needle at 90°, do not withdraw plunger, inject medication slowly. Still holding the bunch of fat, withdraw the needle in same direction; apply pressure, but do **not** rub. A "belly chart" is kept either in the patient's room or in the chart so all injections can be charted. Injections are not made within two inches of the umbilicus or on a scar.

When administering heparin intravenously, a heparin lock is most commonly used. The trap is flushed with a saline-heparin solution (usually 10–100 units of heparin in 1 ml of saline) before and after the heparin is injected. Always aspirate before flushing to ensure that the needle is still properly placed in the vein. Heparin locks can safely be left in place for 48–72 hours.

When continuous IV infusions of heparin are administered, infusion pumps and microdrip regulators are used to carefully titrate the dose. Flow sheets, containing clotting times, the time of medication administration, and the route used, are kept on the patient's chart. IM injection should be avoided in this patient because the continuous heparin drip elevates the clotting levels continually.

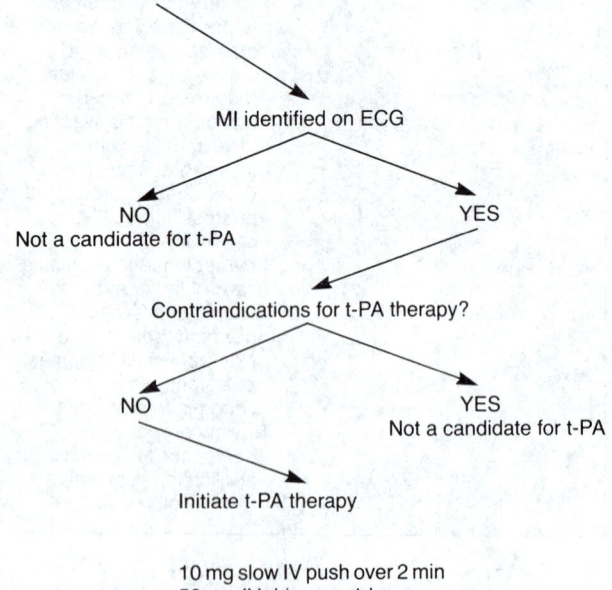

t-PA Administration Algorithm

Patient arrives in ER with severe chest pain, 6 hr of onset

ER physician identifies as t-PA candidate
Obtain 12 lead ECG
Challenge with SL NTG
Obtain initial labs (CBC, CPK, SAM 6, PT, PTT, fibrinogen)
Establish at least 2 IVs

MI identified on ECG

NO
Not a candidate for t-PA

YES

Contraindications for t-PA therapy?

NO

YES
Not a candidate for t-PA

Initiate t-PA therapy

10 mg slow IV push over 2 min
50 mg IV drip over 1 hour
20 mg/hr drip times 2 hours

100 mg total.

Figure 33–3. t-PA Administration Algorithm. (Courtesy of Mary Lamb, Sacred Heart Hospital, Pensacola, FL.)

Heparin is often used as a "flush" to clear central lines such as subclavian lines. The line is generally flushed with 1.5–2.0 ml of 100 units/ml heparin. Peripheral lines can be flushed with 10 units/ml heparin. If the lines are flushed more than four times per day, then a less concentrated solution is used to prevent changing the patient's clotting times.

The antagonist for heparin—protamine sulfate—is always available. If a medication error is made and the patient is given too much heparin, the protamine is used carefully for the first four hours after a dose.

Oral anticoagulants are started three to five days prior to discontinuing heparin. To obtain an accurate prothrombin time, at least four to six hours must elapse after the last IV dose and 12–24 hours after the last subcutaneous dose.

To initiate oral anticoagulant therapy, patients are often started above maintenance dosage levels, typically 10 mg/day for two to four days. Daily prothrombin times are taken prior to subsequent dosing, until stabilization is achieved within therapeutic range. After stabilization, prothrombin times can be performed every one to four weeks. Any additions or deletions of concomitant medications requires a prothrombin time to be done after 48 hours.

Thrombolytic Enzymes

When the nurse is administering a thrombolytic enzyme (streptokinase, urokinase, recombinant alteplase), it is generally an acute emergency situation in which clot dissolution is required to preserve organ or limb func-

tion. Acute necrosis begins in about 15 minutes and continues until all tissue becomes necrotic, about four to six hours. Reperfusion must be performed before irreversible necrosis occurs. There is evidence that early reperfusion limits necrosis. Patient selection is most important and the nurse is often in a position to assist with early detection of vascular occlusion. Figure 33–3 includes a tPA administration algorithm. Candidates for thrombolytic therapy include:

Pulmonary embolism:

1. Acute, massive or severe life-threatening pulmonary embolism
2. Two-thirds or more of a main branch of the pulmonary artery is obstructed
3. Accompanied by acute right-sided heart failure with or without shock
4. Unstable circulatory status

Evolving myocardial infarction:

1. Chest pain for at least 30 minutes but less than four hours
2. S–T elevation of at least 0.1 mV in two leads
3. No relief of pain with nitroglycerin

Generally, the potential benefits should outweigh the dangers, such as the increased risk of bleeding.

The thrombolytic enzymes are mixed carefully according to manufacturer's direction found in the package inserts. They are administered through microdrip tubing with an automatic IV control pump, and a filter is used. Tables 33–7 and 33–8 include a currently used

---

Table 33–7. tPA ADMINISTRATION

If the patient is a tPA candidate the following procedure must be followed:

1. Mix 2 50-mg vials of tPA with the 100 ml sterile water supplied with the tPA vials.
2. Further dilute this solution with 100 ml normal saline (100 mg tPA in 200 ml)
3. Give a 10-mg bolus IV push **over 2 min**
4. Give 50 mg tPA by **IV infusion** over **1 hr**
5. Start nitroglycerin drip at 10 μg/min (6 ml/hr) and titrate for pain.
6. Give 50 mg Lidocaine bolus IV push. Repeat in 10 min × 2.
7. Start Lidocaine drip at 2 mg/min.
8. Give Heparin, 5000 units, IV push toward the end of the above tPA infusion.
9. Then give 20 mg tPA per hour for **2 hours.** This is a total of 100 mg over a 3-hour period.
10. At the same time as #8 give heparin, 1000 units/hr by IV infusion (20,000 units heparin in 500 ml D$_5$W run at 25 ml/hr).

NOTE: a total of 3 peripheral lines will be needed: one of tPA infusion, one for nitroglycerin and lidocaine (piggyback), and one for heparin infusion.

Dosage:
No patient will receive a dosage of more than 100 mg. Patients weighing less than 65 kg will have a reduced dosage as follows (doses are rounded to the nearest 5 mg):

Weight	Total Dose	=	Bolus Dose	+	Dose Given Over Hour 1 @ Rate ×	+	Dose Given Over Hours 2 & 3
60 kg (132 lb)	75 mg		5 mg		40 mg (40 mg/hr)		30 mg (15 mg/hr)
55 kg (121 lb)	70 mg		5 mg		35 mg (35 mg/hr)		30 mg (15 mg/hr)
50 kg (110 lb)	65 mg		5 mg		35 mg (35 mg/hr)		25 mg (13 mg/hr)
45 kg (99 lb)	55 mg		5 mg		30 mg (30 mg/hr)		20 mg (10 mg/hr)
40 kg (88 lb)	50 mg		5 mg		25 mg (25 mg/hr)		20 mg (10 mg/hr)

Courtesy of Mary Lamb, Sacred Heart Hospital, Pensacola, FL.

Table 33–8. tPA ADMINISTRATION CHECKOFF SHEET

Time	Initial	
_____	_____	1. Nitroglycerin challenge done. (nitroglycerin ⅟₁₅₀ gr sublingual q 5 min × without pain relief.)
_____	_____	2. Contraindication sheet filled out and checked by physician.

The following medications must be given as quickly as possible. A total of at least 3 peripheral IVs will be needed. One should already be in place from the initial assessment and treatment of the patient.

Time	Initial	
_____	_____	3. Mix tPA 100 mg (2 vials) in 100-ml diluent. Transfer tPA into a 100-ml bag of normal saline to make 100 mg tPA in 200 ml solution. Draw 20 ml (10 mg) out of bag and give IV push over 2 min.
_____	_____	4. Start tPA IV drip at 50 mg/hr for 1 hour immediately after above bolus. [After 1 hour change rate to 20 mg/hr for 2 hours. Place time for rate change on line 10.]
_____	_____	5. Nitroglycerin drip 10 μg/min (6 ml/hr) and titrate for pain. [Start in second peripheral IV.]
_____	_____	6. Lidocaine 50 mg IV bolus. Repeat every 10 min × 2. Place time for repeat doses on lines 8 and 9.
_____	_____	7. Lidocaine drip at 2 mg/min. [may piggyback this with nitroglycerin drip].
_____	_____	8. Second Lidocaine 50-mg IV bolus.
_____	_____	9. Third Lidocaine 50-mg IV bolus.
_____	_____	10. Change tPA drip to infuse at 20 mg/hr [40 ml/hr].
_____	_____	11. Heparin 5000 units IV push (at end of first hour of tPA therapy).
_____	_____	12. Heparin drip 20,000 units in 500 ml D₅W at 25 ml/hr (third peripheral IV).
_____	_____	13. At the end of 2 hours when the tPA infusion is in, add 50 ml normal saline to the empty IV bag and continue to infuse at 40 ml/hr to clear the tPA from the IV tubing.

Courtesy of Mary Lamb, Sacred Heart Hospital, Pensacola, FL.

tPA administration procedure and tPA administration checkoff sheet.

The National Conference of Antithrombotic Therapy, co-sponsored by the American College of Chest Physicians and National Institutes of Health—National Heart, Lung, and Blood Institute recently suggested antithrombotic therapy for various conditions. They suggest that a patient with a diagnosis of an anterior transmural myocardial infarction (MI) should receive full doses of heparin followed by coumadin therapy for one to three months. After an anterior MI, patients are at high risk for embolic complications because there is an associated incidence of developing mural thrombus (33%). When mural thrombus is present in anterior MI and anticoagulants are not administered, the risk of stroke or embolism ranges from 20%–43%. In comparison to MIs at other locations, anterior MI carries double the risk of stroke.

Patients who survive an MI and have atrial fibrillation, previous systemic embolism, or congestive heart failure should also receive full doses of heparin followed by coumadin for at least three months. Patients with uncomplicated MI should receive aspirin for an unknown duration. And patients with unstable angina should receive 325 mg/day for two years.

PATIENT TEACHING

Clotting disorders may be idiopathic or due to a determined cause. It is important to teach the patient about the causative factors so action can be taken to prevent recurrence. Deep-vein thrombosis with pulmonary emboli may be related to venous stasis, wearing of garters or panty girdles, varicose veins, trauma, or prolonged immobilization. The patient and family should know and understand these factors and how to prevent recurrence. Clotting disorders such as pulmonary embolism or cerebral vascular diseases may be life threatening.

Often patients are discharged on anticoagulants. The nurse, as teacher, must ensure that the patient knows and understands the information in Table 33–9 to safely administer his or her own medication at home.

Uncooperative patients, patients of advanced age, and patients with hypertension, unexplained anemia, a history of peptic ulcer, or neoplastic disease are considered at high risk, and must be monitored very closely. Some authorities suggest that these groups of patients should not receive anticoagulants at all because of the related side effects. (Incidence of hemorrhage may approach 50%, whereas in the normal population it ranges from 7% to 15%.) The physician weighs the benefits of therapy against the risk of adverse or serious reactions. All elderly patients at home are followed closely. Relatives are encouraged to check frequently for compliance and overcompliance.

Statistics show that 10% of all patients on long-term anticoagulants bleed at some time during the course of their therapy. However, fatalities are rare. Patients are taught to go to the emergency room for definitive treatment.

Dietary counseling and teaching is important when the patient is going home on coumarin products. Patients need to understand the natural sources of vitamin

Table 33–9. PATIENT TEACHING INFORMATION—ANTICOAGULANTS

Dear Patient:
This drug has been ordered for you. This is what you should know about your drug to get the most from your therapy.

1. The anticoagulant _____ is taken to thin your blood to prevent further clotting.
2. Anticoagulant therapy is often long term. (Most patients take anticoagulants for at least 6 months and some need them for a lifetime.)
3. You may take your anticoagulant with or between meals.
4. Many drug interactions can occur with anticoagulants. Always check with your druggist or doctor before taking any new medication, whether prescribed or over the counter.
5. If you forget your drug for a whole day, **do not** take it. **Do not** catch up.
6. Do not stop the drug without your doctor's approval.
7. If you note any bleeding from the gums, contact your doctor. Use a soft toothbrush to prevent gum injury.
8. If you note any dark brown or red urine, dark or tarry stools, slight bruising resulting in large black and blue areas, nose bleeds, excessive menstrual flow, and prolonged oozing from any injury, report these to your doctor.
9. Shave with an electric razor to avoid scraping your skin.
10. Do not eat large amounts of foods rich in vitamin K, such as green leafy vegetables (cabbage, spinach, kale, lettuce, cauliflower), tomatoes, fish, liver, cheese, egg yolks, and fats from red meats. Avoid alcohol intake because of its effect on the liver. Drinking even 2 or 3 oz of liquor may increase your tendency to bleed. If you require nutritional supplements such as Ensure, Vital, or Nutramigen, you may have difficulty with coumarin product regulation because of their high vitamin K content. Consult your doctor.
11. When traveling to a hot climate from a cold one, the dose of your drug may need to be reduced. Consult with the doctor before traveling to any area where a change in climate is expected.
12. Carry an identification card or wear a piece of jewelry that states the drug you are taking and the doctor's name and telephone number.
13. Always inform all other doctors and dentists that you are taking anticoagulants before any treatments are started.
14. Store anticoagulants in a tight, moisture-resistant container, since they can lose their potency when exposed to air.

K and to limit their intake of these foods (see Table 33–9).

EVALUATION

The evaluation of the effectiveness of medications that affect coagulation is based on a predetermined list of evaluation outcome criteria that are developed on an individual basis through discussion among the nurse, patient, and family, and based on the nursing diagnoses.

The information from the data base, obtained in the original assessment, is used to formulate the criteria for evaluation. Typical outcome evaluation criteria are included in Table 33–5.

It is extremely important to work with the patient and family to ensure their complete assistance and support. The majority of patients, once they understand the importance of their continued medical treatment, are compliant. The primary reason for noncompliance is forgetting the medication. Overcompliance is occasionally a problem in the elderly or emotionally ill patient, who may use overdosing on anticoagulants as an attention-getting mechanism. These patients must be followed very closely; usually a family member must assume responsibility for the administration of the medication.

The patient should know about the adverse effects of the medications. The patient is taught to call the physician if he or she notes any unusual symptom. The adverse effect most often experienced is bleeding of the gums or nasal mucosa, bleeding into the urine, bleeding under the skin when lightly bruised, and/or bleeding in the gastrointestinal tract. The actual incidence of bleeding associated with careful follow-up is estimated to be 4% or less. The physician evaluates the situation and decides whether the patient is to withhold medication, have a clotting study performed, take a dose of vitamin K, or come in to be further evaluated. Oral anticoagulation generally provides maximum benefit at a minimum risk.

The more the patient and family are involved with health-care planning, the more likely they are to comply. The nurse must stress the importance of continued medical care. All other evaluation criteria are also assessed and evaluated before the patient leaves the health care facility. All previously taught material is reviewed and updated, if necessary, to ensure that the patient's knowledge base remains accurate.

SUMMARY

Numerous drugs are available that affect blood coagulation. Anticoagulants prevent or retard clotting; hemostatics hasten clotting; antifibrinolytics prevent the dissolution of the clot; and enzymes actually dissolve the clot.

Heparin is the drug of choice to treat and prevent venous thromboembolism. The antagonist for heparin is protamine sulfate. The oral coumarin products are the choice for long-term management of patients with or at risk for thromboembolism. The antagonist for the coumarins is vitamin K. The thrombolytic agents are used to dissolve deep-vein thrombosis, pulmonary embolism, arterial thrombosis and embolism, coronary thrombosis, and clotted arteriovenous catheters. Aminocaproic acid (Amicar) may be used as an antidote, although this use is not well documented.

The nurse obtains a history and baseline bleeding and

clotting studies before administering these drugs. The nurse must be aware of the proper method of administering these products. Patient teaching is important when the patient is going home on anticoagulants.

There are many drug interactions that can occur. Therefore, the nurse teaches the patient always to check with the physician or pharmacist before taking other medications.

SITUATION 33–1

Madeline Grabel, a 60-year-old, is admitted to the medical unit with complaints of severe calf pain. Her right lower leg is red, tender, and swollen.

1. Ms. Grabel is to be started on intravenous heparin therapy for thrombophlebitis of the right leg. If Ms. Grabel weighs 80 kg, the approximate initial dosage would be:
   a. 16,000 units
   b. 8,000 units
   c. 800 units
   d. 1,600 units

2. After the bolus dose, Ms. Grabel is to begin an intravenous (IV) infusion of heparin at 1,000 units per hour. A nursing action related to this situation is to:
   a. monitor IV drip without infusion pump
   b. use macrotubing to regulate flow
   c. avoid intramuscular injections
   d. protect tubing and bottle from light

3. In planning nursing care for Ms. Grabel, the following drug should be available in case of heparin overdose:
   a. aminocaproic acid
   b. vitamin K
   c. protamine sulfate
   d. tranexamic acid

4. To evaluate therapeutic effectiveness of heparin therapy, the nurse will note the following:
   a. fibrinogen
   b. prothrombin time (PT)
   c. partial thromboplastin time (PTT)
   d. fibrin split products

5. After four days of intravenous heparin therapy, Ms. Grabel is to be switched to subcutaneous heparin therapy. She is to receive 10,000 units every 12 hours. When giving heparin by this method, the nurse will:
   a. apply pressure to site after injection
   b. withdraw plunger to check for flash-back of blood
   c. insert the needle at a 45-degree angle
   d. massage the site after injection of heparin

6. Ms. Grabel complains of a headache and requests medication. Which of the following would be most appropriate for her?
   a. aspirin
   b. acetaminophen
   c. ibuprofen
   d. indomethacin

SITUATION 33–2

Arnold Campbell, a 45-year-old, presents to the emergency room with severe crushing chest pain, unrelieved with nitroglycerin, which began 30 minutes earlier. A 12-lead EKG reveals elevated ST segments consistent with an acute anterior myocardial infarction.

1. Mr. Campbell is to receive streptokinase via peripheral infusion. The nurse is aware that the standard dosage is:
   a. 3 million units over 1 hour
   b. 50,000 units over 1 hour
   c. 1.5 million units over 1 hour
   d. 20,000 units over 1 hour

2. During and after streptokinase infusion, the nurse will pay particular attention for signs of:
   a. peripheral edema
   b. dysphagia
   c. headache
   d. urticaria

3. After successful treatment with streptokinase followed by heparinization, Mr. Campbell is started on coumadin 10 mg daily. The nurse will check the following laboratory data daily:
   a. prothrombin time (PT)
   b. partial thromboplastin time (PTT)
   c. Lee-White clotting time (LWCT)
   d. activated clotting time (ACT)

4. Medical plans for Mr. Campbell include continuing daily coumadin (2.5 mg) after discharge from the hospital. The nurse will include the following in patient teaching:

   a. Take two pills in one day if a daily dose is missed.
   b. Avoid drinking liquor, beer, or wine.
   c. Eat a diet high in leafy green vegetables.
   d. Take over-the-counter medications as needed.

5. The nurse observes that Mr. Campbell has hematuria and gingival bleeding. After reporting these signs to the physician, the nurse will plan to administer:
   a. Dextran
   b. platelets
   c. protamaine sulfate
   d. vitamin K

6. Which of the following statements by Mr. Campbell indicates successful patient teaching regarding coumadin therapy?
   a. "I need to include plenty of fish and cheese in my diet."
   b. "It is better for me to use an electric razor for shaving."
   c. "If I notice any bruising, I should stop taking the pills."
   d. "I am taking this drug to dissolve the clots in my heart."

Please refer to the Appendices for correct answers and additional reveiw questions with answers.

BIBLIOGRAPHY

Alerman, EL, Jutzy, KR, Berte, LE, et al: Randomized comparison of intravenous versus intracoronary streptokinase for acute myocardial infarction. Am J Cardiol 54:14–19, 1984.

AMA Drug Evaluation, WB Saunders, Philadelphia, 1986.

Bodnar, AG, Hutter, AM: Anticoagulation in valvular heart disease preoperatively and post-operatively. Cardiovasc Clin 14(247), 1984.

Brewer, CC, et al: Streptokinase and TPA in acute myocardial infarction. Heart Lung 15(6):552–8, November 1986.

Brooks–Brunn, J: Formulating appropriate nursing diagnoses for patient receiving TPA. Heart Lung 16(6):787–791, November 1987.

Camesas, AM: Anticoagulation and cardiovascular disease: Determining therapeutic options. Hosp Formul 20(12):1238–1246, December 1985.

Chang, JC: White clot syndrome associated with heparin–induced thrombocytopenia: A review of 23 cases. Heart Lung 16(4):403–407, 1987.

Cunliffe, MT, Rolomano, RC: How to clear catheter clots with urokinase. Nursing 86 16(12):40–43, 1986.

Cyganski, JM, et al: The case for the heparin flush. Am J Nurs 87(6):796–7, 1987.

Gilman, AG, Goodman, LS, and Gilman, A (eds): Goodman and Gilman's The Pharmacological Basis of Therapeutics. Macmillan, New York, 1985.

Grau, E et al: Erythromycin-oral anticoagulants interaction. Archives of Internal Medicine 146:1639, August 1986.

Gruppo Italiano per lo studio della streptochinasi nell' infarto miocardio (GISSI). Effectiveness of IV thrombolytic treatment in acute myocardial infarction. Lancet 86(2):397–401, February 1986.

Kennedy, JW, Ritchie, JL, Davis, KB, et al: The western Washington randomized trial of intracoronary streptokinase in acute myo-

cardial infarction: A 12-month follow-up report. N Engl J Med 312:1073–1078, 1985.

Leser, DR: Synthetic blood: A future alternative. Am J Nurs 82:452–459, March 1982.

Low-dose heparin and postoperative wound hematoma. Nurses Drug Alert 11(2):11, 1987.

Masorli, ST and Piercy, S: A step by step guide to trouble-free transfusions. RN 44:34–42, May 1984.

Muller Camesas, A: Anticoagulation and cardiovascular disease determining therapeutic options. Hosp Formul 20(12):1238–1246, December 1985.

Sheehan, FH, Braunwald, E, Canner, P, et al: The effect of intravenous thrombolytic therapy on left ventricular function: A report on tissue-type plasminogen activator and streptokinase from the Thrombolysis in Myocardial Infarction (TIMI Phase I) trial. Circulation 75:817–829, 1987.

Strauss, E, Rudy, EB: Tissue plasminogen activatory: A new drug in reperfusion therapy. Crit Care Nurse 6(3):30+, 1986.

The Thrombolysis in Myocardial Infarction (TIMI) trial: Phase I findings. N Engl J Med 312:932–936, 1985.

Tissue-type plasminogen activator for acute coronary thrombosis. Med Lett 29(754):107–109, December 4, 1987.

Topol, E: Clinical use of streptokinase and urokinase therapy for AMI. Heart Lung 16(6):760–773 part 2, November 1987.

Valentine, RP, Brooks–Brunn, JA, Williams, JG, et al: Intravenous versus intracoronary streptokinase in acute myocardial infarction. Am J Cardiol 55:309–312, 1985.

VanDeWerf, F, Ludbrook, PA, Bergmann, SR, et al: Coronary thrombolysis with tissue-type plasminogen activator in patients with evolving myocardial infarction. N Engl J Med 310:609–613, 1984.

Verstraete, M, Bory, M, Collen, D, et al: Randomized trial of intravenous recombinant tissue-type plasminogen activatory versus intravenous streptokinase in acute myocardial infarction. Lancet 85(4):842–847, April 1985.

Wescott, BL: TPa a new advancement in fib therapy. Focus Crit Care 13(6):22–26, December 1986.

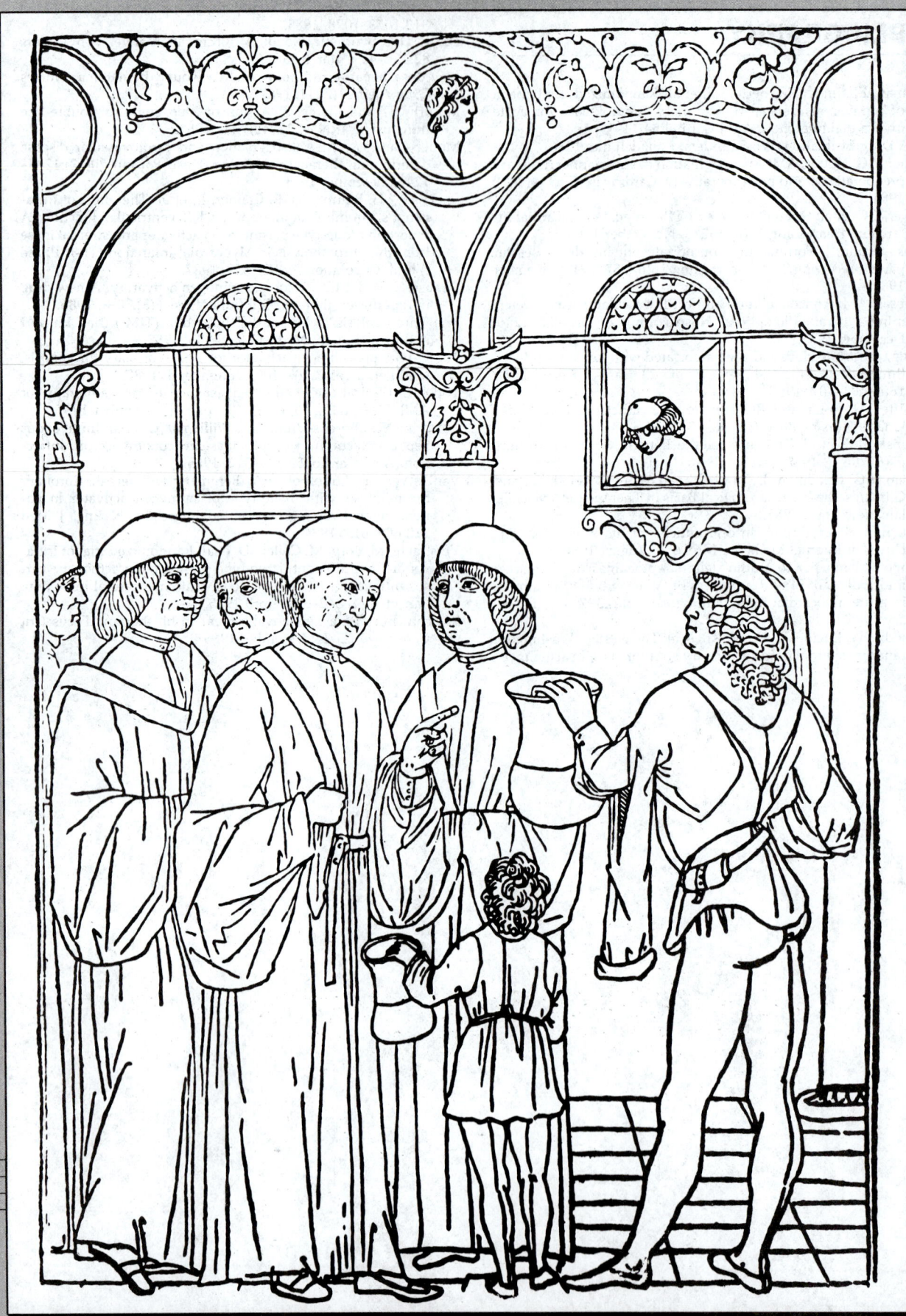

Discussing disease and body fluids, 1522. The Bettmann Archive.

5

DRUGS AFFECTING THE RESPIRATORY SYSTEM

GLOSSARY TERMS IN THIS CHAPTER

Adenoids
Airway resistance
Alveolus
Bronchi
Bronchioles
Bronchospasm
Carina
Chemoreceptors
Compliance
Cyclic 3,5-AMP
Cyclic 3,5-GMP
External intercostals
Larynx
Mucociliary escalator
Mucous membrane
Muscarinic receptor
Surfactant
Tonsils
Turbinates
Ventilation

34
CHAPTER

OVERVIEW OF FUNCTIONAL ANATOMY OF THE RESPIRATORY SYSTEM

ROBERT HIRNLE, M.S., R.R.T.

LEARNING OBJECTIVES

After reading this chapter, the student will be able to:

1. Identify the major structures of the respiratory system.

2. Describe the primary functions of those structures of the upper and lower airways.

3. Discuss four means by which the airways are protected against trauma, obstruction, and infection.

4. Explain a simple model for bronchial smooth muscle control.

5. Describe the role of the central and peripheral nervous system in the control of ventilation.

6. Explain basic factors that contribute to the work of breathing.

THE RESPIRATORY SYSTEM

The primary function of the respiratory system is gas exchange. The airways and the lungs provide a route for oxygen to enter the blood and for carbon dioxide to leave it. In order to accomplish this, neural pathways and muscles of the chest work in concert to cause the movement of air through the respiratory system.

The upper airway consists of the nose, mouth, and throat. The structures of the upper airway serve as air conditioners and as protectors of the lung. The lower airway contains the many conducting passages that bring air to the alveoli. This is where gas exchange takes place. The extrapulmonary portion of the respiratory system includes the structures that affect the mechanical act of breathing (Fig. 34–1).

THE UPPER AIRWAY

The mouth and the nose provide the entryway into the respiratory system. In addition to this obvious function, these cavities are responsible for filtering, humidifying, and warming the incoming air. They also help to prevent aspiration of foreign bodies into the lower airways, and to control germ growth in the airways.

The nostrils are lined with short hairs that trap dust and other particulate matter. They provide the first filtration mechanism of the respiratory system.

The nostrils lead into the nasal cavity. This chamber is divided into two passages by the nasal septum. The walls of the nasal cavity are convoluted. These prominent folds are called the *turbinates*. These structures are lined with a highly vascular epithelium containing many mucous and serous glands. Because of the many folds of the turbinates, this *mucous membrane* presents a very large surface area to the air being drawn in through the nose. The uneven surface of the nasal passages causes the air to slow down, allowing it to fully contact the mucous membrane. Warmth from the rich blood flow and moisture from the secretory glands are thus imparted to the air. This ''air conditioning'' is necessary to prevent drying of the lower airways, and to keep the delicate lower structures from becoming hyperreactive.

The mucous membrane of the nasal cavity also protects the lower airway by acting as a second filter. Particles that are not successfully trapped by the hairs of the nostrils may become stuck in the layer of mucus that lines the nasal passages. Dust settling in the nose may be sufficient to stimulate a sneeze, which helps to protect the airways by clearing these particles from the nose. The trapped particles may also be removed when the nose is blown.

Immediately behind the nasal passages is a chamber called the pharynx. This cavity is the common connection between the nose, mouth, and throat. The uppermost portion of the pharynx contains lymphoid tissue known as the *adenoids*. The *tonsils* are similar tissues found in the middle, or oropharynx. These lymphoid

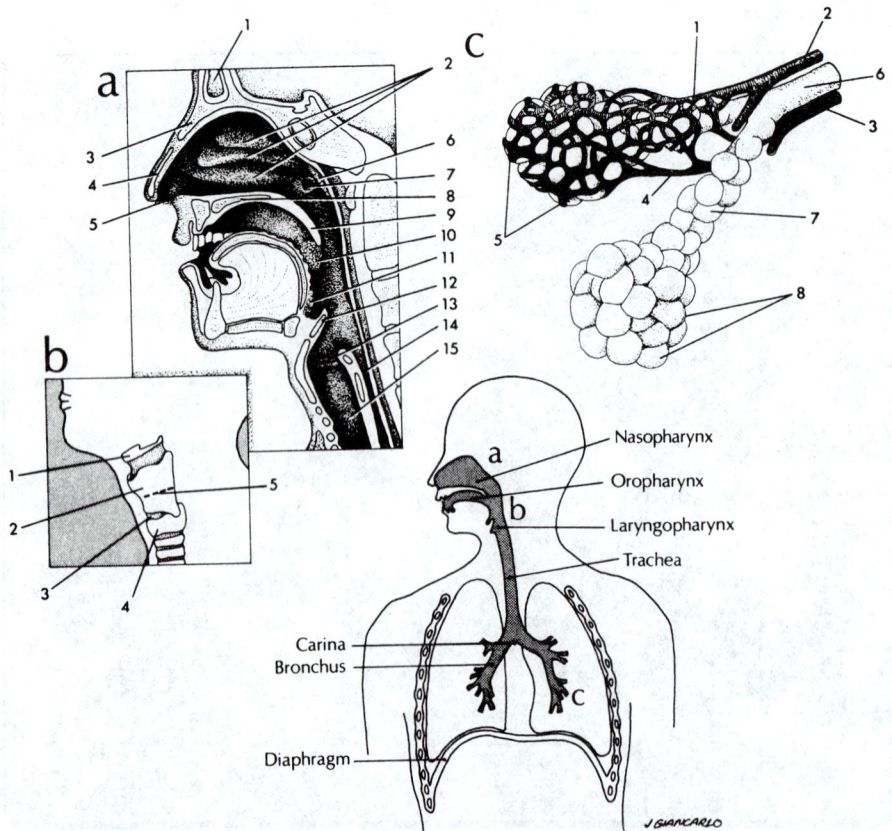

Figure 34–1. Anatomic landmarks of the pulmonary system. **a)** 1. Frontal bone and sinuses; 2. turbinates; 3. bony structure to upper third of nose; 4. cartilaginous structure to lower two thirds of nose; 5. vibrissae and nasal vestibule; 6. pharyngeal tonsils (''the adenoids''); 7. eustachian tube stoma (taurus tubarus); 8. hard palate; 9. soft palate; 10. faucial tonsils (''the tonsils''); 11. lingual tonsils; 12. epiglottis; 13. vocal cords; 14. esophagus; and 15. trachea. **b)** 1. Hyoid bone; 2. thyroid cartilage; 3. cricothyroid membrane; 4. cricoid cartilage; and 5. area of vocal cords. **c)** 1. Pulmonary venule; 2. small pulmonary vein; 3. small pulmonary artery; 4. pulmonary arteriole; 5. pulmonary capillaries; 6. terminal respiratory bronchiole; 7. alveolar duct; and 8. alveolar sacs. (From Shapiro, B. et al: Applications of Respiratory Care, ed 3. Year Book Medical Publishers, Inc, Chicago, 1985, with permission.)

structures trap bacteria and are thus an important line of defense against respiratory infection. In addition, the oropharynx is the common passageway for food and air. The lowest portion of this chamber, the laryngopharynx, contains the epiglottis and a rich nerve supply. These structures protect the airway from aspiration of foreign matter into the lungs. They help to keep the airway closed during swallowing.

The *larynx* marks the transition of the upper airway to the lower airway. Commonly called the "voice box," the larynx is the organ of speech. The vocal cords are located here, as are other structures that help to protect the lower airways from aspiration. Complex neural reflexes cause the larynx to close tightly when food or liquids enter the oropharynx. This ability of the larynx to seal itself is also essential for the proper operation of another major defense mechanism: the cough reflex.

THE LOWER AIRWAY

By the time air has traveled through the upper airway it has been warmed to near body temperature. It has also become almost saturated with water vapor, and has been very efficiently cleaned of all but the minutest particles. It is the job of the trachea, the *bronchi,* and their many branches to complete the filtration of inspired air. These passages also serve as the conduits for air to the alveoli where gas exchange takes place.

The trachea is a flexible tube approximately 10–12 cm long and 1.5–2.5 cm in diameter. It branches at the *carina* to become the bronchi. These tubes branch further into progressively smaller bronchi. The trachea and bronchi are structurally similar in that they are made of three layers. The outermost layer consists of supportive C-shaped cartilaginous rings. The median layer is made of smooth muscle, and lining the innermost portion of these tubes is an epithelial mucous membrane. The mucosal layer contains mucus-producing cells and glands. It also contains ciliated cells that play an important role in airway clearance.

The bronchi continue to branch, treelike with successively smaller tubes growing from larger ones to deliver air to the more distal areas of the lung. At about the ninth generation of branching the bronchial tubes become *bronchioles.* These tubes differ from the larger bronchi in that they have no cartilage to support them. They remain open as a result of smooth muscle tone. The diameter of each bronchiole is 1 mm or less.

As the branching of the "tracheobronchial tree" continues, smaller and more numerous bronchioles arise from their precedents. By the 17th generation of branches alveolar sacs can be found sprouting from the walls of the bronchioles. These units are called respiratory bronchioles because respiration can take place here. These bronchioles have no smooth muscle. Instead they are simple epithelial tubes, and their lumens are held open by the subatmospheric pressure of the thoracic cavity.

Respiratory bronchioles branch finally into the alveolar ducts, from which arise the majority of alveolar sacs. The alveolar sacs are thin-walled epithelial spheres. Each alveolus is normally matched with a multichan-

neled pulmonary capillary. The tremendous number of alveoli (approximately 300 million in the adult lung) provides a huge surface for gas exchange to occur.

Since the lung is a very elastic organ, its natural tendency is to collapse. Adding to this tendency is the surface tension exerted by the fluid lining within the alveoli. If this "elastic recoil" were not kept in check, the alveoli would collapse and the gas exchange capability of the lung would suffer. In addition, each breath would require a great deal of effort. However, collapse of the alveoli is prevented by the presence of *surfactant.* This phospholipid substance is manufactured by specialized alveolar cells. With surfactant lining the alveolar sacs the subatmospheric pressure within the chest is sufficient to keep them open.

EXTRAPULMONARY PORTIONS OF THE RESPIRATORY SYSTEM

The lungs and airways are the most important structures of the respiratory system because they are responsible for gas exchange. For gas exchange to occur, however, air must enter the lungs. This happens as a result of breathing, and with regard to breathing the lungs are passive. In order to accomplish the mechanical act of breathing, muscle groups and neural mechanisms must be operating harmoniously.

Muscles of Respiration

The primary muscles of respiration are the diaphragm and the *external intercostals.* A secondary "accessory" group of muscles of the neck and upper chest may also be used at times to assist breathing. Normally these are used by healthy persons only during periods of heavy exercise. Persons with chronic lung disease sometimes must rely entirely upon the accessory muscles for breathing because of pathologic changes in the lungs and chest.

Ventilation, or the movement of air into and out of the lungs, occurs when the respiratory muscles contract. The diaphragm drops downward, and the intercostals (and/or the accessory muscles) pull the ribs upward and outward. This enlarges the chest, which in turn causes the pressure within the chest to become less than atmospheric. This "suction effect" pulls the lung outward with the chest. As the lung increases in size, the pressure within the airways decreases, and air rushes in.

Exhalation occurs passively as the respiratory muscles relax. The volume of the thorax and lung decreases, which causes a rise in the pressure within them. Air thus flows out as a result of the reversing pressure gradient.

All of the muscles of ventilation are striated muscle and are innervated by the somatic nervous system. As such, they are therefore affected by skeletal muscle relaxants (also called neuromuscular blocking agents). This is extremely important to remember when this type of agent is being used, since the patient will be unable to breathe spontaneously.

Neural Control of Ventilation

Ventilatory control mechanisms arise from the central and peripheral nervous systems. Some control mechanisms have inherent rhythmicity, whereas others become operative only with changes in blood chemistry.

In the medulla of the brain stem are specialized neurons that regularly discharge impulses to the respiratory muscles. When signaled by these neurons, the respiratory muscles contract, and inspiration occurs. A group of inhibitory neurons turns off the inspiratory neurons, thus causing exhalation. The medullary neurons are automatic in their function, but they are influenced by impulses from several sources, including other centers in the brain (particularly in the pons), and from peripheral neurons that are sensitive to physical and chemical stimuli.

Other highly specialized neurons, called *chemoreceptors*, are found in the arch of the aorta and at the bifurcation of the carotid arteries, as well as in the medulla. These nerves are highly sensitive to changes in blood levels of carbon dioxide and to blood pH. The aortic and carotid bodies are additionally sensitive to changes in blood oxygen levels.

The chemoreceptors respond to a minute rise in blood carbon dioxide by sending impulses to the inspiratory neurons. This results in an increase in ventilation, which continues until the level of carbon dioxide returns to normal. The same effect occurs with a decrease in the pH of the blood, or when oxygen levels fall substantially. These latter two stimuli generate weaker responses, however, than does alteration of carbon dioxide levels. The net effect of the chemoreceptors is to adjust ventilation to maintain relatively constant levels of oxygen and carbon dioxide in the blood, as well as to regulate blood pH.

All of the neural control mechanisms can be influenced by different drugs. The medullary and pontile neurons can be depressed by alcohol, barbiturates, and narcotics. They can be stimulated by the methylxanthines (such as theophylline), analeptic agents, and certain hormones. The central and peripheral chemoreceptors can be either stimulated or depressed by oxygen or carbon dioxide therapy. They are also affected by agents that alter the acid–base balance of the blood.

AIRWAY DEFENSE MECHANISMS

The respiratory system has several built-in safeguards that help to keep the airways open and free from infectious or inflammatory agents. The nose has the nostril hairs and nasal mucosa. The tonsils and adenoids trap germs while the epiglottis and other structures prevent aspiration of foreign matter. In addition, the upper airway protects the lungs by means of the sneeze and cough reflexes.

When any of these mechanisms fails, potentially injurious material can enter the lung. However, two major mechanisms operate within the lower airway to keep the lungs practically sterile.

The *mucociliary escalator* is the name applied to the mobile mucus blanket which lines the trachea and bronchi. Sticky mucus secreted by the glands of the bronchial epithelium traps most of the dust and bacteria that get past the upper airways. The mucus lies atop the cil-

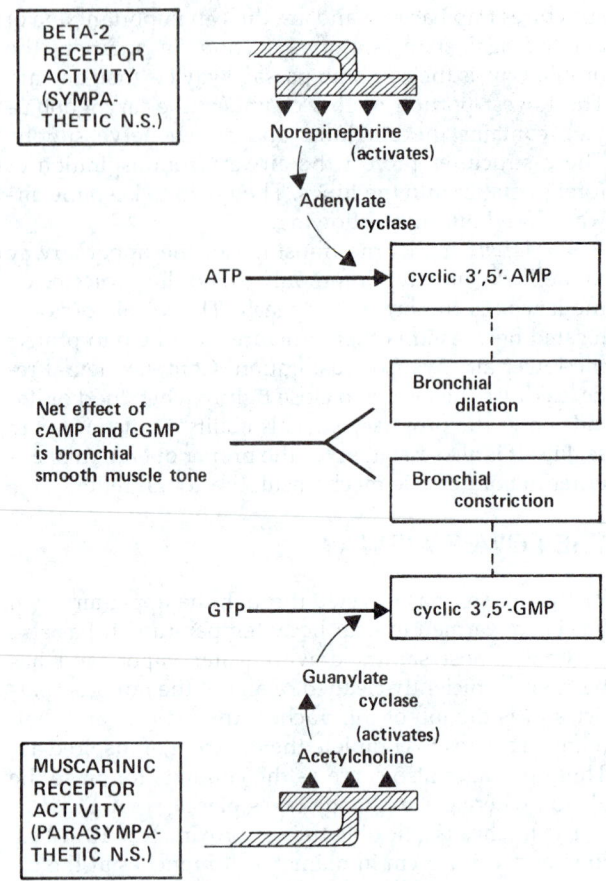

Figure 34–2. Autonomic control of bronchial smooth muscle.

iated cells of the epithelium. The hairlike projections of these cells beat in one direction, always upward toward the throat. This propels the mucus layer with its trapped particles up and out of the lung. When a bolus of mucus reaches the larger airways, it can be coughed into the mouth and then expectorated or swallowed.

The mucociliary escalator normally moves debris upward at a rate of an inch a minute. Thus, it is a highly effective cleansing mechanism. Certain conditions can decrease its effectiveness, though. Smoking, lung disease, infection, and dehydration all can slow the movement of the mucus layer. Mucous stasis can block airways, thereby decreasing gas exchange, as well as predisposing the lung to infection.

Alveolar macrophages provide a second line of defense in the lower airways. These are freely moving scavenger cells whose function is to clean the alveolar epithelium. They phagocytize bacteria or dusts that may have escaped the mucociliary escalator. The macrophages enter lymph channels, where they undergo lysis, or they become trapped in the mucus layer and are removed by ciliary action.

Table 34–1. SPECIFIC RECEPTORS OF THE AUTONOMIC NERVOUS SYSTEM

Type	Where Found	Effect of Stimulation
SYMPATHETIC BRANCH		
α	Bronchial mucosa	Mucosal decongestion
	Systemic arterioles	Increased blood pressure
β_1	Heart	Increased heart rate
β_2	Bronchial smooth muscle	Bronchial dilation
PARASYMPATHETIC BRANCH		
Muscarinic	Bronchial smooth muscle	Bronchial constriction; increased mucus secretion

(The autonomic receptors are also found in other tissues. The receptors listed here are the ones most affected by respiratory pharmacologic agents.)

WORK OF BREATHING

The respiratory system must provide the body with a steady supply of oxygen every minute of every day. It must also cleanse the blood of its primary metabolic waste product, carbon dioxide. Regardless of the effort required, the respiratory system attempts to breathe sufficiently to meet these metabolic demands.

Under normal conditions breathing is an almost effortless activity. However, when any component of the respiratory system is malfunctioning because of disease, the work involved in breathing can be tremendous. When the work of breathing increases, it can become an oxygen-robbing activity, depriving other vital organs of the oxygen they require. It can exhaust the sufferer and lead to respiratory failure.

Causes of increased work of breathing include decreased *compliance* of the lung or chest wall, muscular weakness, or increased *airway resistance*.

Compliance is a measure of how easily the lungs or chest can be expanded. When both are easily expanded, compliance is high. Decreased compliance means that the lungs or chest is stiffer than normal. Thus, in low compliance more work is needed to breathe. Many of the causes of low compliance are chronic in nature, but one of the most common causes for this condition is infection. If the patient has pneumonia, the lung will not expand easily because it will be filled with inflammatory exudate. In such a case antimicrobial therapy will be indicated. Successful treatment with the appropriate agents should clear the infection and reduce the work of breathing.

Muscular weakness will also limit the ability of the patient to ventilate his lungs. To get the amount of air needed to meet metabolic demands, the patient will need to work harder for each breath. If the weakness is caused by myasthenia gravis, anticholinergic agents may strengthen the patient, thereby decreasing the patient's work.

INCREASED AIRWAY RESISTANCE

By far the most important reason for an increase in the patient's work of breathing is an increase in airway resistance. Because of this, and because the majority of respiratory pharmacology is aimed at minimizing airway resistance, it deserves special attention.

Airway resistance is a measure of the difficulty encountered by air as it flows through the bronchial tubes. When resistance is low, air can flow freely. High airway resistance greatly obstructs airflow. This adds tremendously to the effort needed to draw a breath. Airway resistance increases whenever the lumen of the airway is decreased in diameter. Physical obstructions, such as a tumor or an aspirated foreign body, are obvious causes of increased airway resistance. More commonly, however, airway obstruction results from excessive mucus production, edematous inflamed tissue, or spasm of the bronchial smooth muscle.

Excessive mucus production is a feature of several diseases, most notably chronic bronchitis, cystic fibrosis, and asthma. It can result from irritation of the airways, or from pathologic changes in the epithelium, which results in hypersecretion of mucous glands. Airway edema can occur in any of the same disorders. It is the result of an inflammatory response to tissue damage in the airways. Mucus that lines the inner aspect of the airway, or edema that swells epithelial tissue can result in complete airway obstruction.

Bronchospasm is a complex process that occurs primarily in asthma, but also in bronchitis, emphysema, and some other diseases. When this occurs, the smallest airways constrict, and thus airflow to the alveoli is severely limited. The cause of this constriction is increased bronchiolar smooth muscle tone, which is usually due to hyperactivity of the bronchioles.

Normal bronchial smooth muscle tone is thought to be maintained by autonomic nervous system control. The autonomic nervous system's two major components, the sympathetic nervous system (SNS) and the parasympathetic nervous system (PNS), exert opposing effects on bronchial smooth muscle. The effects of these two systems are the results of biochemical changes that occur at specific receptors (Table 34–1).

Stimulation of the *muscarinic receptors* of the PNS results in constriction of bronchial smooth muscle. Neural impulses from the PNS cause activation of an enzyme, guanylate cyclase, which catalyzes the formation of *cyclic 3,5-guanosine monophosphate (cyclic 3,5-GMP)*. This substance causes the smooth muscle fibers to contract, and thus increases airway resistance (Fig. 34–2).

Table 34–2. BIOCHEMICAL MEDIATORS INVOLVED IN BRONCHIAL OBSTRUCTION

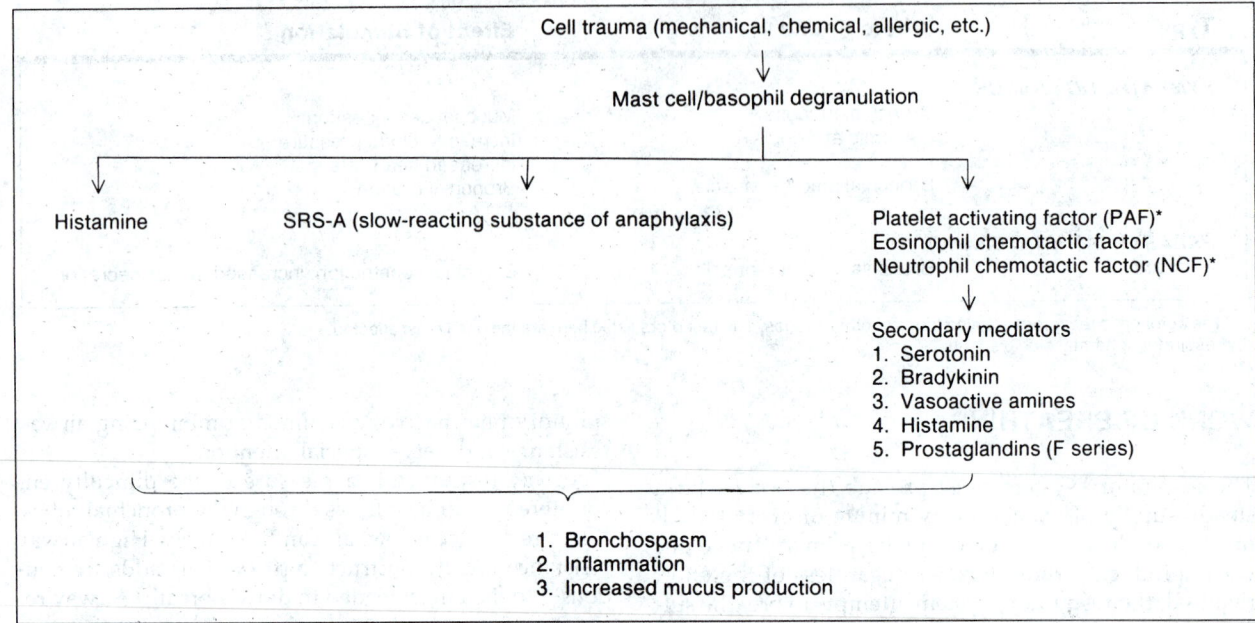

*PAF and NCF contribute to bronchospasm by degranulation of platelets and neutrophils. This causes further release of histamine by these cells.

Stimulation of the adrenergic receptors of the SNS causes bronchial dilation. Specific β_2 receptors receive impulses from the SNS. The impulses cause the activation of adenylate cyclase. This enzyme catalyzes the production of *cyclic 3,5-adenosine monophosphate (cyclic 3,5-AMP)* from the high-energy compound adenosine triphosphate (ATP). Cyclic 3,5-AMP relaxes the bronchial smooth muscle; thus, airway lumen size is increased and airway resistance is decreased.

Under normal conditions the autonomic receptors are believed to receive regular stimulation from their respective nervous system branches. The force of constriction caused by the PNS is countered by the relaxing effects of the SNS. The net result of both receptors being continually stimulated is bronchial smooth muscle tone.

This balance of opposing forces can be upset, and the result is bronchospasm. Humoral mediators released from mast cells and basophils may cause overstimulation of PNS receptors. They may also inhibit or block the actions of the SNS on the β_2 receptors. In either case, bronchial constriction occurs. These mediators are released as a consequence of allergy, physical or chemical trauma to the lung, exercise, or infection. A list of these bronchoactive mediators can be found in Table 34–2.

SUMMARY

The respiratory system consists of the airways and the lungs. The large upper airways conduct air to the small lower airways; in the process of conducting air, the upper airways also filter, warm, and humidify inspired air. The small airways, whose caliber is controlled by the autonomic nervous system, are an important factor in determining the effort required for breathing.

Ventilation is the result of a complex interaction of neural impulses and muscular movements. Chemoreceptors, which are influenced by blood levels of carbon dioxide, oxygen, and hydrogen ion, provide impulses to the brain, which in turn regulates breathing rate and depth. Gas exchange occurs by diffusion, which takes place in response to pressure gradients of oxygen and carbon dioxide on both sides of the alveolar-capillary membrane.

BIBLIOGRAPHY

Cherniack, R and Cherniack, L: Respiration in Health and Disease, ed 3. WB Saunders Co, Philadelphia, 1983.

Murray, J: The Normal Lung, ed 2. WB Saunders Co, Philadelphia, 1986.

Rau, J: Respiratory Therapy Pharmacology, ed 2. Year Book Medical Publishers, Chicago, 1984.

Shapiro, B, Harrison, R, Kacmarek, R, and Cane, R: Clinical Applications of Respiratory Care, ed 3. Year Book Medical Publishers, Chicago, 1985.

Slonim, N and Hamilton, L: Respiratory Physiology, ed 4. CV Mosby Co, St Louis, 1986.

Soffer, A, ed: Neurohumoral mechanisms in obstructive airway disease. Chest (suppl) 91(5), May 1987.

35
CHAPTER

AGENTS USED TO TREAT BRONCHIAL OBSTRUCTION

35
CHAPTER

AGENTS USED TO TREAT BRONCHIAL OBSTRUCTION

ROBERT W. HIRNLE, M.S., R.R.T.

LEARNING OBJECTIVES

After reading this chapter the student will be able to:

1. Describe three primary causes of bronchial obstruction.

2. Identify medications commonly used to treat bronchial obstruction.

3. Describe the mechanism of action, routes of administration, pharmacokinetics, adverse effects, contraindications, and potential interactions of agents used to treat bronchial obstruction.

4. Identify specific areas to assess in the patient who requires antibronchial obstruction medications for the purpose of formulating appropriate nursing diagnoses.

5. Plan nursing intervention needed to administer antibronchial obstruction medications and choose appropriate teaching strategies to gain patient compliance.

6. Evaluate the patient at various stages of treatment to gauge nursing interventions.

Bronchial obstruction occurs as a result of bronchospasm, airway edema, or excessive bronchial secretions. These problems make breathing difficult for the respiratory patient and may hinder gas exchange. Each of these problems may occur in varying degrees in a wide variety of respiratory diseases.

THERAPEUTIC AGENTS

BRONCHODILATING AGENTS

A sudden increase in bronchial smooth muscle tone is called *bronchospasm*. This condition, which severely narrows the airways, can be caused by allergy, exercise, infection, and emotional factors. It has been postulated that in each case the autonomic control mechanism for bronchial smooth muscle has been unbalanced. (Chapter 34 outlines bronchial smooth muscle control in detail.) When bronchospasm is present, *bronchodilators* are administered. Major categories of bronchodilators include *sympathomimetics, xanthines,* and *anticholinergics.* These drugs are described in Table 35–1.

Sympathomimetic Drugs

Sympathomimetic agents imitate (or mimic) the effects of the sympathetic nervous system. In the lung, sympathetic stimulation of specialized β_2 receptors results in bronchodilation. Activation of the enzyme adenylate cyclase by the sympathetic neurotransmitter causes cyclic 3',5'-adenosine monophosphate (cAMP) to be formed from adenosine triphosphate (ATP). Cyclic

AMP relaxes the bronchial smooth muscle, causing the bronchioles to open fully and allowing air to flow freely through them (see Fig. 35–1).

Sympathomimetic drugs directly stimulate the β_2 receptors of the lung. Thus, they cause bronchodilation by increasing the amount of cAMP in bronchial smooth muscle.

Catecholamine compounds have been used for many years as bronchodilators because of their sympathomimetic activity. Epinephrine, isoproterenol (Isuprel), and isoetharine (Bronkosol) are examples of catecholamines which are still commonly prescribed. Although these drugs are highly effective bronchodilators, their popularity and usefulness have decreased in recent years because of their short duration of action and adverse cardiovascular effects. Catecholamines are gradually being replaced by a newer generation of sympathomimetic bronchodilators. Among the newer drugs are metaproterenol (Alupent), terbutaline (Brethine, Brethaire, Bricanyl), albuterol (Proventil, Ventolin), femoterol, and bitolterol (Tornalate). Because of decreased susceptibility to the enzymes that metabolize catecholamines, these "new bronchodilators" provide longer relief from bronchospasm. These agents also have less affinity for the sympathetic receptors of the cardiovascular system. Thus, they cause problems such as tachycardia, palpitations, and blood pressure fluctuations much less often and less severely than their catecholamine counterparts.

PHARMACOKINETICS. Catecholamines are generally deactivated in the small intestine and metabolized by the liver. For this reason these agents are not available for oral use. Monoamine oxidase (MAO) and catechol-O-methyltransferase (COMT) are enzymes that also inactivate these compounds at bronchial smooth

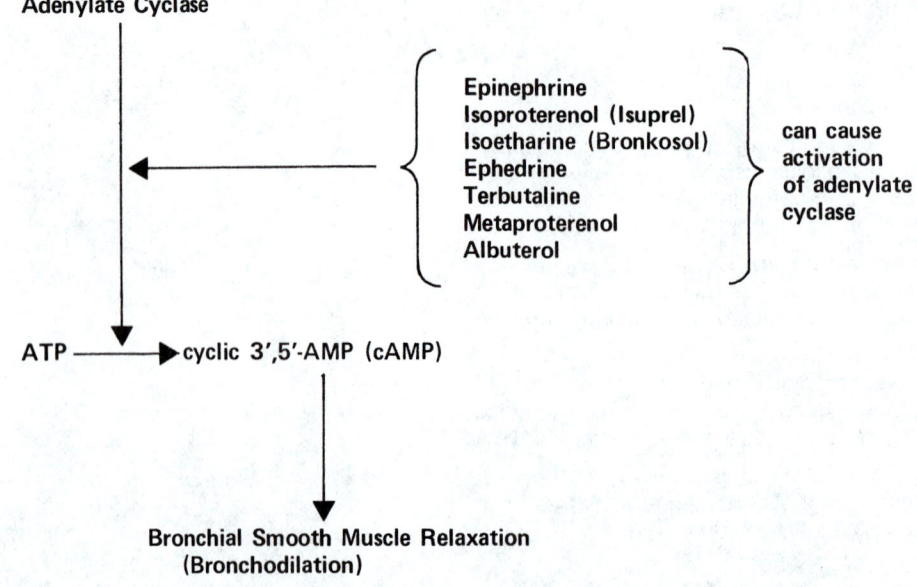

Figure 35–1. Action of sympathomimetic bronchodilators. Sympathomimetic bronchodilators act by increasing conversion of ATP to cAMP.

muscle. The newer, noncatecholamine agents are extensively metabolized in the liver.

Most of the sympathomimetics are thoroughly and rapidly absorbed. All are widely distributed throughout the body's tissues. They freely enter the breast milk and cross the placental and blood–brain barriers. These agents are excreted in the urine.

Because may sympathomimetics are administered as aerosols, drug absorption is affected by such factors as patient breathing pattern, amount of bronchial secretions, and efficiency of the aerosol device used.

CONTRAINDICATIONS AND PRECAUTIONS. The use of sympathomimetics is contraindicated for anyone with known hypersensitivity to any of the ingredients in these medications. Otherwise, there are no absolute contraindications to their use in treating bronchospasm. All sympathomimetics can increase heart rate, myocardial contractility, and blood pressure. These drugs may exacerbate hypertension, precipitate angina attacks, cause or aggravate dysrhythmias, or cause extension of acute myocardial infarction. For these reasons sympathomimetics are used with caution in patients with these disease states. Sympathomimetics can exacerbate the symptoms of hyperthyroidism, such as anxiety, agitation, and tachycardia. Thus, these drugs are used with caution in the patient with thyroid dysfunction. Because of their ability to stimulate the liver to increase glucose synthesis, sympathomimetics are used cautiously in the diabetic patient.

ADVERSE EFFECTS. The major adverse effects caused by sympathomimetics are central nervous system (CNS) stimulation, cardiovascular stimulation, nausea and vomiting, and (occasionally) urinary retention. These responses are thought to be mediated through the receptors of the sympathetic system.

Because α, β_1, and β_2 receptors are found in many tissues of the body, the sympathomimetic agents produce widespread systemic effects. The extent of these side effects and adverse reactions, however, depends largely upon the selectivity of each agent. The older catecholamine agents generally have a relatively low degree of receptor selectivity. Because they have affinity for several types of receptors, they initiate a wider range of biologic activity than do the newer, more β_2-selective drugs. Thus, the side effects of the older agents are generally more pronounced.

Virtually all sympathomimetics are capable of causing an increase in heart rate and in myocardial contractility. Stimulation of β_1 receptors has been cited as the cause of this action, although recent research has indicated that β_2 stimulation may also play a part. This may account for the fact that even the so-called selective β_2 agonists may cause cardiac stimulation. Because an increase in cardiac action results in increased myocardial oxygen demand, the diseased heart is prone to dysrhythmias. Certain patients may be hypersensitive to drugs in this class and develop dysrhythmias despite the lack of previous cardiac problems.

Epinephrine and ephedrine are capable of stimulating α receptors as well as β receptors. This causes vasoconstriction, which may result in elevated blood pressure.

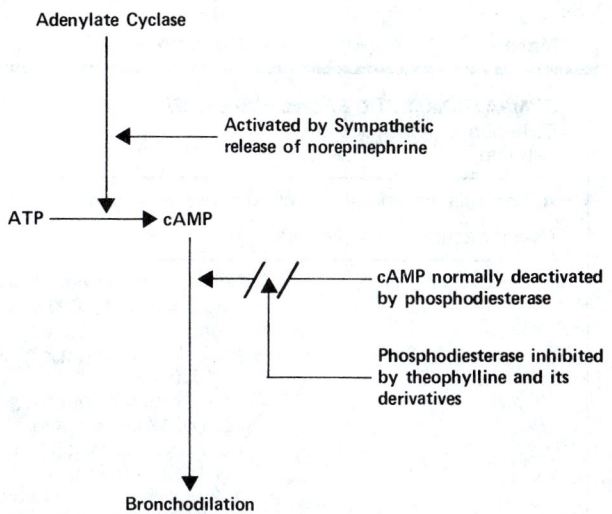

Action of Methylxanthine Bronchodilators

Figure 35–2. Action of methylxanthine bronchodilators. Methylxanthine bronchodilators act by inhibiting the deactivation of cAMP by phosphodiesterase. Other mechanisms by which methylxanthines help to achieve bronchodilation may include prostaglandin antagonism, enhancement of epinephrine release, and alterations in adenosine or calcium transport in bronchial smooth muscle.

The sympathomimetics are also strong CNS stimulants. Thus, they cause nervousness, agitation and restlessness, insomnia, hyperactive reflexes, and irritability. Nausea and vomiting may be the result of local gastric irritation, or they may be caused by stimulation of the areas of the brain stem that control those sensations. Tremors caused by sympathomimetics may be due to central nervous stimulation, or they may be a result of the stimulation of β receptors in striated muscle. This side effect (and to a lesser degree the other effects noted here) is dose related and will abate with a reduction in dose. Some patients develop a tolerance to this side effect (and occasionally to the others).

INTERACTIONS. Sympathomimetics are antagonized by β-blocking agents such as propranolol. Concomitant use of these drugs results in diminished effectiveness of both agents. Use of sympathomimetics with other bronchodilator agents (including xanthines, anticholinergics, and other sympathomimetics) can result in potentiation of therapeutic and adverse effects. Antidepressants such as MAO inhibitors, some tricyclic compounds, thyroid hormone, and some antihistamines, can increase the tachycardia or the blood pressure effects of the sympathomimetics.

Theophylline and Its Derivatives

A second approach to treating bronchospasm is with the use of theophylline. Classified as a xanthine, this drug causes bronchial smooth muscle relaxation by indirectly contributing to cAMP production (Fig. 35–2). Because of

TEXT RESUMES ON PAGE 940

Table 35–1. DRUGS USED TO TREAT BRONCHIAL OBSTRUCTION

Name	Dosage	Mode of Administration	Pharmacokinetics
SYMPATHOMIMETIC BRONCHODILATORS Epinephrine (Adrenalin, Sus-Phrine)			

Action: relaxes smooth muscle via adrenergic stimulation.

Use: for acute asthma attacks.

	Children: 0.1 mg/kg, max 0.5 mg q 4 hr of 1:1000 solution.	SC	O: 1–10 min P: 10–20 min D: 1–1.5 hr
	Adult: 0.2–0.5 mg q 2 hr of 1:1000 solution.	SC	½L: UA PB: UA
	Children: 0.005 ml/kg q 4 hr prn of 1:200 solution.	IM	B: liver E: urine, breast milk
	Adult: 0.1–0.3 ml q 4 hr prn of 1:200 solution.	IM	
	1–2 puffs with 1 min between puffs (0.1–0.2 mg/puff) q 4 hr.	MDI	

Racemic epinephrine (Vaponefrin)

Action: local decongestant via adrenergic stimulation.

Use: reduce subglottic edema (as occurs in croup or post-extubation).

	Adult, children: 1–4 inhalations 4–6 times/day approximate 0.3 mg q 2–4 hr.	MDI solution for inhalation	Same as epinephrine

Key to Abbreviations in the *Pharmacokinetics* column O-onset; P-peak; D-duration; PB-protein bound; B-biotransformed in; E-excreted in; ½L-halflife.
  *Within the column listing adverse effects, underlines indicate the most common effects; CAPITALS indicate life-threatening effects.

Contraindications/ Precautions	Adverse Effects*	Interactions	Nursing Implications
Contraindicated for patients with known hypersensitivity to sympathomimetics or any ingredients in the preparation (many forms contain metabisulfites). May cause or aggravate cardiac arrhythmias; monitor ECG in patients with known or suspected heart disease. May cause sharp increase in blood pressure in most patients; monitor blood pressure in patients with hypertension, congestive heart failure, or myocardial infarction. Variable vasopressor activity may aggravate shock in some hypotensive patients (except anaphylaxis). May cause increased urinary retention in some patients with renal disease; use with caution. Epinephrine may elevate blood sugar levels in diabetics; use with caution. Use this drug and all sympathomimetics cautiously in patients receiving theophylline preparations.	CNS: nervousness, restlessness, tremor, insomnia, headache, (rarely) psychosis CV: hypertension, angina, palpitations, arrhythmias. Resp: occasional rebound bronchospasm GI: nausea, vomiting GU: urinary retention	Antagonized by β-blocking agents (e.g., propranolol, nadolol, timolol). Some antidepressants (e.g., MAO inhibitors, tricyclic agents), thyroid hormone, and some antihistamines may increase tachycardia and hypertension effect. Synergizes action of theophylline and its derivatives, as well as other sympathomimetics (including decongestants).	ASSESSMENT: Auscultate chest for wheezing and general movement of air. Monitor blood pressure and pulse. Check for possible interactions. Observe for possible overdose or hypersensitivity (dysrhythmias, chest pain, hyper- or hypotension, headache, nervousness). INTERVENTION: Check dose and route carefully. Administer second dose as ordered 20–30 min after initial dose. Avoid gluteal IM injection to prevent abscess. Discard any discolored solution. Discourage overuse of inhalers. EVALUATION: Effectiveness of this drug can be demonstrated by increased air movement in lungs, relief of respiratory distress, and improvement in wheezing.
Same as epinephrine	Same as epinephrine, but generally much milder; also drying of mucous membranes	Same as epinephrine	ASSESSMENT: Listen for stridor or crowing inspiratory sounds and observe for respiratory distress in croup patient. (In postextubation patients these signs

CONTINUED ON THE FOLLOWING PAGE

Drugs for Bronchial Obstruction

Table 35–1. DRUGS USED TO TREAT BRONCHIAL OBSTRUCTION–*CONTINUED*

Name	Dosage	Mode of Administration	Pharmacokinetics
Racemic epinephrine–*Continued*			
Ephedrine sulfate			
Action: same as epinephrine			
Use: same as epinephrine			
	15–50 mg qid	PO	O: 15–60 min P: rapid/variable D: 1–4 hr ½L: UA PB: UA B: some deactivation by liver E: large amount unchanged in urine
Isoproterenol (Isuprel)	Adult: 1–4 inhalations q 3–4 hr up to 2.5 q 3–4 hr. Children: 1–4 inhalations q 3–4 hr up to 1.25 mg q 3–4 hr.	Metered aerosol solution for inhalation	O: rapid P: almost immediate D: 1–2 hr ½L: UA PB: UA B: liver E: urine

Key to Abbreviations in the *Pharmacokinetics* column O-onset; P-peak; D-duration; PB-protein bound; B-biotransformed in; E-excreted in; ½L-halflife.
*Within the column listing adverse effects, underlines indicate the most common effects; CAPITALS indicate life-threatening effects.

Contraindications/ Precautions	Adverse Effects*	Interactions	Nursing Implications
			indicate laryngeal edema.) Observe for epinephrine-like adverse reactions (rare). INTERVENTION: Deliver aerosol spray to back of throat. EVALUATION: Effectiveness of this drug is demonstrated by a reduction in patient stridor, and by relief of respiratory distress.
Contraindicated in patients with severe bronchospasm, hypertension, cardiac disease, or glaucoma. May aggravate diabetes and hyperthyroidism. May cause serious dysrhythmias when used with digitalis.	CNS: anxiety, irritability, tremors, apprehension, insomnia, rarely psychosis CV: cardiac irritability, hypertension CU: urinary retention	Antagonized by β blockers. Use with MAO inhibitors may cause drastic rise in blood pressure. Synergistic with theophylline preparations.	ASSESSMENT: Observe for wheezing and determine severity. Monitor HR and BP. Assess for possible interactions (preparations often are combinations with barbiturates and/or theophylline). Watch for tolerance and for adverse CV and CNS reactions. INTERVENTION: Administer as ordered; if ordered QD, administer in morning to avoid insomnia. Teach patient to avoid increasing dose if tolerance develops, and to inform physician. If bronchospasm is severe, consult physician (since drug is effective for only milder forms of bronchospasm). EVALUATION: Effectiveness of this drug is demonstrated by relief of bronchospasm.
Contraindicated in coronary arteriosclerosis, and in known hypersensitivity. Safe use in pregnancy and lactation not established. Use cautiously in hypertension, coronary insufficiency, renal dysfunction, hyperthyroidism, diabetes, glaucoma, and tuberculosis. Contraindicated for use by patients with arrhythmias associated with tachycardia.	CNS: nervousness, restlessness, tremors, insomnia, headache CV: hypertension, palpitations, tachycardia, DYSRHYTHMIAS, angina GI: nausea, vomiting CU: rarely, urinary retention Endo: hyperglycemia Resp: paradoxical bronchospasm, decreased PaO_2	Synergistic with theophylline preparations and other sympathomimetics. Use with cyclopropane or halothane anesthesia agents increases chance of arrhythmias. Potentiated by tricyclic antidepressants.	ASSESSMENT: Listen to breath sounds for wheezing. Watch for aggravation of hypoxemia. Monitor pulse closely, especially in cardiac patient. Observe for signs of tolerance or paradoxical bronchospasm. Assess sulfite sensitivity (many asthmatics are allergic to this preservative, which may be used in preparations of this drug). Determine patient progress through periodic pulmonary function testing. INTERVENTION: Use oxygen to treat hypoxemia as needed. If HR increases by

CONTINUED ON THE FOLLOWING PAGE

Table 35-1. DRUGS USED TO TREAT BRONCHIAL OBSTRUCTION-*CONTINUED*

Name	Dosage	Mode of Administration	Pharmacokinetics
Isoproterenol-*Continued*			
Isoetharine (Bronkosol, Bronkometer)	Adult, children: 2-10 mg qid, 1-4 inhalations q 3-6 hr.	Metered aerosol solution for inhalation	O: rapid (1-5 min) P: 5-15 min D: 1-4 hr ½L: UA PB: UA B: liver E: urine
Albuterol (Proventil, Ventolin)	Adults, children >12 yr: 2-4 mg 3-4 times per day. 4 mg BID. 2 puffs q 4-6 hr (90 μg/puff) 0.5 ml of 0.5% in 2-3 ml saline q 4-6 hr (solution for inhalation; also in unit dose packaging).	PO Tabs, extended release. MDI	O: 5-15 min (inhaled) O: 30 min (PO) P: ½-2 hr D: 3-6 hr ½L: 4-6 hr PB: UA B: liver E: urine
Metaproterenol (Alupent)	Adults, children >9 yr and 27 kg: 20 mg 3-4 times daily. Children 6-9 yr <27 kg: 10 mg 3-4 times daily. Adult, children >12 yr: 2-3 puffs q 3-4 hr up to 12 puffs/day (650 μg/puff). Inhalation solution: 0.2-0.3 ml of 5% in 2.0-2.5 ml NSS 3-4 times daily (also available as 0.6% solution in 2.5 ml unit dose packages, used 3-4 times daily).	PO PO MDI	O: 1-15 min P: ½-1 hr D: 1-5 hr ½L: UA PB: UA B: liver E: urine
Terbutaline sulfate (Bricanyl, Brethine, Brethaire)	Adult: 2.5-5.0 mg 3 times daily q 6 hr. Children 12-15 yr: 2.5 mg 3 times daily q 6 hr. Adult: 0.25 mg, repeat as needed in 15-30 min (do not exceed 0.5 mg in 4 hr). Adult, children >12 yr: 2 puffs q 4-6 hr (0.2 mg/puff).	PO PO SC MDI	O: 5-30 min P: ½-2 hr D: 3-6 hr (inhaled) D: 4-8 hr (PO) D: 1.5-4 hr (SC) ½L: 13-18 hr PB: UA B: liver E: urine
XANTHINE BRONCHODILATORS: THEOPHYLLINE PREPARATIONS Aminophylline			
Action: dilates bronchial smooth muscle by indirectly increasing cAMP.			
Use: to relieve bronchial constriction in asthma and COPD.			
	Adult: loading dose 5.6 mg/kg over 30 min. Maintenance dose 0.2-0.9 mg/kg/hr by continuous infusion as	IV	O: rapid (15-60 min) P: maintenance drug (peak effects depend on peak serum levels)

Key to Abbreviations in the *Pharmacokinetics* column O-onset; P-peak; D-duration; PB-protein bound; B-biotransformed in; E-excreted in; ½L-halflife.

*Within the column listing adverse effects, underlines indicate the most common effects; CAPITALS indicate life-threatening effects.

Contraindications/ Precautions	Adverse Effects*	Interactions	Nursing Implications
			20%, discontinue use and notify physician. If using with inhaled anti-inflammatory agent, wait 15 min between ''puffs'' to avoid toxic effects of propellant. EVALUATION: Same as epinephrine.
Same as isoproterenol	Same as isoproterenol	Same as isoproterenol	ASSESSMENT: Same as isoproterenol. INTERVENTION: Explain pink sputum is result of drug exposure to air. EVALUATION: Same as isoproterenol.
Same as isoproterenol	Same as isoproterenol	Same as isoproterenol	ASSESSMENT: Same as isoproterenol. INTERVENTION: Avoid contact with eyes. Take oral preparations with meals to minimize gastric irritation. Not recommended for use by children under 12. EVALUATION: Same as isoproterenol.
Same as isoproterenol	Same as isoproterenol	Same as isoproterenol	Same as isoproterenol
Same as isoproterenol	Same as isoproterenol	Same as isoproternol	ASSESSMENT: Same as isoproterenol. INTERVENTION: Reduced dose will cause tremors to subside. EVALUATION: Same as isoproterenol.
Contraindicated in patients with uncon-	CNS: nervousness, anxiety, tremor, SEIZURES, head-	CV and CNS effects increased by adrenergic	ASSESSMENT: Monitor breath sounds for wheezing

CONTINUED ON THE FOLLOWING PAGE

Drugs for Bronchial Obstruction

Table 35–1. DRUGS USED TO TREAT BRONCHIAL OBSTRUCTION–*CONTINUED*

Name	Dosage	Mode of Administration	Pharmacokinetics
Aminophylline–*Continued*	determined by serum levels. Children: loading dose (age 6 mo–16 yr) 6 mg/kg over 20 min. Maintenance dose (age 6 mo–16 yr) 1 mg/kg/hr by continuous infusion.	IV	D: 6–12 hr, depending on preparation used. ½L: varies with age and preparation used (3 hr in young children, 8 hr adults).
	Adult: 500 mg followed by 250–500 mg q 6–8 hr. Children: 7.5 mg/kg followed by 3–6 mg/kg q 6–8 hr.	PO and rectal solution	PB: 50% (avg) B: liver E: urine
Dyphylline	Adult: 15 mg/kg q 6 hr up to 4 times daily (up to 800 mg/ dose).	PO	O: within 1 hr P: 1 hr D: short
	Children: 4.4–6.6 mg/kg/day in divided doses (up to 15 mg/kg q 6 hr).	PO	½L: 2 hr PB: UA B: liver
	Adult: 250–500 mg q 6 hr. Children: not recommended.	IM	E: urine

Key to Abbreviations in the *Pharmacokinetics* column O–onset; P–peak; D–duration; PB–protein bound; B–biotransformed in; E–excreted in; ½L–halflife.
*Within the column listing adverse effects, underlines indicate the most common effects; CAPITALS indicate life-threatening effects.

Contraindications/ Precautions	Adverse Effects*	Interactions	Nursing Implications
trolled dysrhythmias or tachycardia, uncontrolled hyperthyroidism, or uncontrolled seizure disorder. Use with caution in patients with congestive heart failure and liver disease, elderly patients ($>$60 yr), patients with gastric ulcers. Concomitant use of other bronchodilators may lead to synergistic effects; use both with caution. Rapid infusion can cause tachyarrhythmias, seizures, and cardiovascular collapse; solutions should be no stronger than 25 mg/ml and infused at a rate no faster than 25 mg/min to avoid these extreme reactions.	ache, insomnia, dizziness, flushing, faintness CV: tachycardia, palpitations, arrhythmias, angina, hypotension, rarely hypertension GI: nausea, vomiting, cramps, diarrhea, anorexia, indigestion; rarely, reactivation of ulcer Other: rarely, anaphylaxis, hematuria, hypokalemia	bronchodilators, anticholinergics, and cardiac glycosides. Antagonized by β blockers; also antagonizes their effects. May reduce the duration of effects of lithium. Rate of clearance is increased by smoking (tobacco and marijuana), barbiturates, phenytoin, rifampin, carbamazepine. Rate of clearance is decreased by β blockers, allopurinol, cimetidine, erythromycin, troleandomycin, clindamycin, lincomycin. Use with diuretic agents may lead to increased level of diuresis. Incompatible in solution with: calcium salt preparations, acidic solutions, potassium penicillin, tetracyclines, cephalothin, erythromycin, chloramphenicol, levarterenol, hydrocortisone, methylprednisolone, insulin, ACTH, epinephrine, isoproterenol. Because of the many incompatibilities, admixing of infusion is not recommended. Caffeine-containing beverages may enhance stimulant and diuretic effects of aminophylline.	and air movement. Check for factors that could influence drug clearance and therefore dosage (such as smoking or certain diseases—see list). Monitor blood pressure and HR closely; monitor ECG in patients with history of cardiac problems. Monitor serum levels regularly. Watch for toxicity symptoms (e.g., nausea, restlessness, tachycardia, insomnia, arrhythmias, seizures) and for interactions. Check for concurrent use of OTC theophylline products. Check infusion rate of IV solutions frequently. INTERVENTION: Keep infusion rate slower than 25 mg/min (for intermittent dosing) or 0.3–1.2 mg/kg/hr (continuous infusion). Adjust dose as ordered if patient smokes (smokers require up to 100% larger dose than usual), if interacting drugs are part of regimen, or if serum level is not within therapeutic range 10–20 μg/ml). If toxicity signs occur, slow infusion and inform physician (NOTE: stop infusion immediately if arrhythmias or seizures occur.) Encourage patient receiving rectal solution to retain for ½ hr for best result. Do not admix aminophylline with other drugs in IV solution because of many incompatibilities. When administering IV, flush main IV line before administering the drug. Give this drug around the clock as ordered. EVALUATION: Effectiveness of this drug can be demonstrated by relief of dyspnea, improved distribution of air in lung fields, and improved quality of breath sounds.
Same as aminophylline	Same as aminophylline	Same as aminophylline	ASSESSMENT: Generally the same as aminophylline. However, serum levels are unavailable. Assess for need for more frequent or larger doses (because of shorter duration and lower

CONTINUED ON THE FOLLOWING PAGE

Table 35–1. DRUGS USED TO TREAT BRONCHIAL OBSTRUCTION–*CONTINUED*

Name	Dosage	Mode of Administration	Pharmacokinetics
Dyphylline–*Continued*			
Theophylline anhydrous	Adult: 3–6 mg/kg initially, 100–200 mg q 6 hr maintenance.	PO	O: rapid P: same as aminophylline D: 4–15 hr depending on preparation used. ½L: same as aminophylline PB: same as aminophylline B: liver E: urine
	Children: 3–6 mg/kg initially, 50–100 mg q 6 hr maintenance.	PO	
	Adult: 250–500 mg q 6–12 hr.	Rectal	
	Children: 10–12 mg/kg/day to be given no more often than q 6 hr.	Rectal	
Oxtriphylline (Choledyl)	Adult: 200 mg 4 times daily, or 400–600 mg sustained action tabs q 12 hr.	PO	O: slow, variable P: UA D: UA (generally long) ½L: 3.5–10 hr. PB: same as aminophylline B: same as aminophylline E: same as aminophylline
	Children: 3.6 mg/kg 4 times daily.	PO	
Theophylline sodium glycinate (Synophylate)	Adult: 330–660 mg q 6–8 hr.	PO	O: slow P: UA D: long ½L: UA PB: same as aminophylline B: same as aminophylline E: same as aminophylline
	Children 6–12 yr: 220–330 mg q 6–8 hr.	PO	
	Children <6 yr: 55–165 mg q 6–8 hr.		
ANTI-INFLAMMATORY AGENTS Beclomethasone (Vanceril, Beclovent, Beconase)			

Action: decrease local airway inflammation by inhibiting effects of histamine and other mediators.

Use: in asthma, COPD, to decrease airway edema.

	Adult: 336 µg/day (1–2 puffs 4 times daily; dosage may be higher initially, not to exceed 20 inhalations daily).	MDI	O: very gradual (maintenance) P: UA D: used for long-term effects ½L: UA PB: UA B: locally, by lung tissues E: feces
	Children 6–12 yr: half the adult dose.	MDI	

Key to Abbreviations in the *Pharmacokinetics* column O-onset; P-peak; D-duration; PB-protein bound; B-biotransformed in; E-excreted in; ½L-halflife.
*Within the column listing adverse effects, underlines indicate the most common effects; CAPITALS indicate life-threatening effects.

Drugs for Bronchial Obstruction

Contraindications/ Precautions	Adverse Effects*	Interactions	Nursing Implications
			potency than other theophylline products). INTERVENTION: May administer IM as ordered (this is the only theophylline product suitable for IM injection). If signs of toxicity or hypersensitivity occur, stop use of drug and notify physician at once. EVALUATION: Same as aminophylline.
Same as aminophylline	Same as aminophylline	Same as aminophylline	ASSESSMENT: Generally same as aminophylline. Since many forms and dosages are available, check drug orders carefully. Monitor patient response to sustained-release preparations (absorption of these products may be erratic, and some patients may not obtain continuous relief from once- or twice-daily dosaging). Do not crush timed-release tablets, since this releases the theophylline immediately. EVALUATION: Same as aminophylline
Same as aminophylline	Same as aminophylline	Same as aminophylline	Same as aminophylline
Same as aminophylline	Same as aminophylline	Same as aminophylline	Same as aminophylline
This drug is contraindicated in cases of acute bronchospasm. Use with caution in	Resp: hoarseness, throat irritation, rhinitis, reflex bronchospasm; fungal infections GI: nausea, vomiting, diarrhea, upset	With recommended doses, no major interactions noted.	ASSESSMENT: Check for sore throat, and for signs of oral candidiasis. Monitor for changes in sputum color or viscosity, which may indi-

CONTINUED ON THE FOLLOWING PAGE

Table 35–1. DRUGS USED TO TREAT BRONCHIAL OBSTRUCTION–*CONTINUED*

Name	Dosage	Mode of Administration	Pharmacokinetics
Beclomethasone–*Continued*			
Triamcinolone acetonide (Azmacort)	Adult: 800 μg/day (2 puffs 4 times daily) not to exceed 16 inhalations daily.	MDI	Same as beclomethasone
	Children 6–12 yr: 400 μg/day (1 puff 4 times daily) not to exceed 12 inhalations daily.	MDI	
Flunisolide (AeroBid)	Adult: 1–2 mg/day (2–4 puffs twice daily).	MDI	Same as beclomethasone
	Children 6–15 yr: half the adult dose.	MDI	

Key to Abbreviations in the *Pharmacokinetics* column O-onset; P-peak; D-duration; PB-protein bound; B-bio-transformed in; E-excreted in; ½L-halflife.
*Within the column listing adverse effects, underlines indicate the most common effects; CAPITALS indicate life-threatening effects.

Contraindications/ Precautions	Adverse Effects*	Interactions	Nursing Implications
patients with bron- chiectasis or puru- lent bronchitis. Aerosol may cause reflex broncho- spasm in some patients. Not recommended for use in children under 6 yr.	CNS: headache CV: palpitations Other: menstrual distur- bances. May cause steroid dependence and general steroid side effects in excess doses		cate infection. If using inhaler as replacement for systemic steroid therapy, watch for signs of adrenal crisis. Observe for new development of systemic steroid side effects in long- term user. Listen to breath sounds regularly to deter- mine severity of wheezing and to follow patient prog- ress. Monitor serum glu- cose and sodium for increases and serum cal- cium and potassium for decreases. Monitor patient for harsh cough and burn- ing sensation in lungs when breathing. INTERVENTION: Instruct patient to rinse mouth thor- oughly to avoid *Candida* overgrowth. Instruct patient to take on a regular (not prn) basis. When changing patient from systemic ste- roid regimen to aerosol reg- imen, administer both forms as ordered until patient has gradually been weaned completely to aerosol. At first signs of adrenal crisis inform physician and initiate systemic steroid therapy as ordered. Bronchodilators, if ordered, should be used 15 min prior to use of beclo- methasone inhaler to pro- mote distribution in airways and to minimize potentially toxic effects of propellants. Use during acute wheezing attack may exacerbate symptoms. Warn patient not to exceed prescribed dos- age. Instruct patient to clean inhaler daily. EVALUATION: Effectiveness of this drug is demonstrated by increased comfort in patient's breathing (de- creased burning in chest, less harsh coughing), and by decreased severity of wheezing attacks.
Same as beclometha- sone	Same as beclomethasone	Same as beclomethasone	Same as beclomethasone
Same as beclometha- sone	Same as beclomethasone	Same as beclomethasone	Same as beclomethasone

CONTINUED ON THE FOLLOWING PAGE

Table 35–1. DRUGS USED TO TREAT BRONCHIAL OBSTRUCTION–*CONTINUED*

Name	Dosage	Mode of Administration	Pharmacokinetics
Cromolyn sodium (Intal)			

Action: stabilizes mast cells in airways, inhibiting histamine release.

Use: prevention of allergic and exercise-induced asthma attacks.

	Dosage	Mode of Administration	Pharmacokinetics
	Adult, children: 20 mg 4 times daily (via Spinhaler or as solution for nebullization). 2 puffs 4 times (800 μg/puff).	Spinhaler MDI	O: 2–4 wks P: UA D: used as maintenance drug for long-term effects ½L: UA PB: UA B: excreted unchanged E: bile, urine

MUCOKINETIC AGENTS
Acetylcysteine (Mucomyst)

Action: aerosol breaks disulfide bonds in respiratory mucus; taken orally, acetylcysteine alters metabolic pathway of acetaminophen

Use: to decrease viscosity of secretions in COPD, cystic fibrosis; taken orally to protect liver from acetaminophen overdose

	Dosage	Mode of Administration	Pharmacokinetics
	Adult, children: 3–5 ml of 20% solution (or 6–10 ml of 10% solution) 3–4 times daily. Up to 10 ml of 20% or 20 ml of 10% solution can be given q 2–6 hr.	Inhalation, direct instillation. Oral (for acetaminophen overdose).	O: rapid P: UA D: brief ½L: UA PB: UA B: local-acting, small amts metabolized by liver E: in respiratory mucus and urine

Key to Abbreviations in the *Pharmacokinetics* column O-onset; P-peak; D-duration; PB-protein bound; B-biotransformed in; E-excreted in; ½L-halflife.
*Within the column listing adverse effects, underlines indicate the most common effects; CAPITALS indicate life-threatening effects.

Contraindications/ Precautions	Adverse Effects*	Interactions	Nursing Implications
Contraindicated in cases of acute bronchospasm. May cause reflex bronchospasm. Safety for use in pregnancy and long-term toxicity have not been established. Patients with impaired liver or kidney function may require decreased dosages.	CNS: headache Derm: rash Resp: cough, dry throat, bronchospasm Misc: unpleasant taste, allergy, rash, urticaria, erythema, worsening of asthma	No significant interactions known.	ASSESSMENT: Maintain log of frequency and severity of asthma attacks to evaluate efficacy. Monitor pulmonary function prior to start of therapy. Assess breath sounds periodically throughout the course of therapy. Check for dry throat and hoarseness. INTERVENTION: Instruct patient in use of Spinhaler (if ordered, capsules are not to be taken orally). Instruct patient to take drug for 2–4 wk as ordered before expecting results. Rinsing of mouth after administration will prevent dry throat. Instruct patient not to take cromolyn during asthma attack, since it can exacerbate symptoms. If using bronchodilator, cromolyn should be administered 20–30 min afterward for optimal inhalation of drug. EVALUATION: The effectiveness of this drug is demonstrated by eventual (within 4 wk) decrease in the number and intensity of asthma attacks, and by a reduction in the need for other asthmatic medications.
Contraindicated in hypersensitivity. Use with caution in patients with asthma or respiratory insufficiency. May precipitate bronchospasms in susceptible patients. Safety for use in pregnancy or lactation not established.	CNS: drowsiness, headache GI: nausea, vomiting EENT: stomatitis, rhinorrhea, tracheitis, laryngitis	May deactivate amphotericin, erythromycin, or ampicillin, but only when these are mixed as one solution with Mucomyst. Alters metabolic pathway of acetaminophen overdosage.	ASSESSMENT: Assess character of patient's cough (productive?, sputum volume?, sputum viscosity?, difficulty in raising sputum?). Watch for sensitivity or adverse reactions. INTERVENTION: To prevent irritation of oral and pharyngeal tissues, have patient rinse mouth after treatment. When 25% of the drug remains in nebulizer, dilute with an equal amount of

CONTINUED ON THE FOLLOWING PAGE

Table 35–1. DRUGS USED TO TREAT BRONCHIAL OBSTRUCTION-*CONTINUED*

Name	Dosage	Mode of Administration	Pharmacokinetics
Acetylcysteine–*Continued*			
EXPECTORANTS Guaifenesin (contained in various products)			

Action: stimulates bronchial mucus glands to secrete less viscous mucus.

Use: symptomatic management of coughs associated with colds.

Name	Dosage	Mode of Administration	Pharmacokinetics
	Adult: 200–400 mg q 4 hr. Children 6–11 yr: 100–200 mg q 4 hr (1200 mg/day max.). Children 2–5 yr: 50–100 mg q 4 hr (600 mg/day max).	PO PO	O: rapid (30 min) P: UA D: 4–6 hr ½L: UA PB: UA B: liver E: urine
Terpin hydrate (various products)	Adult: 300 mg q 6 hr. Children 6–12 yr: 125 mg q 6 hr.	PO PO	O: rapid (<30 min) P: UA D: 4–6 hr ½L: UA PB: UA B: UA E: urine

Key to Abbreviations in the *Pharmacokinetics* column O-onset; P-peak; D-duration; PB-protein bound; B-biotransformed in; E-excreted in; ½L-halflife.
*Within the column listing adverse effects, underlines indicate the most common effects; CAPITALS indicate life-threatening effects.

Contraindications/ Precautions	Adverse Effects*	Interactions	Nursing Implications
			normal saline solution to minimize reconcentration. Have suction apparatus available for patients with ineffective cough. If wheezing occurs after treatment, inform the physician and suggest possible concurrent use of bronchodilator. Unused portion should be capped tightly and discarded after 4 days (although purple discoloration does not affect potency). Other uses for acetylcysteine include oral administration for loosening inspissated intestinal contents in cystic fibrosis patients, and as antidote for acetaminophen overdose. Encourage adequate hydration to decrease sputum viscosity. EVALUATION: Effectiveness of this drug is demonstrated by increased sputum productivity and decreased sputum viscosity.
Contraindicated in hypersensitivity. If cough persists for a week, or is accompanied by fever, headache, or rash, consult a physician. Safety in pregnancy is not firmly established, but adverse effects have not been reported.	GI: nausea, vomiting	None significant.	ASSESSMENT: Note character of cough and sputum. Watch for sensitivity. INTERVENTION: Withhold fluids for up to 30 min after administering to promote demulcent effects. Instruct patient not to chew capsules. Instruct in proper cough techniques. Contact physician if cough persists for a week or more. EVALUATION: The effectiveness of this drug is demonstrated by increased sputum clearance.
Contraindicated for patients undergoing therapy for alcoholism.	CNS: headache GI: nausea	May increase effects of barbiturates in large doses.	Same as guaifenesin

CONTINUED ON THE FOLLOWING PAGE

Table 35–1. DRUGS USED TO TREAT BRONCHIAL OBSTRUCTION–*CONTINUED*

Name	Dosage	Mode of Administration	Pharmacokinetics
Iodide preparations (various products)	Adult: 300–600 mg 4 times daily of SSKI (saturated solution of potassium iodide). Adult: 60 mg 4 times daily of iodinated glycerol. Children: half adult dose.	PO as elixir, solution, tabs	O: UA P: UA D: UA ½L: UA PB: UA B: UA E: urine, also breast milk

Key to Abbreviations in the *Pharmacokinetics* column O-onset; P-peak; D-duration; PB-protein bound; B-biotransformed in; E-excreted in; ½L-halflife.
*Within the column listing adverse effects, underlines indicate the most common effects; CAPITALS indicate life-threatening effects.

its ability to decrease the activity of the enzyme that inactivates cAMP, theophylline has been called a phosphodiesterase inhibitor. For years this action has been used to explain its effectiveness as a bronchodilator. Recently, however, evidence has pointed to theophylline's action on either intracellular calcium or adenosine (or perhaps both) as a more likely explanation for its bronchodilation properties.

Aminophylline is the main therapeutic derivative of theophylline. This drug is often regarded as the most important agent in the treatment of the hospitalized asthmatic. The many forms of theophylline are listed in Table 35–2, and many specific theophylline products are listed in Table 35–3.

PHARMACOKINETICS. Absorption of theophylline is dependent upon its mode of administration. Oral preparations are generally well absorbed from the gastrointestinal tract. Sustained-release products have become widely prescribed during the past few years. These preparations absorb as completely as the shorter-acting agents, but the rate at which they are absorbed is slower. This results in a wide range of peak serum blood levels for theophylline. Oral aminophylline reaches peak blood levels in one to two hours, while sustained-release products such as TheoDur or Slo-Bid may not peak for three to four hours. Theo-24, designed for once-daily dosing, reaches peak serum levels in 10–15 hours.

Rectal solutions are generally well absorbed when they are retained for a sufficient amount of time. However, rectal suppositories are absorbed erratically and are not recommended for use.

Intramuscular injection of aminophylline is effective, but because it is very painful it is also not recommended. Intravenous infusion is the most reliable and predictable route of administration.

Different theophylline preparations contain varying amounts of theophylline. Determination of proper dosage and the level of therapeutic response depends upon the percentage of theophylline in each compound. For a listing of many theophylline preparations and their theophylline content, see Tables 35–1 and 35–2.

Theophylline is widely distributed. Approximately 50% is bound to plasma proteins. It can cross the pla-

Table 35–2. THEOPHYLLINE PREPARATIONS AND VARIOUS SALTS

Name	% Theophylline	Common Trade Names
Theophylline anhydrous	100	Aerolate, Elixophylline, TheoDur, Slo-Phyllin, Theobid, Theo-24, Theolair, Respbid, Sustaire
Theophylline ethylenediamine	78–86	Aminophylline, Aminodur, Phyllocontin, Somophyllin, Truphylline
Theophylline sodium glycinate	49	Synophylate
Oxtryphylline	64	Choledyl, Brondecon
Dyphylline	0*	Asminyl, Dilin, Dilor, Dyflex, Lufyllin, Neothylline, Droxine

*Dyphylline (dihydroxypropyl theophylline) is a chemically related derivative of theophylline. It is *not* metabolized to free theophylline. Thus, it cannot be measured by normal serum theophylline assays. Equivalent to approximately 70% theophylline by weight.
Adapted from IV dosing guidelines for theophylline products. FDA Drug Bull 10:4–6, 1980.

Contraindications/ Precautions	Adverse Effects*	Interactions	Nursing Implications
Contraindicated in hypersensitivity to organic iodides. Not recommended for use in pregnancy or lactation. Discontinue use if rash or other signs of sensitivity appear. Cystic fibrosis patients may be more susceptible to goitrogenic effects. Do not use in patients with known thyroid dysfunction.	GI: GI upset Other: parotitis, thyroid gland enlargement, rash, hypersensitivity	May alter radioactive iodine tests indefinitely following iodide therapy.	ASSESSMENT: Same as guaifenesin. INTERVENTION: Administer with fruit juice or milk to disguise bitter taste. (Gastric irritation is decreased by giving drug with a whole glass after meals.) EVALUATION: Same as guaifenesin.

centa and enter breast milk, where concentrations are about half those of serum concentrations. It does not seem to enter adipose tissue; for this reason dosages are calculated on the basis of lean body weight. Once absorbed, theophylline is extensively metabolized in the liver to several inactive metabolites. These are excreted in the urine.

For nearly all patients a serum concentration of 10–20 $\mu g/ml$ provides therapeutic effects. Several factors can affect serum concentrations of theophylline. Half-life of the drug in nonsmoking adults is seven to ten hours. Metabolism of theophylline is accelerated by tobacco or marijuana smoking, as well as by several drugs. Clearance of the drug also occurs more rapidly in young children than in adults. Conversely, theophylline metabolism is slowed by several pharmacologic agents (as discussed below), and by a number of pathologic conditions. Patients with hepatic failure, congestive heart failure (CHF), viral illnesses, or pneumonia will have a prolonged serum half-life of theophylline. Neonates and elderly patients also have a decreased rate of metabolism of theophylline.

Because theophylline toxicity can be life threatening, and because so many factors can affect the rate of me-

Table 35–3. TIMED-RELEASED PRODUCTS

Product	Manufacturer	Dose (mg)	Dose Interval (hr)
THEOPHYLLINE PRODUCTS			
Aerolate (III, JR, SR)	Fleming	65,130,260	Q12
Bronkodyl S-R	Breon	300	Q12
Choledyl SA	Parke–Davis	400,600	Q12
Constant-T	Geigy	200,300	Q12
Elixophyllin SR	Berlex	125,250	Q12
LABID	Norwich–Eaton	100,250	Q12
Quibron-T/SR	Mead Johnson	300	Q12
Respbid	Boehringer–Ingelheim	250,500	Q6–8
Slo-Bid Gyrocaps	Rorer	100,200,300	Q12
Somophyllin-CRT	Fisons	50,100,250	Q12
Sustaire	Roerig	100,300	Q12
Theo24	Searle	300,600	Q24
Theobid Duracaps	Glaxo	130,260	Q12
Theoclear L.A. Cenules	Central	130,260	Q6–8
TheoDur	Key Pharm.	100,200,300	Q12
Theolair-SR	Riker	250,500	Q8–12
Theospan SR	Laser	130,260	Q12
Theophyl-SR	McNeil	125,250	Q12
Theovent	Schering	125,250	Q12
Slophyllin Gyrocaps	Rorer	60,125,250	Q8–12
Uniphyl	Purdue Frederick	200,400	Q12
AMINOPHYLLINE PRODUCTS			
Phyllocontin	Purdue Frederick	225	Q12
Aminodur Duratabs	Berlex	300	Q8–12

Table 35–4. DOSING GUIDELINES OF ACUTE ADMINISTRATION OF AMINOPHYLLINE

Group	Loading Dose	Maintenance Dose for Next 12 hr	Maintenance Dose Beyond 12 hr†
Patients with congestive heart failure, liver disease	6 mg/kg *(5)	0.5 mg/kg/hr *(0.4)	0.1–0.2 mg/kg/hr *(0.1)
Older patients and patients with cor pulmonale	6 mg/kg *(5)	0.6 mg/kg/hr *(0.5)	0.3 mg/kg/hr *(0.26)
Otherwise healthy nonsmoking adults	6 mg/kg *(5)	0.7 mg/kg/hr *(0.6)	0.5 mg/kg/hr *(0.43)
Children 9–16 yr and young adult smokers	6 mg/kg *(5)	1.0 mg/kg/hr *(0.85)	0.8 mg/kg/hr *(0.7)
Children 6 mo–9 yr	6 mg/kg *(5)	1.2 mg/kg/hr *(1.0)	1.0 mg/kg/hr *(0.85)
Preterm infant <40 weeks post-conception		1 mg/kg q 12 hr	‡
Term infant		1–2 mg/kg q 12 hr	‡
Infant 4–8 wk		1–2 mg/kg q 8 hr	‡
Infant 8 wk–6 mo		1–3 mg/kg q 6 hr	‡

*Based on estimated lean (ideal) body weight. Equivalent anhydrous theophylline dose indicated in parentheses.

†If theophylline levels are not available, the maintenance infusion rate beyond 12 hours needs to be reduced so that adverse effects associated with drug accumulation may be minimized.

‡These dosages are based upon clinical reports; because of widely variant theophylline clearance in infants, theophylline is not recommended for use in children less than 6 months of age. If used, serum theophylline levels must be monitored scrupulously.

tabolism of this drug, strict guidelines concerning its administration have been established. These dosage recommendations, listed in Table 35–4, should be strictly followed to ensure patient safety.

CONTRAINDICATIONS AND PRECAUTIONS. Patients with known hypersensitivity to ethylenediamine (also a component of the steroid/antibiotic cream Mycolog) should not receive aminophylline products. Because it increases heart rate and force of myocardial contraction, and reduces the heart's ventricular fibrillation threshold, theophylline is contraindicated in patients with uncontrolled cardiac dysrhythmias. It must be given with caution to patients with any cardiovascular disease. Since it can cause seizures, patients with seizure disorders should receive theophylline only if their bronchospasm is unresponsive to other treatment approaches, and only with extreme caution. Patients with hyperthyroidism will experience exacerbation of their symptoms with theophylline, and for this reason should not receive the drug. Finally, theophylline increases gastric acid secretion. This may aggravate the conditions of patients with esophageal reflux, or with active gastric or duodenal ulcers.

ADVERSE REACTIONS. Adverse effects associated with theophylline products are very similar to those seen with sympathomimetics. In general, however, toxic reactions caused by theophylline are much more severe, so great caution must be exercised in its administration. When serum levels are maintained within the therapeutic range of 10–20 μg/ml, serious adverse reactions are rare. As the serum level increases beyond this range, potentially dangerous toxic effects appear.

Patients receiving theophylline complain most frequently of caffeine-like symptoms, including nervousness, insomnia, jitteriness, headache, frequent urination, and palpitations. These can be very mild, appearing even when the patient's serum level is relatively low. Mild symptoms usually disappear in a short period of time. These same symptoms may be the first

indication of serious toxicity, however, so they must not be ignored.

More serious side effects are related directly to serum levels of the drug. With concentrations of 15–25 μg/ml, severe nausea, vomiting, and anorexia occur. Tachycardia is common. More intense CNS effects, such as agitation, tremors, and anxiety, also appear when serum levels are within this range. As the serum level rises above 30 μg/ml, dangerous cardiac effects are likely. Atrial and ventricular dysrhythmias, including ventricular fibrillation, can occur suddenly, with fatal results. Cardiovascular collapse occurs when aminophylline is infused too rapidly. For this reason aminophylline must be administered no faster than 25 mg/min in concentrations no stronger than 25 mg/ml.

Although seizures can occur at lower serum levels, they are most common when serum levels exceed 40 μg/ml. Seizures caused by theophylline toxicity are usually refractory to treatment and can be fatal.

Because of the potentially lethal nature of theophylline's adverse effects, it is essential that patient response to therapy be monitored closely, and that serum levels be monitored regularly.

INTERACTIONS. The stimulatory effects of theophylline are increased by sympathomimetic agents, anticholinergics, and cardiac glycosides. When used together, each drug potentiates both the therapeutic and adverse effects of the other. Use of theophylline with β-blockers results in mutual antagonism of effects. Theophylline also seems to enhance the effectiveness of some diuretic agents and to decrease the therapeutic effect of lithium.

Several drugs known to be enzyme inducers increase metabolism of theophylline. Among these drugs are phenytoin, rifampin, barbiturates, and carbamazepine. Use of these agents with theophylline results in a decrease in the duration of theophylline's action. The same effect occurs in patients who are smokers.

Drugs that decrease the rate of metabolism of theophylline include allopurinol, β-blockers, and cimetidine. Several antibiotics, notably erythromycin, clindamycin, troleandomycin, and lincomycin, also decrease the clearance of theophylline. Patients receiving these drugs with theophylline are thus at greater risk of developing toxicity.

Numerous drugs are incompatible in solution with theophylline. These are listed in Table 35–1. Because there are so many drugs that can react with theophylline, mixing of this drug with other IV medications is not recommended.

Beverages and foods that contain caffeine may accentuate some of the stimulatory effects of theophylline preparations. Patients who use these together report increased diuresis and nervousness. A full stomach does not alter the extent of oral theophylline absorption, but it does slow the rate at which it is absorbed. Sustained-release theophylline products are administered twice or three times daily, although dosages must be individualized on the basis of serum levels.

Anticholinergic Bronchodilators

Some patients who demonstrate only limited response to sympathomimetics or theophylline may benefit from the use of aerosolized anticholinergic agents. Although bronchospasm seems to result more often from a lack of cAMP, it can also occur from excessive parasympathetic nervous stimulation. When the vagus nerve is stimulated, bronchial smooth muscle tone can increase because of increased manufacture of a cyclic nucleotide called cyclic 3′,5′-guanosine monophosphate (cGMP). This substance opposes the action of cAMP, constricting bronchial smooth muscle. Together, cGMP and cAMP maintain bronchial tone.

Patients in whom vagal tone is increased, such as patients with gastric reflux and some patients with asthma and chronic bronchitis, may benefit from anticholinergic medications. These drugs competitively antagonize the activity of acetylcholine, which is secreted from parasympathetic nerve endings. By blocking the action of this neurotransmitter, anticholinergics decrease the production of cGMP. This allows the cAMP in the bronchial smooth muscle to exert greater influence, resulting in bronchial relaxation (Fig. 35–3).

Atropine, versatile in so many areas of medicine, has been used with some success in patients with refractory bronchospasm. Ipratropium bromide (Atrovent) is a newer, related medication that has shown much promise as a bronchodilator. It seems to cause fewer and less

severe adverse reactions than does atropine, and is gaining widespread popularity.

PHARMACOKINETICS. When anticholinergics are given by aerosol, their systemic effects occur less readily than when other routes of administration are used. This indicates less than complete absorption by this route. Atropine is more thoroughly absorbed than is ipratropium, as evidenced by the fewer and less pronounced side effects of the latter. Atropine crosses the blood–brain barrier and enters the placenta and breast milk. The extent of ipratropium's absorption is not well known.

Both drugs are metabolized by the liver. Up to 50% of atropine is excreted unchanged by the kidney.

CONTRAINDICATIONS AND PRECAUTIONS. The use of either bronchodilator is contraindicated in patients with hypersensitivity to atropine. In addition, atropine is not used by the patient with narrow-angle glaucoma, because it dilates the pupil and decreases visual accommodation. Patients with acute hemorrhage, or with tachycardia caused by cardiac insufficiency or thyrotoxicosis, should not use atropine because it increases heart rate significantly. Because ipratropium can cause many of the same effects as atropine, it is used with caution in any of these patients.

Atropine and ipratropium are used with caution in patients with prostate hypertrophy, bladder-neck obstruction, or any chronic renal, cardiac, pulmonary, or liver disease. The elderly and the very young are more susceptible to adverse effects caused by these agents.

ADVERSE REACTIONS. Like theophylline or sympathomimetics, anticholinergics stimulate the heart. Tachycardia and palpitations are reported occasionally and occur more frequently with atropine than ipratropium. Nausea and gastrointestinal upset occur occasionally with inhaled anticholinergics.

Unlike the other bronchodilators, anticholinergics are not normally CNS stimulants. Headache, drowsiness, and even confusion are more often encountered, although some patients have reported experiencing nervousness following use of these drugs. Atropine has been known to cause urinary hesitancy and retention, as well as constipation. These effects are probably a result of atropine's antispasmodic activity. Because it decreases sweat gland secretion, atropine has caused increases in some patients temperature.

Both of these agents can cause blurred vision, especially if they are inadvertently sprayed in the eyes. Dry mouth, irritated throat, and rash have also been re-

Figure 35–3. Action of anticholinergic bronchodilators. Anticholinergic bronchodilators such as atropine and ipratropium compete with acetylcholine for muscarinic site. By occupying this site, these agents prevent acetylcholine from activating guanylate cyclase, thus decreasing production of cyclic GMP, a potent bronchoconstrictor.

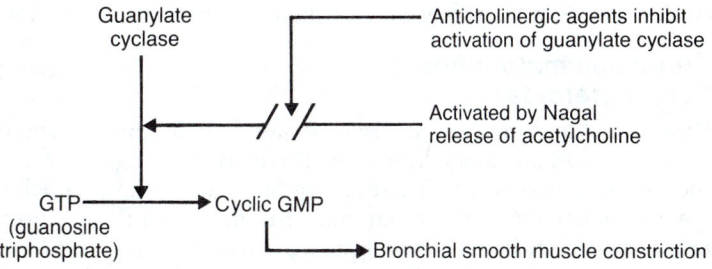

ported. Since both agents tend to dry mucus gland secretions, the potential exists for causing increased airway resistance due to mucus plugging. With adequate hydration, however, this should not be a problem for most patients.

INTERACTIONS. Additive effects can occur when atropine is used with other anticholinergic medications such as quinidine, antihistamines, disopyramide, and tricyclic antidepressants. In larger doses or in patients receiving long-term atropine by aerosol, gastrointestinal motility may be slowed. This causes slowed absorption of other oral medications.

There are no documented drug interactions with ipratroprium bromide.

OTHER AGENTS USED TO DECREASE BRONCHIAL OBSTRUCTION

While bronchospasm is the most important cause of bronchial obstruction, inflammation and excessive mucus secretions can also decrease air flow through the bronchial tubes. Inflammation is caused by allergy, chemical or physical irritation of the airways, or viral or bacterial infection. Accompanying inflammation is cell damage. When cells are injured, histamine and other mediators are released. These cause airway edema, as well as bronchospasm and abundant secretions. Inflammation is a common feature of asthma and chronic bronchitis. Regardless of its cause, the edema of inflammation swells the bronchial tubes, thereby decreasing their lumen size.

For patient comfort, as well as to ensure adequate ventilation, airway inflammation must be controlled. Corticosteroids can be highly effective in treating both acute and chronic airway inflammation. For many patients, large doses of oral or IV steroids are needed to control airway inflammation. Once under control, however, many patients can be maintained on aerosolized steroids, thus minimizing their systemic adverse effects. This chapter discusses the use of aerosolized steroids. For a complete discussion of the use and effects of corticosteroids, see Chapter 42.

In some patients, airway inflammation is preventable. Cromolyn sodium decreases the sensitivity of some asthmatics' airways to allergens, thereby reducing the number and intensity of asthma attacks.

Excessive mucus secretions are usually the result of airway irritation or inflammation. Patients with chronic obstructive pulmonary disease (COPD), bronchiectasis, cystic fibrosis, and pneumonia can have copious amounts of mucus. The manner by which they are controlled varies, depending upon the patient's clinical circumstances. Several approaches are discussed below.

Anti-inflammatory Agents: Corticosteroids

Prednisone and methylprednisolone are among the major anti-inflammatory agents available for treating the respiratory patient. These powerful agents can greatly change the course of an exacerbation of COPD or an asthma attack, but their systemic adverse effects

can be extreme. To avoid these effects, locally acting inhaled steroids are used. Beclomethasone (Beclovent, Vanceril), betamethasone (Valisone), triamcinolone acetonide (Azmacort), and flunisolide (AeroBid) are examples of corticosteroids that are available as aerosol medications.

Inhaled steroids act locally to suppress the inflammatory response in the lung. The precise mechanism by which this is accomplished is unknown. They evidently decrease the release and the effects of inflammatory mediators from injured tissues. Capillaries are stabilized, resulting in decreased airway edema. The usual effects of mediator action in the lung, including bronchospasm and increased mucus production, are countered by corticosteroids.

PHARMACOKINETICS. Virtually all of the steroids available in metered-dose inhalers act almost exclusively in the airways. Absorption across the alveolar–capillary membrane is minimal at recommended doses, and systemic effects are unlikely. Because some of the drug is swallowed and because the potential for systemic absorption exists, the long-term use of aerosol steroids may increase the patient's risk of some toxic effects.

Because the aerosolized steroids are not distributed beyond the airways, their clearance is accomplished through the mucociliary escalator, the cough reflex, and alveolar macrophages. The amounts that are swallowed or otherwise absorbed systemically are rapidly metabolized and are excreted in the feces.

CONTRAINDICATIONS AND PRECAUTIONS. Patients with known or suspected hypersensitivity to the propellants used in metered-dose inhalers should not use these agents. Patients who have received long-term oral steroid therapy for breathing problems must be gradually weaned from systemic therapy. This is necessary to allow the patient's suppressed adrenal cortex to resume normal function. Failure to decrease the systemic dose gradually while initiating inhaled steroid therapy may result in Addisonian crisis.

Use of inhaled steroids at doses higher than those recommended may lead to systemic absorption. This can cause the systemic side effects described in Chapter 42.

These agents are not primarily bronchodilators. They should not be used in patients experiencing an acute episode of bronchospasm, because their use may delay the use of more appropriate medications. They may even exacerbate bronchospasm.

ADVERSE REACTIONS. The most significant adverse effect noted with the use of inhaled steroids has been death due to adrenal insufficiency. This may occur if oral steroids are discontinued abruptly and replaced by inhaled drugs.

Patients have experienced mainly minor side effects from the use of inhaled steroids. Complaints most commonly offered are oropharyngeal irritation and cold-like symptoms. Sore throat, sinusitis, and oral fungal infections may occur, but these can be minimized by thorough mouth rinsing after each dose.

Some patients experience diarrhea, nausea and vomiting, and stomach upset. Headache, fever, dizziness, angioedema, rash, urticaria, and paradoxical bronchospasm are rare but not unknown.

INTERACTIONS. Inhaled steroids have no significant interactions when they are administered within the therapeutic dosage range.

Inflammation Prophylaxis: Cromolyn Sodium

In recent years cromolyn sodium (Intal) has become an important part of asthma treatment. This agent is reputed to stabilize mast cell membranes. Mast cells, which contain high concentrations of histamine, are found in great abundance in the airways. In allergic asthma, antibody–allergen complexes cause degranulation of the mast cell. They spill their contents, resulting in bronchospasm, inflammation, and irritation. Cromolyn apparently alters the mast cell's permeability to calcium ions. This inhibits their degranulation and prevents mediator release. Many patients with allergic asthma, and some with exercise-induced asthma, have benefited from cromolyn by having fewer and less severe attacks.

Cromolyn sodium is also available as nasal spray and optic solution. It is used with great success as a preventive against hay fever symptoms.

PHARMACOKINETICS. Cromolyn is one of the rare drugs that is effective only when it is administered by means of inhalation. It is poorly absorbed, with a limited ability to cross membranes. Of the small amount that is absorbed, most is rapidly excreted unchanged in urine and bile. The remainder is excreted in feces or removed by means of the mucociliary escalator.

Because so little of the drug is absorbed into the cell membranes, a several-week regimen of daily dosing is required before therapeutic effects are noticeable.

CONTRAINDICATIONS AND PRECAUTIONS. Cromolyn is contraindicated for use in patients with hypersensitivity to the drug. The metered-dose inhaler is used with caution in patients with cardiac dysrhythmias, since the fluorocarbon propellant may have cardiotoxic effects. Patients with impaired renal or hepatic function may require lowered dosages.

Cromolyn is an asthma-preventive agent. It does not reverse bronchospasm and can aggravate it. This drug is not given during an acute asthma attack.

ADVERSE REACTIONS. Side effects from cromolyn are mild and relatively rare. The reactions most frequently reported include dry or irritated throat, cough, wheeze, unpleasant taste, and headache. Other reported adverse reactions are rash, urticaria, erythema, allergic response, nausea, swollen parotid glands, and bronchospasm.

INTERACTIONS. Cromolyn is not known to interact significantly with any drug.

Mucokinetic Agents

Obstruction of bronchial tubes by mucus is certainly one of the most common problems of the respiratory patient. In many cases secretion control is easily accomplished. However, for the patient who is unable to cough effectively, or whose mucus is extremely thick

and viscous, mucus plugging of airways is a serious problem. Like bronchospasm or inflammation, mucus in airways hinders gas exchange and greatly increases the work of breathing. It also fosters bacterial growth and thus predisposes the patient to pneumonia. For all these reasons, it is important to facilitate the removal of mucus from airways.

The most effective means of mobilizing mucus from airways is a strong cough. Secretions that are thin are easiest to raise, so hydration of the patient is essential. When mucus is dried and thick, rehydration can most often be accomplished by ensuring adequate fluid intake. When this is not feasible, the use of aerosols may help to decrease mucus viscosity. Water or saline aerosols delivered via a large-volume nebulizer are usually sufficient to promote *mucokinesis.*

When mucus is very viscous and wetting agents are unable to loosen it, an aerosolized *mucolytic* may be used. Acetylcysteine (Mucomyst) may help to dissolve mucus by breaking specific bonds in the mucoprotein molecules. This drug has been used by patients with cystic fibrosis and COPD with varying results. It may precipitate bronchospasm in some patients, so it is usually administered with a bronchodilator.

Some physicians prescribe *expectorants* to aid in secretion control. These agents, such as guaifenesin, terpin hydrate, and iodide preparations, stimulate mucus-producing glands, causing them to secrete a thinner, more fluid mucus. The use of these drugs actually increases mucus volume but supposedly makes it easier for the patient to expectorate the secretions. Expectorants are typically administered as elixirs rather than aerosols. Their most significant adverse effects are nausea, headache, and allergic response. Patients with thyroid problems should not receive iodide products because of their ability to further alter thyroid function.

Mucolytics and expectorants play a minor role in the treatment of bronchial obstruction. Major points concerning their administration can be found in Table 35–1.

USING THE NURSING PROCESS

ASSESSMENT

The nurse assesses the causes and the extent of bronchial obstruction, as well as the effects of therapeutic intervention. Often bronchial obstruction occurs suddenly, and prompt treatment is necessary. The nurse must recognize the primary signs and symptoms of bronchial obstruction so that proper therapy can be initiated. Assessment data collected are featured on Table 35–5.

The patient's work of breathing increases in direct proportion to the degree of obstruction. Use of accessory muscles, tachypnea, diaphoresis, and prolonged expiration are signs of dyspnea caused by bronchial obstruction. Cyanosis may or may not be evident. The patient

Table 35–5. NURSING PROCESS FOR PATIENT REQUIRING BRONCHODILATOR THERAPY

Assessment

Assess respiratory pattern, noting use of accessory muscles/pursed lip breathing, tachypnea, diaphoresis, and prolonged expiration.
Auscultate breath sounds.
Note history of seasonal allergies.
Assess respiratory status in presence of increasing anxiety.
Review history for presence of hypertension, angina, dysrhythmias, thyroid dysfunction, narrow-angle glaucoma, diabetes.

Nursing Diagnosis	Nursing Actions	Rationale	Desired Actions/ Evaluation Criteria
Airway Clearance ineffective/Gas Exchange, impaired related to bronchial obstruction, increased amount and viscosity of secretions, altered oxygen supply as evidenced by inability to move secretions, presence of crackles/wheezes, changes in rate/depth of respiration, dyspnea, restlessness.	Maintain airway, elevate head of bed/position patient appropriately. Provide airway adjuncts and suction as indicated	Promotes adequate ventilation.	Demonstrates improved ventilation and adequate oxygenation with ABGs within patient's normal ranges and absence of symptoms of respiratory distress.
	Encourage deep breathing/use of "pursed lip" breathing, coughing exercises; splint chest/incision while coughing.	Promotes passage of air through narrowed bronchioles. Splinting maximizes effort while minimizing associated discomfort.	
	Increase fluid intake to 2000 ml/day within level of cardiac reserve.	Liquifies secretions enhancing expectoration.	
	Provide more warm fluids, than cold.	Decreases spasms, facilitates expectoration.	
	Administer medications as indicated, e.g., metaproterenol, theophylline.	Bronchodilators relieve bronchospasm to enhance passage of air and expectorations of secretions.	
	Schedule/carefully time administration of intermittent drugs with aerosol therapy.	Provides for more sustained drug effect, maximizing effectiveness and minimizing potentiation of side effects.	
	Administer supplemental oxygen as indicated.	Provides additional oxygen for cellular uptake.	
	Review laboratory findings, e.g., ABGs, pulmonary function tests.	Identifies therapeutic needs, evaluates effectiveness of therapy.	
Anxiety, (specify level) related to perceived threat of death (difficulty breathing) as evidenced by apprehension, restlessness, increased muscle tension and focus on self.	Encourage "pursed lip" breathing.	Assists patient to "take control" of respiratory situation.	Reports anxiety reduced to a manageable level, and able to sleep/rest appropriately.
	Provide quiet environment, maintain calm confident manner.	Promotes rest/relaxation to enhance breathing.	
	Coordinate interventions/activities to allow for periods of undisturbed rest.	Activity increases O_2 requirements and may heighten anxiety.	
	Stay with patient during acute episodes of dyspnea.	Provides reassurance that help is immediately available should it be needed.	
	Acknowledge reality of situation and other concerns that may be present.	Physiologic anxiety is fearful and it is helpful to let the patient know it is all right to express feelings. Other anxieties are overshadowed by breathing problem.	
Knowledge deficit related to lack of information/misinterpretation, unfamiliarity with resources as evidenced by questions, statement of concern,	Explain function, use, storage and side effects of drugs as well as results of omitting medication.	Knowledge/understanding may enhance cooperation with therapeutic regimen and reduces frequency of problems/attacks.	Verbalizes understanding of condition/disease process and treatment. Initiates lifestyle changes as indicated.
	Demonstrate use of and provide written instructions	Maximizes deposition of the drug in the lungs. Provides	

Table 35–5. NURSING PROCESS FOR PATIENT REQUIRING BRONCHODILATOR THERAPY-*CONTINUED*

Nursing Diagnosis	Nursing Actions	Rationale	Desired Actions/ Evaluation Criteria
inaccurate follow through of instructions, development of preventable complications.	outlining correct use of aerosol delivery devices.	post-discharge reinforcement of inpatient instruction.	
	Develop medication schedule to meet individual needs.	Promotes optimal therapeutic effect and enhances cooperation with regimen.	
	Differentiate between expected/nuisance side effects versus untoward or toxic drug effects.	Promotes patient awareness/independence. Provides for timely intervention and prevention of complications.	
	Discuss importance of restricting use of OTC drugs, caffeine.	Many drugs are stimulants which increase catecholamine release in the body, accentuating stimulation effects of prescribed medications.	
	Identify non-caffeinated beverage choices to meet daily fluid needs.	May require up to 3000 cc/day to maintain hydration, liquify secretions and offset diuretic effects of theophylline.	
	Review relaxation techniques/stress management program.	Stress reduction can strengthen coping abilities and may help reduce/minimize asthma attacks.	
	Review diet and stress reduction needs to support the immune system.	Poor nutrition as well as stress in general may weaken the immune system, contributing to exacerbation of asthma attacks.	
	Identify environmental risks/pollutants affecting respiratory function.	Provides opportunity to control these factors as possible.	

often assumes an upright posture to maximize comfort and accessory-muscle efficiency. When bronchial obstruction is severe, the chest becomes hyperinflated and the patient moves little air with each breath. Panic and anxiety increases as breathing difficulty increases, giving way to fatigue in the extremely obstructed patient. Tachycardia and a rise in blood pressure accompany dyspnea.

The patient's breath sounds confirm the presence of airway obstruction, as well as indicate their cause and extent. Bronchial obstruction caused by bronchospasm results in wheezing. Almost always these high-pitched sounds occur bilaterally during exhalation. Mild to moderate bronchospasm causes relatively loud wheezing, whereas severe bronchospasm causes higher-pitched, quieter wheezes. A silent chest is an ominous sign, indicating very little air movement. A patient who is wheezing often describes his chest as feeling "tight."

Rumbling or gurgling sounds heard on auscultation indicate the presence of mucus in airways. This can be confirmed by an accompanying moist or productive cough. Since inflamed airways are narrower than normal, this condition also is heralded by wheezing. The patient with inflamed airways has a harsh, burning cough. When such a cough accompanies an elevated temperature, a bronchial infection is strongly suggested.

Laboratory tests and various measures of pulmonary function can be helpful. Infection can be confirmed by an elevated white blood cell count. Sputum samples can be cultured to identify the specific organisms causing the infection. Eosinophilia of the sputum or blood is common in asthma. Arterial blood gases can indicate whether obstruction is severe enough to impede oxygenation or ventilation.

Bronchial obstruction diminishes the flow of air from the lungs. Thus, prolonged exhalation time, decreased peak expiratory flow rate, and diminished vital capacity all indicate the presence of airway obstruction. Signs and symptoms of bronchial obstruction are outlined in Table 35–6.

NURSING DIAGNOSES

Possible nursing diagnoses for the patient who requires agents to counter bronchial obstruction include: (1) ineffective airway clearance, (2) ineffective breathing pattern, and (3) impaired gas exchange.

Table 35–6. SIGNS AND SYMPTOMS OF BRONCHIAL OBSTRUCTION

	Degree of Obstruction		
	Mild	**Moderate**	**Severe**
Breath sound	Wheezing on auscultation	Wheezing may be audible without stethoscope	All breath sounds greatly diminished
Use of accessory muscles	Minimal	Marked	Maximal
Dyspnea	Mild	Moderate	Severe
Respiratory pattern	Slightly elevated rate	Elevated rate, prolonged exhalation	Elevated rate, prolonged exhalation
Heart rate and pulse	Slightly elevated, strong pulse	Tachycardia, usually accompanied by bounding pulse	Tachycardia, pulse may be weak, thready
Mental status	Alert, may be anxious	Alert, often anxious and irritable	May be somnolent and/or disoriented

INTERVENTION

Once bronchial obstruction is recognized and its cause established, drug therapy is planned and implemented. Possible goals for nursing intervention are included in Table 35–5.

NURSING IMPLICATIONS

The nurse plays a pivotal role in determining the effectivenss of respiratory drug therapy. It is essential that the nurse be familiar with all routes of drug administration, including inhalation. This unique method of drug delivery has often been the duty of the respiratory therapist, but in many hospitals nurses are now administering aerosol medications. The advantages and disadvantages of aerosol therapy are listed in Table 35–7.

There are many types of aerosol delivery devices, but the nurse is likely to encounter metered-dose inhalers, small volume nebulizers, and the Spinhaler (Fig. 35–4). Metered-dose inhalers (MDIs) are compact, self-contained units powered by a small gas canister. They can be carried in a purse or pocket and are designed for self-administration of medication. They are very convenient, but do require good coordination of hand action with breathing. Use of a spacer or aerosol chamber can make MDI devices more effective. They deliver highly concentrated doses of medication, which makes overdosing relatively easy. And, because the medication they carry is so readily available, these units are prone to abuse. The uncooperative patient, the one who cannot inhale fully, or who is unable to coordinate inspiration with the compression of the MDI gas cartridge will not benefit from this device. Still, the MDI is very effective, and is appropriate for many patients.

Small-volume nebulizers (also called updraft or hand-held nebulizers) are powered by a wall oxygen flow-meter or small compressor. They are less portable than the MDI but far more effective for the patient with limited coordination. Unlike the MDI, which produces one short "puff" of medication at a time, these nebulizers provide a steady stream of aerosol medication. The medication is usually diluted so that overdosage is less likely to occur.

The Spinhaler is a specialized device used only to administer cromolyn sodium. This drug is supplied in capsules as a powder. Two small pins in the Spinhaler pierce the capsule. The patient's inhalation activates a propeller, which blows the cromolyn powder into the airways.

Regardless of the type of delivery system used, the primary goal of aerosol therapy is to maximize deposition of the drug in the patient's lungs. When administered improperly, aerosol medications will do little or no good. Shallow inspiration causes the medication to be deposited in the oropharynx. The drug will then be swallowed and will have no therapeutic effect. For maximal deposition of the drug the patient must inhale deeply, hold the breath for several seconds, and exhale slowly. Table 35–8 lists several points concerning delivery of aerosol medications.

It is essential that the nurse be familiar with the ef-

Table 35–7. MAJOR ADVANTAGES AND DISADVANTAGES OF AEROSOL MEDICATIONS

Advantages	**Disadvantages**
Administration route is relatively safe and convenient.	Imprecise method of administration, actual amount of drug delivered to lung varies.
Rapid onset of drug action.	
Self-medication is economical.	Patient cooperation and coordination are necessary for successful administration.
Relatively simple to administer.	
Local effects predominate and systemic side effects are minimized.	Some aerosol equipment is very expensive, requires specially trained personnel to operate.
	High potential for overuse due to availability.

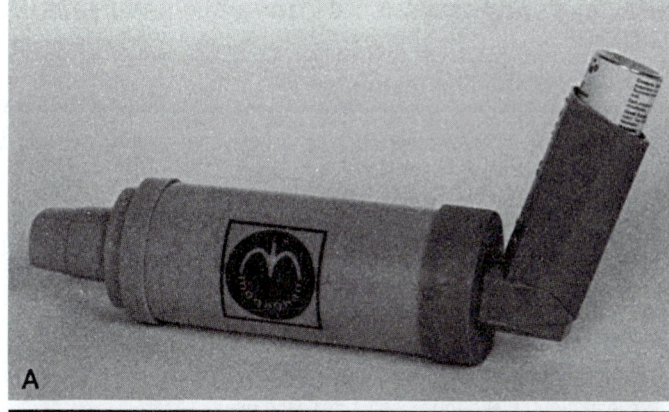

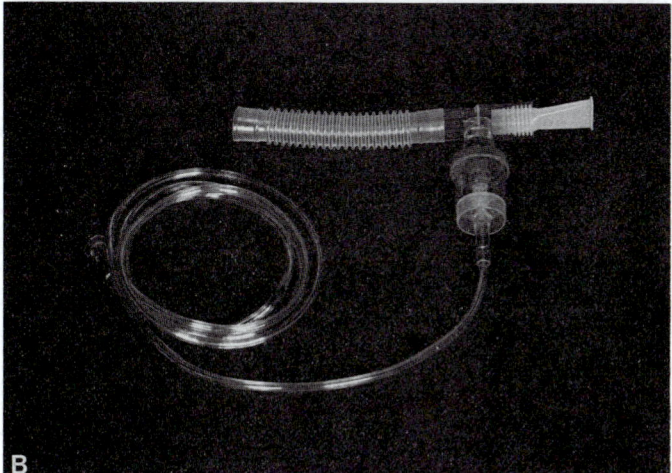

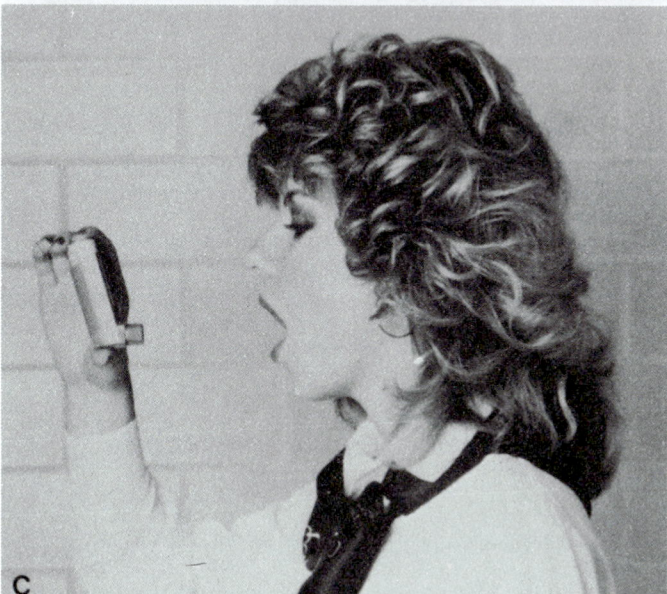

Figure 35–4, (A–C.) Delivery systems for aerosol medications. (A and B from Hess, D: Aerosolized drug delivery: Technical aspects. In Kacmarek, RM and Stoller, JK (Eds): Current Respiratory Care, BC Decker, Toronto, 1988, p 58, with permission. C from Petty, TL, and Nett, LM: Enjoying Life with Emphysema, ed. 2, Lea & Febiger, Philadelphia, 1987, p 45, with permission.)

fects of the bronchodilators. Despite different modes of action, these powerful agents are similar in their major side effects. All bronchodilators, regardless of type, can cause a substantial increase in heart rate. This is undesirable and potentially dangerous in the patient with cardiac problems. These patients can develop dysrhythmias that may be life-threatening. The nurse must closely monitor the pulse when administering any bronchodilator. An increase of 20% or greater is significant and may indicate a hypersenstive reaction to the drug. Patients with known cardiovascular problems who require bronchodilator therapy (especially theophylline) should be monitored for electrocardiogram abnormalities. This may require that the patient be treated in an

Table 35–8. AEROSOL MEDICATION DELIVERY SYSTEMS: INSTRUCTING THE PATIENT

Patient Should be Instructed to	Remarks/Rationale
I. GENERAL RULES FOR THE USE OF ALL TYPES OF AEROSOL MEDICATION DELIVERY SYSTEMS	
Sit upright, using good posture.	Good posture allows for most efficient use of diaphragm.
Keep chin level or pointed slightly upward.	This provides a direct route for medication to enter airways.
Hold nebulizer upright an inch from mouth; open mouth wide.	Ideally, this minimizes deposition of drug in mouth.
Exhale fully.	This allows for deeper inspiration.
Inspire deeply and slowly until lungs are full.	Steady inspiratory flow enhances even distribution of aerosol.
Hold breath for several seconds.	This helps maximize absorption of medication.
Clean mouthpiece thoroughly after each use.	This minimizes risk of infection and maximizes nebulizer efficiency (dirt in nebulizer diminishes its ability to produce proper aerosol).
II. SPECIAL INSTRUCTIONS FOR THE USE OF METERED-DOSE INHALER (MDI)	
Patient should be instructed to shake nebulizer cartridge.	This maximizes dispersion of medication in propellant; ensures uniform dosage delivery.
Begin deep and slow inspiration through mouth, depress cartridge fully.	''Puff'' of medication must be delivered at beginning of inspiration to ensure deposit of aerosol in distal airways; full depression of cartridge ensures delivery of complete dose; coordination of effort is vital for maximum effectiveness.
Wait 1–2 min before taking a second inhalation.	This allows medication from first puff to distribute; also, any reflex airway narrowing from first puff will have disappeared.
Take no more than 2 puffs.	Drugs in MDIs are highly concentrated—overdose occurs easily.
If the Patient Uses a Spacer (Aerosol Chamber)	
Shake canister well just before attaching it to the spacer.	Use of aerosol spacer simplifies administration of metered-dose aerosol medication. MDI is not easy to shake once it is attached.
Exhale into room while pressing the canister once to spray medication into the spacer.	Aerosol will be momentarily suspended in the chamber.
Inhale deeply from the spacer mouthpiece, hold inspiration for several seconds.	The chamber reduces the need for close coordination of manual efforts and inhalation. More aerosol is available for deposit in the distal airways, and less will be swallowed.
III. IF THE NEBULIZER IS POWERED BY COMPRESSOR, OR BY OXYGEN	
Use thumb regulator or tilt nebulizer on side for delivery of aerosol during inspiration only.	This will prevent wasting of medication.
Turn on compressor (if using oxygen from wall outlet) set flowmeter at 5–7 liters/min.	Sufficient flow is required to provide adequate nebulization.
IV. IF PATIENT IS USING A SPINHALER (FOR USE WITH CROMOLYN SODIUM)	
Insert cromolyn capsule into Spinhaler; puncture capsule only once by sliding the sleeve up and back; hold Spinhaler upright.	Puncturing the capsule more than once can cause powder to spill, as can holding Spinhaler improperly.
Hyperextend neck.	This allows patient to keep Spinhaler upright and provides a more direct route for inhaled powder.
Exhale fully into room, then place lips around Spinhaler and inhale sharply.	Do not exhale through Spinhaler; this causes powder to stick to the sides and decreases efficiency. Quick, but deep, inhalation propels power most efficiently.
Maintain inspiratory hold 3–4 sec; repeat until capsule is empty.	Inspiratory hold allows optimal deposition of cromolyn in airways; several inhalations may be needed to empty capsule.

intensive care setting. Other effects common to all types of bronchodilators include palpitations, nervousness, tremors, and occasionally nausea. The nurse monitors the patient for these signs.

Because of these side effects, special attention must be given to scheduling of drug doses. The nurse must adhere to a rigid schedule to minimize the potential of toxic effects, as well as to maximize the effectiveness of therapy. Observations the nurse makes after the first few doses serve as the basis for recommending dosage or schedule changes.

Bronchodilators may be given alone or in combination with other bronchodilators. Often theophylline is ordered along with a sympathomimetic or anticholinergic aerosol. Although this type of therapy may provide the patient with more effective bronchodilation, it greatly increases the risk of toxicity. If the patient is receiving aminophylline by continuous infusion, the dosage can be regulated on the basis of the serum level and observed effects. Often a lowered infusion rate can be used if the patient is also receiving aerosolized bronchodilators. If aminophylline is administered intravenously by intermittent infusion, the nurse must take special care to avoid administering the aerosol too soon after aminophylline. Ideally, the aerosolized bronchodilator should not be given any sooner than three hours after a bolus of aminophylline to minimize the possibility of severe cardiac side effects.

Although many bronchodilators are available in unit dose packages, most are also available in stock solutions. Because each drug is manufactured in different concentrations, the nurse must pay close attention to dilution specifications for each drug. Sympathomimetics are degraded by air and light, so containers are stored tightly capped in a dark place. Discolored solution should not be used.

The actions of bronchodilators are the most profound of the respiratory medications. The actions of inhaled corticosteroids are usually subtle and benign. They have been useful in allowing many patients to decrease their intake of systemically acting oral steroids. The nurse must be aware that although these agents help to open airways they are not the same as bronchodilators. It can be easy to mistake an MDI containing a steroid for one that contains a bronchodilator. During an attack or bronchospasm, the inhaled steroid will be useless and it may aggravate the condition, so care must be exercised when selecting the proper MDI for the patient.

Proper secretion removal is essential for effective mucokinetic therapy. Unless the airway is cleared, mucokinetic therapy is worthless; indeed, it is potentially harmful. Secretions that are liquefied can swell and coalesce, blocking airways and hindering gas exchange. The nurse best encourages mucokinesis by ensuring the patient is well hydrated and is coughing effectively. Often the patient who receives hydrating aerosols or a mucolytic will be unable to expectorate mucus immediately after a treatment. The nurse should return within a half-hour to encourage further coughing. Some patients may require further therapy, such as chest percussion, postural drainage, or suctioning, to facilitate secretion removal.

PATIENT TEACHING

The nurse plays an important role in helping the patient to obtain the greatest benefit from therapy. Table 35–9 lists several items the nurse educator should include in the teaching plan for each respiratory patient.

The nurse is responsible for helping the patient understand the disease and its treatment. The predisposing factors of the disease, reasons for changes in breathing, early signs of exacerbation, avoidance of deleterious substances or activities, and nonpharmacologic therapy are explained to the patient by the nurse. In addition,

---

Table 35–9. PATIENT TEACHING INFORMATION: AGENTS USED TO TREAT BRONCHIAL OBSTRUCTION

Dear Patient:
  This drug has been prescribed for you. This is what you should know about your drug to get the most from your therapy:

1. Bronchodilators are generally taken by adults for their entire lifetime. Children who use these drugs often outgrow the need for them before reaching adulthood.
2. Take your pulse before and after using a bronchodilator. If your pulse rises by more than 20–30 beats/min, tell your doctor.
3. Taking theophylline with meals may minimize stomach upset. Other bronchodilators can be taken with or without food.
4. If you are taking prescribed β-blockers or calcium-channel blockers, consult your doctor if your wheezing increases.
5. Do not use over-the-counter medications for breathing relief unless specifically authorized by your doctor. These medications have many undesirable side effects.
6. Stick to a strict dosage schedule; if you miss a dose of bronchodilator, **do not** double the next dose. Instead, take the missed dose and readjust the dosage schedule accordingly.
7. Do not stop taking your bronchodilator without the authorization of your doctor.
8. The side effects of nearly all bronchodilators include increased heart rate, palpitations, nervousness, tremors, and sweating.
9. If you must mix drugs, be sure to mix precisely according to your prescription.
10. Liquid mixtures of bronchodilators should be stored in the refrigerator.
11. Inhaled steroids or cromolyn sodium are not bronchodilators and are **not** to be used during an acute attack of wheezing. They may aggravate your symptoms.
12. Drink plenty of fluids to keep mucus easy to expectorate.

---

the nurse informs the patient of the basic actions and adverse effects of the prescribed medications. The nurse discusses fully the importance of a regular dosing schedule, anticipated interactions and their effects, the proper use of prn orders, and appropriate actions after side effects or interactions have been identified. This information helps to ensure patient safety in the hospital and after discharge.

EVALUATION

The goals of nursing intervention form the basis for the establishment of evaluation criteria. These criteria, which may be used to measure the effectiveness of therapy, are included in Table 35–5.

Compliance with the prescribed regimen is imperative for successful treatment of the respiratory patient. In the hospital the nurse is the primary locus of control for drug therapy. However, many hospitals allow some self-medication by patients. This makes it difficult for the nurse to determine with precision how fully the patient is complying with the medication plan. This is also a problem with the home-care patient. The complexity of the medication orders for these patients can cause confusion, frustration, and finally noncompliance. To ensure patient compliance with the prescribed regimen, and thereby maximize the medications' benefits, the nurse continually teaches and encourages the patient to take medications properly.

Many factors are considered in the evaluation of respiratory drugs' effectiveness. One of the best indicators of the success of therapy is the patient's subjective response. Many of the drugs that treat bronchial obstruction provide almost immediate relief of symptoms. The bronchodilator patient should be able to state quickly whether or not the drug has improved breathing. The patient using anti-inflammatory aerosol steroids will require a couple of doses to feel less burning in the chest. Mucokinetic agents should increase sputum volume and the ease with which it is expectorated.

Observations and objective measures of drug effectiveness are also used. With effective therapy, patient anxiety decreases. Other obvious indicators of respiratory distress, such as gasping, cold sweats, and use of accessory muscles, should decrease. Breath sounds improve: more air movement is heard and wheezing is diminished. Drier breath sounds, with fewer crackles and rhonchi, indicate effective mucokinesis. The volume of expectorated sputum increases.

If hypoxemia was present prior to therapy, the PaO_2 should increase significantly. If respiratory failure was evident, the patient's $PaCO_2$ should decrease toward the 35–45-mmHg range and arterial blood pH should be within the 7.35–7.45 range. Spriometric tests should improve: the patient's timed vital capacity, forced exhaled volume in one second (FEV_1), and peak expiratory flow should all increase.

Serum theophylline levels must be monitored if the patient is at added risk for developing toxicity, if the patient requires larger or more frequent doses for relief of bronchospasm, or if toxicity is suspected. A level of 10–20 μg/ml will usually provide adequate bronchodilation. Periodic assessment of serum theophylline levels and close observation of the patient for early signs of toxicity ensure safe drug administration. If signs of toxicity are evident, or if the serum level exceeds 20 μg/ml, the nurse withholds a dose. The physician is then notified and adjustments are made to the dosing schedule.

Since all bronchodilators can elevate heart rate, the nurse monitors the pulse closely. Hypersensitivity to the drug being administered or incipient toxicity raises the pulse 20 or more beats/min. In most patients an increase in heart rate from 80 to 100 beats/min is harmless. However, the added cardiovascular work could be dangerous to a patient with congestive heart failure or coronary artery disease. If a significant increase in pulse is noted, the treatment should be temporarily discontinued. The patient should be allowed to rest so the heart rate can return to its initial pace. If the patient's pulse rises abnormally after the treatment is resumed, the treatment should be stopped completely. The nurse notes the untoward reaction and the episode is discussed with the physician, who may be able to order an alternative medication.

Nausea may be an indicator of theophylline toxicity or it may be caused by local gastric irritation. Some patients with safe serum levels who complain of nausea may better tolerate the drug with food. In severe cases of nausea not caused by toxicity, an antiemetic can be given one half-hour before theophylline is administered.

The nurse also assesses other side effects of bronchodilatory therapy. Agitation, tremors, and flushing are relatively common minor effects. The nurse should become familiar with these and other expected side effects of these drugs. Recognition of serious adverse reactions is essential so that appropriate intervention can be instituted.

SUMMARY

Of major concern in respiratory pharmacology is the maintenance of airway patency. Breathing difficulty can result from bronchial smooth muscle spasm, edema caused by airway inflammation, or excessive mucus secretions. Bronchodilators are used to treat bronchospasm, aerosolized steroids can reduce airway edema, and mucokinetic agents can reduce the volume and viscosity of mucus.

The most important pharmacologic agents for the treatment of respiratory disorders are the bronchodilators. Inhaled agents—such as isoetharine, metaproterenol, terbutaline, or albuterol—and oral and parenteral preparations of theophylline are powerful drugs with a wide variety of systemic effects. Because several of these are potentially dangerous, the nurse administers these agents with great care and recognizes early signs of toxicity.

BIBLIOGRAPHY

Barnes, P: Using anticholinergics to best advantage. J Respir Dis 8:84–95, May 1987.
Byrd, R: A practical approach to nocturnal asthma. J Respir Dis 8:54–57, July 1987.
Drugs for asthma. Med Lett Drugs Ther 29(732) January 30, 1987.
Fanta, C: Corticosteroid therapy in asthma: The double-edged sword. J Respir Dis 8:75–86, November 1987.
Garrity, E and Gross, N: Prompt management for status asthmaticus. J Respir Dis 8:21–32, May 1987.
Shafouri, M, Patil, K, and Kass, I: Sputum changes associated with the use of ipratroprium bromide. Chest 86:387–393, September 1984.
Holgate, S: Role of mediators and inflammation in asthma. J Respir Dis 8:20–37, April 1987.
Jenne, J (ed): Rationale for the use of theophylline in COPD: Bronchodilation and beyond. Chest (Suppl) 92(1) July 1987.
McFadden, E: Cromolyn: First-line treatment for chronic asthma? J Respir Dis 8:39–48, January 1987.
O'Bryne, P, Hargreave, F, and Kirby, J: Airway inflammation and hyper-responsiveness. Am Rev Respir Dis (Suppl) 136(4 part 2):535–537, October 1987.

Petty, T: Drug strategies for airflow obstruction. Am J Nurs 87:180–184, February 1987.

Soffer, A (ed): Neurohumoral mechanisms in obstructive airway disease: Role of inhaled anticholinergic agents. Chest (Suppl) 91(5) May 1987.

Svedmyr, N: Theophylline. Am Rev Respir Dis (Suppl) 136(4 part 2):568–570, October 1987.

Tashkin, D, et al: Comparison of the anticholinergic bronchodilator ipratroprium bromide with metaproterenol in chronic obstuctive pulmonary disease: A 90-day multi-center study. Am J Med 81:59–68, November 1986.

Tattersfield, A: Effect of beta-agonists and anticholinergic drugs on bronchial reactivity. Am Rev Respir Dis (Suppl) 136(4 part 2):564–567, October 1987.

Wilson, M and Larsen, G: Gaining control over the late asthmatic response. J Respir Dis 7:51–60, August 1986.

Ziment, I and Au, J: Making the best use of aminophylline in the ICU. J Crit Illness 1:21–32, November 1986.

Zwillich, C: Asthma therapy: An update. Respir Ther 16:13–17, March/April 1986.

SITUATION   35–1

Teruyo Sakamoto, aged 45, has a history of asthma. He presents to the emergency with shortness of breath.

1. An aminophylline infusion has been ordered for Mr. Sakamoto, and plans are to admit him to the medical unit. After a loading dose, the maintenance infusion dose of aminophylline should be:
   a. 10 to 20 mcg/kg/hr
   b. 0.2 to 0.9 mg/kg/hr
   c. .8 to 15 mcg/kg/min
   d. 1.0 to 5.0 mg/kg/hr

2. Twenty-four hours later, Mr. Sakamoto is breathing easier. A serum theophylline level is drawn. Which of the following values represents a therapeutic level?
   a. 18 mcg/ml   c. 4 mcg/ml
   b. 25 mcg/ml   d. 30 mcg/ml

3. Mr. Sakamoto begins theophylline anhydrous and is weaned off of intravenous aminophylline. The nurse will be aware of the following precaution or oral theophylline:
   a. glaucoma
   b. pseudomembranous colitis
   c. gastric bleeding
   d. photosensitivity

4. When administering oral theophylline, the nurse will observe Mr. Sakamoto for the following side effect:
   a. difficulty voiding
   b. drowsiness
   c. palpitations
   d. confusion

5. Mr. Sakamoto is to be discharged on Theodur 200 mg orally twice a day. Patient teaching for him will include the following information:
   a. Limit intake of caffeine.
   b. Increase intake of high calcium foods.
   c. Take only on an empty stomach.
   d. Reduce oral fluid intake.

6. The dosage of theophylline may need to be altered if Mr. Sakamoto:
   a. take steroids
   b. operates machinery
   c. lifts weights
   d. smokes cigarettes

SITUATION   35–2

Pierre St. Phillip is a 62-year-old with chronic bronchitis, who has undergone a colon resection for cancer. Postoperatively he complains to the nurse of "tightness" in his chest.

1. When assessing Mr. St. Phillip for evidence of bronchial obstruction, the nurse would observe for:
   a. bronchial breath sounds
   b. use of accessory muscles
   c. slowed pulse
   d. prolonged inspiration

2. Mr. St. Phillip is to receive terbutaline sulfate inhaler 2 puffs every 4 to 6 hours. After administration of this drug, the nurse will monitor:
   a. muscle strength
   b. pupil reaction
   c. reflexes
   d. heart rate

3. Which of the following nursing interventions is most appropriate for Mr. St. Phillip concerning terbutaline therapy?
   a. Restrict oral fluids.
   b. Monitor arterial blood gases.
   c. Measure abdominal girth.
   d. Check pupils every 1 hour.

4. Bronchoconstriction improves, and two days later, Mr. St. Phillip is scheduled to receive beclomethasone (Vanceril) 1 puff four times a day (qid). In order to safeguard against side effects of this drug, the nurse will instruct him to:

   a. rinse mouth after each dose
   b. take benadryl before each dose
   c. cough with force after using
   d. avoid inhaling deeply after using.

5. When administering the inhalants to Mr. St. Phillip, the nurse will see that he:
   a. lies in a semi-Fowler's position
   b. holds chin in a downward position
   c. holds breath for several seconds after instilling medication
   d. places nebulizer directly to lips and closes mouth tightly

6. Which of the following statements by Mr. St. Phillip indicates the need for further teaching concerning the use of beclomethasone via metered-dose inhaler?
   a. "I should fully inhale before depressing the cartridge."
   b. "I should wait 1 to 2 minutes before taking a second inhalation."
   c. "It is best to use only one to two puffs at a dosage schedule."
   d. "The nebulizer cartridge should be shaken well before using."

Please refer to the Appendices for correct answers and additional review questions with answers.

GLOSSARY TERMS IN THIS CHAPTER
Analeptic
Antitussive
Atelectasis
Crackles
Cyanosis
Dead space
Hypoxemia
Hypoxia
Minute volume
Oxygen toxicity
Oxygen-induced hypoventilation
Rales
Retrolental fibroplasia
Rhonchi
Tidal volume
Wheeze

MISCELLANEOUS RESPIRATORY AGENTS

ROBERT W. HIRNLE, M.S., R.R.T.

LEARNING OBJECTIVES

After reading this chapter the student will be able to:

1. Identify medications that have been used as respiratory stimulants.

2. Differentiate the various mechanisms of action, routes of administration, pharmacokinetics, adverse effects, contraindications, and interactions among medications that affect the respiratory system.

3. Identify specific areas to assess in the patient who requires respiratory system medications in order to formulate appropriate nursing diagnoses.

4. Plan the nursing interventions necessary to administer respiratory system medications and choose appropriate teaching strategies to gain patient compliance.

5. Evaluate the patient at appropriate intervals during treatment to gauge nursing interventions.

THERAPEUTIC AGENTS

Perhaps the broadest category of respiratory therapy medications are those that affect the patency of the bronchial tubes. There are, however, a number of therapeutic agents that affect the respiratory system in other ways. These are discussed in this chapter. Among the most important are respiratory stimulants, oxygen, and antitussives (cough medicines).

RESPIRATORY STIMULANTS

Through the years medicine has sought ways to help persons who are unable to breathe sufficiently. Many pharmacologic agents have been used for the purpose of stimulating a more effective breathing pattern in these people. While a few of these agents have shown some degree of efficacy, their adverse effects have made them undesirable for general use. Some of these drugs have been relatively safe, but their short duration of action and their expense have made them impractical. In addition, nonpharmacologic methods of maintaining breathing (such as mechanical ventilation and adjunctive support of cardiovascular function) are safer and more effective. For these reasons the use of respiratory stimulants has been limited to a few specific clinical conditions. (See Table 36–1 for a summary of the respiratory stimulants.)

Respiratory stimulants may be used occasionally in the recovery room to counteract the depressant effects of anesthesia on the respiratory center. They can also be used to counter respiratory depression caused by narcotics, barbiturates, carbon monoxide, electroshock therapy, or severe heart failure. They have been used with some success in cases of oxygen-induced hypoventilation, and certain agents have been useful in treating apnea of the premature newborn. In some cases respiratory stimulants have helped to increase ventilatory capability of patients with COPD. Oral preparations of these compounds have proved ineffective; thus, they are useful only in a short-term critical care situation.

There has been no agreement about the value of these agents, although it seems a tendency toward their obsolescence may have begun. Their use in major hospitals appears to be declining, but many physicians still prescribe them regularly.

For a discussion on assessment, intervention, and evaluation of therapy in barbiturate overdose, see Chapter 13. Oxygen-induced hypoventilation is discussed in this chapter.

The majority of the most significant respiratory stimulants are classified as *analeptics*. Included in this category are doxapram and xanthines such as caffeine and theophylline. These agents exert a "restorative" effect to the respiratory system. They act primarily upon the central nervous system (CNS). The respiratory centers of the pons and medulla are stimulated by these drugs, but only as a secondary effect of this action. The exact mode of action by which analeptics operate is not yet known. The clinical response is related directly to the size of the dosage received. Because analeptics are potentially capable of precipitating seizures, great care must be taken in the administration of these substances. Other adverse reactions associated with the use of these drugs are hypertension, tachycardia, tremors, vomiting, arrhythmias, flushing, and diaphoresis. The undesirable CNS effects may be counteracted by concurrent administration of diazepam. Doxapram and phosphodiesterase inhibitors such as caffeine or theophylline are presently used as analeptic respiratory stimulants. Analeptic drugs are **not** to be used to reverse narcotic overdose. When used to counteract narcotics, analeptics can cause convulsions.

CARBON DIOXIDE. The primary nonanaleptic respiratory stimulant is carbon dioxide. This gas causes increased ventilation by activating the chemoreceptors. These specialized nerves are directly sensitive to the level of carbon dioxide in the blood and to alterations in blood pH caused by changes in $Paco_2$. A slight elevation in $Paco_2$ or drop in pH will stimulate the chemoreceptors, which will cause the respiratory centers to increase the rate and depth of ventilation.

Uses. Carbon dioxide is administered by means of a mask in combination with oxygen. The most common mixture is 95% oxygen with 5% carbon dioxide. Possible uses for carbon dioxide therapy include postanesthesia hypoventilation, severe anxiety reaction, and hiccoughs. Treatments should be no longer than six minutes, and the patient should be monitored closely. The treatment should be discontinued as soon as ventilation increases. If the patient becomes nauseated, dyspneic, dizzy, or hypertensive, the treatment should be stopped immediately.

Carbon dioxide should not be used for the patient who has oxygen-induced hypoventilation. Nor should it be used for any patient who is a known carbon dioxide retainer. Many such patients have become gradually desensitized to carbon dioxide as a breathing stimulant, and in these patients this gas acts as a depressant. Additional carbon dioxide will contribute to their hypoventilation and will further aggravate any acidosis.

Because it is expensive and inconvenient to administer, carbon dioxide is rarely used as a treatment to stimulate breathing. A simple paper bag for rebreathing exhaled air is much cheaper and usually just as effective.

Miscellaneous Respiratory Stimulants

Several hormones have been studied for their ventilatory effects, including adrenocorticotropic hormone (ACTH), thyroxine, and catecholamines. The hormone which has demonstrated the most interesting effect has been progesterone. Oral medroxyprogesterone acetate (Provera) has been used to stimulate the respiratory drive. This hormone seems to act by increasing the responsiveness of the respiratory center to carbon dioxide, as well as by decreasing its excitability threshold. It may also cause a heightened response of the peripheral chemoreceptors to hypoxemia. The hormone has been used with some success in the treatment of alveolar hypoventilation, particularly when caused by metabolic alkalosis or morbid obesity.

Finally, methylxanthine agents such as caffeine and theophylline have been used to treat pathologic apnea in the newborn. It is not uncommon for newborns, especially premature babies, to breathe with periodic episodes of apnea. However, when apnea becomes prolonged or occurs frequently, it must be treated. Theophylline has proved to be more easily regulated than caffeine, and is thus more frequently administered. It is thought that theophylline can stimulate diaphragmatic contraction, which may account for its ability to increase ventilation in the baby.

Using the Nursing Process

ASSESSMENT OF THE PATIENT WHO REQUIRES A RESPIRATORY STIMULANT. Inadequate ventilation is indicated by both subjective and objective signs. The patient with slow, shallow breathing who is difficult to rouse and reacts slowly and who is known to be at risk for hypoventilation should be closely monitored. A respirometer is used to measure *minute volume.* Adults normally breathe between five and eight liters of air each minute, depending upon their size. A minute volume that is lower than normal indicates possible hypoventilation. This is confirmed by arterial blood gas analysis. If the patient's $Paco_2$ has risen and pH has fallen, hypoventilation is present. If the decision is made to attempt to stimulate respiration pharmacologically, provisions are also made for initiating mechanical ventilation should the attempt fail.

NURSING DIAGNOSES. A possible nursing diagnosis for a patient who requires a respiratory stimulant is ineffective breathing pattern.

Intervention. The primary goal of intervention with respiratory stimulants is an increase in the patient's minute volume. Hypoventilation can cause severe acid–base disturbances, hypoxia, cardiac dysrhythmias, and possible cardiorespiratory arrest. Other intervention goals are stated in Table 36–2.

These little-used agents should be administered in an intensive care setting. Because many adverse effects are associated with these drugs, the nurse must monitor the patient closely and frequently for signs of toxicity.

EVALUATION. Criteria for evaluating the effectiveness of respiratory stimulant therapy are included in Table 36–2. By measuring the patient's minute volume the nurse is able to determine whether the patient is breathing more deeply or more rapidly. The patient's *tidal volume* (the amount of air moved with each breath) and the total minute volume should be greater than they were before drug therapy was initiated. It is important that both be larger, because an increase in minute volume alone would probably be insufficient to increase alveolar ventilation. A faster breathing frequency may contribute only to *dead space* ventilation (or, the delivery of air to non–gas exchanging areas of the lung). This increased frequency is undesirable because it simply adds to the work of breathing without improving gas exchange.

There are many adverse effects associated with analeptics, so the patient receiving them must be closely monitored. Hyperexcitability, dysrhythmias, hyperten-

sion, and seizures may occur with these drugs. When the patient is being treated for barbiturate overdose, close and prolonged observation is needed. The nurse must see that the effects of the overdosed drug have actually vanished, and have not only been masked by the analeptic.

The nurse remains with the patient who is receiving inhalation therapy with carbon dioxide gas. If success in increasing tidal and minute volume is achieved, the treatment should be stopped. Signs of toxicity, including disorientation, dyspnea, nausea, and tremors, indicate that the treatment should be stopped immediately, whether successful or not. If the patient does not exhibit toxic effects, the treatment can be continued for up to ten minutes.

OXYGEN

Regardless of how one defines the terms "medication" and "drug," oxygen most certainly qualifies as both. It is administered to achieve specific therapeutic goals, it causes identifiable physiologic effects, it should be administered in precise doses, and it can cause potentially fatal side effects. Nonetheless, oxygen administration is too often treated casually by nurses and physicians. Oxygen is a drug, and the nurse should be knowledgeable about its purpose, its limitations, and its safe delivery.

Oxygen is essential for life. It enters the blood through the millions of respiratory units of the lung. Oxygenated blood is pumped from the lungs to all the body's tissues. The oxygen diffuses from the blood into the tissues, where it is used in the mitochondria of cells for the oxidation of glucose.

The amount of oxygen that is available to the tissues is indicated by its partial pressure in arterial blood, or Pao_2. Healthy persons normally have a Pao_2 between 80 and 100 mmHg. If the Pao_2 is lower than this, *hypoxemia* is said to be present. This condition is potentially dangerous, since it can result in *hypoxia,* or tissue oxygen deprivation. The purpose of oxygen therapy is to treat acute or chronic hypoxemia.

A number of lung diseases can cause hypoxemia. If the airways are narrowed and a sufficient flow of air cannot be maintained in the lungs, then oxygen availability to the alveoli is limited and hypoxemia occurs. The obstructive diseases, such as emphysema, asthma, or bronchitis, can cause hypoxemia in this fashion. If alveolar tissues become thickened through inflammation or exudation, oxygen is unable to pass readily into the blood. Smoke inhalation, pneumonia, and pulmonary fibrosis are conditions that cause hypoxemia by this mechanism.

Supplemental oxygen therapy for these problems can provide the oxygen required for homeostasis. Room air contains 21% oxygen; when the amount of oxygen inspired by the patient is increased, more oxygen is available to enter the blood. The resulting rise in Pao_2 can reverse hypoxemia, and thus guard against hypoxia.

While oxygen is used most often to treat hypoxemia,

TEXT RESUMES ON PAGE 960

Table 36–1. RESPIRATORY STIMULANTS

Name	Dosage	Mode of Administration	Pharmacokinetics
Caffeine			
Action: stimulation of CNS, including respiratory centers of brain stem.			
Use: for treatment of alveolar hypoventilation and/or apnea secondary to respiratory center depression.			
	Neonatal: Loading dose: 10 mg/kg. Maintenance: 2.5 mg/kg. once daily Adults - 500 mg IV (not rec- ommended)	PO, IM, IV	O: rapid P: 1–2 hr D: depends on serum level ½L: 3.5 hr (adults) PB: <20% B: liver E: urine
Doxapram (Dopram)			
Action: same as above.			
Use: same as above.			
	0.5–2 mg/kg (IV injection) or 1.0–3.0 mg/min by IV infu- sion. (maximum dose 3 g) (repeated doses may be given after a rest period of 30 min to 2 hr).	IV	O: 2 min P: UA D: 5–12 min ½L: UA PB: UA B: liver E: metabolites in urine

Key to Abbreviations in the *Pharmacokinetics* column O-onset; P-peak; D-duration; PB-protein bound; B-bio-transformed in; E-excreted in; ½L-halflife.
*Within the column listing adverse effects, underlines indicate the most common effects; CAPITALS indicate life-threatening effects.

Contraindications/Precautions	Adverse Effects*	Interactions	Nursing Implications
Doses in excess of 1 g may accentuate adverse effects; in preterm infants paradoxical depression of respiration may occur.	CNS: restlessness, insomnia, tremors, headache Resp: increased rate and depth of breathing CV: tachycardia, palpitations, hypertension GI: nausea EENT: tinnitus GU: diuresis	Antagonizes barbiturates, narcotics, alcohol; potentiates theophylline.	ASSESSMENT: Closely observe respiratory pattern. Frequent apneic periods that are 20 sec long are pathologic. Monitor for CNS hyper-reactivity. INTERVENTION: Ensure patency of airway. Maintain cardiac and respiratory monitoring. Have equipment for intubation and mechanical ventilation available. EVALUATION: Effectiveness of this drug as a respiratory stimulant is evaluated in terms of a decrease in frequency and length of apneic periods.
Contraindicated in epilepsy, head injury, CVA, acute asthma, pulmonary embolus, pneumothorax, heart failure, neuromuscular disorders, coronary artery disease, extreme dyspnea, airway obstruction. Monitor blood pressure closely to prevent overdose. Infuse slowly to prevent possible hemolysis. Overdosage may result in convulsions.	CNS: hyperexcitability, flushing, paresthesias, dizziness, tremors, SEIZURES, headache, disorientation, hyper-reflexia CV: hypertension, tachycardia, chest pain, arrhythmias Resp: cough, bronchospasm, laryngospasm, hiccoughs, dyspnea GI: nausea, vomiting, diarrhea Other: decreased Hg and Hct, urinary retention, incontinence	Anesthetic agents such as halothane or enflurane may enhance the dysrhythmia-inducing capability of doxapram. May potentiate effects of MAO inhibitors and sympathomimetics. Adverse effects may be potentiated by other CNS stimulants. May potentiate CNS effects of amantadine.	ASSESSMENT: Closely monitor heart rate and blood pressure, deep tendon reflexes, and ECG pattern. Ensure patent airway. Monitor arterial blood gases at regular intervals. Check infusion rate frequently. Signs of toxicity, including tachycardia, hyper- or hypotension, tremors, or spasticity. INTERVENTION: Discontinue drug if sudden dyspnea or obvious toxicity occurs. Delay use of doxapram for 15 min after halothane or enflurane have been stopped. Stop IV immediately if extravasation occurs to avoid thrombophlebitis. If respiratory efforts increase but Paco₂ rises, consider intubation and mechanical ventilation. Mix only with saline or dextrose in water to avoid precipitation. Observe for at least 1 hr after infusion to prevent hypoventilation after effects wear off.

CONTINUED ON THE FOLLOWING PAGE

Respiratory Stimulants

Table 36–1. RESPIRATORY STIMULANTS–*CONTINUED*

Name	Dosage	Mode of Administration	Pharmacokinetics
Doxapram–*Continued*			
Carbon Dioxide (CO_2, Carbogen)			

Action: stimulates central and peripheral chemoreceptors, increasing efferent impulses to respiratory centers.

Use: same as above.

Name	Dosage	Mode of Administration	Pharmacokinetics
	Up to 7% CO_2 in oxygen mixture for 5–10 min.	Inhalation by snug-fitting non-rebreathing mask.	O: immediate P: UA D: primarily throughout treatment ½L: UA PB: 0 B: carried as dissolved gas and as bicarbonate E: lungs

Key to Abbreviations in the *Pharmacokinetics* column O-onset; P-peak; D-duration; PB-protein bound; B-biotransformed in; E-excreted in; ½L-halflife.
  *Within the column listing adverse effects, underlines indicate the most common effects; CAPITALS indicate life-threatening effects.

it is also useful in the treatment of a number of other conditions. Supplemental oxygen can help to reduce the work of the myocardium; thus, it is valuable in the treatment of patients with cardiac conditions. It is also able to reduce the work of breathing in certain dyspneic patients. Many of the conditions that are improved by oxygen therapy are listed in Table 36–3.

For most patients, routine oxygen therapy presents relatively few risks. However, besides the fire hazard posed by oxygen, there are a number of dangers involved in its use. High oxygen concentrations administered for long periods are toxic, and lung damage can result *(oxygen toxicity)*. Premature infants who require intensive oxygen therapy are at risk for development of

retrolental fibroplasia, which can result in blindness. And, if certain patients with chronic obstructive pulmonary disease (COPD) receive too much oxygen, they may experience *oxygen-induced hypoventilation*, which can lead to respiratory and cardiac arrest. These and other adverse effects are discussed further in the Evaluation section of this chapter.

Using the Nursing Process

ASSESSMENT OF THE PATIENT WHO REQUIRES OXYGEN THERAPY. Each of the conditions listed in Table 36–3 is often treated successfully with oxygen. Although milder forms of these diseases may resolve with-

Contraindications/ Precautions	Adverse Effects*	Interactions	Nursing Implications
			EVALUATION: The effectiveness of this drug as a respiratory stimulant is evaluated in terms of increased tidal volume and respiratory rate. ADDITIONAL NOTES: Although seldom used, doxapram is regarded as the safest and most effective of the respiratory stimulants.
Contraindicated in patient with head injury (carbon dioxide dilates cerebral vessels). Carbon dioxide must never be given to patient with unresponsive respiratory center. Fatal acidosis and hypercapnia may result. It is thus not recommended for COPD patients.	CNS: headache, dizziness, mental depression, paresthesias, flushing, disorientation, CONVULSIONS, RESPIRATORY DEPRESSION WITH OD CV: hypertension, ARRHYTHMIAS, HYPOTENSION, and CARDIAC ARREST WITH OD Resp: dyspnea GI: nausea	Barbiturates may prevent CO_2 from stimulating respiration (respiratory depression effects may be enhanced).	ASSESSMENT: Note breathing rate and depth. Note skin color, and observe closely for toxic effects. Check gas contents: mixture must have no less than 93% oxygen. INTERVENTION: Discontinue treatment as soon as respiratory efforts increase, or as soon as toxicity is apparent. Discontinue treatment if $Paco_2$ rises above 45 mm Hg without additional respiratory effort. EVALUATION: Effectiveness of CO_2 as a respiratory stimulant is evaluated in terms of increased rate and depth of breathing. Effectiveness of CO_2 as a treatment for hiccoughs is evaluated in terms of cessation of hiccoughs.

out supplemental oxygen, it is important to minimize the danger of hypoxia. Used judiciously, oxygen can help to prevent hypoxia.

The nurse is often the first person to recognize the need for oxygen therapy in a patient. It is therefore essential that the nurse be skilled in assessment of the patient's oxygenation status. The need for supplemental oxygen can be determined by a systematic evaluation of clinical signs and by an understanding of the patient's underlying disease.

The most obvious indicator of oxygenation status is the patient's respiratory pattern. Hypoxemia is usually accompanied by shortness of breath, rapid and shallow breathing, and dyspnea on exertion. The simple presence of any or all of these signs is insufficient reason to begin oxygen therapy, but it does indicate that further investigation is needed. *Cyanosis,* or a bluish coloration of the skin and mucous membranes, is a sign of severe hypoxemia, but it may be absent in mild or moderate cases, or in the anemic patient. The hypoxemic patient may exhibit pallor of the skin, and may be diaphoretic.

Other indicators of possible hypoxemia include cardiovascular, pulmonary, and neurologic changes:

1. Cardiovascular effects:
   a. Pulse: initially, tachycardia will occur with bounding pulse in early, mild to moderate hypoxemia; severe hypoxemia will cause bradycardia with weak "thready" pulse
   b. Blood pressure: mild or moderate hypoxemia may result in a slight elevation of blood pressure; hypotension will occur when hypoxemia is severe
   c. Rhythm: premature ventricular contractions (PVCs) may occur with increasing frequency as

Table 36–2. NURSING PROCESS FOR PATIENT REQUIRING RESPIRATORY STIMULANTS

Assessment

Auscultate chest for character of breath sounds, presence of secretions.
Note type of breathing pattern: tachypnea, Cheyne-Stokes, other irregular patterns.
Determine underlying cause for breathing difficulty, e.g., depressant effects of anesthesia, narcotics, barbiturates, carbon monoxide, electroshock therapy, or severe heart failure.
Review laboratory findings, e.g., ABGs, drug screen, and respiratory vital capacity/tidal volume.

Nursing Diagnosis	Nursing Actions	Rationale	Desired Outcomes/ Evaluation Criteria
Breathing pattern ineffective related to decreased lung expansion, tracheo-bronchial obstruction, alteration of normal O_2/ CO_2 ratio as evidenced by shortness of breath, dyspnea, cyanosis, nasal flaring, tachypnea, use of accessory muscles, altered chest excursion.	Administer analeptic drugs, e.g., doxapram and xanthines such as caffeine and theophyl-line. Observe response to drug, development of adverse effects, e.g., seizures, hypertension, tachycardia, tremors, vomiting, dysrhythmias, and diaphoresis.	These respiratory stimu-lants exert a so-called "restorative" effect to the respiratory system and act primarily on the central nervous system. Analeptic drugs are not used to reverse narcotic overdose.	Establishes a normal/ effective respiratory pat-tern. Free of cyanosis and other signs and symptoms of hypoxia with AGBs within patient's normal range.
	Administer carbon dioxide via mask with oxygen as indicated.	This non-analeptic respi-ratory stimulant causes increased ventilation by activating the chemore-ceptors.	
	Monitor infusion of dox-apram solutions closely.	Rapid administration may cause hemolysis, while extravasation can lead to thrombophlebitis.	
	Remain with patient and note signs of toxicity, e.g., disorientation, dys-pnea, and tremors. Stop treatment immediately if these signs appear.	Provides opportunity to observe success or fail-ure of treatment and to stop if tidal and minute volume is achieved, or if toxic effects are noted.	
	Assist patient to take slower/deeper respira-tions.	Promotes individual "con-trol" of the situation.	
	Have patient breathe into a paper bag.	Usually this method satis-factorily reverses hyper-ventilation.	
	Measure minute volume as indicated.	Determines whether patient is breathing more deeply or rapidly.	

severity of hypoxia increases; dysrhythmias will occur as cardiac hypoxia worsens

2. Pulmonary effects:
   a. Adventitious breath sounds such as *rales (crackles), rhonchi* (rumbles), or *wheezes* (whistles) may be indicative of lung problems that can cause hypoxemia

3. Neurologic effects:
   a. Restlessness and agitation, confusion, sleep disturbances, euphoria, slurred speech, lassitude, and intellectual impairment occur in varying degrees with mild to moderate hypoxemia; depression and paranoia may occur with chronic oxygen lack. Severe hypoxemia will cause obtundation and coma.

It must be noted that these signs and symptoms may occur without hypoxemia—or hypoxia—being present. It may also be true that either or both of these problems may be present without obvious signs. The nurse sometimes needs to rely upon knowledge of the patient's overall condition and upon clinical judgment to determine the need for further evaluation. If it appears to be warranted, an arterial blood sample is drawn and analyzed.

Arterial blood sampling, when performed by trained personnel, is a relatively safe and reliable means for assessing the patient's oxygenation status. However, it should be judiciously ordered since it is also an invasive procedure which is moderately uncomfortable and is not inexpensive for the patient. In addition to providing

Table 36–3. INDICATIONS FOR OXYGEN THERAPY

Cardiovascular Problems

Congestive Heart failure
Cardiac Dysrhythmias
Myocardial Infarction
Shock
Hemorrhage
Tachycardia
Unstable blood pressure

Oxygen Transport Problems

Severe anemia
Hemoglobinopathies (such as sickle-cell crisis, methemo-globinemia)
Carbon Monoxide poisoning
Cyanide poisoning
Decreased Pa_{O_2}
Evidence of hypoxia, such as pallor, cyanosis, restless-ness, and confusion

Pulmonary Problems

Obstructive disorders (such as asthma, emphysema, COPD)
Restrictive disorders (such as severe pneumonia, fibrosis, inhalation pneumonitis)
Pulmonary embolism
Pulmonary edema
Respiratory failure
Adventitious lung sounds

information about oxygen levels, an arterial blood sample can show acid–base and ventilation status.

Severity of hypoxemia can be classified by Pa_{O_2}. Table 36–4 shows the range of values associated with mild, moderate, and severe hypoxemia. These ranges are always interpreted in light of the patient's underlying condition. For example, while mild hypoxemia may be easily tolerated by a young, otherwise healthy patient, it can seriously endanger the patient who has had a myocardial infarction.

Table 36–4. CLASSIFICATION OF HYPOXEMIA

Degree	Pa_{O_2} Range
Normal (no hypoxemia)	80–100 mmHg*
Mild	60–80 mmHg
Moderate	40–60 mmHg
Severe	<40 mmHg

*Deduct 1 mmHg per year over age 60; eg — normal Pa_{O_2} for a 70-year-old is 70–100 mmHg
NOTE: Interpretation of hypoxia must not be based solely upon Pa_{O_2}, but also on the patient's overall clinical status. Other data, such as acid-base status, hemoglobin/hematocrit, oxygen saturation, and temperature all must be considered.
(Adapted from *Clinical Application of Respiratory Care*, 3rd ed., by Barry Shapiro, Ronald Harrison, Robert Kacmarek, and Roy Cane; Year Book Medical Publishers, Co. Chicago; 1985 with permission.)

NURSING DIAGNOSES. A possible nursing diagnosis for the patient who requires oxygen therapy is impaired gas exchange.

INTERVENTION. Nursing goals related to oxygen therapy are included in Table 36–5. Oxygen therapy can be initiated for any patient for short periods provided reasonable precautions are taken. Table 36–6 shows general rules for safe oxygen administration.

Caution must be observed for any patient with known or suspected carbon dioxide retention. This may include patients with status asthmaticus, cystic fibrosis, or COPD. For these patients, only low concentrations of oxygen (24 to 28 percent by venturi type mask, or one to three liters per minute via nasal cannula) should be given for distress. If this is insufficient to relieve distress, the patient's arterial blood gas status is evaluated. If a higher oxygen concentration is required for maintenance of reasonable blood gas values, the patient may need to be more closely monitored in an intensive care setting.

Patients without chronic lung disease are able to tolerate higher oxygen concentrations, although the general rule for all patients should be "as little as possible for as brief a time as possible." Obviously, severe respiratory distress should always be treated with oxygen while a thorough assessment is being conducted. Once the patient's actual oxygenation status has been determined, oxygen therapy can be adjusted accordingly. While it is perhaps ideally preferable to be able to obtain a "room-air baseline" blood gas, the nurse must be able to judge whether the withholding of oxygen for this purpose is safe and justified. If there is any question about the stability of the patient's condition, then it is better to begin oxygen without the benefit of baseline values. Acting upon the side of safety can avert a potential crisis.

Table 36–7 shows the capabilities of several oxygen administration devices. Some of these devices are shown in Figures 36–1 through 36–4.

EVALUATION. Criteria for evaluating the effectiveness of the nursing intervention are included in Table 36–5. The effectiveness of oxygen therapy can be determined by close monitoring of the patient's clinical status. There should be improvement in the physical signs of respiratory distress. Among the objective indicators of improved oxygenation are a stable and decreased heart rate, decreased breathing rate, and improved color. The patient's subjective feeling of lessened anxiety and a more relaxed appearance also indicate improvement.

Effective oxygen therapy should eliminate dangerous hypoxemia. As long as the patient is not a chronic carbon dioxide retainer, a major goal of oxygen therapy is to restore Pa_{O_2} to within normal limits for the patient's age. There is no advantage to maintaining a Pa_{O_2} of greater than 100 mmHg in the adult patient, and to do so can eventually be harmful. If the patient is capable of maintaining Pa_{O_2} above 80 mmHg without supplemental oxygen, it is unlikely that further oxygen therapy is needed.

For the CO_2-retaining patient, the Pa_{O_2} is kept in the

Table 36–5. NURSING PROCESS FOR PATIENT REQUIRING OXYGEN

Assessment

Assess respiratory rate; note use of accessory muscles, presence of adventitious breath sounds.
Observe color of mucous membranes.
Evaluate degree of anxiety.

Nursing Diagnosis	Nursing Actions	Rationale	Desired Outcomes/ Evaluation Criteria
Gas exchange, impaired related to altered oxygen supply (e.g., narrowing of airways by secretions, bronchospasm), alveolar-capillary membrane changes (e.g., fibrosis, injury) as evidenced by dyspnea, restlessness, inability to move secretions, abnormal ABG values (hypoxia and hypercapnea), confusion/somnolence.	Elevate head of bed, assist patient to assume position of comfort. Encourage deep, slow or pursed-lip breathing as individually needed/ tolerated. Encourage expectoration of sputum; suction when indicated.	Oxygen delivery may be improved by upright position and breathing exercises to decrease airway collapse, dyspnea, and work of breathing. Thick, tenacious copious secretions are a major source of impaired gas exchange in small airways. Deep suctioning may be required when cough is ineffective for removal of secretions.	Demonstrates improved ventilation and adequate oxygenation of tissues by ABGs within patient's normal range and absence of symptoms of respiratory distress.
	Monitor color of skin and mucous membrane.	Duskiness and central cyanosis indicate advancing hypoxemia.	
	Administer supplemental oxygen at appropriate rate and method as indicated.	Maximizes oxygen delivery with minimal effort. Low concentrations of oxygen are indicated in conditions, such as COPD, status asthmaticus, cystic fibrosis where the level of carbon dioxide drives respiratory function.	
	Review laboratory studies, i.e., ABGs.	Useful in determining therapy needs/effectiveness.	
Anxiety, moderate/Fear related to threat of death/change in health status, physiologic factors as evidenced by increased tension, apprehension, statements of inability to breathe.	Acknowledge reality of situation and encourage expression of feelings.	Being unable to "catch one's breath" is an anxiety-producing situation. Knowing that others are aware helps to allay tension. Expression of feelings identifies them and provides opportunity for effective coping.	Appears relaxed, able to sleep/rest appropriately. Reports anxiety is reduced to a manageable level.
	Review current situation and measures being taken to remedy the problems.	Provides reassurance. Explanations need to be short and repeated frequently because the patient may have a reduced attention span.	
	Discuss current coping skills being used.	Identifies effectiveness of these skills and promotes opportunity to acquire new ways of handling difficult situation.	
	Develop activity program within limits of physical ability.	Provides a healthy outlet for energy generated by feelings.	
	Be alert for out-of-control behavior or escalating cardiopulmonary dysfunction, e.g., worsening dyspnea and tachycardia.	Development of incapacitating anxiety requires further evaluation and intervention because increased activity increases demand for oxygen.	

Table 36–5. NURSING PROCESS FOR PATIENT REQUIRING OXYGEN–*CONTINUED*

Nursing Diagnosis	Nursing Actions	Rationale	Desired Outcomes/ Evaluation Criteria
Knowledge deficit related to lack of information/ unfamiliarity with resources, misinterpretation as evidenced by questions, request for information, statements of concern, inaccurate follow-through of instructions, development of preventable complications.	Explain/reinforce explanation of individual disease process. Encourage patient/SO to ask questions. Instruct/reinforce rationale for breathing exercises as well as general conditioning exercises.	Decreases anxiety and can lead to improved participation in treatment plan. Pursed-lip and abdominal breathing exercises strengthen muscles of respiration, helps minimize collapse of small airways and provides a means to control dyspnea.	Verbalizes understanding of condition/disease process and treatment. Identifies relationship of current signs/symptoms to the disease process and correlates with causative factors. Initiates lifestyle changes as indicated.
	Provide information about the harmful effects of smoking on the lungs, and encourage cessation of smoking by both patient and SO.	Even when patient wants to stop smoking, support groups and medical monitoring may be needed. "Side-stream" of "second-hand" smoke has been shown to be detrimental as well as actual smoking.	
	Review oxygen requirements/dosage for patient who is discharged on supplemental oxygen.	Reduces risk of misuse (too little/too much) and resultant complications.	
	Instruct in safe use of oxygen and refer to supplier.	Promotes environmental/ physical safety.	
	Refer to/encourage participation in support groups.	May need additional support to manage depression, anxiety which often accompany a chronic disease/treatment which may interfere with desired lifestyle.	

Table 36–6. RULES FOR OXYGEN ADMINISTRATION

Post "DO NOT TOUCH" sign on oxygen flowmeter and instruct patient not to adjust flow rate.
Prevent fire hazards.
  Instruct patient not to smoke.
  Remove cigarettes, matches, etc., from room.
  Do not allow patient to use electric razor while using oxygen.
  Use no oils (e.g., mineral oil, hair dressings) or flammable liquids (alcohol) on patient.
  Post "NO SMOKING" sign on door.
Ensure proper humidification to prevent drying of respiratory tract mucosa.
Change equipment daily to prevent infection.
Monitor patient status:
  Avoid giving in excess of 60% O_2 for more than two days.
  Evaluate Pa_{O_2} and maintain between 60 and 80 mmHg.
  If possible, avoid 100% oxygen (Note: Even 95% oxygen will help in preventing atelectasis).
  Beware of diminishing hypoxic drive in susceptible COPD patients.
Monitor cardiac status in unstable hypoxic patient.

60–70 mmHg range. It is essential to avoid overoxygenating these patients because this could result in oxygen-induced hypoventilation. In some patients chronic hypercarbia results in gradual desensitization of the chemoreceptors to carbon dioxide as a breathing stimulus. The hypoxic drive, normally a secondary mechanism, then becomes the primary breathing stimulus in these patients. Thus, as long as the patient is hypoxemic, chemoreceptors continually stimulate the respiratory centers and he or she will breathe. However, if too much oxygen is given and hypoxemia is eliminated, the patient's chemoreceptors will not be stimulated. Breathing then decreases because the patient's reason for breathing, a low Pa_{O_2}, has been overly corrected. With the resulting hypoventilation, the patient's carbon dioxide level rises and acidemia develops. Respiratory and cardiac arrest follows unless mechanical ventilation is started immediately. Signs of oxygen-induced hypoventilation include lethargy, obtundation, a decrease in depth or rate of breathing, and pink flushed skin. If these signs are apparent, an arterial blood sample is drawn and analyzed. Respiratory depression causes a significant rise in Pa_{CO_2} above the patient's usual level

Table 36–7. COMMONLY USED OXYGEN DELIVERY SYSTEMS

Device	Approximate Oxygen Delivery Capability	Comments
Nasal cannula	24% @ L/min 28% @ 2 L/min 32% @ 3 L/min 35%–45% @ 4–6 L/min	Suitable for most hypoxemic patients; comfortable; oxygen concentration varies widely with patient breathing pattern; not suited for high oxygen concentrations.
Simple oxygen mask	30% @ 4 L/min 40% @ 6 L/min 50% @ 8 L/min Up to 60% @ 10–12 L/min	Less comfortable than cannula; oxygen concentration varies widely with patient breathing pattern; provides better humidification.
Venturi mask	24% @ 4–6 L/min 28% @ 4–6 L/min 35% @ 8–10 L/min 40% @ 8–10 L/min 50% @ 8–10 L/min	Very precise oxygen concentration delivered; expensive; noisy and uncomfortable.
Reservoir mask	60%–100% @ 8–12 L/min	High-concentration delivery for critically hypoxemic patient; uncomfortable; short-term use only.
Oxygen tent/croup tent	40%–50% @ 15 L/min	Oxygen concentration higher, variable; cooling mechanism required to maintain patient comfort; strict fire precautions necessary; high oxygen flow needed to flush out carbon dioxide of patient's exhaled air.

of hypercarbia, along with a sizable drop in pH. When this occurs, the patient is placed in an intensive care unit with provisions available for respiratory support.

When high concentrations of oxygen (40% or greater) are administered for extended periods of time, it may exert toxic effects upon the lung itself. *Atelectasis*, pulmonary infiltrates, and interstitial pneumonitis may all be effects of oxygen toxicity. Early signs of this syndrome include cough, nasal congestion, sore throat, pain on inspiration, burning in the chest, and increasing dyspnea. The lungs stiffen and are more difficult to fill. The patient's work of breathing increases, and a further reduction in the oxygen supply of the blood occurs.

Oxygen toxicity has been cited as one of the causes of adult respiratory distress syndrome (ARDS). Whenever high concentrations of oxygen are used, the dangers of

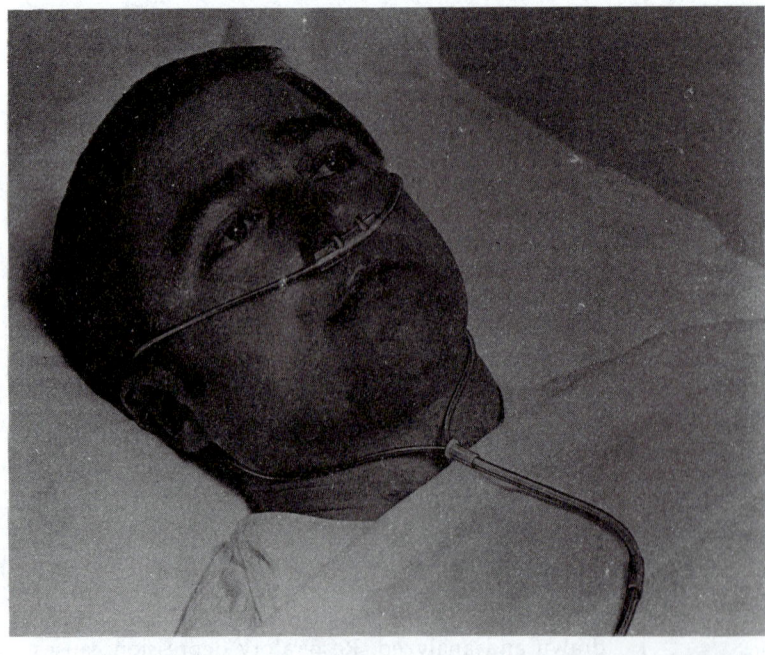

Figure 36–1. Nasal cannula. (Courtesy of Hudson Oxygen Therapy Sales Company, Temecula, CA)

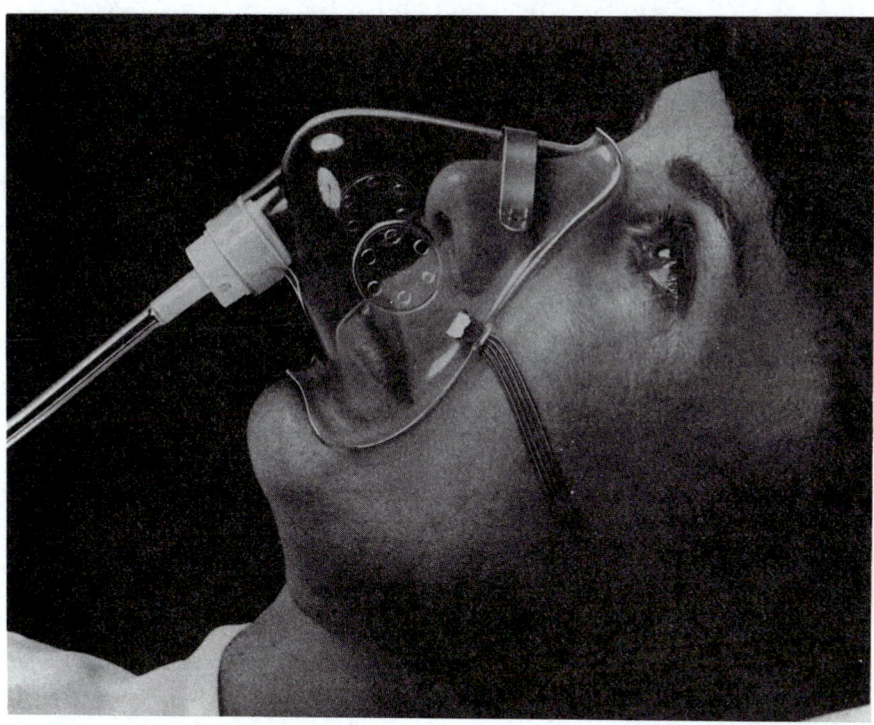

Figure 36–2. Simple mask. (Courtesy of Hudson Oxygen Therapy Sales Company, Temecula, CA)

oxygen toxicity must be weighed against the possibly life-saving benefits of oxygen therapy. It is generally agreed that in acute cases of respiratory failure, tissue hypoxia must be prevented at all costs.

Finally, a word must be mentioned about the administration of oxygen to infants. Premature babies are especially at risk for retrolental fibroplasia. In these babies the blood vessels of the retina are extremely delicate. They are also highly sensitive to the effects of oxygen. When the premature infant's Pa_{O_2} rises excessively, the dissolved oxygen of the blood can cause the retinal vessels to spasm. The result can be partial or total blindness as retinal tissue dies from lack of nourishment. The problem may be avoided by close monitoring of the infant's Pa_{O_2}. Oxygen is administered in concentrations sufficient to prevent hypoxemia, but not in amounts that would raise the Pa_{O_2} above 80 mmHg. Many clinicians agree that the premature infant can be maintained with a Pa_{O_2} between 50 and 80 mmHg. New noninvasive methods of oxygen monitoring, such as transcutaneous electrodes and vastly improved oximeters, hold promise as means by which retrolental fibroplasia may be prevented.

Chronic lung damage may also result from prolonged

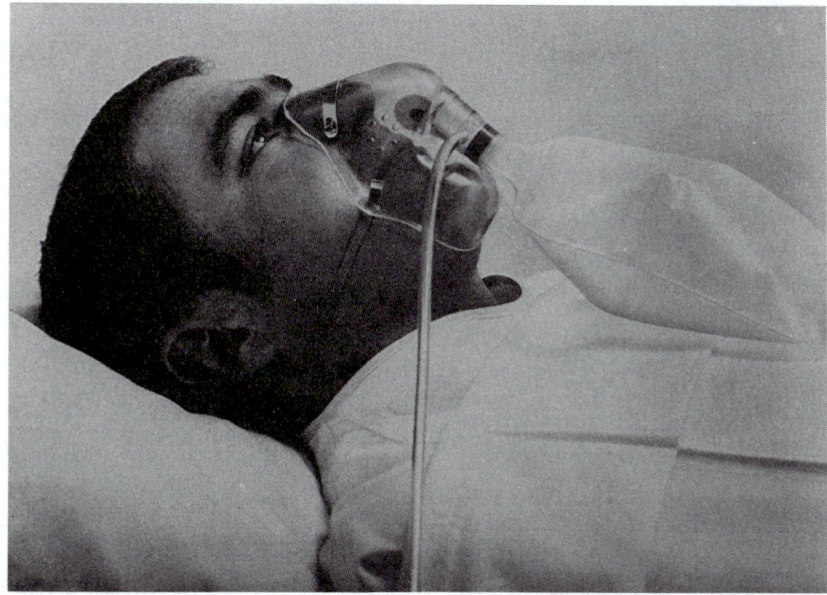

Figure 36–3. Nonrebreathing mask. (Courtesy of Hudson Oxygen Therapy Sales Company, Temecula, CA)

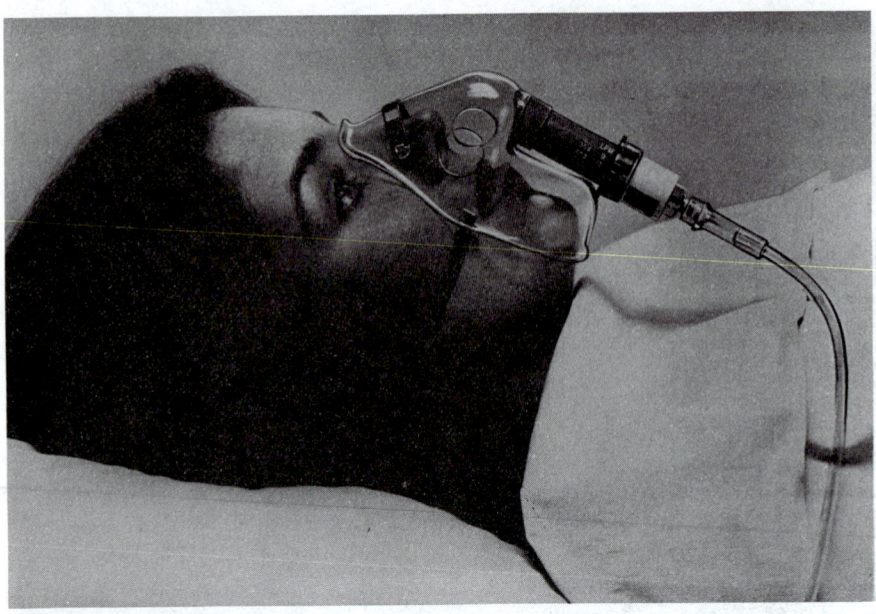

Figure 36–4. Venturi mask. (Courtesy of Hudson Oxygen Therapy Sales Company, Temecula, CA)

Table 36–8. THERAPEUTIC GAS

Name	Dosage	Mode of Administration	Pharmacokinetics
Oxygen (O₂)			

Action: Increases saturation of hemoglobin and amount of oxygen dissolved in blood, making more oxygen available to tissues.

Use: Treatment of hypoxemia, decrease work of breathing, and decreasing work of the heart.

Name	Dosage	Mode of Administration	Pharmacokinetics
	22%–100% depending on underlying condition	Inhalation by various devices (see Table 36–7)	O: immediate P: UA D: continuous ½L: NA PB: 0 B & E: carried on hemoglobin and dissolved in plasma; through lungs as carbon dioxide

Key to Abbreviations in the *Pharmacokinetics* column O-onset; P-peak; D-duration; PB-protein bound; B-biotransformed in; E-excreted in; ½L-halflife.

*Within the column listing adverse effects, underlines indicate the most common effects; CAPITALS indicate life-threatening effects.

oxygen therapy. Full-term infants are less likely to develop these problems, but the same precautions as for the premature baby should be observed.

Table 36–8 provides a summary of oxygen as a therapeutic agent.

ANTITUSSIVE AGENTS

The cough reflex is a protective mechanism. Its function is to keep the airway clear of excessive mucus and foreign material. It occurs as a response to irritation, but although it is a "normal response" there is no such thing as a normal cough. The presence of a cough is an indication that the lung is being provoked by noxious stimuli.

The cough reflex is initiated by the stimulation of irritant receptors in the larger airways. Physical irritation, such as dryness or hot or cold, can stimulate these receptors. Mechanical irritants (such as dusts and foreign bodies) and chemical irritants (gases, histamine and other biochemical mediators, aspirated liquids that are dissimilar to respiratory mucus in pH or tonicity, etc.) can also stimulate the irritant receptors. Impulses are thus generated and transmitted from the receptors

through neural pathways to the cough center in the medulla. The cough center in turn sends impulses through efferent nerves to the respiratory muscles. These contract forcefully against a closed glottis. As the glottis opens, the rapid expulsion of air from the lungs helps to propel the irritant upward out of the airway.

Antitussives are used to decrease the intensity and frequency of coughing episodes. These agents modify the cough reflex in one of two ways. Centrally acting antitussives suppress the cough center by decreasing its threshold for stimulation. It is thus rendered less sensitive to the impulses sent to it from the irritant receptors. Other antitussives act peripherally to decrease the sensitivity of the irritant receptors to stimulation.

"Cough medicines" are among the most commonly sold types of medication. There are literally hundreds of prescription and over-the-counter preparations available in the United States. The more important narcotic and non-narcotic antitussive agents are listed in Table 36–9. Expectorants, a related group of medications are discussed in Chapter 35.

Contraindications/ Precautions	Adverse Effects*	Interactions	Nursing Implications
Use only low concentrations of oxygen for COPD patient with unresponsive respiratory centers. COPD patients who require high concentrations of oxygen should be in an intensive care unit and monitored continuously. Excessive oxygenation can induce hypoventilation in some COPD patients. Higher concentrations (over 60%) for extended periods (more than 2 days) may predispose patient to development of oxygen toxicity syndromes. Use with extreme caution in infants, especially premature babies. They are at risk for eye damage (retrolental fibroplasia) and lung damage (bronchopulmonary dysplasia).	CNS: respiratory depression (only in patients whose respiratory chemoreceptors are unresponsive to carbon dioxide), headache CV: tachycardia, hypotension Resp: bronchitis, pneumonitis, atelectasis, alveolar damage (in toxicity syndrome) EENT: sinusitis, ear discomfort, dried mucosa, BLINDNESS from retrolental fibroplasia (in premature infants)	In general, oxygen is not interactive with other drugs. However, certain agents may increase the potential for the development of oxygen toxicity in patients receiving long-term, high concentrations of oxygen. Among these are dextroamphetamine, carbon dioxide inhalation, aspirin, atropine, insulin, ACTH, thyroid preparations.	ASSESSMENT: Check patient's breathing pattern by noting rate and volume, dyspnea. Determine presence of hypoxemia by Pao_2 less than 80 mmHg. Check for cyanosis, abnormal breath sounds, tachycardia, arrhythmias: all are indicative of oxygen deficit. Assess $Paco_2$ level in known COPD patients. INTERVENTION: Administer prescribed oxygen concentration or flow according to delivery device specification; see Table 36–7. EVALUATION: Effectiveness of oxygen administration as a treatment for hypoxia is evaluated in terms of increased Pao_2, reduction of dyspnea, and stable heart rate.

Table 36–9. ANTITUSSIVE AGENTS

Name	Dosage	Mode of Administration	Pharmacokinetics
Action: Suppress cough mechanism centrally or locally			
Use: Symptomatic relief and treatment of coughs due to various causes			
NARCOTIC ANTITUSSIVES Codeine, codeine phosphate, codeine sulfate.	Adults: 10–20 mg q 3–6 hr (120 mg/day max). Children: 6–12 years: 5–10 mg q 4–6 hr, 60 mg/day max. 2–5 yr: 1.4–5.0 mg q 4–6 hr, 30 mg/day max.	PO	O: rapid (under 30 min) P: 60–90 min D: 4–6 hr ½L: 3 hr PB: 30%–35% bound B: liver E: urine, feces
Hydrocodone (Dihydrocodeinone)	Adults: 5–10 mg tid or qid. Children: 2–12 yr: 2.5 mg tid or qid. 1–2 yr: 1.25 mg tid or qid.	PO	O: rapid P: 30–90 min D: 4–8 hr ½L: 4 hr PB: 30%–35% B: liver E: urine, feces
Methadone (Dolophine)	2.5–10 mg q 3–4 hr, up to 5–20 mg q 6–8 hr.	PO, IM, SC	O: 10–15 min P: 1–2 hr D: 3–5 hr; up to 48 hr in patients on methadone maintenance ½L: 25 hr

Key to Abbreviations in the *Pharmacokinetics* column O-onset; P-peak; D-duration; PB-protein bound; B-biotransformed in; E-excreted in; ½L-halflife.

*Within the column listing adverse effects, underlines indicate the most common effects; CAPITALS indicate life-threatening effects.

Contraindications/ Precautions	Adverse Effects*	Interactions	Nursing Implications
Hypersensitivity reactions noted in patients with allergy to opiates. Not recommended for use in pregnancy and in adults with asthma. Caution needed in patients with head trauma, severe renal or liver disease, hypothyroid or adrenal insufficiency.	CNS: sedation, confusion, headache, euphoria, dysphoria, hallucinations CV: HYPOTENSION, BRADYCARDIA Resp: RESPIRATORY DEPRESSION GI: constipation, nausea, vomiting EENT: blurred vision Other: physical and/or psychologic dependence, sweating, flushing	Potentiated by MAO inhibitors, alcohol, anticholinergics, sedatives, and tranquilizers. Antagonized by narcotic antagonists.	ASSESSMENT: Check cough and sputum produced to ensure secretions are not inspissated. Check for nausea and vomiting and abdominal pain before administering. Check for bowel function. INTERVENTION: Inform patient of drowsiness effects, caution against driving or operating machinery. Ensure adequate hydration to assist in mucokinesis. Inform patient to avoid alcohol or other depressants. EVALUATION: Effectiveness of this drug as a cough suppressant is evaluated in terms of decrease in frequency and intensity of cough. ADDITIONAL NOTES: Addiction potential is mild but considerable. Patient should be observed for constipation. Codeine is contained in many preparations, including Cheracol, Coseadin, Cosanyl, Endotussin-C, Histadyl EC, Robitussin AC, Sedatole. Prescription required for preparations containing more than 200 mg/100 ml (or 1 g/fl oz). Driving and operating machinery not recommended since drowsiness may occur.
Same as codeine plus not recommended for children less than 1 yr of age.	Same as codeine.	Same as codeine.	Same as codeine, plus, ADDITIONAL NOTES: More potent than codeine regarding side effects and addiction potential. Preparations include Codone, Dicodid, Hycodan, Hycomine, Pseudo-Hist, S-T Forte, Triaminic Expectorant DH, Tussanil DH, Tussend, Tussionex. Prescription required.
Extremely high addiction potential. Contraindicated in head trauma, convulsive dis-	Same as codeine, but of generally greater magnitude; overdose may lead to cardiovascular collapse.	Same as codeine.	Same as codeine; plus, ADDITIONAL NOTES: Methadone is a powerful antitussive useful in cases where

CONTINUED ON THE FOLLOWING PAGE

Table 36–9. ANTITUSSIVE AGENTS–*CONTINUED*

Name	Dosage	Mode of Administration	Pharmacokinetics
Methadone–*Continued*			PB: high B: liver E: urine, bile
NON-NARCOTIC ANTITUSSIVES			
Benzonatate (Tessalon)	100 mg tid, 600 mg/day max.	PO	O: 15–20 min P: UA D: 3–8 hr ½L: UA PB: UA B: UA E: UA
Dextromethorphan	Adults: 15–30 mg tid or qid. Children: 6–12 yr: 5–10 mg q 4 hr. 2–6 yr: 2.5–5.0 mg q 4 hr.	PO	O: 15–30 min P: UA D: 3–6 hr ½L: UA PB: UA B: liver E: UA

Key to Abbreviations in the *Pharmacokinetics* column O-onset; P-peak; D-duration; PB-protein bound; B-biotransformed in; E-excreted in; ½L-halflife.*
*Within the column listing adverse effects, underlines indicate the most common effects; CAPITALS indicate life-threatening effects.

Contraindications/ Precautions	Adverse Effects*	Interactions	Nursing Implications
orders, Addison's disease, asthma, thyroid dysfunction. Use with extreme caution in patients with inadequate respiratory reserve, or hypotensive patients.			extreme pain is aggravated by coughing (lung cancer, chest trauma). Long duration of opiate-like effects (up to 18 hr) make overdosing a very distinct possibility. Overdose may require ventilatory support due to respiratory depression. See Chapter 21 for additional information.
Overdose may cause CNS stimulation and convulsions, followed by CNS depression. Safe use in pregnancy not yet established.	CNS: drowsiness, headache, dizziness CV: numbness in the chest GI: constipation, nausea, GI upset EENT: nasal congestion, burning eyes Integ: skin eruptions and pruritis	CNS stimulants potentiate its actions.	ASSESSMENT: Check cough and sputum produced to ensure secretions are not inspissated. Check for nausea and vomiting, and abdominal pain before administering. Check bowel function. INTERVENTION: Inform patient of possible drowsiness, caution against driving or machinery operation. Ensure adequate hydration to assist in mucokinesis. Suggest use of hard candies to help in cough control. EVALUATION: Effectiveness of this drug as a cough suppressant is evaluated in terms of decrease in frequency and intensity of cough. ADDITIONAL NOTES: Inform patient that drug should be swallowed rapidly: local anesthesia (numbness) of tongue and pharynx can result.
Use with caution in patients with liver disease, diabetes, thyroid disease, or hypotension. Not established as safe for use in pregnancy. Do not use in patient using MAO inhibitors. Consult physician if cough persists more than 1 wk.	CNS: drowsiness, dizziness GI: nausea	Use with MAO inhibitors can cause nausea, coma, hypotension, hyperpyrexia, and death. CNS depressants may potentiate sedation effects.	ASSESSMENT: Check cough and sputum produced to ensure secretions are not inspissated. INTERVENTION: Inform patient of possible drowsiness, caution patient against driving or machinery operation. Ensure adequate hydration to assist in mucokinesis. Suggest use of hard candies to help in cough control. Do not give water for 30 min following administration to optimize antitussive effect. Tablet preparations should be chewed for maximal effect.

CONTINUED ON THE FOLLOWING PAGE

Table 36–9. ANTITUSSIVE AGENTS-*CONTINUED*

Name	Dosage	Mode of Administration	Pharmacokinetics
Dextromethorphan–*Continued*			
Chlophedianol hydrochloride (Ulo) (Not on U.S. market)	Adults: 25 mg tid or qid. Children: 6–12 yr: 12.5–25 mg tid or qid. 2–6 yr: 12.5 mg tid or qid.	PO	O: 30–60 min P: UA D: 4–8 hr ½L: UA PB: UA B: UA E: UA
Diphenhydramine hydrochloride (Benalyn)	Adults: 25–50 mg tid or qid. Children: 12.5 mg tid or qid.	PO	O: 15–60 min P: 1–2 hr D: 4–8 hr ½L: 2.4–9.3 hr PB: 80–85% B: liver E: urine
Levopropoxyphene (Novrad) (Not on U.S. market)	Adults: 100 mg q 4 hr, max dose 600 mg. Children: 25 lb: 75 mg, 50 lb: 150 mg, 75–100 lb: 200 mg.	PO	O: moderate P: UA D: UA ½L: UA PB: UA B: liver E: urine

Key to Abbreviations in the *Pharmacokinetics* column O-onset; P-peak; D-duration; PB-protein bound; B-biotransformed in; E-excreted in; ½L-halflife.*
*Within the column listing adverse effects, underlines indicate the most common effects; CAPITALS indicate life-threatening effects.

Contraindications/ Precautions	Adverse Effects*	Interactions	Nursing Implications
			EVALUATION: Effectiveness of this drug as a cough suppressant is evaluated in terms of decrease in frequency and intensity of cough. ADDITIONAL NOTES: Most reliable of nonnarcotic antitussives. Available in dozens of prescription and nonprescription formulas. Effectiveness of this drug as a cough suppressant is evaluated in terms of in frequency and intensity of cough.
Not for use in children less than 2 yr. Pregnant or nursing women and elderly most prone to developing adverse response.	CNS: stimulation including irritability, excitation, possible hallucinations, vertigo GI: nausea, vomiting, constipation Other: hypersensitivity, dry mouth, visual disturbance	May potentiate either CNS stimulants or CNS depressants.	Same as dextromethorphan, plus, ADDITIONAL NOTES: Available by prescription as Ulo (US) or Ulone (Canada). Potency is comparable to narcotic antitussives, but has slower onset and longer duration of action.
Do not use for cough resulting from asthma attack. Not for use during pregnancy or by nursing mothers. Use with caution in elderly, patients with liver disease, glaucoma, seizure disorders, or prostatic hypertrophy.	CNS: drowsiness, excitation (in children), dizziness, headache CV: palpitations, hypotension Resp: dried respiratory secretions GI: dry mouth, anorexia, constipation, diarrhea Renal: frequency, dysuria, urinary retention Integ: photosensitivity EENT: blurred vision, tinnitus	Potentiated by MAO inhibitors. Additive CNS effects when used with other CNS depressants (alcohol, sedatives, narcotics). Diphenhydramine hinders GI absorption of para-amino-salicylic acid.	ASSESSMENT: Check cough and sputum produced to ensure secretions are not inspissated. Check for nausea and vomiting and abdominal pain before administering. INTERVENTION: Inform patient of drowsiness effects, caution against driving or machinery operation. Ensure adequate hydration to assist in mucokinesis. Sunscreen or long clothing will protect against photosensitivity reaction. Inform patient to avoid alcohol or other depressants. EVALUATION: Effectiveness of this drug as a cough suppressant is evaluated in terms of decrease in frequency and intensity of cough.
Safe use in pregnancy not established.	CNS: sedation, dizziness, nervousness GI: nausea, epigastric distress Integ: rashes	None known.	Same as dextromethorphan, plus, ADDITIONAL NOTES: Reportedly equivalent in potency to codeine without opiate side effects. Available as Novrad by prescription.

CONTINUED ON THE FOLLOWING PAGE

A
n
t
i
t
u
s
s
i
v
e
s

Table 36–9. ANTITUSSIVE AGENTS–_CONTINUED_

Name	Dosage	Mode of Administration	Pharmacokinetics
Noscapine (Tusscapine) (Not on U.S. market)	Adults: 15–30 mg tid or qid, max 130 mg/day. Children: 6–12 yr: 15 mg tid or qid, max 60 mg/day. 2–6 yr: 7.5–15 mg tid or qid, no more than 4 doses/day.	PO	O: rapid P: UA D: UA ½L: UA PB: UA B: UA E: UA

Key to Abbreviations in the _Pharmacokinetics_ column O-onset; P-peak; D-duration; PB-protein bound; B-biotransformed in; E-excreted in; ½L-halflife.*

*Within the column listing adverse effects, <u>underlines</u> indicate the most common effects; CAPITALS indicate life-threatening effects.

Using the Nursing Process

ASSESSMENT OF THE PATIENT WITH A COUGH. A cough can be described in many ways, but there are two essential categories of coughs. A productive cough is one that raises mucus, whereas a nonproductive cough does not. The productive cough is useful: it helps to keep the airways clean. The patient with a productive cough is kept well hydrated and allowed to cough. It is desirable to help the postoperative patient maintain clear lungs by assisting him or her to cough regularly. If the cough is loose or productive, the patient is encouraged to cough until the lungs are clear.

By contrast, a nonproductive cough generally serves no purpose. When the airways are very dry or inflamed, a cough can be almost continual. Problems such as acute bronchitis or gas inhalation injuries are characterized by repeated episodes of nonproductive, often harsh coughing. This type of cough can disrupt the patient's sleep pattern and lead to general discomfort. The surgical patient who has a nagging cough experiences pain at the incisional site, and the patient with fractured ribs feels severe pain with each cough. Dry, hacking spasms of coughing, burning in the chest caused by coughing, and even the dry, annoying "tickle in the throat" are reasons for considering antitussive therapy. Antitussives are justified in any such cases to allow these patients some periods of uninterrupted rest.

When the patient has little or no mucus evident in his lungs, antitussives can provide relief from disruptive coughing. Excessive mucus is apparent as audible gurgling or "clicking" sounds. Most often mucus in the airways can be detected by auscultation with a stethoscope. Crackles (also called rales, which are heard primarily on inspiration) and rhonchi (rumbling expiratory sounds) are the main signs of excessive respiratory secretions.

NURSING DIAGNOSES. Possible nursing diagnoses for the patient who requires antitussive therapy are ineffective airway clearance and alteration in comfort due to coughing.

INTERVENTION. The primary goal of nursing intervention is to restore the patient's comfort by suppressing the disruptive cough. Once this is accomplished the nurse can plan the patient's schedule to allow for additional rest as necessary. Procedures are grouped whenever possible to allow the sleep-deprived patient to sleep undisturbed for long periods.

There are several considerations about the administration of antitussives of which the nurse must be aware.

Table 36–10. PATIENT TEACHING: ANTITUSSIVES

Dear Patient:

This drug has been prescribed for you. This is what you should know about your drug to get the most from your therapy.

1. Antitussives are used for the harsh, irritating nonproductive cough. The patient whose cough produces sputum should continue to cough and should not take antitussives unless the cough disrupts sleep patterns.
2. Antitussive therapy is normally of short duration. When the cough diminishes in intensity and frequency, antitussive therapy is no longer needed. If a harsh cough persists for several days, the patient should seek medical advice.
3. No liquids or food are to be taken for ½ hr following administration of cough medicine. This allows the medication to provide the benefit of soothing local tissues.
4. If the antitussive contains narcotics or antihistamines, do not consume alcohol during the course of therapy. Also, use barbiturates only as prescribed by the physician.
5. Do not exceed single-dose or 24-hr prescribed dosage of antitussives.
6. Major side effects include drowsiness, decreased coordination, constipation, and potential for abuse.
7. Use caution when driving or operating machinery, since many antitussives may diminish alertness.
8. Keep antitussives away from children.

Contraindications/ Precautions	Adverse Effects*	Interactions	Nursing Implications
Use with caution in patients with hypertension, heart disease, diabetes, or hyperthyroidism, since additional ingredients in preparations may aggravate these.	CNS: drowsiness (rarely) GI: nausea	None known.	Same as dextromethorphan, plus, ADDITIONAL NOTES: As with Novrad, this drug is equal to codeine in antitussive potency. Available as Tusscapine and various proprietary mixtures. In experimental animals this agent has caused histamine release, resulting in bronchoconstriction.

These include:

1. Preparations containing codeine tend to cause constipation. Thus, nursing measures to prevent constipation are employed.
2. Cough syrups and lozenges exert a local soothing effect on the throat. The patient should not take liquids for a half hour after taking them.
3. The patient with a dry hacking cough is encouraged to take fluids freely to promote thin, easily raised secretions.
4. Coughs caused by allergies or by postnasal drip may be more effectively treated by antihistamines or decongestants.
5. Drowsiness is a side-effect common to many cough preparations. The patient should be aware of this and warned of the danger of driving or operating machinery.
6. Narcotic antitussives carry with them the risk of habituation. Recommended doses should not be exceeded, since this does not appreciably increase the drug's cough suppression effect. The potential for abuse, however, is increased with an increase in dosage.
7. Narcotic side effects are potentiated by alcohol, so the patient taking these types of antitussives is cautioned against drinking alcoholic beverages while using them. Alcohol content of some preparations may be as high as forty percent.
8. Sometimes effective cough control can be achieved with minimal pharmacologic intervention. Time honored remedies such as the use of a vaporizer and sucking on hard candies can decrease coughing without danger of any serious side effects.

A list of patient teaching information can be found in Table 36–10.

EVALUATION. The criterion for evaluating the effectiveness of antitussive therapy is a decrease in the frequency and intensity of the patient's cough. If the patient appears more comfortable and is coughing less, then the cough medicine has been effective.

The nurse must be cautious in evaluating the patient's need for antitussives. Since many of these drugs have abuse potential, it is the nurse's duty to minimize this risk. The patient who requests cough medicine more frequently than it is ordered may be a potential or actual abuser. This should be further evaluated by the patient's physician.

Table 36-11 describes the nursing process as it applies to the patient who requires antitussive therapy.

Table 36–11. NURSING PROCESS FOR PATIENT REQUIRING ANTITUSSIVES

Assessment			
Assess cough for quality and frequency (including time of day), whether productive or nonproductive as well as amount and color of sputum. Note complaints of pain, difficulty sleeping. Determine level of knowledge regarding treatment regimen.			
Nursing Diagnosis	**Nursing Actions**	**Rationale**	**Desired Outcomes/ Evaluation Criteria**
Pain related to biologic injuring agents (irritated mucosa with dry, hack-	Administer antitussives, e.g., narcotic (codeine preparations, dolophine)	These drugs decrease the force and frequency of nonproductive cough-	Reports pain is relieved/ minimized.

CONTINUED ON THE FOLLOWING PAGE

Table 36–11. NURSING PROCESS FOR PATIENT REQUIRING ANTITUSSIVES–
CONTINUED

Nursing Diagnosis	Nursing Actions	Rationale	Desired Outcomes/ Evaluation Criteria
ing, nonproductive cough) as evidenced by complaints, guarding behavior.	or nonnarcotic (tessa-lon). Provide room humidification. Encourage increased fluid intake.	ing and promote comfort. Soothes dry mucosa, thins secretions if present, to aid expectoration.	
	Promote use of hard candy, throat lozenges, cough drops as indicated.	Exerts a local soothing effect on the throat, decreasing irritating "tickle," dryness, discomfort.	
Sleep pattern disturbance related to presence of consistent/recurrent cough as evidenced by interrupted sleep, irritability, verbalizations of not feeling well-rested.	Administer medications as ordered at HS.	Promotes suppression of cough to allow for increased length/quality of sleep.	Reports improvement in sleep/rest pattern with increased sense well-being and feeling rested
	Provide comfort measures, e.g., back rub, warm bath.	Promotes relaxation and improves quality rest.	
	Encourage adequate balance between activity/rest. Provide interrupted periods for sleep/rest.	Conserves energy, prevents undue fatigue, promotes general well-being.	
Knowledge deficit related to lack of recall/misinterpretation, unfamiliarity with information resources as evidenced by questions, verbalization of concerns, inaccurate follow-through of instruction, development of preventable complications.	Review actions, dosage, and side effects of cough medications.	Enhances safe use and may promote cooperation with treatment regimen.	Identifies relationship of signs/symptoms to disease process. Correctly manages medications and explains reasons for actions.
	Discuss special considerations regarding the use of these drugs, e.g., codeine preparations may cause constipation; liquids should not be taken for half an hour after use of syrups/lozenges; drowsiness may be a side effect of some drugs; narcotic-containing preparations can potentiate other substances such as alcohol and barbiturates.	Maximizes drug effectiveness while reducing potential risks, uptoward effects.	
	Encourage use of other measures, e.g., vaporizer, rest.	May reduce problems of cough with minimal pharmacologic intervention.	

SUMMARY

Patients who are unable to maintain adequate ventilation because of anesthesia or prematurity may benefit from the use of respiratory stimulants. These agents can increase ventilation in some patients, but because of potentially severe side effects are not often used.

Oxygen and antitussives ("cough medicine") are commonly prescribed. Oxygen administered via specialized delivery devices increases blood oxygen levels so that tissue oxygenation can be maintained. The nurse is alert to signs of hypoxia and is aware of safety considerations in administering oxygen. Antitussives are prescribed for the patient whose cough disrupts sleep routines or who experiences discomfort without coughing. Various preparations require different safety considerations.

BIBLIOGRAPHY

Clark, J, Queener, S, and Karb, V: Pharmacological Basis of Nursing Practice, ed 2. CV Mosby, St Louis, 1986.

Clinical news—transtracheal oxygen: The nose knows the difference. Am J Nurs 87:421, 1987.

Daily, D: Home oxygen therapy for infants with bronchopulmonary dysplasia: Growth and development. Respir Management 17(3):13, 1987.

Geller, R and Fisher, J: The role of symptomatic treatment for the common cold. J Respir Dis 8(1):20, 1987.

Gilman, A, Goodman, L, and Gilman, A: The Pharmacological Basis for Therapeutics, ed 6. Macmillan, New York, 1985.

Hahn, A, Oestreich, S, and Barkin, R: Mosby's Pharmacology in Nursing, ed 16. Macmillan, New York, 1980.

Herman, J: New oxygen delivery systems: Gaining patient compliance. Respir Management 17(3):30, 1987.

Hunt, C, Inwood, R, and Shannon, D: Respiratory and nonrespiratory effects of doxapram in congenital central hypoventilation syndrome. Am Rev Respir Dis 119(2):263, 1979.

Johnson, G and Hannah, K: Pharmacology and the Nursing Process, ed 2. WB Saunders, Toronto, 1987.

Lugliami, R, Whipp, B, and Wasserman, K: Doxapram hydrochloride: A respiratory stimulant for patients with primary alveolar hypoventilation. Chest 76(3):414, 1979.

Malseed, R: Drug Therapy and Nursing Considerations. JB Lippincott, Philadelphia, 1985.

Petty, T: New developments in home oxygen therapy. Respir Management 17(3):24, 1987.

Rau, J: Respiratory Therapy Pharmacology, ed 2. Year Book Medical Publishers, Chicago, 1984.

Rodman, M, Karch, A, Boyd, E, and Smith, D: Pharmacology and Drug Therapy in Nursing, ed 3. JB Lippincott, Philadelphia, 1985.

Wiener, M and Pepper, G: Clinical Pharmacology and Therapeutics in Nursing, ed 2. McGraw–Hill, New York, 1985.

Ziment, I: Respiratory Pharmacology and Therapeutics. WB Saunders, Philadelphia, 1977.

SITUATION 36–1

Clifford Sifert, a 72-year-old with chronic bronchitis, is admitted to the emergency department in mild respiratory distress. His Pao_2 is 50 mmHg.

1. The nurse will plan to monitor oxygen therapy. Which of the following oxygen concentrations would be most appropriate for Mr. Sifert?
   a. 100 percent per non-rebreather mask
   b. 28 percent per Venturi mask
   c. 60 percent per aerosol mask
   d. 80 percent per reservoir mask

2. An expected outcome of oxygen treatment for Mr. Sifert would be the following:
   a. Pao_2 of 96 mmHg
   b. Pao_2 of 86 mmHg
   c. Pao_2 of 70 mmHg
   d. Pao_2 of 56 mmHg

3. The nurse will monitor Mr. Sifert closely for the following:
   a. lethargy
   b. pallor
   c. poor skin turgor
   d. sore throat

4. A nursing responsibility which applies in Mr. Sifert's case is:

   a. Teach him how to adjust the flow rate.
   b. Ensure humidification of the oxygen delivered.
   c. Keep lips moistened with petroleum jelly.
   d. Change oxygen equipment every two days.

5. Mr. Sifert tells the nurse that he is "breathing easier." Arterial blood gases reveal appropriate Pao_2 levels. Oxygen is ordered per nasal cannula at 24 percent. The nurse will set the flow rate of oxygen at:
   a. 1 L/min
   b. 2 L/min
   c. 3 L/min
   d. .5 L/min

6. When assessing Mr. Sifert, which of the following would indicate a sign of potential impaired gas exchange?
   a. photosensitivity
   b. warm flushed skin
   c. wheezes
   d. unequal hand grips

Please refer to Appendices for correct answer and additional review questions with answers.

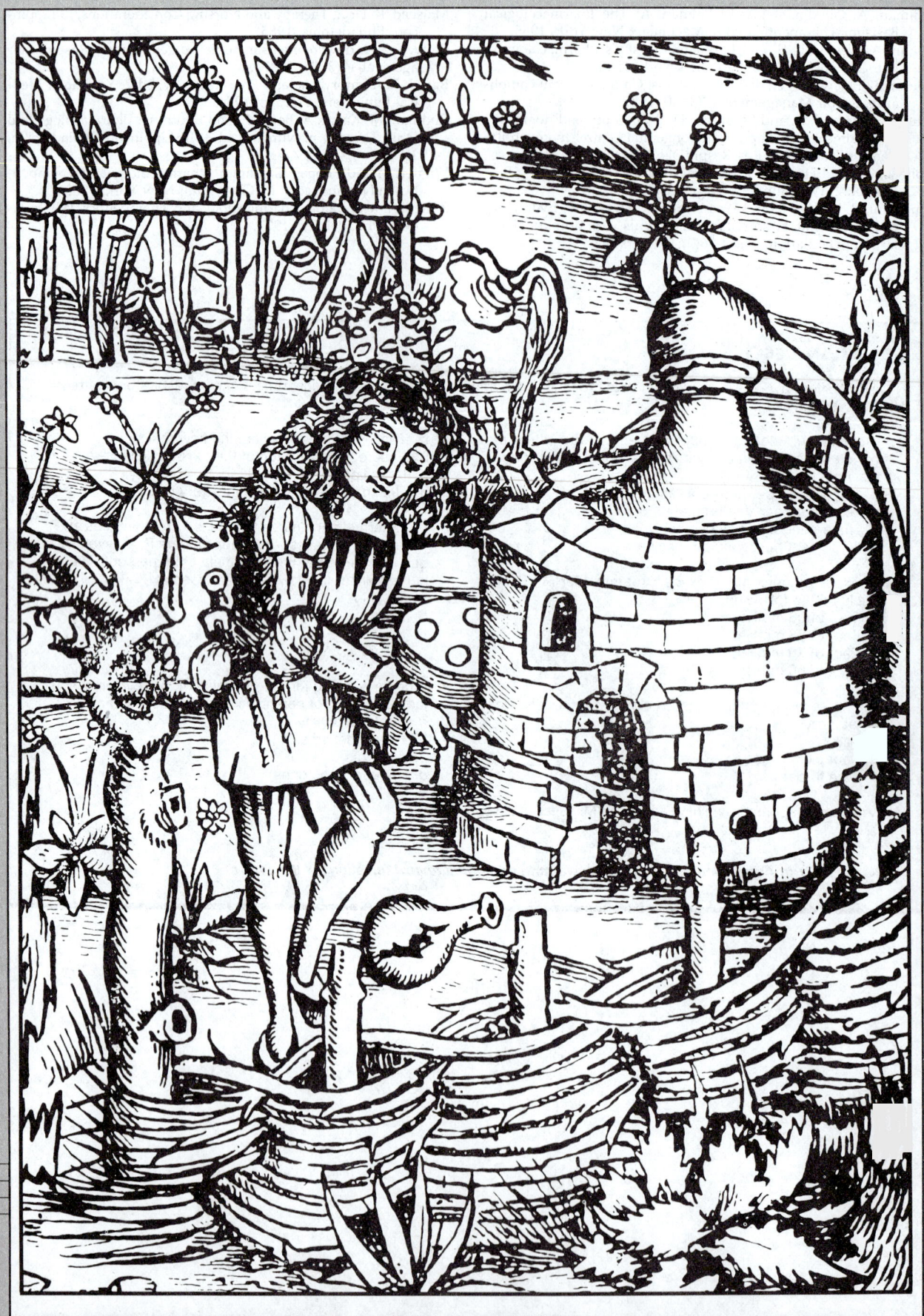

Garden with distilling stove for preparing medicinal herbs, 1521. The Bettmann Archive.

6
UNIT

DRUGS AFFECTING THE URINARY SYSTEM

ANATOMY AND PHYSIOLOGY OF THE URINARY SYSTEM

MERRILY MATHEWSON KUHN, R.N.C., Ph.D., CCRN

LEARNING OBJECTIVES

After reading this chapter, the learner will be able to:

1. Label a diagram of the anatomy of the kidney.

2. Identify the functions of the various parts of the nephron.

3. Identify the functions of the kidney that contribute to homeostasis.

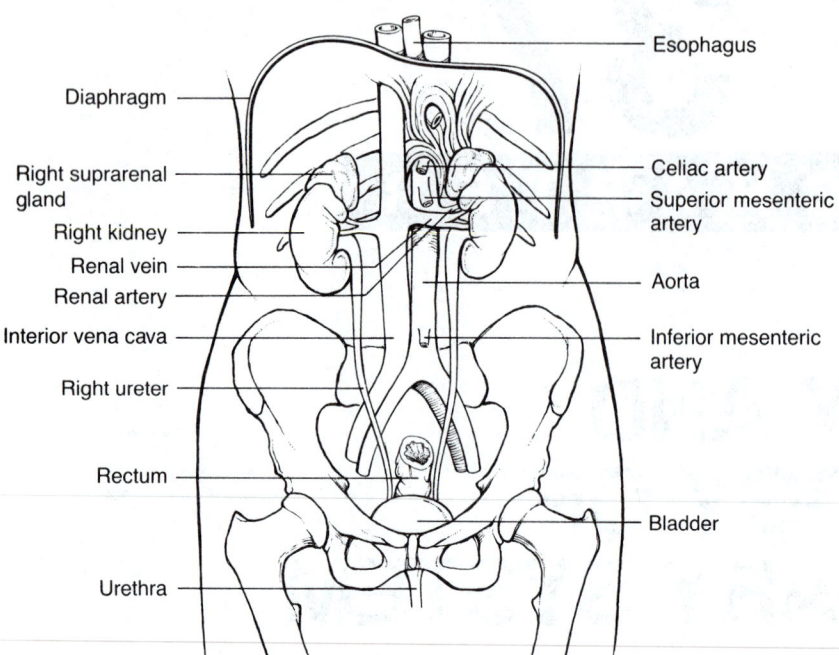

Figure 37–1. Anatomic drawing of urinary system.

ANATOMY AND PHYSIOLOGY

The kidneys are two bean-shaped structures located in the back of the abdominal cavity (Fig. 37–1). Blood vessels and nerves enter and leave the kidney at the central concave area called the *hilus*. The ureters, which connect the kidney with the bladder, also enter the kidney in the hilus.

The outer portion of the kidney is the cortex (Fig. 37–2). The inner portion, the medulla, contains 6 to 12 cone-shaped masses known as renal pyramids. The free ends of the pyramids form the *renal papillae* which open into the *renal pelvis.* The renal pelvis is composed of *calyces* (plural of *calyx*) which drain the upper and lower parts of the kidney. The calyces unite with the renal pelvis at the upper end of the ureter.

The nephron is the basic functional unit of the kidney, with each kidney containing approximately one million nephrons. The nephrons filter the blood, return vital body constituents to the circulation, and excrete waste as the final product called urine.

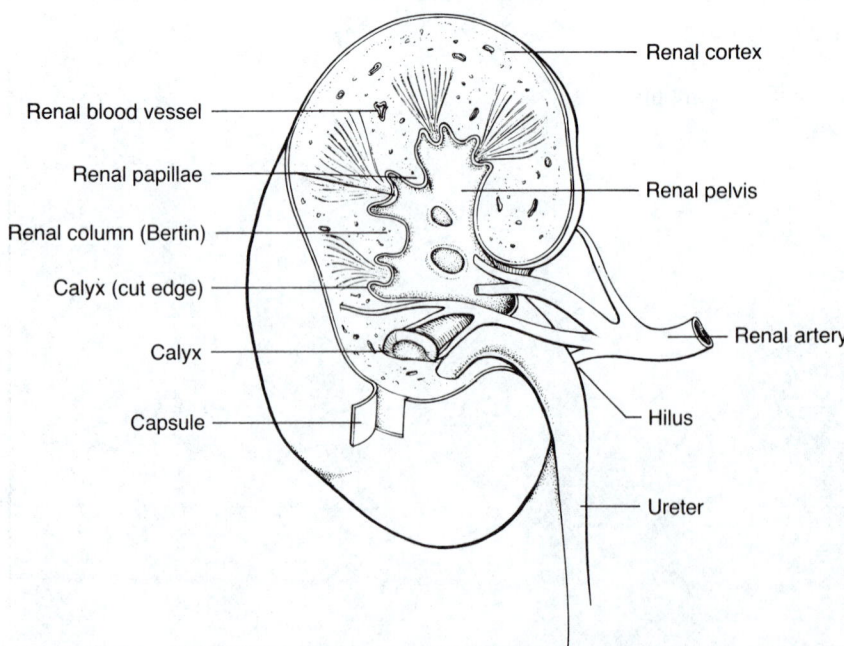

Figure 37–2. Anatomy of the internal structures of the kidney.

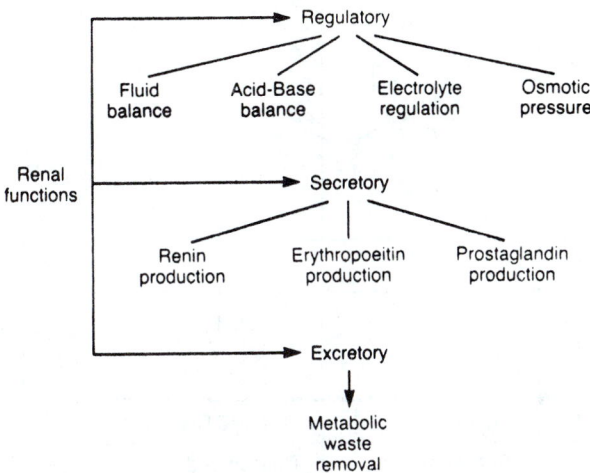

Figure 37–3. Schematic representation of general renal functions.

cium, and hydrogen ions must remain at a relatively constant rate. Through metabolic processes like the consumption of oxygen and glucose and the production of waste products, this environment is in a constant state of change.

Most body systems are in some way involved with homeostasis. However, the kidneys are the main excretory organs and are critically important in maintaining the balance within the internal environment of the body. The kidneys eliminate a variety of metabolic products such as urea, uric acid, and creatinine from the body. In addition, the kidneys regulate water and electrolyte balance. The kidneys also act as endocrine structures by either producing or activating *renin, erythropoietin,* and vitamin D. All these functions are discussed in this chapter and are featured in Figure 37–3.

Each cell in the body is surrounded by a stable environment in order for it to survive and carry out its function. The maintenance of this environment is called *homeostasis.* To preserve homeostasis, the concentration of water and electrolytes such as sodium, potassium, cal-

GLOMERULAR FILTRATION

The filtration of blood occurs at the glomerulus, a tuft of interwoven capillaries that derive from an afferent arteriole (Fig. 37–4). The rate that blood is filtered by the glomerulus is called the *glomerular filtration rate* (GFR).

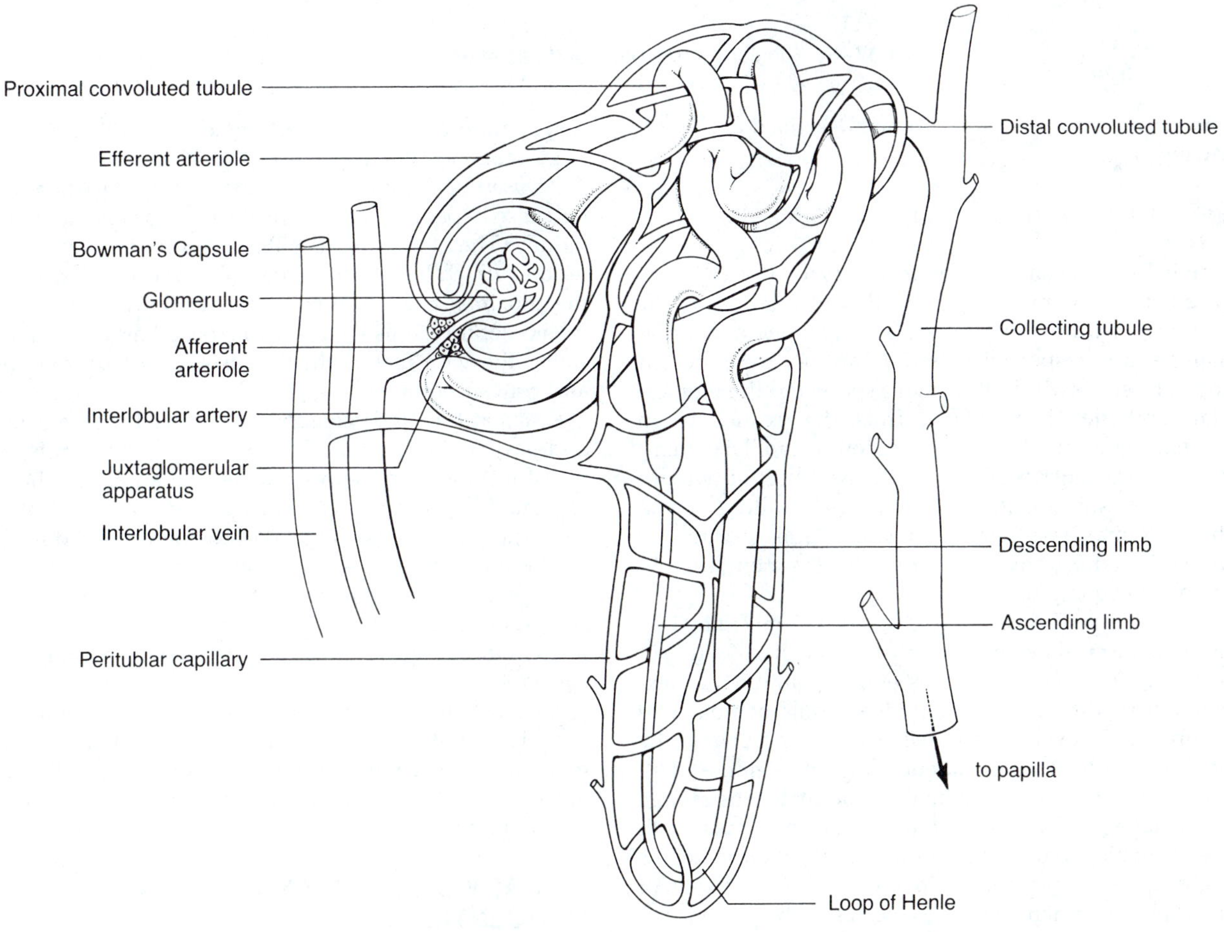

Proximal convoluted tubule

Efferent arteriole

Bowman's Capsule

Glomerulus

Afferent arteriole

Interlobular artery

Juxtaglomerular apparatus

Interlobular vein

Peritublar capillary

Distal convoluted tubule

Collecting tubule

Descending limb

Ascending limb

to papilla

Loop of Henle

Figure 37–4. Anatomy of the nephron.

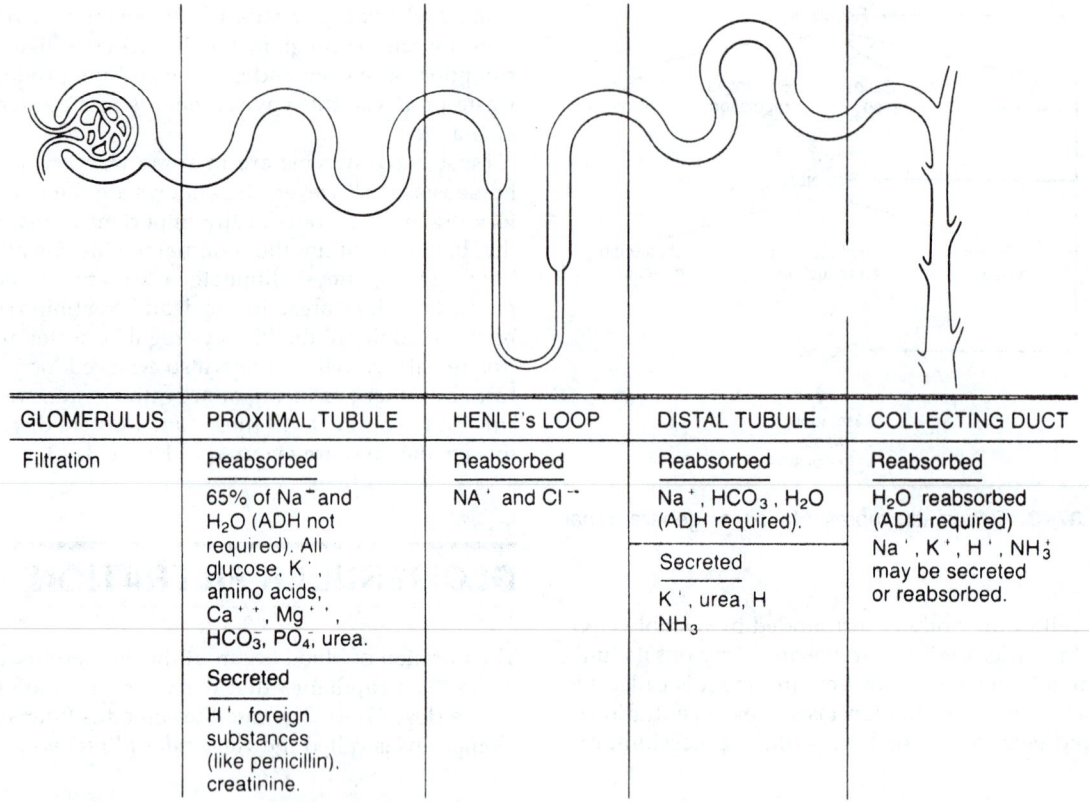

GLOMERULUS	PROXIMAL TUBULE	HENLE's LOOP	DISTAL TUBULE	COLLECTING DUCT
Filtration	**Reabsorbed**	**Reabsorbed**	**Reabsorbed**	**Reabsorbed**
	65% of Na⁻ and H_2O (ADH not required). All glucose, K⁺, amino acids, Ca⁺⁺, Mg⁺⁺, HCO_3^-, PO_4, urea.	NA⁺ and Cl⁻	Na⁺, HCO_3, H_2O (ADH required).	H_2O reabsorbed (ADH required) Na⁺, K⁺, H⁺, NH_3^+ may be secreted or reabsorbed.
			Secreted	
	Secreted		K⁺, urea, H NH₃	
	H⁺, foreign substances (like penicillin), creatinine.			

Figure 37–5. Tubular reabsorption and secretion along the nephron.

The factors governing the GFR are described in the following equation:

$$GFR = K_f[(P_{glom} + \pi_{bs}) - (P_{bs} + \pi_{glom})] \quad \text{(eq. 1)}$$

where K_f represents the permeability of the capillary basement membrane; P_{glom} and P_{bs} are the hydrostatic pressures within the glomerular capillaries and Bowman's space, respectively; and π_{bs} and π_{glom} are the oncotic pressures within Bowman's space and the glomerular capillaries, respectively. Thus, the creation of an *ultrafiltrate* of plasma is the function of capillary membrane characteristics as well as the net effect of two opposing pressures, *hydrostatic* and *oncotic*. Alterations in the GFR may result from numerous disease states or drugs that affect any or all of the factors mentioned in the above equation.

The average GFR is approximately 125 ml/min/1.73 m², which translates into a daily volume of 180 liters of ultrafiltrate. Obviously, if this entire quantity were excreted from the body, an individual would be unable to survive. To prevent this imbalance from occurring, the nephron exhibits a phenomenon known as glomerular–tubular balance. The proximal tubule reabsorbs a large percentage (70% to 80%) of the filtrate and returns it to the systemic circulation. The proximal tubule owes its reabsorptive capabilities to numerous invaginations of the tubular epithelial lining as well as to the presence of microvilli that increase the surface area in contact with the filtrate. The proximal tubule reclaims large quantities of sodium (with water), potassium, chloride, glu-

cose, amino acids, and bicarbonate in fulfilling its role in glomerular-tubular balance (Fig. 37–5).

Reabsorption from the *secretion* into the proximal tubule also depends on the intricate vascular system of the kidney. The glomerular capillaries form the efferent arteriole, which leaves the glomerulus and winds around the proximal and distal convoluted tubules. Juxtamedullary nephrons also have a microcapillary circulation called the vasa recta, which assists in urinary dilution and concentration.

Reabsorption and secretion take place by both *active* and *passive transport* mechanisms. A mechanism is active if it transports a substance against an electrochemical gradient, that is, against a gradient of electrical or chemical potential, or both. Work is performed directly on the substance and energy is expended in the process. Passive transport occurs when the substance being reabsorbed or secreted moves down an electrochemical gradient. No energy is directly expended in moving the substance.

Through the selective processes of reabsorption and secretion, water balance and acid-base balance are maintained. Several hormones, including antidiuretic hormone (ADH) and aldosterone, regulate the tubular reabsorption and secretion of solutes and water.

URINARY DILUTION AND CONCENTRATION

Fluid leaving the proximal tubule has a similar osmolality to plasma (i.e., isotonic) as it enters the loop of

Henle. However, depending on the needs of the individual, excretion of an isotonic urine may not permit the maintenance of body homeostasis. For example, elimination of excess water (i.e., creation of hypotonic urine) may be essential in certain situations, whereas conservation of as much water as possible (i.e., creation of hypertonic urine) may be needed in other settings. Thus, the need to alter the osmolality of fluid entering the loop of Henle is evident, and an interesting physiologic mechanism has evolved that allows the nephron to accomplish this task, the *countercurrent mechanism.*

The countercurrent mechanism (Fig. 37–6) alters urine osmolality as a result of membrane permeability differences within the loop of Henle, the distal convoluted tubule, and the collecting duct. The thin descending limb of the loop of Henle is permeable to water but not to sodium chloride (NaCl) or urea. As the nephron progresses deeper into the renal medulla, the tonicity of the surrounding tissue increases, which draws water out of the tubular lumen. The removal of water without solute increases the concentration of NaCl and urea within the lumen.

As the nephron approaches the renal papilla, it enters into a hairpin turn and begins to go back toward the cortex. The thin segment of the ascending limb of the loop of Henle is impermeable to water but permits NaCl and urea to diffuse out of the lumen into the medullary interstitium along the concentration gradient. The thick segment of the ascending loop of Henle is also impermeable to water and, in addition, contains an active

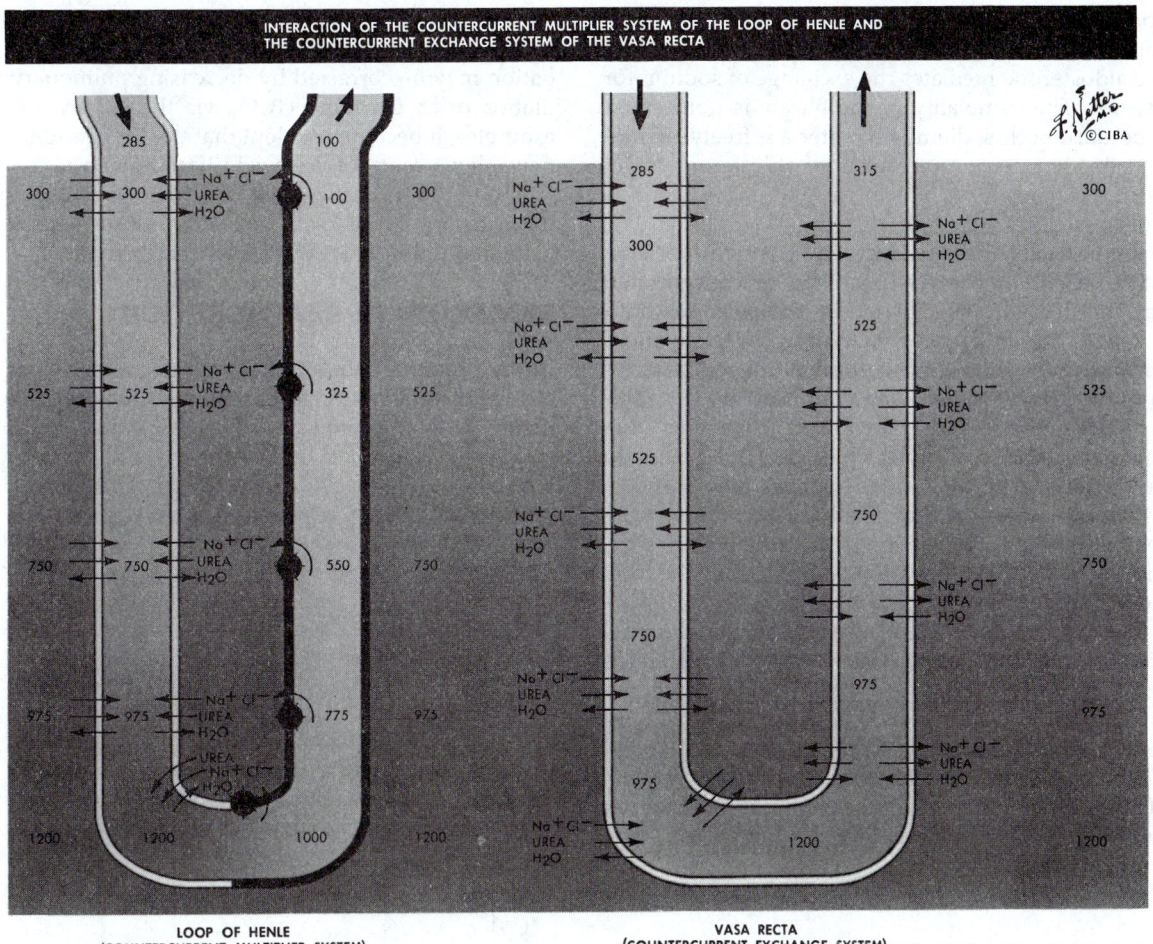

Figure 37–6. The countercurrent mechanism. See text for explanation. (From Netter, FH: The Ciba Collection of Medical Illustrations Volume 6—Kidneys, Ureters, and Urinary Bladder, pg 55. Summit, NJ, CIBA Pharmaceutical Company, 1973.)

chloride pump. This pump transfers chloride (sodium follows) from the lumen to the medullary interstitium, thus increasing the tonicity of the surrounding tissue. As will be discussed in Chapter 38, this chloride pump is the primary site of action for the "loop diuretics." In summary, the removal of osmotically active particles (i.e., Na^+, Cl^-, urea) from the ultrafiltrate as it progresses through the loop of Henle creates a hypotonic fluid. The ultrafiltrate that left the proximal tubule was isotonic, thus the first step in the alteration of urine osmolality has been reached.

Fluid entering the distal convoluted tubule has been diluted by the removal of NaCl in the loop of Henle. This next segment of the nephron is impermeable to water and urea, but contains a sodium-pumping mechanism. The removal of sodium (with chloride) further dilutes the filtrate. As will be discussed in Chapter 38, this pump is the primary site of action for the "thiazide" diuretics. Farther along the distal nephron is the area where aldosterone mediates the exchange of sodium for potassium. The osmolality of the filtrate is not altered here because both sodium and water are freely permeable in this segment. Antagonism of aldosterone is yet another mechanism of inducing a mild diuresis and is also discussed in Chapter 38.

In the cortical collecting duct, an important decision is made: whether to excrete a dilute or concentrated urine. The decision is facilitated by the posterior pituitary gland, which secretes ADH into the circulation. ADH acts on the cells of the cortical and medullary collecting ducts to alter their water permeability. In addition, ADH enhances the medullary collecting duct permeability to urea. The net effect of ADH is thus to enhance removal of only water from the filtrate and to allow urea to move into the medullary interstitium. The increased osmolality of the interstitium then causes extraction of water from the descending limb of the loop of Henle, initiating the sequence again.

In summary, isotonic fluid leaves the proximal tubule and enters the descending limb of the loop of Henle where water is extracted (see Fig. 37–5). The ascending limb of the loop of Henle removes solutes without water, creating a hypotonic fluid. The presence or absence of ADH determines the fate of the hypotonic fluid. If ADH is present, a concentrated urine is excreted; in the absence of ADH, a dilute urine is eliminated.

THE ROLE OF THE KIDNEY IN ACID–BASE HOMEOSTASIS

Acid-base homeostasis refers to the maintenance of the extracellular pH within the range of 7.35 to 7.45. The homeostatic mechanism is best illustrated by examining the bicarbonate (HCO_3^-)/carbon dioxide (CO_2) buffering system:

$$H^+ + HCO_3^- \rightleftharpoons H_2CO_3 \rightleftharpoons H_2O + CO_2 \quad \text{(eq. 2)}$$

At equilibrium, equation 2 can be expressed by the law of mass action, as follows:

$$[H^+] = 24 \times P_{CO_2}/[HCO_3^-] \quad \text{(eq. 3)}$$

and if expressed in terms of the Henderson–Hasselbach equation:

$$pH = 6.10 + \log [HCO_3^-]/0.03\ P_{CO_2} \quad \text{(eq. 4)}$$

The significance of the relationship expressed in equation 2 is that the $[H^+]$ is a function of the ratio of P_{CO_2} to bicarbonate concentration. The P_{CO_2} is regulated by the rate of pulmonary ventilation, whereas the bicarbonate concentration is controlled by renal H^+ excretion. Close inspection of equation 2 reveals that an increase in H^+ shifts the equilibrium to the right, decreasing HCO_3^- and increasing CO_2. Therefore, addition of H^+ can be counteracted by increasing pulmonary ventilation (to eliminate CO_2) or by generation of HCO_3^- by the kidney. When the H^+ decreases, the situation may be corrected by decreasing pulmonary ventilation or by excreting HCO_3^- via the kidney. In these examples, it becomes evident that the lungs and the kidneys play a central role in acid-base homeostasis.

The nephron participates in acid-base regulation by the reabsorption of HCO_3^- from the ultrafiltrate and by generation of new HCO_3^- through H^+ excretion.

BICARBONATE REABSORPTION

In the proximal tubule, fluid and electrolyte balance is intimately related to acid-base homeostatis, as shown in Figure 37–7. A proton, H^+, and HCO_3^- from the blood

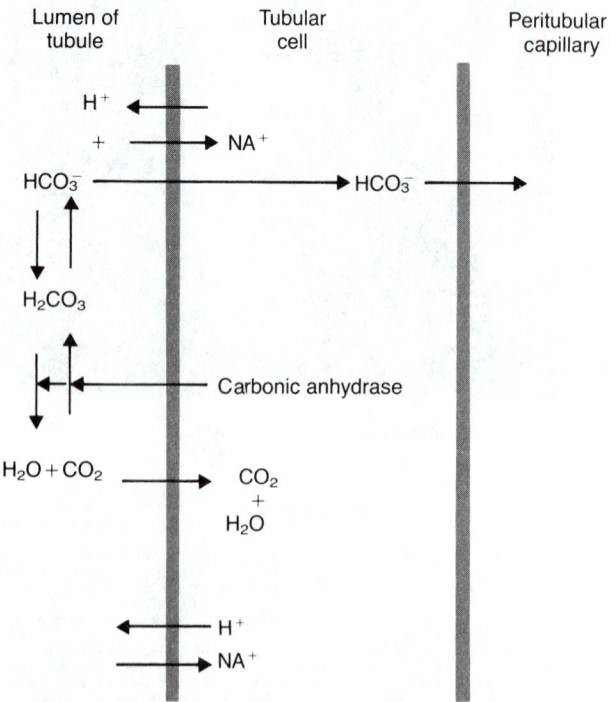

Figure 37–7. Model for renal tubular HCO_3^- reabsorption.

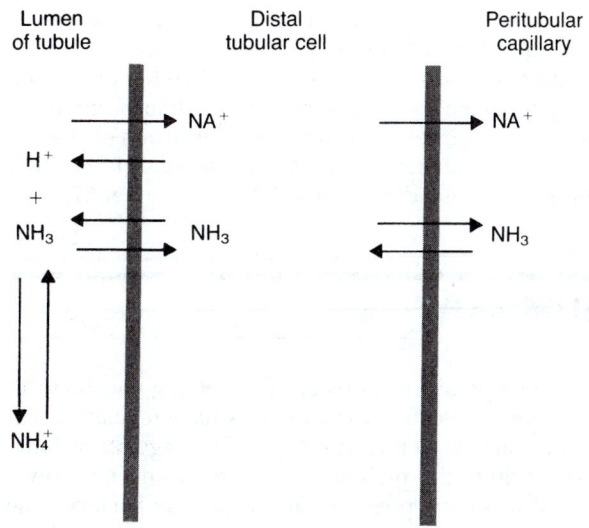

Figure 37–8. Formation of NH_4^+ in the tubule.

stream combine to form carbonic acid (H_2CO_3) in the proximal tubular cell. The reaction is catalyzed by the enzyme carbonic anhydrase located in the tubular cell. In the tubular cell, H_2CO_3 dissociates into HCO_3^- (which is reabsorbed into the peritubular capillaries) and H^+ (which is then available to be exchanged for Na^+). Sodium is then reabsorbed from the tubular fluid. In this manner, sodium reabsorption is achieved, and bicarbonate is returned to the circulation to prevent alterations in systemic pH.

HYDROGEN ION EXCRETION AND BICARBONATE GENERATION

The nephron also regulates acid-base balance by forming ammonia in the cells of the distal tubule. As shown

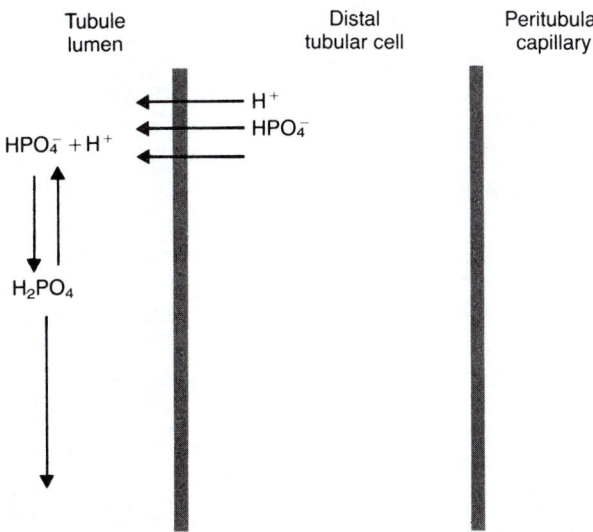

Figure 37–9. Formation of titratable acidity.

in Figure 37–8, ammonia (NH_3) diffuses into the lumen and combines with H^+ to form ammonium ion (NH_4^+):

$$NH_3 + H^+ \rightarrow NH_4^+$$

Ammonium ion then passes out in the urine, and the net result is elimination of H^+. H^+ is also eliminated in the urine by combining with sulfate or phosphate that has been filtered by the glomerulus:

$$HPO_4^- + H^+ \rightarrow H_2PO_4$$
$$HSO_4^- + H^+ \rightarrow H_2SO_4$$

When H^+ combines with HPO_4^- or HSO_4^-, it is referred to as *titratable acidity* (Figure 37–9). The formation of ammonia and of titratable acidity are the two primary mechanisms by which the nephron can eliminate unwanted H^+ from the body. For every H^+ the nephron can excrete, an HCO_3^- is generated and returned to the extracellular space, as illustrated in Figure 37–7.

THE ENDOCRINE FUNCTION OF THE KIDNEY

SECRETORY FUNCTIONS

The secretory functions of the kidney consist of releasing both renin and erythropoietin. When blood pressure is low, the juxtaglomerular cells secrete renin. Renin is an enzyme that combines with angiotensinogen, a circulating plasma protein, to form angiotensin I, which is subsequently converted to angiotensin II by an enzyme found almost entirely in the small vessels of the lungs. Angiotensin II is one of the most potent vasoconstrictors known; it also stimulates the adrenal cortex to secrete aldosterone, causing increased sodium reabsorption and increased ECF volume, resulting in increased blood pressure. Excessive renin production may be important in the etiology of some forms of hypertension.

Erythrocytes transport oxygen and carbon dioxide and buffer the acid-base system. In the healthy adult, erythrocyte production takes place in the bone marrow. This production is stimulated by erythropoietin, a protein formed primarily in the kidneys. Although the role of the kidney in erythropoietin production is not fully understood, it is believed that the kidney responds to hypoxia by producing erythropoietin. As a result, patients with chronic hypoxia (congestive heart failure, chronic obstructive pulmonary disease) often have increased red blood cell levels due to increased erythropoietin levels. On the other hand, patients with renal disease have a reduction to erythropoietin production and thus are chronically anemic.

The kidneys are concerned with the degradation of insulin. About 20% of the insulin produced by the pancreas is degraded by the renal tubular cells. Consequently, diabetic patients with renal disease may require less insulin.

The kidneys are also involved with the production of a group of compounds of possible endocrine significance, the *prostaglandins*. Prostaglandins (PG) are unsaturated fatty acid hormones which are present in many body tissues. The renal medulla produces PGA_2 and PGE_2, which are potent vasodilators. In the kidney, prostaglandins may play a role in the regulation of renal blood flow, renin release, and sodium reabsorption. Prostaglandins also do many other activities in the body. They are discussed in detail in Chapter 47.

CALCIUM AND PHOSPHATE HOMEOSTASIS

Calcium and phosphate regulation within the human body is a delicate balance of dietary intake, bone metabolism, and kidney excretion. Most of the body calcium and phosphate is found in bone. Calcium is also located in other intracellular and extracellular locations, whereas phosphorus is an essential component within cell membranes and other important biochemicals. The plasma calcium concentration, although a small percentage of total calcium, is finely modulated by hormonal control. Both calcium and phosphorus are discussed in greater detail in Chapter 57.

Parathyroid hormone (PTH), also called parathormone, is secreted by the parathyroid glands when the plasma calcium concentration decreases below the desired range (8.5–10.5 mg/dL). PTH elevates plasma calcium by working with vitamin D to enhance bone resorption, increase intestinal calcium absorption, and decrease renal calcium excretion. PTH also promotes phosphate resorption from bone and increases renal elimination of phosphate. The net result of PTH is to elevate plasma calcium and to decrease plasma phosphate concentrations.

Vitamin D (cholecalciferol) is a steroid compound that is ingested in the diet and synthesized in the skin. Vitamin D circulates to the liver where it is converted to 25-hydroxycholecalciferol (25-D). Further metabolism in the kidney forms 1,25-dihydroxycholecalciferol (1,25-D). The conversion of 25-D within the kidney is stimulated by PTH and hypophosphatemia.

Vitamin D acts to increase the availability of calcium and phosphate by enhancing intestinal absorption and increasing their release from bone. The action of vitamin D on bone is dependent on the presence of PTH. Vitamin D is discussed in greater detail in Chapter 57.

SUMMARY

The kidneys are responsible for helping the body to maintain homeostasis. The kidneys have regulatory, excretory, and secretory functions. The regulatory functions include the maintenance of fluid and electrolyte balance, osmotic pressure, and acid-base balance. The excretory functions include the elimination of metabolic waste products. The secretory functions include the release of renin, erythropoietin, and several prostaglandins.

BIBLIOGRAPHY

Abels, L: Critical Care Nursing: A Physiological Approach. CV Mosby, St. Louis, 1986.

Dossey, B: Acute renal failure. In Kenner, C, Guzzetta, C, and Dossey, B (eds): Critical Care Nursing: Body–Mind–Spirit. Little, Brown & Co, Boston, 1985.

Guyton, AC: Human Physiology and Mechanisms of Disease Control. WB Saunders, Philadelphia, 1988.

Kaye, WA: Understanding kidney disease. Diabetes Forcast 40(11):24, 1987.

Lancaster, LE: Renal and endocrine regulation and water and electrolyte balance. Nurs Clin North Am 22(4):761, 1987.

Maree, SM: The renal system. Am Ass Nephrol J 55(3):269, 1987.

Roberts, SL: Physiologic Concepts and the Critically Ill Patient. Prentice-Hall, Englewood Cliffs, NJ, 1985.

38
CHAPTER

DIURETICS

38

DIURETICS

GLOSSARY TERMS IN THIS CHAPTER

Anasarca
Ascites
Cirrhosis
Diuretic resistance
Edema
Fluid challenge
Hepatic encephalopathy
Hydrostatic pressure
Hyperglycemic hyperosmolar nonketotic coma
Hypoalbuminemia
Interstitial
Nephrogenic diabetes insipidus
Nephrotic syndrome
Oncotic pressure
Peripheral edema
Pitting edema
Pulmonary edema
Step therapy
Venodilation

38

DIURETICS

MERRILY MATHEWSON KUHN, R.N.C., Ph.D., CCRN

LEARNING OBJECTIVES

After reading this chapter, the learner will be able to:

1. Identify common pathophysiologic conditions that lead to the development of edema.

2. Differentiate among the diuretics based on site and mechanism of action, as well as relative potency.

3. Identify pharmacokinetics, pharmacodynamics, contraindications and precautions, adverse reactions, and interactions related to diuretic therapy.

4. Identify specific areas of assessment in the patient requiring diuretic therapy in order to formulate nursing diagnoses.

5. Plan appropriate nursing interventions and patient teaching for diuretic therapy.

6. Evaluate therapeutic response and revise assessment, diagnoses, and nursing interventions accordingly.

PATHOPHYSIOLOGY OF EDEMATOUS STATES

The ultimate goal of the circulatory system is to transport nutritional elements to living cells and remove the waste products of cellular metabolism and thus preserve an optimal environment in which the cells function. The exchange of nutrients and waste products is facilitated by transfer across the blood vessel membrane, as well as the active and passive transport processes across the cell membrane.

The distribution of water and electrolytes throughout the human body is maintained by a complex interaction between hydrostatic and oncotic forces. *Hydrostatic pressure* is generated by the contraction of the heart, whereas *oncotic pressure* is a result of the amount of protein within the body compartments. If the body is considered as a series of separate compartments, it is easier to understand the movement of fluid and electrolytes.

Figure 38–1 illustrates the dynamic equilibrium that exists between fluid within the extracellular space, which includes both the intravascular and *interstitial* fluid compartments, and the intracellular space. The hydrostatic pressure within the blood vessels is greater than that within the interstitial space. Therefore, the tendency is for water to be forced out of the vascular space. The oncotic pressure within the vessels is primarily caused by albumin (the major blood protein) and tends to pull water into the vessels. The net effect is that nutrients move out of the blood at the arterial end due to hydrostatic pressure (and diffusion), and water and waste products are transferred into the blood due to oncotic pressure (and diffusion) at the venous end. Thus, the arteries supply the cell's metabolic requirement, while the veins remove waste products and transport them away from the cellular environment.

This system works very well in the healthy individual. However, in the presence of certain diseases, the equilibrium is not maintained and fluid accumulates in the interstitial space ("third space"). In examining Figure 38–1, it becomes clear that diseases that increase intravascular hydrostatic pressure, decrease intravascular oncotic pressure, or alter capillary permeability, lead to accumulation of fluid within the interstitial space. The increased volume of salt and water within space is called *edema*. Edema may accumulate in the peritoneal cavity—*ascites*, or generally in all body tissues—*anasarca*.

The major disease states causing edema are cardiac failure, cirrhosis of the liver, and the nephrotic syndrome (Fig. 38–2). In other situations, the edema may be of idiopathic, or unknown, origin or may be associated with pregnancy.

EDEMA OF CARDIAC FAILURE

When the heart begins to fail as a pump, the body responds in many ways to maintain an effective blood pressure. The ineffective pumping action is "compensated" for by an enhanced tone of the sympathetic nervous system, resulting in an increased heart rate, increased cardiac contractility, and peripheral artery constriction. Sympathetic stimulation is also important in causing the release of vasopressin from the posterior pituitary. Although hyponatremia is generally the clinical hallmark which causes the release of vasopressin, the vasoconstriction properties of the hormone may represent the evolutionary basis for the release of this hormone in response to diminished cardiac output.

The arterial constriction decreases peripheral blood flow and thus, kidney perfusion declines. The kidneys respond by releasing renin, an enzyme that enhances conversion of circulating angiotensin I precursor to angiotensin I. Angiotensin I circulates in the blood to the lungs, where it is converted to angiotensin II, a powerful vasoconstrictor. Angiotensin II travels to the adrenal gland, where it stimulates aldosterone release. Aldosterone then proceeds to the kidney where it stimulates Na^+ and water reabsorption. The net effect is to maintain the blood pressure by constricting the blood vessels (i.e., angiotensin II), by increasing intravascular volume (i.e., aldosterone), and by decreasing glomerular filtration rate, resulting in a decreased elimination of Na^+ and H_2O.

Heart failure occurs in stages, with each successive decrease in cardiac output eliciting further compensatory responses as described above. At some point, the failing pump elicits a response from the kidneys, which, in an attempt to restore normal circulation, begin to overload the capacity of the blood vessels. As heart failure worsens, the overloaded circulatory system develops increased hydrostatic pressure, leading to edema. As the left ventricular pumping action fails, the back pressure induces excessive pressure within the blood

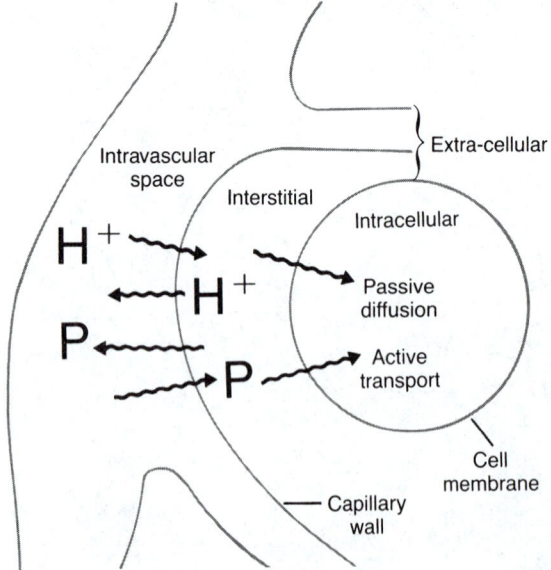

Figure 38–1. The various "spaces" within the human body. Hydrostatic pressure (H) and oncotic pressure (P) are greater within the blood vessels than within the interstitial space in a normal healthy person.

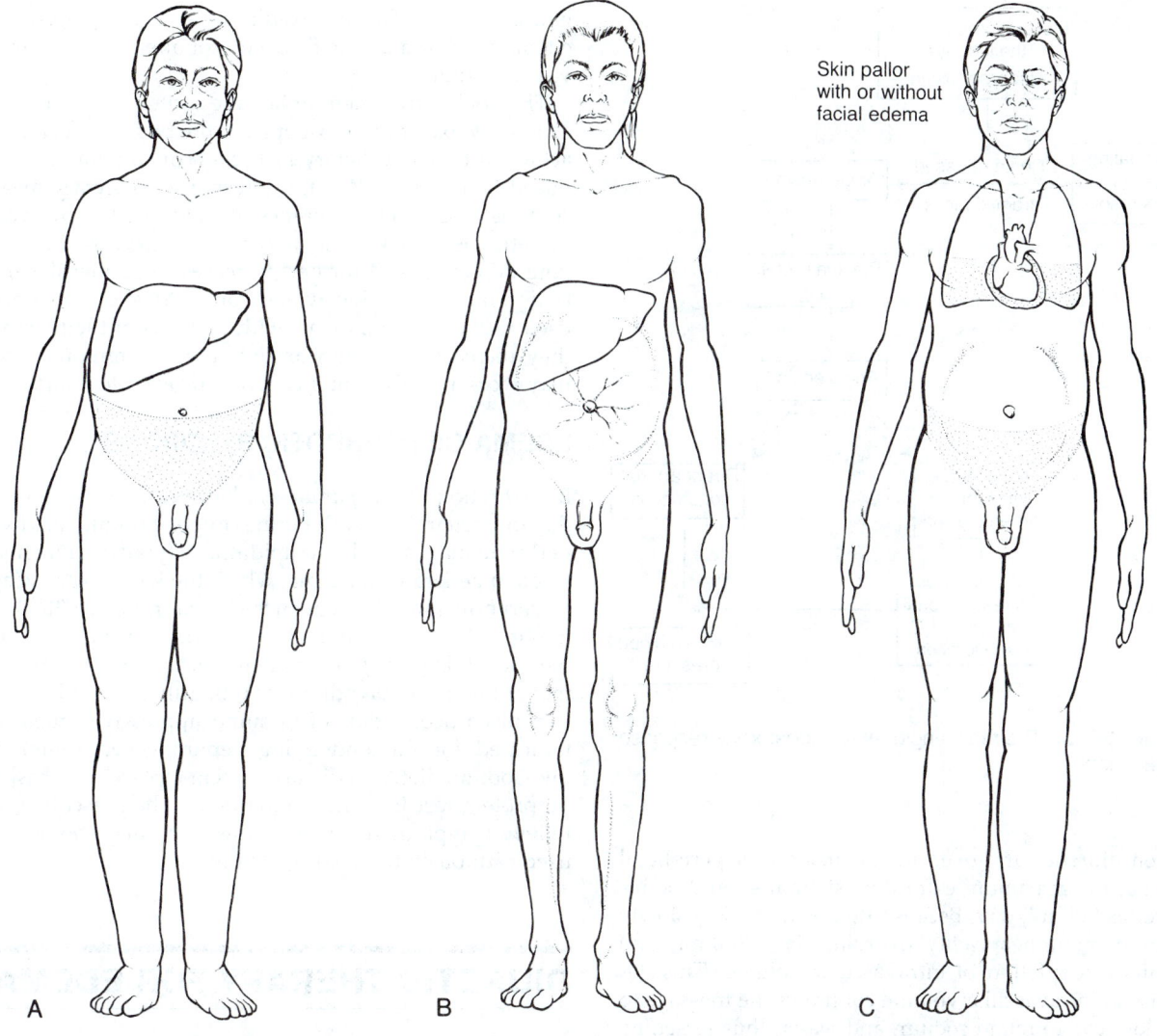

Skin pallor
with or without
facial edema

A   B   C

Figure 38–2. Comparison of the different forms of edema. (A) Cardiac edema may be peripheral as with RHF or in the lungs with LHF. (B) Liver edema is primarily found in the form of ascites. (C) Renal edema may be peripheral but also occurs in the face—Potter's face.

vessels of the lungs, causing *pulmonary edema.* The failure may eventually involve the right ventricle, and then the pressure within the venous system increases, leading to generalized *peripheral edema.* This is evidenced by edema of the lower extremities that responds to pressure by forming a depression in the tissue called *pitting edema.*

Treatment of cardiac edema includes bed rest and decreased dietary sodium intake which decreases total body sodium, a cardiac inotrope to enhance pumping activity, and diuretics to eliminate Na⁺ and water and decrease intravascular volume.

EDEMA OF LIVER FAILURE

Patients with *cirrhosis* of the liver also develop an abnormality in the way their kidneys reabsorb sodium and water. High pressures within the portal vein and low serum albumin due to decreased synthesis in liver failure combine to increase hydrostatic pressure and decrease plasma oncotic pressure. The net effect is the accumulation of fluid within the peritoneal cavity, called ascites. As ascites develops, there is often hypovolemia; the patient's kidneys sense underperfusion, and the sequence of events described in Figure 38–3 is initiated. In addition, the metabolism of aldosterone is also decreased. The kidney responds by retaining sodium and water, which contributes to further accumulation of ascitic fluid. Patients with cirrhosis often have generalized, peripheral edema related to *hypoalbuminemia.* The presence of peripheral edema is an important factor to consider when diuretics are prescribed for these patients (Fig. 38–4). Patients with hypoalbuminemia are generally treated with protein replacement as well as diuretics.

Diuretics are administered with the ultimate goal of decreasing ascites, because large amounts of ascitic fluid may lead to cardiovascular and pulmonary problems.

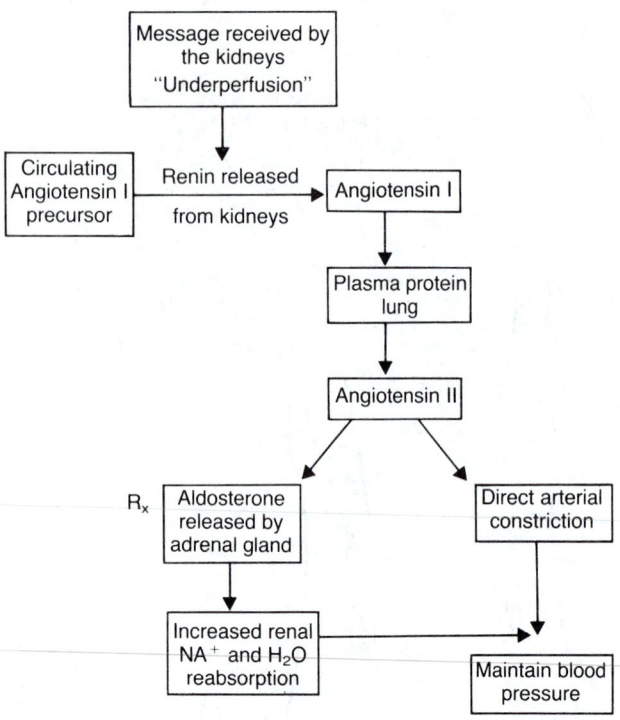

Figure 38–3. The renin-angiotensin-aldosterone response by the kidneys.

When diuretics are given in the absence of peripheral edema, the maximum extra diuresis that should be induced is 900 ml/day. Because fluid is mobilized slowly from the peritoneal cavity, overdiuresis (>900 ml/day) results in depletion of intravascular volume. This decrease in intravascular volume continues the message to the kidneys to retain sodium and water, thus lessening the diuretic effects.

When diuretics are administered to mobilize ascitic fluid and the patient has peripheral edema, the amount of diuresis that can be tolerated is greater. This is because the peripheral edema fluid is mobilized faster than is ascitic fluid. The net result is decreased peripheral edema fluid and ascitic fluid but not alteration of intravascular volume.

The goal of treatment of hepatic ascites is weight loss caused by excretion of water from the body. This can be achieved by strict dietary restriction of sodium and reduced fluid intake. When the response to dietary measures is insufficient, diuretics are indicated. However, diuretics used excessively may lead to intravascular volume depletion and further decreases in glomerular filtration rate, as previously mentioned. Most diuretics are used cautiously in patients with cirrhosis of the liver as they increase the hemoconcentration of ammonia and may worsen the symptoms of *hepatic encephalopathy.*

EDEMA OF NEPHROTIC SYNDROME

By definition, the *nephrotic syndrome* consists of >3 g/day of protein loss in the urine, hypoalbuminemia, hyperlipidemia, and hyperlipiduria. Hypoalbuminemia leads to generalized edema, which the kidneys sense as underperfusion. The sequence shown in Figure 38–3 is initiated and sodium and water reabsorption is enhanced, thus perpetuating edema formation. The treatment of nephrotic syndrome is primarily the administration of corticosteroids of immunosuppressive drugs (if indicated for the underlying nephrotic syndrome), a low-sodium diet, and dietary protein replacement based on protein lost in urine. Diuretics may be prescribed to relieve symptomatic edema; however, they should be used cautiously to avoid overdiuresis.

DIURETIC THERAPY FOR EDEMA

As described previously, the edematous patient exhibits enhanced reabsorption of sodium and water by the kidney. This leads to intravascular volume expansion and eventually an increase in edema (see Fig. 38–4). The clinical use of diuretics in these patients is meant to pre-

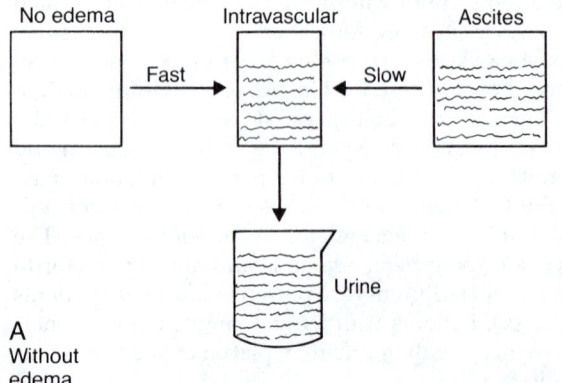 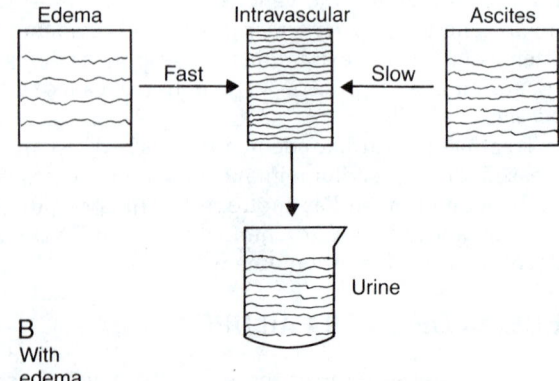

Figure 38–4. (A) Mobilization of ascitic fluid in the absence of edema after diuretic administration. (B) Mobilization of fluid in the presence of both ascites and peripheral edema.

vent reabsorption of sodium and water, thus increasing urinary sodium excretion. If successful, diuretics cause sodium excretion to exceed sodium intake, resulting in negative sodium balance and reduction of edema. The loss of sodium is essential for the anti-edema effect and for at least one major component of the antihypertensive effect. Unfortunately, when sodium is lost, it is inevitable to lose other ions such as potassium, magnesium, and calcium.

The selection of a particular diuretic for therapy of edema depends upon how well the kidneys are being perfused with blood. In situations where the glomerular filtration rate (GFR) is greater than 30 ml/minute, thiazide-type diuretics or an aldosterone antagonist may be effective. When the GFR drops below 30 ml/minute, diuresis may be achieved only with the more powerful loop diuretics. At times, combinations of different diuretics may be more effective than single-agent therapy (i.e., additive diuretic effects). The toxicities associated with diuretic therapy for edematous patients are the same as for other diuretic indications and are discussed in the section under diuretic pharmacology.

SITE OF ACTION

Most of the true diuretics have a direct effect on the kidney, rather than an indirect action via the heart or the circulation. In general, diuretics work by inhibiting sodium or chloride reabsorption by the tubular epithelial cells of the nephron. Sodium that is not reabsorbed remains in the urinary lumen and retains water within the lumen by osmosis. The increased volume of urine passes out of the nephron, resulting in diuresis. Diuretics work at various locations along the nephron (Fig. 38–5).

DIURETIC PHARMACOLOGY

The mainstay of diuretic therapy in the early 1950s was the mercurial diuretics. These agents have been pre-empted by newer, more effective, less toxic diuretics. The diuretics are featured in Table 38–1. All drug dosage information can be found in this table.

Carbonic Anhydrase Inhibitors

ACTION. Carbonic anhydrase inhibitors (CAIs) such as acetazolamide (Diamox, Ak-Zol, and others) methazolamide (Neptazane), and dichlorphenamide (Daranide) are derived from sulfonamide antibiotics and are able to bind to carbonic anhydrase, the enzyme found in the brush border of the proximal tubule epithelial cells. This enzyme catalyzes the following reaction: $CO_2 + H_2O \leftrightarrow H_2CO_3$. H_2CO_3 then dissociates into H^+ and HCO_3^-. As described in Chapter 37, this reaction is essential for acid–base homeostasis. When carbonic anhydrase activity is depressed, the net result is that Na^+ and HCO_3^- are excreted in the urine, initiating an alkaline diuresis. However, the diuretic effects are limited because of the resulting acid–base disturbance that develops—a systemic hyperchloremic acidosis.

As bicarbonate is excreted in the urine, it leads to systemic acidosis. In fact, this is the basis for using acetazolamide in certain patients with metabolic alkalosis. Carbonic anhydrase inhibitors also increase potassium excretion and may cause hypokalemia.

The CAI also noncompetitively inhibit carbonic anhydrase in the eye. This action reduces the rate of aqueous humor formation, which ultimately decreases intraocular pressure (IOP).

USES. Because of the tolerance that develops rapidly to CAIs, these drugs have limited usefulness as diuret-

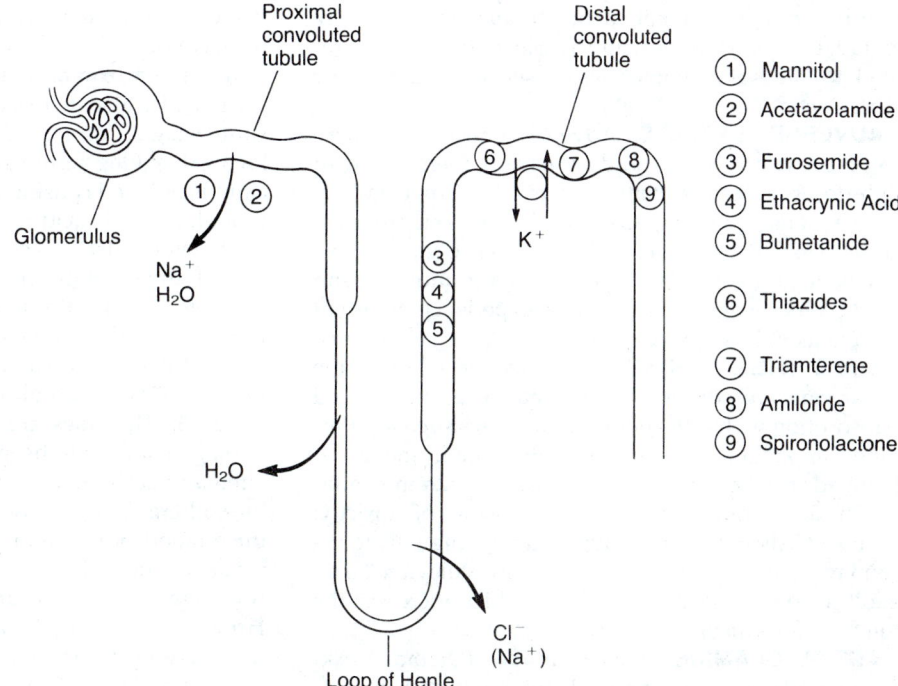

Figure 38–5. Sites of action of diuretics. The primary site of action is presented. Many of these drugs have multiple sites of action.

Proximal convoluted tubule

Distal convoluted tubule

1. Mannitol
2. Acetazolamide
3. Furosemide
4. Ethacrynic Acid
5. Bumetanide
6. Thiazides
7. Triamterene
8. Amiloride
9. Spironolactone

Glomerulus

Na^+
H_2O

K^+

H_2O

Cl^-
(Na^+)

Loop of Henle

ics. Today, they are mainly used for the adjunctive treatment of chronic simple (open-angle) glaucoma and secondary glaucoma. Acetazolamide is also used for the prevention and treatment of acute mountain sickness. Since acetazolamide does not prevent the life-threatening complications of pulmonary and cerebral edema, it should not be used routinely as a substitute for gradual ascent to higher elevations. Acetazolamide is also used as adjunctive therapy to treating congestive heart failure, drug-induced edema, and generalized absence seizures.

PHARMACOKINETICS. The CAIs are well absorbed following oral administration. The CAIs are not metabolized by the liver and are primarily excreted by the kidneys. The onset, peak, and duration of action of the CAIs varies from drug to drug. Onset ranges from one to four hours, peak effect occurs between two and eight hours, while the duration of action ranges from six to eighteen hours. For specific drug information see Table 38–1.

CONTRAINDICATIONS AND PRECAUTIONS. The CAIs are contraindicated in persons hypersensitive to these products. In addition, patients who have fluid and electrolyte imbalance such as hyponatremia, hypokalemia, and hyperchloremic acidosis are not given these products because all of these conditions would be worsened. CAIs are also contraindicated in patients with severe pulmonary obstruction because the resulting acidotic state would increase the respiratory rate.

CAIs are also contraindicated in patients with chronic noncongestive angle-closure glaucoma. Organic closure of the angle may occur. While the use of CAIs causes worsening glaucoma, the symptoms are masked by the lowered IOP.

Safety during pregnancy and lactation has not yet been established.

The CAIs are used with caution in patients with respiratory acidosis or emphysema because the CAI may aggravate or worsen the acidosis. Since the CAIs are related to the sulfonamides, cross sensitivities may be experienced.

ADVERSE EFFECTS. Adverse effects of these agents are relatively rare and are usually seen only with high doses. Certain patients may exhibit hypersensitivity reactions including fever, rash, or bone marrow suppression. Patients may also experience gastrointestinal complaints such as nausea, vomiting, anorexia, and constipation. Some patients may experience transient myopia as IOP is reduced.

DRUG INTERACTIONS. Alkalinization of the urine by carbonic anhydrase inhibitors may lead to enhanced reabsorption within the nephron for drugs such as quinidine, amphetamine, ephedrine, flecainide, and pseudoephedrine. Patients receiving these agents in combination are monitored closely for signs of toxicity. Because CAIs may induce hypokalemia, digitalis toxicity may occur. Combined therapy with salicylates may result in severe metabolic acidosis, which increases the potential for salicylate toxicity.

ACETAZOLAMIDE. Acetazolamide (Diamox, Ak-Zol, and others) is administered to patients with chronic simple glaucoma in oral doses of 250 mg/day to 1 g/day, usually in divided doses. To treat mountain sickness, oral doses of 500–1000 mg/day are administered. Sustained-release capsules are also available, but should only be used in glaucoma and acute mountain sickness. The dosage is 500 mg, once daily. Acetazolamide is available for parenteral administration; however, intravenous administration is preferred because the alkaline solution is painful when given intramuscularly.

METHAZOLAMIDE. Methazolamide (Neptazane) is administered orally in a dosage of 50–100 mg, two or three times daily.

DICHLORPHENAMIDE. Dichlorphenamide (Daranide) is administered in initial doses of 100–200 mg, followed by 100 mg every 12 hours until the desired response is obtained. The maintenance dosage is then 25–50 mg, one to three times daily. Dichlorphenamide is most effective in reducing IOP when used concurrently with miotics and osmotic agents.

Thiazides and Thiazide-like Diuretics

The thiazide diuretics were discovered during attempts to modify the structure of various carbonic anhydrase inhibitors. The results led to a new class of compounds, which have their primary diuretic actions at the cortical diluting segment of the nephron. They were first introduced in 1958. A number of derivatives and four similarly-acting nonthiazide agents have been subsequently developed. The thiazides exhibit a flat dose-response curve; that is, the toxic and therapeutic levels never meet. Therefore, they have a wide margin of safety.

ACTION. The thiazide-type diuretics increase the urinary excretion of sodium chloride and water by directly inhibiting sodium reabsorption in the early distal tube (see Fig. 38–5). Thiazides lose their efficacy as the GFR decreases below 30 ml/minute because insufficient quantities of sodium reach this site of the nephron. The decreased sodium reaching the distal nephron is a result of decreased filtration and increased sodium reabsorption in the proximal tubule.

Thiazides also increase the urinary excretion of potassium, magnesium, and, to a small extent, bicarbonate ions. After long-term therapy, urinary excretion of calcium is reduced causing increased serum calcium levels. In addition, uric acid retention may occur.

Thiazides also have an antihypertensive action, although the exact mechanism is unknown. During initial therapy, cardiac output decreases and blood volume diminishes. With chronic therapy, cardiac output normalizes but peripheral vascular resistance falls, which may be due to inhibition of the intracellular Na^+–K^+ pump.

USES. Thiazides are used as adjunctive therapy to manage congestive heart failure, hepatic cirrhosis, and edema of early renal disease. Thiazides may be used as monotherapy or in association with other drugs to reduce blood pressure in patients with relatively normal renal function. They are also helpful in reversing the fluid retention that occurs with some antihypertensives. However, the full therapeutic antihypertensive effect may take up to one month, so that a common error is premature upward movement in *step therapy*; that is, going on to the next step too soon. Diuretics may be the initial agent of choice in salt-sensitive patients such as the elderly, blacks, some diabetics, and the obese. They are also often used in combination with other antihypertensive drugs because they tend to potentiate these drugs by one third to one half.

As renal function decreases, the thiazides have diminished efficacy, probably because of impaired delivery of the drug to the active site. In addition, due to alterations in functioning of the nephrons, the thiazides have a decreased ability to produce diuresis.

Thiazides are the only drugs available to reduce urinary volume in patients with *nephrogenic diabetes insipidus* and may do so by 30% to 50%.

PHARMACOKINETICS. The thiazides are well absorbed following oral ingestion, and a diuretic effect is initiated within one hour. These agents are distributed throughout extracellular fluid. The members of this group vary in their peak and duration of effect. In general, their effects are related to their rate of elimination through the kidneys. All of the thiazides are primarily excreted by the kidneys, with little hepatic metabolism. The half-life varies from one to twenty-five hours depending on the product. For specific drug information see Table 38–1. Administration for three to four weeks is generally required to obtain optimal therapeutic effect.

The primary difference between the thiazides is their duration of action. Chlorothiazide (Diuril) and hydrochlorothiazide (Esidrix) are short acting—12 hours or less; bendroflumethiazide (Naturetin), benzthiazide (Aquatag), and hydroflumethiazide (Diucardin) are intermediate acting—18 hours or less; while chlorthalidone (Hygroton), polythiazide (Renese), and trichlormethiazide (Naqua) are long acting—24 hours or more.

CONTRAINDICATIONS AND PRECAUTIONS. Thiazides are contraindicated in patients with renal decompensation, anuria, or hypersensitivity to thiazides. Thiazides are administered cautiously to persons with impaired renal function since these agents may precipitate azotemia. When a patient experiences a rising blood urea nitrogen (BUN) level, therapy should be discontinued. When creatinine clearance falls below 40–50 ml/minute, the kidney is unresponsive to thiazides and a loop diuretic is more effective.

Thiazides can be administered during pregnancy when edema is due to pathologic causes. Safety and efficacy in children has not been established.

ADVERSE EFFECTS. Hypersensitivity reactions such as dermatitis, photosensitivity, bone marrow suppression, and vasculitis have been reported. Patients may also complain of dizziness, weakness, fatigue, orthostatic hypotension, and leg cramps. Orthostatic hypotension generally disappears, especially when therapy is cotinued. The leg cramps may be associated with electrolyte imbalances.

In clinical practice, a primary concern of thiazide therapy is the abnormalities in biochemistry that may result. Thiazides may cause hypokalemia, hypomagnesemia, hyponatremia, and hypochloremia. For this reason, clinical chemistry values are monitored closely when patients are taking diuretics. The serum potassium level often falls to 3.0–3.5 mEq/liter during long-term therapy. Hypokalemia can lead to diarrhea, vomiting, and anorexia. Corrective measures should be taken to return the potassium level to normal limits. Patients who are concurrently receiving digitalis may experience myocardial irritability as the potassium levels fall.

Thiazides increase fasting blood glucose levels and decrease glucose tolerance during long-term therapy. Thiazide-induced glucose intolerance is sometimes attributed to potassium loss. Generally, the effect on blood glucose is not clinically important except in patients with diabetes or predisposition to the disease. These patients may require some alteration in their drug regimens.

The thiazides may also cause an elevation of blood urea nitrogen or prerenal azotemia. This prerenal azotemia is related to a decrease in renal blood flow and glomerular filtration rate due to the reduction in blood volume. Prerenal azotemia is reversible when the thiazides are discontinued.

Hyperuricemia may develop because there is a decreased secretion of uric acid by the tubular cells and/or an increased renal reabsorption of uric acid. This increased uric acid level rarely causes symptoms unless the patient has a hereditary predisposition to gout or has chronic renal failure. Patients may continue to take the thiazides if they take colchicine, another uricosuric agent, or allopurinol.

Hypercalcemia can also occur in patients receiving the thiazides due to an increased protein-bound fraction of calcium. This elevation of calcium levels rarely causes symptoms. Thiazides have also been reported to reduce libido and to cause impotence.

Thiazides have been reported to be associated with elevating serum cholesterol, triglycerides, and LDL cholesterol levels. The rationale for this elevation is not clearly understood but obesity, glucose intolerance, and hyperuricemia has been suggested. A concurrent lipid-lowering diet may be beneficial. Thiazides may also induce an allergic interstitial nephritis, resulting in a decrease in renal function. Thiazides have also been shown to be a possible link to the development of gallstones, particularly in women.

INTERACTIONS. Thiazides may increase serum lithium levels by reducing renal excretion of lithium. It is thought that volume depletion secondary to thiazides increases proximal tubular reabsorption of sodium (and lithium). When thiazides are added to the therapy of patients who are stabilized on lithium, the patients are monitored closely for signs of lithium intoxication such as tremors and gastrointestinal disturbances. Lithium serum concentrations are also followed during thiazide treatment.

Thiazides may induce hypokalemia and potentiate digitalis toxicity. Anion-exchange resins (cholestyramine, colestipol) may bind thiazides, thus preventing their absorption.

Thiazide diuretics have been reported to induce ele-

TEXT RESUMES ON PAGE 1014

Table 38–1. DIURETICS

Name	Dosage	Mode of Administration	Pharmacokinetics
CARBONIC ANHYDRASE INHIBITORS:			
Action: Nonbacteriostatic sulfonamides that noncompetitively inhibit the enzyme carbonic anhydrase.			
Use: Chronic simple and secondary glaucoma, to reduce intraocular pressure.			
Acetazolamide (Diamox, Ak-Zol, and others)			
Use: Same as for all plus prevention and treatment of acute mountain sickness. Adjunct for treating congestive heart failure.			
	250 mg–1 g/day	Oral, IV	O: Oral, 1–2 hr; IV, 2 min P: Oral, 2–4 hr; IV, 15 min D: Oral, 8–12 hr; IV, 4–5 hr ½L: 2.4–5.8 hr PB: UA B: excreted unchanged E: kidneys
	500 mg daily S-R	Oral	O: 2 hr P: 8–12 hr D: 18–24 hr
Dichlorphenamide (Dara-nide)	Initial: 100–200 mg followed by 100 mg every 12 hr Maintenance: 25–50 mg, 1–3 times daily	Oral	O: within 1 hr P: 2–4 hr D: 6–12 hr ½L: UA PB: UA B: liver E: kidneys
Methazolamide (Neptazane)	50–100 mg, 2–3 times daily	Oral	O: 2–4 hr P: 6–8 hr D: 10–18 hr ½L: UA PB: UA B: liver E: kidneys

Key to Abbreviations in the *Pharmacokinetics* column O-onset; P-peak; D-duration; PB-protein bound; B-biotransformed in; E-excreted in; ½L-halflife.
*Within the column of adverse effects, <u>underlines</u> indicate the most common effects; CAPITALS indicate life-threatening effects.

Contraindications/ Precautions	Adverse Effects*	Interactions	Nursing Implications
For all CAI diuretics: CONTRAINDICATIONS: Hypersensitivity to sulfonamide derivatives, hyponatremia or hypokalemia, marked kidney or liver disease, acidosis, electrolyte imbalance, adrenocortical insufficiency or failure. PRECAUTIONS: Increasing dose does NOT increase diuresis and may lead to drowsiness or paresthesias. Adequate/balanced electrolyte intake is essential. Use in impaired hepatic function may precipitate coma.	**For all CAI diuretics:** Sulfonamide cross-sensitivity may occur. *Neuro:* convulsions, weakness, fatigue, paresthesias, sedation, drowsiness, depression, dizziness *GI:* melena, anorexia, nausea, vomiting, constipation, hepatic insufficiency *Hemo:* BONE MARROW DEPRESSION, THROMBOCYTOPENIA, HEMOLYTIC ANEMIA, AGRANULOCYTOSIS *Renal:* hematuria, glycosuria, urinary frequency, renal colic, calculi, polyuria, electrolyte loss (K$^+$), acidosis *Derm:* urticaria, pruritis, STEVENS-JOHNSON SYNDROME, rash	**For all CAI diuretics:** Alkaline urine decreases excretion of quinidine, amphetamines, pseudoephedrine, ephedrine, and flecainide, and may lead to toxicity. Concurrent salicylates may result in severe metabolic acidosis, increasing potential of salicylate toxicity.	**For all CAI diuretics:** ASSESSMENT: Assess level of motor function during therapy. Assess gastrointestinal side effects of therapy. INTERVENTION: Instruct patient not to drive or operate machinery while taking these diuretics. Instruct patient to take with food if GI upset occurs. Also, do not stop taking drugs unless instructed to do so. EVALUATION: Evaluate therapy frequently for efficacy. Evaluate for sore throat, fever, unexplained bleeding or bruising, tingling or tremor, or rash and report to physician.
Same as for all.	Same as for all.	Same as for all.	Same as for all.
Same as for all.	Same as for all.	Same as for all.	Same as for all.
Same as for all.	Same as for all.	Same as for all.	Same as for all.

CONTINUED ON THE FOLLOWING PAGE

Table 38-1. DIURETICS–*CONTINUED*

Name	Dosage	Mode of Administration	Pharmacokinetics
DIURETICS ACTING IN THE DISTAL TUBULE THIAZIDE AND THIAZIDE-LIKE DIURETICS:			
Action: Inhibit tubular reabsorption of Na^+ and Cl^- by direct action on distal tube.			
Use: Edema, hypertension.			
Thiazide Diuretics Chlorothiazide (Diuril, Diachlor, and others)	0.5–2.0 g/day *Pediatric:* under 6 mo: 33 mg/kg/day in 2 doses; over 6 mo: 22 mg/kg/day in 2 doses	Oral, IV	O: 1–2 hr; IV, 15 min P: 4 hr; IV, 90 min D: 6–12 hr; IV, 2 hr ½L: 1–2 hr PB: UA B: unchanged E: kidneys
Hydrochlorothiazide (Esidrix, HydroDiuril)	For edema: *Initial:* 25 mg daily *Maintenance:* 25–100 mg daily up to 200 mg For hypertension: *Initial:* 25 mg daily *Maintenance:* 25–100 mg daily *Pediatric:* under 6 mo: 3.3 mg/kg in 2 doses; 6 mo–2 hr: 12.5–37.5 mg/day in 2 doses; 2 yr–12 yr: 37.5–100 mg/day in 2 doses	Oral	O: 2 hrs P: 4–6 hr D: 6–12 hr ½L: 5.6–14.8 hr PB: UA B: 5% liver E: kidneys
Bendroflumethiazide (Naturetin)	For edema: *Initial:* 2.5 mg daily *Maintenance:* 2.5–5.0 mg daily For hypertension: *Initial:* 2.5 mg daily *Maintenance:* 2.5–15.0 mg daily	PO	O: 2 hr P: 4 hr D: 6–12 hr ½L: 3.0–3.9 hr PB: UA B: unchanged E: kidneys

Key to Abbreviations in the *Pharmacokinetics* column O-onset; P-peak; D-duration; PB-protein bound; B-biotransformed in; E-excreted in; ½L-halflife.
*Within the column of adverse effects, underlines indicate the most common effects; CAPITALS indicate life-threatening effects.

Contraindications/ Precautions	Adverse Effects*	Interactions	Nursing Implications
For all thiazide diuretics: CONTRAINDICATIONS: Hypersensitivity, sulfonamide cross-sensitivity, anuria, lactation. PRECAUTIONS: Use with caution in renal or severe hepatic disease. Jaundice or thrombocytopenia may be noted in newborns of mothers treated with thiazides.	**For all thiazide diuretics:** *Neuro:* dizziness, vertigo, headache, drowsiness, fatigue, depression, diuretic-induced hypokalemia may potentiate digitalis-glycoside toxicity, orthostatic hypotension *Resp:* respiratory distress, cough, sinus congestion *GI:* anorexia, nausea, vomiting, pancreatitis, gastric irritation *Renal:* electrolyte imbalances (hypokalemia, hypomagnesemia, hyponatremia, hypochloremia, hyperglycemia, hypercalcemia) *Musc-Skel:* muscle cramps/ spasm, joint pain, acute gouty attacks *CV:* increases serum cholesterol	**For all thiazide diuretics:** Additive hypotension when given with antihypertensives. Increased K^+ loss when given with the following: glucocorticoids, amphotericin B, azlocillin, carbenicillin, mezlocillin, piperacillin, ticarcillin. Decreased excretion of lithium which may lead to toxicity. Cholestyramine and colestipol decreases absorption of thiazides.	**For all thiazide diuretics:** ASSESSMENT: Assess serum electrolytes, uric acid, and blood glucose. Weigh daily and record. Assess cardiac activity carefully for dysrhythmias when on digitalis. INTERVENTION: Take with food to avoid GI upset. Administer early in day to avoid sleep disruption. Best not to administer after 3 PM. Diet counseling regarding foods high in potassium and sodium. Hyperglycemia may affect diabetes mellitus. Hypoglycemic dose may need to be adjusted. EVALUATION: Monitor therapy for efficacy. Renal insufficiency may increase after long-term thiazide therapy. Evaluate weight pattern and input and output. Notify physician of muscle cramps, nausea, vomiting, diarrhea, or dizziness.
Same as for all.	Same as for all.	Same as for all.	Same as for all.
Same as for all.	Same as for all.	Same as for all.	Same as for all.
Same as for all.	Same as for all.	Same as for all.	Same as for all.

CONTINUED ON THE FOLLOWING PAGE

Table 38–1. DIURETICS–*CONTINUED*

Name	Dosage	Mode of Administration	Pharmacokinetics
Cyclothiazide (Anhydron)	For edema: *Initial:* 1–2 mg in AM *Maintenance:* 1–2 mg q OD or 2–3 times weekly For hypertension: 2–6 mg daily	PO	O: within 6 hr P: 7–12 hr D: 18–24 hr ½L: UA PB: UA B: UA: E: kidneys
Methychlothiazide (Enduron, Ethon, others)	For edema: 2.5–10.0 mg daily For hypertension: *Initial:* 2.5–5.0 mg daily; if blood pressure not controlled after 8–12 wk, add another drug	PO	O: 2 hr P: 6 hr D: 24 hr ½L: UA PB: UA B: UA E: kidneys
Benzthiazide (Aquatag, Hydrex, and others)	For edema: *Initial:* 50–200 mg daily; if over 100 mg, administer in 2 doses *Maintenance:* 50–150 mg/day For hypertension: *Initial:* 25–100 mg daily *Maintenance:* individualized up to 200 mg/day	PO	O: 2 hr P: 4–6 hr D: 12–18 hr ½L: UA PB: UA B: UA: E: kidneys
Hydroflumethiazide (Saluron, Diucardin)	For edema: *Initial:* 50 mg 1–2 times daily *Maintenance:* 25–200 mg/day; if over 100 mg, give in divided doses For hypertension: *Initial:* 50 mg, 2 times/day *Maintenance:* 50–100 mg/day, not to exceed 200 mg/day	PO	O: 2 hr P: 4 hr D: 12–24 hr ½L: 17 hr PB: UA B: UA E: kidneys
Trichlormethiazide (Metahydrin, Naqua, and others)	For edema: 1–4 mg daily For hypertension: 2–4 mg daily	PO	O: 2 hr P: 6 hr D: 24 hr ½L: 2.3–7.3 hr PB: UA B: UA E: kidneys
Polythiazide (Renese)	For edema: 1–4 mg daily For hypertension: 2–4 mg daily	PO	O: 2 hr P: 6 hr D: 24–36 hr ½L: 25.7 hr PB: UA B: 80% liver E: kidneys
Thiazide-like Diuretics: Quinethazone (Hydromox)	50–100 mg daily	PO	O: 2 hr P: 6 hr D: 18–24 hr ½L: UA PB: UA B: UA E: kidneys

Key to Abbreviations in the *Pharmacokinetics* column O-onset; P-peak; D-duration; PB-protein bound; B-biotransformed in; E-excreted in; ½L-halflife.
*Within the column of adverse effects, underlines indicate the most common effects; CAPITALS indicate life-threatening effects.

Contraindications/ Precautions	Adverse Effects*	Interactions	Nursing Implications
Same as for all.	Same as for all.	Same as for all.	Same as for all.
Same as for all.	Same as for all.	Same as for all.	Same as for all.
Same as for all.	Same as for all.	Same as for all.	Same as for all.
Same as for all.	Same as for all.	Same as for all.	Same as for all.
Same as for all.	Same as for all.	Same as for all.	Same as for all.
Same as for all.	Same as for all.	Same as for all.	Same as for all.
Same as for all.	Same as for all.	Same as for all.	Same as for all.

CONTINUED ON THE FOLLOWING PAGE

Table 38–1. DIURETICS–*CONTINUED*

Name	Dosage	Mode of Administration	Pharmacokinetics
Metolazone (Diulo, Zaroxolyn) (Microx)	For hypertension: 2.5–5.0 mg daily For edema of renal disease: 5–20 mg daily For edema of cardiac disease: 5–10 mg daily For hypertension: 0.5–1.0 mg daily	PO	O: 1 hr P: 2 hr D: 12–24 hr ½L: 8 hr PB: 33% B: 10–20% liver E: kidneys
Chlorthalidone (Hygroton)	For edema: *Initial:* 50–100 mg daily *Maintenance:* 50–200 mg daily For hypertension: *Initial:* 25 mg daily *Maintenance:* 25–100 mg daily	PO	O: 2 hr P: 2–6 hr D: 24–72 hr ½L: 40 hr PB: UA B: UA E: kidneys
Indapamide (Lozol)	2.5–5.0 mg/day	PO	O: 1–2 hr P: within 2 hr D: up to 36 hr ½L: 14 hr PB: 71–79% B: 93% liver E: kidneys

LOOP DIURETICS:

Action: Inhibit reabsorption of Na$^+$ and Cl$^-$

Use: Edema.

Key to Abbreviations in the *Pharmacokinetics* column O-onset; P-peak; D-duration; PB-protein bound; B-biotransformed in; E-excreted in; ½L-halflife.
*Within the column of adverse effects, underlines indicate the most common effects; CAPITALS indicate life-threatening effects.

Contraindications/ Precautions	Adverse Effects*	Interactions	Nursing Implications
Same as for all.	Same as for all.	Same as for all.	Same as for all.
Same as for all.	Same as for all.	Same as for all.	Same as for all.
Same as for all.	Same as for all.	Same as for all.	Same as for all.

For all loop diuretics:
CONTRAINDICATIONS: Hypersensitivity, anuria, pregnancy or lactation, bumetanide contraindicated in hepatic coma. PRECAUTIONS: Use with caution in severe liver disease, electrolyte depletion, or diabetes mellitus. Ethacrynic acid and furosemide should be used with extreme caution in progressive azotemia.

For all loop diuretics:
Neuro: hearing loss
CVR: hypotension, hypovolemia, dehydration
GI: abdominal discomfort and pain
Hemo: AGRANULOCYTOSIS, LEUKOPENIA, THROMBOCYTOPENIA
Renal: hyponatremia, hypokalemia, hypomagnesemia
Derm: rashes, photosensitivity

For all loop diuretics:
Additive hypotension when given with antihypertensives or nitrates. Diuretic-induced hypokalemia may increase digitalis glycoside toxicity. Decreases lithium excretion, which may lead to toxicity. Ethacrynic acid and furosemide may increase the effect of oral anticoagulants. Concurrent aminoglycosides and cisplatin increases incidence for ototoxicity. Concurrent indomethacin decreases natriuretic and antihypertensive effect.

For all loop diuretics:
ASSESSMENT: Assess baseline urinary output. Assess for alkalosis and electrolyte imbalance. Assess daily weight and report rapid weight changes. Assess for development of orthostatic hypotension.
INTERVENTION: Instruct to take with meals to avoid GI upset. Administer early in day so sleep is not interrupted. Do not administer after 3 PM. Weigh and measure input and output daily. Instruct patient regarding foods high in potassium. Instruct patient regarding OTC drug use, especially sodium-containing products. Administer IV products slowly over several minutes. Administer furosemide no faster than 4 mg/minute. Administer furosemide deep IM at a maximum dose of 40 mg to minimize irritation. Do not use discolored solutions.

CONTINUED ON THE FOLLOWING PAGE

Table 38–1. DIURETICS–*CONTINUED*

Name	Dosage	Mode of Administration	Pharmacokinetics
LOOP DIURETICS–Continued			
Furosemide (Lasix, Fumide, Luramide, and others)			
Use: As for all plus hypertension.			
	For edema: *Initial:* 20–80 mg/day or alternate days; increase by 20–40 mg; maximum dose of 600 mg/day For hypertension: *Adult:* 20 mg qd, reduce dose as blood pressure falls *Pediatric:* 2 mg/kg; increase 1–2 mg/kg at 6–8 hr intervals; maximum dose 6 mg/kg.	PO, IM	O: Oral, within 60 min; IV, within 5 min; IM, 30 min P: Oral, 60–120 min; IV, 30 min D: Oral, 6–8 hr; IV, 2 hr ½L: 30–120 min PB: 96–98% B: 30–40% liver E: kidneys
	For edema: 20–40 mg given slowly over 1–2 min, not to exceed 4 mg/min; increase by 20 mg after 2 hr For acute pulmonary edema: *Adult:* 40 mg, if no response double *Pediatric:* 1 mg/kg; increase by 1 mg/kg after 2 hr	IV	
Ethacrynic Acid (Edecrin)			
Use: As for all, plus malignant edema, lymphedema.			
	Adult: 50–200 mg daily or on alternate days; adjust dose in 25–50 mg increments *Pediatric:* 25 mg/day; 0.5–1.0 mg/kg given slowly over several min up to 100 mg	Oral, IV	O: Oral, within 30 min; IV, within 5 min P: Oral, 120 min; IV, 15–30 min D: Oral, 6–8 hr; IV, 2 hr ½L: 60 min PB: 95% B: liver E: 35–45% bile, 55–65% kidneys
Bumetanide (Bumex)	0.5–2.0 mg/day; up to maximum dose of 10 mg/day	Oral	O: Oral, 30–60 min; IM, 40 min; IV, within minutes P: Oral, 6–120 min; IM/IV, 15–45 min D: 4–6 hr; IV, 2–3 hr ½L: 60–90 min PB: 94–96% B: 45% liver E: kidneys
	0.5–1.0 mg over 1–2 min up to a maximum daily dose of 10 mg	IV, IM	

Key to Abbreviations in the *Pharmacokinetics* column O-onset; P-peak; D-duration; PB-protein bound; B-biotransformed in; E-excreted in; ½L-halflife.

*Within the column of adverse effects, underlines indicate the most common effects; CAPITALS indicate life-threatening effects.

Contraindications/ Precautions	Adverse Effects*	Interactions	Nursing Implications
			EVALUATION: Evaluate therapy for efficacy. Evaluate lithium and digitalis levels for toxicity. Evaluate diabetics for hyperglycemia, glycosuria, and electrolyte disturbances. Evaluate coagulation studies.
Same as for all.	Same as for all.	Same as for all.	Same as for all.
Same as for all.	Same as for all.	Same as for all.	Same as for all.
Same as for all.	Same as for all.	Same as for all.	Same as for all.

CONTINUED ON THE FOLLOWING PAGE

Table 38-1. DIURETICS–*CONTINUED*

Name	Dosage	Mode of Administration	Pharmacokinetics
POTASSIUM-SPARING DIURETICS			

Spironolactone (Aldactone, Alatone)

Action: Competitively inhibits aldosterone; therefore, interferes with sodium reabsorption. Weak diuretic and antihypertensive action when used alone.

Use: Primary hyperaldosteronism, edema, hypertension, hypokalemia.

	For hyperaldosteronism: 100–400 mg daily For edema: 25–200 mg daily For hypertension: 50–100 mg daily For hypokalemia: 25–100 mg daily	PO	O: 24–48 hr P: 48–72 hr D: 48–72 hr ½L: 1.3–2 hr (13–24 canrenone) PB: 98+% B: liver, to canrenone and other active metabolites E: urine and bile

Amiloride (Midamor)

Action: Inhibit Na$^+$ reabsorption induced by aldosterone, not aldosterone antagonist.

Use: Congestive heart failure, hypertension.

	5–20 mg/day	Oral	O: 2 hr P: 6–10 hr D: 24 hr ½L: 6–9 hr PB: 23% B: 10% liver E: 50% unchanged by kidneys, 40% unabsorbed drug in feces

Key to Abbreviations in the *Pharmacokinetics* column O-onset; P-peak; D-duration; PB-protein bound; B-biotransformed in; E-excreted in; ½L-halflife.

*Within the column of adverse effects, underlines indicate the most common effects; CAPITALS indicate life-threatening effects.

Contraindications/ Precautions	Adverse Effects*	Interactions	Nursing Implications
			For all potassium-sparing diuretics: ASSESSMENT: Assess baseline potassium level. Assess blood pressure regularly during therapy. Assess intake and output and weight. INTERVENTION: Teach patient to avoid potassium supplements. Counsel regarding foods high in potassium. Weigh daily. Record intake and output. Rise slowly to avoid orthostatic hypotension. Avoid excessive, strenuous exercise. EVALUATION: Evaluate therapy for efficacy. If GI cramping, diarrhea, headache, skin rash, or breast enlargment occur, notify physician.
CONTRAINDICATIONS: Anuria, hypersensitivity, renal insufficiency, pregnancy, and lactation. PRECAUTIONS: Use with caution in elderly or debilitated patients, and hyperkalemia.	*Neuro:* headache, drowsiness, lethargy, confusion *GI:* nausea, vomiting, anorexia, diarrhea *Renal:* hyperkalemia, hyponatremia, dehydration, metabolic acidosis *Endo:* gynecomastia in males, menstrual disturbance in females, hirsutism	Additive hypotension when given with antihypertensives or nitrates. With captopril, enalapril, or K^+ supplements, hyperkalemia may result. Diuretic effect may be decreased with concurrent salicylates.	Same as above plus INTERVENTION: Store in dark container away from light.
CONTRAINDICATIONS: Hypersensitivity, anuria. PRECAUTIONS: Use with precaution in hyperkalemia, diabetes, acutely ill respiratory patient. Safety in pregnancy, lactating women, and children not established.	*Neuro:* headache, dizziness, tremors, vertigo, visual disturbances *CVR:* orthostatic hypotension, dysrhythmias *Resp:* cough, dyspnea *GI:* nausea, vomiting, diarrhea, abdominal pain *Renal:* hyperkalemia *Musc-Skel:* weakness, muscle cramps	Additive hypotension when given with antihypertensives or nitrates. With captopril, enalapril, or K^+ supplements, hyperkalemia may result. Reduces renal clearance of lithium.	Same as for all.

CONTINUED ON THE FOLLOWING PAGE

Table 38–1. DIURETICS–*CONTINUED*

Name	Dosage	Mode of Administration	Pharmacokinetics
Triamterine (Dyrenium)			
Action: Edema associated with congestive heart failure, hepatic cirrhosis, and nephrotic syndrome.			
Use: Edema			
	200–300 mg daily	Oral	O: 2 hr P: 6–8 hr D: 12–16 hr ½L: 100–150 min PB: 50–67% B: liver 95% to hydroxytriamterene sulfate E: kidneys (3%–5% unchanged)
OSMOTIC DIURETICS:			
Action: Elevate osmolarity of glomerular filtrate, thereby hindering the tubular reabsorption of water.			
Use: Prophylaxis of acute renal failure, reduction of intracranial and intraocular pressure.			
Mannitol (Osmitrol)	For acute renal failure: 50–100 g as a 5%–25% solution For oliguria: 300–400 mg/kg as a 20%–25% solution; up to 100 g of a 15%–20% solution For increased ICP: 1.5–2.0 g/kg as a 15%–25% solution over 30–60 min For increased IOP: 1.5–2.0 g/kg 20–25% solution over 30 min, 1 to 1½ hr before surgery	IV	O: 30–60 min P: 1–3 hr D: 6–8 hr ½L: 100 min PB: UA B: 7–10% liver E: 90% kidneys

Key to Abbreviations in the *Pharmacokinetics* column O-onset; P-peak; D-duration; PB-protein bound; B-biotransformed in; E-excreted in; ½L-halflife.

*Within the column of adverse effects, underlines indicate the most common effects; CAPITALS indicate life-threatening effects.

Contraindications/ Precautions	Adverse Effects*	Interactions	Nursing Implications
Same as amiloride	*GI:* diarrhea, nausea, vomiting, dry mouth *Biliary:* jaundice *Hemo:* thrombocytopenia, megaloblastic anemia *Renal:* azotemia, increased blood urea nitrogen level, hyperkalemia *Integ:* photosensitivity	Same as above	Same as amiloride plus INTERVENTION: Take with meals to avoid GI upset. Protect skin from sun. EVALUATION: Notify physician of fever, sore throat, nausea, or dry mouth.
For all osmotic diuretics. CONTRAINDICATIONS: Anuric renal disease, severe pulmonary congestion or frank pulmonary edema, active intracranial bleeding, severe dehydration, increasing oliguria and azotemia. PRECAUTIONS: Carefully evaluate cardiac status as sudden ECF expansion may exacerbate CHF.	For all osmotic diuretics. *Neuro:* headache, blurred vision, convulsions, dizziness *CVR:* transient volume expansion, edema, thrombophlebitis, hypotension, hypertension, tachycardia, angina-like pain *Resp:* congestion *GI:* nausea, vomiting, diarrhea, dry mouth, thirst *GU:* marked diuresis and urinary retention; fluid and electrolyte imbalance—hyponatremia, hypernatremia, hypokalemia, hyperkalemia; acidosis; dehydration *Other:* rhinitis, arm pain, skin necrosis, chills, fever, urticaria	For all osmotic diuretics. None known	For all osmotic diuretics. ASSESSMENT: Assess for fluid rebound. Assess IV sites (very irritating on infiltration). Assess intake and output—if less than 30 ml/hr, assess for circulatory overload. Assess daily weight. Assess baseline electrolyte levels. INTERVENTION: Use large venous sites and monitor patency. Do NOT administer through same IV set as blood or blood products. Administer reconstituted solutions within 48 hr. Provide good mouth care and provide ice chips frequently. EVALUATION: Evaluate therapy frequently for efficacy.
Same as above.	Same as above.		Same as above. INTERVENTION: If crystals form in IV bottle, warm it in hot water bath and shake vigorously. Allow to return to room temperature before administering. Do not administer solutions with crystals. Administer through an inline IV filter (5 microns or less). Store mannitol at 59–86°F. Do NOT give free mannitol with blood. 20 mEq of NaCl should be added to each liter of mannitol to avoid pseudoagglutination.

CONTINUED ON THE FOLLOWING PAGE

Table 38–1. DIURETICS–*CONTINUED*

Name	Dosage	Mode of Administration	Pharmacokinetics
Urea (Ureaphil)			
Use: Reduction of both intracranial and intraocular pressure.			
	30% solution *Adult:* 1.0–1.5 g/kg daily *Pediatric:* 0.5–1.5 g/kg; DO NOT EXCEED 120 g/day	IV	O: 30–45 min P: 1–2 hr D: 5–6 hr ½L: UA PB: UA B: excreted unchanged; some hydrolyzed in gut E: kidneys
Glycerin (Glyrol, Osmoglyn)			
Use: Short-term use for reduction of intraocular pressure.			
	1.0–1.5 g/kg 1–1½ hr before surgery	Oral only	O: 10–30 min P: 0.5–2 hr D: 4–8 hr ½L: 30–45 min PB: UA B: 80% liver, 10–20% kidney E: kidney
Isosorbide (Ismotic)			
Use: Short-term use for reduction of intraocular pressure.			
	1–3 g/kg	Oral only	O: 10–30 min P: 1.0–1.5 hr D: 5–6 hr ½L: 5–9.5 hr PB: UA B: excreted unchanged E: kidneys

Key to Abbreviations in the *Pharmacokinetics* column O-onset; P-peak; D-duration; PB-protein bound; B-biotransformed in; E-excreted in; ½L-halflife.

*Within the column of adverse effects, underlines indicate the most common effects; CAPITALS indicate life-threatening effects.

vations of blood glucose in certain patients. Patients who are stabilized on oral hypoglycemic agents may experience hyperglycemia if thiazides are added to their therapy and are therefore at risk for *hyperglycemic hyperosmolar nonketotic coma.*

THIAZIDE   DIURETICS. *Chlorothiazide.* Chlorothiazide (Diuril, Diachlor, and others), a thiazide diuretic, is used to treat edema in adults either orally or intravenously in a dosage of 0.5–2.0 g once or twice daily. Chlorothiazide is more effective when administered in a dosage of 250 mg every six to twelve hours than when given in large doses once daily. To treat hypertension, oral chlorothiazide is administered in doses ranging from 0.5 to 2.0 g per day. Pediatric dosing is featured in Table 38–1.

Hydrochlorothiazide. Hydrochlorothiazide (Esidrix, Hydro-T, Diaqua, and others) is a thiazide diuretic used to treat both edema and hypertension. The initial dose for edema is 25 mg/day until a dry weight is obtained,

when the maintenance dose is 25–100 mg daily or every other day. Above doses of 100 mg, there is usually no added diuretic or antihypertensive effect. To treat hypertension, the dose is 25–100 mg daily. Pediatric dosing is featured in Table 38–1.

Recent research has indicated that current coadministration of nonsteroidal anti-inflammatory drugs (NSAIDs) with hydrochlorothiazide attenuated the antihypertensive effect in approximately half of the patients. Although additional documentation is needed to confirm this potential interaction, careful monitoring of blood pressure should be done when NSAIDs are added to hydrochlorothiazide therapy.

Bendroflumethiazide. Bendroflumethiazide (Naturetin) is used to treat edema initially in a single dose of 20 mg or divided into two doses. Maintenance dose is 2.5–5.0 mg/day. To treat hypertension, the initial dose is 5–20 mg/day with a maintenance dose of 2.5–15.0 mg/day.

Contraindications/ Precautions	Adverse Effects*	Interactions	Nursing Implications
Same as above.	Same as above.	May increase excretion of lithium.	Same as above.
Same as above.	Same as above.	Same as above.	Same as above.
Same as above.	Same as above.	Same as above.	Palatability is improved if the medication is poured over cracked ice and sipped.

Cyclothiazide. Cyclothiazide (Anhydron) is used to treat edema in initial doses of 1–2 mg in the morning. Once dry weight has been obtained, the maintenance dose is 1–2 mg every other day or two to three times weekly. For hypertension, the daily dose is 2–6 mg.

Methyclothiazide. Methyclothiazide (Enduron, Ethon, and others) is a long-acting thiazide diuretic used to treat both edema and hypertension. In adults, the oral dose for treating edema ranges between 2.5 and 10.0 mg once daily; for hypertension, the adult dose is 2.5–5.0 mg. If blood pressure is not controlled at a satisfactory level in 8 to 12 weeks with 5 mg, then another antihypertensive drug should be added.

Benzthiazide. Benzthiazide (Hydrex, Aquatag, and others) is also used to treat edema and hypertension. To treat edema, the initial dose is 50–200 mg daily for several days or until dry weight is obtained. If it is necessary to give more than 100 mg daily, the drug should be administered in two doses, one in the morning and one in the evening. The maintenance dose range is 50–150 mg/day. To treat hypertension, the initial dose is 50–100 mg/day, generally administered twice daily—after breakfast and after lunch. The maintenance dose is individualized with a maximal effective dose of 200 mg/day.

Hydroflumethiazide. Hydroflumethiazide (Saluron, Diucardin, and others) is administered to treat both edema and hypertension. The initial dose to treat edema is 50 mg once or twice daily. The maintenance dose is 25–200 mg/day. Divided doses are administered when the daily dose exceeds 100 mg. The initial dose to treat hypertension is 50 mg twice a day. The maintenance dose is 50–100 mg/day, not to exceed 200 mg/day.

Trichlormethiazide. Trichlormethiazide (Naqua, Diurese, and others) is a long-acting thiazide diuretic used to treat both edema and hypertension. Trichlormethiazide is administered in doses of 1–4 mg/day to treat edema and 2–4 mg/day to treat hypertension.

Polythiazide. Polythiazide (Renese) is a long-acting thiazide diuretic used to treat edema and hypertension. To treat edema, the daily dose is 1–4 mg. To treat hypertension, the daily dose is 2–4 mg.

THIAZIDE-LIKE DIURETICS. _Quinethazone._ Quinethazone (Hydromox) is a thiazide-like diuretic used to treat edema. The usual adult dose is 50–100 mg/day. However, 150–200 mg/day may be necessary.

Metolazone. Metolazone (Diulo, Zaroxolyn, Microx) is a thiazide-like diuretic that is used to treat hypertension, and edema secondary to congestive heart failure, hepatic disease, or renal disease. Metolazone is used to treat mild to moderate essential hypertension in daily doses of 2.5–5.0 mg. When this drug is used to treat edema of renal disease, the daily dose is 5–20 mg. Metolazone may also be used to treat the edema of cardiac failure with a daily dose of 5–10 mg. Microx, compounded in a different way, is used to treat mild to moderate hypertension. It is usually administered in a 0.5-mg single daily dose taken in the morning; however, doses up to 1 mg/day may be administered. An important additional property of metolazone is that it appears to be effective even in patients with reduced renal function, thus it resembles the loop diuretics. Metolazone has a duration of action of 24 hours and can be used in conjunction with loop diuretics.

Chlorthalidone. Chlorthalidone (Hygroton, Thalitone) is a long-acting thiazide-like diuretic that is used to treat edema and hypertension. When treating edema, the initial dose is 50–100 mg/day or 100 mg on alternate days. Dosage may be increased to 150–200 mg/day. The initial dose to treat hypertension is 25 mg/day. Doses can be increased to 100 mg once a day. When daily doses are above 25 mg/day, they are likely to potentiate potassium excretion, but appear to have no other benefit in sodium excretion or blood pressure reduction.

Indapamide. Indapamide (Lozol) is a long-acting thiazide-like diuretic primarily used to treat hypertension and edema of congestive heart failure. The initial dose is 2.5 mg/day. If response is not satisfactory after one week, the dose can be increased to 5 mg/day. In general, doses above 5 mg do not provide any additional effects on blood pressure or on heart failure.

Loop Diuretics

The loop diuretics—furosemide (Lasix), bumetanide (Bumex), and ethacrynic acid (Edecrin)—are diuretics that act primarily in the loop of Henle. These agents are also referred to as high-ceiling diuretics because of their greater range of diuresis-inducing properties. Furosemide and bumetanide are sulfonamide derivatives, whereas ethacrynic acid is structurally different. Overall, these agents may be classified together and their diuretic actions discussed as a group.

ACTION. The loop diuretics inhibit the reabsorption of Na^+ and Cl^- in the proximal and distal tubule but primarily in the loop of Henle. The loop diuretics have a much greater diuretic effect than the thiazides largely due to their unique site of action. These drugs remain effective even in the presence of electrolyte and acid-base disturbances.

Ethacrynic acid inhibits the reabsorption of sodium, so it may be more effective in patients with renal insuf-

ficiency. Bumetanide inhibits more chloride than sodium. It also does not appear to act on the distal tubule.

USES. The loop diuretics are used primarily to treat edema associated with congestive heart failure, hepatic or renal disease, and the nephrotic syndrome. These drugs can be administered intravenously when rapid diuresis is necessary, such as in acute pulmonary edema. The loop diuretics promote *venodilation*, preload reduction, and afterload reduction.

A particular advantage of loop diuretics is that increasing the dose exerts an increasing diuresis before the ''ceiling'' is reached.

The loop diuretics, particularly furosemide, are used concurrently with other drugs to control hypertension. They should be reserved for hypertensive patients with fluid retention refractory to thiazides or for patients with impaired renal function. Since they have a different site of action, the loop diuretics may be effective for such patients when thiazides are not. Furosemide is also used with mannitol to manage cerebral edema. Bumetanide and furosemide are used for the short-term management of ascites due to malignancies, lymphedema, nephrogenic diabetes insipidus, and hypercalcemia.

In the oliguric patient, furosemide and bumetanide are used for diagnosis and prophylaxis of acute renal failure. Excessive diuresis should be avoided because of the danger of precipitating shock.

PHARMACOKINETICS. The loop diuretics are absorbed rapidly from the gastrointestinal tract, and their onset of action occurs within one hour after oral ingestion. Food slows the rate of absorption but does not alter the total amount absorbed. Absorption is also slowed in patients with congestive heart failure. In patients with severe edema of the gastrointestinal tract, absorption may be erratic and intravenous administration may be required. When given intravenously, the onset of diuresis may be as fast as 10 minutes. All of the loop diuretics are greater than 90% protein bound. The duration of action ranges from two hours for intravenous administration to four to six hours after oral administration. The loop diuretics are primarily excreted by the kidney via glomerular filtration and tubular secretion. (For specific information on each drug, see Table 38–1.)

CONTRAINDICATIONS AND PRECAUTIONS. The loop diuretics are contraindicated in patients with a history of hypersensitivity to the products and in patients with anuria. Bumetanide is also contraindicated in patients with hepatic coma or severe electrolyte depletion. Ethacrynic acid is contraindicated in infants.

The loop diuretics are administered cautiously to the elderly and to patients with cardiovascular disease because the diuresis may induce an acute hypotensive episode along with hemoconcentration that could lead to thromboembolic episodes. The loop diuretics are also administered cautiously to cardiac patients receiving digitalis. The diuresis and the associated loss of potassium may precipitate digitalis toxicity and dysrhythmias.

Cautiously administer furosemide and bumetanide to pregnant women only when the potential benefits outweigh the risks. Furosemide does appear in breast milk and should not be administered to nursing women. It is unknown whether ethacrynic or bumetanide are transferred through breast milk. Safety for bumetanide and ethacrynic acid in children under 18 years of age has not been established. When administering intravenous furosemide, particularly to children, diarrhea may occur secondary to the sorbitol present in the furosemide solution.

The loop diuretics are administered cautiously to patients with severely impaired renal function and dehydration.

ADVERSE EFFECTS. The major complication associated with loop diuretic therapy is the development of fluid and electrolyte imbalances. Loss of sodium and chloride as well as potassium occurs secondary to the potent effects of these diuretics within the loop of Henle. Certain patients may experience abnormal glucose tolerance while on these agents.

Hypersensitivity reactions may occur and present as gastrointestinal disturbances, skin rashes, and hepatic dysfunction. Patients with a history of sulfonamide allergy may cross-react when furosemide or bumetanide are ingested. Rapid intravenous administration of large doses of these agents may induce transient but rarely permanent deafness. For this reason, the manufacturer of furosemide recommends infusing large doses at a rate no greater than 4 mg/minute.

Photosensitivity may also occur. Patients need to be taught to wear protective clothing until tolerance can be determined.

DRUG INTERACTIONS. Indomethacin (Indocin) and other nonsteroid anti-inflammatory drugs may reduce sodium and water excretion and the antihypertensive effects caused by loop diuretics. Patients receiving loop diuretics for hypertension may lose the hypotensive effect if started on indomethacin. Both of these effects are due to the inhibition of prostaglandins. Sulindac has a similar effect on bumetanide.

Patients who receive concurrent therapy with loop diuretics and aminoglycoside antibiotics may experience additive ototoxicity from these agents. Hearing ability and vestibular function are followed closely in patients who receive this combination. Patients with renal failure appear to be at greater risk for this drug interaction.

Loop diuretics commonly cause excessive loss of potassium, leading to hypokalemia. The toxic effect of digitalis is potentiated by hypokalemia; therefore, serum electrolyte levels should be monitored in patients who receive loop diuretics and digitalis.

Concurrent administration of cisplatin may increase the potential for ototoxicity. Loop diuretics may increase levels of lithium. It is important to monitor serum lithium levels carefully to avoid toxicity.

Ethacrynic acid may increase the hypoprothrombinemic effect of warfarin. Furosemide and bumetanide do not appear to interact with warfarin.

FUROSEMIDE. Furosemide (Lasix, Fumide, Luramide, and others) was the first loop diuretic to be released. It is the preferred loop diuretic because it: causes fewer gastrointestinal effects, is more convenient for intravenous use, has a broader dose-response curve, is less ototoxic, and is available in an oral solution.

Oral furosemide is usually effective in patients with congestive heart failure who do not respond to the thiazides. It is also effective in treating edema of renal disease as it is effective even when glomerular filtration is greatly reduced.

For edema, the initial oral dose is 20–80 mg in the morning. If there is inadequate response, the dose can be increased. The maximum dose should be no more than 600 mg/day. Dosage is individualized. Some patients may need daily doses, others may benefit with alternate-day dosing.

The initial oral dose to treat hypertension is 20 mg/day. If there is no response, another antihypertensive drug should be added. When furosemide is added to another agent, it may be necessary to decrease the dose of the first drug by as much as 50% to prevent an excessive decrease in blood pressure.

For acute conditions, the initial intravenous dose of furosemide is 40 mg; this dose can be repeated in 60–90 minutes. The dose can be increased to a total of 1 g in a 24-hour period until a diuretic response is obtained. Large intravenous doses should not be administered faster than 40 mg/minute. When large doses are administered, fluid losses are replaced every two to four hours to maintain adequate plasma volume and renal perfusion.

ETHACRYNIC ACID. Ethacrynic acid (Edecrin) is a short-acting diuretic with short onset and duration of action. To treat edema, ethacrynic acid is given orally in doses of 50–200 mg daily or on alternate days. Dosage is adjusted by 25–50 mg increments. The chloruretic effect of ethacrynic acid may cause bicarbonate retention and metabolic alkalosis. Chloride can be administered to correct this condition.

Parenterally, only intravenous administration is used as subcutaneous or intramuscular injections cause local pain and irritation. Ethacrynic acid is a powder that is mixed with 50 ml of 5% dextrose or sodium chloride. Fifty milligrams of ethacrynic acid is infused slowly over several minutes as a test dose, then 50 mg more. If no results are obtained, ethacrynic acid is discontinued. If the solution becomes hazy or opalescent, it should not be used.

BUMETANIDE. Bumetanide (Bumex) can be used when the patient has hypersensitivity to furosemide. The striking difference between furosemide and bumetanide is the much greater bioavailability and potency of bumetanide allowing the use of smaller doses. Because the major difference between furosemide and bumetanide is dose equivalency, an average dose of 40–80 mg of furosemide is equivalent to 1–2 mg of bumetanide. The incidence of side effects and the therapeutic effectiveness of the two drugs are similar. Orally, 0.5–2.0 mg/day is administered up to a maximum daily dose of 10 mg. When intravenous administration is needed, 0.5–1.0 mg is administered intravenously or intramuscularly. If there is no response, a second or third dose can be administered in two to three hours. The 24-hour dose should not exceed 10 mg.

Potassium-Sparing Diuretics

USES. The potassium-sparing diuretics are most commonly used to counteract potassium loss induced by other diuretics. They are most often given concurrently with thiazides or loop diuretics to increase the serum potassium level. They are most useful in patients with increased renal mineralocorticoid activity or primary or secondary aldosteronism. These abnormalities may occur in hepatic cirrhosis, congestive heart failure, renal artery stenosis, Cushing's syndrome, and during chronic prednisone use. When used for increased mineralocortical activity, the potassium-sparing diuretics are usually given alone. Potassium-sparing diuretics counter the tendency for increased potassium secretion in these patients.

ALDOSTERONE ANTAGONISTS. *Spironolactone*. *Action.* Knowledge of the adrenal hormone aldosterone and its role in sodium and water regulation led to the development of the aldosterone-antagonist diuretics. Spironolactone (Aldactone) is the only member of this group available in this country. The actions of aldosterone-antagonists are to compete with aldosterone and to prevent the reabsorption of sodium in the distal portion of the nephron. Only a small percentage (3%–5%) of the fluid filtered by the glomerulus reaches this segment of the nephron; thus, only mild diuretic actions are noted with these agents. It is effective in lowering both systolic and diastolic blood pressure in both hyperaldosteronism and essential hypertension. Additionally, spironolactone interferes with testosterone synthesis, which may permit a relative increase in estrogen activity; this action may be responsible for endocrine dysfunctions which are occasionally seen during therapy.

Spironolactone is the logical therapy for patients who develop hypertension in the presence of elevated mineralocorticoid levels. It is also chosen when diabetes or gout may be present or when there is fear of their precipitation, or when it is important to avoid potassium or magnesium loss and thiazide combinations are contraindicated. Spironolactone has antihypertensive activity but does cause more troublesome adverse effects.

Pharmacokinetics. Spironolactone is well absorbed, about 70%, following oral administration, and a mild diuresis ensues. Food promotes absorption; however, it is not known at this time if there are changes in biotransformation. Spironolactone is more than 90% bound to plasma proteins. The duration of action increases with multiple doses. Spironolactone has extensive first-pass metabolism in the liver. It is metabolized to its active metabolite, canrenone, by the liver, and its duration of effect is related to the amount of endogenous aldosterone present. The half-life ranges from three to twelve hours.

Contraindications and Precautions. Spironolactone is contraindicated in hypersensitivity, anuria, and acute renal impairment. It is not used during pregnancy or lac-

Table 38–2. FOODS THAT CONTAIN HIGH AMOUNTS OF POTASSIUM OR SODIUM

HIGH-POTASSIUM FOODS		
Avocados	Grapefruit	Prunes
Apricots	Lima beans	Rhubarb
Bananas	Navy beans	Spinach
Cantaloupe	Nuts	Sunflower seeds
Dried fruits	Oranges	Tomatoes
HIGH-SODIUM FOODS		
Barbecue sauce	Canned soups	Macaroni and cheese
Butter, margarine	Canned spaghetti sauce	Parmesan cheese
Buttermilk	Catsup	Pickles
Most cheeses	Cured meats	Potato salad
Canned chili	Dry soup mixes	Pretzels, potato chips
Canned seafood		

tation because its safety in such cases has not been established. The drug is contraindicated in patients with hyperkalemia as it causes decreased potassium excretion and may lead to toxicity.

Adverse Effects. Inhibition of the exchange of sodium for potassium by spironolactone may induce hyperkalemia. This should be remembered when administering this agent to patients with renal insufficiency who have impaired potassium elimination. Other problems with spironolactone therapy are associated with this compound's estrogenic effects (i.e., gynecomastia). Spironolactone may also produce central nervous system symptoms such as drowsiness, ataxia, and mental confusion.

Interactions. Spironolactone may cause additive hypotension when used with antihypertensives or nitrates. Use of spironolactone with the angiotensin-converting enzyme (ACE) inhibitors—captopril, lisinopril, enalapril—or potassium supplements may lead to hyperkalemia. Aspirin may decrease the diuretic response to spironolactone. Spironolactone may decrease the vasopressor response to norepinephrine. Ingestion of large amounts of potassium-rich foods (Table 38–2) may also lead to hyperkalemia.

Dosage. Spironolactone is administered to treat hyperaldosteronism in doses of 100–400 mg/day. To treat edema of congestive heart failure, cirrhosis, or nephrotic syndrome, the usual dose is 25–200 mg/day. If there is inadequate response after five days, a second diuretic should be added. Spironolactone is administered to treat hypertension in doses of 50–100 mg/day and to treat hypokalemia in doses of 25–100 mg/day.

OTHER POTASSIUM-SPARING DIURETICS. Although these agents—triamterene (Dyrenium) and amiloride (Midamor)—have mild diuretic effects, their primary use is related to preventing potassium loss. These compounds impair exchange of sodium and potassium at the same site as spironolactone but do not work by competing with aldosterone. Both of these drugs have the duration of action increased with multiple doses and prolonged therapy.

Interactions. The pharmacologic effect of these drugs is to enhance sodium excretion and decrease potassium secretion. As a result of this, patients receiving potassium supplements with these drugs may develop hyperkalemia. Hyperkalemia may induce central nervous system (CNS) depression, cardiac dysrhythmias, and other effects. This interaction is especially significant in patients with renal failure, who have an inability to excrete excess potassium.

Triamterene. Triamterene (Dyrenium, Maxzide) is a pteridine derivative that is chemically related to folic acid. It interferes with Na$^+$ reabsorption and K$^+$ and H$^+$ ion secretion in the cortical collecting tubule by a direct action. Triamterene is not an effective antihypertensive agent when used alone, but is often used in combination with other diuretics and antihypertensives. Triamterene is also used to treat edema associated with congestive heart failure, cirrhosis, and nephrotic syndrome as well as idiopathic and steroid-induced edema, as well as edema of hyperaldosteronism. Triamterene is absorbed (50%) after oral administration. It is extensively metabolized and rapidly eliminated by both hepatic metabolism and by the kidneys. The majority of a dose can be found as metabolites in the urine within two hours after administration.

Triamterene elicits minor problems such as nausea, vomiting, leg cramps, and dizziness in certain patients. The major concern is the development of hyperkalemia when triamterene is prescribed for patients with impaired renal function. This situation may be made worse if patients are also given potassium supplements. Triamterene-containing kidney stones have also been reported. Triamterene is a weak folic acid–antagonist which may cause the development of megaloblastic anemias. Triamterene is generally administered in a dosage of 100 mg orally twice daily after meals. The maximum dose per day should not exceed 300 mg.

Amiloride. Amiloride (Midamor) has a mild diuretic effect similar to that of spironolactone. Like triamterene, amiloride is a pteridine compound which inhibits Na$^+$ reabsorption and K$^+$ and H$^+$ ion secretion in the distal tubule and cortical collecting tubule by a direct action. This agent also appears to prevent potassium loss in a similar fashion to triamterene. Amiloride is primarily used to treat hypertension or edema associated with congestive heart failure and to assist in restoring normal serum potassium levels in patients with hypokalemia. Amiloride is usually administered in combination with other diuretics, such as the thiazides or loop diuretics.

Amiloride has a more rapid onset of action than spironolactone. Amiloride is only 25% absorbed when administered orally. The peak diuretic effect occurs in 6 hours and lasts 12–16 hours. Amiloride is excreted unchanged in the urine, with minimal hepatic metabolism.

The development of hyperkalemia, as discussed under triamterene, is also a concern during amiloride therapy.

Amiloride is generally administered in oral doses of 5–10 mg daily up to a maximum dose of 20 mg/day.

Osmotic Diuretics

The osmotic diuretics are low–molecular-weight substances that increase plasma osmolarity, glomerular filtrate, and tubular fluid by remaining in high concentration in the renal tubules. Osmotic diuretics include mannitol (Osmitrol), urea (Ureaphil), glycerin (Glyrol, Osmoglyn), and isosorbide (Ismotic).

ACTION. Osmotic diuretics cause diuresis by increasing the osmolarity of the glomerular filtrate, which inhibits the reabsorption of water. The excretion of both sodium and chloride is also enhanced by these drugs. All osmotic agents share three characteristics: (1) they are freely filtered at the glomerulus; (2) their reabsorption by the renal tubule is limited; and (3) they are relatively inert, pharmacologically. The activity of osmotic diuretics is a function of their concentration in solution.

USES. The main indication for the osmotic diuretics, primarily mannitol, is prophylaxis of acute renal failure in patients with varying conditions including cardiovascular surgery, trauma, surgery in the presence of hepatic injury, and in management of hemolytic transfusion reaction. The early use of osmotic diuretics protects the kidney by insuring adequate flow of relatively dilute urine. These agents are also used to reduce the pressure and volume of cerebrospinal fluid in patients with elevated intracranial pressure; this is accomplished by increasing the osmolality of plasma, which draws fluid from the cerebrospinal fluid back into plasma. Osmotics are used for short-term reduction of increased intraocular pressure (IOP), particularly pre- and post-operatively in patients requiring ocular surgery; this reduction operates by increasing osmolality of plasma, which draws fluid into plasma from ocular fluid.

PHARMACOKINETICS. Following intravenous administration, the osmotic diuretics are absorbed either into the extracellular fluid or total body water. Mannitol is only slightly metabolized by the liver, with the balance being excreted unchanged in the urine. Glycerin is largely metabolized by the liver (80%), with the balance being metabolized by the kidney. Neither urea nor isosorbide are metabolized to any great extent and are excreted largely unchanged by the kidney.

CONTRAINDICATIONS AND PRECAUTIONS. Osmotic diuretics are contraindicated in hypersensitivity. These agents are also not indicated for use in anuric renal failure, dehydration, or active intracranial bleeding as rapid expansion of the extracellular fluid may further compromise these patients. This effect limits the use of osmotics in patients with cardiac decompensation. The safety of these drugs during pregnancy and lactation has not been established.

ADVERSE REACTIONS. The most common adverse reactions are transient volume expansion, hyponatremia, and hypokalemia, all due to rapid expansion of the extracellular fluid, which dilutes ionic concentrations. Hypernatremia may occur due to administration of mannitol in hypertonic solution. Headache and confusion may occur with rapidly changing intracranial pressure.

INTERACTIONS. The osmotic diuretics have few drug-drug interactions. Urea is known to increase the excretion of lithium; the enhanced excretion may decrease the effectiveness of lithium therapy in bipolar disorder.

MANNITOL. Mannitol (Osmitrol) is used as follows: to treat oliguria in acute renal failure; to reduce intracranial and intraocular pressure; and to treat drug intoxication from aspirin, carbon tetrachloride, secobarbital, and imipramine. Mannitol can also be used in combination with sorbitol as a urogenital irrigation.

To prevent acute renal failure, mannitol is administered in doses of 50–100 g as a 5%–25% solution. To treat oliguria, the dose is 300–400 mg/kg of a 20% or 25% solution, up to a maximum dose of 100 g of a 15% or 20% solution. To reduce intracranial pressure, the usual dose of mannitol is 1.5–2.0 g/kg as a 15%–25% solution, which is infused over 30 to 60 minutes. Generally, a reduction in cerebrospinal fluid (CSF) pressure will be observed within 15 minutes after starting the infusion. To reduce intraocular pressure, 1.5–2.0 g/kg is administered as a 20%–25% solution over a period of 30 minutes. This is generally administered 1.0–1.5 hours before surgery to achieve maximal effect.

Solutions of mannitol frequently form crystals during storage; any solution with crystals is rewarmed gently in a water bath to reincorporate the crystals. Additionally, solutions of mannitol require filtering during administration.

UREA. Urea (Ureaphil) is indicated to reduce intracranial and intraocular pressure. The usual adult dose is 1.0–1.5 g/kg, while the dose for children is 0.5–1.5 g/kg.

GLYCERIN. Glycerin (Glyrol, Osmoglyn) is used to treat acute attacks of glaucoma and to reduce pressure before ocular surgery. The adult dose is 1.0–1.5 g/kg 1.0–1.5 hours before surgery.

ISOSORBIDE. Isosorbide (Ismotic) can be used for the interruption of acute attacks of glaucoma as well as for short-term reduction of intraocular pressure before and after surgery. The initial dose is 1.5 g/kg and the dose range is 1–3 g/kg two to four times a day. This product is for oral use only and palatability is improved if the medication is poured over cracked ice and sipped.

Combination of Diuretics

Diuretics are often combined to obtain greater diuresis in edematous states such as congestive heart failure, nephrotic syndrome, and cirrhosis. Because there is altered kidney function in these conditions, it is often necessary to use drugs that act at sequential sites along the tubule to sustain diuresis.

A common example is to combine a loop diuretic (e.g., furosemide) with a thiazide-like diuretic (e.g., metolazone). Furosemide delivers more sodium to the distal tubule than a thiazide, but without a thiazide such as metolazone, the distal tubule absorbs more of that salt and reduces the net effects of the diuresis.

OTHER USES OF DIURETICS

Diuretics are used most commonly in the treatment of edema, hypertension, congestive heart failure, and renal failure. Recently, diuretics have also been studied in management of the following: bronchoconstriction; near drowning; hyperparathyroidism; hirsutism; chronic macula edema; and Reye's syndrome.

NONPRESCRIPTION DIURETICS

Nonprescription diuretics are used to alleviate menstrual discomfort. When taken four to six days before the onset of menses, they may help relieve symptoms related to water retention including temporary weight gain, bloating, puffiness, painful breasts, cramps, and tension. The most frequently used products are pamabrom (Fluidex with Pamabrom) and combinations of ammonium chloride and caffeine (Aqua-Ban).

Pamabrom is a theophylline derivative and has weak diuretic properties when taken alone. It is often combined with analgesics and antihistamines for relief of symptoms associated with menses or premenstrual syndrome.

Ammonium chloride is an acid-forming salt which has limited value in terms of diuresis. It is often used in combination with caffeine for adjunctive effects. Large doses may cause gastrointestinal irritation and central nervous system toxicity. Ammonium chloride is contraindicated for individuals with impaired renal or hepatic function. Metabolic acidosis may occur with large doses of ammonium chloride.

Caffeine promotes diuresis by inhibiting reabsorption of both sodium and chloride. It may alleviate the mental and physical fatigue associated with fluid retention. Doses above 100 mg may cause gastrointestinal irritation. The calculation of total caffeine intake should include drinking coffee, tea, or caffeine-containing soft drinks, as well as eating chocolate or taking other caffeine-containing products.

USING THE NURSING PROCESS

ASSESSMENT

Assessment of the patient requiring diuretics begins with a thorough nursing history. Multiple symptoms indicating the need for diuretic therapy may be present and are elicited during both the history and the physical assessment. Typical information to assess is featured in Table 38–3. The patient's self-consciousness may be ev-

TEXT RESUMES ON PAGE 1022

Table 38–3. NURSING PROCESS FOR PATIENT REQUIRING DIURETIC THERAPY

Assessment

Auscultate breath sounds, note presence of cough.
Assess for jugular venous distention, hepatojugular reflux, S3.
Palpate abdomen for hepatomegaly, hepatic pulsations, ascites, splenomegaly.
Examine for dependent, generalized or periorbital edema.
Determine weight, note recent changes.
Determine dietary intake of potassium and sodium.

Nursing Diagnosis	Nursing Actions	Rationale	Desired Actions/ Evaluation Criteria
Knowledge deficit related to unfamiliarity with information resources/ misinterpretation as evidenced by questions, request for information, inaccurate follow-through of instructions, development of preventable complications.	Review pathophysiology of condition and need for diuretic therapy.	Provide opportunity for patient/SO to ask questions, clarify misconceptions and make informed choices.	Verbalizes understanding of illness/condition and treatment. Identifies signs/symptoms or side-effects requiring medical attention.
	Discuss medications, dosage, schedule, and side effects.	Understanding function of the medication in own terms can help patient to manage own regimen, promote sense of control.	
	Stress importance of followup and reporting of side-effects.	Provides for timely intervention to prevent occurrence of drug-related complications.	
	Discuss importance of sodium limitation, signs/symptoms of imbalance.	Dietary intake of sodium above 3 g daily will offset diuretic effect.	
	Provide list of foods high in sodium that are to be avoided/limited. Encourage reading of labels on food and drug packages.		
	Recommend taking diuretic early in morning.	Provides adequate time for drug effect before bedtime to prevent/limit interruption of sleep.	
	Suggest patient weigh regularly.	Documents changes in fluid overload/ edema in response to therapy.	
	Encourage discussion of situation and treatment and how it affects lifestyle.	Provides insight about how patient/ SO view condition and are coping with needed changes.	
Fluid Volume Excess related to altered glomerular filtration increased ADH production, excess intake or retention of sodium/ water as evidenced by orthopnea, S3 heart sound, oliguria, edema, weight gain, hypertension, respiratory distress.	Calculate 24-hour intake and output balance. Compare with weight.	Aids in identifying therapeutic needs/ effectiveness, and potential complications. Diuretic therapy may result in sudden/excessive fluid loss (circulating hypovolemia) even though edema/ascites	Demonstrates stabilized fluid volume with balanced intake and output, breath sounds clear/clearing, vital signs within acceptable range, stable weight, and absence of edema.

CONTINUED ON THE FOLLOWING PAGE

Table 38–3. NURSING PROCESS FOR PATIENT REQUIRING DIURETIC THERAPY–*CONTINUED*

Nursing Diagnosis	Nursing Actions	Rationale	Desired Outcomes Evaluation Criteria
	Maintain chair or bed-rest in semi-Fowler's position.	Recumbency increases glomerular filtration and decreases production of ADH, thereby enhancing diuresis.	
	Establish fluid intake schedule, incorporating beverage preferences when possible. Give frequent mouth care.	Involving patient in therapy regimen may enhance sense of control and cooperation with restrictions.	
	Monitor laboratory studies, e.g., Hgb/Hct, electrolytes	Evaluates response to therapy and identifies additional therapeutic needs to prevent complications.	

ident during discussions of urinary patterns and changes. The following specific questions are asked:

1. Is there any change in amount, color, or odor of the urine?
2. Is there any change in urinary pattern—dysuria, frequency, hesitation, incontinence?
3. Do you wake during the night to void?
4. Do you notice any unusual swelling or puffiness of the hands or feet, or around the eyes?
5. Has there been an unexplained weight change?
6. Are shoes, rings, or wrist watches too tight? Terminology and phrasing are directed to the patient's educational and knowledge level.

A thorough history includes any known electrolyte imbalances, hepatic or renal dysfunction, diabetes history, pregnancy and lactation, as well as a history of drug allergies, such as an allergy to sulfonamides (loop diuretics are related to sulfonamides) and specific allergic symptoms. A medication history of drugs currently taken, including nonprescription drugs, is also required.

Physical assessment of patients requiring diuretic therapy includes several areas: neurologic, cardiovascular, respiratory, renal, skin, and nutrition. Each area is assessed to detect pre-existing or potential problems that may compromise diuretic therapy. It is essential to establish a baseline assessment in each area to evaluate effectiveness of therapy and to monitor any potential detrimental effects. The neurologic examination is composed of reflexes, orientation and mental status, cranial nerve testing, muscle strength, and hearing. Cardiovascular assessment, at minimum, encompasses pulses, baseline electrocardiogram (ECG), blood pressure (lying, sitting, and standing), and the presence of edema. The respiratory exam considers respiratory rate and pattern, and any adventitious breath sounds (crackles, wheezes, or rubs). Skin assessment is composed of peripheral perfusion exams (such as capillary refill and color and temperature observations), and assessment of skin turgor for level of hydration, lesions, and the presence of peripheral edema. Nutritional assessment includes dietary history, obesity or emaciation, and nutritional deficits.

Once the patient has been placed on diuretic therapy, the nurse needs to be alert to signs of electrolyte imbalance. Early warning signs of electrolyte imbalances include: dryness of the mouth, thirst, anorexia, weakness, lethargy, drowsiness, restlessness, paresthesias, muscle pain or cramps, hypotension, oliguria, tachycardia, dysrhythmias, and gastrointestinal symptoms such as nausea and vomiting. Since many diuretics enhance electrolyte excretion along with fluid, these patients may become sodium-, potassium-, magnesium-, or chloride-depleted.

Hypokalemia is a potentially life-threatening condition. Because potassium is necessary for proper neuromuscular and cardiac function, patients with hypokalemia may exhibit cardiac dysrhythmias, muscle weakness and cramps, abdominal distention, and mental status changes such as confusion, apathy, drowsiness, and irritability. Very often family members notice changes in the patient's mental status, so the nurse should be alert to any of their statements reflecting changes. Patients with underlying cardiac disease who are receiving digitalis and thiazide therapy run an increased risk of developing digitalis toxicity from potassium depletion. Also patients with ischemic heart disease, congestive heart failure treated with digitalis, or hypertension with left ventricle hypertrophy are at higher risk for developing dysrhythmias. Using a potassium- and magnesium-retaining diuretic, or cotherapy with an angiotensin-converting enzyme (ACE) inhibitor or calcium channel blocker may be beneficial for these patients. When ACE inhibitors are used, potassium supplements should be avoided.

NURSING DIAGNOSIS

Based on the information gained during the history and physical assessment, nursing diagnoses for the patient requiring diuretic therapy are formed. Typical nursing diagnoses are shown in Table 38–3.

PLANNING AND INTERVENTION

Nursing diagnoses direct the plan of care for patients receiving diuretic therapy. Nursing goals are derived from the nursing diagnoses. Typical goals for intervention are included in Table 38–3. In all cases, the plan of care is individually tailored to the needs of each patient. Cooperation cannot be achieved if patients do not see the total picture in regard to therapy. An empathetic nurse can help establish a relationship that encourages the patient to ask questions about treatment.

The nurse, patient, and family members must also have some understanding of the underlying pathology. Diuretics are usually part of long-term therapy, and often this is difficult for both the patient and family to accept. Unfortunately, the overnight "cure" is rarely available. Table 38–4 reviews the numerous conditions that can be treated with diuretics and the usual choice of agents. Today, when prescribing medication, the physician often looks at the benefit-risk ratio. The benefit-risk ratio of diuretics is very high in congestive heart failure. However, in contrast, the benefit-risk ratio of diuretics in the therapy of mild hypertension is increasingly being questioned.

Nursing Responsibilities

The use of diuretics in cardiac, hepatic, or renal disease has an effect on a number of body systems. Decreased muscle tone and generalized weakness may be observed

Table 38–4. DISEASE AND CHOICE OF DIURETIC

| Disease | Agent Selection | |
	First Choice	Second Choice
Congestive heart failure	Thiazide	Loop
Acute pulmonary edema	Loop	
Cirrhosis	Spironolactone	Thiazide
Nephrotic syndrome	Thiazide	Loop
Hypertension	Thiazide	Loop
Hypercalcemia	Loop	
Acute renal failure	Loop	
Nephrogenic diabetes insipidus	Thiazide	
Syndrome of inappropriate antidiuretic hormone	Loop	

along with signs and symptoms of dehydration. Any number of electrolyte imbalances may occur and must be carefully assessed in each patient. Dietary adjustments also need to be made in order to compensate for electrolyte imbalances. Sodium restrictions often accompany diuretic therapy to improve diuresis and decrease high blood pressure. Planning and teaching include potassium replacement and limitations on sodium intake. (Foods that contain high amounts of potassium and sodium are listed in Table 38–2.)

Decreased muscle tone and generalized weakness, along with signs of dehydration, are observed by the nurse and the patient. Hypokalemia (decreased serum potassium level) is a potentially life-threatening condition. Replacement of potassium can be accomplished by increasing the dietary intake of potassium-rich foods. Foods especially high in potassium content include bananas, oranges, orange juice, and dried fruits. One six-inch banana or one eight-ounce glass of orange juice contains 25–50 mEq of potassium, which is one-third to one-half more than the minimum daily requirement (MDR).

When administering diuretics, the nurse must understand when and how to administer them. Most diuretics are administered with meals to avoid gastrointestinal upset. All diuretics are best given in the morning as soon as the patient wakes up. At times, patients may be able to take diuretics on alternate days or several times per week, rather than on a daily basis. When intravenous administration is used, diuretics, particularly the loop diuretics, are administered slowly. Large doses of furosemide are administered at a rate no faster than 4 mg/minute. Slow administration will decrease the risk of ototoxicity.

Patient Teaching

Guidelines for patient teaching are shown in Table 38–5. In all patient situations, teaching is geared to the patient's knowledge level and level of understanding.

Patients should understand the function of their medication in their own terms (a diuretic or a "fluid pill,") and its clinical use in the body. Patients should also be taught the appropriate dosage and schedule to ensure their compliance with the therapeutic regimen. Signs and symptoms of potential problems are also vital parts of patient education. Patients need to be taught how to avoid orthostatic hypotension. Patients should change positions, from lying down to sitting to standing, slowly. Patients should limit their alcohol intake since alcohol also acts as a mild diuretic. During warm weather, patients should be careful to avoid strenuous exercise and heavy sweating to prevent the possibility of fluid and electrolyte imbalances.

EVALUATION

Evaluation is an ongoing process of review that gives rise to changes in assessment, nursing diagnoses, and/or the interventions being used in patient care. It is a dynamic, rather than static, view of therapy and nursing

---

Table 38–5. PATIENT TEACHING INFORMATION—DIURETICS

Dear Patient:

The drug that has been ordered for you is called a *diuretic*, or a fluid pill. This drug helps to reduce the amount of fluid in your body by causing the kidneys to pass a large amount of water and salt from your blood. Removing this fluid helps to decrease the work on your heart and to decrease the edema, or swelling, in your body. This is what you need to know about this drug:

1. The name of your drug is _____.
2. Diuretics may be needed for the rest of your life.
3. Change positions slowly to avoid dizziness.
4. Limit the amount of sodium that you take in. (High sodium foods are listed in Table 38–2.)
5. You may need to replace potassium in your body. Be guided by instructions from your nurse or physician. (High potassium foods are listed in Table 38–2.)
6. Always check with your physician or pharmacist about possible interactions between nonprescription drugs and diuretics.
7. Do not take this drug after 3 PM unless otherwise directed by your doctor. If you do, you will be awake during the night to go to the bathroom.
8. Do not stop taking this drug without checking with your physician or nurse.
9. Be aware of signs of dehydration, such as increased thirst or dry, scaly skin, and report these to the nurse or physician.
10. Report signs of potassium loss, such as muscle weakness or irritability, to the nurse or physician.
11. Check your weight daily and record it. If you lose or gain more than 3 pounds in 1 day, report it to the nurse or physician.
12. Store your medication in a tight, light-resistant container.

---

care. Guidelines for evaluation of the patient receiving diuretic therapy are included in Table 38–3.

Evaluation of the effectiveness of diuretic therapy is based on outcome criteria which are determined beforehand. In most cases, the goals of nursing intervention become the evaluation criteria. As a general rule, these criteria include: (1) an informed client and family who understand the disease process and both the medical and nursing regimens; (2) a reduction in uncomfortable symptoms due to medication compliance; (3) dietary controls; and (4) minimum side effects related to diuretic therapy.

Diuretics are used in conditions that present with a variety of clinical manifestations; therefore, both the patient and the nurse must be aware of the underlying pathology. Many of these conditions are chronic problems in which the patient may have to make major lifestyle adjustments. The patient needs a clear understanding of the consequences of any action that he or she may take or refuse to take. Compliance may become a problem if the patient expects an overnight cure.

The decrease in uncomfortable symptoms such as swollen feet and ankles, puffy hands, or dyspnea on exertion may be sufficient incentive for patient compliance. Reinforcement of the need for the medication and the therapeutic regimen is necessary with each patient contact.

During therapy of edematous states, excessive diuresis may occur. The result is a reduction in venous pressure and ventricular filling so that cardiac output drops and tissues become underperfused. Over-diuresis is most frequently seen during hospital admissions when a rigid policy of regular administration of diuretics is carried out. Excessive diuresis is most commonly seen when intravenous loop diuretics are used. It may be necessary to cautiously administer a *fluid challenge* with a saline solution or a colloid preparation while checking the patient's cardiovascular status. If the resting heart rate falls, renal function improves and blood pressure stabilizes, the ventricular filling pressure has been inadequate.

Chronic diuretic administration can also lead to leveling off of the effect or *diuretic resistance*. In the face of a shrunken intravascular volume, the part of the tubular system not affected by the diuretic reacts by reabsorbing more sodium. It is important to evaluate the following: Is there compliance with the dietary salt restriction? Is the optimal agent being used? Is complete bed rest required? Is the optimal dose being used? Are there any electrolyte disturbances that need to be corrected? Has the general cardiovascular status been made optimal by judicious use of unloading or inotropic drugs? To achieve ideal metabolic hormonal status, an ACE inhibitor may have to be added to thiazide or loop diuretics. Sometimes fewer drugs work better. A prime example are potassium supplements requiring several tablets per day which are not taken by the patient.

Other causes of apparent diuretic resistance include: excessive circulating catecholamines frequently seen in congestive heart failure which can be corrected by increased inotropic support; interfering drugs like the NSAIDs; activation of the renin-angiotensin-aldosterone system, often seen in congestive heart failure and corrected by ACE inhibitors; and incorrect use of diuretics. Incorrect use of diuretics may include use of two drugs in the same group, use of thiazides when the glomerular filtration rate is low, excessive dosing, and poor patient compliance.

Patient teaching includes alternative actions that may be taken to relieve unpleasant medication side effects should they occur. Often patients discontinue therapy due to unpleasant side effects without realizing that there are dosage and medication alternatives to minimize problems. The nurse-patient relationship facilitates communication of these concerns.

In ideal diuretic therapy, the patient's urine output increases, electrolyte imbalances are corrected, and edema decreases. If all of these goals are not possible, realistic goals, within the limits of illness, must be set by the patient and the family. The nurse provides the encouragement to overcome anxieties and lifestyle adjustments.

SUMMARY

As described previously, the patient with edema exhibits enhanced reabsorption of sodium and water by the kidney. This leads to intravascular volume expansion and eventually, an increase in edema. The clinical use of diuretics in these patients is intended to prevent this pathophysiology. If successful, diuretics cause sodium exchange to exceed sodium intake, resulting in a negative sodium balance and reduction in edema.

The selection of a particular diuretic agent for therapy of edema is dependent upon type of edema, patient tolerance, and degree of renal damage. Because they are so widely used, the diuretics are one of the most important classes of drugs. Knowledge of how the renal system functions and the specific action of diuretics are essentials of nursing. The variety of disorders that are treated with diuretic therapy virtually ensure that nurses will have daily contact with these agents. This knowledge plays a vital role in patient education, patient compliance, and nursing intervention to prevent or treat response to illness.

BIBLIOGRAPHY

Acute drug reactions in the elderly. Emerg Med 19(14):79, 1987.

Abels, L: Critical Care Nursing: A Physiological Approach. CV Mosby, St Louis, 1986.

AMA Department of Drugs: AMA Drug Evaluations, ed 6. PSG Publishing, Littleton, MA, 1986.

Barth, JH: Alopecia and hirsuties: Current concepts in pathogenesis and management. Drugs 35:83, 1988.

Bianco, S, et al: Prevention of exercise-induced bronchoconstriction by inhaled furosemide. Lancet 2:252, 1988.

Connor, PA, et al: Nursing implications of renal pelvis irrigation of chemolysis. J Urologic Nursing 7(1):350, 1988.

Cox, SN, et al: Treatment of chronic macular edema with acetazolamide. Arch Ophthalmol 106:1190, 1988.

Culpepper, RM: Which diuretic for which patient? Patient Care 21(20):103, 1987.

Ede, RJ: Reye's syndrome in adults. Br Med J 296:517, 1988.

Ferry N, et al: Influence of renal insufficiency on the pharmacokinetics of cicletanine and its effects on the urinary excretion of electrolytes and prostanoids. Br J Clin Pharmacol 25(3):359, 1988.

Gever, LN: Bumetanide: the latest loop diuretic. Nursing 87 17 (4):115, 1987.

Gilman, AC, Goodman, LS, and Gilman A (eds): Goodman and Gilman's The Pharmacological Basis of Therapeutics. Macmillan, New York, 1985.

Hill, MW: Diuretics for mild high blood pressure: Still the best choice? Nursing 87 17(9):62, 1987.

Jacobson, HR: Diuretics: Mechanism of action and uses. Hosp Pract 15(22):129, 1987.

Kakar, F, et al: Thiazide use and the risk of cholecystectomy in women. Am J Epidemiol 124:428, September, 1986.

Koopmans, PP, Thien, TH, and Bribnau, FWJ: The influence of ibuprofen, diclofenac and sulindac on the blood pressure lowering effect of hydrochlorothiazide. Eur J Clin Pharmacol 31:553, 1987.

Lamy, PP: Hypertension, diuretics, and the elderly. Caring 6(2):58, 1987.

Langford, H, et al: Is thiazide-produced uric acid elevation harmful? Arch Intern Med 147:645, April, 1987.

Margolis, S, et al: Pharmacokinetics excretion elimination. Emerg Med Serv 16(8):65, 1987.

Martin, B and Milligan, K: Diuretic-associated hypomagnesemia in the elderly. Arch Intern Med 147:1768, October, 1987.

Maxwell, MH, et al: Secondary high blood pressure: Treatable entities. Hosp Med 31(1):47, 1987.

Morganroth, J, et al: Cardiovascular Drug Therapy. Year Book Medical Publishers, Chicago, 1986.

Narins, RG and Chusid, P: Diuretic use in critical care. Am J Cardiol 57:26A, 1986.

Olin, B (ed): Facts and Comparisons: JB Lippincott, St Louis, MO, 1989.

Overdiek, HW, Merkus, FW: Influence of food on the bioavailability of spironolactone. Clin Pharmacol Ther 40:531, 1986.

Papademetriou, V: Diuretics, hypokalemia, and cardiac arrhythmias: A critical analysis. Am Heart J 111:1217, June, 1986.

Pett, WA, et al: Influence of furosemide on parathyroid hormone levels in hyperparathyroidism. N Engl J Med 318:644, 1988.

Puschett, JB: Diuretic therapy update. Comprehensive Therapy 11(10):50, 1985.

Rasch, DK: Near drowning in children: Management and outcome. NY State J Med 28:427, 1988.

Schrier, RW: Pathogenesis of sodium and water retention in high-output and low-output cardiac failure, nephrotic syndrome, cirrhosis, and pregnancy. N Engl J Med 319(16):1065, 1988.

Smith, S: How drugs act: Diuretic agents. Nursing Times 83(23):53, 1987.

Stein, JH: Hypokalemia: Common and uncommon causes. Hosp Pract 23(3A):55, 1988.

USP Dispensing Information—Drug Information for the Health Care Provider. Vol 1. United States Pharmacopeial Convention, Rockville, 1986.

Valle, GA, et al: Electrolyte imbalance in cardiovascular diseases: The forgotten factor. Heart Lung 17(3):324, 1988.

SITUATION   38–1

Duncan McKeough is admitted to the medical-surgical unit with symptoms of shortness of breath and peripheral edema. Mr. McKeough is 52 years old and has a history of ETOH abuse and recurrent congestive heart failure.

1. An IV is started, and Mr. McKeough is to receive furosemide (Lasix) 40 mg IV. Because of his history, the nurse will assess the following with regard to diuretic therapy:
   a. T_3, T_4
   b. 12-lead ECG
   c. albumin levels
   d. neurological status

2. The nurse will observe for the following side effect of intravenous furosemide by assessing for:
   a. blurred vision
   b. rhinitis
   c. drowsiness
   d. hearing loss

3. Mr. McKeough is started on oral furosemide 40 mg twice a day. The nurse will check lab values daily because of the potential for:
   a. hyponatremia
   b. hyperchloremia
   c. hypermagnesemia
   d. hypophosphatemia

4. Mr. McKeough is to continue furosemide (Lasix) 20 mg daily after discharge. The nurse will teach him to:

CONTINUED ON THE FOLLOWING PAGE

SITUATION 38–1–*CONTINUED*

a. take the medication on an empty stomach
b. eat foods high in calcium
c. weigh daily and report rapid changes
d. take medication in the evening

5. The nurse will teach Mr. McKeough to include the following in his daily diet while taking furosemide:
a. milk
b. red meats

c. dried fruits
d. grains

6. When evaluating Mr. McKeough for the effects of diuretics, which of the following factors might be noted:
a. elevated clotting time
b. reduced BUN levels
c. acidosis
d. hypoglycemia

SITUATION 38–2

Margaret Roberts, aged 47 years, is recovering from a craniotomy. The nurse monitors the intracranial pressure (ICP) and reports an elevated reading.

1. The physician orders mannitol (Osmitrol) to be given via intravenous infusion. The nurse is aware that the usual dosage for a 25 percent solution would be:
a. 5 to 6 gms per kg
b. 600 to 1000 mg per kg
c. 200 to 300 mg per kg
d. 1.5 to 2.0 gms per kg

2. The nurse will expect to observe Ms. Roberts for a reduction in the ICP within:
a. 2 hours
b. 5 minutes
c. 15 minutes
d. 1 hour

3. A nursing responsibility associated with administration of mannitol to Ms. Roberts is to:
a. discard the solution if crystals are present
b. use only specially prepared tubing for administration
c. rewarm the solution if crystals are present
d. cover the solution with foil to prevent deterioration

4. Which of the following nursing diagnostic categories is *most* applicable to Ms. Roberts' situation in relation to mannitol therapy?
a. Alteration in Oral Mucous Membrane
b. Alteration in Bowel Elimination: constipation
c. Sleep Pattern Disturbance
d. Hypothermia

5. When planning Ms. Roberts' care, the following interventions apply regarding mannitol therapy:
a. weigh every third day
b. give with blood products if necessary
c. use a 21-gauge needle for infusion
d. use an inline IV filter

6. Which of the following outcomes *best* represents therapeutic effects of mannitol therapy for Ms. Roberts?
a. improved neurological status
b. increased intracranial pressure
c. decreased peripheral edema
d. enhanced creatinine clearance

Please refer to the Appendices for correct answers and additional review questions with answers.

39
CHAPTER

DRUG THERAPY FOR THE PATIENT WITH RENAL DISEASE

CHAPTER OUTLINE

GLOSSARY TERMS IN THIS CHAPTER

Anuria
Chronic ambulatory peritoneal dialysis (CAPD)
Continuous cycling peritoneal dialysis (CCPD)
Dialysis
Furosemide threshold
Kaluretic
Manual peritoneal dialysis
Moderate renal failure
Oliguric
Osteitis fibrosa
Osteomalacia
Osteoporosis
Prerenal azotemia
Severe renal failure
Uremic frost

DRUG THERAPY FOR THE PATIENT WITH RENAL DISEASE

KENNETH A. KELLICK, PHARM.D.

LEARNING OBJECTIVES

After reading this chapter, the learner will be able to:

1. Assess the hyperkalemia of renal failure and understand the treatment modalities.

2. Understand the use of diuretics and vasoactive substances in ameliorating the excretory and cardiovascular aberrations associated with renal failure.

3. Understand the role of the kidney in regulation of acid-base balance and how to treat acid-base abnormalities.

4. Discuss the use of various agents to control calcium and phosphate imbalances in renal failure.

5. Recommend the various dietary restrictions necessary to the homeostasis of the patient in renal failure.

INTRODUCTION

The kidney is one of our most vital organs. As explained in the previous chapter, it is responsible for homeostasis of our fluid and electrolyte balance. In addition, it is one of two major elimination routes for drugs, the other being the liver. The clinical problems presented by renal failure, therefore, are: restoring renal function if possbile; compensating where necessary for the imbalances caused during renal failure; and finally, considering dosage adjustment of various drugs whose main elimination route is through the kidneys.

The focus of this chapter will be to discuss the clinical problems associated with renal failure and drug regimens used to modify these situations. Renal failure may be stratified into acute renal failure and chronic renal failure. Electrolyte imbalances, oliguria, hypertension, anemia, hyperuricemia, and acid-base disturbances are among the hallmarks of renal failure to be covered in the ensuing pages. Upon reading this information, the nurse will have a good understanding of problem management in renal failure and knowledge relative to drug dosing in renal dysfunction.

ACUTE RENAL FAILURE

In approaching the patient with acute renal failure, the nurse must understand several clinical factors. Acute renal failure is loosely described as the sudden onset of parenchymal damage. If the loss of renal function is due to a sudden injury or illness, it may be termed acute tubular necrosis (ATN), which is a temporary condition. Acute tubular necrosis may last from several days to a few weeks and is terminated by a rapid return to normal or near normal renal function. Precise measurements of urine output, blood urea nitrogen (BUN), creatinine and other waste products must be obtained before making a proper diagnosis.

OLIGURIA

When the urine output is <20 ml/hour (500 ml/day), the patient is said to be *oliguric*. A worsening of renal function may result in *anuria*, the absence of urine output. Blood urea nitrogen (BUN) and creatinine measurements often help establish a cause for acute renal failure. Elevation in BUN greater than the rise in serum creatinine early on in the oliguric process is termed *prerenal azotemia*. This may be caused by hypovolemia, hypotension, or severe congestive heart failure. To determine prerenal azotemia, a urinary sodium and creatinine must be measured. A ratio of urine to plasma creatinine greater than 20 generally points to pre-renal causes for acute renal failure.

A urine specific gravity should be obtained to access tubular concentrating functions. A value of ≥1.010 in-dicates loss of concentrating ability and may be due to parenchymal damage as suggested by the presence of red blood cells in the urine. Serum electrolytes should be monitored closely as abnormal electrolyte profiles often accompany acute renal failure, and must be dealt with appropriately.

DIURETICS

The goal of initial therapy for oliguria associated with renal failure is to increase urine flow. If volume depletion is suspected, a fluid challenge with 500–1000 ml of 0.9% NaCl may be administered intravenously over 30–60 minutes. If unsuccessful, an osmotic diuretic such as mannitol may be given. Osmotic diuretics increase the osmolarity of the glomerular filtrate, drawing more water into the nephron, thereby increasing the urine flow. Mannitol may be particularly effective since it easily passes through the glomerulus of the nephron, but is not reabsorbed into the interstitial tissues. The use of mannitol is discussed in greater detail in Chapter 38. All mannitol infusions should be administered through an inline filter (5 μm or a blood set) to prevent injection of microcrystals. Multiple boluses or a constant infusion may be warranted in different clinical settings.

Large doses of a loop diuretic, such as furosemide (Lasix), are often used in the treatment of acute renal failure. The initial dose range of furosemide is 200–400 mg. Doses should be given via controlled infusions at rates no greater than 4 mg/minute. Faster infusion rates may cause an acute hypotensive state or ototoxicity. One may have to slowly increase the doses every hour until the *furosemide threshold* for the patient has been established. This is the minimum number of milligrams of the drug necessary to produce an adequate urinary response. If patients are not responsive to furosemide, concurrent administration of metolazone (Zaroxolyn, Diulo) may be of value. The initial total daily dose of 2.5–10.0 mg may be doubled until desired effects are achieved.

Patients who demonstrate a rare hypersensitivity to furosemide may be tried on bumetanide (Bumex). This is a more potent diuretic and is dosed using a 1:40 ratio, where 1 mg of bumetanide is equivalent to 40 mg of furosemide. It is administered slowly over one to two minutes and the total daily dose is not to exceed 10 mg.

CARDIOVASCULAR STATUS

The patient with acute renal failure may demonstrate signs of hypotension or shock. In this situation, the use of a vasopressor such as dopamine may be indicated. Dopamine is an endogenous catecholamine precursor of norepinephrine. It acts on alpha, beta, and dopaminergic receptors. In the lower dosage ranges, such as 2–5 μg/kg/minute, dopamine dilates the renal and mesenteric vessels, producing a corresponding increase in glomerular filtration rate (GFR). Because of profound cardiotonic effects, dopamine is only given in emergency situations or in intensive care monitoring environments. Larger doses are possbile; however, in the larger dosage ranges the beneficial effects on GFR are obliterated, and the effects are predominantly cardiotonic and vasoconstrictive.

Often in acute renal failure, maximal cardiac output is insufficient to improve the clinical picture. The administration of cardiotonic agents such as digoxin, dobutamine, or amrinone may be warranted to improve the hemodynamic status and, thus, increase GFR. Digoxin must be administered cautiously, due to the fact that it is primarily excreted by the kidney and toxicity may rapidly develop.

Hypertension is common in acute renal failure. The etiology is either hypervolemic or idiopathic. Several antihypertensives can be used with reducing renal blood flow. Traditionally, hydralazine, clonidine, and prazosin have played an important role. Recent literature and clinical trials have shown the angiotensin-converting enzyme (ACE) inhibitors and calcium channel blockers as being preferred agents in this situation. There is postulated to be a calcium channel receptor in the kidney which may improve GFR in response to therapy with the calcium channel blockers. The calcium channel blockers include diltiazem, verapamil, and nicardipine. In those patients with decreased renal perfusion secondary to bilateral renal artery disease, the ACE inhibitors may decrease glomerular filtration rate. Sodium restriction (2 g/day) may also play an important role in the management of hypertension associated with acute renal failure.

HYPERKALEMIA

Hyperkalemia very often accompanies acute renal failure and is dealt with by one of several measures. In addition to the use of sodium bicarbonate to combat renal tubular and metabolic acidosis, it is also an accepted therapy for treating hyperkalemia. Using bolus injections of 50 ml (44.6 mEq) of bicarbonate in patients who are not volume overloaded is a rapid method of lowering serum potassium. Using an intravenous solution containing dextrose and regular insulin will also ameliorate hyperkalemia. The drawback with both of these methods is that the potassium is merely driven intracellularly. It can re-emerge at any time, starting the problem all over again. The most sound method of treating hyperkalemia is by using sodium polystyrene sulfonate (Kayexalate). Additional information on Kayexalate may be found in Chapter 58. This is an orally or rectally administered cation-exchange resin, exchanging sodium for potassium in the lumen of the intestine or colon. The oral dose is one to four tablespoonfuls daily. Polystyrene is very constipating and should generally be given as a slurry with 70% sorbitol. The sorbitol is an osmotic laxative which will prevent intestinal obstruction. If the patient is obtunded, then the rectal route may be preferred. An enema is made up of 30–50 g of resin in an appropriate mixture of water and sorbitol. The slurry should be thick enough to suspend the resin, but not so viscous as to form a paste. Using a gravity-fed enema bag, the solution is introduced with the patient lying on his/her left side. Retention, often aided by a clamp or

rectal tube, should be for 30 minutes. Irrigation with a tap water solution is recommended before evacuation. The procedure may be repeated as often as necessary or as the patient tolerates. Maximal results from one enema may lower the serum potassium by 0.5–1.0 mEq/liter.

GLOMERULONEPHRITIS

One of the etiologies of acute renal failure may be glomerulonephritis. This is often a rapidly progressing pathology involving degeneration of the subcellular fabric of the glomerulus. The glomerulonephritis may result from an autoimmune process or an infectious process. Drug treatment of glomerulonephritis may require large doses of glucocorticoids, such as methylprednisolone (Solu-Medrol) or prednisone. Immunosuppressive therapy with cyclophosphamide (Cytoxan) or azathioprine (Immuran) is also used pending the findings of renal biopsy. In addition, appropriate antibiotic therapy with drugs such as cotrimoxazole (Septra, Bactrim), ampicillin, or ciprofloxacin (Cipro) may be necessary.

CHRONIC RENAL FAILURE

Many of the management problems heretofore mentioned become intensified in the setting of chronic renal failure (CRF). Prolonged injury and stress cause hypertrophy of previously healthy nephrons in an attempt to normalize the patient's fluid and electrolyte balance. Often the acute phase of renal failure is overlooked due to the similarity of the malaise to other infectious processes. Upon ultrasound or radiologic examination, the kidneys in chronic renal failure appear small in size. Exceptions to this rule include the renal failure of the following: diabetic nephropathy, multiple myeloma, amyloidosis, and malignant hypertension. Congestive heart failure (CHF), protein restriction, and fluid and salt restriction are commonalities in the pathogenesis of both acute and chronic renal failure. The previously discussed use of diuretics, Kayexalate, antihypertensives, and anti-infectives also play a role in the therapy of the patient with chronic renal failure.

CALCIUM AND PHOSPHATE METABOLISM

The autoregulation of serum calcium and phosphate is greatly affected during renal dysfunction. As serum phosphate rises due to decreased excretion, calcium phosphate crystals begin to precipitate in soft tissue. These changes in serum levels trigger the release of parathormone from the parathyroid gland. This causes a biphasic effect on calcium metabolism. Mobile calcium stores in the epiphysis of long bones are shifted to increase serum calcium at the same time there is increased excretion of renal phosphate. Normally, the kidney converts 25-hydroxyvitamin D into 1,25-hydroxyvitamin D, the active moiety. The latter substance increases gas-

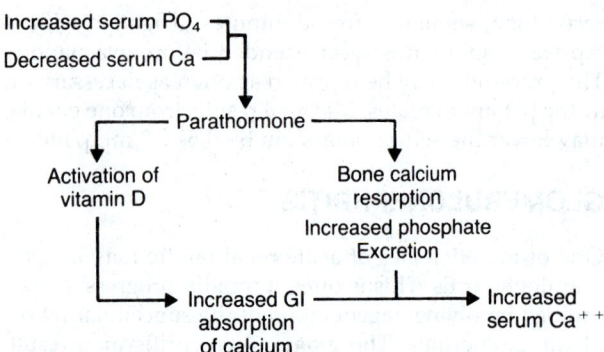

Figure 39–1. Hypocalcemia increases parathormone activity, which can cause increased activation of vitamin D and lead to increased GI absorption of calcium, or mobilize pooled bone stores of calcium.

trointestinal absorption, thereby increasing serum calcium (Fig. 39-1). As renal failure progresses, 1,25-hydroxyvitamin D levels fall and serum phosphate levels continue to rise, both of which reduce serum Ca^{++} and lead to a secondary hyperparathyroidism. Continued resorption of bone leads to *osteomalacia, osteoporosis,* or *osteitis fibrosa.*

Early therapy is aimed at reducing the absorption of phosphate from the gastrointestinal tract. Aluminum-containing antacids bind with phosphate creating a nonabsorbable complex. Products containing aluminum hydroxide include Amphojel, Basaljel, Alternagel, and Alu-Caps. The usual dose is 30–60 ml or one to three capsules before meals. Once the phosphate has been lowered to acceptable levels (5–6 mg/dL), then calcium carbonate (650-mg tablets) may be used in an attempt at normalizing the serum calcium. If unsuccessful, therapy with exogenous vitamin D may be useful. There are currently four vitamin D products available: vitamin D_2 (ergocalciferol); 25 (OH)-D_3 (calcifediol, Calderol); dihydrotachysterol (DHT, Hytakerol); and 1,25(OH)$_2$-D_3 (calcitrol, Rocaltrol). These products are discussed in greater detail in Chapter 57. Calcitrol and DHT are approved for the hyperparathyroidism of renal failure and are generally administered as one dose daily.

ANEMIA

Anemia is a common occurrence in acute and chronic renal failure. Erythrocyte survival time is shortened. Blood shunting and gastrointestinal bleeding all contribute to the decrease in hemoglobin. The anemia is generally normocytic and normochromic. Transfusions are generally not indicated, due to the possibility of volume overload. If required, the newly developed "super-packed" products should be selected. Androgens, iron, folic acid, and B vitamins are also used to combat the anemia of renal failure.

A new advance in genetic engineering has given us erythropoietin (Epogen). Renal hypoxia stimulates erythropoietin release from the kidney. The polypeptide acts on erythroid tissues in the bone marrow accelerating maturations of red blood cell precursors. The rHU-EPO (recombinant human erythropoietin) has been shown to produce an increase in erythrocyte count from seven to fourteen days following initial intravenous injection.

The major indication for rHU-EPO has been to reverse the anemia of chronic renal failure. Doses vary among patients at 5–500 U/kg, three times weekly posthemodialysis. Anemia reversal has decreased the need and risk of transfusions and has improved physical endurance pre- and post-dialysis. Limb tenderness or pain following intravenous injection has been a common side effect. Chills and sweats without an accompanying febrile response have been reported. Hypertensive episodes, seizures, and a hypertensive encephalopathy have also been noted.

ACID-BASE BALANCE

The homeostatic mechanism regulating acid-base balance is like a teeter-totter. The metabolic component is well balanced on the other side by the respiratory mechanisms. The major factor in the metabolic control of pH is renal function. The excretion of titratable acid, secretion of ammonia, and the process of hydrogen ion secretion results in a net excretion of 50–70 mEq H^+/day. The bicarbonate reabsorption pathways, although dependent on hydrogen ion excretion, do not affect the net acid-base balance. The enzyme carbonic anyhydrase is responsible for the recovery of most of the filtered bicarbonate.

METABOLIC ALKALOSIS

Increases in arterial P_{CO_2} correspond to an up-regulation of the bicarbonate reabsorptive mechanisms, hence the teeter-totter effect. Respiratory acidosis (increased P_{CO_2}, decreased pH) often leads to a compensatory metabolic alkalosis (increased HCO_3^-, increased pH). Renal function is not the only controller for acid-base balance; it may be affected by vomiting or nasogastric suctioning.

In the early treatment of metabolic alkalosis, a saline infusion may be tried. This is used with caution in patients with CRF because of the possiblility of pre-existing volume overload. If hypokalemia is the primary etiology, administration of oral or intravenous potassium chloride preparations will be therapeutic. If the serum potassium is not below 2.5 mEq/liter, then the total deficit is in the range of 100–200 mEq. If the blood level is less than 2.5 mEq, then it will take 200–400 mEq of potassium to raise this level by 1.0 mEq/liter. Interestingly, as the blood pH rises there is also a shift of potassium into the intracellular fluid; and as one corrects the pH, the serum potassium may be greater than originally predicted based upon the shift of this anion out of the cells. For moderate deficits, intravenous potassium concentrations should not exceed 30 mEq/liter and the flow rate should be ≤ 10 mEq/hour. With these precautions, ECG monitoring is not required. In situations where the deficit is greater, or the need for replacement more urgent, potassium concentrations may be up to 60 mEq/liter and flow rates may approximate 40 mEq/hour via peripheral line. ECG monitoring as well as serial potassium measurements are warranted in the latter. Oral potassium supplements are used where appropriate. When potassium supplements are used, the chloride salt is always preferred. Some of the older, perhaps more tasty, citrate and bicarbonate salts of potassium have been used, but do little to correct hypochloremic alkalosis.

In severe metabolic alkalosis, direct administration of a 0.1 N (100 mEq/liter) solution of hydrochloric acid may be chosen. The solution, always made extemporaneously, cannot be guaranteed for sterility. It must be given cautiously via large vein. Often excessive nasogastric suction obviates the need for such a therapy. Older alternatives included administration of ammonium chloride intravenously. This is generally not done because of the danger of increased ammonia levels in hepatic or renal failure.

METABOLIC ACIDOSIS

In renal tubular acidosis, the renal mechanisms for acid excretion fail, leading to the development of systemic acidosis. There are two distinct forms of renal tubular acidosis: proximal, and distal. Proximal renal tubular acidosis is caused by a defect in the bicarbonate reabsorptive mechanism. A "dumping" of bicarbonate occurs into the distal tubule. This causes an increased excretion of HCO_3^- and competition with distal tubular acidification mechanisms. The result is decreased formation of ammonia and titratable acid from phosphate and other buffers. In distal tubule acidosis, the bicarbonate conservation is normal; however, there is impaired ability to acidify the urinary buffers (HPO_4^{-2} and NH_3). In both situations, secretion of potassium is markedly elevated.

Usually the picture is a mild acidosis with pH = 7.35 and serum $HCO_3^- = 18\text{--}23$ mEq/liter; however, as the clinical picture worsens, so can these values. Sodium bicarbonate is given chronically to prevent osteomalacia in a dose of 1.8–4.8 g/day (24–64 mEq). The drug is generally available in 325 mg (5 grain) oral tablets. Caution is advised with regard to sodium administration in those patients with a secondary cardiac condition, as excess salt intake may cause an increase in blood volume and increased preload. Schol's solution (Bicitra) is a more palatable form providing 1m Eq $NaHCO_3$/ml.

Hypoxic or lactic acidosis occurs when the serum concentration of lactate rises to > 5 mmol/liter. Type A lactic acidosis occurs when there is poor tissue oxygenation such as in sepsis, hypovolemia, or cardiogenic shock. Type B lactic acidosis refers to those situations where lack of tissue oxygenation is not the primary picture including: diabetic ketoacidosis; tumor; status epilepticus; and chemical poisonings, such as salicylate, ethanol, methanol, and ethylene glycol. Treatment of lactic aci-

dosis may be considered a medical emergency as the condition rapidly fulminates. Large amounts of intravenous sodium bicarbonate are required. Care is taken not to overshoot the deficit as this clinical condition is quite labile. As to renal involvement, the kidney is generally not able to excrete the tremendous load of lactate presented to the glomerulus. Fluid challenges coupled with diuretic therapy often help, but are used cautiously in patients with an underlying component of renal failure. It goes without saying, that the underlying cause of the condition must be promptly addressed.

RESPIRATORY ACIDOSIS AND ALKALOSIS

As previously stated, renal and extrarenal mechanisms often compensate or result in compensated respiratory acidosis or alkalosis. Acute depression of respiration leads to respiratory acidosis and is managed by assisting the patient with a mechanical respirator. Chronically impaired pulmonary function is usually compensated for by HCO_3^- retention by the kidneys. Treatment of chronic respiratory acidosis is directed toward enhancing lung function with bronchodilators, steroids, oxygen, and other conventional measures. As airway resistance decreases and better alveolar gas exchange occurs, the carbon dioxide content of the blood will decrease and the pH should return to normal. Acute respiratory alkalosis occurs when ventilation increases rapidly and excessive carbon dioxide is blown off (decreased P_{CO_2}). Various stimuli such as hypoxemia (low P_{CO_2}), fever infection, and salicylate intoxication, may result in rapid ventilation and respiratory alkalosis. Therapy is directed toward removing the underlying cause.

MISCELLANEOUS PROBLEMS

Gastrointestinal bleeding may be a problem in the uremic patient. Gastritis due to an altered mucosal lining is not uncommon, and bleeding may reflect altered platelet function. Acute therapy with an H_2-receptor antagonist or sucralfate is suggested if these symptoms occur.

Hyperuricemia is a common sequelae of acute renal failure. Uric acid is a breakdown product of protein metabolism via the enzyme xanthine oxidase. Hyperuricemia often accompanies the administration of cytotoxic therapy due to rapid cell lysis. Intraluminary sludging is often a common cause of acute renal failure. Therapy includes alkalinization of the urine with sodium bicarbonate or acetazolamide (Diamox). Allopurinol (Zyloprim), a xanthine oxidase inhibitor, may be necessary to decrease the production of uric acid. Initial dosage is 600 mg/day for several days, followed by maintenance doses of 300 mg/day.

Nonsteroidal anti-inflammatory drugs (NSAIDs) such as ibuprofen (Motrin, Advil), naproxen (Naprosyn), sulindac (Clinoril), and diclofenac (Voltaren) should be avoided in *severe renal failure*. They have been reported to cause abrupt and sustained reductions in renal plasma flow and GFR. The mechanism of action is inhibition of vasodilatory prostaglandin release and thereby, reduction in renal hemodynamics. Manufacturers have claimed various NSAIDs to be superior over others in the patient with reduced renal function; however, current information does not clearly substantiate major differences among agents. Caution is advised when NSAIDs are to be used in this patient population.

DIALYSIS

Various methods of dialysis have been developed since the turn of the century. *Dialysis* is the process by which small molecules are passed through a semipermeable membrane, leaving the large molecules behind. The two distinct methods of dialysis are hemodialysis and peritoneal dialysis. In the first method, arterial blood is passed across an artificial membrane and the uremic toxins and excess electrolytes are collected in the dialysate as the blood is recirculated to a vein (Fig. 39–2). In the second method, the dialysate is infused directly into the peritoneal cavity, and the abdominal viscera acts as the semipermeable membrane (Fig. 39–3). There are several techniques used for peritoneal dialysis. *Manual peritoneal dialysis* refers to the use of a "Y" tubing attached to the patient's peritoneal catheter. One end of the tubing enters the dialysis solution, and the other ends in a collection device. The fluid is infused and is allowed to dwell in the abdomen for generally 30 minutes, then it is drained. With *chronic ambulatory peritoneal dialysis (CAPD)*, the patient performs the exchanges himself at home, three to four times a day. Generally,

three of the exchanges use a 1.5% glucose solution; for the last one, a 4.25% glucose solution is selected. These exchanges are performed each and every day, seven days/week; usually before breakfast, lunch, dinner, and bedtime. The exchanges may include small amounts of heparin (500 IU/liter) to prevent clotting of the catheter. In *continuous cycling peritoneal dialysis (CCPD)*, the patient is connected to an automated machine and is given three exchanges (dwell time = three hours) at night. When he wakes in the morning, the last exchange (4.25% glucose) is made. It is left in the peritoneal cavity throughout the day, freeing the patient so that normal daily activities can be performed.

While both peritoneal dialysis and hemodialysis use exchange fluids, the major difference between the two is the glucose content of the peritoneal solutions. In hemodialysis, an ultrafiltration system produces a positive pressure within the blood path or another system produces a low pressure gradient around the blood path in the dialysis fluid (negative pressure). Peritoneal solutions need a minimum concentration of about 1.5% glucose to cause the small molecular particles (urea, potassium) to move from within the peritoneal circulation across a membrane into the dialysate. The larger the glucose content, the greater the osmotic gradient, and the more waste products can be removed.

As illustrated in Table 39–1, the dialysis solutions available in the United States contain glucose concentrations of 1.5%, 2.5%, and 4.25%. The pH of the solutions is about 5.5 to prevent carmelization of the sugar during the sterilization processes. The normal blood pH is 7.4, so the difference in acidity may cause some discomfort as the dialysate is first infused. The solutions contain no potassium; however, this may be added extemporaneously to offset a hypokalemia. The sodium content is generally less than 140 mEq/liter, which apparently prevents a potential hypernatremia by pulling off some free sodium with water. Calcium contents are

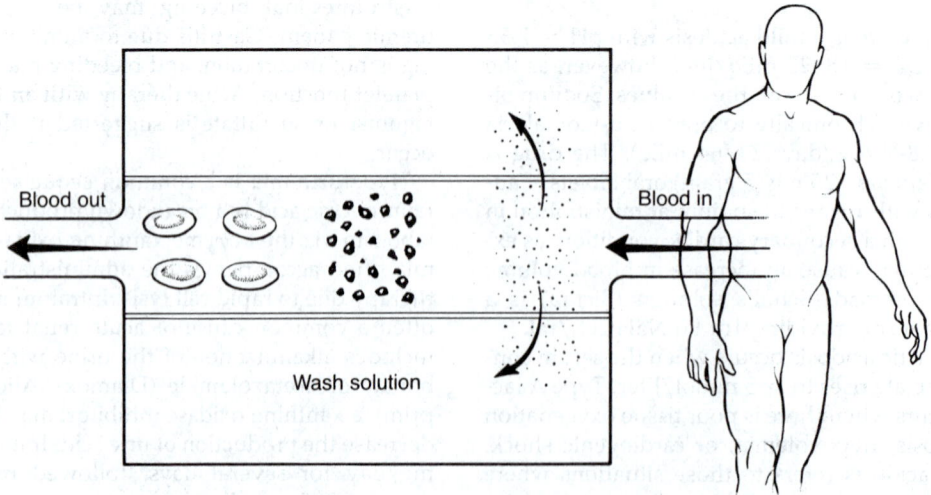

Figure 39–2. Hemodialysis. A schematic diagram of the inner workings and mechanisms of some hemodialysis machines.

Blood out

Wash solution

Blood in

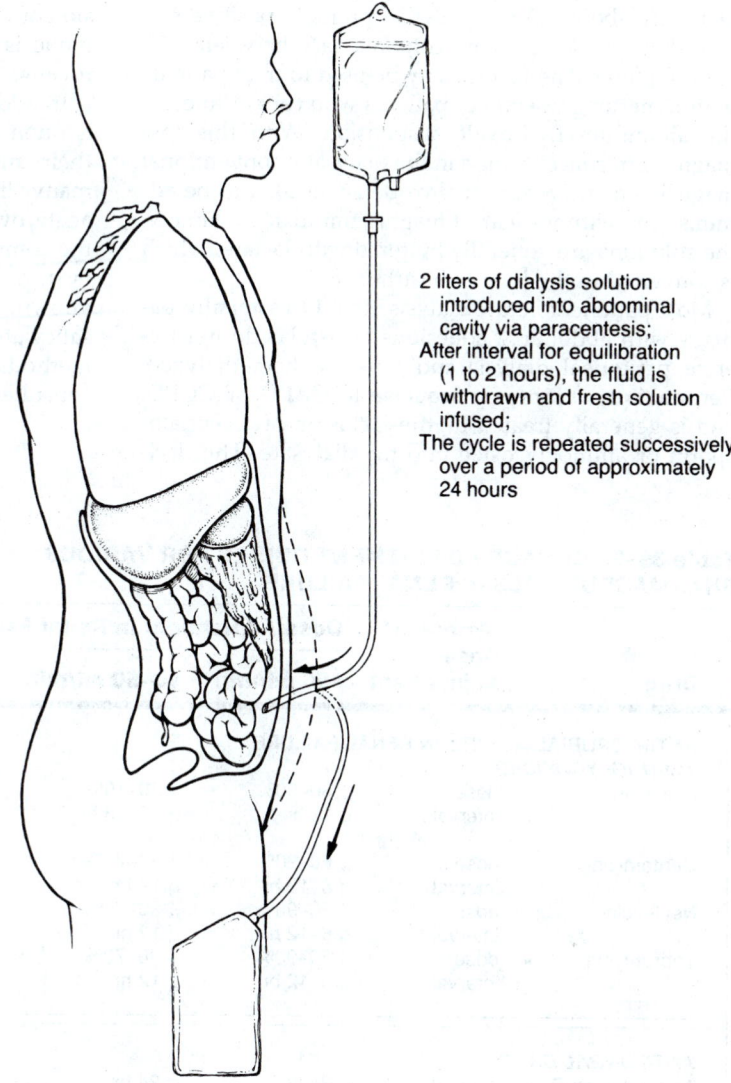

2 liters of dialysis solution
   introduced into abdominal
   cavity via paracentesis;
After interval for equilibration
   (1 to 2 hours), the fluid is
   withdrawn and fresh solution
   infused;
The cycle is repeated successively
   over a period of approximately
   24 hours

Figure 39–3. Peritoneal dialysis. A diagram of a typical peritoneal dialysis setup for CAPD or CCPD.

Table 39–1. CONTENTS OF REPRESENTATIVE DIALYSIS SOLUTIONS

Solution	Glucose (g/liter)	Na (mEq/liter)	Ca (mEq/liter)	Mg (mEq/liter)	Cl (mEq/liter)	Lactate	Osmolarity (mosm/liter)
Dianeal with 1.5% Dextrose	15	141	3.5	1.5	101	45	364
Impersol LM with 1.5% Dextrose	15	132	3.5	0.5	96	40	346
Impersol with 2.5% Dextrose	25	132	3.5	0.5	96	40	396
Dianeal with 4.25% Dextrose	42.5	141	3.5	1.5	101	45	503

generally about 3.5 mEq/liter to promote positive calcium balance. Magnesium contents vary between 0.5–1.5 mEq/liter. The former may be used to treat patients with hypermagnesemia or patients who cannot tolerate the aluminum hydroxide suspension. With this low magnesium concentration in the dialysate, conventional magnesium/aluminum hydroxide anatacids can be administered without fear of magnesium toxicity. Finally, the solutions are generally buffered with lactate, which is converted in the liver to bicarbonate.

Most patients tolerate dialysis well. Occasionally patients with abdominal adhesions or fistulas do not tolerate peritoneal dialysis and must be hemodialyzed. Peritonitis is a common sequelae to CAPD or CCPD, and is generally treated by the inclusion of a cephalosporin or aminoglycoside into the dialysate. The deci-

sion of which patient is qualified for which dialysis technique is complicated and is beyond the scope of this review.

In addition to the treatment of ARF or CRF, dialysis is often used to treat drug intoxication. Depending on their metabolism, structure, and pharmacokinetics, many drugs are suitable for dialysis in the face of an acute overdose. As illustrated in Table 39–2, many of the common pharmaceuticals are well dialyzable; however, many are not or their ability to be dialyzed is not known. Agents such as phenobarbital, chloral hydrate, salicylates, methanol, and others respond to various methods of dialysis. The individual literature should be consulted in each and every case of poisoning.

TEXT RESUMES ON PAGE 1042

Table 39–2. DOSAGE ADJUSTMENT GUIDES FOR VARIOUS PHARMACEUTICALS IN RENAL FAILURE

Drug	Method of Dose Adjustment	Dose Adjustment in Renal Failure by CrCl			Dialysis	Toxicity
		>50 ml/min	10–50 ml/min	<10 ml/min		
ANTIMICROBIAL AGENTS IN RENAL FAILURE						
AMINOGLYCOSIDES						
Amikacin	dose	↓ 60–90%	↓ 30–70%	↓ 20–30%	H,P	All are oto-toxic and nephrotoxic
	interval	q 12 hr	q 12–18 hr	q 24 hr		
Gentamicin	dose	↓ 60–90%	↓ 30–70%	↓ 20–30%	H,P	
	interval	q 8–12 hr	q 12 hr	q 24 hr		
Netilmicin	dose	↓ 60–90%	↓ 30–70%	↓ 20–30%	H,P	
	interval	q 8–12 hr	q 12 hr	q 24 hr		
Tobramycin	dose	↓ 60–90%	↓ 30–70%	↓ 20–30%	H,P	
	interval	q 8–12 hr	q 12 hr	q 24 hr		
ANTIFUNGAL DRUGS						
Amphotericin B	interval	q 24 hr	q 24 hr	q 24–36 hr	No	Nephrotoxic acidosis ↓ K
Flucytosine	interval	q 6 hr	q 12–24 hr	q 24–48 hr	H,P	↑ LFT
	dose	↓ 50%	↓ 30–50%	↓ 20–30%		↓ WBC
Ketoconazole	dose	unchanged	unchanged	unchanged	No	
Miconazole	dose	unchanged	unchanged	unchanged	No	↓ Na
CEPHALOSPORINS						
First Generation						
Cephalexin	interval	q 6 hr	q 6–8 hr	q 6–12 hr	H	All are cross allergic with Penicillin G
Cefadroxil	interval	q 8 hr	q 12–24 hr	q 24–48 hr	H	
Cephradine	dose	unchanged	↓ 50%	↓ 25%	H,P	
Cephapirin	interval	q 6 hr	q 6–8 hr	q 12 hr	H,P	
Cefazolin	interval	q 8 hr	q 12 hr	q 24–48 hr	H	
Second Generation						
Cefaclor	dose	unchanged	↓ 50%	↓ 33%	H	
Cefamandole	interval	q 6 hr	q 6–8 hr	q 8 hr	H	
Cefoxitin	interval	q 8 hr	q 8–12 hr	q 24–48 hr	H	
Cefuroxime	interval	q 8–12 hr	q 24–48 hr	q 48–72 hr	H,P	

Interval: dosing interval is adjusted in renal failure with adjustment given as interval in hours; e.g., q 8 h = every 8 hours.

Dose: dose is adjusted in renal failure with adjustment given as percentage; e.g., ↓ 50% = new adjusted dose is 50% (0.5) times normal dose.

H: removed by hemodialysis; P: removed by peritoneal dialysis.

Table 39–2. DOSAGE ADJUSTMENT GUIDES FOR VARIOUS PHARMACEUTICALS IN RENAL FAILURE-*CONTINUED*

Drug	Method of Dose Adjustment	Dose Adjustment in Renal Failure by CrCl			Dialysis	Toxicity
		>50 ml/min	10–50 ml/min	<10 ml/min		
Cefonicid	dose	↓ 50%	↓ 20–50%	↓ 10–20%	H	
Ceforanide	interval	q 24 hr	q 48 hr	q 48–72 hr	H	
CEPHALOSPORINS						
Third Generation						
Cefoperazone	interval	unchanged	unchanged	unchanged	H	
Moxalactam	interval	q 8 hr	q 12 hr	q 12–24 hr	H	
Cefotaxime	dose	↓ 50–75%	↓ 50%	↓ 25%	H	
Ceftizoxime	dose	↓ 50–100%	↓ 15–50%	↓ 10–15%	H	
Ceftriaxone	dose	unchanged	unchanged	unchanged	No	
Cefotetan	interval	q 12 hr	q 24 hr	q 48 hr	H	
Ceftazidime	interval	q 8–12 hr	q 8–12 hr	q 18–24 hr	H	
Imipenem-Cilastin	interval	q 6–8 hr	q 8 hr	q 12 hr	H	Phlebitis
TETRACYCLINES						
Doxycycline	interval	q 12 hr	q 12–18 hr	q 18–24 hr	No	
Minocycline	dose	unchanged	unchanged	unchanged	No	
Tetracycline	interval	q 8–12 hr	q 12–24 hr	q 24 hr	No	
FLUOROQUINOLONES						
Nalidixic acid	dose	unchanged	DO NOT USE	DO NOT USE	?	
Norfloxacin	interval	unchanged	q 24 hr	q 24 hr	H,P	GI symptoms
Ciprofloxacin	interval	unchanged	q 12 hr	q 24 hr	H,P	
Nitrofurantoin	dose	unchanged	DO NOT USE	DO NOT USE	H	GI symptoms
PENICILLINS						
Amoxicillin	interval	q 6 hr	q 6–12 hr	q 12–16 hr	H	All are cross allergic
Ampicillin	interval	q 6 hr	q 6–12 hr	q 12–16 hr	H	Diarrhea, rash
Ampicillin + Sublactam	interval	q 6–8 hr	q 12 hr	q 24 hr	H	
Azlocillin	interval	q 4–6 hr	q 6–8 hr	q 8 hr	H	
Carbenicillin	interval	q 8–12 hr	q 12–24 hr	q 24–48 hr	H,P	
Cloxacillin	dose	unchanged	unchanged	unchanged	No	
Dicloxacillin	interval	unchanged	unchanged	unchanged	No	
Mezlocillin	interval	q 4–6 hr	q 6–8 hr	q 8 hr	H	
Nafcillin	dose	unchanged	unchanged	unchanged	No	↓ in liver failure
Oxacillin	dose	unchanged	unchanged	unchanged	No	
Penicillin G	dose	unchanged	↓ 75%	↓ 25–50%	H	Maximum dose 6 million U/day in severe renal failure
	interval	q 6–8 hr	q 8–12 hr	q 12–16 hr		
Piperacillin	interval	q 4–6 hr	q 6–8 hr	q 8 hr	H	1.7 mEq Na/g
Ticarcillin	interval	q 8–12 hr	q 12–24 hr	q 24–48 hr	H,P	
Ticarcillin-Clavulanate	interval	q 4 hr	q 8 hr	q 12–24 hr	H	↓ in liver failure
Cotrimoxazole (SMZ–TMP)	interval	q 12 hr	q 18 hr	q 24 hr	H	

CONTINUED ON THE FOLLOWING PAGE

Interval: dosing interval is adjusted in renal failure with adjustment given as interval in hours; e.g., q 8 h = every 8 hours.

Dose: dose is adjusted in renal failure with adjustment given as percentage; e.g., ↓ 50% = new adjusted dose is 50% (0.5) times normal dose.

H: removed by hemodialysis; P: removed by peritoneal dialysis.

Table 39–2. DOSAGE ADJUSTMENT GUIDES FOR VARIOUS PHARMACEUTICALS IN RENAL FAILURE–*CONTINUED*

Drug	Method of Dose Adjustment	Dose Adjustment in Renal Failure by CrCl			Dialysis	Toxicity
		>50 ml/min	**10–50 ml/min**	**<10 ml/min**		
ANTIMICROBIAL AGENTS IN RENAL FAILURE–*Continued*						
Vancomycin	interval	q 24–72 hr	q 72–240 hr	q 240 hr	No	Ototoxic, nephrotoxic
Chloramphenicol	dose	unchanged	unchanged	unchanged	H	Caution in ↓ liver function
Clindamycin	dose	unchanged	unchanged	unchanged	No	Colitis
Erythromycin	dose	unchanged	unchanged	unchanged	No	
Methanamine	dose	unchanged	DO NOT USE	DO NOT USE		↓ effect in renal failure
Metronidazole	interval	q 8 hr	q 8–12 hr	q 12–24 hr	H	Neurotoxic, GI symptoms
ANTI-TUBERCULOSIS DRUGS						
Ethambutol	interval	q 24 hr	q 24–36 hr	q 48 hr	H,P	Peripheral neuritis
	dose	unchanged	↓ 50%	↓ 30–50%		
Isoniazid	dose	unchanged	unchanged	↓ 66–75%	H,P	Peripheral neuritis
Rifampin	interval	unchanged	unchanged	unchanged	No	Acute renal failure
ANTIVIRAL AGENTS						
Acyclovir	interval	q 8 hr	q 24 hr	q 48 hr	H	CNS toxicity
Amantadine	interval	q 12–24 hr	q 48–72 hr	q 168 hr	No	
MISCELLANEOUS ANTIBIOTIC						
Aztreonam	dose	unchanged	↓ 50–75%	↓ 25%		
ANTIADRENERGIC DRUGS						
Methyldopa	interval	q 6 hr	q 9–18 hr	q 12–24 hr	H,P	
Clonidine	dose	unchanged	unchanged	↓ 50–75%	No	
Guanfacine, Guanabenz	dose	unchanged	unchanged	unchanged	No	
Reserpine	dose	unchanged	unchanged	DO NOT USE	No	
Guanethidine	interval	q 24 hr	q 24 hr	q 24 hr	No	
Prazosin, Terazosin	dose	unchanged	unchanged	unchanged	No	
VASODILATORS						
Hydralazine	interval	8 hr	q 8 hr	q 12–17 hr	No	
Diazoxide, Minoxidil, Nitroprusside	dose	unchanged	unchanged	unchanged	H,P	
ACE INHIBITORS						
Captopril, Enalapril, Lisinopril	dose	unchanged	unchanged	↓ 50% for CrCl <30 ml	H	
ANTIARRHYTHMICS						
Amiodarone	dose	unchanged	unchanged	unchanged	No	
Bretylium	dose	unchanged	↓ 25–50%	DO NOT USE	?	

Interval: dosing interval is adjusted in renal failure with adjustment given as interval in hours; e.g., q 8 h = every 8 hours.

Dose: dose is adjusted in renal failure with adjustment given as percentage; e.g., ↓ 50% = new adjusted dose is 50% (0.5) times normal dose.

H: removed by hemodialysis; P: removed by peritoneal dialysis.

Table 39–2. DOSAGE ADJUSTMENT GUIDES FOR VARIOUS PHARMACEUTICALS IN RENAL FAILURE-*CONTINUED*

Drug	Method of Dose Adjustment	Dose Adjustment in Renal Failure by CrCl			Dialysis	Toxicity
		>50 ml/min	10–50 ml/min	<10 ml/min		
Disopyramide	dose	unchanged	↓ 12–24%	↓ 24–40%	H	
Encainide	dose	unchanged	unchanged	unchanged	?	
Flecainide	dose	unchanged	unchanged	↓ 50–75%	No	
Lidocaine	dose	unchanged	unchanged	unchanged	No	
Mexiletine	dose	unchanged	unchanged	↓ 50–75%	?	
Procainamide	interval	q 4 hr	q 6–12 hr	q 8–24 hr	H	
Quinidine	dose	unchanged	unchanged	unchanged	H,P	
Tocainide	dose	unchanged	unchanged	unchanged	H	
BETA-BLOCKERS						
Acebutolol	dose	unchanged	↓ 50%	↓ 30–50%	No	
Atenolol	dose	unchanged	↓ 50%	↓ 25%	H	
Labetalol, Pindolol, Propranolol, Timolol	dose	unchanged	unchanged	unchanged	No	
Metoprolol	dose	unchanged	unchanged	unchanged	H	
CALCIUM CHANNEL BLOCKERS						
Diltiazem	dose	unchanged	unchanged	unchanged	?	
Nifedipine, Nicardipine	dose	unchanged	unchanged	unchanged	No	
Verapamil	dose	unchanged	unchanged	↓ 50–75%	No	
CARDIAC GLYCOSIDES						
Digoxin	dose	unchanged	↓ 25–75%	↓ 10–25%	No	↑ level with quinidine
	interval	q 24 hr	q 36 hr	q 48 hr		
Digitoxin	dose	unchanged	unchanged	↓ 50–75%	No	
DIURETICS						
Bumetanide, Furosemide, Indapamide, Metolazone, Thiazides	dose	unchanged	unchanged	unchanged	No	
Chlorthalidone	interval	q 24 hr	q 24 hr	q 48 hr	?	
Ethacrynic acid	interval	q 24 hr	q 24 hr	DO NOT USE	No	Ototoxic
Spironolactone	interval	q 6–12 hr	q 12–24 hr	DO NOT USE	?	
ANTIPYRETICS						
Acetaminophen	interval	q 4 hr	q 6 hr	q 8 hr	H	Overdose, neprotoxic
Aspirin	interval	q 4 hr	q 4–6 hr	DO NOT USE	H,P	Overdose, neprotoxic
NARCOTIC AGONISTS/ANTAGONISTS						
Codeine, Fentanyl, Meperidine, Morphine,	dose	unchanged	unchanged	unchanged	generally not dialyzed	
Naloxone,					H	

CONTINUED ON THE FOLLOWING PAGE

Interval: dosing interval is adjusted in renal failure with adjustment given as interval in hours; e.g., q 8 h = every 8 hours.

Dose: dose is adjusted in renal failure with adjustment given as percentage; e.g., ↓ 50% = new adjusted dose is 50% (0.5) times normal dose.

H: removed by hemodialysis; P: removed by peritoneal dialysis.

Table 39–2. DOSAGE ADJUSTMENT GUIDES FOR VARIOUS PHARMACEUTICALS IN RENAL FAILURE–*CONTINUED*

Drug	Method of Dose Adjustment	Dose Adjustment in Renal Failure by CrCl			Dialysis	Toxicity
		>50 ml/min	10–50 ml/min	<10 ml/min		
CNS DRUGS IN RENAL FAILURE						
Nalbuphine						
Pentazocine						
Methadone	dose	unchanged	unchanged	↓ 50–75%	No	
Propoxyphene	dose	unchanged	unchanged	↓ 25%	No	
BARBITURATES						
Hexobarbital, Pentobarbital Secobarbital	dose	unchanged	unchanged	unchanged	No	
Phenobarbital	dose	unchanged	unchanged	↓ 12–15%	H,P	
BENZODIAZEPINES						
Chloral hydrate	dose	unchanged	DO NOT USE	DO NOT USE	H	
Alprazolam, Chlordiazepoxide, Clonazepam, Diazepam, Flurazepam, Triazolam	dose	unchanged	unchanged	unchanged	No	
Lorazepam, Oxazepam	dose	unchanged	unchanged	unchanged	No	
MISCELLANEOUS SEDATIVES						
Droperidol, Haloperidol	dose	unchanged	unchanged	unchanged	No	
Ethchlorvynol, Glutethemide	dose	unchanged	DO NOT USE	DO NOT USE	No	
Lithium Carbonate	dose	unchanged	↓ 50–75%	↓ 25–50%	H,P	
PHENOTHIAZINES						
Chlorpromazine and others	dose	unchanged	unchanged	unchanged	No	
TRICYCLIC ANTIDEPRESSANTS						
Amitriptyline and others	dose	unchanged	unchanged	unchanged	No	
ANTINEOPLASTICS						
Azathioprine	dose	unchanged	unchanged	↓ 75%	H	
Bleomycin, Busulfan, Cyclosoporine, Cytarabine, 5-Fluorouracil, Vinblastine, Vincristine	dose	unchanged	unchanged	unchanged	? or No	
Cisplatin	dose	unchanged	↓ 75%	↓ 50%	H	
Cyclophosphamide, Ifosfamide	dose	unchanged	unchanged	↓ 50–75%	H	
Doxorubicin	dose	unchanged	unchanged	↓ 75%	?	
Hydroxyurea	dose	unchanged	unchanged	↓ 50%	?	

Interval: dosing interval is adjusted in renal failure with adjustment given as interval in hours; e.g., q 8 h = every 8 hours.

Dose: dose is adjusted in renal failure with adjustment given as percentage; e.g., ↓ 50% = new adjusted dose is 50% (0.5) times normal dose.

H: removed by hemodialysis; P: removed by peritoneal dialysis.

**Table 39–2. DOSAGE ADJUSTMENT GUIDES FOR VARIOUS
PHARMACEUTICALS IN RENAL FAILURE**-*CONTINUED*

Drug	Method of Dose Adjustment	Dose Adjustment in Renal Failure by CrCl			Dialysis	Toxicity
		>50 ml/min	10–50 ml/min	<10 ml/min		
CNS DRUGS IN RENAL FAILURE-*Continued*						
Methotrexate	dose	unchanged	↓ 50%	DO NOT USE	H	May be neprotoxic
Mithramycin	dose	unchanged	↓ 75%	↓ 50%	?	
Mitomycin C	dose	unchanged	unchanged	↓ 75%	?	
Methyl CCNU	dose	unchanged	unchanged	DO NOT USE	?	Neprotoxic
Streptozocin	dose	unchanged	↓ 75%	↓ 50%	?	
ANTICOAGULANTS						
Alteplase (TPA)	dose	unchanged	unchanged	unchanged	No	
Heparin						
Streptokinase						
Urokinase						
Warfarin						
ANTIHISTAMINES						
Chlorpheniramine	dose	unchanged	unchanged	unchanged	Yes	
Astemizole	dose	unchanged	unchanged	unchanged	?	
Terfenadine						
Diphenhydramine	interval	q 6 hr	q 6–9 hr	q 9–12 hr	?	
ANTILIPEMIC DRUGS						
Cholestyramine	dose	unchanged	unchanged	unchanged	No	
Colestipol						
Gemfibrozil	dose	unchanged	↓ 50%	↓ 25%	?	
Lovastatin	dose	unchanged	unchanged	unchanged	?	
Nicotinic acid	dose	unchanged	↓ 50%	↓ 25%	?	
Probucol	dose	unchanged	unchanged	unchanged	?	
ARTHRITIS/GOUT DRUGS						
Allopurinol	dose	unchanged	↓ 75%	↓ 50%	?	
Colchicine	dose	unchanged	unchanged	↓ 50%	?	
Diflunisal	dose	unchanged	unchanged	↓ 50%	?	
Diclofenac,	dose	unchanged	unchanged	usually unchanged (see note to right)	No	In severe renal failure small dose decrease may be needed
Flubiprofen						
Fenoprofen						
Ibuprofen						
Meclofenamate						
Mefenamic acid						
Ketoprofen						
Naproxen						
Piroxicam						
Sulindac						
Indomethacin						
CORTICOSTEROIDS						
Cortisone,					No	
Dexamethasone					?	
Hydrocortisone	dose	unchanged	unchanged	unchanged	?	
Methylprednisolone					H	
Prednisolone					No	

CONTINUED ON THE FOLLOWING PAGE

Interval: dosing interval is adjusted in renal failure with adjustment given as interval in hours; e.g., q 8 h = every 8 hours.

Dose: dose is adjusted in renal failure with adjustment given as percentage; e.g., ↓ 50% = new adjusted dose is 50% (0.5) times normal dose.

H: removed by hemodialysis; P: removed by peritoneal dialysis.

Table 39–2. DOSAGE ADJUSTMENT GUIDES FOR VARIOUS PHARMACEUTICALS IN RENAL FAILURE–*CONTINUED*

Drug	Method of Dose Adjustment	Dose Adjustment in Renal Failure by CrCl			Dialysis	Toxicity
		>50 ml/min	10–50 ml/min	<10 ml/min		
HYPLOGLYCEMIC DRUGS						
Acetohexamide	interval	q 12 hr	DO NOT USE	DO NOT USE	No	
Chlorpropamide	interval	q 24 hr	DO NOT USE	DO NOT USE	No	
Glyburide, Glipizide, Tolbutamide, Tolazamide	dose	unchanged	unchanged	unchanged	? or No	
NEUROLOGIC DRUGS						
Bromocriptine	dose	unchanged	unchanged	↓ 75%	?	
Carbamazepine	dose	unchanged	unchanged	↓ 75%	No	May cause SIADH
Carbidopa-Levo-dopa	dose	unchanged	unchanged	unchanged	?	
Ethosuximide	dose	unchanged	unchanged	unchanged	?	
Phenytoin	dose	unchanged	unchanged	unchanged	No	
Primidone	interval	q 8 hr	q 8–12 hr	q 12–24 hr	H	
Trihexyphenidyl	dose	unchanged	unchanged	unchanged	?	
Valproic acid	dose	unchanged	unchanged	unchanged	No	
H₂ ANTAGONISTS						
Cimetidine	dose	unchanged	↓ 75%	↓ 50%	No	
Ranitidine	dose	unchanged	↓ 75%	↓ 50%	H	
Famotidine	interval	unchanged	unchanged	q 36–48 hr	?	
Nizatidine	interval	unchanged	q 48 hr	q 72 hr	?	
OTHER DRUGS						
Methimazole	dose	unchanged	↓ 75%	↓ 50%	?	
Metoclopramide	dose	unchanged	↓ 75%	↓ 50%	?	
Penicillamine	dose	unchanged	DO NOT USE	DO NOT USE	?	
Propylthiouracil	dose	unchanged	unchanged	unchanged	?	
Terbutaline	dose	unchanged	↓ 50%	DO NOT USE	?	
Theophylline	dose	unchanged	unchanged	unchanged	H,P	

Interval: dosing interval is adjusted in renal failure with adjustment given as interval in hours; e.g., q 8 h = every 8 hours.
Dose: dose is adjusted in renal failure with adjustment given as percentage; e.g., ↓ 50% = new adjusted dose is 50% (0.5) times normal dose.
H: removed by hemodialysis; P: removed by peritoneal dialysis.

DRUG DOSING IN RENAL FAILURE

The kidney is one of two elimination routes for most drugs, the other being the liver. During renal failure, those drugs that use the kidney as the major route of elimination will probably require an adjustment in dose. As a patient's creatinine clearance falls below 50 ml/minute, there is a need to understand which drugs may require such a modification in dose. Table 39–2 includes dose adjustment guides to many of the pharmaceuticals used today. Drugs like digoxin have a narrow therapeutic index and patients may quickly become toxic in the face of renal failure. To use these tables, the nurse must assess the patient's creatinine clearance. A popular formula for estimating creatinine clearance (CrCl) is the Cockroft-Gault equation:

$$CrCl_{(males)} = \frac{(140 - Age)\ (Weight)}{(72)\ (SrCr_{ss})}$$
$$CrCl_{(females)} = (0.85)\ (CrCl_{males})$$

Normal creatinine clearances are 140 ± 27 ml/minute for men, and 112 ± 20 ml/minute for women.

Alterations in dosing interval are given for some of the drugs and decreases in the actual dose administered are listed for others. A 60-kg patient who might normally receive 80 mg of gentamicin every eight hours for infection has an estimated CrCl of 10 ml/minute. The patient might, therefore, receive 80 mg of gentamicin every 24 hours or alternatively, 16 mg every eight hours.

Many of these dose alterations can be confirmed by serum drug samples. The use of steady-state or peak/trough levels is an important tool for the prescriber to use in monitoring the drug therapy of a renal failure patient. The nurse should recognize those drugs that might require a dose or interval adjustment and use Table 39–2 or other reference sources to calculate the correct dose for the patient.

USING THE NURSING PROCESS

ASSESSMENT

While the monitoring of renal function is essential to maintaining homeostasis, it is incumbent on the professional nurse to review the body as a whole. Limiting measurements and observations to one organ system is not always in the best interests of the patient. Table 39–3 contains a valuable flow plan for assessment.

The patient history is an important fact-sorting tool. Although renal failure is generally of insidious onset, certain pre-existing symptomatologies often help in proper assessment. In general, early features of renal failure include decreased mental acuity, fatigue, and general malaise. While the patient may be unaware of these changes, friends or family members should be questioned to illicit an accurate history.

Nervous disorders such as coarse muscular twitches, tics, and cramps may be present. The patient may suffer from tactile abnormalities, peripheral neuropathies, and other various motor disorders as a result of poor kidney function. If present, seizures should be dealt with appropriately (see Chapter 22 for treatment of epileptic disorders).

The patient's general appearance is assessed. Malnutrition leading to tissue wasting is often common in uremia. The sclerae may be discolored and the skin may be similarly discolored, often to a yellow-brown. *Uremic frost* is characterized by the presence of topical yellow-white crystals which come from the excess urea contained in sweat. Patients with uremic frost may very often complain of mild to severe pruritis.

Many of these patients possess underlying cardiac or pulmonary problems. The nurse auscultates the chest for fluid changes in the lungs. Crackles or rhonchi are appropriately noted in addition to any suggestion of dyspnea or othopnea. Screening for abnormal heart sounds or a pericardial friction rub is also performed.

A clear, concise dietary history often discovers early GI manifestations of renal failure. Symptoms of stomatitis, unpleasant tastes, halitosis, anorexia, nausea, and vomiting are documented. More severe symptoms may include coffee-ground, heme-positive stools as signs of active GI bleeding. Proper dietary counseling as to nitrogen and sodium intake is essential to chronic maintenance of these patients.

Daily weights are important to determine if the patient is retaining fluids. Often, edema is insidious and weight gain may be the first symptom (the usual rule is 1 kg of weight gain equals one liter of fluid). Monitoring fluid intake and output is often an underrated tool for assessment. Any patient who shows discrepancies between intake and output is assessed further to determine if renal function has been compromised. This is especially important if for some reason blood flow to the kidneys may have been affected, for example, by hemorrhage or dehydration.

The nurse accurately records blood pressure in both the supine and standing positions routinely in these patients. Extra fluid can cause an increase in blood pressure when the patient assumes a supine position. Also, if the patient is receiving antihypertensive drugs, he or she may be susceptible to orthostasis.

Labortory evaluations are made and levels are closely followed. While a 24-hour creatinine clearance is one of the best indicators of renal function, collection may not always be possible or feasible. Assessment of the creatinine clearance may be made by nomogram or by equation. The level of blood urea nitrogen is another measure of renal function, increasing as the kidneys are unable to secrete nitrogenous byproducts. However, this number is often vague in its clinical significance, and creatinine clearances remain the most valuable indicator of renal status. A creatinine clearance of 30 ml/minute may be broadly classified as *moderate renal failure,* while a creatinine clearance of 10 ml/minute or less is termed severe renal failure. Accurate estimation or determination of creatinine clearance is essential for establishing doses for various drugs in the patient with renal failure (see Table 39–2 for more information). In addition to the values discussed above, urine specific gravities and sodium/potassium excretion values often give valuable information.

Serum electrolytes, bicarbonate, and hemoglobin values must be part of the rational assessment process. The use of diuretics as well as other agents to reduce high serum sodium or potassium concentrations has been discussed. In assessing anemia, the dilutional phenomena of renal failure must constantly be taken into account.

NURSING DIAGNOSIS AND INTERVENTION

The nurse establishes the nursing diagnoses based upon the information obtained in the initial assessment. From these nursing diagnoses, the goals of intervention and evaluation are developed. Typical nursing diagnoses for a patient with renal disease are included in Table 39–3.

TEXT RESUMES ON PAGE 1046

Table 39–3. NURSING PROCESS FOR PATIENT WITH RENAL DISEASE

Assessment
Determine history of past and present illness. Evaluate heart rate, blood pressure and CVP (if available.) Note fluid intake/output, current weight and pattern of weight gain/loss. Ascertain dietary intake, especially in relation to sodium. Note general appearance, presence of nervous disorders. Assess effectiveness of individual/family coping mechanisms. Identify behaviors indicative of failure to follow treatment program.

Nursing Diagnosis	Nursing Actions	Rationale	Desired Outcomes/ Evaluation Criteria
Fluid Volume, excess related to compromised regulatory mechanism (renal failure) with retention of water as evidenced by intake greater than output, oliguria, changes in urine specific gravity, generalized tissue edema, weight gain.	Monitor heart rate, blood pressure (supine and standing) and CVP.	Tachycardia and hypertension can occur because of failure of the kidneys to excrete urine, excessive fluid resuscitation and/or changes in the renin-angiotensin system. Orthostatic hypotension and tachycardia can occur if hypovolemia develops in response to excessive diuretic-induced fluid losses.	Displays appropriate urinary output with special gravity/laboratory studies near normal, stable weight and absence of edema.
	Record accurate intake and output. Calculate 24 hour balance.	Necessary for determining renal function, fluid replacement needs and reducing risk of fluid overload	
	Monitor urine specific gravity.	Measures the kidney's ability to concentrate urine.	
	Weigh daily on the same scale.	Daily weight is the best monitor of fluid status although muscle wasting may affect accuracy.	
	Note presence/degree of edema.	Useful in noting progression/resolution of fluid imbalance and effectiveness of therapy.	
	Observe for dry mucous membranes, thirst, dulled sensorium, peripheral vasoconstriction.	Indicators of fluid and electrolyte imbalances e.g., dehydration/sodium depletion.	
	Explain dietary modifications, i.e., sodium, potassium, protein, fluid.	Restrictions are based on severity of condition to prevent worsening of failure/dangerous accumulation of waste products.	
	Plan oral fluid replacement, spacing desired beverages and varying choices.	Helps avoid periods without fluids, minimizing boredom of limited choices and reducing sense of deprivation and thirst.	
	Provide hard candy or saliva substitute as appropriate.	Use in relieving discomfort associated with dryness of mouth and may help limit desire for additional fluids.	
	Administer diuretics (furosemide, mannitol);	Given to flush the tubular lumen, reduce hyperkalemia, and promote adequate urine volume.	
	antihypertensives (clinidine, methyldopa).	May be given to treat hypertension by counteracting effects of decreased renal blood flow, and/or circulating volume overload.	

Table 39-3. NURSING PROCESS FOR PATIENT WITH RENAL DISEASE-*CONTINUED*

Nursing Diagnosis	Nursing Actions	Rationale	Desired Outcomes/ Evaluation Criteria
	Monitor laboratory studies, e.g., BUN, creatinine, urine sodium and creatinine, serum sodium/potassium, Hb/Hct, chest x-rays.	Assess progression and management of renal dysfunction/failure and need for additional therapies.	
Adjustment, impaired related to disability requiring change in lifestyle, assault to self-esteem, altered locus of control as evidenced by verbalization of nonacceptance of health status change, lack of involvement in problem-solving.	Listen to patient's perception of difficulty adapting to situation.	Identifies individual needs/concerns and appropriate interventions.	Demonstrates increasing interest in active and passive participation in self-care. Initiates lifestyle changes that will permit adaptation to present life situation.
	Encourage expression of feelings, e.g., fear, anger.	Promotes awareness and allows patient to begin to deal with them realistically.	
	Review previous life situations and role changes which have occurred.	Helps patient to identify coping skills already been developed	
	Develop a plan of action to meet immediate needs.	Promotes sense of control and gives direction to care.	
	Identify resources which may be useful, e.g., vocational rehabilitation, employment services, psychosocial support services.	May need assistance to make identified changes.	
	Refer to other resources as indicated.	May need additional help with resolution of adjustment to chronic illness/dialysis.	
Knowledge deficit related to cognitive limitation, lack of exposure/recall, information misinterpretation as evidenced by questions/request for information, statement of concern inaccurate follow through of instructions/development of preventable complications.	Review disease process/prognosis and future expectations.	Provides knowledge base on which patient can make informed choices.	Verbalizes understanding of condition/disease process and treatment. Correctly performs necessary procedures and explains reasons for the actions
	Discuss drug therapy, including use of calcium supplements, phosphate binders (with meals), and avoidance of magnesium antiacids.	Prevents serious complications, e.g., reduces risk of bone demineralization/fractures, tetany; osteodystrophy; hypermagnesemia.	
	Identify peak action time of diuretics.	Allows patient to schedule medication and still maintain usual activities, adequate sleep.	
	Stress importance of reading all product labels and not taking medications without prior approval of health care provider.	Exogenous intake of electrolytes must be factored into dietary restrictions to maintain appropriate balances.	
	Review dietary restrictions, including sodium, phosphorus, (e.g., milk products, poultry, peanuts) and magnesium, (e.g., whole grain products, legumes).	Sodium potentiates fluid retention, increasing edema, hypertension and risk of cardiac complications. Retention of phosphorus stimulates the parathyroid glands to shift calcium from bones and accumulation of magnesium can impair neuromuscular function and mentation.	
	Instruct in home monitoring of BP, including scheduling rest period before taking pressure, using same arm/position.	Incidence of hypertension is increased in CRF, often requiring management with antihypertensive drugs, necessitating close observation of treatment effects.	

CONTINUED ON THE FOLLOWING PAGE

Table 39–3. NURSING PROCESS FOR PATIENT WITH RENAL DISEASE–*CONTINUED*

Nursing Diagnosis	Nursing Actions	Rationale	Desired Outcomes/ Evaluation Criteria
	Review measures to prevent bleeding/hemorrhage, e.g., use of soft toothbrush, electric razor; avoidance of constipation, forceful blowing of nose, strenuous exercise/contact sports.	Reduces risks related to alteration of clotting factors/decreased platelet count.	
	Caution against exposure to external temperature extremes, e.g., heating pads/snow.	Peripheral neuropathy may develop, especially in lower extremities, impairing peripheral sensation and potentiating risk of tissue injury.	
Noncompliance, potential related to patient value system, health beliefs, cultural influences, changes in mentation; complexities, costs, side effects of therapy.	Ascertain patient/SO's perception/understanding of situation and consequences of behavior.	Provides insight into how they view illness and treatment regimen and aids in understanding problems patient/SO are encountering.	Verbalizes accurate knowledge of disease and understanding of therapeutic regimen. Participates in the development of goals and treatment plan to meet individual needs.
	Determine value system.	Therapeutic regimen may be incongruent with patient's social/cultural life-style and perceived role responsibilities.	
	Listen/Active-listen to complaints and comments.	Conveys message of concern, belief in individual's capability to resolve situation in a positive manner.	
	Accept patient's choice/ point of view, even if it appears to be detrimental.	Patient has the right to make own decisions/ choices, and acceptance may give a sense of control, which will help patient to look more clearly at consequences of choice.	
	Establish graduated goals with patient; modify regimen as necessary/possible.	When patient has participated in setting of goals, a sense of investment encourages cooperation and willingness to adhere to/work with program as established.	
	Encourage self-monitoring of BP and weight. Provide copies of laboratory reports.	Provides a sense of control, enables patient to follow own progress and to make informed choices.	
	Provide positive feedback for efforts/involvement in therapy.	Promotes sense of self-esteem, encourages continued participation in regimen.	

PLANNING AND INTERVENTION

Both the patient and family should demonstrate to the nurse their understanding of the implications of renal disease. If the renal condition is a chronic one, both must understand that this means a modification in lifestyle. The goals of the nursing intervention are based on the nursing diagnoses previously established. Typical goals of intervention for a patient with renal disease are included in Table 39–3.

There are many barriers to patient education including: preformed ideas of disease processes, educational level and capacity of the patient, reading ability, language barriers, motivation, previous compliance, and more. Psychological depression with the underlying realization that their problem will not disappear after a routine course of drug therapy needs to be addressed with patients. In this setting, education is not a matter of one 30–60 minute intervention session, but rather days and weeks of repeat encounters. The professional nurse should: plan educational goals for each patient; access the patient's knowledge; establish a teaching plan using formalized sessions; periodically evaluate the patient's response and re-evaluate the teaching plan; and finally, provide ongoing patient support and follow-up.

DIET

Dietary and fluid restrictions depend upon the degree of renal impairment. Early in therapy, sodium and fluids may require moderate restriction. As the patient gradually loses more renal function, diet is severely modified in relation to sodium, potassium, protein, and fluid intake.

Dietary and fluid restrictions are often the most difficult adjustments that the patient and family must make. The patient's first introduction to this may be totally overwhelming, and they may react by rejecting the idea completely. The nurse must allow the patient and family members to express any negative feelings that they have and, in conjunction with a dietitian, work to fit the dietary and fluid restrictions to their lifestyle. Having the patient bring a list of the dietary intake for a few days can give the nurse an idea of his or her eating habits. Many patients really understand the need for the four basic food groups. The patient must learn to weigh and measure portions accurately and not guess or estimate amounts.

Salt restrictions often pose the biggest problem because the average American diet is too high in salt. Salting food before it is even tasted is a common habit. By removing the salt shaker from the table and using herbs or spices for flavoring, salt intake can be drastically reduced. Common salt substitutes, while advisable, should be used in small quantities as they are high in potassium content.

An accurate way for the patient to measure fluid restrictions is as follows: If the patient is restricted to one liter of fluid, he should use a quart container as a measuring device and every time the patient consumes any fluid, the same amount of water must be placed in the container. When the container is full, the patient has used up the allotted fluid intake allowance.

The nurse must be sure that the patient understands that all fluids must be considered when measuring intake. This includes soups, ice cubes, and the liquid used to take medications. Hard candy or a saliva substitute can help to relieve dryness in the patient's mouth instead of drinking fluids.

MEDICATIONS

If the patient is receiving aluminum hydroxide gel, he or she should remember to take it along with meals. The phosphate-binding effect is best when it is taken with food. The liquid preparations are superior because they have a larger surface area. If the tablets are used, they should be chewed well before swallowing. Aluminum-containing antacids are constipating, and a stool soft-ener or additional bulk-type laxative may be necessary to relieve this uncomfortable side effect. The antacid may be left at the bedside to be taken as "a dessert."

Patients taking diuretics at home are instructed not to take them in the evening. The peak action of the drug should not be during the night if the patient is to have a restful sleep. If these are taken for hypertension alone or with other medications, their effect is greatest in the morning, at the ebb of the diurnal cycle. Even if the diuretic is a potassium-losing (kaluretic) diuretic, the patient's dietary intake of potassium may have to be limited because of renal failure. Orange juice, bananas, and dried fruits are rich sources of K^+. Potassium-sparing diuretics are usually not indicated for the patient with renal failure. ECG changes are prevalent with both hyperkalemia and hypokalemia.

If the patient is on daily antihypertensive therapy, it might be helpful for the nurse to devise a chart to record blood pressure and medication. By helping the patient to establish a routine, there is less chance of forgetting a dose. And, by having each dose time written down, the patient has a tangible way to check the administration. Similar results can be achieved or augmented by use of specially divided pill boxes available from most pharmacies. These contain either daily time divisions or day by day separators. High-tech "alarm" pill boxes are also available.

Both the family and the patient are given instruction on how to take a blood pressure. Automatic blood pressure reading and recording devices are now available at nominal cost to the patient. Patients should practice under the supervision of the nurse until they feel competent. They should use the same device from reading to reading to establish consistency.

EVALUATION

As the evaluation phase begins, the evaluation criteria are developed through dialogue among the nurse, patient, and family. Typical evaluation outcome criteria for a patient with renal disease are included in Table 39–3.

The nurse and patient are observant of any changes in urine characteristics or quantity. Any changes that are related to specific medications are explained at the time the patient is given the medication. Table 39–4 provides a listing of drugs that may color the urine. Any blood or unusual odor to the urine should also be reported. Explaining to the patient the importance of accurate reporting is tantamount to a good treatment plan.

The nurse also evaluates the signs of fluid retention. If the patient is on diuretic therapy, edema should decrease. If renal disease is worsening, edema will increase. Does the patient notice tight rings, tight sʰ swollen ankles, or difficulty breathing? Thᵉ should also know what to expect so thaᵗ ' give accurate information and seek ⌐ intervention while symptoms arᵉ

The psychologic implications often the most frustrating for the nurse. Some people undergo an alʰ

Table 39–4. DRUGS THAT COLOR URINE

Drug	Color
Amitriptyline	Blue-green
Cascara	Brown (acid urine)
	Pink (alkaline urine)
Chlorzoxazone	Red-purple, orange
Indomethacin	Green
Levodopa	Red-tinged
Methocarbamol	Brown, black
Methyldopa	Red, brown-black
Nitrofurantoin	Brown or rust yellow
Phenazopyridine	Orange, red
Phenolphthalein	Orange, rust (acid urine)
	Pink, red, purple (alkaline urine)
Phenothiazines	Pink, purple, orange, rust
Phenytoin	Pink, red, red-brown
Primaquine	Rust yellow, brown
Quinine	Brown
Riboflavin	Yellow
Rifampin	Red-orange
Senna	Yellow-brown (acid urine)
	Yellow-pink (alkaline urine)
Sulfonamides	Rust yellow, brown
Triamterene	Blue, green

sonality change. They become easily irritated and lack the ability to remember details and to concentrate. The exhibited symptoms are not always consistent with uremia, but may generally improve as the creatinine clearance improves, or after the patient has undergone dialysis.

The nurse also needs to evaluate the patient to see if the desired effects of the medication regimen are occurring. Diuretics should produce diuresis and loss of weight. Evaluation of patient compliance is of great importance to the evaluation of any therapeutic regimen. Patients are often too busy to correctly take their medications, but yet are quick to chastise the ineffectiveness of therapy. Patients are cautioned not to discontinue the medications as soon as they are feeling better, or not to take the medications as needed for symptomatic relief.

In this age of new and expensive wonder drugs, cost is often a barrier to proper compliance. If patients are not privy to prescription plans, a re-evaluation of therapy may be needed. The use of less costly, but equally effective, generic medications may be possible in some instances.

If the patient has a chronic condition, compliance may not be good because he or she sees no reason to live within the restrictions (see Chapter 8). These patients and families need to be helped to set realistic goals. As they begin to respond to treatment and feel better, patients may decide that a modification in lifestyle is not the threat it may first have seemed. The nurse has the responsibility to make the patient aware of the alternatives if he or she does not comply with the prescribed regimen; but the ultimate responsibility for compliance belongs to the patient, as long as he or she is alert and coherent.

SUMMARY

To properly manage the patient with renal failure, the nurse must be familiar with the measurements of renal function. In acute renal failure, using osmotic or potent loop diuretics may restore some urine flow. Patients may require the use of vasoactive agents, such as dopamine, in an attempt to increase glomerular flow. Potassium concentrations may be severely elevated, often necessitating acute and chronic treatment modalities. With appropriate evaluation, therapy, and intervention, acute renal failure should be short lived.

While many of the problems in acute renal failure are the same as those in chronic renal failure, they often become great in magnitude. Problems such as hypocalcemia and hyperkalemia become daily occurrences and need to be dealt with appropriately. The anemia of renal failure may become severe and the patient may require often dangerous transfusions. Problems such as acidosis or alkalosis may also cause difficulty. Patients on potentially toxic drugs such as aminoglycosides or digoxin require constant therapeutic drug monitoring as well as dosage adjustments.

With appropriate medical and nursing management, patients with renal failure can lead a long and healthy life. The nurse should listen closely to these patients, and not view them merely as a chart full of graphs and numbers. Proper assessment, education, and intervention will spot potential problems early, before they become serious in nature. The health management team concept needs to be the main operative. Interfacing with the dialysis technician, social worker, dietitian, physician, pharmacist, and most importantly, the patient, will provide the nurse with truly rewarding experiences that ultimately can improve the care of the patient.

BIBLIOGRAPHY

Anderson, S and Brenner, BM: Therapeutic implications of converting-enzyme inhibitors in renal disese. Am J Kidney Dis 10:87, 1987.
Bennett, WM: Guide to drug dosage in renal failure. Clin Pharmacokinet 15:326, 1988.
Brenner, BM and Lazarus MJ: Acute Renal Failure, ed 2. Churchill-Livingston, New York, 1988.
Fine, RN: Chronic Ambulatory Peritoneal Dialysis (CAPD) and Chronic Cycling Peritoneal Dialysis (CCPD) in Children. Martinus Nijhoff, New York, 1987.
Maxwell, MH, Kleeman, CR, and Narins, RG: Clinical Disorders of Fluid and Electrolyte Metabolism, ed 4. McGraw-Hill, New York, 1987.
Plawecki, HM, Brewer, S, and Plawecki, JA: Chronic renal failure. J Gerontol Nurs 13:14, 1987.
Schrier, RW and Gottschalk, CW: Disease of the Kidney, ed 4. Little, Brown & Co, Boston, 1988.
Stuart, G: Peritoneal dialysis. Nursing Times 83:40, 1987.
Van Stone, JC: Dialysis and the Treatment of Renal Insufficiency. Grune & Stratton, New York, 1983.

SITUATION   39–1

Maude McKeever is a 49-year-old, transferred to the intensive care unit for management of acute tubular necrosis (ATN) related to hypovolemia secondary to an anaphylactic reaction.

1. Ms. McKeever is to be started on a continuous furosemide (Lasix) infusion. The nurse will expect to infuse the drug no greater than:
   a. 5 mg/min
   b. 2 mg/min
   c. 6 mg/min
   d. 4 mg/min

2. The nurse will check Ms. McKeever's urine for specific gravity every eight hours. Which of the following values corresponds with a diagnosis of ATN?
   a. 1.011
   b. 1.001
   c. 1.009
   d. 1.003

3. Ms. McKeever has a urine output of 22 cc/hour on the furosemide infusion. In addition, the physician orders a dopamine drip at renal (dopaminergic) dosage. The nurse will begin the infusion at the following rate:
   a. 8 mcg/kg/min
   b. 10 mcg/kg/min
   c. 2 mcg/kg/min
   d. 15 mcg/kg/min

4. Ms. McKeever is taking calcium channel blockers for management of elevated blood pressure. In addition, the nurse will expect to:
   a. restrict dietary sodium
   b. encourage high protein diet
   c. restrict fluid intake
   d. encourage high fat intake

5. Ms. McKeever's serum potassium is reported to be 7.0 mEq/L. A sodium polystyrene sulfonate (Kayexalate) enema is ordered to be given. The nurse will mix the drug with sorbitol for administration. The nurse is aware that the sorbitol reduces the potential for:
   a. Kayexalate tolerance
   b. allergic reaction
   c. diarrhea
   d. intestinal obstruction

6. An expected outcome for Ms. McKeever following two Kayexalate enemas would be a serum potassium of:
   a. 5.5 mEq/L
   b. 4.5 mEq/L
   c. 4.0 mEq/L
   d. 3.5 mEq/L

SITUATION   39–2

Hung Vu is a 52-year-old with chronic renal failure, admitted for placement of an A-V fistula for the purpose of hemodialysis. In addition to hemodialysis, he is to be managed medically for renal dysfunction-related problems and congestive heart failure.

1. Mr. Vu is to take an aluminum-containing antacid (Basagel) three times a day. The nurse is aware that the purpose of this antacid is to correct:
   a. hyperphosphatemia
   b. hypokalemia
   c. hypomagnesemia
   d. hypercalcemia

2. The nurse will plan to administer the Basagel to Mr. Vu at the following times:
   a. between meals
   b. with meals
   c. an hour before meals
   d. an hour after meals

3. Mr. Vu is currently taking Schol's solution (Bicitra) daily. An adverse effect of this agent may be demonstrated by:
   a. acidosis
   b. fluid excess
   c. sedation
   d. reduced urine output

4. Mr. Vu complains of pain in the right big toe. It is red, swollen, and warm to touch. He is to be started on allo-

purinol (Zyloprim) 600 mg daily for three days. When evaluating benefit of this therapy, the nurse will assess which laboratory value?
   a. ammonia
   b. calcium
   c. BUN
   d. uric acid

5. The nurse reports that Mr. Vu is pale and complains of weakness. His hematocrit is 22.8. The nurse is aware that, when assessing anemia in the renal failure patient, the following must be taken into account:
   a. iron intake
   b. kidney size
   c. dilutional factors
   d. activity level

6. Mr. Vu is to begin treatment with rHU-EPO (recombinant human erythropoietin) following hemodialysis three times weekly. An outcome of this type of therapy would be:
   a. decreased BUN levels
   b. elevated platelet count
   c. reduced creatinine levels
   d. elevated red blood cell count

Please refer to the Appendices for correct answers and additional review questions with answers.

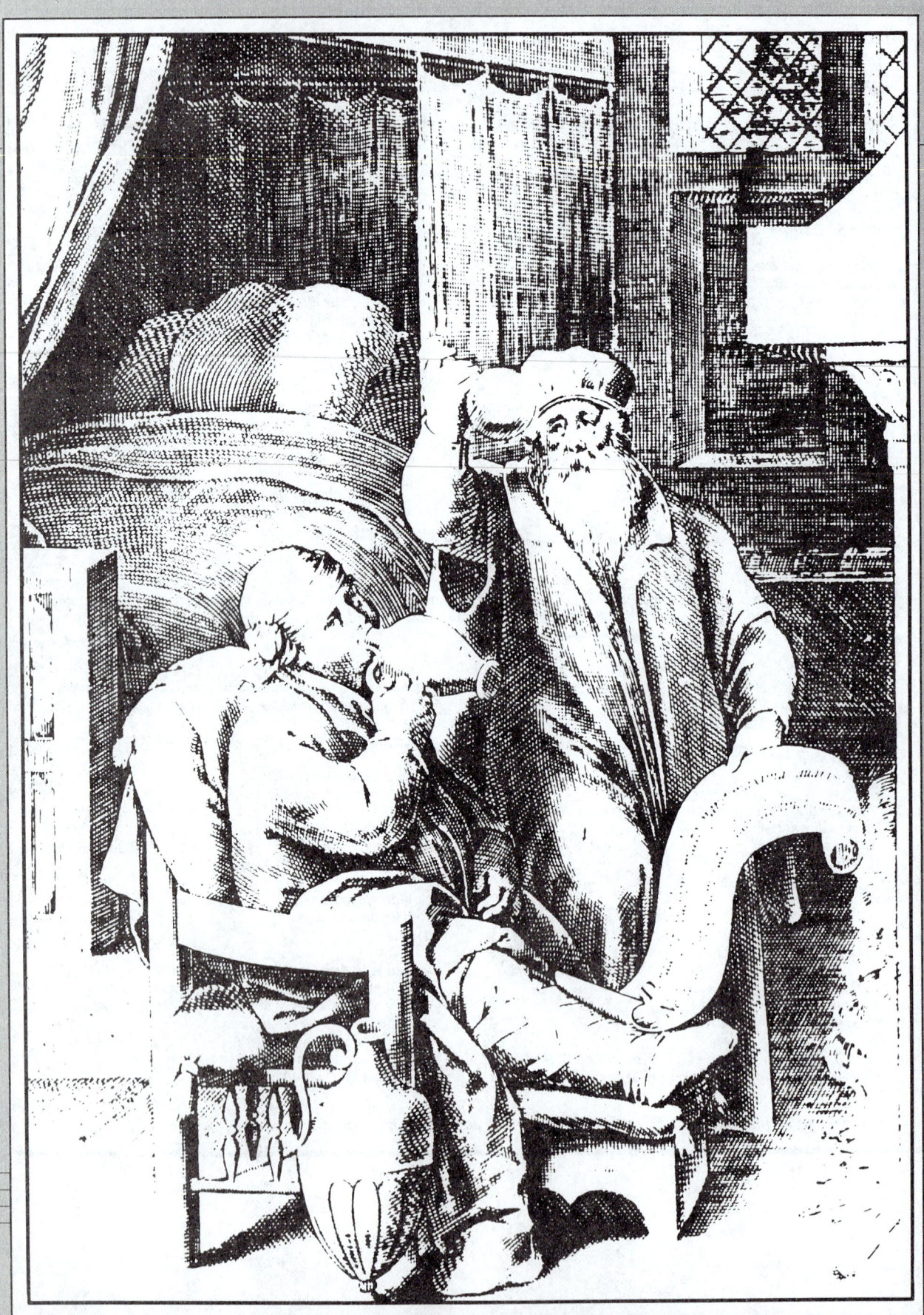

Treating a gouty patient, 1607. The Bettmann Archive.

7
UNIT

DRUGS AFFECTING THE ENDOCRINE SYSTEM

GLOSSARY TERMS IN THIS CHAPTER
Adenohypophysis
Anabolism
Calcitonin
Circadian
Corticotropin
Diabetes insipidus
Hormones
Hypophyseal gland
Lipolysis
Negative feedback mechanism
Neurohypophysis
Somatotropin
Syndrome of inappropriate ADH (SIADH)
Thyrotropin
Thyroxine (T_4)
Triiodothyronine (T_3)

OVERVIEW OF ANATOMY AND PHYSIOLOGY OF THE ENDOCRINE SYSTEM

MERRILY MATHEWSON KUHN, R.N.C., Ph.D., CCRN

LEARNING OBJECTIVES

After reading this chapter, the student will be able to:

1. Identify all parts of the endocrine system, and the specific hormones they secrete.

2. Describe the functions of the various endocrine hormones.

3. Explain the regulatory functions of the endocrine system.

4. Describe the feedback loops within the endocrine system.

OVERVIEW OF THE ENDOCRINE SYSTEM

Along with the central nervous system, the endocrine system is responsible for maintaining the constant internal environment of the body via production of chemical substances called *hormones*. Specifically, the endocrine system helps to regulate and maintain: (1) response to stress and injury; (2) growth, development, and reproduction; (3) fluid and electrolyte balance; and (4) energy metabolism (Fig. 40–1).

The endocrine system is composed of several glands capable of synthesizing hormones and releasing them directly into the bloodstream for transport to their target organs. Exocrine glands, such as the pancreas with its digestive enzymes, secrete their substances via ducts to an epithelial surface. The endocrine glands include the pituitary, thyroid, parathyroid, pancreas (which functions as both an exocrine and endocrine gland), adrenals, ovaries, and testes (Fig. 40–2). Researchers have now identified that hormone synthesis is not exclusive to endocrine glands but occurs in diverse tissue. Estrogen, for example, can be formed from testosterone and androstenedione in ovary, brain, adipocytes, and hair follicles.

All glands within the endocrine system have the potential for hypo- or hyperfunction. Table 40–1 reviews the endocrine glands, their function and dysfunction, and the hormones they produce.

HORMONES

Hormones are defined as chemical substances secreted by one group of cells that exert physiologic effects on other cells. Hormonal function involves four broad domains: (1) reproduction; (2) growth and development; (3) maintenance of the internal environment; and (4) production, utilization, and storage of energy. The quantity of hormones in the body is normally very small compared with the quantity of other substances such as electrolytes. Structurally, hormones are either steroids or proteins. Secretions from the gonads and adrenal cortex are steroids; the rest are proteins or small peptides.

Compounds classified as steroids are complex molecules containing carbon atoms in interlocking rings; these include, in addition to the gonadal and adrenocortical hormones, sterols, bile acids, and vitamin D. Steroid hormones and catecholamines are synthesized from small–molecular-weight precursors. Steroid hormones work directly inside the cell by binding to intracellular receptors. Ultimately, steroid hormones affect the transcription of deoxyribonucleic acid (DNA) to initiate protein synthesis, activating cell function.

Protein hormones bind with specific receptors on the cell membrane, activating the conversion of adenosine triphosphate (ATP) into cyclic adenosine 3',5'-monophosphate (cAMP). Cyclic AMP then moves to other structures within the cell to produce changes in the rate of protein synthesis and to activate cell function.

Water-soluble hormones are transported in plasma in solution and require no specific transport mechanism. The more insoluble hormones (thyroid, testosterones, and cortisol hormones) require carrier proteins. When the hormone is bound to protein, it is inactive. When the hormone leaves its protein carrier, it can then enter its target cell. Therefore, the protein acts as a reservoir for hormones.

Hormones are deactivated in the liver, and the end products are excreted by the kidneys. Alterations in hepatic and renal function may change the rate at which hormones are metabolized and excreted, thereby influencing their function.

FEEDBACK RELATIONSHIPS

The distinguishing characteristic of the endocrine system is the feedback control of hormone production. In most instances, the control is through a negative feedback mechanism (Fig. 40–3). The following factors must be discussed to understand this mechanism: (1) The endocrine glands have a natural tendency to oversecrete hormones. (2) Because of this oversecretion, the hormone exerts more and more control on the target organ. (3) The target organ performs its normal function. (4) When the target organ is stimulated too much, some factor about the function then feeds back to the original endocrine gland and causes a negative effect on the gland to decrease its secretory rate (Guyton, 1986). This is known as a *negative feedback mechanism*. The main factor in this system is the degree of activity of the target organ. Only when the target organ's activity rises to an appropriate level will the feedback to the gland become

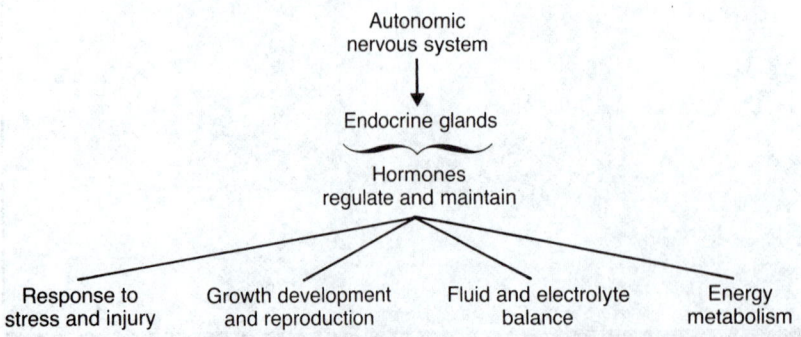

Figure 40–1. The endocrine system is regulated by the autonomic nervous system. In turn, the endocrine glands produce hormones which regulate and maintain the response to stress and injury; growth, development, and reproduction; fluid and electrolyte balance; and energy metabolism.

ENDOCRINE SYSTEM

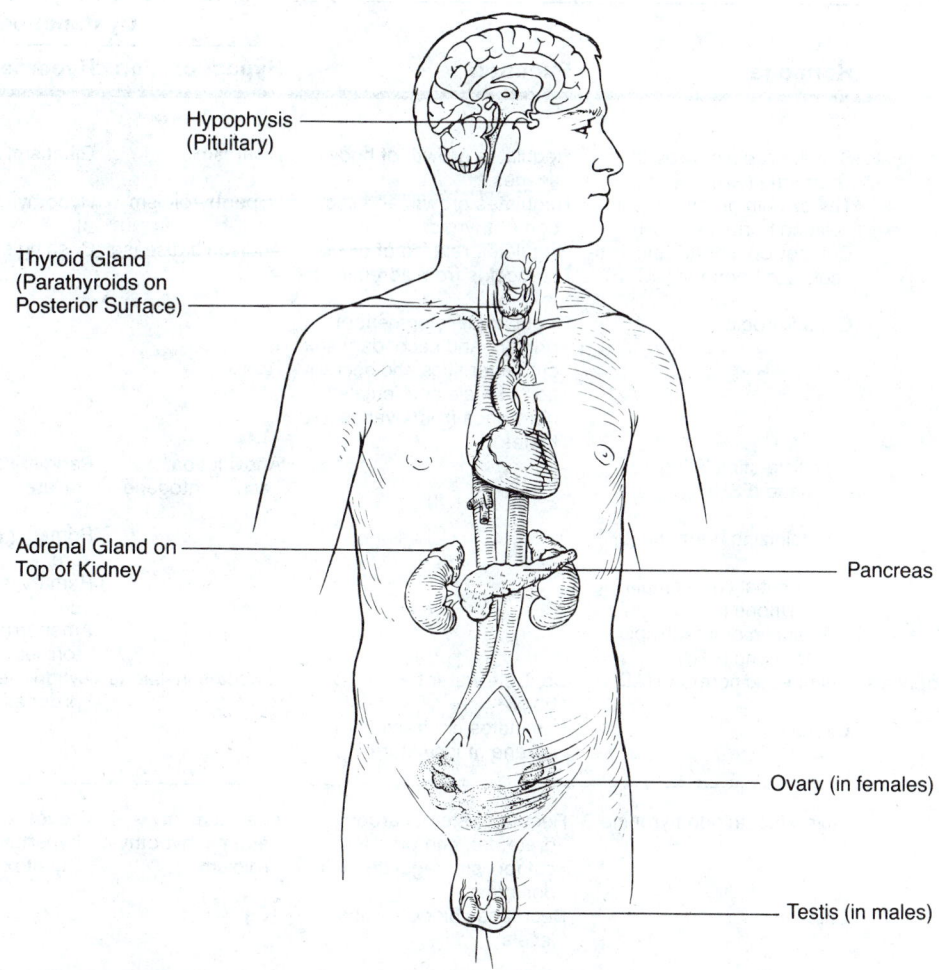

Hypophysis
(Pituitary)

Thyroid Gland
(Parathyroids on
Posterior Surface)

Adrenal Gland on
Top of Kidney

Pancreas

Ovary (in females)

Testis (in males)

Figure 40–2. The endocrine glands secrete hormones directly into the blood stream. The illustration shows the glands and the hormones they produce. (From Taber's Cyclopedic Medical Dictionary, ed 16, FA Davis Co, Philadelphia, 1989, p 589.)

powerful enough to slow further secretion of the hormone. If the target organ responds poorly to the hormone, the endocrine gland will continue to secrete the hormone in increasingly large quantities.

All hormones are under feedback control, some by cations (calcium or parathyroid hormone), some by metabolites (glucose or insulin and glucagon), some by other hormones (somatostatin of insulin and glucagon), and some by osmolality or extracellular fluid volume (vasopressin, renin, aldosterone) (Fig. 40–3).

BIORHYTHMS

The endocrine glands have various rhythms of production that can vary from hours (luteinizing hormone and testosterone) to a day (*circadian* rhythm of cortisol, Fig. 40–4), weeks (menstrual cycle), or even longer, such as seasonal variation with thyroxine. These cycles are regulated by sleep-associated alterations, light-dark cycles,

and environmental factors. The mechanism by which these rhythms operate and the physiologic ramifications of the rhythms are poorly understood at this time.

PITUITARY

The pituitary or *hypophyseal gland,* a round structure about 1.27 cm in diameter and weighing about 0.5–0.7 g, is located in the sella turcica of the sphenoid bone and is attached to the hypothalamus by the infundibular stem. It is composed of two major lobes: a larger anterior lobe called the *adenohypophysis,* and a smaller posterior lobe sometimes referred to as the *neurohypophysis.*

Anterior Pituitary

The anterior pituitary synthesizes polypeptide and glycoprotein hormones in response to the secretion of releasing factors and inhibitory factors from the hypothalamus. The polypeptide hormones include growth

Table 40–1. SUMMARY OF ENDOCRINE GLANDS, HORMONES, AND THEIR FUNCTIONS

Gland	Hormone	Function	Dysfunction	
			Hyposecretion	**Hypersecretion**
Pituitary				
Adenohypophysis	Somatotropin or growth hormone (GH)	Regulates growth of body tissues	Dwarfism	Giantism, acromegaly
	Thyrotropin or thyroid-stimulating hormone (TSH)	Regulates growth and secretion of thyroid	Hyperthyroidism	Hypothyroidism
	Corticotropin or adrenocorticotropic hormone (ACTH)	Regulates release of glucocorticoids from adrenal cortex	Addison's disease	Cushing's disease
	Gonadotropins:	Regulate development of primary and secondary sex characteristics and secretion of male and female hormones from ovaries and testes		
	Follicle-stimulating hormone (FSH)		Anovulation, aspermatogenesis	Parimary gonadal failure
	Luteinizing hormone (LH)			Primary gonadal failure
	Interstitial cell–stimulating hormone (ICSH)			Primary gonadal failure
	Prolactin or luteotropic hormone (LTH)			Amenorrhea, galactorrhea
Neurohypophysis	Antidiuretic hormone (ADH)	Controls water balance of body	Diabetes insipidus	Syndrome of inappropriate ADH
	Oxytocin	Stimulates contraction of uterine musculature		
Thyroid	Thyroxine, triiodothyronine	Regulate rate of carbohydrate, fat, and protein catabolism; regulate metabolic rate	Cretinism, myxedema, hypothyroidism	Graves' disease, hyperthyroidism, thyrotoxicosis
	Calcitonin	Decreases blood calcium levels	↑Ca	↓Ca
Parathyroid	Parathormone	Increases blood calcium levels	↓Ca	↑Ca
Pancreas	Glucagon	Increases blood glucose levels	Hypoglycemia	
	Insulin	Decreases blood glucose levels	Diabetes mellitus, ketoacidosis	Hypoglycemia, insulin shock
Adrenals				
Cortex	Mineralocorticoids (aldosterone)	Maintain fluid and electrolyte balance	Addison's disease	Hyperaldosteronism
	Glucocorticoids (cortisol)	Promote positive response to stress by affecting carbohydrate, fat, and protein metabolism	Addison's disease, acute adrenal crisis	Cushing's syndrome
	Sex hormones (androgens, estrogens, progestins)	Influence secondary sex characteristics ONLY in certain disorders; normally, their levels are too low for physiologic activity		Adrenogenital syndrome
Medulla	Epinephrine, norepinephrine	Provide for response to stress	Severe hypotension, cardiovascular collapse	Pheochromocytoma
Gonads				
Ovaries	Estrogen	Regulates development of secondary sex characteris-	Sexual dysfunction, infertility	Sexual dysfunction, precocious puberty

Table 40–1. SUMMARY OF ENDOCRINE GLANDS, HORMONES, AND THEIR FUNCTIONS–*CONTINUED*

Gland	Hormone	Function	Dysfunction	
			Hyposecretion	Hypersecretion
		tics and sexual maturation and functioning		
	Progesterone	Regulates preparation for and maintenance of pregnancy		
Testes	Testosterone	Regulates development of secondary sex characteristics and sexual maturation and functioning	Delayed male puberty, male hypogonadism	Hirsutism in women, genetic female pseudohermaphroditism

hormone (GH), prolactin (PRL), and corticotropin (ACTH). The glycoprotein hormones include thyrotropin (TSH), luteinizing hormone (LH), and follicle-stimulating hormone (FSH). The following releasing and inhibiting factors have been identified: growth hormone–releasing factor (GH-RF) and growth hormone–inhibiting factor (GH-IF), thyrotropin–releasing factor (TRF), corticotropin–releasing factor (CRF), follicle-stimulating hormone–releasing factor (FRF), luteinizing hormone–releasing factor (LH-RF), prolactin–releasing factor (PRF), prolactin–inhibiting factor (PIF), melanocyte-stimulating hormone–releasing factor (MRF), and melanocyte–inhibiting factor (MIF).

Growth hormone, also called *somatotropin* or soma-

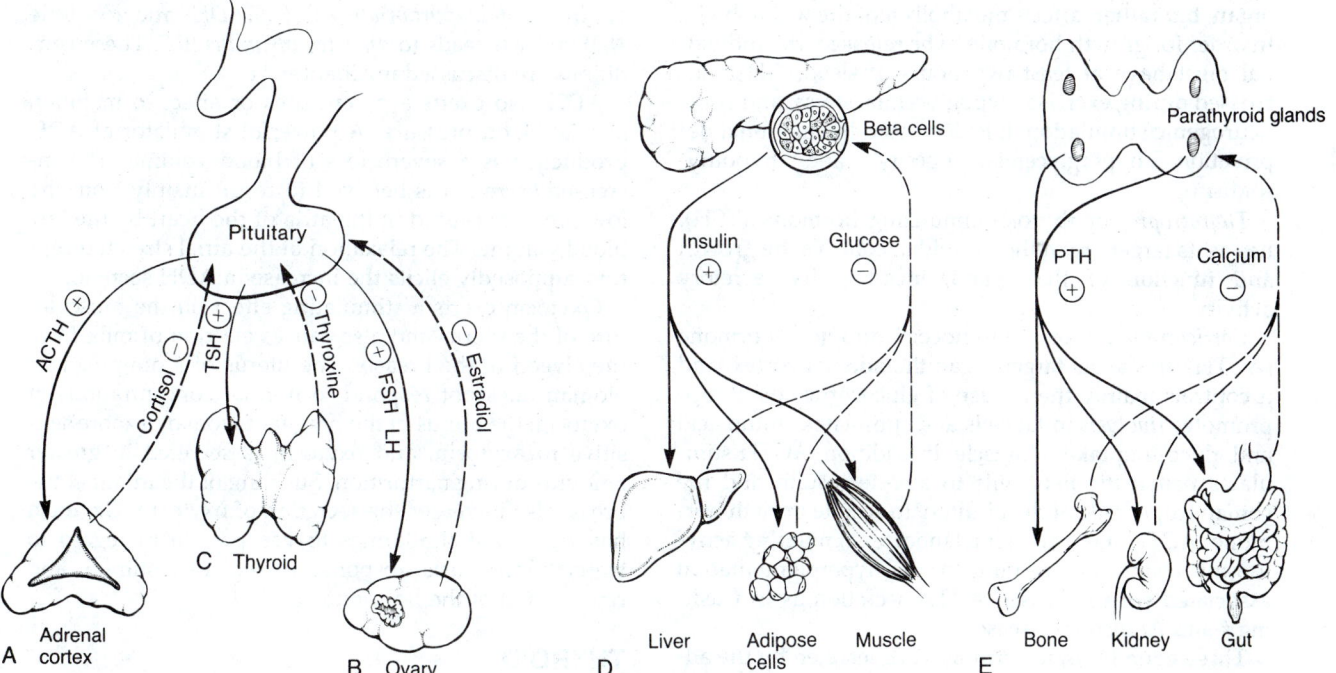

Figure 40–3. A diagramatic representation of several feedback systems. A, B, and C represent the feedback control in which the hormonal product of the target gland acts on the release of the corresponding pituitary hormone.
A. ACTH stimulates the adrenal cortex to secrete cortisol. Cortisol feeds back to the hypothalamic-pituitary axis and inhibits CRF-ACTH release.
B. FSH and LH stimulate the ovaries to release estradiol. Estradiol feeds back to the hypothalamic-pituitary axis and inhibits GNRH-FSH/LH release.
C. TSH stimulates the thyroid to secrete thyroxine. Thyroxine feeds back to the hypothalamic-pituitary axis and inhibits TRH/TSH release.
D and E illustrate feedback control in which the metabolic substance controlled by the hormone acts directly upon its release.
D. Insulin release is controlled by glucose in the blood. If glucose increases, insulin is secreted. If glucose decreases, insulin is inhibited.
E. The parathyroid gland regulates serum calcium. A drop in serum calcium stimulates parathormone secretion. Conversely, an increase in calcium shuts off parathormone production.

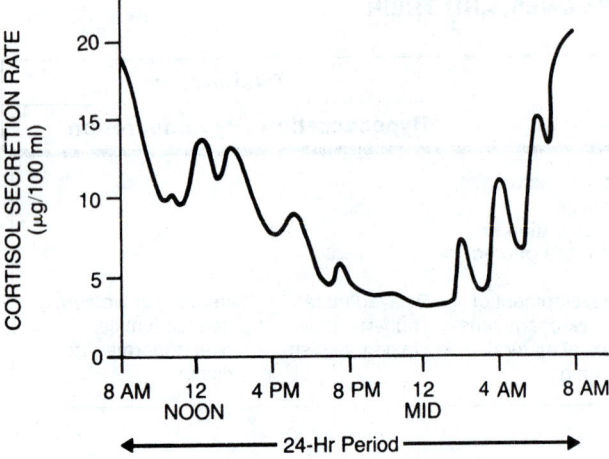

Figure 40–4. The circadian rhythm of cortisol. Cortisol peaks daily at approximately 8:00 AM, and troughs daily at approximately 12:00 midnight.

totropic hormone (STH), regulates growth of bone, muscles, and viscera. It also affects the metabolism of carbohydrates, proteins, and fats; it has no specific target organ, but rather, affects metabolism of the whole body. In order for growth hormone to be released, the individual must have at least two hours of sleep. GH is increased during exercise, hypoglycemia, stress, and some neurogenic stimulation; it is decreased in emotional deprivation, hyperglycemia, obesity, and hypothyroidism.

Thyrotropin, or thyroid-stimulating hormone (TSH), has as its target organ the thyroid; it controls the growth and function of that gland, incuding its secretory activity.

Corticotropin, or adrenocorticotropic hormone (ACTH), has as its target organ the adrenal cortex, and it controls mainly the release of glucocorticoids. It also promotes *lipolysis* in fat cells and stimulates amino acid and glucose uptake in muscle. In addition, ACTH stimulates pancreatic beta cells to secrete insulin and the somatotropic cells of the pituitary to secrete growth hormone. ACTH has a weak melanocyte-stimulating activity; this action may account for the hyperpigmentation associated with increased ACTH secretion as in Cushing's and Addison's disease.

Three gonadotropic hormones are secreted by the adenohypophysis: (1) Follicle-stimulating hormone (FSH) has as its target organs the ovaries and testes. (2) Luteotropic hormone (LTH) or prolactin has the breast as its target organ and is responsible for initiation and maintenance of lactation. (3) Luteinizing hormone (LH) is important in the female ovary for follicular rupture or interstitial cell–stimulating hormone (ICSH), and has as its target organs the testes. As a group, these hormones are necessary for the development of the primary and secondary sex characteristics, as well as for the functioning of the male and female reproductive systems.

There is a small intermediate lobe of the pituitary that contains melanocyte-stimulating hormone (MSH), which is secreted in response to MSH-releasing factor (MRF) and MSH-inhibiting factor (MIF). The function of MSH in humans is unclear at present, and it may represent an evolutionary vestige. It may also play a part in the regulation of skin pigmentation.

Posterior Pituitary

The posterior pituitary stores and secretes two chemically related hormones that are produced in the hypothalamus: (1) antidiuretic hormone (ADH), or vasopressin, and (2) oxytocin. In the hypothalamus, these hormones are produced in the supraoptic nucleus and are transported by axons to the posterior pituitary.

ADH functions to control water balance in the body by increasing the permeability of the cells of the distal tubules in the kidney to water, thus decreasing the formation of urine. Osmolality, volume of the blood, and thirst regulate the secretion of ADH, with a rise in osmotic pressure or a decrease in volume increasing the secretion of ADH. Other factors influencing vasopressin release include: a decreased blood pressure; atrial stretch receptors; baroreceptors in the carotid, aortic, and pulmonary arteries; nausea; and emotional stress. Too much ADH release leads to the development of a *syndrome of inappropriate ADH (SIADH)* and too little ADH release leads to *diabetes insipidus (DI).* These conditions are discussed in Chapter 41.

ADH also exerts a potent pressor effect to maintain arterial blood pressure. A powerful stimulator of ADH production is a severe loss of blood volume. The increased secretion is believed to result mainly from the low pressure caused in the atria of the heart by the low blood volume. The relaxation of the atrial stretch receptors supposedly elicits the increase in ADH secretion.

Oxytocin exerts a stimulating effect on the musculature of the uterus and also causes ejection of milk from the alveoli of the breasts. The uterus of a nonpregnant woman does not respond to normal concentrations of oxytocin; the uterus of the pregnant woman is more sensitive to oxytocin, and oxytocin is secreted in greater amounts during parturition. Suckling of the infant at the breast also increases the secretion of oxytocin. Oxytocin has significant similarities to vasopressin in regard to water homeostasis, response to secretory stimuli, and renal action of the hormone.

THYROID

The thyroid, measuring about 5 cm by 3 cm and weighing 30 g, has two lobes situated at the sides of the trachea and connected by a bridge of thyroid tissue ventral to the trachea called the isthmus. Three hormones are produced and secreted by the thyroid: (1) thyroxine, (2) triiodothyronine, and (3) calcitonin.

Thyroxine (T_4) and *triiodothyronine* (T_3) are stored in the thyroid in combination with proteins as thyroglobulin and serve to maintain many metabolic functions by regulating the rate of carbohydrate, protein, and fat metabolism. Other functions include the regulation of body heat production and the rate of glucose utilization by the cells. Thyroid hormones also have an effect on cardiac output, heart rate, and arterial pressure. An increase in thyroid hormone leads to hyperthyroidism or thyrotoxic crisis, while a decrease results in hypothyroidism or myxedema.

Calcitonin, or thyrocalcitonin, functions in the regulation of calcium and phosphorus levels in the body. It is released in response to hypercalcemia and serves to inhibit bone resorption, reduces calcium absorption in the intestine, and increases kidney excretion of calcium. Calcitonin causes inhibition of parathyroid hormones.

PARATHYROIDS

The parathyroid glands, usually four in number, are most often located on the dorsal surface of the thyroid and measure about 6–7 mm in length and 2–3 mm in width. The hormone produced by these glands is parathyroid hormone (PTH) or parathormone, which functions in the regulation of calcium and phosphorus levels in the body, causing calcium levels to rise and phosphorus levels to fall. Hypocalcemia is the stimulus for its release. Upon release, PTH stimulates calcium absorption in the gastrointestinal tract; stimulates bone resorption of calcium; and increases a reabsorption of calcium in the proximal tubule of the kidney. The metabolism of calcium in the body is jointly regulated by calcitonin, parathormone, and vitamin D.

PANCREAS

The pancreas lies below and behind the stomach and is about 15 cm long and 3.8 cm wide. The endocrine function of the pancreas is contained in a specialized group of cells called the islets of Langerhans. Islet tissue contains alpha, beta, and delta cells.

The alpha cells produce and secrete the hormone called glucagon. Glucagon functions to increase blood glucose levels by causing glycogenolysis (the conversion of glycogen to glucose) in the liver. Hypoglycemia serves as the stimulus for glucagon secretion.

The beta cells produce and secrete the hormone called insulin. Insulin has a half-life of six mintues and is mainly cleared from the plasma in 10–15 minutes. Insulin functions to decrease blood glucose levels by promoting the utilization of glucose in tissue cells, especially skeletal muscle and adipose tissue, and by promoting glycogen formation and storage. The rate of insulin secretion is regulated by the concentration of glucose in the plasma; thus, hyperglycemia serves as a stimulus for increased insulin secretion. Insulin and glucagon, together with other hormones, serve to maintain the normal ranges of blood glucose.

Insulin also affects fat metabolism, enhancing fat synthesis; enhancing protein synthesis and protein metabolism; promoting amino acid uptake; and inhibiting protein degradation.

The delta cells secrete a hormone called somatostatin, which has an extremely short half-life of two minutes.

Ingestion of food stimulates somatostatin, which is responsible for slowing the assimilation of food from the gut. Somatostatin also depresses insulin and glucagon secretion, which further decreases the utilization of the absorbed nutrients by the tissues. This action prevents the rapid exhaustion of nutrients and makes them available for a longer period of time.

The pancreas also serves as an exocrine gland, secreting several digestive enzymes. Trypsin and chymotrypsin aid in the digestion of protein; pancreatic amylase aids in the digestion of carbohydrates; and pancreatic lipase aids in the digestion of fat.

ADRENALS

The two adrenal glands lie at the superior poles of the kidneys and weigh about 5–9 g each. Each gland is composed of: a cortex secreting mineralocorticoids, glucocorticoids, and gonadal hormones; and a medulla secreting the catecholamines, epinephrine and norepinephrine. As a whole, the adrenals give the individual the capacity to respond to stress of any kind in a positive manner.

Adrenal Cortex

The mineralocorticoids produced by the adrenal cortex are concerned with the maintenance of fluid and electrolyte balance. Aldosterone is the major hormone of this group; it functions to stimulate reabsorption of sodium and chloride in the renal distal tubule. Water, too, is reabsorbed, serving to maintain the normovolemic state. On the other hand, the reabsorption of potassium is decreased. Aldosterone secretion is regulated by the renin-angiotensin-aldosterone mechanism, by extracellular fluid volume.

The glucocorticoids, produced in response to pituitary ACTH, are primarily concerned with carbohydrate, protein, and fat metabolism. Cortisol (hydrocortisone) is the major hormone of this group, and it has many functions: (1) It maintains blood glucose levels by stimulating gluconeogenesis in the liver and decreasing the rate of glucose utilization by cells. (2) It decreases the rate of protein anabolism and alters fat metabolism by either mobilizing fatty acids or promoting storage of fat as the need arises. (3) Cortisol also exerts effects on lymph and blood tissue and is necessary for the normal functioning of the central nervous system. Cortisol secretion has a diurnal pattern, with secretion being highest in the early morning and lowest in the evening (Fig. 40–4). Psychological or physical stress causes an increase in adrenal stimulation. Too much of the glucocorticoids can result in Cushing's syndrome, while too little results in Addison's disease.

The adrenal cortex also secretes, in minute amounts, a number of gonadal hormones, among them androgens, estrogens, and progestins. These function in the same manner as the hormones produced by the gonads; the extremely small amount produced by the adrenals makes them insignificant in terms of sexual functioning. They may, however, assume more significance if they

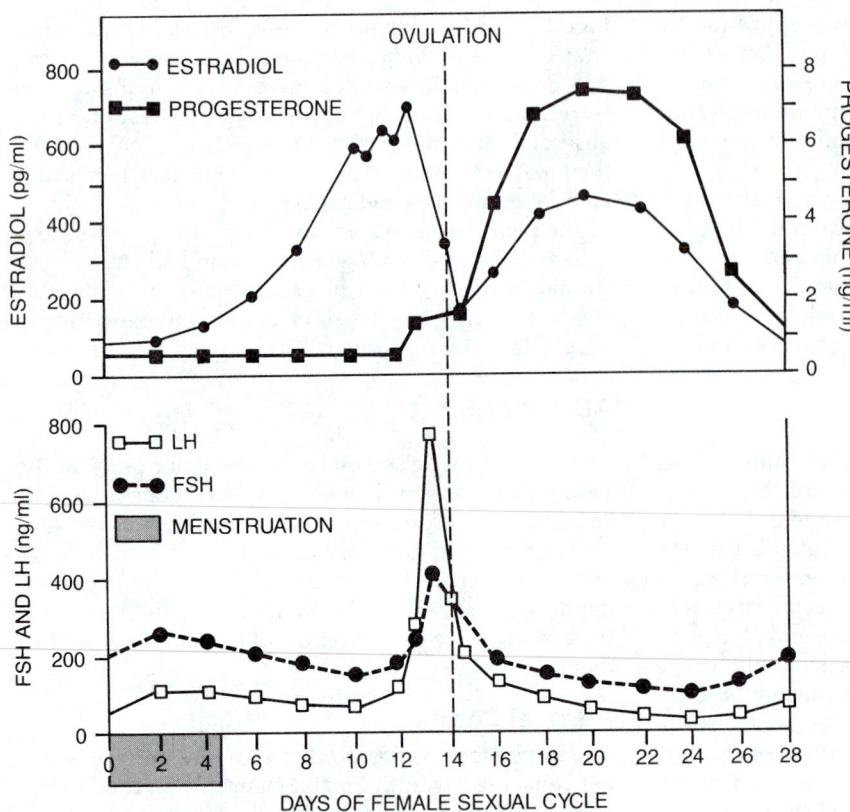

Figure 40–5. Monthly cyclic release of FSH and LH in normally-menstruating women.

are produced in abnormally large amounts, as may occur in certain disease states or if the gonads are nonfunctional.

Adrenal Medulla

The adrenal medulla is functionally related to the autonomic nervous system (ANS), and its hormones epinephrine and norepinephrine are known as sympathomimetic amines because their effects are the same as the physiologic effects of the sympathetic branch of the ANS.

Basically, epinephrine and norepinephrine are short-acting hormones that serve to stimulate gluconeogenesis and glycogenolysis and to stimuluate the release of free fatty acids in order to provide fuel for the body during periods of stress. These hormones also cause vasoconstriction, increase of the heart rate and myocardial strength, elevation of blood pressure, and bronchial relaxation.

Epinephrine is located almost exclusively in the chromaffin cells of the adrenal medulla, where it is stored in high concentrations. The amounts of epinephrine in the brain and sympathetic ganglia are small. On the other hand, norepinephrine is widely distributed; in addition to the adrenal medulla, it is found in the peripheral sympathetic nerves, the central nervous system (CNS), and in small amounts in extra-adrenal chromaffin cells. Since virtually all of the norepinephrine outside the CNS and the adrenal gland is located in the sympathetic

nerve endings, the norepinephrine content of a particular tissue reflects the extent of its sympathetic innervation.

Differences between the two hormones are related to their ratios of alpha- and beta-receptor activity. Epinephrine has a greater beta effect than does norepinephrine, whereas their alpha effects are similar in most tissues (Chapters 17 and 19).

GONADS

Ovaries

The ovaries, located in the pelvic cavity of the female on either side of the uterus, weigh about 2.0–3.5 g; they produce and secrete two classes of hormones, estrogens and progesterone.

Three major estrogens are produced: 17-beta-estradiol (the most important), estrone, and estriol. The estrogens cause cellular proliferation and growth of the sexual organs. Specifically, they increase the size of the vagina and uterus, cause proliferation of the endometrium, cause proliferation of glandular and ciliated cells in the epithelium of the fallopian tubes, and increase fat deposits in the breast and growth of the breasts' ductile tissue. The estrogens also increase osteoblastic activity; cause retention of calcium, sodium, and water; increase the vascularity of the skin; and increase the deposition of fat in the subcutaneous tissues.

Progesterone is secreted by the corpus luteum during

the latter half of the menstrual cycle. It promotes secretory changes in the uterine epithelium and decreases the frequency of uterine contractions. Thus, it assists in implantation of the fertilized ovum, should fertilization occur. Progesterone also promotes secretory changes in tubal mucosa; promotes development of lobules and alveoli of the breasts; and causes some sodium, chloride, and water reabsorption.

Rather than being secreted at continuous levels, estrogen and progesterone are secreted in a cyclic fashion, and in this manner govern the female menstrual cycle (Fig. 40–5).

The ovaries also secrete a small amount of testosterone and androgenic precursors, which are thought to contribute to sexual development in the female.

Testes

The testes, located in the scrotum in the male and weighing about 10.5–14 g, produce and secrete testosterone. This production is in response to ICSH from the pituitary. Testosterone is produced in the cells of Leydig.

Testosterone is essential for the development of the primary sex characteristics, causing enlargement of the penis, scrotum, and testes at puberty. Testosterone is also essential for the maturation of spermatozoa. It is responsible for the development of the secondary sex characteristics as well, including the male pattern of hair growth, voice changes, increased secretions of seba-

ceous glands, and calcium retention; it also has a positive effect on protein *anabolism.*

SUMMARY

This chapter has presented a brief overview of normal anatomy and physiology of the endocrine system, including the function of the various hormones produced. This material is basic to the student's understanding of how various medications affect the endocrine system.

BIBLIOGRAPHY

Goodman, AG, Goodman, L, and Gilman, A (eds): Goodman & Gilman's The Pharmacological Basis of Therapeutics, ed 7. Macmillan, New York, 1985.

Guyton, A: Textbook of Medical Physiology. WB Saunders, Philadelphia, 1986.

Price, SA and Wilson, LM: Pathophysiology: Clinical Concepts of Disease Processes. McGraw-Hill, New York, 1985.

Tepperman, J and Tepperman, H. Metabolic & Endocrine Physiology. Year Book Medical Publishers, Chicago, 1987.

Wilson, J and Foster, D: Textbook of Endocrinology. WB Saunders, Philadelphia, 1985.

GLOSSARY TERMS IN THIS CHAPTER

Craniophyaryngioma
Diabetogenic effect
Hemophilia A
Ketogenic effect
Somatomedins
von Willebrand's disease

41

CHAPTER

PITUITARY DRUGS

MERRILY MATHEWSON KUHN, R.N.C., Ph.D., CCRN

LEARNING OBJECTIVES

After reading this chapter, the student will be able to:

1. Identify those medications commonly used as pituitary drugs.

2. Differentiate among the pituitary drugs as to mechanisms of action, route of administration, pharmacokinetics, adverse effects, contraindications, and interactions.

3. Identify specific areas to assess in the patient requiring pituitary drugs in order to formulate appropriate nursing diagnoses.

4. Plan the nursing interventions necessary to administer pituitary drugs and choose appropriate teaching strategies to gain patient compliance.

5. Evaluate the patient at various stages of treatment to gauge nursing interventions.

THERAPEUTIC AGENTS

Many medications are used to treat dysfunction of the pituitary. Those discussed in this chapter are growth hormone (GH), secreted from the anterior pituitary; and antidiuretic hormone (ADH), secreted from the posterior pituitary. Other anterior pituitary hormones are discussed in other chapters: ACTH, Chapter 24; TSH, Chapter 45; and oxytocin, Chapter 15. Pituitary drugs are reviewed in Table 41–1. Figure 41–1 reviews the anatomy of the pituitary gland. Figure 41–2 summarizes the specific action for each pituitary hormone.

Table 41–1. PITUITARY DRUGS

Name	Dosage	Mode of Administration	Pharmacokinetics
ANTERIOR PITUITARY			
Action: Replacement of natural growth hormone, produces increased number of muscle cells and increases connective tissue metabolism.			
Use: To treat linear growth failure from hormonal insufficiency.			
Somatrem (Protropin)	Individualized maximum dose 0.1 mg/kg (0.2 IU/kg) 3 times a week	IM	UA
Somatropin (Humatrope)	0.06 mg/kg 3 times a week; if growth does not exceed 2.5 cm in 6 months, dose is doubled for 6 months	IM	UA
POSTERIOR PITUITARY			
Action: Vasopressor activity by stimulating smooth muscle contraction, particularly in the hepatic and splanchnic beds; acts in the kidney in the distal tubules and collecting ducts to increase the cellular permeability to water, thus decreasing urine output and increasing water absorption.			
Use: For all neurogenic diabetes insipidus; GI bleeds associated with esophageal varices, and stomach bleeds.			
Vasopressin (Pitressin, synthetic)	5–10 U bid/tid; *Pediatric:* individualized	IM,SC	O: UA P: UA D: 2–8 hr ½ L: UA PB: UA B: UA E: UA
Vasopressin tannate (Pitressin tannate)	1.5–5.0 U repeated as required q 2–3 days; *Pediatric:* 1.25–2.5 U q 1–3 days	IM	O: UA P: UA D: 24–96 hr ½ L: UA PB: UA B: UA E: UA

Key to Abbreviations in the *Pharmacokinetics* column O-onset; P-peak; D-duration; PB-protein bound; B-biotransformed in; E-excreted in; ½ L-halflife.
*Within the column listing adverse effects, underlines indicate the most common effects; CAPITALS indicate life-threatening effects.

ANTERIOR PITUITARY HORMONES

Growth Hormone

Growth hormone (GH), also known as somatotropin or somatotropic hormone (STH), is a protein secreted in response to growth hormone–releasing and growth hormone–inhibiting factors released from the hypothalamus. GH is a polypeptide which has growth-promoting and anabolic properties.

ACTION. Growth hormone has no specific target gland; rather, many tissues are affected, leading to increased cellular size and increased rates of growth. Spe-

TEXT RESUMES ON PAGE 1068

Contraindications/ Precautions	Adverse Effects*	Interactions	Nursing Implications
CONTRAINDICATIONS: Closed epiphyses.	*Hemo:* antibody formation *Endo:* increased blood glucose	Glucocorticoids may inhibit somatropin.	ASSESSMENT: Establish true pituitary deficiency. Assess glucose at onset and periodically. Assess thyroid function and treat as needed. INTERVENTION: Reconstitute with sterile water only. Do not shake. Solution should be clear with no particles. Inject into muscle. EVALUATION: Evaluate growth every 6 months or more often.
CONTRAINDICATIONS: Hypersensitivity. PRECAUTIONS: Use cautiously in pregnancy, congestive heart failure, elderly persons.	*Neuro:* sweating, tremor, pounding head *CVR:* circumoral pallor, hypertension, anginal pain, overhydration *GI:* abdominal camps, nausea, diarrhea *Renal:* water intoxication	Increased antidiuretic response with chlorpropamide, carbamazepine, and clofibrate.	ASSESSMENT: Assess urinary output and weight at onset and periodically. Assess baseline ECG. Assess GI function. INTERVENTION: Warm ampule and shake vigorously to disperse tannate uniformly. Administer with 1–2 glasses of water to minimize side-effects. Advise patient to carry medication card, bracelet, or necklace if condition is chronic. EVALUATION: Be alert for signs of water toxicity and withdraw drug and restrict fluid intake until at least a 1.015 urine specific gravity is obtained.

CONTINUED ON THE FOLLOWING PAGE

Table 41–1. PITUITARY DRUGS–*CONTINUED*

Name	Dosage	Mode of Administration	Pharmacokinetics
Lypressin (Diapid)			

Action: Mainly antidiuretic activity as above.

Use: Diabetes insipidus.

	Adult and pediatric: 1–2 sprays in each naris qid; do not use more than 3 sprays	Intranasal	O: quickly P: 30–60 min D: 3–8 hr ½ L: UA PB: UA B: UA E: UA

Desmopressin acetate

Action: Antidiuretic effect, increase Factor VIII levels.

Use: Neurogenic diabetes insipidus, hemophilia A, von Willebrand's disease.

(DDVAP)	For diabetes insipidus: *Adult:* 0.1–0.4 ml (4–40 mEq)/day in divided doses	Intranasal	O: 30 min P: 90–120 min D: 8–20 hr ½ L: biphasic 7.8/75.5 min PB: UA B: UA E: UA
(Stimate)	*Pediatric:* 3 mo–12 yr, 0.05–0.3 mg/day Hemophilia A and von Willebrand's Disease: 0.3 μg/kg diluted in normal saline. 10 kg or less: 10 ml. More than 10 kg: 50 ml slowly over 30 min. Administer 30 min prior to surgery.	Intranasal IV infusion	

Posterior Pituitary Injection (Pituitrin)

Action: Antidiuretic effect, stimulates GI peristalsis, possesses oxytoxic effects.

Use: Control postoperative ileus, stimulates expulsion of gas prior to pyelography, diabetes insipidus. Near term, it can provide prolonged stimulation of uterine tonus. Assists uterine contractions after complete placental expulsion.

	5–20 U	SQ IM	O: UA P: UA D: UA ½ L: UA PB: UA B: UA E: UA

Key to Abbreviations in the *Pharmacokinetics* column O-onset; P-peak; D-duration; PB-protein bound; B-biotransformed in; E-excreted in; ½ L-halflife.

*Within the column listing adverse effects, <u>underlines</u> indicate the most common effects; CAPITALS indicate life-threatening effects.

Contraindications/ Precautions	Adverse Effects*	Interactions	Nursing Implications
No known contraindications. PRECAUTIONS: Use with caution in coronary artery disease, allergic rhinitis, and URI.	Infrequent and mild *Neuro:* headache, conjunctivitis *Resp:* rhinitis, rhinorrhea, nasal congestion, and local irritation *GI:* heartburn	Same as vasopressin.	ASSESSMENT: Assess urinary output and weight at onset and periodically. INTERVENTION: Drug should not be inhaled. Allergic rhinitis or upper respiratory infections may affect absorption. Hold bottle upright and patient should be in a vertical position with head upright. Do not use more than 3 sprays. EVALUATION: If unusual drowsiness, headache, shortness of breath, nausea, or severe nasal congestion occur, call physician.
CONTRAINDICATIONS: Nephrogenic diabetes insipidus, hypersensitivity. PRECAUTIONS: Use with caution in coronary artery disease. Safety in pregnancy, lactation, and children less than 3 months old not established.	Infrequent *Neuro:* transient headache *CVR:* slight increase in blood pressure, facial flushing *Resp:* rhinitis, local irritation *GI:* nausea, mild abdominal pain	Same as vasopressin.	Same as above.
CONTRAINDICATIONS: Toxemia of pregnancy, cardiac disease, hypertension, coronary insufficiency, dysrhythmias. PRECAUTIONS: Use with caution in persons with decreased cardiac output.	*Neuro:* tinnitus, anxiety, unconsciousness *CVR:* facial pallor *GI:* increased activity, diarrhea *GU:* uterine cramps, proteinuria *Ophth:* mydriasis, BLINDNESS	Chlorpropamide, clofibrate, and carbamazepine potentiate posterior pituitary injection. Concurrent barbiturates may increase likelihood of coronary insufficiency and dysrhythmia.	ASSESSMENT: If used in obstetric patients, use a fetal monitor to assess for fetal distress. Assess vital signs closely. INTERVENTION: Administer SC or IM. EVALUATION: Evaluate for presence of angina and decreased cardiac output. These may necessitate discontinuation.

CONTINUED ON THE FOLLOWING PAGE

Table 41–1. PITUITARY DRUGS–*CONTINUED*

Name	Dosage	Mode of Administration	Pharmacokinetics
Posterior Pituitary Intranasal (Posterior Pituitary)			

Action: Antidiuretic effect, stimulates GI peristalsis, possesses oxytoxic effects.

Use: Diabetes insipidus.

	Dosage	Mode of Administration	Pharmacokinetics
	1 cap 3–4 times a day	Intranasal	O: UA P: UA D: UA ½ L: UA PB: UA B: UA E: UA

Key to Abbreviations in the *Pharmacokinetics* column O-onset; P-peak; D-duration; PB-protein bound; B-biotransformed in; E-excreted in; ½ L-halflife.

*Within the column listing adverse effects, <u>underlines</u> indicate the most common effects; CAPITALS indicate lifethreatening effects.

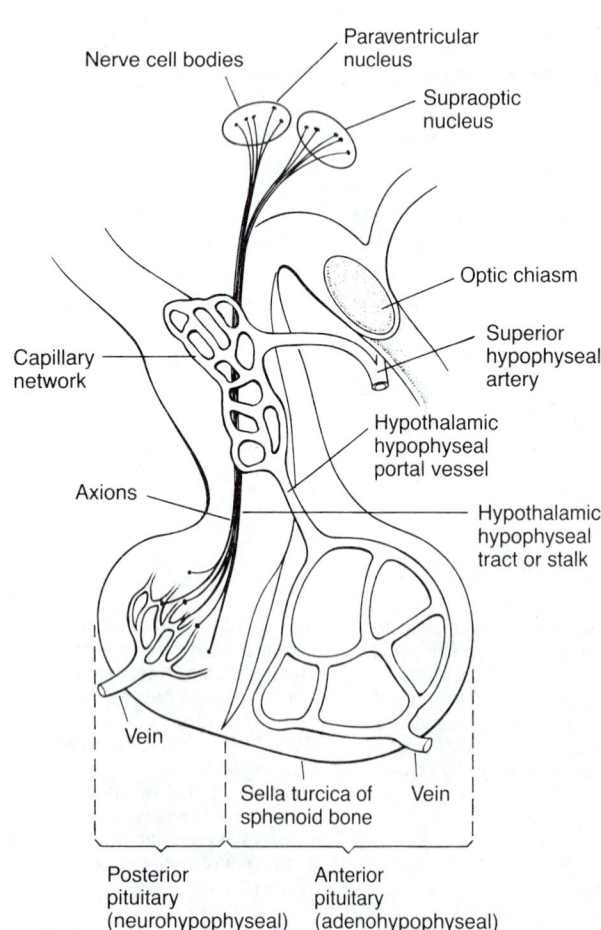

Nerve cell bodies

Paraventricular nucleus

Supraoptic nucleus

Optic chiasm

Superior hypophyseal artery

Capillary network

Hypothalamic hypophyseal portal vessel

Axions

Hypothalamic hypophyseal tract or stalk

Vein

Sella turcica of sphenoid bone

Vein

Posterior pituitary (neurohypophyseal)

Anterior pituitary (adenohypophyseal)

Figure 41–1. The pituitary gland. (From Mathewson, M: Antidiuretic hormone. Critical Care Nurse 6(5):88–93, 1986, with permission.)

cifically, it facilitates transport of amino acids across cell membranes, thereby stimulating a protein-building cycle. This increases nitrogen balance and decreases urea production. GH also decreases the transport of glucose into the cells and decreases glucose utilization, causing what is known as the *diabetogenic effect* of growth hormone. It also facilitates the release of free fatty acids from adipose tissues, leading to an increased fat storage in the liver and an increased availability of fatty acids for energy needs. This latter effect is referred to as the *ketogenic effect* of growth hormone, since it results from fat lipolysis and leads to the conversion of fatty acids to ketone bodies. Many of these actions are mediated by substances synthesized in the liver (and probably synthesized in the kidney, muscle, and other tissues also) called *somatomedins.* Somatomedins, under the regulation of growth hormone, promote growth of cartilage and bone. Somatomedin levels increase with age up to the second decade of life. In children, growth hormone is essential to stimulate linear bone growth.

Although levels of GH are high in the neonate, it does not appear to be a requisite for either fetal or neonatal growth. After two to four weeks, this level falls, with rises occurring after activity, during sleep, and during adolescence and pregnancy. Stress, emotional excitement, and hypoglycemia also can increase the secretion of GH. Secretion of GH is suppressed by glucocorticoid drugs.

USE. Presently, the sole medical use for GH, or somatotropin, is to stimulate linear growth in patients with documented growth failure caused by a deficiency of endogenous GH, a condition called pituitary dwarfism. (Pituitary dwarfism is reviewed in Table 41–2.) In order to accomplish its goal, the drug must be administered before the closure of the bone epiphyses. Epiphyseal closure, occurring during adolescence and sooner in females than males, varies considerably from individual to individual and is usually determined by studying radiographs of the hands and wrists. In terms of attainment of a normal adult height, the best results are ob-

Contraindications/ Precautions	Adverse Effects*	Interactions	Nursing Implications
CONTRAINDICATIONS: Contraindicated in known sensitivity. May cause abortion. PRECAUTIONS: Use with caution in cardiovascular disease.	*Resp:* nasal irritation, cough, transient dyspnea *CVR:* substernal tightness	None known.	Same as above plus INTERVENTION: Use special inhaler. Follow specific directions on package insert.

tained when the hormone administration is begun in early childhood.

PREPARATIONS. Somatotropin obtained from cadaver pituitaries was recently removed from the market because of possible contamination. Two new GHs, somatrem (Protropin) and somatropin (Humatrope), produced in bacteria by recombinant DNA technology, have recently become available. Somatropin has the same amino acid sequence as endogenous growth hormone, while somatrem has an extra methionine group.

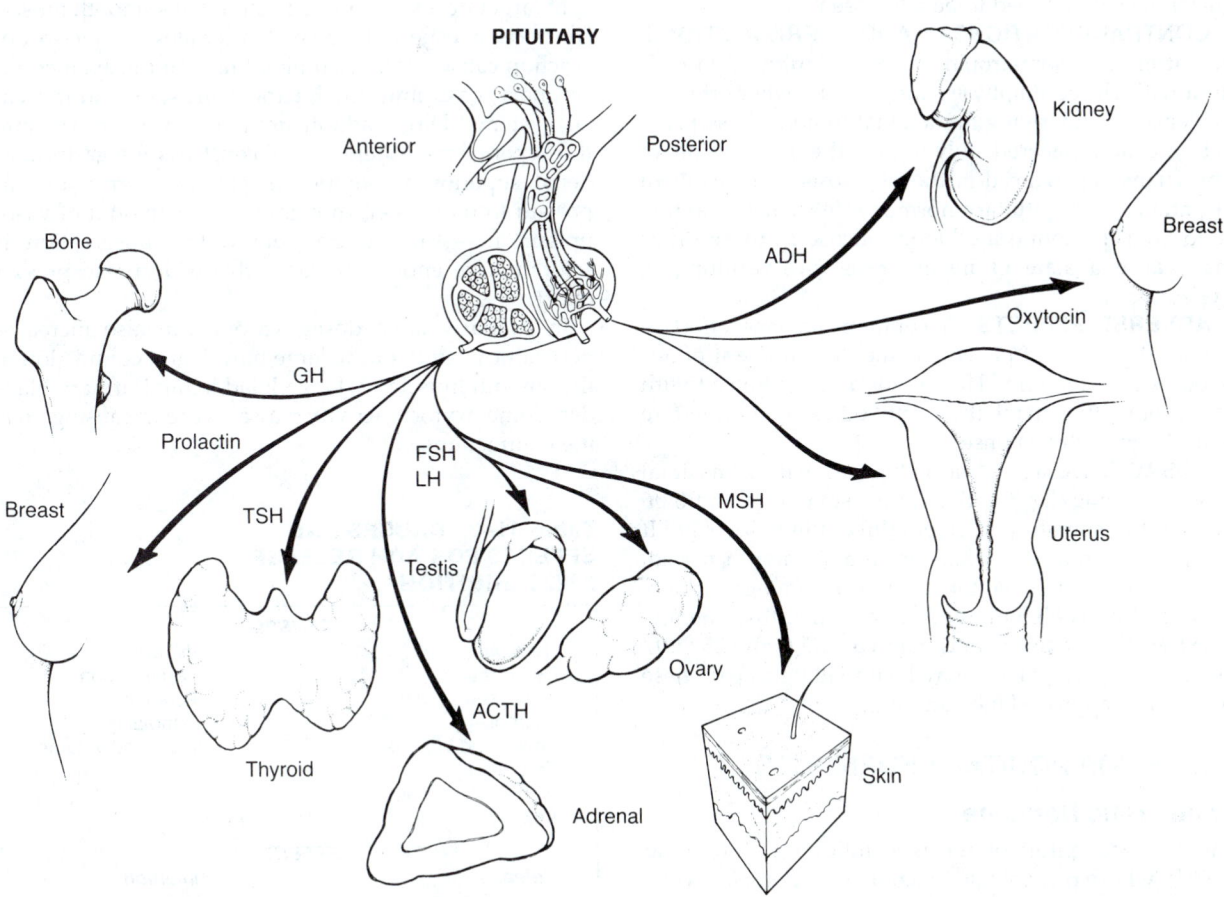

Figure 41–2. A summary of the pituitary hormones and the target organs involved with each hormone. The anterior pituitary hormones include: GH which controls body growth and metabolism; prolactin which controls breast growth and milk production; TSH which regulates the thyroid gland; FSH and LH which affect function of the gonads; ACTH which regulates the adrenal cortex; and MSH which controls pigmentation. The posterior pituitary hormones include: ADH which affects water balance in the body and oxytocin which affects the breast and uterus.

Table 41–2. PITUITARY DWARFISM

> **DEFINITION:**
> Lack of linear bone growth in childhood due to deficiency of growth hormone and resulting in abnormally short stature.
>
> **ETIOLOGY:**
> 1. Idiopathic
> 2. Rarely, tumors such as craniopharyngiomas
>
> **SYMPTOMS:**
> OBJECTIVE:
> 1. Retardation of linear growth usually noted by 1 year of age
> 2. Linear growth rates below normal for child's age and sex
>
> **MEDICAL MANAGEMENT:**
> Replacement of growth hormone

Many ethical questions are raised with the soon to be unlimited supplies of GH. Should GH be available to children with genetic short stature in the normal range; or for persons who consider a short stature to be a functional handicap; or to children whose parents focus on athletic or business advantage for a taller child? These questions will all need to be addressed.

CONTRAINDICATIONS AND PRECAUTIONS. Somatrem and somatropin are contraindicated in children with closed epiphyses and persons where there is evidence of underlying intracranial tumor. These products are administered only under the supervision of physicians experienced in the diagnosis and treatment of patients with pituitary hormone deficiency. Caution is advised in monitoring blood glucose as these drugs may cause a state of insulin resistance resulting in hyperglycemia.

ADVERSE EFFECTS. A common adverse effect in about 30 percent of patients is the development of antibodies to somatrem. This is not as pronounced with somatropin. In general, these antibodies do not interfere with the growth response.

DOSAGE. Dosage is individualized with a maximal dose of 0.1 mg/kg (0.2 IU/kg) for somatrem and 0.06 mg/kg for somatropin given three times weekly. If growth does not exceed 2.5 cm in a six-month period, dosage may be doubled for six months. If no growth occurs, therapy is discontinued after six months. Therapy is extremely expensive and may cost $5,000–$25,000/year. Third-party payers may be unwilling to pay these costs for unapproved indications.

POSTERIOR PITUITARY HORMONES

Antidiuretic Hormone

The posterior pituitary releases antidiuretic hormone (ADH), whose physiologic function is that of water conservation. Pharmacologic amounts (much larger than those required for antidiuretic effect) of ADH also serve to cause widespread vasoconstriction, thus, its synonymous name of vasopressin. ADH can either be inhibited or released by the body in response to certain physio-logic parameters. These conditions are reviewed in Table 41–3.

ACTION. Vasopressin is synthesized in the hypothalamus in the supraoptic nuclei. It is stored in the posterior pituitary to be released as needed, as the rate of hypothalamic synthesis and transport are too slow to meet immediate needs for water conservation. The primary stimuli for secretion of vasopressin are: an increase in plasma osmolality as detected by osmoreceptors in the supraoptic nuclei, and a decreased blood volume as detected by baroreceptors in the vasculature. Hemorrhage and circulatory shock probably are the most potent stimuli for release of vasopressin. Vasopressin secretion is also stimulated by pain; anxiety; and certain drugs such as nicotine, barbiturates (in large doses), chlorpropamide (Diabinese), and the tricyclic antidepressants. Other drugs inhibit vasopressin release, including alcohol, phenytoin (Dilantin), glucocorticoids, chlorpromazine (Thorazine), and reserpine (Serpasil) (Table 41–4).

In physiologic doses, vasopressin acts in the kidneys in the distal tubules and collecting ducts to increase the cellular permeability to water, thus increasing the amounts of water reabsorbed by the kidney and decreasing urine output.

In larger doses, vasopressin stimulates smooth muscle contraction, especially in small arterioles. This vasoconstriction causes decreased blood flow to the splanchnic, coronary, gastrointestinal, pancreatic, skin, and muscular systems. Direct administration of vasopressin into the superior mesenteric artery constricts the gastroduodenal, superior mesenteric, and splenic arteries. It is important to remember, though, that the amount of vasopressin necessary to promote water conservation is seldom large enough to cause this widespread pressor effect.

In similarly large doses, vasopressin also increases peristaltic activity of the large bowel, and contraction of the smooth muscle of the gallbladder and urinary bladder. Some oxytocic activity may also occur, causing uterine contractions.

Table 41–3. CAUSES AND EFFECTS FOR ADH RELEASE AND INHIBITION

CAUSES	
Release	**Inhibition**
Dehydration	Overhydration
Increased serum osmolality	Decreased osmolality
Low blood volume	High blood volume
Trauma	
Pain	
Anxiety	
EFFECTS	
Release	**Inhibition**
Less urine	More urine
Hypertonic urine	Hypotonic urine
Body water retention	Body water loss

From Mathewson, M: Antidiuretic hormone. Critical Care Nurse 6(5):88, 1986, with permission.

**Table 41–4. DRUGS THAT
AFFECT ADH LEVELS***

DECREASING ADH LEVEL/ACTION	INCREASING ADH LEVEL/ACTION
Demeclocycline	Acetaminophen
Ethanol	Morphine
Glucocorticosteroids	Meperidine
Lithium	Most anesthetics
Morphine antagonists	Antipsychotic tranquilizers
Norepinephrine	Cancer drugs especially vincristine
Phenytoin	Clofibrate
Reserpine	Isoproterenol
Chlorpromazine	Phenobarbital
Amphotericin B	Tricyclic antidepressants
Colchicine	Nicotine
	Diabinese
EFFECTS ON URINE FLOW	
Increased urine	Decreased urine
More hypotonic	More hypertonic

*Modified from Porth, C: Pathophysiology. JB Lippincott, Philadelphia, 1982, p 290. From Mathewson, M: Antidiuretic hormone. Critical Care Nurse 6(5):88, 1986, with permission.

As with other hormones, the action and adverse effects of exogenous vasopressin, either natural or synthetic, are the same as those of the endogenous hormone.

USE. Vasopressin or antidiuretic hormone (in either natural or synthetic form) is used primarily in the control of hypothalamic diabetes insipidus. Table 41–5 compares and contrasts diabetes insipidus, too little ADH, with syndrome of inappropriate ADH (SIADH), too much ADH. Vasopressin is not effective in treating nephrogenic diabetes insipidus, a condition in which the kidneys are unable to respond appropriately to this hormone. Vasopressin injection is also used as an intravenous or intra-arterial infusion in the emergency management of massive gastrointestinal bleeding. Intra-arterial infusion is via the superior mesenteric artery. Intravenous and intra-arterial infusion have been found to be equally effective; therefore, the intravenous route is preferred. Vasopressin decreases portal blood pressure and reduces blood loss. Vasopressin is also used to relieve postoperative intestinal gaseous distention and to dispel gas shadows appearing before abdominal roentgenography.

PHARMACOKINETICS. Vasopressin, in natural or synthetic form, is destroyed by enzyme activity (notably trypsin) in the gastrointestinal tract and, therefore, cannot be administered orally.

Vasopressin products, isolated from swine or synthetic, have been shown to be distributed in extracellular fluids following administration with no evidence of plasma protein binding. They are metabolized in the kidney and liver, and small amounts are excreted unchanged in the urine. During pregnancy, circulating enzymes such as oxytocinase are capable of inactivating vasopressin in the plasma.

Vasopressin

The commercially available preparations vasopressin (Pitressin) and vasopressin tannate (Pitressin Tannate) are prepared from bovine and porcine pituitaries and have pressor and antidiuretic activity. Vasopressin tannate possesses longer duration of action, approximately 48–96 hours.

Vasopressin injection is used in the initial treatment of diabetes insipidus and also for short-term treatment of the disease. It is not recommended for chronic therapy; its short duration of action (two to eight hours), along with the need to administer it via injection, make it impractical to use on a long-term basis.

Vasopressin tannate in oil is useful as an adjunct to other agents in treatment of severe diabetes insipidus. With vasopressin tannate, cumulative effects are more likely to occur, and water intoxication may result. Vasopressin tannate must be administered intramuscularly; it is not used intravenously.

Vasopressin has a vasopressor effect that results from a contraction of smooth muscle in the vascular bed. The vasoconstriction is seen in the portal and splanchnic vessels and, to a lesser degree, in peripheral, coronary, cerebral, pulmonary, and intrahepatic vessels. Vasopressin is used to control gastrointestinal bleeds associated with esophageal varices. Vasopressin also enhances the mobility and tone of the gastrointestinal tract.

ADVERSE EFFECTS. Adverse effects of vasopressin and vasopressin tannate are usually mild with small dosages. The most common side effects are: circumoral pallor, sweating, tremor, pounding in the head, abdominal cramps, and nausea. Uterine cramping and diarrhea may occur because of the oxytocic and smooth muscle–stimulant effects of vasopressin. Since shifts in fluid volumes occur with initial therapy, patients who may have difficulty tolerating this, such as those with congestive heart failure, should be treated carefully with small doses.

In larger doses, cardiovascular effects such as an increase in blood pressure, anginal pain, dysrhythmias, and even myocardial infarction may be evident. The pressor effects of vasopressin are not usually evident with the amounts used to control polyuria. However, in patients with coronary artery disease, even small doses of these drugs have been found to precipitate angina, especially in the elderly. Vasodilators such as nitroglycerin may be helpful in controlling the angina.

Overhydration and water intoxication are adverse effects that may occur with the use of vasopressin tannate because of its cumulative effects. In addition, some patients may experience allergic effects from the oil used for this suspension.

DOSAGE. Vasopressin and vasopressin tannate are administered parenterally. Vasopressin is given intramuscularly or subcutaneously in a dose of 5–10 units, two to three times daily. Vasopressin tannate (a peanut oil suspension)) is given intramuscularly in a dose of 1.5–5.0 U, repeated as required every two to three days. Vasopressin tannate needs prolonged rotation and shaking of the ampule to ensure that all the particles are included in the suspension. Failure to shake the ampule thoroughly can result in inaccurate dosage and, conse-

Table 41–5. COMPARISON OF DIABETES INSIPIDUS AND SIADH

COMPARISONS	Diabetes Insipidus	SIADH
Etiology*	Tumor of hypothalamus Tumor of hypophysis Head trauma, brain tumor, drugs	Bronchogenic carcinoma (oat cell) Head trauma, brain abscess/ tumor, drugs
ADH level	Decreased	Increased
Thirst	Yes	No
Serum osmol (270–290 mosm/L)	Over 300 mosm/L	Under 280 mosm/L
Serum Na normally (135–145 mEq/L)	Over 150–160 mEq/l	Under 130 mEq/L
Urine (65–1200 mosm/L)	Under 200 mosm/kg	Over 1400 mosm/L
Specific gravity (1.010–1.020)	1.002–1.006	Over 1.020
Urine output	4–15 L/day	Low
Dehydration	Yes (may be severe)	No
Overhydration	No	Yes (may be severe)

Other symptoms	Polydipsia
	No sweat/saliva
		Fatigue, headache, weakness,
		  confusion, personality changes,
		  nausea, vomiting, seizures

Diagnosis	Serum and urine studies Dehydration test Hypertonic saline infusion test X-rays	Serum and urine studies Water-loading test
Complications	Dehydration Hypovolemic shock Dilatation of bladder and/or ureters	Seizures Brain damage Coma

Treatment	Maintain water and electrolyte bal-
	  ance
	Vasopression
	Na restriction
		Maintain water and electrolyte bal-
		  ance
		Restrict fluids
		Diuretics
		Demeclocyline HCl
		Lithium

NURSING CARE:	Diabetes Insipidus Identify patient at risk Administer fluid, electrolytes Monitor fluid and electrolyte balance Monitor intake and output closely Monitor level of consciousness Daily weight Good skin and oral care Administer medications as ordered Provide patient teaching as necessary	SIADH Identify patient at risk Administer electrolytes as needed Maintain fluid restriction Monitor intake and output closely Monitor level of consciousness Daily weight Maintain seizure precautions Monitor bowel activity Prevent constipation Administer medications as ordered Reorient patient frequently Provide patient teaching as neces- sary

*Most common etiologies shown here; other causes exist.
From Mathewson, M: Antidiuretic hormone. Critical Care Nurse 6(5):88, 1986, with permission.

quently, inadequate therapeutic response. Pediatric dosages are individualized. Absorption of vasopressin tannate is often erratic.

Synthetic Preparations

Analogs of vasopressin, either natural or synthetic, differ in antidiuretic potency as well as in their vasopressor potency. Lypressin (Diapid), prepared synthetically, possesses antidiuretic properties similar to those of vasopressin, but has fewer pressor and oxytocic effects. Lypressin is useful in patients who have become unresponsive to other therapy or who experience local or systemic reactions, allergic reactions, or other undesirable effects from preparation of animal origin. Desmopressin acetate (DDAVP), a synthetic product, causes a greater antidiuretic effect than either vasopressin or lypressin, while producing only minimal pressor and smooth muscle–contraction effects. Desmopressin is often the preferred drug in the treatment of mild to moderate diabetes insipidus for a number of reasons. It has a relatively long duration of action as opposed to aqueous vasopressin injection, it can be administered intranasally, and it is relatively free of adverse effects. Duration of action also differs with desmopressin, offering the longest duration of action (8–20 hours) of the synethetic preparations. Duration of action of lypressin is three to eight hours. Desmopressin produces a dose-related increase in Factor VIII levels. This increase begins in 30 minutes and peaks in 90–120 minutes. Desmopressin is used to maintain hemostasis during surgery and postoperatively in patients with *hemophilia A* and classic *von Willebrand's disease.*

When a nasal spray is used, rhinitis and gastric irritation may occur from the postnasal drip. Local erythema and burning pain can also occur. Additional adverse effects are featured in Table 41–1.

DOSAGE. Desmopressin and lypressin are both administered intranasally as sprays; desmopressin is administered in a dosage of 0.1–0.4 ml/day (or 4–40 mEq/day) in divided doses. The pediatric dose is 0.05–0.3 ml/day. Lypressin is administered in a dosage of one to two sprays in each naris every four hours. Absorption of these two drugs may be decreased by conditions causing nasal congestion, such as allergic rhinitis or upper respiratory infections. In such instances, dosages may need to be increased.

The dosage of both lypressin and desmopressin are adjusted to maintain a urine volume of 1.5–2.0 liters/day. Patients usually require two or, occasionally, three sprays/day to control their symptoms. Small doses are administered initially and doses are increased to effectively control polyuria. The smallest effective dose is used.

When desmopressin (Stimate) is administered to patients with hemophilia A and von Willebrand's disease, the dosage is 0.3 μg/kg, diluted in normal saline, infused slowly IV over 15–30 minutes. When used preoperatively, administer 30 minutes before surgery.

Posterior Pituitary Injection

Posterior pituitary injection (Pituitrin) is used to control postoperative ileus and stimulate the expulsion of gas prior to pyelography. It is also useful in treating the enuresis of diabetes insipidus, but it is not curative. (See Table 41–1 for more information.)

Posterior Pituitary, Intranasal

Posterior pituitary, intranasal (Posterior Pituitary) is used to control the symptoms of diabetes insipidus. It is used with a special inhaler. The patient should follow the directions on the inhaler for proper use.

USING THE NURSING PROCESS

Assessment of the patient requiring pituitary drugs begins with a thorough nursing history to establish the data base (Tables 41–6 and 41–7).

Table 41–6. NURSING PROCESS FOR THE PATIENT REQUIRING SOMATOTROPIC HORMONES

Assessment
Determine linear bone growth, weight and height comparisons. Assess plasma levels of growth hormone (by immunoassay) and x-ray for bone age to determine epiphyseal closure. Evaluate effect of condition on child's self-esteem. Note concomitant/previous use of glucocorticoids, thyroid preparations. Review family history for presence of diabetes mellitus.

Nursing Diagnosis	Nursing Action	Rationale	Desired Outcomes/Evaluation Criteria
Knowledge deficit related to lack of information/misinterpretation, unfamiliarity with resources as evidenced by questions, verbalization of the problem, inaccurate follow-through of instruction, development of preventable complications.	Provide oral and written information about somatropin, including action, use, adverse effects, and interactions. Demonstrate correct drug reconstitution and injection techniques and site rotation. Emphasize importance of examining sites prior to injection; stress need to report presence of lumps, redness, swelling, sponginess, and pain at injection site or development of thirst, decreased energy level, fatigue, sudden changes in behavior.	Promotes understanding of treatment regimen. May prevent development of serious complications, e.g., renal calculi, increased blood glucose levels/decreased sensitivity to exogenous insulin. Ensures correct administration, reduces risk of tissue damage, and limits pain at the injection sites. Prompt evaluation and intervention may prevent adverse effects/complications.	(Parents and child) Verbalizes understanding of condition and treatment. Correctly performs necessary procedures and explains reasons for actions.

CONTINUED ON THE FOLLOWING PAGE

Table 41–6. NURSING PROCESS FOR THE PATIENT REQUIRING SOMATOTROPIC HORMONES–*CONTINUED*

Nursing Diagnosis	Nursing Action	Rationale	Desired Outcomes/ Evaluation Criteria
	Encourage balanced dietary intake.	Supports normal growth.	
	Discuss necessity of continued medical followup.	Provides for evaluation of growth, thyroid, and pancreatic function.	
Growth and development, altered related to deficiency of growth hormone as evidenced by altered physical growth.	Administer somatropin as ordered.	Used to stimulate linear growth in patients documented to have growth failure caused by a deficiency of endogenous GH or pituitary dwarfism.	Verbalizes understanding of developmental deviation and plans for intervention.
	Discuss administration, safety factors and possible adverse side effects with both parents and child.	Understanding of the pituitary function and need for continued therapy and monitoring helps the family to cooperate with treatment regimen.	
	Request parent to accurately measure and record height at regular intervals.	Indicator of success of treatment/need to alter or discontinue therapy.	
	Discuss importance of annual evaluation of bone age.	Monitors the effectiveness of therapy and determines epiphyseal closure.	
Body image/self-esteem disturbance, potential related to failure to develop at an expected rate, size, which is smaller than peers.	Discuss child/parent perceptions of condition/threat to self.	Provides base on which to decide appropriate interventions. Identifies depth of concern.	Verbalizes increased sense of self-esteem in relation to individual situation. Demonstrates adaptation to changes as evidenced by setting of realistic goals and active participation in play/relationships.
	Stress need to avoid comparing self with others. Active-Listen to expressions of concern. Use I-messages to provide information and give positive feedback.	Helps patient to focus on own concerns/abilities. Conveys sense of caring, support, promoting belief in patient's own ability to manage situation.	
	Support patient's need to progress at own rate.	Adaptation to change depends on its significance to individual, how disruptive it is, and degree/length of debility.	

ASSESSMENT—GROWTH HORMONE

The assessment of the child with growth hormone deficiency begins early in his or her development. Repeated physical examination of the child yields important information relative to growth patterns.

Plasma levels of growth hormone are detected by immunoassay; but since normal levels are very small, it is common to use a stimulation test in order to increase the levels of somatotropin. Insulin, arginine, or levodopa may be used in these tests. In normal individuals, somatotropin levels should rise after administration of these substances. Patients with growth hormone deficiency show no such increases.

Two important points in relation to diagnostic testing are made. First, almost one half of the children with growth hormone deficiency have deficiencies of other tropic hormones (TSH, ACTH); therefore, careful evaluation for other hormone deficiencies is necessary. (See Chapters 42 and 45 for information on testing related to adrenal and thyroid hormones.) Second, careful assessment for any signs and symptoms of *craniopharyngioma* is carried out. This may include skull radiography and computerized axial tomography. It is important to question the parents about any history of nausea, vomiting, headache, loss of vision, or increase in head circumference, all indicative of increased intracranial pressure.

ASSESSMENT—ANTIDIURETIC HORMONE

In assessing the patient suspected of having diabetes insipidus, the nurse must be aware that the signs and symptoms of this disease can be either sudden or insid-

Table 41-7. NURSING PROCESS FOR THE PATIENT REQUIRING ANTIDIURETIC DRUGS

Assessment

Note history of cardiovascular disease, hypertension.
Assess presence of irritability and general weakness.
Obtain accurate baseline measurement of body weight.
Review serum and urine osmolality and results of water deprivation test.

Nursing Diagnosis	Nursing Actions	Rationale	Desired Outcomes/ Evaluation Criteria
Fluid volume deficit, Actual 1 related to failure of regulatory mechanisms as evidenced by large urinary output, dehydration and weight loss.	Provides information relating to condition and treatment.	Provides for early assessment and intervention to prevent serious complications, death.	Demonstrates improved fluid balance as evidenced by individually appropriate urinary output, stable vital signs and weight, moist mucous membranes, good skin turgor.
	Record intake, output, and specific gravity. Calculate 24-hr fluid balance.	Useful for identifying therapy needs/effectiveness.	
	Observe for excessive thirst, poor skin turgor, dry skin/mucous membranes.	Signs of dehydration indicating need for prompt intervention/changes in therapy.	
	Administer vasopressin, lypressin, or desmopressin acetate as ordered, e.g., by injection, subcutaneous, or intranasal administration.	Antidiuretic effect promotes water reabsorption and more appropriate rate urine output.	
	Review laboratory studies, e.g., urine/serum sodium, potassium, osmolality.	Rapid depletion of electrolytes may occur in diabetes insipidus requiring prompt intervention.	
Knowledge deficit related to lack of exposure/unfamiliarity with information resources, misinterpretation as evidenced by questions, statement of concern, inaccurate follow-through of instructions/development of preventable complications.	Provide information about antidiuretic drugs, including action, use, adverse effects, and interactions.	Understanding of medication/ treatment regimen allows patient to make informed choices and participate knowledgeably in treatment.	Verbalizes understanding of condition and treatment needs. Correctly performs necessary procedures and explains reasons for the actions.
	Review side effects of antidiuretic drugs.	Helps patient to recognize problems that might indicate onset of water intoxication (e.g., nausea, vomiting, confusion, drowsiness and headaches), or hypovolemia (e.g., weight loss, dizziness, and lightheadedness).	
	Demonstrate correct preparation and administration technique. Discuss site rotation.	Maximizes therapeutic effect and avoids problems of lipodystrophy.	
	Instruct patient to contact physician if nasal congestion occurs, e.g., allergic rhinitis, URI.	Can impair absorption of drug when administered intranasally, possibly requiring an increase in dosage.	
	Show patient how to monitor intake, output, and specific gravity. Stress importance of adequate fluid replacement.	Promotes sense of control, accurate measure to prevent development of untoward complications.	
	Encourage wearing of a medical identification bracelet.	Identifies problem immediately in case of an emergency situation, avoiding possibility of complications.	
	Discuss necessity of abstaining from alcohol and reading of OTC drug labels.	Alcohol may alter therapeutic response to drug even in smaller amounts as may be found in OTC products.	
	Review need for further medical followup.	Provides opportunity to identify problems and adjust therapy if needed.	

ious in onset. Signs of dehydration such as dry skin and mucous membranes, irritability, and weakness are noted on physical examination.

Careful, accurate measurements of body weight also reflect the water losses of diabetes insipidus. Measurements of serum and urine osmolality and serum sodium are used in assessing the patient for diabetes insipidus. Typical laboratory findings are featured in Table 41–5.

Other laboratory tests are used to determine whether the patient can produce endogenous antidiuretic hormone and whether the kidneys are responsive to it. In the water deprivation test, fluids are withheld until two to five percent of body weight is lost. A hypotonic saline infusion may be used to stimulate antidiuretic hormone secretion. In normal individuals, the ensuing increase in serum osmolality causes a diminished urine output because of the effects of elevated antidiuretic hormone levels. The patient with diabetes insipidus continues to produce large amounts of urine and may become profoundly dehydrated. During the test, hourly measurements of urine output and specific gravity are made.

In an adaptation of this test, after the period of dehydration, a small amount of aqueous vasopressin is administered. In one hour, another urine output and specific gravity are determined. In hypothalamic diabetes insipidus, urine volumes should decrease; in the nephrogenic type of diabetes insipidus, the vasopressin has no effect.

NURSING DIAGNOSES

Following assessment, nursing diagnoses are established. Tables 41–6 and 41–7 list some typical nursing diagnoses for patients with growth hormone deficiency and diabetes insipidus.

INTERVENTION

The nurse develops the goals for nursing intervention from the nursing diagnoses. Nursing goals in caring for the patient requiring pituitary drugs are included in Tables 41–6 and 41–7.

NURSING RESPONSIBILITIES WHEN ADMINISTERING PITUITARY DRUGS

In order for the nurse to administer pituitary drugs safely, specific information related to administration, patient safety, and patient teaching must be remembered. These points can be found in the column headed "Nursing Implications" in Table 41–1. Since diabetes insipidus can occur secondary to neurologic injuries (head trauma, brain surgery) affecting levels of consciousness, certain patients might be unable to monitor their own signs and symptoms. For these patients, it is vital for the nurse to obtain accurate body weights, intake and output measurements, and urine specific gravities.

When administering vasopressin tannate by intramuscular injection, the ampule is warmed by rotating it between the palms of the hands. After it is warmed, shake it vigorously to mix. The patient is instructed to drink one or two glasses of water after taking the drug to help minimize side effects.

PATIENT TEACHING

Nursing intervention for the patient with growth hormone deficiency necessitates education for the child as well as the parents. Complex explanations are, of course, unsuitable for the young child, but the parents should be educated about pituitary function and the need for growth hormone. Parents should understand the need for continued therapy with somatropin, and should be aware of the possibility of adverse effects. Specific teaching points are listed in Table 41–8.

Nursing intervention for the patient requiring antidiuretic drugs necessitates educating the patient about the disease process, the medication, and the possible occurrence of adverse effects. Patients are taught to avoid alcohol when taking antidiuretic drugs as they can alter therapeutic response. Information for the nurse to use in the teaching plan is included in Table 41–9.

EVALUATION

During the evaluation phase, the nurse determines the effectiveness of the nursing interventions and achievement of goals. This evaluation is based on the goals for nursing intervention determined by the nurse, patient, and family and is included in Tables 41–6 and 41–7.

Evaluation—Growth Hormone

For the child requiring somatropin therapy, growth rates should average about 7 cm (2.8 in)/year. An annual

---

Table 41–8. PATIENT TEACHING INFORMATION—SOMATOTROPIC HORMONES

Dear Patient:
This drug has been prescribed for you/your child. This is what you should know about the drug to get the most from therapy.

1. Somatropin is taken to help your growth.
2. Drugs will be taken until you are 5 feet tall or until your bones stop growing.
3. Reconstitute (mix) somatropin with sterile water. Gently roll the vial between your hands. Do not shake. Inject deep into muscle.
4. Drugs are administered by a shot in your muscle.
5. Drugs are usually given 3 times per week, and 48 hours should pass between shots.
6. Drugs must be given as prescribed; do not stop the drug without first consulting with your doctor.
7. If side effects occur, consult with your doctor. These might include less than expected growth rates, tiredness, and infection.
8. You should not give a shot in the same place 2 times in a row. Keep a record of the sites. This will help to decrease soreness at the sites.
9. Record your (child's) height regularly.
10. Test your (child's) urine for glucose regularly.

Table 41–9. PATIENT TEACHING INFORMATION—ANTIDIURETIC DRUGS (VASOPRESSIN, LYPRESSIN, DESMOPRESSIN)

Dear Patient:

This drug has been prescribed for you. This is what you should know about your drug to get the most from your therapy.

1. Antidiuretic hormone is taken to _____.
2. Antidiuretic drugs will often be taken indefinitely.
3. Antidiuretic drugs are generally taken at the following times:
   a. Vasopressin tannate at bedtime.
   b. Desmopressin in the morning and evening.
   c. Lypressin 4 times a day.
4. Lypressin and desmopressin are taken by spraying the solutions into one or both nostrils. DO NOT INHALE the drugs. The head may be tilted back slightly while a short spray is given. Pinching the nose for a few seconds afterward may help. Practice is necessary. If nasal congestion is present, a decongestant should be given first.
5. Vasopressin tannate is given by intramuscular shot.
   a. Before giving, warm the ampule by rotating between your palms and shake it vigorously to mix.
   b. Drink 1 or 2 glasses of water after taking the drug. This helps to decrease side effects.
6. Do not drink much alcohol (beer, wine, whiskey) as these can change your response to antidiuretic drugs. Also, some liquid medicines are mixed with alcohol (cough syrups). Do not take these medicines.
7. Do not stop taking antidiuretic drugs without first talking to your doctor.
8. Call your doctor if you begin to experience side effects. These include (fill in from Table 41–1).
9. If you experience increased urination or thirst, notify your doctor; your dosage may need to be altered.

evaluation of bone age is necessary to monitor the effectiveness of therapy and to determine epiphyseal closure.

The nurse should know the adverse effects of somatropin and should evaluate the patient's and family's understanding of them. In particular, the nurse emphasizes to the patient those side effects that require immediate medical attention. Although discomfort at injection sites is fairly common, adverse effects of therapy with somatropin are infrequent. Antibodies are found in approximately 30 percent of patients. With only one exception, the antibodies did not interfere with growth stimulation. There is also a need to monitor blood glucose, particularly in the diabetic, as somatropin is diabetogenic.

Evaluation—Antidiuretic Hormone

For the patient requiring vasopressin, the nurse determines whether the patient is experiencing polyuria, nocturia, or increased thirst. The nurse asks the patient to briefly review medication schedules and, if the patient has not obtained a medication card or necklace, the nurse takes time to reinforce the importance of this type of identification.

The nurse knows the adverse effects of the antidiuretic drugs and evaluates the patient's knowledge and understanding of them, especially those that, should they occur, require medical attention.

Adverse effects of antidiuretics occur with greater frequency when larger doses are used; usually, adverse effects are not pronounced. Headaches, nasal congestion, abdominal cramps, nausea, and diarrhea can occur. Very large doses can give rise to cardiovascular symptoms such as increased blood pressure, anginal pain, and dysrhythmias. A worsening of polyuria or signs of dehydration are reported immediately, as they indicate a need for alteration in dosage.

The majority of patients taking these pituitary drugs comply with their medication regimens, as the drugs alleviate their symptomatology.

Throughout the nursing interaction, the nurse continually stresses the need for medical follow-up care and periodically reviews all previously taught information with the patient and family to ensure that the patient's knowledge remains accurate and current.

SUMMARY

The pituitary gland is divided into two lobes. The pituitary hormones are available as natural products or synthetic analogues. The anterior pituitary is responsible for producing growth hormone (GH) and several other hormones discussed in other chapters. GH has many target issues and stimulates increases in cellular size and rate of growth. GH accomplishes this activity through many mechanisms.

The nurse is often involved with the initial assessment of the child and then follow-up studies as the child is treated with GH. Growth rates should average about 7 cm (2.8 in)/year. The nurse frequently evaluates the child for the development of antibodies.

The posterior pituitary releases antidiuretic hormone (ADH). Diabetes insipidus (DI) develops from a deficiency of ADH production or release. To treat DI, ADH, also known as vasopressin, is administered. Vasopressin acts in the kidneys in the distal tubules and collecting ducts to increase the cellular permeability to water, thus increasing the amount of water reabsorbed by the kidney and decreasing urine output. In large doses, vasopressin also has a vasopressor effect resulting from contraction of smooth muscle in the vascular bed. Therefore, vasopressin is effective in managing gastrointestinal bleeds.

The nurse assesses the symptoms associated with DI and monitors daily intake and output carefully. Patients are encouraged to drink one to two glasses of water after taking their medication to help minimize side effects. Various forms of vasopressin are available for intramuscular, subcutaneous, and intranasal administration. The nurse must be knowledgeable about the administration techniques for each of these products. The nurse continually assesses the patient for side effects which include symptoms of fluid overload.

BIBLIOGRAPHY

AMA Department of Drugs: AMA Drug Evaluations, ed 4. PSG Publishing, Littleton, MA, 1986.

Drug Newsletter: New Drugs: Somatropin (Humatrope by Lilly). Facts and Comparisons, St. Louis, MO, 6(7):56, July 1987.

Gilman, AG, Goodman, LS, and Gilman, A: Goodman and Gilman's The Pharmacological Basis of Therapeutics, ed 6. Macmillan, New York, 1985.

Hamilton, H: Nursing84 Books: Endocrine System. Springhouse Corp, Springhouse, PA, 1984.

Mathewson, M: Antidiuretic Hormone. Crit Care Nurse 6(5):88, 1986.

Medical Letter: A New Biosynthetic Human Growth Hormone. The Medical Letter on Drugs and Therapeutics, New Rochelle, NY, 29(745):73, 1988.

SITUATION 41–1

Inez Greenberg, aged 47 years, is admitted to the intensive care unit after a craniotomy for removal of a pituitary tumor.

1. On the second postoperative day, the nurse notes that Ms. Greenberg's urine output for 3 consecutive hours is >300 cc per hour. The nurse informs the physician and is aware that this sign is related to:
   a. diabetes mellitus
   b. acute renal failure
   c. nephrogenic diabetes insipidus
   d. hypothalamic diabetes insipidus

2. The nurse is to administer vasopressin tannate to Ms. Greenberg. The expected route of administration of this drug is:
   a. oral
   b. intramuscular
   c. intravenous
   d. intranasal

3. A nursing action associated with vasopressin tannate therapy for Ms. Greenberg includes:
   a. taking the blood pressure before administration
   b. keeping the patient on bed rest
   c. shaking the medication to mix well
   d. storing the medication away from light

4. Two hours after administration of vasopressin, Ms. Greenberg complains of a throbbing headache. This symptom most probably relates to:
   a. subtherapeutic dose of vasopressin
   b. adverse effects of vasopressin
   c. allergic reaction to vasopressin
   d. toxic effects of vasopressin

5. An expected outcome for Ms. Greenberg would be a urine output of:
   a. 1.5 to 2 liters per day
   b. 200 cc/hour for 24 hours
   c. 3 to 3.5 liters per day
   d. 150 cc/hour for 24 hours

6. In monitoring Ms. Greenberg, the nurse will report the following subjective symptom:
   a. tremors
   b. nasal congestion
   c. sore throat
   d. thirst

Please refer to Appendices for correct answers and additional review questions with answers.

42
CHAPTER

ADRENAL CORTICAL DRUGS

GLOSSARY TERMS IN THIS CHAPTER
Bradykinins
Catabolism
Corticosteroid
Glucocorticoid
Gluconeogenesis
Interleukin
Lipogenesis
Lipolysis
Mineralocorticoid
Prostaglandins
Pulse therapy

42
CHAPTER

ADRENAL CORTICAL DRUGS

MERRILY MATHEWSON KUHN, R.N.C., Ph.D., CCRN

LEARNING OBJECTIVES

After reading this chapter, the student will be able to:

1. Identify those medications commonly used as adrenal cortical drugs.

2. Differentiate among the adrenal cortical drugs as to mechanisms of action, route of administration, pharmacokinetics, adverse effects, contraindications, and interactions.

3. Identify specific areas to assess in the patient requiring adrenal cortical drugs in order to formulate appropriate nursing diagnoses.

4. Plan the nursing interventions necessary to administer adrenal cortical drugs and choose appropriate teaching strategies to gain patient compliance.

5. Evaluate the patient at various stages of treatment to gauge nursing interventions.

THERAPEUTIC AGENTS

The adrenal medulla secretes the sympathetic amines epinephrine and norepinephrine (see Chapter 19); the adrenal cortex produces steroids, including mineralocorticoids—aldosterone, glucocorticoids—hydrocortisone, and gonadal hormones (see Chapter 43). *Corticosteroids* are synthesized in the adrenal cortex from cholesterol; they regulate water and electrolyte balance, and carbohydrate, protein, and fat metabolism.

The discussion in this chapter is limited to the adrenal cortex and its secretions, specifically the mineralocorticoids and glucocorticoids. Both of these groups are indicated for the treatment of primary adrenocortical insufficiency (Addison's disease). These products are featured in Table 42–1. The adrenal cortex does not store appreciable amounts of these hormones.

CORTICOTROPIN

Corticotropin (ACTH) is the pituitary hormone that stimulates the adrenal cortex. If the adrenal cortex needs to be stimulated, corticotropin can be administered either intravenously, intramuscularly, or subcutaneously. Corticotropin is given intramuscularly as 20 U/24 hours, or subcutaneously as 40–80 units every 24–72 hours. The onset of action is 5 minutes after intravenous administration.

MINERALOCORTICOIDS

Mineralocorticoid is the term applied to those steroids that have their major effects on water and electrolyte balance. Aldosterone secretion is primarily controlled by potassium and angiotensin. Aldosterone is the prototypic drug in this group; but its use is limited by its high cost, limited availability, and requirement of parenteral administration.

Action

Mineralocorticoids act primarily on the kidney's distal tubules, enhancing the reabsorption of sodium and chloride ions and the excretion of potassium and hydrogen ions. The retention of sodium and chloride in turn causes an increase in water absorption from the tubules. By extension, these compounds then help to maintain cardiac output and blood pressure by maintaining extracellular fluid volumes.

Use

The synthetic mineralocorticoids desoxycorticosterone pivalate (Percorten Pivalate) and fludrocortisone (Florinef) are used in replacement therapy for treatment of primary and secondary adrenocortical insufficiency (see Table 42–2 for a review of this condition) and for treatment of salt-losing adrenogenital syndrome. Fludrocortisone is also used in some patients with renal failure to assist with potassium balance. These products are also used empirically for primary orthostatic hypotension.

Pharmacokinetics

The mineralocorticoids are all well absorbed and distributed to all tissues. The onset, peak, and duration of action vary widely with the product. The liver is the major metabolic site. The mineralocorticoids are excreted as inactive metabolites by the kidney.

Contraindications and Precautions

The mineralocorticoids are contraindicated in patients hypersensitive to these products. The mineralocorticoids are contraindicated in persons with hypertension, congestive heart failure, and cardiac disease, as they may increase sodium and water retention, worsening these conditions. Safety in pregnancy and in children has not been established.

Adverse Effects

The major adverse effects of the mineralocorticoid drugs are sodium retention and the subsequent water retention. In certain individuals, this increase in blood volume could lead to increases in blood pressure. These effects are dose-related and are generally not problematic at replacement levels.

Hypokalemia, secondary to the potassium loss associated with the sodium-retaining activity of the mineralocorticoids, can also occur. It generally can be avoided by encouraging the patient to maintain a diet high in potassium-rich foods.

Frontal and occipital headaches, probably caused by the sodium and water retention, have been reported. Arthralgias and hypersensitivity reactions are less common adverse effects of mineralocorticoid therapy.

DESOXYCORTICOSTERONE ACETATE. Desoxycorticosterone acetate (DOCA) has pure mineralocorticoid activity. If desoxycorticosterone acetate is being used to treat primary deficiency of the adrenal gland (Addison's disease), glucocorticoids are also administered.

Pharmacokinetics. Desoxycorticosterone acetate is only available in parenteral forms as it is destroyed by the gastrointestinal tract. When given IM, the pivalate form is slowly absorbed over a month. When implanted into subcutaneous tissue, desoxycorticosterone acetate pellets are slowly released over 8–12 months. Desoxycorticosterone acetate is metabolized in the liver and excreted by the kidneys.

Dosage. Desoxycorticosterone acetate is available in two forms: acetate, given in doses of 2–5 mg in 24 hours; and pivalate, given in doses of 25–100 mg monthly. Both are available in injectable forms only.

DESOXYCORTICOSTERONE PIVALATE. Desoxycorticosterone pivalate (Percorten Pivalate) is used for maintenance therapy for patients with salt-losing adrenogenital syndrome. Desoxycorticosterone pivalate is also used concurrently with glucocorticoids to treat adrenocortical insufficiency.

Desoxycorticosterone pivalate is administered intramuscularly in doses of 25–100 mg every four weeks.

FLUDROCORTISONE. Fludrocortisone (Florinef) has mineralocorticoid activity and also has a modest glucocorticoid effect; however, it is used only for its mineralocorticoid effects.

Pharmacokinetics. Fludrocortisone is readily absorbed from the gastrointestinal tract and reaches peak concentrations in 1.7 hours. The plasma half-life is 3.5 hours and the biologic half-life range is 18–36 hours. Fludrocortisone is metabolized in the liver and excreted by the kidneys.

Dosage. For mineralocorticoid activity, a fludrocortisone dose of 0.1–0.2 mg is administered once daily. If hypertension develops, this dosage must be adjusted.

GLUCOCORTICOIDS

Glucocorticoids are those corticosteroids that have the most pronounced effect on carbohydrate, protein, and fat metabolism. Glucocorticoid regulation is mediated by corticotropin (ACTH), which is secreted by the anterior pituitary gland or adenohypophysis. The ACTH-secreting cells of the anterior pituitary are, in turn, regulated by corticotropin-releasing hormones (CRH) from the hypothalamus. When glucocorticoids are needed, ACTH stimulates the adrenal gland and within minutes glucocorticoids are released. Secretion of ACTH is inhibited by a negative feedback effect of glucocorticoids. Stress (e.g., trauma, anxiety, severe infection, hypoglycemia, and surgery) is one of the most potent stimulators of ACTH production.

Numerous synthetic analogs of cortisol have been developed. The significant differences between the synthetics and the parent compounds, cortisol and cortisone, are: (1) the synthetics have a greater anti-inflammatory potency; and (2) often, the synthetic analogs have a longer duration of action. In addition, the sodium-retaining potential is lessened or eliminated.

It is important to point out that although glucocorticoids may be administered only for their anti-inflammatory effects, the catabolic effects of these drugs will also occur. This fact explains many of the adverse effects that are seen with glucocorticoid therapy.

Action

Glucocorticoids exert three important therapeutic actions: anti-inflammatory, anti-allergic, and anti-stress.

Glucocorticoids inhibit the inflammatory response. They inhibit local edema formation (probably by decreasing capillary permeability and dilation), fibroblast proliferation, and deposition of fibrin and collagen. Glucocorticoids suppress signs of inflammation, such as heat and redness, by preventing synthesis or release of vasodilator substances such as *bradykinins, prostaglandins,* and histamine. Furthermore, they inhibit the migration of macrophages and leukocytes toward areas of inflammation. Cortisol also functions to stabilize the lysosomal membranes within the cells and prevents the release of hydrolyzing enzymes. Corticosteroids interfere with the movement of polymorphonuclear leukocytes from the blood to the site of injury or irritation. Glucocorticoids also have an effect on fibroblast formation and other substances that take part in the late healing phase. This interference tends to prevent scar tissue formation that may damage delicate structures like the eye.

Anti-allergic actions of glucocorticoids are similar to their anti-inflammatory actions. Immediate hypersensitivity reactions are suppressed by the interference of histamine release. Delayed hypersensitivity reactions are suppressed by decreasing activity of cellular mediators of immune reactions such as macrophages, monocytes, and T- and B-lymphocytes. Glucocorticoids also suppress or prevent cell-mediated immune reactions such as: reduce the concentration of thymus-dependent leukocytes, monocytes, and eosinophils; inhibit *interleukin* synthesis; and decrease the binding of immunoglobulins to cell surface receptors.

The specific anti-stress action of glucocorticoids is still uncertain. However, glucocorticoids do improve cardiovascular function by several mechanisms. First, the natural hormones have a salt- and water-retaining effect which can prevent hypovolemia in patients with adrenocortical insufficiency and improve cardiovascular performance. Second, glucocorticoids increase the responsiveness of the heart, blood vessels, and other tissues to circulating catecholamines such as epinephrine and norepinephrine. The improved cardiovascular function increases cardiac output and local perfusion pressure. Ultimately, there is improved blood flow to the brain and other vital organs. This may be why glucocorticoids are helpful in preventing and treating circulatory collapse in persons with acute adrenal crisis and shock associated with septicemia.

In terms of carbohydrate metabolism, the glucocorticoids exert an effect opposite to that of insulin, that is, they stimulate *gluconeogenesis* (formation of glucose from noncarbohydrate sources such as protein or fat), decrease utilization of glucose by many body cells, and promote glucose storage as glycogen.

The increase in glucose production is at the expense of protein stores, and protein *catabolism* occurs with high, nonphysiologic levels of glucocorticoids. Particularly affected are bone matrix, muscle tissue, vascular tissue, skin, and lymphatic tissue. This protein catabolism, which serves to mobilize amino acids, provides substrate for the increased production of glucose in the liver. The increase in protein catabolism leads to poor wound healing, muscle wasting, and scanty hair growth.

Fat, or lipid, metabolism is also affected by exogenous glucocorticoid therapy. These drugs enhance the breakdown of triglycerides in the body's fat deposits to fatty acids *(lipolysis)*. Glucocorticoids can also indirectly increase the formation of fat and its storage in adipose tissue. This *lipogenesis* occurs as a result of the action of insulin which is released from the pancreas. This rise in blood sugar is secondary to the effect of glucocorticoids on carbohydrate metabolism. The fat distribution changes are discussed later in this chapter.

Glucocorticoids affect other aspects of body functioning, too. Central nervous system and emotional functioning is, in part, maintained by the glucocorticoids.

TEXT RESUMES ON PAGE 1088

Table 42–1. ADRENAL CORTICAL DRUGS

Name	Dosage	Mode of Administration	Pharmacokinetics
MINERALOCORTICOIDS			
Action: Enhance reabsorption of sodium and chloride and enhance excretion of potassium and hydrogen in distal tubule of kidney.			
Use: Primary adrenocortical insufficiency, salt-losing adrenogenital syndromes.			
Desoxycorticosterone acetate (DOCA)	Actetate: 2–5 mg/24 hr; Pellets: q 8–12 months	IM Implanted	O: slowly P: UA D: 24–48 hr ½L: UA PB: yes B: liver E: urine
Desoxycorticosterone pivalate (Percorten Pivalate)	25–100 mg q 4 wk	IM	O: slowly P: UA D: 4 wk ½L: UA PB: yes B: liver E: urine
Fludrocortisone (Florinef)	0.01–0.2 mg/24 hr	PO	O: rapid P: 1.7 hr D: 24–48 hr ½L: 3.5 hr; 18–36 hr PB: yes B: liver E: urine
GLUCOCORTICOIDS			
Action: Suppress normal immune response and inflammation. Suppresses natural adrenal function with doses greater than 20 mg/day of cortisone or its equivalent.			
Use: Adrenal insufficiency, inflammatory diseases, allergic diseases.			
			For all glucocorticoids: Onset of action, peak, and duration depend on dose being administered and condition being treated.
Hydrocortisone (Cortef, Hydrocortone)	*Adult:* 20–240 mg/day; 5–120 mg in 2 divided doses	PO, IM, intra-articular, intralesional, topical, ophthalmic	O: slow P: UA D: 12 hr ½L: 8–12 hr For all PB: highly For all B: liver For all E: urine
	Pediatric: 0.56–8.0 mg/kg/24 hr, PO; ⅓–½ the PO dose	PO IM	
Hydrocortisone sodium succinate (Solu-Cortef, Cortisol, Hydrocortone)	*Adult:* 100–500 mg; *Pediatric:* approximately 80% of adult dose	IM or IV	O: rapid P: UA D: 1–1.5 days ½L: 8–12 hr
Cortisone acetate (Cortone)	*Adult:* 25–300 mg/day; 25–300 mg/24 hr in 4 doses *Pediatric:* 2.5–10 mg/kg/24 hr divided q 6–8 hr	PO IM	O: rapid P: 2 hr O: slow P: 20–48 hr D: 1.24–1.5 days ½L: 8–12 hr

Key to Abbreviations in the *Pharmacokinetics* column O-onset; P-peak; D-duration; PB-protein bound; B-biotransformed in; ½L-halflife.
*Within the column listing adverse effects, underlines indicate the most common effects.
†Little sodium retention.
‡No sodium retention.

A
d
r
e
n
a
l

C
o
r
t
i
c
a
l

D
r
u
g
s

Contraindications/ Precautions	Adverse Effects*	Interactions	Nursing Implications
For all mineralocorticoids: CONTRAINDICATIONS: Hypersensitivity, hypertension, cardiac disease, and congestive heart failure. PRECAUTIONS: Safety in pregnancy and children not established.	For all mineralocorticoids: *Neuro:* frontal/occipital headaches *CVR:* increased blood volume, hypertension, congestive heart failure, dysrhythmias, hypokalemia *Renal:* sodium retention *Resp:* hypersensitivity *Musculoskeletal:* arthralgias, extreme weakness	For all mineralocorticoids: Other drugs that cause sodium and water retention.	For all mineralocorticoids: ASSESSMENT: Assess blood pressure, weight at onset and periodically. INTERVENTION: Monitor salt intake to avoid edema, weight gain, hypertension. Eat potassium-rich foods. Store in airtight, light-resistant containers. Inject into dorsal gluteal or ventrogluteal areas of buttock, not deltoid, due to risk of subcutaneous atrophy. Use 23-gauge needle. Take missed dose as soon as possible. Do not double dose the next time. EVALUATION: Notify physician if persistent dizziness, headache, or weight gain occur.
For all glucocorticoids: CONTRAINDICATIONS: Hypersensitivity, fungal infections, tuberculosis, viral diseases, Cushing's syndrome. PRECAUTIONS: Use cautiously in active or latent peptic ulcer, ocular herpes simplex, diverticulitis, hypertension, osteoporosis, and infectious diseases.	For all glucocorticoids: *Neuro:* convulsions, increased intracranial pressure with papilledema, steroid psychoses, depression *CVR:* cardiac dysrhythmias, congestive heart failure, hypotension *GI:* nausea, vomiting, increased appetite, weight gain, peptic ulcer, pancreatitis *Renal:* sodium and fluid retention, hypokalemia, hypocalcemia *Reprod:* amenorrhea, postmenopausal bleeding *Integ:* petechiae, impaired wound healing, thin fragile skin, suppression of skin tests, striae, hyperpigmentation *Endo:* buffalo hump, moon face, decreased growth in children, hyperglycemia *Ophth:* cataracts, glaucoma, exophthalmos	For all glucocorticoids: Barbiturates, phenytoin, and rifampin increase glucocorticoid metabolism. Concomitant use of salicylates or any NSAIDs may increase risk of GI ulceration. Glucocorticoids may decrease blood levels of salicylates. Potassium-depleting diuretics and amphotericin B enhance potassium-wasting effect. Cholestyramine delays absorption of hydrocortisone. Insulin and oral hypoglycemic agents may need to be increased. Oral contraceptives and troleandomycin may inhibit metabolism of steroids. Lab: Urine glucose and serum cholesterol and triglycerides may increase. K, T_3, T_4, may decrease.	For all glucocorticoids: ASSESSMENT: Assess for signs of adrenal insufficiency throughout therapy. Obtain baseline CBC, electrolytes, eye exams, vital signs, and weight. Obtain TB test before long-term therapy. INTERVENTION: Never discontinue abruptly or without checking with physician. Obtain an order for parenteral form if unable to take PO. Carry identification card or wear a bracelet or necklace if on long-term therapy. Weigh regularly, and check urine for glucosuria. Take antacids as prescribed. Avoid aspirin, alcohol, and caffeine. Take oral drugs with food. Teach patient at what time of day drug is to be taken. Teach patient that dose will need to be increased with physiologic

CONTINUED ON THE FOLLOWING PAGE

Table 42–1. ADRENAL CORTICAL DRUGS—*CONTINUED*

Name	Dosage	Mode of Administration	Pharmacokinetics
Prednisone (Deltasone, Meticorten)	*Adult:* 5–60 mg/24 hr in 1–4 doses *Pediatric:* 0.1–0.15 mg/kg/24 hr	PO	O: hours P: UA D: 1.25–1.5 days ½L: 18–36 hr
Prednisolone (Delta-Cortef, Sterane)	*Adult:* 5–60 mg/24 hr in 1–4 doses *Pediatric:* 0.14–2.0 mg/kg/24 hr in 3 doses, PO; ⅓–½ the PO dose for IM	PO, IM	O: slow P: 1–2 hr D: 1.25–1.5 days ½L: 18–36 hr
Prednisolone acetate (Key-Pred 25, Predcor 50)	4–60 mg/day 5–100 mg	IM Intralesion, intra-articular, soft tissue	O: slowly P: UA D: up to 4 wk ½L: 18–36 hr
Prednisolone sodium phosphate (Hydeltrasol, Predicort RP, Pediapred)	4–60 mg/day 2–30 mg	IM, IV Intralesional, intra-articular, soft tissue	O: rapid P: 1 hr D: UA ½L: 18–36 hr
Methylprednisolone (Medrol)†	*Adult:* 4–48 mg in 2–4 divided doses *Pediatric:* 0.117–1.167 mg/kg/24 hr in 3 doses	PO PO	O: hours P: 1–2 hr D: 1.25–1.5 days ½L: 18–36 hr
Methylprednisolone acetate (Depo-Medrol)†	*Adult:* 40–120 mg/wk 20–60 mg *Pediatric:* same as for methylprednisolone	IM, intra-articular Intralesional	O: 6–48 hr P: 4–8 day D: 1–4 wk ½L: 18–36 hr
Methylprednisolone sodium succinate (Solu-Medrol)†	*Adult:* 10–250 mg q 4–6 hr; 30 mg/kg over 10–20 min, repeat q 4–6 hr for 48–72 hr only *Pediatric:* same as for methylprednisolone	IV, IM IV	O: rapid P: UA D: UA ½L: 18–36 hr
Triamcinolone (Aristocort, Kenalog)†	*Adult:* 4–60 mg/24 hr *Pediatric:* 1–2 mg/kg	PO	O: UA P: 1–2 hr D: 2.25 day ½L: 10–36 hr
Triamicinolone diacetate (Aristocort Forte)	40 mg/wk 5–40 mg 5–48 mg; not more than 12.5 mg/injection site	IM Intra-articular, intrasynovial Intralesional	O: slow P: UA D: 4 days–4 wk ½L: 200+ min
Betamethasone (Celestone)†	*Adult:* 0.6–7.2 mg/24 hr 0.5–9 mg/day *Pediatric:* 17.5–200 µg/kg/24 hr in 3 doses	PO IM intra-articular, intrasynovial	O: rapid P: UA D: UA ½L: 36–54 hr

Key to Abbreviations in the *Pharmacokinetics* column O-onset; P-peak; D-duration; PB-protein bound; B-biotransformed in; E-excreted in; ½L-halflife.
*Within the column listing adverse effects, <u>underlines</u> indicate the most common effects.
†Little sodium retention.
‡No sodium retention.

Contraindications/ Precautions	Adverse Effects*	Interactions	Nursing Implications
	Musculoskeletal: muscle weakness, steroid myopathy, osteoporosis, spontaneous fracture *Misc:* increased susceptibility to infection		stress and that doctor should be consulted. Store in a dry, tightly closed container; protect from light. Massage topical drugs into area thoroughly and gently. Apply sparingly. Wear gloves when applying. Apply occlusive dressing only if ordered. Inject IM deeply into dorsal gluteal or ventrogluteal of buttock. Rotate injection sites and record. Dilute IV solutions according to package directions. EVALUATION: Disease symptoms should lessen. Notify physician if unusual weight gain, swelling of lower extremities, vomiting, GI distress, prolonged sore throat, fever, or cold.

CONTINUED ON THE FOLLOWING PAGE

Table 42–1. ADRENAL CORTICAL DRUGS–*CONTINUED*

Name	Dosage	Mode of Administration	Pharmacokinetics
Paramethasone acetate (Haldrone)	Initial: 2–24 mg/day	PO	O: rapid P: UA D: UA ½L: 18–36 hr
Dexamethasone acetate (Decadron-LA)‡	8–16 mg, repeat in 1–3 wk 0.8–1.6 mg 4–6 mg	IM Intralesional Intra-articular D: 6 days	O: rapid P: 8 hr ½L: 36–54 hr
Dexamethasone (Decadron)‡	*Adult:* 0.75–9.0 mg/24 hr in 2–4 doses	PO	O: rapid P: 1–2 hr D: 2.75 days
	Pediatric: 23.3–333.3 μg/kg/ 24 hr in 3 doses	PO	½L: 36–54 hr
Dexamethasone sodium phosphate (Decadron Phosphate, Decadrol, Dexone)	0.5–9.0 mg/day 2–4 mg 0.8–1.0 mg 10 mg for cerebral edema	IM/IV Intra-articular, large joints Intra-articular, small joints IV	O: rapid P: UA D: UA ½L: 36–54 hr

ADRENOCORTICOTROPIC HORMONE

Action: Stimulates adrenal cortex to produce and secrete adrenocortical hormones.

Use: Diagnostic testing, several endocrine diseases, acute exacerbation of multiple sclerosis, numerous miscellaneous conditions.

Corticotropin (ACTH)	*Adult:* 10–25 U in 500 ml over 8 hr (diagnostic testing) 20–80 U q 4 hr 40–80 U q 24–72 hr (respository injection) *Pediatric:* 1.6 U/kg/24 hr divided q 6–8 hr	IV IV, IM, SC IV, IM, SC IV, IM, SC	O: rapid P: UA D: 2 hr ½L: 15 min

Key to Abbreviations in the *Pharmacokinetics* column O-onset; P-peak; D-duration; PB-protein bound; B-biotransformed in; E-excreted in; ½L-halflife.
*Within the column listing adverse effects, <u>underlines</u> indicate the most common effects.
†Little sodium retention.
‡No sodium retention.

Exogenous glucocorticoid administration has been shown to increase brain excitability.

Corticosteroid drugs exert pharmacologic actions that are on a continuum, with sodium retention and anti-inflammatory actions being on opposing ends (Fig. 42–1). That is, many drugs that we think of as glucocorticoids have significant mineralocorticoid activity. Cortisol, for example, causes sodium and water retention. The terms mineralocorticoid and glucocorticoid are used to delineate at which end of the continuum of action certain corticosteroids are found, and which activity is predominant.

Use

Aside from their use in replacement therapy for adrenocortical insufficiency (see Table 42–2 for a review of Addison's disease), the glucocorticoid drugs are most often used for their anti-inflammatory effects. Glucocorticoids are used for their anti-inflammatory effect to treat a variety of disorders such as rheumatic fever, osteoarthritis, rheumatoid arthritis, nephrotic syndrome, inflammatory bowel disease, chronic obstructive pulmonary disease, and collagen diseases. The glucocorticoids may cause a rapid and marked reduction in symptoms but do not alter the course of the disease. The

Contraindications/ Precautions	Adverse Effects*	Interactions	Nursing Implications
CONTRAINDICATIONS: Same as glucocorticoids plus contraindicated in scleroderma, recent surgery. PRECAUTIONS: Use cautiously in sensitivity to porcine proteins, acute gouty arthritis, mental disturbances, diabetes, renal insufficiency.	Same as glucocorticoids	Increases serum salicylate level and salicylate toxicity. Increases requirements of insulin and oral hypoglycemics. Enhances electrolyte loss with diuretics.	Same as glucocorticoids.

glucocorticoids are used for their anti-lymphocytic effect to treat leukemias, lymphomas, myelomas, and multiple sclerosis. The glucocorticoids are also used to reduce or prevent cerebral edema associated with neoplasms, neurosurgery, and trauma. The glucocorticoids suppress the inflammatory response and relieve hypersensitivity reactions in patients with asthma, bee stings, hay fever, contact and exfoliative dermatitis, ulcerative colitis, and vasculitis. Glucocorticoids are commonly used to decrease ocular inflammatory processes. Glucocorticoids are also combined with other immunosuppressants to prevent or manage transplant rejection.

Glucocorticoids are also used to suppress adrenocortical hyperfunction in patients with adrenogenital syndrome. The glucocorticoids increase calcium excretion and are used for treatment of hypercalcemia in patients with the following conditions: cancer with bone metas-

tases such as breast cancer; multiple myeloma; and vitamin D intoxication.

Glucocorticoids may be administered via a variety of different routes, dependent on the desired use of the glucocorticoids. Most can be given orally, intramuscularly, and intravenously. The intravenous route allows a faster onset of action and is preferred in emergencies.

Local use of glucocorticoids may be preferred over systemic routes. The advantage of these routes is that they avoid much of the systemic adverse effects. Topical administration, for example, is a mainstay of much dermatologic therapy. However, it should be noted that even topical application of glucocorticoids can cause hypothalamic-pituitary-adrenal (HPA) suppression. Other adverse effects can also occur when glucocorticoids are applied over a large area of body surface, especially if the skin is more permeable such as when inflamed, and

Table 42–2. ADRENAL CORTEX HYPOFUNCTION

DEFINITION
Reduced function of adrenal cortex leading to decreased production of glucocorticoids, androgens, and (in Addison's disease) mineralocorticoids.

TYPES
1. Primary (Addison's disease)
2. Secondary

ETIOLOGY
1. Primary
   a. Idiopathic (probably autoimmune)
2. Secondary
   a. Administration of exogenous corticosteroids (causes suppression of ACTH secretion)
   b. Hypopituitarism
   c. Bilateral adrenalectomy

SYMPTOMS
1. Objective
   a. Fluid and electrolyte imbalances (sodium, water loss; potassium retention)
   b. Hypoglycemia
   c. Emotional disturbances
   d. Bronze coloration to skin
   e. Decreased response to stress
2. Subjective
   a. Weakness
   b. Fatigue
   c. Emotional disturbances

MANAGEMENT (Hormone Replacement)
1. Cortisone is used to replace glucocorticoids.
2. Fludrocortisone is used to replace mineralocorticoids.

---

if occlusive dressings are used. When intralesional injections of glucocorticoids are used in treating severe forms of skin disorders such as acne, systemic absorption may occur.

Intra-articular injections of glucocorticoids are a useful form of local therapy for patients with inflammatory joint problems. Rectal administration via enemas or foams for the treatment of inflammatory bowel disorders is another example of local use.

Glucocorticoids may also be administered to the respiratory tract via inhalation. Beclomethasone (Vanceril) is used via this route in the treatment of asthma that does not respond to conventional therapy with bronchodilators. Beclomethasone is discussed in detail in

Chapter 35. Again, it must be noted that when this route of administration is properly used, systemic adverse effects are minimal; however, abuse or overuse may in fact cause some HPA suppression.

In 1972, clinical trials began that evaluated the usefulness of antenatal glucocorticoids in preventing neonatal respiratory distress syndrome (RDS). Betamethasone (Celestone) or dexamethasone (Decadron) administered to mothers parenterally at least 24 hours before delivery has been shown to decrease the incidence of RDS in premature infants of less than 32 weeks gestation.

In the treatment of septic shock, the use of extremely large doses of glucocorticoids administered within the first 24–48 hours of the onset of shock can be beneficial in reducing the inflammation associated with the infection. However, ongoing research indicates that the cause may be ultimately worsened. Use of glucocorticoids in treating shock of other etiologies is not beneficial.

Pharmacokinetics

The majority of glucocorticoids are effective by mouth but are also used for parenteral administration. The glucocorticoids are highly protein-bound to corticosteroid-binding globulin or transcortin- and corticosteroid-binding albumin. It is the unbound, or free, fraction of cortisol that is pharmacologically active. These products are distributed to all body tissues and several also cross the placenta. Glucocorticoids are metabolized by the liver and excreted in the urine. Biologic half-life varies with the specific drug and ranges from 8 to 54 hours (see Table 42–1 for specific information on each drug).

Contraindications and Precautions

Glucocorticoids are contraindicated in systemic viral infection and active or arrested tuberculosis as these conditions may worsen with glucocorticoid therapy. Before patients are started on long-term therapy, a tuberculosis test is always done to determine the presence of inactive disease. Arrested tuberculosis may reactivate when steroids are administered. Patients are usually given prophylactic isoniazid (INH).

Because of their effects on numerous body systems and because they interfere with inflammatory response,

ACTIVITY	PRODUCTS	USES
Highest mineralocorticoid activity, no glucocorticoid activity	Desocycorticosterone Fludrocortisone	Replacement in Addison's
Equal mineralocorticoid and glucocorticoid activities	Cortisone, Cortisol, Hydrocortisone	Replacement in adrenocortical insufficiency, anti-inflammatory, immunosuppression
	Prednisone, prednisolone, methylprednisolone	Autoimmune disorders, antiinflammatory, immunosuppression
Highest glucocorticoid activity, no mineralocorticoid activity	Dexamethasone Betamethasone	Increased intracranial pressure, anti-inflammatory

Figure 42–1. Continuum of adrenocorticoids. Several steroids are represented on the continuum with their uses.

glucocorticoids need to be given cautiously to patients who have certain disease conditions, as they may be exacerbated. Some conditions worsened by the use of glucocorticoids are: active or latent peptic ulcer, ulcerative colitis, diverticulitis, ocular herpes simplex, hypertension, and osteoporosis.

Adverse Effects

The occurrence of adverse effects from glucocorticoid administration is related to the alterations in physiologic function that the adrenal hormones naturally cause. Generally, the pharmacologic doses of glucocorticoids cause adverse effects, not the physiologic, or replacement, doses; and the occurrence of adverse effects is related to the amounts of the medications used and the length of therapy. The adrenal cortex generally produces about 20–30 mg of glucocorticoids per day and in acute stress situations can produce ten times as much. Pharmacologic doses are greater than 30 mg/day.

The onset of acute adrenal insufficiency is a life-threatening complication that occurs most often when patients are abruptly withdrawn from long-term therapy. Chronic glucocorticoid treatment suppresses HPA activity and leads to adrenal cortical atrophy. Since HPA responsiveness may take many months to return to normal, the patient is closely observed for this complication for the year following the termination of therapy. General muscular weakness, nausea, anorexia, hypotension, and syncope are indicative of this complication. Supplemental amounts of glucocorticoids are administered to alleviate these symptoms of insufficiency and to prevent vasomotor collapse. These additional glucocorticoids are withdrawn gradually over a period of several days until the maintenance dose is reached.

The catabolic effect of glucocorticoids on protein metabolism leads to many changes. "Steroid myopathy," muscular weakness involving all extremities, especially the lower extremities, can occur. Myopathy is mainly a result of negative nitrogen balance, which develops despite the fact that these drugs increase the patient's appetite. Triamcinolone, a synthetic steroid, is said not to stimulate appetite and lead to weight gain (unlike other steroids) and, therefore, may be more likely to cause muscle wasting. Protein catabolism may also appear as osteoporosis, largely due to wasting of the bone matrix from calcium depletion (most noticeable in the vertebrae). Decreased calcium absorption by the gastrointestinal tract combined with enhanced renal excretion of calcium is also involved. Some studies have indicated that the risk of osteoporosis is most pronounced in patients with certain predisposing factors, such as decreased calcium intake, immobility, and menopause.

The protein component of skin and vascular walls is also affected. The patient on long-term glucocorticoid therapy may bruise readily, related to capillary fragility; and have a very "thin," delicate skin, related to decreased protein.

In children, the skeletal system may be markedly affected, and a decrease in growth rate is often noted, since glucocorticoids impair cell division and increase bone demineralization. After steroid therapy is discontinued, most children experience a growth spurt, although large doses given for long periods of time may cause irreversible growth retardation.

The hematopoietic system also suffers from the protein catabolism induced by nonphysiologic doses of glucocorticoids. Eosinophils and lymphocytes decrease in numbers. Although lymphoid tissue may atrophy, reduction of antibody production usually does not occur unless large amounts of corticosteroids are used over long periods of time. Nevertheless, delayed hypersensitivity responses may be altered. For example, skin sensitivity to tuberculin, as in the Mantoux test, may be lost. In addition, neutrophils may actually increase. A modestly high white blood cell count of 10,000–15,000 may be the result of steroids as opposed to infection.

Wound healing is also decreased by glucocorticoids since they decrease fibroblast proliferation and collagen deposition. Patients receiving glucocorticoids who require surgery will need an increase in dosage due to the increase in physiologic stress. Patients receiving glucocorticoids postoperatively need to be monitored closely for increases in blood pressure secondary to salt and water retention, particularly if the natural glucocorticoids are administered.

Another effect to consider is that although patients on glucocorticoids are more susceptible to infection, the anti-inflammatory action of the medications tends to hide, or mask, the more common signs of inflammation such as fever, redness, swelling, and pain.

Carbohydrate metabolism is profoundly affected by the use of exogenous glucocorticoid therapy. In fact, the normal physiologic role of these hormones is to provide for glucose production during periods of decreased carbohydrate intake. As glucose synthesis is increased, glucose utilization is at the same time decreased. This may lead to an increase in blood glucose, sometimes referred to as adrenal diabetes or steroid-induced diabetes. Patients treated with high doses of glucocorticoids over prolonged periods may eventually develop signs and symptoms of diabetes mellitus. Other patients, at risk of developing diabetes mellitus, may develop clinically evident disease during treatment.

Fat metabolism is affected as well. Redistribution of fat stores occurs. This results in the typical cushingoid appearance (Fig. 42–2) of patients on long-term therapy: a cervicodorsal fat pad ("buffalo hump"), obesity of the torso, "moon" face, and decreased fat deposits in the extremities (see Table 42–3 for a review of Cushing's syndrome). These changes can occur with doses of 25 mg/day of prednisone or its equivalent for two weeks. Glucocorticoid therapy is also associated with hyperlipidemia, with increases in triglycerides being most notable.

In addition to these metabolic effects, several other important adverse effects need to be reviewed. Significant changes in fluid and electrolyte balance can occur when either mineralocorticoids or glucocorticoids with pronounced mineralocorticoid activity, such as hydrocortisone, are used. Sodium retention and the subsequent water retention may be great enough to produce hypertension in some patients. Potassium-depleting effects can lead to hypokalemia.

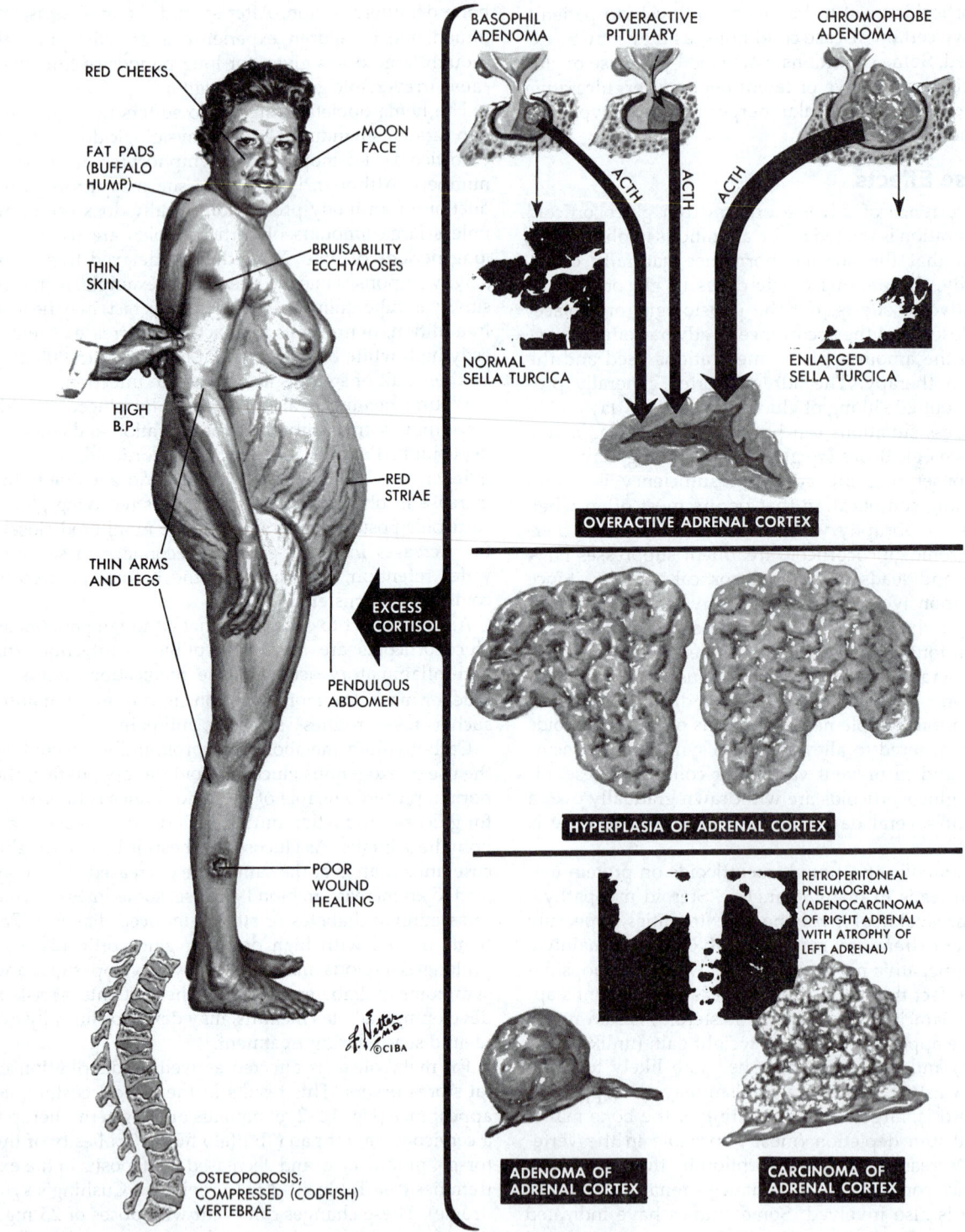

RED CHEEKS

FAT PADS (BUFFALO HUMP)

MOON FACE

THIN SKIN

BRUISABILITY ECCHYMOSES

HIGH B.P.

RED STRIAE

THIN ARMS AND LEGS

EXCESS CORTISOL

PENDULOUS ABDOMEN

POOR WOUND HEALING

OSTEOPOROSIS; COMPRESSED (CODFISH) VERTEBRAE

BASOPHIL ADENOMA

OVERACTIVE PITUITARY

CHROMOPHOBE ADENOMA

ACTH

ACTH

ACTH

NORMAL SELLA TURCICA

ENLARGED SELLA TURCICA

OVERACTIVE ADRENAL CORTEX

HYPERPLASIA OF ADRENAL CORTEX

RETROPERITONEAL PNEUMOGRAM (ADENOCARCINOMA OF RIGHT ADRENAL WITH ATROPHY OF LEFT ADRENAL)

ADENOMA OF ADRENAL CORTEX

CARCINOMA OF ADRENAL CORTEX

N12-61 VOLUME 4 - ENDOCRINE SYSTEM CUSHING'S SYNDROME I D

Figure 42–2. Cushingoid appearance often seen in patients on long-term steroid therapy. Typical moon face and buffalo hump are seen (Ciba Collection Endocrine System Vol. 4 p. 85, 1965, with permission).

The occurrence of peptic ulcer in glucocorticoid therapy has been the topic of much discussion and research. Currently, it is believed that glucocorticoids are ulcerogenic. Evidence exists that gastric mucus production is decreased and mucosal cell renewal is affected. These factors alter the mucosal defense mechanisms and potentiate the development of gastric ulcers when other factors, such as aspirin intake, are introduced. In addition, the anti-inflammatory effects of the medications may hide the symptoms of ulceration, and perforation can occur with little outward evidence.

One other less common adverse effect on the gastrointestinal system is the occurrence of pancreatitis. The mechanisms by which glucocorticoids cause this is

Table 42–3. CUSHING'S SYNDROME

DEFINITION
A clinical condition caused by excessive amounts of corticosteroids.

ETIOLOGY
1. Adrenal tumors
2. Pituitary tumors (Cushing's disease)
3. Ectopic ACTH secretion
4. Administration of exogenous glucocorticoids

SYMPTOMS
1. Objective
   a. Hyperglycemia
   b. Hypokalemia
   c. Sodium and water retention
   d. Edema
   e. Muscle wasting
   f. Altered distribution of body fat: "moon" face, obesity of torso, "buffalo hump"
   g. Osteoporosis
   h. Striae, bruising, fungal infections
2. Subjective
   a. Emotional changes

MANAGEMENT
Dependent on cause:
1. Surgical excision of tumors
2. Stoppage of exogenous administration of glucocorticoids
3. Administration of aminoglutethimide (Cytadren) to inhibit cortisol synthesis

unknown; again, the clinical signs and symptoms may be masked by the medications.

Increases in intraocular pressure can occur with either ocular or systemic use of glucocorticoids. Glaucoma may occur in high-risk patients, such as those genetically predisposed or those with diabetes. Cataracts can also develop from long-term use of topical ophthalmic agents.

Lastly, central nervous sytem and psychiatric disturbances can occur. As noted previously, glucocorticoids do cause an increase in brain excitability. Cases of spontaneous seizure activity have been noted with large doses. Psychiatric reactions are usually reversible but vary widely. Some evidence suggests that they are less common with the use of the more potent synthetic analogs. Many researchers feel that these reactions are most common in individuals who have a history of personality disorders. Changes that may occur include: insomnia; nervousness; euphoria; and depression, sometimes suicidal in severity.

Interactions

Corticosteroids can interact with a number of other drugs. The concurrent use of potassium-depleting diuretics, such as thiazides or furosemide, amphotericin B can lead to severe hypokalemia. Concurrent use of salicylates or indomethacin (Indocin) may increase the risk of peptic ulceration. Steroids may also reduce salicylate levels by increased metabolism or clearance. Use of barbiturates, phenytoin (Dilantin), or rifampin (Rifadin) increases glucocorticoid metabolism. Concurrent use of corticosteroids may inhibit the response of coumarin anticoagulants, making it necessary to check pro-

thrombin times (PTs) frequently. Anion-exchange resins decrease the effectiveness of steroids because of the fact that their absorption is decreased. Oral contraceptives and troleandomycin may inhibit steroid hepatic metabolism. The diabetic may need more insulin or oral agents while taking steroids concurrently because of their effect on carbohydrate metabolism.

Steroids may also cause urine glucose and serum cholesterol and triglyceride levels to rise due to their action in the body. Decreases in potassium and T_3 levels, and minimal decreases in T_4 may also be seen.

Dosage

Dosages of various glucocorticoids vary widely, depending on the agent used and the particular reason for giving the drug. Maintenance doses are generally at the low end of the dosage range given in Table 42–1.

Because of the potential for serious adverse effects, glucocorticoids prescribed for anti-inflammatory activity generally are given in the smallest doses possible for the shortest possible period of time. For patients with chronic conditions, glucocorticoids may not be given in amounts to completely suppress all symptomatology.

In general, in adrenal insufficiency, replacement of the normal amount of cortisol produced by the body (approximately 20–30 mg/day) is the goal. Usually, 10–25 mg/day of hydrocortisone or an equivalent analog will suffice for this purpose.

For anti-inflammatory activity, a pharmacologic dose is used; 25–50 mg of cortisone (Cortone) or the equivalent amount of an analog is often prescribed. For acute life-threatening illnesses, as much as 75–300 mg/day might be used. The relative anti-inflammatory effect of steroids is based on hydrocortisone, which is given a value of one (Table 42–4).

Frequently, glucocorticoid therapy is adjusted to mimic, as closely as possible, the normal diurnal pattern of cortisol secretion in the body. As described in Chapter 40, cortisol secretion is highest in the early morning (6–9 AM) and lowest later in the day (9 PM to 12 midnight). Therefore, replacements may be administered in

Table 42–4. GLUCOCORTICOD POTENCY

Glucocorticoid	Comparative Anti-Inflammatory Potency	Equivalent Dose (mg) (Approximate)
LONG ACTING		
Betamethasone	25	0.6–0.75
Dexamethasone	25–30	0.75
Paramethasone	10	2
INTERMEDIATE-ACTING		
Methylprednisolone	5	4
Prednisolone	4	5
Prednisone	4	5
Triamcinolone	5	4
SHORT-ACTING		
Cortisone	0.8	25
Hydrocortisone	1	20

divided doses, with two thirds given in the morning and one third given in the early afternoon. Or the entire daily dose might be administered early in the morning (7–8 AM). If the entire dose is administered in the morning, the adrenal gland may be suppressed. If suppression of gland activity is not desired, the entire dose may be administered in the early afternoon. This allows the gland to function normally, plus giving the patient a second peak of hormone to manage current symptoms.

For patients who need long-term glucocorticoid therapy, it has been found that alternate-day therapy is helpful in reducing the incidence of some adverse effects, especially the cushingoid appearance and adrenocortical suppression, by giving the HPA axis a chance to recover. (Normal adrenal activity can be minimally suppressed with alternate-day therapy). Alternate-day therapy is of particular value in the pediatric patient, where numerous studies have shown that, in most cases, growth retardation can be avoided. Growth was not impaired in asthmatic children treated with alternate-day therapy. However, children with renal disease such as nephrotic syndrome treated with alternate-day therapy, still may have some growth retardation.

In alternate-day therapy, a single dose of a glucocorticoid, such as prednisone or prednisolone, with an intermediate duration of action (24–36 hours) is administered on alternate mornings in an amount equal to that needed for a 48-hour period.

Two points concerning this therapy regimen should be kept in mind. First, patients are not initially treated with this regimen. It is used for maintenance after the desired anti-inflammatory action has been achieved. Second, certain patients may have an exacerbation of their symptoms on the "off" day. For this reason, some patients may be unsuited for alternate-day therapy, such as those with ulcerative colitis or rheumatoid arthritis. If flare-ups of symptoms do occur, treatment with other drugs may be helpful. For example, the patient with arthritis might benefit from the use of analgesics on the "off" day.

Corticosteroid Products

Chemists have worked for many years to develop synthetic corticosteroids. The synthetic corticosteroids are more potent than cortisone and hydrocortisone. In addition, the therapeutic actions of the synthetic steroids have been partially separated from the adverse effects that limit their usefulness.

The first synthetic steroids to be developed were prednisone and prednisolone. These products are four to five times more potent than cortisone and hydrocortisone. More recently, dexamethasone and betamethasone were developed. A 1-mg dose of these products has the same anti-inflammatory effects as 25 mg of cortisone and hydrocortisone, without causing the sodium-retaining effects.

These potent synthetic products also have a long duration of action, which can suppress the HPA axis. This suppression can be beneficial, but can also be detrimental. Alternate-day dosing of intermediate-acting products like prednisone and prednisolone can be used if HPA axis suppression is not required.

NATURAL PRODUCTS. *Hydrocortisone.* Hydrocortisone (Cortef, Hydrocortone) is the principal natural glucocorticoid secreted by the adrenal cortex. It is administered in oral doses of 20–240 mg for replacement therapy and for other conditions. In acute situations, it is not a preferred drug because of its slow onset of action. It can also be given intramuscularly in doses of 5–120 mg/day. When needed, hydrocortisone is also administered via the intra-articular, intralesional, topical, and ophthalmic routes. Hydrocortisone is metabolized to cortisone.

Hydrocortisone Sodium Succinate. Hydrocortisone sodium succinate (Solu-Cortef), an ester of hydrocortisone, is one of the most commonly administered parenteral glucocorticoids. Hydrocortisone sodium succinate is administered in doses of 100–500 mg. It is primarily used to treat adrenocortical insufficiency and severe inflammation.

Cortisone Acetate. Cortisone acetate (Cortone) is usually the drug of choice for replacement therapy in patients with adrenocortical insufficiency. It has both glucocorticoid and mineralocorticoid properties. It is administered orally as a replacement in 25- to 300-mg doses. Intramuscularly, it is administered in four doses of 25–300 mg within 24 hours. Cortisone acetate is also administered as ophthalmic drops.

SYNTHETIC PRODUCTS. *Prednisone.* Prednisone (Deltasone, Meticorten) is the most commonly administered synthetic oral glucocorticoid. It is generally administered in one to four doses of 5–60 mg each in 24 hours. Prednisone is inactive and must be metabolized to prednisolone in the liver. It is also used in alternate-day therapy. Pediatric dosage is 0.1–0.15 mg/kg bid. Prednisone is primarily used for its anti-inflammatory or immunosuppressant effects.

Prednisolone. Prednisolone (Cortalone, Delta-Cortef, Fernisolone-P), a synthetic steroid, is administered orally in one to four doses of 5–60 mg in 24 hours. It is also used in alternate-day therapy. Prednisolone is used primarily as an anti-inflammatory or immunosuppressant agent.

Prednisolone Acetate. Prednisolone acetate (Key-Pred 25, Predcor 50) is the synthetic acetate salt of prednisolone and is administered intramuscularly, intra-articularly, intralesionally, topically, or ophthalmically. The initial dose is 4–60 mg/day intramuscularly; or 5 mg up to 100 mg intralesionally, intra-articularly, or into soft tissue. It is used primarily for its anti-inflammatory or immunosuppressant effect.

Prednisolone Sodium Phosphate. Prednisolone sodium phosphate (Hydeltrasol, Predicort RP, Pediapred) is a water-soluble, rapid-acting, short-duration product used for its anti-inflammatory or immunosuppressant effects. It is given in doses of 4–60 mg/day either intramuscularly or intravenously. It can also be injected intralesionally, intra-articularly, or into soft tissue in doses of 2–30 mg. Pediapred is a liquid steroid that is free of alcohol, sugar, and dye, and provides readily available prednisolone in a palatable form. This product is especially useful in children who require long-term, high-dose steroids for chronic inflammatory disease.

Methylprednisolone. Methylprednisolone (Medrol)

is used primarily as an anti-inflammatory or immuno-suppressant agent. It is not used alone in adrenocortical insufficiency because it has minimal mineralocorticoid activity. Methylprednisolone is administered in doses of 4–48 mg orally. It is available as a 21 Dosepak for acute inflammatory conditions. The 21 Dosepak is designed for one week of therapy. A large first dose is taken and each of the next days a smaller dose is consumed. The patient is taught to follow the manufacturer's directions. It is also suitable for alternate-day therapy.

Methylprednisolone Acetate. Methylprednisolone acetate (Depo-Medrol) is the acetate salt of methylprednisolone and is used for its anti-inflammatory properties. Methylprednisolone acetate is administered intramuscularly in doses of 40–120 mg weekly. It has a low solubility and, therefore, a sustained effect. It can also be given through the intra-articular, intralesional, and topical routes.

Methylprednisolone Sodium Succinate. Methylprednisolone sodium succinate (Solu-Medrol) is a commonly used corticosteroid. Methylprednisolone sodium succinate is used with prednisone and prednisolone in *pulse therapy* for patients with severe lupus nephritis or incapacitating rheumatoid arthritis. If "pulse therapy" is effective, the patient has a temporary remission. Methylprednisolone sodium succinate is given either intramuscularly or intravenously in doses of 10–250 mg every four to six hours. In emergency situations, doses up to 30–40 mg/kg may be given during the first 48–72 hours. It is infused intravenously over a 10–20 minute period and repeated every four to six hours.

Triamcinolone. Triamcinolone (Aristocort, Kenacort) is used primarily as an anti-inflammatory or immuno-suppressant drug. It has minimal mineralocorticoid activity, so it is not used alone to treat adrenocortical insufficiency. Triamcinolone is administered in doses of 4–60 mg in 24 hours. It is administered orally, in either tablets or syrup.

Triamcinolone Diacetate. Triamcinolone diacetate (Aristocort Forte) is used for its anti-inflammatory or immunosuppressant properties. Triamcinolone diacetate is administered in doses of: 40 mg/week, intramuscular; 5–40 mg, intra-articular or intrasynovial; and 5–48 mg, intralesional. Do not use more than 12.5 mg/injection site.

Betamethasone. Betamethasone (Celestone) is a synthetic product with potent anti-inflammatory and immunosuppressant properties. It has minimal mineralocorticoid activity, so it is not used alone to treat adrenocortical insufficiency. Betamethasone is given in doses of 0.6–7.2 mg PO or 0.5–9.0 mg IM in 24 hours. It may be injected into inflamed joints or bursas.

Paramethasone Acetate. Paramethasone acetate (Haldrone) is used primarily for its anti-inflammatory and immunosuppressant properties. It is not used alone to treat adrenocortical insufficiency because of its minimal mineralocorticoid activity. The initial dose is 2–24 mg/day PO and dosage is then individualized to meet patient needs.

Beclomethasone Dipropionate. Beclomethasone dipropionate (Vanceril, Beclovent) is a synthetic glucocorticoid used to control bronchial asthma in patients re-

quiring chronic treatment with corticosteroids in conjunction with other therapies. The use of an inhaler makes it possible to provide effective local steroid activity with minimal systemic effect. Beclomethasone dipropionate is discussed in more detail in Chapter 35.

Dexamethasone. Dexamethasone (Decadron, Hexadrol) is used systemically and locally for a wide variety of acute and chronic inflammatory, allergic, hematologic, neoplastic, and autoimmune diseases. Dexamethasone is also useful in the acute early management of cerebral edema and septic shock. Dexamethasone is used as a diagnostic aid to test for Cushing's syndrome and depression. Dexamethasone is given in two to four doses of 0.75–9.0 mg/day. It is available in tablets for oral use. Dexamethasone phosphate, a salt of dexamethasone, is available for intramuscular and intravenous use in doses of 0.5–9 mg/day. Dexamethasone phosphate can also be injected into joints.

TOPICAL STEROIDS. Topical steroids are available as creams, ointments, gels, aerosols, lotions, solutions, and drug-impregnated tape. They are used to treat numerous inflammatory and proliferative skin diseases. The numerous preparations available have similar action and can cause similar adverse effects. These products are reviewed in Chapter 63.

USE OF STEROIDS TO DETECT HORMONE DYSFUNCTION. Numerous tests of adrenal cortical function are used clinically if adrenal dysfunction is suspected. Electrolyte determinations, especially sodium and potassium levels, may point to disturbances in adrenal function, as may blood glucose concentration. Blood levels of ACTH and cortisol may be measured by radioimmunoassay.

Several urine tests may be employed. In these tests, the metabolic end products of the corticosteroids are measured in 24-hour urine collections. These tests include analysis for 17-ketosteroids (17-KS), 17-ketogenic steroids (17-KGS), and 17-hydroxycorticosteroids (17-OHCS).

Diagnostic tests can be used to either stimulate or suppress adrenal function to help diagnose hormone dysfunction. In the intravenous ACTH stimulation test, baseline 24-hour urine samples for 17-KS, 17-KGS, and 17-OHCS are collected. Then dexamethasone and ACTH are administered to stimulate gland activity. Following this, a second 24-hour urine sample is collected. In normal individuals, the urinary steroid levels increase threefold to fivefold. In primary adrenal insufficiency, the levels do not increase; in adrenal cortical hyperplasia, the levels increase up to tenfold.

In the test of plasma cortisol response to ACTH, a fasting baseline plasma cortisol level is determined. Then ACTH is administered and in 30 minutes, a second plasma sample is drawn. In healthy persons, the cortisol level should rise. If it fails to increase above 10 μg/dL, primary adrenal insufficiency is suspected.

In the dexamethasone suppression test, a 24-hour urine sample for 17-OHCS is collected for baseline data. Then dexamethasone is administered for two days, after which a second urine collection is obtained. Normally, 17-OHCS levels should drop, since dexamethasone suppresses pituitary secretion of ACTH. In adrenal cortical hyperplasia due to a pituitary tumor, less of a decrease in 17-OHCS levels occurs.

USING THE NURSING PROCESS

ASSESSMENT

Assessment of the patient requiring adrenal drugs begins with a careful nursing history in order to establish the data base. Information the nurse obtains is depicted in Table 42–5. One very important component of the history is to identify whether or not the patient is currently taking any type of corticosteroid and the condition for which he or she is taking it. It is equally important to know if the patient has taken corticosteroids at any time within the past year.

The nurse also assesses for a current and past history of gastrointestinal upset, ulcers, or epigastric pain. Steroids may cause or activate an ulcer. During therapy, the nurse also assesses the patient for any gastrointestinal complaints one to three hours after meals; and for nau-

Table 42–5. NURSING PROCESS FOR PATIENT RECEIVING ADRENAL CORTICAL DRUGS (GLUCOCORTICOIDS)

Assessment
Determine current/past drug history. Assess dietary/nutritional and weight control history. Review baseline laboratory data, e.g., ECG, chest and spinal x-rays, glucose-tolerance test, Mantoux, CBC, fluid and electrolyte balance, and ocular pressure. Record BP, body weight, and hypothalamic-pituitary-adrenal axis function. Evaluate for muscle weakness/wasting, redistribution of fat deposits, changes in hair growth, presence of edema.

Nursing Diagnosis	Nursing Actions	Rationale	Desired Outcomes/ Evaluation Criteria
Knowledge deficit related to information misinterpretation, unfamiliarity with resources as evidenced by questions, statement of concern, inaccurate follow-through of instruction/ development of preventable complications.	Review pathophysiology of disease process/condition and therapeutic regimen.	Understanding of need for therapy helps patient to make informed decisions/cooperate with therapy.	Verbalizes understanding of condition/disease process, administration and side effects of steroid therapy.
	Provide information about hormone replacement therapy (adrenal drugs) and necessity of adherence to drug schedule.	Promotes effective therapy, reducing risk of adverse effects.	Initiates necessary lifestyle changes and participates in treatment regimen.
	Stress need to wear an identification bracelet and to carry emergency drugs, e.g., IM or IV dexamethasone sodium.	Assists with prompt/ appropriate intervention in case of emergency and prevents abrupt withdrawal from drug.	
	Define and problem-solve ways to limit/control stressors, e.g., infection, dental work, personal/family crises, increased activity.	Dosage of glucocortocoids may need to be adjusted (doubled/or tripled) during periods of stress.	
	Stress importance of avoiding exposure to infection or trauma/irritation of skin that may result in dermal injury. Recommend prompt reporting of signs of infection.	Suppression of the inflammatory response increases risk of infection and possibility of progression to a life-threatening situation.	
	Discuss necessity of regular medical checkup.	Facilitates control of chronic condition and prevention of complications.	
	Recommend limiting use of caffeine and alcohol, products containing aspirin.	Increasing secretion of gastric acid, irritation of gastric mucosa potentiates risk of GI bleed.	
Fluid volume deficit, Actual 1 related to failure of regulatory mechanisms (aldosterone deficit) as evidenced by nausea, vomiting, weakness, thirst, weight loss, diarrhea,	Determine duration/ intensity of present symptoms, e.g., vomiting, excessive urination. Measure intake/output. Weigh patient daily.	Assists in estimation of total volume depletion. Provides ongoing estimate of volume replacemnt needs/ effectiveness of therapy.	Demonstrates improved fluid balance, as evidenced by individually adequate urine output, stable vital signs, palpable peripheral pulses, good skin turgor and capillary refill, moist mucous membranes.

Table 42–5. NURSING PROCESS FOR PATIENT RECEIVING ADRENAL CORTICAL DRUGS (GLUCOCORTICOIDS)–*CONTINUED*

Nursing Diagnosis	Nursing Action	Rationale	Desired Outcomes/ Evaluation Criteria
excessive urination, dilute urine, weak/ thready pulses.	Monitor vital signs, noting postural changes, strength of peripheral pulses.	Postural hypotension is due in part to hypovolemia that results from aldosterone deficiency and from reduced cardiac output that results from cortisol deficiency.	
	Promote bedrest, assist with position changes and self-care activities. Caution patient not to change position too quickly.	Minimizes orthostatic hypotension, reducing risk of loss of consciousness and injury.	
	Administer fluids as indicated, e.g., 0.9% saline, glucose solutions.	May require up to 4–6 liters of fluid to achieve homeostasis.	
	Administer medications, e.g., cortisone or hydrocortisone; mineralocorticoids.	Drugs of choice to replace cortisol deficits and promote sodium reabsorption, which may reduce fluid losses and maintain cardiac output.	
	Monitor laboratory findings.	Elevated Hct levels reflect hemoconcentration; elevated BUN/Cr may reflect cellular breakdown; serum osmolality may be elevated due to dehydration; hyponatremia reflects urinary loss due to impaired tubule reabsorption; decreased aldosterone levels may result in hyperkalemia.	
Nutrition, Less than body requirements, Altered potential related to glucocorticoid deficiency; abnormal fat, protein, and carbohydrate metabolism.	Auscultate bowel sounds and assess for abdominal pain, nausea or vomiting.	Cortisol deficit can cause GI symptoms, affecting ingestion and absorption of nutrients.	Reports relief of nausea and vomiting. Demonstrates stable weight or weight gain toward desired goal with absence of presenting signs and normalization of laboratory values.
	Monitor dietary intake and weigh daily.	Aids in identifying nutritional needs and effectiveness of therapy.	
	Increase sodium in diet, e.g., meats, fish, poultry, milk, eggs.	May help to prevent/correct hyponatremia.	
	Administer medications, e.g., glucocorticoids;	Corrects hypoglycemia, provides energy source for cellular function. Stimulates gluconeogenesis, decreases utilization of glucose and promotes glucose storage as glycogen.	
	androgens;	May be useful in debilitated/malnourished patient to improve appetite, foster a positive nitrogen balance.	
	IV glucose as indicated. Perform finger-stick glucose testing as indicated.	Provides fluid replacement when needed. Evaluates serum glucose level/therapy needs.	
Adjustment, impaired, potential related to disability requiring change in lifestyle, assault to self-esteem, altered locus of control.	Arrange short periods of uninterrupted time and encourage patient to express feelings about effects of condition.	Fosters rapport and promotes openness on the part of the patient. Helps to evaluate how much of a problem the various changes are to the patient.	Verbalizes understanding of condition and need for treatment. Participates in treatment regimen. Initiates lifestyle changes that will permit adaptation to present life situation.

CONTINUED ON THE FOLLOWING PAGE

Table 42–5. NURSING PROCESS FOR PATIENT RECEIVING ADRENAL CORTICAL DRUGS (GLUCOCORTICOIDS)–*CONTINUED*

Nursing Diagnosis	Nursing Actions	Rationale	Desired Outcomes/ Evaluation Criteria
	Review possible side effects, e.g., redistribution of body fat, moon face, etc.	Cushingoid appearance may be very distressing and may affect patient's willingness to comply with drug regimen. Knowing that these changes are reversible when the drug is discontinued may be reassuring.	
	Discuss probability of mood swings occurring.	Provides anticipatory guidance so patient/SO can deal effectively with emotional lability.	
	Encourage participation of SO in problem-solving and planning.	Involvement of SO fosters understanding and adjustment to situation. Participation of SO helps patient to feel supported.	Improves present life situation.
	Encourage patient to make choices and participate in care.	May help to increase confidence level, improve self-esteem, decrease preoccupation with the changes and enhance sense of control.	
	Point out improvements that are occurring with treatment.	These comments may lift patient's spirits and promotes self-esteem/ adjustment to situation.	

sea, vomiting, bloody stools, hematemesis, and coffee-ground vomitus.

Baseline laboratory data is also obtained before the patient begins long-term glucocorticoid therapy. This data includes an ECG, chest and spinal x-rays, glucose tolerance test, Mantoux test for tuberculosis, CBC, and fluids and electrolyte balance. Measurement of ocular pressure is also performed. The nurse records baseline blood pressure, body weight, and hypothalamic-pituitary-adrenal axis function.

Physical examination of the patient with suspected adrenal cortical dysfunction may reveal some typical changes in physical appearance related to either an increase or a decrease in production of the hormones of the adrenal cortex. Table 42–6 summarizes the metabolic effects of adrenocortical dysfunction.

Diet, nutrition history, and history of weight control are also important items to assess. A nutrition consultation is often necessary, and baseline data is important. Also, a discussion of emotional stability is important.

Table 42–6. SUMMARY OF METABOLIC EFFECTS OF ADRENAL CORTEX DYSFUNCTION

	Hyperfunction (Cushing's Syndrome)	Hypofunction (Addison's Disease)
Carbohydrate	Hyperglycemia	Hypoglycemia
Protein	Protein wasting affecting skin, skeletal muscles, bone matrix, etc. Scanty hair growth Ecchymosis Poor wound healing Muscle weakness	
Fat	Redistribution of fat deposits Obesity of torso Cervicodorsal fat pad "Moon" face	
Fluid and electrolyte	Sodium retention Potassium loss Edema Hypertension	Sodium loss Potassium retention Hypovolemia Hypotension Muscle weakness

Often the patient on glucocorticoids has frequent mood swings and it is important to determine pretreatment patterns.

Because patients receiving glucocorticoids are more susceptible to infection, the patient is assessed carefully before and during therapy for signs of delayed wound healing, infection, and fever.

NURSING DIAGNOSES

When the patient assessment is complete, the nurse establishes the nursing diagnoses to facilitate the next step, planning of interventions. Some typical nursing diagnoses for a patient with adrenal cortical dysfunction are illustrated in Table 42–5.

INTERVENTION

Goals for nursing interventions are developed from the list of nursing diagnoses. Typical goals in caring for the patient requiring adrenal corticosteroids are included in Table 42–5.

NURSING RESPONSIBILITIES WHEN ADMINISTERING ADRENAL DRUGS

Safe administration of adrenal corticosteroid drugs depends on the nurse knowing specific information related to administration, patient safety, and patient teaching. This information is summarized in Table 42–1 in the column headed Nursing Implications.

Patients receiving glucocorticoids for inflammation are those most likely to experience adverse effects. These adverse effects generally result from the intensification of the basic functions of the hormones in the body (see Table 42–6). Although not all of these effects are preventable, careful nursing interventions are invaluable in detecting and managing these patient problems.

The nurse stresses to the patient that medications are taken exactly as prescribed. This is especially important to emphasize for patients who are on alternate-day therapy. Extra doses of medications are never taken nor is the dosage altered in any way; and medications are never stopped without first checking with the physician.

Patients who have been on long-term therapy (the equivalent of greater than 20 mg of hydrocortisone per day for longer than one to two weeks) are never abruptly withdrawn from corticosteroids. Rather, their dose is tapered off gradually. A reduction of 5–10 mg every three to seven days, as tolerated, may be employed.

Patients who have adrenocortical insufficiency need to increase corticosteroid dosage when subjected to physiologic stress. They should follow their physician's guidelines in these instances. Carrying a card or wearing a bracelet or necklace identifying their condition could be lifesaving in these circumstances.

As a rule, corticosteroids are taken with food or at mealtimes. Administration of the medications in the morning mimics the normal diurnal secretion of cortisol, which is highest in the early morning. If antacids are prescribed, the patient is encouraged to take these faithfully. Many physicians order the concomitant administration of a nonabsorbable antacid for patients on corticosteroids; although some feel that antacids are not helpful unless given on a very frequent basis, that is, hourly. Cautioning patients to restrict their intake of caffeine and alcohol is also necessary, as these substances increase gastric secretions, which can lead to the development of a peptic ulcer. Excessive use of aspirin or aspirin-containing compounds are avoided since the additional gastric irritation may initiate ulcer development. Testing the stools for occult blood at regular intervals to detect a bleeding ulcer is another important intervention in the care of the patient.

If sodium retention or potassium loss occurs, dietary sodium restriction or potassium supplementation, or both, may be helpful. Patients should follow their physician's orders in this regard.

Regular measurements of serum glucose levels are also performed. Known diabetics frequently need to have their insulin or oral hypoglycemic therapy altered to assist them in adapting to increases in blood glucose, and the nurse should anticipate this.

Skin testing for infectious diseases such as tuberculosis may be done prior to the institution of glucocorticoid therapy. If a patient has inactive or encapsulated tuberculosis, the administration of glucocorticoids may cause the tuberculosis to become active. Patients with encapsulated tuberculosis may need prophylactic antituberculosis therapy, usually isoniazid (INH), while concurrently taking their glucocorticoids.

The anti-inflammatory effects of the glucocorticoids may cause a delay in wound healing. The nurse is particularly alert to this in patients who undergo surgical procedures while on glucocorticoid therapy. The nurse must use meticulously sterile technique when dressing wounds and handling tubes and catheters. Also, white blood cell counts are performed routinely on patients receiving large doses and/or long-term therapy.

Since increases in intraocular pressure can occur, the nurse encourages patients to have regular tonometry testing.

Glucocorticoid administration can cause psychologic disturbances in some patients. The nurse must be alert to subtle changes in behavior such as restlessness, insomnia, and nightmares, as these may precede more serious disturbances.

Nursing interventions must also include well-defined emergency indicators for the patient, and instructions as to what to do should they occur. For example, the patient with Addison's disease who is subjected to stress needs to increase the dosage of corticosteroids according to the physician's guidelines. The occurrence of a sudden weight gain, weakness or undue fatigue, change in sleep patterns, black or tarry stools, injuries, or infections are reported to the physician.

PATIENT TEACHING

Table 42–7 summarizes the information concerning adrenal drugs that the nurse educator should include in the teaching plan for each patient.

Table 42–7. PATIENT TEACHING INFORMATION—ADRENAL CORTICAL DRUGS

Dear Patient:

This drug has been prescribed for you. This is what you should know about your drug to get the most from your therapy.

Adrenal drugs are used for many conditions. They are being used for you to _____.

1. Adrenal drugs (corticosteroids) are to be taken exactly as prescribed.
2. Extra doses of medication are NEVER to be taken, nor should you change your dose in any way. *Exception:* Patients who have adrenocortical insufficiency will need to increase corticosteroid dosage when subjected to physiologic stress; you should follow your doctor's instructions for times of stress.
3. Corticosteroids are taken with food to avoid stomach upset.
4. If your doctor prescribes it, be sure to faithfully take your antacids or anti-ulcer drugs while you are taking corticosteroids.
5. Check with your doctor or pharmacist before taking other drugs. Generally, you should not take aspirin or aspirin-containing drugs.
6. You should not drink much coffee, tea, or alcohol while taking corticosteroids (1 cup coffee or tea per day; 1 or 2 beers, 5 glasses of wine or shots of whiskey per week).
7. NEVER stop taking your corticosteroids without first talking to your doctor. *IMPORTANT:* If you have been taking corticosteroids for longer than 1–2 weeks, you MUST NOT stop taking them abruptly; your doctor will taper you off.
8. If you experience side effects from corticosteroids, check with your doctor. Common side effects include swelling of feet and hands, weight gain, nausea, and vomiting.
9. If you have an injury that does not heal or you develop an infection, call your doctor.
10. Have your blood pressure checked every week, as corticosteroids may increase it.
11. If you are taking corticosteroids for a long period of time, you should carry a bracelet or card with this information on it.
12. Store your corticosteroids in a light-resistant, tightly closed bottle.

EVALUATION

During the evaluation phase of the nursing process, the nurse determines the effectiveness of the adrenal corticosteroid medications. This evaluation is based on outcomes determined by the nurse and patient. Typical outcomes for a patient requiring adrenal corticosteroids are included in Table 42–5.

The nurse is familiar with the adverse effects of the adrenal corticosteroids and evaluates the patient's understanding of them. Sodium retention, potassium loss, hypertension, muscle wasting, and peptic ulceration can occur with long-term use. See Table 42–1 for a listing of other adverse effects.

The majority of patients requiring adrenal corticosteroids comply with their medication regimen since they note improvements in their symptomatology. Occasionally, a few "over comply," rationalizing that if some amount of corticosteroid makes them feel better, taking more will cause an even greater improvement. Patients on alternate-day therapy may need a great deal of encouragement and support to stay on their medication schedule.

The cushingoid appearance, caused by long-term glucocorticoid use, can be very disturbing to patients and may interfere with compliance for some. Again, nursing support and encouragement are important for these patients. The knowledge that the cushingoid changes reverse themselves on discontinuance of therapy may be helpful.

The nurse stresses the need for continued medical follow-up and should periodically review his or her teaching with the patient in order to ensure that the patient's knowledge is accurate, complete, and up to date.

SUMMARY

Several adrenal cortical hormones are secreted by the adrenal gland including the mineralocorticoids, the glucocorticoids, and the gonadal hormones. The natural mineralocorticoid—aldosterone— is the prototype, but it is not used due to its high cost and limited availability.

The mineralocorticoids act primarily on the kidney to enhance reabsorption of sodium and chloride ions and, thus, water absorption. Therefore, these products help to maintain cardiac output and blood pressure. The synthetic mineralocorticoids are used in replacement therapy for patients with adrenocortical insufficiency and for salt-losing adrenogenital syndromes.

Glucocorticoids are available as both natural and synthetic products. They are used for replacement therapy as well as for their anti-inflammatory, and anti-lymphocytic effects. Glucocorticoids are also used to decrease transplant rejection. The glucocorticoids have many adverse effects.

As the nurse administers glucocorticoids, he or she must assess current and past history of gastrointestinal upset, ulcers, or epigastric pain, as steroids may cause or activate an ulcer. The nurse also carefully assesses for signs of infection and delayed wound healing. Patient teaching is very important as it is imperative for the patient to take these products specifically as ordered. Several different dosing schedules are possible, including daily or alternate-day regimens. Patients are taught the side effects to be expected and what can be done about them.

BIBLIOGRAPHY

American Medical Association Department of Drugs, Division of Drugs and Technology: Drug Evaluation, 6th ed. WB Saunders, Philadelphia, 1986.

Covington, TR: Topical steroids—Guidelines for use. Drug Newsletter 7(5):38, 1988.

Covington, TR: Adrenal corticosteroids—glucocorticoids. Drug Newsletter 8(7):52, 1989.

Facts and Comparisons: Glucocorticoid Equivalencies. St. Louis, MO, June 1986.

Gilman, AG, Goodman, LS, and Gilman, A: Goodman and Gilman's The Pharmacological Basis of Therapeutics, ed 7. Macmillan, New York, 1985.

Petersdorf, RG, et al (eds): Harrison's Principles of Internal Medicine, ed 10. McGraw-Hill, New York, 1987.

Segarneck, DJ: Steroids. American Association of Head Nurses 35(6):286, June 1987.

Tepperman, J and Tepperman, H: Metabolic & Endocrine Physiology, ed 5. Year Book Medical Publishers, Chicago, 1987.

SITUATION   42–1

Mac Rubin is a 55-year-old undergoing diagnostic testing for suspected Addison's disease. He is being cared for on a medical floor.

1. After obtaining baseline 24-hour urine samples for 17-KS, 17-KGS, and 17-OHCS, the nurse administers dexamethasone and ACTH as ordered. A second 24-hour urine specimen is obtained for the same values. The nurse is aware that the following results correlate with a diagnosis of primary adrenal insufficiency:
   a. increase in urinary steroid levels threefold
   b. decrease in urinary steroid levels threefold
   c. no increase in urinary steroid levels
   d. increase in urinary steroid levels tenfold

2. Mr. Rubin is to receive desoxycorticosterone acetate (DOCA) 5 mg intramuscularly. After giving the drug, the nurse will monitor the following:
   a. attention span
   b. fine motor movement
   c. deep tendon reflexes
   d. blood pressure

3. In planning care for Mr. Rubin after initiating therapy DOCA, the nurse will include the following nursing measure:
   a. Maintain the patient NPO until two days past first dose.
   b. Force oral fluids at 73000 cc per day.

   c. Reduce protein and sodium intake.
   d. Encourage a diet high in potassium.

4. For discharge, Mr. Rubin is to begin cortisone acetate (Cortone) 25 mg orally three times a day. Patient teaching should focus on:
   a. taking the drug on an empty stomach
   b. stopping the medication if drowsiness occurs
   c. using aspirin-containing products as needed
   d. avoiding excessive intake of coffee and alcohol

5. An anticipated outcome of therapy for Mr. Rubin would be:
   a. less fatigue
   b. increased cardiac output
   c. increased urine output
   d. altered consciousness

6. When providing follow-up care for Mr. Rubin, the nurse will check the following laboratory result, which tends to elevate due to steroid therapy:
   a. cholesterol
   b. T_3
   c. potassium
   d. T_4

SITUATION   42–2

Ralph Kuper is a 62-year-old admitted to the emergency room in acute respiratory distress related to status asthmaticus.

1. In addition to respiratory inhalation treatments, Mr. Kuper is to receive methylprednisolone sodium succinate (Solu-Medrol) intravenously. Prior to administering this drug, the nurse will assess for the following condition, which represents the need for cautious administration:
   a. coronary artery disease
   b. chronic lung disease
   c. peptic ulcer disease
   d. urinary retention

2. When administering 1 gram of solu-Medrol intravenously to Mr. Kuper, the nurse will infuse the medication over:
   a. 60 minutes
   b. 20 minutes
   c. 2 hours
   d. 4 hours

3. After initial emergency treatment, Mr. Kuper is transferred to a telemetry unit. A nursing history reveals that he has adult onset diabetes which is controlled by oral medication. Because he is receiving glucocorticoids, the nurse is aware of the potential for:
   a. reduced blood glucose levels
   b. increased effect of hypoglycemic agents
   c. reduced effectiveness of Solu-Medrol
   d. increased blood glucose levels

4. Before Mr. Rubin begins long-term therapy with steroids

as anti-inflammatory agents, the nurse will anticipate the following test:
   a. Tensilon
   b. tuberculosis
   c. ACTH stimulation
   d. creatinine clearance

5. Mr. Rubin is to use a beclomethasone (Vanceril) inhaler prn for asthma attacks. Which statement indicates adequate understanding of its use?
   a. "Since it is habit forming, I shouldn't use it every day."
   b. "If I have to use the drug more often than prescribed, I will call the doctor."
   c. "Nausea and vomiting are side effects to be expected with this drug."
   d. "I should keep the inhaler in a dry, warm place when it is not in use."

6. Mr. Rubin will be discharged on prednisone 5 mg po q d. The nurse will plan the following goal for him:
   a. maintenance on short-term therapy at lowest dose possible
   b. elimination of all symptoms associated with asthma
   c. maintenance on long-term glucocorticoid therapy
   d. elimination of all side effects associated with prednisone

Please refer to Appendices for correct answers and additional review questions with answers.

43

HORMONES: MALE AND FEMALE

MERRILY MATHEWSON KUHN, R.N.C., Ph.D., CCRN

LEARNING OBJECTIVES

After reading this chapter, the student will be able to:

1. Identify those medications commonly used as male and female hormones and those used to treat disorders of the reproductive systems.

2. Differentiate among the male and female hormones as to mechanisms of action, route of administration, pharmacokinetics, adverse effects, contraindications, and interactions.

3. Identify specific areas to assess in the patient requiring male and female hormones in order to formulate appropriate nursing diagnoses.

4. Plan the nursing intervention necessary to administer male and female hormones and choose appropriate teaching strategies to gain patient compliance.

5. Evaluate the patient at various stages to determine the effectiveness of nursing interventions.

This chapter deals with several widely used drugs. Male hormones are discussed, both as androgenic and anabolic therapies. Female hormones are also discussed, again related to their variety of uses, including that of contraception.

This chapter also reviews other medications that in some manner affect the female reproductive system. Drugs that are used to treat infertility and to treat premenstrual syndrome are discussed in the following pages.

THERAPEUTIC AGENTS—MALE HORMONES

ANDROGENS

The testes, the male sex organs, produce and secrete *androgens*, the male sex hormones. *Proandrogens* are also synthesized in the ovaries and adrenal glands. Cholesterol is the common precursor of the biosynthesis of the androgens. Testosterone, the principal androgen, is synthesized in the greatest amounts in the male testes by the interstitial cells of Leydig in response to stimulation by the gonadotropic hormones (interstitial cell–stimulating hormone) of the adenohypophysis. A negative feedback system involving the hypothalamus, the anterior pituitary, and the testes controls hormone secretion.

Action

Although concentrations of testosterone are high in male infants, prepubertal levels are low (0–20 ng/dL). In the adult male, concentrations range from 350 to 1000 ng/dL, with about 2.5–10 mg (average 8–9 mg) of testosterone being produced each day. In men, approximately 98 percent of circulating testosterone is bound to protein.

In most body tissues, with the exception of skeletal muscle and bone marrow, testosterone is converted to dihydrotestosterone (DHT), the active form of the hormone. At the cellular level, DHT binds to cytoplasmic protein receptors and is transferred to the nucleus; eventually, through increased synthesis of RNA, an increase in protein synthesis occurs.

In the male fetus, testosterone is necessary for the differentiation, growth, and development of the male sexual organs. During puberty, testosterone is necessary for the development of the primary sex characteristics of the male, causing increased growth of the penis, scrotum, and testes. The male secondary sex characteristics are also influenced by the action of testosterone. The male pattern of hair growth, enlargement of the larynx leading to a deepening of the voice, increased thickness of the skin, and increased activity of the sebaceous glands are all caused by the action of testosterone.

In women, androgens are responsible for the growth of pubic hair and, possibly, for stimulation of libido. They also act as estrogen precursors, particularly after menopause. Excessive production of androgens leads to masculinizing effects such as acne, hirsutism, hoarseness, menstrual irregularities, permanent deepening of the voice, and clitoral enlargement.

Testosterone also has anabolic activity. By increasing the rate of amino acid transfer into the cells, it produces several changes. A positive nitrogen balance is achieved, an increase in musculature occurs, and an increase in bone thickness and calcium deposition leads to greater length and size of the bones. In the presence of testosterone, basal metabolic rate and red blood cell production are both increased. Finally, testosterone has some salt- and water-retaining properties, causing men to have a greater blood and extracellular fluid volume than women. During administration of exogenous androgens, endogenous testosterone release is inhibited through feedback inhibition of pituitary luteinizing hormone. Large doses of androgens may suppress spermatogenesis through feedback inhibition of pituitary follicle-stimulating hormone.

Uses

There are several indications for the use of androgens in clinical practice. Basically, testosterone and similar compounds are administered for their androgenic properties or for their anabolic properties. Although several anabolic steroids with minimal androgenic properties have been developed, it is important to remember that all of these drugs have both effects to some extent. Androgens may be used to replace androgen deficiencies in states of *hypogonadism* or decreased testosterone production.

The longer-acting esters of testosterone, testosterone cypionate (Depo-Testosterone) or testosterone enanthate (Delatestryl), are usually preferred for therapy and need to be administered intramuscularly, on a regular basis, until the sexual characteristics have developed. Following this, one of the shorter-acting oral preparations, such as fluoxymesterone (Halotestin) or methyltestosterone (Metandren), can be substituted.

The postpubertal male may be treated with the oral androgen preparations as replacement therapy. In the adult male, replacement of testosterone should supply approximately 10 mg/day. All products need to be administered on a lifelong basis, with dosages adjusted to the individual.

Cryptorchidism (undescended testes) is another condition where testosterone therapy is used. Administration of exogenous testosterone to boys with undescended testes may prompt descent of these organs into the scrotum. Human chorionic gonadotropin, a natural polypeptide hormone produced by the human placenta, can also be used for this purpose.

Several disorders in the female are often treated by androgen administration. *Endometriosis*, a condition in which ectopic endometrial tissue implants occur, is treated with androgens. Androgens antagonize the effects of estrogen and cause suppression of gonadotropin secretion. Endometriosis can be treated with a synthetic androgen, danazol (Danocrine). Danazol has mild androgenic properties and causes pituitary suppression of follicle-stimulating hormone (FSH) and luteinizing hormone (LH), leading to anovulation, amenorrhea, and involution of endometrial implants. However, danazol is very expensive to use. For most patients, the use of progestins or combined oral contraceptives is just as effective, with the added advantage of having no androgenic effects. Danazol is also used to partially or completely relieve the breast pain, tenderness, and nodularity in women with fibrocystic breast disease.

Androgens may also be used in the treatment of postpartum breast engorgement. Administered for 1 to 4 days postpartum, these medications cause minimal side effects; however, there is no satisfactory evidence that they prevent or suppress lactation.

In females, androgens may also be utilized in the palliative therapy of metastatic breast malignancies in postmenopausal women. Testolactone (Teslac) possesses little androgenic activity in therapeutic doses and has been found to be effective in the treatment of some patients with estrogen-responsive tumors. However, masculinizing side effects occur frequently at the dosages needed to interfere with tumor growth. The effects, such as deepening of voice or altered hair growth, that occur in women on androgen therapy are often permanent and do not reverse with termination of the drug. In the treatment of breast cancer, many clinicians prefer to use the shorter-acting oral preparations rather than the sustained-acting parenteral preparations. In this way, should adverse effects occur, the drug can be withdrawn quickly. Tamoxifen (Nolvadex), an estrogen antagonist, offers an alternative to androgen therapy causing no distressing masculinizing effects.

Senile or postmenopausal osteoporosis may be treated with anabolic steroids, taking advantage of the fact that the androgens increase calcium deposition in bones. These drugs may also be administered to offset the osteoporosis that can occur with long-term use of glucocorticoid therapy. However, because there is no objective evidence that they are superior to estrogens and because of their masculinizing effects, these agents are not commonly used for this indication. Estrogen therapy may be preferred.

Anabolic steroids also are used in the treatment of mild to moderate aplastic and hemolytic anemias, as well as those anemias associated with chronic renal failure, lymphoma, and leukemia. It is believed that androgens stimulate the production of erythropoietin by the kidney, leading to an increase in red blood cell production.

The anabolic effects of androgens make them useful in a variety of other conditions, and there are a number of preparations available, administered either orally or parenterally. Although the androgenic effects of these preparations are minimal, they are still present, especially if large dosages are employed. The use of anabolic steroids to improve athletic performance is "contrary to the ethical principles of athletic competition and is deplored" (American College of Sports Medicine, 1984). Even with conflicting results from numerous studies, many athletes feel that they benefit from ingesting large quantities of these agents. The use of anabolic steroids in athletes is apparently widespread due to the per-

ceived beneficial effects such as: increased muscular strength, heightened aggressive tendencies, more energy, and the ability to train more intensively. Serious adverse effects associated with large doses include: altered liver function tests and liver cancer in both sexes; deepening of the voice, decreased libido, and altered hair growth in women; and decreased testicular size and depressed spermatogenesis in men. Retention of salt and fluid may cause hypertension, while blood cholesterol levels may rise.

Lastly, the anabolic steroids are used in many debilitating diseases to improve appetite, foster a positive nitrogen balance, cause weight gain, and promote a feeling of well-being. These drugs may be used in patients recovering from extensive surgery, burns, trauma, or infection and in emaciated, debilitated patients. In these instances, it has been found that beneficial effects of the anabolic steroids are related to an adequate dietary intake of calories and protein by the patient. Although there are no adequate clinical trials proving efficacy, use of anabolic agents as adjunctive or supportive therapy in such conditions, particularly in terminal patients, may be helpful.

Pharmacokinetics

As with many of the other medications affecting the endocrine system, exogenous administration of testosterone causes the same physiologic effects as the endogenous hormone. Synthetic forms of the hormone vary somewhat in their potencies, durations of action, and absorption following oral administration. Synthetics may also vary in their ratios of androgenic activity to anabolic activity. Currently, no preparation is available that provides anabolic effects without the androgenic effects.

Testosterone is readily absorbed from the gastrointestinal tract; however, it is also relatively ineffective given orally, since most of it is metabolized by the liver (high first-pass effect) before reaching the systemic circulation. The synthetic androgens are less extensively metabolized by the liver and have longer half-lives. Parenteral administration is often used. Testosterone may be administered intramuscularly or via the use of slow-release subcutaneous pellets implanted beneath the skin surface, usually in the thigh. The effects of esters of testosterone, testosterone cypionate (Depo-Testosterone), and testosterone enanthate (Delatestryl), last two to four weeks; testosterone and testosterone propionate (Oreton Propionate) must be administered several times a week. Methyltestosterone (Metandren) may also be administered as buccal tablets.

In the blood, 98 to 99 percent of testosterone is bound to proteins: sex hormone–binding globulin, cortisol-binding globulin, and albumin. Only about one percent of testosterone is free, or available for use. The serum half-life of testosterone is about 10–20 minutes. Synthetic androgens have a longer half-life ranging from two and a half hours to eight days. Testosterone is inactivated in the liver, where it is converted to androsterone and androstenedione. The metabolites are excreted mostly into the urine (90 percent) as 17-ketosteroids and also are eliminated into the feces (6 percent).

Contraindications and Precautions

There are several conditions in which androgen use is contraindicated including: pregnancy and lactation, as the use of androgens may lead to precocious puberty in males and masculinization in females; carcinoma of the prostate or male breast, which may be stimulated by androgens; hepatic disease, which may be exacerbated (see Adverse Effects below); prostatic hypertrophy, which is increased; and coronary artery disease, because of the retention of fluids and alteration of cholesterol levels.

Androgens are given cautiously to patients who have experienced allergic reactions during previous androgen therapy and to elderly males as their risk of developing prostatic hypertrophy and prostatic carcinoma are increased.

Adverse Effects

As with other hormones, the administration of androgens is not without problems. The occurrence of adverse effects is related to dosage and length of administration. Given at replacement doses to men with hypogonadism, adverse effects are usually minimal. The woman requiring androgen therapy in the treatment of metastatic breast cancer, on the other hand, will probably experience many distressing and often permanent adverse effects, such as masculinization.

In both sexes, nausea, vomiting, gastric irritation, and diarrhea may occur with the administration of oral preparations. Taking the oral preparations with food may decrease these symptoms. The use of buccal tablets may irritate the oral mucosa, and stomatitis can occur. Local inflammation and induration can follow administration of intramuscular preparations. Inflammation at the site of pellet implantation can also occur, in severe cases causing skin sloughing and subsequent loss of the pellets. The pellets are usually implanted as an outpatient procedure.

In both sexes, some nervous system changes may be noted. Sleeplessness and excitation may occur, as may changes in libido. Psychotic symptoms, including hallucinations, delusions, and manic episodes have all been reported as adverse effects of anabolic steroids in large doses.

Sodium and water retention may occur, leading to edema, especially in the elderly patient or in the patient with cardiovascular disease. This occurs most often with larger doses of androgens and can usually be controlled with dietary salt restriction or diuretic therapy.

Allergic reactions to testosterone or its salts are rather rare, but may range from urticaria to frank anaphylaxis. For this reason, it is important to ascertain in the medical history whether or not the patient has ever experienced an allergic reaction to previous androgen therapy.

In both sexes, hepatic dysfunction can occur during androgen therapy. Cholestatic hepatitis has been noted

and tends to occur in greater frequency with larger doses. Patients need to understand the importance of reporting such signs and symptoms as darkened urine, pruritus, and color changes in the skin and sclera. Liver tests (bilirubin, LDH, SGOT, alkaline phosphatase) are monitored regularly, and increases in these levels may warrant termination of therapy. Hepatic carcinoma has developed in some patients on prolonged (one to seven years) therapy.

Androgen therapy may alter serum cholesterol levels; therefore, patients with coronary artery disease are monitored carefully and cholesterol levels are determined periodically during therapy.

Androgen therapy may alter the results of diagnostic tests. Creatinine levels may increase as well as T_3 uptake. Excretion of 17-ketosteroids, and the production of clotting factors II, V, VII, and X may be decreased.

In boys being treated with androgens, determinations of bone maturation are vital in order to prevent early epiphyseal closure prompted by androgens. In addition, signs and symptoms of precocious puberty may occur, including phallic enlargement and growth of facial and body hair. *Priapism* may occur in the initial stages of therapy but usually subsides with continued treatment.

Adult males being treated with androgens may develop breast tenderness and, occasionally, gynecomastia. Impotence and azoospermia may also develop, as prolonged androgen therapy tends to inhibit gonadotropin secretion. Administration of 25 mg of testosterone propionate daily for six weeks has been shown to decrease spermatogenesis.

Women requiring androgen therapy, especially those receiving it for disseminated breast cancer, tend to develop virilizing effects. Hoarseness, or deepening of the voice, and changes in libido are early indications of this and are watched carefully. Growth of facial hair, acne, baldness, decreased breast size, and menstrual irregularities can occur. Unfortunately, some of the masculinizing changes may be permanent and will not reverse with the discontinuation of therapy. The benefits of androgen therapy as opposed to adverse effects must be carefully weighed.

Another adverse effect of androgen therapy that occurs most often in women with breast cancer and bone metastases is hypercalcemia. Therefore, the onset of the representative symptoms of nausea, vomiting, anorexia, constipation, polyuria, and muscle weakness should be reported immediately. Generally, these will necessitate termination of androgen therapy.

Interactions

Androgens can interact with other medications. Sensitivity to oral anticoagulants is increased, as are the hypoglycemic effects of insulin and the oral hypoglycemic agents. Concomitant use of androgens with adrenal corticosteroids may tend to enhance the occurrence of edema, since both have a tendency to cause water retention.

Androgens, both androgenic and anabolic, are summarized in Table 43–1.

Androgenic Steroids

TESTOSTERONE. In men, testosterone (Andro 100) is used primarily for its androgenic effects to treat *eunuchism* and male climacteric symptoms. Testosterone is used to treat breast cancer in postmenopausal women and breast engorgement in postpartum women. Testosterone is administered in intramuscular doses of 25–50 mg, two to three times weekly. Palliation of mammary cancer is treated with 50–100 mg, three times weekly.

TESTOSTERONE PROPIONATE. Testosterone propionate (Testex) is used for the same purposes as testosterone. Testosterone propionate is administerd in intramuscular doses of 25–100 mg, two to four times weekly.

TESTOSTERONE ENANTHATE AND TESTOSTERONE CYPIONATE. Both testosterone enanthate (Delatestryl) and testosterone cypionate (Depo-Testosterone) are used for the same purposes as testosterone. In addition, testosterone enanthate is used to treat oligospermia (insufficient sperm in the semen). Testosterone enanthate and testosterone cypionate are adiministered intramuscularly every four to six weeks in doses of 50–400 mg. They have a duration of action of two to four weeks. Crystals may dissolve with warming or shaking of vial.

METHYLTESTOSTERONE. Methyltestosterone (Metandren) is used for the same purposes as testosterone. In addition, methyltestosterone is also used to treat postpubertal cryptorchidism. Methyltestosterone is administered orally in dosages of 10–80 mg in divided doses. Buccal tablets are also available and are given in dosages of 5–20 mg/day. Up to 200 mg/day may be given for the treatment of breast cancer.

FLUOXYMESTERONE. Fluoxymesterone (Halotestin) is used primarily to treat hypogonadism and impotence caused by testicular deficiency. It can also be used in women to treat postpartum breast engorgement and as a pallative treatment for breast cancer. Fluoxymesterone is administered orally in doses of 2.5–20 mg/day.

DANAZOL. Danazol (Danocrine) is a synthetic androgen which, like other androgens, suppresses the pituitary-ovarian axis by inhibiting the output of pituitary gonadotropins. Danazol also depresses the output of follicle-stimulating hormone and luteinizing hormone. Danazol is primarily used in women to treat endometriosis and fibrocystic breast disease. Danazol is administered orally in doses of 400 mg twice a day and is continued for three to six months.

Anabolic Steroids

Anabolic steroids reserve catabolic processes and promote bodybuilding processes. These products can be used in patients who are underweight due to a recent illness; in patients with senile or illness-produced osteoporosis; and in patients with certain types of anemias.

These are the products that are often abused by athletes. Although a small number of athletes may derive some benefit with anabolic steroids, the serious side effects minimize any real or perceived gain in performance.

ETHYLESTRENOL. Ethylestrenol (Maxibolin) promotes weight gain and combats tissue depletion from refractory anemias, corticosteroid therapy, osteoporosis, prolonged immobilization, and various debilitated states. Therapy should not exceed 6 weeks, but after a four-week interval, therapy can be continued again for six weeks. Ethylestrenol is administerd orally in doses of 4–8 mg/day.

NANDROLONE PHENPROPIONATE. Nandrolone phenpropionate (Durabolin) is used primarily to control metastatic breast cancer. Nandrolone phenpropionate is available as an intramuscular injection with a dose range of 50–100 mg/week.

NANDROLONE DECANOATE. Nandrolone decanoate (Deca-Durabolin) is primarily used to treat refractory anemia and to build tissue. Nandrolone decanoate is administered intramuscularly in doses of 50–100 mg/ week.

OXANDROLONE. Oxandrolone (Anavar) is used to promote weight gain after excessive surgery, chronic infection, trauma, or other causes of weight loss. It is also used to offset bone pain of osteoporosis. Oxandrolone is administered orally in dosages of 2.5–20 mg/day in divided doses.

OXYMETHOLONE. Oxymetholone (Anadrol) is used to treat anemias caused by deficient red cells, acquired or congenital aplastic anemia, myelofibrosis, and myelotoxic drugs. Oxymetholone is administered orally in doses of 1–5 mg/kg/day.

STANOZOLOL. Stanozolol (Winstrol) is used to treat hereditary angioedema. Stanozolol is administered daily in oral dosages of two to six mg divided in several doses.

Combination androgen and anabolic steroids are presented in Table 43–2.

USING THE NURSING PROCESS

ASSESSMENT

Assessment of the patient requiring male sex hormones for either their androgenic or their anabolic properties can be complex. An accurate health history, as part of the data base, is helpful for the nurse in determining for what conditions the patient requires androgen therapy, and in preparing the nursing care plan. Table 43–3 summarizes the information the nurse obtains.

Hypogonadism may be suspected when a male has not reached puberty at the expected age. Since variances in developmental rates are normal, it is not uncommon to wait until the patient is in his late teens to carefully assess his endocrine function. These patients often have characteristic body features, which, when noted in the physical examination, can point toward a hypogonadal state. Excessive growth of long bones, high-pitched

TEXT RESUMES ON PAGE 1110

Table 43–1. MALE HORMONES

Name	Dosage	Mode of Administration	Pharmacokinetics
ANDROGENIC STEROIDS:			
Action: Differentiation, growth, and development of male sexual organs, increases muscle and bone growth.			
Use: Replacement therapy, cryptorchidism, endometriosis, postpartum breast engorgement, breast cancer.			
			For all androgenic steroids: O: rapid P: UA D: UA ½L: UA PB: 98% B: liver E: urine, feces
Testosterone (Andro 100)	25–50 mg, 2–3 times/wk	IM	½L: 10–100 min
Testosterone propionate (Testex)	25–100 mg, 2–4 times/wk	IM	½L: 10–100 min
Testosterone enanthate (Delatestryl)	50–400 mg q 4–6 wk	IM	½L: 10–100 min D: 2–4 wk
Testosterone cypionate (Depo-Testosterone)	50–400 mg q 4–6 wk	IM	½L: 8 days D: 2–4 wk
Methyltestosterone (Metandren)	10–80 mg/day in divided doses	PO	½L: 2.5–3.0 hr
	5–20 mg/day	Buccal	
Fluoxymesterone (Halotestin)	2.5–20.0 mg/day	PO	½L: 9.2–10.0 hr
SYNTHETIC ANDROGENS			
Danazol (Danocrine)	400 mg, 2 times daily, 3–6 months	PO	O: UA P: UA D: UA ½L: 4.5 hr B: liver E: UA

Key to Abbreviations in the *Pharmacokinetics* column O-onset; P-peak; D-duration; PB-protein bound; B-bio-transformed in; E-excreted in; ½ L-halflife.
*Within the column listing adverse effects, underlines indicate the most common effects.

Contraindications/ Precautions	Adverse Effects*	Interactions	Nursing Implications
For all androgenic steroids: CONTRAINDICATIONS: Pregnancy, lactation, cancer of prostate or male breast, liver disease, prostatic hypertrophy, and coronary artery disease. PRECAUTIONS: Use cautiously in persons who have experienced previous allergic reactions and in elderly patients.	For all androgenic steroids: *Neuro:* sleeplessness, excitation, psychotic symptoms, headache, anxiety, depression *CV:* Sodium and water retention, elevated serum cholesterol *GI:* nausea, vomiting, diarrhea, gastric irritation, (buccal—stomatitis) *Biliary:* hepatitis *Hemo:* suppression of clotting factors *Reprod:* Female: amenorrhea, deepening voice, clitoral enlargement; Male: gynecomastia, excessive penile erections, testicular atrophy, acne, facial hair *Integ:* pellet—skin irritation, sloughing, hirsutism	Androgens: Increased sensitivity to oral anticoagulants. Increased hypoglycemic effects of insulin or oral hypoglycemics. Concomitant use with adrenal steroids increases edema. Lab: Suppresses clotting factors II, V, VII, X; increases creatinine levels, decreases 17-ketosteroid excretion.	ASSESSMENT: Obtain baseline weight and blood pressure. INTERVENTION: *Oral:* Take shortly before or with meals. Protect from light. Store in dry, tightly closed containers. *IM:* Inject deeply into gluteal muscles. Rotate injection sites. Shake vials to disperse medication evenly. Store at room temperature. *Buccal:* Place under tongue or between gums and cheek. Change location with each dose. Do not chew or swallow. Do not eat, drink, or smoke until tablet is absorbed. *All routes:* Check weight regularly. Carry an identification card or wear jewelry to identify the drug use. EVALUATION: Report weight gain, nausea, vomiting, priapism, or jaundice to physician.
CONTRAINDICATIONS: Undiagnosed abnormal genital bleeding; impaired hepatic, renal, or cardiac function; pregnancy and lactation. PRECAUTIONS: Use with caution in patients with edema.	*CVR:* flushing, weight gain *GI:* nausea, vomiting *Biliary:* hepatic dysfunction *Reprod:* clitoral hypertrophy, testicular atrophy, changes in libido, decreased breast size *Integ:* acne, mild hirsuitism, oily skin/hair *EENT:* deepening of voice	Insulin requirements may increase. Prolonged PT with concurrent warfarin.	ASSESSMENT: Determine method of birth control. A nonhormonal method needs to be used. Needs to be discontinued if pregnancy occurs. EVALUATION: Notify physician if masculinizing effects occur.

CONTINUED ON THE FOLLOWING PAGE

Table 43–1. MALE HORMONES–*CONTINUED*

Name	Dosage	Mode of Administration	Pharmacokinetics
ANABOLIC STEROIDS			
Action: Promotes body tissue building process.			
Use: For weight gain, osteoporosis, certain anemias.			
Ethylestrenol (Maxibolin)	*Adult:* 4–8 mg/day	PO	O: UA
	Pediatric: average 2 mg/day	PO	P: UA
Nandrolone phenpropionate (Durabolin)	50–100 mg/wk	IM	D: UA
Nandrolone decanoate (Deca-Durabolin)	*Adult:* 50–100 mg/wk	IM	
	Pediatric: 2–13 yr: 25–50 mg q 3–4 wk	IM	
Oxandrolone (Anavar)	*Adult:* 2.5–20.0 mg/day in divided doses	PO	½L: UA
			PB: UA
	Pediatric: 2–13 yr: 0.1–0.25 mg/kg/day		B: UA
			E: UA
Oxymetholone (Anadrol)	1–5 mg/kg	PO	
Stanozolol (Winstrol)	2–6 mg/day in divided doses	PO	

Key to Abbreviations in the *Pharmacokinetics* column O-onset; P-peak; D-duration; PB-protein bound; B-biotransformed in; E-excreted in; ½ L-halflife.
*Within the column listing adverse effects, underlines indicate the most common effects.

voice, poor musculature, absence of male pattern hair growth, and small external genitalia are termed eunuchoid features.

In a sexually mature male, the features of hypogonadism differ. Some feminization occurs in physical appearance. The beard thins, there is an increased accumulation of subcutaneous fat, muscle strength declines, gynecomastia may occur, and external genitalia atrophy. In addition, libido declines and impotence and sterility occur.

Often men come for a medical examination because of complaints of decreased libido and impotence. It is important for the nurse who is doing a sexual history to be open and empathetic. Patients are often confused and embarrassed about their lack of desire or their lack of arousal even though desire is present.

Important factors that affect sexual function include: the individual's own self-worth or self-esteem, his general health and age, his partner's ability and interest, and the environment. It is also important to take a drug history. Many drugs can affect sexuality or sexual functioning. Drugs may do this as a direct or indirect effect or as an adverse effect. Drugs can directly reduce sexual desire by making it difficult to produce or maintain an erection. Indirectly, drugs can cause depression, drowsiness, mental confusion, or nausea, all of which affect sexuality. Adverse effects of drugs can also cause difficulties with erection and ejaculation, or cause crooked erections due to hardening of tissue within the penis. Table 43–4 features commonly used drugs and their possible sexual side effects.

Various diagnostic tests are used to determine whether the hypogonadal state is primary, due to testicular dysfunction, or secondary, due to pituitary disorders. Buccal smears may be taken in the young male to rule out chromosomal abnormalities leading to testicu-

Table 43–2. COMBINATION DRUGS FOR ANDROGENS AND ANABOLIC STEROIDS

Combination Drug	Basic Products (mg)*						
	A	B	C	D	E	F	G
Deladumone Injection	90	4					
Depo-Testadiol Injection	50	2					
Ditate-DS Injection	180	8					
Duo-Cyp Injection	50	2					
Premarin with Methyl-testosterone Tablets						1.250	10
						0.625	5
Halodrin tablets			0.02	1			
Estratest					1.25		2.5

*Basic products: A = testosterone enanthate; B = estradiol valerate; C = ethinyl estradiol; D = fluoxymesterone; E = esterified estrogen; F = conjugated estrogens; G = methyltestosterone.

Contraindications/ Precautions	Adverse Effects*	Interactions	Nursing Implications
For all anabolic steroids: CONTRAINDICATIONS: Hypersensitivity, males with prostatic or breast cancer, females with breast cancer, nephrosis, history of myocardial infarction, hepatic dysfunction, pregnancy. PRECAUTIONS: Use with caution in patients with congestive heart failure and elderly patients.	For all anabolic steroids: *Neuro:* excitation, insomnia, chills *CVR:* increased serum cholesterol, ankle swelling *GI:* nausea, vomiting, diarrhea, abdominal fullness *Bilary:* hepatic necrosis, neoplasm *Renal:* sodium retention *Reprod:* Females: hirsutism, clitoral enlargement; Males: inhibition of testicular function	Potentiates anticoagulants. Insulin and oral hypoglycemics may need to be decreased. Steroids may increase tendency toward edema.	ASSESSMENT: baseline blood glucose should be obtained in diabetic patients and checked periodically during therapy. INTERVENTION: Take with food, may cause GI upset. EVALUATION: Notify physician if nausea, vomiting, change in skin color, or ankle swelling occur.

lar dysfunction. Testicular biopsies may also be done to rule out possible anatomic abnormalities of the testes. Testosterone levels, measured by immunoassay, are also determined. The hypogonadal male has testosterone deficiency. Measurement of urinary excretion of the metabolites of the androgens is also used in the clinical assessment, as the testicular androgens comprise about one third of the total 17-ketosteroid excretion in adult males. Collection of a 24-hour urine sample is required for this test.

To assess pituitary function in suspected hypogonadism, blood and urine levels of the gonadotropins are measured by immunoassay. Low levels of these are found when the testosterone deficiency is related to pituitary dysfunction. It is important for the nurse to remember that gonadotropin deficiency may signal more widespread pituitary dysfunction; ideally, this finding in patients should prompt a workup for pituitary disease which may include skull x-rays, visual examinations, and determination of levels of other pituitary hormones.

Assessment of patients requiring anabolic steroids focuses on their nutritional status and includes body weights, both past and current; serum protein determinations to give a picture of nitrogen and protein balance; and a complete blood count. The physical examination may show a patient who is underweight to varying degrees and weak, with a poor appetite and poor food intake.

NURSING DIAGNOSES

Once initial assessment is complete, nursing diagnoses are established. Typical nursing diagnoses for a patient requiring androgen replacement are depicted in Table 43–3.

INTERVENTION

After compiling a data base and establishing the nursing diagnoses, the nurse begins to determine with the patient, goals for nursing intervention. Goals for patients requiring androgen medications are included in Table 43–3.

NURSING RESPONSIBILITIES WHEN ADMINISTERING MALE HORMONES

The safe administration of androgenic medications depends on the nurse being familiar with specific information related to administration, patient safety, and patient teaching. This information can be found in Table 43–1.

Instructions for the patient on self-administration of androgen medications are clear and simple. Patients receiving anabolic androgen medications need to understand the importance of high-quality nutrition as part of their therapy. The nurse may need to request the assistance of the dietitian to assist the patient and family in planning dietary modifications.

PATIENT TEACHING

General information concerning male hormones that the nurse educator includes in the teaching plan is found in Table 43–5.

EVALUATION

The nurse, with the assistance of the patient, determines the effectiveness of the nursing interventions based on evaluation criteria. Typical patient outcome criteria are

Table 43–3 NURSING PROCESS FOR PATIENT REQUIRING ANDROGENS

Assessment

Determine developmental level, noting excessive growth of long bones, high-pitched voice, poor musculature, absence of male pattern hair growth, and small external genitalia in late teens.

In the sexually mature male, some feminization in physical appearance may be noted, with thin beard, accumulation of subcutaneous fat, decline in muscle strength, gynecomastia, and atrophy of external genitalia.

Evaluate libido (may be decreased), note problem with impotence and presence of sterility.

Assess drug history.

Review findings of diagnostic tests of endocrine function.

Nursing Diagnosis	Nursing Actions	Rationale	Desired Outcomes/ Evaluation Criteria
Sexual dysfunction related to altered body function as evidenced by change in physical appearance, decreased libido, impotence, inability to achieve desired satisfaction, failure to develop at puberty.	Provide information about reasons for lack of growth, inability to function sexually. Discuss how drugs can be expected to correct the problem.	Understanding of condition and treatment provides opportunity for patient to make informed choices and cooperate with treatment.	Verbalizes understanding of disease and effect on sexual functioning. Reports improvement and expresses satisfaction with sexual functioning. Develops normal pubescent growth.
	Determine degree of impairment according to patient's perception.	Provides base for identification of individual interventions.	
	Encourage expression of feelings and concerns about lack of development, lack of ability to perform, father a child.	The teenager in need of male hormone treatment has concerns about his appearance and if he will grow up "normal". The adult male may feel embarrassed about his virility and question his ability to function as a man.	
	Active listen patient concerns and assist with problem-solving.	Provides opportunity for patient to be actively involved in planning and maintain a sense of control.	
	Note onset of conditions such as priaprism, reduced ejaculatory volume, impotence.	Reduction of dosage/temporary drug holiday may reverse/control these problems when they are the result of drug side-effects.	
Knowledge deficit related to information misinterpretation, unfamiliarity with information resources as evidenced by questions, statement of concern, inaccurate follow-through of instructions/ development of preventable complications.	Provide information about pathophysiology of condition and reasons for treatment.	Understanding will help patient to make informed decisions and cooperate with treatment regimen.	Verbalizes understanding of condition/illness and treatment regimen. Correctly performs necessary procedures and explains reasons for the actions.
	Discuss administration of drug, possible side-effects.	Facilitates safety and prompt identification of undesired side-effects.	
	Discuss and demonstrate rotation of injection sites.	Drug absorption is slow and inflammation or abscess may occur.	
	Demonstrate proper placement of buccal tablets when used.	Use of four possible locations reduces chance of mucosal ulceration.	
	Take oral medications with food.	Minimizes GI upset.	
	Stress importance of regular checkup with health care provider.	Early identification of damaging side-effects or premature epiphyseal closure provides opportunity to reassess comparison of risks versus benefits of continued medication.	
	Recommend daily weight and observance for swelling, changes in fit of jewelry/clothing	Fluid retention may occur requiring medical evaluation.	
	Review signs/symptoms of vomiting, lethargy, constipation, muscle weakness, increased urinary output.	Early detection and prompt intervention may prevent serious side effects, e.g., hypercalcemia and renal calculi may develop, especially in the bedfast patient.	

Table 43–4. DRUGS AFFECTING SEXUAL FUNCTION

Drug	Possible Sexual Dysfunctions*					
	A	B	C	D	E	F
Aldactone	x	x	—	x	—	—
Aldomet	x	x	x	x	x	—
Amphetamines	x	x	x	—	—	—
Antidepressants	x	x	x	x	—	—
Apresoline	—	x	—	—	—	—
Atromid-S	x	x	—	—	—	—
Aventyl	x	x	—	—	—	x
Barbiturates	x	—	—	—	—	—
Catapres	x	x	—	x	x	—
Compazine	—	—	x	—	—	—
Dexedrine	x	x	x	—	—	—
Diamox	x	x	—	—	—	—
Digoxin	x	x	—	—	—	—
Dilantin	x	—	—	—	—	—
Donnatal	—	x	—	x	—	—
Estrogen	x	—	—	x	—	—
Inderal	x	x	—	—	x	—
Ismelin	—	x	x	—	—	—
Librax	x	—	—	—	—	x
Librium	x	—	—	—	—	x
Lithium	—	x	—	—	—	—
Mellaril	—	x	x	x	x	—
Minipress	—	x	—	—	—	—
Naprosyn	—	x	x	—	—	—
Preludin	x	x	—	—	—	x
Pro-Banthine	—	x	—	x	—	—
Stelazine	—	x	—	x	—	—
Tagamet	x	x	—	x	—	—
Thorazine	x	x	x	x	—	—
Timoptic	x	x	—	—	—	—
Valium	x	x	—	x	—	—

*A = decreased sexual drive; B = impotence; C = impaired orgasm; D = hormonal alterations; E = erection or lubrication difficulties; F = increased sexual drive.

Table 43–5. PATIENT TEACHING INFORMATION—MALE HORMONES

Dear Patient:
   This drug has been prescribed for you. This is what you should know about your drug to get the most from your therapy.
   Androgens (_____) are used for a number of reasons. You are taking them because

_____

1. Male hormones will be taken for varying lengths of time; your doctor will tell you what is best for you.
2. For women: You should NOT take male hormones if you are pregnant or are breastfeeding.
3. Take your drugs exactly as ordered.
4. Take your oral (by mouth) male hormones shortly before or with meals.
5. Buccal tablets:
   a. Place under tongue or between gum and cheek.
   b. Change location of tablet with each dose.
   c. Do not chew or swallow tablet.
   d. Do not eat, drink, or smoke until tablet is absorbed.
6. Do not stop taking your male hormones without first checking with your doctor.
7. Report any side effects to your doctor; some examples are:
   Buccal tablets: soreness in mouth
   Subcutaneous (under the skin) pellets: soreness or redness at site
   All preparations: weight gain, edema, nausea, vomiting, jaundice (yellowing of eyes and skin).
8. Check your weight weekly at the same time of day. Report a weight gain or loss of _____ pounds/day or week.
9. Carry an identification card or other similar identification.
10. Store your drugs in light-resistant, dry, tightly closed containers.

included in Table 43–3. A reduction in the signs and symptoms of the disorder for which he or she is being treated and, for the patient receiving anabolic medications, objective signs of improvement, such as increased appetite and weight gain, may be anticipated with androgen therapy.

The nurse also evaluates the patient for the occurrence of adverse effects. The use of androgenic medications is associated with side effects such as nausea, vomiting, diarrhea, sodium and water retention, edema, and change in libido in both sexes. Males may develop an enlarged prostate and increased sex drive. In women, virilization can occur, including hair growth, reduced breast size, hoarseness, menstrual irregularities, and hypercalcemia with all its attendant problems. (See Chapter 57 for information on hypercalcemia.) Refer to Table 43–1 for further information.

Changes in body image in both men and women may possibly lead to noncompliance with medication regimens. These patients need a great deal of support and encouragement from their families and the nurse during this therapy.

Throughout the nursing intervention, the nurse continually stresses to the patient the need for regular medical follow-up. The nurse also periodically reviews his or her teaching with the patient to ensure that the patient's information remains current and accurate.

THERAPEUTIC AGENTS— FEMALE HORMONES

ESTROGENS AND PROGESTOGENS

Three estrogens are secreted by the ovary: about 100 to 600 μcg per day of 17-beta-estradiol, the most potent and the major product (about 100 to 600 μcg per day) and estrone—about one-half as potent as estradiol, and estriol—the weakest estrogen. Progesterone is the naturally occurring hormone and is also produced by direct secretion from the ovary. Estrogens and progestogens are summarized in Table 43–6.

Action

The estrogens are formed in the ovary from androstenedione, an androgen precursor, where it is converted to testosterone, which in turn is converted to estrogen. Es-

TEXT RESUMES ON PAGE 1116

Table 43–6. FEMALE HORMONES

Name	Dosage	Mode of Administration	Pharmacokinetics
ESTROGENS:			
Action: Cause the development of female secondary sex characteristics.			
Use: Prevent complication of menopause, prevention of pregnancy, palliation for breast cancer.			
			For all estrogens O: rapid P: UA D: varies ½L: UA PB: 80% B: liver E: bile, urine
Diethylstilbestrol (DES, Stilbestrol)	0.2–1.0 mg/day 0.1–0.5 mg/day	PO Intravaginal	
Conjugated estrogens (Premarin)	0.3–1.25 mg qd or bid, cyclically	PO, intravaginal, IV, IM	
Estradiol (Estrace)	1–2 mg/day	PO, vaginal cream	
Estradiol cypionate (Depo-Estradiol)	1–5 mg q 3–4 wk	IM	D: 2–3 wk
Estradiol valerate (Delestrogen)	5–30 mg q 2–3 wk	IM	D: 2–3 wk
Estradiol, transdermal (Estraderm)	0.05 mg/24 hr, 0.10 mg/24 hr, applied 2 times/week	Patch for skin	D: 3–4 days
Ethinyl estradiol (Estinyl)	0.02–0.05 mg daily in 21-day cycle for 3–6 months followed by 2 months off therapy	PO	D: UA
Estrone (Bestrone, Kestrone-5)	0.1–0.5 mg 2–3 times weekly for menopause; 0.1–0.2 mg weekly for female hypogonadism	IM IM	D: 2–3 days
Quinestrol (Estrovis)	100 mcg/day for 7 days, no drug for 7 days, followed by maintenance of 100–200 mcg/week	PO	

Key to Abbreviations in the *Pharmacokinetics* column O-onset; P-peak; D-duration; PB-protein bound; B-biotransformed in; E-excreted in; ½ L-halflife.
*Within the column listing adverse effects, underlines indicate the most common effects.

Contraindications/ Precautions	Adverse Effects*	Interactions	Nursing Implications
For all estrogens: CONTRAINDICATIONS: Thrombophlebitis, thromboembolism, history of cerebrovascular accident, history of mammary or genital malignancy, impaired liver function, and pregnancy. PRECAUTIONS: Use cautiously in cardiac or renal disease, hypertension, mental depression.	For all estrogens: *Neuro:* headache, migraine, dizziness *CV:* edema, thromboembolism, hypertension, myocardial infarction *GI:* nausea, vomiting, abdominal cramps, bloating, colitis, weight gain *Biliary:* gallbladder disease, jaundice *Reprod:* Female: breakthrough bleeding, dysmenorrhea, changed libido, breast tenderness; Male: gynecomastia, impotence *Integ:* rash, loss of scalp hair, hirsutism, urticaria, acne, oily skin *Ophth:* change in corneal curvature, intolerance to contact lens	For all estrogens: Effects decreased by barbiturates, tetracycline, antituberculosis drugs, antifungals. Decreased effects of oral anticoagulants, anticonvulsants, antidiabetic drugs. Increased effects of hydrocortisone, meperidine, and tricyclic antidepressants.	For all estrogens: ASSESSMENT: Assess weight regularly, once or twice a week. Practice regular breast self-examination. Obtain regular Pap test and pelvic examinations. Assess blood pressure regularly. INTERVENTION: All products: Teach patient not to smoke during therapy. Obtain Pap smears every 6–12 months and do breast self-exam monthly. *PO:* Take after meals. Protect from light. Store in dry, tightly closed containers. *IM:* Inject deeply into gluteal muscles. Rotate injection sites and record. Shake vial to assure uniform dispersion. *Intravaginal:* Administer at bedtime to enhance absorption. Use a sanitary napkin to protect clothing. EVALUATION: Notify physician if pain in calf occurs, suspected pregnancy, lumps in breast, or severe headache.

CONTINUED ON THE FOLLOWING PAGE

Table 43–6. FEMALE HORMONES–*CONTINUED*

Name	Dosage	Mode of Administration	Pharmacokinetics
PROGESTINS			
Action: Prepares the uterus for pregnancy and the breast for lactation.			
Use: Prevention of contraception, treatment of menopause, amenorrhea, abnormal uterine bleeding.			
Hydroxyprogesterone caproate (Delalutin)	250–375 mg	IM	D: 9–17 days
Medroxyprogesterone acetate (Provera, Amen)	2.5–5.0 mg qd 100–400 mg/wk	PO IM	D: prolonged and variable
Norethindrone (Norlutin)	5–20 mg qd	PO	D: UA
Norethindrone acetate (Norlutate)	2.5–10.0 mg qd	PO	D: UA
Progesterone (Femotrone, Progelan)	5–10 mg qd or qod	IM	D: UA

Key to Abbreviations in the *Pharmacokinetics* column O-onset; P-peak; D-duration; PB-protein bound; B-biotransformed in; E-excreted in; ½ L-halflife.
*Within the column listing adverse effects, underlines indicate the most common effects.

trogens are also produced in much smaller amounts in the adrenals and testes, and in some peripheral tissues. Large amounts of estrogen are produced by the placenta during pregnancy.

Development of the sexual organs of the female and development of the secondary sex characteristics are regulated by the presence of estrogen. In addition, estrogen in varying concentrations gives rise to many of the characteristics of the normal menstrual cycle: proliferation of vaginal and uterine mucosa, increased cervical secretions, and breast fullness. Increasing amounts of estrogen inhibit follicle-stimulating hormone (FHS) released by the pituitary, which again contributes to the cyclic nature of the female reproductive system.

Progesterone, like the estrogens, is synthesized in the ovary. During the latter half of the menstrual cycle, progesterone is synthesized in the corpus luteum. Also, as with the estrogens, progesterone is produced in the testes and adrenals, and by the placenta during pregnancy from precursors derived from cholesterol. During the luteal phase of the menstrual cycle, 10–20 mg of progesterone are secreted daily; several hundred milligrams are secreted during pregnancy. Progesterone has a *thermogenic* effect and may affect basal body temperature.

The net effects of progesterone in the female are to prepare the uterus for pregnancy and the breasts for lactation. Thus, the uterine endometrium becomes secretory, cervical secretions become viscid, and the acini of the mammary glands proliferate. Progesterone is a requisite for the maintenance of pregnancy, because of the aforementioned changes. Progesterone has also been shown to decrease uterine contractility, thus preventing spontaneous abortion. Research also indicates that this hormone, by suppressing T-lymphocyte activity, prevents immunologic rejection of the fetus by the mother's body. Progesterone also influences the menstrual cycle;

the declining levels of progesterone give rise to the onset of menses.

Progesterone, when administered orally, undergoes extensive first-pass metabolism in the liver. To overcome this disadvantage, researchers developed synthetic *progestins* which remain active after oral administration.

Although not as potent as the adrogens in terms of anabolic effects, the estrogens do cause some salt, water, and nitrogen retention. At the cellular level, similarly to the androgens, estrogens and progesterone are bound to cytoplasmic receptor proteins, which are transferred to the cell nucleus. The end result is an increase in protein synthesis.

Secretion of the ovarian hormones is regulated by the gonadotropic hormones of the anterior pituitary; production of the gonadotropins is in turn regulated by the plasma levels of estrogen and progesterone. The normal female menstrual cycle can be summarized as follows: Beginning at day one (onset of menses), FSH stimulates follicular growth in the ovary; within six days, estrogen levels begin to rise and continue to do so until ovulation; at ovulation, a rise in FSH and LH secretion occurs, leading to an increase in progesterone secretion by the corpus luteum, which reaches its maximum at about the 22nd day (of a 28-day cycle); the corpus luteum then begins to involute, leading to a decrease in the secretion of estrogen and progesterone, which in turn leads to the onset of menses and the beginning of another cycle (Fig. 43–1).

Uses

Estrogens and progestogens are used clinically to treat hormonal deficiency states that may result from a failure of ovarian development, as in hypopituitarism, or from declining ovarian function, as in menopause. Combinations of estrogens and progestins (progesterone-like

Contraindications/ Precautions	Adverse Effects*	Interactions	Nursing Implications
Same as estrogens.	Same as estrogens.	For all progestins: Affects laboratory results of hepatic and endocrine tests. Possible decrease in glucose tolerance test results.	Same as estrogens plus INTERVENTION: If GI upset occurs, take with food.

drugs) are more widely used as contraceptive agents because of the fact that administration of these suppresses levels of FSH and LH, thus leading to an anovulatory state. (Oral contraceptives will be discussed later in this chapter.) Estrogen, most commonly diethylstilbestrol, is also used as a postcoital, or "morning after," pill. This method of contraception is recommended only for isolated incidents of unprotected intercourse, and treat-ment must commence within 72 hours of intercourse. Usually, 25 mg of diethylstilbestrol is administered twice a day for five days. Dysmenorrhea, endometriosis, and dysfunctional uterine bleeding are two other indications for the combined use of estrogens and progestogens. Most of the agents used therapeutically are synthetic or naturally-occurring analogs of endogenous hormones. Estrogens, progesterone, and progestins

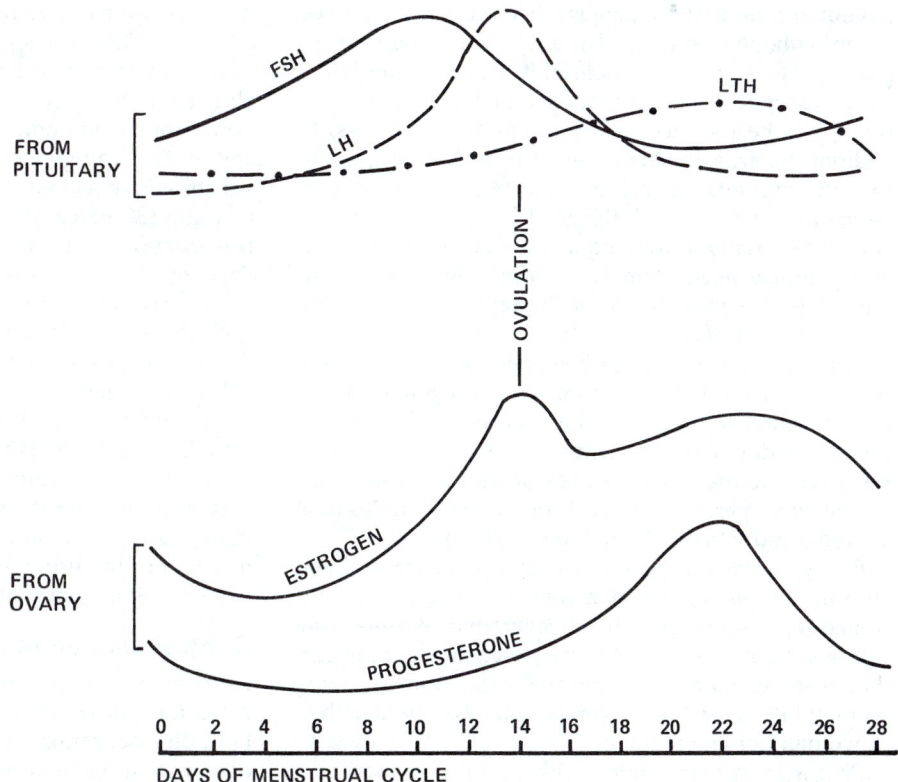

Figure 43–1. Relative relationship of gonadotropins, female hormones, to the menstrual cycle (Redrawn from Guyton, AC: Textbook of Medical Physiology, ed. 7. WB Saunders, Philadelphia, 1986, with permission.)

FROM PITUITARY

FROM OVARY

FSH

LH

LTH

OVULATION

ESTROGEN

PROGESTERONE

0 2 4 6 8 10 12 14 16 18 20 22 24 26 28

DAYS OF MENSTRUAL CYCLE

(synthetic compounds possessing progestational activity) are available in a variety of preparations for oral, parenteral, or topical administration.

Estrogens alone are used in the pharmacologic management of menopause and are effective in controlling hot flushes due to vasomotor instability, and atrophic vaginitis. For women requiring long-term therapy with estrogens, cyclic therapy is usually recommended in order to avoid continuous stimulation of the breasts and uterus. In general, the goal of menopausal estrogen therapy is to relieve specific symptoms with the lowest effective dosage. Not all target organs are restored to the normal premenopausal condition, but most symptoms can be controlled by conjugated estrogens, 0.625 mg or the equivalent daily. Conjugated estrogens contain the three natural estrogens. Bone loss and fractures are also prevented by this amount of estrogen. A combined regimen is often used: estrogen administered daily for three weeks, with progestin administered daily for 10–13 days of each estrogen cycle, and one week of no hormonal therapy during which withdrawal bleeding occurs. This combination therapy has recently been shown to reduce the incidence of endometrial hyperplasia, which can occur with estrogen therapy alone.

By altering the hormonal milieu, estrogen has been shown to offer some palliation in the treatment of breast cancer, especially in postmenopausal patients. Estrogen, specifically diethylstilbestrol, is frequently used to treat prostatic cancer in men. (See Chapter 49 for a discussion of hormonal therapy in cancer.)

Estrogen is particularly effective in preventing osteoporosis both in women who have undergone oophorectomy before natural menopause, and in women who have had a natural menopause. Estrogens are believed to inhibit bone resorption. The addition of progestin appears to be even more beneficial by not only inhibiting bone resorption, but also adding to bone mass. This therapy is best started before significant bone loss. In addition to drug therapy, weight-bearing exercise and calcium supplements are encouraged. Premenopausal women in their 30s and 40s need to have 1 gm of calcium intake daily. Postmenopausal women treated with estrogen also need 1 gm of calcium daily, while postmenopausal women not receiving replacement therapy require 1.5 gm of calcium daily.

In the past, estrogen has been used in the treatment of acne, since estrogen suppresses androgen secretion (which tends to stimulate the sebaceous glands) and thereby reduces the severity of the acne. Currently, however, the preferred methods of treatment are: topical benzoyl peroxide; topical antibiotics; intralesional steroids; and vitamin A, tretinoin, or both.

Estrogen was once advocated as a prophylactic measure in the prevention of myocardial infarction. Controlled studies have shown, however, that administering estrogen to men results in an increased incidence of cardiac disease. Rates of myocardial infarction in young women taking oral contraceptives are also higher than in women not taking them.

Progestin in combination with estrogen is used as a contraceptive. Used in this context, sometimes referred to as "minipills," the progestins do not reliably block ovulation; they probably exert their contraceptive action through their effects on the endometrium and cervical mucus, causing these to be unfavorable for sperm transport and implantation. The "minipills" are taken once daily for all 28 days of the menstrual cycle. When taken as directed, these drugs offer approximately 97 percent protection from pregnancy. The progestin minipills do have a higher incidence of breakthrough bleeding and spotting. However, they do not cause the more serious toxicities associated with the use of estrogen.

Oral progestins are used, with success, in the treatment of endometriosis and premenstrual syndrome (PMS). Long-term use results in regression of endometrial growths, giving symptomatic relief in about 80 percent of cases and a return of fertility in about 50 percent. Danazol (previously discussed) is also used to treat endometriosis. Progestins also are useful in the palliative treatment of endometrial carcinomas.

Pharmacokinetics

The administration of exogenous estrogens or progestins causes the same physiologic responses as the endogenous hormones. Synthetic versions of these hormones vary in duration and intensity of action. Female hormones are featured in Table 43–6.

Natural estrogens and their esters are rapidly absorbed from the gastrointestinal tract. However, they are metabolized by the liver too rapidly to be effective orally. Nonsteroidal estrogens may be administered orally but are also metabolized rapidly, and frequent (usually daily) administration is required. Aqueous or oil suspensions of estrogen are administered parenterally; absorption takes place over a period of days. Subcutaneous implantation of estrogen-containing pellets allows for absorption over a period of months. Absorption through skin and mucous membranes is also good and, in fact, can give rise to systemic effects.

Estrogens circulate in the blood bound to globulin and albumin (80 percent). The greatest concentration of estrogen appears in fat deposits. Estrogens are metabolized by the liver and are excreted primarily into the urine. Excretion of estrogens averages 25–100 μg at midcycle, 5–10 μg after menopause, and about 30 μg during the later stages of pregnancy.

Like estrogen, progestin is not very effective when given by mouth, and parenteral administration is preferred. Even so, metabolism is still rapid, necessitating frequent (daily) administration. Synthetic progestins may be administered orally as well as parenterally. Progestins are metabolized by the liver and excreted primarily into the urine, in part as pregnanediol (12 to 15 percent). Small amounts are stored in fat tissue.

Contraindications and Precautions

Estrogen and progestin therapy is generally contraindicated for the patient who has a history of thromboembolic disease, genital or mammary malignancies, hepatic dysfunction, or hypertension, or one who is pregnant.

This rationale is based directly on the adverse effects produced by the drugs. Estrogen treatment has been associated with an increased incidence of thromboembolism, genital malignancy, and hypertension. Therefore, estrogen use in the patient with these conditions preexisting or with a history of these conditions is unacceptable because of the increased risk. Because of the increased incidence of thromboembolism occurring in women who smoke, a current history of smoking may either be a contraindication or a caution. Since estrogens are metabolized by the liver, the function of that organ should be unimpaired; and since estrogen is teratogenic, it should not be given during pregnancy or a suspected pregnancy.

In addition, these drugs should be used cautiously in patients with histories of cardiac or renal disease, or epilepsy. These cautions are related to retention of salt and water.

Adverse Effects

Female hormones given at replacement levels (physiologic levels) for a short duration may not cause the appearance of bothersome adverse effects; when given over extended periods of time, the risk of adverse effects is increased.

Use of estrogen frequently gives rise to gastrointestinal symptoms such as nausea, vomiting, abdominal cramps, and bloating. The nausea usually does not interfere with nutrition and can be minimized by instructing the patient to take the drug after meals. The patient may be encouraged to know that the nausea usually subsides with one to two weeks of continued therapy.

Dermatologic effects can be especially distressing for patients. The occurrence of skin rash, pruritus, acne, loss of scalp hair, hirsutism, and chloasma is not rare.

Effects on the nervous system may be reflected in the onset of headaches, migraine, vertigo, mental depression, malaise, or irritability.

Estrogen therapy can induce many changes in the metabolic function of the body. Edema and sodium retention can occur, leading in some instances to hypertension. Blood glucose levels may increase, a factor of special concern in the care of the diabetic patient. The occurrence of cholestatic jaundice reflects estrogen's effects on the biliary system. Endocrine changes are reflected in the possible occurrence of breakthrough bleeding and spotting, breast enlargement, increased cervical mucus production, and changes in menstrual flow. (In males, gynecomastia, testicular atrophy, feminization, and reversible impotence can occur with estrogen administration.)

Perhaps the most serious adverse effects of estrogen therapy are related to its effect on the vascular system. The occurrence of thromboembolism in women receiving estrogen therapy is well documented. Men who receive estrogen therapy are at the same increased risk. The higher the dose of estrogen, the higher the risk. The risk of thromboembolic disorders related to estrogen increases with age, beginning at about 30 years, and increasing even more after 40 years of age. In addition, even women who discontinue long-term estrogen use also have a higher incidence of thromboembolic complications. Women who use estrogen-containing oral contraceptives for five years or more have a 1000 percent (tenfold) increase in the risk of death from thromboembolic disorders in contrast to women who have not used these products.

Peripheral thrombophlebitis is not the only concern, however, as the incidence of cerebral and coronary thromboses also increases.

Estrogen used in pregnancy may result in fetal deformities; therefore, if pregnancy is suspected, use of these drugs should be discontinued until a pregnancy test can either confirm or discount the possibility.

Therapeutic administration of estrogen has been shown to be carcinogenic in certain instances. Increased incidences of nonmalignant genital changes and vaginal and cervical cancers are noted in female offspring and testicular tumors in male offspring of women treated with diethylstilbestrol (DES) during the first trimester of pregnancy. Estrogen therapy in postmenopausal women has given rise to increased incidence of endometrial cancers, although, as yet, use in premenopausal women has not shown the same carcinogenic effect. Most recent studies show no correlation with estrogen use and breast cancer. Benign liver tumors occur with greater-than-anticipated frequency in young women using estrogen-containing oral contraceptives.

Progestin administration also can cause adverse effects, most of which are similar to those caused by estrogen. In fact, when the two hormones are used in combination, as in the oral contraceptives, it is not always possible to tell which effects are due to which hormone. When progestins are administered during pregnancy, masculinization of the female fetus can occur. Eye changes can occur suddenly with progestin therapy; the nurse should inform the patient to immediately report such changes as loss of vision, diplopia, or *proptosis*. Medication should be withheld until these can be investigated.

Interactions

The effect of estrogen may be decreased by the concurrent use of tetracycline-type antibiotics, the anti-tuberculosis antibiotic rifampin, the antifungal agent griseofulvin, and anticonvulsant drugs like phenytoin, primidone, and barbiturates, as hepatic breakdown is enhanced. Women taking oral contraceptives concurrently with these products need to use another method of birth control for that cycle, as they may not have full protection. Estrogens can alter the effectiveness of many drugs. They decrease the effect of: oral anticoagulants, through increasing the action of selected clotting factors; anticonvulsants, by depressing breakdown of anticonvulsant; and antidiabetic drugs, by decreasing glucose tolerance. Conversely, estrogen increases the effects of: hydrocortisone, by potentiating anti-inflammatory effect; meperidine, by decreasing hepatic breakdown; and the tricyclic antidepressants. Ascorbic acid may increase the effects of estrogen.

Estrogens

DIETHYLSTILBESTROL. Diethylstilbestrol (Stilphostrol, DES), a synthetic estrogen, is administered to relieve vasomotor symptoms of menopause and to treat atrophic vaginitis, kraurosis vulvae, female hypogonadism, surgical castration, primary ovarian failure, and postpartum breast engorgement. Diethylstilbestrol can also be used as a postcoital contraceptive.

Diethylstilbestrol is administered orally in a dose range of 0.2–1.0 mg/day, or as intravaginal suppositories in a dosage of 0.1–0.5 mg, once or twice a day.

CONJUGATED ESTROGENS. Conjugated estrogens (Premarin), a naturally occurring estrogen, is used to relieve the vasomotor symptoms of menopause and to treat atrophic vaginitis, kraurosis vulvae, female hypogonadism, surgical castration, primary ovarian failure, postpartum breast engorgement, and abnormal uterine bleeding from hormone imbalance. Conjugated estrogen is a short-acting preparation administered orally in a dose range of 0.3–1.25 mg once or twice daily. They are administered cyclically—three weeks on and one week off—for menopausal symptoms, abnormal uterine bleeding, and atrophic vaginitis or kraurosis vulvae. For abnormal uterine bleeding caused by hormone imbalance, 25 mg is administered IM or IV and can be repeated in six to twelve hours if needed. It can also be administered as an intravaginal cream.

ESTRADIOL. Estradiol (Estrace), a natural estrogen, is used for the same conditions as diethylstilbestrol. Estradiol is administered orally in doses of 1–2 mg/day. Estrace is also available as a vaginal cream that is used to treat atropic vaginitis or kraurosis vulvae.

ESTRADIOL (TRANSDERMAL). Transdermal estradiol (Estraderm) is available as a patch in two dosage forms—0.05 mg/24 hours and 0.10 mg/24 hours. The patches may minimize the problems and maximize the benefits of hormone replacement because the hormone is released in small amounts continually for the time it is worn. The patch includes a reservoir that contains the estradiol, a membrane that controls the drug's release, and a nonallergenic adhesive that keeps the unit on the skin. The patch is applied twice weekly.

ESTRADIOL CYPIONATE. Estradiol cypionate (DepoEstradiol) is a long-lasting preparation administered intramuscularly in doses of 1–5 mg every three to four weeks for primary ovarian failure, surgical castration, or menopausal symptoms. In female hypogonadism, 1.5–2.0 mg is given intramuscularly at monthly intervals.

ETHINYL ESTRADIOL. Ethinyl estradiol (Estinyl, Feminone), a synthetic oral estrogen, is administered in doses of 0.02–0.05 mg daily in a 21-day cycle for menopausal symptoms. For female hypogonadism, ethinyl estradiol is administered as a 0.05-mg dose, three times a day for two weeks per month. It is followed by two weeks of progesterone therapy. This series is continued for three to six months, followed by two months off therapy.

ESTRADIOL VALERATE. Estradiol valerate (Delestrogen) is another sustained-action preparation with effects lasting two to three weeks and is used for primary ovarian failure, surgical castration, or menopausal symptoms. It is administered intramuscularly in doses of 5–30 mg.

ESTRONE. Estrone (Bestrone, Kestrone-5, Theelin) is a naturally occurring estrogen. It is administered intramuscularly two to three times per week in doses of 0.1–0.5 mg for menopausal symptoms, atrophic vaginitis, and kraurosis vulvae. For female hypogonadism and primary ovarian failure, it is administered weekly in doses of 0.1–0.2 mg.

QUINESTROL. Quinestrol (Estrovis), a long-acting synthetic estrogen, is used to treat female hypogonadism, primary ovarian failure, atrophic vaginitis, and kraurosis vulvae; and to relieve menopausal symptoms. The usual dosing schedule for all uses is 100 μg/day for seven days, then no drug for seven days, followed by a maintenance dose of 100 μg/week. If needed, the dose may be increased to 200 μg/week.

EQUIVALENT DOSING OF ESTROGEN. Occasionally, the patient may need to move from one estrogen product to another. Approximate dosing equivalents for estrogen are: 1 mg diethylstilbestrol = 0.5 mg estradiol = 5 mg conjugated or esterified estrogen = 0.8 mg mestranol.

Progestins

HYDROXYPROGESTERONE CAPROATE. Hydroxyprogesterone caproate (Delalutin) is a long-acting synthetic progestin administered intramuscularly in doses of 250–375 mg. Hydroxyprogesterone caproate is used to treat amenorrhea and abnormal uterine bleeding caused by hormonal imbalance.

MEDROXYPROGESTERONE. Medroxyprogesterone (Provera, Amen, Curretab) is a synthetic progestin that can be administered orally, in doses of 2.5–5.0 mg daily to treat amenorrhea or abnormal uterine bleeding caused by hormonal imbalance; or intramuscularly (Depo-Provera), in doses averaging 100–400 mg/week. Since the injectable form has a long duration of action, it is only recommended for cancer treatment.

NORETHINDRONE AND NORETHINDRONE ACETATE. Synthetic products norethindrone (Norlutin) and norethindrone acetate (Norlutate), which is twice as potent, are administered orally in doses of 5–20 mg/day and 2.5–10.0 mg/day, respectively. They are used to treat amenorrhea, abnormal uterine bleeding caused by hormonal imbalance, and endometriosis.

PROGESTERONE. Progesterone (Femotrone, Progelan), a natural progestin product, is available for intramuscular injection in doses varying from five to ten mg daily or every other day. Progesterone is used to treat amenorrhea, abnormal uterine bleeding caused by hormonal imbalance, and premenstrual syndrome. It is also available as an intrauterine contraceptive device (Progestasert), inserted once yearly, which delivers approximately 65 μg/day. For premenstrual syndrome, progesterone is available as a 200–400 mg suppository, inserted either rectally or vaginally, once or twice daily.

Table 43–7. COMBINATION ESTROGEN/ANTIANXIETY PRODUCTS

Combination Drug	Basic Products (mg)*			
	A	**B**	**C**	**D**
Menrium 5-2	5	0.2	—	—
Menrium 5-4	5	0.4	—	—
Menrium 10-4	10	0.4	—	—
Milprem-200	—	—	0.45	200
Milprem-400	—	—	0.45	400
PMB 200	—	—	0.45	200
PMB 400	—	—	0.45	400

*Basic products: A = chlordiazepoxide; B = esterified estrogens; C = conjugated estrogens; D = meprobamate.

ESTROGENS COMBINED WITH OTHER DRUGS. Sometimes the symptoms of menopause—hot flushes, atrophic vaginitis—lead to increased anxiety that does not seem to respond to estrogen alone. Several products which combine estrogen and anatianxiety agents are available. They are featured in Table 43–7. These products are used for short-term therapy only, and only if the combination of drugs has been found to be beneficial when used individually.

DRUGS FOR PREMENSTRUAL SYNDROME. Premenstrual syndrome (PMS) affects 9–12 million (30 to 40 percent of all women in the United States. Premenstrual syndrome may occur in any menstruating woman, but the incidence increases in those over 30 years of age. PMS has been implicated in work absenteeism, criminal behavior, marital discord, and billions of dollars worth of business loss.

The etiology remains obscure, but symptoms generally begin about seven to ten days before the onset of menses, and resolve within 24 hours after menstruation begins. The typical symptoms reported include: mood swings, abdominal bloating, irritability, depression, crying, food cravings, and sleep disorders.

Several drugs for relief of the symptoms of PMS are

being studied, including alprazolam (Xanax) and danazol (Danocrine)—a synthetic androgen discussed previously. In separate studies, both of these drugs have significantly reduced symptoms of PMS. Alprazolam is reviewed in detail in Chapter 24. In addition, progesterone has been used in the treatment of severe PMS. Its use is based on the theoretical premise that a relative progesterone deficiency or an increased estrogen:progesterone ratio causes PMS. Diuretics are also used in the treatment of PMS to relieve symptoms related to fluid retention.

Contraception

Ever since the relationship between coitus and pregnancy became known, efforts have been made to limit the number of pregnancies. Various methods of contraception are currently available. Table 43–8 compares the therapeutic effectiveness and adverse effects of the various methods. A brief overview of oral contraceptives, vaginal spermicides, and intrauterine devices follows. For a more detailed review, please see an obstetrical nursing text.

ORAL CONTRACEPTIVES. Oral contraceptives (Table 43–9) are highly effective in preventing pregnancy. Oral contraceptives have different actions dependent on the product being used. The combination oral contraceptives inhibit ovulation through a negative feedback effect on the hypothalamus. The cervical mucous thickens, rendering it unfavorable to penetration by sperm. In addition, the endometrial lining is unfavorable for implantation. The progestin-only minipills do not inhibit ovulation, but cause the formation of a thick cervical mucus that is relatively impenetrable to sperm.

The oral contraceptives are available in low-, medium-, or high-estrogen doses (Table 43–10). The preparation chosen should closely mimic the balance of the patient's endogenous hormones or minimize problems

TEXT RESUMES ON PAGE 1124

Table 43–8. COMPARISON OF EFFECTIVENESS AND ADVERSE EFFECTS OF VARIOUS METHODS OF CONTRACEPTION

Method	% Theoretical Effectiveness	% Use Effectiveness	Adverse Effects
Oral contraceptives Fixed ratio (estrogen and progestin)	100	97–98	Nausea, edema, increased weight gain, fatigue, leukorrhea, thromboembolic disorders, increased incidence of gallbladder disease, teratogenesis in pregnancy
Minipill (progestin only)	99	96–97.5	
Intrauterine devices	96–99	90–94	Dysmenorrhea, alterations in menstrual flow, pelvic inflammatory disease
Condom	97	80–97	None
Diaphragm	97	80	Possible allergies to rubber or irritation from spermicides
Spermicidal foams	97	70–98	Local irritation
Rhythm	95	70–75	None
Contraceptive sponge	—	73–91	Local irritation, toxic shock syndrome

Table 43–9. ORAL CONTRACEPTIVES

Name	Dosage (All PO, qd)	
Action: Prevent conception by several different methods (see text).		
Use: Prevention of pregnancy.		
PROGESTINS		Progestin only:
Norethindrone (Micronor)	0.35 mg	O: rapid
Norgestrel (Ovrette)	0.075 mg	P: 0.5–4.0 hr
		D: UA
		½L: 5–45 hr
		PB: to albumin
		B: liver
		E: bile, urine
		Estrogen only:
		O: rapid
		P: 1–2 hr
		D: UA
		½L: 6–20 hr
		PB: 97%–98%
		B: liver
		E: bile, urine
COMBINATIONS	Progestin/Estrogen	
Norethindrone/mestranol		
(Norinyl)	1 mg/0.08 mg	
(Ortho-Novum)	1 mg/50 μg	
(Ortho-Novum 2)	2 mg/100 μg	
(Norinyl 2)	2 mg/100 μg	
(Norinyl 1 + 80)	1 mg/80 μg	
Norethindrone/ethinyl estradiol		
(Loestrin)	1.5 mg/30 μg	
(Norlestrin)	1 mg/50 μg	
	5 mg/75 μg	
Norethynodrel/mestranol	9.85 mg/150 μg	
(Enovid)		
Ethynodiol/mestranol (Ovulen)	1 mg/100 μcg	

Key to Abbreviations in the *Pharmacokinetics* column O-onset; P-peak; D-duration; PB-protein bound; B-biotransformed in; E-excreted in; ½ L-halflife.
*Within the column listing adverse effects, underlines indicate the most common effects; CAPITALS indicate life-threatening effects.

Contraindications/ Precautions	Adverse Effects*	Interactions	Nursing Implications
For all oral contraceptives: CONTRAINDICATIONS: Thromboembolic disorders, cerebral vascular disease, myocardial infarction, coronary artery disease, known or suspected breast cancer, liver tumors, known or suspected pregnancy. PRECAUTIONS: Use with caution in women who smoke, over 30 years of age, family history of hypertension, hepatic dysfunction.	For all oral contraceptives: *Neuro:* migraine, mental depression, CEREBROVASCULAR ACCIDENT *CV:* edema, THROMBOEMBOLIC PHENOMENA, MYOCARDIAL INFARCTION, hypertension *GI:* nausea, vomiting, abdominal cramps, bloating, weight gain *Biliary:* gallbladder disease, liver tumors *Reprod:* breakthrough bleeding, spotting, dysmenorrhea, breast tenderness *Integ:* rash *Ophth:* change in corneal curvature	For all oral contraceptives: Reduced efficacy with barbiturates, phenylbutazone, phenytoin, primidone, rifampin, isoniazid, penicillin V, tetracycline, chloramphenicol, griseofulvin, sulfonamides, analgesics, tranquilizers, antihistamines. Insulin and pyridoxine requirements may be increased. Oral contraceptives may impair metabolism of caffeine, diazepam, metoprolol, corticosteroids, imipramine, phenytoin, phenylbutazone. (See Table 43–11 for additional information.)	For all oral contraceptives: ASSESSMENT: Assess blood pressure, weight, pregnancy status, and liver function before starting oral contraceptives. INTERVENTION: Take as directed. For missed table information, see text. Caution patient about not smoking during therapy. EVALUATION: If breakthrough bleeding occurs second month, notify physician.

Table 43–10. ESTROGEN CONTENT OF BIRTH CONTROL PILLS

Brand Name	Estrogen Dose (μg)	Progestin Component (mg)					
		A	B	C	D	E
HIGH DOSE						
Enovid 5	75	—	—	5	—	—
Norinyl 1 + 80	80	—	1	—	—	—
Norinyl 2	100	—	2	—	—	—
Ortho-Novum 1/80	80	—	1	—	—	—
Orhto-Novum 2	100	—	2	—	—	—
Ovulen	100	—	—	—	1	—
MEDIUM DOSE						
Demulen	50	—	—	—	1	—
Norinyl 1 + 50	50	—	1	—	—	—
Norlestrin 1/50	50	1	—	—	—	—
Norlestrin 2.5/50	50	2.5	—	—	—	—
Ortho-Novum 1/50	50	1	—	—	—	—
Ovcon-50	50	—	1	—	—	—
Ovral	50	—	—	0.5	—	—
LOW DOSE						
Brevicon	35	—	0.5	—	—	—
*Demulen 1/35	35	—	—	—	1	—
Levlen	30	—	—	—	—	0.15
*Loestrin 1/20	20	1	—	—	—	—
Loestrin 1.5/30	30	1.5	—	—	—	—
*Lo/Ovral	30	—	—	0.3	—	—
Modicon	35	—	0.5	—	—	—
Nordette	30	—	—	—	—	0.15
*Norinyl 1 + 35	35	—	1	—	—	—
*Ortho-Novum 1/35	35	—	1	—	—	—
*Ortho-Novum 10/11	35	—	0.5, 1.0	—	—	—
*Ortho-Novum 7/7/7	35	—	0.5, 0.75, 1.0	—	—	—
*Ovcon-35	35	—	0.4	—	—	—
Tri-Levlen	30–40	—	—	—	—	0.05, 0.075, 0.125
*Tri-Norinyl	35	—	0.5, 1.0, 0.5	—	—	—

A = Norethindrone acetate; B = Norethindrone; C = Norgestrel; D = Ethynodiol diacetate; E = Levonorgestrel.

with her specific hormone sensitivities. For example, a woman with symptoms of estrogen sensitivity (vomiting, fluid retention, increased menstrual flow) should be given low-dose estrogen products. Patients with androgen sensitivity (oily skin and scalp, acne) or progestin sensitivity (depression, noncyclic weight gain) should be given a product low in both androgenic and progestational activities.

COMBINATION ORAL CONTRACEPTIVES. Several types of oral contraceptives are available: monophasic, biphasic, and triphasic products. These products are graphically represented in Figure 43–2.

Monophasic Oral Contraceptive Products. The monophasic oral contraceptives are the most common and provide a fixed dose of estrogen and progestin throughout a 21-day cycle.

Biphasic Oral Contraceptive Products. Biphasic products, introduced in 1982, stimulate a woman's normal hormonal pattern. Low-dose estrogen (35 mcg) is kept constant throughout the cycle, while the progestin is increased (0.5–1.0 mg) from day 11 through day 21. The biphasic pill is intended to reduce total steroid exposure,

while alleviating problems with breakthrough bleeding and spotting common with lower-dose pills.

The benefits of decreasing progestin include a possible reduction in: hypertension, pelvic congestion, depression, fatigue, headache, and high-density lipoprotein levels. However, there may also be a loss of some noncontraceptive benefits of progestins such as: protection against pelvic inflammatory disease, less dysmenorrhea and menstrual blood loss, and protection against endometrial cancer and fibrocystic breast disease.

Triphasic Oral Contraceptive Products. The newest oral contraceptive, the triphasic product, appeared in 1985. Its design approximates the normal female cycle even more closely. Both low-dose estrogen and progestin change in a "low-higher-low" pattern. Estrogen is constant, while progestin rises at midcycle and falls before the onset of bleeding. The triphasic pill reduces the total steroid exposure, while providing greater protection at midcycle. Breakthrough bleeding is also reduced. The triphasic products are available in a 28-day cycle with seven inert tablets, or a 21-day cycle with the inert pills omitted.

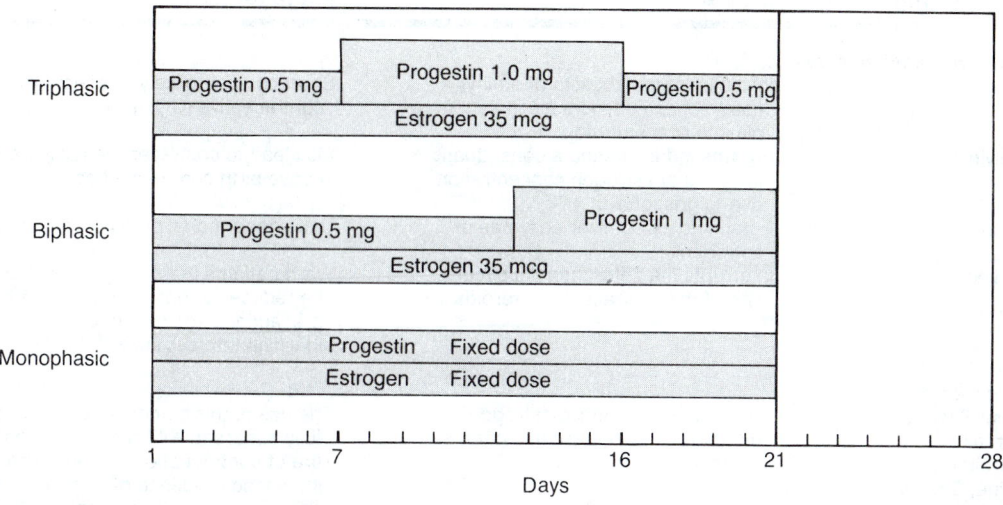

Figure 43–2. Represents the three types of oral contraceptives. Monophasic products contain fixed amounts of estrogen and progestin throughout the 21-day cycle. Biphasic products contain a fixed low-dose of estrogen (35 μg) and progestin that increases from 0.5 mg to 1 mg at day 11. The triphasic products also contain a fixed dose of estrogen (35 μg) and progestin in a ''low-high-low'' pattern.

ADVERSE EFFECTS. During the 1970s, a large number of studies reported on increased risk of disease or death among women using oral contraceptives. This created widespread controversy and resulted in modification of the formulation of oral contraceptives. Since then, there have been few reports regarding the effects of the newer formulations. A recent study encompassed 300,538 women-years, and found a calculated mortality of 25.5/100,000 women-years for users and 20/100,000 women-years for nonusers. These results suggest that women who use oral contraceptives have dramatically fewer risks with the newer formulations than with earlier preparations.

The primary risk factors involved in complications of oral contraceptive use appear to be: (1) the estrogen dose, (2) the age of the woman, (3) tobacco smoking, and (4) the duration of therapy.

Women using oral contraceptives who smoke 15 or more cigarettes/day have a 500 percent (fivefold) increase in risk of having a fatal myocardial infarction (MI), in comparison with women who are also taking oral contraceptives but do not smoke. In addition, these women who are taking oral contraceptives and smoke have a 1000 to 1200 percent (tenfold to twelvefold) increased risk of having a fatal myocardial infarction, in comparison with women who neither use oral contraceptives nor smoke.

Clotting disorders such as stroke, pulmonary embolism, retinal vein thrombosis, and thrombophlebitis have occurred more frequently in women using oral contraceptives. There is more rapid fibrin formation with increased clot firmness among pill users than among nonusers. There is also an increase in certain blood factors associated with coagulation, an increase in platelet count with changes in electrophoretic mobility of platelets, and an increase in vascular lesions and venous stasis. The incidences of complications are dose re-

lated. There is a significant difference between women taking pills with less than 50 μg estrogen/day and those taking dosages above 50 μg estrogen/day.

If a woman develops deep vein thrombosis while taking oral contraceptives, the contraceptive should be stopped and not restarted. Also, caution is used when oral contraceptives are used after any surgical procedure, as the incidence of deep vein thrombosis is almost twice as high as that for nonusers.

Hypertension has been observed in about five percent of all contraceptive users. While the increase in blood pressure is usually gradual, it may be quite severe. Generally, the hypertension is reversible within several months of discontinuation of medications. These effects probably result from the retention of sodium and water secondary to the increased circulating concentration of renin and angiotensin.

Various ocular conditions have also been reported, including corneal sensitivity, retinal thrombosis, optic neuritis, diplopia, and others. Women wearing contact lenses may experience intolerance to their lenses due to a change in corneal curvation. Women wearing contact lenses are encouraged to have periodic eye exams.

Many other minor disturbances have been attributed to oral contraceptives. Some symptoms, including depression of mood, easy fatigue, and lack of initiative, have been attributed to progestin tablets. An increase in female-initiated sexual activity that is said to be present at the time of ovulation is suppressed or absent in women using oral contraceptives.

Women frequently complain of mild side effects including nausea, occasional vomiting, dizziness, headache, discomfort in the breasts, and gain in weight. These symptoms are all found in early pregnancy and are the direct result of estrogen in the preparation. Most times these symptoms are present during the first or second cycle and then disappear. Irregular menstrual

Table 43–11. DRUG INTERACTIONS OF ORAL CONTRACEPTIVES

Interacting Drug	Interaction	Management
Antibiotics and Antibacterials		
Co-Trimoxazole	Inhibition of metabolism of ethinyl estradiol and an increase in its plasma concentration.	Short course unlikely to effect long-term oral contraceptive (OC) user.
Griseofulvin	Enzyme induction and a consequent lowering of estrogen concentration due to griseofulvin.	May lead to contraceptive failure. Use alternative birth control method.
Rifampicin	Potent inducer of liver enzymes of estrogen.	Use nonhormonal birth control method.
Tetracycline	Interrupts the enterohepatic circulation of the contraceptive steroids.	Warn patients that the efficacy of OCs may be reduced and that they should take extra precautions against conceiving in any cycle in which tetracycline is given.
Anticonvulsants		
Phenytoin, Phenobarbital, Primidone, Butobarbital, Carbamazepine, Ethosuximide, Mephobarbital (alone or combined)	Anticonvulsants induce estrogen metabolism by hepatic microsomal enzymes.	The use of this combination has to be carefully assessed with respect to possible failure of contraception and, in some cases, increased incidence of seizures (Combined OCs may cause fluid retention which may precipitate seizures in epileptics; cases of OC-induced exacerbation of epilepsy have been reported). Paradoxically, the combination may also cause an increase in serum phenytoin concentrations and this could lead to enhanced phenytoin toxicity. There are 3 possible methods of management: (1) change to a nonhormonal method of contraception; (2) change the antiepileptic medication from phenytoin to sodium valproate (which does not seem to affect contraceptive efficacy); or (3) increase the OC dosage by prescribing two types of OC preparations simultaneously to bring the total estrogen dosage up to 80 μg/day, although this may be undesirable because of the increased risk of side effects which cannot as yet be quantified. Where possible, it would be better to advise alternative methods of contraception.
Antifibrinolytic Agents		
Aminocaproic acid	OCs augment blood levels of clotting factors due to their estrogen content. Blood clotting factors increased are Factors VII, VIII, IX, and X.	Aminocaproic acid and OCs should not be given together.
Analgesics		
Acetaminophen	Data suggest that increased clearance of acetaminophen from plasma in women taking OCs results from increased glucuronidation of the drug.	The clinical significance of this interaction has not been established, but women taking OCs may require larger doses of the analgesic than those used by women not taking OC steroids.
Aspirin	Induces metabolism by OCs.	Any clinical significance of this interaction is unlikely, although the reduction in half-life for aspirin may warrant a higher or more frequent dosage in women on OCs for a short period. That may not be necessary with long-term OC use.
Meperidine	Possible increased analgesia and CNS depression due to inhibition of metabolism of meperidine.	Use this analgesic with caution in women taking OCs.
Anticoagulants		
Coumarin products Heparin	Oral contraceptives increase the synthesis of specific blood coagulation factors; this may impair the efficacy of anticoagulant therapy.	Any patient who requires anticoagulants should not take OCs.

Table 43–11. DRUG INTERACTIONS OF ORAL CONTRACEPTIVES-*CONTINUED*

Interacting Drug	Interaction	Management
Antidiabetic Agents (oral products)	Impairment of glucose tolerance with development of overt diabetes mellitus, and an increase in insulin requirements have been reported in women taking OCs.	The use of other methods of contraception may be required for some diabetics. If this is not practical, the patient should be carefully monitored for decreased diabetic control; existing antidiabetic treatment may have to be modified. The risk of cardiovascular complications and microangiopathic changes in diabetic patients is increased when OCs are used.
Antihypertensive Agents Cyclopenthiazide, Guanethidine, Methyldopa, Metoprolol	Reduced efficacy is probably due to contraceptive-induced sodium and fluid retention. The OC has an inhibitory effect on hepatic microsomal oxidase.	OCs may have to be stopped in order to treat hypertension adequately. Clinical importance of this interaction is likely to be small because the patient population taking beta-blockers overlaps very little with that taking OCs.
Caffeine	Mechanism of interaction is OC inhibition of hepatic metabolism of caffeine.	Impairment of caffeine elimination by OCs suggests that it would be reasonable to advise women taking OCs to moderate their intake of caffeine.
Clofibrate	Unknown	The interaction has not been confirmed, but caution is suggested in the use of this combination.
Corticosteroids	Plasma cortisol concentrations were elevated approximately two-fold in OC users compared to control subjects.	The addition of OCs to the treatment regimen of patients receiving corticosteroid therapy may result in potentiation of both beneficial and adverse effects of corticosteroids.
Hypnotics, Sedatives, or Other CNS Depressants Diazepam	Volume of distribution of diazepam 10 mg IV did not differ between OC users and nonusers, but the apparent elimination half-life was longer and the total metabolic clearance was significantly less in the OC users.	Increased effects diazepam should be anticipated and reduction in diazepam dosage may be required.
Phenothiazines	Estrogen-containing OCs may potentiate phenothiazine-stimulated prolactin secretion, resulting in mammary hypertrophy and galactorrhea.	OCs can potentiate an adverse effect caused by other agents.
Theophylline	OC users had a significantly lower total plasma clearance of theophylline.	OC users may require lower than normal doses of the bronchodilator.
Drugs Potentiating Side Effects of Oral Contraceptives Allopurinol Aminosalicyclic acid Aspirin Chloramphenicol Cimetidine Disulfiram Hydrocortisone Isoniazid Methandrostenolone Methylphenidate MAOI antidepressants Phenothiazines Phenyramidol Sulfaphenazole Triparanol and other drugs causing inhibition of microsomal enzymes, also influenza and BCG vaccines.	All these drugs are reported to cause liver enzyme inhibition. Concomitant administration with OCs could, theoretically, be expected to potentiate the actions of OCs by delaying the hepatic metabolism of both the estrogen and progestogen components.	These drugs should be used with care in women taking OCs.

(Adapted from D'Arcy, PF: Drug interactions with oral contraceptives. Drug Intelligence and Clinical Pharmacy 20(5) 353, May, 1986.)

bleeding, so-called breakthrough bleeding, is also more frequent at first. It appears to be less troublesome with preparations containing larger amounts of estrogen.

Oral contraceptives also may cause intolerance to carbohydrates, resulting in elevations of blood glucose and insulin. If notable alteration in blood sugar occurs, oral contraceptives should be discontinued. Oral contraceptives may also alter lipoprotein levels.

INTERACTIONS. Oral contraceptives may interact with other drugs through various mechanisms. Table 43–11 features drugs that reduce the efficacy of oral contraceptives. It is possible for oral contraceptives to be potentiated by displacement from protein-binding sites by other drugs such as phenylbutazone or barbiturates. There is also the potential for decreased absorption of oral contraceptives from the gastrointestinal tract with concurrent use of antibiotics such as penicillins.

Women taking these medications should be advised to use some other method of birth control instead of, or in addition to, oral contraceptives. Spotting or bleeding that takes place between menstrual periods may be a sign that the contraceptive is not working well enough to inhibit ovulation. It is likely that current knowledge of these types of interactions is far from comprehensive and that other drugs, not yet identified, can enter into such interactions.

SPERMICIDES. Vaginal spermicides containing nonoxynol 9, such as creams, gels, foams, suppositories, and sponges (Table 43–12), are inexpensive and available for topical vaginal application. All these products are available over the counter and are easy to use. These products are applied minutes to 1 hour before coitus and are reapplied before each ejaculation. Douching is avoided for the next 6–8 hours. Vaginal spermicides are one of the safest methods of contraception, particularly when combined with barrier contraceptives.

CONTRACEPTIVE SPONGE. The contraceptive sponge, the newest type of vaginal contraceptive approved by the FDA in 1983, is a disposable polyurethane sponge containing a spermicide (1 gm of nonoxynol 9). It acts as a mechanical barrier to sperm, absorbs seminal fluid, and releases the spermicide that is incorporated into the sponge. The sponge has several advantages in that it is not messy, the spermicide is readily available, and it may be left in place for multiple coital encounters over a 24–30 hour period. No additional spermicide is needed for repeated intercourse. Vaginal sponges offer some advantages common to barrier contraceptives, such as protection from sexually transmitted diseases, and possible protection against cervical neoplasia. General complaints about diaphragms and vaginal spermicides, such as their messiness and distastefulness, are avoided with use of sponges. However, some women find sponges make the vagina dry by absorbing vaginal lubrication.

INTRAUTERINE DEVICES. Only one intrauterine device (IUD) remains on the market in the United States today—the Progestasert system. This device contains progesterone and must be replaced annually. IUDs prevent implantation of the blastocyst by altering the biochemical milieu of the endometrium. The progesterone (65 μg/day) that is continually released into the endometrial cavity causes a reaction which makes the conditions for implantation unfavorable. Progesterone may also inhibit the metabolism, capacitation, and swimming speed of sperm. IUDs are not recommended as a contraceptive method until a woman has completed her family.

Table 43–12. VAGINAL SPERMICIDES (NONPRESCRIPTION)*

PRODUCT AND MANUFACTURER
Creams Conceptrol (Ortho) Orth-Creme (Ortho)
Gels Conceptrol Disposable Gel (Ortho) Gynol II (Ortho) Koromex Gel (Youngs) Koromex II A Jelly (Youngs) Ramses Vaginal Jelly (Schmid)
Foams Delfen Foam (Ortho) Emko (Schering) Emko Because (Schering) Koromex (Youngs)
Sponge Today (VLI)
Suppositories Encare (Thompson Medical) Intercept Inserts (Ortho) Semicid (Whitehall)

*The active ingredient in all these products is nonoxynol 9, in various concentrations.

USING THE NURSING PROCESS

ASSESSMENT

Assessment of the patient requiring female hormones or other drugs affecting the female reproductive system can be very complex, depending on individual circumstances. Information the nurse needs to obtain is featured in Table 43–13.

Various diagnostic tests can be used to determine the specific cause of decreased ovarian function. Urinary levels of estrogens and progesterone and their metabolites can be measured. The three principal estrogens that are measured are 17β-estradiol, estrone, and estriol. The metabolite of progesterone, pregnanediol, is a specific metabolite and its urinary level is an accurate indicator of serum progesterone levels. Radioimmunoassays are also used to measure levels of ovarian hormones. In primary ovarian insufficiency, the levels are low.

Blood and urine measurements of the gonadotropic hormones are also useful in determining whether the hypogonadal state is due to a primary or secondary ovarian insufficiency. Low levels of the gonadotropins are characteristic of secondary insufficiency, whereas

Table 43–13. NURSING PROCESS FOR PATIENT REQUIRING FEMALE HORMONES

Assessment

Assess history of menstrual function, including presence of dysmenorrhea, dysfunctional bleeding or menopausal symptoms, PMS. Note history of other endocrine and genitourinary problems.
Determine previous/current medications patient is taking, including oral contraceptives and OTC/street drugs, use of tobacco.
Note exercise habits.
Review laboratory studies, e.g., urinary levels of estrogens, progesterone and their metabolites; blood and urine measurements of the gonadotropic hormones;
Examine vaginal epithelium for estrogenic effect, cornification of epithelial cells, secretory changes characteristic of progesterone stimulation of endometrial tissue and hormone influences on endocervical mucus.
Review radioimmunoassay reports which measure levels of ovarian hormones

Nursing Diagnosis	Nursing Actions	Rationale	Desired Outcomes/ Evaluation Criteria
Knowledge deficit related to information misinterpretation, unfamiliarity with information resources as evidenced by questions, statement of concern, inaccurate follow-through of instructions, development of preventable complications.	Provide information about condition/disease and treatment regimen. Discuss action, use, dose, storage, and side effects of hormones. Discuss ways to minimize GI upset, reduce discomfort and improve sexual relations.	Understanding helps patient to make informed choices and participate in treatment. Promotes correct use of medications to maximize effectiveness and minimizes adverse reactions. While transient side effects may disappear with continued use of estrogen, simple measures may reduce others, e.g., taking drug with meals, use of mild antidiarrheal drugs, use of a vaginal lubricant.	Verbalizes understanding of condition/disease process and need for treatment. Identifies relationship of signs/symptoms to the disease process. Participates in treatment regimen.
	Instruct patient to monitor for significant side effects, e.g., fluid retention, increased blood pressure, vaginal candidiasis, thromboembolism, jaundice or depression.	Early identification allows for appropriate intervention to avoid complications.	
	Recommend cessation of smoking.	Smoking increases risk of thromboembolic side-effects of these drugs.	
	Stress importance of routine follow-up.	Because of increased risk of thromboembolic and cardiovascular problems, checkups may detect early signs and promote preventive actions.	
	Discuss necessity of contacting physician if taking oral contraceptives and pregnancy is suspected.	Estrogen and progesterones can cause fetal abnormalities and medication needs to be discontinued.	
Sexual Patterns, altered/Sexual Dysfunction, Potential related to altered body structure/function, illness, fear of pregnancy.	Provide privacy and have patient describe problem(s) in own words. Discuss pathophysiology of condition/illness, e.g., menopause, hypogonadism, avoidance of pregnancy.	Promotes identification and clarification of problems and defines interventions. Promotes understanding and informed choices.	Verbalizes understanding of individual reasons for sexual difficulties/changes that have occurred. Follows treatment regimen. Identifies and uses appropriate method of contraception.
	Encourage open discussion with SO.	Clarifies problems and provides opportunity to resolve misunderstandings/improve the relationship.	

Table 43–14. SIGNS OF ESTROGEN/PROGESTIN EXCESS AND DEFICIT

Sign	Estrogen Excess	Progestin Excess	Estrogen Deficit	Progestin Deficit
Abdominal distention	x	—	—	—
Breast tenderness	x	x	—	—
Cystic breasts	x	—	—	—
Dysmenorrhea	x	—	—	x
Edema	x	—	—	—
Hypermenorrhea	x	—	—	x
Increased breast size	x	x	—	—
Migraine headache	x	—	—	—
Nervousness	x	—	x	—
Uterine cramping	x	—	—	—
Weight gain	x	x	—	—
Change in libido	—	x	—	—
Depression	—	x	—	—
Fatigue	—	x	—	—
Hypomenorrhea	—	x	x	—
Vaginal infection	—	x	—	—
Amenorrhea	—	—	x	x
Cystocele, rectocele	—	—	x	—
Irritability	x	—	x	—
Decreased breast size	—	—	—	x
Weight loss	—	—	—	x

high gonadotropin levels are consistent with primary ovarian dysfunction. (Since low gonadotropin levels may be indicative of widespread pituitary dysfunction, this finding should be followed up with a thorough assessment of pituitary function.)

Ovarian function can also be evaluated indirectly by assessing for the effects of the hormones. Vaginal epithelium may be examined for the estrogenic effect, cornification of the epithelial cells. Endometrial tissue may be examined for secretory changes characteristic of progesterone stimulation. Endocervical mucus also reflects hormonal influences. Women may experience both an estrogen or progestin excess or deficit. Table 43–14 features common signs associated with these hormonal disturbances.

A careful nursing history of menstrual function also helps in the diagnosis of ovarian dysfunction as well as in the diagnosis of other conditions such as dysmenorrhea, dysfunctional bleeding, or menopausal symptoms. Patients are questioned about medications they may be taking, since disruption of the menstrual cycle can be due to pharmacologic influences. Specific questions to ask include age at menarche, interval and duration of menstrual periods, amount of flow, occurrence of pain, and dates of onset of the last one or two periods.

As menopause approaches, the menstrual cycles come closer together. Women often experience hot flushes and excessive perspiration due primarily to hypothalamic imbalances induced by decreased release of ovarian steroids. Hormonal therapy may be helpful in alleviating these symptoms.

When oral contraceptives are being taken, it is important to obtain a recent sexual history as well as a recent drug history to look for drugs which might decrease the efficacy of oral contraceptives. The reasons for using this birth control method are disucssed. Also, it is important to determine how well the patient will comply with therapy.

Baseline weight, blood pressure, and eye exams—particularly for contact lens wearers—are obtained. These items must be reassessed periodically during therapy. Also a current smoking history is obtained. If the patient smokes, it is important to do health teaching during the intervention phase to help her quit. There is an increased incidence of complications in women on estrogen therapy who continue to smoke.

NURSING DIAGNOSES

When assessment is completed, nursing diagnoses are established. Typical nursing diagnoses for patients requiring estrogen and progestogens are included in Table 43–13.

INTERVENTION

Goals for nursing interventions are developed from the list of nursing diagnoses. Table 43–13 illustrates nursing goals for intervention.

NURSING RESPONSIBILITIES WHEN ADMINISTERING FEMALE HORMONES

The nurse encourages all patients taking estrogen, progestins, or oral contraceptives to practice preventive health measures. Regular gynecologic examinations with Pap tests are important. The nurse makes sure that the patient understands how to practice breast self-examination and encourages this on a monthly basis. Body weight and blood pressure are also monitored regularly.

Other safety implications are featured in Table 43–5 in the column headed "Nursing Implications."

PATIENT TEACHING

Patient teaching information may be found in Table 43–15.

In teaching patients about the use of oral contraceptives, additional information should include the recommended use of an additional method of birth control during the first week of the initial cycle, and instructions for dealing with "missed" pills. The following serves as a guideline only:

1. *One omitted pill:* The missed tablet can be taken as soon as remembered or taken the next day with regular dose (double up).
2. *Two consecutive omitted pills:* Use another contraceptive method for the next seven days, then take two tablets daily for two days, and resume regular schedule.
3. *Three consecutive omitted pills:* Cycle should be resumed seven days after the last tablet was taken; another method of contraception should be used during this period and for seven days into the cycle.

Table 43–15. PATIENT TEACHING INFORMATION—FEMALE HORMONES

Dear Patient:
This drug has been prescribed for you. This is what you should know about your drug to get the most from your therapy.
Female hormones are used for several reasons. For you they are being used for _____.

1. Female hormones are taken for an indefinite time; your doctor will tell you what is best for you.
2. Take your drugs exactly as ordered.
3. Do not take female hormones if you have a history of blood clots, stroke, cancer (breast or genitalia), or liver disease.
4. Do not take female hormones if you are pregnant or breastfeeding.
5. Take oral female hormones after meals to decrease feeling "sick to your stomach."
6. Do not stop taking your female hormones without first checking with your doctor.
7. Report any side effects to your doctor. Some side effects are weight gain, or jaundice (yellowing of skin or eyeball).
8. Immediately report any pain, redness, or swelling in your legs; these could be signs of a blood clot.
9. Immediately report sudden, partial, or complete loss of vision; double vision; or migraine. DO NOT continue to take your drugs until you talk with your physician.
10. Check your weight weekly at the same time of day. Report a gain/loss of weight of more than _____ pounds/week.
11. Practice regular breast self-examination and have regular PAP exams.
12. Stop smoking.
13. Carry a Medic Alert card or other similar identification.
14. Store your drugs in tightly closed containers.

If pregnancy is suspected, the woman should contact her physician. Estrogen and progesterones can cause fetal abnormalities and, therefore, need to be discontinued.

Another common method of birth control today is the use of condoms. Condoms also are a means of preventing the spread of sexually transmitted disease (STD), particularly human immunodeficiency virus (HIV). Due to the 10 to 15 percent contraceptive failure rate of condoms and the potential for slippage and rupture during intercourse, a backup virucidal chemcial barrier may be beneficial. The spermicide, nonoxynol 9, inhibits the growth of organisms responsible for STDs and HIV. The spermicides featured in Table 43–10 all contain nonoxynol 9 in various concentrations. Women are encouraged to use both a spermicide and a condom for better protection.

Female condoms will be on the market in 1989. They are held in place by two flexible rings. The one-size-fits-all top ring is inserted like a diaphragm, snug against the cervix, while the bottom ring prevents the condom from "riding up" in the vagina. Connecting the two rings is a polyurethane sheath. One advantage is that the condom can be inserted hours before intercourse, permitting sexual spontaneity.

Diaphragms are another frequently used method of birth control. The diaphragm, a dome-shaped rubber cap with a size range of 7–10 cm, is inserted into the vagina and over the anterior vaginal wall and cervix prior to intercourse. Some diaphragms are inserted with the help of an "inserter." It is used with a spermicidal gel or cream that is placed in the diaphragm between it and the cervix. It can be inserted up to two hours before sex. If intercourse occurs a second or third time, additional spermicide is inserted for added protection. The diaphragm is left in place for six hours after intercourse. A douche is recommended after removal to cleanse the remaining gel or cream.

EVALUATION

During this phase of the nursing process, the nurse determines the effectiveness of the nursing interventions. The expected outcomes for patients requiring drugs affecting the female reproductive system are included in Table 43–13.

The patient using female hormones for contraception should be expected to have an understanding of her reproductive cycle, how the oral contraceptives function within that cycle, side effects and potential risks associated with them, and the necessity for consistent use in order to achieve maximum effectiveness.

The nurse should know the adverse effects of these drugs and should determine that the patient understands them as well. Adverse effects of the estrogens and progestins include nausea, vomiting, diarrhea, skin rashes, irregular menstrual bleeding, and headache.

Compliance with medication regimens is somewhat dependent on the circumstances that initiate therapy. For example, patients taking fertility drugs are usually very conscientious about their medication, as it reflects yet another in a series of interventions designed to achieve pregnancy. Once pregnant, the patient is cautioned about taking all medications. (Refer to a maternal text for more information.) Compliance by patients taking oral contraceptives is related to the strength of their desire to avoid pregnancy and to their feelings regarding pregnancy or a termination of pregnancy should it result.

A large number of unplanned pregnancies continue to occur in the adolescent. A recent study (Emans, et al, 1987) evaluated 209 unmarried sexually active adolescents initiating use of oral contraceptives. Predictors of compliance include white race, older—over 18 years of age, history of prior contraceptive use, older sexual partner, and satisfaction with the pill. Additional predictors of compliance include having a private suburban health care provider, married parents, and suburban residence. Much health teaching is required to gain compliance in the nonwhite group.

Throughout, the nurse stresses the need for continuous medical follow-up and should periodically review teaching with the patient to ensure that the patient's information is accurate and up-to-date.

FERTILITY MEDICATIONS

Infertility is generally defined as the inability to conceive after one year or more of unprotected, regular sexual intercourse. About 10 to 15 percent of American couples are estimated to be involuntarily infertile. Depending on the etiology of the infertility problem, medications may be prescribed to bring hormone levels to normal or to enhance ovarian function—the so-called fertility drugs. Four drugs are currently used to stimulate ovulation in the anovulatory infertile woman. Three are gonadotropins: human chorionic gonadotropin (HCG, Follutein), prepared from the urine of pregnant women; menotropins or human menopausal gonadotropin (HMG, Pergonal); and urofollitropin (Metrodin), a preparation of FSH and LH extracted from the urine of postmenopausal women. Chorionic gonadotropin is secreted by the placenta during pregnancy and functions to sustain the corpus luteum. The fourth drug is clomiphene (Clomid), which is often classified as an antiestrogen, but has weak estrogenic properties as well.

The use of menotropins and urofollitropin stimulates growth and maturation of ovarian follicles due to the FSH and LH activities. Clomiphene competes for estrogen-binding sites, leaving fewer receptors available for endogenous estrogen attachment. This interferes with the normal feedback mechanism, and the body (hypothalamus) interprets this as a low level of estrogen. Consequently, there is an increased secretion of gonadotropins. Clomiphene is most effective in women who have adequate amounts of estrogen and follicular function, but who lack effective stimulation from the pituitary gonadotropins.

In many treatment regimens for infertility, clomiphene is employed initially, particularly when inadequate gonadotropic stimulation exists. Starting on the second or fifth day of the menstrual cycle, 50 mg is administered daily for five days. The majority of women who respond to clomiphene will ovulate after the first course of therapy. Dosage may be increased to 100 mg in a second 5-day cycle of therapy. Generally, no more than three courses of therapy are recommended if there is no response to the drug.

If ovulation still has not occurred, HCG in a dose of 10,000 IU can be administered in conjunction with the clomiphene during that cycle. HCG is given at midcycle to induce ovulation within approximately 18–48 hours. If this therapy, too, proves ineffective, menotropins can be administered during the next cycle. Initial dosage is 75 IU of FSH and LH intramuscularly for 9–12 days. Then, chorionic gonadotropin is given in a dose of 10,000 IU intramuscularly when optimal estrogen levels have been reached. Two to five such treatment cycles may be required for success. A 90 percent ovulation rate and a 50 to 70 percent pregnancy rate has been attained. The cost of menotropins may range from $150 to $750 per cycle. The use of menotropins necessitates almost daily ultrasound to determine follicle size and to strictly monitor estradiol levels.

Therapy with fertility drugs is not without problems. The most common reactions to clomiphene administration include hot flushes, breast discomfort, headache, nausea and vomiting, abdominal distention, and pain related to ovarian enlargement. Visual disturbances, such as blurred vision, sparkling visual sensations, ghosting, and photophobia, can also occur.

The use of chorionic gonadotropin and menotropins is associated with an increased risk of thromboembolic disease. Headache, irritability, and restlessness can occur when HCG is administered to pregnant women. Both drugs can also induce the ovarian hyperstimulation discussed in relation to clomiphene.

The possibility of multiple births increases with the use of the fertility drugs. Clomiphene administration is associated with a 10% chance of multiple births (usually twins); use of mentotropins and HCG is associated with a five percent chance of having three or more babies. Fertility drugs are featured in Table 43–16.

USING THE NURSING PROCESS

ASSESSMENT

Assessment of clients for infertility problems includes all of the information listed in the section on female hormones, along with further specialized testing. Disorders that are at least partly amenable to drug therapy include unfavorable cervical mucus, anovulation, luteal phase defect, and endometriosis. Since infertility can be due to factors affecting the male as well as the female, both partners are assessed. A thorough sexual history (including, but not limited to: frequency of intercourse, timing in relation to ovulation, and use of contraceptives) is obtained from both partners and is essential to begin formation of the data base. Assessment of the male includes an endocrine evaluation and semen analysis. Assessment of the female includes the previously mentioned tests of ovarian function as well as: regular measurements of basal body temperature (progesterone has a thermogenic effect), endometrial biopsy, and the tubal insufflation of Rubin test. Endoscopic procedures such as culdoscopy or laparoscopy may also be utilized.

NURSING DIAGNOSES

Following data collection, nursing diagnoses are established. Some typical nursing diagnoses for the woman requiring fertility medications might be: Family process, alteration in, related to: infertility; or Self-concept, alterations in, related to: infertility.

INTERVENTION

Based on the nursing diagnoses, specific nursing interventions are planned. For the infertile patient electing use of ovulatory medications, the nurse must again emphasize the teaching aspects of care, giving the client and her partner necessary information about the drugs she is taking and the expected results. Psychologic support for these clients is an important aspect of nursing care, as the process of diagnosis and treatment for the infertility can be a long, frustrating one in which the anticipated outcome (pregnancy) cannot be guaranteed.

The timing of administration of the fertility drugs is crucial to their successful use. Menotropins are administered on the 7th through the 14th day of the menstrual cycle. Chorionic gonadotropin is administered seven to ten days following clomiphene therapy or when optimal estrogen levels (as measured by 24-hour urinary estrogen secretion or plasma estradiol) have been reached with menotropins. Both menotropins and HCG must be administered via intramuscular injection. Following HCG administration, couples should be directed to have intercourse within 12–18 hours and daily for the next two days.

The ovarian enlargement that can occur with clomiphene use can pose serious problems. The hyperstimulated ovaries are enlarged, fragile, and often cystic. Strenuous physical activity, a pelvic examination, or intercourse can, at this time, cause rupture of ovarian cysts. Symptoms of enlargement to caution the patient about include unilateral pelvic discomfort aggravated by walking, and/or abdominal distention. Should these occur, the nurse encourages the patient to minimize her activity, avoid intercourse, and notify her physician. Other indicators of distress include sudden weight gain, abdominal pain, vaginal bleeding, and dyspnea.

TEXT RESUMES ON PAGE 1136

Table 43–16. FERTILITY DRUGS

Name	Dosage	Mode of Administration	Pharmacokinetics
Clomiphene (Clomid)			
Action: Nonsteroidal agent which increases output of pituitary gonadotropins.			
Use: May induce ovulation in selected anovulatory women.			
	50 mg/day × 5 days starting on fifth day of cycle; if no ovulation occurs, increase to 100 mg/day × 5 days	PO	O: rapid P: UA D: 6 wk ½L: UA PB: UA B: liver E: feces
Human Menopausal Gonadotropin (HMG)			
Action: Produces ovarian follicular growth in women who do not have primary ovarian failure.			
Use: Induction of ovulation and pregnancy.			
Menotropins (Pergonal)	75–150 IU qd × 9–12 days	IM	UA
Urofollitropin (Metrodin)			
Action: Produces ovarian follicular growth in women who do not have primary ovarian failure.			
Use: Induction of ovulation and pregnancy.			
	75 IU/day for 7–12 days plus 2 more courses	IM	

Key to Abbreviations in the *Pharmacokinetics* column O-onset; P-peak; D-duration; PB-protein bound; B-biotransformed in; E-excreted in; ½ L-halflife.
*Within the column listing adverse effects, underlines indicate the most common effects.

Contraindications/ Precautions	Adverse Effects*	Interactions	Nursing Implications
CONTRAINDICATIONS: Pregnancy, liver dysfunction, and abnormal bleeding. PRECAUTIONS: Use with caution in enlarged ovaries or pelvic discomfort.	Generally mild effects. *Neuro:* nervousness, insomnia, depression, fatigue, headache *GI:* abdominal distress, bloating, nausea, vomiting *Renal:* increased urination *Reprod:* vasomotor flushes, breast tenderness, ovarian enlargement *Integ:* urticaria *Eye:* flashes, ghosting	May increase BSP levels, plasma thyroxine, and thyroid-binding-globulin.	For all Fertility drugs: ASSESSMENT: Take sexual history. Daily measurement of basal body temperature. EVALUATION: Report side effects. Same as for all. INTERVENTION: Take exactly as prescribed for 5 consecutive days. Do not administer if history of ovarian cysts exists.
CONTRAINDICATIONS: Ovarian cysts, thyroid or adrenal dysfunction, pregnancy, abnormal bleeding.	*CV:* arterial thromboembolism *Reprod:* ovarian enlargement, hemoperitoneum	None significant.	Same as for all. INTERVENTION: Administer 7th to 14th day of cycle. The dose is dependent on estradiol levels and follicle size determined by ultrasound. Administer deep IM. Prepare by diluting with 1–2 ml of sterile normal saline solution. Administer immediately after preparation. Do not administer if history of ovarian cysts exists. Couple should have intercourse every other day starting with last day of therapy.
CONTRAINDICATIONS: Primary ovarian failure, thyroid/adrenal dysfunction, pituitary tumor, abnormal bleeding, ovarian cysts or enlargement, and pregnancy.	*Neuro:* headache *CV:* arterial thromboembolism *GI:* abdominal pain, nausea, vomiting, diarrhea, abdominal cramps, bloating *Reprod:* ovarian enlargement, breast tenderness *Integ:* rash *Misc:* febrile reactions, muscle aches and pains, malaise, fatigue	None significant.	Same as for all. INTERVENTION: Administer for 7–12 days. Dose is dependent on estradiol levels and follicle size as determined by ultrasound. Couple should have intercourse daily starting with last day of therapy. Dissolve ampule in 1–2 ml saline and administer immediately. Discard unused medication. Protect from light.

CONTINUED ON THE FOLLOWING PAGE

Table 43–16. FERTILITY DRUGS–*CONTINUED*

Name	Dosage	Mode of Administration	Pharmacokinetics
Human chorionic gonadotropins (HCG, Follutein)			
Action: Stimulates production of gonadal steroid hormones.			
Use: Prepubertal cryptorchidism, induction of ovulation, stimulate spermatogenesis in males.			
	Males: 500–5000 U qd or qod *Females:* single dose of 10,000 U	IM	UA

Key to Abbreviations in the *Pharmacokinetics* column O-onset; P-peak; D-duration; PB-protein bound; B-biotransformed in; ½ L-halflife.
*Within the column listing adverse effects, <u>underlines</u> indicate the most common effects.

EVALUATION

Evaluation criteria are developed by the nurse after discussion with the patient. Although the patient may feel that the only successful outcome of treatment with fertility drugs is a pregnancy, that cannot be guaranteed.

Criteria should include a patient who is knowledgeable about her therapy and her drugs and who experiences minimal side effects. The nurse should make certain that the patient is aware of side effects to anticipate. Adverse effects of the fertility drugs include nausea and vomiting, headache, and ovarian enlargement.

SUMMARY

Male hormones are necessary in men for the differentiation, growth, and development of male sexual organs. Testosterone also has anabolic activity which causes an increase in musculature. Male hormones can be used for a variety of disorders in both men and women.

Female hormones, estrogens and progestogens, are necessary for the secondary sex characteristics in women. Estrogens and progestogens are used clinically to treat hormonal deficiencies, as contraceptive agents, to treat dysmenorrhea, and estrogen alone can be used to treat symptoms of menopause.

When the nurse is administering either male or female hormones, a thorough history is obtained. Blood and urine measurements of the gonadotropic hormones may be done. Weight, body size, sexual history, and for women a menstrual history are all obtained. Once started on these products, patient teaching is important. The patient needs to understand the importance of taking these medications as prescribed as well as reporting side effects to the physician.

BIBLIOGRAPHY

After 10 years on the IUD, what should I use instead? Patient Care 21(8):81, 1987.
Contraception choices now. Changing Times 40(11):121, 1986.
Covington, TR: Contraception: Spermicidal foams, creams and gels. Facts & Comparisons Drug Newsletter, 6(10):77, October, 1987.
D'Arcy, PF: Drug interactions with oral contraceptives. Drug Int Clin Pharm 20(5):353, May, 1986.
Dirubbo, NE: The condom barrier. Am J Nurs 87(10):1306, 1987.
Drug abuse in athletes. JAMA 259(11):1703, 1988.
Durie, B: Drugs and sexual function. Nurs Times 83(32):34, 1987.
Emans, SJ, et al: Adolescents' compliance with the use of oral contraceptives. JAMA 257:3377, 1987.
Gambrell, RD: Banishing the shadow of menopause. Emerg Med 18(19):24, November, 1986.
Gilman, AG, Goodman, LS, and Gilman, A: Goodman and Gilman's The Pharmacological Basis of Therapeutics, ed 6. Macmillan, New York, 1985.
Goldzieher, JW, et al: Medical aspects of contraception. Hosp Pract 22(3):93, 1987.
Hatcher, RA, et al: Contraceptive Technology, ed 13. Irvington Public, New York, 1986.
Hospital Formulary. American Society of Hospital Pharmacists, Washington, DC, 1986.
Orshan, S: The pill, the patient, and you. RN 88(7):49, 1988.
Pope, H and Katz, D: Bodybuilder's psychosis (letter). Lancet 1:863, April 11, 1987.
Porter, JB, Jick, H, and Walker, AM: Mortality among oral contraceptive users. Obstet Gynecol 70:29, 1987.
Prevention and treatment of postmenopausal osteoporosis. The Medical Letter 29(746):75, August 14, 1987.
Rietmeijer, CAM, et al: Condoms as physical and chemical barriers against human immunodeficiency virus. JAMA 259:1851, 1988.

Contraindications/ Precautions	Adverse Effects*	Interactions	Nursing Implications
CONTRAINDICATIONS: Hypersensitivity, prostatic carcinoma, precocious puberty. PRECAUTIONS: Use cautiously in patients with epilepsy, migraine, asthma, cardiac or renal disease.	*Neuro:* headache, irritability, restlessness, depression, fatigue *CV:* edema *Reprod:* precocious puberty, gynecomastia	None significant	Same as for all. INTERVENTION: Administer at optimal estrogen levels to stimulate ovulation. Administer deep IM. Reconstitute with diluent supplied by manufacturer. Stable for 1–3 months after reconstitution under refrigeration.

Sarno, AP, Miller, EJ, and Lundblad, EG: Premenstrual syndrome: Beneficial effects of periodic low-dose danazol. Obstet Gynecol 70:33, 1987.

Smith, S, et al: Treatment of premenstrual syndrome with alprazolam: Results of a double-blind placebo controlled randomized crossover clinical trial. Obstet Gynecol 70:37, 1987.

Vessey, M, et al: Oral contraceptives and venous thromboembolism: Findings in a large prospective study. Br Med J 292:526, February 22, 1986.

Weintraub, M and Evans, P: Transdermal estradiol: Technology and theory integrated for patient care. Hosp Formul 21:1001, October, 1986.

When technology takes over manipulating women's fertility. Nurs Times 83(20), 1987.

Willis, J: The pill may not mix well with other drugs. FDS Consum 21(2):26, March, 1987.

SITUATION   43–1

Johathan Stance, an 18-year-old, has been evaluated for hypogonadism and is to be treated through the health clinic.

1. During the nursing assessment the nurse will check Johathan for:
   a. excessive growth of long bones
   b. decreased subcutaneous fat
   c. heavy growth of facial hair
   d. increased muscle strength

2. Jonathan is to begin treatment with testosterone cypionate (Depo-testosterone). The nurse will expect that this drug will be given by the following route:
   a. intravenous
   b. subcutaneous
   c. intramuscular
   d. buccal

3. The nurse will plan for Jonathan's medication schedule of testosterone cypionate based on the following length of drug effectiveness:
   a. 2 months
   b. 2 to 4 weeks
   c. 5 days
   d. 24 to 48 hours

4. The nurse will teach Jonathan about side effects related to testosterone therapy. The following side effect is included
   a. insomnia
   b. high-pitched voice
   c. weakness
   d. photosensitivity

5. On a follow-up visit, Jonathan is to begin oral therapy with fluoxymesterone (Halotestin) after evidence of sexual characteristics develops. The nurse will instruct him to:
   a. use antacids regularly
   b. force oral fluids
   c. reduce protein intake
   d. take the drug with meals

6. When evaluating Jonathan, an important aspect to monitor would be:
   a. tuberculin skin test
   b. liver function tests
   c. creatinine clearance
   d. cardiac enzyme levels

CONTINUED ON THE FOLLOWING PAGE

SITUATION 43–2

Lauren Mann, aged 46, presents to the health clinic with symptoms of postmenopausal syndrome. She complains of excessive perspiration, hot flashes, and fatigue.

1. Ms. Mann will be placed on 1 mg of conjugated estrogens (Premarin). The nurse will anticipate the following schedule of administration of Premarin:
   a. every other day
   b. every third day
   c. fourteen days on/fourteen days off
   d. three weeks on/one week off

2. When taking Ms. Mann's history, the nurse will report the following, which represents a contraindication to estrogen therapy:
   a. osteoporosis
   b. chronic asthma
   c. coronary artery disease
   d. liver disease

3. The nurse will include the following in a teaching session with Ms. Mann:
   a. avoid strenuous activity
   b. check weight regularly
   c. report any nausea immediately
   d. take as needed for hot flashes

4. Which of the following activities reported by Ms. Mann warrants immediate attention by the nurse?
   a. voracious reading
   b. gourmet cooking
   c. jogging
   d. cigarette smoking

5. Additional teaching information relative to Ms. Mann's care would include:
   a. reducing intake of citrus juices
   b. avoiding large meals
   c. taking medication after meals
   d. preventing excess sun exposure

6. The nurse takes a diet history of Ms. Mann and will encourage a high dietary intake of:
   a. potassium
   b. sodium
   c. calcium
   d. Vitamin C

Please refer to Appendices for correct answers and additional review questions with answers.

44
CHAPTER

AGENTS USED TO TREAT DIABETES MELLITUS

GLOSSARY TERMS IN THIS CHAPTER

Diabetes mellitus
Disulfiram-like reaction
Endogenous insulin
Exogenous insulin
Gluconeogenesis
Glycogenolysis
Glycosuria
Glycosylated hemoglobin
Hyperglycemic hyperosmolar nonketotic coma
Ketoacidosis
Ketosis
Lipoatrophy
Lipohypertrophy
Neuropathy
Normoglycemia

44
CHAPTER

AGENTS USED TO TREAT DIABETES MELLITUS

CHRISTINE M. BELLARI, M.S., R.N., CDE

LEARNING OBJECTIVES

After reading this chapter, the student will be able to:

1. Identify those medications commonly used in the treatment of diabetes mellitus.

2. Differentiate between insulin and oral hypoglycemic agents as to the mechanism of action, route of administration, pharmacokinetics, adverse effects, contraindications, and interactions.

3. Identify specific areas to assess in the patient requiring antidiabetic agents in order to formulate appropriate nursing diagnoses.

4. Plan the nursing interventions necessary to administer antidiabetic medications and choose appropriate teaching strategies to gain patient compliance.

5. Evaluate the diabetic patient at various stages of treatment to gauge effectiveness of nursing interventions.

THERAPEUTIC AGENTS

Diabetes mellitus is a disease characterized by an absolute or relative deficiency of insulin, resulting in an elevated level of sugar in the blood. This leads to abnormalities of carbohydrate, protein, and fat metabolism and to eventual complications of the eye, kidney, blood vessels, and nervous system. More than 11 million Americans have diabetes and the overall incidence is increasing each year. Diabetes, along with its complications, is a major cause of morbidity and mortality in the United States.

There are two major types of diabetes, Type I and Type II. Type I, or insulin-dependent diabetes mellitus (IDDM), is characterized by an absolute deficiency of insulin, abrupt onset of symptoms, and proneness to *ketosis*. This type of diabetes most commonly occurs in youth, but may occur at any age.

Type II, or non–insulin-dependent diabetes mellitus (NIDDM), frequently occurs without any symptoms. The individual is able to produce some insulin and therefore is not prone to ketosis. In many cases, the individual produces an above normal amount of insulin and the hyperglycemia is due to the body cells being resistant to the insulin. Type II diabetes is most frequently seen after the age of forty, but may occur at any age. Usually, the individual has a family history of diabetes and is overweight. For a more detailed comparison of Type I versus Type II diabetes, refer to Table 44–1.

There is no known cure for diabetes. However, it can be controlled. The major goals of management are to: restore cellular utilization of glucose, prevent ketosis, abolish symptoms indicative of hyperglycemia, attain normal growth and development for a child, and maintain the blood glucose at a near normal level without frequent episodes of hypoglycemia. Normalization of blood glucose levels is desired in an effort to prevent, postpone, or reverse the chronic complications of diabetes.

INSULIN

Diabetes was recognized as early as 1500 B.C. From that time until the discovery of insulin, there was no successful mode of treatment. The individual with diabetes was destined to a short uncomfortable life, succumbing to the acute complication of *ketoacidosis*. In 1921, insulin was discovered by Banting and Best. Since then, the extraction of insulin from animal pancreas has made replacement therapy possible. The life expectancy of the individual with diabetes increased tremendously, and the major cause of death changed from acute complications of the disease to chronic complications, developing years after diagnosis.

Insulin is classified biochemically as a protein, composed of 51 amino acids and having a molecular weight of approximately 6,000. It is composed of two amino acid chains, chain A (acidic) and chain B (basic), linked together by two disulfide bridges. Both of these chains

Table 44–1. DIABETES MELLITUS

DEFINITION
A chronic disorder of carbohydrate metabolism, resulting from the overproduction and underutilization of glucose due to the lack of or inactivity of insulin.

TYPES
Only major types are listed.

Type I, or Insulin-Dependent Diabetes Mellitus (IDDM): Individual has an absolute deficiency of insulin from the beta cells of the pancreas.

Type II, or Non–Insulin-Dependent Diabetes Mellitus (NIDDM): Individual has a relative lack of insulin or a resistance to its effect.

ETIOLOGIES

Type I (IDDM)	*Type II (NIDDM)*
More frequently found in HLA types B8, BW15, DW3, and DW4. Viral insult may trigger beta cell damage, possibly via an autoimmune reaction. Islet cell antibodies can frequently be found.	Serum insulin levels may be depressed, normal, or elevated. Inability to utilize insulin may be due to fewer receptor sites, increased circulating insulin antibodies, or receptor defects that impair insulin binding to cells of the body. Often related to obesity or stress.
Onset most commonly before the age of 20 but can occur in the adult as well.	Onset after the age of 40 with gradual onset.

OBJECTIVE SYMPTOMS	**TYPE I**	**TYPE II**
Elevated blood glucose	x	x
Glycosuria	x	x
Polyuria	x	x
Ketonuria	x	
Weight loss	x	x
Susceptibility to infection	x	x
Poor wound healing	x	x

SUBJECTIVE SYMPTOMS		
Fatigue	x	x
Thirst	x	x
Hunger	x	x
Blurred vision	x	x
Dry, itchy skin	x	x

MANAGEMENT		
Insulin	x	x
Diet management	x	x
Oral hypoglycemics		x
Urine and/or blood testing	x	x
Weight loss		x
Exercise program	x	x
Patient education	x	x

are formed from a single-chain precursor, namely, proinsulin. Insulin is primarily extracted from beef and pork pancreas. The insulin obtained from beef pancreas differs from human insulin by three amino acids, whereas the insulin obtained from a pig differs by only one amino acid. Until 1980, the insulin manufactured was a combination of beef and pork insulin with small amounts of proinsulin (10,000 ppm). Proinsulin is an impurity that can result in antibody formation, leading to a loss of insulin effectiveness. Advanced technology has enabled manufacturers to decrease the amount of proinsulin to ≤10 ppm for standard insulins and ≤1 ppm for purified insulins.

A concurrent change to decrease antibody formation also occurred at that time. As mentioned previously, beef and pork insulin differ structurally from human insulin. As a result of this difference, diabetics taking beef and pork insulin form some insulin-blocking antibodies that will delay the activity of *exogenous insulin*. Since pork insulin most closely resembles human insulin, it is

less immunogenic than beef insulin. It is upon this premise that purified pork insulin was introduced to the market. Then in 1983, insulin manufacturers went one step further to develop "human insulin." The Eli Lilly company introduced a biosynthetic human insulin developed by recombinant DNA technology using *Escherichia coli* bacteria. The Squibb-Novo and Nordisk companies created a semisynthetic human insulin by replacing the amino acid alanine in pork with theonine, the amino acid necessary to change the pork insulin to the structure of human insulin. Currently there are over thirty different insulin products available in the United States. Table 44–2 provides a listing of insulin products, species, and manufacturers.

Table 44–2. INSULIN PRODUCTS CURRENTLY AVAILABLE IN THE UNITED STATES

Product (Manufacturer)	Concentration (IU)	Species	Onset (hours)	Peak (hours)	Duration (hours)
RAPID-ACTING INSULINS					
Standard					
Regular, Iletin I (Lilly)	40, 100	Beef/pork mixture	0.5	2–4	6–8
Regular (Squibb-Novo)	100	Pork	0.5	2–4	6–8
Semilente, Illetin I (Lilly)	40, 100	Beef/pork mixture	1–2	3–8	10–16
Semilente (Squibb-Novo)	100	Beef	1.5–4	5–10	11–16
Purified					
Regular, Iletin II (Lilly)	100	Pork or beef	0.5	2–4	6–8
Regular, Iletin II Concentrated (Lilly)	500	Pork	0.5	2–4	6–8
Regular, Purified (Squibb-Novo)	100	Pork	0.5	2.5–5	5–8
Velosulin (Nordisk)	100	Pork	0.5	1–3	8
Semilente, Purified (Squibb-Novo)	100	Pork	1.5–4	5–10	11–16
Human					
Humulin R (Lilly)	100	Human, biosynthetic	0.5	2–4	6–8
Humulin BR (Lilly)*	100	Human, biosynthetic	0.5	2–4	6–8
Novolin R (Squibb-Novo)	100	Human, semisynthetic	0.5	2.5–5	6–8
Velosulin, Human (Nordisk)	100	Human, semisynthetic	0.5	1–3	8
INTERMEDIATE-ACTING INSULINS					
Standard					
NPH, Iletin I (Lilly)	40, 100	Beef/pork mixture	1–2	6–12	18–26
Lente, Iletin I (Lilly)	40, 100	Beef/pork mixture	1–3	6–12	18–26
NPH (Squibb-Novo)	100	Beef	1.5–4	4–12	12–24
Lente (Squibb-Novo)	100	Beef	2.5–5.5	7–15	16–24
Purified					
NPH, Iletin II (Lilly)	100	Pork or beef	1–2	6–12	18–24
Lente, Iletin II (Lilly)	100	Pork or beef	1–3	6–12	18–26
NPH, Purified (Squibb-Novo)	100	Pork	1.5–4	4–12	12–24
Lente, Purified (Squibb-Novo)	100	Pork	2.5–5.5	7–15	16–22
Insulatard NPH (Nordisk)	100	Pork	1.5	4–12	24
Human					
Humulin N (Lilly)	100	Human, biosynthetic	1–2	6–12	18–24
Humulin L (Lilly)	100	Human, biosynthetic	1–3	6–12	18–24
Novolin N (Squibb-Novo)	100	Human, semisynthetic	1.5	4–12	24
Novolin L (Squibb-Novo)	100	Human, semisynthetic	2.5	7–15	22
Insulatard NPH, Human (Nordisk)	100	Human, semisynthetic	1.5	4–12	24

CONTINUED ON THE FOLLOWING PAGE

Table 44–2. INSULIN PRODUCTS CURRENTLY AVAILABLE IN THE UNITED STATES– *CONTINUED*

Product (Manufacturer)	Concentration (IU)	Species	Onset (hours)	Peak (hours)	Duration (hours)
MIXTURES					
Purified					
Mixtard; 70% NPH: 30% Regular Premix (Nordisk)	100	Pork	0.5	4–12	24
Human					
Novolin 70/30; 70% NPH: 30% Regular Premix (Squibb-Novo)	100	Human, semisynthetic	0.5	2–12	24
Mixtard, Human; 70% NPH: 30% Regular Premix (Nordisk)	100	Human, semisynthetic	0.5	4–12	24
LONG-ACTING INSULINS					
Standard					
Ultralente, Iletin I (Lilly)	40, 100	Beef/pork mixture	4–6	14–24	28–36
PZI, Iletin I (Lilly)	40, 100	Beef/pork mixture	4–6	14–24	26–36
Ultralente (Squibb-Novo)	100	Beef	4–9	10–30	30–36
Purified					
PZI, Iletin II (Lilly)	100	Pork or beef	4–6	14–24	26–36
Ultralente, Purified (Squibb-Novo)	100	Beef	4–9	10–30	30–36
Human					
Humulin U (Lilly)	100	Human, biosynthetic	4–6	8–20	24–28

*For patients on infusion pumps.
Note. Onset, peak, and duration can vary widely with different dosages and different patients.

Action

Insulin plays an important role in carbohydrate, protein, and fat metabolism. The majority of the body's cells require insulin to allow the entry of glucose. Exceptions are the brain, liver, epithelium of the kidney, and retina.

In the muscle, insulin transports glucose inside to be used as energy if the individual is exercising. However, if the individual is sedentary, the glucose is converted to muscle glycogen for later use. Insulin also stimulates the uptake of amino acids and their conversion to protein in the muscle.

In the adipocyte cells, insulin allows glucose to enter and be converted to free fatty acids. Although the liver itself does not require insulin to utilize glucose, insulin facilitates the conversion of glucose to glycogen. This glycogen is then converted to glucose when the body is in a fasting state to prevent hypoglycemia and to provide cell nourishment. Insulin also decreases the rate of *gluconeogenesis* in the liver.

In the absence of insulin, there is an underutilization of glucose, since it is no longer readily transported into the cells. Protein synthesis ceases and wasting of the muscle cells begins. Large amounts of amino acids are released into the plasma. Since gluconeogenesis is no longer suppressed, these amino acids are converted to glucose. This combination of effects leads to hyperglycemia, resulting in *glycosuria*. In the absence of insulin, there is an increase in the metabolism of fat stores to free fatty acids and glycerol. These fragments of fatty acid metabolism are referred to collectively as "ketone bodies" and consist of acetone, beta-hydroxybutyric acid, and acetoacetic acid. Their presence in large quantities in the body fluids is called ketosis, and since two of the three compounds are acids, the term ketoacidosis also applies. Accumulation of these acids can cause coma and death.

Additionally, the lack of insulin increases the amount of stored triglycerides in the liver, resulting in a fatty liver. The excess of fatty acids in the liver promotes conversion of some of the fatty acids into phospholipids and cholesterol. Along with triglycerides, these substances are discharged into the blood stream as lipoproteins. This can lead to rapid development of atherosclerosis. Figure 44–1 is a pictorial representation of the function of insulin or its lack.

Biochemically, insulin works by binding with receptors on the cell membrane. This activates a "second messenger," guanidine monophosphate (cyclic GMP), which serves to activate the cell's metabolic processes to utilize glucose as a source of energy.

Although the pharmacologic action of all insulins is the same, different preparations have been developed (Regular, Semilente, NPH, Lente, Ultralente, and PZI) with varying onsets, peaks, and durations of action to provide the diabetic individual with individualized control. Regular insulin was the first insulin preparation available. Insulins with longer onset, peak, and duration were created by adding a protein such as protamine, globin, or zinc to regular insulin. It is important to note that the onset, peak, and duration of the different types

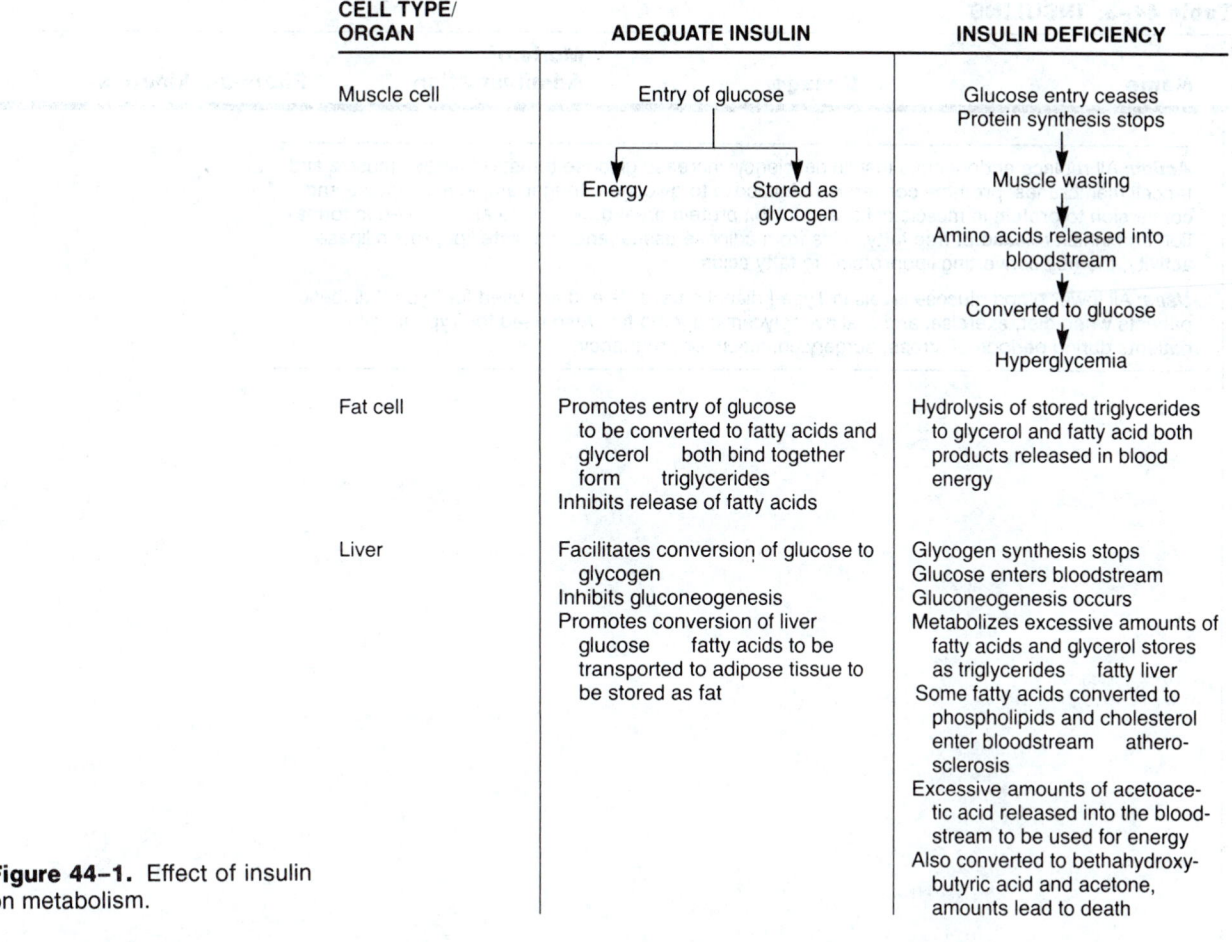

Figure 44–1. Effect of insulin on metabolism.

of insulin have been derived through many laboratory studies and that the diabetic individuals chosen for the study were often volunteers who were in optimal health. In any patient these times can be altered by an individual's specific metabolism and diabetic pathology.

As mentioned earlier, there are over thirty insulin products currently available. Most diabetic patients use the standard insulins. These are least expensive to the individual. The purified pork and human insulins are more costly, and are generally equal to each other in price. Since the human insulins cause less antibody formation than the purified pork insulin, they are becoming the insulins of choice for individuals with special needs. Human insulin is recommended for patients using insulin intermittently since these individuals are more likely to develop an insulin allergy and/or increased antibody formation if they require insulin therapy at a later time. Patients who fall into this category include: individuals with gestational diabetes; those with Type II diabetes who need close regulation during surgery or during an infectious process; and nondiabetic individuals who are receiving parenteral nutrition. A pregnant woman with Type I diabetes should be given human insulin because the insulin antibodies that may form are passed to the fetus. Some diabetologists believe that all newly diagnosed diabetic patients should be started on human insulin. For a complete listing

all insulins and the nursing process for administration of insulin, see Table 44–3.

Uses

Insulin therapy is indicated in the treatment of all patients with Type I, insulin-dependent diabetes. It is also used for the Type II, non–insulin-dependent diabetic patient who is pregnant, or for the gestational diabetic patient, to achieve diabetic control. Insulin may be used for the Type II diabetic patient during periods of stress, surgery, or infection. Insulin may also be used for the Type II diabetic individual who has failed to achieve glycemic control by following a diet, exercise regimen, and oral hypoglycemic therapy.

Types of Insulin

RAPID-ACTING INSULINS. Rapid- or short-acting insulins are insulins with the quickest onset, peak, and duration of activity. It is important for the patient to eat within one-half hour after administration of rapid-acting insulin in order to prevent a hypoglycemic reaction.

Regular Insulin. Regular insulin is a rapid-acting insulin, which begins to act 15 minutes to one hour after administration. Its peak activity is between two to four hours. During this time, the patient should be observed

TEXT RESUMES ON PAGE 1150

Table 44–3. INSULINS

Name	Dosage	Mode of Administration	Pharmacokinetics

Action: All replace endogenous insulin deficiency: increase glucose transport across muscle and fat cell membranes; promote conversion of glucose to glycogen; trigger amino acid uptake and conversion to protein in muscle cells, and inhibit protein breakdown; stimulate triglyceride formation and inhibit release of free fatty acids from adipose tissue; and stimulate lipoprotein lipase activity, thereby converting lipoproteins to fatty acids.

Uses: All lower blood glucose levels in Type I diabetic patients and are used for Type II diabetic patients when diet, exercise, and oral hypoglycemic agents fail. Also used for Type II diabetic patients during periods of stress, surgery, infection, or pregnancy.

Key to Abbreviations in the *Pharmacokinetics* column O-onset; P-peak; D-duration; B-biotransformation; PB-protein bound; E-excreted by; ½L-half-life.
*Within the column listing adverse effects, underlines indicate the most common effects; CAPITALS indicate life-threatening effects.

Contraindications/ Precautions	Adverse Effects*	Interactions	Nursing Implications
For All Insulins: Do not administer when blood sugar level is below 70 mg/dL or when the signs of hypoglycemia are present. Check serum potassium levels for hyperkalemia or hypokalemia resulting from glucose fluctuations. Dysrhythmias may occur. Patients should remain on the type of insulin prescribed by their physician and only change types or species under the guidance and recommendation of the physician. Human insulin should be used for patients who are on insulin therapy intermittently. This decreases the occurrence of allergy if the patient is placed on the insulin at another time. Humulin BR is to be used with the insulin pump only. Regular U-100 insulin is the only insulin that may be given IV.	*For All Insulins:* *Neuro:* hypoglycemia—most likely to occur at peak time of insulin activity; symptoms include diaphoresis, pallor, confusion, hunger, tremors, weakness, or seizures *Integumentary:* delayed localized reaction—rash, itching at injection site 3–6 hours after administration SYSTEMIC ALLERGIC REACTION: rare occurrence; rash develops at injection site moments after insulin is administered; may lead to anaphylaxis *Lipohypertrophy:* excess fat at injection site *Lipoatrophy:* loss of fat at injection site (both lipohypertrophy and lipoatrophy result from frequent injections in the same site) *Endocrine:* insulin resistance—situation in which the patient requires more than 200 units of insulin each day	*For All Insulins:* Refer to Table 44–4 for a listing of medications that augment or antagonize the effect of insulin. Numerous OTC medications contain sugar. Always read labels.	*For All Insulins:* *ASSESSMENT:* Obtain baseline and periodic assessments of blood glucose levels; blood cell counts; potassium, triglyceride, and cholesterol levels. Assess glycosylated hemoglobin (Hb A$_{lc}$) level. If patient has DKA, monitor ECG and assess for cardiac dysrhythmias. Assess the patient's present knowledge of diabetes and basics of care including meal pattern, hyperglycemia, hypoglycemia, role of exercise, blood glucose monitoring and/or urine testing, and skin and foot care. If patient is on insulin therapy, assess injection technique. Assess injection sites for lipohypertrophy. If patient is on pump therapy, assess abdomen for abcesses at the catheter insertion sites. Assess knowledge of blood glucose testing and urine testing, as well as performance of the above mentioned skills. Assess insulin injection sites for localized or delayed allergy. Continually assess for hyperglycemia and hypoglycemia. *INTERVENTION:* Administer insulin as ordered. Double check type and dosage with another nurse before administration. When administering insulin intravenously, do not mix insulin with any other medication in an IV bag. Some insulin adheres to the IV bottle as well as the IV tubing. Flush 50 ml of the solution through the tubing to minimize further adherence. IV pumps or controllers should be used to safely monitor intermittent or continuous insulin infusions.

CONTINUED ON THE FOLLOWING PAGE

Table 44–3. INSULINS–*CONTINUED*

Name	Dosage	Mode of Administration	Pharmacokinetics
RAPID-ACTING INSULINS			
Regular: Regular Iletin I & II, Regular Purified, Velosulin Humulin R, Novolin R, Velosulin Human	The dosage is individualized according to the patient's blood glucose values. When given SC, usually given 15–30 minutes a.c. meals.	IV SC	O: 0.5 hr P: 1–4 hr D: 8 hr ½L: UA PB: not bound B: mainly in the liver, to a lesser extent in the kidney and muscle tissue E: kidney
Humulin BR *Semilente:* Semilente Iletin I, Semilente Purified	Same	Insulin Pump SC	O: 1.5 hr P: 3–10 hr D: 10–16 hr PB: same B: same E: same
INTERMEDIATE-ACTING INSULINS			
NPH: NPH Iletin I & II, NPH Purified, Insulatard NPH, Humulin N, Novolin N, Insulatard NPH Human	Individualized for patient based on blood glucose levels. Usually given 30 minutes before breakfast. General dosage is 0.5–1.0 U/kg of body weight.	SC	O: 1–4 hr P: 4–12 hr D: 12–24 hr ½L: UA PB: same B: same E: same
Lente: Lente Iletin I & II, Novolin L, Lente Purified, Humulin L	Same	SC	O: 1.5–5 hr P: 6–15 hr D: 16–22 hr ½L: UA PB: same B: same E: same
MIXTURES			
Mixtard (70% NPH: 30% regular pork)	Individualized for patient based on blood glucose levels.	SC	O: 0.5 hr P: 2–12 hr D: 24 hr

Key to Abbreviations in the *Pharmacokinetics* column O-onset; P-peak; D-duration; B-biotransformation; PB-protein bound; E-excreted by; ½L-half-life.
*Within the column listing adverse effects, underlines indicate the most common effects; CAPITALS indicate life-threatening effects.

Contraindications/ Precautions	Adverse Effects*	Interactions	Nursing Implications
			Serum potassium levels must be monitored. The patient should receive insulin and meals on time. Educate patient according to needs determined through needs assessment. Determine if there is a need for follow-up care at home. *EVALUATION:* Evaluate the patient's blood glucose level and urinary glucose and ketones. Evaluate patient's knowledge of diabetes and basics of treatment. Evaluate all technical skills that will be performed in the home setting. Evaluate the patient's desire to adhere to the prescribed regimen, using verbal and nonverbal cues.

CONTINUED ON THE FOLLOWING PAGE

Table 44–3. INSULINS–*CONTINUED*

Name	Dosage	Mode of Administration	Pharmacokinetics
MIXTURES–*Continued* Novolin 70/30 (70% NPH human: 30% regular human) Mixtard Human (70% NPH human: 30% regular human)	Usually given 15–30 minutes before breakfast if a single dose. If given twice daily, give before breakfast and supper.		½L: UA PB: same B: same E: same
LONG-ACTING INSULINS *Ultralente:* Ultralente Iletin I, Humulin U	Individualized for patient, often given in combination with regular insulin to achieve tight diabetic control.	SC	O: 4–9 hr P: 8–24 hr D: 26–36 hr ½L: UA PB: same B: same E: same
PZI: PZI Iletin I & II	Usually given before breakfast or at bedtime. Acts as a basal dose.		O: 4–6 hr P: 2–24 hr D: 26–36 hr PB: same B: same E: same

Key to Abbreviations in the *Pharmacokinetics* column O-onset; P-peak; D-duration; B-biotransformation; PB-protein bound; E-excreted by; ½L-half-life.

*Within the column listing adverse effects, <u>underlines</u> indicate the most common effects; CAPITALS indicate life-threatening effects.

closely for an insulin reaction. However, it is important to note that a reaction may occur at any time. The duration of action of regular insulin is five to eight hours.

Regular insulin is a clear solution without any added modifying agent and, therefore, is the only insulin that may be used intravenously when the diabetic patient is out of control. Regular insulin is also given subcutaneously in the hospital setting to regulate the blood glucose. The dosage of regular insulin to be given is often a sliding scale dependent upon blood glucose levels. Regular insulin may be used in combination with intermediate- or long-acting insulins to obtain better diabetic control.

Regular insulin is the only insulin that may be used in the insulin pump. A buffered insulin, Humulin-BR, was recently developed specifically for pump therapy. The addition of disodium phosphate to regular insulin has been found successful in reducing insulin crystallization that often occurs in the catheter, and therefore lessens the chance of catheter obstruction.

Semilente Insulin. Semilente insulin (prompt insulin zinc suspension) is a cloudy solution which begins to act in one to four hours after administration. The peak activity range is three to ten hours, and the effects last from ten to sixteen hours. Semilente insulin may be used in combination with lente or ultralente insulin to achieve optimal control for the patient with diabetes.

INTERMEDIATE-ACTING INSULINS. Intermediate-acting insulins are commonly administered once or twice daily before breakfast and/or supper to achieve diabetic control. Regular insulin may be added to these insulins if additional control is necessary. The most likely time for an insulin reaction to occur in a patient who takes an intermediate-acting insulin in the morning is before supper; whereas, the most likely time for a reaction to occur in a patient taking an intermediate-acting insulin before supper would be around midnight. Afternoon and evening snacks incorporated into the meal plan can help prevent these reactions.

NPH Insulin. NPH insulin (Isophane Insulin Suspension) is a cloudy suspension that begins to act 1–2 hours after administration and peaks in 6–12 hours. The duration of activity range is 12–26 hours.

NPH insulin is often used in combination with regular insulin, since it takes some time for the NPH insulin to have a measurable effect.

Lente Insulin. Lente insulin (Insulin Zinc Suspension) is a cloudy suspension with an onset, peak, and duration similar to NPH insulin. Lente insulin may be used in combination with semilente insulin or regular insulin to achieve tight diabetic control.

LONG-ACTING INSULINS. Long-acting insulins are rarely used alone. They are most frequently combined with rapid-acting insulins to provide control throughout the day and night. At low doses, these insulins mimic physiologic insulin release by supplying a basal level of insulin to suppress *glycogenolysis* and gluconeogenesis. Then, regular insulin is added before meals to cover the intake. If long-acting insulins are given in large doses, reactions may occur during the night since these insu-

Contraindications/ Precautions	Adverse Effects*	Interactions	Nursing Implications

lins peak in 10–30 hours after administration. This may be dangerous since the patient may not waken. Irritability, nightmares, and diaphoresis during the night may signal a hypoglycemic reaction.

PZI Insulin. PZI (Protamine Zinc Insulin Suspension) has an onset of 4–6 hours following administration and has a duration of 26–36 hours. It peaks in 14–24 hours.

Ultralente Insulin. Ultralente insulin is a long-acting insulin with properties similar to PZI.

Concentrations of Insulin

Insulin is available in the United States in three different concentrations: U-40, U-100, and U-500. The concentration indicates how many units (U) of insulin are contained in each cubic centimeter (cc) or milliliter (mL). For example, U-100 insulin provides the patient with 100 units of insulin per milliliter. Corresponding insulin syringes of the same calibration must be used with each specific concentration of insulin.

Since the introduction of U-100 insulin in 1973, there have been various educational campaigns to change patients from U-40 and U-80 insulin to U-100 insulin. This was done in an attempt to prevent dosage error. Since that time, U-80 insulin has been withdrawn from the market. U-500 insulin is available to patients with insulin resistance and may be purchased with a prescription.

Determining Insulin Dosage

DETERMINING THE INITIAL INSULIN DOSAGE. Several methods can be used to determine the initial amount of insulin necessary for the patient with diabe-tes. Many physicians will start with an average dose of an intermediate-acting insulin for the individual being treated. The initial dosage range is usually 15–30 U of insulin per day, with the obese patient requiring the greater amount. The dosage is then adjusted to meet the patient's individualized insulin requirement. Some physicians may hospitalize the patient who needs insulin therapy and administer rapid-acting insulin on a sliding scale according to blood sugar elevations. This would give the physician an idea of the patient's daily requirements. A new method of determining insulin requirements is to attach the patient to a closed loop infusion device. An example of this type of device is the Biostator (Fig. 44–2). This machine checks blood glucose and administers the amount of insulin necessary to keep the blood glucose at a previously determined level. The amount of daily insulin required can be determined by analyzing the 24-hour requirement on the machine. Traditionally, most patients with diabetes were managed on one injection of an intermediate-acting insulin daily before breakfast. This would abolish the problem of ketosis and the symptoms of hyperglycemia. However, with research indicating that *normoglycemia* may prevent, delay, or reverse some of the chronic complications of the disease, today's management is to maintain a blood glucose as close to that of the nondiabetic as possible, without undue risks of hypoglycemia. This may include a regimen of self glucose-monitoring, administration of split and mixed insulin dosages, intensified insulin therapy using the insulin pump, or multiple injections of regular insulin daily combined with an intermediate- or long-acting insulin. To achieve this re-

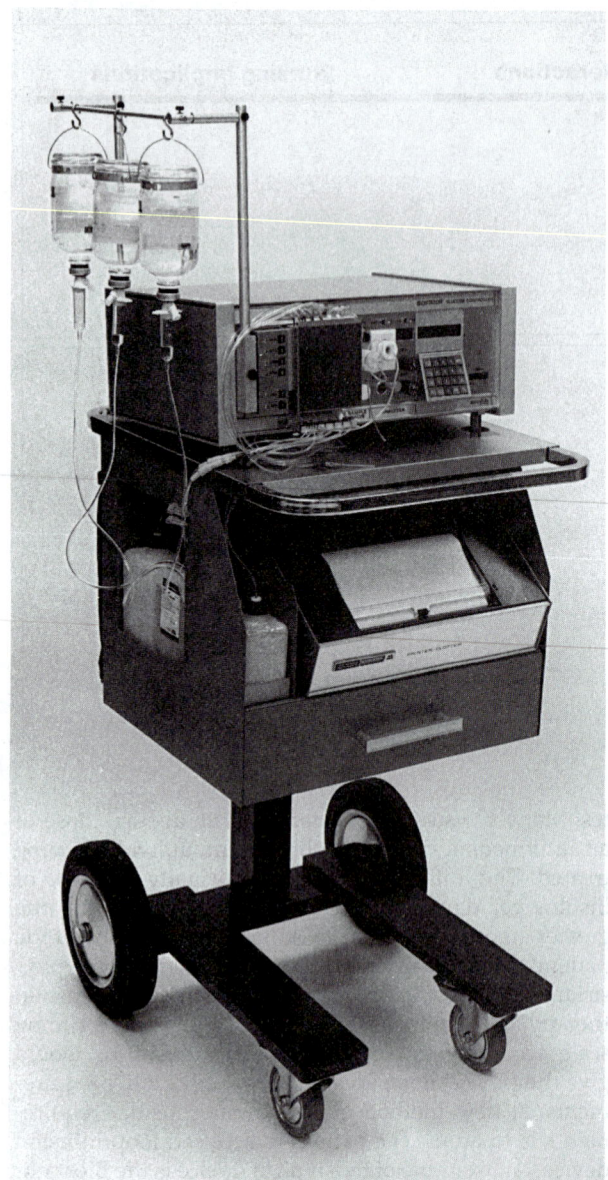

Figure 44–2. The Biostator. (Courtesy of Miles, Inc., Diagnostic Division, Mishawaka, IN.)

quires collaboration between the physician and patient, as well as the motivation and commitment of both parties.

GENERAL INSULIN DOSING. Once the amount of daily insulin requirements is determined, intermediate-acting insulin is initiated. Usually a single dose of the intermediate-acting insulin does not provide optimal control, since the individual receiving it may achieve adequate control during the day but be hyperglycemic at night. Therefore, one daily injection is often limited to the Type II diabetic patient, over the age of 60, who requires insulin. In this case, advancing age diminishes the value of strict control of blood glucose levels in preventing or delaying complications of diabetes. Also, hy-

poglycemia may be a greater risk for this patient. The majority of patients begin control with .66 to .75 of the intermediate-acting insulin dose given before breakfast, and the rest given before supper. Blood glucose levels are then determined before breakfast, two hours after breakfast, before supper, two hours after supper, and at bedtime, to assess the results of the intermediate-acting insulin and to determine if rapid-acting insulin is necessary. For example, if the blood glucose level is elevated before supper, it would indicate that the morning intermediate-acting insulin dosage would have to be increased. However, if the blood glucose level is elevated two hours after breakfast, rapid-acting insulin would be indicated along with the morning's intermediate-acting insulin. Refer to Figure 44–3 for a pictorial diagram of the course of action for split and mixed insulin regimens.

INTENSIFIED INSULIN THERAPY. Intensified insulin therapy is designed to enable the patient with diabetes to achieve a daily blood glucose profile that mimics a physiologically normal glucose profile. This has only been made possible through the development of home blood glucose monitoring devices. The patient usually has to monitor his or her blood sugar four times daily and adjust his own insulin dosage according to a scale provided by his physician.

Intensified insulin therapy is indicated for the pregnant diabetic patient, where normoglycemia is essential in order to prevent fetal morbidity and mortality. It is also indicated for highly motivated individuals with Type I diabetes who desire to reduce their blood glucose, *glycosylated hemoglobin*, and lipid levels in order to possibly prevent, postpone, or reverse the chronic complications of diabetes. Additionally, some patients believe that this type of therapy promotes a flexibility in lifestyle that they did not previously have, especially with meal timing. Two forms of intensified insulin therapy exist: the insulin pump, and multiple injections of regular and intermediate- or long-acting insulin daily.

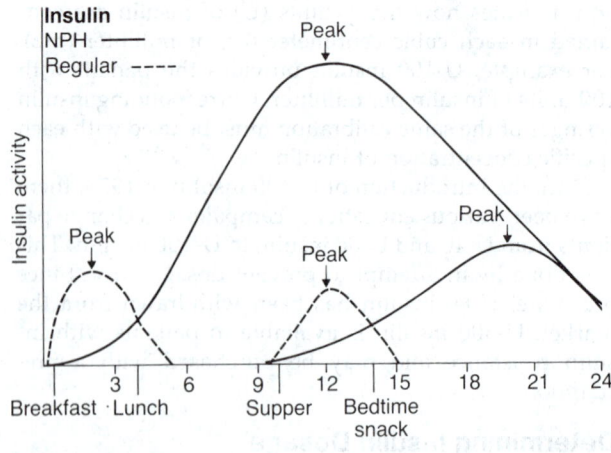

Figure 44–3. Time and activity of split and mixed dosages of insulin.

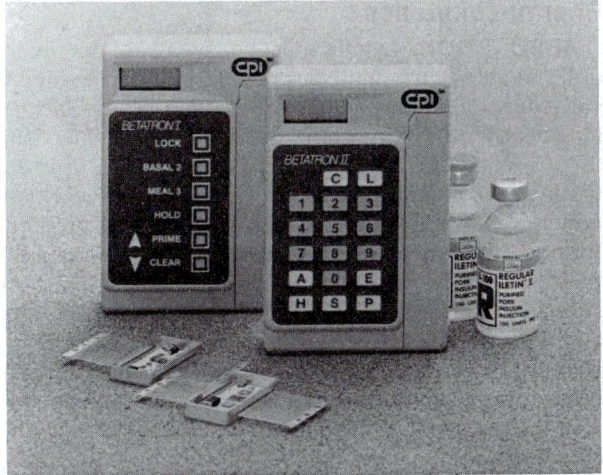

Figure 44–4. The insulin infusion pump. (Courtesy of CPI Lilly, St. Paul, MN.)

Insulin pump therapy began in 1974 and since then, many studies have been done on patients using the pump to determine the benefits of strict glycemic control. The results have been noteworthy in the outcome of diabetic pregnancies, lipid profiles, and nerve conduction studies.

The typical pump consists of a small programmable battery-operated box, about the size of a calculator. Inside, it contains a syringe filled with regular insulin. The insulin is delivered to the body through a plastic catheter that is attached to a fine needle placed subcutaneously in the abdomen (Fig. 44–4).

A basal dose or continuous small pulsations of insulin is given over a 24-hour time period. This amount is predetermined, usually as units per 24 hours. The basal insulin dose is supplemented by a bolus dosage of insulin which is given approximately 30 minutes before each meal. The bolus dosage is dependent upon the blood glucose reading at the time, taking into account the size of the meal to be ingested, as well as anticipated exercise. Generally, the patient uses a sliding scale. It must be noted that this is an open loop system in which frequent blood glucose monitoring is an essential requirement for pump use. Patients must demonstrate ability and willingness to adhere to the intense regimen. They must be reliable and competent.

Regular insulin must be used in the insulin pump. Recently, due to a problem with the catheters becoming clogged, Humulin BR, a buffered human insulin, was developed for use in the insulin pumps.

The most common problems with pump therapy are the acute effects of hyperglycemia and hypoglycemia. If the catheter is blocked or if it malfunctions, an individual may experience hyperglycemia and diabetic ketoacidosis in a short period of time, since there is no intermediate- or long-acting insulin circulating in the blood stream. An alarm system indicates when the pump is malfunctioning; however, to check the system the patient must remove the needle from his or her skin, pro-

gram a bolus dose, and then assume that the same insulin is being delivered in the subcutaneous tissue.

Additionally, many patients do not experience the less severe symptoms of hypoglycemia and, therefore, may have severe reactions. There have also been some catheter-related problems such as blocking by aggregated insulin, as well as abscesses at the site of needle injection. Lastly, some patients find the pump troublesome due to cosmetic appearance and the constant external reminder that they have diabetes.

Another method of achieving tight control of blood glucose levels is through multiple or bolus injections of regular insulin before meals, and a basal dose of an intermediate-acting or long-acting insulin, usually at bedtime. The benefits of this type of approach are similar to those achieved through pump therapy. The patient is able to have tight control of his/her blood glucose levels and have flexibility in meal timing and size. Blood glucose monitoring is mandatory for this system since the bolus amount of insulin that is taken before meals is dependent upon the blood glucose level. The inconvenience and discomfort of multiple injections can be minimized by using a device such as the Button Infusor or the Novo Pen system. The Button Infusor is a device inserted subcutaneously into the abdomen and taped so doses of insulin can be inserted through the opening at the top. The device must be changed every 2–3 days to prevent infection. The Novo Pen system (Figure 44–5) is a pen-like insulin injection device that is equipped with replaceable, multiple-dose cartridge reservoirs of Novolin R. It has a single-use needle and a needle cover, which are disposable. When full, the Pen Fill Cartridge holds 150 units of rapid-acting Novolin R. It is convenient since the patient may take it with him and administer his insulin by depressing a push button on top of the apparatus. Thus, the patient does not have to carry insulin bottles throughout the day.

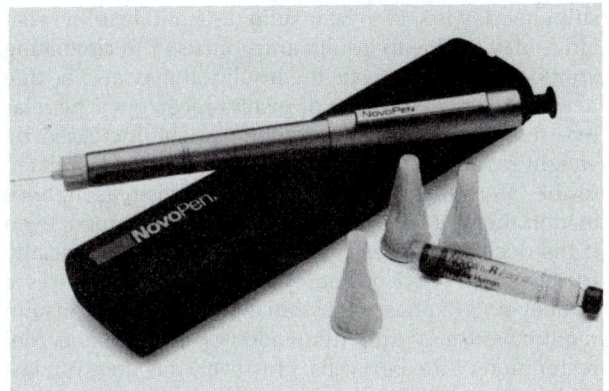

Figure 44–5. The Novo Pen System. (Courtesy of Squibb-Novo, Princeton, NJ.)

The patient using multiple daily injections of insulin is not as likely to develop ketoacidosis as the patient using the insulin pump since there is some long- or intermediate-acting insulin circulating in the blood stream. However, similar to the individual using the insulin pump, the patient may have insulin reactions. Despite the new devices to minimize the discomfort of multiple injections, the patient still has to administer the insulin.

The patient, physician, and diabetes nurse educator must discuss the pros and cons of both systems and determine which system would best fit into the patient's lifestyle, if intensified insulin therapy is desired.

Factors that Alter Insulin Requirements

Regardless of the diabetic regimen the patient is following, it must be recognized that numerous factors can affect insulin requirements. Initially, if the patient begins insulin therapy in the hospital setting, the dosage will most likely have to be altered once he/she returns to his/her normal surroundings and activity level.

Fluctuations in food intake may necessitate adjustments in insulin dosage. Stress, either physiologic or emotional, causes the release of epinephrine, which elevates blood glucose levels. This is especially common when the patient develops an infection. Other hormones including glucagon, cortisol, and growth hormone can elevate blood glucose levels. Exercise lowers blood glucose by oxidizing carbohydrates after facilitating their transport into cells. A good daily exercise program can decrease the amount of insulin a patient needs to take. However, sporadic, unplanned exercise can result in episodes of hypoglycemia. The amount of insulin prescribed for a patient can vary on different days if the schedule is very erratic in terms of exercise. For example, a construction worker who physically works very hard Monday through Friday may need only 10–20 units of insulin on those days. The insulin requirement may increase to 40–50 units of insulin on weekend days when he is sedentary.

Any individual requiring more than 200 units of insulin per day is said to be insulin resistant. Insulin resistance may be due to insulin antagonists or to circulating antibodies that inactivate the insulin. It may also be due to an inadequate number of insulin receptors. The relative number of insulin receptors can be increased by weight reduction. Insulin resistance may also be related to the intermittent use of insulin. For this reason, once insulin therapy is begun it generally is continued, even if the dosage requirements are small. This is especially true in the Type I diabetic patient who experiences a "honeymoon" phase after initial diagnosis. The insulin requirement may drop tremendously as there is partial restoration of the beta cells. However, this does not last and within a few weeks or several months, the patient requires insulin again.

If it is known that therapy will be intermittent, such as in a woman with gestational diabetes or a Type II diabetic patient experiencing an infection or undergoing surgery, a human form of insulin is utilized.

Pharmacokinetics

ABSORPTION. Insulin must be given parenterally in order to avoid enzymatic destruction in the intestine. A variety of factors may affect absorption. These factors include: the site of injection, the depth of the injection, the presence of *lipohypertrophy* (accumulation of extra tissue at the insulin injection site), and increased blood flow to the injection site through massage or exercise.

Some sites where insulin is given absorb more rapidly than others. The order of absorption speed for injection sites from highest to lowest is the abdomen, arm, leg, and buttock, respectively. The depth of the injection is also an important consideration. Intravenous administration is the most direct way in which to administer insulin, followed by intramuscular injection, then subcutaneous administration. Lipohypertrophy at the injection site may cause erratic absorption; therefore, it is essential that insulin injection sites be systematically rotated so this condition does not occur. A problem with the development of lipohypertrophy is that patients continue to inject in these sites since many report less pain than at other sites. With the purer preparations of insulin available today, this condition does not occur as frequently as it did in the past.

Massaging the site immediately after injection will increase the blood flow to the area and, therefore, speed up absorption. If an individual exercises, the absorption of insulin is quicker if it is injected into the area that is heavily exercised. For example, if an individual jogs, insulin injected into the legs absorbs more rapidly than insulin injected into the arms or abdomen.

DISTRIBUTION. Insulin does not bind significantly with plasma proteins. Primarily, it circulates in the blood and lymph as a free hormone.

BIOTRANSFORMATION. The plasma half-life of insulin injected intravenously is less than nine minutes in man. However, as a result of antibody binding, the half-life may be extended up to 13 hours. Insulin is primarily metabolized in the liver by an enzyme called glutathione-insulin transhydrogenase. It is metabolized to a lesser extent in the kidneys and muscle tissue.

ELIMINATION. In the kidney, insulin is filtered at the glomerulus and is 98% reabsorbed in the proximal tubules. About 40% of the reabsorbed insulin returns to the venous blood, and 60% is metabolized in cells lining the proximal tubule. In patients without renal impairment, less than 2% of the filtered insulin dose is excreted unchanged in the urine.

Commonly, as a result of vascular insufficiency, the patient with diabetes experiences renal dysfunction. Renal damage reduces the amount of insulin required since there will no longer be excretion of normal quantities of the drug. Severe impairment of renal function appears to affect the rate of disappearance of circulating insulin to a greater extent than hepatic disease.

Contraindications and Precautions

Administration of the rapid-acting insulins is contraindicated if the blood glucose level is below 70 mg/dL or if the signs of hypoglycemia are present. Regular insulin is the only insulin that may be given intravenously because it does not have a modifying agent. Humulin BR is an insulin developed for use with the insulin pump only.

Patients should remain on the type of insulin prescribed by their physician. If a patient is switched to a more purified product, a slight change in the insulin dosage may be necessary. Human insulins have a more rapid onset and a shorter duration than the insulins derived from animal sources. Patients, therefore, may have to ingest their meal more promptly when taking a regular human product than if they were taking an animal source product. Also, patients switching to human insulins from animal sources may not experience the usual warning symptoms of hypoglycemia and, therefore, should be aware of this. If an individual is placed on insulin therapy for a short period of time, he or she should be given a human insulin since use of human products involves less chance of insulin antibody formation.

Adverse Reactions

The most serious adverse effect of insulin therapy is hypoglycemia. The patient is carefully monitored to avoid this and taught the symptoms of hypoglycemia to facilitate early recognition. Often hypoglycemic reactions can be avoided by carefully balancing dietary intake, meal times, exercise, and insulin dosage. If the patient is aware, he or she may notice early symptoms of hypoglycemia which include: headache; difficulty thinking or concentrating; development of cool, clammy sweat; intense hunger; nervousness; weakness; and tachycardia. These manifestations are the result of epinephrine release as the body tries to elevate blood glucose levels through normal compensatory mechanisms. As hypoglycemia worsens, blurred vision, disorientation, unconsciousness, and convulsions may result. If this occurs while the patient is asleep, he or she may awaken with a nightmare and notice a cool, clammy, profuse sweat. Some individuals do not feel the sensation of hypoglycemia. These individuals include patients who have had diabetes for numerous years in whom the lack of sensation is due to neuropathy, patients taking beta-blockers, and patients whose blood sugar is dropping very slowly. Since the brain is dependent upon a constant supply of glucose to function, rapid treatment of hypoglycemia is essential to prevent brain damage. Ten grams of a fast-acting carbohydrate such as one-half cup of regular soda pop or two sugar cubes can be administered if the patient is able to tolerate food or fluid. Otherwise, glucagon or IV dextrose is given to patients who are unconscious.

Other adverse effects may occur such as insulin *lipoatrophy*, lipohypertrophy, delayed local reactions at the injection site, and systemic allergic reactions. Lipoatrophy is a benign condition in which a loss of subcutaneous fat occurs at the injection site. The cause of this problem is unknown. However, the immune response to insulin contaminants is thought to be involved. The treatment for lipoatrophy involves injecting a purer insulin into the depressed area to allow the reaccumulation of the fatty tissue.

Insulin-induced lipohypertrophy can also be considered to be an adverse effect of insulin therapy resulting from repeated injections in the same spot. Avoidance of these areas for future injection may result in the disappearance of this extra tissue. The patient must also be taught a systematic method of site rotation.

Delayed localized reactions are an adverse effect in patients receiving insulin. These reactions occur in about 50% of patients receiving insulin for the first time. Lesions appear three to six hours after an injection. These lesions are reddened and itchy, and last for several days. They are often preceded by a stinging or burning sensation at the time of injection. These reactions are self-limiting and usually disappear in one to three months. No treatment is indicated. However, switching to a purer form of insulin may resolve the problem.

A systemic insulin allergy or true insulin allergy is a rare occurrence. This complication begins as an immediate reaction at the injection site and quickly spreads all over the body. Anaphylactic shock may occur. This situation is more common in patients with a history of interrupted insulin therapy. The manifestations of insulin allergy are usually seen one to two weeks after the resumption of insulin therapy. Since the patient seems to be allergic to the insulin molecule itself, desensitization is the only effective treatment.

Insulin resistance may also be considered an adverse effect of insulin therapy. This is a situation where the individual requires more than 200 units of insulin per day. A history of intermittent insulin use is common in these patients. Switching from beef or beef-pork mixtures to purified pork or human insulin is often helpful. It is important to note that insulin resistance may abruptly cease and the patient may become hypoglycemic from the large doses of insulin. Patients must be monitored closely.

Interactions

Many medications affect blood glucose levels by promoting either hyperglycemia or hypoglycemia. Less interactions occur with insulin when compared with the oral hypoglycemic agents (see Table 44–4).

Some medications antagonize the effect of insulin. Epinephrine works to mobilize glycogen to increase the blood glucose level. Glucocorticoids increase hepatic glucogenesis and gluconeogenesis. Thiazide diuretics and, to a lesser extent, furosemide and ethacrynic acid also elevate the blood glucose, possibly through potassium depletion or inhibition of insulin secretion. Other agents that cause hyperglycemia include ACTH, amphetamines, asparaginase, carbonic anhydrase inhibitors, decongestants, diazoxide, glucagon, marijuana, nicotinic acid, phenytoin, and thyroid preparations.

Some medications have been found to augment the effect of insulin and, therefore, cause hypoglycemia. Fenfluramine increases the uptake of glucose by the muscles and may have intrinsic hypoglycemic activity. Monoamine oxidase inhibitors also have a hypoglyce-

Table 44–4. MEDICATIONS THAT AFFECT BLOOD GLUCOSE

Hypoglycemia	Hyperglycemia
Acetaminophen*	ACTH
Alcohol	Amphetamines
Allopurinol*	Asparaginase
Anabolic Steroids	Carbonic Anhydrase Inhibitors
Beta-Blockers	Decongestants (i.e., Sudafed)
Clofibrate*	Diazoxide
Chloramphenicol*	Epinephrine
Fenfluramine	Estrogens
Guanethidine	Furosemide
Isoniazid	Glucagon
MAO Inhibitors	Glucocorticoids
Oral Anticoagulants*	Marijuana
Oxyphenbutazone*	Nicotinic Acid
Oxytetracycline	Phenytoin
Phenylbutazone*	Thiazide Diuretics
Salicylates*	Thyroid Hormones
Sulfonamides*	

*These medications interact with the sulfonylurea agents only.
Adapted from Blevins, DR: The Diabetic and Nursing Care.
McGraw-Hill, New York, 1979, p 203.

mic effect since they inhibit hepatic gluconeogenesis. Alcohol has also been found to suppress gluconeogenesis and, therefore, potentiate a hypoglycemic reaction. Concurrent use of insulin with oral hypoglycemic agents in the treatment of Type II diabetes decreases the blood glucose level.

Beta-adrenergic blocking agents may cause hyperglycemia or hypoglycemia. These medications also mask some of the warning symptoms of hypoglycemia.

Some medications may contain varying amounts of "hidden" dextrose. Often, the sugar base is an attempt to make the medication more palatable. The sugar content may be classified as an "inactive" ingredient, and thus not listed on the label. It is also important to avoid diluting medications with a dextrose solution, to avoid the hyperglycemic effect.

ORAL HYPOGLYCEMIC AGENTS

Oral hypoglycemic agents are indicated for the Type II diabetic patient when diet and exercise fail to control hyperglycemia. These agents are useful to the patient who can produce some *endogenous insulin*. A general guideline used by many physicians is that oral agents may be tried in the Type II diabetic patient receiving insulin if they can be controlled on a daily dosage of 30 units of insulin or less. The oral hypoglycemic agents currently available on the market are classified as sulfonylureas. They are divided into four "first generation" agents that were released in the late 1950s and two "second generation" agents released in 1984. The classification of oral agents known as biguanides (DBI and DBI-TD; Meltrol) have been banned for use in the United States by the FDA, owing to reports of increased incidence of lactic acidosis and hepatic damage among users. However, these medications are still available in

some European countries. For a listing of sulfonylureas currently available in the United States, see Table 44–5.

Action

The exact mechanism in which oral hypoglycemic agents work is not completely understood. Initially, these agents stimulate the beta cells of the pancreas to produce insulin. However, this effect tends to last for only two to three weeks after initiation of therapy. The oral agents have also have been found to suppress hepatic glucose production, which would account for lower blood glucose levels found in individuals on oral hypoglycemic therapy. Also, oral hypoglycemic agents are thought to lower the blood glucose by increasing the number of insulin receptors on the cell and may influence events within the cell after glucose has been transferred inside.

Uses

Oral hypoglycemic agents may be used in the treatment of the Type II or non–insulin-dependent diabetic. They are to be used only after therapy with diet and exercise fail. The oral hypoglycemic agents may be tried as the sole treatment for Type II diabetic patients on less than 30 units of daily insulin. They may also be used concurrently with insulin in the treatment of a Type II diabetic patient who requires a large amount of insulin. The type of patient who may benefit from combination therapy usually weights over 300 pounds, requires 300 or more units of insulin daily, and still has a blood glucose level above 300 mg/dL. The oral hypoglycemic agents are thought to increase the number of insulin receptors on the cells and, therefore, would decrease the patient's daily insulin requirement.

Specific Oral Hypoglycemic Agents

FIRST GENERATION SULFONYLUREAS. The first generation sulfonylureas differ according to onset, peak, and duration of activity, as well as adverse reactions. Therefore, therapy must be individualized to the patient's needs.

Acetohexamide. Acetohexamide (Dymelor) begins its action in 0.5–1 hour after administration. Its peak activity occurs approximately six hours after administration and it has a duration of 12–24 hours. Since acetohexamide breaks down to an active metabolite called L-hydroxyhexamide, which is excreted in the urine, it may have a prolonged effect in individuals with kidney disease; therefore, it would not be the oral hypoglycemic agent of choice for this type of patient. The usual dosage range of acetohexamide is 150 mg to 1.5 g daily.

Chlorpropamide. Chlorpropamide (Diabinese) is a long-acting sulfonylurea. Its activity begins one hour after administration. Its peak activity occurs 12 hours later, and it lasts 36–90 hours. Due to its long duration of activity, chlorpropamide is not recommended for the elderly diabetic or the diabetic with renal failure since a hypoglycemic reaction may last for several days. Caution is used when using chlorpropamide with this population since it may cause water dilutional hyponatremia. Although *disulfiram-like reactions* may occur with other first generation sulfonylureas, they most frequently occur with chlorpropamide therapy. Therefore, chlorpropamide is not used for the patient who routinely ingests alcohol. Despite these adverse reactions, this medication is frequently prescribed. Generally, only one daily dose is necessary and it is, therefore, convenient for many patients. The usual dosage range is 100–500 mg.

Tolazamide. Tolazamide (Tolinase) begins its action four to six hours after administration. Its peak activity is approximately six hours and its duration of action range is 12–24 hours. The usual dosage of tolazamide ranges from 100 mg to 1 g daily.

Tolbutamide. Tolbutamide (Orinase) is the weakest sulfonylurea and generally must be taken at least twice daily to achieve diabetic control. Its onset of action range is 0.5–1 hour. Its peak activity occurs three to five hours after administration and its duration is 6–12 hours. Due to this short duration of activity and its metabolism to inactive metabolites, tolbutamide may be useful for the patient with kidney disease. The usual dosage of tolbutamide ranges from 500 mg to 3 gm daily.

SECOND GENERATION SULFONYLUREAS. The second generation sulfonylureas have a higher potency than the first generation agents. Therefore, the therapeutic effective dose is lower for these agents; however, this has no clinical relevance. Also, these agents have fewer drug interactions and adverse reactions than the first generation agents. However, if a patient has been successfully managed on a first generation agent, it is not recommended to switch to these agents.

Glipizide. Glipizide (Glucotrol) begins its action 0.5–1.5 hours after administration. Its peak activity range is one to three hours and its effects last 12–24 hours. The usual dosage range is 2.5–40 mg/day. This is the only agent that must be taken on an empty stomach.

Glyburide. Glyburide (DiaBeta, Micronase) begins its activity two to four hours after administration. Its peak activity occurs approximately six hours later and its effects last 24 hours. The usual dosage range is 2.5–20 mg.

For the equivalent therapeutic dosage of the above sulfonylureas, refer to Table 44–6.

Pharmacokinetics

ABSORPTION. The sulfonylureas are administered orally and are rapidly absorbed from the gastrointestinal tract, with the exception of tolazamide (Tolinase), which is absorbed at a slower rate. Glipizide (Glucotrol) is the only oral hypoglycemic agent that must be taken on an empty stomach. Food delays absorption of glipizide by approximately 40 minutes.

DISTRIBUTION. Once absorbed, the sulfonylureas are widely distributed throughout the body. Chlorpropamide (Diabinese) and tolbutamide (Orinase) have been found to be excreted in breast milk. All of the oral hypoglycemic agents are highly bound to plasma proteins, which accounts for their differences in duration of action. The first generation agents have ionic binding and the second generation agents have nonionic bind-

ing. Therefore, the second generation agents are thought to have less displacement reactions from other ionic-binding drugs and, thus, should have fewer drug interactions.

METABOLISM. All of the sulfonylureas are metabolized in the liver. Acetohexamide (Dymelor) is reduced to an active metabolite which has about three times the half-life of the parent drug. Originally, it was thought that chlorpropamide was not metabolized and remained bound to plasma proteins until it was excreted in the urine, which would account for its long duration. Today, a urinary metabolite has been found. Glipizide and tolbutamide are metabolized to inactive metabolites. Tolazamide is metabolized to a mildly active metabolite and glyburide is metabolized to several compounds, one of which may be weakly active. Due to the metabolism of these agents in the liver, individuals with hepatic dysfunction are monitored carefully for hypoglycemia since the action of the drug may be prolonged.

ELIMINATION. The majority of the sulfonylureas are eliminated from the body through the kidneys. Therefore, individuals with impaired renal function may have a prolonged effect of the drug. This is especially true with chlorpropamide, which has a long duration, and with acetohexamide, which has active metabolites. Glyburide is the only agent that is excreted in bile as well as urine.

Contraindications and Precautions

Oral hypoglycemic agents are contraindicated for use in the Type I, insulin-dependent diabetic patient since they do not work for these patients and the individual may develop ketoacidosis. They are also contraindicated for the Type II diabetic patient when the diabetes is complicated by fever, severe infections, severe trauma, or major surgery. Precise blood glucose control, which may only be achieved through insulin therapy, is necessary in the preceding situations. Oral hypoglycemic agents are not indicated for the pregnant diabetic patient, strict control is necessary during pregnancy to prevent fetal abnormalities and fetal mortality. Oral hypoglycemic agents do not provide the strict control that is desired. Chlorpropamide and tolbutamide have been found in breast milk and it is assumed that other oral agents may be passed to the infant by this route. Therefore, oral hypoglycemic agents are not recommended for the lactating woman since hypoglycemia of the nursing infant may occur.

Oral hypoglycemic agents are contraindicated in patients with severe hepatic or renal disease due to prolonged metabolism and excretion. They are also contraindicated in individuals allergic to other sulfonylureas.

Caution is advised for patients who have a history of allergy to sulfa medications since cross-sensitivity may occur. Cross-sensitivity may occur in individuals allergic to tartrazine; however, the incidence of this is low. Often people who are allergic to aspirin possess this sensitivity.

TEXT RESUMES ON PAGE 1160

Table 44–5. ORAL HYPOGLYCEMIC AGENTS (SULFONYLUREAS)

Name	Dosage	Mode of Administration	Pharmacokinetics

Action: All stimulate insulin release from the beta cells of the pancreas and reduce glucose output from the liver. They also increase peripheral sensitivity to insulin.

Uses: All are used to lower blood glucose levels for the Type II diabetic patient when diet and exercise fail. May also be used concurrently with insulin therapy in the Type II diabetic patient when oral hypoglycemic agents or insulin do not work sufficiently alone.

Key to Abbreviations in the *Pharmacokinetics* column O-onset; P-peak; D-duration; B-biotransformation; PB-protein bound; E-excreted by; ½L-half-life.

*Within the column listing adverse effects, underlines indicate the most common effects; CAPITALS indicate life-threatening effects.

Contraindications/ Precautions	Adverse Effects*	Interactions	Nursing Implications

For All Sulfonylureas:
CONTRAINDICATIONS:
Contraindicated for use in: patients with known hypersensitivity to sulfonylureas; Type I, insulin-dependent diabetic patients; and pregnant or lactating diabetic patients. Also contraindicated in diabetes complicated by severe infections, major surgery, or ketosis. Contraindicated in the diabetic patient with serious impairment of hepatic, thyroid, renal, or endocrine function, as well as patients with primary renal disease exhibiting glycosuria.
PRECAUTIONS:
Use cautiously in patients who have allergies to sulfa drugs or aspirin. Caution should be used when using chlorpropamide with the elderly—it may cause prolonged hypoglycemia. Withhold if the patient is hypoglycemic and unable to eat food.

For All Sulfonylureas:
Neuro: hypoglycemia
CVR: possible increased incidence of cardiovascular disease
GI: gastrointestinal disturbances (anorexia, nausea, vomiting, diarrhea)
Bilary: HEPATOTOXIC (rare occurrence—may see jaundice, rash, eosinophelia; liver biopsy may show intrahepatic cholestasis with minimal cellular damage)
Hematologic: blood dyscrasias, hemolytic anemia
Renal: inappropriate antidiuretic hormone secretion (chlorpropamide)
Integumentary: allergic skin rashes, photosensitivity

For All Sulfonylureas:
Certain medications when used in combination with sulfonylureas may enhance or prolong their effect and others may produce hyperglycemia and loss of diabetic control. Refer to Table 44–4. Beta-adrenergic agents may decrease the effectiveness of sulfonylureas. They may also disguise the typical manifestations of hypoglycemia. Concurrent use of the oral hypoglycemic agents with anticoagulants, coumarin, or indandione derivatives may result initially in increased plasma concentration of both, then decreased plasma concentration and effectiveness of the anticoagulant. Concurrent use of oral hypoglycemics with antithyroid agents may increase the risk of agranulocytosis.
Asparaginase has been found to alter diabetic control.

For All Sulfonylureas:
ASSESSMENT:
Obtain baseline and periodic assessments of: blood glucose levels; blood cell counts; glycosylated hemoglobin levels; and liver function tests, especially, bilirubin, cholesterol, SGOT, and SGPT. Before initiation of treatment, assess whether the patient has any allergies to sulfa drugs. Ask the patient if he or she is taking any other medications and determine if they interact with the sulfonylureas. If the female patient is of childbearing age, ask if she is planning a pregnancy in the near future. Assess the patient's present knowledge of diabetes care including meal pattern, role of exercise, medication, hypoglycemia, blood glucose or urine testing, and skin and foot care.

INTERVENTION:
Provide sulfonylureas po ½ hour before breakfast. If divided doses are ordered, administer second dosage ½ hour before supper. Continually assess for hypoglycemia. Monitor blood and urinary glucose levels. Keep medication away from heat and direct light. If patient complains of GI upset, inquire whether divided dosages may be used.

EVALUATION:
Evaluate the patient's blood and urinary glucose levels. Evaluate the patient's knowledge of diabetes and the basics of treatment. Evaluate all technical skills that will be performed in the home setting. Evaluate the patient's desire to adhere to the prescribed regimen, using verbal and nonverbal cues.

CONTINUED ON THE FOLLOWING PAGE

Oral Hypoglycemic Agents

Table 44–5. ORAL HYPOGLYCEMIC AGENTS (SULFONYLUREAS)–*CONTINUED*

Name	Dosage	Mode of Administration	Pharmacokinetics
FIRST GENERATION SULFONYLUREAS			
Acetohexamide (Dymelor, Dimelor)	*Initial dosage:* 250 mg once per day; adjust gradually until diabetic control is reached *Maximum dosage:* 1.5 g/day	PO	O: 0.5–1 hr P: 6 hr D: 12–24 hr ½L: parent, 1.5 hr; metabolite, 6 hr PB: very highly bound B: liver E: kidney
Chlorpropamide (Diabinese, Apo-Chlorpropamide, Glucamide, Novopropamide)	*Initial dosage:* 100–200 mg/ day; dosage may be increased by 50–125 mg at 1 week intervals until diabetic control is achieved *Maximum dosage:* 750 mg/ day	PO	O: 1 hr P: 12 hr D: 36–90 hr ½L: 35 hr PB: very highly bound B: liver E: kidney
Tolazamide (Tolinase, Ronase)	*Initial dosage:* 100–250 mg/ day until diabetic control is reached; when more than 500 mg is required, the dosage should be divided and given before morning and evening meals *Maximum dosage:* 1.0 g/day	PO	O: 4–6 hr P: 6 hr D: 12–24 hr ½L: 7 hr PB: very highly bound B: liver E: kidney
Tolbutamide (Orinase, Apo-Tolbutamide, Mobenol, Novobutamide, Oramide, SK-Tolbutamide)	*Initial dosage:* 0.5 g 1–2 times daily until diabetic control is reached *Maximum dosage:* 3 g/day	PO	O: 0.5–1 hr P: 3–5 hr D: 6–12 hr ½L: 7 hr PB: 95% B: liver E: kidney
SECOND GENERATION SULFONYLUREAS			
Glipizide (Glucotrol)	*Initial dosage:* 5 mg daily (elderly 2.5 mg); increase by 2.5–5 mg at weekly intervals to achieve diabetic control; if dosage reaches 15 mg or more per day, divide dose at breakfast and at supper *Maximum dosage:* 40 mg/ day	PO	O: 0.5–1.5 hr P: 1–3 hr D: 12–24 hr ½L: 4 hr PB: 92–99% B: liver E: kidney
Glyburide (Diabeta, Micronase)	*Initial dosage:* 2.5–5 mg daily (elderly 1.25 mg); Increase dosage by 2.5 mg weekly if necessary to achieve diabetic control; when 10 mg or more is required per day, the dosage should be divided and given before morning and evening meals *Maximum dosage:* 20 mg/ day	PO	O: 2–4 hr P: 6 hr D: 24 hr ½L: 10 hr PB: >99% B: liver E: kidney and bile

Key to Abbreviations in the *Pharmacokinetics* column O-onset; P-peak; D-duration; B-biotransformation; PB-protein bound; E-excreted by; ½L-half-life.

*Within the column listing adverse effects, underlines indicate the most common effects; CAPITALS indicate life-threatening effects.

Patients with thyroid or endocrine disorders may be difficult to control with oral hypoglycemic agents and, therefore, may benefit from insulin therapy.

These medications are used with caution in geriatric patients and patients with renal insufficiency. These patients may be more sensitive to the effects of the medication due to prolonged metabolism and excretion. For these patients, dosage is initiated at a lower level and adjusted very cautiously. Additionally, hypoglycemia is more difficult to recognize in the elderly and causes

Contraindications/ Precautions	Adverse Effects*	Interactions	Nursing Implications
Same as for all.	Same as for all.	Same as for all.	Same as for all.
Same as for all.	Same as for all.	Same as for all.	Same as for all.

Oral Hypoglycemic Agents

more neurologic symptoms. Therefore, it is advisable to avoid oral hypoglycemic agents with prolonged duration in these patients.

Adverse Reactions

One of the major adverse effects of the oral hypoglycemic agents is hypoglycemia. This occurs most frequently in the elderly, debilitated, or malnourished individual. It may also occur in a patient with impaired renal or hepatic function due to delayed metabolism or excretion of the drug. Hypoglycemic episodes may occur if a meal is omitted or if exercise is performed erratically. Therefore, it must be emphasized that the patient on oral hypoglycemic agents follow a regular meal pattern and ex-

Table 44–6. EQUIVALENT THERAPEUTIC DOSAGES OF SULFONYLUREAS

Sulfonylurea	Dosage (mg)
Acetohexamide (Dymelor)	500
Chlorpropamide (Diabinese)	250
Tolazamide (Tolinase)	250
Tolbutamide (Orinase)	1000
Glipizide (Glucotrol)	10
Glyburide (Diabeta, Micronase)	5

ercise regimen. The hypoglycemia that occurs from sulfonylureas requires treatment over a period of days due to the prolonged action of the medication.

One of the most frequent adverse effects of all sulfonylureas is gastrointestinal upset. If this occurs, all of the agents with the exception of glipizide may be taken with food. The gastrointestinal upset is related to dosage. Therefore, reducing the dosage or splitting it into two doses to be taken twice a day can be helpful. In time, symptoms often disappear on their own.

Chlorpropamide and tolbutamide interact with alcohol causing a disulfiram-like reaction. This reaction may occur with other sulfonylureas, but to a lesser extent, especially with the second generation oral hypoglycemic agents.

Inappropriate antidiuretic hormone secretion may occur when a patient is taking chlorpropamide, and to a lesser extent if taking tolbutamide. These drugs may stimulate the antidiuretic hormone release from the hypothalamus and potentiate its effect in water retention. Serum sodium levels fall and the patient may present with headache, lethargy, and swelling. This may progress to stupor, seizures, and coma. Prompt medical attention is necessary for this situation. All of the other sulfonylureas possess a mild diuretic effect.

Hematological conditions (leukopenia, agranulocytosis, thrombocytopenia, pancytopenia, and hemolytic anemia) have been reported rarely in patients taking the oral hypoglycemic agents. Cutaneous manifestations such as photosensitivity and rashes may also occur. Hepatic manifestations such as elevated serum alkaline phosphatase levels and cholestatic jaundice are infrequent adverse effects. These conditions can be reversed by discontinuation of the drugs.

The University Group Diabetes Program (UGDP) study results suggest another adverse reaction for the patient taking oral hypoglycemic agents. This study found a higher incidence of cardiovascular disease in patients taking tolbutamide than in those following a regimen of diet alone or diet and insulin therapy. Today, the study results are still referred to on all oral hypoglycemic agent package inserts. Yet, there are many questions regarding the actual validity of the study and whether or not the results should be generalized to other oral hypoglycemic agents, since the study had several flaws. One of the major flaws of this study was the fact that the prevalence of baseline cardiovascular risks was higher in the tolbutamide group than in the

other test groups. The increase in cardiovascular mortality was restricted to patients who were taking tolbutamide, but whose diabetes remained out of control. Ordinarily, the therapy would have been changed in these patients because uncontrolled diabetes itself is a cardiac risk factor. In light of the above information and several other concerns, the American Diabetes Association (ADA) has withdrawn its endorsement of the study. Since the UGDP study, several other studies of tolbutamide have been undertaken. These have not demonstrated higher rates of cardiovascular mortality in patients using tolbutamide. The physician, pharmacist, or nurse should discuss the UGDP study, its flaws, and other studies with the patient before initiating sulfonylurea therapy.

Some patients do not respond to oral hypoglycemic agents from the time therapy is initiated. This is called primary failure. Other patients respond to the oral agents for a while, then lose their responsiveness and experience a rise in blood sugar levels. This is called secondary failure. In some cases, this is due to the patient's failure to adhere to the prescribed diet.

Interactions

The function of the sulfonylureas or oral hypoglycemic agents can be affected by the same medications that interact with insulin (refer to the section on interactions with insulin). However, some medications only interact with oral hypoglycemic agents and, therefore, alter diabetic control. Salicylates and other nonsteroidal anti-inflammatory agents may displace sulfonylureas from protein-binding sites, resulting in enhanced hypoglycemic activity. Anabolic steroids inhibit the metabolism of the oral hypoglycemic agents. Allopurinol, chloramphenicol, and dicumarol inhibit the metabolism of the oral agents, giving them an increased half-life.

Oral hypoglycemic agents may enhance the metabolism of digoxin by microsomal enzyme induction.

With regard to laboratory test values, the only interaction that may occur is a false urine test for albumin when a patient is taking tolbutamide.

Table 44–4 provides a listing of medications that interact with the sulfonylureas as well as insulin to raise or lower the blood glucose level.

USING THE NURSING PROCESS

The diagnosis of diabetes is often a crisis for the patient. The individual is suddenly faced with a chronic illness that alters his or her lifestyle. It is a condition in which the patient must take control in order to successfully manage. The physician, nurse, dietitian, and other members of the health care team provide care when the patient is hospitalized and acutely ill. However, once the patient is out of the controlled hospital environment, the health care professionals become mere consultants in helping the patient achieve diabetic control. The patient is the one who must follow the prescribed meal pattern, omitting foods that previously were enjoyed, and eating at designated times whether hungry or not. The patient must also: monitor blood and/or urinary glucose levels; balance exercise and medication with meal patterns; inject insulin; know the causes, symptoms, and treatment of hyperglycemia and hypoglycemia; and take meticulous care of the skin and feet. The patient must know how to manage diabetes during illness and travel. This requires tremendous motivation and commitment.

ASSESSMENT

Assessment of the patient with diabetes requires an understanding of his or her medical history and laboratory blood and urine values, especially glucose, ketone, and glycosylated hemoglobin levels.

The nurse may assess the patient in a variety of settings. The patient may be acutely ill with ketoacidosis or *hyperglycemic hyperosmolar nonketotic coma*. The nurse basically assesses the patient and initially intervenes by caring for the patient during these life-threatening situations. The nurse waits to do a complete diabetes educational assessment until the patient is physically stable and able to answer questions. Patients who are not acutely ill are often assessed by the nurse in a clinic or in a medical-surgical unit in a hospital.

During the initial patient assessment, the nurse must work toward developing a nonthreatening, trusting relationship with the patient. When this occurs, the patient feels free to discuss previous diabetes management if any with her, as well as his or her fears and concerns. The patient must not be made to feel that he or she was erroneous in their management. Throughout the assessment, the nurse points out positive aspects of the past regimen.

In addition to the information obtained in a general nursing history, the nurse must collect a more detailed information base regarding the individual with diabetes. The nurse asks the patient about daily routines, meal times, dietary preferences, and previous medical management. Open-ended questions are asked to allow the patient to explain situations. A patient may be asked if he or she follows a 1200 calorie ADA diet and the patient may say yes. However, if open-ended questions are asked and the patient's daily routine is explored, the nurse may find that the patient consumes all of the calories at suppertime. Assessment of the patient's knowledge of the medication he or she is receiving is essential. Sometimes patients taking oral hypoglycemic agents will stop the therapy due to shakiness and dizziness if a meal is missed. Frequently, these patients are unaware of the meal plan and the importance of eating on time. If the patient is taking insulin, the nurse assesses the measurement and injection technique by having the patient draw up and inject the dosage at least once while in the hospital. In the clinic setting, this may be done after a fasting blood sugar is drawn on a routine visit. The nurse can assess the pattern of site rotation by inquiring about the method and then inspecting the sites for lipohypertrophy. The nurse inquires about urinary

and blood glucose testing. If the patient does this, the nurse assesses the technique using the equipment the patient uses at home. The nurse collects information on how the patient feels when he or she is experiencing hyperglycemia or hypoglycemia, and what action the patient takes if these situations occur. The nurse also inquires about how the patient feels about having diabetes.

Assessment of the patient's anxiety level is important since learning is less productive when a patient is highly anxious. Learning may not take place despite excellent teaching. Due to the anxiety of diagnosis, and the large volume of information the patient will need to learn in order to control diabetes, often only survival information is provided during a newly diagnosed diabetic patient's hospitalization. This information is expanded over time through outpatient education, future clinic visits using one-on-one consultations, or diabetes classes. For the housebound individual, the visiting nurse continues the education in the home setting.

Literacy as well as cognitive functioning is also assessed. Many patients are unable to read or understand the literature available regarding diabetes. By assessing the patient's reading level, the nurse can provide appropriate literature that will be understood. The nurse may also use a film or a slide and tape presentation for the illiterate individual.

Physical limitations, especially in the areas of physical dexterity, visual impairment, and sensory defects are important to assess. Often, the diabetic patient who has been out of control cannot see the written literature or the numbers on an insulin syringe due to the osmotic changes in the eye as a result of glucose fluctuation. The changes generally stabilize in about five weeks. However, it is frustrating for the patient since his or her vision is too poor to draw up the insulin dosage or read any material about the condition. Modifications in management may be necessary for the individual with poor vision or poor fine motor coordination. These problems most frequently occur in the elderly patient who suffers from other medical conditions and in the patient who has had diabetes for numerous years. These modifications may include using prefilled insulin syringes, having a public health nurse monitor blood or urinary glucose levels, or using a "meals on wheels" service.

Cultural and religious preferences are also important to note. The Jewish patient may prefer not to use pork insulin or consume pork in the diet due to dietary codes. Protein sources other than meat are explored for the vegetarian patient. Some patients may have difficulty with dietary restrictions of carbohydrates if their diet contained much pasta and bread. Holiday feasting in any culture or religion has social significance that makes traditions difficult to change.

The cost of changes in diet, medications, syringes, blood glucose monitoring equipment, urine testing equipment, and frequent physician visits can impose a financial burden on the patient, especially if he or she is on a fixed income. The nurse must investigate the financial situation of the patient and the patient's medical insurance coverage. Low-income individuals may subsist on a high-carbohydrate diet because that is all they can afford. They may try to test their urine twice with a reagent testing strip cut in half or thirds to economize, and obtain inaccurate results. Food stamps, Medicare eligibility, and other financial assistance should be explored.

The nurse continually assesses the daily blood glucose levels. These levels are often determined by venous blood samples and analyzed in a laboratory. Home blood glucose monitoring equipment is also being used in clinics and on hospital units, as well as in the home setting. The home monitoring products provide a blood glucose value within two to three minutes and allow prompt regulation of blood glucose levels. Often a sliding scale of regular insulin is used to lower the blood glucose level. The amount of regular insulin the patient receives depends upon the results of the blood test.

If the nurse works in a clinic and the patient is monitoring blood glucose levels at home, the nurse encourages the patient to bring in testing records so the nurse can carefully assess the overall control. Home blood glucose testing products that are often used are Chemstrip bG and Glucostix.

Blood glucose levels are monitored frequently when the patient is in the hospital or is out of control. If the patient is stabilized and is not monitoring blood glucose levels at home, blood glucose may be tested every one to two months at the physician's office.

Urine glucose and ketone testing is generally done before every meal for the hospitalized diabetic. This provides the health care team with a "reflection" of the patient's diabetic control. Before home blood glucose monitoring products were available, a sliding scale of regular insulin based on urine glucose readings was used to lower the blood glucose level before meals. In some facilities, this method is still used. However, the urinary glucose method is becoming less common and capillary blood glucose is being used instead since it is much more accurate. When testing the urinary glucose, it is important to remember that spillage of glucose in the urine only occurs when the blood glucose levels exceed an individual's renal threshold for glucose (usually 160–180 mg/dL). Therefore, two individuals could have the same blood glucose level, yet yield different urine test results if their renal thresholds differ. Elderly individuals often have a high renal threshold, and they may not begin to demonstrate glycosuria until blood glucose levels approach 200 mg/dL. The renal threshold is generally lower than normal in children and pregnant women. Despite the fact that urine testing is not as accurate as blood glucose testing, it is less expensive and easy to perform. Many patients test their urine at home. The nurse in the clinic assesses diabetic control by checking the patient's urine test record.

NURSING DIAGNOSES

Following a thorough assessment, the nurse is able to identify specific nursing diagnoses for the diabetic patient and develop a plan of care. Continual reassessment and evaluation are necessary to note any need for changes in the patient's nursing diagnoses. The changes can be quickly incorporated into the written plan of care

so that communication with all the health team members is smooth. Typical nursing diagnoses for the diabetic patient receiving insulin are included in Table 44–7.

INTERVENTION

Many of the following interventions are performed by the nurse if the patient is hospitalized and acutely ill. As the patient recovers, these interventions are taught to the patient so he or she can manage the diabetes at home.

Meal Pattern

Dietary management is of the utmost importance in achieving control of diabetes. Unless the patient follows the prescribed diet, control is unattainable. The physician prescribes a specific calorie value American Diabetes Association (ADA) diet, based upon individual need. The diet generally ranges from 1,000 to 2,000 calories. The diet is arranged around a system of exchanges determined by the number of calories prescribed. The exchanges include starches, proteins, fats, vegetables, and fruits.

In the hospital setting, the nurse is responsible for assuring that the patient receives meals on time and that the entire meal is consumed. The dietitian, along with the nurse, helps the patient understand the system of exchanges and the dietary regulations.

Eating the prescribed food at the prescribed time is important for diabetic control. Generally, lunch is consumed four to five hours after breakfast, and supper is consumed five to six hours after lunch. An evening snack is necessary for the diabetic patient receiving oral hypoglycemic agents or insulin therapy to prevent hypoglycemia during the night. Mid-morning and mid-afternoon snacks may also be incorporated into the diet. The nurse and dietitian discuss the use of alcohol with the patient. Alcohol is discouraged since it can block gluconeogenesis and, thus, induce a hypoglycemic reaction for individuals taking insulin or oral hypoglycemic agents. The patient is taught that if a drink is desired on occasion, it must be taken immediately before or with a meal in order to prevent a hypoglycemic reaction. Alcohol also contains additional carbohydrates. If alcohol consumption is a regular occurrence, it is incorporated into the meal pattern. The nurse and dietitian also discuss dining out guidelines with the patient.

Blood Glucose Monitoring

As mentioned earlier, blood glucose monitoring may be used in the hospital setting to help the diabetic patient regain control. The nurse or laboratory technician may perform this procedure on the nursing unit and receive a capillary blood glucose reading within two to three minutes. The result usually differs by 10% from a venous sample analyzed in the laboratory. The capillary blood glucose tests using home glucose monitoring equipment are simple to perform and provide more information about diabetic control than a urine test. The products used vary, so it is crucial to read the information packet and follow the procedure precisely. For all

Table 44–7. NURSING PROCESS FOR THE INSULIN-DEPENDENT DIABETIC PATIENT

Assessment

Note duration/intensity of present symptoms, e.g., vomiting, excessive urination.
Assess peripheral pulses, capillary refill, skin turgor, and mucous membranes.
Ascertain usual dietary pattern and intake.
Review drug history.

Nursing Diagnosis	Nursing Actions	Rationale	Desired Outcomes/ Evaluation Criteria
Fluid Volume deficit, Actual 1 related to failure of regulatory mechanisms, osmotic diuresis, excessive gastric losses (diarrhea, vomiting), restricted intake as evidenced by increased urine output, dilute urine, weakness, thirst, dry skin/mucous membranes, hypotension.	Monitor vital signs, note orthostatic changes; changes in respiratory pattern, (e.g., Kussmaul respirations, periods of apnea, use of accessory muscles, presence of acetone breath, cyanosis. Measure intake and output, note specific gravity. Obtain weight daily. Maintain fluid intake of at least 2500 ml/day within cardiac tolerance. Review laboratory studies, e.g., Hg/Hct, serum osmolality, electrolytes, BUN/Cr.	Hypovolemia may be manifested by hypotension and tachycardia. Lungs remove carbonic acid through respirations, producing a compensatory respiratory alkalosis for ketoacidosis. Provides ongoing estimate of volume replacement needs, kidney function, and effectiveness of therapy. Maintains hydration/circulating volume. Useful in evaluating level of hydration and effectiveness of therapy as well as additional needs.	Demonstrates adequate hydration as evidenced by stable vital signs, palpable peripheral pulses, good skin turgor and capillary refill, individually appropriate urinary output and electrolyte levels within normal range.
Nutrition, Less than body requirements, Altered related to insulin deficiency, anorexia, hypermetabolic state as evidenced by reported inadequate food intake, recent weight loss, diarrhea, increased ketones.	Perform finger-stick glucose testing. Administer insulin as ordered based on blood glucose readings. Consult with dietician. Provide appropriate diet as tolerated. Weigh daily or as indicated.	Analysis of serum glucose displays current levels, indicating therapy needs. Meets individually determined needs. Useful in calculating and adjusting diet to meet individual needs. Oral route is preferred when patient is alert and bowel is functioning. Assesses adequacy of nutritional intake.	Ingesting appropriate amounts of calories/ nutrients. Displays usual energy level. Demonstrates stabilized weight or gain toward usual/ desired range with normal laboratory values.
Knowledge deficit related to lack of exposure/ recall, information misinterpretation, unfamiliarity with information resources as evidenced by questions, statement of concern, inaccurate follow-through of instructions, development of preventable complications.	Discuss normal blood glucose level and compare with patient's, type of diabetes mellitus patient has, relationship between insulin deficiency and a high glucose level. Discuss acute and chronic complications of the disease. Demonstrate fingerstick testing.	Provides knowledge base on which patient can make informed lifestyle choices. Awareness helps patient to be more consistent with care and may prevent/delay onset of complications. Self-monitoring of blood glucose (SMBG) four or more times a day allows flexibility in self-care, promotes tighter control of serum levels and may prevent/delay development of long-term complications.	Verbalizes understanding of disease process. Identifies relationship of signs/symptoms to the disease process and correlates symptoms with causative factors. Correctly performs necessary procedures and explains reasons for the actions. Initiates necessary lifestyle changes and participates in treatment regimen.

CONTINUED ON THE FOLLOWING PAGE

Table 44–7. NURSING PROCESS FOR THE INSULIN-DEPENDENT DIABETIC PATIENT– *CONTINUED*

Nursing Diagnosis	Nursing Actions	Rationale	Desired Outcomes/ Evaluation Criteria
	Review medication regimen, including onset, peak, and duration of prescribed insulin.	Understanding all aspects of drug usage promotes proper use.	
	Review self-administration of insulin and care of equipment. Have patient demonstrate procedure.	Identifies understanding and correctness of procedure or potential problems so that alternate solutions can be found if necessary.	
	Discuss factors that play a part in diabetic control, e.g., exercise, stress, surgery. Review Sick-day rules.	Promotes diabetic control and can greatly reduce the occurrence of ketoacidosis.	
	Identify symptoms of hypoglycemia, e.g., weakness, dizziness, lethargy, hunger, irritability, diaphoresis, pallor, tachycardia, tremors, headache, changes in mentation and explain causes.	May promote early detection and treatment, preventing occurrence.	
	Review signs/symptoms requiring medical evaluation.	Prompt intervention may prevent development of more serious/lifethreatening complications.	
	Identify community resources, e.g., American Diabetic Association, VNA, weight loss/ stop smoking clinic, and a contact person/diabetic instructor.	Continued support is usually necessary to sustain lifestyle changes and promotes well-being.	

products, a small drop of blood is required, taken from the outer aspect of the finger by a lancet. The blood is dropped on a reagent paper, timed for a specific amount of time, wiped off, timed again, and then the results are read by comparing the strip to a color chart. The results are as good as the technique and the vision of the individual performing the test. Some institutions prefer to use a meter such as the Glucometer II (Fig. 44–6) or the Accu-Chek II to perform the reading. The procedure is basically the same for the meter readings as for visual readings, with the exception that an electronic eye reads the blood glucose level with the meter and gives a digital value instead of the individual's visual interpretation. There are also some new meters on the market in which the blood does not have to be wiped off the strip prior to insertion into the meter for a glucose reading. Once again, it must be stressed that proper technique and care of the equipment is necessary to attain accurate results.

The nurse or diabetes nurse educator teaches the patient how to use home blood glucose monitoring, if this is included in the regimen. The nurse demonstrates several visual and meter methods and allows the patient to decide which product is preferred. The nurse assists the patient in receiving insurance coverage for these products. People that benefit from home blood glucose monitoring include Type I diabetic patients, diabetic patients with poor color vision, pregnant diabetic patients, diabetic patients that have difficulty recognizing hypoglycemia, and virtually any diabetic patient who wishes to achieve strict control of the diabetes. Home blood glucose monitoring is required for any individual on intensified insulin therapy. The major drawbacks of home blood glucose testing are the cost and that the patient must pierce the skin with a lancet.

Urine Testing

The nurse tests the patient's urine for glucose and ketone bodies during the hospitalization. The nurse can compare the urine tests with the blood tests to determine the approximate renal threshold. It can be utilized as a reference guideline for the patient who tests urine at home. In the hospital setting, the nurse may administer regular insulin according to the results of the urine tests. The nurse must do this cautiously, remembering that renal thresholds vary.

The nurse teaches the Type II, non–insulin-dependent diabetic patient to test for glucose in the urine. The

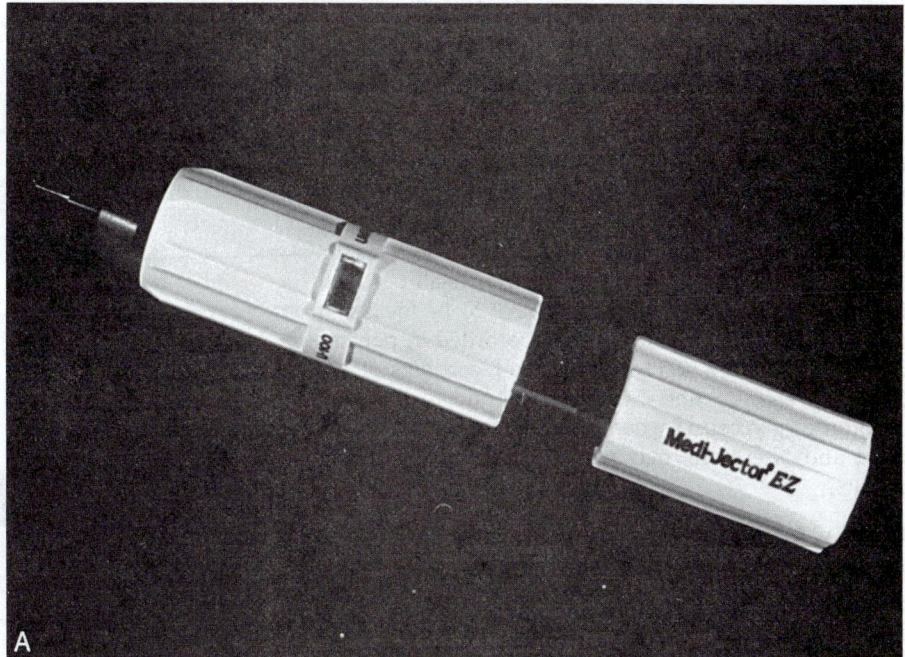

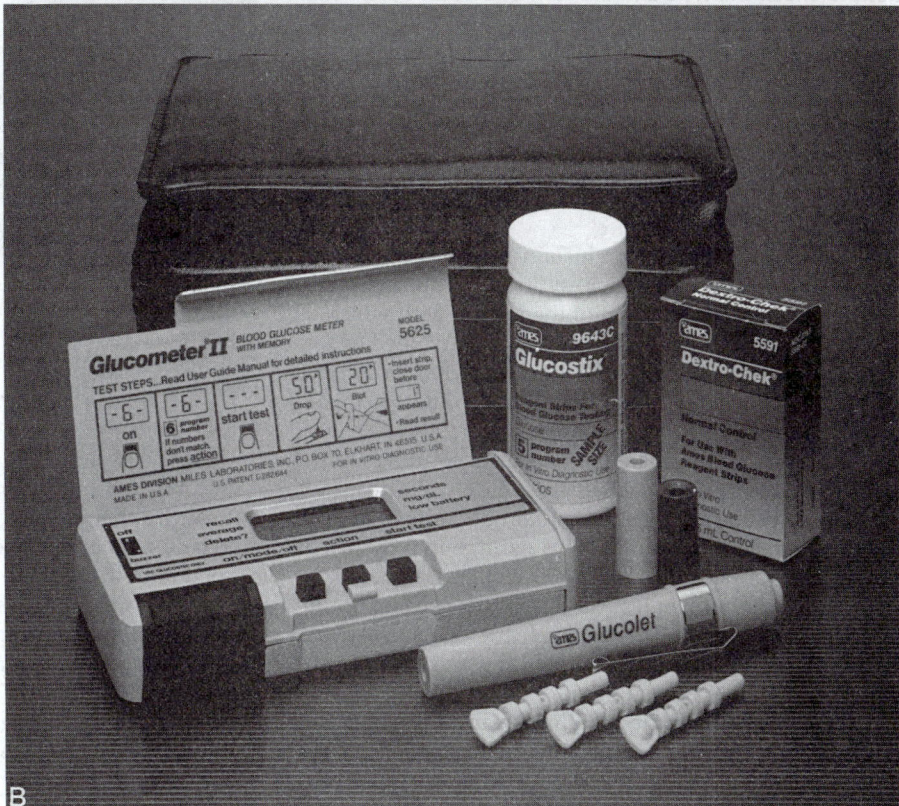

Figure 44–6. *A*, The Medi-Jector EZ (courtesy of Derata Corporation, Minneapolis, MN). *B*, The Glucometer II blood glucose monitoring meter (courtesy of Ames Div. of Miles Laboratories, Inc., Elkhart, IN).

Type I, insulin-dependent diabetic patient is taught to test the urine for both ketones and glucose. Even if the Type I diabetic patient uses home blood glucose monitoring, the patient is advised to test for ketones if the blood glucose reading exceeds 250 mg/dL. The nurse helps the patient choose the appropriate method for urine testing. Products often used are Keto-Diastix, Ketostix, Tes-Tape, and Diastix.

Urine is routinely tested before meals and at bedtime. Ketonuria without glycosuria usually indicates starvation rather than poor diabetic control. Double-voided urine samples are often used in the hospital setting, especially if the patient's urinary glucose is being covered with regular insulin, since it was thought that the second-voided urine sample most accurately reflected the patient's blood sugar. However, nursing research has indicated that double-voided specimens may not be necessary, as they do not show any significant differences from the first-voided specimens in most cases. Additionally, some sources advocate first-voided specimens to get a clearer picture of diabetic control. Eventually, blood glucose testing using a home blood glucose testing product will replace a urine test for glucose.

In the hospital, the nurse records the urine test results on a flow sheet and instructs the patient to do the same thing when at home. Such a record allows all pertinent information regarding diabetic control to be located in the same place. All urine tests are recorded in percentages (0.1%, 0.25%, 0.5%, etc.), since recordings of 1+, 2+, 3+, etc., do not always correspond to the same amount of glycosuria when different testing agents are used and, therefore, may lead to misinterpretation of results.

Insulin Administration

In providing the patient with insulin, it is the nurse's responsibility to draw up the correct type and dosage of insulin. It is generally recommended that another nurse double check the type and amount of insulin before the first nurse administers the insulin to the patient.

INJECTION TECHNIQUE. The exact technique for insulin injection may vary slightly from institution to institution, but the goal remains the same. Subcutaneous insulin is injected between the fat and muscle layer to ensure proper absorption. This may be accomplished by lightly pinching a large fold of skin and inserting the needle at a 90-degree angle.

Hypodermic syringes for insulin injection are either disposable or reusable. Each syringe is calibrated according to the concentration of the insulin with which it is used. U-100 syringes provide 100 U/ml. Needles for injection are usually 27–28-gauge and vary in length from ⅜- to ⅝-inch. Often, this length is too short to inject insulin properly for the obese patient. Needles are changed to an appropriate length by substituting an insulin syringe with a detachable needle. A "lo-dose syringe" has been calibrated to contain 50 units of U-100 insulin in a 0.5-ml volume. This syringe may be used when less than 50 units of U-100 insulin is ordered. It is especially helpful for less than 20 units. Because of the decreased diameter of the syringe, the calibrations are farther apart, permitting easier reading and more accurate measurement of insulin.

Before drawing up the insulin, the insulin vial is inspected. Intermediate- and long-acting insulins are rolled and appear uniformly cloudy after mixing. They are not to be shaken. The vials are not used if insulin material remains at the bottom of the bottle, if clumps are floating in the insulin after mixing, or if particles on the bottom or wall of the bottle have a frosted appearance. The expiration date of the insulin is also checked.

When drawing up insulin, it is important to be exact in measuring the number of units that the physician has prescribed. Avoidance of bubbles is important. The volume of the bubble can easily displace a few units of insulin, which can make a substantial difference in dosage.

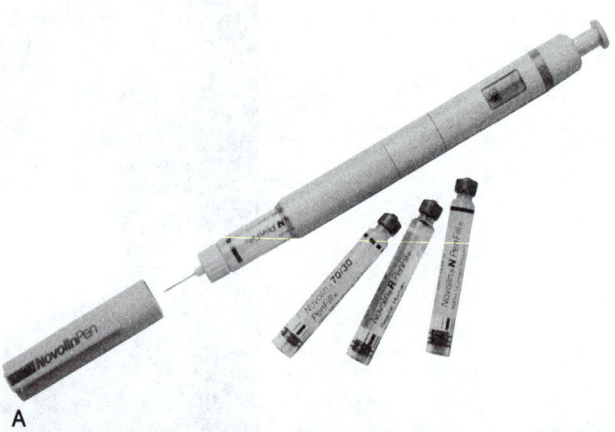

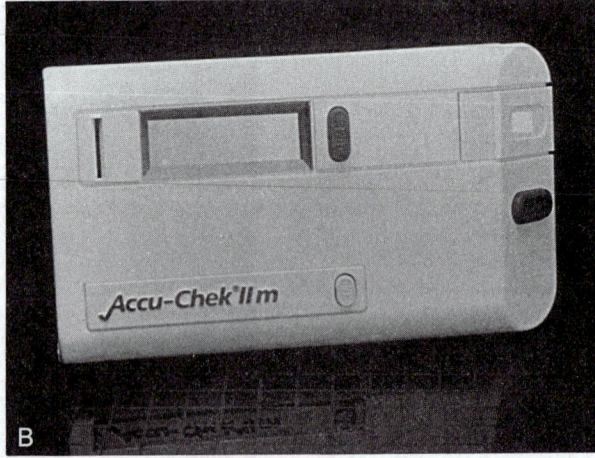

Figure 44–7. *A,* The Novolin Pen, an aid to insulin administration (courtesy of Squibb-Novo, Princeton, NJ). *B,* The Accu-Chek II blood glucose monitoring meter (courtesy of Boehringer-Mannheim Diagnostics, Indianapolis, IN).

Accurate measurement of insulin may be especially difficult for the visually impaired patient. Aids are commercially available to help the blind or visually handicapped patient draw up and administer insulin. Magnifying glasses that clip directly on the insulin syringe can enlarge the numbers so the visually impaired patient can see them. An example of this would be the B-D Magni-Guide (Fig. 44–7). Guides can assist the blind individual in filling syringes.

Injection aids that can be used with standard syringes may be a help to some patients. Using these aids, a standard syringe is filled with insulin and placed in the device. The device is placed against a desired site and a button is pushed or the device is pressed against the skin to release a spring mechanism that pushes the needle automatically into the skin. All the patient has to do is push the plunger to inject the insulin. Some devices even push the plunger. Examples of these devices are the Autojector, Diamatic, Inject-Ease, and Robinject. Injection pens are also available. A cartridge containing insulin is stored in a device about the size of a ballpoint pen. A disposable needle is used at one end of the pen and there is a push button or turn knob on the other end. The pen is held and the needle is inserted into the skin like an ordinary injection. These pens are convenient since the patient does not have to carry syringes and bottles of insulin in order to give the prescribed dose. The pens also have audible clicks and enlarged numbers that help the visually impaired patient determine how much insulin is being injected. Some examples of these injection pens are the Novo Pen, Novolin Pen (Fig. 44–7), and Accupen. For individuals who dislike injecting insulin or fear needles, "no-needle" injectors or "jet" injectors are an alternative. These injectors deliver a tiny stream of insulin under pressure directly through the skin. Often there is little or no sensation at the time of injection. Examples of these "no-needle" insulin injectors include the Preci-Jet 50, Vitajet, Medi-Jector EZ (Fig. 44–6), and Medi-Jector II.

Often, to obtain optimum control, the physician orders two types of insulin to be administered at the same time. Some insulins may be combined in the same syringe provided that they are given within five minutes after mixing, other insulins may be given any time after being combined in the syringe, and others may not be combined at all. Refer to Table 44–8 for guidelines regarding the mixing of two different types of insulin. If the desired insulins may be mixed, it is important that the patient always draw up the insulins in the same order. Air should be added to each vial, then the proper amount of rapid-acting insulin drawn into the syringe, followed by the proper amount of intermediate-acting insulin. This prevents contamination of the rapid-acting insulin with the intermediate-acting insulin.

If the patient is unable to safely draw up two different types of insulin in the same syringe, alternatives are available. A family member can be taught to prefill the syringes with the designated amount of insulin, so that the patient will have a week's supply for injection. It is important that the patient wait at least 15 minutes after NPH and regular insulin are mixed and at least 24 hours after Lente and regular insulin are mixed before using prefilled syringes, so the therapeutic results remain consistent on a day-to-day basis. The prefilled syringes should be stored in the refrigerator and gently rotated before injection. Several mixtures of NPH and regular insulin are commercially available. Examples of these include Mixtard, which is 70% NPH and 30% regular pure pork insulin; and Novolin 70/30 which is 70% NPH human and 30% regular human insulin. These premixed insulins are desirable for the individual who can fill the syringe, but cannot master the technique of mixing, and for the patient who happens to require a 70/30 ratio of doses.

In addition to instructing the patient on insulin injection technique, the nurse also instructs the patient regarding injection site rotation in order to prevent lipohypertrophy. As mentioned previously, lipohypertrophy is an adverse reaction to insulin therapy that occurs when insulin is injected frequently into the same area. The patient should be taught to systematically rotate injection sites using areas of the upper thighs, upper arms, back, abdomen, and buttocks. The patient should be

Table 44–8. GUIDELINES FOR MIXING TWO TYPES OF INSULIN IN THE SAME SYRINGE

1. Use the same procedure each time you prepare an insulin mixture.
2. Mix insulins produced by the same manufacturer only.
3. Semilente, Lente, and Ultralente insulins may be combined in any ratio desired.
4. NPH–regular insulin mixtures should be given within 5 minutes of preparation to achieve the same clinical response as separate injections of each product. Within 5–15 minutes, the NPH and regular insulin mixture undergoes a stabilization process. During that time, binding occurs and some regular insulin is lost to yield more NPH insulin. The greater the ratio of NPH to regular insulin, the more binding will take place. After 15 minutes, the mixture is stable. To achieve a consistent clinical response, the NPH–regular insulin mixture should be given within 5 minutes of mixing or 15 minutes after mixing. Therefore, if a patient will be going home from the hospital with prefilled syringes, the NPH–regular insulin given in the hospital should be given 15 minutes after mixing.
5. Lente–regular insulin mixtures should be administered immediately after preparation to achieve the same clinical effect as each separate product. The Lente–regular insulin mixture undergoes a stabilization process that occurs during the first 24 hours after mixing. During that time, binding occurs and some regular insulin is lost to yield more Lente insulin. The greater the ratio of Lente to regular insulin, the more binding occurs. After 24 hours, the mixture is stable. Therefore, if a patient will be going home from the hospital with prefilled syringes, the Lente–regular insulin administered in the hospital should be given 24 hours after mixing.
6. PZI–regular insulin mixtures are unstable and the insulins should be given as separate injections.
7. Ultralente–regular insulin mixtures decrease the rapid-acting effect of the regular insulin and should not be mixed in the same syringe.
8. Formulations of buffered insulins (all brands of NPH and PZI insulins, Humulin BR, and all Nordisk insulins) should not be mixed with any lente family insulins. The phosphate buffer will precipitate the zinc from one suspension, converting the extended insulin to a "regular" line insulin.

taught to avoid areas around old scars, varicosities, and the immediate area around the navel. One method that may be used is to choose a general area and select sites one inch or two fingers apart. Then, after approximately 15 days of using one area, the patient should choose a different site (Figure 44–8). Other systems have been developed that have the patient change injection sites from area to area. When using this system, it is important to not return to the previously used site too soon.

STORAGE OF INSULIN. The insulin the patient is using does not need to be refrigerated, but it must be protected from extremes of temperature. Freezing or excessive heat can affect the potency of the insulin. Insulin products remain stable at room temperature (68–75°F) for one month. When traveling, insulin can be protected from extremes of temperature by carrying it in a vacuum bottle. Bottles of insulin that are not in use should be stored in the refrigerator.

Injection Sites

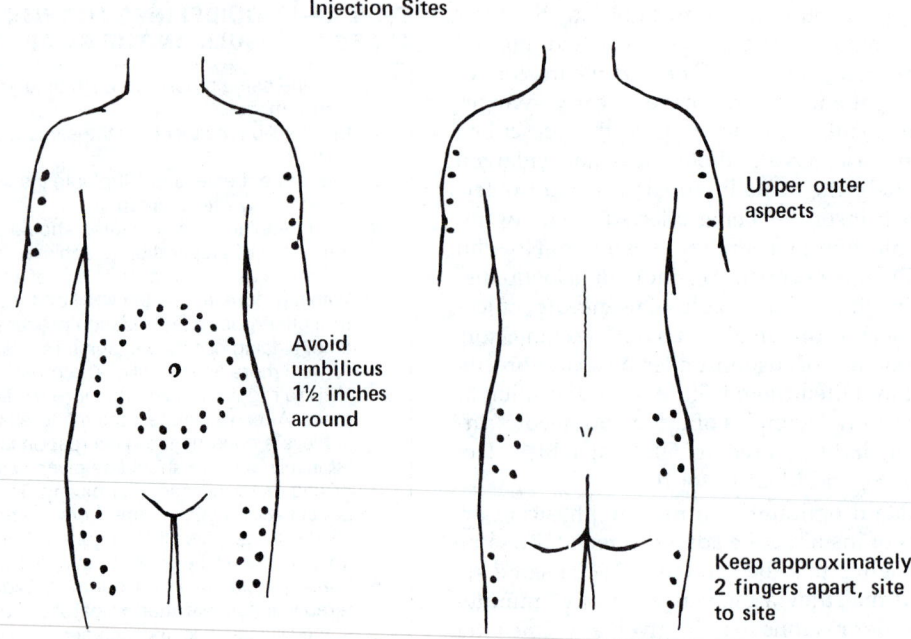

Upper outer
aspects

Avoid
umbilicus
1½ inches
around

Keep approximately
2 fingers apart, site
to site

Figure 44–8. Injection sites. (Redrawn with permission of Deborah G. Smith, MS, RN, Diabetes Clinical Specialist, Buffalo, NY, 1985.)

Exercise

The nurse originally assessed the patient's general exercise regime. During instruction the nurse stresses that planned exercise is helpful in lowering the blood glucose level, increasing cardiovascular fitness, increasing circulation, and promoting a feeling of well-being. The nurse suggests that exercise is done preferably after a meal and not at a time when a meal is due because of the risk of hypoglycemia. If the patient wishes to exercise before a meal, the nurse suggests that the patient test his or her blood sugar; if it is low normal, the patient should eat two peanut butter crackers or half of a sandwich and half a cup of milk, the amount of food depending upon the amount of exercise that is planned. Generally, if the blood sugar level is greater than 250 mg/dL, or if the patient is spilling ketones, he or she is advised not to exercise.

Oral Hypoglycemic Agents

The nurse administers the oral hypoglycemic agent that is prescribed for the patient. At the time of administration, the nurse identifies the medication, describes its use, and the time of administration.

Management of Hyperglycemia and Hypoglycemia

In caring for the diabetic, it is essential that the nurse have knowledge of the causes, symptoms, and treatment of hyperglycemia as well as hypoglycemia (see Table 44–9). The patient must be taught how to recognize when diabetes is out of control and to take appropriate action.

HYPERGLYCEMIA. The patient with hyperglycemia often experiences glycosuria, increased urine output,

thirst, hunger, and fatigue. It is important to try to detect the cause of the hyperglycemia, so that it may be treated. For example, if an infection has elevated the blood sugar level, the infection must be treated, rather than just increasing the insulin dosage.

Hyperglycemia can be treated with sliding scale insulin coverage. This procedure involves the testing of urine or blood glucose levels at specific intervals and the administration of regular insulin based on test results indicating glycosuria or hyperglycemia. Sliding scale coverage can be administered along with or instead of the usual insulin dosage, either at home or during hospitalization. An order for sliding scale coverage may resemble the following:

	Blood Glucose Values
180 mg/dL	No insulin
180–240 mg/dL	10 units of regular insulin
240–400 mg/dL	20 units of regular insulin
400 mg/dL	Call physician

	Urine Glucose Values
0 or 0.25%	No insulin coverage
0.5%	10 units of regular insulin
1%	15 units of regular insulin
2%	20 units of regular insulin

Add 5 additional units of regular insulin for any degree of ketonuria.

If an individual has a daily insulin order and is on sliding scale coverage, it is important that both orders be followed.

KETOACIDOSIS. If the patient is admitted to the hospital with ketoacidosis, treatment consists of hydration and insulin therapy. Hydration is begun with a nor-

Table 44–9. COMPARISON OF HYPOGLYCEMIA, KETOACIDOSIS, AND HYPERGLYCEMIC HYPEROSMOLAR NONKETOTIC COMA (HHNK)

	Hypoglycemia	Ketoacidosis	HHNK
DIABETES TYPE	Either	IDDM, usually young	NIDDM, usually over age 50
ONSET	Rapid: mintues to hours	Slow: hours to days (usually <2 days)	Insidious (>5 days), then rapid
CAUSES	Delayed or skipped meal; increased exercise without additional food; too much insulin; Somogyi effect; gastroenteritis	Undetected diabetes; stress (physical or emotional); illness or infection; excessive food intake; inadequate insulin or dosage errors; drugs such as thiazides or corticosteroids; reduced exercise	May be first indication of diabetes; usually adult-onset with enough insulin production to prevent ketosis; steroid therapy; stress states; hyperalimentation; dialysis, especially with solutions high in dextrose; pancreatic disease
SIGNS AND SYMPTOMS			
Neurologic	Weak, lightheaded, drowsy, trembly, headache, numbness of the mouth and tongue, anxious, memory loss, seizures, primitive reflexes (Babinski present)	Early: irritable, tired, headache, weakness; progressively more listless, decreased sensation until coma No focal symptoms Hyporeflexia	Focal symptoms (aphasia, homonymous hemianopsia, hemiparesis, hemisensory defects, unilateral hyperreflexia and Babinski, hallucinations and psychic disturbances)
Respiratory	Bradypnea; in shock, respiratory rate may increase	Kussmaul respiration (deep and rapid); sweet (acetone) odor to breath	Increased respiratory rate; no Kussmaul respirations or sweet odor to breath
Cardiovascular	Increased blood pressure and heart rate	Lower blood pressure, especially orthostatic; weak, rapid pulse	Lower blood pressure; weak, rapid pulse
Renal	Asymptomatic	Early: great increase in urine output; later, as shock develops: oliguria or anuria	Great increase in urine output, causing massive dehydration and hyperosmolarity; progresses to decreased output as shock develops
Gastrointestinal	Nausea, hunger, stomachache, vomiting	Nausea and vomiting, thirst, abdominal cramping, decreased bowel sounds, acute abdomen symptoms, weight loss	Nausea and vomiting, thirst, hunger, less acute abdomen symptoms
Skin	Diaphoretic, cold, clammy, pale; circumoral pallor	Hot, flushed, and dry; low body temperature	Flushed, very dry; elevated body temperature
Mucous Membranes	Normal	Very dry	Extremely dry
CLINICAL DATA			
Blood Sugar Level	Below 60 mg/dL or when a sudden drop occurs (for example, a drop from 400 mg/dL down to 200 mg/dL)	Above 200 mg/dL; usually, 400–800 mg/dL, sometimes higher	Usually above 600 mg/dL; up to 3000 mg/dL
Urine Glucose Level	Negative	2% or higher	2% or higher
Urine Ketone Bodies	Negative	Positive	Negative
Other Laboratory Tests	Essentially normal, except for low blood sugar levels	Falling pH (below 7.3); increased BUN and serum creatine; increased Hct, Hb, and total protein; initially increased, normal, or decreased K; normal or	Normal or decreased pH due to lactic acidosis not ketosis; increased BUN; increased, normal, or decreased K; normal or decreased Na; increased

CONTINUED ON THE FOLLOWING PAGE

Table 44–9. COMPARISON OF HYPOGLYCEMIA, KETOACIDOSIS, AND HYPERGLYCEMIC HYPEROSMOLAR NONKETOTIC COMA (HHNK)–*CONTINUED*

	Hypoglycemia	Ketoacidosis	HHNK
		decreased Na; increased WBC, SGOT, SGPT, and LDH; increased osmolarity, <350 mOsm/kg	WBC; serum osmolarity increased, >350 mOsm/kg
Treatment	Validate blood sugar level; administer 10 g fast-acting carbohydrate, followed by slow-acting carbohydrate. If patient is unable to swallow, give glucagon, 0.5–1.0 mg (IV, IM, or SC); repeat in 15 minutes, if needed. If no response, give 25–50 ml 50% dextrose; follow with a slow-acting carbohydrate meal when patient is alert.	Validate blood sugar level; monitor blood sugar, urine glucose, and acetone levels; hydration, first with normal saline, then dextrose solution as blood sugar level approaches normal; give regular insulin, IV or IM. Monitor vital signs and urine output; give K$^+$ supplements, if needed, after insulin is administered and when urine output is adequate.	Hydration; give small doses of regular insulin; very sensitive to insulin, blood sugar level may drop suddenly with only small amounts of insulin; give K$^+$ supplements.

mal saline solution, followed by a dextrose solution when blood glucose levels approach 250 mg/dL. Regular insulin is given either subcutaneously or intravenously, based on blood glucose values. If the patient is in shock, poor peripheral perfusion prevents adequate absorption when the insulin is administered subcutaneously. Rebound hypoglycemia can then occur when the shock is reversed and the insulin is absorbed. Rehydration, as well as insulin administration will lower serum potassium. Hypokalemia, as well as hyperkalemia, can have a detrimental effect on the cardiovascular and respiratory status. Therefore, it is essential to monitor serum potassium values and the ECG. Potassium is given only in the presence of adequate urine output.

Continuous low-dose infusion of insulin is the preferred treatment in managing ketoacidosis, since intravenous delivery of insulin rapidly establishes effective blood glucose levels which can be maintained or altered quickly. An IV bolus of 0.1 U per kg of body weight is often given, followed by an infusion of 6–10 U/hour. The insulin infusion is kept separate from the fluids being used to replace volume. An insulin concentration of 1 U/10 mL may be obtained by adding 50 units of regular insulin to 500 mL of normal saline. If the blood glucose is unchanged after two hours, the infusion rate is doubled. Insulin adheres to glass and plastic IV bottles, as well as IV tubing. The problem can be minimized by flushing the tubing with the insulin preparation before connecting it to the patient. This is not a major problem when the patient's blood sugars are monitored closely and insulin adjustments can be made.

HYPERGLYCEMIC HYPEROSMOLAR NONKETOTIC COMA. Hyperglycemic hyperosmolar nonketotic coma (HHNK) is a metabolic disorder that may occur in the diagnosed or undiagnosed Type II diabetic patient. The mortality rate is 50%–70%. In HHNK, the patient's blood sugar level becomes elevated. Since the Type II diabetic patient produces some insulin, ketosis is prevented. Therefore, the blood glucose level rises dramatically, often above 1000 mg/dL. The osmotic pull of the serum glucose is great, which causes profound dehydration in the body's cells and tissues and a fluid shift in the bloodstream. This fluid is rapidly eliminated by the kidney. The treatment of HHNK focuses on hydration to reverse shock, and small doses of insulin to counteract hyperglycemia (see Table 44–9). The emergency room nurse must be especially aware of this condition, since many patients are admitted to the hospital to rule out a stroke when it is really HHNK. Prompt determination of the blood glucose levels is, therefore, imperative.

HYPOGLYCEMIA. Hypoglycemia is a medical emergency and must be treated promptly to avoid brain damage. The nurse must be alert to recognize hypoglycemic symptoms and initiate prompt treatment. Hypoglycemic reactions most likely occur when the patient's insulin dose is peaking. The patient must be taught the causes, symptoms, and treatment of hypoglycemia, as well as how to prevent it from occurring.

If the patient is conscious, he or she takes 10 g of a fast-acting carbohydrate. This is about four to six ounces of juice without sugar added. This is followed by a slowly digested carbohydrate such as bread or milk. If a reaction immediately precedes a meal, the meal contains the slowly digested carbohydrate. If the diabetic patient is unconscious, oral foods or fluid should not be given. Instead, glucagon (0.5–1.0 mg IV, IM, or SC), IV dextrose (10%–15%), or 50% dextrose IV push can be used to elevate the blood sugar level. Relatives, along with the patient, are taught special administration procedures. Glucose products prepared in a synthetic base with a gel-like consistency are also available. Products such as Instant Glucose can be squeezed into the mouth from a tube. Cake-decorating icing can also be used in this manner.

Illness

When the diabetic patient becomes ill, control is more difficult. It is important for the nurse to give the patient guidelines to follow when illness occurs. Insulin is not omitted. If the patient is unable to eat regular meals, liquid carbohydrates such as soda pop or juices are substituted to fulfill daily caloric needs. The blood glucose or urine glucose levels are tested at least four times a day to detect hyperglycemia. The urine is also tested for the presence of ketones. If the illness progresses past two days, or if vomiting or diarrhea occurs, the physician is notified.

Infection is more common among patients with diabetes, and healing occurs more slowly than among nondiabetic persons. Infections cause blood glucose levels to rise and, if untreated, can cause diabetic ketoacidosis. For this reason, it is important for the diabetic patient to notify the physician immediately when signs of infection are present. A good program of skin care is encouraged to lessen the incidence of local infection.

Foot Care

The patient with diabetes is taught a regimen of proper foot care. Often as a result of *neuropathy* (chronic complication affecting the nervous system), a patient loses the ability to feel discomfort or pain in the feet and legs. Therefore, if the patient develops an injury, he or she will not recognize it; the injury then worsens and the blood glucose goes out of control. The nurse must enforce good foot care habits such as encouraging the patient to wear slippers at home as well as in the hospital. The nurse teaches the patient how to inspect the feet and perform care of the feet at home.

Considerations for the Pregnant Woman with Diabetes

The nurse often cares for the pregnant diabetic patient in the hospital or a clinic. Teaching is extremely important in this situation since pregnancy is a time period in which strict diabetic control is necessary in order to prevent abnormalities and mortality of the fetus. For a known diabetic, this requires home blood glucose monitoring, and mixed and split doses of insulin or insulin pump therapy. It is advisable that the blood glucose level remain around 100 mg/dL.

Oral hypoglycemic agents are not recommended during pregnancy since they do not control the blood sugar level as precisely as insulin therapy. Also, the effect of the oral hypoglycemic agent on the fetus is unknown. The insulin that is used is purified pork or human insulin since insulin antibodies are passed to the fetus.

Generally, during the first trimester of pregnancy, the patient who previously received insulin requires the same amount or the dose may have to be decreased. Nausea and vomiting during early pregnancy may make the meal pattern more difficult to follow and the diabetes more difficult to control. As the pregnancy progresses, the patient requires increasing amounts of insulin since the placenta produces hormones (cortisol, human placental lactogen, estrogens, progesterones, and prolactin) which elevate blood glucose levels. An insulin-degrading enzyme, insulinase, also increases insulin requirements during this time period.

The above situation often produces a glucose intolerance in some pregnant women, commonly referred to as gestational diabetes. This type of diabetes generally begins in the 26th to 28th week of pregnancy when the hormones are elevated, and frequently disappears as soon as the baby is born. The woman may have to take insulin during this time period, like the woman who has had diabetes prior to conception. Normoglycemia is a goal for the gestational diabetic patient.

Traditionally, women with diabetes were hospitalized during the last trimester of pregnancy to achieve strict control of blood glucose levels. Today, with home blood glucose monitoring, the woman can monitor her blood glucose levels and adjust her insulin dosage according to her physician's specified guidelines. Blood glucose testing is generally done before breakfast and two hours after meals.

During the postpartum period, the mother's insulin requirement returns to her prepregnancy level. Frequently, the infant of a diabetic mother is large for gestational age. The infant is placed in a special care nursery and monitored for hypoglycemia, which frequently occurs.

Considerations for the Patient Having Surgery

The major goals for good management of the diabetic patient during surgery are prevention of diabetic ketoacidosis, and prevention of severe fluid loss and hypoglycemia, especially during the period of anesthesia.

Specific orders for the patient undergoing a surgical procedure must be obtained before the day of surgery. If the patient is managed on an oral hypoglycemic agent, it is generally discontinued 24 hours before surgery except for chloropropamide, which may have to be stopped 48 hours before surgery. The patient is then placed on a low dose of an intermediate-acting insulin, or blood glucoses are covered with regular insulin on a sliding scale. For the patient who was on insulin therapy, half of the usual daily dose of intermediate-acting insulin is given subcutaneously during the morning and one or two liters of 5% glucose and water is given during the surgical procedure. Every four to six hours after the initial insulin dosage was administered, additional regular insulin may be given depending upon the degree of hyperglycemia. Another method that may be used is providing a continuous infusion of insulin preoperatively, which is continued during the period of anesthesia and into the postoperative period. One or two units of regular insulin per hour is given intravenously.

Regardless of the specific medical management of the diabetic patient undergoing surgery, the nurse must make frequent assessments of diabetic control. The nurse monitors continually for hyperglycemia and hypoglycemia. The nurse also strives to prevent infection since infection further compromises diabetic control for the patient.

PATIENT TEACHING

A thorough assessment of each patient with diabetes is essential in order to develop an individualized teaching plan. The nurse assesses the patient's knowledge of diabetes and its management, psychomotor skills such as insulin administration and urine testing, psychological factors such as stress and anxiety, physical limitations such as arthritis and retinopathy, sociological factors, support system, and economic factors. The nurse also assesses motivation and what diabetes means to the individual. Teaching is essential since the patient must learn how to manage the condition in order to live a long, productive life. Through assessment the nurse determines the appropriate method and materials to be used for instruction, and the rate at which the information is to be delivered. The nurse determines if survival or very basic information is all that the patient can comprehend or if a more detailed explanation of the disease process is necessary. The nurse teaches the patient what he or she needs to know and does not reteach material the patient has verbalized or demonstrated competency in.

The teaching plan, therefore, differs according to whether the patient's diabetes is controlled by diet alone, diet and oral hypoglycemic agents, or diet and insulin therapy. The teaching plan for the patient solely on dietary management consists of instruction regarding physiology of diabetes and treatment of hyperglycemia, dietary management, urine or blood glucose testing, exercise, and foot and skin care. The patient is advised to contact the nurse for further instructions if the treatment routine changes.

If the patient is managed on diet and oral hypoglycemic agents, all of the previously stated information is taught. In addition, teaching includes: information regarding the type, dosage, and action of the oral hypoglycemic agent; causes, symptoms, and treatment of hypoglycemia; and travel and sick day management. The patient is not taught about insulin therapy unless it is going to be used within a few days. The patient is encouraged to attend follow-up classes if he or she does not respond to the oral hypoglycemic agents and insulin therapy is warranted.

The patient who is on dietary management and insulin therapy requires all of the previously stated information except the teaching regarding oral agents. The patient also needs specific information regarding: the type, dosage, and action of the insulin; drawing up and injection technique; site rotation; and storage of insulin.

All patients should understand the basic function of the pancreas in terms of insulin production. It is important for the patient to understand the function of insulin in lowering the blood glucose by transporting it into the cell to provide energy. Pamphlets and visual aids are helpful in explaining what is occurring in the body. Understanding the way in which the body functions allows the patient to understand the symptoms of the disease and why they occur.

The teaching plan for the diabetic patient must be specific (see Table 44–10). Minor changes in technique, which are all within acceptable nursing practice, can be confusing for the patient who is trying to learn. Since

---

Table 44–10. PATIENT TEACHING INFORMATION FOR THE DIABETIC PATIENT TAKING INSULIN

Dear Patient:

This drug has been prescribed for you. This is what you should know about your drug to get the most from your therapy:

1. Insulin is a medication that will lower your blood sugar level. It takes the sugar from your bloodstream and brings it into the muscle cells in your body to give you energy. The insulin you are taking will make up for the insulin your body is not able to produce.
2. You will be taking insulin for the rest of your life.* The dosage and the times you administer the insulin may change over the course of time.
3. The amount of insulin you will be taking depends upon your doctor's orders. Obtain the correct vial of insulin and insulin syringe. Rotate the vial slowly between the palms of your hands to mix the solution thoroughly. Do not shake the vial. Take the insulin syringe and, using sterile technique, measure an amount of air equal to the amount of insulin you need and inject it into the vial. Turn the vial upside down and withdraw the correct number of units of insulin from the vial. Inject the insulin under the skin in a place that is ½" away from the previous place that you have used in the past 30 days. Follow the injection pattern of site rotation that you learned in the hospital. If you are using 2 types of insulin, draw the insulin up in the same order each day.
4. Many prescription as well as nonprescription medications may raise or lower your blood sugar level. Before taking any over-the-counter medications (i.e., cold and cough preparations, laxatives, antacids, and other medications you can get without a prescription), consult with your physician, pharmacist, or diabetes nurse educator about medications that do not contain sugar. If you are placed on any prescription medications, ask your doctor about the medication's effect on your blood sugar level.
5. If you forget to take your insulin, your blood sugar level will go up. Take the usual dosage of insulin if you remember, and it is 2 hours or less after the scheduled dosage was omitted. If more time elapses, consult your doctor to obtain the amount of insulin you should take. If you can't remember whether you took your insulin or not, do not take it.
6. Do not stop taking your insulin. High blood sugar levels, diabetic ketoacidosis, and even death can result from not taking your medication.
7. Your insulin dosage may change over time. You may be given a specific dosage by your doctor, or you may adjust your insulin dosage according to a scale based upon your blood glucose monitoring results. **Do not** adjust your insulin dosage without your doctor's advice.

Table 44–10. PATIENT TEACHING INFORMATION FOR THE DIABETIC PATIENT TAKING INSULIN–*CONTINUED*

8. You should not drink alcoholic beverages (beer, wine, whiskey) since they may lower your blood sugar level and cause an insulin reaction. If you have an "occasional" drink, it should be consumed before a meal. If you plan to drink alcoholic beverages on a regular basis, contact your doctor and dietitian in order to incorporate it into your meal pattern.

9. If you take too much insulin, skip or delay a meal, or exercise too hard, you may develop low blood sugar, which is a side effect of the medication. You will suddenly feel tired, dizzy, shaky, nervous, weak, and irritable, and break out into a cold clammy sweat. Immediately, take 2 sugar cubes, half a cup orange juice, or half a cup of sweetened soft drink to reverse these symptoms. It is important that your family learn how to give you glucagon in case you pass out and are unable to eat or drink. Wear a Medical Alert bracelet so emergency care can be given if you are unconscious. Another side effect of insulin therapy is a painless hardened area or lump in the skin area where you inject your insulin. Contact your doctor or nurse to review site rotation with you. If you notice any reddened areas around the insulin injection site, notify your doctor. Generally if the reddened areas occur several hours after the injection, this problem will disappear on its own. If it occurs within 1 hour of the injection, this could be an insulin allergy that requires prompt medical attention.

10. Insulin may be stored at room temperature for up to 1 month. However, it must be protected from extremes of temperature, which can alter its potency. It is stable in the refrigerator for 3 months. Do not use your intermediate- or long-acting insulin if the insulin material remains at the bottom of the bottle after mixing, or if particles on the bottom or wall of the bottle give it a frosted appearance.

*The Type II diabetic patient may not require insulin for the rest of his or her life and this must be discussed.

Table 44–11. RESOURCES FOR INFORMATION REGARDING DIABETES

American Association of Diabetes Educators
Suite 1400
500 North Michigan Avenue
Chicago, IL 60611

American Diabetes Association
National Service
1660 Duke Street
P.O. Box 25757
Alexandria, VA 22313
1-800-232-3472

Canadian Diabetes Association
National Office
78 Bond Street
Toronto, Ontario M5B2J8

Juvenile Diabetes Foundation
432 Park Avenue South, 16th floor
New York, NY 10016
1-800-223-1138 (In New York state, 212-889-7575)

National Diabetes Information Clearinghouse
Box NDIC
Bethesda, MD 20205

patient to feel that he or she is not alone with this disease. Family members and friends should be encouraged to take part in diabetes instruction.

The patient with Type II, non–insulin-dependent diabetes, on diet alone or receiving oral agents, may have a more lax attitude than the diabetic patient receiving insulin. Sometimes the patient feels that the diabetes is less serious or that he or she just has a "touch" of diabetes. It must be stressed that control is as important for this person as for the person on insulin. The individual's weight may increase over time from poor dietary adherence, and the diet and oral hypoglycemic agents may fail. The individual then may be placed on insulin. In this case, it is essential for the nurse to explain that insulin is not a lifelong sentence. The nurse should inform the patient that weight reduction brings the blood glucose levels back to normal and, although the patient still has diabetes, insulin or even oral hypoglycemia agents may no longer be required.

The changes in diet and lifestyle are often more difficult for the elderly patient with diabetes. The elderly patient may live alone and find it difficult to prepare three meals daily. The elderly patient may forget to take medication. Elderly patients may also have other health problems such as arthritis, poor vision, or poor motor coordination, which affect how well they are able to accomplish new tasks. Also, the added expense that diabetes imposes can be stressful for the elderly patient who is on a fixed income. The nurse can assist the elderly patient by seeing if he or she is eligible to receive Meals on Wheels (if they are unable to cook) and/or by arranging for a public health nurse or nurse's aide to help with care.

there are various insulin syringes available as well as urine and blood testing products, the nurse must be consistent in using the same product and communicate what products the patient is using with other nurses. For information regarding diabetes education material available and publications, see Table 44–11.

Diabetes teaching should proceed slowly and begin with simple instruction before the presentation of complex information. Teaching must focus on individual need. For example, if an individual is highly anxious regarding insulin therapy with numerous questions, and the nurse planned on teaching urine testing that day, the nurse should switch the agenda and discuss insulin therapy. Otherwise, the patient will not be listening to the discussion of urine testing.

Teaching that occurs in the hospital is reinforced and expanded in follow-up classes after discharge. Generally, after discharge the patient is less anxious and has questions based upon problems that arose while at home. The classes also provide support in allowing the

Table 44–12. DIABETES TEACHING RECORD

Topic	Not Applicable	To Whom—Specify Pt or SO	Date	Initials of Professional	Evaluation Date	Pt or SO is able to Verbalize or Demonstrate Knowledge of Topic	Initials of Professional	Comments
Diet								Type:
Booklet: What Is Diabetes Mellitus? (Causes, Symptoms, Rx, Hyperglycemia)								
Blood Glucose Monitoring								Product:
Urine Testing								Product:
Oral Agent								Type:
Insulin:								Type:
Measuring								
Injecting								
Mixing Two Types								
Hypoglycemia (Causes, Symptoms, Rx, Prevention)								
Foot and Skin Care								
Exercise								
Sick Day Management								
Travel Guidelines								
Dining Out Guidelines								

Initial	Name	Title

EVALUATION

During the evaluation phase of the nursing process, the nurse evaluates the patient to determine the effectiveness of the interventions. Some examples of evaluation criteria are included in Table 44–7.

Evaluation of the patient's knowledge of and compliance with the treatment plan is essential. Evaluation is an ongoing process in order to update and reuse the teaching plan as needed. A form that may be helpful in accomplishing this is shown in Table 44–12. Such a form can be placed in the front of the patient's chart on admission to assist the nurse in developing and evaluating a teaching plan. For patients who were previously diagnosed with diabetes, the form can be used to evaluate their knowledge-base and learning needs. It is important to evaluate the knowledge-base by having the patient verbalize knowledge or demonstrate a technique previously taught.

Even though the patient may be able to verbalize knowledge of the diabetes regimen and demonstrate techniques appropriately, compliance may not occur. Objective data such as blood glucose values, urine testing, and glycosylated hemoglobin tests must be analyzed in order to evaluate diabetic control.

The patient's urine test record is a valuable reflection of diabetic control. Glycosuria is to be avoided and evidence of its existence may indicate failure to adhere to the diabetic regimen, underlying infection, or a need for increased diabetic medication.

Blood glucose levels are important in evaluating the effectiveness of the diabetes regimen. The timing of these tests are just as important as the actual results. All of the blood sugars are done to ascertain that the blood glucose levels are close to the levels of the individual without diabetes. Generally, when a person is on insulin therapy, the fasting blood sugar is done to determine whether the intermediate-acting insulin given the day before is still effective. Blood sugar samples taken before lunch are used to evaluate the need for, or effectiveness of the rapid insulin given before breakfast. Blood sugar samples drawn in the evening (8:00–9:00 PM) are used to determine the need or effectiveness of rapid-acting insulin given before supper. Samples drawn during the night might indicate the need for giving a dose or adjusting a dose of intermediate-acting insulin before supper.

Another laboratory test that is helpful in evaluating diabetic control over a long period of time is the glycosylated hemoglobin level. This test reflects the mean blood glucose level over a period of three to eight weeks.

This test avoids the problem of evaluating the patient who adheres to the recommended diet for two to three days before the physician's visit so that he or she appears to be well controlled. It also can aid in determining if the extremely elevated blood glucose levels that prompted a hospitalization were part of a singular event or if the elevated levels have been occurring for a while. For example, a previously well-controlled insulin-dependent diabetic patient may arrive at a hospital with a blood sugar level of 500 mg/dL and be labeled as noncompliant. However, a normal glycosylated hemoglobin level leads the physician to investigate further to find other causes for hyperglycemia, such as a recent infection.

The normal glycosylated hemoglobin level for the well-controlled patient is 8% or less. Certain conditions such as hemolytic anemia, severe hemorrhage, and pregnancy can invalidate the results obtained for this test.

Diabetes Out of Control

Improper diabetic control, leading to diabetic ketoacidosis, hyperglycemic hyperosmolar nonketotic coma, or insulin shock (all previously discussed), can be very dangerous. Every diabetic patient has fluctuations of blood glucose levels, but severe fluctuations must be detected and treated promptly. It is important for the nurse to realize that poor diabetic control is not always a result of noncompliance. An infection or differing metabolic demands can create severe problems in diabetic balance.

Following prompt treatment, assessment of the underlying causes is important in preventing recurrent episodes of hypoglycemia or hyperglycemia. Modifications in insulin, diet, or exercise may be necessary.

Somogyi Effect

When a patient's insulin requirements seem to be steadily increasing without any apparent cause (e.g., infection) and fluctuations between hypoglycemia and hyperglycemia occur, the Somogyi effect should be suspected. This asymptomatic phenomenon is a rebound hyperglycemia, directly resulting from the hormonal response to hypoglycemia induced by excessive insulin administration. Hypoglycemia is overcompensated for by a slow prolonged release of glucose from the liver. When the patient's blood sugar level is again tested, it is high. Thus, the physician prescribes more insulin, which only contributes to a more severe hypoglycemia. Usually, rebound hyperglycemia occurs 6–12 hours after periods of hypoglycemia. Blood samples drawn around 4:00 or 5:00 AM often reflect this hypoglycemia. For patients experiencing the Somogyi effect, a decrease in insulin dosage will control rebound hyperglycemia and promote better control.

Chronic Complications of Diabetes

Diabetes, especially if poorly controlled, can lead to numerous complications. Most of these complications result from inadequate circulation, either within the arteries due to atherosclerosis, or within the capillaries due to increased basement membrane thickness.

In evaluating the diabetic patient for atherosclerosis (macrovascular changes) it is important to consider cerebral effects (transient ischemic attack, cerebrovascular accident), cardiac effects (angina, myocardial infarction), and peripheral vascular disease. Peripheral vascular occlusive disease can eventually lead to gangrene and necessitate the amputation of limbs. Meticulous care of the feet is therefore essential for the diabetic patient.

Interference with capillary blood flow (microvascular changes) affects three major areas for the patient with diabetes: the retina, which can lead to blindness; the kidney, which can lead to renal failure; and the nerves, which results in neuropathy. Neuropathy leads to a variety of symptoms: decreased cutaneous sensation that may result in injury or trauma; decreased nerve function in the bladder that can lead to neurogenic bladder and urinary retention; decreased nerve function to the gastrointestinal tract that can lead to delayed gastric emptying, diarrhea, constipation, or malabsorption of food; and decreased capillary blood flow to the sex organs that can result in impotence in the male patient with diabetes.

Infections are also much more common among persons with diabetes. Poor circulation limits the number of antibodies and lymphocytes that can reach an infected area, thus decreasing the individual's effective immune response. Also, high glucose levels provide an excellent medium for bacterial growth.

Evaluation Criteria

Specific appropriate data are collected systematically in all of the above areas. Such data give the nurse a clear picture of the patient's diabetic status. Sudden deterioration in a specific area can be due to poor diabetic control. The following can be used as criteria for good control in the patient with diabetes:

1. Blood glucose and urine testing values are within normal limits specified by the physician.
2. The patient experiences few episodes of hypoglycemia or hyperglycemia.
3. The patient demonstrates the ability to perform the technical skills necessary for managing diabetes in the home setting. This may include insulin injection, home blood glucose testing, urine testing, and foot care.
4. The patient is able to follow the ADA diet and incorporate the diet into his or her lifestyle.
5. The patient verbalizes a willingness to comply with the medical management of the diabetes.
6. The patient is able to recognize when to seek the guidance of a professional for follow-up care or additional information regarding diabetes.

SUMMARY

Diabetes mellitus is a chronic disease that can affect nearly every part of the body. Good control of diabetes can prevent, postpone, or reverse some of the chronic complications associated with the disease. Two different groups of medications, namely insulin or oral hypoglycemic agents (sulfonylureas) may be used to help achieve diabetic control. Insulin is used for the Type I, insulin-dependent diabetic patient whose pancreas is unable to produce insulin, or for the Type II non–insulin-dependent diabetic patient who is unable to achieve diabetic control through diet, exercise, and oral hypoglycemic therapy. Oral hypoglycemic agents are used for the Type II diabetic patient who is able to produce some insulin, when diet and exercise fail to control hyperglycemia. These agents stimulate the cells of the pancreas to produce more insulin and suppress hepatic glucose production. They also increase the number of insulin receptors on the cells so the patient can utilize the insulin that he or she produces. Additionally, the sulfonylureas influence events within the cell after glucose is transferred inside. Occasionally, oral hypoglycemic agents and insulin therapy may be used in combination for the Type II diabetic patient who is unable to control the diabetes with oral hypoglycemic agents or insulin alone.

Important nursing implications in administering insulin or oral hypoglycemic agents include: determination of the patient's blood glucose levels; provision of the correct meal pattern; administration of the antidiabetic medication; assessment and evaluation of the patient's response to the medication including blood glucose monitoring, urine testing, observation for hypoglycemia, and assessment for allergy; and awareness of the many drug interactions. Education of the patient and his or her family is of utmost importance since the patient is the primary manager of the disease.

BIBLIOGRAPHY

Anderson, JH: Personal communication, Lilly Research Laboratories, August 1987.

Baker, DE and Campbell, RK: The second-generation sulfonylureas: Glipizide and glyburide. The Diabetes Educator 11:29, 1985.

Basso, LV: Management of the diabetic patient undergoing surgery. Practical Diabetology 1:1, 1982.

Bonar, JR: Diabetes: A Clinical Guide. Medical Examination, New York, 1977.

Campbell, RK: Diabetes Management: Insulin, Oral Agents and Intensified Insulin Therapy. American Association of Diabetes Educators Continuing Education, Chicago, 1985.

Davidson, MB: Diabetes Mellitus: Diagnosis and Treatment. John Wiley & Sons, New York, 1981.

Drug Information American Hospital Formulary Service. Authority of the Board of Directors of the American Society of Hospital Pharmacists, Bethesda, MD, 1987.

Evaluations of Drug Interactions. American Pharmaceutical Association, Washington, DC, 1986.

Facts and Comparisons: Drug Information. Facts and Comparisons, St. Louis, MO, 1987.

Feinstein, AR: Clinical biostatistics: XXXV. The persistent clinical failures and fallicies of the UGDP study. Clin Pharmacol Ther 19:78, 1976.

Fies, LM and Campbell, RK: Insulin, sulfonylureas or both? Practical Diabetology 7:15, 1988.

Gilman, AG, Goodman, LS, and Gilman, A. (eds): The Pharmacological Basis of Therapeutics, ed 7. Macmillan, New York, 1985.

Guyton, AC: Textbook of Medical Physiology, ed 6. WB Saunders, Philadelphia, 1981.

Haire-Joshu, D, Flavin, K, and Santiago, J: Intensive conventional insulin therapy. Am J Nurs 86:1251, 1986.

Katcher, BS, Young, LY, and Koda-Kimble, MA (eds): Applied Therapeutics The Clinical Use of Drugs. Applied Therapeutics, San Francisco and Spokane, 1983.

Ramsey, PN: Hyperglycemia at dawn. Am J Nurs 87:1424, 1987.

Robertson, C. The new challenges of insulin therapy. RN May:34, 1989

Roth, J: Injections made easier. Diabetes Self-Management May–June:40, 1988.

Saudek, CD: Update on insulin pumps. Practical Diabetology 4:1, 1985.

Sabo, C and Rush-Michael S: Managing DKA—and preventing a recurrence. Nursing 89 19:50, 1989.

Szabo, AJ: Diabetic ketoacidosis: Practical guide to emergency treatment. Practical Diabetology 2:1, 1983.

Thatcher, G: Insulin injection: The case against random rotation. Am J Nurs 85:690, 1985.

University Group Diabetes Program: A study of the effects of hypoglycemic agents on vascular complications in patients with adult-onset diabetes. I. Design, methods and baseline results. Diabetes 19:747, 1970.

University Group Diabetes Program: A study of the effects of hypoglycemic agents on vascular complications in patients with

adult-onset diabetes. II. Mortality results. Diabetes 19:789, 1970.

Vorce-Tish, H: Independent living for the visually impaired. Diabetes Self-Management May–June:21, 1988.

SITUATION 44–1

Karen, a six-year-old, has just been diagnosed with Type I diabetes (IDDM). She is being cared for on the pediatric unit.

1. Karen is to receive Regular Humulin Insulin 10 units and NPH Humulin Insulin 30 units subcutaneously before breakfast (7:30 AM). The nurse will anticipate the onset of insulin action in approximately:
   a. three hours
   b. 30 minutes
   c. 1½ hours
   d. two hours

2. At what time of the day would the nurse be alert to the potential for a hypoglycemic reaction?
   a. after breakfast
   b. at midnight
   c. before bedtime
   d. before supper

3. When teaching Karen's mother about signs and symptoms of hypoglycemia, the nurse will include the following sign:
   a. sweating
   b. polyuria
   c. polydipsia
   d. "fruity" breath

4. The nurse will teach Karen's mother to administer insulin. The following information should be included:

   a. Intermediate-acting insulins should be clear in color.
   b. The vial of insulin should be shaken well before drawing up the dose.
   c. Regular insulin is drawn up before NPH insulin in the same syringe.
   d. An air bubble should remain in the syringe for proper injection.

5. A potential nursing diagnosis category which *best* fits Karen's situation would be:
   a. Alteration in Growth and Development
   b. Self Care Deficit
   c. Anxiety
   d. Sleep Pattern Disturbance

6. Which of the following statements by Karen's mother indicates a need for further education?
   a. "It is important to accurately prepare the dosages of insulin."
   b. "The insulin should be injected at a 90-degree angle."
   c. "Some kind of sugar should always be available in case of a reaction."
   d. "Periods of increased exercise will mean Karen will need more insulin."

SITUATION 44–2

Bernard Wallace is a 50-year-old with a history of obesity and congestive heart failure. His blood sugars have not been well controlled by diet, and he is to begin therapy with an oral hypoglycemia agent.

1. Before starting treatment with chlorpropamide (Diabinese), Mr. Wallace will have complete blood work and assessment performed. The nurse will be aware that the following result indicates a contraindication to treatment with this drug:
   a. elevated prothrombin time
   b. low hemoglobin
   c. elevated creatinine
   d. reduced calcium

2. Additional data which is important to assess prior to beginning therapy with chlorpropamide is that of allergy history. Mr. Wallace should not take this agent if he is allergic to:
   a. iodine
   b. insulin
   c. sulfa
   d. caffeine

3. Laboratory data are within normal limits, and Mr. Wallace is started on 250 mg of chlorpropamide (Diabinese) daily. Patient teaching about this agent will include the following information:
   a. Report headache and feelings of lethargy promptly.
   b. Take the medication with an antacid.

   c. Sporadic mealtimes are allowed with this agent.
   d. Avoid exercising, since this can potentiate the drug's effect.

4. Additional patient teaching regarding chlorpropamide should include listing medication which should be avoided while taking this drug. An example would be:
   a. cimetidine
   b. prednisone
   c. penicillin
   d. aspirin

5. Mr. Wallace has been taking digoxin 0.25 mg po daily. Aware of the interaction between chlorpropamide and digoxin, the nurse will observe for signs of:
   a. hyperglycemia
   b. digoxin toxicity
   c. hypoglycemia
   d. subtherapeutic digoxin levels

6. If Mr. Wallace takes chlorpropamide at 8:00 AM, he should expect the drug's peak activity to be at:
   a. 12:00 midnight
   b. 8:00 PM
   c. 4:00 PM
   d. 10:00 PM

Please refer to the Appendices for correct answers and additional review questions with answers.

GLOSSARY TERMS IN THIS CHAPTER
Azotemia
Carpopedal spasm
Cerebration
Chvostek's sign
Euthyroid
Exophthalmos
Hyperkinesis
Myopathy
Ophthalmopathy
Trousseau's sign

45
CHAPTER

THYROID AND PARATHYROID DRUGS

MERRILY MATHEWSON KUHN, R.N.C., Ph.D., CCRN

LEARNING OBJECTIVES

After reading this chapter, the student will be able to:

1. Identify those medications used in thyroid and parathyroid disorders.

2. Differentiate among the thyroid and parathyroid medications as to mechanism of action, route of administration, pharmacokinetics, adverse effects, contraindications, and interactions.

3. Identify specific areas to assess in the patient requiring thyroid or parathyroid medications in order to formulate appropriate nursing diagnoses.

4. Plan the nursing interventions necessary to administer thyroid or parathyroid medications and choose appropriate teaching strategies to gain patient compliance.

5. Evaluate the patient at various stages of treatment to determine the effectiveness of nursing interventions.

THYROID HORMONES

Three hormones are produced by the thyroid gland; thyroxine (T_4), triiodothyronine (T_3), and thyrocalcitonin. Thyroid hormone secretion is primarily controlled by thyroid-stimulating hormone (TSH), secreted by the anterior pituitary, which is in turn stimulated by thyrotropin-releasing hormone (TRH), secreted by the hypothalamus. Decreased serum levels of T_3 and T_4 stimulate TRH secretion, which in turn stimulates the pituitary gland to secrete TSH, which in turn releases the thyroid hormones from thyroglobulin. Thyroxine and triiodothyronine are synthesized in the thyroid gland and are stored as thyroglobulin. The storage and secretion of these hormones is dependent on circulating thyroid and iodine levels. The ratio of T_4 to T_3 is normally about 4:1, with T_3 being the more potent form of thyroid hormone. T_4 is converted to T_3 by peripheral tissues. Both of these hormones function to control the metabolic rate of tissues by accelerating chemical reactions, oxygen consumption, and heat production. Various theories are being explored to explain this action. Thyrocalcitonin or calcitonin regulates calcium levels by opposing parathyroid hormone. Calcitonin decreases serum calcium levels, while parathyroid hormone increases serum calcium levels. The function of the thyroid is featured in Table 45–1.

Iodine is the major component of T_3 and T_4. In the United States and Canada, the average daily iodine intake is 200–500 μg. The average daily requirements range from 100 to 300 μg. Iodine is found in iodized salt, iodine-rich foods such as shellfish, and foods such as milk that have been stablized with iodine. The gastrointestinal tract reduces two thirds of the iodine and it enters the circulation as iodide. The remaining one third is taken up by the thyroid. The ratio between iodide in the thyroid gland to that in the serum is referred to as the T/S ratio. The normal T/S ratio is 20:1, but if the gland is hyperactive, the T/S ratio is 250:1; if the gland is hypoactive, the T/S ratio may be 10:1.

Once the thyroid gland has concentrated iodide, thyroglobulin is synthesized first. Thyroglobulin contains tyrosine, an amino acid. The iodide combines with tyrosine to form monoiodotyrosine (MIT) and diiodotyrosine (DIT). MIT and DIT then join to form T_3 and T_4. T_3 and T_4 are stored in the follicles of the thyroid gland for later release. A main constituent of the thyroid mass is stored thyroglobulin, which stores enough thyroid hormone to last 2–3 months (Fig. 45–1).

ACTION

The principal action of thyroid hormones is to increase the metabolic rate of body tissues. Thyroid hormones serve to: increase the rate and depth of respiration; strengthen the rate and force of contraction of the heart; increase heat production; accelerate the metabolism of foodstuffs for energy; increase the rate of protein synthesis and catabolism; regulate growth in children; stimulate lipid synthesis, mobilization, and degradation; lower the concentration of cholesterol in plasma; and maintain nervous system development and *cerebration*. Normal daily production of thyroxine is about 70–90 μg; triiodothyronine, 15–30 μg. In the presence of adequate iodide substrate, the thyroid stores more T_4 than T_3 and releases about 1% of its stores daily. Both T_3 and T_4 are transported in the serum bound to protein, specifically, thyroxine-binding globulin. These protein storage molecules can store T_3 and T_4 for up to several months. This long-term storage helps to explain why patients do not exhibit symptoms of hypothyroidism until several months after thyroid production has ceased.

Thyrocalcitonin, or calcitonin, functions in regulating calcium metabolism. Thyrocalcitonin is released in response to a high serum calcium level. It exerts its effects: on bone, preventing resorption by decreasing osteoclastic activity; on the gastrointestinal tract, to decrease absorption of calcium; and on the renal tubule, to increase calcium excretion.

Thyroid hormones for use as medication are available as natural or synthetic products. The natural products are derived from beef or pork. Synthetic forms of thyroid hormone exert the same physiologic effects as T_3 and T_4; they vary from the natural compounds in their potency, in the ratio of T_3 and T_4 contained within them, or both.

USE

Thyroid hormone, either natural or synthetic, is used to replace deficient hormone in cases of inadequate thyroid production (Table 45–2 reviews hypothyroidism) and to

Table 45–1. FUNCTIONS OF THE THYROID

BODY SYSTEM	T_3/T_4
Gastrointestinal	Increases metabolic activities of all body tissue.
	Affects all aspects of carbohydrate metabolism.
	Affects all aspects of fat metabolism.
	Increases protein synthesis/breakdown.
	Increases appetite and weight.
	Increases growth.
	Affects cholesterol, phospholipids, and triglyceride levels.
Neurologic	Maintains cerebration.
Respiratory	Increases oxygen consumption.
Cardiovascular	Directly excites the heart.
Metabolic	Increases activity of cellular enzyme systems (such as Na-K-ATPase).
	Increases mitochondrial numbers and activity.
	Regulates female sexual function.
BODY SYSTEM	**THYROID CALCITONIN**
Skeletal	Inhibits bone resorption.

From Mathewson, MK: Functions of the thyroid. Crit Care Nurse 7(1):75, January/February 1987, with permission.

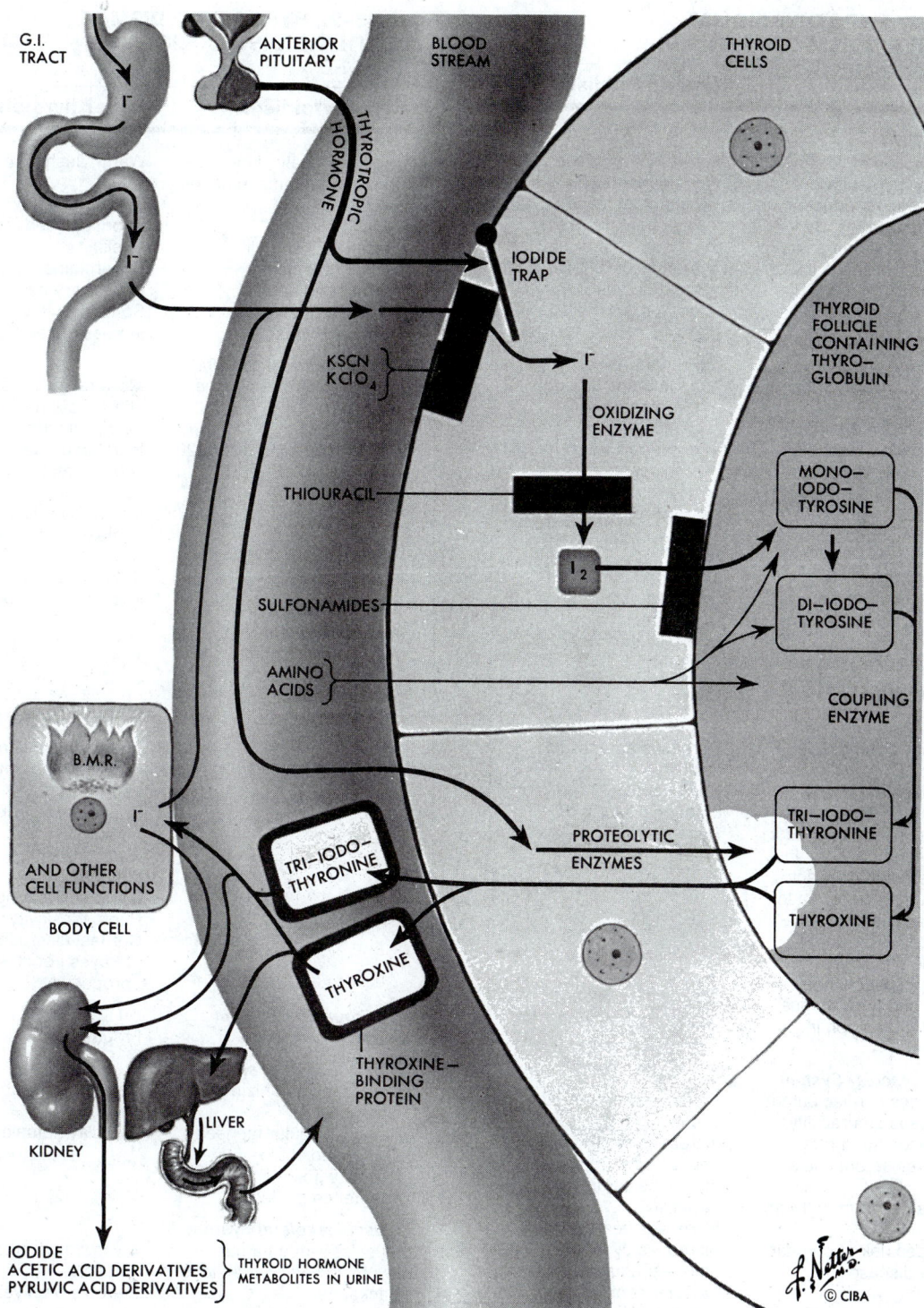

Figure 45–1. Thyroid Hormone Storage and Release. Iodine is consumed in the diet. The gastrointestinal tract reduces ⅔ of the iodine to iodide. The remaining ⅓ of the iodine is taken up by the thyroid. Once iodine is in the thyroid, thyroglobulin is synthesized. Thyroglobulin contains the amino acid thyrosine. The iodide combines with tyrosine to form monoiodotyrosine (MIT) and diiodotyrosine (DIT). MIT and DIT join to form T_3 and T_4. T_3 and T_4 are stored in the follicles of the thyroid gland for later release. Approximately 30 percent of the thyroid mass is stored thyroglobulin (courtesy of Ciba-Geigy, with permission).

**Table 45–2. HYPOTHYROIDISM/
HYPERTHYROIDISM COMPARISON**

Hypothyroidism	Hyperthyroidism
DEFINITION:	
Hypofunction of the thyroid gland with resultant decrease in production of thyroid hormone. Synonyms: myxedema, in adult; cretinism, in infant.	Hyperfunction of the thyroid gland with resultant increase in production of thyroid hormone. Synonyms: thyrotoxicosis, toxic goiter, Graves' disease.
ETIOLOGY:	
1. Primary	1. Primary
a. Chronic lymphocytic thyroiditis (autoimmune disorder)	a. Immune defect
b. Iodine excess (impairs secretion of thyroid hormone)	b. Hyperplastic disease
c. Iodine deficiency	c. Neoplastic disease
d. Prolonged lithium therapy	d. Iodine excess (rare)
2. Secondary	2. Secondary
a. Pituitary dysfunction	a. Metastasizing tumor
b. Hypothalamic dysfunction	b. Pituitary tumor
c. Metastasizing tumor	
SYMPTOMS:	
Central Nervous System	
Decreases adrenergic activity	Increases adrenergic activity
Decreases blood flow to brain, including slow mental functioning, poor short-term memory, loss of interest in daily activity, tiredness, sleeping a lot, and flat affect	Nervousness Emotional liability *Hyperkinesis* Tremors
Increases infiltrates in tongue and larynx, slowed speech, hoarseness, and thick tongue	
Mental retardation in infants	
Cardiovascular System	
Decreases cardiac output	Enhances adrenergic activity
Decreases contractility	Increases cardiac output activity
Decreases heart rate	Increases cardiac contractility
Increases serum cholesterol	Increases heart rate
Increases serum triglycerides	Increases dysrhythmia—premature ventricular contractions, atrial fibrillation, paroxysmal atrial tachycardia
Increases risk of coronary artery disease	Increases tendency to develop CHF
	Increases blood pressure
Cutaneous Symptoms	
Decreased body temperature	Increased body temperature
Cold intolerance	Heat intolerance

**Table 45–2. HYPOTHYROIDISM/
HYPERTHYROIDISM COMPARISON–**
CONTINUED

Hypothyroidism	Hyperthyroidism
Cool, dry, scaly skin	Warm, flushed, moist skin
Nonpitting edema in hands and feet	Separation of fingernail from nail bed (onycholysis)
Facial puffiness	Hyperpigmentation
Coarse broken hair	Palmar erythema
Thick, brittle nails	Soft, easily broken hair
Poor wound healing	Increased hair loss
Yellowing of skin	
Night blindness	
Gastrointestinal System	
Prolonged GI transit time	More rapid GI transit time—diarrhea, nausea, vomiting
Anorexia	
Constipation	Increased rate of glucose metabolism from GI system
Weight increased by 10–20 pounds	Increased rate of uptake of glucose into cells
	Decreased weight
	Mild fat malabsorption
Immune System	
May have autoimmune diseases, such as pernicious anemia	
Ocular System	
None	Irreversible infiltrative *ophthalmopathy* in 50%
	Poor convergent vision
	Exophthalamos
	Lid edema
	Increased tearing
	Photosensitivity
	Corneal ulceration due to eyes not closing properly
Genitourinary System	
None	Frequent urination
Reproductive System	
Decreased luteinizing hormone level	Decreased or absent menses
Heavy, irregular menses	Infertility (females)
Decreased libido	
Infertility (females)	
Impotence (males)	
Musculoskeletal System	
Muscles—edematous, with slowed contractions	*Myopathy* in proximal muscles
Backache	Periodic paralysis
Goiter	
Endemic	Exophthalmic
MANAGEMENT:	
Replacement of thyroid hormone	Antithyroid drug therapy
	Surgical resection
	Radioactive iodine

treat simple goiter. The pituitary hormone, thyrotropin, is used primarily in the diagnosis of hypothyroidism and to enhance radioactive iodine uptake in the treatment of metastatic thyroid carcinoma.

PHARMACOKINETICS

Absorption and Distribution

The various thyroid preparations (Table 45–3) are effectively absorbed from the gastrointestinal tract and are given via the oral route for maintenance therapy. Patients are advised to take their medication in the morning, preferably on an empty stomach, to facilitate absorption. Absorption of T_3 is 95% and absorption of T_4 is 48%–79%.

In the blood, 99.94% of thyroid hormone becomes bound with protein, especially thyroxine-binding globulin (TBG), which is synthesized in the liver. In addition, thyroxine-binding prealbumin (TBPA) and albumin (TBA) also carry small amounts of thyroid hormones. It is the very minute, unbound portion of the hormone that is pharmacologically active. Protein binding serves to protect the hormones from immediate metabolism and excretion and gives them a longer half-life in circulation. TBG levels increase during pregnancy, after the administration of estrogen, and in viral hepatitis. They decrease after administration of androgens or excessive amounts of glucocorticoids, and in conditions resulting in protein wasting.

Biotransformation and Excretion

The half-life of thyroxine is about 6–7 days; triiodothyronine, about two days. The maximum effect of T_4 is not reached for several weeks; T_3 achieves full effect in 4–8 days.

The liver degrades the thyroid hormones and excretes them in bile into the intestine, where some is reabsorbed and returned to the liver. About 20%–40% of thyroxine is eliminated in the feces, primarily unchanged. Thyroxine is also partly excreted in the urine.

CONTRAINDICATIONS AND PRECAUTIONS

Use of thyroid hormones is contraindicated in patients with: diagnosed thyrotoxicosis, acute myocardial infarction uncomplicated by hypothyroidism (as these conditions may be worsened), and where hypersensitivity exists.

Thyroid hormones are used with great caution in patients with cardiac disease, including coronary artery disease and hypertension, as these drugs increase the metabolic demands on the heart. These products are not administered to persons with uncorrected adrenal insufficiency, as thyroid agents increase tissue demand for adrenal hormones. This increased demand may precipitate an acute adrenal crisis.

ADVERSE EFFECTS

The adverse effects of these drugs are primarily due to overdosage and are essentially the occurrence of the signs and symptoms of hyperthyroidism (see Table 45–2 for a review of hyperthyroidism). The cardiovascular system is commonly affected. The onset of tachycardia is often an early sign of overdosage; consequently, patients are taught to monitor their pulse rates, particularly during initial therapy. The occurrence of anginal pain or symptoms of congestive heart failure are usually related to the increased cardiac workload resulting from the increase in metabolism. The elderly patient is especially at risk for these adverse effects. In addition, patients may experience increased blood pressure and dysrhythmias.

Sweating and intolerance to heat may develop. Diarrhea and abdominal cramping may occur, and weight loss may ensue related to the increased metabolic rate. Regular weight monitoring helps to detect this at an early stage. Adverse effects relating to the central nervous system include tremors, headache, nervousness, and sleep disturbances; these are all related to the increased metabolic rate.

The occurrence of any of the adverse effects is reported immediately to the physician. Reduction of the dosage of the thyroid drug usually resolves these problems.

INTERACTIONS

The use of thyroid hormones concurrently with other drugs can lead to various interactions. Aspirin may compete for protein binding of T_3 and T_4. Patients who are hyperthyroid should not be given aspirin as this releases more T_3 and T_4 into circulation. Phenytoin (Dilantin) tends to potentiate the effects of the thyroid hormones. Cholestyramine (Questran) decreases the effects of thyroid hormones by interfering with their absorption.

Thyroid hormone can also alter the effects of other drugs. Concurrent use tends to increase the effects of stimulants, epinephrine, ephedrine (due to the stimulatory effects), oral anticoagulants (by enhanced metabolism of clotting factors), tricyclic antidepressants, and imipramine (by increasing receptor sensitivity and enhancing antidepressant activity). The therapeutic effectiveness of digitalis products may be decreased with possible exacerbations of cardiac dysrhythmias or congestive heart failure. Antidiabetic medications may need to be increased when thyroid hormones are given concurrently.

Numerous drugs have a tendency to interfere with accurate testing of T_3, T_4, and serum TSH levels. Several of these drugs are featured in Table 45–4.

DOSAGE

Dosages of the thyroid preparations vary from patient to patient, depending on individual needs and on the specific preparation used. Generally, patients are started on small doses of thyroid hormones and gradually given increasing doses until the signs and symptoms of hy-

TEXT RESUMES ON PAGE 1188

Table 45–3. THYROID/ANTITHYROID DRUGS

Name	Dosage	Mode of Administration	Pharmacokinetics
THYROID HORMONES			
Action: Increase metabolic activity in body.			
Use: Hypothyroidism.			
T_3 and T_4: Thyroid desiccated (Thyroid)	*Initial dosage:* 15 mg/day for 2 weeks then increase to 30 mg/day for 2 weeks; increase up to 60 mg/day *Maximum dosage:* 180 mg/day	PO	*For All Thyroid Hormones:* O: slow P: 1–2 wk D: 3 wk ½L: 2–7 days PB: 99% B: liver E: bile, urine
	Pediatric dosage: 4 mg/kg/day; for cretinism, 60 mg/day		
Thyroglobulin (Proloid)	*Initial dosage:* 32 mg/day, increase q 2–3 wk *Maintenance dosage:* 65–200 mg/day No pediatric dose	PO	
Liotrix (Euthroid— 60 μg T_4 and 15 μg T_3; Thyrolar— 50 μg T_4 and 12.5 μg T_3)	Equivalent to 15–30 mg/day No pediatric dose	PO	
T_4: Levothyroxine (Synthroid)	*Initial dosage:* 0.2–0.5 mg as a solution containing 0.1 mg/ml	IV	
	Maintenance dosage: 50–200 μg daily	PO	
	Pediatric dosage: 0–6 mo, 8–10 μg/kg; 6–12 mo, 6–8 μg/kg; 1–5 yr, 5–6 μg/kg; 6–12 yr, 4–5 μg/kg; over 12 yr, 2–3 μg/kg	PO	
T_3: Liothyronine (Cytomel)	*Initial dosage:* 25 μg/day *Maintenance dosage:* 25–75 μg/day	PO	
	Pediatric dosage: 5–50 μg/day	PO	
ANTITHYROID MEDICATIONS			
Action: Inhibit synthesis of thyroid hormones.			
Use: Hyperthyroidism, preparation for thyroid surgery.			
Propylthiouracil (PTU)	*Adult dosage: Initial:* 30 mg/day q 8 hr; *Maintenance:* 50–200 mg/day *Pediatric dosage: Initial:* 6–10 yr, 50–150 mg/day; 10 yr and over, 150–300 mg/day	PO	O: 10–21 days P: 6–10 wk D: weeks ½L: 1–2 hr PB: 75–80% B: liver E: urine
Methimazole (Tapazole)	*Adult dosage: Initial:* 15–60 mg in 3 equal doses; *Maintenance:* 5–15 mg/day in divided doses *Pediatric dosage: Initial:* 0.4 mg/kg/day in divided doses; *Maintenance:* half the initial dose	PO	O: 1 wk P: 4–10 wks D: weeks PB: 0% ½L: 3–5 hr B: liver E: urine, 10% unchanged

Key to Abbreviations in the *Pharmacokinetics* column O-onset; P-peak; D-duration; ½L-half-life; PB-protein bound; B-biotransformation; E-elimination.
*Within the column listing adverse effects, underlines indicate the most common effects; CAPITALS indicate life-threatening effects.

Contraindications/ Precautions	Adverse Effects*	Interactions	Nursing Implications
For All Thyroid Hormones: CONTRAINDICATIONS: Thyrotoxicosis, acute myocardial infarction uncomplicated by hypothyroidism, hypersensitivity. PRECAUTIONS: Use cautiously in cardiac disease, hypertension, and angina.	**For All Thyroid Hormones:** *Neuro:* tremors, headache, nervousness, insomnia, irritability *CVR:* palpitation, increased blood pressure, tachycardia, dysrhythmias, angina, fever, CARDIOVASCULAR COLLAPSE *GI:* change in appetite, nausea, vomiting, weight loss *Reprod:* menstrual irregularities *Integ:* allergic skin reaction (rare) *Misc:* heat intolerance	**For All Thyroid Hormones:** Increases effects of stimulants and epinephrine. Potentiates anticoagulants. Enhances antidepressant effect of tricyclic antidepressants and imipramine. Decreases effectiveness of digitalis. May increase need for antidiabetic medications. Cholestyramine decreases effects.	**For All Thyroid Hormones:** *ASSESSMENT:* Baseline thyroid studies and weight. *INTERVENTION:* Avoid excessive use of aspirin. Do not take this medication for the purpose of weight loss. Protect from light. Store in dry, tightly closed container. Carry Medic Alert card. Check pulse rate; if above 100 beats per minute, check with physician before taking medication. Do not decrease this medication without physician approval. *EVALUATION:* Notify physician of severe headache, diarrhea, excessive sweating, heat intolerance, or chest pain.
For All Antithyroid Medications CONTRAINDICATIONS: Contraindicated in lactation and hypersensitivity. PRECAUTIONS: Use cautiously in concomitant use of anticoagulants, and in setting of hematologic disorders.	**For All Antithyroid Medications:** *Neuro:* paresthesias, neuritis, headache, vertigo, drowsiness *GI:* nausea, vomiting, epigastric distress, loss of taste *Bilary:* jaundice, hepatitis *Hemo:* AGRANULOCYTOSIS, thrombocytopenia, bleeding, hypoprothrombinemia, leukopenia *Renal:* nephritis *Integ:* skin rash, urticaria, exfoliative dermatitis	**For All Antithyroid Medications:** May enhance anticoagulants.	**For All Antithyroid Medications:** *ASSESSMENT:* Assess baseline vital signs and weight. *INTERVENTION:* Carry identification card. Take medication at regularly spaced intervals, e.g., q 8 hr. Take medication with food to minimize gastric distress. Protect drug from light. Store in dry, tightly closed container.

CONTINUED ON THE FOLLOWING PAGE

Table 45–3. THYROID/ANTITHYROID DRUGS–*CONTINUED*

Name	Dosage	Mode of Administration	Pharmacokinetics
ANTITHYROID MEDICATIONS–Continued			
RADIOACTIVE IODINES			
Action: Concentrates in thyroid and destroys follicular cells through beta radiation.			
Use: Hyperthyroidism in older persons.			
Sodium Iodide-131 (Iodotope-131, Oriodide-131)	*Hyperthyroidism:* 4–10 mCi *Cancer of thyroid:* 50 mCi	PO	O: rapid P: UA D: UA ½L: 8.06 days PB: UA B: UA E: urine
IODIDES			
Action: Prevent thyroid hormones synthesis.			
Use: Hyperthyroidism, expectorant.			
Strong Iodine Solution (Lugol's solution)	2–6 drops tid	PO	O: 24–48 hr P: 10–15 days D: 6 wk ½L: UA
Potassium Iodide (KI, SSKI)	*Adult dosage:* 300–600 mg 3 times a day or 5 gtts 3 times a day *Pediatric dosage:* 25–35 mg/ kg/day in 3–4 doses	PO	PB: UA B: UA E: UA
Sodium Iodide	2 g/day	IV	

Key to Abbreviations in the *Pharmacokinetics* column O-onset; P-peak; D-duration; ½L-half-life; PB-protein bound; B-biotransformation; E-elimination.
   *Within the column listing adverse effects, underlines indicate the most common effects; CAPITALS indicate life-threatening effects.

pofunction disappear. This may take up to six weeks, depending on the product used. In the treatment of simple goiter, complete response may not occur for several months. Full therapeutic doses are not begun initially; this could impose a severe strain on the cardiovascular system because of cardiac stimulation. Older patients and those with a history of arteriosclerotic disease need to be carefully assessed in this regard; they are especially prone to the occurrence of angina pectoris, dysrhythmias, and congestive heart failure.

Therapeutic equivalents include: 60–65 mg of thyroid USP; 65 mg of thyroglobulin; 100 μg of levothyroxine; or 25 μg of eiothyronine.

Thyroid Desiccated

Thyroid USP (Thyroid) is used to treat hypothyroidism and to suppress excessive thyrotropin hormone in patients with simple goiter or chronic lymphocytic thyroiditis. Thyroid desiccated is given in oral doses of 15–180 mg/day. It is a natural product derived from domesticated animals such as pigs, sheep, and cattle, with the active hormones available in their natural state and ratio.

Thyroglobulin

Thyroglobulin (Proloid), obtained from hog thyroid glands, is used primarily for replacement in hypothy-

Contraindications/ Precautions	Adverse Effects*	Interactions	Nursing Implications
			EVALUATION: Notify physician if fever, sore throat, unusual bleeding or bruising occur.
CONTRAINDICATIONS: Contraindicated in pre-existing vomiting and diarrhea. *PRECAUTIONS:* Use cautiously in acute hyperthyroidism, patients younger than 18 years, during childbearing years, and in impaired renal function.	*Hemo:* bone marrow depression (with large doses), anemia, blood dyscrasias *Integ:* thinning of hair for 2–3 months *Misc:* radiation sickness	Uptake of ^{131}I will be affected by recent intake of stable iodine and thyroid and antithyroid drugs.	*INTERVENTION:* Antithyroid drugs need to be discontinued 3–4 days before therapy. Isolate patient. Urine, saliva, and prespiration is radioactive for 3 days. Use disposable eating utensils. Save all urine in a lead container for 24–48 hours. Drink as much fluid as possible for 48 hours after medication administration to facilitate excretion. Limit patient contact with visitors: day 1, 30 minutes; day 2, 1 hour.
CONTRAINDICATIONS: Contraindicated in hypersensitivity, pulmonary edema, pulmonary TB. *PRECAUTIONS:* Use cautiously in laryngeal edema, swelling of salivary glands.	*Resp:* productive cough *GI:* unpleasant taste, burning in mouth, sore mouth and throat, diarrhea *Integ:* acne, other rashes	Lithium causes increased potential for development of hypothyroidism.	*INTERVENTION:* Avoid use of OTC cough and cold remedies containing iodides. Dilute liquids in milk or fruit juice. Take medication after meals. Limit intake of iodine-rich dietary products.

roidism. It has no clinical advantage over thyroid USP. Thyroglobulin is given in oral maintenance doses of 65–200 mg/day. It contains T$_4$ and T$_3$ in an approximate ratio of 2.5:1.

Liotrix

Liotrix (Euthroid, Thyrolar) is a synthetic product used primarily as replacement for hypothyroidism. However, its use is controversial because of its higher level of T$_3$. Liotrix is a mixture of physiologic proportions of T$_4$ and T$_3$ in a ratio of 4:1. It is administered in maintenance oral doses of 15–30 mg. Liotrix contains tartrazine yellow dye, which may produce bronchial asthma and other allergic conditions in susceptible persons.

Levothyroxine

Levothyroxine (Synthroid, Levothroid), which is synthetic T$_4$, is available in parenteral as well as oral forms, and may be used intravenously in the treatment of myxedema coma. Levothyroxine is also used to treat primary hypothyroidism and cretinism. Levothyroxine contains tartrazine yellow dye which, again, can cause bronchial asthma and other allergic conditions in susceptible persons. An initial dose of 0.2–0.5 mg IV as a solution containing 0.1 mg/ml raises the T$_4$ level within 6–8 hours. Oral doses range from 50 to 200 μg/day. The pediatric dose (Table 45–3) range is 2–10 μg/kg given once daily.

Table 45–4

Effects of Drugs on Thyroid Function Tests[1]					
▲ Increased △ Slightly increased ▼ Decreased ▽ Slightly decreased 0 No effect blank space signifies no data	Serum T_4	T_3 Uptake Resin	Free thyroxine Index (FTI)	Serum T_3	Serum TSH
p-aminosalicylic acid	▼		▼		
Aminoglutethimide	▼				▲
Anabolic steroids/androgens	▼	▲	0		
Antithyroid (PTU, methimazole)	▼	▼	▼	▼	0/▲
Asparaginase	▼	▲			
Barbiturates	▼		▼	0/▽	
Contraceptives, oral	▲	▼	0	▲	0
Corticosteroids	0/▼	0/▲	0/▼	▼	▼
Danazol	▼	▲	0/△	▼	0/▼
Diazepam	▼		▽		
Estrogens	▲	▼	0/△	▲	0
Ethionamide	▼				
Fluorouracil	▲	▼	0	▲	0
Heparin (IV)	▼	0/▲	▲	0	
Insulin	▲				
Lithium carbonate	0/▼	0/▼	0/▼	0/▼	0/▲
Methadone	▲	▼	0	▲	0
Mitotane	▼	0			
Nitroprusside	▼				
Oxyphenbutazone/phenylbutazone	0/▼	▲	▼		
Perphenazine	▲	▼	▼	▲	
Phenytoin	▼	0/△	0/▽	▼	0
Propranolol	0/▲		△	▼	0
Resorcinol (excessive topical use)	▼	▼	▼	▼	▲
Salicylates (large doses)	▼	△		▼	
Sulfonylureas	▼	0	0		
Thiazides	0			▲	

[1]*Adapted from Medical Letter on Drugs and Therapeutics 1981; 23:30-32 with permission from The Medical Letter, Inc.*

Liothyronine Sodium

Liothyronine sodium (Cytomel) is used to treat hypothyroidism. It has a rapid onset and short duration of action. It is also used in the T_3 suppression test to differentiate hyperthyroidism from euthyroidism in patients with borderline to high values on the ^{131}I thyroid uptake test. Liothyronine sodium is given in oral maintenance doses of 25–75 µg/day. Liothyronine sodium is a synthetic form of T_3. It can be used in persons allergic to thyroid extract from pork or beef.

Combination Products

Combination drugs are also available. Several thyroid combination drugs are featured in Table 45–5.

ANTITHYROID MEDICATIONS

ACTION

The antithyroid drugs featured in Table 45–3 include propylthiouracil (PTU), methimazole (Tapazole), and sodium iodide (I-131). These drugs inhibit the synthesis of thyroid hormones. Propylthiouracil also partially inhibits the peripheral conversion of T_4 to T_3.

USES

The antithyroid medications are used to treat hyperthyroidism (see Table 45–2 for a review of hyperthyroid-

Table 45–5. COMBINATION DRUGS FOR THYROID HORMONES

Combination Drug	Basic Products*	
	A	**B**
Euthroid-½	30	7.5
Euthroid-1	60	15
Euthroid-2	120	30
Euthroid-3	180	45
Thyrolar-¼	12.5	3.1
Thyrolar-½	25	6.25
Thyrolar-1	50	12.5
Thyrolar-2	100	25
Thyrolar-3	150	37.5

*Basic products: A = levothyroxine sodium, μg (T_4); B = liothyronine sodium, μg (T_3).

ism). They are also used, along with certain iodides, to bring the patient to an euthyroid state before thyroid surgery. These drugs are also used in conjunction with radioactive iodine therapy to hasten recovery and to control the signs and symptoms of hyperthyroidism until the radioactive iodine therapy becomes effective.

PHARMACOKINETICS

Propylthiouracil and methimazole are effectively absorbed via the gastrointestinal tract. They are not available in parenteral forms. Their half-lives are short (propylthiouracil, about 1–2 hours; methimazole, 3–5 hours), thus necessitating frequent, regularly spaced administration. Their metabolites appear mostly in the urine.

CONTRAINDICATIONS AND PRECAUTIONS

Use of antithyroid drugs is generally contraindicated during lactation, as they cross the placental barrier and can cause hypothyroidism in the fetus. Thyroid is often given concomitantly throughout pregnancy to minimize fetal and infant thyroid dysfunction. Propylthiouracil is excreted partly in breast milk, and mothers on this therapy should bottle-feed their infants. These drugs are given cautiously in persons with hematologic diseases such as agranulocytosis, leukopenia, and thrombocytopenia, as these conditions may be worsened, and in patients receiving anticoagulants, as propylthiouracil may cause hypoprothrombinemia.

ADVERSE EFFECTS

Adverse effects of propylthiouracil and methimazole are relatively rare; only 3% of patients experience them. Adverse effects are similar for both drugs and include arthralgias, nausea and vomiting, headache, abnormal hair loss, hyperpigmentation, and paresthesias. Severe skin rashes may necessitate switching to another antithyroid drug; milder rashes may be treated symptomatically with antihistamines.

The most serious adverse effects of propylthiouracil and methimazole are relatively rare. About 1 in 500 patients develops agranulocytosis during the first few months of therapy. It is vital, therefore, that the patient understand the importance of reporting the onset of a fever or any sign of infection, especially a sore throat, immediately. If laboratory tests confirm the presence of agranulocytosis or granulocytopenia, the drug is discontinued. Recovery is usually the rule. Thrombocytopenia and hypoprothrombinemia, with subsequent bleeding, can also occur with antithyroid therapy. The nurse teaches the importance of regular observation for petechiae, ecchymosis, or other unexplained bleeding. Prothrombin time may be monitored regularly, along with cell counts. Patients are also directed to avoid the excessive use of aspirin or aspirin-containing compounds. The use of anticoagulants or drugs that might suppress cell counts should be undertaken only with close medical supervision.

The nurse is also aware that with continued antithyroid therapy, clinical manifestations of goitrogenic hypothyroidism may appear. To prevent this, thyroid hormone may be added to the treatment regimen once the patient has reached an *euthyroid* state. Since hypothyroidism may occur very insidiously, the nurse alerts the patient to watch for such signs and symptoms as intolerance to cold, increased weight gain, goiter, and decreased cardiac rate.

INTERACTIONS

The concomitant use of antithyroid drugs with heparin or oral anticoagulants may enhance the anticoagulant effects.

Propylthiouracil

Propylthiouracil (PTU), the prototype of the antithyroid drugs, is used primarily to manage hyperthyroidism, to prepare hyperthyroid persons for surgery, and to treat thyrotoxic crisis. Its rapid onset of action makes it well suited to treat hyperthyroid states. It is also used in pregnant patients as it is safer for the fetus. Propylthiouracil inhibits the synthesis of thyroid hormones by preventing the iodination of tyrosine residue in thyroglobulin.

Propylthiouracil is generally administered in three equal doses at 8-hour intervals. An initial dose begins at 30 mg/day with maintenance doses of 50–200 mg/day.

Methimazole

Methimazole (Tapazole) has the same actions and indications as propylthiouracil, but its onset of action is slower. It is approximately 10 times more potent. The dosage varies from 15 to 60 mg/day, depending on the severity of the hyperthyroidism.

Sodium Iodide I-131

Radioactive iodine (Idotope, Oriodide) is administered by mouth in doses of 4–10 μCi for hyperthyroidism and 50 μCi for malignancies. It passes quickly into the circulation where it concentrates in the thyroid gland. It destroys follicular cells through the effects of ionizing beta radiation. Much smaller doses (1–100 μCi) are used for diagnostic tests. It has a half-life of eight days, and most of it is excreted in the urine. Propranolol is often administered following radioactive iodine therapy since it causes a temporary increase in circulating thyroid hormone.

Immediate adverse effects of radioactive iodine therapy are relatively uncommon, but a radiation thyroiditis may occur 1–2 weeks after therapy. Clinical manifestations to observe for include fever, malaise, headache, and pain. On a long-term basis, a majority of patients who receive radioactive iodine eventually develop hypothyroidism and then require replacement therapy.

Iodine/Iodides

Iodides are also used as antithyroid drugs and serve to: reduce the vascularity of the thyroid gland; increase the quantity of bound, and therefore inactive, hormone; and inhibit release of the hormones into the circulation.

Iodides, however, are no longer used as the sole form of treatment in hyperthyroidism. Although they are associated with a rapid response, they often do not completely control the signs and symptoms. In addition, their beneficial effects are not sustained over long periods of time. Iodides are useful, though, in the immediate preoperative preparation of the patient undergoing thyroid surgery and also in the treatment of thyroid crisis. Oral administration is generally used, with parenteral therapy being reserved for treatment of crisis.

Adverse effects from the use of iodides are generally those of iodism. They include a brassy taste, increased salivation, gingival soreness, skin lesions, and burning sensations in the mouth and throat. In addition, signs and symptoms resembling the common cold occur, such as coryza, sneezing, eye irritation, and headache. These are usually treated by reducing the dosage or stopping the administration of iodides until the signs of iodism abate. When given concurrently with lithium, the iodides may potentiate the development of hypothyroidism.

STRONG IODINE SOLUTION. Strong iodine solution (Lugol's Solution) is primarily used to prepare the thyroid gland for surgery. Strong iodine solution causes the thyroid to become firm and reduces its vascularity. Strong iodine solution is also used to treat hyperthyroidism. It begins to be effective within three days. Strong iodine solution is administered three times daily in oral doses of 2–6 drops. Lugol's solution contains 5 g iodine and 10 g of potassium iodide per 100 ml of solution, yielding 6 mg iodine/gtt.

POTASSIUM IODIDE. Potassium iodide (KI, SSKI) is administered three times daily in doses of 5 drops. SSKI contains 100 g of potassium iodide per 100 ml of solution and yields 50 mg iodide/gtt. It tastes terrible, and needs to be mixed in a diluent, then followed by a glass of liquid.

SODIUM IODIDE. Sodium iodide is available as a parenteral form of iodide. It is used as adjunctive management of thyroid crisis. It is administered intravenously in doses of 2 g/day.

OTHER DRUGS TO TREAT HYPERTHYROIDISM

PROPRANOLOL

Propranolol is commonly used in the treatment of thyroid crisis to minimize manifestations of catecholamine activity by decreasing heart rate and metabolic activity (Chapter 19). Thyroid crisis or thyroid storm can be fatal because of excessive cardiac stimulation. In these instances, propranolol can protect the heart from stimulation. Intravenous administration may be used in this situation. Propranolol administered before and after radioactive iodine controls the symptomatology associated with this therapy. Propranolol must be used cautiously in the patient with hyperthyroidism who exhibits indications of congestive heart failure.

PARATHYROID AND ANTIHYPOCALCEMIC DRUGS

The parathyroid glands secrete parathyroid hormone (PTH), also known as parathormone, a principal regulator of calcium and phosphate metabolism. Parathormone affects bone, causing bone resorption; the kidney, increasing the excretion of phosphate and decreasing the excretion of calcium and magnesium; and the gastrointestinal tract, promoting calcium absorption. Vitamin D also affects calcium absorption, as it facilitates the

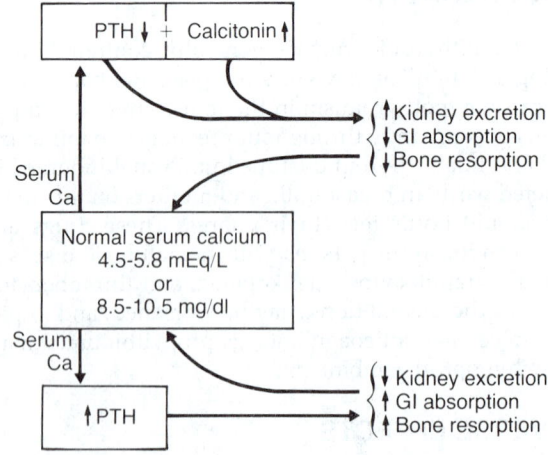

Regulation of serum calcium

Figure 45–2. Regulation of Serum Calcium. Normal serum calcium is regulated by PTH and calcitonin. As serum calcium rises, PTH is inhibited by calcitonin. In turn, the kidney excretes more calcium, the GI system absorbs less, and there is a reduction in bone resorption. As serum calcium falls, PTH is secreted, and in turn, raises the calcium level by decreasing the amount of calcium lost in the kidney, increasing the amount absorbed in the GI tract, and decreasing bone resorption.

transfer of calcium from the intestinal lumen into the cells. Vitamin D appears to be an essential cofactor for PTH. In effect, PTH serves to increase serum calcium concentration and to decrease serum phosphate concentration (Fig. 45–2). Other hormones (glucocorticoids, growth hormone, thyroid hormone, insulin, androgens, estrogens) also affect calcium balance and bone metabolism, either directly, or by influencing the secretion and/or action of the primary regulators.

Parathyroid injection is no longer used therapeutically (since antibodies form against the extract), but it is still employed to distinguish pseudohypoparathyroidism from idiopathic and postsurgical hypoparathyroidism.

HYPOCALCEMIA

Hypocalcemia results from numerous etiologies (Table 45–6), but regardless of the etiology, treatment is necessary to prevent complications such as convulsions, tetany, laryngospasm, respiratory spasms, and other muscle spasms. The initial treatment of severe symptomatic hypocalcemia is intravenous infusion of a rapidly available calcium product, such as calcium gluconate. This is followed by oral calcium salts (calcium gluconate—9%, calcium carbonate—40%). Vitamin D may also be administered.

Table 45–6. HYPOCALCEMIA

DEFINITION
Low serum calcium levels
Normal ranges: 8.5–10.5 mg/dL
4.5–5.8 mEq/L

ETIOLOGY
Parathyroid hypofunction
Vitamin D deficiency
Pancreatitis
Renal failure
Massive blood transfusion
Alcoholism
Chemotherapy
Chronic liver disease
Osteoporosis

SYMPTOMS
Objective:
1. Lethargy
2. Personality disturbances
3. Tetany
4. Dysphagia
5. Laryngeal spasm
6. Convulsions
7. Vomiting
8. Diarrhea or constipation

Subjective:
1. Paresthesias
2. Headache
3. Abdominal pain
4. Nausea

MANAGEMENT
Supplemental calcium
Supplemental vitamin D
Parathyroid injection

ANTIHYPOCALCEMIC DRUGS

CONTRAINDICATIONS AND PRECAUTIONS

Use of the antihypocalcemic drugs is contraindicated for patients with pre-existing hypercalcemia or vitamin D toxicity, as these drugs would worsen these conditions. These drugs are used cautiously in individuals with renal or cardiac disease, especially patients requiring digitalis preparations, as cardiac activity may be enhanced.

ADVERSE EFFECTS

The adverse effects of the antihypocalcemic drugs used in the treatment of hypocalcemia are, for the most part, those of hypercalcemia, and they affect many organ systems. Renal symptoms include polyuria, nephrolithiasis, and the potential development of *azotemia* and renal failure. The gastrointestinal system is affected in a variety of ways. Anorexia, nausea, vomiting, constipation, and abdominal pain are common signs of hypercalcemia. Bone demineralization can occur, resulting in pathologic fractures or skeletal deformities. The central nervous system is affected, as evidenced by the occurrence of disorientation, delirium, confusion, lethargy, and, in severe hypercalcemia, coma. Decreased neuromuscular irritability appears, causing muscle weakness, hypotonia, and depressed reflexes. Bradycardia and other cardiac dysrhythmias may occur.

The occurrence of any of these signs or symptoms should be reported to the physician immediately. Discontinuation of vitamin D and a low-calcium diet may serve to remedy mild cases of hypercalcemia. In instances where the serum calcium levels have risen greatly, other interventions may be required, such as hydration with isotonic saline, the administration of oral phosphates, and the use of calciuretic diuretics (furosemide and ethacrynic acid).

Calcium Salts

The various calcium salts can be used to treat hypocalcemia over a long period of time and are effectively absorbed via the oral route. The calcium products are discussed in detail in Chapter 58. Acute episodes of hypocalcemia are treated with calcium salts given intravenously. Most calcium preparations are excreted in feces or urine.

Vitamin D Preparations

Vitamin D is obtained through ingestion of vitamin D_2 (ergocalciferol) or vitamin D_3 (cholecalciferol), or by ultraviolet irradiation of vitamin D_3 in the skin. Vitamin D_3 is hydroxylated first to 25-hydroxycholecalciferol and then to 1,25-dihydroxycholecalciferol (the most active form) in the kidney. Vitamin D preparations are featured in Table 45–7.

TEXT RESUMES ON PAGE 1196

Table 45–7. ANTIHYPOCALCEMIC AND ANTIHYPERCALCEMIC DRUGS AND VITAMIN D PRODUCTS

Name	Dosage	Mode of Administration	Pharmacokinetics
VITAMIN D PRODUCTS			
Action: Increase serum calcium levels.			
Use: Hypocalcemia, hypophosphatemia, and hypoparathyroidism.			
Calcitriol (Rocaltrol)	*Adult dosage:* 0.25–2 µg/day *Pediatric dosage:* 1–5 yr, 0.25–0.75 µg/day	PO	O: 15 min P: UA D: 3–5 days ½L: 1–2 days PB: UA B: liver E: bile
Dihydrotachysterol (Hytakerol)	*Adult dosage:* 0.25–1.25 mg/day *Pediatric dosage: Initial:* 0.01 mg/day	PO	O: several hours P: hypercalcemic effect, 1–2 wk D: 2 wk ½L: UA PB: UA B: none E: feces
Vitamin D₂ (Ergocalciferol, Calciferol, Drisdol)	*Adult dosage: Initial:* 50,000–200,000 IU/day; *Maintenance:* 25,000–100,000 IU/day *Pediatric dosage:* 10,000–25,000 IU/day	PO	O: 10–14 days P: UA D: long ½L: UA PB: UA B: liver E: bile
ANTIHYPERCALCEMIC DRUGS			
Action: Reduce bone resorption.			
Use: Paget's disease, postmenopausal osteoporosis, multiple myeloma.			
Calcitonin, Salmon (Calcimar)	50–200 IU/day	SC, IM	O: 15 min P: 4 hr D: 8–24 hr ½L: 1.02 hr PB: UA B: kidney E: urine
Calcitonin, Human (Cibacalcin)	0.25–0.5 mg/day 2–3 times a week.	SC	O: 15 min P: 4 hr D: 8–24 hr ½L: 1.02 hr PB: UA B: kidney E: urine

Key to Abbreviations in the *Pharmacokinetics* column O-onset; P-peak; D-duration; ½L-half-life; PB-protein bound; B-biotransformation; E-elimination.
*Within the column listing adverse effects, underlines indicate the most common effects; CAPITALS indicate life-threatening effects.

Contraindications/ Precautions	Adverse Effects*	Interactions	Nursing Implications
For All Vitamin D Products: CONTRAINDICATIONS: Contraindicated in hypercalcemia, vitamin D toxicity, hypersensitivity, and hyperphosphatemia. PRECAUTIONS: Use cautiously in pregnant or lactating patients, and patients who are taking digitalis.	*Neuro:* headache, somnolence *CV:* dysrhythmias, increased blood pressure *GI:* nausea, vomiting, dry mouth with metallic taste, polydipsia, anorexia, weight loss *GU:* polyuria, nocturia	**For All Vitamin D Products:** Mineral oil interferes with absorption. Cholestyramine may impair absorption. Hypermagnesemia may occur with concurrent use of magnesium-containing antacids. Barbiturates and phenytoin may decrease effects.	**For All Vitamin D Products:** ASSESSMENT: Assess calcium level and dietary intake of calcium. INTERVENTION: Patient should carry identification card. Add sources of calcium to diet: milk products, green leafy vegetables, clams, oysters, sardines. Store in tightly closed, light-resistant container. Do not refrigerate. Do not crush or chew. EVALUATION: Notify physician if weakness, headache, anorexia, weight loss, nausea, vomiting, diarrhea, constipation, or excessive urinary output occur.
Same as above.	*Neuro:* headache, somnolence *CV:* weakness *GI:* nausea, vomiting, dry mouth, constipation, metallic taste, polydipsia, anorexia, weight loss *Renal:* polyuria, nocturia *EENT:* conjunctivitis, photophobia	Same as above.	Same as above.
CONTRAINDICATIONS: Contraindicated in pregnancy, lactation, hypersensitivity, and allergy to salmon.	*CV:* facial flushing *GI:* nausea, vomiting *Renal:* nocturia *Integ:* inflammation at injection site, pruritis, rashes *EENT:* eye pain *Misc:* ANAPHYLAXIS	None significant.	INTERVENTION: Rotate injection sites. Dilute with supplied diluent. Refrigerate reconstituted solution.
CONTRAINDICATIONS: Contraindicated in pregnancy, lactation, and hypersensitivity.	Same as for salmon calcitonin plus: *Neuro:* weakness, headache, paresthesias *CV:* chest pressure *Resp:* shortness of breath *GI:* metallic taste *Renal:* urinary frequency	Same as above.	INTERVENTION: Protect medication from light. Adverse effects may be minimized if administered at bedtime.

CONTINUED ON THE FOLLOWING PAGE

Table 45–7. ANTIHYPOCALCEMIC AND ANTIHYPERCALCEMIC DRUGS AND VITAMIN D PRODUCTS–*CONTINUED*

Name	Dosage	Mode of Administration	Pharmacokinetics
Etidronate disodium (Didronel) (Didronel IV)	5–10 mg/kg qd	PO	O: rapid P: UA
	7.5 mg/kg for 3 days diluted in 250 ml saline and run over 2 hr	IV	D: 8–9 hr ½L: 3–6 hr PB: UA B: not metabolized E: urine

Key to Abbreviations in the *Pharmacokinetics* column O-onset; P-peak; D-duration; ½L-half-life; PB-protein bound; B-biotransformation; E-elimination.
*Within the column listing adverse effects, underlines indicate the most common effects; CAPITALS indicate life-threatening effects.

PHARMACOKINETICS. In general, the onset of action of vitamin D is slow and the duration is long. The half-life of vitamin D is several days.

CONTRAINDICATIONS, PRECAUTIONS, AND ADVERSE EFFECTS. The vitamin D preparations are contraindicated in hypervitamin D states, hypercalcemia, hypersensitivity, and hyperphosphatemia. They are given cautiously to patients who are taking digitalis as the resultant hypercalcemia may precipitate dysrhythmias.

Vitamin D products are potentially harmful with serious renal complications and even death resulting. In addition, the gastrointestinal system, central nervous system, and soft tissues are affected, resulting in calcification.

INTERACTIONS. Mineral oil given concurrently with vitamin D decreases its absorption.

Dihydrotachysterol

Dihydrotachysterol (Hytakerol), a derivative or analog of vitamin D, elevates serum calcium levels by stimulating calcium absorption in the intestine and mobilization of calcium from bones, in the absence of PTH. Dihydrotachysterol is used primarily in the treatment of hypocalcemia associated with hypoparathyroidism and pseudohypoparathyroidism, and to treat renal osteodystrophy in chronic uremia. It is well absorbed following oral administration in doses of 0.25–1.25 mg/day. This form is hydroxylated in the liver, but does not require renal activation.

Calcitriol

Calcitriol (Rocaltrol), a synthetic active form of vitamin D_3, elevates serum calcium levels by the same mechanisms as those described above. It is more potent and more expensive than dihydrotachysterol. Calcitriol is the most active vitamin D metabolite. Calcitriol is used primarily to treat hypocalcemia in patients undergoing chronic dialysis and in patients with hypoparathyroidism and pseudohypoparathyroidism.

Calcitriol is used primarily to treat patients with chronic renal failure or tubular disease, but it is also used in other hypocalcemic conditions. The usual oral dose of calcitriol is 0.25–2 µg/day.

Vitamin D₂

Vitamin D_2 (Ergocalciferol) is generally administered in maintenance doses of 25,000–100,000 IU/day.

ANTIHYPERCALCEMIC MEDICATIONS

Antihypercalcemic drugs lower serum calcium levels in patients with a variety of conditions leading to hypercalcemia (see Table 45–8 for a review of hypercalcemia). Several drugs are available to lower serum calcium levels. Mithramycin (Mithracin), an antineoplastic agent, is used to lower serum calcium levels in patients who have hypercalcemia associated with malignancies (see Chapter 49 for more information). Furosemide (Lasix), a diuretic, reduces the serum calcium concentration by increasing calcium excretion (see Chapter 38 for more information). Calcitonin and etidronate disodium are further discussed in this chapter and are featured in Table 45–7.

CALCITONIN

Calcitonin (Calcimar) is primarily produced in C cells of the thyroid, but it is also produced in small amounts by the parathyroid and thymus glands. Calcitonin for therapeutic use is obtained from salmon or derived from pigs. Salmon calcitonin lasts longer and is more potent than calcitonin derived from pigs. Calcitonin is generally antagonistic to PTH. Salmon calcitonin, which prevents bone resorption, is the most potent form and is administered parenterally in 50–200 MRC (Medical Research Council) IU several times a day. Calcitonin is used in patients with Paget's disease and postmenopausal osteoporosis, and as an adjunct to chemotherapy and anabolic steroids to treat multiple myeloma. It has a relatively rapid action (15 minutes) and low toxicity; however, it has a short duration of action (8–24 hours).

Calcitonin use is contraindicated in pregnancy and lactation. Antibody formation has occurred after 2–18 months of therapy.

Contraindications/ Precautions	Adverse Effects*	Interactions	Nursing Implications
CONTRAINDICATIONS: Contraindicated in pregnancy, lactation. *PRECAUTIONS:* Use cautiously in impaired renal function, entercolitis.	GI: metallic taste, nausea, diarrhea *Integ:* angioedema, urticaria, rash, pruritis.	None significant.	*ASSESSMENT:* Assess intake of calcium and vitamin D. *INTERVENTION:* Take on an empty stomach 2 hr before meals. Take with a full glass of water. May cause GI upset.

Few adverse effects occur with calcitonin therapy. Transient nausea and vomiting (10%) can occur, but usually subside with continued therapy. Facial flushing (2%–5%) may also appear, as well as tingling and tenderness in the hands. Local inflammation may occur at the injection site following intramuscular or subcutaneous administration (10%). Although no cases have yet been reported, hypocalcemia is a potential adverse effect of calcitonin therapy. Indicators of hypocalcemia to be alert for include nervousness and irritability, muscle cramps, paresthesias, and tetany as evidenced by *carpopedal spasms*. The nurse may observe for latent tetany by inducing *Chvostek's sign* and *Trousseau's sign*.

Human calcitonin (Cibacalcin) is also available and may be used when patients have developed resistance to nonhuman or pig calcitonin (Table 45–7).

ETIDRONATE DISODIUM

Etidronate disodium (Didronel), a synthetic compound, acts primarily by inhibiting calcium crystal resorption from bone. Etidronate disodium is the drug of choice for Paget's disease as it ultimately reduces bone turnover and the associated bone pain. Etidronate disodium is also used to treat a nonmalignant overgrowth of bone— heterotopic ossification. Heterotopic ossification may occur after total hip replacement or spinal cord injury. Following oral administration of 5–10 mg/kg/day, about 1% of the drug is absorbed. It is not metabolized, and the absorbed drug is excreted in the urine.

This medication is used cautiously in patients with enterocolitis. It is contraindicated in pregnancy and lactation, and in the setting of impaired renal function.

Adverse effects of etidronate disodium include a metallic taste in the mouth (5%), nausea and diarrhea (6.7%), and skin reactions (Table 45–7).

Etidronate disodium (Didronel IV) is a parenteral form of etidronate. It is the drug of choice for treating hypercalcemia of pregnancy. Etidronate disodium is administered in a dosage of 7.5 mg/kg/day for three days. Each dose is diluted in at least 250 ml of sterile normal saline and run in a time interval of at least two hours. Retreatment may be necessary, but there should be at least 7 days between courses of treatment.

Table 45–8. HYPERCALCEMIA

DEFINITION High serum calcium levels Normal ranges: 8.5–10.5 mg/dL 4.5–5.8 mEq/L
ETIOLOGY Hyperparathyroidism Malignancies Vitamin D intoxication Milk-alkali syndrome
SYMPTOMS *Objective:* 1. Polyuria 2. Renal calculi 3. Hypertension 4. Vomiting 5. Constipation 6. Bradycardia 7. Pathologic fractures 8. Personality disturbances 9. Muscle weakness 10. Diminished reflexes *Subjective:* 1. Anorexia 2. Nausea 3. Abdominal pain 4. Bone pain 5. Headache
MANAGEMENT Surgical excision if due to hyperparathyroidism Antihypercalcemics

USING THE NURSING PROCESS

ASSESSMENT—THYROID DISEASE

Assessment of the patient with possible thyroid dysfunction can be a difficult problem since the signs and symptoms of hypothyroidism and hyperthyroidism often appear insidiously and over long periods of time. This is especially true in hypothyroidism. In addition, the signs and symptoms often vary in intensity from patient to patient and from time to time. Tables 45–9 and

TEXT RESUMES ON PAGE 1200

Table 45–9. NURSING PROCESS FOR PATIENT REQUIRING THYROID/ANTITHYROID DRUGS

Assessment

Determine onset and duration of symptoms/illness, recent stress situations (emotional/physical).
Note family history of thyroid problems.
Assess history for hypothyroidism, recent partial thyroidectomy, use of thyroid/antithyroid drugs, premature withdrawal of antithyroid drugs.
Note recent weight loss/amount.

Nursing Diagnosis	Nursing Actions	Rationale	Desired Outcomes
Cardiac output decreased, potential related to decreased venous return, vasodilation, and tachycardia.	Monitor vital signs, obtain BP lying/sitting and standing, if able.	General/orthostatic hypotension may occur as a result of excessive peripheral vasodilation and decreased circulating volume. Pulse is typically elevated and even at rest, tachycardia may be noted.	Maintains adequate cardiac output for tissue needs as evidenced by stable vital signs, palpable peripheral pulses, good capillary refill, usual mentation and absence of dysrhythmias.
	Investigate complaints of chest pain/angina.	May reflect increased myocardial oxygen demands/ischemia.	
	Monitor temperature, provide cool environment, limit bed linens/clothes, administer tepid sponge baths.	Fever may occur as a result of excessive thyroid levels and can aggravate diuresis and dehydration and cause increased peripheral vasodilation, venous pooling, and hypotension.	
	Record intake/output. Note urine specific gravity. Weigh daily.	Significant fluid losses can lead to profound dehydration, concentrated urine, and weight loss.	
	Observe signs/symptoms of severe thirst, dry mucous membranes, weak/thready pulse, poor capillary refill, decreased urine output, and hypotension.	Rapid dehydration can occur, which reduces circulating volume and compromises cardiac output.	
	Administer thyroid hormone.	Blocks thyroid hormone synthesis and inhibits peripheral conversion of T_4 to T_3.	
	Sodium iodine IV or supersaturated potassium iodide (SSKI) by mouth.	Temporarily acts to prevent release of thyroid hormone into circulation by increasing the amount of thyroid hormone stored within the gland.	
	Beta-blockers (Inderal, Tenormin).	Given to control thyrotoxic effects of tachycardia, tremors, and nervousness and is first drug of choice for acute storm.	
	Monitor patient response to administration of thyroid, Proloid, Synthroid, etc.	Initial treatment of a hypothyroid state can cause a tachycardia, increasing cardiac workload with possibility of a resultant cardiac decompensation.	
Fatigue related to hypermetabolic state with	Provide quiet environment; cool room,	Reduces stimuli that potentiate hyperactivity/	Verbalizes increase in level of energy. Displays

Table 45–9. NURSING PROCESS FOR PATIENT REQUIRING THYROID/ANTITHYROID DRUGS–*CONTINUED*

Nursing Diagnosis	Nursing Actions	Rationale	Desired Outcomes
increased energy requirements; irritability of CNS; altered body chemistry as evidenced by verbalization of overwhelming lack of energy to maintain usual routine, decreased performance, emotional lability/irritability; nervousness, impaired ability to concentrate.	decreased sensory stimuli, quiet music. Encourage patient to restrict activity and rest in bed as much as possible. Assist with self-care activities. Provide routine comfort measures, (e.g., judicious touch/massage, cool showers) and diversional activities that are calming. Discuss with SO reasons for fatigue and emotional lability.	and insomnia, promotes rest. Helps to counteract effects of increased metabolism. Conserves energy, prevents undue fatigue. May decrease nervous energy, promoting relaxation. Allows for use of nervous energy in a constructive manner and may reduce anxiety. Understanding that the behavior is physically based may enhance coping with current situation and encourage SO to respond more positively and provide support for the patient.	improved ability to participate in desired activities.
Nutrition, altered Less than body requirements, potential related to inadequate intake for increased metabolism, relative insulin insufficiency.	Note complaints of anorexia, generalized weakness/aches, abdominal pain; presence of nausea/vomiting, polydipsea/uria, changes in respiratory rate/depth. Compare daily food intake with daily weight. Provide diet high in calories, protein, carbohydrates and vitamins. Increase number of meals and snacks. Consult with dietician as indicated.	Increased adrenergic activity can cause impaired insulin secretion/resistance, resulting in hyperglycemia. Continued weight loss in face of adequate caloric intake may indicate failure of antithyroid therapy. Aids in keeping caloric intake high enough to keep up with rapid expenditure of calories caused by hypermetabolic state. Useful for determining adequacy of intake, identifying appropriate supplements and readjusting diet when medication reduces hypermetabolic state.	Demonstrates stable weight with normal laboratory values and no signs of malnutrition.
Knowledge deficit related to lack of exposure/recall, information misinterpretation, unfamiliarity with information resources as evidenced by questions, requests for information, inaccurate follow-through of instructions/development of preventable complications.	Review disease process and future expectations. Provide information appropriate to individual situation. Identify stressors and discuss precipitators of thyroid crises, e.g., personal/social and job concerns, infection and pregnancy. Provide information about signs/symptoms of	Provides knowledge base on which patient can make informed choices. Severity of condition (hyper/hypothyroidism), cause, age, and concurrent complications determines course of treatment. Psychogenic as well as physical factors are often of prime importance in occurrence/exacerbation of this condition. The patient who has been treated for hyperthyroid-	Verbalizes understanding of disease process and treatment. Identifies relationship of signs/symptoms to the disease process and correlates symptoms with causative factors. Initiates necessary lifestyle changes and participates in treatment regimen.

CONTINUED ON THE FOLLOWING PAGE

Table 45–9. NURSING PROCESS FOR PATIENT REQUIRING THYROID/ANTITHYROID DRUGS–*CONTINUED*

Nursing Diagnosis	Nursing Actions	Rationale	Desired Outcomes
hypothyroidism and the need for continuing follow-up care.		ism needs to be aware of possible development of hypothyroidism which can occur immediately after treatment or as long as 5 years later. To prevent this, thyroid hormone may be added to therapeutic regimen to maintain euthroid state.	
	Discuss drug therapy, including need for adhering to regimen, and expected therapeutic side effects.	Requires adherence to a medical regimen over an extended period of time to inhibit/supplement hormone production.	
	Identify signs/symptoms requiring medical evaluation, e.g., fever, sore throat, and skin eruptions.	Early identification of toxic reactions (thiourea therapy) and intervention are important in preventing development of agranulocytosis.	
	Stress necessity of continued medical follow-up.	Important for monitoring effectiveness of therapy and prevention of potentially fatal complications.	

45–10 summarize the information the nurse obtains for the data base.

A careful health history is necessary in order to establish a data base and begin the nursing care plan. It is especially important to determine whether the patient has been treated for any thyroid disease in the past. Patients being treated for hypothyroidism may, if their medication regimen is not well controlled, exhibit indications of hyperthyroidism. Likewise, the patient who has been treated for hyperthyroidism may go on to develop hypofunction of the thyroid gland. To illustrate, after antithyroid therapy, 5%–10% of patients develop hypothyroid conditions; after surgical intervention, 15%–20%; and after radioactive iodine therapy, 30%–50% of patients eventually develop hypothyroidism.

It is important to assess current weight and recent pattern of weight loss or gain. Level of nutrition and dietary intake is also important to evaluate, as teaching may be necessary.

Various laboratory tests can be used to measure thyroid function. Direct measurement of thyroid function can be done by evaluating the gland's uptake of radioactive ^{131}I (RAIU test). T_3, T_4, and TSH can be measured directly by radioimmunoassay. The resin T_3 uptake test (RT$_3$U) measures the degree to which thyroid-binding globulin is saturated, thus indirectly indicating the level of circulating hormone. It is important to note that many of these tests may be interfered with by the use of common drugs. The T_3 resin uptake can be distorted by use of birth control pills, estrogen, androgens, and phenytoin.

ASSESSMENT—PARATHYROID DISEASE

Assessment of the patient with hypoparathyroidism or hyperparathyroidism is dependent on the nurse's ability to assess the effects of either increased or decreased serum calcium levels on the body systems. As with many other endocrine disorders, signs and symptoms of parathyroid dysfunction can be variable from patient to patient; chronicity of the disorders may also determine the degree of symptomatology.

A thorough health history, necessary for the data base, may identify some factors that relate to the etiology and course of parathyroid dysfunction. A history of previous neck surgery (for example, thyroidectomy) is noted, as inadvertent removal of the parathyroids is a cause of parathyroid insufficiency.

Diagnostic tests used in the assessment of parathyroid function include measurement of serum calcium and inorganic phosphorus levels and assessment of urinary calcium excretion. Radiologic examinations of the skeletal system give an indication of bone status in the face of excessive parathyroid activity, with osteoporosis, pathologic fractures, and skeletal deformities appearing in severe cases. PTH can be measured directly by radioimmunoassay.

NURSING DIAGNOSES

After assessment, nursing diagnoses are established. Some typical nursing diagnoses are illustrated in Tables 45–9 and 45–10.

Table 45–10. NURSING PROCESS FOR PATIENT REQUIRING ANTIHYPERCALCEMIC/ ANTIHYPOCALCEMIC DRUGS

Assessment

Note previous history of neck surgery, (e.g., thyroidectomy), alcohol abuse (pancreatitis, chronic liver disease), renal failure, osteoporosis, chemotherapy, massive blood transfusions.
Review laboratory studies, e.g., serum calcium and inorganic phosphorus levels and assessment of urinary calcium excretion.
Determine nutritional history.
Examine skeletal system for indication of bone status (osteoporosis, pathologic fractures, and skeletal deformities).

Nursing Diagnosis	Nursing Actions	Rationale	Desired Outcomes/ Evaluation Criteria
Injury, potential for, related to increased nervous and muscular excitability/tetany (Hypoparathyroidism).	Administer medications to gain optimal effect, e.g., IV, IM or orally.	Severity of symptoms will dictate choice of route to provide adequate availability of the drug.	Verbalizes understanding of individual factors that contribute to possibility of tetany/convulsions. Reports absence of muscle spasms/tetany.
	Give calcium salts slowly when using IV method.	This drug is highly irritating to veins, may cause thrombosis and too rapid administration can cause cardiac arrest.	
	Give Rocaltrol, Ergocalciferol, or Drisdol.	Vitamin D products increase the absorption of the calcium.	
	Encourage use of antacids as appropriate.	Aluminum hydroxide gel binds phosphate and decreases intestinal absorption.	
	Observe for complaints of renal colic.	May have stone formation if too much calcium accumulates.	
	Identify signs/symptoms which need to be reported to health-care provider, e.g., anorexia, nausea and vomiting, diarrhea, polyuria, polydipsia, headache, muscle cramps/spasms.	Indicators of hypercalcemia which requires alteration/discontinuation of therapy.	
	Monitor laboratory results of serum/urine calcium, inorganic phosphorus, PTH levels.	Evaluates therapeutic needs/effectiveness.	
Fluid volume, deficit, potential related to excessive losses from vomiting, diarrhea and polyuria (Hyperparathyroidism).	Promote oral intake.	Route of choice for fluid replacement if possible.	Maintains fluid balance and is free of signs of dehydration.
	Measure intake/output. Observe mucous membranes, skin turgor and capillary refill.	Reflects effectiveness of therapy/therapeutic needs.	
	Administer glucose, isotonic IV fluids, electrolytes. Give inorganic phosphate.	Replacement necessary to provide adequate hydration, promote calciuria. Reduces calcium levels when hypercalcemia is life-threatening.	
	Monitor BP, note complaints of dizziness with changes in position.	Administration of phosphate may potentiate hypotension if present.	
	Review serial serum calcium levels.	Decreasing level indicates dehydration is being corrected/renal clearance of calcium is progressing.	
Urinary Retention Potential related to presence of obstructive renal calculi. (Hyperparathyroidism)	Encourage limiting dietary intake of calcium and alkalies, such as milk and dairy products.	These foods potentiate stone formation.	Maintains appropriate urinary output free of signs of stone formation.

CONTINUED ON THE FOLLOWING PAGE

**Table 45–10. NURSING PROCESS FOR PATIENT REQUIRING ANTIHYPERCALCEMIC/
ANTIHYPOCALCEMIC DRUGS**–*CONTINUED*

Nursing Diagnosis	Nursing Actions	Rationale	Desired Outcomes/ Evaluation Criteria
	Promote increased oral fluid intake. Administer medications, e.g.:	Flushes calcium from system helping to reduce stone formation.	
	Calcitonin/cibacalcin;	Antagonistic to PTH, prevents bone resorption.	
	Didronel;	Synthetic compound inhibits resorption of calcium from the bone.	
	Diuretics, and IV saline;	Promotes renal clearance of calcium (avoid thiazides which decrease renal excretion of calcium).	
	Oral phosphate.	Inorganic phosphate can decrease serum calcium.	
	Monitor serum calcium and BUN daily.	Identifies changes in renal clearance/developing complications.	
Knowledge deficit related to information misinterpretation, unfamiliarity with information resources as evidenced by questions, statement of concern, inaccurate follow-through of instruction/development of preventable complications.	Discuss condition/disease process and therapy.	Provides knowledge base for patient to make informed choices and may enhance cooperation with therapeutic regimen.	Verbalizes understanding of condition/disease process and treatment. Identifies relationship of signs/symptoms to the disease process and correlates symptoms with causative factors. Initiates necessary lifestyle changes and participates in treatment regimen.
	Review drug purpose, dosage, administration, proper storage, adverse effects, and possible interactions.	Maximizes therapeutic effects of drug, minimizes side effects.	
	Recommend avoidance of mineral oil.	May interfere with absorption of vitamin D.	
	Identify dietary sources of calcium, e.g., milk, green leafy vegetables, clams, oysters.	Use will be encouraged/ limited based on individual need.	
	Encourage patient to carry wallet card/wear identification tag.	Provides for prompt intervention in emergency situations.	

PLANNING AND INTERVENTION

Goals for nursing interventions are developed from the nursing diagnoses. Typical goals when caring for patients requiring thyroid or parathyroid medications are included in Tables 45–9 and 45–10.

Learning the importance of carrying a medication card or other similar identification is added to the list of nursing goals for the patient.

NURSING RESPONSIBILITIES WHEN ADMINISTERING THYROID AND PARATHYROID MEDICATIONS

In order to administer thyroid and parathyroid medication safely, the nurse must be aware of specific information related to administration guidelines, patient safety, and patient teaching. These are summarized in Tables 45–3 and 45–7.

Nursing intervention for the patient requiring thyroid drugs or antithyroid drugs focuses on educating the patient about the disease process, the medications being taken, and the potential occurrence of adverse effects.

A concept mentioned earlier in this chapter deserves re-emphasis. In treatment of hypothyroidism, replacement hormones are introduced gradually because of the increase in the overall metabolism they cause. Once a maintenance dose is established, patients are educated to the fact that the need for thyroid replacement will ordinarily be a lifelong one. Although missing medication for one or two days may not lead to the recurrence of symptoms, discontinuance of the drug certainly will.

PATIENT TEACHING

Information that is included in the nurse educator's plan for teaching patients about thyroid and parathyroid

Table 45–11. PATIENT TEACHING INFORMATION—THYROID DRUGS

Dear Patient:
  This drug has been ordered for you. This is what you should know about your drug to get the most from your therapy:

1. Thyroid drugs replace the hormones in your body and bring your blood levels of these hormones back to normal.
2. Thyroid drugs are generally taken for the rest of your life. Most are slow-acting and full effect may not be felt for a few weeks.
3. Take your thyroid drugs exactly as ordered.
4. Check your pulse; if it is greater than 100 beats per minute, don't take your drug for that day.
5. Take your thyroid drug in the morning on an empty stomach.
6. Do not use more than 2 aspirin per day while taking thyroid drugs.
7. If you forget a day's dose, do not try to "make it up."
8. Do not stop your thyroid drug without first asking your doctor.
9. Notify your doctor if you have any adverse effects. Some common side effects are: skin rash, headache, chest pain, increased nervousness, or increased pulse rate.
10. Carry a medication card or other similar identification.
11. Store your thyroid drug in a light-resistant, dry, tightly closed container.

Table 45–12. PATIENT TEACHING INFORMATION—ANTITHYROID DRUGS

Dear Patient:
  This drug has been ordered for you. This is what you should know about your drug to get the most from your therapy:

1. Antithyroid drugs, such as _____, are ordered to reduce the level of thyroid hormone in your body.
2. Antithyroid drugs are taken for different lengths of time; your doctor will tell you how long you will need to take this drug.
3. Take your drugs exactly as ordered.
4. Antithyroid drugs should be taken with food. Exceptions: liquid iodides are diluted in milk or fruit juice and taken after meals.
5. Avoid the use of over-the-counter cough and cold remedies that contain iodides. Ask your pharmacist if you have any questions about which over-the-counter drugs you may take.
6. Limit your intake of iodine-rich foods, such as iodized salt and seafood.
7. Do not stop taking your antithyroid drug without consulting with your doctor.
8. Report any adverse effects to your doctor. Some adverse effects are: skin rash, unexplained bleeding, sore throat, and fever. If you are taking iodides, adverse effects may include runny nose, headache, increased salivation, and a "brassy" taste in your mouth.
9. Carry a medication card or other similar identification.
10. Store your drugs in a light-resistant, tightly closed container.

Table 45–13. PATIENT TEACHING INFORMATION—ANTIHYPOCALCEMIC DRUGS

Dear Patient:
  This drug has been ordered for you. This is what you should know about your drug to get the most from your therapy:

1. Antihypocalcemic drugs, such as _____, are ordered to elevate your serum calcium level.
2. Antihypocalcemic drugs are taken for an indefinite amount of time; your doctor will tell you how long you will need to take this drug.
3. Take your drugs daily, exactly as directed.
4. Take your drugs 1 to 1.5 hours after meals; you may take them with milk.
5. Avoid use of mineral oil as a laxative, because it decreases vitamin D absorption. Vitamin D is needed to work with your drug.
6. Avoid eating too much spinach, rhubarb, brain, or whole-grain cereals, because they decrease calcium absorption.
7. Eat more foods that have calcium in them. Good dietary sources of calcium are milk products, dark green leafy vegetables, clams, oysters, sardines, and orange juice with calcium.
8. Do not stop your drug without first consulting your doctor.
9. Report adverse effects to your doctor. Some of these effects are: loss of appetite, constipation, nausea, vomiting, increased urination, thirst, and flank pain.
10. Carry a medication card or other similar identification.
11. Store your drugs in a light-resistant, tightly closed container.

drugs is summarized in Tables 45–11, 45–12, 45–13, and 45–14.

EVALUATION

In order to evaluate the patient's care and response to therapy, the nurse, with the patient, determines the effectiveness of the nursing interventions. Evaluation criteria are included in Tables 45–9 and 45–10.

  The nurse ensures that the patient fully understands the potential for adverse effects of the medications he or she is taking. Adverse effects of thyroid medications are generally dose-related and include tachycardia, nervousness, increased sweating, and heat intolerance. These symptoms are reported at once, in order that dosage may be adjusted.

  Pruritus and urticaria are the most common adverse effects of the antithyroid drugs. More serious adverse effects occur less frequently; agranulocytosis, thrombocytopenia, and hypoprothrombinemia necessitate immediate discontinuance of the medications. Patients must fully understand the need to report fever, sore throat, or unexplained bleeding immediately, as these may indicate the presence of blood dyscrasias.

  Treatment with antihypocalcemic drugs is associated with adverse effects caused by hypercalcemia such as

Table 45–14. PATIENT TEACHING INFORMATION—ANTIHYPERCALCEMIC DRUGS

Dear Patient:

This drug has been ordered for you. This is what you should know about your drug to get the most from your therapy:

1. Antihypercalcemic drugs, such as _____, are ordered to reduce your blood level of calcium.
2. Antihypercalcemic drugs are taken for varying lengths of time; your doctor will tell you how long you will need to take this drug.
3. Calcitonin is taken in subcutaneous injections (shots).
   a. Be sure to rotate injection sites to minimize inflammation.
   b. Do not inject more than .5 mL of solution; check label for mixing instructions.
4. Take your etidronate disodium (Didronel) on an empty stomach (approximately 2 hours before meals). Take with a full glass of water to reduce stomach upset.
5. If your doctor wants you to eat less food that contains calcium, you should not eat as much leafy green vegetables and dairy products.
6. Do not stop taking your drugs without asking your doctor.
7. Report signs of low calcium levels to your doctor. They include: headache, numbness or tingling, nausea or vomiting, diarrhea or constipation, and abdominal pain.
8. Carry a medication card or other similar identification.
9. Refrigerate reconstituted calcitonin.

nausea, vomiting, constipation, anorexia, headache, abdominal pain, and polyuria.

The use of calcitonin for hypercalcemia is associated with transient nausea and vomiting, facial flushing, tingling and tenderness of the hands, and local inflammation at the injection site. Adverse effects noted with etidronate disodium include diarrhea, nausea, and bone pain.

The majority of patients, if carefully instructed, follow their therapy program since it corrects their problem. Since treatment for thyroid and parathyroid disorders can cause the opposite disorder to occur, the nurse ensures that patients are familiar with indications of both hypofunction and hyperfunction of these organs.

The nurse continuously stresses the need for regular medical follow-up and periodically reviews all previous teaching with the patient, adding or revising information in order to keep the patient's knowledge current and accurate.

SUMMARY

The thyroid glands secrete T_3, T_4, and calcitonin; while the parathyroid gland secretes PTH. T_3 and T_4 help regulate metabolism and calcitonin helps to regulate the serum calcium level. PTH also acts as a calcium regulator.

Both natural and synthetic thyroid products are currently available. These products have various onsets, peaks, and durations. However, they are all used to replace inadequate levels of thyroid hormone.

Patients that are to receive these products should have a thorough baseline assessment including lab tests, weight, and cardiovascular assessment. Most of the drugs will be taken for a lifetime and the patient is taught to recognize the symptoms of both hypo and hyperthyroidism.

Various products, natural and synthetic, are available to help regulate calcium. Natural products are more rapidly metabolized and have a shorter duration of action. These products have various onsets, peaks, and durations. There are products to increase serum calcium levels, such as vitamin D analogs, and products to decrease calcium levels, such as calcitonin and etidronate disodium.

Baseline assessment begins with a history of the presenting symptoms, weight, presence of bone pain, and a history of recent neck injury or surgery. Patients are taught how to administer these drugs and how to recognize the symptoms of both hypo and hypercalcemia.

BIBLIOGRAPHY

AMA Division of Drugs: AMA Drug Evaluations, ed 6. John Wiley & Sons, New York, 1986.

American Society of Hospital Pharmacists: Hospital Formulary Service. American Society of Hospital Pharmacists, 1987.

DeGroot, L, et al: The Thyroid and Its Diseases, ed 5. John Wiley & Sons, New York, 1984.

Evancer, D: Look for these clues to thyrotoxicosis. Patient Care 17:143, April 1983.

Evangelisti, J: Thyroid storm: A nursing crisis. Heart Lung 12(2):184, March/April 1983.

Gilman, AG, Goodman, LS, and Gilman, A: Goodman and Gilman's The Pharmacological Basis of Therapeutics. Macmillan, New York, 1986.

Mathewson, MK: Thyroid disorder. Crit Care Nurse 7(1):74, 1987.

Rosenbaum, RL: Levothyroxine replacement dose for primary hypothyroidism decreases with age. Ann Intern Med 96:53, 1982.

Will surgery complicate your patient's drug therapy? Emerg Med 19(18):56, 1987.

SITUATION 45–1

Mr. Emile Haus is a 50-year-old admitted to the Medical Unit with a history of weight loss, nervousness, and insomnia. A diagnosis of hyperthyroidism is made.

1. The nurse may note the following sign of hyperthyroidism when assessing Mr. Haus:
   a. constipation
   b. anorexia
   c. dry skin
   d. exophthalmos

2. Mr. Haus' blood pressure elevates to 210/150, and heart rate increases to 150 beats per minute. He is transferred to the Intensive Care Unit for management of athyrotoxic crisis. Propylthiouracil (PTU) 30 mg has been ordered. The nurse will expect to give this drug by the following route:
   a. intramuscularly
   b. orally
   c. subcutaneously
   d. intravenously

3. A drug of choice for Mr. Haus' cardiac symptoms related to thyroid crisis would be:
   a. atropine
   b. digoxin
   c. epinephrine
   d. propranolol

4. In addition to PTU administration, Mr. Haus will receive sodium iodide 2 gms IV. The nurse will monitor him for the following side effects of iodide therapy:
   a. increased salivation
   b. urinary hesitancy
   c. dizziness
   d. tinnitis

5. After successful treatment of thyroid crisis, Mr. Haus is transferred back to the Medical Unit. He is to be discharged on PTU 50 mg per day and Lugol's solution .3 ml tid. Which of the following foods should be eliminated from his diet?
   a. seafood
   b. alcohol
   c. green vegetables
   d. citrus fruits

6. Mr. Haus will need to be monitored regularly for effects of PTU therapy. This includes checking:
   a. prothrombin time
   b. serum protein electrophoresis
   c. serum calcium levels
   d. 2-hour urine amylase

Please refer to the Appendices for correct answers and additional review questions with answers.

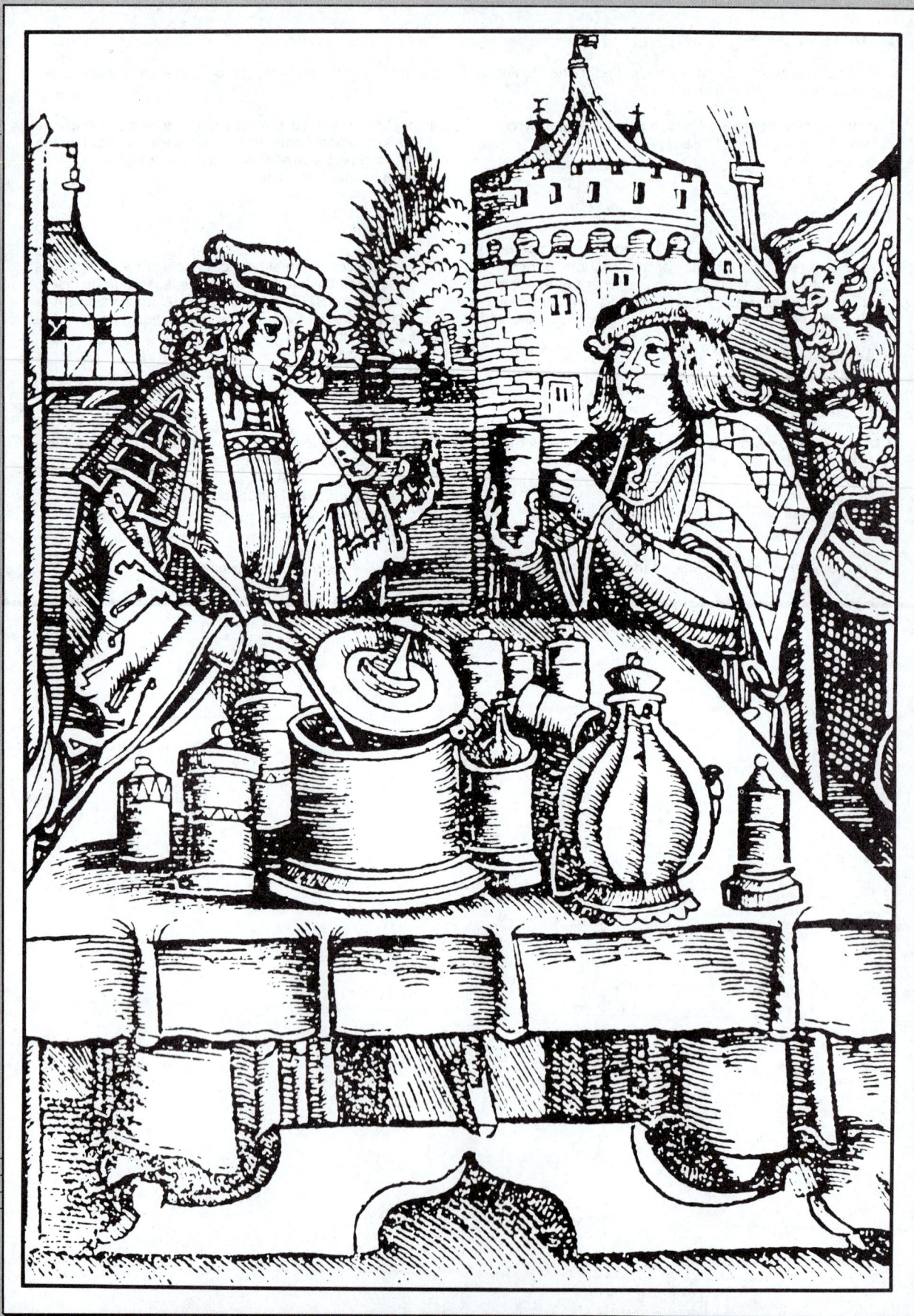

The preparation of medicine, circa 1500. Free Library of Philadelphia Print Collection.

8
UNIT

ANTI-INFECTIVE/ANTI-INFLAMMATORY MEDICATIONS

GLOSSARY TERMS IN THIS CHAPTER

Acetylation
Aerobic organisms
Anaerobic organisms
Antibiotic-associated colitis
Bacterial resistance
Bactericidal
Bacteriostatic
Beta-lactamase
Beta-lactamase inhibitor
Beta-lactam
Broad-spectrum
Chlamydia
Chromosomal mutation
Colonization
Conjugation
Crystalluria
Cytomegalovirus (CMV)
Cytoplasmic membrane
Disulfiram-like reaction
DNA gyrase
DNA polymerase
Enterohepatic recirculation
Eosinophilia
Epstein-Barr virus (EBV)
Facultative anaerobes
Fungicidal
Fungistatic
Glucose-6-phosphate dehydrogenase deficiency
Gray baby syndrome
Hemolytic anemia
Host defenses
Interstitial nephritis
Lipoproteins
Livedo reticularis
Microorganisms
Monobactam
Mycoplasma
Normal flora
Obligate anaerobes
Optic neuritis
Para-aminobenzoic acid
Pathogens
Penicillinase
Penicillin-binding proteins (PBP)
Penicillinase-resistant penicillins
Peptidoglycan
Peripheral neuritis
Plasmids
Protozoa
Pseudomembranous colitis
Pseudotumor cerebri
Ribosomes
Rickettsiae
RNA polymerase
Serum sickness
Sterols (ergosterol)
Superinfection
Synergy
Teratogenic
Tetrahydrofolic acid reductase
Thymidine kinase
Transduction
Translocation
Transpeptidase
Virucidal
Virostatic

46
CHAPTER

ANTI-INFECTIVES

STEVEN F. KOWALSKY, Pharm. D.

LEARNING OBJECTIVES

After reading this chapter, the student will be able to:

1. Identify those antimicrobial agents commonly used in the treatment of infectious diseases.

2. Differentiate among the antimicrobial agents as to mechanism of action, spectrum of activity, route of administration, absorption, distribution, metabolism, excretion, adverse effects, and drug interactions.

3. Identify specific areas to assess in the patient requiring antimicrobials and choose appropriate nursing diagnoses.

4. Evaluate the patient at various stages of treatment to ascertain the effectiveness of nursing interventions.

NORMAL FLORA OF THE HUMAN BODY

The population of *microorganisms* inhabiting internal and external surfaces of healthy human beings is often referred to as the *"normal flora."* Important anatomic locations populated by various bacteria, fungi, and *protozoa* include the oropharynx, upper and lower intestine, lower genitourinary tract, conjunctiva, and skin.

Normal bacterial flora functions to prevent *pathogens* from causing infection. It is probably easier to examine this protective role by considering the consequences suffered when the normal flora are altered. Patients who experience viral respiratory tract infections often develop secondary bacterial infections. In this situation, the initial viral infection is believed to alter the epithelial cells lining the oropharynx, thus allowing pathogenic bacteria to colonize the area. These pathogenic bacteria can invade the host and cause a secondary bacterial infection.

The most dramatic alterations of the normal flora come about as a result of administering antibiotic agents. A common example is the occurrence of vaginal yeast infections in patients taking *broad-spectrum* antibiotics (e.g. tetracyclines, cephalosporins). The mechanism is thought to be elimination of the normal vaginal flora by the broad-spectrum antibiotic with subsequent overgrowth of yeast causing clinical vaginitis. This phenomenon is called *superinfection.*

Another example of the protective role of normal flora is seen in patients who experience *antibiotic-associated colitis.* The colitis is due to a toxin that is produced by *Clostridium difficile.* Under antibiotic-free conditions, the intestinal growth of this organism is limited by the presence of normal flora. When patients receive antibiotics that suppress the normal intestinal flora (e.g., ampicillin, cephalosporins, clindamycin, etc), *Clostridium difficile* begins to multiply and produce toxin.

Finally, the administration of potent, broad-spectrum antibiotics to hospitalized patients can result in *colonization* and infection with organisms resistant to numerous antibiotics, including the antibiotic being prescribed. Colonization and infection with multi–drug–resistant bacteria is most often seen in patients who have received prolonged courses of antibiotics (e.g., burn patients). For this reason, antibiotic therapy should prescribe narrow-spectrum agents whenever possible, and for only the appropriate duration of treatment.

BACTERIAL RESISTANCE TO ANTIBIOTICS

Bacterial resistance to antibiotics occurs when bacteria alter genetic material that codes for biochemical changes within their cells. These biochemical changes inhibit the therapeutic effects of anti-infective agents and allow the bacteria to continue to grow. The mechanisms by which bacteria alter their genetic material include chromosomal mutation, recombination of DNA, and transfer of plasmids (small pieces of DNA containing genetic information).

Chromosomal mutation occurs spontaneously among a given population of bacteria. Suppression of the non-mutant bacteria by antibiotics allows the mutant organisms to multiply. Chromosomal mutation usually increases bacterial resistance by causing the bacteria to produce an enzyme that inactivates the antibiotic. Mutation may also induce changes in bacterial membranes preventing antibiotic penetration, as well as by altering the target site of the antibiotic, thus preventing attachment.

Transfer of plasmids may be achieved by numerous bacterial mechanisms such as *conjugation* and *transduction.* Plasmids contain instructions for the bacteria. These genetic instructions give the bacterial cell the ability to synthesize enzymes that inactivate antibiotics or to alter membrane permeability, preventing antibiotic entry into the cell. The most common example of plasmid-mediated resistance is the elaboration of β-lactamases (e.g., penicillinase, cephalosporinase) by various bacteria.

BACTERIAL CELL WALL SYNTHESIS

Bacteria elaborate a biochemically complex cell wall, which provides a supportive architecture for the organism and protects the cell membrane. The synthesis of the cell wall depends on elaboration of *peptidoglycan*— a cross-linked lattice work structure consisting of strands of complex sugar molecules cross-linked by peptide chains.

The intricate process of cell wall synthesis can be divided into three phases.

Phase I: During this phase, cell wall precursors are being manufactured within the cytoplasm.

Phase II: The precursors are incorporated into more complex molecules (sugar-pentapeptides), which are bound to lipid components of the cell membrane.

Phase III: Sugar-pentapeptides are joined in the presence of an enzyme, *transpeptidase,* resulting in the essential cross-linking of molecules.

Knowledge of bacterial cell wall synthesis is important because many antibiotics inhibit cell growth by altering cell wall construction.

GENERAL PRINCIPLES OF ANTI-INFECTIVE THERAPY

Frequently, the selection of appropriate antibiotic therapy must be made without the results of culture and sensitivity data. In other words, antibiotic therapy is often empiric in nature and these factors are considered when antibiotic therapy is being considered:

1. The infecting organism (suspected or confirmed).
2. Sensitivity of the organism to antibiotics.

3. Site of infection.
4. Status of host defenses.
5. Antibiotic pharmacokinetics.
6. Status of the patient's renal and hepatic function.
7. Monitoring of therapy.

The following sections will briefly discuss each of these important considerations.

THE INFECTING ORGANISM

In most clinical situations where infection is suspected, the pathogen is not identified within the first 24–48 hours. This lag period requires that initial treatment be empiric and directed against the most likely bacteria that may be responsible for the infectious process. For this reason, knowledge of the normal flora, the status of host defenses, and underlying disease is important. If an organism is identified or documented, antimicrobial therapy may then be directed against the specific pathogen(s).

ANTIBIOTIC SENSITIVITY TESTING

Collecting various body fluids or tissues for routine culture and antibiotic sensitivity testing is very important when infection is suspected. Initial or empiric "broad-spectrum" coverage may be narrowed or "streamlined" based on test results.

SITE OF INFECTION

Although an organism may be identified, it is important to consider the site of infection. Antibiotics may not reach the necessary body compartment in sufficient concentrations (e.g., aminoglycosides or selected cephalosporins in bacterial meningitis) to eradicate the infecting organism, therefore, alternative dosing regimens or routes of administration need to be considered.

HOST DEFENSES

An awareness of the patient's *host defenses* is important. Patients may be immunocompromised because of underlying diseases (e.g., cancer) or drug therapy (e.g., corticosteroids). In these cases, the infecting organism may not be the usual bacterial pathogen, but instead may be fungus (e.g., *Candida albicans*), a virus (e.g., *cytomegalovirus*), or a parasite (e.g., *Pneumocystis carinii*). In addition, these patients may require broader spectrum antibiotics and more aggressive management because of their decreased ability to fight infection.

ANTIBIOTIC PHARMACOKINETICS

Antibiotics are absorbed, distributed, metabolized, and excreted in a variety of ways. Knowledge of the severity of infection, the site of infection, etc., help guide in the selection of appropriate antibiotics.

RENAL AND HEPATIC FUNCTION

The primary organ of elimination for most antibiotics is the kidney and/or the liver. In patients with impaired renal or hepatic function, the dose of most antibiotics must be reduced or the interval of drug administration increased. Antimicrobial agents for which no reduction in dose is necessary in patients with renal insufficiency are chloramphenicol, nafcillin, oxacillin, cloxacillin, dicloxacillin, clindamycin, cefoperazone, ceftriaxone, erythromycin, and metronidazole. In addition, hemodialysis and peritoneal dialysis can have a major impact on antibiotic removal from the body.

MONITORING OF THERAPY

Clinical evaluation of antibiotic effectiveness will be discussed in later sections. A number of antibiotics (e.g., aminoglycosides, vancomycin) are now monitored by measuring drug concentrations in blood at various times during therapy. Knowledge of the antibiotic concentration may avoid underdosing, as well as avoid potential toxicities (i.e., maximize therapy and minimize toxicity). Laboratory values (as discussed in each antibiotic section) should be followed regularly during therapy.

THERAPEUTIC AGENTS

BETA-LACTAM ANTIBIOTICS

Mechanism of Action

Antibiotics with the *beta-lactam* structure are able to bind transpeptidase and prevent Phase III cross-linking of peptidoglycan (see section on bacterial cell wall synthesis). Beta-lactams may also bind to other enzymes regulating various aspects of bacterial cell division. Ultimately, defective cell wall synthesis leads to cell lysis and destruction of the organism.

Penicillins

Penicillins are natural or synthetic antibiotics produced by or derived from species of the mold *Penicillium* and other fungi. Penicillin was discovered in 1896 by Ernest Duchesne, however, this important finding was ignored at that time. In 1928, Alexander Fleming noticed the inhibitory effects of a mold growing in one of his bacterial cultures. The mold belonged to the genus *Penicillium*, and so the substance was named penicillin.

CLASSIFICATION. In the following sections, penicillin G and the other members of the penicillin family will be classified into the following categories:

(1) Natural penicillins: the original penicillins, including penicillin G (Pfizerpen, Pentids), penicillin V (Pen Vee K, V-Cillin K, Veetids).

(2) Antistaphylococcal penicillins: the penicillinase-resistant penicillins such as methicillin (Staphcillin), nafcillin (Nafcil, Unipen), oxacillin (Prostaphlin), cloxacillin (Tegopen), dicloxacillin (Dynapen, Pathocil).

(3) Broad-spectrum penicillins: ampicillin (Amcil, Omnipen, Polycillin), ampicillin/sulbactam (Unasyn), amoxicillin (Amoxil, Polymox, Trimox), amoxicillin/ clavulanic acid (Augmentin), hetacillin, bacampicillin (Spectrobid), cyclacillin (Cyclapen-W).

(4) Antipseudomonal penicillins: the extended spectrum penicillins such as carbenicillin (Geocillin, oral tablets: Geopen, injection), ticarcillin (Ticar), ticarcillin/ clavulanic acid (Timentin), mezlocillin (Mezlin), piperacillin (Pipracil), azlocillin (Azlin).

The usual dosages of the various penicillins are listed in Table 46–1. Natural penicillins are produced by the process of fermentation. Synthetic penicillins are produced by chemical modification of the natural penicillin structure.

SPECTRUM OF ACTIVITY. In general, the penicillins are active against gram-positive cocci and bacilli (rods), and some gram-negative cocci. Certain derivatives (e.g., ampicillin, mezlocillin) are active against gram-negative bacilli (Table 46–1).

Natural Penicillins. Penicillin G and penicillin V are active against aerobic, gram-positive organisms. However, penicillin G is five to ten times more active against gram-negative cocci and certain *anaerobic organisms.* Natural penicillins are active against various species of streptococci (including enterococci) and staphylococci (except penicillinase-producing staphylococci). They are the drugs of choice for infections due to *Neisseria gonorrhoeae* and *Neisseria meningitidis*. These agents are not indicated as primary therapy for serious gram-negative bacillary infections because most of these pathogens are resistant to the natural penicillins. Most anaerobes (except *Bacteroides fragilis*) are susceptible to the natural penicillins. In addition, *Corynebacterium diphtheriae, Actinomyces israelii, Streptobacillus moniliformis, Pasteurella multocida, Listeria monocytogenes*, and *Treponema pallidum*, are highly sensitive.

Antistaphylococcal Penicillins. This class of penicillins was created in response to an ever-increasing population of staphylococci that had developed resistance to the natural penicillins. Bacterial resistance is related to the ability of various strains to synthesize *penicillinase*. This enzyme destroys the beta-lactam nucleus and renders the penicillin molecule microbiologically inactive. Antistaphylococcal penicillins have been structurally modified to prevent penicillinase inactivation. Penicillins in this category are primarily indicated for the treatment of *Staphylococcus aureus* infections. These drugs are less active than penicillin G against other penicillin-G–sensitive organisms. There is an increasing incidence of "methicillin-resistant *Staphylococcus aureus*" (M-RSA) which are also resistant to the other members of the category. In addition to *Staphylococcus aureus*, this group of penicillins is active against *Staphylococcus epidermidis*; however, this organism may also be "methicillin-resistant" (MRSE).

Broad-Spectrum Penicillins. These agents are active against most organisms sensitive to penicillin G and are also active against some gram-negative bacilli. An advantage gained by this category is enhanced activity against common urinary tract pathogens (*Escherichia coli, Proteus mirabilis*) and *Streptococcus faecalis* (enterococci). *Hemophilus influenzae* type b (non–penicillinase-producing strains) is also susceptible to this group of penicillins.

Resistance to these penicillins is primarily via production of penicillinase (*beta-lactamase*). For example, it is recommended that pediatric meningitis, commonly caused by *H. influenzae*, be treated initially with either a combination of ampicillin and chloramphenicol or a second generation cephalosporin (e.g., cefuroxime) to avoid the possibility of inadequately treating a beta-lactamase strain of *H. influenzae*.

The recent addition of clavulanic acid and sulbactam to selected broad-spectrum penicillins (amoxicillin/clavulanic acid, Augmentin; ampicillin/sulbactam, Unasyn) has coupled both penicillins with a *beta-lactamase inhibitor* drug and "broadened" the spectrum of these penicillin derivatives to now include penicillinase-producing microorganisms (e.g., *Staphylcoccus aureus*).

Antipseudomonal Penicillins. Further modification of the basic penicillin structure has led to enhanced activity against gram-negative bacilli (especially *Pseudomonas aeruginosa*), while retaining activity similar to that of the broad-spectrum penicillins. The major advantage of carbenicillin and ticarcillin is activity against *Pseudomonas aeruginosa* and ampicillin-resistant *Proteus* species. The combination of ticarcillin and clavulanic acid has recently been marketed. Mezlocillin, piperacillin, and azlocillin have activity against *P. aeruginosa* and other enteric gram-negative rods. Mezlocillin has consistently superior microbiologic activity against *Klebsiella* species. These agents are often combined with an aminoglycoside antibiotic (e.g., gentamicin, tobramycin, or amikacin) to enhance bactericidal activity.

PHARMACOKINETICS. *Oral Absorption.* Penicillin G is rapidly inactivated within the acidic environment of the stomach, resulting in variable and inconsistent absorption. Food in the stomach enhances penicillin G destruction. Its only use orally is for the prevention of rheumatic fever (200,000 units twice daily). Penicillin VK (the K stands for the potassium salt), a phenoxymethyl derivative, was synthesized to overcome this gastric inactivation problem. Penicillin VK is resistant to acid hydrolysis and is able to pass through the stomach to the upper portion of the small intestine, where absorption occurs. Food intake has minimal effect on the breakdown of penicillin VK.

Methicillin is rapidly destroyed by gastric contents and therefore, it is not available as an oral preparation. Nafcillin is available for oral administration; however, the oral route is not recommended because of variable absorption from the gastrointestinal tract. Oxacillin, cloxacillin, and dicloxacillin are rapidly but incompletely absorbed following oral administration. Absorption is less variable when they are taken on an empty stomach.

Ampicillin is stable in gastric contents and is well absorbed following oral administration, but food intake may result in altered absorption. Amoxicillin is absorbed more rapidly and to a greater extent than ampicillin. This excellent absorption pattern is unaffected by food intake. Other antibiotics in this category (hetacillin, bacampicillin, cyclacillin) exhibit less reliable absorption than ampicillin. Amoxicillin/clavulanic acid combination (Augmentin) has absorption characteristics similar to that of amoxicillin alone.

Of the antipseudomonal penicillins, only carbenicillin is available orally, and must be taken as the indanyl ester. The ester form is acid stable and allows carbenicillin to reach the small intestine, where it is absorbed. Following absorption, the ester is removed by hydrolysis, delivering free carbenicillin to the systemic circulation.

Intramuscular Absorption. Intramuscular penicillins are designed for deep intramuscular (IM) injection. IM administration results in lower peak serum concentrations (in comparison to IV) and can be uncomfortable. In many clinical situations (e.g., meningitis, endocarditis), where high serum penicillin concentrations are desired, the intravenous route is preferred. The primary indication for IM administration is when compliance with an oral regimen is inconvenient or the patient's compliance behavior is in question. Long-acting preparations of penicillin G (aqueous procaine penicillin G and benzathine penicillin G) are available for these situations. Benzathine penicillin G is very slowly absorbed following IM injection and provides the longest antibiotic effect of all long-acting penicillin preparations (average: 26 days). Aqueous procaine penicillin G provides a source of penicillin for up to twenty-four hours. Procaine has local anesthetic properties, which make injections less painful. Patients with a history of hypersensitivity reactions to procaine should receive an intradermal skin test (0.1 ml of a 1% procaine solution) before administration of aqueous procaine penicillin G.

Distribution. Following administration, all penicillins distribute out of blood vessels and into interstitial fluids. Penicillins do not penetrate cell membranes easily because of their polar characteristics at physiologic pH. When inflammation is present, membrane permeability increases and a greater amount of penicillin can cross physiologic membranes. For example, penicillin penetration is enhanced during meningitis (meningeal inflammation), but progressively decreases as the inflammatory process subsides.

Metabolism and Excretion. Natural penicillins are predominantly excreted by the kidney via glomerular filtration and proximal tubular secretion in the unchanged form. When tubular secretion is blocked by another compound (e.g., probenecid), the serum concentration of penicillin is maintained for a longer period of time. This method is used in situations where elevated blood concentrations are desired, as well as in situations where compliance is doubtful (gonorrhea).

Penicillin G is metabolized to a limited extent in the liver and also actively secreted into the bile. The plasma half-life of penicillin G is three hours in neonates; it is decreased to 0.7 hour in adults and prolonged to five to ten hours in patients with severe renal dysfunction. In patients with reduced renal function (decreased creatinine clearance), the dosage of penicillins may need to be reduced to prevent toxicity.

Antistaphylococcal penicillins are secreted in the bile (40%–50%) and do not require extensive dosage alterations in patients with renal failure.

ADVERSE REACTIONS. *Hypersensitivity Reactions.* The penicillin molecule itself is too small to elicit an immunologic response. However, penicillin breakdown products may bind to proteins within the body, and this complex may induce antibody production. Penicillin hypersensitivity may present as anaphylactic reactions, *serum sickness*, contact dermatitis, or local injection reactions. Anaphylactic reactions occur in previously sensitized patients and are rare. Immediate treatment includes epinephrine, corticosteroids, saline or plasma expanders, and other resuscitative measures. Serum sickness usually occurs seven to ten days after treatment is initiated. The clinical presentation may include fever, arthritis, urticaria, lymphadenopathy, and generalized edema.

Neurotoxicity. Extremely high doses of penicillins may induce convulsions or coma secondary to direct central nervous system irritation. Neurotoxicity is more likely to occur in patients receiving large doses, patients with renal impairment, and/or patients with an underlying CNS disease.

Nephropathy. *Interstitial nephritis* (inflammation of renal tissue) may occur in patients receiving parenteral penicillin therapy. The onset is usually within two to four weeks after initiating therapy. A rising serum creatinine level and blood urea nitrogen (BUN) level may indicate decreased renal function, while blood and urinary eosinophils (*eosinophilia* and eosinophiluria, respectively) suggests that a possible drug-induced reaction has occurred. Fever and rash may also occur. This reaction usually subsides when the penicillin is discontinued; however, in some cases, corticosteroids may be administered in an attempt to correct the deterioration in renal function.

Hematologic Effects. A fall in hemoglobin concentration and laboratory evidence of hemolysis in a patient receiving high-dose intravenous penicillin may indicate the presence of penicillin-induced immune *hemolytic anemia.* The proposed mechanism is that penicillin binds to erythrocyte membrane proteins, forming a "coating." Immunoglobulin G, directed at the penicillin-RBC complex, binds to the erythrocyte. Activation of complement initiates the sequence of events leading to RBC lysis. This adverse effect can be life-threatening if the penicillin is continued. Withdrawal of penicillin usually results in a return of the hemoglobin level to a normal value. Similarly, a dose-related bone marrow suppressive effect may decrease the white blood cell count. The onset is approximately three weeks after the initiation of therapy and is reversible upon penicillin withdrawal. Penicillins (primarily carbenicillin and ticarcillin) may induce platelet dysfunction (inhibit platelet

TEXT RESUMES ON PAGE 1220

Table 46–1. PENICILLINS

Name	Dosage	Mode of Administration	Pharmacokinetics
ALL PENICILLINS			
Action: Inhibits cell wall synthesis of susceptible microorganisms.			
Use: Treatment of infections caused by gram-positive cocci and rods and anaerobic bacteria.			
Natural Penicillins Penicillin G (Pentids)	*Adults and children over 12:* 200,000–500,000 units q 6 hr;	PO	P: 1–2 hr A: 15%–30% PB: 60%
	Children under 12: 25,000–90,000 U/kg/day in 4–6 doses	PO	½L: 0.7 hr E: renal, 15%–30%; hepatic, 19%
	Adults dosage: 4–24 million units daily	IM, IV	P: 0.5–1 hr
	Pediatric dosage: 50,000–250,000 U/kg/day in 4–6 divided doses	IM, IV	
Penicillin VK (V-Cillin K)	*Adults and children over 12 yr:* 125–500 mg q 6 hr	PO	P: 0.5–1 hr A: 60%
	Children under 12 yr: 15–50 mg/kg/day in 4–6 divided doses	PO	PB: 80% ½L: 0.5 hr E: renal, hepatic
Antistaphylococcal Penicillins			
Action: Same as for all penicillins.			
Uses: Primarily for treating aerobic gram-positive infections secondary to staphylococci.			
Cloxacillin (Tegopen)	*Adults and children 20 kg and over:* 250–500 mg q 6 hr	PO	P: 1–2 hr A: 49% PB: 93%
	Children under 20 kg: 12.5–25 mg/kg q 6 hr	PO	½L: 0.5 hr E: renal, hepatic

P-peak; A-absorption; PB-protein bound; ½L-serum half-life; E-excretion.
*Within the column listing adverse effects, underlines indicate the most common effects; CAPITALS indicate life-threatening effects.

Contraindications/ Precautions	Adverse Effects*	Interactions	Nursing Implications
Simultaneous use with bacteriostatic agents (e.g., tetracycline, chloramphenicol, erythromycin) should be avoided. Consider dosage adjustment in renal insufficiency.	*Neuro:* CONVULSIONS, COMA, fever *CVR:* ANAPHYLAXIS, HYPOTENSION, sodium overload, edema *Resp:* SHORTNESS OF BREATH *GI:* diarrhea, hepatitis *Hemo:* hemolytic anemia, eosinophilia, leukopenia, thrombocytopenia, inhibition of platelet aggregation and prolongation of bleeding time, SERUM SICKNESS *Renal:* interstitial nephritis, hypokalemia *Integ:* rash, URTICARIA (HIVES), swollen glands	Aspirin increases blood levels. Probenecid blocks tubular secretion in kidneys and increases the blood levels. Concomitant use of bacteriostatic agent (e.g., chloramphenicol, erythromycin, tetracycline) decreases activity of penicillin.	*ASSESSMENT:* Full course of therapy is required; medication should be taken around the clock; administering IM injections can be painful. *INTERVENTION:* Tell patient to avoid administering concomitantly with food and that medication should be taken around the clock. *EVALUATION:* Check for fever and presence of symptoms. WBC count should return to normal. Adverse reactions must be reported.
CONTRAINDICATIONS: Contraindicated in patients with penicillin or cephalosporin allergy. Oral administration contraindicated in serious infections, nausea or vomiting.	Same as for all penicillins.	Same as for all penicillins.	Same as for all penicillins.
See penicillin G.	Same as for all penicillins.	Same as for all penicillins.	Same as for all penicillins.
Use cautiously in penicillin or cephalosporin allergy. Safe use in newborns and during pregnancy not established.	Same as for all penicillins.	Same as for all penicillins.	Same as for all penicillins.
Same as for all penicillins.	Same as for all penicillins.	Same as for all penicillins.	Same as for all penicillins.

CONTINUED ON THE FOLLOWING PAGE

Table 46–1. PENICILLINS–*CONTINUED*

Name	Dosage	Mode of Administration	Pharmacokinetics
Dicloxacillin (Dynapen)	*Adults and children over 40 kg:* 125–250 mg q 6 hr *Children under 40 kg:* 3–6 mg/kg q 6 hr	PO PO	P: 1–2 hr A: 56% PB: 96% ½L: 0.8 hr E: renal, hepatic
Methicillin (Staphcillin)	*Adults:* 1–2 g q 4–6 hr *Children:* 25 mg/kg q 6 hr	IM, IV IM	P: 0.5–1 hr A: minimal PB: 40% ½L: 0.4 hr E: renal
Nafcillin (Unipen)	*Adults:* 500 mg–1 g q 4–6 hr *Infants and children:* 50–100 mg/kg/day in 4 divided doses *Neonates:* 10 mg/kg 2–4× daily	PO, IM, IV PO, IM, IV PO, IM	P: PO 1–2 hr P: IM 0.5–1 hr P: IV, immed A: low PB: 80% ½L: 0.5–1 hr E: biliary
Oxacillin (Prostaphlin)	*Adults and children >40 kg:* 500 mg–2 g q 4–6 hr *Children <40 kg:* 50–100 mg/kg q 6 hr *Neonates:* <14 days old, <2000 g: 25 mg/kg q 12 hr; >2000 g: 25 mg/kg q 8 hr; 15–30 days old, <2000 g: 25 mg/kg q 8 hr; >2000 q: 25 mg/kg q 6 hr	PO, IM, IV PO, IM, IV PO, IM, IV	P: PO, 1–2 hr; IV, 0.5–1 hr A: 33% PB: 90% ½L: 0.4–0.7 hr E: renal, hepatic

Broad-Spectrum Penicillins

Action: See all penicillins.

Use: Same as natural penicillins including urinary tract pathogens.

Name	Dosage	Mode of Administration	Pharmacokinetics
Amoxicillin (Amoxil)	*Adults and children 20 kg and over:* 20–40 mg/kg/day in equally divided doses q 8 hr *Gonorrhea:* 3 g single dose plus 1 g probenecid	PO PO	P: 1–2 hr A: 80% PB: 20% ½L: 1–1.3 hr E: renal, hepatic
Amoxicillin/Clavulanic Acid (Augmentin)	*Adults:* 250–500 mg q 8 hr *Children:* 20–40 mg/kg/day divided into 3 doses	PO PO	(see amoxicillin)
Ampicillin	*Patients >20 kg:* 250–500 mg q 6 hr *Patients <20 kg:* 50–100 mg/kg/day in 4 equally divided doses *Patients >40 kg:* 250–1000 mg q 6 hr *Patients <40 kg:* 25–50 mg/ kg/day in 4 equally divided doses	PO PO IM, IV IM, IV	P: PO, 1–2 hr A: 50% PB: 20% ½L: 1–1.3 hr E: renal, 43%; hepatic, 26% P: IM, 0.5–1 hr P: IV, immed

P-peak; A-absorption; PB-protein bound; ½L-serum half-life; E-excretion.
*Within the column listing adverse effects, underlines indicate the most common effects; CAPITALS indicate life-threatening effects.

Contraindications/ Precautions	Adverse Effects*	Interactions	Nursing Implications
Same as for all penicillins.	Same as for all penicillins.	Same as for all penicillins.	Same as for all penicillins.
Same as for all penicillins.	Same as for all penicillins.	Same as for all penicillins.	Same as for all penicillins.
Same as for all penicillins.	Same as for all penicillins.	Same as for all penicillins.	Same as for all penicillins.
Same as for all penicillins.	Same as for all penicillins.	Same as for all penicillins.	Same as for all penicillins.
Same as for all penicillins.	Same as for all penicillins.	Same as for all penicillins.	Same as for all penicillins.
Same as for all penicillins.	Same as for all penicillins.	Same as for all penicillins.	Same as for all penicillins.
CONTRAINDICATIONS: Prior hypersensitivity reaction to beta-lactamase inhibitors.	Same as for all penicillins.	Concomitant use with allopurinol may predispose patient to ''ampicillin rash.''	Same as for all penicillins.
Same as for all penicillins.	Same as for all penicillins.	Same as for all penicillins.	Same as for all penicillins.

CONTINUED ON THE FOLLOWING PAGE

Table 46–1. PENICILLINS–*CONTINUED*

Name	Dosage	Mode of Administration	Pharmacokinetics
Ampicillin/Sulbactam (Unasyn)	*Adults:* 1.5–3.0 g q 6 hr	IM, IV	(see ampicillin)
Bacampicillin (Spectrobid)	*Patients >25 kg:* 400–800 mg q 12 hr *Children and infants <25 kg:* 25–50 mg/kg q 12 hr *Gonorrhea:* 1600 mg single dose plus 1 g probenecid	PO PO PO	(see ampicillin) A: 90%

Antipseudomonal Penicillins

Action: See all penicillins.

Use: Same as broad-spectrum penicillins including *Pseudomonas aeruginosa.*

Name	Dosage	Mode of Administration	Pharmacokinetics
Azlocillin (Azlin)	*Adults:* 200–300 mg/kg/day in divided doses q 4–6 hr *Children:* 50–200 mg/kg/day q 4–12 hr	IV	P: immed A: 0% PB: 30% ½L: 0.8 hr E: renal, biliary
Carbenicillin (Geopen, Geocillin)	*Adults:* 1–2 tablets (382–764 mg) q 6 hr *Adults:* 1–2 g q 6 hr *Children:* 50–200 mg/kg/day in divided doses q 4–6 hr *Adults:* 300–500 mg/kg/day in divided doses q 4–6 hr *Children:* 400–600 mg/kg/day in divided doses	PO IM IM IV IV	P: PO, 1–2 hr; IM, 0.5–1 hr A: 30% PB: 50% ½L: 1 hr E: renal
Mezlocillin (Mezlin)	*Adults:* 100–300 mg/kg/day q 4–6 hr *Children:* 50–225 mg/kg/day q 8 hr	IM, IV IM, IV	P: 0.5–1 hr (IM) A: 0% PB: 30% ½L: 0.8–1.3 hr E: renal, biliary
Piperacillin (Pipracil)	*Adults:* 100–300 mg/kg/day q 4–6 hr *Children:* 50–300 mg/kg/day q 8 hr	IM, IV IM, IV	P: 0.5–1 hr (IM) A: 0% PB: 30% ½L: 0.6–1.2 hr E: renal, 70%; biliary, 30%

P-peak; A-absorption; PB-protein bound; ½L-serum half-life; E-excretion.
*Within the column listing adverse effects, underlines indicate the most common effects; CAPITALS indicate life-threatening effects.

Contraindications/ Precautions	Adverse Effects*	Interactions	Nursing Implications
See amoxicillin/clavulanic acid. Safe use in pregnancy not established. Safety and efficacy in children not established.	Same as above.	Same as above.	Same as above.
Same as for all penicillins.	Same as for all penicillins.	Same as for all penicillins.	Same as for all penicillins.
PRECAUTIONS: Use cautiously in patients allergic to penicillins and/or cephalosporins. Safe use during pregnancy not established. Hypokalemia may be seen with these agents. Use cautiously in patients on sodium restricted diet. Platelet aggregation inhibition may be seen with these agents.	Same as for all penicillins.	Concomitant use with oral anticoagulants may put patient at risk for bleeding. Synergistic effect when using aminoglycosides. Physical mixing with aminoglycosides will cause precipitation.	*ASSESSMENT:* Avoid physically mixing penicillins and aminoglycosides in same syringe or IV bag. *INTERVENTION:* See all penicillins. *EVALUATION:* See all penicillins.
Same as for all penicillins.	Same as for all penicillins.	Same as for all penicillins.	Same as for all penicillins.
Same as for all penicillins.	Same as for all penicillins.	Same as for all penicillins.	Same as for all penicillins.
Same as for all penicillins.	Same as for all penicillins.	Same as for all penicillins.	Same as for all penicillins.
Same as for all penicillins.	Same as for all penicillins.	Same as for all penicillins.	Same as for all penicillins.

CONTINUED ON THE FOLLOWING PAGE

Table 46–1. PENICILLINS–*CONTINUED*

Name	Dosage	Mode of Administration	Pharmacokinetics
Ticarcillin (Ticar)	*Adults and children >40 kg:* 150–300 mg/kg/day in divided doses q 4–6 hr	IV	P: 0.5–1 hr A: 0% PB: 50%
	Children <40 kg: 150–200 mg/kg/day q 4–6 hr	IV	½L: 1.2 hr E: renal
	Neonates: 1–7 days of age, <2000 g: 75 mg/kg q 8 hr; 1–7 days of age, >2000 g: 75 mg/kg q 6 hr; >7 days of age: 75 mg/kg q 4 hr For uncomplicated UTI:	IV	
	Adults and children >40 kg: 1 g q 6 hr	I,M IV	
	Children <40 kg: 50–100 mg/kg/day q 6–8 hr		
Ticarcillin/Clavulanic Acid (Timentin)	*Adults >60 kg:* 3 g q 4–6 hr *Adults <60 kg:* 200–300 mg/ kg/day in divided doses q 4–6 hr *Children <12 yr:* 200–300 mg/kg/day q 4–6 hr	IV	(see ticarcillin)

P-peak; A-absorption; PB-protein bound; ½L-serum half-life; E-excretion.
*Within the column listing adverse effects, underlines indicate the most common effects; CAPITALS indicate life-threatening effects.

aggregation), resulting in a prolonged bleeding time. The effects may be exaggerated in patients with pre-existing coagulation abnormalities (such as uremia or hepatic disease). Platelet function returns to baseline after the drug is discontinued.

Electrolyte Disturbances. Antipseudomonal penicillins (carbenicillin and ticarcillin) are administered as the disodium salts. Patients with underlying renal or cardiac disease may not tolerate the excess sodium load. Newer members of this category (mezlocillin, piperacillin, azlocillin) are monosodium salts and may be useful alternatives in these patients. All penicillins, if given in high doses, may induce hypokalemia. Renal distal tubular secretion of potassium is enhanced because the penicillin is a negatively charged molecule (anion) that is not reabsorbed with sodium within the nephron. To maintain electrical neutrality, potassium is secreted in exchange for sodium. In clinical situations where high doses of penicillins are indicated, supplemental potassium may be required.

Hepatotoxicity. Certain penicillins (e.g., oxacillin, carbenicillin) have been associated with an elevation in levels of serum enzymes that are of hepatic origin (e.g., AST). The onset of this particular adverse effect is approximately three weeks after therapy is initiated, however, serum enzyme levels return to normal upon withdrawal of the offending agent.

DRUG INTERACTIONS. Chloramphenicol, Erythromycin, Tetracyclines. Penicillins are *bactericidal* agents active against dividing bacterial cells. When penicillins are administered concurrently with *bacteriostatic*

(inhibit bacterial growth) antibiotics (e.g., chloramphenicol, erythromycin, tetracyclines), the possibility exists that the activity of the penicillin will be decreased. The clinical significance of this interaction is questionable.

Anticoagulants. Carbenicillin and ticarcillin may impair normal platelet function. Patients who are on anticoagulants (warfarin, heparin) for therapeutic reasons may be at a risk for bleeding when high doses of penicillins are prescribed concurrently.

Aminoglycosides. High concentrations of penicillins (200 μg/ml) may microbiologically inactivate aminoglycoside antibiotics. Because of this interaction, penicillins and aminoglycosides are not to be admixed in the same intravenous fluid. From a clinical standpoint, this interaction is relevant in patients with poor renal function where elevated concentrations of both agents may be present, or when both are added to the same intravenous fluid. Inactivation of aminoglycosides by penicillins is dependent on the penicillin concentration, temperature of the blood samples, and the duration of time the two antibiotics are in contact. In some institutions, penicillinase is added to the blood collection tube to destroy penicillin within the sample. When penicillinase is not available, the sample should be kept on ice while transported to the laboratory for aminoglycosides concentration measurement.

Probenecid. Probenecid inhibits the renal tubular secretion of penicillins, resulting in elevated penicillin concentrations. This interaction is used therapeutically to sustain penicillin concentrations in patients with gonorrhea.

Contraindications/ Precautions	Adverse Effects*	Interactions	Nursing Implications
Same as for all penicillins.	Same as for all penicillins.	Same as for all penicillins.	Same as for all penicillins.
Same as for all antipseu- domonal penicillins.	Same as for all penicillins.	Same as for all penicillins.	Same as for all penicillins.

Cephalosporins

The cephalosporins were first isolated by Brotzu in 1948 from *Cephalosporium acremonium,* a fungus growing in the sewer near the Sardinian coast. The basic structure for cephalosporins has been modified chemically to provide a large number of derivatives that have activity against many microorganisms.

CLASSIFICATION. Although not an absolute classification system, the following nomenclature may be a convenient method for recalling the large number of cephalosporins (see Table 46–2):

(1) First Generation: cephalothin (Keflin, Seffin), cefazolin (Ancef, Kefzol), cephapirin (Cefadyl), cephalexin (Keflex), cephradine (Velosef, Anspor), cefadroxil (Duricef, Ultracef).
(2) Second Generation: cefamandole (Mandol), cefoxitin (Mefoxin), cefaclor (Ceclor), cefuroxime (Zinacef, Ceftin), cefonocid (Monocid), ceforanide (Precef), cefotetan (Cefotan), cefixime (Suprax).
(3) Third Generation: cefotaxime (Claforan), moxalactam (Moxam), cefoperazone (Cefobid), ceftizoxime (Cefizox), ceftriaxone (Rocephin), ceftazidime (Fortaz, Tazicef, Tazidime).

MECHANISM OF ACTION. The mechanism of action of cephalosporins is similar to that of penicillins (see Mechanism of Action under Beta-Lactam Antibiotics) and includes binding to transpeptidase enzymes and prevention of Phase III cross-linking of peptidoglycan.

SPECTRUM OF ACTIVITY. *First Generation.* The members of the first generation cephalosporins all have similar antimicrobial activity. They inhibit the growth of most gram-positive cocci including penicillinase-pro-

ducing staphylococci. These cephalosporins are effective against certain gram-negative bacilli, including *Escherichia coli, Klebsiella pneumoniae, Proteus mirabilis, Salmonella* species, and *Shigella* species. Resistant gram-negative bacilli include most strains of *Hemophilus influenzae, Enterobacter aerogenes, Enterobacter cloacae,* incole-positive *Proteus, Pseudomonas aeruginosa, Serratia marcescens, Acinetobacter* species, and *Bacteroides fragilis.* Group D streptococci (including enterococci) and *Listeria monocytogenes* are also resistant.

Second Generation. The second generation cephalosporins offer a broadened antimicrobial spectrum, particularly the gram-negative spectrum, in comparison with first generation agents. In general, these cephalosporins are more active against the gram-negative bacilli mentioned above, as well as, strains of indole-positive *Proteus, E. cloacae, E. aerogenes,* and *Hemophilus influenzae.* Cefoxitin, although less active against *H. influenzae* than cefamandole and cefuroxime, has greater activity versus anaerobic bacteria, including *Bacteroides fragilis.* Cefotetan is comparable to cefoxitin in terms of anaerobic activity.

Third Generation. Third generation cephalosporins broaden the spectrum a little further to include antipseudomonal activity. In comparison to the other two generation agents, the third generation agents are more potent against selected gram-negative organisms and anaerobic pathogens. Against *Pseudomonas aeruginosa,* ceftazidime and cefoperazone are the most active. Cefotaxime, moxalactam, ceftizoxime, and ceftriaxone are intermediate in their antipseudomonal activity. Against

TEXT RESUMES ON PAGE 1226

Table 46–2. CEPHALOSPORINS

Name	Dosage	Mode of Administration	Pharmacokinetics
CEPHALOSPORINS			
Action: Inhibits cell wall synthesis of susceptible microorganisms.			
Use: For gram-positive and gram-negative infections including *Pseudomonas aeruginosa* (some third generation agents).			
First Generation Agents Cephalexin (Keflex)	*Adults:* 250–500 mg q 6 hr *Children:* 25–50 mg/kg/day in 4 equally divided doses	PO PO (Pediatric suspension is available)	A: 90% PB: 14% ½L: 0.6–0.9 hr E: renal
Cephalothin (Keflin, Seffin)	*Adults:* 500 mg–2 g q 4–6 hr *Children:* 80–160 mg/kg/day	IM, IV IM, IV	A: none PB: 62%–65% ½L: 0.65 hr E: renal
Cephapirin (Cefadyl)	*Adults:* 500 mg–2 g q 4–6 hr *Children: >3 mo:* 40–80 mg/ kg/day in 4 equally divided doses	IM, IV IM, IV	A: none PB: 44%–50% ½L: 0.6 hr E: renal, liver, plasma
Cefazolin (Ancef, Kefzol)	*Adults:* 0.5–2 g q 6–8 hr *Children and Infants >1 mo:* 25–50 mg/kg/day, divided into 3–4 doses	IM, IV IM, IV	A: none PB: 84% ½L: 1.8 hr E: renal
Cefadroxil (Duricef, Ultracef)	*Adults:* 1–2 g/day in 1 or 2 divided doses *Children:* 15 mg/kg q 12 hr	PO PO (Oral suspension is available)	A: >90% PB: 15%–20% ½L: 1.1–2 hr E: renal
Cephradine (Velosel, Anspor)	Same as Cephalexin *Adults:* 0.5–1g q 6 hr *Children:* 50–100 mg/kg/day in 4 doses	PO IV, IM	A: >90% PB: 6%–20% ½L: 0.7–2 hr E: renal

A-absorption; PB-protein binding; ½L-half-life; E-excretion.
*Within the column listing adverse effects, underlines indicate the most common effects; CAPITALS indicate life-threatening effects.

Contraindications/ Precautions	Adverse Effects*	Interactions	Nursing Implications
For All Cephalosporins: PRECAUTIONS: Use cautiously in patients allergic to other beta-lactam antibiotics (e.g., penicillins, cephalosporins, carbapenems). Use cautiously in pregnant and lactating women. Adjust dose in renal insufficiency.	**For All Cephalosporins:** CVR: ANAPHYLAXIS, HYPOTENSION Resp: SHORTNESS OF BREATH GI: diarrhea, PSEUDOMEMBRANOUS COLITIS, nausea, vomiting Renal: nephrotoxicity Integ: rash, fungal overgrowth	**For All Cephalosporins:** Probenecid decreases renal clearance. Interferes with the following lab test results: Coomb's test, Clinitest.	**For All Cephalosporins:** ASSESSMENT: A full course of therapy is required. INTERVENTION: Administering IM injections can be painful; inject deep into muscle. EVALUATION: Check to see if fever and symptoms have disappeared. Check WBC count. Adverse effects must be reported.
Same as for all cephalosporins.	GI: diarrhea, PSEUDOMEMBRANOUS COLITIS, nausea, vomiting Integ: rash, fungal overgrowth	Same as for all cephalosporins.	ASSESSMENT: See Cephalosporins. INTERVENTION: Patient should avoid taking with food. EVALUATION: See Cephalosporins.
Same as for all cephalosporins.	Neuro: fever CVR: phlebitis GI: diarrhea Biliary: liver dysfunction Hemo: SERUM SICKNESS Renal: nephrotoxicity Integ: URTICARIA, rash, pain on IM administration, abscess formation	Same as for all cephalosporins.	ASSESSMENT: See Cephalosporins. INTERVENTION: See Cephalosporins. EVALUATION: See Cephalosporins.
Same as for all cephalosporins. Safe use in children <3 months not established.	GI: diarrhea, PSEUDOMEMBRANOUS COLITIS, nausea, vomiting Integ: rash, fungal overgrowth	Increased AST, ALT, alkaline phosphatase bilirubin, and BUN levels. Same as for all cephalosporins.	Same as for all cephalosporins.
Same as for all cephalosporins. Safe use in infants <1 month not established.	CVR: phlebitis GI: diarrhea, PSEUDOMEMBRANOUS COLITIS, nausea, vomiting Integ: rash, fungal overgrowth, pain and tenderness at IM injection site	Same as for all cephalosporins.	Same as for all cephalosporins.
Same as for all cephalosporins.	Neuro: dizziness, headache GI: diarrhea Integ: fungal overgrowth	Same as for all cephalosporins.	Same as for all cephalosporins. INTERVENTION: Patient may take with food.
Same as for all cephalosporins.	Same as for all cephalosporins.	Same as for all cephalosporins.	Same as for all cephalosporins.

CONTINUED ON THE FOLLOWING PAGE

Table 46–2. CEPHALOSPORINS–*CONTINUED*

Name	Dosage	Mode of Administration	Pharmacokinetics
Second Generation Agents Cefaclor (Ceclor)	*Adults:* 250–500 mg q 8 hr *Children ≥ 1 mo of age:* 20–40 mg/kg/day in 3 equally divided doses	PO PO	A: very good PB: 25% ½L: 0.6–0.9 hr E: renal
Cefamandole (Mandol)	*Adults:* 0.5–2 g IM, IV q 4–6 hr *Children ≥ 1 mo of age:* 50–100 mg/kg/day in divided doses q 4–8 hr	IM, IV IM, IV	A: none PB: 74% ½L: 0.78 hr E: renal
Cefonocid (Monocid)	*Adults:* 0.5–2 g q 24 hr	IM, IV	A: none PB: 98% ½L: 4.5 hr E: renal
Ceforanide (Precef)	*Adults:* 0.5–1 g q 12 hr *Children:* 20–40 mg/kg/day in equally divided doses every 12 hr	IM, IV IM, IV	A: none PB: 80% ½L: 2.9 hr E: renal
Cefotetan (Cefotan)	*Adults:* 0.5–2 g q 12 hr	IM, IV	A: none PB: 88% ½L: 3–5 hr E: renal
Cefoxitin (Mefoxin)	*Adults:* 1–2 g q 4–8 hr *Children >3 mo of age:* 80–160 mg/kg/day in equally divided doses q 4–6 hr	IM, IV IM, IV	A: none PB: 73% ½L: 0.7–1.1 hr E: renal
Cefuroxime Axetil (Ceftin)	*Adults and children ≥ 12 yr of age:* 125–500 mg twice daily *Infants and children <12 yr of age:* 125–250 mg twice daily	PO PO	A: 36%–52% PB: 33%–50% ½L: 1–2 hr E: renal
Cefuroxime, sodium (Zinacef)	*Adult:* 750 mg–1.5 g q 6–8 hr *Infants and children >3 mo of age:* 50–240 mg/kg/day in equally divided doses q 6–8 hr	IM, IV IM, IV	A: none PB: 33%–50% ½L: 1–2 hr E: renal
Cefixime (Suprax)	*Adult and Children >12 years or older:* 400 mg daily or 200 mg every 12 hr *Children >12 years old and < 50 ks:* 8 mg/kg/day of suspension	PO PO (Oral suspension)	A: 40%–50% PB: 65% ½L: 3–4 hr E: renal

A-absorption; PB-protein binding; ½L-half-life; E-excretion.
*Within the column listing adverse effects, underlines indicate the most common effects; CAPITALS indicate life-threatening effects.

Contraindications/ Precautions	Adverse Effects*	Interactions	Nursing Implications
Same as for all cephalosporins.	*GI:* diarrhea, nausea, vomiting, anorexia *Integ:* rash, fungal overgrowth	Same as for all cephalosporins.	Same as for all cephalosporins.
Same as for all cephalosporins. Safety in children <1 mo of age not established. Prolongation of prothrombin time may occur.	*CVR:* phlebitis, BLEEDING *GI:* diarrhea *Integ:* fungal overgrowth, pain at IM injection site	Disulfiram (Antabuse)-like reaction with ethanol.	*ASSESSMENT:* Use lidocaine to decrease pain at IM injection site. *INTERVENTION:* Same as for all cephalosporins. *EVALUATION:* Monitor for signs of bleeding.
Same as for all cephalosporins. Safe use in children has not been established.	Same as for all cephalosporins.	Same as for all cephalosporins.	Same as for all cephalosporins.
Same as for all cephalosporins.	Same as for all cephalosporins.	Same as for all cephalosporins.	Same as for all cephalosporins.
Same as for all cephalosporins. Safety in children has not been established. Prolongation of the prothrombin time may occur.	Same as for all cephalosporins.	Disulfiram (Antabuse)-like reaction with ethanol.	Same as for all cephalosporins. *EVALUATION:* Monitor the patient for signs of bleeding.
Same as for all cephalosporins. Safe use in children <3 mo of age has not been established.	*CVR:* phlebitis at IV site *GI:* diarrhea, nausea *Integ:* pain, tenderness, induration at IM injection site	Same as for all cephalosporins.	Same as for all cephalosporins. *ASSESSMENT:* Mix IM injections with 0.5% lidocaine to minimize pain.
Same as for all cephalosporins.	*GI:* diarrhea, nausea *Integ:* superinfection	Same as for all cephalosporins.	*ASSESSMENT:* Administer with food to increase absorption *INTERVENTION:* Crushed tablets have strong, persistent bitter taste. *EVALUATION:* Same as for all cephalosporins.
Same as for all cephalosporins.	Same as for all cephalosporins.	Same as for all cephalosporins.	Same as for all cephalosporins.
Same as for all cephalosporins. Safe use in children <6 months not established	*GI:* diarrhea, PSEUDOMEMBRANOUS COLITIS, nausea, vomiting *Integ:* rash, fungal overgrowth	Increased AST, ALT, alkaline phosphatase. Same as for all cephalosporins	Same as for all cephalosporins

CONTINUED ON THE FOLLOWING PAGE

Table 46–2. CEPHALOSPORINS–*CONTINUED*

Name	Dosage	Mode of Administration	Pharmacokinetics
Third Generation Agents Cefoperazone (Cefobid)	*Adults:* 2–4 g q 12 hr	IM, IV	A: none PB: 82%–93% ½L: 1.6–2.6 hr E: dual (renal/biliary)
Cefotaxime (Claforan)	*Adults and children ≥50 kg:* 1–2 g q 4–12 hr *Neonates:* 50 mg/kg q 8–12 hr *Infants and children ≤12 yr of age, <50 kg:* 50–180 mg/kg q 4–6 hr	IM, IV IM, IV	A: none PB: 13%–38% ½L: 0.9–1.7 hr E: renal, liver (active metabolites)
Ceftazidime (Fortaz, Tazicef, Tazidime)	*Adults and children >12 yr of age:* 1–2 g q 8–12 hr *Infants and children (1 mo–12 yr):* 30–50 mg/kg q 8 hr *Neonates (≤1 mo):* 30 mg/kg q 12 hr	IM, IV IV	A: none PB: 17% ½L: 1.7 hr E: renal
Ceftizoxime (Cefizox)	*Adults:* 500 mg–4 g q 8–12 hr *Children ≥6 mo of age:* 50 mg/kg q 6–8 hr	IM, IV IM, IV	A: none PB: 30% ½L: 1.7 hr E: renal
Ceftriaxone (Rocephin)	*Adults:* 0.5–2 g q 12–24 hr *Children:* 50–100 mg/kg/day in divided doses every 12 hr	IM, IV	A: none PB: 95% ½L: 5.8–8.7 hr E: dual (renal and biliary)
Moxalactam (Moxam)	*Adults:* 2–12 g/day administered in divided doses every 8–12 hrs *Neonates:* ≤1 wk of age: 50 mg/kg q 12 hrs; ≤4 wk of age: 50 mg/kg q 8 hr *Infants:* 50 mg/kg q 6 hr *Children:* 50 mg/kg q 6–8 hr	 IM, IV IM, IV	A: none PB: 40%–51% ½L: 1.7 hr E: renal, small amounts via bile

A-absorption; PB-protein binding; ½L-half-life; E-excretion.
*Within the column listing adverse effects, underlines indicate the most common effects; CAPITALS indicate life-threatening effects.

Serratia marcescens, ceftazidime, moxalactam, ceftizoxime, cefotaxime, cefoperazone, and ceftriaxone have excellent in vitro activity. Finally, against *Bacteroides fragilis*, moxalactam demonstrates the greatest activity followed by ceftizoxime. The other third generation agents are less active than cefoxitin versus *B. fragilis*.

In general, as the gram-negative activity of cephalosporins has been enhanced, their activity against gram-positive cocci has decreased. As a result, patients receiving third generation cephalosporins with minimal gram-positive activity may be at increased risk of developing superinfection with gram-positive cocci.

PHARMACOKINETICS. *Absorption.* First generation agents available for oral administration are cephalexin, cephradine, and cefadroxil. Second generation agents available are cefaclor, cefixime, cefuroxime axetil. There are no third generation cephalosporins currently available for oral use. Cephalexin and cephradine ab-

Contraindications/ Precautions	Adverse Effects*	Interactions	Nursing Implications
Same as for all cephalosporins. Prolongation of prothrombin time may occur. Safety in children has not been established.	*CVR:* phlebitis at IV site, BLEEDING *GI:* diarrhea, nausea *Integ:* Pain and irritation at IM injection site	Disulfiram (Antabuse)-like reaction with ethanol.	Same as for all cephalosporins. *EVALUATION:* Monitor the patient for signs of bleeding.
Same as for all cephalosporins.	Same as for all cephalosporins.	Same as for all cephalosporins.	Same as for all cephalosporins.
Same as for all cephalosporins.	Same as for all cephalosporins.	Same as for all cephalosporins.	Same as for all cephalosporins.
Same as for all cephalosporins.	Same as for all cephalosporins.	Same as for all cephalosporins.	*ASSESSMENT:* When administering a 2 g IM dose, give in 2 different large muscle masses. *INTERVENTION:* Same as for all cephalosporins. *EVALUATION:* Same as for all cephalosporins.
Same as for all cephalosporins.	*GI:* diarrhea	Same as for all cephalosporins.	Same as for all cephalosporins. *EVALUATION:* Monitor the patient for signs of bleeding.
Same as for all cephalosporins. Prolongation of prothrombin time may occur.	*CVR:* phlebitis at IV site, BLEEDING *GI:* nausea, diarrhea	Disulfiram (Antabuse)-like reaction with ethanol.	*ASSESSMENT:* Patient should receive supplemental Vitamin K 3 times weekly. *INTERVENTION:* Same as for all cephalosporins. *EVALUATION:* Monitor the patient for signs of bleeding.

sorption differs only from the standpoint of the effect of food on the absorption process in infants and children. In adults, the rate of absorption, but not the extent of absorption, is reduced. This holds true for cephradine absorption in infants and children but not for cephalexin. It appears that in addition to the rate of absorption, the extent of cephalexin absorption is also reduced. Cefadroxil is well absorbed from the gastrointestinal tract and even less affected by the presence of food in the stomach when compared to cephalexin and cephradine.

Cefaclor is well absorbed from the gastrointestinal tract and unaffected by the presence of food. Cefuroxime axetil is likewise well absorbed and unaffected by food in the gastrointestinal tract. Absolute bioavailability in the presence of food is 52% for cefuroxime. It is rapidly hydrolyzed by nonspecific esterases in the intestinal tract and blood to release cefuroxime into the circulation. Cefixime is approximately 40%–50% absorbed with or without food. However, food does delay the time to reach peak plasma concentrations by about one hour. The suspension formulation of cefixime produces 25%–40% greater plasma concentrations for all doses given, when compared to the tablets. Cephalosporins

Table 46–3. MONOBACTAMS AND CARBAPENEMS

Name	Dosage	Mode of Administration	Pharmacokinetics
MONOBACTAMS			
Action: Inhibits bacterial cell wall synthesis.			
Use: For aerobic gram-negative rod infections.			
Aztreonam (Azactam)	*Adults:* 500 mg–2 g every 6–12 hr *Children:* 30–50 mg/kg q 6–12 hr	IM, IV	A: 0% PB: 56% ½L: 1.7 hrs. E: renal, liver
CARBAPENEMS			
Action: Inhibits bacterial cell wall synthesis.			
Use: For aerobic and anaerobic gram-positive and gram-negative infections.			
Imipenem/Cilastatin (Primaxin)	*Adults:* 250–500 mg every 6–8 hr; rarely, up to 4 g may be used *Children:* 15–25 mg/kg/q 6 hr	IV	A: 0% PB: 20% ½L: 1 hr E: renal, 75%; nonrenal, 25%

A-absorption; PB-protein binding; ½L-half-life; E-excretion.
*Within the column listing adverse effects, <u>underlines</u> indicate the most common effects; CAPITALS indicate life-threatening effects.

can be administered intramuscularly and are well absorbed from the site of injection. Large volumes (>2 ml) may be painful when injected.

Distribution. The first generation cephalosporins (oral and parenteral) distribute throughout the body fluids but do not penetrate cells to a great extent. These drugs do not penetrate the cerebrospinal fluid (CSF) and should not be used for the treatment of bacterial meningitis. Members of the second generation have similar distribution properties, however, cefuroxime does penetrate the CSF. Third generation cephalosporins distribute in a similar manner; however, these agents do attain higher concentrations in the CSF in the presence of meningitis.

Metabolism and Excretion. Members of the first generation cephalosporins, with the exception of cephalothin and cephapirin, both of which are deacetylated in the liver, are primarily eliminated from the body by the kidneys. Biliary excretion of any of the first generation agents is minimal. Second generation cephalosporins are mainly excreted by the kidneys and to a lesser extent in the bile. Sixty percent or more of an administered dose of cefotaxime, moxalactam, ceftizoxime, and ceftazidime are excreted by the kidneys. Cefoperazone

and ceftriaxone are 40% or more metabolized by the liver and excreted in the bile. With the exception of cefoperazone and ceftriaxone, major dosage modifications are necessary in the presence of renal insufficiency.

ADVERSE REACTIONS. *Hypersensitivity Reactions.* As with penicillins, hypersensitivity reactions are the most common adverse reaction of cephalosporins. A small percentage of patients with penicillin allergy will be cross-sensitive to the cephalosporins (probably because of their structural similarities). (See penicillin toxicity.)

Coagulation Disorders. When high doses are given, cephalosporins may alter the coagulation mechanism and expose patients to a risk of bleeding. Cephalosporins may inhibit normal platelet function as well as depress the hepatic synthesis of prothrombin leading to prolongation of the prothrombin time (PT). Bleeding episodes have been reported with cefamandole, cefoperazone, and moxalactam. Patients at risk for this adverse effect are those with malnutrition or renal insufficiency, patients receiving prolonged antibiotic therapy, and patients receiving relatively high dose therapy with one of the above mentioned agents. Platelet effects do not influence the prothrombin time but rather prolong the

Contraindications/ Precautions	Adverse Effects*	Interactions	Nursing Implications
CONTRAINDICATIONS: Prior hypersensitivity reactions. PRECAUTIONS: Use cautiously in patients with impaired renal or hepatic function. Safe use in pregnancy and during lactation not established. Safety and efficacy not established in children.	Neuro: SEIZURES CVR: phlebitis, ANAPHYLAXIS Resp: SHORTNESS OF BREATH GI: diarrhea, nausea, vomiting Biliary: hepatitis Hemo: pancytopenia, neutropenia, thrombocytopenia Integ: rash	Elevations in AST, ALT and alkaline phosphatase levels. Prolongation of the partial thromboplastin time and prothrombin time. Increases in serum creatinine.	ASSESSMENT: Full course of therapy is required; administering IM injections can be painful. INTERVENTION: None. EVALUATION: Evaluate for fever and symptoms. Check WBC count. Adverse reactions need to be reported.
CONTRAINDICATIONS: Prior hypersensitivity reactions. PRECAUTIONS: Safe use in pregnancy or during lactation not established. Safe and effective use in children not established. Use cautiously in patients with underlying CNS disorders (e.g., seizures).	Neuro: SEIZURES, fever CVR: phlebitis at IV site, hypotension GI: nausea, diarrhea, vomiting Integ: rash		ASSESSMENT: No IM dosage form is available. Nausea, vomiting, hypotension may be the result of too rapid an IV infusion (i.e., <60 min). INTERVENTION: None. EVALUATION: See Aztreonam.

bleeding time. Patients with preexisting platelet dysfunction (such as is seen in renal failure) are probably at increased risk.

Gastrointestinal System. Patients receiving oral cephalosporins may experience diarrhea, nausea, or vomiting. In some, these side effects may be alleviated by taking the drug with food. Antibiotic-associated colitis or *pseudomembranous colitis* (PMC) is another complication of the cephalosporins. This adverse effect may be seen after therapy has been initiated or following a course of therapy. It may present as fever, abdominal cramping, watery diarrhea, and mucus in the stool. The stool may or may not contain blood. This may be a life-threatening side effect and therapy should be discontinued and/or alternative agents selected. If necessary, metronidazole 500 mg every six hours orally or vancomycin 250–500 mg every six hours orally may be administered.

Neurotoxicity. High doses of cephalosporins, administered to patients with impaired kidney function, may induce seizures. For this reason, cephalosporins which are primarily excreted by the kidneys should have their dosage adjusted when renal failure is present.

Nephrotoxicity. Early reports of nephrotoxicity were common with cephaloridine. In patients with preexisting renal disease, cephalosporins and aminoglycosides

have additive toxicity on the kidneys. This direct toxicity is relatively rare; however, these agents may induce interstitial nephritis like that seen with penicillins.

DRUG INTERACTIONS. Patients receiving cefamandole, moxalactam, and cefoperazone may experience a *disulfiram-like reaction* if they ingest ethanol. Patients may experience headache, flushing, dizziness, nausea, and vomiting within thirty minutes of ethanol ingestion.

Concurrent administration of cephalosporins (e.g., cephalothin) with nephrotoxic antibiotics such as aminoglycosides may have additive toxic effects, however, this interaction is questionable.

Recently, newer cephalosporins (e.g., cefamandole, moxalactam, cefoperazone) have been associated with suppression of vitamin-K–dependent clotting factor synthesis. It is recommended that patients receiving any of these agents also be given vitamin K to prevent prothrombin time prolongation.

Monobactams

AZTREONAM (AZACTAM). Aztreonam is the first of a new class of beta-lactam antibiotics and differs from penicillins and cephalosporins in that it is structurally a monocyclic antibiotic. It is known as a *monobactam*, is totally synthetic, and is currently the only one in its class (see Table 46–3).

Mechanism of Action. Like the penicillins and the cephalosporins, aztreonam disrupts bacterial cell wall synthesis and binds primarily to penicillin-binding protein 3 (PBP 3).

Spectrum of Activity. The spectrum of activity of this monobactam is limited to *aerobic* gram-negative rods (e.g., *Escherichia coli, Klebsiella pneumoniae, Proteus mirabilis,* indole-positive *Proteus* species, *Enterobacter* species, and *Pseudomonas aeruginosa*). In addition, it is active against *Neisseria gonorrhoeae* and a *Hemophilus influenzae.* It has no activity against gram-positive organisms or against anaerobic microorganisms.

Pharmacokinetics. Absorption. Only available in parenteral form, aztreonam is rapidly and completely absorbed following intramuscular administration with serum concentrations being very similar to those achieved following intravenous administration.

Distribution. Distribution is rapid following administration with 56% of the drug bound to serum proteins. Penetration into the cerebrospinal fluid in patients with meningitis is similar to that of the penicillin antibiotics.

Metabolism and Excretion. The drug does undergo some extrarenal metabolism to a microbiologically inactive metabolite; however, the majority of aztreonam is eliminated by the kidney in the unchanged form. Approximately 1% of a dose appears unchanged in the feces, therefore, some biliary excretion may occur. The half-life of aztreonam is 1.7 hours. The dose of aztreonam must be altered in patients with renal insufficiency and because hemodialysis does remove the drug from the serum, postdialysis dosing is recommended.

Adverse Reactions. Aztreonam has the same toxicity profile as many of the penicillin and cephalosporin antibiotics. Structurally, the drug is dissimilar enough so that cross-allergenicity with other beta-lactam drugs is minimal to nonexistent.

Carbapenems

IMIPENEM/CILASTATIN (PRIMAXIN). A new class of antibiotics structurally similar to the penicillins was introduced early in 1986. Substitution of the sulfur molecule with a carbon atom in the ring has created this class of compounds known as carbapenems. Imipenem is the only carbapenem currently on the market.

Mechanism of Action. Imipenem interferes with synthesis of the bacterial cell wall (see Table 46–3). It binds to *penicillin-binding protein* 2 (PBP 2) and penicillin-binding protein 1 (PBP 1), which results in elongation and subsequent lysis of the microorganism. It is a bactericidal antibiotic for the majority of susceptible bacteria.

Spectrum of Activity. Imipenem has the broadest antibacterial spectrum of any beta-lactam antibiotic currently on the market. It is extremely potent against gram-positive cocci (e.g., *Staphylococcus aureus, Staphylococcus epidermidis, Streptococcus pneumoniae, Streptococcus pyogenes,* and viridans streptococci). Activity against the enterococci is variable. It has no activity against methicillin-resistant staphylococci. Imipenem is active against enterobacteriaceae (e.g., *Escherichia coli, Klebsiella* species, *Enterobacter* species, *Proteus mirabilis,*

indole positive *Proteus*) and *Pseudomonas aeruginosa.* In addition, it maintains activity against *Hemophilus influenzae, Neisseria meningitidis,* and *Neisseria gonorrhoeae.* Its anaerobic activity is also very broad and includes *Bacteroides fragilis, Peptostreptococcus* and *Peptococcus* organisms, as well as *Fusobacterium.*

Pharmacokinetics. Absorption. Imipenem is not absorbed by the oral route and is only available for intravenous administration. When 500–1000 mg are administered, resultant serum concentrations are in the range of 35–70 μg/ml.

Distribution. The drug is well distributed into most tissues and fluids with 20% binding to serum proteins. It does penetrate the inflamed meninges and concentrations of active drug above the minimum inhibitory concentration (minimum concentration of antibiotic necessary to inhibit growth of a microorganism) of many central nervous system bacterial pathogens can be achieved.

Metabolism and Excretion. Approximately 50% of a dose of imipenem is excreted by the kidneys via glomerular filtration, 25% by tubular secretion, and approximately 25% by nonrenal routes. An extremely unique feature of imipenem is that it is inactivated in the kidney by the enzyme dihydropeptidase, which is found in the brush border of the proximal tubular cells of the kidney. This postexcretory metabolism can be prevented by coadministering the enzyme inhibitor cilastatin. Cilastatin has virtually no antibacterial activity. By inhibiting the dihydropeptidase enzymes in the proximal tubule, the amount of antibacterially active imipenem which is excreted in the urine is markedly increased. The half-life of imipenem is one hour. Dosage adjustments are necessary in patients with renal insufficiency. In addition, both imipenem and cilastatin are removed by hemodialysis, therefore, postdialysis dosing is necessary.

Adverse Reactions. Allergic Reactions. Patients allergic to penicillin antibiotics should be considered allergic to imipenem. Infrequent reactions have included drug fever, urticaria, pruritis, and other rashes.

Local Reactions or Infusion-Related Reactions. Phlebitis, thrombophlebitis, and erythema (redness) have been reported following the intravenous administration of imipenem. Severe nausea and vomiting (which may or may not occur with episodes of hypotension, dizziness, and sweating) have been attributed to infusions of imipenem. This effect is unpredictable and may occur inconsistently in the same patient. Slowing the infusion may be the only intervention necessary; however, the drug may need to be discontinued in selected situations.

Seizures. Seizures have been reported in up to 1.5% of patients receiving imipenem. This adverse effect appears to be more common in elderly patients with renal insufficiency and other predisposing factors such as head injury, intracranial neoplasm, and/or a history of seizures or alcohol abuse. The dose of imipenem also appears to be of importance with respect to this particular adverse effect and should not exceed 2 g/day in the patient at risk.

Drug Interactions. Because of its ability to block the tubular secretion of beta-lactam antibiotics, concomitant administration of probenecid with imipenem will result in increased serum concentrations (and possible toxicity) of imipenem.

AMINOGLYCOSIDES

The inability of penicillin G to inhibit the growth of gram-negative organisms prompted researchers to investigate new antimicrobial agents with activity against these organisms. In 1944, streptomycin a product of *Streptomyces griseus*, was discovered. At first clinically useful, streptomycin resistance has limited its usefulness. Subsequently, neomycin (1949) and kanamycin (1957) [Kantrex] were introduced, but their usefulness was limited by toxicity and the development of resistance. Currently, gentamicin (1964) [Garamycin], tobramycin (1967) [Nebcin], amikacin (1972) [Amikin], and netilmicin (1984) [Netromycin] are the aminoglycosides used for the treatment of gram-negative bacillary infections. Table 46–4 presents the aminoglycosides.

Mechanism of Action

After transport across cell membranes, aminoglycosides act at the 30S bacterial ribosome to interrupt protein synthesis. Although other antibiotics that alter protein synthesis may be bacteriostatic, the effects of aminoglycosides are bactericidal. Bacterial resistance to aminoglycosides may be related to failure to cross or penetrate the cell membrane, altered binding to *ribosomes*, or inactivation by microbial enzymes. When penicillin is added to aminoglycoside therapy, the cell wall is altered (by the penicillin), thus allowing the aminoglycoside to more easily penetrate the cell. This is an excellent example of antibiotic synergy.

Spectrum of Activity

The primary indication for the aminoglycosides is for the treatment of infection caused by aerobic gram-negative bacilli (e.g., enterobacteriaceae). In general, the aminoglycosides have similar activity against gram-negative bacilli; however, certain strains of *Pseudomonas aeruginosa* are more sensitive to tobramycin than to gentamicin. On the other hand, strains of *Serratia marcescens* are more sensitive to gentamicin than to tobramycin. Organisms resistant to gentamicin may be sensitive to netilmicin because of its resistance to bacterial enzyme inactivation. Bacteria resistant to gentamicin, tobramycin, and netilmicin are usually sensitive to amikacin, again because of its structural modification and resultant resistance to bacterial enzyme inactivation. Anaerobic bacteria are resistant to aminoglycosides because the uptake process into the cell is an active process which requires oxygen.

Pharmacokinetics

ABSORPTION. Aminoglycosides are positively charged polar molecules and are poorly absorbed after oral administration. This property is employed clinically when neomycin is prescribed to sterilize the bowel be-

fore surgery. Neomycin is also used to eliminate urease-producing bacteria in patients with hepatic encephalopathy, and thus prevent the absorption of ammonia (the product of urease activity on intestinal urea). Aminoglycosides are absorbed rapidly after intramuscular injection. However, in many situations, aminoglycosides are prescribed for seriously ill patients and IM administration may not produce reliable serum concentrations. In these patients, the intravenous route is preferred.

DISTRIBUTION. Aminoglycosides do not penetrate cell membranes. In the clinical setting, this poor penetration means low aminoglycoside concentrations in bronchial secretions (sputum), cerebrospinal fluid (CSF), and eye fluids. Low CSF concentrations following parenteral administration may require direct injection of these antibiotics into the CSF (intrathecally or intraventricularly). Similarly, in serious eye infections, periocular injections may be indicated. Despite the low concentrations described in the above fluids, aminoglycosides achieve concentrations in peritoneal fluid (e.g., ascites) that are useful for treating peritonitis. Aminoglycoside administration during pregnancy may result in amniotic fluid and fetal plasma exposure to these agents.

METABOLISM AND EXCRETION. Aminoglycosides are eliminated from the body almost entirely by glomerular filtration. There is little if any tubular secretion and no hepatic metabolism. The significant toxicity (ototoxicity and nephrotoxicity) resulting from prolonged tissue accumulation of these agents is the primary reason aminoglycoside dosing must be altered in patients with decreased renal function. The serum half-life of these agents is approximately two hours in patients with normal renal function and may be prolonged up to 50–60 hours in the absence of renal function. In patients with cystic fibrosis, the elimination of aminoglycosides is remarkably fast and the serum half-life is often <2 hours.

Adverse Reactions

PREFERENTIAL OTOTOXICITY. Auditory and vestibular symptoms may occur in patients receiving aminoglycoside therapy. Risk factors for aminoglycoside ototoxicity are impaired renal function, prolonged therapy, and/or concomitant treatment with other ototoxic drugs such as ethacrynic acid (Edecrin) or furosemide (Lasix). High serum concentrations (>10 μg/ml) immediately following an intravenous dose are thought to provide a gradient that drives these agents into ear tissue. This effect is reversible in many patients if recognized early in treatment.

NEPHROTOXICITY. Although there may be substantial differences among the nephrotoxic potentials of the various aminoglycosides used in clinical practice, aminoglycoside serum concentrations and renal function should be monitored closely during therapy. These antibiotics cause injury to the proximal tubular cells of the nephrons and may lead to acute renal failure. Risk factors for nephrotoxicity appear to be age, shock (hypotension), dehydration, preexisting renal disease, or

TEXT RESUMES ON PAGE 1234

Table 46–4. AMINOGLYCOSIDES

Name	Dosage	Mode of Administration	Pharmacokinetics
AMINOGLYCOSIDES			
Action: Inhibit protein synthesis by irreversibly binding to the 30S ribosomal subunit.			
Use: For aerobic gram-negative infections.			
Amikacin (Amikin)	*Adults, children, and older infants:* 7.5 mg/kg q 12 hr	IM, IV	A: none PB: 4%
	Neonates: loading dose 10 mg/kg × 1; maintenance dose, 7.5 mg/kg q 12 hr	IV	½L: 2–3 hr E: renal
Gentamicin (Garamycin)	*Adults:* loading dose, 2 mg/kg × 1; maintenance dose, 1.5 mg/kg q 8 hr	IM, IV	A: none PB: <10% ½L: 2–3 hr.
	Neonates (≤1 wk): 2.5 mg/kg q 12 hr	IM, IV	E: renal
	Older neonates and infants: 2.5 mg/kg q 8 hr	IM, IV	
	Children: 2–2.5 mg/kg q 8 hr.	IM, IV Also available as an: ophthalmic solution (3 mg/ml); ophthalmic ointment (2 mg/g); topical ointment or cream (0.1%); intrathecal injection preparation without preservatives (2 mg/ml).	
Kanamycin (Kantrex)	*Adults and children:* 7.5 mg/kg q 12 hr	IM, IV	A: none PB: <10%
	Hepatic coma: 8–12 g/day in divided doses	PO (500-mg capsules)	½L: 2–3 hr E: renal
	Adjunct to mechanical bowel prep: 1 g q 1hr × 4 hr followed by 1 g q 6 hr × 36–72 hr	PO (500-mg capsules)	
Netilmicin (Netromycin)	*Adults:* 1.3–2.2 mg/kg q 8–12 hr.	IM, IV	A: none PB: 10%
	Infants and children (6 wk–12 yr): 1.8–2.7 mg/kg q 8 hr	IM, IV	½L: 2.3 hr E: renal
	Neonates (<6 wk): 2–3.25 mg/kg q 12 hr	IM, IV	

A-absorption; PB-protein binding; ½L-half-life; E-excretion.
*Within the column of adverse effects, underlines indicate the most common effects; CAPITALS indicate life-threatening effects.

Contraindications/ Precautions	Adverse Effects*	Interactions	Nursing Implications
PRECAUTIONS: Use with caution in patients allergic to aminoglycosides. Use with caution in patients with preexisting renal disease; myasthenia gravis, and/or receiving concomitant renal toxic agents (e.g., amphotericin B, vancomycin)	*Neuro:* auditory and vestibular; NEUROMUSCULAR BLOCKADE *Renal:* NEPHROTOXICITY (e.g., RISING BUN AND SERUM CREATININE) *Integ:* rash	Interferes with SGOT (AST), SGPT (ALT) LDH, bilirubin, calcium, magnesium, sodium, and potassium levels. Causes possible respiratory depression following inhalation anesthetics (e.g., cyclopropane, halothane, nitrous oxide), neuromuscular blocking agents (e.g., tubocurarine, succinylcholine). Increased potential for ototoxicity after ethacrynic acid or furosemide.	ASSESSMENT: Full course of therapy is required; should not be administered by IV push; monitor drug levels. INTERVENTION: None. EVALUATION: check for fever symptoms. WBC count should return to normal. Adverse reactions need to be reported. Monitor BUN and serum creatinine levels; check hearing and balance.
Same as for all aminoglycosides.	Same as for all aminoglycosides.	Same as for all aminoglycosides. Interaction with carbicillin is minimal.	ASSESSMENT: See Aminoglycosides. INTERVENTION: See Aminoglycosides. EVALUATION: Monitor drug levels: peak, <30 μg/ml; trough, <10 μg/ml.
Safe use during pregnancy not established.	Same as for all aminoglycosides.	Microbiologic activity decreased when administered simultaneously with carbenicillin. May be inactivated when coadministered with heparin.	ASSESSMENT: See Aminoglycosides. INTERVENTION: See Aminoglycosides. EVALUATION: Monitor drug levels: peak <10 μg/ml; trough, <2 μg/ml.
Same as for all aminoglycosides.	Same as for all aminoglycosides.	Same as for all aminoglycosides.	ASSESSMENT: See Aminoglycosides. INTERVENTION: See Aminoglycosides. EVALUATION: Monitor drug levels: peak, <30 μg/ml; trough <10 μg/ml.
Same as for all aminoglycosides.	Same as for all aminoglycosides.	Same as for all aminoglycosides.	ASSESSMENT: See Aminoglycosides. INTERVENTION: See Aminoglycosides. EVALUATION: Monitor drug levels: peak <10 μg/ml; trough <2 μg/ml.

CONTINUED ON THE FOLLOWING PAGE

Table 46–4. AMINOGLYCOSIDES–*CONTINUED*

Name	Dosage	Mode of Administration	Pharmacokinetics
Streptomycin	*Tubercular adults:* 1 g/day *Children:* 20–40 mg/kg/day *Bacterial endocarditis:* 0.5–1 g twice daily *Tularemia:* 1–2 g/day *Plague:* 2–4 g/day in divided doses	IM only IM only IM only IM only IM only	A: none PB: 30% ½L: 2–3 hr E: renal
Tobramycin (Nebcin)	*Adults:* loading dose, 2 mg/kg × 1; maintenance dose, 1–1.5 mg/kg q 8 hr *Children:* 2–2.5 mg/kg q 8 hr or 1.5–1.9 mg/kg q 6 hr *Premature or full-term infants (≤4 wk):* 2 mg/kg q 12 hr	IM, IV IM, IV IM, IV Also available as an ophthalmic solution (3 mg/ml); ophthalmic ointment (3 mg/ml).	A: none PB: <10% ½L: 2–3 hr E: renal

A-absorption; PB-protein binding; ½L-half-life; E-excretion.
*Within the column of adverse effects, <u>underlines</u> indicate the most common effects; CAPITALS indicate life-threatening effects.

concurrent administration of other nephrotoxic drugs (e.g., amphotericin B, vancomycin).

NEUROMUSCULAR BLOCKADE. This toxic effect occurs rarely and is thought to be secondary to aminoglycoside-induced inhibition of acetylcholine release. Although uncommon, this effect should be acknowledged, especially in patients with myasthenia gravis, who may be particularly sensitive. In addition, patients receiving neuromuscular blocking agents (e.g., pancuronium bromide) may have prolongation of their paralysis when these agents are used concomitantly with aminoglycosides.

Monitoring Aminoglycoside Therapy

As mentioned previously, the toxicity of aminoglycosides is a primary impetus for close surveillance during treatment. Serum creatinine is the usual marker for detecting changes in a renal function. Damage caused by these agents is usually reflected by an increase in serum creatinine level three to four days later. Therefore, a rising serum creatinine level reflects damage that has already occurred. In many institutions, aminoglycoside serum concentrations are measured routinely. The goal is to obtain a peak serum concentration in the range of 4–10 μg/ml for gentamicin, tobramycin, and netilmicin, and 30–40 μg/ml for kanamycin and amikacin, depending on the pathogen and site of infection. Trough serum concentrations (concentrations before the next dose) should drop below 2 μg/ml for gentamicin, tobramycin, and netilmicin, and below 10 μg/ml for kanamycin and amikacin. Peak serum concentrations should be obtained approximately fifteen minutes after the aminoglycoside infusion has finished and the trough serum concentration should be obtained immediately before the aminoglycoside infusion is started.

Drug Interactions

Concurrent administration of aminoglycosides with high doses of loop diuretics (furosemide, ethacrynic acid, bumetanide) is believed to have additive ototoxic potential. Patients receiving this combination should be monitored by audiometry and for altered vestibular function (e.g., dizziness, lightheadedness).

Clinically, the neuromuscular blocking effects of aminoglycosides are not usually a problem. However, when these agents are administered concurrently with neuromuscular blocking agents (e.g., succinylcholine, pancuronium bromide) the effects may be additive, and respiratory paralysis may occur. Treatment with calcium salts may reverse the impaired respiratory function.

As discussed earlier, penicillins have the potential to inactivate aminoglycosides in certain situations (see the section on drug interactions of penicillins for details of the inactivation process).

SULFONAMIDES

The sulfonamides were the first effective group of antibiotics used for the treatment of bacterial infections in man. Although the azo dye sulfanilamide was discovered in 1908, it was not until 1935 that the first sulfonamide of clinical importance, "prontosil rubrum," was used as an anti-infective agent.

Classification

The sulfonamides are often categorized into groups based upon their rate of absorption and excretion. While not limited to the groups below, some of the more commonly used agents can be classified as:

(1) Short-acting: rapid absorption, rapid excretion; sulfisoxazole (Gantrisin), sulfadiazine.

A
m
i
n
o
g
l
y
c
o
s
i
d
e
s

Contraindications/ Precautions	Adverse Effects*	Interactions	Nursing Implications
Same as for all aminoglycosides. Safe use in pregnancy has not been established.	Same as for all aminoglycosides.	Same as for all aminoglycosides.	*ASSESSMENT:* For IM administration only. *INTERVENTION:* See Aminoglycosides. *EVALUATION:* See Aminoglycosides.
Same as for all aminoglycosides.	Same as for all aminoglycosides.	Same as for all aminoglycosides.	*ASSESSMENT:* See Aminoglycosides. *INTERVENTION:* See Aminoglycosides. *EVALUATION:* Monitor drug levels: peak <10 μg/ml; trough, <2 μg/ml.

(2) Medium-acting: rapid absorption, slow excretion; sulfamethoxazole (Gantanol).

(3) Ultra–long-acting: used in combination with pyrimethamine for the treatment of malaria; sulfadoxine (Fansidar).

The dosage recommendations for the various sulfonamides are listed in Table 46–5.

Mechanism of Action

Bacterial and human cells use folic acid derivatives to build purines, which are essential components in the synthesis of DNA. Human cells are able to use folic acid present in the diet, whereas bacteria must synthesize folate from *para-aminobenzoic acid* (PABA). The biochemical conversion of PABA to folate involves a sequence of steps, each catalyzed by the enzyme dihydrofolic acid synthetase. Because sulfonamides are structurally similar to PABA, they compete for this enzyme. The net result of this competition is a decrease in the synthesis of folic acid and suppression of purine synthesis. Without the building blocks of DNA, the bacterial cell is unable to survive and death ensues. Sulfamethoxazole, has been combined with another antibiotic, trimethoprim. Trimethoprim is able to compete with another enzyme, *tetrahydrofolic acid reductase*, in the chain of events leading up to the synthesis of folic acid. This "sequential" inhibition of the folic acid pathway has markedly enhanced the activity of each component of the drug combination.

Spectrum of Activity

The sulfonamides were originally very effective antibiotics; however, their clinical value presently is limited by the development of bacterial resistance. The mechanism of resistance to these agents is probably through a modification of the enzyme sequence leading to folic acid production. Gram-positive cocci such as *Streptococcus pyogenes* and *Streptococcus pneumoniae* are usually sensitive, but enterococci are resistant. Of the gram-positive bacilli, *Bacillus anthracis* and *Clostridium perfringens* are sensitive. Enteric gram-negative bacilli such as *Escherichia coli, Enterobacter, Klebsiella, Proteus, Salmonella,* and *Shigella* species are sensitive. *Hemophilus influenzae* (type b), *Pseudomonas pseudomallei*, and some strains of *Pseudomonas aeruginosa* are also sensitive. The pathogenic *Neisseria* species (gonococci and meningococci) are inhibited by sulfonamides, but because of increasing resistance, sulfonamides are not recommended for these infections.

Sulfonamides are active against *Chlamydia trachomatis* (the causative organism of lymphogranuloma venereum, trachoma, and inclusion body conjunctivitis) but not against *C. psittaci*, which causes psittacosis.

Pharmacokinetics

ABSORPTION. There are a group of poorly absorbed sulfonamides (e.g., sulfaguanidine), which are used for their local antibacterial effect in the lower gastrointestinal tract. These drugs are rarely used. All other sulfonamides are well absorbed (70%–100%) after oral administration.

DISTRIBUTION. Following absorption, they are distributed throughout all body fluids with good penetration into pleural, peritoneal, synovial, and ocular fluids. Sulfonamides also diffuse into the cerebrospinal fluid, cross the placenta, and reach the fetal circulation.

METABOLISM AND EXCRETION. Sulfonamides are eliminated from the body by hepatic metabolism, as well as, by renal excretion. The largest percentage of sulfonamide is excreted by the kidney, therefore, dosage adjustments must be made in patients with renal insufficiency. In addition, the possibility of sulfonamide crystal formation in the urinary tract exists and patients should be encouraged to drink at least 1000 ml of water each day during treatment.

Table 46–5. SULFONAMIDES

Name	Dosage	Mode of Administration	Pharmacokinetics
SULFONAMIDES			
Action: Act as PABA antagonists and inhibit susceptible microorganisms.			
Use: For treating urinary tract infections due to common gram-negative rods.			
Sulfadiazine	*Adults:* 2–4 g/day in 3–6 divided doses	PO	A: 70%–100%
	Children >2 mo: 150 mg/kg/day in 4–6 divided doses	PO	P: 3–7 hr PB: 20% ½L: 13 hr M: liver
	Children ≤2 mo: 100–150 mg/kg/day in 4–6 divided doses	PO	E: kidney
Sulfadoxine (only available in combination with pyrimethamine—Fansidar)			
Sulfamethoxazole (Gantanol)	*Adults:* 1 g 2–3 times daily *Children >2 mo:* 25–30 mg/kg morning and evening	PO PO (Also available as a suspension, 500 mg/5 ml)	A: 70%–100% P: 3–7 hr PB: 65% ½L: 9 hr M: liver E: kidney
Sulfisoxazole (Gantrisin)	*Adults:* 4–8 g/day in 4–6 divided doses *Children and infants >2 mo:* 150 mg/kg/day in 4–6 divided doses	PO PO (Also available as syrup/suspension, 500 mg/5 ml)	A: 70%–100% P: 2–4 hr PB: 90% ½L: 5–6 hr M: liver (30%) E: kidney
Trimethoprim/Sulfamethoxazole (Bactrim, Septra)	For UTI, shigellosis, acute otitis media: *Adults:* 160 mg TMP/SMZ q 12 hr or 8–10 mg/kg TMP/SMZ q 6–12 hr *Children >2 mo:* 8 mg/kg/day TMP/SMZ q 12 hr For *Pneumocystis carinii* pneumonia: *Adults and children >2 mo:* 15–20 mg/kg/day in 4 divided doses (doses as TMP component)	 PO PO, IV PO, IV	A: 70%–100% P: 1–4 hr PB: TMP, 50%; SMZ, 65% ½L: TMP, 10 hr; SMZ, 9 hr M: TMP, liver; SMZ, liver E: kidney

A-absorption; PB-protein binding; ½L-serum half-life; M-metabolism; E-excretion; UA-unavailable.
*Within the column of adverse effects, underlines indicate the most common effects; CAPITALS indicate life-threatening effects.

Sulfonamides

Contraindications/ Precautions	Adverse Effects*	Interactions	Nursing Implications
CONTRAINDICATIONS: Sulfonamide allergy or previous toxicity (e.g., bone marrow, kidney, liver). Avoid in newborns and during pregnancy or during breast feeding. *PRECAUTIONS:* Use with caution in patients with decreased renal function.	*Neuro:* fever *GI:* nausea, vomiting *Biliary:* hepatitis *Hemo:* anemia, agranulocytosis, thrombocytopenia, eosinophilia *Renal:* crystalluria *Integ:* joint pains, arthritis, rash, photosensitivity	May interfere with BSP, PSP, thyroid function, urine glucose, and protein tests. Interactions with oral anticoagulants, hypoglycemic agents, and phenytoin.	*ASSESSMENT:* Fluid intake should be high; CBC should be done every 2 weeks. *INTERVENTION:* Patient should avoid sunlight or ultraviolet light. *EVALUATION:* Evaluate for fever and symptoms. Check WBC count. Adverse reactions should be reported.
Same as for all sulfonamides.	Same as for all sulfonamides.	Same as for all sulfonamides.	Same as for all sulfonamides.
Same as for all sulfonamides.	Same as for all sulfonamides.	Same as for all sulfonamides.	Same as for all sulfonamides.
Same as for all sulfonamides.	Same as for all sulfonamides.	Same as for all sulfonamides.	Same as for all sulfonamides.
Same as for all sulfonamides.	Same as for all sulfonamides.	Same as for all sulfonamides.	Same as for all sulfonamides.
Same as for all sulfonamides.	Same as for all sulfonamides.	Same as for all sulfonamides including interactions with methotrexate, thiazide diuretics, and cyclosporine.	Same as for all sulfonamides.

Adverse Reactions

HYPERSENSITIVITY REACTIONS. Rashes are common during sulfonamide treatment and may be life-threatening. The most common rashes are maculopapular or urticarial; however, more serious reactions like erythema nodosum or exfoliative dermatitis may also occur. The most serious form of cutaneous hypersensitivity is the Stevens-Johnson Syndrome, consisting of erythema and ulceration of the mucous membranes (eyes, mouth, and urethra). This syndrome has been described with all sulfonamides. Serum sickness and drug fever are also noted during treatment with these agents. It should be pointed out that patients with the acquired immunodeficiency syndrome (AIDS) are more likely to develop rashes secondary to sulfonamide therapy than are patients without AIDS.

HEMATOPOIETIC DISORDERS. Acute hemolytic anemia may occur in patients whose red blood cells are sensitized due to a lack of a specific enzyme, *glucose-6-phosphate dehydrogenase* (G-6-PD deficiency). Agranulocytosis or aplastic anemia can occur during sulfonamide therapy because of a direct toxic effect on bone marrow. Both of these reactions are uncommon; however, if they occur, prompt discontinuation of the offending drug is essential.

URINARY TRACT ABNORMALITIES. The deposition of the sulfonamide crystals within the tissue of the urinary tract is a concern during treatment with these agents. Maintenance of adequate fluid intake (>1000 ml/day) and in certain situations, alkalinization of the urine (to increase solubility), will prevent *crystalluria*.

HEPATITIS. Rarely, focal or diffuse necrosis of the liver secondary to direct toxicity or hypersensitivity may occur. Immediate drug withdrawal is recommended.

Drug Interactions

Patients receiving oral anticoagulants who have trimethoprim-sulfamethoxazole added to their therapy may experience a further prolongation of the prothrombin time and increased risk of bleeding. This interaction is thought to occur because the trimethoprim-sulfamethoxazole inhibits the metabolism of warfarin, thus potentiating the anticoagulant effect.

The combination of sulfonamides and oral hypoglycemic agents (e.g., tolbutamide and chlorpropamide) may lead to excessive decreases in blood sugar. The exact mechanism and incidence of this interaction are unclear, but patients taking these agents should be monitored closely.

Patients who are stabilized on anticonvulsant therapy with phenytoin may experience signs of phenytoin toxicity (e.g., nystagmus, ataxia) when sulfonamides are prescribed concurrently. Close observation for phenytoin toxicity is important when these agents are used together.

Trimethoprim-Sulfamethoxazole

This combination of a sulfonamide (sulfamethoxazole) and a folic acid antagonist (trimethoprim) has been available in the United Kingdom since 1968 as co-trimoxazole. The combination was introduced into the United States in 1974 as Bactrim or Septra. While fixed combination products should generally be avoided, this combination of two antibacterial agents was developed to promote the synergistic effect against certain bacteria (see Table 46–4).

SPECTRUM OF ACTIVITY. Trimethoprim (TMP) is more active than sulfamethoxazole (SMZ) against most

bacteria and, for the most part, TMP/SMZ is aimed at aerobic gram-negative bacteria (e.g., enterobacteriaceae); however, gram-positive organisms (*S. aureus, S. epidermidis, S. pneumoniae, S. pyogenes, Listeria monocytogenes), Nocardia asteroides*, and the protozoal organism *Pneumocystis carinii*, are also susceptible. When present in combination, TMP and SMZ will frequently inhibit organisms at much lower concentrations of each drug than would be inhibitory individually. For most organisms the ratio of the two drugs that produces maximum *synergy* is equal to 1:20 (TMP:SMZ) in plasma.

Mechanism of Action. The combination of trimethoprim and sulfamethoxazole can be bacteriostatic against certain organisms (e.g., *Hemophilus influenzae*) or bactericidal (e.g., *E. coli, P. mirabilis, Morganella morganii*). The sequential action of sulfonamides and trimethoprim explains the synergistic actions of this combination against sensitive bacteria. The ultimate target of chemotherapy with TMP/SMZ is the pool of tetrahydrofolic acid cofactors in the microbial cell. The objective is to reduce the size of this pool to a level that is inadequate for the functions essential to the growth and survival of the bacteria. The mechanisms of action of the sulfonamides is discussed above and the mechanism of action of trimethoprim is to competitively inhibit the conversion of dihydrofolic acid to tetrahydrofolic acid by the enzyme dihydrofolic acid reductase. The combination of TMP/SMZ is superior to either component alone in several important ways. It is more potent and has a broadened spectrum of activity, it is more widely bactericidal, and it is less susceptible to the emergence of resistant organisms.

PHARMACOKINETICS. *Absorption.* Both components are well absorbed from the gastrointestinal tract and peak serum concentrations are reached in two hours for TMP and four hours for SMZ. The administration of these drugs in a 1:5 ratio (TMP:SMZ) results in serum concentration ratios of approximately 1:20 (TMP:SMZ). After an oral dose of TMP/SMZ (160 mg/800 mg), peak serum concentrations of 1–2 μg/ml and 30–50 μg/ml are reached for TMP and SMZ, respectively. After a 1-hour intravenous infusion of TMP/SMZ (160 mg/800 mg), peak serum concentrations of 3–4 μg/ml and 45–50 μg/ml are reached for TMP and SMZ, respectively.

Distribution. Once absorbed, TMP and active SMZ are 50% and 65% protein bound, respectively. TMP is much more widely distributed than SMZ and cerebrospinal fluid (CSF) studies have found 50% and 30% of the serum level of TMP and SMZ, respectively, are achieved in the CSF. Therapeutic concentrations of both drugs are found in other body fluids such as bile and sputum.

Metabolism and Excretion. The liver metabolizes approximately 5%–15% of TMP and 25%–30% of SMZ to microbiologically inactive metabolites. The half-life of each component is ten hours for TMP and nine hours for SMZ. The kidneys are the major elimination organ for this drug combination. Since both drugs are eliminated to a large extent by the kidneys, dosage reductions are necessary in renal insufficiency. TMP/SMZ is removed by hemodialysis and patients should receive a normal dose after each dialysis procedure.

ADVERSE REACTIONS. See under Sulfonamides.

DRUG INTERACTIONS. See under Sulfonamides.

ERYTHROMYCINS

Erythromycin (E-Mycin, Erythrocin, Ilosone, Ilotycin, Pediamycin) is a member of the macrolide group of antibiotics and was first isolated from *Streptomyces erythraeus* in 1952. Other members of the macrolide group of antibacterial agents are carbomycin, oleandomycin, troleandomycin, and spiramycin; these agents will not be the focus of this discussion (see Table 46–6).

Mechanism of Action

Erythromycin penetrates the cell wall of sensitive bacteria and reversibly binds to the 50S ribosomal subunit, thereby inhibiting *translocation,* a step in polypeptide chain formation. A single molecule of erythromycin attaches to each ribosomal fragment. This ribosomal binding fails to occur in resistant bacteria. Both bacteriostatic and bactericidal activity can be seen with erythromycin and depends upon the microorganism and the drug concentration.

Spectrum of Activity

The antimicrobial activity of erythromycin is similar to that of penicillin G, with some notable exceptions. Erythromycin is active against most gram-positive microorganisms; however, its gram-negative activity is much less impressive, particularly against aerobic gram-negative rods. In fact, erythromycin is not active against most aerobic gram-negative rods. While staphylococci are usually sensitive to erythromycin, one must realize that hospital-acquired *Staphylococcus aureus* are frequently more erythromycin-resistant. Both *Streptococcus pneumoniae* and Group A, B, C, and G streptococci are quite sensitive to erythromycin; however, resistant strains have been reported. Approximately 90% of *Streptococcus faecalis* (enterococcus, Group D) strains are sensitive to erythromycin. Several other gram-position microorganisms are sensitive to this drug including *Clostridium perfringens* and *Listeria monocytogenes.* Moderate activity can be demonstrated against *Hemophilus influenzae* and *Neisseria meningitidis.* Excellent activity against *Neisseria gonorrhoeae* has been shown. Erythromycin has variable activity against anaerobic gram-negative bacteria and concentrations required to effectively treat infections secondary to such pathogens need to be high and are only attained by parenteral administration. Erythromycin is very active against *Mycoplasma pneumoniae, Legionella pneumophilia, Treponema pallidum, Campylobacter fetus* subspecies *jejuni,* and *Chlamydia trachomatis.*

Pharmacokinetics

ABSORPTION. Erythromycin base and stearate are susceptible to inactivation by gastric acid resulting in decreased absorption following oral administration. To overcome this problem, modifications of the drug have proceeded in two directions. One involves protecting the base with an enteric coating and the other involves altering the chemical structure to decrease acid inactivation by preparing an ester (ethylsuccinate) and the lauryl sulfate of the propionyl ester (estolate). Intramuscular administration results in erratic absorption and pain.

DISTRIBUTION. Erythromycin derivatives diffuse into all tissues well except the brain and cerebrospinal fluid, where therapeutic concentrations are barely achieved even in the presence of inflammation. The drug is concentrated in the liver and excreted in bile in concentrations greater than those in serum. Penetration into the prostate is on the order of approximately 40% of a simultaneous serum concentration. Bronchial secretions, and middle ear and sinus fluids achieve levels of erythromycin which are in excess of the inhibitory concentrations of several pathogens causing community-acquired pneumonias, otitis media, or acute sinusitis. Protein binding is approximately 65%. This agent crosses the placental barrier and attains a fetal plasma concentrations up to 20% of those in maternal circulation.

METABOLISM AND EXCRETION. The serum half-life of erythromycin is approximately 1.4 hours. Concentrations of erythromycin are high in the feces but are quite variable in the urine (2.5%, oral administration; 12%–15%, intravenous administration). Because of its minimal dependence on the kidney for elimination, dosage alterations are usually unnecessary in patients with renal insufficiency. Hemodialysis and peritoneal dialysis have no effect on erythromycin elimination. Depending upon the extent of liver dysfunction, the erythromycin dosage may require reduction in patients with both renal and hepatic disease.

Adverse Reactions

GASTROINTESTINAL EFFECTS. Gastrointestinal symptoms such as nausea, vomiting, epigastric distress, and diarrhea are dose-related side effects often experienced with erythromycin.

PHLEBITIS. Other dose-related side effects are phlebitis and a burning sensation at the site of intravenous infusion. This adverse reaction can be prevented by diluting erythromycin in at least 100 ml of diluent (e.g., normal saline or 5% dextrose) and infusing the dose over one hour or more.

HYPERSENSITIVITY REACTIONS AND HEPATITIS. Side effects unrelated to the dose of erythromycin include hypersensitivity reactions (e.g., skin rash, drug fever, eosinophilia) and hepatotoxicity (e.g., cholestatic jaundice). The hepatotoxicity occurs with the estolate and the ethylsuccinate forms of the drug. It can occur in both adults and children in approximately 10–20 days after initial exposure and within hours after subsequent exposures to erythromycin. Clinically, abdominal pain, nausea and vomiting, jaundice, acholic (clay-colored) stools, dark urine, right upper quadrant tenderness and

TEXT RESUMES ON PAGE 1242

Table 46–6. MISCELLANEOUS ANTIBIOTICS

Name	Dosage	Mode of Administration	Pharmacokinetics
ERYTHROMYCINS			
Action: Inhibits protein synthesis by irreversibly binding to 50S ribosomal subunit.			
Use: For treating gram-positive infections in penicillin-allergic patients; drug of choice for Legionnaire's disease and *Mycoplasma* pneumonia.			
Erythromycin base	*Adults:* 250–500 mg q 6–12 hr (up to 4 g/day) *Children:* 30–50 mg/kg/day in divided doses.	PO (tablets)	A: 60% P: 1–4 hr PB: 65% ½L: 1.4 hr E: bile, kidney
Erythromycin Ethylsuccinate (EES)	*Adults:* 400 mg q 6 hr *Children:* 30–50 mg/kg/day	PO (Also available as chewable tablets, oral suspension)	
Erythromycin Estolate	*Adults:* 250 mg q 6 hr *Children:* 30–50 mg/kg/day	PO (Also available as a chewable tablet, drops, or suspension)	
Erythromycin Gluceptate and Lactobionate	*Adults:* 500–1000 mg q 6 hr *Children:* 30–50 mg/kg/day	IV	
Erythromycin Stearate	*Adults:* 250–500 mg q 6–12 hr *Children:* 30–50 mg/kg/day	PO	
Clindamycin (Cleocin)			
Use: Primary antibiotic for treating anaerobic infections.			
	Adults: 150–450 mg q 6 hr; 300–900 mg q 6–8 hr. *Children:* 8–20 mg/kg/day in 3–4 divided doses 15–40 mg/kg day in 3–4 divided doses	PO IM, IV PO IM, IV, topical application	A: 90% P: 45–60 min PB: 93% ½L: 2–3 hr E: liver, feces, bile, urine
Chloramphenicol (Chloromycetin)			
Use: Broad-spectrum antibiotic for aerobic and anaerobic gram-positive and gram-negative infections.			
–Sodium Succinate	*Adults and children:* 50–100 mg/kg/day in divided doses q 6 hrs *Newborns:* 25–50 mg/kg/day in divided doses q 6 hr	IV IV	A: rapid and complete PB: 60% ½L: 1.5–3.5 hr E: liver, urine

A-absorption; PB-protein binding; ½L-half-life; E-excretion.
*Within the column listing adverse effects, underlines indicate the most common effects; CAPITALS indicate life-threatening effects.

Contraindications/ Precautions	Adverse Effects*	Interactions	Nursing Implications
CONTRAINDICATIONS: Prior history of allergy. PRECAUTIONS: Safe use in pregnancy and lactation not established. Use cautiously in hepatic dysfunction.	*Neuro:* hearing loss *GI:* nausea, vomiting, dyspepsia *Biliary:* hepatitis	Erythromycin derivatives may decrease the metabolism of theophylline, corticosteroids, carbamazepine, phenytoin, digoxin.	*ASSESSMENT:* Avoid IM injections as they are very painful. *INTERVENTION:* Patient should avoid taking medication with food. *EVALUATION:* Check for fever and symptoms. Check WBC count. Adverse reactions must be reported.
Same as for all erythromycins.	Same as for all erythromycins.	Same as for all erythromycins.	See above.
Same as for all erythromycins.	Same as for all erythromycins.	May interfere with ALT. Causes false increase in urinary steroids and catecholamines.	See above.
Same as for all erythromycins.	Same as for all erythromycins.	Has cross-resistance with clindamycin.	See above.
Same as for all erythromycins.	Same as for all erythromycins.	Same as for all erythromycins.	See above.
CONTRAINDICATIONS: Prior allergic reactions. *PRECAUTIONS:* Safety in pregnancy and lactation not established.	*GI:* nausea, vomiting, diarrhea, PSEUDOMEMBRANOUS COLITIS (e.g., abdominal cramping, fever, mucus in stool, watery diarrhea)	Increases serum alkaline phosphatase, bilirubin, CPK, ALT, AST levels. Enhances neuromuscular blocking action.	*ASSESSMENT:* Observe for severe diarrhea. *INTERVENTION:* Patient should be instructed to report first signs of severe diarrhea. *EVALUATION:* Evaluate for fever and symptoms. Check WBC count. Adverse reactions should be reported.
CONTRAINDICATIONS: Prior hypersensitivity. *PRECAUTIONS:* Safety during pregnancy not	*Neuro:* optic neuritis, blurred vision *CVR:* GRAY BABY SYNDROME *Resp:* GRAY BABY SYNDROME	False-positive urine glucose (Clinitest). May interfere with urine steroid determination and urobilinogen	*ASSESSMENT:* Avoid IV infiltration; watch for signs of agranulocytosis (fever, sore throat).

CONTINUED ON THE FOLLOWING PAGE

Table 46–6. MISCELLANEOUS ANTIBIOTICS–*CONTINUED*

Name	Dosage	Mode of Administration	Pharmacokinetics
Sodium Succinate–*Continued*	*Neonates:* <2 kg, 25 mg/kg once daily; >7 days of age, >2 kg—50 mg/kg/day in divided doses q 12 hr; ≤7 days of age, >2 kg—50 mg/kg once daily	IV	
–Palmitate	Dosage as above	PO (oral suspension, 150 mg/5 ml)	
	Capsules: dosage as above	PO (250 mg, 500 mg)	
	Ophthalmic ointment	Topical	
	Otic drops	Topical (0.5%)	
	Cream	Topical (1%)	
Vancomycin (Vancocin, Vancoled, Lyphocin)			
Use: For treating *S. aureus, S. epidermidis*, methicillin-resistant *S. aureus*, and enterococcal infections. Orally, for treating *C. difficile* diarrhea only.			
	Adults: 125–500 mg q 6–8 hrs	PO	A: <1% P: UA
	Children: 40 mg/kg/day in 4 divided doses	PO	PB:52%–56% ½L: 6 hr
	Neonates: 10 mg/kg/day in divided doses	PO	E: renal
	Adults: 500 mg–1 g q 6–12 hr	IV	
	Children >1 mo: 10–15 mg/kg q 6 hr	IV	
	Infants: ≤7 days: 10 mg/kg q 12 hr	IV	
	Infants ≤1 mo: 10 mg/kg q 8 hr	IV	
Metronidazole (Flagyl)			
Use: Anaerobic bacterial infections.			
	Adults: 500 mg–1 g q 6 hr	IV	A: 80%–100%
	For amebiasis: *Adults:* 750 mg 3 times daily for 10 days	PO	P: 1–3 hr PB: 20%
	For trichomoniasis: *Adults:* 2 g × 1 (single dose regimen) or 250 mg 3 times daily × 7 days	PO (tablets)	½L: 6–8 hr E: liver

A-absorption; PB-protein binding; ½L-serum half-life; E-excretion.
*Within the column of adverse effects, underlines indicate the most common effects; CAPITALS indicate life-threatening effects.

an enlarged liver are present. Laboratory abnormalities include increased white blood cells, increased number of eosinophils (eosinophilia), and elevated bilirubin, alkaline phosphatase, SGOT, and SGPT levels. This is a reversible adverse reaction.

OTOTOXICITY. Erythromycin has been reported to cause tinnitus, vertigo, and transient hearing loss. The majority of cases of hearing loss have occurred follow-

ing intravenous administration. The time of onset is within thirty-six hours to one week and recovery occurs within twenty-four hours to two weeks after discontinuation of the drug. Recovery time is not dose-related. All reported cases of ototoxicity secondary to erythromycin have been reversible. Patients receiving large doses, patients with renal and/or hepatic dysfunction, the elderly, and women seem to be at greatest risk. The

Contraindications/ Precautions	Adverse Effects*	Interactions	Nursing Implications
established. Use cautiously with impaired hepatic function, newborns and children, and G-6-PD deficiency.	*GI:* nausea, vomiting *Biliary:* jaundice *Hemo:* APLASTIC ANEMIA, reversible anemia (bone marrow depression can be irreversible) *Integ:* rash, superinfections	excretion. May prolong half-life of: coumadin; oral hypoglycemic agents (e.g., chlorpropamide, tolbutamide); phenytoin. Phenobarbital may increase the metabolism of chloramphenicol. May decrease response to vitamin B_{12}.	*INTERVENTION:* Report any signs of fever or sore throat while taking medication. *EVALUATION:* Evaluate for fever and symptoms. Check WBC count. Report any adverse reactions.
CONTRAINDICATIONS: Prior history of hypersensitivity reactions. *PRECAUTIONS:* Safe use during pregnancy not established. Do not administer by intramuscular route.	*Neuro:* ototoxicity *CVR:* red neck syndrome (hypotension, flushing); phlebitis *Hemo:* leukopenia, eosinophilia *Renal:* nephrotoxicity *Integ:* rash, superinfections	Additive toxicity with other nephro-/ototoxic drugs (e.g., aminoglycosides, furosemide, ethacrynic acid).	*ASSESSMENT:* Avoid IV infiltration. Do not administer IM. Infuse drug over at least 60 minutes. *INTERVENTION:* Remind patient to report any signs of rash. *EVALUATION:* Evaluate for fever and symptoms. Check WBC count. Report any adverse reactions.
CONTRAINDICATIONS: Prior hypersensitivity reactions. *PRECAUTIONS:* Use cautiously during pregnancy and in nursing mothers. Avoid the concomitant use of alcohol-containing products.	*Neuro:* dizziness, vertigo, numbness or tingling in extremities *CVR:* ECG changes *GI:* nausea, metallic taste *Hemo:* neutropenia *Renal:* dark urine *Integ:* rash	Disulfiram (Antabuse)-like reaction with ethanol. Coumadin metabolism may be inhibited.	*ASSESSMENT:* Give with food to decrease GI distress; do not give IV bolus. *INTERVENTION:* Instruct patient to take medication with food. *EVALUATION:* Evaluate for fever and symptoms. Check WBC count. Report any adverse reactions.

concomitant administration of other ototoxic agents (e.g., furosemide, aminoglycosides) also contribute to the ototoxic potential of erythromycin.

Drug Interactions

The common setting for the interaction between erythromycin and theophylline is in a patient with chronic lung disease receiving theophylline therapy who develops acute bronchitis or pneumonia and has erythromycin added to the drug regimen. Erythromycin inhibits the metabolism of theophylline and may precipitate

signs of theophylline toxicity (e.g., tachycardia, nervousness, nausea). Patients stabilized on theophylline and requiring erythromycin should be monitored clinically and/or with theophylline serum concentrations.

Erythromycin may also decrease the metabolism of corticosteroids, resulting in enhanced steroid effects. The dosage of the steroid may need to be reduced when erythromycin is prescribed concurrently.

Likewise, erythromycin inhibits the breakdown of phenytoin and carbamazepine and toxicity may be precipitated by the addition of this antibiotic. Patients receiving both of these agents may experience nausea, vomiting, nystagmus, or ataxia, and require dosage reduction of carbamazepine or phenytoin.

Digoxin is partially metabolized by bacteria in the gastrointestinal tract. When the normal flora are altered by erythromycin ingestion, the amount of digoxin that is absorbed may increase. This increased amount of digoxin may induce toxicity depending on the patient's status before antibiotic administration. When a patient who is stabilized on digoxin requires erythromycin, the patient should be observed for signs of digoxin toxicity (anorexia, nausea, vomiting, green-yellow vision, bradycardia).

CLINDAMYCIN AND LINCOMYCIN

Lincomycin (Lincocin) is produced by *Streptomyces lincolnensis* and was first isolated in soil collected near Lincoln, Nebraska. Subsequently, chemical modification produced clindamycin (7-chloro-7-deoxy-lincomycin), a microbiologically more active antibiotic with fewer side effects. There are only limited indications for lincomycin; therefore, only clindamycin (Cleocin) will be discussed in the following section (see Table 46–6).

Spectrum of Activity

Clindamycin, like erythromycin, has activity against most gram-positive organisms including *Staphylococcus aureus, Staphylococcus epidermidis, Streptococcus pneumoniae, Streptococcus pyogenes,* and *Streptococcus viridans.* Organisms resistant to erythromycin are usually resistant to clindamycin. Clindamycin is inactive against *Streptococcus faecalis* and has virtually no activity against *Neisseria meningitidis, Neisseria gonorrhoeae,* or *Hemophilus influenzae.* The anaerobic spectrum of clindamycin is its major strong point. Anaerobic microorganisms (gram-positive and gram-negative, cocci and rods) above (respiratory tract) and below (abdomen and pelvis) the diaphram are usually susceptible to clindamycin. Most *Bacteroides* species (e.g., *B. fragilis*) are inhibited by clindamycin; however, resistance in up to 7% of clinical isolates have been reported. *Peptostreptococcus, Eubacterium, Propionobacterium, Bifidobacterium* species, and *Actinomyces israelii* are usually sensitive. Most strains of *Clostridium perfringens* and peptococcus are susceptible, although occasional isolates are resistant. It is important to emphasize that clindamycin is not active against aerobic, gram-negative bacilli (e.g., *E. coli, Proteus mirabilis*).

Mechanism of Action

Clindamycin inhibits bacterial protein synthesis by binding to the 50S ribosomal subunit (site of action similar to erythromycin and chloramphenicol).

Pharmacokinetics

ABSORPTION. Clindamycin may be administered orally as the hydrochloride salt (capsules) and the ester suspension (palmitate) or parenterally as the phosphate ester. Oral absorption is complete with peak serum concentrations attained within one to two hours of inges-

tion. Food does not significantly interfere with drug absorption. The palmitate ester suspension is inactive and must be activated (hydrolyzed) *in vivo.* Absorption is similar to that of the hydrochloride salt. Parenteral administration is usually well tolerated and like the palmitate ester, the phosphate ester must be activated in vivo (i.e., before microbiological activity can be exerted, both the phosphate and palmitate constituents must be removed from the parent drug). Peak serum concentrations following intramuscular administration are reached in three hours (one hour in children).

DISTRIBUTION. Significant concentrations of clindamycin can be found in pleural and peritoneal fluid; however, in the absence of inflammation, penetration into the cerebrospinal fluid is poor. High biliary concentrations can be seen; however, in the presence of common bile duct obstruction, no drug can be detected. The drug readily crosses the placental barrier.

METABOLISM AND EXCRETION. Clindamycin is metabolically altered in the liver to two major (microbiologically active) metabolites. Both of these metabolites and the parent drug are eliminated in bile and urine. Only about 10% of an administered dose is excreted unchanged in the urine with a small percentage (<5%) appearing in the feces. Since the half-life of clindamycin (two to three hours) is minimally prolonged in patients with renal insufficiency, alterations in dosage are only necessary in anuric individuals. Patients with liver disease have prolonged serum half-lives and dosage reductions may be indicated for individuals with severe hepatic disease.

Adverse Reactions

THROMBOPHLEBITIS. Local thrombophlebitis may occur following intravenous administration, and skin rash is noted in 10% of patients receiving clindamycin.

DIARRHEA AND PSEUDOMEMBRANOUS COLITIS. The most notable problem associated with clindamycin therapy is antibiotic-associated diarrhea and pseudomembranous colitis. These complications are not unique to clindamycin and are seen with numerous broad-spectrum antibiotics (e.g., ampicillin, cephalosporins). The effects of an antibiotic on normal colonic flora are to allow overgrowth of *Clostridium difficile,* which produces a powerful toxin. If significant diarrhea or colitis persists, the offending antibiotic should be discontinued. More serious cases may require administration of oral metronidazole or vancomycin.

CHLORAMPHENICOL

Chloramphenicol (Chloromycetin), first identified as a natural product of *Streptomyces venezuelae,* was discovered by Burkholder and coworkers in 1947. In 1948, its structure and a method of chemically synthesizing the drug were elucidated. The drug is marketed under the name of Chloromycetin because its structure contains a chlorine atom and is produced by an actinomycetes (Table 46–6). Chloramphenicol proved to be extremely useful for certain bacterial and rickettsial infections. In 1950, reports of fatal blood disorders induced by chloramphenicol began to appear. This agent is still prescribed in various clinical settings, with its primary indications related to infections caused by ampicillin-resistant strains of *Hemophilus influenzae* or by *Bacteroides fragilis*.

Mechanism of Action

Chloramphenicol is primarily a bacteriostatic agent which enters bacterial cells and blocks protein synthesis by reversible inhibition of the peptidyl transferase reaction at the 50S ribosomal subunit. It is generally accepted that chloramphenicol does not inhibit protein synthesis in mammalian cells by the same mechanism as in bacterial cells. While bacteriostatic for many bacteria, it is bactericidal against *Hemophilus influenzae*, *Neisseria meningitidis*, and *Streptococcus pneumoniae*. Resistance occurs when bacteria produce enzymes (e.g., acetyl transferase) which inactivate chloramphenicol.

Spectrum of Activity

Chloramphenicol is a broad-spectrum antibiotic that has activity against both aerobic and anaerobic gram-positive and gram-negative microorganisms as well as *Rickettsia*, *Chlamydia*, and *Mycoplasma* species. Microorganisms considered almost "always susceptible" are *Streptococcus pneumoniae*, Group A beta-hemolytic streptococci, *Streptococcus viridans*, *Streptococcus faecalis* (enterococcus), *Neisseria* species, *Hemophilus* species, *Listeria monocytogenes*, and virtually all obligate (strict) anaerobes. The organisms that display variable sensitivity to chloramphenicol are certain strains of staphylococci, and the enterobacteriaceae (gastrointestinal flora). *Pseudomonas aeruginosa* is resistant to this agent.

Pharmacokinetics

ABSORPTION. Chloramphenicol is well absorbed when given orally, and peak serum concentrations are comparable to those following intravenous administration of chloramphenicol succinate. The oral formulations of chloramphenicol include a tasteless, palmitate ester suspension and chloramphenicol base in capsular form. The suspension is not microbiologically active until the palmitate ester is removed from the parent drug (this hydrolytic reaction occurs in the duodenum) and the "free" chloramphenicol is than absorbed into the blood stream. Intramuscular injection of the succinate form of the drug is accompanied by slow, erratic absorption and is not recommended.

DISTRIBUTION. Chloramphenicol distributes into most body tissues and fluids. Chloramphenicol penetrates ocular fluid and the cerebrospinal fluid ($\geq$50%), even in the absence of inflammation. Chloramphenicol crosses the placental barrier and also enters breast milk. Protein binding is approximately 44%.

METABOLISM AND EXCRETION. Elimination of chloramphenicol is primarily through metabolism in the liver to the more water-soluble glucuronide derivative. Only a small percentage (<10%) is excreted unchanged by the kidneys. Dosage adjustments are unnecessary in patients with renal insufficiency; however, chloramphenicol dosage must be adjusted in patients with he-

patic disease to avoid accumulation of the parent drug. The serum half-life of chloramphenicol ranges from 1.5 to 3.5 hours. It is only slightly prolonged in patients with renal failure, but it is markedly lengthened in patients with compromised hepatic function. The therapeutic range for chloramphenicol serum levels is 10–20 μg/ml.

Adverse Reactions

HEMATOLOGIC TOXICITY. Chloramphenicol has two major effects on the bone marrow. The first is a hypersensitivity (idiosyncratic and irreversible) reaction. Fatal aplastic anemia (complete suppression of all bone marrow blood components) is reported to occur in 1:40,000 courses of therapy. This reaction is unpredictable, independent of serum chloramphenicol levels, not dose-related, and may occur more often during prolonged drug administration or in patients who have had previous exposure. While most cases of chloramphenicol-induced aplastic anemia have been reported following oral administration, there are cases reported following intravenous or topical administration. The other effect which chloramphenicol has on the blood system is anemia with a normal-appearing bone marrow. This effect is predictable, reversible, correlates with blood chloramphenicol concentrations, and is a dose-related adverse effect. It can be minimized by maintaining chloramphenicol serum concentrations below 25 μg/ml. Patients who develop anemia, leukopenia, or thrombocytopenia during chloramphenicol administration should be suspected of having chloramphenicol-related toxicity. In these patients, a dosage reduction should be considered.

GASTROINTESTINAL EFFECTS. Patients receiving chloramphenicol orally may experience nausea and vomiting. Because it is a broad-spectrum antibiotic, bacterial or fungal superinfection can occur and diarrhea may result. An unpleasant taste or perineal irritation may also occur.

NEUROTOXICITY. *Optic neuritis* may develop in 3%–5% of patients receiving chloramphenicol chronically. Blurred vision and *peripheral neuritis* have also been described.

GRAY BABY SYNDROME. Chloramphenicol, administered to newborn babies in high doses (>100 mg/kg), has been implicated in the *gray baby syndrome* or "toddler syndrome," which is characterized by abdominal distention, cyanosis (gray discoloration), and circulatory collapse. Repeated administration of chloramphenicol to neonates who have both immature hepatic and kidney function leads to accumulation of large amounts of chloramphenicol, which appears to interfere with tissue respiration.

Drug Interactions

The addition of chloramphenicol to the treatment of a patient who is stabilized on phenytoin may result in the development of phenytoin toxicity. Chloramphenicol appears to inhibit the metabolism of phenytoin, resulting in decreased elimination of the drug from the body. Patients who develop nystagmus, ataxia, or other signs of phenytoin intoxication should have serum phenytoin concentrations measured and the dose reduced until chloramphenicol is discontinued. Phenobarbital increases the metabolism of chloramphenicol, which may lead to subtherapeutic serum concentrations of chloramphenicol.

Chloramphenicol decreases the metabolism of warfarin and may lead to an increased risk of bleeding (prothrombin time may be markedly prolonged). Patients who are on anticoagulants should have their prothrombin time monitored closely if chloramphenicol is prescribed. Observe the patient for bleeding gums, blood in the urine, and other signs of bleeding.

A decrease in the hepatic metabolism of sulfonylureas is thought to be the mechanism whereby chloramphenicol may induce hypoglycemia. Patients are observed for signs of hypoglycemia and monitored by determinations of blood glucose levels.

Patients receiving vitamin B_{12} for treatment of anemia may demonstrate a decreased response. Chloramphenicol seems to inhibit optimal use of vitamin B_{12} within the bone marrow during red blood cell production.

VANCOMYCIN

Vancomycin (Vancocin, Vancoled) is a narrow spectrum bactericidal glycopeptide antibiotic produced by the soil microorganism *Streptomyces orientalis*. Vancomycin enjoyed widespread use in the 1950s; however, by the 1960s, reports of toxicities and the introduction of the safer antistaphylococcal penicillins limited its use. Recently, interest in vancomycin as an antistaphylococcal agent has been rekindled because of the development of methicillin-resistant *Staphylococcus aureus* (M-RSA) and *Staphylococcus epidermidis* (M-RSE) (see Table 46–6).

Mechanism of Action

The primary mechanism of action of vancomycin is to inhibit cell wall synthesis at a point distinct from that of penicillins and cephalosporins. Specifically, it binds or complexes with UDP-N-acetylmuramylpentapeptide, a precursor of peptidoglycan. In addition, vancomycin also has been shown to inhibit ribonucleic acid (RNA) synthesis and to alter bacterial cell wall permeability.

Spectrum of Activity

Vancomycin primarily inhibits growth of gram-positive bacteria and is considered to be a narrow-spectrum bactericidal antibiotic. It is considered the drug of choice for methicillin-resistant *Staphylococcus aureus* or *S. epidermidis*. However, against *Streptococcus faecalis* (enterococcus), it is only bacteriostatic, and combination therapy with an aminoglycoside is usually necessary for treating infections secondary to this particular organism. Vancomycin is active against most strains of streptococci and staphylococci. Vancomycin is also active against *Clostridium difficile*, the responsible organism in antibiotic-associated colitis. It is inactive against gram-negative bacteria (e.g., enterobacteriaceae).

Pharmacokinetics

ABSORPTION. Vancomycin is poorly absorbed when administered orally (<1%), with most of the dose appearing in the feces. This is the basis for prescribing vancomycin when *Clostridium difficile* is the cause of antibiotic-associated colitis. For systemic infections, vancomycin is administered intravenously. Intramuscular administration results in muscle necrosis and should be avoided.

DISTRIBUTION. Vancomycin distributes throughout various body fluids and enters the cerebrospinal fluid only in the presence of inflammation. Vancomycin is about 52%–56% bound to serum proteins.

METABOLISM AND EXCRETION. Approximately 90% of an intravenous dose of vancomycin is excreted by the kidneys. It is imperative that dosage be decreased in patients with renal dysfunction to avoid toxicity. The elimination half-life of vancomycin in individuals with normal renal function is approximately six hours. In patients without kidney function, the half-life of the drug is remarkably prolonged (up to 240 hours) and once weekly dosing may be appropriate. Hemodialysis does not remove vancomycin from the body.

Adverse Reactions

OTOTOXICITY. Hearing loss may occur in patients receiving vancomycin. Deafness may be preceded by ringing in the ears and is associated with elevated serum concentrations of vancomycin. Prolonged, high serum concentrations of vancomycin are usually seen in patients with decreased renal function in whom the dosage has not been reduced.

NEPHROTOXICITY. Kidney damage was more common when vancomycin was prescribed without a true appreciation for its toxic potential and dependence on normal renal function for elimination. More recent experience suggests that nephrotoxicity is rare. However, combined use of vancomycin with other nephrotoxic agents (e.g., aminoglycosides) may result in additive nephrotoxicity.

RED NECK SYNDROME. A side effect unique to vancomycin is that related to the rapid infusion of large doses of vancomycin. It is characterized by fever, chills, paresthesias (numbness), and erythema (reddening) at the base of the neck and the upper back, and may be followed by hypotension. It usually begins ten minutes after the start of the infusion and resolves 15–20 minutes after the infusion has stopped. The reaction seems to be related to histamine release and not a hypersensitivity (or immunologic) reaction.

OTHER REACTIONS. Patients receiving intravenous vancomycin may experience thrombophlebitis, neutropenia (decreased number of white cells), and thrombocytopenia (decreased number of platelets).

Drug Interactions

Vancomycin may have an additive toxic effect with other agents that induce nephrotoxicity or ototoxicity (e.g., aminoglycosides, furosemide, ethacrynic acid).

METRONIDAZOLE

Metronidazole (Flagyl), a derivative of azomycin, was synthesized in 1959. Metronidazole provided the first effective therapy of trichomoniasis and is also recommended for amebiasis and giardiasis. More recently, it has been promoted as an excellent drug for treating anaerobic infections (see Table 46-6).

Mechanism of Action

It is thought that metronidazole is "reduced" to microbiologically active intermediary metabolites. It is these reduction products that react with bacterial DNA, disrupting transcription and replication.

Spectrum of Activity

Metronidazole is active against obligate (strict) anaerobes. *Facultative anaerobes*, microaerophilic bacteria, and *obligate aerobes* are usually not susceptible. Metronidazole has activity against *Trichomonas vaginalis, Entamoeba histolytica, Giardia lamblia, Campylobacter fetus*, and *Gardnerella vaginalis*.

Pharmacokinetics

ABSORPTION. Metronidazole is completely absorbed from the gastrointestinal tract. An intravenous formulation has also been developed for treatment of systemic infection. There is no intramuscular formulation.

DISTRIBUTION. Metronidazole distributes into body fluids and penetrates the cerebrospinal fluid. It crosses the placental barrier and is found in breast milk. Protein binding is less than 20%.

METABOLISM AND EXCRETION. This agent is extensively metabolized by the liver with less than 10% excreted unchanged in the urine. The serum half-life is approximately eight hours.

Adverse Reactions

TERATOGENICITY. Evidence from animal and human studies indicate that metronidazole is not *teratogenic* or embryotoxic. While it does cross the placental barrier, its use during pregnancy should be carefully considered.

CARCINOGENICITY. Data collected over a ten-year period have not revealed increases in cancer attributable to metronidazole.

GASTROINTESTINAL EFFECTS. The most common gastrointestinal effects are nausea, anorexia, cramping, and diarrhea. An unpleasant metallic taste and dry mouth have also been described.

NEUROTOXICITY. Patients may experience neurotoxicity during metronidazole treatment. These neurologic effects include dizziness, vertigo, and numbness or tingling in the extremities.

OTHER SIDE EFFECTS. Darkened urine has been noted and attributed to a metabolite of metronidazole. Rashes (e.g., erythematous, maculopapular, and pruritic) and reversible neutropenia have also been described.

Thrombophlebitis may be one of the most frequent effects seen with the intravenous form of the drug.

Drug Interactions

When metronidazole and disulfiram are administered concurrently, an acute toxic psychosis may occur, although the mechanism is not understood. A disulfiram-like reaction may occur if patients ingest ethanol while taking metronidazole. Flushing, dizziness, sweating, and nausea are the clinical manifestations of this response.

Metronidazole may inhibit the hepatic metabolism of anticoagulants (warfarin), thus increasing the risk of bleeding. Clinical signs of bleeding, as well as, prothrombin time prolongation are monitored closely when this combination is prescribed.

TETRACYCLINES

The tetracyclines, a family of compounds with a four-ringed structure in common, were discovered in 1948. They are: Chlortetracycline (Aureomycin), Oxytetracycline (Terramycin), Tetracycline (Achromycin, Sumycin), Demeclocycline (Declomycin), Methacycline (Rondomycin), Doxycycline (Vibramycin), and Minocycline (Minocin). The tetracyclines are featured in Table 46-7. although the various members of the tetracycline family possess a few specific differences, the group will be discussed as a whole.

Mechanism of Action

The site of action of the tetracyclines is the 30S ribosome with access depending upon both a passive diffusion process, as well as an active process which is energy-dependent. This last step is responsible for pumping all tetracyclines through the cytoplasmic membrane and may require a periplasmic protein carrier. Once inside the bacterial cell wall, tetracyclines inhibit protein synthesis and are bacteriostatic antibiotics. Resistance to tetracyclines appears to occur by three mechanisms: alteration in the ribosome; production of an inactivating enzyme; and permeability changes in the organism.

Spectrum of Activity

As a class, tetracyclines can be considered broad-spectrum antibiotics. In addition, they demonstrate clinical efficacy against organisms frequently resistant to other agents (e.g., *Rickettsiae, Mycoplasma*, and *Chlamydia* organisms. In general, tetracyclines are more active against gram-positive organisms than gram-negative organisms; however, resistance has significantly limited their usefulness. Minocycline is clearly more active than other derivatives against *Staphylococcus aureus. Streptococcus pneumoniae* resistance to tetracyclines may be as high as 15%–20% in some geographic areas. *Streptococcus pyogenes* is generally sensitive; however, Group B, C, and G streptococci demonstrate variable susceptibilities. *Neisseria meningitidis* and *Neisseria gonorrhoeae* are

TEXT RESUMES ON PAGE 1250

Table 46–7. TETRACYCLINES

Name	Dosage	Mode of Administration	Pharmacokinetics
TETRACYCLINES			
Action: Inhibit protein synthesis by binding to the 30S ribosomal subunit.			
Use: For treating infections in penicillin-allergic patients; drug of choice for rickettsial infections.			
Chlortetracycline (Aureomycin)	Ophthalmic ointment Ointment (3%)	Topical (10 mg/g) Topical	
Oxytetracyline (Terramycin)	*Adults:* 250–500 mg q 6–12 hr *Children: >8 yr:* 25–50 mg/kg/day in 2 or 4 divided doses 10–20 mg/kg/day	PO, IV PO IV	A: 58% P: 1.5–4 hr PB: 10%–40% ½L: 8–10 hr E: renal
Tetracycline HCL (Achromycin)	*Adults:* 250–500 mg q 6–12 hr *Children: >8 yr:* 25–50 mg/kg/day in 2 or 4 divided doses 10–20 mg/kg/day	PO, IV IV	A: 77% P: 1.5–4 hr PB: 20%–67% ½L: 8–10 hr E: renal
Demeclocycline (Declomycin)	*Adults:* 150–300 mg 4 × daily *Children: >8 yr:* 6–12 mg/kg/day divided into 2 or 4 doses	PO PO	A: 66% P: 1.5–4 hr PB: 36%–91% ½L: 15 hr E: renal
Doxycycline (Vibramycin)	*Adults and children (>8 yr, >45 kg):* 200 mg × 1 followed by 100 mg q 12 hr *Children: (>8 yr, <45 kg):* 4.4 mg/kg × 1 followed by 2.2 mg/kg divided into 2 doses per day *Adults and children: (>8 yr, >45 kg):* 200 mg × 1 followed by 100–200 mg q 24 hr *Children: (>8 yr, <45 kg):* 4.4 mg/kg × 1 followed by 2.2–4.4 mg/kg q 24 hr	PO PO IV IV	A: 93% P: 1.5–4 hr PB: 25%–93% ½L: 14–24 hr E: hepatobiliary, renal

A-absorption; PB-protein binding; ½L-serum half-life; E-excretion; NA-not available.
*Within the column of adverse effects, underlines indicate the most common effects; CAPITALS indicate life-threatening effects.

Contraindications/ Precautions	Adverse Effects*	Interactions	Nursing Implications
CONTRAINDICATIONS: Prior hypersensitivity reactions. Avoid use during pregnancy and in young children (<8 yr)	*GI:* nausea, vomiting, dyspepsia, diarrhea, stomatitis *Biliary:* hepatitis, pancreatitis *Integ:* rash, PHOTO-SENSITIVITY	May increase ALT, AST, and BUN levels. Absorption inhibited by antacids, calcium or iron supplements, magnesium. Increased nephrotoxicity with methoxyflurane. May decrease the efficacy of oral contraceptives.	*ASSESSMENT:* Milk and antacids should not be administered concomitantly. Administer with large volume of water (240 ml). *INTERVENTION:* Patient should avoid taking medication with dairy products or antacids. Protect skin from sunlight (ultraviolet) with sunscreen or protective clothing. *EVALUATION:* Evaluate for fever and symptoms. Check WBC count. Report any adverse reactions.
Same as for all tetracyclines.	Same as for all tetracyclines.	Same as for all tetracyclines.	See above.
Same as for all tetracyclines.	Same as for all tetracyclines.	Same as for all tetracyclines.	See above.
Same as for all tetracyclines.	Same as for all tetracyclines.	Same as for all tetracyclines.	See above.
Same as for all tetracyclines.	Same as for all tetracyclines.	Same as for all tetracyclines.	*ASSESSMENT:* Do not inject IM or SC. *INTERVENTION:* See above. *EVALUATION:* See above.

CONTINUED ON THE FOLLOWING PAGE

Table 46–7. TETRACYCLINES–*CONTINUED*

Name	Dosage	Mode of Administration	Pharmacokinetics
Methacycline (Rondomycin)	*Adults:* 600 mg daily in 4 divided doses	PO	A: 60%–80% P: 1.5–4 hr
	Children >8 yr: 6–12 mg/kg/ day in 2 or 4 divided doses per day	PO	PB: 75%–90% ½L: 7–15 hr E: renal
Minocycline (Minocin)	*Adults:* 200 mg × 1 followed by 100 mg q 12 hr	PO, IV	A: 90%–100% P: 1.5–4 hr
	Children >8 yr: 4 mg/kg × 1 followed by 2 mg/kg q 12 hr	PO, IV	PB: 55%–88% ½L: 15–20 hr E: liver, renal (5%–10%)

A-absorption; PB-protein binding; ½L-serum half-life; E-excretion; NA-not available.
*Within the column of adverse effects, <u>underlines</u> indicate the most common effects; CAPITALS indicate life-threatening effects.

both inhibited, although 50% of the former strains may be resistant. Against aerobic gram-negative rods (e.g., *E. coli, Klebsiella pneumoniae, Enterobacter aerogenes, Proteus mirabilis*) the activity of the tetracyclines is variable. Activity against *Hemophilus influenzae* is poorest with oxytetracycline and tetracycline. Indole-positive *Proteus* species (e.g., *Proteus vulgaris*) and pseudomonas are resistant.

The anaerobic spectrum is most impressive with doxycycline and includes *Bacteroides fragilis*.

Pharmacokinetics

ABSORPTION. Oral absorption of tetracyclines is incomplete and can be enhanced by taking these agents without food or other medications. Concomitant administration of milk, milk-containing products, antacids (aluminum hydroxide), sodium bicarbonate, calcium and magnesium salts and iron preparations impair absorption. Food appears to interfere less with the absorption of doxycycline and minocycline. Alterations in gastric pH (as after antacid administration) may also decrease absorption of tetracyclines. Intramuscular injections are slowly and erratically absorbed and are not recommended.

DISTRIBUTION. Lipid solubility plays an important role in the distribution of tetracycline congeners. Doxycycline and minocycline are the most lipid-soluble and thus penetrate into various tissues (e.g., spinal fluid) the best. Also, minocycline demonstrates exceptionally good penetration of saliva, which makes it an ideal agent for the treatment of the meningococcal carrier state. Distribution is also dependent upon protein binding. Tetracyclines cross the placenta and umbilical cord, and fetal plasma concentrations have been reported to reach 60% of the level in the maternal circulation. These agents are also found in breast milk. Dosage information can be found in Table 46–7.

METABOLISM AND EXCRETION. The members of the tetracycline family are excreted in the urine and feces to varying degrees. Chlortetracycline, doxycycline, and minocycline are all primarily eliminated by non-renal routes, whereas demeclocycline, tetracycline, and oxytetracycline are mainly excreted in the urine. Doxycycline exhibits the most unusual mode of elimination since it is secreted into the intestinal lumen, bound by the feces, and finally eliminated. Tetracyclines, as a class of antibiotics, are actively secreted into the bile and undergo *enterohepatic recirculation*. Minocycline and doxycycline require minimal dosage adjustment in patients with reduced renal function. The other tetracyclines should be dosage-adjusted in patients with renal disease. The serum half-life of these agents vary from six to nine hours for oxytetracycline, chlortetracycline, and tetracycline; to 16 hours for demeclocycline; and up to 17–22 hours for doxycycline and minocycline.

Adverse Reactions

GASTROINTESTINAL EFFECTS. Tetracyclines have the potential to cause gastrointestinal irritation following oral administration. Patients may complain of epigastric burning, nausea, vomiting, or diarrhea. These problems are more common with large doses, and certain patients may require smaller doses at more frequent intervals. Taking these agents with food may help in certain cases; however, absorption is compromised.

PHOTOTOXICITY. Of the tetracyclines, demeclocycline is most commonly associated with a "sunburn" reaction. Patients taking any tetracycline should avoid direct sunlight or sunlamps. This "phototoxic" reaction may occur in patients who also develop fever and eosinophilia (increase in blood eosinophil count). Minocycline appears to be the tetracycline derivative least likely to cause phototoxic reactions.

HEPATOTOXICITY. All tetracyclines have the potential to induce acute hepatic injury (fatty liver). It appears that high doses (>2 g/day), intravenous administration, and pregnancy may be associated with developing a toxic hepatic reaction.

NEPHROTOXICITY. A possible association has been suggested between tetracycline treatment and decreased kidney function. Although not a well described toxicity, the effect of tetracyclines on renal function should be

Contraindications/ Precautions	Adverse Effects*	Interactions	Nursing Implications
Same as for all tetracyclines.	Same as for all tetracyclines.	Same as for all tetracyclines.	Same as for all tetracyclines.
Same as for all tetracyclines.	*Neuro:* disequilibrium syndrome or dizziness	Same as for all tetracyclines.	See above.

considered, especially in patients with preexisting renal insufficiency.

Demeclocycline has been reported to antagonize the effect of antidiuretic hormone (ADH), leading to a situation of drug-induced diabetes insipidus (excessive thirst and urination). This toxic effect has been used for therapeutic benefit in patients with the syndrome of inappropriate ADH (SIADH) secretion, where excess ADH is present.

EFFECTS ON CALCIFIED TISSUE. Tetracyclines bind to calcium found in teeth and bones. The patients most susceptible to this effect are neonates and infants before their first dentition. Brown discoloration of teeth has been described in children from birth until the age of eight. These effects can also appear in the child when tetracycline is given during pregnancy from midpregnancy to delivery.

Skeletal deposition of tetracyclines can also occur in the fetus and young child. Bone growth can be depressed up to 40% after prolonged tetracycline exposure.

THROMBOPHLEBITIS. Tetracyclines are very irritating to blood vessels when administered intravenously. Injection sites may have to be rotated and infusion solutions diluted in some patients.

CATABOLIC EFFECTS. Tetracyclines may induce a catabolic effect in human cells because of inhibition of protein synthesis. The effect is dose-related and may induce a negative nitrogen balance and elevations in blood urea nitrogen (BUN) levels.

HYPERSENSITIVITY REACTIONS. Hypersensitivity to tetracyclines is uncommon. Patients may present with various skin reactions, angioedema, anaphylaxis, or burning eyes. These reactions may last for weeks or months after the tetracycline is discontinued. When a patient displays hypersensitivity to one tetracycline, it should be assumed the patient will be hypersensitive (allergic) to all members of the tetracycline family.

HEMATOLOGIC TOXICITY. Long-term administration of tetracyclines has been associated with leukocytosis, atypical lymphocyte formation, and thrombocytopenia.

OTOTOXICITY. Minocycline has been reported to induce vestibular toxicity. The patient may complain of dizziness, ataxia, nausea, or vomiting. This effect is dose-related and subsides when minocycline is discontinued or the daily dose decreased.

INTRACRANIAL PRESSURE ELEVATIONS. Increased intracranial pressure *(pseudotumor cerebri)* has been described in infants primarily and in adults. The symptoms of headache and blurred vision disappear once the drug is discontinued.

SUPERINFECTIONS. Broad-spectrum antibiotic therapy can lead to resistant organisms which may overgrow the respiratory and gastrointestinal tract. Staphylococcal enterocolitis; pseudomembranous colitis; and vaginal, oral, pharyngeal yeast infections are all examples of the results of altering the normal host bacterial flora.

Drug Interactions

Tetracycline absorption may be decreased when administered orally with various compounds containing divalent (Mg^{2+}, Ca^{2+}, Ba^{2+}) or trivalent (Fe^{3+}, Al^{3+}) cations. Common examples include magnesium-, calcium-, or aluminum-containing antacids; dairy products (Ca^{2+}); and iron (Fe^{3+}) preparations. The net effect is a decrease in the antibacterial effect of tetracycline.

Tetracyclines are reported to decrease the efficacy of oral contraceptives. Synthetic estrogens (e.g., oral contraceptive agents) are excreted in the bile almost exclusively as glucuronide or sulfate conjugates. These conjugates, on reaching the gut, are hydrolyzed by enzymes present in intestinal microorganisms to liberate the unchanged drug (oral contraceptive agent) which is then reabsorbed. Treatment with tetracyclines, which undergo the same type of enterohepatic recirculation, could be expected to interfere with this oral contraceptive hydrolytic process by eliminating the gut microorganisms and thus reducing or abolishing the reabsorption of the active oral contraceptive drug. The risk of pregnancy could be significant and alternative methods of contraception should be recommended until the next menstrual period.

As described in detail for penicillin, the concurrent administration of a bacteriostatic agent may decrease the efficacy of a bactericidal agent (see penicillin discussion for details).

Table 46–8. URINARY TRACT ANTI-INFECTIVES

Name	Dosage	Mode of Administration	Pharmacokinetics
Methenamine (Mandelamine, Hiprex)			
Use: For treating urinary tract infections secondary to gram-negative organisms.			
	Adults and children > 12 yr: 1 g qid	PO	A: 70% PB: NA
	Children 6–12 yr: 0.5–1 g qid	PO (Also available as a suspension, 0.5 g/5 cc; as granules, [1 g/packet])	½L: 4 hr E: renal
Nitrofurantoin (Macrodantin)			
Use: For treating urinary tract infections secondary to gram-negative organisms.			
	Adults: 50–100 mg 4 times daily	PO	A: well absorbed PB: 20%–60%
	Children: 4–7 mg/kg/day given in 4 divided doses	PO (Also available as oral suspension, 25 mg/5 ml)	½L: 20 min E: renal, liver

A-absorption; PB-protein binding; ½L-serum half-life; E-excretion; NA-not available.
*Within the column of adverse effects, underlines indicate the most common effects; CAPITALS indicate life-threatening effects.

URINARY TRACT ANTI-INFECTIVES

These anti-infective drugs provide an effective "local" antibacterial effect within the urinary tract because they are highly concentrated in the urine. They are ineffective as treatment for systemic infections because of the low serum concentrations achieved (Table 46–8).

Methenamine

MECHANISM OF ACTION. When placed in an acid aqueous environment, methenamine (Hiprex, Mandelamine) decomposes to form formaldehyde. The decomposition is negligible at the pH found in blood. For maximum formation of formaldehyde, urinary pH must be below 6.0.

SPECTRUM OF ACTIVITY. Bacteria causing urinary tract infections (both gram-positive and gram-negative) and fungi are sensitive to formaldehyde. However, bacteria able to raise urinary pH (e.g., *Proteus* species) are not inhibited by methenamine.

PHARMACOKINETICS. *Absorption.* Methenamine is absorbed when given orally, but about 25% decomposes in the stomach. That which decomposes in the gastrointestinal tract also liberates ammonia. Ammonia may be detrimental to patients with hepatic disease, therefore, methenamine is not prescribed for these patients.

Metabolism and Excretion. Various methods have been tried to lower the urinary pH, with the hope of increasing formaldehyde formation. About 20% of methenamine excreted in the urine is converted to formaldehyde at a urine pH of 5. Antibacterial activity can be detected in the urine within thirty minutes of administration. Methenamine is available in combination with mandelic acid and hippuric acid, both of which acidify the urine. Patients may also be advised to take methenamine with cranberry juice, which also acidifies the urine. An important aspect of treatment with this compound is that it must reside in the urinary bladder for conversion to formaldehyde. Patients with foley catheters (continuous urinary drainage) will not benefit from the antibacterial activity of this drug under the above circumstances. Patients with moderate to severe renal function should not be given this drug.

Contraindications/ Precautions	Adverse Effects*	Interactions	Nursing Implications
CONTRAINDICATIONS: Avoid in the presence of renal impairment, hepatic disease, or dehydration. *PRECAUTIONS:* Safe use in pregnancy not established.	*Neuro:* tinnitus *GI:* nausea, vomiting, diarrhea, abdominal discomfort *Integ:* muscle cramps	Increases urinary catecholamines and steroids. False urine glucose results with Benedict's test. Interferes with urobilinogen and urinary VMA.	*ASSESSMENT:* Administer after meals to decrease GI distress. Maintain adequate fluid intake. Maintain an acid urine to achieve antibacterial benefit of the drug. *INTERVENTION:* Patient should take medication after meals. *EVALUATION:* Evaluate for fever and symptoms. Check WBC count. Report any adverse reactions.
CONTRAINDICATIONS: Prior hypersensitivity; renal impairment, G-6-PD deficiency; infants <3 mo. *PRECAUTIONS:* Safe use in women of childbearing age and during pregnancy or lactation is not established.	*Neuro:* PERIPHERAL NEURITIS, headache, dizziness *Resp:* PULMONARY FIBROSIS (e.g. cough, fever) *GI:* nausea, vomiting *Biliary:* hepatitis *Hemo:* HEMOLYTIC ANEMIA	False positive urine glucose with Benedict's test. Drugs that increase urinary pH decrease effectiveness of nitrofurantoin. Antacids delay absorption. Concomitant administration of probenecid and sulfinpyrazone raises levels of nitrofurantoin in blood to toxic levels.	*ASSESSMENT:* Administer with meals. Dilute oral suspension to prevent tooth staining. Do not crush the tablets. *INTERVENTION:* Instruct patient to take medication with meals. *EVALUATION:* See methenamine above.

ADVERSE REACTIONS. Gastrointestinal distress, painful urination, increased frequency of urination, blood in the urine, and rash may result after methenamine administration.

Nitrofurantoin

Nitrofurantoin (Furadantin, Macrodantin) is another synthetic antibiotic used to prevent and treat urinary tract infections.

MECHANISM OF ACTION. The mechanism of action of nitrofurantoin is unknown.

SPECTRUM OF ACTIVITY. Nitrofurantoin is active against *E. coli;* however, many other gram-negative bacilli are resistant. The action of this agent is enhanced when the urinary pH is acidic.

PHARMACOKINETICS. *Absorption.* Nitrofurantoin is well absorbed from the small intestine following oral administration.

Distribution. Serum concentrations are minimal because the drug is eliminated so rapidly and therapeutic serum concentrations are not attained in most body fluids or tissues.

Metabolism and Excretion. Little is known about the metabolic fate of nitrofurantoin. It is speculated that inactivation occurs in all body tissues including the liver. The plasma half-life is approximately twenty minutes, and approximately 30% of the dose is excreted by the kidneys in the active form. The dosage of nitrofurantoin should be reduced in patients with decreased renal function.

ADVERSE REACTIONS. *Gastrointestinal Effects.* When given orally, nausea, vomiting, and diarrhea are common.

Hypersensitivity Reactions. Nitrofurantoin may rarely cause chills, fever, decreased blood count, or jaundice. Pulmonary symptoms (cough, chest pain) may result within days after nitrofurantoin is started and require discontinuation of the drug.

Neurotoxicity. One of the most serious side effects of nitrofurantoin may be peripheral neuritis. The mechanism of the toxicity appears to be the accumulation of the drug in neural tissue and interference with anaerobic glycolysis. This adverse effect may occur within the first forty-five days of treatment, although it may occur two months after therapy has been discontinued. The clinical course is usually that of an ascending sensorimotor neuropathy. It has been most commonly described in patients with renal insufficiency; however, it can occur

Table 46–9. QUINOLONES

Name	Dosage	Mode of Administration	Pharmacokinetics
Ciprofloxacin (Cipro)			
Action: Inhibits the enzyme DNA gyrase.			
Use: For treating gram-positive and gram-negative infections.			
	Adults: 250–750 mg q 12 hr	PO (tablets)	A: 70% P: 1–2 hr PB: 20% ½L: 3–4 hr E: renal and nonrenal
Nalidixic Acid (NegGram)			
Action: Inhibits DNA gyrase.			
Use: For the treatment of urinary tract infections only.			
	Adults: 1 g 4 times daily *Children > 12 yr:* 55 mg/kg/day in 4 equally divided doses	PO (tablet) PO (Also available as a suspension, 250 mg/5 ml)	A: 100% P: 1–2 hr PB: 95% ½L: 6–7 hr E: renal and hepatic
Norfloxacin (Noroxin)			
Action: Inhibits DNA gyrase.			
Use: For the treatment of urinary tract infections.			
	Adults: 400 mg twice daily	PO (tablets)	A: 30%–50% P: 1–2 hr PB: 10%–15% ½L: 3–4 hr E: hepatic and renal

A-absorption; PB-protein binding; ½L-serum half-life; E-excretion.
*Within the column of adverse effects, <u>underlines</u> indicate the most common effects; CAPITALS indicate life-threatening effects.

in individuals with normal kidney function. Despite discontinuing the drug, it may take several months for the neuritis to disappear and in some patients, it may be irreversible. Other toxicities associated with nitrofurantoin may be headache and dizziness.

Pulmonary Reactions. The pulmonary side effects of nitrofurantoin can be acute, subacute, or chronic in nature. The first of these reactions is most likely allergic in nature and eosinophilia (elevated blood levels of eosinophils) should be present. The onset is within hours to weeks after the drug has been started and is usually accompanied by the sudden onset of fever, cough, chills, myalgias and dyspnea (difficulty breathing). It may occur more frequently in elderly patients. If the

drug is discontinued, the acute reaction is completely reversible. The subacute form of this adverse effect usually develops after one month of drug exposure and is characterized by persistent and progressive cough, dyspnea, and fever. The patient recovers rapidly once the drug is discontinued. The chronic form of nitrofurantoin-induced pneumonitis is insidious in onset (6 months after the start of drug treatment). A nonproductive cough and dyspnea are common, whereas fever is not. Usually, there is regression of the diffuse interstitial, fibrotic lung picture; however, this may not be the case in some patients.

Other Side Effects. Hepatotoxicity has been rarely reported with nitrofurantoin administration. Hemolytic

Contraindications/ Precautions	Adverse Effects*	Interactions	Nursing Implications
CONTRAINDICATIONS: Prior hypersensitivity reactions. *PRECAUTIONS:* Use with caution in patients with history of CNS disease. Avoid alkalinization of urine. Avoid use during pregnancy and lactation. Safe use in children has not been established.	*Neuro:* dizziness, lightheadedness, insomnia, SEIZURES, blurred vision *GI:* diarrhea, nausea, vomiting *Integ:* rash, joint or back pain, cartilage abnormalities	Antacids will impair the absorption of ciprofloxacin. Ciprofloxacin will inhibit the metabolism of theophylline.	*ASSESSMENT:* Maintain good hydration. Do not give concomitantly with antacids. *INTERVENTION:* Instruct patient not to take medication with antacids. *EVALUATION:* Evaluate for fever and symptoms. Check WBC count. Report any adverse reactions.
Same as for ciprofloxacin.	Same as for ciprofloxacin.	May exaggerate the anticoagulant effect of coumadin. May interfere with urine glucose testing by Benedict's method.	See above.
Same as for ciprofloxacin.	Same as for ciprofloxacin.	Probenecid can decrease the urinary elimination of norfloxacin. Concomitant administration of nitrofurantoin can antagonize the antibacterial activity of norfloxacin. Antacids may impair the absorption of norfloxacin.	See above.

anemia, especially in patients with a G-6-PD deficiency, has been well documented.

QUINOLONES

Nalidixic Acid

MECHANISM OF ACTION. Nalidixic acid (Neg-Gram) is thought to inhibit bacterial growth by interfering with *DNA gyrase*, an enzyme instrumental in the stranding of bacterial DNA synthesis (see Table 46–9).

SPECTRUM OF ACTIVITY. Nalidixic acid is active against most gram-negative urinary tract pathogens (e.g., *E. coli, Proteus mirabilis, Klebsiella* species, *Enterobacter* species, *Serratia* species). *Pseudomonas aeruginosa* is always resistant. Nalidixic acid has minimal action against gram-positive bacteria such as *Staphylococcus aureus, Streptococcus pneumoniae,* and *Streptococcus fae-*

calis (enterococcus). The rapid development of resistance has significantly limited the overall clinical use of nalidixic acid.

PHARMACOKINETICS. Absorption. Nalidixic acid is available as an oral dosage form and is completely absorbed.

Distribution. The drug is not highly tissue bound and primarily concentrates in kidney tissue and the urine. It is 95% protein bound.

Metabolism and Excretion. Nalidixic acid and its active metabolite (hydroxynalidixic acid) are both conjugated in the liver to antibacterially inactive monoglucuronides which are then rapidly excreted in the urine. Approximately 85%–90% of the drug is excreted as the monoglucuronide conjugates; however, the remainder is excreted as the microbiologically active parent drug. The serum half-life of nalidixic acid is 8 hours in patients with normal renal function, but may be prolonged up to twenty-one hours in the presence of renal dysfunction. In patients with liver impairment, the drug should be administered cautiously.

ADVERSE REACTIONS. Gastrointestinal Effects. Nalidixic acid is usually well tolerated; however, nausea, vomiting, or abdominal pain and diarrhea may occur after ingestion.

Neurotoxicity. An uncommon complication of therapy with nalidixic acid, neurotoxocity may occur after prolonged administration and may include headache, drowsiness, dizziness, visual disturbances, and, rarely, seizures.

Allergic Reactions. Itching, hives, rashes, and photosensitivity may occur.

DRUG INTERACTIONS. Because of its highly protein bound nature, nalidixic acid may compete for binding sites with anticoagulants, resulting in an exaggerated anticoagulant effect. Patients stabilized on coumadin should be carefully monitored for bleeding episodes when nalidixic acid is added to their regimen.

In addition, nalidixic acid conjugates can interfere with urine glucose testing methods (e.g., Clinitest or Benedict's test). Diabetic patients should be made aware of this if they are placed on nalidixic acid.

Norfloxacin

MECHANISM OF ACTION. See Nalidixic Acid.

SPECTRUM OF ACTIVITY. Norfloxacin (Noroxin) has excellent activity against most urinary tract pathogens including enterobacteriaceae, enterococci, *Staphylococcus saprophyticus*, and *Pseudomonas aeruginosa*. It is also active against those organisms responsible for enteritis such as *Salmonella, Shigella, Campylobacter jejuni, Yersinia enterocolitica, Escherichia coli*, and *Vibrio*.

PHARMACOKINETICS. Absorption. Norfloxacin is rapidly absorbed from the gastrointestinal tract; however, food does interfere with absorption. It is only available as an oral dosage form.

Distribution. Norfloxacin is widely distributed to many tissues including the prostate. Protein binding is in the range of 14%–30%.

Metabolism and Excretion. Metabolism of norfloxacin is limited with only 15%–30% of the drug appearing in the urine as metabolites. Metabolism probably occurs in the liver. Excretion is by the kidney (both glomerular filtration and tubular secretion) and in the bile. The half-life range is three to four hours. Dosage adjustment is necessary when the creatinine clearance drops below 30 ml/minute.

ADVERSE REACTIONS. See Nalidixic Acid.

DRUG INTERACTIONS. Norfloxacin will not be absorbed from the gastrointestinal tract if it is coadministered with antacids; therefore, these drugs should not be administered concomitantly and should be separated by at least two hours.

The antibacterial activity of norfloxacin can be antagonized by the concomitant administration of nitrofurantoin.

The urinary elimination of norfloxacin is decreased in the presence of probenecid; therefore, urine levels of norfloxacin may be subtherapeutic.

Ciprofloxacin

MECHANISM OF ACTION. See Nalidixic Acid.

SPECTRUM OF ACTIVITY. Unlike nalidixic acid, ciprofloxacin (Cipro) has broad-spectrum activity encompassing both gram-positive (e.g., *Staphylococcus aureus, Staphylococcus epidermidis, Streptococcus faecalis*) and gram-negative (e.g., enterobacteriaceae, *Pseudomonas aeruginosa*) microorganisms. In addition, ciprofloxacin is active against methicillin-resistant *Staphylococcus aureus* and *S. epidermidis*. However, its activity against anaerobic pathogens is limited.

PHARMACOKINETICS. Absorption. Currently, ciprofloxacin is only available in an oral dosage form. Bioavailability is approximately 70%. The drug is best taken on an empty stomach and patients should be instructed to avoid concomitantly administered antacids.

Distribution. Unlike nalidixic acid, ciprofloxacin is widely distributed throughout body fluid and tissues. Protein binding is approximately 20%.

Metabolism and Excretion. Ciprofloxacin is partially metabolized in the liver to microbiologically less active metabolites. The half-life of ciprofloxacin is about three to four hours. Excretion is by both renal and nonrenal routes.

ADVERSE REACTIONS. See Nalidixic Acid.

Cartilage Toxicity. Bone and cartilage toxicities have been shown in animals; however, they have not been shown in humans. Until further studies are conducted, it would seem prudent to avoid this drug in patients whose skeletal growth is incomplete.

DRUG INTERACTIONS. Ciprofloxacin will not be absorbed from the gastrointestinal tract if it is coadministered with magnesium- or aluminum-containing antacids; therefore, these drugs should not be administered concomitantly and should be separated by at least two hours.

Because of its effect on hepatic cytochrome P-450 enzymes (enzymes responsible for metabolizing theophylline), ciprofloxacin has been reported to increase serum concentrations of theophylline, resulting in toxicity. This drug should be added cautiously to the regimen of any patient receiving theophylline derivatives.

Although speculative at this time, there may be an interaction between ciprofloxacin and iron in the gastrointestinal tract. This interaction may only occur in patients taking iron supplements several times daily (three times daily) and may result in poor absorption of ciprofloxacin.

ANTIMICROBIAL AGENTS FOR TUBERCULOSIS

As is true for many modes of medical treatment, the approach to the therapy of tuberculosis has evolved a great deal since the discovery of isoniazid (isonicotinic acid hydrazine; INH) in 1952. Patients are no longer committed to long-term institutions, but rather basic concepts in the management of communicable diseases have been employed (Table 46–10). Two important features distinguish the treatment of tuberculosis from other therapies for infections. First, effective treatment of tuberculosis requires anti-infective administration for a prolonged period (9–24 months). Second, because of the necessity for prolonged antibiotic administration, the development of bacterial resistance is an important consideration.

Antitubercular drugs may be thought of as either first-line or second-line agents. Drugs considered first-line provide the most effective antituberculous activity with an acceptable degree of toxicity. Second-line agents provide adequate antimicrobial activity, but have excessive toxicities.

First-Line Antitubercular Agents

ISONIAZID. Isoniazid (INH) is the primary choice for therapy against *Mycobacterium tuberculosis.*

Mechanism of Action and Resistance. Tubercle bacilli sensitive to INH possess a mechanism for transportation of the compound intracellularly. After entry into the cell, the drug interferes with the formation of an essential metabolite for the organism. In addition, the drug also inhibits the synthesis of mycolic acid. Whatever the mechanism of action, INH is bactericidal against *M. tuberculosis.* Resistance to isoniazid is thought to occur because mutant organisms prevent penetration of the antibiotic into the cell.

Spectrum of Activity. Isoniazid is active against *Mycobacterium tuberculosis* and is bactericidal.

Pharmacokinetics. Absorption. Isoniazid is rapidly absorbed from the gastrointestinal tract with peak serum concentrations achieved within one to two hours after administration. Aluminum-containing antacids may interfere with absorption.

Distribution. The drug penetrates into all body tissues and fluids, with cerebrospinal fluid concentrations approximately 20% of simultaneous plasma concentrations. INH is not bound to serum protein. INH is secreted in breast milk.

Metabolism and Excretion. INH is extensively metabolized in the liver by a process known as *acetylation.* This metabolic pathway is catalyzed by the enzyme N-acetyl transferase. A patient's rate of acetylation (either fast or slow) is genetically determined and dependent on race, not on sex or age. Ninety percent or more of Orientals are fast acetylators, whereas only 45%–50% of Caucasians are considered to be fast acetylators. For this reason, the serum half-life is variable (1.1 hours, fast acetylator; 3.1 hours, slow acetylator). More than 75% of INH is excreted in the urine within 24 hours as metabolites. The kidneys do not contribute significantly to the elimination of the parent drug (INH); however, the drug is hemodialyzable and the usual dose should be given following the dialysis procedure.

Adverse Reactions. Hypersensitivity Reactions. Fever and maculopapular rashes have been described with INH.

Gastrointestinal Effects. While nausea, vomiting, and diarrhea have been reported, they are uncommon.

Hepatotoxicity. This is a well known side effect of INH and most likely the result of a "toxic" metabolite of the drug. It is possible that rapid acetylators are more likely to develop INH-induced hepatitis because they metabolize more INH to acetylhydrazine. While the reaction can occur in a patient receiving only INH, it may be even more likely in someone taking both INH and rifampin. INH frequently (10%–20%) causes a rise in liver enzymes levels (e.g., ALT, AST) which occurs one week to months after the start of therapy. It may persist without progression or resolve spontaneously. In most patients, it disappears once the drug is discontinued. One of the more notable side effects of INH may be an overt and sometimes fatal hepatitis, indistinguishable from viral hepatitis. The overall incidence seems to be approximately 1%; however, there is an association with age (i.e., the older the patient the more likely this type of hepatitis). Hepatitis is rare under the age of 20 years. While hepatitis can occur anytime during INH therapy, it is more likely during the first two months of treatment. Alcohol (especially daily consumption) can increase the likelihood of hepatitis, as can the concomitant administration of rifampin.

Hematologic Effects. Various blood elements may be altered during INH treatment, and agranulocytosis, eosinophilia, thrombocytopenia, and anemia have been reported. For this reason, it is important to monitor complete blood counts when a patient receives INH.

Neuropathies. INH interferes with the normal action of pyridoxine (vitamin B_6), an essential component in nerve function. As a result, peripheral neuritis may develop. This common toxicity (seen in 20% of patients) can be prevented by the prophylactic administration of pyridoxine (25–50 mg/day). Additional neurotoxicities reported are convulsions, optic neuritis, muscle twitching, dizziness, ataxia, and toxic encephalopathy. Mental status changes may appear during INH treatment, and patients may manifest euphoria, memory loss, loss of self-control, and psychoses.

Drug Interactions. INH may inhibit the hepatic metabolism of phenytoin, leading to phenytoin toxicity. Patients may exhibit nystagmus, ataxia, and confusion following addition of INH to the anticonvulsant therapy. A reduction of phenytoin dosage may be required until the INH is discontinued. Symptoms of carbamazepine intoxication have been reported in patients who have had INH prescribed. The mechanism appears to be via impaired hepatic metabolism of carbamazepine and may require a dosage reduction.

Corticosteroids may stimulate enzymes in the liver that metabolize INH, thus, decreasing the antitubercular activity. This interaction may require higher doses of INH.

RIFAMPIN OR RIFAMPICIN. Rifampin (Rimactane) is a semisynthetic derivative of rifamycin B, an antibiotic produced by *Streptomyces mediterranei.*

Mechanism of Action. DNA-dependent *RNA polymerase*, a crucial enzyme in RNA synthesis, is inhibited by the presence of rifampin. These effects are limited to bacteria, and mammalian cells are unaffected. Bacterial resistance develops when a modification of the DNA-dependent RNA polymerase is made, enabling the enzyme to escape binding to rifampin.

Spectrum of Activity. Rifampin is an extremely broad-spectrum antibacterial agent with activity against many gram-positive and gram-negative microor-

TEXT RESUMES ON PAGE 1260

Table 46–10. ANTITUBERCULOUS DRUGS

Name	Dosage	Mode of Administration	Pharmacokinetics
Isoniazid (INH)	*Adults:* 5 mg/kg/day (up to 300 mg/day); give once daily	PO, IM, IV	A: rapid P: 1–2 hr PB: 0%
	Infants and children: 10–20 mg/kg/day given once daily	PO, IM, IV	½L: 1.1 hr (FA); 3.1 hr (SA) E: liver
Rifampin (Rifadin, Rimactane)	*Adults:* 600 mg given once daily	PO	A: well absorbed P: 2–4 hr
	Children; 10–20 mg/kg/day	PO	PB: 84%–91% ½L: 1.5–5 hr E: liver, urine
Ethambutol (Myambutol)	*Adults:* 15 mg/kg as a single oral dose given once daily		A: 80% P: 2–4 hr PB: 8%–22% ½L: 3–4 hr E: kidney, liver
Streptomycin (see Table 46–4)			
Pyrazinamide	*Adults:* 30–35 mg/kg/day given once daily	PO	A: rapid and complete P: 2 hr PB: 50% ½L: 9 hr E: liver and kidneys
Ethionamide (Trecator-SC)	*Adults:* 15–30 mg/kg/day in 1 or 2 divided doses	PO	A: 80% P: 3 hr PB: 10% ½L: 2–3 hr E: renal, liver, urine

A-absorption; PB-protein binding; ½L-serum half-life; E-excretion; NA-not available.
*Within the solumn of adverse effects, <u>underlines</u> indicate the most common effects; CAPITALS indicate life-threatening effects.

Contraindications/ Precautions	Adverse Effects*	Interactions	Nursing Implications
CONTRAINDICATIONS: Prior hypersensitivity reaction, hepatic disease, or renal disease.	*Neuro:* PERIPHERAL NEURITIS, OPTIC NEURITIS, MUSCLE TWITCHING AND PARESTHESIAS, CONVULSIONS, ATAXIA, TOXIC ENCEPHALOPATHY, euphoria, memory loss, psychosis, fever *Biliary:* HEPATITIS *Integ:* rash	INH may inhibit the metabolism of carbamazepine and phenytoin. Corticosteroids may enhance the metabolic breakdown of INH.	*ASSESSMENT:* Coadminister Vitamin B₆ (pyridoxine); compliance with medication regimen must be reinforced. *INTERVENTION:* Patient must be instructed to continue medication for the entire treatment course. *EVALUATION:* Evaluate for fever and symptoms. Report any adverse reactions.
CONTRAINDICATIONS: Prior hypersensitivity reaction. *PRECAUTIONS:* Avoid during pregnancy. Use cautiously in hepatic or renal disease.	*Biliary:* hepatitis *Hemo:* decrease in platelets *Integ:* reddish-orange discoloration of secretions, flushing and pruritis	Rifampin may induce the metabolism of anticoagulants, oral contraceptives, oral hypoglycemic agents, and corticosteroids.	*ASSESSMENT:* If given concomitantly with INH, additive liver damage may occur. *INTERVENTION:* Tell patient that bodily secretions may be discolored. Patients taking oral contraceptive agents should use alternative methods of birth controls. *EVALUATION:* See above.
CONTRAINDICATIONS: Use in children <13 yr not recommended. Prior hypersensitivity reactions. *PRECAUTIONS:* Use with caution in patients with renal impairment.	*Neuro:* malaise, headache, mental confusion, RETROBULBAR NEURITIS, fever *GI:* nausea, vomiting *Hemo:* elevated serum uric acid levels *Integ:* dermatitis, pruritis, joint pain	See INH.	See INH.
CONTRAINDICATIONS: Contraindicated in hepatic disease and in children. *PRECAUTIONS:* Use cautiously in the presence of gout, diabetes mellitus, renal impairment, and peptic ulcer disease.	*Neuro:* headache *GI:* anorexia, nausea, vomiting *Biliary:* hepatitis, jaundice *Hemo:* elevated serum uric acid levels *Integ:* PHOTOSENSITIVITY, arthralgias	Increases protein-bound iodine. Decreases 17-ketosteroid production.	See INH.
PRECAUTIONS: Use cautiously in patients with diabetes mellitus, pregnant patients, and children.	*Neuro:* drowsiness, depression, CONVULSIONS, PERIPHERAL NEURITIS, blurred vision, OPTIC NEURITIS *GI:* nausea, vomiting *Hemo:* decrease in platelets *Reprod:* gynecomastia, impotence *Integ:* rash, alopecia, acne	See INH.	See INH.

CONTINUED ON THE FOLLOWING PAGE

Table 46–10. ANTITUBERCULOUS DRUGS–*CONTINUED*

Name	Dosage	Mode of Administration	Pharmacokinetics
Para-aminosalicylic acid (PAS)	*Adults:* 14–16 g/day in 2–3 divided doses	PO	A: well absorbed. P: 3–4 hr
	Children: 150 mg/kg/day in 3–4 divided doses	PO	PB: 60%–70% ½L: 1 hr E: kidneys, liver, intestine
Cycloserine (Seromycin)	*Adults:* 500 mg–1 g daily in divided doses	PO	A: 70%–90% P: 3–4 hr
	Children 2–10 yr: 250–500 mg daily in divided doses	PO	PB: 0% ½L: 10 hr
	Children <2 yr: 125–250 mg daily in divided doses	PO	E: kidneys, feces

A-absorption; PB-protein binding; ½L-serum half-life; FA-fast acetylator; SA-slow acetylator; NA-not available; E-excretion.
*Within the column of adverse effects, underlines indicate the most common effects; CAPITALS indicate life-threatening effects.

ganisms, as well as *Mycobacterium tuberculosis*. Rifampin is less active than penicillin G against gram-positive cocci, but it is very active against *Staphylococcus aureus*. It is also very active against *Neisseria meningitidis*, *Neisseria gonorrhoeae*, and *Hemophilus influenzae*. While the activity is variable, this agent also inhibits the growth of *Escherichia coli*, *Enterobacter* species, *Pseudomonas aeruginosa*, *Proteus* species, and *Klebsiella* species. The primary clinical use for rifampin is, however, in the treatment of tuberculosis and selected staphylococcal infections. Against *Mycobacterium tuberculosis*, rifampin is bactericidal, and is often used in combination with INH and/or streptomycin to increase the effectiveness of treatment and prevent emergence of resistance. Against staphylococcus, it is frequently used in combination with an antistaphylococcal penicillin (e.g., nafcillin).

Pharmacokinetics. *Absorption.* Following oral administration, rifampin is well absorbed. Food has been shown to delay absorption, as well as decrease peak plasma concentrations. Rifampin enters the systemic circulation and is eventually excreted in bile and into the small intestine. Reabsorption of rifampin from the gastrointestinal tract occurs and the drug returns to the systemic circulation. This phenomenon is known as enterohepatic recirculation.

Distribution. Rifampin is distributed throughout body fluids, including the cerebrospinal fluid. The extent of distribution is evident from the orange-red color change imparted to the urine, feces, saliva, sputum, tears, and sweat. Patients should be made aware of this color change so as not to be alarmed. Rifampin may also tint contact lenses orange-red. Although the teratogenic

potential is unknown, the drug has been measured in the fetal circulation and is secreted into breast milk. Rifampin also penetrates phagocytic cells and can kill intracellular organisms. Rifampin is about 80% bound to serum proteins.

Metabolism and Excretion. Rifampin is excreted in the bile and undergoes enterohepatic recirculation. As the drug passes through the liver, it is also metabolized to a microbiologically less active deacetylated compound. The metabolite is not reabsorbed and is eliminated in the feces. The parent compound (rifampin) is eventually excreted in the feces (approximately 60%). The plasma half-life of rifampin range is 1.5–5 hours and is prolonged in patients with hepatic disease. Minimal rifampin is excreted through the kidneys, therefore, dosage alteration is not required in patients with renal disease. The effects of dialysis on rifampin serum concentrations are insignificant.

Adverse Reactions. *Hypersensitivity Reactions.* Hypersensitivity reactions to rifampin are rare; however, a "cutaneous syndrome" has been described in patients receiving daily or intermittent therapy with rifampin. Typically, this reaction occurs early in the course of therapy and is manifested by flushing and pruritis (itching), with or without a rash. Areas most often involved are the face and scalp, with watering and redness of the eyes also occurring.

Hepatotoxicity. Rifampin-induced hepatitis is not an uncommon side effect of the drug; however, it is usually asymptomatic in nature and transient with mild elevation in transaminase enzyme levels (e.g., ALT). A more serious and symptomatic form of hepatitis has been described and patients at particular risk are the elderly pa-

Contraindications/ Precautions	Adverse Effects*	Interactions	Nursing Implications
CONTRAINDICATIONS: Prior hypersensitivity reactions. *PRECAUTIONS:* Use cautiously in patients with impaired renal and hepatic function.	*Neuro:* fever, malaise *GI:* nausea, vomiting, epigastric pain, peptic ulceration *Hemo:* HEMOLYTIC ANEMIA *Renal:* crystalluria *Integ:* conjunctivitis, pruritis, rash, joint pain	Interferes with urine urobilinogen. False positive urine protein and VMA. Increased blood levels with probenecid, phenytoin, salicylates, and sulfinpyrazone. Impaired absorption when given with rifampin or diphenhydramine.	*ASSESSMENT:* Give with or immediately after meals. Maintain fluid intake *INTERVENTION:* Instruct patient to take with meals or immediately after meals. *EVALUATION:* See INH.
CONTRAINDICATIONS: Prior hypersensitivity reactions. *PRECAUTIONS:* Use cautiously in patients with CNS disorders, renal impairment, and during pregnancy. Use cautiously in children.	*Neuro:* psychosis, somnolence, headache, tremor, virtigo, confusion and depression, aggression, visual disturbances, insomnia, SEIZURES *Biliary:* hepatitis *Integ:* rash		See INH.

tient, the patient with preexisting liver disease, or the alcoholic patient. There may be additive toxicity when rifampin is used in combination with other antitubercular agents known to cause liver injury (e.g., INH, pyrazinamide).

Hematologic Toxicity. Rifampin is known to induce thrombocytopenia more often when it is used intermittently, as opposed to when daily therapy is used.

Drug Interactions. Rifampin is a potent inducer of liver enzymes and has been reported to increase the metabolism of anticoagulants, oral contraceptives, methadone, quinidine, oral hypoglycemic agents, and corticosteroids. The increased metabolic capability results in a decreased pharmacologic effect of these agents and, therefore, higher dosages may be required. In the case of oral contraceptive agents, patients receiving rifampin should be instructed to use an alternative method of birth control.

ETHAMBUTOL. ***Mechanism of Action.*** The mechanism of action of ethambutol (Myambutol) is not precisely known; however, it probably acts as an antimetabolite and inhibits mycobacterial RNA synthesis.

Spectrum of Activity. Ethambutol is active (bacteriostatic) against *Mycobacterium tuberculosis*. Against other atypical mycobacterial species (e.g., avium-intracellulare) the drug is active in vitro; however, combination therapy with INH is often necessary for effective clinical results.

Pharmacokinetics. *Absorption.* Ethambutol is well absorbed after oral administration (80%) and unaffected by food.

Distribution. Ethambutol distributes to most body tissues including the lung and is localized within pulmonary alveolar macrophages. In the presence of inflammation, cerebrospinal fluid penetration is seen. The drug is approximately 10% serum protein bound.

Metabolism and Excretion. The majority (80%) of an oral dose of ethambutol is excreted unchanged in the urine. Approximately 15% of absorbed drug is metabolized by the liver to inactive metabolites and unabsorbed drug is excreted in the feces (20%). The elimination half-life of ethambutol in subjects with normal renal function is three to four hours. Dosage alteration in patients with reduced renal function is necessary. Ethambutol is hemodialyzed and the daily dose should be administered after the dialysis procedure.

Adverse Reactions. *Hypersensitivity Reactions and Hepatitis.* Ethambutol is generally well tolerated and these reactions are rare.

Retrobulbar Neuritis. This is considered the major toxicity of ethambutol and is clearly a dose-related phenomenon. If the dose of ethambutol is 15 mg/kg/day or less, this adverse effect is extremely uncommon. This effect is readily reversible if it is recognized early and the drug is discontinued; however, optic atrophy and blindness may result if therapy is continued. Symptoms include blurring of vision, central blind spots or constriction of the visual fields, and/or alterations in red/ green color perception. Patients should be made aware of this toxicity and be instructed to report any changes in visual function.

Hyperuricemia. Because of its ability to decrease the renal clearance of uric acid, ethambutol can induce an elevation in serum uric acid concentrations. However, it seldom causes acute gouty attacks.

STREPTOMYCIN. Streptomycin was first isolated from *Streptomyces griseus* in 1944 and belongs to the aminoglycoside family of antibiotics. While considered by many to be a primary antitubercular agent (bacteriostatic), it also has activity against other microorganisms and continues to be used in combination with penicillin G for the treatment of selected streptococcal infections (e.g., infective endocarditis). Refer to the section on aminoglycosides for a general discussion of the pharmacology and pharmacokinetics of streptomycin.

Second-Line Antitubercular Agents

PYRAZINAMIDE. Pyrazinamide, a derivative of nicotinamide, was synthesized in 1952.

Mechanism of Action. The manner in which pyrazinamide suppresses the growth of the tubercle bacillus is unknown. It is inactive against other bacteria and is bacteriostatic against *Mycobacterium tuberculosis*. As with other antitubercular drugs, resistance may develop during prolonged treatment, particularly if the drug is used alone.

Pharmacokinetics. Absorption. Pyrazinamide is rapidly and completely absorbed following oral ingestion with peak plasma concentrations occurring in two hours.

Distribution. The drug penetrates well into the liver, lungs, and kidney, and into the cerebrospinal fluid of patients with tuberculous meningitis. Pyrazinamide enters cells that have phagocytized tubercle bacilli.

Metabolism and Excretion. Pyrazinamide is metabolized in the liver by hepatic microsomal enzymes (deaminidase), as well as excreted in its original form by glomerular filtration (3%). Its half-life is approximately nine hours. The dosage of pyrazinamide is adjusted accordingly in patients with impaired hepatic or renal function.

Adverse Reactions. Gastrointestinal Effects. Patients may experience mild degrees of anorexia and nausea. Vomiting is much less common.

Hepatotoxicity. The incidence of hepatotoxicity secondary to pyrazinamide is variable and ranges from 2% to 20% of patients. It is often felt that because patients who receive pyrazinamide failed on prior therapy with hepatotoxic drugs (such as INH or rifampin), this agent may only contribute to previous hepatic damage. Patients should be monitored closely for signs of hepatic injury (jaundice or altered liver function tests) while on pyrazinamide.

Hyperuricemia. One of the metabolites of pyrazinamide (pyrazinoic acid), like ethambutol, inhibits the tubular secretion of uric acid. Early studies reported certain patients who developed clinical gout secondary to elevations of serum uric acid levels. The significance of this toxicity has been questioned; however, patients with a previous history of abnormalities of uric acid metabolism should be monitored closely during pyrazinamide treatment.

Arthralgias. This may be the result of elevated serum uric acid levels; however, unlike gout, the joint pain usually involves both large and small joints (most commonly the shoulders, knees, and fingers) and often involves more than one type of joint. The onset is usually during the first couple of months after treatment has been initiated. This condition is usually self-limiting, and responds readily to symptomatic therapy (e.g., aspirin).

ETHIONAMIDE. Ethionamide (Trecator-SC), a derivative of isonicotinic acid, was discovered in France in 1956 and was subsequently shown to be an effective antitubercular drug.

Mechanism of Action. The mechanism of action of ethionamide is unknown.

Pharmacokinetics. Absorption. The absorption of ethionamide following oral administration has been reported to be variable depending on the dosage formulation. The absorption pattern of coated tablets may be erratic; however, when uncoated tablets are prescribed, absorption is good.

Distribution. Ethionamide is distributed into various body organs. This agent penetrates the cerebrospinal fluid of patients with or without tuberculous meningitis.

Metabolism and Excretion. Metabolism of ethionamide is presumed to be in the liver and six metabolites have been identified. The half-life of ethionamide is approximately two hours. It appears that the only metabolite with demonstrable antitubercular activity is ethionamide sulphoxide. Less then 1% of the parent compound is eliminated in the urine in the unchanged form.

Adverse Reactions. Gastrointestinal Effects. These are the major adverse effects which limit the use of ethionamide. Patients receiving the drug may complain of excessive salivation, nausea, vomiting, anorexia, diarrhea, abdominal pain, or a metallic taste. In some patients, these effects are severe enough to require discontinuation of therapy. Gastrointestinal side effects may be more common in women than in men.

Hepatotoxicity. Liver damage is uncommon with this agent; however, it has been reported and patients should be monitored for hepatic dysfunction.

Psychiatric and Neurologic Side Effects. In the clinical setting, patients ingesting ethionamide may experience mental status changes. Giddiness and headache are common. In addition, depression, acute psychoses, and dizziness may be reported. Patients may experience visual alterations or peripheral nerve abnormalities (tingling fingers).

Teratogenicity. Ethionamide is teratogenic in animals and should be avoided during pregnancy.

PARA-AMINOSALICYLIC ACID. In 1946, Lehmann and coworkers observed that para-aminosalicylic acid (PAS) had a tuberculostatic effect. Clinical usage of this agent has decreased with newer, less toxic antitubercular agents on the market.

Mechanism of Action. PAS is similar in structure to para-aminobenzoic acid (PABA) and is thought to interfere with folate metabolism much like that seen with the sulfonamides. The effects of PAS are limited to the tubercle bacillus.

Pharmacokinetics. Absorption. PAS is well absorbed from the gastrointestinal tract, however, it may cause significant gastrointestinal irritation, increase peristalsis, and lead to a decrease in overall absorption. With this in mind, the drug is best administered with food or antacids to decrease irritation.

Distribution. PAS distributes into most cells of the body, but does not attain high concentrations in the cerebrospinal fluid. Serum protein binding is approximately 60%–70%.

Metabolism and Excretion. Approximately 80% of PAS is excreted in the urine (both glomerular filtration and tubular secretion) of which half is in the acetylated form. Hepatic metabolism plays a significant role in the detoxification of the drug and the elaboration of several metabolites with antitubercular activity. The serum half-life is approximately 0.75 hours. Patients with severe renal dysfunction do not eliminate this agent efficiently, therefore, the drug is not recommended in renal failure.

Adverse Reactions. *Gastrointestinal Effects.* PAS is a gastrointestinal irritant and the large doses commonly used to treat tuberculosis (10–20 g/day) may be associated with anorexia, nausea, diarrhea, and abdominal discomfort in many patients.

Hypersensitivity Reactions. These reactions are common and may present as fever, malaise, joint pain, skin eruptions, pruritis, and conjunctivitis. The hepatitis which may occur with this agent is felt to be a hypersensitivity reaction and becomes apparent within the first two to three months of therapy.

Hematologic Side Effects. Rarely, neutropenia or acute hemolytic anemia may occur; the latter occurring in patients with glucose-6-phosphate dehydrogenase deficiency (G-6-PD deficiency).

CYCLOSERINE. Cycloserine (Seromycin) is a broad-spectrum antibiotic produced by *Streptomyces orchidaceus* and *Streptomyces garyphalus.* Although cycloserine is active against other microorganisms, its primary clinical indication is as a second-line antituberculous agent.

Mechanism of Action. Cycloserine is a cell wall active antibiotic; however, it appears to work at a site different from that of other cell wall active agents (e.g., penicillins). Specifically, cycloserine competitively inhibits the linking of D-alanine molecules early in the formation or synthesis of the bacterial cell wall.

Pharmacokinetics. *Absorption.* Cycloserine is well absorbed when given orally and peak serum concentrations are reached in three to four hours.

Distribution. The drug is not appreciably bound to serum protein, therefore, it has a large volume of distribution throughout the body. The cerebrospinal fluid is extremely accessible to cycloserine with concentrations comparable to serum concentrations.

Metabolism and Excretion. Cycloserine is primarily eliminated by the kidneys (65%) by glomerular filtration. Approximately 35% is metabolized. The dosage of cycloserine should be decreased in patients with reduced renal function.

Adverse Reactions. *Neuropsychiatric Side Effects.* The most common reactions to cycloserine are related to the central nervous system. The excellent penetration of cycloserine into the cerebrospinal fluid may result in psychosis, somnolence, headache, tremor, vertigo, confusion and depression, aggression, visual disturbances, slurred speech, insomnia, seizures, and hyperreflexia. All these reactions appear to be dose-related and are less likely to occur with lower daily doses (e.g., 0.5 g/day). The drug should be avoided in patients with a history of epilepsy or psychiatric illness.

Other Side Effects. Hypersensitivity reactions and hepatitis are rare.

ANTIFUNGAL AGENTS

Amphotericin B

Amphotericin B (Fungizone) is a product of a soil organism, *Streptomyces nodesus,* and was discovered in 1956. Antifungal agents are featured in Table 46–11.

MECHANISM OF ACTION. The antifungal activity of amphotericin B is related to its ability to bind to ergosterol, which is the principal *sterol* on the fungal cell membrane. As a result of this binding phenomenon, pores appear in the cell membrane and life-sustaining cellular materials "leak" out of the organism, ultimately causing the death of the fungus. Amphotericin B has a greater affinity for components of fungal membranes than for human membranes. However, toxicity of this agent is thought to be caused by altered membrane permeability of human cells. Resistance is associated with fungal alteration of cell membrane components to resist amphotericin B binding and also reduced penetration of amphotericin B through the membrane.

SPECTRUM OF ACTIVITY. Amphotericin B is either *fungistatic* (inhibits fungal growth) or *fungicidal* (kills fungi), depending upon the concentration attained and the sensitivity of the fungus. It is active against many of the fungi seen commonly in hospitalized patients such as *Candida* species, *Cryptococcus neoformans, Aspergillus fumigatus,* and others. The antifungal activity of amphotericin B is enhanced (synergy) when administered together with tetracyclines, rifampin, or 5-flucytosine. The alteration in the membrane permeability induced by amphotericin B makes it easier for the other agent (e.g., 5-flucytosine) to penetrate the fungal cell wall.

PHARMACOKINETICS. *Absorption.* Amphotericin B is not absorbed from the gastrointestinal tract, therefore, the intravenous route of administration is most often used for the treatment of systemic fungal infections.

Distribution. Following intravenous administration, approximately 95% of amphotericin B is bound to *lipoproteins.* Penetration into the cerebrospinal fluid is poor; however, it is effective in the treatment of fungal infections of the central nervous system (e.g., cryptococcal meningitis).

Metabolism and Excretion. The plasma half-life of amphotericin B is approximately twenty-four hours. Less than 5% of a dose is excreted by the kidneys. The remainder is inactivated in the body, but the site and existence of metabolites is unclear. Renal failure does not affect elimination of amphotericin B and dosage need not be altered. The drug is not hemodialyzed.

ADVERSE REACTIONS. *Toxicity Associated with Intravenous Administration.* During and after intravenous administration, patients may experience thrombophlebitis, fever, chills, headache, anorexia, nausea, and vomiting. The reactions may represent toxic effects of the drug and/or hypersensitivity on the part of the patient. Amphotericin B solutions should be at room temperature and the solution thoroughly mixed (shaken) before the infusion begins. For infusions longer

TEXT RESUMES ON PAGE 1266

Table 46–11. ANTIFUNGAL AGENTS

Name	Dosage	Mode of Administration	Pharmacokinetics
Amphotericin B (Fungizone)			
Action: Bind to fungal cell wall sterols and cause "leakage" of intracellular material.			
Use: For treating systemic fungal infections.			
	Adults: test dose, 1 mg; if tolerated, 0.25–1 mg/kg/day as tolerated	IV infusion over 4–6 hr	A: 0% PB: 95% ½L: 24 hr E: nonrenal
Clotrimazole (Mycelex)			
Action: Effects the fungal cell wall and causes "leakage" of intracellular material.			
Use: For treating local fungal infections.			
	Adults: 1 troche 5 times daily	PO (Troche, 10 mg)	A: 0%
	Adults: 1 tablet or full applicator daily	Vaginal (tablet: 100 mg, 500 mg; cream, 1%)	PB: NA ½L: NA E: NA
	Adults: apply to affected area twice daily	Topical (cream, solution, and lotion, 1%)	
Flucytosine (Ancobon)			
Action: Disrupts protein synthesis of fungal organisms.			
Use: Treatment of systemic fungal infections.			
	Adults: 50–150 mg/kg/day at 6 hourly intervals	PO	A: 75%–90% PB: 2–4% ½L: 3–4 hr E: kidneys
Miconazole (Monistat IV)			
Action: See clotrimazole.			
Use: Treatment of systemic fungal infections.			
	Adults: 200 mg test dose followed by 200–3600 mg/day in 3 equally divided doses	IV	A: 50% PB: 95% ½L: 24 hr E: hepatic
	Children: 20–40 mg/kg/day	IV	
	Adults: 1 tablet daily	Vaginal tablet (100 mg or 200 mg)	

A-absorption; PB-protein binding; ½L-serum half-life; E-excretion; NA-not available.
*Within the column of adverse effects, underlines indicate the most common effects; CAPITALS indicate life-threatening effects.

Contraindications/ Precautions	Adverse Effects*	Interactions	Nursing Implications
CONTRAINDICATIONS: Prior hypersensitivity reactions. *PRECAUTIONS:* Safe use in pregnancy not established.	*Neuro:* fever, chills, head-ache *CVR:* HYPOTENSION, thrombo-phlebitis, arrhythmias *GI:* nausea, vomiting, anorexia *Hemo:* ANEMIA, hypokalemia, hypomagnesemia *Renal:* NEPHROTOXICITY, META-BOLIC ACIDOSIS	Synergistic nephrotoxicity with other drugs (e.g., ami-noglycosides, cis-platinum, ethacrynic acid, furose-mide).	*ASSESSMENT:* Monitor for phlebitis; IV infusion should be 4–6 hr in length. Monitor for signs of decreased serum potassium (e.g., muscle cramps, fatigue). IV solution should be thor-oughly mixed before infu-sion is begun. *INTERVENTION:* Patient should report any fever, chills, shaking, dizziness (hypotension), flushing dur-ing infusion. Premedicate with diphenhydramine (Ben-adryl) and acetaminophen (Tylenol).
CONTRAINDICATIONS: Prior hypersensitivity reactions.	Minimal adverse effects.		*ASSESSMENT:* Patient should be instructed to suck and not swallow. *EVALUATION:* Evaluate for signs of clearing of local fungal infection.
PRECAUTIONS: Safe use during pregnancy not established. Use cau-tiously in patients with impaired renal function.	*GI:* diarrhea, nausea, vomit-ing *Hemo:* leukopenia, thrombo-cytopenia, anemia	Elevations in alkaline phos-phatase levels. Increased ALT, AST, BUN, and serum creatinine levels.	*ASSESSMENT:* Lower initial doses may decrease GI upset. *EVALUATION:* Evaluate for fever and symptoms. Check WBC count. Report any adverse reactions.
CONTRAINDICATIONS: Prior hypersensitivity reactions. *PRECAUTIONS:* Safe use in pregnancy and in chil-dren under 1 year of age has not been estab-lished.	*CVR:* thrombophlebitis *GI:* nausea, vomiting, diar-rhea *Hemo:* anemia	Miconazole may enhance the action of coumadin and oral hypoglycemic agents.	*ASSESSMENT:* Administer via large vein. *EVALUATION:* See ampho-tericin B.

CONTINUED ON THE FOLLOWING PAGE

Table 46–11. ANTIFUNGAL AGENTS–*CONTINUED*

Name	Dosage	Mode of Administration	Pharmacokinetics
Ketoconazole (Nizoral)			
Action: See miconazole.			
Use: Treatment of systemic fungal infections.			
	Adults: 200–400 mg once daily	PO	A: variable PB: >90%
	Children >2 yr: 3.3–6.6 mg/ kg/day as a single dose	PO	½L: 8 hr E: kidney, bile, urine
Nystatin (Mycostatin)			
Action: Binds to fungal cell membrane and induces alterations in cell permeability.			
Use: Treatment of local fungal infections.			
	Adults: 500,000–1,000,000 units 3 times daily	PO (tablets)	
	Adults and children: 400,000–600,000 units 4 times daily	PO (Oral suspension, 100,000 U/ml)	A: 0% PB: NA ½L: NA
	Infants: 200,000 units 4 times daily	PO (Oral suspension, 100,000 U/ml)	E: NA
	Adults and children: 200,000–400,000 units 4 or 5 times daily		
	Adults: 1 tablet daily	Vaginal tablet (100,000 U)	
	Adults: apply 2–3 times daily	Topical (cream or oint- ment, 100,000 U/g)	
Griseofulvin (Grifulvin, Fulvi- cin U/F)			
Action: Interferes with fungal DNA replication.			
Use: Treatment of deep-seated mycotic infections.			
	Adults: 500 mg–1 g once daily, microsize; 330–750 mg, ultramicrosize	PO (Capsules/tablets)	A: 25%–70% PB: NA ½L: 10–24 hr
	Children >2 yr: 11 mg/kg/ day, microsize; 7.3 mg/kg/ day, ultramicrosize	PO (Also available as an oral suspension, 125 mg/5 ml)	E: hepatic

A-absorption; PB-protein binding; ½L-serum half-life; E-excretion; NA-not available.
*Within the solumn of adverse effects, underlines indicate the most common effects; CAPITALS indicate life-threatening effects.

than four hours, the intravenous bag should be period-ically mixed during the infusion. The addition of hepa-rin or hydrocortisone, as well as a prolonged duration of infusion (four to six hours) may overcome these re-actions. Premedication with diphenhydramine (Bena-dryl) and acetaminophen (Tylenol) can decrease the adverse effects associated with amphotericin B administration.

Contraindications/ Precautions	Adverse Effects*	Interactions	Nursing Implications
CONTRAINDICATIONS: Prior hypersensitivity reactions. *PRECAUTIONS:* Safe use in children <2 yr not established	*GI:* nausea, vomiting *Biliary:* HEPATITIS *Reprod:* gynecomastia, impotence *Integ:* hair loss	Antacids and H$_2$-antagonists (e.g., cimetidine, ranitidine, famotidine, nizatidine) may decrease the absorption of ketoconazole. The half-life of cyclosporin may be prolonged. Rifampin may increase the metabolism of ketoconazole. The anticoagulant effects of coumadin may be exaggerated by ketoconazole.	*ASSESSMENT:* Avoid concomitant use of antacids or H$_2$-antagonists (e.g., cimetidine, ranitidine, famotidine, nizatidine) *INTERVENTION:* Patient may take medication with meals to minimize GI distress. *EVALUATION:* Evaluate for fever and symptoms. Report any adverse reactions.
CONTRAINDICATIONS: Prior hypersensitivity reactions.	*GI:* nausea, vomiting		*ASSESSMENT:* Patient should swish then swallow oral suspension. *INTERVENTION:* Instruct patient on proper oral hygiene for infected areas. *EVALUATION:* Same as for clotrimazole.
CONTRAINDICATIONS: Prior hypersensitivity reactions. *PRECAUTIONS:* Safe use in pregnancy not established. Use cautiously in penicillin-allergic patients.	*GI:* nausea, vomiting, diarrhea, flatulence, heartburn *Integ:* PHOTOSENSITIVITY REACTIONS	Griseofulvin may decrease the anticoagulant effect of warfarin. Barbiturates enhance the metabolic breakdown of griseofulvin. Griseofulvin can enhance the effects of alcohol.	*ASSESSMENT:* Give with meals to decrease GI distress. Concomitant administration with food will enhance absorption. *INTERVENTION:* Instruct patient to use a sunscreen when going outdoors. Avoid concomitant alcohol use. Take medication with meals. *EVALUATION:* See amphotercin B.

Nephrotoxicity. Most patients experience a decrease in renal function during amphotericin B therapy. The decreased renal function is monitored clinically by changes in the serum creatinine concentration. When the serum creatinine level reaches 2.5 mg/dL, the drug is usually discontinued and then resumed again after two to three days, or an every-other-day administration regimen is followed.

Anemia. Patients receiving amphotericin B usually develop mild anemia because of suppression of red blood cell production in the bone marrow. This effect is reversible when the drug is discontinued.

Electrolyte and Acid-Base Imbalance. As a result of amphotericin-B–induced renal dysfunction, the kidneys may excrete excess potassium, leading to severe hypokalemia. Patients are monitored closely and given potassium supplements when indicated. Hypomagnesemia may also occur and require magnesium supplementation. Metabolic acidosis, which is due to altered renal acidifying mechanisms, can also occur during amphotericin B administration.

DRUG INTERACTIONS. Concurrent administration of amphotericin B with other nephrotoxic agents (e.g., aminoglycosides, cis-platinum, ethacrynic acid, furosemide) may have additive toxic effects on the kidneys.

Flucytosine

Flucytosine (Ancobon), also known as 5-flucytosine or 5-FC, is a synthetic antimetabolite of the fluoropyrimidine series.

MECHANISM OF ACTION. 5-FC penetrates fungal cells with the help of an enzyme known as cytosine permease. Once inside the cell, 5-FC is converted, with the help of another enzyme (cytosine deaminase), to 5-FU (5-fluorouracil), which is then incorporated into RNA, disrupting protein synthesis and resulting in cell death. Part of the selective action of 5-FC is the fact that human cells do not contain the enzyme cytosine deaminase. Fungi may develop resistance to 5-FC as a result of a deficiency of permease activity, therefore, 5-FC will not penetrate the fungal cell. Resistance to 5-FC develops rapidly when it is prescribed alone.

SPECTRUM OF ACTIVITY. 5-FC has been prescribed in combination with other antifungals for the treatment of infections caused by *Candida albicans, Cryptococcus neoformans, Torulopsis glabrata,* and *Aspergillus* species.

PHARMACOKINETICS. *Absorption.* This agent is administered via the oral route, and is well absorbed after ingestion. Peak serum concentrations are reached within two to four hours after a dose.

Distribution. The drug is distributed widely throughout the body tissues with levels in the cerebrospinal fluid being 75% of simultaneous serum concentrations. The drug is 48% protein bound.

Metabolism and Excretion. 5-FC is primarily (>90%) eliminated unchanged by glomerular filtration. The serum half-life is three to four hours. Patients with impaired renal function must have their dose reduced.

ADVERSE REACTIONS. *Gastrointestinal Effects.* Patients receiving 5-FC may develop nausea, vomiting, or diarrhea and may require a dosage reduction.

Hematologic Effects. 5-FC–induced bone marrow suppression may lead to neutropenia (decrease in the number of neutrophils), thrombocytopenia (decrease in the number of platelets), or anemia. Patients at risk for this particular side effect appear to be individuals with decreased renal function.

Miconazole

Miconazole (Monistat IV) another imidazole antifungal agent, was synthesized in 1969 by Godefrol and co-workers in Belgium. In addition to its use as a topical antifungal, it is also available for intravenous administration.

MECHANISM OF ACTION. Miconazole has a similar mechanism of action to clotrimazole.

SPECTRUM OF ACTIVITY. Miconazole inhibits the growth of *Candida albicans, Cryptococcus neoformans, Blastomyces dermatitidis, Histoplasma capsulatum, Coccidioides immitis, Aspergillus* species, *Trichophyton* species, and *Epidermophyton* species. This agent also has activity against gram-positive cocci and bacilli; however, it is not used as an antibacterial agent.

PHARMACOKINETICS. *Absorption.* Miconazole is poorly absorbed when given orally, therefore, therapy for systemic infections requires intravenous administration. Oral formulations are not available in the United States; however, both topical and parenteral products are available.

Distribution. Miconazole is approximately 95% protein bound and diffuses poorly into the cerebrospinal fluid. It does penetrate synovial (joint) fluid and vitreous fluid.

Metabolism and Excretion. Miconazole is rapidly metabolized in the liver by oxidation, hydrolysis, and conjugation.

Approximately 10% of an administered dose is excreted in the urine as inactive metabolites. The plasma half-life of the drug is approximately twenty-four hours. While minimal amounts are excreted by the kidneys, the dose of miconazole need not be altered in patients with renal disease. Hemodialysis has no effect on elimination of the drug.

ADVERSE REACTIONS. *Hematologic Effects.* Following intravenous administration miconazole appears to suppress red blood cell production. This effect is dose-related and disappears when miconazole is discontinued.

Gastrointestinal Effects. Oral and intravenous dosing may result in symptoms such as nausea, vomiting, or diarrhea.

Thrombophlebitis. Intravenous infusions in miconazole may cause thrombophlebitis when given through peripheral veins. This problem is avoided by administering the drug via larger, central veins.

DRUG INTERACTIONS. While the exact mechanism of this drug-drug interaction is not known, concomitant administration of anticoagulants may result in prolongation of the prothrombin time (PT) and an increased risk of bleeding.

Concomitant administration of hypoglycemic agents may result in hypoglycemia. The exact mechanism of this drug-drug interaction is unknown.

Ketoconazole

Ketoconazole (Nizoral) is another imidazole antifungal agent, similar in structure to miconazole.

MECHANISM OF ACTION. The mechanism of antifungal action is similar to that of miconazole in that ergosterol biosynthesis is impaired and there is alteration in the cell membrane which leads to cell death. In addition, ketoconazole may affect oxidative and peroxidative systems within fungal organisms resulting in the intracellular accumulation of toxic endoperoxides.

SPECTRUM OF ACTIVITY. See discussion of spectrum of activity for miconazole.

PHARMACOKINETICS. *Absorption.* Ketoconazole is active orally and is water-soluble at pH <3. Peak serum concentrations are reached two to four hours after the dose. Absorption may be variable and may be impaired by the administration of agents known to increase gastric pH (e.g., antacids, H_2-antagonists). Its absorption may be enhanced when given with food.

Distribution. Ketoconazole is highly protein bound (>90%) and diffusion into the cerebrospinal fluid is poor.

Metabolism and Excretion. Ketoconazole is extensively metabolized in the liver and excreted as inactive drug in the bile. It has a half-life of eight hours. Less than 1% of the drug is excreted unchanged in the urine, therefore, the dosage need not be altered in patients with renal disease.

ADVERSE REACTIONS. *Gastrointestinal Effects.* Following oral doses of 400–600 mg/day of ketoconazole, patients may complain of mild nausea and occasional vomiting. These symptoms may be alleviated by taking the drug with meals.

Hepatotoxicity. Although symptomatic hepatic disease is rare, asymptomatic elevations in transaminase enzyme levels has been reported in 2%–5% of patients.

Other Side Effects. The ability of ketoconazole to inhibit testosterone and adrenocorticotropic hormone synthesis can explain some of the observed side effects such as sexual impotence, hair loss, and gynecomastia. These effects may only occur after high doses and/or prolonged dosing.

DRUG INTERACTIONS. The solubility of ketoconazole and subsequent absorption of the drug is dependent upon an acidic environment. Agents which increase the pH of the stomach will affect the absorption of ketoconazole.

The plasma half-life of cyclosporin is reported to be prolonged by ketoconazole, however, the mechanism of this interaction is not known.

Rifampin is a known enzyme stimulator and can increase the metabolism of ketoconazole resulting in a decrease in the clinical effect of the antifungal agent.

Prolongation of the prothrombin time has been reported with the concomitant administration of ketoconazole and oral anticoagulants. The precise mechanism of this interaction is unknown; however, patients receiving both agents should be monitored for potential bleeding episodes.

Nystatin

Nystatin (Mycostatin) is a polyene antifungal agent (like amphotericin B) isolated from *Streptomyces noursei* in 1950. Because of toxicity it is not used parenterally; it is used primarily for topical therapy of superficial fungal infections.

MECHANISM OF ACTION. Nystatin binds to fungal cell membranes (specifically sterols) and induces an alteration in cell permeability, which results in cell death.

SPECTRUM OF ACTIVITY. Nystatin inhibits the growth of various fungi including: *Candida albicans; Cryptococcus neoformans; Histoplasma capsulatum; Blastomyces dermatitidis; Coccidioides immitis;* and *Aspergillus, Trichophyton, Epidermophyton,* and *Microsporum* species. However, this agent is too toxic when administered systemically, and so is of little use for serious fungal infections.

PHARMACOKINETICS. *Absorption.* Nystatin is administered orally (swish and swallow) and vaginally, but it is not absorbed systemically.

ADVERSE REACTIONS. Minimal toxicity is associated with topical administration of nystatin; however, following oral ingestion of large doses, nausea and diarrhea may occur.

Clotrimazole

Clotrimazole (Lotrimin, Mycelex) was synthesized in Germany in 1967; however, gastrointestinal toxicity has limited its clinical application to topical treatment of superficial fungal infections.

MECHANISM OF ACTION. Like other imidazole antifungal agents (e.g., miconazole, ketoconazole), clotrimazole appears to effect the fungal cell wall which leads to "leakage" of vital cellular elements and ultimately to cell death. Although it works by altering the permeability of the fungal membrane, it appears to do so at a site different from the polyene antifungal agents.

SPECTRUM OF ACTIVITY. See discussion of spectrum of activity for nystatin.

PHARMACOKINETICS. *Absorption.* Presently, clotrimazole is administered topically (both orally and vaginally) and systemic absorption is minimal.

ADVERSE REACTIONS. When administered topically or vaginally, minimal toxicity is encountered.

Griseofulvin

Griseofulvin (Fulvicin), first isolated in 1939, is a metabolic product of *Penicillium griseofulvium.*

MECHANISM OF ACTION. The mechanism of antifungal activity is likely to be interference with fungal DNA replication.

SPECTRUM OF ACTIVITY. Griseofulvin is used primarily for its activity against various dermatophytes (ringworm fungi) including *Microsporum, Trichophyton,* and *Epidermophyton* species.

PHARMACOKINETICS. *Absorption.* Griseofulvin has been manufactured in various oral dosage forms to enhance absorption. It has been noted that if the drug is taken with a fatty meal, absorption is approximately doubled. Peak serum concentrations are reached approximately 4 hours following an oral dose.

Distribution. Griseofulvin is widely distributed throughout body tissue and fluids and is highly concentrated in liver, fat, and skeletal muscle. It is also concentrated in skin, hair, and nails.

Metabolism and Excretion. Griseofulvin is metabolized in the liver by dealkylation to a microbiologically inactive metabolite which is then excreted in the urine. The elimination half-life range is 10–24 hours. Very little (<1%) of the parent drug (griseofulvin) is eliminated unchanged in the urine and dosage adjustment in the presence of renal disease is unnecessary.

ADVERSE REACTIONS. *Gastrointestinal Effects.* Unabsorbed griseofulvin may induce nausea, diarrhea, heartburn, or flatulence in certain patients. Prescribing a different oral preparation may help to alleviate these problems.

Hypersensitivity Reactions. Photosensitivity and skin rashes have been described during griseofulvin treatment and may require discontinuation of the medicine.

DRUG INTERACTIONS. Griseofulvin may reduce the anticoagulant effect of warfarin by enhancing the hepatic metabolism of this agent. Barbiturates enhance the metabolic breakdown of griseofulvin, resulting in a diminished effect of the antifungal agent. Griseofulvin can enhance the effects of alcohol when the two drugs are used concomitantly.

ANTIVIRAL AGENTS

Acyclovir

An acyclic nucleoside analogue of guanosine, acyclovir (Zovirax) is the first antiviral compound which requires a viral enzyme (thymidine kinase) for activation (see Table 46-12).

MECHANISM OF ACTION. Acyclovir requires enzyme (thymidine kinase) activation before it becomes *virucidal*. Acyclovir binds much more avidly to viral thymidine kinase than to host (human) cell thymidine kinase. This enzyme phosphorylates acyclovir to acyclovir monophosphate, which is subsequently phosphorylated to acyclovir triphosphate by cellular enzymes such as guanosine monophosphate kinase. It is acyclovir triphosphate which inhibits viral *DNA polymerase*. Another mechanism of action of acyclovir probably exists for viruses which lack thymidine kinase (e.g., cytomegalovirus and *Epstein-Barr virus*). In this situation, acyclovir triphosphate can be incorporated into a growing DNA chain by the action of viral-induced DNA polymerase. Once incorporated, there is termination of the DNA chain.

Three mechanisms of resistance to acyclovir have been proposed and documented with herpes simplex and varicella-zoster virus: (1) the resistant virus lacks adequate thymidine kinase activity; (2) there is a decrease in DNA polymerase sensitivity to acyclovir; and (3) the enzyme *thymidine kinase* has a decreased specificity for acyclovir.

SPECTRUM OF ACTIVITY. The spectrum of activity of acyclovir is limited to herpes viruses, with activity against: herpes simplex type 1 (HSV 1), herpes simplex type 2 (HSV 2), and varicella zoster virus (VZV). Other herpes viruses (e.g., cytomegalovirus and Epstein-Barr virus) are less susceptible. Combining acyclovir with other antiviral agents (e.g., human leukocyte interferon, vidarabine) has demonstrated enhanced activity against HSV 1 and HSV 2. Similar combinations have shown additive and, in some cases, synergistic activity against VZV.

PHARMACOKINETICS. *Absorption.* Absorption from the gastrointestinal tract is slow and dose-dependent. Absolute bioavailability is 20%; however, bioavailability decreases with increasing dose. Systemic absorption from topical administration of 5% acyclovir in a polyethylene glycol (PEG) base is minimal.

Distribution. Acyclovir distributes extensively into lung, heart, liver, kidney, and cerebrospinal fluid (CSF). Approximately 50% of the serum concentration is achieved in the CSF. It is also found in saliva and vaginal secretions in concentrations well above the susceptibility level of most HSV. Plasma protein binding is in the range of 9-33%.

Metabolism and Excretion. Most of the drug is eliminated unchanged by both glomerular filtration and tubular secretion. The only significant metabolite is 9-carboxymethoxyguanine. The half-life of acyclovir is two to three hours in subjects with normal renal function; however, in the presence of renal insufficiency, the half-life is markedly prolonged (e.g., 20 hours in the absence of renal function). Acyclovir is approximately 60% hemodialyzed.

ADVERSE REACTIONS. *Nephrotoxicity.* Adverse effects in the kidneys have been reported when patients receive large intravenous doses of acyclovir. At high doses, solubility may cause acyclovir to crystallize within the kidney, causing renal damage. This toxicity is avoided by infusing acyclovir slowly (over a period of at least 1 hour) and keeping the patient well hydrated.

Thrombophlebitis. Irritation or inflammation may occur at the injection site during acyclovir administration. Slow infusion and rotation of injection sites may alleviate this problem.

Neurotoxicity. Certain patients may experience central nervous system toxicity such as lethargy, delirium, tremulousness, or seizures, while receiving acyclovir.

DRUG INTERACTIONS. Although anecdotal at this point in time, concomitant administration of acyclovir and zidovudine (AZT) may result in "incapacitating drowsiness and lethargy."

Probenecid blocks the renal tubular secretion of acyclovir and prolongs the serum half-life of the drug.

Vidarabine

Vidarabine (Adenine Arabinoside, Ara-A, Vira-A) was developed in the early 1960s during a search for anti-cancer drugs. It was later found to inhibit viral growth and has been primarily used for its antiviral effects.

MECHANISM OF ACTION. Despite deamination to a less active derivative, vidarabine is transported into cells where mono-, di-, and tri-phosphate derivatives are formed. It is the triphosphate form that acts as a competitive inhibitor of viral DNA polymerase. In addition, this active form of vidarabine is incorporated into the growing DNA molecule at terminal positions, preventing completion of the DNA chains.

SPECTRUM OF ACTIVITY. The antiviral activity of vidarabine is limited to DNA viruses such as herpes simplex virus (HSV) types 1 and 2, varicella-zoster virus (VZV), and cytomegalovirus (CMV). HSV 1 is the most sensitive to vidarabine. Next most sensitive is HSV 2, followed by VZV; the least sensitive virus is CMV.

PHARMACOKINETICS. *Absorption.* Vidarabine must be administered intravenously, due to poor oral absorption. It is a poorly soluble compound and, therefore, requires dissolution in large volumes of fluid. Intraocular penetration of topically applied vidarabine (3% ophthalmic ointment) is extremely poor. The human cornea deaminates vidarabine to vidarabine hypoxanthine and, therefore, use of topical vidarabine to treat deep herpetic ocular infections would be pointless.

Distribution. Distribution of vidarabine is extensive with concentrations highest in kidney, liver, and spleen, and somewhat lower concentrations in brain (50%–60% of plasma).

Metabolism and Excretion. Metabolic conversion of vidarabine to a less active hypoxanthine derivative occurs quickly within the erythrocyte. Plasma level monitoring of vidarabine over a 12-hour infusion period indicates that most of the drug is in the form of the hypoxanthine derivative extracellularly and only a small percentage exists as parent drug (vidarabine triphosphate). Vidarabine is cleared from the body by the kidney, with nearly 60% of a dose appearing in the urine, primarily as vidarabine hypoxanthine. The plasma half-life (about three hours) is extended somewhat in subjects with renal insufficiency and dosage adjustments may be necessary. Dosing is necessary following hemodialysis.

ADVERSE REACTIONS. *Local Side Effects.* Burning and stinging from topical application has been described.

Neurotoxicity. Neurotoxicity is the most serious toxicity associated with vidarabine treatment. The neurologic abnormalities include tremors, ataxia, and tingling extremities. Encephalopathy may also develop during therapy and may be difficult to distinguish from worsening encephalitis. Patients at risk may be those with impaired hepatic or renal function.

Zidovudine

Zidovudine (AZT; Retrovir), a dideoxynucleoside analog of thymidine, has recently been approved by the FDA for the treatment of acquired immune deficiency syndrome (AIDS). The virus that is associated with AIDS is known as the human immunodeficiency virus (HIV). It is currently the only antiviral agent approved for this disease.

MECHANISM OF ACTION. As a thymidine analog, zidovudine is phosphorylated to zidovudine monophosphate (ZIDO-MP) by cellular thymidine kinase. Subsequent phosphorylation to zidovudine diphosphate, and then zidovudine triphosphate, results in a *virostatic* agent. In the life cycle of HIV, the virus duplicates itself once it is inside the host cell (T-lymphocyte); however, because of the unique feature of retroviruses, whose genetic material is RNA, viral reverse transcrip-

tase changes RNA to DNA. It is this step in viral replication that is inhibited by zidovudine.

SPECTRUM OF ACTIVITY. Zidovudine is primarily active against retroviruses, such as the virus responsible for AIDS.

PHARMACOKINETICS. *Absorption.* Zidovudine absorption from the gastrointestinal tract is rapid with peak serum concentrations achieved in 0.5–1 hour after administration. Zidovudine is approximately 65% bioavailable.

Distribution. Distribution to the cerebrospinal fluid (CSF) occurs with peak concentrations achieved in approximately two hours following oral doses of 200 mg every four hours. Levels in the CSF are about 50% of those in the serum. Zidovudine is approximately 36% protein bound.

Metabolism and Excretion. The drug is extensively metabolized by the liver to an inactive glucuronide metabolite, which is then excreted by the kidneys. The serum half-life of the parent compound is one hour.

ADVERSE REACTIONS. *Hematologic Effects.* The side effect profile of zidovudine is primarily related to bone marrow toxicity (anemia and leukopenia). Approximately 50% of patients receiving 1200 mg/day of zidovudine will have suppression of red blood cell production. Approximately 30% of these patients will require blood transfusions. An increase in the mean corpuscular volume (MCV), reflecting megaloblastic changes, is often an early sign of these toxic effects.

Other Side Effects. Dermatologic reactions are rare with zidovudine; however, black discoloration of the fingernails after prolonged treatment can occur.

DRUG INTERACTIONS. These drugs are known to interfere with the glucuronidation of many drugs and may potentially interfere with glucuronidation of zidovudine. This can lead to increased serum concentrations of zidovudine and subsequent toxicity.

The excretion of zidovudine can be blocked by coadministration of probenecid, resulting in increased serum concentrations of zidovudine and enhanced toxicity.

Although anecdotal at this point in time, concomitant administration of acyclovir and zidovudine (AZT) may result in "incapacitating drowsiness and lethargy."

Amantadine

Amantadine (Symmetrel), a chemically synthesized compound, was approved in 1966 for prevention of influenza A viral infections. However, for various reasons, the clinical usefulness of this agent has remained unclear, as has its potential for toxicity.

MECHANISM OF ACTION. Amantadine prevents uncoating of the virus once it (the virus) has attached to the cell membrane of the host. In addition, amantadine has a slight effect on influenza A virus penetration into the host cell. Resistance to amantadine appears to be a genetically determined property and amantadine-resistant strains of influenza virus can be selected out.

TEXT RESUMES ON PAGE 1274

Table 46–12. ANTIVIRAL AGENTS

Name	Dosage	Mode of Administration	Pharmacokinetics
Acyclovir (Zovirax)			
Action: Inhibits viral DNA polymerase.			
Use: Treatment of viral infections secondary to herpes viruses.			
	Adults: 5 mg/kg q 8 hr	IV infusion only	A: 20%
	Children <12 yr: 250 mg/m^2 q 8 hr	IV infusion only	P: 1.5–2.5 hr
			PB: 9%–33%
	Adults: 200 mg 3–5 times daily	PO (capsules	½L: 2–3 hr
	Apply to all lesions q 3 hr	Topical (ointment, 5%)	E: kidneys
Amantadine (Symmetrel)			
Action: Prevents viral uncoating.			
Use: Treatment or prophylaxis of influenza infections.			
	Adults: 200 mg once daily; 100 mg twice daily		A: 100%
			P: 1–4 hr
	Children 1–9 yr: 4.4–8.8 mg/ kg/day; given once daily or divided into 2 doses daily	PO (Also available as syrup, 50 mg/5 ml)	PB: NA
			½L: 15–20 hr
			E: kidneys
Zidovudine (AZT, Retrovir)			
Action: Inhibits viral reverse transcriptase enzyme.			
Use: Treatment of human immunodeficiency virus infections.			
	Adults: 200 mg q 4 hr around the clock	PO (Capsules)	A: 65%
			P: 0.5–1.5 hr
			PB: 36%
			½L: 1 hr
			E: liver
Vidarabine (Ara-A, Vira-A)			
Action: Competitive inhibitor of viral DNA polymerase.			
Use: Treatment of viral infections secondary to herpes viruses.			
	Adults and children: 15 mg/ kg over a 12–24 hr period	IV infusion only	A: poor
			P: NA
	Apply approximately ½ inch into the lower conjunctival	Topical (Ophthalmic ointment, 3%)	PB: 20%–30%
			½L: 1.5–3.3 hr

A-absorption; PB-protein binding; ½L-serum half-life; E-excretion; NA-not available.
*Within the column of adverse effects, underlines indicate the most common effects; CAPITALS indicate life-threatening effects.

Contraindications/ Precautions	Adverse Effects*	Interactions	Nursing Implications
CONTRAINDICATIONS: Prior hypersensitivity reactions. *PRECAUTIONS:* Use cautiously in patients with renal impairment, pregnant patients, and children.	*Neuro:* lethargy, delirium, SEI-ZURES, tremulousness *CVR:* thrombophlebitis *GI:* nausea, anorexia, diarrhea *Renal:* NEPHROTOXICITY *Integ:* rash	Zidovudine (AZT) and probenecid block the renal tubular secretion of acyclovir.	*ASSESSMENT:* Monitor for phlebitis; IV infusion should be over 1 hour. Use a finger cot or rubber glove to apply ointment. Maintain adequate hydration. *INTERVENTION:* Patient should be instructed to use a finger cot or rubber gloves when applying ointment. *EVALUATION:* Evaluate for fever and symptoms. Report any adverse reactions.
CONTRAINDICATIONS: Prior hypersensitivity reactions. *PRECAUTIONS:* Use cautiously in patients with renal impairment, congestive heart failure, during pregnancy or lactation, and in children and infants.	*Neuro:* depression, nervousness, dizziness, lightheadedness, insomnia *CVR:* congestive heart failure, edema *Integ:* livedo reticularis (purplish discoloration of the skin)		*ASSESSMENT:* Make certain patient completes full course of therapy *INTERVENTION:* Remind patient to take all medication until it is gone. *EVALUATION:* Report any adverse reactions.
CONTRAINDICATIONS: Prior hypersensitivity reaction. *PRECAUTIONS:* Use cautiously in patients with hepatic or renal impairment. Avoid use during pregnancy, lactation, or in children.	*GI:* anorexia, nausea, vomiting diarrhea *Hemo:* anemia, leukopenia *Integ:* rash, black discoloration of fingernails	Acetaminophen and sulfonamides may impair the metabolism of AZT. Probenecid blocks the excretion of AZT. Acyclovir, if given concomitantly with AZT, may cause incapacitating drowsiness and lethargy.	*ASSESSMENT:* Drug must be administered every 4 hours around the clock; do not double-up on missed doses. *INTERVENTION:* Patient should be instructed to take the drug around the clock; doubling up on doses should be avoided. *EVALUATION:* Evaluate for signs and/or symptoms of drug toxicity.
CONTRAINDICATIONS: Prior hypersensitivity reactions.	*Neuro:* burning and stinging from topical application,		*ASSESSMENT:* IV infusion should be administered

CONTINUED ON THE FOLLOWING PAGE

Table 46–12. ANTIVIRAL AGENTS–*CONTINUED*

Name	Dosage	Mode of Administration	Pharmacokinetics
Vidarabine–*Continued*	sac 5 times daily at 3-hr intervals		E: liver, kidney
Idoxuridine (Herplex, Stoxil)			
Action: Inhibits DNA polymerase.			
Use: Treatment of local viral infections.			
	Adults: 1 drop into each infected eye q hr during the day and q 3 hr during the night	Topical (Ophthalmic solution, 0.1%)	NA
	Adults: 5 instillations daily	Topical (Ophthalmic ointment 0.5%)	
Ribavirin (Virazole)			
Action: Inhibits herpes viruses.			
Use: Treatment of respiratory syncytial virus infections.			
	20 mg/ml concentration administered as aerosol for 12–18 hr/day	Aerosol administration only (SPAG-2 units)	A: 45% after oral administration; 70% after aerosol administration PB: 0% ½L: 9.5–35 hr E: liver, kidney

A-absorption; PB-protein binding; ½L-serum half-life; E-excretion; NA-not available.

*Within the column of adverse effects, underlines indicate the most common effects; CAPITALS indicate life-threatening effects.

SPECTRUM OF ACTIVITY. Amantadine is primarily active against only influenza A viruses.

PHARMACOKINETICS. *Absorption.* Amantadine is well absorbed (100%) following oral administration with peak serum concentrations occurring 1–8 hours after a dose.

Distribution. Amantadine distributes to the cerebrospinal fluid (approximately 60% of a simultaneous serum concentration) and is also found in saliva, nasal secretions, and breast milk.

Metabolism and Excretion. Amantadine is excreted by the kidneys (90%) in the unchanged form, therefore, dosage adjustment in the presence of renal insufficiency is necessary. Accumulation occurs after chronic dosing, even in patients with normal renal function. The half-

life of elimination is 15–20 hours in individuals with normal kidney function.

ADVERSE REACTIONS. *General.* Most of the adverse reactions to amantadine are not severe in the dosage range of 200–300 mg/day. Most are transient and rapidly reversible upon discontinuation (e.g., gastrointestinal complaints, edema, rash, and dryness of the mouth).

Central Nervous System Effects. Patients may experience nervousness, difficulty in concentration, dizziness, lightheadedness, slurred speech, ataxia, drowsiness, and insomnia. In addition, blurred vision, dry mouth, and palpitations have been reported.

Livedo Reticularis. A diffuse, rose-colored mottling of the skin, usually confined to the lower extremities,

Contraindications/ Precautions	Adverse Effects*	Interactions	Nursing Implications
PRECAUTIONS: Use cautiously in patients with renal impairment, pregnant patients or during lactation.	TREMORS, ATAXIA, tingling extremities *CVR:* phlebitis *GI:* diarrhea, nausea, vomiting, anorexia *Hemo:* leukopenia, thrombocytopenia, anemia		over 12–24 hours. Monitor fluid intake. Cooling of IV solution may cause precipitation of durg. *INTERVENTION:* Instruct patient to report any symptoms of burning or stinging. *EVALUATION:* Evaluate for fever and symptoms. Report any adverse reactions.
CONTRAINDICATIONS: Prior hypersensitivity reactions.	*Eye:* corneal defects; allergic reactions or inflammation		*ASSESSMENT:* Monitor for any signs of corneal changes. *INTERVENTION:* Bright lights may become unbearable while drug is being administered. *EVALUATION:* Report any adverse reactions.
CONTRAINDICATIONS: Prior hypersensitivity reactions. *PRECAUTIONS:* Pregnant women or women of childbearing age should avoid exposure to ribavirin.	*CVR:* HYPOTENSION, CARDIAC ARREST *Resp:* DYSPNEA, PNEUMOTHORAX, APNEA *Integ:* rash		*ASSESSMENT:* Drug solution should be changed every 24 hr. Monitor ventilation tube for crystal formation. Nursing personnel should avoid inhaling the aerosol during the treatment period. *EVALUATION:* Report any adverse reactions.

has been described with amantadine. This condition is called *livedo reticularis.* Mild ankle edema is usually present and most noticeable when the patient is standing or is exposed to cold. It is reversible in two to six weeks upon discontinuation of the drug and is relatively benign clinically, even when the drug is continued.

Idoxuridine

Idoxuridine (Stoxil, Herplex), a synthetic compound structurally similar to thymidine, was discovered in 1959. The primary use of idoxuridine is for the topical treatment of herpes simplex virus keratitis.

MECHANISM OF ACTION. Idoxuridine functions in a method similar to that of divarabine. It is phosphorylated intracellularly into an active antiviral compound that competes with thymidine and inhibits DNA synthesis. This antiviral activity can be reversed by thymidine.

SPECTRUM OF ACTIVITY. Idoxuridine is considered a broad-spectrum antiviral compound with activity against DNA viruses (e.g., herpes simplex virus, varicella-zoster virus, and cytomegalovirus).

PHARMACOKINETICS. Idoxuridine is used topically as an ophthalmic ointment and systemic absorption is minimal.

ADVERSE REACTIONS. Following instillation of idoxuridine into the eye, allergic or inflammatory responses may occur with pain and itching in the eye or eyelids. Frequent administration may induce small corneal defects. Patients should avoid soaking their eyes with boric acid solution because additive irritant effects may result.

Ribavirin

Ribavirin (Virazole), 1-beta-D-ribofuranosyl-1H-1,2,4-triazole-3-carboxamide, is a new nucleoside analog that has shown in vitro activity against a number of DNA and RNA viruses.

MECHANISM OF ACTION. Like most of the other antiviral drugs already discussed, ribavirin must first be activated to the triphosphorylated form (ribavirin triphosphate). The mechanism of action of ribavirin is understood only for the influenza viruses. There are three possible mechanisms of action: (1) ribavirin decreases the intracellular concentrations of GTP (guanosine triphosphate); (2) ribavirin inhibits 5'-cap formation of mRNAs (messenger RNA); and (3) ribavirin inhibits the function of virus-coded RNA polymerases necessary to initiate and elongate viral mRNAs.

SPECTRUM OF ACTIVITY. Ribavirin is a broad-spectrum virostatic antiviral compound with activity against a number of RNA and DNA viruses. It has shown clinical efficacy against both influenza A and B viruses, respiratory syncytial virus (RSV), parainfluenza virus infections, and Lassa fever. Its major indication, however, is for the treatment of severe lower respiratory tract infections secondary to RSV.

PHARMACOKINETICS. *Absorption.* Ribavirin is currently available for aerosol administration only via the Viratek Small Particle Aerosol Generator (SPAG-2) into a face mask or oxyhood. Small-particle aerosol administration deposits approximately 70% of the inhaled drug onto the respiratory epithelium. Oral and intravenous formulations of the drug are currently being investigated. Current information on the oral absorption of ribavirin shows that it is incompletely absorbed (45%).

Distribution. Ribavirin appears to be widely distributed with most of the drug existing in the plasma as free drug (i.e., protein binding 0%).

Metabolism and Excretion. Metabolism is probably the major method of elimination of ribavirin with renal excretion playing a minor role. Following intravenous administration, approximately 30% of a dose is recovered unchanged in the urine. The half-life of elimination is approximately 35 hours.

ADVERSE REACTIONS. *Pulmonary Effects.* Worsening of the patient's respiratory status, as well as the development of bacterial pneumonia and/or pneumothorax have been reported.

Cardiovascular Effects. Cardiac arrest, hypotension, and digitalis intoxication have all been reported in patients treated with ribavirin.

Other Side Effects. Rash and conjunctivitis have been reported with the aerosol use of ribavirin. Anemia, while reported with the intravenous and oral forms of the drug, has not been seen following aerosol administration. Recent data (Morbidity Mortality Weekly Report 37:560, 1988) suggest that health care personnel should minimize their exposure to ribavirin, particularly if the drug is administered by oxygen tent.

ANTIPROTOZOAL AGENTS

Pentamidine

Pentamidine isethionate (Pentam 300), an aromatic diamidine derivative, was discovered in 1938. It has since been found to be effective in the treatment of pro-

tozoal infections such as *Trypanosoma gambiense, Trypanosoma rhodesiense, Leishmania donovani,* and *Pneumocystis carinii.* Until recently, the use of pentamidine has been limited. It has been only since the epidemic of acquired immunodeficiency syndrome (AIDS), and its associated high rate of *P. carinii* pneumonia, that interest in this drug has been renewed.

MECHANISM OF ACTION. The mechanism of action of pentamidine appears to vary depending on the protozoan it is being used to treat. Against *Pneumocystis carinii*, a likely mechanism of action is that the drug interferes with oxidative phosphorylation and synthesis of nucleic acids. In addition, pentamidine may alter the ability of *P. carinii* organisms to use extracellular nutritional constituents and impair their ability to metabolize glucose.

SPECTRUM OF ACTIVITY. While the spectrum of activity of pentamidine includes trypanosomal organisms, its major use in the United States is for the treatment and prophylaxis of *Pneumocystis carinii* infections.

PHARMACOKINETICS. *Absorption.* Because of its poor absorption from the gastrointestinal tract, pentamidine is not available for oral administration. Following intramuscular administration, the drug is well absorbed with peak plasma concentrations reached in approximately one hour. The drug may also be administered by intravenous infusion or by aerosol.

Distribution. The drug is widely distributed in the body with tissue concentrations highest in the kidneys, followed by the liver, and then other tissues (e.g., lungs). Very little of the drug is found in the brain. The volume of distribution in humans is approximately 3 liters/kg of body weight.

Metabolism and Excretion. Pentamidine undergoes no biotransformation and is eliminated virtually unchanged by the kidney. The half-life of the drug in patients with normal renal function is approximately six hours. Dosing alterations need to be made in the patient with decreased kidney function since drug accumulation does occur. Hemodialysis and peritoneal dialysis apparently have no effect on the removal of pentamidine from the plasma.

ADVERSE REACTIONS. *Immediate Reactions.* These adverse reactions may be seen more frequently following intravenous administration of pentamidine and include hypotension, tachycardia, nausea and/or vomiting, facial flushing, pruritis (itching), unpleasant taste, hallucinations, and syncope (fainting). Hypotension is the most frequently seen immediate reaction and may appear to be related to the infusion rate. If the dose of pentamidine (4 mg/kg/day) is infused over a period of at least 60 minutes, this reaction is minimized.

Local Reactions. Following intramuscular administration, moderate-to-severe pain at the injection site, sterile abscess formation, and/or dermal necrosis of the overlying skin have been reported. Following intravenous infusions of pentamidine, urticaria occurring at the infusion site, phlebitis, and thrombosis may occur.

Systemic Reactions. Mild and reversible nephrotoxicity is the most frequent adverse systemic reaction to pentamidine. In addition, leukopenia (decrease in white blood cells) or neutropenia (decrease in polymorphonuclear leukocytes), anemia, and thrombocytopenia are also seen. Abnormalities in glucose metabolism with resultant hypoglycemia has been described, and up to 5% of patients receiving pentamidine may develop insulin-dependent diabetes. Pancreatitis is another reported adverse effect. Liver function test abnormalities (e.g., transaminase enzyme level elevations) have been reported. Other less frequent systemic adverse reactions include skin rashes, alopecia, hypocalcemia, decreased folic acid levels, and fever.

DOSAGE AND ADMINISTRATION. The dose of pentamidine may be given by either the intramuscular or intravenous route. The daily dose of the drug is based on the total body weight of the patient and renal function. In general, patients with normal renal function should receive 4 mg/kg/day of pentamidine. If the intramuscular route is used, the site of injection should be rotated daily. Intravenous doses of pentamidine should be diluted in 50–100 ml of diluent and infused over a period of at least 60 minutes, so as to minimize immediate adverse effects. For patients with renal insufficiency, the dose of pentamidine may be reduced and/or the interval of administration extended. This is probably necessary only for patients with a creatinine clearance of less than 35 ml/minute. Aerosolized pentamidine has recently been used in an attempt to deliver greater concentrations of drug to the site of the infection (lungs) and to decrease systemic adverse reactions. By this route of administration, doses of 60, 120, and 300 mg have been given over a 20–30 minute period. Bronchospasm and a metallic taste in the mouth have been reported as an adverse reaction to aerosolized pentamidine.

ANTIPARASITIC AGENTS

Agents used for the treatment of amebiasis, helminthiasis, cryptosporidiosis, giardiasis, isosporiasis, lice, malaria, scabies, strongyloidiasis, toxoplasmosis, and trichinosis are featured in Table 46–13.

NURSING PROCESS FOR PATIENTS RECEIVING ANTI-INFECTIVE THERAPY

ASSESSMENT

The nurse plays an important role in the management of patients with infection. Essential clues to the nature of the infection may be identified as the nurse obtains a history of the illness (Table 46–14). In addition, a knowledge of previous history of drug allergies is important when antibiotics are to be prescribed. A detailed description of the type of allergic reaction the patient experienced is imperative since many patients may have experienced a side effect (such as nausea or vomiting) and mistakenly labeled the response a "drug allergy."

An awareness of the patient's current disease states and drug therapy is important because many antibiotics may interact with other medications the patient is receiving (see drug interaction sections under each anti-infective agent).

Initial assessment of the patient begins with the determination of the vital signs (temperature, blood pressure, pulse, respiratory rate). An elevated body temperature (fever) is a cardinal sign of the presence of inflammation and/or infection. The cardiovascular response to infection may present as a rapid heart rate or as a drop in blood pressure. For every degree of elevation in temperature, there is an increase in heart rate by approximately 8–10 beats/minute. Metabolic acidosis secondary to infection often elicits a compensatory increase in respiratory rate.

Clinical signs and symptoms related to infection may be present when the patient is examined. General signs and symptoms may be malaise, arthralgias, myalgias, or drowsiness. In other situations, clinical findings may be more specific to the site of infection. For example, a patient may describe a productive cough, shortness of breath (pneumonia); burning upon urination, frequency, urgency (urinary tract infection); or a stiff neck (meningitis).

A complete patient history and physical examination are essential to fully understand the possible causes of infection. A complete blood count with a differential count is an important diagnostic tool when infection is suspected. An increase in the number of leukocytes including an increased number of immature neutrophils or bands ('shift to the left") is a common finding in bacterial infections.

Analysis of body fluids that are thought to be infected is also an important diagnostic aid. In addition, body fluids (urine, sputum, peritoneal fluid, cerebrospinal fluid, joint fluid) are examined for the presence of cells (leukocytes, RBCs), and changes in pH, glucose, and protein. Body fluids suspected of being infected should be gram-stained and cultured in the laboratory to determine the presence of bacteria. Accurate sample collection and rapid transportation to the laboratory are important aspects of this process. If an organism is grown from a body fluid, it is tested against a battery of antibiotics to determine sensitivity patterns.

Patients suspected of having infection often require radiographic confirmation. A common example is the use of a chest x-ray to document pneumonia. More complex testing may be done, depending on the site of infection (bone scan, computerized tomography).

NURSING DIAGNOSES

The nurse completes the initial assessment and then develops nursing diagnoses, which become the basis for all nursing care delivered to the patient. Typical nursing diagnoses for a patient requiring anti-infective therapy are featured in Table 46–14.

TEXT RESUMES ON PAGE 1287

Table 46–13. DRUGS USED TO TREAT PARASITIC INFECTIONS

Parasitic Infection/ Drug Name	Dosage	Mode of Administration	Pharmacokinetics
AMEBIASIS			
Entamoeba histolytica Metronidazole (Flagyl)			
Action: Inhibits bacterial DNA, leads to cell disruption and death.			
	Adults: 750 mg 3 times daily for 10 days, followed by Idoquinol	PO (Tablets)	
	Children: 35–50 mg/kg/day in 3 doses for 10 days, followed by iodoquinol	PO (Tablets)	See Table 46–6.
Iodoquinol (Diiodohydroxy- quin, Yodoxin)			
Action: Unknown.			
	Adults: 650 mg 3 times daily for 20 days	PO (Tablets)	A: NA PB: NA
	Children: 30–40 mg/kg/day in 3 doses for 20 days		½L: 11–14 hr E: NA
ASCARIASIS			
Ascaris lumbricoides, roundworm Mebendazole (Vermox)			
Action: Direct toxic action on worms; causes immobilization and death.			
	Adults: 100 mg twice daily for 3 days	PO (Chewable tablets)	A: 5%–10% PB: highly
	Children >2 yr: 100 mg twice daily for 3 days	PO (Chewable tablets)	½L: 2.8–9 hr E: liver, urine
CRYPTOSPORIDIOSIS			
Cryptosporidium species Spiramycin (Rovamycin) (not commercially available in USA)			
Action: Unknown.			
	Adults: 1 g 3 times daily for 14 days or longer	PO	A: good PB: NA ½L: 4–8 hr E: nonrenal (bile)
Pyrantel Pamoate (Antiminth)			
Action: Causes spastic paralysis of the worm.			
	Adults and children: 11 mg/ kg once (maximum of 1 g)	PO (Oral suspension, 50 mg/ml)	A: poor PB: NA

A-absorption; PB-protein binding; ½L-serum half-life; E-excretion.
*Within the column of adverse effects, underlines indicate the most common effects; CAPITALS indicate life-threatening effects.

Contraindications/ Precautions	Adverse Effects*	Interactions	Nursing Implications
See Table 46–6.	See Table 46–6.	See Table 46–6.	See Table 46–6.
CONTRAINDICATIONS: Prior hypersensitivity reactions to iodine. *PRECAUTIONS:* Avoid using in patients with hepatic damage. Safe use in pregnancy and during lactation has not been established. Use with caution in patients with thyroid disease.	*Neuro:* OPTIC NEURITIS, visual disturbances, peripheral neuropathy *GI:* nausea, diarrhea, abdominal cramps, rectal itching *Endo:* thyroid enlargement *Integ:* rash, acne	Interference with thyroid function test may occur (e.g., protein–bound iodine).	*INTERVENTION:* Patient should be instructed to complete full course of therapy. *EVALUATION:* Evaluate for symptoms. Report any adverse reactions.
CONTRAINDICATIONS: Prior hypersensitivity reactions. *PRECAUTIONS:* Avoid use during the first trimester of pregnancy. Safe use during lactation and in children <2 yr has not been established.	*Neuro:* fever *GI:* abdominal pain, diarrhea *Hemo:* leukopenia *Reprod:* hypospermia		*ASSESSMENT:* Tablets should be crushed and administered with food. *INTERVENTION:* Patient should be instructed to maintain strict hygiene during infestation. *EVALUATION:* Evaluate for signs and/or symptoms of drug toxicity.
	GI: nausea, vomiting, dry mouth, abdominal pain *Integ:* rash		
PRECAUTIONS: Experience with this drug in	*Neuro:* fever, headache, dizziness		*ASSESSMENT:* Give the entire dose of the drug.

CONTINUED ON THE FOLLOWING PAGE

Drugs to Treat Parasitic Infections

Table 46–13. DRUGS USED TO TREAT PARASITIC INFECTIONS–*CONTINUED*

Parasitic Infection/ Drug Name	Dosage	Mode of Administration	Pharmacokinetics
Pyrantel Pamoate–*Continued*			½L: NA E: feces
***Enterobius vermicularis* (pinworm)**			
Pyrantel Pamoate (Antiminth)	*Adults and children:* 11 mg/ kg once (maximum 1 g); repeat after 2 weeks	PO (Oral suspension, 50 mg/ml)	See above.
Mebendazole (Vermox)	*Adults and children >2 yr:* 100 mg as a single dose; repeat after 2 weeks	PO (chewable tablet)	See above.
GIARDIASIS			
Giardia lamblia Quinacrine (Atabrine)			
Action: Unknown.			
	Adults: 100 mg 3 times daily after meals for 5 days	PO (Tablets)	A: very good PB: high
	Children: 2 mg/kg 3 times daily after meals for 5 days; maximum dose 300 mg/day	PO (Tablets)	½L: NA E: urine
Metronidazole (Flagyl)	*Adults:* 250 mg 3 times daily for 5 days	PO	See Table 46–6.
	Children: 5 mg/kg 3 times daily for 5 days	PO	
HOOKWORM			
Ancylostoma duodenale, Necator americanus Mebendazole (Vermox)	*Adults and children >2 yr:* 100 mg 2 times daily for 3 days	PO (Chewable tablets)	See above.
Pyrantel Pamoate (Antiminth)	*Adults and children:* 11 mg/ kg for 3 days; maximum dose 1 g/day	PO (Oral suspension, 50 mg/ml)	See above.
ISOSPORIASIS			
Isospora belli Trimenthoprim/Sulfamethox- azole (Bactrim, Septra)	*Adults:* 160 mg TMP/800 mg SMZ 4 times daily for 10 days, then twice daily for 3 weeks	PO (tablets)	See Table 46–5.

A-absorption; PB-protein binding; ½L-serum half-life; E-excretion; NA-not available.
*Within the column listing adverse effects, underlines indicate the most common effects; CAPITALS indicate life-threatening effects.

Contraindications/ Precautions	Adverse Effects*	Interactions	Nursing Implications
pregnancy is limited. Safe and effective use in children <2 yr has not been established. Use cautiously in patients with hepatic disease.	*GI:* nausea, vomiting *Integ:* rash		*INTERVENTION:* Patient should be instructed to complete full course of therapy. Medication may be taken with food. Strict hygiene must be observed. Warn the patient that the drug will stain clothing. *EVALUATION:* Evaluate for symptoms. Report any adverse reactions.
See above.	See above.	See above.	See above.
PRECAUTIONS: Avoid use during pregnancy. Avoid use in patients with a history of psychosis. Use cautiously in patients with impaired liver function, porphyria, or psoriasis.	*Neruo:* headache, dizziness, psychosis, CONVULSIONS *Eye:* visual halos, focusing difficulties, blurred vision, RETINOPATHY *GI:* anorexia, nausea, vomiting, abdominal cramps *Biliary:* hepatitis *Hemo:* aplastic anemia *Renal:* imparts intense yellow color to urine *Integ:* may impart intense yellow color to skin, rash	Quinacrine increases the toxicity of primaquine. Disulfiram (Antabuse)–like reaction with ethanol.	*ASSESSMENT:* Administer with meals and a full glass of water. *INTERVENTION:* Patient should be warned that the drug may turn the urine and/or skin yellow. Take drug with meals and a full glass of water; report any visual disturbances. *EVALUATION:* Evaluate for signs and/or symptoms of drug toxicity.
See Table 46–6.	See Table 46–6.	See Table 46–6.	See Table 46–6.
See above.	See above.	See above.	See above.
See above.	See above.	See above.	See above.
See Table 46–5.	See Table 46–5.	See Table 46–5.	See Table 46–5.

CONTINUED ON THE FOLLOWING PAGE

Drugs to Treat Parasitic Infections

Table 46–13. DRUGS USED TO TREAT PARASITIC INFECTIONS–*CONTINUED*

Parasitic Infection/ Drug Name	Dosage	Mode of Administration	Pharmacokinetics
LICE			
Pediculus humanus capitis, Phthirus pubis Permethrin 1% (Nix)			
Action: Unknown.			
	Adults and children: use after hair has been washed with shampoo, rinsed with water, and towel dried; apply a sufficient volume to saturate the hair and scalp; allow to remain on the hair for 10 minutes before rinsing off with water	Topical application (Liquid)	See Table 46–5.
Lindane 1% (Kwell, G-Well, Kwildane, Scabene)			
Action: Unknown.			
	Adults and children: apply a sufficient amount to affected area and leave in place 8–12 hr, followed by thorough washing; for shampoo, apply a sufficient amount and work into lather; allow to remain in place for 4 min; rinse hair thoroughly and towel dry briskly; comb with tooth comb to remove any remaining nit shells	Topical application (Lotion, shampoo, cream)	See Table 46–5.
MALARIA			
Plasmodium vivax, P. ovale, P. malariae, and chloroquine-susceptible P. falciparum Chloroquine (Aralen)			
Action: Interacts with DNA and kills the parasite.			
	TREATMENT: *Adults:* 600 mg of base (1000 mg of phosphate tablets) initially followed by 300 mg of base in 6 hr and again on days 2 and 3	PO (Tablets)	A: rapid and complete PB: 55% ½L: 4–7 days E: nonrenal
	Adults: 2.5 mg/kg of base every 4 hr or 3.5 mg/kg every 6 hr; total dose not to exceed 25 mg/kg	IM	
	Adults: 10 mg/kg of base over 4 hr, followed by 5 mg/kg every 12 hr; total dose not to exceed 25 mg/kg PROPHYLAXIS:	IV	
	Adults: 300 mg of base (500 mg of phosphate tablet) per week; begin 1 week prior to exposure; continue during vacation and for 6 weeks after vacation	PO	

A-absorption; PB-protein binding; ½L-serum half-life; E-excretion; NA-not available.
*Within the solumn of adverse effects, underlines indicate the most common effects; CAPITALS indicate life-threatening effects.

Contraindications/ Precautions	Adverse Effects*	Interactions	Nursing Implications
CONTRAINDICATIONS: Prior hypersensitivity. *PRECAUTIONS:* Use in pregnancy, during lactation, or in children <2 yr should be avoided. Itching, redness, and edema may be temporarily aggravated.	*Neuro:* numbness of scalp *Integ:* rash, redness, itching, burning/tingling		*ASSESSMENT:* Avoid getting in eyes; one application is usually sufficient. *INTERVENTION:* Instruct the patient to avoid getting medication in the eyes. Repeat administrations should only be done with doctor's permission. *EVALUATION:* Evaluate for signs and/or symptoms of infestation. Report any adverse reactions.
CONTRAINDICATIONS: Prior hypersensitivity reactions. *PRECAUTIONS:* Avoid in premature neonates, infants, and patients with a history of seizure disorders. Use cautiously during pregnancy, lactation, or in children. Avoid contact with eyes	*Neuro:* dizziness, CONVULSIONS *Integ:* eczematous eruptions		See above.
CONTRAINDICATIONS: Prior hypersensitivity reactions. *PRECAUTIONS:* Use cautiously in patients with psoriasis or porphyria. Use cautiously during pregnancy and lactation. Children are especially sensitive to this class of drugs. (Do not give more than 10 mg/kg of base to infants or children). Use with caution in patients with liver disease.	*Neuro:* headache, agitation *Eye:* IRREVERSIBLE RETINAL CHANGES *CVR:* hypotension *GI:* nausea, vomiting, anorexia, diarrhea *Hemo:* agranulocytosis *Integ:* rash, pruritis		*ASSESSMENT:* The treatment regimen must be followed precisely. *INTERVENTION:* Patient should be instructed to complete full course of therapy. *EVALUATION:* Evaluate for symptoms. Report any adverse reactions.

CONTINUED ON THE FOLLOWING PAGE

Table 46–13. DRUGS USED TO TREAT PARASITIC INFECTIONS–*CONTINUED*

Parasitic Infection/ Drug Name	Dosage	Mode of Administration	Pharmacokinetics
Chloroquine–*Continued*	*Children:* 5 mg/kg of base per week; up to 300 mg of base; follow regimen above	PO	
SCABIES			
Sarcoptes scabiei Lindane 1% (Kwell, G-well, Kwildane, Scabene)	*Adults and children:* apply a thin layer to affected area and rub in thoroughly; leave on 8–12 hr and then remove by thorough washing	Topical application	
STRONGYLOIDIASIS			
Strongyloides stercoralis Thiabendazole (Mintezol)			
Action: Primary mechanism is unknown.			
	Adults and children: 25 mg/ kg twice daily for 2 days; maximum dose of 3 g/day	PO (Chewable tablets; also available as an oral suspension, 500 mg/5 ml)	A: rapid PB: NA ½L: NA E: renal
TOXOPLASMOSIS			
Toxoplasma gondii Pyrimethamine (Daraprim)			
Action: Inhibits plasmodial dihydrofolate reductase.			
	Adults: 25 mg/day for 3–4 weeks	PO	A: very good PB: NA
	Children: 2 mg/kg/day for 3 days, then 1 mg/kg/day for 4 weeks; maximum dose 25 mg/day	PO	½L: 4 days E: nonrenal
PLUS Sulfadiazine	*Adults:* 2–4 g/day in 3–6 divided doses for 3–4 weeks	PO	See Table 46–5.
	Children: 150 mg/kg/day in 4–6 divided doses for 3–4 weeks	PO	
TRICHINOSIS			
Trichinella spiralis Steroids for severe symptoms *PLUS* Thiabendazole (Mintezol)	*Adults and children:* 25 mg/ kg twice daily for 5 days; maximum dose of 3 g/day	PO (Chewable tablets; also available as an oral suspension, 500 mg/5 ml)	See above.

A-absorption; PB-protein binding; ½L-serum half-life; E-excretion; NA-not available.
*Within the solumn of adverse effects, underlines indicate the most common effects; CAPITALS indicate life-threatening effects.

Contraindications/ Precautions	Adverse Effects*	Interactions	Nursing Implications
See above.	See above	See above.	See above.
CONTRAINDICATIONS: Prior hypersensitivity reactions. *PRECAUTIONS:* Avoid use during times when mental alertness is necessary. Safe use during pregnancy or lactation has not been established.	*Neuro:* dizziness, tinnitus, hyperirritability, fever, chills *GI:* anorexia, nausea, vomiting, diarrhea *Integ:* rash, pruritis *GU:* urinary odor	-	*ASSESSMENT:* Tell patient that urine may have an unusual odor related to use of the drug. *INTERVENTION:* Instruct the patient to chew the tablets before swallowing. *EVALUATION:* Evaluate for signs and/or symptoms. Report any adverse reactions.
PRECAUTIONS: Use cautiously during pregnancy and lactation. May precipitate hemolytic anemia in G-6-PD–deficient patients.	*GI:* nausea, vomiting *Hemo:* megaloblastic anemia, leukopenia, thrombocytopenia *Integ:* severe skin rash	-	*ASSESSMENT:* Administer with a full glass of water. *INTERVENTION:* Patient should be warned that the drug may cause a severe skin rash. Take drug with meals and a full glass of water. *EVALUATION:* Evaluate for signs and/or symptoms of drug toxicity.
See Table 46–5.	See Table 46–5.	See Table 46–5.	See Table 46–5.
See above.	See above.	See above.	See above.

Table 46–14. NURSING PROCESS FOR ADMINISTRATION OF ANTI-INFECTIVES

Assessment

Note previous/current use of prescription drugs (especially antibotics, glucocorticoids), history of drug sensitivity/allergic reactions.
Assess nutritional status.
Determine presence/history of liver, kidney or gastrointestinal disorders, pregnancy/nursing.
Describe infection site; associated signs/symptoms, e.g., presence of temperature elevation, tachycardia, malaise, arthralgias, myalgias.

Nursing Diagnosis	Nursing Actions	Rationale	Desired Outcomes/ Evaluation Criteria
Knowledge deficit related to lack of information/ misinterpretation, unfamiliarity with resources as evidenced by questions, statement of concern, inaccurate follow-through of instructions/ development of preventable complications.	Provide information about disease process and future expectations.	Understanding allows the patient to make informed choices and participate in treatment regimen.	Identifies relationship of signs/symptoms to the disease process and correlates symptoms with causative factors. Correctly performs necessary procedures and explains reasons for the actions.
	Demonstrate correct administration of prescribed drug.	Ensures safe administration and desired therapeutic effect. IV, IM, oral (tablet and liquid) may be used.	
	Discuss foods to avoid while on antibiotics.	Certain foods can interfere with the optimal therapeutic level of the drug.	
	Determine financial circumstances of the patient/family.	Patient may not be able to afford drug but be afraid to ask for assistance/or know what resources are available.	
	Identify signs/symptoms that require physician notification, e.g., continued fever, chills, diaphoresis, rash.	Provides for prompt evaluation and intervention to alter treatment.	
	Encourage intake of nutritionally balanced diet, adequate rest periods.	Promotes healing and general wellness.	
	Review necessity of personal hygiene and environmental cleanliness.	Helps to control environmental exposure by diminishing the number of pathogens present.	
Infection, potential for spread related to absence of or inadequate/ inappropriate drug therapy.	Obtain culture/sensitivities from site of infection.	Identifies organism and determines most appropriate drug.	Achieves timely wound healing, free of purulent drainage or erythema, and afebrile.
	Administer antiinfective agent.	Specific choice usually determined by results of culture and sensitivities. Prompt treatment of infection can prevent progression to life threatening situations, e.g., septicemia.	
	Emphasize importance of taking drug exactly as prescribed and completing entire amount.	Patient may think that s/he is well when symptoms abate and believe the drug is no longer needed.	
	Monitor signs/symptoms of infection, noting reduction of temperature, decreased WBC count, reduced pain, and swelling, redness.	Should subside within 48 hours and be resolved within 7–10 days.	
	Stress proper handwashing techniques.	First-line defense against infection.	

**Table 46–14. NURSING PROCESS FOR ADMINISTRATION OF
ANTI-INFECTIVES**–CONTINUED

Nursing Diagnosis	Nursing Actions	Rationale	Desired Outcomes/ Evaluation Criteria
	Maintain aseptic technique when inserting invasive lines, administering IV fluids/medications, changing IV bottles.	Prevents cross-contamination, introduction of bacteria.	
	Cleanse incisions/insertion sites daily/prn with appropriate solutions.	Prevents introduction of bacteria/contamination of the site.	
	Monitor appropriate laboratory studies, e.g., CBC, liver/renal function.	Depending on history or drug used, tests can monitor for adverse effects.	
	Demonstrate proper handling/disposal of infective or soiled material, e.g., dressings, tissues.	Reduces risk of contamination, limits spread of airborne organisms.	
	Recommend avoidance of crowds, contact with infected persons.	Reduces risk of secondary infection.	

PLANNING AND INTERVENTION

The nursing diagnoses are used by the nurse as the goals of intervention are established. The nurse consults with the patient and family as the goals are planned. The goals of nursing intervention are included in Table 46–14.

Constant observation of the patient allows the nurse to follow the outcome of anti-infective therapy. Normalization of body temperature and laboratory tests, as well as sterilization of body fluids, often provides evidence of antibiotic efficacy. However, the nurse must be keenly aware of signs and symptoms of treatment failure or drug toxicity. Also, accurate timing of sample collections is extremely important when antibiotic concentrations are measured in the blood.

In most institutions, a single nurse cares for many patients. In this setting, awareness of those patients who are infected and attention to appropriate handwashing techniques will prevent the spread of microorganisms among patients.

It is obvious from the discussion in the preceding section that the nurse plays a pivotal role in providing health care to patients with infection.

NURSING RESPONSIBILITIES WHEN ADMINISTERING ANTI-INFECTIVES

The nurse in the hospital situation has several nursing responsibilities when administering anti-infective agents. These are featured in the column marked Special Implications for Nurse and Patient in each of the drug tables.

The proper timing of antibiotic administration must be emphasized. Consideration must be given to the effect that food or antacids may have on the rate and extent of antibiotic absorption. In certain cases (e.g., tetracyclines) the patient may have to avoid the use of aluminum-containing or magnesium-containing antacids and schedule antibiotic administration around other maintenance medications. Meals can effect the absorption of many anti-infective agents; therefore, patients may have to be instructed on the appropriate timing of their antibiotics in relationship to meals.

Frequently, intravenous antibiotics must be administered because of the severity of the infection and/or because of a nonfunctioning gastrointestinal tract. Intravenous anti-infectives are administered over a 30–60 minute period using intravenous equipment—partial fills, burettes, or piggybacks. Phlebitis may frequently be a problem associated with the route of administration and the nurse needs to evaluate the intravenous site daily for complications.

When the nurse administers intramuscular anti-infectives, the sites are always rotated to enhance absorption. The site is massaged by either the nurse or the patient for a full two minutes after each injection to improve circulation. Intramuscular injections should be avoided in patients with small muscle mass, decreased circulation, or sepsis, because absorption is erratic and unreliable.

PATIENT TEACHING

During the intervention phase, the nurse is responsible for patient teaching (Table 46–15). The nurse teaches the patient that a full course of therapy is extremely important to adequately treat the underlying infection. Often the patient is treated as an outpatient or released from the hospital before therapy is concluded. There-

Table 46-15. PATIENT TEACHING INFORMATION—ANTI-INFECTIVES

Dear Patient:
This drug has been prescribed for you. This is what you should know about your drug to get the most from your therapy.

1. Anti-infectives will be taken until all symptoms have been eliminated to prevent reinfection.
2. Do not stop taking your anti-infective without consulting with your physician. Take the medication until it is all gone.
3. All anti-infectives should be taken as prescribed. Do not save any medication "until the next time."
4. Take your anti-infective one hour before, with, or one to two hours after meals as indicated by your nurse, pharmacist, or physician.
5. Always check with your physician or pharmacist before taking other medications, as interactions may occur.
6. If you forget to take your anti-infective for a period of time, eliminate that dose. DO NOT try to catch up by taking two doses at the same time. Take all the medication as prescribed.
7. If you experience any side effects from your anti-infectives, consult your physician or pharmacist. Common side effects include: (a list of side effects specific for each drug the patient is on should be included).
8. Store your medication in a tight and moisture-resistant container to prevent deterioration.
9. Anti-infectives may also be taken prophylactically (to prevent infection) for tooth extractions and other minor surgical procedures as prescribed by your physician. Again, take all these medications as ordered.

fore, the patient is educated to continue treatment and take all of the medication prescribed. Patients are cautioned about the dangers of saving a few tablets "till next time." The nurse needs to educate the patient in the use of handwashing techniques, proper food preparation (washing hands before and after preparation), and proper disposal of waste products (sputum, urine, stool) to limit the further spread of infection.

The patient also needs to be taught the importance of proper nutrition with adequate protein, vitamins, and minerals, and of getting enough rest during the acute and recovery phases of infection.

EVALUATION

During the evaluation phase, the nurse evaluates the effectiveness of treatment through outcome evaluation criteria. Outcome evaluation criteria are included in Table 46-14. A successful therapy is indicated by a reduction in the severity of the condition or a complete loss of symtomatology. In most cases, an effective treatment begins to reduce symptoms within two days. However, several infections, such as tuberculosis or fungal infections, may take weeks to months to resolve.

The nurse evaluates the patient's response to therapy. The infection should be brought under control with the patient experiencing no adverse drug reactions. The most common adverse reaction is gastrointestinal complaints (nausea, vomiting, and diarrhea). Nausea and vomiting can be minimized by decreasing the dose of the anti-infective agent or scheduling the doses to coincide with meals, assuming meals do not interfere with drug absorption. Diarrhea is generally self-limited and subsides when the anti-infective agent is discontinued. When diarrhea occurs, increasing the bulk in the diet and taking *Lactobacillus* cultures (yogurt, buttermilk, or Lactinex tablets) will help to restore the normal intestinal flora and reduce diarrhea. The possibility of pseudomembranous colitis must always be considered in the setting of broad-spectrum antibiotic therapy and profuse diarrhea. Females may experience vaginitis secondary to antibiotic therapy. Vaginitis may require specific treatment.

When the patient is receiving intravenous or intramuscular antibiotics, the nurse evaluates the site for inflammation, phlebitis, and sterile abscess formation. Rotation of the intravenous site every forty-eight hours may help to reduce these side effects.

Before the patient leaves the nursing intervention, all previously taught material is reviewed and updated to ensure that the patient's knowledge base remains accurate.

SUMMARY

Learning the plethora of antimicrobial agents is merely a matter of identifying the various categories of agents and memorizing each of the specific antibiotics. However, the real objective to "learning" antibiotics should be to understand the reasons antibiotics are prescribed and the thought process of antibiotic selection. This chapter has provided a list of commonly used anti-infective agents with focus on the mechanism of action, spectrum of activity, pharmacokinetics, adverse reactions, drug interactions, and dosage recommendations.

Controversy will always surround the clinical use of antimicrobial agents. Knowing the most appropriate antibiotic to use for a given infectious disease (i.e., the right drug for the right bug) can only come from a basic understanding of the concepts of antibiotic pharmacotherapy. Coupled with clinical experience, the knowledge of antibiotic pharmcotherapy will make the rationale for antibiotic selection more apparent to the nurse.

BIBLIOGRAPHY

Abramowicz, M (ed): Antimicrobial prophylaxis in surgery. Med Lett Drugs Ther 29:91, 1987.
Abramowicz, M (ed): Safety of antimicrobial drugs in pregnancy. Med Lett Drugs Ther 29:61, 1987.
Abramowicz, M (ed): The choice of antimicrobial drugs. Med Lett Drug Ther 30:33, 1988.

Abramowicz, M (ed): Treatment of sexually transmitted diseases. Med Lett Drugs Ther 30:5, 1988.

Abramowicz, M (ed): Drugs for parasitic infections. Med Lett Drugs Ther 30:15, 1988.

Barza, M: Imipenem: First of a new class of beta-lactam antibiotics. Ann Intern Med 103:552, 1985.

Childs, SJ and Bodey, GP: Aztreonam. Pharmacotherapy 6:138, 1986.

Drouhet, E and Dupont, B: Evolution of antifungal agents: Past, present, and future. Rev Infect Dis 9(Suppl 1):S4, 1987.

Gilman, AG, et al (eds): Goodman and Gilman's The Pharmacological Basis of Therapeutics, ed 7. Macmillan, New York, 1985.

Hooper, DC and Wolfson, JS: The fluoroquinolones: Pharmacology, clinical uses, and toxicities in humans. Antimicrob Agents Chemother 28:716, 1985.

Shalit, I and Marks, MI: Chloramphenicol in the 1980s. Drugs 28:281, 1984.

Vogt, M and Hirsch, MS: Prospects for the prevention and treatment of infections with human immunodeficiency virus. Rev Infect Dis 8:991, 1986.

Washington, JA and Wilson, WR: Erythromycin: A microbial and clinical perspective after 30 years of clinical use. Mayo Clin Proc 60:189, 1985.

Wolfson, JS and Hooper, DC: The fluoroquinolones: Structure, mechanisms of action and resistance, and spectra of activity in vitro. Antimicrob Agents Chemother 28:581, 1985.

SITUATION 46–1

Leonard Olds is a 34-year-old who is admitted to the medical unit with episodes of fever, night sweats, and a persistent cough. The preliminary diagnosis is respiratory tuberculosis.

1. Mr. Olds is to begin isoniazide (INH) orally 350 mg per day. The nurse will be alert to adverse side effects of the drug, such as:
   a. photosensitivity
   b. crystalluria
   c. muscle twitching
   d. pseudomembranous colitis

2. Due to INH therapy, the nurse will expect to administer the following nutritional supplement:
   a. B₆ (pyridoxine)
   b. Vitamin C
   c. Vitamin A
   d. folic acid

3. Along with INH therapy, Mr. Olds is to take rifampin 600 mg orally daily. Assessment of Mr. Olds may reveal the following in relation to rifampin therapy:
   a. "butterfly" rash
   b. discoloration of teeth
   c. cherry red lips
   d. reddish-orange urine

4. When teaching Mr. Olds about his drug regimen, the nurse will plan to include the following information:
   a. Rifampin should be taken on an empty stomach.
   b. INH therapy is usually two weeks in length.
   c. Rifampin interacts with milk and should only be taken with water.
   d. The drugs may be discontinued when symptoms subside.

5. The nurse will monitor the following lab values while caring for Mr. Olds:
   a. magnesium level
   b. urinary amylase
   c. liver enzymes
   d. urine osmolarity

6. The nurse performs discharge teaching for Mr. Olds and his wife. Which of the following statements by Mrs. Olds indicates successful teaching?
   a. "If one dose is missed, he should take two doses the next day."
   b. "I should report mental changes promptly."
   c. "Hearing loss is expected with this medication."
   d. "He must measure his urine output daily."

SITUATION 46–2

Mary Greco is a 57-year-old who suffered a ruptured appendix. Following surgery, she has been admitted to the surgical unit with orders including gentamycin (Garamycin) 80 mg IVPB every 8 hours.

1. While caring for Ms. Greco, the nurse will carefully monitor the following lab value relative to therapy with gentamycin:
   a. urinary amylase
   b. creatinine
   c. serum albumin
   d. phosphorus

2. After the third IV dose of gentamycin, Ms. Greco is to have a serum peak level drawn. Which of the following results indicates a therapeutic gentamycin peak level?
   a. 8 μg/ml
   b. 3g/ml
   c. 12 μg/ml
   d. 20 μg/ml

3. On the third post-operative day, Ms. Greco's chest x-ray shows consolidation of the left lower lobe, consistent with pneumonia. An additional antibiotic, ticarcillin/clavulanic acid (Timentin) 3.1 grams is started IVPB every 12 hours. The nurse will include the following intervention:
   a. Infuse the two antibiotics together in the same IV solution.
   b. Discontinue the gentamycin before starting the penicillin agent.
   c. Monitor white blood cell (WBC) count daily.
   d. Obtain sputum cultures after two doses of Timentin are given.

4. Which of the following nursing diagnostic categories applies to Ms. Greco?
   a. Noncompliance
   b. Potential for Injury: Bleeding
   c. Alteration in Cardiac Output
   d. Fluid Volume Excess

CONTINUED ON THE FOLLOWING PAGE

SITUATION 46–2–*Continued*

5. Considering penicillin therapy, which of the following electrolytes may need to be supplemented:
   a. calcium
   b. chloride
   c. sodium
   d. potassium

6. Because of aminoglycoside therapy, the nurse will assess Ms. Greco daily for the presence of:
   a. crystalluria
   b. hearing loss
   c. diarrhea
   d. tetany

Please refer to the Appendices for correct answers and additional review questions with answers.

47
CHAPTER

ANTI-INFLAMMATORY MEDICATIONS

GLOSSARY TERMS IN THIS CHAPTER

Ceiling effect
De-esterification
Kinins
Lysosomal enzymes
Monoamines
Pentagastrin
Prostaglandins

CHAPTER 47

ANTI-INFLAMMATORY MEDICATIONS

MERRILY MATHEWSON KUHN, R.N.C., Ph.D., CCRN

LEARNING OBJECTIVES

After reading this chapter, the student will be able to:

1. Identify those drugs commonly used as anti-inflammatory medications.

2. Differentiate among the anti-inflammatory medications as to mechanism of action, route of administration, pharmacokinetics, adverse effects, contraindications, and interactions.

3. Identify specific areas to assess in the patient requiring anti-inflammatory medications in order to formulate appropriate nursing diagnoses.

4. Plan the nursing interventions necessary to administer anti-inflammatory medications and choose appropriate teaching strategies to gain patient compliance.

5. Evaluate the patient at various stages of treatment to gauge nursing interventions.

THERAPEUTIC AGENTS

Inflammatory diseases range from rheumatoid arthritis and degenerative joint disease to connective tissue disorders such as lupus erythematosus and scleroderma. Therapeutic agents for treating inflammatory diseases (Table 47–1 and Fig. 47–1) include salicylates, nonsteroidal anti-inflammatory drugs, salicylate-like medications, gold products, antimalarials, cytotoxic medications, and antigout drugs. Salicylates, nonsteroidal anti-inflammatory drugs (NSAIDs), and salicylate-like medications provide symptomatic relief of the disease, but it is unknown at this time whether they actively alter the course of disease. Gold products and antigout products suppress the destructive course of the disease, while antimalarials and cytotoxic drugs may or may not have this effect. Research is ongoing.

The choice of drug is dependent on the acuteness and the severity of the disease. Patients often have remissions and exacerbation of symptoms. During early treatment, conservative therapy is used such as rest, exercise, physical therapy, avoidance of activities which activate discomfort, and maintenance of normal weight and emotional stability. Salicylates are often the first drugs used as they are inexpensive and usually produce rapid results.

Each group of medications are reviewed briefly as to action, uses, dosage, contraindications, precautions, and adverse effects. The common anti-inflammatory drugs are classified in Table 47–2 and featured in Table 47–3.

ACTION

In general, these agents act, at least in part, by inhibiting prostaglandin synthesis. In addition, the majority are thought to have an analgesic effect either by acting peripherally, or by displacing certain peptides from their protein-binding sites to exert a protective effect on the tissues. Some agents such as salicylates also have an antipyretic effect, which may aid in decreasing warmth of the affected area, as well as in decreasing swelling.

Table 47–1. INFLAMMATORY DISEASES

> **ARTHRITIS**
>
> **Definition:** A group of conditions or disorders resulting from the body's own antigen-antibody reaction.
>
> **Classification of Arthritis by the American Rheumatic Association and Arthritis Foundation:**
>   I. Polyarthritis of unknown origin (includes rheumatoid arthritis)
>   II. Connective tissue disorders (includes lupus erythematosus)
>   III. Rheumatic fever
>   IV. Degenerative joint diseases (includes osteoarthritis)
>   V. Nonarticular rheumatism
>   VI. Diseases with which arthritis is frequently associated
>   VII. Associated with known infectious agents
>   VIII. Traumatic and/or neurogenic disorders
>   IX. Associated with known biochemical or endocrine disorders (includes gout)
>   X. Tumor and tumor-like conditions
>   XI. Allergy and drug reactions
>   XII. Inherited and congenital disorders
>   XIII. Miscellaneous disorders (including amyloidosis)

Condition	Pathologic Process	Sex Preference/ Onset Age (yr)	Symptoms
Rheumatoid arthritis	Chronic, systemic, inflammatory	F, 20–40	Joints swollen, painful, and inflamed, leading to calcification, immobility, and deformity (Fig. 47–1)
Osteoarthritis	Chronic, localized, degenerative	F, 45–55	Slow degeneration of spine and weight-bearing joints
Gouty arthritis	Acute, familial, metabolic disorder of purine metabolism	M, 35 +	Joint or joints become swollen, painful, and inflamed; can lead to chronic deformity (may be precipitated by certain medications)
Juvenile arthritis	Systemic inflammatory disease affecting one or more joints	Undetermined	Joint swollen, painful and inflamed; 75% have remission without joint damage

Table 47–1. INFLAMMATORY DISEASES–*CONTINUED*

CONNECTIVE TISSUE DISEASES

Definition: Conditions that affect and destroy connective tissue.

Types: Lupus erythematosus
Polyarteritis nodosa
Scleroderma

Condition	Pathologic Process	Sex Preference/ Onset Age (yr)	Symptoms
Lupus erythematosus	Chronic, systemic, produce antibodies that attack own nucleoproteins	F, 15 +	Swollen joints, skin rash, organ damage, generalized alopecia, photosensitivity
Polyarteritis nodosa	Chronic, diffuse, inflammatory, and necrosis of small arteries	F, 25 +	Damage to small to medium-sized arteries in major organs of body leading to organ damage
Scleroderma	Chronic, diffuse	M, 35 +	Skin thickens and has pigmentation changes; respiratory impairment

Treatments Include:
Medications including salicylates and nonsteroidal anti-inflammatory drugs, gold compounds, steroids, cytotoxic agents, and antigout preparations.
Minimization of functional limitation, discomfort, infection, and deformity.
Education regarding self-help devices (Self-Help Devices Office, Institute of Physical Medicine and Rehabilitation, 400 East 34th Street, New York, NY 10016).
Helping patient develop support system to maintain independence as long as possible.
Establishment of realistic goals.
Maintenance of prescribed exercise and/or rest program to improve circulation, promote relaxation, relieve pain, improve range of motion, including heat and cold application.
Maintenance of routine schedule of sleep (firm mattress is recommended).

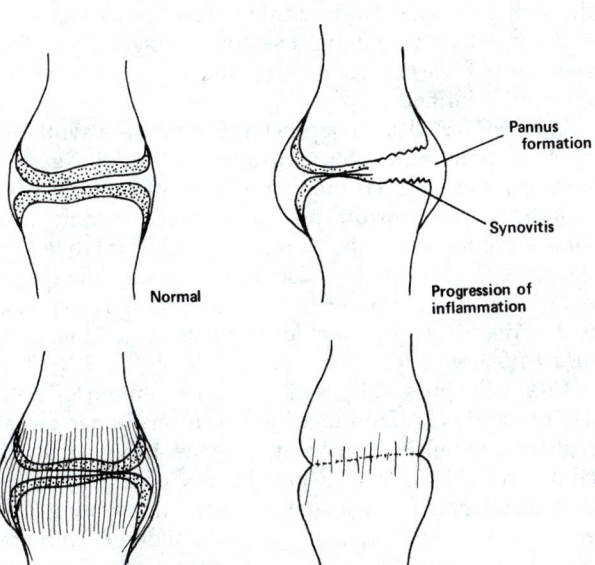

Figure 47–1. Joint changes associated with arthritis.

USES

In general, anti-inflammatory drugs are used to treat autoimmune diseases, including certain types of arthritis.

The anti-inflammatory drugs are used for both short- and long-term therapy. The medications developed for short-term therapy are normally used for 1–4 weeks. Short duration of use is required because of severe adverse effects that can develop.

When the long-term medications are prescribed, the patient is evaluated by the physician at the end of 1–2 weeks to ascertain if the medication is effective.

SALICYLATES, NSAID, SALICYLATE-LIKE MEDICATIONS

Prostaglandins

The *prostaglandins*, first discovered in the 1930s, have been detected in almost every tissue and body fluid, and take part in almost every biologic function. They are not stored in the body, but are produced and released under certain conditions, such as cell damage (injury, inflammation, or tumor).

Several groups of prostaglandins, synthesized from essential fatty acids through the arachidonic acid cas-

Table 47–2. ANTI-INFLAMMATORY CLASSES

Agent	OTC	Rx
I. Group I Agents: Salicylates and Nonsteroidal Anti-Inflammatory Agents		
A. Salicylates		
1. Aspirin	X	
2. Choline salicylate (Arthropan)	X	
3. Choline magnesium trisalicylate (Trilisate)	X	X
4. Diflunisal (Dolobid)	X	X
B. Propionic Acid Derivatives		
1. Fenoprofen (Nalfon)		X
2. Flurbiprofen (Ansaid)		X
3. Ibuprofen (Motrin, Rufen)	X	X
4. Ibuprofen (Datril)	X	
5. Naproxen (Naprosyn, Anaprox)		X
6. Ketoprofen (Orudis)		X
7. Carpofen (Rimadyl)		X
C. Indoles		
1. Indomethacin (Indocin)		X
2. Sulindac (Clinoril)		X
3. Tolmetin (Tolectin)		X
D. Pyrazolones		
1. Phenylbutazone (Butazolidin)		X
2. Oxyphenbutazone (Tandearil)		X
E. Fenamates		
1. Mefenamic Acid (Ponstel)		X
2. Meclofenamate sodium (Meclomen)		X
F. Oxicams		
1. Piroxicam (Feldene)		X
II. Group II Agents		
A. Gold		
1. Gold sodium thiomalate (Myochrysine)		X
2. Aurothioglucose (Solganal)		X
3. Auranofin (SKF's investigational oral gold preparation; not on the market yet)		X
B. Penicillamine (Cuprimine)		X
C. Hydroxychloroquine (Plaquenil)		X
D. Levamisole—an immune stimulant; not as yet available in United States		X
III. Group III Agents (oral and intersynovial; see Chapter 42)		
IV. Group IV Agents—Cytotoxic Agents (last-ditch effort; unapproved use at this time; see Chapter 49)		
1. Cyclophosphamide (Cytoxan)		X
2. Azathioprine (Imuran)		X
3. Methotrexate		X

cade, have been recognized, and are referred to by the letters A, B, C, D, E, F, H, I, and nonPG (thromboxane). A numerical subscript 1 to 3 may be added, indicating the prostaglandin series (PGI_2). The prostaglandins PGE and PGF are currently best known. PGE and PGF are stable in blood, but are rapidly metabolized (80%–90%) on a single pass through either the kidneys or the liver. Once synthesized, prostaglandins are released locally, where they may act as local mediators of cellular action leading to a wide variety of functional changes followed by a local metabolism or secondary "overflow" release into the venous circulation for eventual metabolism. The prostaglandins have been described as having an "awesome and bewildering" diversity of actions, which include:

1. Vasodilation.
2. Increased cardiac output.
3. Increased capillary permeability.
4. Stimulation of uterine contractions.
5. Either vasodilation or constriction of bronchioles (PGE_1 and PGE_2 dilate, PGF_2 constricts).
6. Possible pain production.
7. Interruption of early pregnancy, causing abortion.
8. Stimulation of adrenal and pituitary secretion.
9. Release of lysosomal enzymes.
10. Inhibition of platelet aggregation.
11. Stimulation of erythropoietin production.
12. Suppression of the immune response by inhibiting both T- and B-lymphocyte activity.
13. Inhibition of gastric acid secretion and stabilization of the gastric mucosa.
14. Prevention of release of histamine from sensitized leukocytes.
15. Elevation of body temperature.
16. Vascular dilatation in kidney to help regulate renal vascular resistance.

Research has demonstrated that nonsteroidal anti-inflammatory agents inhibit prostaglandin synthesis and, thereby, help to relieve pain. There is great promise for the potential use of currently known prostaglandins, as well as their derivatives, and for drugs that work through prostaglandin inhibition. Table 47–4 lists several current and potential uses of prostaglandins. The spectrum of uses for such compounds has yet to be defined and clarified.

MISOPROSTOL. Misoprostol (Cytotec) is a synthetic prostaglandin E_1 analog. Misoprostol inhibits gastric acid secretion and has mucosal protective properties.

Action. Misoprostol can increase bicarbonate and mucus production in the stomach, which is inhibited by the NSAIDs. Misoprostol also inhibits basal and nocturnal gastric acid secretion and acid secretion in response to a variety of stimuli including meals, histamine, *pentagastrin*, and coffee.

Use. Misoprostol is used in the prevention of both aspirin- and NSAID-induced gastric ulcers in persons at high risk for ulcer formation. Persons at high risk include: individuals with a past history of ulcer, the elderly, and patients with concomitant debilitating diseases. Misoprostol is taken for the duration of aspirin or NSAID therapy. Misoprostol does not prevent duodenal ulcers in patients on NSAIDs.

Pharmacokinetics. Misoprostol is rapidly absorbed after oral administration and reaches a peak concentration in 12 ± 3 minutes. It has a terminal half-life of 20–

40 minutes. Misoprostol undergoes rapid *de-esterification* and 80% is excreted in the urine.

Contraindications and Precautions. Misoprostol is contraindicated in patients with previous allergy to the prostaglandins. It is also contraindicated in pregnant patients. Misoprostol has abortifacient properties and actually produces uterine contractions that may endanger pregnancy. It should only be administered to women who are capable of complying with effective contraceptive measures.

Misoprostol is used cautiously in persons with renal impairment as it is 80 percent excreted in the urine. Dosage may need to be decreased for patients with renal disease. Safety has not been established in children under the age of 18 years. Misoprostol should not be administered to nursing mothers as misoprostol is excreted in milk and could cause significant diarrhea in nursing infants.

Adverse Effects. The most common adverse effect is diarrhea occurring in 13–40 percent of patients. Diarrhea is dose-related and usually develops early in the course of therapy (after thirteen days). The diarrhea is generally self-limiting and resolves within eight days. If diarrhea continues, it may necessitate discontinuation of misoprostol. Diarrhea, as well as other gastrointestinal symptoms, such as abdominal pain (7%–20%), nausea (3.2%), flatulence (2.9%), dyspepsia (2%), and vomiting (1.3%), can be reduced by administering misoprostol after meals and at bedtime, and by avoiding coadministration with magnesium-containing antacids.

Additional adverse effects can occur in female patients including spotting, cramps, hypermenorrhea, menstrual disorders, and dysmenorrhea.

Interactions. Antacids—particularly magnesium-containing antacids—reduce the total availability of misoprostol. This does not appear to be clinically important since misoprostol acts locally in the stomach. Plasma concentrations are also diminished when misoprostol is taken with food.

Dosage. Misoprostol is administered orally four times daily with food or meals and at bedtime. The usual dose is 200 μg. If this dose cannot be tolerated, 100 μg can be used.

Kinins, Monoamines, and Lysosomal Enzymes

Along with prostaglandins, other substances play a role in inflammation, including *kinins, monoamines,* and *lysosomal enzymes.* Kinins, including bradykinin, are biologically active polypeptides formed as a result of injury or inflammation; they are powerful vasodilators. Vasodilation is also accompanied by increased permeability of the vessels, resulting in local redness, edema, burning, and throbbing pain. In the lung, bradykinin causes bronchospasm and bronchoconstriction when it is released following a stimulus.

The monoamines (including histamine and serotonin) are stored in the mast cells in the lung and in other body cells, and are released as a result of bodily injury. Both bradykinin and histamine encourage the phagocytic cells to migrate from the bloodstream to the place of injury. The lysosomal membrane surrounding the cell is damaged when phagocytic cells are broken down as they attempt to engulf foreign particles. As a result of lysosomal breakdown, several lysosomal enzymes, including proteases and hydrolases, are released. These begin to clean up the damaged phagocytes and their original prey (for example, uric acid crystals); however, they also begin to break down the collagenous connective tissue within the arthritic joint. This leads to the development of more prostaglandins, bradykinin, and histamine, causing the inflammation to worsen (Fig. 47–2).

Salicylates

Salicylates, the most extensively employed analgesic, antipyretic, and anti-inflammatory chemical group used today, are most commonly prescribed for the control of arthritic pain. The salicylates are believed to inhibit prostaglandin synthesis in the body, resulting in a decrease in the development of pain and deformity in the person with arthritis.

The salicylates affect the composition, biosynthesis, and metabolism of connective tissue, providing a barrier for the spread of infection, and inflammation. Salicylates are thought to stabilize the lysosomal membrane, thereby preventing it from releasing substances that cause inflammation. Also, salicylates inhibit formation of excessive amounts of prostaglandins in the brain, which may possibly account for their effectiveness in the treatment of headaches. Some researchers believe that salicylates have a central site of action, within the brain. Aspirin also retards platelet aggregation, allowing it to be used as an adjunct to therapy in cardiovascular and neurologic disorders. This effect can be dangerous in patients with clotting abnormalities or other bleeding disorders. Salicylate levels (15–30 mg/dL) are often used to monitor dosing. Salicylates are discussed in detail in Chapter 20.

ASPIRIN. Aspirin or acetylsalicylic acid is the most common salicylate used for arthritic pain. It is available OTC and is one of the most widely taken and prescribed drugs. The usual adult dose is 650 mg (10 gr). Many OTC products contain aspirin for its analgesic, antipyretic, and anti-inflammatory effects.

Adverse effects of aspirin are minimal with normal doses. Some patients may complain of gastrointestinal upset (10–30%), which may be decreased by taking aspirin with food or by taking enteric-coated aspirin. Toxic effects are most common with accidental ingestion of high doses and include gastrointestinal bleeding (70%), ringing in the ears, profuse sweating, weakness, slowed respirations and heart rate, and cyanosis. These effects can be serious and the patient may need medical attention and discontinuation of drug for some time (more information may be found in Chapter 20).

Nonsteroidal Anti-Inflammatory Drugs

The nonsteroidal anti-inflammatory drugs (NSAIDs) are classified into several groups:

1. Propionic acid derivatives including ibuprofen (Motrin, Rufen), fenoprofen (Nalfon), naproxen (Naprosyn), carprofen (Rimadyl), and ketoprofen (Orudis);

TEXT RESUMES ON PAGE 1312

Table 47–3. ANTI-INFLAMMATORY MEDICATIONS

Name	Dosage	Mode of Administration	Pharmacokinetics
PROSTAGLANDINS Misoprostol (Cytotec)			
Action: Inhibits gastric acid secretion; mucosal protective properties; can increase bicarbonate and mucus production in the stomach.			
Use: To decrease or prevent the incidence of gastric irritation and ulceration when NSAIDs are administered concurrently.			
	100–200 µg 4 times daily	PO	O: rapid P: 12 ± 3 min D: 3 hr ½L: 20–40 min PB: less than 90% B: liver E: 80% urine
NONSTEROIDAL ANTI-INFLAMMATORY DRUGS (NSAIDs)			
Action: Anti-inflammatories; reduce joint swelling, stiffness, specific action unknown; analgesic and antipyretic properties.			
Use: Rheumatoid arthritis, osteoarthritis, mild to moderate pain, primary dysmenorrhea.			
Proprionic Acid Derivatives Ibuprofen (Motrin)			
Use: Same as with all plus with tetracycline to treat resistant acne vulgaris.			
	200–800 mg 3–4 times daily; maximum daily dose 3200 mg	PO	O: 30–60 min P: 1–2 hr D: 2–4 hr ½L: 1.8–2.5 hr PB: 99% B: liver E: urine (5%–10% unchanged), liver

Key to abbreviations in *Pharmacokinetics* column: O-onset; P-peak; D-duration; ½L-half-life; PB-protein bound; B-biotransformation; E-elimination.

*Within the column of adverse effects, underlines indicate the most common effects; CAPITALS indicate life-threatening effects.

Contraindications/ Precautions	Adverse Effects*	Interactions	Nursing Implications
CONTRAINDICATIONS: Contraindicated in persons with previous allergy to prostaglandins and in pregant women. Do not administer to nursing mothers. *PRECAUTIONS:* Use with caution in patients with renal impairment. Safety in children under 18 not established.	*GI:* diarrhea, abdominal pain, nausea, flatulence, dyspepsia, vomiting, constipation *Neuro:* headache *Reprod:* spotting, cramps, menstrual disorders, miscarriage in pregnant women	Antacids reduce availability. Maximal plasma concentrations are reduced when taken with food.	*ASSESSMENT:* Pregnancy test. *INTERVENTION:* Therapy is begun after a negative pregnancy test 2 weeks before. It is then started on 2nd or 3rd day of the next menstrual period. Administer after meals and at bedtime. Do not give concurrent magnesium-containing antacids. Teach patient not to give this medicine to anyone else. *EVALUATION:* Evaluate for diarrhea and gynecological disorders. Report these to the physician.
For All NSAIDs: *CONTRAINDICATIONS:* Contraindicated in GI lesions, hypersensitivity, allergy to aspirin or iodides, symptoms of asthma, rhinitis, urticaria, angioedema or bronchospasm. *PRECAUTIONS:* Use with caution in previous history of GI ulceration, renal/hepatic disease, cardiac disease.	*For all NSAIDs:* *Neuro:* tinnitis, headache, dizziness, blurred vision *Resp:* asthmatic bronchospasm *GI:* nausea, vomiting, heartburn, GI BLEED, ulceration *Biliary:* HEPATITIS-LIKE SYNDROME *Hemo:* BONE MARROW DEPRESSION *Renal:* decreased glomerular filtration, hyperkalemia *Integ:* skin eruptions, hives *Misc:* allergic reactions, ANAPHYLAXIS, salt, water retention	*For all NSAIDs:* Increased ulcerogenic effects with corticosteroids and salicylates. Increased bleeding with anticoagulants. Concurrent aspirin decreases anti-inflammatory effects. Decreased antihypertensive effect with beta-adrenergic blockers and captopril. NSAIDs may displace hydantoins, sulfonamides, and sulfonylureas from albumin.	*For all NSAIDs:* *ASSESSMENT:* Obtain baseline blood studies and thorough GI history. *INTERVENTION:* Avoid aspirin and alcoholic beverages while taking medication. If GI upset occurs, take with food, milk, or antacids (except for Tolmetin—use only antacids). Caution when driving or operating heavy equipment. *EVALUATION:* Notify physician if persistent rash, itching, black stools, edema, or weight gain occur.
Same as for all plus: Safety in children not established	*Integ:* rash, dermatitis	*Same as for all plus:* Reduces the effectiveness of antihypertensives.	*Same as for all plus:* *INTERVENTION:* Do not administer with aspirin. Give lowest possible dose to decrease side effects. *EVALUATION:* When taking concurrent antihypertensives, evaluate blood pressure frequently.

CONTINUED ON THE FOLLOWING PAGE

Anti-Inflammatory Medications

Table 47–3. ANTI-INFLAMMATORY MEDICATIONS–*CONTINUED*

Name	Dosage	Mode of Administration	Pharmacokinetics
Naproxen (Naprosyn)			
Use: Same as for all plus ankylosing spondylitis, tendonitis, bursitis, acute gout, juvenile rheumatoid arthritis.			
	Adult: 250–750 mg 2 times daily; maximum daily dose 1500 mg *Pediatric:* total dose 10 mg/kg in 2 doses	PO	O: 1–2 hr P: 2–4 hr D: 7 hr ½L: 12–15 hr PB: 99% B: liver E: urine (70% unchanged)
Fenopren (Nalfon)	300–600 mg 3–4 times daily (30 min ac or 2 hr pc is best); maximum dose 3200 mg/day	PO	O: 0.5 hr P: 1–2 hr D: 5 hr ½L: 2–3 hr PB: 90% B: liver E: urine (70% unchanged)
Ketoprofen (Orudis)	150–300 mg/day, single or divided daily dose; maximum dose 300 mg/day	PO	O: rapid P: 0.5–2 hr D: UA ½L: 2–4 hr PB: 99% B: liver E: urine
Flurbiprofen (Ansaid)	200–300 mg 2–4 × daily	PO	O: rapid P: 1.5 hr D: UA ½L: 5.7 hr PB: 99% B: liver E: urine
Indole Analogs Indomethacin (Indocin)			
Use: Same as for all plus moderate to severe ankylosing spondylitis, painful shoulders, short-term therapy only.			
	25–50 mg 2–4 times daily; maximum dose 200 mg/day S-R capsules, 75 mg qd or bid (do not crush S-R capsules)	PO	O: 0.5–2 hr P: 3 hr D: 5–6 hr ½L: 4.5–6 hr P: 2–4 hr D: 8–12 hr ½L: 4.5–6 hr PB: 90% B: liver E: urine (10%–20% unchanged), feces

Key to abbreviations in *Pharmacokinetics* column: O-onset; P-peak; D-duration; ½L-half-life; PB-protein bound; B-biotransformation; E-elimination.

*Within the column of adverse effects, underlines indicate the most common effects; CAPITALS indicate life-threatening effects.

Contraindications/Precautions	Adverse Effects*	Interactions	Nursing Implications
Same as for all plus: Safety in pregnancy not established.	*Same as for all plus:* *Neuro:* somnolence/drowsiness *Resp:* dyspnea, hemoptysis, pharyngitis, rhinitis, pulmonary infiltrates *GI:* dyspepsia, constipation *Integ:* rash, dermatitis	*Same as for all plus:* Methotrexate may cause fatal reaction. Diflunisal decreases renal excretion of naproxen, so decrease naproxen dosage. *Lab:* May increase urine 17-ketosteroids. May interface with 5-hydroxy-indoleacetic acid	*Same as for all plus:* INTERVENTION: Do not give with ASA. Symptomatic relief may not occur for 2 weeks.
Same as for all plus: Use cautiously in patients with genitourinary tract disease. Safety in children and persons with auditory problems not established.	*Same as for all plus:* *Neuro:* somnolence/drowsiness *GI:* dyspepsia, constipation *Renal:* dysuria, cystitis, hematuria, interstitial nephritis	*Same as for all plus:* Phenobarbital may decrease half-life of fenoprofen.	*Same as for all plus:* INTERVENTION: Give with food or milk, not ASA. EVALUATION: Evaluate for excessive bleeding with concurrent anticoagulants.
Same as for all plus: Safety in children and pregnant women not established.	*Same as for all plus:* *Neuro:* headache	*Same as for all plus:* Methotrexate may cause fatal reaction. Concurrent hydrochlorothiazide reduces urinary excretion of K. *Lab:* May prolong bleeding time by 3–4 minutes.	*Same as for all plus:* INTERVENTION: Reduce dose in renal disease.
Same as for all.	Same as for all.	Same as for all.	Same as for all. INTERVENTION: Food decreases absorption and peak plasma levels.
Same as for all plus: Use cautiously in patients with impaired renal and hepatic function, individuals with psychiatric illness, and elderly patients.	*Same as for all plus:* *Neuro:* headache, dizziness, psychiatric disturbances *GI:* GASTRIC BLEEDS, rectal irritation with suppositories, ulcerative stomatitis, anorexia, dry/sore mouth	*Same as for all plus:* Concurrent use with diflunisal decreases renal clearance of indomethacin. Increases serum levels of lithium.	*Same as for all plus:* ASSESSMENT: Obtain complete eye exam at onset of therapy and periodically.

CONTINUED ON THE FOLLOWING PAGE

Table 47–3. ANTI-INFLAMMATORY MEDICATIONS–*CONTINUED*

Name	Dosage	Mode of Administration	Pharmacokinetics
Indomethacin–*Continued*			
Sulindac (Clinoril)			
Use: Same as for all plus ankylosing spondylitis, acute painful shoulder.			
	150–200 mg 2 times daily, maximum dose 400 mg/day	PO	O: 1 hr P: 2 hr D: 7–16 hr ½L: 7–8 hr PB: 90% B: liver E: urine
Tolmetin (Tolectin)			
Use: Acute/long-term rheumatoid arthritis, and osteoarthritis, and juvenile rheumatoid arthritis.			
	Adult: Initial dosage: 200–400 mg 3–4 times a day; *Maintenance dosage:* 600–1800 mg daily in divided doses; maximum dose 2000 mg/day *Pediatric:* Children 2 years and older: *Initial dosage:* 20 mg/kg/day in 3–4 divided doses; *Maintenance dosage:* 15–30 mg/kg/day in 3–4 divided doses	PO	O: rapid P: 0.5–1 hr D: UA ½L: 1–1.5 hr PB: 99% B: liver E: urine (5%–10% unchanged)
Oxicam Products Piroxicam (Feldene)			
Use: Rheumatoid arthritis, osteoarthritis.			
	Adult: 10–20 mg daily or in divided doses	PO	O: rapid P: 3–5 hr D: long ½L: 30–86 hr PB: 99% B: liver E: urine (2%–5% unchanged), feces

Key to abbreviations in *Pharmacokinetics* column: O-onset; P-peak; D-duration; ½L-half-life; PB-protein bound; B-biotransformation; E-elimination.

*Within the column of adverse effects, underlines indicate the most common effects; CAPITALS indicate life-threatening effects.

Contraindications/ Precautions	Adverse Effects*	Interactions	Nursing Implications
			INTERVENTION: Twice-daily medications are best taken on arising in the morning and at bedtime. If stomach distress arises, give with food, milk, or antacid. Complete physical examination and laboratory studies are recommended before and during therapy. Monitor stool for bleeding, and monitor intake and output. Older patient may need lower dose.
Same as for all plus: Safety in children not established.	Same as for all.	*Same as for all plus:* Diflunisal decreases plasma levels of sulindac by one third. Dimethyl sulfoxide reduces efficacy of sulindac. May decrease serum lithium levels.	*Same as for all plus:* Food delays peaks of action.
Same as for all.	*Same as for all plus:* *GI:* decreased appetite, weight increase/decrease *Hemo:* increases K, decreases Na *Endo:* hyper/hypo-glycemia	*Same as for all plus:* *Lab:* False-positive protein-uria.	*Same as for all plus:* *INTERVENTION:* If GI distress, give with food or antacid. Milk decreases bioavailability. Do not give with aspirin. *EVALUATION:* Improvement should occur within a few days to weeks
Same as for all plus: Safety in children not established	*Same as for all plus:* *GI:* pancreatitis *Integ:* photosensitivity	Same as for all.	Same as for all.

CONTINUED ON THE FOLLOWING PAGE

Table 47–3. ANTI-INFLAMMATORY MEDICATIONS–*CONTINUED*

Name	Dosage	Mode of Administration	Pharmacokinetics
Pyrazolone Derivatives			
Action: Unknown but thought to inhibit prostaglandin synthesis, leukocyte migration, lysosomal enzyme release.			
Use: Acute short-term therapy only, acute gouty arthritis, acute rheumatoid arthritis, active ankylosing spondylitis, painful shoulder.			
Phenylbutazone (Butazolidin, Azolid)	100 mg 3–4 times daily; maximum dose 400 mg/day; should be administered for 7 days only	PO	O: 30–60 min P: 2.5 hr D: 3–5 days ½L: 77 hr PB: 98% B: liver E: urine (2% unchanged), feces
Fenamates/Salicylate–Like Medications			
Mefenamic acid (Ponstel)	250 mg 3–4 times daily; maximum dose 1000 mg/day	PO	O: 1–2 hr P: 2–4 hr D: 6 hr ½L: 2–4 hr PB: 90% B: liver E: urine (5%–100% unchanged)
Meclofenamate sodium (Meclomen)	200–400 mg/day in 3–4 divided doses; maximum dose 400 mg/day	PO	O: 0.5–1 hr P: 0.5–2 hr D: 6 hr ½L: 2 hr PB: 99% B: liver E: urine, feces

Key to abbreviations in *Pharmacokinetics* column: O-onset; P-peak; D-duration; ½L-half-life; PB-protein bound; B-biotransformation; E-elimination.
*Within the column of adverse effects, <u>underlines</u> indicate the most common effects; CAPITALS indicate life-threatening effects.

Contraindications/ Precautions	Adverse Effects*	Interactions	Nursing Implications
CONTRAINDICATIONS: Contraindicated in allergic reactions to aspirin or other NSAIDs, GI lesions, pregnancy, nursing mothers, and children under age 14 years. PRECAUTIONS: Use cautiously in impaired renal and hepatic function, glaucoma, and patients over age 40 years.	Neuro: headache, drowsiness, agitation, hearing loss, tinnitus, blurred vision CVR: edema, congestive heart failure GI: abdominal discomfort, nausea, dyspepsia, vomiting, abdominal distention, GI BLEEDS, constipation, diarrhea Hemo: APLASTIC ANEMIA, AGRANULOCYTOSIS, anemia, leukopenia, BONE MARROW DEPRESSION Renal: hematuria, proteinuria, ATN, glomerulonephritis Integ: rash, pruritis Misc: STEVENS-JOHNSON SYNDROME	Increased activity of other anti-inflammatories, oral antidiabetics, sulfonamides, and phenytoin. Decreased levels of dicoumarol, digitoxin, cortisone. Half-life decreases with concurrent barbiturate, promethazine, rifampin, corticosteroids. Cholestyramine decreases enteral absorption. Methylphenidate increases half-life. Potentiates methotrexate, insulin, sulfonylureas, and sulfonamides. Enhances the effects of oral anticoagulants. Lab: Interferes with thyroid function tests.	Same as for all plus: INTERVENTION: Persons over age 60 should not receive the drug for more than 1 week. Monitor CBC closely during therapy. Improvement should occur within 2–3 days. If no improvement occurs, discontinue after 1 week. Take with food or milk. Observe caution while operating heavy equipment. Refrain from alcohol. EVALUATION: Notify physician of sore throat, unusual bleeding, fever, swelling of hands and feet
Same as for all plus: CONTRAINDICATIONS: Contraindicated in sensitivity, aspirin allergy, active peptic ulcer, compromised renal function, pregnancy, and children under age 14 years. PRECAUTIONS: Use cautiously in patients with GI ulceration, hepatic disease, or cardiac disease.	Same as for all.	Concurrent warfarin increases PT. Concurrent aspirin decreases plasma levels of mefenamic acid.	For all salicylate-like medications: ASSESSMENT: GI system, obtain baseline blood work. INTERVENTION: Administer with food or an antacid to reduce GI complications. Medications are used for acute treatment. Therapeutic effects are generally noted within 24–36 hours. Aspirin is not given concurrently because it will potentiate the ulcerative effects of these medications. After the acute flareup is over, the medication should be reduced and discontinued. Patients over 40 should be placed on these medications for 1 week only. EVALUATION: If rash or diarrhea occur, notify physician.
Same as above plus: Safety in pregnant women, lactating women, and children not established.	Neuro: headache, dizziness GI: GI distress, diarrhea, nausea, vomiting, pyrosis, flatulence Integ: rash	Same as above.	Same as above plus: INTERVENTION: Not recommended as initial drug because of GI side effects.

CONTINUED ON THE FOLLOWING PAGE

Table 47–3. ANTI-INFLAMMATORY MEDICATIONS–*CONTINUED*

Name	Dosage	Mode of Administration	Pharmacokinetics
Phenylacetic Acid Derivatives Diclofenac sodium (Voltaren)	*Adult:* 100–200 mg/day in divided doses *Pediatric:* 2–3 mg/kg/day	PO	O: 1 hr P: 2–3 hr D: 4–6 hr ½L: 1.2–1.8 hr PB: over 90% B: liver E: kidney

REMISSION-INDUCING DRUGS

Gold Products

Action: Inhibit phagocytosis, inhibit lysosomal enzymes, decrease immunoglobulins.

Use: Rheumatoid arthritis.

Name	Dosage	Mode of Administration	Pharmacokinetics
Gold sodium thiomalate (Myochrysine—contains 50% gold)	Highly individualized; 10 mg at first, to 50 mg by 16–20 injections. *Maintenance dosage:* 50 mg q 1–2 wk × 4; 50 mg q 3 wk × 4; 50 mg monthly to total dose of 0.8–1.0 g (see text)	IM	O: slow P: 2–6 hr D: 6 mo ½L: 3–27 hr* PB: 95%–99% B: none E: urine (70% unchanged), feces

*Single dose; 14–40 hr by third dose; up to 168 hr after 11th dose.

Name	Dosage	Mode of Administration	Pharmacokinetics
Aurothioglucose (Solganal—contains 50% gold)	1st dose: 10 mg; 2nd and 3rd dose: 25 mg; 4th and other doses: 50 mg. Continue until 0.8–1.0 g has been given and evaluate; if improvement, give 50 mg q 3–4 weeks	IM	O: slow P: 4–6 hr D: 6 mo ½L: 3–27 hr PB: 95%–99% B: none E: urine

Key to abbreviations in *Pharmacokinetics* column: O-onset; P-peak; D-duration; ½L-half-life; PB-protein bound; B-biotransformation; E-elimination.

*Within the column of adverse effects, underlines indicate the most common effects; CAPITALS indicate life-threatening effects.

Contraindications/ Precautions	Adverse Effects*	Interactions	Nursing Implications
Same as for all.	Same as for all.	Enhances nephrotoxicity of cyclosporine. Increases plasma levels of digoxin. Decreases lithium clearance. Increases hypotensive effects of hydrochlorothiazide.	Same as for all.
CONTRAINDICATIONS: Contraindicated in toxicity to heavy metals, renal or hepatic disease, congestive heart failure, uncontrolled diabetes, hepatitis, and hypertension. *PRECAUTIONS:* Safety in pregnant women, lactating women, and children not established.	*For All Gold Products:* *Neuro:* neuropathy, headache, dizziness *CVR:* vasomotor reaction *Resp:* pneumonitis, bronchitis, shortness of breath, cough *GI:* stomatitis, colitis, metallic taste in mouth, nausea, vomiting *Biliary:* hepatitis, jaundice *Hemo:* THROMBOCYTOPENIA, LEUKOPENIA, APLASTIC ANEMIA, AGRANULOCYTOSIS *Renal:* proteinuria, nephrotic syndrome *Integ:* rashes, pruritis, exfoliative dermatitis, chrysiasis (blue/grey skin color) *EENT:* IRITIS, CORNEAL ULCERS, corneal gold deposits *Misc:* ANAPHYLAXIS, sweating	None known.	*For All Gold Products:* *ASSESSMENT:* Baseline CBC, BUN, and creatinine are obtained before the start of therapy and at regular intervals thereafter. *INTERVENTION:* Exposure to the sun may aggravate dermatitis, so patient should wear hats and long-sleeved clothing for protection. Therapeutic effects may not be seen for 6–8 weeks. May continue to improve for as long as 1 year. When administering, agitate the bottle before medication is withdrawn into syringe to ensure a uniform suspension. Use a 20–21-gauge needle. Then inject the medication deep intragluteally with the patient in a recumbent position. It is best if the patient can remain recumbent for 30 minutes. (Transient side effects, such as dizziness, facial flushing, and vertigo, may be experienced.) Medication should be preserved in a tightly closed, light-resistant container and should not be used if it is darker in color than pale yellow. *EVALUATION:* Notify physician for continued rash, sore mouth, indigestion, and diarrhea.
Same as above.	Same as above.	Same as above.	*Same as for all plus:* *INTERVENTION:* Use an 18-gauge needle. Keep patient lying flat for 15 minutes.

CONTINUED ON THE FOLLOWING PAGE

Table 47–3. ANTI-INFLAMMATORY MEDICATIONS–*CONTINUED*

Name	Dosage	Mode of Administration	Pharmacokinetics
Auranofin (Ridaura—contains 29% gold)	*Initial dose:* 6 mg/day; if no response in 6 months, increase to 9 mg/day; if no response in 3 months, discontinue	PO	O: rapid P: 1–2 hr D: 6 mo ½L: 26 days PB: 60% B: UA E: urine (85% unchanged), feces

Other Medications
D-Penicillamine (Cuprimine)

Action: Unknown but has immunosuppressive activity.

Use: Rheumatoid arthritis.

	Adult: 125–250 mg daily; up to 750 mg/day, with increases every several months *Pediatric:* 5 mg/kg/day; up to 10–15 mg/kg/day	PO	O: 2–3 mo P: 130 min D: months to years ½L: 60 min PB: UA B: UA E: urine, feces

ANTIGOUT AGENTS

Action: Unknown but may affect leukocytes in synovial cells.

Use: Acute gouty arthritis.

Colchicine	*For acute gout:* 0.5–1.2 mg/hr × 10 doses or until GI side effects occur; maximum dose 4–8 mg *For chronic gout:* 0.5–1.2 mg/day	PO	O: 20 min P: 1–2 hr D: 9 days ½L: 20 min (plasma); 60 hr (WBC) PB: UA B: liver E: urine
	1–3 mg to start, then 0.5 mg q 6 hr; maximal dose 4 mg in 1 course of therapy	IV	

Key to abbreviations in *Pharmacokinetics* column: O-onset; P-peak; D-duration; ½L-half-life; PB-protein bound; B-biotransformation; E-elimination.
*Within the column of adverse effects, underlines indicate the most common effects; CAPITALS indicate life-threatening effects.

Contraindications/ Precautions	Adverse Effects*	Interactions	Nursing Implications
Same as above plus: Contraindicated in bone marrow aplasia, pulmonary fibrosis, exfoliative dermatitis.	*GI:* diarrhea, oral ulceration *Renal:* proteinuria *Integ:* rashes	Increased phenytoin levels.	Same as above.
CONTRAINDICATIONS: Contraindicated in pregnancy, blood dyscrasias, and renal insufficiency. If fever develops, discontinue.	*GI:* anorexia, epigastric pain, nausea, vomiting, diarrhea, alteration in taste *Hemo:* THROMBOCYTOPENIA, LEUKOPENIA, AGRANULOCYTOSIS, APLASTIC ANEMIA *Renal:* proteinuria, hypoalbuminemia, NEPHROTIC SYNDROME *Integ:* pruritis, rash	Should not be given concurrently with salicylates, nonsteroidal anti-inflammatory drugs, or corticosteroids.	*ASSESSMENT:* Assess patient before and during therapy for skin, blood, renal, and hepatic problems. Assess temperature daily (may be the first sign of allergy). Routine CBC and renal studies are done q 2 weeks for 6 months, then monthly. *INTERVENTION:* Administer on an empty stomach (30–60 minutes before, or 2 hours after, meals). Separate other medications by 1 hour. Capsules may be opened and mixed with juice. Patient may need supplemental vitamin B$_6$.
CONTRAINDICATIONS: Contraindicated in hypersensitivity, and in GI, renal, hepatic, or cardiac disease, and blood dyscrasias. *PRECAUTIONS:* Use cautiously in elderly or debilitated patients and in early GI disease. Safety in pregnant women, lactating women, and children not established.	*Neuro:* peripheral neuritis *GI:* vomiting, diarrhea, abdominal pain, nausea *Hemo:* BONE MARROW DEPRESSION, AGRANULOCYTOSIS, APLASTIC ANEMIA *Integ:* hair loss, dermatosis	Inhibited by acidifying agents. Potentiated by alkalating agents. Increases sensitivity to CNS depressants. Inhibits vitamin B$_{12}$ absorption. *Lab:* May increase alkaline phosphatase and SGOT levels. False positive in urine tests for RBCs and hemoglobin.	*For All Antigout Medications:* *ASSESSMENT:* Baseline uric acid levels as well as CBC are obtained and periodically checked during therapy. *INTERVENTION:* Administer immediately before, during, or after meal to limit gastric irritation. Increase fluid intake to at least 3000 ml/day (assuming there are no contraindications to increased fluid intake) to prevent the formation of uric acid stones by the kid-

CONTINUED ON THE FOLLOWING PAGE

Table 47-3. ANTI-INFLAMMATORY MEDICATIONS-*CONTINUED*

Name	Dosage	Mode of Administration	Pharmacokinetics
Colchicine-*Continued*			
Probenecid (Benemid)			

Action: Inhibit tubular reabsorption of uric acid in kidney.

| | 250 mg 2 times daily; increased to 1 g/day over many weeks to control symptoms | PO | O: 30 min
P: 2–4 hr
D: 8 hr
½L: 4–9 hr
PB: highly
B: liver
E: urine |
| Sulfinpyrazone (Anturane) | *Initial dosage:* 100–200 mg 2 times daily; up to 200–400 mg 2 times daily
Maintenance dosage: 200–800 mg/day | PO | O: 30 min
P: 1–2 hr
D: 4–6 hr (maybe 10 hr)
½L: 1–3 hr
PB: highly
B: metabolized
E: urine (unchanged) |

Key to abbreviations in *Pharmacokinetics* column: O-onset; P-peak; D-duration; ½L-half-life; PB-protein bound; B-biotransformation; E-elimination.

*Within the column of adverse effects, underlines indicate the most common effects; CAPITALS indicate life-threatening effects.

Contraindications/ Precautions	Adverse Effects*	Interactions	Nursing Implications
			ney. Activity of the affected joint is limited during the acute attack. May begin exercise, warmth, and physical therapy when pain and swelling subside, generally about 24–72 hours from the onset of therapy. Understand and follow diet limitations. Patients may be encouraged to test their urinary pH with nitrazine paper. A highly acidic urine tends to occur during a gout attack. If urinary pH is decreasing, patients should notify the physician and begin their medication immediately. Lifelong therapy may be required to control symptoms. The patient should not take aspirin or aspirin-containing medications without consulting physician. If an analgesic is required, acetaminophen is recommended. Patient should not experiment with drug dosage but should take the prescribed dose. *EVALUATION:* Notify physician if rash, sore throat, fever, or unusual bleeding, bruising, or weakness occur, Discontinue as soon as gout pain is relieved.
CONTRAINDICATIONS: Contraindicated in hypersensitivity, blood dyscrasias, uric acid kidney stones, and children under age 2 years. *PRECAUTIONS:* Use cautiously in history of peptic ulcer, renal disease. Use in pregnancy not established.	*Neuro:* headache, dizziness *GI:* anorexia, nausea, vomiting, sore gums *Hemo:* HEMOLYTIC ANEMIA, APLASTIC ANEMIA *Renal:* urinary frequency, uric acid stones	Salicylates inhibit uricosuric effects. Increases plasma levels of sulfonamides, sulfonylureas, indomethacin, rifampin, methotrexate, clofibrate, and aminosalicylic acid. *Lab:* Interferes with laboratory tests for urinary 17-ketosteroids. Interferes with BSP urinary secretion test.	*Same as Above Plus:* *INTERVENTION:* Take with food or antacid.
CONTRAINDICATIONS: Contraindicated in hypersensitivity, active peptic ulcer, concurrent use of aspirin, and blood dyscrasias. *PRECAUTIONS:* Use in pregnancy not established.	*GI:* GI disturbances *Hemo:* BLOOD DYSCRASIAS *Renal:* renal failure *Integ:* rash	Potentiates hypoglycemic effects of tolbutamide. Increases hypoprothrombinemic effect of warfarin. Potentiates sulfonamides. Salicylates inhibit uricosuric effects.	*Same as Above Plus:* *INTERVENTION:* Give with meals. Drink at least 10–12 glasses of fluid per day.

CONTINUED ON THE FOLLOWING PAGE

Table 47–3. ANTI-INFLAMMATORY MEDICATIONS–*CONTINUED*

Name	Dosage	Mode of Administration	Pharmacokinetics
Allopurinol (Zyloprim)			
Action: Inhibits conversion of xanthine to uric acid.			
	200–800 mg 1–2 times daily; maximum dose 800 mg/day	PO	O: 30–60 min P: 1.5–4.5 hr D: 18–30 hr ½L: 1–2 hr (metabolite, 15 hr) PB: UA B: liver E: urine

Key to abbreviations in *Pharmacokinetics* column: O-onset; P-peak; D-duration; ½L-half-life; PB-protein bound; B-biotransformation; E-elimination.
*Within the column of adverse effects, <u>underlines</u> indicate the most common effects; CAPITALS indicate life-threatening effects.

2. Indole analogs such as indomethacin (Indocin), sulindac (Clinoril), and tolmetin (Tolectin);
3. Oxicam drugs such as piroxicam (Feldene);
4. Pyrazolone derivatives such as phenylbutazone (Butozolidin);
5. Fenamates such as meclofenamate (Meclomen) and mefenamic acid (Ponstel); and
6. Phenylacetic acid drugs—diclofenac sodium (Voltaren).

ACTION. Most of the NSAIDs presumably act by inhibiting the enzyme cyclo-oxygenase, thus blocking the synthesis of prostaglandins E_2 which, due to their potent vasodilator effect, increase vascular permeability and increase the inflammatory process. In addition, NSAIDs may also affect T-cell function, stabilize lysosomal membranes, inhibit chemotaxis of inflamed cells, and decrease release of superoxide radicals (which also contribute to inflammation). These agents differ from narcotic analgesics in that they have a *ceiling effect*. In addition, they do not produce tolerance, or physical or psychological dependence.

USES. All of the nonsteroidal anti-inflammatory drugs are effective in alleviating symptoms of rheumatoid arthritis and osteoarthritis, such as swelling, pain,

Table 47–4. THERAPEUTIC APPLICATIONS OF THE PROSTAGLANDINS

Prostaglandins	PG Synthesis Inhibition
Current Applications	
Midtrimester abortion	Rheumatoid arthritis
Peripheral vascular disease	Fever and headache
	Bartter's syndrome
Hemodialysis	Patent ductus arteriosus
Induction of labor	
Potential Applications	
Hypertension	Hypercalcemia of malignant disease
Congestive heart failure	Periodontal inflammation
Infertility	Cholera and certain diarrheal states
Coronary and deep thrombosis	Burns
Peptic ulceration	Lupus erythematosus
Gastric hyperacidity	Glaucoma
Bronchial asthma (PGE)	Migraine headache
Nasal congestion	Bronchial asthma (leukotriene)

From Wilson, J and Foster, D: Textbook of Endocrinology. WB Saunders, Philadelphia, 1985, with permission.

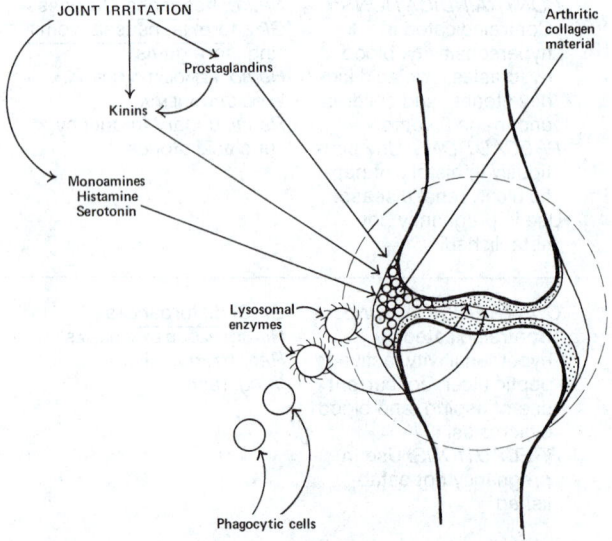

Figure 47–2. As a result of joint injury, prostaglandins, kinins, and monoamines are released, along with lysosomal enzymes released by the damaged phagocytic cell, and more inflammation and pain occur.

Contraindications/ Precautions	Adverse Effects*	Interactions	Nursing Implications
CONTRAINDICATIONS: Contraindicated in hypersensitivity, in pregnancy, and in children. *PRECAUTIONS:* Use cautiously in patients with hepatic or renal disease.	*Neuro:* headache, peripheral neuropathy, paresthesias, cataracts *GI:* nausea, vomiting, diarrhea, abdominal pain *Biliary:* hepatitis *Hemo:* BLOOD DYSCRASIAS *Integ:* rash, exfoliative urticaria, or purpuric lesions *Other:* acute attack of gout	Thiazides enhance allopurinol toxicity. Reduce allopurinol dose when concurrently administering 6-MP or azathioprine. Allopurinol prolongs the half-life of oral anticoagulants and chlorpropamide. Increases tendency for skin rash with ampicillin and amoxicillin.	*Same as Above Plus:* *INTERVENTION:* Take with meals. Do not take excessive vitamin C as there is increased risk of kidney stone formation. *EVALUATION:* Observe caution when performing tasks requiring alertness. Notify physician of skin rash.

stiffness, and tenderness. They are also effective in relieving mild to moderate pain of dental extractions, postsurgical episiotomy pain, and soft tissue athletic injuries. Primary dysmenorrhea is also relieved with these drugs. NSAIDs are especially effective for bone pain due to tumor metastasis. However, caution is used when administering NSAIDs to oncology patients because the antipyretic effect that these drugs have may mask infection. In addition, because of their effect on platelet function, these drugs may promote hemorrhage.

PHARMACOKINETICS. *Absorption and Distribution.* All of these medications are rapidly absorbed from the gastrointestinal tract, so the effects are quickly enjoyed by the patient. Food can delay absorption, but it does not significantly affect the total amount of drug absorbed. Approximately 90%–99% of the medications are tightly bound to specific plasma proteins. This binding ability is often responsible for the displacement of other highly protein-bound medications when they are given in combination.

The nonsteroidal and anti-inflammatory drugs cross the placental barrier and are found in breast milk. They should not be given to either pregnant or lactating women, because their effects on the fetus are unknown.

Biotransformation and Excretion. NSAIDs have varying half-lives ranging from one to two hours for ibuprofen to 35+ hours for piroxicam. Table 47–3 lists the half-life of the NSAIDs. Generally, the longer the elimination half-life, the more toxic the drug. Toxicity is not determined solely by slow elimination. However, sustained high concentration of the drug in the tissues probably tends to maximize any toxic effects that occur. The varying half-lives also account for the differences of

duration of analgesic effect that these drugs have. Anti-inflammatory drugs are almost completely metabolized in the liver and excreted in the urine. Table 47–3 lists the percentage of drug excreted changed and unchanged in the urine and feces.

Unlike the other medications in this group, ibuprofen (Motrin) is also partially excreted by the biliary system. This preparation can be administered, with care, to individuals with renal disease. All other medications should be given very cautiously to individuals with renal disease or used at reduced dosage with careful monitoring.

CONTRAINDICATIONS AND PRECAUTIONS. The nonsteroidal anti-inflammatory drugs are contraindicated in: patients with gastrointestinal lesions; patients sensitive to these or similar drugs; patients who are allergic to aspirin or iodides; and patients in whom these drugs have induced symptoms of asthma, rhinitis, urticaria, angioedema, or bronchospasm. These conditions may be exacerbated by NSAIDs. They are given cautiously to: persons with a previous history of gastrointestinal ulceration, as bleeding may occur; patients with renal or hepatic disease, as serum levels may be elevated, increasing the possibility of toxicity; and individuals with cardiac disease, as fluid retention may occur, compromising cardiac function. Because the NSAIDs impair platelet aggregation and prolong bleeding time, they are given cautiously to persons with bleeding disorders. These medications are generally stopped 24–48 hours before surgery. Specific contraindications and precautions can be found in Table 47–3.

ADVERSE EFFECTS. Many adverse effects may result from these drugs including gastrointestinal irritation leading to nausea, vomiting, heartburn, gastrointestinal bleeding, and ulceration. Gastrointestinal bleeding is a significant problem in the elderly. The gastric ulcer may be a silent condition, detectable only by gastrostomy. The relative gastrointestinal toxicity of the following NSAIDs is shown in descending order: phenylbutazone, indomethacin, mefenamic acid, sulindac, tolmetin sodium, naproxen, fenoprofen, and ibuprofen. Many medications are best administered with food or milk to avoid gastrointestinal irritation. Antacids and food do not interfere with the extent of absorption, but do decrease the rate of absorption. Other adverse effects include: bone marrow depression effects, such as anemia and decreased WBC; renal effects such as decreased glomerular filtration rate, and decreased renal blood flow mediated by inhibition of prostaglandin synthesis; hepatitis-like syndrome (rare), which is reversible and often accompanied by abnormal liver function tests; skin eruptions; CNS symptoms such as tinnitus, headache, dizziness, and blurred vision; and allergic reactions manifested as hives, anaphylaxis, and asthmatic bronchospasm. There is often a cross-sensitivity to other NSAIDs and yellow food dye. Specific adverse effects are listed in Table 47–3.

Frequent blood counts are performed in patients taking drugs such as phenylbutazone and indomethocin. If changes occur, the medication is discontinued and other therapies are instituted. These agents inhibit platelet aggregation and, therefore, bleeding may occur.

INTERACTIONS. Interactions include an increase in ulcerogenic effects when nonsteroidal anti-inflammatory drugs are given concurrently with corticosteroids or salicylates. NSAIDs are given cautiously with anticoagulants, as they increase the incidence of bleeding. Also, concurrent aspirin administration may decrease anti-inflammatory effects. The antihypertensive effects of beta-adrenergic blockers and captopril may be decreased if NSAIDs are taken concurrently. Probenecid may increase the plasma level and the half-life of most of these agents.

PROPIONIC ACID DERIVATIVES. These drugs include ibuprofen, naproxen, fenoprofen, ketoprofen, and carprofen.

Ibuprofen. Ibuprofen (Motrin) is administered in doses of 300–800 mg, three to four times daily. Dosage should not exceed 3.2 g/day. Therapeutic effect usually takes two weeks to occur, so the patient needs to be encouraged to keep taking the medication. Ibuprofen is also available over the counter in doses of 200 mg and is safe for long-term therapy.

Ibuprofen is also used in the treatment of dysmenorrhea that is believed to be caused by prostaglandin production, and to reduce fever.

Naproxen. Naproxen (Naprosyn) is a nonsteroidal anti-inflammatory agent of the propionic acid class that is used for various types of arthritis, tendonitis, bursitis, acute gout, and primary dysmenorrhea. Naproxen is administered in doses of 250–750 mg twice daily with a maximum dose of 1.5 g/day. Naproxen is safe for acute and long-term therapy.

Fenoprofen. Fenoprofen (Nalfon) is administered in doses of 300–600 mg, three to four times daily, with a

maximum dose of 3200 mg/day. Fenoprofen is safe for acute and long-term therapy.

Ketoprofen. Ketoprofen (Orudis) is administered as a dosage of 150–300 mg in single or three to four divided doses. Dosages should be reduced in the elderly or individuals with renal dysfunction. The maximum daily dose is 300 mg. It is safe for both acute and long-term therapy.

Flurbiprofen. Flurbiprofen (Ansaid) is used for both acute and long-term treatment of the signs and symptoms of rheumatoid arthritis and osteoarthritis. The usual oral dose is 200 to 300 mg administered two to four times daily.

INDOLE ANALOGS. These agents include indomethacin, sulindac, and tolmetin.

Indomethacin. Indomethacin (Indocin) is a potent anti-inflammatory analgesic with antipyretic properties belonging to the indole analog group. It is a potent prostaglandin inhibitor. Indomethacin is considered for use only in acute active disease processes because of its potential for adverse effects.

Indomethacin is administered in doses of 25–50 mg, two to three times daily, up to a maximum dose of 200 mg/day. Also available are 75-mg sustained-release capsules given once a day, or twice daily if needed.

Indomethacin shares the same adverse effects as the other nonsteroidal anti-inflammatory drugs but with increased frequency and severity. Also, because of these adverse effects, it is given cautiously to patients with impaired renal or hepatic function, individuals with psychiatric illness, and the elderly. Laboratory studies are done routinely when patients are on indomethacin to check for abnormalities. It is titrated to the lowest possible effective dosage to prevent these major complications.

Sulindac. Sulindac (Clinoril) is an anti-inflammatory agent of the indole analog group. It is effective in the treatment of ankylosing spondylitis, acute painful shoulder (tendonitis/bursitis), and acute gouty arthritis. The usual dosage of sulindac is 150–200 mg twice daily, with a maximum dose of 400 mg/day. Sulindac is safe for both acute and long-term therapy.

Tolmetin. Tolmetin (Tolectin) is an indole analog anti-inflammatory agent similar to the others in its action; however, it differs chemically. It shares the same uses as the other anti-inflammatory agents, and is used in both short- and long-term management of juvenile rheumatoid arthritis. Tolmetin is administered in doses of 200–400 mg, three to four times daily, with a 2 g maximum daily dose.

OXICAM PRODUCTS. *Piroxicam.* Piroxicam (Feldene) is a nonsteroidal anti-inflammatory agent used for acute or long-term treatment of osteoarthritis and rheumatoid arthritis. It has a half-life of 30–86 hours, which allows once-daily administration. The usual dose is 10–20 mg/day. The therapeutic effects are evident early in the treatment of both diseases and progress over 8–12 weeks. It may be administered concurrently with fixed doses of gold salts and corticosteroids.

Pyrazolone Derivatives. *Phenylbutazone.* The pyrazolone derivative, phenylbutazone (Butazolidin), is one of the oldest anti-inflammatory medications. Phenylbutazone exhibits antipyretic, analgesic, anti-inflammatory, and mild uricosuric activity, which provides symptomatic relief but leaves the disease process unchanged. But, because of its many and severe adverse effects, phenylbutazone is used only for short-term therapy. The exact mechanism of its effect is unknown, but it is thought that it inhibits prostaglandin synthesis, leukocyte migration, and lysosomal enzymes.

Uses. Phenylbutazone is used most effectively for the treatment of bursitis, traumatic tenosynovitis, ankylosing spondylitis, acute gout, and acute rheumatoid arthritis.

Pharmacokinetics. Phenylbutazone is rapidly absorbed after oral administration and reaches a peak plasma concentration in 2.5 hours (± 1.4 hours). It is 98% bound to plasma proteins. Phenylbutazone is biotransformed in the liver and excreted in the urine. The half-life is 77 hours.

Contraindications and Precautions. Phenylbutazone is contraindicated in persons with hypersensitivity, senile patients, and in children under the age of 14 years. It is given cautiously to patients with gastrointestinal disease, as ulceration and bleeding may occur, and patients with hepatic disease, as liver abnormalities may progress. Safety for its use in pregnant and lactating women has not been established.

Adverse Effects. The most serious adverse effects of phenylbutazone are aplastic anemia and agranulocytosis, while the most common adverse effects are abdominal discomfort and edema (3%–9%), nausea, dyspepsia, and rash. Numerous other adverse effects occur and are listed in Table 47–3. Because of these possible side effects, patients are assessed frequently during therapy.

Interactions. Phenylbutazone has many interactions with other drugs. It can enhance oral anticoagulants. Concurrent use with anticoagulants may increase the incidence of bleeding. Additional interactions are featured in Table 47–3.

Dosage. Phenylbutazone is administered in doses of 100 mg, three to four times daily. The maximum dosage is 400 mg/day. This drug is recommended to be first given for a seven-day trial period. It can be used for more than seven days if it is effective, but a less toxic drug is preferred. As improvement occurs, the dosage is decreased. It is best given with meals, milk, or antacids to prevent gastrointestinal upset. Phenylbutazone may also be used for short-term therapy of degenerative disease of hip and knee joints that is unresponsive to other therapy.

FENAMATE DRUGS. The fenamate drugs or the salicylate-like medications include mefenamic acid (Ponstel) and meclofenamate sodium (Meclomen). Both have antipyretic, analgesic, and anti-inflammatory effects. These drugs are indicated for mild to moderate pain relief for short-term use. They are both prostaglandin inhibitors.

Contraindications and Precautions. These salicylate-like medications are contraindicated in patients sensitive to aspirin, in patients with active peptic ulcer disease, during pregnancy, and in children under the age of 14 years (because a significant amount of research has not been done in this population). They are given cautiously to persons with a previous history of gastrointestinal ulceration, and individuals with renal, hepatic, or cardiac disease, as all these conditions may be worsened.

Interactions. Several drug interactions can occur with these products. They are by themselves ulcerogenic, but the ulcerogenic effects are potentiated when they are given concurrently with corticosteroids, phenylbutazone, or salicylates. Aspirin may decrease the plasma level of these drugs. When anticoagulants are given concurrently, the dose of warfarin may need to be reduced to prevent bleeding.

Mefenamic Acid. Mefenamic acid (Ponstel) is indicated for short-term pain relief, for which it generally should be used for no longer than one week. It is administered in doses of 250 mg, three-to-four times daily, with a maximum dose of 1000 mg/day. It is best administered with food or milk to prevent gastrointestinal upset.

Meclofenamate Sodium. Meclofenamate sodium (Meclomen) is used in the management of acute and chronic rheumatoid arthritis and osteoarthritis. It appears to be as effective as aspirin in relieving the symptoms of arthritis. Although it is less likely than aspirin to cause tinnitus, it causes more gastrointestinal side effects, especially diarrhea. For some patients (4%), diarrhea is so severe that the drug must be discontinued. Some patients have developed peptic ulcer while taking meclofenamate sodium, especially those with a history of ulcer disease, or those taking other anti-inflammatory drugs concurrently.

The usual dosage is 200–400 mg/day, administered in three or four equal doses. It may be administered with food, milk, or antacids to minimize gastrointestinal side effects. Patients should not exceed the prescribed dosage, even if full therapeutic benefit is not achieved for several weeks.

PHENYLACETIC ACID DRUGS. *Diclofenac Sodium.* Diclofenac sodium (Voltaren) is indicated for the management of both acute and chronic rheumatoid and osteoarthritis, and ankylosing spondylitis. Diclofenac is a phenylacetic acid derivative with both analgesic and antipyretic activity. Its exact mechanism of action is unknown; however, it is thought to decrease synthesis of prostaglandins, prostacyclin, and thromboxane.

Diclofenac sodium is rapidly absorbed after oral use. Peak plasma levels are reached in 2.5–12.0 hours after oral dosing. Diclofenac sodium undergoes a high first-pass effect in the liver. The half-life range is 1.2–1.8 hours. Approximately 40%–60% of diclofenac sodium is excreted in the urine. Neither renal nor hepatic impairment appears to affect the pharmacokinetics of diclofenac sodium.

Adverse effects are similar to the other NSAIDs, with the most frequent side effect being gastrointestinal complaints. The dosage range is 100–200 mg/day in divided doses.

REMISSION-INDUCING DRUGS

The remission-inducing drugs—gold products, antimalarials, penicillamine, and cytotoxic drugs—may produce partial or complete remission. These drugs are all slow-acting and require six weeks to six months of treatment before benefits can be recognized.

Gold Preparations

Rheumatoid arthritis has been treated with parenteral gold salts for more than 50 years. (An oral preparation is now also available.) Studies suggest that about 50% of patients will have a positive clinical response to gold therapy.

The exact mechanism of action of gold preparations has not yet been determined. It is thought that they may inhibit the formation of abnormal proteins (such as bradykinin) by retarding the formation of disulfide bonds, or they may stabilize the collagen fibers, making them less susceptible to inflammation. Gold preparations may also act through a combination effect.

Gold seems to alter the progression of the disease by suppressing synovial inflammation and inhibiting the activity of lysosomal enzymes, reducing lymphocyte proliferation, and lessening phagocytic activity within the joint. However, therapy is often necessary for three to four months before any response can be noted.

Gold products have beneficial effects in approximately 80%–90% of patients when a cumulative dosage of 200–400 mg has been reached. Parenteral gold—gold sodium thiomalate—is 50% gold, while oral gold—auranofin—is 29% gold.

PHARMACOKINETICS. *Absorption and Distribution.* Both oral and parenteral gold are similar in their pharmacokinetic behavior. Gold preparations are readily absorbed following intramuscular injections and become highly concentrated in the kidneys, liver, spleen, and synovial fluid. The highest concentration of parenteral gold is found in the reticuloendothelial system. The highest concentration of oral gold is found in the red blood cells.

Biotransformation and Excretion. Gold compounds are primarily excreted in the urine (60%–70%), with a small amount excreted in the feces (30%, parenteral form; 85%, oral form). As the period of treatment lengthens, so does the excretion time. After a course of treatment has been terminated, traces of gold are found in the tissues for as long as 6 months.

GOLD SODIUM THIOMALATE. *Contraindications and Precautions.* Contraindications for the use of gold sodium thiomalate include toxicity to heavy metals, renal or hepatic disease, congestive heart failure, hypertension, uncontrolled diabetes, and acute hepatitis; all of these conditions may be worsened from gold deposits in tissues. Oral gold is also contraindicated in persons with bone marrow aplasia, pulmonary fibrosis, or exfoliative dermatitis. Safety in pregnant or lactating women, and children has not been established.

Adverse Effects. The most common adverse effects occur secondary to the deposits of gold in the tissues and include pruritus, dermatitis, alopecia, skin pigment changes (gray to blue coloration), metallic taste, stoma-

titis, nephrotic syndrome and proteinuria, allergic reactions, and thrombocytopenia. Adverse effects most generally appear when the cumulative dose is 400–800 mg of parenteral gold. These adverse effects are experienced by about 40% of the population receiving gold compounds. Less commonly, anemias, hepatitis, and gold deposits in the eyes are experienced.

Dosage. The dose of gold sodium thiomalate (Myochrysine) is highly individualized, usually starting with 10 mg and increasing weekly up to 25 mg in the second week; 25–50 mg in the third week; and, in subsequent weeks, up to 1 gm, or until clinical improvement. The maintenance dose is: 50 mg twice a week for four weeks; followed by 50 mg every three weeks for four weeks; then 50 mg monthly, to a total of 1000 mg. If a remission has occurred, the dosage is reduced to 50 mg every other week for four doses, then every three weeks for four doses, and then every four weeks for a year. Therapy can then be discontinued or maintenance therapy begun (four weeks without therapy, then four weeks of therapy). The gold preparations are very thick. To aid administration, the medication is brought to body temperature and shaken vigorously. A 21-gauge 1.5-inch needle is used to draw up and administer the preparation. It is administered deeply into the ventral gluteal region. Until the gold therapy becomes effective, penicillamine, chloroquine, or hydroxychloroquine should also be given.

AUROTHIOGLUCOSE. Aurothioglucose (Solganal), like gold sodium thiomalate, contains approximately 50% gold. It is administered only intramuscularly in the gluteal muscle. It is administered weekly: the first dose is 10 mg; second and third doses, 25 mg; fourth and subsequent doses, 50 mg. Continue this schedule until 0.8–1.0 g has been administered. If improvement occurs, continue the 50 mg dose every three to four weeks. If there is no improvement when large doses have been administered, aurothioglucose is discontinued.

AURANOFIN. Auranofin (Ridaura) is an oral gold product for adult rheumatoid arthritis. This drug is indicated for patients who have not responded to or cannot tolerate the NSAIDs.

Therapeutic response to auranofin takes at least three to four months. The usual dose is 6 mg daily. In controlled studies, fewer patients dropped out of therapy because of side effects due to auranofin than because of those due to injectable gold. Therapeutic effects may start in three to four months but may not be seen for six months. If response is inadequate after six months, dosage can be increased to 9 mg/day in three divided doses. If there is inadequate response in three months, auranofin should be discontinued.

D-Penicillamine

D-Penicillamine (Cuprimine) is a chelating agent recommended for the removal of excess copper in patients with Wilson's disease. In numerous studies in England, it has been shown to be effective in suppressing disease activity in rheumatoid arthritis. Its direct action in rheumatoid arthritis is still under investigation; but it does reduce serum immunoglobulins (IgM and IgG) and, with prolonged use, it also reduces titers of the rheumatoid factor (RF) and decreases erythrocyte sedimentation rate (ESR). D-Penicillamine helps to control the symptoms of rheumatoid arthritis, but complete remissions are rare.

CONTRAINDICATIONS AND PRECAUTIONS. D-Penicillamine is contraindicated in pregnancy, blood dyscrasias, and renal insufficiency. If fever develops, the drug is discontinued.

It should be given cautiously to individuals who are allergic to penicillin because of the possibility of hypersensitivity, and in patients who are currently using or have taken gold salts within the past four months.

ADVERSE EFFECTS. D-Penicillamine has many dangerous adverse effects, so the patient must remain under medical supervision during therapy. The adverse effects include gastrointestinal complaints, allergic reactions, bone marrow depression, alopecia, and increased skin friability. This drug should not be given concurrently with salicylates, nonsteroidal anti-inflammatory drugs, or corticosteroids because of the increased incidence of serious gastrointestinal side effects.

DOSAGE. The dose is started low at 125–250 mg/day, and increased every several months up to 750 mg/day, until the effects are noted. The minimal effective dose appears to be 500–750 mg/day. Like gold, it may take two to three months before any effects, such as reduction in pain, swelling, and tenderness, are recognized. The duration of action may be months or years after the medication is discontinued.

CYTOTOXIC MEDICATIONS USED AS ANTI-INFLAMMATORY DRUGS

Three very potent cytotoxic medications that are most commonly used to treat cancer, cyclophosphamide (Cytoxan), azathioprine (Imuran), and methotrexate, can also be used as anti-inflammatory agents. These medications depress lymphocyte activity. The lymphocytes are primarily responsible for the damage to the connective tissue.

Gastrointestinal complaints and hair loss are common with cyclophosphamide, whereas hematologic complications are more common with azathioprine. See Chapter 49 for more information on these drugs.

ANTIMALARIAL MEDICATIONS USED AS ANTI-INFLAMMATORY AGENTS

The antimalarials, chloroquine (Aralen), quinacrine (Atabrine), and hydroxychloroquine (Plaquenil), can be used as anti-inflammatory agents in both rheumatoid arthritis and lupus erythematosus (for more information on these drugs see Chapter 47). These preparations are rapidly absorbed from the gastrointestinal tract. A patient receiving these preparations for long-term therapy should have his or her eyes evaluated frequently for macular degeneration, a common complication.

OTHER INVESTIGATIONAL DRUGS

Sulfasalazine is currently under investigation for treatment of rheumatoid arthritis. It appears to have efficacy

similar to that of both gold and D-penicillamine. Captopril (Capoten), an antihypertensive drug, is also currently being investigated as a treatment for rheumatoid arthritis.

ANTIGOUT AGENTS

Gout is a metabolic disorder of purine metabolism. Gout, resulting in hyperuricemia, is classified as primary or secondary. Primary hyperuricemia results from either overproduction of uric acid or decreased renal excretion of uric acid. Secondary hyperuricemia develops during the course of another disease or secondary to chemotherapy.

The symptoms of gout appear when the serum uric acid level is above 6 mg/dL. Urate crystals are deposited in synovial fluid, which eventually precipitates an acute attack. Before therapy is started, it is important to definitively diagnose acute gout, as the symptoms may resemble several other types of arthritis.

There are three primary agents used in the treatment of gout. The first and primary treatment for gout is the administration of colchicine which, if started immediately after the attack begins, is effective in about 90% of all cases. If started later, it is less effective. The mechanism of action of colchicine is not known, but it may involve an action on leukocytes or synovial cells in the area of inflammation.

The second group of antigout agents is the uricosurics, which inhibit the tubular reabsorption of uric acid in the kidney. Consequently, uric acid is excreted and serum levels are decreased. This group includes both probenecid (Benemid) and sulfinpyrazone (Anturane).

The third type of drug used in the treatment of gout is allopurinol (Lopurin, Zyloprim), which inhibits the conversion of xanthine to uric acid by inhibition of the enzyme xanthine oxidase. Ultimately, there is a reduced serum uric acid level, which begins in about 24–48 hours. See Figure 47–3 for the site of action of each of these agents.

Colchicine

As previously mentioned, the exact mechanism of action of colchicine is unknown, although it may inhibit leukocyte activity in the joint. Colchicine can relieve pain, but it is not an analgesic.

PHARMACOKINETICS. Colchicine is rapidly absorbed after oral administration. Colchicine is only partially metabolized by the liver and then secreted back into the gastrointestinal tract via the bile. Thus, the metabolic unchanged drug can then go through the cycle again, essentially acting as new drug. This often results in adverse effects for the patient after several doses have been administered. Colchicine is concentrated in the white blood cells.

CONTRAINDICATIONS AND PRECAUTIONS. Colchicine is contraindicated in persons hypersensitive to it, and in those with gastrointestinal and hepatic disease and blood dyscrasias, as these conditions may be aggravated or worsened. It is given cautiously to the elderly or to debilitated patients. Use in pregnant women, lactating women, and children has not been established.

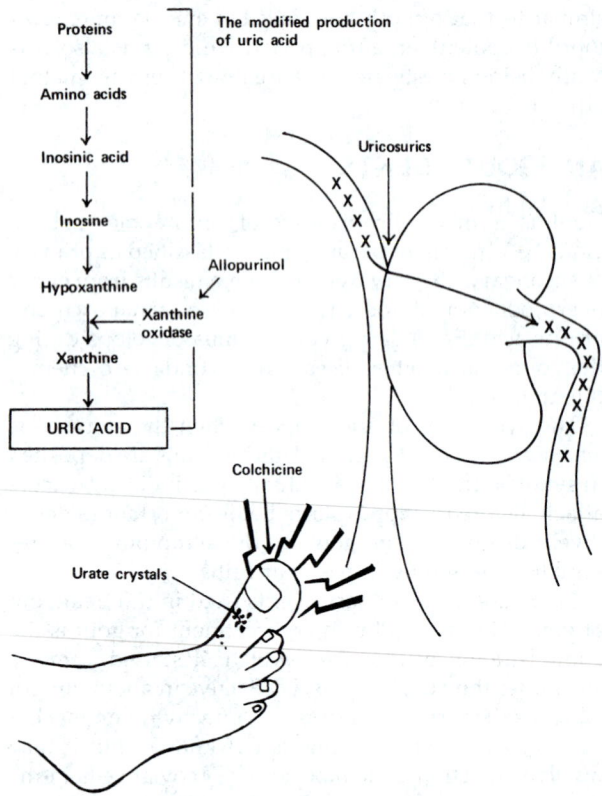

Figure 47–3. Three different mechanisms of action of antigout medications. Colchicine opposes leukocyte phagocytosis, which inhibits further deposits: uricosurics interfere with tubular reabsorption of uric acid; and allopurinol interferes with xanthine oxidase, an enzyme necessary for uric acid production.

ADVERSE EFFECTS. The most common adverse effects include bone marrow depression and peripheral neuritis. Gastrointestinal symptoms, especially diarrhea, are also common, particularly with maximal doses.

INTERACTIONS. Colchicine is inhibited by urinary acidifying agents and potentiated by urinary alkalinizing agents. Colchicine may increase sensitivity to CNS depressants. Vitamin B_{12} absorption may be affected by colchicine as it may alter the intestinal mucosa. Colchicine can increase alkaline phosphate and SGOT levels and may give false positives in tests of urine for RBCs and hemoglobin.

DOSAGE. Colchicine is administered in an initial oral dose of 0.5–1.2 mg; then, 0.5–1.2 mg is given hourly during the acute stage until, the pain is relieved, the patient experiences diarrhea, or the total of 4 mg in 24 hours has been reached. Colchicine can also be used prophylactically to reduce the frequency and severity of gouty attacks. The usual dose ranges from 0.5 to 1.2 mg daily.

Colchicine may also be given intravenously in 1- to 3-mg doses to start, and then 0.5 mg every six hours. Maximal dose is 4 mg in one course of therapy.

Probenecid

Probenecid (Benemid) is started only after the initial attack has subsided, since its administration may make the acute symptoms worse. Probenecid is not an anti-inflammatory drug; it is classed as a uricosuric agent. It increases renal excretion of uric acid by blocking tubular reabsorption.

PHARMACOKINETICS. Probenecid is well absorbed after oral administration and reaches peak plasma levels in 2–4 hours. It is highly bound to plasma proteins with a serum half-life of 4–9 hours. Probenecid is biotransformed in the liver and excreted as metabolites in the urine.

CONTRAINDICATIONS AND PRECAUTIONS. Probenecid is contraindicated in children under two years of age and in patients with hypersensitivity, blood dyscrasias, or kidney stones. It is given cautiously to persons with a history of peptic ulcer, as ulcers may be activated; and in persons with renal disease, as renal failure may be worsened. Use during pregnancy has not been thoroughly studied.

ADVERSE EFFECTS. The most common adverse effects of probenecid include diarrhea, headache, anorexia, sore gums, anemia, dermatitis, and uric acid kidney stones. Exacerbations of gout and uric acid stones can also occur.

INTERACTIONS. Probenecid inhibits the renal excretion and, therefore, may increase the plasma levels of sulfonamides, sulfonylureas, indomethacin, rifampin, methotrexate, clofibrate, and aminosalicylic acid. Concurrent therapy with salicylates inhibits its uricosuric effects. Probenecid interferes with laboratory test results such as urinary 17-ketosteroids and BSP, by inhibiting excretion of the steroid compounds and the dye BSP.

DOSAGE. The dosage begins at 250 mg twice daily, and may be increased to 1 g/day over many weeks to control symptoms.

OTHER USES OF PROBENECID. As well as being used as an antigout medication, probenecid is also used as an adjunct to therapy with penicillin or other short-acting penicillin preparations. It inhibits the tubular secretion of penicillin and increases the penicillin plasma levels two to four times. It is frequently given to prolong the effectiveness of penicillin when treating gonorrhea or gonococcal infections in both men and women.

Sulfinpyrazone

ACTION. Sulfinpyrazone (Anturane) has little anti-inflammatory effect; thus, it is not recommended for acute gout attacks, but only for chronic prophylaxis or for intermittent gout attacks. It also inhibits platelet aggregation and is currently used investigationally for the prophylactic treatment of recurrent myocardial infarction.

PHARMACOKINETICS. Sulfinpyrazone is well absorbed and is 98%–99% protein bound. Serum half-life is about two to three hours. It is readily metabolized by the liver and excreted 50% unchanged in the urine.

CONTRAINDICATIONS AND PRECAUTIONS. Contraindications include hypersensitivity, active peptic ulcer, concurrent salicylate therapy, and blood dyscrasias. Sulfinpyrazone is given cautiously to persons with renal dysfunction, individuals with a history of ulcer disease, and pregnant women.

ADVERSE EFFECTS. The most common adverse effects include gastrointestinal disturbances, blood dyscrasias, and skin rash.

DOSAGE. Sulfinpyrazone is administered in doses of 100–200 mg, up to 200–400 mg twice daily. Daily maintenance dosage ranges from 200 to 800 mg. Since sulfinpyrazone aids in the excretion of uric acid, adequate fluid intake (8–10 glasses of fluid per day) is necessary to prevent renal calculi.

Allopurinol

Allopurinol (Zyloprim) inhibits xanthine oxidase, thus reducing the production of uric acid. It is the preferred drug in the treatment of tophaceous gout. It is also used in patients who are receiving cytotoxic agents that break cellular nucleic acid, leading to acute uric acid nephropathy. If allopurinol is given during acute attacks, colchicine or another NSAID is also given to treat the attack.

PHARMACOKINETICS. Allopurinol is rapidly absorbed and distributed in all extracellular fluid. Peak plasma levels are achieved in 1.5–4.5 hours. Half-life is one to two hours and half-life of a pharmacologically active metabolite (oxypurinol) is 15 hours. The majority of the drug is rapidly oxidized to oxypurinol, which inhibits xanthine oxidase. It is then slowly excreted in the urine.

CONTRAINDICATIONS AND PRECAUTIONS. Allopurinol is contraindicated in patients who are hypersensitive to its ingredients. In pregnant women and children, its safety has not been established. It is given cautiously to persons with hepatic and renal disease, as it is biotransformed in the liver and excreted by the kidney.

ADVERSE EFFECTS. The most common adverse effects include rash, dermatitis, gastrointestinal complaints, diarrhea, drowsiness, and, less commonly, hepatotoxicity and peripheral neuritis.

DOSAGE. Allopurinol is given in doses of 200–800 mg, once or twice daily. The maximal dose is 800 mg/day. Because of its long duration of action, it is normally given only once daily. To lessen the possibility of urate stone formation, at least 8–10 glasses of fluid should be consumed daily while taking the drug.

USING THE NURSING PROCESS

ASSESSMENT

Assessment of the patient requiring anti-inflammatory drugs for the control of inflammation always begins with a thorough nursing history to develop the data base. Additional information is found in Table 47–5.

All the information is used later when preparing the nursing care plan. The patient requiring anti-inflammatory drugs may be acutely ill in a hospital or relatively healthy, with the condition being treated on an outpatient basis. The course of most of these conditions is variable. A group of patients will have one acute attack and then completely remit; another group will have re-

peated remissions and exacerbations; and another group will have inexorable progression of the disease that is unresponsive to therapeutic modalities. It is important for the nurse to assess the activity level of the patient and to identify what assistance is needed with activities of daily living. Both the patient and family should understand that fatigue or malaise present with these diseases is not laziness, but a disease symptom that could disappear as therapy progresses. Assessment of ability to do household work, on-the-job and specific activities such as climbing stairs, and personal hygiene is made. It is often useful to ask the patient which specific activities are most impaired by the disease and to follow this as an indicator of improvement.

Dietary assessment is also important. Recent research indicates that there is a connection between nutrition and arthritis. Most of these research findings will need to be replicated in larger groups of patients. Currently, eliminating milk, cheese, and yogurt can reduce joint stiffness, pain, and swelling in certain patients. Cereal grains (wheat, oat, rye), shrimp, and sodium nitrate (food preservative) can trigger joint problems in some arthritics. Patients should eliminate one food at a time from their diets. If symptoms improve, the food should be eliminated permanently.

One food substance—eicosopentanoic acid—a fatty acid found in fish such as salmon, mackerel, tuna, rainbow trout, and sardines, may alleviate symptoms of arthritis.

Laboratory tests, such as CBC, sedimentation rate, uric acid levels, immunoglobulin or rheumatoid factor levels, and x-rays may also be performed to develop the baseline data as well as periodically to monitor treatment and assess for adverse effects of medication.

Psychological assessment is also important as the diagnosis of anti-inflammatory disease may cause great anxiety in both the patient and family. During the intervention phase, teaching emphasis is placed on the broad spectrum of disease manifestations and multiple options for therapy.

NURSING DIAGNOSES

As the initial assessment is completed, the nurse begins to develop the nursing diagnoses, which become the framework for the nursing intervention. Typical nursing diagnoses for a patient requiring anti-inflammatory medications are included in Table 47–5.

PLANNING AND INTERVENTION

From the nursing diagnoses, the goals of nursing intervention are developed. Typical goals of nursing intervention when caring for the patient requiring anti-inflammatory drugs are shown in Table 47–5; they include reducing pain and inflammation, maintaining joint mobility, and preventing deformity. Different drugs and dosages are tried to determine the optimum regimen. Aspirin is the preferred drug for the initial management of rheumatoid arthritis and osteoarthritis. Aspirin has both an analgesic effect, which benefits osteoarthritis patients, and an anti-inflammatory effect,

Table 47–5. NURSING PROCESS FOR PATIENTS RECEIVING PROSTAGLANDINS AND ANTI-INFLAMMATORIES

Assessment

Note past history/presence of inflammatory disease, e.g., rheumatoid arthritis, gout.
Assess level of activity and ability to maintain activities of daily living.
Determine nutritional status.
Review laboratory studies, e.g., CBC, sedimentation rate, uric acid, immunoglobulin or rheumatoid factor levels.
Assess psychologic state and determine how illness has affected life.

Nursing Diagnosis	Nursing Actions	Rationale	Desired Outcomes/ Evaluation Criteria
Pain related to distention of tissues by accumulation of fluid/inflammatory process.	Investigate complaints of pain, noting location, and intensity (scale of 1–10). Note precipitating factors and nonverbal pain cues.	Helpful in determining pain management needs and effectiveness of therapy.	Reports pain is relieved/ controlled. Appears relaxed, able to sleep/ rest and participate in activities appropriately. Incorporates relaxation skills and diversional activities into pain control program.
	Have patient assume position of comfort while in bed or sitting in chair.	In severe disease/acute exacerbation, total bed-rest may be necessary to limit pain/injury to joints.	
	Maintain neutral position of affected joints with pillows, sandbags, trochanter rolls, splints, braces.	Rests painful joints.	
	Encourage frequent changes of position. Assist as needed.	Prevents general fatigue and joint stiffness.	
	Encourage use of stress management techniques, e.g., progressive relaxation, Therapeutic Touch, biofeedback, visualization, guided imagery, self-hypnosis and controlled breathing.	Promotes relaxation, provides sense of control and may enhance coping abilities.	
	Administer medications as indicated, e.g., acetylsalicylates, nonsteroidal anti-inflammatory drugs, e.g., ibuprofen, naproxen, misoprostol.	ASA exerts an anti-inflammatory and mild analgesic effect decreasing stiffness and increasing mobility. Used when patient does not respond to aspirin or to enhance effects of aspirin. Given to decrease or prevent the incidence of gastric irritation and ulceration when NSAIDs are administered concurrently. (Contraindicated in pregnant women/nursing mothers).	
	Discuss taking drugs with food, milk, or antacids.	Minimizes gastric upset and irritation.	
Mobility, impaired physical related to skeletal deformity, pain/discomfort, intolerance to activity as evidenced by reluctance to attempt movement/inability to purposefully move, limited range of motion, decreased muscle strength.	Evaluate/continuously monitor degree of joint inflammation/pain.	Level of activity/exercise is dependent on progression/resolution of inflammatory process.	Maintains position of function and absence of contractures. Displays increased strength and function of affected and/ or compensatory body part. Demonstrates techniques/behaviors that enable resumption/ continuation of activities.
	Maintain bed/chair rest when indicated.	Systemic rest is mandatory during acute exacerbations and throughout the course of the disease.	

Table 47–5. NURSING PROCESS FOR PATIENTS RECEIVING PROSTAGLANDINS AND ANTI-INFLAMMATORIES–*CONTINUED*

Assessment

Note past history/presence of inflammatory disease, e.g., rheumatoid arthritis, gout.
Assess level of activity and ability to maintain activities of daily living.
Determine nutritional status.
Review laboratory studies, e.g., CBC, sedimentation rate, uric acid, immunoglobulin or rheumatoid factor levels.
Assess psychologic state and determine how illness has affected life.

Nursing Diagnosis	Nursing Actions	Rationale	Desired Outcomes/ Evaluation Criteria
	Assist with active/passive ROM as well as resistive exercises and isometrics when able.	Maintains/improves joint function, muscle strength and general stamina.	
	Demonstrate use of pillows, sandbags, trochanter rolls, splints and braces for positioning.	Promotes joint stability and maintains proper joint position and body alignment, minimizing contractures.	
	Provide safe environment, e.g., raised chairs/ toilet seat, use of handrails in tub/shower and toilet, proper use of mobility aids/wheelchair safety.	Avoids accidental injuries/ falls.	
	Consult with physical/ occupational therapists.	Helpful in formulating exercise/activity program based on individual needs and in identifying mobility devices/ adjuncts.	
	Administer medications as indicated, e.g., antirheumatic agents, e.g., gold, myochrysine or auranofin; or	Chrysotherapy (gold salts) may produce dramatic/sustained remission but may result in rebound inflammation if discontinued or if serious side effects occur, e.g., nitritoid crisis with dizziness, blurred vision, flushing, progressing to anaphylactic shock.	
	steroids.	May be necessary to suppress acute systemic inflammation.	
Body image disturbance/ Role performance related to disfigurement, changes in ability to perform usual tasks, increased energy expenditure, as evidenced by change in structure/ function of affected parts, negative self-talk, feelings of helplessness, hopelessness.	Encourage verbalization about concerns of disease process, future expectations.	Provides opportunity to identify fears/misconceptions and deal with directly.	Verbalizes increased confidence in ability to deal with illness, changes in lifestyle, and possible limitations. Makes realistic goals/plans for future.
	Discuss meaning of loss/ change to patient/SO. Ascertain how patient views self as a man/ woman in usual lifestyle functioning, including sexual aspects. Discuss patient's perception of how SO perceives limitations.	Identifying how illness affects perception of self and interactions with others will determine need for further intervention/counseling. Verbal/nonverbal cues from SO may have a major impact on how patient views self.	
	Acknowledge and accept feelings of grief, hostility, dependency.	Constant pain is wearing, and feelings of anger and hostility are common. Acceptance provides feedback that feelings are normal.	

CONTINUED ON THE FOLLOWING PAGE

Table 47–5. NURSING PROCESS FOR PATIENTS RECEIVING PROSTAGLANDINS AND ANTI-INFLAMMATORIES–*CONTINUED*

Nursing Diagnosis	Nursing Actions	Rationale	Desired Outcomes/ Evaluation Criteria
	Involve patient in planning care and scheduling activities.	Enhances feelings of competency/self-worth, encourages independence, and participation in therapy.	
Knowledge deficit related to lack of exposure/ recall, information misinterpretation as evidenced by questions, statement of concern, inaccurate follow-through of instruction/ development of preventable complications.	Review disease process, prognosis, and future expectations. Review drug purpose, dosage schedule, expected/adverse reactions. Discuss patient's role in management of disease process through diet, medication, and balanced program of exercise and rest. Stress importance of continued pharmacotherapeutic management.	Provide knowledge base on which patient can make informed choices. Promotes understanding of and enhances cooperation with treatment regimen. Goal of disease control is to suppress inflammation in joints/other tissues to maintain joint function and prevent deformities. Benefits of drug therapy are dependent on correct dosage, e.g., aspirin must be taken regularly in order to sustain therapeutic blood levels of 18–25 mg.	Verbalizes understanding of condition/prognosis, treatment. Develops a plan for self-care, including lifestyle modifications consistent with mobility and/or activity restrictions.
	Recommend use of enteric coated/buffered aspirin or nonacetylated salicylates, e.g., choline salicylates or choline magnesium trisalicylate.	Coated/buffered preparations ingested with food, etc. minimize gastric irritation, reducing risk of bleeding. Nonacetylated products have a longer half-life, requiring less frequent administration in addition to producing less gastric irritation.	
	Suggest ingestion of medications with meals, milk products, or antacids and at bedtime.	Limits gastric irritation. Reduction of pain at HS enhances sleep and increased blood level decreases early morning stiffness.	
	Identify adverse drug effects, e.g., tinnitus, gastric intolerance, GI bleeding, purpuric rash.	Prolonged, maximal doses of aspirin may result in toxicity. Tinnitus usually indicates high therapeutic blood levels and need for adjustment of dosage.	
	Stress importance of reading labels and refraining from OTC drug usage without prior medical approval. Discuss necessity of medical follow-up/laboratory studies, e.g., ESR, salicylate levels, prothrombin time.	Many products contain hidden salicylates that increase risk of drug overdose/harmful side effects. Drug therapy requires frequent assessment/ refinement to assure optimal effect and to prevent overdose/dangerous side effects.	

which is especially important for treating rheumatoid arthritis. While pain relief can often be obtained from 7 regular strength aspirin (2300 mg) per day, the anti-inflammatory effect is only achieved with 4000–6000 mg/day. Aspirin must be taken at regular intervals to maintain a stable blood level. Time-release aspirin products can be used to maintain serum levels throughout the night.

When aspirin is not helpful, other drugs are tried for two to four weeks each to evaluate their efficacy. If there is insufficient improvement with one drug, another drug is substituted. NSAIDs and salicylates are generally not used together because of the increased risk of interaction and decreased anti-inflammatory effect.

Juvenile arthritis varies from adult disease in that children frequently have more joint deformity. The prognosis for the majority of children is good if treatment is begun immediately. Drug therapy is similar to that for adults, with aspirin being the mainstay of therapy.

The families should also be involved in the patient's education. The more they know, the more likely the patient and family are to be compliant with the treatment program.

PATIENT TEACHING

The nurse must understand as well as teach the patient several important points about the anti-inflammatory drugs. This information is summarized in Table 47–6.

Table 47–6. PATIENT TEACHING INFORMATION FOR PATIENT REQUIRING ANTI-INFLAMMATORY AGENTS

Dear Patient:
This drug has been ordered for you. This is what you should know about your drug to get the most from your therapy. Anti-inflammatory drugs are used to decrease redness and soreness in diseases such as arthritis and bursitis.

1. Drugs will be taken (until your symptoms disappear; for _____ days; for several months until your symptoms are controlled; for the rest of your life).
2. Drugs should be taken (with meals; between meals—see Table 47–3 for specific information).
3. Interactions with other drugs are possible with your medication. Do not take any drug without first checking with your doctor or pharmacist.
4. If you forget your drug until your next dose time, forget it. Do not try to "catch up."
5. Do not stop your drug without talking to your doctor first.
6. Side effects can occur from your drug. They might include upset stomach and headache. Additional side effects include (fill in from Table 47–3). If any of these occur, tell your doctor.
7. Take your weight every week. Call your doctor if you have a change of more than 5 lb in a week.
8. Check your stool for presence of blood. Stools may appear black or have actual blood in them.
9. Keep all drugs out of the reach of small children.
10. Store your medication in a tight, moisture-resistant container.

All the NSAIDs cause gastrointestinal side effects, including irritation and bleeding. To reduce the risk of bleeding, the drugs are administered with food or milk. Enteric-coated aspirin may be helpful. Misoprostol may be administered concurrently with NSAIDs or aspirin to prevent gastric ulcer formation. The best way to monitor gastrointestinal bleeding is to have a baseline CBC done before therapy begins, then perform follow-up testing every four to six months.

When NSAIDs do cause upper gastrointestinal bleeding, the blood that reaches the colon is usually digested and is, therefore, unlikely to react with the hemoccult reagent. For this reason, a positive hemoccult test in an NSAID-treated patient should not be attributed to upper gastrointestinal bleeding. This patient needs to have a thorough colorectal workup.

Relief of pain is a separate goal that can be difficult to manage. NSAIDs may not adequately control pain with active disease. If additional pain medications are needed, the use of codeine or propoxyphene may be justified. Patients need to be taught not to take alcohol, tranquilizers, sedatives, or other central nervous system depressants along with their pain medication. Nondrug alternatives to pain medication may also be tried, such as relaxation techniques, biofeedback, or transcutaneous electrical nerve stimulation (TENS). Acute exacerbation may also be treated with low-dose, short-term steroids. When administering corticosteroids, the lowest effective dose is the most desirable. However, the longer the drug is administered, the higher the dose needed to obtain therapeutic results. Side effects of corticosteroids include gastrointestinal ulcers, osteoporosis, hyperglycemia, fluid retention, skin lesions, infection, thrombi, and psychosis. Patients with acute joint flare-up may receive the corticosteroids directly into the joint. This injection usually brings relief in 24–48 hours. Adjunctive therapies such as splints and physical therapy may also be helpful.

The nurse may also teach the patient about dietary limitations when he or she is diagnosed as having gout. The diet usually includes placing the patient on a purine-limited diet (see Table 47–7 for purine-rich foods); increasing fluid volume daily; and limiting beer, ale, or wine, as they may precipitate a gout attack. The patient should not take aspirin or aspirin-containing medications without consulting the physician. If an analgesic is required, acetaminophen is recommended.

Patients should not experiment with their drug dosages; they should take the prescribed dose. For example, taking a subtherapeutic dose of sulfinpyrazone can precipitate an acute gout attack.

EVALUATION

The evaluation of the effectiveness of anti-inflammatory drugs is based on a predetermined list of outcome evaluation criteria. These evaluation criteria are developed on an individual basis through discussion among the nurse, patient, and family. The data base information obtained in the original assessment is used to formulate the criteria for evaluation. Typical outcome evaluation criteria are included in Table 47–5.

Table 47–7. PURINE CONTENT OF FOODS

High Purine Content	Moderate Purine Content
Organ meats	Other meats
Meat extracts	Fish
Gravy	Fowl
Broth	Vegetables: asparagus, spinach, leeks
Wild game	Dried legumes
Goose	
Anchovies	
Herring	
Sardines	
Mackerel	
Scallops	

It is extremely important for the nurse to work with the patient and family to ensure complete assistance and support. Once they understand the importance of their continued medical treatment, the majority of patients usually are compliant. The primary reasons for noncompliance are forgetting the medication, stopping it because all the symptoms have been eliminated, and stopping it because of side effects. Education for the patient with arthritis must stress that stopping the medication for any period of time only causes a flare-up of the symptoms, possibly with more damage resulting. In gout, the average patient may have only four to five attacks in a lifetime, even if he or she is on no medication.

The nurse also determines whether or not the patient can open the medication bottles. Childproof tops may be impossible to open for the individual with arthritic hands. Upon request, the pharmacist can put a regular cap on the prescription bottle. The patient can also ask for a large bottle with a regular cap to store aspirin or related OTC preparations. The nurse stresses the importance of properly labeling and storing these medications out of the reach of children since they do not have childproof caps.

The nurse teaches the patient about the adverse effects of the medications. If an unusual symptom is noted, the patient is encouraged to call the physician or nurse.

The salicylate-like medications—indomethacin, phenylbutazone, and oxyphenbutazone—have many serious adverse effects and should be prescribed only for short-term therapy. The incidence of adverse reactions is high, particularly in the elderly. Gastrointestinal complications are most common, including ulcerative stomatitis, gastric or duodenal ulceration, often leading to bleeding, and, rarely, perforation. Patients are encouraged to report even minor gastrointestinal symptoms to the physician. Other symptoms that should be reported at once include sore throat, onset of fever, skin rashes, blurred vision, unusual weight gain, or the presence of edema. If the patient complains of blurred vision, he or she should have a thorough ophthalmic examination. While the patient is taking anti-inflammatory drugs, systemic infections may be masked. A complete blood count is performed approximately every four weeks to evaluate the presence of infection as well as the presence of leukopenia, thrombocytopenic purpura, agranulocytosis, and anemia.

When placed on the nonsteroidal anti-inflammatory drugs, ibuprofen, naproxen, fenoprofen, tolmetin, or mefenamic acid, or the antimalarials, the patient is encouraged to report any visual changes immediately. Also, because of the central nervous system effects of dizziness, drowsiness, and lightheadedness, the patient is cautioned about operating a car or heavy equipment. The patient also monitors his or her weight and reports any unusual weight gain or edema. All medications are discontinued promptly if the patient complains of diarrhea, skin rash, or bleeding from any body area.

In general, these medications enhance the ulcerogenic effects of other anti-inflammatory agents, such as corticosteroids and salicylates, and, therefore, are not given concurrently. In addition, although they do not enhance anticoagulant activity, they may increase the patient's bleeding time.

The majority of the nonsteroidal anti-inflammatory drugs cause abnormal liver enzyme levels on laboratory tests. Baseline tests are obtained whenever these medications are to be used for long-term therapy.

The antigout medications, colchicine, probenecid, sulfinpyrazone, and allopurinol, generally cause diarrhea as one of their first toxic side effects. They can be discontinued until the gastrointestinal complaints disappear and are then reinstituted. Antidiarrheal medication may be administered to control mild diarrhea that occurs with low maintenance doses.

Gold salts may cause many adverse effects including pruritus and dermatitis from deposition in the skin. Stomatitis and a metallic taste in the mouth are also common. Adverse reactions may occur any time during therapy or after therapy has been discontinued. They are most likely to occur when the dose has reached 250–500 mg at one time. Any rapid improvement in joint swelling usually indicates that the patient is closely approaching drug tolerance levels. Treatment is then usually interrupted for a short period of time and reinstituted.

The more patient and family are involved with the planning of care, the more likely they are to comply. The nurse stresses the importance of continued medical care. During a remission, the dosages are usually reduced; during an exacerbation, they are increased. The nurse is always alert for possible drug interactions. In addition, all other evaluation criteria are evaluated before the patient finishes the care plan. All previously taught material is reviewed and updated, if necessary, to ensure that the patient's knowledge base remains accurate.

As long as there is no cure for arthritis, new drugs will continually be developed to treat the symptoms. As they are released, the media will herald them as the latest miracle cure, often raising false hopes for the millions of arthritis sufferers. These patients need continued education that nurses can provide concerning the benefits of these new therapies.

SUMMARY

Inflammatory diseases range from rheumatoid arthritis and degenerative joint disease to connective tissue disorders. Therapeutic agents for treating these disorders include salicylates, NSAIDs, salicylate-like medications, gold products, antimalarials, cytotoxic medications, and antigout drugs. Salicylates, NSAIDs, and salicylate-like medications provide symptomatic relief of the disease by inhibiting prostaglandin synthesis. It remains unknown whether these drugs actually alter the course of the disease. Gold products, and antigout products suppress the destructive course of the disease, while antimalarials and cytotoxic drugs may or may not have this effect.

It is important for the nurse to assess the patient's level of activity before therapy is instituted as well as the presence of any past or current gastrointestinal complaints. Medications are generally tried for two to four weeks to determine their effectiveness. If there is insufficient improvement with one drug, another drug is substituted. Since most of the drugs are continued at home, patient teaching is important.

BIBLIOGRAPHY

Adams, S: Non-steroidal anti-inflammatory drugs, plasma half-lives, and adverse reactions (letter). Lancet 2:1204, 1987.

AMA Drug Evaluations. PSG Publishing, Littleton, MA, 1986.

Butler, CD: Preventing peptic ulcer disease resulting from NSAIDs. Facts & Comparisons Drug Newsletter 6(11):81, November, 1987.

Cerrato, PL: What diet can do for your arthritic patient. RN 87(9):69, 1987.

Clegg, DO and Ward, JR: Slow-acting anti-rheumatic drug therapy for rheumatoid arthritis. The Nurse Practitioner 12(3):44, March, 1987.

Connell, S: Metabolites of the arachidonic acid cascade. Facts & Comparisons Drug Newsletter 6(12):89, December, 1987.

Drugs for rheumatoid arthritis. The Medical Letter 29(734), February 27, 1987.

Dugowson, C and Gilliland, B: Management of rheumatoid arthritis. Disease of the Month 32(1):14, January 1, 1986.

Foley, JJ, et al: Selecting an appropriate NSAID. Hosp Pract 22(4):54, April 15, 1987.

Fuller, E: Aggressive drug therapy for rheumatoid arthritis. Patient Care 21(5):22, March 15, 1987.

Gilman, AG, Goodman, LS, and Gilman, A (eds): Goodman and Gilman's The Pharmacological Basis of Therapeutics, ed 7. Macmillan, New York, 1985.

Harris, ED Jr: Wider options for rheumatoid arthritis. Emerg Med 18(19):74, November 15, 1986.

Kuncl, RW, et al: Colchicine myopathy and neuropathy. N Engl J Med 316:1562, 1987.

Nonsteroidals in the GI tract. Emerg Med 19(9):55, 1987.

Pye, G, et al: Influence of non-steroidal anti-inflammatory drugs on the outcome of faecal occult tests in screening for colorectal cancer. Brit Med J 294:1510, 1987.

Radack, KL: Ibuprofen interferes with the efficacy of antihypertensive drugs. Ann Intern Med 107(5):628, 1987.

Relative GI toxicity of seven NSAIDs. Facts & Comparisons Drug Newsletter 6(8):59, August, 1987.

Riskin, WG and Gottlieb, NL: Gold therapy for rheumatoid arthritis: Use of injectable and oral preparations. Hosp Formulary 20:1232, 1985.

Wilson, J and Foster, D: Textbook of Endocrinology. WB Saunders, Philadelphia, 1985.

SITUATION 47-1

Marvin Ungerman, aged 50, has rheumatoid arthritis for which he is being treated through the health clinic.

1. Mr. Ungerman has been placed on drug therapy with ibuprofen (Motrin) 200 mg three times a day. The clinic nurse will provide the following information when teaching him about this drug:
   a. Wear a hat outdoors to reduce sun exposure.
   b. Expect water retention and weight gain.
   c. Use in conjunction with aspirin for relief of pain.
   d. Take with food to reduce gastric irritation.

2. When evaluating Mr. Ungerman on return visits to the clinic, the nurse will monitor the following with regard to ibuprofen therapy:
   a. potassium level
   b. bleeding time
   c. T_3 T_4 levels
   d. urine amylase

3. Three months later, Mr. Ungerman continues to experience arthritic pain despite ibuprofen therapy. His physician plans to place him on gold therapy with gold sodium thiomalate (Myochrysine). Prior to therapy, Mr. Ungerman will be assessed for the following contraindication to its use:
   a. aspirin allergy
   b. peptic ulcer disease

   c. narrow angle glaucoma
   d. congestive heart failure

4. In order to administer gold sodium thiomalate correctly to Mr. Ungerman, the nurse will plan to:
   a. agitate the vial to ensure uniform suspension
   b. keep the patient NPO before giving
   c. use any subcutaneous site for injection
   d. keep medication cool for injection

5. The nurse will teach Mr. Ungerman about adverse side effects of gold therapy, which include:
   a. seizures
   b. angina
   c. rashes
   d. hypertension

6. Which of the following statements by Mr. Ungerman indicates successful patient teaching?
   a. "The medication should be used only if it is a dark yellow."
   b. "Getting direct sunlight will help relieve side effects."
   c. "It may take 6 to 8 weeks for benefits to be felt."
   d. "It is best to walk for 30 minutes after the gold injection."

Please refer to the Appendices for correct answers and additional review questions with answers.

9
UNIT

CHEMOTHERAPY AND IMMUNOTHERAPY OF NEOPLASTIC DISEASE

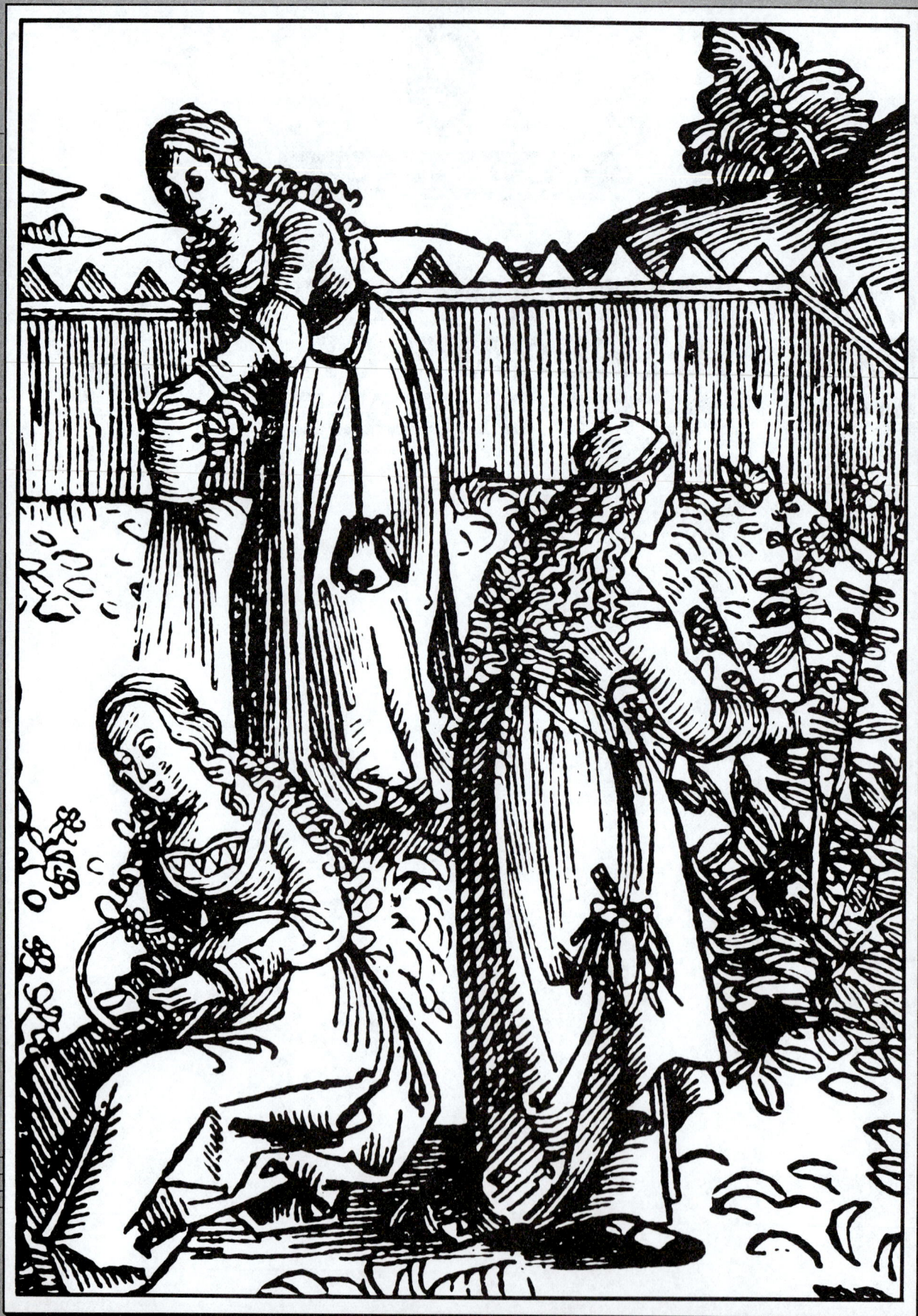

Tending medicinal plants in a medieval herb garden, 1512. The Bettmann Archive.

UNIT 9

CHEMOTHERAPY AND IMMUNOTHERAPY OF NEOPLASTIC DISEASE

48

CHAPTER

THE PRINCIPLES OF ANTINEPLASTIC CHEMOTHERAPY

ANNE MORACA-SAWICKI, RN, MSN

LEARNING OBJECTIVES

After reading this chapter, the student will be able to:

1. Identify major historical events in the development of chemotherapeutic agents.

2. Explain what differentiates the growth of a cancerous cell from that of a normal cell.

3. Identify the principles of antineoplastic chemotherapy.

4. Explain the stem cell theory.

5. Differentiate among the five phases of the cell life cycle.

6. Compare and contrast the uses of antineoplastic chemotherapy.

7. Define the terms cell cycle-specific and cell cycle-nonspecific. Explain how each achieves its antineoplastic effects.

8. Recognize the mechanisms by which drugs can produce their antineoplastic effects.

SCOPE OF THE CANCER PROBLEM

Approximately 800,000 new cases of cancer are diagnosed each year in the United States. Cancer deaths are second only to cardiovascular deaths and are approaching 400,000 per year in the United States (Fig. 48–1 shows the relative frequencies of cancer). In 1984, the Centers for Disease Control confirmed that lung cancer deaths in women had surpassed those of breast cancer, thereby making the lung the leading site of cancer incidence and mortality in both men and women.

The term *neoplasm* is taken from the Greek words meaning "new formation" and means any new tissue growth in which the growth is uncontrolled or progressive. Neoplasms may be benign or malignant. Malignant neoplasms differ from benign neoplasms in that they generally show a greater degree of anaplasia (loss

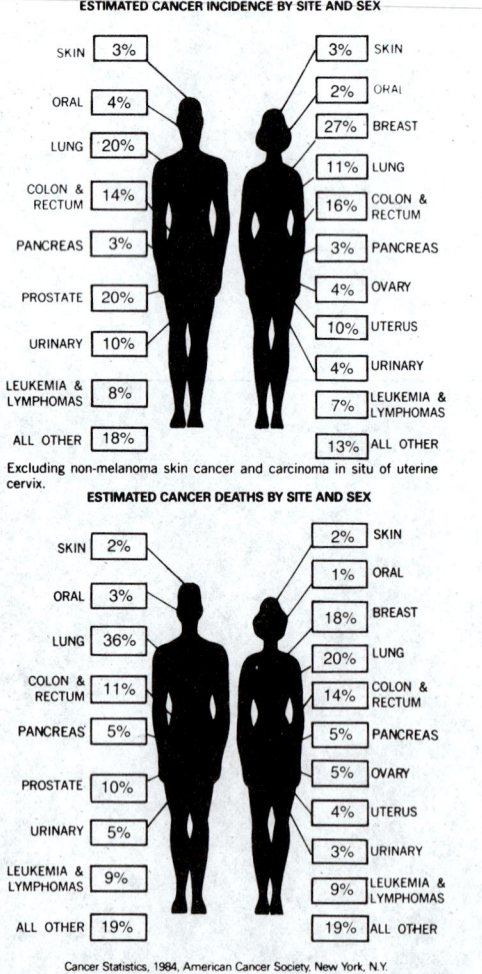

ESTIMATED CANCER INCIDENCE BY SITE AND SEX

Excluding non-melanoma skin cancer and carcinoma in situ of uterine cervix.

ESTIMATED CANCER DEATHS BY SITE AND SEX

Cancer Statistics, 1984, American Cancer Society, New York, N.Y.

Figure 48–1. Cancer incidence and deaths by site and sex—1987 estimates. Based on Cancer Statistics, 1987, American Cancer Society, New York, NY. (From Thomas, CL [Ed.]: Taber's Cyclopedic Medical Dictionary, ed. 16. FA Davis, Philadelphia, 1989, p. 275, with permission.)

Table 48–1. HUMAN CANCERS OF POSSIBLE VIRAL ORIGIN

Cancer	Virus
Breast	B-type
Burkitt's Lymphoma	Epstein-Barr
Leukemia	C-type
Liver Cancer	Hepatitis-B Virus
Nasopharyngeal	Herpes Simplex Type I
Uterine Cervix	Herpes Simplex Type II

of cell differentiation) and also have the properties of invasion and metastasis. Although neoplasms can be benign or malignant, this term is frequently misinterpreted as being synonymous with cancer.

The term cancer does not refer to one disease but is used as a collective term to refer to a group of diseases that share the common feature of unrestrained cell growth resulting in tumors that invade and destroy normal tissue. Cancer may arise in any organ or tissue in the body. The cancer process is the end result of a series of complex interactions at the chemical, biochemical, cellular, tissue, organ, and organism levels. There are three major categories of factors implicated as being able to initiate the cancer process. These are viruses such as herpes and Epstein-Barr as initiating agents; chemical carcinogens such as asbestos; and physical carcinogens such as chronic irritation, radiation, radionuclides, and the mechanism of radiation carcinogenesis (see Tables 48–1 and 48–2).

STEM CELL THEORY

It is possible for many different cell types to undergo malignant change. In some cases, the primary tumor arises from a single cell and is thus said to be of *clonal* origin. According to the *stem cell theory*, only a small number of cells are clonogenic. It is this clonogenic (stem cell) population that has the potential for division and the ability to reproduce the entire tissue from its genetic storehouses. It is believed that neoplastic tumors may arise from a single aberrant stem cell. In some neoplastic tumors, it is possible to prove that all the tumor cells have a common origin, and this supports the theory of a single aberrant stem cell origin. Not all members of a stem cell population are involved in cell division at the same time. Research indicates that a certain percentage of stem cells in a given population are in the resting (G_0) phase. This percentage of stem cells at rest remains constant in tissues. Certain stimuli can encourage the resting cells to enter the cell cycle and begin the division process. For example, a break in the skin will cause some at-rest skin stem cells to enter the cell cycle and repair the wound. Once repair is complete, the stimulus ends and the G_0 skin stem cell population returns to its constant level. Thus, normal growth and repair of tissue occur. Normal cells grow logarithmically until they reach critical mass, when their growth rate is altered by hormonal and cellular factors. Cancer cells lack

Table 48–2. SOME ENVIRONMENTAL CARCINOGENS LINKED TO HUMAN CANCERS

Chemical Carcinogen	Type of Cancer Associated with
Arsenic	Skin, lung
Asbestos	Lung, pleura
Benzene	Bone marrow
Beta-naphthalene	Urinary bladder
Carbon tetrachloride	Liver
Diethylstilbestrol (DES)	Vaginal adenocarcinoma (in daughters of women treated with drug during pregnancy; sons of such women may have increased risk of testicular tumors)
Dioxin	Various tumors
Estrogens	Uterus, vagina
Polycyclic hydrocarbons (present in tobacco smoke)	Lung
Rubber Industry Chemicals	Lung, urinary bladder
Vinyl chloride	Angiosarcoma of the liver

Radiant Energy	Type of Cancer Associated with
Atomic radiation (bombs)	Leukemia, lung, breast, thyroid
Ionizing radiation (radium, x-rays)	Leukemia, bone cancers

these normal control factors and continue to multiply past the critical mass state, although growth is at a slower-than-logarithmic rate. This growth rate of cancer cells is referred to as *Gompertzian kinetics.*

Malignant tumors have their own population of stem cells. Although it is true that malignant tumors somehow escape normal growth controls, not all malignant cells are involved in division at a given time. This can make antineoplastic therapy difficult, because many drugs do not affect resting cells. Total kill of the stem cell population in solid tumors such as lung cancer is difficult; however, chemotherapy of other tumors such as leukemia has shown that cure is possible. Thorough knowledge of cell kinetics makes it possible to measure tumor growth and thereby evaluate the effectiveness of the therapeutic regimen.

A BRIEF HISTORY OF ANTINEOPLASTIC CHEMOTHERAPY

Chemotherapy is the use of a drug to weaken or kill an unwanted organism or cell without undue harm to the host (patient). The use of pharmacologic agents dates back to the Egyptian use of aloes, herbs, and opium. However, the use of drugs for antineoplastic chemotherapy is a science in its infancy.

Antineoplastic chemotherapy had its beginning in 1919 with the discovery of nitrogen mustard's leukopenic activity in man. Administration of chemotherapeutic agents began about 50 years ago. In 1940, Huggins demonstrated that patients with prostatic cancer improved following the administration of estrogens. The drug mechlorethamine (Mustargen) was first ad-

ministered to patients in 1942. The 1950s brought the introduction of the first antimetabolic agents. In the 1960s, the metaphase inhibitors and agents such as hydroxyurea, procarbazine, L-asparaginase, and dacarbazine (DTIC) were added to the list of chemotherapeutic drugs. Introduction of the antibiotics Adriamycin and bleomycin occurred during the 1970s.

In the 1980s, the greatest progress in chemotherapy of neoplastic diseases has not been the discovery of new drugs, but rather more effective regimens for the use of existing drugs and other conceptual advances that have made chemotherapy more successful. Advances in knowledge of how antitumor drugs act have resulted in new methods to prevent or minimize drug toxicity and the increased use of *adjuvant chemotherapy.* Adjuvant chemotherapy is the administration of chemotherapeutic agents to destroy micrometastasis and prevent the development of secondary tumors following the removal or destruction of a primary tumor. This therapy is done before any evidence of overt metastasis in order to prevent recurrence. The discovery of the role of *oncogenes* in carcinogenesis has opened a new avenue of study that, it is hoped, will lead to more effective methods of cancer chemotherapy. Oncogenes are activated forms of normal cellular proto-oncogenes that have been altered by mutations or chromosomal translocation. Oncogenes are introduced into cells by retroviruses. Certain proteins encoded by viral oncogenes are related to cellular growth factors or their receptors. Research is continuing to study this process for new clues on how cancer develops and how it can be treated. Study of the retrovirus HIV in AIDS may lead to significant advances for both chemotherapy of cancer and AIDS.

What advances in chemotherapy do the 1990s hold? Scientists are exploring the ramifications of interferon therapy and likening it to that of Alexander Fleming's 1929 observation that penicillium mold exerted antibiotic activity against *staphylococcus*. Early clinical trials with interferon are encouraging scientists to think that this drug will be an important clue in unlocking a whole new era of chemotherapeutic advances. The discovery of the role of oncogenes in carcinogenesis will hopefully lead to the discovery of more effective use of chemotherapy to kill cancer cells.

Selective toxicity is the ultimate goal in chemotherapy. The cytotoxic agent should destroy cancer cells without doing irreversible damage to normal cells. To date, there is no agent so selective that it destroys cancer cells only.

The timing of chemotherapy doses can be critical. Intermittent high-dose (pulse) therapy with cell cycle-specific and cell cycle-nonspecific agents has been shown to achieve better therapeutic results with less toxic side effects than more frequent divided doses. This is true with several types of tumors. It allows the host to achieve better recovery of normal cells, such as those in bone marrow and the gastrointestinal tract, during the drug-free interval. Timing drug doses in relation to another drug can allow for cell synchronization to yield greater cell kill with the second drug's administration. However, this principle applies to the normal cells also.

Combinations of antineoplastic agents can be more effective against malignancies and have been highly effective against certain tumors such as Hodgkin's disease. Although tumor effectiveness is additive, host toxicity need not be, due to the pairing of drugs with different side effects.

THE CELL CYCLE

In order for the nurse to understand the activity of chemotherapeutic agents, a somewhat detailed knowledge of cell growth and division is necessary. The normal cell cycle consists of several distinct phases of biochemical activity. There are essentially five phases in the cell cycle (Fig. 48–2). These phases are the same in both normal and malignant cells.

Following cell division, the daughter cells enter the resting phase (G$_0$), indicating that the cell is out of the cycle, yet not actively committed to replication. The cell remains thus dormant until a yet-to-be-determined biochemical stimulus triggers the onset of the replication process. Once this process is triggered, the cell enters interphase, where several activities occur. The postmitotic Gap 1 (G1) phase begins with the manufacture of enzymes necessary for DNA synthesis to occur.

During the next phase of the cell cycle, actual DNA synthesis occurs. This S phase can take the cell from 10–20 hours to double its DNA complement, needed to ready the chromosomes for division. Each strand of nucleotides in the DNA double helix is joined by base pairings between a purine and a pyrimidine base. In order for DNA replication to occur, the strands separate, allowing the exposed bases to become templates (patterns) with which free nucleotides can base pair. Triphosphates containing one of the four bases—adenine, cytosine, guanine, or thymine—and the sugar deoxyribose are the free nucleotides that form the DNA strands. Once the DNA replicates itself, there are two identical molecules, each with one original strand and a newly synthesized strand copied from the original. Once this process has been completed, there are two molecules of DNA, one for each cell, resulting from the division process.

Most of the cell cycle-specific agents exert their greatest activity during the S phase of the cell cycle, thereby blocking the DNA replication process. Although the S phase is relatively long, the time spent in this DNA replication phase is only about 10–20 hours. Many chemotherapeutic agents affect only dividing cells and only during certain phases of the cell cycle. Thus, the number of tumor cells involved in the cell division process (often referred to as the "growth fraction") is a crucial factor in the effectiveness of drug therapy.

The second gap (G2) is a short, premitotic phase. Specialized protein and RNA synthesis occur, as well as

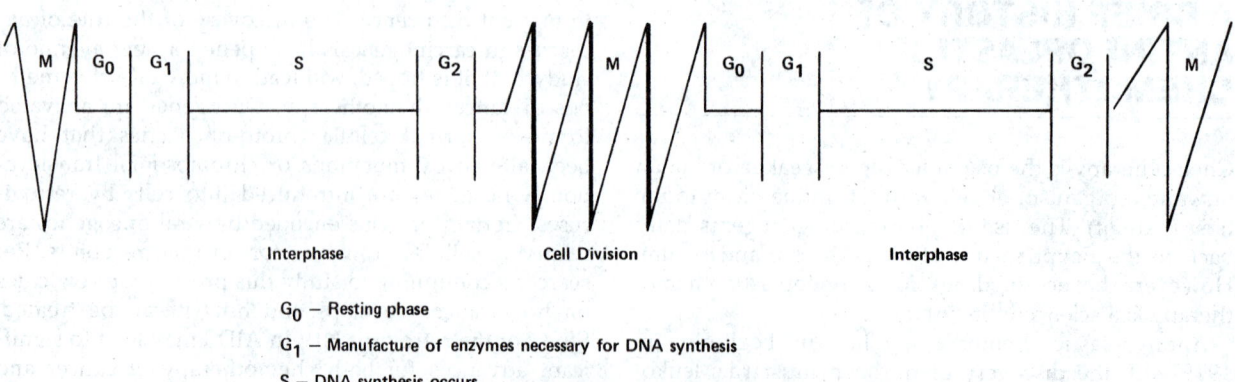

G$_0$ — Resting phase

G$_1$ — Manufacture of enzymes necessary for DNA synthesis

S — DNA synthesis occurs

G$_2$ — Specialized protein and RNA synthesis occurs; manufacture of mitotic spindle apparatus

M — Mitotic cell division occurs

Figure 48–2. The cell cycle.

manufacture of the mitotic spindle apparatus. Also synthesized is a special DNA necessary for cell division to occur. The G2 phase may take from 2–10 hours.

Once the cell completes the G2 phase, it enters the mitosis (M) phase, which is the actual cell division process. This is a brief phase and generally lasts an hour or less. The mitotic phase of the cell cycle consists of four distinct phases in itself. The phases of mitosis are prophase, metaphase, anaphase, and telophase. The nuclear membrane breaks down and chromosome "clumping" begins in the prophase. Metaphase follows, with the chromosomes lining up in the middle of the cell. This phase is followed by anaphase, which sees the chromosomes segregate to the *centrioles.* In telophase, the last phase of mitosis, actual division yields two cells, one being a daughter cell identical to the original. Following mitosis, the daughter cells differentiate into functioning cells of the parent cell's tissue type. Most cells then enter a resting phase (G_0) not actively involved in cell division. A portion of the cells retain proliferative abilities in order to maintain the necessary complement of stem cells.

CELL CYCLE-SPECIFIC AGENTS

Antineoplastic agents that affect the cell during only one phase of the cell life cycle are called cell cycle-specific. Actually, a more technically correct designation is cell cycle phase-specific, because these agents are active only in a specific phase of the cell cycle. Cell cycle-specific drugs are most often described as being antimetabolic. Each drug of this type works by causing a biochemical blockade of a reaction or reactions occurring in a specific phase of the cell cycle. Most often, these chemical blockades occur because of the drugs' structural similarity to vitamins, coenzymes, or normal cell intermediary products essential for growth and division. The antineoplastic agent is an impostor that the cell takes in to use during the life cycle. Once the antineoplastic agent binds within the cell, the normal metabolic pathway is interrupted, causing a halt to the growth and division process. This ultimately leads to cell death.

The antineoplastic agents mercaptopurine, methotrexate, fluorouracil, procarbazine, bleomycin, and vincristine are all examples of cell cycle-specific agents. Many of these drugs are also referred to as being "schedule dependent," because they produce a greater cell kill when given in multiple, repeated fractions rather than in a single large dose or bolus.

CELL CYCLE-NONSPECIFIC AGENTS

Antineoplastic agents that exert their effects during more than one phase of the cell cycle are termed cell cycle-nonspecific agents. These drugs are effective against large tumors where the growth fraction and mitotic index are low. Drugs contained in this group are the alkylating agents. Tumors that the alkylating agents are typically used to treat include hematopoietic tissue malignancies; neuroblastoma; and disseminated carcinomas of the breast, ovaries, testes, and lungs. Drugs belonging to this cell cycle-nonspecific class are not schedule-dependent, but rather are dose-dependent. Dose-dependency indicates that the degree of cell kill is directly proportional to the amount of drug given. Therefore, these agents are typically administered in a bolus fashion. Examples of drugs in this cell cycle-nonspecific class include the alkylating agents melphalan and mechlorethamine, the nitrosoureas carmustine and lomustine, the anthracyclines doxorubicin and daunorubicin, as well as dacarbazine and cisplatin.

Technically, the agents listed above are cell cycle-nonspecific; however, their activities do depend on the cell at some point either attempting division or repair of drug-induced damage. It is at this point that the drug-induced intracellular lethal effects become apparent and cell death ensues. Some drugs in this class, such as nitrogen mustard and the nitrosoureas, have an uncharacteristically nonselective effect on normal and malignant cells, which has prompted some experts to classify these agents as nonselective, phase-nonspecific drugs.

CELL KINETICS

The study of cell kinetics has led to the development of the principles of cancer chemotherapy and enhanced the development of new antineoplastic agents. It is as important for the nurse to understand the relationship between cell kinetics and chemotherapeutic strategy as it is to know the relationship between the cell cycle and drug mode of action.

In order to enhance understanding of chemotherapeutic principles and drug actions, an explanation of various terms is essential. The phrase *"mitotic index"* (MI) refers to the fraction of cells in mitosis at a given time. The term *"growth fraction"* (GF) describes the overall number of proliferating neoplastic cells in the system. *"Doubling time"* is the length of time required for a tumor cell population to double itself. The doubling time of a neoplastic tumor varies according to the type of tissue involved. The term *"cell loss"* refers to the loss of neoplastic cells from the tumor mass. Cell loss can occur in a variety of ways, including metastasis and cell death. Advanced tumors typically have a high cell loss rate.

The most important factor in determining the relative specificity of antineoplastic agents is the growth fraction. In general, neoplastic cells have a higher growth fraction than do normal cells. A higher growth fraction (more cells actively dividing) correlates with a greater cell kill from both cell cycle-specific and cell cycle-nonspecific agents. Unfortunately, certain normal tissue types—the bone marrow, hair follicles, and cells of the gastrointestinal tract—also have very high growth fractions. It is not surprising that these rapidly dividing cellular populations suffer the most toxicity when chemotherapeutic agents are administered.

CURRENT STATUS OF ANTINEOPLASTIC CHEMOTHERAPY

Historically, chemotherapy was not a primary treatment for malignant disease. In the past, chemotherapy was used in a last-ditch effort to palliate metastatic disease. In the early days of antineoplastic chemotherapy, the drugs were not as specific or refined as they are today. Drug side effects were more difficult to manage because of the lack of rapid, sophisticated blood analysis techniques. Thus, the major uses of cytotoxic agents were for treatment of hematologic and metastatic tumors.

Current use of antineoplastic agents is much more expansive. Sophisticated serum and blood cell analysis coupled with modern drugs have produced excellent response rates in treatment of many tumors. Chemotherapy is no longer a treatment given when all else fails, but is actually the primary treatment or treatment of choice for many malignancies such as inflammatory carcinomas of the breast, acute leukemias, and Hodgkin's disease (Table 48–3). Chemotherapy makes normal life expectancy possible in at least ten different malignancies. In advanced cancers, it may be combined with surgery, radiotherapy, or immunotherapy in order to achieve the highest possible cell kill. Another application of chemotherapy that is becoming increasingly used is adjuvant chemotherapy. The rationale for adjuvant chemotherapy is to administer the cytotoxic agents before the onset of clinically apparent disease in order to prevent recurrent disease. The drugs are administered to eradicate any residual tumor cells or micrometastases that may remain following reduction of tumor burden by surgery, radiation, or other therapy. Studies of breast cancer patients with two or more lymph nodes positive for tumor cells at the time of surgery show increased five-year survival and disease-free intervals for patients who received adjuvant chemotherapy. The benefits of adjuvant chemotherapy in patients with colon cancer and non–small-cell lung cancer are currently being studied. Initial results appear encouraging. Since these are common cancers, even modest gains can save many lives.

BASIC PRINCIPLES OF ANTINEOPLASTIC CHEMOTHERAPY

The ultimate goal of antineoplastic chemotherapy is to achieve total cell kill. Several principles make this a difficult task. First of all, the presence of a single clonogenic malignant cell may yield sufficient offspring to kill the human host. A second factor is the negligible contribution of host immune mechanisms and defenses in augmenting therapy. Another principle is that cell kill produced by the cytotoxic agent occurs according to *first-order kinetics*. This means a specific dose of a specific drug kills a constant percentage of the body burden of cancer cells, rather than a specific number of cells. For example, if your patient had a tumor composed of approximately 1 kg of cells and you administered a 99.9% effective drug, your patient would still have about 1 g of cancer cells in the body. A way of dealing with this residual body burden of tumor cells to try and achieve total cell kill is to administer drugs in combination or sequences. This combination chemotherapy approach has been highly successful in the treatment of diseases such as acute lymphocytic leukemia.

Cell cycle-specific and cell cycle-nonspecific agents have already been discussed. However, it is important to remember that cytotoxic drugs are generally more effective against dividing cells than resting cells. Also, patients tolerate chemotherapy better when tumor cell burden is low and is associated with less organ impairment. Reductive therapy to decrease the body burden of cancer cells may be done before chemotherapy. This can

Table 48–3. REMISSION RATES IN SELECTED CHEMOTHERAPY-TREATED TUMORS

Type of Cancer	CR* Rate (%)	10-Year Survival CR (%)	5-Year Survival CR (%)
Acute childhood lymphoblastic leukemia	90	50	70
Acute myelocytic leukemia	60	20	
Hodgkin's disease	80	—	70
Burkitt's lymphoma	90	60 (for those treated in early stages of disease) 50 (for later stages)	—
Choriocarcinoma	90	90 (cure for those treated in early disease stages) 75 (cure in metastatic stages)	—
Ewing's sarcoma	†	—	66
Ovarian cancer	33	40	—
Wilm's tumor	†	—	80

*Complete remission (CR) is defined as complete regression of all evidence of cancer by physical, radiologic, and biochemical criteria and a return to normal performance status. Remissions are always expressed in terms of duration.

†Chemotherapy is used as part of multidisciplinary treatment approach to this disease. Surgery and/or radiotherapy are used in conjunction with combination chemotherapy.

be accomplished through surgery, radiotherapy, or other therapy.

The use of adjuvant therapy prior to clinical signs of recurrent disease has been discussed. It is hoped that this therapy will reduce tumor burden to levels more likely to be handled by the host's immunologic mechanisms. One must remember that cytotoxic therapy in itself can be immunosuppressive and teratogenic.

RESISTANCE TO CHEMOTHERAPY

The effectiveness of chemotherapy can be diminished by cell resistance. There are three types of resistance:

1. Type I resistance, in which permanently resistant tumor cells cannot be affected by the drug at all;
2. Type II resistance, in which temporarily resistant tumor cells can be affected through a combination of therapies including radiation or surgery; and
3. Type III resistance, which occurs when the tumor cells receive less than adequate drug exposure due to tumor site or local conditions. Once these conditions are overcome by using different administration techniques, this resistance is overcome.

Antineoplastic chemotherapy may be administered orally, intramuscularly, intravenously, intrathecally, by intra-arterial infusion, or by perfusion pump. Specific nursing measures relative to each type of administration depend upon the drug and its properties (for example, photosensitivity). Actual approaches and interventions relative to nursing goals with respect to chemotherapy are covered in depth in Chapter 49. The nursing process remains the vehicle for the application of good nursing care. The nursing process is discussed in detail in Chapter 49.

SUMMARY

The science of antineoplastic chemotherapy is relatively new. Although the use of medicines to treat illnesses dates back to ancient times, the use of drugs to treat cancer began shortly after the discovery of nitrogen mustard's leukopenic effect on humans. Thus, out of the wartime use of mustard gas came a useful and beneficial discovery. The drug Mustargen (derived from nitrogen mustard) was first administered in 1942. Estrogen ther-

apy to treat patients with prostate cancer also began in the 1940s. In the 1950s, the first antimetabolic drugs were used. The 1960s and 1970s brought other antineoplastic drugs into the treatment picture. The development of new drugs slowed in the 1980s as researchers began to concentrate on the development of more effective drug regimens and combinations of available drugs.

Research that began in the 1980s helped oncology researchers gain new insight into the spread of cancer, the role of oncogenes, and the relationship of these to antineoplastic drug therapy. Research continues today not only in the development of new drugs but on the more effective use of existing drugs to treat cancer. The use of pulse therapy and new combination chemotherapy, as well as perfusion therapy techniques, have helped improve survival rates for many cancers. Chemotherapy is no longer a treatment of last resort, but in many cases is the primary treatment for certain cancers. Chemotherapy can offer many cancer patients extended, meaningful, disease-free lives.

BIBLIOGRAPHY

Bakemeir, R (ed): Clinical Oncology. The University of Rochester School of Medicine and Dentistry, American Society Publishers, Rochester, NY, 1980.

Ballentine, R: Nursing implications of cancer chemotherapy. Nursing83 13(7):56A, 1983.

Burns, N: Nursing and Cancer. WB Saunders, Philadelphia, 1982.

Calabresi, R and Parks, E: Chemotherapy of Neoplastic Diseases. In Gilman, AG, Goodman, LS, and Gilman, A (eds): Goodman and Gilman's The Pharmacological Basis of Therapeutics, ed 7. Macmillan, New York, 1986.

Chabner, B: Pharmacologic Principles of Cancer Treatment. WB Saunders, Philadelphia, 1982.

Clinical Oncology Alert: Adjuvant therapy for colon cancer—Yes or no? 3(3):9, 1988.

Clinical Oncology Alert: Oncogene amplification and prognosis in breast cancer. 2(4): 13, 1987.

Clinical Oncology Alert: Recent studies on treatment of related toxicities. 2(9):33, 1987.

Moraca, A: Nursing Management of the Client With Breast Cancer. State University of New York at Buffalo, Buffalo, NY, 1977.

Pinedo, HM, Longo, DL, and Chabner, BA: Cancer Chemotherapy and Biological Response Modifiers. Annual 19. Elsevier, New York, 1987.

Shimkin, M: Science and Cancer. US Department of Health and Human Services, National Institutes of Health, Washington, DC, 1984.

Simonson, GM: Caring for patients with acute myelocytic leukemia. Am J Nurs 88(3):304, 1988.

49

ANTINEOPLASTIC CHEMOTHERAPY

ANNE MORACA-SAWICKI, MSN, RN

LEARNING OBJECTIVES

After reading this chapter, the student will be able to:

1. Identify those medications commonly used as antineoplastic agents.

2. Differentiate among the antineoplastic medications as to mechanism of action, route of administration, absorption and fate, adverse effects, contraindications, and interactions.

3. Identify specific areas to assess in the patient requiring antineoplastic medications in order to formulate appropriate nursing diagnoses.

4. Plan the nursing interventions necessary to administer antineoplastic medications and choose appropriate teaching strategies to gain patient compliance.

5. Evaluate the patient at various stages of treatment to gauge nursing interventions.

THERAPEUTIC AGENTS

Therapeutic agents are classified by their probable mode of action and the phase of the cell cycle on which they act. Knowledge of the cell cycle and neoplastic cell growth, as discussed in the preceding chapter, is essential to the understanding of information in this chapter. The therapeutic agents are featured in Table 49–1. It should be noted that dosages for all antineoplastic drugs are given in milligrams per square meter (body surface area) or milligrams per kilogram of body weight. Dosing by body surface area is the most accurate means of dose calculation. To ascertain the patient's surface area, refer to pediatric (see Chapter 14) and adult nomograms, which are widely available. Unless otherwise specified, all drug dosages cited in this chapter are for adults.

GUIDELINES FOR WORKING WITH ANTINEOPLASTIC DRUGS

There has been increasing concern recently about the handling of antineoplastic drugs. Many antineoplastic drugs are themselves capable of producing mutagenic or carcinogenic effects, in addition to causing direct injury to eyes, skin, or mucous membranes on contact. The handling of antineoplastic drugs is currently considered to be an "occupationally hazardous" task necessitating specific safety precautions to protect the health and safety of all health care personnel who may be exposed to these drugs.

Research studies have shown that the major hazard in the mixture and administration of chemotherapeutic agents is from droplet contamination. This results from aerosol exposure of the skin and mucous membranes during drug preparation and administration. For those who handle these drugs regularly, this is a particular problem. Such regular, low-level exposure, even in the absence of symptoms, may produce long-term effects.

The National Institutes of Health, National Cancer Institute, Centers for Disease Control, Occupational Safety and Health Administration, and the International Agency for Research on Cancer have proposed guidelines for the safe handling of antineoplastic drugs. The basic principles surrounding the handling of these drugs deal with protective equipment and safety precautions. Mixing and transfer procedures involving chemotherapeutic drugs should occur in a Class II Biological Safety Cabinet (vertical flow laminar hood); otherwise, a face mask and protective clothing must be worn to protect the preparer from airborne particles or aerosolization of the drug. Oral pipetting is prohibited; pharmacy work and storage areas where chemical carcinogens are present must be posted as such; and materials contaminated by these drugs must be labeled as biohazards and disposed of as such. Additional guidelines and procedures for management of spills or exposure to carcinogenic chemicals have also been proposed. Owing to the hazards inherent in handling these drugs, they should not be prepared on patient care units or in poorly ventilated medication rooms. Each institution should have definite protocols established for handling, preparation, and administration of chemical therapeutic drugs, and the disposal of equipment used in handling these drugs. Such protocols should comply with recently published guidelines of The Office of Occupational Medicine, Department of the Occupational Safety and Health Administration (OSHA).

CLASSIFICATION OF CHEMOTHERAPEUTIC AGENTS

ALKYLATING AGENTS

Alkylating agents were derived from the sulfur mustard gases used in the World Wars. They are so named because their primary mode of action is the alkylation of nucleic acids, which results in the inactivation of DNA, thereby halting cell replication processes. They act by forming electrophilic bonds in the guanine of DNA. The resultant cross-linking and abnormal base pairing prevent DNA replication. Alkylating agents also react with amino, phosphate, and sulfhydryl groups to cause multiple lesions in both dividing and nondividing cells. This ability to act on both dividing and nondividing cells means these drugs are non–cell cycle-dependent. These agents affect cells in the same way that radiation exposure does and are often referred to as being radiomimetic. Several alkylating agents have been developed since the initial use of mechlorethamine, in an attempt to increase antineoplastic activity and decrease the toxic effects to normal cells.

Most alkylating agents are similar in effect. The drugs included in this category are: (1) the nitrogen mustards mechlorethamine (nitrogen mustard, NH2), cyclophosphamide (Cytoxan), melphalan (Alkeran), and chlorambucil (Leukeran); (2) the alkyl sulfonate busulfan (Myleran); (3) ethylenimine thiotepa (Thiotepa); (4) the triazene dacarbazine (DTIC); (5) the nitrosoureas carmustine (BCNU), lomustine (CCNU), and semustine (Methyl-CCNU); and (6) streptozocin (SZN, Zanosar R). Alkylating agents are used primarily in treatment of hematopoietic tissue malignancies, neuroblastoma, and disseminated carcinomas of the breasts, ovaries, testes, and lungs.

Pharmacokinetics

The absorption, distribution, metabolization, and excretion of drugs in the alkylating agent class are similar. Busulfan, chlorambucil, cyclophosphamide, lomustine, melphalan, and semustine are all absorbed from the gastrointestinal tract following oral administration. The other alkylating agents must be administered parenterally. All alkylating agents are widely distributed to body tissues. Carmustine, lomustine, and thiotepa cross the blood–brain barrier. All the alkylating agents except thiotepa are metabolized in the liver and excreted in the urine. Thiotepa is excreted unchanged by the kidneys.

Adverse Effects

As a class, the alkylating agents share the common side effects of *alopecia*, bone marrow depression, nausea, and vomiting. These drugs can also cause impaired spermatogenesis in males. Busulfan can also cause an irreversible pulmonary fibrosis, which is also termed "busulfan lung."

Interactions

The significant drug interactions in this group of drugs occur with cyclophosphamide. Concomitant administration of corticosteroids or chloramphenicol causes reduced activity of cyclophosphamide; therefore, these drugs are used together cautiously. Succinylcholine administration can cause apnea and should be avoided.

Dosage

All dosages of antineoplastic drugs are highly individualized and dependent on many conditions, including the patient's degree of bone marrow depression, concurrent illnesses, past response to therapy, and current condition. Dosages are based on ideal or actual body weight, whichever is less. Refer to Table 49–1 for usual dosages of the alkylating agents.

Pretreatment with a small dose of an alkylating agent can protect against the toxicity of subsequent doses of the same or other alkylating agents if given within a precise period. This mechanism is referred to as *priming*. The exact mechanism of this priming phenomenon is not clear, although several different pathways or mechanisms have been proposed. The study of the priming phenomenon is complicated by the fact that alkylating agents cause different organ toxicities at different dose levels. Studies are in progress to help determine which drugs provide this priming effect best. There are also investigational agents being studied as priming agents. Cyclophosphamide is effective in protecting against alkylating agent–induced bone marrow damage.

Cyclophosphamide

ACTION AND USE. Cyclophosphamide (Cytoxan) is the most commonly used drug in the alkylator group. It has the widest spectrum of activity of the alkylating agents. Cyclophosphamide is not active itself; rather, it requires multistep metabolic activation. The first steps are in the liver, but the final step to the active antineoplastic compound phosphoramide mustard and a side product, acrolein, occurs within target cells. Since tumor cells contain large quantities of the converting enzymes, cyclophosphamide was originally thought to be a tumor-specific antimetabolite. However, this has not proven to be the case, and the active moiety phosphoramide mustard is capable of cross-linking DNA in many normal cells, causing considerable toxicity.

ADVERSE EFFECTS. The adverse effects of cyclophosphamide include hematologic, gastrointestinal, and

urologic toxicity, as well as alopecia. The hematologic toxicity is generally dose-limiting. Cyclophosphamide can cause cardiotoxicity when given in high doses or when given in combination with doxorubicin (Adriamycin). Gonadal suppression and sterility can also occur with administration of this drug.

Cyclophosphamide is thought to be relatively platelet-sparing, since platelets or thrombocytes are devoid of the enzymes necessary for activation. The side product of activation, acrolein, is thought to cause two unusual urologic toxicities: hemorrhagic cystitis and syndrome of inappropriate antidiuretic hormone (SIADH), also known as water intoxication. Hemorrhage cystitis is especially common in high-dose intravenous or long-term oral therapy. The patient may develop microscopic or gross hematuria. The best treatment is prevention by hydration and patient education. Patients are told to drink plenty of fluids, empty their bladders frequently, and not to take oral cyclophosphamide at night. However, with SIADH, the effect is on the distal tubule rather than the bladder. The patient may become water overloaded, hyponatremic, and even develop seizures. The syndrome is reversible and usually treated with only water deprivation.

DOSAGE. The usual adult dose of cyclophosphamide is 40–50 mg/kg by mouth or intravenously as a single dose or in two to five daily doses, then adjust for maintenance. It may also be given in a dose of 2–4 mg/kg by mouth for ten days, then adjusted for maintenance. The maintenance dose is 1.5–3 mg/kg daily by mouth or 10–15 mg/kg intravenously every seven to ten days, or 3–5 mg/kg intravenously twice weekly.

Nitrosoureas

The alkylating nitrosoureas carmustine, lomustine, and the investigational semustine have the unique ability to cross the blood–brain barrier, a capability linked to their lipid solubility. Thus, they are especially useful against primary and metastatic brain tumors. Alkylating agents are curative only in the treatment of Burkitt's lymphoma. However, long-term remissions have occurred in the treatment of acute lymphoblastic leukemia (90% remission with combination chemotherapy, 70% five-year survival according to American Cancer Society statistics) and stages IIIB and IV of Hodgkin's disease (70% response with 40% five-year survival according to American Cancer Society statistics). As a class, these agents share the common side effects of alopecia, bone marrow depression, nausea, vomiting, and impaired spermatogenesis in males. There are no significant interactions with any of the nitrosourea alkylating agents. The usual dose of carmustine is 100 mg/m^2 by slow intravenous infusion for two days, repeated every six weeks if the white blood cell count remains above 4,000/mm^3 and platelets above 100,000/mm^3. The usual dose of lomustine is 130 mg/m^2 repeated every six weeks, with dose adjustments based on patient level of bone marrow depression. Ideal dosage for the investigational semustine have yet to be determined.

TEXT RESUMES ON PAGE 1366

Table 49–1. ANTINEOPLASTIC AGENTS

Name	Dosage and Route	Uses	Precautions
Action: All antineoplastic agents interfere with cell growth or division of cancer cells either directly or indirectly. **Use:** All are used to treat neoplastic diseases, rarely used to treat other disease because of the severity of adverse effects.			

ALKYLATING AGENTS

Action: Cross-link strands of DNA leading to growth imbalance and cell death.

Name	Dosage and Route	Uses	Precautions
Mechlorethamine (Mustargen)	0.4 mg/kg or 6 to 10 mg/m^2 in single or divided doses in IV. Dosages decreased to 0.2–0.4 mg/kg following prior radiotherapy or chemotherapy. For neoplastic effusions, 10–20 mg intracavitarily.	Hodgkin's lymphoma; cancer of ovary, breast; bronchogenic cancer; and control of neoplastic effusions.	Severe tissue damage if infiltrated or spilled on skin.
Cyclophosphamide (Cytoxan)	Adults: 40–50 mg/kg/day PO or IV as single dose, or up to 5 divided doses daily; or 2–4 mg/kg PO qd for 10 days. Children: 2–8 mg/kg or 60–250 mg/m^2 PO or IV for 6 days	Acute lymphocytic leukemia; Hodgkin's disease; lymphosarcoma; many solid tumors; Wilm's tumor; rabdomyosarcoma.	Dehydrated patients may develop hemorrhagic cystitis due to drug concentration in kidneys and bladder. Not to be taken during pregnancy or while nursing.
Melphalan (Alkeran)	6 mg PO daily for 2–3 wk; then stop drug 4 wk before resuming cycle. 2–4 mg/day maintenance	Myeloma; cancer of breast, ovary, and testes; osteogenic sarcoma; malignant melanoma; and reticulum cell sarcoma.	Dose may need to be decreased if patient has renal impairment. Not to be taken during pregnancy (risk to fetus is significant) or while nursing.

*Within the column listing adverse effects, <u>underlines</u> indicate the most common effects; CAPITALS indicate life-threatening effects.

Interactions	Acute Toxic Signs	Adverse Effects*	Nursing Implications
None significant.	Nausea and vomiting.	Neuro: Vertigo. GI: Anorexia, nausea, vomiting. Hemo: BONE MARROW DEPRESSION. Integ: Corrosive to tissues if extravasation occurs. Metabolic: Hyperuricemia. Other: Alopecia, tinnitis, metallic taste, deafness in high doses.	INTERVENTION: Monitor IV sites carefully for signs of infiltration. Monitor CBC and platelets carefully. Solution is unstable; use within 15 minutes after preparation. Administer antiemetics as needed. EVALUATION: Determine effectiveness of antinausea and nutritional enhancement actions.
Corticosteroids and chloramphenicol can reduce activity of cyclophosphamide, use together cautiously. Succinylcholine—don't use together, may cause apnea.	Bone marrow depression, nausea and vomiting, hemorrhagic cystitis, anaphylaxis, cardiotoxicity (with high doses and in combination with adriamycin).	GI: Anorexia, nausea, vomiting, stomatitis. Hemo: BONE MARROW DEPRESSION. CV: CARDIOTOXICITY (high doses). GU: Gonadal suppression, hemorrhagic cystitis, sterility, nephrotoxicity. Metabolic: Immunosuppression, liver dysfunction, S.I.A.D.H. Other: Alopecia, ANAPHYLAXIS, PULMONARY FIBROSIS (in high doses).	ASSESSMENT: Assess respiratory status, breath sounds. Assess oral cavity for stomatitis. INTERVENTION: Monitor CBC, platelets, and liver enzymes. Push fluids, and monitor intake. Promote good oral care and bland diet to decrease oral irritation. EVALUATION: Determine effectiveness of antinausea and nutritional enhancement actions. Adequate hydration is achieved, cardiopulmonary status is unimpaired. Health teaching is successful.
Antigout drugs: may decrease antigout effect. Other antineoplastic drugs: may increase effect of all drugs (this can be beneficial for patient.)	None.	GI: Nausea, vomiting, stomatitis. Hemo: BONE MARROW DEPRESSION (AGRANULOCYTOSIS, LEUKOPENIA, THROMBOCYTOPENIA). GU: May cause sterility. Other: Pneumonitis, rare PULMONARY FIBROSIS.	ASSESSMENT: Assess respiratory status, breath sounds. Assess oral cavity for stomatitis. INTERVENTION: Monitor CBC and platelets. Promote good oral care and bland diet to decrease oral irritation. Administer drug on an empty stomach since food delays absorption. EVALUATION: Same as Mechlorethamine.

CONTINUED ON THE FOLLOWING PAGE

Table 49–1. ANTINEOPLASTIC AGENTS–*CONTINUED*

Name	Dosage and Route	Uses	Precautions
Chlorambucil (Leukeran)	0.1–0.2 mg/kg/day PO for 3–6 wk. 2–12 mg/day maintenance.	Chronic lymphocytic leukemia; Hodgkin's disease; lymphosarcoma; cancer of breast, ovary, or testes.	Do not give full dose less than 4 wk after a full dose of radiation. Bone marrow depression. Not to be taken during pregnancy (risk to fetus significant) or while nursing.
Carmustine (BCNU)	100 mg/m² by slow IV infusion for 2 days; repeat q 6 wk if WBC above 4,000/mm³ and platelets above 100,000/mm³.	Primary/secondary CNS tumors; lymphomas; multiple myeloma; and malignant melanoma.	Skin contact causes brown staining.
Thiotepa (Thiotepa)	0.2 mg/kg/day IV ×5 days. Maintenance 0.2 mg/kg IV q 1–3 wk. For bladder instillation: 60 mg in 60 ml sterile water q wk ×4. For malignant effusions: 10–15 mg intracavitarily prn.	Cancer of breast, ovary, lungs, or bladder; lymphomas; Hodgkin's disease; control of malignant effusions.	Potential anaphylactic reactions.
Busulfan (Myleran)	4–6 mg/day PO, up to 8 mg PO qd until WBC drops from 100,000/mm³ to 20,000/mm³.	Chronic myelocytic (granulocytic) leukemia.	Do not give if WBC below 10,000/mm³.

*Within the column listing adverse effects, underlines indicate the most common effects; CAPITALS indicate life-threatening effects.

Interactions	Acute Toxic Signs	Adverse Effects*	Nursing Implications
Same as Melphalan.	None.	GI: Nausea, vomiting. Hemo: Bone marrow depression (severe neutropenia.) GU: May cause sterility. Metabolic: Hyperuricemia. Other: Allergic febrile reactions, rare PULMONARY FIBROSIS.	ASSESSMENT: Assess respiratory status, breath sounds. INTERVENTION: Monitor CBC, platelets, uric acid levels, and nutritional status. EVALUATION: Same as Cytoxan.
None significant.	Nausea and vomiting.	GI: Nausea, vomiting. Hemo: Cumulative bone marrow depression (up to 6 weeks after drug.) Other: Mild hepatotoxicity, intense pain at infusion site, rare PULMONARY FIBROSIS.	ASSESSMENT: Assess respiratory status, breath sounds. INTERVENTION: Nausea and vomiting occur approximately 6 hours after administration; give antiemetics. Local vein discomfort and flushed sensation frequently occur after administration; explain to patient. Explain to patient that the bone marrow depression occurs 3–6 weeks after dose. EVALUATION: Same as Cytoxan.
None significant.	None.	Neuro: Headache, dizziness. GI: Tightness in throat, nausea, vomiting, rare GI perforation. Metabolic: Hyperuricemia, fever. Hemo: Bone marrow depression (anemia, leukopenia, neutropenia, and thrombocytopenia.) GU: Amenorrhea, decreased, spermatogenesis. Integ: Hives Other: Pain at administration site, ANAPHYLAXIS.	INTERVENTION: Monitor CBC, platelets, and renal enzymes, since drug used with caution in patients with pre-existing renal, hepatic, or bone marrow dysfunction. Appropriate health teaching. EVALUATION: Adequate nutritional status maintained. Health teaching successful.
None significant.	None.	GI: Nausea, vomiting, diarrhea. Hemo: Bone marrow, depression (anemia, pancytopenia, thrombocytopenia.) GU: Amenorrhea, testicular atrophy, impotence. Integ: transient hyperpigmentation. Metabolic: Profound hyperuricemia, Addison-like wasting syndrome. Other: Alopecia, gynecomastia, IRREVERSIBLE PULMONARY FIBROSIS ("BUSULFAN LUNG") possible up to 10 years after therapy.	ASSESSMENT: Assess respiratory status, breath sounds. INTERVENTION: Monitor CBC (WCB continues to fall for 2 weeks after therapy), platelets, urinary output. Explain side effects of amenorrhea, gynecomastia, and skin changes so patient is prepared if they occur. EVALUATION: Same as Cytoxan.

CONTINUED ON THE FOLLOWING PAGE

Table 49–1. ANTINEOPLASTIC AGENTS–*CONTINUED*

Name	Dosage and Route	Uses	Precautions
Dacarbazine (DTIC)	2–4.5 mg/kg or 70–160 mg/m² IV qd ×10 days and repeat q 4 wk.	Hodgkin's disease, metastatic malignant melanoma, neuroblastoma, sarcomas.	Infuse over 20-minute period. May burn on infusion and cause metallic taste in mouth. Drug is photosensitive.
Lomustine (CCNU)	130 mg/m² PO q 6 wk; reduce dose according to bone marrow depression.	Hodgkin's disease; primary and secondary CNS tumors; gastric, renal, and bronchogenic cancers. Multiple myeloma.	Do not repeat dose unless WBC is over 4,000/mm³ and platelets over 100,000/mm³.
Streptozocin (Zanosar)	500 mg/m² IV for 5 consecutive days q 6 wk until maximum benefit or toxicity occurs. Maximum single dose 1500 mg/m².	Pancreatic islet cell cancer.	Toxic to tissues if infiltration occurs. Use cautiously with other nephrotoxic drugs such as aminoglycosides. Drug is photosensitive (light-sensitive).

*Within the column listing adverse effects, underlines indicate the most common effects; CAPITALS indicate life-threatening effects.

Interactions	Acute Toxic Signs	Adverse Effects*	Nursing Implications
None significant.	Nausea and vomiting	GI: Severe nausea, vomiting (90% of patients.), anorexia. Hemo: Leukopenia, thrombocytopenia. Integ: Phototoxicity. Corrosive to tissues if infiltration occurs. Other: Flu-like syndrome (headache, myalgia, malaise) lasting several days, alopecia, pain at infusion site, mild hepatotoxicity.	ASSESSMENT: Assess IV site frequently for signs of infiltration. INTERVENTION: Explain to patient that nausea and vomiting generally decrease after several doses. Infection and bleeding precautions necessary due to bone marrow depression. Protect drug from light. Patient should avoid sunlight and sunlamps for first 2 days after treatment. EVALUATION: Antinausea and nutritional enhancement actions successful. No extravasation at IV sites. Infection/bleeding precautions successful.
None significant.	Nausea and vomiting.	GI: Nausea, vomiting, stomatitis. Hemo: Leukopenia (may be delayed 6 wks.), thrombocytopenia (delayed up to 4 wks.) GU: Nephrotoxicity. Other: Alopecia.	ASSESSMENT: Assess oral mucosa for lesions, stomatitis. INTERVENTION: Give 2–4 hours after meals. Give antiemetic before chemotherapy. Nausea and vomiting occur 2–6 hours after dose. Warn patient that bone marrow depression can occur 4–6 weeks after dose; infection and bleeding precautions necessary. Teach appropriate oral care that minimizes trauma to oral tissues. EVALUATION: Antinausea and nutritional enhancement actions successful. Health teaching effective. Infection/bleeding precautions successful.
Other potentially nephrotoxic drugs such as aminoglycosides: additive nephrotoxicity—use cautiously. Phenytoin: may decrease the effects of streptozocin. Monitor carefully.	Nausea and vomiting.	GI: Nausea, vomiting, diarrhea, stomatitis, cramps. Hemo: APLASTIC ANEMIA, mild drop in hematocrit levels. Hepatic: Elevated liver enzymes. Metabolic: Hyperglycemia, hypoglycemia. Renal: RENAL TOXICITY (symptoms azotemia, glycosuria, and renal tubular acidosis.)	ASSESSMENT: Assess IV site frequently for signs of infiltration. Assess oral cavity for lesions and stomatitis. INTERVENTION: Test urine for glycosuria. Avoid extravasation; check vein patency before administering. Tell patient drug often burns on administration and this sensation will pass. Give IV infusion slowly. Store drug in refrigerator. Drug is photosensitive; protect from light. EVALUATION: Antinausea and nutritional enhancement actions successful. No extravasation at IV sites. Nephrotoxicity avoided.

CONTINUED ON THE FOLLOWING PAGE

Antineoplastic Agents

Table 49–1. ANTINEOPLASTIC AGENTS–CONTINUED

Name	Dosage and Route	Uses	Precautions
Cisplatin (Platinol)	20 mg/m^2 IV qd ×5; repeat q 3 wk for metastatic testicular cancer. 100 mg/m^2 IV q 4 wk as adjunct in metastatic ovarian cancer.	Metastatic ovarian or testicular cancer; bladder cancer.	Do not use aluminum needles when preparing drug—a black precipitate will form.

ANTIMETABOLITES

Action: All antimetabolites interfere with DNA metabolism.

Name	Dosage and Route	Uses	Precautions
Methotrexate (MTX, Mexate)	3.3 mg/m^2 PO, IM, or IV daily for 4–6 wk or until remission occurs. Doses vary greatly, depending on disease being treated and patient status. High-dose therapy (over 100-mg IV doses) must be followed by leucovorin rescue.	Acute leukemia; choriocarcinoma; lymphosarcoma; solid tumors; osteogenic sarcomas; head, neck, lung, breast, and ovarian tumors. Also for severe adult psoriasis, and rheumatoid arthritis.	Used cautiously in hepatic or renal dysfunction and in bone marrow depression.
Floxuridine (FUDR)	0.1–0.6 mg/kg/day by intra-arterial infusion pump, or 0.4–0.6 mg/kg/day into hepatic artery.	Breast, brain, liver, gallbladder, or bile duct tumors; head and neck tumors.	Stop drug if WBC falls below 3,500/mm^3 or platelets below 100,000/mm^3. Drug used cautiously in impaired renal or hepatic function.

*Within the column listing adverse effects, underlines indicate the most common effects; CAPITALS indicate life-threatening effects.

Interactions	Acute Toxic Signs	Adverse Effects*	Nursing Implications
Aminoglycoside antibiotics: Additive nephrotoxicity. Renal studies should be carefully monitored.	None.	GI: Severe nausea & vomiting, diarrhea. CNS: Peripheral neuritis. GU: Chances of renal toxicity increases with repeat courses of therapy. Other: ANAPHYLAXIS, ototoxicity.	INTERVENTION: Prehydration and mannitol-induced diuresis may significantly decrease ototoxicity and nephrotoxicity. Do not repeat dose of drug unless WBC above 4000/mm^3, BUN less than 25 mg/dl, and creatinine less than 1.5 mg/dl. Metoclopramide is useful in treating nausea and vomiting associated with platinol. Reconstituted drug stable 24 hours at room temperature. EVALUATION: Antinausea and nutritional enhancement actions successful. Nephrotoxicity avoided.
Alcohol: increased hepatotoxicity, warn patient to avoid alcoholic beverages. Probenecid, phenylbutazone, salicylates (including aspirin), sulfonamides, tetracyclines: increases methotrexate toxicity.	Elevated SGOT, SGPT, alkaline phosphatase may indicate hepatotoxicity. Skin rash, oral ulcers, or pulmonary side effects can indicate serious problems.	Neuro: ARACHNOIDITIS after intrathecal administration; subacute neurotoxicity weeks later; demyelinating leukoencephalopathy years later. GI: Nausea, vomiting, stomatitis, diarrhea, HEMORRHAGIC, ENTERITIS AND INTESTINAL PERFORATION. Hemo: Dose-related bone marrow depression (anemia, leukopenia, thrombocytopenia.) GU: TUBULAR NECROSIS. Metabolic: Hyperuricemia. Integ: Photosensitivity, rash. Other: Alopecia, PULMONARY INTERSTITIAL INFILTRATES.	ASSESSMENT: Assess oral mucosa for lesions, stomatitis. INTERVENTION: Monitor CBC, platelets, and liver and renal enzymes. Effects of drug toxicity increased by salicylates, sulfonamides, phenylbutazone, and PABA. Tell patient to avoid use of self-administered vitamins. If possible, avoid giving with tetracyclines, chloramphenicol, and phenytoin. Patient should abstain from alcohol while on this drug, as it can cause increased hepatotoxicity. Teach appropriate oral care. EVALUATION: Same as Platinol.
None significant.	None	Hemo: Bone marrow depression (anemia, leukopenia, thrombocytopenia.) Neuro: Cerebellar ataxia, vertigo, depression, lethargy, hemiplegia. GI: Cramps, nausea, vomiting, stomatitis, diarrhea, bleeding, enteritis. Other: Blurred vision, erythema, dermatitis, pruritis.	INTERVENTION: Monitor intake and output, CBC, and renal and hepatic functions. Reconstitute with sterile water and add to 5% dextrose in water or 0.9% sodium chloride solution for IV infusion. Observe and care for arterial line appropriately. Teach appropriate oral care. EVALUATION: Antinausea and nutritional enhancement actions successful. Hepatic and renal toxicity avoided. Health teaching successful.

CONTINUED ON THE FOLLOWING PAGE

Table 49–1. ANTINEOPLASTIC AGENTS–*CONTINUED*

Name	Dosage and Route	Uses	Precautions
Fluorouracil (5-FU)	12.5 mg/kg/day ×3–5 days. Smaller doses 1–2×/wk for maintenance. May also be given intra-arterially or topically.	Cancer of GI tract, breast, uterus, lung, ovary, liver, skin, bladder, and oropharynx.	Used cautiously in presence of serious infections, bone marrow depression, impaired hepatic or renal function, cachexia.
Cytarabine (Cytosine arabinoside, Cytosar)	200 mg/m^2 qd by continuous IV infusion for 5 days. May also be given SC and intrathecally. Intrathecal dose range 10–30 mg/m^2 up to 3×/wk.	Acute granulocytic leukemia, lymphocytic leukemia.	Infuse slowly, usually over 24 hours, by continuous infusion pump. Stop drug if polymorphonuclear granulocyte count is 1,000/mm^3 or platelets below 50,000/mm^3.
Mercaptopurine (6-MP, Purinethol)	80–100 mg/m^2 PO qd as single dose, up to 5 mg/kg daily. Children given slightly lower doses: 70 mg/m^2 qd. Maintenance dose for adults and children is 1.5–2.5 mg/kg/day.	Acute lymphoblastic leukemia in children; chronic myelocytic leukemia.	Contraindicated in alcoholics and in liver dysfunction. Decrease dose to ⅓ or ¼ of normal dose if allopurinol is given concurrently. Used with caution following radiotherapy or other chemotherapy. Avoid drug if pregnant or nursing.
Thioguanine (6-TG)	Adult and pediatric: 2 mg/kg/day PO. Dose may be increased to 3 mg/kg/day if no toxic effects occur.	Acute leukemia; chronic granulocytic leukemia.	
Hydroxyurea (Hydrea)	80 mg/kg PO every 3 days, or 20–30 mg/kg PO qd.	Chronic granulocytic leukemia; malignant melanoma; recurrent, metastatic, or inoperable ovarian cancer.	Give with caution to patients with liver or kidney impairment. Drug is synergistic with radiotherapy. Stop drug if WBC falls below 2,500/mm^3 or platelets below 100,000/mm^3.

*Within the column listing adverse effects, underlines indicate the most common effects; CAPITALS indicate life-threatening effects.

Interactions	Acute Toxic Signs	Adverse Effects*	Nursing Implications
None significant.	Stomatitis and diarrhea. (Stomatitis is precursor of bone marrow depression.)	**Neuro:** Rare cerebellar dysfunction. **GI:** Nausea, vomiting, stomatitis, GI ulcer may precede leukopenia. **Hemo:** Anemia, leukopenia, thrombocytopenia. **Integ:** Dermatitis, hyperpigmentation, nail changes. **Other:** Alopecia, weakness, malaise.	INTERVENTION: Monitor CBC and platelets. Drug most effective in mildly toxic range. Give frequent oral care; administer antiemetics before fluorouracil therapy. Stop drug if WBC drops below 3,500/mm³ or platelets below 100,000/mm³. EVALUATION: Antinausea and nutritional enhancement actions successful. Bone marrow toxicity minimized.
None significant.	Nausea and vomiting.	**Hemo:** Anemia, leukopenia, MEGALOBLASTOSIS, reticulocytopenia, thrombocytopenia. **GI:** Dysphagia, nausea, vomiting, stomatitis, diarrhea. **Hepatic:** Mild hepatotoxicity. **Metabolic:** Hyperuricemia. **Integ:** Rash. **Other:** Flu-like syndrome	INTERVENTION: Give antiemetics (start before cytarabine), as nausea and vomiting are common with high doses of drug. Good oral hygiene and bland diet should be promoted. Monitor CBC, platelets, and liver enzymes. Store unreconstituted drug in refrigerator. Once mixed, drug is stable for 48 hours in refrigerator. EVALUATION: Same as fluorouracil.
Acetaminophen and Isoniazid: increased likelihood of liver toxicity. Allopurinol: may increase toxic effect of mercaptopurine, reduce mercaptopurine dose by ⅔ to ¾ of normal dose. Other antineoplastic drugs: increased effect of both (may be desirable) or increased toxicity of each drug.	None.	**Hemo:** Decreased RBC, anemia, leukopenia, thrombocytopenia. **GI:** Anorexia, nausea, vomiting, stomatitis. **Hepatic:** Jaundice, HEPATIC NECROSIS. **Metabolic:** Hyperuricemia.	ASSESSMENT: Observe oral mucosa for lesions, stomatitis. INTERVENTION: Monitor CBC, platelets, uric acid, and liver enzymes. Push fluids. Give antiemetics as needed. Teach oral care that minimizes trauma to oral tissues. EVALUATION: Antinausea and nutritional support actions successful. Bone marrow and hepatic toxicity avoided.
None significant.	None.	**Hemo:** Bone marrow depression—anemia, leukopenia, thrombocytopenia. **GI:** Stomatitis, nausea, vomiting, diarrhea, anorexia. **Hepatic:** Jaundice, hepatic dysfunction. **Metabolic:** Hyperuricemia. **Other:** Rash.	ASSESSMENT: Observe oral mucosa for lesions, stomatitis. INTERVENTION: Monitor CBC, platelets, & liver enzymes. Teach appropriate oral care. EVALUATION: Same as Mercaptopurine.
None significant.	None.	**Hemo:** Anemia, leukopenia, MEGALOBLASTOSIS, thrombocytopenia.	ASSESSMENT: Observe oral mucosa for lesions, stomatitis.

CONTINUED ON THE FOLLOWING PAGE

Table 49–1. ANTINEOPLASTIC AGENTS–_CONTINUED_

Name	Dosage and Route	Uses	Precautions
Hydroxyurea–_Continued_			

NATURAL PRODUCTS

Plant Alkaloids

Action: Vinca alkaloids arrest mitosis in metaphase to block cell division.

Name	Dosage and Route	Uses	Precautions
Vincristine (Oncovin, VCR)	Adults: 1–2 mg/m² IV weekly. Children: 1.5–2 mg/m² IV weekly. Maximum single dose is 2 mg (adults and children). Children <10 kg: 0.05 mg/kg.	Acute lymphoblastic leukemia; other leukemias; lymphoma; neuroblastoma; Wilm's tumor; rhabdomyosarcoma; cancer of the testes, lung or breast; reticulum cell, osteogenic and other sarcomas.	Very toxic to skin if infiltrated. Used with caution in patients with pre-existing neuropathies, hepatic dysfunction.
Vinblastine (Velban, VLB)	0.1 mg/kg or 3.7 mg/m² IV per wk or q 2 wk. Dose may be increased to maximum of 0.5 mg/kg or 18.5 mg/m² IV q wk for adults.	Hodgkin's and other lymphomas; breast or testicular malignancies; lymphosarcoma; neuroblastoma; mycosis fungoides.	Causes corneal ulceration if splashed in eye. Very toxic to skin if infiltration occurs. Has cumulative toxicity.

*Within the column listing adverse effects, underlines indicate the most common effects; CAPITALS indicate life-threatening effects.

Interactions	Acute Toxic Signs	Adverse Effects*	Nursing Implications
		Neuro: Drowsiness, hallucinations. GI: Anorexia, nausea, vomiting, diarrhea, stomatitis. GU: Elevated BUN and creatinine levels. Integ: Pruritis and rash. Metabolic: Hyperuricemia.	INTERVENTION: Monitor CBC, platelets, liver, and renal enzymes. Give antiemetics as needed. Push fluids. Teach oral care that minimizes trauma to tissues. EVALUATION: Same as Mercaptopurine.
None significant.	None.	Neuro: Peripheral neuropathy, paresthesias, loss of deep tendon reflexes, ataxia, cranial nerve palsies (jaw pain), cramps, muscle weakness, NEUROTOXICITIES MAY BE PERMANENT. GI: Constipation, cramps, anorexia, nausea, vomiting, stomatitis, paralytic ileus. Hemo: Mild anemia, leukopenia. GU: Urinary retention. Other: Diplopia, phlebitis, cellulitis, alopecia. Integ: Corrosive to tissue on infiltration.	ASSESSMENT: Assess oral mucosa. Assess infusion site. INTERVENTION: Monitor CBC and platelets. Do frequent neurologic checks. Watch for signs of neurotoxicity. Give drug direct IV or into tubing of running IV after determining that needle is placed in vein. Give antiemetics as needed. Teach good oral care. Monitor for constipation (may be early sign of neurotoxicity.) EVALUATION: Antinausea and nutritional support actions are successful. No extravasation at IV sites occurs. Bone marrow and neurotoxicities are avoided.
None significant.	Nausea, vomiting, stomatitis.	Neuro: Peripheral neuropathies, paresthesias, neuropathy, neuritis, loss of deep tendon reflexes, muscle pain, and weakness. GI: Nausea, vomiting, stomatitis, weight loss, anorexia, paralytic ileus. Hemo: Leukopenia, thrombocytopenia. Integ: Corrosive to tissue on infiltration. GU: Aspermia, urinary retention. Other: Alopecia, pain in tumor site.	ASSESSMENT: Assess oral mucosa. Assess IV infusion site. INTERVENTION: Monitor CBC and platelets. Do frequent neurologic checks. Watch for IV site infiltration—Phlebitis, cellulitis, and tissue necrosis can occur if drug extravasates. Monitor for leukopenia, thrombocytopenia, constipation, and urinary retention. Teach good oral care. EVALUATION: Same as Vincristine.

CONTINUED ON THE FOLLOWING PAGE

Table 49–1. ANTINEOPLASTIC AGENTS–*CONTINUED*

Name	Dosage and Route	Uses	Precautions

Antibiotics

Actions: Dactinomycin, daunorubicin and doxorubicin interfere with DNA-dependent RNA synthesis. Bleomycin inhibits DNA synthesis. Mitomycin cross-links strands of DNA causing growth imbalance and cell death. Plicamycin inhibits osteocytic activity. Procarbazine inhibits DNA, RNA, and protein synthesis.

Name	Dosage and Route	Uses	Precautions
Dactinomycin (Cosmegen, Actinomycin D)	Adults: 500 μg IV/day $\times$5; wait 2–4 wk, then repeat. Children with Wilm's tumor: 15 μg/kg IV qd $\times$5 days. Maximum dose 500 μg/day.	Wilms' tumor, choriocarcinoma; testicular cancer; rhabdomyosarcoma; melanoma; Ewing's sarcoma.	Corrosive to tissue if infiltrated. May reactivate radiation site if given after radiation therapy. Used cautiously in combination with chlorambucil or methotrexate therapy. Contraindicated in presence of renal, hepatic or bone marrow impairment; viral infections; or herpes zoster or chicken pox.
Daunorubicin (Cerubidine)	60 mg/m^2 IV qd on days 1–3 of 3- or 4-wk cycle when used as sole induction agent. In combination chemotherapy, dose is 45 mg/m^2 IV qd, days 1–3 of first chemotherapy cycle and days 1 and 2 of subsequent cycles. Maximum total lifetime dose is 450–550 mg/m^2 due to cumulative cardiotoxicity.	Acute nonlymphocytic leukemia; acute myeloid leukemia.	Cardiac toxicity at cumulative doses over 550 mg/m^2 (25 mg/kg). Avoid extravasation; severe tissue necrosis may result.
Doxorubicin (Adriamycin)	60–75 mg/m^2 in single or divided doses q 3 wk IV. Or 30 mg/m^2 single daily dose IV, days 1–3 of 28-day cycle. Maximum life-time dose is 550 mg/m^2.	Sarcomas; Hodgkin's disease; acute leukemia; breast, genitourinary, thyroid, and lung cancers; neuroblastoma; lymphomas; Wilms' tumor; head, neck, and ovarian tumors.	Drug very toxic if infiltrated. May cause cardiomyopathy.

*Within the column listing adverse effects, underlines indicate the most common effects; CAPITALS indicate life-threatening effects.

Interactions	Acute Toxic Signs	Adverse Effects*	Nursing Implications
None significant.	Nausea and vomiting.	GI: Anorexia, nausea, vomiting, stomatitis, diarrhea. Hemo: Anemia, leukopenia, pancytopenia, thrombocytopenia. Integ: Erythema, hyperpigmentation, "acne-like" eruptions, phlebitis, corrosive to tissues on infiltration. Other: Alopecia.	ASSESSMENT: Assess oral mucosa. Assess IV infusion site. INTERVENTION: Watch IV site carefully for infiltration. Promote good oral care and bland diet. Monitor CBC, platelets, and renal hepatic functions. Avoid extravasation; give via a well-running IV. Use sterile water without preservatives for reconstitution. Do not expose solution to direct sunlight. EVALUATION: Antinausea and nutritional support actions are successful. No extravasation at IV sites occurs. Bone marrow toxicity avoided. Health teaching successful.
Heparin; don't mix, may form a precipitate.	Severe nausea and vomiting, fever, congestive heart failure, cardiomyopathy.	GI: Anorexia, nausea, vomiting, stomatitis, esophagitis. CV: DOSE-RELATED CARDIOMYOPATHY, EKG changes, ARRHYTHMIAS, pericarditis. Renal: Nephrotoxicity. Hepatic:Hepatotoxicity. Integ: Rash, tissue corrosive if extravasated. Other: Alopecia, fever, chills.	ASSESSMENT: Assess oral mucosa. Assess IV infusion site. INTERVENTION: Monitor CBC, platelets, cardiac enzymes, and ECG. A high resting pulse rate may indicate cardiac side effects. Urine turns red due to drug, not hematuria; warn patient of this harmless side effect. Inject drug into free-flowing IV. Never give drug IM or SC. Do not mix with heparin; a precipitate will form. EVALUATION: Same as Dactinomycin plus cardiotoxicity, nephrotoxicity and hepatotoxicity are avoided.
Streptozocin: increased and prolonged blood levels of doxorubicin can occur. Dose may need adjusting.	Nausea, vomiting, cardiac depression, arrhythmias.	GI: Nausea, vomiting, stomatitis. CV: CARDIAC TOXICITY (dose-related.) EKG changes, ARRHYTHMIAS. Hemo: Agranulocytosis, leukopenia, thrombocytopenia. Integ: Tissue corrosive if infiltrated, hyperpigmentation of skin, nails. Other: Alopecia.	ASSESSMENT: Assess oral mucosa. Assess IV infusion site. INTERVENTION: Monitor CBC, platelets, liver enzymes, ECG, and cardiac enzymes. Observe for signs of cardiac decompensation. Forewarn patient that drug causes red urine (not hematuria). Avoid extravasation—inject into free-flowing IV. Teach good oral care.

CONTINUED ON THE FOLLOWING PAGE

Table 49–1. ANTINEOPLASTIC AGENTS–*CONTINUED*

Name	Dosage and Route	Uses	Precautions
Doxorubicin–*Continued*			
Bleomycin (Blenoxane)	10–20 units/m² IV, IM or SC 1–2×/wk. Maximum total dose is 300–400 units. For adults with Hodgkin's disease, follow same dosing schedule and after patient response, give maintenance dose of 1 unit IM or IV qd or 5 units/wk.	Hodgkin's disease; lymphomas; testicular and urinary tract carcinomas; head and neck tumors; skin and cervical cancer; mycosis fungoides.	Test dose given before therapeutic dose, as occasional anaphylaxis can occur in 1%–6% of patients. First 2 doses should be 5 units (or less) of drug in order to test for anaphylaxis.
Mitomycin (Mutamycin)	Adults: 20 mg/m² IV as a single dose. Repeat cycle q 6–8 wk. Can also be given by bladder instillation (20 mg drug per 20 ml diluent) or by intra-arterial administration via hepatic artery.	Gastric, breast, cervical, head, and neck carcinoma; malignant melanoma; lung, colon and pancreatic cancers; chronic myelogenous leukemia; bladder and some hepatic tumors.	Toxic to tissues; avoid extravasation.
Procarbazine (Matulane)	100–150 mg/m² PO for 10 days until WBC drops below 4,000/mm³. Maintenance dose 50–100 mg PO qd.	Hodgkin's disease; non-Hodgkin's lymphoma; bronchogenic carcinoma; multiple myeloma; malignant melanoma; polycythemia vera; and brain tumors.	Drug inhibits monoamine oxidase (MAO) and is used cautiously with other MAO inhibitors, tricyclic antidepressants, and phenothiazines. Use with alcohol causes disulfiram reaction—headache, diaphoresis, nausea, vomiting, hyperventilation, chest pain, syncope, anxiety, weakness. Drug crosses blood–brain barrier. Dispose of used drug administration equipment to prevent

*Within the column listing adverse effects, underlines indicate the most common effects; CAPITALS indicate life-threatening effects.

Interactions	Acute Toxic Signs	Adverse Effects*	Nursing Implications
			EVALUATION: Same as Dactinomycin plus cardiotoxicity avoided.
None significant.	Allergic reactions 3–5 hours after initial dose. Pulmonary fibrosis: dose-related and seen with cumulative doses greater than 400 units.	Neuro: Hyperesthesia of fingers and scalp. GI: Anorexia, nausea, vomiting, stomatitis, diarrhea. Hemo: Bone marrow depression (rare). Integ: Hyperpigmentation, acne, erythema, vesiculation and hardening of plantar and palmar skin. Other: PULMONARY FIBROSIS occurs in 10% of pts., pulmonary side effects (dyspnea, fever, rales cough.) Alopecia. ANAPHYLAXIS 1–6% of pts.	ASSESSMENT: Assess oral mucosa. Assess respiratory status. INTERVENTION: Fever generally occurs only on first day of therapy and subsides with acetaminophen. Watch patient for signs of pulmonary fibrosis. Monitor CBC, platelets, uric acid levels, blood gasses, and pulmonary function studies. Teach good oral care. EVALUATION: Antinausea and nutritional support actions successful. Pulmonary side effects avoided. Health teaching effective.
None significant.	Nausea and vomiting.	Neuro: Paresthesias, CNS toxicity. GI: Anorexia, nausea, vomiting, stomatitis. Hemo: Leukopenia, thrombocytopenia. Integ: Pain at infusion site; corrosive to tissue on infiltration, purple bands in nails. Other: Alopecia, renal damage, hepatic damage, can be teratogenic.	ASSESSMENT: Assess oral mucosa. Assess IV site. INTERVENTION: Monitor CBC, platelets, and renal and hepatic enzymes. Take care not to allow drug to infiltrate tissues. Teach pt. bland diet and oral care to help reduce discomfort of stomatitis. Give antiemetics before drug. Stop drug if WBC drops below 4,000/mm³ or platelets below 75,000/mm³. EVALUATION: Antinausea and nutritional support actions are successful. No extravasation at IV sites occurs. Renal, hepatic, bone marrow and neurotoxicities are avoided. Health teaching is effective.
Alcohol: Antabuse-type reaction. Also avoid: tricyclic antidepressants, phenothiazines; and foods high in tyramines.	Nausea and vomiting.	CNS: Confusion, insomnia, hallucinations, mental depression, mild CNS toxicity. GI: Anorexia, nausea, vomiting, stomatitis. Hemo: Anemia, leukopenia, thrombocytopenia, bleeding tendency. Integ: Dermatitis. Other: Alpecia, photophobia, pleural effusion.	ASSESSMENT: Assess oral mucosa. Assess IV site. INTERVENTION: Teach appropriate oral care. Give antiemetics but no phenothiazines for nausea and vomiting. Drug is an MAO inhibitor, so tell patient to avoid alcohol, sedatives, narcotics, tricyclic antidepressants (check with physician before taking any medication). Also, patient should avoid foods with high tyramine content. Mon-

CONTINUED ON THE FOLLOWING PAGE

Antineoplastic Agents

Table 49–1. ANTINEOPLASTIC AGENTS–*CONTINUED*

Name	Dosage and Route	Uses	Precautions
Procarbazine–*Continued*			unnecessary human exposure; drug is known carcinogen.
Plicamycin (Mithracin)	25 μg/kg IV daily ×3–4 days for treatment of hypercalcemia secondary to cancer. Or 25–50 μg/kg IV qd for 3–8 doses.	Greatest antitumor effect is against disseminated embryonal carcinoma of the testes. Greatest clinical use is in treatment of hypercalcemia of malignancy unresponsive to other therapy.	Toxic to tissues if infiltrated. Use gentle rotation of vial to reconstitute drug. Avoid admixture with solutions containing trace elements as drug rapidly chelates.

ENZYME

Action: Asparaginase destroys the amino acid asparagine which is needed for protein synthesis of leukemic cells leading to cell death of leukemia cells.

L-Asparaginase (Elspar)	Acute lymphocytic leukemia (in combination therapy): 1000 IU/kg/day IV for 10 days. Give over 30 min in 0.9% NaCl solution. As sole induction agent: 200 IU/kg/day IV for 28 days.	Acute lymphocytic leukemia.	Shaking vial harms enzyme.

*Within the column listing adverse effects, <u>underlines</u> indicate the most common effects; CAPITALS indicate life-threatening effects.

Interactions	Acute Toxic Signs	Adverse Effects*	Nursing Implications
			itor CBC, platelets, and liver enzymes. Observe patient for signs of bleeding. Warn patient that alcohol intake can produce acute illness (disulfiram-like reaction). EVALUATION: Health teaching of food/fluid restrictions effective and adverse reactions are avoided. Antinausea interventions are effective. Severe bone marrow depression is avoided.
None significant.	Nausea, vomiting, hemorrhagic syndrome.	GI: Anorexia, nausea, vomiting, stomatitis, diarrhea. Hemo: Bleeding, thrombocytopenia. Renal: Renal toxicity, proteinuria. Integ: Hyperpigmentation of skin, corrosive to tissues on infiltration. Metabolic: Decreased serum calcium, potassium, phosphorus. Other: Hepatotoxicity.	ASSESSMENT: Assess oral mucosa. Assess IV site. INTERVENTION: Monitor CBC, platelets, liver and kidney functions, prothrombin bleeding and clotting times, and calcium and potassium levels. Prevent IV infiltration. Infuse over 4 to 6 hours in large-volume dilutions or over 20 to 30 minutes in small-volume dilutions. Observe patient for signs of hypocalcemia, muscle weakness, and signs of bleeding. Teach pt. oral care. Give antiemetics as needed. EVALUATION: Health teaching is effective. Extravasation at IV sites is avoided. Renal, hepatic, and bone marrow toxicities are avoided.
None significant.	Nausea, vomiting, anorexia, fever, hypersensitivity reactions.	Neuro: Lethargy, somnolence. GI: Anorexia, nausea, vomiting, weight loss, HEMORRHAGIC PANCREATITIS. GU: Azotemia, renal failure, polyuria. Integ: Rash, urticaria. Metabolic: Hyperglycemia, increased serum ammonia. Other: ANAPHYLAXIS, hepatotoxicity (reversible).	ASSESSMENT: Assess oral mucosa for lesions, stomatitis. INTERVENTION: Monitor CBC, platelets, renal and pancreatic enzymes, clotting studies, uric acid, glucose, and serum albumin levels. Do not shake vial. Administer clear solutions only. Risk of hypersensitivity increases with each dose. Test dose administration can identify patients at risk. Teach patient oral care. Give antiemetics as needed.

CONTINUED ON THE FOLLOWING PAGE

Table 49–1. ANTINEOPLASTIC AGENTS–*CONTINUED*

Name	Dosage and Route	Uses	Precautions
L-Asparaginase–*Continued*			
HORMONES			
Action (in Neoplastic Diseases: To render environment inhospitable to growth of cancer cells by changing hormonal environment within patient.			
Steroids Prednisone (Deltasone, Orasone)	1–100 mg/day PO	All steroids: leukemia; lymphoma; breast, ovary and prostate cancers; multiple myeloma.	All steroids: Given with caution to patients with herpes simplex, keratitis, acute infections, or acute psychosis.
Prednisolone (Delta-Cortef) Methylprednisolone succinate (Solu-Medrol)	2.5–15 mg PO bid, tid, or qid; 2–30 mg IM. Adults: 2–60 mg PO in 4 divided doses daily; 10–250 mg IM q 4 hr. Children: 117 μg–1.66 mg/kg IM.		
Estrogens Diethylstilbestrol (DES)	15 mg qd PO for breast cancer; 1 mg/day for prostate cancer.	Prostatic and breast carcinomas.	Mental depression, liver dysfunction.
Ethinyl estradiol (Estinyl)	1.0 mg tid PO for breast cancer; 0.15–2 mg/day for prostate cancer.		

*Within the column listing adverse effects, underlines indicate the most common effects; CAPITALS indicate life-threatening effects.

Interactions	Acute Toxic Signs	Adverse Effects*	Nursing Implications
			EVALUATION: Antinausea interventions are effective. Renal, hepatic, and pancreatic toxicities are avoided.
Barbiturates, phenytoin, rifampin: decreases corticosteroid effect. Indomethacin, aspirin: increased risk of GI distress/bleeding. Same as Prednisone. Same as Prednisone.	All steroids: None with any steroid when given in therapeutic doses.	All steroids Neuro: Euphoria, insomnia, psychosis (rare). GI: Gastric bleeding, ulcer, increased appetite. Hemo: CHF, hypertension, edema. Integ: Acne, delayed healing. Metabolic: Possible hyperglycemia, hypokalemia. Other: Muscle weakness, increased risk of infections. Long-term causes body changes such as "moon face," purpura, striae, trunk obesity, and rarely psychosis. Can also cause adrenal atrophy. SUDDEN CESSATION OF STEROIDS AFTER LONG-TERM THERAPY MAY BE FATAL.	ASSESSMENT: Assess patient for mood swings, changes in psychological status. INTERVENTION: All steroids: Monitor electrolytes; patient should have electrolyte levels done regularly during therapy. Observe diabetics carefully, as steroid administration makes diabetes more difficult to manage. Encourage intake of foods high in potassium. Monitor blood pressure. Have patient avoid aspirin and take drug with milk or antacid. Report any dramatic mood swings to physician. EVALUATION: Health teaching is effective. Serious GI effects are avoided.
None significant. None significant.	Occasional nausea and vomiting.	All estrogens Neuro: Anxiety, headache, vertigo, insomnia. GI: Nausea, weight changes, vomiting. CV: THROMBOEMBOLISM, phlebitis, edema, hypertension. GU: Uterine bleeding, libido changes. Metabolic: Changes in calcium, phosphorus, and folic acid metabolism. In Males: Feminization—gynecomastia, testicular atrophy, impotence.	ASSESSMENT: Assess males for signs of feminization. Assess for signs of phlebitis. INTERVENTION: All estrogens: monitor calcium and phosphorus levels. Give antiemetics for nausea and vomiting. Encourage low-salt diet. Monitor weight. For male patients, warn of feminizing effects and decreased libido, and explain that these effects abate when drug is discontinued. Use during pregnancy causes vaginal cancer in some female offspring and testicular tumors in some male offspring. EVALUATION: Health teaching is effective. Serious vascular problems are avoided. Males do not suffer severe self-esteem problems due to feminizing effects of drugs.

CONTINUED ON THE FOLLOWING PAGE

Table 49–1. ANTINEOPLASTIC AGENTS–*CONTINUED*

Name	Dosage and Route	Uses	Precautions
Androgens Fluoxymesterone (Halostestin)	NOTE: doses vary according to drug preparation being used and patient need. 10–45 mg PO qd individual doses	Breast cancer postmenopausal or postcastration (in females).	Liver disease, nephritis, nephrosis.
Testosterone (Andronaq, Malogen)	100 mg IM 3 times per week		
Estrogen Antagonist Tamoxifen citrate (Nolvadex)	10–20 mg PO bid	Advanced premenopausal and postmenopausal breast cancer.	
Progestins Hydroxyprogesterone	1–5 g IM/wk.	Endometrial carcinomas.	All progestins: History of depression, porphyria, cardiac or renal disease.
Methylhydroxyprogesterone (Provera)	400–1,000 mg IM/wk.	Endometrial, renal cell, and breast carcinomas.	
Megestrol acetate (Megace)	40 mg PO qid (breast cancer.) 40–320 mg/day PO (endometrial cancer.)	Breast and endometrial carcinomas.	

*Within the column listing adverse effects, <u>underlines</u> indicate the most common effects; CAPITALS indicate life-threatening effects.

Interactions	Acute Toxic Signs	Adverse Effects*	Nursing Implications
None significant.	None with any androgen when given in therapeutic doses.	**All androgens (in Females)** GI: Nausea, vomiting, weight gain. CV: Edema and fluid retention. GU: Vaginal dryness, itching, menstrual irregularities. Integ: Acne, oily skin, hirsutism. Metabolic: Hypercalcemia if bone lesions present. Other: Pain at IM injection sites. Masculinization of Females—clitoral enlargement, libido changes, hirsutism, menstrual irregularities.	ASSESSMENT: Assess patient for masculinizing effects. INTERVENTION: All androgens: Monitor weight, encourage low-salt diet, and observe for edema. Restrict fluids if necessary. Give antiemetics if needed. Give psychologic support and explain that masculinizing effects abate when drug is discontinued. Monitor blood pressure. EVALUATION: Health teaching is effective. Patient's self-image does not suffer unduly from masculinizing effects of drugs.
None significant. None significant.			
None significant.	None	GI: Anorexia, nausea. Hemo: Temporary drop in WBC. Integ: Rash. GU: Vaginal discharge, bleeding. Other: Hot flashes, temporary bone pain (at metastases), temporary tumor pain.	ASSESSMENT: Ask patient if she is pre- or post-menopausal. INTERVENTION: Monitor WBC and platelets. Side effects are generally minor. Short-term therapy causes ovulation in premenopausal women—mechanical contraception is recommended. Appropriate Health teaching. EVALUATION: Health teaching is effective.
None significant.	None with any progestin given in therapeutic doses.	Neuro: Depression, dizziness, headache, lethargy. GI: Nausea, vomiting, cramps. GU: Amenorrhea, breakthrough bleeding, dysmenorrhea, cervical erosions, vaginal candidiasis. CV: Edema, PULMONARY EMBOLISM, phlebitis, hypertension. Integ: Rash, pain at injection site. Metabolic: Hyperglycemia. Other: Breast tenderness, enlargement, discharge. Decreased libido. Methylhydroxyprogesterone: Same as hydroxyprogesterone. Megestrol: Carpal tunnel syndrome, thrombophlebitis.	ASSESSMENT: Assess for signs of phlebitis. INTERVENTION: All progestins: Encourage low-salt diet. Monitor weight. Caution if hypertension or cardiac disease is present so patient complies with follow-up care needed. Observe for signs of hypercalcemia. EVALUATION: Health teaching is effective. Serious vascular problems are avoided.
None significant None significant			

CONTINUED ON THE FOLLOWING PAGE

Antineoplastic Agents

Table 49-1. ANTINEOPLASTIC AGENTS-*CONTINUED*

Name	Dosage and Route	Uses	Precautions
Drugs Altering Hormone Balance			
Mitotane (Lysodren)	9–10 g PO qd in 3–4 divided doses.	Inoperable adrenocortical cancer.	
Aminoglutethimide (Cytadren)	1 g/day PO in divided doses (at 6-hr intervals). Dose may be increased q 1–2 wk to maximum of 2 g.	Cushing's syndrome, adrenal cancer, hormone-responsive metastatic breast cancer.	A high percentage of patients treated with this drug will initially manifest an allergic skin rash. This rash is self-limiting and generally subsides in 5–8 days. It is not an indication for discontinuing therapy unless it persists.
RADIOACTIVE ISOTOPES			
Action (All): To disrupt growth activity of cells resulting in cell death.			
Radiogold (^{198}Au)	35–100 μCi intrapleurally or intraperitoneally.	To treat pleural effusions and ascites caused by cancer.	All radioisotopes: For radiation protection, observe all precautionary practices required by law and institutional policy.
Sodium radioiodine (^{131}I) Sodium radiophosphate (^{32}P, Phosphotope)	50–150 μCi PO. NOTE: All doses of radisotopes are highly individualized.	Thyroid cancer. Polycythemia vera, metastatic lesions.	

*Within the column listing adverse effects, underlines indicate the most common effects; CAPITALS indicate life-threatening effects.

Interactions	Acute Toxic Signs	Adverse Effects*	Nursing Implications
Spironalactone should not be taken by patients on mitotane since it interferes with the adrenal suppression produced by mitotane.	Nausea and vomiting.	Neuro: Depression, dizziness, tremors may affect coordination. GI: anorexia, severe nausea and vomiting, diarrhea, GI toxicity. Integ: Dermatitis. Metabolic: Altered steroid metabolism and adrenal insufficiency.	INTERVENTION: Give antiemetics. Warn patient to use care when operating vehicles or doing anything requiring coordination and concentration. Monitor liver enzymes. EVALUATION: Health teaching is effective. Antinausea measures are effective.
None significant.	Persistent skin rash (longer than 8 days' duration) generally requires discontinuation of therapy. Severe lethargy.	Neuro: Dizziness, drowsiness, headache, ataxia. GI: Anorexia, nausea. Hemo: Severe pancytopenia, transient leukopenia. CV: Hypotension. Integ: Rash, pruritus, myalgia, facial flushing, hirsutism. Other: Fever adrenal insufficiency, masculinization. Symptoms generally decrease or abate with slight reduction in dosage.	ASSESSMENT: Assess knowledge gaps to determine needed health teaching. INTERVENTION: Appropriate health teaching to patient/family since drug produces medical adrenalectomy in inhibiting synthesis of glucocorticoids, mineralocorticoids, and other steroids. Many patients may require hydrocortisone and mineralocorticoid replacement therapy while receiving aminoglutehimide. Monitor blood pressure regularly. Also monitor thyroid studies, CBC. Warn patient that drug can cause drowsiness, orthostatic hypotension. Tell patient to report persistent skin rash (more than 5–8 days in duration). EVALUATION: Health teaching is effective.
Unknown. Lithium carbonate—hypothyroidism. Unknown.	All radioisotopes: None when given in therapeutic doses.	All radioisotopes Hemo: Bone marrow depression. Other: Rare radiation sickness. Theoretical increased risk of leukemia in later life due to therapy, also possible increased risk of birth defects in offspring. ^{131}I—Feeling of fullness in neck—"radiation mumps"—until drug is excreted.	INTERVENTION: All radioisotopes: Explain to patient/family that patient is on isolation until sufficient quantities of the isotope have been excreted. All urine is collected for 24–48 hours so the amount of radioisotope excreted can be measured. Follow hospital protocol carefully to prevent unnecessary exposure of self, staff, patient visitors to radiaiton. Carefully explain to patient/family any restriction following discharge (some trace amounts of radioactive elements may be excreted for several days after discharge so patient should avoid extended close contact with small children/infants for several days. (Example: should not hold infant or small child on lap for extended periods.)

Antineoplastic Agents

Cisplatin

ACTION AND USE. Cisplatin (Platinol) inhibits DNA synthesis by cross-linking. It is the first inorganic compound successfully used to treat cancer. The cis-isomer of this heavy metal is the only part that is therapeutically active. The drug has an alkylating-like action and is effective in all phases of the cell cycle. Cisplatin is excreted primarily unchanged in the urine. It is most effective in the treatment of germinal cell neoplasms of the testes, especially when used in combination with bleomycin (Blenoxane) and vinblastine (Velban). Cisplatin has also shown antitumor activity against lymphoma, ovarian cancer, bladder cancer, and squamous cell tumors of the head and neck.

ADVERSE EFFECTS. The adverse effects include nausea, vomiting, ototoxicity, and nephrotoxicity. Concomitant adminsitration of aminoglycoside antibiotics causes additive nephrotoxicity. Nausea and emesis are particularly troublesome adverse effects with this drug. It has been called the most emetogenic drug known to medical science. Almost 100% of patients experience nausea and vomiting, which may be severe and protracted. Metoclopramide hydrochloride (Reglan) is especially helpful in relieving cisplatin-induced emesis.

DOSAGE. Adult dosage of cisplatin is 20 mg/m² intravenously daily for five days. This is repeated every three weeks for three cycles or longer.

ANTIMETABOLITES

Action

Antimetabolites are structurally similar to vitamins, coenzymes, or normal cell intermediary products needed for growth and division of both normal and neoplastic cells. They interfere with the metabolic pathways of dividing cells and exert their greatest effect in the S phase of the cell cycle. A drug-induced block of DNA synthesis occurs when the antimetabolic agent is taken into the cell rather than the necessary nutrient or enzyme. This is the major cause of cell death from antimetabolite therapy. The antimetabolic antineoplastic agents are most effective against rapidly growing tumors such as breast, head, and neck tumors, and leukemias. However, the same properties that render them so effective against rapidly growing neoplasms also make them highly toxic to rapidly proliferating normal tissues such as the hair and lining of the gastrointestinal tract.

Use

Antimetabolites are often used in combination to treat acute and chronic leukemia, breast, head, and neck tumors. Colon, ovarian, and bronchogenic carcinomas, trophoblastic tumors, and liver metastases may also be treated by antimetabolites alone or in combination with other agents. Azothioprine is used to suppress rejection following renal transplants and for treatment of severe, active rheumatoid arthritis unresponsive to other therapy.

The antimetabolites include: (1) the folic acid antagonist methotrexate (MTX, Mexate); (2) the pyrimidine antagonists floxuridine (FUDR), fluorouracil (5-FU), and cytarabine (Cytosar, Ara-C); (3) the purine antagonists mercaptopurine (MP, Purinethol), thioguanine (6-TG), and azathioprine (Imuran); and (4) hydroxyurea (Hydrea). Allopurinol (Zyloprim), an antigout medication, is frequently used in conjunction with thioguanine to prevent the formation of uric acid crystals. Although allopurinol was originally developed as an adjunct for cancer treatment, its primary usage now is in the management of non-neoplastic diseases.

Pharmacokinetics

The antimetabolite drugs are absorbed, distributed, metabolized, and excreted as follows: Azathioprine, hydroxyurea, mercaptopurine, methotrexate, and thioguanine are well absorbed following oral administration. Cytarabine, floxuridine, and fluorouracil are given parenterally since they are not well absorbed from the gastrointestinal tract. Fluorouracil is sometimes given orally and topically for the local treatment of some gastrointestinal tumors. The antimetabolites are all widely distributed in body tissues and fluids, metabolized in the liver, and excreted in the urine.

Adverse Effects

The antimetabolites are effective during the S and G2 phases of the cell cycle. As a group, these drugs share the common adverse effects of myelosuppression and gastrointestinal disturbances. Mercaptopurine causes fewer gastrointestinal problems than methotrexate, and thioguanine causes fewer than mercaptopurine.

Folic Acid Antagonist

ACTION. The folic acid antagonist methotrexate is the prototype antimetabolite. This B-complex impostor was the first of its class to demonstrate effective antineoplastic activity. Its use in children with acute leukemia during the 1940s induced many remissions and sparked the hope that chemotherapy would eventually lead to more dramatic results.

USE. Methotrexate is used to treat acute leukemia, Burkitt's lymphoma (stage I or II), lymphosarcoma (stage III), mycosis fungoides, and the trophoblastic tumors choriocarcinoma and hydatidiform mole. Methotrexate is curative for choriocarcinoma, a rare, rapidly growing placental tissue tumor. This drug is also used in small doses (10–25 mg orally or intravenously weekly) to treat severe cases of adult psoriasis (a non-neoplastic disease characterized by abnormally rapid proliferation of the epidermal cells), asthma, and rheumatoid arthritis.

PHARMACOKINETICS. Methotrexate is a potent antimetabolite whose cytotoxic effect is achieved by binding with the enzyme dihydrofolate reductase and blocking conversion of folic acid and dihydrofolate to tetrahydrofolic acid, the active form of folic acid. Tetrahydrofolate is essential for protein synthesis. Methotrexate is cell cycle-specific and arrests DNA synthesis at the G1-S interphase of the cell cycle. High doses of folic acid analogs like methotrexate can have severe, potentially fatal toxic effects owing to the death of bone marrow and other rapidly proliferating normal cells deprived of tetrahydrofolate. Administration of folic acid cannot reverse the damage to normal cells. This is because the methotrexate-produced enzyme inhibition would prevent folic acid from being converted to the necessary active metabolite. Normal cells suffering the toxic effects of methotrexate can be saved by the administration of an antidote called leucovorin (folinic acid, citrovorum factor). This substance provides a tetrahydrofolate derivative that can be used in protein synthesis by the normal cells. The cancer cells are not able to use the leucovorin. Use of this antidote several hours after a massive dose (up to 15 g/m^2) of methotrexate has made it possible to kill tumors previously resistant to safe doses of methotrexate (MTX). The toxic effects of methotrexate on normal cells can be greatly diminished with leucovorin administration after the methotrexate has had sufficient time to kill resistant tumor cells, such as is done in osteogenic sarcoma. Thus, the leucovorin is used to "rescue" the normal cells from the toxic effects of methotrexate. This is often called *leucovorin rescue* therapy.

ADVERSE REACTIONS. The adverse reactions following methotrexate administration include: dose-related leukopenia and thrombocytopenia; nausea; vomiting; diarrhea; stomatitis; renal tubular necrosis; hepatic dysfunction; hyperuricemia; photosensitivity; alopecia; and pulmonary interstitial infiltrates. Intrathecal administration can cause arachnoiditis within hours after administration.

INTERACTIONS. Patients should avoid alcoholic beverages, since this can cause increased hepatoxicity. Concurrent administration of phenylbutazone, probenecid, and salicylates can cause increased methotrexate toxicity and should be avoided if possible.

DOSAGE. Dosages of methotrexate vary according to the type of tumor being treated. The adult and pediatric dose for patients with acute lymphoblastic and lymphatic leukemia is 3.3 mg/m^2 orally, intramuscularly, or intravenously daily for four to six weeks or until remission, then 20–30 mg/m^2 orally or intramuscularly twice weekly. For patients with stage I or II Burkitt's lymphoma, 10–25 mg orally daily for four to eight days, with 1-week rest intervals between dose cycles, is given. The dose for stage III lymphosarcoma patients is 0.625–2.5 mg/kg daily orally, intramuscularly, or intravenously. The dosage for patients with mycosis fungoides is 2.5–10.0 mg orally daily or 50 mg intramuscularly weekly, or 25 mg intramuscularly twice weekly. The dosage of methotrexate for patients with trophoblastic tumors is 15–30 mg orally or intramuscularly daily for five days, then repeat after one or more weeks, depending on response or toxicity. High-dose therapy (over 100 mg intravenous doses) must be followed by leucovorin rescue.

Pyrimidine Antagonists

ACTION. The antimetabolite pyrimidine analogs fluorouracil (5-FU), cytarabine (Ara-C, Cytosar), and floxuridine (FUDR) work by inhibiting pyrimidine synthesis in DNA synthesis. Fluorouracil and cytarabine inhibit

thymidylate synthetase to prevent DNA synthesis during the S phase of the cell cycle. Floxuridine is apparently catabolized to fluorouracil and produces the same toxic and antimetabolic effects as doses of fluorouracil.

USE. The pyrimidine antagonists may be used to treat a wide variety of solid tumors. Temporary remissions can be obtained for patients with cancer of the colon, rectum, stomach, and pancreas through the administration of fluorouracil. Although all antineoplastic drugs are immunosuppressive to a certain degree, cytarabine is especially immunosuppressive, particularly when given by a continuous infusion.

PHARMACOKINETICS. Cytarabine, floxuridine, and fluorouracil are given parenterally since they are poorly absorbed from the gastrointestinal tract. Once administered, these drugs are widely distributed to body tissues and fluids before being metabolized by the liver and excreted in the urine.

FLUOROURACIL AND FLOXURIDINE. *Action.* The antimetabolite pyrimidine antagonists fluorouracil and floxuridine have been in clinical use for about 25 years. These drugs are currently creating new interest because of developments that make it possible to follow the drug's uptake in both normal and malignant cells. In addition, biomechanical modulation of fluorouracil in combination with leucovorin has led to an apparent enhancement in its clinical activity. This is an example of how research and technology are enabling therapists to devise newer, more effective cancer treatments, not with new drugs, but with new regimens using existing drugs.

Use. Fluorouracil is used to treat bladder, breast, cervical, colon, liver, ovarian, pancreatic, and rectal cancers. Floxuridine is used to treat bile duct, bladder, brain, breast, head and neck, gall bladder, and liver cancers.

Pharmacokinetics. Floxuridine and fluorouracil are administered parenterally. Fluorouracil can be administered orally for the local treatment of some gastrointestinal carcinomas. Both drugs are widely distributed to body tissues and fluids, metabolized in the liver, and excreted in the urine, largely as inactive metabolites.

Adverse Reactions. Adverse effects associated with floxuridine include: leukopenia; anemia; thrombocytopenia; ataxia; vertigo; nystagmus; convulsions; depression; hemiplegia; lethargy; stomatitis; nausea and vomiting; erythema; and pruritus. Fluorouracil-associated adverse effects include: leukopenia; thrombocytopenia; anemia; stomatitis; gastrointestinal ulcers; nausea; vomiting; dermatitis; hyperpigmentation (especially in blacks); alopecia; and malaise.

Interactions. There are no significant interactions seen with either floxuridine or fluorouracil.

Dosage. Floxuridine is designed for special administration techniques. Floxuridine dose ranges are 0.1–0.6 mg/kg daily by *intra-arterial* infusion via pump for uniform dose administration rate. Floxuridine is also administered in doses of 0.4–0.6 mg/kg daily into the hepatic artery. Fluorouracil doses are based on lean body weight. Fluorouracil is administered in doses of 12.5 mg/kg intravenously daily for three to five days every four weeks or 15 mg/kg weekly for six weeks. Oral administration of fluorouracil has been used for local treatment of some gastrointestinal tumors.

Many of the antineoplastic agents have a narrow therapeutic index. Individual factors may vary, and patients require close supervision or observation to preserve a margin of safety, especially patients receiving drugs that cause bone marrow depression. Due to fluorouracil's narrow margin of safety, the patient's blood count must be carefully monitored for signs of severe bone marrow depression and dangerously low white blood count. Systemic toxicity of fluorouracil and its derivative floxuridine can also be minimized by injecting the drug directly into the arteries supplying blood to the involved organs. This technique of *intra-arterial chemotherapy* (IAC) has been useful in the treatment of liver metastasis with floxuridine injected into the hepatic artery. Damage to normal cells is greatly reduced because most of the drug is metabolized by the liver before entering the systemic circulation. Some patients receiving IAC may have an intra-arterial catheter permanently inserted so they can manage their own chemotherapy on an outpatient basis. There is, however, some degree of morbidity associated with the catheter itself. This approach may not be suitable or desirable for all patients, and some may require periodic hospitalization for their IAC therapy.

CYTARABINE. Cytarabine works by inhibiting pyrimidine synthesis. Cytarabine is used to treat acute myelocytic and other acute leukemias. Pharmacokinetically, cytarabine is well absorbed following parenteral administration, widely distributed to all body tissues, metabolized in the liver, and excreted by the kidneys. Adverse effects following cytarabine administration include: leukopenia; anemia; thrombocytopenia; megablastosis; nausea; vomiting; reversible hepatoxicity; hyperuricemia; rash; and flu-like symptoms. Adult and pediatric dose of cytarabine is 200 mg/m² daily by continuous intravenous infusion for five days; or 10–30 mg/m² intrathecally up to three times weekly. There are no significant interactions with cytarabine.

Purine Antagonists

USE. The antabolite purine analogs mercaptopurine (6-MP, Purinethol) and thioguanine (6-TG, Thioguanine) are useful alone or in combination therapy to treat acute and chronic leukemia. Mercaptopurine was the first clinically effective antipyrine and remains the most important and widely used of this group. In addition to their antileukemic activity, drugs of this class also have immunosuppressive activity. Azathioprine (Imuran), a derivative of mercaptopurine, is used to prevent rejection of transplanted kidneys. Azathioprine is also used to treat severe acute rheumatoid arthritis not responsive to other therapy.

MERCAPTOPURINE. Mercaptopurine is a hypoxanthine analog that acts against tumor cells through interference with purine biosynthesis and the interconversions necessary for nucleic acid synthesis. Pharmacokinetically, mercaptopurine is well absorbed after oral administration, distributed widely throughout body tissues, metabolized in the liver, and excreted via the kidneys.

Patients receiving mercaptopurine therapy must be monitored carefully for signs of bone marrow depression. Other adverse effects of mercaptopurine include: anorexia, nausea, vomiting, stomatitis, hepatic necrosis, and hyperuricemia. The only significant interaction with mercaptopurine is with allopurinol. Purines are released when cells are destroyed following mercaptopurine administration. Xanthine oxidase converts these excess purines to uric acid, which can lead to precipitation of uric acid crystals with resultant kidney damage. Allopurinol, the antigout medication, is often prescribed to prevent this. Allopurinol inhibits the enzyme xanthine oxidase, thus preventing crystal formation. However, this same enzyme is necessary for breaking down mercaptopurine, so use of allopurinol can prolong and potentiate mercaptopurine's cytotoxic effects on bone marrow. Therefore, patients receiving both allopurinol and mercaptopurine for treatment of leukemia require only one third to one fourth of the normally prescribed antimetabolite dose. Dosage of mercaptopurine is 80–100 mg/m² orally daily as a single dose, up to 5 mg/kg daily. Pediatric dose is 70 mg/m² daily. Maintenance dose for adults and children is 1.5–2.5 mg/kg daily.

THIOGUANINE. Thioguanine is an antimetabolite purine antagonist. Thioguanine is similar to and used to treat the same diseases as mercaptopurine. It is one of the most effective agents against acute granulocytic leukemia, but is not very effective against solid tumors. Pharmacokinetically, thioguanine is well absorbed after oral administration, widely distributed to body tissues, metabolized in the liver, and excreted by the kidneys. Adverse effects seen with thioguanine include: leukopenia, anemia, thrombocytopenia, nausea, vomiting, stomatitis, anorexia, hepatotoxicity, and hyperuricemia. There are no significant interactions with thioguanine; however, as with mercaptopurine, this drug also causes increased uric acid levels, so concomitant administration of allopurinol is often a part of chemotherapy. Unlike mercaptopurine, thioguanine activity is not affected by allopurinol, so therapeutic doses remain the same. Adult and pediatric dosages of thioguanine start at 2 mg/kg orally daily (calculated to nearest 20 mg) and gradually increased to 3 mg/kg daily if no toxic effects occur.

Hydroxyurea

Hydroxyurea acts as an antimetabolite; however, it cannot be assigned to any of the previous antimetabolite subgroups. Hydroxyurea inhibits DNA synthesis through its action on the enzyme ribonucleotide diphosphate reductase. The action of this drug is specific for the S phase of the cell cycle. The primary use of hydroxyurea at the present time is in the management of busulfan-resistant chronic granulocytic leukemia. Hydroxyurea is sometimes used in combination with radiation to treat cancers of the head and neck. It is also used to treat melanoma and metastatic ovarian cancers. Pharmacokinetically, hydroxyurea is well absorbed from the gastrointestinal tract following oral administration. It is then widely distributed to body tissues, metabolized in the liver, and excreted via the kidneys. There are no significant interactions with hydroxyurea. Bone marrow depression is the major toxic effect and subsides rapidly when the drug is discontinued for several days. Adverse effects also include gastrointestinal disturbances, mild dermatologic reactions, and rarely, stomatitis, alopecia, and neurologic manifestations. Dosage for hydroxyurea is 80 mg/kg orally every third day or 20–30 mg/kg orally daily.

NATURAL PRODUCTS

Drugs in this group include (1) the vinca alkaloids vincristine (Oncovin) and vinblastine (Velban); (2) the antibiotics actinomycin D (dactinomycin, Cosmegen), daunorubicin (Daunomycin, DAU), doxorubicin (Adriamycin, ADRIA), bleomycin (blenoxane), mitomycin C, and mithramycin (Mithracin); (3) procarbazine hydrochloride (Matulane); (4) the enzyme L-asparaginase; and (5) the recently marketed mitoxantrone (Novantrone). Unlike the alkylating agents and antimetabolites, which are classified in terms of their mode of action, the natural products are classified together because of their sources as naturally occurring vinca alkaloids, antibiotics, and enzymes. So although these drugs may be classed together, their modes of action differ significantly.

Vinca Alkaloids

ACTION. The vinca alkaloids vinblastine, vincristine, and vindesine are derivatives of the plant *Vinca rosea* (periwinkle) and differ structurally from each other only by one ring substituent. They are cell cycle-specific, active only when the cell is in the mitotic (M) phase of division. Their mechanism of action is to interfere with the microtubule assembly in the miotic spindle formation. Although similar in mode of action and metabolism, they differ strikingly in antitumor spectrum, dose, and toxicity. Vindesine is a soon-to-be-marketed semisynthetic vinca alkaloid derivative.

USE. The major uses for the vinca alkaloids is in the palliative chemotherapy of leukemias, lymphomas, sarcomas, and such carcinomas as breast and testicular tumors.

PHARMACOKINETICS. The vinca alkaloids are administered intravenously only. They are widely distributed to body tissues but penetrate the blood–brain barrier poorly. These drugs are metabolized in the liver and eliminated in both the urine and feces.

ADVERSE EFFECTS. Adverse effects common with the vinca alkaloids are numbness and tingling of the extremities (paresthesias), loss of deep tendon reflexes, and ataxia. All the vinca alkaloids can produce tissue necrosis if intravenous infusions containing these agents are allowed to extravasate (infiltrate) (see Tables 49–2 and 49–3).

VINBLASTINE. *Action.* Vinblastine interferes with microtubule assembly by binding to or crystallizing microtubule proteins necessary for the formation of the mitotic spindle. It can also bind to other types of microtubules to affect the function of phagocytes and neurons.

Use. Vinblastine is used to treat breast, choriocarcinoma, histiocytosis, Hodgkin's and non-Hodgkin's lymphomas, lymphosarcoma, mycosis fungoides, neuro-

Table 49–2. ANTINEOPLASTIC DRUGS DAMAGING TO TISSUES ON EXTRAVASATION

Drug	Effect
Carmustine (BCNU)	Can cause intense pain on infusion
Dacarbazine (DTIC)	Corrosive to tissues on infiltration
Actinomycin D (Dactinomycin, Cosmegen)	Extravasation can cause phlebitis, severe soft tissue damage
Daunorubicin (Cerubidine)	Severe cellulitis and tissue sloughage if drug extravasates
Doxorubicin (Adriamycin, ADRIA)	Severe cellulitis and tissue sloughage if drug extravastes
Mechlorethamine/nitrogen mustard (Mustargen)	Corrosive to tissue on contact
Mithramycin (Mithracin)	Extravasation causes irritation, cellulitis
Mitomycin (Mutamycin)	Extravasation causes cellulitis, necrosis, tissue sloughage
Vinblastine (Velban)	Extravasation can cause irritation, phlebitis, cellulitis, or necrosis
Vincristine (Oncovin)	Can cause local cellulitis, phlebitis
Vindesine (DAVA, Eldesine)	Extravasation can cause phlebitis, necrosis

blastoma, and testicular cancers. In the treatment of Hodgkin's disease, vinblastine is probably the most effective single drug used and is often used in combination chemotherapy.

Pharmacokinetics. Vinblastine is widely distributed to body tissues after intravenous administration. Metabolism of vinblastine is accomplished extensively by the liver, and excretion occurs in the bile.

Adverse Effects. Unlike vincristine, vinblastine has bone marrow depression as a dose-limiting side effect. Nausea, vomiting, and stomatitis are also frequent. Neurotoxicity has been reported, but is less common with vinblastine. Paresthesias, peripheral neuropathy, numbness, and loss of deep tendon reflexes can occur. This drug is corrosive to tissues and can cause cellulitis, phlebitis, and tissue necrosis if infiltration into subcutaneous tissues occurs. There are no significant interactions with vinblastine.

Table 49–3. GUIDELINES FOR TREATMENT OF EXTRAVASATION OF VESICANT CHEMOTHERAPEUTIC AGENTS

GENERAL

If extravasation is suspected, the IV should be discontinued immediately. With needle or catheter still in place, an attempt to remove the material from the vein should be made with a syringe fixed to the catheter (remove catheter or needle afterwards).

If ice packs are used, they should be used on and off intermittently for half-hour periods for 18–24 hours.

Topical corticosteroid creams spread in the area of extravasation and covered with gauze may also help reduce cutaneous reactions.

SPECIFIC ANTIDOTES

It is generally recognized that 50–100 mg hydrocortisone (Solu-Cortef) or 4–12 mg dexamethasone (Decadron) subcutaneously injected in a series of small punctures in the area of extravasation followed by ice packs for 24 hours is an effective means to deal with most cases (TB or insulin syringe).

Specific antidotes MAY be needed for the following drugs:

DRUG	*SPECIFIC ANTIDOTE*	*DOSE*
Carmustine	Sodium Bicarbonate 7–8.5%	3–5 ml SC
Doxorubicin	Sodium Bicarbonate 7–8.5%	3–5 ml SC
Daunorubicin	Sodium Bicarbonate 7–9.5%	3–5 ml SC
DTIC (Dactinomycin)	Sodium Thiosulfate 10% 4 ml plus sterile H_2O 6 ml (to make 10 ml)	3–5 ml SC
Etoposide	No specific antidote	
Fluorouracil	No specific antidote	
Mithramycin	Sodium Edetate 150 mg/ml	1 ml SC
Nitrogen Mustard	Sodium Thiosulfate 10% 4 ml plus sterile H_2O 5 ml (to make 10 ml)	3–5 ml SC
Streptozocin	No specific antidote	
Vincristine	No specific antidote	
Vinblastine	No specific antidote	
Vindesine	No specific antidote	

From Kelly, 1984, with permission.

Dosage. Adult and pediatric dosage is 0.1 mg/kg or 3.7 mg/m² intravenous weekly or every two weeks. Adults may be increased to a maximum dose of 0.5 mg/kg or 18.5 mg/m² intravenous weekly, depending on response to therapy. Dose should not be administered if white blood count drops below 4000/mm³.

VINCRISTINE. Action. Vincristine has similar chemistry, biologic effects, and mechanism of action to vinblastine. One remarkable feature is the lack of cross-resistance between these two drugs that are so similar in chemical structure.

Use. Vincristine is effective in the treatment of Hodgkin's disease and other lymphomas. Although somewhat less effective against Hodgkin's disease when used alone, vincristine is considered the drug of choice for combination chemotherapy in stages III and IV of the disease. The combination therapy most useful in Hodgkin's disease is the MOPP regimen, which groups vincristine (Oncovin) with mechlorethamine, prednisone, and procarbazine. Vincristine is extremely effective in the treatment of acute leukemia in children. It has also shown significant activity against Wilms' tumor, neuroblastoma, melanoma, and breast cancer.

Pharmacokinetics. Vincristine is widely distributed to body tissues following intravenous administration. It is metabolized in the liver and excreted in both the urine and feces.

Interactions. There are no significant interactions with vincristine.

Adverse Effects. The major adverse effect of vincristine is neurotoxicity, which limits the maximum single dose to 2 mg. Gastrointestinal side effects are common, especially nausea, vomiting, and constipation due to autonomic neuropathy, causing paralytic ileus. Vincristine is bone marrow–sparing, which makes it an attractive drug to use in combination with bone marrow–toxic agents. Urinary retention, diplopia, and alopecia can also occur. Vincristine is corrosive to tissues and can cause cellulitis and tissue necrosis if infiltration into subcutaneous tissues occurs.

Dosage. The usual dose is 1–2 mg/m² intravenously weekly, with the maximum single dose being 2 mg.

VINDESINE SULFATE. Action and Use. A recent addition to the vinca alkaloids is the semisynthetic alkaloid derivative vindesine sulfate. Vindesine sulfate (Eldesine, DAVA) works by producing metaphase arrest during mitosis to prevent cell division. It is used to treat acute lymphoblastic leukemia, breast cancer, malignant melanoma, and lymphosarcoma. This investigational drug will soon become available.

Pharmacokinetics. Like the other vinca alkaloids, vindesine is administered intravenously and is widely distributed to body tissues. Vindesine is metabolized in the liver and excreted in the urine and feces.

Adverse Effects and Interactions. Vindesine sulfate shares adverse effects similar to those of the other vinca alkaloids, but has both bone marrow and neurotoxic effects. Vindesine is corrosive to tissue if extravasation occurs: severe tissue necrosis can occur. There are no significant interactions with vindesine.

Dosage. The usual dose of vindesine is 3–4 mg/m² intravenously every 7–14 days or by continuous intravenous infusion of 1.2–1.5 mg/m² daily for five days every three weeks.

ANTIBIOTICS

Certain antibiotics have been found to be useful antineoplastic agents. Although originally developed for the treatment of bacterial infections, these drugs were found to be too toxic for that purpose. Most antibiotics affect the function and synthesis of nucleic acids, although cytotoxicity does not always correlate directly with altered DNA functions.

Antibiotics have different types of effects on the cancer cell. Actinomycin D combines with deoxyguanine residues to inhibit DNA-directed RNA synthesis. It is useful in the treatment of Wilms' tumor, rhabdomyosarcoma, and methotrexate-resistant choriocarcinoma in women, and in combination therapy for Ewing's sarcoma and testicular tumors. Bone marrow depression, gastrointestinal disturbances, and local inflammation of parenteral sites are common side effects of therapy with this drug.

The drugs daunorubicin, doxorubicin, bleomycin, and mitomycin-C all act as alkylating agents, although the exact mechanism of action is not completely understood with all of these agents.

Anthracycline Antibiotics

Doxorubicin and daunorubicin are important antineoplastic drugs obtained from the fermented products of different Streptomyces species. Both of these anthracycline antibiotics were first isolated in the 1960s. Both of these drugs are called anthracyclines because the anthracycline portion of their molecules produces the antineoplastic effect. Although only slightly different in chemical structure, both drugs display markedly different antitumor activity. Both drugs act by reacting with DNA to form complexes that block DNA-directed RNA and DNA transcription. Current evidence suggests that both drugs are probably effective during all phases of the cell cycle and therefore are cell cycle-nonspecific.

DAUNORUBICIN. *Action and Use.* Daunorubicin is an anthracycline antibiotic. It achieves its antineoplastic action by interfering with DNA-dependent RNA synthesis by *intercalation*. The effectiveness of daunorubicin is limited to acute nonlymphocytic leukemia (myelogenous, monocytic, and erythroid).

Pharmacokinetics. Daunorubicin is widely distributed to body tissues following intravenous administration. It is then metabolized by the liver, and the inactive metabolites are eliminated in the urine and feces.

Adverse Effects and Interactions. Many of the adverse effects of daunorubicin are similar to the effects produced by the alkylating agents. Adverse effects common to both are myelosuppression, alopecia, and gastrointestinal disturbances. Cardiotoxicity is one unique and potentially fatal side effect associated with administration of high doses of either of the anthracyclines. There is a well-documented chronic, cumulative, dose-dependent cardiomyopathy that presents like congestive heart failure. This syndrome is usually rapidly pro-gressive and may be unresponsive to therapy. In order to lessen the risk of cardiotoxic effects, the maximum cumulative dose of daunorubicin is limited to 550 mg/m². However, patients who have received other cardiotoxic drugs (i.e., cyclophosphamide) or radiation to the chest or who have pre-existing cardiomyopathy may tolerate a much lower cumulative dose. Special monitoring techniques such as echocardiography can be used to determine if cardiac effects are occurring. Daunorubicin should not be mixed with heparin, as a precipitate may form.

Dosage. Daunorubicin dosage and indications may vary depending on patient's protocol: when used as a single agent, 60 mg/m² daily intravenously on days 1, 2, and 3 of chemotherapy cycle every three to four weeks; when used in combination with cytosine arabinoside, 45 mg/m² intravenous daily on days 1, 2, and 3 of first chemotherapy cycle and then days 1 and 2 of subsequent courses. Daunorubicin dosages are reduced for patients with impaired liver function. Maximum cumulative dose is 550 mg/m².

DOXORUBICIN. *Action and Use.* Doxorubicin is a DNA intercalator that causes unwinding of the double helix structure by positioning itself between the base pairs of DNA. Doxorubicin has a much broader spectrum of activity than daunorubicin and is particularly useful in treating sarcomas; breast, ovarian, cervical, and testicular carcinomas; neuroblastoma; Wilms' tumor; lymphomas; and acute leukemia. It is frequently used in combination chemotherapy to treat various solid tumors.

Pharmacokinetics. Doxorubicin is widely distributed to body tissues following intravenous administration. Metabolization is done by the liver, and the drug is excreted in both the urine and feces.

Adverse Effects. The major adverse effects following doxorubicin administration are: leukopenia, thrombocytopenia, cardiac depression, arrhythmias, cardiomyopathy, nausea, vomiting, stomatitis, hyperpigmentation of skin, and enhancement of cyclophosphamide-induced bladder injury. Doxorubicin causes severe cellulitis and tissue necrosis if infiltration into subcutaneous tissues occurs.

Interactions. The only significant interaction with doxorubicin is with streptozocin, which can cause increased and prolonged levels of doxorubicin in the blood. Doxorubicin dose may need to be adjusted. Usual doxorubicin dose is 60–75 mg/m² intravenously as a single dose once every three weeks. There is a maximum cumulative dose of 550 mg/m² for this drug because of its potential cardiotoxic effects.

Bleomycin

ACTION AND USE. Bleomycin is an antibiotic isolated from *Streptomyces verticillus*. It inhibits DNA synthesis by scission of the DNA strands, although the exact mechanism of this action is not completely understood at present. Bleomycin is cell cycle-specific for the mitosis and G2 phases of the cell cycle. This drug is useful in the treatment of squamous cell carcinomas of the head and neck, vulva, vagina, penis, and skin, as well as lymphomas, testicular carcinoma, and mycosis fungoides.

PHARMACOKINETICS. Pharmacokinetically, bleomycin is widely distributed to body tissues following parenteral administration. It is then metabolized by the liver and excreted. There are no significant interactions with bleomycin.

ADVERSE EFFECTS. The adverse effects of bleomycin include: fever, anaphylaxis, alopecia, skin and nail changes, and acute pulmonary edema in patients hypersensitive to the drug. Pulmonary fibrosis has been reported in 10% of patients, especially those receiving high doses of the drug, and this limits the cumulative bleomycin dose to 400 units. Bleomycin produces only minimal bone marrow depression and is, therefore, useful in combination with bone marrow–toxic agents.

DOSAGE. Dosages vary according to tumor being treated, patient status (used cautiously in presence of renal or pulmonary impairment), and clinical protocol. For treatment of cervical, esophageal, head, neck, and testicular cancers, the dose is 10–20 units/m^2 intramuscularly, intravenously, or subcutaneously once or twice a week to 300–400 units total dose administered. In Hodgkin's disease, 10–20 units/m^2 intravenously, intramuscularly, or subcutaneously once or twice weekly is administered. After a 50% response occurs, the dose is reduced to 1 unit intramuscularly or intravenously daily or 5 units weekly for maintenance.

Mithramycin

ACTION AND USE. Mithramycin (Plicamycin) is an antibiotic produced by *Streptomyces plicatus* and acts by inhibition of RNA synthesis. This drug's use is limited almost exclusively to embryonal cell carcinoma of the testes. Mithramycin inhibits osteocytic activity, limiting calcium and phoshorus resorption from the bones. Thus, mithramycin administration can produce a dramatic drop in elevated serum calcium levels and has been used to treat hypercalcemias of malignancy unresponsive to other therapies.

PHARMACOKINETICS AND INTERACTIONS. Mithramycin is widely distributed to body tissues and fluids. Mithramycin is the only antibiotic antineoplastic drug that crosses the blood–brain barrier in significant amounts. There are no significant interactions with mithramycin.

ADVERSE REACTIONS. Adverse reactions following mithramycin administration include: bone marrow depression, hepatotoxicity, renal toxicity, and possible decreased serum levels of calcium, potassium, and phosphorus. A unique toxic effect of this drug is a hemorrhagic syndrome, which may initially manifest itself as facial flushing, epistaxis, or hematemesis.

DOSAGE. Drug dosage in testicular cancer is 25–30 μg/kg by intravenous administration daily for up to eight to ten days. Dosage is based on ideal body weight or actual weight, whichever is less. Dosage for hypercalcemia is 25 μg/kg intravenously daily for one to four days.

Mitomycin

ACTION AND USE. Mitomycin is an antibiotic that is isolated from *Streptomyces caespitosus* and acts by inhibiting DNA synthesis through alkylation. It reacts with DNA through covalent bonding, alkylating the DNA and forming cross-links that prevent the unwinding of the DNA double helix, to cause cell death. Like most of the antineoplastic drugs, mitomycin produces chromosomal aberrations and is teratogenic. It is generally used in combination with fluorouracil or the nitrosoureas against gastric and breast carcinomas. It has also been used to treat head and neck, lung, malignant melanoma, pancreatic, colon, and selected hepatic tumors.

PHARMACOKINETICS AND INTERACTIONS. Mitomycin is widely distributed to body tissues following intravenous administration. Adverse effects of mitomycin are myelosuppression, nausea, anorexia, cellulitis, and ulceration at intravenous administration sites on infiltration, renal and hepatic damage, nail changes, alopecia, and fever. There are no significant interactions with mitomycin.

DOSAGE. The usual dosage is 2 mg/m^2 intravenous daily for five days, stop for two days, then repeat for five days; or it may be given 20 mg/m^2 as a single dose. The cycle is repeated every six to eight weeks. The drug is not given if white blood cells drop below 4,000/mm^3 or when platelets fall below 75,000/mm.^{3} Mitomycin is sometimes given topically or by bladder instillation and can also be given intra-arterially via the hepatic artery.

Procarbazine

ACTION AND USE. Procarbazine is substituted hydrazine with monoamine oxidase (MAO)-inhibiting qualities, originally synthesized as a potential antidepressant. It was unsuitable for that purpose because of its bone marrow–depressing effects. However, it subsequently proved useful as an antineoplastic agent. Although procarbazine is not an antibiotic, it acts in a similar manner. The exact mechanism of cytotoxic activity is uncertain at present, however, it does inhibit DNA, RNA, and protein synthesis. It may damage RNA through peroxide formation. Procarbazine has a plasma half-life of only seven minutes. Its greatest clinical effectiveness has been as a component of the MOPP regimen in the treatment of Hodgkin's disease. It may also be used as a single agent in the treatment of lung cancer and for brain tumors, since it is a highly lipophilic drug.

PHARMACOKINETICS. Pharmacokinetically, procarbazine is well absorbed following oral administration and is widely distributed to body tissues.

ADVERSE EFFECTS. Adverse effects include: bleeding tendencies, nausea, stomatitis, myelosuppression, alopecia, central nervous system depression, insomnia, confusion, hallucinations, pleural effusion, and MAO-inhibiting effects similar to MAO-inhibiting antidepressants.

DOSAGE AND INTERACTIONS. The usual dose of procarbazine is 100–150 mg/m^2 by mouth for ten days until the white blood cells drop below 4,000/mm^3 or platelets drop below 100,000/mm^3. Maintenance dose of 50–100 mg per day is begun when bone marrow recovers. This drug inhibits MAO and should be avoided or used with caution in patients receiving sympathomimetics, tricyclic antidepressants, or phenothiazines. (See section on MAO-inhibiting drugs in Chapter 26.) Patients should limit intake of foods with high tyramine content. A significant interaction can occur if a patient on procarbazine drinks any alcohol-containing beverage. Therefore, patients must also abstain from alcohol while on this drug, since a disulfiram-like reaction may occur.

ENZYME—ASPARAGINASE

Action and Use

Asparaginase (also called L-asparaginase) represents a unique development in the field of cancer chemotherapy, as it is the first enzyme to be successfully used to treat cancer. This drug was first isolated from the bacterium *Escherichia coli* and is primarily used in the treatment of acute lymphoblastic leukemia. It is especially useful in inducing remissions in patients who are beginning to show resistance to other drugs. Its antitumor effect is achieved by depriving tumor cells of the necessary amino acid L-asparagine, which results in the inhibition of protein synthesis and death of the leukemic cells. The administration of asparaginase causes serum asparagine to be broken down into nonfunctional aspartic acid and ammonia, thus depriving tumor cells of this required amino acid. Many normal cells are not as sensitive to the effects of this drug enzyme because they can synthesize their own supply of asparagine, which the tumor cells cannot do. Antitumor effects of this drug occur primarily in the G1 phase of the cell cycle. Tissues of the body usually affected adversely by chemotherapy (gastrointestinal mucosa, bone marrow, hair follicles) are not affected by asparaginase.

When asparaginase was first introduced into chemotherapy, it was believed that this drug was almost nontoxic to normal cells. Researchers believed that a distinct biochemical difference had been discovered between normal cells and certain specific cancer cells. Although this drug is useful in the treatment of acute lymphoblastic leukemia, it is now known that many normal tissues are sensitive to the effects of asparaginase. Toxic effects can result from the impairment of synthesis of secreted proteins such as insulin, prothrombin, and other clotting factors. Unfortunately, asparaginase has not lived up to the expectations of early researchers, who anticipated high tumoricidal activity with minimal toxicity in the treatment of human cancers. The main role of asparaginase in antineoplastic therapy is currently limited to combination chemotherapy in acute lymphoblastic leukemia when other drugs have failed to induce remission.

Pharmacokinetics

Asparaginase is well absorbed after intramuscular injection. It can also be administered intravenously. Metab-

olization and excretion routes of asparaginase are unknown; only trace amounts are present in the urine.

Adverse Effects

Asparaginase is a foreign protein that can produce hypersensitivity and anaphylactic reactions. Skin sensitivity testing and desensitization, if necessary, should be done before drug administration. Fever, anorexia, nausea, and vomiting are all signs of acute toxic reaction. Elevated BUN and ammonia levels can result from enzyme action. Liver function is often impaired and can increase the toxicity of other antileukemic drugs. Toxic effects have also been noted in the kidney, pancreas, central nervous system, and the clotting mechanism. Some patients suffer a temporary decrease in insulin production during treatment, which may be due to toxic effects of L-asparagine on the pancreas.

Interactions

There are no significant interactions with this drug.

Dosage

Asparaginase dose for patients receiving combination chemotherapy is 1000 IU/kg/day for ten days by intravenous infusion. When used as a sole induction agent, the dose is 200 IU/kg/day intravenously for 28 days.

ORPHAN DRUG—MITOXANTRONE

Mitoxantrone hydrochloride (Novantrone) was recently approved for use by the Food and Drug Administration. It was approved for intravenous use in combination with other approved drug(s) for use in initial therapy of acute nonlymphocytic leukemia in adults (ANLL). Acute nonlymphocytic leukemia is a type of cancer that includes myelogenous, promyelocytic, monocytic, and erythroid leukemias. It is estimated that about 8000 patients in the United States might be eligible for treatment with this drug. Because of this relatively limited number of potential patients, this drug is one of the few to be designated as an "orphan drug" under the terms of the "Orphan Drug Act," which was passed by Congress in 1983. Mitoxantrone was approved for use in 1988.

The mechanism of action of mitoxantrone is not fully known at present, although it is a DNA-reactive agent. It has a cytocidal effect on both proliferating and nonproliferating cultured human cells, suggesting a non–cell cycle specificity.

The major toxic adverse effects of mitoxantrone are myelosuppression and cardiac problems, including ECG changes, dysrhythmias, chest pain, and tachycardia.

HORMONES AND HORMONE ANTAGONISTS

Hormones have a wide range of therapeutic uses not limited to achieving antineoplastic effects. However, in this chapter, discussion is limited to their antineoplastic effects. The use of hormones in the treatment of neoplasms has the major advantage of not causing bone marrow depression, as do many other cytotoxic agents. The exact mechanism of antitumor action is not completely clear at present. However, it is known that for some tumors sensitive to hormonal growth controls, giving the opposite sex hormone changes the hormonal input to the cell, thereby creating an unfavorable setting for tumor growth. For this to occur, the tumor cells must have retained hormone receptors. These receptors are what cause the tumor cell's sensitivity to hormones. Hormonal treatment is most frequently used to treat breast cancer and is also useful in treating cancer of the endometrium of the uterus and in prostatic cancer.

Steroids and antisteroid compounds are found in this class of drugs. They are: (1) the corticosteroids, most notably prednisone; (2) the estrogens; (3) the antiestrogen tamoxifen (Nolvadex); (4) the androgens; and (5) the progestins.

Corticosteroids

ACTION. The lympholytic effect of the glucocorticoids is presumed responsible for their therapeutic effect in acute lymphoblastic leukemia, chronic lymphocytic leukemia, and the malignant lymphomas. Prednisone is the most commonly used preparation because it has 4–5 times the anti-inflammatory effect of cortisol. Prednisone is a component of the MOPP regimen, long considered the most effective means of producing remissions in advanced Hodgkin's disease.

USE. The corticosteroids are occasionally useful in treating breast cancer and are a necessary replacement hormone for the patients who have had adrenalectomy for metastatic breast disease. Their anti-inflammatory effects may be useful in reducing some sequelae of neoplastic activity. Corticosteroids help reduce cerebral edema secondary to cranial tumor growth or radiation therapy. Corticosteroids are sometimes used to combat the general debility, fever, and anorexia so commonly seen in cancer patients, because they can produce euphoria that tends to decrease patient perception of these symptoms. Although the patient may feel better, tumor growth may not be significantly inhibited.

PHARMACOKINETICS. Pharmacokinetically, corticosteroids are well absorbed from the gastrointestinal tract following oral administration; they are then rapidly distributed to all body tissues, metabolized by the liver, and excreted in the urine. Corticosteroids are also available in parenteral form for injection.

ADVERSE EFFECTS. The major adverse effects with corticosteroid therapy include: muscle weakness, increased appetite, euphoria, and with long-term therapy, changes in body fat distribution, increased risk of infection, potassium loss, and rarely psychosis. Long-term use can also result in adrenal atrophy and gastric bleeding.

INTERACTIONS. Interactions with barbiturates, phenytoin, and rifampin can occur and result in a decreased corticosteroid effect. Interaction can occur with indomethacin and aspirin, increasing the risk of gastrointestinal distress, ulcers, and bleeding.

DOSAGE. Dosages are highly individualized and also depend upon the type of cortisone preparation used. Prednisone (Deltasone, Orasone) dose ranges from 1–100 mg/day.

Drugs Altering Hormone Balance

ESTRAMUSTINE PHOSPHATE. *Action and Use.* Estramustine phosphate, or emustine (Emcyt) is used for the treatment of prostatic carcinoma. This drug has been found to be especially effective against metastatic prostate cancer in patients resistant to estrogen. It is a combination of nitrogen mustard and a derivative of estradiol, and as such combines hormone therapy with cytotoxic therapy. It was designed to achieve selective transport of the cytotoxic agent to the prostate gland and has been described by researchers as one of the most effective drugs studied in patients with hormone-resistant prostatic cancer. Estramustine was found to be superior to diethylstilbestrol (DES), producing a longer disease-free interval, better control of pain, higher response rate, and less cardiovascular toxicity than DES. However, there was no significant difference in the overall survival rates between the two drugs.

Pharmacokinetics. Pharmacokinetically, estramustine is well absorbed after oral administration, metabolized in the liver, and excreted in the urine.

Adverse Effects. The most commonly seen adverse effects are gynecomastia (due to the estrogenic nature of this compound), fluid retention, nausea, and occasional diarrhea.

Interactions. There are no significant interactions with estramustine.

Dosage. The usual dose of estramustine phosphate is 10–16 mg/kg/day in three divided oral doses. Doses above 15–20 mg/kg/day can cause a delayed, intractable nausea as a result of cumulative gastrointestinal toxicity. This drug is generally well tolerated.

MITOTANE. *Action and Use.* Mitotane is an adrenocortical suppressant closely related to the insecticide chlorophenothane (DDT). Its high lipid solubility is the reason for its localization in the adrenal cortex and central nervous system. Mitotane is selectively toxic to adrenocortical tissue. In addition to destroying adrenal tissue, mitotane hinders the extra-adrenal metabolism of cortisol. Currently, the only clinical indication for the use of this drug is the palliation of metastatic or inoperable adrenal cortical carcinoma. Due to the action of this drug, adrenal insufficiency can occur; thus, administration of adrenocorticosteroids is necessary.

Pharmacokinetics. Mitotane is partially absorbed (about 40%) after oral administration. It is metabolized in the liver and excreted in the urine.

Adverse Effects. Adverse effects include hypoadrenalism, dermatitis, visual disturbances, lethargy, and somnolence, all of which abate with decreased dosage of the drug. Nausea and vomiting are generally dose limited, and there is no liver, kidney, or bone marrow toxicity with this drug.

Interactions. Spironolactone should not be taken by patients on mitotane, since it interferes with the adrenal suppression produced by the mitotane.

Dosage. The usual dose of mitotane is 9–10 g orally daily divided into three or four doses.

AMINOGLUTETHIMIDE. Although not a hormone, aminoglutethimide alters hormonal balance by suppressing adrenal function in adrenal cancer and Cushing's syndrome. It may also be used to produce medical adrenalectomy in patients with metastatic cancer of the breast.

Pharmacokinetics. Pharmacokinetically, aminoglutethimide is well absorbed following oral administration and excreted mainly unchanged in the urine or feces.

Dose and Interactions. The usual dose of aminoglutethimide is 250 mg four times per day at six-hour intervals. The dosage may be increased in increments of 250 mg daily every one to two weeks until a maximum daily dose of 2 g is achieved. There are no significant interactions with aminoglutethimide.

Adverse Effects. Adverse effects of aminoglutethimide therapy include adrenal and thyroid hypofunction, especially under stressful conditions, transient *leukopenia*, severe *pancytopenia*, drowsiness, hypotension and tachycardia, nausea, anorexia, morbilliform skin rash, and masculinization and hirsutism in female patients. Skin rash usually subsides after the first week of therapy. Drowsiness, anorexia, and nausea generally diminish within two weeks after initiation of therapy.

Estrogen Therapy

ACTION AND USE. Estrogen therapy is useful in the treatment of postmenopausal women with metastatic breast carcinoma and in men with metastatic prostate cancer. Although tumor regression may not be evident for six to ten weeks in breast carcinoma, subjective responses in patients with prostatic carcinoma are often rapid. Positive estrogen therapy response in breast cancer patients rises with increasing patient age to a high of approximately 30%. Response rate in prostatic cancer patients is approximately 80%. The most commonly used estrogens are diethylstilbestrol (DES), ethinyl estradiol (Estinyl), and the conjugated estrogens (e.g., Premarin), which are more expensive than DES but produce less nausea.

PHARMACOKINETICS. Pharmacokinetically, the estrogens are well absorbed from the gastrointestinal tract following oral administration, widely distributed to all body tissues, and metabolized in the liver. Estrogens are primarily excreted in the urine, although small amounts are also eliminated through the bile in feces.

ADVERSE EFFECTS AND INTERACTIONS. Adverse effects common to estrogen therapy include some nausea and vomiting, fluid retention, polydipsia, polyuria, muscle weakness, lethargy, and feminization and changes in libido in men. Use during pregnancy causes later development of vaginal cancer in some female offspring. Current data also links DES use in pregnancy to later appearance of testicular tumors in some male offspring. However, since the chemotherapeutic use of DES is limited to postmenopausal women, the latter two effects have not been a problem. There are no significant interactions with the estrogens.

DOSAGE. Estrogen doses cited relate specifically to their use in treatment of neoplastic diseases. Diethylstilbestrol (DES) dose for men and postmenopausal women with breast cancer is 15 mg by mouth daily. The DES dose for prostate cancer is 1 mg/day. Ethinyl estradiol dose for postmenopausal women with breast cancer is 1.0 mg/day, and for prostate cancer, 0.15–2 mg/day.

Anti-Estrogen Therapy

Hormonal therapy for breast cancer was revolutionized in recent years by the discovery that the presence of estrogen-binding receptors in breast cancer tissue was highly correlated with likelihood of response to endocrine manipulative therapy. The presence of estrogen receptors indicates that an estrogen-dependent tumor is present; that is, the tumor requires estrogen for growth. Thus, if an estrogen impostor is present and taken into the cancer cell instead of the needed hormone, growth of the tumor cell will be blocked. This is what occurs when the estrogen antagonist tamoxifen is taken into cancer cells.

TAMOXIFEN. *Action and Use.* Tamoxifen (Nolvadex) is a synthetic anti-estrogen quite useful in the treatment of breast cancer. Action occurs by two mechanisms. First, tamoxifen produces a simple blockade of the estrogen receptors in the cytosol of the cell; and second, the estrogen receptor–tamoxifen complex is translocated to the cell nucleus, where it inhibits messenger RNA synthesis. Thus, nucleic acid synthesis is blocked by the false messenger of estrogen receptor tamoxifen. This competitive inhibitor of estrogen can achieve therapeutic effects similar to those of androgen therapy in women with advanced breast cancer, without the masculinizing effects seen with androgen use.

Pharmacokinetics. Pharmacokinetically, tamoxifen is well absorbed following oral administration, widely distributed to body tissues, metabolized in the liver, and excreted in the urine.

Adverse Effects. Tamoxifen has the minor adverse effects of nausea, vomiting, hot flashes, and occasional vaginal spotting. However, these reactions, although annoying, rarely require discontinuation of therapy. Bone marrow depression, renal, and hepatic toxicity are rare. Some patients report an "initial flare" of bone pain at metastatic lesion sites or erythema of skin lesions. This can be frightening to patients, who may think it means disease progression. However, these reactions may be an indicator of positive response to therapy. They are not indications for discontinuation of therapy.

Dosage. The usual dose of tamoxifen is 10–20 mg orally twice a day.

Androgens

Androgen therapy can produce response in about 20% of women with disseminated breast cancer. Androgens are favored over estrogens in women with premenopausal onset of disease who responded favorably to oophorectomy in the past. It can also be useful to treat early postmenopausal women with breast cancer.

PHARMACOKINETICS. The androgens are well absorbed following oral ingestion, widely distributed to body tissues, metabolized by the liver, and excreted in the urine. Some androgens, such as testolactone, can be administered parenterally.

ADVERSE EFFECTS. Adverse effects seen with androgen therapy include: nausea, vomiting, anorexia, myalgia, fluid retention, libido changes, and virilization in women. Although the virilizing effects of androgens such as testosterone propionate cease when the drug is discontinued, most physicians now prescribe synthetic substances that exert little or no masculinizing effects. Fluoxymesterone (Halotestin, Ora-Testryl) is a commonly used synthetic androgen.

INTERACTIONS. There are no significant interactions with these drugs.

DOSAGE. The usual fluoxymesterone dose is 15–30 mg orally daily. The usual testosterone dose is 100 mg injected deeply into a large muscle mass three times per week.

Progestins

ACTION AND USE. Progestins are useful in the treatment of carcinomas of the endometrium and in some cases of advanced breast cancer. Approximately 30% of women with disseminated endometrial disease respond to progestin therapy, as do occasional patients with prostatic or renal tumors. Drugs of this type most commonly used include hydroxyprogesterone caproate (Delalutin), medroxyprogesterone acetate (Provera), and the synthetic hormone megestrol (Megace). These drugs act by altering the hormonal environment so it becomes less favorable to tumor growth.

PHARMACOKINETICS. These drugs are all well absorbed from the gastrointestinal tract, distributed to all body tissues, metabolized in the liver, and excreted in the urine. Provera and Delalutin can also be administered by intramuscular injection.

ADVERSE EFFECTS. There are no acute toxic effects with progestin use. Adverse effects include minimal fluid retention and thrombotic disorders (drug is discontinued with the latter). When used in combination with estrogen, adverse effects can include nausea and vomiting, anorexia, changes in libido, breast tenderness, and breakthrough bleeding.

INTERACTIONS. There are no significant interactions with these drugs.

DOSAGE. Dosage of hydroxyprogesterone caproate for endometrial carcinomas is 1–5 g intramuscularly per week. Dosage of medroxyprogesterone acetate for endometrial, renal, and breast cancers is 400–1000 mg/week intramuscularly. Dosage of megestrol for breast and endometrial cancers is 40–320 mg/day orally.

RADIOACTIVE ISOTOPES

Certain neoplasms respond to treatment by radioactive isotopes. Theoretically, the radioactive element selectively destroys cancer cells without harm to normal tissues. In actuality, such selective toxicity does not occur. Neoplastic and some normal cells are destroyed by these substances. Presently, three radioactive elements are employed in cancer therapy. They are sodium ra-diophosphate (^{32}P), radiogold (^{198}Au), and sodium radioiodine (^{131}I).

All three radioactive isotopes employed in the treatment of cancer emit beta particles that damage normal as well as neoplastic cells. Although beta particles travel only short distances, it is possible for anyone in prolonged close contact with the patient so treated to experience some potentially damaging effects from radiation. For this reason, patients undergoing such therapy are placed on protective isolation precautions until this hazard is past. Isotope half-life, radioactive materials, regulations and laws, and drug excretion determine when precautions are no longer necessary. All dosages of radioactive isotopes are highly individualized.

Sodium Radiophosphate

Sodium radiophosphate (^{32}P) is available as a solution for oral use and in sterile form for injection. Its half-life is 14.3 days. When given orally, approximately 25% of the drug is excreted unabsorbed in the feces. Renal elimination of the absorbed dose begins rapidly, excreting 25%–50% in the first four to six days, then slowing to 1%/day. The isotope concentrates in the bones, regardless of the initial distribution of the drug. Dose is 6 μCi by mouth.

Radioactive phosphate was once the therapy of choice in chronic leukemias because of its affinity for bones. However, more effective chemotherapeutic regimens have replaced its use in leukemia treatment. It is occasionally used to palliate metastatic bone pain in ovarian cancer. Because of its potentially serious adverse effects, such as an increased risk of leukemia to the patient, and availability of more effective chemotherapeutic agents, current use of sodium radiophosphate is rare. Interactions with this drug are unknown.

Radiogold

Radiogold (^{198}Au), with a half-life of 2.7 days, emits both gamma and beta particles. Average effective life of particle emissions is approximately four days. It has been used in the treatment of pediatric brain tumors and also has been instilled locally in doses from 35–100 μCi as a treatment for metastatic peritoneal and pleural effusions. Use of this element is rare for several reasons, including high cost of patient therapy, potential hazard to hospital personnel, and the availability of the more effective and far less hazardous alkylating agents for the treatment of malignant effusions. Interactions with this drug are unknown.

Sodium Radioiodine

Sodium radioiodine (^{131}I) is the most effective of the radioisotopes used in cancer therapy. It has a half-life of 8.8 days. This element is used in the treatment of well-differentiated follicular and papillary thyroid carcinomas to achieve complete thyroid ablation (destruction) after thyroidectomy. Since iodine is readily absorbed and trapped by thyroid tissue, sodium radioiodine is successful in destroying the neoplastic as well as normal thyroid tissue. Thus, it is also used to treat hyperthyroidism.

Pharmacokinetically, it is well absorbed following oral administration and, since it has an affinity for thyroid tissue, it is "trapped" in thyroid tissue wherever it is located in the body. The isotope is excreted mainly in the urine, although scant amounts are present in the saliva and perspiration. About 80% of the isotope is excreted in the urine in 24–48 hours.

In order to achieve adequate uptake of the isotope and optimum benefit from the therapy, patients are deprived of thyroid hormone for several weeks prior to therapy in order to induce mild hypothyroidism. Most thyroid cancers respond well to this therapy, although two to three courses of treatment several months apart may be necessary to achieve total thyroid ablation.

Patients receiving sodium radioiodine are placed in isolation, and all urine is collected for radioactive assay for 48 hours to determine when sufficient amounts of the drug have been excreted. Once 80% has been excreted (usually 24–48 hours), the patient is removed from isolation. It generally takes seven to ten days for the rest of the radiation to dissipate. Close contact for extended periods (for example, sleeping in the same bed or holding an infant for an extended period) during that interval is not recommended, as this increases the risk of thyroid cancer to individuals so exposed. Linens and clothing are handled with care, as some of the isotope may be excreted in the perspiration.

The dose of sodium radioiodine for treatment of thyroid cancer is highly individualized and dependent on estimated malignant thyroid and metastatic tissue present. Dose range is 50–150 mCi by mouth. The only significant interaction with ^{131}I involves lithium carbonate, which may result in hypothyroidism if used together. Since thyroid ablation (destruction) is the goal in cancer treatment and lifetime thyroid hormone replacement will be necessary, this interaction is more problematic for patients with hyperthyroidism who may receive this therapy.

Adverse effects with this treatment are transient and mild. Patients may report sensations of fullness in the neck, may experience transient swelling of the neck area ("radiation mumps"), or may experience a metallic, sweet taste in the mouth. Women experience the latter more frequently than men. There is a theoretical increased risk of developing leukemia in later life after receiving sodium radioiodine therapy.

COMBINATION THERAPY

Often, several different drugs are used to treat cancer, as their effect may be stronger together than separately. Table 49–4 reviews several common drug combinations and the types of tumors that they are used in treating. Researchers are continually updating combination regimens to devise new and more effective therapies.

INVESTIGATIONAL DRUGS

Drugs in this class are not yet commercially available for use but are expected to be available in the near future, as soon as clinical trials are completed. The Food and Drug Administration grants drug approval once data from all phases of clinical trials have been completed (see Table 49–5). These drugs are all approved for use in certain neoplastic diseases and are available to oncologic physicians for the treatment of patients with specific neoplasms. These drugs may be obtained through the National Cancer Institute (NCI) by any qualified oncology physician willing to submit the required study forms to the NCI. Among the drugs in this class are hexamethylmelamine (HMM), 5-azacytidine, iproplatin (CHIP), and new forms of interferon (IFN).

Hexamethylmelamine

Hexamethylmelamine is a triazene derivative. The exact mechanism of its antitumor activity is unknown at present. It is structurally similar to an alkylating agent, and it has been suggested that it is activated into an alkylating agent in the body. Hexamethylmelamine is well absorbed from the gastrointestinal tract after oral administration, metabolized largely in the liver, and excreted in the urine and feces. There are no significant interactions with this drug. Dosage is 4–8 mg/kg/day continuously, or 240–320 mg/m^2 daily for 21 days, with this cycle repeated every six weeks. This drug is clinically useful in treating malignant lymphoma, cancer of the ovary, and bronchogenic cancer.

Clinical activity and toxicity resemble those of the alkylating agents, although the drug may have some antimetabolite activity. Adverse effects of hexamethylmelamine include: mild leukopenia, paresthesias, numbness, confusion, seizures, ataxia, and severe gastrotoxicity including anorexia, nausea, and vomiting.

Azacytidine

Azacytidine is useful in treatment of cytarabine-resistant acute myelogenous leukemia. Researchers hope it will become a drug of choice for this disease. This drug may also be useful in the treatment of melanoma, breast, and colon cancers. Azacytidine acts as an antimetabolite disrupting the translation of nucleic acid sequences into protein. Pharmacokinetically, this drug is well distributed following intravenous administration, metabolized mostly by the liver, and excreted in the urine and feces. Adult and pediatric dosage is 200–400 mg/m^2 intravenously daily for five to ten days. This cycle can be repeated as needed every two to three weeks. There are no significant interactions with this drug. Adverse effects include nausea, vomiting, diarrhea, hypotension, and fever. Rarely, hepatotoxicity occurs. Toxic bone marrow hypoplasia is the desired effect in treating acute myeloblastic leukemia with this drug, although severe leukopenia is usually the dose-limiting adverse effect with this drug.

Iproplatin

Iproplatin (CHIP) is a second generation cisplatin derivative. Preclinical antitumor studies show that iproplatin has a spectrum of activity similar to that of cisplatin. Further phase I and phase II clinical trials are currently in progress, so ideal dosages have yet to be determined.

Myelosuppression is the dose-limiting toxicity asso-

Table 49–4. EXAMPLES OF COMBINATION CHEMOTHERAPY REGIMENS

Type of Cancer	Therapy	Components of Therapy Regimen
Advanced bladder cancer	CMV	Cisplatin, methotrexate, and vinblastine
Breast	FAC	5-Fluorouracil, doxorubicin (Adriamycin), cyclophosphamide (Cytoxan)
	CMF	Cyclophosphamide, methotrexate, and 5-fluorouracil
	Cooper's Regimen (CVFMP)	5-fluorouracil, methotrexate, vincristine (Oncovin), Cytoxan, prednisone
Colon (adjuvant therapy)	MOF	Semustine (methyl-CCNU), vincristine (Oncovin), 5-fluorouracil
Hodgkin's disease	MOPP	Mustargen (mechlorethamine), Oncovin (vincristine), procarbazine, prednisone
	ABVD	Doxorubicin (Adriamycin), bleomycin (Blenoxane), vinblastine (Velban), and dacarbazine (DTIC)
Hodgkin's disease salvage (for patients who relapse)	PCVP	Vinblastine, procarbazine, cyclophosphamide, and prednisone
Leukemia	OAP	Oncovin, Ara-C (cytarabine), and prednisone
	COAP	Cyclophosphamide, Oncovin, Ara-C, and prednisone
	Ad-OAP	Adriamycin, Oncovin, Ara-C, and prednisone
	DAT	Daunorubicin, Ara-C, and thioguanine
Lung (incompletely resected non–small cell lung cancer)	CAP	Cytoxan, Adriamycin, cisplatin (Platinol)
Multiple myeloma	VBAP	Vincristine, BCNU (carmustine), Adriamycin, and prednisone
	VCAP	Vincristine, Cytoxan, Adriamycin, and prednisone
Non-Hodgkin's lymphoma	CHOP	Cytoxan, doxorubicin,* Oncovin, prednisone
	COP	Cytoxan, Oncovin, prednisone
Stomach	FAM	5-Fluorouracil, Adriamycin, Mitomycin-C
Testicular tumors	VB-3	Vinblastine, bleomycin

*The H in this regimen refers to hydroxyldaunorubicin, a chemical synonym for doxorubicin.

ciated with this drug. The myelosuppression appears to be cumulative in some patients, especially those receiving six or more courses of therapy. Gastrointestinal toxicity with nausea and vomiting are common and seen in more than half of the patients receiving this drug, although the nausea and vomiting are readily relieved with antiemetic therapy. No neurotoxicity has been observed to date in patients receiving iproplatin. Further phase I and phase II studies are underway, including studies of iproplatin in combination with other antineoplastic drugs.

Aclacinomycin A

Aclacinomycin A is an investigational anthracycline being used in the treatment of acute leukemias. This drug is a pyrimidine antagonist that produces less cardiotoxicity and mutagenicity than the well-known anthracycline doxorubicin. Although several investiga-

tional anthracyclines are currently being studied, researchers feel that aclacinomycin A has the most therapeutic potential for patients.

Interferon

Interferon (IFN) is the drug that scientists hope holds the most promise for the 1990s. Researchers hope this drug will do for certain cancers what penicillin did for infections. Although first discovered in 1957 by virologists Alick Isaacs and Jean Lindenmann, few researchers have been involved in interferon work until recent years because of its scarcity and expense, and the difficulties of producing pure enough substance with which to work. Interferon is a protein that inhibits viruses. Although one type of interferon, interferon alpha-2a (Roferon) is now available for use, several other types of interferons are still under investigation. It is discussed in depth in Chapter 50.

**Table 49-5. PHASES OF
CLINICAL TRIALS**

A new drug is screened for antitumor effectiveness according to rigorous standards established by the National Cancer Institute (NCI). New compounds are tested extensively in the laboratory against cultures of different types of animal and human tumors. Those showing promising antitumor effects are tested on animals next in an effort to predict toxicity in humans. Only 1 in 5000 compounds reaches the phase of human trials. The NCI has established a series of three progressive phases of human trials. The purpose of each phase of study are:

Phase I	to establish the maximum tolerated human dose to establish an optimum dosing schedule to try and determine clinical pharmacology of drug action to determine toxicity levels to normal organs
Phase II	to identify antitumor activity against specific human cancers to establish documentation of patient response in relation to drug dose and schedule to validate drug toxicity data generated by Phase I trials
Phase III*	to compare the new drug against a standard treatment to evaluate the effect of the new drug on patient survival to evaluate the effect of the new drug on the quality of survival for the patient

*Note that only in Phase III trials does treatment of individual disease processes become the focus of the study.

UNPROVEN SUBSTANCES

It is unfortunate that, in a text devoted to recognized and proven therapeutic agents, space must be used to discuss unproven, unrecognized, and potentially dangerous substances. The most unfortunate aspect of these unorthodox methods of cancer treatment is that they rob the cancer patient of precious time in which conventional therapy could effect a remission or cure. Most proponents of these therapies—which include drugs, diets, energy therapies, devices, and vitamins—have professional-looking offices, run clinics dedicated to their form of treatment, and offer the desperate patient and family psychologic support. These actions easily influence many people. Often, the therapist is an expert salesperson who tells the patient what he or she wants so desperately to hear—that there is a cure for cancer that is easy and painless, without the side effects of traditional surgery, radiation, or chemotherapy. All that has to be done is stick to the "prescribed" regimen of diet and/or drugs and various methods of purifying the body to remove environmental and chemical "poisons." Even in the face of obvious therapeutic failure, many patients are convinced that the method did not work because of some failure on their part. They may blame a late or missed pill, eating a forbidden food, or their failure to believe as the cause of therapeutic failure rather than the fact the treatment itself is worthless.

The most widely known of the unproven substances is laetrile, produced from apricot pits. The postulated theory behind this substance is that when the amygdalin in the laetrile comes in contact with beta-glucuronidase produced by tumor cells, cyanide is released. Allegedly, the cyanide then chokes off and kills the tumor cells. In actuality, this does not happen; amygdalin has no effect on tumor cells that can be demonstrated in the laboratory or clinical trials. Cyanide is toxic to humans and has been responsible for deaths in children who ingested laetrile. In an attempt to bypass the Food and Drug Administration's requirements in regard to marketing new drugs, laetrile producers gave this substance the generic name of vitamin B_{17} several years ago. There is no evidence that laetrile is an essential nutrient, so the term "vitamin" in reference to this substance is a misnomer. The attempt to legalize laetrile by claiming it was a vitamin failed, and it is illegal in most states. However, there are more than a dozen states that allow patients to buy laetrile for personal use.

There has been increased activity on the part of laetrile-supporting organizations such as the Cancer Control Society and the Committee for Freedom of Choice in Cancer Therapy, clamoring for human trials of this substance. Although there have been some animal studies in the past, there were no controlled studies in humans until 1981 because the animal studies showed the substance to be of no value. Several institutions, including the Mayo Clinic and M. D. Anderson Hospital, did conduct double-blind studies with laetrile, not because of any scientific justification but in response to the political and social controversy surrounding this substance. Results of these initial phase I and phase II clinical trials have shown laetrile to be of no value in the prolongation of life in cancer patients. It produced no cures and no remissions. Therefore, no further studies were indicated. Phase III studies are not planned.

Patients or their families often question nurses about unproven therapies that receive publicity in the lay press. It is important that the nurse understand the psychologic needs of those who ask and not merely dismiss the whole question. Stress the fact that the best treatment for the patient is one that has proven results. Even when comfort and palliation are the only alternatives available, it is important that emotional needs be met. Remember this is how the unorthodox therapists gain converts—they play on the psychologic and emotional needs of people. Protect your patients by meeting these needs.

Despite the nurse's best efforts, a patient may ultimately decide on an unproven method of therapy. The nurse should not feel a sense of failure if every effort to motivate patient compliance has been tried. Some people must try everything for themselves. Ultimately, the individual, not the health care team, controls what will happen to him or her in this case.

USING THE NURSING PROCESS

The nurse plays a vitally important role in the care of the patient receiving antineoplastic chemotherapy. The nurse is the practitioner with the most direct patient contact. Nurses often administer chemotherapy and are responsible for anticipating side effects and working to prevent, reduce, or alleviate them. Many patients receive chemotherapy as outpatients or take the drugs themselves at home. The nursing implications for such patients center mainly on anticipatory care and health teaching. It is essential to view the patient as a holistic being, greater than the sum of the parts. It is only for the purpose of assessing needs that categories are established. Once the patient is systemically assessed, the information can be put together in order to help the whole patient—physically and psychologically.

ASSESSMENT

Assessing the patient is the initial step of the nursing process. The assessment is essential for the identification of patient problems. Identified patient problems are termed nursing diagnoses. The focus of the assessment and interventions discussed in this chapter is specifically in relation to chemotherapy and the cancer patient. A comprehensive nursing history is an essential component of the assessment process. Areas of patient assessment relative to chemotherapy are highlighted in Table 49–6.

Physical assessment of the patient is a vitally important step in this phase of the nursing process and is essential in establishing a pretherapeutic data base. Good assessment of physical status prior to the initiation of therapy allows for more accurate evaluation of the patient's response to therapy. It also assists in recognizing changes that may warn of impending drug toxicity.

Observation of lesions is important in the objective evaluation of patient's response to chemotherapy. Direct, accurate measurement is essential. Photographs may be taken or whole-body diagrams included in the chart. The nurse may have to map lesions and record measurements in addition to the photographic record made.

Indirect methods of tumor measurement are more common. The accuracy of indirect methods is increasing as new and increasingly sophisticated testing methods are developed. Whole body CT scans, magnetic resonance imaging, sonograms, and x-ray scans are becoming increasingly accurate in the detection and measurement of lesions. The PET (positron emission tomography) is the newest and most accurate scanning method to date. It produces a unique metabolic portrait of how the tissue or organ is functioning.

The prechemotherapy laboratory work-up may be extensive in order to establish as complete a data base as possible. Acid and alkaline phosphatase levels, carcinoembryonic antigen (CEA), CBC, electrolytes, and renal, liver, and cardiac enzymes are a few of the important serum chemistry values monitored. Throughout a patient's course of therapy, regular evaluation of blood chemistry is essential, as many drugs have wide dosage ranges, dependent on patient response and toxic effects such as those seen in the bone marrow, liver, and kidneys. Drug doses are adjusted accordingly. This is why it is imperative for the outpatient to return to the hospital or clinic for regular blood testing throughout the course of therapy.

Assessment of the patient's sexual status relative to receiving chemotherapy should be made. Since psychologic factors play a strong role in sexuality, many patients will experience some changes in this area because of the anxiety and stress of their disease and its treatment. Some drugs do produce libido changes and may temporarily produce physical changes such as gynecomastia in men receiving estrogens. Women on androgen therapy may experience virilization. Patients should be told of the possibility of these effects occurring. Since physical appearance is so strongly linked to sexual desirability, any changes to the physical self can have a dramatic impact on the patient's self-concept. Decreased self-esteem can precipitate depression, with its resultant physical problems such as anorexia and insomnia. Assess patient understanding of antineoplastic drugs relative to parenthood, since most of these drugs can be teratogenic. Males receiving alkylating agents usually develop sterility as a result of their treatment. Since females are born with a fixed number of oocytes (reproductive cells), the risk of sterility is much less. A young male patient should be discreetly counseled and may decide to freeze some sperm should he later desire a family. It requires sensitivity and empathy to deal with this area of the patient's life. If the patient or a family member perceives the nurse as empathetic and understanding, they are more likely to bring up topics of such important concern.

Most of the drugs used in antineoplastic chemotherapy will be present in breast milk; therefore, nursing of infants is generally not recommended while undergoing chemotherapy. Likewise, many of these drugs are teratogenic. Therefore, pregnancy can be risky to the fetus. Women should discuss these issues with their oncologist as well as obstetrician. In some cases, a fertility specialist may be consulted. In addition, there are also concerns for patients who have received chemotherapy for childhood leukemia. Many of these patients who have survived are now of childbearing age themselves and now have concerns about the possible effect such therapy may have on their children.

Assessment of hydration and nutritional status is an important nursing task. Anorexia and *cachexia* are often observed in cancer patients. This altered nutritional status can be the result of drug toxicity, adverse effects, tumor involvement, emotional stress, or effects of radia-

Table 49–6. NURSING PROCESS FOR THE PATIENT RECEIVING ANTINEOPLASTIC CHEMOTHERAPY

Assessment

Note type of cancer present, length of illness, prognosis, previous chemotherapy. Determine nutritional/hydration status. Assess signs/symptoms of chemotherapy/radiation side effects, e.g., stomatitis, edema, hypertension, signs of bone marrow depression. Assess respiratory status. Assess cardiac status via EKG/telemetry reading as appropriate. Assess urinary output.
Assess dental health and oral hygiene. Note if lesions are present. Assess lymph node areas. Assess knowledge level regarding illness and chemotherapy to determine gaps.

Nursing Diagnosis	Nursing Actions	Rationale	Desired Outcomes/ Evaluation Criteria
Altered Nutrition, Less than Body requirements related to consequences of treatment, as evidenced by reported inadequate food intake, altered taste sensation, loss of interest in food, loss of weight, sore/inflamed buccal cavity.	Monitor daily food intake. Encourage patient to eat high-calorie nutrient-rich diet, with adequate fluid intake. Provide supplements and frequent/smaller meals spaced throughout the day. Time chemotherapy doses to interfere least with meals. Administer antiemetic on a regular schedule before/during and after administration of antineoplastic agent as appropriate Review laboratory studies as indicated, e.g., total lymphocyte count, serum transferrin, and albumin. Recommend use of viscous lidocaine as appropriate for oral lesions. Refer to dietician/nutritional support team.	Useful in identifying nutritional needs. Metabolic tissue and fluid needs are increased. Supplements can play an important part in maintaining adequate caloric and protein intake. The effectiveness of diet adjustment is very individualized in relief of post-therapy nausea. Patients need to experiment to find best solution/combination. Nausea/vomiting are frequently the most disabling and pychologically stressful side effects of chemotherapy. Helps identify the degree of biochemical imbalance/ malnutrition and influences choice of dietary interventions May be given to relieve oral pain associated with stomatitis to improve oral intake. Provides for specific dietary plan to meet individual needs and reduce problems associated with protein-calorie malnutrition and micronutrient deficiences.	Demonstrates stable weight or progressive weight gain toward goal with normalization of laboratory values and free of signs of malnutrition. Participates in specific interventions to stimulate appetite/increase dietary intake. Antinausea medications are effective.
Potential noncompliance with dietary restrictions of chemotherapy e.g. no alcohol while on methotrexate, no foods high in tyramines while on procarbazine.	Teach patient the reasons for any restrictions. Also inform family.	Health teaching stressing the reasons for restrictions and the temporary nature of these should promote compliance.	Compliance with dietary restrictions results in no preventable adverse effects, e.g. no Disulfira like reactions while on procarbazine and no hepatotoxicity while methotrexate.
Potential Fluid volume, deficit, related to excessive losses through vomiting, diarrhea, wounds, or impaired oral intake.	Record intake/output, including all sources. Measure specific urine gravity.	Continued negative fluid balance, decreasing renal output/concentration of urine suggests developing dehydration and need for increased fluid replacement	Displays adequate fl ance as evidence ble vital signs, m mucous membr pt good skin turg vid capillary refill, y ually adequat output.

CONTINUED ON THE FOLL PAGE

Nursing Diagnosis	Nursing Actions	Rationale	Desired Outcomes/ Evaluation Criteria
	Weigh as indicated.	Sensitive measure of fluctuations in fluid balance.	
	Monitor vital signs. Evaluate peripheral pulses, capillary refill.	Reflects adequacy of circulating volume.	
	Encourage increased fluid intake to 3000 ml/day as individually appropriate/ tolerated.	Assists in meeting fluid requirements and reduces risk of harmful side effects, e.g., hemorrhagic cystitis in patient receiving Cytoxan.	
	Administer antiemetics as indicated.	Alleviation of nausea/vomiting decreases gastric losses and allows for increased oral intake.	
	Provide IV fluids as ordered.	Given for general hydration as well as to dilute antineoplastic drugs and reduce adverse side effects such as nephrotoxicity or cystitis.	
Oral Mucous Membranes Altered potential related to side effects of chemotherapeutic agents (e.g., antimetabolites).	Inspect oral cavity daily, noting changes in mucous membrane integrity.	The range of response extends from mild erythema to severe ulceration, which can be very painful, inhibit oral intake, and be potentially life-threatening. Early identification enables prompt treatment.	Displays moist mucous membranes, which are free of inflammation/ulcerations. Verbalizes understanding of causative factors. Demonstrates techniques to maintain/ restore integrity of oral mucosa.
	Discuss/demonstrate methods for good oral hygiene care with soft toothbrush/ toothette, flossing or cautious use of WaterPik.	Good care is critical during treatment to control stomatitis complications prevent oral trauma, inhibit bacterial growth.	
	Avoid use of commercial mouthwashes, lemon-glycerine swabs.	Products containing alcohol or phenol may exacerbate mucous membrane dryness/irritation.	
	Suggest use of mouthwash made from warm saline, dilute solution of hydrogen pyroxide or baking soda and water.	May be soothing to the membranes.	
	Administer analgesics, topical xylocaine jelly, and/or antimicrobial mouthwash preparation, e.g., nystatin.	Patient will be more likely to eat if mouth is free from discomfort/pain.	
Impaired Potential Skin/Tissue Integrity, related to effects of chemotherapy, immunologic deficit, altered nutritional state/ anemia, or presence of lesions, drug extravasation.	Inspect skin frequently for side effects of cancer therapy, e.g., breakdown, early signs of infection.	Skin reactions may occur with some chemotherapy agents.	Identifies interventions appropriate for specific condition. Participates in techniques to prevent complications/promote healing as appropriate.
	Bathe with lukewarm water and mild soap.	Maintain cleanliness without irritating the skin.	
	Encourage patient to avoid scratching and to pat skin dry instead of rubbing.	Helps prevent skin friction/ trauma.	
	Turn/reposition frequently.	Promotes circulation and prevents undue pressure on skin/tissues.	
	Review expected dermatologic side effects seen with chemotherapy, e.g., rash, hyperpigmentation, alopecia and peeling of palms with 5FU.	Anticipatory guidance may help adjustment to/ decrease concern if side effects do occur.	
	Advise patients receiving 5FU and methotrexate to avoid sun exposure. Report to physician if sun-	Sun can cause exacerbation of burn spotting or can cause a red "flash" area with methotrexate,	

Nursing Diagnosis	Nursing Actions	Rationale	Desired Outcomes/ Evaluation Criteria
	burn is present as he/she may order drug to be withheld.	which can exacerbate adverse drug effect.	
	Ascertain that IV is infusing well, dilute anticancer drug per protocol.	Reduces risk of tissue irritation/injury.	
	Instruct patient to notify caregiver promptly of discomfort at IV insertion site.	Development of pain at infusion site indicates need for prompt determination of cause. If due to drug infiltration/extravasation prompt intervention to prevent more serious reaction is essential. IV site or flow rate may need changing.	
	Observe skin/IV and vein for erythema, edema, tenderness, weltlike patches, itching/burning or swelling, soreness, blisters.	Presence of phlebitis, vein flare or extravastion requires immediate discontinuation of antineoplastic agents and medical intervention.	
	Wash skin immediately with soap and water if antineoplastic agents are spilled on unprotected skin. Wear gloves, protective eye covering (glasses, goggles) if drawing up drug, starting or discontinuing IV. Dispose of drug contaminated waste properly.	Dilutes drug to reduce risk of skin irritation/burn.	
	Administer appropriate antidote per protocol and physician's orders if extravasation should occur.	Reduces local tissue damage. Injection of antidotes is a controversial therapy, however some studies show that it is beneficial.	
	Hyaluronidase;	Injected subcutaneously for vincristine.	
	Sodium bicarbonate;	Injected IV and/or into surrounding tissues for Carmustine.	
	⅙th molar sodium thiosulfates;	Injected subcutaneously for nitrogen mustard.	
	Apply topical ointment, e.g., silver sulfadiazine as ordered.	May be used to prevent infection/facilitate healing if chemical burn occurs.	
	Apply icepack/warm compresses as ordered.	Controversial intervention is dependent on type of agent used to restrict blood flow, keeping drug localized, or to enhance dispersion of antidote.	
Potential Impaired, Gas Exchange related to alveolar-capillary membrane thickening (pulmonary fibrosis), altered blood flow/decreased circulation or altered oxygen-carrying capacity (anemia).	Elevate head of bed, assist patient to assume position of comfort. Promote adequate rest periods, assist with self care needs.	Eases work of breathing and promotes maximal inspiration. Prevents undue fatigue/excessive oxygen demands which could comprise cardio-respiratory function.	Demonstrates adequate oxygenation of tissues by ABGs within patient's normal range and free of symptoms of respiratory distress.
	Auscultate breath sounds routinely. Note presence of crackles/rhonchi or dyspnea.	Early detection of respiratory compromise may indicate development of toxic effects such as pulmonary fibrosis (Busulfan, Carmustine, Melphalan, Bleomycin) or cardiomyopathy (Daunorubicin).	

CONTINUED ON THE FOLLOWING PAGE

Table 49–6. NURSING PROCESS FOR THE PATIENT RECEIVING ANTINEOPLASTIC CHEMOTHERAPY–*CONTINUED*

Nursing Diagnosis	Nursing Actions	Rationale	Desired Outcomes/ Evaluation Criteria
	Evaluate heart rate/rhythm.	High resting pulse or dys-rhythmias may be early signs of decreased oxygenation, cardiotoxicity.	
	Administer supplemental oxygen as appropriate. Review serial ABG results.	Maximizes oxygen available for tissue uptake. Evaluates therapeutic needs/effectiveness.	
Fear/Anxiety (specify level) related to situational crisis, threat to/change in health/socioeconomic status, role functioning, interaction patterns, threat of death, separation from family as evidenced by increased tension, shakiness, apprehension, restlessness, expressed concerns regarding changes in life events, feelings of helplessness/hopelessness.	Review previous experience with cancer. Determine what the doctor has told patient/SO and what conclusion patient has reached.	Assists in identification of fear(s) and misconceptions based on past experience with cancer.	Displays appropriate range of feelings. Appears relaxed and reports anxiety is reduced to a manageable level. Demonstrates use of effective coping mechanisms and active participation in treatment regimen.
	Encourage patient to share thoughts and feelings.	Provides opportunity to examine realistic fears as well as misconceptions about diagnosis.	
	Maintain frequent contact with patient. Talk with and touch patient as appropriate.	Provides assurance that the patient is not alone or rejected; conveys respect for and acceptance of the person, fostering trust.	
	Assist patient/SO in recognizing and clarifying fears.	Coping skills are often impaired after diagnosis and during early phase of treatment. Support and counseling are often necessary to enable individual to recognize and begin to deal with fear and to realize control.	
	Provide accurate, consistent information regarding prognosis.	Can reduce anxiety and enable patient to make decisions/choices based on realities.	
Knowledge deficit related to lack of exposure/recall, information misinterpretation, myths, unfamiliarity with resources as evidenced by questions/ request for information, inaccurate follow-through of instructions/development of preventable complications.	Review with patient/SO understanding of specific diagnosis, treatment alternatives, and future expectations.	Validates current level of understanding. Identifies learning needs, and provides base on which patient can make informed decisions.	Verbalizes accurate information about diagnosis and treatment regimen. Correctly performs necessary procedures and explains reasons for the actions. Initiates necessary lifestyle changes and participates in treatment regimen.
	Provide anticipatory guidance with patient/SO regarding treatment protocol, length of therapy, expected results, possible side effects.	Accurate and concise information helps to dispel fears and anxiety, helps clarify the expected routine, and enables patient to maintain some degree of control.	
	Review specific medication regimen and use of OTC drugs.	Enhances ability to manage self care and avoid potential complications, drug reactions/interactions.	
	Identify signs and symptoms requiring medical evaluation, e.g., drug reactions, delayed healing, increased pain (dependent on individual situation), infection.	Early identification and treatment may limit severity of complications.	
	Stress importance of continuing medical follow-up.	Provides ongoing monitoring of progression/resolution of disease process and opportunity for timely diagnosis and treatment of complications.	

tion or surgery. Poor nutrition and hydration status can lead to systemic problems such as poor uptake of the antineoplastic drugs by cancer cells, thereby increasing systemic toxicity of these agents. Also, poor nutritional status may prevent normal cells from recovering from chemotherapeutic effects. Insufficient fluid intake can cause increased toxicity of the urinary tract, as the kidneys excrete many antineoplastic agents. The use of certain agents such as cyclophosphamide in poorly hydrated patients can lead to hemorrhagic cystitis. Other drugs increase uric acid levels, and poor hydration can predispose to obstructive uropathy in these individuals.

Nutrition and hydration assessment is fairly easy to ascertain. Key factors to observe include weight, tissue turgor, complexion, coloring, and condition of mucous membranes, hair, and nails. The nurse should also inquire about food likes and dislikes. It is important to ascertain deficiencies perceived by the patient and family in these areas.

Oxygenation status plays an important role in chemotherapy. Poor oxygenation may result from tumor growth or extension, concurrent diseases such as emphysema, or the toxic effects of drugs such as bleomycin. Poor oxygenation can result in poor uptake of antineoplastic agents by tumor cells, again leading to increased systemic toxicity and decreased antitumor effect.

Some patients may exhibit pyrexia. If this happens, infection should be ruled out before the initiation of chemotherapy. It is important to remember that fever can also be the result of tumor-produced toxins, other disease processes, or attendant to the use of certain chemotherapeutic or other drugs.

Because of the systemic effects produced by most antineoplastic drugs, a waiting period of four to eight weeks between courses of chemotherapy is customary. Most chemotherapeutic agents cannot effect an adequate tumor cell kill without at the same time causing the destruction of many normal cells. Thus, the toxic and therapeutic effects of these drugs overlap. The cells most susceptible to chemotherapeutic agents are those cell populations that are rapidly proliferating, as are tumor cells. Unfortunately, certain normal tissue populations are also rapidly growing: gastrointestinal mucosa, hair, bone marrow stem cells, immunologic cells, and gonadal cells. Some of the gastrointestinal effects can be minimized by the use of pharmacologic agents such as antiemetics; however, others such as anorexia and *stomatitis* may be unavoidable. In a similar way, judicious scheduling of dosing of bone marrow-toxic agents may minimize, but not prevent, bone marrow suppression. Alopecia results from the chemotherapeutic effect on the hair-cell protein coating and must be dealt with in a nonmedical manner. Patients must be made to understand that their treatment is not benign and the adverse effects may be considerable. Anticipation of the aforementioned effects and careful monitoring by nursing staff are mandatory to prevent further complications. However, the only "cure" for the adverse effects on these rapidly growing cellular popula-

tions is time to recover from drug effects as new, healthy cells begin to develop.

Blood chemistry studies should reflect adequate hepatic, renal, and bone marrow function prior to the initiation of further chemotherapy and are assessed regularly.

The presence of concurrent illness complicates but does not rule out chemotherapy. Active infections, bleeding, and serious illness may be aggravated by chemotherapy. This is due to the antineoplastic agent decreasing immune resistance and affecting the speed of the healing processes. Use of certain agents may aggravate or exacerbate serious emotional illnesses, so it is important to assess psychosocial as well as physical status.

Assessment of lymph nodes in certain body areas is important because of tumor affinity to spread via this route. Observation and palpation of the lymph node areas the particular tumor may extend to are essential. For the breast cancer patient, assessment of axillary lymph nodes is vital. Often, it is the nurse who first becomes aware of enlarged nodes in the course of giving care such as bathing. Other lymph areas to assess are the supraclavicular, sternocleidomastoid, and groin area.

Assessing the patient's psychological status is as important as assessing physical status, as it is this psychological status that determines his or her overall sense of well-being. The importance of the psychologic status of the individual has been stressed by nursing theorists such as Callista Roy in her Adaptation Theory. Both the patient and family need to have their understanding of the illness and its treatment assessed. Concurrent assessment of anxiety levels is also essential for appropriate anticipatory guidance and care. So fundamental is this interpersonal nurse–patient relationship that Peplau used it as the core of her nursing theory. The establishment of patient trust is especially important in motivating compliance with chemotherapeutic regimens. Because of the seriousness of cancer, most patients are highly motivated to comply with therapy regimens, despite adverse drug effects. However, some patients may decide that the adverse effects of palliative chemotherapy are more debilitating than their disease symptoms and discontinue therapy. This is the patient's right as long as he or she understands the ramifications of stopping treatment. This concept is referred to as *informed refusal.*

NURSING DIAGNOSES

The nursing diagnosis is derived from the assessment data. Possible nursing diagnoses relative to chemotherapy appear in Table 49–6. Planning nursing intervention for each diagnosis is the next step of the nursing process. Individual patient needs may vary according to their level of understanding, therapy schedule, disease stage, and ability to cope with their illness. It is not uncommon for nursing diagnoses to center on health teaching about chemotherapy because of patient/family knowledge deficits. Altered oral mucous membranes is another common nursing diagnosis relative to chemotherapy because of the frequency of adverse drug effects on the oral mucosa.

INTERVENTIONS

Nursing interventions are based on nursing diagnoses resulting from assessment. The nurse needs to consider the patient's feelings and goals in determining long- and short-range goals consistent with the therapeutic objectives of the health team. Possible courses of action are considered, and actions best meeting individual needs are implemented. Nursing interventions associated with assessment data relative to chemotherapy follow. They are also featured in Table 49–6.

Lesion-associated interventions include knowledge of x-ray, scan, and test results, and recordkeeping appropriate to the type of lesion and institutional policies. The nurse is often responsible for regular direct measurement of visible lesions and documentation using diagrams or photographs as appropriate. Measurement of lesions is especially important in the use of investigational agents to determine objective remissions. For this reason, often times, lesions are photographed.

Hydration and nutritional interventions can have a dramatic impact on the patient's overall physical status. Weigh the patient regularly. Many drugs are calculated according to patient weight. Weight differences of as little as 1 kg may require dose recalculation. Fluids are encouraged, forced if necessary, in order to prevent urinary tract problems. Frequent oral care is essential to minimize stomatitis and promote healing. These patients are also encouraged to eat soft, bland types of food in an effort to decrease the mechanical irritation of chewing and the possibility of bleeding gums.

For patients receiving drugs that cause gastrointestinal irritation, the bland diet is also useful. These drugs may be administered with antacids in order to help decrease gastritis. Nausea and vomiting are the two most common side effects of chemotherapy, and, along with stomatitis, they contribute the most to poor hydration and nutrition. Appropriate nursing interventions are the use of antiemetics and the scheduling of drug doses for the least interference with mealtime. For example, if the patient receives one dose of the medication per day, it is sometimes helpful to schedule the dose a couple hours after dinner. The concurrent administration of antiemetics and/or central nervous system depressants with chemotherapy may decrease nausea and vomiting (refer to Chapter 53 for information on specific antiemetic drugs to treat nausea and vomiting). Patients suffering the effects of nausea-related anorexia are encouraged to eat in any way possible, including the use of elemental diets and supplements, such as Vivonex (refer to Chapter 56 for further information on nutritional support therapy).

Some patients have reported decreased nausea and vomiting due to marijuana smoking prior to chemotherapy. Studies on the antiemetic effects of tetrahydrocannabinol (THC) show significant antiemetic effects and low side effects. Nabilone, a close chemical congener of THC, is useful as an antiemetic. Adverse effects of these agents include euphoria (more associated with THC), increased appetite, drowsiness, and postural hypotension. The phenothiazines are the most commonly used antiemetics. As a class, they have been studied the most thoroughly and have shown both efficacy and safety. They may, however, not be effective against strongly emetic agents. High-dose metoclopramide (Reglan) therapy has been successful in combating the severe nausea and vomiting associated with cisplatin therapy. Adverse effects of metoclopramide are minor, with mild sedation being the most common. Rarely, transient extrapyramidal effects may occur. Ativan and Decadron can also be used to treat severe nausea and vomiting due to cisplatin therapy. For further information on antiemetics, see Chapter 53.

Stomatitis is a common side effect of many chemotherapeutic agents, especially the antibiotics and antimetabolites. The inflammation and ulceration of the oral mucosa result from the effect of chemotherapeutic drugs on rapidly proliferating cells of the oral cavity. Nursing interventions promote patient comfort, maintain adequate hydration and nutritional status, and help reduce the chance of bleeding or secondary infections of the oral cavity. It is important for the patient to prevent trauma to irritated oral mucosa. Patients receiving chemotherapeutic drugs that cause stomatitis are prone to secondary infections with candida, pseudomonas, herpes simplex, and *Escherichia coli*. Medicated mouth rinses like nystatin suspension may be ordered for the patient with candidiasis. Likewise, viscous lidocaine may be ordered to relieve oral pain.

The infiltration of irritating chemotherapeutic drugs into subcutaneous tissues can cause cellulitis, phlebitis, necrosis, or tissue sloughage. The best interventions for this problem are those aimed at prevention. The nurse always tests the intravenous line for placement in the vein by checking for blood return before administering a chemotherapeutic drug. If inserting a new intravenous line for the administration, do not probe excessively with the needle, as this may create a tract along which the drug can infiltrate. Throughout the infusion of an intravenous chemotherapeutic drug, frequently check the site so that, if infiltration does occur, it will be recognized quickly so corrective measures can be instituted. If infiltration does occur, follow institution protocol for treatment of infiltration of corrosive drugs. Prompt treatment can minimize or prevent tissue damage. Some drug manufacturers recommend a specific antidote if infiltration occurs. For example, hyaluronidase (Wydase) is recommended for vincristine infiltrations. When injected around the infiltration site within 1 hour of occurrence, this enzyme reduces or prevents tissue damage by temporarily breaking down tissue cement. This causes the extravasated drug to rapidly diffuse through the tissues and increases the absorptive surfaces, resulting in an increased rate of drug resorption. In order for the hyaluronidase to be effective, it must be injected subcutaneously or intradermally at the infiltration site. The recommended method is to surround the leading edge of the site with approximately five injections of 0.2 ml each. A separate fine-gauge needle is used for each injection. Infiltration treatment with a ⅙ molar sodium thiosulfate solution is recommended for the extravasation of mechlorethamine. For infiltration of anthracycline-type antineoplastic drugs (doxorubicin, daunorubicin, etc.), the simple injection of corticosteroids and/or specific antidote may not be sufficient to control severe, prolonged tissue damage due to latent, local drug activity. Tissue destruction can occur for up to nine months after the extravasation. Many researchers currently recommend that the patient with an extravasation of these products be seen by a qualified cosmetic surgeon as well as having periodic surveillance of the affected area for several weeks afterward.

Nursing assessment and intervention to alleviate respiratory problems is another crucial area of care for the chemotherapy patient. In addition to its effect on perfusion of tissues to maximize chemotherapeutic effects, respiratory status is an indicator of toxic effects such as pulmonary fibrosis, which can accompany the use of certain agents such as busulfan, carmustine, melphalan, or bleomycin. Monitor the patient for signs of crackles and rhonchi. In addition, obtain arterial blood gas specimens as ordered and monitor reports closely so the physician can be informed of any significant changes in the patient's respiratory status. Observe for skin and nail bed color changes, and for central cyanosis. Oxygen may be administered prior to the administration of the chemotherapeutic agent. Encourage the patient to rest for specific intervals during the day.

Helping the patient and family cope with the psychologic impact of cancer is a major nursing responsibility. The psychologic impact of cancer, along with the sometimes drastic changes treatment effects in body image, represent a major life crisis to patient and family. Other problems such as the presence of concurrent illnesses, pre-existing marital and family problems, and financial worries add to their burden considerably. The nurse fails to give adequate care if these areas are ignored. Psychologic stress and depression can contribute to immune system depression, making it more difficult for the patient to resist infections and disease/drug effects.

Nursing tasks such as the routine taking of vital signs can help to establish a trusting therapeutic relationship, so that areas of great concern to the patient can be broached. Monitoring the patient for progression or problems with concurrent illnesses also conveys to the patient and family the message that all aspects of the patient's care are being addressed. Situational emotional support is the single most important nursing intervention in this area. At this time of severe stress, the nurse's role as teacher, support system, and role model can be extremely valuable.

For the cancer patient receiving chemotherapy, emotional ups and downs are the rule rather than the exception. However, it is important that the nurse not dismiss important changes in patient emotional stress, but report them as noted. Drastic mood changes, euphoria, and signs of impending psychosis or depression may be drug related and should be brought to the attention of the physician.

It is necessary for the nurse to maintain an attitude of realistic hope when dealing with the cancer patient and family. Even when cure goals must be changed to comfort goals, it is psychologically uplifing for the patient and family to know that continuing efforts are being made on the patient's behalf.

A final nursing intervention in the area of psychologic support is in the area of allaying patient fears. Many times, the patient has fears founded in outdated knowledge, misinformation, or just plain fear of the unknown. The honest approach of explaining usual drug effects can do much to allay fears. It is a fact that some patients are highly suggestible, and too descriptive an explanation of drug effects will predispose them to these. The use of good nursing judgment tempered with experience works best in determining the best way to educate the patient without adding to their anxiety or expectation of adverse effects.

The extended hospitalizations sometimes necessitated by cancer therapy can have a dramatic effect to the patient's expression of sexuality. Sensitivity to patient concerns is again important. Sexual expression is not limited to intercourse; it also includes kissing, hugging, and caressing. Allowing the patient and his or her partner times of privacy is important. Closing the patient's door or drawing the curtains for a few minutes may allow for kissing or shared embraces, which reinforce to the patient that he or she is still loved and desired by the partner. Parenthood during chemotherapy needs to be discussed with the physician. All chemotherapeutic agents cross the placenta and are capable of producing fetal abnormalities. Most physicians prefer that patients wait until chemotherapy is completed to father or bear children. Consultation with the physician will be necessary to determine the best method of birth control. Use of birth control pills may not be appropriate for all female patients because of their hormonal composition. Some drugs or treatments may impair fertility or increase the risk of birth defects in offspring. For these reasons, patients may consult fertility specialists when planning parenthood following cancer treatment.

The final group of nursing interventions deals with health teaching. Anticipatory guidance and health teaching are becoming increasingly important, since more patients than ever before are continuing chemotherapy in the home. Patient and family members must be taught the appropriate dose and handling of the drug, as well as what adverse effects are normal and what adverse effects signal toxicity. See Table 49–7 for an example of a patient drug information card.

As with any teaching situation, learning will not occur in times of severe anxiety or stress. If there is such stress, it is best to use supportive techniques and approach the patient when the anxiety has lessened. Begin teaching where assessed deficiencies exist. Write instructions out so they are not forgotten or misinterpreted. Use lay terminology rather than medical jargon to explain things. The advent of intra-arterial chemotherapy using implanted Silastic catheters such as the Hickman catheter

Table 49–7. PATIENT TEACHING FOR PATIENTS TAKING ANTINEOPLASTIC DRUGS

Patients taking antineoplastic drugs at home need to know about potentially serious drug adverse effects and which symptoms require prompt medical attention. A card or form with the following information is a helpful summary for patients/family. The information below is on the drug procarbazine (Matulane®).

Dear Patient:

The drug procarbazine (Matulane) has been prescribed to treat your cancer. This drug works by inhibiting the DNA and RNA and interfering with protein synthesis in cells to cause cell death.

How Long to take drug: Follow doctors' orders.

WHEN TO TAKE: At same time each day. Best taken after light meal. Drink extra fluids between meals.

WHEN ON DRUG DON'T USE: Alcoholic beverages, marijuana, cocaine—serious adverse effects can occur.

OTHER FOOD/FLUID RESTRICTIONS: Avoid foods with high tyramine content—such as homemade breads with lots of yeast; sour cream; strong cheeses; crackers containing cheese; aged game meats; robust red wines; beer.

POSSIBLE DRUG SIDE EFFECTS: Decreased white blood cell count (you will be more prone to infections, so avoid contact with sick persons); decreased red blood cell count (anemia); decreased platelets; mouth ulcers; fatigue; dizziness; insomnia.

OTHER PRECAUTIONS: Avoid pregnancy if possible. Consult physician before breast feeding as safety not yet established (drug may pass to milk). Avoid tanning salons, prolonged sunbathing as drug can cause photophobia. Avoid driving, piloting, or operating hazardous machinery until you learn how medicine affects you (it can cause dizziness.)

Storage: Keep out of reach of children.

How supplied: tablets or capsules.

IF YOU FORGET A DOSE: Take as soon as you remember but DO NOT double up on doses ever.

POSSIBLE INTERACTIONS WITH OTHER DRUGS: Amphetamines, anticonvulsants, tricyclic antidepressants, diuretics, guanethidine, Levodopa. Always consult with oncologist before taking any new medication, even over the counter drugs while on Procarbazine.

ANY LIFE-THREATENING SIDE EFFECTS: None expected.

CONTACT PHYSICIAN RIGHT AWAY IF YOU EXPERIENCE ANY OF THE FOLLOWING:

1. Fever = 102° F with or without shaking chills.
2. Unusual bleeding, bruising, chest pain.
3. Extreme weakness/fatigue.
4. Mouth sores.
5. Continued vomiting.
6. Severe headaches.

OVERDOSE/POISONING EMERGENCY:

Symptoms: Restlessness, agitation, fever, convulsions, bleeding.

Call ambulance, transport patient to hospital. *Do not induce vomiting.* If patient is unconscious and not breathing give mouth-to-mouth resuscitation; if no breathing or heartbeat give CPR until ambulance arrives.

has made it possible for many patients to continue their therapy at home. For patients who can master drug administration and catheter care, this allows them to maintain a more nearly normal lifestyle.

EVALUATION

The evaluation step of the nursing process should never be underestimated. It is this step that determines the effectiveness of intervention and modifies or reformulates nursing diagnoses based on patient responses. It is this important step that makes the nursing process cyclic and dynamic rather than linear.

Meaningful evaluation is based on objective data. For example, if the patient with anorexia induced by nausea begins to eat better and shows a weight gain, then this is objective proof of successful nursing intervention. Patients with sufficient output of normal urine after dehydration interventions are likewise showing progress. Monitoring laboratory data and vital signs provides the best objective evaluative data.

Although the nursing goal may have been to improve respiratory status and evaluation after intervention does show improvement, the nurse is remiss if he or she does not take the evaluation one step further. Determining which interventions were the most helpful in solving the patient problems and sharing this information with other members of the health care team will ensure prompt, appropriate intervention on the patient's behalf the next time the problem recurs. Modify intervention when appropriate.

In the area of health teaching, the nurse has a specific responsibility in evaluating the effectiveness of interventions taken. The best means of determining the effectiveness of health teaching is to have the patient or family member demonstrate the pouring of the medication or care of the Hickman catheter and describe actions taken to minimize drug side effects. Knowledge of when and which side effects to report to the physician is also essential. Have the patient or responsible family member describe these signs in his or her own words so you are certain there is understanding. Medic Alert identification is a good idea for the patient on chemotherapy. Refer to the sample nursing process in Table 49–6 for specific health teaching information on the various chemotherapeutic drugs.

Since bone marrow depression is an adverse effect of many agents and it often lasts several weeks after therapy, it is most appropriately discussed with the patient in the context of health teaching for discharge planning. Leukopenia may produce an increased susceptibility to infections. Patients are warned of this and told to report signs of fever and any wound redness or swelling to the physician. They should also avoid contact with ill persons. During chemotherapy, the ability to resist colds, viruses, and other infections is reduced.

For patients who may experience thrombocytopenia, explain the increased bleeding tendency and have them avoid aspirin. Any petechiae or increased tendency to bruising is reported to the physician. Diabetics who take insulin should use extra care when administering insulin injections. Pressure is applied for three to five minutes after insulin injection to prevent bleeding, bruising, or hematoma formation.

The importance of follow-up blood work and checkups must also be stressed to the patient and family. Cancer patients receiving chemotherapy are usually the most cooperative in terms of follow-up care. However, these aspects of therapy must still be stressed lest their importance be forgotten.

Other important side effects for the patient to be aware of are the endocrinologic effects of hormone therapy, neurologic effects, signs of cardiac toxicity, and the psychologic impact of the disease, its sequelae, or therapeutic adverse effects such as altered body image or alopecia. Those patients receiving hormone-manipulative therapy need to know what effects that this will have and especially that these effects, no matter how upsetting, are only temporary and will regress following discontinuation of the drug(s). In terms of neurologic effects, it is necessary that the patient be warned if the drug will interfere with coordination and concentration, and to notify the physician if numbness of fingers, toes, or limbs occurs. Seizure activity should also be reported. The nurse may have to teach seizure precautions if appropriate. Patients may need to be informed of adverse effects peculiar to certain drugs. For example, doxorubicin can cause the urine to become bright red. This is not hematuria. The patient who knows what effects to expect is usually less anxious and more compliant with the therapeutic regimen.

Patients are told to notify the physician if swelling in the feet, heart palpitations, dizziness, or difficulty breathing occurs when cardiac toxicity is associated with the drug they are taking. It is important for the nurse to educate without frightening the patient.

One distressing side effect for patients to bear is alopecia. Even though they know that this is temporary, it can be extremely demoralizing for some people. Although use of a scalp tourniquet and ice caps may be of some help in lessening this effect, it is not possible to use these devices in the presence of blood-borne tumors. Following chemotherapy, the patient may experience a generalized thinning out of hair. The physical problem can be disguised by temporary use of wigs, hairpieces, scarves, or turbans for several weeks or months until hair growth returns. In some instances, the alopecia is actually more disturbing to the family than to the patient. Because this is generally a temporary effect, most patients adjust quite well.

Nursing intervention in discharge planning is vitally important in the home care chemotherapy of the cancer patient. As more hospitals develop minimal care units and lengthen patient passes from the hospital, nursing intervention via health teaching will assume greater responsibilities in patient and family education. If current trends in health care continue, more patients than ever before will be taught how to manage care in the home. For patients who can continue therapy at home, this will mean less disruption of the family unit and may diminish some of the feelings of loneliness and isolation that occur in hospitalization.

SUMMARY

Antineoplastic chemotherapy is a relatively new avenue of pharmacologic disease therapy that traces its origins to the sulfur mustard gases used in the World Wars. It was noted that these agents produced leukopenia in humans. The first antineoplastic drug used, mechlorethamine, was a derivative of the mustard gases used for chemical warfare. It became the prototype antineoplastic alkylating agent. There are several groups of drugs that produce antineoplastic activity in humans, including alkylating agents, antimetabolites, natural products such as the vinca alkaloids and antibiotics, hormones and hormone antagonists, and radioactive isotopes. Antineoplastic drugs destroy cancer cells by one of two means: they interfere with either cell growth or division (replication). These drugs achieve their actions by blocking the cell's ability to obtain or use essential growth nutrients; or they interfere with cell division in the cell cycle to prevent the cancer cell from reproducing.

Nursing activities for patients receiving antineoplastic chemotherapy center around proper drug administration; observation and assessment of the patient for adverse effects; and appropriate patient teaching relative to drug therapy, early recognition of adverse effects, and developing appropriate measures for coping with chemotherapy effects. In order for antineoplastic drugs to kill cancer cells, these drugs must be relatively cytotoxic. Thus, normal as well as cancer cells can be affected by these drugs. Usually the normal cells at greatest risk of toxic effects are those which are rapidly growing such as those of the oral cavity, gastrointestinal tract, skin, hair, bone marrow, and fetal tissue. The benefits of chemotherapy are generally worth the risks of the adverse or toxic effects. Through the use of appropriate assessment, nursing diagnoses, and interventions, you can prevent or help minimize many of chemotherapy-associated adverse effects for your patients. Oncologic nursing is one of the fastest-growing specialities in the nursing profession today. Although every nurse will not want to enter this area of care exclusively, cancer patients can be found on every unit of the hospital. Thus, knowledge of the basics of chemotherapy is essential for every nurse.

BIBLIOGRAPHY

Bacteremia in patients with cancer. Nurse's Drug Alert: Am J Nurs 12(3): 1988.

Bruera, E, et al: Managing chemotherapy-induced emesis. Am J Nurs 88(3):367, 1988.

Bubela, N: Technical and psychological problems and concerns arising from the outpatient treatment of cancer with direct intra-arterial infusion. Cancer Nurs 4(4):305, 1981.

Calabresi, P and Parks, E: Alkylating agents and drugs used for immunosuppression. In Goodman, AG, Gilman, LS, and Gilman, A (eds): The Pharmacological Basis of Therapeutics, ed 7. Macmillan, New York, 1986.

Cancer recurrence curbed. Am J Nurs 86(11):1217, 1986.

Cisplatin neurotoxicity. Nurse's Drug Alert: Am J Nurs 10(11), 1986.

Dana, BW: Treating malignancies with curative intent: Understanding growth and differentiation. Hematol Oncol Clin North Am 2(3):337, 1988.

Dorr, RT and Fritz, WL: Cancer Chemotherapy Handbook. Elsevier, New York, 1980.

FDA Drug Bulletin: Designated Orphan Approvals Total 24. 18(1):April 1988.

Filicetti, J: Unproven methods of cancer treatment. American Association of Occupational Health Nursing Journal, April 1987.

Intra-arterial therapy for head and neck cancer. Clinical Oncology Alert 3(8):32, 1988.

Kelly, W: Hamot Medical Center Chemotherapy Information Manual. Hamot Medical Center, Erie, PA, 1984.

Kolata, G: Predicting cancer's course: New findings: Examination of oncogenes ushers in new era of research. Cancer News 41(3):16, 1987.

Larson, D: Treatment of tissue extravasation by antitumor agents. Cancer 49(5):1796, 1982.

Lippman, ME, Lichter, AS, and Danforth, DN: Diagnosis and Management of Breast Cancer. WB Saunders, Philadelphia, 1988.

Moraca, AM: Nursing management of the client with breast cancer. State University of New York at Buffalo, 1977.

Pinedo, HM, Longo, DL, and Cabner, BA: Cancer Chemotherapy and Biological Response Modifiers, Annual 19. Elsevier, New York, 1987.

Riehl, JP and Roy, C: Conceptual Models for Nursing Practice, ed 2. Appleton-Century-Crofts, New York, 1980.

Rogers, B: Work practices of nurses who handle antineoplastic agents. American Association of Occupational Health Nursing April 1987.

SITUATION   49–1

Hannah Berry is a 52-year-old with disseminated breast cancer. She has been admitted to the oncology unit for chemotherapy.

1. Prior to administration of fluorouracil (5FU) to Ms. Berry, the nurse will check the following lab data:
   a. sodium and potassium
   b. sedimentation rate and sodium
   c. white blood cell count and platelets
   d. liver enzymes and amylase

2. Ms. Berry begins a three-day course of intravenous fluorouracil. The nurse will plan to include the following intervention:
   a. restrict fluid intake
   b. perform frequent oral care
   c. limit meat exercise
   d. monitor thyroid studies

3. When the nurse teaches Ms. Berry about drug therapy, the following information will be included:
   a. Eliminate foods high in tyramine.
   b. Report dark, tarry stools.
   c. Avoid antiemetics.
   d. Eat foods high in fiber.

4. After successful administration of fluorouracil, Ms. Berry is to be discharged home on cyclophosphanide (Cytoxan) orally. Discharge teaching will include:
   a. taking Cytoxin with meals
   b. doubling doses if one is missed
   c. taking Cytoxan at bedtime
   d. drinking plenty of fluids

5. The nurse will monitor the following lab value on a routine basis while Ms. Berry is on Cytoxan:
   a. liver enzymes
   b. uric acid levels
   c. calcium
   d. potassium

6. Which of the following statements by Ms. Berry indicates the need for further patient teaching?
   a. "I may lose my hair due to this chemotherapy."
   b. "Soft toothbrushes will reduce bleeding gums."
   c. "Red urine means that I am getting rid of the medicine."
   d. "I should weigh myself and report unexpected weight gain."

Please refer to the Appendices for correct answers and additional review questions with answers.

SITUATION   49–2

Randolph Alvin, aged 49, continues to receive chemotherapy for multiple myeloma. Medication therapy includes doxorubicin and carmustine. He is being cared for on the Medical Oncology Unit.

1. While Mr. Alvin is receiving doxorubicin (Adriamycin) via peripheral intravenous infusion, the nurse will monitor:
   a. 12 lead ECGs
   b. uric acid levels
   c. potassium levels
   d. abdominal films

2. Mr. Alvin complains of burning and swelling at the IV site through which Adriamycin is infusing. The nurse's best action would be to discontinue the IV and:
   a. place hot packs over the site for at least 24 hours
   b. medicate with morphine sulfate as needed for pain
   c. elevate the extremity and apply pressure at the site
   d. inject sodium bicarbonate subcutaneously at the site

3. In addition, Mr. Alvin is to receive carmustine (BCNU) via slow infusion for two days. The nurse will expect to give the following along with this agent:
   a. antigout medication
   b. leucovorin rescue
   c. antiemetics
   d. Vitamin B12

4. When evaluating Mr. Alvin for bone marrow depression related to BCNU therapy, the nurse will do so:
   a. 2 days after the dose
   b. 3–6 weeks after the dose
   c. 1–2 weeks after the dose
   d. 1 month after the dose

5. Two weeks after discharge from the hospital, Mr. Alvin is readmitted with symptoms related to hypercalcemia. He is to be treated with mithramycin (Mithracin) via intravenous infusion. The nurse will monitor Mr. Alvin for acute toxic signs of this drug, which include:
   a. facial flushing and epistaxis
   b. confusion and stomatitis
   c. purple bands in nail beds
   d. breast tenderness

6. With regard to mithramycin therapy, the nurse selects the nursing diagnostic category Potential for Injury for Mr. Alvin. This nursing diagnosis is related to:
   a. seizures
   b. bleeding tendencies
   c. psychotic reactions
   d. ataxia

Please refer to the Appendices for correct answers and additional review questions with answers.

50
CHAPTER

IMMUNOTHERAPY AND BIOLOGIC RESPONSE MODIFIERS

ANNE MORACA-SAWICKI, RN, MSN

LEARNING OBJECTIVES

After reading this chapter, the student will be able to:

1. Differentiate between cell-mediated and humoral immunity.

2. Identify host antitumor immune mechanisms.

3. Identify and discuss methods by which tumors may escape host immune system detection.

4. Compare and contrast the types of immunity when presented with a list of immunologic terms.

5. Identify which administration routes are used with each drug discussed.

6. Distinguish between side effects common to immunotherapeutic agents and chemotherapeutic agents.

7. Discern from a list of assessment measures those most appropriate for the patient receiving immunotherapy.

8. List nursing diagnoses appropriate to the immmunotherapy patient receiving immunologic drugs.

9. Plan intervention essential to the safe administration of immunologic drugs and teach the patient relevant information about the therapy and its side effects.

10. Correlate appropriate teaching strategies useful in patient/family understanding of immunologic drugs.

11. Compare and contrast the various methods of evaluation of the nursing process and select those most appropriate to the administration of immunologic drugs.

The homeostatic mechanism of immunity is essential for human survival in a world teeming with potentially pathogenic organisms. Cancer researchers hope to augment this complex physiologic function in order to cause the body's own defense system to destroy malignant cells. This chapter discusses basic principles of immunity and immunotherapy. It then focuses on the nurse's role in the assessment, planning, intervention, and evaluation of nursing care relative to patients undergoing these therapies.

IMMUNITY

HISTORICAL PERSPECTIVES

The first use of immunotherapy was in ancient India and China, where attempts were made to prevent smallpox by injecting live nonattenuated organisms from disease pustules into healthy individuals. Needless to say, this treatment caused more disease than it prevented. The first successful use of immunotherapy did not come for several hundred years when, in 1798, Edward Jenner used cowpox organisms to vaccinate people against smallpox.

The first antibodies were discovered in the late 19th century. In 1895, Hericourt and Richet became the first to document tumor immunotherapy in humans. Their sample population contained 50 melanoma patients injected with animal antisera. Although their results were no better than those achieved with other forms of therapy, immunotherapy was looked on with great hope.

Antigen–antibody reactions were studied intensely at the turn of the century. A flurry of early enthusiasm in tumor immunology, created when tumor tissues were transplanted between different strains of laboratory animals, turned to disappointment when researchers realized that tissue rejection occurred because of histoincompatibility between animals, not because of immunologically stimulated antineoplastic effects. Results of many similar tests led to a decreased interest in cancer immunology from the early 1930s to the 1950s. However, advances in the understanding of immunity during those years provided a sufficient data base on which to build modern immunotherapy. Although there is much yet to learn, the basic knowledge of how the immune system functions has provided a good starting point. Immunotherapy is a science still in its infancy, with therapies still in the investigational stage. Today, in the realm of cancer therapy, immunotherapy is often referred to as the fourth major treatment modality (surgery, chemotherapy, and radiotherapy are the other three).

Acquired Immune Deficiency Syndrome (AIDS) has sparked intense interest in finding a cure or means to arrest this disease. At present, researchers are concentrating on drugs that either augment the patient's overwhelmed immune system or arrest the effects of the virus. Drugs that are useful against the opportunistic infections such as *Pneumocystis carinii* pneumonia often seen in AIDS patients are under investigation. The intense research into finding drugs that halt or reverse the AIDS process is enhancing knowledge about the immune system and cancer immunotherapy.

The FDA has recently approved the investigational use of various *biologic response modifiers* to determine their effects on various cancers. The use of *interleukin-2*, *tumor necrosis factor*, and *monoclonal antibodies* are being studied as anticancer agents. Alpha-interferon is the first biologic response modifier to be marketed for use as an anticancer therapy. It is hoped that these new therapies will enable cancer patients to live longer, more productive lives. The National Cancer Institute's Surveillance, Epidemiology, and End Results (SEER) Program reports that 48% of cancer patients can now be cured. It is hoped that breakthroughs with new therapeutic agents can increase this rate even more.

The science of organ transplantation has spurred research into immunity and the process of rejection. The development of immunosuppressive drugs such as Atgam and cyclosporine has made it possible to suppress the immune response of organ transplant recipients. Such immunosuppressive therapy has increased the success rate of organ transplants. Such therapy is a lifelong part of the transplant patient's life; the antirejection drugs must be taken daily for life in order to supress rejection of the transplanted organ(s).

Human monoclonal antibodies are another type of biologic response modifier that are being researched. Monoclonal antibodies are antibodies derived from the fusion of an antibody-producing cell such as a lymphocyte and another cell such as a cancer cell. The hybrid cell is capable of producing a continuous supply of antibody. These antibodies are of exceptional purity and specificity and useful in the identification of antigens on certain viruses, in blood and tissue typing, as well as in the diagnosis of infectious diseases and identification of tumor antigens. Extensive study of monoclonal antibodies is underway in an effort to try and generate human antitumor antibodies. The first cancer study involving monoclonal antibodies and cancer was with multiple myeloma. Studies of monoclonal antibodies and other cancers such as breast, lung, colorectal, and lymphomas are underway in an effort to develop antitumor antibodies.

IMMUNE SYSTEM

The major function of the human immune system is to protect the body from foreign biologic and chemical products, whether they emanate from within or without. Lymphocytes occur in two forms, each with a specific function in the process of immunity. The T cells initiate cell-mediated (cellular) immunity and the B cells initiate antibody-mediated (humoral) immunity.

T Cells

During fetal development, lymphoid stem cells are produced. From these primitive lymphocytes, the *T cells* and *B cells* develop via different mechanisms. Those that will become T cells migrate to the thymus gland, where they mature under its influence, hence their designation as T cells. The T cells become the initiators of the cellular immune response, which yields delayed hypersensitivity reactions, such as positive skin tests, contact dermatitis, homograft rejection, and killer T cell activity. The cytodestructive activity of the killer T cells can occur without antibody or complement. The killer T cells establish membrane contact with the foreign cell so that chemicals produced in the T cells are able to diffuse through the adjacent membranes to destroy the foreign cell (Fig. 50–1).

T cells also play a "helper" role, assisting the B cells in the synthesis of antibody, although they do not produce any antibody or antibody-like proteins. Thus, their exact role in this process remains a mystery for the present time.

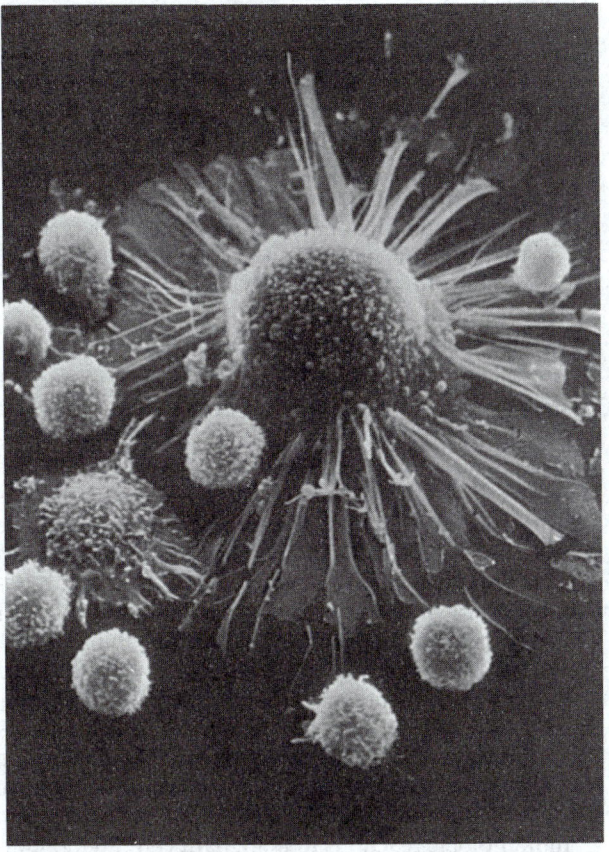

Figure 50–1. A squad of killer T cells surround a large cancerous cell. The T cells are attracted to the cancer cell by its surface antigens, which indicates that it is an abnormal cell. They will take lethal action against the cancer cell by surrounding it and engulfing it. The killer T cells will break down the cell wall of the cancer cell by chemical means. Once the cell wall of the cancer cell is ruptured by the killer T cells, it will die. (Courtesy of Bonnier Fakta, Stockholm, Sweden, with permission.)

B Cells

Bursa cells (B cells), found in the bursa of Fabricius in certain animals, arise from the same primitive lymphocyte cells as do the T cells. However, they mature in a different area. In humans, the B cells mature in bursa-equivalent areas located in Peyer's patches in the intestines, the appendix, and other gut-associated lymph tissue, and possibly the bone marrow itself.

B cells initiate antibody synthesis (humoral immunity). When a mature B cell encounters an antigen (protein foreign to the body), it is stimulated to divide into a plasma cell. The plasma cell begins production of antibodies specific to the offending antigen. Several results can occur when antibodies combine with antigens. Among these responses are toxin neutralization, bacteria lysis, antigen agglutination, or antigen precipitation.

Not all sensitized T and B cells are involved in the sensitizing or immune response. Some of these cells return to the lymphoid tissue and serve as memory cells, lying in wait to respond to future contact with the same antigen. A secondary immune response occurs rapidly on re-exposure to the offending antigen. The severest secondary immune response that may occur is anaphylaxis.

Effector Cells

Within the body's immune system, there are four types of cells that are *effector cells* (cells that kill cancer). These cells are: the killer T cell; the macrophage; the natural killer (NK) cell; and the lymphokine-activated killer (LAK) cell.

A person's complete blood count (CBC) contains the white count and its differential. The granulocytes, lymphocytes, and monocytes are a part of this differential. Monocytes are circulating macrophages. As the monocytes pass from the bloodstream into tissues, they become macrophages, one type of effector cell.

Lymphocytes fall into three categories: B cells and T cells, which are previously discussed; and *null cells*. Most of the lymphocytes in peripheral blood, about 70%–75% are T cells. About 15%–20% are B cells and about 5% are null cells. Null cells lack the markers for both B and T cells, hence their designation as null. The T cells are classified into three groups: helper cells; killer cells; and suppressor cells. It is the second group, the killer T cells, that are effector cells and act against cancer cells. The null cell population contains the other two types of cells that act against cancer. They are the lymphokine-activated killer (LAK) and the natural killer (NK) cells. The helper T cells secrete substances that stimulate B cells to make antibodies or immunoglobulins. One of these substances is interleukin-2, which also stimulates the killer T cells to secrete substances such as gamma interferon.

The macrophage plays an important dual role in the immune system's response to foreign cells. First of all, the macrophage recognizes various antigen/antibody complexes and presents these complexes to the T cell. When this T cell comes in contact with the macrophage, it is able to transmit this information to other effector cells. The macrophage is also capable itself of acting as an effector cell that can secrete substances that can both affect the helper T cells and directly attack cancer cells. The substances that the macrophages can secrete include interleukin-1 and tumor necrosis factor (TNF).

Natural killer cells are cells that without previous exposure to a cancer, are able to kill the cancer without needing complement or antibody. Natural killer cells are stimulated by both interferon and interleukin-2.

The other major cell stimulated by interleukin-2 is the lymphokine-activated killer (LAK) cell. Lymphokine-activated killer cells are different from both natural killer cells and classic killer T cells. Unactivated LAK cells are null cells. However, when activated by interleukin-2, the LAK cells exhibit the same surface markers as do killer T cells. Thus, there is some controversy as to whether these LAK cells are truly null cells or if they are just unactivated T cells.

Human Immunologic Surveillance

Researchers in the 1950s discovered the existence of tumor-specific immunity in neoplastic tumors caused by viruses and chemicals. It was found that most chemically induced tumors have unique individual surface antigens (tumor-specific antigens) and that virally induced tumors have common antigens (tumor-associated antigens) that can produce immunologic cross-reactions. The tumor-specific antigens are often referred to as tumor-specific transplantation antigens (TSTA) because they were first identified in transplantation experiments with *syngeneic* animal tumor systems. It is believed that virtually all human cancers have antigens and these antigens are capable of eliciting an immune response.

Immunologic surveillance is the ability of the body to protect itself against mutant cells arising from within. Thousands of body cells are dividing constantly; thus a cell may make the transformation to being malignant spontaneously or following exposure to carcinogenic substances such as drugs, chemicals, or radiation. Once this transformation has occurred, the malignant cell can be recognized by the immune system as foreign by the presence of new antigens on the surface of the cells. When appropriate immune responses are activated, the malignant cell may be destroyed. This host defense mechanism destroys malignant growths in their preclinical stage. If this immune surveillance system is impaired, suppressed, or bypassed, then malignant cells proliferate to the stage of clinical recognition.

There is evidence that supports this concept of immunosurveillance in humans. The following clinical examples are often cited: (1) Incidence rates of neoplastic tumors are highest in childhood and old age, when the immune system is weak; (2) there is an increased tumor incidence in individuals with immunodeficiency diseases; (3) use of immunosuppressive drugs in organ transplant patients results in a much higher than normal tumor incidence, up to 100 times higher than the controls in one such study; and (4) organ recipients who accidentally receive transplanted malignancies develop gross tumor growth due to immunosuppressive drug therapy to prevent organ rejection. Once these drugs are discontinued, the patient's own cells destroy the invading tumor as well as the transplanted organ.

Host Defense Mechanisms in Malignancy

Host defense mechanisms play a role even in clinically evident malignancy. How successful these mechanisms are can ultimately influence the spread of the tumor, its response to treatment, and the patient's prognosis as well. Examples of hose defense mechanisms follow:

1. Spontaneous tumor regression has occurred, especially in patients with small tumor burdens, which suggests that the immune system may be abe to deal with certain tumor loads.
2. Cancerous tumors heavily infiltrated by lymphocytes generally have a better prognosis than those without such infiltration, especially cancers of the breast, bladder, cervix, stomach, and malignant melanoma. Women with lymphocyte-predominant breast tumors have a well-documented improved prognosis over their counterparts with lymphocyte-depleted cancers.
3. Likewise, patients who demonstrate immunocompetence via an intact cell-mediated immune response at the time of initial treatment will respond better to drug therapy.
4. A final example of host defense mechanisms involves the loss of, or failure of, the immune system. Researchers feel that the appearance of metastatic disease in some patients 15–30 years after removal of a primary tumor represents a failure of the host to maintain control over aberrant cells.

Host Antitumor Immune Mechanisms

Earlier in this chapter, general aspects of the immune system were discussed. More specific aspects of these processes now follow. Recall the function of the T cells in the initiation of the cellular immune response. Once T-lymphocyte cells become sensitized by the foreign antigens of tumor cells, the killer T cell response may be initiated. The effects of these sensitized cells are enhanced by the release of soluble factors called lymphokines. Lymphotoxin and migration inhibitory factor (MIF) are two such substances. Migration inhibitory factor is thought to be responsible for the activation and recruitment of tissue macrophages at T-lymphocyte–tumor cell reaction sites. Such activated macrophages have increased lysosome enzyme content and increased mitotic rates, and they demonstrate more aggressive phagocytic behavior.

Immunologic reactions to malignant cells are not limited to the T cells. The B cells and their humoral products have an active role also. Several antibody-dependent mechanisms against tumor cells are mediated by the B-lymphocytes. For example, tumor-specific IgM antibody will have directly cytotoxic effects on tumor cells in the presence of complement. Antibody-dependent lymphotoxicity is the result of IgG antibodies. (There are five immunoglobulins produced by the B cells—IgM, IgG, IgA, IgD, and IgE.)

Tumor Escape from Host Immune Responses

Such detailed explanations of immunologic surveillance and immune reactions cannot help but lead to one question. In the midst of such elaborate defense mechanisms, how does cancer arise and proliferate? Although no definite answer has yet been found, several factors are thought to contribute to the escape of tumors from host immune responses.

Age as a factor in tumor escape from host immune mechanisms has already been discussed. Some other "escape mechanisms" from host immune mechanisms are thought to be:

1. Mechanical factors, which may interfere with lymphocyte accessibility to the tumor, thereby limiting or preventing its destruction.
2. Circumvention of the immune response by production of a tolerance to the foreign antigen so the tumor antigens go unrecognized as foreign.
3. Drug cytotoxicity, which may decrease tumor antigen production that would sensitize the host to tumor presence.
4. The "sneaking through" phenomenon, in which the tumor does not immunize the host until too large a tumor burden for the immune system to handle is established.
5. The "biphasic" nature of some antitumor responses, which may actually foster malignant growth. For example, when a tumor elicits a strong immune response, the tumor may be destroyed; but if a weak immune response is triggered, then the tumor may actually be stimulated.
6. Weakly antigenic tumors, which may not stimulate sufficient immunologic defense mechanisms, and tumor growth in "immunologically privileged" sites with poor lymphatic connections, which would also fail to muster an immune response capable of effectively dealing with the malignant assault.
7. The presence of "blocking factors" or "blocking antibodies," which can be found in many human tumors. This can occur if antibody or tumor antigen–antibody complexes cover the antigenic sites on the cancer cells, or when large tumor burdens overwhelm the host's immune system with antigen. Some patients exhibit an "unblocking" ability in their serum, and this is associated with a better patient prognosis.

GOALS AND PRINCIPLES OF IMMUNOTHERAPY IN NEOPLASTIC DISEASE

Immunity is a homeostatic function essential to human survival. Yet certain disease states suppress or circumvent this sophisticated survival system, cancer being the most notable example. As knowledge of these immune processes increases, so too have hopes for their application. Much is yet to be learned about immune mechanisms and how to augment them. Many hope that immunotherapy will become a major cancer treatment in the near future, although as a science immunology is still in its infancy and its treatments experimental.

GOALS

There are three basic goals in cancer immunotherapy. They are: 1) to stimulate immunocompetence by active or passive means in the cancer patient; 2) to promote tumor-specific immunity; and 3) as an adjunct to other treatments, to produce tumor regression in the cancer patient.

PRINCIPLES

The basic principles of immunotherapy are often used as criteria to determine patient eligibility for this therapy, since not all patients will benefit from a particular treatment. The following considerations are important:

1. Tumor reduction—Reduction of tumor body burden is achieved by removing as much of the tumor as possible, since large tumor burdens depress the immune system.
2. Tumor type—Patients with hairy cell leukemia; malignant melanoma; AIDS-related Kaposi's sarcoma; chronic myelocytic leukemia; superficial bladder cancer; and follicular lymphomas respond best to immunotherapy. Patients who derive the most benefit from therapy have disease that has not progressed beyond stage II and are not severely immunosuppressed.
3. Immunocompetence—Assessment of immune response mechanisms can be done by delayed hypersensitivity skin testing with such agents as purified protein derivative of tuberculin (PPD), mumps vaccine, and Candida. There is a better prognosis for patients able to mediate sufficient immune response, as demonstrated by these and other qualitative examinations. Quantitiative assessment of immune function is made by peripheral blood counts, immunoglobulin assays, and bone marrow aspiration.
4. Treatment scheduling—Treatment should be timed carefully in regard to surgery, chemotherapy, and radiotherapy, so the patient's immune system can recover from the depressive effects of these modalities.

The major advantage of immunotherapy is that it is not a severely debilitating treatment. Side effects are usually mild and consist of localized skin reactions with self-limiting symptoms such as pruritus. Occasionally, patients may experience flu-like symptoms. About the only reason for discontinuance of therapy is severe hypersensitivity reactions (anaphylaxis), which is a rare occurrence.

TYPES OF IMMUNOTHERAPY

Immunotherapy is divided into two major categories: active and passive. These two categories consist of specific and nonspecific treatments. There is also a third classification of passive immunotherapy called *adoptive immunotherapy*. Immune therapies are described only in the context of their use in cancer treatment.

ACTIVE SPECIFIC IMMUNOTHERAPY

Active immunotherapy can be achieved by use of specific and nonspecific techniques. In *active specific immunotherapy*, the tumor cell and its products or antigens are reinjected into the original host after they have been *attenuated*. This process is termed autoimmunization. This technique uses *autologous* tumor cells. This therapy is in a preliminary stage of development.

ACTIVE NONSPECIFIC AUGMENTATION OF IMMUNITY

Active nonspecific immunotherapy is the stimulation of the immune system by administration of attenuated live bacteria or their products, or chemical agents. The major agents used for this purpose are bacillus Calmette-Guerin (BCG) vaccine, *Corynebacterium parvum (C. parvum)* organisms, levamisole, and dinitrochlorobenzene (DNCB). This therapy has been applied in the treatment of malignant melanoma, bladder cancer, metastatic breast cancer, mycosis fungoides, and multiple basal cell carcinoma. This form of immunotherapy is the oldest approach. The use of BCG, *C. parvum*, and DNCB fell into disfavor because therapeutic efficacy was extremely limited. Also, newer and more potent immunoregulatory agents such as interferon and interleukin-2 were discovered.

PASSIVE IMMUNOTHERAPY

Passive immunotherapy can be achieved by any of the following methods: injecting antitumor sera into the host; administering lymphocyte transfusions to the cancer patient from healthy individuals; or removing immunosuppressive substances from the cancer patient through techniques such as plasmapheresis. In general, passive immunotherapy has not been a very successful means of generating tumor remission.

Passive Specific Immunotherapy

Passive specific immunotherapy is the injection of specific serum into patients with active disease in an attempt to stimulate antitumor antibody formation. Researchers have had moderate success in the treatment of some Burkitt's lymphoma tumors using this technique. Patients with active disease were immunized with serum from patients in remission.

Passive Nonspecific Immunotherapy

Passive nonspecific immunotherapy is the collection of serum from healthy individuals for injection into cancer patients. This treatment is usually employed in the treatment of patients with chronic lymphocytic leukemia, who lack ability to produce normal amounts of effective antibodies. It also may be used in the treatment of nonmalignant conditions that produce an inability to resist infection.

ADOPTIVE IMMUNOTHERAPY

Adoptive immunotherapy is the transfer of live immunocompetent lymphocytes for their effect on substances from a compatible donor to the cancer patient to provide passive immunity. The donor's lymphocytes are incubated *in vitro* with tumor cells from the patient to sensitize the lymphocytes. They are then infused into the patient. It is hoped that the patient's immunologic defense system will accept and use these new immune cells. Administration of *transfer factor* is one example of this therapy. Use of this therapy in the treatment of malignant melanoma and other tumors has produced some remissions. Early study results are encouraging, and researchers believe this therapy to be of good potential value. Much further research in this area is needed.

IMMUNORESTORATIVE IMMUNOTHERAPY

This type of immunologic therapy uses agents that increase patient immune response, especially the number of mature, functioning T-lymphocytes. Substances that would augment the patient's immune system in this manner could be called immunologic stimulants. One such type of immunologic stimulant is *interferon* (IFN).

Preliminary research is beginning to show some promising aspects of interferon's activity. Alpha interferons have shown excellent tumor response rates

Table 50–1. CLINICAL ACTIVITIES OF SELECTED BIOLOGICAL RESPONSE MODIFIERS

Biological Response Modifier	Disease	Response Rate (%)
Alpha Interferons	Chronic myelocytic leukemia	70
	Epidemic Kaposi's sarcoma	20–80
	Follicular lymphomas	35–55
	Hairy cell leukemia	80–100
	Malignant melanoma	0–23
	Renal cell carcinoma	0–27
Interleukin-2	Colon cancer	10
	Malignant melanoma	30
	Renal cell cancer	30

against hairy cell leukemia (80%–100%) and renal cell carcinomas (up to 27% response rates) (see Table 50–1 for other examples of clinical activity). Much further research is needed into the clinical applications of interferons.

Other substances are currently being studied to determine their usefulness as immunologic stimulants. Other agents being investigated for their value as immunorestorative agents include lymphokines, thymic hormones, and levamisole.

IMMUNOTHERAPEUTIC AGENTS

Many agents have been tested for their value in immunotherapy, and others are currently under investigation. The agents most frequently studied in the 1980s were bacillus Calmette-Guerin (BCG), *C. parvum,* and methanol-extracted residue of BCG (MER). Although these agents may be used to evaluate a patient's immunocompetence, they are rarely used as nonspecific cancer immunologic adjuvants today. The advent of molecular biologic techniques has brought superior substances such as interferons and lymphokines into the forefront of immunology research. Interferons, cytokines, and lymphokines are felt to be more specific agents for immune stimulation than the earlier substances. Agents currently under study as cancer immunologics are: transfer factor, Immune RNA (I-RNA), interleukin-2, and tumor necrosis factor (TNF). The therapeutic agents are featured in Table 50–2. Since most immunotherapeutic agents discussed are still being investigated for their effect in cancer therapy, all dosages cited are based on investigational data and are therefore subject to change. For agents still in early Phase I and Phase II trials, therapeutic dosage levels have yet to be determined.

BACILLUS CALMETTE-GUERIN

Although BCG was first isolated in 1910 at the Pasteur Institute by Calmette and Guerin, it was not clinically tested until 1921, when it was used as a tuberculosis vaccine. Its use as a cancer therapy did not come until nearly half a century later. Bacillus Calmette-Guerin is an attenuated live bacterium. Its use in cancer therapy is still under study. The nonspecific immunologic-stimulating effect of BCG is believed to be responsible for the antitumor activity of this agent. The exact mechanism by which BCG achieves its antitumor effects is not completely clear at present. Use of BCG or its derivative BCG-MER has been studied in many cancers. However, the only significant results have been in the use of BCG for bladder cancer. It appears that repeated contact of the bladder mucosa with instilled BCG solution somehow augments the immune system to produce antitumor effects. Prolonged disease-free intervals in bladder cancer patients also occurs with intravesical BCG therapy with or without concurrent intradermal BCG. An-

other use of BCG was in intralesional therapy of cutaneous metastatic melanoma and head and neck tumors. However, other established therapies yield superior results, so intralesional therapy is now rare. Use of adjuvant BCG therapy in breast, ovarian, colon cancers, and leukemias has been all but abandoned due to lack of positive long-term results.

Bacillus Calmette-Guerin may be administered in several ways, although the dermal scarification and intradermal techniques are the most common routes. Bacillus Calmette-Guerin also may be administered by the following methods: instillation, intralesional, intrapleural, and oral. The following precautions should be observed in handling and administration of BCG: When preparing to administer BCG, do not prepare the skin with alcohol, as this will destroy the live organisms present in the vaccine. The vaccine should be protected from light when stored and only the supplied diluent used for reconstitution. Discarded injection materials must be autoclaved and/or incinerated in order to destroy the bacilli.

Lyophilized BCG preparations will retain potency for prolonged periods when stored under refrigeration and protected from light. The number of viable organisms present in each vial varies from supplier to supplier and from lot to lot within the same supplier's stock. Because of this biologic variability, doses are commonly listed in acceptable ranges. Bacillus Calmette-Guerin dosage for cancer therapy is 3×10^7 organisms. Adjustments in dose can be made by serial dilutions. The lyophilized suspensions come with a vial of diluent solution to be used for reconstitution and resuspension of the vaccine. Diluents with chemical preservatives, such as bacteriostatic water or normal saline, are not used to reconstitute BCG vaccine.

Side effects seen in BCG therapy depend on the route of administration used. Most patients experience influenza-like symptoms within 12–24 hours of therapy, which subside within 48 hours. Intralesional administration of BCG can cause abscess formation. Rarely, a generalized infection can occur following BCG administration. Anaphylaxis and death, although rare, may also occur. Since BCG is a live bacterium, it should not be administered to patients who are severely immunocompromised.

The only known drug interaction with BCG at present is with isoniazid (INH). Isoniazid inhibits multiplication of BCG. Therefore, concurrent use of these two agents should be avoided.

LEVAMISOLE

Levamisole is an enantiomer of the antihelmintic agent tetramisole. It has only been in investigational use as a cancer agent since 1971. Consequently, it is still a phase II drug. Levamisole apparently partially restores the functions of macrophages and T cells. Cell-mediated immunologic reactions are augmented, although the biochemical basis of this activity is not yet known. Levamisole has a higher chemical purity and lower toxicity than BCG and C. parvum.

Name	Dosage and Route	Uses	Precautions
Action (All Immunotherapeutic Agents): *To augment immune system so as to help the body's immune system kill cancer cells.*			
Bacillus Calmette-Guerin (BCG)	0.1 ml intradermally	Bladder cancer.	Vaccine precautions (use diluent provided; do not agitate violently; autoclave or incinerate discarded injection materials before discarding).
ALPHA INTERFERONS Alpha-2A Inteferon (Roferon); Alpha-2B Interferon (Intron-A); Alpha-N1 Interferon (Wellferon)	All doses cited are guidelines only and subject to change. Hairy cell leukemia: 2–3 million units IV/day. AIDS-related Kaposi's sarcoma: 30–50 million units IV/day. Renal Cell Carcinoma: 10–20 million units IV/day or 3 times per week.	Hairy cell leukemia; AIDS-related Kaposi's sarcoma; renal cell carcinoma. Non-malignant use: venereal warts.	
Interleukin-2 (IL-2)	Maximum tolerated dose: 10 million units/m^2 IV 3 times per week in clinical trials. (Optimum therapeutic doses yet to be determined.)	Clinical trials underway in treatment of renal cell cancer; melanoma; and colon cancer.	None.
Tumor Necrosis Factor (TNF)	Optimum therapeutic doses yet to be determined.	Studies still underway. Initial studies show the greatest use may be in combination with other biologic response modifiers or chemotherapeutic agents.	None.
Zidovudine (AZT)	AIDS and Advanced ARC: 200 mg PO Q4 hrs around the clock.	AIDS and advanced ARC.	Patients on AZT are still capable of transmitting AIDS virus so all AIDS-related precautions still apply.

Interactions	Acute Toxic Signs	Major Adverse Effects	Nursing Implications
Isoniazid (INH)—inhibits the multiplication of BCG, concurrent use not advised.	None	Local Integ: Pruritus, redness, swelling; warmth, scab formation, and discomfort at site; scarring; lymph node tenderness. Other: flu-like symptoms for 24–48 hrs. (low-grade fever, headache, myalgia, malaise); ANAPHYLAXIS.	INTERVENTION: Do not use alcohol to prepare skin since it can kill organisms in vaccine. Read intradermal injection sites & observe scarification sites at appropriate intervals. Have epinephrine 1:1,000 on hand in order to treat anaphylaxis. EVALUATION: Intradermal sites are properly monitored. Serious allergic reactions are avoided.
None significant.	Unknown	CV: Rare—hypertension, arrhythmias, palpitations. Other: Flu-like symptoms; chronic fatigue; depression.	ASSESSMENT: Assess patient's emotional status. Assess for signs of flu-like symptoms. INTERVENTION: Observe AIDS precautions and proper disposal of all injection materials following treatment of AIDS patients. Instruct patient/family about drug adverse effects, stress that they are generally milder than those associated with chemotherapy drugs. Offer appropriate emotional support. EVALUATION: Health teaching measures are effective.
Undetermined.	Superventricular tachycardias; myocardial infarction.	CV: SUPERVENTRICULAR TACHY-CARDIA: MYOCARDIAL INFARCTION. Musculoskeletal: arthritic symptoms. Other: flu-like symptoms; respiratory impairment; chronic adverse effects include anorexia and depression.	ASSESSMENT: Monitor cardiac status, respiratory status. INTERVENTION: Careful documentation of patient response important for all drugs in early trials and initial release. EVALUATION: Serious cardiac effects are avoided.
Actinomycin D: concurrent administration may enhance the cytotoxicity of cells to TNF.	Undetermined.	CV: hypotension (may be dose limiting). Musculoskeletal: arthralgia. GI: anorexia; diarrhea. Other: fever and chills (may be profound); headaches. Chronic effects: fatigue and malaise.	INTERVENTION: Careful documentation of patient response. Encourage proper rest/diet. EVALUATION: Health teaching effective.
Acetaminophen, aspirin, indomethacin, and probenecid: Concurrent use may increase toxic effects of AZT, so patient should consult physician before using.	Severe bone marrow depression.	GI: nausea; anorexia; vomiting; strange aftertaste after taking drug. Hemo: anemia; leukopenia. Neuro: severe headaches; dizziness; numbness of hands and feet. Integ: skin rash; myalgia. Other: insomnia; sweating; fever; dyspnea. GU: drug passes to breast milk. Effects on developing fetus unknown.	INTERVENTION: AIDS precautions necessary for caregivers giving injections or handling body secretions. Health teaching patient/significant others that drug does not prevent transmission of AIDS virus and precautions still necessary. EVALUATION: Health teaching measures are effective.

Levamisole is available in 50-mg film-coated tablets and is stable at room temperature. Since studies are in the initial stages, optimum dose schedules have not yet been determined. However, doses of 100 mg/m^2 po for two to three days every two weeks have been utilized in studies. Doses of up to 750 mg po three times per week have been generally well tolerated by patients, although the optimum beneficial dose appears to be in a lower range. Preliminary study results of lung cancer patients indicate benefit with levamisole occurred at dose levels less than 2 mg/kg/day (80 mg/m^2/day) for three days every two weeks.

Levamisole has been studied as an adjuvant to help prevent recurrent lung, breast, and renal cancer with some encouraging initial results, especially in breast cancer. However, the most significant use of this drug was recently announced by the Mayo Clinic where it was used in combination therapy with 5FU against colon cancer. Their preliminary study reported that there was a significant decrease in the death rate from colon cancer when Levamisole was used in combination with 5FU. The therapy was started three–five weeks following surgery for colon cancer and therapy continued for one year. This type of adjuvant therapy was found to work best in patients who did not have extensive metastatic disease. Since Levamisole is currently available for other approved uses, it will require FDA approval to add this use as a newly approved indication for drug use and not require the same time consuming process as a new drug would. Research is continuing with Levamisole, as well as other currently available drugs, to find new applications which will help patients.

Adverse effects with Levamisole are generally transient and mild, with mild gastrointestinal complaints being the most common. Granulocytopenia is the only apparent toxic effect and this occurs in approximately 20% of patients, mostly those with arthritis.

INTERFERONS

Interferon (IFN) was the first biologic therapy to be approved by the FDA. Researchers hope that interferons and other biologic response modifiers will do for cancer what the discovery of penicillin did for infections. Although first discovered by virologists Alick Isaacs and Jean Lindenmann in 1957, few researchers were involved in interferon work until recent years because of its scarcity and expense. It was also extremely difficult to obtain pure enough interferon with which to work. The name interferon was originally coined due to the ability of this substance to interfere with the ability of a virus to replicate. The term interferon does not refer to a single substance, but rather to an entire class (group) of substances. Interferons are quantified by their antiviral activity.

Types of Interferons

Three types of interferons were originally identified by researchers: leukocyte; fibroblast; and immune interferon. Alpha and beta interferons were called type 1 interferons in earlier nomenclature, and gamma interferon was called type 2. Alpha interferon was known as leukocyte interferon because it came from leukocytes. Beta interferon was known as fibroblast interferon because of its origin from the fibroblasts of fetal foreskins. Gamma interferon originates from immune T-lymphocytes.

The major drawback in early interferon research was the minute quantities of these substances that are produced in the human body. However, the technology of recombinant gene production now enables us to produce cloned interferons. This has enabled several companies to develop recombinant alpha interferons that have been approved by the FDA. Roferon is the alpha-2 interferon produced by Roche. Intron-A is the alpha-2 interferon produced by Schering. Both preparations are different clones of the same interferon. The alpha-2A was called leukocyte-A interferon in earlier nomenclature and this is the Roferon. Alpha-2B was called alpha-2 interferon and is the Intron-A. The only difference in these two preparations is a single amino acid substitution. Although each company claims that this different amino acid makes their product more effective, the data do not support these claims. Both substances seem to work equally. Burroughs-Wellcome Laboratories also produces an interferon called Wellferon. This product is a lymphoblastoid interferon called alpha-N1. This product shows no significant differences from the previous two interferons discussed. All three have the same therapeutic activity and adverse effects. Therefore, they will be discussed as a unit.

Uses of Alpha Interferons

Alpha interferons have been approved for the treatment of hairy cell leukemia patients who have not responded to splenectomy (the standard therapy). Response rates of 80%–100% have been reported with alpha interferon therapy. Ironically, hairy cell leukemia was first identified in 1958, the year after interferon was discovered. This type of leukemia is a monoclonal neoplastic proliferation of B cells that produces chronic disease. Hairy cell leukemia occurs in men five times more frequently than in women. Its onset is generally in the fifth decade of life, and it takes its name from the many fine projections that appear on the surface of the reticulum cells. The disease is characterized by anemia, fatigue, pancytopenia, and marked splenomegaly. Death generally occurs from infection or bleeding. If splenectomy and chemotherapy fail to help the patient, then they are a candidate for alpha interferon therapy. Patient response to the interferon therapy is seen regardless of the alpha interferon used. Although complete remissions occur in only about 5% of patients, the overwhelming majority have long-term remissions. Therapy lasts up to 18 months.

Alpha interferons are currently being studied as treatment for a number of other neoplastic diseases including renal cell carcinoma; AIDS-related Kaposi's sarcoma; malignant melanoma; follicular lymphomas; and chronic myelocytic leukemia (CML). It is believed by many researchers that the most promising future use of alpha interferons will be in the treatment of CML. There is no curative treatment currently available for CML.

Early trials show that aggressive alpha interferon therapy in CML can eradicate the neoplastic clone that causes oncogene expression of CML in about 20% of patients. Further studies and long-term patient follow-up are continuing. Studies of combination therapy of interferon and chemotherapy have shown some initially encouraging results in some neoplastic diseases. Interferons are also useful in non-neoplastic diseases. The first non-neoplastic disease treatment approved by the FDA is venereal warts. The use of interferons is being studied in other diseases as well. Since the adverse effects associated with interferons are much less severe than seen with other chemotherapeutic agents such as the alkylating agents or anti-metabolies, they may eventually be used to treat many other illnesses.

Action

Interferon directly inhibits cell growth. Interferon induces changes in the cell cycle, inhibits cellular differentiation, and interferes with oncogene expression. The immune system effects of interferon include the regulation of cytotoxic effector cells, especially the natural killer cells. Interferon alters the cells' surface antigen expression and effects antibody production. It brings the cells from the resting phase (G_0) of the cell cycle into the growth phase (G_1) of the cell cycle, thereby causing them to be killed. The exact mechanism by which interferon produces cell death is not completely clear at present. It is hoped that the combination of interferon therapy with chemotherapy can result in augmentation of cell kill and enhance response rates in many cancers. This avenue of therapy is being extensively studied.

Adverse Effects

The adverse effects seen in interferon therapy are proportionate to the dose of interferon adminstered. Adverse and toxic effects increase dramatically as the dose increases. Interferon-associated adverse effects can be acute or chronic. Commonly seen acute adverse effects include: flu-like symptoms of fever (98% of patients), chills (64%), myalgia (73%), fatigue (89%), and headache (71%). These effects tend to diminish with continued therapy. The chronic adverse effects are the dose-limiting effects; they are chronic fatigue and depression.

Interactions

At present, no undesirable interactions have been identified. It is hoped that a synergistic effect can occur when interferon is administered with chemotherapy that will augment patient response.

Dosages

Dosages of interferon vary according to the disease being treated. For those diseases that are in early phase or clinical trials with interferon, it must be remembered that the optimum therapeutic dosages have yet to be determined. Thus, all dosages cited herein are guidelines only. Always double-check dosage with current recommendations and/or protocols. Doses cited are for intravenous infusions, unless otherwise specified.

Treatment of hairy cell leukemia was the first approved use for the alpha-2a interferon drugs. The second approved use was the intralesional treatment of venereal warts. Studies of interferons in the treatment of other diseases are underway.

Hairy cell leukemia is treated with 2–3 million units of alpha-interferon per day. Treatment can last up to 18 months. Patients being treated for AIDS-related Kaposi's sarcoma require doses of 30–50 million units per day. Response rates range from 20%–80% against this cancer. Interferon is probably the only available drug that has any effect on renal cell carcinoma. Intermediate doses that range from 10–20 million units daily or three times a week appear to be the most effective. Higher doses are no more effective and response rates of up to 27% can occur. Intralesional treatment of venereal warts requires the following dosage: 1 million units per lesion, three times per week for up to three weeks.

GAMMA INTERFERON. Gamma interferon is similar in clinical activity, adverse effects, and toxicity to both alpha and beta interferons. There are some significant differences, though. Gamma interferon does have somewhat different functions in the immune system. Gamma interferon originates in a different cell than other interferons and has an important role in stimulating macrophages. Alpha and beta interferons share the same receptor on their cells. Gamma interferon has a different receptor. This difference causes gamma interferon to have a synergistic effect when given with either of these other interferons. If alpha and beta interferon were given together, they would have to compete for the same receptor in order to kill a disease cell. This would not increase cancer cell kill, and there would be no advantage to giving both substances at the same time. However, since gamma interferon has a different receptor, if it is given with either alpha or beta interferon the result is synergistic enhancement of therapeutic effect.

Gamma interferon produces synergistic effects when used with interleukin-2 and tumor necrosis factor (TNF) as well. Researchers believe that the most promising use of gamma interferon in the future will be in combination with other substances to synergistically improve therapeutic response. Phase I and early phase II studies of gamma interferon in combination with other substances are currently underway.

INTERLEUKIN-2

The biological response modifier interleukin-2 was discovered about ten years ago. It is primarily made by helper T cells. Preliminary phase I studies of this substance are especially encouraging. Presently, interleukin-2 is the only true immune-enhancing agent that shows consistent efficacy.

Action

Interleukin-2 (IL2) has several important activities in the immune system. It stimulates activated lymphocytes, induces gamma interferon, and enhances the generation of both LAK cells and natural killer cells. Interleukin-2 regulates its own receptor expression, thereby causing production of more IL2 via this feedback mechanism.

Interleukin-2 also supports the growth of macrophages as well as both B and T cells.

Uses

Interleukin-2 is being studied in several different cancers as a single agent and in combination with other immunotherapeutic substances. It is being used to treat colon cancers (10% response rate); renal cell cancer (30% response rate); and melanoma (30% response rate). In addition to these trials, phase 2 clinical trials are underway with combination therapy of IL2 and beta interferon in the following cancers: AIDS-related Kaposi's sarcoma; colon cancer; malignant melanoma; non–small cell carcinoma of the lung; and renal cancer. Phase 1 results of this combination therapy have been encouraging; actual LAK cell activation *in vivo* in some patients with objective responses was observed. Some studies are using IL2 in combination with LAK cells. Other studies are in progress with IL2 and low-dose cyclophosphamide.

Adverse Effects

The adverse effects seen in IL2 therapy are similar to those seen with interferon and other biologic response–modifying therapies. Acute adverse effects of IL2 are fever, nausea, vomiting, and violent chills. High doses of IL2 can cause supraventricular tachycardias and even lead to myocardial infarction. Chronic adverse effects of IL2 therapy are anorexia and depression. Interleukin-2 can also cause arthritis, diarrhea, and respiratory impairment.

Interactions

At the present time and stage of clinical trials, no undesirable interactions with IL2 have been identified.

Doses

When used as a single agent, the maximum tolerated dose of IL2 is 10 million units/m^2 given three times per week via intravenous infusion. Since phase I and II studies and clinical trials are still underway with IL2, the optimum therapeutically effective dose for each disease entity has yet to be established.

TUMOR NECROSIS FACTOR

In 1975, Carswell and associates discovered a factor in the sera of mice that had been primed with BCG, *C. parvum,* or *zymosan* and subsequently challenged with bacterial endotoxin (lipopolysaccharide). This substance was able to induce hemorrhagic necrosis, growth inhibition, or regression in a variety of human and mouse tumors both *in vivo* and *in vitro*. Thus, this substance was named tumor necrosis factor (TNF). It was later discovered that the major source of TNF is macrophage monocyte cells. Recombinant gene technology has also made it possible for TNF to be cloned and mass produced. Following the discovery of TNF, researchers identified a molecule they called cachectin associated with the weight loss seen in patients with cancer. They also discovered that this cachectin was structurally the same as TNF.

Actions

Tumor necrosis factor is more than just an antitumor-effector molecule. It mediates a number of events, which suggest that it plays an important role in host response to inflammatory insults. Tumor necrosis factor appears to be closely integrated with the complexities of the body's response to inflammation, which requires interaction among TNF, interleukin-1, interleukin-2, and the interferons. Tumor necrosis factor stimulates macrophage-mediated antitumor activity, endothelial cells, granulocytes, and seems to be selective for certain types of tumors. Cachectin (TNF) is felt to be the central mediator of the wasting and weight loss often seen in chronic diseases such as cancer. The exact role of TNF is not completely understood at present; however, it does seem to have an enhancing effect on interferon therapy.

Research has also shown that TNF-induced effector molecules are responsible for the cytotoxic activities of natural cytotoxic (NC) cells, which are distinctly different from natural killer (NK) cells. Natural cytotoxic cells lyse different target cells than do NK cells. It is apparent that the different cells involved in natural immunity act by producing different effector molecules that are closely related. These molecules, besides causing tumor cell lysis, can initiate a cascade of events leading to an immune response to an invading stimulus. What remains to be determined is how the cells in the individual's natural immune system are able to recognize malignant cells as abnormal or different and exactly what events initiate the production of the effector molecules.

There seems to be a marked synergy between TNF and gamma interferon. Initial research shows that the administration of actinomycin D enhances the cytotoxicity of cells to TNF; even cells that were resistant to TNF alone are killed when treated with this combination. As with other biologic response modifiers, the major use of this substance in the future may not be as a single agent but rather as a part of a combination therapy against cancer.

Use

Tumor necrosis factor is still in the early phases of development, so no significant antitumor activities have been reported as yet. However, researchers believe that the major use of this substance in the future will be in combination with other biologic response modifiers or chemotherapeutic drugs in order to produce the highest possible cell kill of malignant cells.

Adverse Effects

As with other biologic response modifiers, the adverse effects that occur can be categorized as acute and chronic. Acute adverse effects include: fever and chills, which can be profound; headaches; hypotension; arthralgia; anorexia; and diarrhea. Chronic fatigue and malaise have been reported also. The hypotension appears to be a dose-limiting problem.

Dose

Since TNF is still in the early phases of development and not all phase 1 and phase 2 data complete, there has yet to be determined a therapeutic dose range for this substance (The purpose of early phase trials is to establish a maximum tolerated dose of a drug.). After this happens, therapeutic doses are determined. Different routes of administration are being studied, including arterial therapy and intraperitoneal administration.

ZIDOVUDINE

Zidovudine (AZT; Retrovir) works by exerting an antiviral effect against the AIDS virus by preventing virus replication. Since the AIDS virus effectively cripples the hosts' immune system, leading to the development of a variety of opportunistic infections and cancers, the desired effect of AZT is restoration of the host's immune function. Thus, although AZT is an antiviral agent, its effect on the immune system and use against diseases and cancers dependent on loss of immunocompetence make inclusion of this drug in this chapter essential. Zidovudine (AZT), also called azidothymidine, was first shown to be active against HIV (AIDS) virus *in vitro* in 1985. Several months later, intensive phase 1 trials began in order to determine the pharmacokinetic activity of AZT. The drug was well absorbed when given orally and levels that inhibited HIV replication *in vitro* could be achieved in patients. The half-life of AZT was found to be about one hour, with much of the drug being cleared by the liver and renal tubular secretion. Thus, the drug must be taken every four hours around the clock in order to achieve and maintain therapeutic drug levels. Zidovudine crosses the blood–brain barrier.

Patients in the above phase 1 trial had partial restoration of immune function after six weeks of therapy. They also gained weight and exhibited other signs of clinical improvements. To determine if AZT increased the survival time of patients with AIDS or AIDS-related complex (ARC), phase 2 clinical trials were begun in February 1986 in several medical and cancer centers in the United States.

The phase 2 clinical trials had about 280 patients enrolled, some of whom had AIDS with *Pneumocystis carinii* pneumonia within 90 days of entry and some who had ARC. Patients received 250 mg of AZT (or a placebo) every four hours around the clock. By September 1987, there had been 20 deaths among the study participants—19 deaths occurred among the placebo group and only one in the AZT group. Due to this dramatic difference in the mortality rates between the two groups, an independent data safety-monitoring board analyzed the double-blind data of the study and elected to prematurely end the study and give AZT to all the patients who had been receiving placebos.

Use

Beginning in September 1986 under the mechanism of a Treatment IND (Investigational New Drug), AZT was made widely available to AIDS patients with *Pneumocystis carinii* pneumonia (PCP) who met other criteria as well. In an unprecedented move on March 20, 1987, the Food and Drug Administration approved AZT for use in patients with symptomatic HIV infections (AIDS and advanced ARC) with a history of cytologically confirmed PCP or an absolute CD4 lymphocyte count of less than $200/mm^3$ in the peripheral blood before therapy is initiated.

Pharmacokinetics

Zidovudine (AZT; Retrovir) is well absorbed orally, with a bioavailability of about 60%. The half-life of AZT is about one hour, although any factor that affects hepatic blood flow or liver function could affect AZT metabolism and its toxicity.

Adverse Effects

The major AZT-associated toxicity is bone marrow depression. The bone marrow depression is generally more pronounced in patients with AIDS than those with ARC. Anemia and leukopenia are the most frequently seen results of this bone marrow depression. If bone marrow depression becomes too severe, AZT therapy may need to be stopped. Other common adverse effects of AZT therapy are severe headaches, nausea, and insomnia. Less frequent adverse effects include sweating, fever, anorexia, vomiting, myalgia, dizziness, numbness of hands/feet, dyspnea, skin rash, and strange taste sensations after ingestion.

The effect of AZT on the developing fetus is not known at present. The drug does pass into the breast milk; thus the patient should consult with her physician about whether or not to continue breast-feeding while on AZT.

Interactions

Zidovudine has only been on the market a short time, so the safety and effectiveness of this substance are not fully known. The concurrent use of acetaminophen, aspirin, indomethacin, or probenecid may increase the toxic effects of AZT. Therefore, the patient should consult with the physician before taking any of these drugs while on AZT. The effects or interaction of alcohol, cocaine, marijuana, and other recreational drugs of abuse is not known. Thus, the patient taking AZT should avoid these substances.

Other Warnings

The use of AZT does not reduce the risk of transmitting the virus to others. AIDS and ARC patients are still capable of transmitting the virus to others while on AZT; therefore, precautions against the virus must be maintained. Zidovudine does not *cure* the disease; however, it does inhibit virus replication and has helped prevent disease progression in some patients (Figs. 50–2 and 50–3).

Dose

For AIDS and advanced ARC, the dose of AZT is 250 mg orally every four hours around the clock. Several weeks of therapy may be needed before the effects of the drug are evident.

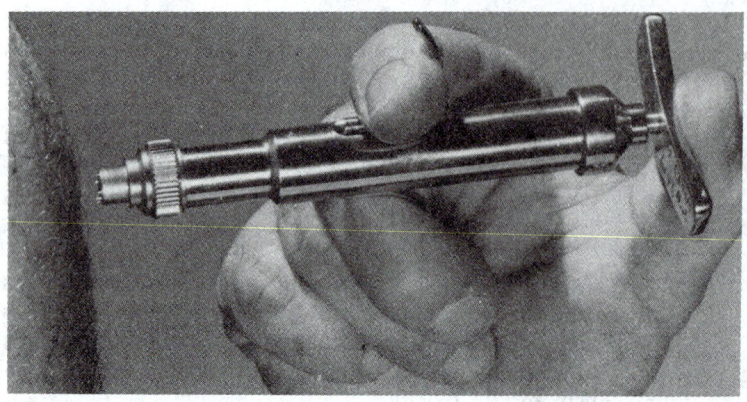

Figure 50–2. The Heaf gun. (From White, DS: Cancer Nursing. CV Mosby, St Louis, 1981, with permission.)

VAXSYN-HIV-1

The Food and Drug Administration has approved VaxSyn-HIV-1 only for investigational use. This is the first substance approved in the United States for study as a possible vaccine against the human immunodeficiency virus (HIV), the causative virus in AIDS. Although intensive research is underway on this and other possible vaccines, an AIDS vaccine is probably 10–20 years away.

VaxSyn-HIV-1 was created through the use of recombinant DNA technology. The vaccine duplicates an HIV envelope protein and should stimulate production of so-called neutralizing antibodies. Researchers believe that these antibodies block the viral proteins that usually bind to the T cell receptor, thus locking out the virus. Researchers speculate that if denied its port of entry into the cell, the HIV virus cannot infect T-lymphocytes and cause diffuse HIV infection.

Phase 1 studies are underway to determine the vaccine's toxicity at various doses and dose schedules. Phase 2 trials will determine the optimum dose. Phase 3 efficacy trials involving large populations may begin in the early 1990s.

TRANSFER FACTOR

Transfer factor is a dialyzable extract of stimulated lymphocytes. Transferring delayed hypersensitivity reactivity from one individual to another is being studied as a way of transferring antitumor immunity. This is a highly specific agent whose only source is patients who have been in long-term remission from their tumors. Transfer factor has been used for treatment of colon cancer, malignant melanoma, breast cancer, Hodgkin's disease, and sarcomas with suggestive antitumor effects. Further study of this type of adoptive immunotherapy is continuing. Optimal dosage and administration schedules

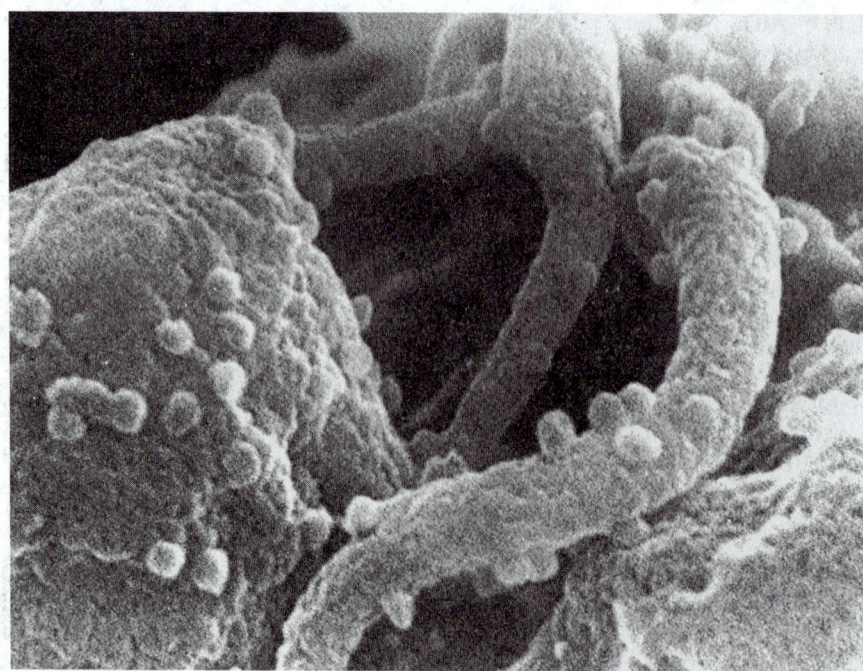

Figure 50–3. AIDS virus (Courtesy of Discover Syndication Department of Time & Life, New York, NY, with permission).

have not yet been determined. Since this is an investigational agent, contraindications and precautions have not yet been fully determined.

THYMOSIN

The thymus produces a number of important polypeptides with immunoregulatory effects. Tymosin fraction-5, an extract produced from bovine thymus glands, is also being used investigationally as an immunotherapy agent, although its usefulness is not certain at this time. The hormone thymosin is essential for the maturation of T cells, which initiate cell-mediated immunity. This substance has been used investigationally to treat leukemia and melanoma. Thymosin is administered intramuscularly or subcutaneously, with optimum therapeutic doses yet to be determined. Initial studies have not shown significant responses with thymosin as the sole therapeutic agent. However, significant activity occurs when it is combined with chemotherapy.

IMMUNE RIBONUCLEIC ACID

Immune ribonucleic acid (I-RNA) is produced by injecting animals with tumor cells from the cancer patient. An immune RNA extract is then prepared from the animal's lymphocytes and injected into the same patient intradermally in lymph node areas such as the groin, axilla, and chest. Immune RNA is an investigational form of passive adoptive immunotherapy used to treat breast cancer, melanoma, and sarcoma. The only notable side effect of this therapy is local inflammation at the injection site. To date, no significant systemic side effects have been noted from this therapy. Since this is an investigational agent, contraindications and precautions have not yet been fully determined.

IMMUNOSUPPRESSIVE THERAPY

ANTITHYMOCYTIC GLOBULIN EQUINE

The goal of cancer immunotherapy is to augment patient immunocompetence. However, there are times when it is desirable to administer immunosuppressive drugs, such as when the renal transplant patient is experiencing allograft reaction. Antithymocytic globulin equine (Atgam) is a lymphocyte-selective immunosuppressant. Following intravenous administration, Atgam reduces the number of circulating thymus-dependent lymphocytes that form rosettes with sheep erythrocytes. It is believed that the antilymphocytic effect of Atgam results in an altered function of the T-lymphocytes, which have a major role in cell-mediated immunity and a minor role in humoral immunity. Atgam also contains low concentrations of other antibodies capable of acting against other formed blood elements. Although Atgam reduces the number of circulating lymphocytes, it does not cause severe lymphopenia. The current use of Atgam is limited to patients experiencing renal allograft rejection.

Intradermal skin testing is recommended before IV administration of this drug. If the skin test results in wheal and/or erythema formation greater than 10 mm, Atgam is administered cautiously. Any systemic reaction (rash, tachycardia, hypotension, dyspnea, or anaphylaxis) precludes further administration of this drug. A negative skin test does not exclude the possibility of allergic reaction to Atgam. Atgam is contraindicated for patients who have had prior severe systemic reactions to Atgam or any other equine gamma globulin preparations.

Adverse Effects

Atgam is usually administered in conjunction with other immunosuppressive drugs such as antimetabolites and corticosteroids. Adverse reactions to Atgam include fever, chills, leukopenia, thrombocytopenia, dermatologic reactions, diarrhea, dyspnea, headache, stomatitis, herpes simplex infection, pulmonary edema, laryngospasm, clotting IV tubing, and anaphylaxis. Safe use of Atgam in pregnant and lactating women has not yet been established.

Dosage

The usual adult dosage of Atgam is 10–15 mg/kg/day for 14 days. Additional alternate-day doses can be given to a total of 21 doses. Atgam is administered intravenously and should be diluted in sterile saline solution to a concentration of 1 mg/ml of saline. The drug should then be infused for four to six hours. Dilution with dextrose solutions causes precipitate formation.

CYCLOSPORINE

Uses and Action

Successful organ transplantation of the kidneys, lungs, heart, and liver is being aided with the immunosuppressive agent cyclosporine (Sandimmune). The newly transplanted organ contains foreign antigens that trigger an immune response in the recipient. A major component of the immune response is activation of T-lymphocytes, which attack and destroy the newly transplanted organ. Cyclosporine selectively acts on the T-lymphocytes to prevent their production and response to interleukin-2. Interleukin-2 is released by helper T cells (regulator cells), which activates activity in the killer T cells (effector cells). If the process is already activated—that is, interleukin-2 is being released—cyclosporine is ineffective.

Pharmacokinetics

The absorption of cyclosporine is variable on a day-to-day basis. Peak and trough blood levels drawn and evaluated through radioimmunoassay testing are inconclusive at this time in determining the relationship of blood levels to graft rejection. Cyclosporine is metabolized in the liver.

Adverse Effects

Nephrotoxicity is a common adverse effect, and is relatively common when the IV route is used for drug administration. Careful renal assessments are made to detect this effect. Additional side effects include hirsutism, gum hyperplasia, tremors, increased risk of infection, and increased risk of malignancies, especially lymphomas.

Dosage

The dosage is highly individualized, ranging from 14–25 mg/kg/day. It is available in oral and IV forms. The oral form is in corn oil and is mixed with some diluent (fruit juice/milk) in a 1:10 ratio, and is best administered before meals, as food delays its absorption. When the IV route is used, the kidneys are watched closely for renal toxicity, resulting in a lower urinary output.

USING THE NURSING PROCESS

The science of cancer immunotherapy is still in the developmental stage, with virtually all forms of immunotherapy investigational in nature. Since this is a new form of therapy, a new role for the nurse has emerged—that of the immunotherapy nurse. The effectiveness of the nurse's role on an immunotherapy team is largely dependent on how successfully the nursing process is employed. Since this is such a new area of expertise, the immunotherapy nurse is a pioneer who must rely on an understanding of the treatment process coupled with internal problem-solving methods (the nursing process) in order to deliver optimum patient care. Nursing care efforts center on educating the patient, family members, and staff members about the immune process, as well as assessing patients prior to and throughout therapy. Planning and implementation of nursing care are dependent on the results of assessment. Due to the investigational nature of most immunotherapy, scrupulous recordkeeping is essential in order to achieve valid data interpretation of therapeutic results. It is also the nurse's responsibility to understand the method of administration, usual dosages, mechanism of drug action, and potential side effects of each drug administered.

ASSESSMENT

Detailed information on the assessment of the cancer patient is included in Chapter 49, Antineoplastic Chemotherapy. Refer to that section of the text for basic information on use of the nursing process in the cancer patient, since much of that information is also relevant for these patients. Nursing process examples for the patient receiving cancer immunotherapy are summarized in Table 50–3.

One important assessment relative to immunotherapy that the nurse can make is the observation of skin reactions to the drugs administered. Delayed hypersensitivity skin testing is sometimes a precursor to immunotherapy. Often the nurse is responsible for preparing and/or administering these agents as well as assessing the resultant skin reactions. Careful, accurate descriptions of local reactions including measurements, diagrams, and photographs are essential. These assessments continue at regular intervals throughout the patient's therapy.

Psychologic factors are especially important for the nurse to consider in these patients. Immunotherapy requires many follow-up visits to the hospital or clinic. Once patients have recovered from their initial surgery or chemotherapy and have begun to feel better, they may dislike returning so often, since each visit reminds them of their diagnosis and they may fear disease progression will be discovered. This can be psychologically draining for many patients. Those receiving adjuvant therapy may lose their motivation as a defense against confronting feelings about their cancer. During the initial assessment of the patient, and with each subsequent visit, the nurse carefully assesses the patient's psychologic and emotional status. Motivating compliance in these patient's can be an ongoing challenge.

Remember to include the patient's family in the assessment. Observe and determine their understanding of the patient's treatments, the need for follow-up visits, and their feelings about the patient's illness. The family can be an important ally in motivating continued patient compliance. Alterations in family dynamics can occur with any disease process. When a serious or life-threatening illness such as cancer or AIDS exists, family dynamics and interactions are affected, coping mechanisms tested, and roles within the family structure are altered. Family members and the patient's significant others are extremely important in helping the patient cope with the anxiety, isolation, alterations in body image, and grief associated with these illnesses.

Patients receiving immunologic assessment and immunotherapy are often immunologically depressed and at risk for developing infection. A major nursing role is the assessment of risk potential for infection and also prevention of infection. Observe and screen visitors of hospitalized patients if necessary to prevent anyone with infection from coming into close contact with the patient. Exposure to people with colds or cold sores can pose a serious threat to the patient with a severely depressed immunologic system. Also remember to assess the patient's environment carefully for any potential reservoirs of disease such as standing water found in flower arrangements and suction equipment as well as fomites (blankets, equipment, newspapers, backrub lotion, etc.).

Carefully assess the patient's skin and mucous membranes, since an intact skin best performs its job as the body's first line of defense against invading organisms. Good nutrition and adequate rest are just as important for these patients, as malnutrition and fatigue also can contribute to a lack of immunocompetency. Assess these areas frequently, as patient needs change according to changes in condition.

Table 50–3. NURSING PROCESS FOR THE PATIENT RECEIVING CANCER IMMUNOTHERAPY

Assessment

Observe skin testing/drug administration sites for reactions. Observe, measure, and record skin lesions.
Assess psychologic and emotional status, noting verbal and nonverbal cues.
Evaluate for signs of infection, e.g., temperature elevation, flu/cold symptoms.

Nursing Diagnosis	Nursing Actions	Rationale	Desired Outcomes/ Evaluation Criteria
Skin Integrity impaired related to skin testing and administration of immunotherapeutic drugs or disease process as evidenced by presence of: pruritis; redness; swelling; warmth; scab formation; scarification; or skin lesions.	Prepare and administer skin tests/drugs. Observe and measure reaction(s).	Correct preparation and administration technique can minimize adverse effects. Incorrect preparation can kill organisms prior to administration and impair treatment.	Verbalizes understanding of condition, treatment protocols and side effects. Demonstrates behaviors/ techniques to promote healing and prevent complications.
	Assess skin daily, noting color, turgor, circulation and sensation. Note breakdown/delayed wound healing.	Establishes baseline with which changes in status can be compared. Interference with healing can occur with immunosuppression.	
	Remind patient not to scratch the treatment area or apply alcohol-containing lotions.	Interference with the area can spread the organisms and/or increase scarring. Alcohol can kill the live virus contained in the vaccine.	
	Show patient/SO how to measure test sites if necessary. Review signs of adverse reactions.	Accurate information is essential so the reactions can be read accurately and treatment can progress.	
Infection, potential for related to inadequate secondary defenses and immunosuppression, malnutrition, chronic disease.	Promote good handwashing procedures. Screen/ limit visitors and staff. Place in reverse isolation as indicated.	Protects patient from sources of infection, such as URI/influenza, cold sores. Severe immunocompromise (e.g., bone-marrow suppression) necessitates increased protection and vigilance.	Identifies and participates in interventions to prevent/reduce risk of infection. Remains afebrile and achieves timely healing as appropriate.
	Assess all systems (e.g., skin, respiratory, genitourinary) for signs/symptoms of infection on a continual basis.	Early recognition and intervention may prevent progression to more serious situation/sepsis.	
	Emphasize personal hygiene.	Limits potential sources of infection and/or secondary overgrowth.	
	Promote adequate rest/ exercise periods.	Limits fatigue, yet encourages sufficient movement to prevent stasis complications, e.g., pneumonia, decubitus, and thrombus formation.	
	Assess environment for and eliminate potential hazards, e.g., standing water	Reduces exposure to pathogens and risk of acquired illness.	

CONTINUED ON THE FOLLOWING PAGE

Table 50–3. NURSING PROCESS FOR THE PATIENT RECEIVING CANCER IMMUNOTHERAPY–*CONTINUED*

Nursing Diagnosis	Nursing Actions	Rationale	Desired Outcomes/ Evaluation Criteria
	(flower arrangements), fomites (blankets, backrub lotion, newspapers).		
Knowledge deficit related to lack of exposure, information misinterpretation, unfamiliarity with resources as evidenced by questions, statement of concern, inaccurate followthrough of instruction/development of preventable complications.	Provide information (verbal and written) about disease process and immunotherapeutic treatment/agents, expected results, side effects and adverse reactions. Assess extent of care and support available from family/SO and need for other care givers. Review modes of transmission of infectious diseases. Review dietary needs (high-protein and calorie) and ways to improve intake when anorexia, diarrhea, weakness, depression interfere with intake. Identify signs/symptoms requiring medical evaluation.	Provides knowledge base on which patient can make informed decisions. Treatments are often experimental but side effects are usually mild and self-limiting. Identifies resources to plan and carry out treatment. Corrects myths and misconceptions, promotes safety for patient/others. Promotes adequate nutrition necessary for healing and support of immune system, enhances feeling of well-being. Early recognition of developing complications and timely interventions may prevent progression to serious adverse effects.	Verbalizes understanding of condition/disease process and treatment. Identifies relationship of signs/ symptoms to the disease/ treatment process and correlates symptoms with causative factors. Correctly performs necessary procedures and explains reasons for actions.
Alterations in family dynamics due to patient illness and treatment.	Observe patient/family interactions. Question patient/SO about coping methods. Assess verbal and non-verbal cues on patient feelings/fears.	Once problems are identified/verbalized solutions can be devised. Ineffective coping impedes the problem solving process. Both verbal and non-verbal cues are important in determining actual patient feelings/fears. Psychological depression contributes to depression of immune system.	Patient/SO demonstrate positive adaptation through use of adequate coping mechanisms.

NURSING DIAGNOSES

Following careful assessment of the patient and family, the nurse makes nursing diagnoses relative to what has been observed. This statement of patient problems is essential for the next step of the nursing process to take place. Nursing diagnoses generally center on the patient's nutritional, psychologic, rest, elimination, and pain status, as well as on objective observational findings. It is at this point that the nurse usually determines which of the patient problems are most immediate and require intervention first.

Patients experience both physical and emotional responses to their disease. Nursing diagnoses specific to patients receiving immunotherapy can include knowledge deficit regarding immunotherapy and follow-up care; fear of disease progression or death; alterations in family dynamics due to illness; potential impairment of skin integrity due to delayed hypersensitivity reactions following skin tests; disturbances in self-concept due to illness; and self-care deficits related to the physical status. The psychologic status of these patients is especially important to their overall physical and emotional well-being. The nursing diagnoses relating to self-image changes, problems in affiliative relationships, and changes in family process are as important as those dealing with the patient's physical problems.

PLANNING AND INTERVENTION

Patients may receive immunotherapy while hospitalized or on an outpatient basis, depending on their condition and the type of treatment to be administered. The planning of nursing care often involves the coordination of immunotherapy around radiation treatments, chemotherapy, and/or surgery. Since patients derive the most benefit from treatment when the immune system is at its best, it is important that immunotherapy be scheduled carefully around other therapy. Thus, the patient should be able to receive maximum benefits from all the treatments.

Psychologic factors are also important. Cancer is a serious and potentially fatal illness, and many patients experience depression. Since emotional depression can contribute to a depression of the immune system, this is an important symptom to observe for. Because immunotherapy is largely investigational, some patients may also feel that they are being experimented on. If this is the case, reinforce the known benefits of therapy.

Keep alert to changes in the patient's blood count. Notify the physician of leukopenia, since severe bone marrow depression may necessitate an order for protective reverse isolation in such patients.

Nursing intervention for the patient centers around the administration of immunotherapeutic agents, accurate recordkeeping of patient response to treatment, and appropriate patient and family teaching.

Immunotherapeutic agents such as BCG may be administered in a variety of techniques including intradermal, scarification, multiple puncture, intralesional, intraabdominal, and intravenous. The nurse will not be injecting drugs intralesionally or intra-abdominally, although assisting with these procedures is common. Depending on the drug to be administered, institutional policy, and patient's tumor, the nurse may use one or more of the other administration techniques.

The scarification technique is a commonly used method of BCG administration. This is done by making multiple scratches on the patient's arm or thigh with a beveled cutting edge instead of the point of a needle. To correctly administer drugs in this manner, the skin is carefully prepared and an area 5 cm² is marked off. Eight horizontal and vertical lines are etched about ½ cm apart in the square to form a grid or checkerboard pattern. The scratches made should be deep enough to produce serum oozing but not bleeding. The appropriate vaccine is applied in drops to the scarified area, rubbed in with the flat of the needle, and allowed to dry. Sometimes a hair dryer (hand-held, blower type) is used to speed the drying process. However, do not use the heat settings of the dryer, as this will kill the organisms in the vaccine. When dry, a slight glaze will form over the site. The area is covered with a small inverted petri dish or similar object for 24 to 48 hours to protect the site. After that time, the area can be left uncovered. Remind the patient not to scratch the treatment area or apply alcohol-containing lotions.

Multiple puncture injections of immunotherapeutic agents may be administered by Tine technique or by the use of the Heaf gun. The Tine technique uses a magnet to hold a 36-prong metal disc, which applies pressure to skin onto which the immunotherapeutic agent has been dropped. The pressure makes small punctures in the epidermis and the drug thus enters the system (Fig. 50–4). The Heaf gun is another means of administering BCG intradermally (Fig. 50–5). It was used extensively in the past for mass tuberculous screenings. Scarification and intradermal injection (with a syringe) are presently more widely used than Heaf or Tine techniques.

It is important to remember several things about handling, preparing, and administering immunologic agents. First and foremost, these drugs may contain live organisms and must be protected from heat. When preparing solutions for injection, use only the diluent provided. Use of other solutions for dilution may be incompatible with the vaccine or render it nonviable. Sterile water and normal saline with preservatives both contain small amounts of alcohol, which can kill the organisms in the vaccine. Remember not to use alcohol for skin preparation, as alcohol on the skin surface can also kill vaccine organisms. Acetone is effective for skin preparation. When mixing the drugs preparatory to drawing

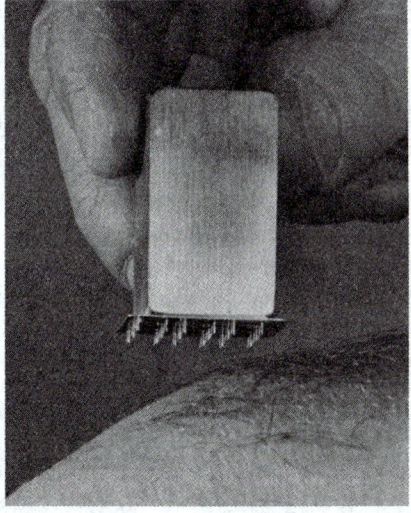

Figure 50–4. The Tine Technique—36-prong disc and magnet (From White, DS: Cancer Nursing. CV Mosby, St Louis, 1981, with permission).

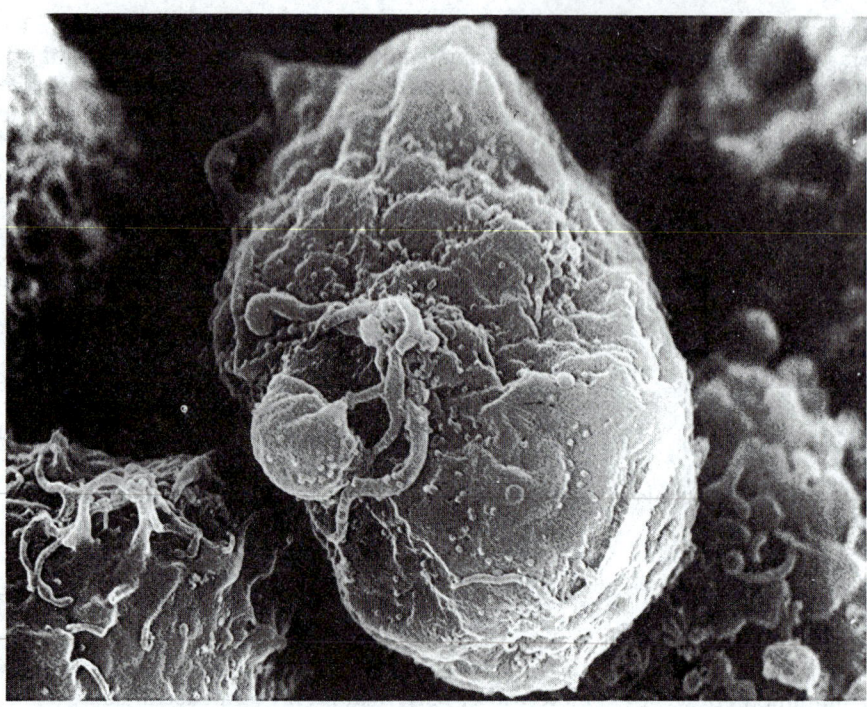

Figure 50–5. AIDS virus (Courtesy of Discover Syndication Department of Time & Life, New York, NY, with permission).

up solutions, do not agitate the vial. Gently roll the vial between the hands to achieve a uniform dilution. Excessive agitation of the vial can damage vaccine organisms.

EVALUATION

This final step of the nursing process is used to determine the effectiveness of the assessment and diagnosis-generated plan. Those interventions that were successful in dealing with identified problems may be successfully used in the future.

Unsuccesful interventions may be modified or discarded, depending on the circumstances. Evaluate patient/family compliance with therapeutic regimen. Evaluate patient/family understanding of health teaching given. Evaluate patient/family coping mechanisms to determine if successful adjustment is being achieved.

Adverse effects experienced by patients receiving immunotherapy are usually limited to flu-like symptoms such as fever, chills, or malaise. However, patients may experience serious adverse effects such as bone marrow depression while taking drugs such as AZT. Patients who are successfully taught about which symptoms require the prompt contacting of their physician will experience less severe sequelae.

Patients receiving immunotherapy for the first time who may have experienced chemotherapy side effects should be reassured that usually only mild side effects will be experienced while receiving this type of therapy. Those receiving treatment on an outpatient basis should be reminded not to take aspirin or over-the-counter medications (many contain aspirin), or drink alcoholic beverages during the treatment period, as these substances have immunosuppressive properties.

Immunotherapy of neoplastic disease is a relatively new modality of cancer treatment. Many investigational studies are currently underway to determine the value of different types of immunotherapy. Undoubtedly, studies will continue in the near future since the advent of monoclonal antibodies, interferon, interleukin-2, and increasing knowledge of the immune process have rekindled interest in both immunology and immunotherapy. Understanding immunity is integral to the understanding of immunotherapy and the drugs used to stimulate the immune system in various ways.

SUMMARY

The concept of immunization against disease has been with mankind for centuries. Successful development of preventative immunizations against specific diseases did not begin until Jenner vaccinated against smallpox in 1798. The concept of harnessing the immune system or augmenting its ability to destroy invading organisms from without (bacteria; viruses; microbes) or within (cancer) is a relatively recent phenomenon. Although scientific knowledge about the function and interrelationships of the immune system are still incomplete, during the 1970s and 1980s there has been a tremendous increase in our understanding of the complexities of the immune system. The discovery of an entire new class of substances called biologic response modifiers has resulted in great increases in immunotherapeutic research. Interferon, the first biologic response modifier, as well as newer discoveries such as interleukin-2, tumor necrosis factor, and monoclonal antibodies are all being studied as anticancer agents. It is hoped that the use of these agents can harness the individual's immune system to rid the body of cancer. Technology has spurred great medical developments in the last twenty-five years, one of the most dramatic being organ transplantation. Unfortunately, technical surgical skill developed more quickly than the ability to deal with the ultimate nemesis of transplants—rejection. However, in recent years newer, more effective drugs have been developed that supress the immune system and thus help prevent rejection of the transplanted organ(s). Atgam and cyclosporine are both used to help prevent organ rejection.

Immunotherapy seeks to alter the patient's immune response, either to augment or enhance it, such as in cancer, or to suppress it following organ transplants. In the case of augmentation of the immune system for cancer or AIDS treatment, the role of the nurse centers around patient/family health teaching and observation of the patient for response to drug therapy. Since cancer immunotherapy is a relatively new science, most of the agents used are in the various developmental stages of investigational study. The role of the nurse for patients receiving investigational therapy includes adhering to study protocol and keen observation of patients for adverse effects or sensitivity reactions. Often patients participating in such investigational studies are those for whom conventional therapies have been exhausted. Therefore, patients may be more anxious, debilitated, or depressed. The nurse must be sure to include psychologic support and stress management as needed for such patients. Likewise, those patients for whom immunosuppression is desired following organ transplants must also be assessed for psychosocial needs and anxiety level. Both groups of patients are more susceptible to infection because of lowered immunocompetence. Both groups of patients may require careful screening of visitors and/or reverse isolation precautions. Inclusion of family members/significant others in planning patient care and setting realistic goals is especially important in these patient groups, since the patients may be severely ill and not able to independently carry out activities of daily living. As investigational immunologic agents develop into accepted therapies, we can expect to see the science of cancer immunotherapy become a more important mode of treatment.

BIBLIOGRAPHY

AIDS File. Am J Nurs 88(3):282, 1988.

Calabresi, P and Parks, RE: Antiproliferative agents and drugs used for immunosuppression. In Goodman and Gilman (eds): The Pharmocological Basis of Therapeutics, ed 7. Macmillan, New York, 1986.

FDA Drug Bulletin: Alpha Interferon for Venereal Warts, Vol. 18, No. 2, August 1988.

FDA Drug Bulletin: Special AIDS Issue, Vol 17, No 2, September 1987.

FDA Drug Bulletin: Treatment IND for AIDS Drug, Vol 18, No 1, April 1988.

Gong, V: AIDS Facts and Issues. Rutgers University Press, New Brunswick, NJ, 1987.

Investigational AIDS Vaccine. Am J Nurs 87(12):1540, December 1987.

Jaroff, L: Stop That Germ. Time Magazine 131(21):56, May 23, 1988.

Kolata, G: Predicting cancers course: New findings—Examination of oncogenes ushers in a new era in research. Cancer News, Autumn 1987.

Krigel, R: Interleukins, interferons, and tumor necrosis factor in cancer treatment. AAOHN Journal, April 1987.

Lippman, M, Lichter, A, and Danforth, D: Diagnosis and Management of Breast Cancer. WB Saunders, Philadelphia, 1988.

Lymphokine-activated killer cells and interleukin-2 redux. Clinical Oncology Alert 2(6), June 1987.

Moertel, Charles, MD: Interview on new application of Levamasol treatment of colon cancer, October 4, 1989 from Mayo Clinic, Rochester, MN.

Oncogene amplification and prognosis in breast cancer. Clinical Oncology Alert 2(4), April 1987.

Pinedo, HM, Longo, DL, and Chabner, BA (eds): Cancer Chemotherapy and Biological Response Modifiers, Annual 9. Elsevier Science Publications, New York, 1987.

Sherry, P: Cancer update for the occupational health nurse. AAOHN Journal, April 1987.

Which is better: More IL-2 or less? Clinical Oncology Alert 3(5), May 1988.

SITUATION 50–1

Carl Pazos is a 33-year-old recently diagnosed with AIDS. He is being treated through a public health clinic specializing in immune altered patients.

1. Mr. Pazos is to begin therapy with Zidovudine (AZT) 250 mg orally. The nurse will anticipate the following dosage schedule:
   a. every 8 hours
   b. twice a day
   c. every 4 hours
   d. four times a day

2. The nurse will teach Mr. Pazos about the side effects to be expected with AZT, including:
   a. photosensitivity
   b. alopecia
   c. fever and chills
   d. nausea

3. Upon his return visits to the clinic, the nurse will evaluate Mr. Pazos' response to AZT therapy. Which of the following lab values would be especially important to note?
   a. complete blood count (CBC)
   b. creatinine and BUN
   c. calcium and phosphorus
   d. potassium and magnesium

4. Should Mr. Pazos experience severe headaches, he should be instructed to:
   a. take indomethacin
   b. contact the physician
   c. take acetaminophen
   d. drink extra fluids

5. While providing care for Mr. Pazos after six months of AZT therapy, the nurse will be mindful of which of the following?
   a. respiratory protection
   b. AIDS transmission precautions
   c. isolation precautions
   d. no precautions necessary

6. Additional assessment of Mr. Pazos which should be employed on a routine basis would be to:
   a. expect patient to be depressed and withdrawn
   b. observe for serious systemic side effects
   c. check mucous membranes and skin for areas of breakdown
   d. monitor cardiac rhythm prior to drug administration

10
UNIT

DRUGS AFFECTING THE GASTROINTESTINAL SYSTEM

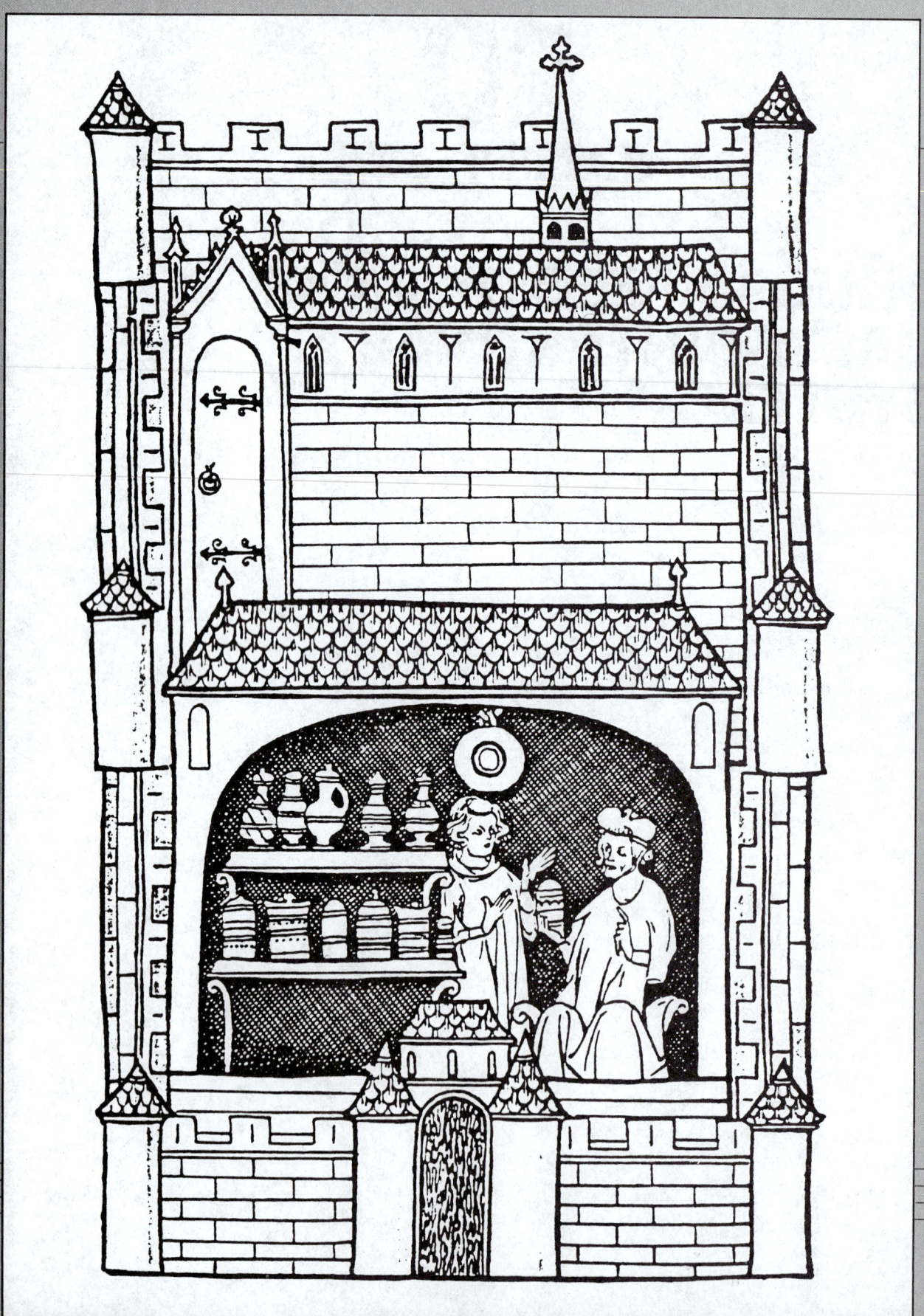

DRUGS AFFECTING THE GASTROINTESTINAL SYSTEM

GLOSSARY TERMS IN THIS CHAPTER

Alimentary canal
Bolus
Chyme
Deamination
Hydroxylation
Interconverts
Mastication
Peristalsis
Segmental contractions
Tonus waves

OVERVIEW OF ANATOMY AND PHYSIOLOGY OF THE GASTROINTESTINAL SYSTEM

MERRILY MATHEWSON KUHN, R.N.C., Ph.D., CCRN

LEARNING OBJECTIVES

After reading this chapter, the student will be able to:

1. Identify the major parts of the gastrointestinal system, and the specific secretions and hormones they generate and require for function.

2. Describe the movement of nutrients from the mouth to the anus, and how those nutrients are transformed within the digestive system.

3. Explain the regulatory functions of the gastrointestinal system.

THE ALIMENTARY CANAL

The gastrointestinal system, containing the *alimentary canal* or digestive tract, the biliary system, and the pancreatic gland, is responsible for processing the fluids, nutrients, and electrolytes entering the body (Fig. 51–1). As the raw materials of food and fluids are consumed by the individual, they undergo many chemical changes, which permit them to be used for maintenance of body functions, as energy, for tissue production, and for repairs in the body. The digestive tract, open at both ends, is normally the only port of entry in the body for nutrients.

The gastrointestinal system is responsible for a unique series of functions that allows food to be utilized by the body. The anatomy and physiology of each part of the system is discussed individually.

The alimentary canal, often called the digestive tract, is the site of major digestive activities in the body and is responsible for the elimination of residues from digestion.

The structures located between the mouth and the anus constitute the alimentary canal. These include the mouth; the esophagus, which is about 25 cm long; the stomach; the small intestine, which is about 4 m long and is composed of duodenum, jejunum, and ileum; the large intestine, which is about 1.5 m long and is composed of the cecum and the ascending, transverse, descending, and sigmoid colons; and, finally, the rectum.

The alimentary canal has five primary functions: it (1) moves ingested products through the system; (2) digests food substances; (3) secretes electrolytes and enzymes along the route to assist with digestion; (4) allows for the final absorption of nutrients into the blood stream (Fig. 51–2); and (5) excretes the indigestible residues.

The alimentary canal is responsible for moving the ingested food and fluids through the system by combining mixing movements (*segmental contractions*) and propulsion waves (*peristalsis*) (Fig. 51–3). Both movements are

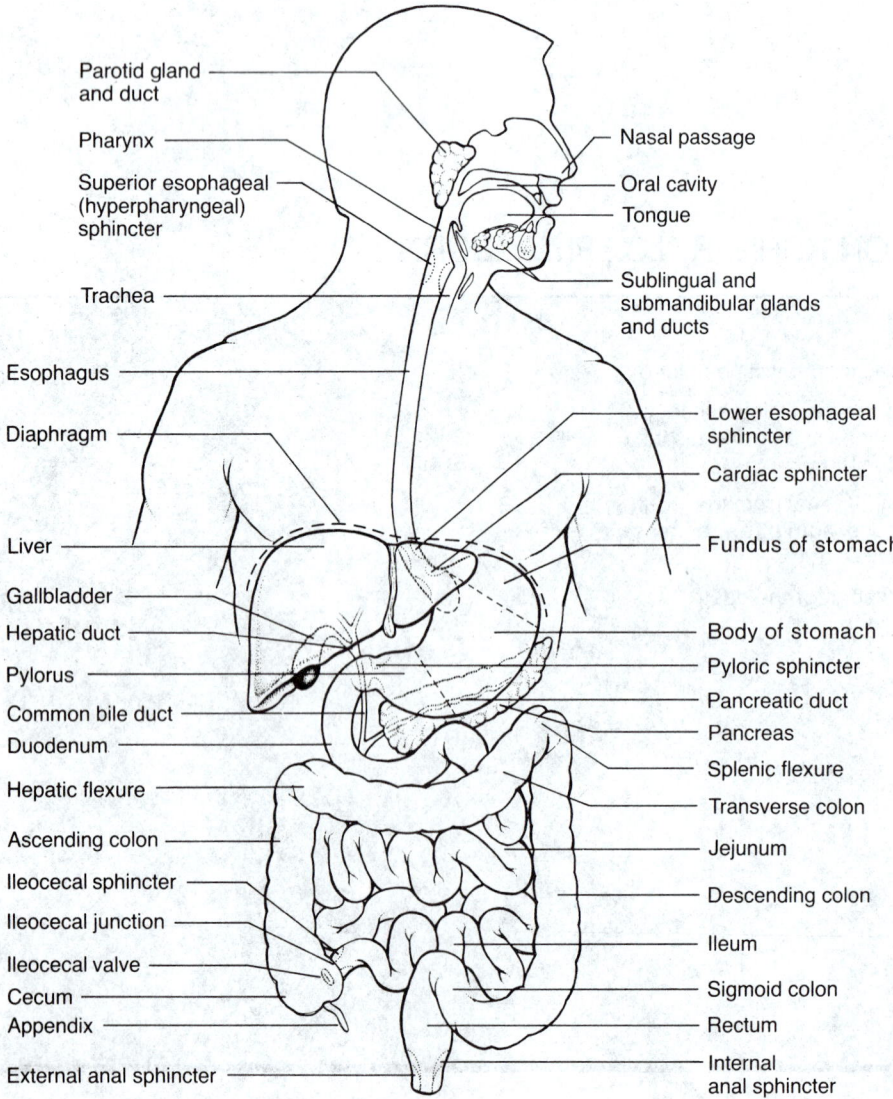

Figure 51–1. Diagram of the entire digestive system.

Parotid gland and duct
Pharynx
Superior esophageal (hyperpharyngeal) sphincter
Trachea
Esophagus
Diaphragm
Liver
Gallbladder
Hepatic duct
Pylorus
Common bile duct
Duodenum
Hepatic flexure
Ascending colon
Ileocecal sphincter
Ileocecal junction
Ileocecal valve
Cecum
Appendix
External anal sphincter

Nasal passage
Oral cavity
Tongue
Sublingual and submandibular glands and ducts
Lower esophageal sphincter
Cardiac sphincter
Fundus of stomach
Body of stomach
Pyloric sphincter
Pancreatic duct
Pancreas
Splenic flexure
Transverse colon
Jejunum
Descending colon
Ileum
Sigmoid colon
Rectum
Internal anal sphincter

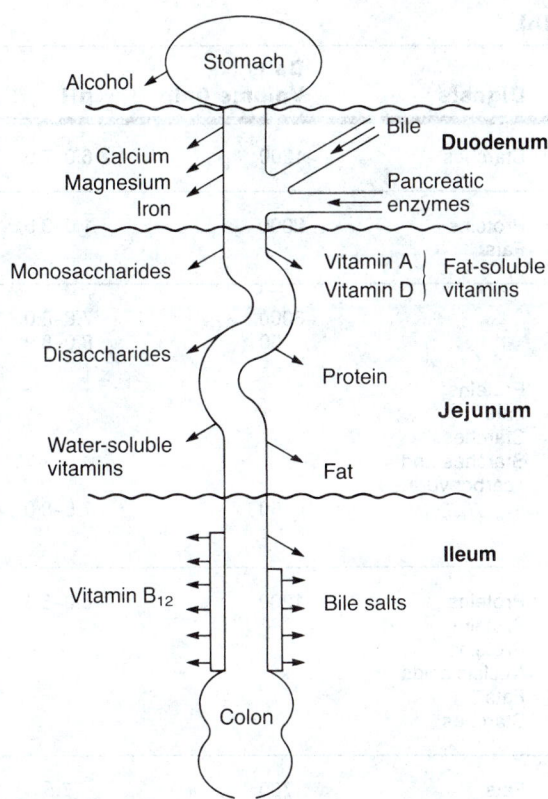

Figure 51–2. The sites of absorption of products within the gastrointestinal system.

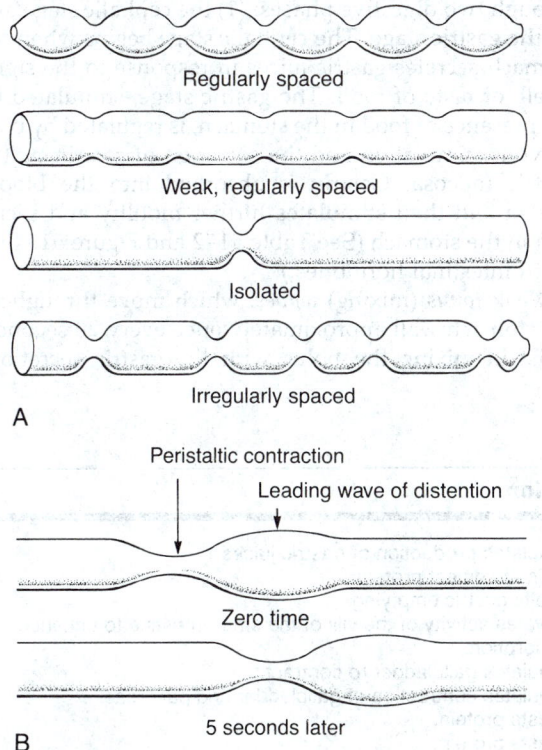

Figure 51–3. Two types of movements occur within the alimentary canal to move food and fluids. *A*, segmental contractions are mixing movements, and *B*, peristaltic waves are propulsion movements.

produced by rhythmic contractions of the smooth muscle fibers that surround the canal. These movements usually progress from the mouth to the anus. Reverse peristalsis may occasionally occur, resulting in vomiting.

As the ingested food is propelled through the canal, digestion occurs. Digestion is the breaking down of food substances by digestive juices into absorbable chemical compounds. The digestive juices secreted by the mouth, stomach, small intestine, biliary system, and pancreas contain electrolytes and enzymes that are responsible for the digestive process. Most of the electrolytes are later reabsorbed by the body for reuse. All nonabsorbable residues are excreted.

MOUTH AND ESOPHAGUS

The first stage of digestion, chewing, begins as soon as food enters the mouth. The fifth cranial nerve controls this reflex activity. Chewing *(mastication)* is of prime importance to mix solid and semisolid food thoroughly with saliva to form a *bolus* capable of being swallowed. The fibrous coverings of certain foods are also broken down by the activity of the teeth, tongue, walls of the cheeks, and the hard and soft palates. The extent of digestion of the food occurring later in the small intestine depends on the amount of surface area that is exposed to digestive enzymes. Digestive enzymes act only on the surfaces of food particles. Therefore, thorough chewing is the first step in proper digestion.

Saliva, secreted by the submaxillary, parotid, and sublingual glands, as well as by the many small buccal glands in the mouth, lubricates and softens the food. The saliva contains the enzyme ptyalin (amylase), produced by the parotid glands, which begins the breakdown or hydrolysis of starches. Approximately 1000–1500 ml of saliva—with a pH of 6.0–7.0—is secreted each day (Table 51–1 summarizes the digestive secretions of the alimentary canal).

The food, now called a *bolus*, is ready for swallowing (deglutition). Swallowing is a complex process that has three phases: (1) the voluntary stage, (2) the pharyngeal stage, and (3) the esophageal stage.

The voluntary stage is that stage in which the bolus is squeezed and rolled posteriorly by the tongue against the palate into the pharynx. The pharynx also contains the trachea, the main air passage to the lungs. In the pharyngeal stage of swallowing, the epiglottis closes over the trachea, the esophagus opens, and a fast peristaltic wave forces the bolus into the upper esophagus. The voluntary and pharyngeal processes take one to two seconds. The esophageal stage conducts food from the pharynx through the lower esophageal sphincter and into the stomach by means of both primary and secondary peristaltic waves. The waves pass from the pharynx to the stomach in about five to ten seconds; however, the food arrives faster, usually in four to eight seconds, because of the additional assistance of gravity.

The motor impulses from the swallowing center to the pharynx and upper esophagus that cause swallowing are transmitted by the fifth—trigeminal, ninth—glossopharyngeal, tenth—vagus, and 12th—hypoglossal cranial nerves.

Table 51–1 DAILY SECRETION OF THE ALIMENTARY CANAL

Source	Secretion	Enzyme	Digests	Daily Volume (ml)	pH
Mouth	Saliva	Ptyalin	Starches	1200	6.0–7.0
Gastric secretions	Mucus Hydrochloric acid	Pepsin Gastric lipase	Proteins Fats	2000	1.0–3.5
Intestinal secretions	Small intestine: Mucus (Brunner's gland)			3000 50	7.8–8.0 8.0–8.9
		Peptidases Lipase Maltase Lactase, sucrase, isomaltase	Proteins Fats Starches Starches and carbohydrates		
	Large intestine: Mucus			60	7.5–8.0
Pancreatic secretion		Trypsin Chymotrypsin Carboxypeptidase Nucleases Lipase Amylase	Proteins Proteins Proteins Nucleic acids Fats Starches	1200	8.0–8.3
Liver	Bile		Fats	700	7.8

The esophagus has mucus-secreting glands along its length, which further lubricate the bolus and protect the esophageal mucous membrane from damage from partially chewed food.

STOMACH

The stomach is a muscular, distensible pouch capable of holding 1500–2000 ml. The stomach has a threefold function: (1) it stores large quantities of food directly after a meal; (2) it mixes the bolus with gastric secretions like pepsin, mucus, and hydrochloric acid to form a semisolid mixture called *chyme*; and (3) it regulates delivery of chyme to the intestine.

Partial digestion of food in the stomach is carried on through two digestive phases: (1) the cephalic stage and (2) the gastric stage. The cephalic stage begins when the stomach secretes gastric juices in response to the sight, smell, or taste of food. The gastric stage, stimulated by the presence of food in the stomach, is regulated by both nervous stimulation and the secretion of gastrin by the gastric mucosa. Gastrin is absorbed into the bloodstream and then stimulates further motility and secretion in the stomach (See Table 51–2 and Figure 51–4 for gastrointestinal hormones.).

Weak *tonus* (mixing) *waves,* which move throughout the stomach wall approximately once every 20 seconds, assist in mixing the bolus with the gastric secretions

Table 51–2. GASTROINTESTINAL HORMONES

Hormone	Source	Action
Gastrin	Mucosa of stomach	Stimulates production of gastric juices.
Pepsin	Mucosa of stomach	Begins to digest protein.
Enterogastrone	Small intestine	Inhibits gastric emptying.
Villikinin	Small intestine	Activates activity of the villi of the small intestine to enhance absorption.
Cholecystokinin	Duodenum	Stimulates gallbladder to contract.
Secretin	Duodenum	Stimulates contraction of gallbladder and pancreas.
Trypsin	Pancreas	Digests protein.
Chymotrypsin	Pancreas	Digests protein.
Carboxypolypeptides	Pancreas	Digests protein.
Ribonuclease	Pancreas	Digests protein.
Deoxyribonuclease	Pancreas	Digests protein.
Amylase	Pancreas	Digests starch.
Lipase	Pancreas	Hydrolyzes neutral fats into glycerol and fatty acids.

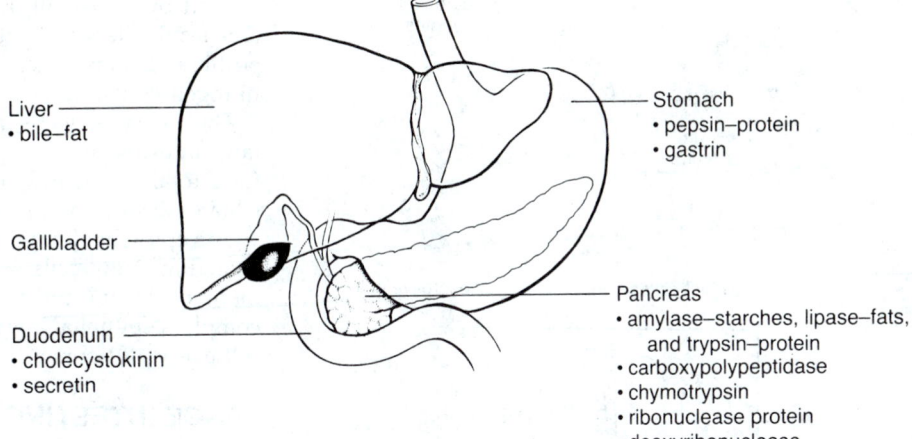

Figure 51–4. Diagram illustrates hormones and enzyme secretion within the gastrointestinal tract. The action of the enzyme is also reviewed.

until it is liquefied. In addition, strong peristaltic waves spread across the stomach to assist with mixing and emptying of the stomach. The waves are approximately six times more powerful than the usual mixing waves.

On occasion, a third type of contraction, hunger contractions, may be felt. These are normal rhythmic contractions that occur about every two minutes when the stomach has been empty for 12–24 hours. These waves may become very strong and form a tetanic contraction lasting two to ten minutes.

In the stomach, gastric glands produce secretions that assist in digestion (HCl, pepsinogen, and mucus); and the pyloric and a few cardiac glands (found in the cardiac portion of the stomach) produce mucus, which protects the gastric mucosa. The pyloric glands also produce pepsinogen and gastrin. Pepsinogen is converted into pepsin in the presence of gastric acid or pepsin itself. The gastric glands, located throughout the entire stomach wall, contain three different types of cells. The mucous neck cells produce mucus identical to that produced by the pyloric and cardiac glands. The chief cells produce the digestive enzyme pepsin that begins protein digestion. The parietal cells produce intrinsic factor, necessary for absorption of vitamin B_{12} later in the digestive tract. The oxyntic cells produce hydrochloric acid, which provides the medium in which pepsin works.

Peristaltic waves generated by the stomach cause gastric emptying. The pyloric sphincter allows chyme to exit the stomach slowly, at a rate of approximately 10–15 ml/minute, depending on the volume and on the degree of fluidity of the chyme, and the small intestine's receptivity to it. As the highly acidic chyme moves into the duodenum, enterogastrone, a hormone produced in the small intestine, is secreted and absorbed into the blood stream. Enterogastrone helps regulate the rate at which the stomach empties. If the duodenum is receiving a highly acidic chyme, enterogastrone inhibits gastric emptying, thereby protecting the duodenal walls and ensuring the alkalotic optimum necessary for intestinal enzymes. At the same time, the duodenum activates the enterogastric reflex to slow down peristalsis in the stomach. This action prevents the duodenum from becoming too full. The enterogastric reflex is also activated if the pH of the chyme falls below 3.5–4.0, if there

is distention of the duodenum, if there is excessive protein breakdown or hypotonicity or hypertonicity of the chyme, or if there is irritation of the mucosa. Activation of this reflex when the chyme is either hypotonic or hypertonic prevents the body from developing water and electrolyte disturbances.

The time required to empty the stomach also varies with the type of food ingested. Fats have the greatest inhibition, sometimes delaying emptying for as long as three hours. This is why a fatty meal provides a greater sense of satiation. Proteins have an intermediate effect, and carbohydrates have a mild effect, exiting the stomach very quickly. Ethyl alcohol is absorbed through the epithelial wall of the stomach, entering the bloodstream almost immediately.

After all food has left the stomach, the pH falls to 2.0 or lower, inhibiting gastric secretions. This prevents the emptying of large quantities of hydrochloric acid and pepsin into the duodenum.

SMALL INTESTINE

The small intestine is composed of the duodenum, jejunum, and the ileum. As chyme enters the small intestine, it is pushed along slowly, with regular peristaltic waves occurring at the rate of about 11 per minute. These contractions are segmental and appear to "chop" the chyme as it moves along. The chyme is also rotated in a clockwise direction as it passes along the gut to better expose it to the intestinal secretions as well as the many microvilli (Fig. 51–5) in the intestinal wall where absorption occurs. Villikinin, a hormone secreted by the intestinal wall, acts as a catalyst, exciting the villi to produce more villikinin, which, in turn, allows the villi to absorb more nutrients through the process of active transport and passive diffusion.

Mucus is produced in large quantities by both the Brunner's glands, located just inside the duodenum, and goblet cells, found extensively over the intestinal mucosa wall, to protect the wall of the small intestine from breakdown by the strongly acidic chyme. In the presence of anxiety, fear, and stress, the Brunner's glands are strongly inhibited by the sympathetic nervous system. When this inhibition occurs, the duodenum is left

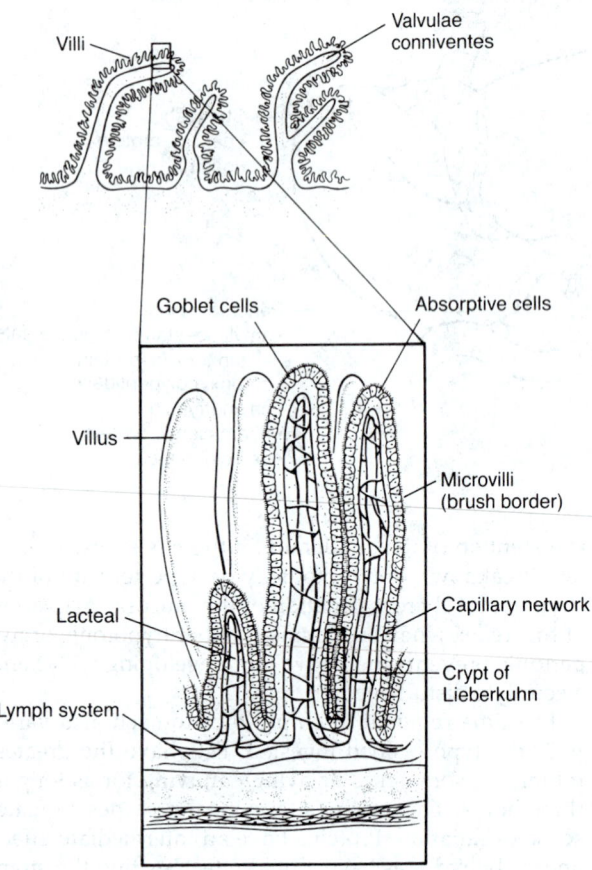

Figure 51–5. The mucous membrane of the small intestine including the numerous villi on a circular fold. (Adapted from Guyton, AC: Textbook of Medical Physiology. WB Saunders, 1986, p 791, with permission.

totally unprotected from the gastric secretions; this has been suggested as a possible cause of duodenal ulcers.

Small tubular glands called crypts of Lieberkühn are located within the entire surface of the small intestine and secrete about 2000 ml of alkaline secretions daily. These secretions contain peptidases for splitting small peptides into amino acids; lipase for splitting neutral fats into glycerol and fatty acids; and four additional enzymes for splitting disaccharides into monosaccharides—sucrase, maltase, isomaltase, and lactase. All of these secretions enable final digestion of the food before absorption. Bacteria found in the small intestine also take part in digestion by helping to split food by-products.

When the digestive functions are complete, the following transformations have occurred; carbohydrates have been converted to disaccharides and monosaccharides; proteins have become amino acids; and fats have been converted to fatty acids and to triglycerides (90%), diglycerides, and monoglycerides. The end products are absorbed along with electrolytes by both passive diffusion and active transport, while water is absorbed by osmosis. Both digestion and absorption are efficiently performed by the small intestine. By the time the chyme reaches the ileocecal valve, the chyme contains little digestible carbohydrates, few lipids, and only 15%–17% nitrogen-containing substances.

The ileocecal valve allows the chyme to enter the large intestine at a rate of only 4 ml per peristaltic wave, for a total of about 750 ml/day. This delay further facilitates absorption in the terminal ileum.

The epithelial lining of the small bowel is continually changing. New cells are being created near the basement membrane and move upward toward the villi. The complete epithelial layer of the small bowel replaces itself every 48 hours.

LARGE INTESTINE

The large intestine completes absorption and acts as a storage area for fecal matter until it can be expelled. Water absorption in the large intestine is critical to normal elimination. If water absorption is increased or decreased, constipation or diarrhea ensues. The fecal material is rolled, pushed, and squeezed, very much as in the small intestine. This movement gradually exposes the material to the surface of the large intestine, where fluid is progressively absorbed until only about 80 ml of chyme remains of the initial 750 ml. The propulsive movements in the large intestine are called mass movements. In most people, these are strongest early in the morning after eating breakfast. When a mass of feces has been pushed into the rectum, a person feels the desire to defecate.

Defecation occurs when a nerve impulse relaxes the normally tonic internal and external anal sphincters and the person simultaneously contracts the muscles of the abdominal wall and pelvic floor and takes a deep breath to pull the diaphragm downward. As pressure greatly increases in the abdominal cavity, the feces are pushed out of the rectum through the anus.

NERVE CONTROL OF THE ALIMENTARY CANAL

The autonomic nervous system, acting through both the parasympathetic and sympathetic nervous systems, controls the functioning of the alimentary tract. The parasympathetic nervous system, primarily through the vagus nerve, is responsible for proper functioning of the gastrointestinal tract, including swallowing, gastric secretion, intestinal motility, and defecation. Any psychologic stimulation of the parasympathetic nervous system, as with aggression, anger, resentment, and prolonged worry, increases activity of the alimentary canal and possibly results in digestive disturbances such as indigestion and diarrhea.

In general, the sympathetic nervous system slows or stops completely all gastrointestinal tract function. Therefore, any stimulation of the sympathetic nervous system, such as fear or excitement, can alter function of the gastrointestinal tract. Also, the protective stimulation of mucus is inhibited, such that prolonged sympathetic stimulation may lead to ulcer formation.

BILIARY SYSTEM

The biliary system is composed of the liver and gall-bladder, both of which actively function in the digestion of food.

LIVER

The liver, weighing about 1500 g, is the largest gland in the body. The liver is essential for the maintenance of normal metabolic function of the body; using only 10%–20% of its tissue, it performs more than 500 individual functions. The liver, unlike other organs, has impressive regenerative abilities; if part is removed or destroyed, the liver will, in most cases, initiate rapid regeneration of healthy liver tissue.

The liver's major function in digestion is to process the bile formed from old and defective red cells, cholesterol, phospholipids, bilirubin, and electrolyes. The hepatic ducts transport bile to the gallbladder, which rests directly beneath the liver, for storage. Bile assists with the alkalinization of intestinal contents and plays a role in the emulsification, absorption, and digestion of fat. The liver produces about 15 ml of bile per hour during a person's sleeping hours and about 22 ml per hour during waking hours. Most of the bile salts secreted in bile are reabsorbed by the intestines and then resecreted by the liver over and over again.

The liver is a very vascular organ and receives all of the venous blood flow from the intestinal tract. Blood flow through the portal vein is approximately 1000–1500 ml/min. This means that the liver has the first opportunity to absorb nutrients and drugs from the blood stream after the blood leaves the intestine.

The liver also plays an active role in metabolism. The liver is active in carbohydrate metabolism—it synthesizes and stores glycogen (which helps regulate blood sugar), converts galactose and fructose to glucose, takes part in gluconeogenesis, and forms many intermediate products of carbohydrate metabolism. The liver is active in fat metabolism—it converts fatty acids to acetoacetic acid; forms lipoproteins, cholesterol, and phospholipids; and converts large quantities of carbohydrates and proteins to fats. The liver is also active in protein metabolism—it *deaminates* amino acids, forms urea to remove ammonia from the body, forms plasma proteins, and *interconverts* amino acids and other compounds important to metabolic processes in the body. The liver stores vitamins A, D, and B_{12}, as well as iron in the form of ferritin, and releases it when iron stores in the body reach a low level.

The liver synthesizes cholesterol, and the clotting factors fibrinogen, prothrombin (II), and Factors V, VII, VIII, IX, and X. Vitamin K, normally absorbed only in the presence of bile in the small intestine, is needed by the liver to synthesize prothrombin and clotting Factors VII, IX, and X. The liver further acts as a sponge or blood chamber reservoir to absorb blood in congestive states. The liver removes bacteria from the blood through the action of the Kupffer's cells. Other metabolic capabilities of the liver include inactivating, altering, and excreting thyroxine and steroids such as aldosterone, glucocorticoids, estrogens, progesterone, and testosterone.

The liver is the chief organ of biotransformation of drugs. The active chemical medium of the liver is capable of metabolizing or excreting many different drugs into the bile. Drug metabolism can be depressed in starvation, obstructive jaundice, hepatic disease, severe cardiovascular disease, and immaturity, which depresses the microsomal drug-metabolizing system. Drug metabolism can also be stimulated by substances such as certain central nervous system depressants, xanthines, pesticides, food preservatives, and dyes that activate the microsomal drug-metabolizing enzymes (See Chapter 4 for more information.).

The liver has long been recognized as the major site of drug biotransformation, but only recently has this mechanism been clarified. A substance known as cytochrome P-450 has been identified as bearing paramount importance for the deactivation and detoxification of medications and other substances. Cytochrome P-450 is a pigment in hepatic microsomes found in the oxidase system of the liver, and it is responsible for biotransforming literally hundreds of endogenous compounds, such as steroids and fatty acids, and exogenous compounds, such as drugs and other chemicals. Its fundamental action is to *hydroxylate* water-soluble compounds (steroids and other substances), making them more water-soluble so they can more readily be excreted. This process occurs in the microsomal oxidase system.

Research has demonstrated that many compounds, such as phenobarbital, a sedative and hypnotic, can enhance the rates of their own biotransformation as well as those of others. These compounds increase hepatic levels of cytochrome P-450 and the microsomal oxidases, which subsequently increase the hepatic smooth endoplasmic reticulum and thereby enhance their own biotransformation as well as enhancing biotransformation of other substances. This logically explains why patients develop a tolerance to certain medications and need to have dosage increased to achieve therapeutic effects. This same effect results from chronic alcohol ingestion and probably accounts for the altered tolerance alcoholics have for sedatives, hypnotics, anticoagulants, and many other medications.

Recent research has found that when cytochrome P-450 detoxifies and biotransforms some substances that are relatively benign, other substances that may be toxic or even carcinogenic are released. As an example, benzpyrene, found in city smog, cigarette smoke, and charcoal-cooked foods, although not a toxic substance itself, yields substances that ultimately can act as carcinogens in the body after biotransformation. Cytochrome P-450 is also responsible for the serious and sometimes fatal liver and kidney injuries that are produced by an overdose (10 g or more) of acetaminophen (Tylenol) (Refer to Chapter 20 for more information on acetaminophen.).

Understanding cytochrome P-450 activity is basic to

understanding how other factors such as host genetic composition, nutritional status, and ingestion of alcohol or other medications enhance drug toxicity.

GALLBLADDER

The gallbladder, a pear-shaped organ located below the liver, is about one inch wide and three to four inches long. It collects and concentrates bile produced in the liver and stores it until it is needed for digestion. It is capable of holding about 45 ml of bile. After water and inorganic salts are absorbed into the bloodstream, gallbladder bile remains about ten times more concentrated than the unconcentrated hepatic bile. Bilirubin, the main bile pigment, is a metabolic end product from the processing of hemoglobin. Bile salts are essential for digestion and absorption of fats and fat-soluble vitamins (A, D, E, and K) in the intestine. At intervals, the gallbladder contracts and empties the bile into the common bile duct, which, in turn, carries the bile to the relaxed sphincter of Oddi, and into the duodenum. The normal stimulus for contraction of the gallbladder is the acid chyme in the duodenum; however, the strongest stimulus is the presence of fatty foods in the chyme. This contraction is mediated by the hormone cholecystokinin.

PANCREAS

The pancreas is located behind the stomach and is composed of a head, body, and tail. It resembles a bunch of grapes, each grape represented by a gland, with branches formed by ducts that terminate in the main duct (the pancreatic duct or the duct of Wirsung). The pancreatic duct traverses the entire length of the pancreas and carries the pancreatic juice into the common bile duct and then into the duodenum.

The pancreas is both an exocrine and endocrine gland; it produces enzymes and hormones that are released into the gastrointestinal system as well as into the bloodstream in response to the hormone secretion. As an exocrine gland, the pancreas produces the most potent digestive juice, which contains trypsin, chymotrypsin, and carboxypeptidases, all of which digest proteins; nucleases (ribonuclease and deoxyribonuclease), which digest nucleic acids; lipase, which digests fats; and amylase, which digests starches. It is important that the proteolytic enzymes of the pancreatic juice not become activated until they have been secreted into the intestine, for the trypsin and other enzymes would digest the pancreas itself. The same cells that secrete the proteolytic enzymes into the acini of the pancreas simultaneously secrete another substance called trypsin inhibitor. This substance is stored in the glandular cells surrounding the enzyme granules, and it prevents activation of trypsin both in the cells and in the ducts of the pancreas. When the pancreas becomes severely damaged, large quantities of pancreatic secretions become pooled into these damaged areas, and may overwhelm trypsin inhibitor. The pancreatic secretion then becomes rapidly activated and begins to literally digest the entire pancreas. This is called acute pancreatitis.

Pancreatic secretions are also high in bicarbonate and low in chloride. As sodium bicarbonate enters the duodenum, it combines with hydrochloric acid, with an end result of NaCl and carbonic acid. The carbonic acid immediately dissociates into carbon dioxide and water. The carbon dioxide is absorbed into body fluids, leaving a neutral sodium solution behind. This reaction neutralizes the acidic stomach contents and consequently protects small intestinal walls. The change in pH is also necessary for the activation of pancreatic enzymes. These enzymes help to complete the digestive process.

As an endocrine gland, the pancreas produces insulin and glucagon. Insulin is necessary for several processes, including active transport of glucose into the muscle cells where it is used; uptake and storage of glucose in the liver; conversion of liver glucose into fatty acids; inhibition of gluconeogenesis; and active transport of amino acids into the cells. Glucagon, often referred to as a counter-regulatory hormone, causes conversion of glycogen, stored in the liver and muscle tissue, to glucose.

SUMMARY

This brief overview of the normal anatomy and physiology of the gastrointestinal system demonstrates the role each part of the gastrointestinal system plays in providing the body with nutrients and digestive actions the body needs to process energy. The chapters that follow explore the effects of medications on all of the elements of the gastrointestinal system.

BIBLIOGRAPHY

Guyton, A: Medical Physiology. WB Saunders, Philadelphia, 1986.
Luckman, J and Sorensen, K: Medical-Surgical Nursing. WB Saunders, Philadelphia, 1986.
Netter, F: The Ciba Collection of Medical Illustrations: Gastrointestinal System, Vols 3, 4, and 5. Ciba Pharmaceutical, New York, 1959.
Price, S and Wilson, L: Pathophysiology: Clinical Concepts of Disease Process. McGraw-Hill, New York, 1985.

52

MEDICATIONS TO TREAT GASTRIC HYPERACIDITY

52

CHAPTER

MEDICATIONS TO TREAT GASTRIC HYPERACIDITY

MERRILY MATHEWSON KUHN, R.N.C., Ph.D., CCRN

LEARNING OBJECTIVES

After reading this chapter, the student will be able to:

1. Identify medications commonly used to treat gastric hyperacidity.

2. Differentiate among the medications to treat gastric hyperacidity as to mechanism of action, route of administration, pharmacokinetics, adverse effects, contraindications, and interactions.

3. Identify specific areas to assess in the patient requiring medications to treat gastric hyperacidity in order to formulate appropriate nursing diagnoses.

4. Plan the nursing interventions necessary to administer medications for gastric hyperacidity and choose appropriate teaching strategies to gain patient compliance.

5. Evaluate the patient at various stages of treatment to gauge nursing interventions.

PEPTIC ULCER DISEASE

Peptic ulcers (esophageal, gastric, duodenal) occur in areas of the gastrointestinal tract that are exposed to acid and pepsin. The gastrointestinal walls are no longer protected by the mucosal defense system. The etiology of peptic ulcers is unclear, but may be related to genetic factors, environmental factors, and psychologic factors. Recent research indicates that there might be an infectious origin of peptic ulcer disease. More research is needed to determine the direct cause of ulcer disease. It is estimated that approximately 10%–15% of the world's population has peptic ulcers (Table 52–1). There are over 400,000 hospitalizations/year, with about 9000 deaths.

Ulcers appearing in the stomach or esophagus are called *gastric ulcers;* those appearing within the duodenum are *duodenal ulcers;* and those appearing as a result of severe stress, trauma, sepsis, burns, or head injuries are called *stress ulcers* (Figs. 52–1 and 52–2). Ulcers can occur at any age, although rarely in children under the age of ten years.

Goals of treating peptic ulcers include to decrease symptoms, to hasten healing, to prevent complications (hemorrhage, perforation, and obstruction), and to prevent recurrences. These goals can usually be achieved through a combination of dietary measures (often bland diet and avoidance of spices, alcohol, and caffeine), avoidance of irritating drugs (aspirin and nonsteroidal anti-inflammatory drugs [NSAIDs]), avoidance of smoking, control of emotional factors, and a combination of drugs.

Traditionally, therapy for peptic ulcer has been a combination of products to protect the gastroduodenal mucosa. Within the last few years, there has been an explosion of new products that offer patients many alternatives. Therapeutic agents are aimed today at modifying gastric acidity either by neutralizing (antacids) or by inhibiting acid secretion (anticholinergics, H_2 receptor antagonists, and the still experimental inhibitors of the H^+-K^+ ATPase system).

The most common medications used to treat peptic ulcers include antacids to neutralize acidity, such as aluminum hydroxide gel (Amphojel); magnesium hydroxide gel ($MgOH_2$) combined with aluminum hydroxide (Maalox, Gelusil, Mylanta); anticholinergics to inhibit gastric motility and hydrochloric acid secretion, such as propantheline bromide (Pro-Banthine); the histamine-blocking agents (H_2 inhibitor) cimetidine (Tagamet); ranitidine hydrochloride (Zantac), famotidine (Pepcid), and nizatidine (Axid), which prevent the production of hydrochloric acid by the stomach. In addition, a new group of drugs enhance the resistance of the gastroduodenal mucosa to peptic digestion and protect the mucosa against injurious agents acting together with gastric acid (sucralfate and prostaglandins). Each group of medications is reviewed individually. Other medications used to treat patients with hyperacidity include antianxiety medications (see Chapter 26) and hypnotics (see Chapter 24). Both groups are discussed completely in the corresponding chapters.

Table 52–1. ULCER DISEASE

Ulcer Disease

DEFINITION:
A peptic ulcer is a circumscribed break in the continuity of the mucosa generally due to its exposure to hydrochloric acid, pepsin, gastric juices, or drugs, and can occur in the esophagus, stomach, duodenum, and jejunum. Marginal ulcers can occur whenever an abnormal opening, that is, a gastrojejunostomy, is made between a portion of the small intestine and the antral area of the stomach.

TYPES:
Esophageal
Gastric
Duodenal
Stress

ETIOLOGY
Personality type (hard-driving, time-oriented, aggressive individual, typical type A behavior patterns); type O blood (35% more susceptible than other blood types); genetic factors; eating patterns; stress, both internal and external; medications (aspirin, corticosteroids, alcohol, caffeine, bile salts).

SYMPTOMS
Gastric Ulcer—Gnawing, burning pain in the upper quadrant of the abdomen, pain-food-pain syndrome, hyperacidity, indigestion, frequent eructations (burping).

Duodenal Ulcer—Dull, gnawing, burning pain in the upper quandrant of the abdomen, pain-food-relief syndrome, indigestion.

TREATMENT:
Antacids, H_2 inhibitors, anti-ulcer drugs, anticholinergics, dietary modification, psychologic counseling.

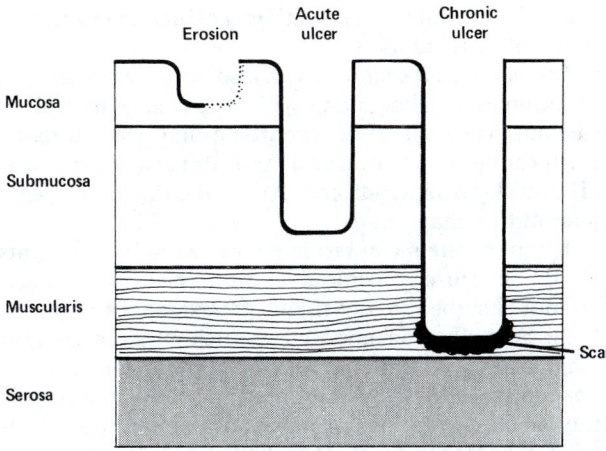

Figure 52–1. Peptic ulcers, illustrating an erosion, acute ulcer, and chronic ulcer. Both acute and chronic ulcers may penetrate the entire stomach wall. (From Price, S, and Wilson, L: Pathophysiology. McGraw Hill, New York, 1978, with permission.)

THERAPEUTIC AGENTS

ANTACIDS

The pH of the gastric contents is 1.0—a very highly acidic medium. Hyperacidity (too much acid in the stomach), also called hyperchlorhydria, is a common physiologic sign. The pain and discomfort associated with hyperchlorhydria are frequent complaints of patients diagnosed as having peptic ulcers.

Antacids, a complex group of medications, are one of the mainstays for the treatment of peptic ulcers because of their ability to effectively reduce acidity, at relatively low cost, and with low incidence of side effects. Unfortunately, these largely OTC preparations are frequently abused by many consumers who use them habitually and improperly to treat self-diagnosed hyperacidity, heartburn, indigestion, or discomfort resulting from overindulgence in food or alcohol. All medication should be used by a knowledgeable consumer.

Action

Antacids interact with gastric secretions, releasing anions that partially neutralize gastric hydrochloric acid and thereby increase the gastric pH. They do not absorb the acid—a popular misconception. Normally, the pH of the stomach is approximately 1.0. Antacid therapy generally raises the pH to above 4.0. Pepsin, a proteolytic enzyme, is suppressed with a pH above 2–3 and inactivated with a pH above 7–8. If a patient is bleeding, the pH has to be above 6.5 for blood to clot. Also, pepsin needs to be inactivated in this person. Pepsin and hydrochloric acid are the two primary causes for inflammation and erosion of the gastric mucosa.

Acid-neutralizing capacity (ANC) is a primary consideration in selecting an antacid. It is expressed in milliequivalents per milliliter (mEq/ml). Milliequivalents of antacid is defined by the mEq of hydrochloride required to keep an antacid suspension at pH 3.0 for two hours *in vitro*. The higher the ANC, the more effective the antacid.

Uses

Antacids are effective in treating conditions such as acid indigestion, heartburn, *reflux esophagitis*, and both active and chronic peptic ulcers, and in preventing stress ulcers. Antacids may also be effective in relieving pain from ulcers and are especially effective in binding bile salts that reflux into the stomach. When antacids are appropriately prescribed, they may be administered every one to two hours during waking hours for the first two weeks, and subsequently one and three hours after meals and at bedtime during the healing stage.

Aluminum antacids can also be used to treat individuals who are prone to the development of phosphate kidney stones or treatment of hyperphosphatemia associated with chronic renal failure. Aluminum hydroxide antacids (Amphojel, Gelusil) bind with phosphate in the bowel, causing an insoluble precipitate to be excreted in the feces. Therefore, phosphate does not enter the bloodstream. Since phosphate and calcium have an inverse relationship, as serum phosphate increases, serum calcium falls and the needed calcium is reabsorbed from the bone reservoir. Again, by administering aluminum hydroxide antacids (Amphojel), phosphate is bound in the intestine to the aluminum, forming aluminum phosphate, and is excreted in the feces. Plasma phosphate levels fall and calcium levels in the serum rise. Since a large quantity of phosphate is found in saliva, antacids are best given after meals. Prolonged use of these antacids can create hypophosphatemia with symptoms of anorexia, malaise, and muscle weakness.

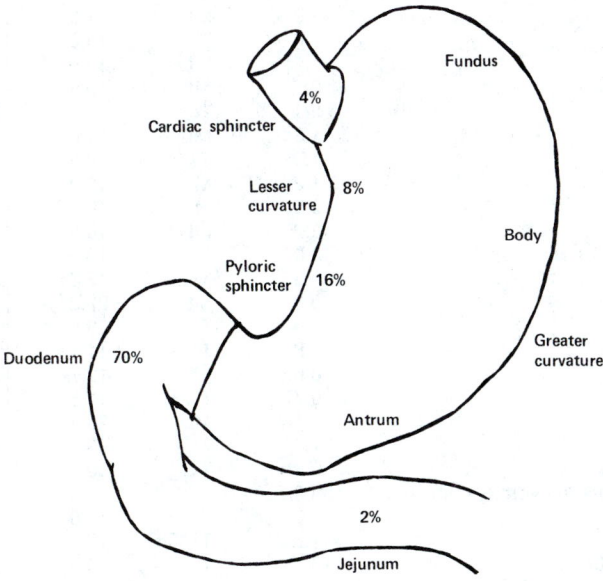

Figure 52–2. The distribution of peptic ulcers.

Patients must be monitored closely. Patients with renal disease also hold on to the aluminum, and increased brain and liver aluminum levels have been found.

Antacid Classification

There are two general classifications of antacids—systemic and nonsystemic. The systemic antacids are soluble in gastric contents and are capable of being absorbed systemically, and therefore may alter electrolyte balance and precipitate metabolic alkalosis. The most commonly used systemic antacid is sodium bicarbonate, USP (baking soda). It is rarely prescribed by the physician but is frequently taken by the public because it is readily available in the home. Sodium bicarbonate is also contained in many effervescent over-the-counter drugs such as Alka Seltzer, Soda Mint, and Instant Metamucil.

Sodium bicarbonate may be taken as a powder or in tablet form, and readily produces a gastric pH of 8.5. This rapid rise in pH inactivates and overneutralizes the gastric contents. Owing to the overneutralization and short duration of action, a rapid return of pH to the acidic side occurs, which necessitates retaking sodium bicarbonate at more frequent intervals. As sodium bicarbonate enters the stomach, it combines with hydrochloric acid and liberates water and carbon dioxide. This carbon dioxide may cause gastric distention or may cause the patient to eructate (burp), which seems to give relief (of distention).

The *milk-alkali syndrome* can also occur when sodium bicarbonate is taken along with or mixed with milk or calcium. The milk-alkali syndrome may lead to tissue calcification (with calcium) and urinary crystalluria. (The milk-alkali syndrome is described in more detail later in this chapter.)

The nonsystemic antacids neutralize gastric contents but do not cause systemic alkalosis because the products are not absorbed to any significant extent. The nonsystemic antacids are composed of calcium, aluminum, or magnesium, or some combination of those agents. Magnesium is the best overall antacid, while aluminum is the weakest antacid. Calcium and aluminum products have a tendency to cause constipation, whereas magnesium products cause diarrhea. The ideal antacid is a combination product that would not alter the patient's bowel activity. However, most patients experience some bowel alteration. Calcium carbonate has high neutralizing capabilities, followed by magnesium hydroxide and aluminum hydroxide. All three products have a duration of action of 30 minutes in a fasting patient, and two to four hours when there is food in the stomach.

The most common antacid preparations are listed in Table 52–2, with a comparison of their ingredients, neutralizing capacity, and sodium content.

Table 52–2. COMMON ANTACIDS WITH THEIR INGREDIENTS

	A	B	C	D	Other Ingredients	Sodium (mg)	Form	ANC (mEq)
Aludrox	—	x	x	—		1.3	T	9.5
Amphojel	—	x	—	—		2.2	ML	12.0
Amphojel	—	x	—	—		3.1	T	16.0
Basaljel	—	x	—	—		2.7	T	12.5
Basaljel	—	x	—	—		2.9	ML	11.5
Camalox	x	x	x	—		1.0	T	18.0
Camalox	x	x	x	—		1.2	ML	18.0
Di-Gel	—	x	x	x		8.5	ML	10.5
Gelusil II	—	x	x	x		2.1	T	21.0
Gelusil II	—	x	x	x		1.3	ML	24.0
Gelusil M	—	x	x	x		1.3	T	12.5
Gelusil M	—	x	x	x		1.2	ML	15.0
Alternagel	—	x	—	—		<2.5	ML	16.0
Kolantyl	—	x	x	—		2.2	ML	10.5
Kolantyl	—	x	x	—		2.0	T	10.8
Maalox	—	x	x	—		1.35	ML	13.3
Maalox concentrate	—	x	x	—		0.8	ML	27.2
	—	x	x	—		0.5	T	28.0
Maalox Plus	—	x	x	x		0.8	T	11.4
Mylanta	—	x	x	x		0.68	ML	12.7
Mylanta	—	x	x	x		0.77	T	11.5
Mylanta II	—	x	x	x		1.14	ML	25.4
Mylanta II	—	x	x	x		1.3	T	23.0
Riopan	—	—	—	—	Magaldrate	0.3	T	30.0
Rolaids	—	—	—	—	Na carbonate, dihydroxyaluminum	53.0	T	7.5
Tums	x	—	—	—		<3.0	T	10.0
Wingel	—	x	x	—		<2.5	T	12.2
Gaviscon	—	x	—	—	Mg trisilicate	19.0	T	0.5
Gaviscon	—	x	—	—	Alginic acid	39.1	ML	3.8

Form: T = Tablet, ML = Liquid; ANC: Acid-neutralizing capacity for therapeutic dose of 5 ml or tablet. A = calcium carbonate; B = aluminum hydroxide; C = magnesium; D: simethicone.

Contraindications and Precautions

In general, the antacids are contraindicated in individuals with sensitivities to the component's properties. Antacids are contraindicated in patients with renal dysfunction because of the possibility of producing urinary calculi if the renal output is reduced. In addition, in patients with renal impairment, metal ions may accumulate in the compromised kidney, leading to additional kidney impairment, systemic alkalosis, and fluid and electrolyte imbalance. In particular, increased magnesium ion may create neurologic, cardiovascular, and neuromuscular dysfunction; whereas excessive calcium may result in hypercalcemia, weakness, and mental confusion. Additional symptoms of hypercalcemia include nausea, vomiting, anorexia, weakness, headache, dizziness, and a change in mental status.

Precautions are used when administering aluminum antacids in patients with gastric outlet syndrome, as aluminum inhibits smooth muscle contraction and thus inhibits gastric emptying.

Patients with cardiovascular and renal disease must be given antacids low in sodium to help prevent the retention of water, which could worsen their condition. The majority of antacids today have low sodium contents. Sodium content is more a "marketing tool" rather than a true chemical hazard today.

Adverse Effects

In general, the majority of antacids are nontoxic. The most common complaint from patients is a change in bowel habits. Aluminum and calcium products generally cause constipation, whereas magnesium products attract and retain water, creating an osmotic effect leading to diarrhea. The diarrhea can result in an increased risk of potassium depletion and acidosis. This condition can usually be eliminated by using combination products or by alternating aluminum and calcium products with magnesium products during the day. However, calcium products may stimulate rebound gastric acid secretion and are usually not recommended in a patient with ulcer disease.

Many antacids can lead to electrolyte disturbances, such as hypermagnesemia, hypophosphatemia, and hyperphosphatemia. It is important to stress that the use of magnesium-containing antacids can result in hypermagnesemia (5%–10% absorption) in patients with renal insufficiency or renal failure, due to the decreased clearance. An elevated magnesium could result in hypotension and respiratory arrest. Therefore, it is recommended that magnesium-containing products be avoided in this subgroup of patients. Calcium products may promote positive phosphate balance. Sodium bicarbonate along with calcium carbonate are implicated as the culprits in the development of the milk-alkali syndrome characterized by hypercalcemia, alkalosis, and renal failure. Patients at high risk for developing milk-alkali syndrome are those receiving: hydrochlorothiazide, which decreases the renal excretion of calcium carbonate; and 0.5–10 g of calcium antacids a day. Patients prone to the development of these problems need to have occasional electrolyte studies performed.

Rebound hyperacidity may be an adverse effect in some patients receiving calcium carbonate. Levant, Walsh, and Isenberg in 1973 demonstrated that 2 g of calcium carbonate orally causes significant stimulation of acid secretion and a small increment in serum gastrin. The magnitude of the acid rebound may be as high as one third the maximal gastric secretory capacity. This is probably mediated by increased serum calcium, although there is no relationship between serum calcium levels and the stimulation of acid secretion. Acid rebound does not seem to be related to significant increases in serum gastrin. Because of the rebound effect, calcium carbonate and all calcium products including milk are recommended less frequently. Renal calculi may also develop in patients receiving calcium carbonate. The patient needs to be encouraged to drink at least two liters of fluid daily in order to prevent stones from forming. Chronic ingestion of aluminum-containing antacids in patients with chronic renal failure can result in accumulation of aluminum in serum, bone, and the central nervous system and may cause decreased absorption of fluoride. Additional adverse effects can be found in Table 52–3.

Drug Interactions

Drug interactions occur because of increased absorption, delayed gastric emptying, renal elimination (change in urinary pH), and formation of insoluble complexes. Drug interactions are covered in detail in Table 52–4.

Antacids, because they change the pH of the stomach, are not given concurrently with enteric-coated tablets. The acid-resistant enteric coating is broken down in an alkaline medium, causing the drug to be released in the stomach rather than in the alkaline duodenum. This can irritate the stomach and change the absorption characteristics of the medication.

In general, antacids decrease the absorption of digitalis products, iron products, and tetracycline antibiotics. The antacid compounds tend to bind with either digitalis or tetracycline products to form complexes that are not easily absorbed. Their administration is separated by at least two to three hours.

Because aluminum products also inhibit the absorption of isoniazid (given for tuberculosis), and the phenothiazine tranquilizers, give these medications one hour before the antacids.

Magnesium products, alone or in combination, decrease the absorption of the phenothiazines and digoxin. Kayexalate, a binding agent used to lower serum potassium, may also bind magnesium antacids.

Dosage

Dosage of antacids must be adjusted to achieve a pH of at least 3.5 in the gastric contents. Usually, the manufacturers' suggested doses are far too low to effect the neutralization. The production of acid in a patient with a duodenal ulcer is 50–80 mEq/hr, while acid production is 25–40 mEq/hr in a patient with a gastric ulcer. In order for any antacid to be effective, it must be ca-

TEXT RESUMES ON PAGE 1440

Table 52–3. MEDICATIONS TO TREAT HYPERACIDITY

Name	Dosage	Mode of Administration	Pharmacokinetics
ANTACIDS			
Action: neutralize or reduce gastric acidity.			
Use: hyperacidity, peptic ulcer disease, hiatal hernia, prophylaxis of gastrointestinal bleeding, and stress ulcers.			
Calcium Compounds Calcium carbonate (Alka-2, Chooz, Amitone, Tums, Dicarbosil, Equilet)	0.5–1 g (liquid, tablets) every 2–4 hrs.	PO	O: rapid D: 30–60 min
Aluminum Compounds Aluminum hydroxide gel USP (Amphogel, Alu-Cap, Dia-lume)	Adult: 5–30 ml 3–6× daily with or after meals or hs. Children: 2–5 ml every 4–6 hr.	PO	O: rapid D: 30–60 min (not absorbed)
Aluminum carbonate, basic (Basaljel)	10–15 ml, 2 caps or tabs q 2 hr, up to 12×/day. To prevent phosphate stones: 2–6 caps or tabs 1 hr pc and hs. Extra strength = 5–15 ml.	PO in water or fruit juice.	O: rapid D: 30–60 min (not absorbed)
Aluminum phosphate gel, NF (Phosphaljel)	15–30 ml q 2 hr, between meals and hs.	PO	O: slow D: 30–60 min (not absorbed)
Dihydroxyaluminum sodium carbonte NF (Rolaids)	334 mg/T (1–2 tabs), chewing required.	PO tabs, chewable	O: slow D: moderate
Magnesium Products Magnesium hydroxide NF (Milk of Magnesia)	650 mg (1–2 tablets) qid Children 2–6 yrs laxative dose: 5–15 ml single dose. Children 6–12 yrs laxative dose: 15–30 ml single dose.	PO	O: rapid D: prolonged
Magnesium oxide USP (Par Mag Maox)	280 mg–1.5 g with water or milk qid.	PO caps, tabs	O: rapid

Key to Abbreviations in the *Pharmacokinetics* column O-onset; P-peak; D-duration; PB-protein bound, B-biotransformed in; E-excreted in; ½ L-halflife.
*Within the column listing adverse effects, underlines indicate the most common effects; CAPITALS indicate life-threatening effects.

Contraindications/ Precautions	Adverse Effects*	Interactions	Nursing Implications
For All: Contraindicated in renal dysfunction and in renal calculi, sensitivity to component preparation, and abdominal pain of unknown origin. Use cautiously in cardiovascular or renal disease in relation to sodium content.	*For All:* GI: change in bowel habit Renal: hypermagnesemia, hyperphosphatemia	*For All:* For detailed interactions of antacids see Table 52–4.	For All: ASSESSMENT: Assess pain, food history. INTERVENTION: Take between meals, 1 hour before or 3 hours after meals, or both. Note any changes in bowel habits. If constipation occurs, alternate with other preparations. Antacids should be given cautiously to patients on a low-sodium diet. Chew tablets thoroughly and take with full glass of water. Take other drugs 1 hour before or 2 hours after antacids. EVALUATION: Notify physician if continued pain or tarry stools.
Same as for all.	Same as for all plus GI: nausea, vomiting, rebound hyperacidity Renal: milk-alkali syndrome	Same as for all.	Same as for all plus INTERVENTION: Patient should be aware of the symptoms of milk-alkali syndrome if drug is being used chronically. These include headache, confusion, nausea, vomiting, distaste for food, abdominal pain, and hypercalcemia.
Same as for all plus Use cautiously in gastric outlet syndrome.	Same as for all plus Neuro: dialysis dementia in dialysis patient, accumulation of aluminum in serum bone and CNS, headache, weakness GI: constipation, nausea, vomiting Renal: alkalosis	Same as for all plus Inhibit absorption of isoniazid (give 1 hour before antacid), quinine, phenothiazines, iron salts, digoxin (separate by 2 hours), warfarin and quinidine; complexes with tetracyclines.	Same as for all plus INTERVENTION: Aluminum hydroxide interferes with the absorption of phosphates from the intestine and in the presence of a low-phosphate diet, may cause deficiencies. When administering aluminum products continuously through a nasogastric tube, dilute them 1:2 or 1:4 with water.
Same as for all.	Same as for all.	Same as for all.	Same as for all plus INTERVENTION: Long-term use is not advisable. Note consistency of stools daily. Tell physician that you are taking magnesium products when other medications are prescribed. Store in tightly covered container.

CONTINUED ON THE FOLLOWING PAGE

Medications for Hyperacidity

Table 52–3. MEDICATIONS TO TREAT HYPERACIDITY–*CONTINUED*

Name	Dosage	Mode of Administration	Pharmacokinetics
Mixtures			
Aluminum hydroxide and magnesium hydroxide USP (Aludrox, Maalox, Wingel)	300–600 mg	PO suspension, tablets	O: rapid
Aluminum hydroxide and magnesium trisilicate USP (Triconsil, Parviscon)	300–600 mg	PO suspension, tablets	O: rapid

HISTAMINE H₂ ANTAGONISTS

Action: competitively inhibits histamine release and therefore decreases gastric acidity.

Use: peptic ulcer, prophylaxis for stress ulcer, pathologic hypersecretory conditions.

Cimetidine (Tagamet)	300 mg 4×/day, 400 mg bid, 800 mg hs. Liquid: 300 mg/5 ml.	PO	O: 30 min P: 1 hr D: 4–5 hr ½L: 2 hr PB: 13%–25% B: liver E: urine (48% unchanged)
	300 mg diluted with any IV solution to 1.2–5.0 mg/ml administered over 15–30 min	IV drip	O: 10 min P: 30 min E: urine (50%–75% unchanged)
	300 mg mixed with 20 ml administered over 5 min.	IV bolus	

Key to Abbreviations in the *Pharmacokinetics* column O-onset; P-peak; D-duration; PB-protein bound; B-biotransformed in; E-excreted in; ½ L-halflife.
*Within the column listing adverse effects, underlines indicate the most common effects; CAPITALS indicate life-threatening effects.

Contraindications/ Precautions	Adverse Effects*	Interactions	Nursing Implications
Same as for all.	Same as for all.	Same as for all.	Same as for all.
Contradicted in hypersensitivity. Use cautiously in pregnancy, nursing mothers, and in impaired renal or hepatic function.			*For all:* ASSESSMENT: Check for signs and symptoms of occult bleeding, assess stool color and vital signs daily. INTERVENTION: Antacids are given concurrently but not at the same time. Monitor gastric pH whenever possible. A pH of 3.5 or higher is desirable and for stress ulcers a pH above 7.4 is desirable. Check for reduced dosages in the elderly or in patients with reduced renal function. Advise the patient to avoid all products that increase gastric acid secretion, like smoking. EVALUATION: Notify physician of diarrhea, dizziness, black tarry stools.
Same as for all	Neuro: somnolence, dizziness; and in elderly particularly confusion, agitation, drowsiness, and even coma. CV: bradycardia, sinus and cardiac arrest after rapid IV administration. GI: nausea, diarrhea, abdominal pain Hemo: depression of immune system, AGRANULOCYTOSIS, APLASTIC ANEMIA Reprod: gynecomastia in men and breast pain and enlargement in both men and women, reduction of libido and impotence. Integ: rash Misc: arthralgia	Concurrent administration will increase serum levels of warfarin-type anticoagulants, theophylline, phenytoin, beta blockers, quinidine, caffeine, diazepam, ethanol, and calcium channel blockers and others. Concurrent use of antacids may decrease cimetidine absorption. Digoxin levels may decrease.	INTERVENTION: Cimetidine can be administered IV by slow bolus or drip every 4–6 hours during the 24-hour period. Bolus of 300 mg should be diluted with normal saline solution to a total volume of 20 ml and given over 5 minutes. IV drip of 300 mg should be diluted in at least 50 ml of any solution and given over 15–20 minutes. Cimetidine is given with meals and at bedtime when it is given orally and the patient is eating.

CONTINUED ON THE FOLLOWING PAGE

Table 52–3. MEDICATIONS TO TREAT HYPERACIDITY–*CONTINUED*

Name	Dosage	Mode of Administration	Pharmacokinetics
Ranitidine hydrochloride (Zantac)	150 mg q 12 hr 300 mg hs.	PO	O: rapid P: 1–3 hr D: 8–12 hr ½L: 2–3 hr PB: 15% B: liver E: urine (30% unchanged)
	50 mg q 6–8 hr, dilute to 20 ml and give over 5 minutes.	IV	O: 0.25 hr E: urine (70% unchanged)
Famotidine (Pepcid)	40 mg hs or 20 mg q 12 hr. liquid 40 mg/5 ml	PO	O: 1 hr P: 2–4 hr D: 10–12 hr ½L: 2.5–4 hr PB: 15%–20% B: liver E: urine (IV: 70% unchanged; Oral: 30% unchanged)
	20 mg in 10 ml over 2 min.	IV bolus	
	20 mg with 100 ml over 15–30 min.	IV drip	
Nizatidine (Axid)	300 mg hs. 150 mg bid.	PO	O: 0.5–1 hr P: 0.5–3 hr D: 3–10 hr ½L: 2–3 hr PB: 35% B: liver E: urine 90% (60% unchanged)

ANTI-ULCER DRUGS

Action: forms an ulcer-adherent complex with protein exudates at ulcer site.

Use: short-term therapy for duodenal ulcers, prophylaxis of stress ulcers, provides pain relief for oral ulcers and mucosal pain associated with chemotherapy and radiation.

Sucralfate (Carafate)	1 g 4×/day ac and hs.	PO	O: 30 min P: UA D: 6 hr ½L: 6–20 hr PB: UA B: liver E: stool (90%)
	Oral suspension	PO	

Key to Abbreviations in the *Pharmacokinetics* column O-onset; P-peak; D-duration; PB-protein bound, B-biotransformed in; E-excreted in; ½ L-halflife.
*Within the column listing adverse effects, underlines indicate the most common effects; CAPITALS indicate life-threatening effects.

Contraindications/ Precautions	Adverse Effects*	Interactions	Nursing Implications
Same as for all plus Use cautiously in renal impairment. Safe use in children not established.	Neuro: headache, malaise, confusion, blurred vision, change in lens accommodation CV: tachycardia, bradycardia, PVCs Resp: hypersensitivity reactions GI: constipation, diarrhea, nausea, vomiting, abdominal discomfort Bilary: reversible hepatitis Hemo: leukopenia, granulocytopenia, thrombocytopenia Reprod: gynecomastia Integ: rash Musculoskel: arthralgia	Antacids may decrease absorption. Ranitidine decreases renal clearance of warfarin.	Same as for all plus INTERVENTION: May be administered before, during, or after meals. Therapy is usually for 4 weeks.
Contraindicated in hypersensitivity. Use cautiously in renal disease. Safety in pregnant and lactating women and children not established.	Neuro: headache, dizziness, tinnitus Resp: bronchospasm GI: diarrhea, constipation, nausea, vomiting, taste disorder Integ: rash	None	As above.
Same as for all plus Safe use in children not established.	Neuro: somnolence GI: increased liver enzymes Hemo: THROMBOCYTOPENIA Renal: hyperuricemia Integ: sweating, urticaria, rash	Increases serum salicylates.	Same as for all
Contraindicated in hypersensitivity. Safety in pregnancy, nursing mothers, and children is unknown.	Minor Effects. Neuro: dizziness, sleepiness, vertigo GI: constipation, diarrhea, nausea, gastric discomfort, indigestion, dry mouth. Integ: rash, pruritis	May decrease bioavailability of tetracycline, cimetidine, phenytoin, and warfarin. Separate by 2 hours.	INTERVENTION: Do not administer antacids concurrently within ½ hour before meals or ½ hour after sucralfate. Administer on empty stomach 1 hour before or 2 hours after meals and hs.

CONTINUED ON THE FOLLOWING PAGE

Table 52–3. MEDICATIONS TO TREAT HYPERACIDITY–*CONTINUED*

Name	Dosage	Mode of Administration	Pharmacokinetics
GASTROINTESTINAL STIMULANT			
Action: increases gastrointestinal motility; appears to sensitize tissues to the action of acetylcholine			
Use: diabetic gastroparesis, gastroesphogeal reflux, nausea secondary to cancer chemotherapy, pregnancy and labor, gastric ulcer, and anorexia nervosa.			
Metoclopramide (Reglan)	10 mg 30 min before meals and bedtime for 2–8 wks.	PO	O: 30–60 min P: 60 min D: 1–2 hr ½L: 3–6 hr PB: 13%–22% B: liver (minimal) E: urine (80% unchanged), bile
	Facilitation of intubation: 10 mg over 1–2 min	IV	O: 1–3 min. P: immediate D: 1–2 hr
	Nausea secondary to chemotherapy: 1–2 mg/kg over 1–2 min. If over 10 mg, mix in 50 ml and administer in not less than 15 min.	IV	
	Gastric stasis: 10 mg 30 min. before meals and hs.	IM	O: 10–15 min P: UA D: 1–2 hr

Key to Abbreviations in the *Pharmacokinetics* column O-onset; P-peak; D-duration; PB-protein bound, B-biotransformed in; E-excreted in; ½ L-halflife.
*Within the column listing adverse effects, underlines indicate the most common effects; CAPITALS indicate life-threatening effects.

pable of neutralizing that amount of acid per hour. Magnesium hydroxide preparations have the greatest neutralizing or buffering capacity. In patients with acute disease, this neutralization can occur through a continuous drip in a nasogastric tube. The dosage for acute ulcer is usually 15–30 ml every two hours for two weeks, which maintains the pH at about 3.4. During the healing stage, the dosage is 15–30 ml one to three hours after meals and at bedtime; and for occasional pain, the dosage is usually 15 ml, as needed.

Antacids are available as liquid suspensions, chewable tablets, tablets to be swallowed, capsules, and powders. Liquid suspensions are the preparation of choice because of the large surface area covered and quick onset of action, and they are most cost effective. Liquid preparations may not be palatable, and may, therefore, decrease the patient's compliance and desire for food and drink. Chewable tablets are another alternative, but they must be thoroughly chewed, as their neutralizing capacity is related to the surface area of the particles. They must be taken with a full glass of water. Also, numerous tablets must be taken to achieve the same neutralizing ability of a liquid. The patient is encouraged to use several different preparations concurrently to avoid "taste fatigue."

CALCIUM PREPARATIONS. Calcium carbonate, once regarded as the agent of choice for its long action, insolubility, and low cost, has recently fallen into disfavor and is no longer recommended. Research has indicated that about 10% of the calcium may be absorbed and cause electrolyte disturbances. The amount absorbed probably depends on the amount of gastric acid present, as 2% is absorbed if the patient is achlorhydric, 9%–16% is absorbed if the patient has normal hydrochloric acid, and 11%–37% can be absorbed in peptic ulcer disease. Ingestion of large quantities of calcium carbonate may result in metabolic alkalosis or the milk-alkali syndrome. The alkalosis is presumed to develop because the net loss of hydrogen ions in the stomach is no longer balanced by the binding of bicarbonate ions in the upper small intestine by unabsorbed calcium. Calcium carbonate is the only antacid that causes acid-rebound; that is, acid hypersecretion after neutralization of the gastric content.

ALUMINUM PRODUCTS. The aluminum products available as liquids, solid forms, and gels are the most commonly used group today and vary in their neutralizing ability. Aluminum absorbs and temporarily inactivates pepsin, which may contribute to healing of peptic ulcers. They also relax gastric smooth muscles and delay gastric emptying, which prolongs their duration of action. Aluminum hydroxide (Amphojel, Alternagel, Basaljel Extra Strength), the most common preparation, has demulcent (soothing), absorbent, and astringent properties and is sometimes used in soothing and treating skin excoriations such as decubitus. Aluminum

Contraindications/ Precautions	Adverse Effects*	Interactions	Nursing Implications
Contraindicated in GI hemorrhage, GI obstruction, pheochromocytoma, hypersensitivity. Use cautiously in hypoglycemia, pregnancy, lactating women, and children.	Neuro: restlessness, drowsiness, fatigue, extrapyramidal effects CV: transient hypertension GI: nausea, diarrhea	Anticholinergics and narcotics antagonize metoclopramide. Additive effect with alcohol, sedatives, hypnotics, narcotics, and tranquilizers. Extrapyramidal effects are increased with phenothiazines, butyrophenol, and thioxanthine drugs.	INTERVENTION: Dosage of insulin may require adjustment as food reaches intestine more quickly. Take medication 30 minutes before meals and at hs. Observe caution while operating heavy equipment.

products readily react with hydrochloric acid in the stomach to form aluminum chloride. This reacts with bicarbonate and phosphate in the intestine to form insoluble aluminum salts. The aluminum products commonly cause constipation by binding with bile salts, but are generally nontoxic. Aluminum can be combined with sodium carbonate to form dihydroxyaluminum sodium carbonate (Rolaids, Camalox, Gaviscon), which combines the assets of both aluminum and sodium carbonate to neutralize rapidly (see Table 52–2).

MAGNESIUM PRODUCTS. Magnesium is found as an antacid in combination with carbonate, oxide, hydroxide, trisilicate, or phosphate salts. Since magnesium causes diarrhea (by an osmotic effect), it is often combined with aluminum or calcium products to avoid this side effect. Magnesium hydroxide (milk of magnesia) is used mainly as a laxative. It has a rapid onset of action and somewhat prolonged duration of action. Some of the magnesium is absorbed and may cause hypermagnesemia in patients with renal impairment. The magnesium combines in the stomach with hydrochloric acid to form magnesium chloride and water.

Magnesium hydroxide and magnesium oxide have a high neutralizing capacity with a rapid onset of action. These preparations hydrolyze to water and magnesium salts in the stomach after combining with hydrochloric acid. The dose is determined by the number of substitutions with either aluminum or calcium products, which results in normal stools in the patient.

Magnesium carbonate is similar to the above preparations, but it liberates carbon dioxide rather than water. It has a high neutralizing capacity.

Magnesium phosphate has a neutralizing capacity just below that of magnesium carbonate. Magnesium trisilicate is a poor acid buffer and has a slow onset of action because of its slow solubilization.

COMBINATION PRODUCTS. Since each of the antacid ingredients—calcium, aluminum, and magnesium—has an effect on bowel activity, the best antacid is achieved by combining these products into mixtures containing, most commonly, aluminum and magnesium.

Magaldrate (Riopan), a complex molecule of aluminum hydroxide and magnesium hydroxide, is not absorbed and therefore is unlikely to cause acid–base imbalances.

Simethicone, an antifoaming agent (not an antacid), breaks down gas bubbles to relieve flatulence, and can be added to various antacids: Mylanta, Mylanta II, Gelusil, Gelusil II, Gelusil M, and Maalox Plus. In addition, Mylicon (40- and 80-mg chewable tablets) and Silain (50-mg tablets) are available as 40–mg/0.6-ml drops (sugar-free), containing only simethicone. The gas bubbles do not disappear, but may form one large gas mass that is potentially more easily eliminated. These medications are taken four times daily, after meals and at bedtime, and as needed for control of flatulence. The efficacy of simethicone at this time is doubtful.

Other combinations are prepared by combining calcium carbonate and both aluminum hydroxide and magnesium hydroxide (see Table 52–2).

Another specific additive to antacids is alginic acid (not an antacid itself), which is added to Gaviscon. This causes a viscous solution to float on top of the gastric contents and protects the esophageal mucosa of patients with esophageal reflux of ulcers, or hiatus hernias.

Table 52–4. INTERACTION OF ANTACIDS

Increased absorption due to increased gastric pH
Pseudoephedrine (Sudafed and others)
—absorption rate increased in first 4 hours
—total absorption not changed
—chemical significance unknown
Dicumarol—depends on antacid
1 dose = 50% increase in absorption with MgOH (not noted with AlOH)
Naproxen—depends on specific antacid
sodium bicarbonate—some increase in rate of absorption
Mg-oxide > AlOH—delayed absorption
Clinical significance unknown
Other Drugs—Salicylates and Sulfas
usually decrease absorption (they are weak acids because ionizations decrease)

Drug adsorption
Antacids may bind or adsorb other drugs to their surfaces
Mg-Trisilicate and Mg-Hydroxide have greatest adsorption potential
Calcium carbonate, $AlOH_3$ intermediate potential
i.e., digoxin: adsorption documented *in vitro* and *in vivo*.
Because of variable bioavailability of digoxin and potential for altered patient response, should not take concurrently
Indomethacin, peak concentration is delayed, bioavailability is reduced,? clinical significance.
Nitrofurantoin, Mg-trisilicate, decreased rate and extent of absorption

---

Decreased Drug Absorption
Digoxin—see above
Isoniazid—decreased absorption probably 20% to decrease gastric emptying time, caused by aluminum. Also—some reports of adsorption (by magnesium oxide)
Diazepam—reported to
a. Absorption reported to be increased by aluminum hydroxide
b. Other studies—decreased rate of absorption but NOT extent of absorption (with AlMg hydroxide gel)

Urinary pH
Readily absorbed antacids (i.e., bicarbonate), most pronounced effects
Aluminum hydroxide—"qid"—no effect on urine pH
Mg-Hydroxide—increased pH = 0.4 units
Calcium carbonate—increased pH = 0.5 units
Mg-aluminum hydroxide gel—increased pH = 0.9 units
Dose 15–30 ml of MgAl hydroxide, significantly different than 5 ml; 30 ml not a significantly greater effect than 15 ml
Effect lasts for one day after antacid regimen (qid) stopped
Urine pH can effect drug excretion and reabsorption through renal system; i.e., if urine pH is made alkaline with antacid therapy, can increase salicylate excretion by 30%–70%.
Clinically—serum levels fall; loss of control when used on chronic conditions such as rheumatoid arthritis
Plan—Monitor urine pH, serum levels.
Other drugs:
1. Quinidine if urine pH increased (as with antacids), excretion decreased. Levels increase in body. Cases of quinidine toxicity 20% urine pH change.
2. Amphetamine in an alkaline urine, excretion is decreased, increased retention in the body.

Complex Formation
Tetracycline—Chelation occurs with polyvalent cations—calcium, aluminum, magnesium up to 90% reduction in tetracycline when given with MgAl antacid.
Iron—Similar rationale

Other Reports
Valproic Acid −AlMgOH = increased total absorption
In vitro oral contraceptive—Mg-Trisilicate = adsorbs estrogen and progesterone
Clinical significance—?

ANTICHOLINERGICS

The anticholinergic antispasmodics, including the belladonna alkaloids, their derivatives, and numerous synthetic preparations, are questionable adjuncts in the management of peptic ulcers. Anticholinergics are used much less frequently in modern ulcer management. The most common anticholinergics used to treat peptic ulcers are featured in Table 52–5. Because they are classified as adjunctive medications, they should only be given in combination with other drugs, not alone. These drugs are discussed more fully in Chapter 18.

Table 52–5. ANTICHOLINERGICS USED TO TREAT PEPTIC ULCERS

Preparation	Dose	Form		Times Per Day	Usual Dose
Anisotropine methylbromide (Valpin)	50 mg	T	B	tid	50 mg
Dicyclomine hydrochloride (Bentyl, Di-Spaz)	10 mg	C	Q	qid/tid	10–20 mg
Glycopyrrolate (Robinul) (do not use in children < 12 yr)	1–2 mg	T	Q	bid/tid maintenance 1 mg bid	PO 1 mg tid 2 mg bid-tid
	0.2 mg/ml (inj.)	IM		q 4 hr × 1 dose	IM 0.1–0.2 mg
Isopropamide iodide (Darbid) (do not use in children < 12 yr)	5 mg	T	Q	q 12 hr bid	5 mg or 10 mg
Methantheline bromide (Banthine)	50 mg	T	Q	q 6 hr	50–100 mg no elixir, pharm. compounds
Oxyphencyclimine (Daricon)	10 mg	T	Q	bid	5–10 mg
Oxyphenonium bromide (Antrenyl)	5 mg	T	Q	qid	10 mg
Propantheline bromine (Pro-Banthine)	7.5 + 15 mg	T	Q	.5 hr ac	15 mg or 25 tid hs 30 mg
Tridihexethyl chloride (Pathilon)	25 mg	T	Q	tid/qid	25–50 mg
Belladonna extract	15 mg	T	B	tid	15 mg
Belladonna tincture	30 mg belladonna alkaloids/100 ml		B		Adult: 0.6–1.0 ml 3–4×/day
Levohyoscyamine sulfate (Anaspaz) Tabs = 0.125, 0.15 (Cysto-spaz-M) TR = 0.375 cap (Levsin) Drops Solution = 0.125/ml (Levsin) Elixir = 0.125 (Levsin) Inj = 0.5 mg/ml	0.125 mg/5 ml	T TR, IM SQ, IV	B	q 4 hr q 3–4 hr inj = 0.25–0.5 mg 3–4×/day	0.125–0.25 mg
Hexocyclium methylsulfate (Tral Filmtabs)	25 mg	T TR	Q	ac/hs bid	25 mg 50 mg
Clidinium bromide (Quarzan)	2.5, 5 mg	C	B	tid/qid	2.5–5.0
Mepenzolate bromide (do not use in children)	25 mg	T	Q	tid/qid	25–50 mg

T = tablet; C = capsule; TR = timed-release; B = belladonna alkaloid; Q = quaternary.

Anticholinergics relieve pain by inhibiting motility and secretions and possibly by exerting a local anesthetic action. These agents block acetylcholine at the postganglionic parasympathetic neuroeffector sites in smooth muscle and secretory glands. This reduces both the secretion of hydrochloric acid and gastric and intestinal motility. A full dose of anticholinergic also blocks gastric cells, which stops pepsin and mucus production. To achieve this result, it is often necessary to elevate the dose to just below the level of adverse effects. Because they delay gastric emptying time by decreasing motility, they may ultimately stimulate gastric production and even increase gastric ulceration.

Contraindications and Precautions

Anticholinergics are contraindicated in pre-existing narrow-angle glaucoma, paralytic ileus, obstructive disease of the gastrointestinal tract, acute ulcerative colitis, myasthenia gravis, intestinal atony (generally in elderly or debilitated patients), and obstructive uropathy, as all these conditions are worsened. Patients should inform

physicians of their medications and why they were prescribed so that if a new medical condition is diagnosed, such as glaucoma, the medication can be altered or discontinued as necessary. Several combination anticholinergic medications are available and are featured in Table 52–6.

Adverse Effects

Unfortunately, the action of anticholinergics is not limited to gastric sites but is generalized to postganglionic nerve transmission throughout the body, such as in the heart, bladder, pupil, and mucous membranes. This gives rise to the many adverse effects that occur.

The majority of untoward effects of anticholinergics are manifestations of their pharmacologic action, such as dryness of the mouth, cycloplegia, tachycardia, constipation, and acute urinary retention. Large doses of both the belladonna alkaloids and the synthetic preparations can cause central nervous system stimulation including tremor, irritability, restlessness, delirium, and hallucinations. Children and elderly persons are more

Table 52–6. COMBINATION DRUGS FOR GASTROINTESTINAL ANTICHOLINERGICS

| Combination Drugs | Basic Products | | | | | | | |
---	A	B	C	D	E	F	G	Other
Barbidonna Elixir/5ml	0.034	21.6	0.174	0.01	15			Apricot flavor
Barbidonna Tablets	0.025	32	0.1286	0.0074				
Barbidonna #2 Tablets	0.025	16	0.1286	0.0074				
Belladenal Tablets		50						0.25 H
		15			19			
		15						
Butibel Elixir/5 ml					7			15 J
								15 K
Butibel Tablets								15 J
								15 K
Chardonna-2		15						15 J
Daricon PB Tablets		15						5 O
Donnatal Elixir/5 ml	0.0194	16.2	0.1037	0.0065	23			
Donnatal Extentabs	0.0582	48.6	0.3111	0.0195				
	0.0194	16.2	0.1037	0.0065				
Donnatal #2 Tablets	0.0194	32.4	0.1037	0.0065				
Hybephen Tablets	0.0233	15	0.1277	0.0094				
Kinesed Tablets	0.02	16	0.1	0.007				
Librax Capsules								2.5 Q
								5 R
Pathibamate 200 Tablets						25	200	
Pathibamate 400 Tablets						25	400	
Vistarex 10								25 P

Basic products: A = atropine sulfate, mg; B = phenobarbital, mg; C = hyoscyamine hyrochloride or sulfate, mg; D = scopolomine, mg; E = alcohol, %; F = tridihexethyl chloride, mg; G = meprobamate, mg; H = L-alkaloids of belladonna, mg; J = belladonna extract, mg; K = butabarbital sodium, mg; O = oxyphencyclimine hydrochloride, mg; P = hydroxyzine hydrochloride, mg; Q = clidinium bromide, mg; R = chlordiazepoxide hydrochloride, mg.

susceptible to these toxic effects than are young and middle-aged adults.

The belladonna alkaloids (belladonna, atropine, hyoscyamine hydrobromide, and hyoscyamine sulfate) are readily absorbed from the gastrointestinal tract and readily cross the blood–brain barrier. Large doses, by leaving the adrenergic system unopposed, stimulate the central nervous system; toxic doses depress the central nervous system.

The synthetic anticholinergics (all the medications in Table 52–5 except belladonna and hyoscyamine) are less readily absorbed and, in normal doses, do not readily cross the blood–brain barrier. Therefore, they exert relatively less effect on the central nervous system. Most of their pharmacologic actions can be attributed to their antimuscarinic effects (see Chapter 18).

HISTAMINE H$_2$ ANTAGONISTS

The histamine H$_2$ antagonists, including cimetidine (Tagamet), ranitidine (Zantac), famotidine (Pepcid), and nizatidine (Axid), are a relatively new group of medications that are competitive blockers of histamine at the H$_2$ receptors. Histamine stimulates contractions of the smooth muscles of the gastrointestinal tract and bronchi. This effect can be suppressed by antihistamines such as mepyrimine. These receptor sites have been named H$_1$ receptors to differentiate them from those in the parietal cell that cannot be blocked by mepyrimine and related compounds. These drugs are potent inhibitors of secretions caused by histamine, muscarinic agonists, and gastrin, inhibiting all phases of gastric acid secretion from the parietal and oxyntic cells, labeled H$_2$

receptors. Secretions are inhibited during fasting (day and night) as well as those normally produced by food, insulin, and caffeine.

Uses

The histamine H_2 antagonists are all effective in alleviating symptoms and preventing complication of peptic ulcer disease; also to prevent stress ulcers and recurrence of all ulcers; and to treat pathologic hypersecretory disorders such as Zollinger-Ellison syndrome.

Cimetidine

For many years, researchers have tried to develop a drug that would suppress gastric secretions. Finally in the mid-1970s, cimetidine (Tagamet), the first commercially available histamine H_2 receptor antagonist, was placed on the market in the United States. The exact mechanism of action is unknown; however, the potentiating interactions theory has been postulated. This theory states that isolated parietal cells have specific receptors for gastrin, acetylcholine, and histamine. A background concentration of histamine may be responsible for potentiating the action of gastrin and acetylcholine; therefore, H_2 antagonists inhibit acid secretion by blocking the effects of histamine on its receptors and thus eliminating the potentiating effect of histamine on gastrin and acetylcholine. Histamine is located in the lamina propria of the parietal cell. The mast cell (a connective tissue cell) contains granules filled with histamine, heparin, and lysosome. Cimetidine occupies the receptor site in the parietal cells and does not allow it to be stimulated by incoming histamine; thus it is called an H_2 receptor antagonist. Three hundred milligrams of cimetidine is capable of reducing hydrochloric acid production by 50% for the first two hours, by 75% for the next two hours, and by 90% for four hours. Cimetidine is effective in preventing acid release when the stomach is stimulated by food, histamine, insulin, caffeine, and pentagastrin. The mean gastric pH for the first hour after cimetidine is 3.1, the second hour, 3.5; the third hour 3.8; and the fourth hour, 6.1.

USES. Cimetidine is currently being used to treat all of the conditions previously reviewed. In addition, cimetidine has recently been demonstrated to be effective in reducing the pain and improving the clinical course of peptic ulcer, decreasing the incidence of new lesions, and accelerating healing. Recent research indicates that cimetidine is of limited value in treating or preventing NSAID-induced gastrointestinal distress or ulcers. Cimetidine has been used in both the United States and other countries in the treatment of upper gastrointestinal hemorrhage. However, conflicting research is available. Large numbers of publications compared antacids and cimetidine and concluded that patients receiving high doses of antacids bleed less than those who receive cimetidine. From this it seems fair to conclude that antacids appear to be more effective than cimetidine in preventing bleeding from stress ulcers in acutely ill patients. Therefore, the routine prescription of cimetidine

instead of antacids in all patients admitted to intensive care units does not seem to be justified.

PHARMACOKINETICS. *Absorption and Distribution.* Cimetidine is well absorbed by mouth even in the presence of antacids, although absorption may be slowed. Therapeutic levels can be achieved after both oral and intravenous bolus or drip infusion. It starts to work in ten minutes after intravenous administration and 30 minutes after oral administration. Its peak action occurs in 30 minutes after intravenous administration and 1 hour after an oral dose. Both modes of administration have a half-life of about two hours. It is distributed to all body tissues. Protein binding is 13%–25%.

Biotransformation and Excretion. Cimetidine is biotransformed in the liver (30%–40%). Most drugs are metabolized in two phases: phase 1 is mediated through the microsomal enzyme oxidase system of cytochrome P-450 and is accomplished by oxidation, reduction, and hydrolysis, and is where compounds are made more water soluble; and phase 2 is where drugs are eliminated by conjugation. Cimetidine reversibly inhibits microsomal metabolism in either a competitive or noncompetitive manner. This action of cimetidine accounts for numerous drug interactions that occur with cimetidine, to be discussed later. Cimetidine clearance will be decreased in liver disease. Approximately 48% of the oral drug is excreted unchanged in the urine, while 75% is found in the urine following intravenous or intramuscular injection. The half-life is two hours. Therefore, a patient with renal disease should have the dosage reduced.

CONTRAINDICATIONS AND PRECAUTIONS. There are no contraindications at this time, but cimetidine should be given cautiously in pregnant and nursing women, and in persons with impaired renal or hepatic function, as clearance may be reduced.

ADVERSE EFFECTS. Cimetidine has been one of the most thoroughly tested drugs in recent years. Many adverse effects occur including endocrine effects, renal and hepatic effects, central nervous system effects, effects on the immune and cardiovascular systems, and several miscellaneous effects.

Cimetidine displaces testosterone from its receptor site and causes gynecomastia in men. Cimetidine may also cause breast pain and breast enlargement in both men and women. These effects are generally dose- and duration-dependent and usually disappear when treatment is discontinued. Also, prolonged high-dose cimetidine may reduce libido and cause impotence.

Small increases in serum creatinine have been noted but are not usually associated with significant changes in renal function. Acute interstitial nephritis is a rare complication and is thought to be an idiosyncratic reaction to cimetidine.

Some patients receiving cimetidine experience a rise in their liver transaminase levels, which return to normal after discontinuation of cimetidine.

Elderly patients in particular with decreased renal or hepatic function may develop confusion, agitation, drowsiness, and even coma after receiving cimetidine.

Mental changes improve with discontinuation of cimetidine.

Histamine and H_2 receptors are found in leukocytes and in suppressor T-lymphocytes. Therefore, cimetidine may depress the immune system.

The cardiovascular system is also affected, particularly following rapid intravenous administration of cimetidine. Patients may develop bradycardia, sinus, and cardiac arrest.

Patients may also experience mild and transient gastrointestinal symptoms, including nausea, diarrhea, and abdominal pain. Central nervous system signs such as dizziness, somnolence, and headache have also been reported. Patients may also complain of rash, myalgia, and arthralgia.

INTERACTIONS. As previously discussed, cimetidine reversibly inhibits hepatic microsomal metabolism of the enzyme oxidase system of cytochrome P-450. Thus, because of these actions, cimetidine decreases the clearance of antipyrine, caffeine, meperidine, chlordiazepoxide, diazepam, ethanol, phenytoin, quinidine, theophylline, and warfarin. Cimetidine also decreases the formation of toxic metabolites from acetaminophen. The effect of cimetidine on drug metabolism can be detected 24–48 hours after initiation of its administration and usually disappears 48 hours after cimetidine is discontinued. The doses of the above listed drugs need to be adjusted in order to prevent toxic plasma levels of the associated drug.

If cimetidine is given concurrently by mouth with antacids in a fasting state, cimetidine absorption may be slowed. Therefore, oral cimetidine and antacids are always separated by one hour.

Serum digoxin levels may decrease during co-administration with cimetidine.

DOSAGE. Cimetidine is administered in 300-mg doses by mouth, slow intravenous bolus, or four times day with meals or at bedtime, or 400 mg bid, or 800 mg at bedtime. If the patient is receiving nothing by mouth, the medication is spaced at even intervals around the clock.

Cimetidine is compatible with all of the common IV solutions such as 5% and 10% dextrose, dextrose and sodium chloride, dextrose and Ringer's lactate, either plain sodium chloride, Ringer's lactate, or total parenteral nutrition (TPN). It can be run piggyback with most antibiotics, insulin, and potassium chloride. It should not be mixed with barbiturates and aminophylline. Once mixed, cimetidine is stable at room temperature for at least 24 hours. Following dilution with most IV infusion fluids, cimetidine solutions containing 1.2–5 mg/ml have been reported to be stable for at least three days at room temperature.

Ranitidine Hydrochloride

Ranitidine hydrochloride (Zantac) is a competitive, reversible inhibitor of histamine that works at the histamine receptors, including those of the gastric cells. Ranitidine is a second generation H_2 receptor antagonist with a slightly different structure than cimetidine. For this reason, ranitidine lacks some of the adverse effects and drug interactions that are common to cimetidine. Ranitidine in a molar basis is 13 times more potent in inhibiting pentagastrin-stimulated acid secretion and ten times more potent than cimetidine in inhibiting pepsin secretion. Ranitidine hydrochloride inhibits both daytime and nocturnal basal gastric acid secretion, as well as gastric acid secretions stimulated by food and histamine from 3–13 hours after a dose (the 13 hours is for nocturnal suppression).

USES. Ranitidine is indicated for short-term treatment of active duodenal and gastric ulcer, gastroesophageal reflux disease, and pathologic hypersecretion syndromes. Ranitidine has recently been shown to offer some protection against pulmonary aspiration of gastric secretions during anesthesia, particularly in ambulatory surgery patients.

Ranitidine is also currently being studied in patients being treated for theophylline toxicity. Ranitidine decreases the vomiting so that these patients can retain the antidote, charcoal, in their stomach. Ranitidine is thought to control the patient's vomiting by reducing the secretion of gastric acid—an effect of the theophylline.

PHARMACOKINETICS. *Absorption and Distribution.* Ranitidine hydrochloride is absorbed well after oral administration and reaches a peak in one to three hours. Its absorption is slightly impaired by concurrent administration of food or antacids. Serum concentrations remain elevated for up to 12 hours after a single 150-mg dose. Protein binding is about 15%.

Biotransformation and Excretion. Ranitidine is metabolized by the liver. The principal route of excretion is the urine, with approximately 30% of the dose being actively excreted unchanged by the tubules in 24 hours. The half-life is two to three hours. Ranitidine is removed through both hemodialysis and peritoneal dialysis.

CONTRAINDICATIONS AND PRECAUTIONS. Ranitidine hydrochloride has no known contraindications at this time. Precautions include administration to pregnant and lactating women. Ranitidine hydrochloride is secreted in human milk and therefore is not administered to lactating women. The safety and effectiveness in children have not yet been established. Caution is also advised in patients with kidney disease, since the drug is excreted through renal action.

ADVERSE EFFECTS. Ranitidine appears to be a safe drug, with less than 2% of patients complaining of general adverse effects. The most common adverse effect of ranitidine hydrochloride is headache. Additional symptoms have been reported but at a very low frequency, including malaise, dizziness, constipation, nausea, abdominal pain, and rash. There have been several instances of decreases of white blood cells and platelet count, although no cases of agranulocytosis and aplastic anemia have been reported. Ranitidine does not affect the immune system as does cimetidine. A few cases of bradycardia have been reported after both intravenous infusion and oral administration of ranitidine.

INTERACTIONS. Ranitidine does not avidly bind to the drug-metabolizing hepatic microsomal P-450 system and therefore does not appear to impair the hepatic metabolism of drugs such as diazepam or aminophylline, although it has been observed to decrease warfarin clearance. Several studies indicate that the hypoglycemic effect of glipizide may be increased by ranitidine.

DOSAGE. The recommended adult dosage of ranitidine hydrochloride for duodenal ulcer is 150 mg twice daily with an alternate dosage of 300 mg at bedtime. In patients with conditions of pathologic hypersecretion, dosage is again 150 mg twice a day, but doses of up to 6 g/day have been employed in these individuals. Antacids are given concurrently as needed for the relief of pain and do not interfere with the absorption of ranitidine hydrochloride. The intravenous dosage is 50 mg every six to eight hours. Dilute to a total volume of at least 20 ml and inject over five minutes. Ranitidine is stable in most intravenous solutions and is stable for at least 24 hours.

Famotidine

Famotidine (Pepcid) is another H_2 receptor antagonist. It is similar to cimetidine and ranitidine. A dosage of 5–10 mg of famotidine inhibits gastric acid secretion similarly to a dosage of 300 mg of cimetidine. Its inhibitory effect is also more prolonged than that of cimetidine and it does not seem to have antiandrogenic properties. The daytime pH range is about 5.0 and the nighttime pH range is 5.0–6.4.

PHARMACOKINETICS. *Absorption and Distribution.* Famotidine is incompletely absorbed and begins its effect in one hour, peaks in one to three hours, and persists for 10–12 hours. Plasma protein binding is 15%–20%.

Biotransformation and Excretion. Famotidine is eliminated by both metabolic (30%–35%) and renal routes (65%–70%), with a large percentage of drug being recovered in the urine unchanged. The half-life is two to three hours.

CONTRAINDICATIONS AND PRECAUTIONS. The only known contraindication is hypersensitivity to any component of the drug. Safety in pregnancy, lactating women, and children has not been established. It is given cautiously in renal disease, as this is the primary organ of metabolism and excretion.

INTERACTIONS. Famotidine does not affect the microsomal enzyme oxidase system of cytochrome P-450 in the liver. No drug interactions have yet been identified.

ADVERSE EFFECTS. Few adverse effects have been reported: headache (4.7%), diarrhea (1.7%), dizziness (1.3%), and constipation (1.2%). Other adverse effects have been reported, but as yet a causal relationship has not been established.

DOSAGE. Famotidine may be administered orally once daily 40 mg at bedtime or 20 mg every 12 hours. Dosage up to 160 mg/day can be administered for hypersecretion syndromes. For intravenous bolus administration, dilute 2 ml of famotidine in solution (compat-ible with most solutions) to a volume of at least 10 ml and inject over at least two minutes. As a drip, it is mixed with 100 ml and infused over 15–30 minutes.

Nizatidine

Nizatidine (Axid) is the newest H_2 receptor antagonist. Nizatidine appears to be as effective as the other H_2 inhibitors already discussed. Like famotidine, nizatidine does not appear to interfere with hepatic metabolism of other drugs. The long-term safety of nizatidine remains to be determined.

USES. Nizatidine is currently being used for active duodenal and gastric ulcer treatment for up to eight weeks. After ulcer healing, nizatidine can be used for maintenance therapy at reduced dosages at bedtime for up to one year. Consequences of therapy with nizatidine for longer than one year are not known.

PHARMACOKINETICS. Nizatidine is well absorbed after an oral dose. Absorption is enhanced by about 10% with food but may be decreased with aluminum or magnesium hydroxide antacids. Peak plasma levels occur in 0.5–3 hours. Approximately 35% of nizatidine is bound to plasma proteins. The elimination half-life is one to two hours. Nizatidine is metabolized by the liver and 65%–90% of each dose is excreted unchanged in the urine. Renal impairment will prolong the half-life.

CONTRAINDICATIONS AND PRECAUTIONS. Nizatidine is administered cautiously to persons hypersensitive to the other H_2 receptor antagonists. Also, administer cautiously to elderly persons, as they are likely to have reduced renal clearance. Administer cautiously to persons with hepatic dysfunction. Use during pregnancy and lactating women and children has not been established.

ADVERSE EFFECTS. The most common adverse effects include somnolence (2.4%), sweating (1%), and urticaria (0.5%). Blood dyscrasias have been reported, but rarely. Hepatocellular injury evidenced by elevated liver enzyme tests has also been reported. Like famotidine, there is no evidence of antiandrogenic activity, although gynecomastia has been reported rarely.

INTERACTIONS. Nizatidine does not inhibit the cytochrome P-450 system, so drug interactions mediated by inhibition of hepatic metabolism are not expected to occur. Nizatidine may increase serum salicylate concentrations when given concurrently with high doses of aspirin.

DOSAGE. Nizatidine is administered orally in 150-mg doses twice daily or 300 mg on retiring. Maintenance dosage for healed ulcers is 150 mg at bedtime. Therapy is generally continued for one year.

CHOICE OF DRUG

The decision to use one H_2 receptor antagonist rather than another is based on a multiplicity of factors: efficacy, cost, compliance, safety, interactions with other drugs, and physician's own experience. The efficacy of all H_2 receptor antagonists is similar for the treatment of duodenal ulcer and for maintenance. The cost of most products is similar, with cimetidine being the least expensive and famotidine being the most expensive.

OTHER ANTI-ULCER DRUGS

Sucralfate

Sucralfate (Carafate) (see Table 52–3) exerts its effect through a local, rather than a systemic, action to heal ulcers. Sucralfate forms an ulcer-adherent complex with protein exudates (albumin and fibrinogen) at the ulcer site. This complex covers the ulcer site and protects it against further attack by acid, pepsin, or bile salts. Sucralfate has a negligible acid-neutralizing capacity, but does inhibit pepsin activity in gastric juice by 32%. Sucralfate also blocks the diffusion of gastric acid across the protective barrier and limits proteolytic activity of pepsin. Sucralfate also appears to stimulate synthesis of prostaglandins by the mucosa of the stomach and duodenum. Healing of ulcers begins in two weeks and proceeds through eight weeks.

Several clinical trials have compared cimetidine and sucralfate as to healing rate after four to eight weeks. The healing rate after four weeks was 76% with cimetidine and 80% for sucralfate, and after eight weeks was 86% with cimetidine and 90% for sucralfate. The relapse rate after 6–12 months was significantly lower for patients treated with sucralfate.

USES. Sucralfate is indicated for short-term therapy of duodenal ulcers and prophylaxis of stress ulcers. Sucralfate appears effective on spontaneous and aspirin-induced gastric microbleeding. Sucralfate is also being used to provide relief for oral ulcers and mucosal pain associated with chemotherapy and radiation. Sucralfate may also have a beneficial effect in the treatment of reflux esophagitis and bile reflux gastritis, as well as recurrent ulcer post-gastric surgery. A sucralfate suspension is swished in the mouth for two minutes up to six times per day. Sucralfate deposits a pasty protective layer over the mucosa, reduces pain, and promotes healing.

CONTRAINDICATIONS AND PRECAUTIONS. There are no known contraindications to sucralfate at this time. Safety and effectiveness in pregnant and nursing women and children have not been established.

ADVERSE EFFECTS. Adverse effects of sucralfate are minor as it is not a systemic drug, with the most frequent being constipation (2.2%). Additional adverse effects include diarrhea, nausea, gastric discomfort, indigestion, dry mouth, rash, dizziness, and vertigo.

INTERACTIONS. Cimetidine, phenytoin, warfarin, and tetracycline may bind in the stomach and have decreased bioavailability. They are given two hours before or after sucralfate.

DOSAGE. Sucralfate is administered orally in 1-g doses four times a day (one hour before meals and at bedtime). If the drug is to be placed down a nasogastric tube, dissolve it, do not crush it. A liquid product should be on the market soon. Antacids may also be given to control pain, but are not administered within one half hour before or after sucralfate.

GASTROINTESTINAL STIMULANTS

Metoclopramide

Metoclopramide (Reglan) is structurally similar to procainamide but has a different spectrum of activity. Metoclopramide stimulates motility of the upper GI tract and increases the rate of gastric emptying, without stimulating gastric, biliary, or pancreatic secretions. Its exact mode of action is unknown, but it does appear to sensitize tissues to the action of acetylcholine.

USES. Metoclopramide is used to relieve the symptoms of acute and recurrent diabetic gastroparesis, gastroesophageal reflux, and to prevent nausea and vomiting associated with cancer chemotherapy. Metoclopramide is also being used to treat nausea and vomiting of pregnancy and labor, gastric ulcer disease, and anorexia nervosa. Metoclopramide is featured in Table 52–3.

PHARMACOKINETICS. Metoclopramide is well absorbed after oral administration, having an onset of action in 30–60 minutes. Effects persist for one to two hours. Metoclopramide has a high first pass effect. It is weakly bound to plasma proteins and rapidly distributed to most tissues. The half-life of metoclopramide is three to six hours. Metoclopramide is excreted in the bile (up to 25%) and urine (80%). With hepatic and renal dysfunction, the dose is reduced.

CONTRAINDICATIONS AND PRECAUTIONS. Metoclopramide is contraindicated in patients with known sensitivity, also in patients where stimulation of gastrointestinal motility may be dangerous, such as in mechanical obstruction or perforation or gastrointestinal hemorrhage. In patients with pheochromocytoma, metoclopramide may precipitate hypertensive crisis due to the release of catecholamines from the tumor. Extrapyramidal symptoms may occur in some patients. The incidence may be increased in persons taking drugs likely to cause extrapyramidal symptoms.

Metoclopramide may cause drowsiness, so caution is advised when driving. Safety during pregnancy and lactation has not been clearly documented, so it is used only when the potential benefits outweigh the risks.

ADVERSE EFFECTS. Approximately 20%–30% of all patients receiving metoclopramide experience side effects that are usually mild and transient. Since metoclopramide is widely distributed to all tissues, there is a high incidence of central nervous system effects (12%–24%). These effects include restlessness, drowsiness, fatigue, extrapyramidal reactions, parkinsonism-like reactions, dizziness, insomnia, and headache. Metoclopramide does increase the release of prolactin and may cause galactorrhea, reversible amenorrhea, nipple tenderness, and gynecomastia in males.

INTERACTIONS. Metoclopramide interacts with numerous drugs. Anticholinergics and narcotic analgesics antagonize metoclopramide. Alcohol, sedatives, hypnotics, narcotics, and tranquilizers have an additive effect. Drug absorption in the stomach may be diminished while drug absorption in the small bowel may be accelerated. Concurrent use of phenothiazines, butyrophenone, and thioxanthene drugs may potentiate extrapyramidal effects.

DOSAGE. Metoclopramide is available for oral, intramuscular, intravenous, or rectal administration. The oral dose ranges from 10–15 mg. Intravenous administration should be at 2 mg/kg over a one- to two-minute period. If the dose is to be over 10 mg, it is diluted in 50 ml of diluent and infused slowly over not less than 15 minutes.

Prostaglandins

Prostaglandins are potent inhibitors of gastric acid secretion and have a stabilizing effect on the gastric mucosa. (For more information see Chapter 47.) Prostaglandin E, PGA, and PGI inhibit basal acid secretion by food, histamine, pentagastrin, and cholinergic agents. Two synthetic analogs—PGE_2 and PGE_1—have been developed. Antisecretory effects of these agents last longer than the actual natural product and they can be given orally. Prostaglandins being studied investigationally today may be more effective than H_2 antagonists or sucralfate in treating peptic ulcers in refractory patients, especially in smokers and patients on chronic NSAIDS. The first prostaglandin drug, misoprostol (Cytotec) that is used to prevent ulcer formation in patients taking NSAIDs is discussed in Chapter 47. The major adverse effects of the prostaglandins in treating peptic ulcers is diarrhea.

USING THE NURSING PROCESS

ASSESSMENT

Assessment of the patient requiring medications to reduce gastric hyperacidity always begins with a thorough nursing history to develop the data base. Information to be obtained from the patient is included in Table 52–7. The nurse will use all this information when preparing the nursing care plan.

The patient requiring medications to reduce gastric hyperacidity may be acutely ill in a hospital or relatively healthy, with this condition diagnosed or treated as an outpatient. Therefore, the locus of control may be with the nurse, the patient, or both. Any patient who continually self-medicates with antacids is encouraged to seek medical attention as he or she may be treating the symptoms, and not the problem.

A complete medication history is most important in these patients. Determine what medications are taken, including prescription and over-the-counter, to determine if any of these will cause or aggravate current symptoms. There is evidence that nonsteroidal anti-inflammatory drugs aggravate mucosal damage, delay healing, and/or predispose to bleeding. Therefore, they are avoided in patients with peptic ulcer. Determine when and how they take their medication—with food or in between meals on an empty stomach. Determine

how long it takes them to use a bottle of antacid. As an example, if the patient says he or she uses a bottle (12 oz.) a week, then he or she takes less than 2 oz./day, which is less than a 15-ml dose four times daily. This dose is probably less than effective. Also determine if patients substitute tablets for liquid. Since tablets are less effective than liquids, their dosing, again, may not be adequate.

It is important to assess eating habits, including the types, quantities, and time food is consumed. There is little evidence that any single dietary factor influences the healing of peptic ulcers, and the so-called "ulcer diet" consisting of bland soft foods with milk or cream does not affect the rate of healing or recurrence. However, foods, spices, and liquids that provoke or worsen symptoms should be avoided, and patients should eat three meals a day that constitute a balanced diet of their choosing. Eating small meals every two or three hours may minimize variations in intragastric pH, but may not be necessary in patients receiving anti-ulcer medications. Alteration of dietary pattern may be part of the nursing intervention phase.

It is important to assess any emotional factors that may contribute to the development of peptic ulcers. The resolution of problems that contribute to emotional distress may reduce the extent and frequency of pain. Reassurance by the nurse can often reduce anxiety and promote compliance with the medical regimen. It is also important to assess for smoking, since cigarette smoking delays healing and may increase recurrence as it increases gastric secretions. In addition, smoking may decrease the effectiveness of cimetidine and other anti-ulcer medications.

The nurse also obtains laboratory data such as complete blood count (CBC), electrocardiogram (ECG), fluid and electrolyte levels, and stool specimens to assess for the presence of melena. Melena is caused by bleeding from a level above the ileocecal valve. A blood urea nitrogen (BUN) is also obtained. Transient elevation of BUN without corresponding increases in serum creatinine concentration occurs regularly in patients with upper gastrointestinal bleeding and restricted renal perfusion. Lower gastrointestinal bleeding is usually typified by a normal BUN. Patients may also be prepared for x-rays or endoscopic exam.

NURSING DIAGNOSIS

The nurse begins the nursing intervention by developing the nursing diagnoses, which become the goals of intervention and later the evaluation process. Typical nursing diagnoses for a patient requiring medications to reduce gastric acidity are included in Table 52–7.

PLANNING AND INTERVENTION

From the nursing diagnoses, the nurse establishes the goals of nursing intervention. When caring for the patient requiring medications to reduce gastric acidity, typical goals of nursing intervention are included in Table

Table 52–7. NURSING PROCESS FOR PATIENT REQUIRING DRUGS TO REDUCE GASTRIC ACIDITY

Assessment

Note history of current illness, including pain and dietary patterns (types, quantities, and time food is consumed); alcohol, caffeine use; and smoking habits.
Determine medication use (prescription and OTC), including when, how, and amount of antacids taken.
Assess emotional/stress factors (financial, relationship, job-related).
Review laboratory studies, e.g., CBC, electrolytes, BUN, stool specimens, and ECG.
Review bowel habits (diarrhea/constipation) and relationship to current problems.

Nursing Diagnosis	Nursing Actions	Rationale	Desired Outcomes/ Evaluation Criteria
Pain (acute)/ chronic, related to physical response, e.g., reflex muscle spasm in the stomach wall, chemical burn of gastric mucosa as evidenced by complaints, abdominal guarding, rigid body posture, facial grimacing, autonomic reponses.	Note complaints of pain, including location, duration, intensity (1–10 scale).	Pain is not always present, but if present, should be compared with previous pain symptoms, to assist in diagnosis of etiology/ development of complications.	Verbalizes relief of pain. Demonstrates relaxed body posture and is able to sleep/rest appropriately.
	Review factors that aggravate or alleviate pain.	Helpful in establishing diagnosis and treatment needs.	
	Provide small frequent meals as indicated for individual patient. Identify and limit foods that create discomfort.	Has an acid neutralizing effect, as well as diluting the gastric contents. Small meals prevent distention and the release of gastrin.	
	Administer antacids.	Decreases gastric acidity by absorption or by chemical neutralization. Evaluate type of antacid in regard to total health picture, e.g., sodium restriction.	
	Administer anticholinergics.	May be given at bedtime to decrease gastric motility, suppress acid production, delay gastric emptying, and alleviate nocturnal pain associated with gastric ulcer.	
Knowledge deficit related to lack of information, unfamiliarity with information resources as evidenced by questions, statement of concern, inaccurate followthrough of instructions/development of preventable complications.	Provide/review information regarding etiology/pathophysiology of illness, cause/effect relationship of lifestyle behaviors and ways to reduce risk/contributing factors.	Provides knowledge base on which patient can make information choices/decisions about future and control of health problems.	Verbalizes understanding of illness, cause, treatment, and prognosis. Begins to discuss own role in preventing recurrence. Indentifies necessary lifestyle changes and participates in treatment regimen
	Review drug regimen and possible side effects. Problem-solve solutions to side-effects as appropriate.	Helpful to patient's understanding of reason for taking drugs, and what symptoms are important to report to health care giver. Although dry mouth or photophobia may be annoying, drowsiness/dizziness encountered with initial anticholinergic therapy may increase risk of injury if not anticipated/planned for.	

Table 52–7. NURSING PROCESS FOR PATIENT REQUIRING DRUGS TO REDUCE GASTRIC ACIDITY–*CONTINUED*

Nursing Diagnosis	Nursing Actions	Rationale	Desired Outcomes/ Evaluation Criteria
	Discuss common side-effects, e.g., constipation/diarrhea.	Anticipation of problems and taking appropriate action can prevent untoward complications.	
	Caution against use of other OTC products/ antacids.	Combinations of antacids may potentiate development of milk-alkali syndrome, rebound acidity, sodium retention.	
	Review signs of electrolyte disturbance for particular drug patient is taking.	Electrolyte imbalance can be a serious side-effect of antacid use and prompt identification can prevent complications.	
	Encourage patient to follow diet as prescribed.	Modifications are based on individual needs. Avoiding late-night snacks, eating smaller, more frequent meals each day, eliminating caffeine, limiting milk and dairy products and eliminating foods that cause problems for the patient have been found to be helpful.	
	Encourage cessation of smoking. Discuss use of alcohol.	Nicotine increases gastric secretions. Consumption of alcohol on an empty stomach may delay healing but moderate use with food intake does not seem to aggravate symptoms.	
	Stress importance of returning for regular medical checkup.	Monitoring for/early identification of developing complications can prevent untoward results, (e.g., hypercalcemia).	

52–7. The overall goals of peptic ulcer therapy are to decrease or abolish symptoms, to hasten healing, to prevent serious complications such as hemorrhage, perforation, or obstruction, and to prevent recurrences. These goals can usually be achieved by eliminating precipitating or aggravating factors and with drug therapy.

NURSING RESPONSIBILITIES

Patients that are acutely ill with nasogastric tubes may require antacids. The nurse often administers aluminum products through a nasogastric tube; they are diluted either 1:2 or 1:4 with water. Aluminum hydroxide interferes with the absorption of phosphates from the intestine, and in the presence of a low-phosphate diet may cause deficiencies.

When administering anticholinergic medication, the nurse must know that the optimum time for administration is 30 minutes before meals and at bedtime. This allows the peak action of the anticholinergic to occur at the time of peak acid secretion from eating. All anticholinergics are preserved in tight, light-resistant containers away from excessive heat. The nurse prepares parenteral medications immediately before administering, and the patient's urinary output is observed for symptoms of urinary retention, as sphincter control is increased. Patients are encouraged to avoid excessive heat because anticholinergics suppress perspiration and therefore may precipitate heat stroke. Patients are encouraged to stay indoors during times of high temperatures and high humidity.

When administering H_2 receptor antagonists, the nurse administers antacids concurrently but not at the same time. These products are available in various forms; the best form is chosen for each patient.

PATIENT TEACHING

The patient requires medications to reduce gastric acidity while in the hospital, as well as administration at home. He or she may need them only for a few weeks or months, or for a lifetime. The patient is made aware of the general information relevant to safe antacid administration included in Table 52–8, and in Table 52–3 included in the column marked Nursing Implications.

When the patient is ready to be discharged, the nurse must ensure that the patient has an adequate level of knowledge about the medication and disease. The pain pattern that the patient exhibits and strategies for alleviating some of the discomfort with diet or behavior modification are reviewed with the patient.

Patients are also encouraged to follow the diet prescribed for them. Much research has been done recently on diet therapy for patients with ulcers. Today they are cautioned to avoid late-night snacks, as this increases nocturnal gastric secretions; eat smaller, more frequent meals each day, because this has been shown to decrease gastrin production; although this may not be necessary if the patient is receiving anti-ulcer medications; eliminate caffeine, not only in coffee, but also in tea and cola beverages; limit milk and dairy products because recent evidence has shown that the calcium and protein in milk may even increase gastric secretion (this information may contradict the information the patient believed or was given several years ago); and eliminate any foods that cause problems for the patient such as spicy foods, gas-producing vegetables or legumes, onions, and others. In addition, the patient is encouraged to decrease or, if possible, stop smoking. The nicotine in cigarette and tobacco smoke increases gastric secretions. However, cessation of smoking may cause increased anxiety and tension for the patient, which can also increase gastric secretions. Consumption of alcohol on an empty stomach may delay healing and is not recommended, but moderate alcohol intake with meals does not aggravate symptoms or delay healing.

When administering calcium preparations, the patient must know that serum calcium levels will be measured frequently to assess for hypercalcemia. The nurse and patient should be aware of the symptoms of hypercalcemia, including nausea, vomiting, abdominal pain, polyuria, cloudy memory, loss of muscle tone, and muscle and joint pain. In addition, the patient with renal impairment should take calcium carbonate cautiously because of the possible development of renal calculi. All patients should be aware of the symptoms of milk-alkali

---

Table 52–8. PATIENT TEACHING INFORMATION—ANTACIDS

Dear Patient:
 This drug has been prescribed for you. This is what you should know about your drug to get the most from your therapy.

1. Antacids make your stomach less acidic.
2. You will take antacids until your current medical problem is resolved, that is, pain is relieved and/or ulcer is healed (4–6 weeks).
3. Shake all liquids well before taking them, so they are well mixed. Refrigerating them may make them taste better. Chew tablets well (the smaller the particles, the faster it works) and take with a full glass of water.
4. Antacid tablets are not equal to liquid. Do not substitute without your doctor's OK.
5. Carry a small bottle of liquid in order to have doses available away from home.
6. Always measure your antacid dose; do not drink from the bottle.
7. Make sure you take your antacid on time. Antacids are taken either 1 or 3 hours after eating and at bedtime.
8. In general, the following drugs interact with antacids and are given 1 hour before or 1–2 hours after the antacids. These include tetracycline antibiotics, phenothiazine tranquilizers, cardiac glycosides (lanoxin, digoxin), iron salts, isoniazid (INH), propranolol (Inderal), diazepam (Valium), amphetamines, all enteric-coated tablets (Ecotrin), and salicylates. In addition, antacids help your body rid itself of aspirin products. You may have to increase the amount of aspirin product you take to keep pain and inflammation under control. Talk to your doctor about adjusting your aspirin dose.
9. Observe the number of bowel movements and what they look like daily; if diarrhea or constipation develops, the antacid preparation may be changed. If stools get loose, substitute aluminum hydroxide products every other dose or so; and if constipation occurs, substitute milk of magnesia.
10. The age of the antacid is important. Aluminum hydroxide gel does not work as well when it is old.
11. It is best not to take other medications within 1–2 hours of your antacid. A general rule is to take all drugs before meals.
12. Antacids are stored in tight, light-resistant bottles.

---

syndrome if calcium products and sodium bicarbonate are being used chronically (Table 52–9).

Patients are cautioned against using sodium bicarbonate and "fizzy-type" antacids not prescribed by the physician as an antacid because of the rebound acidity, systemic absorption, and high sodium content.

When the nurse cares for the patient with a peptic ulcer, teaching always includes the signs and symptoms of occult bleeding, which are increasing fatigue, light-headedness, dizziness, and a change in the color of the stool.

It is always important to discuss the interactions that occur with other medications. The patient should always carry the medication profile card to the physician's office or to the pharmacy when filling a prescription or buying an over-the-counter preparation.

Stress, anxiety, and tension may be predisposing fac-

Table 52–9. ACUTE SYMPTOMS OF THE MILK-ALKALI SYNDROME, A POSSIBLE COMPLICATION OF ANTACID THERAPY

Central	GI
Headache	Nausea
Confusion	Vomiting
Hypercalcemia	Distate for food
Hyperphosphatemia	Abdominal pain
Renal insufficiency	
Metabolic alkalosis	
Irritability	

Note: The acute form develops within 2–30 days after calcium alkali ingestion.

tors to ulcer formation. The nurse shares with the patient methods of stress reduction or behavior modification methods that may be beneficial. As additional problems are identified by the nurse during the intervention, the nurse may need to develop new nursing diagnoses and then plan and implement additional nursing care.

Peptic ulcers may be a chronic, recurring problem for the patient and family. By increasing the knowledge level about the cause of peptic ulcers, the patient can evaluate his or her behavior and lifestyle and modify them as necessary if he or she wishes. This change ultimately rests within the patient's locus of control. The nurse and medical staff can encourage and support the patient toward these changes. Because antacids are available OTC, nurses may have a tendency to disregard the importance of these medications in the treatment of peptic ulcer. Antacids are a major modality in controlling gastric ulcer disease.

EVALUATION

The nurse evaluates the effectiveness of medications to reduce gastric acidity based on a list of evaluation criteria that have been developed in relation to the goals determined by the nurse, patient, and family. The data base that was obtained in the original assessment and used to formulate the nursing diagnoses provides helpful criteria for measuring the treatment's effectiveness. Typical outcome evaluation criteria are included in Table 52–7.

It is extremely important to work with the patient and family to ensure their complete assistance and support. The majority of patients, once they understand and believe in the importance of their continued medical treatment, usually are compliant. The primary reason for noncompliance is forgetting the medication or experiencing an unpleasant adverse effect that causes the patient to discontinue medication.

The nurse teaches the patient about potential adverse effects so that a patient taking this medication at home is more likely to report any unusual symptom to the physician or nurse. The most common complaint from patients taking antacids is a change in bowel habits,

which can usually be corrected by altering the dose or type of antacid used.

If the patient experiences adverse effects from anticholinergics, such as dry mouth and photophobia due to mydriasis, the nurse can suggest frequent ingestion of ice chips or sucking on hard candy (sugarless candy works best because it causes fewer dental problems) for dry mouth; and for the photophobia, shading the eyes or wearing sunglasses or photosensitive lenses in the bright light. Accommodation to light generally becomes better as therapy is continued. Postural hypotension and tachycardia may develop during early therapy, so patients are instructed to change body positions slowly to avoid fainting. Drowsiness and dizziness may also be experienced, so care must be taken in operating heavy equipment or driving an automobile.

The physician may wish to evaluate the patient for ulcer healing through endoscopic examinations. The patient and family need to know the importance of this procedure. Also, the patient is encouraged to keep the scheduled clinic or physician visits, even though he or she is feeling better.

The more the nurse involves the patient and family with the planning and care, the more likely they are to comply. The nurse must stress the importance of continued medical care. All previously taught material is reviewed and updated with patient and family, if necessary, to ensure that their knowledge base remains accurate.

SUMMARY

Considerable progress has been made in the treatment of peptic ulcer disease during the last decade with the introduction of numerous new drugs. The histamine H_2 receptor antagonists are very effective drugs in treating diseases related to gastric acid secretion. Additional anti-ulcer drugs such as sucralfate and metoclopramide enhance the protective mechanisms of the gastroduodenal mucosa. These drugs provide a new therapeutic modality for those patients who do not respond to the acid suppression drugs. In addition, there are alternative choices for treating patients, considering their pathology, incidence of side effects, cost of the drug, and patient compliance.

As the nurse begins to administer drugs to treat peptic ulcer disease, a thorough history is obtained that includes drug and dietary history. Patient teaching is a priority. The nurse must ensure that the patient has an adequate level of knowledge about the medication and the disease. The patient's pain pattern and strategies for alleviating some of the discomfort with food, antacids, other drugs, or behavior modification are reviewed with the patient.

Peptic ulcers may be a chronic, recurring problem for both the patient and family. By increasing the knowledge level about the cause of peptic ulcers, the patient can evaluate his or her behavior and lifestyle and modify them as necessary.

SITUATION 52–1

Artie Simon is a 24-year-old who is on the telemetry unit following a motor vehicle accident during which he suffered a head injury. He has a tracheostomy, nasogastric tube, and a central line.

1. Mr. Simon is receiving cimetidine (Tagamet) 300 mg IVPB every 6 hours to reduce the risk of gastric ulcer formation. The nurse will avoid rapid intravenous infusion due to the potential for:
   a. hyperthermia
   b. hypertension
   c. bradycardia
   d. seizures

2. The nurse will monitor Mr. Simon for which of the following side effects related to cimetidine therapy?
   a. tetany
   b. abdominal pain
   c. visual disturbances
   d. cough

3. Mr. Simon also receives aluminum hydroxide (Amphojel) 30 cc via nasogastric tube every 4 hours. The nurse will plan to check him for:
   a. hypersensitivity reaction
   b. oral thrush
   c. milk-alkali syndrome
   d. constipation

4. Mr. Simon is receiving continuous tube feeding. Assessment reveals abdominal distention. He is to begin metoclopramide (Reglan). The nurse is aware of the following contraindication to its use:
   a. bowel obstruction
   b. glaucoma
   c. cardiovascular disease
   d. pulmonary fibrosis

5. When administering metoclopramide, the nurse will monitor Mr. Simon for the following adverse effects:
   a. nausea and vomiting
   b. photosensitivity reactions
   c. restlessness
   d. tachycardia

6. An appropriate outcome for Mr. Simon would be:
   a. gastric residual >150 cc
   b. stools negative for occult blood
   c. at least 3 formed stools per day
   d. evidence of tube feeding around trach site

BIBLIOGRAPHY

AMA Department of Drugs: AMA Drug Evaluations, ed 5. PSG Publishing, Littleton, MA, 1986.

Amitai, Y, et al: Repetitive oral activated charcoal and control of emesis in severe theophylline toxicity. Letter to the Editor. Ann Intern Med 105(3):386, 1986.

Are aluminum-containing antacids safe in pregnancy? Nurses Drug Alert 11(5):33, 1987.

Aronoff, GR, et al: Nizatidine. Clin Pharmacol Ther 43:688, 1988.

Cimetidine plus warfarin = ?. Emerg Med 19(6):109, 1987.

Connell, SI: Metabolites of the arachidonic acid cascace. Facts and Comparisons Newsletter 6(12):89, 1987.

D'Arcy, PF, et al: Drug-antacid interactions: Assessment of clinical importance. Drug Intell Clin Pharm 21(7/8):607, 1987.

DiPalma, J: Drill's Pharmacology in Medicine. McGraw-Hill, New York, 1985.

Gilman, AG, Goodman, LS, and Gilman, A: Goodman and Gilman's The Pharmacological Basis of Therapeutics, ed 7. Macmillan, New York, 1985.

Gonzalez, ER, et al: Cimetidine versus ranitidine: Single-dose, oral regimen for reducing gastric acidity and volume in ambulatory surgery patients. Drug Intell Clin Pharm 21:192, 1987.

Konturek, SJ, et al: Double blind controlled study on the effect of sucralfate on gastric prostaglandin formation and microbleeding in normal and aspirin treated man. Gut 27:1450, 1986.

Levant, JA, Walsh, JH, and Isenberg, JI: Stimulation of gastric secretion and gastrin release by single oral dose of calcium carbonate in man. N Engl J Med 289:555, 1973.

Maronde, R: Topics in Clinical Pharmacology and Therapeutics. Springer-Verlag, New York, 1985.

Marshall, BJ, and Warren, JB: Unidentified curved bacilli in the stomach of patients with gastritis and peptic ulceration. Lancet 1:1311, 1984.

Medical Letter. Famotidine. 29(733):17, Feb. 13, 1987.

Nizatidine (Axid). The Medical Letter 30(772):77, 1988.

Rand, KH, et al: Antibodies to herpes simplex type I in patients with active duodenal ulcer. Arch Intern Med 143:1917, 1983.

Roth, SH, et al: Cimetidine therapy in nonsteroidal anti-inflammatory drug gastropathy. Double-blind long-term evaluation. Arch Intern Med 147:1798, 1987.

Solomon, MA: Oral sucralfate suspension for mucositis. Letter to the Editor. N Engl J Med 315:459, 1986.

Sloan, RW: Antiulcer treatment in the elderly: Update on drug therapy for maximum benefits. Consultant 27(8):59, 1987.

GLOSSARY TERMS IN THIS CHAPTER
Akathisia
Antiemetic
Antiserotonergic
Chemoreceptor trigger zone
Dystonia
Extrapyramidal symptoms
Gynecomastia

53
CHAPTER

ANTIEMETIC AND EMETIC MEDICATIONS AND ANTIHISTAMINES

MERRILY MATHEWSON KUHN, R.N.C., Ph.D., CCRN

LEARNING OBJECTIVES

After reading this chapter, the student will be able to:

1. Identify those medications commonly used as antiemetic and emetic medications.

2. Differentiate among the antiemetic and emetic medications as to mechansim of action, route of administration, pharmacokinetics, adverse effects, contraindications, and interactions.

3. Identify specific areas to assess in the patient requiring antiemetic and emetic medications in order to formulate appropriate nursing diagnoses.

4. Plan the nursing interventions necessary to administer antiemetic and emetic medications and choose appropriate teaching strategies to gain patient compliance.

5. Evaluate the patient at various stages of treatment to gauge the success of nursing interventions.

NAUSEA AND VOMITING

Nausea, vomiting, and vertigo are not diseases in themselves but are symptoms of some underlying problem. Nausea and vomiting may occur secondary to drugs, radiation, metabolic disorders, surgery, motion, pregnancy, gastrointestinal disorders, food intolerances, and the list could go on forever (Table 53–1).

In general, nausea and vomiting occur after the *chemoreceptor trigger zone* (CTZ) (in the medulla of the brain) is stimulated by ascending efferent messages (Fig. 53–1) and in turn stimulates the vomiting center (VC), also located in the medulla. Consequently to this stimulation, there is increased activity of central neurotransmitters—dopamine in the CTZ and acetylcholine in the VC—which are the major mediators for the induction of vomiting. Excitatory messages are then transmitted through efferent fibers to the salivary glands and the muscles of the diaphragm, anterior abdominal wall, gastric antrum, and duodenum, and vomiting ensues (Fig. 53–2).

Since nausea and vomiting are symptoms of disease, it is always a priority to determine the underlying cause so it can be corrected. If vomiting is occurring, medications are best administered parenterally or by suppository. Generally, drug therapy is more effective for prophylaxis than for actual treatment of vomiting. Oral forms of medications are used for prophylaxis. Patients undergoing cancer chemotherapy often experience nausea and vomiting and are treated with antiemetics before chemotherapy is received.

Postoperative vomiting is due to many causes and is often difficult to predict and prevent. Numerous medi-

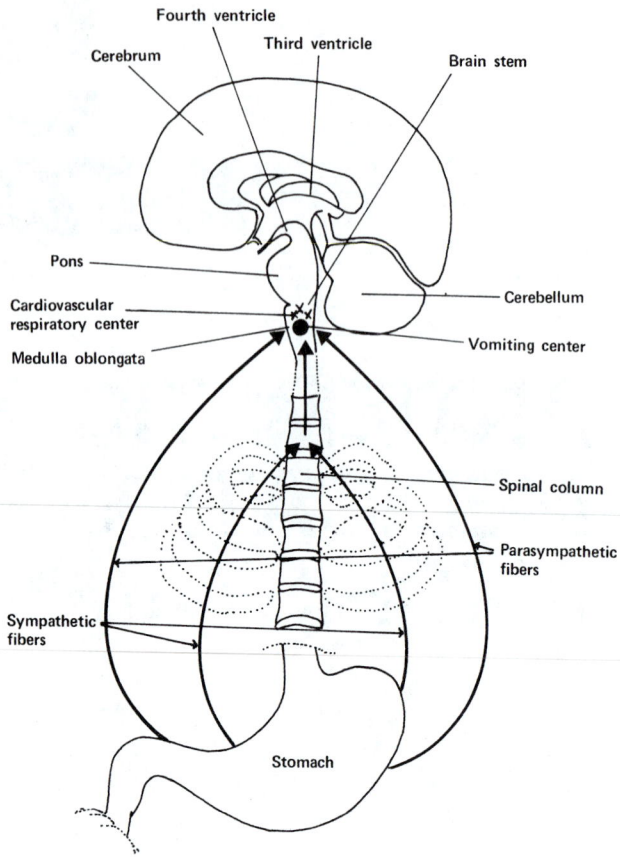

Figure 53–1. Efferent impulses travel to the diaphragm, glottis, stomach, and anterior abdominal muscle, and vomiting occurs.

cations are used to manage nausea and vomiting once it has occurred.

Nausea and vomiting associated with motion sickness, such as air, car, boat, amusement rides, etc., is a common complaint. The prophylactic use of drugs, one to two hours prior to the event, is an effective treatment.

Nausea and vomiting are also common complaints (50%–80%) during pregnancy from the 6th through the 14th week of gestation. In general, drugs are not recommended to treat vomiting of pregnancy unless absolutely necessary. All drugs cross the placenta and many affect the fetus adversely. Non–drug therapy is tried before antiemetics are prescribed.

Table 53–1. NAUSEA AND VOMITING

Causes and Mechanism
CAUSES:
Excess food and drink
Medication side effects (antineoplastic medication)
Medication toxic effects (digoxin, theophylline)
Radiation
Metabolic disturbances
Food intolerances (fatty foods in gall bladder diseases)
Infection
Pregnancy
Trauma
Anxiety, tension, fear
Motion sickness
Vertigo (due to middle ear disease)
Electrolyte imbalance
Disease states (stomach and intestinal condition, increasing intracranial pressure, etc.)
MECHANISM:
Psychologic
Abdominal organ abnormalities
Stimulation of vestibular organs
Chemical

THERAPEUTIC AGENTS

ANTIEMETICS

Antiemetics prevent or relieve the symptoms of nausea and vomiting by action on one or several of the following areas: the chemoreceptor trigger zone within the vomiting center of the medulla, the cerebral cortex, or the aural vestibular apparatus in the ear. It is important

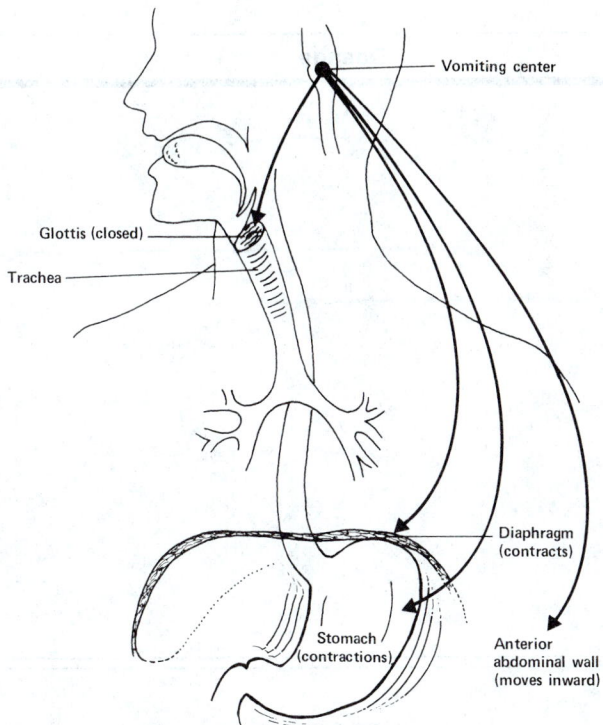

Figure 53–2. Stimuli leave the stomach or other sensory centers and follow the afferent parasympathetic fibers or the sympathetic fibers, and travel via the spinal column to the vomiting center in the medulla oblongata.

to understand the cause of the nausea and vomiting and to administer a medication with the correct site of action to rectify the condition. In general, antiemetics are more successful in preventing vomiting than in treating it. They are best administered as prophylaxis before actual vomiting has occurred.

Antiemetics may be either locally-acting or centrally-acting. The locally-acting antiemetics include topical mucosal anesthetics, adsorbents and demulcents, antacids, protective agents, and medications that reduce distention by eliminating retained gases. The drugs effective as antiemetics include the antidopaminergic agents such as the phenothiazines, chlorpromazine (Thorazine) and promethazine (Phenergan), and metoclopramide; the anticholinergic antihistamines like diphenhydramine (Benadryl), dimenhydrinate (Dramamine), and others, discussed in more detail later in this chapter; and the miscellaneous agents such as benzquinamide (Emete-Con) and trimethobenzamide (Tigan).

Locally-Acting Antiemetics

Vomiting caused by local irritation of the gastric mucosa can be treated with locally acting agents. In general, vomiting caused by local irritation is self-limiting: when the stomach rids itself of the irritant, the sensations are relieved. However, an individual with acute or chronic inflammations of the gastrointestinal tract, such as gastritis or gastroenteritis, may have prolonged symptoms.

Locally acting medications soothe the receptors or reduce the reactivity of the irritants. These are temporary measures that can be used while the patient's gastrointestinal tract heals.

Topical anesthetics, such as viscous lidocaine, can be taken orally. These agents raise the threshold of the receptor reactivity to irritants; consequently, nausea and vomiting are relieved.

Antacids (Chapter 52), adsorbents and demulcents (Chapter 54), and medications that reduce distention (Chapter 54) all act on the stomach mucosa or the receptor centers, or both, to make them less sensitive. These preparations are given between meals. Other protective agents are phosphorylated carbohydrate solution (Emetrol) and cola syrup, which are both taken as undiluted liquid. These substances are believed to relax gastrointestinal muscle spasms and thereby permit fewer afferent impulses to reach the vomiting center.

Centrally-Acting Antiemetics

The centrally acting antiemetics inhibit or depress the afferent nerve impulses in the brain pathways, consequently preventing nausea and vomiting. Each of the various groups of medications used as centrally-acting antiemetics affects different sites; some act on the chemoreceptor trigger zone in the vomiting center, others on the cerebral cortex or the aural vestibular apparatus. Table 53–2 features the various groups of medications used as centrally-acting antiemetics, their specific site of action, their common antiemetic dose, their common indications, and adverse reactions. The majority of these medications, excluding the miscellaneous group, are used for other purposes but possess antiemetic qualities. Only their antiemetic use is reviewed here, as they are discussed fully in other chapters.

Contraindications and Precautions. Antiemetics, in general, are contraindicated in pregnancy because of possible teratogenic effects. Caution is always required with all antiemetics, as they mask the symptoms of organic disease or the toxic effects of other drugs. Antiemetics are not recommended for uncomplicated vomiting in children. Although there is no confirmatory evidence, antiemetics may contribute, in combination with viral illness, to the development of Reye's syndrome.

Adverse Reactions. Antiemetics are not without adverse effects. Most commonly, drowsiness occurs so patients need to be cautioned about performing activities that require alertness. Patients also need to avoid alcohol and other CNS depressants that could further depress their CNS.

ANTIDOPAMINERGICS. ***Phenothiazines.*** The phenothiazines, major tranquilizers or antipsychotic agents, are currently the most effective antiemetics. Their antiemetic effect occurs with very low doses. However, because of their relative toxicity, they are administered only when vomiting cannot be controlled by other means or when no more than a few doses will be needed. This approach is important when medicating

TEXT RESUMES ON PAGE 1464

Table 53–2. CENTRALLY ACTING ANTIEMETICS

Name	Site of Action	Dosage
ALL ANTIEMETICS:		
ANTIDOPAMINERGICS		
Phenothiazines (Aliphatic Compounds):		
Chlorpromazine (Thorazine)	Chemoreceptor trigger zone, vomiting center.	Adult: PO: 10–25 mg q 4–6 hr prn. R: 50–100 mg q 6–8 hr prn. IM: 25–50 mg q 3–4 hr prn. Pediatric: do not use less than 6 months old. O: 0.55 mg/kg q 4–6 hr. R: 1.1 mg/kg q 6–8 hr. IM: 0.55 mg/kg q 6–8 hr.
Triflupromazine (Vesprin)	Same as above.	Adult: IM: 5–15 mg q 4 hr. IV: 1 mg. Pediatric over 2½ years: IM: 0.2–0.25 mg/kg, may last 12 hrs.
Promethazine (Phenergan)	Chemoreceptor trigger zone (?), labyrinth.	IM: 12.5–25 mg q 4–6 hr. Supp: 12.5–50 mg. Tab: 25–50 mg

*Within the column listing adverse effects, underlines indicate the most common effects.

General Uses	Adverse Effects*	Nursing Implications
		ASSESSMENT: Assess cause of nausea and vomiting.
		INTERVENTION: Intramuscular injection sites should be rotated, and medication given deep IM. Drowsiness may occur, so the individual needs to be encouraged not to operate heavy equipment or drive a car. Hard candy, gum, or sips of water may be taken to moisten the mouth. Will have an additive effect if taken with alcohol and many other drugs. When these medications are taken to prevent motion sickness, they are administered 30 minutes to 1 hour before beginning to travel. If meal time nausea is a problem give before meals.
		EVALUATION: Evaluate for drowsiness.
Chemotherapy, radiation, other.	All phenothiazine compounds: Neuro: sedation, drowsiness, moderate extrapyramidal effects, ocular changes (only with prolonged treatment). CV: orthostatic hypotension Resp: nasal congestion Misc: strong anticholinergic effects.	All phenothiazines: ASSESSMENT: Assess blood pressure before and during therapy to assess for orthostatic hypotension. INTERVENTION: Caution patient to slowly change body position. Also, wearing elastic stockings and/or elevating feet may help in preventing hypotension. Do not mix these medications with other medications in the same syringe. Monitor urinary output carefully for urinary retention. Phenothiazines may have an additive or cumulative effect either alone or when given with alcohol, tranquilizers, and other medications that depress the central nervous system. The patient should be cautioned about drinking alcohol. Impaired mental or physical abilities may occur after administration. The patient must be cautioned about driving a car or working with heavy equipment. EVALUATION: Carefully evaluate the patient for occurrence of any extrapyramidal adverse effects.
Postoperative, chemotherapy, radiation.	Same as above.	Same as above.
Motion sickness, postoperative, chemotherapy, radiation.	Same as above.	Same as above.

CONTINUED ON THE FOLLOWING PAGE

Centrally Acting Antiemetics

Table 53–2. CENTRALLY ACTING ANTIEMETICS–*CONTINUED*

Name	Site of Action	Dosage
Promazine (Sparine)	Same as chlorpromazine.	PO: 25–50 mg q 4–6 hr IM: 50 mg q 4–6 hr.
Phenothiazines (Piperazone Compounds): Prochlorperazine (Compazine)	Chemoreceptor trigger zone, vomiting center.	Adult: PO, IM: 5–10 mg 3–4×/day. Sustained-Release: 10 mg q 12 hr or 15 mg qd. Sol. 5 mg/5 ml. Supp: 2.5–25 mg. Pediatric: PO: 2.5 mg. 1–3× daily. IM: 0.13 mg/kg 1–2× daily.
Fluphenazine (Permitil, Prolixin)	Chemoreceptor trigger zone, vomiting center.	PO tabs: 0.5–10 mg. Elix: 2.5 mg/5 ml. Sol: 5 mg/ml Inj: 25 mg/ml (long-lasting); decanoate or enanthate: 2.5 mg/ml (regular acting).
Perphenazine (Trilafon)	Chemoreceptor trigger zone, vomiting center.	Adult: PO tabs: 4–16 mg 2–3× daily. Concentrated sol: 16 mg/5 ml. Repetabs: 8 mg. Inj: 5–10 mg.
Thiethylperazine (Torecan)	Chemoreceptor trigger zone, vomiting center.	PO tabs: 10 mg 1–2× daily. Inj: 5 mg/ml. Supp: 10 mg.
Miscellaneous Antidopaminergics: Metoclopramide (Reglan)	Chemoreceptor trigger zone, increases GI motility.	IV: 0.75–1 mg/kg diluted in 50 ml over 15 min, 30 min before and after chemotherapy as necessary. PO: 0.5 mg/kg 4–6× day.
Anticholinergics: Scopolamine (Hyoscine)	Central nervous system aural vestibular apparatus, chemoreceptor trigger zone, labyrinth, increased esophageal tone, decreased retrograde motility.	PO: 0.25 mg 1 hr before travel.
Scopolamine (Transderm-Scop)	Same as above.	1.5 mg transdermal (delivers 0.5 mg over 3 days). Apply 4 hours antiemetic effect is desired.
ANTIHISTAMINES: Dimenhydrinate (Dramamine)	Vomiting center, chemoreceptor trigger zone (?), increased gastroesophageal sphincter tone.	Adult: PO 50 mg q 4–6 hr. IV, IM: as needed. Pediatric: PO: 2–6 yrs, 25 mg q 6–8 hr; 6–12 yrs, 25–50 mg q 6–8 hr; <2 yrs, 1.25 mg/kg q 6–8 hr.
Buclizine (Bucladin-S Softabs)	Decreased retrograde motility, labyrinth, central nervous system.	PO: 5mg 2×/day.

*Within the column listing adverse effects, <u>underlines</u> indicate the most common effects.

General Uses	Adverse Effects*	Nursing Implications
Postoperative.	Same as above.	Same as above.
Postoperative, chemotherapy, radiation.	All piperazines: Neuro: blurred vision, moderate sedative effects, strong extrapyramidal effects GI: dry mouth Renal: urinary retention Misc: weak anticholinergic effects.	Same as above plus do not crush or chew sustained-action tablets.
Postoperative, chemotherapy, radiation.	Misc: Hypersensitivity reactions.	Same as all.
Postoperative, chemotherapy, radiation.	Neuro: drowsiness Endo: gynecomastia, hyperglycemia Renal: glycosuria	Same as all plus do not crush or chew repeat action tablets.
Postoperative, chemotherapy, radiation.	Same as above.	Same as above.
Chemotherapy, gastric stasis due to narcotics, diabetic gastroparesis.	Neuro: sedation, parkinsonian symptoms GI: diarrhea	
Motion sickness.	Neuro: dizziness, drowsiness, dilated pupils GI: dry throat Renal: urinary retention Misc: fatigue	INTERVENTION: Observe patient closely for excitement, delirium, and disorientation, which may occur shortly after drug is administered.
Motion sickness.	Same as above plus Integ: skin irritation	Same as above, plus: INTERVENTION: Patients should wash site after removing transdermal patch and hands after touching patch.
Motion sickness, vertigo.	All antihistamines: Neuro: Drowsiness, blurred vision, headache, hypotension, palpitations, tachycardia. GI: dryness of mouth	INTERVENTION: Administer 30–60 min before activity is to begin. Care should be taken about operating heavy equipment.
Motion sickness, vertigo.	Same as all.	Same as above plus INTERVENTION: Do not administer when allergy to tartrazine is present. Take without swallowing water. Allow tablet to dissolve, or chew it, or swallow it whole.

CONTINUED ON THE FOLLOWING PAGE

Centrally Acting Antiemetics

Table 53–2. CENTRALLY ACTING ANTIEMETICS–*CONTINUED*

Name	Site of Action	Dosage
Cyclizine hydrochloride (Marezine)	Vomiting center, central nervous system, labyrinth	Adult: PO: 50 mg (OTC) q 4–6 hr. IM: 50 mg. Pediatric 6–12 yrs: 25 mg 3× daily
Hydroxyzine (Atarax, Vistaril)	Central nervous system, subcortical; decreased GI motility.	PO, IM: 25–50 mg
Diphenhydramine (Benadryl)	Same as dimenhydrinate.	Adult: PO: 25–50 mg, tabs; 12.5 mg/ml elixir (14% ETOH) 3–4x/day. IV, IM: 10–50 mg 3–4x/day Pediatric: PO: 12.5–25 mg q 3–4x/day. IV, IM: 5 mg/kg 4x/day.
Meclizine (Antivert, Bonine)	Labyrinth; central nervous system; decreased conduction in vestibular/cerebellar pathways.	PO: 10–50 mg tabs 1 hr prior to travel.
MISCELLANEOUS AGENTS: Benzquinamide (Emete-Con)	Chemoreceptor trigger zone, vomiting center.	IM: 50 mg or 0.5–1 mg/kg. IV: 25 mg or 0.2–0.4 mg/kg. slowly 1 ml/minute, give subsequent doses IM.
Diphenidol (Vontrol)	Aural vestibular apparatus, chemoreceptor trigger zone (?), labyrinth.	PO tabs: 25–50 mg q 4 hr. Pediatric over 6 yrs: 0.9 mg/kg.
Trimethobenzamide (Tigan)	Chemoreceptor trigger zone.	Adult: PO: 250 mg 3–4×/day. IM: 200 mg 3–4×/day. Supp: 200 mg 3–4×/day. Pediatric: PO: 4–5 mg/kg q 6–8 hr.

*Within the column listing adverse effects, <u>underlines</u> indicate the most common effects.

patients with acute presurgical conditions or neurologic syndromes because the phenothiazine may mask diagnostic symptoms. They are used most commonly to control postoperative nausea and vomiting, radiation sickness, nausea and vomiting from cancer chemotherapy, and the nausea and vomiting secondary to the ingestion of toxins. They have also proven effective in controlling intractable vomiting in patients with terminal uremia. With the exception of promethazine (Phenergan), they are relatively ineffective in treating motion sickness.

Action. The phenothiazines act mainly by decreasing the sensitivity to stimulation of the chemoreceptor trigger zone in the vomiting center to the central neurotransmitter dopamine. This decrease in sensitivity probably accounts for a wide range of effectiveness.

Adverse Effects. The aliphatic phenothiazine compounds, including triflupromazine (Vesprin), promethazine (Phenergan), promazine (Sparine), and chlor-promazine (Thorazine), generally cause adverse effects of sedation, drowsiness, dizziness, and orthostatic hypotension. Other adverse effects include nasal congestion; anticholinergic side effects, such as blurred vision, dry mouth, and urinary retention; and *extrapyramidal symptoms.* Usually the extrapyramidal side effects seen with all phenothiazines appear when high dosages are used. However, three types of extrapyramidal side effects can be seen within days of initiating therapy, even at low dosages. Acute *dystonia* can occur after the first dose and up to one to five days after starting treatment and is characterized by spasms of the tongue, face, neck, and back. Dystonia is more common in younger patients. This syndrome may be mistaken for a hysterical reaction or seizure. Parkinson-like symptoms can appear anywhere within the first week to the first month. These symptoms include an expressionless face, akinesia (slowing of voluntary movement), rigidity, and

General Uses	Adverse Effects*	Nursing Implications
Motion sickness, vertigo, postoperative, pregnancy.	Same as all.	Same as above.
Motion sickness; postoperative, vertigo.	Same as all.	Same as above.
Motion sickness, vertigo, chemotherapy, pregnancy.	Same as all.	Same as above.
Motion sickness, vertigo, radiation, pregnancy.	Same as all.	Same as above.
Postoperative, chemotherapy, radiation, vertigo.	Similar to phenothiazines. Neuro: excitation, nervousness CV: increased CO, increased blood pressure. IV—increased blood pressure and transient dysrhythmias Resp: increased respirations	Same as for all.
Postoperative, chemotherapy, radiation, vertigo, other.	Neuro: drowsiness, confusion, auditory and visual hallucinations GI: dry mouth	Same as for all plus ASSESSMENT: Assess for allergy to tartrazine.
Postoperative, vertigo, radiation, motion sickness.	Neuro: extrapyramidal reactions, drowsiness, vertigo, blurred vision CV: hypotension GI: diarrhea Misc: hypersensitivity	Same as for all.

tremor at rest. These adverse effects can be mistaken for depression. *Akathisia* (motor restlessness and anxiety) can be mistaken for agitation because this side effect is characterized by a patient's need to be in constant motion. This can be demonstrated by pacing back and forth or by the constant nonpurposeful movement of an extremity (restless foot sign). The aliphatic phenothiazine group is the least likely to cause these extrapyramidal symptoms.

The piperazine phenothiazine compounds, such as prochlorperazine (Compazine), fluphenazine (Prolixin), perphenazine (Trilafon), and thiethylperazine (Torecan), tend to cause more serious adverse effects earlier in treatment but are less sedating as a group. These drugs do cause extrapyramidal side effects. Other adverse effects include hypersensitive reactions, drowsiness, *gynecomastia,* hyperglycemia and hypoglycemia, and glycosuria. Because of the severe side effects, these medications are administered with great caution. More information can be found on the phenothiazines in Chapter 25.

Metoclopramide. Metoclopramide (Reglan), like the phenothiazines, has an antidopaminergic effect at the chemoreceptor trigger zone, but also increases gastrointestinal motility. Metoclopramide is used to combat the nausea and vomiting associated with antineoplastic agents, to reverse the gastric stasis induced by narcotics, and to treat diabetic gastroparesis.

ANTICHOLINERGICS. Scopolamine hydrobromide (Hyoscine) is one of the most effective medications to prevent motion sickness, but it has limited usefulness orally, because of side effects of blurred vision and dryness of mouth. It has a very short duration time, so it may be used if only a one-time dose is needed. Repeated doses may have a cumulative effect.

Scopolamine is also available as a newly released skin patch (Transdermscop) that is applied to a hairless area of the skin behind the ear. Transdermscop is applied four hours before the antiemetic effect is required. It is available by prescription only. This form allows for a continuous release of scopolamine for up to three days. The Transdermscop system is a 0.2-mm thick film, with four layers containing a drug reservoir of scopolamine, mineral oil, and polyisobutylene, which controls the rate of delivery, on an adhesive patch.

The adult dose is one Transdermscop system, which delivers 0.5 mg of scopolamine over three days. The hands should be washed before applying the medication. When the patch is removed, the area behind the ear and the hands are washed thoroughly to prevent any residue of the medication from remaining. If more than 72 hours of therapy are needed, the first patch is removed and the area cleaned, and a second patch is applied to a new postauricular location.

Scopolamine is used with caution in persons with glaucoma, pyloric obstruction, and urinary obstruction because of its anticholinergic effects. Safety in nursing mothers has not yet been established. This system should not be used in children.

The most frequent adverse effect, occurring in about two thirds of the patients, is dryness of the mouth and drowsiness. Blurred vision is less common, but may also occur. Infrequently, hallucinations, confusion, disorientation, memory disturbances, restlessness, and dizziness occur. Persons are cautioned about operating heavy equipment.

Antihistamines. The antihistamines are generally considered the best group of drugs for the alleviation of motion sickness and vestibular-induced vomiting. Dimenhydrinate (Dramamine), diphenhydramine (Benadryl), and meclizine (Bonine) are sold over the counter for the prevention of motion sickness. Buclizine (Bucladin-S), loratadine (Claritin) and hydroxyzine (Atarax, Vistaril) are also effective antiemetics but are available by presciption only. Antihistamines are also used to modify symptoms of the common cold or allergic rhinitis. They are effective alone in managing mild to moderate symptoms when sneezing and rhinorrhea predom-

inate and nasal congestion is minimal. However, it must be remembered that antihistamines do not prevent or cure a cold, nor do they shorten the course of the cold. Patients who take antihistamines for long periods may become refractory. Switching from one class to another may restore individual response. Antihistamines are featured in Table 53–2 with the other central-acting antiemetics and also in Table 53–3.

Histamine is a naturally occurring chemical found throughout the body in tissues and organs such as the skin, lungs, and gut. Histamine is stored in the basophils of the blood, in mast cells, and in other body tissues. In the gut, histamine is stored in the mucosal layer. Once histamine is released from storage sites, it can act on receptors known as histamine receptors to produce various effects (Fig. 53–3). The effects are mediated by two different histamine receptor types designated H_1 and H_2. Stimulation of H_1 receptors by histamine produces constriction of the smooth muscle of the bronchioles and gut. Stimulation of the H_2 receptors causes an increase in gastric secretions. Both receptors are involved in producing vasodilation in vascular smooth muscle.

When tissue is injured, histamine release causes a triple response—redness, flare, and a wheal. Itching or pain may also occur due to the action of histamine on the nerve endings.

Histamine, along with other endogenous substances such as renins, slow-reacting substance of anaphylaxis (SRS-A), and prostaglandins, are mediators of immediate allergic reactions (allergic rhinitis to anaphylaxis). When an individual is allergic to an agent, contact causes release of histamine and these other endogenous substances to produce the allergic reaction. Allergic reactions can range from mildly irritating to life-threatening.

Antihistamines do not bind with histamine to inacti-

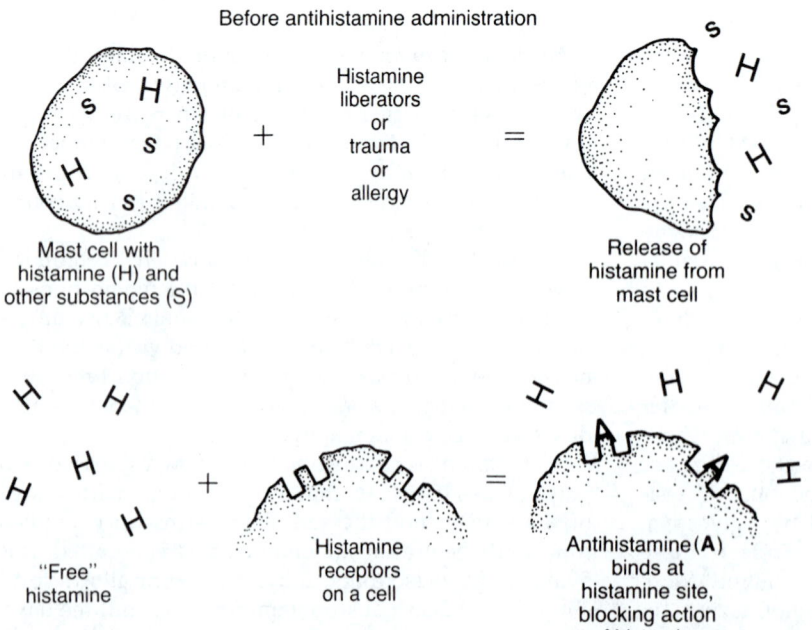

Before antihistamine administration

Mast cell with histamine (H) and other substances (S)

Histamine liberators or trauma or allergy

Release of histamine from mast cell

"Free" histamine

Histamine receptors on a cell

Antihistamine (A) binds at histamine site, blocking action of histamine

Figure 53–3. Histamine release and antihistamine receptor theory.

vate it but rather competitively antagonize histamine at the H_1 receptor site. Terfenadine, the most specific H_1 antagonist, binds preferentially to peripheral rather than central H_1 receptors. Antihistamines antagonize most of the pharmacologic effects of histamine, including the triple response, but do not block histamine release, antibody production, or antigen–antibody interactions.

Action. Antihistamines act by inhibiting transmission of impulses along the vestibular portion of the eighth cranial nerve, as it passes through the cerebellum and chemoreceptor trigger zone. This depression accounts for their special effectiveness in combating nausea and vomiting due to middle ear disorders such as Ménière's disease or labyrinthitis. Antihistamines also act on the vomiting center to reduce stimulation and may also work on the chemoreceptor trigger zone. Antihistamines also have drying (anticholinergic), antipruritic, and sedative effects.

Contraindications and Precautions. The antihistamines are contraindicated in patients sensitive to their ingredients. As a group, they are generally not used in pregnant women. In studies with rates, the antihistamines have caused teratogenic effects; however, no large scale studies have been carried out in humans. Safety in children under twelve has also not been established. Antihistamines are also contraindicated in persons on monoamine oxidase inhibitor (MAOI) therapy.

Antihistamines are used with caution in conditions that might be aggravated by their anticholinergic effect such as prostatic hypertrophy, narrow-angle glaucoma, bronchial asthma, and cardiac dysrhythmias.

Adverse Effects. The adverse effects of antihistamines include drowsiness and, because of their action on the vomiting center, dizziness, as well as dry mouth, blurred vision, urinary retention, and headache. Additional adverse effects include hypotension, palpitations, and tachycardia.

Drug Interactions. All the antihistamines produce an additive effect when given concurrently with alcohol and CNS depressants. Patients need to be cautioned about drinking alcohol concurrently with antihistamines. Antihistamines may diminish the activity of oral anticoagulants and heparin and may enhance the effects of epinephrine.

Cyclizine and Meclizine. Cyclizine (Marezine) and meclizine (Antivert, Bonine) have antiemetic, anticholinergic, and antihistamine properties. Antivert requires a prescription, while Bonine is available over the counter. Both contain 25 mg of meclizine. These products depress the vomiting center by their actions on both the chemoreceptor trigger zone and peripheral pathways.

Both drugs have their onset of action in 30–60 minutes and a duration of four to six hours for cyclizine and 12–24 hours for meclizine. Cyclizine and meclizine are both excellent drugs for postoperative nausea and vomiting and motion sickness. As a prevention of motion sickness, cyclizine and meclizine are taken 30–60 minutes before travel begins and then every 4–6 hours as necessary.

Buclizine Hydrochloride. Buclizine hydrochloride (Bucladin-S), a piperazine antihistamine, acts centrally to suppress nausea and vomiting. Buclizine contains tartrazine, which can result in allergic reactions in persons sensitive to it. Persons hypersensitive to aspirin may also have a cross-sensitivity to tartrazine. Buclizine is taken without swallowing water; the tablet is allowed to dissolve, or chewed, or swallowed hole.

Loratadine. Loratadine (Claritin) is a long-acting antihistamine with minimal central nervous system and anticholinergic effects. It is a selective H_1 receptor antagonist which works peripherally rather than centrally and therefore is non-sedating. Loratadine is used for seasonal and allergic rhinitis. Usual dose is 10–20 mg per day. Loratadine reaches a peak in 1.5 hours and has a half-life of 14.4 hours. Loratadine undergoes extensive first pass metabolism in the liver.

Dimenhydrinate. Dimenhydrinate (Dramamine), a chemical combination of diphenhydramine (Benadryl) and chlorotheophylline, depresses the labyrinth, and is therefore useful in treating vertigo due to motion sickness and Ménière's disease. Dimenhydrinate can be used in children.

Diphenhydramine Hydrochloride. Diphenhydramine hydrochloride (Benadryl) is similar to cyclizine and very effective in preventing and treating vertigo, motion sickness, and nausea and vomiting of pregnancy. When administered IV, diphenhydramine is very effective in treating the extrapyramidal reactions induced by dopaminergic blocking agents. The primary side effect is drowsiness. Patients have to understand that driving or operating equipment may be dangerous.

Hydroxyzine Hydrochloride. Hydroxyzine hydrochloride (Vistaril) has antianxiety, antihistamine, and antiemetic properties. Hydroxyzine is particularly useful in treating motion sickness and vertigo and postoperative nausea. Drowsiness is minimal.

Miscellaneous Antiemetics

The miscellaneous antiemetics are specifically designed to be used as antiemetics. Several of these products are available—benzquinamide hydrochloride (Emete-Con), diphenidol hydrochloride (Vontrol), trimethobenzamide hydrochloride (Tigan), astemizole (Hismanal) and the cannabinoids—dronabinol (Marinol) and nabilone (Cesamet). The cannabinoids are the principle psychoactive component of marijuana. The drugs are reviewed in both Tables 53–2 and 53–4.

BENZQUINAMIDE HYDROCHLORIDE. Benzquinamide hydrochloride (Emete-Con) has antiemetic, antihistaminic, anticholinergic, *antiserotonergic*, and antisedative effects. Due to this combination of actions, it is thought to depress the vomiting center and inhibit stimuli from entering the chemoreceptor trigger zone. Its unique action increases cardiac output, blood pressure, and respiration, and therefore may be particularly effective in patients with central nervous system depression.

Pharmacokinetics. Benzquinamide hydrochloride is rapidly absorbed after intramuscular administration and is distributed to most tissues of the body, with the high-

TEXT RESUMES ON PAGE 1470

Table 53-3. ANTIHISTAMINES

Name	Dosage	Mode of Administration	Pharmacokinetics
Action: For all: inhibit transmission along the eighth cranial nerve (vestibular portion), reduce stimulation of vomiting center. **Use:** For all: combat nausea and vomiting, mild sedation, alleviate motion sickness.			
Cyclizine (Marezine)	Adult: 50 mg q 4–6 hr. 50 mg 4–6 hr Pediatric: 6–12 yrs, 25 mg 3×/day. 1 mg/kg q 8 hr	PO IM PO IM	O: 30 min D: 4–6 hr B: liver E: urine
Meclizine (Antivert, Bonine, Dizmiss) (OTC product)	25–50 mg 1 hr before travel and q 24 hr after.	PO	O: 1 hr D: 12–24 hr ½L: 6 hr B: liver E: urine
Buclizine hydrochloride (Bucladin-S Softabs)	50 mg 30 min before travel and 4–6 hr later	PO	O: 30 min D: 4–6 hr
Dimenhydrinate (Dramamine, Marmine)	Adult: 50–100mg q 4–6 hr. 50 mg as needed 50 mg in 10 ml over 2 min. Pediatric under 2 yrs: 1.25 mg/kg q 6–8 hr. 2–6 yrs: 25 mg q 6–8 hr. 6–12 yrs: 25–50 mg q 6–8 hr.	PO IM IV IM PO PO	O: 30 min D: 4–6 hr B: liver
Diphenhydramine (Benadryl)	Adult: 25–50 mg 3–4×/day. Elixir 12.5 mg/5 ml has 14% alcohol. 10–50 mg 3–4× day. Pediatric: 12.5–25 mg q 3–4× day. 5 mg/kg 4× day.	PO IV, IM PO IV, IM	O: 30 min D: 4–6 hr P: 1–4 hr PB: 80%–88% ½L: 2.4–9.3 hr B: liver E: urine

Key to Abbreviations in the *Pharmacokinetics* column O-onset; P-peak; D-duration; PB-protein bound; B-biotransformed in; E-excreted in; ½ L-halflife.
*Within the column listing adverse effects, underlines indicate the most common effects.

Contraindications/ Precautions	Adverse Effects*	Interactions	Nursing Implications
For all: Contraindicated in hypersensitivity. Use with caution in lactating women, glaucoma, prostatic hypertrophy, asthma.	For all: Neuro: drowsiness, restlessness, excitation, nervousness, blurred vision, diplopia, vertigo, tinnitis. CV: hypotension, palpitations, tachycardia GI: dry mouth, diarrhea, constipation Renal: urinary frequency, difficulty in urination Integ: rash	For all: Additive effect with alcohol and CNS depressants	For all: ASSESSMENT: Assess history of current symptoms to determine cause of nausea and vomiting. Assess for pregnancy. INTERVENTION: Administer 30–60 minutes before activity is to begin. Care should be taken about operating heavy equipment.
Same as for all.	Same as for all	Same as for all	Same as for all
Same as for all.	Same as for all.	Same as for all.	Same as for all.
Same as for all plus: Contraindicated in tartrazine allergy.	Same as for all plus: Neuro: drowsiness, headache, jitteriness GI: dry mouth	Same as for all.	Same as for all plus: ASSESSMENT: Assess for tartrazine allergy. INTERVENTION: Do not swallow water with tablet. Either chew, allow to dissolve, or swallow tablet whole.
Same as for all plus: Contraindicated in neonates.	Neuro: drowsiness, confusion, headache, insomnia, heaviness in hands, vertigo, dizziness, blurred vision, diplopia CV: palpitation, hypotension, tachycardia. Resp: wheezing, thick bronchial secretions GI: dry mouth, nausea, vomiting, diarrhea, constipation, anorexia Renal: painful, difficult urination. Integ: urticaria, rash, photosensitivity	Same as for all plus may mask signs of ototoxicity and cause irreversible eighth cranial nerve damage when given with ototoxic antibiotics.	Same as for all.
Same as for all	Same as for all.	Same as for all.	Same as for all.

CONTINUED ON THE FOLLOWING PAGE

Table 53–3. ANTIHISTAMINES–*CONTINUED*

Name	Dosage	Mode of Administration	Pharmacokinetics
Hydroxyzine hydrochloride (Vistaril)	25–50 mg 4–6×/day.	PO, IM	O: 30 min D: 4–6 hr.
Antagonizer H₁ Receptors			
Use: seasonal rhinitis and chronic idiopathic urticaria			
Astemizole (Hismanil)	Day 1: 30 mg Day 2: 20 mg, Each day thereafter: 10 mg.	PO	O: UA P: UA D: 4 mon. after several wks of therapy. ½L: 9 days PB: UA B: liver E: urine & feces
Loratadine (Claritin)	10–20 mg/day	PO	O: rapid P: 1.5 hr ½L: 14.4 hr

Key to Abbreviations in the *Pharmacokinetics* column O-onset; P-peak; D-duration; PB-protein bound; B-biotransformed in; E-excreted in; ½ L-halflife.
*Within the column listing adverse effects, underlines indicate the most common effects.

est concentrations appearing in the liver and kidneys. Approximately 58% of the medication is bound to protein. It is rapidly metabolized in the liver and then excreted in the urine and feces with a half-life of 40 minutes. Less than 10% of benzquinamide is excreted unchanged in the urine.

Contraindications and Precautions. Contraindications include hypersensitivity to the agent, and cardiovascular disease because of the cardiac adverse effects. Safety in pregnancy, lactating women, and children has not been established.

Adverse Effects. Established adverse effects are similar to those of the aliphatic phenothiazine compounds and include drowsiness, dizziness, orthostatic hypotension, and sometimes excitation and nervousness.

Dosage. Benzquinamide hydrochloride is administered either intramuscularly or intravenously. It is available in 2-ml vials containing 50 mg of base. Reconstitution is done using 2.2 ml of sterile water to produce a solution containing 25 mg/ml. The initial intramuscular injection is 50 mg or 0.5–1 mg/kg, which may be repeated in one hour and every three to four hours as necessary. Intramuscular injections should be given deeply into the muscle tissue. For intravenous injection, 25 mg or 0.2–0.4 mg/kg is given over a 30-second to one-minute time span. Additional doses, when needed, are administered intramuscularly. Intravenous administration has been associated with sudden increase in blood pressure and transient cardiac dysrhythmias.

DIPHENIDOL HYDROCHLORIDE. Diphenidol hydrochloride (Vontrol) inhibits the vestibular–cerebellar pathways and possibly the chemoreceptor trigger zone

in the medulla. It is rapid-acting and best used to combat nausea and vomiting secondary to surgery, radiation, and chemotherapy; motion sickness; and middle ear disease.

Contraindications and Precautions. Diphenidol hydrochloride is contraindicated in infants, pregnant and lactating women, persons who have low blood pressure, and those with known sensitivity. It is also contraindicated in persons with renal failure and anuria, since 90% is excreted in the urine. It should be administered cautiously to persons with glaucoma, or when pyloric stenosis and spasm are present because of its weak peripheral anticholinergic effect. Diphenidol contains tartrazine, which may cause allergic reactions.

Adverse Effects. Adverse effects include drowsiness, sleep disturbances, dry mouth, confusion, and auditory and visual hallucinations. It is therefore reserved for hospitalized patients who can be observed.

Dosage. Diphenidol hydrochloride can be administered orally in doses of 25–50 mg every four hours as needed.

TRIMETHOBENZAMIDE HYDROCHLORIDE. Trimethobenzamide hydrochloride (Tigan) has both an antiemetic effect and an antihistaminic effect. It inhibits activity of the chemoreceptor trigger zone. It is generally less effective than the phenothiazine antiemetics.

Contraindications and Precautions. Trimethobenzamide is contraindicated in persons with known hypersensitivity. It may potentiate central nervous system medications as well as the phenothiazines, so it should be given cautiously to patients receiving these medications. Safety in pregnant and nursing women has not been established.

Contraindications/ Precautions	Adverse Effects*	Interactions	Nursing Implications
Same as for all.	Same as for all.	Same as for all.	Same as for all.
Contraindicated in hypersensitivity.	CV: increased QT interval on ECG. GI: increased appetite, weight gain.	Unknown.	Same as for all.
Same as for all.	Few side effects.	Same as for all.	ASSESSMENT: Assess for cause of seasonal and allergic rhinitis

Adverse Effects. Adverse effects are similar to those of the phenothiazine antiemetics but much less severe. They include allergic reactions, extrapyramidal symptoms, hypotension (parenteral), drowsiness, headache, diarrhea, and blurred vision.

Dosage. The usual adult parenteral dose is 200 mg intramuscularly given three to four times daily. It is not recommended for children. Oral and rectal doses are available; however, they are somewhat unpredictable.

ASTEMIZOLE. ***Action and Use.*** Astemizole (Hismanal) is a potent histamine H_1-receptor antagonist with a high affinity for H_1 receptors; however, it does not readily cross the blood-brain barrier to reach H_1 receptors in the brain so it does not cause sedation. In addition, a single daily dosage is recommended. Astemizole is indicated for the treatment of seasonal allergic rhinitis and chronic idiopathic urticaria.

Pharmacokinetics. Astemizole is readily absorbed in the gastrointestinal tract. Food does markedly decrease absorption so it should be taken on an empty stomach. Astemizole undergoes extensive first-pass metabolism in the liver and is excreted in the urine and feces. It does not appear to be dialyzable. The elimination half-life is about nine days while the elimination half-life at steady-state, which is achieved after four to eight weeks of daily use, is 18 to 20 days.

Dosage. The usual dose of astemizole is 10 mg daily. The initial dose of astemizole is 30 mg on the first day, 20 mg on the second day, and 10 mg thereafter.

CANNABINOIDS. Two cannabinoids are currently available: dronabinol (Marinol) the principle psychoactive substance present in *Cannabis sativa L* (marijuana) and nabilone (Cesamet), a synthetic cannabinoid. Both are controlled substances. These drugs are featured in Table 53–4. These products are indicated in persons receiving cancer chemotherapy who have not responded or have developed a tolerance for other antiemetics. These products are most effective when given with methotrexate and high-dose cisplatin (Chapter 49). Since these products are related to marijuana, they may alter the mental state and are used only in persons who will be closely supervised.

Pharmacokinetics. Both of these products are rapidly absorbed after oral administration, with peak plasma levels being obtained in 60–90 minutes for dronabinol and 60–120 minutes for nabilone. Both drugs undergo an extensive first pass effect in the liver and are excreted in the bile, with small amounts being found in the urine. Both drugs exhibit diphasic kinetics with an alpha half-life of four hours for dronabinol and two hours for nabilone and a terminal half-life of 25–36 hours for dronabinol and 35 hours for nabilone.

Contraindications and Precautions. The cannabinoids are contraindicated in nausea and vomiting from any cause other than cancer chemotherapy and in persons hypersensitive to marijuana or to sesame oil. They are given cautiously to persons with increased blood pressure and heart disease, as they may cause transient tachycardia and in large doses may produce orthostatic hypotension. Safety in children, pregnancy, and lactating women has not been established. Both drugs have high abuse potential and are not administered to persons with previous psychiatric disorders where abuse may become a problem.

Interactions. The cannabinoids are not administered with alcohol or other CNS depressants like sedatives and hypnotics because of the possible combined effect.

Adverse Effects. The cannabinoids cause numerous adverse effects within the central nervous system, including drowsiness (48%–66%), a high or heightened

TEXT RESUMES ON PAGE 1474

Table 53–4. MISCELLANEOUS ANTIEMETICS

Name	Dosage	Mode of Administration	Pharmacokinetics
Action: depress the vomiting center			
Use: prevention of postoperative vomiting.			
Benzquinamide hydrochloride (Emete-Con)	50 mg q 3–4 hr. 25 mg over 10 min.	IM IV	O: 15 min P: 30 min D: 3–4 hr ½L: 40 min PB: 58% B: liver E: urine, bile
Trimethobenzamide hydrochloride (Tigan)	200 mg q 3–4 hr.	IM PO Supp.	O: 10–50 min PO; 15–35 min IM D: 3–4 hr PO; 2–3 hr IM ½L: UA PB: UA B: liver E: urine
Diphenidol (Vontrol)	25–50 mg q 3–4 hr.	PO	O: 15 min D: 3–4 hr P: 1.5–3 hr ½L: 4 hr PB: UA B: liver E: urine
Cannabinoids			
Use: only nausea and vomiting from cancer chemotherapy.			
Dronabinol (Marinol)	5 mg/m² 1–3 hr prior to chemotherapy then 2–4 hr after chemo for a total of 4–6 doses/day. Increase dose by 2.5 mg/m² increments to max. of 15 mg/m².	PO	O: rapid P: 60–90 min D: 2–3 hr ½L: 4 hr (25–36 hr metabolites) PB: 97%–99% B: liver E: feces 50%, urine 10%–15%
Nabilone (Cesamet)	1–2 mg 2× day, max daily dose is 6 mg divided 3× day.	PO	O: rapid P: 60–120 min ½L: 2 hr (35 hr, metabolites) PB: UA B: liver E: bile 65% urine 20%

Key to Abbreviations in the *Pharmacokinetics* column O-onset; P-peak; D-duration; PB-protein bound; B-biotransformed in; E-excreted in; ½ L-halflife.
*Within the column listing adverse effects, <u>underlines</u> indicate the most common effects.

Contraindications/ Precautions	Adverse Effects*	Interactions	Nursing Implications
			ASSESSMENT: Assess vital signs, causes of vomiting. INTERVENTION: Administer 15 minutes before vomiting is expected. IM injection should be well into the muscle mass. Do not use the deltoid unless well developed. Drowsiness is a major adverse effect, along with cardiovascular effects of hypotension. Reconstituted solutions should not be refrigerated and remain potent for 14 days at room temperature.
Contraindicated in hypersensitivity and in cardiovascular disease. Safety in pregnancy, lactating women, and children not established.	Neuro: drowsiness, fatigue, restlessness, headache, excitement, sweating, shivering, tremors. CV: hyper/hypotension, atrial fibrillation, premature beats GI: dry mouth, anorexia, nausea Integ: hives/rash, urticaria	Reduce dose of benzquinamide when concurrent pressors and epinephrine-like drugs are given.	Same as for all plus: INTERVENTION: reconstitute in 2.2 ml solution for injection.
Contraindicated in hypersensitivity. Use cautiously in patients receiving CNS drugs. Safety in pregnancy and lactating women not established.	Neuro: Parkinson-like syndrome, blurred vision, convulsions, coma, dizziness, drowsiness CV: hypotension Resp: hypersensitivity GI: diarrhea Bilary: jaundice Hemo: blood dyscrasias Integ: rash	Avoid alcohol. Cautiously use CNS depressants.	Same as for all.
Contraindicated in hypersensitivity, children, pregnancy, lactating women, anuria, and renal failure. Use cautiously in glaucoma, pyloric stenosis and/or spasm.	Neuro: auditory and visual hallucinations, disorientation, confusion, drowsiness, sleep disturbances CV: lowered blood pressure GI: dry mouth, nausea, indigestion Bilary: jaundice Integ: rash	Unknown	Same as for all.
Contraindicated in hypersensitivity, nausea, and vomiting from any other cause than cancer chemotherapy. Use with caution in increased blood pressure, heart disease, epilepsy, and with patients with psychiatric disturbances. Safety in children, pregnancy, and lactating women not established. CAUTION: high potential for abuse.	Neuro: drowsiness, dizziness, concentration difficulties, headache, visual distortions, weakness GI: dry mouth	Do not give in combination with any other CNS depressant or alcohol.	ASSESSMENT: Assess vital signs. INTERVENTION: Administer 1–3 hours prior to chemotherapy. Avoid alcohol and other CNS depressants. May cause drowsiness. Caution about driving or doing activities requiring mental alertness. Patients should remain under the control of a responsible adult. EVALUATION: Behavioral changes may occur. Patient and family should be alert to these.

awareness (24%–38%), dizziness (14%–21%), muddled thinking, concentration difficulties (12%–25%), depression (7%–14%), and weakness (6%–12%), all due to their complex CNS effect.

Dronabinol. Dronabinol (Marinol) is administered orally in 5 mg/m^2 doses one to three hours prior to the administration of chemotherapy, followed by every two to four hours for a total of four to six days. If ineffective, the dosage can be increased by 2.5 mg/m^2 to a maximal dose of 15 mg/m^2.

Nabilone. Nabilone (Cesamet) is administered orally in 1- to 2-mg doses twice daily. Maximal dose is 6 mg daily divided into two to three daily doses.

EMETICS

The emetics are used to induce vomiting when poisons or toxins that have been ingested are still in the stomach. Before emetics are administered, the substances that were taken MUST BE KNOWN. For example, emetics are not administered if the individual swallowed a strong acid or alkali such as those found in many household cleaners. The poison may have already burned the throat and esophagus, and would do so again were vomiting induced. In all cases, where possible, the local poison control center is notified before any intervention

is begun. Emesis is more effective than gastric lavage in removing the substance from the stomach.

Emetics induce vomiting by acting in several locations in the reflex arc. They irritate the stomach and stimulate the vomiting center, promoting vomiting about 15–60 minutes after they are ingested by mouth or given subcutaneously. The most common emetics are ipecac syrup, available OTC in the pharmacy, and apomorphine hydrochloride (Table 53–5).

Contraindications and Precautions

Emetics are contraindicated when strong alkaline, acidic, strychnine, or petroleum distillate poisons have been consumed. Other treatment modalities must be used in these patients, such as nasogastric suction or dialysis. Emetics are further contraindicated for any patient who is not alert. In a comatose, semicomatose, inebriated, or sedated patient, there is increased risk of aspiration if vomiting is induced. Emetics are also contraindicated in patients who have taken central nervous system stimulants. The emetic will cause further CNS stimulation, which may result in convulsion. Nasogastric suction is the best treatment with overdoses of CNS stimulants.

IPECAC SYRUP. Ipecac syrup acts on both the stomach and the chemoreceptor trigger zone and induces

Table 53–5. EMETIC MEDICATIONS

Name	Dosage	Mode of Administration	Pharmacokinetics
Action: produce vomiting.			
Use: to induce vomiting when ingested known substances.			
Ipecac syrup USP	15–30 ml (over 1 year old)	PO	O: 20–30 min
Apomorphine hydrochloride	Adults: 2–10 mg Infants and children: 0.1 mg/kg in 1 dose. DO NOT REPEAT.	SC (IM, IV rarely used)	O: 5–15 min

Key to Abbreviations in the *Pharmacokinetics* column O-onset· P-peak; D-duration; PB-protein bound; B-biotransformed in; E-excreted in; ½ L-halflife.
*Within the column listing adverse effects, underline indicates the most common effect.

vomiting only if medullary centers are responsive. It also has an expectorant action, which lowers sputum viscosity. It is available without a prescription for emergency use.

Dosage. Ipecac syrup is administered orally in doses of 15 ml, or one tablespoonful, to anyone over one year of age. At least eight ounces of water should accompany ipecac syrup to increase the fluid volume in the stomach. The dose may be repeated in 20–30 minutes if vomiting has not occurred. If vomiting has still not occurred, ipecac syrup should be removed from the stomach via nasogastric suction or its absorption minimized by the administration of activated charcoal. If ipecac syrup is not removed through vomiting and is absorbed systemically, it may provoke bleeding in the intestinal tract and cause bloody diarrhea. Its absorption may also cause convulsions, dysrhythmias, and coma. Ipecac syrup becomes outdated within 1 year after the bottle is opened.

APOMORPHINE HYDROCHLORIDE. Apomorphine hydrochloride stimulates the chemoreceptor trigger zone (CTZ) to induce vomiting only when medullary centers are responsive. In the CTZ, apomorphine combines with dopamine receptors to produce emesis; thus, apomorphine is a dopaminergic agonist. It is also classified as a narcotic, has a mild sedative effect, and may depress the respiratory center. After vomiting occurs, in

about 15 minutes after a subcutaneous injection, the sedative effects begin and last about two hours. If the central nervous system depression is too great, the narcotic antagonist naloxone hydrochloride (Narcan) must be administered intramuscularly to counteract the central nervous system depression. Naloxone hydrochloride may also help antagonize the violent and protracted vomiting often seen with the use of apomorphine. The dopaminergic effects result in lacrimation, salivation, nausea, and perspiration.

USING THE NURSING PROCESS

ASSESSMENT

Assessment of the patient requiring either antiemetic or emetic medications for the control or promotion of vomiting always begins with a thorough nursing history to develop the data base. This information may be obtained from the family if the patient is comatose or too young to supply it. The information obtained is included in Table 53–6. A thorough drug history is important in

TEXT RESUMES ON PAGE 1478

Contraindications/ Precautions	Adverse Effects*	Interactions	Nursing Implications
Contraindicated for treatment of strong alkalis or acids, strychnine, petroleum distillates, and in comatose or semicomatose, inebriated, or sedated patients.	If medicine is absorbed and not vomited: Neuro: convulsions, coma CV: dysrhythmia GT: bloody diarrhea	Not to be administered for overdose of CNS stimulant. Charcoal, milk, carbonated beverages inactivates ipecac. Not given concurrently with antiemetic.	ASSESSMENT: Assess baseline pulse and rhythm. INTERVENTION: Follow ipecac with 1 glass of lukewarm water. Walking induces emesis more quickly. Obtain pulse 1 hour after administration. EVALUATION: If vomiting does not occur, repeat in 20–30 minutes. If still no vomiting, give activated charcoal or remove through gastric suctioning.
Contraindicated in narcosis due to opiates, barbiturates, ethyl alcohol; coma; shock; convulsions; allergy to morphine; poisonings due to corrosive alkali (lye) and petroleum products. Use cautiously in children and in elderly patients and in persons with cardiovascular disease.	Neuro: sedation, syncope, weakness, perspiration, euphoria, tremor CV: pallor, tachycardia, dysrhythmia GI: increased salivation, violent emesis	Acts synergistically with CNS sedatives. Not to be given concurrently.	ASSESSMENT: Assess baseline vital signs. INTERVENTION: Administer 1 glass milk or lukewarm water to enhance vomiting. Walking induces vomiting more quickly. Monitor vital signs q 15 minutes for 2 hours. EVALUATION: If prolonged vomiting occurs, administer narcotic antagonist.

Table 53–6. NURSING PROCESS FOR PATIENT REQUIRING ANTIEMETIC AND EMETIC MEDICATIONS

Assessment
Determine medication history, including recent change of medication, chemotherapy, current antiemetic therapy. Note history of current illness, pregnancy, drug overdose (poisoning), motion sickness. Note use/effectiveness of home remedies.

Nursing Diagnosis	Nursing Actions	Rationale	Desired Outcomes/ Evaluation Criteria
Antiemetics Fluid Volume, deficit, Potential related to excessive losses through vomiting, reduced oral intake/absorption of fluids.	Record intake and output, including emesis. Measure urine specific gravity.	Useful in evaluation of fluid needs.	Verbalizes individual risk factors and appropriate interventions. Demonstrates adequacy of fluid balance with moist mucous membranes, good skin turgor, stable vital signs, individually appropriate urinary output.
	Weigh daily as appropriate.	Sensitive indicator of fluid volume shifts.	
	Evaluate mucous membranes, skin turgor, strength/rate of peripheral pulses. Monitor vital signs.	Indicators of additional therapy needs/effectiveness.	
	Administer antiemetics, e.g., benzquinamide hydrochloride, trimethobenzamide hydrochloride.	Given to eliminate nausea/vomiting.	
	Evaluate effectiveness of drug.	Prolonged use may result in tolerance requiring increased dosage/change of drug.	
	Encourage increased oral intake of bland beverages, gelatin, sherbet, etc. in small/frequent amounts.	Replaces losses, small amounts may be retained/absorbed better.	
	Recommend changing body position slowly as appropriate.	Parenteral administration of antiemetics may result in othostatic hypotension.	
	Discuss strategies for dealing with unpleasant results of vomiting, e.g., eliminate noise and unpleasant odors; provide clean environment, removing vomitus promptly; provide frequent oral care.	These measures can contribute to lessening of the vomiting reflex.	
Knowledge deficit related to lack of information/information misinterpretation, unfamiliarity with resources as evidenced by questions, statement of concern, inaccurate follow-through of instruction/ development of preventable complications.	Provide information about pathophysiology of illness and relationship of vomiting.	Understanding of reasons for vomiting and treatment required provides base for making decisions/cooperation with treatment required.	Verbalizes understanding of underlying cause of vomiting and treatment regimen. Identifies relationship of vomiting to disease process. Participates in treatment regimen.
	Discuss action, dose, timing of drug, and possible side-effects.	Helps patient to manage use of antiemetics effectively, e.g., give drug on an empty stomach or before activity which may cause nausea (chemotherapy).	
	Suggest use of hard candy or gum.	Reduces discomfort of dry mucous membranes.	

Table 53–6. NURSING PROCESS FOR PATIENT REQUIRING ANTIEMETIC AND EMETIC MEDICATIONS–*CONTINUED*

Nursing Diagnosis	Nursing Actions	Rationale	Desired Outcomes/ Evaluation Criteria
	Review "safe" handling of transdermal drug patch if used.	Washing skin site/ hands after handling or removal of patch reduces irritation/removes drug residue.	
	Caution patient not to drive when taking antiemetic drugs.	Side effects of these medications include drowsiness, dizziness, vertigo, and hypotension.	
Emetics Poisoning, Potential related to large supplies of drugs in home, dangerous products/ drugs placed or stored within reach of children or confused persons, presence of poisonous vegetation.	Review safe storage of medications and household products, coding medicines for the visually impaired. Encourage discarding outdated/unused drugs.	Reduces likelihood of accidental poisoning.	Verbalizes understanding of dangers of poisoning. Identifies hazards that could lead to accidental poisoning. Corrects environmental hazards as identified. Demonstrates necessary action to promote safe environment.
	Provide information about when and how to use emetic drugs. Stress importance of contacting the poison control center/local hospital before administering medication.	Supports safe/ appropriate use of drug, reducing risk of additional injury to patient. Promotes cooperation with treatment.	
	Administer emetics with water/milk:	Drug effects are enhanced when given on a full stomach.	
	Ipecac syrup (po);	Exerts emetic effect by direct irritant action on the GI tract and on the CTZ.	
	apomorphine (injection).	Apomorphine acts centrally at the level of CTZ.	
	Discuss side-effects to be reported, e.g., severe continued vomiting, restlessness, tachypnea, fibrillation.	Awareness of what to expect and which symptoms are of concern allows for early intervention to avoid serious complications.	
	Monitor vital signs and do not leave patient alone following drug administration (especially Apomorphine).	Drowsiness occurs following vomiting and respiratory depression may occur increasing risk of aspiration.	
	Instruct parents to discard any left-over Ipecac syrup.	Once opened, efficacy of drug will diminish.	
	Stress necessity of medical follow-up if drug is administered at home.	Important to observe and evaluate effectiveness of treatment and adverse reaction of poisonous substance.	

ruling out serious causes of nausea and vomiting, such as side effects of medications. Antiemetics are resorted to only when no other therapy is available, especially in children. When administering an antiemetic, it is important to assist the physician in determining the cause of the vomiting. If the vomiting is associated with motion, there are numerous OTC products available. The patient will have to be taught how to take the medication for effective use.

A woman in her first trimester of pregnancy or just starting on birth control pills may experience nausea and vomiting early in the morning or on the sight or smell of certain foods. This is usually transient, but the woman still needs to be assessed for dehydration, fluid and electrolyte derangements, and acid–base imbalances.

When the patient requires emetics, he or she is generally experiencing an emergency either at home or in the emergency room of a hospital or clinic. The health team must always determine what was swallowed before evoking emesis, in order to prevent further damage to the mucous membranes during vomiting. The poisoning could be deliberate, as with a drug overdose (see Chapter 13), or accidental, as in the case of a child who has swallowed an improperly stored household preparation not meant for oral ingestion or a medication. In general, the patient is hospitalized for observation for at least 24 hours after the acute poisoning incident.

NURSING DIAGNOSES— ANTIEMETICS

The nurse develops nursing diagnoses for the patient as he or she develops the plan of care. Possible nursing diagnoses for a patient requiring antiemetics are included in Table 53–6.

PLANNING AND INTERVENTION— ANTIEMETICS

The nurse develops the goals of intervention from the nursing diagnoses. When caring for the patient requiring antiemetic medication, typical goals are included in Table 53–6. The locus of control may be either with the nurse or the patient when these medications are being administered.

The nurse may administer antiemetics, or they may be self-administered by the patient at home. The nurse and patient must know specific information about the antiemetics to ensure their safe administration. This information is summarized in Tables 53–2 and 53–3 in the column headed "Nursing Implications."

NURSING RESPONSIBILITY— ANTIEMETICS

The nurse, in general, must always rotate injection sites when administering antiemetics intramuscularly, in order to prevent irritation of the tissues. Since all anti-

emetics dry mucous membranes, particularly of the mouth, the nurse might suggest that patients employ hard candy or gum to moisten their mouths.

A nauseated postoperative patient who vomits may need additional treatments, such as insertion of a nasogastric tube or IV therapy. Violent retching could put undue pressure on the suture line, as well as further agitating the patient. A patient who vomits for any length of time may become dehydrated or develop a fluid, electrolyte, or acid–base imbalance. Therefore, the nurse must continue to observe laboratory reports and report any significant finding to the attending physician.

In general, when a patient is taking antiemetics to control the nausea and vomiting that accompany radiation or chemotherapy, many helpful suggestions may be given to the patient and family. They are outlined in Chapter 49.

PATIENT TEACHING—ANTIEMETICS

Patients may take their own antiemetics at home for various conditions. General teaching measures are included in Table 53–7.

EVALUATION—ANTIEMETICS

During the evaluation phase, the nurse evaluates the effectiveness of antiemetic medications. This evaluation is

---

Table 53–7. PATIENT TEACHING INFORMATION—ANTIEMETICS

Dear Patient:
This drug has been prescribed for you. This is what you should know about your drug to get the most from your therapy.

1. Antiemetic, such as _____, has been specifically ordered for you to reduce your nausea and vomiting associated with

   _____
2. Antiemetic drugs will be taken until your current health problem is resolved.
3. Antiemetic medications are taken about 30 to 60 minutes before the activity or the event that may lead to nausea and vomiting.
4. Antiemetics are taken on an empty stomach (at least 2 hours after a meal).
5. Antiemetics react with other medications; therefore, always check with your pharmacist or doctor before taking other medications with your antiemetic.
6. Antiemetic medications may also worsen the effects of alcohol (beer, wine, liquor) or other central nervous system depressants (tranquilizers, sleeping pills); therefore, DO NOT take these products together.
7. All antiemetics tend to cause sleepiness or slowed mental or physical abilities, so you should avoid driving a car or operating heavy equipment for several hours after taking these medications.
8. Medications are stored at room temperature away from heat and in light-resistant containers. Suppositories are stored below 77°F, below room temperature.

based on a list of outcome evaluation criteria that has been developed in relation to the goals determined by the nurse, patient, and family. The information from the data base obtained in the original assessment is used to formulate the criteria for evaluation. Typical patient outcome evaluation criteria are included in Table 53–6.

It is extremely important to work with the patient and family to ensure their complete assistance and support. Patients who understand the importance of their continued medical treatment are usually compliant. The nurse should teach the patient about potential side effects so that a patient taking these medications at home will report any unusual symptoms to the physician or nurse. In general, the side effects of the antiemetics include drowsiness, dizziness, vertigo, and hypotension. Patients who receive parenteral antiemetics should change their body position slowly to prevent the occurrence of orthostatic hypotension. When the phenothiazine group and several miscellaneous antiemetics are administered, the patient may experience extrapyramidal effects (such a masklike face, tremors, dystonia, akathisia [inability to sit still], and tardive dyskinesia [involuntary rhythmic movements of the face]—see Chapter 25). Dosage is decreased or the medication discontinued to prevent these side effects from becoming permanent.

NURSING DIAGNOSES—EMETICS

The nurse develops the nursing diagnoses, which become the basis for the goals and priorities of the nursing care. Typical nursing diagnoses for a patient requiring emetics are included in Table 53–6.

PLANNING AND INTERVENTION— EMETICS

The nurse develops the goals of the nursing intervention from the nursing diagnoses. Goals for the patient requiring emetics are included in Table 53–6.

Depending on the location of care, the nurse calls the poison control center, physician, or local hospital for immediate advice before instituting treatment. In most cases, emesis is preferred over stomach lavage. However, emetics should never be administered in the following cases:

1. Patients with significant central nervous system depression who may have lost their gag reflex and there is a risk of aspiration.
2. Patients at high risk of seizures, since emetics may produce or worsen seizures.
3. Patients who have ingested petroleum distillates, as there is a potential for lipid droplet aspiration.
4. Patients who have ingested caustics, as this will reexpose the already damaged mouth and esophagus to the caustic substance again.
5. Patients who have ingested drugs with antiemetic activity, as their effectiveness is reduced.

The nurse lends psychologic support to the patient and family during the treatment, and assists them in obtaining further psychologic help if needed. The nurse also counsels the family about placing bottles and jars out of the reach of small children, if such misplacement caused the incident. Suggest safety locks on kitchen cupboards and high, locked cabinets in the garage for outdoor pesticides and fertilizers. Families with small children should keep syrup of ipecac on hand. The parents are instructed not to use it without first checking with the poison control center. Also, parents and guardians are encouraged to learn the current first aid treatment for poisonings and to keep a first aid reference handy. Many old "universal antidotes" have proven useless. Do not use them!

In general, most emetics' effects are enhanced if given on a full stomach. Therefore, they are generally given along with water or milk. Vomiting usually occurs in 30–60 minutes. The emetic effect can also be enhanced by walking an adult or bouncing a child.

EVALUATION—EMETICS

The nurse is primarily concerned with getting the patient to vomit. The medication can be repeated once, but if vomiting does not occur, some other means of emptying the stomach must be used, such as gastric lavage.

The medications all have side effects, and the nurse or family must be familiar with those specific to the agent being administered. All sedate the patient after the vomiting episode, so the nurse needs to evaluate the patient's vital signs and the amount of central nervous system depression. Also, prevent aspiration to reduce the risk of aspiration pneumonia. If the patient is too sedated, particularly when apomorphine is used, a narcotic antagonist may be needed.

SUMMARY

The patient and family are likely to comply with instructions and treatment procedures to the extent that they are involved with the planning of patient care. The nurse must stress the importance of continued medical care whenever necessary. The nurse reviews and updates all previously taught material with the patient and family, if necessary, to ensure that the patient's knowledge base remains accurate.

BIBLIOGRAPHY

AMA Drug Department: AMA Drug Evaluations, ed 6. PSG Publishing, Littleton, MA, 1986.

Gilman, AG, Goodman, LS, and Gilman, A (eds): Goodman and Gilman's The Pharmacological Basis of Therapeutics, ed 7. Macmillan, New York, 1985.

Olin, B (ed): Facts and Comparisons. JB Lippincott, St. Louis, 1989.

SITUATION   53–1

Edgar Randazzo, aged 50 years, is receiving chemotherapy for cancer of the stomach. To reduce the nausea and vomiting related to the treatment, various antiemetics are being tried.

1. Mr. Randazzo is to receive prochlorperazine (Compazine) 10 mg IM 30 minutes before the scheduled chemotherapy. Prior to administration, the nurse will check the:
   a. pupillary response
   b. blood pressure
   c. complete blood count
   d. age of patient

2. While Mr. Randazzo is on prochlorperazine therapy, the nurse will provide the following intervention:
   a. restrict oral fluids
   b. encourage large meals
   c. frequent oral care
   d. provide distractions

3. The nurse will monitor Mr. Randazzo for side effects of prochlorperazine, which include:
   a. urinary frequency
   b. alopecia
   c. blurred vision
   d. insomnia

4. For discharge home, Mr. Randazzo is given a prescription for diphenidol (Vontrol) po 50 mg q 4 hours prn nausea/vomiting. The nurse will instruct him about the following side effect related to this drug:
   a. auditory hallucinations
   b. diarrhea
   c. abdominal pain
   d. photosensitivity

5. Which of the following statements by Mr. Randazzo indicates the need for further discharge teaching?
   a. "I should get up slowly from a lying position."
   b. "It would be okay to have wine with my dinner."
   c. "I should avoid driving a car while taking my medication."
   d. "If I have difficulty voiding, I should call the doctor."

6. When evaluating Mr. Randazzo for effectiveness of antiemetic therapy, the following outcome is important:
   a. mild hypotension
   b. central nervous system depression
   c. output greater than intake
   d. acid-base balance

54

MEDICATIONS FOR COMMON DIGESTIVE PROBLEMS (DIGESTANTS AND INTESTINAL PREPARATIONS)

MEDICATIONS FOR
COMMON DIGESTIVE
PROBLEMS (DIGESTANTS
AND INTESTINAL
PREPARATIONS)

CHAPTER OUTLINE

THERAPEUTIC AGENTS
    Digestants
    Antidiarrheals
    Laxatives
USING THE NURSING PROCESS
    Assessment
    Nursing Diagnoses
    Planning and Intervention
    Patient Teaching
    Evaluation
SUMMARY

TABLES

Nursing Process

Patient Teaching

Drug Tables

GLOSSARY TERMS IN THIS CHAPTER

Achlorhydria
Antiperistalsis
Auerbach's plexus
Hypochlorhydria
Pernicious anemia
Vermifuge

MEDICATIONS FOR COMMON DIGESTIVE PROBLEMS (DIGESTANTS AND INTESTINAL PREPARATIONS)

MERRILY MATHEWSON KUHN, R.N.C., Ph.D., CCRN

LEARNING OBJECTIVES

After reading this chapter, the student will be able to:

1. Identify those agents commonly used as digestive system medications.

2. Compare the digestive system medications as to mechanism of action, route of administration, pharmacokinetics, adverse effects, contraindications, and interactions.

3. Identify specific parameters to assess in the patient requiring digestive system medications in order to formulate appropriate nursing diagnoses.

4. Plan the nursing interventions necessary to administer digestive system medications, monitor effects, and choose appropriate teaching strategies to gain patient compliance.

5. Evaluate the patient at various stages of treatment to gauge the success of nursing interventions.

THERAPEUTIC AGENTS

The gastrointestinal tract is responsible for the digestion of food substances, and ultimately, absorption of nutrients. Difficulties with the digestion of food or maladies affecting the bowel disrupt proper functioning of the tract and ultimately affect the digestion and absorption of nutrients. This chapter discusses the pharmacologic management of problems of digestion and the bowel, including both diarrhea and constipation. The nursing process section discusses nursing interventions.

DIGESTANTS

Carbohydrates, fats, and protein must be broken down into their simplest form before they are available to the body. These products are broken down by gastric acids and enzymes. Products designed to aid digestion are known as digestants.

Digestants (Table 54–1) include hydrochloric acid (as glutamic acid HCl), stomach enzymes (such as pepsin), pancreatic enzymes (such as pancrelipase and pancreatin), and the bile salts.

Hydrochloric Acid

Individuals can have either a decrease in the amount of hydrochloric acid produced (*hypochlorhydria*), or an al-

Table 54–1. DIGESTANTS

Name	Dosage	Mode of Administration	Pharmacokinetics
Acidifiers/Digestive Enzymes:			
Action: replace hydrochloride missing from the stomach.			
Use: pernicious anemias, achlorhydria, gastric carcinoma.			
Glutamic acid hydrochloride (Acidulin) 340-mg cap.	1–3 capsules tid ac.	PO	Unavailable
Pancreatic Enzyme:			
Action: helps digest and absorb protein, fat, and CHO.			
Use: deficient pancreatic enzymes, cystic fibrosis, chronic pancreatitis, and others			
Precrelipase (Cotazym, Ilozyme, Kuzyme HP, Pancrease, Viokase)	1–3 tab or cap with meals and snacks, or 1–2 packets with meals or snacks.	PO	Unavailable
Pancreatin (Elzyme 303, Pancreatin, Enseals) (All of these are OTC)	18 g ac or with meals. Pediatric: 0.3–0.6 g 3× daily.	PO	
Bile Salts:			
Action: aids normal digestion and absorption of fat			
Use: laxative			
Bile extract (Ox bile extract, Enseals, Bilron-Pulvules)	150–600 mg; enteric coated tabs: 325 mg. Pediatric: 150–600 mg.	PO	Unavailable
Hydrochloretics:			
Action: increase amount of high water content, low viscosity bile.			
Use: temporary constipation			
Dehydrocholic acid	1–2 tabs 3×/day.	PO	Unavailable

*Within the column listing adverse effects, underlines indicate the most common effects; CAPITALS indicate life-threatening effects.

most complete absence of hydrochloric acid *(achlorhydria)*. Achlorhydria is most likely to occur in elderly patients and those with gastric cancer. *Pernicious anemia* occurs with achlorhydria and leads to peripheral neuritis, and possibly death. Surprisingly, patients with hypochlorhydria have more gastric complaints than do those with achlorhydria.

Hydrochloric acid can be administered in capsule form as glutamic acid hydrochloride (Acidulin), which provides 1.8 mEq of hydrochloric acid. The very small amount of free hydrochloric acid is usually sufficient to relieve symptoms. The capsules release their hydrochloric acid when in contact with water and therefore are administered with an 8-ounce glass of water.

Hydrochloric acid preparations may precipitate, or worsen, existing metabolic acidosis by decreasing the body supply of bicarbonate ion. As bicarbonate decreases, the kidneys respond by retaining chloride. Therefore, these preparations are not recommended for administration in patients with metabolic acidosis.

Digestive Enzymes

The digestive enzymes are secreted by the gastrointestinal tract and enhance the chemical digestion of food substances. The mouth, stomach, small intestine, pancreas, and liver each secrete one or more digestive enzymes. The absence of enzymes in the stomach or pancreas, or of bile in the gallbladder, causes major digestive disturbances. As an example, lack of bile results in the inability to digest fats.

Contraindications/ Precautions	Adverse Effects	Interactions	Nursing Implications
Contraindicated in hyper- acidity and peptic ulcer.	Metabolic acidosis, fall in bicarbonate, rise in serum chloride.		INTERACTION: Give with 8 ounces of water.
Contraindicated in allergy to pig protein. Contraindicated in allergy to pig, ox, or beef pro- tein.	GI: anorexia, nausea, vomit- ing, diarrhea.		INTERVENTION: Take with or before meals. Packets may be sprinkled on food, capsules may be opened, or tablets crushed and sprinkled on food. Do not take milk or antacid within 1 hour of pancreatic enzymes. Do not chew cap- sule contents. Avoid inhala- tion of powder.
Contraindicated in severe jaundice.	GI: diarrhea, cramping.		INTERVENTION: Swallow table whole, do not chew.
Contraindicated in abdominal pain.	Allergic reactions, diarrhea.		INTERVENTION: Take with or after meals.

Pancreatic Enzymes

The pancreatic enzymes include amylase to digest starches, lipase to digest fats, and trypsin (a protease) to digest protein. Pancreatic secretion also includes bicarbonate, which protects the enzymes from denaturation by acid and pepsin. Pancreatic secretions may be impaired following chronic pancreatitis, pancreatectomy, cystic fibrosis, pancreatic duct obstruction, and carcinomas of the pancreas.

Pancreatic enzymes enter the digestive system through the common bile duct in the duodenum. Products containing pancreatic enzymes are extracted from pig and beef pancreas. The most commonly used are pancrelipase (Cotazym), extracted only from porcine pancreas, and pancreatin, extracted from beef or porcine sources. All patients treated with these enzymes must be reminded to eat a well-balanced diet including fat, protein, and starch to avoid indigestion. Steatorrhea (fatty stools) is a major finding in pancreatic enzyme deficiency, and this symptom is an important sign of treatment success or failure.

PANCRELIPASE. Pancrelipase is used for the symptomatic treatment of malabsorption syndromes due to cystic fibrosis and other conditions associated with exocrine pancreatic insufficiency. Each of the trade name products have different combinations of lipase, ranging from 4000–8000 U, protease ranging from 13,000–70,000 U, and amylase ranging from 20,000–70,000 U. Pancrelipase is the most potent of all the pancreatic replacement enzymes, being highest in its lipase content. The high lipase content makes it most beneficial for treating *steatorrhea.* Pancrelipase is available in capsule, tablet, or packet form. The usual adult dose is one to three capsules or tablets, or one to two packets, before or with each meal or snack. For children, the dosage is one to two capsules or tablets with each meal. The tablets or capsules, because of their enteric coating, resist gastric inactivation and begin to break down in the duodenum. Enteric-coated tablets should not be chewed or crushed, but swallowed whole, to avoid being destroyed by gastric secretion.

The adverse effects of pancrelipase include anorexia, nausea, vomiting, and diarrhea. Since it is synthesized from pig pancreas, it is contraindicated in persons allergic to pig protein. Persons allergic to pig protein will have digestive disturbances when pork is ingested.

PANCREATIN. Pancreatin is obtained from both porcine and bovine origin. It also includes all pancreatic enzymes—lipase, amylase, and protease. The usual dose for adults is 4 g (as high as 18 g/day may be prescribed in divided doses) taken before or during meals. Adverse effects and contraindications are the same as for pancrelipase.

Bile Salts

Bile salts are digestive aids that are produced by the liver, stored and concentrated in the gallbladder, and released into the duodenum through the common bile duct. Bile salts are responsible for aiding in the digestion of fats through their detergent action, and are necessary for the absorption of the fat-soluble vitamins A, D, K, and E. Without vitamin K, prothrombin and other vitamins K–dependent clotting factors cannot be synthesized by the liver, resulting in bleeding disorders. (It is necessary to monitor the prothrombin time to notice vitamin K deficiency before it manifests as clinical bleeding.) However, there is no evidence of efficacy in replacement therapy for bile deficiencies. The major indication today is as a laxative. The usual dosage of bile extract is 150–600 mg/day in capsules or tablets.

An individual with a partial biliary obstruction, biliary fistulas, or who is recovering from liver or gallbladder surgery may need bile supplements. *Hydrochloretics* are agents that increase the amount of high–water content, low-viscosity bile. These agents do not increase the amount of bile produced, and are not as effective as natural bile in promoting normal bile functions. Hydrochloretics (ketocholanic acids and dehydrocholic acid) are indicated for temporary relief of constipation and as adjunctive therapy in the conditions mentioned above (See Table 54–1 for dosing information).

Digestants in combination with other preparations are also available. Combination digestants are featured in Table 54–2.

ANTIDIARRHEALS

A common malady is diarrhea, a term used to describe an acute or chronic condition of excess water elimination from the bowel. It is difficult to conceive of an older or more universal scourge than diarrhea. The average normal weight of the stool passed each day usually ranges from 200–400 g, of which 60%–65% is water. If diarrhea is present, the stools increase in water content, increasing the number of stools each day. When the number of liquid stools approaches ten per day, perianal irritation causes the patient discomfort. Associated with diarrhea is cramping from intermittent spasm of the intestine, as well as distention from gas production caused by rapid fermentation occurring in the bowel. Hyperactive bowel sounds are usually present. The nature and consistency of the stool, and the presence of blood and mucus, are determined, particularly when the diarrhea is severe.

Acute diarrhea can result from infection, gastrointestinal disease, a change in diet, nervousness and anxiety, allergic reaction, intoxication, or as the side effect of a medication. In the United States, the most common causes of brief acute episodes of diarrhea are probably viruses, protozoa, or enterotoxin-producing *E. coli.* Symptoms associated with acute diarrhea often include fever, headache, anorexia, vomiting, malaise, myalgia and can persist for one to three days. Diarrhea can be chronic, as part of a malabsorption syndrome, inflammation of the bowel, endocrine dysfunction, or, periodically, certain rare hormone-producing neoplasms. Any episode of diarrhea causes water and electrolyte depletion, which can lead to dehydration and electrolyte imbalance. The very young and the very elderly are more likely to develop these symptoms quickly, and the effects may become life-threatening because of the body's inability to compensate.

Table 54–2. COMBINATION DRUGS FOR DIGESTANTS

Combination Drugs	Basic Products							
	A	B	C	D	E	F	G	Other
Cholan-HMB Tablets					8			250 V 2.5 W
Cotazym-B Tablets	4,000	15,000	15,000	2				65 H
Donnazyme Tablets					8.1	300	150	150 N 0.0518 X 0.0097 Y 0.0033 LL
Entozyme Tablets						300	250	150 N
Festalan Tablets	6,000	30,000	20,000					1 DD
Kanulase Tablets	1,000	1,000	12,000	9			150	100 K 200 EE
Phazyme Tablets (enteric coated)					8.1	300	150	60 FF 0.2885 W 0.0519 X 0.0033 LL
Phazyme-PB Tablets (enteric coated)	240	2,000	3,000		15			60 FF

Basic products: A = lipase, units; B = amylase, units; C = protease, units; D = cellulose, mg; E = phenobarbital, mg; F = pancreatin, mg; G = pepsin, mg; H = mixed conjugated bile salts, mg; K = ox bile extract, mg; N = bile salts, mg; V = dehydrocholic acid, mg; W = homatropine methylbromide, mg; X = hyoscyamine sulfate, mg; Y = atropine sulfate, mg; DD = atropine methylnitrate, mg; EE = glutamic acid hydrochloride, mg; FF = simethicone, mg; LL = scopolamine HBR, mg.

Diarrhea is usually a self-limiting condition. Diagnostic testing is rarely necessary if diarrhea lasts less than three days. However, if symptoms persist beyond three days, a diagnostic work-up should be done to determine the cause. Treatment for acute diarrhea is optional and in some cases may even prolong the course of an enteric infection. Symptomatic treatment of severe acute or chronic diarrhea is justified to provide temporary relief until the cause is identified.

Diarrhea can be treated with antidiarrheal preparations, which act either locally in the bowel, or systemically to decrease the number, consistency, and fluidity of the stool. To date, there is no absolute clinical evidence that substantiates antidiarrheals' threapeutic effect in curing the underlying disease causing diarrhea. However, these drugs do reduce the number of stools and, therefore, reduce the interference with daily activities. Antidiarrheals are useful for symptomatic control of both acute and chronic diarrhea, and diarrhea secondary to radiation or gastrointestinal surgery, or to decrease the volume of intestinal discharge in patients with ileostomies and colostomies. If symptoms of acute diarrhea have not improved, or fever persists, or blood or mucus appears in the stool, antidiarrheals should be discontinued. Local antidiarrheals include adsorbents, astringents, and intestinal flora modifiers, which help replace the normal bacterial flora. The bacterial flora modifiers, adsorbents, and astringents are of questionable benefit as antidiarrheals. The majority of these preparations are OTC drugs easily obtainable by the general public and safe, but their effectiveness is debatable; most researchers feel that a patient experiencing diarrhea would improve even if left untreated by these preparations. Table 54–3 features the common local-acting antidiarrheals.

The systemically acting antidiarrheals are generally more effective than locally acting agents, having both antispasmodic and antiperistaltic properties. These include the opiates (opium, paregoric, and codeine); synthetic opiate products diphenoxylate (Lomotil) and loperamide (Imodium), and the natural belladonna alkaloid anticholinergics (Donnagel and Donnagel PG).

Another group of medications that can be used in the treatment of diarrhea includes antibiotics, generally used in acute infectious diarrhea. Antibiotics are discussed in Chapter 46.

Locally Acting Antidiarrheals

Locally acting antidiarrheals act locally on the bowel wall to soothe and reduce irritation of the mucous lin-

Table 54–3. LOCALLY ACTING ANTIDIARRHEALS

Medication	Dosage	Type	Interactions	Comments
Kaolin with pectin (Kaopectate) Components: 5.85 g kaolin; 139 mg pectin/ml.	60–120 ml after each bowel movement.	A,D	For all antidiarrheals: Many medications are absorbed by antidiarrheals when given concurrently, including digoxin, quinidine, and antibiotics. This can be eliminated by separating the doses by 2 hours.	Decrease fluidity but total water loss seems unchanged. Given in large doses after each loose bowel movement.
Kaopectate Concentrate	45–90 ml	A,D	Same as above.	Same as above.
Bismuth subsalicylate (Pepto-Bismol)	30 ml or 2 tabs.	A,As	Same as above.	Contraindicated in people allergic to salicylates or taking coumarin products. Dose is 30 ml or 2 tablets dissolved or chewed every 30 min to 1 hour up to 8 doses.
Cholestyramine	4 g (pc)	A	Same as above.	Must be diluted with fruit juice and administered not less than 2 hours before meals to lessen the chance of it binding with fat-soluble vitamins and other minerals.
Lactobacillus acidophilus (Bacid) Components: 100 mg Na and carboxymethylcellulose	2 caps bid–qid	R	Same as above.	Fruity odor may be apparent in stools during administration. Should be administered with milk.
Lactinex	1 packet or 4 tablets tid-qid	R	Same as above.	Tablets or granules need to be refrigerated. Can be sprinkled on food.
Activated attapulgite (Rheaban)	750 mg/tablet	A	Same as above.	Administer 2 tablets after each bowel movement.
Psyllium (Metamucil, Cillium, Correctol, Konsyl, and many others)	1 rounded tsp in water, 1–3× daily.	A	Same as above.	Bulk-producing laxative absorbs excess fluid and ultimately controls diarrhea. Comes as plain or flavored. Mix in 8 oz. of water; follow with 8 oz. of water. Drink immediately. May be more palatable if mixed with milk or juice. Has 14 calories/dose.
Methylcellulose (Cologel, Citrucel) Components: 450 mg methylcellulose in 5 ml 5% EDTH.	5–20 ml tid with water	D	Same as above.	Take with a full glass of water. Citrucel is less gritty, good taste. High in calories.

Table 54–3. LOCALLY ACTING ANTIDIARRHEALS–*CONTINUED*

Medication	Dosage	Type	Interactions	Comments
Polycarbophil	1–1.5 mg	A	Same as above.	Safe and effective for treating mild diarrhea; absorbs water and bile salts. Safe and effective for treating constipation also as it opposes the dehydrating forces of the bowel.

A = adsorbent; D = demulcent; R = intestinal flora modifiers; As = astringent.

ing. There are two forms: adsorbents, which may also have a soothing (*demulcent*) effect on the irritated mucous membrane, and intestinal flora replacements. All of these preparations can be purchased OTC.

ADSORBENTS. These agents have the nonspecific ability of binding to gas, toxins, and irritants. Thus, adsorbents inactivate toxins and bind them until they are excreted. Adsorbents also adsorb normal enzymes and nutrients from the bowel. Adsorbents contribute to the adhesion of the stool but do not necessarily stop or control diarrhea. The most commonly used adsorbents not requiring a prescription include kaolin and pectin, activated charcoal, salts of bismuth, and attapulgite. All have the advantage of being nontoxic and inexpensive. Some adsorbents have an additional demulcent effect, including the salts of bismuth, and kaolin and pectin. Because of the large amounts of adsorbents that are taken after each loose bowel movement, constipation is often a side effect of these agents.

All of the medications that act as adsorbents have a tendency to also absorb other concurrently administered medications such as digoxin, quinidine, and antibiotics. This possible drug interaction can be made less likely by separating the administration of any drug and the antidiarrheal adsorbent by at least two hours.

Adsorbents currently are thought to cause more fluid and electrolyte loss than if the diarrhea was not treated at all. Research has also indicated that adsorbents can cause bowel obstructions. Adsorbents may also give both the patient and medical personnel a false sense of security by increasing the fecal mass. At this time, there is little literature to support their effectiveness or use.

Kaolin and Pectin. Kaolin, a natural aluminum silicate clay, has been used for hundreds of years to treat diarrhea. Kaolin (5.85 g) is often mixed with pectin (130 mg) in every 30 ml of Kaopectate, which acts as both an adsorbent and a demulcent. Kaopectate must be given in large doses after each loose bowel movement. Often, constipation results from the use of Kaopectate. The usual dose of Kaopectate is 60–120 ml after each loose bowel movement. A variant preparation is Kaopectate Concentrate, a mint-flavored liquid that combines 8.78 g kaolin and 195 mg pectin in each 30 ml; the dosage is 45–90 ml after each loose bowel movement. Currently,

kaolin and pectin are not recognized as effective by the FDA.

Activated Charcoal. Activated charcoal, a powder, is probably the most effective adsorbent of toxins and irritants, but it does not necessarily control diarrhea. It is used mostly as an antidote for certain types of poisonings.

Bismuth Subsalicylate. The bismuth salts are relatively insoluble compounds with adsorbent, demulcent, astringent, and weak antacid properties. Research suggests that the bismuth salts remove gas, toxins (*E. Coli* and *Vibrio cholerae*), bacteria, and viruses from the intestinal tract by adsorption. The bismuth salts can be used to treat diarrhea, enteritis, dysentery, and ulcerations of the bowel, and sometimes as a local protectant for the skin.

Bismuth subsalicylate (Pepto-Bismol) is hydrolyzed to liberate salicylate and is contraindicated in patients allergic to them and in patients taking coumarin products as anticoagulants. A 2-ounce dose of bismuth salts can produce the same salicylate blood level as one 5-gr aspirin tablet.

Attapulgite. Some research claims attapulgite (Reabon, DiarKote) to be superior to kaolin in its absorptive abilities for bacteria, viruses, and toxins. Prolonged use of attapulgite may interfere with intestinal adsorption of nutrients, resulting in constipation. Several OTC products are available and are described in Table 54–3.

Cholestyramine. Cholestyramine (Questran) has a direct affinity for acidic materials such as bile acids and the toxin *Clostridium difficile*. Cholestyramine relieves diarrhea due to excessive bile salts and may be effective for antibiotic-induced pseudomembranous colitis. It is administered most commonly to patients with high cholesterol levels. The powder is diluted in juice or mixed with fruit and administered not less than two hours before meals or ingestion of drugs, to lessen the chances of binding with fat-soluble vitamins and other materials. It is described in more detail in Chapter 32.

INTESTINAL FLORA MODIFIERS. The bowel is filled with many different bacteria, which help to break down and digest food. Often, in patients receiving antibiotic therapy (ampicillin particularly), many of these bacteria are destroyed, causing diarrhea. The growth of normal intestinal flora can be encouraged when the patient ingests *Lactobacillus acidophilus* found in Bacid or Lactinex, both OTC preparations, or acidophilus tablets, sweet acidophilus milk, or unpasteurized yogurt. The presence of this bacillus also allows the growth of *Escherichia coli*, another normal bacterium found in the bowel. Well-controlled studies to support the use of these products are needed.

To assist in the treatment of diarrhea, particularly secondary to antibiotic therapy, the diet can also be increased in carbohydrates containing lactose and dextrose—milk, buttermilk, and yogurt, all of which are equally effective in recolonizing the intestine. However, some antibiotics may cause a lactose intolerance. Recent research has indicated that diet therapy may be more effective than actual ingestion of the Lactobacillus organism. Diarrhea secondary to antibiotic therapy is often difficult to control during the time the patient is receiving the antibiotic. However, when the antibiotics are discontinued, the diarrhea subsides in several days.

Lactinex. Lactinex (*Lactobacillus acidophilus* and *bulgaricus*) is available as both tablets and granules, which can be sprinkled on food. Lactinex is stored in the refrigerator. The usual dosage is one packet of granules or four tablets taken three to four times daily.

Bacid. Bacid contains *Lactobacillus acidophilus* in sodium carboxymethylcellulose. Bacid capsules are administered two to four times daily, and a fruity odor may be apparent in the stool while the patient is taking Bacid.

Systemically Acting Antidiarrheals

The systemically acting antidiarrheals are much more effective than the locally acting preparations in treating and controlling diarrhea (Table 54–4). These have both antispasmodic and antiperistaltic properties and are available only with a physician's prescription. Systemically acting diarrheals are derivatives of either opium or belladonna—both natural and synthetic preparations. Opium is habit-forming and is used only for short-term therapy; generally, the prescription is not refillable.

OPIUM PRODUCTS. Opium products (Chapter 20) directly act on the gastrointestinal system to decrease intestinal motility, thus leading to constipation. Opiates also increase tone of smooth muscles and sphincters in the gastrointestinal tract. Because there is a delay in transit time, intestinal contents are permitted greater contact time with the intestinal mucosa, which permits an increase in the reabsorption of water and electrolytes, and thus interacts with central opiate receptors that regulate intestinal motility. Opiates also reduce the cramping associated with diarrhea. Most opiates are used to control pain, but a major adverse effect is constipation. This adverse effect is advantageously used to treat an individual with diarrhea. Morphine is very effective in treating severe cases of diarrhea, but because of its potential for additional effects, it is not commonly used. The opium preparations in current general use include paregoric tincture and codeine.

It is recommended that opioids be avoided in acute diarrhea caused by antibiotics, poisons, infectious organisms, or exotoxins until it can be assumed that the toxic material has been eliminated.

Paregoric Tincture. Paregoric contains 2 mg morphine per 5 ml and 45% alcohol. It is administered to adults in 5- to 10-ml doses. Children receive 0.25–0.5 ml/kg of body weight. By itself, it is a class III controlled substance; but when mixed with other products (Parepectolin, Parelixir, DIA-Quel), it becomes a class V product. (See Chapter 2 for more detail on drug classification.)

Parepectolin Suspension. Parepectolin suspension, a class V medication, is a combination of 15 mg of opium (equivalent to 3.7 mg paregoric/30 ml), kaolin (5.5 gm), pectin (162 mg), and alcohol (0.69%). The usual dose is 15–30 ml after each loose stool.

Parelixir. Parelixir, a class V medication, combines 0.2 ml tincture of opium/30 ml with pectin (4.8 mg/ml) in an alcohol elixir (18%) and is fruit-flavored. The usual dose is 15–30 ml three or four times daily.

DIA-Quel. A class V medication, DIA-Quel, combines 18 mg of opium, homatropine (0.9 mg), pectin (144 mg), in an alcohol (10%) base for every 30 ml of cherry-flavored DIA-Quel. The usual dose is 15–30 ml three or four times daily.

Codeine. Codeine has effective antidiarrheal properties. It is administered four times daily in 15- to 60-mg doses.

SYNTHETIC OPIATES. Two derivatives of the synthetic opiate meperidine (Demerol)—diphenoxylate hydrochloride (Lomotil) and loperamide (Imodium)—are less addictive, while still retaining the antidiarrheal effect common to the opiates. Lomotil also contains a small amount of atropine, which in high doses causes undesirable side effects such as nausea, vomiting, dry mouth, and blurred vision. Atropine, therefore, discourages potential abuse of diphenoxylate, arising from the morphine-like euphoria that results. However, even with atropine sulfate, habituation can still occur. These preparations are as effective as paregoric. Because both Lomotil and Imodium are available in tablet/capsule form and are less addictive, they have almost totally replaced paregoric as an antidiarrheal preparation. Lomotil and Imodium are classified as class V drugs. Both agents act directly on the intestinal smooth muscle to decrease transit time.

These products, as well as narcotics, should not be administered to patients with infectious diarrhea caused by bacteria (*E. coli, Salmonella,* or *Shigella*), parasites (*Giardia lambia*), or viruses (parvovirus or reovirus), because these causative agents should be eliminated in the feces. These agents should also not be used with antibiotic-induced pseudomembranous colitis (especially clindamycin and lincomycin) because the irritating agent *Clostridium difficile* and its toxins will be retained in the bowel.

Diphenoxylate Hydrochloride with Atropine. Diphenoxylate hydrochloride with atropine (Lomotil, Logen, Low-Quel, Lonox, and many others) limit peristalsis by inhibiting mucosal receptors which abolishes the local mucosal peristaltic reflex.

Pharmacokinetics. Diphenoxylate has a short duration of action, a half-life of 12–14 hours. Half of the total daily dose of diphenoxylate is excreted as metabolites (some are active metabolites) in the urine within 96 hours. An additional 49% is found in the feces. The liver metabolizes as well as recycles this medication. Trace amounts are found in breast milk.

Contraindications and Precautions. Diphenoxylate is contraindicated in any patient hypersensitive to its ingredients, obstructive jaundice, glaucoma (because it contains atropine), or diarrhea associated with pseudomembranous enterocolitis. It should be given cautiously to patients with abnormal liver function studies (as this is the site of metabolism), to addicted persons, and to patients with ulcerative colitis. Safety has not been established in pregnancy. Administer with caution to children and nursing mothers. Since diphenoxylate may cause drowsiness, patients are cautioned about driving or performing tasks requiring alertness.

Adverse Effects. Adverse effects of diphenoxylate include nausea, vomiting, sedation, and vertigo. Since it also contains atropine, such adverse effects as dry mouth and blurred vision may occur, although these are rare in the low doses that are used. Diphenoxylate also can contribute to the development of paralytic ileus.

Interactions. Diphenoxylate may potentiate the CNS-depressant effects of alcohol, barbiturates, and tranquilizers when given concurrently. The patient taking these products needs to be closely observed. Long-term use has resulted in dependence. Opiate dependence can be by the CNS, as seen with heroin addicts, or by the gastrointestinal system, as seen with loss of bowel regularity without opiates. There is great potential for serious intoxication in children, from as few as six tablets. Parents must keep this medication out of the reach of children.

Dosage. Diphenoxylate is administered to adults in tablet or liquid form in dosage of about 5 ml or 1 2.5-mg tablet four times a day. In children, the dosage is generally a 2-mg tablet, or 4 ml, administered from three to five times daily (see Table 54–4). A tablet or liquid dose contains 2.5 mg diphenoxylate and 0.025 mg atropine sulfate and is equivalent to the antidiarrheal effect achieved from 4 ml of paregoric.

Loperamide Hydrochloride. Loperamide hydrochloride (Imodium) is a synthetic opioid for oral antidiarrheal use. It is similar in chemical structure to haloperidol (Haldol) and diphenoxylate. This product has both a direct cholinergic effect and other effects on the neuronal pathways in the intestine, which slow intestinal motility and improve absorption of water and electrolytes.

Pharmacokinetics. Research indicates that peak plasma levels are achieved five hours after the initial dose. Plasma half-life ranges from 9.1–14.4 hours. Elimination ocurs in both the feces (25%) and the urine (1.3%).

Contraindications and Precautions. Loperamide hydrochloride is contraindicated in persons hypersensitive to its ingredients, and should also be given cautiously to pregnant and lactating women and to children under two years.

Adverse Effects. The adverse effects of loperamide hydrochloride are generally minor and self-limiting and include abdominal pain, drowsiness, dry mouth, constipation, gastrointestinal irritation, nausea, and vomiting,

and central nervous system depression. Naloxone (Narcan), a short-acting narcotic antagonist, may be administered to reverse these effects. Due to loperamide hydrochloride's long duration of action, the nurse must closely monitor the patient for at least 24 hours.

Dosage. The initial dose of loperamide hydrochloride for acute diarrhea is 4 mg, with an additional 2 mg administered after each loose stool, not to exceed 16 mg (eight capsules) per day. Once the acute diarrhea has been controlled, the medication is administered twice daily. For pediatric dosing, see Table 54–4.

ANTICHOLINERGIC PREPARATIONS. The belladonna alkaloids, classified as anticholinergic agents, include atropine, hyoscine, and hyoscyamine. There is no conclusive evidence that medications in this class actually exert a selective effect on the gastrointestinal system to control diarrhea, but they do prevent the spasms and cramping frequently associated with acute or chronic diarrhea if a sufficient dose is given. Extreme caution must be taken in administering these preparations to patients sensitive to anticholinergic effects. The patient with ulcerative colitis receiving the belladonna alkaloids may develop paralytic ileus or toxic megacolon when treated with doses large enough to control motility.

Donnagel and Donnagel PG. Donnagel and Donnagel PG are antidiarrheal mixtures containing absorbents and protectants. Donnagel and Donnagel PG are frequently prescribed by physicians and used by lay people to provide some degree of symptomatic relief. Since there are so many ingredients in these products, the patient may be exposed to added expense and combined adverse effects. Single-ingredient drugs are still recommended to control specific symptoms.

Donnagel contains alcohol 3.8%, kaolin 6 g, pectin 142.8 mg, atropine 0.194 mg, hyoscyamine sulfate 0.1037 mg, and scopolamine hydrobromide 0.065 mg in each 30 ml. Donnagel is administered in a 30-ml dose after the first loose stool and then 15–30 ml after each loose bowel movement.

Donnagel PG contains 24 mg powdered opium, 6 g kaolin, 142.8 mg pectin, 0.0137 mg hyoscyamine, 0.0194 mg atropine, 0.0065 mg scopolamine in a 5% alcohol base in each 30 ml. The usual dose is 30 ml after the first loose stool and 15 ml every three hours thereafter as needed for the loose stools.

Because of the addition of atropine and hyoscyamine sulfate, both medications are contraindicated in narrow-angle glaucoma and intestinal obstruction as these conditions are worsened and in persons hypersensitive to their ingredients. Both are given cautiously to patients with urinary tract obstruction because of their ability to cause obstructive uropathy; and to patients with cardiac and respiratory diseases.

ANTIBIOTICS. Antibiotic medications used for the specific treatment of acute infectious diarrhea include antibacterial agents—sulfonamides, neomycin, chloramphenicol, ampicillin, and tetracyclines; and antiprotozoal agents—metronidazole (Flagyl) and chloroquine (Aralen). It is important to obtain a stool culture to iso-

TEXT RESUMES ON PAGE 1494

Table 54–4. SYSTEMIC ACTING ANTIDIARRHEALS

Name	Dosage	Mode of Administration	Pharmacokinetics
Action: slow GI motility prolonging transient time **Use:** diarrhea			
Paregoric	Adults: 5–10 ml qid. Children: 0.25–0.5 ml/kg body weight qid.	PO	O: 15–20 min P: 0.5–1 hr D: 4–5 hr ½L: 3 hr PB: UA B: UA E: UA
Diphenoxylate hydrochloride and atropine sulfate (Lomotil)	5 ml (tablet or liquid) qid. Children: 13–20 kg = 2 mg tid; 20–27 kg = 2 mg qid; 27–36 kg = 2 mg 5×/day.	PO	O: 45–60 min P: 2 hr D: 3–4 hr ½L: 2.5 hr (3–14 hr active metabolites) PB: UA B: liver E: feces 49%, urine 14%
Loperamide (Imodium)	4 mg initially, then 2 mg after each loose bowel movement, up to 16 mg/day. Children: 20 kg or less 1 mg tid; 21 kg or more 2 mg bid-tid.	PO	O: 1 hr P: 4–5 hr (capsules); 2.5 hr (liq) D: 10 hr ½L: 9.1–14.4 hr PB: UA B: liver E: feces 25%, urine 13%
Donnagel	30 ml initially, with 15–30 ml after each loose stool. Children: 10 ml initially, with 5–10 ml after each loose stool.	PO	O: 15–20 min P: NA D: NA ½L: NA PB: NA B: NA E: NA
Donnagel PG	30 ml, then 15 ml every 3 hr. Children up to 6 yr: dosage must be individualized by a physician. Children over 6 yr: 10 ml initially, followed by 5–10 ml q 3 hr, up to 4 doses/24 hr.	PO	O: 15–20 min P: NA D: 3–4 hr ½L: UA PB: UA B: UA E: UA

Key to Abbreviations in the *Pharmacokinetics* column O-onset; P-peak; D-duration; PB-protein bound; B-biotransformed in; E-excreted in; ½ L-halflife.
*Within the column listing adverse effects, <u>underlines</u> indicate the most common effects; CAPITALS indicate life-threatening effects.

Contraindications/ Precautions	Adverse Effects*	Interactions	Nursing Implications
Contraindicated in hypersensitivity to opiates, diarrhea caused by poisons. Use cautiously in asthma, hepatic disease, severe prostatic hypertrophy. Safety during pregnancy and in infants less than 1 month has not been established.	Neuro: dizziness, CNS depression CV: sweating RESP: respiratory depression GI: nausea, vomiting, constipation Misc: physical dependence	Potentiates all other CNS depressants.	**For all antidiarrheals:** ASSESSMENT: Determine cause of diarrhea. Assess number and color of stools. Assess fluid and electrolyte balance and daily weights. INTERVENTION: Give with sufficient water to allow medication to enter the stomach. If relief is not obtained within 48 hours, medication should be discontinued and patient hospitalized to determine cause of diarrhea.
Contraindicated in hypersensitivity, obstructive jaundice, glaucoma, and children under age 2. Use cautiously in abnormal liver function, addicted persons, and ulcerative colitis. Safety has not been established in pregnancy.	Neuro: dizziness, drowsiness, sedation, headache, malaise, lethargy, restlessness CV: tachycardia GI: dry mouth, anorexia, nausea, vomiting, abdominal discomfort, PARALYTIC ILEUS, TOXIC MEGACOLON, swelling gums Biliary: pancreatitis Integ: pruritis, urticaria	Potentiates CNS side effects of barbiturates, tranquilizers.	Same as above plus. INTERVENTION: Caution patient about performing tasks requiring alertness. May cause drowsiness. EVALUATION: Notify physician if diarrhea persists.
Contraindicated in hypersensitivity. Administer cautiously to pregnant and lactating women, and children under age 2.	Minor and self-limiting. Neuro: drowsiness, dizziness GI: abdominal pain, distension, constipation, dry mouth, nausea, vomiting Integ: rash	None known.	Same as above.
Contraindicated in narrow-angle glaucoma, intestinal obstruction, hypersensitivity. Use cautiously in urinary tract obstruction and prostatic hypertrophy.	Neuro: blurred vision GI: dry mouth Integ: flushing, dry skin	None known.	Same as above.
Same as above.	Same as above.	None known.	Same as above plus: INTERVENTION: Donnagel PG contains opium and is a class V drug.

late the causative agent before any of these medications is prescribed, especially to the very young and the elderly patient. Often, while waiting for the results of the culture, broad-spectrum antibiotics such as tetracyclines are prescribed. The most common causes of acute infectious diarrhea include *Salmonella* species, *Shigella* species, *Vibrio parahaemolyticus*, and certain strains of *Escherichia coli*. For short-term diarrhea secondary to *Salmonella*, anti-infectives may not actually be necessary and in fact may increase the amount of time the individual "carries" *Salmonella*; *Salmonella* organisms usually cause a self-limiting infection, which usually clears in several days with fluid and electrolyte replacement. However, more prolonged, systemic, or severe infections call for anti-infective therapy. Appropriate therapy to prevent dehydration and electrolyte imbalance is always undertaken.

Travelers' diarrhea, often associated with ingestion of the food and water in a foreign country, may be caused by certain strains of *E. coli*. It frequently is accompanied by cramps, nausea, vomiting, headache, and fever of several days' duration, which can be relieved by prophylactic antibiotics such as trimethoprim/sulfamethoxazole (Bactrim) once daily, doxycycline (Vibramycin) once daily, ciprofloxacin hydrochloride 500 mg every 12 hours, or bismuth subsalicylate (Pepto-Bismol) 60 ml four times daily; or a simple antispasmodic and antiperistaltic agent.

Specific causes of infective diarrhea are generally treated with the specific medications (Table 54–5). Consult the Index to locate more detailed coverage of these medications in this text.

Antidiarrheal agents are often combined with other preparations. Table 54–6 features combination antidiarrheals. Polycarbophil should be included as an antidiarrheal. Indeed, it is one of only two agents (along with opiates) that the FDA recognizes as effective in the management of diarrhea.

POLYCARBOPHIL. Polycarbophil (FiberCon, Mitrolan) is a hydrophilic agent that actually retains free water within the intestinal lumen, indirectly opposes dehydration, and promotes well-formed stool when the patient has constipation. When the patient has diarrhea, polycarbophil absorbs free fecal water, forming a gel, and produces a formed stool. Thus, polycarbophil can be used to manage both constipation and diarrhea.

Dosage is individualized, with the average adult dose ranging from 1–6 g within a 24-hour period.

LAXATIVES

Daily bowel movements may not be normal for everyone. Whereas some may evacuate their bowels daily, for others every two, three, or even four days is normal regularity. Constipation is the occurrence of hard, dry stool that lacks sufficient water to allow it to be passed easily. The majority of laxatives are self-prescribed for treatment of what individuals perceive to be constipation. Some people become neurotically preoccupied with bowel habits and use laxatives habitually. Because laxatives are generally available over the counter, laxative abuse is a major health problem.

Table 54–5. COMMON INFECTIVE DIARRHEA AND SPECIFIC MEDICATIONS

Type or Causative Organism	Medication
Escherichia coli	Neomycin Ciprofloxacin Colistin sulfate (Coly-mycin S) Trimethoprim/sulfamethoxazole (Bactrim)
Shigella	Ampicillin Erythromycin
Pseudomonal enterocolitis	Gentamicin Polymyxin B
Coagulase-positive staphylococcal enterocolitis	Vancomycin (Vancocin) Ciprofloxacin
Acute amebic dysentery	Metronidazole (Flagyl) Tetracyclines
Travelers' diarrhea	Ciprofloxacin Doxycycline (Vibramycin) Ampicillin Trimethoprim/sulfamethoxazole (Bactrim)
Salmonellae	Ampicillin

Uses

Laxative, or cathartic, medications, available both OTC and by prescription, accelerate the passage of feces through the bowel. Their use may be necessary to treat constipation; to prepare patients for diagnostic tests (see Chapter 9) or surgery; to prevent or decrease colonic absorption of ammonia in patients with hepatic encephalopathy; to hasten the excretion of various parasites or poisons from the intestinal tract; in children with congenital or acquired megacolon; in geriatric patients with poor muscle tone; to provide fresh stool for parasitologic exam; to empty bowel before surgery, colonoscopy, or barium enema; and to modify the effluent in patients with an ileostomy or colostomy. Physicians, in full recognition of dependency formation, may order laxatives for patients with congenital decreased bowel activity, or for geriatric clients with chronic atonic constipation.

Formerly, laxatives were classified according to the consistency of stool resulting from their use:

1. Laxatives at one time were limited to those that caused a few formed stools with no cramping;
2. Cathartics were drugs that caused a few more stools than laxatives; and
3. Purgatives were medications that caused many liquid stools with frequent cramping.

Table 54–6. COMBINATION DRUGS FOR ANTIDIARRHEALS

Combination Drugs	A	B	C	D	E	F	G	Other
Corrective Mixture with Paregoric	10	22	85	45	2/5 ml			85Q 1.8H
Donnagel Suspension					3.8/30 ml	6	142.8	0.1037 I 0.0194 J 0.0065 K
Donnagel-PG					5/30 ml	6	142.8	0.1037 I 0.0194 J 0.0065 K 24 L
Kapectolin						5.85	130	
Kenpectin-P						5.85	195	16.27 M 650/30 ml N
Parepectolin					0.69/30 ml	5.5	162	15 M
Polymagma							45	500 O
Rheaban								750 O
Diar-Aid							150	750 O

Basic products: A = zinc sulfocarbolate, mg; B = phenyl salicylate, mg; C = bismuth subsalicylate, mg; D = pepsin, mg; E = alcohol, %; F = kaolin, g; G = pectin, mg; H = paregoric, ml; I = hyoscyamine sulfate, mg; J = atropine sulfate, mg; K = scopolamine hydrobromide; O = attapulgite, mg; Q = subsalicylate, mg.

A more manageable and useful classification system in use today is based on the mechanism of action: a contact laxative or stimulant, bulk-forming agents, saline, or osmotic cathartics, lubricants, and mineral oil; and several miscellaneous agents (Table 54–7 and Fig. 54–1). All of these groups of medications are discussed individually in the following sections and are featured in Table 54–8.

Action

Laxatives promote bowel evacuation by promoting net fluid accumulation within the bowel lumen by a hydrophilic effect, an osmotic action, and/or a direct action on mucosal cells to decrease absorption and/or enhance secretion of water and electrolytes.

Contraindications and Precautions

Laxatives are contraindicated in persons hypersensitive to any ingredient, in patients who have acute symptoms of appendicitis, acute abdomen, intestinal obstruction, or undiagnosed abdominal pain, and in patients suspected of having a fecal impaction. Administer laxatives cautiously to persons who may develop fluid and electrolyte imbalances such as the elderly, small children, and persons that are acutely ill. Preparations containing sodium are given cautiously to patients with cardiac or

Table 54–7. CLASSIFICATION OF LAXATIVES BY MECHANISM OF ACTION

Types of Laxatives
Contact Laxative Stimulant Bisacodyl (Dulcolax) Castor oil Cascara sagrada Docusate calcium (Surfak) Docusate potassium (Dialose) Docusate sodium (Colace) Senna products
Bulk-Forming Agents Plantago seed (psyllium seed) Psyllium hydrophilic mucilloid (Metamucil)
Saline or Osmotic Cathartics Magnesium salts Sodium salts Potassium salts
Lubricants Mineral oil

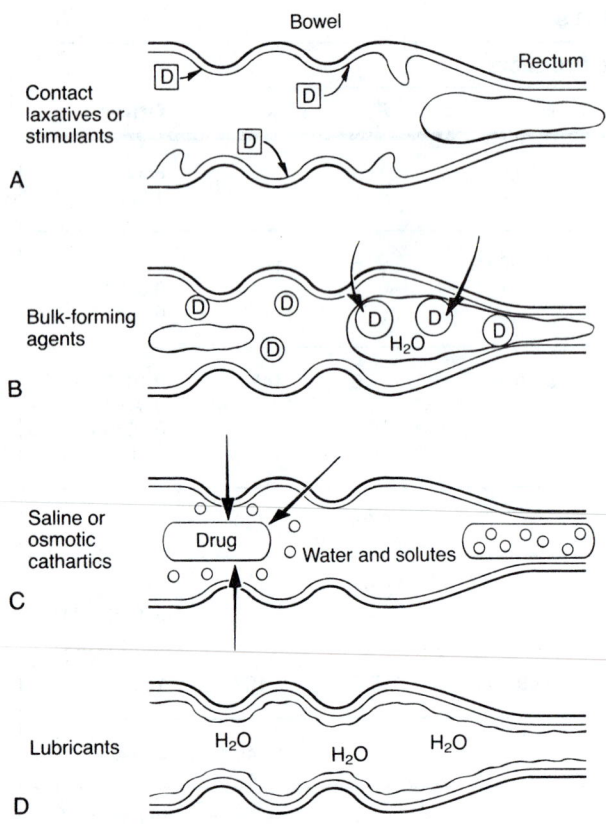

Figure 54–1. Mechanism of action of laxatives. *A*, Contact laxatives stimulate the intestinal wall thus producing an increase in peristalsis. *B*, Bulk-forming agents absorb water into the fecal contents, giving more bulk to the stool. *C*, Saline or osmotic cathartics are osmotically active and pull solutes and water into the bowel, thus increasing intestinal contents and bulk. *D*, Lubricants lubricate and soften the intestinal contents as well as retard water absorption.

renal diseases due to the possibility of sodium retention. Products containing magnesium or calcium are also administered cautiously to patients with renal disease, as these electrolytes may be retained.

Adverse Effects

All laxatives are capable of causing excessive bowel activity such as diarrhea, nausea, and vomiting. The frequent stools may cause perianal irritation. Patients may also experience abdominal cramps, bloating, and flatulence. Specific adverse effects for each drug can be found in Table 54–7.

CONTACT/STIMULANT LAXATIVES. The contact/stimulant laxatives are all obtained from the bark, seed pods, leaves, and roots of a number of plants including cascara, senna, rhubarb, and aloe. Rhubarb and aloe are rarely used today because of their excessive irritating properties. Contact/stimulant laxatives produce an increase in peristalsis when either the laxative itself or its breakdown products come in contact with the wall of the small or large intestine. The contact/stimulant ca-

thartics also release prostaglandins and cause an increase in the mucosal concentration of cyclic 3',5'-adenosine monophosphate (cAMP), which in turn increases secretion of electrolytes and may contribute to the total cathartic effect. Specifically, bisacodyl (Dulcolax, Dacodyl, Deficol, and others), phenolphthalein, and three anthraquinone-containing laxatives, cascara, and senna, are believed to stimulate the submucosal and mysenteric plexus. Caster oil directly stimulates small intestine smooth muscle and inhibits water and electrolyte reabsorption from the intestinal lumen. It also acts as a hypertonic fluid within the bowel by drawing more water into the feces and providing a bulk-forming function. Glycerin suppositories stimulate the rectal mucosa. Docusate salts are presumed to soften the feces by an emollient action that reduces surface tension, thus permitting penetration of the fecal mass by intestinal fluids. These products may also inhibit water absorption in the jejunum and colon.

The contact/stimulant laxatives are often abused; therefore, they should not be used regularly for longer than one week. The continuous use of these laxatives can produce irritable bowel–like diarrhea that is often severe enough to cause fluid and electrolyte imbalances.

Contraindications and Precautions. Castor oil is contraindicated in pregnancy as its irritant effect may induce premature labor. Castor oil is also contraindicated in infestations of fat soluble *vermifuge.* Stimulant laxatives are given cautiously to persons with anal and rectal fissures. The anthraquinone-containing product, cascara, should not be given to lactating mothers, because this medication is excreted in breast milk. The contact/stimulant laxatives are rarely used in children.

Adverse Effects. The adverse effects of the stimulant laxatives include mild cramping, nausea, vomiting, diarrhea, and even dehydration in certain individuals. Patients receiving bisacodyl (Dulcolax) in rectal suppositories may also complain of rectal burning. Phenolphthalein can cause a mild to severe skin rash in susceptible patients, and severe systemic allergic reactions have been reported as well.

Bisacodyl. Bisacodyl (Dulcolax) is a synthetic contact/stimulant laxative. Because less than 5% is systemically absorbed and it is relatively nontoxic, it is widely used to treat various types of constipation, and to evacuate the colon before endoscopy, surgery, and radiologic examinations. Bisacodyl, an enteric-coated tablet, is soluble in neutral or alkaline solutions. It is not administered within 1 hour of an antacid, milk, or dairy products because it will then be released in the stomach where it causes severe cramping. The tablets are never chewed, and bisacodyl is administered only with water.

The oral dose is generally 10–15 mg, with as much as 30 mg given for a special procedure. The tablets take six to ten hours to act. A rectal suppository is available in 10-mg doses, and the suppositories act within 15–60 minutes. The suppositories may cause burning and itching as well as proctitis with repeated doses.

Phenolphthalein. Phenolphthalein is similar to bisacodyl in its pharmacologic properties and it acts mainly on the colon. Onset of action is within six to ten hours, with little associated pain or colic. Approximately 15% of this drug is absorbed and resecreted into the bile, which may prolong the cathartic effect for three to four days. If urine and feces are alkaline, they will turn pink-red in color. Because of its mild action and pleasant taste, it is found in many over-the-counter products such as Ex-Lax and Feen-A-Mint. The usual adult dose is a 60-mg tablet (tablets are available in two sizes, 60 and 130 mg).

Castor Oil. Castor oil, obtained from the seeds of the castor bean, is a bland, colorless, emollient glyceride. Castor oil is not as frequently used today as it was in the past because of its many adverse effects.

Because castor oil, given orally, inhibits gastric emptying as do other fatty substances, it is always administered when the stomach is empty. Upon entering the small intestine, castor oil is hydrolyzed by pancreatic lipase to glycerol and a fatty acid, ricinoleic acid. This fatty acid is thought to cause the irritation of the bowel, which, in turn, causes a rapid propulsion of contents through both the small and large intestines. Ricinoleic acid may further stimulate motor activity in the small intestine and inhibit *antiperistalsis* in the colon, also preventing normal fluid absorption from the intestinal contents. A single therapeutic dose results in several copious semiliquid stools within two to six hours, emptying the bowel completely. Because of this short action time, castor oil is administered early in the day.

Most commonly, castor oil is used to prepare the bowel for radiographic studies of the colon, and to evacuate irritants and poisons from the intestinal tract. Castor oil is generally not recommended for the relief of constipation. On occasion, castor oil can be used as a emollient and applied locally to the skin.

Castor oil should not be administered to persons with lesions in the bowel or an irritable bowel because they may be made very ill due to the oil irritating the lesions in the bowel. Castor oil is also excreted in breast milk. Castor oil is, therefore, contraindicated in persons with ulcerative colitis and in nursing mothers.

The usual adult dose is 15–60 ml. In children, 5–15 ml is given. Since the natural oil is very irritating to the stomach and is nauseating, fruit juices may be mixed with castor oil.

Cascara Sagrada. Cascara sagrada, an anthraquinone cathartic obtained from the bark of the buckthorn tree *(Rhamnus purshiana)*, is one of the most popular cathartics. Cascara sagrada is partially absorbed in the small intestine and reaches the large intestine via the blood stream as well as by passage along the gastrointestinal tract. Cascara sagrada causes propulsive movements of the colon by direct chemical irritation, which evacuates the bowel in approximately eight hours. The anthraquinone-containing stimulants, absorbed in the small intestine, circulate through the body and are excreted in bile, urine, saliva, colonic mucosa, and in the milk of lactating mothers. Because anthraquinone-containing stimulant laxatives are excreted in the urine, the patient may note a change in urine color; cascara, in particular, may tint acid urine a yellow-brown color, and alkaline urine a reddish color.

Cascara sagrada is available in three forms: as an extract, as a fluid extract, and as tablets.

Cascara sagrada extract is a powder with starch added. The usual dose is 300 mg; the range of dose is 200–400 mg.

Cascara sagrada fluid extract has alcohol added as a preservative, which gives it a very bitter taste. The usual dose is 0.5–1.5 ml.

Aromatic cascara fluid extract is treated with magnesium oxide to make it less bitter and more palatable. In addition, flavoring agents, sweeteners, and alcohol (18%) are added. Patients who are alcoholics and taking disulfiram for control should not take this medication or any other medication with alcohol added. The usual dose in adults is 5 ml (range, 5–15 ml), in children 2.5 ml, and in infants 1–2 ml. Aromatic cascara fluid extract is often mixed with milk of magnesia.

Cascara is also available as 325 mg tablets.

Senna Products. Senna products are anthraquinone derivatives prepared from the dried leaflets of *Cassia acutifolia.* They are similar to cascara sagrada, but with more potent action. Senna products are converted in the colon to active aglycones, which stimulate *Auerbach's plexus* to induce peristalsis. Senna products are available as crude drugs (Black Draught) and standardized senna concentrations (Senokot). The senna products produce bowel evacuation in six to ten hours, which may be accompanied by abdominal pain and colic.

Docusate Sodium. Docusate sodium (Dioctyl sodium sulfosuccinate) (Colace) is available as a capsule, tablet, syrup, or solution. Besides being a contact/stimulant laxative, all the docusate products are also fecal softeners. The electrolyte component of docusate—the sodium, calcium, or potassium—is not absorbed from these products. One or two days or more may be needed before a softened fecal bolus reaches the rectum. The adult (12 years and over) dosage is 50–500 mg, with a dose of over 300 mg most often being effective; and children 6–12 years 40–120 mg; 3–6 years, 20–60 mg; and under 3 years, 10–40 mg. A half glass of milk or fruit juice may be administered after the syrup or solution to help mask the taste.

Docusate sodium is also available as a disposable enema. Therevac Plus contains 283 mg of docusate sodium and 20 mg of benzocaine in a soap base.

Docusate Calcium. Docusate calcium (Surfak) is claimed to be superior to the sodium product. It is indicated in patients where only the prevention of constipation is indicated and no cathartic effect is desired. The usual dosage is one capsule (240 mg) daily.

Docusate Potassium. Docusate potassium (Dialose) is administered to adults in doses of 100–300 mg daily and to children six years and up 100 mg at bedtime.

BULK-FORMING LAXATIVES. Bulk-producing agents, including natural and semisynthetic cellulose derivatives, are made from agar, natural bran, plantago seed (psyllium seed), and methylcellulose and polycarbophil, which absorb water into the fecal contents and expand, giving more bulk to the stool. This increased

TEXT RESUMES ON PAGE 1504

Table 54–8. LAXATIVES

Name	Dosage	Onset of Action (O) Site of Action Type of Stool
Action: promote bowel evacuation by promoting net fluid accumulation with bowel lumen by a hydrophilic effect, or a direct action on the mucosal cells to decrease absorption or enhance secretion of water and electrolytes. *Use:* to treat constipation, to prepare bowel for diagnostic tests, to decrease absorption of ammonia, to hasten excretion of various parasites or poisons, and to treat megacolon or poor muscle tone in the bowel.		
Contact/Stimulant Laxatives: Bisacodyl (Dulcolax, Fleet Bisacodyl, Theralax, Dacodyl, Deficol, and others)	PO: 10–15 mg; R: 10 mg.	O: 6–10 hr C SS
Castor oil (Neoloid, Purge, Emulsoil)	Adult: 15–60 ml. Children: 5–15 ml.	O: 2–6 hr SM W
Cascara sagrada	Extract: 200–400 mg; Fluid-extract: 0.5–1.5 ml; Tablets: 1–2.	O: 6–10 hr C SS
Phenolphthalein (Modane, Ex-Lax, Feen-a-mint, Correctol)	60–130 mg.	O: 6–10 hr C SS

SM-small intestine; LG-large intestine; C-colon; S-soft formed, 1–3 days; W-watery, 2–6 hours; SS-semisoft, semifluid, 6–12 hours.
*Within the column listing adverse effects, underlines indicate the most common effects.

Contraindications/ Precautions	Adverse Effects*	Interactions	Nursing Implications
For all laxatives: Contraindicated in hypersensitivity to ingredients, patients with symptoms of acute abdomen, appendicitis, intestinal obstruction, and in patients suspected of having a fecal impaction. Use cautiously in elderly and children where there is a risk of fluid and electrolyte imbalance and in persons acutely ill. Administer sodium preparations cautiously to renal and cardiac patients. Administer magnesium and calcium products cautiously to renal patients.	**For all laxatives:** GI: diarrhea, nausea, vomiting, abdominal cramps, bloating, flatulence		**For all laxatives:** ASSESSMENT: History of bowel activity. Fluid and electrolyte balance. Assess dietary patterns, fiber and fluid intake. INTERVENTION: Take all with a full glass of water or juice. Teach about proper diet—fiber and fluids, and daily exercise. Laxatives are only a temporary measure and should not be used long-term in most patients. Some products may discolor urine. EVALUATION: Notify physician of persistent constipation, rectal bleeding, or of signs of fluid and electrolyte imbalance (muscle pain, dizziness, weakness).
Same as for all plus: Contraindicated in ulcerative lesions in colon and children under 10 years old.	Same as for all plus: GI: suppositories cause proctitis and rectal burning.	Concurrent milk and antacids cause enteric coat to dissolve.	Same as for all plus: INTERVENTION: Enteric-coated tablets should not be taken within 1 hour of drinking milk or ingesting an antacid, because the enteric coating will be broken down in the stomach and the medication may cause gastric irritation. Administer with water only.
Same as for all plus: Contraindicated in infestation of fat-soluble vermifuge, pregnancy, nursing mothers.	Same as for all.	None known.	Same as for all plus: INTERVENTION: Administer on an empty stomach, chilled, with fruit juice or a carbonated beverage.
Same as for all plus: Use cautiously in lactating women.	Same as for all plus: Renal: change in the color of urine: acid urine yellow-brown; alkaline urine: reddish.	None known.	Same as for all.
Same as for all plus: Cautious use in skin hypersensitivity.	Renal: change in color of urine to pink-red which may last 3–4 days. Integ: dermatitis	None known.	Same as for all.

CONTINUED ON THE FOLLOWING PAGE

Table 54–8. LAXATIVES–*CONTINUED*

Name	Dosage	Onset of Action (O) Site of Action Type of Stool
Senna (Senokot, Black Draught, Senexon)	Standardized Adults: 1–4 tablets. Children: 1–2 tablets.	O: 6–10 hr C SS
Docusate calcium (Surfak)	Adult: 240 mg/day. Children over 6 yrs: 50–150 mg/day.	O: 24–72 hr SM & LG S
Docusate potassium (Dialose, Kasof)	Adult: 100–300 mg/day. Children over 6 yrs: 100 mg at hs.	O: 24–72 hr SM & LG S
Docusate sodium (Colace, Doss, Modane Soft)	Adult: 50–500 mg. Children 6–12 yrs: 40–120 mg; 3–6 yrs; 20–60 mg; under 3 yrs: 10–40 mg.	O: 24–72 hr SM & LG S
Docusate sodium (Therevac-SB)	Adult: 1 enema	O: immediate
Docusate sodium (Therevac Plus)	Adult: 1 enema	O: immediate
Bulk-Forming Laxatives: Plantago seed (Psyllium seed)	Range 25–30 g, dose 4–7 g.	O: 12–24 hr SM & LG S
Psyllium hydrophilic mucilloid (Metamucil, Konsyl, Fiberall, Correctol, and many others)	7 g or 1 packet or 1 rounded teaspoonful	O: 12–24 hr SM & LG S
Polycarbophil (Mitrolan, FiberCon)	Tablets chewed thoroughly and followed with 8 oz water. Adults: 12 tabs in 24 hr. Children 6–12 yr: 3–6 tabs/24 hr; 3–6 yr: 1–3 tabs/24 hr.	O: 12–24 hr SM & LG S
Methycellulose (Cologel, Citrucel)	Adult: 4–6 g daily. Children 6 and over: 1.0–1.5 g or Adult: 5–20 ml with 1 glass water daily.	O: 12–24 hr SM & LG S
Osmotic/Saline Laxatives: Magnesium sulfate (Epsom Salt)	10–30 g	O: 0.5–3 hr SM & LG W
Magnesium hydroxide (milk of magnesia, Magnesia Magma)	15–60 ml	O: 0.5–3 hr SM & LG W
Magnesium citrate solution	200 ml	O: 0.5–3 hr SM & LG W
Phospho-soda Fleet	10–20 ml	O: 0.03–0.25 hr C W

SM-small intestine; LG-large intestine; C-colon; S-soft formed, 1–3 days; W-watery, 2–6 hours; SS-semisoft, semifluid, 6–12 hours.
*Within the column listing adverse effects, <u>underlines</u> indicate the most common effects.

Contraindications/ Precautions	Adverse Effects*	Interactions	Nursing Implications
Same as for all.	Same as cascara.	None known.	Same as for all.
Same as for all plus: Contraindicated with concurrent mineral oil.	Same as for all.	None known.	Same as for all.
Same as for all.	Same as for all.	Concurrent administration of salicylates, digitalis, and other cardiac glycosides not recommended.	Same as for all plus: INTERVENTION: For all bulk-forming laxatives: All are slow acting and may need to be repeated for 2–3 days to achieve satisfactory results. Powders are diluted in 1 full glass of water, milk, fruit juice, or other liquid and mixed thoroughly before drinking. Another full glass of liquid should then be consumed. Do not take before bedtime, to prevent intestinal obstruction.
Same as for all.	Same as for all.	Impaired absorption of tetracycline. Administer at least 2 hours apart.	Same as for all and for all bulk-forming laxatives.
Same as for all plus: Contraindicated in persons with edema or congestive heart failure or on low-sodium diets. Use cautiously in renal impairment, digitalized patients, and patients receiving CNS depressants, and with seizures.	Same as for all.	None	Same as for all plus: INTERVENTION: For all osmotic/saline laxatives: Take with at least 240 ml of fluid in the morning or early afternoon before eating any food or drinking any liquid. The fluid ensures the medication reaches the bowel. All liquid preparations are shaken well before being poured. Magnesium sulfate has a bitter taste and is best served chilled and mixed with cold fruit juice or ice chips.

CONTINUED ON THE FOLLOWING PAGE

Table 54–8. LAXATIVES–*CONTINUED*

Name	Dosage	Onset of Action (O) Site of Action Type of Stool
Potassium phosphate	4 g	O: 0.03–0.25 hr C W
Potassium sodium tartrate (Rochelle Salt)	5–10 g	O: 0.03–0.25 hr C W
Sodium phosphate	3.6–7.2 g	O: 0.5–3 hr SM & LG W
Sodium phosphate effervescent	10 g	O: 0.5–3 hr SM & LG W
Sodium phosphate solution	7.5–10 ml	O: 0.5–3 hr SM & LG W
Seidlitz Powders	Contents of 1 blue & 1 white paper mixed with 60 ml water.	O: 0.03–0.25 hr C W
Polyethylene Glycol-Electrolyte Solute (Colyte, Golytely)	4 L of solution—250 ml every 10 minutes.	O: 30–60 min SM & LG W
Lubricants: Mineral oil (Kondremul, Petrogalar plain, white mineral oil, Fleet Mineral Oil Enema, Agoral Plain, Zymenol)	PO Adult: 15–45 ml. R: 90–120 ml. PO Children over 6 yrs: 10–15 ml.	O: 6–8 hr C SS
Miscellaneous Laxatives: Glycerin suppositories	Adult: 1.5–3 g. Children under 6 yr: 1–1.5 g.	O: 0.25–0.5 hr C S
Lactulose (Cephulac, Chronulac)	Adult: 15–30 ml, 3–4× day, up to 60 ml/day. Children: 10–30 ml/day. Enema: 300 mL in 700 ml water, retain for 30–60 min.	O: 24–48 hr C S

SM-small intestine; LG-large intestine; C-colon; S-soft formed, 1–3 days; W-watery, 2–6 hours; SS-semisoft, semifluid, 6–12 hours.
*Within the column listing adverse effects, underlines indicate the most common effects.

Contraindications/ Precautions	Adverse Effects*	Interactions	Nursing Implications
Same as for all.	Same as for all plus: Resp: lipid pneumonia GI: nutritional deficiencies of fat-soluble vitamins.	May decrease absorption of fat-soluble vitamins or drugs.	INTERVENTION: Best administered at bedtime on an empty stomach. Best administered cold or mixed with orange juice, or patient may suck on a lemon or orange slice after drinking the medication. Prolonged use of lubricants can interfere with absorption of fat-soluble vitamins A, D, E, and K. A mineral oil retention enema should always be followed 30–60 minutes later with a cleansing enema. Should be taken regularly at the same time each day to promote normal bowel activity.
Same as for all.	Same as for all.	None known.	Same as for all.
Contraindicated in low-galactose diet. Use cautiously in pregnancy and in persons with diabetes.	GI: gaseous distention, abdominal distention, diarrhea, nausea	Concurrent neomycin and other anti-infectives may prevent lactulose action.	Same as for all plus: ASSESSMENT: Assess blood glucose levels in the patient with diabetes. INTERVENTION: Maintain adequate fluid volume. In the elderly, periodically measure electrolytes. May be mixed with fruit juice or milk to increase palatability. DO NOT take other laxatives at same time. EVALUATION: Notify physician if diarrhea ensues.

bulk occurs naturally and promotes peristalsis and natural elimination about 12–24 hours after administration, but may take one to three days to be effective. These laxatives are the least harmful and do not interfere with the absorption of food. The bulk-forming laxatives may need to be administered for several consecutive days before they achieve their maximal effect. They are less likely to be habit-forming than other types of laxatives because of their slower action time, and because they evacuate only the descending, sigmoid colon, and rectum, rather than emptying the whole bowel, as contact/stimulants do. Some physicians recommend bran or dried fruits, rather than bulk-forming laxatives, as they have the same effect. Dietary fiber should be 6–10 g/day to prevent or treat constipation.

The bulk-forming laxatives contain sugar, salt, and potassium. Patients may need to restrict their intake of sugar and salt when they are taking these agents.

Often, the bulk-forming laxatives are combined with other products such as fecal softeners or stimulant laxatives, or emulsified with liquid petroleum (Petrogalar, Agoral), cascara, phenolphthalein, and magnesium hydroxide.

Uses. The bulk-forming laxatives are generally used in treating chronic, atonic (in the elderly), or spastic constipation. Currently, the bulk-forming laxatives are used to treat patients with diverticulosis, irritable bowel syndrome, and to relieve painful defecation in patients with hemorrhoids.

The bulk-forming laxatives are generally contraindicated in patients with suspected bowel obstruction, dysphagia, or intestinal ulceration. They are always administered with a full glass of liquid and should be followed by 8 ounces of water to prevent the likelihood of either esophageal or intestinal obstruction or impaction.

Plantago Seed (Psyllium Seed). Plantago seed is the dried fruit of the plantago psyllium. The seed itself swells in the presence of moisture to form an indigestible, jellylike mass. The seeds have a sharp end, which may irritate the bowel; therefore, gum extracts are available, which have the same pharmacologic effect.

Psyllium hydrophilic mucilloid (Metamucil, Konsyl, Correctol, and many others) is a mixture of 50% powdered plantago seeds and 50% dextrose or a sugar-free variety in a cream-colored powder. It is effective in about 12–72 hours and also has a demulcent effect on an inflamed bowel. The usual daily adult dosage (one rounded teaspoonful or one packet instant mix) is 7 g mixed in 8 ounces of water and followed by 8 ounces of water administered one to three times daily. Psyllium hydrophilic mucilloid can be administered as many as three times a day.

Calcium Polycarbophil. Calcium polycarbophil (Mitrolan) is recommended for treating both constipation and diarrhea. Its effectiveness as a stool normalizer comes from its ability to bind up to 60 to 100 times its weight of water. This is three times as much as is possible with previously available hydrophilic substances obtained from psyllium seeds.

When calcium polycarbophil is used to manage constipation, it keeps free water from being absorbed out of the intestine, which in turn converts dry, hard, scanty stools into a soft, bulky mass. When calcium polycarbophil is used to manage acute diarrhea that results when water rushes out of the intestine at abnormally rapid rates, this drug binds with excessive fluid. This helps to stop the frequent liquid bowel movements.

Calcium polycarbophil is especially useful for symptomatic relief of gastrointestinal disorders in which diarrhea and constipation alternate, as in irritable bowel syndrome and diverticulosis.

Polycarbophil calcium tablets (vanilla or citrus flavor) are chewed thoroughly before swallowing and followed by 8 ounces of fluid. Adults should receive 8–12 tablets in 24 hours; children 6–12 years, no more than 6 tablets in 24 hours; and children 3–6 years, no more than 3 tablets in 24 hours. The even spacing of these small doses overcomes abdominal fullness.

Methylcellulose. Methylcellulose (Cologel) is a hydrophilic semisynthetic cellulose derivative. Oral preparation of 4–6 g (two to four times daily) swells on contact with water and forms a demulcent nonabsorbable gel that facilitates passage of stool and reflexly stimulates stool. Methylcellulose is also available as 500-mg tablets; these should not be chewed, to avoid the risk of esophageal obstruction. These preparations should either be mixed in eight ounces of fluid or followed by eight ounces of fluid.

OSMOTIC/SALINE LAXATIVES. The most rapid-acting and powerful of all laxatives, the osmotic/saline laxatives, usually a salt of nonabsorbable anions or cations, act by increasing the bulk of the intestinal contents. Consequently, peristalsis occurs more quickly than with bulk laxatives. Their cathartic action can occur within two to six hours after administration. Osmotic laxatives include magnesium citrate and sulfate, sodium phosphate, and magnesium hydroxide (milk of magnesia).

The greater the concentraion of the salt, the greater the osmotic ability once the salt enters the bowel. A hypertonic saline solution causes diffusion of fluid from the plasma into the intestine in order to dilute the solution to isotonic. The magnesium salts cause an increase in the secretion of cholecystokinin from the duodenum, which is thought to increase the secretion and motility of the small intestine and colon and may contribute to the cathartic effect. The greater their concentration, the more likely the osmotic laxatives are to cause nausea. Therefore, a hypertonic saline solution is made isotonic by adding water when administering it. All preparations are accompanied by at least 8 ounces of water. The water also assists the laxative to leave the stomach. A nonsaline osmotic cathartic, lactulose (Cephulac), has a mechanism of action that is slightly different. It will be discussed later in this section.

Uses. Because of their short action time, the osmotic/saline laxatives are often used to cleanse the entire intestinal tract for diagnostic tests, to flush poisons, or to remove parasites. These laxatives provide a liquid stool but do not rupture the egg capsules of the parasites.

Contraindications and Precautions. All the osmotic/saline laxatives are contraindicated in abdominal pain, fecal impaction, nausea, vomiting of unknown origin, and intestinal obstructions. The magnesium and potassium salts are contraindicated in renal disease, as these electrolytes may be retained. They are given cautiously to a patient with renal disease due to their sodium content. Also, they are given cautiously to patients receiving central nervous system depressants, as there may be a significant drop in serum calcium that could precipitate more seizure activity.

Magnesium Citrate. Magnesium citrate is flavored and carbonated. It is not very soluble; therefore, relatively large doses need to be administered. Magnesium citrate is more palatable when served chilled. The usual adult dose is 200 ml, which results in a bowel evacuation in 30 minutes to three hours.

Magnesium Sulfate. Magnesium sulfate (Epsom Salt) occurs as a glassy, sharp crystal or as a white powder, both of which are readily soluble in water. The usual adult dose is 15 g (.5 ounce), with a range of 10–30 g, mixed in water. It has a bitter taste.

Sodium Phosphate. Sodium phosphate is readily dissolved in water and has a more agreeable taste than other compounds. The usual adult dose is 3.6–7.2 g.

Effervescent Sodium Phosphate. Effervescent sodium phosphate contains sodium bicarbonate and citric and tartaric acids. The usual dose is 10 g.

Fleet Phospho-Soda. Fleet Phospho-Soda is a concentrated aqueous solution of sodium biphosphate and sodium phosphate. The usual oral dose is 10–20 ml. Fleet Phospho-Soda is also available as a disposable enema unit but should be administered cautiously to persons on a low-sodium diet.

Polyethylene Glycol-Electrolyte Solution. Polyethylene Glycol-Electrolyte Solution (Colyte, Golytely) is used prior to gastrointestinal exams. After oral administration, the solution induces diarrhea within 30–60 minutes and rapidly cleanses the bowel, usually within four hours. Polyethylene glycol-electrolyte solutions are nonabsorbable solutions that act as an osmotic agent. The patient should fast three to four hours prior to ingestion of the solution. The patient must drink four liters of this solution—240 ml every ten minutes until the four liters are consumed. The solution is more palatable when chilled.

Magnesium Hydroxide Mixture. In the stomach, magnesium hydroxide (milk of magnesia) reacts with hydrochloric acid to form magnesium chloride, which then becomes the laxative. It is available in liquid form, with 15–60 ml being the usual dose.

LUBRICANTS—MINERAL OIL. Mineral oil, the only lubricant in use today, is used for temporary relief of constipation, to prevent tearing of hemorrhoids or fissures, and to prevent straining at stool for patients with recent surgery or cardiac disease. It lubricates and softens the intestinal contents as well as retarding water absorption, and takes effect six to eight hours after administration.

Mineral oil is minimally absorbed from the intestinal tract, with distribution to the liver, spleen, mesenteric lymph nodes, and intestinal mucosa.

Adverse Effects. The adverse effects of mineral oil include anorexia, nausea, vomiting, and nutritional deficiencies. Also, lipid pneumonia may occur if accidentally aspirated. Small children and the elderly are at highest risk for aspiration. Chronic use may decrease the absorption of vitamins (particularly the fat-soluble vitamins A, D, E, and K), food, and bile salts. Some researchers believe that only the precursor of vitamin A (carotene) is affected, and that natural vitamin A is absorbed in the intestine in the presence of mineral oil.

Dosage. The usual adult dose of mineral oil ranges between 15 and 45 ml; for children over the age of six years, between 10 and 15 ml. Mineral oil retards the emptying of the stomach, so it should not be administered after meals. To relieve the oily taste in the mouth, a slice of citrus fruit or a glass of citrus fruit juice can be administered after the mineral oil. Mineral oil can also be found as a primary ingredient in several oil-retention enemas (Fleet-mineral oil enema).

MISCELLANEOUS LAXATIVES. *Glycerin Suppositories.* Glycerin suppositories promote peristalsis through local irritation of the mucous membranes of the rectum. Glycerin suppositories are safe for temporary use to re-establish proper bowel habits in patients who have lost the rectal reflex. Glycerin suppositories are often helpful in bowel retraining regimens and in individuals with intermittent constipation. Glycerin suppositories are effective in 15 minutes to one hour. The usual adult dose is 3 gr; for children under six years the dose is 1.15 gr.

Lactulose. Lactulose syrup (Cephulac) is a synthetic disaccharide analog of lactose that increases the number of bowel movements daily. Lactulose is primarily used in patients with hepatic dysfunction to decrease blood ammonia levels and to reduce hepatic encephalopathy, and in patients with renal failure. Lactulose is metabolized in the colon by bacteria to short-chain organic acids (lactic, acetic, and formic acids). These acids have osmotic activity and increase the net fluid in the colon.

Contraindications and Precautions. Lactulose is contraindicated in patients on a low-galactose diet, since it contains galactose. It is given cautiously to pregnant women and to patients concurrently receiving neomycin. Neomycin and other nonabsorbable antibiotics may reduce or destroy enough colonic bacteria to interfere with the effective action of lactulose syrup. Lactulose syrup, because of its sugar content, is given to diabetic patients with caution; changes in blood sugar have been noted. Also, elderly patients receiving lactulose syrup for six months or longer should have periodic measurements of their serum electrolytes including potassium and chloride.

Adverse Effects. The adverse effects include flatulence, intestinal cramps, gas, and belching. Excessive doses may produce diarrhea with hypokalemia and nausea, because of its sweet taste. Since it acts on the colon, there is no interference with absorption of secretion in the small intestine.

Table 54–9. COMBINATION DRUGS FOR LAXATIVES

| Combination Drugs | Basic Products | | | | | | | |
	A	B	C	D	E	F	G	Other
Agoral	28	200						
Dialose-Plus				100	30			
Dorbantyl				50		25		
Doxidan		65		60				
D-S-S Plus				100	30			
Gentlax S							326.1	1 Z
Haley's M-O	25							M
Kondremul with Phenolphthalein	55	150/15 ml						P
Peri-Colace (Capsules)				100	30			10% alcohol
Peri-Colace (Syrup)				60	30/15 ml			
Senokot-S					50		187	
Syllamalt			3					4 W

Basic products: A = mineral oil, %; B = white phenolphthalein, mg; C = psyllium husk powder, g; D = docusate sodium, mg; E = casanthranol, mg; F = danthron, mg; G = standardized senna concentrate, mg; M = magnesium hydroxide; P = irish moss; W = malt soup extract, g; Z = guar gum, g.

Dosage. Lactulose syrup (15 ml) contains lactulose 10 gr, galactose 2.2 g, lactose 1.2 g, and less than 1.2 g of other sugars. There are 60 calories in the 15-ml dose, with less than 18 calories in absorbable sugars. This same dose contains 0.4–0.7 mg sodium.

The usual adult dose ranges from 15–30 ml per day and may be increased to 60 ml per day for chronic and acute diarrhea. In portal encephalopathy, the initial dose is 30–45 ml, three times daily, and is then adjusted to produce a fecal pH of 5–5.5 and two to three soft, formed stools daily.

COMBINATION PRODUCTS. The combination products combine ingredients from two or more classes of laxatives. Table 54–9 features combination laxatives and their specific additives. Sufficient evidence is not available as yet to confirm the effectiveness of combination preparations.

USING THE NURSING PROCESS

ASSESSMENT

Assessment of the patient requiring medications that affect the digestive system always begins with a thorough nursing history to develop the data base. The patient requiring these medications may be acutely ill in the hospital, or relatively healthy and self-treating a digestive problem with OTC preparations. Typical information obtained from the patient is included in Table 54–10.

If the patient's chief complaint is diarrhea, the nurse learns whether or not the patient traveled recently, particularly to areas where hygiene is poor or has had altered normal dietary habits. In order to implement the correct treatment of diarrhea later on, it is important to discover the cause of the malady. In general, antidiarrheals are not chosen to treat acute diarrhea associated with organisms that penetrate the intestinal mucosa, such as viruses, *E. coli*, *Salmonella*, or *Shigella*. A nurse who suspects the presence of these organisms always requests a stool sample for culture. The nurse assesses the character, frequency, and odor (foul-smelling feces is indicative of a need for increased digestive enzymes); notes the number of stools per day; and detects the presence of mucus, blood, and fat. The very young or old need to have close assessments to prevent dehydration and electrolyte imbalances. Patients found to have chronic diarrhea that appears as a reaction to stress, excessive alcohol consumption, or improper dietary habits will need counseling during the implementation phase to help them correct the problem.

When a patient complains of constipation, the nurse always determines the cause before planning and starting treatment. This assessment begins with the patient describing, in detail, what he or she perceives as constipation and how much time is spent defecating. Often, by increasing the time allowed for defecating, the patient can avoid constipation. The nurse also assesses dietary patterns and may suggest that the patient add fresh fruits, vegetables, and whole grains to the diet, to provide bulk; and drink eight to ten glasses of water daily to assure adequate hydration. This may help to regulate bowel activity. The nurse also assesses the amount of daily exercise; increased physical activity can stimulate peristalsis. The nurse also assesses the cardiovascular status of the patient; a patient with cardiovascular impairment is encouraged during the intervention phase to avoid straining at stool, which activates the vagus nerve (Valsalva maneuver) and slows the heart rate. In most instances, laxatives are used only as a temporary measure.

The nurse assesses bowel sounds, and establishes the absence of fecal impaction, nausea and vomiting, abdominal pain, and bowel obstruction before administering cathartics. Cathartics are contraindicated for patients who exhibit these symptoms.

Table 54–10. NURSING PROCESS FOR PATIENTS REQUIRING DRUGS FOR DIGESTIVE DISORDERS

Assessment

Note current complaints of diarrhea, constipation, nausea/vomiting, abdominal pain; frequency of bowel movement and odor of stool.
Auscultate bowel sounds.
Review history for fecal impaction, bowel obstruction, chronic disease/conditions, cardiovascular impairment.
Determine dietary patterns, noting fluid intake and amount of daily exercise.
Ascertain medication history, alcohol, laxative and enema use/abuse and patient perception of what constipation is.
Review laboratory studies, e.g., stool specimen.

Nursing Diagnosis	Nursing Actions	Rationale	Desired Outcomes/ Evaluation Criteria
Constipation related to altered dietary intake, inadequate bulk, chronic use of laxatives/enemas, some medications, changes in level of activity possibly evidenced by frequency less than usual pattern, hard-formed stool, straining at stool, decreased bowel sounds.	Administer laxatives (e.g., Dulcolax, fleet enema) as indicated. Remove fecal impaction if present.	Promotes bowel evacuation and relieves constipation. Impaction needs to be removed before regular bowel function can be reestablished.	Reestablishes normal patterns of bowel functioning. Verbalizes understanding of factors and appropriate interventions/solutions related to individual situation. Demonstrates changes in lifestyle, as necessitated by causative, contributing factors.
	Discuss use of stool softeners (Surfak), bulk-forming products (metamucil, fiberall).	Useful in preventing constipation based on individual need.	
	Encourage intake of a well-balanced diet, (including fresh fruits/ vegetables) and to increase fluid intake to at least 3000 ml/day as tolerated.	May be sufficient to correct situation by promoting more normal amount and consistency of stool.	
	Establish regular exercise program.	Increased activity promotes increased bowel motility and regularity.	
Diarrhea related to toxins, contaminants, medications, dietary intake, inflammation/irritation, or malabsorption of bowel as evidenced by abdominal pain, urgency, cramping, increased frequency, loose, liquid stools.	Administer antidiarrheal (e.g., Paregoric, Lomotil, Imodium) or digestive enzymes (e.g., bile salts and pancreatic enzymes) as indicated.	Slows GI motility prolonging transit time to reduce frequency of stools; promotes normal digestive process and absorption of fat.	Reestablishes and maintains normal pattern of bowel functioning. Verbalizes understanding of causative factors and rationale of treatment regimen. Demonstrates appropriate behavior to assist with resolution of causative factors, e.g., proper food preparation and avoidance of irritating foods.
	Monitor vital signs as appropriate. Observe mucous membranes, skin turgor.	Indicators of degree of dehydration.	
	Restrict foods/fluids as indicated.	Promotes intestinal rest and may prevent precipitation of further diarrhea.	
	Encourage patient to drink fluids (boiled/bottled water if indicated), eat bland food and get extra rest.	Maintains hydration and helps to regain homeostasis.	
	Suggest intake of whole grains and additional bulk (e.g., bran, cereal fibers).	Aids in promoting firm, soft stool which is more easily passed.	
	Stress importance of medical follow-up.	Further evaluation and treatment may be required when diarrhea continues for an extended period of time.	
	Discuss side-effects. Advise patient not to drive and to report untoward reactions.	Dry mouth and drowsiness are expected and dependent on the dose and individual response. More serious reactions may require change of dose or choice of drug.	

CONTINUED ON THE FOLLOWING PAGE

Table 54–10. NURSING PROCESS FOR PATIENTS REQUIRING DRUGS FOR DIGESTIVE DISORDERS–*CONTINUED*

Nursing Diagnosis	Nursing Actions	Rationale	Desired Outcomes/ Evaluation Criteria
	Suggest use of ointment, skin barrier preparations.	Provides relief for irritated anal tissue, helps protect skin from excoriation.	
	Discuss preventive use of antidiarrheal drugs.	May be helpful in preventing diarrhea when traveling in a foreign country.	
Knowledge, deficit related to lack of exposure/ recall, information misinterpretation, unfamiliarity with information resources possibly evidenced by questions, statement of concern, inaccurate followthrough of instruction/ development of preventable complications.	Review usual bowel activity and underlying reasons for individual situation.	Understanding of pathophysiology of problem helps patient to make informed choices and cooperate with treatment regimen.	Verbalizes understanding of condition/disease process and treatment. Initiates necessary procedures and explains reasons for the actions.
	Discuss beliefs patient may have about bowel functioning. Clarify myths/misconceptions and provide accurate information.	Patients often believe they must have a daily bowel movement and taking laxatives to promote this goal can create a dependence which is both physiologic and psychologic. Interrupting this cycle enables normal bowel activity to be resumed. In addition, patient may believe that several loose-formed stools indicate diarrhea although this may actually be normal.	
	Discuss action, dose, safe use of medications, e.g., importance of not taking antidiarrheal when viral infection or food poisoning are suspected; not taking enteric coated laxative pills within 1 hour of ingesting milk or antacids.	Since most of these medications are readily obtained over the counter, it is important to know when, how, and why to take drugs to promote optimal effect.	
	Instruct patient to report changes in bowel habits.	May be a symptom of a more serious problem such as bowel obstruction and/or malignancy.	

NURSING DIAGNOSES

Typical nursing diagnoses for a patient with digestive problems are included in Table 54–10.

PLANNING AND INTERVENTION

The nurse develops the goals of nursing intervention from the nursing diagnoses. When caring for the patient requiring medications for common problems of the digestive system, typical nursing goals are included in Table 54–10.

Dietary modification may be a long-term solution to digestive problems. The nurse always encourages the patient to eat a well-balanced diet. The addition of fresh fruits and vegetables may prevent constipation, whereas the addition of whole grains and additional bulk (bran, fresh fruits and vegetables, cereal fibers) may prevent diarrhea. Patients should drink sufficient water to prevent dehydration and to soften the stool. Exercise is also important to restore normal bowel activity.

The nurse emphasizes to the patient that diarrhea is often a symptom of disease, not a disease in itself. Patients are encouraged not to self-treat immediately because diarrhea can be a defense mechanism to rid the body of a toxin or other causative agent. If treatment is started too early, this normal defense may be hindered.

The nurse counsels a patient traveling to a foreign country where travelers' diarrhea is likely to occur to choose hotels and restaurants with good sanitary conditions and to drink only bottled water with no ice cubes unless the restaurant makes ice cubes from boiled water.

Salad, cold sandwiches, and uncooked vegetables should also be avoided. Fruits and vegetables should be eaten only after they are peeled or washed in chlorinated water. Buffet-table foods, which may have spent hours away from proper refrigeration, should be avoided. If travelers' diarrhea does occur, the individual should rest, keep warm, drink only boiled or bottled water, and eat bland, cooked foods. It is important to avoid dehydration and to provide an easily digestible energy source.

Various drugs taken prophylactically can prevent travelers' diarrhea, but for most people, the risks of such use probably outweigh the benefits. Typical drugs that could be ordered by the physician and taken include doxycycline (Vibramycin), trimethoprim-sulfamethoxazole (Bactrim DS), trimethoprim (Proloprim), norfloxacin (Noroxin), and also the nonprescription Pepto-Bismol.

Patients who are seeking advice about laxatives because of their increased need are encouraged to consult with their physician. Most constipation is due to poor dietary or living conditions; however, a change in bowel habits can also be a symptom of a more serious problem such as bowel obstruction and/or a malignancy. The physician will rule out such organic problems, then the patient can be helped to normalize their bowel habits.

Often patients believe that they must evacuate the bowel on a daily basis; if they do not have a bowel movement, they take a laxative. The laxative empties their lower bowel, which in turn prevents a normal bowel movement the following day. Instead of the laxative restoring "normal regularity," the continued use of cathartics soon makes it difficult for the laxative abuser to ever achieve a natural movement. This dependence can become both physiologic and psychologic. This cycle must be interrupted if normal bowel activity is to return.

Often, constipation may be a side effect of other medications such as opiates, antacids, iron, phenothiazines, sedatives, multiple vitamin complexes, and tricyclic antidepressants. Patients having constipation secondary to these drugs are encouraged to modify their diet to include extra fluid and bulk. Often, these additions may eliminate the constipation.

Chronic constipation can cause numerous problems for the patient, including hemorrhoids or diverticulosis, and may even predispose an individual to cancer of the colon. Therefore, the nurse encourages the patient to prevent constipation on a daily basis.

PATIENT TEACHING

In order for the nurse to safely administer medications affecting the digestive tract, the nurse must remember to teach patients the information found in each drug table in the column marked Nursing Implications. Additional information for patient teaching can be found in Tables 54–11, 54–12, and 54–13.

Patients who have experienced chronic constipation may be placed on a bowel retraining program. The first step of any retraining program is to ensure that the diet

is high in fluid and bulk, particularly breakfast. Breakfast should also be consumed at approximately the same time each day. The patient is then placed on the toilet or commode for 15–30 minutes after the meal. If reflex defecation does not occur, a lubricated glycerin suppository is inserted into the rectum. If defecation still does not occur, a Fleet enema is generally administered. Within a short period, the patient begins to defecate on a regular schedule following breakfast without the use of the suppository or enema. The importance of diet, exercise, and adequate fluids are stressed to each patient.

Table 54–11. PATIENT TEACHING INFORMATION—DIGESTANTS

Dear Patient:
This drug has been prescribed for you. This is what you should know about your drug to get the most from your therapy.

DIGESTANTS:

1. Digestants such as _____ are taken to help in the digestion of food you eat.
2. Digestants will usually be taken for the rest of your life.
3. Digestants are taken with meals to make sure that the drug is present when the food enters the stomach and bowels. They are best sprinkled on the food.
4. Check your stools daily for the presence of fat, an increasing foul smell, or bulky or foamy stool. Both an increase in fat and foul smell may mean that your dose may need to be changed.

Table 54–12. PATIENT TEACHING INFORMATION—ANTIDIARRHEALS

Dear Patient:
This drug has been prescribed for you. This is what you should know about your drug to get the most from your therapy.

1. Antidiarrheals such as _____ are taken to control diarrhea and reduce the number of stools daily.
2. Many locally acting antidiarrheals are available as OTC preparations. Do not take them when fever is present, or for more than 3 days if the symptoms are not stopped. The diarrhea may mean you have a more serious problem that needs medical attention. Systemically acting antidiarrheals should also not be taken for longer than 2 days if symptoms are not stopped.
3. During the acute attack, you may be asked to not eat anything for a few days, or drink a clear liquid or a bland diet and not eat any milk products (ice cream, pudding, etc.), to rest the bowel for a few days.
4. You may also have other medications such as anti-infectives, antiemetics, digestive enzymes, narcotics or their derivatives, and steroids added to control diarrhea.

Table 54–13. PATIENT TEACHING INFORMATION—LAXATIVES
Dear Patient: This drug has been prescribed for you. This is what you should know about your drug to get the most from your therapy. 1. Laxatives such as _____ are taken to soften and make the passage of stool easier. 2. Take your laxatives either at bedtime or before breakfast to allow for the peak action to occur at a convenient time. 3. Often, laxatives are best taken with milk or fruit juice. Many types of laxatives need to be taken with a full glass of water or liquid. 4. Enteric-coated tablets are not taken within 1 hour of drinking milk or taking an antacid, because their enteric coating is broken down in the stomach and may lead to stomach upset.

EVALUATION

During the evaluation phase, the nurse evaluates the effectiveness of the medications that alter the digestive system. This evaluation is based on a list of outcome evaluation criteria that has been developed in relation to the goals determined by the nurse, patient, and family. The data base obtained in the original assessment and used to formulate the nursing diagnoses provides helpful criteria for measuring the treatment's effectiveness. Typical outcome evaluation criteria are included in Table 54–10.

It is extremely important to work with the patient and family to ensure their complete assistance and support. Patients who understand the importance of their continued medical treatment are usually compliant. The primary reasons for noncompliance are forgetting to take the medication, or not liking the unpleasant side effects. The nurse teaches the patient about potential common side effects so that a patient who takes medication at home reports any unusual symptoms to the physician or nurse. Patients with renal or hepatic disease need to be watched more closely for side effects. Adverse effects are included in each drug table.

Constipation is often a complication of antidiarrheal medication; therefore, frequent evaluation of bowel activity is performed. Encouraging the patient to drink plenty of liquids may help to prevent constipation.

The more the nurse involves the patient and family with the planning of the care, the more likely they are to comply. The nurse must stress the importance of continued medical care. Evaluation always focuses on patient results and on compliance. The majority of these problems will be managed at home by the patient, so compliance is most important. All previously taught material is reviewed and updated with the patient and family, if necessary, to ensure that the patient's knowledge base remains accurate.

SUMMARY

The gastrointestinal tract is responsible for the digestion of food substances, and ultimately, the absorption of nutrients. Digestants such as hydrochloric acid, pancreatic enzymes, and bile salts aid in the breakdown of nutrients. Antidiarrheals are useful for the symptomatic control of both acute and chronic diarrhea, diarrhea secondary to radiation or gastrointestinal surgery, or to decrease the volume of intestinal discharge in patients with ileostomies and colostomies. Local antidiarrheals include absorbents, astringents, and intestinal flora modifiers that help replace the normal bacteria flora. Most of these products are available over the counter. Systemic-acting antidiarrheals are more effective than local acting agents. The opiates, synthetic opiates, and the natural belladonna alkaloid anticholinergics have both antispasmodic and antiperistaltic properties. Laxatives are available as both OTC and prescription to accelerate the passage of feces through the bowel. Numerous types of laxatives are available, including the contact or stimulant laxatives, bulk-forming agents, saline or osmotic cathartics, and several miscellaneous agents.

As the nurse prepares to administer any of these medications, it is important to obtain a thorough history to determine the onset of symptoms and any precipitating factors. Diet history and normal eating patterns are also obtained. Dietary modification may be a long-term solution to digestive problems. Patients are also encouraged to drink sufficient water and exercise regularly. Since most of these medications are readily available over the counter, patient teaching is stressed.

BIBLIOGRAPHY

Advice For Travelers. The Medical Letter 29(741):53, June 5, 1987.

AMA Department of Drugs: AMA Drug Evaluations, ed 6. PSG Publishing, Littleton, MA, 1986.

Bitterman, RA: Getting the bowel under control sufferers of diarrhea. Emerg Med 19(5):68, 1987.

Covington, TR: Management of diarrhea. Facts and Comparisons Drug Newsletter 7(1):1, January 1988.

Gilman, AG, Goodman, LS, and Gilman, A (eds): Goodman and Gilman's The Pharmacological Basis of Therapeutics, ed 7. Macmillan, New York, 1985.

Johnson, PC, DuPont, HL, and Ericsson, CD: Travelers' diarrhea, strategies to help decrease the odds. Consultant 87(5):102, 1987.

New pharmaceuticals and medicinal products. Antidiarrheal Diasorb. US Pharm 12:88, 1987.

Olin, B, et al: Antidiarrheals. Facts and Comparisons. JB Lippincott, St. Louis, 1987.

Olin, B (ed): Facts and Comparisons. JB Lippincott, St. Louis, 1989.

SITUATION 54–1

Ida Vinnett is a 70-year-old who has been cared for in a nursing home since a massive stroke two years earlier.

1. According to the nurse's notes, Ms. Vinnett has not had a stool in four days. Prior to giving her a laxative, the nurse will check for evidence of:
   a. confusion
   b. fecal impaction
   c. anxiety
   d. urinary incontinence

2. Ms. Vinnett is to receive bisacodyl (Dulcolax) orally. It is best to administer this drug with:
   a. water
   b. milk
   c. an antacid
   d. food

3. After bowel evacuation, Ms. Vinnett is to begin taking psyllium hydrophilic mucilloid (Metamucil) daily. The nurse will include the following intervention in her plan of care:
   a. Administer at least 8 oz of fluid with medication.
   b. Mix medication with evening meal.
   c. Add all of the patient's medications to the Metamucil.
   d. Discontinue Metamucil if no bowel movement noted in four hours.

4. Metamucil should be given with caution if Ms. Vinnett has:
   a. arthritis
   b. glaucoma
   c. hepatic dysfunction
   d. diabetes mellitus

5. The nurse will expect to see results of Metamucil:
   a. after one week
   b. within 1 to 3 days
   c. after 2 weeks
   d. within 12 hours

6. Ms. Vinnett is to receive magnesium hydroxide (Milk of Magnesia) prn every evening. The nurse will assess for evidence of renal disease because this agent contains a high concentration of:
   a. purine
   b. iron
   c. potassium
   d. sodium

Please refer to the Appendices for correct answers and additional review questions with answers.

MEDICATIONS USED IN HEPATIC AND BILIARY DISEASE

MERRILY MATHEWSON KUHN, R.N.C., Ph.D., CCRN

LEARNING OBJECTIVES

After reading this chapter, the student will be able to:

1. Identify medications commonly used to manage hepatic and biliary disease.

2. Differentiate among the various types of medications used to manage hepatic and biliary disease in reference to mechanisms of action, routes of administration, pharmacokinetics, contraindications, adverse effects, and interactions.

3. Identify specific areas to assess in the patient requiring management of complications of hepatic and biliary disease in order to formulate appropriate nursing diagnoses.

4. Plan the nursing interventions necessary to administer medications used in the management of complications of hepatic and biliary disease safely and choose appropriate teaching strategies to gain patient compliance.

5. Evaluate the patient at various stages to gauge nursing interventions.

The hepatic and biliary systems are a major part of the digestive system, contributing many digestive enzymes. The biliary system includes the gallbladder and the pancreas (which is also an endocrine gland, producing insulin). The normal functioning of the hepatic and biliary systems in digestion has been described in Chapter 51.

THERAPEUTIC AGENTS

The patient with any type of hepatic or biliary disease (Table 55–1) is acutely ill and must be continually ob-

served and evaluated. The majority of the medications used to treat the patient with hepatic or biliary disease are covered elsewhere in this text, and therefore only a brief overview is presented.

MEDICATIONS FOR HEPATIC CELL NECROSIS

The cytochrome P-450 (Fig. 55–1) mixed-function oxidase system normally processes minor amounts of acetaminophen (Tylenol) into reactive metabolites that are normally bound to *glutathione*. Glutathione normally carries oxygen to the liver and is fundamentally impor-

Table 55–1. HEPATIC DISEASE

Hepatic Diseases
HEPATITIS
Definition: A highly contagious viral disease of the liver; it can also be noncontagious, due to alcohol, other drugs, biliary obstruction, etc.
Types: Several types: (1) hepatitis A (HA); (2) hepatitis B (HB), (3) hepatitis non-A, non-B (HAV-HBV, sometimes called hepatitis C), and (4) Delta hepatitis.
Etiology: All are of viral origin.
Symptoms: Jaundice, pruritis, loss of appetite, fever, chills, abdominal discomfort, reduced liver function, bleeding tendencies, skin rash, pain in right upper quadrant of abdomen, reduced metabolism of foodstuffs.
Management: Decreased activity until liver is near normal size, diet (increased calories, 5 g carbohydrate, 75–100 g protein, moderate- to low-fat diet).
CIRRHOSIS
Definition: Chronic condition of the liver, where normal liver tissue is replaced with fibrous tissue. More than three fourths of the liver must be involved before symptoms appear.
Etiology: Chronic alcoholism, postnecrotic causes, secondary to hepatitis or certain drugs (see Table 55–5); or obstructive, secondary to biliary obstruction.
Symptoms: Jaundice, gastrointestinal disturbances, vitamin deficiencies, clotting disorders, red palms, ascites, weight loss, fatigue, loss of body hair, *caput medusae,* and in men testicular atrophy and *gynecomastia.*
Management: Treated symptomatically with primary removal of the precipitating cause; rest, adequate nutrition, diuretics, and medication to relieve itching.
LIVER DAMAGE SECONDARY TO DRUGS AND POISON
Substances Causing Injury: Hepatotoxic drugs and poisons such as carbon tetrachloride, phosphate-containing compounds, arsenicals, certain mushrooms, lead, and similar compounds.
Incidence: Accounts for 5% of jaundice in all patients and as high as 20% in the elderly. Mortality may be as high as 10%–50%. Obesity enhances susceptibility to hepatic injury.
Symptoms: Acute poisoning: symptoms include nausea, vomiting, malaise, abdominal pain, fever, hypoprothrombinemia, jaundice, and hepatomegaly. Chronic poisoning: although less noticeable, symptoms include weight loss, pallor, hematemesis, jaundice, hypoprothrombinemia, ascites, and a cirrhotic liver.
Management: Bedrest, elimination of the causative agent, and supportive care.
HEPATIC ENCEPHALOPHY
Definition: Neuropsychiatric syndrome due to liver disease and usually associated with portal-systemic shunting of venous blood.
Etiology: Fulminating hepatitis due to viruses, drugs, or toxins; cirrhosis; following portacaval shunt or similar anastomoses; chronic liver disease.
Symptoms: Personality changes, impaired consciousness, constructive apraxia, fetor hepaticus, hyper-reflexia agitation, mania, seizures, localizing neurologic signs.
Management: Eliminate precipitating causes when possible; bedrest; reduce or eliminate dietary protein; oral neomycin; oral lactulose; prevention of infection.

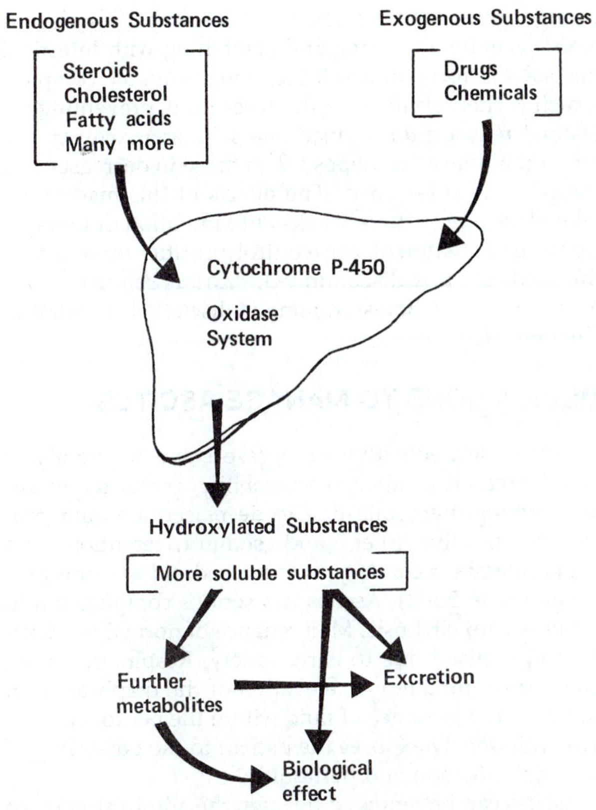

Figure 55–1. The action of cytochrome P-450 in the oxidase system of the liver. Both endogenous and exogenous substances are biotransformed with the help of cytochrome P-450.

Table 55–2. HEPATIC ENCEPHALOPATHY PHASES

Phase	Symptoms
I	Personality change, vacant stare, agitation, difficulty in performing calculations and writing legibly
II	Confusion, abnormal sleep patterns, lethargy, asterixis
III	Stupor, accentuated disturbances in thought processes, sleepiness, asterixis
IV	Coma

tant in cellular respiration. When large doses of acetaminophen are ingested, glutathione is depleted. This allows the active metabolites of acetaminophen to accumulate and bind to hepatocellular proteins, which results in cell death.

It is important to obtain the time and amount of acetaminophen that was ingested. If more than 7.5 g or 140 mg/kg was ingested, it is important to begin prophylactic antidotal therapy with N-acetylcysteine (Mucomyst). Nausea and vomiting are the usual side effects of N-acetylcysteine. Administering by a nasogastric tube or coadministering an antiemetic such as droperidol may help reduce vomiting. N-acetylcysteine, a mucolytic agent, is described in Chapters 6 and 36, provides additional glutathione and thereby prevents cell injury and necrosis.

MEDICATIONS TO PREVENT HEPATITIS

Several medications are now available to prevent the development of hepatitis. All these medications and their uses are discussed more fully in Chapter 64. They are reviewed briefly in Table 55–2. Hepatitis B vaccine (Heptavax-B) is inactivated human hepatitis B surface antigen (HBsAg) obtained by plasmapheresis from healthy chronic carriers of the HBsAg antigen. Recombinant vaccine (Recombivax-HB) is derived from HBsAg

produced in yeast cells. These vaccines provide pre-exposure protection against hepatitis. Hepatitis B immune globulin (HBIG) is administered immediately after exposure to hepatitis B.

Hepatitis B Vaccine

Hepatitis B vaccine (Heptavax, Recombivax-HB) is recommended for pre-exposure prevention in susceptible individuals of all ages who are or will be at increased risk for contracting hepatitis B. It is designed for healthy individuals as well as those who are immunosuppressed. It produces *active immunization* against hepatitis B virus only and will not work against other hepatitides like hepatitis A, non-A, non-B, or hepatitis C.

CONTRAINDICATIONS AND PRECAUTIONS. Hepatitis B vaccine is contraindicated in people who are hypersensitive to the components of the vaccine such as thimerosol and aluminum. Persons may also be allergic to yeast, which is used to produce recombinant vaccine. General precautions include administration to pregnant females and nursing mothers. Care is taken when administering hepatitis B vaccine to individuals with severely compromised cardiopulmonary status or to those in whom a febrile or a systemic reaction could pose a significant risk.

ADVERSE EFFECTS. No serious adverse reactions have been attributed to hepatitis B vaccine. Since hepatitis B vaccine is obtained from human serum, the AIDS antibodies can be transmitted. The AIDS virus is NOT. Persons having an AIDS test (ELISSA) performed shortly after receiving hepatitis B vaccine may test positive. The antibodies are generally gone within six months and the AIDS test will be negative. See Chapter 64 for more information.

The most common mild adverse effect is pain and soreness at the injection site. Less commonly, adverse effects include erythema, swelling, warmth, and induration, which may result from hypersensitivity to thimerosal, the preservative. Thimerosol is also found in contact lens solutions and often precipitates allergic reaction. A low-grade fever (less than 101°F) frequently follows the injection for the first 48 hours. Additional complaints that have been reported include malaise, fatigue, headache, nausea, vomiting, dizziness, myalgia, arthralgia, and *acute radiculoneuropathy* including *Guillain-Barré syndrome.*

DOSAGE. Hepatitis B vaccine is administered intramuscularly (the preferred site in adults is the deltoid; the anterior thigh is recommended for infants and young children), in three doses. An initial adult dose of 1 ml is administered followed by two additional 1-ml doses at one and six months. Hepatitis B is more effective when given in the arm than in the buttocks. In a recent hospital study, almost 90% of the patients vaccinated in the arm developed protective antibody, while only 73% of those who received injection in the buttocks were protected. This occurs because the vaccine may be inadvertently administered intralipomatously rather than intramuscularly. Each 1 ml of Heptavax-B contains 20 μg of hepatitis surface antigen, which is formulated in an alum adjuvant, and thimerosal (mercury derivative), which is added as a preservative. After injection is complete, it is important to assess anti-HB to determine if the person has immunity. If immunity has not been achieved, another dose is necessary. The most common reason for nonresponse is that the medication did not reach the muscle.

MEDICATION TO MANAGE PRURITUS

Cholestyramine

The pruritus associated with hepatic disease can often be alleviated by prolonged administration of the ion-exchange resin cholestyramine (Questran). Cholestyramine acts by adsorbing and combining with intestinal bile salts to form an insoluble, nonabsorbable complex, which is then excreted in the feces, thus preventing intestinal reabsorption. Since bile salts are excreted, the amount of bile acids deposited in the skin decreases and the pruritus is lessened. The effects of this medication take place one to three weeks after initiation of therapy. Continued treatment can control pruritus for years. If the medication is discontinued, pruritus returns in one to two weeks. Cholestyramine is discussed in detail in Chapter 54.

MEDICATIONS TO MANAGE ASCITES

Ascites associated with liver disease is due to several factors: increased capillary permeability, portal hypertension, hypoproteinemia due to decreased albumin production in the liver, and sodium retention and hypervolemia secondary to increased aldosterone production (Fig. 55–2). Ascites is a serious complication in patients with cirrhosis. Maintenance of normal nutrition is compromised due to early satiety. Respiratory function is also impaired by elevation of the diaphragm. In addition, the presence of fluid within the peritoneal cavity continuously exposes the patient to the possibility of bacterial infection and peritonitis.

Ascites can be removed through the administration of diuretics or by treatment called *paracentesis* (mechanical removal of fluid from the abdomen), although paracen-

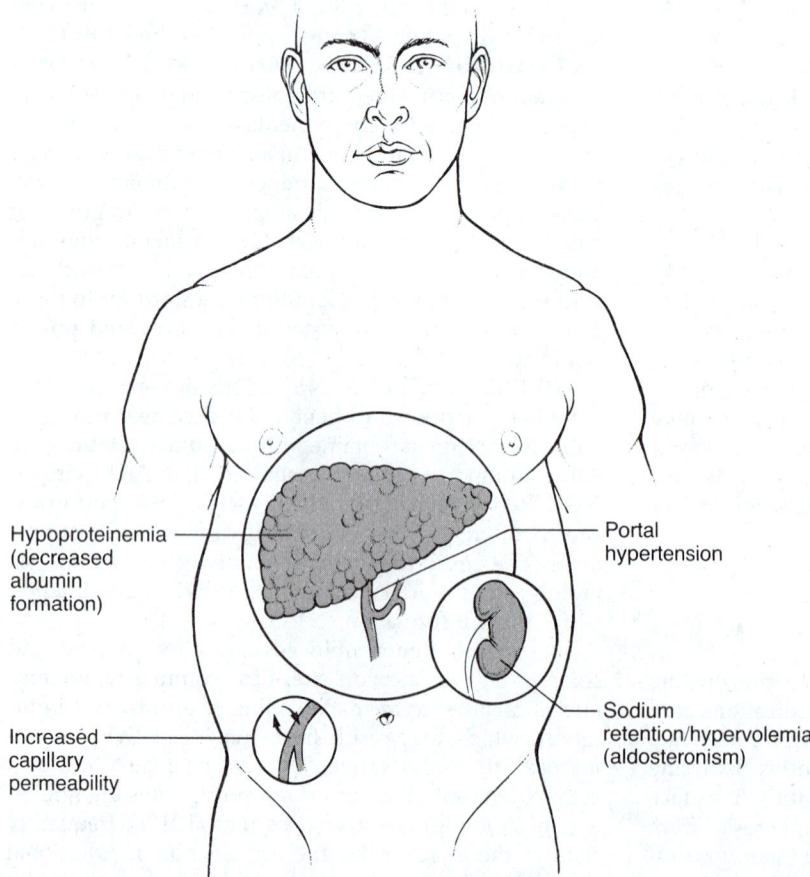

Hypoproteinemia (decreased albumin formation)

Portal hypertension

Sodium retention/hypervolemia (aldosteronism)

Increased capillary permeability

Figure 55–2. Contributing factors for development of ascites.

tesis is no longer recommended because it removes the protein-rich fluid from the abdominal cavity. Paracentesis decreases the patient's protein level, and rebound ascites generally develops due to the loss of intravascular oncotic pressure. Since there is increased aldosterone production and decreased aldosterone metabolism in the liver, the level increases in the body and promotes fluid retention. Therefore, aldosterone antagonists are often helpful in treatment. The drug of choice is spironolactone (Aldactone). When spironolactone, in doses of 100–600 mg/day, is combined with a 10–20 mEq sodium diet, 70%–80% of patients have a satisfactory diuresis. If spironolactone is not effective, the thiazide diuretics are added. Furosemide is clearly inferior to either spironolactone used alone or the combination of spironolactone and furosemide. For more information on diuretics, see Chapter 38.

MEDICATIONS FOR ENCEPHALOPATHY

Hypoprothrombinemia, if severe, can be treated with platelet transfusions and injections of vitamin K to prevent further bleeding. Vitamin and iron deficiencies can be treated with vitamins including iron supplements (Chapter 57) and folic acid supplements (Chapter 32). Ammonia is a key intermediate in the excretion of nitrogenous residues from the body. The major sites of ammonia production are the intestine and the kidney. Within the intestine there are two major substrates for ammonia production: nitrogenous substances, including blood and dietary protein, and urea, which is converted by bacteria in the colon into ammonia. The kidney produces ammonia in the tubular cell by deamidization of glutamine. Ammonia combines with excess hydrogen ion in the renal tubule to form ammonium, which is then excreted. The liver is the sole site for conversion of ammonia to urea. Reduced liver function and shunting of blood around the liver due to portal hypertension are the probable causes of ammonia intoxication.

The brain normally removes small amounts of ammonia from the blood. As the blood levels rise, the brain responds by removing larger amounts. As ammonia levels rise, it is postulated that there is a diminished cerebral metabolism or that there is an accumulation of "false neurotransmittors." Both of these hypotheses need to be proven through research.

The diagnosis of *hepatic encephalopathy* is based on a number of clinical symptoms and laboratory studies. Hepatic encephalopathy is often grade I to IV (Table 55–2).

The goals of treatment of hepatic encephalopathy are to decrease the amount of ammonia and other toxins in the brain and the reverse precipitating factors. All sedatives and narcotics are discontinued and any infection treated with medication. Renal function is maintained to prevent urea accumulation and acid–base balance is normalized to prevent exaggerated movement of ammonia and ammonium ion, normally found in the blood and tissues.

In treating encephalopathy, protein is eliminated from the diet during the acute stage and added slowly as the patient recovers. Special enteral and parenteral diets are available for patients with hepatic disease. These are discussed in detail in Chapter 56. Other treatments include oral administration of neomycin (see Chapter 46) to reduce the ammonia-producing organisms in the gastrointestinal tract; lactulose, given orally, is metabolized by intestinal bacteria into end products that acidify the colonic contents, which converts reabsorbable, nonionic ammonia (NH_3) to nonabsorbable, ionic ammonium (NH_4^+), which is excreted; administration of laxatives (see Chapter 54) to increase transit time of the feces, thereby allowing less ammonia to be reabsorbed by the intestine; and administration of levodopa (see Chapter 23), which is experimental at this time for liver failure but is thought to improve brain function in hepatic encephalopathy.

Neomycin

Neomycin, or other aminoglycosides such as kanamycin or paromomycin, can be used to reduce the number of colonic bacteria that normally convert urea and the amino acids of proteins into ammonia and other toxic metabolites. These medications are capable of reaching high antibacterial concentrations in the colon without causing systemic toxicity. Neomycin is useful for short-term management of severe disease. Neomycin is also used as a preoperative bowel preparation.

When treating hepatic encephalopathy, aminoglycosides, such as neomycin, are given only orally or via the nasogastric tube and only 1%–3% of the dose is absorbed. In someone with normal renal function, this small amount of drug is easily excreted via the kidneys, so no toxicity occurs.

A patient with hepatic disease and resultant encephalopathy may have altered renal function due to the hepatorenal syndrome. The abnormally functioning liver suppresses kidney function, through an unknown process. If kidneys are removed from patients with the hepatorenal syndrome and transplanted, they function normally.

If the patient with hepatic disease, such as encephalopathy, has altered renal function, the small amount of absorbed neomycin will not be excreted and can accumulate. This can lead to further kidney damage. Whether or not neomycin is used in patients with impaired renal function depends on the treatment goals. Chapter 46 provides more information on neomycin and the aminoglycosides.

Lactulose

Lactulose (Cephulac) is a synthetic derivative of the sugar lactose. It is effective in reducing ammonia levels in most patients with portal-systemic encephalopathy, including those not helped by neomycin or other aminoglycosides. Lactulose also improves protein tolerance in patients with advanced hepatic cirrhosis.

Lactulose is administered orally in the form of a syrup. It is not changed or absorbed, and reaches the lower digestive tract intact, where the colonic bacterial enzymes convert it to lactic and acetic acids, which lower the colon's pH. This acidification of the colon's contents converts ammonia (NH_3) to ammonium ion (NH_4^+), thus reducing the concentration of ammonia, allowing more ammonia to diffuse from the blood to the colon, where the ammonium ion can then be evacuated in the feces. The laxative action of lactulose speeds this evacuation.

Lactulose is classified as a nonosmotic cathartic and is described in greater detail in Chapter 54.

MEDICATION TO TREAT CHOLELITHIASIS

Cholelithiasis affects approximately 10% of the general population in the United States and 20% of those over 40. Peak occurrence is seen in obese women who are past the age of forty. The most common precipitating factors include overconsumption of cholesterol and calories, metabolic as well as genetic factors, inadequate exercise, and medications such as birth control pills. Patients generally complain of fat intolerance and experience nausea and vomiting, which eventually may be complicated with biliary colic and jaundice.

The major constituents of normal bile are water, various inorganic ions, bile salts, cholesterol, lecithin, and conjugated bilirubin. Cholesterol and lecithin are insoluble in water and are rendered soluble in bile water by the action of bile salts. The cholesterol found in bile has no known function; it is assumed to be a byproduct of

bile salt formation, and its presence is linked to the excretory function of bile. Many bile salt ions join with cholesterol and lecithin molecules to form water-solute complexes. Specific etiology is unknown, but a change in the nature of bile permits low-solubility bile components to come out of solution. They are said to precipitate out of the bile. As they do, they form small crystals on the gallbladder mucosal surface. Over time, they gradually increase in size. Three substances usually precipitate to form gallstones: cholesterol, calcium salt of bilirubin (calcium bilirubinate), and calcium carbonate.

In many cases, the presence of stones in the gallbladder produces no symptoms; in fact, many are first discovered in x-rays of the abdomen taken for reasons unrelated to their presence. The major complication of cholelithiasis follows the movement of a stone into the duct system where it obstructs bile flow.

Surgery is still the preferred treatment, but there are several approved products to treat gallstones medically—chenodiol [Chenodeoxycholic acid] (Chenix), monoctanoin (Moctanin), and ursodeoxycholic acid ("urso," Actigall)—and there are several experimental substances undergoing controlled trials in the United States and other countries to determine their efficacy in treating gallstones nonsurgically. Researchers are currently attempting either to inhibit the synthesis of cholesterol by inhibiting the activity of the enzyme 3-hydroxy-3-methyl-glutaryl CoA reductase (HMG CoA reductase) with preparations of bile acids such as chenodeoxycholic acid (CDCA) or ursodeoxycholic acid

Table 55–3. MEDICATIONS USED TO TREAT HEPATIC AND BILIARY TRACT DISEASE

Name	Dosage	Mode of Administration	Pharmacokinetics
Hepatitis B Vaccine:			
Action: produces protective anti-HBs			
Uses: persons exposed or susceptible to the development of hepatitis B			
Hepatitis B vaccine (Heptavax-B)	Adult: 1 ml initially IM in deltoid, then 1 ml at 1 and 6 months. Children birth to 10 yrs: 0.5 ml initially in anterolateral thigh followed by 0.5 ml at 1 and 6 months. Immunosuppressed patient: 2 ml initially and 2 ml at 1 and 6 months.	IM	UA
Hepatitis B Immune Globulin (HBIG)	Adult: 0.06 ml/kg as soon as possible after exposure. Children at birth: 0.5 ml.	IM / IM	UA

("urso," Actigall), or to enhance the hydroxylation of cholesterol by increasing the activity of enzyme 7-alpha-hydroxylase with experimental substances such as beta-glycerophosphate, a precursor of lecithin, phenobarbital, and certain terpene compounds. These drugs are featured in Table 55–3.

Radiopaque or large calculi are relatively resistant to dissolution by bile acids, as are cholesterol stones containing more than 4% calcium. These agents are used only in selected patients. Some dissolution of stones occurs in 40%–80% of patients within about two years. Although 25%–75% of patients experience recurrences within five years, retreatment is usually successful.

Regardless of the choice of therapy: surgery, medical dissolution, or lithotripsy, patients are encouraged to return to their ideal body weight and consume a high-fiber diet.

Chenodiol (Chenodeoxycholic Acid)

Many gallstones are composed of cholesterol and occur when the cholesterol content of the bile becomes greater in proportion to the bile salt and phospholipid content. Chenodiol is a natural bile salt that decreases cholesterol saturation of bile by decreasing the secretion of cholesterol and perhaps by increasing the secretion of bile salts. Chenodiol is administered for 9–12 months and is given in doses of 13–16 mg/kg in two divided doses. Adverse effects include diarrhea and possible hepatotoxicity from its breakdown products. More information can be found in Table 55–3.

Monoctanoin

Monoctanoin is a semisynthetic esterified glycerol (vegetable oil) that can be used when stones of calcium bilirubinate and calcium soaps are resistant to dissolution by oral chenodiol. Monoctanoin is administered through a T-tube, nasobiliary catheter, or percutaneous transhepatic catheter, and is considered a contact solvent. It is only effective when it is in contact with the stone. Monoctanoin is generally well tolerated if the rate is slow (3–5 ml/hour). Monoctanoin is continued for 7–21 days with diagnostic studies such as T-tube cholangiograms taken every three to four days to assess the process of dissolution. If the number or size of the stones has not changed in seven days, treatment is discontinued. The major adverse effects include diarrhea, nausea, and abdominal pain.

Ursodiol (Ursodeoxycholic Acid) (Actigall)

Ursodiol (Ursodeoxycholic Acid) (Actigall) is a naturally occurring bile salt. It suppresses hepatic synthesis and secretion of cholesterol and inhibits intestinal absorption of cholesterol. After repeated dosing, steady state is achieved in three weeks. Gallstone dissolution with ursodiol requires months of therapy. The usual dosage is 8–10 mg/kg/day given in two or three divided doses. Ultrasound images of the gallbladder are obtained within six months. If partial stone dissolution has not occurred within 12 months, the likelihood of success is greatly reduced.

Contraindications/ Precautions	Adverse Effects*	Interactions	Nursing Implications
Hypersensitivity to any component of vaccine. Precautions: delay vaccine if serious infection present. Administer cautiously in severely compromised cardiopulmonary status or when febrile reaction could cause risk. Safety in pregnancy and lactating women not established.	Neuro: earache, optic neuritis, Guillain-Barré syndrome, Bell's palsy, herpes zoster. Resp: URI, rhinitis GI: nausea, vomiting, diarrhea, abdominal pain, decreased appetite Integ: local site soreness, erythema, swelling, induration, pain, ecchymosis, pruritis, rash, pharyngitis Musculoskel: arthralgia, myalgia, back/neck/shoulder pain, fatigue, weakness	None known	ASSESSMENT: For current infection and cardiovascular status. INTERVENTION: Adults: administer deep IM into deltoid. Children: administer deep IM into anterolateral thigh. Agitate thoroughly—vaccine is slightly opaque. Store in refrigerator. EVALUATION: Vaccine is 80%–90% effective in producing immunity. Check anti-HB to see if immunity has developed. Some may need an additional dose.
Same as above.	CV: chest tightness GI: emesis, nausea Hemo: ANAPHYLAXIS Integ: tenderness, muscle stiffness at injection site, urticaria	Same as above.	Same as above. INTERVENTION: Very painful.

Table 55–3. MEDICATIONS USED TO TREAT HEPATIC AND BILIARY TRACT DISEASE–*CONTINUED*

Name	Dosage	Mode of Administration	Pharmacokinetics
Gallstone Solubilizing Agents:			
Chenodiol [chenodeoxycholic acid] (Chenix)			
Action: naturally occurring bile salt which suppresses hepatic production of cholesterol.			
Use: gradually reduces the size of radiolucent cholesterol gallstones.			
	13–16 mg/kg in 2 divided doses daily increased weekly by 250 mg until maximal tolerated dose is reached.	PO	O: rapid P: UA D: UA ½L: UA PB: UA B: liver E: bile
Monoctanoin (Moctanin)			
Action: semi-synthetic esterified glycerol that dissolves gallstones by acting as a contact solvent.			
Uses: gradually reduces calcium-based gallstones.			
	3–5 ml/hour daily for 2–10 days—average 5 days.	Into T-tube	UA
Ursodiol (ursodeoxycholic acid) (Actigall)			
Action: decreases cholesterol secretion into bile, alters the cholesterol/phospholipid ratio of lipid vesicles secreted in bile, increases bile flow			
Use: dissolution of gallbladder stones and decreases incidence of new gallstone formation.			
	8–10 mg/kg/day in 2–3 divided doses with meals.	PO	O: UA P: steady state 3 wks D: UA ½L: UA PB: highly B: liver E: bile

Key to Abbreviations in the *Pharmacokinetics* column O-onset; P-peak; D-duration; PB-protein bound; B-biotransformed in; E-excreted in; ½ L-halflife.
*Within the column listing adverse effects, underlines indicate the most common effects; CAPITALS indicate life-threatening effects.

Contraindications/Precautions	Adverse Effects*	Interactions	Nursing Implications
Contraindicated in hepatocyte dysfunction, primary biliary cirrhosis, biliary obstruction, pregnancy, or in women who may become pregnant. Safety in children not established. Used infrequently due to expense, limited usefulness, and incidence of adverse effects.	CV: elevate serum cholesterol (LDL) and triglyceride levels GI: diarrhea, cramps, nausea, vomiting, flatulence, dyspepsia, constipation Biliary: increased SGPT levels, pain, HEPATOXICITY Hemo: decreased WBC	Bile acid sequestering agents and aluminum antacids reduce absorption. Estrogens, oral contraceptives, and clofibrate counteract effectiveness of chenodiol.	ASSESSMENT: Baseline liver function studies and CBC and periodically during therapy. INTERVENTION: Take as directed EVALUATION: Contact physician if nonspecific abdominal pain and sudden RUQ pain, nausea, vomiting all associated with gallstone complications.
Contraindicated in clinical jaundice, significant biliary infection, recent history of duodenal ulcer. Use cautiously in pregnant and lactating women and impaired renal function.	CV: hypokalemia GI: abdominal pain, nausea, vomiting, diarrhea, anorexia Biliary: increased serum amylase Misc: fever, fatigue	None known	ASSESSMENT: Liver and gallbladder function. INTERVENTION: Warm to 70–80 degrees F before perfusing into T-tube. Perfusion pressure should not exceed 15 cm. Water pump is needed to maintain pressure. EVALUATION: If no dissolution occurs in 72 hours, stop therapy.
Contraindicated in chronic liver disease or allergy to bile acids.	Neuro: headache, anxiety, depression, sleep disorder Resp: cough, rhinitis GI: nausea, vomiting, dyspepsia, metallic taste, abdominal pain with stomatitis. Integ: pruritis, rash, urticaria, dry skin	Concurrent cholestyramine, colestipol, or aluminum antacids may interfere with absorption. Estrogen, oral contraceptives, and clofibrate may decrease effectiveness.	ASSESSMENT: Assess baseline liver function and SGOT and SGPT. Follow stones by ultrasound q 6 months. INTERVENTION: After complete dissolution of stones, continue for 1–3 months. Stones may recur in 50% of patients within 5 years. More common in persons with multiple stones originally.

Table 55–4. NURSING PROCESS IN HEPATIC DISEASE

Assessment

Note history of current illness, medication use (prescription, OTC, alcohol/street drugs).
Assess respiratory status, noting increased respiratory rate, dyspnea.
Ascertain dietary patterns.
Note exposure to hepatitis, or household/commercial cleaning agents which might be hepatotoxic.
Review laboratory studies, e.g., serum bilirubin, glucose, LDH, SGOT, albumin, total protein, ammonia levels.

Nursing Diagnosis	Nursing	Rationale	Desired Patient/ Evaluation Criteria
Fluid Volume, excess related to compromised regulatory mechanism (e.g., SIADH, decreased plasma proteins, malnutrition) as evidenced by edema/anasarca, weight gain; intake greater than output, oliguria, changes in urine specific gravity, dyspnea, pleural effusion, elevated blood pressure.	Administer diuretics (e.g., spironolactone); potassium; positive inotropic drugs and arterial vasodilators. Measure intake/output, noting positive balance (intake in excess of output). Weigh daily and note gain greater than 0.5 kg/day. Inspect dependent tissues routinely. Measure abdominal girth as indicated. Monitor blood pressure and CVP. Note jugular/abdominal vein distention. Auscultate lungs, noting diminished/absent breath sounds and developing adventitious sounds.	Used to control edema and ascites, block effect of aldosterone and increase water excretion while sparing potassium. Serum and cellular potassium are usually depleted because of liver disease as well as urinary losses. Given to increase cardiac output/improve renal blood flow and function, promoting reduction of fluid volume. Reflects circulating volume status, developing/resolution of fluid shifts, and response to therapy. Positive balance/weight gain reflect continuing fluid retention. Useful in monitoring development/resolution of edema/ascites. Blood pressure elevations are usually associated with excess in circulating volume, but may occur because of fluid shifts out of the vascular space. Indicative of pulmonary congestion/edema, which may result in consolidation, impaired gas exchange, and respiratory distress.	Demonstrates appropriate fluid volume with balanced intake and output, stable weight, vital signs within patient's normal range, and absence of edema.
Nutrition, altered, Less than body requirements related to inadequate diet; inability to process/digest nutrients, anorexia, nausea, abnormal bowel function as evidenced by weight loss, changes in bowel sounds, abdominal cramping, aversion to eating/lack of interest in food.	Record daily intake by calorie count. Assist and encourage patient to eat; explain reasons for type of diet. Consider individual food preferences in food choices. Provide mouth care frequently and prior to meals. Weigh as indicated. Compare changes in fluid status, recent weight history, triceps skin measurement.	Provides information about intake needs/deficiencies. Proper diet is vital to recovery. May eat better when preferred foods are included. Patient is prone to sore and/or bleeding gums and bad taste in mouth, which adds to anorexia. It may be difficult to use weight as a direct indicator of nutritional status in view of edema/ascites. Triceps skinfold	Demonstrates increased muscle mass/progressive weight gain toward goal with normalization of laboratory values and free of signs of malnutrition.

Table 55–4. NURSING PROCESS IN HEPATIC DISEASE–*CONTINUED*

Nursing Diagnosis	Nursing	Rationale	Desired Patient/ Evaluation Criteria
		measurement is useful in assessing changes in muscle mass and subcutaneous fat reserves.	
	Recommend cessation of smoking, as appropriate.	Reduces excessive gastric stimulation and risk of irritation/bleeding.	
	Consult with dietician as indicated.	Useful in determining individual needs.	
Thought Processes altered, potential related to physiologic changes (increased serum ammonia level, inability of liver to detoxify certain enzymes/drugs).	Observe for changes in behavior and mentation, e.g., lethargy, confusion, drowsiness, slowing/ slurring of speech, and irritability. Arouse patient at intervals.	Ongoing assessment is important because of fluctuating nature of impending hepatic coma.	Maintains usual level of mentation/reality orientation. Demonstrates behaviors/lifestyle changes to prevent/minimize changes in mentation.
	Note development/presence of asterixis, fetor hepaticus, tremors/seizure activity.	Suggest elevating serum ammonia levels, increased risk of progression to encephalopathy.	
	Reorient to time, place, person as needed.	Assists in maintaining reality orientation, reducing confusion/anxiety.	
	Investigate temperature elevations. Monitor for signs of infection.	Infection may precipitate hepatic encephalopathy due to tissue catabolism and release of nitrogen.	
	Avoid use of narcotics or sedatives, tranquilizers, and limit/restrict use of medications metabolized by the liver.	Certain drugs are toxic to the liver while other drugs may not be metabolized quickly because of cirrhosis, causing cumulative effects that affect mentation, mask signs of developing encephalopathy, or precipitate coma.	
	Monitor laboratory studies, e.g., ammonia, electrolytes, pH, BUN, glucose, CBC with differential.	Elevated ammonia levels, hypokalemia, metabolic alkalosis, hypoglycemia, anemia, and infection can precipitate or potentiate development of hepatic coma.	
	Administer antibiotics, e.g., (neomycin, p.o.)	Reduces ammonia-producing organisms in the gastrointestinal tract.	
	lactulose;	Metabolized by intestinal bacteria into end products that acidify colonic contents to convert NH_3 to NH_4^+ which is then excreted.	
	laxatives;	Increase transit time of feces, thereby allowing less ammonia to be reabsorbed by the intestine.	
	levadopa.	Experimentally thought to improve brain function.	

CONTINUED ON THE FOLLOWING PAGE

Table 55–4. NURSING PROCESS IN HEPATIC DISEASE–*CONTINUED*

Nursing Diagnosis	Nursing	Rationale	Desired Patient/ Evaluation Criteria
Knowledge deficit related to lack of recall, information misinterpretation, unfamiliarity with resources as evidenced by questions, statement of concern, inaccurate follow-through of instruction/development of preventable complications.	Review disease process/ prognosis and future expectations.	Provides knowledge base on which patient can make informed choices.	Verbalizes understanding of disease process/ prognosis. Correlates symptoms with causative factors. Initiates necessary lifestyle changes and participates in care.
	Inform patient of altered effects of medications with cirrhosis and the importance of using only drugs prescribed or cleared by a physician who is familiar with patient's history.	Altered metabolism of drugs affects action, half-life. In addition, some drugs are hepatotoxic (especially narcotics, sedatives, and hypnotics).	
	Stress importance of avoiding alcohol.	Alcohol is the leading cause in the development of cirrhosis.	
	Discuss restriction of sodium, use of salt substitutes, and necessity of reading food/OTC drug labels.	Minimizes ascites and edema formation. Overuse of substitutes may result in other electrolyte imbalances.	
	Encourage scheduling activities with adequate rest periods.	Decreases metabolic demands on the body and increases energy available for tissue regeneration.	
	Recommend avoidance of persons with infections, especially URI.	Altered nutritional status, impairs immune response, potentiates risk of infection.	
	Identify environmental dangers, e.g., carbon tetrachloride type cleaning agents, exposure to hepatitis.	Can precipitate recurrence.	
	Discuss use of vaccines as appropriate.	May be indicated to provide pre-/postexposure protection against hepatitis.	
	Stress necessity of follow-up care.	Chronic nature of disease has potential for life-threatening complications.	
	Instruct SO to notify health care providers of any confusion, untidiness, night wandering, tremors, or personality change.	Changes (reflecting deterioration) may be more apparent to SO, although insidious changes may be noted by others with less frequent contact with patient.	

USING THE NURSING PROCESS

ASSESSMENT

To develop the data base for a patient with liver or biliary disease, the nurse obtains from the patient or the family a nursing history. Typical items to be included are featured in Tables 55–4 and 55–5. The patient's recent use of cleaning agents such as oven cleaners, toilet cleaners, or commercial cleaners is determined; hepatic injury has been known to occur from the mixing of sev-

eral commercial cleaners together and from breathing vapors of any or all of them in a poorly ventilated area for a prolonged period. If, as is often the case, an interaction of medications has precipitated the hepatic injury, the causative medication may not be identified when hepatic injury is first diagnosed. Therefore, all medications are stopped immediately while supportive care is instituted. Medications that can adversely affect liver function may be found in Table 55–6.

The nurse obtains specimens for laboratory tests as ordered, including lactate dehydrogenase (LDH) and serum glutamic-oxaloacetic transaminase (SGOT), to assess hepatocellular damage, and other laboratory tests

Table 55–5. NURSING PROCESS FOR THE PATIENT WITH BILIARY DISEASE

Assessment

Assess dietary pattern and intolerances.
Review current medical history, e.g., recent pregnancy, inflammatory bowel disease, blood dyscrasias.
Ascertain characteristics of urine/stool.
Review diagnostic studies, e.g., abdominal x-ray, CT scan, ultrasound; serum bilirubin, amylase and liver enzyme levels.

Nursing Diagnosis	Nursing Actions	Rationale	Desired Outcomes/ Evaluation Criteria
Pain related to biologic injurying agents (obstruction/ductal spasm, inflammatory process, tissue ischemia/necrosis) evidenced by complaints, facial mask of pain, guarding behavior, autonomic responses.	Administer chenodeoxycholic acid (Chenic acid), chenodiol (Chenix);	A natural bile acid that decreases cholesterol synthesis, reducing size of gallstones.	Reports pain is relieved/ controlled. Follows prescribed pharmacologic regimen. Demonstrate use of relaxation skills as indicated for individual situation.
	hyperlipidemic agents, e.g., cholestyramine (Questran);	Reduces itching (pruritis) from bile salts in the skin.	
	anticholinergics, e.g., atropine, propantheline (Pro-Banthine) as indicated.	Relieves reflex spasm/ smooth muscle contraction and assists with pain management.	
	Observe and document location, severity (1–10 scale), and character of pain (steady, intermittent, colicky).	Assists in differentiating cause of pain and provides information about disease progression/ resolution, development of complications, and effectiveness of interventions.	
	Promote bedrest in position comfort.	Bedrest in low Fowler's position reduces intraabdominal pressures, however, patient will naturally assume least painful position.	
	Encourage use of relaxation techniques.	Promotes rest, redirects attention, may enhance coping.	
	Use soft/cotton linens, calamine lotion, oil bath (e.g., Alpha-Keri), cool/ moist compresses as indicated.	Reduces irritation/dryness of the skin and itching sensation.	
	Instruct patient to avoid food/fluids high in fats, gas-producers, or gastric irritants.	Prevents/limits recurrence of gallbladder attacks.	
Knowledge defict related to lack of exposure/recall, unfamiliarity with information resources/misinterpretation evidenced by questions, statement of concern, inaccurate follow-through of instructions/development of preventable complications.	Review disease process/ prognosis and future expectations.	Provides knowledge base on which patient can make informed choices.	Verbalizes understanding of condition/disease process and treatment. Identifies relationship of signs/symptoms to the disease process and correlates symptoms with causative factors. Initiates necessary lifestyle changes and participates in treatment regimen.
	Review drug regimen, possible side-effects.	Gallstones often recur, necessitating long-term therapy. Development of diarrhea/cramps during chenodiol therapy may be dose related/correctable.	
	Discuss weight reduction programs if indicated.	Obesity is a risk factor associated with cholecystitis and weight loss is beneficial in medical management of chronic condition.	
	Review signs/symptoms requiring medical evaluation, e.g., recurrent fever, persistent nausea, vomiting and pain, jaundice, dark urine, evidence of bleeding.	Indicative of progression of disease process/ development of complications requiring further intervention.	

Table 55–6. MEDICATIONS ADVERSELY AFFECTING THE LIVER

Anesthetics:
Halothane

Anti-inflammatory and Anti-Muscle Spasm Agents:
Allopurinol
Colchicine
Fenoprofen
Gold salts*
Indomethacin*
Oxyphenbutazone
Phenylbutazone*
Probenecid*
Steroids, C-17-alkyl

Antimicrobials:
Aminosalicylic acid (PAS)
Antifungal agents
Cephalosporins—rare, very rare
Chloramphenicol
Erythromycin estolate* (occurs most frequently with estolate, but all salts and bases have been implicated)
Griseofulvin
Isoniazid (INH)
Nitrofuran derivatives
Organic arsenicals
Penicillins*—rare, considering the number of milligrams administered every day
Procarbazine
Pyrazinamide (PZA)
Rifampin
Streptomycin
Sulfonamides*
Tetracyclines, IV

Antineoplastics:
Azathioprine*
Chlorambucil*
L-Asparaginase†
Mercaptopurine (6-MP)
Methotrexate
Mithramycin
Nitrogen mustard
Nitrosoureas

Cardiac Drugs:
Chlorothiazide
Methyldopa (Aldomet)
Papaverine*
Procainamide (Pronestyl)
Propranolol (Inderal)
Quinidine

Hormones—Derivatives:
Acetohexamide*
Chlorpropamide*
Contraceptives, oral
Methimazole
Methyltestosterone
Oral hypoglycemics
Oxymetholone (Anadrol)
Propylthiouracil*
Tolbutamide

Tranquilizers, Hypnotics, Pain Medications:
Acetaminophen—only when ingested in large amounts
Benzodiazepine derivatives
Chlorpromazine* (Thorazine)
MAO inhibitors
Phenobarbital
Phenothiazines
Phenytoin (Dilantin)
Salicylates
Tricyclics

Miscellaneous
Ethyl alcohol
Ethyl chloride
Fat emulsion
Ferrous salts
Heavy metal antagonists
Levodopa
Niacin (nicotinic acid)
Phenacetamide (Phenurone)
Vitamin A

NOTE: The medications listed in this table have been identified as possibly affecting adversely the functions of or being directly toxic to the liver. The medications marked with an asterisk (*) may affect the liver in some persons through an idiosyncratic reaction that is not entirely understood. The medications marked with a dagger (†) cause liver toxicity in many patients, and persons receiving these preparations must be watched very closely. The nurse must also remember that when the patient has hepatic disease, medications normally biotransformed by the liver will need the dosage modified or the patient will develop toxic effects.

to assess liver function. A serum bilirubin (indirect and direct) test is often used in cases of jaundice to determine the presence of an elevated serum bilirubin.

Whenever a patient has any hepatic problem—cirrhosis, hepatitis, or chronic alcoholism—the nurse must be very alert to the medications prescribed for and administered to the patient. Any medication that is biotransformed in the liver to inactive metabolites is given at lower dosage levels or is withheld altogether. The nurse must continually assess the patient for toxic drug effects and report them as soon as they are suspected. Table 55–7 identifies common drugs and their routes of excretion.

It is important to assess all current symptoms and how they have changed over time such as intolerance to fatty meals, change in stool or skin color, or itching. Symptoms of the current condition are assessed and they are then treated during the intervention phase.

NURSING DIAGNOSIS

From the outcomes of the assessment, the nurse develops the nursing diagnoses. Typical nursing diagnoses for patients with hepatic and/or biliary disease are included in Tables 55–4 and 55–5.

PLANNING AND INTERVENTION

From the nursing diagnoses, the nurse determines the goals of nursing intervention, which are included in Tables 55–4 and 55–5.

Table 55–7. MEDICATIONS AND WHERE THEY ARE EXCRETED

Drug	Site of Excretion*	Drug	Site of Excretion
ANTIBIOTICS:		***CENTRAL NERVOUS SYSTEM DRUGS:***	
Aminoglycosides		*Barbiturates*	
Amikacin	Renal	Pentobarbital	Hepatic
Gentamicin	Renal	Phenobarbital	Hepatic (renal)
Tobramycin	Renal	Secobarbital	Hepatic
Kanamycin	Renal	*Benzodiazepines*	
Neomycin	Renal	Chlordiazepoxide (Librium)	Hepatic
Streptomycin	Renal	Diazepam (Valium)	Hepatic (renal, GI)
Cephalosporins		Flurazepam (Dalmane)	GI (renal)
Cephalexin	Renal	Haloperidol	Hepatic (renal, GI)
Cephalothin	Renal (hepatic)	*Phenothiazines*	
Cefazolin	Renal	Chlorpromazine	Hepatic
Choloramphenicol	Hepatic (renal)		
Clindamycin	Hepatic (renal)	***CARDIOVASCULAR DRUGS:***	
Colistimethate	Renal	*Antiarrhythmic agents*	
Erythromycin	Hepatic	Lidocaine	Hepatic (renal)
Lincomycin	Hepatic (renal)	Procainamide	Renal (hepatic)
Penicillins		Propranolol	Hepatic
Amoxicillin	Renal	Quinidine	Nonrenal (renal)
Ampicillin	Renal (hepatic)	*Antihypertensive agents*	
Carbenicillin	Renal (hepatic)	Diazoxide	Renal (nonrenal)
Cloxacillin	Hepatic (renal)	Hydralazine	Hepatic (renal, GI)
Dicloxacillin	Renal (hepatic)	Methyldopa	Renal (hepatic)
Methicillin	Renal (hepatic)	Minoxidil	Nonrenal
Nafcillin	Hepatic	Nitroprusside	Nonrenal
Oxacillin	Renal (hepatic)	Prazosin	Hepatic (renal)
Penicillin	Renal (hepatic)	*Cardiac glycosides*	
Ticarcillin	Renal	Digitoxin	Hepatic (renal)
Sulfisoxazole	Renal	Digoxin	Renal (nonrenal)
Tetracyclines		*Diuretics*	
Tetracycline	Renal (hepatic)	Chlorthalidone	Renal (nonrenal)
Doxycycline	Renal (hepatic)	Ethacrynic acid	Hepatic
Minocycline	Hepatic	Furosemide	Renal
		Metolazone	Renal
ANALGESICS (NON-NARCOTIC):		Thiazides	Renal
Acetaminophen (Tylenol)	Hepatic		
Acetylsalicylic acid	Renal (hepatic)	***MISCELLANEOUS AGENTS:***	
Phenazopyridine (Pyridium)	Renal	*Anticoagulants*	
		Heparin	Nonrenal
		Neurologic drugs	
NARCOTICS AND NARCOTIC ANTAGONISTS:		Diphenylhydantoin	Hepatic (renal)
Codeine	Hepatic (renal)	(Dilantin)	
Meperidine (Demerol)	Hepatic (renal)	Neostigmine	Nonrenal
Methadone	Hepatic (renal)	*Hypoglycemic agents*	
Morphine	Hepatic (renal, GI)	Insulin, regular	Hepatic (renal)
Naloxone (Narcan)	Hepatic	*Neuromuscular blocking agents*	
Pentazocine (Talwin)	Hepatic (renal)	Gallamine	Renal
		Succinylcholine	Nonrenal
		Tubocurarine	Renal

*First organ is primary organ of excretion. Organ in parentheses is secondary organ of excretion.

Patients with hepatic or biliary diseases are managed with a nutritional diet usually high in proteins, carbohydrates, and vitamins. However, a patient in hepatic coma would have a reduced-protein diet to help eliminate the ammonia from the body. Numerous specialized nutritional products are available, such as Hepatic Aid and Hepatamine. These products are described in detail in Chapter 56. Fluid and electrolyte balance is also monitored carefully, particularly in the patient with vomiting or diarrhea.

HEPATOTOXICITY FROM OTHER DRUGS

If the hepatotoxicity is found to be drug induced, typical nursing goals might include (1) identification of the causative agent if possible, and (2) education of the patient to discourage further exposure to or ingestion of the causative agent or a chemically similar agent.

During the acute phase, all previous medications are stopped and only supportive therapy, such as corticosteroids or exchange transfusions, is used. Both therapies are still controversial but should not be omitted. A few days could be crucial to any patient this acutely ill. Constant nursing supervision includes close monitoring of all body systems, including the neurologic, cardiovascular, renal, respiratory, and gastrointestinal systems. Any change in these systems signals the need for immediate interventions to prevent further deterioration of the patient's condition.

Treatment of a patient with drug-induced hepatotoxicity is managed similarly to that of a patient in hepatic coma. If the causative agent or agents have been identified, the patient and family need to be educated about the danger of further use of it or similar drugs.

EVALUATION

The evaluation process is ongoing. The nurse evaluates every nursing intervention to determine if the goals are being achieved. The goals of nursing intervention become the outcome criteria for evaluation. Typical evaluation criteria are included in Tables 55–4 and 55–5.

Whether or not the patient comes through the illness with chronic hepatic dysfunction can only be determined through liver function studies. If it becomes necessary to administer supportive medications to the patient during the acute phase, these medications must be evaluated closely to prevent further hepatic toxicity. Some drugs remain active until they are biotransformed by the liver's microsomal system; if this system is injured, the medications remain active longer and result in the development of adverse effects or toxic effects. All medications being administered to the patient are reviewed closely to determine if they cause more hepatic damage. When possible, medications that are totally excreted by the kidney are used.

Patients are evaluated to determine whether the medications being administered are effective. If the medication is ineffective, or adverse or toxic effects are being experienced, the medication is discontinued. Often, patients are discharged from the acute care setting on medications to control chronic symptoms. Patient compliance and knowledge level are evaluated. Adequate knowledge about the disease condition and medications often helps patients comply with their medical and nursing regimen.

Patient symptoms of jaundice, pruritis, hypoprothrombinemia, ascites, and vitamin and iron deficiencies are evaluated to determine if they are being brought under control. The treatment regimen is then modified as necessary.

SUMMARY

The hepatic and biliary systems are a major part of the digestive system, contributing many digestive enzymes. This chapter briefly discusses drugs that are used to: treat hepatic cell necrosis—N-acetylcysteine; prevent hepatitis—hepatitis B vaccine and recombinant hepatitis vaccine; manage ascites—spironolactone; manage pruritis—cholestyramine; treat hepatic encephalopathy—neomycin and lactulose; and treat cholelithiasis—chenodiol, monoctanoin, and ursodeoxycholic acid.

Assessment of the patient with hepatic and biliary disease always begins with a thorough nursing history including precipitating symptoms, alcohol intake, drug history, and dietary patterns. Laboratory data is obtained to determine the extent of dysfunction. All drugs are administered cautiously to persons with hepatic/biliary disease.

BIBLIOGRAPHY

AMA Department of Drugs: AMA Drug Evaluations, ed 5. PSG Publishing, Littleton, MA, 1986.

Bishop, ML, et al: The influence of hepatic disease on drug disposition. J Med Tech 42(2):60, 1987.

Gilman, AG, Goodman, LS, and Gilman, A (eds): Goodman and Gilman's The Pharmacological Basis of Therapeutics, ed 7. Macmillan, New York, 1985.

Medical Letter. Ursodiol for dissolving cholesterol gallstones. The Medical Letter 30(773):81, 1988.

Middleton, D: Epidemiology watch. Diagnosis 7:19, 1985.

Monoctanoin for gallstones. The Medical Letter, 29(740):52, 1987.

Olin, B (ed): Facts and Comparisons. JB Lippincott, St. Louis, 1989.

Slawson, M and Slawson, S: The hidden alcohol in drugs. RN 43:54, April 1983.

SITUATION   55–1

Albert Shinn is a 56-year-old with alcoholic cirrhosis. He is admitted to the telemetry unit for care. Mr. Shinn is lethargic and confused. His abdomen is distended and firm; pitting edema is noted of the lower extremities.

1. A nasogastric tube is inserted, and Mr. Shinn is to receive lactulose (Cephulac) via n/g tube every 4 hours. The nurse will anticipate the following effect of this drug:
   a. nausea and vomiting
   b. frequent stools
   c. tremors and muscle spasms
   d. skin rash

2. When evaluating Mr. Shinn for the effectiveness of lactulose therapy, the nurse will check the following:
   a. complete blood count
   b. total serum protein
   c. ammonia levels
   d. stools for occult blood

3. Mr. Shinn is scheduled to receive neomycin for short-term management of acute cirrhosis. The nurse will expect to administer this medication via:
   a. subcutaneous injection
   b. intravenous administration
   c. intramuscular injection
   d. nasogastric tube

4. While Mr. Shinn is on neomycin therapy, the nurse will check the daily lab work for elevation of:
   a. amylase
   b. creatinine
   c. white blood cells
   d. $T_3 T_4$

5. The nurse notes alteration in skin integrity related to the pruritus associated with hepatic dysfunction. Mr. Shinn is started on cholestyramine (Questran) via nasogastric tube. The nurse will anticipate reduced pruritus within:
   a. 1 to 3 weeks
   b. 2 to 4 days
   c. 24 hours
   d. 5 days

6. During the acute phase of hepatic encephalopathy, the nurse will plan to eliminate the following from Mr. Shinn's diet:
   a. protein
   b. sodium
   c. potassium
   d. fats

Please refer to the Appendices for correct answers and additional review questions with answers

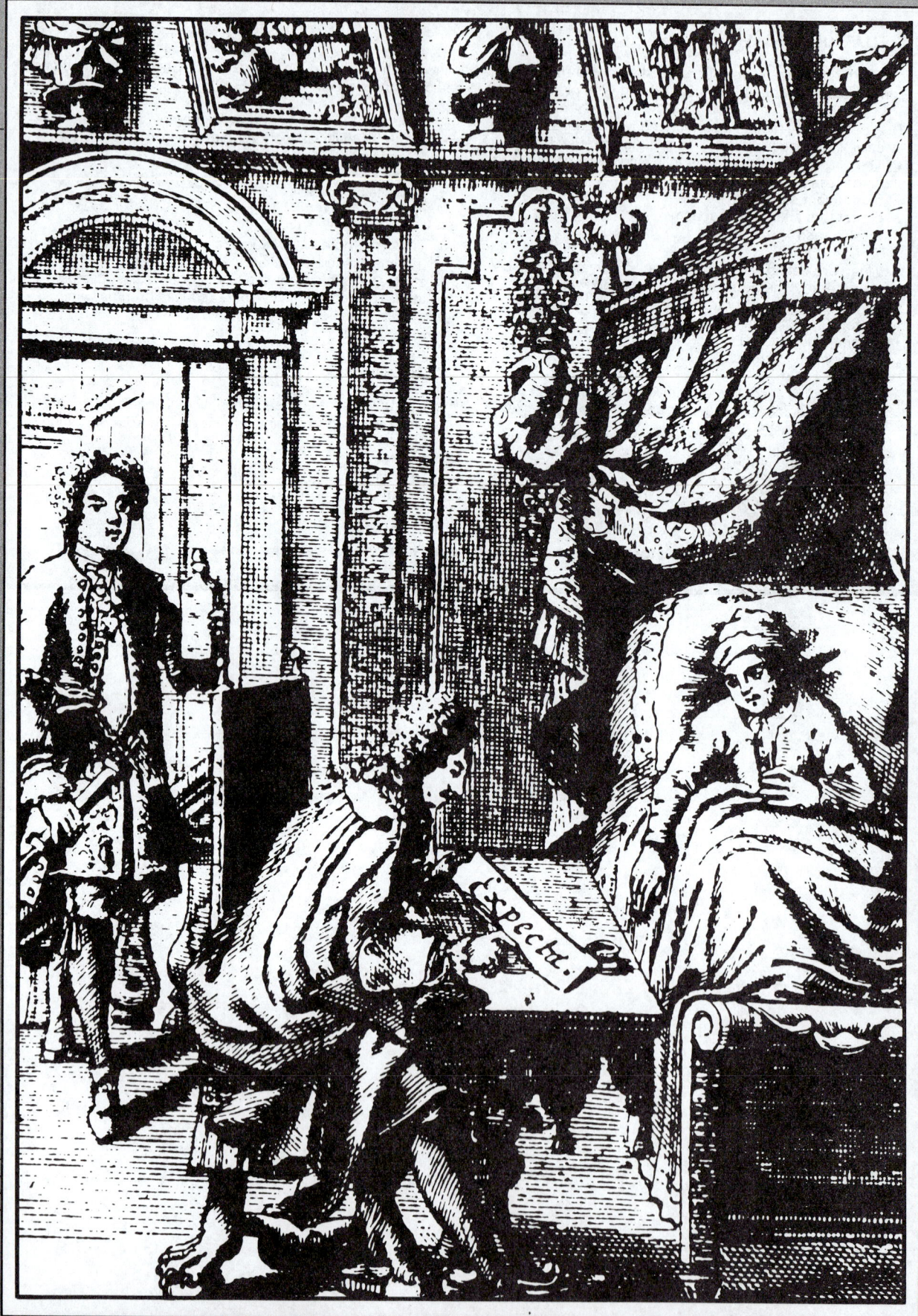

Writing prescriptions for a patient, circa 1700. The Bettmann Archive.

11
UNIT

NUTRITIONAL AGENTS

56 CHAPTER

ENTERAL AND PARENTERAL AGENTS

MERRILY MATHEWSON KUHN, R.N.C., Ph.D., CCRN

LEARNING OBJECTIVES

After reading this chapter, the student will be able to:

1. Identify those agents commonly used as enteral and parenteral products.

2. Identify specific areas to assess in the patient requiring enteral and parenteral agents in order to formulate appropriate nursing diagnoses.

3. Plan the nursing interventions necessary to administer enteral agents and choose appropriate teaching strategies to gain patient compliance.

4. Evaluate the patient at various stages of treatment to gauge nursing interventions.

NUTRITION

Nutrition is an important aspect of patient care. Today, even with increased knowledge of nutrition, large numbers of patients in hospitals and nursing homes suffer from *malnutrition*. Fifty percent of all hospitalized patients are malnourished and 5%–10% of these persons suffer from severe protein–calorie malnutrition (Farley, 1988). A well-nourished patient can usually tolerate three to four days of fasting, provided standard intravenous fluids are infused to maintain hydration. However, acutely ill patients have increased energy needs and may even double their normal calorie requirements. If a patient enters the hospital in a malnourished state, he/she will require nutritional support immediately.

Malnutrition is associated with increased length of hospital/nursing home stay due to poor wound healing, muscle atrophy, impaired immunocompetence, reduced lymphocyte count, sepsis, and even death. A reduction in plasma proteins leads to dry, flaky skin, peripheral edema, and even noncardiac pulmonary edema. The stress of illness or surgery increases the likelihood of becoming malnourished.

Nutritional requirements vary according to a person's age, weight, activity, and hormone metabolic activities within the body. These factors need to be taken into consideration when determining nutritional support. A patient may have nutritional needs met either by the *enteral* routes, through the mouth or into the gastrointestinal tract, or by *parenteral* routes, through the vascular system. Enteral and parenteral nutrition are discussed in this chapter.

In order to survive, people need a daily supply of nutrients—including carbohydrates, fats, and proteins. These complex products are transformed, through the chemical process of metabolism, into simpler products, along with the production of heat and energy.

The goals of nutrition support therapy are derived from the processes of the metabolic response to injury. The goals include:

1. to support current organ function and structure
2. to prevent malnutrition from developing
3. to treat malnutrition when and where present
4. to do no harm.

METABOLISM

There are two main phases of metabolism—catabolism and anabolism (Table 56–1). *Catabolism* is the breaking down of complex cellular materials into simpler constituents for use in energy production or excretion. *Anabolism* is the synthesis of cellular materials for growth, maintenance, and repair of body tissues, during which simple substances are combined to form more complex substances, with a net result of new cellular material and the storage of energy. When anabolism exceeds catabolism, lean body mass (LBM) and fat are produced,

Table 56–1. ANABOLISM VS. CATABOLISM

Anabolism	Catabolism
NITROGEN BALANCE	
+	−
Simple > Complex	Complex > Simple
HORMONES:	
Insulin	Epinephrine
Growth Hormone	Glucocorticoids
Anabolic steroids	Glucagon
Testosterone	
17-Keto-steroids	
ACTIVATED BY:	
Puberty	Fever
	Illness
	Stress
	Trauma
	Burns
RESULTS IN:	
Weight gain	Weight loss
Growth and repair	Decreased wound healing
	Anemia
	Leukopenia
	Decreased immune function
	Muscle wasting
	Decreased mentation

and growth occurs. When catabolism exceeds anabolism, tissue is lost and the body loses substance and weight. In a healthy state, a balance exists between catabolism and anabolism, so body weight and substance are maintained at a constant level.

The intake of food directly relates to metabolism. If food intake is increased above metabolic demands, anabolism occurs and weight is gained. Conversely, if food intake is decreased below metabolic demands, catabolism occurs and weight is lost. Other factors influencing metabolism include change in physical activity and endocrine function. Hormones favoring anabolism include insulin, growth hormone, testosterone, and 17-ketosteroids (see Table 56–1). Insulin is the major anabolic hormone, facilitating entry of glucose into cells and cellular uptake of amino acids for protein synthesis. Growth hormone and testosterone stimulate nitrogen, phosphorus, and potassium retention, resulting in an increase in lean body and visceral protein mass. Another example of anabolism occurs during puberty, when there is an increased release of growth hormone from the pituitary, stimulating tissue growth.

The catecholamine epinephrine, the glucocorticoids, corticotropin, and glucagon favor catabolism by mobilizing substrates to provide energy (see Table 56–1). This results in *glycogenolysis, gluconeogenesis*, augmented *lipolysis*, and inhibition of protein synthesis. Factors influencing the release of these hormones, resulting in catabolism, include stressors such as fever, fractures, burns, bacterial or other infections, and surgery.

When food is consumed and metabolized, the energy produced is measured in calories. Calorie is the common word for the proper term *kilocalorie* (kcal). The kcal is the easily determined standard measure of heat resulting from the generation of energy: the heat energy required to raise the temperature of 1 kg of water 1°C. These terms, kcal and calorie, are used interchangeably.

Food products produce energy at various levels: 1 g of protein produces 4.0 calories; 1 g of fat—9.45 calories; and 1 g of carbohydrate—3.4 calories. The gram-equivalents used are 4 g for protein, 9 g for fat, and 3.4 g for carbohydrate. Under normal situations, all three substrates contribute to the caloric needs of the body. Carbohydrates are completely oxidized to carbon dioxide and water. Fats are broken down into two components, glycerol, which is used by the liver to make glucose, and fatty acids. A portion of the fatty acids is converted to ketone bodies. Certain tissues can utilize fatty acids and ketone bodies for energy. Proteins are converted to amino acids; some are then oxidized to urea, creatinine, uric acids, and other compounds, whereas others are used for gluconeogenesis.

The food groups—carbohydrates in the form of glucose, fats as fatty acids, and proteins as amino acids—react with enzymes and oxygen within the cell. The energy produced forms adenosine triphosphate (ATP), composed of nitrogen phosphate and a sugar, which can be stored by the body for later use or can be released instantly for mechanical work such as muscle contraction or movement of substances across cell membranes (active transport).

The normal daily intake of nutrients for a healthy adult between the ages of 20 and 50 years is 1500–3000 calories. This intake is divided into 45%–60% or 380–504 g carbohydrate; 20% or 45–55 g protein (about 8–9 g of nitrogen); and 20%–35% or 56–100 g fats. These nutrients, along with the necessary vitamins and minerals, must be consumed on a daily basis to maintain normal body activities and constant body weight.

Carbohydrates

Carbohydrates are sugars composed of carbon, hydrogen, and oxygen. Carbohydrates are oxidized through the process of *glycolysis* into saccharides. Polysaccharides include sucrose, lactose, and maltose, and the simplest monosaccharides include glucose, fructose, and galactose. Fructose and galactose can also be converted to glucose. Glucose in the presence of oxygen is converted to pyruvate, which can move into the mitochondria of the cell to be converted to energy. When oxygen is not available, as in periods of stress or severe exercise, pyruvate is reduced to lactate in the cell. When oxygen becomes available, lactate, which has built up in muscle and blood, is reconverted to pyruvate for oxidation.

Extra carbohydrate in the body is stored as glycogen in the liver and muscle. From these sites, glucose is immediately available for maintenance of blood sugar (liver) and anaerobic glycolysis for exercise (muscle). The amount of glycogen stored in the body is about 300 g.

Lipids

Lipids, or fats, are composed of fatty acids and triglycerides containing carbon, hydrogen, and oxygen. Triglycerides transport and are the storage forms of fatty acids. Triglycerides are *hydrolyzed* to form glycerol and fatty acids, which then are available for oxidation for energy. Fatty acids serve as a very important substrate for *energy trapping* in the body.

During starvation, fatty acid oxidation rates are high and the liver produces large quantities of ketones. Ketones can be oxidized for energy in most tissues.

Fat is the principal form of energy storage in the body. Fat is anhydrous and, therefore, can be stored without water. Fatty acids are stored in adipose tissue mostly as triglycerides. The amount of fat a person can store is unlimited. When energy intake exceeds expenditure, energy can be stored in the form of fat.

Protein

Protein consists of amino acids that are unique in that they contain nitrogen along with carbon, hydrogen, and water. Many body components, such as enzymes, muscle fibers, collagen, and antibodies, are protein. All proteins in the body perform some structural or functional role. There is no storage form of protein like with other nutrients. Therefore, protein must be consumed on a daily basis. Protein consumed in excess of body requirements is converted to fat for storage.

There are two types of amino acids: essential and nonessential. Essential amino acids must be supplied by the diet, whereas nonessential can be manufactured by the body from other amino acids. If a single amino acid is missing, synthesis of any protein containing that amino acid will not occur. Amino acids undergo *deamination* or *transamination*, which requires pyridoxine (vitamin B$_6$). Through this process, the nitrogen is removed and incorporated into urea or ammonia for excretion. The remaining carbon skeletons, through the process of gluconeogenesis in the liver, form glucose.

Branched-chain amino acids (valine, leucine, and isoleucine) may be oxidized directly in skeletal muscle. This oxidation is a potential energy source for muscle. Patients who are suffering from stress or trauma have greater branched-chain oxidation. When this disproportionate increase occurs, the body must then dispose of other amino acids, since an incomplete mixture of amino acids is useless for protein synthesis. The excess nitrogen is lost in the urine. Therefore, patients who are severely stressed, traumatized, or septic may receive supplemental branched-chain amino acids.

Patients with liver disease ultimately have a change in the normal plasma amino acid profile, with an increase in the *aromatic amino acids*, compared with the branched-chain amino acids. A diet high in branched-chain amino acids and low in aromatic amino acids may be beneficial in the nutritional support of patients with liver disease. However, research data are not available to support this fact.

RESPIRATORY QUOTIENT

The respiratory quotient (RQ) is the ratio of carbon dioxide production to oxygen utilization by the body. Carbon dioxide is a byproduct of metabolism that is eliminated by the lung. When carbohydrates are metabolized in the body, an average of 100 carbon dioxide molecules are formed for each 100 molecules of oxygen consumed. Therefore, the RQ for carbohydrates is 1.0. Using this same formula, the RQ for fat is 0.7 and the RQ for protein is 0.8. The reason for the lower RQ with fat and protein is that a large share of the oxygen metabolized with these foods is required to combine with the excess hydrogen ions present in them instead of forming carbon dioxide. The average RQ for a well-balanced diet is approximately 0.8.

NUTRITION IN ILLNESS

At times, individuals are unable to consume or digest food in the normal fashion. Persons may have difficulty digesting, absorbing, or metabolizing food, as with recent bowel surgery, a type of malabsorption syndrome like sprue, or a decreased number of teeth. Persons may have allergic reactions to food and be unable to digest, absorb, or metabolize specific nutrients like wheat or milk products. Persons may also develop intolerances to food because of a lack of enzymes for digestion. As an example, lactase is required for the digestion of milk. Intolerances to milk can occur as lactase levels decrease with aging. In addition, persons may become undernourished with chronic illness—like cancer, acute trauma, or severe burns. In each of these instances, catabolism is accelerated, and the individual loses weight and lacks energy for even normal metabolic functions. Signs and symptoms that can be observed in a patient in a catabolic state are featured in Table 56–2. At this point, the patient must receive additional nutrients either through tube feedings or via the parenteral route if the oral route is impossible or inadequate.

Starvation begins when nutrients are not supplied to

Table 56–2. SIGNS AND SYMPTOMS OF A CATABOLIC STATE

Increased temperature
Increased pulse and respiration
Decreased level of consciousness
Poor skin turgor
Lesion of skin and mucous membranes
Dehydration
Changes in bowel activity (number and character of stools)
Decreasing body weight
Tissue edema
Eczema (fatty acid deficiencies)

the body in adequate amounts. A normal adult has about 200 g of glycogen (900 kcal) stored in the liver, 6000 g of protein (24,000 kcal) found in muscles and viseral proteins, and 15,000 g of fat (141,000 kcal) in storage, with fat content varying the most among individuals. When food no longer enters the body, these stores are used for energy production. Glycogen stores are used first, with primary glycogenolysis occurring in the liver to increase blood glucose. The glycogen stores are usually exhausted in eight to ten hours. Glucose requirements are then met by the initiation of gluconeogenesis. Although various substances are shuttled to the liver and kidneys for conversion to glycogen, amino acids derived from muscle and visceral proteins are the major substrate for this process. The protein must have the nitrogen (N) removed before it can be converted into glucose; the nitrogen is then excreted in the urine (1 g N = 6.25 g of protein). Therefore, as urinary nitrogen increases, a negative nitrogen balance (catabolism) develops.

In the first few days of starvation, the body may break down up to 75 g of protein daily to meet energy requirements. At this rate of protein breakdown, a third of the body protein would be depleted in several weeks, leading to death. In addition, protein, although calorically important, is not accumulated or stored in humans purely as a nutritional reservoir. Each protein molecule serves a nonfuel function—as an enzyme, or a contractile, structural, or carrier protein. Since each molecule is already serving some nonfuel function, an adaptive process occurs to spare protein. Protein catabolism diminishes with prolonged starvation due to a change in fuel utilization. When food is consumed and glucose is available, the body, particularly the brain and nervous system, preferentially uses glucose for energy. In starvation, the body adapts to the lack of glucose and begins to break down fats (adipose tissue) to fatty acids and ketone bodies for energy in order to spare protein.

This adaptive process occurs through hormone-mediated changes. The amount of insulin secreted by a normal individual decreases during starvation. This decrease triggers the lipolytic release of fatty acids and glycerol from adipose tissue to be used either directly or indirectly as metabolic fuel. The oxidation of adipose tissue is also associated with a sharp rise in ketone bodies, as the body gradually enters a state described as "starvation ketosis." This ketosis is characterized by a decrease in endogenous protein catabolism as a fuel source and a conversion of the CNS to ketone body metabolism. Once this adaptive process occurs, protein breakdown decreases to 20–25 g daily, and urinary nitrogen excretion also decreases.

A feedback mechanism exists to prevent a pathologic ketosis from occurring, as is seen in diabetes. As ketone levels rise, insulin production is stimulated, and the lipolytic process is temporarily decreased.

With the adaptation to starvation ketosis, the fasting state can be prolonged, depending on the amount of body fat an individual has. Seventy percent of the brain's energy needs can be supplied by the oxidation of ketones, with glucose from amino acids supplying the rest. When fat stores are depleted, muscle and organ tissue is then sacrificed for energy. A normal healthy individual will not tolerate a loss of more than 35%–45% of his or her body weight.

A totally fasting healthy person adapts to an economical utilization of body fat and a conservation of body protein to the greatest possible extent. The person who is stressed (burns, surgery, trauma, infection, or shock) does not adapt as well to starvation. Starvation begins to occur as early as 24 hours after the initial stress when the patient has no oral intake, and is being supported only with regular IV fluids such as dextrose and water, or Ringer's lactate, or normal saline solutions.

When stress of disease or injury occurs, catabolism begins just after the onset. Research has indicated that there is a 13% rise in metabolic rate for each 1°C or 2.2°F rise in temperature. Energy demands may be 60% above normal and higher. In addition to a negative nitrogen balance, deficiencies of potassium, magnesium, phosphate, sulfate, and zinc and other trace elements occur, and can persist through convalescence. Stress, from any cause, enhances the catabolism of glycogen, muscle, and fat due to the increased energy demands. Stress, then, causes dramatic alterations in nutrient metabolism as the normal adaptive processes that occur in starvation are prevented.

Glucose requirements increase as the body responds to the stress situation. A relative insulin resistance occurs, as the tissues are not as responsive to insulin in the uptake of glucose. This leads to greater production of insulin, which in turn decreases lipolysis. Because the body has only minimal glycogen stores and fat is not easily mobilized in this situation, protein catabolism increases to provide a substrate for gluconeogenesis. Protein catabolism also supplies the amino acids needed to synthesize blood cells, structural proteins, and enzymes. In addition to the body's need for more nutrients during fever or infection, there are usually greater losses such as through vomiting or diarrhea, hemorrhage, transudation and exudation, wound drainage, and intestinal losses.

After several days, sufficient ketone bodies become available to decrease the demand on endogenous protein. However, the catabolism of protein continues with detrimental effects on the immune system, wound healing, the respiratory system, and lean body mass in general.

Malnutrition

Two major classifications of malnutrition can occur: protein-calorie or *marasmic* type and protein or *kwashiorkor* malnutrition. Elements of both types may occur in a nutritionally compromised patient.

Protein-calorie malnutrition or marasma is a manifestation of *somatic* or lean-muscle protein deficiency. Patients who are at risk for this type of malnutrition have generally experienced a recent unplanned weight loss of 10% or more in less than two weeks. As this condition progresses, subcutaneous fat stores decrease and muscle

mass atrophies. These patients experience diarrhea and usually a diminished appetite or anorexia. A patient with marasmic type malnutrition does not usually experience edema.

Protein or kwashiorkor malnutrition has depressed *visceral* or endogenous protein synthesis. (See Table 56–3 for comparison of somatic and visceral proteins.) Visceral proteins are divided into three groups: group I proteins include the actual gut mass; group II includes proteins of homeostasis such as albumin, prealbumin, transferrin, and total protein; and group III includes the acute phase proteins such as fibronectin, C-reactive proteins, globulins, and *opsonic proteins*. To measure visceral proteins, total protein and the effectiveness of the immune system are assessed. Visceral proteins are within normal range during health and are depressed during illness, especially infection. However, the acute phase proteins (fibronectin, C-reactive protein, and opsonic proteins) are low during health and rise during illness such as infection.

Albumin is responsible for maintaining plasma colloid osmotic pressure (COP). Fluid and metabolic flow from the interstitial fluid into the blood stream depends on COP. When protein or kwashiorkor malnutrition are present, edema and muscle wasting are usually present. The patient is generally apathetic and may claim to have an appetite, yet often the foods that are eaten are high in carbohydrate and low in protein.

Patients with either type of malnutrition have a compromised muscle endurance and a decreased efficiency of the diaphragm, intercostal, and accessory muscles of respiration. Loss of strength occurs in both inspiration and expiration. Studies have shown that chronically starved persons lack the periodic sighs that automati-

Table 56–3. COMPARISON OF SOMATIC AND VISCERAL PROTEINS

Somatic Proteins	Visceral Proteins
Types of Proteins:	
Muscle proteins	**Group I:** Gut mass protein **Group II:** Homeostasis protein Albumin Transferrin Total protein **Group III:** Acute phase proteins Fibronectin C-Reactive proteins Globulins Opsonic proteins
Measurement	
Estimated by measuring muscle bulk.	Estimated by measuring blood proteins and measuring immune function.

cally provide for reinflation of atelectatic areas. If it is necessary to increase respiratory effort, respiratory failure may ensue.

Patients who are going to have surgery need to be carefully assessed for the presence of either type of malnutrition. Surgical patients with malnutrition are at high risk for poor wound healing, which in turn increases the threat of infection and dehiscence.

The goal of nutritional support is to decrease the catabolic effects on the body by supplying adequate amounts of calories and protein. Significant advances in nutritional support in recent years now provide for the support of all patients who are unable to eat, unable to eat enough, should not eat, or will not eat. The preferred route of nutritional support is, of course, via the gastrointestinal tract (GIT) with abundant, nutritious, and frequent meals and supplements or with aggressive tube feedings. Tube feedings should be used when the patient is unable to increase his or her nutritional intake, and may be required because of oral or gastrointestinal surgery, esophageal or stomach obstructions, or a semicomatose or comatose state. When the GIT cannot or should not be used, parenteral nutrition is used as soon as possible.

THERAPEUTIC AGENTS— ENTERAL

Enteral nutrition is designed for patients who are unable to consume sufficient calories to maintain normal metabolic processes but who have a functional alimentary tract. Enteral nutrition may comprise part or all of the daily diet. Enteral nutrition allows the body to use nutrients efficiently and causes few metabolic problems. Enteral nutrition is also inexpensive, averaging about one tenth the cost of parenteral nutrition.

Enteral feedings would not be appropriate in various situations. In patients with a total bowel obstruction or persistent vomiting, enteral feeding would not be used. Also, patients who were experiencing malabsorption disease or severe diarrhea would not be appropriate candidates.

Enteral formulas differ in many ways. Products contain minimally altered foods or processed or chemically isolated foods with various amounts of residue. Products also differ in their fat or protein content, viscosity, and osmolarity. Products may contain high or low levels of lactose (milk sugar) or be lactose free. Enteral products that contain intact proteins are more palatable than those made of crystalline amino acids or hydrolyzed protein.

TUBE FEEDINGS

A tube feeding is a method of administering adequate nutrition in a form that is easily digestible to the patient. Tube feedings (Fig. 56–1) may be inserted into the stomach through a nasogastric tube; gastrostomy tube, or percutaneous endoscopic gastrostomy tube; into the duodenum through a nasoduodenal tube; or into the jejunum through a nasojejunal tube or a jejunostomy tube. The nasoduodenal and nasojejunal tubes are usually placed under fluoroscopy. However, they may also be placed like a nasogastric tube, then allowed to pass by peristaltic action into the duodenum or jejunum. The percutaneous endoscopic gastrostomy tube (PEG) is placed under gastroscopic visualization. Both the gastrostomy and jejunostomy tubes are inserted through a surgical incision in the abdominal wall and sutured in place. Patients with either of these tubes may experience skin excoriation and infection. These complications are avoided with a cervical esophagostomy. This tube is passed through a surgically created, skin-lined canal from the lower neck border extending to below the cervical esophagus. Whenever a feeding is placed into the stomach, there is a higher risk of aspiration. Therefore, nasogastric tubes have the highest risk while the jejunostomy tube has the lowest risk for aspiration.

Tube-feeding diets can be made from a mixture of foods served in an adequate normal diet, finely homogenized in a mechanical blender and strained to ensure passage through the tube, or from food combinations planned to meet specific therapeutic needs. Commercial products contain varying amounts of electrolytes, vitamins, and trace elements and contain a known quantity of protein, carbohydrate, and fat, which may not always be the case with a blenderized meal. Many formulas are tailored to meet specific nutrient needs, for example, high-nitrogen formulas for stressed patients, and low-fat formulas for patients with fat malabsorption. Commercial preparations have predominantly replaced blenderized diets.

Types of Tubes

When it is necessary to administer feedings via feeding tubes, the size of the tube is determined first. A smaller tube is more comfortable for transnasal feedings, but may require the use of a food pump to administer more viscous formulas. During the past several years, many types of feeding tubes have been developed.

Tubes used for these feedings are made from polyvinyl chloride (PVC) (Salem or Levin sump), polyurethane (Dobbhoff and Flexiflo), or silicone rubber (Keofeed), and come in various diameters ranging from a # 5 to a #16, with a different number of holes at the end of the tube (1–4), with holes of different sizes, different tip contents (tungsten or mercury), and different means of introduction into the patient (stiffer outer tube or a stylet). The weighted tip is supposed to assist the movement of the tube through the pylorus into the duodenum within 24 hours. Polyvinyl chloride tubes are larger bore nasogastric tubes, are more uncomfortable, and increase the risk of aspiration and other complications such as ulceration, fistulas, and tissue necrosis. Therefore, they should not be used for tube feedings.

The polyurethane and silicone rubber tubes have a mercury- or tungsten-weighted tip, and many have a

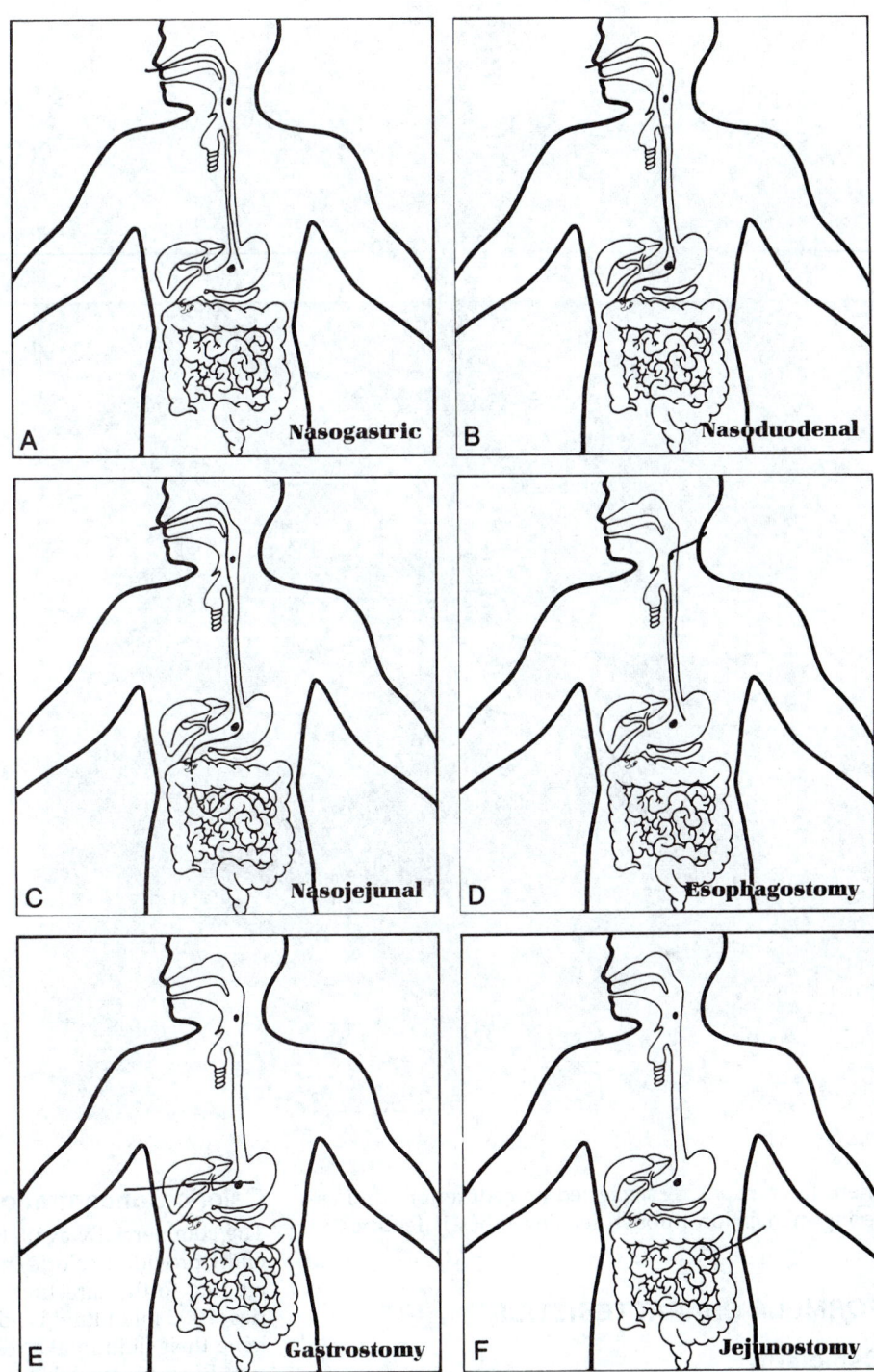

Figure 56–1. Enteral feedings can be administered via various routes. For short-term therapy a nasogastric (*A*), nasoduodenal (*B*), or nasojejunal (*C*) tube may be used. For long-term therapy a esophagostomy (*D*), gastrostomy (*E*), or jejunostomy (*F*) tube may be used. (continues pg. 1040)

Figure Continues Opposite

guide-wire included to aid in insertion. The silicone rubber and polyurethane tubes are better tolerated and produce fewer complications than the more rigid Levin tubes. These tubes do not harden in the presence of gastric juice, nor do they need to be changed as frequently as PVC tubes. They are available as #5 or #16 French tubes and vary in length from 36–45 inches. The type of administered diet and its consistency may determine the tube size. For example, a home-prepared blenderized diet, because of its large particle size or consistency, can

only be inserted through a #16 tube. Patients using an esophagostomy or gastrostomy tube can be given any consistency formula because these tubes are generally of a large diameter. The silicone rubber and polyurethane tubes can be used with any of the commercially prepared formulas. Feeding tubes may also be used to administer medications. Liquid forms of medication should be used with these tubes whenever possible. Also, avoid mixing medications with the formula, as they may lead to curdling of the formula or drug–nu-

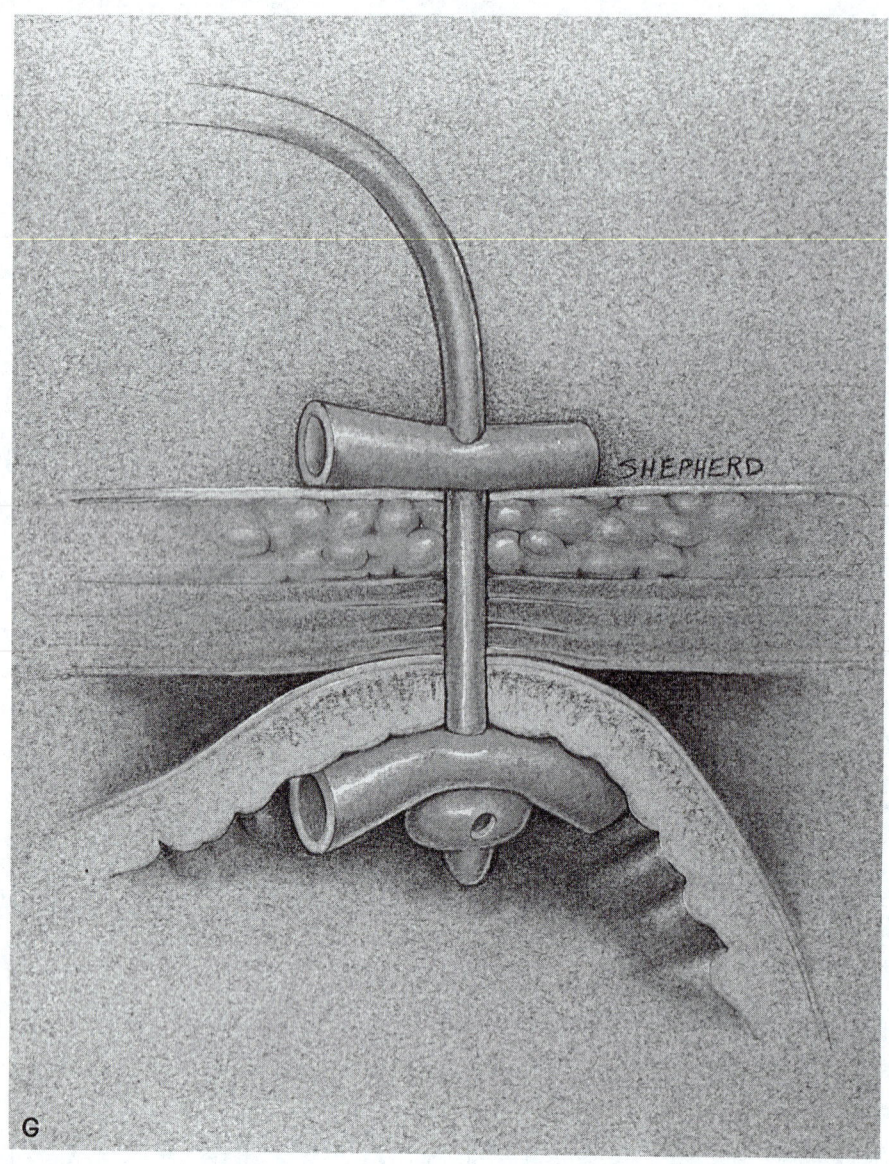

Figure 56–1. *Continued* (*G*) A percutaneous endoscopic gastrostomy (*G*) tube—this tube does not require general surgery or laparotomy. It is inserted under endoscopic visualization. (*A–F*, Courtesy of Ross Laboratories, Columbus, OH.)

trient interactions. A suggested procedure for administering medication through feeding tubes is featured in Table 56–4.

FORMULA CHARACTERISTICS

Osmolarity

Osmolarity is a measure of the osmotically active particles dispersed in solution, most often water. The osmolarity of normal body fluids is about 275–298 milliosmoles (mOsm). Solutions having osmolarity greater than this are hyperosmolar and have a tendency to draw water into the area where the solution is located. Solutions with lesser osmolarity are hypo-osmolar and have a tendency to give up water. Some tube-feeding products are hyperosmolar and have a tendency to draw water into the gastrointestinal tract, so initially, as feedings are started, the preparations must be administered slowly to prevent diarrhea. Isotonic formulas are available and may be better tolerated by some patients.

Caloric Concentration

The commercially available tube-feeding products generally provide 1 calorie/ml when mixed full strength according to the directions; therefore, to give 1000 calories, 1000 ml of fluid is administered. Since some clients have their fluid intake restricted, formulas, such as Ensure Plus, are available to give 1000 calories in only 676 ml, or to provide 2000 calories in 1000 ml, such as Magnacal and Two-Cal. These high-caloric/low-volume formulas may also be helpful for the severely debilitated patient.

Protein Content

The protein content, as well as the source, varies among products. Protein content ranges from 9%–24% of the calories. Protein source may originate from milk protein, beef, egg albumin, skim milk powder, soy, hydrolyzed casein, or amino acids. The protein may be complete, partially hydrolyzed into peptides and amino acids, or administered as amino acids for easier digestion and ab-

Table 56–4. SUGGESTED PROCEDURE FOR ADMINISTERING MEDICATIONS THROUGH FEEDING TUBES

1. Obtain drugs in liquid form if possible.
2. If the drug is not commercially available in liquid form consult the pharmacy for extemporaneous formulations provided by American Society of Hospital Pharmacists in *Pediatric Extemporaneous Formulation List* or manufacturer's suggestions.
3. Calculate equivalent liquid dose carefully. Many liquid dosage forms are intended for pediatric use and the dose of the drug must be adjusted appropriately for adults.
4. Administer crushed tablets only when no other alternatives are available.
5. If crushed tablets are administered, crush the tablet to a fine powder and mix in water. Do not crush any tablet on the list of oral drugs that should not be crushed or drugs with enteric coatings or sustain release action. If in doubt check with the pharmacy.
6. Administer each drug separately. Do not mix all the medications for 1 dosing time in 1 container. Flush with at least 5 ml of water between each medication.
7. Flush the tube with at least 30 ml of water prior to giving the medication and before reinstituting the tube feeding.
8. Drugs that are hypertonic or irritating to the gastric mucosa such as potassium chloride should be diluted in at least 30 ml of water before administering to avoid gastric irritation and diarrhea.
9. If the medication is ordered to be added to the feeding such as sodium chloride, observe the feeding after the addition for any reaction or precipitation. Shake the solution thoroughly. Label the feeding with at least the name and amount of the drug added.
10. Drugs that are usually administered with meals to avoid gastric irritation, such as indomethacin, should also be diluted with water prior to administering.
11. Slow release or sustained formulation of drugs that are used for once-daily dosing may need to have divided dosing schedules when administered in a liquid form. An example is phenytoin. If you are uncertain about dosing schedule, contact the pharmacy.

From Wright, B, and Robinson, L: Enteral feeding tubes as drug delivery systems. Nutritional Support Services 6(2), 1986, p. 37, with permission.

sorption. The latter are generally necessary only for patients with certain malabsorption problems. Many formulas use a milk-based preparation, with casein as the primary protein source, because it is completely and easily digested. Formulas that contain whole proteins are generally more palatable than those containing hydrolyzed protein or amino acids. Hydrolyzed protein and amino acids also increase the osmolality of the solution.

Fat Content

The fat content in most commercial formulas is obtained from soy, corn, or safflower oil. Depending on the formula, it may be 1%–47% of the total calories. Fats increase the calorie content of the formulas without increasing the osmolarity. Fat also gives the patient a feeling of satiety. Several formulas contain medium-chain triglycerides, which are easier to digest. These are often used in persons with fat malabsorption syn-

dromes. Fat-free formulas are also available. When fat-free formulas are used, small amounts of fat (10 g/liter) can be added to the feeding each day in order to increase fat intake gradually.

Electrolytes

Enteral feedings contain varying amounts of phosphorus, 0–1250 mg; sodium, 0–1915 mg; and potassium, 0–1670 mg.

Carbohydrate Content

Carbohydrates can be obtained from many sources, including pureed fruits and vegetables, corn syrup, and sugars such as fructose, sucrose, and lactose. Fructose is a monosaccharide sugar already in its simplest form. It is the sweetest sugar and is found in honey and fruit. Sucrose, ordinary table sugar, and lactose, the sugar found in milk, are disaccharides or double sugars. Both sucrose and lactose are hydrolyzed by digestive enzymes to the constituent monosaccharides before absorption into the body. (Sucrose equals glucose and fructose; lactose equals glucose and galactose.) Many individuals are lactase deficient, which leads to lactose intolerance and diarrhea. Thus, most enteral feeding formulas do not contain lactose. The carbohydrate source greatly affects the palatability of the formulas, with pureed fruits and vegetables being the best in taste. The amount and type of carbohydrates in the formulas also affect the osmolarity.

Vitamin and Mineral Content

The majority of commercially prepared formulas are fortified with vitamins and minerals. These usually meet the recommended daily allowances (RDA) when a specific volume is administered. The RDAs are designed for healthy individuals; therefore, requirements may be increased in an ill person, sometimes necessitating the administration of both supplemental vitamins and minerals. Home-prepared or institutionally prepared formulas generally need to have supplemental vitamins and minerals added, since this content depends on the choice of food selected. Some patients may also need added electrolytes.

ENTERAL FORMULAS

There are a wide variety of commercially prepared enteral formulas. All enteral diets can have additional proteins, carbohydrates, or fat added to improve healing and promote tissue growth. Since there is little chance of sepsis with tube or oral formulas, they are safer for the individual than parenteral forms of nutrition. Patients have been maintained on these products for months, both in the hospital and at home, with no side effects. In general, all tube feedings in the catabolic patient are clinically effective in restoring a positive nitrogen balance.

Commercially available feeding formulas vary in osmolarity, caloric concentration, protein, carbohydrate, fat, and vitamin composition. Commercially available products and their compositions are listed in Table 56–5.

Table 56–5. NUTRITIONALLY COMPLETE ENTERAL FORMULATIONS

Preparations	Per 1000 Kcal					
	Protein (g)	Fat (g)	Carbohydrate (g)	Phosphorus (mg)	Sodium (mg)	Potassium (mg)
LACTOSE-CONTAIN-ING FORMULATIONS						
Compleat-B (Sandoz Nutrition)	40	40	120.4	1250	1187	1314
Meritene Liquid (Sandoz Nutrition)	60	33.3	115	1250	1915	1670
LACTOSE-FREE FOR-MULATIONS						
(1 kcal/ml, standard protein content)						
Criticare HN (Mead Johnson)	38.0	3.1	222	500	630	1320
Enrich (Ross)	36.2	33.8	147.3	654	770	1538
Ensure (Ross)	35.2	35.2	137.2	500	800	1480
Ensure HN (Ross)	42.0	33.6	133.6	716	880	1480
High Nitrogen Vivonex (Norwich Eaton)	44.4	0.9	210	333	529	1173
Jevity (Ross)	43.7	36.1	149	716	915	1539
Osmolite (Ross)	36.6	37.8	142.6	500	624	998
Osmolite-HN (Ross)	42.0	34.8	133.6	716	880	1480
Precision High Nitrogen (Sandoz Nutrition)	43.9	1.3	216	333	980	910
Precision Isotonic (Sandoz Nutrition)	30	31.3	150	667	801	1001
Precision LR (Sandoz Nutrition)	23.7	1.4	223.2	526	632	790
Standard Vivonex (Norwich Eaton)	21.8	1.5	230.7	556	469	1173
Travasorb (Travenol)	33	35	136.4	500	699	1204
Travasorb HN (Travenol)	45	13.3	175	500	920	1173
Vital High Nitrogen (Ross)	41.7	10.8	184.7	667	467	1333
Vivonex T.E.N. (Norwich Eaton)	38.2	2.8	206	500	460	782
(1.5 kcal/ml)						
Ensure Plus (Ross)	36.6	35.5	133.2	470	761	1408
Ensure Plus HN (Ross)	61.5	49	196.7	704	1164	1788
Sustacal HC (Mead Johnson)	40	38	125	560	552	977
Traumacal (Mead-Johnson)	55	46	95	500	782	938
Travasorb MCT (Travenol)	50	34	125	500	529	1001
(2 kcal/ml)						
Isocal HCN (Mead Johnson)	38	45	113	330	414	704
Magnacal (Cheseborough-Pond's)	35	40	125	500	499	626

Type of Formula*	mOsm/kg	Volume to Supply 1000 Kcal (ml)	Flavor	Kcal to Supply 100% of RDA for Vitamins	Comment
B	405	938	Natural	1500	Tube feeding, moderate residue
M	505–570†	1042	Varied	1255	Oral and tube feeding, low residue (3.8 g fiber/liter)
D	650	943	Unflavored	2000	Fat free, low residue
M	480‡	909		1530	Contains fiber, moderate residue— 14.4 g fiber/liter (oral & tube feeding)
M	450‡	943	Varied	2000	Low residue
H	470‡	943	Vanilla	1400	Low residue
D	810§	1000	Varied	3000	Oligomeric, fat free, low residue
D	300	943	Unflavored	2000	Isotonic, low residue
H	310	943	Unflavored	1400	Isotonic, low residue
D	525	950	Citrus & vanilla	3030	Oligomeric, fat free, low residue
D	300	1040	Vanilla & orange	1500	Isotonic, low residue
D	480–510¶	890	Varied	1900	Oligomeric, fat free, low residue
D	550§	1000	Varied	1786	Oligomeric, fat free, low residue
M	486	1000	Varied	2000	Low residue
H	560	1000	Unflavored	2000	Oligomeric, low fat, low residue
D	500	1000	Vanilla	1500	Oligomeric, low fat, low residue
D	630	1000	Varied	2000	Oligomeric, fat free, protein content is high in branched-chain amino acids (33% of total amino acids)
D	310	943	Unflavored	1400	Gluten-free, high fiber (14.4 g/liter) / 1,400 kcal, isotonic, provides trace minerals.
H	690	666.7	Varied	2130	Oral and tube feeding, low residue
H	650‡	666.7	Vanilla	1420	Oral and tube feeding, low residue
H	650	654	Vanilla & egg nog	1785	Oral and tube feeding, low residue
H	550	667	Unflavored	3000	Oral and tube feeding, high protein, low residue
M	312	670	Unflavored	2000	High protein, oral and tube feeding, low residue, isotonic
H	690	500	Unflavored	3000	Tube feeding, low residue
H	590	500	Vanilla	2000	Oral and tube feeding, low residue

CONTINUED ON THE FOLLOWING PAGE

Table 56–5. NUTRITIONALLY COMPLETE ENTERAL FORMULATIONS–*CONTINUED*

Preparations	Per 1000 Kcal					
	Protein (g)	Fat (g)	Carbohydrate (g)	Phosphorus (mg)	Sodium (mg)	Potassium (mg)
SPECIALIZED FORMU- LAS						
Renal Failure Formu- las						
Amin-Aid (American McGaw)	19	46	366	0	169	<3
Travasorb Renal (Travenol)	22.9	17.7	271	0	<321	0
Hepatic Encephalopa- thy Formulas						
Hepatic-Aid II (American McGaw)	44	36	168	0	<338	3
Travasorb Hepatic (Travenol)	29.4	14.7	215	435	235	882
Formulas for Trauma Patients						
Stesstein Powder (Sandoz Nutrition)	70	28	170	417	650	1100
Traum-Aid HBC (American McGaw)	66.6	14.7	197.5	400	618	1380
MISCELLANEOUS FORMULAS						
Pulmocare (Ross)	61.5	90.6	104	704	1289	1872
ProMod	3.0**	<0.48**	<0.54**	<20.8	<12	<52
Polycose powder	—	—	5.6**	<13.4	<6.6	<0.6
Moducal	—	—	23**	—	—	—
Sumacal	—	—	4.8**	—	—	—
Lipomul	—	4**	—	—	—	—
BLENDERIZED FOR- MULAS						
Vitaneed	35	40	125	—	—	—
Compleat-Modified	43	37	131	—	—	—

Adapted from AMA Drug Evaluations, ed. 6. PSG Publishing, Littleton, MA, 1986, p. 878, with permission.
*Type of Formula: †Depending on flavor
B = blenderized diet,   ‡Add 15 to 30 mOsm/kg per flavor packet
D = defined or elemental;   §Add 45 mOsm/kg per flavor packet
S = specialized;   ¶30 kcal/30 ml
H = high calorie, high protein;   **All these measures are per tablespoon. < = Does Not Exceed.
M = modular.

Type of Formula*	mOsm/kg	Volume to Supply 1000 Kcal (ml)	Flavor	Kcal to Supply 100% of RDA for Vitamins	Comment
D	700	500	Varied	—	2 kcal/ml, oral and tube feeding, protein content is 100% essential amino acids
D	590	750	Apricot & strawberry	—	1.33 kcal/ml, oral and tube feeding, protein content is 100% essential amino acids
D	560	850	Varied	—	1.2 kcal/ml, oral and tube feeding, protein content is high in branched chain amino acids and low in aromatic amino acids and methionine
D	600	926	Apricot & strawberry	2270	1.1 kcal/ml, oral and tube feeding. Protein content is high in branched chain amino acids and arginine, low in aromatic amino acids and methionine
D	910	850	Unflavored	2400	1.2 kcal/ml, tube feeding, high protein content consisting of 44% branched chain amino acids
D	760	1000	Lemon, cream	3000	1 kcal/ml, oral and tube feeding, high protein content is 50% branched chain amino acids
D	490	500	Vanilla	1420	1.5 kcal/ml, oral and tube feeding, low carbohydrate, high fat. For patients with impaired pulmonary function
M	—	—		NA	Protein modular component.
M	—	—		NA	CHO modular component.
M	—	—		90**	CHO modular component.
M	—	—		19**	CHO modular component.
M	—	—		36**	Fat modular component.
B	310	1000	Natural		Low sodium, lactose-free, requires digestion.
B	300	1000	Unflavored		High protein, lactose-free, low sodium, requires digestion.

Enteral formulas are categorized as: polymeric or monomeric formulas, specialized formulas, and modular formulas.

Polymeric Formulas

Polymeric or nonelemental formulas contain protein, fat, and carbohydrate in high molecular weight form. They are low in osmolality and generally lactose free. These formulas can be used for the majority of patients, providing the patient has normal lipolytic and proteolytic ability. Polymeric formulas include blenderized diets and meal replacement formulas. Blenderized diets are generally high in residue, highly viscous, with intact proteins. Meal replacement formulas may either be milk based, that is, nutritionally complete and palatable for oral ingestion, or lactose free, which are also nutritionally complete, well tolerated by lactose-deficient persons, low in residue, and fairly palatable for oral ingestion.

BLENDERIZED DIETS. The blenderized diet is adequate for patients with an intact digestive and absorptive capacity. Commercially prepared formulas are made with intact food products such as meat, vegetables, milk, cereal, and fruit products, and are higher in residue than some of the other formulations. For home patients, a blenderized diet can be achieved using a normal diet. For hospitalized patients, a commercial product is preferred.

MEAL REPLACEMENT FORMULAS. These formulas can be divided into two types—milk based and lactose free. In milk-based formulas, the protein source is milk with or without soy protein. These are nutritionally complete, containing the RDA of vitamins and minerals, and are generally used for oral ingestion. Because they are high in lactose, these formulas should be avoided in patients known to be lactose intolerant.

Lactose-free formulas contain casein, soy, or egg albumin as the protein source, plus complex carbohydrates. They vary in caloric content from the standard 1 kcal/ml to the newer higher-density formulas, with 1.5–2 kcal/ml. The high-density formulas are ideal for patients who are fluid restricted or catabolic and need additional calories and protein. The osmolality of these formulas ranges from 300–700 mOsm. The lactose-free formulas also contain the RDA for vitamins and minerals in calorically adequate volumes. They are low in viscosity and may be administered through small-bore feeding tubes. Some of these formulas are flavored and can be administered orally.

Monomeric Formulas

Monomeric, elemental, or so-called chemically defined formulas provide nutrients in a form that requires little or no digestion. These formulas are generally incomplete and designed specifically for patients with gastrointestinal disorders (limited or impaired gastrointestinal function) or metabolic disorders. They are considered clear liquid, low-residue, lactose-free diets. The protein source is either crystalline amino acids and/or peptides. The main calorie source in most of these formulas is carbohydrate, which may be a problem in patients with respiratory insufficiency.

Monomeric formulas are generally low in fat. Some contain only minimal amounts of long-chain fatty acids and may require supplementation. Because they are low in fat, stomach emptying is not delayed. Many of these formulas are designed to be administered directly into the small intestine. Even though flavor packets are available to improve taste, they are generally unpalatable and best suited for tube feeding. When given in calorically adequate volumes, the RDAs for vitamins and minerals are met or exceeded. These formulas are higher in osmolality than meal replacement formulas and, if started at full-strength concentration, generally produce

diarrhea. The osmolalities range from 450–900 mOsm. Thus, they should be gradually increased in strength and rate when initiating feeding.

Monomeric diets are ideal for patients with digestive problems such as malabsorption syndromes, short-bowel syndrome, and antibiotic- or radiation-induced damage. Additionally, there is minimal stimulation of digestive secretions, which makes the formulas useful in treating chronic pancreatitis. Monomeric formulas are more expensive than polymeric formulas.

Specialized Formulas

Specialty formulations are designed for patients with specific needs such as renal failure, hepatic failure, pulmonary disease, sepsis, burns, or hypermetabolic states. Because these formulas are designed for specific disease states, they are, in some cases, nutritionally incomplete and require vitamin and mineral supplementation.

The diets for renal failure, hepatic failure, and pulmonary disease contain crystalline amino acids (CAA) as the protein source, are hyperosmolar, and are available in various flavors. The renal-failure formulas contain only the eight essential amino acids plus histidine. The renal failure formulas have a high osmolality ranging from 590–1095 mOsm. The hepatic-failure formulas are high in branched-chain amino acids and low in aromatic amino acids. The hepatic failure formula has a high osmolality ranging from 560–690 mOsm. The pulmonary formula is given to patients with pulmonary disease but who have normal absorptive and digestive capabilities. The formula is high in fat and low in carbohydrates. Because the metabolism of fat results in a lower respiratory quotient than the metabolism of carbohydrates, the use of this formula results in less carbon dioxide production and therefore less stress to the respiratory system. The osmolality is 490 mOsm and this product is lactose free.

The formulas for hypermetabolic states contain CAA as the protein source. Although they are flavored, the taste of the amino acids is difficult to camouflage. These formulas generally have increased amounts of branched-chain amino acids, are also hyperosmolar (470–740 mOsm), and vary in electrolyte and vitamin content. They are also lactose free.

Modular Formulas

Modules or supplements are also available to supply a single nutrient and yield a higher calorie density. These are sources of fat, carbohydrate, or protein and can be used alone or mixed with food or enteral formulas. Modular formulas are not designed to serve as a sole source of nutrition. Protein modules can be added to other products to help meet the extra nitrogen needs of a patient with burns or a severe trauma. Fat modules can be added to the formula of a ventilator-dependent patient to increase the ratio of fat-to-carbohydrate kilocalories and, thus, decrease the respiratory quotient. Carbohydrate modules can be added to enteral formulas or foods to increase caloric intake.

THERAPEUTIC AGENTS— PARENTERAL NUTRITION

For hospitalized patients who are unable to eat or drink for longer than three days, some method of prolonged nutritional support must be maintained. This can be accomplished through enteral feedings, if the intestinal tract is intact, or parenteral nutrition, if there is a dysfunction within the intestinal tract. Parenteral nutrition is also called *total parenteral nutrition (TPN)* or intravenous *hyperalimentation* because of the number of calories that can be provided via this method. Total parenteral nutrition is a technique that can provide sufficient calories, amino acids, and other nutrients intravenously to achieve or maintain a positive nitrogen balance indefinitely. It may be administered peripherally or centrally, depending on the hypertonicity of the solution. Prior to the development of TPN in the early 1970s, patients who became debilitated and malnourished and who could not take oral nutrients had little hope for recovery. Today, they can be supported with TPN, which promotes growth of tissue, improves wound healing, and often results in a weight gain of as much as a pound per day.

Total parenteral nutrition is also indicated for individuals who have lost 10% or more of their normal body weight, and are unable to obtain adequate nutrition orally, or by tube enteral nutrition, or by peripheral intravenous fluids; and for those who have a caloric need of greater than 50% over normal. A patient receiving TPN may receive 3000 calories, or more, per day. Individuals who are unable to eat, digest, and absorb ingested nutrients usually become debilitated or malnourished. Conditions such as Crohn's disease, ulcerative colitis, burns, diverticulitis, hypermetabolic states, or cancer; severe gastrointestinal side effects from surgery, chemotherapy, or radiation; acute hepatic or renal failure; or prematurity may cause a need for nutritional support, often for months. Sepsis is also a unique use for TPN. In sepsis, there is increased breakdown of muscle tissue that is used for energy *(proteolysis)*. There is also a decrease in glucose utilization due to an increase in insulin resistance. Septic patients are often allowed nothing by mouth for prolonged periods, which also increases their nitrogen imbalance. Septic patients are placed on TPN solution to prevent further nitrogen imbalance, to supply an available energy source, and to improve their recovery time. Total parenteral nutrition provides carbohydrates, protein, and lipids all in various concentrations, as well as electrolytes, vitamins, and trace elements.

TOTAL PARENTERAL NUTRITION

Parenteral nutrition is available in three forms: protein sparing, peripheral vein total parenteral nutrition (PTPN), and central venous hyperalimentation.

Protein-Sparing Nutrition

Protein-sparing nutrition is essentially a 3%–5% solution of isotonic amino acids, both essential and nonessential, mixed with other carbohydrate-free fluids, vitamins, minerals, and electrolyte additives that is administered through any peripheral vein. This solution provides approximately 400–600 kcal/day. The body meets its energy requirements by the use of free fatty acids and ketone bodies derived from endogenous adipose tissue as the fuel substrate, preserving the protein compartment. Depending on the amount of calorie supplementation, the protein solutions provide a substrate for protein synthesis or anabolism or enhance conservation of existing body protein, which is a protein-sparing effect. It can be of significant value in the treatment of the patient who has minimal protein deficits and adequate fat stores. Numerous amino acid solutions are available today. They are reviewed in Table 56–6.

Peripheral Vein Total Parenteral Nutrition

Peripheral vein total parenteral nutrition (PTPN) is indicated in patients when central access cannot be obtained or is not appropriate. It is also used to supplement enteral feedings and for temporary use when the length of starvation is unpredictable.

The major development in PTPN is the use of lipid as a nonprotein calories source. Lipids (to be discussed later) are used to increase the caloric density of the formula, to decrease the osmolarity, and to "buffer" the vein. A crystalline amino acid solution is mixed with dextrose to supply protein and energy requirements. However, the final dextrose concentration must be limited to 10% since the peripheral vein will sclerose at higher concentrations. Vitamins, electrolytes and trace elements are added to this solution. This admixture is infused with the lipid emulsion continuously through a Y connector. Some centers mix all the hyperalimentation components into one bag, which allows infusion of the mixture without the need for a Y connector. The concentration of potassium and calcium must be limited to prevent sclerosis and irritation to the vein. A PTPN solution usually contains about 200 nonprotein calories, 35–50 g of protein per liter, and may contain lipids.

When possible, it is advantageous to administer peripheral TPN because there is less risk of catheter placement, care of the infusion site is simpler, and the complications associated with a hyperosmolar solution are avoided. The limitations associated with PTPN include the need for several peripheral veins, as the catheter is rotated on a regular basis. The veins must also be adequate size to accommodate the catheter. In addition, in a stressed or hypermetabolic patient, calorie requirements may exceed those that can be delivered by PTPN. Another limitation is the patient's inability to utilize lipids as an energy source. If the patient has a disorder of lipid metabolism, hypertonic dextrose through a central line may be necessary.

Table 56–6. AMINO ACID SOLUTIONS

Amino Acid Concentration:	Aminosyn (Abbott)						FreAmine III (Kendell-McGaw)	
	3.5%	3.5%*	5%	7%	8.5%	10%	8.5%	10%
NORMALIZED AMINO ACID CONTENT (mg/1%)								
Essential (% Nitrogen)								
Isoleucine (10.7)	72	252	72	73	73	72	69	69
Leucine (10.7)	94	329	94	94	95	94	91	91
Lysine (19.2)	72	252	72	73	73	72	73	73
Methionine (9.4)	40	140	40	40	40	40	53	53
Phenylalanine (8.5)	44	154	44	44	45	44	56	56
Threonine (11.8)	52	182	52	53	54	52	40	40
Tryptophan (13.7)	16	56	16	17	18	16	15	15
Valine (12.0)	80	280	80	80	80	66	66	66
Nonessential (% Nitrogen)								
Alanine (15.7)	128	448	128	129	129	128	71	71
Arginine (32.2)	98	343	98	99	100	98	95	95
Histidine (27.1)	30	105	30	30	31	30	28	28
Proline (12.2)	86	300	86	87	88	86	112	112
Serine (13.3)	42	147	42	43	44	42	59	59
Tyrosine (7.7)	9	31	9	6	5	4	—	—
Glycine (18.9)	128	448	128	129	129	128	140	140
Cysteine (11.6)	—	—	—	—	—	—	<3	<3
ELECTROLYTES (mEq/ liter)								
Sodium	7	47	—	—	—	—	10	10
Potassium	—	13	5.4	5.4	5.4	5.4	—	—
Magnesium	—	3	—	—	—	—	—	—
Chloride	—	40	—	—	35	—	<3	<3
Acetate	46	58	86	105	90	148	72	89
Phosphate (mmol/L)	—	3.5	—	—	—	—	10	10
OSMOLARITY (mOsm/liter)	357	477	500	700	850	1000	810	950
Administration Route:								
Peripheral	x	x	—	x†	—	—	x†	x†
Central	—	—	x	x	x	x	x	x

Adapted from AMA Drug Evaluations, ed. 6. PSG Publishing, Littleton, MA, 1986, p 868, with permission.
*Amino acid solution with electrolyte.
†Before peripheral administration, these products must be diluted.

Central Hyperalimentation

Central hyperalimentation is the administration through a central vein of both crystalline amino acids and nonprotein calories (given as dextrose and lipid emulsion). A central TPN solution is a hypertonic, concentrated solution. In general, the nitrogen-to-calorie ratio is 1:150 to 1:200, which is ideal for normal patients for maximum utilization, anabolism, and protein synthesis. Highly stressed patients require 1:80–1:100 nitrogen-to-calorie ratio. The usual dosage of TPN varies from 1–5 liters/day, depending on the patient's needs, with 1–3 liters/day being most common. Few patients require more than 3 liters/day.

The caloric source for central TPN ranges between 12.5% and 50% dextrose in water, usually in a volume of 500–1000 ml. This solution is a concentrated calorie source of relatively small volume. Hypertonic concentrations greater than 12.5% necessitate that the TPN infusion be given through a central line at a regular rate.

Total parenteral nutrition solutions are composed of a carbohydrate source—dextrose, fructose, or alcohol—and a protein source. Vitamins and minerals are added to the preparation to meet all the daily nutritional requirements.

CARBOHYDRATES. The most common carbohydrate source is dextrose derived from corn starch. Dextrose is an inexpensive and readily available source that provides 4 kcal/g. If patients are allergic to dextrose, which is rare, invert sugars, derived from beet or cane sugar, are available. Fructose is also available, but it can intensify existing metabolic acidosis, deplete liver adenine nucleotides, and dehydrate due to its osmotic diuretic effect.

PROTEIN. In the majority of TPN solutions used today, the protein source is crystalline amino acids (CAA). Crystalline amino acid solutions have a defined amount of essential and nonessential amino acids, although it is different among brands and different among

ProcalAmine* (Kendell-McGaw) 3%	* 5.5%	Travasol (Travenol) 5.5%	8.5%	10%	Novamine (KabiVitrum) 8.5%	11.4%
210	48	263	48	60	49	50
270	62	340	62	73	69	69
220	58	318	58	58	79	79
160	58	318	58	40	49	50
170	62	340	62	56	69	69
120	42	230	42	42	49	50
46	18	99	18	18	16	17
200	46	252	46	58	65	64
210	207	1140	207	207	146	145
290	103	570	104	115	99	98
85	44	241	44	48	59	60
340	42	230	42	68	59	60
180	—	—	—	50	40	39
—	4	22	4	4	2	3
420	207	1140	207	103	69	69
20	—	—	—	—	—	—
35	—	70	—	—	—	—
24	—	60	—	—	—	—
5		10				
41	22	70	35	—	—	—
47	48	102	73	87	88	114
3.5	—	30	—	—	—	—
735	575	850	890	1000	785	1049
x	x†	x	x†	x†	x†	x†
	x	x	x	x	x	x

concentrations within a brand; the nitrogen content is completely utilizable and does not vary from one manufacturing lot to the next.

Essential amino acids are those that cannot be synthesized by the body. There are eight essential amino acids, including valine, lysine, threonine, leucine, isoleucine, tryptophan, phenylalanine, and methionine. Nonessential amino acids can be synthesized from a nitrogen source such as amino acids, urea, or ammonium salts. In addition, there are two semi-essential amino acids that cannot be synthesized in adequate amounts during growth periods. Therefore, ten amino acids are considered essential in children.

Most patients require 2–3 liters of TPN per day to meet their protein requirements, which are 0.5–1.5 grams per kilogram of body weight. Severely stressed patients may require 2–2.5 g/kg. Infants require at least 2.5 grams per kilogram of body weight.

ELECTROLYTES. The crystalline amino acid solutions contain small amounts of sodium, potassium, phosphate, chloride, and acetate. Additional electrolytes are added according to patient need to prevent deficiencies. Potassium, phosphate, and magnesium are particularly important, as requirements of each increase as the patient enters the anabolic state. Potassium and phosphate also move intracellularly due to the effect of the hypertonic glucose. Potassium is important in protein synthesis. Phosphate is an essential component in the production of ATP, phospholipids, and nucleic acids. Magnesium is needed for a number of enzyme reactions. Calcium is added to balance the phosphate infusion as well as to meet body needs for calcium. Sodium, chloride, sulfate, and acetate are also needed to help maintain normal serum levels and to maintain acid–base balance.

VITAMINS. For those patients whose only nutritional intake is the TPN solution, adequate vitamin supplementation is also important. Vitamins such as A, C, D, E, K, B complex, and folic acid may be added to the TPN solution, or administered intramuscularly or intravenously or through another IV line. The addition of vitamins can be made by daily alternating the administration of 5 ml of a multiple vitamin infusion (MVI) with 2 ml of a product containing B and C vitamins. The patient receives adequate amounts of fat- and water-soluble vitamins without the risk of excess administration of fat-soluble vitamins. This regimen provides vitamin A 10,000 IU, vitamin D 1000 IU, vitamin E 5 IU, thiamine 50 mg, riboflavin 10 mg, pyridoxine 15 mg, niacin 100 mg, pantothenic acid 25 mg, and vitamin C 100 mg. With this method, folic acid, vitamin B_{12}, and vitamin K are not included. Folic acid (1 mg/day) and vitamin K (5–10 mg/week) can be added daily to the TPN solution or given weekly intramuscularly. Vitamin B_{12} (1000 μg) should be given intramuscularly monthly.

The preferred method for providing adequate vitamins is to use an MVI-12 product daily. Fat- and water-soluble vitamins are provided in smaller amounts on a daily basis. MVI-12 contains vitamin A 3300 IU, vitamin D 200 IU, vitamin E 10 IU, thiamine 3.0 mg, riboflavin 3.6 mg, pyridoxine 4.0 mg, vitamin B_{12} 5 μg, niacin 40 mg, pantothenic acid 15 mg, biotin 60 μg, folic acid 400 μg, and vitamin C 100 mg. Vitamin K must be administered separately. Iron dextran can be used to prevent iron deficiency from occurring. Iron is administered intramuscularly by Z-track method and not added to the bottle.

When TPN is given for prolonged periods, trace elements such as copper, zinc, manganese, iodine, chromium, and others also have to be administered to prevent deficiency syndromes. Several commercially available products can be used.

SPECIAL TPN FORMULATIONS. Three special formulations are available for patients with renal failure, hepatic failure, or hypermetabolic states. These formulations are similar to their enteral counterparts.

Renal-failure formulas are generally mixed with 70% dextrose and 250–300 ml of amino acid solution to provide a high-calorie, low-protein feeding. Vitamins, trace elements, and electrolytes are added as needed. Generally, this formula is infused at a low rate according to the patient's fluid tolerance.

The hepatic-failure formula contains all the amino acids but has increased amounts of branched-chain and smaller amounts of aromatic amino acids. The amino acid solution (500 ml) is mixed with dextrose 50% (500 ml), depending on the patient's needs. Electrolytes, vitamins, and minerals are added as needed. Depending on protein and fluid tolerance, 1–3 liters/day may be infused.

The hypermetabolic formula is similar to the hepatic-failure formula but does not have decreased amounts of osmotic amino acids. This amino acid solution (750 ml) is mixed with 250 ml of 70% dextrose to form a high-protein, low-carbohydrate formula. Again, electrolytes, vitamins, and minerals are added as needed. Administration depends on fluid tolerance (see Table 56–7).

PARENTERAL FAT EMULSIONS

Parenteral fat emulsions (PFE) are prepared from either soybean, safflower oil, or a combination of both and provide a mixture of neutral triglycerides and unsaturated fatty acids. Fat emulsions also contain 1.2% egg yolk phospholipids as an emulsifier and glycerol to adjust tonicity. Fat emulsions are isotonic and may be given intravenously either centrally or peripherally. Fat emulsions are featured in Table 56–8.

Of the total daily calories, 4%–8% need to be endogenous fatty acids (EFA) to prevent EFA deficiency. Patients maintained on TPN without fat for longer than two weeks are at risk for developing this deficiency. Parenteral fat emulsions are used in conjunction with TPN as a source of essential fatty acids or as a calorie source. Most studies indicate 20%–40% of the total daily calories should be fat. Minimal fat requirements can be met with two or three 500-ml bottles of 10% fat/week. Infants have substantially less essential fatty acid stores than adults and often require supplemental fat administration at the onset of parenteral therapy. Parenteral fat emulsions are also used as a calorie source in patients who do not tolerate the large amount of dextrose used in central TPN solutions. This intolerance is seen as hyperglycemia, as the development of fatty liver from increased glycogen deposits, or as an increased production of carbon dioxide. The emulsions may also be used as a calorie source to provide a more balanced feeding regimen and to provide additional calories in peripheral vein TPN.

Pharmacokinetics

It is thought that PFE are handled by the body in the same manner as ingested fats are metabolized. As the PFE enters the blood stream, the protein in blood acts as an emulsifier. The fat particles are coated with a hydrophilic layer, forming lipid–protein complexes. These complexes are carried to the liver, adipose tissue, muscle, and other cells, where they are hydrolyzed to fatty acids and glycerol, transported into cells, resynthesized as triglycerides, and stored. When needed for energy, the triglycerides are mobilized and oxidized. The PFE have a "protein-sparing" effect like that of dextrose and may be administered concurrently with amino acid–dextrose solutions to ensure that the amino acids are utilized properly.

Contraindications and Precautions

Parenteral fat emulsions are contraindicated for patients with disturbances in normal fat metabolism, such as acute pancreatitis associated with hyperlipemia, because they tend to augment the dysfunction. They are administered with caution when there is a risk of fat embolism, as in a patient with long bone fractures, and when the patient has severe hepatic damage, anemia, or blood coagulation disorders. Parenteral fat emulsions are administered with extreme caution to premature and low–birth weight infants. Such administration has been the cause of death in several infants because they have poor clearance of lipids and increased serum levels of free fatty acids after infusion. Because egg yolk phospholipids are used to stabilize the PFE, a history of severe egg allergy precludes their use. Safe use in pregnancy has not been established.

Table 56–7. SPECIAL TPN FORMULATIONS

Solution	Amino Acid Concentration	Composition	Indications
Nephramine	5.4%	EAA Sodium Acetate Chloride	Renal failure
Aminosyn RF	5.2%	EAA Acetate Potassium	Renal failure
HepatAmine	8.0%	EAA/NEAA (Inc. BCAA, Dec. AAA and methionine) Sodium Chloride Acetate Phosphate	Liver failure
FreAmine HBC	6.9%	EAA/NEAA (Inc. BCAA) Sodium Chloride Acetate	Hypercatabolic, stressed patients
RenAmin	6.5%	EAA/NEAA Acetate Chloride	Renal failure

EAA = essential amino acids; NEAA = nonessential amino acids; BCAA = branched-chain amino acids;
AAA = aromatic amino acids.

Adverse Effects

Acute adverse effects that can develop from the administration of any of the PFE include chills, fever, flushing, diaphoresis, dyspnea, cyanosis, allergic reactions, chest and back pain, nausea, vomiting, headache, a feeling of pressure over the eyes, dizziness, and sleepiness that may be related to an allergy to the egg protein in the fat emulsion. Signs of thrombophlebitis at the injection site can also occur. Most acute reactions necessitate discontinuation of the PFE solution. Adverse effects seen on chronic administration include deposition of IV fat pigment in Kupffer's cells of the liver and a decrease in hemoglobin concentration. These effects are reversible on

Table 56–8. IV FAT EMULSIONS

Product: Manufacturer: Fat Source:	Intralipid (Clintec) Soybean Oil	Nutrilipid (Kendall-McGaw) Soybean Oil	Soyacal (Alpha Therapeutic) Soybean Oil	Liposyn II (Abbott) Safflower Oil
Percent Linoleic	50	49–60	49–60	65.8
Percent Linolenic	9	6–9	6–9	4.2
Percent Oleic	26	21–26	21–26	17.7
Percent Palmitic	10	9–13	9–13	8.8
Percent Stearic	3.5	3–5	3–5	3.4
Percent Egg phospholipids	1.2	1.2	1.2	1.2
Percent Glycerin	2.25	2.21	2.21	2.5
Osmolarity (mOsm/liter)	260 (10%) 260 (20%)	280 (10%) 315 (20%)	280 (10%) 315 (20%)	276 (10%) 258 (20%)
Calorie content	1.1 cal/ml (10%) 2.0 kcal/ml (20%)	1.1 kcal/ml (10%) 2.0 kcal/ml (20%)	1.1 kcal/ml (10%) 2.0 kcal/ml (20%)	1.1 kcal/ml (10%) 2.0 kcal/ml (20%)

discontinuation of the PFE. Men may experience priapism (persistent painful erection). Blood becomes entrapped within the penis because fat emulsions can increase thrombin production and shorten coagulation time. Priapism is a rare occurrence.

Dosage

The usual dose of PFE in adults is 500 ml/day of a 10% formula two to three times weekly for the prevention of treatment of EFA deficiency. As a calorie source, these emulsions may be used daily in infants and adults, providing up to 60% of the total daily caloric needs. The remaining calories are supplied by carbohydrates. It is recommended that the daily dose of PFE not exceed 2 g/kg body weight in an adult. These emulsions are relatively expensive compared with the cost of dextrose and therefore may not be routinely used in adults on short-term (less than three weeks) parenteral therapy.

Fat emulsions are available as either 10% or 20% emulsions. The 10% emulsion is infused initially at a rate of 1 ml/minute for the first 15–30 minutes. If there are no adverse effects, the rate is increased to 50 ml/hour. Usually, only 500 ml is infused the first day. If a 20% emulsion is used, the initial rate is 0.5 ml/minute for the first 15–30 minutes. If there are no adverse effects, the rate can be increased to 50 ml/hour. The first day, patients should receive only 250–500 ml. Fat emulsions can be administered alone. Heparin (1–2 U/ml) is the only medication added to the emulsions. The nurse follows specific guidelines (described later) in order to administer fat emulsions safely. Fat emulsions can also be mixed with TPN and administered slowly over a 24-hour period. This technique is discussed later.

USING THE NURSING PROCESS

ASSESSMENT

Assessment of the patient requiring enteral and parenteral feedings always begins with a thorough nursing history to develop a data base. Information that is obtained from the patient and/or family is featured in Table 56–9. Patients requiring these feedings may be in the hospital or may be maintained on these therapies at home.

The nurse also assesses for the presence of underlying diseases of the heart, kidney, or liver, which may limit the type or the amount of the feedings, or the amount of weight the patient can safely gain. Often the current symptoms of malnutrition are produced by medications or other forms of therapy, such as radiation therapy for cancer treatment. If the malnourished state is due to current therapy, there may be no additional need for supplemental feeding after therapy is discontinued. If, however, the reason for the malnutrition is found to be a lack of understanding about proper nutrition or poor nutritional habits, this problem will have to be resolved during the intervention phase. Additional causes of a poor nutritional state may be psychologic, sensory deficits, chronic conditions such as cancer, drug or alcohol dependence, abuse of cathartics, or increases in metabolism. All underlying conditions need to be carefully assessed and treated to prevent further recurrences.

The nurse needs to assess for food allergies. Enteral products are derived from real food; thus, if the patient has food allergies, care must be taken to ensure that those foods are not part of the feeding.

The nurse also assesses for a history of lactose intolerance. Blacks, Orientals, American Indians, and Jews are particularly prone to lactase deficiencies. Lactase is found in the intestinal brush border and is necessary for lactose (milk sugar) absorption. If a lactose intolerance is present, the patient experiences varying degrees of diarrhea, abdominal cramps, bloating, and flatulence after consuming milk or milk products. Many enteral formulas are lactose free and are used for this patient. Actually, it is wise to use lactose-free formulas for all patients, as it is not often evident from patient history that a lactose intolerance is present.

Nursing assessments include observations of objective symptoms of a catabolic state (see Table 56–1). The nurse assesses daily weight at the same time every morning. The patient's weight may provide a means of assessing whether calorie and fluid needs are being met or exceeded (tissue gain vs. edema). It may also be beneficial to discuss calorie needs with other members of the health team, such as the registered dietitian. The registered dietitian will use formulas that take into account age, weight, diagnosis, and stressors to help determine caloric needs. If the patient continues to lose weight after several days of nutritional support, the formula will need to be adjusted, possibly by increasing the protein and calories.

The nurse also needs to evaluate other fluid balance indicators, including jugular vein distention, dependent edema, lung sounds, mucous membrane moisture, presence of thirst, and skin turgor.

The nurse also assesses for the presence of subjective symptoms such as thirst, fatigue, and anorexia. Thirst may be one of the first signs of impending dehydration from the administration of hyperosmolar enteral preparations. In addition, the nurse may also assist with determining how the patient is to receive the additional nourishment, such as through supplemental oral feedings between meals, through tube feedings, or through TPN.

Patients receiving TPN alone for prolonged periods are assessed for essential fatty acid deficiency. The signs to observe for include thrombocytopenia; increased hemolysis; impaired wound healing; light, flaky, and reddened skin lesions often appearing on the scalp, arms, and legs; and growth retardation in infants and children. The dermatologic signs are usually noted first.

The nurse should see to it that frequent laboratory tests are ordered and evaluated by the physician on a regular basis to assess the objective status of nutrition

Table 56-9. NURSING PROCESS FOR PATIENTS REQUIRING ENTERAL/PARENTERAL NUTRITION

Assessment

Review nutritional history, note cultural, economic and religious variables; housing and cooking facilities; where meals are taken; likes and dislikes of food; allergies.
Note history of illness/treatment (e.g., cancer/chemotherapy, renal or liver failure), extent of weight loss.
Determine psychological status.

Nursing Diagnosis	Nursing Actions	Rationale	Desired Outcomes/ Evaluation Criteria
Nutrition, altered Less than body requirements related to conditions that interfere with nutrient intake or increase nutrient need/metabolic demand (massive burns, cancer and associated treatments, surgical procedures, dysphagia/ difficulty swallowing, depressed mental status/level of consciousness) as evidenced by body weight 10% or more under ideal, decreased subcutaneous fat/muscle mass, changes in gastric motility and stool characteristics.	Consult with dietician/ nutritional support team. Document oral intake by use of 24 hour recall, food history, calorie counts as appropriate. Administer nutritional solutions at prescribed rate via infusion control device. Adjust rate to prescribed hourly rate but never "catch up". Be familiar with electrolyte content of nutritional solutions. Schedule activities with adequate rest periods. Promote relaxation techniques. Monitor nutritional status routinely. Weigh daily and compare with admission weight. Monitor for development of diarrhea with enteral feedings.	Useful in calculating individual needs and appropriate formula/product. Identifies imbalance between estimated nutritional requirements and actual intake. Nutrition support prescriptions are based on estimated caloric and protein requirements. A consistent rate of nutrient administration will assure proper utilization with fewer side effects. Metabolic complications of nutritional support often result from a lack of appreciation of changes that can occur as a result of refeeding. Conserves energy/ reduces calorie needs. Provides the opportunity to observe deviations from normals/patient baseline and influences choices of interventions. Establishes baseline, aids in monitoring effectiveness of therapeutic regimen and alerts nurse to inappropriate trends in weight loss/gain. Changes in intestinal flora, hyperosmolar solutions, or lactose intolerance may necessitate changes in drug therapy or type of formula/rate of administration to improve patient tolerance.	Demonstrates stable weight or progressive weight gain toward goal with normalization of laboratory values and free of signs of malnutrition.
Injury, potential for, multifactors related to catheter-related complications, aspiration, effects of therapy/drug interactions.	Administer appropriate TPN solution via peripheral or central venous route. Maintain a closed central intravenous system using LuerLok connections and taping all connections.	Solutions containing high concentrations of dextrose must be delivered via a central vein, because they will result in chemical phlebitis when delivered through small peripheral vein. Inadvertent disconnection of central IV system can result in lethal air emboli or exsanguination.	Free of complications associated with nutritional support. Modifies environment/corrects hazards to enhance safety.

CONTINUED ON THE FOLLOWING PAGE

Table 56–9. NURSING PROCESS FOR PATIENTS REQUIRING ENTERAL/PARENTERAL NUTRITION–*CONTINUED*

Nursing Diagnosis	Nursing Actions	Rationale	Desired Outcomes/ Evaluation Criteria
	Elevate head of bed 30–45 degrees during, and for at least 1 hour after enteral feeding.	Aspiration of enteral formula is irritating to the lung parenchyma and may result in pneumonia and respiratory compromise.	
	Check gastric residual per protocol and verify position of tube periodically/before bolus feedings are begun.	Delayed gastric emptying increases risk of regurgitation; migration or malposition of feeding tube may alter gastric tolerance, cause aspiration or lead to leakage into the abdominal cavity.	
	Monitor for potential drug/nutrient interactions.	For example, digoxin, in conjunction with diuretic therapy, can cause hypomagnesemia.	
	Consult with pharmacist in regard to site/time of delivery of drugs whose action might be adversely affected by enteral formula.	Absorption of vitamin D is impaired by administration of mineral oil and by neomycin. Aluminum-containing antacids bind with the phosphorus in the feeding solution, potentiating hypophosphatemia.	
Fluid volume, deficit, (potential) related to active loss and/or failure of regulatory mechanisms, complications of nutrition therapy, e.g. high-glucose solutions, hyperglycemia, inability to obtain/ingest fluids.	Incorporate knowledge of caloric density of enteral formulas into assessment of fluid balance. Provide additional water/flush tubing as indicated.	Enteric solutions are usually concentrated and do not meet free water needs. With higher calorie formula, additional water is needed to prevent dehydration/HHNC.	Displays moist skin/ mucous membranes, stable vital signs, individually adequate urinary output, and is free of edema and excessive weight loss/inappropriate gain.
	Record intake and output, calculate fluid balance. Measure urine specific gravity.	Excessive urinary losses may reflect developing hyperglycemia. Specific gravity is an indicator of hydration and renal function.	
	Monitor laboratory studies, e.g., serum potassium/phosphorus;	Hypokalemia/phosphatemia can occur due to intracellular shifts during initial refeeding and may compromise cardiac function if not corrected.	
	Hct;	Reflects hydration/circulating volume.	
	Serum albumin.	Hypoalbuminemia/ decreased colloidal osmotic pressure leads to decreased circulating volume as fluid shifts into the tissues.	
Knowledge deficit related to lack of exposure/recall, information misinterpretation, cognitive limitation as evidenced by questions/statement of concern, inaccurate follow-through of instructions/develop-	Discuss reasons for use of parenteral/enteral nutrition support.	May experience anxiety regarding inability to eat and may not comprehend the nutritional value of the prescribed TPN/tube feedings.	Verbalizes understanding of condition/disease process and individual nutritional needs. Correctly performs necessary procedures and explains reasons for the actions.
	Provide adequate time for patient/SO teaching when patient is going home on enteral/parenteral feedings.	Generally 3–4 days is sufficient to become proficient with tube feedings. Parenteral therapy is more complex and may	

Table 56-9. NURSING PROCESS FOR PATIENTS REQUIRING ENTERAL/PARENTERAL NUTRITION-*CONTINUED*

Nursing Diagnosis	Nursing Actions	Rationale	Desired Outcomes/ Evaluation Criteria
ment of preventable complications.		require a week or longer for patient/SO to feel comfortable and ready for home management. Usually requires follow-up in the home.	
	Identify signs/symptoms requiring medical evaluation, e.g., nausea/vomiting, abdominal cramping/bloating, diarrhea; rapid weight changes; erythema, drainage/foul odor at tube insertion site; fever/chills; coughing/choking or difficulty breathing during enteral feeding.	Early evaluation and treatment of problems may prevent progression to more serious complications.	
	Recommend frequent oral care, intake of water if able, use of hard candy, chewing gum.	Helpful in relieving sense of thirst, deprivation of taste.	
	Refer to nutritional support nurse, home health care agency. Provide with immediate access phone numbers.	Patient/SO need ready support persons to assist with home therapy, equipment problems, and emotional adjustments in long-term therapy.	

and endocrine function. Laboratory tests should examine various hormones, total proteins, albumin, blood urea nitrogen, electrolytes, minerals, and vitamins. All individuals will have frequent assessments of their blood glucose level, as hyperglycemia can precipitate osmotic diuresis and hyperosmolar dehydration.

The patient may also have various laboratory and x-ray tests ordered by the physician to assess endocrine, renal, and hepatic function before therapy is begun. Patients in need of nutritional support need to have their serum protein levels assessed often. When malnutrition is present, the liver's ability to synthesize albumin is reduced. Nitrogen balance studies—the balance between nitrogen intake and output—may also be obtained. This is done by assessing a 24-hour urine for urea, the major form of nitrogen loss. All urine for the 24-hour period is saved for this analysis. Nitrogen balance can be calculated using the following formula:

$$\text{N balance} = \frac{\text{Protein Intake (g)}}{6.25}$$
$$- \text{(urinary urea nitrogen} + 4)$$

A value below 0 indicates negative nitrogen balance.

During both TPN and tube enteral nutrition (TEN) therapy, the following laboratory tests may be ordered daily until a constant volume of TPN is being delivered, and then reduced to three times a week: hematocrit, sodium, potassium, chloride, carbon dioxide, calcium, phosphate, albumin, total protein, creatinine, blood sugar, and BUN. Additional laboratory tests are generally ordered weekly, including magnesium level, complete blood count, prothrombin time, and liver function tests.

Nutritional assessment may also be based on *anthropometric parameters*, biochemical data, physical findings, medical or surgical interventions, diet, drug, and socioeconomic histories. It may be necessary to estimate the patient's ideal weight. This can be done from weight charts or by estimation:

Men: 106 pounds (48 kg) for first 5 feet (150 cm) + 6 pounds (2.7 kg)/inch (2.5 cm) over 5 feet ($\pm$ 10%)

Women: 100 pounds (45 kg) for first 5 feet + 5 pounds (2.2 kg)/inch over 5 feet ($\pm$ 10%)

More complex methods such as the Harris-Benedict (Long, CL, et al, 1979) equation are available for calculation of precise energy requirements. The Harris-Benedict equation is as follows:

Men: (66.47 + 13.75 weight in kilograms + 5.0 height in centimeters − 6.76 age in years) × (activity factor*) × (injury factor*).

Women: (655.10 + 9.56 weight in kilograms + 1.85 height in centimeters − 4.68 age in years) × (activity factor*) × (injury factor*)

*Activity factor and injury factor are featured in Table 56-10.

Table 56–10. ACTIVITY AND INJURY FACTORS AND VALUES FOR ESTIMATING CALORIC REQUIREMENTS

Factor	Value
Activity:	
Confined to bed	1.2
Ambulatory	1.3
Injury*:	
Surgery:	
Minor	1.1
Major	1.2
Trauma:	
Skeletal	1.35
Head injury with steroid therapy	1.6
Blunt	1.35
Infection:	
Mild	1.2
Moderate	1.4
Severe	1.8
Burns:	
40% BSA†	1.5
100% BSA	1.95

Reprinted with permission of Ross Laboratories, Columbus, OH 43216, from Tube Feedings: Clinical Application, 1986.
*The magnitude of the injury factor decreases as metabolic responses return to normal, nonstressed levels during recovery.
†BSA = body surface area.

Another method to determine caloric requirements is use of a simple "rule of thumb" relation. For the most part, patients experiencing little stress require 25–35 kcal/kg per day, those with moderate stress require 30–40 kcal/kg per day, and those with severe stress 40–45 kcal/kg per day. The degree of stress can be estimated from the clinical setting or from collection of a 24-hour urine with determination of nitrogen excretion. Patients excreting less than 10 g nitrogen a day can be classified as having mild stress; those with 10–15 g/day, moderate stress; and those with greater than 15 g/day, as severe stress.

NURSING DIAGNOSIS

The nurse develops the nursing diagnoses from the problems identified in the assessment. Typical nursing diagnoses for a patient requiring enteral and parenteral feedings are included in Table 56–9.

PLANNING AND INTERVENTION— ENTERAL NUTRITION

The nurse plans the nursing interventions and establishes the goals of care based on the nursing diagnoses. When caring for a patient requiring enteral feedings, the typical goals of nursing intervention are included in Table 56–9. Three modalities of intervention that the nurse frequently uses for patients in states of malnutrition are education, nutritional modifications, and medications. The nurse, as part of the health team, will share these responsibilities with the dietitian and physician.

Patients may require nutritional support both in the hospital and at home. Patients may require only supple-mental support through administration of between-meal high-protein or high-calorie preparation, or may need to be totally maintained with tube feedings. In general, most patients will be hospitalized if they need tube feeding; but when long-term feedings are required, the patient may be discharged with the tubes in place.

NURSING RESPONSIBILITIES FOR ADMINISTERING SPECIAL FEEDING

Supplemental Feedings

When the nurse administers supplemental feedings between meals, he or she records the exact amount of formula taken. It is very important that these supplemental feedings be administered between meals so they do not interfere with normal food intake.

Patients often need encouragement to take this formula, as they may not feel well or do not have big appetites. Enteral feedings are available in various flavors—strawberry, vanilla, chocolate, and others—and only those appealing to the patient, assuming an absence of allergy, are ordered. In general, formulas taste like milkshakes and are best served very cold. In order to calculate the amount of supplement feeding the patient needs, the following calculation is used:

1. Determine patient's total caloric need.
2. Determine amount of calories the patient is actually eating.
3. Provide enough calories to make up the difference between need and intake.

Tube Feedings

The nurse may be responsible for inserting the feeding tube or for teaching the patient how to insert his/her own tube. All necessary equipment should be gathered, including the feeding tube of appropriate length and diameter, a 30- to 50-ml syringe, towel, hypoallergenic tape, stethoscope, glass of water, straw, emesis basin, and—if the tube is not prelubricated—water-soluble lubricant.

The following guidelines can be used for tube insertion (Ross Laboratories, 1986):

1. Explain the procedure to the patient.
2. Wash hands.
3. Elevate the head of the bed 90° or have the patient sit up at the side of the bed. A side-lying position is less desirable but may be necessary for a patient who is unable to sit up. Intubation should not be performed with the patient lying supine unless the head is elevated (Fig. 56–2A).
4. Examine the nasal passages for possible obstructions. Have the patient alternately close each nostril and breathe. The more patent nostril should be used for insertion.
5. Examine the tube for such flaws as rough or sharp edges on the distal end and closed or clogged outlet holes.
6. Determine the approximate depth of insertion. The traditional method for nasogastric insertion involves measuring the distance from the tip of the

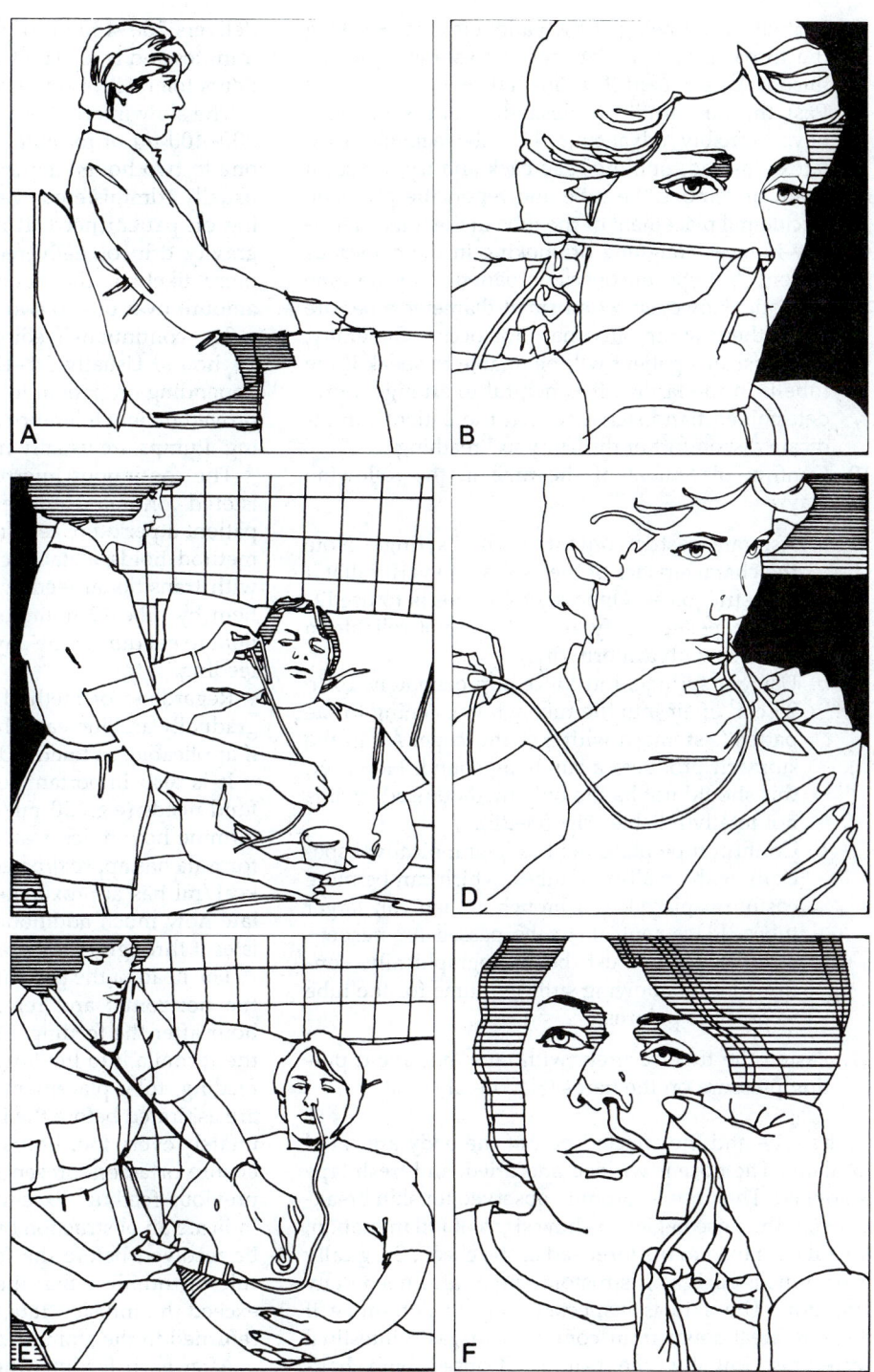

Figure 56–2. Insertion of feeding tube. (See narrative for procedure.) (Courtesy of Ross Laboratories, Columbus, OH.)

nose to the earlobe to the xiphoid process of the sternum. However, Hanson (1979) suggests that a more accurate method is to mark the 50-cm point on the nasogastric tube, then take the usual nose-to-ear-to-xiphoid (NEX) measurement. Tube insertion length is the midway point between the 50-cm measurement and the NEX measurement. Whichever method is used, mark the distance with tape or pen. When nasoenteric placement is desired, an ad-

ditional length of tubing must be passed (Figs. 56–2B and C).

7. Lubricate the tube, if necessary, with water-soluble lubricant along the first 10 cm, or follow the manufacturer's directions for prelubricated tubes.

8. Ease the tube gently through the nares, aiming down and back toward the ear. When the tube reaches the nasopharynx, rotate the tube 180° and instruct the patient to swallow. Sipping water will

facilitate swallowing, if the patient is able. Stroking the throat may stimulate reflex swallowing in the unconscious patient (Fig. 56–2D).

9. Pass the tube until the desired length is inserted, never forcibly advancing the tube against resistance. Instead, pull the tube back and try to pass it again or remove the tube and report the problem. Accidental placement of the tube in the trachea usually induces coughing or choking in the conscious patient, but the unconscious patient may become cyanotic. However, when small-diameter tubes are used, these symptoms may not occur. Generally, the conscious patient will be unable to speak if the tube is in the larynx. It is helpful to arrange a predetermined hand signal so that the patient can indicate discomfort or difficulty in breathing.

10. Confirm placement of the tube in the following ways:

    a. Aspirate gastric contents with a syringe. Note the characteristics of the aspirate to verify that it is gastric juices. One way to do this is to use litmus paper to verify an acid pH (not reliable in patients with achlorhydria).

    b. Using a syringe, introduce approximately 10 to 25 cm^3 of air into the tube while listening to the patient's stomach with a stethoscope. Air in the stomach produces a rumbling sound. However, this should not be the only method used, as it is not totally reliable (Fig. 56–2E).

    c. Confirm tube placement radiographically, especially with small-bore tubes, which can be more easily misplaced in a bronchus than can larger tubes. Placement of a tube passed for nasoenteric feedings must be radiographically confirmed after allowing sufficient time for the tube to pass the pylorus.

11. Fasten the tube securely with tape, but avoid putting pressure on the nares (Fig. 56–2F).

The tube and the affected part of the body are cared for daily. The nose is washed and dried, and fresh tape is applied. The nose is carefully observed for skin breakdown; if the nose begins to show signs of inflammation, the tube is taped to the forehead or the cheek. Surgically placed tubes such as gastrostomy tubes also need daily attention. The skin is inspected daily to determine if there is breakdown from contact with gastrointestinal secretions. Initially, the skin is cleansed with half-strength hydrogen peroxide daily. Once healing has occurred, soap and water is sufficient. A dressing is avoided if possible. If a dressing is used, it must be changed immediately if it becomes wet. If there is gastric leakage around the tube, the skin must be protected with a skin barrier (ointment or commercial disk). An enterostomal therapist can be most helpful in determining the cause of the leakage as well as in providing suggestions for skin care.

Tube feedings can be administered by several different methods: intermittent feeding, including bolus or slow intermittent feeding; continuous feeding; or continuous interrupt or cyclic feeding. The bolus method delivers 200–400 ml of feeding by gravity over several minutes and is repeated every four to six hours. Few patients tolerate this method, and it is rarely used today.

The slow intermittent feeding delivers approximately 200–400 ml of formula over a period of 20 minutes to one to two hours, depending on patient tolerance. It is usually administered every three to four hours, depending on patient need. It may be administered either by gravity drip or delivered by pump. Pump delivery is more likely if the patient must receive a prescribed amount over one to two hours.

The continuous feeding method is administered over 24 hours. Usually 50–125 ml/hour are administered, depending on patient tolerance and needs. There is improved patient tolerance especially when initiating feeding. Pumps are usually necessary.

The continuous interrupt or cyclic feeding is administered continuously over 12–16 hours. This allows the patient a period of rest from the feeding. Some feel this method holds metabolic advantages. It is also helpful with transitional feeding, for example, feeding the patient by tube 12 hours overnight and allowing the patient to eat during the day to wean the patient from tube feeding.

Regardless of method used, there is a need to start gradually and increase the rate and strength of formula, if applicable, as tolerated by the patient.

It is also important to determine the patient's total fluid needs (e.g., 30 ml/kg of body weight) and to determine how much water is in formula (e.g., 1 kcal/ml formula has approximately 840 ml water/liter, while 1.6 kcal/ml has approximately 770 ml water/liter). Calculate how much additional water is needed and administer it throughout the day.

The head of the patient is elevated to at least 45° from the horizontal and remains elevated for at least one hour after the feeding. This helps prevent aspiration of the formula into the lungs. Before administering a tube feeding, tube placement is checked. Stomach contents are aspirated before the intermittent feeding, or approximately every four hours during continuous feedings, to ensure or assess presence of minimal residue from the previous feeding. Excessive residue (over 100 ml) may indicate an obstruction or digestive problem that should be resolved before the feeding is continued. A general rule of thumb is that the volume aspirated should not exceed the infusion rate. The gastric aspirate should be returned to the stomach, not discarded.

After each feeding, the tube is carefully rinsed with about 30 ml of water to prevent a source of contamination and plugging of the tube. Protein in the feedings has a tendency to coagulate when it comes in contact with hydrochloric acid in the stomach. Flushing the tubing every four hours or each time the feeding is interrupted with 20–30 ml of water helps keep the tube patent.

During the tube feeding, the respiratory rate and status of the patient need to be closely monitored. Respiratory distress may indicate the feeding was given too quickly, pushing the stomach up into the chest cavity and compromising chest expansion, or that the patient has aspirated.

For hospitalized patients, continuous drip feedings may be preferable. With the use of small-bore feeding tube and a pump (to be discussed later), there are fewer complications. The patient receives more intake (up to 3 liters/day), and nursing time is reduced. The problems of aspiration, diarrhea, and cramping are greatly reduced, a constant rate is maintained, and the GIT does not suddenly have to contend with a large amount of solution.

A continuous administration of about 50–125 mg/hour is ideal; more solution, and therefore more calories and nitrogen, can be administered. This does restrict the patient's activity. It is necessary for the feeding bag and pump to be moved with the patient and may require movement of the food pump.

At the onset of the tube feeding, a hypertonic formula is administered half-strength at a rate of 50 ml/hour for eight hours. Critically ill patients may need a slower rate of 20–30 ml/hour. The rate is then increased to 75 ml/hour of half strength or three-quarter strength for eight hours. If there are no complications (diarrhea, nausea, vomiting, or glucosuria), the rate is increased to full strength 100–125 ml/hour. This half-strength administration helps the patient develop a gradual tolerance to the hyperosmolarity of the formula. Hyperosmolar solutions draw water into the intestinal tract, and patients are likely to complain of cramping or diarrhea or both. Debilitated patients, patients with gastrointestinal disorders, patients who have not had food for a long time, and patients who are being fed via gastrostomy and jejunostomy tubes are more likely to be intolerant of hyperosmolar formulas. When patients are fed half-strength or reduced-strength formulas because of problems with cramping or diarrhea, they are not receiving the full supply of nutrients, vitamins, and minerals. Supplemental intravenous preparations may have to be administered to ensure proper nutrition. Isotonic solutions can be started and run at full strength.

Patients who are alert and being tube-fed by the nurse can be encouraged to help with the feeding. If the patient is receiving several administrations of tube feedings daily, feedings should arrive at normal meal times in an attractive container on a clean, neat tray. When caring for a patient with enteral feedings, there are many items to check and monitor. Table 56–11 briefly reviews the monitoring summary and check list.

Use of Enteral Pumps

Today, numerous enteral pumps are available. Ideally, pumps should have the following characteristics: The pump should have enough force to push the solution through the tubing even in the presence of small twists in the tubing. There should be alarms for an empty bag, obstruction, and low battery. Obstruction is measured by an increased resistance in the tubing. The pump should be light so it can easily be carried over a shoulder and there should be a similar carrying device for the bag. Flow accuracy should be within 10%. Rate should be controllable in increments of at least 5.0 ml, to optimize flow and adjust for changes in rate-prescription. The pump should be sturdy, resist bumps, and be easily cleaned. A rechargeable battery should last several

Table 56–11. MONITORING SUMMARY AND CHECKLIST

Monitoring Summary	Checklist
When initiating a new or intermittent feeding:	Check tube placement. Check amount of residual. If greater than 100 ml, delay feeding for approximately 0.5–1 hour. Consider possible reasons for delayed gastric emptying.
Every half hour and prn—Intermittent feeding:	Check gravity drip rates and patient response.
Every hour and prn—Continuous pump feeding:	Check pump functioning and patient response.
Every 2–4 hours of continuous feeding:	Check residual.
Every 4 hours:	Check vital signs, including blood pressure, temperature, pulse, and respiration. Check blood sugar. (In nondiabetic patient, checks can be discontinued after 48 hours if consistently negative.)
Every 8 hours:	Check fluid intake and output. Check specific gravity of urine. Hang new formula for continuous feeding. Chart.
Every day:	Change feeding container and pump or gravity tubing. Check patient's weight. Check electrolytes, blood urea nitrogen, and blood glucose until stabilized.
Every 7–10 days:	Repeat nutrition assessment.
prn:	Observe patient for any negative response to tube feeding (e.g. nausea, vomiting, diarrhea). Check tube placement (nasogastric). Calculate nitrogen balance. Conduct delayed hypersensitivity skin testing. Check laboratory data as ordered by physician. Change feeding tube. Clean pump.

Reprinted with permission of Ross Laboratories, Columbus, OH. 43216, from Tube Feeding: Clinical Application, 1986.

hours. And, finally, the pump should be simple to operate. A study reviewing several pump features is found in Table 56–12. Several enteral pumps are featured in Figure 56–3.

Table 56–12. SUMMARY OF PUMP FEATURES

Product	Maximum Bag Size (ml)	Leaks	Maximum Pump Pressure (psi)	Easy to Wash	Battery (hr)	Weight (lb)
Flexiflo II	1000	Quite often	7.7	Yes	8	5
Kangaroo	1000	Sometimes	12	Yes	3†	5.5
Travenol 2000	1300	No	Over 12*	Yes	6	6
Biosearch	1000	Yes	Over 12*	No	*	*
IVAC 3000	1500	*	10–30	Yes*	*	8
Corpak VTR 300	1500	No*	12	Yes*	3	7.5

*These were judged from drawings (not tested).

Note: The following pumps could not be tested at this time: Travenol 2000, Corpak VTR 300, IVAC 3000. Overall, the new pumps appear to be quite nice for a hospital environment but poorly designed for ambulatory care. This is unfortunate because it would be easy to attach at least a shoulder strap to many of these pumps.

From Siquel, EN: Use of pumps for enteral alimentation. Nutritional Support Services, 6(2a), 1986, p. 42, with permission.

Complications of Enteral Feedings

One of the most common complications of enteral feedings is diarrhea. Diarrhea may be associated with too rapid an infusion rate, lactose intolerance, osmolarity intolerance, low serum albumin levels, vitamin B deficiencies, change in intestinal bacterial, concurrent antibiotic administration, lack of fiber, fat intolerance, or too much fluid.

Infusion rates can easily be slowed to a maximum of 100–125 mg/hour. A lactose-free feeding is also an easy solution. Osmolarity intolerance can be cured by either switching to a low-osmolarity formula or by diluting the current formula and gradually working back to a full-strength solution. Serum albumin levels should be kept near normal to prevent malabsorption in the intestine due to edema of the villi. Some clinical investigations have found that the administration of albumin is helpful to prevent this type of diarrhea. Some investigations have also found that the temporary use of elemental formulas is helpful. Vitamin B deficiencies can result in scaly, dry skin, difficulties in swallowing, mental confusion, and diarrhea. Supplement vitamin B alleviates this problem.

Often diarrhea is due to the change in bacterial flora of the intestine. This may be due to drugs like antibiotics. Decreasing or discontinuation of the drug may decrease the diarrhea. If the intestinal flora has been reduced, the administration of lactobacillus (Lactinex) may help restore intestinal flora. Lactobacillus can also be found in sweet milk and yogurt with the fresh culture.

Lack of fiber may also cause diarrhea. Switching to Jerity, Enrich, or similar high-fiber products adds bulk to help form soft rather than liquid stools.

Fat intolerance may also result in diarrhea. Patients who are acutely ill, or who have pancreatic disease or recent gastric surgery may not be able to tolerate fat. Several products are available that are low in fat.

Finally, too much fluid can easily be eliminated by decreasing the flow rate.

Cramping and diarrhea may also be associated with cold feedings. Research has recommended that room temperature feedings be administered. If feedings must be refrigerated, they should be brought to room temperature before administering. But never heat a formula!

Another common complication of enteral feeding is nausea. This may be related to the odor of the enteral feeding. Using flavored feedings may be helpful; however, large volumes of flavorings increase the osmolarity of the feeding, which may in turn lead to diarrhea. Nausea may also indicate a slowed gastric emptying time. A residual should be checked. Other causes of nausea may be too rapid administration, lactose, or fat intolerance. All of these problems are easily eliminated.

A possible complication can occur when aluminum antacids are combined with high-protein enteral formulas. The aluminum in the antacid and the protein in the formula can interact, causing gastric obstruction.

Aspiration pneumonia is a potentially lethal complication requiring special precautionary measures. Large-bore tubes decrease the competency of the gastroesophageal sphincter, increasing the risk of gastric reflux and aspiration. Thus, small-bore tubes are preferred. Once the location of the tube is confirmed, proper taping is important to prevent movement. Positioning the patient in an upright position (minimum 30°–45°) during the feeding also prevents aspiration. When possible, the use of nasoduodenal or nasojejunal tubes are preferred over nasogastric tubes, as the risk of aspiration is reduced. Some institutions may also evaluate the tracheal aspirate every three to six hours with glucose oxidase reagent strips. Since glucose is not normally found in the sputum, its presence in the tracheal aspirate may indicate aspiration. If there is blood present in the aspirate, it will also give a positive glucose reaction.

Constipation may be a problem in patients maintained on long-term tube feedings. Many of the commercial products are low in residue, which decreases bowel movements. This should not be confused with constipation. If constipation is a problem, the use of a high-fiber product may be indicated. In addition, sufficient fluids and adequate exercise (if possible) are helpful.

A final complication of enteral feedings may be bacterial contamination of the enteral feeding. This may

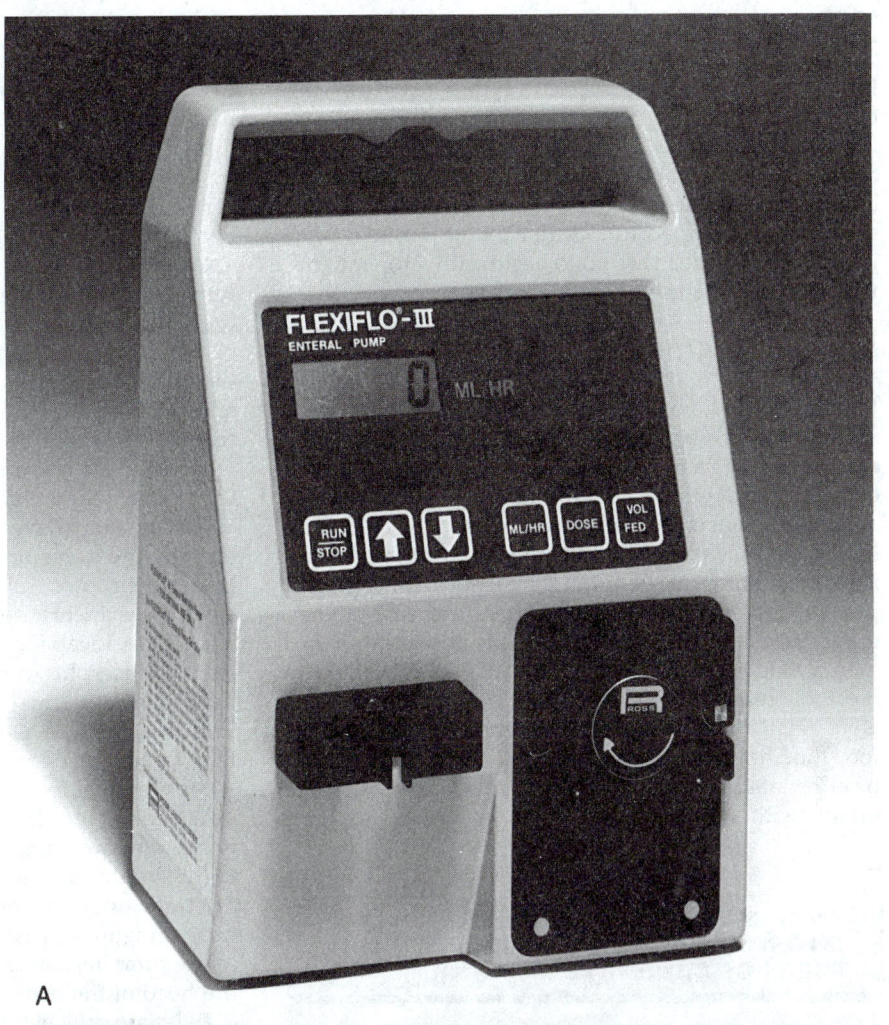

A

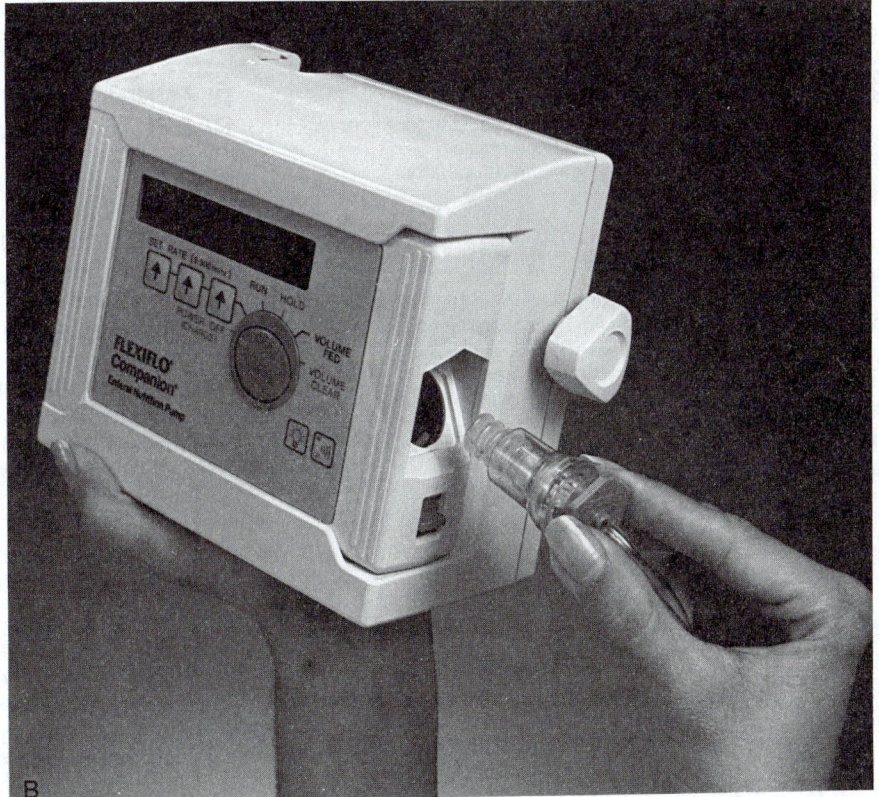

Figure 56–3. Two enteral feeding tube pumps: *A*, the Flexiflo III, and *B*, the Flexiflo companion enteral pump. (Courtesy of Ross Laboratories, Columbus, OH.)

B

lead to diarrhea or other gastric symptoms. This contamination can occur during mixing or hanging. It has been suggested in a few studies that the feeding container and tubing be changed daily, that fresh feeding be hung every four to eight hours, and that new formula should not be added to any remaining formula. Most important are a clean set-up to begin with, proper handwashing, and the use of aseptic technique.

PATIENT TEACHING

Patients going home on tube feedings need to have the information presented in Table 56–13 included in their teaching plan. Patients being fed via a tube are deprived of the personal gratification of the act of eating. Patients and families need to have the opportunity to discuss their feelings. Patients are encouraged to join their family at meal times for the social interactions. If the patient prefers not be present when others are eating, then other provisions for social activities is important.

In a study, Padilla, GV, et al (1979) found that the most distressing experiences of tube-feeding patients were related to thirst, being deprived of the taste of food, and having an unsatisfied taste for food. Thirst can be eliminated by providing additional water, rinsing the mouth with water, chewing gum, or sucking on hard

candy. Lubricating the lips with petroleum jelly also enhances comfort.

Patients and families both have to understand the rationale for the feeding, the proposed length of time that this method will be necessary, and what is to be expected from these feedings.

Patients are taught how to prepare their feedings and how to administer them. Also, they are taught about the type of tube present and how it is best cared for. Both patients and their families have to learn what to do if the patient aspirates, what to do if the tube comes out, and what to do in case of any other complications already discussed. Patients need to know who to call and what is, and is not, an emergency. Both verbal and written instructions are given to the patient and family.

Patients may have permanent feeding tubes changed only by the nurse or physician, or may be educated to insert their own tubes. Several manufacturers make small (size French #6 to #8) diameter, flexible tubes, which are ideal for this purpose. Having the patient learn to insert his/her own feeding tube allows the patient to look "normal" when going to work or shopping. The feeding tube is inserted each evening when the feeding will be done.

Most enteral formulas are thick and if spilled act as a very strong glue. They are very difficult to clean up. Patients who are going to receive tube feeding during the night should tape all the connections and place papers or plastic under the bottles. Also, to allow the patient to turn at night, suggest that he/she tape the feeding tube to their forehead and place the feeding and the pump at the head of the bed.

Poles are difficult to push around in most homes, particularly up and down stairs, so all apparatus should be wearable.

PLANNING AND INTERVENTION— PARENTERAL NUTRITION

Patients may need parenteral nutritional support both in the hospital and at home. In general, most patients are hospitalized during the initial stage of parenteral nutrition. Later, they may be discharged to home with the feedings. Patients and their families need a great deal of education and support to continue parenteral nutrition at home.

The intervention phase can be divided into four stages: (1) product preparation, (2) preparation of the patient and insertion of the catheter (for TPN) or peripheral IV line (for PTPN), (3) the administration of the solution, and (4) the care of the catheter line. Each step is described.

Preparing the Solution

All TPN solutions are mixed in sterile conditions under a laminar flow hood, and according to written hospital protocols. Ideally, the solution is prepared in the pharmacy and then sent to the nursing unit. The ambient air found on a busy nursing unit does not provide a satisfactory environment for preparing sterile TPN solutions. Contamination rates of 10%–18% have been reported

---

Table 56–13. PATIENT TEACHING INFORMATION—PATIENTS REQUIRING FEEDINGS AT HOME

Dear Patient:

Supplemental Feedings:

1. You will have to use supplemental feedings for
   _____.
2. Mix the feeding just like the hospital staff told you.
3. Take the extra feeding between meals.
4. Keep any leftover feeding in the refrigerator.

Tube Feedings:

1. You will have to use tube feedings for
   _____.
2. Mix the feeding just like the hospital staff told you.
3. Administer the tube feeding as taught in the hospital.
4. Sit up when receiving the tube feeding.
5. If you have a change in bowel habits (diarrhea or constipation), notify your doctor.
6. Keep any leftover feeding in the refrigerator.

Parenteral Feedings:

1. You will have to use parenteral feedings for
   _____.
2. Make the feeding just like the hospital staff told you, or use ready-made solution.
3. Administer the parenteral feeding as taught in the hospital.
4. Care for the IV line as you were taught by the nurse.
5. If you see any redness or swelling at the site, or you get a fever, notify your doctor.
6. Keep you TPN solution in the refrigerator after mixing, and use it within 24 hours.

when TPN is mixed without a laminar flow environment. No substances are added to the solution once it is on the nursing unit.

Most pharmacies use commercially prepared TPN solutions. These contain a dextrose bottle and bottle of amino acid solution, which are mixed together. The exact mixing of TPN solutions is done according to individual institutional policies. Some general policies, however, are always maintained, and may include some of the following. Prior to preparation, the pharmacist inspects commercially prepared bottles for cracks and precipitates. If present, the bottle is discarded. The bottle is then cleansed with 70% isopropyl alcohol. The collar seals are removed from both bottles, and the latex seal is removed from the protein. Any additives are generally introduced to the dextrose bottle. Each additive may change the pH of the TPN solution and possibly inactive another additive. To avoid this, additives are introduced in a particular sequence (Table 56–14). Not all additives are added all the time. Insulin may be added to control hyperglycemia, and it can be added at any time. Many authorities today recommend that insulin not be placed in the bottle. Instead, the urine should be assessed for sugar, and insulin administered every six hours as needed. Some medications are incompatible with TPN solution and should never be administered through the same central line.

The spike end of the transfer tubing is inserted into the protein bottle and the needle inserted into the dextrose bottle, and the transfer of protein to dextrose bottle is begun. The transfer tubing is closed before the protein bottle is completely empty. The transfer tubing is removed and the bottle is recapped with a metal or plastic cover included in the package. The label is affixed to the bottle, identifying all components of the solution, its expiration date and time, and the name of the patient.

The TPN solution is administered immediately after mixing or stored in refrigerator at 4°–8°C. The solution must generally be used within seven days of its preparation, although home IV suppliers give a 30-day expiration date.

When PFE is used, it is the nurse's responsibility to maintain stability of the lipid emulsion before and during the infusion. The PFE has an unconventional, milk-like appearance. The bottle is never agitated because the fat globules may aggregate. Lipid emulsions may be stored at room temperature. The bottle is inspected carefully before infusion for cracks and any signs of altered stability. It should not be used if the oil has separated out or if there is an inconsistent texture or color. Unused portions are discarded within 30 minutes. Nothing except heparin, 1–2 units/ml, is ever added to a lipid emulsion.

Inserting the Lines

Before the catheter is inserted, the nurse explains the entire procedure to the patient. The patient should understand what is going to be done, where the catheter is to be inserted (the subclavian vein is most common), why this particular form of therapy was selected, and the approximate duration of the therapy. Before the procedure begins, the patient, if alert, is also taught how to do the Valsalva maneuver (unless it is contraindicated) and allowed to practice. A properly timed Valsalva maneuver prevents air from entering the catheter and vascular system during the threading maneuver. (See a procedure manual for proper insertion technique.) Whenever possible, the catheter insertions are performed in the operating room to maintain sterility.

Hickman, Broviac, Portacath, or Groshong catheters are central lines for long-term use that can be used for infusion of drugs, parenteral feedings, or other therapies (Fig. 56–4). These catheters are designed so that the ends may be capped between infusions. The Hickman has a dacron cuff that is placed under the skin in a tunnel. This decreases the risk of infection and prevents the catheter from becoming dislodged. If this catheter is severed or cut, repair kits are available. The Broviac catheter has a small diameter and it is particularly suitable for children. The Groshong catheter has 1, 2, or 3 lumens and also has a dacron cuff that is tunneled under the skin. An advantage of the Groshong is that a heparin flush is required only once weekly. When the patient is to receive PFE, a peripheral line may be used with any needle size greater than 20-gauge. For short-term use, a double- or triple-lumen central catheter is preferred.

Administering the Solution

The solutions are administered steadily, always with an infusion pump. The infusion is never speeded up or slowed down. Patients receiving TPN solutions need to be checked at least hourly to observe the infusion rate and to prevent changes in the drip rate, which may be caused by changes in body position or kinked tubing. Since TPN solutions contain great quantities of glucose, the balance between insulin release and glucose infusion is best achieved by a constant infusion rate. If a TPN solution containing over 20% dextrose must be suddenly interrupted, it is recommended that a 5% dextrose solution with appropriate electrolytes be substituted, either through the central catheter or via a peripheral vein to run at the same rate as the previous TPN solution.

The nurse initiates the TPN solution slowly at a rate

Table 56–14. PROPER SEQUENCE OF SOLUTION MIXING

1. Multivitamin solution
2. Folic acid
3. Ascorbic acid
4. Sodium chloride
5. Sodium lactate and acetate
6. Potassium phosphate and acetate
7. Potassium
8. Calcium
9. Magnesium sulfate
10. Heparin
11. Regular insulin
12. Albumin
13. Trace elements

From Kaminski, MV: Hyperalimentation: A Guide for Clinicians. Marcel Dekker, New York, 1985, page 141, with permission.

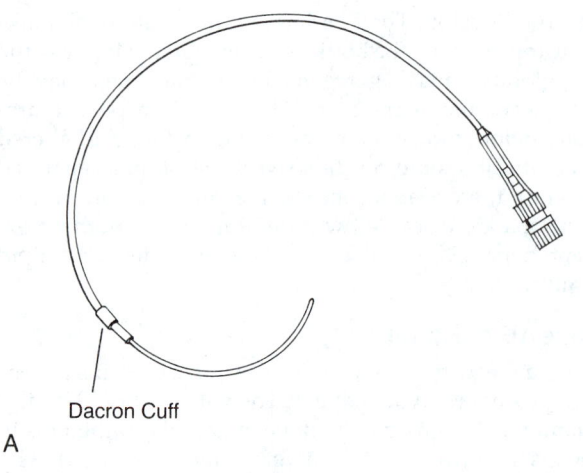

Dacron Cuff

A

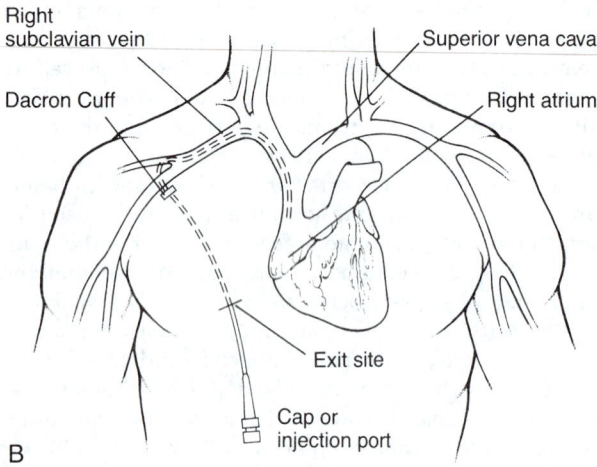

Right subclavian vein

Superior vena cava

Dacron Cuff

Right atrium

Exit site

Cap or injection port

B

Figure 56–4. Hickman catheter (*A*) and insertion (*B*). The hickman catheter has a dacron cuff which is placed in a tunnel under the skin. This cuff prevents the catheter from becoming dislodged as well as preventing infection.

of 40–50 ml/hour and increases the rate over a 24-hour period until the desired rate is reached. The solution is started slowly to allow for the stimulation of the microsomal proteins within the body to utilize the TPN products. In addition, the pancreas is stimulated slowly to increase its release of insulin. To avoid the possibility of contamination and degradation of vitamins, TPN solutions should be changed at least every 24 hours. Tubing is changed daily or with the addition of each new bottle. In-line filters may be used to prevent infection, although their effectiveness has not as yet been conclusively substantiated by research. The filter, if used, is changed daily. If a TPN administration is interrupted for more than one hour, the remaining solution is discarded.

Before starting the first lipid emulsion, baseline vital signs are taken. The initial administration should be no more than 1.0 ml/minute for the first 30 minutes, be-

cause initial adverse reactions are possible. Vital signs are monitored every ten minutes during this period, and the patient is observed for the presence of chills, fever, flushing, diaphoresis, chest or back pain, nausea, vomiting, or any other signs of an allergic reaction. If problems do arise, the infusion is stopped and the physician is notified.

If there are no ill effects from the initial 30.0 ml, the rate of infusion can then be increased. In general, fat emulsions are infused in a 8- to 12-hour period. Continuous observation is necessary during the entire infusion. The majority of adverse reactions occur within the first 30 minutes; however, reactions are possible later.

It is recommended that the lipid emulsion be inserted into a Y connector or sterile stopcock of the primary tubing closest to the catheter insertion site. This reduces the length of time the PFE is in contact with a foreign substance, which may affect its stability. Because the lipid particles are very large, an in-line filter is *never* used with PFE. Heparin may be given to the patient during the PFE to help speed clearance of the lipids from the patient's plasma.

When the PFE is completed, the bottle is removed and a bottle of 5% dextrose solution is added and the tubing is flushed. This part of the Y line can then be turned off; but it is left intact until the next lipid infusion, tube, or dressing change. Blood, IV fluids, and some medications are administered through a separate site to avoid contamination of the TPN catheter. Routine blood work should not be done until two to six hours after a PFE, so the extra fat in the bloodstream will not distort results. During an infusion of a PFE, a patient should not be moved anywhere, as this will cause agitation of the bottle.

Care of the Catheter or Line

Special care of the TPN line must always be taken to ensure its sterility. Infection at the insertion site can progress to colonization of the catheter tip, and cause sepsis. Care should consist of either daily or alternate-day site care, which may be performed by either the nurse or a physician, depending on institutional policy. Transparent dressings are often used once the site has been cleaned according to institutional policies. A TPN line is generally left in place until it is no longer needed. However, if a patient has some distant infection in the body, the line may be changed routinely every one to two weeks to prevent spread of the local infection; although unless the line is clearly the source of infection, it is better to leave the line in place than to expose the patient to risks of reinsertion.

A line used for PFE is cared for like any other peripheral line.

Nutritional Admixtures

Currently, 3-in-1 or all-in-one total nutritional admixtures are being used. This mixture is a 24-hour supply of dextrose, crystalline amino acids, and lipids in one container. By mixing these three products, all are absorbed evenly over the 24-hour period. Since the lipid is in the combination, piggy-back attachments and additional peripheral lines are not necessary. Less frequent manipulation of the lines may reduce the possibility of infection. Only one container is hung every 24 hours, so mixing time is saved. And, fewer administration sets are used. This combination admixture is opaque, which prevents the nurse from visually checking for suspended particles, fine precipitates, or microbial growth. Also, because of the fat, an in-line filter cannot be used.

Infusion Interrupts

As the patient becomes stabilized on the parenteral feeding, better utilization of nutrients occurs if the infusion is interrupted for a period each day. The infusion interrupt is started for two hours. The IV that is hung during the interrupt can be 5% dextrose/water with half of all the additives in the TPN bottle. The interrupt time is gradually increased to eight hours.

Interruption of the TPN allows for better utilization of nutrients and allows any fat that has accumulated in the liver to be utilized.

Home Care

Patients requiring TPN and PFE are generally in the hospital at the initiation of the therapy. However, because of the prolonged duration of the therapy, patients without other problems are sent home with a TPN line in place. Policies differ among institutions concerning the discharge care of the individual. Three distinct policies are common. First, some hospitals may send a nurse with the premixed TPN solution daily to the home. The nurse continues to care for the line and observe the patient for complications. Or secondly, a public health nurse assumes responsibility for visiting the patient, mixing the solution, and changing the dressings. Or thirdly, the patient and family are taught how to mix the solutions, how to administer them, how to care for the line(s), what side effects to observe for, and how to handle complications. If the third option is chosen, the nurse has the responsibility of ensuring that the patient's level of knowledge is adequate to care for him- or herself at home. Patient teaching information is included in Table 56–13. Patients on home TPN may infuse their feedings only at night. This technique enhances patient mobility during the day.

Complications of TPN

As with enteral nutrition, patients receiving parenteral nutrition can experience complications. Patients can experience substrate intolerance, often demonstrated by hepatic dysfunction. Hepatic dysfunction is recognized by an increase in liver enzymes. The hepatic dysfunction is generally reversible. Fluid and electrolyte problems can also occur. Patients need to have frequent laboratory analysis to monitor sodium, potassium, phosphate, magnesium, and calcium. Adequate fluids are also monitored through daily weights and urinary output. Dehydration and hypovolemia can develop secondarily to the high osmolarity of these solutions.

Identifying infection of the catheter in an acutely stressed patient with multiple sources of fever is often difficult. Patients should have blood cultures drawn. If the TPN solution is suspect, it is discontinued. The line may also be removed and a new one inserted in a new location when the patient has been afebrile for 48 hours.

Patients receiving large amounts of dextrose (15%–25%) may experience hyperglycemia and will need to have insulin administered. Insulin is generally not placed in the TPN bottle but administered every six hours as needed. Patients receiving less than 25% dextrose solutions will generally not require insulin after one to two days. Diabetics are monitored carefully throughout TPN therapy and insulin adjustments are made as needed.

Drug incompatibilities can also occur with TPN solutions. The field of compatibilities is complex and confusing. As administration systems and solutions change, so do the medications that can be safely mixed with them. In the early 1980s, TPN solutions were mixed with only vitamins and minerals. Now admixtures of dextrose, amino acids, fats, and vitamins are becoming more common. Also, TPN solutions are known to be compatible with medications like aminophylline, cimetidine, albumin, cyanocobalamin, cyclophosphamide, cytarabine, dopamine, fluorouracil, furosemide, heparin, hydrocortisone, insulin, iron dextran, isoproterenol, levarterenol, lidocaine, metaraminol, methyldopa, methylprednisolone, and polymyxin B. Frequent updating on drug compatibilities is necessary.

EVALUATION

During the evaluation phase, the nurse evaluates the effectiveness of the enteral and parenteral feedings. This evaluation is based on a list of evaluation criteria that has been developed in relation to the goals determined by the nurse, patient, and family. The data base obtained in the original assessment and use to formulate the nursing diagnoses provides useful criteria for measuring treatment effectiveness. The typical goals of enteral and parenteral feedings are included in Table 56–9.

The nurse also evaluates all objective symptoms of the patient to ensure they are returning to normal. Skin turgor, the presence of abnormal thirst, the presence of edema, growth (in infants), changes in weight, urine characteristics—such as amount and specific gravity, and the conditions of the mucous membranes (dry, moist, pink, etc.)—indicate changes in hydration level. The older, unconscious, semicomatose, confused, sedated, or intubated patient requires closer evaluation because he or she is unable to convey the presence of thirst.

The nurse also evaluates the patient's psychologic response to therapy. Does the patient accept the therapy? How does the patient plan on coping with not eating regular foods (if therapy is long-term)? Will the patient comply with the therapy?

As TPN is started, the nurse evaluates blood glucose levels on a routine basis, usually every six hours. The patient may be receiving insulin in the TPN solution or be covered with insulin injections. A nurse must stress to the patient that he or she will probably not be permanently diabetic. After TPN is stopped, blood and urinary glucose levels usually fall to normal levels within several days.

Frequent laboratory tests are performed to evaluate electrolytes, and to detect the presence of infection. If infection at the insertion site, or due to the catheter, is suspected, all lines are removed and their tips cultured. New lines are inserted in different locations. If a patient complains of sudden chills, fever, or chest or back pain, suspect that the TPN solution has been contaminated. Other sources of infection should also be ruled out. Suspected TPN solution should be sent to the laboratory for culture.

The nurse also evaluates subjective symptoms such as anorexia, pain, discomfort, and any emotional complications. Patients receiving parenteral nutrition for long periods may need much skilled emotional support. "Food" is normally associated with eating, and not eating can have major psychologic effects on some people, even to the point of hallucinating about food. Patients need to be reassured that their appetites, which are suppressed by parenteral nutrition, will return to normal when this form of feeding is discontinued; and that their bowel activity will return to normal after parenteral feedings have been stopped. Patients will have very few, small stools, possibly only once a week while TPN is being used.

The nurse should know the side effects of TPN as well as teaching the patient and family what to look for if the patient is being discharged on TPN. The most common side effects of TPN include reactions of the patient to the solution manifested by fever or allergic reactions such as itching and hives; metabolic abnormalities noted by glucose intolerance with a blood sugar over 200 mg/100 ml or urine glucose to 3–4+, or hyperosmolar hyperglycemic nonketotic coma (HHNK); electrolyte disorders, or elevated blood urea nitrogen or ammonia; mineral deficiencies, including hypocalcemia, hypophosphatemia, and hypomagnesemia, trace mineral deficiencies; and sepsis, where no other source of contamination can be identified, which necessitates removal of the catheter. The most common side effects of PFE include fever, chills, shivering, vomiting, a sensation of warmth, and pain in the chest and back.

Patients requiring enteral and parenteral feedings need a great deal of encouragement. Often, feedings are given for an indefinite period. Patients and their families are supported psychologically through their adaptation and maintenance phases. Parenteral hyperalimentation is a new mode of therapy; research is still ongoing as to its effectiveness and long-term effects. Total parenteral nutrition has been shown to lower both morbidity and mortality, and to shorten hospitalization, convalescence, and rehabilitation in the severely debilitated patient. Many patients survive serious illnesses today because of TPN.

SUMMARY

Nutritional support is part of the therapeutic armamentarium for managing patients safely and effectively after surgery, trauma, or sepsis. Nutritional support is available through both the enteral and parenteral routes to meet the specific needs of the patient. The timing of the start of nutrition is important. Ideally, nutrition support is started in patients previously well nourished after three days when it becomes apparent that nutrient intake will not resume in a reasonable period. Malnourished patients need to have nutritional support started immediately.

As the nurse prepares to administer enteral and parenteral nutrition, a thorough assessment is obtained, including history of current illness, recent weight changes, and food allergies or intolerances. Solutions are administered according to institutional policies. Patients are evaluated to ensure that the nutritional support is effective. Protein levels and fluid and electrolyte balances should return to normal and weight should increase. If this does not occur, the patient and the nutritional regimen is evaluated.

BIBLIOGRAPHY

AMA Drug Evaluations, ed 6. PSG Publishing, Littleton, MA, 1986.

Anderson, BJ: Tube feeding: Is diarrhea inevitable? Am J Nurs 86(6):705, 1986.

Bernard, M, Jacobs, D, and Rombeau, J: Nutritional and Metabolic Support of Hospitalized Patients. WB Saunders, Philadelphia, 1986.

Birdsall, C: Do total nutritional admixtures benefit your patients? Am J Nurs 87(1):14, 1987.

Cerrato, PL: What diet does for wound healing. RN 88(6):73, 1988.

Cerrato, PL: The special nutritional needs of a COPD patient. RN 87(11):7576, 1987.

Cerrato, PL: Will IV feeding endanger your patient? RN 86(12):59, 1986.

Davis, J: A handy guide for TPN. AJN 88(1):103, 1988.

Dickerson, RN, and Brown, RO: Hypomagnesemia in hospitalized patients receiving nutritional support. Heart Lung 14(6):561, 1985.

Doizaki, KK and Weber, JN: Restoring patency to occluded venous access ports. Am J Hosp Pharm 43:880, 1986.

Dougherty, S: The malnourished respiratory patient. Critical Care Nurse 8(4):13, 1988.

Ekstrom, B and Olsson, AM: Priapism in patients treated with total parenteral nutrition. Br J Urol 59:170, 1987.

Farley, JM: Current trends in enteral feeding. Critical Care Nurse 8(4):23, 1988.

Flynn, KT, Norton, LC, and Fisher, RL: Enteral tube feeding: Indications, practices and outcomes. Image 19(1):16, 1987.

Holmes, R, et al: Combating pressure sores—nutritionally. Am J Nurs 87(10):1301, 1987.

Horbal-Shuster, M and Irwin, M: Keeping enteral nutrition on track. Am J Nurs 87(4):523, 1987.

Irwin, M: Managing leaking gastrostomy sites. Am J Nurs 88(3):359, 1988.

Kaminski, MV: Hyperalimentation: A Guide for Clinicians. Marcel Dekker, New York, 1985.

Kennedy-Caldwell, C: Clinical Triads: Water Metabolism, the NPO Patient, and Parenteral Nutrition. Critical Care Nurse 6(3):63, 1986.

Kittelberger-Bockus, SB: Tube Feedings: Clinical Applications. Ross Laboratories, Columbus, OH, 1986.

Krause, M and Mahon, K: Food Nutrition and Diet Therapy, ed. 8. WB Saunders, Philadelphia, 1986.

Long, CL: Energy and protein requirements in stress and trauma part 2. Crit Care Nurs Clinics 2:7, 1984.

Long, CL: Nutritional Support in Critical Care. Aspen Publishing, Rockville, MD, 1987.

Long, CL, et al: Metabolic response to injury and illness: Estimation of energy and protein needs from indirect calorimetry and nitrogen balance. JPEN 3:452, 1979.

Mackinnon, C: Total parenteral nutrition for patients with respiratory insufficiency. Intensive Care Nurse 2(4):166, 1987.

Miller, LS, et al: Enteral and parenteral nutrition in the critically ill patient. Hosp Formul 21:672, 1986.

Moore, MC: Do you still believe these myths about tube feeding? RN 50(5):51, 1987.

Noller, C and Mobarhan, S: Enteral feeding in patients with advanced chronic obstructive pulmonary disease. Nutritional Support Services 6(2a):37, 1986.

Openbrier, DR and Covey, M: Ineffective breathing pattern related to malnutrition. Nurs Clin North Am 22(1):225, 1987.

Pagana, KD: Preventing complications in jejunostomy tube feedings. Dimensions of Critical Care Nursing 6(1):28, 1987.

Rombeau, JL and Caldwell, MD: Enteral and Tube Feeding. WB Saunders, Philadelphia, 1986.

Siquel, EN: Use of pumps for enteral alimentation. Nutritional Support Services 6(2a):40, 1986.

Starkey, JF, Jefferson, PA, and Kirby, DF: Taking care of percutaneous endoscopic gastrostomy. Am J Nurs 88(1):42, 1988.

Steinbaugh, M and Sauls, H: The gastrointestinal response to injury, starvation, and enteral nutrition. Ross Laboratories, Columbus, OH, 1988.

Stranz, MH and Barfoot, KS: Total parenteral nutrition compatibility of antibiotic admixtures. Journal of Intravenous Nursing 11(1):43, 1988.

Valli, C, et al: Interaction of nutrients with antacids: A complication during enteral tube feeding. Lancet 1:747, 1986.

Walter, J: Which of your patients is starving to death? RN 87(7):45, 1987.

Weinmann-Winkler, S and Dudrick, SJ: Enteral nutrition history: Past, present, future. Nutritional Support Services 6(2a):7, 1986.

Wills, JS, et al: Percutaneous gastrostomy: A safe, cost-effective alternative to surgical gastrostomy and intravascular hyperalimentation. Nutritional Support Service 6(2):10, 1986.

Wolk, RA and Swartz, RD: Nutritional support of patients with acute renal failure. Nutritional Support Services 6(2):38, 1986.

Wright, B and Robinson, L: Enteral feeding tubes as drug delivery systems. Nutritional Support Services 6(2):33, 1986.

Zimmaro, DM: Diarrhea associated with enteral nutrition. Focus on Critical Care 13(5):58, 1986.

GLOSSARY TERMS IN THIS CHAPTER

Ariboflavinosis
Avitaminosis
Cones
Keratomalacia
Kwashiorkor
Mineral
Nyctalopia·
Osteomalacia
Provitamin
Refractory rickets
Rickets
Rods
Tetany
Vitamin
Xerophthalmia

57
CHAPTER

VITAMINS AND MINERALS

MERRILY MATHEWSON KUHN, R.N.C., Ph.D., CCRN

LEARNING OBJECTIVES

After reading this chapter, the student will be able to:

1. Identify commonly used vitamins and minerals.

2. Differentiate among the various vitamins and minerals as to their function, routes of administration, pharmacokinetics, deficiency states, common sources, and interactions.

3. Identify specific areas to assess in the patient requiring vitamins and minerals in order to formulate appropriate nursing diagnoses.

4. Plan the nursing interventions necessary to administer vitamins and minerals and choose appropriate teaching strategies to gain patient compliance.

5. Evaluate the patient at various stages of treatment to gauge nursing interventions.

In order to maintain normal metabolic function, the human body needs a daily intake of both vitamins and minerals. It is estimated that 40% of adults in the United States take vitamin and mineral supplements. A *vitamin* is defined as a biologically active, organic compound, a controlling agent essential for human health and growth (its absence causing a deficiency disease or disorder). Vitamins are carried in small concentrations via the circulatory system and act on target organs or tissues. Vitamins include both the four fat-soluble vitamins A, D, E, and K; and the nine water-soluble vitamins including vitamin C, folic acid, pantothenic acid, niacin (nicotinic acid), biotin, and the B-complex vitamins—B_1, B_2, B_6, and B_{12}.

A *mineral* is defined as any naturally occurring nonorganic homogenous solid substance, essential for human health and growth (its absence causing a deficiency disease or disorder), neither synthesized nor produced within the body, but available in the diet in small amounts. Minerals are carried in small amounts via the circulatory system and act on target organs or tissues. Minerals are electropositive (cations) or electronegative (anions). There are 15 minerals. Ten minerals are cations: calcium (Ca), magnesium (Mg), sodium (Na), potassium (K), iron (Fe), copper (Cu), manganese (Mn), zinc (Zn), chromium (Cr), and cobalt (Co); five minerals are anions: phosphorus (P), idoine (I), selenium (Se), molybdenum (Mo), and fluorine (F). Three of the anions are most commonly found as oxide complexes: phosphorus oxide (PO_4), selenium oxide (SeO_4), and molybdenum oxide (MoO_4).

Of the 15 minerals, five are considered macro (bulk essential) elements—Ca, Mg, Na, K, P—and are needed daily by the body to maintain health. The remaining ten minerals (Fe, Cu, Mn, Zn, I, Se, Mo, Cr, Co, and F) are termed micro (trace) elements. As yet, not all of these have been proven essential for life. Se, Mo, Mn, Cr, and F will probably be determined to be essential for human life in the near future. (Cr, Mn, and Se deficiencies have been reported.)

Minerals carry one or more charges in solution. They may be univalent (carrying one charge) such as Na^+, K^+, F^-, and I^-; or bivalent (carrying two charges) such as Ca^{2+}, Mg^{2+}, Fe^{2+}, Cu^{2+}, Co^{2+}, Mn^{2+}, Zn^{2+}, SeO_4^{2-}, MoO_4^{2+}, and PO_4^{2-}. There is also one trivalent mineral element, Cr^{3+}.

Mineral elements are capable of interacting with each other in solution. The majority of the ions are soluble in the acid pH of the stomach. However, as the pH turns alkaline in the intestine, most of the divalent positive ions (Mg^{2+}, Co^{2+}, Fe^{2+}, Cu^{2+}, Mn^{2+}, and Zn^{2+}) become insoluble. This is especially true of the trace minerals, making it more difficult for metallic ions to be absorbed and necessitating special mechanisms for absorption, such as active transport, vitamin D, and bile salts. Toxic excesses of metal ions are thus more difficult to absorb, but these mechanisms make it also difficult to absorb needed trace mineral elements.

This chapter discusses the 13 fat- and water-soluble vitamins. It also reviews the bulk minerals; discusses the four trace mineral elements—Zn, Cu, I, Co—known to be essential for life at this time; and discusses Cr and Mn deficiency.

VITAMINS

Vitamins are essential for a healthy, normal life and must be consumed daily. However, vitamins are frequently misused; and if taken in large doses, may cause disease. The body is capable of synthesizing only a few vitamins; for example, vitamin K and biotin are synthesized from bacteria in the small intestine, and vitamin D is produced by the skin on exposure to ultraviolet light.

In general, the body needs only small quantities of vitamins, which can be easily obtained from a well-balanced diet. All vitamins are obtained primarily from plant sources. The sale of vitamins in the United States is a 3 billion dollar business. Because of successful advertising, many individuals unnecessarily take supplemental vitamins, thinking that they will improve normal health. It is important to understand the difference between vitamins used as prophylactic supplements to prevent a deficiency and therapeutic use to treat a deficiency. It is relatively rare for vitamin deficiencies to be found in people living in the United States and Canada, although mild forms of deficiencies may be seen. It is also unusual for pronounced deficiencies such as pellagra, *rickets*, scurvy, and beriberi—found in underdeveloped or developing countries—to occur. Vitamin supplements are useful during periods of increased demand (Table 57–1).

The fat-soluble vitamins require fat or bile salts for absorption. A patient with a biliary obstruction that prevents bile from entering the duodenum will have difficulty absorbing these vitamins. They are stored in large quantities in both the liver and fatty tissues, and are metabolized and excreted slowly. For this reason, a person develops deficiency states from lack of fat-soluble vitamins only after a long period of deprivation. Con-

Table 57–1. CONDITIONS WHERE VITAMIN SUPPLEMENTS ARE APPROPRIATE

Adults	Children
Pregnancy	Acute/chronic illness
Lactation	Rapid growth phase
Acute/chronic illness	Malabsorption
Malabsorption	Regular, strenuous
Regular, strenous	physical activity
physical activity	Neglect of diet
Neglect of diet	Breast-fed infants
Drug ingestion that	Premature infants
increases vitamin	Vegetarian children
requirements	Children receiving non-fortified skim milk

versely, excessive intake of the fat-soluble vitamins can lead to toxicity.

The water-soluble vitamins, including the B-complex vitamins and vitamin C (ascorbic acid), are dissimilar in structure but similar in action to the fat-soluble vitamins. They all have a coenzyme action, which means they function mainly as substances that activate the protein portion of enzymes. They assist in catalyzing the reactions of protein, fat, and carbohydrate metabolism. A very small quantity of vitamin as coenzyme is capable of catalyzing a great deal of biochemical activity. Chemically, folic acid, pantothenic acid, and biotin are substituted amino acids; whereas vitamins B_1, B_2, B_6, and B_{12}, and nicotinic acid are amines (nucleotides) acting as coenzymes. Vitamin C is totally different from those listed above and is a hexose sugar derivative acting as an oxidation-reduction and electron-transfer agent. The water-soluble vitamins are not stored in the body in large quantitites, so short periods of inadequate intake can result in deficiency states. Because these vitamins are not stored in the body, overdoses are not as much a problem as with the fat-soluble vitamins.

Toxic states from too much vitamin intake—generally vitamins A and D, and limited toxicity for E, K, niacin, C, and B_6—can occur. Education of the patient is important to prevent toxic vitaminosis. The body not only needs vitamins in the correct amount in the body, but also needs correct amounts of minerals and hormones to function in a healthy, normal way.

The Food and Drug Administration has developed a minimum daily requirement (MDR), which represents the minimum daily dietary requirement needed to prevent the development of deficiency symptoms. Another list, the Recommended Daily Dietary Allowances (RDA) list, established and periodically revised by the Nutrition Board of the National Academy of Sciences—National Research Council, indicates the quantity of nutrients needed to keep most people healthy. This list of requirements is higher than the MDR list. Table 57–2 presents the MDR list for both vitamins and minerals. Table 57–3 lists the estimated and adequate dietary intakes of additional vitamins and minerals, where less information is available on which to base allowance.

Vitamin requirements and dosages are measured in several ways. Vitamins A, D, and E are measured in units (either USP units or international units [IU]); biotin and vitamin B_{12} are measured in micrograms (μg); and the remaining vitamins are measured in milligrams. All vitamins can be found in Table 57–4.

FAT-SOLUBLE VITAMINS

Vitamin A

Vitamin A, also referred to as retinol, is the major naturally occurring form, A_1, A_2, or the anti-infective vitamin. It is essential for growth in children and adolescents and is needed particularly for development and maintenance of epithelial tissues and bone. Vitamin A is needed to produce visual purple and to maintain function of both *rods* and *cones*. If vitamin A is lacking,

night blindness ensues. Vitamin A is also needed to maintain the integrity of the skin and epithelial cells, helping to promote resistance to infection. In addition, vitamin A is necessary in the maintenance of the adrenal cortex and the synthesis of steroid hormones.

USES. Vitamin A is indicated only for treatment or prevention of vitamin A deficiency. It is still also prescribed to treat or prevent hyperkeratotic dermatoses, including psoriasis, lichen planus, ichthyosis, and pityriasis rubra pilaris, even though vitamin A has not been proven effective for treatment of many of these conditions. Vitamin A cream is available in the form of tretinoin or retinoic acid (Retin-A). Isotretinoin (Accutane), an isomer or retinoic acid, is available as an oral capsule. Both are available to treat acne vulgaris and are described in detail in Chapter 62.

ABSORPTION,   SOURCES,   AND   STORAGE. Carotenoid pigments, especially beta-carotene, the precursor of vitamin A, are found in organ meats (liver and kidneys), carrots, and green leafy vegetables such as spinach, parsley, turnip, dandelion and beet greens, lettuce, and broccoli, as well as in dairy products. Once the carotenoid pigments are consumed by the human body, only about one sixth to one third are converted to vitamin A. Vitamin A is an unsaturated fat-soluble alcohol, which requires dietary fat in order to be effectively absorbed. Proteins are also necessary for absorption and for the mobilization of reserves to be stored in the liver. Current research also suggests that adequate amounts of zinc are necessary for mobilization of vitamin A. Orally ingested vitamin A is absorbed in the upper gastrointestinal tract, especially in the duodenum. This is also the primary site of conversion of carotene to vitamin A. If mineral oil is ingested simultaneously, marked inhibition of vitamin A and carotene absorption occurs due to vitamin A's complexation with the mineral oil. Absorption is also inhibited in the presence of diarrhea, bile salt depletion, sprue, cystic fibrosis of the pancreas, ileitis, and in patients recovering from subtotal gastrectomy. Absorbed vitamin A is transported by the lymphatic system to the bloodstream and is primarily stored in the liver. A major portion of vitamin A is excreted in bile, with a small amount excreted in the urine.

DEFICIENCY STATES. Varying degrees of vitamin A deficiency can develop. Deficiencies may arise because of interference with absorption or storage (celiac syndrome, sprue, cystic fibrosis, ulcerative colitis, operations that bypass the duodenum, congenital partial obstruction of the jejunum, giardiasis, obstructions of the bile ducts, cirrhosis of the liver, lack of dietary fat, and excessive use of oil-type laxatives), inadequate dietary intake, interference with the conversion of carotene to vitamin A (associated with diabetes and hypothyroidism), or rapid loss of vitamin A from the body (infectious processes such as pneumonia, rheumatic fever, appendicitis). An *avitaminosis* may develop in premature infants who may have low liver reserves of vitamin A, or in infants fed unfortified skin milk or milk-free formulas.

The initial symptom of vitamin A deficiency is *nyctal-*

Table 57–2. RECOMMENDED DIETARY ALLOWANCES, REVISED 1980.*
DESIGNED FOR THE MAINTENANCE OF GOOD NUTRITION OF PRACTICALLY ALL HEALTHY PEOPLE IN THE U.S.A.

| Age and Sex Group | Weight | | Height | | Protein | Fat-Soluble Vitamins | | | Water-Soluble Vitamins | | |
	kg	lb	cm	in		Vitamin A (I Units)	Vitamin D (I Units)	Vitamin E (α T.E.)§	Vitamin C (mg)	Thiamin (mg)	Riboflavin (mg)
Infants											
0.0–0.5 yr	6	13	60	24	kg × 2.2	420	10	3	35	0.3	0.4
0.5–1.0 yr	9	20	71	28	kg × 2.0	400	10	4	35	0.5	0.6
Children											
1–3 yr	13	29	90	35	23	400	10	5	45	0.7	0.8
4–6 yr	20	44	112	44	30	500	10	6	45	0.9	1.0
7–10 yr	28	62	132	52	34	700	10	7	45	1.2	1.4
Males											
11–14 yr	45	99	157	62	45	1000	10	8	50	1.4	1.6
15–18 yr	66	145	176	69	56	1000	10	10	60	1.4	1.7
19–22 yr	70	154	177	70	56	1000	7.5	10	60	1.5	1.7
23–50 yr	70	154	178	70	56	1000	5	10	60	1.4	1.6
51+ yr	70	154	178	70	56	1000	5	10	60	1.2	1.4
Females											
11–14 yr	46	101	157	62	46	800	10	8	50	1.1	1.3
15–18 yr	55	120	163	64	46	800	10	8	60	1.1	1.3
19–22 yr	55	120	163	64	44	800	7.5	8	60	1.1	1.3
23–50 yr	55	120	163	64	44	800	5	8	60	1.0	1.2
51+ yr	55	120	163	64	44	800	5	8	60	1.0	1.2
Pregnancy					+30	+200	+5	+2	+20	+0.4	+0.3
Lactation					+20	+400	+5	+3	+40	+0.5	+0.5

*The allowances are intended to provide for individual variations among most normal persons as they live in the United States under usual environmental stresses. Diets should be based on a variety of common foods in order to provide other nutrients for which human requirements have been less well defined.

§α-tocopherol equivalents: 1 mg d-α-tocopherol = 1 α-TE

¶1 N.E. (niacin equivalent) = 1 mg niacin or 60 mg dietary tryptophan.

**The RDA for vitamin B_{12} in infants is based on average concentration of the vitamin in human milk. The allowances after weaning are based on energy intake (as recommended by the American Academy of Pediatrics) and consideration of other factors, such as intestinal absorption.

††The increased requirement during pregnancy cannot be met by the iron content of habitual American diets or by the existing iron stores of many women; therfore, the use of 30–60 mg supplemental iron is recommended. Iron needs during lactation are not substantially different from those of nonpregnant women, but continued supplementation of the mother for 2–3 months after parturition is advisable in order to replenish stores depleted by pregnancy.

From National Academy of Sciences—National Research Council, Washington, DC, 1980.

opia (night blindness), which may progress, particularly in children, to *xerophthalmia* (inflammation of the eye) and *keratomalacia* (softening of the cornea). Xerophthalmia is a manifestation of severe vitamin A deficiency. Corneal softening, if untreated, can lead to perforation and blindness. The skin may become dry and keratinized, leading to a decrease in the ability of the skin and mucous membranes to protect the body from infection. Diarrhea may develop following changes in the intestinal wall. Kidney stones are also likely to occur, as the kidney is damaged, shedding groups of epithelial cells that later collect crystals. In infants and children, growth and development are slowed.

TOXIC EFFECTS. Recent research has shown that megadoses of vitamin A are not effective in preventing or treating infections, or treating sunburn, cutaneous ulcerations of the skin, or acne vulgaris. In fact, because toxic side effects can develop from higher-than-therapeutic blood levels, vitamin A should be taken only in diagnosed deficiency conditions.

Vitamin A toxicity may occur in a few months in an infant or child, but may take years to manifest in an adult. The half-life of vitamin A is very long, weeks to months. The target tissues include the retina, skin, bone, liver, and adrenals. Toxic side effects include increased intracranial pressure, diplopia, papilledema, skin changes, psychiatric symptoms, hepatic dysfunction, alopecia, and brittle nails. Fatigue, malaise, lethargy, anorexia, irritability, and severe headaches also occur. Most symptoms disappear when the vitamin is discontinued, but permanent retardation of growth and premature epiphyseal closure may occur in children.

TEXT RESUMES ON PAGE 1582

Water-Soluble Vitamins			Minerals			
Niacin (mg N.E.)¶	Vitamin B₆ (mg)	Vitamin B₁₂ (µg)	Magnesium (mg)	Iron (mg)	Zinc (mg)	Iodine (µg)
6	0.3	0.5**	50	10	3	40
8	0.6	1.5	70	15	5	50
9	0.9	2.0	150	15	10	70
11	1.3	2.5	200	10	10	90
16	1.6	3.0	250	10	10	120
18	1.8	3.0	350	18	15	150
18	2.0	3.0	400	18	15	150
19	2.2	3.0	350	10	15	150
18	2.2	3.0	350	10	15	150
16	2.2	3.0	350	10	15	150
15	1.8	3.0	300	18	15	150
14	2.0	3.0	300	18	15	150
14	2.0	3.0	300	18	15	150
13	2.0	3.0	300	18	15	150
13	2.0	3.0	300	10	15	150
+2	+0.6	+1.0	+150	††	+5	+25
+5	+0.5	+1.0	+150	††	+10	+50

57–3. ESTIMATED SAFE AND ADEQUATE DAILY DIETARY INTAKES OF ADDITIONAL SELECTED VITAMINS AND MINERALS*

	Vitamins			Trace Elements†					
Age Group	Vitamin K (mg)	Biotin (mg)	Panto-thenic Acid (units)	Copper (units)	Manganese (units)	Fluoride (units)	Chromium (units)	Selenium (mg)	Molyb-denum (units)
Infants									
0.0–0.5 yr	12	35	2	0.5–0.7	0.5–0.7	0.1–0.5	0.01–0.04	0.01–0.04	0.03–0.06
0.5–1.0 yr	10–20	50	3	0.7–1.0	0.7–1.0	0.2–1.0	0.02–0.06	0.02–0.06	0.04–0.08
Children and adolescents									
1–3 yr	15–30	65	3	1.0–1.5	1.0–1.5	0.5–1.5	0.02–0.08	0.02–0.08	0.05–0.1
4–6 yr	20–40	85	3–4	1.5–2.0	1.5–2.0	1.0–2.5	0.03–0.12	0.03–0.12	0.06–0.15
7–10 yr	30–60	120	4–5	2.0–2.5	2.0–3.0	1.5–2.5	0.05–0.2	0.05–0.2	0.1–0.3
11+ yr	50–100	100–200	4–7	2.0–3.0	2.5–5.0	1.5–2.5	0.05–0.2	0.05–0.2	0.15–0.5
Adults	70–140	100–200	4–7	2.0–3.0	2.5–5.0	1.5–4.0	0.05–0.2	0.05–0.2	0.15–0.5

*From Recommended Dietary Allowances, Revised 1980. Food and Nutrition Board, National Academy of Sciences—National Research Council. Because there is less information on which to base allowances, these figures are not given in the main table of the RDAs and are provided here in the form of ranges of recommended intakes.

†Since the toxic levels for many trace elements may be only several times usual intakes, the upper levels for the trace elements given in this table should not be habitually exceeded.

Table 57–4. VITAMIN SOURCE CHART

Vitamin	Synonyms	Physiologic Functions	Deficiency/ Disease/ Disorders	Storage Site and Half-Life	Target Tissue	Dietary Sources	Mode
Vitamin A	A_1, A_2, retinol, anti-infective vitamin	Growth, produces visual purple; maintenance of skin and epithelial cells; resistance to infection; bone development; maintenance of adrenal cortex, and steroid hormone synthesis	Night blindness, hyperkeratosis, xerophthalmia, corneal softening	Liver Weeks or months	Retina, skin, bone, liver, adrenals	Liver, carrots, green leafy vegetables, dairy products	PO IM
Vitamin D	D_2 (ergocalciferol), cholecalciferol (D_3)	Normal bone growth, Ca^{2+} and PO_4 absorption in gut, and maintenance of serum levels	Rickets, osteomalacia, hypoparathyroidism	Liver Calcifediol: 16 days; Calcitriol: 3–8 hr; Ergocalciferol: 19–48 hr.	Kidney, bone, intestine, liver	Liver oils, egg yolk, butter, oily fish	PO IM Topical

Dose	Toxic Effects	Contraindications and Precautions	Interactions	Nursing Implications
Adults: RDA 4,000–5,000 IU PO. Children: RDA 1300–2300 IU PO. Vitamin A (Retinol, Retinyl Palmitate, Retinyl Acetate, Aquasol A) for topical use. Severe deficiency, oral: over 8 years old 100,000 IU/day for 3 days; 50,000 IU/day for 2 weeks; 10,000–20,000 IU/day for 2 months. Severe deficiency IM for 10 days: Infants: 5,000–10,000 IU; Children 1–8 years: 5,000–15,000 IU; Adults: 50,000–100,000 IU for 3 days and 50,000 IU/day for 2 weeks. Betacarotene (Solatene) PO: Adult: 30–300 mg/day; Children 30–150 mg/day. Cod liver oil, halibut liver oil, halibut liver capsule; A & D ointment	Malaise, slow growth, headache, retarded growth, dry cracked skin. Anaphylactic reaction from bolus IV administration.	Contraindicated in hypersensitivity and in malabsorption syndromes. IV forms are contraindicated except for special water-miscible forms used in large parenteral volumes. Use cautiously in pregnancy, nursing mothers, children.	Mineral oil, antacids, sucralfate, neomycin, cholestyramine, colestipol decreases absorption of vitamin. Contraceptives may increase vitamin A levels. Anticoagulants and vitamin A may precipitate hypoprothrombinemia.	ASSESSMENT: Assess for vitamin A deficiency. Assess for vitamin A intake in food and other multivitamins. INTERVENTION: Administer with meals to stimulate bile secretion, which aids absorption and reduces nausea. Teach patient to avoid mineral oil and protect vitamin A from light and heat. Also, do not megadose vitamin A. Vitamin A is never administered intravenous push because of possibility of anaphylaxis or anaphylactoid reactions. IV vitamin A is mixed in a large volume of fluid. EVALUATION: Evaluate for signs of vitamin A toxicity and report to physician.
Adults and Children: RDA Adult 200 IU, RDA Children 400 IU, RDA pregnant and lactating women 400–500 IU. Ergocalciferol (Vitamin D_2) 12,000–500,000 IU. Calciferol 50–100 µg/day. Cholecalciferol (D_3) 400–1000 IU day. Calcitriol (Rocaltrol) 0.25–2 µg/day. Dihydrotachysterol (DHT, Hytakerol) 0.2–2.4 mg/day.	Hypercalcemia, fatigue, nausea, vomiting, nephrotoxicity, mental retardation, decreased growth.	Contraindicated in hypersensitivity, hypercalcemia, vitamin D toxicity, and hyperphosphatemia. Use with caution in pregnant and nursing mothers. Use with caution in patients receiving digitalis products because hypercalcemia may precipitate dysrhythmias.	Mineral oil, antacids, sucralfate, neomycin, cholestyramine, colestipol decreases absorption of vitamin. Anticonvulsants, hydantoin, barbituates, or primidone may reduce the effectiveness of vitamin D. Vitamin D may potentiate digitalis products.	ASSESSMENT: Assess for vitamin D deficiency. Assess for intake of vitamin D in foods and other multivitamins. Assess serum and urine calcium, serum phosphorus, magnesium, and BUN before therapy and periodically during therapy. INTERVENTION: Take with food to avoid GI upset. Administer IV vitamin D in large volume of IV fluid only. Teach about importance of increased vitamin D foods in the diet. EVALUATION: Evaluate for toxic signs (dry mouth, nausea, vomiting, metallic taste in mouth, diarrhea, constipation) and report to physician.

CONTINUED ON THE FOLLOWING PAGE

Table 57–4. VITAMIN SOURCE CHART–*CONTINUED*

Vitamin	Synonyms	Physiologic Functions	Deficiency/ Disease/ Disorders	Storage Site and Half-Life	Target Tissue	Dietary Sources	Mode
Vitamin E	Antisterility vitamin (Aquasol E, Alfacol)	Biologic antitoxin, normal maintenance of growth, fertility, and gestation; maintain normal muscle metabolism; protects unsaturated fatty acids and membrane structure	Skin collagenosis, red cell hemolysis, xanthomatosis, cirrhosis, steatorrhea, creatinuria	Muscle, adipose tissue, liver 2 wks.	Kidneys, genital organs, muscle, liver, lung, bone marrow	Oil, margarine, mayonnaise, wheat germ, grains, seeds, nuts	PO Topical IM
Vitamin K	Prothrombin factor, menadiol sodium (K_4 Synkayvite), phytonadione (K_1; Mephyton— PO; Konakion—IM; Aqua-MEPHYTON—IM, IV)	Prothrombin synthesis in liver, blood clotting mechanism	Hypothrombinemia, increased bleeding and hemorrhage, increased clotting time	Liver Limited storage for short time	Liver, vascular system	Most foods, green leafy vegetables, cauliflower, pork, spinach, liver, kidney, dairy products	PO IM IV
Vitamin B_1 (Thiamine)	Antiberiberi factor, thiamine chloride (Betaxin)	Coenzyme in pyruvate metabolism	Beriberi, polyneuritis, cardiac dysrhythmias, edema, Wernicke's encephalopathy.	Heart, liver, kidney, brain. 1 mg/day destroyed in tissues	Heart, liver, kidney, peripheral nerves	Wheat germ, cereal, grains, yeast, meat, peas, vegetables	PO (preferred) IM IV

Dose	Toxic Effects	Contraindications and Precautions	Interactions	Nursing Implications
RDA Adults: 12–15 IU daily. Vitamin E (Aquasol E) 30–75 IU PO daily or 30–100 IU IM daily. 5 IU PO premature or low-birth-weight neonate.	Generally nontoxic but may include fatigue, weakness, nausea, diarrhea, headache, blurred vision.	Not for IV administration.	Mineral oil, antacids, sucralfate, neomycin, cholestyramine, colestipol decreases absorption of vitamin. Large doses of iron may increase daily requirements of vitamin E.	ASSESSMENT: Assess for signs of vitamin E deficiency. Assess for dietary intake of vitamin E. INTERVENTION: Oral—swallow whole, do not crush or chew tablets or capsules. Teach to not take megadoses of vitamin E and store in cool, dry place. EVALUATION: Evaluate for signs of toxicity such as fatigue, weakness, nausea, diarrhea, and report to physician.
RDA not established. Adults: 5–15 mg/day menadiol sodium (Synkayvite, K$_4$). Phytonadione (Mephyton) 2.5–10 mg—PO; Konakion 2.5–10 mg—IM; Aquamephyton undiluted, or diluted in 500–1000 ml should not be infused at a rate exceeding 1 mg/min—IV.	Allergic reactions, gastric upset, prolonged prothrombin time. IV vitamin K can cause severe reactions including anaphylaxis, shock, cardiac and respiratory arrest.	Contraindicated in sensitivity and in pregnancy. Phytonadione is contraindicated with hereditary hypothrombinemia because vitamin K can worsen hypothrombinemia. Oral vitamin K is contraindicated when there is inadequate bile. Use cautiously in depressed liver function and lactating women.	Antagonizes oral anticoagulants. Antibiotics, quinidine, quinine, high dose salicylates may increase vitamin K requirements. Mineral oil and cholestyramine may decrease absorption.	ASSESSMENT: Assess for signs of vitamin K deficiency. Assess for dietary intake of vitamin K. Assess PT before and during therapy. Improvement of PT takes 1–2 hours after IM, or 6–12 hours after PO administration. Assess bilirubin in neonates receiving vitamin K. INTERVENTION: Take PO vitamin K with food to reduce GI upset. Teach patient about increased dietary vitamin K. EVALUATION: Evaluate for continued signs of hypothrombinemia such as continued bleeding, oozing around IV catheters, petechiae, easy bruising.
RDA Adult: 1–1.4 mg. Dietary supplement adults & children: 5–30 mg/day. Thiamine B$_1$ (Betalin S and others): Beriberi: 10–120 mg IM 3 times daily for 2 weeks. Wet beriberi with congestive heart failure: 30 mg IV 3 times daily slowly.	Weakness, labored breathing, feeling of warmth, pruritis, nausea.	Contraindicated in hypersensitivity.	May enhance the effect of neuromuscular blocking agents. Unstable with alkaline solutions.	ASSESSMENT: Assess for thiamine deficiency. Assess for thiamine dietary intake. INTERVENTION: Administer IV slowly. Have epinephrine on hand when giving larger parenteral doses. Take vitamin B$_1$ with food. Store in cool, dry place. Potency diminishes rapidly.

CONTINUED ON THE FOLLOWING PAGE

Table 57–4. VITAMIN SOURCE CHART–*CONTINUED*

Vitamin	Synonyms	Physiologic Functions	Deficiency/ Disease/ Disorders	Storage Site and Half-Life	Target Tissue	Dietary Sources	Mode
Vitamin B₁ (Thiamine)–*Continued*							
Vitamin B₂ (Ribo-flavin)	Vitamin G, lactoflavin (Riboderm)	Constituent of respiratory enzymes, growth and development of fetus, maintenance of mucosal epithelial and ocular tissue	Glossitis, dermatitis, corneal vascularization, stomatitis	Heart, liver, kidneys. 12% of intake excreted in 24 hr.	Heart, liver, kidneys	Liver, yeast, green leafy vegetables, fruit	PO
Vitamin B₆ (Pyri-doxine)	Pyridoxol (Beesix, Hexabetalin, Hydoxin)	Protein, carbohydrate, and lipid metabolism; coenzyme of amino acid metabolism; erythrocyte formation; growth	Convulsions, irritability, nervous disorders, neuritis, edema	Skeletal muscle. 15–20 days	Nervous tissue, liver, lymph nodes, muscle tissue	Liver, grains, yeast, vegetables, meat, fish	PO (pre-ferred) IV SC
Vitamin B₁₂	Cyanocobalamin, pernicious anemia vitamin (Betalin 12, Redisol)	Coenzyme in nucleic acid, protein, and lipid synthesis; maintain growth, maintain epithelial cells and nervous system (myelin sheath); coenzyme in red blood synthesis.	Retarded growth, megaloblastic anemias, sprue, glossitis	Liver (30%–60%), lungs, kidneys, spleen. 1 year	Central nervous system, kidneys, myocardium, muscle, skin	Organ meats, egg yolk, seafood	PO IM

Dose	Toxic Effects	Contraindications and Precautions	Interactions	Nursing Implications
				EVALUATION: Evaluate for toxic effects such as weakness, labored breathing, pruritis, nausea. Report to physician.
RDA: 1.2–1.6 mg. Riboflavin vitamin B_2 deficiency states: Adults: 5–30 mg/day PO. Children: 5–10 mg/ day PO, IM, IV.	None known.	None known.	Antidepressants, phenothiazines, probenecid may increase riboflavin requirements. May cause false elevations of urinary catecholamines. Alcohol inhibits absorption.	ASSESSMENT: Assess for B_2 deficiency. Assess for B_2 intake in diet. Assess for increased need for vitamin B_2 with liver disease. INTERVENTION: Take with food to enhance absorption. Teach patient that vitamin B_2 colors urine bright yellow. Store in light-resistant container. EVALUATION: Evaluate for signs of overdose and notify physician.
RDA Adults: 2–2.2 mg daily. Pyridoxine-B_6 (Pyridoxine hydrochloride, Nestrex, Beesix, Hexa-Betalin) Dietary deficiency: Adults and children: 10–20 mg/day up to 600 mg in acute deficiencies. For INH toxicity: 4 g IV followed by 1 g IV every 30 min until seizures stop.	Rare paresthesias, somnolence, flushing, temporary burning at injection site.	Contraindicated in hypersensitivity. Use with caution in lactating women—may depress lactation through inhibition of prolactin.	When taken in doses of more than 5 mg daily, may enhance metabolism of levodopa. Estrogens may increase requirement of pyridoxine. Chloramphenicol, hydralazine, ACTH, cyclosporine, and isoniazid may interact. Phenobarbital and phenytoin biotransformation may be accelerated.	ASSESSMENT: Assess for symptoms of deficiency. INTERVENTION: Store in light-resistant container.
RDA Adults: 3 μg. Deficiency states: B_{12} (Cyanocobalamin) 25–250 μg PO daily with normal intestinal absorption. B_{12} (Cobex, Crystamine, Betalin 12, and many others) 100–1000 μg IM monthly.	Mild transient diarrhea, itching, rash, peripheral vascular thrombosis, congestive heart failure.	Contraindicated in hypersensitivity to cobalt and hereditary optic atrophy. Use cautiously in pregnant and lactating women.	Vitamin B_{12} absorption is increased by prednisone. Chloramphenicol may cause poor therapeutic response to vitamin B_{12}. Concurrent use of antibiotics, methotrexate, and pyrimethamine produce invalid tests of vitamin B_{12} and folic acid.	ASSESSMENT: Assess for symptoms of deficiency. Assess blood folate levels before and during therapy with large doses (10 μg or more) as folate deficiency may occur. Assess serum potassium level during therapy. INTERVENTION: Teach importance of monthly B_{12} injection for persons with pernicious anemia as neurologic damage can occur. EVALUATION: Evaluate for signs of toxicity such as hematologic, cardiovascular, and respiratory complication and report to physician.

CONTINUED ON THE FOLLOWING PAGE

Table 57–4. VITAMIN SOURCE CHART–*CONTINUED*

Vitamin	Synonyms	Physiologic Functions	Deficiency/ Disease/ Disorders	Storage Site and Half-Life	Target Tissue	Dietary Sources	Mode
Folic acid	Antianemic factor, pter-oylglutamic acid, vitamin M (Folvite)	Synthesis of nucleic acid, coenzyme in purine metabolism. Important for red blood cell division.	Anemia, glossitis, diarrhea, malabsorp-tion syndromes, spure	Liver, spinal fluid, 75% excreted in 24 hrs.	Liver, bone marrow, lymph nodes, kidneys	Liver, wheat, yeast, beans, green veg-etables, nuts, fruits	PO SC IM IV
Vitamin C (Ascorbic acid)	Antiscorbutic vitamin (Cetaine, Ce-vi-sol)	Oxidation-reduction processes, mainte-nance of normal con-nective tissue, cold tol-erance, growth, wound healing, maintenance of capillaries.	Scurvy, megaloblastic anemia of infancy	Adrenal cortex, liver. 16 days	Adrenal cortex, pituitary, ovary, connec-tive tis-sue	Fruits, fresh green veg-etables, rose hips	PO Paren-teral IM SC
Panto-thenic acid	Antidermatitis factor	Functions as coenzyme A in carbohydrate, lipid, and protein metabolism	Neurologic disorder, irritability, fatigue; dry, scaly skin; adre-nal hypofunction, muscle cramps	Possible liver, heart, kid-ney. Esti-mated 25% daily.	All, espe-cially brain, heart, kidney	Liver, eggs, wheat germ, wal-nuts, salmon	PO Paren-teral
Niacin (Nico-tinic acid)	Antipellagra factor, B$_3$ (Nicobid, Nicolar)	Functions as a control agent in coenzyme system that converts fats, proteins, and car-bohydrates to energy through oxidation-reduction	Pellagra, dermatosis	Liver, heart. 45 min.	Liver, heart, muscle, kidney.	Liver, pea-nuts, poul-try, yeast, beans, nuts, fish, meat	PO Paren-teral
Biotin	Vitamin H pro-tective factor x	As a coenzyme, growth, maintenance of skin, nerves, bone marrow	Dermatitis	Liver. 3–4 wk.	Skin, ner-vous tis-sue	Yeast, liver, royal jelly, grains	PO Paren-teral

Dose	Toxic Effects	Contraindications and Precautions	Interactions	Nursing Implications
RDA 0.4 mg daily. Deficiency states: Folic Acid (Folate, Vitamin B$_9$, Folvite). Adults: 100–400 μg/day. Leucovorin calcium (Wellcovorin): doses vary.	Relatively nontoxic.	Contraindicated alone in treatment of pernicious anemia as may mask neurologic damage.	False low folic acid levels in patients receiving tetracyclines. Some anticonvulsants and oral contraceptives may decrease folate metabolism.	ASSESSMENT: Assess for signs of folic acid deficiency. Assess dietary intake. INTERVENTION: Teach—may need increased folic acid during pregnancy.
RDA: 60 mg daily. Vitamin C—ascorbic acid (Cevalin, Cevita, and many others). Deficiency states to treat scurvy: Adults: 50–2000 mg/day ascorbic acid, PO. Children: 100–300 mg/day. To acidify urine: 4–12 gm daily in divided doses.	Hemolytic anemia in patients with G6PD deficiency, diarrhea, high acidification of urine, crystalluria	Use cautiously in gout, crystalluria, pregnancy, and lactating women.	Enhances salicylates. Decreases effects of amphetamines and tricyclic antidepressants. Increased crystalluria when taking aminosalicylic acid and sulfonamidies. False-negative or false-positive glucose tests depending on type of test used. Possible false-positive test for occult blood in stool.	ASSESSMENT: Assess for signs of vitamin C deficiency. Assess for aspirin or tartrazine allergy. Give test dose of ascorbic acid to determine if allergic to this product. INTERVENTION: Teach patients with diabetes or history of renal calculi that intake should be limited. Ascorbic acid can interfere with urine testing for glucose. Store in closed container away from heat and light. EVALUATION: Evaluate for signs of toxicity and report to physician.
RDA not established. Pantothenic acid (Calcium Pantothenate B5). Adults and Children: 5–20 mg in multivitamin preparation.	None known.	None known.	None known.	ASSESSMENT: Assess for symptoms of deficiency. INTERVENTION: Administer with food.
RDA: 13–18 mg/day. Nicotinic acid, Niacin, vitamin B$_3$ (Nicobid, Nicolor, many others). Daily supplement: 10–20 mg/day. To treat pellegra: PO 300–500 mg daily; PO time-release 125–250 mg; IV 25–100 mg 2 or more times daily; IM 50–100 mg 5 or more times daily. Hyperlipidemia: 1–2 g/day in divided doses. Nicotinamide or niacinamide pellegra treatment only 50 mg 3–10 times daily.	Flushing face, tingling, dryness of skin, headache, diarrhea, anorexia, heartburn, impaired liver function.	Contraindicated in hypersensitivity, severe hypotension, and hepatic dysfunction. Use cautiously in pregnancy, lactation, glaucoma, gout, peptic ulcer, diabetes, and liver disease.	Potentiates vasodilation and hypotension when taken with adrenergic-blocking drugs. May inhibit uricosuric effects of probenecid and sulfinpyrazone.	ASSESSMENT: Assess for symptoms of niacin deficiency. Assess liver function, blood glucose, and serum uric acid levels before and during therapy. Assess for aspirin or tartrazine sensitivity. INTERVENTION: Start all oral doses in small doses and gradually increase. Administer with meals to minimize GI complaints. Administer IV slowly to reduce vasodilitation effects. EVALUATION: Evaluate for signs of toxicity and report to physician.
Adults: 100–200 μg/day. Children: 65–120 μg/day	None known.	None known.	None known.	ASSESSMENT: Assess for signs of biotin deficiency.

CONTRAINDICATIONS AND PRECAUTIONS. Vitamin A is contraindicated in hypersensitivity. Oral administration of vitamin A is contraindicated in patients with malabsorption syndrome; if malabsorption is the result of inadequate bile secretion, the oral route may be used with concurrent administration of bile salts. Fetal abnormalities, growth retardation, and early epiphyseal closure have been reported in children whose mothers took excessive amounts (above 6000 IU) during pregnancy. Caution is recommended in nursing mothers, as vitamin A is excreted in breast milk and in children who are more sensitive to high doses of vitamin A. Use with caution in persons with impaired renal function, as vitamin A toxicity and elevated plasma calcium and alkaline phosphatase can occur.

INTERACTIONS. A patient taking mineral oil as a laxative on a regular basis or antacids, sucralfate, neomycin, cholestyramine, or colestipol will have decreased absorption of vitamin A. Contraceptives may increase the plasma level of vitamin A.

DOSAGE. The daily RDA dose in an adult is between 4000 and 5000 IU orally. In deficiency states, larger doses can be given both orally and intramuscularly.

Many vitamin A preparations are made from fish oils such as cod liver oil, halibut liver oil, or a combination of fish oils. Vitamin A is often combined with vitamin D, in both oral and topical forms. A and D Ointment is an OTC preparation in a lanolin base, used to treat skin irritations such as diaper rash, superficial burns, or minor excoriations. (Recent research has indicated that A and D Ointment has little therapeutic effect.) Large doses of vitamin A are currently under investigation for treatment of diarrhea associated with Crohn's disease.

Vitamin A (Aquasol A). Vitamin A (as retinol, retinyl palmitate, or retinyl acetate) (Aquasol A) is used to prevent and/or treat vitamin A deficiencies. Oral doses in severe deficiency for adults and children over 8—100,000 IU daily for three days, followed by 50,000 IU for two weeks, and 10,000–20,000 IU daily for two months. During deficiency states, the following doses can be administered daily intramuscularly for approximately ten days: infants 5,000–10,000 IU; children one to eight years, 5,000–15,000 IU; and adults 50,000–100,000 IU for three days, and then 50,000 IU daily for two weeks. When a severe vitamin A deficiency alone with xerophthalmia is present, the adult dose is 500,000 IU per day for three days, followed by 50,000 IU/day for two weeks.

Betacarotene. Betacarotene (Solatene) is used to reduce the severity of photosensitivity reactions associated with erythropietic protoporphyria (an inherited condition associated with increased amounts of porphyrins in blood-forming tissue of the bone marrow). Betacarotene is best administered with meals. Adults receive 30–300 mg orally per day, while children receive 30–150 mg orally per day.

Vitamin D

Vitamin D is a natural vitamin derived from fish liver oils or other *provitamins* and is also considered to be a hormone. Vitamin D, also referred to as D_2 or ergocalciferol (D_3), is essential (along with parathyroid hormone) in regulating the absorption and excretion, in the gut and kidney, of both calcium and phosphate. It accomplishes this by increasing the intestinal absorption of calcium, and probably by directly influencing bone mineralization; it also increases the rate of reabsorption of phosphate by the renal tubules. Since calcium and phosphate are inversely controlled by the body, vitamin D indirectly affects phosphate absorption and mobilization in the bone as well.

ABSORPTION, STORAGE, AND SOURCES. Vitamin D is a sterol compound similar to cholesterol. It accumulates in the skin as the inactive form, 7-dehydrocholesterol. On exposure to sunlight, vitamin D is produced (D_3, or cholecalciferol) and is transported to the liver to be hydroxylated. Then this product is converted into its active form (1,25-dihydroxycholecalciferol) in the kidney and released into the bloodstream. It has a half-life of days to weeks in the normal adult.

Vitamin D is obtained mainly from ultraviolet-irradiated skin and dietary sources. It is found only in animal and fish products, such as liver oils, egg yolks, and butter. Once vitamin D is consumed, absorption is dependent on the presence of bile and fats in the intestine and takes place in the jejunum and ileum. Vitamin D is passively absorbed into the intestinal mucosal cells, incorporated into chylomicrons, and transferred by the lymphatics to the blood. If there is biliary obstruction or faulty fat metabolism, deficiency states can occur. Bile also appears to be the major pathway of excretion of vitamin D metabolites.

There is no indication that dietary supplements are necessary in the normal adult on an average diet, as many foods are fortified with vitamin D and he or she is exposed to sunlight for reasonable periods.

USES. Vitamin D is used to treat hypocalcemia, hypophosphatemia, and osteodystrophy. Vitamin D is also used to prevent and treat rickets, tetany, and vitamin D deficiency. Vitamin D is also used in the management of metabolic bone disease or hypocalcemia in patients on chronic renal dialysis.

DEFICIENCY STATES. The primary symptoms of avitaminosis are *osteomalacia* in adults, rickets in children, and infantile tetany. These disorders are ultimately due to disturbances of calcium and phosphorus metabolism. Low serum calcium and phosphate levels and elevated alkaline phosphatase concentrations are seen. These conditions generally respond rapidly to adequate doses of vitamin D, when due to dietary deficiencies.

These conditions may also be due to malabsorption syndromes in the bowel, chronic pancreatitis, and renal disease. In bowel disease, such as ulcerative colitis or malabsorption, and in pancreatitis, vitamin D cannot be adequately absorbed. Since the kidney converts inactive vitamin D to its active counterpart, any condition that affects kidney function may have an effect on the conversion of vitamin D. Renal diseases include renal tubular acidosis, renal osteodystrophy, and Fanconi's syndrome, as well as any crushing injuries to the kidneys. When the kidney is diseased, massive doses of vitamin

D may have to be administered at the same time that electrolyte disturbances are being corrected.

ADVERSE EFFECTS. As with other medications, when large doses of vitamin D (1000–3000 IU for a few weeks to months) are administered for long periods, toxic symptoms can occur. Target tissues for vitamin D include the kidney, bone, intestine, and liver. When toxic levels develop, the patient may have symptoms resembling hyperparathyroidism (anorexia, nausea and vomiting, headache, drowsiness, diarrhea, or constipation, polyuria, polydipsia, generalized weakness, stiffness, vague aches, and mild weight loss). Serum calcium and phosphate levels are increased, and correspondingly high concentrations are found in the urine, leading eventually to irreversible renal damage. Osteoporosis occurs with the simultaneous deposition of calcium in the heart, large blood vessels, lungs, renal tubules, and other soft tissues. Discontinuation of vitamin D is usually sufficient to control the symptoms. If irreversible kidney damage has occurred, the patient needs supportive treatment for this condition.

CONTRAINDICATIONS AND PRECAUTIONS. Vitamin D is contraindicated in hypersensitive patients, hypercalcemia, and hyperphosphatemia. It is used cautiously in pregnant women, as it may suppress parathyroid function in the fetus. Safety in children, above RDA requirements, has not been established.

INTERACTIONS. A patient taking mineral oil as a laxative on a routine basis, or antacids, sucralfate, neomycin, cholestyramine, and colestipol, has a decreased amount of vitamin D absorbed in the gut. Anticonvulsants, hydantoins, barbiturates, or primidone may reduce the effectiveness of vitamin D. Also, vitamin D may potentiate digitalis products. Vitamin D may antagonize calcium channel blockers by increasing calcium levels.

DOSAGE. Dosage is highly individualized and dependent on what is being treated. Vitamin D is swallowed whole, never crushed or chewed. The oral dose for normal maintenance is 400 IU/day; for nutritional rickets, it increases to 4000 IU daily; for vitamin D–resistant rickets, 12,000–500,000 IU may be needed daily. As soon as symptoms are relieved, vitamin D should be reduced to RDA recommendations, as hypercalcemia and renal damage may result. The FDA is attempting to place all vitamin D supplements containing over 400 IU/dosage unit on a prescription-only status.

Several forms of vitamin D are available today.

CHOLECALCIFEROL. Cholecalciferol (D_3, Delta-D) is used as a daily vitamin D supplement or to treat vitamin D deficiency. Dosage ranges from 400–1000 μg intravenously daily. A dose of 1 mg of cholecalciferol provides 40,000 IU of vitamin D activity.

CALCIFEDIOL. Calcifediol (Calderol) is a hydroxylated form of cholecalciferol used primarily in the management of metabolic bone disease or hypocalcemia in patients with chronic renal disease. Calcifediol increases serum calcium levels and decreases alkaline phosphatase, prevents bone resorption, and decreases parathyroid hormone levels. Initial dosage is 300–350 μg/week administered daily or on alternate days. If adequate response is not obtained, dosage can be increased at four-week intervals. If hypercalcemia is found, calcifediol is discontinued until a normal calcium returns. After therapeutic results are obtained, maintenance dose is generally 50–100 μg/day or 100–200 μg on alternate days.

ERGOCALCIFEROL. Ergocalciferol (D_2, Drisdol, Calciferol, others) is used to treat familial hypophosphatemia, or *refractory rickets*. A dose of 1.25 mg of ergocalciferol provides 50,000 IU of vitamin D activity. Dosage ranges between 12,000 and 500,000 IU daily.

CALCITRIOL. Calcitriol (Rocaltrol), also called 1,25-dihydroxycholecalciferol, is used to manage hypocalcemia in patients with chronic renal failure. Daily doses range from 0.25–2 μg/day.

DIHYDROTACHYSTEROL. Dihydrotachysterol (Hytakerol, DHT) is used to treat *tetany*, in either acute or chronic forms, and hypoparathyroidism. A dose of 1 mg of dihydrotachysterol is approximately equivalent to 3 mg (120,000 IU) of vitamin D_2. Daily dose ranges from 0.2–2.4 mg/day.

Vitamin E

Today, Vitamin E is perhaps the most mysterious of all known major vitamins. Vitamin E actually refers to a group of naturally occurring fat-soluble substances known as tocopherols (alpha, beta, gamma, and delta). Alpha-tocopherol is the most active and abundant of the tocopherols present in animal tissue. Some of its functions have been identified only recently. Vitamin E, along with the mineral selenium, functions as a tissue antioxidant that protects polyunsaturated fatty acids from oxidative deterioration. It also appears to influence heme and porphyrin synthesis and, indirectly, the synthesis of several heme proteins. It also retards the hemolysis of red blood cells. Other functions of vitamin E include the enhancement of vitamin A utilization, stimulation of essential cofactors produced in steroid metabolism, and maintenance of normal muscle metabolism. Vitamin E also inhibits prostaglandin production and stimulates an essential cofactor in steroid metabolism. Vitamin E is believed to be needed for fertility and gestation; much of the research on vitamin E has taken place in rats, which have been found to be unable to conceive or carry a fetus to term when vitamin E is deficient. Some research has linked vitamin E with aging. Confirmation with controlled experiments is still needed.

USES. Vitamin E is indicated for prevention and treatment of vitamin E deficiency. It is also necessary in patients receiving total parenteral nutrition or who are undergoing rapid weight loss. Vitamin E has been found to be therapeutically useful in actual dietary deficiencies and in certain anemias (macrocytic, megaloblastic anemia often associated with the protein and calorie malnutrition of *kwashiorkor* and hemolytic anemia in premature infants). It can also be used topically to moisten dry and chapped skin, and to relieve temporary skin irritation. Although many claims have been made, vitamin E has not been proven effective to treat inflammatory skin disorders, loss of hair, habitual abortion, heart disease, impotence, bursitis, liver spots, deterioration from aging, or to increase physical endurance or sexual ability.

ABSORPTION, STORAGE, AND SOURCES. Vitamin E is readily absorbed passively but relatively inefficiently from the gastrointestinal tract and incorporated into chylomicrons for lymphatic transfer. Vitamin E, being a fat-soluble vitamin, depends on the presence of bile and fats in the gut for efficient absorption. Vitamin E accumulates slowly in the muscle, liver, and fatty tissue, but can be stored for long periods, up to four years. If vitamin E is not stored, it has a half-life of about two weeks in the body and is primarily excreted in the bile and feces.

In general, a normal diet supplies vitamin E in adequate amounts. The RDA in adults is 12–15 IU. Foods high in vitamin E include vegetable oils; margarine; shortening; whole grains such as wheat germ, alfalfa, and barley; certain seeds including apple, poppy, and sesame seeds; nuts; fruits; vegetables, eggs; and whole milk.

DEFICIENCY STATES. Vitamin E deficiency may occur in malabsorption syndromes (celiac disease, tropical sprue, gastrointestinal resections), in patients who abuse oil-type laxatives, or in other conditions characterized by malabsorption of fats (hepatic cirrhosis, biliary obstruction, cystic fibrosis, pancreatitis). Clinical indications of vitamin E deficiency can be a low serum vitamin E level or increased fragility of the red blood cells, which may lead to hemolytic anemias, although a causal relationship is not well established. Iron supplementation can greatly increase hemolysis in the presence of vitamin E deficiency. With prolonged or severe depletion, ceroid (fatty pigment) material is deposited in smooth muscle. Lesions in skeletal muscles, resembling muscular dystrophy, are seen, and anemia may become marked. Requirements for vitamin E may increase in individuals who increase their intake of unsaturated fats.

In animals, degeneration of the reproductive system, as well as sterility and inability to carry a fetus to term, can occur. These symptoms are still under investigation in humans.

ADVERSE EFFECTS. Vitamin E appears to be relatively nontoxic at therapeutic doses. When excessive doses are administered for prolonged periods, the patient may develop skeletal muscle weakness, fatigue, disturbances in the reproductive system, and gastrointestinal upset. Symptoms generally subside within a few weeks after excessive doses are discontinued.

INTERACTIONS. Possible interactions of vitamin E include decreased absorption when administered concurrently with mineral oil, antacids, sucralfate, neomycin, cholestyramine, and colestipol. Also, large doses of iron may increase the daily requirements of vitamin E.

DOSAGE. The prophylactic dose of vitamin E is 30–75 IU daily by mouth. Therapeutic doses can range from 30–100 IU and can be administered by mouth or parenterally. Vitamin E is administered in premature and low–birth–weight neonates to prevent vitamin E deficiencies in doses of 5 IU by mouth daily. Vitamin E is swallowed whole and not crushed or chewed. Topical preparations are also available for skin disorders.

Vitamin E (Aquasol E, E-Vital, E-vitamin Succinate, Solucap E) is available for both oral and intramuscular administration. It is not administered intravenously. When vitamin E deficiencies are present, water-miscible oral products are preferred. Several forms of vitamin E are available with varying potencies. They are all standardized into international units (IU). For example:

1 mg/dl alpha-tocopherol acetate = 1 IU
1 mg/dl alpha-tocopherol = 1.1 IU
1 mg/dl alpha-tocopherol acetate = 1.36 IU
1 mg/dl alpha-tocopherol = 1.49 IU
1 mg/dl alpha-tocopherol acid succinate = 1.21 IU
1 mg/dl alpha-tocopherol acid succinate = 0.89 IU

Free tocopherols are easily oxidized and destroyed when exposed to air and light. The ester acetate and succinate forms are more stable.

Vitamin K

Vitamin K was discovered accidentally in 1935 while studying newly hatched chicks with a fatal hemorrhagic condition, and was identified as a compound needed for clotting factor synthesis. Vitamin K occurs naturally in two forms, K_1 and K_2. In the normal human, intestinal bacteria can synthesize adequate amounts to meet daily requirements. These forms are fat soluble. Synthetic vitamin K_3 is similar in structure and is water soluble.

Orally ingested or bacteria-derived vitamin K is absorbed by the intestinal wall in the presence of bile and pancreatic juice. Since 50% of vitamin K is synthesized by bacterial flora of the intestine, when the patient is allowed nothing by mouth and is on antibiotics, vitamin K synthesis may cease. Vitamin K is needed by the body to synthesize prothrombin, and factors IV, IX, X, and VII in the liver, although the exact mechanism of its action still remains unknown.

USES. Vitamin K is used to treat hypoprothrombinemia due to vitamin K deficiency. Vitamin K can also be used when a deficiency has occurred secondary to administration of one or more of the other fat-soluble vitamins in excessive doses. Newborn infants, especially those that are premature, have a low level of vitamin K–dependent clotting factors that decrease for a few days after birth. To prevent this occurrence, small doses of vitamin K are administered at birth.

Vitamin K is also effective in patients with bleeding disorders due to a low prothrombin level or bleeding disorders secondary to large doses or overdoses of salicylates, quinine, sulfonamides, arsenicals, or barbiturates. It is also the antidote for the oral anticoagulants, such as warfarin.

ABSORPTION, STORAGE, AND SOURCES. Vitamin K is unique in that it is the only vitamin that is supplied almost totally by resident bacteria in the intestine. Like the other fat-soluble vitamins, vitamin K is passively absorbed (with carrier mediation—bile salts), incorporated into chylomicrons, and transferred to lymph and blood. It has its peak effect six to ten hours after oral administration and one to two hours after parenteral administration. If vitamin K is being administered to control hemorrhage, cessation of bleeding generally occurs within three to six hours.

Vitamin K is stored in the liver for only a short time; therefore, a continued intake is necessary. The target tissues are the liver and the vascular system.

Vitamin K is widely distributed in foods, including vegetables, meats, organ meats, and seeds and nuts. A true dietary deficiency rarely occurs.

DEFICIENCY STATES. In general, vitamin K deficiencies result from malabsorption syndromes and long-term total parenteral nutrition, such as obstructive jaundice, sprue, bowel shunts, regional ileitis, or secondary ulcerative colitis; other fat-soluble vitamin excesses; prolonged antibiotic therapy; or chronic hepatic disease. Vitamin K deficiencies lead to increased bleeding tendency, increased clotting time, and hypoprothrombinemia.

ADVERSE EFFECTS. Toxic effects include gastric upset, mild allergic reactions, and headache. When large doses are administered to a patient with liver disease, liver function may be depressed. When excessive amounts of vitamin K are administered to infants, particularly premature infants, hyperbilirubinemia, kernicterus, brain damage, and even death have been noted.

CONTRAINDICATIONS AND PRECAUTIONS. Vitamin K is contraindicated in persons hypersensitive to its components as well as pregnant women, particularly during the last few weeks of pregnancy or during labor, as hemorrhagic diseases of the newborn may occur. In addition, vitamin K crosses the placenta; and as yet, there is no information concerning teratogenic or other adverse effects on the fetus. Vitamin K is excreted in breast milk, so vitamin K is administered cautiously to nursing women. Vitamin K is administered cautiously to persons with impaired liver functions. Generally, the hypoprothrombinemia due to hepatocellular damage is not corrected with administration of vitamin K and, paradoxically, may even be worsened.

INTERACTIONS. Since vitamin K is fat soluble, less vitamin K will be absorbed in the gut if the patient is taking mineral oil routinely as a cathartic or cholestyramine. Also, vitamin K antagonizes oral anticoagulants to the extent that the patient cannot become anticoagulated again for about a week. A patient receiving supplemental vitamin K may have a falsely elevated urinary steroid level.

DOSAGE. Several forms of vitamin K are available for administration.

MENADIOL SODIUM DIPHOSPHATE. Menadiol sodium diphosphate (MSD, K4, Synkayvite) can be administered orally, subcutaneously, intravenously, or intramuscularly in doses of 5–10 mg for children and 5–15 mg in adults either once or twice daily. Menadiol sodium diphosphate is used to treat hypoprothrombinemia secondary to liver disease, antibacterials, or salicylates. Menadiol sodium diphosphate is a synthetic, water-soluble form of vitamin K_3.

PHYTONADIONE. Phytonadione (Phytonadione K_1, Konakion, AquaMEPHYTON) is a derivative identical to the naturally occurring vitamin K_1. Phytonadione is administered orally as AquaMEPHYTON in 5-mg tablets or intramuscularly as Konakion in doses from 2.5–20 mg. To prevent hypoproteinemia associated with vitamin K deficiency in patients on prolonged TPN, 5–10 mg intramuscularly weekly is generally administered.

PHYTONADIONE SOLUTION. Phytonadione solution (Aquamephyton) is given subcutaneously, intramuscularly, or by slow intravenous administration. When AquaMEPHYTON is to be administered intravenously, the rate should not exceed 1 mg/minute. Slower rates are safer. The drug is also diluted in either dextrose or saline solution and NEVER administered by intravenous bolus or undiluted. Severe reactions including fatalities have been reported after intravenous administration.

WATER-SOLUBLE VITAMINS

Vitamin B_1

Vitamin B_1, or thiamine, is a water-soluble vitamin and a member of the B-complex group. It functions as a coenzyme in pyruvate metabolism, which is necessary for carbohydrate metabolism, nerve conduction, energy production, and aerobic metabolism.

Vitamin B_1 requirements are increased in untreated hyperthyroidism, heavy manual labor, malabsorptive syndromes, prolonged diarrhea, biliary disease, in alcoholism, and in pregnancy. The normal RDA for adults is 1.0–1.5 mg.

Vitamin B_1 requirements are proportional to the number of calories ingested and the metabolic rate; therefore, as carbohydrate intake increases, so does the need for vitamin B_1. A total absence of vitamin B_1 in the diet produces symptoms in about three weeks.

USES. Thiamine is indicated only in the treatment of a thiamine deficiency.

ABSORPTION, STORAGE, AND SOURCE. Vitamin B_1 is absorbed in only small amounts from the jejunum by active transport and is stored in small amounts in the heart, liver, kidney, and brain. It is excreted rapidly in the urine with as much as 1 mg being destroyed by the tissues daily. The target tissues are the heart, liver, kidneys, and peripheral nerves.

The primary sources of vitamin B_1 are wheat germ, cereal grains, nuts, yeast, meat (beef, pork, liver), and vegetables. Much vitamin B_1 is lost from processed cereals and grains; therefore, individuals consuming only these foods may need vitamin B_1 supplements.

DEFICIENCY STATES. The most common overt symptoms of vitamin B_1 deficiency are related to the nervous system. Mild deficiency is associated with a peripheral neuropathy, characterized by symptoms such as burning, tingling, and motor nerve disabilities, which may lead to muscle weakness. Muscles become tender and may atrophy. Fatigue, decreased attention span, and an impaired capacity for work are seen. Central nervous system irritability, depression, and loss of memory are also often associated with vitamin B_1 deficiencies. With increasing thiamine deficiency, neurologic symptoms become more severe, and cardiovascular symptoms also arise, leading to congestive heart failure with edema, dyspnea, and tachycardia. Gastrointestinal complaints include vomiting, chronic diarrhea, and loss of appetite. These symptoms are found more often in the alcoholic than in other individuals.

Prolonged thiamine deficiency can lead to Wernicke's encephalopathy. This is characterized by disturbed consciousness ranging from mild confusion to coma, paralysis of the extraocular muscles, nystagmus, tremor, ataxia, and impaired vestibular function. In severe cases, damage to the cerebral cortex may result in Korsakoff's psychosis. In this psychosis, retentive memory and cognitive function are severely impaired. Both Wernicke's encephalopathy and Korsakoff's psychosis are common to the extreme alcoholic because of the likelihood of nutritional neglect.

Thiamine deficiency causes beriberi, which is recognized by its neurologic symptoms of peripheral neuritis, fatigue, decreased attention span, and so on. This is referred to as "dry" beriberi. The cardiovascular symptoms such as increased cardiac output are referred to as "wet" beriberi. Beriberi is most common in alcoholics, in pregnant women with inadequate diets, or in persons with malabsorption syndromes, prolonged diarrhea, or hepatic disease, all of which cause defective utilization of thiamine.

Nutritional deficiencies of thiamine are common. Adequate thiamine may be lacking in a fairly good diet due to its limited distribution in food, and it is certainly lacking in many fad diets. Prolonged antacid therapy may also lead to a deficiency by destroying the vitamin in the bowel. Antacids raise the pH of the gastrointestinal tract, and thiamine is unstable in the alkaline environment. Patients on prolonged parenteral nutrition are prone to the development of thiamine deficiency. These patients are often malnourished and stressed and are receiving a high carbohydrate load—all of which increase thiamine requirements. Alcoholics are the group of people most likely to develop a deficiency, especially when they have been drinking to the exclusion of eating for several weeks. Vitamin B_1 deficiencies may also be found on occasion during pregnancy.

ADVERSE EFFECTS. In general, the incidence of adverse effects to thiamine is relatively low. Patients may complain of weakness or difficulty in breathing and may experience a slight fall in blood pressure. There are reports of anaphylactic reactions when vitamin B_1 is administered intravenously. Most likely, this is due to an allergic reaction to the preparation rather than to the vitamin B_1. Patients have also experienced a feeling of warmth, pruritis, urticaria, and nausea.

DOSAGE. The normal RDA in adults varies from 1.0–1.5 mg. In normal, healthy individuals consuming a normal diet, 5 mg/day is the most that is ever needed as a dietary supplement.

THIAMINE. Thiamine (B_1, Betalin S, thiamine hydrochloride, Bramine) may be administered orally (preferred), intramuscularly, or intravenously. In persons with a true vitamin B_1 deficiency, as much as 100 mg can be administered daily. Once vitamin B_1 levels return to normal, the dosage is reduced. Beriberi with cardiac failure is an emergency and should be treated with 30 mg slowly intravenously three times a day. Rapid administration may cause anaphylactic reaction. Beriberi alone can be treated with 10–20 mg intramuscularly three times a day for two weeks. This is followed with 5–10 mg orally daily for one month. For Wernicke's encephalopathy, 100 mg of thiamine is administered intravenously.

Vitamine B₂

Vitamin B_2, or riboflavin, is a water-soluble vitamin that has few tissue stores in the body. It functions primarily as a coenzyme in various steps in cellular respiration. For energy to be produced in the mitochondrial energy system, vitamin B_2 is needed by the respiratory proteins. Vitamin B_2 is also concerned with fetal growth and development, and with the maintenance of external tissues in the eyes and skin.

The RDA of vitamin B_2 for adults ranges from 1.2–1.6 mg. Human requirements are proportional to energy expenditures.

USES. Vitamin B_2 is used primarily to treat and prevent riboflavin deficiencies.

ABSORPTION, STORAGE, AND SOURCES. Vitamin B_2 is readily absorbed from both the GI tract (through facilitated diffusion) and parenteral sites. It is not stored in the body to any great extent and is excreted rapidly; approximately 12% of the intake is excreted in the urine within 24 hours and colors the urine a bright yellow. The target organs are the heart, liver, and kidneys, where it is also stored. Vitamin B_2 is bound to plasma proteins.

Rich dietary sources of vitamin B_2 include liver from all animals, yeast, green leafy vegetables, and fruits. It is also found in most types of meat and in eggs and dairy products.

DEFICIENCY STATES. *Ariboflavinosis* is not uncommon in the United States because of the low concentration of vitamin B_2 in common foods, and because it is easily destroyed by ultraviolet light and alkaline conditions. However, a diet containing milk and the usual portions of meat is not likely to be deficient. Special conditions that may necessitate dietary supplementation include pregnancy and lactation, high energy expenditure, fevers, antibiotic treatment, stress, hyperthyroidism, hepatic malfunction, and alcoholism.

Lack of vitamin B_2 does not cause deficiency disease, but rather a group of symptoms, which include photophobia, increased tearing, and itching and burning of the skin. The cornea of the eye may show an increased growth in capillaries (vascularization). The mucous membranes, particularly of the mouth, may develop deep fissures, resulting in stomatitis or glossitis.

Vitamin B_2 deficiencies rarely occur alone, but rather in combination with other B-complex deficiencies.

ADVERSE EFFECTS. Vitamin B_2 is relatively nontoxic in normal and megadose quantities.

INTERACTIONS. Antidepressants, phenothiazines, and probenecid, when given concurrently, may increase requirements for riboflavin. Alcohol inhibits absorption of riboflavin. Riboflavin may cause false elevations of urinary catecholamines.

DOSAGE. The RDA is 1.2–1.6 mg/day.

RIBOFLAVIN. Riboflavin (Vitamin B_2, riboflavin) is used to prevent or treat riboflavin deficiency. The adult dose to treat deficiencies is about 5–30 mg orally daily. The pediatric dose is 3–10 mg orally, sucutaneously, intramuscularly, or intravenously. There are no valid reports of any benefits derived from megadose treatment. Riboflavin may cause a yellow-orange discoloration of the urine.

Vitamin B₆

Vitamin B₆ (pyridoxine) is a water-soluble B-complex vitamin. It functions as a coenzyme for a number of reactions associated with nitrogen metabolism. Vitamin B₆ also aids in the metabolism of tryptophan and enhances the transport of amino acids and potassium into cells.

Vitamin B₆ is needed in the formation of the heme part of erythrocytes. It also participates in the transfer of energy both in the brain and in nervous tissue. Vitamin B₆ is a complex of three closely related compounds—pyridoxine, pyridoxal, and pyridoxamine. Pyridoxine is found in plants, while pyridoxal and pyridoxamine are found in animals. All of these compounds are converted to physiologically active forms of vitamin B₆—pyridoxal phosphate (codecarboxylase) and pyridoxamine phosphate.

The RDA for vitamin B₆ in adults is 1.8–2.2 mg and is closely proportional to the protein intake of individuals. (Approximately 0.02 mg/g of protein compound).

USES. Pyridoxine is indicated in pyridoxine deficiency, which is associated with inadequate diet, drug-induced deficiencies (isoniazid, oral contraceptives) causing peripheral neuritis, and inborn errors of metabolism.

ABSORPTION, STORAGE, AND SOURCES. Vitamin B₆ is readily absorbed after both oral and parenteral administration. Vitamin B₆ is absorbed throughout the intestine by simple diffusion. It is biotransformed in the liver and excreted in the urine. Its target tissues include nervous tissue, liver, lymph nodes, and muscle tissue. Very little is stored in the body in skeletal tissue. It has a half-life of 15–20 days.

Vitamin B₆ is obtained from both plant and animal sources, although in small amounts. The greatest dietary sources are liver, grains, yeasts, vegetables, meat, and fish. It is rapidly destroyed in cooking. It is synergistic with most other vitamins and minerals; maintaining adequate levels is sometimes difficult.

DEFICIENCY STATES. A lowered vitamin B₆ level is seen in individuals with an inadequate dietary intake, and during pregnancy and lactation. Drug-induced deficiencies related to concurrent use of isoniazid (INH) or oral contraceptives are further causes, as are inborn errors of vitamin B₆ metabolism, which may result in convulsions and anemias. Convulsive disorders have been reported in infants and children deficient in vitamin B₆; whereas in adults seborrheic dermatitis, lesions of the mucous membranes, and peripheral neuritis are most common. A clinical syndrome associated with vitamin B₆ deficiency in humans has also been described. Symptoms seen are personality changes, with irritability, depression, and a loss of a sense of responsibility. There may be a tendency to develop infections. A sideroblastic anemia may develop after prolonged deficiency.

ADVERSE EFFECTS. Adverse effects rarely occur in normal or even therapeutic doses. However, paresthesia, somnolence, flushing, and a feeling of warmth have been reported after large parenteral injections.

Temporary burnings or a stinging pain have also been reported after injections.

INTERACTIONS. Vitamin B₆, when taken in doses of greater than 5 mg daily concurrently with levodopa (L-Dopa), enhances the peripheral metabolism of levodopa. This prevents it from having a therapeutic effect and may necessitate increasing the dose of levodopa. Special pyridoxine-free multivitamin preparations are available for those taking levodopa. Doses over 80 mg daily enhance hepatic metabolism of phenobarbital or phenytoin by 40%–50%. Isoniazid and penicillamine increase the urinary excretion of pyridoxine.

DOSAGE. Dosage varies depending on the condition being treated.

PYRODOXINE B₆. Pyridoxine B₆ (pyridoxine hydrochloride, Nestrex, Beesix, HexaBetalin) is used to treat a dietary deficiency, in doses of 10–20 mg daily for two to three weeks, followed by 2–5 mg for several additional weeks. If the patient has a vitamin B₆ deficiency syndrome, he or she may need 600 mg/day for several weeks followed by a lifetime maintenance dose of 25–50 mg daily. Requirements are higher if the patient is concurrently taking INH or oral contraceptives. If treating seizures induced by INH toxicity, give an equal amount of pyridoxine, 4 g intravenously, followed by 1 g intramuscularly every 30 minutes until seizures stop.

Vitamin B₁₂ and Folic Acid

Vitamin B₁₂ and folic acid are included in Table 57–2 and are discussed in detail in Chapter 32.

Vitamin C

Vitamin C (ascorbic acid) is a naturally occurring water-soluble vitamin. Vitamin C cannot be synthesized by the human body; it must be provided exogenously. It is probably the most controversial vitamin, because of the research of Linus Pauling that claims that megadoses relieve cold symptoms. In addition, other research claims that vitamin C can treat cancer, heat rash, thrombophlebitis, emotional illness, and enhance wound healing. Primarily, vitamin C functions as an antioxidant, which is essential in many enzymatic activities, particularly those of cellular respiration. It is also essential for the synthesis and maintenance of both collagen and intercellular substances, which ultimately are needed for wound healing. Vitamin C is also necessary for carbohydrate metabolism, the conversion of folic acid to folinic acid, the formation of serotonin, and the maintenance of vascular tone.

The current RDA is 60 mg, with greater doses indicated for larger individuals. The megadose advocates say we need 10,000 mg. Environmental stress (trauma, surgery, burns, temperature extremes) and smoking cigarettes increase the daily requirements of vitamin C by 300% and 50%, respectively.

USES. Vitamin C is indicated for the prevention and treatment of scurvy. Vitamin C, in large doses, acts as a urinary acidifier. Doses of vitamin C can be beneficial to bedridden patients with infectious diseases. Patients with severe infectious diseases such as tuberculosis, rheumatic fever, and pneumonia have an increased need for vitamin C. Failure to receive adequate vitamin

C can result in delayed soft-tissue healing and disruption of the body's immune response. Most patients with infectious diseases should take a daily supplement of 100–300 mg/day.

ABSORPTION, STORAGE, AND SOURCES. Vitamin C is readily absorbed after both oral and parenteral administration. Vitamin C is absorbed from the terminal ileum by active transport. It is distributed to many tissues, particularly the adrenal cortex, pituitary, ovaries, and connective tissue. There is limited body storage in the adrenal cortex and liver. The half-life is approximately 16 days. Excessive amounts are excreted in the urine.

Vitamin C, when combined with iron-rich foods like spinach, broccoli, eggs, and raisins, enhances the body's absorption of iron.

Vitamin C is found primarily in citrus and other fruits, fresh green vegetables, and rose hips.

DEFICIENCY STATES. The major deficiency state is scurvy. Symptoms of scurvy include anemia, joint pain, and hemorrhage from mucous membranes of the mouth and gastrointestinal tract. A less severe deficiency is thought to result in slow healing of wounds, decreased ability to fight infections, and decreased ability to metabolize amino acids. A deficiency of vitamin C can also produce megaloblastic anemia in infants.

ADVERSE EFFECTS. With excessive oral doses, the patient may experience diarrhea (due to direct irritation of the intestinal mucosa), or strong acidification of the urine with possible precipitation of crystals of vitamin C. Hemolytic anemia may develop in patients who have a deficiency of glucose-6-phosphate dehydrogenase (G6PD). After intravenous administration, mild soreness, dizziness, and faintness may be experienced.

CONTRAINDICATIONS AND PRECAUTIONS. Vitamin C is administered cautiously in persons with gout and crystalluria, as the acidification of the urine from vitamin C may worsen these conditions. Vitamin C is contraindicated in pregnancy, as there are no studies that indicate whether or not fetal harm will occur. Vitamin C is administered cautiously to lactating women, as it is excreted in breast milk. The effects on the infant are unknown at this time.

INTERACTIONS. Large doses of vitamin C, when taken concurrently with aminosalicylic acid and sulfonamides, may increase the possibility of producing urinary crystals of the other drugs, because of urine acidification. The effect of salicylates may be enhanced by increasing the renal tubular absorption, whereas amphetamines and tricyclic antidepressants may have decreased effects due to a decrease in renal tubular absorption.

Vitamin C can interfere with the therapeutic effects of heparin, warfarin, methyldopa, fluphenazine, and aminoglycoside antibiotics.

A patient taking large doses of vitamin C may have a false-negative or false-positive urinary glucose reading, depending on the type of glucose test used. The patient may also have false-positive tests for occult blood in the stool.

DOSAGE. The daily adult prophylactic dosage range is 50–150 mg, generally in divided doses; for children,

it is 30 mg daily, also in divided doses. Vitamin C is available in several forms—ascorbic acid, sodium ascorbate, and calcium ascorbate.

VITAMIN C OR ASCORBIC ACID. Vitamin C (ascorbic acid, Cevalin, Cevita, and many others) is available for oral, intramuscular, or intravenous administration. The therapeutic dose to treat scurvy for adults may range from 300 mg to 2 g or more for two to three weeks; and for children, from 100–300 mg daily for two to three weeks. To acidify the urine, the usual dose is 4–12 g daily in divided doses.

Pantothenic Acid

Pantothenic acid (calcium pantothenate, vitamin B_5) occupies a key role in body metabolism. It is incorporated into coenzyme A, which is involved in a large number of biochemical processes, including metabolism of fats, protein, carbohydrates and the synthesis of steroids, porphyrins, acetylcholine, and other substrates.

Exact human requirements have not been established. An ordinary American diet contains approximately 10 mg of pantothenic acid, which seems to be sufficient to prevent overt deficiencies.

USES. Pantothenic acid is indicated for the prevention and treatment of vitamin B deficiency. Special conditions that may require supplementation include stress, aging, arthritis, malabsorption, weakness, and depression.

ABSORPTION, STORAGE, AND SOURCES. Pantothenic acid is absorbed from the intestine and excreted fairly rapidly. Target organs include all tissues, but especially the brain, heart, and kidneys. Research is still being conducted to determine in what quantities pantothenic acid is stored. It is believed to be stored in the liver, heart, and kidneys. It is estimated that approximately 25% of the daily intake is excreted within 24 hours after ingestion.

Pantothenic acid is widely distributed in natural foods; large quantities can be found in liver, eggs, wheat germ, yeast, walnuts, and salmon.

DEFICIENCY STATE. Specific deficiencies are unlikely to occur. Experimentally provoked deficiencies have produced neurologic disorders, irritability, fatigue, dry scaly skin, muscle cramps, and adrenal hypofunction.

DOSAGE. Evidence indicates that dietary supplementation in a normal, healthy individual is not necessary. Pantothenic acid is considered suitable for inclusion in multivitamin preparations in amounts of 5–20 mg.

Niacin

Niacin (nicotinic acid) is a water-soluble derivative of pyridine, formerly called vitamin B_3. Niacin occurs in two physiologically active forms that take part in many oxidation-reduction reactions: NAD (nicotinamide adenine dinucleotide), formerly known as DPN (diphosphopyridine nucleotide); and NADP (nicotinamide adenine dinucleotide phosphate). These substances act as hydrogen acceptors, which ultimately help to convert protein, carbohydrate, and fat into energy through oxidation-reduction. At this time, there is no known biologic role for niacin other than this coenzyme function.

High niacin doses have a positive effect on lipid metabolism and may lower plasma cholesterol, triglycerides, and free fatty acids.

The adult RDA for niacin is 13–19 mg.

USES. Niacin is indicated for treatment of pellagra. It is also used as adjunctive therapy in patients with significant hyperlipidemia who do not respond adequately to diet and weight loss.

ABSORPTION, STORAGE, AND SOURCES. Niacin is readily absorbed after both oral and parenteral administration. Niacin is absorbed in the proximal jejunum through active transport. It is metabolized by the liver, with small doses excreted as metabolites and large doses unchanged in the urine. Approximately one third of the daily intake is excreted in 24 hours.

The target tissues include the liver, heart, muscle, and kidney, although niacin is found in most body tissues. Interestingly, there is minimal storage in the liver and heart.

Niacin is widely distributed in food, with rich sources in liver, nuts (particularly peanuts), yeast, poultry, fish, and meats.

DEFICIENCY STATES. The primary deficiency state is pellagra, which affects the skin, digestive tract, and nervous system. Patients with pellagra usually experience red patch skin eruptions that closely resemble sunburn, a red swollen tongue, and mental changes including mental confusion, memory loss, and depression. Severe deficiency is characterized by dementia, dermatitis, and diarrhea. Occasionally, a subclinical form of niacin deficiency can be found in persons with chronic alcoholism, who experience headache, insomnia, itching and burning skin, and GI upset.

ADVERSE EFFECTS. Many adverse effects can be experienced, including flushing of the face and neck (as niacin may stimulate histamine release), pruritus, dry skin, headache, dizziness, heartburn, anorexia, activation of peptic ulcer, vomiting, mild hypotension, impaired liver function, and allergic reactions. Flushing and itching reactions usually subside after about three days of therapy.

CONTRAINDICATIONS AND PRECAUTIONS. Niacin is contraindicated with hepatic dysfunction and in active peptic ulcer, as histamine release may activate bleeding. Caution is advised in patients with gout, as elevated uric acid levels do occur, and in patients with gallbladder disease. Diabetics may have a decreased glucose tolerance and may need to have dietary or hypoglycemic therapy modification.

INTERACTIONS. When niacin is given concurrently with adrenergic blocking drugs—particularly the ganglionic blockers—the vasodilating and hypotensive effects may be potentiated.

DOSAGE. Nicotinic acid and nicotinamide are used to prevent and treat nicotinic acid deficiency and pellagra. Nicotinic acid is also used as an adjunct to dietary therapy for the treatment of hyperlipidemia.

NICOTINIC ACID. Nicotinic acid, niacin, vitamin B$_3$ (Nicobid, Nicolar, and many others) is administered to relieve the symptoms of pellagra. Niacin is administered orally in doses of 300–500 mg daily, or in timed-release forms of 125–250 mg each morning or evening. For intravenous administration, 25–100 mg are administered two or more times daily. For intramuscular injections, administer 50–100 mg five or more times daily. For hyperlipidemia, 1–2 g are administered orally three times a day. Dosage should not exceed 6 g/day. As a daily supplement, 10–20 mg is given daily. Orally, nicotinic acid is started in small doses and increased gradually to avoid the vasodilating reactions. If the intravenous route is required, 25–100 mg are administered two or more times daily.

NICOTINAMIDE OR NIACINAMIDE. Nicotinamide or niacinamide is used by the body as a source of niacin. Nicotinamide does not have hypolipidemic or vasodilating effects. It is used for the prophylaxis and treatment of pellegra. Therapeutic dose is 50 mg three to ten times daily.

Biotin

Biotin is slightly water soluble, and its major function is as a coenzyme in the metabolism of proteins, fats, and carbohydrates. Biotin is also important for the maintenance of skin, hair, nerves, and sex glands. Although it is still a little-known vitamin, it seems to have an important role in human growth.

The adult RDA for biotin is 100–200 μg.

ABSORPTION, STORAGE, AND SOURCES. Biotin is absorbed well after both oral and parenteral doses. Its target tissues include the skin and the nervous tissue. It is stored in the liver and excreted slowly over three to four weeks. Much of the daily requirement of biotin is synthesized by intestinal flora and supplements oral intake.

The dietary sources include yeast, liver, royal jelly, and most grains.

DEFICIENCY STATES. Deficiency states are rare in humans who have a normal intake of nutrients. Primarily, patients deprived of biotin experience skin lesions, dermatitis, partial memory loss, and mental depression.

DOSAGE. Therapeutic dose for adults is 100–200 μg daily for deficiency. Special conditions that may require dietary supplementation include certain cutaneous lesions, antibiotic and sulfa therapy, pregnancy, and excessive egg white ingestion. Egg whites contain avidin, a protein, which binds orally ingested and bacteria-produced biotin and prevents its absorption in the intestine.

Megadose therapy has been experimentally used to aid hair growth; no conclusive evidence as to its efficacy exists at this time.

MINERALS

The bulk minerals calcium, magnesium, sodium, potassium, and phosphorus are discussed in Chapter 58. They are included in Table 57–5 for reference. The trace elements include iron (described in detail in Chapter

TEXT RESUMES ON PAGE 1594

Table 57–5. MINERALS

Mineral	Excretion	Physiologic Function	Deficiency Symptoms	Excesses	Dietary Sources
Ca (Calcium)	Feces, small amount in urine	Excites heart, inhibits ADH, necessary for nerve transmission, needed for muscle contraction, constituent of bone, blood clotting	Rickets, tetany, osteoporosis, hypocalcemia	Hypercalcemia, hyperparathyroidism	Seafood, organ meats, egg yolk, nuts/seeds, dairy products
Mg (Magnesium)	Feces, small amount in urine	Maintenance of cardiac function and neuromuscular transmission, bone structure, clotting	Poor growth, hyperirritability, convulsions, tetany	Purgative, nausea, malaise, muscular and cardiovascular weakness	Nuts, seeds, soybeans, grains, yeast, cocoa, kelp
Na (Sodium)	Urine	Maintenance of fluid volume, cell permeability, nerve irritability, blood osmolarity, cellular contraction	Anorexia, nausea, muscle atrophy, weight loss, poor growth	Hypernatremia, hypertension	Salt, seafood, organ meats, dairly products, preservatives
K (Potassium)	Urine, small amount in feces	Maintenance of acid–base balance, RBC transport, blood osmolarity	Muscle weakness, cardiac dysrhythmias, bone fragility	Convulsions, CNS paralysis, cardiac and CNS depression	Seafood, nuts, seeds, fruits, grains, yeast
P (Phosphorus)	Urine, feces	RBC oxygen release, calcium excretion, component of bones and teeth	Rickets, osteomalacia, respiratory muscle weakness	Tetany, laxative effect, hypocalcemia, hypomagnesemia, bone reabsorption	Seafood, organ meats, nuts/seeds, legumes, dairy products, yeast.
Fe (Iron)	Feces, small amount in urine, skin.	Heart muscle, hemostasis, oxygen transport, hemoglobin production	Hypochromic anemia	Hypotension, death from cardiac failure, prolonged clotting time	Organ meats, nuts/seeds, wheat germ, yeast, bone meal

Half-Life	Tissue	Storage	Adverse Effects	Contraindications and Precautions	Interactions
Not available	All	Bone	PO: Constipation, increased serum calcium, anorexia, nausea, decreased excitability of nerves, mental confusion, renal calculi IV: Tingling or "heatwave" sensation over body; chalky taste, cardiac irritability and arrest	Use cautiously in patients receiving cardiac glycosides.	Enhances digitalis products. Decreases effect of tetracyclines. False decline in serum and urine magnesium.
Not available	Connective, skin	Skeletal muscle, red blood cells	Flushing, thirst, increased blood pressure, muscle weakness, dehydration, decreased reflexes, decreases labor	Contraindicated in myocardial infarction, heart block, abdominal pain, and for 2 hr before delivery. Use cautiously in decreased renal function, heart disease.	Enhances neuromuscular blockade with neuromuscular blocking agents. Enhanced CNS depression with narcotics, barbiturates, and anesthetics.
Not available	All	Extracellular fluid; small amount in bones	Muscle weakness, CNS restlessness, increased metabolic activity	Contraindicated in renal and cardiac disease.	Causes water absorption.
Not available	All (intracellular)	No storage	Nausea, vomiting, GI distress, heart block, muscle weakness	Contraindicated in renal impairment, crushing injuries, high digitalis levels. Use cautiously in cardiac disease and acidosis.	Elevated potassium level with potassium-sparing diuretics spironolactone and triamterene. Lowered potassium level with other diuretics.
Not available	All	Skeleton	Mild laxative effect	Contraindicated in Addison's disease. Use cautiously in sodium- and potassium-restricted diets.	None significant.
Not available	Liver, spleen, bone marrow	Liver, spleen, bone marrow, muscle	Constipation, diarrhea, dark stools, GI distress, staining and pain at IM sites	Contraindicated in hypersensitivity and peptic ulcer. Use cautiously in GI distress and renal of hepatic dysfunction.	Inhibited absorption of tetracyclines (separate doses by 2–3 hours). False-positive test for occult blood in stool.

CONTINUED ON THE FOLLOWING PAGE

Table 57–5. MINERALS–*CONTINUED*

Mineral	Excretion	Physiologic Function	Deficiency Symptoms	Excesses	Dietary Sources
Cu (Copper)	Feces, bile	Maintenance of hemostasis, stabilization of hemoglobin content, required for function of various enzymes involved in cellular respiration, maintains myelin on spinal cord	Hypochromic anemia, bone disease	Nausea, vomiting, diarrhea, epigastric pain, malaise, hemolysis, renal tubular disorders	Seafood, organ meats, nuts/seeds, grains, yeast
Zn (Zinc)	Feces	Needed by enzymes essential in cellular metabolic processes (carbonic anhydrase is a zinc-containing enzyme); arterial wall homeostasis, brain development, appetite, taste, smell, maintenance of sex gland function.	Growth failure, asexual infantilism, dermatitis	Lassitude, slow tendon reflexes, bloody enteritis, diarrhea, leukopenia, CNS depression	Oysters, organ meats, sunflower seeds, cheeses, wheat germ, yeast
I (Iodine)	Urine	Necessary for synthesis of T_4 and T_3	Cretinism, myxedema, goiter (simple), hypothyroidism	Graves' disease (thyrotoxicosis), goiter (exophthalmic)	Seafood, kelp, cod liver oil, mushrooms, sunflower seeds
Co (Cobalt)	Urine, feces, bile	Essential for production of vitamin B_{12}	Same as vitamin B_{12}, glottitis, sprue, anemias	Polycythemia, cardiomyopathy, goiter	Seafood, liver, peanuts, butter, grains
Cr (Chromium)	Urine	Maintenance of normal glucose utilization; may stabilize tertiary structures of proteins and nucleic acids	Glucose intolerance	Not reported	Seafood, organ meats, peanuts, American cheese, wheat, wheat germ
Mn (Manganese)	Bile, pancreatic juices	Activates many enzymes involved in synthesis of protein and central nervous system function	Weight loss, transient dermatitis, nausea, vomiting, reduced growth, change in hair color	Not reported	Snails, peanuts, pecans, blueberries, olives, corn, corn germ, wheat, wheat germ, tea
Se (Selenium)	Urine, feces, lungs, skin	Part of glutathiane peroxidase in RBCs which protects cell components from oxidative damage due to peroxides produced in cellular metabolism	Muscle pain or tenderness, cardiomyopathy, kwashiorkor	Hair loss, weak nails, dermatitis, GI disorders	Grains, onions, meats, milk, vegetables

Half-Life	Tissue	Storage	Adverse Effects	Contraindications and Precautions	Interactions
3–7 days	Liver, kidney, GI tract, brain	Liver, kidneys	Not available	Not available	Not available
Less than 3 hours	Liver, choroid, prostate, skin	Bones, spleen, kidney	Nausea, vomiting, gastric ulceration.	Do not exceed prescribed dosage. Will cause emesis.	Zinc will impair absorption of tetracyclines. Bran and dairy products may decrease zinc absorption.
Possibly 6–7 hr	Thyroid	Thyroid	Not available	Not available	Not available
Possibly 3 days	All	Kidney, liver, bone marrow	Not available	Not available	Not available
Few days	All	Skin, muscles, fat, testes, bone, liver, spleen	Not available	Not available	Not available
<1 hr	Tissues rich in mitochondria	Brain, kidneys, pancreas, liver	Unlikely	Hypersensitivity	Not applicable
Unknown	RBCs	Kidney, liver	Unlikely	Hypersensitivity	None known

33), copper, zinc, iodine, cobalt, chromium, and manganese.

COPPER

Copper is required for many functions in the body. Copper is an essential component of a number of proteins (erythrocuprein, hepatocuprein) and enzymes (lysyl hydroxylase, dopamine beta-hydroxylase). It is necessary for hemostasis, for stabilization of hemoglobin in the red blood cell, and for the normal function of various enzymes involved in cellular respiration, and it helps to maintain the integrity of the myelin sheath on the spincal cord.

The RDA for adults ranges from 2.0–3.0 mg. Copper is richly present in foods such as seafood, organ meats, nuts and seeds, grains, and yeast. Virtually all soft water supplies contain large amounts of copper because of current use of copper piping. Therefore, copper deficiencies rarely occur, but may be found in infants and adults receiving copper-deficient parenteral nutrition. Copper deficiency is associated with hypochromic anemia, leukopenia, hypoproteinemia, and bone disease. Copper excess is possible in an American diet. An excess of copper antagonizes the effect of both iron and zinc, thereby resulting in deficiencies. Elevated copper levels may be produced by drugs such as estrogens, thyroid, and corticotropin. Acute toxicities are manifested by nausea and vomiting, epigastric pain, diarrhea, malaise with hemolysis, and renal tubular disorders occurring in severe toxicity.

Copper is optimally absorbed and has a half-life of three to seven days. Target tissues include the liver, kidney, GI tract, and brain, and copper is stored in both the liver and kidneys. It is excreted in the feces and in the bile.

Copper (Coppertrace, cupric sulfate, and others) is administered intramuscularly to adults in doses of 0.5–1.5 mg/day and to children in doses of 20 μg/kg/day.

ZINC

Zinc is essential for normal growth and development. It is an essential cofactor needed for the proper functioning of over 100 enzymes essential for metabolic processes. Zinc is involved within ribonucleic acid and protein metabolism, acts as a stabilizer of cell membranes, and interacts with insulin. Zinc is also essential for maintenance of arterial wall hemostasis, for brain development, and for stimulation of appetite, taste, and smell. It is also important for the maintenance of the sex glands, particularly the prostate. Zinc is also necessary for the metabolism of carbohydrates.

The RDA for an adult is 15 mg, and in lactating women it increases to 25 mg. Other conditions that increase need for zinc include high stress, sepsis, and increased intestinal losses. Zinc can be found in oysters, organ meats, sunflower seeds, all cheeses, wheat germ, and yeast. Some current research indicates that a normal American diet may not contain sufficient zinc. This can be eliminated by merely increasing the intake of foods high in zinc.

Zinc is absorbed from the intestinal tract via active transport. Of the zinc consumed, only about 20%–30% is absorbed and this is dependent on a number of factors, including the source of zinc. Zinc from animal sources is generally better absorbed than from plant sources. Absorption is also enhanced by pregnancy, corticosteroids, endotoxin, and leukocyte endogenous mediation (interleukin 2). It has a half-life of less than three hours. The target tissues include the liver, choroid, prostrate, and skin; zinc is stored in the bones, spleen, and kidneys. Zinc is excreted in the feces.

Deficiencies of zinc include growth failure, particularly in children; dermatitis; and sexual infantilism. With research indicating that zinc is responsible for maintenance of the sense of taste, deficiencies could be a cause of a child's poor eating habits and consequent poor growth. Zinc replacement is also important in wound healing. Zinc should be added to parenteral nutrition and to dialysate solutions to prevent deficiencies from occurring.

Zinc Sulfate

Zinc sulfate (Zinc 15, Orazinc, and many others) is 23% zinc and used primarily to treat zinc deficiencies. The average adult dose of zinc is 25–50 mg daily. When a zinc deficiency exists, 200–220 mg orally three times a day is administered. This is equal to nine times the RDA for zinc or 135–150 mg of elemental zinc. Zinc may be added to TPN solutions, with the usual dose being 2.5–6 mg intravenously daily.

Zinc Gluconate

Zinc gluconate (Z-Pro-C) is 14.3% zinc. It is also administered in 25–50-mg doses for therapeutic use and 200–220 mg for zinc deficiency.

IODINE

Iodine, biologically inactive alone, is required by the body to produce the thyroid hormones T_3 and T_4, and is therefore essential for regulation of body metabolism.

The RDA for adults is approximately 150 μg. Iodine is efficiently absorbed in the intestinal tract; its target and storage organ is the thyroid. Iodine is excreted in the urine.

Iodine exists in all plants and animals, with large sources in seafood, kelp, cod liver oil, mushrooms, and sunflower seeds. Iodine may be lacking in inland geographic areas, but adequate amounts of iodine can be obtained from iodized salt. In general, the average American diet does not need iodine supplementation.

If iodine deficiency exists, the patient may develop poorly as a child (cretinism). Adults may develop myxedema, hypothyroidism, with or without a simple endemic goiter. If iodine is excessive, the patient may develop signs of hyperthyroidism, including exophthalmic goiter or Graves' disease (thyrotoxicosis).

Iodine (SSKI solution) is used to treat goiter and hypothyroidism secondary to iodine deficiency; to suppress mild forms of hyperthyroidism and thyroid crisis in doses of 250–500 mg intravenously daily or 50–100 mg orally; to prepare patients for thyroidectomy in doses of two to six drops three times a day for ten days before surgery; as an expectorant in doses of one to two drops three to four times daily. It can also be placed in TPN solutions in doses of 1–2 $\mu g/kg/day$.

Iodine (Iodopen) is an injectable form of iodine that is administered to stable adults in doses of 1–2 $\mu g/kg/day$ and to pregnant and lactating women and growing children in doses of 2–3 $\mu g/kg/day$.

COBALT

Cobalt is essential for the production of vitamin B_{12} and thus for all of the functions of vitamin B_{12}. (See vitamin B_{12} in Chapter 32.) The daily requirements are easily obtained from a normal diet.

Cobalt is absorbed well in the intestine. The target tissues are all tissues in the body; and cobalt is stored in the kidney, liver, and bone marrow. It is excreted in the urine, feces, and bile.

The deficiencies that develop are those related to vitamin B_{12} deficiency. If supplemental cobalt must be administered, cobalt salts should be avoided because they are absorbed readily, and exert a competitive effect on the absorption of iron and manganese. Vitamin B_{12} should be administered instead.

An excessive cobalt level causes the development of polycythemia (because excessive erythropoietin is excreted by the kidney), cardiomyopathies, and thyroid hyperplasia.

CHROMIUM

Normal glucose utilization in humans requires chromium, which affects the sensitivity of peripheral tissues to insulin. A diabetes-like syndrome has been observed in chromium-deficient laboratory rats and in humans. Chromium may also act to stabilize the tertiary structures of proteins and nucleic acids, and it apparently stimulates hepatic synthesis of fatty acids and cholesterol from acetate.

Only about 0.5% of ingested chromium is absorbed through the gastrointestinal tract. It is excreted almost exclusively via the urine except for small amounts lost through the gastrointestinal tract.

For chromium (Chrometrace, chromic chloride) the minimum oral requirement is 0.29 mg/day. Suggested daily intravenous intake in patients receiving TPN is 10–20 μg of chromium. The oral dose is 50–200 μg daily.

MANGANESE

Manganese is an essential mineral for humans because it is an activator of several enzymes, such as liver arginase and serum alkaline phosphatase. It is also involved in the synthesis of protein and in central nervous system function.

Manganese is poorly absorbed from the gastrointestinal tract. It is distributed throughout the body, with highest concentrations in the pituitary gland, brain, kidney, pancreas, liver, and bones. It is excreted almost exclusively through the gastrointestinal tract, with bile and pancreatic juices contributing large amounts. Almost no manganese is excreted in the urine.

Symptoms of manganese deficiency include weight loss, transient dermatitis, occasional nausea and vomiting, slow growth, and changes in hair color. In animals, a diabetes-like glucose tolerance curve is seen in manganese deficiency.

The estimated RDA for manganese is 0.7–2.2 mg.

Manganese (Chelated Manganese) is administered as a dietary supplement only. The usual oral doses are 5–50 mg daily.

Manganese (Mangatrace, manganese sulfate) is administered parenterally to adults in doses of 0.15–0.8 mg/day and to children in doses of 2–10 $\mu g/kg/day$. It is also added to TPN solutions in doses of 0.15–0.8 mg/day.

USING THE NURSING PROCESS

ASSESSMENT

Patients suspected of having vitamin or mineral excesses or deficiencies need to have careful assessments. The information obtained is featured in Table 57–6. The dietary history includes the intake of fortified foods, style of eating (one or several meals daily), special diets (whether prescribed by physician, or followed through religious or personal preference, such as kosher or vegetarian regimen), cultural background, economic status, the patient's personal views about nutrition, and the patient's smoking history. Information on current use of self-administered or prescription vitamins and minerals including reasons for use, length of time used, dosage, and frequency of administration; who prescribed them; other medications used; and other dietary supplements used is also obtained. As an example, women taking oral contraceptives tend to have higher plasma levels of vitamin A. If they were to take large supplemental doses of vitamin A, they might have a tendency to develop symptoms of vitamin A toxicity. Also, oral contraceptives can deplete vitamin C stores.

Since many people know what they should eat even though they may not eat correctly, the nurse must take care during the diet history to assume a nonjudgmental attitude and to avoid leading questions, so that the information will be as accurate as possible. Vegetarian diets utilizing multiple food sources can provide essential nutrients if milk products or eggs are added to supply vitamin B_{12}. As vegetarian diets become more restrictive, the risk of nutritional inadequacies increases

Table 57–6. NURSING PROCESS FOR PATIENTS REQUIRING VITAMINS AND MINERALS

Assessment

Assess nutrition history, including style of eating, special diets (e.g., vegetarian), cultural eating patterns, personal food preferences.
Determine socioeconomic status.
Note current drug history and use of self-administered/prescribed vitamins/minerals and other medications used (including oral contraceptives).
Evaluate presence of deficiency states.
Review laboratory studies specific to the deficiency.

Nursing Diagnosis	Nursing Actions	Rationale	Desired Outcomes/ Evaluation Criteria
Nutrition, altered Less than body requirements related to inability to ingest/digest food or to absorb nutrients because of biologic, psychologic or economic factors as evidenced by reported inadequate food intake, altered taste sensation, poor muscle tone, sore/ inflamed buccal cavity, capillary fragility.	Administer prescribed supplements as appropriate. Review usual daily dietary intake/patterns. Discuss dietary sources of specific deficient vitamins/minerals. Recommend patient record weight weekly.	Provides for more rapid correction of identified deficiencies or may be used to prevent deficiency (e.g., prenatal). Useful for identifying strengths/deficiencies within diet. In most cases, once deficiency is corrected, ingestion of a balanced diet (possibly with an OTC daily product) will prevent recurrence and reduce likelihood of side-effects/adverse reactions related to drug therapy. Useful in monitoring adequacy of nutritional intake.	Verbalizes understanding of causative factors and necessary interventions. Demonstrates change of nutritional habits to regain/maintain positive nutritional status and is free of signs of deficiency.
Knowledge deficit related to lack of exposure/ recall, information misinterpretation, unfamiliarity with information resources as evidenced by questions, statement of concern, development of preventable complications.	Provide information (verbal and written) concerning patient's individual deficiencies and treatment needs. Discuss specific factors for safe vitamin/mineral administration, e.g., some may be taken with food to enhance absorption or reduce gastric irritation; some may potentiate or interfere with other medications, laboratory tests; or cause urinary stone formation. Review methods of food preparation. Stress importance of reading expiration dates on OTC products and avoid buying in "bulk" or several months' supply. Discuss current beliefs of patient/SO about vitamins/minerals, and provide objective information.	Accurate information helps patient control own situation and prevents complications from inappropriate use. Helps to get the most from medication regimen and prevent untoward effects. Preparing food properly can preserve vitamins/ minerals (e.g., use small amount of water, microwave/steam). Vitamins lose potency as they age (up to 80% in 6 months) and although buying in bulk may reduce price, it may also reduce benefit. Many individuals believe that most illness/conditions can be treated and cured with vitamin/mineral therapy and correcting myths and misconceptions helps patient to deal with own situation more effectively.	Verbalizes understanding of condition/disease process and treatment. Takes vitmain/mineral supplements correctly and explains reasons for individual regimen.

greatly, especially deficiencies of protein, vitamin B_{12}, calcium, vitamin D, and riboflavin. The Zen macrobiotic diets can endanger health. In particular, infants fed KoKoh, a zen macrobiotic food mixture for infant feeding, grow poorly, and become protein malnourished, which may lead to death.

The cause of deficiency states is clearly identified. The majority of deficiency states develop from poor dietary habits; therefore, during the intervention phase, dietary management must be stressed.

A patient who develops a deficiency of the fat-soluble vitamins A, D, E, and K is assessed for possible abuse of laxatives, particularly mineral oil. Oily laxatives prevent absorption of the fat-soluble vitamins in the intestine. Also, a patient who is allowed nothing by mouth and is on antibiotics needs to be carefully assessed for vitamin K deficiencies.

Nurses often do not think of assessing patients for vitamin deficiencies. But often the older, critically ill adult is a candidate for vitamin deficiencies. Patients experiencing gum disease and loose teeth, bone pain, respiratory infections, spontaneous hemorrhages, and anemia may be exhibiting a vitamin C deficiency or other deficiency that needs to be assessed and treated.

The nurse also assesses the patient's need for supplemental vitamin or mineral therapy. Infants and children generally need supplemental therapy, as do pregnant and lactating women. In general, the physician prescribes vitamin or mineral supplements for these age groups. However, the physician may suggest a multivitamin and mineral preparation, and the patient may then ask the nurse's assistance in choosing an appropriate product. The pharmacist or registered dietitian may also be of help in selecting vitamin and mineral supplements. The nurse needs to be aware of the common OTC vitamin and mineral preparations and their primary ingredients to effectively suggest a preparation during the intervention phase. When recommending a preparation, this table should be compared with the RDAs in Tables 57–2 and 57–3 to ensure that the patient receives an adequate supplement.

The Federal Food and Drug Administration divides vitamin and mineral products into three groups:

1. Supplemental—all ingredients are within established limits.
2. OTC proprietary—the vitamin–mineral content is above standard limits, but not excessive.
3. Prescription status—contents exceed OTC proprietary limits and are available by prescription only.

The nurse also needs to assess for hypersensitivity to aspirin, aspirin-like products, and tartrazine before administering certain vitamins. Also, patients who will be receiving iodine need to be assessed for an allergy to seafood.

The nurse continues to assess during each of the remaining phases of the nursing process and modifies or changes the nursing management as necessary.

NURSING DIAGNOSIS

As nursing care begins, the nurse develops the nursing diagnoses, which are the basis for all nursing care given, as well as for the evaluation process. Possible nursing diagnoses for a patient with vitamin and mineral disorders are included in Table 57–6.

PLANNING AND INTERVENTION

From the nursing diagnoses, the nurse develops the goals of the nursing intervention, which will, in turn, become the evaluation criteria. Typical goals when caring for a patient with a vitamin or mineral deficiency or excess are included in Table 57–6. The more the patient and family are involved with the planning process, the more likely they are to comply with the treatment regimen.

NURSING RESPONSIBILITIES IN ADMINISTERING VITAMINS AND MINERALS

The nurse may have to administer vitamins and minerals in the hospital situation to patients who cannot receive sufficient oral nourishment. Many vitamins and minerals can be administered both intramuscularly and intravenously. Iron preparations (e.g., Imferon) are to be administered using the Z-track method. This is explained in Chapter 32. Intravenous vitamins and minerals should not be mixed with other preparations in the same IV bottle unless it is known to be safe, since there may be drug interactions within the intravenous solution between some drugs and vitamins and minerals. As an example, mixing vitamins B and C in the same IV bottle with antibiotics will generally cause the antibiotic to be destroyed. The nurse does not mix any vitamin or mineral with another drug before checking with a pharmacist or other reliable reference to be sure no interaction will occur. The nurse also needs to check the expiration date to ensure that the vitamin or mineral preparation is effective. All parenteral vitamins and minerals need to be well diluted to decrease vessel irritation. Solutions of vitamins and minerals are discarded after 24 hours if they are not used.

Vitamin mixtures, particularly A, B_1, B_2, and B_6 are particularly light sensitive. Some authorities suggest that all IV bottles containing vitamin products should be covered with a UVF cover so the vitamins are not degraded by light (Kaminski, MV, 1985).

In order to administer vitamins and minerals to the patient safely, the following specific points must be followed by the nurse. Mineral oil should be avoided in all patients taking any of the fat-soluble vitamins. The margin of safety of vitamin D is quite narrow; therefore, individuals receiving therapeutic doses of vitamin D need close medical supervision and frequent laboratory work (serum calcium, phosphate, and urea; urinary calcium and albumin; and checks for the presence of casts and red blood cells in the urine every two weeks or more frequently). Patients need to be monitored to ensure they obtain sufficient amount of calcium to enhance the effectiveness of vitamin D. Vitamin D is best taken with food to avoid gastrointestinal upset and promote better absorption.

When the patient receives vitamin K, prothrombin activity of the blood must be measured frequently. The dosage of vitamin K is generally determined as a result of the laboratory work. Patients with biliary deficiencies who require oral vitamin K also require concomitant administration of bile salts to promote absorption of the vitamin. The nurse must be aware that some medications, including salicylates, oral antibiotics, quinidine, quinine, and sulfonamides, either inhibit or interfere with vitamin K activity. Vitamin K is taken with food to promote absorption and decrease gastrointestinal upset.

When a patient receives vitamin B_1 (thiamine), intradermal testing is recommended prior to intravenous administration to prevent anaphylactic reaction, although this is rarely done. When vitamin B_1 is given IM, sites are rotated and ice applied to reduce the pain associated with the injections. Thiamine is not mixed in alkaline or neutral solution, because it is unstable.

When vitamin B_2 (riboflavin) is being administered, the nurse informs the patient that large doses may color the urine an intense yellow.

Vitamin A is best taken with food, which helps stimulate bile secretion, thereby aiding absorption and reducing nausea. Also, patients are taught about foods high in vitamin A. Proper storage of foods prevents vitamin A loss; 5%–10% of vitamin A activity is lost when frozen foods are stored for twelve months at −23°C.

Niacin is generally administered with or shortly after meals to reduce the incidence of GI symptoms. Also, the nurse suggests to the patient that he or she sit down for approximately 30–60 minutes after receiving the medication to help eliminate dizziness and faintness, which are secondary to its vasodilating effect.

Mineral products are best taken immediately after meals to prevent gastrointestinal upset, except for zinc. Zinc is not taken concurrently with diary products; and in addition, zinc is not taken concurrently with a high-fiber diet, as fiber interferes with absorption. Liquid preparations are diluted well before administration to improve taste and decrease gastric irritation.

Fluoride rinses or gels used for dental prophylaxis are most effective if used immediately after brushing teeth and before bed time. The patient should not eat or drink for ½-hour after rinsing with fluoride.

PATIENT TEACHING

Many individuals have come to believe that just about any malady—from sexual difficulties to cancer—can be treated and cured with vitamin and mineral therapy. One has only to look at the growth of health food stores and current vitamin and mineral advertisements to see evidence of these beliefs. Just about every processed food is enriched with vitamins and minerals, from breakfast cereals to frozen dinners. Some individuals may begin self-treatment with megadose vitamins and minerals to cure a problem that should have medical attention. Approximately 75% of the public believes that vitamins will provide extra energy; however, no vitamin will produce a rapid burst of energy. Vitamin supplements are also not effective in protecting against emotional stress.

As an educator, the nurse has a responsibility to be aware of the various claims for vitamin therapy, to evaluate the existing research, and then to disseminate objective information to patients. During the intervention phase, the nurse emphasizes that diet is the treatment of choice—the four basic food groups—for vitamin and mineral deficiencies. Vitamins and minerals are best preserved by cooking foods in the smallest amount of water possible. Microwave cooking is an excellent way to preserve vitamins and minerals. Vitamins should not be used in place of a balanced diet. Additional patient teaching information appears in Table 57–7. Vitamins and minerals are taken until the initial deficiency is

---

Table 57–7. PATIENT TEACHING—VITAMINS AND MINERALS

Dear Patient:

This drug has been ordered for you. This is what you should know about your drug to get the most from your drug.

1. Vitamins and minerals are taken to return your own body levels to normal and to maintain that level.
2. Vitamins and minerals are taken until the initial deficiency is treated. Daily multivitamin/mineral products may then be taken for the rest of your life.
3. Vitamins and minerals can be taken with or between meals. Taking them with meals may prevent stomach upset. Mix liquids well to improve taste.
4. Vitamins and minerals can interfere with other medications. Check with your doctor or pharmacist before taking extra vitamins and minerals.
5. Vitamins and minerals can interfere with laboratory tests. Tell your doctor that you are taking vitamin and mineral products before blood or urine tests are done.
6. If you forget a dose, do not take it, but move on to the next dose.
7. Do not stop taking your vitamins and minerals without checking with your doctor.
8. Very large doses of vitamin C may cause stones to form in the urine.
9. Vitamins lose stability and become less potent as they age. Vitamins may lose as much as one third of their potency in 1 month and as much as 80% in 6 months. Look at expiration dates on vitamin bottles and do not buy large numbers of vitamins that will not be taken until many months later.
10. Read vitamin labels and buy the most inexpensive product that meets your needs. The Food and Drug Administration requires that all vitamin labels identify the amount of each ingredient and the amount of the Minimum Daily Requirements (MDR) in each tablet.
11. Megadoses, those that far exceed the MDR, have as yet not been proven to be helpful and may even be harmful.
12. Store vitamins and minerals in tight, light-resistant, dry containers.

treated. Daily multivitamin/mineral supplements may then need to be taken for life. Vitamins and minerals can be taken with or between meals. Vitamins and minerals can interfere with other medications, such as vitamin A and oral contraceptives; and 5 mg/day or more of vitamin B_6 (pyridoxine) may enhance the metabolism of levodopa (L-dopa), making it less effective in treating Parkinson's disease. Vitamins and minerals can interfere with laboratory tests. For example, vitamin K can falsely elevate urinary steroids; vitamin B_2 can cause false elevations of urinary catecholamines; and vitamin C may give false-positive glucose readings (proving dangerous for patients with diabetes). If a dose is forgotten, the patient should skip it and move on to the next dose. Medication should not be stopped without checking with the physician. Megadoses of vitamin C may enhance crystal formation in the urine, which may cause dysfunctions for the patient, including hypervitaminosis and hypermineralosis. Vitamins lose stability and become less potent as they age. Vitamins may lose as much as one third of their potency in one month and as much as 80% in six months. Expiration dates on vitamin bottles should be checked, and old vitamins should be discarded.

Vitamin labels should be read and the most inexpensive product that meets current dietary needs purchased. The Food and Drug Administration requires that all vitamin labels identify the amount of each ingredient and the proportion of the Minimum Daily Requirements (MDR) in each tablet.

The natural versus synthetic vitamin controversy continues to rage. Getting "back to nature" can be an expensive trip. For example, vitamin C derived from rose hips, acerola, cherries, or other "natural sources" (that are often fertilized and sprayed with pesticides) consistently costs at least five times more than synthesized molecules. Formulations containing "natural vitamins" generally contain synthetically derived fillers, binders, preservatives, dyes, and other products to stabilize the pill. Finally, the body cannot tell the difference between a molecule derived from a natural source and one that was synthesized; they are identical. Only the pocketbook will know for sure.

Megadoses, those that far exceed the MDR, have as yet not been proven to be helpful and may even be harmful. Vitamins that are the same as or only slightly higher than the RDA should be purchased.

All vitamins and minerals should be kept out of the reach of children. They should be stored in tight, light-resistant containers and protected from heat to prevent deterioration.

EVALUATION

The nurse bases the evaluation of the effectiveness of vitamin and mineral therapy on a predetermined list of evaluation criteria. These evaluation criteria are developed on an individual basis through discussion among the nurse, patient, and family during the planning phase. The nurse uses the information from the data base, obtained in the original assessment, to formulate the criteria for evaluation. Typical outcome criteria are included in Table 57–6.

The nurse evaluates the patient to determine if the patient is taking the proper dosage of vitamins and minerals. Several vitamins are commonly abused. For example, because the fat-soluble vitamins accumulate in the liver and adipose tissue, there is a far greater risk of overdosing on them than on the water-soluble vitamins. Vitamin A in large doses (over 25,000 IU/day for many months) eventually saturates the retinol stores and the patient begins to complain of nausea and headache. Pediatric clients are also more likely to develop toxicity.

Vitamin D in doses of 60,000 IU daily can cause toxicity with associated signs of hypercalcemia. In pediatric clients, vitamin D can result in supravalvular aortic stenosis.

Vitamin B_6 in massive doses (over 2,000 mg/daily) can cause reversible neurologic damage. Vitamin C, even in large doses, rarely causes toxicities in persons with normal renal function. However, if renal function is depressed, oxalate kidney stones may develop. Vitamin C, in any dose, can cause complications in persons taking anticoagulants.

The patient should know the side effects of his or her medications. If the patient notes an unusual symptom, he or she is encouraged to call the physician or nurse.

Before the patient leaves the nurse's care, all previously taught material is reviewed and updated, if necessary, to ensure that the patient's knowledge base remains accurate.

SUMMARY

A vitamin is a biologically active, organic compound. A mineral is a naturally occurring nonorganic homogenous solid substance. Both vitamins and minerals are essential for human health and growth. Vitamins and minerals, generally needed by the body in only small quanitites, are easily obtained from a well-balanced diet. Vitamins are either water-soluble, which are not stored as long in the body, or fat-soluble, which are stored in the body. Both vitamins and minerals are used to prevent and treat deficiency states.

When the nurse is going to administer vitamins and minerals, a thorough dietary and smoking history is obtained. Also, it is important to determine if vitamins and minerals supplements are being taken; and if so, in what dosage. There are specific implications for administering vitamins and minerals that the nurse needs to be aware of. For example, vitamin A is best administered with food; niacin is generally administered with or shortly after meals; minerals are best taken after meals; and zinc is not taken concurrently with a high-fiber diet. Vitamins lose stability and become less potent as they age. Natural vitamins are much more costly than synthetic vitamins, but the body does not know the difference. Megadosing, although a popular fad, has not as yet been proven to be helpful and may even be harmful.

BIBLIOGRAPHY

American Pharmaceutical Association: Handbook of Nonprescription Drugs, ed 7. American Pharmaceutical Association, Washington, DC, 1986.

Cerrato, PL: When to worry about vitamin overdose. RN 85(10):69, 1985.

Cerrato, PL: Would you miss these clues to a vitamin C deficiency? RN 86(9):69, 1986.

Cerrato, PL: Could you spot the other anemia? RN 86(11):63, 1986.

Cerrato, PL: Vitamin C: Who needs it? And when? RN: 85, 1985.

Cerrato, PL: Does the patient need extra vitamins? RN 87(10):123, 1987.

Covington, TR: Vitamins: Part I: Common myths. Facts and Comparisons Drug Newsletter 6(7):54, 1987.

Covington, TR: Vitamins: Part II: The fat-soluble vitamins. Facts and Comparisons Drug Newsletter 6(8):60, 1987.

Covington, TR: Vitamins: Part III. The water-soluble vitamins. Facts and Comparisons Drug Newsletter 6(9):68, 1987.

Gilman, AG, Goodman, LS, and Gilman, A (eds): Goodman and Gilman's The Pharmacological Basis of Therapeutics, ed 7. Macmillan, New York, 1985.

Goodhart, RS and Shils, ME (eds): Modern Nutrition in Health and Disease. Lea & Febiger, Philadelphia, 1986.

Hazards of nature's drugs vitamin and herbal preparations. Emerg Med 18(20):20, 1986.

Holmes, P: The value of vitamins. Nursing Times 83(16):31, 1987.

Kaminski, MV: Hyperalimentation. Marcel Dekker, New York, 1985.

Kee, JL: Fluids and Electrolytes With Clinical Applications: A Programmed Approach, ed 3. John Wiley & Sons, New York, 1982.

Kutsky, R: Handbook of Vitamins, Minerals and Hormones, ed 2. VanNostrand Reinhold, New York, 1981.

Nutritional Disorders. Nurses Reference Library, Springhouse Co, Springhouse, PA, 1983.

58 CHAPTER

MAJOR BODY ELECTROLYTES

GLOSSARY TERMS IN THIS CHAPTER

Active transport
Anion
Cation
Chvostek's sign
Electrolyte
Facilitated diffusion
Hypertonic
Hypotonic
Isotonic
Osmolality
Osmolarity
Oxalates
Passive transport
Phytates
Rhabdomyolysis
Trousseau's sign

58
CHAPTER

MAJOR BODY ELECTROLYTES

MERRILY MATHEWSON KUHN, R.N.C., Ph.D., CCRN

LEARNING OBJECTIVES

After reading this chapter, the student will be able to:

1. Identify major body electrolytes commonly used as medications and select those specific to the patient requiring electrolyte medications.

2. Identify specific areas to assess in the patient requiring electrolytes in order to formulate appropriate nursing diagnoses.

3. Determine the nursing interventions necessary to administer electrolytes and choose appropriate teaching strategies to gain patient compliance.

4. Evaluate the patient at various stages of treatment to gauge nursing interventions.

THERAPEUTIC AGENTS

Electrolytes are substances capable of dissociating in water into their component parts. Each part carries either a positive *(cation)* or a negative *(anion)* charge. Other substances in the body not capable of dissociating are nonelectrolytes. Table 58–1 lists the major body cations, anions, and nonelectrolytes.

Electrolytes are found in varying concentrations inside and outside the cell (Fig. 58–1). Substances are capable of moving from one location to another through two types of diffusion: (1) *passive transport*, which occurs when a substance moves by itself from an area of greater concentration to an area of lesser concentration; and (2) *facilitated diffusion*, which takes place with the help of a carrier substance, as when glucose moves into the cell with the assistance of insulin. Another way in which electrolytes move is by *active transport*, which occurs when a substance moves against a concentration gradient (toward an area of greater concentration). An example of active transport is cellular uptake of potassium.

This chapter reviews briefly the major electrolyte products and their nursing management. Electrolytes, their action, location, normal values, body regulation, dietary requirements, and other comments are reviewed in Table 58–2. Electrolyte imbalances, their etiologies, assessable clinical symptoms and pathophysiology, and their goals of management are featured in Table 58–3.

All electrolyte solutions are combination products; that is, they contain one cation for every anion. In order to prepare a solution, a stable solid composed of a combination salt such as KCl, $MgSO_4$, or NaCl is diluted in a vehicle. In order to make the solid stable, all of the cations must be neutralized by all of the anions.

SODIUM

Sodium is the major cation in the extracellular fluid (ECF). Normal serum sodium is 135–145 mEq/liter. Sodium maintains osmotic pressure and serum osmolarity; helps to maintain acid–base and water balance; contributes to nerve conduction and neuromuscular function; and plays a role in grandular secretions.

Table 58–1. MAJOR ELECTROLYTES AND NONELECTROLYTES

Electrolytes		
Cations	**Anions**	**Nonelectrolytes**
Sodium (NA$^+$)	Chloride (Cl$^-$)	Glucose
Potassium (K$^+$)	Phosphate	Proteins
Calcium (Ca^{+2})	(HPO$_4^-$)	Urea
Magnesium	Bicarbonate	Organic acid
(Mg^{2+})	(HCO$_3^-$)	Carbonic acid
	Sulfate (SO$_4^{-2}$)	

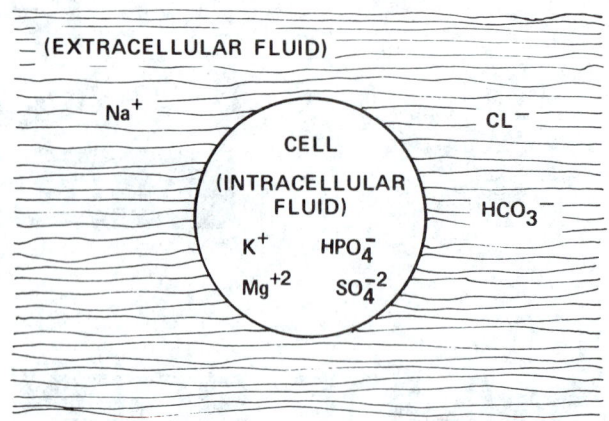

Figure 58–1. Electrolytes are found both inside and outside the cell in varying concentrations. The diagram shows where the major concentrations of each electrolyte are found.

Sodium, when taken orally, is readily absorbed in the small intestine. Small amounts are excreted through the kidneys and the skin. Sodium is regulated in the kidney by several hormones: aldosterone, ADH, and the third factor—a kidney tubular enzyme.

Sodium replacement is necessary when there is rapid loss of fluid in the body such as in diarrhea, vomiting, trauma, adrenal insufficiency, cirrhosis, inappropriate ADH secretion, and burns.

The most commonly used sodium preparation is sodium chloride. It is often used to correct an extracellular volume depletion. If oral intake is possible, table salt or sodium bicarbonate can be used for replacement. If IV replacement is necessary, several forms of sodium chloride are available.

Sodium Chloride

Solutions of sodium chloride are available as 0.45% *hypotonic* solution, 0.9% *isotonic* solutions, or as *hypertonic* solutions of 3% (513 mEq sodium/liter) or 5% (855 mEq sodium/liter). For discussion of these terms, refer to Chapter 11. Hypotonic solutions are administered (often with dextrose) for maintenance therapy in patients unable to take anything by mouth for three days or less. Isotonic solutions are infused when both sodium and water have been depleted in isotonic proportions. Isotonic solutions are used to maintain effective extravascular fluid volume and a stable circulation in many conditions. Hypertonic solutions are reserved for the treatment of severe symptomatic hyponatremia (serum sodium less than 120 mEq/liter) and only during the acute phase. In general, the hypertonic saline solutions are administered slowly to prevent fluid overload and the development of pulmonary edema. For additional information on IV solutions, see Chapter 11.

Sodium Bicarbonate

Sodium bicarbonate (Neut) is used as a systemic alkalizer to correct metabolic acidosis, which may occur secondary to diabetic ketoacidosis, shock, cardiac arrest,

Table 58–2. ELECTROLYTES

Electrolyte	Action in Body	Regulated by	Normal Values (mEq/liter)/ Location*	Daily Requirements	Comments
Sodium (Na^+)	Maintains osmotic pressure, and serum osmolarity. Helps to maintain acid–base balance, along with bicarbonate ion. Regulates fluid volume. Controls muscle contraction.	Kidney through aldosterone, ADH, glomular filtration rate, 3rd factor in kidney, tubular enzymes	135–145 E	500 mg	Na^+ competes with H^+ and K^+ in the renal tubule for excretion and absorption. 99% filtered Na^+ is reabsorbed in the kidney.
Potassium (K^+)	Maintains cellular osmolarity. Necessary for transmission of nerve impulses and for muscle contraction. Helps transform CHO into energy. Assists with reassembling amino acids into proteins. Maintains acid–base balance.	Kidney through glomular filtration rate, aldosterone	3.5–5.0 I	50–125 mEq	Kidney cannot conserve K^+, so it must be consumed daily. K^+ and H^+ move together in the kidney. If cellular K^+ is lowered, Na^+ enters the cell, making it more irritable.
Calcium (Ca^{+2})	Serves as framework for bones and teeth. Essential for blood clotting, for normal functioning of the central nervous system, and for muscle contraction and neuromuscular stability. Stabilizes cell membranes.	Parathyroid hormone, thyrocalcitonin, vitamin D, kidney function	8.5–10.0 total; 4.5–5.5 unbound. E	800 mg	Major concentration is in the bone. 50% of serum Ca^{+2} is bound to protein. Normal gastric acidity is necessary for absorption of Ca^{+2} in the gut. Acts as a sedative on body.
Magnesium (Mg^{+2})	Acts as coenzyme in metabolism of CHO and proteins. Regulates neuromuscular excitability and phosphate level, acts as a co-factor in ATPase maintenance.	Kidney function, parathyroid hormone	1.7–2.3 I	250 mg	Has a higher concentration in cerebrospinal fluid than in serum. 35% is bound to protein. Stored in bone, muscle, and soft tissue.
Chloride (Cl^-)	Regulates acid–base balance through chloride shift. Maintains resting membrane potential.	GI tract	95–106 I	6–15 mg	Chloride loss follows a Na^+ loss. Loss of Cl^- leads to increase in bicarbonate. Chloride is a functional acid.
Phosphate (HPO_4^-)	Acts as buffering agent for urine. Responsible for bone growth. Interacts with Hg in the red blood cell so as to promote oxygen release to tissues. Essential for metabolic processes such as ATP production. Promotes white blood cell's phagocytic action. Important in platelet structure and function.	Kidney function, parathyroid hormone, vitamin D	2.5–4.5 I	800–1300 mg	Stored in bone. Calcium and phosphate have a reciprocal relationship.
Bicarbonate (HCO_3^-)	Regulates acid–base balance. Acts as a buffer.	Pancreas, kidney, RBC, and lung function	22–26 E	—	Bicarbonate is produced in RBC, liberated through exchange with chloride, and then excreted by the kidney.

*E = extracellular; I = intracellular.

Table 58–3. MAJOR ELECTROLYTE DISTURBANCES

Imbalance	Laboratory Findings	Etiology	Assessable Clinical Symptoms	Pathophysiology	Goals of Nursing Management
Hyponatremia (sodium deficit and H_2O deficit = extra-cellular volume depletion)	Less than 137 mEq/liter serum Na. High specific gravity of urine, serum osm. normal	Excessive sweating, diarrhea, vomiting, gastric suction, potent diuretics, burns, decreased intake, ascites	Anorexia, nausea, mental confusion, giddiness, reduced blood volume, apprehension, increased blood viscosity, convulsions, decreased renal flow, pallid clammy skin, low blood pressure.	Vascular and cellular dehydration account for the symptoms observed.	Restore sodium concentration to normal levels.
Hyponatremia (sodium deficit and H_2O overload = hypoosmolar imbalance)	Less than 137 mEq/liter serum Na, Low specific gravity of urine, decreased serum osm.	Excessive ADH production (SIADH), renal disease	Headache, weakness, hyporeflexia, increased blood pressure, edema, hemodilution, abdominal cramps.	Decreased serum osm. causes H_2O to move into body cells, causing them to swell, resulting in listed symptoms.	Decreased ECF volume, diuretics, H_2O restriction, demeclocycline or lithium for SIADH. Hypertonic (3%–5%) saline solutions slowly if severe.
Hypernatremia (sodium excess and H_2O excess = extracellular volume excess)	Greater than 147 mEq/liter serum Na, less than normal specific gravity of urine	Impaired renal function, Cushing's syndrome, inhalation or ingestion of sea water	Increased urine output, increased temperature, edema, increased blood pressure, weight gain.	Extracellular fluid becomes hypertonic in relation to intracellular fluid, H_2O is thus pulled out of cells including skin & mucous membranes. Neural function is impaired due to cellular dehydration.	Diuretics, limit fluids.
Hypernatremia (sodium excess and water loss = hyperosmolar imbalance)	Greater than 147 mEq/liter serum Na, greater than normal urine specific gravity	Fever, decreased H_2O intake, diabetes mellitus or insipidus	Decreased urine, flushed skin, decreased blood pressure, thirst.	Same as above.	Restore sodium concentration to normal levels by: —diluting electrolyte concentration excess with balanced solution (5% or 10% Travert's with electrolytes) —administering D_5W if there is a true water deficit with no real change in electrolyte concentration.
Hypokalemia (potassium deficit)	Less than 3.5 mEq/liter	Excessive loss of K^+ from body, diuretic therapy, surgical intervention, trauma, metabolic disease, renal disease, intestinal tract diseases, excessive perspiration, excessive use by body, healing of burns, recovery from diabetic ketoacidosis, hyperinsulinism, and decreased intake of K^+	Skeletal muscle: weakness, fatigue, decreased reflexes. Heart muscle: weak pulse, low voltage T waves, S-T depression, predominant U waves, faint heart sounds, dysrhythmias. GI disturbances: vomiting. Shortness of breath, depression, mental clouding.	As extracellular K is lowered, intracellular K leaves the cells depressing cellular activity	Return serum potassium level to normal by administering: —diet high in potassium —special potassium replacement solutions (10% Travert's, KCl in 0.45% NaCl) —prophylactic potassium solutions (Lactated Ringer's solution) —K concentrates into any IV solution (available as KCl in a single-dose vial, or as KHPO$_4$ with 30 mEq of K in a single-dose vial).

Table 58–3. MAJOR ELECTROLYTE DISTURBANCES–*CONTINUED*

Imbalance	Laboratory Findings	Etiology	Assessable Clinical Symptoms	Pathophysiology	Goals of Nursing Management
Hyperkalemia (potassium excess)	Greater than 5.5 mEq/liter	Massive crushing injuries, early burns, hemolysis, renal disease, adrenal insufficiency, too much intake of K	Intestinal colic, diarrhea, irritability, nausea, dizziness, muscle weakness, cramps and pain, flaccid muscle paralysis, high peaked T waves on ECG, wide QRS. Seriously elevated serum potassium constitutes a medical emergency. Cardiac arrest may be imminent.	As extracellular K increases, more K moves into the cell causing increased irritability	Return serum potassium level to normal by: —reducing K intake —giving oral or IV hydrating solutions—giving dextrose and insulin infusions (20% dextrose solution with 1 unit of insulin for each 2 g of dextrose) —using extrarenal dialysis —giving binding resins (e.g., Kayexalate) —giving osmotic diarrheal (Sorbitol).
Hypocalcemia (calcium deficit)	Less than 8.5 mEq/liter	Hypoparathyroidism, acute pancreatitis, peritonitis, dietary lack of Ca, deficiency of vitamin D, burns, renal failure, hyperphosphatemia, osteomalacia, diuretic therapy	Abdominal cramps, muscle cramps, tetany, tingling of fingertips and circumoral area, numbness, laryngeal stridor, positive Chvostek's and Trousseau's signs, confusion, coarse dry skin, alopecia, tetany, ECG changes—prolonged Q-T interval.	As serum ionized calcium is lowered, there is increased neuromuscular activity (Ca^{2+} has a sedative effect on the body, producing hyperaction of motor and sensory nerves to stimuli.)	Return calcium level to normal by administering: —isotonic 0.9% NaCl solution with calcium additives (calcium gluconate, calcium chloride —oral Ca with additional vitamin D —parathyroid hormone 100–200 units given every 4–6 hr during acute episode.
Hypercalcemia (calcium excess)	Greater than 10.5 mEq/liter	Hyperparathyroidism, renal disease, immobilization, vitamin D intoxication, neoplastic disease of bone, breast, and lungs, Paget's disease, Addison's disease, milk-alkali syndrome, sarcoidosis	Anorexia, nausea, weight loss, bone loss resulting in deep bone pain, kidney stones, muscle hypotonicity, lethargy, azotemia, EKG—AV block.	As serum calcium rises, there is depression of all neuromuscular activity and increased myocardial irritability. Excess serum levels cause nephrolithiasis and kidney loses its ability to concentrate urine. Increased calcium ions in sympathetic ganglia impedes transmission of impulses within GI system	Return calcium level to normal through administration of: —isotonic 0.9% NaCl solution to cause saline diuresis and flush excess Ca from kidney (assess for fluid overload) —phosphate (PO, rectal, IV) to bind with Ca and move it back to bone— corticosteroids (150–200 mg IV hydrocortisone or 20–80 mg PO prednisone), which antagonize vitamin D, causing more Ca to be lost in gut (takes about 7 days to work) —EDTA (disodium salt) 50 mg/kg IV over 4–6 hr, which binds with calcium and excreted by kidneys (works immediately) —calcium-free solutions like Plasmalyte if other fluid imbalances are being corrected.

CONTINUED ON THE FOLLOWING PAGE

Table 58–3. MAJOR ELECTROLYTE DISTURBANCES–CONTINUED

Imbalance	Laboratory Findings	Etiology	Assessable Clinical Symptoms	Pathophysiology	Goals of Nursing Management
Hypomagnesemia (magnesium deficit)	Less than 1.5 mEq/liter	Impaired absorption or intake—alcoholism, small bowel bypass, malnutrition, increased loses, diabetic ketoacidosis, diuretic therapy, renal disease	CNS agitation, positive Chvostek's and Trousseau's signs, tachycardia, increased BP, ventricular dysrhythmias, EKG changes, depressed ST, prolonged QT.	As intracellular Mg^{+2} decreases, its ability to act at the neuromuscular junction like acetylcholine is reduced leading to increased irritability throughout the body. There is also decreased cardiac muscle function	Increase magnesium-containing foods (chlorophyll foods), IV magnesium (Mg sulfate).
Hypermagnesemia (magnesium excess)	Greater than 2.5 mEq/liter	Renal disease, overuse of magnesium-containing antacids	Hypoflexia, hypotension, cardiac dysrhythmias, weakness, coma, respiratory arrest.	As extracellular Mg^{+2} increases, activity at the neuromuscular synapse like acetylcholine is increased and acts as a sedative particularly on the respiratory system	Return serum level to normal by: —peritoneal or hemodialysis —elimination of magnesium-containing antacids. For magnesium toxicity, administer 10% calcium gluconate slowly IV.
Hypophosphatemia (phosphate deficit)	Less than 2.5 mEq/liter	Familial disease, prolonged hyperalimentation with phosphate-free solution, osteomalacia, rickets, alcoholism, alkalosis	Hemolytic anemia; lethargy; weakness, especially respiratory muscles; mental confusion.	As extracellular HPO_4^- is reduced, there is less formation of nucleic acid within cells and diminished ATP and 2,3-DPG	Return serum phosphate level to normal by administering phosphate in combination with sodium or potassium.
Hyperphosphatemia (phosphate excess)	Greater than 4.5 mEq/liter	Renal failure, acute/chronic poisoning with insecticides, rodent poison, or fertilizers	Abdominal cramps, muscle cramps, tetany, tingling of fingertips and circumoral area, numbness, laryngeal stridor, positive Chvostek's and Trousseau's signs, confusion, coarse dry skin, alopecia, tetany, ECG changes—prolonged Q-T interval.	As HPO_4^- increases, extracellularly, there is a lowering of serum Ca^{+2}, which precipitates symptoms associated with hypocalcemia	Return phosphate level to normal by administering: —aluminum or calcium antacids to bind with phosphate —gastric lavage with 0.1% copper sulfate solution, which binds with phosphate if it is done within 5 hrs of ingestion of phosphate.
Bicarbonate deficit (metabolic acidosis, primary alkali deficit)	Less than 20 mEq/liter bicarbonate; less than 7.35 pH blood; less than 6 pH urine	Renal disease, diabetic acidosis, lactic acidosis, administration of acidifying acids, Addison disease, diarrhea, shock, salicylate poisoning	Weakness, stupor, shortness of breath, deep, rapid breathing (Kussmaul).	Due to increased concentration of acids in the serum, HCO_3^- is used as a buffer and levels decrease causing an acidotic state to occur. Also, as acidosis occurs, more Ca^{+2} becomes ionized; therefore symptoms of hypercalcemia occur	Return bicarbonate level to normal by: —correcting underlying pathology —administering bicarbonate IV (1 amp for every —5 Base Excess the bicarbonate is below normal) (Base excess is the base not neutralized by acid).
Bicarbonate excess (metabolic alkalosis, primary alkali excess)	Greater than 29 mEq/liter bicarbonate; greater than 7.45 pH blood; greater than 7.0 pH urine, less than 4 mEq/liter potassium	Excessive ingestion of bicarbonate, GI suction, vomiting, potent diuretics, K^+ deficit	Hyperactive reflexes, tetany, convulsions, depressed breathing.	The increased HCO_3^- level causes more Ca^{+2} to be bound; therefore, there is a lowering of serum Ca^{+2}, resulting in associated hypocalcemia symptoms. As alkalosis develops, more K^+ is lost in the urine and therefore an associated hypokalemia results	Return bicarbonate level to normal by: —correcting underlying pathology —providing nonbicarbonate ions (Cl), which can be retained in place of bicarbonate.

and vascular collapse. Sodium bicarbonate is rarely administered today unless the pH is less than 7.1–7.0. An intravenous bolus of 200–300 mEq as a 7.5%–8.4% solution can be administered rapidly; or, an intravenous infusion of 2–5 mEq/kg over four to eight hours can be administered. Sodium bicarbonate is featured in Table 58–4.

POTASSIUM

Potassium is the most important intracellular cation. Ninety-eight percent of all potassium is found in intracellular fluid while only 2% is found in extracellular fluid. Normal plasma concentrations range from 3.5–5.0 mEq/liter. Potassium has many functions. Potassium assists with the regulation of intracellular osmolality and is necessary for cellular growth and metabolism. Potassium helps to maintain acid–base balance and enzyme action necessary to change carbohydrates into energy and to reassemble amino acids into protein. Potassium is also necessary for proper function of skeletal, cardiac, and smooth muscle.

Normally, 40 mEq of potassium is required each day; potassium cannot be stored in the body, so it must be consumed each day. Eighty percent to 90% of the ingested potassium is excreted in the urine under the influence of aldosterone. Ten percent to 20% is excreted in the stool. The kidney can conserve potassium to some degree when cellular potassium becomes depleted.

Potassium is moved into the cells when glucose is metabolized, during beta-adrenergic stimulation, and during alkalosis. Potassium moves out of the cells during strenuous exercise, when cellular metabolism is impaired, when cells die, and during acidosis. When potassium is lost from cells, sodium and hydrogen ion shift into the cells to replace the lost potassium. This makes the cells more acid while the extracellular fluid becomes more alkaline.

Hypokalemia

Potassium deficits are likely to occur when there is inadequate intake of potassium through the diet, such as in patients with nausea, anorexia, extreme dieting, or in acute alcoholism. Also, potassium deficits can occur in patients maintained on intravenous therapy with low potassium levels. Potassium deficits can also occur when potassium utilization is increased during the healing phase of burns. Potassium deficits may also occur secondary to excessive loss of potassium such as in vomiting, diarrhea, fistulas, or secondary to therapies such as diuretics, antibiotics, corticosteroids, or nasogastric suction.

A host of symptoms threatens when the patient's potassium level deviates from the normal range. The variety of potential problems reflects the importance of potassium. As the potassium is decreased, the symptoms include weakness, speech changes, flaccid paralysis, shallow respirations, decreased intestinal motility, abdominal distention, anorexia, and paralytic ileus all due to decreased neuromuscular irritability. Dysrhythmias, a slow, weak, irregular pulse, hypotension, low flat T

waves, and U waves on the ECG (Fig. 58–2), and cardiac arrest are all related to weakness of the cardiovascular smooth muscle and prolongation of myocardial repolarization. Polyuria and nocturia are related to the inability of the kidney to concentrate urine.

Potassium Preparations

CONTRAINDICATIONS AND PRECAUTIONS. Potassium products are contraindicated in severe renal impairment, such as with early postoperative oliguria, anuria, and oliguria; acute crushing injuries; Addison's disease; and acute dehydration, as all these conditions are prone to developing hyperkalemia. All potassium products are given cautiously to persons with cardiac disease, particularly digitalized patients, as there is increased risk of hyperkalemic adverse effects.

ADVERSE EFFECTS. Potassium products may cause adverse effects including nausea, vomiting, gastrointestinal disturbances, cardiac dysrhythmias, and muscle weakness. The local gastrointestinal effects can be reduced by diluting oral potassium products even further or by taking them with meals. Local tissue necrosis can also occur if extravastion occurs. Local infiltration of the affected area with 1% procaine hydrochloride with hyaluronidase will often reduce venospasm and dilute the potassium remaining in the tissues locally. Local application of heat may also be helpful.

INTERACTIONS. Potassium products are not given concurrently with potassium-sparing diuretics such as spironolactone, triamterene, or amiloride, as hyperkalemia can result. Captopril and enalapril may cause potassium retention due to lowering circulating aldosterone levels. Hyperkalemia can result in one to two days. Concurrent administration with anticholinergics, which slow gastrointestinal motility, can increase the likelihood of gastrointestinal erosion when solid potassium products are administered concurrently. In addition, there are drugs (anorexiants, flecainide, mecamylamine, quinidine, quinine, and sympathomimetics) that decrease the excretion of potassium and thus increase the pharmacologic effects. There are also drugs (chlorpropamide, lithium, methotrexate, salicylates, and tetracyclines) that increase the excretion of potassium and thus decrease its pharmacologic effects.

DOSAGE. Several salts of potassium are available for administration. These products vary in the amount of potassium they contain. Potassium preparations can be given orally, either for prevention of hypokalemia, as in a patient receiving diuretics, or for the actual treatment of hypokalemia (see Table 58–4). Potassium salts come in liquid form, as tablets—both enteric-coated and wax matrix, in fizz tablets, or as powders that can be dissolved in water. Tablets are coated to prevent irritation to the stomach. Time-release products are also available (Table 58–5).

Potassium preparations for IV use come in vials of 10, 20, 30, 40, 60, 90, and 120 mEq per single-dose vial. These vials are diluted in IV solution and given slowly into a large vein to prevent irritation. (A large vein,

TEXT RESUMES ON PAGE 1614

Table 58–4. PREPARATIONS AVAILABLE FOR USE IN TREATING SODIUM AND POTASSIUM IMBALANCES

Name	Dosage	Mode of Administration	Pharmacokinetics
Sodium bicarbonate (Neut)			
Action: essential electrolyte for maintaining serum osmolality and acid–base balance.			
Use: treatment of metabolic acidosis.			
	200–300 mEq as 7.5–8.4% solution.	IV bolus	O: rapid
	2–5 mEq/kg over 4–8 hr.	IV infusion.	P: 15 min
			D: 1–2 hr
			½L: UA
			PB: UA
			B: UA
			E: urine
Tromethamine (Tham, Tham E)			
Action: acts as a proton acceptor, combines with H^+ ion to form HCO_3, acts as osmotic diuretic.			
Use: prevention or correction of systemic acidosis.			
	0.5–0.9 ml/kg	IV	
FOR HYPOKALEMIA:			
Potassium Products			
Action: essential electrolyte for maintaining intracellular tonicity, muscle contraction, and renal function.			
Use: prevention and/or correction of moderate to severe potassium deficiency.			
Potassium Chloride USP (for specific listing of oral products see Table 58–5) (1 gm KCl = 13.41 mEq K)	Adults: 20 mEq/day. Adults: 40–100 mEq/day. Children: 1–3 mEq/kg/day. Adults: 40–300 mEq/day.	PO (prevention) PO (treatment) PO (treatment) IV	
Potassium gluconate, NF (Kalinate, Kaon) 1 gm potassium gluconate = 4.27 mEq K)	Adults: 5–20 mEq 2–4 × daily. Children: 20–40 mEq/m² in divided doses.	PO	
Potassium bicarbonate (K-lyte)	25–50 mEq daily. 1–2 times daily.	PO	
Potassium phosphate (Neutra-Phos-K)	1 cap mixed with 75 ml water.	PO	

Key to Abbreviations in the *Pharmacokinetics* column O-onset; P-peak; D-duration; PB-protein bound; B-bio-transformed in; E-excreted in; ½ L-halflife.

*Within the column of adverse effects, underlines indicate the most common effects; CAPITALS indicate life-threatening effects.

Contraindications/ Precautions	Adverse Effects*	Interactions	Nursing Implications
Contraindicated in severe vomiting and patients receiving diuretics known to produce hypochoremic alkalosis; metabolic and respiratory alkalosis; hypocalcemia. Use with caution in impaired renal function, congestive heart failure, edematous states.	Neuro: headache, dizziness GI: abdominal cramps, nausea, vomiting Renal: fluid retention Misc: alkalosis, tetany, hypokalemia	Do not mix with calcium, dopamine, dobutamine as precipitation may occur. Increases renal clearance of tetracyclines and doxycyline. Increases half-life of quinidine, amphetamines, ephedrine, and pseudoephedrine.	ASSESSMENT: Assess serum sodium level before and during therapy. INTERVENTION: Administer slowly IV. If extravasation occurs, infiltrate area with lidocaine or hyaluronidase.
Contraindicated in anuria, uremia. Use with caution in patients with respiratory depression and impaired renal function.	Resp: depression Misc: febrile response, infection and phlebitis at injection site	None known.	Same as sodium bicarbonate
Contraindicated in renal impairment, crushing injuries, and increased digitalis levels. Use cautiously in cardiac disease and acidosis.	CV: hyperkalemia, dysrhythmia GI: nausea, vomiting, abdominal pain, diarrhea, ulcers Integ: local tissue necrosis	Concurrent administration of K penicillin, ACE inhibitors, NSAIDS, and amloride may cause hyperkalemia. Anorexiants, flecainide, mecamylamine, quinidine, quinine, and sympathomimetics may increase effects of potassium. Chlorpropamide, lithium, methotrexate, salicylates, and tetracyclines may decrease effects of potassium.	ASSESSMENT: Assess baseline potassium level, urine output, and EKG and then periodically during therapy. INTERVENTION: Administer PO with meals, may be irritating to GI tract. Dilute products well in ½–1 glass of water and sip over 5–10 minutes. Do not chew or crush tablets. Teach patient that the wax-matrix tablet may be found in the stool but that the medication has been absorbed. Teach patients about foods high in potassium. Do not give until urine flow is re-established in postoperative period. Give IV into large vein slow. Never give IV push or IM. Always dilute before IV administration. Administer

CONTINUED ON THE FOLLOWING PAGE

Table 58–4. PREPARATIONS AVAILABLE FOR USE IN TREATING SODIUM AND POTASSIUM IMBALANCES

Name	Dosage	Mode of Administration	Pharmacokinetics
Potassium Products–Continued			
FOR HYPERKALEMIA: Sodium polystyrene sulfo- nate (Kayexalate)			
Action: exchange sodium for potassium in the intestine.			
Use: lowers serum potassium levels in 2–24 hours.			
	Adults: 15–60 g/day (4 level tsp 1–4 ×/day in 20–100 ml sorbitol). Children: 1 mEq/g of resin.	PO, rectal enema	

Key to Abbreviations in the *Pharmacokinetics* column O-onset; P-peak; D-duration; PB-protein bound; B-bio-transformed in; E-excreted in; ½ L-halflife.

*Within the column of adverse effects, underlines indicate the most common effects; CAPITALS indicate life-threatening effects.

Contraindications/ Precautions	Adverse Effects*	Interactions	Nursing Implications
			no faster than 10 mEq/ hour. Always add to new IV, not in a hanging position. Do not mix potassium in an IV solution that contains calcium or magnesium as a precipitate will occur. EVALUATION: Evaluate for signs of hyperkalemia, increased fatigue, muscle weakness, cramps, nausea, vomiting, or black stools. Evaluate ECG and serum potassium periodically. Evaluate T and QRS wave changes on the ECG. These herald potassium toxicity and impending cardiac arrest.
Contraindicated in sodium restriction. Use cautiously in congestive heart failure, renal disease, edema, and the elderly.	CV: hypokalemia, hypocalcemia, sodium retention GI: gastric irritation, anorexia, nausea, vomiting, constipation, diarrhea, fecal impaction	Concurrent use of antacids containing mg/calcium causes binding and may result in metabolic alkalosis.	ASSESSMENT: Assess potassium and sodium serum level frequently. INTERVENTION: Watch for sodium overload. Use only fresh suspensions. Stir before use. Mix with water or syrup. Check for constipation. Do not expose to heat. For retention enema: Use warm fluid to prepare emulsion. Keep particles in suspension by continuous stirring. Flush suspension with 50–100 ml of fluid, then clamp tube and leave it in place. Urge patient to retain enema for 30–60 minutes or longer if possible. If leakage occurs, elevate hips on pillow or place patient temporarily in knee-chest position. After enema has been expelled, irrigate colon with 1–2 quarts of flushing solution. Allow drainage to return constantly through a Y tube connection.

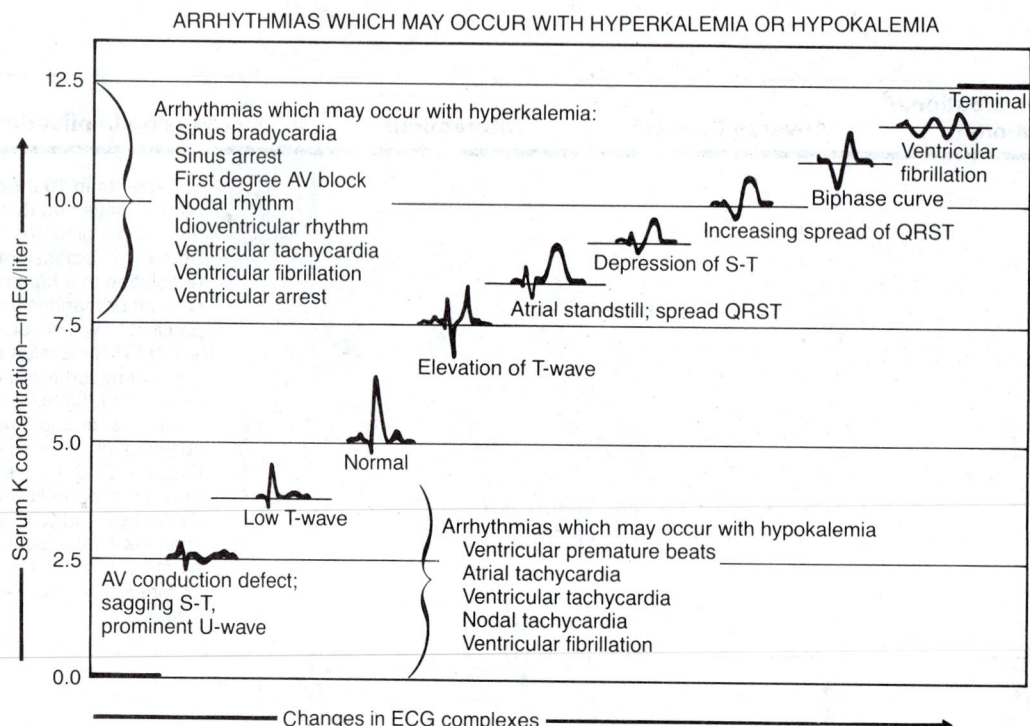

Figure 58–2. ECG changes at various levels of serum potassium concentration. (Used with permission from Krupp, MA, Chatton, MJ (eds): Current Medical Diagnosis and Treatment. Lange Medical Publications, Los Altos, CA, 1974.)

while not absolutely necessary, is recommended.) The usual maintenance dose is 20 mEq/day, while the treatment dose can be 40–100 mEq/day. Generally, the maximum IV concentration is 40 mEq/liter at a rate of 10 mEq/hour, except in life-threatening hypokalemia, when an ECG can be taken continuously and concentrations of up to 40 mEq/hour can be administered.

While administering potassium products, the patient is monitored closely for changes in heart rate and urinary output. Potassium is not administered until urinary output is established. When hypokalemia is associated with alkalosis, use potassium chloride products. When acidosis is present, use bicarbonate, acetate, or gluconate potassium salts.

POTASSIUM CHLORIDE. Since chloride depletion often occurs along with a potassium loss, these substances are frequently administered together as potassium chloride (Kaochlor, Slow K, and many others). These products are most often used concurrently when patients are taking potassium-depleting diuretics. Potassium chloride as an intravenous product contains 13.4 mEq/g. It is generally used for intravenous replacement of potassium with 40 mEq/liter administered at a rate of 10 mEq/hour. Potassium chloride products are available as liquids, soluble powders, and effervescent tablets (Table 58–5). Effervescent tablets should be diluted with a full glass of water or juice and drunk slowly. Tablets are not chewed or crushed but swallowed whole. Potassium is also available as a wax-matrix tablet. The tablet is not absorbed and is found in the stool.

POTASSIUM BICARBONATE. Potassium bicarbonate (K-lyte) has 10 mEq of potassium per gram. Potassium bicarbonate is available as an oral solution or as effervescent tablets. An oral dose of 25–50 mEq is dissolved in one half to a whole glass of cold water either one or two times daily.

POTASSIUM GLUCONATE. Potassium gluconate (Kaon) has 4.3 mEq of potassium per gram and is used to replace potassium levels. Usual dose is 5–20 mEq two to four times daily.

POTASSIUM PHOSPHATE. Potassium phosphate (Neutra-Phos-K) has either 14.25 mEq of potassium and 250 mg of phosphate for the oral form or 14.5 mEq of potassium and 935 mg of phosphate for the intravenous form. Potassium phosphate can be used to treat both potassium and phosphate deficiencies. The oral capsule is emptied and mixed with 75 ml of cold water.

Hyperkalemia

Hyperkalemia is indicated when the serum potassium level is above 5.5 mEq/liter. Hyperkalemia has three major etiologies: retention of potassium within the body primarily due to poor renal function or adrenocortical insufficiency; excessive release of potassium from the cells such as in patients with serious burns, traumatic injuries, infection, and acidosis; and excessive intravenous infusion of potassium-containing fluids even with normal renal function.

Assessment findings of hyperkalemia include intestinal colic, diarrhea, muscle twitching proceeding to

Table 58–5. ORAL POTASSIUM AND CHLORIDE PREPARATIONS

Trade Name	Potassium (mEq)*	Chloride (mEq)*
Liquid Products		
Kaochlor 10% Liquid†‡	20	20
Kaochlor S-F 10% Liquid†‡	20	20
Kaon-Cl 20%†	40	40
Kay Ciel†	20	20
Klorvess 10%†	20	20
Rum-K	30	30
SK-Potassium Chloride†	20	20
Effervescent Products§		
Klorvess Effervescent Granules	20	20
Klorvess	20	20
K-Lyte/Cl	25	25
K-Lyte/Cl 50	50	50
Time-Release Products¶		
Kaon Cl‡	6.7	6.7
Kaon Cl-10	10	10
Klotrix	10	10
K-Tab	10	10
Micro-K	8	8
Micro-K 10	10	10
Slow-K**	8	8

*Per 15 ml, packet, or tablet.
†Contains alcohol.
‡Contains tartrazine, which may cause allergic reactions.
§Most effervescent formulas are sugar-free. Completely dissolve and allow "fizzing" to stop, then sip slowly over a 5–10-minute period.
¶Time-release products reduce the danger of bowel ulceration and potential complications.
**Slow K uses a wax matrix as a carrier for the crystals. After absorption, the tablet carcass appears in the stool. There is no cause for alarm.

skeletal muscle weakness, flaccid paralysis, and cardiac dysrhythmias. These are related to increased neuromuscular irritability in mild hyperkalemia and reduced neuromuscular irritability in more severe hyperkalemia. There is also altered cardiac muscle function.

PRODUCTS TO MANAGE HYPERKALEMIA. When the potassium level rises above 6.5 mEq/liter or there are significant ECG changes (See Fig. 58–2), treatment is instituted. Several treatment modalities are available. A 5%–10% dextrose IV solution with 10–15 units of regular insulin redistributes potassium from the plasma to the cells. The insulin causes potassium to enter the cells, while glucose prevents hypoglycemia caused by the insulin. The addition of sodium bicarbonate elevates blood pH, causing alkalosis, which in turn promotes potassium movement into the cells in exchange for hydrogen ion. The additional amount of sodium also promotes potassium excretion.

Sodium Polystyrene Sulfonate. The exchange resin—sodium polystyrene (Kayexalate)—given orally or by rectum (Table 58–4) promotes the excretion of potassium by acting as an exchange resin. Oral therapy takes several hours to work, but an enema effectively lowers the serum potassium level in about one hour.

CALCIUM

Calcium, the fifth most common element in the body, is primarily stored in the bones. The normal serum calcium level is rather narrow, 8.6–10.5 mEq/dl. Calcium is necessary to support neuromuscular transmission, to promote muscle cell and cardiac contraction, to provide a component for coagulation, to promote normal neuromuscular irritability, to build bones and teeth, to assist with the secretion of many hormones, and to strengthen cell membranes.

The daily adult requirement for calcium is at least 0.8 g. Infants and children require 0.17–1.4 g/day, while pregnant and lactating women require 1.3–1.5 g/day. Calcium is primarily supplied in the American diet by milk and milk products, with a small amount being supplied by vegetables and fruit. Dietary calcium is absorbed in the gut in the presence of vitamin D. Calcium is controlled by parathyroid hormone (PTH). When serum calcium levels are increased, PTH is decreased, causing increased excretion of calcium in the urine and decreased gastrointestinal absorption. When serum calcium levels are decreased, PTH is increased, causing a decreased calcium loss in the urine and increased bone resorption.

Hypocalcemia

Hypocalcemia can occur when there is excessive loss or removal of calcium from the body, which can result from acute pancreatitis, hypoparathyroidism, and renal disorders. Hypocalcemia can also occur secondary to damage or removal of the thyroid, resulting in parathyroid dysfunction. Hypocalcemia can also occur when there is inadequate intake of vitamin D, following the correction of acidosis, or during alkalosis as more calcium is bound to protein.

Assessment findings in hypocalcemia include tingling and numbness of the fingers and circumoral region; painful tonic muscle spasms; fatigue; a positive *Trousseau's* and *Chvostek's* sign; facial spasms; laryngospasm; and convulsions. All these symptoms are related to increased neuromuscular irritability producing hyperaction of motor and sensory nerves to stimuli. Changes in the ECG and dysrhythmias occur due to altered cardiac muscle function.

Calcium Preparations

Calcium products are available orally or intravenously for prevention or treatment of hypocalcemia, and to relieve hypocalcemic tetany. Calcium products are often administered as nutritional supplements during pregnancy and lactation and for postmenopausal osteoporosis (Table 58–6).

PHARMACOKINETICS. Oral calcium is readily absorbed from the duodenum and proximal jejunum in the presence of PTH and vitamin D. Absorption is also dependent on dietary factors. Calcium can bind to fiber, *phytates, oxalates,* and fatty acids to form insoluble non-

Table 58–6. CALCIUM PRODUCTS

Name	Dosage	Mode of Administration
Action: maintains functional integrity of nervous and muscular systems.		
Use: to treat hypocalcemia, overdose of magnesium and potassium.		
Calcium gluconate (Kalcinate)	Adults: 5–20 ml daily in 10% solution, not to exceed 0.5 ml/min.	IV
	Children: 500 mg/kg/day, in divided doses.	IV
	Tablets: (9% Ca^{2+}) 11 g/day in divided doses, best after meals.	PO
Calcium chloride USP	Adults: 500 mg–1 g in 0.5% solution slowly, not to exceed 1 ml/min.	IV
	Children: 25 mg/kg administered slowly.	
Calcium lactate USP	(13% Ca^{2+}) 325–650 mg 3–4 × daily.	PO with meals, dissolved in hot water
Calcium gluceptate	5–20 ml, 1 ml or less/min.	IV
	2–5 ml	IM
Calcium glubionate	Syrup: (6.5% Ca^{2+}) 5 ml 3–4 times daily with full glass of water.	PO
Calcium citrate (Citracal)	(21% Ca^{2+}) 1–2 tablets 3–4 times daily 1–2 hr after meals.	PO
Calcium carbonate (Calci-Chew, OsCal, BioCal, and others)	500 mg 2–4 times daily 1–2 hrs after meals.	PO

*Within the column of adverse effects, underlines indicate the most common effects; CAPITALS indicate life-threatening effects.

absorpable soaps. Calcium is excreted primarily (80%) in the feces and the rest in the urine.

CONTRAINDICATIONS AND PRECAUTIONS. Calcium products are given cautiously to patients with renal disease and to patients receiving cardiac glycosides, as they potentiate the therapeutic and toxic effects of digitalis. Intravenous calcium is contraindicated in ventricular fibrillation occurring during cardiac resuscitation.

ADVERSE EFFECTS. Adverse effects caused by calcium products include constipation, decreased excitability of the nerves and muscles, and mental confusion, as calcium acts as a sedative on the body, and kidney stones, as excess calcium is filtered and excreted by the kidney. Rapid IV administration can cause peripheral vasodilation and a local burning sensation. Local severe tissue necrosis, sloughing, and abscesses may occur following intramuscular or subcutaneous injection of calcium.

INTERACTIONS. The combination of calcium and digitalis products or administration of calcium to the digitalized patient may precipitate dysrhythmias. Calcium may antagonize the effects of verapamil. However, intravenous calcium chloride has been used as an antidote for verapamil-induced hypotension. Phenytoin and iron salts have decreased absorption when given concurrently with calcium. Calcium carbonate increases urinary pH, which can increase the pharmacologic effect of quinidine and decrease the pharmacologic effects of salicylates. Oral tetracycline levels are decreased with concurrent calcium. Thiazide diuretics may precipitate hypercalcemia, especially in persons with abnormal calcium metabolism. Dietary fiber decreases absorption by complexing with calcium and decreasing transit time in the gastrointestinal tract.

ORAL PRODUCTS. The oral forms of calcium are usually administered three to four times daily. They are best administered during or after meals or with milk to

Contraindications/ Precautions	Adverse Effects*	Interactions	Nursing Implications
For all: Contarindicated in hyper-calcemia, renal calculi, and in ventricular fibrilla-tion during cardiac resuscitation. Use cau-tiously in patients receiv-ing cardiac glycosides (such as digoxin) and in those with renal disease.	For all: Neuro: heat waves in body CV: bradycardia, peripheral vasodilatation, hypotension GI: metallic taste, constipa-tion Renal: calculi Integ: mild local reactions, severe tissue necrosis, phlebitis at IV site	For all: Enhance effects of digoxin; decrease effects of tetracy-cline (these drugs should not be given orally together). Antagonized cal-cium channel blockers. Incompatible in solution with carbonates, phos-phates, sulfates, and tar-trates. Phenytoin and iron salts have decreased absorption. Calcium car-bonate increases urinary pH, which increases phar-macologic effect of quini-dine and decreases phar-macologic effect of salicylates. Increased dietary fiber decreases absorption.	For all: ASSESSMENT: Assess baseline EKG (QT interval), serum calcium level, muscle tone, and presence of Chvostek's and Trous-seau's signs and monitor throughout therapy. INTERVENTION: Carefully monitor IV to avoid infiltra-tion. If infiltration occurs, infiltrate area with 1% pro-caine and hyaluronidase and apply warm, moist compresses. Monitor digi-talized patient carefully when giving calcium, as cal-cium increases risk of digi-talis toxicity. Do not put cal-cium in same IV bottle with bicarbonate, as a precipi-tate may form. Teach patient who is hypocalcemic to increase intake of foods rich in calcium and vitamin D to enhance calcium absorption. Inject calcium gluceptate IM into gluteal region in adults or lateral thigh in children. After injecting calcium, keep patient recumbent for 15 minutes. EVALUATION: Evaluate ECG for QT changes and for signs of hypercalcemia.

avoid gastric upset. Many over-the-counter products are marketed today with various concentrations of calcium to prevent osteoporosis. Recent research indicates that calcium in any form, alone, does not prevent osteopo-rosis, but that co-administration of estrogen during and after menopause does help prevent osteoporosis.

Calcium Glubionate. Calcium glubionate (Neo-Cal-glucon) contains 6.5% calcium in a syrup that contains 115 mg of calcium in every 5 ml. It is best taken with a full glass of water.

Calcium Gluconate. Calcium gluconate (Calcet, Kal-cinate) is 9% calcium. Tablets are best administered after meals.

Calcium Lactate. Calcium lactate contains 13% cal-cium. Calcium lactate tablets are best used as a supplement.

Calcium Citrate. Calcium citrate (Citracal) is 21% calcium. Calcium citrate is better absorbed from the gas-trointestinal tract than calcium carbonate. Tablets are administered one to two hours after meals three to four times daily.

Calcium Carbonate. Calcium carbonate (Calci-Chew, OsCal, BioCal, and many others) is 40% calcium. Calcium carbonate is the most efficient form of calcium available as both a regular and a chewable tablet. Five hundred milligrams is generally administered two to four times daily one to two hours after meals.

INTRAVENOUS PRODUCTS. When administering intravenous calcium products, care must be taken that the needle does not slip out of the vein. If calcium salts infiltrate, they may cause serious tissue irritation. The IV preparations begin their action immediately and con-tinue for one to two hours. The most potent calcium re-placement preparations are calcium chloride (1 g = 13.6 mEq calcium), calcium gluceptate (1 g = 4.5 mEq), and calcium gluconate (1 g = 4.5 mEq).

Calcium Chloride. Calcium chloride is administered slowly, not to exceed 1 ml/minute.

Calcium Gluceptate. Calcium gluceptate can be administered either intravenously in doses of 5–20 ml or intramuscularly in doses of 2–5 ml in the gluteal region in adults or in the lateral thigh in infants.

Calcium Gluconate. Calcium gluconate (Kalcinate) is administered slowly at a rate not to exceed 0.5 ml/minute. Adults may receive 1–15 g/day while children are given 500 mg/kg/day in divided doses. Calcium gluconate can also be given to treat magnesium toxicity in doses of 4.5–10 mEq intravenously slowly.

Hypercalcemia

Serum calcium acts as a sedative on the body. As serum calcium rises above 11 mg/dl, there is a depression of neuromuscular irritability. Hypercalcemia is most often associated with overactivity of the parathyroid gland, but may also occur secondary to immobilization and neoplastic disease where there is increased movement of calcium out of the bones. Decreased renal excretion of calcium in renal disease can also account for hypercalcemia.

Hypercalcemia can also occur secondary to excessive ingestion of calcium or vitamin D, or administration of thiazide diuretics, which decrease calcium excretion. Persons who have ulcers and who drink large amounts of milk and take various alkaline medications may also develop hypercalcemia as part of the *milk-alkali syndrome.*

Assessment findings in a patient with hypercalcemia include flank pain, kidney infection, kidney stones, and polyuria due to increased deposits of calcium in the renal pelvis and parenchyma, which results in the kidney's inability to concentrate urine. Lethargy, confusion, exhaustion, and loss of interest in surroundings occur due to neurologic hypofunction. Bone pain, osteoporosis, *osteomalacia*, and pathologic fractures occur due to *decalcification* of the bones. Hypercalcemia also causes an increase in calcium ions in sympathetic ganglia, which impedes the transmission of stimuli, resulting in diarrhea, constipation, atony of the intestinal tract, peptic ulcer, anorexia, nausea, and vomiting.

Hypercalcemia is treated with several different modalities. First, the cause is eliminated whenever possible and renal excretion of calcium is increased. Intravenous saline solutions can be used to inhibit tubular reabsorption of calcium. Phosphate supplements are used to enhance calcium deposits in the bone and soft tissues and to reduce intestinal absorption of calcium. Glucocorticosteroids decrease calcium absorption from the intestinal tract and are often used to help control symptoms of lymphomas and multiple myeloma. Mithramycin, a cytotoxic antibiotic discussed in detail in Chapter 49, is used when the hypercalcemia is due to malignancy. Calcitonin, a thyroid hormone discussed in detail in Chapter 45, is used when the hypercalcemia is related to excessive parathyroid activity.

MAGNESIUM

Magnesium, primarily found intracellularly, plays a critical role in the maintenance of normal muscle and nerve activity. It promotes regulation of blood phosphorus level and activates many enzyme reactions especially important in carbohydrate metabolism. Normal levels are 1.5–2.5 mEq/liter and symptoms generally present below 1.0 mEq/liter or above 3.0 mEq/liter. Normal adult requirements are 200–300 mg/day. Magnesium is found abundantly in foods such as nuts, soybeans, cocoa, seafood, whole grains, dried beans, peas, and is a vital constituent of chlorophyll.

Approximately 45% of ingested magnesium is absorbed. Parathyroid hormone increases absorption of magnesium in the intestinal tract, while excessive fat, phosphates, calcium, and alkalosis inhibit magnesium absorption. Sixty-six percent is stored in the bone, 1% is found in the plasma and interstitial fluid, and the rest is found within the cells. Magnesium is excreted in both the urine and feces.

Hypomagnesemia

Hypomagnesemia is due to several major causes: poor nutrition and either gastrointestinal or renal losses that were not replaced. Patients prone to magnesium deficiency are more likely to have one or more of the following: chronic and severe malnutrition; chronic renal disease; prolonged severe diarrhea; chronic alcoholism; intestinal malabsorption syndromes; prolonged diuretic therapy; acute renal failure in the diuretic phase; or prolonged intravenous therapy without magnesium replacement.

Assessment findings of hypomagnesemia include a serum level less than 1.5 mEq/liter, hyperactive reflexes, positive Chvostek's and Trousseau's signs, facial twitching, jerking, tetany, and convulsions. These symptoms are all due to increased neuromuscular irritability. Patients can also experience hallucinations, delusions, extreme confusion, and aggressive behavior due to increased stimulation of the central nervous system. Tachycardia and hypotension also occur due to decreased cardiac muscle function.

Magnesium Sulfate

Magnesium is supplied as magnesium sulfate, which comes in both oral and intravenous forms (Table 58–7). Magnesium oxide is also available for oral use (see Chapter 52). Magnesium is used as a supplement in deficiency states, as a laxative, to prevent deficiency in patients receiving hyperalimentation, to control convulsions in toxemia in pregnancy, and to treat preterm labor. When taken in its oral form, it acts as an osmotic cathartic by retaining and drawing water into the bowel. The intravenous form depresses CNS activity as well as activity in smooth, skeletal, and cardiac muscles. In the CNS, it reduces acetylcholine at the neuromuscular junction, thereby producing neuromuscular blockade. In cardiac and other muscle tissue, it slows conduction. Magnesium has been used by some researchers to control ventricular fibrillation and ventricular tachycardia that has not been controlled using antiarrhythmic therapy.

CONTRAINDICATIONS AND PRECAUTIONS. Magnesium is contraindicated in patients with myocardial infarction or heart block, as it may slow cardiac conduction. It is used cautiously in patients with decreased renal function, as this is the organ of excretion, and in patients with heart disease, as peripheral vasodilatation may occur, resulting in hypotension.

ADVERSE EFFECTS. The most common adverse effects of magnesium include flushing, thirst, muscle weakness, dehydration, and hyporeflexia.

INTERACTIONS. Magnesium potentiates the neuromuscular blockade produced by d-tubocurarine, decamethonium, and succinylcholine. Because of the central nervous system effects of magnesium, there may be interactions between magnesium and barbiturates, narcotics, hypnotics, or systemic anesthetics.

DOSAGE. Magnesium can be mixed in TPN solutions. The usual maintenance dose in adults is 8–24 mEq/day and infants 2–10 mEq/day. Magnesium can also be administered intravenously for deficiency. Magnesium solutions should be diluted to a 20% or less solution prior to intravenous administration, and the infusion should not exceed 0.2 mEq/kg/minute. For magnesium deficiencies, the intravenous dosage may range from 32.5–40 mEq/24 hours. When administering intramuscularly, the dose can range from 250 mg/kg every four hours for 24 hours to 1 g of a 50% solution every six hours (to a maximum of four doses in 24 hours).

Hypermagnesemia

Hypermagnesemia, a serum level greater than 2.5 mEq/liter, is generally associated with overdoses of magnesium either orally or parenterally, or poor renal function. Typical assessment findings associated with hypermagnesemia include a warm sensation throughout the body, decreased deep tendon reflexes, flaccid paralysis, hypotension, drowsiness, decreased respirations, dysrhythmias. These symptoms are all related to a pronounced reduction in neuromuscular irritability.

The treatment of hypermagnesemia is aimed at correcting the underlying cause such as renal failure. Patients are placed on dialysis and foods and drugs containing magnesium are withheld. If magnesium toxicity occurs, the patient is given 10% calcium gluconate slowly intravenously. The calcium gluconate slows the action of magnesium on the heart and reverses the symptoms of cardiotoxicity.

PHOSPHORUS

Phosphorus is a critical component of all body tissues and is essential for the proper functioning of muscle, red blood cells, the nervous system, and for the metabolism of carbohydrates, fats, and protein. Eighty percent to 85% of all phosphorus is present in the skeletal system. Phosphorus is a structural part of the phospholipids in cell membranes that are responsible for nutrient transport. Phosphorus is part of the nucleic acids—both RNA and DNA. It is also part of the buffering system that helps to maintain acid–base balance. Normal serum phosphorus is between 2.5 and 4.5 mg/dl and may be as high as 6 mg/dl in children. Phosphorus is higher in children due to the high rate of skeletal growth.

Hypophosphatemia

Hypophosphatemia occurs when the phosphorus level falls below 2.5 mg/dl. The most common cause of hypophosphatemia is severe protein-calorie malnutrition where people are re-fed carbohydrates with inadequate phosphorus. Other causes of hypophosphatemia can include intense hyperventilation, alcohol withdrawal, poor dietary intake, diabetic ketoacidosis, and major thermal burns.

The majority of signs and symptoms that result from hypophosphatemia are as a result of the deficiency of adenosine triphosphate (ATP) and 2,3-diphosphoglycerate (2,3-DPG). Adenosine triphosphate is necessary for production of cellular energy. As ATP declines, muscle weakness, muscle pain and at times *rhabdomyolysis* can occur. Weak respiratory muscles may impair respiratory function. Severe hypophosphatemia is dangerous and requires prompt attention. 2,3-diphosphoglycerate is necessary for oxygen to be unloaded from red blood cells at the tissue level. As 2,3-DPG decreases, tissue anoxia can result.

Phosphate Preparations

Phosphates are obtained as powders or liquids for oral use, or as intravenous solutions (see Table 58–7). Phosphate comes in combination with other electrolytes such as sodium phosphate; sodium phosphate, effervescent, NF; sodium phosphate solution, NF; sodium biphosphate, USP; phosphoric acid, NF; potassium phosphate; diluted phosphoric acid, NF, and many oral phosphate products are also available. The phosphates are used to reduce hypercalcemia, to restore a phosphate depletion syndrome to normal, to bind calcium orally in renal disease, or as effective saline cathartics.

CONTRAINDICATIONS AND PRECAUTIONS. Phosphate is contraindicated in patients with a high phosphorus or a low calcium and in patients with Addison's disease. Also, various products like potassium phosphate are contraindicated in hyperkalemia, while sodium phosphate is contraindicated in hypernatremia. Potassium phosphate is also used cautiously in patients with cardiac disease, particularly the digitalized patient. Both potassium phosphate and sodium phosphate are used cautiously in the renal patient. Sodium phosphate is also used cautiously in any edematous or sodium-retaining state, in cardiac failure, or cirrhosis.

ADVERSE EFFECTS. Typical adverse effects of intravenous phosphate therapy include hypocalcemia and hyperphosphatemia. In addition to these side effects, when oral phosphate is given, diarrhea and gastrointestinal upset may occur.

INTERACTIONS. When oral phosphates are administered, several interactions can occur. Antacids can combine with phosphate preparation and prevent absorption. Calcium and vitamin D products may antagonize the effects of phosphates. Concurrent use of so-

TEXT RESUMES ON PAGE 1622

Table 58–7. MAGNESIUM AND PHOSPHATE PRODUCTS

Name	Dosage	Mode of Administration
MAGNESIUM PRODUCTS:		
Action: maintain neuromuscular excitability and is involved with neurochemical transmission.		
Use: hypomagnesemia, toxemia/eclampsia during pregnancy, preterm labor, dysrhythmia control.		
Magnesium sulfate (Epsom Salts, MgSO$_4$)	5–15 mg/kg/day.	PO
	2–4 g, 25%–50% solution.	IM
	1–5 g, 10%–20% solution, not to exceed 0.2 mEq/kg/min.	IV
PHOSPHATE PRODUCTS:		
Action: helps regulate calcium metabolism, is a buffer to maintain acid–base balance, necessary to make healthy red blood cells, white blood cells, and platelets.		
Use: hypophosphatemia.		
Potassium phosphate (contains 3 mmol PO$_4$/ml; 4.4 mEq K/ml)	Adults in TPN: 10–15 mmol/liter.	IV
	Infants: 1.5–2 mmol/l/kg/day.	IV
Sodium phosphate (contains 3 mmol/liter PO$_4$/ml, 4.0 mEq Na/ml)	1.5 g infused over 6–8 hours.	IV
	TPN: Adults: 10–15 mmol/liter	IV
	Infants: 1.5–2 mmol/kg/day.	
Phosphorus (Uro-KP-Neutral tablets, Neutra-Phos capsules, and many others) (All contain 250 mg phosphorus and varying amounts of potassium or sodium)	1–2 tablets or capsules with meals and at bedtime.	PO

*Within the column of adverse effects, <u>underlines</u> indicate the most common effects; CAPITALS indicate life-threatening effects.

Contraindications/ Precautions	Adverse Effects*	Interactions	Nursing Implications
Contraindicated in myocardial infarction, heart block. Use cautiously in decreased renal function in patients with heart disease.	Neuro: sweating, depressed reflexes, flaccid paralysis, hypothermia, CNS depression CV: flushing, hypotension, circulatory collapse GI: diarrhea	Increases effect of neuromuscular blocking agents, causing excessive blockade. Additional CNS depression with narcotics, anesthetics, barbiturates.	ASSESSMENT: Frequently assess reflexes, serum levels, and vital signs (q 10–15 min) to monitor for hypermagnesemia. INTERVENTION: Oral form is best administered in the morning with a full glass of water or juice. Bitter, salty taste may be disguised by chilling medication or by adding ice chips. It may also be flavored with lemon or orange juice. IM—inject deep IM in gluteal muscle. IV—painful and irritating, so dilute at least 1:20 and do not exceed 0.2 mEq/kg/ minute. EVALUATION: Monitor for signs of hypermagnesemia, profound thirst, feeling of warmth, sedation, depressed deep tendon reflexes, and muscle weakness.
Contraindicated in severe renal impairment, hyperphosphatemia, and alkaline urine as increased risk of stone formation. Contraindicated in hyperkalemia.	For all: CV: hypotension, myocardial infarction Hemo: hypocalcemia, tetany GI: cramping, nausea	For all: Concurrent potassium-sparing diuretics may result in hyperkalemia.	For all: ASSESSMENT: Assess serum calcium, phosphorus and intake and output before & during therapy. INTERVENTION: Do not give postoperatively until urine flow is re-established. Give by IV infusion, never IV push or IM.
Contraindicated in severe renal impairment, hyperphosphatemia, and alkaline urine as increased risk of stone formation. Also contraindicated in hypernatremia.	Same as for all.	Same as for all.	Same as for all.
Same as above.	Same as above.	Same as above.	Same as above.

Magnesium & Phosphate Products

dium phosphate products with antihypertensives or corticosteroids may result in hypernatremia.

DOSAGE. The phosphates (sodium phosphate/potassium phosphate) are ordered and administered as millimoles (mmol). The intravenous products are diluted thoroughly in a large volume of fluid and administered slowly. Phosphate is added to TPN solutions in 10–15-mmol doses, which are the equivalent of 310–465 mg of elemental phosphorus/liter.

PHOSPHORUS REPLACEMENT PRODUCTS. Phosphorus (K-Phos Neutral tablets, Neutra-Phos-K capsules, and many others) is available in both tablets and capsules, which have 250 mg of phosphorus with different combinations of potassium and sodium. These products are best administered after meals and at bed time.

Hyperphosphatemia

Hyperphosphatemia, a serum level above 4.5 mg/dl, is most commonly associated with decreased renal excretion of phosphorus. Other causes include chemotherapy, high phosphorus intake, profound muscle necrosis, and increased phosphorus absorption.

As serum phosphorus levels rise, precipitation of calcium phosphate occurs in nonosseous sites. Also, because of the reciprocal relationship between phosphorus and calcium, a high serum phosphorus tends to lower serum calcium. Tingling sensations around the fingers and mouth and tetany can result.

Treatment is aimed at treating and eliminating the underlying cause. For patients with renal failure, several measures are indicated. These include the administration of phosphate-binding antacids to bind phosphorus in the gut, dietary phosphorus restriction, and dialysis.

USING THE NURSING PROCESS

ASSESSMENT

Assessment of the patient with an electrolyte imbalance always begins with a thorough nursing history to develop the data base. Important information that is obtained is found in Table 58–8. All this information is used later when preparing nursing diagnoses and the nursing care plan.

The nurse may be responsible for obtaining numerous laboratory tests to determine the degree of imbalance. Laboratory tests might include examination of serum electrolytes and serum *osmolarity;* urine for pH, specific gravity, electrolytes, and *osmolality;* and arterial acid–base measurement. When assessing serum calcium levels, it is also important to assess protein levels and pH. Serum calcium levels decrease in alkalosis, as more is bound to protein. In addition, the additional bicarbonate in alkalosis attaches to free calcium and prevents it from fulfilling its normal metabolic function. In acidosis there is more ionized calcium (more free calcium), and serum calcium increases.

It is important that the nurse be able to recognize the signs and symptoms of the various electrolyte imbalances as listed in Table 58–3. General findings include unusual thirst, edema, and alterations in consciousness and muscle activity. The nurse must also assess general parameters on each patient, including daily weight, intake and urine output, urinary pH, number and quality of stools, bowel sounds, and vital signs.

The nurse also needs to be aware of which patients are more susceptible to electrolyte imbalances. These patients include the patient with decreased oral intake from age or debilitation; one with increased fluid losses from nasogastric suction, diarrhea, vomiting, or fistula drainage; one who has an altered metabolism from fever, diabetic ketoacidosis, or adrenal malfunction; the patient receiving diuretics, corticosteroids, IV solutions, or other drugs that may affect electrolyte balance; and finally, the patient with edema. The nurse needs to assess such patients frequently to prevent major complications of electrolyte imbalances, especially since one imbalance rarely occurs in isolation, but precipitates others.

NURSING DIAGNOSIS

Typical nursing diagnoses for a patient with disturbances of major body electrolytes are included in Table 58–8.

PLANNING AND INTERVENTION

The nurse develops the goals of nursing intervention from the nursing diagnoses. When caring for the patient with electrolyte disturbances, typical nursing goals are included in Table 58–8. The data base, developed during the initial health history, is used to achieve these interventions.

Patients who routinely take medications such as diuretics and steroids, which may precipitate electrolyte imbalances, are taught by the nurse how to prevent further episodes of imbalance. (Chapter 38 provides additional important information on diuretics, and Chapter 42 provides more information on steroids.) When the nurse administers diuretics or steroids, a daily record of weight is maintained. The physician is notified if the patient gains or loses more than five pounds per week. If potassium-depleting diuretics are administered, the patient should increase daily intake of foods that are high in potassium (Table 53–9) unless contraindicated.

When administering steroids, patients may need to reduce sodium intake as well as increase intake of potassium-containing foods. When the patient is discharged on either diuretics or steroids, the nurse teaches him or her to monitor weight and diet. In addition, the patient is taught to identify and anticipate expected side effects.

NURSING RESPONSIBILITIES

When administering electrolytes IV to correct imbalances, the nurse always runs electrolyte replacements

Table 58–8. NURSING PROCESS FOR PATIENT REQUIRING MAJOR BODY ELECTROLYTES

Assessment

Assess history of current illness, sources of fluid loss/shifts.
Note complaints of muscle weakness/spasms, lethargy, fatigue.
Review laboratory studies, e.g., serum electrolytes, osmolarity; urine pH, specific gravity.
Identify prescription and OTC drug use (especially diuretics, steroids).

Nursing Diagnosis	Nursing Actions	Rationale	Desired Outcomes/ Evaluation Criteria
Fluid volume, [specify] potential related to active loss and/or failure of regulatory mechanisms (specific to underlying disease process/ trauma), inability to obtain/ingest fluids.	Administer replacement via appropriate route (IV, po) and dilute as indicated.	Corrects imbalance with minimal adverse reactions.	Displays moist skin/ mucous membranes, stable vital signs, individually adequate urinary output; free of edema and excessive weight loss/inappropriate gain.
	Routinely reevaluate for therapeutic response/ adverse reactions.	Replacement may lead to excess and alter neurotransmission, reduced muscle strength or impaired cardiac contractility.	
	Maintain accurate I&O. Calculate fluid balance.	Indicators of fluid balance are important because either fluid excess or deficit can occur.	
	Weigh as indicated.	Sensitive indicator of fluid shifts. Loss/retention of one liter of fluid equals a weight change of 2.2 lb.	
	Monitor vital signs and CVP.	Changes may be indicators of imbalance.	
	Assess skin turgor and mucous membrane moisture.	Water deficit will be manifested by signs of dehydration.	
	Give oral fluids with caution. If fluids are restricted, set up a 24-hour schedule for fluid intake.	Fluid restrictions, as well as extracellular shifts, can cause drying of mucous membranes, and patient may desire more fluids than are prudent.	
	Encourage coughing/ deep breathing exercises.	Pulmonary fluid shifts potentiate respiratory complications.	
Knowledge deficit related to lack of exposure/ recall, information misinterpretation, unfamiliarity with resources as evidenced by questions, statement of concern, inaccurate follow-through of instruction/ development of preventable complications.	Discuss preventive measures to be taken, including adequate dietary intake or measures to replace losses associated with prescription drug use as indicated.	Understanding of these actions can avoid recurrence.	Verbalizes understanding of condition/disease process and treatment. Initiates necessary lifestyle changes and participates in treatment regimen.
	Review proper dosage, safe administration of oral electrolyte preparations.	Helps patient to maintain correct therapy regimen.	
	Stress necessity of strict adherence to therapeutic regimen.	Helps to achieve optimal results.	
	Identify signs/symptoms to be reported to physician, e.g., unusual thirst, edema, changes in mentation or muscle activity.	Prompt evaluation and intervention may prevent serious complications.	

Table 58-9. POTASSIUM-RICH FOODS

Food	mEq of K$^+$
Banana, 1 medium	15
Apricots, 2–3 medium	7
Figs: raw, 2 large	5
dried, 7 small	20
Orange, 1 medium	10
Peaches, dried ½ cup	28
Tomato juice, ½ cup	7
Orange juice, ½ cup	6
Maple syrup, 1 tbsp	7
Instant coffee, 1 tbsp	6

slowly into a large vein and dilutes the electrolyte in the recommended amount of diluent to prevent irritation of vessels. The patient is monitored closely for signs of toxicity. As an example, when electrolytes are given to a patient with hypocalcemia, the patient is observed closely for signs of hypercalcemia. Serum electrolytes, intake and output, daily weight, urine studies, and vital signs are also monitored closely by the nurse.

Potassium Products

Hypokalemia, when mild, can usually be reversed by adding foods that are high in potassium to the diet. Salt substitutes contain a substantial amount of potassium and other electrolytes. Excessive use can be dangerous for the patient who is taking potassium products. Instruct the patient not to use any substitute unless it is specifically ordered by the physician. Co-Salt and Neo-curtasal both deliver 50–60 mEq of potassium and 0.5 mg of sodium per teaspoon, while Morton's Lite Salt delivers 35 mEq of potassium and 1100 mg of sodium per teaspoon. Patients also need to be aware that many over-the-counter products contain potassium, such as antacids (Alka-Seltzer), analgesics (Neocylate), and multiple vitamin preparations.

Patients with moderate hypokalemia, 3.5 mEq/liter or lower, such as those on diuretic therapy, may have oral products ordered. Oral replacements generally prevent the rapid rise of potassium levels that can be associated with IV therapy. If rapid correction is necessary, as in diabetic ketoacidosis, or if the patient is unable to take potassium orally, IV potassium is administered. Potassium chloride solutions are preferred to other salts because, if there is an associated metabolic alkalosis, this salt may correct both the hypokalemia and the metabolic alkalosis.

When administering potassium preparations, the nurse mixes all IV preparations thoroughly before administering and puts a maximum of 40 mEq in each liter. If more is ordered by the physician, mix and run half at a time or place on an IV pump. Administer slowly (10 mEq/hour) through a large vein to prevent irritation to the vein or the development of hyperkalemia. Never give potassium IV push. Intake and output are monitored closely to assess renal function. If urinary

output drops below 0.5 ml/kg/hour for one hour, the nurse reports it immediately to the physician. The potassium is discontinued until urinary output returns to normal. The nurse monitors the electrocardiogram frequently to assess for the dangerous effects of hyperkalemia that can be detected more rapidly on the ECG (See Fig. 58–2) than by measuring serum potassium levels.

If the patient is to go home on potassium products, the nurse is also responsible for patient teaching, which is featured in Table 58–10.

Calcium Products

To prevent hypocalcemia, the high-risk patient should eat plenty of dairy products, sardines, and other foods rich in calcium and vitamin D. Mild hypocalcemia can generally be relieved by dietary management. In addi-

Table 58-10. PATIENT TEACHING FOR POTASSIUM PRODUCTS

Dear Patient:
  This drug has been ordered for you. This is what you should know about your drug to get the most from your therapy.

1. Potassium products have been ordered for you to increase and/or maintain your blood potassium level within normal range.
2. Your potassium product is taken until your imbalance is corrected. (Potassium products may also be taken with certain medications such as digitalis products and diuretics. In this case, take your potassium products as long as your digitalis and diuretics are being taken.)
3. Oral liquids, fizz tablets, or powders are best diluted in 3–4 oz. or more of cold water or juice. Larger doses may be mixed with 6 oz. Potassium salts have a bitter taste and are, therefore, best taken with meals or after meals. Allow the fizz tablets to stop fizzing and then sip over 5–10 minutes. Some potassium products are contained in a wax pill. The drug will be taken up by the body but the wax pill will be found in the stool. This is OK. Potassium tablets should not be taken dry, crushed, or chewed. Whole tablets should be swallowed with a full glass of water or juice.
4. Potassium products are not taken together with potassium-rich foods. Potassium-rich foods are featured in Table 58–9. Also the use of salt substitutes made from potassium salts (Diasal or CoSalt) should be limited, as hyperkalemia may result.
5. If you forget your potassium product through the next dose, do not take it. Do not attempt to catch up.
6. Do not suddenly stop your potassium product without checking with your doctor.
7. If the following side effects occur, contact your doctor: nausea, vomiting, stomach upset, and muscle weakness.
8. Be alert for the following set of symptoms, which may indicate a high potassium level. If these occur, contact your doctor: cramps, diarrhea, irritability, nausea, weakness, and muscle cramps.
9. Store your medication in a tight, moisture-resistant container.

tion, patients should restrict their intake of phosphorus, since it competes with calcium for intestinal absorption.

When oral products are necessary, the nurse administers oral calcium, calcium gluconate, and calcium chloride 1.5 hours after meals with milk, whereas calcium lactate is best administered with meals.

The patient with moderate hypocalcemia receives calcium gluconate (9% calcium) (1 ampule raises the serum calcium level by 1 mEq) or calcium chloride (27% calcium) (1 ampule raises the serum calcium level by 10 mEq) IV slowly. In an emergency, calcium can be delivered by slow IV push.

When administering intravenous calcium preparations, the nurse should not mix calcium products in the same IV bottle with bicarbonate, since this combination forms a precipitate. The nurse carefully monitors the IV to avoid its infiltration, which causes great irritation and possible necrosis of the skin. The physician orders the drip rate low enough to prevent cardiac complications such as a fall in blood pressure or cardiac arrest. During IV administration, the nurse also monitors the ECG to detect Q-T interval and T wave changes that may indicate hypercalcemia. The nurse also assesses both Chvostek's and Trousseau's signs, which indicate the development of hypocalcemia and tetany. The nurse tests Chvostek's sign by lightly brushing the patient's cheek just below the temple. The facial nerve (the seventh cranial nerve) will cause facial twitching if tetany is present. The nurse tests for Trousseau's sign by inflating a blood pressure cuff on the patient's upper arm until the radial pulse has been obliterated for ten seconds. If Trousseau's sign is positive and tetany is present, there will be carpal spasm (Fig. 58–3).

Blood levels drawn to assess serum calcium after calcium infusions are drawn about two hours after finishing the infusion, when the body has had time to distribute the infused calcium. Many patients—most of all with parathyroid deficiencies or dumping syndrome—need repeated calcium infusions.

Calcium products are administered carefully to a patient already receiving digitalis as these may cause an additive effect. In patients who are extremely cardiotoxic and have hyperkalemia, 10–30 ml of calcium gluconate 10% may be injected IV over a three to five-minute period; this dose may be repeated once. The electrocardiogram is constantly monitored.

As calcium is administered, the nurse assesses for signs and symptoms of hypercalcemia, which may include joint pain, conjunctivitis, flaccid paralysis, cardiac arrest, and kidney stones.

The nurse is also responsible for patient teaching. Information to be taught to patients is found in Table 58–11.

Magnesium Products

Mild magnesium deficits can be corrected by increasing intake of meats, fish, dairy products, whole grains, green leafy vegetables, and other magnesium-rich foods. Dietary intake can be supplemented with magnesium-based antacids like Mylanta, Gelusil, or Maalox.

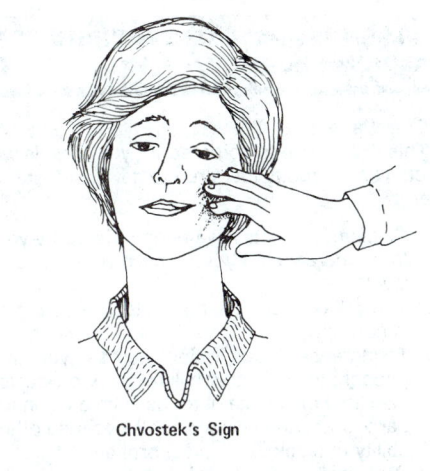

Chvostek's Sign

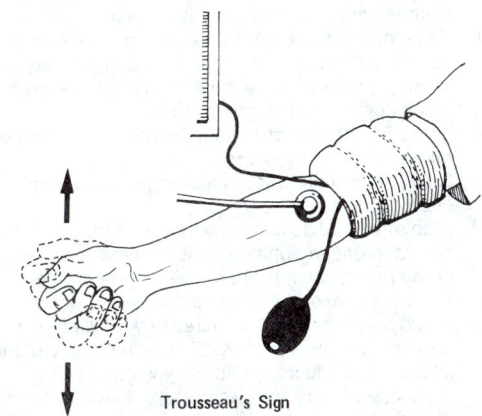

Trousseau's Sign

Figure 58–3. Signs of hypocalcemia. Chvostek's sign is positive when light stroking of the patient's cheek causes seventh cranial nerve stimulation and twitching of the cheek. Trousseau's sign is positive when a blood pressure cuff inflated on the arm for 10 seconds causes carpal spasm.

If oral administration is necessary, magnesium is best administered in the morning in a full glass of ice water or juice to help disguise its bitter taste.

If the patient has a more severe deficit, magnesium sulfate may be given IM (8–16 mEq every eight hours) for five days followed by a maintenance dose (8 mEq/day) until the magnesium levels return to normal. Intramuscular injections should be deep into the gluteal muscle, as they burn and are painful.

Patients who have severe symptoms are treated with IV magnesium sulfate given over one to three hours followed by continuous IV infusion or IM injection. When administering magnesium IV, calcium gluconate is kept near, to reverse the symptoms of potential magnesium toxicity. When the patient is receiving a maintenance dose (between 8 and 24 mEq/day), serum levels are monitored daily. Also monitor blood pressure and respiratory rate, as these may be depressed as a result of therapy.

During the time when magnesium levels are low, the

Table 58–11. PATIENT TEACHING FOR CALCIUM PRODUCTS

Dear Patient:
This drug has been ordered for you. This is what you should know about your drug to get the most from your therapy.

1. Calcium products have been ordered by your doctor to increase and/or maintain your blood calcium level.
2. You will take calcium products until your problem is corrected.
3. To increase GI absorption, increase your intake of phosphate with either milk or dairy products and also limit the intake of foods such as spinach, rhubarb, bran, and whole cereals because of their ability to block calcium absorption.
4. Oral calcium (calcium gluconate and chloride) is best taken 1–1½ hours after meals with milk; calcium lactate is best taken with meals.
5. Calcium products are not taken together with tetracycline antibiotics. Additional interactions may occur. Please check with your physician or pharmacist before taking other drugs.
6. If you forget your drug until the next dose, do not take that dose, do not try to catch up.
7. Do not stop taking your calcium products until your doctor says to.
8. Side effects of calcium products include: constipation, decreased appetite, muscle weakness, and some mental confusion. If these signs or symptoms are present, please contact your doctor.
9. If told by your doctor to increase your dietary intake of calcium, foods high in calcium include milk and dairy products, green leafy vegetables, and certain seafoods such as oysters, sardines, and clams.
10. Store your drug in a tight, moisture-resistant container.

nurse keeps the patient supine to prevent hypotension; gives soft foods to assist with chewing and swallowing, as laryngeal and esophageal spasm may be present; and handles the extremities gently, as muscle spasm may be present.

The nurse needs to be aware of signs of hypermagnesemia (weakness, hypotension, flushed, and hot skin), which occur when serum levels reach 3–5 mEq/liter; or weak, abnormal deep-tendon reflexes, slurred speech, drowsiness, and dysrhythmias, which occur when serum levels reach 5–7 mEq/liter; or flaccid muscle paralysis, respiratory depression, and cardiac arrest, which occur when serum levels reach 10 mEq/liter. The conditions that precipitate hypermagnesemia include chronic renal failure and, less commonly, adrenal insufficiency and overdosing on magnesium products.

EVALUATION

During the evaluation phase, the nurse evaluates the effectiveness of the treatment. The evaluation of electrolyte disturbances is based on a list of outcome evaluation criteria that has been developed in relation to the goals determined through discussion among the nurse, patient, and family. The data base obtained in the original assessment, and used to formulate the nursing diagnoses, provides helpful criteria for measuring the treatment's effectiveness. Typical outcome criteria are included in Table 58–8. The nurse must always listen carefully to what the patient and family are saying; a patient who is not involved with the establishment of these criteria or goals and does not fully understand or agree with them will not comply.

Electrolyte imbalance can be mild or very severe. When the patient is acutely ill and in the hospital, the imbalance is corrected with IV therapy. Patients are often treated by the physician with both oral preparations and diet therapy. The nurse always has the responsibility to evaluate the signs and symptoms of the imbalance and then to observe for signs of improvement (see Table 58–3).

Both overcompliance and undercompliance create problems; therefore, the nurse needs to teach the patient about these hazards. Occasionally, patients develop an imbalance because they self-administer excessive amounts of sodium bicarbonate (baking soda) as an antacid. Sodium bicarbonate has a tendency to produce a rebound acidity, which then prompts the patient to take another dose. This treatment eventually leads to sodium and bicarbonate excess and electrolyte imbalance. Undercompliance can also create a problem if the patient chooses not to follow the prescribed medication or diet regimen.

The evaluation process is continual. If frequent monitoring is not done, the patient with an electrolyte deficit may begin to show signs of an electrolyte excess. Frequent laboratory studies guide the medical staff in their treatment. Studies do not prevent the condition; they calculate the degree of abnormality so the nurse can intervene to correct it.

As the patient is being prepared for discharge, either from the hospital, clinic, or physician's office, all previously taught material is reviewed and updated, if necessary, to ensure that the patient's knowledge base remains accurate. The nurse also encourages the patient to keep all future physician visits. With help from the nurse, physician, and family, the patient can return to and maintain a normal electrolyte balance.

SUMMARY

Electrolytes, such as sodium, potassium, calcium, magnesium, and phosphorus, are essential for proper functioning of cellular function. Electrolytes dissociate into ions, which carry a charge. Electrolytes are primarily absorbed within the gastrointestinal tract and are excreted by the kidneys in varying lengths of time. Kidney disease can precipitate electrolyte disturbances.

When the nurse administers electrolytes, it is important to understand the symptoms of both hypo- and hyper-imbalances. General findings include unusual thirst, edema, alteration in consciousness, and muscle activity. Patients at great risk for developing electrolyte imbalances include the patient with intravenous intake only, decreasing oral intake, increasing fluid losses, altered metabolism, edema, and receiving diuretics, and corticosteroids. Electrolytes may be administered orally or intravenously through a large vein. Dietary modification may also be recommended. Serum levels are drawn frequently to monitor patient progress.

BIBLIOGRAPHY

AMA Department of Drugs: AMA Drug Evaluations, ed 5. PSG Publishing, Littleton, MA, 1986.

Barta, MA: Correcting electrolyte imbalances. RN 87(2):30, 1987.

Calloway, C: When the problem involves magnesium, calcium, or phosphate. RN 87(5):30, 1987.

Luckman, J and Sorenson, K: Medical-Surgical Nursing. WB Saunders, Philadelphia, 1986.

Olin, B (ed): Facts and Comparisons. JB Lippincott, St. Louis, 1989.

Quinlan, M: Solving the mysteries of calcium imbalance: An action guide. RN 45:50, 1983.

Quinlan, M: Would you recognize this dangerous electrolyte imbalance? RN 46:51, 1983.

Toto, KH: When the patient has hypokalemia. RN 87(3):38, 1987.

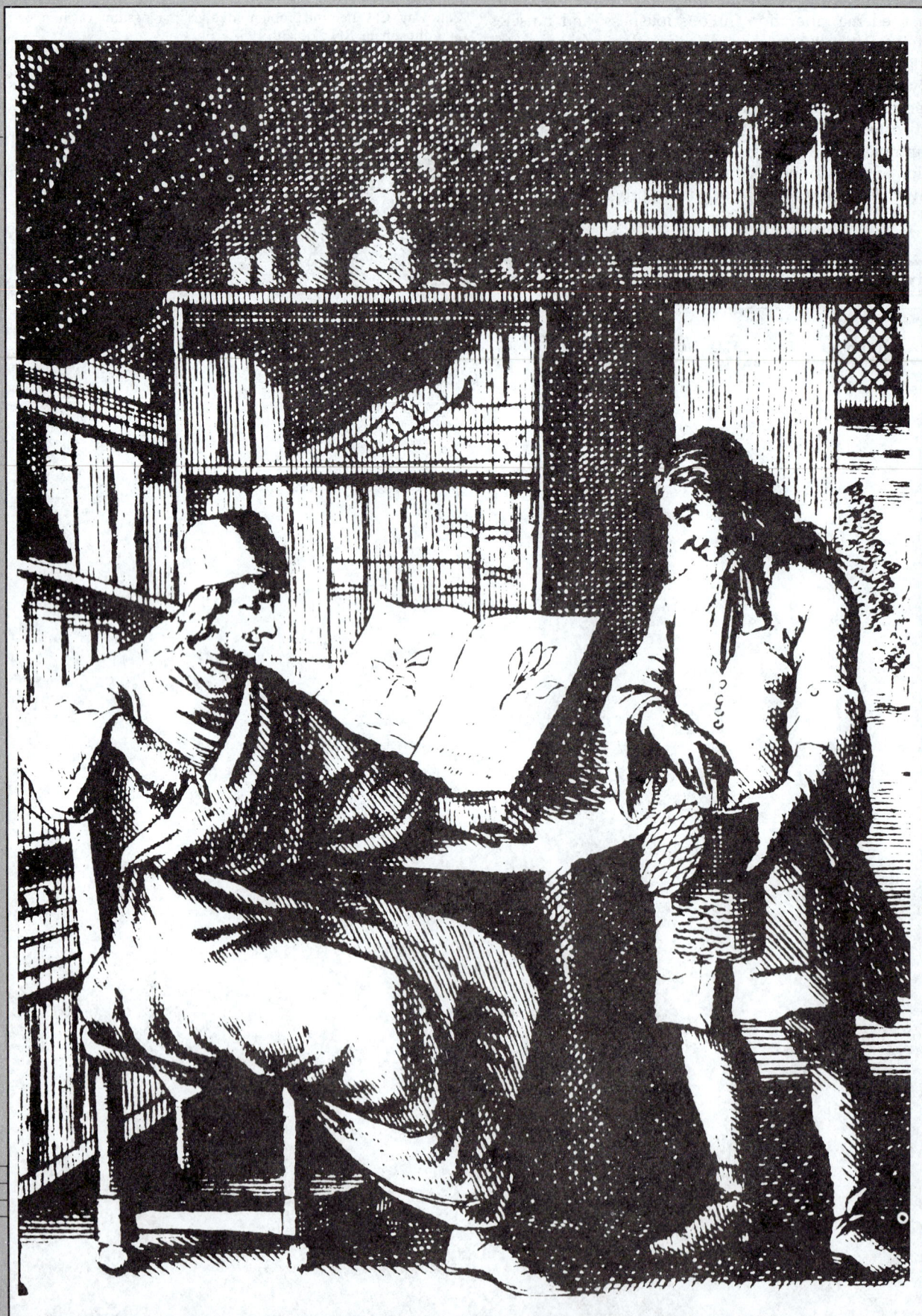

Preparing plants for the sick, circa 1600. The Bettmann Archive.

12
UNIT

EYE AND EAR DRUGS

GLOSSARY TERMS IN THIS CHAPTER

Accommodation reflex
Aqueous humor
Astigmatism
Cerumen
Conjunctiva
Cornea
Fovea centralis
Hypermetropia
Lacrimal apparatus
Macula
Myopia
Optic disc
Proprioception
Sclera
Trabecular meshwork
Tympanic membrane
Vitreous humor

OVERVIEW OF ANATOMY AND PHYSIOLOGY OF THE EYE AND EAR

MERRILY MATHEWSON KUHN, R.N.C., Ph.D., CCRN

LEARNING OBJECTIVES

After reading this chapter, the student will be able to:

1. Identify major anatomic structures of the eye.

2. Explain the function of the refractory media and how vision occurs.

3. Identify major anatomic structures of the ear.

4. Explain the mechanism of hearing.

THE EYE

The eyes, located in the bony cavities or orbits in the anterior cranium, function as the body's organs of vision.

STRUCTURE OF THE EYE

The eye is protected by the bony structure surrounding it, as well as by the eyelids and lashes. The eyelids are lined with a delicate mucous membrane, the *conjunctiva.* The *lacrimal apparatus,* including the lacrimal gland and its ducts and passages, produces tears that wash over the eye with each blink of the lid, lubricating and cleansing away foreign particles. Tears are drained through two small openings in the inner corner of the eye, passing into the lacrimal canaliculus, through the lacrimal sac into the nasolacrimal duct, and finally into the nasal cavity. This route passes near the sinus cavities of the upper face.

The eye is composed of three layers—the outer layer, the cornea and sclera; the middle layer, ciliary body, iris,

and choroid; and the inner layer, the retina (Fig. 59–1). The outer layer consists of the *cornea,* or anterior covering, which is clear and colorless, and the *sclera,* or posterior covering, which is thick and opaque. The highly vascular middle layer is composed of the ciliary body and processes, the iris anteriorly, and the choroid posteriorly. The ciliary muscles, which form the main part of the ciliary body, are the muscles that increase the visual acuity of the eye by changing the size of the lens. The iris, or colored portion of the eye, is a diaphragm with a circular center opening, the pupil, which regulates the amount of light admitted. When a person faces strong light or focuses on a nearby object, the pupil constricts; when the person faces dim light or focuses on a distant object, the pupil dilates to allow more light to enter.

The inner layer of the eye, the retina, has only a posterior portion. It is composed of several layers of nerve cells that translate the light waves to neural impulses; these are then transmitted via the optic nerve to the brain, which interprets them as sight. The retina contains photoreceptive nerve cells of two types: cones (about 100 million), for daylight and color vision, and rods (about 6 million), which allow for vision at low lev-

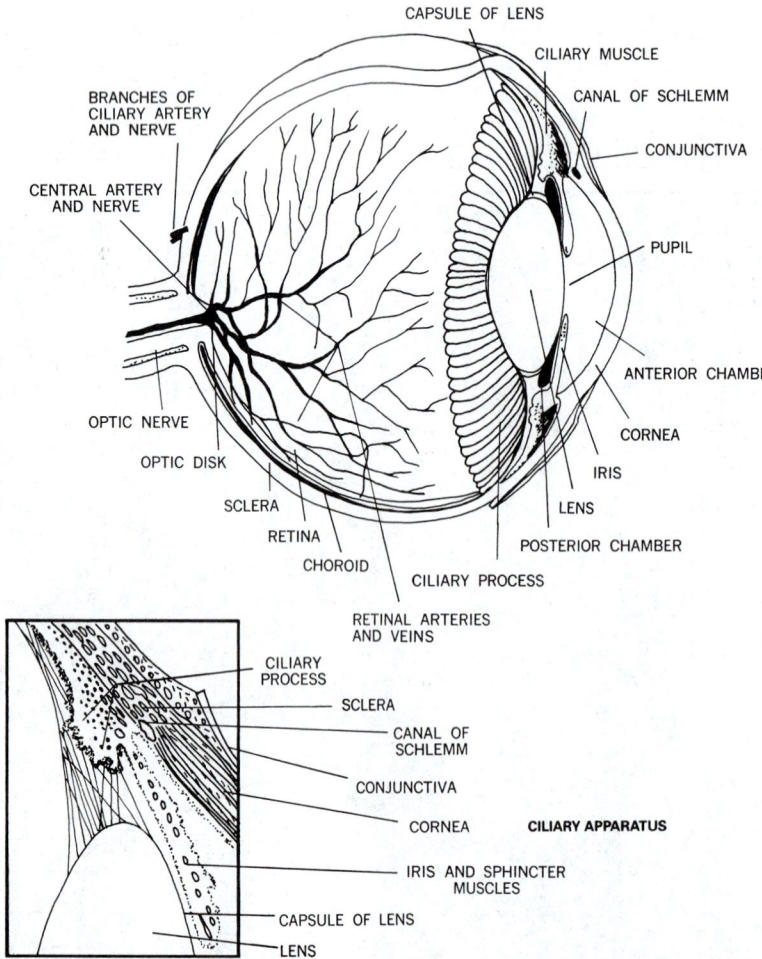

Figure 59–1. Anatomy of eye. (From Thomas, CL [Ed.]: Taber's Cyclopedic Medical Dictionary, ed. 16. FA Davis, Philadelphia, 1989, with permission.)

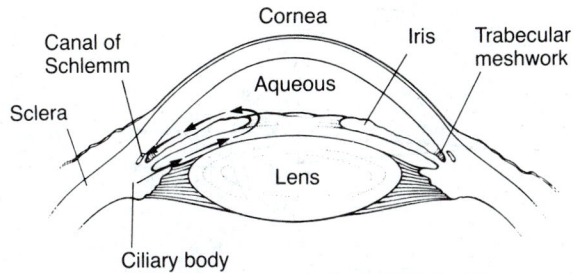

Figure 59–2. Normal flow of aqueous humor. Aqueous humor is produced in the ciliary body and flows through anterior chamber and out the canal of Schlemm.

els of illumination. Cones are most densely concentrated in the *fovea centralis* central depression (a small depression in the center of the *macula* near the center of the retina). The fovea is the portion of the retina where visual acuity is the greatest. The macula is a region located almost exactly at the posterior pole of the eye, and is slightly yellow in appearance. Rods are entirely absent from the fovea and macula, and their number increases in density toward the periphery of the retina. The rods also function as motion detectors.

The anterior chamber of the eye is filled with a watery-clear substance called *aqueous humor*, which is continuously produced by the ciliary body and associated structures at a rate of 2–5 ml/min (Fig. 59–2). Aqueous humor transports nutrients to the eye tissues and carries away cellular debris. Aqueous humor enters the anterior chamber to maintain the shape and intraocular pressure within the chamber (normally 12–25 mmHg). Aqueous humor is formed by the ciliary processes in much the same manner as cerebrospinal fluid is formed by the choroid plexus. The ciliary epithelium actively secretes sodium chloride and bicarbonate ions, which in the presence of carbonic anhydrase (an enzyme that catalyzes the formation of carbonic acid from carbon dioxide and water) promote the osmosis of a large amount of water into the eye. This is the process by which aqueous humor is formed.

It is aqueous humor that furnishes nutritional support to the crystalline (or avascular) lens and cornea. Normally, the same amount of aqueous humor enters the eye as exits it. The aqueous humor flows into the anterior chamber and enters the *trabecular meshwork*—filtering tissue located in the anterior chamber angle between the periphery of the iris and the cornea—and then to the canal of Schlemm. A thin-walled vein that encircles the eye, the canal of Schlemm conveys the aqueous humor into the venous system.

A rise in the rate of aqueous secretion or resistance to humoral outflow can cause intraocular pressure to increase to 60 mmHg or more, leading to the development of glaucoma or to permanent atrophy of the optic nerve and blindness.

The posterior cavity of vitreous body contains *vitreous humor*, which, because of its jelly-like consistency, serves to maintain the inner eye's spherical shape. Vitreous humor allows substances to diffuse through it, but there is no active flow of fluid due to its consistency.

Eye movement is controlled by the oculomotor (third), trochlear (fourth), and abducens (sixth) cranial nerves (Fig. 59–3). The trigeminal nerve (fifth) carries pain, touch, and temperature impulses from the eye and surrounding structures to the brain.

The artery and vein that both supply and drain the retina enter and leave the eye through the *optic disc* or

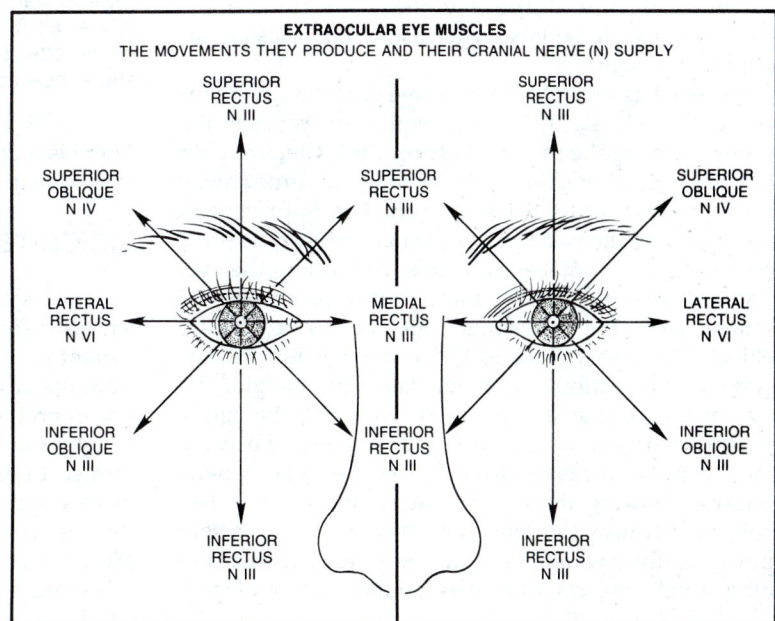

Figure 59–3. Extraocular eye muscles. (From Thomas, CL [Ed.]: Taber's Cyclopedic Medical Dictionary, ed. 16. FA Davis, Philadelphia, 1989, with permission.)

blind spot. These vessels can be examined with an ophthalmoscope and provide valuable information about a person's health. Because these vessels run through the meninges, which cover the brain, the examiner can also determine the presence of increasing intracranial pressure.

THE MECHANISMS OF VISION

The refractory mechanisms transmit the light waves through the eye and focus them on the retina. The image enters the eye through the anterior chamber, which is filled with aqueous humor.

The image is then transmitted through the crystalline lens, suspended in the eye by suspensory ligaments. The lens is 65% water and 35% protein, and changes shape to allow proper focusing of the image. Light rays converge on the lens, are bent, and move into the posterior cavity. In the posterior cavity, the light rays pass through the vitreous humor and are transmitted to the retina.

A normal eye is capable of focusing objects correctly on the retina. However, many eyes have errors in refraction that make them unable to do so. Nearsightedness (*myopia*, or the inability to see distant objects) focuses the image in front of the retina, whereas farsightedness (*hypermetropia*, or the inability to see close objects) focuses the image at a point behind the retina (Fig. 59–4). In addition, *astigmatism* (caused by a difference in curvature in the refractory surfaces of the cornea and/or lens) results in some portions(s) of the image being out of focus with other parts. These conditions can usually be corrected with glasses or contact lenses.

The rods and cones detect light rays and initiate nerve impulses that travel along the optic nerve (the second cranial nerve). In the optic chiasm, impulses from the medial half of each eye cross to the opposite side of the brain, whereas impulses from the lateral half of each retina remain uncrossed. The fibers then travel to either the left or right occipital lobe, whereas the impulses are interpreted as sight.

The eye has several reflexes, some protective and others to assist in sight. Bell's phenomenon protects the eyes by turning the them sharply upward when they are forcibly opened or closed, thus moving the cornea away from direct damage. Bell's phenomenon is present in about 90% of the population. The light reflex causes the pupil to become smaller as light is flashed into the eye. The *accommodation* reflex allows the pupil to become smaller when the gaze shifts from a distant to a closer object. The ciliary muscles controlled by the nervous system also function in accommodation by changing the size of the lens: as a near object is viewed, the ciliary muscles contract, causing the lens to buldge and become more convex; to view a distant object, the ciliary muscle relaxes, allowing the lens to flatten and become less convex. Because the lens can narrow, the refractory power of the eye allows us to see printed matter and other small subjects, as well as large or distant objects.

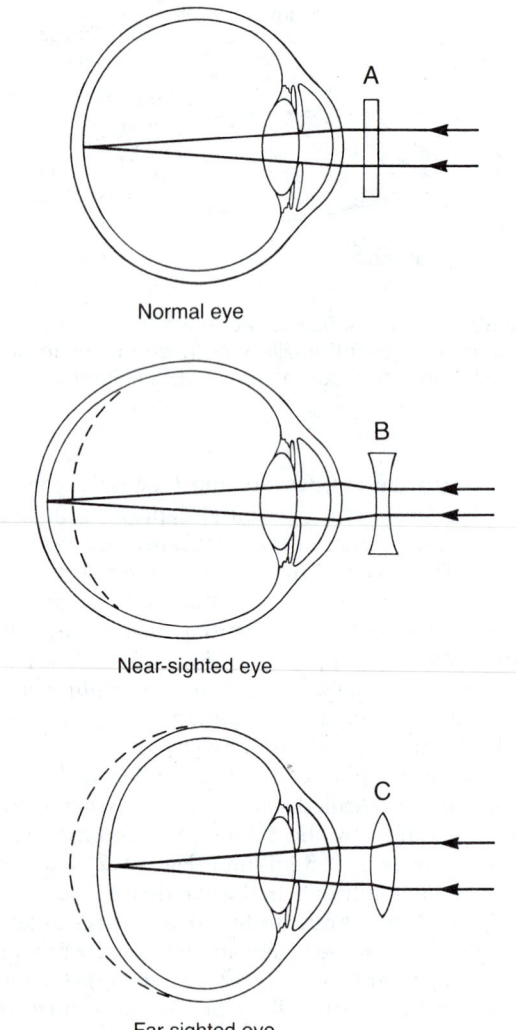

Normal eye

Near-sighted eye

Far-sighted eye

Figure 59–4. The refractory media of the eye. *A*) A normal eye. The image is focused on the retina. *B*) A nearsighted person (myopia) focuses the image before the retina. *C*) A far-sighted person (presbyopia) focuses the image after the retina. Primarily occurs in advancing age and is due to the loss of elasticity of the crystalline lens.

There is a direct and consensual reflex of both eyes, allowing both eyes to see the same object.

VISION TESTING

Several tests are available to test visual acuity. The Snellen test uses an eye chart placed twenty feet from the patient or uses a hand-held card held fourteen inches from the face. The patient then determines the smallest line of print from which he or she is able to identify correctly more than half the figures. Perimetry is also performed to examine the extent of the visual field. Eyedrops (mydriatics and cycloplegics) may be instilled into the eye to assist with further examination of the retina. More information on eye testing can be found in medical–surgical texts.

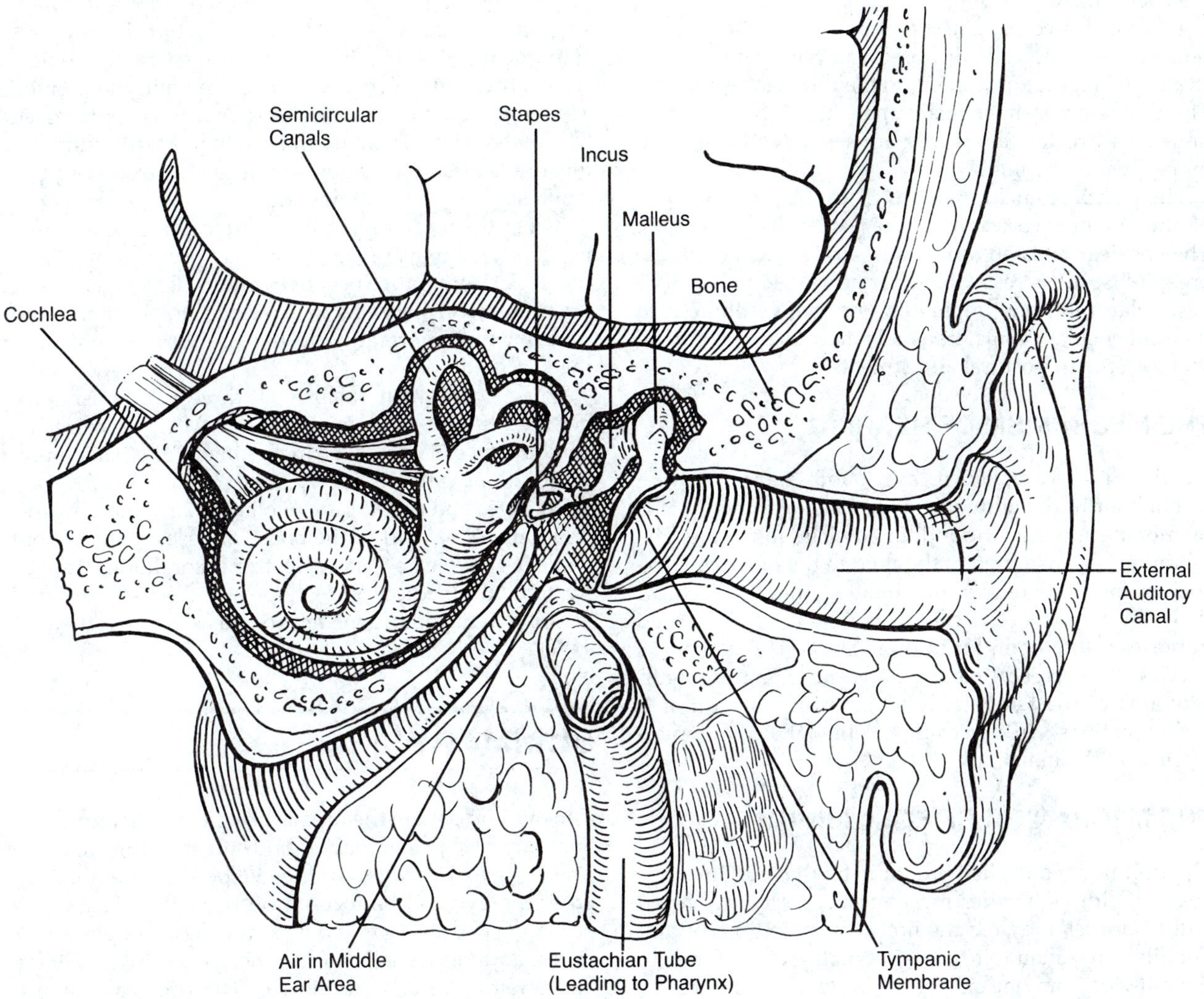

External and Inner Ear

Figure 59–5. External and inner ear. (From Thomas, CL [Ed.]: Taber's Cyclopedic Medical Dictionary, ed. 16. FA Davis, Philadelphia, 1989, with permission.)

THE EAR

The ears are the organs of hearing and assist with maintaining equilibrium. Each ear is composed of three major divisions: external, middle, and inner (Fig. 59–5).

The external ear has two parts, the auricle (pinna) and the external auditory canal (meatus). The auricle, composed of cartilage and skin, is the protrusion on the side of the head that funnels the sound into the external auditory canal. The canal is about 1.25 inches long and travels inward, forward, and downward. Modified sweat glands within the canal secrete *cerumen* (ear wax), which serves to lubricate the canal lining and trap foreign material. Cerumen also helps to prevent bacterial overgrowth. The canal ends at the *tympanic membrane* (eardrum), which stretches across the end of the audi-

tory canal and separates the external ear from the middle ear.

The middle ear, referred to as the tympanic cavity, is a hollowed-out area of the temporal bone that contains auditory ossicles (bones): malleus (hammer), incus (anvil), and stapes (stirrup). The malleus is attached to the tympanic membrane and to the incus. The incus is connected to the stapes which, in turn, fits through the oval window and attaches to a small area in the cochlea. The eustachian tube connects the middle ear area with the nasopharynx and serves to equalize air pressure and provide drainage. The round window, below the oval window, permits the cochlea to bulge slightly into the middle ear area as the stapes vibrates the cochlear membrane.

The inner ear consists of the cochlea, the semicircular canals, and the vestibule. The vestibule contains the suspended utricle and saccule separated by perilymphatic fluid. It opens into the oval and round windows, the cochlea, and the semicircular canals.

The cochlea contains the organ of Corti, the hearing sense organ. The cells of this organ have tiny hairlike strands (cilia) that protrude into the fluid of the cochlea. The three bony semicircular canals house the membranous semicircular canals and are separated from them by perilymphatic fluid.

The eighth cranial nerve travels to the temporal lobe of the cerebral cortex from the ear in two branches. The cochlear division, originating in the cochlea (in the organ of Corti), is responsible for hearing impulses. The vestibular division, originating in the vestibule and the semicircular canals, transmits messages to the brain that assist with postural adjustments.

THE MECHANISM OF HEARING

Hearing is accomplished by sound waves moving through air in the auditory canal, causing the tympanic membrane and then the auditory ossicles to vibrate. The vibration is transmitted to the fluid in the inner ear. The cochlea is stimulated by the vibration, and the cochlear fluid also vibrates. The cilia of the organ of Corti send impulses to the brain for interpretation via the acoustic nerve to the cerebral cortex. Before reaching the auditory area of the temporal lobe, impulses pass through "relay stations" in nuclei in the medulla, pons, midbrain, and thalamus.

THE MECHANISM OF EQUILIBRIUM

Equilibrium is controlled primarily by the vestibular apparatus, although other mechanisms, including vision and *proprioception* from the limbs, assist in this control. Equilibrium is maintained by automatic shifts of tone in the muscles from one side of the body to the other side, or forward and backward, in accordance with various signals arriving from the vestibular apparatus, the eyes, and the proprioceptors.

Inside the vestibular apparatus are many hair cells that are surrounded by fluid and entwined with sensory axons of the vestibular nerve. Bending of the hair cells or tufts to one side activates the axons, causing them to transmit impulses to apprise the central nervous system (CNS) of their relative position. As impulses are transmitted from the hair cells or tufts, indicating, for example, that the body is falling forward, messages are sent by way of the CNS causing the body to lean backward. Leaning backward subsequently changes the position of the hair cells or tufts, which restores equilibrium.

Visual images also help the person to maintain equilibrium by simple visual detection of the upright stance. Any slight linear or angular movement of the body instantaneously shifts the visual images to the retina, which then relays impulses to the equilibrium center. Therefore, optic information is similar to that processed by the semicircular canals and can help equilibrium centers predict that the person will need to correct body position so he or she will not fall.

By far, the most important proprioceptive information needed for the maintenance of equilibrium comes from the neck. Here, proprioceptive centers detect changes in orientation of the head with respect to the body and transmit this information to the equilibrium centers in the CNS.

Thus, to maintain balance, all three mechanisms are needed. If one mechanism is not working correctly, equilibrium can usually be maintained if the person performs all movements slowly.

The eyes and the ears are two important sense organs. As in any other part of the body, diseases occur in both the eyes and ears. Many of these conditions can be treated with medications. Chapter 60 discusses eye and ear disorders and the medications used to treat them.

SUMMARY

The eye and ear are the organs of sight and hearing. The anatomy and physiology of both organs are discussed. The refractory medium of the eye permits the image to enter the eye and be focused on the retina. Hearing is accomplished by sound waves moving through the air in the auditory canal, causing the tympanic membrane and auditory ossicles to vibrate. The cochlea is stimulated by the vibration. The cilia of the organ of Conti send the impulse to the brain along the acoustic nerve to the cerebral cortex for interpretation.

BIBLIOGRAPHY

Guyton, A: Textbook of Medical Physiology. WB Saunders, Philadelphia, 1986.

Luckmann, J and Sorensen, K: Medical–Surgical Nursing. WB Saunders, Philadelphia, 1986.

Pavan–Lanston, D (ed): Manual of Ocular Diagnosis and Therapy. Little, Brown & Co, Boston, 1980.

60
CHAPTER

MEDICATIONS USED IN EYE DISORDERS

CHAPTER OUTLINE

THERAPEUTIC AGENTS
  Diagnostic Aids
  Anti-infective Drugs
  Anti-inflammatory Drugs
  Local Anesthetics
  Lubricants
  Decongestants
  Miotics
  Beta-Adrenergic Blockers
  Carbonic Anhydrase Inhibitors
  Osmotic Agents
  Mydriatics and Cycloplegics
  Miscellaneous Eye Agents
USING THE NURSING PROCESS
  Assessment
  Nursing Diagnosis
  Planning and Intervention
  Patient Teaching
  Evaluation
SUMMARY

TABLES

Nursing Process
Patient Teaching
Drug Tables

GLOSSARY TERMS USED IN THIS CHAPTER

Ciliary body spasm
Conjunctival chemosis
Conjunctivitis
Cycloplegics
Diplopia
Esotropia
Glaucoma
Iontophoresis
Keratopathy
Miosis
Miotic
Mydriasis
Mydriatic
Nystagmus
Ocular palsies
Oculogyric crisis
Optic neuritis
Papilledema
Ptosis
Punctate defects
Retrobulbar Injection
Stevens-Johnson syndrome
Trabeculoplasty
Vagotonia

MEDICATIONS USED IN EYE DISORDERS

MERRILY MATHEWSON KUHN, R.N.C, Ph.D., CCRN

LEARNING OBJECTIVES

After reading this chapter, the student will be able to:

1. Identify those medications commonly used for eye disorders.

2. Differentiate among the medications used for eye disorders as to mechanism of action, route of administration, pharmacokinetics, adverse effects, contraindications, and interactions.

3. Identify specific areas to assess in the patient requiring medications for eye disorders in order to formulate appropriate nursing diagnoses.

4. Plan the nursing interventions necessary to administer medications for eye disorders, and choose appropriate teaching strategies to gain patient compliance.

5. Evaluate the patient at various stages of treatment to gauge nursing interventions.

THERAPEUTIC AGENTS

More than half of the world's population has eye problems. Although many conditions are correctable with eyeglasses or contact lenses, others require medication to control or treat. Antibacterial, anti-inflammatory, antifungal, and antiviral agents are often used to treat inflammatory eye disorders (Table 60–1). Topical anesthetics are used either to allow examination of the eye or to enable surgical operations to be performed on the eye. *Mydriatics* and *cycloplegics*, representing both sympathomimetic and anticholinergic medications, may also be used to dilate the pupil during eye examinations. Lubricants are sometimes needed to replace tears or to prevent damage to the cornea when the ability to blink is absent. *Miotics* (cholinergic drugs), sympathomimetic medications, carbonic anhydrase inhibitors, and osmotic agents are used to treat and control *glaucoma* (Table 60–2). Ocular medications are most often administered topically as sterile solutions, ointments, or conjunctival inserts and are easy to instill into the eye. Although ointments remain in contact with the eye longer than solutions, they leave a film over the eye that may interfere with vision. On the other hand, solutions may be responsible for a higher incidence of contact dermatitis than ointments, as they are most likely to contain preservatives and other common sensitizers. Less frequently, ocular medications may be administered through the application of packs; administered by *iontophoresis*, or subconjunctival or *retrobulbar injection;* or injection directly into either eye chamber.

The majority of eye medications are discussed in other chapters of this book and are reviewed here only briefly with their usual ophthalmic dosages. This chapter discusses in detail the miotics, mydriatics, cycloplegics, lubricants, topical anesthetics, and diagnostic aids.

DIAGNOSTIC AIDS

Several preparations are available for diagnostic purposes. Fluorescein sodium, a nontoxic water-soluble dye, can be applied to the cornea of the eye. The dye stains denuded areas of epithelium, like scratches, a bright green color, while foreign bodies in the eye are surrounded by a green ring. Areas where conjunctiva are absent are stained yellow. The staining of the eye disappears in about 30 minutes. If the nasolacrimal drainage system is patent, the dye that has been instilled in the eye appears in the nasal secretions.

Fluorescein can also be used to fit hard contact lenses, to test lacrimal patency, and to identify defects in retinal pigment epithelium in retinal photography. With the exception of Fuorexan, most fluorescein products are not used to fit soft contact lenses, since the lens absorbs the dye. Fluorexon (Fluoresoft) is available for use with soft contact lenses having less than a 60% water content.

Solutions of fluorescein are easily contaminated with *Pseudomonas aeruginosa*. To prevent this, the dye is impregnated onto strips of dry filter paper. Prior to the instillation of the dye into the eye, the filter paper is moistened with a sterile solution; the filter paper is then gently brought into contact with the conjunctiva, allowing the dye to disperse. Fluorescein products are featured in Table 60–3. Fluorescein can also be administered intravenously as an aid in retinal angiography, including examination of the fundus.

Another diagnostic product is Fluress, a combination of the dye fluorescein and a local anesthtic benoxinate. One drop of a 0.25% solution can be used effectively to facilitate removal of foreign bodies from the eye.

Table 60–1. INFLAMMATORY EYE DISORDERS

Site	Condition	Etiology	Symptoms
Lids	Blepharitis (inflammation of lid margin)	Bacterial infection, seborrhea	Irritation of eye, redness and edema of lid margins, crusting of eye
	Chalazion (inflammation of sebaceous gland [meibomian gland] of eyelid) Hordeolum (sty) (inflammation of eyelash follicle)	Usually not infected initially. Bacterial infections are secondary Bacterial	Cysts of lids. None painful unless associated with secondary infection. Abscess or cyst of lid, red and painful
Conjunctiva	Conjunctivitis	Bacterial, viral "pink eye," fungal, allergy, chemical irritation, environmental irritation	Redness, burning, tearing, edema of eye lids, itching, photophobia, gritty sensation in eye
Cornea	Keratitis	Bacterial, viral (herpes simplex), autoimmune, trauma	Redness, burning

Table 60–2. COMPARISON OF GLAUCOMAS

	Open-Angle Glaucoma	Narrow-Angle Glaucoma
Incidence	Most common.	Least common.
Etiology	Diabetes, severe myopia.	Trauma, inflammation pupillary dilatation.
Pathophysiology	Clogging of trabecular meshwork with tissue debris.	Anterior chamber is too tight for aqueous humor to flow freely through it.
Progression	Slowly, usually in both eyes simultaneously.	Quickly, often a medical emergency, occurs in one eye only.
Vision loss	Peripheral is lost first, followed by precise central vision. Blindness develops in months or years.	Blindness can occur in 3 to 5 days.
Treatment	Medications: miotics, β-blockers, diuretics, mydriatics. Surgery.	Medications: diuretics. Surgery: cryosurgery, laser surgery.

An additional dye used occasionally in diagnosis is rose bengal. It is used for routine ocular examinations or when superficial corneal or conjunctival tissue change is suspected.

When any of these staining agents are used topically, the patient is told that these agents may be irritating and cause discomfort and staining of the eye and skin around the eye for a short period of time. The skin staining can be washed off with mild soap and water.

Other groups of medications are also used in diagnosing problems of the eye, including mydriatics and cycloplegics.

ANTI-INFECTIVE DRUGS

Anti-infective agents may be administered systemically or locally in the form of drops, ointment, packs, corneal baths, or even injections into the anterior chamber. Eye infections require prompt treatment to prevent the spread of infection and damage to the eye resulting in impaired vision.

The causative organisms are identified when possible, but treatment should not be withheld while awaiting results of a culture or smear. Frequently seen causative strains include gram-positive organisms including *Staphylococcus* and *Streptococcus* organisms. Gram-negative causative organisms include *Pseudomonas, Proteus, Klebsiella, Escherichia coli, Neisseria gonorrhoeae* in the newborn, *Haemophilus influenzae* in children, and Koch–Weeks bacillus *(H. aegyptius).* Many inflammatory diseases of the eye are due to viruses or other agents currently not sensitive to antibacterial drugs; the use of antibacterial agents in these situations is usually not warranted.

Table 60-4 features the antibacterial, antifungal, and antiviral agents commonly used in treating eye disorders. The table identifies the general indications and usual doses for topical conjunctival, parenteral, and IV dosages when applicable, as well as general contraindications, precautions, adverse effects, and nursing implications. Although the majority of anti-infectives will not penetrate the eye when given systemically, a few anti-infectives are capable of penetration when the blood–aqueous humor barrier is weakened by inflammation or injury.

Topical application is often the route of choice for ophthalmic drugs. This route is selected because the medication used is rarely or never administered system-

TEXT RESUMES ON PAGE 1646

Table 60–3. DIAGNOSTIC PRODUCTS

Product Name	Manufacturer	Fluorescein	Other Components
Fluorescein sodium	Alcon	2% solution	Phenylmercuric nitrate
Fluorescein sodium	Barnes & Hines	2% solution	Phenylmercuric nitrate
Fluro-I-Strip	Wyeth-Ayerst	9 mg/strip	Chlorobutanol, polysorbate 80, boric acid, potassium chloride, sodium carbonate
Fluro-I-Strip AT	Wyeth-Ayerst	1 mg/strip	Chlorobutanol, polysorbate 80, boric acid, potassium chloride, sodium carbonate
Ful-Glo	Barnes & Hines	0.6 mg/strip	
Fluress	Barnes & Hines	0.25% solution	Boric acid, chlorobutanol, povidone, benoxinate hydrochloride 0.4%
Fluorexon (Fluorexon)	Holles Labs.	0.35% solution	
Rose bengal	Several	1% solution	1% providone, sodium borate, polyethylene glycol, P-isoactylphenol 10, thimerosal 0.01%
Rose bengal	Several	1.3 mg strips	

Table 60–4. ANTIBACTERIAL, ANTIFUNGAL, AND ANTIVIRAL AGENTS USED IN EYE DISORDERS

Medication	Covered	Strength and Dosage*
ANTIBACTERIALS		
Action: interferes with or destroys various pathogens in the eye by inhibiting protein synthesis in micro-organisms.		
Use: gram-positive-negative, fungal or viral infections.		
Bacitracin (AK-Tracin, Bacitracin Ophthalmic)	Gram-positive	**For all:** Not more than 20 ml should be prescribed initially and perscription should not be refilled without consultation with physician. Topical: 1 gtt 10,000 units/ml q 1–4 hr Subconjunctival: 10,000 units in 0.5 ml solution.
Chloramphenicol (Chloromycetin Ophthalmic, Chlorofair, AK-Chlor)	Gram-positive and gram-negative	Topical: ointment 1%, solution 0.5% q 1–4 hr. Subconjunctival: 1.25 mg in 0.5 ml isotonic NaCl.
Erythromycin (AK-Mycin, Ilotycin)	Gram-negative	Subconjunctival: 50 mg in 0.5 ml isotonic NaCl.
Gentamicin sulfate (Gentafair, Gentak)	Gram-positive and gram-negative	Topical: 1 gtt 3–10 mg/ml q 1–4 hr; ointment q 3–4 hr. Subconjunctival: 10–30 mg in 0.5 ml aqueous solution.
Neomycin sulfate (Myciguent)	Gram-positive and gram-negative	Topical: ointment q 3–4 times/day. Subconjunctival: 100–500 mg in 0.5 ml isotonic NaCl.
Polymyxin B sulfate (Aerosporin)	Gram-negative	Topical: solution 1 gtt 5,000–20,000 units/ml. Subconjunctival: 5–10 mg in 0.5 ml isotonic NaCl.
Sulfacetamid sodium (Sulamyd, AK-Sulf)	Gram-positive and gram-negative	Topical: ointment 10%; solution 10% and 30%.

*Within the column listing adverse effects, underlines indicate the most common effects; CAPITALS indicate life-threatening effects.

Contraindications/ Precautions	Adverse Effects*	Interactions	Nursing Implications
Contraindicated in prior hypersensitivity and in epithelial herpes simplex keratitis, vaccinia, varicella, myobacterial infections, and fungal disease.	Ophth: overgrowth of non-susceptible organisms, local irritation, itching Derm: urticaria, vestibular and maculopapular dermatitis	None known	ASSESSMENT: History of symptoms, previous drug hypersensitivity. Carefully assess local (contact dermatitis) and other systemic reactions. INTERVENTION: Tilt head back, place medication in conjunctival sac and close eye. Apply light finger pressure on the lacrimal sac for 1 minute following instillation. Keep medications sterile. Avoid touching applicator tip to reduce contamination. Administer only as directed. Administer the correct vehicle—ointment or liquid. EVALUATION: Notify physician if stinging, burning, or itching become pronounced or if redness, irritation, swelling, or pain persist.
Same as above	Same as for all plus Hemo: BONE MARROW HYPOPLASIA, including APLASTIC ANEMIA	Chloramphenical will inhibit chymotrypsin.	Same as for all
Same as above	Same as for all	Allergic cross-reactions may occur that could prevent further use.	Same as for all
Same as above	Same as for all	None known	Same as for all
Same as above	Integ: Redness, scaling, pruritus. Systemic absorption: NEPHROTOXICITY, NEUROTOXICITY, OTOTOXICITY, neuromuscular blockade, hypersensitivity.	None known	INTERVENTION: May be absorbed through eyes following topical application.
Same as above	Same as for all	None known	Same as for all
Contraindicated in prior hypersensitivity.	Neuro: headache, browache, blurred vision	Local anesthetic will decrease absorption.	ASSESSMENT: Assess for prior hypersensitivity.

CONTINUED ON THE FOLLOWING PAGE

Table 60–4. ANTIBACTERIAL, ANTIFUNGAL, AND ANTIVIRAL AGENTS USED IN EYE DISORDERS–*CONTINUED*

Medication	Covered	Strength and Dosage*
Sulfacetamid sodium–*Continued*		
Sulfisoxazole (Gantrisin)	Gram-negative	Topical: ointment 4%, small amount 1–3 times/day hs; solution 4%, 2–3 gtt tid and prn.
ANTIFUNGAL MEDICATIONS Natamycin (Natacyn)	Yeast and fungi	Topical: 1 gtt of 5% solution q 1–2 hr.
ANTIVIRAL MEDICATIONS For All Antiviral Medications:		**For all:** Not more than 20 ml should be prescribed initially and prescription should not be refilled without consultation with physician.
Idoxuridine (IDU, Herplex, Stoxil, Dendrid)	Herpes simplex keratoconjunctivitis (some strains of herpes simplex resistant to idoxuridine)	Topical: ointment 0.5% q 4 hr; solution 1 gtt 0.1% q 1–2 hr daily and q 2–4 hr nightly.

*Within the column listing adverse effects, <u>underlines</u> indicate the most common effects; CAPITALS indicate life-threatening effects.

Contraindications/ Precautions	Adverse Effects*	Interactions	Nursing Implications
	Hemo: BONE MARROW DEPRESSION Integ: STEVENS-JOHNSON SYNDROME, EXFOLIATIVE DERMATITIS, photo-sensitivity, skin rash Ophth: local irritation, burning, transient stinging		INTERVENTION: May cause sensitivity to bright lights; minimized by wearing sunglasses. EVALUATION: Do not discontinue without consulting physician. Notify physician if no improvement in 7–8 days or if condition worsens.
Same as above.	Same as above.	Same as above.	Same as above.
Contraindicated in prior hypersensitivity. Safe use in pregnancy has been established.	One case reported of conjunctival chemosis and hyperemia.	None known	ASSESSMENT: Carefully note local (contact dermatitis) and systemic reaction. INTERVENTION: Keep medications sterile. Administer only as directed. Administer the correct vehicle—ointment or liquid. Avoid exposure of medication to excessive light and heat. Shake well before use. EVALUATION: If not effective after 7–10 days, the infection is likely not sensitive to this agent.
Contraindicated in prior hypersensitivity. Use cautiously in pregnancy and lactation and in women of childbearing age.	Ophth: Occasional irritation, pain, pruritus, inflammation, edema of lids and eyes, allergic reactions, photophobia, occasional corneal clouding, punctate defects of ephithelium.	Do not administer concurrently with boric acid, as irritation will occur.	For all antiviral medications: ASSESSMENT: Assess for prior hypersensitivity. INTERVENTION: Carefully note local (contact dermatitis) and systemic reactions. Keep medications sterile. Administer only as directed. Administer the correct vehicle—ointment or liquid. Do not mix with other medications. To prevent recurrence of herpes, medication should be administered for 5–7 days after healing has occurred. Improvement usually occurs in 7–8 days and may continue up to 21 days. May cause photosensitivity. Wear dark glasses. EVALUATION: Notify physician if improvement not seen in 7 days or if pain, burning, or irritation occur.
Same as for all.	Same as for all.	Same as for all.	Same as for all.

CONTINUED ON THE FOLLOWING PAGE

Antibacterials/Antifungals/Antivirals for Eyes

Table 60–4. ANTIBACTERIAL, ANTIFUNGAL, AND ANTIVIRAL AGENTS USED IN EYE DISORDERS–*CONTINUED*

Medication	Covered	Strength and Dosage*
Vidarabine (Adenine arabinoside, Ara-A)	Herpes simplex types 1 and 2, idoxuridine-resistant herpes.	Topical: solution 3%
Trifluridine (Viroptic)	Herpes simplex I and II, keratoconjunctivitis, idoxuridine-resistant herpes.	Topical: solution 1%, 1 gtt q 2–4 hr (maximum daily dose 9 gtt)

*Within the column listing adverse effects, <u>underlines</u> indicate the most common effects; CAPITALS indicate life-threatening effects.

ically or because one wants to decrease the risk of systemic side effects and toxicities from a medication. Topical application is more likely to cause local inflammation and can sensitize the patient to that particular preparation.

The most commonly opthalmic antibacterial agents are bacitracin (Baciguent); certain aminoglycosides, including gentamicin sulfate (Garamycin), tobramycin (Tobrex), and neomycin (Myciguent); and sulfonamides such as sulfacetamide (Sulamyd). These agents are effective against most gram-positive and gram-negative organisms. It is important that only ophthalmic solutions be used.

Antifungal agents are also needed on occasion. The most commonly administered antifungals include amphotericin B (Fungizone) and nystatin (Mycostatin).

Antiviral agents are used to treat viral infections such as herpes simplex and viral conjunctivitis. The most common antiviral agents include idoxuridine (IDU), trifluridine (Viroptic), and adenine arabinoside (Ara-A).

Contraindications and Precautions

Antibiotics are contraindicated in persons hypersensitive to a component of the product. Antibiotics are contraindicated in epithelial herpes simplex keratitis, vaccinia, varicella, fungal diseases, and myobacterial infections of the eye. To treat these conditions, systemic antivirals or antifungals are administered.

Adverse Effects

In general, side effects experienced by patients receiving topical anti-infective drugs include local skin and eye ir-

ritation and conjunctivitis. Additional information on anti-infectives can be found in Chapter 46.

Antibiotics

BACITRACIN. Bacitracin (Bacitracin Ophthalmic, AK-Tracin) is most frequently used to treat most gram-positive and *N. gonorrhoeae*, a gram-negative bacterial infection of the eye. It can be administered topically or subconjunctivally in a 10,000 units/ml solution or ointment, every one to four hours.

CHLORAMPHENICOL. Chloramphenicol (Chloromycetin Ophthalmic, Clorofair) is effective against both gram-positive and gram-negative bacteria. It can be topically administered as a 0.5% solution or a 1% ointment every one to four hours; oral or IV use is reserved for severe infections. Chloramphenicol is used systemically only when necessary, in the smallest doses possible, and for the shortest time period, because of the associated risk of aplastic anemia.

NEOMYCIN SULFATE. Neomycin sulfate (Myciguent) is a aminoglycoside antibiotic, generally administered as an ointment three to four times daily for both gram-positive and gram-negative infections. Before beginning administration, a thorough medication history is necessary to determine any previous allergic reactions, since many people are now allergic to this agent. It may cause a local allergic reaction around the eyes. In addition, it is toxic to the kidney when used by injection. (An oral form is not systemically active, since it is poorly absorbed.)

POLYMYXIN B. Polymyxin B (Aerosporin) is effective against most gram-negative bacteria and is particularly useful in treating conjunctivitis. It is generally

Contraindications/ Precautions	Adverse Effects*	Interactions	Nursing Implications
Same as for all.	Ophth: Superficial punctate keratopathy, lacrimation, foreign body sensation, conjunctival infection, burning, irritation, pain, photophobia.	None known	Same as for all.
Same as for all.	Ophth: Transient mild irritation of cornea and conjunctiva, palpebral edema, hypersensitivity reaction, superficial punctate keratopathy, hyperemia, increased intraocular pressure.	Same as for all	Same as for all plus INTERVENTION: Drop medicine on to lower lid while looking up. Release lower lid. Keep eye open and do not blink for at least 30 sec. Apply gentle pressure with fingers to bridge of nose (inside corner of the eye) for about 1 minute. Wait at least 5 minute before using other drops. Do not blink more than usual.

well tolerated. The usual therapeutic dose of topical polymyxin B is one drop of a 5,000–20,000 units/ml solution.

SULFONAMIDES. Sulfacetamide (Sulamyd, AK-Sulf) and sulfisoxazole (Gantrisin) are sulfonamides used widely in eye infections. Before beginning administration, a thorough medication history is necessary to determine any previous allergic reactions to these drugs. Both preparations cause local irritation. Both are available as ointments and solutions in varying strengths. Patients receiving sulfacetamide solution in a stronger concentration may complain of transient eye irritation, which usually subsides with continued use. See Table 60–4 for more information.

Antifungal Agents

NATAMYCIN. Natamycin (Natacyn), an antifungal agent, is used to treat blepharitis, conjunctivitis, and keratitis caused by *Candida, Aspergillus, Cephalosporium, Fusarium,* and *Penicillium.* If improvement has not occurred in seven to ten days, the infection is likely not to be sensitive to this agent. Natamycin is administered as a 5% solution every one to two hours.

Antiviral Agents

Antiviral agents are available against herpes simplex 1 and 2. All products are thought to interfere with DNA synthesis within the virus. Antiviral agents are featured in Table 60–4.

IDOXURIDINE. Idoxuridine (IDU, Stoxil, Herplex, Dendrid) is an antiviral agent that complexes with the DNA of the herpes simplex virus and inhibits DNA replication and cell reproduction. Initial attacks of herpes simplex characterized by dentritic figures and keratitis respond better than stromal infections. Idoxuridine is

administered to the eye as an ophthalmic solution (0.1%) every one to two hours during the day and every two to four hours at night, or as an ointment (0.5%), administered every 4 hours. Side effects include occasional local pain, pruritis, inflammation, edema of the eyes or surrounding area, photophobia, and corneal clouding or ulceration. Idoxuridine is administered cautiously during pregnancy.

VIDARABINE. Vidarabine (Adenine arabinoside, Ara-A) is useful against a broad spectrum of viruses including herpes simplex types 1 and 2, varicella-zoster, and vaccinia viruses and is used as a 3% ophthalmic solution. Vidarabine is a pure analog and not thought to be cross-resistant or antigenic to idoxuridine. For this reason, vidarabine may be effective after idoxuridine has failed to be effective.

TRIFLURIDINE. Trifluridine (Viroptic) is used primarily against herpes simplex 1 and 2 and primary keratoconjunctivitis. It is available in a 1% ophthalmic solution. Specific administration technique is featured in Table 60–4.

Many anti-infectives are also available in combination with each other or other groups of medications. Commonly available ophthalmic combination drugs are included in Table 60–5.

ANTI-INFLAMMATORY DRUGS

The eye structures, because they are delicate, may develop functional damage such as scarring and impaired vision occurring secondarily to inflammation. Anti-inflammatory medications—the adrenal corticosteroids, in particular—are indicated in certain nonpyogenic inflammatory conditions of the eye to control inflammation and ultimately reduce the amount of permanent

Table 60–5. COMBINATION DRUGS FOR OPHTHALMIC ANTI-INFECTIVES

Combination Drugs	Basic Products* A	B	C	D	E	F	Other
AK-Spore				10,000	1.75		0.025 L
Bacticort Suspension				10,000		0.35	1 H
Blephamide Liquifilm Suspension	10	0.2					
Cetapred Ointment	10	0.25					
Chloromycetin Hydrocortisone Ophthalmic							12.5 L
Cor-Oticin Suspension						0.35	1.5 H
Cortisporin Ophthalmic Ointment			400	10,000		0.35	1 J 25 G
Cortisporin Ophthalmic Suspension				10,000		0.35	1 J
Isopto Catpred Suspension	10	0.25					10 K
Maxitrol Ophthalmic Ointment/Suspension				10,000		0.35	0.1 I
Metimyd Ophthalmic Ointment/Suspension	10	0.5					
Neo-Cortef Ophthalmic						0.35	0.5 H
NeoDecadron Ophthalmic Ointment						0.35	0.05 J
Neotal Ophthalmic			400	5,000	5		
Polysporin Ointment			500	10,000			
Vasocidin Ointment	10	0.5					
Vasocidin Solution	10	0.5					0.25 K

*Basic Products: A = sodium sulfacetamide, %; B = prednisolone acetate, %; C = bacitracin zinc, units; D = polymyxin sulfate B, units; E = neomycin sulfate, mg; F = neomycin sulfate, %; G = hydrocortisone acetate, %; H = hydrocortisone, %; I = dexamethasone, %; J = dexamethasone phosphate, %; K = prednisolone phosphate, %; L = gramicidin, mg/ml

scarring and visual loss. It is important to remember that the corticosteroids decrease defense mechanisms and thus reduce resistance to pathogen invasion. Therefore, the eyes are monitored closely for further infection.

Corticosteroids are most commonly used in acute ocular disorders caused by hypersensitivity or allergic reactions. The most commonly used preparations—dexamethasone (Decadron, Maxidex), fluorometholone (FML), hydrocortisone (Eye-Cort, Hydrocortone, Optef), and prednisolone (Econopred, Metraton, Pred)—are featured in Table 60–6. Corticosteroids used in eye disorders may be administered topically, injected into the eye itself, or used systemically. Corticosteroids applied topically increase the potential for fungal infections and, in addition, are related to an increased incidence of glaucoma and cataracts and may delay wound healing. Because of these complications, they are used for short-term therapy only. Additional information on corticosteroids can be found in Chapter 42.

LOCAL ANESTHETICS

Local anesthetics inhibit pain sensation, so the eye can be examined, foreign bodies removed, or superficial surgery performed. The first corneal anesthetic, cocaine hydrochloride, was used as early as 1884. Although the effects of cocaine hydrochloride may last as long as one to two hours, it has generally been replaced with shorter-acting preparations because of its toxicity to the corneal epithelium: with several repeated administrations of cocaine, the cornea may pit and slough, causing severe corneal damage.

All of the normally used topical anesthetics—tetracaine hydrochloride (Pontocaine) and proparacaine hy-

drochloride (Ophthaine, Ophthetic)—produce adequate corneal anesthesia within one minute and generally have a duration of approximately 15 minutes. If longer anesthesia is needed, the application can be repeated. Local anesthetics are listed in Table 60–7.

Action

Local anesthetics stabilize the neuron so it is less permeable to ions, thus preventing the transmission of nerve impulses.

Contraindications and Precautions

Local anesthetics are contraindicated in persons with known hypersensitivity. They are administered cautiously to patients with heart disease as they cause sweating, hypotension, dysrhythmia, and even cardiac arrest. They are also administered cautiously to persons with hyperthyroidism as they can cause restlessness, excitement, nausea and vomiting, twitching, convulsions, and therefore exacerbations of hyperthyroidism. Prolonged use is not recommended since corneal scarring and permanent loss of vision can occur.

Adverse Effects

Patients may complain of temporary stinging, burning, tearing, conjunctival redness, and photophobia due to local irritation. Local anesthetics can also delay wound healing. Permanent corneal opacification and scarring have been reported with prolonged use. Central nervous system (CNS) disturbances occasionally occur and are related to systemic absorption of the topical agent.

PROPARACAINE HYDROCHLORIDE. Proparacaine hydrochloride (Ophthaine, Ophthetic) is available as a 0.5% solution, which starts to work in 20 seconds and

Table 60–6. CORTICOSTEROIDS USED IN EYE DISORDERS

Medication	Topical* Dosage	Contraindications and Precautions	Adverse Effects	Nursing Implications
Action: to exert a topical antiinflammatory effect.				
Use: certain types of conjunctivitis, keratitis, and in corneal injury from chemical, radiation, and thermal burns.				
Dexamethasone (Maxidex)	0.1% suspension	All drugs in group: Contraindicated in fungal infections, acute infections, viral disease, tuberculosis, ocular herpes simplex. Use cautiously in glaucoma, corneal abrasion, pregnant and lactating women. Safety in children has not been established.	All drugs in group: Ophth: Posterior subcapsular cataracts (usually irreversible), increased intraocular pressure, glaucoma, impaired healing, masked symptoms of infections, systemic effects may occur with extensive use.	All drugs in group: ASSESSMENT: Carefully assess local (contact dermatitis) and systemic reactions. INTERVENTION: Keep medications sterile. Administer the correct vehicle—ointment of liquid. Use only for short time periods under close medical supervision. Do not rub eyes, and steroids increase bruisability of delicate eye tissue. Administer only as directed. May cause sensitivity to bright light—wear dark glasses. EVALUATION: Do not discontinue before physician has ordered discontinuation. If improvement has not occured in 7–8 days, or if pain, itching, or swelling occur, notify physician.
Dexamethasone phosphate (AK-Dex, Maxidex)	0.05% ointment			
Hydrocortisone acetate (Cortril A)	0.5% ointment			
Fluoro metholone (FML Forte)	0.25% suspension			
Medrysone (HMS)	0.1% suspension 0.1% ointment 1% suspension			
Prednisolone acetate (Predforte, AK-Tate Ophthalmic)	1% suspension			
(Predmild ophthalmic)	0.12% suspension			

*1–2 gtt into conjunctival sac q 1 hr day, q 2 hr night.
Ointment: apply thin coat to lower conjunctival sac 3–4 times/day.

Table 60–7. ANESTHETICS FOR EYE DISORDERS

Medications	Dose	Contraindications and Precautions	Adverse Effects	Nursing Implications
Action: applied topically to the eye to anesthetize the conjunctiva and cornea. Stabilizes neurons so they are less permeable to ions.				
Use: short surgical procedures, removal of foreign bodies, cataract surgery, and diagnostic procedures.				
Proparacaine hydrochloride (Ophthaine)	0.5% solution 1–2 gtt	For all: Contraindicated in known hypersensitivity. Use cautiously in allergies, hyperthyroidism, cardiac disease, open lesions of eye.	For all: Ophth: Temporary stinging, burning, conjunctival erythema, photophobia, epithelial damage, retardation of healing.	For all: ASSESSMENT: Carefully assess local (contact dermatitis) and systemic reactions. INTERVENTION: Keep medications sterile. Administer only as directed. Try not to blink more than usual. Warm ointment in hand several minutes before use. Administration is short term. Generally not given to patient for home use. Place eye patch over eye to protect it from injury. Corneal reflexes return within 1 hr. Before use of other eye drops wait 5 min. Before use of another ointment, wait 10 min.
Tetracaine hydrochloride (Pontocaine)	0.5% ointment or solution 1–2 gtt			

Table 60–8. LUBRICANTS USED IN THE EYE

1. **Polyvinyl Alcohol** (generally used for moistening hard contact lens):
   Hypotears
   Liquifilm Tears
   Neo-Tears
   Refresh
   Tears Plus
2. **Petrolatum-based Ointments:**
   Artificial Tears
   Duolube
   Duratears
   Hypotears
   Lacrilube
3. **Hydroxypropyl Methylcellulose:**
   Lacril
   Lyteers Isopto Plain
   Muro Tears
   Tears Naturale
   Tearisol
   Ultra Tears
4. **Hydroxpropyl Cellulose Ophthalmic Insert:**
   Lacrisert

has a duration of action of about 15 minutes. Generally, one to two drops are used. The dose may be repeated every five to ten minutes up to five to seven drops.

TETRACAINE HYDROCHLORIDE. Tetracaine hydrochloride (Pontocaine) is available in a 0.5% ophthalmic solution and a 0.5% ointment. Dosage is one to two drops or 0.5–1 inch of ointment that starts to work in 30 seconds and has a duration of action of 10–25 minutes.

LUBRICANTS

Lubricants may be needed by healthy individuals to replace tears or to moisten hard contact lenses or artificial eyes; and by ill patients with keratitis or neuroparalytic keratitis occurring during unconsciousness; or to protect the eye during surgical or diagnostic procedures. Some persons may lose their blink reflex due either to anesthesia or to acute or chronic CNS disorders resulting in unconsciousness. Lubricants or artificial tears contain balanced amounts of salts to maintain ocular tonicity (0.9% sodium chloride); buffers such as boric acid to adjust the pH; viscosity agents such as hydroxpropyl methylcellulose, methylcellulose, or polyvinyl alcohol to prolong eye contact time; and preservatives such as benzalkonium chloride, chlorobutanol, and thimerosal to maintain sterility. Methylcellulose products are nonirritating and can be used for prolonged periods of time to lubricate the eye. Excessive use may cause the lubricant to dry on the eyes and form "sandy" granules. These particles can be washed out with a sterile eye-irrigating solution. Polyvinyl alcohol products are often applied to hard contact lenses to lubricate them before insertion. Often, these lubricants are added to other eye products in order to prolong the contact time of topically applied preparations. Table 60–8 features the most common lubricants. Many of these lubricants are available either as drops or ointments in over-the-counter prepa-

rations. Lacrisert is available as a hydroxpropyl cellulose insert that is placed into the inferior cul-de-sac of the eye. This insert may be inserted once to twice daily and stabilizes and thickens the precorneal tear film and prolongs tear film breakup time. Patients may demonstrate allergies to these products, usually to the preservative, such as redness of the eyes, and should refrain from using them.

DECONGESTANTS

Products contianing adrenergic drugs such as naphazoline (0.01%–0.03%), phenylephrine (0.08%–0.2%), and tetrahydrozoline (0.01%–0.05%) may be used to cause constriction of the conjunctival blood vessels. They are commonly used to relieve conjunctival injection, that is, blood-shot eyes. The percentage following each product is the concentration found to be safe and effective by the FDA Advisory Review Panel on over-the-counter ophthalmic drug products.

These products may temporarily relieve itching and minor irritation caused by chemical or mechanical irritants or by immediate allergic reactions. They are not effective in treating delayed hypersensitivity reaction.

In the concentration present in over-the-counter products, adrenergic drugs rarely cause serious side effects. However, prolonged or indiscriminate use of this product is avoided, since this can lead to neglect of symptoms of serious eye disease, or to rebound vasodilation with increased redness.

Vasoconstrictors are applied topically to the eye (one to two drops every three to four hours or as needed) until symptoms subside.

Local application of decongestant adrenergic drugs may cause browache, headache, blurred vision, irritation, lacrimation, allergic conjunctivitis, and local dermatitis. In patients predisposed to narrow-angle glaucoma, these products may precipitate an acute attack of angle-closure glaucoma.

Naphazoline and tetrahydrozoline are more stable than phenylephrine. The activity of phenylephrine is greatly reduced by oxidation. Table 60–9 features the most commonly used products.

Table 60–9. DECONGESTANTS

	Ingredients*:				
	% A	% B	% C	% D	% E
AK-Con	0.01			0.01	0.01
Clear Eyes	0.012			0.01	0.1
Degest 2	0.012			0.0067	0.02
Vaso Clear	0.02			0.01	
AK-Nefrin		0.12		0.01	
Prefrin		0.12		0.004	
Murine Plus			0.05	0.01	0.1
Soothe			0.15	0.004	0.1
Visine			0.05	0.01	0.1

*A = Naphazoline, %; B = Phenylephrine hydrochloride, % C = Tetrahydrozoline hydrochloride, %; D = Benzalkonium Cl, %; E = Edetate disodium, %

MIOTICS

There are two distinct types of miotics: direct-acting cholinergics and cholinesterase inhibitors. They have the same end result but differ in their pharmacologic mechanisms.

Action

Both types of miotics are capable of penetrating the cornea rapidly and completely. Both groups of drugs induce constriction of the pupil, contraction of the ciliary muscle, and ultimately cause a fall in intraocular pressure that is associated with decreased resistance to the outflow of aqueous humor.

In chronic open-angle glaucoma, miotics lower intraocular pressure by reducing outflow resistances of aqueous humor. This action occurs as a result of contraction of the ciliary muscle and widening of the spaces within the trabecular meshwork.

In angle-closure glaucoma, miotics constrict the pupil, which draws the iris away from the trabecular meshwork. Care must be taken because miotics may close rather than open the angle, aggravating angle-closure glaucoma.

The direct-acting cholinergic medications are chemically related to acetylcholine, the chemical mediator of nerve impulse transmission, and include pilocarpine and carbachol (Miostat). They are used primarily in the treatment of open-angle glaucoma. The cholinesterase inhibitors, isoflurophate (Floropryl), physostigmine (Eserine), demecarium (Humorsol), and echothiopate (Phospholine), are also used in the treatment of open-angle glaucoma and are effective in treating strabismus as well. The miotics are featured in Table 60–10.

The direct-acting cholinergic miotics, when applied topically to the eye, elicit three general effects: they constrict the pupil (miosis) by causing contraction of the sphincter muscle of the iris (Fig. 60–1); they cause spasm of the ciliary muscle controlling accommodation; and they decrease resistance to the outflow of aqueous humor, causing a fall in intraocular pressure.

The cholinesterase-inhibitor miotics inhibit cholinesterase, an enzyme that destroys acetylcholine, thereby leaving acetylcholine free to act on the ciliary muscle and iris sphincter, causing pupil constriction and spasm of accommodation. When cholinesterase is inhibited,

TEXT RESUMES ON PAGE 1656

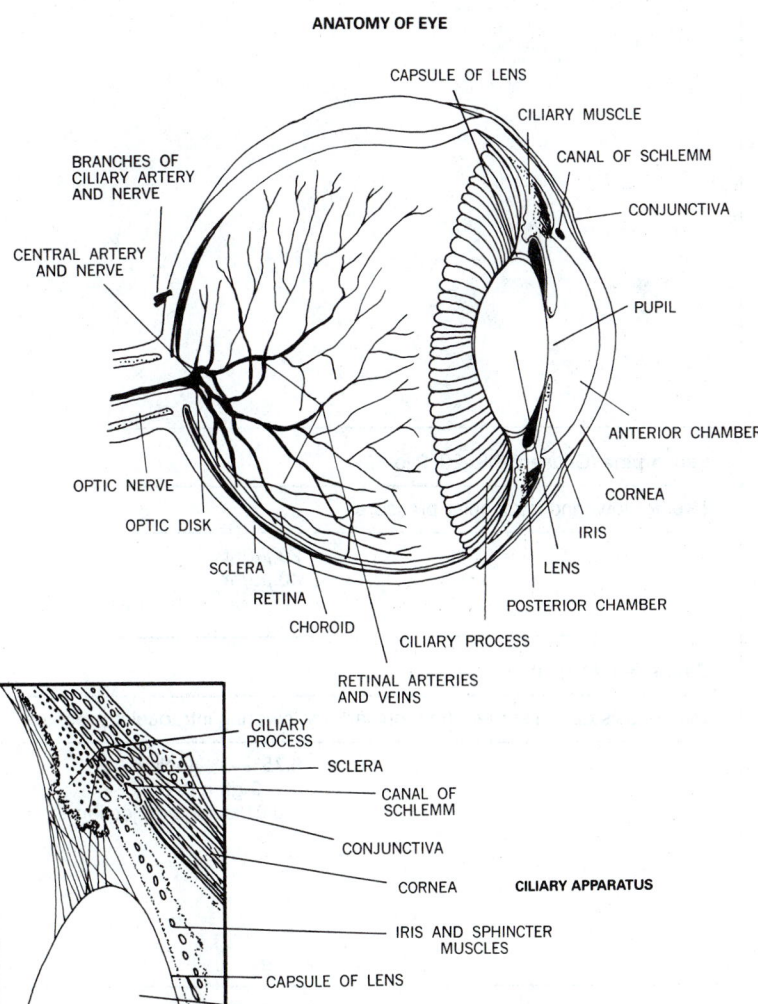

Figure 60–1. Miotics facilitate aqueous outflow by increasing the efficiency of the outflow channels and decreasing pupil size. They pull the iris away from the filtration angle, and this facilitates the outflow of aqueous humor. (From Thomas, C. L. (ed.) Taber's Cyclopedic Medical Dictionary, 16th ed., F. A. Davis, Philadelphia, 1989, with permission.)

Table 60–10. MIOTICS AND BETA-ADRENERGIC BLOCKING MEDICATIONS

Name	Dosage	Pharmacokinetics
DIRECT-ACTING CHOLINERGICS		
Action for all: constricts pupil and contracts ciliary muscle.		
Pilocarpine nitrate or **hydrochloride** (Isopto-carpine)		
Use: chronic simple glaucoma, chronic angle closure glaucoma, to neutralize mydriatics during eye examinations.		
	0.25%–10% sol, 1–2 gtt any solution up to 6 × daily. 4% gel applied at bedtime	O: 10–30 min P: 30 min D: 4–8 hr On lens: 2–3 hr Accommodation: 8 hr Pupillary: 24 hr D: 24 hr
Pilocarpine (Ocusert, Pilo-20, Pilo-40)		
Use: for lowering intraocular pressure		
	20 μg/hr 40 μg/hr	O: 30–60 min P: 1.5–2 hr D: 2–3 days (after removal)
Carbachol (Miostat)		
Use: miosis during surgery (intraocular), for lowering intraocular pressure in glaucoma treatment.		
	0.75%–3% topical sol, 1–2 gtt q 6–8 hr. 0.01% sol for injection	O: 10–20 min D: 4–8 hr O: 2–5 min D: 24 hr

Key to Abbreviations in the *Pharmacokinetics* column O-onset; P-peak; D-duration; PB-protein bound; B-biotransformed in; E-excreted in; ½ L-halflife.

*Within the column listing adverse effects, <u>underlines</u> indicate the most common effects; CAPITALS indicate life-threatening effects.

Contraindications/ Precautions	Adverse Effects*	Interactions	Nursing Implications
Contraindicated in hypersensitivity, secondary glaucoma, acute iritis, and inflammatory disease. Use cautiously in hypertension and bronchial asthma. Safety in pregnancy, lactating women, and children not established.	CV: hypertension, tachycardia Resp: bronchiolar spasm, pulmonary edema GI: salivation, nausea, vomiting, diarrhea Ophth: itching, burning, ciliary spasm, reduced visual acuity in poor illumination, conjunctival and ciliary congestion, ocular and periorbital pain.	None known.	For all drugs in this group: ASSESSMENT: Carefully assess local (contact dermatitis) and systemic reactions. INTERVENTION: Keep medications sterile. Administer only as directed. Administer the correct vehicle—ointment or liquid. Apply gentle pressure to the nasolacrimal canal for 1–2 minutes after administration to prevent drainage of solution from intended area. Avoid hazardous activities such as driving a car or operating heavy equipment because some blurring of vision will occur. May be instilled in both eyes. Patient should not rub or squeeze lids together after administration of medication. Store in tight, lightresistant container away from excessive heat. Patients should wear identification noting they have glaucoma and the medications being taken. EVALUATION: If stinging continues, notify physician.
Same as above.	Ophth: conjunctival irritation, mild erythema	None known.	Same as for all.
Contraindicated in hypersensitivity, secondary glaucoma, acute iritis, and inflammatory disease. Use cautiously in GI spasm, hyperthyroidism,	For all drugs in this group. Neuro: headache CV: syncope, cardiac dysrhythmia, flushing Resp: asthma GI: salivation, GI cramps, vomiting, diarrhea	Concurrent flurbiprofen may cause carbachol to be ineffective.	Same as for all.

CONTINUED ON THE FOLLOWING PAGE

Miotics & Beta-Adrenergic Blockers for Eyes

Table 60–10. MIOTICS AND BETA-ADRENERGIC BLOCKING MEDICATIONS–*CONTINUED*

Name	Dosage	Pharmacokinetics
Carbachol–*Continued*		
CHOLINESTERASE INHIBITORS		
Action: inhibit cholinesterase and thus enhance the effects of endogenous acetylcholine leading to decreased intraocular pressure.		
Physostigmine salicylate (Isopto Eserine)		
Use: Wide-angle glaucoma.		
	0.25% ointment 0.25%–0.5% solution 1–2 gtt 4 × daily.	O: 10–30 min P: UA D: 12–48 hr
Demecarium bromide (Humorsol)		
Use: accommodative esotropia, wide-angle glaucoma		
	0.125%–0.25% solution, 1 gtt q 12–48 hr.	O: 15 min–1 hr P: 2–4 hr D; 3–10 days
Isoflurophate (Floropryl)		
Use: accommodative esotropia, wide-angle glaucoma		
	0.25% ointment; ¼″ strip or less q 8–72 hr.	O: 5–10 min P: 0.5 hr D: 1–4 wk
Echothiophate iodide (Phospholine Iodide)		
Use: accommodative esotropia, wide-angle glaucoma		
	0.03%–0.25% solution, 1 gtt q 12 hr.	O: 10–30 min P: 0.5 hr D: 1–4 wk.

Key to Abbreviations in the *Pharmacokinetics* column O-onset; P-peak; D-duration; PB-protein bound; B-biotransformed in; E-excreted in; ½ L-halflife.

*Within the column listing adverse effects, underlines indicate the most common effects; CAPITALS indicate life-threatening effects.

Contraindications/ Precautions	Adverse Effects*	Interactions	Nursing Implications
Parkinson's disease, heart failure, and bronchial asthma.	Renal: urinary retention Ophth: corneal clouding, persistent bullous keratopathy, retinal detachment, transient ciliary/conjunctival irritation.		
For all drugs in this group. Contraindicated in hypersensitivity, secondary glaucoma, acute iritis, and inflammatory disease. Use cautiously in asthma, GU disease, intestinal or urinary tract obstruction, recent myocardial infarction. Safety in pregnancy and children has not been established. Administer to children with caution.	For all drugs in this group. Resp: difficulties in breathing CV: bradycardia, cardiac irregularities GI: salivation, abdominal cramps, nausea, vomiting, diarrhea Ophth: stinging, burning, lacrimation, eczematoid dermatitis, lid muscle twitching, conjunctival and ciliary redness, browache, headache	For all drugs in this group. Concurrent succinylcholine administration can cause respiratory and cardiovascular collapse. Additive effects occur with concurrent systemic anticholinesterases for myasthenia gravis. Carbamate, organophosphate insecticides, and pesticides may enhance systemic effects.	For all drugs in this group: ASSESSMENT: Assess for local irritation. INTERVENTION: First dose should be administered by a physician and tonometer readings taken at least hourly for 3–4 hours to observe for transient, paradoxic increase in intraocular pressure. Avoid prolonged contact with skin. Bedtime administration may minimize visual side effects. Patients need constant medical supervision while on medication. Ointment is inactivated by water, so the tube should be tightly capped between uses. EVALUATION: Notify physician if nausea, vomiting, cramps or prolonged diarrhea occur.
Same as above.	Same as for all.	Same as above plus chymotrypsin inhibits isofluophate	Same as for all.
Same as above.	Same as for all.	Same as Demecarium.	Same as for all.
Same as above.	Same as for all.	Same as Demecarium.	Same as for all.

CONTINUED ON THE FOLLOWING PAGE

Table 60–10. MIOTICS AND BETA-ADRENERGIC BLOCKING MEDICATIONS–*CONTINUED*

Name	Dosage	Pharmacokinetics
BETA-ADRENERGIC BLOCKING MEDICATIONS		
Action: reduce intraocular pressure; exact mechanism unknown, but does decrease aqueous production.		
Use: lowering intraocular pressure in chronic open-angle glaucoma		
Timolol maleate (Timoptic)	0.25%–0.5% solution 1–2 × daily.	O: 30 min P: 1–2 hr D: 24 hr
Betaxolol (Betoptic)	0.5% solution 1 gtt 2 × daily	O: 30 min P: 2 hr D: 12 hr
Levobunolol (Betagen, Liquifilm)	0.5% solution 1 gtt 1–2 × daily	O: <60 min P: 2–6 hr D: 24 hr

Key to Abbreviations in the *Pharmacokinetics* column O-onset; P-peak; D-duration; PB-protein bound; B-biotransformed in; E-excreted in; ½ L-halflife.
*Within the column listing adverse effects, underlines indicate the most common effects; CAPITALS indicate life-threatening effects.

the destruction of acetylcholine is dependent on the synthesis of new enzyme or eventual diffusion away from the action site. The cholinesterase inhibitors cause more ciliary spasm with discomfort and blurred vision than do the cholinergic miotics. The cholinesterase inhibitors may be short-acting (reversible) or long-acting (irreversible), although even the "irreversible" products eventually wear off.

Use

Miotics are used primarily to lower intraocular pressure in open-angle glaucoma (see Table 60–2). Unless the elevated intraocular pressure in glaucoma is lowered, blood flow to the retina is reduced, resulting in retinal damage and visual field loss.

Contraindications and Precautions

Both types of miotics are contraindicated in hypersensitivity, secondary forms of glaucoma, and acute inflammation of the eye. Safety during pregnancy and lactation and in children has not been established. Both types of miotics are administered cautiously to persons with narrow-angle glaucoma as these drugs may precipitate acute-angle closure. It is suggested that cholinesterase-inhibitor miotics be discontinued prior to surgery, since their action can interfere with the breakdown of succinylcholine, a commonly used muscle relaxant, resulting in prolonged muscle paralysis and apnea.

Direct-Acting Miotics

The direct-acting cholinergic miotics available include pilocarpine nitrate or hydrochloride and carbachol.

PILOCARPINE. Pilocarpine (Isopto-Carpine) is definitely the preferred miotic for both emergency, initial, and maintenance therapy for open-angle glaucoma. In most persons, particularly those over 50 years of age who do not have cataracts, pilocarpine is relatively free of undesirable side effects and is better tolerated than other miotics.

Adverse Effects. Pilocarpine causes side effects in about 80% of all patients. Early local side effects include burning, itching, pain, and ciliary spasm. Reduced visual acuity in poor light also occurs due to pupillary dilatation. Ocular and periorbital pain, additional symptoms of conjunctival and ciliary congestion, rarely persist for more than two weeks. Systemic side effects can also occur, including hypertension, tachycardia, pulmonary edema, salivation, nausea, vomiting, diarrhea, lacrimation, and muscle tremor all related to the direct cholinergic effect on body tissues.

Dosage. Pilocarpine (Isopto-Carpine) is available as an ophthalmic solution in concentrations ranging from 0.25%–10% (usual concentration is 0.5%–4%). The dose is titrated for each patient but often is 1–2 gtt administered up to six times daily. Persons with dark-pigmented eyes are more likely to require higher concentrations.

Contraindications/ Precautions	Adverse Effects*	Interactions	Nursing Implications
For all drugs in this group. Contraindicated in hypersensitivity, bronchospasm, COPD, congestive heart failure, bradycardia, and heart block. Administer with caution in diabetes, cerebral-vascular insufficiency. Use in pregnancy if benefits outweigh risk. Safety in children not established.	For all drugs in this group. Neuro: headache, cerebrovascular accident, depression, insomnia CV: disrhythmias, syncope, heart block, congestive heart failure, palpitation. Resp: bronchospasm GI: nausea Integ: rash Ophth: keratitis, blepharoptosis, visual disturbances, diplopia, ptosis Endo: masked symptoms of hypoglycemia in insulin-dependent diabetic	For all drugs in this group. Digitalis, calcium antagonists, and oral β-blockers have an additive slowing effect on conduction system. Catecholamine-depleting drugs have additive slowing effect on heart and may decrease blood pressure. Concurrent quinidine may cause excessive slowing.	For all drugs in this group: ASSESSMENT: Assess for local (contact dermatitis) and systemic reactions. Keep medications sterile. Administer only as directed. All other antiglaucoma eye medications should be discontinued on the second day of timolol therapy. Frequently monitor vital signs and blood pressure during initial therapy for side effects. EVALUATION: Tolerance has been noted, so follow-up appointment must be kept. Notify physician of severe stinging or discomfort.

Ocusert. Ocusert is a form of pilocarpine currently available as a clear, flexible, elliptical, wafer-like object slightly larger than a hard contact lens, with a white edge for easier visualization. It is inserted into the conjunctival sac for the continuous treatment of open-angle glaucoma. It is available as Ocusert Pilo-20 and Ocusert Pilo-40, releasing pilocarpine at rates of 20 to 40 μg/ hour, respectively. The nurse may instruct patients initially to insert the Ocusert at bedtime. The patient should gently rinse it first with tap water to prevent massive initial release of pilocarpine, which results in severe miosis and *ciliary body spasm* on insertion. The initial releasing dose is approximately equal to one drop of a 1%, 2%, or 3% pilocarpine solution, depending on the dosage being administered. The Ocusert may be moved digitally from the upper to the lower conjunctival sac if irritation begins to occur. It continues to release pilocarpine for about one week, freeing the patient from frequent medication administration and increasing compliance. The patient should always check placement of the product before going to bed and upon arising.

Carbachol. Carbachol (Isopto Carbachol) is a potent synthetic choline ester, similar to acetylcholine, used to treat open-angle and narrow-angle glaucoma and to produce miosis during surgery. It is effective in lowering intraocular pressure in glaucoma patients who have become refractory or allergic to pilocarpine, or when pilocarpine cannot be used. It is more potent and longer acting than pilocarpine because of its slower inactivation by cholinesterase.

Carbachol is available as 0.75%–3% ophthalmic solutions and has a duration of four to eight hours. Because the dose is individually titrated to the patient's response, continued close medical supervision is necessary. It shares the same contraindications as pilocarpine.

Carbachol is also used by single intraocular administration by an ophthalmologist during eye surgery. No more than 0.5 ml of carbachol is instilled into the anterior chamber of the eye before or after securing sutures. Miosis is usually maximal two to five minutes after application.

Cholinesterase Inhibitors

ACTION. The cholinesterase inhibitors inhibit the enzyme cholinesterase and thus enhance the effects of endogenous acetylcholine. The increased cholinergic activity in the eye leads to intense miosis and contraction of the ciliary muscle and loss of accommodation.

USE. The cholinesterase inhibitors are used to treat open-angle glaucoma, following iridectomy, and in convergent strabismus.

CONTRAINDICATIONS AND PRECAUTIONS. The cholinesterase inhibitors are contraindicated with any inflammatory disease of the iris or ciliary body, since there is increased contraction of the ciliary muscle. They are contraindicated in narrow-angle glaucoma (prior or iridectomy) due to the possibility of increasing the angle blockage. Safety in pregnancy and children has not been established. These products can be administered cautiously to children.

The cholinesterase inhibitors are administered cautiously to persons who must drive at night, since accommodation is lost and vision is poor. They are administered cautiously to persons with marked *vagotonia,*

Table 60-11. COMBINATION DRUGS FOR GLAUCOMA THERAPY

Combination Drug	Basic Products		
	Epinephrine Bitartrate (%)	Pilocarpine Hydrochloride (%)	Physostigmin Salicylate (%)
E-Carpine	0.5	1,2,3,4,6	—
E-Pilo (various)	1	1,2,3,4,6	—
Isopto P-ES	—	2	0.25
P1E1	—	—	—
P2E1	—	—	—
P2E1	—	—	—
P4E1	—	—	—
P6E1	1	1,2,3,4,6	—

bronchial asthma, spastic gastrointestinal disturbances, peptic ulcer, and pronounced bradycardia and hypotension, since all these conditions are aggravated by the increased activity of acetylcholine.

ADVERSE EFFECTS. Ocular side effects are most common and include burning and stinging, allergic follicular conjunctivitis, lid muscle twitching, conjunctival and ciliary redness, browache, headache, and myopia with blurred vision. Prolonged use may cause conjunctival thickening. Systemic side effects all are related to increased systemic effects of acetylcholine such as nausea, vomiting, diarrhea, abdominal cramps, urinary incontinence, salivation, bradycardia, or cardiac irregularities.

DRUG INTERACTIONS. Administration of succinylcholine concurrently with cholinesterase inhibitors during surgery may cause respiratory or cardiovascular collapse. Systemic anticholinesterase for myasthenia gravis may cause an additive effect.

PHYSOSTIGMINE. Physostigmine (Eserine) is available as an ointment in a concentration of 0.25% and as a solution in concentrations of 0.25%–0.5%. Both are administered into the conjunctival sac.

Demecarium. Demecarium (Humorsol) is a potent, long-acting quaternary ammonium compound and the most toxic of this group. It is used when patients have become refractory to the less toxic drugs. Besides its use in open-angle glaucoma, it is also used in accommodative *esotropia* (convergent strabismus). Demecarium causes contraction of ciliary muscle. Carbonic anhydrase inhibitors are used frequently in conjunction with demecarium to enhance its action.

Demecarium is available as an ophthalmic solution in concentrations ranging from 0.125%–0.25%.

ISOFLUROPHATE. Isoflurophate (Floropryl) is a potent, long-acting organophosphorus cholinesterase inhibitor. Isoflurophate is available as a 0.025% ointment, which is usually applied in a strip of ¼ inch or less every 8–72 hours to the conjunctival sac.

ECHOTHIOPHATE. Echothiophate (Phospholine) is an extremely potent, long-acting quaternary organophosphorus compound, similar in almost all ways to demecarium. Unlike demecarium, however, the cholinesterase inhibition produced by echothiophate is irreversible until new enzyme is produced.

Echothiophate is available as 0.03%–0.25% solutions and is administered every 12 hours.

Combination miotics are available. These products may combine different miotics or miotics with epinephrine. Common combination miotics are featured in Table 60–11.

BETA-ADRENERGIC BLOCKERS

A newer approach in treating chronic open-angle glaucoma is the use of the β-adrenergic blocking (sympatholytic) agent timolol (Timoptic), betaxolol (Betopic), and levobunolol (Betagon, Liquifilm) (see Table 60–10).

Action

Beta receptors, besides being located in the heart, skeletal muscles, and bronchioles, have been identified in ocular tissue, primarily in the ciliary muscle and in the sphincter muscle of the iris. Beta blockers combine reversibly with these receptors to block the response to sympathetic nerve stimulation or circulating catecholamine. (More detailed information on β-receptor sites can be found in Chapter 19)

Timolol and levobunolol are noncardioselective β_1- and β_2-blockers, whereas betaxolol is a cardioselective β_1-blocker. Intraocular pressure is lowered, although the exact mechanism is unknown. These products may decrease production of aqueous humor, which may lower intraocular pressure.

Use

The β-blockers lower intraocular pressure in patients with chronic open-angle glaucoma.

Contraindications and Precautions

These products produce systemic effects. Therefore, they are contraindicated in patients with bronchial asthma, severe chronic obstructive lung disease, bradycardia, and heart block, as these conditions are aggravated by β-adrenergic blocking agents. Patients with diabetes may experience spontaneous hypoglycemia, and the signs of hypoglycemia may be masked by β blockers. Patients with signs of cerebrovascular insufficiency may have an exacerbation of symptoms related to the decreased blood pressure and pulse. Since betaxolol is a cardioselective β-blocker, these effects are minimal. There are no well-controlled studies in pregnant women, so these products should be used only if the benefits outweigh the risk. Caution is advised when administering to nursing mothers as these products are excreted in milk. Safety in children has not been established.

Adverse Effects

Many side effects can occur from these drugs, including headache, cardiovascular dysrhythmias, nausea, and depression, that are all secondary to the systemic beta effect of these drugs. Additional side effects are found in Table 60–10.

Interactions

Several interactions can occur when administering β-blockers with other medications. Concurrent digitalis and calcium antagonists have an additive slowing effect on the conduction system. Concurrent oral β-blockers can also have an additive effect. Catecholamine-depleting drugs may have an additive slowing effect on the heart and may decrease the blood pressure, leading to vertigo, syncope, and postural hypotension. Additional interactions are found in Table 60–10.

Timolol Maleate

Timolol maleate (Timoptic) is a long-acting nonselective β blocker. When administered as a single agent, timolol does not alter pupillary diameter or reactivity to light, but it enhances the mydriatic effect of epinephrine. Timolol is better tolerated than most miotics in young adults and in older patients with cataracts because it does not cause spasm of accommodation or miosis.

Timolol is available as 0.25%–0.5% solutions and is generally administered twice daily. If it becomes necessary to change from one ophthalmic β-blocker to timolol, the first agent is discontinued after proper dosing on one day and timolol is started on the following day with one drop of 0.25% solution. The dosage can be increased if needed. If it is necessary to change from another antiglaucoma agent to timolol, on the first day continue with the agent being used and add one drop of 0.25% timolol twice daily. The next day discontinue the first agent completely. The dosage of timolol can be increased if needed.

Few adverse effects have been reported, but include ocular irritation, hypersensitivity, and visual disturbances. More recently, sexual dysfunction has been identified as an adverse effect. Various symptoms reported include impotence, decreased libido, and decreased ejaculation volume. In the majority of cases, symptoms reversed when timolol was stopped.

Betaxolol Hydrochloride

Betaxolol (Betopic) is a topical β-blocker acting primarily on β_1- (cardiac) receptors. Betaxolol is as effective as timolol and may be safer in asthmatics and patients with COPD. Betaxolol is available as a 0.5% solution and is administered one drop twice daily.

Levobunolol Hydrochloride

Levobunolol hydrochloride (Betagon) is a long-acting nonselective β-blocker for topical treatment of chronic open-angle glaucoma. It is as effective as timolol. Levobunolol is available as a 0.5% solution and one drop is administered in the affected eye one to two times daily.

CARBONIC ANHYDRASE INHIBITORS

The ciliary body, in order to produce aqueous humor, must have the enzyme carbonic anhydrase present. Carbonic anhydrase inhibitors interfere with the production of carbonic acid, which leads to a reduced level of bicarbonate ion and a systemic acidosis. This is associated with reduced aqueous humor formation and decreased intraocular pressure. The systemic acidosis also adds to the ocular hypotensive effect. These drugs were first developed as diuretics but are now used almost solely for the treatment of glaucoma, particularly when adequate control cannot be achieved with miotics alone. Carbonic anhydrase inhibitors are used in conjunction with miotics and osmotic agents to treat both open-angle and narrow-angle glaucoma as well as angle-closure attacks.

Duration of action is 6–18 hours, depending on the drug, from a single oral therapeutic dose, and aqueous humor production may be reduced by 50%. The effect on carbonic anhydrase does not depend on diuretics. The most commonly prescribed carbonic anhydrase inhibitors are acetazolamide (Diamox), dichlorphenamide (Daranide), and methazolamide (Neptazane).

The most common adverse effects, although usually not severe, include lethargy, anorexia, drowsiness, depression, malaise, diuresis, and numbness and tingling of the face and extremities. The frequency and intensity of these side effects are dose related and some are associated with systemic acidosis. These side effects are often the cause of patient intolerance to these products. When diuresis is produced, potassium depletion can occur. Carbonic anhydrase inhibitors frequently cause gastric distress, nausea, vomiting, and diarrhea. All of these effects are due to a local irritant action that may be alleviated by taking the drug with food. For more information on carbonic anhydrase inhibitors, see Chapter 38. Table 60–12 features the commonly used preparations and their usual doses.

OSMOTIC AGENTS

Osmotic diuretics are administered intravenously or orally for short-term reduction of intraocular pressure and vitreous volume. By increasing the plasma osmolarity, fluid is drawn from the eyeball and pressure is reduced. Osmotic agents are generally effective in patients who do not respond to miotics or carbonic anhydrase inhibitors. They are generally given preoperatively and postoperatively for this reason. (See Chapter 38 for more information on diuretics.)

TEXT RESUMES ON PAGE 1662

Table 60–12. CARBONIC ANHYDRASE INHIBITORS AND OSMOTIC AGENTS USED IN EYE DISORDERS

Name	Dosage	Mode of Administration	Pharmacokinetics
CARBONIC ANHYDRASE INHIBITORS			
Action: block ocular carbonic anhydrase in the ciliary epithelium			
Use: open-angle glaucoma, narrow-angle glaucoma, angle-closure attacks			
Acetazolamide sodium (Diamox)	500 mg cap (time-released)	PO	O: 2 hr P: 8–12 hr D: 18–24 hr ½L: 5 hr PB: 93% B: UA E: urine (unchanged)
	62.5–250 mg tablets 1–2 × daily: 5–30 mg/kg/24 hr.	PO	O: 1 hr P: 2–4 hr D: 8–12 hr ½L: 5 hr PB: 93% B: UA E: urine (unchanged)
Dichlorphenamide (Daranide)	50–200 mg q 6–8 hr.	PO	O: 1 hr P: 2–4 hr D: 6–12 hr ½L: UA PB: UA B: UA E: UA
Methazolamide (Neptazane)	25–50 mg q 6–8 hr	PO	O: 2–4 hr P: 6–8 hr D: 10–18 hr ½L: UA PB: 55% B: UA E: urine, (55% unchanged)
OSMOTIC AGENTS			
Action: by increasing plasma osmolarity, draws fluid from the eye and reduces intraocular pressure			
Use: acute angle-closure glaucoma, pre- and postoperative treatment of chronic glaucoma, also before and after other eye surgeries.			
Glycerin (Glyrol)	50%–75% solution 1–1.5 g/kg 1–1.5 hr prior to surgery.	PO	O: 10–30 min P: 1–1.5 hr D: 4–5 hr ½L: 30–45 min

Key to Abbreviations in the *Pharmacokinetics* column O-onset; P-peak; D-duration; PB-protein bound; B-biotransformed; E-excreted in; ½ L-halflife.
*Within the column listing adverse effects, underlines indicate the most common effects; CAPITALS indicate life-threatening effects.

Contraindications/ Precautions	Adverse Effects*	Interactions	Nursing Implications
For all carbonic anhydrase inhibitors: Contraindicated in sensitivity, renal or hepatic dysfunction. Use cautiously in hypokalemia, hyponatremia, patients with severe respiratory acidosis. Safety in pregnancy, lactating women, and children not established.	For all carbonic anhydrase inhibitors: Neuro: headache, nervousness, paresthesias CV: malaise, fatigue, weakness GI: anorexia, weight loss, nausea, vomiting, diarrhea, constipation Hemo: may increase blood uric acid level, THROMBOCYTOPENIA, LEUKOPENIA, AGRANULOCYTOSIS, APLASTIC ANEMIA Renal: diuresis, hypokalemia, renal colic, hematuria, oliguria Reprod: loss of libido, impotence Ophth: transient myopia	For all carbonic anhydrase inhibitors: None known	For all carbonic anhydrase inhibitors: ASSESSMENT: Assess for dehydration, potassium balance, and vital signs. INTERVENTION: Do not change brands. Take early in day, as it will increase urination. May cause GI upset; take with meals. May increase blood sugar in diabetes; monitor carefully.
	For All Osmotic Agents: Neuro: headache, confusion, dirorientation GI: nausea, vomiting	None known	For all osmotic agents: ASSESSMENT: Carefully assess fluid and electrolyte balance, urinary output, and vital signs. INTERVENTION: Headache may be relieved by having patient lie down during and after oral administration. Flavoring with lemon or lime juice and serving it over cracked ice may reduce nausea and vomiting.
Contraindicated in hypersensitivity. Give cautiously to cardiac patient—may precipitate CHF; to elderly patient—may precipitate dehydra-	Same as for all plus: Thirst, diarrhea	None known	Same as for all

CONTINUED ON THE FOLLOWING PAGE

Table 60–12. CARBONIC ANHYDRASE INHIBITORS AND OSMOTIC AGENTS USED IN EYE DISORDERS–*CONTINUED*

Name	Dosage	Mode of Administration	Pharmacokinetics
Glycerin–*Continued*			
Isosorbide (Ismotic, Alcon)	45% solution I: 1.5 g/kg Range 1–3 g/kg 2–4 × daily.	PO	O: 10–30 min P: 1–1.5 hr D: 5–6 hr ½L: 5–9.5 hr Same as above
Mannitol (Osmitrol)	1–2 g/kg body weight over 30–60 min. Children: 1–2 g/kg	IV IV	O: 30–60 min P: 60 min D: 6–8 hr ½L: 15–100 min Same as above
Urea (Ureaphil)	Adults: 30% solution, 0.5–2 g/kg at 60 gtt/min, not to exceed 4 ml/min. Children: 30% solution, 0.5–1.5 g/kg over 30 min.	IV IV	O: 30–45 min P: 1 hr D: 5–6 hr Same as above

Key to Abbreviations in the *Pharmacokinetics* column O-onset; P-peak; D-duration; PB-protein bound; B-biotransformed; E-excreted in; ½ L-halflife.
*Within the column listing adverse effects, underlines indicate the most common effects; CAPITALS indicate life-threatening effects.

The most commonly used osmotic agents include glycerin (Osmoglyn), isosorbide (Ismotic), mannitol (Osmitrol), and urea (Ureaphil). These agents have an onset of action in 10–60 minutes and a duration of four to eight hours. For specific times, refer to Table 60–12. In general, the side effects include diuresis leading to headache from reduction of cerebrospinal fluid volume, nausea, and vomiting. Other, more specific side effects resulting from use of mannitol and urea include agitation and disorientation.

All osmotic agents are given cautiously to persons with cardiac conditions because of the possible development of pulmonary edema and congestive heart failure due to the osmotic of fluid from the tissues. The weakened heart is unable to pump the added volume and the kidneys are unable to excrete the volume rapidly enough. Osmotic agents are given cautiously to the elderly because of the possible development of dehydration. Glycerin, because it is a carbohydrate, may cause the diabetic patient to develop hyperglycemia and glycosuria. The other osmotic agents are not carbohydrates, so they do not affect blood glucose levels.

Contraindications/ Precautions	Adverse Effects*	Interactions	Nursing Implications
tion; to patient with diabetes—may cause hyperglycemia and glycosuria. Safety in pregnancy, lactating women, and children not established.			
Contraindicated in severe renal disease and dehydration, severe cardiac decompensation. Give cautiously to cardiac patient—may precipitate CHF; to elderly patient—may precipitate dehydration; does not affect blood glucose levels.	Same as glycerin.	None known	Same as for all.
Contraindicated in severe renal disease and dehydration, severe cardiac decompensation. Give cautiously to cardiac patient—may precipitate CHF; to elderly patient—may precipitate dehydration. Safety in pregnancy, lactating women, and children not established.	Same as for all plus: Neuro: disorientation, convulsions GI: thirst, diarrhea	None known	Same as for all.
Contraindicated in severe renal impairment, active cerebral bleeding, marked dehydration, liver failure. Administer cautiously to patients with renal impairment. Safety in pregnancy, lactating women, and children not established.	Same as for all plus: Neuro: dizziness Renal: dehydration	None known	Same as for all plus INTERVENTION: Unstable; must be prepared before each administration. Urea is irritating to tissues and causes pain on injection.

MYDRIATICS AND CYCLOPLEGICS

Mydriatics are used to dilate the pupil, and *cycloplegics* paralyze accommodation (Table 60–13). Two groups of drugs, anticholinergics and α adrenergics, acting by different mechanisms, cause mydriasis.

Action

Anticholinergics, the muscarinic antagonists, inhibit the parasympathetic nervous system, whereas α adrenergics mimic the sympathetic nervous system. (For a review of the autonomic nervous system, see Chapter 19.) At times, both types of medications can be combined to achieve marked mydriasis. However, the anticholinergics alone are capable of producing cycloplegia.

Anticholinergics paralyze the ciliary muscle and the dilator muscle of the iris, causing both dilatation of the pupil and the paralysis of accommodation. This action is achieved through the blockage of acetylcholine. As the anticholinergics relax the ciliary muscle, the lens becomes less convex, and therefore accommodation for close vision becomes more difficult. Alpha adrenergics, on the other hand, contract the dilator muscle of the iris, causing dilation of the pupil, but they have only a slight effect on the ciliary muscle, so that accommodation is not affected.

The adrenergics, besides producing mydriasis and slight relaxation of the ciliary muscle, constrict conjunc-

TEXT RESUMES ON PAGE 1668

Table 60–13. MYDRIATICS AND CYCLOPLEGICS

Medication	Dosage	Onset	Duration
ANTICHOLINERGIC MYDRIATICS AND CLYCLOPLEGICS			
Action: paralyze ciliary muscle and dilator muscle of iris, causing both dilatation of pupil and paralysis of accommodation.			
Use: useful in estimating errors of refraction, intraocular examination, pre- and postoperative mydriasis, malignant glaucoma.			
Atropine sulfate (Atropisol)	Adults: 0.5%–3% solution, 0.5%–1% ointment 1–4 × daily. Children: 0.5% solution, 1–2 gtt 1–3 × daily before examination	M: P: 30–40 min C: P: 1–3 hr	M: 7–12 days C: 6–12 days
Cyclopentolate (Cyclogyl)	0.5%, 1%, and 2% solutions. Adults: 1–3 gtt Children: 1 gtt	M: O: 30–60 min C: P: 25–75 min.	M: 1 day C: 0.25–1 day
Homatropine hydrobromide (Isopto-Homatropine)	2%–5% solution 1–2 gtt q 3–4 hr. Children 1 gtt 2% solution	M: P: 40–60 min. C: P: 30–60 min.	M: 1–3 days C: 1–3 days
Scopolamine hydrobromide (Isopto-Hyoscine)	0.25% solution 1–2 gtt	M: P: 20–30 min. C: P: 30–60 min.	M: 3–7 days C: 3–7 days

Key to abbreviations: M-mydriasis; C-cycloplegia; O-onset; P-peak
*Within the column listing adverse effects, underlines indicate the most common effects; CAPITALS indicate life-threatening effects.

Contraindications/ Precautions	Adverse Effects*	Interactions	Nursing Implications
For all in group: Contraindicated in hypersensitivity and narrow-angle glaucoma. Use cautiously in cardiac conditions and in elderly and debilitated patients.	For all in group: Ophth: increased intraocular pressure, transient stinging, photophobia, allergic lid reactions, blurred vision.	None known	For all in group: ASSESSMENT: Carefully assess local (contact dermatitis) and systemic reactions. Physician should assess intraocular tension before and during use. INTERVENTION: Keep medications sterile. Administer only as directed. Administer the correct vehicle—ointment or liquid. Blurred vision may occur. Wear dark glasses in bright light if photophobia occurs. To avoid systemic absorption, compress lacrimal sac by digital pressure for 1–3 min after instillation. Heavily pigmented eyes may require larger doses. If epinephrine is being administered concurrently with miotics, the miotic is instilled 2–10 min before the epinephrine. Caution patient about driving and performing tasks requiring alertness, as these medications may cause drowsiness. EVALUATION: Notify physician of eye pain.
Same as for all.	Same as for all plus Neuro: ataxic gait, headache CV: tachycardia, dysrhythmia GI: dryness of mouth Renal: bladder distention Integ: flushing, dry skin Misc: fever	Same as for all.	Same as for all.
Same as for all.	Same as for all plus Neuro: psychiatric disturbances in children Neuro: ataxic gait, incoherent speech, restlessness, hallucinations, seizures, disorientation.	Same as for all.	Same as for all.
Same as for all.	Same as for all.	Same as for all.	Same as for all.
Same as for all.	Same as for all.	Same as for all.	Same as for all.

CONTINUED ON THE FOLLOWING PAGE

Table 60–13. MYDRIATICS AND CYCLOPLEGICS–*CONTINUED*

Medication	Dosage	Onset	Duration
Tropicamide (Mydriacyl)	0.5 and 1% solutions, 1–2 gtt.	M: O: 20–40 min C: P: 20–35 min.	M: 0.25–1 day C: 0.25–1 day

ALPHA-ADRENERGIC PREPARATIONS: MYDRIATICS

Epinephrine hydrochloride (Adrenalin Chloride)

Action: contract the dilator muscle of iris, causing dilation of pupil, has only a slight effect on ciliary muscle so accommodation is not affected.

Use: open-angle glaucoma, and glaucoma secondary to uveitis and for ocular examinations.

| | 0.1% solution | Ocular pressure fall:
O: 1 hr,
P: 4 hr
M:
O: few min
P: 30 min | 24 hr

1–3 hr |

Hydroxyamphetamine hydrobromide (Paredrine)

Action: contract the dilator muscle of iris, causing dilation of pupil, has only a slight effect on ciliary muscle so accommodation is not affected.

Use: open-angle glaucoma, and glaucoma secondary to uveitis, and ocular examinations.

| | 1% solution, 1–2 gtt | M: O: not available,
P: 45–60 min | few hours |

OPHTHALMIC VASOCONSTRICTORS

Use: (2.5 to 10% solution): pupil dilitation in uveitis and wide-angle glaucoma and surgery. (0.12%): decongestant to provide temporary relief of eye irritation.

| Phenylephrine hydrochloride (Neo-Synephrine) | 0.12–10% solution.
Adults: 1 gtt any solution | M: O: not availabe,
M: P: 30 min | 0.5–7 hr |

Key to abbreviations M-mydriasis; C-cycloplegia; O-onset; P-peak
*Within the column listing adverse effects, <u>underlines</u> indicate the most common effects; CAPITALS indicate life-threatening effects.

Contraindications/ Precautions	Adverse Effects*	Interactions	Nursing Implications
Same as for all.	Same as for all plus: Neuro: psychiatric disturbances in children	Same as for all.	Same as for all.
For all drugs in this group: Contraindicated in hypersensitivity and narrow-angle glaucoma. Use cautiously in cardiac disease and in elderly. Safety in pregnancy, lactating women, and children not established.	For all drugs in this group: Neuro: headache, browache, subarachnoid hemorrhage, stroke, faintness CV: palpitation, tachycardia, dysrhythmias, hypertension, myocardial infarction, sweating, pallor Resp: pulmonary embolism Integ: transient stinging, blurred vision.	For all in group: Use cycloprone and halothane anesthetics cautiously. When given with or up to 21 days after MAO inhibitors, may exaggerate adrenergic effects. Systemic side effects may be enhanced by beta blockers Pressor effects may be enhanced by tricyclic antidepressants, beta blockers, reserpine, guanethidine, methyldopa, and anticholinergics.	For all in group: ASSESSMENT: Assess local eye irritation. INTERVENTION: Do not use beyond 72 hr without consulting physician. EVALUATION: If severe eye pain, headache, spots before eyes, acute eye redness, discontinue use and consult a physician.
Same as for all.	Same as for all plus: Ophth: adrenochione deposits in conjunctiva and cornea, eye pain, allergic lid reactions.	Same as for all.	Same as for all plus: Do not use while wearing soft contact lenses.
Same as for all.	Same as for all plus Ophth: widely dilated pupils, increased intraocular pressure, photophobia.	Same as for all.	Same as for all.
Same as above plus Contraindicated in long-standing diabetes, advanced ASHD, debilitated or elderly, patient with intraocular lens implants.	Neuro: headache Ophth: rebound miosis	Same as above.	Same as above.

CONTINUED ON THE FOLLOWING PAGE

Mydriatics & Cycloplegics

Table 60–13. MYDRIATICS AND CYCLOPLEGICS–*CONTINUED*

Medication	Dosage	Onset	Duration
Naphazoline (Clear Eyes, Nafazain)			
Use: relief of redness of eye due to minor eye irritation			
	0.012%–0.05% solution OTC. 0.025%–0.1% solution by prescription. 1–2 gtt q 3–4 hr.	minutes	2–3 hr
Tetrahydrozoline (Murine Plus, Visine)	0.05% solution 1–2 gtt 2–4 × daily.	minutes	2–3 hr

Key to abbreviations: M-mydriasis; C-cycloplegia; O-onset; P-peak
*Within the column listing adverse effects, underlines indicate the most common effects; CAPITALS indicate life-threatening effects.

tival blood vessels. They probably also decrease formation of aqueous humor, thereby causing a drop in intraocular pressure. This vasodilation may be the mechanism by which the rate of aqueous humor production is decreased.

Uses

The anticholinergic mydriatics and cycloplegics, such as atropine sulfate, cyclopentolate (Cyclogyl), homatropine (Isopto Homatropine), scopolamine (Isopto Hyoscine), and tropicamide (Mydriacyl) are used in eye examinations for accurate measurement of refractory errors and preoperatively and postoperatively to cause pupillary dilation.

The α-adrenergic mydriatics, such as epinephrine (Epitrate), hydroxyamphetamine (Paredrine), and phenylephrine (Neo-Synephrine), are used to treat open-angle glaucoma and glaucoma secondary to uveitis, and for ocular examinations. These drugs are contraindicated for patients with narrow-angle glaucoma, since further dilation of the pupil will restrict the outflow of aqueous humor and cause an acute attack of glaucoma.

When short-acting anticholinergics such as cyclopentolate, homatropine, or tropicamide are used to produce mydriasis and cycloplegia for eye examinations or refractions, pilocarpine (a cholinergic miotic) may be used to counteract both the mydriasis and cycloplegia.

Adverse Effects

The mydriatics are generally not absorbed systemically after ocular instillation. But if absorption does occur, the anticholinergic drugs can cause side effects. The most commonly observed side effects include dryness of the mouth, flushing, and, rarely, tachycardia, fever, delirium, inhibition of sweating, and coma. In addition, pupillary dilation from either local or systemic administration can precipitate acute glaucoma (angle-closure attack) in those with narrow-angle glaucoma. Although serious systemic side effects are rare with the adrenergic drugs, patients with underlying heart disease should be monitored closely for increases in blood pressure and pulse.

Anticholinergic Mydriatics and Cycloplegics

ATROPINE. Atropine (Atropisol), a tertiary amine derived from Atropa belladonna, is commonly used as a mydriatic and cycloplegic when administered locally, and has many other uses when administered systemically. (See Chapter 18 for more information.) It is frequently used to dilate the pupil in acute inflammations such as anterior uveitis and iritis. In addition, it is used for the initial examination of patients with convergent strabismus and, because of the long duration of action, is the preferred drug for refraction of children with accommodative esotropia.

Atropine is the most potent of all cycloplegic drugs. It is available in both ointment (0.5%–1.0% concentration) and solution (0.5%–3.0% concentration) and is administered one to four times daily. The dosage is adjusted to the severity of the patient's condition. Following ophthalmic administration, mydriasis begins in 30–40 minutes and has a total duration of 7–12 days; cycloplegia is slower in onset, may require several doses over a one to two-hour period to be effective, with peak effect appearing in one to two hours, and may persist for 6–12 days.

Atropine is contraindicated for patients who have demonstrated previous hypersensitivity to the preparation and for patients who have certain cardiac problems, such as tachycardia. It is also contraindicated for patients who have glaucoma, since it may precipitate an attack of narrow-angle glaucoma because of its action of dilation of the pupil and narrowing of the iridocorneal angle, where the canal of Schlemm is located. It is also administered cautiously to elderly and debilitated patients because of its local and systemic side effects. Both local and systemic side effects are similar to those of other anticholinergic preparations. The local effects include photophobia, loss of accommodation, contact der-

Contraindications/ Precautions	Adverse Effects*	Interactions	Nursing Implications
Same as for all.	Same as for all.	Same as for all.	Same as for all.
Same as for all.	Same as for all.	Same as for all.	Same as for all.

matitis, edema around the eye, and conjunctivitis. Patients need to report any of these symptoms as soon as they become evident. Systemic symptoms include tachycardia and dryness of the mouth. If the patient is experiencing systemic side effects at the time of the next scheduled dose, he or she should be instructed to omit that dose. Containers of atropine should always be stored in a safe place out of the reach of children because of the high degree of toxicity.

HOMATROPINE. Homatropine (Isopto-Homatropine) is a synthetic alkaloid with action, contraindications, precautions, and side effects similar to those of atropine. It may be preferred over atropine for certain ophthalmic purposes, since its duration of action is shorter. It is useful in producing mydriasis and cycloplegia for diagnostic purposes. Mydriasis begins 40–60 minutes after administration, while the cycloplegic action begins in thirty minutes to one hour. Both effects have a total duration of one to three days. Homatropine is available in 2%–5% solutions; 2% solutions are usually adequate for mydriasis or ophthalmic examination, whereas 5% solutions are often required for cycloplegia.

CYCLOPENTOLATE. Cyclopentolate (Cyclogyl) is more potent and has a shorter duration of action than homatropine. It is used only as a mydriatic and is available as a 0.5%, 1%, or 2% solution. Mydriasis begins in 30–60 minutes and lasts 24 hours.

SCOPOLAMINE. Scopolamine (Isopto-Hyoscine) is an alkaloid of belladonna similar in most ways to atropine. It is more rapidly acting than atropine sulfate and has a shorter duration of action. Mydriasis peaks in 20–30 minutes after administration and cycloplegia peaks in 30–60 minutes. It is available as a solution of 0.25% concentration. Scopolamine can be used with no side effects in patients who have demonstrated a sensitivity to atropine sulfate.

TROPICAMIDE. Tropicamide (Mydriacyl) is a derivative of tropic acid, with pharmacologic properties similar to those of atropine. It is useful for diagnostic purposes but ineffective for treating inflammatory conditions. It is a rapid-acting, short-duration mydriatic and cycloplegic. Tropicamide is available as 0.5% and 1% solutions which peaks in 20–40 minutes after adminis-

tration and has a duration of action of 6–24 hours. The examination must be completed within 35 minutes of the first administration, or another dose of medication will be needed.

Adrenergic Mydriatics

EPINEPHRINE HYDROCHLORIDE. Epinephrine hydrochloride (Adrenal Chloride, Epifrin, Glaucon) is a naturally occurring or synthetically prepared catecholamine. It lowers intraocular pressure by decreasing aqueous humor production; it therefore is useful in treating glaucoma. During initial therapy for open-angle glaucoma, however, pilocarpine or other miotics may be used along with epinephrine to effect control. Epinephrine prevents the rapid absorption of local ophthalmic anesthetics.

Epinephrine is available as 0.1% solution that is administered according to varying schedules depending on the patient's need and symptoms. Mydriasis begins in a few minutes, peaks in 30 minutes, and lasts one to three hours; a decrease in ocular pressure begins to occur within one hour, peaks in four hours, and has a duration of 24 hours.

More information on all the adrenergic mydriatics can be found in Table 60–13.

HYDROXYAMPHETAMINE. Hydroxyamphetamine (Paredrine) is a sympathomimetic amine used extensively as a mydriatic. It is available as a 1% solution, and when one to two drops are instilled in the eye, produces mydriasis in 45–60 minutes lasting a few hours.

PHENYLEPHRINE. Phenylephrine (Neo-Synephrine) is a potent, noncatecholamine, direct-acting sympathomimetic, similar in most aspects to epinephrine. It is frequently used as a mydriatic and as an aid to produce cycloplegia. It is available as 0.12% and 10% solutions, which are used as decongestants and vasoconstrictors and for pupil dilatation in uveitis, wide-angle glaucoma, and during surgery. A 0.12% solution provides temporary relief of minor eye irritation caused by hay fever, dust, wind, sun, smog, and hard contact lenses. When a 10% solution is administered, care must be taken to prevent systemic absorption of the preparation by pressing gently on the nasolacrimal canal—

Table 60–14. COMBINATION DRUGS FOR MYDRIASIS

Combination Drug	Basic Products*		
	CYCLOPENTOLATE HYDROCHLORIDE (%)	PHENYLEPHRINE HYDRO-CHLORIDE (%)	SCOPOLAMINE HBr (%)
Cyclomydril	0.2	1	
Murocoll-2		10	0.3

tear duct—for one to two minutes after administration. Systemic absorption may cause tachycardia and hypertension. Mydriasis peaks in about 30 minutes and has a duration of 0.50–7 hours, depending on the percentage used.

Several combination mydriatics are also available. These products contain various mydriatics in combination. Table 60–14 features the combination mydriatics.

NAPHAZOLINE. Napazoline (Allerest, Clear Eyes, Muro's Opcon) is available in several over-the-counter (0.012%, 0.02%, 0.03%, and 0.05%) and prescription (0.025% and 0.1%) solutions. Naphazoline is used as a topical ocular vasoconstrictor to soothe, refresh, moisturize, and to remove redness due to minor eye irritation. One to two drops are instilled into the conjunctival sac every 3–4 hours.

TETRAHYDROZOLINE. Tetrahydrozoline (Murine Plus, Visine, Optigene 3) is available as an over-the-counter product in a 0.05% solution. Tetrahydrozoline is used as a topical eye decongestant. One to two drops are used two to four times per day.

MISCELLANEOUS EYE AGENTS

Apraclonidine Hydrochloride

Apraclonidine hydrochloride (Lopidine) is a relatively selective α-adrenergic agonist that does not have local anesthetic properties. It is instilled into the eye to control and reduce intraocular pressure that can occur in patients after argon laser *trabeculoplasty* and iridotomy. Increases in intraocular pressure can lead to visual field loss and optic nerve damage.

Apraclonidine is contraindicated in persons hypersensitive to its components or to clonidine, since it is chemically related to clonidine, the antihypertensive agent. It is used cautiously in persons with severe cardiovascular disease and and hypertension, although it has minimal effect on the heart. Safe use during pregnancy, lactation, and in children has not been clearly established.

Adverse reactions reported when apraclonidine was used during laser surgery included upper lid elevation (in 1.3% of patients), conjunctival blanching (0.4%), and mydriasis (dilation of the pupil, 0.4%). Minimal effect on heart rate or blood pressure was noted during clinical trials.

Apraclonidine is administered in doses of one drop to the operative eye both one hour before and immediately after surgery. Maximal reduction of intraocular pressure

usually occurs three to five hours after a single dose is administered.

USING THE NURSING PROCESS

ASSESSMENT

Assessment of the patient requiring eye medications always begins with a thorough nursing history to develop the data base. The patient who requires eye medications may be acutely ill and hospitalized. Or, the patient may be relatively healthy, with a condition (such as glaucoma) discovered during a routine physical or eye examination. The information obtained is included in Table 60–15. The nurse also investigates for the presence of similar symptoms such as "pink eye" among close friends or relatives. The nurse uses all of this information when preparing the nursing care plan. The nurse examines the eye to assess pupil size and the presence of redness or edema in or around the eye. Visual acuity, peripheral vision, and optic fundi are assessed. Also, determine if there has been a change in visual acuity during the past several months. Laboratory data, such as eye culture results, may be helpful in determining the organisms that cause inflammation and infection.

An accurate current medication history is of vital importance because many eye problems may be precipitated by both prescription and over-the-counter medications. Table 60–16 features commonly used prescription and over-the-counter medications, identifies the way they are likely to affect the eye, and indicates the frequency with which eye examinations should be administered to the patient while the medication is being taken. Some of these medications can cause temporary or permanent damage to the eye. If the patient has been on, or is currently taking, eye medications, it is important to identify specific medications and dosage, the reason they were chosen or prescribed, and how long the patient has been taking them. It is also important to know whether or not the patient has experienced any allergic reaction to eye medications in the past including over-the-counter drugs and contact lens products. The nurse also assesses the activity level of the patient. Does the patient operate heavy equipment or drive a car? Does the patient do many activities at night and there-

Table 60–15. NURSING PROCESS FOR PATIENT WITH EYE DISORDERS

Assessment
Assess pupil size, acuity, peripheral vision and otpic fundi; presence of discharge; redness, edema in or around the eye. Review laboratory data, e.g., eye culture. Determine current medication history.

Nursing Diagnosis	Nursing Actions	Rationale	Desired Outcomes/ Evaluation Criteria
Knowledge deficit related to lack of exposure/ recall, unfamiliarity with information resources/ misinterpretation, cognitive limitation as evidenced by questions, statement of concern, inaccurate follow-through of instructions/ development of preventable complications.	Review information about individual condition, prognosis, type of procedures. Discuss possible effects/ interactions between eye medications and patient's medical problems.	Enhances understanding and promotes cooperation with treatment regimen. Use of topical eye medications, e.g., sympathomimetic agents, β-blockers, anticholinergic agents can cause BP to rise in hypertensive patients; precipitate dyspnea in patients with COPD; mask the symptoms of a hypoglycemic crisis in insulin-dependent diabetics.	Verbalize understanding of condition/disease process and treatment. Correctly performs necessary procedures and explains reasons for the actions.
	Instruct in proper method of instilling eyedrops, counting drops as indicated.	Correction application can limit absorption into systemic circulation, minimizing problems such as drug interactions and unwanted/ untoward systemic effects.	
	Suggest use of dark glasses/reduced room lighting as indicated. Recommend wearing medical identification bracelet if appropriate.	Can reduce discomfort associated with photophobia. Reduces risk that person with glaucoma will receive contraindicated drugs in emergency situation.	
	Identify signs/symptoms requiring prompt evaluation, e.g., sharp/sudden pain, decreased/blurred vision, increased photophobia, flashes of light/ floating particles in visual field, lid swelling, purulent discharge, redness, watering of eyes, photophobia.	Early intervention can prevent development of serious complications, possible loss of vision.	
	Stress importance of routine follow-up care, as indicated.	Periodic monitoring reduces risk of serious complications.	
Infection, potential for spread related to inadequate primary defenses. fenses.	Administer antibacterial, antifungal, or antiviral agent as appropriate. Discuss reasons for infection, how it can be spread, and treatment needs.	Used to treat existing infection. Understanding of how infection is transmitted promotes accurate care and cooperation with treatment regimen.	Verbalizes understand of individual causative/risk factor(s). Identifies interventions to prevent/ reduce risk of spread of infection. Demonstrates proper technique for instillation of eye drops.
	Stress importance of washing hands before and after instilling eye drops.	Prevents possible introduction of other pathogens/spread of infection.	

CONTINUED ON THE FOLLOWING PAGE

Table 60–15. NURSING PROCESS FOR PATIENT WITH EYE DISORDERS–*CONTINUED*

Nursing Diagnosis	Nursing Actions	Rationale	Desired Outcomes/ Evaluation Criteria
	Encourage rest and limit eye activity.	Promotes healing.	
	Discuss ways to prevent reinfection. Recommend abstaining from use of eye makeup during acute infection and routinely discard/replace eye makeup.	Reduces risk of recurrence and spreading infection.	
GLAUCOMA Sensory-perceptual alteration, visual related to altered sensory reception, altered status of sense organ as evidenced by progressive loss of visual field.	Administer appropriate drug, i.g., Diamox, Osmitrol, Timolol. Demonstrate administration of eye drops, e.g., counting drops. Discuss importance of maintaining drug schedule/not missing doses.	Controls intraocular pressure preventing further loss of vision. Helps patient to follow proper procedure. Glaucoma can be controlled, not cured, and maintaining consistent medication regimen is vital to prevent progression of disease.	Maintains current visual field/acuity without further loss.
	Discuss medications that should be avoided, e.g., mydriatic drops, overuse of topical steroids. Monitor vital signs during initial therapy. Reduce environmental clutter, clear travel paths as needed. Encourage expression of feelings about actual/ possible loss of vision.	Some drugs cause pupil dilation, increasing IOP and potentiating additional loss of vision. Blood pressure may drop and pulse may slow with β-adrenergic blocking medications. Reduces safety hazards related to changes in visual fields. While early intervention may prevent blindness, the patient faces the possibility or may already have experienced partial or complete loss of vision.	

fore need good night vision? Can the patient administer his or her own eye drops or ointments?

NURSING DIAGNOSIS

Nursing diagnoses are then developed based on the assessment findings. Typical nursing diagnoses for a patient with eye disorders are included in Table 60–15.

PLANNING AND INTERVENTION

The nurse develops the goals of nursing intervention from the nursing diagnoses. Typical nursing goals when caring for the patient requiring medications for eye disorders are included in Table 60–15.

The hands are always washed thoroughly before administering any eye medication. The tip of the eye dropper or the tube of ointment is not touched to any surface. The container is closed immediately after use. Eye medications are not stored where there is the possibility of extremes of heat such as in a car. Many eye medications may cause temporary stinging or blurred vision.

The guidelines that follow focus on the safe and appropriate use of ophthalmic solutions and ointments.

General Concepts

1. Use medications marked for ophthalmic use only. Antibiotics or steroids for otic or dermatologic use should not be used in the eye.

Table 60–16. OCULAR TOXICITY OF VARIOUS DRUGS

Medications	Ptosis	Miosis	Vision Changes	Mydriasis	Oculogyric Crisis	Optic Neuritis	Nystagmus	Diplopia	Ocular Palsies	Conjunctivitis	Papilledema	Frequency* of Follow-up	Comments
CENTRAL NERVOUS SYSTEM DRUGS													
Barbiturates	X			X			X	X		X		4	
Chloral hydrate (Noctec)								X		X		2	
Chlorpromazine (Thorazine)			X		X							3	Increased pigmentation on all parts of eyes, degeneration of retina
Phenytoin (Dilantin)	X		X				X	X		X		4	
Ethchlorvynol (Placidyl)						X	X					4	
Haloperidol (Haldol)			X	X	X							2	
Levodopa (L-Dopa)				X								2	
Morphine		X	X									2,4	Myopia
Perphenazine (Trilafon)					X	X						2	
Prochlorperazine (Compazine)			X		X							2	Myopia
Thioridazine (Mellaril)			X	X								3	Pigment changes, retina degen.
Tricyclic antidepressants (e.g., Elavil)				X								3	Cycloplegia, aggravation of narrow-angle glaucoma
Diazepam (Valium)			X				X	X				2	Acute glaucoma
Trimethadione (Tridione)			X										Photophobia, hemeralopia
Amphetamines			X	X	X							4	
Cannabis (Marijuana)			X					X				3	
Nasal decongestants			X	X									
CHOLINERGIC AND ANTICHOLINERGIC MEDICATIONS													
Atropine			X	X				X				1	Acute glaucoma, reduced quality of tears
Neostigmine (Prostigmin)	X						X					3	
ANTI-INFECTIVES													
Chloramphenicol (Chloromycetin)			X			X						2	
Piperazine (Antepar)			X									2	
Quinine								X					Optic atrophy, pigment changes
Streptomycin						X						4	
Tetracycline			X								X	3	
Sulfonamides							X						
MEDICATIONS TO TREAT TUBERCULOSIS													
Ethambutol (Myambutol)			X			X						3	Green vision lost
Ethionamide (Trecator)						X						3	
Isoniazid (INH)						X						3	Keratitis

CONTINUED ON THE FOLLOWING PAGE

*1: should be seen at once; 2: if symptoms arise; 3: 3–6 months; 4: 6–12 months.

Table 60–16. OCULAR TOXICITY OF VARIOUS DRUGS–*CONTINUED*

Medications	Ptosis	Miosis	Vision Changes	Mydriasis	Oculogyric Crisis	Optic Neuritis	Nystagmus	Diplopia	Ocular Palsies	Conjunctivitis	Papilledema	Frequency* of Follow-up	Comments
CARDIOVASCULAR MEDICATIONS													
Digitalis preparations									X	X		4	Color vision disturbances especially xanthopsia (yellow vision), halos
Guanethidine (Ismelin)	X											4	
Quinidine			X			X						4	
Reserpine (Serpasil)		X							X			3	Glaucoma
Amiodarone												2	Ocular deposits occur
DIURETICS													
Carbonic anhydrase inhibitors												4	Myopia
Thiazide (Diuril)												4	Myopia, xanthopsia (yellow vision)
Furosemide (Lasix)			X									4	
ANTIRHEUMATOID MEDICATIONS													
Gold salts							X			X		4	Gold deposits in eye
Phenylbutazone (Butazolidin)						X				X		3	Retinal hemorrhages, corneal erosions
Ibuprofen (Motrin)			X									2	Color vision disturbances, changes in tear quality
Indomethacin (Indocin)					X			X				4	Cause corneal deposits
Chloroquine (Aralen)	X											3	Pigment changes, optic atrophy
Salicylates				X		X	X			X		4	Retinal hemorrhages
HORMONAL AGENTS													
ACTH											X	3	Myopia, cataracts
Corticosteroids	X			X							X		Cataracts, retinopahty, myopia, exophthalmia
Oral contraceptives						X	X				X	2,3	Alterations in corneal curvature
Fertility drugs (Clomid)			X										See sparkles and streaks of light and ghosting
OTHER MEDICATIONS													
Vitamin A							X	X	X		X	2,4	Exophthalmia, retinal hemorrhages
Vitamin D												4	Calcium deposits
Nicotinic acid						X						2	Retinal edema
Allopurinol (Zyloprim)												4	Cataracts, macular lesions, both rare
Anticoagulants (Coumadin)												2	Retinal hemorrhages
Chlorambucil (Leukeran)											X	2	
Chlorpropamide (Diabinese)			X			X		X		X		2	
Antihistamines		X	X										Photophobia, reduce lacrimation

*1: should be seen at once; 2: if symptoms arise; 3: 3–6 months; 4: 6–12 months.

2. The normal eye can hold about 10 μl of fluid. Since the average dropper delivers 25 to 50 μl/drop, generally more than one drop is not useful. Due to rapid lacrimal drainage (16%/min) and limited eye capacity, if multiple drop therapy is needed, the best interval between drops is five minutes. This ensures that the first drop is not flushed away by the second or that the second drop is not diluted by the first. Do not use drops that have changed color.

3. It is important to minimize systemic absorption of ophthalmic drops. To do so, compress the lacrimal sac for one to two minutes during, and following, instillation of drops. This retards passage of drops via the nasolacrimal duct into areas of potential absorption such as nasal and pharyngeal mucosa.

4. Certain factors that may increase the absorption of ophthalmic dosage forms include the presence of lax eyelids (usually in elderly patients), which creates a greater reservoir for retention of drops; and hyperemic, or diseased eyes. Topical anesthesia also increases the bioavailability of ophthalmic agents by decreasing the blink reflex and the production and turnover of tears.

5. Use of eye cups is discouraged because of potential contamination and risk of spreading disease.

6. It is important for ophthalmic medications to remain uncontaminated after opening. It is best to use solutions/drops within four weeks and ointments within three months. Monitor expiration dates closely. Do not use outdated medication.

7. Suspensions and solutions remain in the eye longer. Ophthalmic suspensions mix with tears less rapidly and remain in the cul de sac longer than solutions. The clearance rate of ophthalmic ointments from the eye is approximately 0.5% per minute; ophthalmic ointments provide maximum contact between drug and ophthalmic tissues and structures. Ophthalmic ointments may impede delivery of other ophthalmic drugs to the affected site by serving as a barrier to contact. If more than one kind of ointment is needed, wait about 10 minutes before applying the second drug. Ointments may blur vision during the waking hours. Use with caution in conditions in which visual clarity is critical (e.g., operating motor equipment, reading).

8. If the ophthalmic disorder persists or worsens, contact the physician.

Guidelines for Proper Use of Ophthalmic Solutions

1. Wash hands thoroughly before administration.
2. Tilt the head backward or have the patient lie down and gaze upward. Gently pull down lower eyelid to form a pouch. Hold the dropper above the eye and place the prescribed volume of drops inside the lower lid. Avoid contact of the dropper with the eye, finger, or any surface. Release the lid slowly. The patient should try to keep the eye open (not blink) for 30 seconds after administration.
3. Apply gentle pressure with fingers to the bridge of the nose (inside corner of eye) for one to two minutes. This retards drainage of solution from the intended area.
4. Do not rub the eye. Minimize blinking. Do not close the eyes tightly after instillation; this may express medication from the cul-de-sac.
5. In situations in which the instillation of eye drops is difficult (e.g., pediatric patients, adults with particularly strong blink reflex) the closed-eye method may be used. This involves having the patient lying down, placing the prescribed number of drops on the eyelid in the inner corner of the eye, then opening eye so that drops will fall into the eye by gravity.

Guidelines for Proper Use of Ophthalmic Ointments

1. Wash hands thoroughly before administration.
2. When opening the ointment tube for the first time, squeeze out and discard the first 0.25 inch of ointment as it may be too dry. Hold the ointment tube in the hand for a few minutes to warm the ointment and facilitate flow. Gently pull down the lower lid to form a pouch and place 0.25–0.5 inch of ointment inside the lower lid by squeezing the tube gently. Close the eye for one to two minutes and roll the eyeball in all directions. Temporary blurring may occur.
3. Remove excessive ointment around the eye or ointment tube tip with tissue.

PATIENT TEACHING

The patient who requires eye medications will often be self-administering these medications at home. The nurse ensures that the patient knows and understands several basic measures in order to administer eye medication safely. The reasons for the use of the eye medication and the correct way to administer them. Figure 60–2 depicts the proper administration of eye drops, and Figure 60–3 shows the proper administration of eye ointments. Sterile technique must be maintained to prevent contamination of the dropper. Patient teaching information is found in Table 60–17.

The nurse must remember the information found in each drug table in the column marked Nursing Implications to safely administer these medications (or to teach the patient to self-administer them). The nurse may need to repeat directions several times to ensure patient understanding and continued compliance. Eye conditions (particularly glaucoma) associated with possible blindness frequently cause high anxiety levels in patients. Anxious patients may be unable to comprehend simple instructions. Written instructions for reference are helpful to ensure compliance once the patient returns home.

Patients with chronic eye problems, such as glaucoma, are taught the signs and symptoms that would indicate a worsening of the condition or an acute exacerbation of the disease. The nurse must also give the patient specific and individualized instructions, appropriate to the particular situation, on what to do and whom to contact when these symptoms occur.

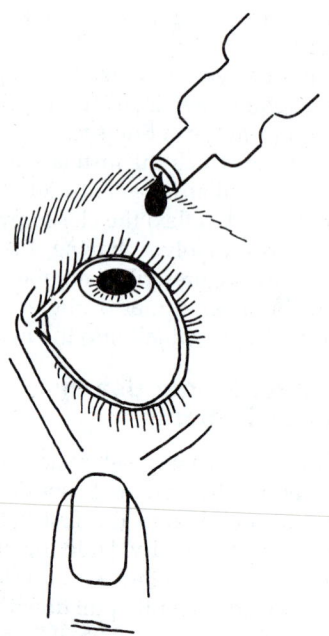

Figure 60–2. Eye drops are administered onto the lower lid, which has been pulled down with the forefinger. The eye is then closed for 30 seconds to allow the medication to flow over the entire eye. The medication applicator approaches the eye from below and outside the patient's field of vision. Do not let dropper tip touch any surface, including eye lashes.

Corticosteroids, when used, are administered to the eyes for short periods of time and only under close supervision. These patients should have frequent tonometry tests for intraocular pressure. The nurse also instructs the patient not to rub the eye vigorously, as

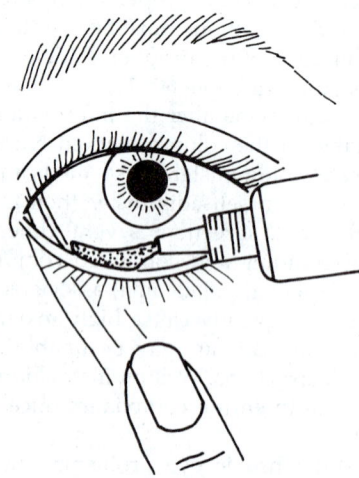

Figure 60–3. Eye ointment is administered onto the lower lid, which is pulled down with the forefinger. Only a small amount (¼ inch) of ointment need be used. The eye is then closed to allow the medication to flow over the entire eye.

Table 60–17. PATIENT TEACHING FOR EYE MEDICATIONS

Dear Patient:

This drug has been ordered for you. This is what you should know about your drug to get the most from your therapy.

1. The drug will be taken for the rest of your life (or until your eye condition is completely cured).
2. Proper handwashing is very important to prevent the passing on your eye infections to others. If only one eye is affected, do not touch or rub your good eye, or share towels or wash clothes with others in your household. This will prevent the spread of the germs.
3. Keep your medication dropper or tube sterile by not touching your eye or any other surface with the tip.
4. If you are taking different kinds of drops or ointments, wait at least 5 min for drops and 10 min for ointments before you put in the next drug.
5. Interactions can occur with eye drugs. These include . . . [include specific information from drug tables].
6. If you forget your drug until it is almost time for your next dose, forget the dose; **do not** try to catch up.
7. Do not stop your drug without your doctor's knowledge.
8. Sometimes side effects may occur from eye drugs. The most usual is irritation and redness around the eye. If redness, itching, or swelling occurs, contact your doctor. Other side effects include . . . [fill in specific information from drug tables].
9. The safety precautions for your particular drug include . . . [fill in information found in drug tables].
10. Store your drugs away from direct heat and freezing and cap them tightly. Do not touch the tip of the applicator. Discard old, discolored, or cloudy solutions.

GUIDELINES FOR PROPER USE OF OPHTHALMIC SOLUTIONS

1. Tilt the head backward or lie down and gaze upward.
2. Gently pull down lower eyelid to form a pouch.
3. Hold the dropper above the eye and place the prescribed volume of drops inside the lower lid.
4. Avoid touching the dropper to the eye, finger, or any other surface.
5. Release the lid slowly.
6. You should try to keep the eye open (not blink) for 30 sec after putting the drug in.
7. Press gently with fingers to the bridge of the nose (inside corner of eye) for 1–2 min. This keeps the drug in the eye and doesn't let it drain out.
8. Do not rub the eye. Do not blink too much. Do not close the eyes tightly after putting the drug in; this may squeeze the medication from the eye lid pouch.
9. Do not rinse the dropper.
10. Prevent freezing of eyedrops.

GUIDELINES FOR PROPER USE OF OPHTHALMIC OINTMENTS

1. When opening the ointment tube for the first time, squeeze out and throw away the first 0.25 inch of ointment as it may be too dry.
2. Holding the ointment tube in the hand for a few minutes will warm the ointment and help it flow better.
3. Gently pull down the lower lid to form a pouch.

Table 60–17. PATIENT TEACHING FOR EYE MEDICATIONS–*CONTINUED*

4. Place 0.25–0.5 inch of ointment inside the lower lid by squeezing the tube gently.
5. Close the eye for 1–2 min and roll the eyeball in all directions.
6. Your eyesight may be blurred for a little while. Do not do things for which you need to see clearly, such as driving, until blurring clears.
7. Remove extra ointment around the eye or ointment tube tip with tissue.

steroid administration may cause the eye tissues to bruise readily.

Topical anesthetics are for short-term therapy only, and are never given to the patient for self-administration. A protective eye patch is recommended to prevent damage to the eye until corneal reflexes are fully restored, usually within one hour after administration.

When administering miotics, the nurse or patient applies gentle pressure to the nasolacrimal canal for one to two minutes after their administration. This prevents the drug from entering the nasal mucosa through the nasolacrimal canal and thus entering the systemic circulation. Some blurring of vision and difficulty of focusing commonly occur, so the nurse instructs the patient to avoid hazardous activities such as driving a car or operating heavy equipment. Constriction of the pupil may cause special problems for the elderly (who already have reduced light adaptation and visual acuity) in adjusting quickly to changes in illumination. Night-time may prove particularly hazardous to these patients. Use of miotics may be specifically ordered at bedtime to avoid a nocturnal elevation of intraocular pressure or disturbing visual effects. The long-acting agents may cause cumulative effects, so the patient needs to report these to the physician. The cholinesterase-inhibitor miotics may cause spasm of the blink reflex, which may be particularly annoying to the patient. Miotics are not stored near excessive heat; they are preserved in tight, light-resistant containers.

When the nurse is administering β-adrenergic blockers such as timolol, all other antiglaucoma medications are discontinued (see earlier discussion for specific information), followed by a check of intraocular pressure. A fall in blood pressure and pulse rate may occur owing to concomitant blockade of β-receptors in the heart and vascular system, so frequent checks on blood pressure and pulse are made during initial and maintenance therapy. Periodic measurement of intraocular pressure is necessary because a tendency toward tolerance has been noted with long-term therapy.

Mydriatics generally produce less effect in persons with heavily pigmented irises; these patients may need to have the dose increased to achieve therapeutic effects. Since these medications do blur vision, they may be administered at bedtime. If photophobia occurs, the patient is instructed to wear dark glasses in bright light. If epinephrine is being given concurrently with a miotic, the miotic is instilled two to ten minutes before the epinephrine.

Cataracts

Cataracts develop most often in the elderly when the crystalline lens develops a greater percentage of protein. Recent research indicates that there are drugs that can increase or decrease the risk of developing cataracts. Drugs known to increase the risk of cataract development include steroids and nifedipine (Procardia). Drugs taken regularly that may reduce the risk of developing cataracts by 50% or more include aspirin, acetaminophen, and ibuprofen (Motrin, Advil). Researchers suspect that analgesics protect against cataracts by lowering levels of plasma glucose, a possible contributor to cataract formation.

Contact Lenses

Several forms of contact lenses are marketed today—hard and soft with the soft available as daily-wear or extended-wear lenses. Contact lenses float on a film of tears and do not actually come in contact with the cornea.

Patients using over-the-counter or prescription antihistamines or anticholinergics should not be fitted for contact lenses while using these products as tear quality may be compromised. Persons who wear lenses and need to use these products should be advised to discontinue contact lens wear until they have stopped using the drugs.

Various drugs, such as the anti-inflammatory sulfasalazine (Azulfidine), stain soft contact lenses a deep yellow color. Routine cleaning removes the stain from daily-wear lenses; however, extended-wear lenses are stained permanently. Therefore, patients who wear extended-wear lenses need to remove their lenses during therapy.

EVALUATION

During the evaluation phase, the nurse evaluates the effectiveness of the medications used for eye disorders as well as other nursing and medical goals. This evaluation is based on a list of outcome evaluation criteria that has been developed in relation to the goals determined by the nurse, patient, and family. The data base obtained in the original assessment and used to formulate the nursing diagnoses provides helpful criteria for measuring the treatment's effectiveness. Typical outcome evaluation criteria are included in Table 60–15.

It is extremely important that the nurse work with the patient and family to ensure their complete assistance and support. A patient who understands the importance of continued medical treatment is usually compliant. No one wants to lose his or her sight; consequently, the person is usually most willing to comply with the treatment regimens. The primary reasons for noncompliance are forgetting to take the medication, discontinuing the medication because of feeling well, or deliberately stopping it because of the uncomfortable side effects. A patient with chronic diseases, such as glaucoma, must understand that the medication controls disease but does not cure it; therefore, lifelong therapy is required. Finally, the nurse makes the patient aware of the importance of continued follow-up for his or her eye condition.

If the patient experiences headache, eye pain, vision changes, continued redness or irritation, or the condition worsens for more than three days, the physician should be notified. The offending product is usually discontinued.

The nurse should teach the patient about potential side effects so that a patient taking medication at home will report any unusual symptoms to the physician or nurse. Antibacterials, when being administered topically to the eye, may interfere with the normal bacterial flora of the eye and thereby encourage the growth of nonsusceptible organisms. Antibacterials may also precipitate contact dermatitis. The preservative in ophthalmic preparations may also be responsible for causing local adverse reactions. A patient who begins to note any signs of redness or irritation should immediately notify the physician. When antibacterials are administered systemically, urticaria and anaphylactic reactions may occur.

When corticosteroids are being topically administered to the eye, they may cause burning, discomfort, and increased lacrimation. Generally, systemic reactions do not occur, but the patient still needs to be evaluated for their occurrence (see Chapter 42). Because corticosteroids lower resistance to infection and modify the inflammatory response, they may sometimes mask serious ocular disease. Corticosteroids, after repeated applications, may reduce the outflow tract for aqueous humor and thus increase intraocular pressure. The nurse needs to assess a patient's eyes at frequent intervals if corticosteroids are to be used for a prolonged period of time.

Miotics are capable of causing many local and systemic side effects. Local effects include twitching of the eyelid, ocular pain, brow or lid pain, increased lacrimation, and local allergic reactions. These effects may become so annoying to the patient that discontinuation of the medication may be necessitated. The patient is encouraged to report any changes in vision because miotics have been associated with the development of cataracts, pupillary margin cysts, and pigment changes, all of which interfere with vision. Following prolonged use of cholinesterase-inhibitor miotics, miosis may persist even after the medication is discontinued, owing to the residual loss of tone of the muscle fibers in the eye.

Occasionally, the patient may complain of systemic side effects from miotics, including sweating, nausea, vomiting, abdominal pain, diarrhea, hypotension, and bradycardia. Pressure applied at the inner canthus for two minutes immediately after instillation of the medication may help to relieve these symptoms by minimizing systemic absorption. The majority of the eye medication then runs down the face.

Farm workers receiving cholinesterase-inhibitor miotics and patients who are exposed to organophosphate insecticides may develop toxic side effects owing to their additive effects. Therefore, careful administration of miotics and follow-up on persons exposed to these insecticides is important. Patients are cautioned about wearing respiratory masks, working carefully, and changing clothes frequently to prevent systemic absorption of farm chemicals.

Timolol has fewer side effects than pilocarpine or epinephrine, and it is generally well tolerated. Although patients may have local reactions, including ocular irritation, allergic reactions, or visual disturbances, the major side effects are due to the systemic absorption and the blockade of β receptors, which lowers blood pressure, slows the pulse, and causes bronchospasm. Timolol has recently been shown to decrease libido in both men and women and lead to impotence and decreased ejaculation volume in men. Since topical ocular timolol is one of the most commonly prescribed drugs in the United States, all patients complaining of sexual dysfunction should be asked if they use timolol eye drops.

Patients who receive carbonic anhydrase inhibitors may experience diuresis, which may be significant at first and generally subsides with continued therapy. However, the patient should have frequent determinations of the serum potassium level to evaluate the presence of hypokalemia, which is particularly dangerous for cardiac patients.

When osmotic agents are used, reduction in volume of cerebrospinal fluid may occur, leading to severe pounding headaches. Also, the sudden shift in body fluids may put an extra burden on the heart and precipitate congestive heart failure. The nurse evaluates fluid and electrolyte balance frequently in order to monitor for disturbances.

The use of mydriatics (anticholinergics and adrenergics) may precipitate an attack of acute angle-closure glaucoma. Patients receiving these medications are encouraged to report any pain, loss of vision, blurring, or loss of visual field to the physician.

Specifically, with the topical use of anticholinergics, the patient may experience systemic side effects including dryness of the mouth, inhibition of sweating, incidences of flushing, tachycardia, fever, delirium, and even coma. The nurse evaluates patients with cardiovascular disease frequently when using either type of mydriatic. In general, mydriatics are discontinued if the patient experiences eye pain, conjunctivitis, palpitations, rapid pulse, or dizziness.

SUMMARY

The nurse will frequently care for persons with disorders of the eye. Many medications are available to treat these conditions including anti-infectives, anti-inflammatories, local anesthetics, lubricants, decongestants, miotics, β-adrenergic blockers, mydriatics, and cycloplegics. These medications have different actions, uses, and pharmacokinetics, which are all discussed within this chapter and its tables.

The majority of patients with eye disorders are treated on an outpatient basis and, therefore, need to be taught the proper technique for administering these medications. Patients need to know that if they experience headache, eye pain, vision changes, or continued redness or irritation, or if the condition worsens for more than three days, their physician should be notified.

BIBLIOGRAPHY

AMA Department of Drugs: AMA Drug Evaluations, ed 5. PSG Publishing, Littleton, MA, 1986.

Covington, TR: Topical Ophthalmic Agents. Facts and Comparisons Drug Newsletter (7(6):46, 1988.

Fraunfelder, F and Meyer, S: Sexual dysfunction secondary to topical ophthalmic timolol (letter). JAMA 253:3092–3093, 1985.

Gilman, AG, Goodman, LS, and Gilman, A (eds): Goodman and Gilman's The Pharmacological Basis of Therapeutics, ed 7. Macmillan, New York, 1985.

Goldstein, J: Ocular side effects of systemic drugs. J Ophthalmic Nurs Techn 5(3):103–105, 1986.

Goldstein, J: Contact lens care products: Uses and action of ingredients. J Ophthalmic Nurs Techn 6(2):70–72, Mar–Apr 1987.

Goldstein, J: Pharmacology of ophthalmic drugs: Anesthetics, mydriatics and cycloplegics and ocular hypotensives. J Ophthalmic Nurs Techn 6(4):146–150, July–Aug 1987.

Nurses Drug Alert. Misuse of steroid eye medications. 11(1):7, Jan 1987.

Osis, M: Drugs and vision: unexplained symptoms: Are they due to eye meds? Gerontion 2(1):14–16, Spring 1987.

Physician's Desk Reference for Ophthalmology. Medical Economics, Oradell, NJ, 1986.

Postsurgery ophthalmic solution. Am J Nurs:841, June 1988.

Radocy, L: What lasers can do for your glaucoma patient. RN 85(10):28–31, 1985.

Riley SA: Contact lens staining due to sulphasalazine (Letter). Lancet 8487:972, April 26, 1986.

Smith, S: How drugs act: Drugs and the eye. Nurs Times 1987 6:24–30, 48–50.

SITUATION   60–1

Inis Cave is a 76-year-old recently diagnosed with open-angle glaucoma. She is being treated at a University Eye Center.

1. Ms. Cave is to begin treatment with pilocarpine .25% 2 gtts every 6 hours. The nurse will caution her about the most common side effects of this drug, which are:
   a. puritis and weakness
   b. sweating and fever
   c. anxiety and tremors
   d. burning and itching

2. When assessing Ms. Cave after administration of pilocarpine, the nurse will anticipate the following:
   a. asymmetrically shaped pupils
   b. constricted pupils
   c. dilated pupils
   d. increased accommodation

3. The nurse will teach Ms. Cave about taking eye drops at home. The following information will be included:
   a. A stinging sensation indicates that the drug is working.
   b. Visual acuity will be reduced in dim light.
   c. Dryness of the mouth and throat is related to pilocarpine.
   d. Eyelids should be massaged after administration.

4. After a month of therapy of pilocarpine, Ms. Cave is to switch to timolol maleate (Timoptic) .25% 1 gtt BID. Prior to administration of this agent, the nurse will check for a history of:
   a. peripheral neuropathy
   b. iodine allergy
   c. asthma
   d. peptic ulcers

5. The nurse will teach Ms. Cave the following schedule for beginning timolol therapy:
   a. Discontinue pilocarpine for three days, then begin timolol.
   b. Continue both agents for one week, then gradually stop pilocarpine.
   c. Continue pilocarpine and timolol for three days, then stop pilocarpine.
   d. Discontinue pilocarpine on the second day of timolol therapy.

6. The nurse will monitor Ms. Cave for the following in relation to timolol therapy:
   a. blood pressure
   b. level of consciousness
   c. reflexes
   d. potassium level

Please refer to the Appendices for correct answers and additional review questions with answers.

61 CHAPTER

MEDICATIONS USED IN EAR DISORDERS

61
CHAPTER

MEDICATIONS USED IN EAR DISORDERS

MERRILY MATHEWSON KUHN, R.N.C., Ph.D., CCRN

LEARNING OBJECTIVES

After reading this chapter, the student will be able to:

1. Identify those medications commonly used for ear disorders.

2. Differentiate among the medications used for ear disorders as to mechanism of action, route of administration, pharmacokinetics, adverse effects, contraindications, and interactions.

3. Identify specific areas to assess in the patient requiring medications for ear disorders in order to formulate appropriate nursing diagnoses.

4. Plan the nursing interventions necessary to administer medications for ear disorders and choose appropriate teaching strategies to gain patient compliance.

5. Evaluate the patient at various stages of treatment to gauge nursing interventions.

THERAPEUTIC AGENTS—EAR

Otic medications are administered locally to prevent or treat conditions of the external ear (Table 61–1) and are generally dissolved or suspended in a liquid vehicle for easier administration in the external ear canal. A few creams or ointments are available to be used on dry, crusted lesions. Generally, the medications used to treat ear conditions are the same preparations commonly used to treat problems in other areas of the body. Examples include anti-infectives, local anesthetics, and combination products containing anti-infectives, adrenal corticosteroids, and/or local anesthetics. Cerumenolytic preparations are used to remove or loosen wax accumulations.

It may be necessary to administer systemic medications when there are severe external infections; when the pain associated with the ear problem cannot be managed with the application of heat or topically applied medications; or when it is preferable or necessary to reach the middle ear via the circulatory system.

Since all of the medications used in otic disorders are discussed in other parts of this text, there is only a brief discussion of the specific action of these preparations.

ANTI-INFECTIVES

External Ear Problems

The anti-infectives (Table 61–2) employed most commonly as otic medications for external use include polymyxin B, colistimethate, and neomycin. Tetracycline, sulfonamides, chloramphenicol, gentamicin, nitrofurazone, neomycin, ampicillin, penicillin G, and nystatin are also used, orally or parenterally, when necessary (see Chapter 46 for more information on anti-infectives). For otitis externa, topical application of polymyxin B, colistimethate, and neomycin alone, or in combination with hydrocortisone, is usually effective. The addition of the hydrocortisone reduces redness, itching, and edema within the ear. Topical therapy should be discontinued after ten days to prevent overgrowth of fungal organisms, or if the infection spreads. Oral products are then used, if necessary.

Another antimicrobial preparation used in external otic diseases is acetic acid as a 2% solution. It is often the drug of choice for several reasons, including

1. a broad spectrum of antimicrobial activity including both fungi and *Pseudomonas*;
2. a lack of bacterial resistance; therefore, there is no chance of the patient developing resistant strains;
3. an absence of toxic or allergic actions;
4. an absence of cross-sensitivity with other medications;
5. low cost; and
6. stability with a long shelf life; therefore, can be used many times.

Ear irrigations may be prescribed in the treatment of otic disorders. Irrigations must be done very gently in order not to damage the tympanic membrane and, therefore, are best performed by direct visualization. The most frequently used irrigating solutions include

Table 61–1. EAR DISEASE

EXTERNAL EAR

Types: External otitis: acute, localized; acute, diffuse; chronic diffuse; progressive, necrotizing.

Age: Most common in infants and young children but can affect all age groups.

Causative Organism: Staphylococcus, Pseudomonas, Proteus, fungi.

Management: (1) Cleansing of the external canal to remove desquamated material, purulent secretions, cerumen (wax), and previously instilled topical medications, often done by irrigation; (2) application of appropriate medications; and (3) alteration of the pH to restore normal bacterial flora, the ear canal being normally acidic.

MIDDLE EAR

Types: Otitis media; acute, chronic.

Etiology: Often follows viral infections of the upper respiratory tract.

Causative Organisms: Streptococcus, Pneumococcus, *Haemophilus influenzae*.

Symptoms: Earache, feeling of fullness and pressure in the ear, loss of hearing, and accumulation of debris behind the tympanic membrane may cause it to perforate or rupture owing to increased pressure.

Management: Systemic antibiotics, systemic analgesics, or a surgical opening of tympanic membrane (myringotomy) to relieve pressure and promote drainage.

MASTOIDITIS

Definition: Inflammation of the mastoid antrum and cells.

Etiology: May follow middle ear infection, sore throat, or respiratory infection.

Symptoms: Earache, ringing in the ears, and painful, swollen mastoid process.

Management: Anti-infectives; and if ineffective, surgery.

Table 61–2. OTIC ANTI-INFECTIVES

Medication	Primary Anti-infectives	Dosage	Contraindications and Precautions	Adverse Effects
Aerosporin Otic Solution	Polymyxin B	3–4 gtt to affected ear 3–4×/day.	Contraindicated in prior hypersensitivity. Safe use in pregnancy not established.	<u>Local irritation</u> and burning.
Chloromycetin Otic	Chloramphenicol	0.5%, 2–3 gtt to affected ear tid at 6–8 hr intervals.	Contraindicated in prior hypersensitivity. Safe use in pregnancy and nursing mothers not established.	Hypersensitivity reactions; BONE MARROW HYPOPLASIA, including APLASTIC ANEMIA; death has been reported following local application; overgrowth of non-susceptible organisms.
Otobiotic Otic Solution	Polymyxin B	4 gtt 3–4× daily.	Contraindicated in prior hypersensitivity and perforated ear drum.	Hypersensitivity, local irritation.
Neosporin	Polymyxin B, bacitracin, neomycin	3–4 gtt q 3–4 hr.	Contraindicated in perforated ear drum and prior hypersensitivity.	Overgrowth of nonsusceptible organisms; hypersensitivity reaction—swelling, dry scaling, itching.
Acetic Acid Solution 2%	Acetic acid	4–6 gtt q 2–3 hr.	Contraindicated in prior hypersensitivity.	Local irritation.
Polycillin, Omnipen, Amcill	Ampicillin	Oral: Over 20 kg: 250–500 mg q 6 hr. Under 20 kg: 50–100 mg/kg/day at 6–8-hr intervals. IM and IV: Over 40 kg: 250–500 mg q 6 hr. Under 40 kg: 25–50 mg/kg/day at 6–8-hr intervals.	Contraindicated in hypersensitivity to penicillin derivatives or cephalosporins. Safe use in pregnancy not established. Use cautiously in history of allergy and in infectious mononucleosis.	GI upset, increased SGOT, superinfection, hypersensitivity, BLOOD DYSCRASIAS, NEUROTOXICITY, ANAPHYLAXIS, INTERSTITIAL NEPHRITIS.
Septra, Bactrim	Sulfamethoxazole and trimethoprim	Oral, children: suspension 1 ml/kg/24 hr. Tablets: 10–20 kg: ½ tab q 12 hr; 20–30 kg: 1 tab q 12 hr; 30–40 kg: 1½ tab q 12 hr.	Contraindicated in hypersensitivity. Use cautiously in pregnancy, lactation, impaired renal and hepatic function, severe allergy or bronchial asthma, and in neonates less than 2 months old. Caution should be used in prophylactic or prolonged administration in otitis media.	BLOOD DYSCRASIAS such as APLASTIC ANEMIA, AGRANULOCYTOSIS. Allergic reactions: urticaria, pruritus, conjunctival infections. Gastrointestinal reactions: nausea, vomiting, abdominal pain, diarrhea. CNS reactions: headache, depression, convulsions, ataxia
Penicillin G, Pentids, V-Cillin, Pen-Vee	Penicillin	Pen G: IM adults: 600,000–1.2 million units daily. Pen G, IM, children: 500,000–1 million units once daily. Pen V, oral, adults: 125–250 mg q 6–8 hr. Pen V, oral, children over 12: 15–50 mg/kg/day in 3–6 divided doses.	Contraindicated in prior hypersensitivity. Use cautiously in history of suspected allergies and in neonates.	Hypersensitivity reactions, GI upset, blood dyscrasias, neuropathy, superinfections.

CONTINUED ON THE FOLLOWING PAGE

*Within the column listing adverse effects, <u>underlines</u> indicate the most common effects; CAPITALS indicate life-threatening effects.

Table 61–2. OTIC ANTI-INFECTIVES–*CONTINUED*

Medication	Primary Anti-infectives	Dosage	Contraindications and Precautions	Adverse Effects
Amoxil, Larotid, Polymox	Amoxicillin	PO, adults: 250–500 mg q 8 hr. PO, children (under 20 kg): 20–40 mg/kg/day in divided doses q 8 hr.	Contraindicated in hypersensitivity. Use cautiously in patients with a history of allergies.	Same as above.
Ceclor	Cefaclor	PO, adults: 250 mg q 8 hr. PO, children: 20 mg/kg/day in divided doses q 8 hr.	Contraindicated in hypersensitivity. Use cautiously in pregnancy and in patients with a previous allergy to penicillin.	Same as above.
Amphotericin B lotion (Fungizone)	Amphotericin B	Adult and children: liberal amount is applied to lesion 2–4× daily.		
Augmentin	Amoxicillin, Clavulonate	Adult: 250 mg q 8 hr. Children over 40 kg: 40 mg/kg/day in divided doses q 8 hr.		Diarrhea common.

aluminum acetate solution (Burow's solution), dilute (10%–20%) ethyl alcohol solution, hydrogen peroxide (3% mixed 1:1 with water), hypertonic (3%) sodium chloride solution, or 1% acetic acid solution (Table 61–3).

Inner Ear Problems

Amoxicillin (Amoxil) and ampicillin (Polycillin) are currently first-line drugs effective for otitis media. Sulfonamides, erythromycin (E-Mycin), trimethoprim and sulfamethoxazole (Bactrim), and amoxicillin and potassium clavulanate (Augmentin), second-line drugs, are used if the first-line drugs are ineffective. The third-line drugs

Table 61–3. EAR MEDICATIONS

Irrigating Solutions*	Local Anesthetic Preparations*
Aluminum acetate solution (Burow's solution) Ethyl alcohol solution 10%–20% Hyrogen peroxide 3% (mixed 1:1 with water) Hypertonic sodium chloride solution 3% Acetic acid solution (Aqueous or Hydro-Alcoholic) 1%	Americaine otic drops Auralgan otic solution Otodyne otic solution Otolgesic otic solution Tympagesic ear drops

*Contraindications for all drugs: prior hypersensitivity and presence of eardrum perforation; side effects for all drugs: local irritation, sensitivity reaction; dosage for all drugs: 1–6 gtt in each ear as ordered.

are of the cephalosporin group, particularly cefaclor (Ceclor). Pneumococcal and streptococcal infections are often treated with a 10-day course of oral penicillin G or penicillin V or with a single injection of penicillin V. Parenteral administration may be ordered when the patient is noncompliant with oral therapy. Penicillin G and penicillin V are not active against *Haemophilus influenzae*; if this is the causative agent, ampicillin is the drug of choice. If patients are allergic to the penicillins, erythromycin (for gram-positive organisms) or sulfonamides (for gram-nevative organisms) are usually effective.

The cephalosporins have a bacterial spectrum similar to that of the penicillins. The cephalosporins may often be administered to persons allergic to penicillin without that person developing a reaction. Only 10% of those allergic to penicillin have a cross-allergy to cephalosporin.

Table 61–2 lists the most common otic anti-infectives with their primary antibiotic ingredients.

ANTIHISTAMINE-DECONGESTANTS

Orally administered antihistamine-decongestant products are an adjunctive therapy, along with anti-infectives, in treating acute otitis media. Research demonstrates that antihistamine-decongestants reduce nasal congestion and middle ear effusion in patients with acute otitis media.

Antihistamine-decongestants are believed to improve eustachian tube patency and to promote resolution of the underlying pathology. As edema around the eustachian tube orifice is reduced, drainage from the middle ear is enhanced.

Table 61–4. ANTIHISTAMINE COMBINATIONS

Combination Drug	Basic Products*								Other
	A	**B**	**C**	**D**	**E**	**F**	**G**	**H**	
Actifed	60	—	—	—	—	—	—	—	2.5 I
Allerest	—	18.7	2	—	—	—	—	—	—
Allergy Relief Medicine	—	37.5	4	—	—	—	—	—	—
Anafed	120	—	8	—	—	—	—	—	—
Bendectin	—	—	—	—	—	—	—	—	10 J 10 K
Chlor-Trimeton Decongestant	—	—	4	60	—	—	—	—	—
Codimal DH	—	—	—	—	5	8.33	—	—	1.66 L 83.3 M 216 N 50 O
Conex D.A.	—	50	—	—	—	—	50	—	—
Co-Pyronil Pulvules	—	—	—	—	—	—	—	—	12.5 Q 15 R
Covanamine Liquid	—	6.25	1	—	3.75	6.25	—	—	—
Demazin Syrup	—	—	1	—	2.5	—	—	7.5	—
Dimetane Decongestant	—	—	—	—	10	—	—	—	4 S
Dimetapp Extentabs	—	15	—	—	15	—	—	—	12 S
Disophrol Chronotab	—	—	—	120	—	—	—	—	6 T
Drixoral	—	—	—	120	—	—	—	—	6 T
Duo-Hist	120	—	—	—	—	—	—	—	12 S
Duphrene	—	—	1	—	5	12.5	—	—	—
Fernhist	—	25	2	—	12.5	—	—	—	—
Histalet Forte	—	50	4	—	10	25	—	—	—
Histalet Syrup	45	—	3	—	—	—	—	0.45	—
Histaspan-D	—	—	8	—	20	—	—	—	2.5 U
Hista-Vadrin	—	40	6	—	5	—	—	—	—
Naldecon	—	40	5	—	10	—	15	—	—
Naldecon Syrup	—	20	2.5	—	5	—	7.5	—	—
Neotep	—	—	9	—	21	—	—	—	—
Nolamine	—	50	4	—	—	—	—	—	24 V
Novafed	120	—	8	—	—	—	—	—	—
Novahistine Elixir	—	18.7	2	—	—	—	—	5/5ml	—
Ornade	—	50	8	—	—	—	—	—	2.5 W
Phenergan-D	60	—	—	—	—	—	—	—	6.25 X
Poly-Histine-D	—	50	—	—	—	—	—	—	16 V 16 Y 16 Z
Relemine	—	25	4	—	15	25	—	—	—
Rhinex D-Lay	—	60	4	—	—	—	—	—	300 AA 300 BB
Rondec	60	—	—	—	—	—	—	—	4 CC
Rondec Tablets	60	—	—	—	—	—	—	—	4 CC
Triaminic Tablets	—	50	—	—	—	25	—	—	25 Z

*Basic products: A = pseudoephedrine HCl, mg; B = phenylpropanolamine HCl, mg; C = chlorpheniramine maleate, mg; D = pseudoephedrine sulfate, mg; E = phenylephrine HCl, mg; F = pyrilamine maleate, mg; G = phenyltoloxamine citrate, mg; H = alcohol, %; I = triprolidine HCl, mg; J = doxylamine succinate, mg; K = pyridoxine HCl, mg; L = hyrocodone bitartrate, mg; M = potassium guaiacolsulfonate, mg; N = sodium citrate, mg; O = citric acid, mg; Q = cylopentamine HCl, mg; R = pyrrobutamine phosphate, mg; S = brompheniramine maleate, mg; T = dexbrompheniramine maleate, mg; U = methscopolamine nitrate, mg; V = phenindamine tartrate, mg; W = isopropamide iodide, mg; X = promethazine HCl, mg; Y = phenyltoloxamine dihydrogen citrate, mg; Z = pheniramine maleate, mg; AA = acetaminophen, mg; BB = salicylamide, mg; CC = carbinoxamine maleate, mg.

Combination antihistamine products are featured in Table 61–4.

The side effects experienced from the antihistamine-decongestants include dry mouth, somnolence, and blurred vision.

LOCAL ANESTHETICS

To control the pain associated with ear infections, local anesthetics are often used topically. They may be used alone or in combination with anti-infective or anti-inflammatory agents, or both. Benzocaine is the most frequently used anesthetic agent. However, it is a known sensitizer and is also not particularly effective because of very poor absorption. Therefore, many clinicians currently oppose its use on the basis that it is minimally useful and, infrequently, harmful.

Pain relief for ear disorders may best be accomplished by using systemic analgesics such as Tylenol or other drugs rather than local agents. Tylenol is recommended, as most ear infections occur in children.

COMBINATION PRODUCTS

The combination products contain anti-infectives and either local anesthetics or anti-inflammatory agents, or both. In general, these combination products are frowned on by much of the medical community, which believes that only the product that is really needed should be used. A steroid, when combined with an anti-infective, may decrease the ultimate effectiveness of the anti-infective. Table 61–5 features a list of the most commonly used combination otic medications.

CERUMENOLYTIC MEDICATIONS

Cerumen (ear wax) is produced by glands in the outer one third of the external canal and has hygroscopic and probably bacteriostatic and fungistatic properties. Normally, cerumen slowly moves toward the external opening of the ear, where it is washed out, and does not cause obstruction or a loss of hearing. However, this mechanism may break down if the individual frequently attempts to remove the cerumen deposits manually.

The type of wax is genetically determined. Persons living in western countries produce moist cerumen, while persons living in eastern countries produce dry cerumen. The ear canal is less effective in clearing dry cerumen than moist cerumen. If the ear canal becomes blocked by cerumen, a significant *conductive hearing loss* may occur and the obstruction may predispose to the development of external otitis.

Gentle irrigation with hypertonic sodium chloride or hydrogen peroxide solutions may be necessary to soften, loosen, and flush out dried cerumen deposits. If the individual has chronic difficulty, the periodic instillation of one to two drops of olive oil, sweet almond oil, mineral oil, glycerin, or hydrogen peroxide will soften the deposits and promote normal removal. The cerumenolytics on the market, triethanolamine poly-peptide oleate-condensate (Cerumenex) and carbamide peroxide (Debrox), are expensive and work no better than the agents listed above. Cerumenex causes more local irritation than does Debrox.

USING THE NURSING PROCESS

ASSESSMENT

Assessment of the patient requiring medications for ear disorders always begins with a thorough nursing history to develop the data base. The patient requiring these medications is generally relatively healthy, and is often treated as an outpatient. The information included in the nursing history is included in Table 61–6. The nurse uses all of this information when preparing the nursing care plan.

At times, medications given for other purposes may cause ear symptoms, such as ringing in the ear *(tinnitus)*, *vertigo*, or hearing loss. During the initial assessment, all medications the patient is taking, both prescription and OTC, are identified. Medications that commonly cause ear symptoms are listed in Table 61–7. At this time, drug regulatory agencies are not required to test new drugs for ototoxic effects. Adverse otologic effects must, therefore, await recognition during general clinical trials. The risk of ototoxicity is greatly increased in patients with impaired renal function and, in general, is more likely in the elderly. The majority of drugs causing ototoxicity also cause nephrotoxicity. For example, the aminoglycosides are excreted unchanged in the urine. Thus, the rate of excretion through the kidney determines the amount of ototoxicity that develops. The use of ordinary doses in patients with renal failure will predictably cause ototoxic effects.

Some drugs, particularly the aminoglycoside antibiotics, have the capacity to damage the eighth cranial

Table 61–5. COMBINATION DRUGS FOR OTICS

Combination Drugs	Basic Products*:							
	A	**B**	**C**	**D**	**E**	**F**	**G**	**Other**
Coly-Mycin S Otic	3.3	—	—	3	1	0.05	—	—
Cortisporin Otic	5	10,000	1	—	—	—	—	—
Otobiotic Solution	—	10,000	0.5	—	—	—	—	—
Otocort Solution	5	10,000	1	—	—	—	—	—
Pyocidin Otic	—	10,000	0.5	—	—	—	—	—
Vosol HC Otic	—	—	1	—	—	—	2	†
Swimear	—	—	—	—	—	—	—	2.75 H & I
Dri/Ear	—	—	—	—	—	—	—	2.75 H & I
Ear-Dry	—	—	—	—	—	—	—	2.75 H & I
Aurocaine 2	—	—	—	—	—	—	—	2.75 H & I

*Basic Products (per ml): A = neomycin SO_4, mg; B = polymyxin B SO_4, units; C = hydrocortisone, %; D = colistin SO_4, mg; E = hydrocortisone acetate, mg; F = thonzonium bromide, %; G = acetic acid, %; H = boric acid, %; I = isopropyl alcohol.
†3% propylene glycol diacetate and 0.02% benzethonium chloride.

Table 61–6. NURSING PROCESS FOR PATIENT RECEIVING EAR MEDICATIONS

Assessment

Note history of current illness/condition, previous occurrence (and frequency) of infection. Ascertain routine care, how often and how ears are cleaned, whether patient is a swimmer. Determine medication use (prescription, and OTC drugs). Assess dizziness.

Nursing Diagnosis	Nursing Actions	Rationale	Desired Outcomes/ Evaluation Criteria
Knowledge deficit related to lack of exposure/ recall, unfamiliarity with information resources/ misinterpretation as evidenced by questions, statement of concern, inaccurate follow-through of instruction/ development of preventable complications.	Provide information about individual condition, treatment rationale and expected outcomes.	Understanding of reasons for ear problems helps patient to make informed choices and cooperate with treatment regimen.	Verbalizes understanding of individual condition/ disease process and treatment. Correctly performs necessary procedures and explains reasons for the actions.
	Review drug dosage, administration schedule, need to continue for specified number of days.	Promotes correct procedure and enhances potential for positive outcome.	
	Instruct in administration of eardrops/medications or irrigations. Have individual return demonstration of procedure.	Provides optimal benefit from medication.	
	Identify possible detrimental side effects (e.g., hypersensitivity) or signs of inadequate treatment (e.g., continuing pain, drainage) and importance of seeking medical attention.	Early identification allows for prompt intervention and prevention of further problems.	
	Demonstrate correct procedure for ear care.	Reduces risk of recurrence.	
	Discuss reasons for infection related to swimming, use of diving hoods, or ear phones.	"Swimmer's ear" is a common summer malady, usually due to *Pseudomonas aeruginosa* or other gram-negative organism.	
	Suggest use of ear plugs, limiting time in the water, and drying ear thoroughly after swimming or showering/shampooing.	Use of barrier/proper care can reduce recurrence of these infections.	
Trauma, potential for related to balancing difficulties.	Monitor complaints of dizziness, swaying gait.	Indicators of vestibular disturbances.	Identifies and corrects potential risk factors in the environment. Demonstrates appropriate actions to reduce risk of injury.
	Note hazards in the environment and take measures to correct.	Can prevent injury from falls related to impaired balance.	
	Assist patient as necessary when walking.	May need help until vertigo is resolved.	
	Determine origin of symptoms and refer for medical evaluation.	Vertigo may be a side effect of drugs such as acetylsalicylic acid, aminoglycosides or a result of the infection.	

nerve, sometimes irreversibly. The onset of hearing loss may not occur until some time after treatment is discontinued, or may continue to progress even when treatment is stopped. Eighth cranial nerve damage may occur to the vestibular portion, causing the patient to complain of vertigo and tinnitus, or to the auditory portion, which often leads to temporary or permanent loss

of high-frequency sound perception. Auditory toxicity is particularly common with kanamycin, neomycin, and streptomycin.

The nurse also assesses how the individual normally cares for his or her ears, since improper hygiene practices may be the source of the problem. If such improper practices are identified, the nurse implements health

Table 61–7. MEDICATIONS ADVERSELY AFFECTING THE EAR

Drug	Tinnitus	Vertigo	Hearing Loss
Gentamicin, tobramycin, kanamy-cin, neomycin	x	x	x (mild to moderate, high frequency)
Streptomycin	x	x	x (moderate to severe)
Loop diuretics (e.g., ethacrynic acid, furosemide, Bumex)	—	—	x (mild to moderate)
Salicylates and other nonsteroidal anti-inflammatory agents	x	x	—
Chloroquine	x	x	—
Platinol	—	—	x (high frequency)
Minocycline	—	x	—

Note: Important to monitor hearing ability when doses are increased, when there is increased duration of treatment, or with decreased renal function.

teaching during the planning and nursing intervention phase in order to inform the patient of proper ear care procedures.

NURSING DIAGNOSES

Possible nursing diagnoses for a patient with ear problems are included in Table 61–6.

PLANNING AND INTERVENTION

The nurse develops the goals of nursing intervention from the nursing diagnoses during the planning phase. When caring for the patient requiring medications for ear disorders, typical nursing actions are included in Table 61–6.

PATIENT TEACHING

The patient requiring medications for ear disorders will normally administer these medications at home. The nurse must therefore make certain that the patient knows and understands the information found in Table 61–8 and Figure 61–1, to ensure the safe administration of medications and the prevention of further ear problems.

Swimmer's Ear

A common malady, particularly during the summer, is "swimmer's ear." It is usually due to *Pseudomonas aeruginosa* or other gram-negative organism. Rarely is the infection fungal. Swimmer's ear may occur when a person's ears have been exposed to prolonged heat or moisture as from swimming or the use of diving hoods or ear phones.

In the earliest, mildest form, of swimmer's ear, which is sometimes called the pre-inflammatory stage, itching and a feeling that the ear is plugged are the most typical complaints. If the canal has been kept dry and free from trauma, the condition rarely needs medical attention. However, if there has been trauma to the skin of the canal from scratching, infection occurs. The canal is red, swollen, and tender. In all but the mildest cases, pushing on the tragus, pulling the auricle up and back, or

exerting gentle outward pressure in the canal with an otoscope speculum causes discomfort. As the infection progresses, the canal fills with varying amounts of cheesy green-blue-gray discharge composed of bacteria, leukocytes, desquamated epithelial cells, and serous

Table 61–8. PATIENT TEACHING FOR EAR MEDICATIONS

Dear Patient:
   This drug has been ordered for you. This is what you should know about your drug to get the most from its use.

1. You must take ear drugs until your ear problem is resolved.
2. To give ear medications correctly you must straighten the ear canal. Tip your head slightly to the opposite side, grasp the top of the ear (auricle) firmly and pull it upward, back, and slightly out. Press gently on the skin flap over the opening after applying the medicine or use an ear wick to move the medication down into the canal. (Cotton plugs do not help the medication move.) (Figure 61–1 shows ear medication instillation.) If you are administering a topical ear medication to a young child, the child should be held securely in order to prevent hurting the ear. A child's ear is pulled down by the ear lobe to open the ear canal.
3. The interactions that may occur with your drugs include: . . .
4. If you forget your ear drug until almost when the next dose is due, forget the dose; do not try to catch up.
5. Typical side effects for your ear medications include:_____.
6. If you usually get ear aches during the warm weather or after swimming, you should try to keep your ear canals dry. After swimming, you can put a few drops of either ethyl or isopropyl alcohol (70%–95%) or isopropyl alcohol mixed with vinegar into the ear to help dry the canal and prevent a ready source of infection.
7. Do not put or poke any foreign objects, such as hairpins, cotton-tipped swabs, match sticks, fingernails, or other small objects into your ear canal for any purpose.
8. Take all of your drugs as ordered by your doctor.
9. Store your drug in a dry, light-resistant container.

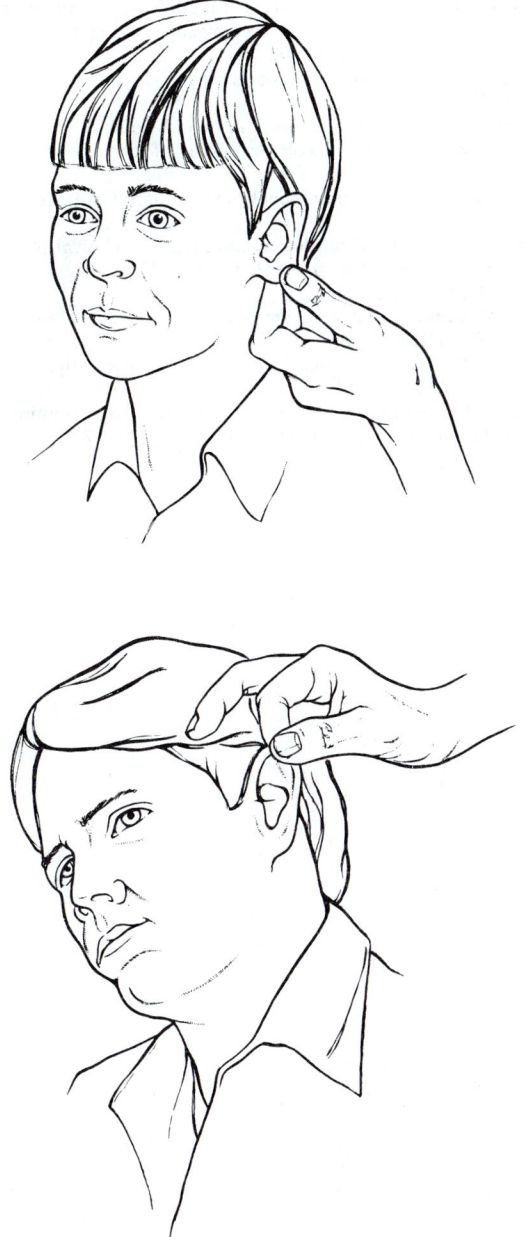

Figure 61–1. To instill ear drops in a child, pull down on the auricle to straighten the external canal. To instill ear drops in an adult, pull up and back on the auricle to straighten the external canal.

fluid. This external otitis is often accompanied by *myringitis.*

The best approach to swimmer's ear is prevention. When teaching the patient, recommend that he or she limit time in the water. The time is determined by trial and error but is generally less than one hour. Shake the head to loosen water and dry the ear with the corner of a towel. The ears should be allowed to dry completely for an hour or two before going back in the water.

In addition, a solution of equal parts of water and vinegar or vinegar and rubbing alcohol can be prepared. A

few drops are put in each ear upon arising in the morning, after each swim, and at bedtime. The solution should remain in the ear for at least five minutes. Nothing should be inserted into the ear canal that could cause injury to the delicate epithelial lining.

If these measures are not effective, medical treatment should be obtained. After treatment begins, the individual should stay out of the water for at least seven days. It is permissible to shower or bathe each day and shampoo the hair every other day if the ear is dried immediately afterwards and ear medications put in. Typical ear medications that are ordered include: local antibiotics, systemic antipruritics, and analgesics. Medications are generally continued for several days after all signs and symptoms have resolved.

EVALUATION

During the evaluation phase, the nurse evaluates the effectiveness of the medications used for ear disorders, based on a list of outcome evaluation criteria that has been developed in relation to the goals determined by the nurse, patient, and family. The data base obtained in the original assessment and used to formulate the nursing diagnoses provides helpful criteria for measuring the treatment's effectiveness.

Typical evaluation criteria are included in Table 61–6.

The patient is made aware of the potential side effects of the medications and instructed to report any unusual symptoms to the physician or nurse. In general, medications applied topically to the ear have few side effects. The most frequent complaint is contact dermatitis. Any local redness or itching should be reported at once and the medication discontinued.

The more the patient and family are involved with the planning of care, the more likely they are to comply. Therefore, it is extremely important for the nurse to work with the patient and family to ensure their complete assistance and support. Since many of the patients with ear disorders are children, the nurse may also elicit assistance from the school or camp nurse in administering the medication. The majority of patients, once they understand the importance of the continued medical treatment, usually comply; the nurse should thus stress the importance of such continued medical care. The primary reason for noncompliance is forgetting medication. It is therefore important to develop a method that the patient and family can use to help them remember the medication schedule and to evaluate its effectiveness.

SUMMARY

The nurse will frequently care for persons with disorders of the ear. Many medications are available to treat these conditions including anti-infectives, local anesthetics, antihistamines, decongestants, and cerumenolytics. These medications have different actions, uses, and pharmacokinetics, which all are discussed within the chapter and tables.

The majority of patients with ear disorders are treated on an outpatient basis and, therefore, need to be taught the proper technique for administering these medications. Patients need to know that if they experience a worsening of their condition or decreased hearing acuity, their physician should be notified.

BIBLIOGRAPHY

AMA Department of Drugs: AMA Drug Evaluations, ed 5. PSG Publishing, Littleton, MA, 1986.

Bickerton, RC, Roberts, C, and Little, JT: Survey of general practitioners' treatment of the discharging ear. Br Med J 296(6637):1649, 1988.

Davis, RH, Leitner, MG, and Russo, JM: Topical anti-inflammatory activity of aloe vera as measured by ear swelling. J Am Podiatr Med Assoc 77(11):610, 1987.

Fireman, P: Newer concepts in otitis media. Hosp Pract 22(11):85, 1987.

Gilman, AG, Goodman, LS, and Gilman, A (eds): Goodman and Gilman's The Pharmacological Basis of Therapeutics, ed 7. Macmillan, New York, 1985.

Ivey, M, et al: Pharmacotherapeutics in Primary Care. New York, Elsevier, 1984.

Minisymposium on "Hyaluronan and its use in clinical otology." Uppsala, December 8–9, 1986. Acta Otolaryngol Supply, Stockholm, Sweden.

Patlak, M: Children's all-too-common ear infections. FDA Consum 21(10):28, Dec 1988.

Richman, E: Swimmer's ear: Timely management tips. Patient Care 21(10):28, 1987.

Richman, E: Swimmer's ear needn't put a stop to swimming: Patient education aid. Patient Care 21(10):82, 1987.

13
UNIT

USING THE NURSING PROCESS WITH DRUGS IN SELECTED MEDICAL DISORDERS

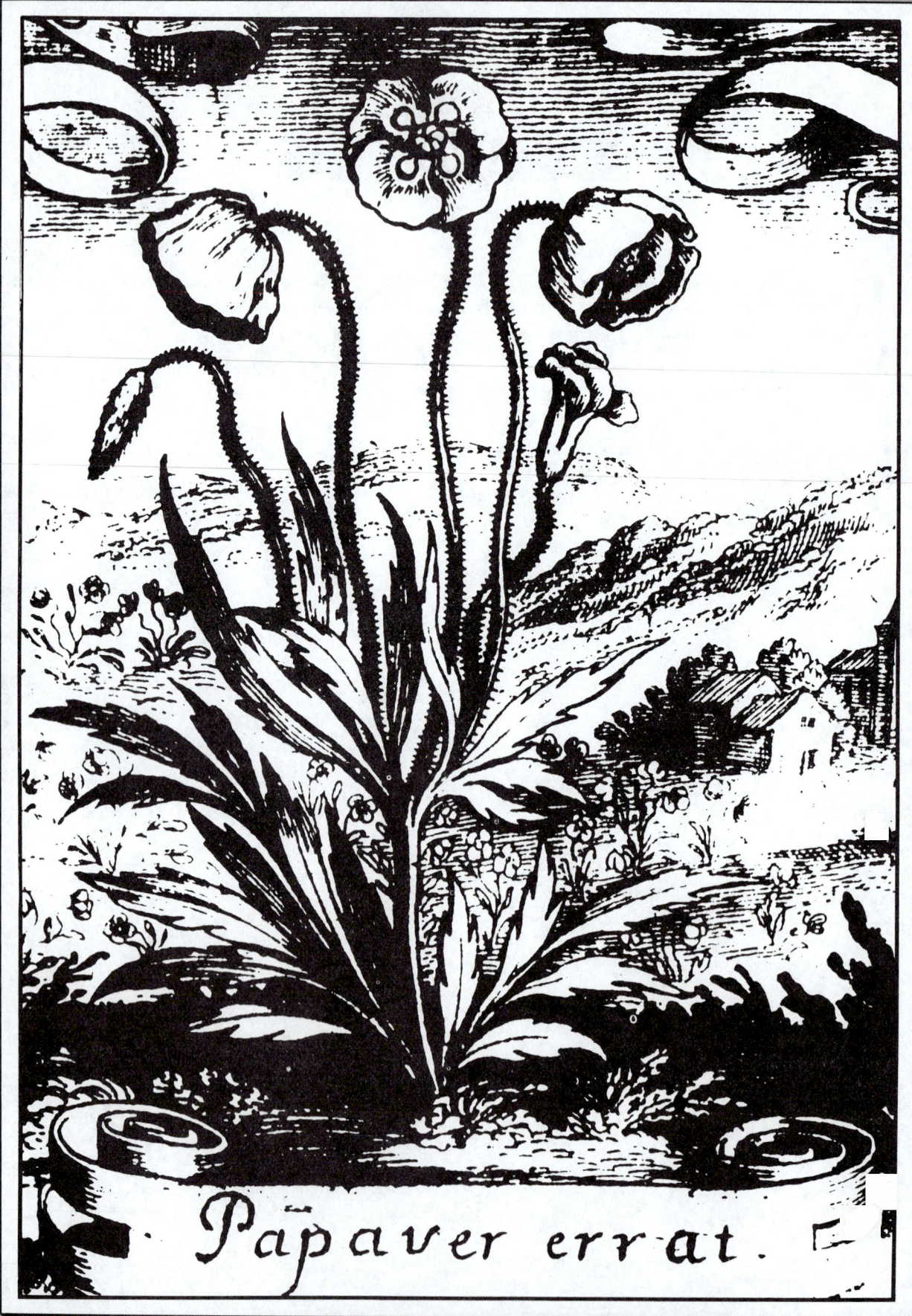

Botanical woodcut of poppies, circa 1550. The Bettmann Archive.

13
UNIT

USING THE NURSING PROCESS WITH DRUGS IN SELECTED MEDICAL DISORDERS

ENZYMES

MERRILY MATHEWSON KUHN, R.N.C., Ph.D., CCRN

LEARNING OBJECTIVES

After reading this chapter, the student will be able to:

1. Identify medications commonly used as enzymes.

2. Differentiate among the enzymes as to mechanism of action, route of administration, pharmacokinetics, adverse effects, contraindications, and interactions.

3. Identify specific areas to assess in the patient requiring enzymes in order to formulate appropriate nursing diagnoses.

4. Plan the nursing interventions necessary to administer enzymes and choose appropriate teaching strategies to gain patient compliance.

5. Evaluate the patient at various stages of treatment to gauge nursing interventions.

THERAPEUTIC AGENTS

Enzymes have many therapeutic uses. They may be used to replace deficient digestive enzymes, to debride skin ulcers, to dissolve clots (see Chapter 54), to promote healing of wounds, and to liquefy tracheobronchial secretions. The majority of enzymes are applied topically as creams or ointments; only a few are available for systemic administration. Table 62–1 lists the currently used enzymes, their usual dosages, the source (bovine, porcine, plant, or bacterial), their contraindications, precautions, adverse effects, and nursing implications.

Enzymes are proteins needed by the body to act as catalysts in chemical reactions. Enzymes mediate the reaction but are not altered or consumed by the reaction. Enzymes act in two ways: on a single substrate (absolute specificity), or on a group of closely related substrates (group specificity). Nearly every step in the metabolism of nutrients, as well as subsequent growth and repair of body parts, is dependent on enzymes. Most all subcellular particles such as mitochondria, microsomes, and lysosomes need enzymes to function properly.

The name of most enzymes contains two parts: the name of the substrate that is acted on, and the suffix "ase." For example, collagenase is an enzyme that breaks down collagen. Enzymes can be divided into two primary groups: *proteolytic*—those that digest protein; and *fibrinolytic*—those that dissolve fibrin.

Many enzymes function only in the presence of *cofactors* such as ions of Ca^{+2}, Cl^-, or nonprotein organic compounds. If these cofactors are missing, the enzymatic reaction does not occur.

Since enzymes are proteins, many cannot be administered orally because destruction by the proteolytic enzymes of the intestinal tract occurs. Replacement enzymes or digestants are an exception. These products are taken orally to replace missing gastric intestinal enzymes. In addition, as foreign protein sources, enzymes are very likely to cause immune reactions within the body.

CONTRAINDICATIONS AND PRECAUTIONS

In general, all of the enzyme preparations are contraindicated in patients sensitive to the original source, such as beef, pork, pineapple, or papaya products. Cross-sensitivity also needs to be evaluated in patients before starting therapy. Since many of the enzymes are fibrinolytic agents, they are contraindicated in patients with bleeding disorders, those currently receiving anticoagulants, or those who have current hemorrhages, as they further increase the anticoagulant effect by dissolving fibrin. In addition, these products are not given to pregnant women or children under 12 years of age.

ADVERSE EFFECTS

The major adverse effect produced by the enzymes is hypersensitivity. Since these agents are foreign proteins that are applied topically or taken orally, immunologic reactions may result. When applied topically, these reactions may result in localized itching, stinging, or tingling. When taken internally, the reactions lead to nausea, vomiting, pruritus, and rash. The patient should be told to notify the physician immediately if these reactions occur, and the enzyme preparation is discontinued until use is reauthorized.

REPLACEMENT ENZYMES

Replacement enzymes most commonly used include pancreatic enzymes, pancreatin, and pancrelipase. These enzymes are used to treat malabsorption syndromes and other digestive disturbances caused by absent or deficient pancreatic enzymes such as cystic fibrosis. Patients, particularly those with steatorrhea (fatty stools) caused by incomplete fat digestion, can benefit from supplemental enzymes. The actions of pancreatic enzymes are to digest proteins with proteases, carbohydrates with amylases, and fats with lipases. Antacids negate the effects of both pancreatin and pancrelipase, so they are not administered concurrently.

Pharmacokinetics

The digestive or replacement enzymes are natural substances of either porcine or bovine origin. They work locally in the gastrointestinal tract, duodenum, and upper jejunum.

Pancreatin

Pancreatin (Dizymes) is a pancreatic replacement enzyme concentrate of bovine or porcine origin containing principally lipase, protease, and amylase in standard amounts. Pancreatin assists in the digestion of starch, protein, and fats. This product is used specifically for enzyme replacement in patients with cystic fibrosis and other pancreatic deficiencies. Pancreatin is administered to adults in doses of one to three tablets with meals, and to children in doses of one to two tablets with meals. In severe deficiency, higher doses may be necessary.

Pancrelipase

Pancrelipase (Cotazym and others), of porcine origin, has about twelve times the lipolytic activity and four times the proteolytic and amylolytic activity as pancreatin. Pancrelipase is administered to adults in doses of one to three tablets or one to two packets prior to or with meals and snacks; or to children in doses of one to two tablets or packets.

ENZYMES TO PROMOTE WOUND HEALING

Enzymes may aid in wound healing. Medications such as papain, hyaluronidase, and bromelains reduce inflammation resulting from trauma and infections. These enzymes also dissolve fibrin clots, which helps to reduce the size of surface hematomas. They may also be used surgically to dissolve fibrin clots in *episiotomies.*

In general, enzyme administration is only adjunctive therapy. The underlying cause is evaluated and often treated with systemic medications. For example, when enzymes are used to debride a large stasis ulcer, other drugs such as peripheral vasodilators and systemic or local antibiotics are also employed. To be effective, the enzyme must be in contact with the affected tissue in adequate concentrations for a sufficient length of time. If necessary, the wound is first surgically debrided. Once the treatment of the wound is completed, enzymes are discontinued because their function is complete. If enzymes are not administered to a clean, debrided wound, healing may be delayed.

Papain

Papain (Papase, Panafil) is a combination of proteolytic enzymes extracted from the papaya plant. It is used topically for enzymatic debridement, promotion of normal healing, and when combined with chlorophyll derivatives, deodorization of surface lesions. Papain does not injure or affect healthy tissue or cells. It is available as a 10% ointment (Panafil) with the addition of urea, which is added to stimulate collagen formation. The ointment is applied twice daily and covered with a dressing. At the time the wound is redressed, all accumulated liquefied necrotic material is removed. Hydrogen peroxide cannot be used to irrigate the wound, because it inactivates the papain. Papain is also available in tablet form (Papase), with two to four tablets being administered orally four times daily for at least five days.

Chymopapain

Chymopapain is a proteolytic enzyme derived from papaya. This agent is used in the treatment of patients with herniated lumbar intervertebral disk who have not responded to an adequate trial of conservative therapy. Although the exact mechanism of action of chymopapain has not been established, the herniated portion of the intervertebral disk is usually absent from its former site following administration directly into the herniated disk.

For intradiskal administration, 5 ml of sterile water for injection is added to a vial labeled as containing 10,000 units of chymopapain to provide a solution containing 2,000 units/ml. The usual adult dose of chymopapain is 2,000–4,000 units/disk as a single injection. Bacteriostatic water for injection must not be used for reconstitution, as it may inactivate the enzyme. Before needles are inserted into the vial of drug, the stopper is cleansed with alcohol; the alcohol is allowed to completely evaporate prior to insertion of the needle, since it may inactivate the chymopapain.

Anaphylaxis, which can be immediate or delayed up to one hour after drug administration, is the most serious adverse effect of chymopapain, occurring in about 1% of patients. Other less severe, but more frequent, adverse effects of chymopapain include back pain, stiffness, and soreness. Patients are instructed that they may experience back pain or involuntary muscle spasm in the lower area of the back for several days after drug administration.

Chymopapain is contraindicated in patients with known sensitivity to the drug, papaya, or papaya derivatives (e.g., meat tenderizers). The drug is also contraindicated in patients who have previously been injected with any form of chymopapain, and in patients with severe *spondylolisthesis*, spinal cord tumor, or cauda equina lesion.

HYALURONIDASE

Hyaluronidase (Wydase), a mucolytic enzyme, is a special type of enzyme. It acts to facilitate the absorption of fluids given by subcutaneous *hypodermoclysis* (the introduction of large quantities of fluids into the subcutaneous tissues). By increasing the rate of fluid absorption in the subcutaneous tissue, the pain and tissue tension caused by the fluid injection are reduced. For hypodermoclysis, the dose of hyaluronidase is injected into the rubber tubing close to the needle of the running clysis solution. Alternatively, the dose of hyaluronidase may be injected under the skin prior to clysis. The amount of fluid administered and the flow rate are no faster than if the fluid were administered intravenously. When administering fluid to children via this route, the nurse is particularly cautious about overhydration.

Another use for hyaluronidase is to inject it subcutaneously into an infiltrated IV site where a potent vasoconstrictor, such as Levophed or Aramine, has infiltrated. This reduces the sloughing of tissue likely to occur secondary to infiltration. It is also used to perform subcutaneous urography.

Hyaluronidase is used in ophthalmic surgery to increase the reabsorption of transudates and edema to prevent damage to the eye.

Hyaluronidase is of bovine origin. The usual dose for clysis is 150 units in 1000 ml of solution. The usual dose for subcutaneous urography is 75 units. In children under the age of three, the volume of a single clysis is limited to 200 ml; in premature infants or during the neonatal period, the daily dosage for clysis should not exceed 25 ml/kg.

ENZYMES TO IMPROVE SURGICAL HEALING

Enzymes also promote rapid healing in certain surgical applications. Both proteolytic and fibrinolytic enzymes are used, including chymotrypsin (Chymar), chymotrypsin alpha (Alpha-Chymar), and trypsin with chymotrypsin (Chymoral, Orenzyme). They are administered both preoperatively and postoperatively to prevent infection and to promote a more rapid and less

TEXT RESUMES ON PAGE 1706

Table 62–1. ENZYMES

Name	Dosage	Source

REPLACEMENT ENZYMES

Action: restore pancreatic enzymes to assist with digestion of fats, CHO, and proteins.

Use: pancreatic enzyme deficiency states.

*Within the column listing adverse effects, underlines indicate the most common effects; CAPITALS indicate life-threatening effects.

For All Enzymes:

ASSESSMENT: Assess for skin reactions and for wound healing.

INTERVENTION: All powders are stored in a cool, dry place and reconstituted just before use. Do not store reconstituted product for more than 24 hours. When mixing, medications are rolled or turned gently, not agitated. This will prevent excessive flocculation. Medications are discontinued at the first sign of sensitivity. Medication may need to be taken every 2 hours during the waking hours, so some schedule to remember the medication may need to be formulated.

EVALUATION: Evaluate for hypersensitivity reactions.

For All Topically Administered Enzymes

ASSESSMENT: Assess within the first 24 hours of treatment, a febrile state often occurs due to the accumulation of leukocytes at the wound site. This may be avoided by frequent aspiration of exudate from the wound. Assess vision when ophthalmic products are used.

INTERVENTION: Enzymes must be in immediate contact with purulent wound material to be most effective. Wounds are cleansed with a prescribed irrigating solution between doses. Wounds are irrigated or cleansed gently to prevent damage to healthy tissue. Itching and stinging often occur after topical application, but they should subside. If symptoms persist, notify the physician. Light dressings and cellophane wrap may be used over the wound to prevent soiling of clothing. Change all dressings frequently to prevent contamination and to remove necrotic debris. Body cavities are drained at least every 6–10 hours and

CONTINUED ON THE FOLLOWING PAGE

Table 62–1. ENZYMES–*CONTINUED*

Name	Dosage	Source
Pancreatin (Dizymes)	Adults: 1–3 tab (300 mg/tab) with or after meals and snacks. Children: 1–2 tabs with meals.	Bovine, Porcine
Pancrelipase (Cotazym and others)	1–3 tab; 1–2 packets prior to or with meals. Children: 1–2 tabs or packets.	Porcine

ENZYMES TO PROMOTE WOUND HEALING

Action: dissolve fibrin clots, which aids in wound healing and provides a clean layer of granulation tissue that serves as a base for epithelialization and optimal healing.

Use: to aid in wound healing.

Name	Dosage	Source
Papain (Papase, Panafil)	PO: 2–4 tabs 4× daily. Topical: 10% ointment 2× daily.	Papaya
Trypsin with chymotrypsin (Chymoral, Orenzyme)	Trypsin 50,000–100,000 units; chymotrypsin 4,000–8,000 units 4×/ day.	Bovine

*Within the column listing adverse effects, underlines indicate the most common effects; CAPITALS indicate life-threatening effects.

Contraindications/ Precautions	Adverse Effects*	Interactions	Nursing Implications
			the enzyme solution replaced. Store between 8–15°C. EVALUATION: Report stinging and burning to physician.
Contraindicated in sensitivity to beef or pork products.	GI: anorexia, nausea, vomiting, diarrhea, buccal and anal soreness. Misc: Hypersensitivity	None known.	ASSESSMENT: Assess quality of stools, particularly fecal fat and nitrogen. Serum carotene and calcium tests are performed to assess response to the medication regimen. INTERVENTION: Tablets are swallowed or chewed and followed by water. If tablets are to be absorbed bucally, mild stinging may occur, which is generally relieved when the tablet is removed. Enteric-coated tablets are swallowed whole, not chewed or crushed. In addition, antacids are not taken concurrently because that will cause them to dissolve in the stomach. Maintain adequate and well-balanced nutrition. Store drugs in tight containers at room temperature. Teach patient that bowel movements will decrease. EVALUATION: Evaluate for hypersensitivity.
Same as above.	Same as above.	Same as above.	Same as above.
Contraindicated in patients with previous hypersensitivity. Use cautiously in blood dyscrasia, current anticoagulant therapy, and renal or hepatic diseases. Not for use in eyes.	GI: nausea, vomiting, diarrhea Integ: stinging, tingling, pruritus, rash	None known.	Same as for all enzymes.

CONTINUED ON THE FOLLOWING PAGE

Table 62–1. ENZYMES–*CONTINUED*

Name	Dosage	Source

Action: proteolytic and fibrinolytic enzyme

Use: preoperatively instilled into eye to soften cataract lens for more easy extraction.

Name	Dosage	Source
Chymotrypsin (Chymar and others)	4,000–40,000 u qid. IM: 2,500–5,000 units.	Bovine
Chymotrypsin ophthalmic (Alpha-Chymar)	150 units.	Bovine

ENZYMES FOR HYPODER-MOCLYSIS

Action: modifies permeability of connective tissue through the hydrolysis of hyaluronic acid.

Use: assists with absorption of hypodermocylsis, and the dispersion of infiltrated vasoconstrictor drugs.

Name	Dosage	Source
Hyaluronidase (Wydase)	Clysis: Adult: 150 units in 1000 ml solution. Children under 3: limit to 200 ml. Premature infants: should not exceed 25 ml/kg daily. 75 units for subcutaneous urography.	Bovine

AGENTS USED FOR SKIN ULCERS

Action: removes purulent exudates in wounds

Use: burns, necrotic ulcers, and wounds.

Name	Dosage	Source
Sutilains (Travase)	Topical: ointment 82,000 u/g, once daily.	Bacteria
Collagenase (Santyl, Bio-zyme-C)	Topical: ointment 250 u/g 1 or more × daily.	Bacteria
Fibrinolysin and desoxyribonuclease (Elase)	Topical: ointment 1 unit fibrinolysin, 666 units desoxyribonuclease 1–3 times daily. Dry powder 25 u fibrinolysin, 15,000 u desoxyribonuclease 1–3 times daily.	Bovine

*Within the column listing adverse effects, underlines indicate the most common effects; CAPITALS indicate life-threatening effects.

Contraindications/ Precautions	Adverse Effects*	Interactions	Nursing Implications
Contraindicated in patients with prior hypersensitivity or severe infection.	GI: GI distress Ophth: transient increase in intraocular pressure, corneal edema	None known.	Same as for all enzymes.
Contraindicated in previous history of hypersensitivity.	Same as Chymotrypsin plus Ophth: temporary glaucoma, moderate uveitis	None known.	Same as for all enzymes.
Not for injection into inflamed, infected, or cancerous areas. Use cautiously in congestive heart failure, hypoproteinemia, during lactation, and in children. Safety in pregnancy not established.	CV: overhydration Integ: hypersensitivity	None known.	Same as for all enzymes.
Contraindicated in wound communicating with major body cavities, neoplastic ulcers, pregnancy. Do not allow medication to come in contact with eyes.	Integ: mild transient pain, contact dermatitis, hemorrhage	Enzyme activity impaired by detergents, antiseptics, and thimerosol.	Same as for all topical enzymes. INTERVENTION: Thoroughly moisten wound with sodium chloride or water and apply loose thin dressing after applying thin film extending ¼ to ½ inch beyond area to be debrided. Refrigerate ointment at 2–8°C.
Contraindicated in known hypersensitivity. Use cautiously in hemorrhage.	Same as Sutilains.	Enzyme activity impaired by detergents and antiseptics and mercury and silver. Avoid Burow's solution because of metal ion and low pH.	INTERVENTION: Apply at least daily with tongue blade directly to deep wound.
Contraindicated with known hypersensitivity. Use cautiously in hemorrhage.	Same as Sutilains.	None known.	INTERVENTION: Clean wound with water, pat dry. Apply thin layer and cover with petrolatum gauze. Flush away necrotic debris with saline.

CONTINUED ON THE FOLLOWING PAGE

Table 62–1. ENZYMES-*CONTINUED*

Name	Dosage	Source
AGENTS USED TO TREAT HERNIATED DISKS:		
Action: proteolytic enzyme that reduces intradiskal pressure and relieves compression symptoms.		
Use: herniated lumbar disks.		
Chymopapain (Chymodiactin, Discase)	2,000–4,000 units/disk.	Papaya

*Within the column listing adverse effects, underlines indicate the most common effects; CAPITALS indicate life-threatening effects.

painful recovery. Chymotrypsin and chymotrypsin alpha are often used in cataract surgery. They are instilled into the eye prior to surgery to soften the lens so it can more easily be removed.

These enzymes are also administered systemically as anti-inflammatory agents, which promote rapid healing after eye or ear surgery. Researchers differ in their opinions of the mechanism of action of these agents. The majority believe that postsurgical inflammation, pain, and edema are due to accumulation of fibrin that occludes capillaries and lymph vessels. Proteolytic and fibrinolytic enzymes dissolve the fibrin clot, thus allowing a greater blood flow to the area for increased healing. Since these enzymes prevent clots from forming, they must be used cautiously postoperatively.

All of these products are derived from bovine tissues, have the same dosage, and are administered four times daily. The usual oral dose is 4000–40,000 u; the intramuscular dose is 2500–5000 u; and the intraocular dose is 150 u.

ENZYMES TO REMOVE EXUDATES

Enzymes also assist in the removal of exudates, although their use is controversial. Many preparations such as sutilains, collagenase, fibrinolysis, and desoxyribonuclease are used to aid in wound debridement. Primarily, these products promote the *depolymerization* (conversion of compounds into smaller molecules) of desoxyribonucleic acid. In addition, since injured tissue cells are protected from further damage by desoxyribonucleic acid, enzymes will alter the previously thick, purulent drainage to become a thin liquid material that can easily be wiped or irrigated off the wound and thus promote wound healing.

To ensure that these products are used properly, the wound is prepared before their application. The wound is cleaned, and cross-hatching of eschar on burns is performed to allow adequate enzyme contact with the wound. Products that interfere with the action of these enzymes, such as cleansers, heavy metals, and antiseptics, are not used concurrently. All the enzyme preparations are designed to be an adjunct to surgical debridement, and not a replacement for surgery.

Sutilains

Sutilains (Travase) is a proteolytic enzyme derived from bacteria. It is particularly useful in removing nonviable or necrotic tissues and purulent exudates from second- or third-degree burns, decubitus ulcers, traumatic injuries, and peripheral vascular disease wounds. This enzyme is virtually inactive on viable tissue. Sutilains is available for topical application in ointment form with 82,000 u/g. The skin is washed with water or isotonic sodium chloride solution and then left moist as a thin layer of the ointment is applied extending 0.25- to 0.5-inch beyond the area to be debrided. Loose wet dressings are then applied to provide the moisture that is needed for the enzymatic action. The entire procedure may be repeated three to four times daily for best results. Sutilains functions best in a pH range of 6.0–6.8. If the wound is not affected after 24–48 hours of use, the medication is discontinued.

Drug interactions are known to occur with sutilains. Concomitant use of metallic ion-containing compounds such as thimerosal (Merthiolate) interferes with its activity. The use of detergents and antiseptics like hexachlorophene, iodine, and nitrofurazone also decreases its effectiveness.

Contraindications/ Precautions	Adverse Effects*	Interactions	Nursing Implications
Contraindicated in prior injection of chymopa-pain, with allergy to papaya, with severe progressive paralysis. Safety not established in pregnancy, in lactating women, or in children.	Neuro: paresis, paresthesias, decreased reflexes GI: temporary loss of bowel control Misc: ANAPHYLAXIS	Halothane and epinephrine increase risk of dysrhythmia.	ASSESSMENT: Assess injection site for pain and swelling. Assess for motor and neurologic function. INTERVENTION: Refrigerate vials. Clean vial with alcohol, allow to dry before injecting needle into vial. EVALUATION: Evaluate for relief of severe back, hip, and leg pain.

Collagenase

Collagenase (Santyl, Biozyme-C) is a proteolytic enzyme derived from bacteria used as a topical debriding agent. It not only acts on the desoxyribonucleic acid, but also on both denatured (changed protein) and undenatured (unchanged) collagen. Other proteolytic enzymes act only on denatured collagen. By acting on both types of collagen, collagenase produces an effective debridement of the collagen tissue at the wound edges where the necrotic tissue is anchored. This encourages the formation of granulation tissue at the edges, and quicker epithelialization of wounds. For this proteolytic activity, a pH range of 6–8 is optimum. Collagenase is available as an ointment containing 250 u/g. It is applied one or more times daily. It should be applied only to the injured area, because healthy tissue may develop a transient erythema. The surrounding tissue can be protected by applying a protectant such as zinc oxide paste. The skin is prepared by washing it with hydrogen peroxide or Dakin's solution, followed by sterile normal saline (all of which are compatible with collagenase), and then patting the area dry. A thin layer of medication is applied over the wound, using a tongue blade for deep wounds. Collagenase does not have any antibiotic properties, so if an infection is present, either topical or systemic anti-infectives are administered concurrently.

Collagenase shares the same interactions with sutilains.

Fibrinolysin and Desoxyribonuclease

Fibrinolysin and desoxyribonuclease (Elase) is a proteolytic and fibrinolytic enzyme product derived from bovine plasma and pancreas, respectively. It acts on both deoxyribonucleic acid and fibrin to debride wounds in-cluding burns, decubitus ulcers, and inflamed or infected lesions. It is available as a dry powder containing 25 units fibrinolysin and 15,000 units desoxyribonuclease, or as an ointment containing 1 u/g fibrinolysin and 666 u/g desoxyribonuclease. It is applied at least once daily, but preferably two to three times. Any of the preparative solutions mentioned above can be used to clean the wound.

Fibrinolysin and desoxyribonuclease are available in combination with the antibiotic Chloromycetin for infected lesions. However, systemic antibiotics may be indicated.

Dextranomer

Dextranomer (Debrisan) is a cross-linked polymer of dextran chains available as beads 0.1–0.3 mm in diameter or as a paste. It is not a debriding agent but is a cleansing agent that actually absorbs peptides and proteins. Dextranomer is effective in wet wounds only.

USING THE NURSING PROCESS

ASSESSMENT

Assessment of the patient requiring enzymes always begins with a thorough nursing history to develop the data base. Typical information obtained from the patient and family is included in Table 62–2. All of this information is used later when preparing the nursing care plan. The patient requiring enzymes may be acutely ill in the hospital or relatively healthy, with this condition being treated on an outpatient basis. The patient may have a

Table 62–2. NURSING PROCESS FOR PATIENT RECEIVING TOPICAL ENZYMES

Assessment
Determine illness/condition requiring enzyme treatment. Note history of allergies to products from which enzymes are produced, e.g., beef, pork, papaya, pineapple, or bacteria. Review current medication use, especially anticoagulants. Note presence of bleeding disorders, current hemorrhage.

Nursing Diagnosis	Nursing Actions	Rationale	Desired Outcomes/ Evaluation Criteria
Skin integrity, impaired related to external (hyper/hypothermia, physical immobilization, trauma, internal altered circulation/nutritional state) excretions/secretions, and edema evidenced by complaints of itching, pain, numbness, pressure, disruption of skin surfaces.	Perform skin testing as indicated. Review importance of skin and measures to maintain proper skin functioning. Discuss factors necessary to improve general health/well-being, e.g., nutrition, cleanliness. Monitor vital signs and evaluate open wound. Cleanse open area, assist with debridement as indicated, apply enzymes (e.g., Papase, Travase) to wound; or apply proteolytic and fibrinolytic agents (e.g., Chymar, Alpha-Chymar) pre and postoperatively as appropriate.	Determines sensitivity to enzyme medication. Helps patient to understand individual situation and enhances cooperation with treatment regimen. Improves body's own ability to heal. Elevation of temperature and pulse may be indicators of infection. Useful for debridement of large stasis ulcers, burns; reduces opportunity for bacterial contamination and enhances healing.	Verbalizes understanding of condition and causative factors. Identifies interventions appropriate for specific condition. Observed improvement in wound/lesion healing.
Knowledge deficit related to lack of exposure/recall, information misinterpretation, unfamiliarity with information resources evidenced by questions, statement of concern, inaccurate follow-through of instruction/development of preventable complications.	Provide information about pathophysiology of condition, treatment regimen, and expected outcomes. Instruct in proper application/use of enzyme medications. Discuss probability of burning sensation at site and measures to take to minimize discomfort. Discuss possible interactions with other drugs. Review indications for medical evaluation.	Understanding of own condition helps patient to make informed decisions and participate fully in treatment regimen. Promotes optimal healing. Common side effect may impair cooperation with treatment regimen. Knowing what to expect can help patient to cope with situation and achieve desired effects. Can prevent negative result from accidental combination(s). Persistent symptoms, indications of infection may indicate need for change in/further treatment.	Verbalizes understanding of condition/disease process and treatment. Correctly performs necessary procedures and explains reasons for the actions.

decubitus ulcer needing care, a necrotic wound after surgery or trauma, or a burn; or may be receiving enzymes to assist with wound healing. Since enzymes are used to treat such a wide variety of conditions, the nursing assessments must be specific for the individual patient's condition. As an example, the wound needs to be assessed daily either in the hospital or at home to determine whether or not therapeutic effects are occurring. When the wound is completely debrided, enzymes need to be discontinued, since they may retard healing.

The nurse assesses the patient for a history of allergies to the products from which enzymes are produced, such as beef, pork, bacteria, papaya, or pineapple. Skin testing (discussed later) may be performed if allergies are suspected.

The nurse also assesses the quality of stools, particularly checking for fecal fat and nitrogen when pancreatic enzymes are being administered. Laboratory tests of serum carotene and calcium are also performed to check the response to the medication regimen. Prothrombin levels are also obtained to assess for bleeding tendencies.

NURSING DIAGNOSES

The nursing diagnoses are developed based on the information obtained in the initial assessment. Typical nursing diagnoses for a patient receiving enzymes are included in Table 62–2.

PLANNING AND INTERVENTION

The goals of nursing intervention are developed from the nursing diagnoses. When caring for a patient requiring enzymes, the goals of planning and intervention are included in Table 62–2. Medication may need to be taken every two hours during the waking hours, so some technique to remember the medication may need to be formulated for the patient at home.

NURSING RESPONSIBILITIES

As the nurse administers these medications, certain basic information should be understood. All powders are stored in a cool, dry place, and reconstituted just before use. Enzymes are not stored for more than 24 hours after reconstitution. When medications are being mixed, they are rolled or turned gently, not agitated. This prevents excessive *flocculation* (the formation of thin translucent fibers) in the preparation. Before enzymes are administered, skin testing, by administering a small amount of medication subcutaneously, is normally performed to assess sensitivity. If a wheal and localized itching occur within five minutes and last for 20–30 minutes, the medication is not used and the patient is informed about the positive allergic reaction. Enzymes are discontinued at the first sign of sensitivity, that is, redness, extreme itching, or other unusual local or systemic reactions.

Wounds are cleansed or irrigated gently to prevent damage to healthy tissue. Itching and stinging often occur after topical application, but generally subside. If symptoms persist, the physician should be notified. Enzymes must be in direct contact with purulent material on the wound to be effective. Light dressings and cellophane wrap may be used over the wound to enhance drug effect and prevent soiling of clothing. Skin surfaces are kept clean and moist with saline solution to ensure enzymatic activity. Dressings are changed frequently to prevent contamination and to remove necrotic debris. Transparent, occlusive, synthetic films such as Op Site, Bioclusive, and Tegaderm may be indicated to minimize bacterial contamination, drying, and pain. Skin grafting

in lesions greater than 3 cm may need to be performed. Antiseptics containing heavy metals such as silver or mercury are not applied to the affected area, because these substances and other detergent antiseptics may inactivate the enzymes. When enzymes are used within body cavities, they are drained at least every six to ten hours and the enzyme solution replaced. Within the first 24 hours of treatment, a febrile state often occurs due to the accumulation of leukocytes at the wound site. This may be avoided by frequent aspiration of exudate from the wound.

PATIENT TEACHING

Patients may administer their own medications at home. The nurse ensures that the patient knows and understands all materials found in Table 62–1 in the column marked Nursing Implications. A teaching guide for enzymes is featured in Table 62–3.

EVALUATION

The evaluation of the effectiveness of enzymes is based on a predetermined list of evaluation criteria. These evaluation criteria are developed on an individual basis through discussion among the nurse, patient, and family. The information from the data base, obtained in the

---

Table 62–3. PATIENT TEACHING INFORMATION—PATIENT REQUIRING ENZYMES

Dear Patient:
   This drug has been prescribed for you. This is what you should know about your drug to get the most from your therapy.

1. Your drug must be taken until your current medical problem is cleared up.
2. Tablets are swallowed (or chewed) and followed by water. If tablets are to be absorbed within the mouth, mild stinging, which is generally relieved when the tablet is removed, may occur. Enteric-coated tablets are swallowed whole, not chewed or crushed. Packets or capsules (after opening) may be sprinkled on food.
3. Your drug can be taken with, between, or after (circle one) meals.
4. Drug interaction can occur with your drug. Check with your pharmacist or doctor before taking any other drug.
5. Antacids are not to be taken with your enzyme because they may decrease the action of your drug.
6. If you forget a dose, do not attempt to "catch up." Take the next scheduled dose at the appropriate time.
7. Do not stop your drug until told to do so by your doctor.
8. Typical side effects of your drug include . . . . If these occur, contact your doctor.
9. If you are applying enzymes to your wound, follow the specific directions taught to you by your nurse, including . . . . Do not use other solutions to wash your wound.
10. Store your drug tightly capped, in a cool dry place.

original assessment, is used to formulate the criteria for evaluation. Typical evaluation criteria are included in Table 62–2.

It is extremely important to work with the patient and family to ensure their complete assistance and support. Once they understand the importance of their continued medical treatment, the majority of patients are usually compliant. The primary reason for noncompliance is usually forgetting the medication or not using it because of the local burning or irritation that may occur. The patient is made aware of the minor side effects to which he or she may have to become accustomed as well as the major side effects, which must be reported to the physician. The presence of side effects is continually evaluated. The dose of the enzyme may be lowered, or the medication changed or stopped completely, depending on the reaction.

The more the patient and family are involved with the planning of care, the more likely they are to comply. The nurse stresses the importance of continued medical care. All previously taught material is reviewed and updated, if necessary, to ensure that the patient's knowledge base remains accurate.

SUMMARY

Enzymes are proteins that are obtained from beef, pork, bacteria, pineapple, or papaya products. Enzymes are used for many purposes, such as: replacement of deficient digestive enzymes, to debride skin ulcers, to promote healing of wounds, to liquefy tracheobronchial secretions, or to dissolve clots. The majority of the products are applied topically as creams or ointments.

As the nurse prepares to administer enzymes, a thorough history is performed, particularly assessing for an allergy to the products from which enzymes are prepared. Since most enzymes are applied to wounds, initial wound assessment is also important. The nurse must understand how to prepare and care for the wound during therapy. Most patients complain of local burning and erythema.

BIBLIOGRAPHY

AMA Department of Drugs. AMA Drug Evaluations, ed 6. PSG Publishing, Littleton, MA, 1986.

Gilman, AG, Goodman, LS, and Gilman, A (eds): Goodman and Gilman's The Pharmacological Basis of Therapeutics, ed 7. Macmillan, New York, 1985.

Forsling, E: Comparison of saline and streptokinase-streptodornase in the treatment of leg ulcers. Eur J Clin Pharmacol 33:637, March 1988.

Olin, B (ed): Facts & Comparisons. St. Louis, JB Lippincott, 1987.

Sussman, B, et al: Injection of collagenase in the treatment of herniated disk. JAMA 245:730, 1981.

Welch, L: "Relatively" painless wound debridement. RN 83(10):39, 1983.

SITUATION   62-1

Stuart Ellsworth is a 78-year-old who is being cared for in a nursing home after several months of hospitalization for a massive CVA. He has a Stage IV sacral decubitus ulcer, 4 inches in diameter.

1. Decubitus wound care for Mr. Ellsworth includes the use of collagenase (Santyl) twice a day with sterile dressing changes. The nurse will monitor the patient within the first 24 hours for:
   a. hypotension
   b. fever
   c. bradycardia
   d. reduced pulses

2. The nurse will report the following persistent side effect of collagenase:
   a. pink moist skin
   b. development of granular tissue
   c. increased exudate
   d. itching and stinging

3. Prior to application of collagenase, the wound should be prepared by washing it with:
   a. soap and water
   b. hydrogen peroxide
   c. Burow's solution
   d. Betadine solution

4. The nurse will plan the following outcome for Mr. Ellsworth relative to collagenase therapy:
   a. wound debridement
   b. elimination of infection
   c. repair of connective tissue
   d. elimination of granulocytes

5. The nurse will implement the following intervention when applying collagenase:
   a. Keep the Okin pH at 5.
   b. Apply to injured as well as healthy tissue.
   c. Put a silver based ointment around wound.
   d. Apply to injured tissue only.

6. Which of the following nursing diagnostic categories applies to Mr. Ellsworth in relation to collagenase therapy?
   a. Decreased Cardiac Output
   b. Sleep Pattern Disturbance
   c. Noncompliance
   d. Potential for Injury: Bleeding

Please refer to the Appendices for correct answers and additional review questions with answers.

63
CHAPTER

MEDICATIONS FOR COMMON SKIN DISORDERS

MERRILY MATHEWSON KUHN, R.N.C., Ph.D., CCRN

LEARNING OBJECTIVES

After reading this chapter, the student will be able to:

1. Identify those medications commonly used in skin disorders.

2. Differentiate among the skin disorder medications as to mechanism of action, route of administration, pharmocokinetics, adverse effects, contraindications, and interactions.

3. Identify specific areas to assess in the patient requiring skin disorder medications in order to formulate appropriate nursing diagnoses.

4. Plan the nursing interventions necessary to administer skin disorder medications and choose appropriate teaching strategies to gain patient compliance.

5. Evaluate the patient at various stages of treatment to gauge nursing interventions.

THE SKIN

ANATOMY AND PHYSIOLOGY

The skin, the largest single organ in the body, acts as a barrier between the environment and the body. The skin is composed of three main layers (Fig. 63–1): the *epidermis*, the *dermis*, and the *hypodermis.* The epidermis, the outer layer, contains several distinct layers. The outside layer, the *stratum corneum,* also called the horny layer, is composed of scaly, *keratinized tissues* (dead) that are constantly shed. The dead cells lost from the outer surface of the epidermis are constantly replaced by new cells generated by other layers of the epidermis. The new cells push the old ones to the surface. During this process, they become flattened, dehydrate, fill with *keratin,* and gradually die. Beneath the horny layer is the granular layer, the *stratum granulosum,* which contains granules of keratohyalin, which are changed to keratin in the outer skin layer.

The next two epidermal layers are involved with the mitotic process of epidermal regeneration and repair. The prickle cells, located beneath the granular layer, contain keratinocytes, which produce *melanin,* the color pigment of the skin. Beneath the prickle cells is the *stratum germinativum,* which is in close association with the second main layer of skin, the dermis. The stratum germinativum contains the columnar/cuboidal epithelial cells.

The second main layer is the dermis, which supports the epidermis and separates it from the lower, hypodermal layer. The dermis contains *collagen, elastin,* and a network of nerves and capillaries. The sublayers of the dermis are the papillary layer closest to the epidermis, which contains small capillary blood vessels and nerve endings, and the reticular layer below. The reticular layer contains coarser tissue and gives the skin its elasticity.

The third main layer of the skin is the hypodermis, which is composed of relatively loose connective tissue of varying thicknesses an provides pliability to the skin. This layer houses an abundance of blood vessels and nerves, as well as a layer of adipose tissue necessary for thermal control, food reserve, and padding.

The skin also has appendages, including hair follicles and sebaceous glands, which produce *sebum* that covers the skin surface. Sebum is a mixture of fatty substances and traces of fat-soluble vitamins. The sebaceous glands are often appendages of the hair follicles but are also found in genital areas, around the nipples of the breast, and on the edges of the lips. Other skin appendages include the sweat glands, which have their secretory components in the hypodermis; and the nails, which are modifications of the keratinized layer of the epidermis.

Function of the Skin

The skin has many functions. Primarily, the skin protects the body from external conditions such as heat and cold and from harmful agents such as organisms and chemicals. The skin is actively involved with temperature control and in regulation of fluid balance, since moisture enters and exits the body through the skin.

The stratum corneum may be greatly affected by water movement. If the body becomes dehydrated, the elasticity of the skin is lost. Returning water to the skin is the only way of reversing this process. Water may be replaced by transfer from the lower layers, or by water accumulation (perspiration) caused by occlusive coverings or pharmacologic agents. Perspiration caused by occlusive coverings lessens the tightness of the stratum corneum and allows molecules of water or medications to penetrate.

Sebum lubricates the skin and acts as a barrier to surface moisture loss because of its lipid nature. Sebum, with a pH of 4.5–5.5, is also weakly acidic. It has antiseptic and antifungal properties, and it prevents penetration of foreign substances.

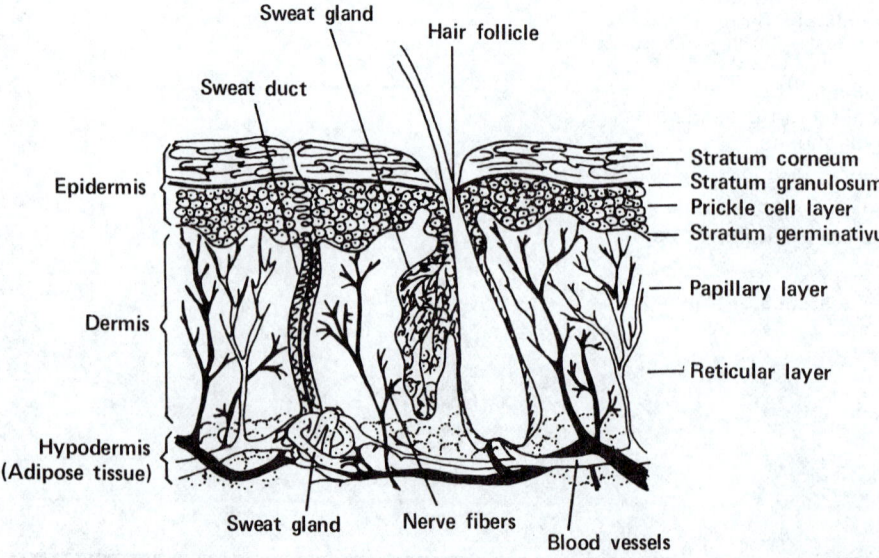

Sweat gland
Hair follicle
Sweat duct
Epidermis
Stratum corneum
Stratum granulosum
Prickle cell layer
Stratum germinativum
Papillary layer
Dermis
Reticular layer
Hypodermis (Adipose tissue)
Sweat gland
Nerve fibers
Blood vessels

Figure 63–1. The three layers of the skin are the epidermis, the dermis, and the hypodermis. The horny, or keratinized, layer is the uppermost layer. Hair, glandular structures, and other organs associated with the skin are found within the dermis.

The surface secretions of the skin house various microorganisms. These bacterial species usually live in an ecologic balance with the host. However, a break in the surface of the skin may have a deleterious effect on the skin's defensive function, allowing pathogenic organisms to be introduced into the inner skin layers.

The skin also contributes to the body's sensory experiences. It is a living tissue and requires a supply of oxygen and nutrients. It produces pigment, giving itself color, and also synthesizes vitamin D.

Diseases of the skin can be classified by the location of their causative agent. These classifications include diseases of the appendages; diseases caused by parasites and insects; bacterial diseases; viral diseases; fungal diseases; eczema and dermatitis; skin conditions caused by sunlight; and malignant tumors of the skin. Each condition has a different and varies widely in its treatment. Table 63–1 identifies the common dermatologic conditions, their assessable characteristics, and their management.

Table 63–1. COMMON SKIN CONDITIONS WITH NURSING INTERVENTIONS

| Condition | Assessable Characteristics | Intervention | |
		Pharmacologic	Nonpharmacologic
DISEASES OF THE APPENDAGES			
Seborrheic dermatitis	Chronic, common, recurrent lesions, which are dry or greasy, scaly red patches, over upper body.	Detergent shampoos, astringents, drying agents, emollients.	Frequent baths and shampooing; well-balanced diet; avoidance of excessive stress.
Acne rosacea	Chronic; common in females in the fourth and fifth decades. Lesions are in middle third of face and appear as areas of vasodilation, with papules and pustules.	Tetracycline.	Avoid facial hyperemia by eliminating alcohol, spicy foods, excessive sun exposure.
Acne vulgaris	Found in 90% of teenagers. Lesions are inflammation of pilosebaceous follicles with formation of cysts.	Frequent washing (2–3×/day) of affected skin with soap; drying agents, keratolytics, irritants, or abrasives. Tetracyclines and other antibiotics (topical and systemic).	Frequent exposure to sunlight when medicine is not used; well-balanced diet.
PARASITES AND INSECTS			
Scabies	Irritation of skin in folds—wrist, between fingers, genitals, buttock, waist. Pruritus varies.	1% Lindane (Kwell, Gamene) cream/lotion. The lotion should be left in place 24 hours. Benzyl benzoate (10%) lotion.	All clothes and bedding thoroughly washed or dry cleaned. Good hygiene. Education.
Pediculosis	Minute, red, noninflamed areas over skin in affected area.	Lindane shampoo.	Same as above.
BACTERIAL DISEASES			
Impetigo	Facial lesions, generally in children. Circular lesions, starting as vesicles and progressing to pustules.	Benzathine penicillin G IM single dose 600,000 units in children 6 years or younger; 1.2 million units in patients over 7 years of age. Or 10 days' therapy with erythromycin 250 mg PO qid or penicillin VK 250 mg PO qid. For staphylococcal impetigo, dicloxacillin 250 mg PO qid.	Washing with mild soaps; warm tap water, saline soaks; washing with bactericidal or bacteriostatic soaps.

CONTINUED ON THE FOLLOWING PAGE

Table 63–1. COMMON SKIN CONDITIONS WITH NURSING INTERVENTIONS– *CONTINUED*

Condition	Assessable Characteristics	Intervention	
		Pharmacologic	Nonpharmacologic
VIRAL DISEASES **Herpes simplex**	Lesions are one-time only or recurrent at same site. Begin as local burning and tingling, followed by multiple, grouped, tiny vesicles on an erythematous base.	Drying agents. Acyclovir topically or IV.	Avoid contact with infected individual.
Warts (verrucae)	Papillary growths anywhere on the skin surface.	Cryotherapy; drying agents; caustics.	Contagious; avoid direct contact with others.
FUNGAL INFECTIONS **Ringworm of the foot (tinea pedis)**	Lesions between toes characterized by cracking and blisters containing a watery liquid.	Topical antibacterial and antifungal agents; antifungal powder.	Keep area clean and dry; wear clogs in any public shower; education on prevention.
ECZEMA AND DERMATITIS **Contact dermatitis**	Lesions occur anywhere on body and appear as reddened, edematous vesicles and bullae, itching usually present.	Wet dressing. Medications to control and relieve itching.	Identify causative agent and prevent further contact.
Atopic dermatitis (allergic eczema)	Lesions most commonly occur on face, neck, scalp, and diaper area shortly after birth. Areas are dry, excoriated, and edematous, and they itch.	Antipruritic, anti-inflammatory agents and lubricants control pruritus. Wet dressings (Burow's solution). Topical steroids.	Mild soaps Dry climate. Avoid irritants.
Pityriasis rosea	Fawn-colored, scaly lesions that appear on trunk and extremities; pruritus.	Most patients require no treatment; however, antihistamines and emollients can be used to control pruritus. Tepid baths (Aveeno oatmeal) 10–15 min daily.	Noninfectious. Limit ultraviolet exposure.
Psoriasis	Lesions are thick, scaly plaques characterized by sharply demarcated lesions of a deep red color covered by a thick overlying silver scales. Emotional stress and anxiety cause exacerbations. Often occurs on elbows, hands, knees, feet, and in genital areas.	Anti-inflammatory agents (potent fluorinated steroids). Antineoplastic drugs (methotrexate). Keratolytics. Coal tar therapy in combination or alternating with corticosteroids. Photoactive drugs (psoralens) in combination with ultravoilet light. Retinoic acid.	Frequent exposure to sunlight. Control stress and anxiety. Avoid cold climates.
Sunburn	First-, second-, and third-degree burns can occur from too much exposure to the sun.	Bland creams. Corticosteroid creams. Aspirin for generalized discomfort.	Cold compresses on burned area. Increase fluid intake.
Skin cancer, basal cell epithelioma	A lesion develops in fair people who have overexposure to the sun; this lesion enlarges peripherally and becomes crusted and bleeds easily.	Antineoplastics (5-fluorouracil).	Surgical removal. x-ray therapy.

THERAPEUTIC AGENTS

Dermatologic agents are so vast in number that it would be difficult to cover them all in this chapter. Many of these preparations are also used to treat other conditions and have been discussed elsewhere in this text. Only a brief review will be given for those groups of products. Dermatologic preparations include emollients to soften or soothe irritated skin; anti-infectives, such as antibacterial, antifungal, or antiparasitic agents; counterirritants to produce mild irritation of the skin to produce healing; keratolytics to soften scales and loosen the horny layer of skin; antipruritics to allay itching; protectives to protect the skin from the outside environment; and cleansers such as soaps and shampoos to clean the skin.

CREAMS, OINTMENTS, EMULSIONS, AND LOTIONS

Emollients are oily or fatty substances that soften or soothe irritated skin by allowing the skin to retain water. They may be found as creams or ointments. *Creams* are emulsions of oil in water or water in oil. Water-in-oil emulsions have a more hydrating effect and provide more lubrication and occlusion, but oil-in-water emulsions are less greasy and more easily removed. When the amount of oil exceeds that of water by a certain proportion, the emulsion changes from a pourable cream to a semisolid *ointment*. Ointments are greasier than creams. In general, unmedicated ointments are not irritating to the skin. Ointments and creams are used as effective vehicles to dissolve active ingredients or medications so that they may be applied to the skin. Creams and ointments are particularly suitable for the chronic inflammatory stage of skin diseases. Dry, scaling, thickened, pruritic, and *lichenified lesions* respond to their softening and lubricating properties.

Emollients may have as a base preparation fixed oils, such as olive, flaxseed, or cottonseed. Glycerin is usually mixed with water or rose water, and often is useful in treating cracked, irritated lips and skin. Petrolatum (petroleum jelly) is a purified, semisolid mixture of hydrocarbons derived from petroleum. Lanolin, a purified hydrous sheep wool fat that can absorb water, is mixed with 25%–30% water. Cold cream is a combination of spermaceti, white wax, and mineral oil. Hydrogenated vegetable oil (Crisco) can also be used as an emollient. Most other emollients are prepared from these bases. Table 63–2 lists the most common ointments and creams.

Lotions are usually liquid suspensions or dispersions that can be prepared by mixing solid ingredients that have been made into a paste consistency with a liquid in which they are insoluble. The suspension requires shaking before application. Medicated lotions are often used as anti-inflammatory agents because they provide a drying, protective, and cooling effect. Lotions are used for subacute inflammatory lesions after the severe exudate phase has ceased. Although lotions are predomi-

Table 63–2. OINTMENTS AND CREAMS

	A*	B*	C*	D*
OINTMENTS				
Rose water ointment (spermaceti wax, white wax, almond oil, sodium borate, rose water, oil of rose, distilled water)	—	x	—	—
Cold cream (same as rose water with mineral oil substituted for almond oil)	—	x	—	—
Yellow ointment (yellow wax and petroleum)	—	—	—	x
Zinc ointment (petroleum, white ointment, 20% zinc oxide ointment)	—	—	x	—
White petroleum	—	—	—	x
Lanolin	—	x	—	—
CREAMS				
Oily cream	x	—	—	—
Aqueous cream	x	—	—	—

*A = oil in water emulsion; B = water in oil emulsion; C = water absorbent ointment; D = water repellent ointment.

nantly water, they have a "drying" effect on the skin when the water evaporates. Lotions are generally not a good vehicle for delivering medications because of this. Table 63–3 lists the most common lotions.

In general, the more chronic and scaly the lesions, the more likely highly hydrating products, such as ointments with oil emulsions, will be used.

ANTISEPTIC AND ANTI-INFECTIVE AGENTS

Anti-infective agents include antiseptic, antibacterial, antifungal, antiparasitic, and antiviral drugs. All the anti-infectives are discussed in detail in Chapter 46.

Several antiseptic solutions are available, and it is important to use the antiseptic solution that best suits the patient's condition. Sodium hypochlorite (Dakin's) is a 0.45% chloride solution that loosens, dissolves, and deodorizes necrotic tissue and blood clots. It kills most common bacteria, spores, amebas, fungi, protozoa, viruses, and yeasts. It is used for irrigating and cleaning necrotic or purulent wounds, or for packing necrotic, not purulent, wounds, since it is inactivated by copious pus. Sodium hypochlorite burns, so it should not be in contact with healing or normal tissue. Recent studies demonstrate that sodium hypochlorite interferes with the body's natural wound-healing process. Sodium hypochlorite loses its potency during storage. Fresh solution should be prepared frequently.

Chlorhexidine gluconate (Hibiclens) is effective for cleansing wounds caused by staphylococci, streptococci, and other gram-positive bacteria. It is used for irrigating and cleansing wounds but not for packing, because it may cause contact dermatitis.

Acetic acid as a 0.25% solution is effective for irrigating, cleansing, and packing wounds infected by *Pseu-

Table 63–3. LOTIONS

General Ingredient	Trade Name	General Use
Calamine lotion (calamine, zinc oxide, glycerin, calcium hydroxide solution)	Caladryl Lotion (has antihistamine included)	Contact dermatitis, poison ivy or oak, insect bites.
Aluminum acetate solution (aluminum subacetate solution 545 ml; glacial acetic acid 15 ml; water 440 ml). Use diluted 1:10 to 1:40 in water.	Burow's solution	Wash for skin, soaks or wet dressings on ulcers, burns.
Potassium permanganate solution 1:4,000–1:10,000 in water	None	Wash for skin, soaks or wet dressings on ulcers, burns.
Zinc stearate (zinc oxide 14%, stearic and palmitic acids) powder or ointment	None	Protective ointment or dusting powder.

domonas aeruginosa. Healthy skin surrounding the wound must be protected with a petrolatum barrier because it excoriates the skin.

Hydrogen peroxide as a 3% solution has effervescent action that releases gas and breaks up necrotic tissue. It is used to irrigate and clean necrotic tissue and pus from open wounds. It is not used to pack wounds because it decomposes too rapidly. When epithelial tissue begins to form, hydrogen peroxide is discontinued, as it inhibits tissue formation.

Alcohol and hexachlorophene (pHisoHex) should not be used for wound care. Alcohol dries and irritates tissues and forms a film that can actually promote infection and it is not a very effective germicide. Hexachlorophene is heavily absorbed through broken skin and can cause neurotoxicity. It should not be used on any type of wound.

When antibacterial drugs are needed, the less absorbable antibiotics such as bacitracin, neomycin, and polymyxin B are generally used. Many experts argue that topical application of these preparations is not effective for acute, superficial, and relatively localized infections. With neomycin in particular, there is risk of drug toxic-

ity. This risk is increased in patients with decreased renal function and increased absorption, such as in extensive burns. In general, side effects related to topical application of antibiotics include local irritation, burning, itching, and vesicular and maculopapular dermatitis. Systemic antibiotics are preferred for more severe, chronic, deep, or generalized infections. Table 63–4 lists the most common antibiotics used in dermatologic conditions and their active ingredients. The skin is generally cleansed prior to application. These products are applied one to five times daily to the infected area and covered if needed.

When antifungal agents are used, the skin is washed at least daily with soap and water and patted dry. The antifungal agents are then rubbed gently into the skin. Friction or trauma to the area should be avoided, including wearing of tight or constricting clothing.

Antifungal agents applied to the skin may cause erythema, stinging, blistering, peeling, pruritis, urticaria, and general skin irritation. Treatment is often protracted, continuing for two to four weeks or longer, depending on the location of the infection. If no results are obtained after four weeks of treatment, the patient is re-

Table 63–4. TOPICAL ANTI-INFECTIVES

Trade Name	Zinc Bacitracin	Neomycin Sulfate	Polymyxin B Sulfate	Bacitracin	Other
Bacitracin Ointment	—	—	—	x	—
Baciguent	—	—	—	x	—
Gentamicin O	—	—	—	—	Gentamicin sulfate
Mity-Mycin	—	x	x	x	Diperodon hydrochloride
Myciguent	—	x	—	—	—
Mycitracin Triple Antibiotic	—	x	x	x	—
Neo-Polycin Ointment	x	x	x	—	—
Neosporin Cream	—	x	x	—	—
Polysporin Powder	x	—	x	—	—
Spectrocin Ointment	—	x	—	—	Gramicidin
Triple Antibiotic	—	x	x	x	—

evaluated. Table 63–5 contains the most common anti-fungal dermatologic agents, their generic and trade names, general uses, and specific comments concerning use.

Antiparasitic agents are used to kill parasitic arthropods, including the causative agents for scabies (mange) and pediculosis (lice). The object of treatment of scabies and pediculosis is elimination of the offending organisms and prevention or treatment of secondary infections. Lindane found in Kwell, Scabene, G-Well, permethrin (Nix), and crotamiton (Eurax) are commonly used prescription antiparasitic agents. They are available as shampoos, creams, or lotions. The drugs are well absorbed through intact skin, and thus may be harmful in young children because of their thinner skin, as well as during pregnancy.

Antiparasitic preparations may irritate the skin, eyes, and mucous membranes, and may even cause allergic reactions. When signs of severe intolerance develop, the medications are discontinued and the inflammation allowed to subside before alternative therapy is substituted. Common antiparasitic agents are listed in Table 63–6.

When treating persons with parasite infections, the clothing must also be cleaned. Two methods may be suggested. Clothes and bedding may be dry cleaned or

Table 63–5. TOPICAL ANTIFUNGAL AGENTS*

Generic Name	Trade Name	General Use	Comments
Haloprogin	Halotex	Superficial fungal infections: tinea pedis, cruris, corporis, manuum.	Available in 1% cream of solution and is applied twice daily for 2–3 weeks.
Miconazole nitrate	Micatin, Monistat-Derm, and others	Tinea pedis, cruris, versicolor; cutaneous candidiasis.	Available as 2% cream, lotion, power, or spray. Applied sparingly twice daily (once daily for tinea versicolor).
Clotrimazole	Lotrimin, Mycelex	Tinea pedis, cruris, corporis, versicolor, candidiasis.	Available as 1% cream, lotion, or solutions. Rub into area twice daily; improvement seen in 1 week.
Ketoconazole	Nizoral	Tinea corporis, cruris, versicolor.	Available as a 2% cream. Apply 1–2 times daily. May need treatment for 2–3 weeks.
Nystatin	Mycostatin, Nilstat, Nystex	Infections due to *Candida albicans.*	Available as ointment, cream, powder. Apply 2–3 times daily.
Tolnaftate	Tinactin, Footwort, and others	Superficial fungus infections.	Available as 1% creams, gels, powder, aerosol, and solution. Apply small quantities only twice daily for 2–3 weeks.
Undecylenic acid and derivatives	Desenex, Kool Foot, many others.	Athlete's foot, ringworm, diaper rash, jock itch.	Available as 2% and 10% powder, 5% and 20% ointment, 20% cream, 10% liquid, 10% foam soap. Ointment, cream, and liquid are used for primary therapy. Cleanse and dry area then apply product.
Iodochlorhydroxyquin	Torofor, Viroform, others.	Eczema, athlete's foot, other fungal infections.	Available as 3% cream or ointment. Apply to affected area 2–3 times daily. Do not use over 1 week.
Econazole nitrate	Spectazole	Tinea pedis, cruris, corporis, & versicolor; cutaneous candidiasis.	Available as 1% cream. Depends on condition: tinea pedis, cruris, corporis, cutaneous candidiasis apply two times daily; tinea versicolor apply once daily.
Ciclopiroxolamine	Loprox	Tinea pedis, cruris, corporis, versicolor; candidiasis.	Available as 1% cream, gently massage into affected area twice daily. Re-evaluate after 4 weeks.
Triacetin	Enzactin, Fungoid	Tinea pedis, superficial fungal infections.	Available as cream, ointment, liquid, and solution. Cleanse area with dilute alcohol and mild soap and water. Apply two times daily. Continue one week after symptoms disappear.
Amphotericin B	Fungizone	Candidiasis	Available as 3% cream, lotion, or ointment. Apply 2–4 times daily for 1–3 weeks.

*Many antifugal combination products are also available.

Table 63–6. TOPICAL ANTIPARASITIC AGENTS

Generic Name	Trade Name	General Use	Product	Specific Directions
Lindane (Gamma benzene hexachloride)	Kwell, Scabene, G-Well, Nix	Scabies, pediculosis.	Cream, Lotion. Shampoo	Apply for 8–12 minutes and then remove by thorough washing. Apply for 4 minutes and then rinse thoroughly. Second application may be necessary 4–7 days later.
Crotamiton	Eurax	Scabies	Cream, Lotion	Thoroughly massage into skin of whole body. Reapply 24 hours later. Change clothing and bed linen the next morning. Take a cleansing bath 48 hours after second application.
Permethrin	Nix	Pediculosis capitis	Liquid	Wash, rinse, and towel dry hair. Apply sufficient volume to saturate hair and scalp. Allow to remain on hair 10 minutes. Rinse with water.

put through the hot cycle of a washer, or they may be sealed in a plastic bag for 30–35 days, which surpasses the life span of lice and nits. All sexual contacts are treated simultaneously.

The primary topical antiviral agent used today is acyclovir (Zovirax). Acyclovir is a synthetic acyclic purine nucleoside analog that has activity against herpes simplex types 1 and 2, varicella-zoster, Epstein-Barr, and cytomegalovirus. Acyclovir inhibits DNA replication in the virus. The major adverse effects include mild pain and transient burning and stinging. Acyclovir is available as a 5% ointment that is applied completely covering the lesion, every three hours six times daily for one week. A rubber glove is used to apply the ointment to prevent the spread of infection.

STIMULANTS AND IRRITANTS

Stimulants and irritants produce a mild irritation to the surface of the skin, causing hyperemia and inflammation, which promote healing. Both mineral and vegetable tars are used. Coal tar, obtained from the destructive distillation of coal, is most widely used. Tars are soluble in most ointment bases, oils, pastes, and alcohols, but not in plain water. Tars, along with topical steroids, are sometimes used in treating psoriasis, seborrheic dermatitis, and atopic dermatitis. They can also act as antiseptics. Tars in general have an unpleasant odor, frequently stain the skin and hair, and cause phototoxicity. Coal tar is available as a cream, emulsion, lotion, oint-

ment, soap, and shampoo. It is also available in combination with steroids.

Compound benzoin tincture, available as a spray-on solution, is a demulcent and stimulant. It is used to protect the skin when the patient has bedsores, ulcers, cracked nipples, and fissures of any orifice such as the lips and anus. The mild irritation that is caused produces increased blood flow and healing.

KERATOLYTICS

Keratolytics, such as salicylic acid (Wart-off, Freezone, many others), resorcinol (Fostex Medicated Bar, Meted 2, Sebulex, and others), podophyllum resin (Pod-Ben), and cantharidin (Cantharone) are preparations that dissolve keratin. These medications soften scales and loosen the horny layer of skin, resulting in minimal peeling or extensive desquamation. Keratolytic preparations are of use in treating superficial fungal infections, seborrheic dermatitis, psoriasis, and localized dermatitis.

Keratolytics are available as gels, ointments, creams, plasters, or *collodions,* which are liquid compounds containing pyroxylin dissolved in ether or alcohol, which dries to a tenacious film.

Salicylic acid is used to treat seborrheic dermatitis, acne, psoriasis, and to thin and remove calluses. Salicylic acid can be absorbed systemically, even from small open lesions. In high enough concentrations, it is slowly excreted in the urine and can cause salicylism, characterized by dizziness and tinnitus. Therefore, salicylic acid is not applied to large surface areas for prolonged periods, particularly in the young. Salicylic acid is not used on open skin lesions, as excessive erythema and scaling could result. Salicylic acid is also available in combination with benzoic acid, marketed as Whitfield's ointment.

Resorcinol is used to treat acne vulgaris, dandruff, seborrheic dermatoses, superficial fungal infections, and diaper dermatosis. Today, more potent and specific keratolytic agents are available and are preferred over resorcinol.

Podophyllum resin is used for various types of skin cancer. Podophyllum resin causes direct degeneration of embryonic or tumor cells. Podophyllum resin is applied daily to the skin. The lesion sloughs off, leaving a superficial ulcer and moderate dermatitis. After the therapy is discontinued, the lesions are dressed with a mild antiseptic ointment. The lesions generally heal within a few days.

Cantharidin is used in treating warts and molluscum contagiosum. Cantharidin has an exfoliation effect only on epidermal cells. The site of application may experience tingling, itching, and burning and may be extremely tender for two to six days.

ANTIPRURITICS

Antipruritics are medications that allay itching of both the skin and mucous membranes. These preparations are applied as wet dressings, pastes, lotions, creams, or ointments. Itching is one of the most frequent complaints of patients with dermatologic conditions and is the one most poorly tolerated. Cornstarch or oatmeal baths, lotions of calamine or phenol applied to the site, or dressings moistened with solutions of potassium permanganate, aluminum subacetate, boric acid, or normal saline are all used to allay itching. See Table 63–7 for commonly used antipruritic medications.

Baths may be used to cleanse or medicate the skin or reduce the temperature. Persons with dry skin should bathe less frequently. Soothing baths have 1–2 ounces/gallon of bran, starch, or gelatin added. Antipruritic baths have 1 ounce/gallon of oilated oatmeal, Alpha-Keri, or Lubath added.

Systemic medication such as antihistamines, diphenhydramine (Benadryl), or some phenothiazine derivatives, in particular trimeprazine (Temaril), may also be administered to reduce itching. Trimeprazine is believed to have an antipruritic activity, largely because of its antihistamine effect, reducing the pruritic action of histamine. Cyproheptadine (Periactin), a drug that blocks both histamine and serotonin (also an itch mediator), is also a very effective antipruritic. Dry skin is a common cause for itching. Emollients may help to rehydrate the skin and prevent further difficulties. Corticosteroids can also be used topically or administered systemically to eliminate itching. These are usually used only as a last resort because of their potential toxic effects, which are discussed later in the chapter.

Table 63–7. ANTIPRURITICS

Preparation	Action
LOTIONS/PASTES	
Phenol 0.5–2%	Local anesthetic
Menthol 0.1–2%	Cooling effect
Camphor 1–3%	Cooling effect
Calamine lotion	Astringent and cooling effect
BATHS (per gallon tub water)	
Cornstarch (1 cup cornstarch with 1 cup baking soda)	Cool and soothe
Oatmeal (1 cup)	Cool and soothe
Aveeno (Colloidal oatmeal—1 cup)	Cool and soothe
WET DRESSING	
Potassium permanganate (dilute to 1:4,000–1:16,000)	Cool and soothe
Aluminum acetate (Burow's solution, dilute 1:10–1:40)	Moderate germicidal activity
Boric acid (1 tbsp in 1 liter of water)	Mild germicidal activity; cool and soothe
Sodium chloride 0.9% (2 tsp in 1 liter of water)	Cool and soothe
Magnesium sulfate (Epsom Salt—8 tsp in 1 liter of water)	Cool and soothe
Silver nitrate 0.25% solution	Good germicidal action

PROTECTIVES

Protectives are either films or preparations that form a film on the skin to protect it from irritations. Ideally, protectives should not further damage the skin when they are applied or removed; also, they protect the skin from light, moisture, air, and dust. Preparations used as protectives include transparent films applied to the skin, such as flexible collodion (Second Skin, and many others); bandages impregnated with special medications, such as zinc oxide paste in an Unna's boot (Dome-Paste, or Gelocast); or preparations that act as sunscreens to protect the skin from ultraviolet light. Protectives are featured in Table 63–8.

The transparent films that are applied to the skin adhere and protect it from further outside injury. This action promotes natural healing without the usual formation of a dry crust over the wound. In some instances they may reduce offensive odors. Some of these products (Tegasorb) are contraindicated on infected wounds or third degree burns. The film is impermeable to odor. The odor that may accumulate under a dressing will be pronounced when the dressing is removed or when leakage occurs. The odor will normally disappear when the wound is cleansed.

Preparations such as Dome-Paste or Gelocast are specially marketed products that are commonly used to im-

Table 63–8. PROTECTIVES

Preparation	Ingredients	Uses
Flexible Collodion	Collodion with 2% camphor and 3% castor oil.	Transparent protective film
Styptic Collodion	20% tannic acid.	As astringent
Tegaderm	Self-adhering transparent polyure-thane dressing, permeable to air and water vapor.	Seals in body's normal defenses against invasion, promotes natural healing without crust formation. To cover pressure sores, skin donor sites, minor abrasions.
DuoDerm	Hydoractive particles embedded in a polymer base, which are soft-ened by wound moisture and act as a protective gel over healing tissue.	Hastens wound healing and prevents contamination of leg ulcers, pres-sure sores, or other open wounds. Can be left in place up to 7 days.
Poly Skin	Self-adhering transparent polyure-thane dressing, gas and oxygen permeable.	To cover central and peripheral IV sites. Change at least every 2–3 days.
Ensure-It	Self-adhering transparent polyure-thane dressing, vapor and gas permeable, that does not stick to itself.	To cover central and peripheral IV sites, pressure sores, and superfi-cial wounds; change every 48 hours.
Op Site	Self-adhering transparent polyure-thane dressing, vapor and gas permeable.	Can be used as an incision drape and sutured through. As backing for split-thickness grafts (change after 10 days), as covering for donor sites, superficial burns, and osto-mies, change at least every 7–10 days.
Tegasorb	Self-adhering, hypoallergenic, hydrocolloid adhesive.	Partial and full-thickness pressure ulcers.
Uniflex	Self-adhering transparent polyure-thane dressing, vapor and gas permeable. Hypoallergenic.	To cover central or peripheral IV sites and pressure sores; change every 2–5 days.
Mediskin and Silver	Silver ions with porcine xenograft (stored at freezer temperatures; must be thawed for 2–3 hours before use).	Used to cover full- or partial-thick-ness burns, skin donor sites, and pressure sores for aggressive anti-bacterial action and pain relief. Change every 2–7 days depending on use.
Zinc oxide paste (Unna's boot) Dome-paste Geolcast	Zinc oxide Zinc stearate	Mechanical support; prevent crusting and trauma; stimulate healing.
PABA	Para-aminobenzoic acid	Sunscreen; filters ultraviolet rays

prove healing in stasis ulcers. These semi-hard casts are impregnated with zinc oxide, zinc stearate, and aluminum silicate product and give mechanical support, which improves healing by preventing further trauma, as well as providing a coating action on the skin.

Sunscreens

The skin must often be protected from the ultraviolet rays of the sun, which can cause acute or chronic injury to the skin. The acute injury is sunburn; the chronic effects include degenerative changes such as wrinkling and pigment alterations, premalignant actitinic keratoses, basal and squamous cell carcinoma, and possible malignant melanoma. Skin cancer is the most common type of cancer by far, accounting for approximately 33 percent of all malignancies. In 1988, approximately 400,000 new cases of basal and squamous cell carcinoma were diagnosed in the U.S. The incidence of malignant melanoma increased 83% between 1982 and 1987. Even on cloudy days, excessive ultraviolet exposure can occur. Ultraviolet exposure is composed of UVB (mid-range ultraviolet is the major cause of sunburn) which peaks in temperate latitudes between 10:00 AM and 3:00 PM, and UVA (long-range ultraviolet), which remains fairly constant throughout the day. Both contribute to chronic skin injury, including aging and skin cancer. After 60 minutes of continuous exposure to UVA, sunburn can also occur.

The best sunscreens contain PABA (para-aminobenzoic acid) or its derivatives. Many commercial products are available containing various percentages of these agents. These products are beneficial only if they are applied before sun exposure to prevent burning. Most suntan lotions now contain a numbering system (Sun Protection Factor or SPF) of 1–50. Preparations with the numeral 1 have minimal protection, whereas those numbered 50 have maximal protection from the sun's rays.

An SPF of 8 to 15 permits little or no tanning. Such products are recommended for very fair people who burn easily and tan very little. For individuals who tan slowly and are prone to burn easily, an SPF of 6 to 8 is recommended. For individuals who tan well and seldom burn or peel, an SPF of 4 to 6 may be appropriate. An SPF of 2 to 4 should only be used by those who rarely burn and are deeply pigmented.

Sunscreens are most effective when applied about 0.5–1.0 hour before exposure to the sun so that they can penetrate the skin. All sunscreens should be reapplied after swimming or sweating. Even sunscreens labeled "waterproof" or "water-resistant" are removed by toweling and perspiration; and such products should still be reapplied often. Reapplication will not extend the period of protection. Environment conditions such as altitude, snow, sand, and water all affect erythema-producing ultraviolet light. The intensity of sunlight at 5,000 feet is about 20% greater than at sea level. Fresh snow and white sand are effective reflectors. Fresh snow may reflect up to 85% of UV light. Water is a variable reflector, depending on the angle of the sun and the presence or absence of waves. Reflected light from any of those sources can cause an additive effect and can strike the skin in previously unexposed areas.

On cloudy days, the skin is also exposed to ultraviolet rays. A bright day with a thin cloud cover has 60%–80% of the ultraviolet radiation present on a bright clear day. Since this day may be cooler, persons may increase their sun exposure, thus increasing their risk.

Researchers currently suggest that by preventing sunburn and by regularly using sunscreens (SPF 15) for the first 18 years of life, it is possible to decrease the incidence of basal and squamous cell carcinoma of the skin by 78%. Even this approach will not totally prevent degenerative skin changes.

Sunscreens are all capable of causing contact dermatitis and photosensitivity reactions. If any of these occur, the product should be discontinued at once.

Sunblocks containing titanium dioxide, talc, or zinc oxide are also available today in many colors. These products prevent all solar radiation from reaching the skin. Sun blocks are particularly useful for the nose, lips, cheeks, and tips of the ears.

CLEANSERS

Cleansers, including soaps and shampoos, are used to clean the surface of the skin. Ordinary soaps are sodium or potassium salts of fatty acids having an alkaline pH. Many different sources of fatty acids can be used, for example, olive oil, coconut oil, and glycerin. Since an alkaline pH can be irritating to injured skin, several soap or soap-like products have a pH of less than 7.5, which is less irritating. Other soaps are superfatted (have large quantities of fat) in order to reduce their alkalinity. Some soaps also contain bacteriostatic agents, providing a deodorant effect. Numerous controlled studies have suggested that bacteriostatic soaps have value in the prophylaxis of cutaneous bacterial infections. Table 63-9 contains a listing of these commonly available products. Other cleansers contain hexachlorophene, available by prescription only. Hexachlorophene has both antiseptic and disinfective qualities. High concentrations applied to extensive body areas can cause local irritation, redness, or burning, and systemic absorption, leading to renal, hepatic, and neuro toxicity. All hexachlorophene products should be well rinsed from the skin after their use to prevent systemic absorption.

The belief that soap is bad for the complexion is incorrect. Clean skin helps promote healthy skin. Soaps used, particularly on the face, should be mild and contain a minimum amount of irritating substances.

Shampoo

Shampoos are liquid soaps or detergents used to wash the hair and scalp, and to relieve pruritus. Several shampoos are available to relieve dandruff. The shampoos containing zinc pyrithione (i.e., Head & Shoulders) or selenium sulfide (i.e., Selsun Blue) are effective in the temporary treatment of dandruff but are usually not cu-

Table 63–9. CLEANSERS, SOAPS, AND SHAMPOOS

SOAPS, NEUTRAL SOAPS, OR SOAP SUBSTITUTES
Acne Aide Detergent Soap
Alpha-Keri
Aveenobar
Caress
Dove
Neutrogena
pHisoDerm
Vel

SUPERFATTED SOAPS
Basis
Camay
Coast
Dermalab Soap
Neutrogena
Nivea Creme Soap
Shield

HEXACHLOROPHENE CLEANSERS
pHisoHex
Pre-op and Pre-op Plus Scrub
Soy-Dome Cleanser

BACTERIOSTATIC AGENTS AND DEODORANT SOAPS
Betadine Skin Cleanser
Dial
Fostex Cake
Ionax
Ionax Scrub
Irish Spring
Jergens Clear Complexion Bar
Lifebuoy
Phase III
Safeguard
Sulfur Soap
Zest

SHAMPOOS
Selenium Sulfide:
   Exsel (2.5% lotion)
   Selsun (2.5% suspension)
   Selsun Blue (1% cream and suspension)
Zinc Pyrithione:
   Breck One Shampoo (shampoo)
   Danex (1% shampoo)
   Head and Shoulders Shampoo (cream or lotion)
   Zincon (1% shampoo)
Selected medicated shampoos:
   Fomac Cream (salicylic acid, colloidal sulfur)
   Fostex Cream (salicylic acid, sulfur)
   Iocon (coat tar, benzalkonium chloride)
   Kwell (gamma benzene hexachloride)
   pHisodan Shampoo (salicylic acid, sulfur)
   Sebulex (salicylic acid, sulfur)
   Tegrin Shampoo (coal tar, allantoin)
   Zetar Shampoo (coal tar, chloroxylenol)

---

rative. They leave a residue on the scalp after shampooing and rinsing that is believed to help control dandruff. Common medicated shampoos are listed in Table 63–9.

SELENIUM SULFIDE SHAMPOO. Preparations of selenium sulfide are temporarily effective for the treatment of dandruff and tinea versicolor. A quantity of 1–2 teaspoons is lathered into the hair and allowed to remain there for two to three minutes, then rinsed and repeated. These products are not used when there is an acute inflammation present, as increased absorption may occur. The 2.5% suspension is available only by prescription, whereas the less potent strength products can be bought without prescription.

ZINC PYRITHIONE. The zinc pyrithione shampoos are widely available nonprescription formulas available for the temporary treatment of dandruff. A quantity of 1–2 teaspoons is lathered into the hair, allowed the remain for two to three minutes, rinsed well, and the process repeated. These products may be used twice weekly if needed.

ENZYMES

Dermatologic conditions are often treated with topical enzyme preparations, although some physicians question the limited data available from clinical studies. These medications are applied sparingly to the skin three to four times daily. Enzyme preparations help to digest necrotic tissue through their proteolytic action (sutilains, fibrolysin, and desoxyribonuclease) or to digest collagenous tissue debriding dermal ulcers or burns (collagenase). Effective enzymatic action is dependent on proper preparation of the skin prior to application. The skin is cleansed thoroughly before use. Crosshatching of eschar may be necessary to ensure the drug's contact with the wound.

Side effects of enzyme preparations include burning at the site and allergic reactions. Sterile dressings are usually applied over the wound and are changed three to four times daily when a new application of enzyme is applied. A more detailed discussion of enzymes can be found in Chapter 62.

CORTICOSTEROIDS

The corticosteroids, when used topically, possess antiinflammatory, antipruritic, and vasoconstrictive actions. Steroids can be used in many dermatologic conditions and come in various strengths, from low to high potency. The relative strength of the topical steroid is determined more by its base or vehicle and the type of lesion treated rather than by the percentage strength. The rate of percutaneous penetration of the skin also influences therapeutic efficacy. Most topical corticosteroids are in suspension, and the addition of a solvent (propylene glycol) enhances dissolution and may improve absorption. Table 63–10 lists the corticosteroids available for skin conditions.

The steroids are available in many forms, including gels, creams, lotions, ointments, solutions, aerosols, and tapes. The vehicle in which the corticosteroid is placed alters the vasoconstrictor property and the therapeutic efficacy. The most effective products are ointments, followed by gels, creams, and lotions. Recent studies indicate that brand-name formulations appear to be more potent that their generic counterparts, but generics may also be more potent than some brand-name products.

Table 63–10. TOPICAL STEROIDS

Steroid	Vehicle
Lowest Potency (May be ineffective for some indications)	
0.1% Dexamethasone (*Decadron Phosphate*—Merck)	Cream
(*Decaderm*—Merck)	Gel
1.0% Hydrocortisone—average generic price	Cream, ointment
	Lotion
average brand-name price	Cream, ointment
	Lotion
(*Cort-Dome*—Miles)	Cream
(*Cortel*—Upjohn)	Ointment
(*Penecort*—Herbert)	Cream
2.5% Hydrocortisone—average generic price	Cream
—average brand-name price	Cream, ointment
(*Penecort*—Herbert)	Cream
(*Synacort*—Syntex)	Cream
(*Hytone*—Dermik)	Lotion
0.25% Methylprednisolone acetate (*Medrol*—Upjohn)	Ointment
1.0% Methylprednisolone acetate (*Medrol*—Upjohn)	Ointment
Lot Potency	
0.01% Betamethasone valerate (*Valisone, Reduced Strength*—Schering)	Cream
0.1% Clocortolone (*Cloderm*—Ortho)	Cream
0.05% Desonide	
(*Desowen*—Owen)	Cream
(*Tridesilon*—Miles)	Cream, ointment
0.01% Fluocinolene acetonide—average generic price	Cream
—average brand-name price	Cream
(*Synalar*—Syntex)	Cream
0.025% Flurandrenolide (*Cordran, Cordran SP*—Dista)	Cream, ointment
0.2% Hydrocortisone valerate (*Westcort*—Westwood)	Cream, ointment
0.025% Triamcinolone acetonide—average generic price	Cream, ointment
—average brand-name price	Lotion, cream
	Ointment
	Lotion
	Cream
(*Aristocort*—Lederle)	Cream
(*Aristocort A*—Lederle)	Cream, ointment
(*Kenalog*—Squibb)	Lotion
Intermediate Potency	
0.025% Betamethasone benzoate	
(*Benisone*—Rydell)	Cream, gel, ointment
	Lotion
(*Uticort*—Parke Davis)	Cream, gel, ointment
	Lotion
0.1% Betamethasone valerate—average generic price	Cream, ointment
	Lotion
0.1% Betamethasone valerate—average brand-name price	Cream, ointment
	Lotion
(*Valisone*—Schering)	Cream, ointment
	Lotion
0.05% Desoximetasone	
(*Topicort LP*—Hoechst-Roussel)	Cream
(*Topicort Gel*—Hoechst-Roussel)	Gel
0.025% Fluocinolone acetonide—average generic price	Cream
	Ointment
—average brand-name price	Cream
	Ointment
(*Fluonid*-Herbert)	Cream
	Ointment
0.05% Flurandrenolide—average generic price	Lotion
(*Cordran, Cordran SP*—Dista)	Cream, ointment
	Lotion

CONTINUED ON THE FOLLOWING PAGE

From The Medical Letter on Drugs and Therapeutics, New Rochelle, NY, Vol 28 (715):58–59, June 6, 1986, with permission.

Table 63–10. TOPICAL STEROIDS–*CONTINUED*

Steroid		Vehicle
Intermediate Potency–*Continued*		
0.025%	Halcinonide (*Halog*—Squibb)	Cream
0.1%	Triamcinolone acetonide—average generic price	Cream, ointment
		Lotion
	—average brand-name price	Cream, ointment
	(*Aristocort*—Lederle)	Cream, ointment
	(*Airstocort A*—Lederle)	Cream, ointment
	(*Kenalog*—Squibb)	Cream, ointment
		Lotion
High Potency		
0.1%	Amcinonide (*Cyclocort*—Lederle)	Cream, ointment
0.05%	Betamethasone dipropionate—average generic price	Cream, ointment
		Lotion
	(*Alphatrex*—Savage)	Cream, ointment
	(*Diprosone*—Schering)	Cream, ointment
	(*Alphatrex*—Savage)	Lotion
	(*Diprosone*—Schering)	Lotion
0.25%	Desoximetasone (*Topicort*—Hoechst-Roussel)	Cream, ointment
		Gel
0.05%	Diflorasone diacetate (*Florone*—Upjohn)	Cream, ointment
	(*Maxiflor*—Herbert)	Cream, ointment
0.2%	Fluocinolone (*Synalar HP*—Syntex)	Cream
0.05%	Fluocinonide (*Lidex, Lidex-E*—Syntex)	Cream, gel, ointment
0.1%	Halcinonide (*Halog, Halog-E*—Squibb)	Cream, ointment
		Solution
0.5%	Triamcinolone acetonide—average generic price	Cream, ointment
	—average brand-name price	Cream
	(*Aristocort A*—Lederle)	Cream
	(*Aristocort*—Lederle)	Cream, ointment
	(*Kenalog*—Squibb)	Cream, ointment
Highest Potency		
0.05%	Betamethasone dipropionate (*Diprolone*—Schering)	Cream, ointment
0.05%	Clobetasol propionate (*Temovate*—Glaxo)	Cream, ointment

From The Medical Letter on Drugs and Therapeutics, New Rochelle, NY, Vol 28 (715):58–59, June 6, 1986, with permission.

The right vehicle is chosen for the area to be treated; for example, lotions can best be applied to hairy areas, while creams and ointments are indicated for dry scaly areas. Sprays, lotions, and gels are suited for the scalp or hairy areas. Sprays have a cooling and antipruritic effect when applied to acute weeping lesions.

Topical steroids are contraindicated in patients demonstrating previous sensitivity to steroids; those with current systemic fungal, viral, or bacterial infections; and those with current complications related to steroid therapy. They should not be used for long periods in pregnant females because of the increased risk to the fetus.

Adverse effects of steroids include hypopigmentation; acneform eruptions; allergic contact dermatitis; burning; dryness; folliculitis; irritation; itching; overgrowth of bacteria, fungi, and viruses; and skin atrophy. Skin atrophy is common and may become clinically significant in three to four weeks when using a potent topical corticosteroid. Atrophy occurs more readily at sites where percutaneous absorption is high. Systemic effects occur rarely but can cause adrenal suppression, Cushing's syndrome, striae, skin atrophy, and ocular effects (glau-

coma and cataracts). These effects occur more frequently when occlusive dressings are used. A more detailed discussion of corticosteroids can be found in Chapter 42.

Patients using these products are taught to apply them sparingly in a light film, rubbing gently. Prolonged contact with the eyes, genital and rectal areas, on the face, and in skin creases is avoided. Washing the area with soap just prior to application may increase drug penetration. The physician is notified if the condition worsens, or if burning, irritation, or infection develops. Corticosteroids may be applied to the skin alone or with a dry occlusive dressing. The occlusive dressing enhances absorption, and there may be a likelihood of toxic reaction, especially in younger patients and in those patients with hepatic dysfunction. If prolonged therapy is needed, plasma cortisol levels may be monitored.

ACNE PRODUCTS

Acne primarily affects adolescents and young adults who are often genetically predisposed. Acne is due to an exaggerated response to androgenic steroids such as testosterone and 17-hydroxyprogesterone. Patients with mild acne have oily skin and closed and open *comedones*. Patients with moderate acne have papules, pustules, and inflammation. These lesions may lead to pitting and hypertrophic scars.

Treatment for acne includes non–drug and drug therapies. Non–drug therapies are aimed at reducing irritating chemical or drugs such as corticosteroids, androgens, and oral contraceptives with a high amount of androgens; humid environments; and heavy occlusive cosmetics. Comedo extraction, dermabrasion, or collagen injection may be useful in a select group of patients.

Acne is associated with development of keratin plugs at the base of the sebaceous follicle; treatment is aimed at: removing the keratin plug; reducing the amount of free fatty acid formation on the skin which, in turn, reduces inflammation; decreasing sebum production; and reducing the number(s) of bacteria that lead to inflammation. By modifying the cause of acne, the patient's appearance is also improved.

Drug therapy includes two major groups: (1) cleansers and drying agents; and (2) antibiotics. The commercial cleansers and drying agents are featured in Table 63–11. These products generally contain a combination of benzoyl peroxide, an antiseptic, drying agent, and keratolytic; sulfur, an antiseptic agent; resorcinol or salicylic acid, keratolytic agents; hexachlorophene, an antiseptic and cleanser; alcohol, a drying agent and antiseptic; and other ingredients to dry, color, and scent the product. Most of these products are available in several forms—lotions, gels, creams, or ointments.

Based on recommendations of an Advisory Panel on OTC Antimicrobial (II) Drug Products, the FDA has published a tentative final monograph on topical acne drug products (Federal Register, January 15, 1985). Benzoyl peroxide, sulfur, and resorcinol with sulfur are considered to be safe and effective for the treatment of acne. Salicylic acid 0.5%–2% is also safe and effective, but data are insufficient to determine the safety of concentrations above 2%. Astringents (aluminum and zinc salts), which promote drying, are classified as ineffective. Antiseptics, which are present in many formulations, are classified as unsafe and/or ineffective. The antimicrobial, povidone-iodine, is considered safe, but data are insufficient to permit its final classification as effective.

Mild acne can be treated with bar soaps, soap-free cakes, liquid cleansers, lotions, gels, and creams. Abrasives remove surface debris and alcohol or acetone promotes drying. For moderate acne, topical anti-inflammatory drugs such as benzoyl peroxide, tretinoin (Retin-A), and antibiotics are useful.

The side effects of acne products can include excessive redness; extreme dryness of the skin, leading to blistering and crusting; temporary pigmentation changes; and peeling of the skin. Patients are cautioned about not overusing these products. The same product should be used each day for a time. If another product is to be tried, the first is discontinued or used only as indicated by the physician.

Benzoyl Peroxide

Benzoyl peroxide is a keratolytic agent that is bacteriostatic and may decrease the production of irritant-free fatty acids in the follicle. The product is applied and left on the skin for 15 minutes the first evening. The length

Table 63–11. COMMERCIAL ACNE PREPARATIONS

Product	Dosage Form	Benzoyl Peroxide	Sulfur	Resorcinol	Salicylic Acid	Alcohol	Hexachlorophene	Other Ingredients
Acne-Aid	Cream Lotion	—	2.5% (cream); 10% (lotion)	1.25% (cream)	—	10%	—	Chloroxylenol 0.375% (cream)
Acne-Aid Detergent Soap	Cleanser	—	—	—	—	—	—	Sulfated surfactants, hydrocarbon hydrotropes 6.3%
Acnycin	Cream	—	5%	2%	—	—	—	Zinc oxide
Aconomel	Cream Cleanser	—	8% (cream); 4% (lotion)	2% (cream); 1% (lotion)	—	—	—	—
	Soap							
Basis	Soap	—	—	—	—	—	—	Tallow
Benoxl	Lotion	5% or 10%	—	—	—	—	—	—
Bensulfoid	Lotion	—	Colloidal 2%	2%	—	12%	0.1%	Zinc oxide 6%, thymol 0.5%, perfume

CONTINUED ON THE FOLLOWING PAGE

Table 63–11. COMMERCIAL ACNE PREPARATIONS–*CONTINUED*

Product	Dosage Form	Benzoyl Peroxide	Sulfur	Resorcinol	Salicylic Acid	Alcohol	Hexachlorophene	Other Ingredients
Betadine	Cleanser	—	—	—	—	—	—	Povidone-iodine 7.5%, detergents
Brade A	Foam	—	—	—	—	—	—	Pumice
Bravisol	Cleanser	—	—	—	—	—	—	Aluminum oxide, neutral soap, detergents
Buf	Soap	—	1%	—	1%	—	—	Sodium, potassium, alcohol sulfate, glycerin
Cenac	Lotion	—	Colloidal 8%	2%	—	30%	—	—
Clearasil Medicated Cleanser	Cleanser	—	—	—	0.25%	43%	—	Allantoin 0.1%
Clearasil (regular tinted)	Cream	—	8%	2%	—	10%	—	Bentonite 11.5%
Clearasil Stick	Stick	—	8%	1%	—	—	—	Bentonite 4%
Clearasil Vanishing Formula	Cream	—	3%	2%	—	10%	—	Bentonite 10%
Cuticura	Ointment	—	Precipitated	—	—	—	—	8-hydroxyquinoline, petrolatum, mineral oil, mineral wax, isopropyl palpitate, beeswax, phenol, pine oil
Cuticura Acne Cream	Cream	5%	—	—	—	1%	—	—
Cuticura Medicated	Liquid	—	—	0.5%	0.5%	28%	—	8-hydroxyquinoline, sulfate, phenol, boric acid, chlorobutanol, camphor, glycerin
Dry and Clear	Lotion	5%	—	—	—	—	—	—
	Cream	10%	—	—	—	—	—	—
Fomac Cream Cleanser	Cleanser	—	Colloidal 2%	—	2%	—	—	Soapless detergents
Fomac-HF	Cleanser	—	—	—	—	—	—	Chloroxylenol 2%
Fostex	Cream	—	2%	—	2%	—	—	—
	Cleanser	—	—	—	—	—	—	—
Fostril	Lotion	—	2%	—	—	4%	—	Laureth-4 6%
Hibiclens	—	—	—	—	—	4%	—	Chlorhexidine gluconate 4%
Ice-O-Derm	Gel	—	—	—	—	—	—	Benzalkonium chloride, alcohol

Table 63–11. COMMERCIAL ACNE PREPARATIONS–*CONTINUED*

Product	Dosage Form	Benzoyl Peroxide	Sulfur	Resor-cinol	Sali-cylic Acid	Alco-hol	Hexachlo-rophene	Other Ingredients
Ionax Foam	Aerosol foam	—	—	—	—	—	—	Benzalkonium chloride 0.2%, polyoxyethylene ethers, soapless surfactant
Ionax Scrub	Paste	—	—	—	—	10%	—	benzalkonium chloride 0.2%, granular polyethylene
Isodine	Cleanser	—	—	—	—	—	—	povidone-iodine 7.5%
Klaron	Lotion	—	Colloidal 5%	—	2%	13.1%	—	—
Komed	Lotion	—	—	2%	2%	22%	—	Sodium thiosulfate 8%; menthol, camphor, colloidal alumina
Liquimat	Lotion	—	5%	—	—	22%	—	Tinted bases
Listerex Herbal	Lotion	—	—	—	2%	—	—	Polyethylene granules, surface-active cleansers
Listerex Regular	Lotion	—	—	—	—	—	—	Thymol 0.16%, polyethylene granules, surface-active cleansers, menthol
Loroxide	Lotion	5.5%	—	—	—	—	—	Chlorhydroxyquinoline 0.25%
Multiscrub	Cream	—	2%	—	1.5%	—	—	Soapless detergents, polyethylene resin granules 26%
Neutrogena	Soap	—	—	—	—	—	—	Tallow, glycerin, coconut oil, stearic acid, triethanolamine, castor oil, NaOH
Noxzema Medicated	Cream Lotion	—	—	—	—	—	—	Phenol 0.5%, menthol, camphor, clove oil, eucalyptus oil, lime water
Oxy-5	Lotion	5%	—	—	—	—	—	—
Oxy-10	Lotion	10%	—	—	—	—	—	—
Oxy-Scrub	Lotion	—	—	—	—	—	—	Sodium tetraborate decahydrate
Oxy-Wash	Cleanser	10%	—	—	—	—	—	—
Pernox	Cleanser	—	2%	—	1.5%	—	—	Polyethylene 26%
Pernox	Lotion	—	2%	—	1.5%	—	—	Polyethylene 26%
Persadox	Lotion Cream	5%	—	—	—	—	—	—
Persadox HP	Cream Lotion	10%	—	—	—	—	—	—

CONTINUED ON THE FOLLOWING PAGE

Table 63–11. COMMERCIAL ACNE PREPARATIONS–*CONTINUED*

Product	Dosage Form	Benzoyl Peroxide	Sulfur	Resor-cinol	Sali-cylic Acid	Alco-hol	Hexachlo-rophene	Other Ingredients
pHisoAc	Cream	—	Colloidal 6%	1.5%	—	10%	—	—
pHisoDerm	Cleanser	—	—	—	—	—	—	Entsulfon sodium petrolatum, lano-lin cholesterols
piSec	Cream	—	3.14%	—	—	—	—	Benzalkonium chloride 0.2%, polyethylene ether
Postacne	Lotion	—	Microsize 2%	—	—	29%	—	—
Propa pH	Cleanser Pads	—	—	—	—	28%	—	Benzalkonium chloride 0.5%, boric acid 0.5%, benzoic acid 0.19%, disodium edetate 0.05%, thymol, chlorothy-mol, eucalyptol
Resulin	Lotion Half-strength Lotion	—	8%	4%	—	32%	—	—
Rezamid	Lotion Cream	—	Microsize 5%	2%	—	28.5%	—	Chloroxylenol 0.5%
Sayman's	Soap	—	—	—	—	—	—	Stannic chloride, sodium cocoate, water, glycerin, coconut oil
Sea-Breeze	Antiseptic breezettes	—	—	—	—	43%	—	Gum camphor, oil of peppermint, oil of cloves, ben-zoic acid, eugenol, oil of eucalyptus, boric acid
Seba-Nil	Solution cleanser	—	—	—	—	49.7%	—	Acetone, polysor-bate-80, polyeth-ylene granules
Stri-Dex	Pads	—	—	—	0.5%	28%	—	Sulfonated alkyl benzenes, citric acid, sodium car-bonate, simethi-cone
Stri-Dex	Cleanser	—	—	—	0.5%	28%	—	Sulfonated alkyl benzenes, citric acid
Sulforcin	Lotion	—	5%	2%	—	11.6%	—	—
Sulfur Soap	Cleanser	—	Precipitated 10%	—	—	—	—	—
Therapads	Pads	—	—	—	1.5%	50%	—	—
Therapads Plus	Wipes	—	—	—	1.5%	70%	—	Sodium alkylaryl polyether sulfo-nate 0.1%
Topex	Lotion	10%	—	—	—	—	—	—
Transact	Cleanser	—	2%	—	—	37%	—	Laureth-4 6%
Vanoxide	Lotion	5%	—	—	—	—	—	Chlorhydroxyqui-noline 0.25%

of time is increased by 15 minutes each day until the product is tolerated for two hours. Eventually, benzoyl peroxide may be left on overnight. Benzoyl peroxide is not applied under an occlusive dressing because of a high incidence of local irritation. Benzoyl peroxide is kept away from the eyes, inside the nose, mucous membranes, hair, and colored fabric.

Tretinoin

Tretinoin (Retin-A) is a vitamin A acid, which is used to treat acne vulgaris, skin cancer, and aging of the skin. Tretinoin decreases cohesiveness of the epithelial cells, increasing cell mitosis and turnover.

Tretinoin is contraindicated in patients hypersensitive to any component. Tretinoin is potentially irritating, particularly when used incorrectly. Within 48 hours, the skin generally becomes red and begins to peel. Temporary hypopigmentation can also occur. Patients using tretinoin should avoid sun exposure, as photosensitivity may occur.

Patients are taught to keep tretinoin away from eyes, mouth and nose, and mucous membranes. Tretinoin is applied lightly once daily at bedtime. The hands are washed thoroughly immediately after applying. Therapeutic results should be seen after two to three weeks, but may not be optimal until after six weeks. Patients may use cosmetics, but the skin needs to be cleansed thoroughly before applying tretinoin.

Isotretinoin

Isotretinoin (Accutane) is also a metabolite of vitamin A. Its use is reserved for persons who have not responded to other therapies, including systemic antibiotics. It is used to treat severe recalcitrant cystic acne.

Isotretinoin has many adverse effects, including xerosis and facial desquamation, palmoplantar desquamation, pruritis, brittle nails, and hair loss. Corneal opacities have been reported. Approximately 25% of patients have an elevated triglyceride level, 15% develop a decrease in high-density lipoprotein (HDL), and about 7% have an increase in cholestrol. Use during pregnancy or in women who could become pregnant is contraindicated because of the increased risk of fetal abnormalities.

Isotretinoin is administered with meals two times daily for 15–20 weeks. If another course of therapy is needed, an eight-week lapse of time should occur. Photosensitivity may occur, so that patient needs to decrease sun and sunlamp exposure. Alcohol consumption should be eliminated during therapy, as alcohol may potentiate the serum triglyceride elevation.

Antibiotics

Local antibiotics are also used to treat acne, the most common being clindamycin (Cleocin-T), erythromycin (many products), tetracycline (Topicycline), and meclocycline (Meclan). These antibiotics are reviewed in Table 63–12. Recent studies indicate that topical blindamycin is as efficacious as oral tetracycline. However, when inflammation is severe, systemic tetracycline is warranted. Therapeutic response generally requires 6–12 weeks of therapy and 250–500 mg/day.

BURNS

Burns may be caused by heat—thermal burns, cauterizing agents—chemical burns, and electricity—electrical burns. Approximately 6000–7000 people die each year across the United States of burns. Usually death is secondary to complications of burns—infection leading to sepsis.

Burns are classified as first, second, or third degree (Fig. 63–2). First degree, also called superficial partial thickness, is characterized by erythema, which is dry and painful. First degree burns involve only the epidermis. They generally heal without complication within five to seven days. A sunburn is an example of a first degree burn.

A second degree burn or deep partial-thickness burn is characterized by thick walled vesicles, which are moist, and very painful. Second degree burns involve the epidermis and part of the dermis. Hair follicles and sebaceous glands may be involved. Second degree burns heal within 7–18 days if they are superficial or may need skin grafting if they are deep second degree.

Table 63–12. ANTIBIOTICS FOR ACNE

Generic Name	Trade Name	Side Effects
Clindamycin phosphate	Cleocin topical solution	Transient burning, irritation, gastrointestinal reactions, staining of skin, contact dermatitis, rashes, erythema
Tetracycline topical solution	Topicycline	Under ultraviolet light, skin will fluoresce, transient stinging, burning
Meclocycline sulfosalicylate cream	Meclan	Acute contact dermatitis, skin irritation
Erythromycin	A/T/S, EryDerm, Staticin, many others.	Erythema, desquamation, tenderness, dryness, pruritus, oiliness, urticaria

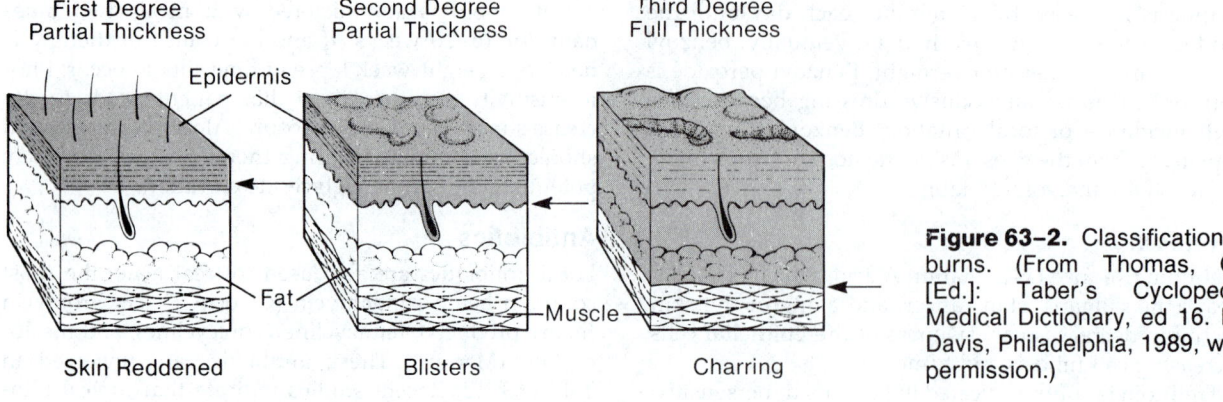

First Degree
Partial Thickness

Second Degree
Partial Thickness

Third Degree
Full Thickness

Epidermis

Fat

Muscle

Skin Reddened

Blisters

Charring

Figure 63–2. Classification of burns. (From Thomas, CL [Ed.]: Taber's Cyclopedic Medical Dictionary, ed 16. FA Davis, Philadelphia, 1989, with permission.)

Table 63–13. BURN PRODUCTS

Name	Dosage	Mode of Administration	Pharmacokinetics

Action: FOR ALL: bactericidal effect against many organisms associated with burns

Use: FOR ALL: second and third degree burns

Name	Dosage	Mode of Administration	Pharmacokinetics
Nitrofurazone (Furacin)	Apply 1/16″ film.	Topical (apply directly to burn)	
Mafenide (Sulfamylon)	Apply 1/16″ film.	Topical	
Silver sulfadiazine (Silvadene, Flint SSD)	Apply 1/16″ film.	Topical	

*Within the column listing adverse effects, underlines indicate the most common effects; CAPITALS indicate life-threatening effects.

Third degree or full thickness burns are characterized by thin walled vesicles, which are open and moist. The skin appears pearly white, charred, or leathery and has thin-walled vesicles. The entire epidermis and dermis are destroyed, including nerve endings, hair follicles, and sebaceous glands. Third degree burns are generally painless because of the destruction of the nerve endings. Most patients having third degree burns will also have some first and second degree burns around the third degree burns, so they will still experience pain.

The first aid for a burn includes immediately cooling the wound to constrict blood vessels and check edema formation. Cold tap water can be used to thoroughly flush the wound and cool hot clothing. The more quickly the wound is cooled, the less tissue damage there is likely to be and thus the quicker the recovery.

The burn may be left exposed or covered with cold wet compresses during transportation to a medical facility.

Electrical burns depend on the amount of voltage received, the condition of the skin, and contraction of flexor muscles, which inhibits release from the power source. Electrical burns may result in several effects in the body: thermal burns associated with electrical arcing, which ignites the patient's clothing; internal injuries along the path of electricity including occlusion thrombosis, or tissue destruction; and a small entrance and large crater-like exit burn. Electrical burns develop more internal tissue necrosis than thermal burns. First aid for an electrical burn involves disconnecting the patient from the electrical source. Cool any thermal burns as previously discussed. Patients are transported as soon as possible to a medical facility for further treatment.

Contraindications/ Precautions	Adverse Effects*	Interactions	Nursing Implications
			For all: ASSESSMENT: Assess degree of burn depth, vital signs, temperature, and urinary output. INTERVENTION: Apply directly to burn with sterile gloved hand. Wash burn daily. EVALUATION: Notify physician of fever, rash, or worsening of burn
Contraindicated in sensitivity to nitrofurans. Cautious use in renal impairment and G-6-PD deficiency. Safety in pregnancy, lactating women, and children not established.	Integ: contact dermatitis, rash, pruritis, local edema	Sutilains enzyme activity may be impaired by nitrofurazone.	Same as for all.
Contraindicated in hypersensitivity. Cautious use in renal disease. Safety in pregnant and lactating women unknown.	Resp: hyperventilation Hemo: BONE MARROW DEPRESSION, HEMOLYTIC ANEMIA Renal: metabolic acidosis Integ: local pain, rash, itching, hives, blisters	None known.	Same as for all plus: ASSESSMENT: Assess burn frequently for development of super infections. INTERVENTION: Keep burn covered with mafenide at all times. EVALUATION: Notify physician if hyperventilation occurs.
Contraindicated in pregnant women near term and premature infants. Cautious use with previous hypersensitivity, G-6-PD deficiency, and during lactation.	Hemo: leukopenia Renal: interstitial nephritis Integ: rash, itching	May inactivate topical proteolytic enzymes.	Same as for mafenide.

Burn Products

Chemical burns are associated with contact from an acid or alkali solution. First aid for a chemical burn is removal of clothing or shoes followed by water irrigation to the part for a minimum of twenty minutes.

BURN PRODUCTS

Several products are available to treat burns. They include nitrofurazone, mafenide, silver sulfadiazine, and silver nitrate. These products are featured in Table 63–13.

Nitrofurazone

Nitrofurazone (Furacin) is applied topically to the burn as a solution, ointment, or a cream. It is a synthetic nitrofuran and has a broad spectrum of antibacterial activity. Nitrofurazone is used in second or third degree burns where bacterial resistance to other agents is a real or potential problem.

Mafenide

Mafenide (Sulfamylon) is a water-soluble cream that is bacteriostatic for both gram-negative and gram-positive organisms. Mafenide is used to treat second and third degree burns to reduce the bacteria present in avascular tissues.

Mafenide diffuses through devascularized areas of the skin and is absorbed, rapidly metabolized, and excreted through the kidneys. Both mafenide and its metabolites are strong carbonic anhydrase inhibitors and, therefore, may precipitate metabolic acidoses usually compensated by hyperventilation. If signs of respiratory embarrassment occur such as rapid or labored respirations, mafenide is washed off the skin.

Mafenide is applied with a sterile gloved hand in a thin film (1/16 inch) once or twice daily. It may cause some local discomfort and burning when first applied.

Silver Sulfadiazine

Silver sulfadiazine (Flint SSD, Silvadene) has a broad spectrum of activity against gram-negative bacteria, gram-positive bacteria, and yeasts. Silver sulfadiazine is released slowly from the cream, which is selectively toxic to bacteria. Silver sulfadiazine is used primarily to prevent sepsis in patients with second and third degree burns.

Silver sulfadiazine is not a carbonic anydrase inhibitor and, therefore, does not cause acidosis. Rash and itching do occur from topical application.

Silver sulfadiazine is applied with a sterile gloved hand in a thin film of 1/16 inch. The burn is kept covered with silver sulfadiazine at all times. If patient activity removes the silver sulfadiazine, it is reapplied.

Silver Nitrate

Silver nitrate as an aqueous solution is used in many burn centers. Silver nitrate is an antiseptic active against gram-negative bacteria. Patients have dressings applied to their burns, which are then kept moist with silver nitrate. Silver nitrate stains anything that it comes in contact with brown or black. This discoloration is usually not permanent.

Silver nitrate, when used for long periods or on extensive burns, may precipitate fluid and electrolyte imbalances. It is important to monitor serum electrolytes frequently for sodium and potassium levels.

SKIN CARE PRODUCTS

Make-up is an integral part of our society. Americans spend about $5 billion annually on make-up and another $2.7 billion on skin care products. Many people believe that beauty can be bottled or canned, whipped into a cream or made into a liquid. To combat aging, the cosmetic industry produces many creams that claim to be anti-aging or anti-wrinkling products. But do the products work?

Some do. But their effectiveness depends on the person's skin type and skill of application. Recently, the United States Food and Drug Administration notified 16 companies to either stop making "anti-aging" claims or to go through the agency's drug approval process to prove their products are safe and effective.

Dr. Barbara Gilchrest, chairperson of the dermatology department at Boston University School of Medicine and senior scientist at the US Department Agriculture's Human Nutrition Research Center on Aging at Tufts University, recently stated that "there are many differences between young skin cells and old ones. What we don't know is, if you took that old cell, which generally doesn't work well, and changed its membrane composition so it was like that a young cell, or changed the number of hormone receptors to match the number on a young cell, would that cell be ready to go again? I'm not aware that any of the materials at present promulgated as useful in cosmetics have met that criterion of effectiveness."

Table 63–14. INGREDIENTS THAT MAY BE HAZARDOUS TO THE FACE
Acetylated Lanolin
Ethoxylated Lanolin
Isopropyl Myristate
Myristyl Myristate
Butyl Stearate
Myristyl Lactate
Isopropyl Isostearate
Isostearyl Neopentanoate
Isopropyl Palmitate
Decyl Oleate
PPG 2 Myristyl Propionate
Laureth-4
Sodium-Lauryl Sulphate
D&C Red No. 9
D&C Red No. 21
D&C Red No. 30
D&C Red No. 36
D&C Red No. 40
Colloidal Sulfer
Sulfated Castor Oil
Cetyl Alcohol
Oleyl Alcohol
Propylene Glycol Monostearate

Reading the ingredients listed on the label also is important. Spotting an allergen or an ingredient that worsens acne can save money and discomfort. A list of ingredients that may be hazardous to the face is featured in Table 63–14. If a problem with a cosmetic is experienced, a dermatologist should be consulted. A recent study examined the causes of contact dermatitis in skin care products. Preservatives were the most likely cause of dermatitis, followed by fragrances and emulsifiers. Then a letter of complaint should be written to the cosmetic company and the Food and Drug Administration.

USING THE NURSING PROCESS

ASSESSMENT

Assessment of the patient requiring medications affecting the skin always begins with a thorough nursing his-tory to develop the data base. The patient requiring these medications may be acutely ill in the hospital or relatively healthy and self-treating a dermatologic problem with OTC preparations. Data to be obtained from the patient are included in Table 63–15. A family history of any serious systemic disease also needs to be obtained. The nurse uses all of this information when preparing the nursing care plan. In addition, any laboratory tests, such as wound cultures or blood counts, may also be performed.

Nurses need to carefully assess all skin conditins. Wearing gloves during the exam may help protect against transmission. However, scabies and lice mites can penetrate cloth and paper isolation gowns. Often scabies and lice can be confused with other less serious conditions. Scabies can be mistaken for eczema, poison ivy, or a scratch, while pediculosis, or lice infestations, look like dandruff. There are two species of lice—head lice (*Pediculus capitis*) and body lice (*Pediculus corporis*). Both types feed by sucking blood. When they bite, the affected area itches. Since adult lice feed five times a

Table 63–15. NURSING PROCESS FOR PATIENT REQUIRING MEDICATIONS FOR THE SKIN

Assessment

Assess current illness/condition, note debilitation, incontinence, presence of allergies.
Inspect skin for reddened areas, decreased sensation, lesions, bites, scratches, patchy excoriations, crusted areas, infection and/or presence of scabies, lice.
Determine source of current infestation.
Note family history of systemic disease.
Ascertain current medication use, including prescribed, OTC, and street drugs.
Review laboratory tests, e.g., wound cultures or blood counts.

Nursing Diagnosis	Nursing Actions	Rationale	Desired Outcomes/ Evaluation Criteria
Skin integrity impaired related to external factors (e.g., chemical substance, physical immobilization), mechanical factors (e.g., pressure, trauma), and internal factors (e.g., medication, altered circulation, nutritional state, excretions/ secretions, edema, skeletal prominence) evidenced by complaints of itching, pain, disruption of skin surface, destruction of skin layers, invasion of body structures.	Administer/apply therapeutic agent, e.g., use of topical sprays, creams, ointment, or soaks. Instruct in aseptic/clean technique for dressing changes and proper disposal of soiled dressings. Maintain strict skin hygiene, using mild, non-detergent soap (if any), drying gently and thoroughly, and lubricating with lotion or emollient. Examine feet and nails routinely and provide foot/nail care as indicated. Change position frequently, in bed and chair. Recommend frequent exercise periods and/or range of motion as indicated.	Promotes healing/alle-viate condition. Prevents spread of bacteria and promotes healing. Cleansing skin and using lubricants can keep it soft/pliable and can protect skin which is susceptible to breakdown. Jagged, rough nails can cause tissue infection by scratching adjacent skin areas. Improves circulation, muscle tone, and joint motion and promotes activity.	Verbalizes understanding of condition and causative factors. Identifies interventions appropriate for specific condition. Verbalizes relief of discomfort/itching. Displays timely healing.

CONTINUED ON THE FOLLOWING PAGE

**Table 63–15. NURSING PROCESS FOR PATIENT REQUIRING
MEDICATIONS FOR THE SKIN**–*CONTINUED*

Nursing Diagnosis	Nursing Actions	Rationale	Desired Outcomes/ Evaluation Criteria
	Provide balanced diet, e.g, adequate protein, vitamins A & E.	A positive nitrogen balance and improved nutritional state can prevent skin breakdown/ promote healing.	
Pain related to injuring agents (biologic, chemical, physical, and psychological) evidenced by complaints, self-focusing, restlessness, autonomic responses.	Administer analgesics as indicated.	Reduces pain and itching.	Reports pain reduced/ controlled. Follows prescribed pharamcologic regimen. Verbalizes methods that provide relief. Sleeps/rests appropriately.
	Keep area clean, dress wounds carefully.	Assists body's natural process of repair and prevents infection.	
	Promotes use of progressive relaxation, breathing exercises, visualization.	Refocuses attention, relieves muscle tension, enhances sense of control and helps to reduce pain and discomfort.	
	Encourage tub baths with Burow's solution, soda.	Soothes skin and promotes relief of itching.	
	Be available to patient for listening and discussion of condition and expected outcome.	Presence of pain/itching can stress individual coping abilitities.	
Knowledge, deficit related to lack of exposure/ recall, information misinterpretation/unfamiliarity with resources as evidenced by questions, statement of concern, inaccurate follow-through of instructions/ development of preventable complications.	Review physiologic importance of skin and measures to maintain skin functioning.	Understanding promotes proper care and helps patient to feel in control of situation.	Verbalizes understanding of condition/disease process and treatment. Identifies relationship of signs/symptoms to the disease process and correlates symptoms with causative factors. Correctly performs necessary procedures and explains reasons for the actions.
	Identify expected actions, side-effects and possible interactions with other drugs.	Helps patient to know what to anticipate and be able to differentiate between expected and potentially dangerous symptoms.	
	Demonstrate appropriate amount of therapeutic agent for application, duration of treatment.	Correct usage reduces likelihood of untoward effects, e.g., inflammation, dermatitis. Condition may be slow to resolve and patient may be tempted to discontinue therapy.	
	Discuss necessity of inspecting skin on a regular basis.	Provides opportunity for early intervention/prevention of recurrence/ complications.	
	Stress importance of adequate fluid intake.	Helps to maintain skin turgor.	
	Review modes of transmission of infectious conditions or infestations as appropriate.	Can prevent spread/ recurrence.	
	Encourage open discussion of patient's attitude toward condition/skin manifestations and expected results.	Some diseases/conditions can be temporarily or permanently disfiguring and may have a negative emotional effect.	

day, each meal lasting 35–40 minutes, they can cause a lot of itching. Lice are very difficult to get rid of. They sometimes fall off injured, but leave voluntarily only if their host becomes too hot, because of fever, or too cold, because of death.

The patient's shoulders, armpits, buttocks, waist, or abdomen are inspected, as these are areas where clothing or bed linen comes in close contact with the body. If lice are present, there will be small bites, scratch marks, and sometimes patchy discolorations, crusted areas, or infection. Lymph nodes may also be enlarged as a result of inflammation and infection. If lice are suspected, the nurse inspects the patient's undergarments, especially the seams, for lice and eggs. If lice or eggs are found, the infection control department of the hospital is notified. Itching can persist even after lice are dead, especially if the skin is already irritated from scratching. A soothing lotion or solution of baking soda and water may help.

The nurse also needs to carefully assess the quality of the skin in ill patients and prevent its breakdown, which can lead to infection. Some of the factors that put a patient at risk for skin breakdown include: incontinence, poor nutritional status, limited mobility, limited or decreased sensation, or redness over a bony prominence that lasts over fifteen minutes. Several types of mattresses are available to prevent at-risk patients from having skin breakdown. The convoluted closed-cell form (egg-crate mattress) is best used in a healthy patient with low risk for breakdown. The static air mattress (Sof-Care) is best used in a patient with a questionable health status at low risk for breakdown or who already has lesions. Low-air-loss therapy (Flexicare, Kinair, Mediscus) is best used in patients at high risk for breakdown who have one or more lesions. Air-fluidized therapy (Clinitron) is best used in patients at high risk for breakdown who will need to be on strict bed rest for a prolonged period of time.

Frequent side effects of medications include skin reactions ranging from photosensitivity to skin eruptions. Medications suspected of causing the skin reaction should be discontinued. These reactions can be mild to very severe. Table 63–16 features medications that are known to cause dermatologic side effects, and Table 63–17 features medications that can cause life-threatening skin eruptions.

Photosensitivity occurs when patients are exposed to sunlight or ultraviolet light during or after receiving certain drugs. This photosensitivity can either be a phototoxic reation (often associated with a nonimmunologic reaction), or a photoallergic reaction (which is associated with an immunologic reaction). These reactions can occur up to a year after discontinuing certain medications, so the nurse must obtain a past medication history. See Table 63–18 for drugs that can cause photosensitivity.

Other reactions secondary to medication include skin eruptions, which may be nonspecific and generalized in nature or may occur in the same site each time the medication is given. Eruptions may appear as either contact dermatitis or exfoliative dermatitis, with either wet or dry lesions. When a nurse observes a rash, it is best to discontinue all topical medication, and the systemic medications that might be causing the rash, if possible, until the rash disappears. Medications are then added to the patient's daily regimen one at a time to determine the offending agent. At times, the causative agent may not be determined. One of the most serious dermatologic reactions to medications is the Stevens-Johnson (S-J) syndrome. The S-J syndrome is a severe form of erythema multiforme in which lesions may involve both the oral and anogenital mucosa. Systemic symptoms may also occur, such as general malaise, fever, headache, arthralgia, and conjunctivitis. The development of the S-J syndrome may be either an allergic or an idiosyncratic reaction. The true mechanism for its development is unknown.

Dermatitis is a complaint of many patients and has various causes. Contact dermatitis can occur following contact with poison oak and ivy, some antibiotics, some over-the-counter analgesics, and certain metals such as gold. Irritant dermatitis is associated with eruptions from direct contact with cosmetics, chemicals, dyes, or detergents. Seborrheic dermatitis is a yellowish-pinkish scaling of the scalp, face, and trunk. Atopic dermatitis has a characteristic distribution in persons with a family history of allergic diseases.

When dermatitis is the problem, skin testing may be able to diagnose the allergen. Emotional stress and food allergies may also be causative agents and may need to be modified during the intervention phase. The reaction can be mild as a slight reddening or as severe with open blisters. Because it is often hard to pin down the source of an allergy, the dermatologist often gets rid of the symptoms without knowing the cause. This can condemn the patient to a life of recurring, frustrating skin problems. Every attempt should be made during the initial assessment to determine the causative agent.

NURSING DIAGNOSES

Possible nursing diagnoses for a patient with dermatologic conditions are included in Table 63–15.

PLANNING AND INTERVENTION

The nurse develops the goals of nursing intervention from the nursing diagnoses. When caring for the patient requiring medications that affect the skin, typical nursing goals are included in Table 63–15.

PATIENT EDUCATION

Patients administering their own medication have a tendency to apply topical preparations more freely and for longer periods than prescribed. Very careful directions are given to patients to prevent the inflammation and dermatitis that can result from overuse of topical agents (Table 63–19).

When patients have acquired infectious dermatologic conditions, the nurse is often responsible for educating the patient and the family about transmission and further prevention of the condition.

Table 63–16. CHARACTERISTIC CLINICAL CUTANEOUS ERUPTIONS AND DRUGS MOST FREQUENTLY CAUSING THESE ERUPTIONS

Acneiform and Pustular:

ACTH	Phenytoin
Bromides	Phenobarbital
Corticosteroids	Isoniazid (INH)
Actinomycin D	Oral contraceptives
Cyanocobalamin	Androgens
Iodides	Ethamubutol
Trimethadione	Ethionamide
Lithium	

Alopecia:

Antithyroid drugs	Thallium
Oral contraceptives	Colchicine
Alkylating agents	Heavy metals
Anticoagulants	Propranolol
Antimetabolites	Retinoids (Toxic doses)
Vitamin A	Levodopa
Allopurinol	Indomethacin
Hypocholesterolemic drugs	Testosterone (in women)
Cytotoxic agents	Valproate
Quinacrine (Atabrine)	

Fixed:

Antipyrine	Phenylbutazone
Barbiturates	Quinidine
Gold	Salicylates
Phenacetin	Sulfonamides
Phenolphthalein	Tetracyclines

Lichenoid and Lichen Planus-like:

Arsenicals	Hydroxychloroquine
Chloroquine (Aralen)	Dapsone
Gold salts	Furosemide
Para-aminosalicylic acid	Methyldopa
Quinidine	Penicillamine
Thiazides	Sulfonylureas
	Chlorothiazide and related drugs

Eczematous:

Arsphenamine	Streptomycin
Chlorpromazine	Sulfonamides
Chlorothiazide	Thiamine
Formaldehyde	Gentamicin
Meprobamate	Kanamycin
Neomycin	Mercurial diuretics
Novobiocin	Chloralhydrates
Penicillin	Iodides
Procaine (and other local anesthetics)	Tolbutamide
	Chlorpropamide
Promethazine	Disulfiram
Quinacrine (Atabrine)	Aminophylline
Resorcin	Hexylresorcinol

Erysipelas-like:

Amidopyrine

Erythema Multiforme:

Chlorpropamide	Sulfonamides
Penicillin	Thiazine derivatives
Phenothiazines	

Erythema Nodosum:

Iodides	Oral contraceptives
Sulfonamides	Penacetin
Penicillin	Salicylates
Sulfones	Antibiotics

Photosensitive:

Griseofulvin	Sulfonamides (chemotherapeutics, antidiabetics, and diuretics)
Phenothiazines	
Tetracycline	
Thiazides	

Pityriasis Rosea-like:

Barbiturates
Bismuth

Exanthematic (Scarlatiniform, Morbilliform):

Aminosalicylic acid	Phenothiazines
Anticonvulsants	Phenylbutazone
Antihistaminics	Quinacrine (Atabrine)
Barbiturates	Streptomycin
Chlorothiazide	Sulfonamides
Chlorpromazine	Sulfones
Gold salts	Thiouracil
Griseofulvin	Ampicillin
Insulin	Allopurinol
Meprobamate	Benzodiazepines
Methaminodiazepoxide	Chloramphenicol
Novobiocin	Tetracyclines
Nitrofurantoin	Pyrazolone derivatives (phenylbutazone, oxyphenbutazone)
Penicillin	
Busulfan	

Pigmentary Changes:

Chloroquine (Aralen)	Busulfan
Chlorpromazine	Doxorubicin
Fluorouracil	Cytoxan
Arsenic	Gold
Silver	Phenytoin
Estrogens	

Porphyria (Exacerbation):

Barbiturates	Estrogens
Chloroquine (Aralen)	Oral contraceptives
Griseofulvin	Sulfonamides
Alcohol	Sulfonylureas
Androgens	

Purpuric:

Barbiturates	Quinidine
Carbamides	Sulfonamides (chemotherapeutics, antidiabetics, and diuretics)
Chlorothiazide	
Chlorpromazine	Phenylbutazone
Gold salts	
Griseofulvin	
Iodides	

Seborrheic Dermatitis:

Gold

Urticarial:

ACTH	Penicillin
Barbiturates	Phenolphthalein
Chloramphenicol	Phenothiazines
Enzymes	Salicylates
Griseofulvin	Streptomycin
Insulin	Sulfonamides
Opiates	Tetracyclines
Indomethacin	

Vesiculobullous:

Aloin	Salicylates
Arsenic	Phenytoin
Bromides	Penicillamine
Iodides	Captopril
Mercury	
Phenolphthalein	

From Moschella, SL, et al.: Dermatology, Vol 1. Drugs and the Skin, p. 1040. WB Saunders, Philadelphia, 1985, with permission.

Table 63–17. LIFE-THREATENING DRUG-INDUCED SKIN ERUPTIONS

Drug Eruptions	Drugs Involved	Reported Sequelae
Exofolitative dermatitis	Aminosalicylic acid (PAS)	Hepatitis, hemolytic anemia
	Antidiabetics, oral	
	Arsenicals	
	Barbiturates	
	Carbamazepine (Tegretol)	
	Chlorpropamide	
	Demeclocycline (Declomycin)	
	Diphtheria and tetanus toxoids and pertussis vaccine, absorbed and Salk poliomyelitis vaccine	Death; probably caused by penicillin in the poliovirus vaccine
	Furosemide (Lasix)	
	Gold	
	Griseofulvin (Grifulvin)	Lymphadenopathy
	Hydroflumethiazide (Saluron)	
	Isoniazid	
	Isosorbide (Isordil)	
	Measles virus vaccine	
	Mercury	
	Methotrimeprazine (Levoprome)	
	Nitrofurans	
	Nitroglycerin	
	Oral antidiabetics	
	Oxyphenbutazone (Tandearil)	
	Penicillin	
	Phenindione (Hedulin)	Hepatitis, nephritis
	Phenothiazines	
	Phenylbutazone (Butazolidin)	
	Phenytoin (Dilantin)	Atypical lymphocytes, hypoproteinemia, hepatosplenomegaly
	Streptomycin	
	Sulfamethoxypyridazine (Midicel)	Death
	Sulfasalazine (Azulfidine)	
	Sulfisomide (Elkosin)	
	Sulfonamides	
	Tetracyclines	
Stevens-Johnson syndrome (erythema multiforme)	Aminophenazone (aminopyrine)	
	Ampicillin	
	Antipyrine	
	Arsenicals	
	Barbiturates	
	Carbamazepine (Tegretol)	
	Chloramphenicol	
	Chlorpropamide (Diabinese)	
	Clindamycin	
	Codeine	
	Cold preparation 666	
	Mephenytoin (Mesantoin)	
	Novobiocin	
	Oxyphenbutazone (Tandearil)	
	Paramethadione	
	Penicillin	
	Phenolphthalein	
	Phenylbutazone (Butazolidin)	
	Phenytoin (Dilantin)	Death
	Phenytoin and trimethadoine (Tridione)	Lupus erythematosus occurred simultaneously
	Rifampin (Rifadin, Rimactane, etc.)	
	Salicylates	
	Sulfamethoxypyridazine (Kynex, Midicel)	Death; 2 out of 14 cases
	Sulfasalazine (Azulfidine)	
	Sulfisomidine (Eikosin)	
	Thiacotazone (Amithiozone)	Death
	Thiazides	

CONTINUED ON THE FOLLOWING PAGE

From Martin, EW, *Hazards of medication,* ed 2, Provest, Inc, Fayetteville, NC, 1978, with permission.

Table 63–17. LIFE-THREATENING DRUG-INDUCED SKIN ERUPTIONS–*CONTINUED*

Drug Eruptions	Drugs Involved	Reported Sequelae
Stevens-Johnson syndrome–*Continued*	Thiouracil Trimethadione (Tridione) and phenobarbital Triple sulfas (Sulphatriad) Tetracycline	Lupus erythematosus with subsequent medication
Toxic epidermal necrolysis (Lyell's syndrome)	Acetazolamide (Diamox) Antihistamines Antipyrine Barbiturates Chenopodium oil Dapsone Diallylbarbituric acid Diphtheria vaccine Ethylmorphine Gold salts Ipecac Methyl salicylate Neomycin sulfate Nitrofurantoin (Furadantin) Opium powder Oxyphenbutazone (Tandearil) Penicillin Pentazocine (Talwin) Phenobarbital Phenolphthalein Phenylbutazone (Butazolidin) Phenytoin (Dilantin) Procaine penicillin, aqueous injection and oral mixed sulfonamide preparation Sulfamethoxypyridazine (Kynex, Midicel) Sulfasalazine (Azulfidine) Sulfathiazole Sulfisomidine (Elkosin) Sulfonamides Tetracycline	Death Death; cause questionable Death; 1 out of 4 cases Death Death
Lupus erythematosus	Aminosalicylic acid Chlorpromazine (Thorazine) Chlortetracycline (Aueromycin) Corticosteroid withdrawal Digitalis (long term) Ethosuximide (Zarontin) Gold compounds (long term) Griseofulvin (Fulvicin) Hydantoin anticonvulsants Hydralazine (Apresoline) Isoniazid (INH) Isoquinazepon Mephenytoin (Mesantoin) Methyldopa (Aldomet) Methysergide Oral contraceptives (mestranol?) Oxyphenbutazone (Tandearil) Para-aminosalicylic acid (PAS) Penicillamine Penicillin Phenobarbital (long term) Phenothiazines Phenylbutazone (Butazolidin) Phenytoin (Dilantin) Practolol Primidone (Mysoline) Propylthiouracil Reserpine (long term)	

From Martin, EW, *Hazards of medication,* ed 2, Provest, Inc, Fayetteville, NC, 1978, with permission.

Table 63–17. LIFE-THREATENING DRUG-INDUCED SKIN ERUPTIONS–*CONTINUED*

Drug Eruptions	Drugs Involved	Reported Sequelae
Lupus erythematosus– *Continued*	Rifampin (Rifadin, Rimactane, Rifampicin) Streptomycin Sulfadiazine Sulfamethoxypyridazine (Kynex) Sulfasalazine (Azulfidine) Sulfonamides (long acting) Tetracycline Thiazides (long term) Trimethadione (Tridione, Troxidone)	

From Martin, EW, *Hazards of medication,* ed 2, Provest, Inc, Fayetteville, NC, 1978, with permission.

Patients with parasitic infections are treated as a family group, with all members of the family group treated at once. All persons having had sexual contact with the patient are also treated simultaneously when patients have pediculosis pubis. All clothing and bed linen are cleaned at the same time.

Many skin lesions are chronic and may lead to psychologic problems, feelings of rejection, and poor body image, which may then further aggravate the symptoms. Much of today's advertising indicates that a smooth, blemish-free skin is a necessity. A patient with a chronic disorder may become overly embarrassed

Table 63–18. DRUG ERUPTIONS (DERMATITIS MEDICAMENTOSA)

Photosensitizing Agents

Drugs
Antidiabetic agents, oral: including carbutamide, tolbutamide, chlorpropamide (Nadisan, Diabinese, Orinase, Orabetic)
Anesthetics: the procaine group of local anesthetics
Antibiotics: including tetracyclines and their derivatives: chlortetracycline (Aureomycin), oxytetracycline (Terramycin), demethylchlortetracycline (Declomycin), and griseofulvin (a penicillium derivative)
Antihistaminics: including diphenhydramine (Benadryl), promethazine (Phenergan), tripyrathiazine (Pyrrolazote), isothipendyl (Theruhistin)
Anticonvulsants: trimethadione (Tridione) and phenytoin (Dilantin)
Arsenicals
Barbiturates
Hormonal substances: including estrone and diethylstilbestrol
Topical antibacterial agents (antiseptics): bithionol, tetrachlorsalicylanilide (TCSA), tribromosalicylanilide (TBS)
Phenothiazine derivatives: including chlorpromazine (Thorazine), prochlorperazine (Compazine), mepazine (Pacatol), perphenazine (Trifalon), trimeprazine (Temaril), triflupromazine (Vesprin), promazine (Sparine), thiopropazate (Dartal)
Psoralens: Furocoumarin derivatives, including 5-methoxypsoralen 8-methoxypsoralen, and others
Sulfonamides: including sulfacetamide, sulfadiazine, sulfaguanidine, sulfamerazine, sulfamethazine, sulfapyridine, sulfathiazole, sulfadimethoxine
Sulfonylureas: see oral antidiabetic drugs above.
Thiazide diuretics (aromatic sulfonamide preparations): chlorothiazide (Diuril) and hydrochlorothiazide (HydroDiuril)
Heavy metals: gold and silver salts
Porphyrins: hematoporphyrin (used experimentally to treat tumors) chlorophyll

Miscellaneous: digalloyltrioleate, monoglycerol paraminobenzoate, *p*-dimethylaminoazobenzene, phenylbutazone, quinine, stilbamidine, salicylates, dicyanine-A, 5-fluorouracil, triethylenemelamine (TEM), 9-aminoacridine

Dyes
Acridine dyes: acridine, trypallavine, and others
"Blankophores" (optical brighteners—mainly sulfa derivatives)
Dibenzypyran derivatives (eosin, fluorescein dyes, rose bengal, and others)
Phenoxazine dyes
Phenazine dyes
Trypan blue

Coal Tar Products and Petroleum Products
Crude coal tar and its derivatives (benzene, anthracene, xylene, naphthalene, toluene, phenanthrene, thiophene, phenolic compounds, puridine, and others)
Pitch and pitch fumes

Essential Oils and Others
Oil of bergamot, oil of cedar, oil of citron, oil of lavendar, lime oil, vanillin oils, other agents included in various perfumes and cologne waters

Plants
Mainly members of the Umbelliferae family: including parsnips, carrots (wild and garden types), celery, yarrow, angelica, fennel, dill, and parsley
Members of the Rutaceae family (rue, bergamot, lime, wafer ash), meadow grass, clover mustards, agrimony, bavachi (corylifolia)
Agave lechiguilla: a perennial flowering plant of Amaryllis family, related to *A. belladonna*
Lantana: a shrub of the Verbenae family
Lady's thumb and smartweed: flower herbs of the buckwheat family

From Moschella, SL, et al.: Dermatology, Volume 1. WB Saunders, Philadelphia, 1985, with permission.

Table 63–19. PATIENT TEACHING FOR DERMATOLOGIC AGENTS

Dear Patient:

This drug has been prescribed for you. This is what you should know about your drug to get the most from your therapy.

1. You will take your drug until your current condition is cleared up.
2. Whenever topical agents are used to treat a skin disorder, the skin is washed daily before each dose of drug with mild soaps and patted dry, before the next dose of drug is applied. If you have a moist lesion, a small amount of medication is gently rubbed into the area. If the lesion is dry or scaly, a thin film is applied over the area. A tongue blade may be helpful in applying the drug. When the lesion is under a hairy area, the hair may have to be parted to ensure the drug is rubbed into the skin.
3. There are several reactions that can occur with your drug. They include: _____. If any of these occur, consult your doctor.
4. Typical side effects from dermatologic agents include staining of the skin, clothes, and nails; local allergic reactions; photosensitivity; and a drying effect. Often, staining of the clothes, photosensitivity, and excessive drying can be eliminated on small areas of the body by placing an occlusive dressing over the area. Check with your doctor to see if this technique is permissible.
5. Occlusive dressing may sometimes be ordered by your doctor to enhance the treatment of psoriasis, and for persistent inflammatory dermatoses. The area is cleaned and shaved (if necessary) before the treatment begins. Any scales or crusts are removed. The drug is applied and is then covered with a plastic wrap (Saran Wrap, Handi-Wrap). A moist gauze may be applied over the skin under the plastic wrap if additional moisture is desired. The edges of the plastic wrap are sealed with tape. It is left in place anywhere from 7–8 hours, to 12–24 hours. (If the dressing is to be worn only part of the day, you may choose to apply it only during the night.) The therapy is continued for several days after the lesion has cleared to prevent a relapse.
6. All tight and constricting clothing is avoided over the affected area. Clothing is washed daily to prevent recontamination. The clothing should also be dry and aerated so that undue moisture does not develop.

about his or her condition. Patients and family may need additional counseling to successfully cope with the condition. The nurse is always careful to avoid showing any sign of rejection to a patient with a skin condition. Offering helpful suggestions such as the use of cosmetic cover-ups like Erase and Covermark or growing a beard may be helpful in camouflaging facial lesions or scarring. However, these may not be appropriate in the patient with active acne. In addition, the nurse educates the consumer to evaluate product advertising intelligently.

EVALUATION

During the evaluation phase, the nurse assesses the effectiveness of the medications for dermatologic condi-

tions. This evaluation is based on a predetermined list of evaluation criteria previously developed in relation to the goals of treatment, as determined by the nurse, patient, and family. The data base obtained in the original assessment used to formulate the nursing diagnoses provides helpful criteria for measuring the treatment's effectiveness. Typical outcome evaluation criteria are included in Table 63–15.

The skin lesions are evaluated daily while the patient is in the hospital, or on each subsequent visit to the clinic or office. Acute conditions generally subside in three to four weeks. Chronic conditions may have periods of remission. Lesions that do not show improvement after four weeks of therapy need to be reevaluated.

It is extremely important to work with the patient and family to ensure their complete assistance and support. Patients who understand the importance of their continued medical treatment are usually more compliant. The primary reason for noncompliance usually is forgetting to take the medication or not liking the unpleasant side effects. The nurse teaches the patient about potential side effects so that when taking the medications at home the patient will report any unusual symptoms to the physician, nurse, or pharmacist.

The more the nurse involves the patient and family with the planning of the care, the more likely they are to comply. The nurse must stress the importance of continued medical care. Often skin conditions are slow to show improvement, and the nurse will frequently be evaluating the lesions for resolution. All previously taught material should be reviewed and updated, if necessary, to ensure that the patient's knowledge base remains accurate.

SUMMARY

The skin is the largest single organ in the body and acts as a barrier between the environment and the body. Many dermatologic agents are available, such as emollients to soften or soothe irritated skin, anti-infectives, irritants that irritate the skin to promote healing, keratolytics to soften scales and loosen the horny layer of skin, antipruritics to allay itching, protectives to protect the skin, and cleansers to clean the skin. It is important for the nurse to understand why the agent is being used and what is the expected outcome of the treatment.

As the nurse prepares to administer dermatologic products, a thorough nursing assessment is obtained. Skin lesions may be associated with medications, so it is important to obtain a current drug history. The skin is washed daily and before each dose of medication with mild soaps and patted dry. If a moist lesion is present, a small amount of medication is gently rubbed into the area. If the lesion is dry and scaly, a thin film is applied over the area. A tongue blade may be helpful in applying the medication. If the lesion is under a hairy area, the hair may have to be parted to ensure the medication is rubbed into the skin.

Acute skin lesions generally subside within three to four weeks. Chronic lesions may have periods of remission.

BIBLIOGRAPHY

AMA Department of Drugs: AMA Drug Evaluations. PSG Publishing, Littleton, MA, 1986.

American Pharmaceutical Association: Handbook of Nonprescription Drugs, ed 6. American Pharmaceutical Association, Washington, DC, 1986.

Arndt, K: Manual of dermatologic therapeutics. Little Brown & Co., Boston, 1983.

Bryant, RA: Saving the skin from tape injuries. AJN 88:189–191, 1988.

Cohen, SR: Barbers, beauticians, ER workers are more susceptible to scabies, lice. Hospital Employee Health 5:87, July 1986.

Coody, D: There is no such thing as a good tan. J. Pediatr Health Care 1(3):125, 1987.

Covington, T: Sunscreens: guidelines for selection & use. Facts & Comparisons Drug Newsletter 8(6): 41–42, Jun 1989.

Cuzzell, JZ and Willey, T: Pressure relief perennials. AJN 87(9):1157, 1987.

Cuzzell, JZ: The new RYB color code. AJN 88(10):1342, 1988.

deGroet, AC: The allergens in cosmetics. Arch Dermatol 124:1525, October 1988.

Fettner, AG: No more wrinkles? Hippocrates 2(1);20, 1988.

Gilchrest, BA: At last? a medical treatment for skin aging. JAMA 259:569–570, 1988.

Gilman, AG, Goodman, LS, and Gilman, A (eds): Goodman and Gilman's The Pharmacological Basis of Therapeutics. New York, Macmillan, 1986.

Hadley, SA and Black, VL: Why use Dakin's solution for wound care? AJN 88(3):284, 1988.

Kozol, R, et al: Effects of sodium hypochlorite (Dakin's solution) on cells of the wound module. Arch Surg 123:420–423, 1988.

Lemmink, JA: Infection control when a surgical wound becomes infected. RN 87(9):24, 1987.

Lund, CA: We made our skin care problems disappear. RN 50(5):18, 1987.

Moschella, SL, et al: Dermatology, Vol 1, Drugs and the Skin, p 1040. Philadelphia, WB Saunders, 1985.

Moser, PW: Search for the wrinkle-free face. Discover 7(8):57, 1987.

Platt, J and Becknall, RA: An experimental evaluation of antiseptic wound irrigation. J Hosp Infec 5:181, 1984.

Preston, KM: Dermal ulcers: simplifying a complex problem. Rehabil Nurs 12(1):17, 1987.

Ross, D: Tackling dermatitis-occupational skin conditions. Occup Health 39(7):220–221, 1987.

Rubin, M: The physiology of bed rest. AJN 88(1):50, 1988.

Sadra, S: Dermatitis: identifying the culprit. Occup Health 39(7):222, 1987.

Stern, RS, et al: Risk reduction for nonmelanoma skin cancer with childhood sunscreen use. Arch Dermatol 122(5):537, 45, 1986.

Stewart, DS: Indoor tanning the nurse's role in preventing skin damage. Cancer Nurs 10(2):93, 1987.

Stroughton, RB in Macbach, HI and Christophers, E (eds) Topical Therapy with Corticosteroids: New Advances. Excerpt Medica, New York, 1988.

Sunscreens. The Medical Letter on Drugs and Therapeutics. New Rochelle, NY, The Medical Letter, Inc, June 17, 1988, Vol. 7 (6):61–63.

Tanzman, E: Long-term tetracycline use in the treatment of acne vulgaris: The role of routine laboratory monitoring. J Am Coll Health 36:272, 1988.

Teutsch, E and Hill, M: Moisture to your life. Am J Nurs 87(3):327, 1987.

Weiss, JS: Topical tretinoin improves photoaged skin. JAMA 259:527, 1988.

Zack, R: What to do if your patient has lice. RN 8(9):30, 1987.

SITUATION   63–1

Joe Terranova is a 17-year-old with moderate to severe acne. He is evaluated in a dermatology clinic for treatment.

1. After washing with an antibacterial soap, Joe is to apply a topical anti-acne agent with benzoyl peroxide. The nurse will instruct him to:
   a. leave on skin for 6 hours initially
   b. apply to oily areas and cover with a dressing
   c. apply to entire face overnight
   d. leave on for 15 minutes initially

2. The nurse will caution Joe about overuse of the benzoyl peroxide cream, which is evidenced by:
   a. dizziness
   b. dry, cracking skin
   c. increased acne
   d. nausea, vomiting

3. After one month of treatment with topical agents, Joe has not demonstrated improvement of acne. He is to begin treatment with tretinoin (Retin-A). The nurse will instruct Joe in the proper use of this product by teaching the following:
   a. Apply a thick layer of tretinoin three times a day.
   b. Expect therapeutic results after one week.
   c. Keep the ointment away from eyes, mouth, and mucous membranes.
   d. Increase sun exposure to aid the healing process.

4. The nurse will check Joe for the following effect of tretinoin:
   a. elimination of wrinkles
   b. permanent pigment changes
   c. oiliness of skin
   d. peeling skin

5. In addition, Joe is to begin therapy with isotretinoin (Accutane). The nurse will instruct him to:
   a. increase sun exposure
   b. eliminate alcohol from diet
   c. take for the rest of his life
   d. take on an empty stomach

6. When evaluating Joe for adverse effects of isotretinoin, the nurse will note the following:
   a. increased triglycerides
   b. decreased cholesterol
   c. increased HDL
   d. decreased CPK

Please refer to the Appendices for correct answers and additional review questions with answers.

64

CHAPTER

VACCINES AND IMMUNIZATIONS

GLOSSARY TERMS IN THIS CHAPTER

Acquired immunity
Active immunity
Antibodies
Antitoxin
Antivenins
Artificially acquired immunity
Attenuated
Immunity
Immunization
Natural immunity
Naturally acquired immunity
Nosocomial
Passive immunity
Plasma cells
Retroviruses
Scarification
Serum
Serum sickness
Toxoid
Vaccine
Virulence

64
CHAPTER

VACCINES AND IMMUNIZATIONS

MERRILY MATHEWSON KUHN, R.N.C., Ph.D., CCRN
CAROLYN SUE B. KIRSCH, M.S.N., R.N.C.

LEARNING OBJECTIVES

After reading this chapter, the student will be able to:

1. Identify medications commonly used as vaccines and immunizations.

2. Differentiate vaccines, serums, and toxoids.

3. Differentiate among the immunizations as to mechanism of action, route of administration, pharmacokinetics, adverse effects, contraindications, and interactions.

4. Identify specific areas to assess in the patient requiring immunizations in order to formulate appropriate nursing diagnoses.

5. Plan the nursing interventions necessary to administer immunizations and choose appropriate teaching strategies to gain patient compliance.

6. Evaluate the patient at various stages of treatment to gauge nursing interventions.

Table 64–1. SELECTED INFECTIOUS DISEASES AND THEIR MANAGEMENT

	Infectious Sources	Entry Site	Infective Organism	Incubation Period	Method of Spread	Therapy*	Prophylaxis
Chickenpox (Varicella)	Human cases	Probably nasopharynx	Varicella-zoster (V-Z) virus	12–17 days	Probably respiratory droplets	Acyclovir (?)	Varicella-zoster globulin (VZIG) primarily for immunocompromised children and certain neonates exposed *in utero*
Diphtheria	Human cases and carriers; fomites; raw milk	Nasopharynx	*Corynebacterium diphtheriae*	2–5 days	Nasal and oral secretions; respiratory droplets	Diphtheria antitoxin; penicillin;	Active immunization with diphtheria toxoid
Influenza	Human cases	Respiratory tract	Virus	24–72 hours	Respiratory	Amantadine; rimantadine	Influenza virus vaccine
Measles	Human cases	Respiratory mucosa	Virus	8–13 days	Nasopharyngeal secretions	None	Measles vaccine
Meningococcal meningitis	Human cases and carriers	Nasopharynx; tonsils	*Neisseria meningitidis*	2–10 days	Respiratory droplets	Penicillin; ampicillin; chloramphenicol	Meningococcal polysaccharide vaccine for persons at risk; rifampin/sufadiazine for carriers or contacts
Mumps	Human cases (early)	Upper respiratory tract	Virus	2–3 weeks (avg. 18 days)	Respiratory droplets	None	Live mumps vaccine
Pneumococcal pneumonia	Human carriers; patient's own	Respiratory mucosa	*Streptococcus pneumoniae*	Variable	Respiratory droplets	Penicillin G; erythromycin	Polyvalent pneumococcal vaccine; control of upper respiratory infections; avoidance of alcoholic intoxication
Poliomyelitis	Human cases and carriers	Gastrointestinal tract	Polioviruses (types I, II, III)	7–14 days	Pharyngeal secretions; fecal-oral	None	Oral polio vaccine (OPV), the live attenuated vaccine containing all 3 strains of poliovirus—produces long-lasting immunity in most recipients
Rubella (German Measles)	Human cases	Respiratory mucosa	Virus	14–23 days	Nasopharyngeal secretions	None	Rubella virus vaccine; immune globulin (human) given to contacts of rubella; rubella in early stages of pregnancy legally recognized as indication for abortion

*Please refer to drug brochures and digests to keep current of changing dosages and uses.

Table 64–1. SELECTED INFECTIOUS DISEASES AND THEIR MANAGEMENT–*CONTINUED*

	Infectious Sources	Entry Site	Infective Organism	Incubation Period	Method of Spread	Therapy*	Prophylaxis
Tetanus	Contaminated soil	Penetrating and crush wounds	*Clostridium tetani*	4–21 days (avg. 10 days)	Horse and cattle feces	Tetanus immune globulin (human—TIG) and tetanus toxoid; penicillin	Wound debridement; toxoid booster injections for patients previously immunized; tetanus toxoid and tetanus immune globulin (separate sites and separate syringes) for non-immune persons
Tuberculosis	Sputum from human cases; milk from infected cows (rare in U.S.)	Respiratory mucosa	*Mycobacterium tuberculosis*	Variable	Sputum; respiratory droplets	Isoniazid; ethambutol; rifampin; streptomycin; pyrazinamide	Early discovery and adequate treatment of active cases; milk pasteurization, BCG vaccine
Whooping cough (pertussis)	Human cases	Respiratory tract	*Bordetella pertussis*	Commonly 7 days	Infected bronchial secretions	Erythromycin; ampicillin	Active immunization with vaccine; case isolation

*Please refer to drug brochures and digests to keep current of changing dosages and uses.

Vaccination or *immunization* is a deliberate attempt to protect humans against disease. Immunization has a long history, but only in the twentieth century has this practice become routine. During the last two hundred years, since the time of Edward Jenner, immunization has controlled nine major diseases at least in parts of the world. These diseases include: smallpox, diphtheria, tetanus, yellow fever, pertussis, poliomyelitis, measles, mumps, and rubella. Smallpox has been completely eradicated from the world. Immunization against influenza, hepatitis B, pneumococci, and *Haemophilus influenza* has made major headways against these infections. But much still remains to be done, even in developed countries.

Immunization has made a major impact on mortality reduction and population growth. With the exception of providing safe water, no other modality has made that impact.

The history of immunization dates to the sixth century in China. However, Edward Jenner's work with cowpox vaccination holds the title to the first scientific attempt to control an infectious disease by means of a deliberate systematic inoculation. Jenner, in 1810, realized that immunity was not lifelong, but did not know why. Later, in the 1880s, Pasteur developed the rabies vaccine. By the end of the 1890s, vaccines were available against typhoid, plague, cholera, and diphtheria.

After World War II, the golden age of immunization began. Numerous immunizations were developed, such as polio, measles, mumps, rubella, and adenovirus, all composed of attenuates (to be described later); polio and rabies composed of killed virus; and pneumococcus, meningococcus, *Haemophilus influenza*, and hepatitis B composed of purified protein.

As the final years of the twentieth century approach, new technologies are available, and the new wave of vaccine development continues.

INFECTIOUS DISEASES AND IMMUNITY

An infectious disease is any disease caused by growth of pathogenic organisms in the body. It may or may not be communicable. Infectious diseases are a major health problem in developing countries. Also, since many people from developed countries like the United States travel abroad, there is increased interest in preventing these diseases. Table 64–1 features a brief review of infectious diseases and how they can be treated.

Immunity is the ability of the body to develop relative resistance to disease after exposure to the agent responsible for causing the disease. Some people are born with the ability to resist invasion by certain types of foreign agents, but the majority of the population have to acquire immunity in some way (Fig. 64–1).

Immunity based on the development of *antibodies* is probably the most efficient and the single most formidable type of immunity. This form of immunity is con-

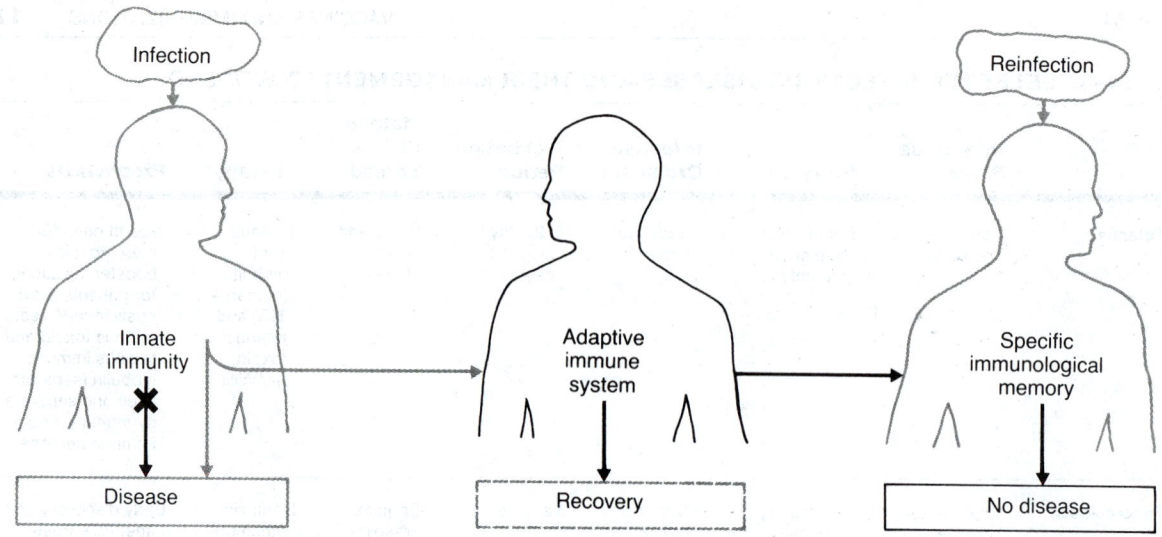

Figure 64–1. Adaptive and innate immunity. When an infectious agent enters the body it first encounters elements of the innate immune system. These may be sufficient to prevent disease but if not, a disease will result and the adaptive immune system is activated. The adaptive immune system produces recovery from the disease and a specific immunological memory is established so that following reinfection with the same agent no disease results; the individual has acquired immunity to the infectious agent.

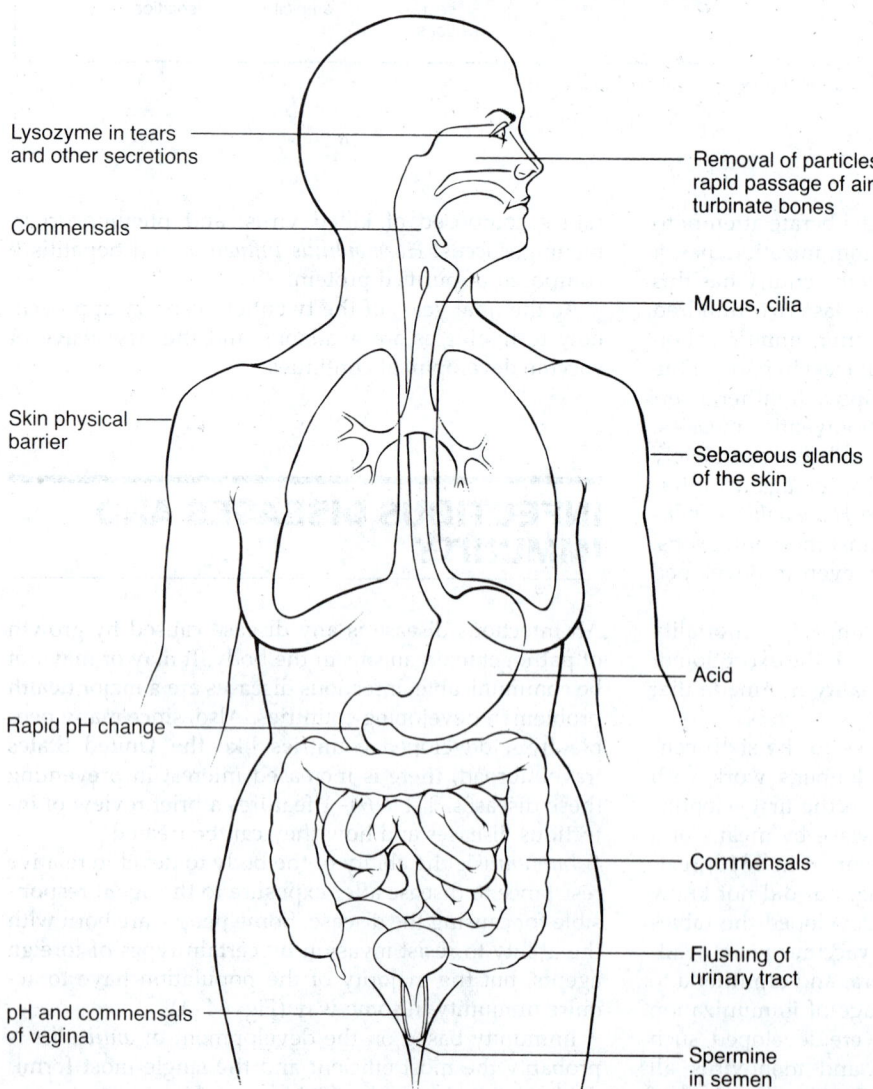

Lysozyme in tears and other secretions

Commensals

Skin physical barrier

Rapid pH change

pH and commensals of vagina

Removal of particles by rapid passage of air over turbinate bones

Mucus, cilia

Sebaceous glands of the skin

Acid

Commensals

Flushing of urinary tract

Spermine in semen

Figure 64–2. Natural body defenses. Most of the infectious agents which an individual encounters do not penetrate the body's surfaces, but are prevented from entering by a variety of biochemical and physical barriers. The body tolerates a number of commensal organisms which compete effectively with many potential pathogens. (1) The intact skin is impenetrable to most bacteria. Additionally, fatty acids produced by the skin are toxic to many organisms. (2) Epithelial surfaces are cleansed, for example, by ciliary action in the trachea or by flushing of the urinary tract. (3) pH changes in the stomach and vagina lead to destruction of many bacteria—both are acidic.

veniently subdivided into that which is actively acquired and that which is passively acquired:

1. Innate or natural immunity
2. Acquired immunity
   a. Actively acquired
      1. Natural
      2. Artificial
   B. Passively acquired
      1. Natural
      2. Artificial

Some humans are born with innate or inherited immunity to certain diseases. This innate immunity, along with immunity acquired from the mother and from exposure to disease, makes up *natural immunity*. Natural immunity provides a nonspecific response to any foreign invader, regardless of the composition of the invader. The basis of these natural defense mechanisms is merely the ability to distinguish between "self" and "nonself." Such natural mechanisms include physical barriers such as intact skin and mucous membranes, and cilia in the respiratory tract; chemical barriers such as gastric juices and enzymes; and biologic response modifiers like interferon (Fig. 64–2). Interferon is a nonspecific viricidal substance naturally produced by the body and capable of stimulating the activity of other components of the immune system (Fig. 64–3). The inflammatory response is also a major component of the natural immune system that is elicited in response to tissue injury or invading organisms. If natural immunity is insufficient to provide the body protection from diseases present in the environment, artificial means must be employed either to provide antibodies or to stimulate their production.

Immunity can be achieved through immunization. The goal of immunization is to render an individual resistant to the occurrence or effects of a particular disease. Throughout the human life cycle, immunizations play a vital role in preventing the spread and contraction of infectious diseases and in promoting the quality of life. Children are at great risk for contracting infectious disease because their limited experiences have given them few opportunities to develop naturally *acquired immunity*, and their lifestyles place them in close proximity to other equally unprotected children. Immunization provides an artificial means of acquiring immunity, and its importance has long been recognized. Many states now require immunizations to be current before a child is allowed into the public school system.

Acquired immunity can be active or passive, natural or artificial. The term *active immunity* refers to those antibodies produced by the body in response to an antigen (the immune system is discussed in detail in Chapter 50). These antigenic substances function to destroy the offending pathogen that has entered the body through disease. Actively acquired immunity is obtained when an antigenic substance—one that has lost its ability to produce illness, but is able to stimulate antibody formation—is injected into the body. Active acquired immunization can be obtained with live *attenuated* organisms,— dead organisms, or toxins. Attenuated vaccines

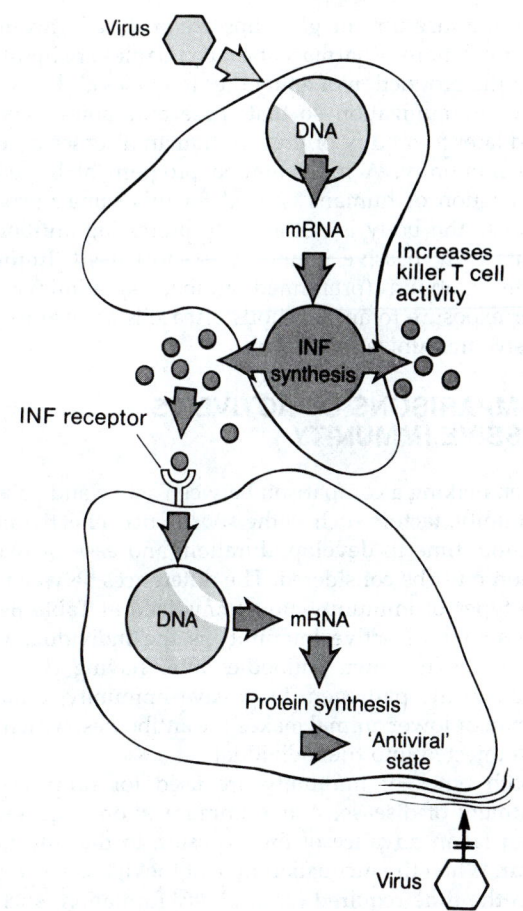

Figure 64–3. The action of interferon. Virus infecting a cell induces the production of interferon (INF). This is released and binds to interferon receptors on other cells. (Interferons are species specific and this is probably determined by the receptor specificity.) The interferon induces production of anti-viral proteins which are activated if virus enters the second cell. Interferon also has other actions.

contain viable but weakened organisms and will produce a mild infection of little danger to the host. It has the advantage, however, of producing a much more permanent form of immunity than killed vaccines. *Toxoids* are detoxified but still antigenically active poisons excreted by certain bacteria. Toxoids are excellent antigens. Antibodies formed against toxoids are fully reactive with the natural toxin and provide an excellent immunity against diseases caused by toxigenic bacteria such as tetanus and diphtheria. Once exposed to an antigenic substance, the body may continue to produce antibodies for an extended period, sometimes for life.

Passive immunity is immunity that is achieved by the introduction of antibodies produced by someone other than the patient. Passive immunity can be achieved through antibody transfer from mother to infant via the placenta or breast milk *(naturally acquired)* and through immunization with antibodies from another human or animal *(artificially acquired)*. Injections of hyperimmune serum, antiserum, or globulins are artificially acquired immunizations. Pharmaceutical companies are involved with the production of antibodies in horses and cows by active immunization so that these antibodies may be used later to modify or prevent human diseases by passive immunity. A more limited program of hyperimmunization of humans is used for this same purpose. Because the body is not actively producing antibodies on its own, passive immunity is short lived. Immune serum globulin (preformed antibodies) administered after exposure to an infectious disease is an example of passive immunization.

COMPARISONS OF ACTIVE VS. PASSIVE IMMUNITY

When making a comparison between active and passive immunity, factors such as the source, use, effectiveness, method, time to develop, duration, and ease of reactivation must be considered. The differences between the two types of immunity are summarized in Table 64–2. The source of active immunity is the individual who makes his/her own antibodies after having been exposed to the pathogen. In passive immunity, another human or lower animal makes the antibodies, which are then injected into the individual.

Both types of immunity are used for prophylactic treatment of disease. Active immunization is generally given far in advance of the exposure to the infectious agent. When the incubation time of the disease is longer than the time required for antibody formation, such as with rabies or smallpox, it is possible for the individual to be immunized after exposure. Passive immunity can also be administered prior to or immediately after exposure. Passive immunity is also used to treat diseases, although this is relatively ineffective.

Active immunity requires 5–14 days to develop after the primary immunization. This is the amount of time it takes for the protective antibodies to appear in the serum. Once active immunity is obtained, it persists for relatively long periods, usually years. This occurs because once the *plasma cells* are activated to produce antibodies, they will continue to do so for the lifetime of the cell. The half-life of a human antibody is about twenty-five days.

Passive immunity provides immediate protection. However, the injected antibodies are removed from the circulation without internal replacement. The half-life of injected antibodies is about seven days. Since these are foreign proteins, the body will make antibodies against the administered foreign antibody, which will hasten its removal.

Active immunity can be restored easily through booster injections. When passive immunity is obtained with foreign species antiserum, because of the already produced antibodies, an anaphylactic reaction of *serum sickness* may occur.

IMMUNIZATIONS

An immunization is often referred to as a vaccination. Any substance that stimulates antibody production or immunity and can be classified as a *serum, vaccine,* or *toxoid.* A serum is used to prevent infectious diseases from occurring or to relieve symptoms of the disease after suspected or actual exposure. Serums are used to produce passive immunity. A vaccine is a biologic agent, whereas a toxoid is a toxin (poisonous substance secreted by a micro-organism) that has been treated to eliminate its toxic properties but retains its ability to stimulate antibodies. Tetanus and diphtheria vaccines are examples of toxoids. Vaccines and toxoids are both used to induce active immunity via the antigen–antibody mechanism. This type of immunity takes days or weeks to develop; however, it is long-term, sometimes lasting for years.

An *antitoxin* provides passive antibodies with destroyed toxins. Antitoxins are used when an individual is suspected of having contracted a micro-organism that secretes toxins. Tetanus antitoxin, botulism antitoxin, diphtheria antitoxin, and rabies antitoxin are examples. Antitoxins can be obtained from animals such as horses. If an individual has a tetanus-prone wound, human tetanus immune globulin (TIG) may be given for passive immunity rather than risking anaphylactic shock from the animal-derived tetanus antitoxin.

Antivenins provide passive immunity and are used to

Table 64–2. COMPARISON OF ACTIVE AND PASSIVE ANTIBODY-MEDIATED IMMUNITY

Factor	Active Immunity	Passive Immunity
Source	Self	Some other human or lower animal
Ease of reactivation	Easy (by booster)	Dangerous, possible anaphylaxis
Use	Prophylactic	Prophylactic and therapeutic
Half-life of antibodies	25 days	7 days
Method	Disease itself, clinical or subclinical; immunization (killed or attenuated vaccines or toxoids)	Administration of antibody by maternal transplacental transfer or injection
Effectiveness	High	Moderate to low
Time to develop	5–14 days	Immediate on injection
Duration	Relatively long, perhaps years	Relatively short, a few days to several weeks

treat symptoms of insect, spider, and snake bites. Antivenins available include: black widow spider antivenin, crotaline antivenin, and *Micrurus fulvius* antivenin.

An immunization made directly from micro-organisms is referred to as an attenuate. In order to protect the recipient, the micro-organisms are killed, inactivated, or altered in such a way that their *virulence* is greatly reduced. The attenuate may contain live micro-organisms and, although they have been altered, they will continue to multiply for a time in the body and can cause reactions. This could be detrimental to a person whose immune system is suppressed, such as a child receiving chemotherapy for a malignancy. The process used to alter the micro-organism in an attenuate may involve neomycin and/or the vaccine may have been grown on chick embryo. It is, therefore, important to carefully assess for allergy of the patient to egg, chicken, or neomycin.

The current immunization for measles is an example of an attenuate. During the years 1963 through 1967, the vaccine consisted of a killed virus, but was later found to be ineffective. Persons immunized between 1963 and 1967 are at risk for contracting the disease unless they have been revaccinated. In 1967, the measles vaccine was changed to an attenuate. The attenuated form of the measles vaccine has been very successful in providing immunity if it is administered after fifteen months of age. Prior to age fifteen months, the child has passive immunity to the disease in the form of maternal antibodies. If immunized with a live vaccine before age fifteen months, the maternal antibodies destroy the micro-organisms before antibody production (active immunity) is stimulated. Occasionally, a younger child who has been exposed to the disease is immunized early. If this happens, the immunization is generally repeated at age fifteen months to assure immunity.

SERUMS

Serums are obtained from humans or animals in which antibodies have been formed against a pathogenic organism. Serum derived from a human source is likely to cause less allergic reaction than that obtained from an animal source. Serums are purified and standardized for injection. Serums are featured in Table 64–3.

Serums provide temporary immunity against disease. They can also prevent formation of active antibodies in an Rh-negative mother carrying or delivering an Rh-positive infant.

There are currently three types of serums available:

1. immune globulin for general use.
2. immune globulin with known antibodies against certain antigens, and
3. animal antitoxins and serums.

Immune globulin preparations are prepared from serum using ethanol fractionation, a process that separates the protein and lipoprotein components. The use of ethanol fractionation inactivates the live human immunodeficiency virus (HIV) (US Center for Disease Control, 1986; Prince, et al, 1986; and Wells, et al, 1986). However, HIV antibodies are passively transmitted.

PHARMOCOKINETICS

Serums are absorbed well after either intramuscular or intravenous administration. Immunity is obtained almost immediately but it is short-term, lasting only one to six weeks.

ADVERSE EFFECTS

The agents used for passive immunity may cause reactions that range from mild local discomfort to severe anaphylaxis, although this is rare. A few patients may experience fever and general malaise, chills, and headache. People receiving immune globulins may develop transient, positive, human immunodeficiency virus (HIV) antibody tests. Passively transmitted antibodies clear from the body within six months of the time immune globulin is received. Thus, patients testing positive to either the enzyme-linked immunosorbent assay (ELISA) or Western Blot confirmation tests for HIV, but who have no identifiable risk factors, should have repeat antibody testing. By the end of six months the test results will become negative if the antibodies were, indeed, passively received from the immune globulin injection.

DOSAGE

The dosage and route of administration for serums are predetermined and are included in the manufacturer's literature accompanying the serum. The usual recommended sites are the anterolateral aspect of the upper thigh and the deltoid muscle of the arm. Either of these sites may be used for intramuscular or subcutaneous injection.

IMMUNE GLOBULIN

Immune globulin is obtained from pooled plasma of approximately 1000 human donors, which contains standardized antibodies to diphtheria, poliomyelitis, measles, hepatitis A, and hepatitis C types. The protection obtained from immune globulin varies from six weeks to several months, depending on the dosage. Immune globulin is primarily used today to treat gamma G immunoglobulin (IgG) deficiency states. See Table 64–3 for additional information.

HEPATITIS B IMMUNE GLOBULIN

Hepatitis B immune globulin (HBIG, HyperHep) is obtained from the pooled plasma of donors with a high titer of antibodies to hepatitis B surface antigen (HBsAg)

TEXT RESUMES ON PAGE 1766

Table 64–3. IMMUNIZATIONS

Name	Dosage	Mode of Administration
SERUMS: Immune Globulin		
Action: For All: provide passive immunity. ***Use:*** immunodeficiency syndromes, exposure to hepatitis A.		
	Hepatitis exposure: 0.02–0.06 ml/kg. IgG deficiency: 1.2 ml/kg followed by 0.6 mg/kg every 3–4 wk, not to exceed 50 ml (adults); 30 ml (children) 100–800 mg/kg every month; dose depends on brand of immune globu- lin and patient response.	IM IM IV
Hepatitis B Immune Globulin (HBIG, HyperHep)		
Use: prophylaxis after exposure to heptatitis B.		
	Adults: Within 7 days of exposure, 0.06 ml/kg and second injection 28– 30 days later. Children, Newborns: 0.5 ml within 24 hr of birth, repeat at 3 & 6 months.	IM IM
Tetanus Immune Globulin (TIG, Hyper-Tet)		
Use: prophylaxis post-exposure to tetanus, treatment of tetanus.		
	Prophylaxis: 250–500 U. For treatment of active Tetanus: 3000–6000 U.	IM IM
Rabies Immune Globulin (RIG, Hyperab, Imogam)		
Use: prophylaxis after exposure to rabies.		
	20 IU/kg: half administered into wound and half IM.	Administered into the wound and IM.

*Within the column listing adverse effects, underlines indicate the most common effects; CAPITALS indicate life-threatening effects.

Contraindications/ Precautions	Adverse Effects*	Interactions	Nursing Implications
Contraindicated in known hypersensitivity or previous anaphylactic reacitons. Safe use in pregnancy not established.	Neuro: headache, faintness CV: chest tightness Resp: dyspnea GI: nausea, vomiting Integ: pain, redness at injection site Misc: malaise, fever, chills	None known	ASSESSMENT: Assess for particles or color change in vial, assess baseline vital signs and temperature. INTERVENTION: Store at 2–8° C. Mix in 5% dextrose in water only. EVALUATION: If chest pain, chills occur, stop IV infusion and notify physician.
IM injection contraindicated in persons with thrombocytopenia. Use cautiously in persons with hypersensitivity reactions to other immune globulins. Safe use in pregnancy not established.	Neuro: dizziness, headache GI: nausea, vomiting Integ: tenderness at site, urticaria, angioedema Misc: fever, malaise	None known	Very expensive. Use only in persons at high risk for developing hepatitis B. ASSESSMENT: Assess baseline vital signs and temperature INTERVENTION: Administer adult dose in deltoid and pediatric dose in vastus lateralis. Asperate carefully before injecting solution. Store at 2–8° C. Teach patient importance of receiving 2 or 3 injections.
Contraindicated in previous hypersensitivity to Ig or thimerosol.	Integ: discomfort at injection site Misc. mild fever	None known	INTERVENTION: Store at 2–6° C, do not freeze.
Contraindicated in previous hypersensitivity. Use caution when administering to patient with concurrent IgA deficiency.	Renal: nephrotic syndrome Integ: tenderness at injection site Misc: mild fever, ANAPHYLACTIC SHOCK	None known	INTERVENTION: Administer IM into deltoid of adults and vastus lateralis in children. Store at 2–8° C, do not freeze. Administer rabies vaccine concurrently.

CONTINUED ON THE FOLLOWING PAGE

Table 64–3. IMMUNIZATIONS–*CONTINUED*

Name	Dosage	Mode of Administration
Antirabies Serum Equine Origin (ARS) (Antirabies Serum)		
Action: for passive protection against rabies.		
Use: pre-exposure of high risk individuals and post-exposure protection.		
	40 IU/g: half administered into wound and half IM. 1000 IU/55#	IM
Varicella-Zoster Immune Globulin (VZIG)		
Use: prevent or treat varicella, provide passive immunity for patient exposed to chickenpox or herpes zoster.		
	Pediatric: up to 10 kg: 125 U; 10.1–20 kg: 250 U; 20.1–30 kg: 375 U; 30.1–40 kg: 500 U; over 40.1 kg: 625 U.	IM
Rho (D) Immunie Globulin (Gamulin Rh, RhoGAM, HypRho-D)		
Action: Effectively suppresses immune response in nonsensitized Rh O negative women who have received Rh O positive blood.		
Use: Rh negative pregnant women carrying an Rh positive fetus.		
	Lab determines fetal packed red blood cell volume. One vial if fetal RBC is 15 ml. If more than 15 ml, administer more than 1 vial. Antepartum: administer at 28 week gestation. Postpartum: administer within 72 hours.	IM
VACCINES		
Action for All: Provide active immunity.		
Bacillus Calmette-Guérin (BCG) Vaccine		
Action: provides active immunity against tuberculosis.		
Use: persons with negative skin test who will be exposed to person with sputum positive for tuberculosis.		
	Adults: 0.1 ml. Children <3 months: 0.05 ml. 0.2–0.3 ml on skin followed by multiple puncture gun. Allow to dry for 24 hours.	Intradermal Intradermal Scarification

*Within the column listing adverse effects, underlines indicate the most common effects; CAPITALS indicate life-threatening effects.

Contraindications/ Precautions	Adverse Effects*	Interactions	Nursing Implications
Contraindicated in allergic reactions to horse serum.	Integ: local pain, erythema, urticaria Misc: SERUM SICKNESS	None known	Same as rabies vaccine
Contraindicated in previous hypersensitivity to immune globulin. Safe use in pregnancy not established.	GI: nausea, vomiting Integ: mild rash, pain, swelling at injection site Misc: mild fever	None known	INTERVENTION: Administer within 72 hours of exposure. Administer deep IM in gluteal muscle. Aspirate carefully to avoid IV administration. Bland diet may reduce GI complaints.
Contraindicated in previous hypersenitivity to immune globulin.	Misc: local tenderness	None known	INTERVENTION: Administer at 28th week of gestation or within 72 hours of delivery or abortion. If 1 vial is needed, inject the entire vial IM. If more than 1 vial is needed, inject at different injection sites but all within 72 hours.
Contraindicated in persons positive for tuberculosis, and persons with impaired immunity from disease or drugs. Avoid use in pregnancy.	Integ: local pain, swelling, LYMPHADENITIS Misc: mild arthralgia, DEATH	Immunosuppressive drugs may interfere with response. Active TB treatment drugs will cause BCG to be ineffective. May impair theophylline excretion.	ASSESSMENT: Assess for presence of TB. Assess immunocompetence.

CONTINUED ON THE FOLLOWING PAGE

Table 64–3. IMMUNIZATIONS–*CONTINUED*

Name	Dosage	Mode of Administration
Bacillus Calmette-Guérin (BCG) Vaccine–*Continued*		

Cholera Vaccine

Action: protective immunity against cholera.

Use: in persons traveling to or residing in country of high cholera incidence.

	6 mon–4 yrs: 0.2 ml.	SC or IM
	5–10 yrs: 0.3 ml.	SC or IM
	Over 10 yrs: 0.5 ml.	SC or IM
	5 yrs & over: 0.2 ml.	Intradermal

Typhoid Vaccine

Action: provide immunity against typhoid fever.

Use: in persons traveling to or residing in country of high typhoid incidence.

	Adults & Children over 10 yrs: 0.5 ml or 0.1 ml.	SC / Intradermal
	Children 6 mos–10 yrs: 0.25 ml or 0.1 ml.	SC / Intradermal

*Within the column listing adverse effects, underlines indicate the most common effects; CAPITALS indicate life-threatening effects.

Contraindications/ Precautions	Adverse Effects*	Interactions	Nursing Implications
			INTERVENTION: Store 2–8° C. Do not expose to light. Add 1 ml sterile water to each ampule. Allow to stand for 1 minute. Do not shake. Withdrawal of solution will yield homogenous suspension. Inject intradermally over the insertion of the deltoid muscle. Keep vaccine site clean until local reaction has disappeared. Keep away from persons with active TB for 6–12 weeks. EVALUATION: Conduct post-vaccine TB test in 2–3 months. If not positive, revaccinate.
Contradicated in acute febrile illness, immuno-suppressed patients, and prior sensitivity.	CV: tachycardia, hypotension Integ: transient soreness, redness, swelling at site Misc: malaise, low-grade fever, flushing	None known	ASSESSMENT: Assess for presence of active infection and symptoms of actual cholera. INTERVENTION: Administer deep SC or IM in deltoid. Store at uniform temperature in refrigerator. EVALUATION: Evaluate signs of reactions and report to physician.
Contraindicated in patients with acute infection or previous systemic reaction. Safety in pregnancy not established.	Neuro: headache Integ: erythema, induration, tenderness Misc: malaise, myalgia, increased temperature	None known	ASSESSMENT: Assess for acute infection. INTERVENTION: Administer SC or intradermal. Store at uniform temperature in refrigerator. EVALUATION: Evaluate for signs of reaction.

CONTINUED ON THE FOLLOWING PAGE

Table 64–3. IMMUNIZATIONS–*CONTINUED*

Name	Dosage	Mode of Administration
Pneumococcal Vaccine Polyvalent (Pneumo-Vax 23, Pnu-Immune 23)		
Action: provides immunity against 23 of the most prevalent pneumococcal sero-types.		
Use: adults and children over 2 years with chronic illness. Adults over 65 years who are otherwise healthy.		
	0.5 ml.	SC or IM
Hemophilus B Polysaccaride Vaccine (Hib-Imune, Hib VAX, B-Capsa 1)		
Action: provides protection against hemophilus b.		
Use: children 10 months to 6 years.		
	0.5 ml	SC, IM
Hemophilus b with diptheria Toxoid Conjugate Vaccine (ProHIBit)		
Action: provides protection against hemophilus b and diptheria.		
Use: children 10 months to 6 years.		
	0.5 ml.	IM
Hepatitis B Vaccine (Recombivax HB)		
Action: plasma derived, inactivated human hepatitis B particles prepared by recombinant DNA technology.		
Use: provide active immunity against hepatitis B; health care personnel who have contact with blood, infants of HBgSAg positive mothers; persons at increased risk due to sexual practices.		
	Infants born to HBgSAg-positive mothers: 0.5 ml.	IM
	Adults: initial 1 ml within 7 days of exposure, 2nd dose in 1 month, 3rd dose in 6 months.	IM

*Within the column listing adverse effects, underlines indicate the most common effects; CAPITALS indicate life-threatening effects.

Contraindications/ Precautions	Adverse Effects*	Interactions	Nursing Implications
Contraindicated in hypersensitivity to pneumococcal vaccine, immunosuppressed patients, and acute infection. Use cautiously in persons with previous history of pneumococcal infection and in persons with severely compromised cardiovascular and respiratory conditions. Safe use in pregnancy and children under 2 not established.	Neuro: paresthesia, GUILLAIN-BARREÉ SYNDROME Integ: local erythema, induration, soreness, rash Misc: low grade fever, arthralgia, ANAPHYLAXIS	None known	ASSESSMENT: Assess for acute infection and prevous history of pneumococcal pneumonia. INTERVENTION: Administer SC or IM preferably in the deltoid or lateral mid-thigh. Refrigerate at 2–8° C. Do not administer IV or intradermal. EVALUATION: Evaluate for local reactions.
Contraindicated in sensitivity to any component, or diphtheria toxoid, or thimeresol. Use cautiously in persons with depressed immune system.	Neuro: seizures GI: anorexia Integ: local erythema, induration, tenderness Misc: fever, irritability	None known	INTERVENTION: Polysaccaride Vaccine: use only diluent provided. INTERVENTION: Conjugate Vaccine: Administer IM in outer aspect of vastus lateralis or deltoid, do not administer IV.
Contraindicated in hypersensitivity. Use cautiously in immunosuppressed patient. Safety in pregnancy and lactating women not established.	Neuro: headache, lightheadedness, vertigo, dizziness, insomnia, GUILLAIN-BARRE Resp: upper respiratory infection GI: nausea, vomiting, diarrhea, abdominal pain, cramps Hemo: thrombocytopenia Integ: soreness, pain, induration, tenderness Misc: fatigue, weakness, arthralgia, myalgia	None known	ASSESSMENT: Assess for acute infection. INTERVENTION: Administer IM in deltoid in adults or anterolateral thigh in infants and children.

CONTINUED ON THE FOLLOWING PAGE

Table 64–3. IMMUNIZATIONS–*CONTINUED*

Name	Dosage	Mode of Administration
Measles (Rubeola) Virus Vaccine (Attenuvax)		
Action: produces a modified measles infection and then immunity for about 8 years.		
Use: children 15 months and older and adults in endemic situation.		
	1000 $TCID_{50}$ (0.5 ml)	SC
Rubella Virus Vaccine (Meruvax II)		
Action: provides immunity against rubella virus for about 6 years.		
Use: children over 12 months, non-pregnant females with negative serologic titers and leukemia patients in remission.		
	1000 $TCID_{50}$ (0.5 ml)	SC
Mumps Virus Vaccine (Mumpsvax)		
Action: induces effective immunity for about 10 years against the mumps virus.		
Use: children over 12 months of age.		
	5000 $TCID_{50}$ (0.5 ml)	SC
Poliovirus Vaccine, live, oral, trivalent (Sabin)		
Action: produces active immunity against poliomyelitis.		
Use: infants from 6 to 12 weeks.		
	0.5 ml	PO

*Within the column listing adverse effects, underlines indicate the most common effects; CAPITALS indicate life-threatening effects.

Contraindications/ Precautions	Adverse Effects*	Interactions	Nursing Implications
Contraindicated in hypersensitivity to neomycin, immunosuppressed persons, and acute infections. Safe use in pregnancy not established. Use cautiously in persons hypersensitive to eggs, chicken, and chicken feathers.	Neuro: FEBRILE CONVULSIONS Hemo: thrombocytopenia Integ: burning, stinging, swelling, redness	None known	ASSESSMENT: Assess for acute infection INTERVENTION: Administer SC in outer aspect of upper arm, use 25-gauge needle. Use only diluent supplied. Discard if not used within 8 hours of mixing. Extremely light- and heat-sensitive. Exposure to light before or after reconstitution kills the live virus.
Contraindicated in hypersensitivity to neomycin, immunosuppressed persons, and acute infections. Safe use in pregnancy not established.	Neuro: ENCEPHALITIS Hemo: thrombocytopenia Misc: arthralgia	None known	Same as measles.
Same as rubella	Neuro: FEBRILE SEIZURES Misc: mild fever	None known	Same as rubella
Contraindications same as rubella. Safety in pregnancy not established.	Neuro: PARALYSIS	None known	ASSESSMENT: Assess for acute infection. INTERVENTION: For PO use only. Keep frozen. If defrosted during transport, 10 freeze–thaw cycles allowed. Once defrosted, vaccine should be used within 30 days. Once opened, vaccine should be used within 7 days.

CONTINUED ON THE FOLLOWING PAGE

Table 64–3. IMMUNIZATIONS–*CONTINUED*

Name	Dosage	Mode of Administration
Poliovirus Vaccine, Inactivated (Salk)		
Action: produces active immunity against poliomyelitis.		
Use: infants from 6–12 weeks.		
	1 ml × 3 at 4 week intervals, 1 ml 6–12 months later.	SC
	1 ml × 2 at 1–2-month intervals, 1 ml 6–12 months later.	SC
Influenza Virus Vaccine (Fluogen, Fluzone)		
Action: produces antibodies against specific strain of influenza.		
Use: children over 6 months of age and adults who may have serious complications if they developed influenza; adults over 45 years; health care workers.		
	0.25–0.5 ml, depending on type.	IM
Rabies Vaccine, Human Diploid Cell Cultures (HDCV) (Imovax, WYVAC Rabies Vaccine)		
Action: produces high titer antibody production.		
Use: pre-exposure of high-risk individuals and post-exposure protection.		
	Pre-exposure 1 ml × 3 on days 7, 21, and 28. Post-exposure 1 ml × 5 on days 0, 3, 7, 14, and 28. (If given intravenously 0.1 ml)	IM
TOXOIDS Tetanus toxoid		
Action: provides active immunity against tetanus.		
Use: all persons from 6 months of age.		
Fluid (0.5 ml contains 4–5 Lf of tetanus toxoid)	0.5 ml × 3 at 4–8 week intervals, 4th dose 6–12 months later, booster 0.5 ml q 10 years.	IM, SC
Adsorbed (0.5 ml contains 5–10 Lf of tetanus toxoid)	0.5 ml × 2 at 4–8-week intervals, 3rd dose 6–12 months later, booster 0.5 ml q 10 years.	IM

*Within the column listing adverse effects, underlines indicate the most common effects; CAPITALS indicate life-threatening effects.

Contraindications/ Precautions	Adverse Effects*	Interactions	Nursing Implications
Contraindicated in persons allergic to streptomycin or neomycin, febrile illness, acute infection. Safe use in pregnancy not established.	Integ: tenderness, rashes, pruritis Misc: fever	None known	ASSESSMENT: Assess for acute infection INTERVENTION: For SC use only.
Contraindicated in hypersensitivity to egg yolk protein, acute infection.	Integ: local soreness, erythema Misc: fever, malaise, myalgia	May inhibit warfarin and theophylline clearance.	ASSESSMENT: Assess for acute infection. INTERVENTION: Do not administer IV. Administer IM in deltoid in adults and anterolateral aspect of thigh in children. Store in refrigerator. Do not freeze as potency is destroyed.
Contraindicated in developing febrile illness.	Neuro: headache, dizziness, NEUROPARALYTIC REACTION GI: nausea, abdominal pain Integ: local swelling, erythema, induration, pain	Corticosteroids and immunosuppresants may interfere with antibody development.	ASSESSMENT: Assess for acute infection, determine source of rabies exposure. INTERVENTION: Administer all doses as recommended.
Contraindicated in prior systemic reaction, active infection, immunosuppressed individuals. Cautious use in infants and children with neurologic disorders.	CV: tachycardia, hypotension Hemo: HYPERSENSITIVITY Integ: local erythema and induration, nodule pruritis Misc: low grade fever, chills, malaise, generalized aches and pains, flushing	None known	ASSESSMENT: Assess for active acute infection. INTERVENTION: Administer in deltoid or vastus lateralis. EVALUATION: Report any severe adverse reaction.

CONTINUED ON THE FOLLOWING PAGE

Table 64-3. IMMUNIZATIONS–*CONTINUED*

Name	Dosage	Mode of Administration
Diphtheria toxoid		
Action: provides active immunity against diphtheria		
Use: in infants and children under 6.		
Adsorbed	0.5 ml × 2 6–8 weeks apart and 3rd dose 1 year later.	IM
Diphtheria and Tetanus Toxoid and Pertussis Vaccine Adsorbed (DTP)		
Action: provides active immunity against diphtheria, tetanus, and pertussis.		
Use: infants 2 months to 6 years.		
	0.5 ml × 3 at 4–8-week intervals. Then, a fourth dose 6–12 mos later.	IM
Diphtheria and tetanus toxoid combined (Td)		
Action: provides active immunity against diphtheria and tetanus.		
Use: children over 7 and adults		
	Pediatric Adsorbed Toxoid Infants: 0.5 ml × 3 at 4-week intervals and at 6–12 months later. Children (1–6 yrs): 0.5 ml × 2 at 4-week intervals and at 6–12 months later. Booster (4–6 yrs): 0.5 ml.	IM
	Adult Adsorbed Toxoid 7 years and older: 0.5 ml × 2 at 4–6-week intervals and 3rd 6–12 months later.	IM

*Within the column listing adverse effects, underlines indicate the most common effects; CAPITALS indicate life-threatening effects.

and then concentrated by cold alcohol fractionation. Hepatitis B immune globulin is indicated only for the postexposure prophylaxis of hepatitis following needle sticks or exposure to blood or other body fluids from patients known to be positive for hepatitis B surface antigen. Additional information is in Table 64–3.

TETANUS IMMUNE GLOBULIN

Tetanus immune globulin (TIG, Hyper-Tet), obtained from human plasma, is effective in producing passive immunity in patients whose wounds may be contaminated with *Clostridium tetani*. Tetanus immune globulin is also used to provide passive immunity for nonimmunized patients and to treat tetanus. Additional information is in Table 64–3.

RABIES IMMUNE GLOBULIN

Rabies immune globulin (RIB, Hyperab, Imogam) is obtained from plasma of hyperimmunized human donors. It is always administered with rabies vaccine. After a bite from an infected animal, half the dose is administered into the wound and the other half is injected intramuscularly. More information is found in Table 64–3.

Contraindications/ Precautions	Adverse Effects*	Interactions	Nursing Implications
Contraindicated in acute active infection and prior hypersensitivity. Cautious use in persons with history of central nervous system disease or convulsions.	CV: tachycardia, hypotension Integ: redness, tenderness, induration, pruritis Misc: transient fever, malaise, flushing	None known	ASSESSMENT: Assess for active infection. INTERVENTION: Administer in vastus lateralis. Do not administer intracutaneously. Do not enter blood vessel. EVALUATION: Report any severe adverse effects.
Contraindicated during acute active infection, prior hypersensitivity. Cautiously use in children with history of convulsions.	GI: anorexia, vomiting Integ: erythema, induration, pain, swelling Misc: fretfulness, drowsiness, SUDDEN INFANT DEATH SYNDROME	None known	Same as above
Same as above	Same as above	Same as above	Same as above

VARICELLA-ZOSTER IMMUNE GLOBULIN

Varicella-zoster immune globulin (VZIG) is obtained from human plasma with high titers of varicella-zoster antibodies. Varicella-zoster immune globulin is used to prevent or ameliorate varicella. It is also used in immunosuppressed patients exposed to chickenpox or herpes zoster. Additional information is found in Table 64–3.

A vaccine has been developed for chickenpox (varicella) but is not available at the time of this writing. Studies indicate the vaccine offers effective immunity with few side effects. Chickenpox may be fatal to a child whose immune system is suppressed.

RHO (D) IMMUNE GLOBULIN

Rho (D) immune globulin (Gamulin Rh, RhoGam) is administered to Rh-negative women who are pregnant or who give birth to Rh-positive infants. Rho (D) immune globulin effectively suppresses the immune response on nonsensitized Rh-negative women who have received Rh-positive blood during fetal–maternal transfer. At the time of delivery, Rho (D) is administered to prevent hemolytic disease of the newborn (*Erythroblastosis fetalis*) in subsequent pregnancies.

Rho (D) is also administered to nonsensitized Rh-negative women after spontaneous or induced abortions, ruptured tubal pregnancies, amniocentesis, abdominal trauma, and any other occurrence of transplacental hemorrhage.

One ample of Rho (D) immune globulin is administered within seventy-two hours of delivery, miscarriage, abortion, or transfusion. If Rho (D) immune globulin is to be administered intramuscularly during pregnancy, one vial is administered intramuscularly at twenty-eight weeks' gestation. More information is found in Table 64–3.

VACCINES

Vaccines provide active immunity for a prolonged period. There are three general types of vaccines:

1. bacterial vaccines prepared from whole or purified capsular polysaccharides of killed bacteria,
2. viral vaccines containing live attenuated or inactive nonliving viruses, and
3. rickettsial vaccines.

The vaccines, unlike immune serum or antitoxin, which contain exogenous antibodies, include specific antigens that induce endogenous production of antibodies. All of the vaccines are featured in Table 64–3.

PHARMACOKINETICS

Vaccines provide long-term or permanent immunity against disease. The onset of action begins in several days to several weeks. The peak action time varies, as does the duration of action. Immunity can vary from one year with influenza vaccine to ten years with tetanus toxoid.

ADVERSE EFFECTS

Adverse effects from immunizations are similar to those experienced from agents that produce passive immunity. Local symptoms at the injection site are most common. Mild systemic symptoms can include mild arthralgia, anorexia, and drowsiness.

DOSAGE

The dosage and route of administration for vaccines are predetermined and are included in the manufacturer's literature accompanying the vaccine. The usual recommended sites are the anterolateral aspect of the upper thigh and the deltoid muscle of the arm. Either of these sites may be used for intramuscular or subcutaneous injection.

BACTERIAL VACCINES

Bacillus Calmette-Guérin (BCG) Vaccine

Bacillus Calmette-Guérin vaccine is available as either the attenuated tubercle bacillus or the live bacillus Calmette-Guérin form. The BCG vaccine provides active immunity for persons who are at high risk of contracting tuberculosis. This vaccine is appropriate for health care workers who will be exposed to tuberculosis patients, and for persons who will be residing in countries where there is an increased incidence of tuberculosis.

The attenuate form is administered intradermally. A small papule should appear over the site of injection within one to three months. Until the individual has a positive skin test (Mantoux or Heaf), they should avoid contact with persons with tuberculosis. The live forms of the BCG are available as either an intradermal administration (injected over the insertion of the deltoid muscle) or for *scarification*.

Cholera Vaccine

Cholera vaccine is available in the United States for cholera prophylaxis in persons traveling to, or residents of, cholera-infested areas. Immunity is brief, only lasting three to six months. A booster is recommended after six months if exposure is to be continued.

Local inflammation and redness may occur at the subcutaneous or intramuscular injection site. In case of allergic reactions, epinephrine and other emergency supplies should be available during administration.

Typhoid Vaccine

Typhoid vaccine, produced from killed *S. typhi*, is about 70%–90% effective in preventing typhoid fever. Protection is short, lasting about three years, but can be overcome by increasing the number of injected organisms. Typhoid vaccine is recommended for persons traveling to areas where typhoid fever is endemic. The most common adverse effect after the subcutaneous injection is local redness and tenderness.

Pneumococcal Vaccine

Pneumococcal vaccine (Polyvalent) contains twenty-three of the most common prevalent or invasive pneumococcal sero types, which account for 85%–90% of all pneumococcal pneumonias. It is useful in adults and children over two years of age with all chronic illnesses, particularly cardiovascular and pulmonary diseases, where there is increased morbidity associated with respiratory infections. The pneumococcal vaccine is also useful in persons over sixty-five who are otherwise healthy. The pneumococcal vaccine can be administered to children, two years and older, with chronic illnesses.

The pneumococcal vaccine is fairly effective in the healthy elderly, but recent research indicates it is far less effective in patients whose capacity for antibody production is impaired by a compromised immune system. Further research may lead to the development of pneumococcal vaccine with greater immunogenicity, which would give reliable protection to higher risk patients.

The pneumococcal vaccine is contraindicated in persons having a prior reaction to any polyvalent pneumococcal vaccine. It is also contraindicated in persons with acute infections until the active infection is passed or in persons who are immunosuppressed.

Local reaction of erythema, induration, and soreness

are common (71%–72%), but last less than three days. Low grade fever may also occur and usually clears within twenty-four hours.

Hemophilus B Vaccine

Hemophilus B vaccine is available as both a Hemophilus B conjugate vaccine, which provides immunity for diphtheria toxoid, and the Hemophilus B polysaccharide V, which provides prophylactic prevention of *Hemophilus influenza* type B and the diseases it causes such as meningitis, epiglottitis, and pericarditis. Hemophilus B conjugated vaccine is prepared from purified capsular polysaccharide covalently bound to diphtheria toxoid.

In 1985, the *Hemophilus influenza* type B (Hib) vaccine was introduced in the United States. The largest group at risk for contracting Hib diseases are children under the age of five years. Approximately 12% of Hib cases occur in children 18–24 months of age. The primary Hib diseases seen in children are epiglottitis, septic arthritis, sepsis, pneumonia, and meningitis. Even with advances in antimicrobial therapy, there remains a 5% mortality rate from *H. influenza* and a high incidence of mental retardation in those who survive meningitis. The initial vaccination should be given at age 24 months. Children who were not vaccinated at 24 months can be given the vaccine up to the age of five years. A physician may decide a child aged 18–23 months should be vaccinated if the child is in a high-risk group such as asplenia, sickle cell anemia, malignancy, immunosuppressed, or attending a day care center. The Hib vaccine can be given at the same time as the DPT vaccine, but a different injection site is used to prevent possible interaction.

In 1988 the FDA approved the first conjugate Hib vaccine for children aged eighteen months to five years. It offers immunity against the same *H. influenza* diseases as the original Hib vaccine, with the advantage of being effective in children aged 18–24 months.

Hib vaccines are contraindicated in persons who are hypersensitive to any component of the vaccine, diphtheria toxoid, or thimerosal. (Thimerosal is a chemical substance used in preparing some vaccines.) Use during pregnancy is not recommended.

Hepatitis B Vaccine

Hepatitis B vaccine (Heptavax B) is a vaccine available to individuals who are at risk of contracting the hepatitis B virus (HBV). Heptavax B is administered in three injections over a six-month period. The highest risk groups are people working with blood and blood products such as dentists, oral surgeons, dental hygienists, health care workers, those involved with dialysis patients, persons at risk due to their sexual practices, and infants born to hepatitis B surface antigen (HBsAg)–positive mothers. If an individual does not have HBV acquired immunity or has not been immunized with Heptavax B and is exposed to HBV, Hepatitis B immune globulin (HBIG) is given, which offers passive immunity. The American Academy of Pediatrics recommends infants of HBsAg-positive mothers be immunized immediately after birth with a combination of Heptavax and HBIG.

Hepatitis B vaccine consists of inactivated human hepatitis B particles obtained by plasmapheresis from healthy chronic HBsAg carriers. The hepatitis B vaccine is 80%–95% effective in preventing acute hepatitis B.

Hepatitis B vaccine is contraindicated in persons with known hypersensitivity and persons who are immunosuppressed. Safe use in pregnancy and lactation has not been established.

Measles, Mumps, and Rubella Vaccines

Measles, mumps, and rubella vaccines are available individually or in combination.

MEASLES VACCINE. Measles vaccine is available as a live, attenuated vaccine that produces a modified infection in susceptible individuals. The vaccine is effective for about eight years. Measles vaccine is primarily used in children fifteen months or older and also in adults in high school or college in epidemic situations.

During early 1989, there were 7000 cases of measles reported to the US Center for Disease Control (CDC), a sharp increase over previous years. Most of these cases were persons under 22 years of age. Because of the changes in the measles vaccine over the past 25 years, it is currently recommended that it is advisable to offer an additional dose of measles vaccine to persons between the ages of 10–22 years. Revaccination appears to be safe.

Measles vaccine is contraindicated in persons hypersensitive to neomycin, with acute active infection, or in persons immunosuppressed. It is given cautiously to persons hypersensitive to eggs, chicken, or chicken feathers, as it is developed on chick embryos.

RUBELLA VIRUS VACCINE. Rubella virus vaccine is a live, attenuated vaccine that gives protection against rubella for about six years. It is recommended for children aged twelve months to puberty, leukemia patients in remission, and nonpregnant females with negative serologic tests. Immunity is indicated by a rubella antibody titer of 1:8 or greater. If a woman becomes pregnant within three months of the vaccination, there is up to a 7% chance of congenital malformations. Rubella virus vaccine has the same contraindications as the measles vaccine.

MUMPS VIRUS VACCINE. Mumps virus vaccine is a live vaccine that induces an effective antibody response in 97% of children and 93% of adults. Immunity persists for about ten years. The mumps virus vaccine is recommended for children aged twelve months or older. Contraindications are similar to those of the measles vaccine.

Poliovirus Vaccine, Live, Oral, Trivalent (Sabin)

The poliovirus vaccine is a live attenuated vaccine that produces active immunity in about 90 percent of persons. The live virus is preferred to inactivated preparations. The live virus multiples in the host and provokes the production of serum antibodies. Live poliovirus is then shed by the host for about three weeks.

The poliovirus vaccine is used for prophylaxis against

poliomyelitis, primarily in childhood. The child receives two to three oral doses with intervals of six to twelve weeks between doses. Simultaneous administration of two or more live virus vaccines should be avoided.

Poliovirus Vaccine, Inactivated (Salk)

Poliovirus vaccine is prepared from inactivated poliovirus and provides active immunity against poliomyelitis. It is currently recommended for persons at risk over eighteen years of age. Persons at risk include travelers to countries where polio is endemic and health care workers. The older poliovirus vaccine contains streptomycin, neomycin, and traces of animal protein, so it is contraindicated in persons allergic to these products. The newer more potent inactivated polio vaccine contains continuous human cell lines. The added potency provides greater antibody response. No adverse effects have been reported with the new vaccine. The newer enhanced-potency inactivated vaccine should make the conventional polio vaccine obsolete. The vaccine is administered subcutaneously into the area of insertion of the deltoid muscle. Three doses at four-week intervals followed by a booster dose six to twelve months later is recommended. Boosters are given after three to five years.

Influenza Virus Vaccine

Influenza is one of the most common viral respiratory infections that affects hundreds of million people yearly. In previous years, influenza has been both endemic and pandemic and caused millions of deaths. Each year the United States Public Health Services Committee on Immunizations Practice recommends which influenza vaccine is to be used, since the antigen components of the influenza strain changes.

The influenza virus vaccine is recommended for persons six months or older who would be at risk if they developed influenza. This group includes people with chronic cardiovascular or pulmonary disorders and all residents (regardless of age) of nursing homes or chronic care facilities. It is also desirable for persons over forty-five years of age and for health care workers. Health care workers are immunized because they are capable of transmitting *nosocomial* infections. About two weeks after the vaccine, antibody levels are usually sufficient to prevent disease.

Rabies Prophylaxis Products

Rabies is endemic throughout the world in animal populations, except in the United Kingdom, Japan, and Antarctica. It is a viral infection that can be transmitted to domestic animals as well as people. Once the virus enters the body it incubates for 10–60 days. The virus travels along afferent sensory nerve pathways to the spinal cord and then on to the brain where it multiplies. The virus then travels down efferent motor nerve pathways to all areas of the body, particularly the salivary glands.

Approximately 25,000 people receive rabies prophylaxis each years. There are two types of immunizing products: vaccines and globulins. Both products are used concurrently for post-exposure prophylaxis. See Table 64–3 for more detailed information.

TOXOIDS

Several toxoids are available today. Toxoids are used for active immunization against tetanus and diphtheria.

TETANUS TOXOID

Tetanus toxoid is used for active immunization against tetanus in both adults and children. The toxin produced by the virulent tetanus bacillus has been treated with formaldehyde to reduce its toxicity. Tetanus immunization is recommended for all persons beginning at age two months. It is particularly important for adults to maintain their immunization if there is an increased risk of lacerations and abrasions such as with firemen, military personnel, farm and utility workers, and people working with horses.

Immunization is generally started in infants by using adsorbed diphtheria, tetanus toxoid, and pertussis vaccine (DTP) or adsorbed diphtheria and tetanus toxoids. The tetanus and diphtheria toxoid is recommended to protect persons over six years of age.

Contraindications to tetanus toxoid include a prior systemic allergic response or an acute active infection. Only healthy persons should be injected.

Tetanus toxoid is administered intramuscularly into the deltoid or midlateral thigh (vastus lateralis).

DIPHTHERIA TOXOID, ADSORBED

Diphtheria toxoid, adsorbed, is used for active immunization against diphtheria in infants and children under the age of six. It is not used in the treatment of actual diphtheria infections.

DIPHTHERIA, TETANUS TOXOIDS AND PERTUSSIS VACCINE, ADSORBED (DTP)

Diphtheria, tetanus toxoids, and pertussis vaccine, adsorbed, contains both the diphtheria and tetanus toxoid, which have been detoxified by formaldehyde with pertussis vaccine. This is the agent of choice for routine immunization of children less than six years of age. It is not recommended for people over seven years of age. The DTP confers protection for at least ten years.

Pertussis contains killed *Bordeteller pertussis* organisms, which provides protection against whooping cough. Only bacteria that possess a capsule are selected for this vaccine, since the capsule presence correlates highly with virulence.

Because of the decline in pertussis-related mortality prior to the institution of wide-spread immunization, some researchers argue that pertussis vaccine is currently superfluous and that it should be abandoned except for certain high-risk groups. In addition, pertussis vaccine may be associated with encephalopathy, infantile spasms, and sudden infant death syndrome.

In spite of these difficulties and uncertainties, it is the consensus of the majority of authorities that the benefits of the vaccine to the individual and to the public far outweigh the risks, even with the current impossibility of providing a precise mathematical estimate of the benefit–risk ratio.

DIPHTHERIA AND TETANUS TOXOID COMBINED (Td)

Diphtheria and tetanus toxoid combined (Td) has both the diphtheria and tetanus toxoids, which are inactivated by formaldehyde. Diphtheria and tetanus toxoid combined is used when the triple vaccine DTP is contraindicated, and in children over seven years of age and adults.

HUMAN IMMUNODEFICIENCY VIRUS

The Acquired Immune Deficiency Syndrome (AIDS) was described in 1981, and the etiologic agent, human immunodeficiency virus (HIV) was identified in 1983–1984. Currently there are two well-characterized subtypes of the virus, HIV-1 and HIV-2, which are both spreading throughout the world. AIDS has already become a leading cause of death in the United States of young adult males. AIDS is also a global health problem, particularly in central Africa, where HIV infection and AIDS are likely to severely test the social and economic resources of all nations.

Human immunodeficiency virus is a member of the lentivirus subfamily of cytopathic *retroviruses*. These viruses are characterized by slow, progressive infections in which the virus escapes host immune defenses (Fig. 64–4). These viruses continue to cause disease after a long latency period (months to years). The viruses are constrained within an envelope glycoprotein that contains reverse transcriptase enzyme and RNA. The virus infects particular cells in the body—lymphocytes (helper T-cells and B-cells), macrocytes, and oligodendrocytes in the central nervous system.

A potential problem in the development of an AIDS vaccine is the geographically divergent envelope glycoprotein. A proposed explanation for this divergence is a high rate of viral mutation.

A vaccine that protected against infection by HIV would be an important tool in the global effort to limit the current epidemic. Human immunodeficiency virus infection evokes a measurable antibody response; however, this does not provide protection from disease once the infection has occurred. The basic premise of vaccine development is that immunity (as manifested by neutralizing antibodies and cell-mediated immunity), if present before exposure, could prevent viral infection. It has also been suggested that a vaccine administered to infected people may restrict disease progression and infection transmission.

AIDS has been identified for less than a decade. Although much is known about the pathogenesis of HIV infection, there are still many questions that must be addressed in the development of an AIDS vaccine. The re-evaluation of vaccines will require patience and persistence. If current technologies are capable of developing a vaccine, studies lasting a minimum of several years and involving thousands of individuals will probably be necessary to assess its safety and efficacy. An effective vaccine appears to be many years away.

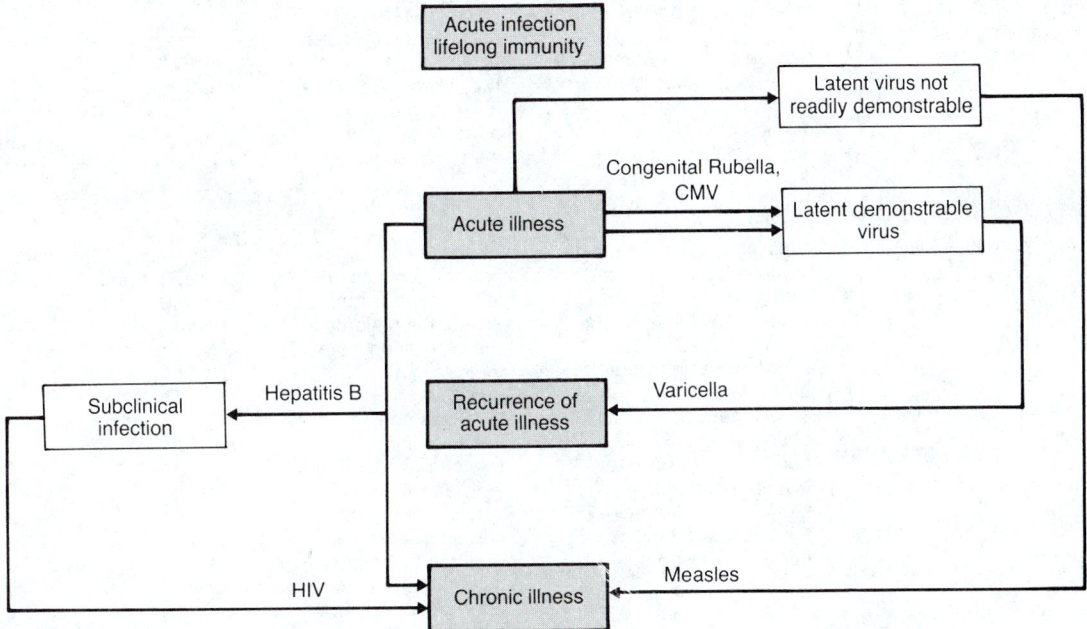

Figure 64–4. Illness and virus infection. The varied pathology of different virus infections is indicated in the dark boxes. While many viruses produce an acute illness followed by sterile lifelong immunity, some are followed by later recurrence, due to virus remaining latent within cells. Examples of different types are given.

USING THE NURSING PROCESS

ASSESSMENT

As the nurse begins the assessment, it is important to determine if the individual has had immunizations before and if there has been an allergic reaction. For certain immunizations it is all important to assess for allergies to animal products and thimerosal. Also, many vaccines should not be given to a patient with an acute infection or anyone who is immunosuppressed. Therefore, an adequate history must be obtained from the patient and family. Typical nursing assessments for patient receiving immunizations are included in Table 64–4.

The majority of immunizations are received during childhood. Tables 64–5 and 64–6 illustrate the recommended immunization schedule. Children and adults at risk of contracting infectious diseases who were not vaccinated in childhood may require further immunization. These risk groups include persons traveling to foreign countries, health care workers, immigrants to this country, the elderly, and the chronically ill.

Vaccines are intended for use by healthy individuals, and the manufacturer usually indicates precautions or contraindications. Minor nonfebrile illnesses in children are not contraindications for inoculation. A vaccine is given at a later date to a child who has a febrile illness.

It is important for the nurse to understand what type of immunizations can be administered together. Immune globulin should not be given for three months before or at least two weeks after a live viral vaccine, although it does not appear to interfere with the immune

Table 64–4. NURSING PROCESS FOR PATIENT REQUIRING IMMUNIZATIONS

Assessment

Determine previous immunization history and reactions which may have occurred.
Note allergies to animal products and thimerosal.
Assess presence of acute infection and/or immunosuppression; pregnancy.

Nursing Diagnosis	Nursing Actions	Rationale	Desired Patient/ Evaluation Criteria
Knowledge deficit related to lack of exposure/ recall, information misinterpretation/unfamiliarity with resources as evidenced by questions, statement of concern, inaccurate follow-through of instruction/ development of preventable complications.	Provide information about diseases and need for protection.	Provides knowledge base for patient to make informed choices. May enhance cooperation with regimen.	Verbalizes understanding of disease process and need for immunizations. Participates in treatment regimen.
	Review expected side effects and potential adverse reactions which need to be reported.	Preparation for normalcy of reaction helps patient cope with minor discomforts and recognize more serious problems.	
	Discuss correct regimen for booster shots.	Full course of immunization promotes optimal protection.	
	Instruct in proper after-care, e.g., do not apply heat or cold to local reaction, use antipyretics to relieve fever.	Improper care can increase reactions.	
Infection, potential related to inadequate acquired immunity.	Administer serum, (e.g., immune globulin, Hyper-Tet); vaccine, (e.g., Mumpsvax, Fluogen); or toxoid, (e.g., DPT), according to individual need.	Although some people are born with innate immunity to certain diseases, the majority of the population have to acquire immunity in some way.	Verbalizes understanding of individual causative risk factor(s). Achieves immunity.
	Discuss need to contact physician/public health department before traveling out of country.	Detrmines need for additional immunizations related to specific area individual is visiting.	
	Instruct patient to maintain record of vaccination/booster shots.	Proof of immunization for certain diseases is required by schools and health departments in an effort to control outbreaks of disease and for determining future health care needs.	

Table 64-5. RECOMMENDED SCHEDULE FOR CHILDHOOD IMMUNIZATIONS

Age	Immunization
2 mos	DPT, OPV
4 mos	DPT, OPV
6 mos	DPT, OPV
12 mos	TB Test*
15 mos	DPT, OPV, MMR
18 mos	Hib
4–6 yr	DPT, OPV
14–16 yr	Td†

KEY:

DPT—Diphtheria and tetanus toxoids with pertussis vaccine.
OPV—Oral, attenuated poliovirus vaccine containing types 1, 2, and 3.
Td—Adult tetanus toxoid (full dose) and diphtheria toxoid (reduced dose) in combination.
Hib—Conjugate *Hemophilus influenza* type b vaccine.
MMR—Live measles, mumps and rubella viruses in a combined vaccine.

*May be repeated every 2 years.
†Repeat every 10 years for life.

Table 64-6. RECOMMENDED IMMUNIZATION SCHEDULES FOR INFANTS AND CHILDREN NOT INITIALLY IMMUNIZED AT USUAL RECOMMENDED TIMES IN EARLY INFANCY

Time of Visit	Immunization
First visit	DPT, OPV, TB test
1 mo after first visit	MMR (not given before age 15 mos) Hib (for children aged 18–60 mos)
2 mo after first visit	DPT, OPV
4 mo after first visit	DPT, OPV
10–16 mos after last dose	DPT, OPV
Preschool	DPT, OPV (may not be necessary if last DPT and OPV given after age 4 years.)
14–16-yr-old	Td—repeat every 10 years

KEY:

DPT—Diphtheria and tetanus toxoids with pertussis vaccine.
OPV—Oral, attenuated poliovirus vaccine contains types 1, 2, and 3.
Hib—Conjugated *Hemophilis influenza* type b vaccine.
MMR—Live measles, mumps and rubella viruses in combined vaccine.
Td—Adult tetanus toxoid (full dose) and diphtheria (reduced dose) in combination.

response to oral poliovirus vaccine or to yellow fever vaccine.

NURSING DIAGNOSIS

Typical nursing diagnoses for a patient receiving immunizations are included in Table 64–4.

PLANNING AND INTERVENTION

During the planning stage, the nurse prepares the immunization. Vaccines are stored according to manufacturers' instructions following their specific recommendations for temperature and light as listed in Table 64–3. Most vaccines should be stored in the refrigerator, not on the door. The temperature is higher on the door. If vaccines are to be transported, ice packs are used to protect vaccines, and they are transported in styrofoam containers. Polio vaccines should be transported with dry ice only.

The nurse is most often responsible for administering the vaccine, so the correct site for injection must be known. Most vaccines are mixed just prior to administration.

Vaccines are often administered on an outpatient basis, so the nurse is responsible for providing the patient with information about potential adverse reactions, home treatment for these reactions, and when to call the physician. If additional injections or boosters are necessary, the nurse teaches the patient about when to return to the clinic or doctor's office. A patient teaching table (Table 64–7) is included with additional information that should be taught to the patient. Many fact sheets are available from the Centers for Disease Control in Atlanta. Figure 64–5 is an example of such a form available about polio vaccine.

EVALUATION

Immunizations are, for the most part, very safe and effective drugs. However, any drug can have side effects or complications. Localized redness and swelling at the injection site and fever are common reactions. Minor symptoms that mimic the disease itself are also common. For example, mild rashes may follow the injection of the measles and rubella vaccine, and minor swelling of the salivary glands may follow the administration of the mumps vaccine. About 5% of the children who get

Table 64-7. PATIENT TEACHING INFORMATION—IMMUNIZATIONS

Dear Patient:
    This drug has been prescribed for you. This is what you should know about your drug to get the most from your therapy.

1. This immunization will protect your from . . . (disease) . . . for approximately . . . (time period) . . . It may then be necessary to receive a booster.
2. Typical side effects from your immunization include redness and soreness and also _____.
    Call your doctor if severe side effects occur.

IMPORTANT INFORMATION ABOUT
POLIO AND ORAL POLIO VACCINE
Please read this carefully

WHAT IS POLIO? Polio is a virus disease that may cause permanent crippling (paralysis) and occasionally death. There used to be thousands of cases and hundreds of deaths from polio every year in the United States. Because of the widespread use of polio vaccines, which became available beginning in the mid-1950's, polio disease has nearly been eliminated from the United States. Although thousands of cases continue to occur each year in the rest of the world, in the United States during the past 5 years there have been only 67 cases of polio reported, an average of 13 cases per year. Our success in preventing the spread of wild polio virus has been so great that most of the recent cases (approximately nine per year) have resulted from the rare side effects of oral polio vaccine (see below). Because of this fact, some people have asked why we should continue to use polio vaccine. The reason is that, even though we may not have much wild polio virus spreading here now, there is so much of it in the rest of the world that there is a great risk of its being reestablished if our children are not vaccinated.

ORAL LIVE POLIO VACCINE: Immunization with oral live polio vaccine (OPV) is one of the best ways to prevent polio. It is given by mouth starting in early infancy. Several doses are needed to provide good protection. Young children should get two or more doses in the first year of life and another dose at about 18 months of age. An additional dose is important for children when they enter school or when there is a high risk of polio, for example, during an epidemic or when traveling to a place where polio is common. The vaccine is easy to take and is effective in preventing the spread of polio. In over 90 percent of people, OPV gives protection for a long time, probably for life. Because OPV viruses live for a time in the intestinal tract of the person who is vaccinated, some of the viruses pass in the stool and can spread from the vaccinated person to those in close contact (usually household members). This may help to immunize these persons and is one of the advantages of OPV. The Immunization Practices Advisory Committee of the Public Health Service and the American Academy of Pediatrics recommend oral live polio vaccine as the preferred polio vaccine for people up to the 18th birthday.

POSSIBLE SIDE EFFECTS FROM THE VACCINE: OPV very rarely (once in about every 8.1 million doses of OPV distributed) causes paralytic polio in the person who is vaccinated. The risk may be slightly higher in adults being vaccinated and substantially higher in persons with abnormally low resistance to infection. Also very rarely (once in about every 5 million doses of OPV distributed) paralytic polio may develop in a close contact of a recently vaccinated person. Even though these risks are very low, they should be recognized. The risk of side effects from the vaccine must be balanced against the risk of the disease, both now and in the future.

(PLEASE READ OTHER SIDE)

PREGNANCY: Polio vaccine experts do not think oral polio vaccine can cause special problems for pregnant women or their unborn babies. However, doctors usually avoid giving any drugs or vaccines to pregnant women unless there is a specific need. Pregnant women should check with a doctor before taking oral polio vaccine.

WARNING—SOME PERSONS SHOULD NOT TAKE ORAL POLIO VACCINE WITHOUT CHECKING WITH A DOCTOR:
- Anyone with cancer, leukemia, or lymphoma.
- Anyone with a disease that lowers the body's resistance to infection.
- Anyone taking a drug that lowers the body's resistance to infection, such as cortisone or prednisone.
- Anyone who lives in the same household with anyone who has one of the conditions listed above.
- Anyone who is sick right now with something more serious than a cold.
- Pregnant women.
- Most persons age 18 and older because adults have a slightly bigger risk of developing paralysis from oral polio vaccine than children (However, if the risk of polio is increased—as may occur, for example, when there is an outbreak in your community—most polio experts recommend that unprotected persons receive oral polio vaccine regardless of age.)

NOTE ON INJECTABLE (KILLED) POLIO VACCINE: Besides the oral polio vaccine (OPV), there is also a killed polio vaccine (IPV) given by injection which protects against polio after several shots. This killed polio vaccine has no known risk of causing paralytic polio. Because OPV may provide lifetime protection, seems to provide stronger immunity in the intestinal tract (where infection first occurs), is simpler to administer, and is more effective in preventing the spread of polio virus than IPV, most polio experts feel that oral vaccine is more effective for controlling polio in the United States. Injectable polio vaccine is recommended for persons needing polio vaccination who have low resistance to serious infections or who live with persons with low resistance to serious infections. It may also be recommended for previously unvaccinated adults who plan to travel to a place where polio is common or for previously unvaccinated adults whose children are to be vaccinated with OPV. It is not widely used in this country at the present time, but it is available. If you would like to know more about this type of polio vaccine, or wish to receive this vaccine, please ask us.

QUESTIONS: If you have any questions about polio or polio vaccination, please ask us now or call your doctor or health department before you sign this form.

REACTIONS: If the person who received the vaccine gets sick and visits a doctor, hospital, or clinic in the 4 weeks after vaccination, please report it to:

Figure 64–5. Important Information About Polio and Oral Polio Vaccine obtained from the Centers for Disease Control, Atlanta, Georgia, or most local health departments.

the rubella vaccine complain of some aching and swelling of the joints. Common side effects should be explained to the client and family before an immunization is given so that they are not surprised or alarmed when they occur. Any unusual reaction is reported immediately to a physician, who will forward this information to the Centers for Disease Control. To prevent possible complications, any woman who is pregnant or planning to become pregnant in the immediate future should consult with her physician before receiving any immunization.

If febrile reactions occur, antipyretics can be used to relieve symptoms. If local reaction occurs, the patient is told not to apply heat or cold because both are likely to increase the local reaction. To reduce local subcutaneous skin reactions, the needle can be changed after the liquid is withdrawn from the vial. This is particularly helpful with DPT.

In past years there have been numerous claims against manufacturers of vaccines because of liability. The 1987 National Childhood Vaccine Injury Act states that all claims are to be submitted to the CDC. The reportable and possible compensable events include:

The DTP, P, DTP/Polio which result in anaphylaxis or anaphylactic shock in 24 hours; encephalopathy (or encephalitis) in seven days; shock-collapse or hypotonic-hyporesponsive collapse in seven days; residual seizure disorder in seven days; or any acute complication or sequela (including death) or above events with no time limit.

The measles, mumps, and rubella; DT, Td, tetanus toxoid which result in anaphylaxis or anaphylactic shock within 24 hours, encephalopathy (or encephalitis) within 15 days for measles, mumps, and rubella vaccines, seven days for DT, Td, and T toxoids; residual seizure disorder with no time limit; or any acute complication or sequela (including death) or above events with no time limit.

Oral polio vaccine which results in paralytic poliomyelitis in a nonimmunodeficient recipient within 30 days, in an immunodeficient recipient within six months; in a vaccine-associated community case with no time limit; or any acute complication or sequela (including death) of above events with no time limit.

Inactivated polio vaccine which results in anaphylaxis or anaphylactic shock within 24 hours; and any acute complication or sequela (including death) of above events with no time limit.

An award to a legitimate claimant includes medical expenses and projected loss of income for a person's lifetime.

The importance of immunization should be stressed to parents. Parental complacency about childhood illnesses or fear of complications or both may result in failure to have their child immunized and could result in contraction of childhood illnesses having very serious, long-term complications.

SUMMARY

Many immunizations are available as serums to produce passive immunity, or toxoids and vaccines to produce active immunity. Immunizations are used to acquire immunity or to protect an individual after exposure to various diseases.

The nurse has an important role in promoting public safety by case finding and disease prevention. The nurse must assess the current immunization history of the individual. Public education is also needed so that people understand the reasons for seeking health care in the case of injury, animal bite, or exposure to various contagious diseases that may require therapeutic treatment or prophylaxis. The nurse also must be knowledgeable about how to store and administer immunizations and the various side effects that can occur.

BIBLIOGRAPHY

A more potent inactivated polio vaccine. The Medical Letter on Drugs and Therapeutics 30(765):50, 1988.

ACIP update: Prevention of *Hemophilus influenzae* type B disease. Texas Preventable Disease News 48(10), 1988.

Adverse events following immunization. Morbidity and Mortality Weekly Report 34(3):43, 1985.

Brunell, PA, et al: *Hemophilus* type B polysaccharide vaccine. Pediatrics 76(2):322, 1985.

Brunell, PA, et al: Recommendations for using pneumococcal vaccine in children. Pediatrics 75(5):1153, 1985.

Cates, KL: *Hemophilus influenzae* type B polysaccharide vaccine. Pediatr Ann 15:461, 1986.

Church, JA and Richards, W: Recurrent abscess formation following DTP immunizations: Association with hypersensitivity to tetanus toxoid. Pediatrics 75(5):889, 1985.

Clements, J: Immunization is not enough. World Health :21, December 1987.

Connaught Laboratories Ltd: Poliovirus vaccine inactivated (drug insert). Willowdale, Ontario, 1986.

Diphtheria, tetanus, and pertussis: Guidelines for vaccine prophylaxis and other preventive measures: Recommendation of the immunization practices advisory committee. Ann Intern Med 103:896, 1985.

Granoff, DM and Cates, KL: *Hemophilus influenzae* type B polysaccharide vaccines. J Pediatr 107(3):330, 1985.

Health Guide for Travelers. Erie County Department of Health, Buffalo, NY.

Kelley, B: To get the shot, or not? Hippocrates 2(6):30, 1988.

Mansell, KA: New immunization against *H influenzae* type B. Ped Nsg 11:433, 1985.

Measles Revaccination. The Medical Letter 31(797):69–70, July 28, 1989.

Minnefor, AB, et al: IV immune globulin: Efficacy and safety. Hosp Pract 22(10):171, 1987.

Pittitteri, A: Child Health Nursing. Little, Brown & Co, 1987.

Prince, AM, et al: Effect of Cohn fractionation conditions on infectivity of the AIDS virus. N Engl J Med 314:386, 1986.

Renn, M: Prevention in triplicate: Three part vaccination for measles, mumps and rubella. Nurs Times 83(44):16, 1987.

Sadler, C: Hepatitis B: Cause for grievance? Nurs Times 83(45):22, 1987.

Salerno, C and Jackson, M: What does the national childhood vaccine injury act require of the nurse? AJN 88(7):1019–1020, July 1988.

Salomon, M, et al: Evaluation of the two-needle strategy for reducing reactions to DPT vaccination. Am J Dis Child 141:796, 1987.

Sims, R, et al: The clinical effectiveness of pneumococcal vaccine in the elderly. Annals of Int Med 108:653–657, May 1988.

Wells, MA, et al: Inactivation and partition of human T-cell lymphotropic virus, type III, during ethanol fractionation of plasma. Transfusion 26:210, 1986.

Whiteman, KF: Why bother about flu shots? Am J Nurs 87(11):1408, 1987.

U.S. Centers for Disease Control: Safety of therapeutic immune globulin preparations with respect to transmission of human T-lymphotropic virus type III/lymphadenopathy-associated virus infection. Morbidity and Mortality Weekly Report, 35:231, 1986.

U.S. Federal Drug Administration: General biological products standards, additional standards for human blood and blood products: Test for antibody to human immunodeficiency virus (HIV). Federal Register 53:111, 1988.

SITUATION 64–1

Evelyn Perez, aged 21 years, has given birth to a healthy baby girl named Alisa. Mrs. Perez is being cared for on the postpartum unit.

1. Mrs. Perez is to receive Rho(D) Immune Globulin. The nurse is aware that:
   a. the mother is Rh negative and daughter Rh positive
   b. the daughter is Rh negative and the mother Rh positive
   c. the daughter is Rh negative and the mother Rh negative
   d. the mother is Rh positive and the daughter is Rh positive

2. The nurse will plan to administer the RhoGAM injection within how many hours of delivery?
   a. 8
   b. 72
   c. 48
   d. 12

3. Mrs. Perez is concerned about when Alisa should begin immunizations. The nurse will explain that the earliest age for beginning immunization is:
   a. 12 days
   b. 1 year
   c. 4 months
   d. 2 months

4. When Mrs. Perez brings Alisa in to the Well Baby Clinic for immunization, which of the following findings would contraindicate immunization at this time?
   a. anemia
   b. malnutrition
   c. active infection
   d. slowed development

5. After Alisa receives the Diptheria and Tetanus Toxoid and Pertussis (DPT) vaccine, the nurse will teach Mrs. Perez about potential side effects, which include:
   a. mild arthralgia and lymphadenitis
   b. abdominal pain and tremors
   c. anorexia and fretfulness
   d. paralysis and hypertension

6. When Alisa is 15 months old, the nurse will plan to administer the following:
   a. DPT and DPV
   b. DPT and TB test
   c. DPT, OPV, and MMR
   d. TB test and OPV

Please refer to the Appendices for correct answers and additional review questions with answers.

65

CHAPTER

EMERGENCY SITUATIONS

GLOSSARY TERMS IN THIS CHAPTER

Cardiac output
Malpractice
Negligence
Pulmonary artery pressure
Systemic vascular resistance

65

CHAPTER

EMERGENCY SITUATIONS

MERRILY MATHEWSON KUHN, R.N.C., Ph.D., CCRN

LEARNING OBJECTIVES

After reading this chapter, the student will be able to:

1. Identify those medications commonly used in emergency situations.

2. Identify specific areas to assess in the patient requiring medications in emergency situations in order to formulate appropriate nursing diagnoses.

3. Plan the nursing interventions necessary to administer medications in emergency situations and choose appropriate teaching strategies to gain patient compliance.

4. Evaluate the patient at various stages of treatment to gauge effectiveness of nursing interventions.

Emergency situations occur at any time and place. The nurse working in an intensive care area, emergency room, or operating room is frequently confronted with emergency situations. However, the nurse working in hospital clinics, industrial locations, nursing homes, public health facilities, or schools can also be confronted with emergencies. In any emergency situation, regardless of its origin, the nurse is expected to function calmly and efficiently.

The terms acute care and critical care are not synonymous, although they are sometimes used that way in hospitals to describe the intensive care unit. Patients in critical care require intensive medical intervention in a life-threatening situation. Acute care is needed when the individual requires hospitalization for emergent or nonemergent intervention.

This chapter briefly summarizes the emergency situations previously discussed in this text in an easy-to-use table. This table can serve as a fast reference source in an emergency situation, as well as to refer the reader to the chapter where more information can be located. Table 65–1 features the emergency condition along with its most common assessable finding, the drug of choice with its primary reason for administration, and its usual dose and route. Each drug is then referenced to the chapter in this text where a more detailed discussion can be found. The majority of these are potent, dangerous medications with many adverse effects, interactions, and contraindications. The nurse must know how these might act and interact within the body before administering them.

CONSIDERATIONS FOR DRUG THERAPY IN THE CRITICAL CARE SETTING

Patients admitted to an intensive care unit (ICU) are most likely to receive multiple drug therapy, experience drug–drug interactions, experience altered pharmacokinetic behavior, and incur drug-induced toxicity. In addition, these patients commonly have multiple disease processes and require supplemental intravenous or enteral nutritional support. The situation is often intimidating to many health-care professionals; however, a sound understanding of pathophysiology and therapeutics often allows one to see past the intravenous lines and various life-support systems and provide appropriate drug therapy.

ALTERED DRUG PHARMACOKINETIC BEHAVIOR

When administering medications to the critically ill, the medical team is concerned with the relationship between the dose of the drug given and the response elicited. The obvious goal is to attain a therapeutic effect

while minimizing toxicity. It is important for the nurse to have an understanding of normal pharmacokinetics so that he/she is able to identify differences in the critically ill. Ultimately, all drugs administered to the critically ill should reach an end point of clinical efficacy, not simply the attainment of a certain blood level.

Absorption

In the acute care setting, the usual route of drug administration, oral ingestion, is inappropriate for various reasons. Patients who are comatose, experiencing gastrointestinal bleeding, or recovering from surgery may not be able to receive medicine orally. In addition, many new medications are not available as oral preparations and so require parenteral (IV or IM) administration.

The intravenous route is generally preferred in acute situations. The medication is placed directly into the vascular system and the onset of action is often within minutes. The nurse must be knowledgeable about mixing and administration of these medications. For example, a bolus of digoxin or lasix is given undiluted over ten minutes; Dilantin is given no faster than at 50 mg/minute and no faster; and protamine sulfate is given over a 10–15-minute period. Administering medications at a faster rate may increase the incidence of adverse effects, including hypotension and dysrhythmia.

Intramuscular administration is another common method of providing drug therapy. However, in this setting, patients who are hypotensive, such as those with septic shock or severe cardiac failure, are not given IM injections. When the blood pressure is lower than normal, blood is shunted away from the peripheral areas of the body. This usually leads to underperfusion of skeletal muscle, and thus erratic drug absorption may occur. In hypotensive patients, the intravenous route is preferred.

When oral administration is possible, certain factors that affect drug absorption must still be considered. Patients with severe edema (congestive heart failure, nephrotic syndrome, cirrhosis, hypoproteinemia) often have fluid accumulation within the intestinal mucosa, which reduces absorption. Also many patients in the ICU receive continuous antacid administration to prevent stress-related ulceration of the gastrointestinal tract. In this situation, the patient's drug therapy is reviewed to identify any medication in which absorption may be altered by concurrent antacid administration (oral digitalis drugs, tetracyclines, quinidine, and salicylates).

The amount of drug absorbed is dependent on its bioavailability. Product formulation and intestinal transit time are important determinants of drug bioavailability. If the formulation dissolves very slowly and the patient has a shortened bowel or rapid intestinal transit because of disease or other drugs, the medications may not spend sufficient time in the intestinal tract for normal absorption to occur. If bioavailability is increased and the ability to metabolize drugs is decreased, such as with liver disease (clearance has decreased), then the overall effect on the serum concentration at steady state has been increased disproportionately to the effect that would occur by changing bioavailability or clearance alone. Thus, critically ill patients may require substantial dosing modifications in order to avoid toxicity from some orally administered drugs.

Rate of absorption can also be affected in the critically ill. Consequently, serum drug levels are obtained to assess clinical end points in individual patients to discern the overall effect of the change in absorption.

Distribution

Following administration, factors controlling drug distribution from the blood to the tissues are complex and often altered in critically ill patients. One of the factors affecting drug distribution from the blood to the tissues is the amount of protein present in plasma. Many drugs (usually acidic drugs) are highly bound to serum albumin, the major serum protein. Only unbound drug in the blood can diffuse or be transported into tissues. In certain disease states (cirrhosis, nephrotic syndrome, malnutrition, and others), the serum albumin concentration is lower than normal and drugs many display altered distribution characteristics. Highly bound drugs like penicillins, cephalosporins, sulfonamides, anticoagulants, nonsteroidal anti-inflammatory drugs, and propranolol, to name just a few, are affected by their relative concentrations in the blood, by changes in circulating protein concentrations, and by diseases such as uremia that can result in accumulation of endogenous competitors for binding and/or alter the binding characteristics. When there is displacement from binding, drug effect is increased. The increased free drug is also available for elimination. The overall result can be a new steady state. Digoxin, although not highly bound, can have clinically relevant changes in drug distribution. In patients with end-stage renal disease, a reduced maintenance dose is required, as there is decreased ability of the kidney to eliminate digoxin, and the drug is distributed into a smaller volume.

Patients with severe cirrhosis or portosystemic shunts do not distribute drugs to the liver well. Since many drugs are metabolized in the liver, this decreased distribution and metabolism can lead to toxic effects.

Another situation affecting drug distribution is seen in patients who have had an acute traumatic injury or major abdominal surgery. In these patients, levels of certain proteins increase in the serum and may bind to drugs and alter their ability to distribute into tissue. This area is relatively new and is currently under intensive research.

Metabolism

The major site of drug metabolism is the liver. In the critical care setting, numerous factors can alter hepatic metabolism of drugs. Drugs absorbed through the gastrointestinal system are delivered to the liver. If drugs have a high first-pass effect or presystemic elimination, like propranolol, their rate of biotransformation can be drastically reduced if liver disease is present. Patients with underlying hepatic disease may be admitted to the ICU for treatment of another medical problem requiring drug therapy with agents that are metabolized by the liver.

The liver has a variety of pathways by which it can metabolize drugs: the microsomal enzyme system; the cytochrome P-450 system; and through reactions that include acetylation, methylation, conjugation, hydrolysis, and reduction. The microsomal enzyme system can be induced with drugs like phenobarbital or phenytoin.

Another factor affecting hepatic metabolism is the addition of an agent that decreases the metabolizing capability of the microsomal enzyme system. Cimetidine (Tagamet) or chloramphenicol (Chloromycetin) for infection is an example of administering drugs that prevent hepatic metabolism of other drugs. Cimetidine and chloramphenicol have been reported to potentiate the effects of drugs such as warfarin (Coumadin), beta-blockers, lidocaine, phenytoin, theophylline, benzodiazepines, and narcotic analgesics. Changes via effects on hepatic metabolism, whether caused by disease or other drugs, must be anticipated to select proper dosing regimens for individual patients.

Half-life may also be affected in the critically ill. The most important use of half-life is to predict how long it takes a dosing regimen to achieve steady state concentration in the blood. When therapy is instituted, if a loading dose is not administered, then it will take four to five half-lives for the drug to reach steady state. Serum levels of drugs must be drawn appropriately to determine steady state. As an example, digoxin has a half-life of approximately 36 hours. Steady state is achieved in a patient with normal kidneys in about one week. If a serum level to determine steady state is drawn in two days, the physician will obtain little insight into the patient's therapeutic drug level. Changing the dosage before the patient has reached steady state can prove confusing and be potentially hazardous for the patient.

In emergency situations, loading doses are usually administered intravenously. They should always be given over three to five minutes to prevent unnecessary complications.

Excretion

Drugs are primarily excreted from the body via the kidneys; however, certain medications are also secreted into the bile and are thus excreted in feces. The kidneys also eliminate the metabolites of drugs that have been metabolized by the liver.

Many critically ill patients may have underperfused kidneys, have pre-existing renal disease, or develop acute renal failure while in the hospital. For this reason, renal function markers (creatinine, BUN) are followed closely, and doses of drugs excreted by the kidneys are adjusted accordingly where indicated.

Finally, many medications administered to critically ill patients may be nephrotoxic, such as aminoglycosides and amphotericin B. All drugs prescribed in this

TEXT RESUMES ON PAGE 1788

Table 65–1. SUMMARY OF EMERGENCY SITUATIONS AND DRUG MANAGEMENT

Condition	Assessment Findings	Drug of Choice	Uses
Acute adrenal insufficiency	Dehydration, hypotension, weakness, fever, lethargy, nausea, vomiting, abdominal pain. Check the following laboratory data: serum sodium, serum glucose, and serum potassium.	Hydrocortisone sodium phosphate (Hydrocortone Phosphate) or hydrocortisone sodium succinate (Solu-Cortef). NOTE: Fluid replacement is also critical and is usually carried out with isotonic sodium chloride or glucose in saline.	Replacement of glucocorticoids.
Acute pulmonary edema	Intense dyspnea, tachycardia, hypotension, crackles, intense anxiety, pink frothy sputum. Laboratory data: ECG changes, chest x-ray changes, acid–base changes.	Digoxin (Lanoxin)	Strengthen and slow cardiac rate.
		Aminophylline	Bronchial dilatation
		Furosemide (Lasix)	Reduce fluid overload.
		Morphine sulfate	Reduce anxiety and tachypnea. Reduces preload.
Cardiac dysrhythmias	Irregular pulse with changes in blood pressure and neurologic status. Laboratory data: ECG changes.	Atropine	Sinus bradycardia, first-degree atrioventricular block.
		Lidocaine (Xylocaine)	Ventricular dysrhythmias: premature ventricular contractions (PVCs), ventricular tachycardia
		Phenytoin (Dilantin)	Paroxysmal atrial tachycardia (PAT) (especially due to digitalis toxicity), ventricular dysrhythmias.
		Procainamide (Pronestyl)	Atrial dysrhythmias; premature atrial contractions (PACs), atrial fibrillation, paroxysmal atrial tachycardia (PAT). Ventricular arrhythmias: premature ventricular contractions (PVCs), ventricular tachycardia.
		Propranolol (Inderal)	Atrial dysrhythmias: atrial fibrillation, atrial flutter, PAT. Ventricular dysrhythmias (associated with digitalis toxicity).
		Quinidine	Atrial dysrhythmias: PACs, atrial fibrillation, atrial flutter, PAT, atrioventricular junctional tachycardia, ventricular dysrhythmias, PVCs.
		Verapamil (Calan)	Supraventricular tachycardia, PAT, atrial flutter, atrial fibrillation.

Dosage	Route	Side and Toxic Effects	Chapter
Adults: 100-mg bolus, then 100 mg q 8 hr or 50–100 mg q 6 hr.	IV	Few side effects on short-term use. Cushing's syndrome; reactivation of ulcer, arrested tuberculosis, or fungal lung infection on long-term, high-dose administration.	42
Adults: 0.125–0.5 mg q 6–8 hr (total 2–3 mg), or 0.25–0.5 mg q 2–4 hr (total 0.75–1.5 mg) Children: 0.03–0.08 mg/kg, or 0.03–0.06 mg/kg.	PO, IV	GI: nausea, vomiting. CNS: nervous irritability, restlessness, blurred vision, alteration in color vision. Cardiac: ventricular bigeminy, ectopic junctional or atrial beats (children), conduction disturbances.	28
Adults, loading dose: 5–7 mg/kg (400 mg average) over 20 min; then 0.5–0.9 mg/kg/hr by continuous infusion (NOTE: no loading dose required for patient who has received oral theophylline regularly).	IV	Ventricular arrhythmias, throbbing, headache, tremor, weakness, reduced renal blood flow.	35
Adults: 20–100 mg bolus repeated q 6–8 hr Children: 2 mg/kg bolus repeated q 6–8 hr	IV	Potassium loss; excess sodium and water loss if overtreated.	38
Adults: 5–15 mg Children: 0.1–0.2 mg/kg	SC	Respiratory depression	20
Adults: 0.4–0.6 mg bolus Children: 0.01 mg/kg bolus	IV	Dryness of mouth; pupillary dilation	18
Adults: 50–100-mg bolus, then 2–4 mg/min infusion after bolus Children: 1 mg/kg bolus; then 1 mg/kg/hr infusion after bolus	IV	Convulsions, sinus arrest.	30
Adults: 50–100 mg bolus q 5 min (up to 1 g)	IV	Hypotension, cardiovascular collapse, CNS depression.	30
Adults: 0.5–1 g q 6 hr Children: 32–50 mg/kg/24 hr	PO, IM	Bitter taste, mental depression, psychosis, hypotension	30
Adults: 250–500 mg/500 ml Children: 2 mg/kg/min	IV	Same as above.	
Adults: 10–40 mg q 6–8 hr	PO	Aggravation of congestive heart failure and bronchial asthma; hypotension.	29, 19
Adults: 0.5–1 mg q 3–5 min (up to 5 mg)	IV		
Adults: 200–400 mg q 6 hr Children: 20–30 mg/kg/24 hr	PO, IM PO, IM	Paradoxical tachycardia, embolism, hypotension, tinnitus.	30
Adults: 10–30 mg Children: 0.1–0.3 mg/kg	PO	Hypotension, peripheral vasodilation	30

CONTINUED ON THE FOLLOWING PAGE

Table 65-1. SUMMARY OF EMERGENCY SITUATIONS AND DRUG MANAGEMENT–*CONTINUED*

Condition	Assessment Findings	Drug of Choice	Uses
Cholinergic crisis	Diplopia, dysarthria, difficulty chewing, dyspnea, generalized weakness, restlessness, anxiety, irritability, salivation, anorexia, nausea, burping, vomiting, abdominal cramps, diarrhea, increased bronchial secretions, lacrimation, perspiration, blurred vision, miosis.	Atropine sulfate	Produces an anticholinergic response to modify cholinergic crisis and improve condition.
Cardiac or respiratory arrest	Absence of pulse and respirations. No response to external stimuli. Brain death develops in 4 min if untreated.	Epinephrine (Adrenalin)	Initiate cardiac rhythm in standstill.
		Sodium bicarbonate	Treat acidosis—pH of less than 7.0
Cardiogenic shock	Hypotension, tachycardia, and tachypnea, increasing fatigue, increasing restlessness, lethargy, cool clammy skin.	Digitalis products	Improve cardiac performance.
		Vasopressors: Dopamine (Intropin)	Improves renal perfusion.
		Norepinephrine (Levophed)	Same as above.
		Inotropics: Dobutamine (Dobutrex)	Improves cardiac performance, improves cardiac output.
		Vasodilators: Isoproterenol (Isuprel)	Counteracts vasoconstriction, increases cardiac output, facilitates AV conduction
		Nitroglycerin	Reduces preload, dilates venous capacitance vessels.
Diabetic ketoacidosis	Kussmaul respirations, flushed dry skin, acetone odor to breath, dehydration, hypotension, shock, coma, or stupor. Laboratory data: elevated blood sugar (over 300 mg/100 ml), acidosis, glycosuria.	Regular insulin	Lowers blood glucose level.
Hemorrhagic shock	Increased anxiety, lethargy, coma, hypotension, cool clammy skin, anorexia, increasing fatigue, tachypnea. Laboratory data: decreased hemoglobin and hematocrit.	Ringer's lactate	Replace volume
		Whole blood and components	Replace volume
		Dopamine (Intropin)	Elevate blood pressure (correct hypovolemia first)
		Norepinephrine (Levophed)	Same as above.
Hypertensive crisis	Sustained blood pressure over 120 diastolic, severe retinopathy, renal impairment, headache, hypertensive encephalopathy.	Diazoxide (Hyperstat IV)	Causes vasodilation of peripheral arterioles.
		Sodium nitroprusside (Nipride)	Potent-acting vasodilator.
		Trimethaphan (Arfonad)	Ganglionic-blocking agent that produces vasodilation.
		Hydralazine (Apresoline)	Causes arteriolar vasodilation, thereby reducing vascular resistance.
		Propranolol (Inderal)	Adrenergic-blocking agent.
		Furosemide (Lasix)	Reduce fluid volume.

Dosage	Route	Side and Toxic Effects	Chapter
Adults: 0.4–0.6 mg; may repeat q 4–6 hr (will need to recheck dosage)	IV, IM	Thirst, headache, dry and flushed skin, fever, drowsiness, vomiting, dizziness, tachycardia and palpitations, urinary hesitancy, constipation, hypertension, restlessness, respiratory depression, death.	18
Adults: 1–2 mg bolus Children: 0.25–1.0 mg bolus Adults and children: 1–2 mg of 1:10,000 solution	IV	Ventricular dysrhythmias, may produce throbbing, headache, tremor, weakness; reduces renal blood flow and glomerular filtration.	19
Adults: 1–2 amp bolus or as indicated by blood gases Children: 1 mEq/kg; repeat as necessary after pH check	IV	Alkalosis.	58
Varies	IV	See acute pulmonary edema.	28
Adults and children: 0.5–5.0 µg/kg/min	IV	Ectopic dysrhythmias; tachycardia, anginal pains, palpitations, tissue sloughing.	19
Adults: 2–4 µg/min Children: 0.1–1 µg/min	IV	Same as above.	19
Adults: 5–15 µg/kg/min	IV	Elevation of blood pressure and cardiac rate.	
Adults: 1–4 mg by drip rate 1–6 µg/min Children: 0.1–0.5 µg/kg/min	IV	Hypotension	19, 35
0.6–12 mg/hr when urgent.	IV	Hypotension, headache, & flushing.	31
Varies, depending on blood glucose level; often between 100 and 200 units.	IV, IM	Insulin shock if overtreated.	44
1000 ml or more	IV	Hypervolemia if overtreated.	11
500 ml or more	IV		12
Adults and children: 2–50 µg/kg/min	IV	Ectopic dysrhythmias, tachycardia, anginal pains, palpitations, tissue sloughing.	19
Adults: 2–4 µg/min Children: 0.1–1 µg/min	IV	Same as above.	19
Adults: 30-mg bolus over 30 sec	IV	Tachycardia, sodium and water retention, hyperglycemia, abdominal discomfort, orthostatic hypotension.	29
Adults: 3 µg/kg/min	IV	Restlessness, agitation, muscle twitching, bone marrow depression.	29
Adults: 1–4 mg/min	IV	Respiratory depression, tachycardia.	29
Adults: 20–40 mg bolus Children: 0.15 mg/kg bolus (not greater than 20 mg)	IV	Headache, palpitations, anxiety, depression, angina, edema, chills, lupus syndrome.	29
Adults 1–3 mg bolus	IV	See cardiac dysrhythmias.	29
Adults: 20–100 mg bolus Children: 2 mg/kg bolus repeated q 6–8 hr	IV	See acute pulmonary edema.	38

CONTINUED ON THE FOLLOWING PAGE

Condition	Assessment Findings	Drug of Choice	Uses
Hypotensive crisis	Blood pressure less than 80 mm Hg systolic, cool clammy skin, tachycardia, tachypnea, lethargy.	Dopamine (Intropin) Norepinephrine (Levophed) Dobutamine (Dobutrex)	Elevate blood pressure (correct hypovolemia first). Same as above. Improve cardiac performance, improves cardiac output.
Insulin shock	Diaphoresis, weakness, nervousness, shakiness, irritability, impaired vision, headache, unconsciousness, convulsions Laboratory data: blood glucose decreases below 50 mg/100 ml.	Glucagon	Elevates blood glucose level.
Myasthenic crisis	Ptosis, diplopia, dysarthria, dysphagia, difficulty chewing, dyspnea, generalized weakness, restlessness, anxiety, irritability.	Edrophonium chloride (Tensilon) Pyridostigmine (Mestinon)	To distinguish between myasthenic and cholinergic crises. To improve myasthenic condition.
Narcotic overdosage (including codeine, hydromorphone, morphine, and meperidine)	Respiratory depression, which may progress to apnea, coma, possible seizures, cardiac arrest, circulatory collapse, miosis with morphine derivatives, mydriasis with meperidine derivatives, cold clammy skin, hypothermia, muscular flaccidity.	Naloxone (Narcan)	Narcotic antagonist.
Overdosage of propoxyphene hydrochloride (Darvon)	Stupor, coma, convulsions, ECG abnormalities, circulatory collapse, miosis, diabetes insipidus, respiratory depression.	Naloxone (Narcan)	Antidote.
Status asthmaticus	Prolonged expiratory time, tachypnea, tachycardia, labored breathing, diaphoresis, wheezing (in severe cases, chest may be silent).	Epinephrine. If no response after second dose of epinephrine, then: Aminophylline	Bronchial dilation. Same as above.
Status epilepticus	Rapid recurrence of seizure activity, generally tonic-clonic in nature; respiratory depression, respiratory acidosis, hyperthermia, cardiac decompensation.	Diazepam (Valium) Phenytoin (Dilantin) Phenobarbital (Luminal) Paraldehyde (Paral)	Control seizure activity. Control seizure activity. Control seizure activity. Control seizure activity.

Dosage	Route	Side and Toxic Effects	Chapter
Adults and children: 2–50 µg/kg/min	IV	Ectopic dysrhythmias tachycardia, anginal pain, palpitations, tissue sloughing.	19
Adults: 2–4 µg Children: 0.1–1 µg/min	IV	Same as above.	19
Adults: 5–15 µg/kg/min.	IV	Elevation of blood pressure and cardiac rate.	19
Adults: 0.5–1 mg or more	IV, SC, IM	Hyperglycemia if overtreated.	44
Adults: 1 mg; may repeat once in 1 min	IV	Muscle weakness, respiratory depression and arrest, hypotension, nausea, vomiting, cramps, sweating, increased bronchial secretions.	23
Adults: 2–6 mg, depending on response	IV or IM	Bradycardia, hypotension, thrombophlebitis, GI side effects, increased bronchial secretions.	23
Adults: 0.4 mg; repeat after 2–3 min, up to 3 times if needed. Children: 0.01 mg/kg, repeated after 2–3 min, up to 3 times if needed.	IV, IM, or SC	May precipitate acute withdrawal in patients physically addicted to narcotics. Excessive dosage: increased blood pressure, tremors, hyperventilation, drowsiness, elevated partial thromboplastin time. Drug given too rapidly: nausea, vomiting, sweating, and tachycardia.	20
Adults: 0.4 mg, repeat in 2–3 min prn Children: 0.01 mg/kg, repeat in 2–3 min prn	IV, IM, or SC	Same as above.	20
Adults: 0.2–1.5 mg, up to twice in 20 min	SC	Ventricular dysrhythmias, throbbing, headache, tremor, weakness, reduces renal blood flow.	19
Adults, loading dose: 5–7 mg/kg (400 mg average) over 20 min, then 0.5–0.9 mg/kg/hr by continuous infusion. (NOTE: no loading dose required for patient who has received oral theophylline regularly.)	IV	Same as above.	35
Adults: 5–10 mg bolus, 1–5 mg/min; may repeat twice at 10–15 min intervals; no more than 100 mg in 24 hr.	IV	Drowsiness, sedation, hypotension, bradycardia, cardiac collapse, pain, thrombosis at injection site.	24
Adults and children: If not on phenytoin previously, can load with 10–15 mg/kg bolus; can repeat 100–150 mg q 30 min for adults, not to exceed 1.5 g in 24 hr. For child, can repeat 1.5 mg/kg q 30 min, not to exceed 20 mg/kg in 24 hr.	IV	Sedation, cardiac dysrhythmias, cardiotoxic reactions, hypotension, apnea.	22
Adults: 150–400 mg, 25–50 mg/min, then repeat 120–240 mg q 20 min, not to exceed 1 g in 24 hr. Children: 6 mg/kg, 25–50 mg/min, then repeat 3 mg/kg q 20 min, not to exceed 12 mg/kg in 24 hr.	IV	Drowsiness, sedation, respiratory depression, hypotension, pain, swelling, thrombophlebitis at site of injection.	24, 22
Adults: 2–4 ml/10 ml of 0.9% NaCl at 0.5 ml/min.	IV	Pulmonary edema, hemorrhage, sedation, circulatory and respiratory failure.	24
Infuse 5 ml/500 ml D5W; titrate rate to control seizures.	IV	Pain, abscess, necrosis at injection site.	
8–10 ml mixed with an equal volume of vegetable oil as a retention enema.	Rectal	Irritation of rectal mucosa.	

CONTINUED ON THE FOLLOWING PAGE

Table 65–1. SUMMARY OF EMERGENCY SITUATIONS AND DRUG MANAGEMENT–*CONTINUED*

Condition	Assessment Findings	Drug of Choice	Uses
Thyrotoxic crisis or thyroid storm	Fever above 100°F, tachycardia, congestive heart failure, restlessness, diaphoresis, tremor, CNS dysfunction, somnolence, coma, psychosis, diarrhea, abdominal pain. Laboratory data: hyperglycemia; elevated T_3, T_4, and T_7 values.	Propranolol (Inderal)	Decreases manifestations of crisis; also blocks conversion of thyroxine to triiodothyronine.
		Acetaminophen (avoid aspirin)	Antipyretic.
		Propylthiouracil	Blocks synthesis of thyroid hormone
		Iodide (Lugol's solution; sodium iodide)	Inhibits release of thyroid hormone.
		Hydrocortisone sodium succinate (Solu-Cortef)	To prevent adrenal insufficiency.

setting are reviewed for their potential to injure the kidneys. When prescribed, these agents are monitored closely and renal function indicators followed closely as well.

DRUG–DRUG INTERACTIONS

It is beyond the scope of this chapter to review all potential drug–drug interactions seen in the critical care setting. The reader is urged to review the particular agents the patient is receiving and to screen for potentially detrimental drug interactions.

Patients in critical care are particularly susceptible to drug interactions. Patients frequently receive multiple drugs that have narrow therapeutic indices and/or are frequently implicated in drug interactions. To compound the potential problems, the patient's primary disease can have a great influence on drug disposition and response.

Patients in intensive care units often require drug therapy to support the cardiovascular system and the lungs, and to fight infection. In addition, certain patients may require anticoagulants, anticonvulsants, or some other form of chemotherapy. Often these patients have multiple organ system failure or senescent organ dysfunction. Because patients may need mechanical ventilation with tracheal intubation and often have central nervous system dysfunction, they are unable to verbalize early symptoms of drug toxicity.

Drug–drug interactions can occur for various reasons: alteration in pharmacokinetics, as with absorption, distribution (protein binding), metabolism, and elimination; or alteration in pharmacodynamics. See Chapter 5 for more specific information on these reactions.

Critical care patients are often so ill that adverse drug effects can easily be misinterpreted as manifestations of the patient's underlying condition. Because of this fact, there is great potential for drug interactions in the critical care setting.

With the increasing numbers of new drugs that are available and the use of multiple drugs in any given patient, the potential for drug interaction is limitless. It is important for the patient to be monitored closely and to have the dosage of drugs altered individually considering age and disease states.

Although drugs are prescribed for their beneficial effects, it is not uncommon for patients to experience drug-induced toxicity. The critical care patient often has multiple disease-associated problems requiring numerous drugs administered concurrently.

PHARMACOKINETIC ALTERATIONS WITH DISEASE

Respiratory Disease

The lungs play an active role in the pharmacokinetics of endogenous compounds and certain drugs. The diseased lung may have an important effect on drug requirements in critical care patients through two mechanisms. First, there may be a direct alteration of lung uptake, distribution, metabolism, or clearance of drugs. And, second, there may be an indirect alteration of pharmacokinetics or drug–receptor response.

The patient with overt or impending pulmonary failure rarely has an isolated disease. There are often other associated organ dysfunctions or infections present. Important drug problems often relate to the secondary effect of hemodynamic changes or other organ alterations involved in drug metabolism. Several examples are cited, but for more detailed information see appropriate chapters in this text.

When beta-adrenergic agents, theophylline drugs, or vasodilators are administered, they may diminish hypoxic pulmonary vasoconstriction, particularly in patients with ventilation–perfusion defects. Consequently, the patient who receives nitroglycerin and other nitrates for the treatment of angina may become hypoxemic because of this or other effects on pulmonary function.

Dopamine infusions may also present a problem for the pulmonary patient. Dopamine blunts the peripheral chemoreceptor's response to hypoxemia. Blood gas monitoring or choice of another inotropic agent is appropriate when a patient has compensated respiratory acidosis.

Dosage	Route	Side and Toxic Effects	Chapter
1–3 mg q 3–4 hr	IV	See cardiac dysrhythmias.	19
20–80 mg q 4–6 hr	PO		
600 mg	PO	Liver damage in overdose; little toxicity in normal doses.	20
900–1200 mg	PO	Blood dyscrasias, especially with long-term use.	45
10 gtt tid Lugol's solution	PO	Excessive inhibition of thyroid activity in large doses. Sensitivity to iodine compounds.	45
1 g tid sodium iodide solution	IV		
300 mg/day	IV	See acute adrenal insufficiency.	42

Parenteral nutrition is often used in patients with acute respiratory conditions to help maintain respiratory muscles and to decrease the possibility of sepsis. Overfeeding or feeding formulas high in carbohydrates increase minute carbon dioxide production by elevating the respiratory quotient. Nutritional therapy needs to be specifically tailored to meet the needs of the acutely ill respiratory and ventilated patient.

Respiratory patients often have fluid retention associated with other concurrent diseases. Diuretic therapy along with fluid restriction can precipitate hypokalemia, hypochloremia, or dehydration alkalosis. Progressive carbon dioxide retention and pulmonary decompensation may complicate the already marginal status of the acutely ill patient. Close monitoring of electrolyte and acid–base balance during diuresis will prevent or control this situation.

Heart Disease

Heart failure, associated with several pathophysiologic states, can lead to important alterations in pharmacokinetics and pharmacodynamics. Associated problems that occur in heart failure that can lead to alteration in drug effect include changes in blood pressure, blood volume, hemodynamics, and heart rate and rhythm.

When it is necessary to administer drugs to a patient with heart failure, the IV route is preferable. Titrable drugs with short half-lives that are rapidly metabolized and excreted are drugs of choice. It is necessary to monitor the effectiveness of the kidney and liver function and acid–base balance. Using drugs that have known blood levels and monitoring those levels can help prevent problems.

Liver Disease

Patients with liver disease are often treated with multiple drugs. This use of potent and often multidrip regimens can lead to the frequent drug problems seen in these patients. The liver is the primary organ of metabolism and excretion for many drugs. When the patient has liver disease, the enzyme systems are less effective, blood flow is depressed, protein production is de-

creased, and many of the hemostatic and metabolic functions are compromised. All will have a negative effect on drug utilization.

There are risks associated with all drugs, but there are three groups of drugs that should be used with extreme caution or, better yet, not at all in patients with liver disease. Group I drugs are those capable of causing hepatic damage, even in a person with a healthy liver, such as acetaminophen, acetylsalicylic acid, chlorpromazine, erythromycin estolate, methotrexate, and methyldopa. Group II drugs are those that are capable of compromising liver function such as anabolic and contraceptive steroids, prednisone, and tetracyclines. Group III drugs are those that may make the complications of liver disease worse, such as indomethacin, diuretics, meperidine, and other central nervous system depressants, morphine, pentazocine, and phenylbutazone. Of all these drugs, diuretics have been found to cause the more adverse drug reactions.

Whenever drug therapy is required in patients with liver disease, it is preferable to use drugs whose disposition is least affected by liver dysfunction.

Numerous references are available that review dosage adjustments for the patient with liver disease. These tables can easily be obtained from the pharmacy department.

Renal Disease

Patients with acute renal disease can be given a one-time dose of most drugs. However, the problem is determining both the maintenance dose and at what intervals the drug is to be administered. Patients with acute renal disease may experience acid–base imbalances, fluid derangements, and alterations in blood pressure, all of which can affect drug effectiveness and elimination.

When dosing patients with renal disease, either the dose should be reduced or the dosing interval prolonged to adjust for impaired elimination. Whenever possible, serum drug levels—peaks and troughs—are used to monitor drug therapy.

Serum creatinine level, which relates inversely to the

elimination rate, is often used but is not really a good estimate of renal function in patients with acute renal failure because equilibrium has not been reached. With chronic renal failure, serum creatinine does correlate directly with prolongation of the half-life and inversely with the elimination rate of many drugs.

Patients with acute renal failure may need to be dialyzed. For a drug to be dialyzable, it must be water soluble. Drugs that are generally removed by the kidneys are removed through dialysis, although at different rates of removal.

Many commonly used drugs will have to have their dose adjusted when administered to patients with acute renal failure. These drugs include penicillin, cephalosporins, aminoglycosides, many other antibiotics, sedatives and analgesics, cardiovascular and antihypertensive drugs, and diuretics.

When drugs are required by the patient with acute renal failure, it is preferable to choose an agent that does not depend mainlly on renal excretion and does not have either active or toxic metabolites.

USING THE NURSING PROCESS

ASSESSMENT

Assessment of a patient in an emergency situation begins with a brief but thorough physical assessment of the patient and his or her symptoms—neurologic, cardiac, renal, respiratory, gastrointestinal, musculoskeletal, immunologic, and hematopoietic. The system with the most presenting symptoms receives the first and most thorough assessment.

The nurse assesses for objective signs and symptoms such as presence of extreme restlessness, orthopnea, or dyspnea; the nature of secretions; lung, heart, and gastrointestinal sounds; level of anxiety; hemodynamic status; urinary output; and muscle strength. Laboratory data are obtained, including electrocardiogram (if needed), blood and urine studies, radiographic studies, and drug levels if poisoning is suspected. Chapter 6 reviews commonly overdosed drugs and toxic agents, along with their most common symptoms and management.

Subjective symptoms are elicited from the patient whenever possible, for example, pain, paresthesia, and numbness anywhere in the body; dizziness; headache; fatigue; dyspnea; change in appetite; urinary frequency; and diarrhea.

If a past medical history can be obtained from either the patient or the family, it is important to learn if the present occurrence is similar to any previous occurrence the patient has had. For example, when a male diabetic child presents in a semicomatose condition, the nurse questions the family about the patient's diabetic control. Is he insulin dependent? Did he receive his insulin this morning? Did he eat adequate food to balance the insulin that was received? Did he have any gastrointestinal symptoms? And, has this happened before? Often, by obtaining a thorough history of the present situation from the family or significant other, the nurse can determine the specific cause of the situation.

The nurse also determines if the patient has any allergies to drugs or food. Cross-sensitivity to medications is common. For example, a patient who is allergic to penicillin may experience allergy to the cephalosporin group of antibiotics as well.

The nurse also questions the patient, family, or significant others about drug ingestion. Does the patient take medications on a daily basis? If so, what are they? Are these drugs prescription, nonprescription, or drugs of abuse (including street drugs such as heroin, cocaine, and marijuana, and legitimate drugs such as amphetamines and barbiturates)? If the patient is suspected of having taken a drug overdose, it is important to determine the specific drug taken, as the treatment will vary.

NURSING DIAGNOSES

The nursing diagnoses are developed based on the information obtained in the initial assessment. From the nursing diagnoses, the goals of the nursing intervention are established, and these later become the criteria for evaluation.

INTERVENTION

The patient in an emergency situation needs to be treated immediately, since speed may be the determining factor in averting death. The goals of the nursing intervention are derived from the nursing diagnoses. Goals vary depending on the causative condition.

In any emergency situation, the patient is transported as quickly as possible to an acute care facility. Intravenous lines are secured, a urinary catheter inserted, and an airway maintained. Intravascular volume is returned to normal as quickly as possible. Fluids that are administered include crystalloids, colloids, or blood products. The nurse continually monitors vital signs, cardiac respiratory, and renal function as fluid resuscitation is performed. Therapy is dictated by the results of the physical assessment and laboratory and radiography data. Therapy may include the administration of emergency medications to manage the situation. Emergency medications include vasopressors to maintain blood pressure; insulin to correct diabetic ketoacidosis; bronchodilators for bronchial dilatation; corticosteroids to reverse symptoms in adrenal crisis; cholinergic drugs to counteract myasthenic crisis; and vasodilators to treat heart disease. The nurse is responsible for knowing the symptoms of these conditions as well as knowing about the drugs being used. The nurse probably is the individual who will be mixing and administering these emergency medications.

When cardiopulmonary resuscitation is necessary, it primarily should restore both cardiac and pulmonary function and maintain vital organ function. Medications are administered concurrently to facilitate the re-establishment of more normal cardiopulmonary functioning.

Medication will be administered to restore cardiac rhythm; maintain both coronary and cerebral perfusion; correct hypoxemia and acidosis; and to improve hemodynamics.

During an emergency situation, intravenous drugs are generally administered through a central line. However, if a central line is not in place, its placement may be time-consuming and requires discontinuation of compressions and ventilations. To alleviate this problem, large catheters are generally inserted through the brachial vein. To enhance delivery to the central circulation, each peripheral venous injection is followed by a bolus of 50 ml of normal saline.

During an emergency situation when there has not been a central line inserted, some drugs may be administered endotracheally. Although endotracheal administration of medications is currently under investigation, drugs that can be used for endotracheal administration include lidocaine, epinephrine, atropine, naloxone, and diazepam. Time to attain a therapeutic blood concentration is five minutes for endotracheal lidocaine, thirty seconds for atropine, and sixty seconds for epinephrine.

Emergency medications are often administered by an IV infusion at a rate of a certain number of micrograms per minute. Table 65–2 presents a simplified approach to complex parenteral infusion administration.

Additional nursing management includes assistance with the placement and aftercare of hemodynamic monitoring lines such as pulmonary artery lines, to measure *pulmonary artery pressures* and *cardiac outputs* (CO); arterial lines to monitor blood pressure; and central venous lines to measure volume. Hemodynamic results are often used to determine proper dosing of vasopressor, vasodilating, or inotropic drugs.

Patients may also be intubated and maintained on ventilators. The nurse inserts a Foley catheter to monitor urinary output, which, in turn, indirectly monitors cardiac output. Fluids are regulated to elicit adequate urinary output of at least 30 ml/hour as well as by blood pressure levels.

Patients in shock are generally managed by left ventricular loading of fluid to increase preload and improve cardiac output; dilators to reduce afterload; and positive inotropics to improve myocardial performance. However, a critically ill patient who has been treated with beta blockers will not respond well to fluid loading to improve a reduced preload. The beta blockers block sympathetic respose to increased volume and the patient may develop congestive heart failure.

Patients with heart disease are often managed with digitalis products, vasodilators, and diuretics, or possibly angiotensin-converting enzyme inhibitors. The goal of vasodilator therapy in treating heart diseases is to improve cardiac output (CO) by reducing unnecessary increases in afterload and to improve elevated ventricular filling pressures by reducing preload. Thus, vasodilator therapy reverses an inappropriate elevated vascular resistance and induces a rise in CO. Vasodilators are most effective in patients with low CO, high left ventricular filling pressures, and elevated *systemic vascular resistance* (SVR). Patients with ischemic heart disease may have their cardiac ischemia worsened when fluids are administered in an attempt to improve preload. The increased vascular volume places pressure on the endocardial layer of the heart and may further compromise blood flow to the heart muscle.

Patients critically ill will also need to be protected from developing stress ulcers and upper GI bleeds. H_2 inhibitors and antacids are generally administered to critically ill patients to stop gastric acid secretion and to raise the gastric pH. By increasing the pH in the upper gastrointestinal system, the environment becomes more favorable for the growth of gram-negative bacilli. This proliferation of bacteria may increase the incidence of gram-negative aspiration pneumonias.

The nurse is also responsible for ensuring that laboratory and radiographic studies are performed on time and results obtained. Patients may need large amounts of fluids, including blood or blood components, so typing and cross-matching of blood is performed.

The nurse emphasizes health teaching to prevent further incidents—keeping medications out of the reach of small children to prevent accidental poisoning, for example. Counseling may also be indicated in certain cases. Patients attempting suicide, alcoholics, or patients with an overdose of "street drugs," are counseled about seeking additional help. The patient is made aware of services and clinics that offer such assistance.

The expansion of the critical care knowledge in the past few years has greatly improved the prognosis and life span for seriously ill patients. Along with knowledge of these advanced technologies come ever-increasing responsibilities that can give rise to numerous legal problems. The critical care or emergency nurse or other practitioner who accepts the responsibility for performing an act is responsible for the consequence of that act. If any act results in injury or damage to the patient, litigation may be brought against the practitioner. The practitioner may be accused of *negligence* or *malpractice*. Many of these legal actions can be prevented when the nurse has a sufficient knowledge base.

EVALUATION

At the conclusion of the nursing intervention, the nurse evaluates his or her actions and the patient's response against the goals of nursing care.

Assuming that the patient lives, actual return to the pre-emergency health state may take from one day to several years. It is important for the nurse to prevent further injury to the patient as well as to prevent complications. Complications of immobility—thrombophlebitis, embolism, kidney stones, muscle wasting—are just examples of complications the nurse attempts to prevent.

Patients are encouraged to keep future appointments for follow-up visits to evaluate their progress. As the patient and family leave the acute care situation, it is important to evaluate all previously taught material to ensure that the patient's and family's knowledge base still remains accurate.

Table 65–2. DRUG INFUSION CHART

IMED RATE (cc/hr)	Epinephrine (Adrenalin) (1mg/250 cc = 4µg/cc) µg/min	(2mg/250 cc = 8µg/cc) µg/min	Dopamine (Intropin) (200mg/250 cc = 800 µg/cc) µg/min	(400mg/250 cc = 1600 µg/cc) µg/min	Sodium Nitroprusside (Nipride) (50mg/250 cc = 200 µg/cc) µg/min	Dobutamine (Dobutrex) (250mg/250 cc = 1000 µg/cc) µg/min	Nitroglycerin (25mg/250 cc = 100 µg/cc) µg/min	(50mg/250 cc = 200 µg/cc) µg/min	Isoproterenol (Isuprel) (1mg/250 cc = 4µg/cc) µg/min	(2mg/250 cc = 8µg/cc) µg/min
1	0.066	0.133	13.33	26.66	3.33	16.66	1.66	3.33	0.066	0.133
2	0.13	0.26	26.6	53.8	6.6	33.3	3.3	6.6	0.13	0.26
3	0.2	0.4	40.0	80.0	10.0	50.0	5.0	10.0	0.2	0.4
4	0.26	0.53	53.3	106.3	13.3	66.6	6.6	13.3	0.26	0.53
5	0.33	0.66	66.6	133.3	16.6	83.3	8.3	16.6	0.33	0.66
6	0.4	0.8	80.0	160.0	20.0	100.0	10.0	20.0	0.4	0.8
7	0.46	0.93	93.3	186.6	23.3	116.6	11.6	23.3	0.46	0.93
8	0.53	1.06	106.3	218.0	26.6	133.3	13.3	26.6	0.53	1.06
9	0.6	1.2	120.0	240.0	30.0	150.0	15.0	30.0	0.5	1.2
10	0.66	1.3	133.3	266.6	33.3	166.6	16.6	33.3	0.66	1.3
12	0.8	1.6	160.0	320.0	40.0	200.0	20.0	40.0	0.8	1.6
14	0.93	1.8	186.6	373.3	46.6	233.3	23.3	46.6	0.93	1.8
16	1.0	2.1	213.3	426.6	53.3	266.6	26.6	53.3	1.0	2.1
18	1.2	2.4	240.0	480.0	60.0	300.0	30.0	60.0	1.2	2.4
20	1.3	2.6	266.6	533.3	66.6	333.3	33.3	66.6	1.3	2.6
25	1.6	3.3	333.3	666.6	83.3	416.6	41.6	83.3	1.6	3.3
30	2.0	4.0	400.0	800.0	100.0	500.0	50.0	100.0	2.0	4.0
35	2.3	4.6	466.6	933.3	116.6	583.3	58.3	116.6	2.3	4.6
40	2.6	5.3	533.3	1066.6	133.3	666.6	66.6	133.3	2.6	5.3
45	3.0	6.0	600.0	1200.0	150.0	750.0	75.0	150.0	3.0	6.0
50	3.3	6.6	666.6	1333.3	166.6	833.3	83.3	166.6	3.3	6.6
55	3.6	7.3	733.3	1466.6	183.3	916.6	91.6	183.3	3.6	7.3
60	4.0	8.0	800.0	1600.0	200.0	1000.0	100.0	200.0	4.0	8.0
65	4.3	8.6	866.6	1733.3	216.6	1083.3	108.3	216.6	4.3	8.6
70	4.6	9.3	933.3	1866.6	233.3	1166.6	116.6	233.3	4.6	9.3
80	5.3	10.6	1066.6	2133.3	266.6	1333.3	133.3	266.6	5.3	10.6
90	6.0	12.0	1200.0	2400.0	300.0	1500.0	150.0	300.0	6.0	12.0
100	6.6	13.3	1333.3	2666.6	333.3	1666.6	166.6	333.3	6.6	13.3

Within the Dopamine (Intropin) columns the regions are labeled BETA (upper), BETA (lower), and ALPHA (bottom).

Infusion Chart Guide (Dosages Based on an Average 70 kg Person)

NOTE: Infusion rate is determined by the formula (IMED Rate) $\times$ (dosage conversion factor) $\times \left(\dfrac{1 \text{ hour}}{60 \text{ min}}\right)$

e.g. $\left(\dfrac{4 \text{ cc}}{\text{hr}}\right) \times \left(\dfrac{4 µg}{\text{cc}}\right) \times \left(\dfrac{1 \text{ hr}}{60 \text{ min}}\right) = \left(\dfrac{4 µg}{60 \text{ min}}\right) = 0.26 \ µg/\text{min}$

Drug		Dosage
Epinephrine (Adrenalin)		Shaded area represents therapeutic dosage.
Dopamine (Intropin)	Beta	2–5µg/kg/min = low dose renal perfusion.
	Alpha & Beta	5–20µg/kg/min = alpha & beta effects of increased heart rate, stroke volume, blood pressure, cardiac output, and renal perfusion.
	Alpha	>20µg/kg/min = decreased renal perfusion.
Sodium nitroprusside (Nipride)		Shaded area represents therapeutic dosage.
Dobutamine (Dobutrex)		Shaded area represents therapeutic dosage.
Nitroglycerin		Dosage is titrated until symptoms are relieved and/or the desired hemodynamic response is noted.
Isoproterenol (Isuprel)		Shaded area represents therapeutic dosage.

From Simone, L and O'Connor, N: A simplified approach to complex parenteral infusion administration. Critical Care Nurse 3(4):82, July/August 1983, with permission.

SUMMARY

Emergency situations can occur at any time and place. The nurse is expected to function calmly and efficiently in any emergency situation. The administration of medications in an emergency situation is generally through the intravenous route. Because the patient is critically ill, the medical team is concerned with the relationship between the dose of the drug given and the response elicited. The pharmacokinetics that occur in the critically ill will be different from those expected in a healthy patient. This chapter briefly reviewed the differences in pharmacokinetics that might be expected in the critically ill.

Before the nurse administers any drug to the critically ill, it is important to perform a thorough assessment. Major organ systems need to be assessed to determine their current function. The nurse must be aware of how to mix and administer emergency drugs and what their expected action will be.

BIBLIOGRAPHY

Barrows, J: Shock demands drugs. Nursing 82 12(2):34, 1982.

Branson, HK: Status epilepticus. Emergency 19(9):22, 1987.

Branson, HK: Defining diabetic emergencies. Emergency 19(7):16, 1987.

Chernow, B: The Pharmacologic Approach to the Critically Ill Patient. Williams & Wilkins, Baltimore, 1988.

Gilman, AG, Goodman, LS, and Gilman, A (eds): Goodman and Gilman's The Pharmacological Basis of Therapeutics, ed 7. Macmillan, New York, 1985.

Hasegawa, EAJ: Endotracheal use of emergency drugs. Heart & Lung 15(1):60, 1986.

Kozloski, G, et al: Guidelines for monitoring parameters for commonly used intravenous drugs in the ED setting. Jr Emergency Nursing 12(6):382, 1986.

Mathewson, M: Autotransfusion. Critical Care Update 9(1):11, 1982.

McAdams, RC and McClure, K: Hypovolemia: How to stop it. RN 86(12):38, December 1986.

Narang, APS, et al: An intensive drug monitoring study suggesting possible clinical irrelevance of impaired drug disposition in liver disease. Br J Clin Pharmacol 15:451, 1983.

Parker, W: Physical compatibilities of critical care medication: What's known. Critical Care Nurse 4(4):70, 1984.

Payne, NR: Emergency care of patients with myxedema coma. JEN 12(6):343, 1986.

Rosequist, CC: Current standards and guidelines for cardiopulmonary resuscitation and emergency cardiac care. Heart & Lung 16(4):408, 1987.

Rudolph, JP: When seconds count endotracheal drug administration. Emergency 17(12):24, 1985.

Sabol, SJ and Ward, DS: Effects of dopamine on hypoxic-hypercapnic interaction in humans. Anesth Analg 67:619, 1987.

Scherer, P: ACLS guidelines: What nurses are saying about the drug changes. Am J Nurs 86(12):1352, 1986.

Simone, L: A simplified approach to complex parenteral infusion administration. Critical Care Nurse 3(4):82, 1983.

Zarowitz, B, Conway, W, and Popovich, J: Adverse interactions of drugs in critical care patients. Henry Ford Hosp Med J 33:48, 1985.

GLOSSARY TERMS IN THIS CHAPTER
Argyrism
Orphan Drug

66 CHAPTER

MISCELLANEOUS AND ORPHAN DRUGS

MERRILY MATHEWSON KUHN, R.N.C., Ph.D. CCRN

LEARNING OBJECTIVES

After reading this chapter, the student will be able to:

1. Identify several miscellaneous medications.

2. Identify orphan drugs.

3. Differentiate among the medications as to mechanism of action, routes of administration, pharmacokinetics, adverse effects, contraindications, and interactions.

4. Identify specific areas to assess in the patient requiring various miscellaneous medications in order to formulate appropriate nursing diagnoses.

5. Identify the nursing interventions necessary to administer various miscellaneous medications and choose appropriate teaching strategies to gain patient compliance.

6. Evaluate the patient at various stages of treatment to gauge nursing interventions.

Table 66–1. MISCELLANEOUS DRUGS

Name	Dosage	Mode of Administration	Pharmacokinetics
ANTIDOTES Dimercaprol (BAL in Oil)			
Action: promotes excretion of arsenic, gold, and mercury by chelation			
Use: antidote in arsenic, gold, mercury poisoning			
	Mild arsenic, or gold poisoning: 2.5 mg/kg 4× /day for 2 days then 2× 3rd day, then OD for 10 days. Severe arsenic and gold poisoning: 3 mg/kg: day 1 and 2—q 4 hr 3rd day—4 times/day, 4–10 day—BID. Mercury poisoning: 5 mg/kg initially; 2.5 mg/kg 1–2 × daily × 10 days.	Deep IM	O: UA P: 30–60 min D: UA ½L: short PB: UA B: complete in 4 hr (liver) E: complete in 4 hr urine, feces
Edetate calcium disodium (Calcium disodium versenate)			
Action: the calcium in this product is readily displaced by heavy metals which then form stable complexes which are excreted in the urine			
Use: acute and chronic lead poisoning and lead encephalopathy; dose is dependant on severity of poisoning			
	1–1.5 g/m^2 diluted in 250–500 ml over 1 hr × 3–5 days, interrupt 2 days, administer × 5 days again.	IV	O: 1 hr P: UA D: 15–20 hr ½L: 20–60 min (IV) PB: UA B: not biotransformed E: 50% urine 1 hr; 95% 24 hr. ½L: 1.5 hr (IM)
	Same as for IV but give in divided doses.	IM	
Pralidoxime chloride (2-PAM, Protopam Chloride, Pralidoxine Chloride)			
Action: reactivates cholinesterase outside central nervous system which has been inactivated by organophosphate pesticide			
Use: antidote in organophosphate pesticide poisoning			
	Organophosphate Poisoning: Adult: 1–2 g in 100 ml of saline over 15–30 min. One hr later 1–2 gm. Child: 20–40 mg/kg as above.	IV IM IV	O: slow PO P: PO, 2–3 hr; IM, 10–20 min; IV, 5–15 min D: short-acting ½L: 1.7 hr PB: not bound B: liver E: urine
	Anticholinesterase Overdose: 1–3 g q 5 hr 1–2 g followed by increments of 250 mg q 5 min.	PO IV	

Key to Abbreviations in the *Pharmacokinetics* column O-onset; P-peak; D-duration; PB-protein bound; B-biotransformed in; E-excreted in; ½ L-halflife.
*Within the column listing adverse effects, underlines indicate the most common effects; CAPITALS indicate life-threatening effects.

Contraindications/ Precautions	Adverse Effects*	Interactions	Nursing Implications
Contraindicated in hepatic or renal insufficiency. Use with caution in G-6PD deficiency. Use in pregnancy only if life-threatening acute poisoning.	Neuro: headache, anxiety, weakness CV: hypertension, tachycardia, chest pain Resp: rhinorrhea GI: nausea, vomiting, burning in mouth and throat, increased salivation, abdominal pain	Do not administer concurrently with iron.	ASSESSMENT: Assess vital signs, liver and renal function, history of poisoning. INTERVENTION: Maintain urine alkalinization as this protects kidneys. EVALUATION: kidney and liver function
Contraindicated in anuria. Use cautiously in patients with renal dysfunction.	Renal: renal tubular necrosis	None known.	ASSESSMENT: Assess fluid volume, avoid excessive hydration. Assess vital signs and do neuro exam. INTERVENTION: For IM injection, add procaine to a 0.5% solution to minimize injection site plan. EVALUATION: Evaluate urinary output and renal function studies frequently.
Contraindicated in hypersensitivity. Use with caution in renal dysfunction, patients with myasthenia gravis. Safety in pregnancy, lactating women, and children not established.	Neuro: dizziness, blurred vision, diplopia, impaired accommodation, headache, drowsiness CV: tachycardia Resp: hyperventilation, LARYNGOSPASM GI: nausea Integ: pain at injection site Misc: elevation of SGOT, SGPT	Potentiates barbiturates. Avoid drugs such as morphine, theophylline, aminophylline, reserpine, phenothiazines.	ASSESSMENT: Assess vital signs, renal function, and respiratory status. INTERVENTION: Maintain patent airway. Administer in appropriate manner. Start therapy without waiting for confirming lab data. Administer slowly IV.

CONTINUED ON THE FOLLOWING PAGE

Table 66-1. MISCELLANEOUS DRUGS-*CONTINUED*

Name	Dosage	Mode of Administration	Pharmacokinetics
URINARY TRACT PRODUCT Cellulose sodium phosphate (Calcibind)			
Action: exchanges sodium ion for calcium ion			
Use: absorptive hypercalciuria Type 1 and 2			
	Initial: 15 g/day in 3 doses with meals, reduce to 10 g/day as calcium falls.	PO	O: immediate P: UA D: UA ½L: UA PB: not bound B: not biotransformed E: feces
SCLEROSING AGENTS			
Action: mild sclerosing drugs, produce effect by irritating the venous intimal endothelium and forming thrombus			
Use: small, uncomplicated varicose veins of lower extremities; esophageal varices			
Sodium tetradecyl sulfate (Sotradecol)	1–3% solution, 0.5–2 ml/injection.	IV	All unknown
Morrhuate sodium (Morrhuate Sodium)	1–5 ml	IV	All unknown
COLLAGEN IMPLANT Zyderm I and II (I = 35 mg/ml; II = 65 mg/ml)			
Action: When introduced into the defect the implanted volume condenses into a soft cohesive network of fibers			
Use: introduced into dermis for correction of contour deficiencies of face and other soft tissues, cosmetic improvements			
	30 ml or less at 1 injection up to 250 ml over several sessions.	Intradermal	All unknown

Key to Abbreviations in the *Pharmacokinetics* column O-onset; P-peak; D-duration; PB-protein bound; B-biotransformed in; E-excreted in; ½ L-halflife.

*Within the column listing adverse effects, <u>underlines</u> indicate the most common effects; CAPITALS indicate life-threatening effects.

Contraindications/ Precautions	Adverse Effects*	Interactions	Nursing Implications
Contraindicated in hyper-parathyroidism. Use with caution in congestive heart failure, ascites. Safety in pregnancy and children not established.	GI: poor taste of drug, loose bowel movement, diarrhea, dyspepsia	None known.	ASSESSMENT: Assess serum calcium levels and renal function. INTERVENTION: Avoid dairy products. Moderate calcium intake. Restrict dietary oxalate and sodium. Encourage fluids.
Contraindicated in hypersensitivity, acute superficial thrombophlebitis, varicosities caused by abdomen and pelvic tumors, uncontrolled diabetes mellitus, sepsis, blood dyscrasias, tuberculosis, asthma, local or systemic infection. Safe use in pregnancy has not been established.	Neuro: dizziness CV: weakness, VASCULAR COLLAPSE Resp: asthma GI: nausea, vomiting Hemo: ANAPHYLACTOID REACTIONS Integ: local burning, urticaria	Evaluate patient carefully when taking oral contraceptives.	ASSESSMENT: Assess for hypersensitivity. Administer 0.5 ml of sodium tetradecyl sulfate or 0.25–1 ml of a 5% morrhuate sodium solution 24 hours prior to use to assess for hypersensitivity. INTERVENTION: Use a small bore needle for injection. Vessel is hard and swollen for 24–48 hours. EVALUATION: Evalute for allergic reaction.
Contraindicated in hypersensitivity. Do not use in breast augmentation or into bone or tendon areas. Use with caution in persons with atopic or allergic reactions or during immunosuppressive therapy. Safety in pregnancy or children not established.	Neuro: headache GI: nausea, vomiting Hemo: ANAPHYLAXIS Integ: erythema, swelling, induration	None known.	ASSESSMENT: To assess for hypersensitivity implant 0.1 ml intradermally 4 weeks before injection. INTERVENTION: Clean area thoroughly with soap, water, and alcohol. Inject with fine needle. 70% of persons require "touch up" implantations at 6–18 month intervals. EVALUATION: Report any incidence of adverse texture change to physician.

CONTINUED ON THE FOLLOWING PAGE

Table 66–1. MISCELLANEOUS DRUGS–*CONTINUED*

Name	Dosage	Mode of Administration	Pharmacokinetics
SMOKING DETERRENTS Nicotine (Nicorette)			

Action: acts as an agonist at nicotinic receptors in both peripheral and central nervous systems.

Use: temporary aid to cigarette smoker giving up smoking

| | Dosage varies: about 10 pieces of gum/day up to maximum of 30/day. | PO | Blood levels of nicotine depend on vigor and duration of chewing.
½L: 30–120 min
B: liver
E: kidneys |

Key to Abbreviations in the *Pharmacokinetics* column O-onset; P-peak; D-duration; PB-protein bound; B-biotransformed in; E-excreted in; ½ L-halflife.

*Within the column listing adverse effects, underlines indicate the most common effects; CAPITALS indicate life-threatening effects.

Contraindications/ Precautions	Adverse Effects*	Interactions	Nursing Implications
Contraindicated in non-smokers, during the immediate postmyocardial infarction period, life-threatening dysrhythmias, severe or worsening angina pectoris, active temporo-mandibular joint disease. Contraindicated in pregnancy and lactating women. Use with caution in persons with dental problems, hypertension, hyperthyroidism, and pheochromocytoma. Safety in children not established.	Neuro: dizziness, headache GI: traumatic injury to oral mucosa or teeth, jaw pain, indigestion, nausea, vomiting, hiccups	Smoking is considered to increase metabolism and lower blood levels of drugs such as caffeine, theophylline, imipramine, and pentazocaine through enzyme induction. Also may reduce diuretic effect of furosemide, and increase blood pressure with propranolol. Smoking cessation may reverse these actions. Smoking and nicotine can increase circulating cortisol and catecholamines.	ASSESSMENT: Assess desire to stop smoking. Assist patient to enter an anti-smoking program. Patient must stop smoking immediately before starting therapy with nicotine gum to prevent overdose. INTERVENTION: Arrange 1-month follow-up visits. Teach patient to chew 1 piece of gum whenever they have urge to smoke. Chew slowly and intermittently for 30 minutes to promote even buccal absorption of nicotine. Chewing gum too rapidly or in too rapid succession may cause an acute nicotine overdose. To prevent gum from sticking: take gum out of mouth when ingesting hot liquids, avoid chewing a piece of gum for more than 45 minutes because it gets stiff. If gum sticks to dental work or dentures, chill with ice or cold water for a few minutes; cold gum is brittle and may easily be removed. Carry a supply of gum at all times. One cigarette can erase all progress in the cessation program, no matter how long abstinence has been maintained. To prevent transference of nicotine dependency from cigarettes to gum, patient is encouraged to gradually decrease number of pieces of gum in 24 hours. Usually a period of 3 months is allowed before patient is advised to taper use of gum. Manufacturers suggest no more than 3 months of gum use. EVALUATION: Assess for symptoms of toxicity. Note return to smoking.

CONTINUED ON THE FOLLOWING PAGE

Table 66–1. MISCELLANEOUS DRUGS–*CONTINUED*

Name	Dosage	Mode of Administration	Pharmacokinetics
Silver acetate (Healthbreak)			
Action: silver acetate clings to the oral mucous membranes and when a cigarette is smoked, an objectionable metallic sweet taste is produced.			
Use: temporary aid to cigarette smoker giving up smoking			
	1 tablet chewed slowly for 10–15 minutes q 4 hr, maximum of 6 tablets/24 hrs.	PO	UA
Lobeline (Bantron)			
Action: produces similar, yet weaker, pharmacologic effect as nicotine. Studies show lobeline has only a placebo effect in decreasing physical craving for cigarettes.			
Use: temporary aid to cigarette smoker giving up smoking			
	1 tablet after meals with half glass of water. Do not use longer than 6 weeks.	PO	UA
VITAMIN PRECURSOR Beta carotene (Max-Caro, Provatene, Solatene)			
Action: provides vitamin A precursor			
Use: reduces severity of photosensitivity reactions in patients with erythropoietic photoporphyria			
	Adult: 30–300 mg/day.	PO	O: 2–4 weeks P: 4–6 weeks D: 1–2 weeks ½L: UA PB: UA B: liver E: feces, urine
	Children under 14 yrs: 30–150 mg/day.	PO	

Key to Abbreviations in the *Pharmacokinetics* column O-onset; P-peak; D-duration; PB-protein bound; B-biotransformed in; E-excreted in; ½ L-halflife.
*Within the column listing adverse effects, underlines indicate the most common effects; CAPITALS indicate life-threatening effects.

Contraindications/ Precautions	Adverse Effects*	Interactions	Nursing Implications
None known. Not recommended during pregnancy or in children. Precautions: Over-use can cause *Argyrism,* a permanent bluish staining of the oral mucous membrane or the skin. May be cosmetically objectionable.	Integ: argyrism	None known.	ASSESSMENT: Assess desire to stop smoking. Assist patient to enter an anti-smoking program. INTERVENTION: Chew product slowly for 10–15 minutes. EVALUATION: Do not use more than 3 weeks. Evaluate color of skin and mucous membranes.
None known. Not recommended during pregnancy or by children.	GI: epigastric pain, nausea, vomiting, heartburn	None known.	ASSESSMENT: Assess desire to stop smoking. Assist patient to enter an anti-smoking program. INTERVENTION: If GI symptoms occur, they may be lessened by an antacid. EVALUATION: Notify physician of nausea, vomiting, palpitations, or convulsion. Do not use more than 6 weeks.
Contraindicated in hypersensitivity to beta-carotene. Use only in pregnancy and lactating women when potential benefit outweighs potential hazard to fetus or infant. Use with caution in renal or hepatic disease.	GI: loose stools Integ: yellow skin, ecchymosis Misc: arthralgia	None known.	ASSESSMENT: Assess for pregnancy and for renal or hepatic disease. INTERVENTION: Capsules may be opened and mixed with juice. Best administered with meals. Protect from sun exposure for 2–6 weeks, then increase sun exposure slowly. Skin may appear yellow while receiving drug. EVALUATION: Evaluate skin effects.

CONTINUED ON THE FOLLOWING PAGE

Table 66–1. MISCELLANEOUS DRUGS–*CONTINUED*

Name	Dosage	Mode of Administration	Pharmacokinetics
RESPIRATORY DRUG: Alpha₁ proteinase inhibitor			

Alpha_1 proteinase inhibitor

Action: replaces alpha₁-antitrypsin necessary for normal lung function

Use: replacement therapy in patients with emphysema who have congenital deficiency of alpha₁ antitrypsin

Name	Dosage	Mode of Administration	Pharmacokinetics
	60 mg/kg once weekly at a rate of 0.08 ml/kg/min.	IV	O: UA P: 6 days D: UA ½L: 4.5–5.2 days PB: UA B: intravascular space E: UA

ANTIHEMOPHILIC FACTOR
Antihemophilic factor (Monoclate, Koate-HT, Koate-HS, Hemofil M)

Action: provides the portion of the Factor VIII complex that is necessary for clotting that is missing or deficient in those patients who have hemophilia A

Use: Hemophilia A.

Name	Dosage	Mode of Administration	Pharmacokinetics
	10–25 AHF/IU/kg, administer at 2–10 ml/minute. (precise dose depends on degree of factor VIII deficiency)	IV	Unknown

Key to Abbreviations in the *Pharmacokinetics* column O-onset; P-peak; D-duration; PB-protein bound; B-biotransformed in; E-excreted in; ½ L-halflife.
*Within the column listing adverse effects, underlines indicate the most common effects; CAPITALS indicate life-threatening effects.

Contraindications/ Precautions	Adverse Effects*	Interactions	Nursing Implications
None known.	Neuro: fever, dizziness Hemo: transient leukocytosis	None known.	ASSESSMENT: Assess lung function, tidal volume and vital capacity. INTERVENTION: Administer within 3 hours after reconstitution. Very expensive drug—general cost is $21,000–22,000/year for 70 kg adult. Administer hepatitis B vaccine before administration as product is prepared from pooled plasma. Store carefully between 2–8° C.
Contraindicated in hypersensitivity to mouse protein. Safety in pregnancy not known.	CV: tightness in chest, hypotension. Resp: wheezing GI: nausea Hemo: ANAPHYLAXIS Integ: hives, urticaria, mild chills, stinging at infusion site Misc: fever	None known.	ASSESSMENT: Assess hematocrit and hemoglobin frequently. Product is obtained from pooled human plasma that is purified and heat treated. INTERVENTION: Should be stored in refrigerator for long-term storage, but may be kept at room temperature for up to 6 months. Warm to room temperature before administering. Test AHF levels to ensure they are adequate. EVALUATION: Report signs of chest tightness to physician.

CONTINUED ON THE FOLLOWING PAGE

Table 66–1. MISCELLANEOUS DRUGS–*CONTINUED*

Name	Dosage	Mode of Administration	Pharmacokinetics
TOPICAL DRUG Minoxidil (Rogaine)			

Action: stimulates vertex hair growth with male pattern baldness, mechanism unknown.

Use: male pattern baldness.

Name	Dosage	Mode of Administration	Pharmacokinetics
	1 ml massaged into scalp 2× daily.	Topical	O: 3–4 mos P: UA D: UA ½L: UA PB: poorly absorbed B: UA E: UA

ABORTIFACIENTS			

Action: stimulate the gravid uterus to contract and produce evacuation

Use: termination of pregnancy: Carboprost 13–20 weeks gestation
Dinoprost 16–20 weeks gestation
Dinoprostone 12–20 weeks gestation

Name	Dosage	Mode of Administration	Pharmacokinetics
Carboprost Tromethamine (Prostin/15M)	Abortion: Initial 250 mcg, then 250 μg at 1.5–3.5 hr intervals depending on contractions. Not to exceed 12 mg in 2 days.	IM	Unavailable

Key to Abbreviations in the *Pharmacokinetics* column O-onset; P-peak; D-duration; PB-protein bound; B-biotransformed in; E-excreted in; ½ L-halflife.
*Within the column listing adverse effects, underlines indicate the most common effects; CAPITALS indicate life-threatening effects.

Contraindications/ Precautions	Adverse Effects*	Interactions	Nursing Implications
Hypersensitivity to any component. Use with precaution in persons with heart disease. Use in pregnant, lactating women and children not established.	CNS: headache, dizziness, lightheadedness, vertigo CV: edema, chest pain, changes in blood pressure, palpitations. Resp: URI, bronchitis, sinusitis GI: nausea, vomiting, diarrhea Hema: lymphadenopathy, THROMBOCYTOPENIA Derm: dermatitis, local erythema, dry skin on scalp, flaking, alopecia.	None known.	ASSESSMENT: Assess level of hair growth and for healthy, normal scalp. INTERVENTION: Hair and scalp should be clean and dry before application. Wash hands after administration. Do not use with other topical drugs. New hair will be soft, downy and colorless. After further treatment, new hair will be same as old hair. Solution contains alcohol which may burn eyes, mucous membranes, or sensitive tissue. Bathe area with large amount of cool tap water. Do not use if scalp becomes irritated or sunburned. EVALUATION: Evaluate for new hair growth. May take 4 months or longer to appear. If treatment is stopped, new hair will be shed.
For all: Contraindications: Hypersensitivity, acute pelvic inflammatory disease, active cardiac, pulmonary, renal, or hepatic disease. Precautions: Cautious use with history of asthma, hyper- or hypotension, anemia, diabetes.			For all: ASSESSMENT: Determine gestational week as calculated from 1st day of last normal menstrual period. Monitor temperature closely for any signs of pyrexia. INTERVENTION: Store all products in refrigerator. EVALUATION: Save contents of the evacuant for examination.
Same as above.	Neuro: headache, anxiety, drowsiness, tinitis, vertigo CV: hypertension, dysrhythmias, chest pain Resp: dyspnea, wheezing, asthma, respiratory distress GI: vomiting, diarrhea, nausea, dry mouth Renal: urinary tract infection Repro: UTERINE RUPTURE Other: flushing, THYROID STORM, increased temperature	Activity of other oxytoxic agents can be augmented by carboprost and dinoprost.	Same as above.

CONTINUED ON THE FOLLOWING PAGE

Table 66–1.   MISCELLANEOUS DRUGS–*CONTINUED*

Name	Dosage	Mode of Administration	Pharmacokinetics
Dinoprost Tromethamine (PGF$_2$) alpha) (Prostin in F$_2$ alpha)	Withdraw 1 ml of amniotic fluid then very slowly inject 40 mg into sac. 10–40 mg additional may be administered.	Transabdominal into amniotic sac	O: 15–30 min P: 22 hr ½L: < 1 min PB: UA B: liver, lung E: UA
Dinoprostone (PGE$_2$) (Prostin E$_2$)	Initial: 1 suppository into vagina, then q 3–5 hr as needed.	Vaginal suppository	O: 10 min D: 2–3 hr B: lung, kidney, spleen E: urine

AGENT FOR PATIENT DUCTUS ARTERIOSUS
Alprostadil (Prostin VR Pediatric)

Action: maintain patency of ductus arteriosus in infants with restricted pulmonary or systemic blood flow by vasodilation and reduction in peripheral vascular resistance.

Use: temporary, palliative therapy to maintain the patency of ductus arteriosus.

	Dosage	Mode of Administration	Pharmacokinetics
	Initial dose: 0.05–0.1 µg/kg/min, then reduce to lowest possible dosage to maintain therapeutic effect.	Continuous IV	Unavailable

Key to Abbreviations in the *Pharmacokinetics* column O-onset; P-peak; D-duration; PB-protein bound; B-biotransformed in; E-excreted in; ½ L-halflife.
*Within the column listing adverse effects, underlines indicate the most common effects; CAPITALS indicate life-threatening effects.

There are several drugs today that do not "fit" in any of the chapters or classifications previously discussed in this text. These drugs are featured in Table 66–1. Some of these drugs are classified as *orphan drugs*. The orphan drug title is applied to drugs and devices that are used to treat or diagnose rare diseases. These include drugs, biologicals (e.g., vaccines), medical devices, and foods for the diagnosis, treatment, or prevention of rare diseases. A major problem related to the development of these products is the financial returns that would be re-

Contraindications/ Precautions	Adverse Effects*	Interactions	Nursing Implications
Same as above.	Neuro: headache, weakness, drowsiness. CV: hypertension, hypotension, CARDIAC ARREST, congestive heart failure Resp: coughing, dyspnea, wheezing, bronchospasm GI: vomiting, diarrhea, nausea Hema: DIC Renal: dysuria, hematuria Repro: uterine pain Integ: pruritis Other: chills, increased temperature	Activity of other oxytoxic agents can be augmented by carboprost and dinoprost.	Same as above.
	Neuro: headache, weakness CV: hypotension. Resp: coughing, wheezing. GI: vomiting, diarrhea, nausea Renal: urine retention. Repro: PERFORATED UTERUS, hot flushes, vaginitis, breast tenderness. Other: chills, backache, joint inflammation, increased temperature.		Same as above, plus: INTERVENTION: Remain supine for 10 min after administration. Store in refrigerator and bring to room temperature before administration.
Contraindications: None Precautions: Use with caution in infants with bleeding tendencies as alprostadil inhibits platelet aggregation.	Neuro: hyperextension of neck, cerebral bleed, lethargy, stiffness. CV: flushing, hypotension, bradycardia, tachycardia, CARDIAC ARREST, congestive heart failure, heart block, dysrhythmias. Resp: apnea, wheezing, hypercapnia, respiratory distress. Hema: DIC, anemia, bleeding, thrombocytopenia. Renal: anuria, hematuria. Musc: cortical proliferation of long bones.	None known.	ASSESSMENT: Assess and monitor continually respiratory status. INTERVENTION: Maintain central or umbilical line for hemodynamic monitoring. Dilute 1 ml of alprostadil with either sodium chloride or dextrose solution. Prepare fresh solution q 24 hours. EVALUATION: Hemodynamic effects.

alized by the manufacturing companies. Drug companies estimate that it costs an average of $125 million to develop a new drug. This may be slightly less for orphan drugs. Most of this cost is incurred during studies in humans; and when studying orphan drugs, the population that is studied is small. The return on the research investment is also small because of the few people using the drug or device. A rare disease or condition affects fewer than 200,000 persons. There are several thousand rare diseases today such as narcolepsy, Wilson's disease, Tourette's syndrome, and Paget's disease.

Table 66–2. PRODUCTS THAT HAVE BEEN GIVEN ORPHAN DRUG APPROVAL

Generic Name (Trade Name)	Application
Acetohydroxamic acid (Lithostat)	Urea-splitting urinary tract infections
Alpha₁-antitrypsin (Prolastin)	Alpha₁-antitrypsin deficiency in the ZZ phenotype population
Amiodarone (Cordarone)	Antidysrhythmic
Amsacrine (Amsidyl)	Acute adult leukemia
Calcitonin-human (Cibacalcin)	Paget's disease
Calcium acetate (Phos-Lo)	Treatment of hyperphosphatemia in end-stage renal disease
Cellulose sodium phosphate (Calcibind)	Hypercalciuria with recurrent calcium oxalate or calcium phosphate nephrolithiasis
Chenodiol (Chenix)	Dissolution of gallstones
Clofazimine (Lamprene)	Antileprosy
Cromolyn sodium (Cromoral)	Magtocytosis vernal keratoconjunctivitis
Cyclosporine (Sandimmune)	Prevention of transplant rejection
Cyclosporine ophthalmic (Optimmune)	Treatment of severe keratoconjunctivitis sicca
Cyproterone acetate (Cyproterone Androcur)	Severe hirsutism
Desmopressin (DDAVP, Stimate)	Diabetes insipidus
Diethyldithiocarbamate (Imuthiol)	Treatment of AIDS
Digoxin-specific antibody fragments (Digibind)	Digoxin antidote
Dronabinol (Marinol)	Antiemetic
Etoposide (VePesid)	Testicular cancer
Factor XIII (Fibrogammin)	Congenital factor XIII deficiency
Gonadorelin (Factrel)	Evaluation of gonadotropic function
Heme arginate (Normosang)	Treatment of symptomatic stage of acute porphyria
Hemin (Panhematin)	Hepatic porphyria
Hexamethylmelamine (Hexastat)	Advanced ovarian adenocarcinoma
Interferon alfa-2a, recombinant (Roferon-A)	Treatment of metastatic renal cell carcinoma
Interferon alfa-2b, recombinant (Intron A)	Treatment of invasive carcinoma of the cervix; treatment of primary brain tumors, treatment of carcinoma in situ of the urinary bladder; treatment of human papillomavirus in patients with recurrent respiratory (laryngeal) papillomatosis; treatment of acute hepatitis B.
Interferon beta, recombinant human (Betaseron)	Treatment of AIDS; treatment of multiple sclerosis
Interferon gamma-1b	Treatment of chronic granulomatous disease

Table 66–2. PRODUCTS THAT HAVE BEEN GIVEN ORPHAN DRUG APPROVAL–CONTINUED

Generic Name (Trade Name)	Application
Interleukin-2, recombinant (Proleukin)	Treatment of metastatic renal cell carcinoma
Iodine I 123 murine monoclonal antibody to human alpha-fetoprotein	Detection of hepatocellular carcinoma and hepatoblastoma; detection of alpha-fetoprotein-producing germ cell tumors
Iodine I 123 murine monoclonal antibody to human chorionic gonadotropin (hCG)	Detection of hCG-producing tumors such as germ cell and trophoblastic cell tumors
Iodine I 131 murine monoclonal antibody to human alpha-fetoprotein	Treatment of hepatocellular carcinoma and hepatoblastoma; treatment of alpha-fetoprotein-producing germ cell tumors
Iodine I 131 murine monoclonal antibody to hCG	Treatment of hCG-producing tumors such as germ cell and trophoblastic cell tumors
L-Carnitine (Carnitor)	Treatment of manifestations of carnitine deficiency in patients with end-stage renal disease who require dialysis
L-carnitine (Carnitor)	Carnitine deficiency
Leucovorin calcium (Wellcovorin)	Treatment of metastatic colorectal cancer
Leucovorin calcium (Leucovorin)	For rescue use after high-dose methotrexate therapy in the treatment of osteosarcoma
Mefloquine hydrochloride (Lariam)	Treatment of acute malaria due to *Plasmodium falciparum* and *Plasmodium vivax;* prophylaxis of *Plasmodium flaciparum* malaria which is resistant to other available drugs
Megestrol acetate (Megace)	Treatment of patients with anorexia, cachexia, or significant weight loss (<10% of baseline body weight) and confirmed diagnosis of AIDS
Metronidazole, topical (MetroGel)	Acne rosacea
Mitoxantrone hydrochloride (Novantrone)	Antineoplastic drug
Monoclonal antibody 17-1A (Panorex)	Treatment of pancreatic cancer
Monoctanoin (Moctanin)	Dissolution of gallstones
Nafarelin acetate	Treatment of central precocious puberty
Naltrexone (Trexan)	Narcotic addiction
Pentamidine (Pentam)	*Pneumocystis carinii* infections
Physostigmine salicylate (Antilirium)	Friedreich's and other inherited ataxias
Pimozide (Orap)	Tourette's syndrome
Potassium citrate (Urocit-K)	Management of renal tubular acidosis with calcium stones, hypocitraturic calcium oxalate nephrolithiasis, uric acid lithiasis

Table 66–2. PRODUCTS THAT HAVE BEEN GIVEN ORPHAN DRUG APPROVAL–*CONTINUED*

Generic Name (Trade Name)	Application
Selegiline hydrochloride (Deprenyl)	Adjuvant in Parkinsonism
Somatostatin (Reducin)	Adjunct to the nonoperative management of secreting cutaneous fistulas of the stomach, duodenum, small intestine (jejunum and ileum), or pancreas
Somatrem (Protropin)	Human growth hormone deficiency
Tranexamic acid (Cyklokapron)	Dental hemostatic in hemophiliacs
Trientine (Cuprid)	Wilson's disease
Trilostane (Modrastane)	Cushing's syndrome
Viloxazine hydrochloride (Vivalan)	Narcolepsy and cataplexy

The Food and Drug Administration established the Office of Orphan Products Development in 1982. It became the responsibility of this office to identify potential new therapies for rare diseases and the possible sponsors for the development of these products. That same year the Orphan Drug Act was passed in both houses of Congress and signed into law in 1983. This law provides both technical assistance and economic incentives to pharmaceutical manufacturers for developing and marketing products for the treatment of people with rare diseases.

Currently, the Office of Orphan Product Development has designated more than 140 orphan drugs for research, and numerous orphan compounds have been approved for marketing (Table 66–2). A number of incentives have been made available to pharmaceutical companies by the government to assist in the development and marketing of drugs for rare diseases.

BIBLIOGRAPHY

AMA Department of Drugs: AMA Drug Evaluations, ed 6. PSG Publishing, Littleton, MA, 1986.

Alpha$_1$-Proteinase Inhibitor for Alpha$_1$-Antitrypsin Deficiency. The Medical Letter on Drugs and Therapeutics 30(761), March 11, 1988.

Guyton, AC: Textbook of Medical Physiology, ed 7. WB Saunders, Philadelphia, 1986.

Olin, B (ed): Facts & Comparisons. JB Lippincott, St. Louis, 1989.

Parks, BR: Orphan drugs. Pediatric Nurse 14(2):152, 1988.

GLOSSARY

—A—

Abortifacient: a drug which causes abortion of a pregnancy. (Ch 15)

Absence epilepsy: petit mal seizures; a seizure disorder characterized by an abrupt, brief loss of consciousness, amnesia, or a period of unawareness. Most commonly afflicts children. (Ch 22)

Absorption: a process of movement of medication from drug administration sites to the vasculature. (Ch 3)

Abuse: misuse or excessive use. Drug abuse is a term commonly used to refer to drug-taking patterns which impact negatively on psychological or social function. (Ch 13, Ch 24)

Accommodation reflex: a reflex that allows the eye to adjust for various distances by changing the sizes of the pupil and the lens. (Ch 59)

Accumulation: a process which occurs when the rate of drug administration exceeds the rate of drug excretion. Accumulation results in the gradual increase in the blood level of a drug. (Ch 4)

Acetylcholine: a neurotransmitter found within the somatic and autonomic nervous systems. (Ch 17)

Acetylcholinesterase: an enzyme which degrades acetylcholine. (Ch 17)

Acetylcholinesterase inhibitor: an agent which inhibits the action of the enzyme acetylcholinesterase. The resultant effect is an increased concentration of acetylcholine at the site of action. (Ch 23)

Achlorhydria: an absence of the gastric production of hydrochloric acid. (Ch 54)

Acid neutralizing capacity: A measure of the effectiveness of an antacid in neutralizing acid. Acid neutralizing capacity is expressed as the number of mEq of acid neutralized for each mL of antacid. (Ch 7, Ch 52)

Acquired defective color vision: a disorder of color perception which results from systemic or ocular disease. (Ch 33)

Acquired immune deficiency syndrome (AIDS): a disease caused by the human immunodeficiency virus which causes the disruption of normal cell-mediated immunity. Patients afflicted with AIDS exhibit various opportunistic infections and certain forms of cancer. (Ch 12)

Acquired immunity: immunity resulting from the development of active or passive immunity as opposed to natural immunity. (Ch 64)

ACTH: see Corticotropin. (Ch 40)

Active immunization: a process of rendering a patient immune to a particular disease by administering an antigen which stimulates the production of antibodies directed against the etiology of that disease. (Ch 55, Ch 64)

Active non-specific immunotherapy: the treatment of cancer via active immunization designed to produce a general stimulation of the immune system. (Ch 50)

Active specific immunotherapy: the treatment of cancer via active immunization utilizing attenuated autologous tumor cells. The immune response is directed specifically at the tumor cells. (Ch 50)

Active transport: a one-way transport process which moves drugs from areas of low concentration to areas of high concentration. Requires the expenditure of energy and the use of carrier proteins. (Ch 4, Ch 37)

Acute pain: pain of a sudden onset and limited duration. Active pain subsides with healing of the injury. (Ch 20)

Acute radiculoneuropathy: an acute disorder of the peripheral nerves, the spinal nerve roots, and the spinal cord caused by viral infection or vaccine. (Ch 55)

Addiction: a condition manifested by the compulsive need to use a drug, evidence of tolerance, and/or withdrawal. (Ch 13, Ch 20, Ch 24)

Additive drug interaction: a form of drug-drug interaction which occurs when each drug has similar clinical effects; the result is the sum of the individual effects. (Ch 5)

Adenohypophysis: the anterior lobe of the pituitary gland. It manufactures and releases growth hormone, prolactin, corticotropin, thyrotropin, luteinizing hormone, and follicle-stimulating hormone. (Ch 40)

Adenoids: lymphatic tissue found in the uppermost portion of the pharynx whose function it is to trap bacteria and prevent respiratory infection. (Ch 34)

ADH: see Antidiuretic hormone. (Ch 22)

Adie's syndrome: a condition characterized by enlargement of the pupil, delayed and slow responses to light, and impaired accommodation. (Ch 18)

Adjuvant chemotherapy: the administration of chemotherapeutic drugs following the removal or destruction of a primary tumor in an attempt to destroy micrometastases. (Ch 48)

Adoptive immunotherapy: the treatment of cancer via passive immunization in which normal lymphocytes of a healthy donor are incubated in vitro with tumor cells from the patient. These lymphocytes are then injected into the patient where they act upon the patient's tumor. (Ch 50)

Adrenaline: see epinephrine. (Ch 17)

Adrenergic: see sympathomimetic effect. (Ch 19)

Adrenergic nerve fibers: nerve which, when stimulated, releases norepinephrine or epinephrine. (Ch 17)

Adrenergic receptors: receptors which bind with norepinephrine or epinephrine. (Ch 17)

Adrenolytic: see sympatholytic effect. (Ch 19)

Adverse drug reaction (adverse effect): any undesired, unintended, and noxious effect of a drug occurring after doses administered for prophylactic, diagnostic, or therapeutic purposes. (Ch 1)

Adverse effect: see adverse drug reaction. (Ch 1)

Aerobic organism: a microorganism that can live and grow in the presence of oxygen. (Ch 46)

Aerosol: a self-contained sprayable product in which the propellant force is supplied by a liquefied gas. (Ch 3)

Afterload: the pressure in the arteries against which the heart must overcome in order for it to eject blood. (Ch 19, Ch 27)

Aged elderly: people 80 years and older. (Ch 16)

Agglutination: the process of cells, such as platelets, sticking together to form a clump. (Ch 30, Ch 50)

Agonist: a drug which complexes with and activates the functional properties of the receptor. (Ch 4)

AIDS: see Acquired immune deficiency syndrome. (Ch 12)

Airway resistance: a measure of the difficulty encountered by air as it flows through the bronchial tubes. High airway resistance increases the effort needed to breathe. (Ch 34)

Akathisia: a condition characterized by motor restlessness and a need to be in constant motion. (Ch 25, Ch 53)

Akinesia: a condition characterized by the inability to make voluntary movements. (Ch 23, Ch 25)

Alimentary canal: digestive tract; the structures located between the mouth and the anus including the mouth, esophagus, stomach, small intestine, large intestine, and rectum. (Ch 51)

Alkylating agent: a drug that introduces an alkyl group, or hydrocarbon radical, into a compound in place of a hydrogen atom. These alkylating agents which act upon nucleic acids destroy normal nucleic acid functions and are therefore useful in treating certain forms of malignancies. (Ch 49)

Alopecia: hair loss, particularly of the head. (Ch 49)

Alpha receptor: a subdivision of adrenergic receptor. Stimulation of alpha receptors will cause vasoconstriction, decreased GI motility, sweat secretion, glycogenolysis, lipolysis, uterine contraction, and ejaculation. (Ch 17)

Alveolus: a thin-walled epithelial sphere located at the final branching of the bronchioles, at which pulmonary capillaries are present and air exchange takes place. (Ch 34)

Ambulatory surgery: outpatient surgery, same-day surgery. Surgery which is performed without admission to a hospital. Following a brief recovery period, the patient is sent home directly from the recovery room. (Ch 10)

Anabolism: the metabolic building of complex substances from more simple compounds; for example, the synthesis of protein from amino acids. (Ch 40, Ch 56)

Anaerobic organism: a micro-organism that can live and grow in the absence of oxygen. (Ch 46)

Analeptic: a central nervous system stimulant, usually utilized to stimulate respiration. (Ch 21, Ch 36)

Anaphylactic: pertaining to anaphylaxis. (Ch 6)

Anaphylactoid: a clinical syndrome resembling anaphylaxis but in which no allergic reaction can be demonstrated. (Ch 6)

Anaphylaxis: a severe allergic reaction manifested by cardiovascular and respiratory collapse, laryngeal edema, hives, and urticaria. Mediated by IgE antibodies. (Ch 6)

Anasarca: edema which is generalized in all body tissues. (Ch 38)

Androgens: male sex hormones. (Ch 43)

Anesthesia: loss of feeling or sensation, particularly the sensation of pain. (Ch 10)

Anesthesiologist: a physician who specializes in the administration of anesthetics. (Ch 10)

Anesthetic: agent which produces a loss of feeling or sensation. (Ch 3)

Anesthetist: a person trained in the administration of anesthetics. Although the term may refer to an anesthesiologist, it more commonly is used in reference to a certified registered nurse anesthetist. (Ch 10)

Angioplasty: a procedure in which an artery which is narrowed due to the deposition of atheromatous placques is catheterized and stretched from within in an attempt to improve blood flow. (Ch 33)

Angiography: x-ray visualization of the vascular system following injection of radiopaque contrast media. (Ch 9)

Anion: particle which carries a negative electric charge. (Ch 11, Ch 58)

Anosmia: absence of the sense of smell. (Ch 21)

Antagonist: a drug which interferes with the action of an agonist. (Ch 4, Ch 13)

Antagonist drug interaction: a drug interaction which results in a lessened pharmacological effect. (Ch 5)

Anterograde amnesia: a side effect produced by hypnotics in which a patient is unable to remember events which occur during a specified period of time following drug administration. Anterograde amnesia may be a desired effect of a drug administered prior to painful or frightful procedures. (Ch 24)

Anthropometric parameters: a measure of nutritional status which evaluates a patient's height, weight, and body proportions in relation to a patient's age and/or population averages. (Ch 56)

Antiadrenergic: see sympatholytic effect. (Ch 19)

Antibiotic: a natural or synthetic compound that inhibits the growth of or destroys microorganisms. (Ch 3)

Antibody: immunoglobulin; serum protein which combines with and destroys antigens. (Ch 6)

Anticholinergic: parasympatholytic; an agent that antogonizes the action of acetylcholine, especially within the parasympathetic nervous system. (Ch 35)

Anticholinesterase: see Acetylcholinesterase inhibitor. (Ch 18)

Anticoagulant: a drug or substance that prevents or retards blood coagulation. (Ch 33)

Antidiuretic hormone: ADH, vasopressin; a hormone normally secreted by the posterior pituitary gland which causes the kidney to retain water and which causes vasoconstriction. (Ch 22)

Antidote: a drug or drug preparation which will counteract the effects of a poison. (Ch 5)

Antiemetic: a drug that prevents or relieves nausea and vomiting. (Ch 53)

Antigen: a substance which can provoke an immune response. (Ch 6, Ch 50)

Antigenic: having the properties of an antigen. (Ch 6)

Antigenicity: potency as an antigen. (Ch 12)

Antihistamine: drug which counteracts the effects of histamine at the H-1 receptor. Commonly used for symptomatic treatment of infectious and allergic rhinitis and other allergic reactions. (Ch 7)

Anti-inflammatory: an agent which reduces or counteracts inflammation. (Ch 3)

Antimetabolite: one of a class of antineoplastic drugs which is structurally similar to vitamins, coenzymes, or other substances essential for growth and division of normal and neoplastic cells. When the antimetabolite is taken up by the cell in lieu of the normal nutrient, DNA synthesis is blocked. (Ch 49)

Antimuscarinic: an anticholinergic effect specifically at the effector cells of the postganglionic fibers of the parasympathetic nervous system. Antimuscarinic effects include dry mouth, blurry vision, urinary retention, slowed GI motility, and tachycardia. (Ch 18)

Antiperistalsis: reverse peristalsis; peristalsis that propels the alimentary contents in a direction from the anus upwards through the alimentary canal. (Ch 54)

Antipsychotic: a drug that modifies psychotic behavior. (Ch 25)

Antipyretic: a drug which will lower a fever. (Ch 7)

Antiseptic: disinfectant, germicide; an agent which kills microorganisms on contact. (Ch 3)

Antiserotonergic: a drug which counteracts the effect of serotonin. (Ch 53)

Antitoxin: an antibody directed against toxins, or the poisonous secretions of certain bacteria. Antitoxins are administered to patients for the purpose of providing passive immunity. (Ch 64)

Antitussive: rough suppressant; a drug which depresses the cough reflex by inhibiting the cough center in the medulla. (Ch 7, Ch 36)

Antivenin: an antibody directed against poisonous insect or animal venom, such as that produced by black widow spiders or certain snakes. Antivenins are administered to patients for the purpose of providing passive immunity. (Ch 64)

Anuria: absence of urine formation. (Ch 39)

Anxiolytic: sedative, tranquilizer; an agent which alleviates anxiety. (Ch 24)

Aortography: angiography of the aorta. (Ch 9)

Aphasia: a complete or partial loss of the ability to comprehend or express language. (Ch 22)

Aqueous humor: a watery substance located within the anterior chamber of the eye which is responsible for bringing nutrients to the eye tissues and removing cellular debris. (Ch 59)

Argyrism: a bluish discoloration of the skin and mucous membranes resulting from the prolonged administration of silver. (Ch 66)

Ariboflavinosis: a deficiency of vitamin B-2 which results in photophobia, increased tearing, itching and burning skin, somatitis, or glossitis. (Ch 57)

Aromatic amino acids: amino acids which contain a benzene ring: phenylalanine, methionine, and tryptophan. Blood vessels of these amino acids are increased in patients with severe liver disease and may contribute to hepatic encephalopathy. (Ch 56)

Arrhythmia: see dysrhythmia. (Ch 30)

Arteriosclerosis: hardening of the arteries; a condition characterized by thickened arterial walls and a loss of elasticity. (Ch 31)

Arthrography: x-ray visualization of a joint. (Ch 9)

Artificially acquired immunity: immunity resulting from the intentional exposure to antigens, antibodies or infectious agents, as in vaccination or in the administration of antibodies. (Ch 64)

Ascites: an abnormal collection of fluid in the abdominal cavity. (Ch 38, Ch 55)

Asthenia: weakness. (Ch 21)

Astigmatism: a vision defect in which some portions of an image are out of focus with other portions. (Ch 59)

Astringent: a medication which causes tissue contraction and toughening. (Ch 3)

Atelectasis: collapse of the lung. (Ch 36)

Atherosclerosis: a condition characterized by the deposition of cholesterol-containing plaque on the inner surface of arterial walls. (Ch 31)

Attenuated: microorganisms or cells which have been rendered less capable of producing disease. Attenuated organisms are sometimes administered to patients for the purpose of stimulating active immunity. (Ch 50, Ch 64)

Auerbach's Plexus: a network of autonomic nerve fibers located in the intestinal wall which, when stimulated, increase peristalsis. (Ch 54)

Aura: a sensation that precedes a seizure, migraine headache, or other recurrent condition. (Ch 22)

Autoimmune disorder: a disease characterized by the body's production of antibodies or lymphocytes directed against other body tissues. (Ch 32)

Autoinduction: a situation in which a drug stimulates the synthesis or action of enzymes responsible for its metabolism. (Ch 22)

Autologous: relating to products derived from a patient for use by that same patient. In an autologous blood transfusion, blood which has been previously collected from a patient is saved and administered to the same person at a later date. (Ch 12, Ch 50)

Automaticity: the ability of a cell to spontaneously develop an action potential. (Ch 27)

Autonomic nervous system: nerves which innervate and regulate cardiac and smooth muscle, glands, and other metabolically active tissue. The autonomic nervous system is subdivided into the sympathetic and parasympathetic systems. (Ch 17)

AV block: atrioventricular block; a delay or blockage in the transmission of impulses from the atria to the ventricles. (Ch 27)

Avitaminosis: a condition caused by a deficiency of a particular vitamin. (Ch 57)

Axon: the portion of the nerve fiber which conducts electrical impulses. (Ch 17)

Azotemia: the presence of excessive concentrations of urea in the blood. (Ch 45)

—B—

Bacterial resistance: the ability of a bacterium to withstand the presence of antibiotics. (Ch 46)

Bactericidal: causing the death and destruction of bacteria. (Ch 3, Ch 46)

Bacteriostatic: inhibiting the growth of bacteria. (Ch 3, Ch 46)

Balanced anesthesia: anesthesia which is achieved with a combination of drugs which are selected to maximize the desired effects and minimize the undesired effects. (Ch 10)

Baroreceptor: sensory nerves located in the carotid arteries, aortic arch, and vena cava which respond to changes in blood pressure. When stimulated by hypotension, the baroreceptors initiate a compensatory mechanism resulting in an increase in heart rate and force of cardiac contraction. (Ch 29)

Basal ganglia: nerves within the cerebrum which are responsible for the control of muscle tone and the initiation and modulation of motor movement. Specific basal ganglia include the amygdaloid body, the corpus striatum, and clasutrum. (Ch 17)

B-cells: lymphocytes which arise in the bone marrow and which serve to produce antibodies. (Ch 50)

Beriberi: a condition caused by thiamine deficiency resulting in anemia, heart failure, and various neurological deficits. (Ch 28)

Beta-lactam: a general description of the chemical structure of the penicillin, cephalosporin, carbapenem, and monobactam antibiotics. Beta-lactam antibiotics work by preventing the cross-linking of peptidoglycan, thereby causing the synthesis of defective cell walls. (Ch 46)

Beta-lactamase: a group of enzymes produced by bacteria which destroy beta-lactam antibiotics. (Ch 46)

Beta receptor: a subdivision of adrenergic receptor. Stimulation of beta receptors will cause an increase in heart rate, cardiac conduction, and cardiac contractility; a relaxation of blood vessels, bronchial muscle, and uterus; gluconeogensis and lipolysis. (Ch 17)

Bifascicular block: an intraventricular conduction defect in which conduction is delayed or blocked through two of the following: the right bundle branch, the anterior portion of the left bundle branch, and the posterior portion of the left bundle branch. (Ch 30)

Bilirubin: an orange-red bile pigment produced by hemoglobin degeneration. High levels of bilirubin are seen in patients with certain forms of liver disease and is the cause of jaundice. (Ch 14)

Bioavailability: the percentage of an administered dose which is absorbed. (Ch 4)

Biological half-life: the amount of time required to reduce the original plasma concentration of a drug by 50 percent. (Ch 4)

Biological response modifiers: a diverse group of substances, including the interleukins, tumor necrosis factor, and monoclonal antibodies, which alter a body's response to disease. (Ch 50)

Biotransformation: metabolism; the enzymatic alteration of a drug molecule. (Ch 4)

Bipolar disorder: a condition characterized by periodic fluctuations between depression and mania. (Ch 26)

Bolus: 1) a mass of food ready to be swallowed. 2) a

dose of drug administered over a very short period of time. (Ch 51)

Botulism: a type of food poisoning caused by a toxin produced by the growth of Clostridium botulinum in improperly canned or preserved foods. (Ch 14)

Bradykinesia: a condition characterized by slow voluntary movements. (Ch 23)

Bradykinin: a polypeptide kinin hormone produced in the blood which acts as a potent vasodilator, promoties smooth muscle contraction, and produces pain when applied to nociceptors. (Ch 42)

Brainstem: the portion of the brain comprised of the mesencephalon, the pons, and medulla oblongata. (Ch 17)

Branched-chain amino acids: valine, leucine, and isoleucine. These amino acids are preferentially metabolized by skeletal muscle and may become depleted in states of trauma, sepsis, or severe stress. (Ch 56)

Brand name: see Trade name. (Ch 3)

Broad-spectrum: a term used to describe antibiotics which are active against a large variety of microorganisms. (Ch 46)

Bronchi: the large cartilagenous air passages located below the trachea but above the bronchioles. (Ch 34)

Bronchioles: small bronchial tubes, of a 1 mm or smaller diameter, which differ from the bronchi in that they are devoid of cartilage. The bronchioles remain open as a result of smooth muscle tone. (Ch 34)

Bronchodilator: an agent that relaxes bronchial smooth muscle thereby decreasing airway resistance. (Ch 35)

Bronchorrhea: excessive discharge of mucus from the bronchi. (Ch 6)

Bronchospasm: abnormal constriction of bronchial smooth muscle with a resultant increase in airway resistance, as is characteristic of bronchial asthma. (Ch 35)

Buccal: a drug dosage form designed to be applied to the mucous membranes of the mouth, most commonly the cheek. (Ch 3)

Bulbar: relating to the medulla oblongata. (Ch 23)

—C—

Cachexia: a state of ill health, malnutrition, and wasting as may occur in cancer, advanced tuberculosis, and various chronic diseases. (Ch 49)

Calcitonin: thyrocalcitonin; a hormone released by the thyroid gland which functions in the regulation of calcium and phosphorus metabolism. (Ch 40)

Calyx: the cup-like portion of the renal pelvis which drains the upper and lower parts of the kidney. pl = calyces (Ch 37)

CAPD: chronic ambulatory peritoneal dialysis. (Ch 39)

Capillary hydrostatic pressure: the force generated by the blood flowing through the capillaries which causes fluid to shift from the capillary to the interstitium. (Ch 27)

Caput medusae: a specific appearance of the abdominal wall caused by stasis of the cutaneous veins around the naval in patients with cirrhosis of the liver. (Ch 55)

Cardiac output: the volume of blood ejected from the left ventricle each minute. (Ch 65)

Cardiotoxicity: having a deleterious effect on the heart. (Ch 16)

Carpopedal spasm: involuntary contraction of the muscles of the wrists and ankles as seen in tetany. (Ch 45)

Carina: an anatomical description of the cartilage located at the lower part of the trachea which divides the air passages into the right and left bronchial trees. (Ch 34)

Catabolism: the metabolic breakdown of complex substances to more simple compounds; for example the catabolism of protein into simple amino acids. (Ch 42, Ch 56)

Cataplexy: sudden loss of muscular tone. (Ch 21)

Catechol-o-methyl transferase (COMT): an enzyme responsible for the degradation of norepinephrine. (Ch 17)

Cation: a particle which carries a positive electric charge. (Ch 11, Ch 58)

CCPD: continuous cycling peritoneal dialysis. (Ch 39)

Ceiling effect: a term referring to an analgesic drug's inherent maximal efficacy. Analgesics which possess a ceiling effect (such as the non-steroidal anti-inflammatory agents) may not be effective in treating severe pain even at progressively higher doses. Analgesics without a ceiling effect (such as most of the narcotics) will have greater efficacy at higher doses and are therefore effective in treating severe pain. (Ch 47)

Cell loss: the loss of neoplastic tissue from the tumor mass via metastasis or cell death. (Ch 48)

Central nervous system: the portion of the nervous system comprised of the brain and spinal cord. (Ch 17)

Centrifugation: a process of separating a mixture of a solid and a liquid or two liquids by rotating the mixture at high speeds. The substance with the higher specific gravity will be forced to the bottom of the container while the other component of the mixture will remain on top. (Ch 12)

Centriole: the portion of a cell in which mitosis occurs. (Ch 48)

Cephalocaudal: proceeding in a direction from the head to the toes. (Ch 14)

Cerebellum: the portion of the brain responsible for the coordination of movements, equilibrium, and posture. (Ch 17)

Cerebral cortex: the thin outer layer of the cerebrum which is rsponsible for awareness and analysis of sensory input, initiation and control of motor activity, and various integrative functions. (Ch 17)

Cerebration: mental action of the brain. (Ch 45)

Cerebrum: the largest part of the brain comprised of the cerebral cortex, corpus callosum, and the medullary center. (Ch 17)

Certified registered nurse anesthetist: a registered nurse specially trained and certified to administer anesthetics. (Ch 10)

Cerumen: ear wax; cerumen functions to lubricate the external ear canal and trap foreign material. (Ch 59, Ch 61)

Chelate: to bind with a metal; a chelating agent is a substance that binds with and removes certain metals from the system. (Ch 32)

Chemoreceptors: 1) neurons located in the aortic arch, the carotid arteries, and the medulla which are sensitive to fluctuations in blood pH, P_{O_2}, and/or P_{CO_2}. These chemoreceptors attempt to normalize these variables by adjusting the rate of ventilation. 2) sensory nerve endings that are stimulated by and react to certain chemical stimuli, such as the taste buds and olfactory cells of the nose. (Ch 34)

Chemoreceptor trigger zone: a section of the medulla that receives sensory information from the stomach and elsewhere and in turn stimulates the vomiting center to initiate emesis. (Ch 53)

Cholecystangiography: x-ray visualization of the gallbladder and bile ducts following injection of radiopaque contrast media. (Ch 9)

Cholelithiasis: the presence of gallstones. (Ch 55)

Cholesterol: a fatty substance found in animal meats and dairy products and manufactured by the liver. Excessive blood levels of cholesterol is a risk factor for the development of atherosclerosis and cardiovascular disease. (Ch 32)

Cholinergic nerve fibers: nerves which, when stimulated, release acetylcholine. (Ch 17)

Cholinergic receptors: receptors which bind with acetylcholine. (Ch 17)

Cholinesterase inhibitor: see acetylcholinesterase inhibitor. (Ch 18)

Cholinomimetic agent: a substance which will elicit a response similar to that elicited by acetylcholine. (Ch 17, Ch 18)

Choreiform: movements that resemble chorea: a variety of involuntary jerky movements. (Ch 21)

Chromatopsia: a condition in which colors are incorrectly perceived. The yellow-green halos around objects in patients with digitalis toxicity is an example of chromatopsia. (Ch 28)

Chromosomal mutation: a mechanism for the development of bacterial resistance in which spontaneous mutation of the organism occurs. Chromosomal mutation usually increases bacterial resistance by causing the bacteria to produce an enzyme that inactivates the antibiotic. (Ch 46)

Chronic ambulatory peritoneal dialysis: CAPD; manual peritoneal dialysis which utilizes an implanted peritoneal catheter and is performed by the patient at home several times daily. (Ch 39)

Chronic pain: pain longer than six months in duration which may persist after the injury has healed. (Ch 20)

Chronobiology: the study of body rhythms or the effect of time on body systems. (Ch 4)

Chronotropic: relating to time or rate, particularly the rate of cardiac contraction. (Ch 28)

Chvostek's sign: a sign of tetany characterized by facial muscle spasm in response to tapping those muscles. (Ch 45, Ch 58)

Chyme: a semisolid mixture of food and gastric secretions which is delivered to the small intestine. (Ch 51)

Ciliary body spasm: abnormal contraction of the ciliary body, or the portion of the eye between the base of the iris and the choroid. May be caused by insertion of pilocarpine via special ocular delivery systems. (Ch 60)

Circadian: daily; circadian rhythm refers to regular, cyclical daily fluctuations in activity. (Ch 40)

Cirrhosis: a chronic liver disease characterized by the loss of functioning liver cells and increased resistance to the flow of blood through the liver. (Ch 38)

Cleansing agent: agent which helps to remove dirt, crusts, secretions, and debris from wherever applied. (Ch 3)

Clearance: a measure of the speed at which a drug leaves the body. (Ch 4)

Clonal cell: a cell which is capable of reproducing in kind; one of a group of identical cells. (Ch 48)

Coarctation: stricture or contracture. (Ch 29)

Co-behavior: enabing behavior patterns of such long standing that the individual is unaware of them. (Ch 13)

Cofactor: a mineral or non-protein organic compound required by an enzyme in order to function. (Ch 62)

Collagen: the main intracellular protein of skin, teeth, cartilage, and other connective tissues. Collagen confers supportive properties to these tissues. (Ch 33, Ch 63)

Collodion: a preparation of pyroxylin dissolved in ether and alcohol. When applied to the skin, it dries to form a strong, thin, transparent film and is useful in sealing the edge of a dressing. (Ch 63)

Colloid: a large molecule dispersed in solution. When administered intravenously, colloidal solutions remain within the vascular space and exert osmotic pressure to pull fluid from the interstitium. (Ch 12)

colloid osmotic pressure: the pressure generated by the presence of large molecules within the blood which causes fluid to shift from the interstitium to the vascular space. (Ch 12, Ch 27)

Colonization: the growth of microorganisms other than the normal flora without the development of disease. (Ch 46)

Comedones: blackheads; discolored dried sebum plugging an excretory duct of the skin. (Ch 63)

Complexation: a drug-drug or drug-food interaction in

which the two substances form a chemical or physical complex that is unable to be absorbed by the gastrointestinal tract. (Ch 5)

Compliance: 1) in keeping with, or in accordance with; act of acquiescing; following direction. 2) a measure of how easily the lungs can be expanded; the higher a lung's compliance, the less work is needed to breathe.

Comprehension: capacity of the mind to understand. (Ch 8)

Compulsion: an abnormal, irresistable, and often irrational impulse to do something. (Ch 24)

COMT: see Catechol-o-methyl transferase. (Ch 17)

Conductive hearing loss: hearing loss resulting from the mechanical inability of sound waves from being transmitted to the auditory nerves. Causes include excessive ear wax and middle ear inflammation. Differs from sensorineural hearing loss in that the latter is secondary to nerve damage and is generally irreversible. (Ch 61)

Conductivity: the ability to conduct impules in an orderly fashion. (Ch 27)

Cones: cells located in the retina of the eye which receive color stimuli. (Ch 57)

Conjunctiva: the mucous membrane lining the inner surface of the eyelids. (Ch 59)

Conjunctivitis: inflammation of the conjunctiva caused by infection, trauma, or allergy. (Ch 60)

Continuous cycling peritoneal dialysis: CCPD; a form of peritoneal dialysis in which the patient, connected to an automated machine, is given 3 dialysis exchanges at night. Another exchange is made upon awakening. This form of chronic dialysis therapy allows the patient to participate in normal daily activities without interruption for dialysis. (Ch 39)

Contractility: the force generated by the heart during contraction. (Ch 27)

Cornea: the clear, colorless anterior covering of the outer layer of the eye. (Ch 59)

Corpora quadrigemina: a portion of the mesencephalon which relays visual and auditory reflexes. (Ch 17)

Corpus callosum: a band of nerve fibers which connects the two hemispheres of the cerebrum. (Ch 17)

Corticosteroid: general term applied to steroid hormones secreted by the adrenal cortex. Corticosteroids are subdivided into glucocorticoids and mineralocorticoids. (Ch 42)

Corticotropin: adrenocorticotropic hormone, ACTH; a hormone released by the anterior pituitary gland which targets the adrenal cortex and regulates the release of glucocorticoids, promotes lipolysis, and stimulates amino acid and glucose uptake in muscle. (Ch 40)

Countercurrent mechanism: in renal physiology, the process which allows the body to alter urinary osmolality in response to the body's need to save or eliminate fluid. (Ch 37)

Coupled premature ventricular beats: a series of two consecutive ventricular beats. (Ch 30)

Crackles: see rales. (Ch 36)

Craniopharyngioma: a tumor of the pituitary gland which is the most common pituitary tumor in children and the most common cause of prepubertal hypopituitarism. (Ch 41)

Craniosacral system: an anatomical description of the parasympathetic nervous system. (Ch 17)

Cream: a topical semi-solid dosage form consisting of an oil in water or a water in oil emulsion. A cream differs from an ointment in that a cream contains a relatively large proportion of water, is easily removable by water, and is relatively non-greasy. (Ch 63)

Criterion reference evaluation: an evaluation in which the patient's performance is compared with a relatively fixed standard that has been decided upon in advance. (Ch 8)

Cross tolerance: a situation in which the development of tolerance to one drug creates a tolerance to other drugs with similar pharmacological effects. (Ch 13, Ch 24)

Cryptorchidism: a condition in which the testes fail to descend into the scrotum. (Ch 43)

Crystalloid: a small molecule dispersed in solution. When administered intravenously, crystalloids readily distribute to the interstitial and extravascular spaces. (Ch 12)

Cyanosis: a bluish skin discoloration caused by severe hypoxemia. (Ch 36)

Cyclic 3,5-AMP: cyclic 3,5-adenosine monophosphate; a substance formed within cells in response to sympathetic stimulation. In the bronchioles, cyclic 3,5-AMP causes relaxation of bronchial smooth muscle. (Ch 34)

Cyclic 3,5-GMP: cyclic 3,5-guanosine monophosphate; a substance formed within cells in response to cholinergic stimulation. In the bronchioles, cyclic 3,5-GMP causes contraction of bronchial smooth muscle. (Ch 34)

Cyclic antidepressant: a chemical description of certain antidepressants in that their chemical structure is comprised of one or more rings. (Ch 26)

Cyclopegic: a drug that paralyzes the ciliary muscle of the eye and prevents accommodation. (Ch 60)

—D—

Deadspace: areas of the lung which are ventilated but do not exchange gas with the blood. (Ch 36)

Deamination: the metabolic removal of an amino group from an amino acid with the consequent formation of ammonia or urea. (Ch 51, Ch 56)

Decubitus ulcer: pressure sore; ulceration of the skin caused by prolonged pressure over a part of the body as might be seen in patients confined to bed for prolonged periods. (Ch 62)

De-esterification: a metabolic process in which an ester portion of a molecule is separated from the remainder of the molecule. (Ch 47)

Delusion: a false belief which is inconsistent with the patient's own knowledge and experience. Delusions are seen most often in psychoses, in which patients cannot distinguish delusions from reality. (Ch 25)

Demulcent: a drug which has a soothing effect on irritated tissue. (Ch 54)

Dependence: see addiction. (Ch 13, Ch 20, Ch 24)

Depolarizing neuromuscular blocking agent: a drug which causes muscle paralysis by blocking the transmission of impulses at the neuromuscular junction. Depolarizing agents accomplish this by stimulating the muscle in a similar fashion as the natural substance acetylcholine; unlike acetylcholine, however, these drugs do not allow normal muscle recovery and therefore do not allow further muscle contraction. (Ch 10, Ch 18)

Depolarizing postsynaptic potential: an action potential produced in a nerve of such a magnitude that it depolarizes the next neuron and allows for conduction. (Ch 21)

Depolymerization: the conversion of large molecules (polymers) into simpler molecules (monomers) of the same or similar chemical structure; for example, the depolymerization of DNA into individual nucleic acids. (Ch 62)

Depression: an emotional state characterized by extreme dejection, gloomy ruminations, and feelings of worthlessness, hopelessness, and apprehension. (Ch 26)

Dermis: the layer of skin between the epidermis and the hypodermis which contains collagen, elastin, nerves, and capillaries. (Ch 63)

Desensitization: down-regulation; a decrease in responsiveness of a receptor caused by continual stimulation. (Ch 4)

Diabetes insipidus: a condition characterized by insufficient production, release, or response to vasopression (antidiuretic hormone) with resultant excessive urination, hypernatremia, and great thirst. (Ch 40, Ch 41)

Diabetes mellitus: a condition characterized by a deficiency in insulin with resultant hyperglycemia. (Ch 44)

Diabetogenic effect: an effect that results in diabetes mellitus. (Ch 41)

Diagnosis related groups (DRGs): a system of hospital reimbursement adopted by the Federal Medicare Program in which a fixed fee is paid to the hospital based upon a patient's diagnosis. (Ch 2)

Dialysis: a process of diffusing blood across a semipermeable membrane to remove toxic materials and to maintain fluid, electrolyte, and acid-base balance in cases of impaired renal function. (Ch 39)

Diastole: the portion of the cardiac cycle during which the heart is at rest. (Ch 27)

Diencephalon: the portion of the brain, just below the telencephalon, which contains the thalamus and hypothalamus. (Ch 17)

Diffusion: movement of molecules from areas of high concentration to areas of low concentration. (Ch 4)

Diplopia: double vision. (Ch 60)

Discovery learning: a learning method in which the principal content to be learned is not presented in final form, but must be independently discovered by the patient before internalization. Used by Ausubel. (Ch 8)

Distribution: the process of delivering a drug to the various tissues of the body. (Ch 4)

Disulfiram-like reaction: a drug interaction between a medication and alcohol with symptoms similar to that elicited when disulfiram interacts with alcohol. Symptoms may include flushing, headache, sweating, vomiting, anxiety, confusion, hyperventilation, tachycardia, hypotension, and blurred vision. (Ch 44)

Diuretic resistance: the inability to respond to diuretics. Diuretic resistance may be caused by compensatory mechanisms resulting from a decreased intravascular volume, hormonal changes, incorrect drug or dose selection, drug interactions, or patient noncompliance. (Ch 38)

Dopamine: an intermediate product in norepinephrine synthesis. In the central nervous system, dopamine regulates emotion and complex movements; in the periphery, dopamine dilates renal and mesenteric arteries, increases cardiac output, and raises blood pressure. (Ch 17)

Dopaminergic receptor: a receptor of the autonomic nervous system which is specifically stimulated by dopamine. (Ch 19)

Doubling time: the length of time required for a tumor cell population to double itself. (Ch 48)

Dromotropic: an effect related to conductivity of a nerve. A drug with a positive dromotropic effect on the heart will increase cardiac conduction. (Ch 19)

Drug: a chemical substance used in humans for diagnosis, prevention, or treatment of disease, pain, or suffering. (Ch 1)

Drug allergy: a form of adverse drug reaction which is precipitated by interaction of the drug and the body's immune system. (Ch 1)

Drug holiday: the prescribed omission of one or more doses of a medication. Drug holidays may be used to treat or minimize an adverse reaction, restore drug effectiveness when tolerance has developed, or to minimize the cost of therapy without compromising efficacy. (Ch 16, Ch 21)

Drug interaction: an interaction between a drug and another drug or a drug and food which results in an increase or decrease in the drug's pharmacological effects. (Ch 5)

Drug toxicity: a form of adverse drug reaction which is an extension of the drug's pharmacological properties and results from excessive drug dosing. (Ch 1)

Dual addiction: simultaneous dependence on two substances which have similar pharmacological effects. (Ch 13)

Duodenal ulcer: peptic ulcer located in the duodenum. (Ch 52)

Dynorphins: a class of endogenous peptides. (Ch 20)

Dyskinesia: a condition characterized by abnormal voluntary movement. (Ch 23, Ch 25)

Dysphagia: difficulty in swallowing. (Ch 25)

Dysphasia: a speech impairment characterized by the inability to arrange words in their proper order. (Ch 22)

Dysrhythmia: a disorder of heart rate and rhythm. (Ch 27, Ch 30)

Dystonia: abnormal muscle tone; acute dystonia is an extrapyramidal reaction to the phenothiazines and is manifested as spasm of the tongue, face, neck, and/or back. (Ch 25, Ch 53)

—E—

Eccrine: exocrine; the external secretion of a gland, such as sweat. (Ch 14)

Eclampsia: severe toxemia of pregnancy characterized by hypertension, oliguria, edema, seizures, and, if untreated, coma. (Ch 15)

Ectopic: at or from an abnormal location. (Ch 27)

Edema: the presence of excess fluid within the body tissues. (Ch 38)

Education: imparting or acquisition of knowledge or skill; systematic instruction or training. (Ch 8)

EEG: electroencephalogram. (Ch 22)

Effective refractory period: see Refractory period. (Ch 30)

Effector cells: natural cells of immunity which in part serve to destroy cancer cells. Included are killer T cells, the macrophage, the natural killer cell, and the lymphokine-activated killer cell. (Ch 50)

Elasticity: the ability of a blood vessel to be stretched. (Ch 27)

Elastin: the main extracellular protein of the skin and other connective tissue. Elastin confers elastic and flexible properties to these tissues. (Ch 63)

Electroencephalogram: EEG; a measurement of brain wave activity. (Ch 22)

Electrolyte: substance which dissociates in water into cations and anions. (Ch 58)

Embryo: the term used to describe a developing baby *in vitro* during the time frame of gestation ranging from implantation until day 60. (Ch 15)

Emollient: bland lipid-containing compound applied locally to soften, sooth, and reduce dryness of the skin. (Ch 3, Ch 63)

Empirical stage of therapeutics: a stage in the development of pharmacotherapeutics which is based upon clinical evidence that a drug is effective, although the mechanism by which it acts is unknown. (Ch 2)

Enabling: behaviors which support an individual's continuing use of a drug by failing to confront the person with the consequences of the addiction and by shielding the person from the realities of the economic and emotional implications of an ongoing addiction. (Ch 13)

Endogenous depression: depression which cannot be related to a specific life event. (Ch 26)

Endogenous insulin: insulin which is manufactured and secreted by a patient's own pancreas. (Ch 44)

Endogenous peptides: endogenous neurotransmitters which bind with opiate receptors and regulate pain. Included are enkephalins, endorphins, and dynorphins. (Ch 20)

Endometriosis: a condition in which ectopic endometrial, or uterine, implants occur. (Ch 43)

Endorphins: a class of endogenous peptides found in the pituitary gland. (Ch 20)

Enkephalins: a class of endogenous peptides found on the brain, spinal cord, adrenal medulla, and intestines. (Ch 20)

Enteral: administration of food or drugs via the gastrointestinal tract. (Ch 56)

Enterohepatic recycling: a situation in which a drug is secreted in the bile into the intestine where it is re-absorbed into the systemic circulation. (Ch 20, Ch 26)

Enzymes: proteins which catalyze chemical reactions but which are not altered or consumed by the reaction. (Ch 62)

Epidermis: the outer layer of the skin containing the stratum corneum, stratum granulosum, prickle cells, and the stratum germinavitum. (Ch 63)

Epidural therapy: administration of a drug directly onto, but not into, the outer membrane of the spinal cord. (Ch 20)

Epilepsy: see seizure disorder. (Ch 22)

Epinephrine: adrenaline; an adrenergic hormone produced by the adrenal medulla. (Ch 17)

Episiotomy: surgical incision of the vulva, usually performed to assist with childbirth. (Ch 62)

Ergotism: Poisoning by excessive quantities of ergot or ergot derivatives. Ergotism is characterized by abdominal complaints, confusion, and circulatory statis. (Ch 19)

Erythromelalgia: a condition characterized by recurrent episodes of peripheral vasodilation accompanied by burning pain, redness, and increased skin temperature. Erythromelalgia is usually most pronounced in the feet. (Ch 23)

Esotropia: cross-eyes, convergent strabismus; marked inward turning of the eye. (Ch 60)

Eunuchism: a condition characterized by the absence of the testes and male hormone. (Ch 43)

Euthyroid: normal thyroid function. (Ch 45)

Excretion: the elimination of drugs, drug metabolites, and bodily wastes from the body. (Ch 4)

Exogenous depression: see reactive depression. (Ch 26)

Exogenous insulin: insulin which is produced outside a patient's body and is administered by injection. (Ch 44)

Exophthalmos: outward bulging of the eyeball. (Ch 45)

Expectorant: drug which decreases the viscosity of bronchial secretions thereby facilitating their removal through coughing. (Ch 7, Ch 35)

Exponential kinetics: a pharmacokinetic model in

which a constant fraction of a drug is eliminated in a set unit of time. (Ch 4)

External intercostals: along with the diaphragm, the primary muscles of respiration. These muscles pull the ribs upward and outward during inspiration. (Ch 34)

Extinction: a behavioral modification approach in which withdrawal of reinforcement results in the extinguishment of the undesired behavior. Used by Skinner. (Ch 8)

Extrapyramidal symptoms: movement disorders that are caused by centrally-acting antidopaminergic drugs such as the phenothiazines. Included are dystonia, akathisia, akinesia, and Parkinson-like symptoms. (Ch 25, Ch 26, Ch 53)

Extravasation: the accidental escape of a drug being administered intravenously into the surrounding tissues. (Ch 16)

—F—

Facilitated Diffusion: movement of drug molecules from areas of high concentration to areas of low concentration using a carrier protein. Requires no energy expenditure. (Ch 4, Ch 58)

Facultative anaerobe: a microorganism that prefers an oxygen-containing environment but which will live and grow in its absence. (Ch 46)

Fasciculation: a small, local, involuntary muscle contraction. (Ch 23)

Fetal period: the time frame during gestation ranging from 60 days after fertilization until the baby is born. (Ch 15)

Fibrinolysis: the dissolution of blood clots. (Ch 33, Ch 62)

Filtration: a passive transport process of removing particles from a solution by allowing the liquid portion to pass through a membrane which contains holes too small for the solid particles to pass. (Ch 4)

First order kinetics: see exponential kinetics. (Ch 4, Ch 48)

First-pass effect: see hepatic first-pass effect. (Ch 3, Ch 26)

First-pass metabolism: see Hepatic first-pass effect. (Ch 26)

Flocculation: the gathering together of fine dispersed particles in a solution into larger visible particles. (Ch 62)

Fluid challenge: a test of over-vigorous diuresis in which a patient is administered a saline solution or colloid preparation. If the fluid challenge results in an improvement in blood pressure, heart rate, and renal function, the patient's blood volume has been inadequate. If these signs fail to correct with the fluid challenge, they are the result of factors other than excessive diuresis. (Ch 38)

Foam: a drug dosage form in which a drug in solution or emulsion is forced through a nozzle and becomes whipped with air. (Ch 3)

Formative evaluation: the process of gathering information about patient performance and providing feedback as soon as possible. (Ch 8)

Formulary: a collection of prescriptions, formulas, and recipes for medicinal products. Modern hospital formularies represent a listing of drugs approved by the medical staff for use in that institution. (Ch 2)

Fovea centralis: a small depression in the center of the macula where cones are most densely concentrated and where visual acuity is the greatest. (Ch 59)

Frank-Starling relationship: a relationship between the degree of stretch of a muscle fiber and the force with which it contracts. Within certain limits, the greater the degree of muscle stretch, the greater the force of contraction. (Ch 31)

Funduscopic exam: examination of the posterior portions of the eye utilizing a special instrument called a funduscope. (Ch 29)

Fungicidal: causing the death and destruction of fungi. (Ch 46)

Fungicide: an agent which destroys fungi. (Ch 3)

Fungistatic: inhibiting the growth of fungi. (Ch 46)

Furosemide threshold: the minimum number of milligrams of furosemide necessary to produce an adequate urinary response. (Ch 39)

—G—

Galenical: a term based upon the prescriptions of the ancient Greek physician Galen which refers to the use of drugs with several active ingredients; crude herb and vegetable medicines. (Ch 2)

Ganglia: a group of nerve fibers which connect autonomic nerves of the spinal cord with other nerves which innervate the effector organs. (Ch 17)

Garrulous: excessive talkativeness. (Ch 21)

Gastric ulcer: peptic ulcer located in the stomach. (Ch 52)

Gel: a colloid which is firm in consistency but which contains a large amount of water. Usually applied topically. (Ch 3)

General anesthesia: the progressive, reversible stage of central nervous system depression that occurs following the administration of drugs used for this purpose. General anesthetics are administered via the intravenous or inhalation route. (Ch 10)

Generalization: in teaching, tells the learner that behavior in a given situation continues to be valid in future learning experiences. (Ch 8)

Generic name: non-proprietary name of a drug substance. Generic names are assigned by the United States Adopted Name Council and are the same regardless of manufacturer. (Ch 3)

Germ cell: a cell which gives rise to specific specialized daughter cells, such as red blood cells. (Ch 32)

GFR: see glomerular filtration rate. (Ch 37)

Glaucoma: a disease of the eye characterized by increased intraocular pressure which, if untreated, results in optic nerve atrophy and blindness. (Ch 60)

Glomerular filtration rate: a measure of renal function which is the rate that blood is filtered by the glomerulus. The average GFR is about 125 ml/min/1.73 m^2. (Ch 37)

Glucocorticoid: steroid hormone secreted by the adrenal cortex that primarily affects carbohydrate, fat, and protein metabolism. (Ch 42)

Gluconeogenesis: the formation of glucose from non-carbohydrate sources, such as protein and fat. (Ch 42, Ch 44, Ch 56)

Glutathione: a tripeptide substance that normally carries oxygen to the liver and is fundamental for cellular respirations. (Ch 55)

Glycogenolysis: the metabolic conversion of glycogen in glucose. (Ch 56)

Glycolysis: the metabolic breakdown of complex carbohydrates into simpler sugars. (Ch 56)

Glycosuria: the presence of abnormally high concentrations of glucose in the urine. (Ch 44)

Glycosylated hemoglobin: hemoglobin which has chemically combined with glucose. Glycosylated hemoglobin levels are a measure of the long-term degree of hyperglycemia and do not fluctuate with day-to-day variations in blood glucose. (Ch 44)

Gompertzian kinetics: a model of the growth rate of cancer cells in which the cells grow faster than normal cells of a similar mass but at a slower-than-logarithmic rate. (Ch 48)

Growth fraction: the fraction of cells which are actively proliferating at a given time. (Ch 48)

Growth hormone: see somatotropin. (Ch 40)

Guillain-Barre syndrome: a syndrome caused by virus or vaccine which is characterized by muscle weakness, absent tendon reflexes, and increased cerebrospinal fluid protein. (Ch 54)

Gynecomastia: abnormal development and enlargement of the male breast. (Ch 25, Ch 53, Ch 55)

—H—

Half-life: see biological half-life. (Ch 4)

Hallucination: a visual, auditory, or olfactory perception having no relation to reality. (Ch 25)

Hapten: molecules that are not normally antigenic which can become antigenic when combined with a carrier protein. (Ch 6)

Health care provider: a person who is extensively trained to provide health care services to the general public. Examples include physician, dentist, optometrist, nurse, pharmacist, and dietitian. (Ch 7)

Hemeralopia: defective vision in bright light. (Ch 22)

Hemophilia A: a defect in blood coagulation in which insufficient quantities of coagulation factor VIII are produced. (Ch 41)

Hemostasis: the process designed to minimize blood loss; hemostasis includes blood coagulation and the formation of platelet plugs. (Ch 33)

Hepatic encephalopathy: abnormal function of the brain caused by the accumulation of toxic substances in patients with severe liver disease. Symptoms range from personality changes, difficulty with mental performance, and confusion to frank coma. (Ch 38, Ch 55)

Hepatic first-pass effect: a phenomenon which occurs whereby a drug which has been absorbed by the gastrointestinal system is extensively metabolized by the liver prior to reaching the systemic circulation. (Ch 3)

Heteroinduction: a form of drug interaction in which one drug stimulates the synthesis or action of enzymes required to metabolize another drug. (Ch 22)

HHNK: see Hyperglycemic hyperosmolar non-ketotic coma. (Ch 44)

Hilus: a recessed site at the entrance or exit of a gland or organ where blood vessels and nerves are connected. (Ch 37)

HIV: see human immunodeficiency virus. (Ch 12)

Homeostasis: stability of the normal body state and internal environment. (Ch 16, Ch 37)

Hormone: a chemical substance secreted by one group of cells that exerts physiologic effects on other cells. (Ch 40)

Host defenses: a term used to describe a patient's natural system to prevent or combat infection. Included are a patient's immune system as well as barrier defenses such as the skin. (Ch 46)

Human immunodeficiency virus (HIV): the virus responsible for the acquired immune deficiency syndrome. (Ch 12)

Humanistic perspective: a teaching model in which the teacher assumes the role of facilitator of learning, the primary requisite of which is to develop a profound trust in the student to develop one's own potentiality for learning. Used by Rogers. (Ch 8)

Hydrocholoretic: an agent that increases the output of bile without increasing the solids secreted in it. The bile secreted has a high-water content and low viscosity. (Ch 54)

Hydrolysis: the metabolic breakdown of a substance by the chemical addition of water molecules. (Ch 56)

Hydrostatic pressure: the pressure exerted by the fluid within a capillary that forces fluid across capillary membranes. (Ch 37)

Hydroxylation: the metabolic addition of a hydroxyl group to a substance in order to increase its water solubility and hasten its elimination. (Ch 51)

Hyperactivity: a level of activity which is excessive for the circumstances; hyperactivity is a common symptom of attention deficit disorder. (Ch 21)

Hyperalimentation: the administration of most or all of a patient's nutritional requirements via the parenteral route. (Ch 56)

Hyperglycemic hyperosmolar non-ketotic coma: a condition usually found in patients with uncontrolled type II diabetes mellitus, characterized by very high blood glucose levels, osmotic diuresis, coma, but without the presence of high levels of ketone bodies. (Ch 38, Ch 44)

Hyperhidrosis: a condition characterized by abnormally excessive sweating. (Ch 18)

Hyperkinesis: a condition characterized by excessive motor function. (Ch 45)

Hypermetropia: far-sightedness; the inability to see close objects clearly. (Ch 59)

Hyperosmotic: containing abnormally high osmolality. A solution which is hyperosmotic will draw water across a membrane until a similar osmolality is present on both sides of the membrane. (Ch 11)

Hyperpolarizing potential: an action potential produced in a nerve of such magnitude that it excessively depolarizes the next neuron and prevents conduction. (Ch 21)

Hyperreactivity: increased sensitivity of a receptor to an agonist. (Ch 4)

Hypertension: high blood pressure; a disorder characterized by persistently elevated systolic and/or diastolic blood pressure. (Ch 29)

Hyperthyroxinemia: excess levels of thyroid hormone in the blood. (Ch 21)

Hypertonic: a situation in which the osmotic pressure is greater on one side of a cell membrane. If a hypertonic solution is administered to a patient, fluid will shift out of the cells. (Ch 11, Ch 14, Ch 58)

Hypnotic: an agent that induces sleep; "sleeping pill." (Ch 24)

Hypoalbuminemia: a serum albumin less than 3.5 g per 100 ml. (Ch 38)

Hypochlorhydria: an abnormal reduction in the gastric production of hydrochloric acid. (Ch 54)

Hypochromic: a cell which has less color or tint than normal; often used to refer to a red blood cell which is deficient in hemoglobin. (Ch 32)

Hypodermis: superficial fascia; loose connective tissue separating the dermis and the underlying tissue which permits free movement and pliability of the skin. (Ch 63)

Hypodermoclysis: the injection of large quantities of fluid subcutaneously. (Ch 62)

Hypogonadism: a condition characterized by reduced activity of the sexual glands (testes or ovaries). (Ch 43)

Hypokinesia: a condition characterized by slow voluntary movements and decreased mobility. (Ch 25)

Hypo-osmotic: containing abnormally low osmolality. A solution which is hypo-osmotic will lose water across a membrane until a similar osmolality is present on both sides of the membrane. (Ch 11)

Hypophyseal gland: the pituitary gland. (Ch 40)

Hypothalamus: the portion of the brain responsible for temperature regulation, water balance, sleep, appetite, and the coordination of autonomic activity. (Ch 17)

Hypotonic: a situation in which the osmotic pressure is lower on one side of a cell membrane. If a hypotonic solution is administered to a patient, fluid will shift into the cells. (Ch 11, Ch 14, Ch 58)

Hypoxemia: a condition characterized by too little oxygen in the blood. (Ch 36)

Hypoxia: a condition characterized by too little oxygen at a given tissue. (Ch 36)

Hysterosalpingography: x-ray visualization of the uterus and uterine tubes following injection of radiopaque contrast media. (Ch 9)

—I—

Ictal: the time frame encompassing an epileptic seizure. (Ch 22)

Idiosyncratic reaction: an unusual and unpredictable reaction to a drug occurring in a small portion of the total population. Often associated with genetic defects. (Ch 1)

Immunity: state of being protected against disease by the presence or development of antibodies or via cell-mediated processes. (Ch 64)

Immunization: vaccination; the administration of antigens, antibodies, or infectious agents in an attempt to protect humans against disease. (Ch 64)

Impairment: a diminished ability to function, e.g. a "professionally impaired person" refers to one who is unable to meet standards of practice because cognitive, interpersonal, and/or psychomotor skills are compromised by the use of drugs or the presence of psychiatric illness. (Ch 13)

Incompatability: chemical or physical reaction that occurs among two or more drugs or between a drug and a delivery device (such as intravenous tubing). (Ch 5)

Induction: in anesthesia, the period from the initial inhalation or injection of an anesthetic drug until optimum level of anesthesia is produced. (Ch 10)

Informal refusal: a situation in which a patient refuses recommended therapy following careful discussion of the potential benefits and risks of both the illness and the treatment. (Ch 49)

Inhalation anesthetic: volatile anesthetic; a general anesthetic in a gaseous or vapor form which is administered by the inhalation route. (Ch 10)

Inotropic: relating to the force of muscle contraction. (Ch 28)

Intercalation: the mechanism of action of the anthracycline antineoplastic agents (daunorubicin, doxorubicin, dactinomycin) whereby the drug forms a complex between itself and DNA base pairs. The result is a disordering of the DNA template and uncoiling of the helix. DNA synthesis, RNA synthesis, and protein synthesis are disrupted. (Ch 49)

Inter-convert: to convert one amino acid into another amino acid. (Ch 51)

Interferon: a protein produced by a cell when exposed to a virus which acts to interfere with the virus' ability to replicate. (Ch 50)

Interleukin: a member of a group of hormones known as lymphokines which are produced by lymphocytes and regulate the immune system. Interleukin-1 is also called lymphocyte-activating factor; interleukin-2 is also known as T-cell growth factor. (Ch 42, Ch 50)

Intermittent claudication: a peripheral vascular disease characterized by progressive weakness and pain in the lower leg during walking. Symptoms are absent during rest. (Ch 31)

Interstitial: referring to the space between cells. (Ch 38)

Interstitial nephritis: a kidney disease characterized by inflammation of the space between the kidney cells. (Ch 6)

Intra-arterial chemotherapy: a method of drug administration in which the chemotherapeutic agent is injected into the artery supplying the involved organ(s). This allows for the delivery of high concentrations of the drug to these tissues without subjecting the rest of the body to potentially toxic levels. (Ch 49)

Intradermal: a parenteral route of drug administration where the medication is injected just under the surface of the skin. (Ch 3)

Intrathecal: injection of a drug directly into the cerebrospinal fluid. (Ch 3, Ch 15, Ch 20)

Intrinsic factor: a substance found in gastric secretions which is necessary for the absorption of vitamin B-12. (Ch 32)

Ionized: polarized molecules; substances which carry an electric charge. Ionized drugs are generally incapable of being absorbed. (Ch 4)

Iontophoresis: administration of drugs via an electrical current. (Ch 60)

Ischemia: a deficiency of blood delivery to a particular site. (Ch 27)

Iso-osmotic: containing a normal osmolality. A solution which is iso-osmotic will neither draw or lose water across a membrane. (Ch 11)

Isotonic: a situation in which the osmotic pressure is the same on both sides of a cell membrane. If an isotonic solution is administered to a patient, no fluid will shift into or out of the cells. (Ch 11, Ch 14, Ch 58)

—J—

—K—

Kaluretic: a drug that causes the loss of potassium in the urine. (Ch 39)

Keratin: an insoluble protein which is the principle constituent of the epidermis, hair, and nails. (Ch 63)

Keratinized tissue: a term referring to tissue whose proteins have been converted to keratin. Keratinized tissues, such as hair and the stratum corneum, are dead. (Ch 63)

Keratolytic: desquamating agent; a drug which dissolves keratin. When applied to the skin, a keratolytic drug will soften scales, loosen the stratum corneum, and cause peeling or shedding of the skin. (Ch 63)

Keratomalacia: softening of the cornea caused by vitamin A deficiency. Untreated, keratomalacia can lead to blindness. (Ch 57)

Keratopathy: a condition characterized by calcium deposition in the cornea. (Ch 60)

Ketoacidosis: a condition, usually found in patients with uncontrolled type I diabetes mellitus, which is characterized by an abnormally low blood pH caused by the buildup of acidic ketone bodies. (Ch 44)

Ketogenic effect: an effect that results in the conversion of fatty acids to ketone bodies. (Ch 41)

Ketosis: a condition characterized by the presence of abnormally high concentrations of ketone bodies. (Ch 44)

Kilocalorie: calorie; the heat energy required to raise the temperature of 1 kilogram of water 1°C; used in nutrition to refer to the energy produced by various foods. (Ch 56)

Kinins: a general group of polypeptide hormones which are formed as a result of injury or inflammation and influence smooth muscle contraction, produce vasodilation, and incite pain. (Ch 47)

Kwashiorkor: protein malnutrition with a depletion of visceral proteins as evidenced by serum level analysis or immune status. (Ch 56, Ch 57)

—L—

Lacrimal apparatus: the structure of the eye that produces tears. (Ch 59)

Lacrimation: tear formation and discharge. (Ch 16)

Larynx: voice box; the organ located at the juncture of the upper and lower airway which contains the vocal cords and assist in the cough reflex and in the prevention of aspiration. (Ch 34)

Learning: act or process of acquiring knowledge or skill. (Ch 8)

Leucovorin rescue: a technique of preventing host toxicity to the antimetabolite methotrexate whereby folinic acid (leucovorin) is administered to a patient soon after the administration of methotrexate. Leucovorin rescue is successful because folinic acid can be utilized by normal tissues but not by cancer cells. (Ch 49)

Leukopenia: abnormal decrease of white blood cells. (Ch 49)

Liability: a legal term denoting responsibility for acts of omission of commission which result in harm to another. (Ch 2)

Lichenified lesion: a general term applied to a variety of skin reactions which are characterized by the presence of papules, or circumscribed red elevations. (Ch 63)

Limbic system: an array of neurons located diffusely around the corpus callosum which is responsible for the expression of mood, feelings, and emotions. (Ch 17)

Linear kinetics: a pharmacokinetic model in which a constant amount of a drug is eliminated in a set unit of time. (Ch 4)

Lipoatrophy: the loss of fatty tissue at the site of insulin injection, possibly caused by an immune reaction to insulin contaminants. (Ch 44)

Lipogenesis: the formation of fat from non-fat sources, such as glucose. (Ch 42)

Lipohypertrophy: accumulation of fatty tissue at the site of insulin injection resulting from repeated injections at the same site. (Ch 44)

Lipolysis: the metabolic breakdown of fat. (Ch 40, Ch 42, Ch 56)

Lipoprotein: combination of triglycerides, phospholipids, and/or cholesterol with a protein. Lipoproteins function to transport lipids which would otherwise be insoluble. (Ch 32)

Lithogenicity: the ability to form mineral deposits or stones, such as gallstones or kidney stones. (Ch 33)

Loading dose: a single large dose of a drug administered to achieve therapeutic serum levels rapidly. (Ch 4)

Local anesthesia: conduction anesthesia; anesthesia confined to one part of the body. Local anesthesia is accomplished by the administration of drugs which prevent the conduction of nerve impulses. (Ch 10)

Local effect: occurs when the effect of a medication is confined to one area of the body. (Ch 3)

Lotion: a liquid suspension or dispersion intended for topical application. (Ch 63)

Lymphography: x-ray visualization of the lymph vessels and lymph nodes following injection of radiopaque contrast media. (Ch 9)

Lysosomal enzymes: enzymes located within the lysosome of a cell which, when released, cause generalized breakdown of proteins and carbohydrates. (Ch 47)

—M—

Macrocytic: referring to a red blood cell which is larger than normal (Ch 32)

Macula: a yellow depression in the center of the retina which contains cones responsible for visual acuity in daylight and for color vision. (Ch 59)

Maintenance dose: a regularly scheduled dose designed to maintain previously established therapeutic serum levels. (Ch 4)

Malnutrition: a state of insufficient, inadequate, or improper intake of food. (Ch 56)

Malpractice: incorrect or negligent treatment of a patient by a health care practitioner. (Ch 65)

Mania: a condition characterized by elevated mood, excessive energy, talkativeness, increased physical activity, flight of ideas, grandiose ideation, and inability to sleep. (Ch 26)

Manual peritoneal dialysis: dialysis across the abdominal viscera which utilizes a Y tubing attached to a peritoneal catheter. The dialysis solution enters the tubing, is allowed to remain in the peritoneum for 0.5 to 2 hours, and is drained into a collection device. (Ch 39)

MAO: see Monoamine oxidase. (Ch 17)

MAOI: see Monoamine oxidase inhibitor. (Ch 26)

Marasmus: protein-calorie malnutrition as evidenced by loss of muscle proteins and low anthropometric parameters. (Ch 56)

Mastication: chewing. (Ch 51)

Mean arterial pressure: the pressure exerted on arterial walls during both the systolic and diastolic phase of the cardiac cycle. (Ch 27)

Meaningful/discovery learning: a learning technique which results when the learner formulates the generalization himself or herself (discovery teaching) and subsequently relates it in a sensible way to existing cognitive structure (meaningful learning). Used by Ausubel. (Ch 8)

Medication: see Drug. (Ch 1)

Medulla oblongata: the portion of the brainstem which is attached to the spinal cord. It is responsible for cardiac, vasogenic, and respiratory regulation as well as vomiting, coughing, sneezing, swallowing, and hiccupping. (Ch 17)

Megaloblastic: referring to a large, immature, nucleated red blood cell. (Ch 32)

Melanin: the color pigment of the skin. (Ch 63)

Mesencephalon: the midbrain; responsible in part for the sensation of pain. (Ch 17)

Metencephalon: the portion of the brain comprised of the pons and cerebellum. (Ch 17)

Metered dose inhalant: an aerosol device which delivers a fixed dose of drug with each spray. (Ch 35)

Michaelis-Menton kinetics: dose-dependent kinetics, non-linear kinetics; a pharmacokinetic model in which higher concentrations of a drug saturate the enzyme systems responsible for their elimination. This results in a slower rate of drug elimination at higher drug concentrations. (Ch 4)

Microcurie (μCi): a measure of radioactivity representing one-millionth of a curie. (Ch 9)

Microcytic: referring to a red blood cell which is smaller than normal. (Ch 32)

Microorganism: minute living body not visible to the naked eye; for example, a bacterium, protozoon, fungus, or virus. (Ch 46)

Milk-alkali syndrome: a syndrome of hypercalcemia, tissue calcification, renal insufficiency, and crystalluria occurring from the chronic administration of sodium bicarbonate with milk or calcium products. (Ch 52)

Millicurie (mCi): a measure of radioactivity representing one-thousandth of a curie. (Ch 9)

Mineral: a naturally occurring non-organic substance necessary for normal metabolism, growth, and development of the body which is available to the body only via dietary intake. (Ch 57)

Mineralocorticoid: steroid hormone secreted by the adrenal cortex that has its major effect on water and electrolyte balance. (Ch 42)

Minute volume: the volume of air breathed each minute. (Ch 36)

Miosis: constriction of the pupil. (Ch 3, Ch 18, Ch 20, Ch 60)

Miotic: a drug that constricts the pupil. (Ch 60)

Mitotic index: the fraction of cells undergoing mitosis at a given time. (Ch 48)

Mixed addiction: simultaneous dependence on more than one substance each of which has different pharmacological effects. (Ch 13)

Mixed angina: a condition characterized by features of both classical and variant angina pectoris. (Ch 31)

Moderate renal failure: renal function which is only 30% of normal; a creatinine clearance less than 30 ml/min. (Ch 39)

Monoamines: substances which contain one amine radical. Included are norepinephrine, epinephrine, serotonin, and histamine. (Ch 47)

Monoamine oxidase: an enzyme responsible for the degradation of norepinephrine, epinephrine, and other monoamines. (Ch 17)

Monoamine oxidase inhibitor: an antidepressant that exerts its effect by inhibiting the enzyme monoamine oxidase. (Ch 26)

Monobactam: a beta-lactam antibiotic group which, in contrast to the penicillins, cephalosporins, and carbapenems, contains only one ring in its basic chemical structure. (Ch 46)

Monoclonal antibodies: antibodies produced by hybridoma cells (a fusion of an antibody producing cell with a multiple myeloma cell). These antibodies are of exceptional purity and specificity and are used to identify antigens in tissue and blood typing. They are currently being studied for their potential for treating cancer. (Ch 50)

Morbilliform: resembling measles. (Ch 22)

Motor neuron: the portion of the somatic nervous system which causes skeletal muscle to contract. (Ch 17)

Mucociliary elevator: the mucus blanket lining the trachea and bronchi which traps bacteria, dust, and other debris and, with the assistance of the motion of epithelial cilia, propels these particles up and out of the lung. (Ch 34)

Mucokinesis: the movement of mucus out of airways. (Ch 35)

Mucolytic: an agent which causes the dissolution of mucus. (Ch 35)

Mucous membrane: a thin tissue that covers a tissue or organ, such as that covering the interior of the mouth, which secretes a slimy substance known as mucus. (Ch 34)

Multifocal ventricular premature beats: a situation in which premature ventricular beats arise from different sections of the ventricle. (Ch 27)

Mural: atrial or ventricular wall. (Ch 27)

Muscarinic receptor: a cholinergic receptor which may also be activated by muscarine. Muscarinic receptors are located on the effector cells of parasympathetic postganglionic fibers, and when activated, cause urination, sweating, bradycardia, and increased gastric motility. (Ch 17, Ch 18, Ch 34)

Mycoplasma: a group of microorganisms responsible for the most common cause of pneumonia in young adults. (Ch 46)

Mydriasis: dilitation of the pupil. (Ch 4, Ch 21, Ch 60)

Mydriatic: a drug that dilates the pupil. (Ch 60)

Myelencephalon: medulla oblongata. (Ch 17)

Myopathy: a general term referring to a muscular disorder. (Ch 45)

Myopia: nearsightedness; the inability to see distant objects clearly. (Ch 59)

Myringitis: inflammation of the eardrum, usually because of infection. (Ch 61)

Mystical stage of therapeutics: a stage in the development of pharmacotherapeutics which was strongly influenced by religion and which employed prayers, surgery, and drugs. (Ch 2)

—N—

Natural immunity: immunity to disease which is inherent to an individual. Natural immunity results from genetic factors, the presence of natural immune substances such as interferon, and the inflammatory response to foreign organisms. (Ch 64)

Naturally acquired immunity: immunity resulting from the natural exposure to infectious agents in the environment or that which is acquired from the mother *in vitro*. (Ch 64)

Nebulizer: a device for producing a spray or mist. (Ch 3)

Negative feedback mechanism: a system that minimizes excessive secretion of a hormone. In this system, exposure to excessive amounts of a hormone causes the target organ to send a message to the secreting organ causing it to slow hormone release. (Ch 40)

Negligence: careless acts of omission or commission. (Ch 65)

Neonatal neurobehavioral scores: a rating evaluation of an infant's neurological and behavioral function shortly after birth. (Ch 15)

Neoplasm: uncontrolled or progresive abnormal growth of new tissue. (Ch 48)

Nephrogenic diabetes insipidus: diabetes insipidus which results when the kidney fails to adequately respond to vasopressin (antidiuretic hormone). (Ch 38)

Nephrotic syndrome: a condition characterized by damage to the capillary wall of the arteries of the glomerulus. Clinically, this leads to the loss of a large amount of protein in the urine, which in turn results in hypoalbuminemia and edema. (Ch 38)

Nephrotoxicity: having a deleterious effect on the kidney. (Ch 16)

Neurohypophysis: the posterior lobe of the pituitary

gland. It manufactures and releases vasopressin and oxytocin. (Ch 40)

Neuroleptic: see antipsychotic. (Ch 25)

Neuroleptic malignant syndrome: a rare syndrome caused by antipsychotic drugs and characterized by muscle rigidity, high fever, altered consciousness, tachycardia, hypertension, and diaphoresis. The mortality rate is about 20%. (Ch 25)

Neuromuscular receptor: the receptor located in the muscle which is activated by neuronal release of acetylcholine. (Ch 18)

Neuropathy: a general term referring to non-specific disorders of the nervous system. (Ch 44)

Neurotransmitter: chemical substance released by a nerve which acts on another nerve or a muscle to initiate or modulate an action potential. (Ch 17)

Neutralizing capacity: see acid neutralizing capacity. (Ch 7)

Nicotinic receptor: a cholinergic receptor which may also be activated by nicotine. Nicotinic receptors are located in the somatic nervous system and in the ganglia of the autonomic nervous system. (Ch 17, Ch 18)

Nociceptors: nerve endings in the skin, tissues, and organs that are stimulated by injury and transmit pain. (Ch 20)

Noncardiac dependent peripheral edema: a form of peripheral edema whose severity and characteristics are independent of cardiac function. (Ch 31)

Noncompliance: not in keeping with; not following direction. (Ch 8)

Nondepolarizing neuromuscular blocking agent: a drug which causes muscle paralysis by blocking the transmission of impulses at the neuromuscular junction. Nondepolarizing agents accomplish this by competing with the natural substance acetylcholine. When the drug binds with the receptor site, the muscle stimulating actions of acetylcholine are blocked. (Ch 10, Ch 18)

Nonionized: non-polarized molecules; substances which do not carry an electric charge. Drugs are absorbed most readily when in a nonionized form. (Ch 4)

Non-linear kinetics: see Michaelis-Menton kinetics. (Ch 4)

Nonpharmacological intervention: therapy without the use of drugs. (Ch 7)

Norepinephrine: levarterenol; a neurotransmitter produced in the brain and adrenal medulla which regulates autonomic activity and blood pressure. (Ch 17)

Normal flora: the usual population of microorganisms which inhabit a particular site. (Ch 46)

Normocytic: referring to a red blood cell of a normal size. (Ch 32)

Normoglycemia: the presence of normal concentrations of glucose in the blood. (Ch 44)

Nuclei: 1.) groups of nerve cells within the central nervous system from which specific nerve fibers originate. 2.) the bodies within a cell which contain chromosomes and other genetic material. (Ch 23)

Null cells: lymphocytes which lack the marker for both T and B cells. Included are the natural killer cells and the lymphokine-activated killer cells. (Ch 50)

Nursing process: a series of planned, logical steps which produce positive patient outcomes. Included are assessment, diagnosis, planning, intervention, and evaluation. (Ch 1)

Nyctalopia: night blindness; a condition in which an individual cannot see well in dim light or at night. (Ch 57)

Nystagmus: constant, involuntary, cyclical movement of the eyeball in any direction. (Ch 60)

—O—

Obligate anaerobe: a microorganism that can live and grow only in the absence of oxygen. (Ch 46)

Obsession: an abnormal pre-occupation with a particular idea, subject, or event. (Ch 24)

Ocular palsy: a condition characterized by the inability to move or control eye movement. (Ch 60)

Oculogyric crisis: a syndrome characterized by hyperextension of the neck and upward fixation of the eyeballs. May be an extrapyramidal side effect of antipsychotic drugs. (Ch 25, Ch 60)

Ocusert system: a proprietary name of a drug delivery system which is placed into the eye and released a consistent amount of drug (pilocarpine) every hour for seven days. (Ch 18)

Ointment: a topical semi-solid form consisting of a pure fatty substance, or an oil in water, or water in oil emulsion. An ointment differs from a cream in that an ointment contains relatively little water, is greasy, and is generally not removable by water. (Ch 63)

Oliguria: a condition of diminished urine formation. (Ch 39)

Oncogenes: genes which lead to tumor formation. Oncogenes are introduced into normal cells by viruses. (Ch 48)

Oncotic pressure: the pressure exerted by large molecules (such as albumin) within a capillary that keeps fluid within the capillary from crossing capillary membranes. (Ch 37)

Opthalmic route: applied to the eye. (Ch 3)

Opthalmopathy: a general term referring to a disease of the eye. (Ch 45)

Optic neuritis: inflammation of the optic nerve resulting in diminished vision. (Ch 60)

Opiate: a substance derived from opium; a drug or substance which mimics the actions of morphine. (Ch 20)

Opiate agonist: a drug or endogenous substance which stimulates opiate receptors. (Ch 20)

Opiate agonist-antagonist: a drug or substance which stimulates certain opiate receptors but antagonizes other opiate receptors. (Ch 20)

Opiate antagonist: a drug which interferes with the action of morphine or other opiates. (Ch 20)

Opiate receptor: a receptor which binds with morphine, endogenous peptides, and other opiates. (Ch 20)

Opisthotonos: a severe muscular spasm characterized by the head and heels being bent backward and the body bent forward so that only the head and heel remain in contact with the ground. (Ch 21)

Opsonic proteins: proteins such as antibodies which are utilized to destroy microorganisms or make them more susceptible to phagocytosis. (Ch 56)

Optic disc: a small white section at the back of the eyeball where the retinal arteries and veins and the optic nerve enter the eye. The optic disc is insensitive to light. (Ch 59)

Orphan drug: a drug which is effective for the treatment of rare diseases but which is not profitable for a manufacturer to produce. The government provides technical assistance and economic incentives to pharmaceutical manufacturers for developing and marketing these agents. (Ch 66)

Orthostatic: relating to standing upright; in orthostatic hypotension, the blood pressure is normal while reclining but low while standing. (Ch 29)

Osmolality: the concentration of free particles, molecules, or ions in solution. (Ch 11, Ch 58)

Osmolarity: the concentration of osmotically active particles in solution. (Ch 11, Ch 58)

Osmotic concentration: osmolality. (Ch 11)

Osteitis fibrosa: a condition resulting from hyperparathyroidism and characterized by decalcification and softening of the bone, nephrolithiasis, increased serum calcium and decreased serum phosphorus. (Ch 39)

Osteomalacia: adult rickets; a condition caused by vitamin D deficiency which is characterized by soft, brittle bones, bone deformities, bone pain, and weakness. (Ch 39, Ch 57)

Osteoporosis: a condition of reduced bone mass sufficient to interfere with the support functic of the bone. Osteoporosis becomes apparent when the bone fractures in situations that would not normally cause damage. (Ch 39)

OTC: see Over-the-counter drug. (Ch 1)

Otic route: applied to the ear. (Ch 3)

Outpatient surgery: see Ambulatory surgery. (Ch 10)

Over-the-counter drug: a drug which may be purchased without a prescription. (Ch 1, Ch 7)

Oxygen-induced hypoventilation: a condition in which the administration of oxygen causes the chemoreceptors to excessively slow the rate of ventilation. This condition occurs most commonly in patients with chronically high pCO_2 values. In these patients, the chemoreceptors are tolerant to the high pCO_2 values and will not cause a compensatory increase in ventilatory drive. (Ch 36)

Oxygen toxicity: lung damage which results from prolonged exposure to high concentrations of oxygen. Characterized by atelectasis, pulmonary infiltrates, and interstitial pneumonitis. (Ch 36)

Oxytocic: a drug which has pharmacological properties similar to oxytocin. Oxytocics are usually used to induce or augment labor, to decrease postpartum hemorrhage, and to assist with lactation. (Ch 15)

—P—

Pancytopenia: abnormal decrease of white blood cells, red blood cells, and platelets. (Ch 49)

Papilledema: edema and inflammation of the optic nerve at its point of entrance into the eyeball. Caused by increased intracranial pressure, papilledema will result in blindness without rapid treatment. (Ch 60)

Paracentesis: mechanical removal of fluid from the abdomen, usually via a needle catheter. (Ch 55)

Paradoxical reaction: a response to a medication which is opposite that which would be predicted by the drug's pharmacology. For example, geriatric or pediatric patients may develop a paradoxical excitation from phenobarbital instead of the expected sedation. (Ch 24)

Parasympathetic nervous system: craniosacral system; the portion of the autonomic nervous system which is responsible for energy conservation. Stimulation of the parasympathetic nervous system results in a slowed heart rate, shunting of blood from muscle to the viscera and kidney, increased food absorption, and glycogen synthesis. (Ch 17)

Paravertebral ganglia: sympathetic ganglia so named for their proximity to the spinal cord. (Ch 17)

Parenteral: injectable route of drug administration, e.g. intradermal, subcutaneous, intramuscular, or intravenous. (Ch 3, Ch 56)

Partial opiate agonist-antagonist: see opiate agonist-antagonist. (Ch 20)

Passive immunity: immunity acquired by the passage of antibodies to the fetus from the mother or via the direct injection of the antibodies. Passive immunization does not stimulate the body's own immune response. (Ch 64)

Passive nonspecific immunotherapy: the treatment of cancer via passive immunization utilizing the serum of normal volunteers. (Ch 50)

Passive specific immunotherapy: the treatment of cancer via passive immunization utilizing the serum of patients who are in remission with the same tumor. (Ch 50)

Passive treatment: a transport process by which drugs move from areas of high concentration to areas of low concentration. Requires no energy expenditure. (Ch 4, Ch 37)

Pathogen: a microorganism which is capable of causing disease. (Ch 46)

Patient package insert: patient education material, developed by the drug's manufacturer and approved by the federal government, designed to be dispensed by the pharmacist with each prescription. (Ch 2)

Penicillinase: a form of beta-lactamase which specifically destroys penicillins. (Ch 46)

Penicillin binding proteins: receptor proteins for beta-lactam antibiotics. (Ch 46)

Pentagastrin: a synthetic form of gastrin which is used to determine the capacity of the stomach to secrete acid. (Ch 47)

Peptic ulcer: an erosion in the mucosal lining of the

walls of the esophagus, stomach, duodenum, or jejunum caused by exposure to the actions of acid and pepsin. (Ch 52)

Peptidoglycan: complex polysaccharide and peptide material that comprise the cell wall of most bacteria. (Ch 46)

Peripheral edema: abnormal accumulation of fluid in the extremities. (Ch 38)

Peripheral resistance: the resistance generated by the arteries and capillaries against the passage of blood. Peripheral resistance is directly related to the tone of the vessel wall and the diameter of the vessel. (Ch 27)

Peristalsis: contractions of the smooth muscles of the alimentary tract that propel food from the esophagus to the anus. (Ch 51)

Pernicious anemia: a megaloblastic anemia characterized by achlorhydrea and a lack of intrinsic factor production. (Ch 54)

Petit mal seizures: see Absence epilepsy. (Ch 22)

Pharmaceutical phase: the stage during which a medication enters the body in one form and changes into another form to be utilized, e.g. a tablet is dissolved into solution in order to be absorbed. (Ch 4)

Pharmaceutical process: see Pharmaceutical phase. (Ch 4)

Pharmacodynamics: the study of the biochemical and physiologic actions and effects of drugs. (Ch 4)

Pharmacokinetics: the study of a drug's absorption, distribution, metabolism, and elimination. (Ch 4)

Pharmacology: the scientific study of drugs including their source, properties, uses, actions, and effects. (Ch 1)

Pharmacopeia: an authoritative book on drugs, drug preparations, drug standards, and formulas for certain mixtures of these substances. (Ch 2)

Pharmacotherapeutics: study of the use of drugs in the treatment of disease. (Ch 1)

Pharyngitis: a syndrome usually infectious in nature characterized by inflammation and pain in the throat, especially upon swallowing. (Ch 7)

Phenochromocytoma: a tumor of the adrenal medulla characterized by episodic or continuous release of excessive quantities of catecholamines. (Ch 19, Ch 26)

Philosopher's stone: a stone, searched for in vain by the 15th century alchemists, which could change base metals into gold and restore health and youth. (Ch 2)

Phobias: a collection of syndromes characterized by an abnormal fear to a particular subject or event. (Ch 24)

Photophobia: abnormal intolerance of light. (Ch 20)

Pinocytosis: a mechanism whereby the cell membrane invaginates, fills with a drug or other substance, breaks off, and moves into the cell. (Ch 4)

Pitting edema: edema, usually of the skin of the extremities, that when pressed firmly with a finger will maintain the depression produced by the finger. (Ch 38)

Placebo: an inactive substance or preparation given to satisfy a patient's symbolic need for drug therapy. (Ch 1, Ch 4)

Placental barrier: a functional activity of the placenta which serves to minimize the passage of certain drugs and other substances from the mother to the fetus. (Ch 15)

Plasma expander: a substance obtained from sources other than blood which has the ability to expand a patient's blood volume. (Ch 12)

Plasmapheresis: a procedure which removes plasma, white blood cells, or platelets from a donor and re-injects the red blood cells. (Ch 12)

Plasmid: genetic material not located in the nucleus of a cell. Transfer of plasmids may occur between bacteria of different species and account for outbreaks of antibiotic resistance in the hospital or nursing home environment. (Ch 46)

Poikilothermia: a condition characterized by abnormal temperature regulation. (Ch 25)

Polypharmacy: the concurrent administration of many drugs; often refers to the concurrent use of many drugs for the same indication. (Ch 16)

Pons: the portion of the brainstem which connects the medulla with the mesencephalon and cerebellum and participates in the regulation of respiration. (Ch 17)

Porphyria: a disorder of porphyrin metabolism characterized by abdominal pain, back pain, peripheral motor deficit, altered mental status, hallucinations, dark urine, tachycardia, and constipation. (Ch 24)

Post-ictal: the time frame beginning at the conclusion of an epileptic seizure to the establishment of full recovery. (Ch 22)

Post-tetanic potentiation: a proposed mechanism of seizure formation which says that repetitive stimulation of the seizure focus results in the release of increasing quantities of neurotransmitters. (Ch 22)

Potency: relationship between the dose of a drug and the intensity of its effect. The more potent a drug is, the smaller the dose is required to achieve a certain effect. (Ch 4)

Potentiation: a synergistic drug interaction in which the effect of one drug is enhanced by the presence of the second drug. (Ch 5)

PPI: see Patient package insert. (Ch 2)

Pre-eclampsia: toxemia of pregnancy; a disorder occurring late in pregnancy characterized by hypertension, edema, and proteinuria. (Ch 15)

Preload: the degree of stretch of the myocardial fibers at the onset of cardiac contraction; the blood volume of the heart at the end of diastole. (Ch 27)

Pre-renal azotemia: an increase in blood urea nitrogen which is greater than the corresponding rise in serum creatinine. Pre-renal azotemia reflects disorders in blood flow to the kidney, such as congestive heart failure, hypotension, or hypovolemia and is not necessarily a reflection of primary kidney disease. (Ch 39)

Priapism: persistent abnormal erection of the penis. (Ch 43)

Priming: in cancer chemotherapy, a technique to prevent host toxicity to an alkylating agent in which a patient is given a small dose of the drug prior to subsequent full dose therapy with the same or a different alkylating agent. The mechanism by which priming protects against drug toxicity is unknown. (Ch 49)

Prinzmetal's angina: see Variant angina. (Ch 31)

Proandrogens: androgen precursors which are secreted by the ovary and adrenal cortex. (Ch 43)

Proarrhythmic: an agent that causes or worsens a cardiac dysrhythmia. (Ch 30)

Progestins: synthetic forms of progesterone. (Ch 43)

Proprietary name: see Trade name. (Ch 3)

Proprioception: the peripheral perception of motion and position which assists in the control of equilibrium. (Ch 59)

Proptosis: downward displacement of the eyeball in exophthalmic goiter or in inflammatory conditions of the orbit. (Ch 43)

Prostaglandins: a large group of cellular hormones derived from essential fatty acids. Prostaglandins are manufactured and released in response to a variety of stimuli and, as a group, affect virtually every organ system. (Ch 42, Ch 37, Ch 47)

Protective: in dermatology, an agent that mechanically protects the skin to which it is applied. (Ch 63)

Proteolysis: the hydrolysis of proteins. (Ch 56, Ch 62)

Protozoa: a division of the animal kingdom that includes the simplest animals. Examples of protozoa include those responsible for malaria (plasmodium), amebic dysentery (entamoeba histolytica), and the African sleeping sickness (trypanosoma). (Ch 46)

Provitamin: an inactive substance which is converted by the body to an active vitamin. (Ch 57)

Proximal-distal: proceeding in a direction from the center of the body to the periphery. (Ch 14)

Pseudoparkinsonism: a condition resembling Parkinson's disease but which is caused by other etiologies, such as drugs or cerebrovascular lesions. (Ch 25)

Psychological dependence: a compulsive incapacitating need to use a drug. Patients who are psychologically dependent on a drug do not necessarily display physiological signs of dependence, such as tolerance or withdrawal. (Ch 13)

Ptosis: drooping of the upper eyelid. (Ch 23, Ch 60)

Pulmonary artery pressure: the pressure as measured directly within the pulmonary artery. This measurement reflects the function of the right side of the heart. (Ch 65)

Pulmonary edema: abnormal accumulation of fluid in the lungs. Pulmonary edema is often a result of congestive heart failure. (Ch 38)

Pulse therapy: the administration of intermittent high doses of a drug. (Ch 42)

Punctate defects: pinpoint punctures or depressions on the surface of the eye or skin. (Ch 60)

Pyrogen: a substance that produces fever. Pyrogens are often of bacterial origin. (Ch 11)

—Q—

—R—

Radioisotope: a chemical element which emits electromagnetic radiation. (Ch 9)

Radionuclide: an atom which emits electromagnetic radiation. (Ch 9)

Radiopaque: description of a substance which does not allow the passage of x-rays or other radiant energy. Radiopaque areas appear white on the exposed film. (Ch 9)

Radiopharmaceutical: a drug which contains a radioisotope or radionuclide which is used systematically for the diagnosis or treatment of disease. (Ch 9)

Rales: abnormal breath sounds usually associated with the presence of fluid in the bronchi. (Ch 36)

Raynaud's disease: see Raynaud's phenomenon. (Ch 31)

Raynaud's phenomenon: a syndrome characterized by recurring attacks of diminished blood supply to the fingers and/or toes. Symptoms may include pain, numbness, tingling, pallor, and cyanosis. Symptoms are often precipitated by exposure to cold or emotional stress. (Ch 29, Ch 31)

Reabsorption: the process of absorbing a substance after it has been filtered, secreted, or otherwise eliminated from a site. It occurs in the kidney when some of the materials filtered out of the blood by the glomerulus are reabsorbed as the filtrate passes through the nephron. opp = secretion. (Ch 37)

Reactive depression: depression which can be related to a specific life event, such as the death of a spouse. (Ch 26)

Readability: the level at which a person is able to read and comprehend the written word. (Ch 8)

Rebound: a situation in which the severity of a disorder is worse shortly after discontinuation of treatment than it was just prior to the initiation of treatment. (Ch 24)

Rebound hypertension: a situation which occurs following the discontinuation of antihypertensive drugs in which the blood pressure becomes higher than it was prior to initiating the drug. (Ch 29)

Reception learning: an educational method of presenting the entire content of what is to be learned in final form to the learner. Used by Ausubel. (Ch 8)

Receptor: a portion of a cell or tissue which can be occupied by a drug and result in a particular effect. (Ch 4, Ch 17)

Re-entry: a mechanism of cardiac dysrhythmia in which the action potential prematurely re-enters and re-excites an area of myocardium. This results in rapid, repetitive depolarization of parts of the cardiac conduction system. (Ch 30)

Reference drug: a formulation of a drug which is the standard for all other drugs of its group for potency, efficacy, and bioavailability. Usually, but not always, the original drug of its kind. (Ch 3)

Reflux esophagitis: inflammation of the esophagus caused by the reflux of acid and pepsin from the stomach into the esophagus. (Ch 52)

Refractory angina: angina pectoris which does not respond to usual therapy. (Ch 31)

Refractory period: the timeframe after cardiac contraction during which the heart is unable to respond, or would respond abnormally, to another cardiac impulse. (Ch 27)

Refractory rickets: rickets which is unresponsive to vitamin D therapy. Refractory rickets is caused by a defect in renal tubular function which results in excessive urinary losses of calcium and phosphorus. (Ch 57)

Reinforcement: the provision of positive rewards in order to strengthen, to augment, or to increase the probability that the behavior occurs again. Used by Skinner. (Ch 8, Ch 24)

Reinforcer: anything that increases the probability of a desired response. (Ch 8)

Relapse: the recurrence of a disease after its apparent cure or remission. (Ch 24)

REM: rapid eye movement; the stage of sleep in which dreaming occurs. (Ch 21, Ch 24)

Renal papilla: the portion of the renal pyramid which delivers urine to the renal pelvis. (Ch 37)

Renal pelvis: the proximal end of the ureter which receives urine through the calyces from the renal papilla. (Ch 37)

Resistance vessels: arteries. (Ch 19, Ch 29)

Reticular activating system: the portion of the reticular formation responsible for alertness and arousal. (Ch 17)

Reticular formation: an array of neurons located throughout the brainstem, diencephalon, and telencephalon which functions to modulate sensory and motor activity, regulate autonomic responses, and produce monoamines. (Ch 17)

Retrobulbar injection: injection of drugs behind the eyeball. (Ch 60)

Retrolental fibroplasia: a condition caused by excessive oxygen administration to premature infants and characterized by the development of fibrous tissue behind the lens with resultant blindness. (Ch 36)

Reverse vegetative symptoms: symptoms often associated with atypical depression and which include afternoon/evening worsening, increased appetite or weight gain, and increased sleep. These symptoms are in contrast to the morning worsening, decreased appetite or weight gain, and decreased sleep patterns more commonly ascribed to the depressive disorders. (Ch 26)

Rhabdomyolsis: rapid muscle breakdown. (Ch 32, Ch 33)

Rhinitis: a syndrome usually caused by a head cold or hay fever which is manifested by nasal dryness and congestion. (Ch 7)

Rhinorrhea: runny nose. (Ch 7, Ch 21)

Rhonchi: abnormal breath sounds usually associated with partial bronchial obstruction. (Ch 36)

Rickets: abnormal bone formation in children caused by vitamin D deficiency. (Ch 57)

Rickettsiae: a group of microorganisms that possess characteristics of both bacteria and viruses. Rickettsia are larger than true viruses but, unlike bacteria, require living cells for growth. (Ch 46)

Rods: cells located in the retina of the eye which are responsible for vision in dim light. (Ch 57)

Rote/Discovery learning: results when the learner discovers the generalization himself or herself (discovery teaching) and subsequently memorizes the new ideas without relating it to other relevant ideas in his or her cognitive structure (rote learning). Used by Ausubel. (Ch 8)

R on T phenomena: a premature ventricular beat which occurs such that the QRS complex is superimposed on the preceeding T wave. R on T phenomena are thought to precipitate ventricular tachycardia or ventricular fibrillation. (Ch 30)

—S—

Same-day surgery: see Ambulatory surgery. (Ch 10)

Sarcoplasmic reticulum: the substance within a cardiac cell. (Ch 27)

Scarification: the process of making numerous superficial scratches on the skin. Scarification is used to administer certain vaccines, such as BCG vaccine. (Ch 64)

Scarlatiniform: resembling scarlet fever. (Ch 22)

Sclera: the thick, white, opaque posterior covering of the outer layer of the eye. (Ch 59)

Sebaceous gland: the glands located in the skin which secrete sebum. (Ch 14)

Sebum: fatty secretion of the skin. (Ch 14, Ch 63)

Second messenger system: biochemical systems which utilize intermediate molecules in order to translate drug-receptor binding interactions into a pharmacological response. (Ch 26)

Secretion: 1) the production of material by a gland. 2) in renal physiology, refers to the transport of substances directly into the proximal tubule of the nephron. (Ch 37)

Sedative: tranquilizer anxiolytic; an agent that produces sedation or calming. (Ch 24)

Segmental contractions: contractions of the smooth muscles of the alimentary tract that cause food and digestive juices to mix. (Ch 51)

Seizure: a sudden, uncontrolled burst of neuronal firing. The specific signs and symptoms of a seizure vary with the nature and location of neuronal firing. (Ch 22)

Seizure disorder: a chronic illness characterized by repeated seizure activity. (Ch 22)

Selectivity: the spectrum of effects that medication precipitates. Highly selective drugs have a narrow spectrum of effects. (Ch 4)

Self-care: prevention or treatment of illness without the direct involvement of a health professional. (Ch 7)

Self-limiting: description of an illness or symptom which will resolve on its own without treatment. (Ch 7)

Sensitizing lymphocytes: white blood cells which, if transfused, can stimulate the recipients immune system. (Ch 12)

Sequestration: a drug interaction which occurs when a drug is surrounded by a lipoid substance and is prevented from coming into contact with the intestinal mucosa. (Ch 5)

Serum: 1) the portion of the blood which does not contain cells or coagulation factors. 2) in immunizations, refers to the serum of an animal or other human immune to a particular disease which is administered to a patient for purposes of providing passive immunity. Examples include immune serum globulin and rabies immune globulin. (Ch 64)

Severe renal failure: renal function which is only 10% of normal; a creatinine clearance less than 10 ml/min. (Ch 39)

SIADH: syndrome of inappropriate antidiuretic hormone. (Ch 40, Ch 41)

Sickle cell anemia: an hereditary form of hemolytic anemia, found mostly in black patients, which is characterized by the presence of an oat-shaped (sickle) red blood cell, abdominal pain, skin ulceration, and priapism. (Ch 32)

Sleep apnea: a condition characterized by the cessation of breathing during sleep. (Ch 24)

Solubility: the ability of a medication to dissolve and form a solution. (Ch 4)

Somatic proteins: the proteins comprising muscle. (Ch 56)

Somatic nerves: the portion of the peripheral nervous system responsible for sensory and motor function. (Ch 17)

Somatomedins: substances that mediate the action of growth hormone on cartilage and bone. (Ch 41)

Somatotropin: growth hormone, somatotropic hormone; a hormone released by the anterior pituitary gland which regulates the growth of tissue and the metabolism of carbohydrates, proteins, and fats. (Ch 40)

Somnambulism: sleep walking. (Ch 24)

Spasticity: a condition characterized by resistance to passive movement of an extremity resulting from excessive muscle tone. (Ch 23)

Specific stage of therapeutics: a stage in the development of pharmacotherapeutics which relies upon the use of simple, specific compounds to treat disease. (Ch 2)

Spondylolisthesis: displacement of one vertebra over another. (Ch 62)

Spray: a liquid form of medication delivered by a jet of air or nebulizer. (Ch 3)

Steady-state: a condition which occurs when the rate of drug administration is equal to the rate of drug excretion. (Ch 4)

Steatorrhea: stools with excessive fat content. (Ch 54)

Stem cell: 1) a cell located in the bone marrow that gives rise to various specialized cells, such as red and white blood cells and platelets. 2) the cell from which a tumor is thought to originate. (Ch 32, Ch 48)

Stem cell theory: the theory of tumor formation which states that a tumor arises from a single aberrant stem cell. (Ch 48)

Step therapy: a treatment modality in which a patient is given a step-wise progression of therapy until the desired results are seen. (Ch 38)

Stevens-Johnson syndrome: a severe allergic reaction characterized by urticaria, a large blister-like rash, fever, and mucous membrane lesions. (Ch 22, Ch 60)

Stimulus-response theory: a theory of learning in which the nurse provides the stimulus experiences and the patient responds. (Ch 8)

Stomatitis: inflammation of the mouth with or without the presence of small ulcers. Stomatitis may be caused by a variety of factors including chemotherapy and results in pain and an inability to eat. (Ch 49)

Stratum corneum: "horny layer" of the skin; the outermost layer of the skin which is comprised by dead cornified cells. (Ch 14, Ch 63)

Stratum germinativum: the innermost layer of the epidermis which contains columnar cells which divide to replace the rest of the epidermis as it wears away. (Ch 63)

Stratum granulosum: the layer of skin just below the stratum corneum so named for the presence of keratohyalin granules. (Ch 63)

Stress ulcer: peptic ulcer that is caused by severe stress such as trauma, sepsis, burns, or head injuries. (Ch 52)

Stroke volume: the volume of blood ejected by the heart with each beat. (Ch 27)

Sublingual: a route of drug administration where the medication is placed under the tongue. (Ch 3)

Superinfection: a new infection caused by an organism different from the original infection and resistant to the antibiotic given to treat the original infection. (Ch 46)

Supersensitivity: see hyperreactivity. (Ch 4)

Suppository: a solid medication intended to be inserted into the rectum or vagina which will then melt or dissolve and release an active drug. (Ch 3)

Surfactant: a phospholipid secreted by specialized alveolar cells which prevents collapse of the alveolar sacs. (Ch 34)

Sympathetic nervous system: thoracolumbar system;

the portion of the autonomic nervous system which is responsible for rapid energy expenditure. Stimulation of the sympathetic nervous system results in an increase in heart rate and contractility, shunting of blood from the skin and viscera to skeletal and cardiac muscle, relaxation of bronchial smooth muscle, and the mobilization of glucose. (Ch 17)

Sympatholytic effect: an effect which is produced by blocking the action of the sympathetic nervous system. (Ch 19)

Sympathomimetic effect: an effect which occurs after stimulation of the sympathetic nervous system. (Ch 17, Ch 19, Ch 35)

Syndrome of inappropriate antidiuretic hormone: a condition characterized by excessive production and release of vasopressin (antidiuretic hormone) with resultant fluid retention and hyponatremia. (Ch 40, Ch 41)

Synergistic drug interaction: a form of drug-drug interaction in which the effects of the two drugs are greater than that of either drug alone. (Ch 5)

Syngeneic: individuals or cells without detectable tissue incompatibility. Strains of mice that are inbred for a great number of generations become syngeneic. (Ch 50)

Systemic effect: occurs when the medication is absorbed, delivered to more than one body tissue, and effects the body as a whole. (Ch 3)

Systemic lupus erythematosus: an autoimmune disease or hypersensitivity reaction characterized by a specific red skin rash. Severe cases may result in destructive arthritis, nephritis, pneumonitis, or cerebritis. (Ch 22)

Systemic vascular resistance: the tone of the vasculature as measured by its resistance to blood flow. Systemic vascular resistance is directly related to blood pressure. (Ch 65)

Systole: cardiac contraction. (Ch 27)

—T—

Tardive dyskinesia: a syndrome caused by the long term administration of antipsychotic medications and characterized by abnormal movements of the mouth, chewing motions, tongue thrusts and sucking, and pursing and blowing movements of the lips. (Ch 25)

T-cells: thymic lymphoid cells; lymphocytes which circulate between the blood and lymph and participate in cell-mediated immunity. (Ch 50)

Teaching-learning: process whereby the nurse imparts knowledge and the patient acquires knowledge. (Ch 8)

Teaching-learning theory: system of rules or principles used in the process of imparting knowledge. (Ch 8)

Telencephalon: the anterior portion of the brain. (Ch 17, Ch 23)

Teratogen: a substance which causes birth defects. (Ch 15)

Teratogenic: relating to causing birth defects. (Ch 15)

Teratogenicity: the ability of a substance to cause birth defects. (Ch 15)

Tetany: a syndrome characterized by intermittent painful tonic spasms of the extremities and occasionally the jaw. Tetany is usually caused by hypocalcemia. (Ch 57)

Thalamus: the portion of the brain responsible for relaying the sensory impulses of pain, touch, pressure and temperature to the cerebral cortex. The thalamus also influences emotions and arousal and coordinates motor movement. (Ch 17)

Therapeutic index: the ratio between the dose of a drug which causes toxic effects and the dose required to produce desired therapeutic effects. (Ch 28)

Thermogenic: an effect which produces heat, thereby raising body temperature. (Ch 43)

Thoracolumbar system: an anatomical description of the sympathetic nervous system. (Ch 17)

Thrombolysis: see fibrinolysis. (Ch 33)

Thyroid-stimulating hormone: see Thyrotropin. (Ch 40)

Thyrotropin: a hormone released by the anterior pituitary gland which controls the growth and function of the thyroid gland. (Ch 40)

Thyroxine: the main thyroid hormone responsible for regulating the rate of carbohydrate, protein, and fat metabolism. (Ch 40)

Tic: twitching; one or several involuntary muscle contractions most commonly involving the face, head, neck, or shoulder muscles. (Ch 23)

Tidal volume: the volume of air moved with each breath. (Ch 36)

Tinnitus: the perception of ringing in the ears. Tinnitus may be caused by neurologic disease or may appear as an adverse reaction to some drugs. (Ch 16, Ch 61)

Titratable acidity: in renal physiology, the elimination of acid by combining hydrogen with sulfate or phosphate. (Ch 37)

Tolerance: a situation in which progressively higher amounts of a drug are necessary to achieve the same effects formerly attained by lesser amounts of the drug. (Ch 13, Ch 20, Ch 24)

Tonsils: lymphatic tissue found in the middle portion of the pharynx whose function it is to trap bacteria and prevent respiratory infection. (Ch 34)

Tonus waves: weak contractions of the stomach muscle which help to mix the food bolus with gastric secretions. (Ch 51)

Torsade de pointe: multiformic ventricular tachycardia or a combination of ventricular tachycardia with ventricular fibrillation. (Ch 30)

Torticollis: a condition characterized by a spasmodic contraction of the neck muscles resulting in the head drawn to one side and the chin pointing to the other side. May be an extrapyramidal side effect of antipsychotic drugs. (Ch 25)

Total parenteral nutrition: see Hyperalimentation. (Ch 56)

Toxicology: the scientific study of the effects of poisons on humans or animals; the aspect of pharmacology that deals with adverse drug reactions. (Ch 6)

Toxoid: a bacterial poison (toxin) which has been detoxified. Although unable to produce toxicity, the toxoid is capable of stimulating active immunity to the toxin. (Ch 64)

TPN: total parenteral nutrition; see hyperalimentation. (Ch 56)

Trabecular meshwork: tissue located in the anterior chamber of the eye which filters aqueous humor before it enters the canal of Schlemm and the systemic circulation. (Ch 59)

Trabeculoplasty: surgical manipulation of the trabecular meshwork of the eye in order to treat glaucoma. (Ch 60)

Trade name: a name of a drug assigned by a manufacturer. Trade names of the same drug are different with each manufacturer. (Ch 3)

Tranquilizer: see sedative. (Ch 24)

Transamination: the metabolic formation of one amino acid from another amino acid by the transfer of an amino group. (Ch 56)

Transdermal: medication which is applied topically in a vehicle which allows for its systemic absorption from the skin. (Ch 3)

Transfer factor: a factor present in lymphocytes that have been sensitized to antigens which can, in man, be transferred to a nonsensitized recipient. The recipient will then react to the same antigen that was originally used to sensitize the lymphocytes of the donor. Use of transfer factor is a form of adoptive immunization. (Ch 50)

Tremor: an involuntary shaking or trembling movement. (Ch 23)

Tricyclic antidepressant: a chemical description of certain antidepressants in that their chemical structure is comprised of three rings. (Ch 26)

Trifascicular block: an intraventricular conduction defect in which conduction is delayed or blocked through the right bundle branch, the anterior portion of the left bundle branch, and the posterior portion of the left bundle branch. (Ch 30)

Triglyceride: a neutral fat which consists of three molecules of fatty acid bound with one molecule of glycerol. Triglyceride is the most common fat stored in humans. (Ch 32)

Triiodothyronine: a thyroid hormone responsible for regulating the rate of carbohydrate, protein, and fat metabolism. Triiodothyronine is less potent than the primary thyroid hormone, thyroxine. (Ch 40)

Troche: lozenge, pastille; a solid candy-shaped tablet containing active medication which is slowly dissolved in the mouth or vagina to liberate the active ingredient. (Ch 3)

Trousseau's sign: a sign of tetany characterized by peripheral muscle spasm in response to pressure applied to that muscle. (Ch 45, Ch 58)

TSH: see Thyrotropin. (Ch 40)

T-tubule: the portion of the cardiac cell through which calcium enters the cell. (Ch 27)

Tumor necrosis factor: cachectin; a substance produced by macrophages which has a complex role in inflammation, the body's response to certain tumors, and the weight loss associated with cancer. (Ch 50)

Turbinates: an anatomical description of the convoluted folds of the nasal cavity. (Ch 34)

Twitch monitor: a device utilized during the administration of skeletal muscle relaxants which assesses the degree of neuromuscular function. Twitch responses which are low or absent indicate excessive muscle relaxation while high responses demonstrate recovery from therapeutic muscle relaxation. (Ch 18)

Tympanic membrane: the eardrum; the membrane that separates the external and middle ear. (Ch 59)

—U—

Ultrafiltrate: the fluid which remains when colloidal particles are separated from crystalloids. In renal physiology, the ultrafiltrate refers to the material that passes across the glomerulus into the nephron following glomerular filtration. (Ch 37)

Unifascicular block: an intraventricular conduction defect in which conduction is delayed or blocked through the right bundle branch, the anterior portion of the left bundle branch, or the posterior portion of the left bundle branch. (Ch 30)

Unstable angina: angina pectoris which is worsening in severity and may lead to a myocardial infarction. (Ch 31)

Uterine inertia: the absence or weakness of uterine contractions during labor. (Ch 15)

Uremic frost: the presence of yellow-white crystals on the skin originating from the excess urea contained in the sweat of patients with severe renal disease. (Ch 39)

Urography: x-ray visualization of the urinary tract following injection of radiopaque contrast media. (Ch 9)

U wave: an electrocardiographic wave, occurring after the T wave, which is secondary to the effects of digitalis. (Ch 28)

—V—

Vaccine: a suspension of live, killed, or attenuated microorganisms or their parts injected for the purpose of achieving active immunization. (Ch 64)

Vagotonia: hyperirritability of the parasympathetic nervous system. (Ch 60)

Variant angina: Prinzmetal's variant; vasospastic angina; a form of angina pectoris in which the attacks occur at rest and in which the ST segment is elevated. Variant angina is thought to be due to coronary vasospasm. (Ch 31)

Vasopressor: a drug which causes constriction of the

arteries, thereby increasing blood pressure. (Ch 19)

Vasospasm: a sudden spasm, or constriction, of a blood vessel. (Ch 31)

Vasospastic angina: see Variant angina. (Ch 31)

Venodilation: dilation of the vein. (Ch 38)

Venography: x-ray visualization of the venous system following injection of radiopaque contrast media. (Ch 9)

Ventilation: the movement of air into and out of the lungs. (Ch 34)

Vermifuge: anthelmintic; a drug that causes the expulsion of intestinal worms. (Ch 54)

Vertigo: disturbed equilibrium characterized by dizziness and lightheadedness. Vertigo is usually caused by middle ear disease or salicylate or aminoglycoside toxicity. (Ch 61)

Vesicant: an agent that causes blistering. (Ch 16)

Vesiculation: the formation of a blister. (Ch 9)

Virucidal: causing the death and destruction of viruses. (Ch 46)

Virulence: the power of a microorganism to produce disease. (Ch 64)

Virustatic: inhibiting the growth of viruses. (Ch 46)

Visceral proteins: proteins required for body function, such as gut mass proteins, albumin, transferrin, globulins, and C-reactive proteins. (Ch 56)

Vitamin: a biologically active organic compound necessary for normal metabolism, growth, and development of the body but which does not supply energy. (Ch 57)

Vitreous humor: the jelly-like material located in the posterior chamber of the eye that serves to maintain the eye's spherical shape. (Ch 59)

Volume of distribution: the size of a compartment necessary to account for the total amount of drug in the body if it were present throughout the body at the same concentration found in the plasma. For practical purposes, the volume of distribution can be calculated by dividing the total body stores of a drug by the measured blood level. (Ch 4)

von Willebrand's disease: a defect in blood coagulation in which coagulation factor VIII activity and platelet function are both abnormal. (Ch 41)

—W—

Wheeze: an abnormal high-pitched breath sound common in patients suffering an acute asthmatic attack. (Ch 36)

Withdrawal: a clinical syndrome which occurs following the cessation of drug taking by the physiologically dependent person. The specific signs and symptoms of withdrawal vary with the specific drug involved. (Ch 13, Ch 24)

—X—Y—Z—

Xanthine: a uric acid precursor. Derivatives of xanthine, including theophylline, theobromine, and caffeine, act as smooth muscle relaxants and are utilized as bronchodilators. (Ch 35)

Xerophthalmia: a condition caused by vitamin A deficiency which is characterized by conjunctival inflammation, atrophy, and dryness. (Ch 57)

Xerostomia: dryness of the mouth caused by reduced secretion of saliva. (Ch 18)

Zero-order kinetics: see Linear kinetics. (Ch 4)

Zymosan: a substance that antagonizes the effects of complement. (Ch 50)

CHAPTER REVIEW QUESTIONS

CHAPTER 1

1. A major responsibility of the nursing profession is to:
   a. discourage the use of over-the-counter medications
   b. teach consumers about the benefits and dangers of medications
   c. control the administration of medications in the hospital setting
   d. alter the consumer's values and beliefs concerning medication use

2. What is the *first* condition which must be met in order for a patient to comply with the medication regime?
   a. adequate knowledge about the disease process
   b. examination of cultural beliefs which may affect compliance
   c. acceptance of the diagnosis
   d. adequate family support

3. For the cognitive domain of learning, teaching involves:
   a. evaluating feedback from the learner about thoughts and feelings
   b. ensuring that the patient can perform a procedure
   c. demonstrating activities necessary for learning
   d. giving factual information

4. Tasks of the affective teaching domain include all of the following except:
   a. analyzing
   b. receiving
   c. valuing
   d. organizing

5. Which of the following is an example of a dermatologic toxic reaction?
   a. mild rash
   b. alopecia
   c. hives
   d. skin pigmentation

6. Symptoms related to anemia and leukopenia are referred to as:
   a. idiosyncratic reactions
   b. adverse effects
   c. allergic reactions
   d. toxic effects

7. During the planning stage of the nursing process:
   a. the patient's actual and potential health problems are identified
   b. nursing actions are based on nursing orders
   c. objective and subjective data are evaluated
   d. goals are established which become the outcomes of nursing care

8. Which statement is *correct* regarding interviewing techniques used by nurses to elicit patient information?
   a. Open-ended questions impose limitations on patient responses.
   b. Loaded questions should be avoided in an information-gathering interview.
   c. Closed-ended questions allow the greatest freedom of response.
   d. Mirror-response questions are evaluative and threatening.

9. In taking a medication history, the nurse knows the following statement to be true:
   a. Heavy smokers may require smaller doeses if taking theophylline, a bronchodilator.
   b. Alcohol consumption decreases the action of tranquilizers and CNS depressants.

The publisher thanks Carol Ann Maull for her preparation of some of these review questions for the first edition of *Pharmacotherapeutics*.

c. Over-the-counter drugs should not be included in a medication history.

d. Patients allergic to fish may also be allergic to contrast dyes used in radiology.

10. All of the following statements are true regarding health teaching, *except:*
    a. The primary aim of health teaching is to ensure patient compliance.
    b. Patients are likely to change behavior if they understand the need and the benefits.
    c. It is inappropriate for the nurse to solicit and evaluate patient feedback to assess learning.
    d. Teaching may involve the cognitive, affective, and psychomotor domains of learning.

CHAPTER 2

1. Early history demonstrates that people of past cultures:
   a. attempted to treat illness through medical intervention
   b. were successful in curing illness through surgical intervention
   c. had few illnesses related to present day forms
   d. had great insight into the causes of disease and related treatments

2. The following statement is true about the early post-Christian era:
   a. Hippocrates was the most famous physician of this era.
   b. Great strides occurred in medicine and pharmacology.
   c. The Catholic Church controlled the knowledge of healing and medicine.
   d. Egyptians were the first to employ the use of belladonna and narcotics.

3. Contributions of the Arabs to the history of pharmacy include all of the following *except:*
   a. established hospitals and medical schools
   b. separated pharmacy from the practice of medicine
   c. introduced the use of decimal notation
   d. popularized the principle of polypharmacy

4. The empirical stage of therapeutics was characterized by:
   a. a lack of detailed record-keeping
   b. clinical evidence that a drug was effective
   c. an understanding of drug action
   d. all of the above

5. The physician-scientist who advocated the use of specific compounds to treat disease was:
   a. Paracelsus
   b. Asclepius
   c. Hippocrates
   d. Dioscorides

6. The mystical stage of the science of therapeutics employed all of the following forms of therapy *except:*
   a. prayer
   b. alchemy
   c. surgery
   d. medication

7. Place the following drugs in order of discovery:
   a. colchicine, digitalis, opium, ether
   b. opium, ether, digitalis, colchicine
   c. ether, opium, digitalis, colchicine
   d. opium, colchicine, ether, digitalis

8. An approved drug label must have all of the following *except:*
   a. the name and business address of the manufacturer
   b. the suggested dose and frequency of use
   c. the date of drug manufacture and distribution
   d. the kind, quantity, and proportion of ingredients

9. Which statement is *not* true regarding the development of the nurse's role in drug administrations?
   a. As early as 1920, the curriculum for student nurses included two courses dealing with medications.
   b. By the late 1920's, nurses were given the authority to administer intramuscular injections.
   c. In the late 1930's, health teaching regarding medications became a more defined nursing role.
   d. At the present time, the nursing process is the scientific framework used by the nurse in medication administration.

10. The Federal Food, Drug, and Cosmetic Act (FFDCA) of 1906 contributed to medication safety by:
    a. empowering state governemnts to enforce official drug standards
    b. requiring only narcotic drugs to comply with standards set by USP and NF
    c. requiring synthetic drugs to list side effects on the label
    d. designating the USP and the NF as official drug standards

CHAPTER 3

1. Local medication preparations may be:
   a. applied to the skin for rapid reabsorption
   b. injected into muscle tissue for altered absorption
   c. injected into a joint cavity
   d. administered safely to all patients

2. Which statement is *true* regarding administration of medications by the oral route?
   a. Gastric upsets rarely occur.

b. Inadvertent aspiration may occur in the seriously ill patient.
c. Water given with the medication retards absorption.
d. Oral administration is best for all patients.

3. Parenteral administration of medications includes all of the following routes *except:*
a. oral
b. intra-articular
c. subcutaneous
d. intrathecal

4. Which of the following nursing actions is *incorrect* relative to medication administration and patient safety?
a. checking the Five Rights of Medication Administration
b. withholding medication if the patient is confused
c. asking the patient to state his or her name
d. checking the patient's ID band

5. In administering a pain-relieving injection, the nurse will implement all of the following actions *except:*
a. select a non-excoriated site
b. insert and remove the needle slowly
c. inject the medicine slowly
d. apply direct pressure to the area afterwards

6. To avoid medication errors, the nurse will:
a. refuse to interpret illegible handwriting
b. question the use of multiple tablets to provide a single dose
c. use the dropper of one medication to administer another
d. decline to investigate atypical drug names

7. One characteristic of generic medications is that they are often:
a. less expensive than brand name drugs
b. not as potent as brand name drugs
c. more difficult to obtain from the pharmacist
d. less regulated by law with respect to drug purity

8. In order to alleviate gastric discomfort associated with taking medication, the nurse should instruct the patient to take the medication:
a. with breakfast
b. in the evening
c. with an antiemetic
d. in divided doses

9. Which of the following statements is *true* regarding a parenteral administration of vitamin B_{12}?
a. It must be injected just under the skin surface.
b. The drug may be destroyed by enzymes in the blood.
c. It must be given by the Z-track method.
d. It must be administered by specially trained individuals.

10. Side effects of a headache associated with nitroglycerin ointment are an example of which type of drug effect?
a. local
b. anaesthetic
c. systemic
d. first-pass

CHAPTER 4

1. Which statement is *true* regarding the pharmacokinetic phase of drug administration?
a. The immature liver or kidneys of the very young may accelerate drug metabolism and excretion.
b. Medications enter the body in sold form and change into solution for absorption and utilization.
c. Medication absorption, distribution to tissues, metabolism and elimination from the body are studied.
d. A therapeutic effect occurs as the medication reaches the target cell.

2. The following statements are concerned with the mechanism of drug absorption. Which statement is *false?*
a. Active transport moves substances against a concentration gradient.
b. Passive transport provides for one-way drug transport into the cell.
c. Energy is not required or utilized during passive diffusion.
d. Protein carriers can only carry specific drugs.

3. Which statement is *true* regarding drug solubility?
a. Medications in aqueous solutions are absorbed more slowly than oil-based products.
b. Lipid-soluble substances are too large to cross the blood brain barrier.
c. Alcohol-based products have a slower absorption rate than oil-based drugs.
d. Only nonionized drug forms are available for absorption.

4. During the phase of drug distribution:
a. most medications are bound in the serum to hormones
b. reduced cardiac output increases tissue drug saturation and concentration
c. tissues such as the bone and middle ear take longer for drug distribution
d. substances pass the placental barrier by an active transport system

5. Which statement is *true* regarding the half-life of medications?
a. Doubling the dose will double the medication half-life.
b. Approximately 6 half-lives are required for a medication to be completely excreted.

c. Patients with renal or hepatic disease usually have decreased drug half-lives.

d. The half-life of a drug determines how often the drug is to be administered.

6. Which statement is *false* regarding medication selectivity?

a. The therapeutic range is the level at which the medication is effective.

b. The margin of safety is the dose with the most therapeutic results and the fewest toxic effects.

c. A medication reference book listing all known adverse and toxic effects is of great use to determine selectivity.

d. Drug selectivity summarizes the pattern and incidence of adverse side effects produced by the therapeutic dose.

7. All of the following are factors which affect patient response to medication, *except:*

a. sex

b. climate

c. weight

d. age

8. The majority of acid drugs are better absorbed in the small intestine, due to the:

a. presence of an acidic medium

b. increased surface area

c. dissociation into ionized forms

d. presence of a basic medium

9. Which of the following processes is associated with passive transport?

a. carrier transport

b. pinocytosis

c. facilitated diffusion

d. one-way transport

10. The following statements refer to plasma drug concentration. Select the statement which is *true*.

a. The plasma concentration is the amount of bound drug in plasma.

b. As the peak concentration is reached, maximal effect usually occurs.

c. The plasma concentration is the amount of free drug in plasma.

d. Peak concentration is reached when all of the drug becomes unbound.

CHAPTER 5

1. A pharmacokinetic drug interaction:

a. Occurs in the drug preparation phase of drug therapy

b. Produces the majority of drug incompatibility reactions

c. May have additive, synergistic, or antagonistic effects

d. Affects the absorption, distribution, biotransformation, and excretion of drugs

2. A pharmacodynamic drug interaction:

a. Occurs when liver function is compromised

b. Refers to a type of drug incompatibility

c. May have additive, synergistic, or antagonistic effects

d. Occurs when plasma protein-binding is modified

3. An antagonistic drug interaction occurs when:

a. Drug absorption is decreased by the presence of food in the stomach

b. A second drug is added to diminish or eliminate the effect of the first

c. A second drug is added that possesses the same overt effect as the first

d. Drug distribution is enhanced by displacement of a protein-bound drug

4. Major mechanisms of drug interaction include all of the following classifications, *except:*

a. incompatibility effects

b. protein-binding changes

c. absorption

d. biotransformation

5. Medications that increase or inhibit liver enzyme activity can affect drug action. Which of the following statements is *true* regarding biotransformation in the liver?

a. Alcohol inhibits liver enzyme activity, resulting in incresed activity of certain drugs.

b. Phenobarbital stimulated liver enzyme activity, resulting in increased metabolism of certain drugs.

c. Cimetidine (Tagamet) stimulates liver enzyme activity, resulting in increased effect of certain drugs.

d. Rifampin inhibits liver enzyme activity, resulting in decreased metabolism of certain drugs.

6. An example of combined toxicity is:

a. warfarin and phenylbutazone

b. quinidine and digoxin

c. acetazolamine (Diamox) and aspirin

d. gentamicin and furosemide (Lasix)

7. Which statement is *true* concerning absorption of oral medications?

a. The faster the drug passes through the intestinal tract, the greater the amount absorbed.

b. Drugs such as morphine and codeine prolong emptying time, increasing drug absorption.

c. Metoclopramide hastens gastric emptying and increases drug absorption in the small intestine.

d. Anticholinergics decrease gastric emptying time and increase drug absorption.

8. Mineral oil inhibits the absorption of fat soluble vitamins. This effect is known as:

a. sequestration

b. antagonism

c. complexation

d. potentiation

9. Patients who are taking phenytoin (Dilantin) or phenobarbital must be observed for:
   a. toxic sodium levels
   b. elevated magnesium levels
   c. decreased calcium levels
   d. decreased phosphorous levels

10. The correct action for the nurse who suspects that a drug interaction is occurring would be to:
   a. withhold all medications until the physician sees the patient
   b. continue the medication and document all reactions in the nurse's notes
   c. give all medications as ordered and inform the physician
   d. withhold the suspected medication and inform the physician

CHAPTER 6

1. Toxicology is concerned with all of the following *except:*
   a. drugs used in therapy
   b. environmental pollution
   c. industrial waste
   d. safety-related injuries

2. Which of the following statements is *true* regarding the adverse effects of drug therapy?
   a. Pharmacologic products should be tested to assure that there are no risks involved.
   b. Toxic effects will occur in all persons given sufficient dosage.
   c. Drug allergies and hypersensitivity reactions are effects which can be predicted.
   d. Adverse reactions to drugs usually take only minutes to manifest.

3. Adverse reactions are more likely to occur in:
   a. male patients
   b. very young patients
   c. patients with nerve damage
   d. patients with renal dysfunction

4. An example of a primary drug reaction would be:
   a. excessive drowsiness from antihistamines
   b. impotence from antihypertensives
   c. excessive lethargy from sedatives
   d. extreme agitation from bronchodilators

5. Which of the following statements is *true* concerning an anaphylactic reaction?
   a. It is a Type III allergic reaction involving the lung and cardiovascular system.
   b. IGE antibodies attach to red blood cells, liberating large amounts of epinephrine.
   c. When the offending drug is administered, mast cells liberate large doses of histamine.
   d. The resulting effect of substrate release includes bronchodilation and peripheral vasoconstriction.

6. The Type II allergic reaction is most often seen in persons receiving:
   a. streptomycin
   b. penicillin
   c. tetracycline
   d. thiazide diuretics

7. The inflammatory process and tissue destruction associated with an auto-immune reaction is mediated by:
   a. activation of complement
   b. increased amounts of IGE
   c. complexation with red blood cells
   d. activation of T-lymphocytes

8. Hemolytic anemia can result secondarily to:
   a. cell-mediated reaction
   b. auto-immune reaction
   c. anaphylaxis
   d. serum sickness

9. Which one of the following statements is *true* concerning chemical poisoning?
   a. In general, substances which are inhaled have a slower onset of action.
   b. Poisoning is the fifth most common cause of accidental death in the United States.
   c. The number of cases involving poisoning has increased over several years.
   d. The signs and symptoms of poisoning are very distinctive, facilitating early diagnosis.

10. Hemodialysis enhances elmination of toxins from the blood. Which one of the following types of toxins is removed by this method?
   a. lipid-bound
   b. protein-bound
   c. low-molecular-weight
   d. high-molecular-weight

CHAPTER 7

1. Over-the-counter drugs are:
   a. categorized as legend drugs
   b. not required to prove effectiveness
   c. defined as safe for use without medical supervision
   d. used for permanent relief of annoying symptoms

2. Which statement is true regarding aspirin?
   a. Gastrointestinal discomfort is the most common adverse effect.
   b. Buffered aspirin products are therapeutically superior to plain aspirin.
   c. Liquid aspirin is preferred for pediatric use.
   d. Enteric-coated aspirin should be administered with an antacid.

3. Which statement is true regarding cough suppressants (antitussives)?
   a. Self-treatment should be limited to 14 days, so

that a serious underlying cause is not overlooked.

b. Antitussives should be used only if a persistent cough causes pain or lack of sleep or is non-productive.

c. The only OTC antitussives recognized as safe and effective are Phenaphren and Tempra.

d. Codeine is not commonly used as a suppressant because of its powerful addiction potential.

4. All of the following are expectorants commonly found in OTC cough remedies, *except:*
   a. ammonium chloride
   b. terpin hydrate
   c. guaifenesin
   d. destromethorphan

5. Of the following drug characteristics, which one is *not* appropriate when selecting a liquid form of an antacid?
   a. potassium content
   b. palatability
   c. volume needed per dose
   d. neutralizing capacity

6. Which of the following OTC medications contains acetaminophen?
   a. Alka-Seltzer
   b. Anacin
   c. Empirin compound
   d. Excedrin

7. Patient guidelines for self-medication include all of the following, *except:*
   a. seeking health care provider if no relief obtained
   b. using non-drug measures to help treat symptoms
   c. selecting a drug which is nonspecific if currently taking prescription drugs
   d. using the OTC medication for only as long as recommended

8. Patients should not self-treat with antacids if the following situation applies:
   a. discomfort associated with sweating and weakness
   b. incompatible diet selection
   c. excessive stress and tension
   d. acute gastritis associated with overeating

9. A disadvantage of acetaminophen is the lack of:
   a. anticoagulant activity
   b. anti-inflammatory activity
   c. analgesic activity
   d. antipyrogenic activity

10. The following statement is *false* regarding self-care measures of a sore throat:
    a. A sore throat due to a streptococcal infecton may lead to serious complications if untreated.
    b. A sore throat related to a common cold may be alleviated with self-care measures and local anaesthetics.

c. A throat culture is needed to definitely establish whether an infection is due to streptococci.

d. Topical antibacterial mouthwashes have been proven effective for mouth and throat infections.

CHAPTER 8

1. In formulating a plan to assess the teaching needs of a patient requiring medication, the nurse knows that the patient's:
   a. cultural traditions have little effect upon the ability to learn
   b. educational level and reading ability must be determined for successful learning to occur
   c. role in the teaching-learning process is one of subordination
   d. self-esteem should be threatened to ensure rapid learning

2. David Ausubel's cognitive/discovery perspective is concerned with all of the following concepts, *except:*
   a. non-observable forms of behavior, thinking, and relationship formation
   b. reception learning where content to be learned is presented in final form
   c. generalizations that tell the learner that behavior in a given situation continues to be true in future learning experiences
   d. how learners solve problems and form concepts

3. In developing nursing diagnoses related to the teaching needs of a patient requiring medication, the nurse educator will:
   a. apply the principles of Ausubel's perspective by developing an interpersonal relationship with the patient
   b. apply Rogers' principles by involving the patient and family in the development of the nursing diagnoses
   c. apply the principles of B. F. Skinner by encouraging questions in an open environment
   d. apply Rogers' principles in dealing with the highly motivated confident learner

4. In developing teaching techniques specific to the learning needs of the patient requiring medication, the nurse educator knows that all of the following facts are *true, except:*
   a. The goals of teaching are achieved the day of patient discharge.
   b. Important information is written down by the patient and checked by the nurse for accuracy.
   c. The patient and family see and handle the medications that will be taken at home.
   d. The patient makes the ultimate decision for medication compliance.

5. Evaluation techniques to assess teaching strategy effectiveness include:
   a. selecting the evaluation criteria as the final step in the evaluation process
   b. spelling out the evaluation conditions in behavioral objective terms

c. determining evaluation techniques and methods during the evaluation phase of the nursing process

d. applying the evaluation process only at the termination of the teaching plan

6. Which of the following statements is *true* regarding the SMOG readability formula?
The SMOG formula is:
   a. based on 90 percent comprehension and is the most accurate way of assessing readability
   b. determined by the square root of the number of polysyllabic words contained within 30 selected sentences
   c. based on dividing the number of complex sentences contained within one paragraph of written material by 3
   d. found to be too complex to be of practical use in the hospital teaching-learning setting

7. Compliance can be defined as:
   a. evidence of comprehension of a medical diagnosis and its lifestyle implications
   b. the ability of the patient to repeat information presented in both verbal and written forms
   c. the extent to which a patient's symptoms can be controlled by medication
   d. the degree to which a patient's behavior regarding the medication plan coincides with medical advice

8. According to B. F. Skinner's conditioning behavioristic perspective, EXTINCTION is achieved by:
   a. punishment measures
   b. withdrawal of reinforcement
   c. rewarding the undesired behavior
   d. refusing to focus on the desired behavior

9. Patients who would be most suited to Ausubel's learning theory would include the:
   a. independent, motivated learner
   b. dependent learner with poor reading skills
   c. anxious, shy, or slow learner
   d. unmotivated learner with low readability level

10. During the assessment phase of the patient's learning needs, the nurse will focus on all of the following *except:*
   a. establishing a trusting and nonthreatening relationship
   b. determining educational level and reading ability
   c. expecting that the patient will demonstrate noncompliance
   d. selecting aspects from all of the learning theories in establishing a data base

CHAPTER 9

1. All of the following medications are used in diagnostic testing *except:*
   a. histamine phosphate
   b. barium sulfate
   c. hypaque sodium
   d. acetylcholine chloride

2. Iodine compounds may be:
   a. administered only by the oral route
   b. administered to all patients without adverse reactions
   c. injected directly into the area to be visualized
   d. limited to use with patients allergic to barium

3. Of the following statements regarding common diagnostic agents, which one is *not* correct?
   a. Radioactive isotopes localize only in abnormal tissue.
   b. The most common side effect following barium use is constipation.
   c. The most serious side effect of iodine testing is anaphylaxis.
   d. The diagnostic dosage of radiopharmaceuticals is higher than the therapeutic dosage.

4. In developing a nursing care plan for the patient undergoing diagnostic testing, the nurse performs all of the following actions *except:*
   a. schedules barium studies last
   b. administers insulin to the NPO diabetic patient
   c. assesses the patient before, during, and after the procedure
   d. explains the procedure at a level the patient can understand

5. Nonradioactive dyes are used to:
   a. detect abnormal tissue
   b. measure organ function
   c. diagnose adrenal insufficiency
   d. delineate soft tissue

6. The following statement is *correct* with regard to agents which stimulate gland secretion:
   a. Agents which stimulate the secretion of enzymes are called tropic hormones.
   b. Secretogogus agents include thyrotropin and adrenocorticotropic hormone.
   c. Pentagastrin stimulates duodenal and pancreatic secretion.
   d. Sincalide stimulates gallbladder contraction and bile release.

7. Diagnostic skin tests are performed for the diagnosis of all of the following *except:*
   a. rheumatoid arthritis
   b. coccidioidomycosis
   c. histoplasmosis
   d. tuberculosis

8. Hypaque Sodium is contraindicated in the following patient situation:
   a. hyperuricemia
   b. intestinal malformations
   c. iodine hypersensitivity
   d. peptic ulcer disease

9. In diagnostic radiology:
   a. particulate radiation is measured
   b. energy is released by stable electrons

c. electromagnetic radiation is measured
d. alpha and beta rays are emitted

10. Which of the following agents might be added with the dye preparation in order to reduce the incidence of allergic reactions?
    a. diphenhydramine
    b. epinephrine
    c. acetominophen
    d. oxygen

CHAPTER 10

1. Which of the following medications is commonly used as an anesthetic?
   a. glycopyrrolate (Robinul)
   b. pentobarbital sodium (Nembutal)
   c. promethazine hydrochloride (Phenergan)
   d. droperidol/fentanyl (Innovar)

2. Methoxyflurane (Penthrane) is an anesthetic that has which of the following properties:
   a. long recovery period
   b. few side effects
   c. good induction properties
   d. high vapor pressure

3. Barbiturates, as intravenously administered anesthetic agents, produce:
   a. good analgesia
   b. respiratory tract irritation
   c. good skeletal muscle relaxation
   d. rapid recovery period

4. Of the following statements, which one is *correct* regarding local anesthesia?
   a. Field block anesthesia involves injecting the agent directly into the area to be desensitized.
   b. Infiltration anesthesia involves infiltrating the tissue around the area to be desensitized.
   c. A nerve block is achieved by injecting the anesthetic agent close to a mixed nerve.
   d. Spinal anesthesia is achieved by injecting a drug into a nerve block in the spinal column.

5. In planning care for the postoperative patient, the nurse knows:
   a. patients receiving spinal anesthesia are kept supine for 2 to 4 hours postoperatively
   b. deep muscle relaxation can result in bladder atony or decreased intestinal motility
   c. if voiding has not occurred within 4 hours postoperatively, the patient is catheterized
   d. immobilization of the patient helps to relieve abdominal distention and pain

6. Depolarizing neuromuscular blocking agents act by depolarization of the:
   a. motor end plate in order to produce muscle paralysis
   b. nerve axon fiber to create desensitization in muscle fibers

c. postsynaptic membrane in order to inhibit muscle movement
d. nerve cell dendrites which then block acetylcholine release

7. Which of the following statements is *correct* regarding anesthesia?
   a. Balanced anesthesia involves utilizing an agent along with its antidote.
   b. Regional anesthesia can be achieved by inhalation of certain drugs.
   c. In order to achieve a painless state, there must be temporary areflexia.
   d. Many drugs are available which meet all of the criteria for an anesthetic.

8. Stage III of anesthesia is characterized by:
   a. minimal muscle relaxation
   b. spinal cord depression
   c. respiratory paralysis
   d. cerebral cortex depression

9. Desirable characteristics of a good local anesthetic drug include all of the following *except:*
   a. action confined to nerve tissue
   b. sufficiently long duration
   c. compatability with vasoconstrictor agents
   d. solubility in high glucose solutions

10. Which of the following local anesthetics is of the ester type?
    a. piperocaine
    b. dibucaine
    c. lidocaine
    d. etridrocaine

CHAPTER 11

1. Of the following statements, which one is *correct* regarding water balance in the human body?
   a. The average adult human body is 80 percent water.
   b. Approximately 15 percent of the body water is intracellular.
   c. Approximately 45 percent of the body water is extracellular.
   d. Lean individuals have a higher percentage of water than fat individuals.

2. All of the following statements are correct regarding the classification of fluid volume imbalances, *except:*
   a. Hyperosmotic contraction occurs when water and solutes are lost from the extracellular compartment.
   b. Hypo-osmotic contraction occurs when there is a loss of solute in excess of water from the extracellular space.
   c. Iso-osmotic contraction occurs when there is an equal loss of fluid volume along with solutes.
   d. Osmolarity describes the concentration of free particles, molecules, or ions in a solution.

3. The hydrating solution of 5 percent dextrose plus 0.45 percent sodium chloride contains:
   a. 38.5 mEq/L of chloride and 38.5 mEq/L of sodium
   b. 51 mEq/L of sodium and 38.5 mEq/L of potassium
   c. 77 mEq/L of sodium and 77 mEq/1 of chloride
   d. 77 mEq/L of chloride and 51 mEq/L of potassium

4. An intravenous replacement solution is:
   a. a combination of water, carbohydrates, and electrolytes used to replace losses from the gastrointestinal tract
   b. available in both 10 and 20 percent dextrose solutions to correct losses due to hemorrhaging
   c. high in potassium and sodium to approximate electrolyte loss through renal excretion
   d. used to promote renal function, when a fluid deficit exists, by using a balance among cations and anions

5. A patient receiving an intravenous feeding of 3000 ml daily of a 10 percent invert sugar in water solution receives approximately:
   a. 1100 calories a day
   b. 2000 calories a day
   c. 510 calories a day
   d. 2800 calories a day

6. Nursing responsibilities in caring for the patient receiving intravenous therapy include to:
   a. examine the intravenous sites at least once every four hours
   b. monitor the patient's intake, output, and body weight daily
   c. prepare the solution and admixture using clean technique
   d. lower the infusion rate if redness or swelling occurs at the intravenous site

7. Body buffers operate in all of the following locations *except:*
   a. body cells through proteins and phosphates
   b. red cells through hemoglobin
   c. intracellular fluid through glucose exchange
   d. extracellular fluid through bicarbonate

8. A primary treatment for respirator acidosis would include:
   a. hemodialysis
   b. mechanical ventilation
   c. sedation for anxiety
   d. rebreather apparatus

9. Lactated Ringers (Hartmann's Solution) is an example of the following type of solution:
   a. hydrating
   b. carbohydrate
   c. balanced
   d. replacement

10. A nursing goal for the patient with fluid volume deficit would be to restore volume to normal by:
    a. administering hypotonic solutions
    b. administering high glucose solutions
    c. monitoring hypertonic solutions
    d. restricting fluid intake

CHAPTER 12

1. Of the following statements, which one is correct with regard to whole blood or its derivatives?
   a. Platelets do not contain the Rh(D) antigen that red cells carry.
   b. White cells must be given within 48 hours after donation.
   c. Whole blood is used to restore a blood loss of greater than 500 ml.
   d. Packed cells contain only red cells in a volume of 250 ml.

2. Plasma expanders are substances which have the ability to expand a depleted blood volume. These substances:
   a. transmit hepatitis and acquired immune deficiency syndrome
   b. are typed and matched with the patient's blood before administration
   c. cause anaphylactic reaction in hypersensitive patients
   d. have oxygen-carrying capacity and contain clotting factors

3. In caring for the patient receiving a blood tranfussion, the nurse:
   a. administers the blood concurrently with a dextrose solution to prevent clumping of red blood cells
   b. monitors the patient at least every 2 hours for signs of a reaction to the blood transfusion
   c. administers the blood using a single tubing with a 170-micron filter
   d. compares the blood group and Rh factor on the label with those of the patient

4. All of the following are usual signs of an anaphylactic reaction *except:*
   a. chills and fever
   b. tingling in toes
   c. change in vital signs
   d. chest and back pain

5. Dextran 40 is a low-molecular weight blood substitute which:
   a. is used as a hemodiluent in the heart-lung machine
   b. increases platelet-aggregation and osmotic pressure
   c. causes sludging of blood in the microcirculation
   d. reduces cardiac output and microcirculatory flow

6. Donated blood is labeled with all of the following information *except:*
   a. the proper name of the component
   b. method by which component was prepared
   c. temperature range for storage
   d. type of antibodies present

7. Which of the following statements is *correct* with regard to the Rh factor system?
   a. Persons with Rh antibodies are considered to have Rh-positive blood type.
   b. Rh-positive mother will develop antibodies when giving birth to Rh-negative child.
   c. Rh-positive persons may receive blood that is Rh-negative.
   d. Type O Rh-negative blood is referred to as the universal recipient.

8. Plasmapheresis is a donor technique with the advantage of:
   a. allowing persons to donate every 48 hours if necessary
   b. retaining plasma platelets or white blood cells
   c. taking only one hour for the process to be completed
   d. returning the plasma and retaining only the red cells

9. Stored whole blood has the following properties:
   a. high pH and calcium levels
   b. low potassium levels
   c. high glucose levels
   d. low 2,3-DPG levels

10. Plasma protein products are contraindicated in all situations *except:*
    a. evidence of repeated infusions
    b. history of allergic reaction to albumin
    c. presence of severe anemia
    d. presence of cardiac failure

CHAPTER 13

1. Which statement is *not* correct regarding the definition of terms related to drug abuse?
   a. Dependency refers to a state in which the person needs a specific drug to maintain abilities to function.
   b. Drug abuse is the use of drugs that create legal, emotional, social, and health problems for the individual.
   c. Tolerance develops when a person requires the drug to experience positive feelings and a sense of self-esteem.
   d. Physical dependence develops when the person experiences physical withdrawal symptoms when the drug wears off.

2. Which statement is *correct* regarding etiologic factors of drug and alcohol dependency?
   a. Physical dependency always has a genetic etiology or causative factor.

   b. Theories exist which adequately explain the causes of drug and alcohol dependency.
   c. Drug and alcohol dependency can be viewed as involving a single factor.
   d. Scientific understanding of dependency is at an early point in development.

3. In the assessment of the patient who abuses drugs, the nurse will:
   a. use the street names for drugs during the information-gathering phase
   b. begin the interview with discussion of sensitive information about drug use
   c. note only verbal responses to questions designed to elicit drug and alcohol usage
   d. utilize indirect questioning in order to make the patient feel more comfortable

4. When providing care for the patient who is withdrawing from the effects of alcohol, the nurse will perform all of the following *except:*
   a. assess mental status
   b. implement seizure precautions
   c. restrict fluid intake
   d. establish a non-stimulating environment

5. Nursing intervention for the patient withdrawing from a hallucinogen includes:
   a. leaving the patient alone in order to reduce environmental stimuli
   b. observing for signs of shock, which include pallor and hypotension
   c. engaging in lengthy conversations in order to decrease patient anxiety
   d. withholding all medications, inlcuding those for medical purposes

6. All of the following statements are correct regarding drug and alcohol abuse, *except:*
   a. The percentage of deaths related to substance abuse has declinded by 10 percent since 1982.
   b. Alcoholism ranks as the third major cause of death in the United States after coronary disease and cancer.
   c. About 20 to 35 percent of persons hospitalized in non-psychiatric settings suffer from alcohol-related illness.
   d. One in four individuals is estimated to have a personal experience with a family member or friend who is substance dependent.

7. Theories on the individual and family suggest that the following characteristic may place the individual at risk for substance-related problems:
   a. resolved psychological conflict
   b. family members with substance problems
   c. increased amount of "free" time
   d. economically advantaged status

8. All of the following statements are correct regarding the impaired nurse *except:*
   a. Nurses develop addictive illness at a higher rate than people in the general population

b. Recognition that addiction is treatable is central to the management of impaired practice.

c. The trend in employing institutions is to treat the impaired nurse before firing.

d. Impaired practice is most readily identified by changes in job performance.

9. The following is correct regarding dual addiction. Dual addiction is:
   a. dependence on more than one substance
   b. tolerance for large amounts of similarly acting drugs
   c. simultaneous dependence on drugs which have similar effects
   d. the combination of physiological and psychological dependence

10. The disease model, articulated by E. M. Jellinek, describes behavior consistent with symptoms of addiction. This model includes all of the following *except:*
    a. loss of control over intake of drug
    b. compulsive need to continue use
    c. psychologic and behavioral change
    d. imitation of family members with substance abuse

CHAPTER 14

1. Which of the following statements is *correct* regarding physiological differences in absorption of oral medications in pediatric patients?
   a. In the newborn, the stomach empties in about three hours.
   b. In the older infant and child, the stomach empties in about two hours.
   c. As an infant matures, the stomach has a less predictable emptying rate.
   d. Conditions such as gastritis cause gastric motility to decrease.

2. With regard to intramuscular injections in the pediatric patient, all of the following statements are correct *except:*
   a. Blood flow and tissue perfusion of the muscle are not fully developed in the neonate.
   b. Drug absorption of intramuscular injections is more unreliable in the neonate than in the child.
   c. Conditions which cause vasoconstriction decrease blood flow to the muscles, inhibiting absorption
   d. As the child grows, tissue perfusion decreases, making absorption of injections less reliable.

3. As drugs enter the blood stream, they bind to plasma protein for distribution. One factor influencing protein binding is the:
   a. amount of fat soluble vitamins available
   b. amount of albumin available for binding
   c. distribution of intracellular fluid and solutes
   d. distribution of enzymes for protein binding

4. Drug absorption via the intestine in the neonate is limited by the following characteristics:
   a. The length of intestinal lumen is short compared to the adult.
   b. There is a relatively small surface area for drug absorption.
   c. Due to neuromuscular immaturity, peristalsis is slowed.
   d. Intestinal peristalsis is rapid and unpredictable.

5. In teaching parents about medication safety and prevention of accidental ingestion of medications, the nurse will include the following information:
   a. Use child proof caps, as they are effective in preventing ingestion errors.
   b. Store medications in a locked container and hide the key.
   c. Store medications in the mother's purse, since it is usually out of reach.
   d. Place all drugs on a high shelf which is beyond the child's reach.

6. The following statement is *correct* regarding gastric acidity during the period immediately following birth:
   a. Gastric acidity in the first week of life is lower than in the adult.
   b. Drugs which are absorbed at a higher rate in a high pH should be withheld.
   c. Serum drug levels may be higher for drugs absorbed at a low pH.
   d. Drugs which are deactivated by a high pH should be given by an alternate route.

7. With regard to topical medication administration in the pediatric patient, which statement is *correct?*
   a. Infants require topical medications for frequent infections due to acidity of the skin.
   b. Children have natural skin barriers which prevent the absorption of topical medications.
   c. Children should not receive topical medication until they are 8 years of age or older.
   d. Infants absorb greater amounts of topical medications, causing potential side effects.

8. The following is *correct* relative to the distribution of fat in the pediatric patient:
   a. A neonate needs a smaller dosage of a fat soluble drug than an older child.
   b. Because the infant has a high fat content, fat soluble drugs are administered with care.
   c. As children grow, fat content decreases, and they require lesser amounts of fat soluble drugs.
   d. To maintain a therapeutic concentration of fat soluble drugs, infants require increased dosages.

9. In the neonate, the proportion of body water varies from the adult in the following way:
   a. A higher proportion of body water is intracellular.
   b. Smaller dosages of water soluble drugs per kg are needed.

c. The proportion of extracellular fluid increases as the infant matures.

d. The neonate exchanges extracellular fluid more rapidly than an adult.

10. For administration of intramuscular drugs, the first muscle of choice for a 4-month-old is the:
    a. deltoid
    b. vastus lateralus
    c. dorsogluteal
    d. ventrogluteal

CHAPTER 15

1. Which of the following statements is *correct* regarding drug distribution and excretion during pregnancy?
    a. As a result of an increase in plasma albumin, pharmacologic drug effects are increased.
    b. An increase in intracellular fluid volume increases the potential for toxic drug effects.
    c. Elimination is increased, creating a potential for reduced drug plasma concentrations.
    d. Drug half-life is prolonged due to the increase in blood flow through the liver.

2. The variables which determine the transfer of drugs across the placenta include all of the following *except:*
    a. physicochemical characteristics
    b. gestational age
    c. placental blood flow
    d. properties of the placenta

3. According to the Federal Drug Administration (FDA), drugs in Category C represent the following risk if taken during pregnancy:
    a. Studies in women have not indicated a risk to the fetus, and harm is remote.
    b. Human studies have not been completed to support the use in women without fetal risk.
    c. Evidence of fetal risk exists, but the drug may be used only if absolutely necessary.
    d. Use in women should be limited, unless the benefit outweighs the risk to the fetus.

4. All of the following may be used for relief of pain during active labor *except:*
    a. barbiturates
    b. analgesics
    c. antiemetics
    d. anesthetics

5. Regarding the use of general anesthesia during delivery, the following statement is *correct:*
    a. General anesthesia potentiates intense uterine contractions which can cause hemorrhaging.
    b. The interval from induction to delivery can be up to one hour before fetal depression is observed.
    c. The risk of aspiration is reduced with the use of general anesthesia in pregnant women.

d. The use of general anesthesia for delivery may result in delayed mother-infant bonding.

6. A risk associated with paracervical block includes:
    a. maternal aspiration
    b. fetal bradycardia
    c. maternal hypoglycemia
    d. fetal hypertension

7. Contraindications for the use of beta sympathomimetic drugs include all of the following *except:*
    a. mild pre-eclampsia
    b. abruptio placenta
    c. pulmonary hypertension
    d. fetal distress

8. A positive oxytocin challenge test (OCT) indicates:
    a. low placental reserve
    b. adequate placental oxygen
    c. prolongation of gestation
    d. placental hemorrhage

9. Oxytocin administration is contraindicated in the following condition:
    a. cardiovascular disease
    b. renal disease
    c. hypertension
    d. placenta previa

10. The following type of drug is known to be excreted in breast milk:
    a. insulin
    b. heparin
    c. diazepam
    d. oxytocin

CHAPTER 16

1. All of the following are correct regarding aging and age-related medication problems *except:*
    a. Some studies suggest that up to 30 percent of older adults suffer adverse drug side effects.
    b. The aging process alters the therapeutic and adverse responses to drug therapy.
    c. The major causes of death among elderly patients are cancer and its related drug therapy.
    d. Some studies have found that 20 percent of the hospitalization of older adults is due to prescription drug effects.

2. The components of drug disposition include all of the following processes *except:*
    a. absorption
    b. adaptation
    c. distribution
    d. metabolism

3. All of the following statements are correct with regard to aging and the drug response *except:*
    a. Often signs of aging are mistaken for side effects of prescription drugs.
    b. In general, medications tend to be overprescribed for the elderly.

c. Drug therapy is often the most risky component of patient care in the elderly.

d. Currently, recommendations are being proposed for medication use in the elderly.

4. The following represents normal physiological changes with aging:
   a. Lean body mass tends to decrease.
   b. Subcutaneous tissue tends to increase.
   c. Total body water in the elderly usually increases.
   d. Muscle mass proportionally increases.

5. In the older adult, fat soluble drugs are:
   a. distributed to a smaller portion of tissue than in young adults
   b. absorbed at a slow rate due to reduced fat stores
   c. released into circulation quickly after being absorbed
   d. associated with increased duration of drug action

6. The least desirable site for intravenous infusion of doxorubicin (Adriamycin) in the older adult would be:
   a. hand
   b. subclavian
   c. forearm
   d. antecubital

7. The following represents the effect of aging on cardiovascular function:
   a. increased cardiac output
   b. reduced arterial wall elasticity
   c. increased renal plasma flow
   d. reduced peripheral vascular resistance

8. The effect of aging on hepatic function results in:
   a. reduced blood levels of drugs
   b. prolonged drug effect
   c. reduced incidence of toxicity
   d. decreased intensity of drug effect

9. Which statement is *correct* regarding sensory changes in the older adult?
   a. Eyesight is not affected by visual changes associated with aging.
   b. All hearing loss in the older adult is due to the aging process.
   c. Sensory changes may affect the elderly person's ability to learn about his medication regime.
   d. Not all senses are affected by aging; for example, olfactory acuity remains stable.

CHAPTER 17

1. The telencephalon consists of both the right and left cerebral hemispheres and the:
   a. substantia nigra
   b. hypothalamus
   c. basal ganglia
   d. thalamus

2. All of the following statements are correct regarding the anatomy and physiology of the brain *except*:

a. The basal ganglia initiate and modulate motor movement.
   b. The limbic system plays a role in musculoskeletal response.
   c. The hypothalamus coordinates complex reflexes.
   d. The cerebellum coordinates activity of the skeletal muscles.

3. Cerebral spinal fluid is formed across the:
   a. pia mater
   b. sulci
   c. dural sinuses
   d. choroid plexus

4. Which of the following statements is *correct* regarding the transmission of nerve impulses?
   a. The action potential crosses directly from nerve to nerve or nerve to muscle.
   b. The action potential releases a chemical substance which diffuses across the nerve synapse.
   c. When a transmitter binds to its antagonist receptor, nerve conduction is elicited.
   d. By occupying transmitter sites, antagonists prevent the appropriate nerve response.

5. The afferent division of the peripheral nervous system is composed of:
   a. cell bodies which lie within the CNS and convey information about voluntary movement
   b. nerves which lie outside the CNS and control involuntary movement
   c. cell bodies which lie outside the CNS and direct messages to the periphery about sensation
   d. nerves which convey sensory information from peripheral receptors to the CNS

6. The sympathetic nervous system:
   a. activates systems which are necessary for rapid energy expenditure
   b. enhances energy conservation and bodily maintenance
   c. activates skeletal or voluntary muscles to contract
   d. facilitates sensory impulses and integrates responses

7. The following statement is *correct* with regard to cholinergic receptors and subtypes:
   a. Muscarinic receptors are located on the ganglia of the sympathetic and parasympathetic systems.
   b. Nicotinic receptors are found only on the effector cell membrane innervated by postganglionic fibers.
   c. Nicotinic antagonists exert effects which block both muscarinic and adrenergic transmission.
   d. Muscarinic antagonists, such as mecamylamine, affect the entire somatic system.

8. Alpha$_1$ adrenergic stimulation causes:
   a. bronchial constriction
   b. vascular vasodilation

c. constriction of intestinal smooth muscle
d. bronchial dilation

9. An example of a drug which possesses both beta$_1$ and beta$_2$ activity is:
   a. atenolol
   b. epinephrine
   c. albutanol
   d. phenylephrine

10. Beta$_1$ receptors are located in all of the following sites *except:*
   a. bronchial smooth muscle
   b. heart
   c. adipose tissue
   d. kidney

CHAPTER 18

1. All of the following statements regarding the classification of parasympathetic medications are correct *except:*
   a. Cholinergic agents mimic the effects of the parasympathetic system.
   b. Indirect-acting parasympathetic agents are cholinesterase inhibitors.
   c. Anticholinergic drugs neutralize the effects of the parasympathetic system.
   d. Depolarizing neuromuscular blockers are reversed by anticholinesterases.

2. Scopolamine, used in the treatment of motion sickness, is contraindicated in patients with:
   a. bradycardia
   b. angle-closure glaucoma
   c. hypersensitivity to cholinergics
   d. excessive salivation

3. A general drug action of a cholinergic agent is:
   a. reduced salivation
   b. increased cardiac conduction
   c. decreased cardiac contractility
   d. relaxation of bronchial glands

4. All of the following conditions contraindicate the use of acetylcholine and its derivatives *except:*
   a. neurogenic bladder
   b. myocardial infarction
   c. asthma
   d. peptic ulcers

5. Carbachol (Miostat) may produce the following side effect:
   a. diarrhea
   b. hypertension
   c. urinary retention
   d. dry skin

6. Neostigmine bromide (Prostigmin) is used to treat all of the following conditions *except:*
   a. myasthenia gravis
   b. esophogeal constriction
   c. urinary obstruction
   d. abdominal distention

7. Ganglionic blocking drugs act by:
   a. preventing the release of norepinephrine from preganglionic nerve endings
   b. stimulating the production of ganglionic cholinesterases
   c. interfering with the breakdown of the norepinephrine
   d. preventing the actions of acetylcholine at the receptor sites

8. An example of a neuromuscular blocking agent is:
   a. curare
   b. mecamylamine
   c. trimethaphan
   d. trihexyphenidyl

9. Which of the following statements is *correct* regarding anticholinesterases?
   a. These drugs block the accumulation of acetylcholine at receptor sites.
   b. Anticholinesterases are only used as agricultural insecticides.
   c. These agents prolong the action of acetylcholine.
   d. Anticholinesterases mimic the effects of acetylcholinesterase (ACHE).

10. Atropine, an anticholinergic drug, is contraindicated in all of the following conditions *except:*
   a. myasthenia gravis
   b. iritis
   c. prostate hypertrophy
   d. glaucoma

CHAPTER 19

1. Drugs acting positively on the beta-adrenergic receptor sites:
   a. decrease cardiac contractility
   b. constrict bronchial smooth muscle
   c. increase cardiac rate
   d. constrict arterioles of skeletal muscle

2. Which statement is *correct* regarding drugs acting as adrenergic stimulants?
   a. Levarterenol bitartrate (Levophed) increases blood flow to the kidney and skeletal muscles.
   b. Isoproterenol hydrochloride (Isuprel) produces bronchial constriction and peripheral vasodilation.
   c. Dobutamine hydrochloride (Dobutrex) causes the release of endogenous norepinephrine from adrenergic fibers.
   d. Epinephrine (Adrenalin) causes vasodilitation in the blood vessels of muscle fibers with mostly beta$_2$ receptors.

3. Which statement is *correct* regarding the interaction of catecholamines and other medications?
   a. Concurrent use of catecholamines with halothane may result in ventricular dysrhythmias.
   b. Tricyclic antidepressant agents antagonize the peripheral effect of catecholamines.

c. Catecholamines' pressor effects are reduced when given with MAO inhibitors.

d. Catecholamine effects are blocked with concurrent use with antihistamines.

4. Adverse effects of indirect and mixed adrenergic agents include all of the following *except:*
   a. drowsiness
   b. palpitations
   c. headache
   d. dysrhythmias

5. Dihydroergotamine mesylate (DHE45) is an alpha-adrenergic blocking agent which:
   a. contains 100 mg of caffeine per dose
   b. constricts cranial blood vessels
   c. prevents serotonin activity
   d. enhances peripheral vascular circulation

6. Which of the following statements is *correct* with regard to the pharmacokinetics of catecholamines?
   a. Most of these drugs are metabolized by cholinesterases in the liver and kidney.
   b. Catecholamines are concentrated at only selected tissue and organ sites.
   c. CNS effects of catecholamines are due to passage across the blood-brain barrier.
   d. Catecholamine drugs are inactivated through uptake at sympathetic nerve endings.

7. In the event of beta-blocker overdose, the following drug has been shown to be useful in reversal of life-threatening complications:
   a. protamine sulfate
   b. phenotolamine
   c. atropine
   d. glucagon

8. Adrenergic drugs work at all of the following receptor sites *except:*
   a. alpha
   b. muscarinic
   c. dopaminergic
   d. beat$_2$

9. An example of an alpha blocking agent is:
   a. atenolol
   b. phentolamine
   c. isoproterinol
   d. dobutamine

10. Which of the following statements is *correct* with regard to dobutamine hydrochloride administration?
    a. This drug is a naturally occurring catecholamine with selective beta$_2$ action.
    b. Even at low doses, dobutamine will increase heart rate significantly.
    c. Dobutamine increases renal and mesenteric blood flow.
    d. This drug is appropriate for management of cardiogenic shock.

CHAPTER 20

1. All of the following are opiate partial antagonists *except:*
   a. palbuphine hydrochloride (Nubain)
   b. butorphanol tatrate (Stadol)
   c. naloxone hydrochloride (Narcan)
   d. pentazocine (Talwin)

2. Propoxyphene hydrochloride (Darvon) 65 mg is:
   a. a Schedule II narcotic used for chronic pain
   b. best suited for the suicidal addiction-prone patient
   c. equivalent to 30 to 45 mg of codeine
   d. recommended for lactating mothers and children

3. All of the following statements regarding methyl morphine (codeine) are correct *except:*
   a. Codeine is contraindicated in patients with high intracranial pressure.
   b. The average adult dosage is 15 to 60 mg four times daily prn.
   c. The drug is classified as a Schedule II controlled substance.
   d. Common side effects include constipation, drowsiness, and nausea.

4. A physiological effect of the opiate kappa receptor is:
   a. dysphoria
   b. respiratory stimulation
   c. miosis
   d. vasomotor stimulation

5. The endorphin peptides are found in the:
   a. adrenal medulla
   b. pituitary
   c. stomach
   d. spinal cord

6. All of the following are correct regarding non-opiate narcotics *except:*
   a. These drugs stimulate the formation of prostaglandins in inflamed tissue.
   b. Non-opiate agents affect the hypothalamus to lower body temperature.
   c. This type of drug is generally well absorbed from the gastrointestinal tract.
   d. The non-opiate analgesics are metabolized in the liver and excreted in the urine.

7. The antidote for an overdose of acetaminophen (Tylenol) is:
   a. syrup of ipecac
   b. sodium bicarbonate
   c. haloxone hydrochloride
   d. acteylcysteine

8. Aspirin interacts adversely with all of the following *except:*
   a. corticosteroids
   b. pyrazolines
   c. synthetic narcotics
   d. sulfonylurea agents

9. Which of the following statements is correct regarding methadone hydrochloride (Dolophine)?
   a. This naturally occurring opiate is used to relieve pain in the terminally ill.
   b. Methadone is administered subcutaneously for detoxification and maintenance.
   c. This synthetic opiate is very effective after oral administration.
   d. Methadone may be administered five days after MAO inhibitor therapy.

10. All of the following are correct with regard to butorphanol (Stadol) *except:*
   a. This drug is less potent than morphine when given IM.
   b. It is a synthetic opiate agonist-antagonist analgesic.
   c. There is less potential for addiction than with morphine.
   d. The recommended IM dose is 2 mg every 3 to 4 hours prn.

CHAPTER 21

1. Central nervous system stimulants produce their pharmacological action by:
   a. decreasing the effect of excitatory neurotransmission
   b. increasing or stimulating inhibitory neurotransmission
   c. enhancing the uptake of catecholamines at adrenergic synapses
   d. modifying neurotransmitter response by altering cAMP

2. The reason for decreased therapeutic use of CNS stimulants is that:
   a. the extremely long duration of action potentiates adverse side effects
   b. more powerful drugs are now used for reversal of CNS depression
   c. the use of these stimulating drugs remains highly controversial
   d. they are ineffective in reducing pharmacologically induced CNS depression

3. Analeptic stimulants produce the following adverse effect:
   a. hypercapnea
   b. clonic-tonic seizures
   c. reduced respirations
   d. severe hypotension

4. Doxapram is contraindicated in the following patient condition:
   a. postanesthesia respiratory depression
   b. chronic pulmonary disease
   c. cerebral vascular accident
   d. drug-induced CNS depression

5. The following statement is *correct* with regard to drug interactions with amphetamines:

a. Acetazolamide increases the amphetamine effect by altering renal excretion.
b. Amphetamines used with quanethidine result in severe hypertension.
c. The use of phenothiazines causes an exaggerated amphetamine response.
d. Tricyclic antidepressants decrease the effects of amphetamines.

6. The combined effect of cocaine used with anticholinergic agents results in:
   a. hypertension and tachycardia
   b. drowsiness and apnea
   c. sweating and nausea
   d. confusion and memory loss

7. Caffeine produces all of the following actions *except:*
   a. exerts a positive chronotropic effect
   b. stimulates pepsin secretion
   c. depresses the cerebral cortex
   d. decreases reabsorption of sodium

8. Important nursing measures when caring for the patient taking cloxapram include:
   a. checking for bradycardia
   b. assessing deep tendon reflexes
   c. noting skin turgor and hydration
   d. palpating peripheral pulses

9. Which of the following statements is *correct* regarding the use of amphetamines?
   a. The overall effect of these drugs on the bladder is sphincter dilation.
   b. These drugs stimulate bronchoconstriction and reduced secretions.
   c. Amphetamines enhance the sense of smell and taste.
   d. Amphetamines cause respiratory stimulation and mydriasis.

CHAPTER 22

1. An agent which blocks enkephalinergic-induced seizures is:
   a. clonazepam
   b. phenobarbital
   c. diazepam
   d. valproic acid

2. Close monitoring during the labor of women on phenobarbital therapy is important because of the potential for:
   a. toxicity
   b. hemorrhage
   c. withdrawal symptoms
   d. febrile seizures

3. Primidone (Mysoline) is similar in chemical composition to the following drug:
   a. phenytoin
   b. phenobarbital
   c. methadone
   d. diazepam

4. Which of the following statements is *correct* with regard to the interaction of phenytoin (Dilantin) and other agents?
   a. Corticosteroid metabolism is decreased when administered with phenytoin.
   b. Isoniazid action inhibits phenytoin, resulting in low serum levels.
   c. Phenytoin serum levels increase when administered with nifedipine.
   d. Alcohol use with phenytoin results in an enhanced anticonvulsant effect.

5. Which of the following is a characteristic of phenobarbital?
   a. Phenobarbital is useful in the control of absence seizures.
   b. Phenobarbital should not be given to comatose patients.
   c. A decrease in drug level occurs with propoxyphene.
   d. The dosage should be increased in the elderly patient.

6. Phenytoin is indicated in the following cardiac-related disorder:
   a. sinus bradycardia
   b. second degree A-V block
   c. Stokes-Adams syndrome
   d. digitalis-induced arrhythmias

7. Carbamazepine (Tegretol) acts by:
   a. increasing the threshold for neuronal firing
   b. decreasing the discharge of nonadrenergic neurons
   c. reducing polysynaptic responses
   d. decreasing the influx of calcium during depolarization

8. An agent which may be used to control myoclonic seizures is:
   a. acetazolamide (Diamox)
   b. ethosuximide (Zarontin)
   c. clonazepam (Klonopin)
   d. mephenytoin (Mesantoin)

9. Which of the following plays a major role in the pharmacokinetics of the benzodiazepines?
   a. availability of glutamate
   b. percentage of extracellular water
   c. degree of plasma acidity
   d. extent of lipid solubility

CHAPTER 23

1. The management of Parkinson's disease is primarily accomplished by:
   a. reducing the dyskinesias through central skeletal muscle relaxants
   b. inhibiting the excitatory action of dopamine at neuron junction
   c. restoring dopamine levels in the central nervous system
   d. stimulating cholinergic activity through the use of dopaminergic drugs

2. Cortical-adrenal autologous transplantation has been performed as a treatment for patients with:
   a. multiple sclerosis
   b. Parkinson's disease
   c. myasthenia gravis
   d. Huntington's chorea

3. The rationale for administering carbidopa with levodopa is that:
   a. carbidopa inhibits the breakdown of levodopa in the peripheral tissue
   b. levodopa reduces the CNS side effects of carbidopa
   c. the drug combination enhances the uptake of pyroxidine for muscular control
   d. carbidopa counteracts the muscarinic effects of levodopa

4. Central skeletal muscle relaxants are *most* effective in relieving muscle spasm caused by:
   a. multiple sclerosis
   b. cerebral palsy
   c. pain receptor stimulation
   d. inflammation or trauma

5. Which of the following is an example of a direct-acting skeletal muscle relaxant?
   a. diazepam (Valium)
   b. methocarbamol (Robaxin)
   c. dantrolene sodium (Dantrium)
   d. carisoprodol (Soma)

6. Which of the following drugs should not be used for patients with myasthenia gravis?
   a. antihistamines
   b. corticosteroids
   c. cytotoxic agents
   d. carbamates

7. In the patients with the neuromuscular disorder myasthenia gravis:
   a. nerve impulses are not present at the neuromuscular junction
   b. destruction of dopaminergic receptors occurs, altering voluntary motor control
   c. reduced availability of receptor sites for acetylcholine results in motor weakness
   d. excess acetylcholine stimulates extrapyramidal tracts, creating dyskinesias

8. Patients on levodopa who demonstrate the "on/off" phenomenon may benefit from:
   a. increased levodopa dosages
   b. corticosteroid therapy
   c. amantadine therapy
   d. antihistamine therapy

9. An initial adverse effect of bromocriptine is:
   a. cardiovascular collapse
   b. erythromelalgra
   c. end-of-dose failure
   d. mottled skin

CHAPTER 24

1. An example of a drug that produces relaxation of skeletal muscles is:
   a. alprazolam (Xanax)
   b. diazepam (Valium)
   c. meprobamate (Equanil)
   d. talbutal (Lotusate)

2. Anxiolytic drugs, such as benzodiazepines, have the following effect:
   a. potentiate effects of other CNS depressants
   b. produce little dependence when given as recommended
   c. are associated with gastritis when given with meals
   d. are absorbed slowly when given orally

3. With regard to the absorption and metabolic fate of barbiturates, the drugs are:
   a. used safely for two months without dependence
   b. absorbed through the colon and may be given rectally
   c. used safely during pregnancy and lactation
   d. excreted as active metabolites via the kidney

4. Barbiturates would be the drug of choice for:
   a. pain
   b. anxiety reaction
   c. hepatic encephalopathy
   d. paradoxical reaction

5. When comparing the use of barbiturates with that of benzodiazepines, the following is correct:
   a. Benzodiazepines cause more dermatitis than barbiturates.
   b. Barbiturates are more economical than benzodiazepines.
   c. Barbiturates cause less drowsiness than benzodiazepines.
   d. Benzodiazepines are less addicting than barbiturates.

6. Chlordiazepoxide (Librium) is:
   a. absorbed rapidly by the intramuscular route
   b. known to have no accumulative effects
   c. used as a treatment for alcohol withdrawal
   d. known to be useful for situational anxiety

7. A sedative/hypnotic associated with a high degree of memory impairment is:
   a. chlorazepate dipotassium (Tranxene)
   b. chloral hydrate (Noctec)
   c. oxazepam (Serax)
   d. triazolam (Halcion)

8. All benzodiazepines are contraindicated if the following condition exists:
   a. coma
   b. senile agitation
   c. alcohol withdrawal
   d. psychosomatic disorders

9. Colorful dreams and nightmares may take place during which sleep stage?
   a. Stage III
   b. Stage II
   c. REM
   d. Stage IV

CHAPTER 25

1. Which of the following statements is *correct* regarding absorption and fate of oral neuraleptics?
   a. Oral concentrates are mixed with 4 ounces of pineapple juice before administration.
   b. Rate of absorption is increased if given concurrently with antacids.
   c. Most oral concentrates are well absorbed from the gastrointestinal tract.
   d. Criteria for oral dosage is dependent on therapeutic serum levels.

2. The antipsychotic drugs have proven to be effective in:
   a. controlling symptoms
   b. reducing side effects
   c. producing a sense of euphoria
   d. preventing psychosis

3. Which of the following statements is *correct* regarding elimination of antipsychotic agents?
   a. The drugs are highly distributed in the extracellular fluid compartments.
   b. Most of the agents have a short half-life which is less than 24 hours.
   c. Hemo-dialysis or peritoneal dialysis is the suggested method for treating overdose.
   d. When discontinued, the drugs may continue to be released from the tissues.

4. Cholinergic sites, which are blocked by neuroleptic drugs, produce the following effect:
   a. akathisia
   b. impaired memory
   c. rigidity
   d. tongue thrusts

5. Tardive dyskinesia, a syndrome associated with antipsychotic drugs, is most likely caused by:
   a. cholinergic receptor blockade
   b. dopamine receptor blockade
   c. short-term drug use
   d. subtherapeutic drug levels

6. Which of the following descriptions is *correct* concerning the extrapyramidal side effects of antipsychotic medications?
   a. Akathisia is characterized by a shuffling gait.
   b. Acute dystonic reactions are characterized by puffing the cheeks.
   c. Pseudoparkinsonism is characterized by motor retardation.
   d. Tardive dyskinesia is characterized by difficulty sitting still.

7. Haloperidol is contraindicated in patients with:
   a. Parkinson's disease
   b. severe anxiety reaction
   c. senile dementia
   d. Alzheimer's disease

8. Which of the following drugs is classified as an aliphatic phenothiazine?
   a. trifluoperazine (Stelazine)
   b. thioridazine (Mellaril)
   c. fluphenazine (Prolixin)
   d. chloropromazine (Thorazine)

9. Which of the following statements is *correct* with regard to drug interactions with antipsychotics?
   a. Amphetamines decrease the effects of neuroleptics.
   b. Alcohol prolongs the effect of neuroleptics.
   c. Neuroleptics prolong the effects of epinephrine.
   d. Antimuscarinics prolong plasma levels of neuroleptics.

CHAPTER 26

1. The action of tricyclic antidepressants is thought to be achieved by:
   a. increasing storage sites of acetylcholine for presynaptic nerves
   b. reducing the levels of dopamine available for receptor transmission
   c. prolonging the presence of norepinephrine within the nerve synapses
   d. inactivating serotonin production at the neurotransmitter

2. Antidepressant drugs are widely distributed because they are predominantly:
   a. inactive metabolites
   b. lipid-soluble
   c. ionized
   d. unbound

3. Which of the following is a common anticholinergic symptom associated with antidepressants?
   a. dysrhythmias
   b. photophobia
   c. blurred vision
   d. diarrhea

4. An example of a monoamine oxidase (MAO) inhibitor is:
   a. trimipramine maleate
   b. doxepin hydrochloride
   c. phenelzine sulfate
   d. zimelidine

4. MAO inhibitors should be given cautiously to patients with the following condition:
   a. pheochromocytoma
   b. asthma
   c. reverse vegetative symptoms
   d. severe anxiety

5. Which of the following statements is *correct* with regard to drug interactions with tricyclic antidepressants?
   a. A decreased effectiveness of antidepressants is seen when given with phenothiazines.
   b. Ammonium chloride increases the effect of tricyclic antidepressants.
   c. Sodium bicarbonate increases the effect of tricyclic antidepressants.
   d. A decreased effectiveness of antidepressants is seen when given with acetazolamide.

6. A symptom of severe lithium toxicity is:
   a. hyperreflexia
   b. vertigo
   c. polydipsia
   d. muscle weakness

7. Which of the following narcotic agents would be contraindicated for patients on MAO inhibitors?
   a. hydromorphone
   b. meperidine
   c. morphine
   d. codeine

8. Some diagnostic tests are altered by tricyclic antidepressants. Which of the following represents a correct example?
   a. reduced serum bilirubin
   b. increased VMA excretion
   c. reduced excretion of catecholamines
   d. increased blood glucose

9. Lithium exerts its therapeutic action by:
   a. stimulating the production of dopamine in the substantia nigra
   b. reducing the release of norepinephrine from synaptic vesicles
   c. inhibiting the breakdown of serotonin at the postsynaptic junction
   d. decreasing the reuptake of norepinephrine by synaptosomes

CHAPTER 27

1. The layer of the heart in which the major blood vessels are located is the:
   a. pericardial sac
   b. epicardium
   c. myocardium
   d. endocardium

2. The tricuspid valve lies between the:
   a. right atrium and right ventricle
   b. right ventricle and pulmonary aratery
   c. left atrium and left ventricle
   d. left ventricle and aorta

3. Which of the following statements is *correct* regarding the action potential curve of the cardiac cell?
   a. During Phase 1, a fast influx of potassium ion moves into the cell.

b. During Phase 4, only a strong stimulus will precipitate an action potential.

c. During Phase 2, a slow influx of calcium ions moves into the cell.

d. During Phase 3, a fast influx of sodium ions moves into the cells.

4. The following description applies to the conduction system of the heart and the EKG pattern:
   a. The P wave reflects atrial repolarization.
   b. The PR interval represents atrial contraction.
   c. The QRS complex represents ventricular depolarization.
   d. The T wave represents ventricular depolarization.

5. Which of the following pacemaker areas initiates a heart rate of 60 to 40 per minute?
   a. AV node
   b. SA node
   c. bundle of His
   d. Purkinje fibers

6. Cardiac output is measured by stroke volume and:
   a. preload
   b. heart rate
   c. conductivity
   d. elasticity

8. The right coronary artery supplies oxygenated blood to the:
   a. SA node in 60 percent of the population
   b. AV node in 10 percent of the population
   c. lateral portion of the left ventrical
   d. posterior leaflet of the mitral valve

9. Which of the following statements is correct regarding capillary pressures?
   a. Capillary hydrostatic pressure ranges from 10 mmHg at the arterial end to 30 mmHg at the venous end.
   b. When capillary hydrostatic pressure is normal and colloid osmotic pressure is low, edema results.
   c. When capillary hydrostatic pressure is normal and colloid osmotic pressure is low, dehydration results.
   d. The higher the colloid osmotic pressure, the higher the gradient of fluid moving into interstitial tissues.

10. Coronary artery perfusion occurs during:
    a. ventricular diastole
    b. atrial repolarization
    c. ventricular systole
    d. ventricular depolarization

CHAPTER 28

1. As a class of drugs, the cardiac glycosides:
   a. are produced from synthetic sources

b. increase the rate of ventricular ejection
   c. are effective within a wide therapeutic range
   d. increase the force of cardiac contraction

2. The overall effect of cardiac glycosides results in:
   a. increased diastolic volume
   b. increased systemic vascular resistance
   c. reduced cardiac preload
   d. reduced sensitivity to acetylcholine

3. The primary site of action by digitalis glycosides is the:
   a. AV node
   b. SA node
   c. Bundle branches
   d. Purkinje fibers

4. Which of the following statements is *correct* regarding the effect of cardiac glycosides?
   a. These agents have an indirect effect on the cardiac conduction system.
   b. Digitalis glycosides have a negative chronotropic effect on the cardiac muscle cells.
   c. The glycosides exert direct action on the heart through the autonomic nervous system.
   d. A greater magnitude of therapeutic effect is seen on the nonfailing heart than on the failing heart.

5. All of the following are outcomes associated with digoxin therapy *except*:
   a. increased heart size
   b. increased urine output
   c. increased afterload
   d. increased stroke volume

6. Which of the following dysrhythmias can be corrected with digitalis preparations?
   a. ventricular tachycardia
   b. sinus bradycardia
   c. first degree AV block
   d. paroxysmal atrial tachycardia

7. Patients on concurrent phenobarbital and digitoxin therapy have the potential for:
   a. reduced phenobarbital levels
   b. elevated digitoxin levels
   c. reduced digitoxin levels
   d. elevated phenobarbital levels

8. When given concurrently with digoxin, which drug will increase the digoxin concentration?
   a. bleomycin
   b. nifedipine
   c. sulfasalazine
   d. procarbazine

9. When adding quinidine therapy to patients who are on digoxin, the following may occur:
   a. ventricular dysrhythmias
   b. reduced digoxin levels
   c. mental status changes
   d. elevated potassium levels

CHAPTER 29

1. All of the following are sympathetic nervous system inhibitors *except:*
   a. clonidine hydrochloride
   b. methyldopa
   c. quanabenz
   d. guanethidine sulfate

2. An antihypertensive drug which has been shown to be useful in opiate withdrawal is:
   a. reserpine
   b. propranolol
   c. clonidine
   d. hydralazine

3. Diazoxide (Hyperstat) is a chlorothiazide derivative which:
   a. has a combined diuretic activity
   b. is used to treat mild hypertension
   c. is useful in ischemic heart disease
   d. inhibits insulin release

4. Reserpine (Serpasil) is contraindicated in the following patient condition:
   a. acute ulcerative colitis
   b. severe hypertension
   c. chronic pulmonary disease
   d. glaucoma

5. Guanethidine sulfate (Ismelin) produces the following effect:
   a. increased cardiac output
   b. decreased contractility
   c. increased venous return
   d. decreased sodium level

6. Minoxodil (Loniten) is a potent oral vasodilator which:
   a. increases cardiac output
   b. reduces glomerular filtration rate
   c. causes reflex bradycardia
   d. reduces fluid retention

7. Which of the following drugs is a ganglionic blocker?
   a. acebutolol hydrochloride
   b. prazosin
   c. mecamylamine hydrochloride
   d. enalapril

8. Which of the following is *correct* regarding methyldopa administration and other concurrent drug use?
   a. The effects of methyldopa are increased when given with amphetamines.
   b. Verapamil may potentiate the effects of methyldopa.
   c. A hyperglycemia effect is seen with methyldopa and Tolbutamide.
   d. Use of methyldopa and propranolol results in paradoxic hypotension.

9. Which of the following drugs is an alpha-adrenergic blocker?
   a. diazoxide
   b. prazosin
   c. hydralazine
   d. diltiazem

10. An example of an antihypertensive agent which competes with epinephrine for available beta-receptor sites is:
    a. sodium nitroprusside
    b. atenolol
    c. terazosin
    d. hydralazine

CHAPTER 30

1. Which of the following statements is *correct* regarding the use of antidysrhythmia agents?
   a. The new antidysrhythmia drugs have few side effects or toxic reactions.
   b. All of the antidysrhythmic medications act by similar mechanisms.
   c. Atrial dysrhythmias are not life-threatening, but usually require therapy.
   d. Treatment of ventricular dysrhythmias does not affect mortality rate.

2. Group IV antidysrhythmia drugs act by the following mechanim:
   a. depressing phase 4 depolarization and lengthening phases 1 and 2 of repolarization
   b. stabilizing the cell membrane and depressing phase 0 of the action potential
   c. prolonging refractoriness, slowing conduction, and decreasing membrane responsiveness
   d. depressing phase 4 of depolarization and prolonging phase 3 of repolarization

3. An example of a Group 1a antidysrhythmia drug is:
   a. amiodarone
   b. tocainide
   c. disopryamide
   d. lidocaine

4. Procainamide (Pronestyl) is contraindicated in the following patient condition:
   a. Wolff-Parkinson-White syndrome
   b. myasthenia gravis
   c. Parkinson's disease
   d. acute myocardial infarction

5. Which of the following statements is *correct* regarding verapamil, a Group IV antidysrhythmia drug?
   a. It is used to treat supraventricular dysrhythmias.
   b. It increases conduction through the heart.
   c. It is used to treat AV nodal blocks.
   d. The drug can be given intravenously with propranolol.

6. An example of an antidyshrythmia drug which interferes with norepinephrine release from sympathatic nerve terminals is:
   a. bretylium
   b. pindolol
   c. propafenone
   d. phenytoin

7. The Group II antidysrhythmia agents are useful in treating:
   a. re-entrant tachycardias involving AV node or accessory pathways
   b. life-threatening ventricular dysrhythmias resistant to lidocaine
   c. ventricular dysrhythmias caused by exercise or excessive catecholamines
   d. ventricular dysrhythmias which arise from conduction delays

8. Which of the following represents an investigational Group I drug?
   a. practolol
   b. sotalol
   c. bepridil
   d. lorcainide

9. Torsade de Pointe can be treated with:
   a. lidocaine
   b. bretylium
   c. propranolol
   d. quinidine

10. Mexiletine hydrochloride is structurally similar to which of the following drugs?
    a. quinidine
    b. lidocaine
    c. propranolol
    d. bretylium

CHAPTER 31

1. As a class of drugs, nitrates have the following action:
   a. constriction of collateral cardiac blood vessels
   b. reduction in systemic venous tone
   c. relaxation of skeletal muscle tissue
   d. constriction of cerebral blood vessels

2. Which of the following represents an outcome of high dose nitrate therapy?
   a. increased left ventricular end-diastolic volume
   b. reduced ventricular outflow resistance
   c. increased myocardial oxygen demand
   d. reduced intracranial pressure

3. Which of the following descriptions is *correct* regarding the pharmacokinetics of nitroglycerin?
   a. readily absorbed via the oral route
   b. dependent on lipids for drug binding
   c. estimated half-life of two hours
   d. extensive first-pass metabolism

4. A drug which can act as a physiological antagonist to nitrates is:
   a. heparin
   b. verapamil
   c. histamine
   d. diltiazem

5. When instructing the patient about use of nitroglycerin translingual (Nitrolingual) for relief of chest pain, the following is stressed:
   a. Inhale deeply after administration of translingual spray.
   b. Shake canister well before using translingual spray.
   c. Swallow immediately after administration of the spray.
   d. Spray 1 or 2 metered doses into the oral mucosa.

6. An expected effect of the use of beta-adrenergic blockers to control angina is:
   a. increased heart rate
   b. reduced force of contraction
   c. increased myocardial demand
   d. reduced tolerance to exercise

7. Verapamil (Isoptin) is contraindicated in patients with the following condition:
   a. cerebral vascular spasm
   b. variant angina
   c. asthma
   d. sick sinus syndrome

8. An example of a beta-adrenergic stimulant is:
   a. phenoxybenzamine
   b. verapamil
   c. erythrityl tetranitrate
   d. nylidrin hydrochloride

9. Which of the following statements is *correct* regarding papaverine (Pavabid)?
   a. As an opium derivative, it is likely to cause habituation, tolerance, and analgesia.
   b. This drug acts directly on vascular smooth muscle to cause vasoconstriction.
   c. Papaverine has been shown to be very effective in treating peripheral vascular disease.
   d. This drug is used primarily for treating peripheral ischemia associated with arterial spasm.

CHAPTER 32

1. Which of the following compounds contains the largest proportion of lipids:
   a. low-density lipoproteins (LDL)
   b. high-density lipoproteins (HDL)
   c. very low-density lipoproteins (VLDL)
   d. intermediate-density lipoproteins (IDL)

2. Normal iron loss through the bowel, skin, and genitourinary tract is:
   a. 1.5 to 3.5 mg/day
   b. 0.1 to 0.3 mg/day

c. 2 to 4.5 mg/day
d. 0.5 to 1 mg/day

3. Which of the following drugs is a chelating agent with a specific affinity for ferric iron?
   a. hydroxocobalamin (Alpharedisol)
   b. ferrous fumarate (Ircon)
   c. deferoxamine (Desferal)
   d. clofibrate (Atromid-S)

4. An example of a simple lipid is:
   a. triglyceride
   b. phospholipid
   c. lipoprotein
   d. cholesterol

5. Type III hyperlipidemia can be treated with diet and:
   a. gemfibrozil
   b. nicotinic acid
   c. lovastatin
   d. colestipol

6. Which of the following drugs reduces serum triglycerides by up to 55 percent?
   a. colestipol
   b. probucol
   c. lovastatin
   d. gemfibrozil

7. Development of cancer of the biliary tract is associated with high doses of which drug?
   a. clofibrate
   b. gemfibrozil
   c. lovastatin
   d. deferoxamine

8. An example of a megaloblastic type of anemia is:
   a. iron deficiency
   b. paroxysmal nocturnal hemoglobinuria
   c. pernicious
   d. aplastic

9. Clofibrate (Atromid-S), an antilipemic medication, has the following action:
   a. inhibits lipolysis in adipose tissue
   b. decreases the hepatic synthesis of LDL
   c. inhibits the hepatic synthesis of cholesterol
   d. decreases biliary excretion of triglycerides

CHAPTER 33

1. In the clotting process, stage II is represented by:
   a. resolution stage of clot formation
   b. formation of active thromboplastin
   c. conversion of fibrinogen to fibrin
   d. conversion of prothrombin to thrombin

2. The intrinsic cascade is activated by:
   a. damage to the endothelium of blood vessels
   b. presence of factors V, VII, and X
   c. damage to surrounding tissue structures
   d. presence of plasminogen and fibrinokinases

3. The use of anticoagulant agents in the clinical setting is to:
   a. stimulate fibrinolysis
   b. dissolve existing clots
   c. retard the clotting process
   d. dissolve clotting factors

4. In the human body, the highest concentration of heparin can be found in the:
   a. brain
   b. pancreas
   c. liver
   d. lungs

5. Oral anticoagulant agents are contraindicated in the following condition:
   a. subacute myocardial infarction
   b. pulmonary embolism
   c. transient ischemic attacks
   d. precordial effusion

6. Which of the following agents inhibits platelet aggregation?
   a. dipyridamole (Persantine)
   b. dicumarol (Dicoumarin)
   c. anisindione (Miradon)
   d. negatol (Negatan)

7. Vitamin K-dependent clotting factors include which of the following?
   a. fibrinogen
   b. prothrombin
   c. thromboplastin
   d. plasma thromboplastin antecedent (PTA)

8. Heparin exerts its therapeutic action by:
   a. antagonizing the production of factors V, VII, and XII
   b. deactivating calcium-dependent clotting factors
   c. blocking the action of plasminogen in stage IV
   d. preventing formation of fibrin in stage III

9. Agents such as streptokinase are contraindicated in the following situation/condition:
   a. arteriovenous cannulae occlusions
   b. chronic asthma
   c. thromboembolic disease
   d. cerebrovascular disease

CHAPTER 34

1. The upper airway is composed of the:
   a. trachea, bronchus, bronchiole
   b. throat, trachea, bronchus
   c. mouth, throat, trachea
   d. nose, mouth, throat

2. The larynx, which marks the transition of the upper airway to the lower airway, has the following function:
   a. plays a role in airway clearance
   b. provides protection to the upper airway

c. humidifies the inhaled air

d. opens when food or liquid enters the oropharynx

3. Which statement is *correct* regarding the operation of airway defense mechanisms?
   a. The mucociliary escalator traps and removes large particles of foreign matter from the alveoli.
   b. Alveolar macrophages are freely moving scavenger cells that regularly clean the tracheo-bronchial tree.
   c. Mucus secreted by the bronchial epithelium holds particles and bacteria that come in contact with it.
   d. The tonsils and the adenoids prevent the aspiration of foreign matter and protect the lungs.

4. Chemoreceptors, located in the arch of the aorta, are sensitive to changes in:
   a. posture
   b. blood pressure
   c. pH levels
   d. temperature

5. Which statement is *correct* regarding neurological control of bronchial smooth muscle?
   a. Parasympathetic stimulation causes bronchial smooth muscle dilation.
   b. Sympathetic stimulation causes bronchial smooth muscle constriction.
   c. The autonomic nervous system stimulates release of Type II surfactant cells.
   d. Humoral mediators released from mast cells cause bronchial constriction.

6. A cause of increased work of breathing is:
   a. increased elastic recoil
   b. increased lung compliance
   c. muscular weakness
   d. decreased airway resistance

7. The most common cause of reduced lung compliance is:
   a. infection
   b. cerebellar injury
   c. myasthenia gravis
   d. musculoskeletal blocking agents

8. Which of the following statements is *correct* concerning airway resistance?
   a. When the lumen of the airway increases, airway resistance increases.
   b. Airway resistance increases as a result of increased mucus production.
   c. Spasms of the bronchial smooth muscle reduce airway resistance.
   d. When airway resistance is high, air moves freely within the system.

9. The specific autonomic receptors found in the bronchial smooth muscle are the:
   a. alpha
   b. muscarinic
   c. $beta_1$
   d. $beta_2$

10. Of the following statements, which is *correct* concerning ventilation control mechanisms?
    a. Rhythmic impulses signaling the ventilatory muscles to contract and relax are found in the reticular activating center.
    b. Peripheral chemoreceptors located in the aortic arch are more sensitive to arterial oxygen levels than CO_2 levels.
    c. The medullary neurons are voluntary in nature and initiate the inhalation phase of ventilation.
    d. Central chemoreceptors in the medulla are extremely sensitive to changes in arterial CO_2 levels.

CHAPTER 35

1. The use of catecholamine compounds has declined due in part to:
   a. prolonged half-life
   b. reduction in bronchial diseases
   c. short duration of action
   d. cost of production

2. Drugs which reduce the effectiveness of sympathomimetics include:
   a. anticholinergics
   b. beta-blocking agents
   c. hypoglycemics
   d. alpha-blocking agents

3. Xanthine agents produce bronchial smooth muscle relaxation by:
   a. directly stimulating $Beta_1$ cells
   b. indirectly stimulating alpha receptor cells
   c. directly contributing to calcium blockade
   d. indirectly contributing to cAMP production

4. An example of a drug which decreases the rate of metabolism of theophylline is:
   a. cimetidine
   b. phenytoin
   c. carbamazepine
   d. furosemide

5. Corticosteroids acts to control bronchospasm by:
   a. direct relaxation of bronchial smooth muscle
   b. stimulation of parasympathetic nervous system
   c. inhibiting the sympathetic nervous system
   d. counteracting bronchial inflammatory processes

6. The following drug is *not* indicated in an acute asthma attack:
   a. theophylline
   b. cromolyn sodium
   c. atropine
   d. epinephrine

7. A side effect of ephedrine is:
   a. generalized vasodilation
   b. premature atrial contractions
   c. hyperglycemia
   d. decreased blood pressure

8. Isoproterenol (Isuprel) has the following adverse effect:
   a. tremors
   b. negative chronotropic effects
   c. decreased myocardial oxygen demand
   d. decreased cardiac contractility

9. Anticholinergic bronchodilators exert their action through:
   a. stimulating production of cAMP
   b. stimulating the activity of acetylcholine
   c. decreasing production of cAMP
   d. decreasing production of cGMP

10. Which statement is *correct* regarding the signs and symptoms of bronchial obstruction?
    a. Wheezing, audible with a stethoscope, is suggestive of mild bronchial obstruction.
    b. All breath sounds are greatly diminished with severe bronchial obstruction.
    c. Evidence of central cyanosis is always present in partial bronchial obstruction.
    d. Tachycardia and a bounding pulse are indicators of mild bronchial obstruction.

CHAPTER 36

1. Which of the following is an example of a respiratory stimulant?
   a. atropine
   b. theophylline
   c. epinephrine
   d. dopamine

2. An early sign of oxygen toxicity is:
   a. tingling in extremities
   b. confusion
   c. cyanosis
   d. cough

3. As a narcotic antitussive agent, methadone (Dolophine) has the following characteristic:
   a. indicated for asthma
   b. low addictive potential
   c. safe for head trauma
   d. rapid onset of action

4. Carbon dioxide acts to increase breathing by:
   a. stimulation of chemoreceptors
   b. stimulation of central nervous system
   c. activation of diaphragm muscles
   d. elevation of the blood pH

5. Medroxyprogesterone acetate (Provera) exerts its action on respirations by:
   a. influencing the pons and medulla oblongata to increase ventilation
   b. increasing responsiveness of respiratory center to carbon dioxide
   c. reducing the level of oxygen, thereby stimulating chemoreceptors
   d. stimulating the chemoreceptors directly, affecting respiratory drive

6. The optimum oxygen range for PaO_2 in premature infants is:
   a. 80 to 100 mmHg
   b. 70 to 90 mmHg
   c. 40 to 60 mmHg
   d. 50 to 80 mmHg

7. An oxygen concentration of 35 percent is best delivered by the following device:
   a. nasal cannula
   b. Venturi mask
   c. simple oxygen mask
   d. reservoir mask

8. Which of the following statements is *correct* regarding oxygen therapy?
   a. It is administered in concentrations of 100 percent for therapeutic effectiveness.
   b. High concentrations can cause toxicity and lung damage when given for long periods of time.
   c. A nasal cannula is the delivery system of choice for patients requiring high concentrations.
   d. Oxygen concentrations of 60 percent are administered to patients with unresponsive respiratory centers.

9. The amount of air moved with each breath is known as the:
   a. tidal volume
   b. minute volume
   c. vital capacity
   d. exhaled volume

CHAPTER 37

1. The process of excreting waste products as urine occurs in the following sequence:
   a. collecting ducts, glomerulus, proximal tubule, loop of Henle
   b. glomerulus, loop of Henle, proximal tubule, collecting ducts
   c. proximal tubule, glomerulus, loop of Henle, collecting ducts
   d. glomerulus, proximal tubule, loop of Henle, collecting ducts

2. The kidney maintains acid-base homeostasis by:
   a. keeping extracellular pH within the range of 7.0 to 7.70
   b. controlling bicarbonate concentration by renal H^+ excretion
   c. forming ammonia in the cells of the proximal tubule
   d. secreting H^+ ions into the proximal tubule in exchange for ammonium ions

3. Parathyroid hormone (PTH) elevates plasma calcium by working with Vitamin D to decrease:
   a. bone resorption
   b. intestinal calcium absorption
   c. renal calcium excretion
   d. renal elimination of phosphate

4. Antidiuretic hormone (ADH) acts on the following renal structure:
   a. collecting ducts
   b. proximal tubule
   c. loop of Henle
   d. glomerulus

5. The exchange of sodium for potassium in the distal convoluted tubule is regulated by:
   a. active chloride pump
   b. aldosterone
   c. posterior pituitary gland
   d. antidiuretic hormone

6. Vitamin D (cholecalciferol) is synthesized in the:
   a. large intestine
   b. stomach
   c. pancreas
   d. skin

7. The kidney produces a substance in response to hypoxia which increases red blood cell levels. This substance is known as:
   a. renin
   b. erythropoietin
   c. prostaglandin
   d. angiotensin

8. Patients with renal disease and diabetes mellitus may require:
   a. additional insulin
   b. less insulin
   c. longer-acting insulin
   d. no insulin

9. The primary site of actions for the triazide diuretics is the:
   a. loop of Henle
   b. proximal tubule
   c. collecting ducts
   d. distal convoluted tubule

10. One method of elimination of acid by the kidneys is accomplished by combining H^+ with:
    a. ammonia
    b. chloride
    c. magnesium
    d. urea

CHAPTER 38

1. Carbonic anhydrase inhibitors:
   a. create an osmotic gradient
   b. result in acidic diuresis
   c. decrease potassium excretion
   d. lead to systemic acidosis

2. Aldosterone antagonists:
   a. produce a potent diuretic action
   b. inhibit the exchange of sodium for potassium
   c. produce severe hypokalemia
   d. have a rapid onset of action

3. The pressure generated by contraction of the heart is referred to as:
   a. hydrostatic
   b. nephrotic
   c. oncotic
   d. osmotic

4. Fluid accumulates in the interstitial space when there exists:
   a. increased intravascular oncotic pressure
   b. decreased intravascular hydrostatic pressure
   c. altered capillary permeability
   d. reduced volume of sodium in third space

5. Angiotensin I is converted to angiotensin II in the:
   a. liver
   b. adrenal glands
   c. lungs
   d. kidneys

6. When treating patients who have ascites but no evidence of peripheral edema, the maximum extra diuresis that should be induced is:
   a. 900 ml/day
   b. 2,000 ml/day
   c. 1,500 ml/day
   d. 1,200 ml/day

7. Carbonic anhydrase inhibitors are contraindicated in the following patient situation:
   a. open-angle glaucoma
   b. pulmonary obstruction
   c. drug-induced edema
   d. absence seizures

8. Which of the following is an example of an osmotic diuretic?
   a. ethacrynic acid (Edecrin)
   b. bumefanide (Bumex)
   c. quinethazone (Hydromox)
   d. urea (Ureaphil)

9. Patients taking triamterene (Dyrenium) should not be given:
   a. aspirin
   b. calcium salts
   c. warfarin
   d. potassium supplements

10. Edema which is generalized in all body tissues is known as:
    a. ascites
    b. anasarca
    c. pitting edema
    d. peripheral edema

CHAPTER 39

1. Patients with chronic renal failure may also exhibit the following condition:
   a. Addison's disease
   b. hyponatremia

c. hypomagnesemia
d. Vitamin D deficiency

2. The body responds to metabolic acidosis (a decrease in arterial pH) by:
   a. decreasing renal ammonia production
   b. increasing ventilation
   c. excreting large amounts of potassium
   d. retaining carbon dioxide

3. Metabolic alkalosis is associated with:
   a. decreased arterial pH
   b. increased plasma HCO_3
   c. increased ventilation
   d. decreased P_{CO_2}

4. A patient is said to be oliguric when the urine output is:
   a. less than 20 ml/hour
   b. greater than 30 ml/hour
   c. less than 10 ml/hour
   d. greater than 200 ml/hour

5. In a patient's chronic renal failure, the regulation serum calcium and phosphate are altered. A result of this dysfunction leads to:
   a. hypothyroidism
   b. hypoparathyroidism
   c. secondary hyperparathyroidism
   d. primary hyperthyroidism

6. For a serum potassium of 2.8 mEq/L, the intravenous potassium supplement flow rate is:
   a. ≤40 mEq/hour
   b. ≤20 mEq/hour
   c. ≤10 mEq/hour
   d. ≤5 mEq/hour

7. Proximal renal tubular acidosis results in:
   a. impaired acidification of buffers
   b. decreased formation of bicarbonate
   c. increased excretion of bicarbonate
   d. increased formation of ammonia

8. A creatinine clearance of 30 ml/min is classified as:
   a. normal renal function
   b. moderate renal failure
   c. mild renal failure
   d. severe renal failure

9. Elevation in the blood urea nitrogen (BUN) greater than the rise in serum creatinine early in the oliguric patient is termed:
   a. severe renal failure
   b. osteitis fibrosa
   c. uremic poisoning
   d. pre-renal azotemia

CHAPTER 40

1. Of the following glands, which one is *not* a part of the endocrine system?
   a. thymus
   b. pancreas
   c. parathyroid
   d. pituitary

2. A polypeptide hormone synthesized by the anterior pituitary gland is:
   a. oxytocin
   b. thyrotropin
   c. prolactin
   d. melanocyte-stimulating hormone

3. Which statement is *correct* regarding the neuroregulation of the endocrine system?
   a. Neuroregulation operates on a positive feedback principle.
   b. Endocrine glands secrete a limited amount of hormone when stimulated.
   c. When the target organ responds strongly, endocrine activity is suppressed.
   d. The main factor in neuroregulation is the strength of the regulating hormone.

4. Which of the following hormones is secreted by the thyroid gland?
   a. thyrotropin
   b. calcitonin
   c. chymotrypsin
   d. growth hormone

5. Somatostatin, secreted by the delta cells of the pancreas, has the following action:
   a. inhibition of insulin secretion
   b. stimulation of glucogon synthesis
   c. inhibition of growth hormone
   d. stimulation of nutrient assimilation

6. Which of the following hormones is secreted by the adrenal cortex?
   a. progesterone
   b. trypsin
   c. epinephrine
   d. aldosterone

7. Which of the following hormones acts to increase serum calcium levels?
   a. calcitonin
   b. oxytocin
   c. parathormone
   d. somatatropin

8. The estrogen hormones have the following action:
   a. increase osteoblastic activity
   b. decrease fat deposits in the breast
   c. increase sodium and water excretion
   d. inhibit endometrial proliferation

9. Cortisol is a hormone which:
   a. stimulates gluconeogenesis in the liver
   b. increasses the rate of glucose utilization
   c. increases the rate of protein anabolism
   d. inhibits fat storage in breast tissue

10. Which of the following hormones requires a protein carrier for transport?
    a. glucogon
    b. insulin
    c. testosterone
    d. antidiuretic hormone

CHAPTER 41

1. Somatotropin hormone produces which of the following effects?
    a. produces a positive nitrogen balance
    b. increases cell size in specific organs
    c. inhibits protein synthesis within the cell
    d. increases glucose transport into the cell

2. The lipolytic effect of growth hormone leads to:
    a. excess low-density lipids in the plasma
    b. reduction of fat storage in the liver
    c. conversion of fatty acids to ketone bodies
    d. decreased availability of fatty acids for energy

3. Certain drugs may stimulate vasopressin release, including:
    a. caffeine
    b. insulin
    c. nicotine
    d. levodopa

4. In large doses, the following effect may occur with vasopressin therapy:
    a. inhibition of peristaltic activity in the large bowel
    b. dilation of the superior mesenteric artery
    c. increased blood flow to the splanchnic system
    d. contraction of smooth muscle in arterioles

5. The agent of choice in maintaining hemostasis during surgery in patients with von Willebrand's disease is:
    a. posterior pituitary injection
    b. desmopressin
    c. lypressin
    d. vasopressin

6. Vasopressin is produced by the:
    a. posterior pituitary
    b. anterior pituitary
    c. hypothalamus
    d. thymus

7. A major disadvantage of somatotropin (Humatrope) therapy is:
    a. cost
    b. side effects
    c. antibody production
    d. contamination

8. The secretion of growth hormone is suppressed by:
    a. stress
    b. emotional excitement
    c. hypoglycemic agents
    d. glucocorticoid drugs

9. Drugs which inhibit vasopressin release include:
    a. tricyclic antidepressants
    b. alcohol
    c. caffeine
    d. barbiturates

CHAPTER 42

1. A sign related to adrenal cortex hypofunction is:
    a. hyperglycemia
    b. electrolyte imbalances
    c. muscle wasting
    d. increased stress response

2. Aldosterone secretion is controlled by potassium and:
    a. antidiuretic hormone
    b. serum osmolality
    c. sodium levels
    d. angiotensin

3. An agent used for maintenance therapy for patients with salt-losing adrenogenital syndrome is:
    a. desoxycorticosterone pivalate
    b. paramethasone acetate
    c. dexamethasone
    d. beclomethasone dipropionate

4. Glucocorticoid regulation is mediated by:
    a. somatotropin
    b. renin
    c. sodium levels
    d. corticotropin

5. The effect of glucocorticoids on protein metabolism results in:
    a. greater coordination, particularly hand-eye coordination
    b. muscular weakness, particularly lower extremities
    c. massive muscular bulk without concomitant strength
    d. marked growth in height and weight in children

6. Which statement regarding glucocorticoid drugs is *correct*?
    a. Physiologic doses usually cause the adverse effects of therapy.
    b. These drugs are most often used for their anti-stress effects.
    c. Therapy is adjusted to mimic the normal diurnal pattern of cortisol.
    d. All glucocorticoids are effective when given by the oral route.

7. Patients who are on long-term glucocorticoid therapy may take on the cushingoid appearance, typified by the following characteristic:
    a. fat deposits in extremities
    b. cervicodorsal fat pad
    c. clubbing of fingernails
    d. exophthalamos

8. When patients are abruptly withdrawn from long-term glucocorticoid therapy, acute adrenal insufficiency may occur. An indicator of this life-threatening complication is:
   a. syncope
   b. palpitations
   c. hypertension
   d. shortness of breath

9. Which statement is *correct* regarding adrenal drugs as a group?
   a. Maintenance doses should be at the high end of the usual adult dosage.
   b. All adrenal cortex agents are among the safest drugs on the market.
   c. The synthetic steroids are more potent than naturally-occurring agents.
   d. The sodium-retaining potential is enhanced in synthetic corticosteroids.

CHAPTER 43

1. Testosterone has anabolic activity and produces:
   a. negative nitrogen balance
   b. decreased red blood cell production
   c. increased musculature
   d. decreased bone thickness

2. Androgen therapy is contraindicated in the following condition:
   a. postpartum breast engorgement
   b. endometriosis
   c. cancer of the prostate gland
   d. metastatic breast cancer

3. Which of the following hormonal agents is classified as an anabolic steroid?
   a. ethylestrenol (Maxibolin)
   b. testolactone (Teslac)
   c. estradiol vallerate (Delestrogen)
   d. norethindrone (Norlutin)

4. Estrogen preparations increase the effect of the following drug when used in combination:
   a. hydrocortisone
   b. phenytoin
   c. tetracycline
   d. rifampin

5. Patients who are taking androgens along with coumadin should be observed for:
   a. elevated clotting times
   b. elevated ptt levels
   c. subtherapeutic pt levels
   d. reduced white blood cells

6. Which of the following signs would indicate the need to discontinue oral contraceptives?
   a. nausea and vomiting
   b. upper quadrant abdominal pain
   c. headache with eyestrain
   d. pain and tenderness in the calf

7. An advantage of triphasic oral contraceptive products is:
   a. reduced risk of vascular effects
   b. reduced breakthrough bleeding
   c. increased protection in the early cycle
   d. increased resistance to infection

8. The following is *correct* regarding the use of spermicidal creams:
   a. Spotting or bleeding is a common side effect.
   b. Douching is avoided for 6 to 8 hours after use.
   c. Contracting the HIV virus is increased with use.
   d. Applying the product two hours before coitus is suggested.

9. At times, a patient may need to change from one estrogen product to another. One milligram of diethylstilbesterol equals:
   a. 1.5 mg conjugated estrogen
   b. 10 mg Estrone
   c. 5 mg mestranol
   d. 0.5 mg estradiol

CHAPTER 44

1. In the absence of insulin:
   a. glucose is readily transported into cells
   b. amino acids are converted to protein
   c. gluconeogenesis is inhibited
   d. free fatty acids are converted to ketone bodies

2. Individuals with diabetes are at risk for atherosclerosis because of:
   a. increased conversion of fatty acids to cholesterol in the absence of insulin
   b. increased cell metabolism of proteins important for maintaining vascular wall structure
   c. reduced ability of the liver to break down cholesterol which is consumed in excess
   d. decreased triglycerides in the liver as a result of ketoacidosis

3. Insulin can be made to be longer acting by the addition of:
   a. lipid
   b. zinc
   c. iron
   d. copper

4. An example of an individual who would benefit from human insulin administration would be:
   a. a gestational diabetic
   b. an older adult with Type I diabetes
   c. the patient without dietary restrictions
   d. a chronic diabetic on pork insulin

5. Which of the following is true of long-acting insulins?
   a. These insulin agents are frequently used alone for chronic diabetics.
   b. Insulin reactions may occur at night since they peak in four to nine hours.

c. An example of a long-acting insulin is NPH, which peaks in 24 hours.

d. At low doses, they suppress glucogenolysis and gluconeogenesis.

6. Which of the following individuals would benefit from a single dose of intermediate-acting insulin per day?
   a. gestational diabetic over 18 years old
   b. Type I newly diagnosed
   c. Type II diabetic over 60 years old
   d. Type I diabetic less than 60 years old

7. The plasma half-life of insulin injected intravenously is usually less than:
   a. 9 minutes
   b. 2 minutes
   c. 90 seconds
   d. 60 seconds

8. Late symptoms of hypoglycemia include:
   a. tachycardia
   b. hunger
   c. blurred vision
   d. headache

9. A medication which antagonizes the effect of insulin is:
   a. fenfluramine
   b. epinephrine
   c. alcohol
   d. acetohexamide

10. Which of the following hypoglycemia agents is best taken on an empty stomach:
    a. tolzamide
    b. glipizide
    c. chlorpropamide
    d. orinase

CHAPTER 45

1. The ratio of T_4 to T_3 is:
   a. 1:1
   b. 4:1
   c. 2:1
   d. 20:1

2. A function of the thyroid hormones (T_3 and T_4) is to:
   a. decelerate chemical reactions
   b. increase oxygen consumption
   c. impede heat production
   d. act as enzymes

3. The ratio between thyroid gland iodine and serum iodine (T/S ratio) is normally:
   a. 20:1
   b. 4:1
   c. 2:1
   d. 10:1

4. Thyrocalcitonin is released from the thyroid gland in response to:
   a. low serum phosphorus

b. low serum calcium
c. high serum calcium
d. high serum phosphorus

5. Parathormone acts on various organs to produce the following:
   a. increasing excretion of calcium
   b. reducing calcium absorption
   c. decreasing excretion of phosphorus
   d. enhancing bone resorption

6. The thyroid hormones:
   a. strenghten rate and force of cardiac contraction
   b. reduce protein synthesis
   c. regulate growth in the adult
   d. increase cholesterol concentration

7. Iodides are used as antithyroid drugs by:
   a. increasing the vascularity of the thyroid gland
   b. decreasing the quantity of bound thyroid
   c. inhibiting the release of T_3 and T_4 into circulation
   d. binding with TSH for thyroid inhibition

8. An action of the antithyroid medication propylthiouracil (PTU) is to:
   a. block TSH production
   b. reduce serum calcitonin levels
   c. inhibit peripheral conversion of T_4 to T_3
   d. block release of TRH

9. Vitamin D derivatives elevate serum calcium by:
   a. stimulating the kidney to reduce excretion
   b. inducing parathyroid hormone production
   c. stimulating calcium absorption in the intestine
   d. inducing the production of calcitonin by the thyroid

10. The most common side effects of antithyroid drugs are:
    a. nausea and vomiting
    b. pruritus and urticaria
    c. diarrhea and weakness
    d. tremor and restlessness

CHAPTER 46

1. "Normal flora," microorganisms inhibiting the internal and external surfaces of healthy human beings, are found in the:
   a. upper genitourinary tract
   b. lymphatic fluid
   c. liver
   d. skin

2. A factor to consider in selection of appropriate antibiotic therapy is:
   a. duration of infection
   b. status of the host's gastrointestinal functioning
   c. sensitivity of the organism to selected antibiotics
   d. presence of a secondary bacterial "super-infection"

3. Which of the following statements is *correct* regarding the absorption of various forms of penicillin?

a. Penicillin G has a highly stable absorption pattern following oral administration.

b. Ampicillin is well absorbed following oral ingestion.

c. Intramuscular injections of procaine penicillin G last up to 26 days.

d. Penicillin G benzathine is rapidly absorbed, providing short-acting effect.

4. An antimicrobial agent for which no reduction in dosage is necessary for patients with renal insufficiency is:
   a. gentamycin
   b. clindamycin
   c. penicillin
   d. tobramycin

5. The addition of clavulanic acid to selected broad-spectrum penicillins has the following effect:
   a. beta-lactamase inhibition
   b. inhibition of plasmid transfer
   c. enhancement of bacterial cell wall destruction
   d. prolongation of penicillin half-life

6. The spectrum of antibiotic activity of aztreonam includes:
   a. fungal microorganisms
   b. aerobic gram-positive cocci
   c. aerobic gram-negative rods
   d. anaerobic microorganisms

7. The action of cilastatin, which is given with imipenem in the form of Primaxin, is to:
   a. inhibit the growth of anaerobic organisms
   b. inhibit dihydropeptidase enzymes
   c. interfere with the action of penicillinase
   d. augment the action of imipenem

8. Sulfonamides act to suppress bacterial growth by:
   a. interfering with folic acid synthesis
   b. inhibiting cell wall structure
   c. translocating the DNA structure
   d. inhibiting beta-lactamase

9. Which of the following statements is *correct* regarding erythromycin drug interactions?
   a. Subtherapeutic digoxin levels may occur with erythromycin.
   b. Erythromycin enhances phenytoin activity.
   c. Corticosteroids enhance erythromycin activity.
   d. Erythromycin inhibits the metabolism of theophylline.

10. The most notable side effect of clindamycin is:
    a. hearing loss
    b. nausea
    c. diarrhea
    d. rash

CHAPTER 47

1. The prostaglandins have a diversity of action which includes:
   a. vasoconstriction

b. decreased cardiac output

c. increased capillary permeability

d. platelet aggregation

2. Prostaglandins have the following effect on the stomach lining:
   a. stimulation of gastric secretions
   b. inhibition of mucous production
   c. histamine release
   d. stabilization of gastric mucosa

3. Misoprostol (Cytotec) is contraindicated in the following patient condition:
   a. pregnancy
   b. gastric ulcers
   c. glaucoma
   d. diabetes mellitus

4. Short-term anti-inflammatory medications are used for:
   a. one to two months only
   b. a temporary cure
   c. pain relief
   d. minimal side effects

5. Which statement is *correct* regarding substances that play a role in inflammation?
   a. Bradykinins cause profound vasoconstriction.
   b. Histamines encourage migration of phagocytic cells.
   c. Protease builds up collagenous connective tissue.
   d. Hydrolases cause bronchospasm in the lung.

6. Salicylates are thought to relieve arthritic pain by:
   a. enhancing platelet aggregation
   b. releasing neurological blockers
   c. stimulating bradykinin synthesis
   d. inhibiting prostaglandin synthesis

7. The nonsteroid anti-inflammatory drugs:
   a. are administered cautiously to patients with renal disease
   b. do not cross the placental barrier and are safe for pregnant women
   c. are used as a substitute for patients allergic to aspirin
   d. are slowly absorbed from the gastrointestinal tract

8. Nonsteroid anti-inflammatory drugs which are used for short-term therapy only include:
   a. piroxicam
   b. fenoprofen
   c. phenylbutazone
   d. ibuprofen

9. While the exact mechanism of action is not known for D-penicillamine (Cuprimine), it is effectively used to treat:
   a. gouty arthritis
   b. rheumatoid arthritis
   c. gastric ulcers
   d. resistant acne vulgaris

10. An adverse side effect of meclofenamate sodium (Meclomen) is:
    a. diarrhea
    b. hair loss
    c. peripheral neuritis
    d. crysiasis

CHAPTER 48

1. In comparing malignant and benign neoplasms, malignant neoplasms are characterized by:
   a. slow, controlled growth
   b. new growth
   c. encapsulation
   d. ability to metastasize

2. During the S phase of cell division, the following activities take place:
   a. resting state
   b. DNA synthesis
   c. specialized protein synthesis
   d. cell mitosis

3. According to the Stem Cell Theory:
   a. all of the cells in a primary tumor are thought to be of clonal origin
   b. the stem cell population has limited ability to reproduce
   c. all members of a stem cell population are involved in cell division at the same time
   d. the primary tumor arises from a clonogenic population

4. The first chemotherapeutic agent, found in 1919, was:
   a. nitrogen mustard
   b. hydroxyurea
   c. dacarbazine
   d. adriamycin

5. Which of the following statements is *correct* regarding adjuvant chemotherapy?
   a. This treatment manages primary tumor growth.
   b. It is the use of agents to destroy micrometastasis.
   c. This group of agents is used to treat overt metastasis.
   d. It is the use of drugs to stimulate viral oncogenes.

6. Cell cycle-specific agents affect the cell during:
   a. the entire cell cycle
   b. mitotic division only
   c. one phase of the cell cycle
   d. resting phase only

7. An example of a cell cycle-nonspecific chemotherapeutic agent is:
   a. cisplatin
   b. bleomycin
   c. vincristine
   d. fluoracil

8. Historically, chemotherapy was used as:
   a. primary treatment for malignant disease
   b. specific agents for particular primary tumors
   c. treatment of hematologic and metastatic tumors
   d. management of side effects of tumor growth

9. Which of the following statements is *true* regarding the history of antineoplastic agents?
   a. The use of chemotherapy dates back to the Egyptians' use of opium.
   b. The first antimetabolic agents were introduced in the 1970s.
   c. The drug Mustargen was first given to patients in 1942.
   d. Introduction of the antibiotics occurred during the 1930s.

10. Cytotoxic drugs are generally more effective:
    a. against resting cells
    b. when tumor burden is high
    c. when there is greater organ impairment
    d. against dividing cells

CHAPTER 49

1. Which of the following is the most accurate means of dose calculation for chemotherapeutic agents?
   a. body surface area
   b. body weight
   c. age
   d. total body fat

2. Guidelines for the preparation of chemotherapeutic agents include utilizing:
   a. patient care units for mixing agents
   b. oral pipetting of certain agents only
   c. disposal of waste in the standard manner
   d. face mask and protective clothing for the preparer

3. In general, alkalizing agents act by:
   a. substituting an enzyme in protein metabolism
   b. inactivating the cell replication process
   c. forming electrophilic bonds in the cytosine of DNA
   d. affecting cells in the GO (resting) phase

4. The alkylating agent cyclophosphamide (Cytoxan):
   a. requires a one-step metabolic activation
   b. crosses the blood-brain barrier
   c. increases activity when given with corticosteroids
   d. acts on both normal and abnormal cells

5. Which of the following agents would be most useful against primary brain tumors?
   a. melphalan
   b. cyclophosphamide
   c. carmustine
   d. cisplatin

6. As a group, the antimetabolites act as antineoplastic agents by:
   a. interfering with the pathways of dividing cells
   b. exerting the greatest effect on GI phase

c. cross-linking RNA replication
d. producing toxic coenzymes

7. The toxic effects of methotrexate on normal cells can be reduced by the administration of:
   a. levorphanol
   b. cytarabine
   c. leucovorin
   d. allopurinol

8. Antineoplastic agents which act by inhibiting pyrimidine synthesis include:
   a. hydroxyurea
   b. thioguanine
   c. cisplatin
   d. fluorouracil

9. For patients on thioguanine therapy, it will be important to monitor the following level:
   a. calcium
   b. uric acid
   c. sodium
   d. potassium

10. The following is *correct* with regard to the vina alkaloids:
    a. cell cycle-nonspecific
    b. derivative of the periwinkle plant
    c. similar in antitumor spectrum
    d. effective in oral doses

CHAPTER 50

1. T-cells play the following role in the immune response:
   a. producing antibody-like proteins
   b. assisting B-cells in antibody synthesis
   c. producing specific antibodies
   d. inhibiting the humoral response

2. In humans, B-cells mature in the:
   a. immature thymus gland
   b. liver and pancreas
   c. epiphysis of long bones
   d. Peyer's patches in the intestines

3. One method by which tumor cells escape detection by the host organism is by:
   a. stimulating a strong host immune response
   b. initiating an early host response
   c. blocking factors which cover the antigenic sites on cancer cells
   d. mechanical obstruction of tumor cells by area leukocytes

4. Passive nonspecific immunotherapy occurs when:
   a. serum from healthy individuals is injected into cancer patients
   b. serum from patients in remission is injected into patients with active disease
   c. immunosuppressive substances from cancer patients are removed
   d. live immunocompetent lymphocytes are transferred to cancer patients

5. Host defenses play a role in retarding tumor growth, spread, or recovery from disease as evidenced by the following example:
   a. Spontaneous tumor regression occurs in patients with large tumor burdens.
   b. Cancers heavily infiltrated by lymphocytes have a better prognosis.
   c. Weak cell-mediated immune response to chemotherapy shows a better prognosis.
   d. Appearance of metastatic disease occurs in all patients in 15 to 30 years.

6. The function of lymphokines is to activate:
   a. tumor-specific antibodies
   b. B-cells
   c. macrophages
   d. killer T-cells

7. A goal of cancer immunotherapy is to:
   a. produce remission as a single agent in cancer therapy
   b. promote tumor-nonspecific immunity
   c. stimulate immunocompetence in cancer patients
   d. bypass side effects of traditional chemotherapy

8. Immunorestorative immunotherapy is utilized to:
   a. replace the patient's immune system
   b. augment the patient's immune response
   c. bypass the patient's effector cell response
   d. prevent overstimulation of the immune response

9. When preparing a BCG injection, the following precaution must be taken:
   a. Prepare skin well with alcohol prep.
   b. Protect the vaccine from light when stored.
   c. Use any diluent for reconstitution.
   d. Store in a dry warm area after reconstitution.

10. Adverse effects of interferon therapy include:
    a. flu-like symptoms
    b. seizures
    c. peripheral neuritis
    d. alopecia

CHAPTER 51

1. The pyloric glands produce:
   a. mucus
   b. ptyalin
   c. hydrochloric acid
   d. pepsin

2. The hormone which regulates the rate of gastric emptying is:
   a. gastrin
   b. pepsinogin
   c. enterogastrone
   d. trypsin

3. Which statement is *correct* concerning the gastrointestinal system?
   a. The esophagus is 2.5 cm long.
   b. The ileum is part of the large intestine.

c. The large intestine is approximately 1.5 meters long.

d. The duodenum is considered a part of the stomach.

4. The primary function of villikinin is to:
   a. allow the villi to absorb more nutrients
   b. stimulate peristaltic activity in the large intestine
   c. inhibit the entrance of chyme into the small intestine
   d. stimulate the production of mucus from the villi

5. Approximately 2000 ml of aklaline secretions are secreted daily by:
   a. Brunner's glands
   b. goblet cells
   c. oxyntic cells
   d. crypts of Lieberkuhn

6. Digestion within the small intestine is dependent on:
   a. peptidases for splitting neutral fats into fatty acids
   b. lipase for splitting peptides into amino acids
   c. lactase for splitting starch into disaccharides
   d. bacteria for splitting food by-products

7. Which statement is *correct* concerning nervous system control of the alimentary canal?
   a. The parasympathetic nervous system decreases gastric secretion.
   b. The sympathetic nervous system slows or stops GI tract function.
   c. The parasympathetic nervous system decreases intestinal motility.
   d. The sympathetic nervous system increases intestinal mucus production.

8. The liver performs the following functions *except:*
   a. producing bile from old defective red blood cells
   b. playing a role in carbohydrate, fat, and protein metabolism
   c. synthesizing Vitamins A, D, and B_{12}
   d. synthesizing cholesterol and clotting factors

9. As an endocrine gland, the pancreas secretes:
   a. trypsin inhibitor
   b. sodium bicarbonate
   c. glucagon
   d. chymotrypsin

10. The primary role of cytochrome P-450, released by the liver, is to:
    a. stimulate steroid release as a stress response
    b. deactivate and detoxify medications and other substances
    c. produce fibrinogen, prothrombin, and factor V
    d. deaminate amino acids, forming urea

CHAPTER 52

1. As a group, antacids act by:
   a. reducing gastric acid secretions
   b. absorbing gastric acid

   c. stimulating an alkaline secretion
   d. raising the gastric pH

2. Sodium bicarbonate and calcium bicarbonate may be responsible for the development of milk-alkali syndrome, characterized by:
   a. hypocalcemia
   b. acidosis
   c. hypokalemia
   d. hypercalcemia

3. Anticholinergics, when administered with other agents:
   a. relieve pain by inhibiting motility and secretions
   b. stimulate the release of acetylcholine at neuroeffector sites
   c. stimulate gastric cells to produce pepsin and mucus
   d. are indicated in the treatment of gastric ulcers

4. Which of the following statements is *correct* regarding antacids and drug interactions?
   a. Antacids increase the absorption of digitalis products.
   b. Antacids decrease the absorption of tetracycline antibiotics.
   c. Aluminum products enhance the absorption of propranolol.
   d. Magnesium products increase the absorption of the phenothiazine.

5. When caring for a patient receiving an anticholinergic drug, a nursing action would be to:
   a. administer the drug with means to enhance effectiveness
   b. observe the patient for symptoms of urinary retention
   c. encourage the patient to avoid excessive heat
   d. prepare parenteral medications at least four hours before administering

6. The belladonna alkaloids, such as belladonna and atropine, have the following characteristic:
   a. are slowly absorbed from the gastrointestinal tract
   b. readily cross the blood-brain barrier
   c. depress the central nervous system in large doses
   d. stimulate the central nervous system in toxic doses

7. Prolonged use of aluminum-containing antacids may cause hypophosphatemia, characterized by:
   a. increased appetite
   b. muscle weakness
   c. irritability
   d. muscle rigidity

8. In addition to their neutralizing ability, aluminum antacids have the following action:
   a. stimulation of peristalsis
   b. increased gastric muscle tone
   c. delayed gastric emptying
   d. reduced number of parietal cells

9. The Acid Neutralizing Capacity (ANC) is defined as the:

a. mEq of HCL required to keep an antacid suspension at a pH of 3.0 for 2 hours
b. ability of the antacid to change the gastric pH to 5.0 and maintain for 2 hours
c. mEq of HCL absorbed by an antacid within a 24-hour period in vitro
d. amount of antacid required to neutralize 10 mEq of HCL to a pH of 4.0

CHAPTER 53

1. As a group of drugs, antiemetics:
   a. are best administered after vomiting occurs
   b. act either locally or centrally
   c. treat rather than prevent vomiting
   d. cause local irritation of gastric mucosa

2. An extrapyramidal side effect which may occur with administration of high doses of phenothiazine drugs is:
   a. spasms of the tongue, face, neck, and back
   b. drowsiness
   c. nasal congestion
   d. rebound hypertension

3. Which of the following statements correctly describes scopolamine hydrobromide (Hyoscine)?
   a. It has a long duration of action.
   b. The drug is most effective for postoperative nausea.
   c. The drug can be used to treat urinary obstruction.
   d. It produces blurred vision and a dry mouth.

4. Antihistamines produce an antiemetic effect by:
   a. enhancing the chemoreceptor trigger zone
   b. stimulating the vestibular portion of the eighth cranial nerve
   c. inhibiting local gastric irritation and secretions
   d. reducing stimulation on the vomiting center

5. An example of an antidopaminergic antiemetic is:
   a. diphenhydramine (Benadryl)
   b. benzquinamide (Emete-Con)
   c. promethazine (Phenergan)
   d. cyclizine (Marezine)

6. Side effects related to phenothiazine use include akathisia, which is characterized by:
   a. expressionless face
   b. hysterical reaction seizures
   c. a need to be in constant motion
   d. forgetfulness about current events

7. A nursing implication associated with the use of the Transderm-Scop system is:
   a. Apply the patch indefinitely for control of nausea.
   b. Place patch on the chest wall for best results.
   c. Apply after the antiemetic effect is needed.
   d. Teach about the side effect of drowsiness.

8. In general, antiemetics are contraindicated in the following patient situation:
   a. glaucoma
   b. pregnancy

   c. gastric ulcers
   d. metastatic cancer

9. An example of a cannabinoid antiemetic is:
   a. dronabinol (Marinol)
   b. fluphenazine (Protixin)
   c. diphenidol (Vontrol)
   d. dimenhydrinate (Dramamine)

CHAPTER 54

1. The pancreatic replacement enzyme pancrelipase (Cotazym) is utilized in the following patient situation:
   a. pernicious anemia
   b. post gallbladder surgery
   c. cystic fibrosis
   d. hypochlorhydria

2. A nursing intervention associated with the administration of antidiarrheal absorbents is to:
   a. hold other medications for 2 hours after administration
   b. give absorbents at least 3 times daily for soothing effect
   c. discontinue if a fruity odor is apparent in the stool
   d. administer absorbents sparingly due to risk of addiction

3. Which of the following statements is correct regarding diphenoxylate hydrochloride (Lomotil)?
   a. It should be given to patients with infectious diarrhea.
   b. The drug is used to control antibiotic-induced pseudo-membranous colitis.
   c. Lomotil is classified as a class III drug.
   d. It contains atropine, causing dry mouth and blurred vision.

4. The primary agent in paregoric tincture which acts as an antidiarrheal is:
   a. meperidine
   b. atropine
   c. morphine
   d. belladonna

5. The intestinal flora modifiers such as lactobacillus acidophilus (Lactinex) have the following action:
   a. destroy diarrhea-producing bacteria in the gut
   b. encourage the growth of normal intestinal flora
   c. build a protective layer of mucus along the gut wall
   d. replace antibiotics in treating certain causes of diarrhea

6. The belladonna preparation Donnagel is contraindicated in the following condition:
   a. diabetes mellitus
   b. Parkinson's disease
   c. peptic ulcer disease
   d. narrow-angle glaucoma

7. Which of the following statements regarding castor oil is correct?
   a. It stimulates gastric emptying.

b. This laxative inhibits water reabsorption from the intestinal lumen.

c. Castor oil should be taken with meals for a cathartic effect.

d. It is the drug of choice for patients with ulcerative colitis.

8. Patients taking cascara sagrada with milk of magnesia should be alert to the following side effect:
   a. foul smelling urine
   b. fruity odor to the breath
   c. oily skin
   d. reddish or yellow-brown urine

9. Which of the following agents stimulates Auerbach's Plexus to induce persitalsis?
   a. senna
   b. calcium polycarbophil
   c. loperamide
   d. docusate calcium

CHAPTER 55

1. The antidotal therapy for acetaminophen overdose is:
   a. naloxone (Narcan)
   b. protamine sulfate
   c. Vitamin K
   d. N-acetylcysteine (Mucomyst)

2. Which of the following drugs is an aldosterone antagonist, useful in the management of ascites?
   a. spironolactone (Aldactone)
   b. furosemide (Lasix)
   c. acetazolamide (Diamox)
   d. ethacrynic acid (Edecrin)

3. Symptoms related to Phase I of hepatic encephalopathy include:
   a. coma and asterixis
   b. stupor and abnormal sleep pattern
   c. agitation and personality change
   d. lethargy and asterixis

4. A side effect of Heptovax B (hepatitis B vaccine) is:
   a. pain and soreness at injection site
   b. fever that may reach 103°F
   c. bleeding tendency
   d. generalized pruritus

5. Which of the following agents improves protein tolerance in patients with advanced heptatic cirrhosis?
   a. Vitamin K
   b. furosemide (Lasix)
   c. lactulose (Cephulac)
   d. folic acid

CHAPTER 56

1. Which of the following statements is *correct* regarding the process of metabolism?
   a. Anabolism is the breaking down of complex cellular materials.
   b. Catabolism is the synthesis of cellular materials for growth.
   c. If food intake exceeds metabolic demands, anabolism occurs.
   d. If food intake is less than metabolic demands, weight is gained.

2. The hormone which favors catabolism is:
   a. insulin
   b. epinephrine
   c. growth hormone
   d. testosterone

3. When nutrients are not supplied to the body in adequate amounts, the following process occurs:
   a. Glycogen stores are used last as the liver acts to increase blood glucose.
   b. Fats are broken down to form fatty acids and ketone bodies.
   c. Visceral proteins are the major substrate for protein anabolism.
   d. As urinary nitrogen increases, a positive nitrogen balance develops.

4. The milk-based meal replacement formulas are:
   a. used in patients with an intact digestive system
   b. low in protein and high in carbohydrate
   c. nutritionally incomplete but high in minerals
   d. used in patients with lactose intolerance

5. A general principle concerning the administration of commercial feeding formulas is that:
   a. hypo-osmolar formulas have a tendency to cause diarrhea
   b. protein content is 50 percent of the total calories
   c. fats increase calories without increasing osmolarity
   d. most formulas provide 10 calories per ml when mixed full strength

6. Parenteral fat emulsions (PFE) are contraindicated in patients with:
   a. peptic ulcer disease
   b. acute renal failure
   c. muscle wasting disease
   d. acute pancreatitis

7. During initial administration of a lipid emulsion, the nurse performs the following intervention:
   a. administers the emulsion at 10 ml/minute for first 30 minutes
   b. observes for signs of an allergic reaction
   c. uses an in-line filter for IV administration
   d. observes for tissue necrosis at administration site

8. When assessing the patient receiving enteral or parenteral feedings, the nurse is aware that:
   a. thirst may be a sign of dehydration from hyperosmolar enteral feedings
   b. light, flaky, reddened skin may indicate impending hyperosmolar shock
   c. patients with food allergies can tolerate enteral feedings without reactions
   d. hyperosmolar-induced edema occurs as a result of fluid overload

9. A possible cause of respiratory distress during administration of continuous tube feeding is:
   a. the feeding tube may be in the duodenum
   b. the patient is allergic to the tube feeding formula
   c. a distended stomach interferes with diaphragmatic excursion
   d. a small bore feeding tube may impede ventilations

10. A nursing intervention for patients receiving central TPN would be to:
   a. initiate the solution slowly at a rate of 40 ml/hour
   b. change the TPN solution every 48 hours
   c. change the TPN IV tubing every 48 hours
   d. hang Ringer's lactate if TPN is interrupted

CHAPTER 57

1. Which of the following minerals is considered to be a macro element (bulk essential)?
   a. iron
   b. zinc
   c. calcium
   d. fluorine

2. A mineral has the following characteristics:
   a. All are electropositive.
   b. All are organic and non-essential.
   c. They are carried by hormones.
   d. They act on target organs.

3. An example of a fat soluble vitamin is:
   a. biotin
   b. niacin
   c. Vitamin K
   d. Vitamin B12

4. Toxic side effects of Vitamin A include:
   a. insomnia
   b. alopecia
   c. tetany
   d. decreased intracranial pressure

5. Vitamin D is used in the treatment of:
   a. hypercalcemia
   b. hypocalcemia
   c. hyperparathyroidism
   d. hypomagnesemia

6. A role of Vitamin E in the maintenance of a healthy state includes:
   a. inhibition of hemolysis of red blood cells
   b. enhances Vitamin K utilization
   c. stimulates prostaglandin production
   d. inhibits steroid metabolism

7. The proper rate for intravenous administration of phytonadione (Aquamephyton) is:
   a. 15 mg/10 minutes
   b. 5 mg/1 minute
   c. 1 mg/minute
   d. 10 mg/2 minutes

8. Which of the following groups of patients are most likely to develop thiamine deficiency?
   a. newborns
   b. teenagers
   c. pregnant women
   d. alcoholics

9. Which of the following statemtents is *correct* regarding drug interactions with Vitamin B6 (pyridoxine)?
   a. B6 enhances the peripheral metabolism of levodopa.
   b. B6 inhibits hepatic metabolism of phenobarbital.
   c. Isoniazid decreases the urinary excretion of B6.
   d. Penicillamine decreases the urinary excretion of B6.

10. Which of the following drugs is associated with elevated copper levels?
   a. nitroglycerin agents
   b. estrogens
   c. prostaglandins
   d. antibiotics

CHAPTER 58

1. Sodium (Na^+) acts in the body to:
   a. inhibit electrical impulses within the cell
   b. maintain serum osmolarity
   c. maintain muscle contraction
   d. regulate intracellular osmolality

2. Administration of potassium is contraindicated for patients taking the following medication:
   a. aspirin
   b. spironolactone
   c. lithium
   d. tetracycline

3. A sign or symptom of hypokalemia is:
   a. muscle weakness
   b. increased reflexes
   c. loud heart sounds
   d. ST elevation on the ECG

4. A nursing intervention associated with administration of sodium polystyrene sulfonate (Kayexalate) is to:
   a. observe the patient for hyponatremia
   b. allow suspension to separate; do not stir
   c. urge patient to retain rectally for 30 to 60 minutes
   d. mix powder with an oil base solution

5. When administering intravenous or oral calcium products, the nurse will monitor the patient for hypercalcemia. A sign of this would be:
   a. tetany
   b. Trousseau's sign
   c. Chvostek's sign
   d. lethargy

6. Intravenous magnesium administration is contraindicated in the following patient situation:
   a. heart block
   b. ventricular tachycardia
   c. pregnancy
   d. constipation

7. In an acidotic state, the following serum electrolyte level occurs:
   a. hypomagnesemia
   b. decreased calcium
   c. decreased potassium
   d. increased calcium

8. Patients taking oral calcium should be taught to:
   a. decrease intake of phosphate-containing foods
   b. take calcium chloride with meals
   c. avoid taking calcium with tetracycline antibiotics
   d. increase intake of spinach, rhubarb, and bran

9. An important action associated with phosphate (HPO_4^-) is:
   a. stabilization of neuromuscular function
   b. regulation of acid-base balance through chloride shift
   c. maintenance of resting membrane potential
   d. promotion of white blood cells' phagocytic action

10. A patient with an electrolyte imbalance demonstrates a high peaked T wave on the ECG. Which electrolyte imbalance does this sign indicate?
    a. hyperkalemia
    b. hyponatremia
    c. hypophosphatemia
    d. hypermagnesemia

CHAPTER 59

1. A structure of the middle layer of the eye is the:
   a. ciliary body
   b. cornea
   c. sclera
   d. retina

2. The inner layer of the eye is composed of:
   a. a diaphragm with a circular opening
   b. muscles which increase visual acuity of the eye
   c. nerve cells that translate light waves to neural impulses
   d. a thick, opaque posterior covering which adjusts to light

3. Which of the following statements is *correct* regarding the fovea centralis?
   a. It contains rods which allow for color vision.
   b. Cones are densely concentrated in the fovea.
   c. The fovea is the area of the eye which adjusts to dim light.
   d. The fovea is composed of nerve cells which are motion detectors.

4. The refractory mechanism occurs through which *correct* sequence to focus light rays on the retina?
   a. lens, cornea, vitreous humor, aqueous humor
   b. aqueous humor, cornea, vitreous humor, lens
   c. cornea, aqueous humor, lens, vitreous humor
   d. cornea, vitreous humor, lens, aqueous humor

5. In myopia, the image focuses:
   a. on the peripheral portion of the retina
   b. in front of the retina
   c. at a point behind the retina
   d. on the macula area of the retina

6. Which of the following statements correctly describes the accommodation reflex?
   a. It protects the cornea from damage by turning the eye upward when forcibly opened.
   b. Accommodation causes the pupil to become smaller when light is flashed into the eye.
   c. Accommodation allows the eyes to move together to focus on a point to the lateral side.
   d. It allows the pupil to become smaller as the gaze shifts from a close to a distant object.

7. The vestibule is a portion of the:
   a. ossicles of the ear
   b. outer ear
   c. middle ear
   d. inner ear

8. Hearing impulses originate in the:
   a. malleus
   b. organ of Corti
   c. semicircular canals
   d. incus

9. The function of the external ear is to:
   a. separate the middle and inner ear
   b. merge with the inner ear
   c. funnel sound through the auditory canal
   d. convert sound waves into vibrations

10. Normal intraocular pressure is:
    a. 12 to 25 mmHg
    b. 50 to 60 mmHg
    c. 2 to 10 mmHg
    d. 30 to 46 mmHg

CHAPTER 60

1. Fluorescein sodium can be used in the eye to:
   a. fit soft contacts
   b. test lacrimal patency
   c. remove foreign bodies from the eye
   d. stain the eye for 60 minutes

2. The antiviral medication idoxuridine (IDU) is administered:
   a. for 5 to 7 days after healing has occurred
   b. concurrently with boric acid solution
   c. in a liquid form only
   d. systemically to treat herpes simplex virus

3. Anti-inflammatory eye medications, such as dexamethasone, are used primarily for:
   a. treatment of fungal infections
   b. management of acute infections
   c. long-term treatment of glaucoma
   d. reduction of permanent scarring

4. The direct-acting cholinergic miotics reduce intraocular pressure by:
   a. relaxing the sphincter muscle of the iris
   b. inhibiting ciliary muscle spasm

c. reducing production of aqueous humor

d. decreasing resistance to outflow of aqueous humor

5. When teaching the patient about insertion of Ocusert (pilocarpine), the following information will be included:
   a. Insert early in the morning initially.
   b. Gently rinse with tap water prior to insertion.
   c. Continue using eye insert if irritation occurs.
   d. Leave insert in place for 14 days.

6. Which of the following agents are cholinesterase inhibitors used to treat open-angle glaucoma?
   a. methazolamide (Neptazane)
   b. carbachol (Isopto Carbachol)
   c. physostigmine (Eserine)
   d. betaxolol (Betoptic)

7. Caution is advised when administering beta-adrenergic blockers, such as timolol maleate (Timoptic), with the following medication:
   a. potassium chloride
   b. digoxin
   c. aspirin
   d. iodine

8. Acetazolamide (Diamox) is used to treat glaucomas due to which of the following actions?
   a. production of systemic alkalosis
   b. interference with production of carbonic acid
   c. production of osmotic diuresis
   d. direct contraction of ciliary muscles

9. Alpha adrenergic ophthalmic agents have the following effect on the eye:
   a. contraction of the constrictor muscle of the iris
   b. complete relaxation of the ciliary muscle
   c. contraction of the dilator muscle of the iris
   d. inhibition of parasympathetic effects on the pupil

10. Osmotic diuretics used to treat eye disorders are used cautiously in the following patient condition:
    a. peptic ulcer disease
    b. increased intracranial pressure
    c. open-angle glaucoma
    d. congestive heart failure

CHAPTER 61

1. A solution which can be used to irrigate the ears is:
   a. 10 percent acetic acid
   b. full strength hydrogen peroxide
   c. 50 percent ethyl alcohol
   d. Burow's solution

2. Which of the following is considered a first line drug for treating otitis media?
   a. cefaclor
   b. ampicillin
   c. erythromycin
   d. Bactrim

3. Antihistamine-decongestant products are utilized along with antibiotics to treat acute otitis media. They work by:
   a. improving eustachian tube patency
   b. resolving infectious process
   c. direct dilation of auditory canal
   d. stimulating ciliary movement in the middle ear

4. When performing a nursing assessment on the patient requiring ear medications, the nurse is aware that:
   a. over-the-counter medications are free of ototoxic effects
   b. patients with renal dysfunction are less prone to ototoxicity
   c. aminoglycoside antibiotics may damage the eighth cranial nerve
   d. vestibular damage causes loss of high-frequency sound perception

5. The agent of choice for patients with otitis media resulting from *Hemophilus influenzae* is:
   a. Novafed
   b. penicillin V
   c. ampicillin
   d. penicillin G

CHAPTER 62

1. As a class of drugs, enzymes are:
   a. given intravenously to aid digestion
   b. synthesized proteins from plants or animals
   c. known to be immunologically neutral
   d. altered by the reactions which they mediate

2. Which of the following statements is *correct* regarding sutilains (Travase) therapy?
   a. This enzyme is active on viable tissue.
   b. Airtight, dry dressings are applied after sutilains.
   c. The skin pH should be kept at a range of 6.0 to 6.8.
   d. The medication is discontinued if no improvement in 7 days.

3. In order to prepare the skin for sutilains (Travase) therapy, the following should be used:
   a. soap and water
   b. isotonic saline
   c. hexachlorophene
   d. iodine

4. Prior to administration of fibrinolysin and desoxyribonuclease (Elase), the nurse will assess for the following allergy:
   a. papaya
   b. iodine
   c. pork
   d. beef

5. The nurse will include the following information when teaching the patient about enzyme replacement therapy:
   a. Enteric-coated tablets are to be chewed, then followed by water.

b. Mild stinging may occur when tablets are absorbed bucally.

c. Bowel movements should increase while on digestive enzymes.

d. Store enzyme tablets in the refrigerator.

CHAPTER 63

1. In addition to blood vessels and nerves, the dermis layer of the skin contains:
   a. collagen and elastin
   b. keratinized tissue and keratohyalin granules
   c. keratinocytes and prickle cells
   d. adipose and loose connective tissue

2. Which of the following is *correct* regarding emollients?
   a. The suspension requires shaking before application.
   b. They have a drying effect on the skin when the water evaporates.
   c. Emollients have fixed oils as a base preparation.
   d. They are predominantly water in base.

3. A common side effect of acyclovir (Zovirax) is:
   a. photosensitivity
   b. hives
   c. mild pain
   d. pigment changes

4. When corticosteroids are used on the skin, they have the following action:
   a. fibrinolytic
   b. vasoconstriction
   c. vasodilation
   d. proteolytic

5. The following information should be included for patients treated with dermatologic agents:
   a. A thick film of medication is applied over dry areas.
   b. Do not use soap and water on affected skin.
   c. A large amount of medication is applied to moist areas.
   d. Any scales or crusts are removed before applying the medication.

6. When evaluating the effectiveness of skin medications, the following is important:
   a. Acute skin lesions should subside in 3 to 4 days.
   b. Skin lesions are often slow to improve and require frequent evaluation.
   c. Noncompliance is a problem due to ineffectiveness of treatment.
   d. Lesions which do not show improvement in 24 hours need to be evaluated.

7. When a patient who is receiving medications for a skin disorder develops a reaction, the nurse will plan to:
   a. discontinue medications one at a time
   b. obtain a complete medication history
   c. assume the rash is due to the current medication(s)

d. continue all medications and document all nursing care

CHAPTER 64

1. An advantage of passive immunity is that it:
   a. stimulates the body to produce antibodies
   b. provides immediate protection
   c. persists for an extended period
   d. treats diseases effectively

2. An example of a toxoid vaccine is:
   a. polio
   b. smallpox
   c. diphtheria
   d. hepatitis A

3. Children should not receive the attenuated measles vaccine before 15 months because:
   a. maternal antibodies destroy the attenuated virus before antibody production occurs
   b. the child's immune system is too young to respond with antibody production
   c. the attenuated virus is too strong and will produce an active form of the disease
   d. antibodies which are produced by a child less than 15 months are immature

4. Before administration of measles vaccine, the nurse should assess for an allergy to:
   a. iodine
   b. yeast
   c. penicillin
   d. neomycin

5. A nursing intervention associated with immunizations is to:
   a. teach patients that unusual side effects are to be expected
   b. mix vaccines at least 6 hours before administration
   c. change the needle before injecting the vaccine
   d. keep vaccines in a dry warm place for storage

6. The pathological organism responsible for chickenpox is:
   a. poliovirus III
   b. varicella-zoster
   c. *Bordetella*
   d. *Mycobacterium*

7. What is the time required for development of active immunity in response to a vaccine?
   a. 6 months
   b. 6 hours
   c. 5 to 14 days
   d. 25 to 75 days

8. The recommended time for *Hemophilus influenza* vaccine (Hib) is at:
   a. 18 to 24 months
   b. 4 to 6 years
   c. 3 years
   d. 8 to 12 months

9. Drug interactions associated with the Bacillus Calmette-Guerin (BCG) vaccine include:
   a. Immunosuppressive drugs enhance BCG response.
   b. BCG may inactivate aminoglycosides.
   c. Active TB treatment drugs inactivate BCG.
   d. BCG facilitates theophylline excretion.

CHAPTER 65

1. A nursing action for drug therapy in the acute care setting is to:
   a. administer drugs intramuscularly if the patient is hypotensive
   b. administer drugs intravenously to patients with severe cardiac failure
   c. monitor cholesterol levels because many acidic drugs are bound to fat
   d. give drugs such as protamine sulfate over 2 minutes intravenously

2. Drugs which may be given endotracheally in an emergency situation include:
   a. epinephrine
   b. bretylium
   c. sodium bicarbonate
   d. dopamine

3. Which of the following emergency drugs is contraindicated in congestive heart failure?
   a. beta blockers
   b. cardiac glycosides
   c. diuretics
   d. vasodilators

4. Patients in pulmonary edema will demonstrate the following sign/symptom:
   a. thick, yellow sputum
   b. abdominal pain
   c. severe dyspnea
   d. poor skin turgor

5. The following agent may be ordered for the patient in cardiogenic shock:
   a. propranolol
   b. dobutamine
   c. atropine
   d. sodium bicarbonate

6. The drug of choice for the patient exhibiting status epilepticus is:
   a. diazepam
   b. epinephrine
   c. propranolol
   d. furosemide

7. The patient with elevated T_3, T_4, and T_7 values with symptoms such as fever, tachycardia, tremor, and restlessness should receive the following agent:
   a. diazepam
   b. phenobarbital
   c. propylthiouracil
   d. paraldehyde

8. In an emergency situation, the nurse's first priority is to:
   a. maintain a patent airway
   b. take blood pressure and pulse
   c. assist with placement of a central line
   d. assess orientation

9. A nursing assessment finding in the patient experiencing acute adrenal insufficiency is:
   a. hypertension
   b. Kussmaul respirations
   c. pink frothy sputum
   d. dehydration

10. The drug of choice in the event of cholinergic crisis is:
    a. lidocaine
    b. epinephrine
    c. atropine
    d. digitalis

CHAPTER 66

1. A nursing intervention associated with administration of dimercaprol (Bal in Oil) is to:
   a. maintain patient in supine position
   b. keep patient awake
   c. avoid excessive hydration
   d. maintain urine alkalinization

2. The use of sclerosing agents such as sodium tetradecyl sulfate (Sotradecol) and morrhuate sodium is contraindicated in patients with:
   a. hyperparathyroidism
   b. asthma
   c. myasthenia gravis
   d. G-6PD deficiency

3. Patient teaching related to nicotine gum (Nicorette) includes the following information:
   a. Continue Nicorette gum for 6 months before tapering.
   b. Smoking cigarettes along with Nicorette is allowed in the first week.
   c. Chew gum slowly and intermittently for 30 minutes.
   d. Chew each piece of gum for 2 hours before discarding.

4. Side effects which are related to therapy with Antihemophilic A factor include:
   a. increased salivation and abdominal pain
   b. chest tightness and wheezing
   c. lymphadenopathy and alopecia
   d. nausea and constipation

5. A nursing intervention which should be planned for patients using minoxidil is to:
   a. wash scalp with strong soap
   b. discontinue if no results in one month
   c. restrict oral fluids
   d. assess blood pressure regularly

ANSWERS, RATIONALES, AND CODES FOR REVIEW QUESTIONS

CHAPTER 1

1. **(b)** Nursing is primarily responsible for patient teaching and for ensuring that patients are adequately informed about the chosen therapy. [CL: KN]

2. **(c)** Answers a, b, and d are important aspects of compliance; however, the nurse must first ensure that the patient accepts the diagnosis and is willing to comply with the treatment. [CL: CO]

3. **(d)** The cognitive domain emphasizes the intellectual aspects associated with learning. Answer a reflects the affective domain, and answers b and c reflect the psychomotor domain. [CL: KN]

4. **(a)** Analyzing involves intellectual or thinking processes and, therefore, is a task of the cognitive domain. [CL: CO]

5. **(c)** Hives represent a toxic dermatologic effect which would require discontinuation of the medication. [CL: CO]

6. **(d)** Anemia and leukopenia can result in harm to the patient and are considered toxic effects. [CL: KN]

7. **(d)** The planning phase of the nursing process involves establishing short-term and long-term goals. [CL: KN]

8. **(b)** Avoid loaded questions, as they tend to be stated in emotional terms and suggest the desired patient response. [CL: KN]

9. **(d)** Cross allergies may occur in patients who are allergic to both fish and x-ray dyes which contain iodine. [CL: KN]

10. **(c)** An important aspect of health teaching involves evaluation of patient feedback in order to assess learning. [CL: CO]

CHAPTER 2

1. **(a)** Through the discovery of ancient artifacts and drawings, it is believed that early cultures attempted to treat illness by medical intervention. [CL: KN]

2. **(c)** The role of the Catholic Church was very influential during the early post-Christian era. [CL: CO]

3. **(d)** The Arabian influence in the history began during the eighth century. Answers a, b, and c represent important contributions. Galen, the Greek physician, popularized the principle of polypharmacy. [CL: CO]

4. **(b)** Empirical therapeutics is based on evidence that a drug is effective, although the mechanism of action may not be understood. [CL: KN]

5. **(a)** Individuals such as Paracelsus (1493–1541) questioned superstitious medicinal beliefs and advocated specific compounds to treat disease. [CL: KN]

6. **(b)** The mystical stage of therapeutics employed prayers, surgery, and drugs as modes of therapy. [CL: KN]

7. **(d)** Opium was discovered in the first century A.D. Colchicine was discovered in the sixth century A.D. Ether was discovered in the sixteenth century A.D., and digitalis was discovered in the eighteenth century A.D. [CL: CO]

Key to [Codes]: CL = Cognitive level; KN = Knowledge; CO = Comprehension; AP = Application; AN = Analysis

B1

8. **(d)** The Federal Food, Drug, and Cosmetic Act (FFDCA) of 1938 established requirements for all drug labels. All but answer d are required. [CL: KN]

9. **(b)** Nurses became responsible for the administration of intramuscular injections during the 1940's. [CL: CO]

10. **(d)** The Federal Food, Drug, and Cosmetic Act of 1906 was the first to designate the USP and NF as the official standards for drugs, thereby providing public protection. [CL: CO]

CHAPTER 3

1. **(c)** An anti-inflammatory effect is produced as the drug is absorbed into the local vasculature. [CL: KN]

2. **(b)** The seriously ill patient may not have adequate control of muscles used in the act of swallowing. [CL: CO]

3. **(a)** Parenteral medications are introduced into the body via a needle. [CL: KN]

4. **(b)** Special care is taken to identify a confused patient, thus properly administering needed medications. [CL: CO]

5. **(b)** Inserting and removing the needle rapidly will decrease the patient's pain sensation. [CL: CO]

6. **(b)** A common cause of medication errors is administering the wrong dose. [CL: AP]

7. **(a)** Generic substitutes reduce the cost of medical care by being less expensive than their brand name equivalents. [CL: KN]

8. **(a)** Administering a medication with meals may decrease a drug's gastrointestinal side effects. [CL: AP]

9. **(d)** Parenteral drugs are those medications introduced into the body via a needle. This type of drug administration requires specialized training and education. [CL: AP]

10. **(d)** A systemic effect such as a headache resulting from vasodilation of cerebral vessels occurs due to absorption of the drug through the skin. [CL: AP]

CHAPTER 4

1. **(c)** The pharmacokinetic phase involves the total process of drug administration from absorption, distribution, and metabolism to elimination from the body. [CL: KN]

2. **(b)** Passive transport is a two-way process allowing drug molecules to move into and out of cells without energy expenditure. [CL: CO]

3. **(d)** Nonionized drugs are lipid soluble and diffusible; therefore, they are available for absorption. [CL: KN]

4. **(c)** Bone, middle ear, skin, and fat are areas with minimal blood supply, and the distribution of medication is slower. [CL: KN]

5. **(d)** Drug dosage schedules are determined according to their biological half-life. The half-life of a drug ultimately determines how often a drug is to be given. [CL: KN]

6. **(c)** The best reference for drug selectivity lists the most and least common toxic drug effects, not all known adverse effects. [CL: CO]

7. **(a)** Individual differences occur in response to medications; these include body weight, age, disease, and psychological states, immune and environmental factors, and the time of administration. Sex is not a factor. [CL: CO]

8. **(b)** Acid drugs return to an ionized form in the small intestine; however, the majority of acidic drugs are absorbed because of increased surface area. [CL: CO]

9. **(c)** Facilitated diffusion is a process of passive transport in which a carrier is needed to cross the cell membrane. This process differs from active transport in that it does not require energy. [CL: KN]

10. **(b)** Peak concentration of a drug is achieved when the maximal amount is absorbed into the target tissue, usually causing the maximal effect. [CL: KN]

CHAPTER 5

1. **(d)** Pharmacokinetic interactions involve reactions where the absorption, distribution, biotransformation, or excretion of one drug is affected by another drug. [CL: CO]

2. **(c)** Pharmacodynamic interactions result from the combined effects of drugs. [CL: KN]

3. **(b)** Antagonism results in a combined effect that is less than either active component alone. [CL: KN]

4. **(a)** Drug incompatibilities are not synonymous with drug interactions, chemical or physical reactions that occur among two or more drugs. [CL: KN]

5. **(b)** Stimulation of microsomal activity in the liver increases the biotransformation of certain drugs, thus decreasing their effect in the body. [CL: CO]

6. **(d)** Combined toxicity occurs when two drugs with toxic effects, such as gentamicin and Lasix, are combined for therapy. Both cause ototoxicity. [CL: CO]

7. **(b)** The longer a drug remains in the gastrointestinal tract, the greater the amount absorbed. Drugs such as morphine and codeine prolong emptying time and increase drug absorption. [CL: KN]

8. **(a)** Sequestration occurs when a drug is surrounded by a lipoid substance and, therefore, cannot be absorbed. [CL: CO]

9. **(c)** Phenytoin and phenobarbital can cause malabsorption of calcium and subsequent development of osteomalacia. [CL: AP]

10. **(d)** The nurse has the legal right to withhold the medication which is suspected to be causing an in-

teraction until the physician evaluates the patient. [CL: CO]

CHAPTER 6

1. **(d)** Toxicology is concerned with drugs used in therapy, as well as with chemicals which are responsible for household, environmental, or industrial intoxication. [CL: CO]

2. **(b)** Toxic effects are dose-related and will occur in all persons who are given a sufficient dosage of a drug. [CL: CO]

3. **(d)** Adverse effects are more likely to occur in patients with impaired renal function. [CL: CO]

4. **(c)** Primary reactions are effects that are extensions of the desired action of the drug, such as an overdose. [CL: CO]

5. **(c)** Anaphylaxis refers to a Type I allergic reaction involving histamine release which causes bronchoconstriction in the lung, peripheral vasodilation, and vascular permeability. [CL: KN]

6. **(b)** The Type III allergic reaction or serum sickness is most often seen in patients receiving penicillin or diptheria and tetanus antitoxin. [CL: KN]

7. **(a)** Local ischemia and necrosis associated with Type III allergic auto-immune reaction results as a consequence of complement activation. [CL: KN]

8. **(d)** Hemolytic anemia, a blood dyscrasia, can result secondarily to a Type II allergic reaction. [CL: CO]

9. **(b)** Poisoning, a common medical emergency, is the fifth most common cause of accidental death in the United States. [CL: KN]

10. **(c)** Hemodialysis exposes blood to a semi-permeable membrane to remove low-molecular-weight toxins. [CL: KN]

CHAPTER 7

1. **(c)** By definition, the FDA has found OTC medications to be safe for use without medical supervision. [CL: KN]

2. **(a)** Aspirin's most common side effect is gastrointestinal discomfort, which includes symptoms such as nausea, indigestion, and heartburn. [CL: KN]

3. **(b)** Cough is often the means by which bronchial congestion is cleared; therefore, suppression of a cough with antitussives is indicated only if the cough is nonproductive, interferes with sleep, or causes pain. [CL: KN[

4. **(d)** Expectorants commonly found in OTC medications include iodides, ammonium chloride, terpin hydrate, and guaifenesin. [CL: CO]

5. **(a)** In choosing an antacid product, sodium content, neutralizing capacity, volume needed per dose, cost, and palatability should be considered. [CL: CO]

6. **(d)** Excedrin is a combination product which contains both aspirin and acetaminophen. [CL: KN]

7. **(c)** Patient guidelines for self-medication include selecting a product which is specific in treating symptoms. Patients should consult a health care provider if taking prescription drugs along with self-care agents. [CL: CO]

8. **(a)** Gastric discomfort associated with weakness or sweating is a situation in which the patient should consult a health care provider. [CL: KN]

9. **(b)** A disadvantage of acetaminophen is the lack of anti-inflammatory activity. [CL: KN]

10. **(d)** Treatment of bacterial infections of the throat and mouth requires systemic medication. None of the OTC topical antibacterials have been proven effective. [CL: CO]

CHAPTER 8

1. **(b)** Comprehension of written information depends upon the ability to read. [CL: CO]

2. **(c)** The concept of generalizations is inherent in Skinner's learning theory. [CL: KN]

3. **(b)** Rogers emphasizes the learner entered educational approach. [CL: AP]

4. **(a)** The goals of teaching should be achieved several days before the patient is ready for discharge. [CL: CO]

5. **(b)** Specific behavioral objectives are easily measurable for the attainment of teaching objectives. [CL: CO]

6. **(b)** The SMOG readability formula is based on the square root of the number of polysyllabic words contained within 30 selected sentences. The number 3 is added to the square root, and this score represents the reading grade that a person must have reached in order to understand the material. [CL: KN]

7. **(d)** Compliance can be defined as the extent to which a patient's behavior with regard to the medication plan coincides with health teaching. [CL: CO]

8. **(b)** Extinction is employed to eliminate undesirable behavior and is achieved by withdrawing reinforcement. [CL: KN]

9. **(a)** Ausubel's learning theory is best suited to the independent, motivated learner. [CL: KN]

Key to [Codes]: CL = Cognitive level; KN = Knowledge; CO = Comprehension; AP = Application; AN = Analysis

10. **(c)** The nurse should initially approach the patient with a positive attitude and expect compliance. The nurse must be aware, however, that noncompliance may be demonstrated. [CL: CO]

CHAPTER 9

1. **(d)** Histamine, barium, and hypaque are all used in diagnostic testing. Acetylcholine chloride is a solution used in cataract surgery to obtain complete miosis. [CL: CO]

2. **(c)** Iodine diagnostic compounds opacify structures and vessels upon contact. These preparations can be administered orally or intravenously. [CL: CO]

3. **(a)** A radiopharmaceutical is chosen because of its affinity to localize in either normal or abnormal tissue. [CL: CO]

4. **(b)** Insulin should be withheld as long as the diabetic patient is NPO. Special scheduling is often necessary for the diabetic patient. [CL: KN]

5. **(b)** Nonradioactive dyes are used to measure organ function. [CL: KN]

6. **(d)** Sincalide is a secretogogus agent which stimulates gallbladder contraction and bile release. [CL: KN]

7. **(a)** Skin tests are administered for the diagnosis of infections such as tuberculosis, coccidioidomycosis, and histoplasmosis. [CL: CO]

8. **(c)** Hypaque Sodium is contraindicated in patients with iodine hypersensitivity. [CL: KN]

9. **(c)** In diagnostic radiology, electromagnetic radiation, the release of gamma or x-rays, is measured. [CL: KN]

10. **(a)** Diphenhydramine (Benadryl) may be given prior to testing if a hypersensitivity reaction is anticipated. [CL: CO]

CHAPTER 10

1. **(d)** Droperidol/fentanyl (Innovar) is the combination narcotic and anesthetic agent which produces a state of neuroleptic analgesia. [CL: KN]

2. **(a)** Methoxyflurane (Penthrane) is a potent inhalation anesthetic with slow induction and recovery times. This drug has numerous side effects and its use is limited. [CL: KN]

3. **(d)** Intravenous barbiturates have a rapid recovery period and are therefore often utilized for short surgical procedures. [CL: KN]

4. **(c)** A nerve block is achieved by injecting the drug close to a mixed nerve in order that the area innervated by the nerve will become insensitive. [CL: CO]

5. **(b)** The state of deep muscle relaxation of general

anesthesia can result in bladder atony or decreased intestinal motility. [CL: KN]

6. **(a)** Depolarizing or noncompetitive neuromuscular blockade is achieved by depolarization of the motor end plate. [CL: KN]

7. **(c)** In order for there to be no pain, there must be an absence of reflexes. [CL: CO]

8. **(b)** Spinal cord depression and true muscle relaxation occur during Stage III of anesthesia. [CL: KN]

9. **(d)** Desirable characteristics of a good local anesthetic drug include solubility in saline solution and water, in addition to long duration, compatability with vasoconstrictor drugs, and action confined to nerve tissue. [CL: CO]

10. **(a)** Piperocaine is a local anesthetic of the ester type. [CL: KN]

CHAPTER 11

1. **(d)** Fat is mostly water free; therefore, the lean individual has more water per kg than the fat individual. [CL: CO]

2. **(a)** Hyperosmotic contraction results when a greater concentration of particles is present in the extracellular compartment due to water loss. Volume then shifts from the intracellular space to the extracellular space by osmosis, resulting in intracellular contraction. [CL: CO]

3. **(c)** The 5 percent dextrose and 0.45 percent sodium chloride solution contains 77 mEq/L of sodium and 77 mEq/L of chloride. [CL: KN]

4. **(a)** Replacement solutions are composed of water, carbohydrates, and electrolytes that are used to replace concurrent losses from the gastrointestinal tract. [CL: KN[

5. **(a)** A 10 percent invert sugar solution has 380 calories per liter. If 3000 ml of the solution is administered daily, the patient will receive approximately 1100 calories per day (3 × 380). [CL: AN]

6. **(b)** With intravenous administration, fluid imbalances may occur; therefore, intake, output, and body weight should be monitored. [CL: KN]

7. **(c)** Buffering occurs in body cells through proteins and phosphates, in red cells through hemoglobin, and in extracellular fluid through bicarbonates. [CL: CO]

8. **(b)** The primary treatment for respiratory acidosis is to improve ventilation, which may be brought about through mechanical means. [CL: KN]

9. **(d)** Lactated Ringers Solution is an example of a replacement solution. [CL: CO]

10. **(a)** In order to achieve proper hydration in patients with fluid volume deficit, hypotonic solutions

should be used to replace extracellular fluid. [CL: AP]

CHAPTER 12

1. **(a)** While platelets share the red blood cell A and B antigens, they do not contain the Rh (D) antigen. [CL: KN]

2. **(c)** Patients receiving plasma expanders need to be monitored closely, due to the possibility of an anaphylactic reaction. [CL: KN]

3. **(d)** To ensure accuracy and compatibility, the nurse compares the blood group and Rh factor of the blood for administration with those of the patient. [CL: KN]

4. **(b)** Signs of a reaction to a blood transfusion include backache, change in vital signs, urticaria, chills and fever, headache, flushing, chest pain, and sudden shock. [CL: CO]

5. **(a)** Because Dextran 40 has a low viscosity and an ability to keep red blood cells from sludging in small vessels, it is sometimes used as a hemodiluent in the heart-lung machine. [CL: KN]

6. **(d)** Donated blood is labeled with information such as proper name of component, method of preparation, and temperature range for storage. [CL: CO]

7. **(c)** An Rh-positive person can receive Rh-negative blood. In the reverse situation, however, the Rh-negative person will produce antibodies when infused with Rh-positive blood. [CL: AN]

8. **(b)** In plasmapheresis, only the plasma platelets or white blood cells are retained; the red cells are returned to the donor. [CL: CO]

9. **(d)** Stored whole blood contains low glucose and 2,3-diphosphoglycerate (2,3-DPG) levels. It is also high in potassium and has a low pH. [CL: KN]

10. **(a)** Plasma protein products contain no cellular elements; therefore, there is no risk of sensitization with repeated infusions. [CL: CO]

CHAPTER 13

1. **(c)** Tolerance is the state in which increased amounts of a substance are necessary to achieve the same effects as previously attained with the use of lesser amounts. [CL: CO]

2. **(d)** Many theories are currently proposed which attempt to explain etiologic factors of drug dependency, but none adequately addresses all aspects of the problem. Scientific understanding of addiction is at an early stage of development. [CL: KN]

3. **(a)** The patient may only know drugs by their street names; therefore, the nurse must be aware of such

terminology in clarification of which drugs the patient takes. [CL: KN]

4. **(c)** In caring for the patient withdrawing from alcohol, the nurse promotes adequate hydration. [CL: CO]

5. **(b)** The patient experiencing withdrawal from hallucinogens needs to be observed for signs of shock. [CL: CO]

6. **(a)** The prevalence of substance abuse and related health problems is widespread and now ranks as the third major cause of death in the United States. [CL: KN]

7. **(b)** Individuals with family members who have substance dependence problems are at risk for the development of a similar dependence. [CL: KN]

8. **(a)** Nurses develop addictive illness at rates comparable to people in the general population. [CL: CO]

9. **(c)** Dual addiction is the simultaneous dependence on psychoactive drugs which have similar effects. [CL: KN]

10. **(d)** The disease model describes addictive behavior as the loss of control over drug use, compulsive need to continue use, and psychological and behavioral change. [CL: KN]

CHAPTER 14

1. **(a)** Gastric emptying time varies within the pediatric population. In the newborn, the stomach empties in two-and-one-half to three hours. [CL: KN]

2. **(d)** Tissue perfusion of the muscles is not fully mature in the neonate. As the child grows, however, tissue perfusion to the muscles increases, making absorption of intramuscular injections more reliable. [CL: CO]

3. **(b)** The amount of albumin available for binding is a factor influencing distribution of medications which bind to protein. Other factors include blood pH, binding capacity, and substances which compete for binding sites. [CL: KN]

4. **(d)** Due to neuromuscular immaturity, the intestinal peristalsis in the newborn is rapid and unpredictable. Contact time for absorption of drugs is reduced. [CL: KN]

5. **(b)** The safest place for medication storage is in a locked container or drawer. The key should then be hidden. [CL: KN]

6. **(c)** In the period immediately following birth, the gastric acidity is high. Therefore, drugs which are absorbed at a higher rate in a low pH may produce elevated serum levels. [CL: CO]

Key to [Codes]: CL = Cognitive level; KN = Knowledge; CO = Comprehension; AP = Application; AN = Analysis

7. **(d)** Because the outer layer of skin (stratum corneum) is thinner in infants than in adults, the infant absorbs greater amounts of topical medications, which may cause undesirable side effects. [CL: KN]

8. **(a)** A small portion of the infant's body weight is fat. Therefore, the infant requires smaller dosages of a fat soluble drug.

9. **(d)** A high proportion of body water in the neonate is extracellular fluid, which the neonate exchanges more rapidly each day than the adult. Therefore, higher doses of water soluble drugs per kg of body weight are necessary to reach desired concentrations. [CL: KN]

10. **(b)** The choice of muscles for intramuscular (IM) injection is limited in the infant, due to small muscle mass. The muscle of choice for IM injections is the vastus lateralis. [CL: AP]

CHAPTER 15

1. **(c)** During pregnancy, elimination is increased, reducing drug concentrations and therapeutic plasma levels. [CL: CO]

2. **(b)** Variables which determine whether drugs will pass through the placental barrier include the physicochemical characteristics of the drug, physiologic properties of the placenta, and maternal and fetal placental blood flow. Gestational age is a factor in determining the effect that the drug will have on the fetus. [CL: CO]

3. **(d)** Category C drugs represent those which may be used in pregnant women only if the benefit of use outweighs the risk to the fetus. [CL: KN]

4. **(a)** Active labor with imminent delivery is a contraindication for barbiturate administration. [CL: KN]

5. **(d)** After general anesthesia, there is a delay in infant and mother contact in the postpartal period. This separation may result in delayed mother-infant bonding. [CL: CO]

6. **(b)** Paracervical blocks are not frequently utilized as a labor anesthetic due to the high incidence of fetal bradycardia. [CL: KN]

7. **(a)** Uterine suppression drugs most frequently used are beta sympathomimetics. These drugs should be used with caution in patients with mild to moderate pre-eclampsia, but are contraindicated if prolongation of labor is deleterious to infant or mother. [CL: CO]

8. **(a)** A positive OCT indicates low placental reserve and the need for termination of the pregnancy. [CL: KN]

9. **(d)** Oxytocin is contraindicated in cases of placenta previa. The dosage should be reduced in patients with cardiovascular, renal, or hypertensive disease. [CL: CO]

10. **(c)** Diazepam should be used with caution in breast-feeding mothers, due to the risk of drug accumulation in the neonate. [CL: CO]

CHAPTER 16

1. **(c)** The number one cause of death continues to be cardiovascular disease, although other illnesses, such as cancer, are associated with aging. [CL: KN]

2. **(b)** The principles of drug disposition involve absorption, distribution, metabolism, and excretion. [CL: CO]

3. **(a)** Many times, side effects of medications are mistaken for symptoms related to the aging process. Most illnesses are treated with drug therapy, but, in the elderly, this can represent a risky component of patient care. [CL: KN]

4. **(a)** Lean body mass and total body water tend to decrease in the elderly. [CL: KN]

5. **(d)** The elderly have increased fat composition and fat soluble drugs are distributed in a greater volume of tissue. After absorption, the drugs are released slowly, resulting in increased duration of effect. [CL: KN]

6. **(a)** Due to the reduction in subcutaneous tissue, intravenous administration of a vesicant drug, such as doxorubicin, should not be administered via veins in the hand. [CL: AP]

7. **(b)** The elastic fibers in the arteries lose about 30 percent of their stretching ability as a person ages. [CL: KN]

8. **(b)** Aging reduces the liver's ability to metabolize certain drugs, resulting in a prolonged effect, due to prolonged concentrations of drug in the system. [CL: KN]

9. **(c)** Sensory and perceptual alterations, such as reduced hearing acuity, may interfere with a person's ability to understand instructions. [CL: CO]

CHAPTER 17

1. **(c)** The basal ganglia are embedded within the cerebral hemispheres. [CL: KN]

2. **(b)** The limbic system is concerned with the expression of mood, feelings, and emotions. It is also involved in the regulation of rhythms, appetite, and learning. [CL: CO]

3. **(d)** Cerebral spinal fluid is formed across the choroid plexus. [CL: KN]

4. **(b)** The action potential does not cross directly from nerve to nerve. As the action potential reaches the nerve ending, it releases a chemical called a transmitter, which diffuses across the nerve synapse and acts on a specific receptor at the post-synaptic membrane. [CL: CO]

5. **(d)** The cell bodies of afferent nerves lie outside the CNS. Action potentials are generated at the receptor end and messages about sensory information are transmitted to the CNS. [CL: KN]

6. **(a)** The sympathetic nervous system enables the body to deal with emergency situations by eliciting the "fight or flight" reaction. [CL: KN]

7. **(c)** Nicotinic receptors are found in the somatic system and in the ganglia of the autonomic system. Ganglionic antagonists which block nicotinic receptors cause both muscarinic and adrenergic blockade. [CL: CO]

8. **(d)** In bronchial and intestinal smooth muscle, alpha$_1$ adrenergic stimulation causes relaxation. In vascular smooth muscle, alpha$_1$ adrenergic stimulation causes vasoconstriction. [CL: CO]

9. **(b)** Epinephrine possesses both beta$_1$ and beta$_2$ activity. [CL: KN]

10. **(a)** Beta$_1$ receptors are located in the heart, kidney, and adipose tissues. Beta$_2$ receptors are located in bronchial smooth muscle. [CL: CO]

CHAPTER 18

1. **(d)** Depolarizing neuromuscular blockers are noncompetitive in that they cannot be reversed by additional acetylcholine. [CL: CO]

2. **(b)** Scopolamine is contraindicated in patients with angle-closure glaucoma, due to the effects of increased intraocular pressure. [CL: KN]

3. **(c)** Direct-acting cholinergic drugs produce decreased cardiac contractility, a negative inotropic effect. [CL: CO]

4. **(a)** Acetylcholine-type drugs are indicated for the patient with neurogenic bladder, due to stimulation of micturation. [CL: CO]

5. **(a)** Systemic effects of carbachol include increased peristalsis, abdominal cramping, and diarrhea. [CL: KN]

6. **(c)** Prostigmin is contraindicated for patients with mechanical obstruction of the urinary tract. [CL: CO]

7. **(d)** One way in which ganglionic blocking agents work is by preventing the action of acetylcholine at the ganglionic receptor sites. [CL: KN]

8. **(a)** Curare is a nondepolarizing neuromuscular blocking agent used to produce muscle relaxation for intubation and anesthesia. [CL: KN]

9. **(c)** Anticholinesterases are agents that interfere with the enzymes which normally destroy acetylcholine at the neuromuscular junctions. This creates a build-up of acetylcholine at the cholinergic receptor sites. [CL: KN]

10. **(b)** Atropine ophthalmic solution is used to treat iritis (inflammation of the iris) by producing mydriasis. [CL: AN]

CHAPTER 19

1. **(c)** An effect of beta-adrenergic stimulation is increased heart rate. [CL: KN]

2. **(d)** Epinephrine causes vasoconstriction in the peripheral vessels and vasodilation of blood vessels of muscles with predominantly beta$_2$ receptors. [CL: KN]

3. **(a)** Ventricular dysrhythmias may develop during surgery if catecholamines are used with halothane anesthetics. [CL: KN]

4. **(a)** Adverse effects of indirect and mixed adrenergic stimulants include nervousness, headache, palpitations, and cardiac dysrhythmias. [CL: KN]

5. **(b)** DHE45 has a direct constricting effect on smooth muscle of peripheral and cranial vessels and is used to prevent or abort vascular headaches. [CL: KN]

6. **(d)** Catecholamine preparations are inactivated through uptake and metabolism at sympathetic nerve endings. The drugs are metabolized by monamine oxidase in the liver, kidneys, and plasma. [CL: KN]

7. **(d)** Glucagon has been shown to enhance myocardial contractility in the event of beta-blocker overdose. [CL: KN]

8. **(b)** Adrenergic drugs work at alpha, beta$_1$, beta$_2$, and dopaminergic receptors. Cholinergic drugs work at muscarinic receptor sites. [CL: CO]

9. **(b)** Phenotolamine hydrochloride is an alpha blocking agent used in the management of secondary hypertension due to pheochromocytoma and in the treatment of extravasation of vasopressors. [CL: KN]

10. **(d)** Dobutamine is an appropriate drug for the treatment of cardiogenic shock, due to its selective ability to increase myocardial contractile force. In low doses, there is little increase in the heart rate. Unlike dopamine, dobutamine does not increase renal or mesenteric blood flow. [CL: KN]

CHAPTER 20

1. **(c)** Narcan is an opiate antagonist without an agonist effect. [CL: CO]

2. **(c)** Propoxyphene hydrochloride 65 mg is equivalent to 30 to 45 mg of codeine. [CL: KN]

Key to [Codes]: CL = Cognitive level; KN = Knowledge; CO = Comprehension; AP = Application; AN = Analysis

3. **(a)** Codeine is the analgesic drug of choice for patients with high intracranial pressure. [CL: CO]

4. **(c)** Miosis is an effect of kappa stimulation, while dysphoria and respiratory and vasomotor stimulation are associated with sigma receptors. [CL: KN]

5. **(b)** The endorphin peptides are found in the pituitary gland. [CL: KN]

6. **(a)** Non-opiate analgesics act peripherally by preventing the formation of prostaglandins in inflamed tissues. This prevents stimulation of pain receptors. [CL: CO]

7. **(d)** Acetylcysteine (Mucomyst) forms an inactive compound with the reactive metabolite of acetaminophen. [CL: KN]

8. **(c)** Aspirin is often combined with synthetic narcotics such as propoxyphene hydrochloride (Darvon). [CL: CO]

9. **(c)** Methadone is a synthetic opiate which is very effective after oral administration. The oral form is preferred for detoxification, but methadone can be given intramuscularly. [CL: KN]

10. **(a)** Stadol is more potent than morphine sulfate. The opiate antagonist properties of Stadol reduce the potential for physical addiction. [CL: CO]

CHAPTER 21

1. **(d)** One way in which CNS stimulants produce their action is to modify the neurotransmitter response by altering cAMP. [CL: KN]

2. **(d)** Because CNS stimulants are nonspecific antagonists of depressant drugs, they are not effective in reducing pharmacologically induced CNS depression. [CL: KN]

3. **(b)** An adverse effect of analeptic stimulants is the production of clonic-tonic seizures. [CL: KN]

4. **(c)** Doxapram is contraindicated in patients who are experiencing stimulation of the CNS, such as those with cerebral vascular accidents. [CL: KN]

5. **(a)** The concurrent use of amphetamines and acetazolamine results in an increased amphetamine effect. This is due to the production of an alkaline urine by acetazolamine which inhibits renal excretion of amphetamines. [CL: CO]

6. **(a)** Using anticholinergic agents with cocaine results in hypertension and tachycardia. [CL: KN]

7. **(c)** Caffeine stimulates the cerebral cortex, reducing fatigue. [CL: CO]

8. **(b)** An adverse effect of doxapram includes increased deep tendon reflexes. Altered deep tendon reflexes may indicate overdose and should be reported immediately. [CL: AP]

9. **(d)** The overall effect of CNS stimulants is respiratory stimulation and mydriasis, in addition to bronchodilation, loss of taste and smell, and constriction of the urinary bladder sphincter. [CL: AP]

CHAPTER 22

1. **(d)** Valproic acid is an anticonvulsant drug which blocks enkephalinergic-induced seizures. The enkephalinergic system is thought to be involved in absence epilepsy. [CL: KN]

2. **(b)** Depression of clotting factors occurs with pregnant women on primidone, phenobarbital, or phenytoin, resulting in a potential for hemorrhage. [CL: KN]

3. **(b)** Primidone is similar in chemical composition to phenobarbital. [CL: KN]

4. **(c)** Drugs, such as nifedipine, which work by enzyme inhibition increase serum phenytoin levels. [CL: KN]

5. **(b)** Due to CNS depression, phenobarbital should not be given to comatose patients. [CL: KN]

6. **(d)** Phenytoin has been shown to be useful in controlling arrhythmias related to digoxin toxicity. [CL: KN]

7. **(c)** Tegretol acts by blocking the post-tetanic potentiation and by reducing polysynaptic responses. [CL: KN]

8. **(c)** Clonozepam (Klonopin) has been shown to be useful in controlling myoclonic seizures. [CL: CO]

9. **(d)** Lipid solubility plays a major role in the rate at which benzodiazepines enter the central nervous system. Drugs with greater lipic solubility have a faster onset of action. [CL: CO]

CHAPTER 23

1. **(c)** Control of symptoms related to Parkinson's disease is dependent primarily on restoring dopamine levels in the brain. [CL: CO]

2. **(b)** The surgical procedure involving transplantation of autologous adrenal cortex tissue to the basal ganglia is performed to treat Parkinson's disease. The adrenal tissue contains dopamine cells which restore dopamine function. [CL: KN]

3. **(c)** Carbidopa inhibits the peripheral breakdown of levodopa, thereby increasing the amount which crosses the blood-brain barrier for conversion to dopamine. [CL: CO]

4. **(d)** Muscle spasms of local origin caused by inflammation or trauma are best treated by central skeletal muscle relaxants. [CL: KN]

5. **(c)** Dantrolene sodium (Dantrium) acts directly on skeletal muscle to produce relaxation. [CL: KN]

6. **(a)** Antihistamines have anticholinergic properties which worsen myasthenia symptoms. [CL: KN]

7. **(c)** In myasthenia gravis, receptor sites for acetylcholine are blocked by antibody complexes, reducing the

nerve impulses generating muscle contraction. [CL: CO]

8. **(c)** Amantadine therapy may prove useful in controlling the "on/off" phenomenon associated with long-term levodopa therapy. [CL: KN]

9. **(a)** Patients taking bromocriptine may demonstrate a "first-dose phenomenon" manifested by sudden cardiovascular collapse. [CL: CO]

CHAPTER 24

1. **(b)** In addition to promoting sleep and reducing anxiety and tension, diazepam produces skeletal muscle relaxation. [CL: CO]

2. **(a)** When benzodiazepines are combined with other CNS depressants, the result is increased CNS depression. [CL: CO]

3. **(b)** In addition to oral absorption, barbiturates are absorbed through the colon and may be given rectally. [CL: KN]

4. **(b)** Barbiturates are useful for daytime management of anxiety. These agents should not be used for the patient in pain because they increase the reaction to painful stimuli. [CL: CO]

5. **(d)** The barbiturates have an even greater potential for dependency than the benzodiazepines. [CL: CO]

6. **(c)** Because of the prolonged half-life, chlordiazepoxide (Librium) is useful in patients with alcohol withdrawal. [CL: KN]

7. **(d)** Memory impairment has been very frequently reported by patients taking triazolam (Halcion). [CL: KN]

8. **(a)** Because of central nervous system depression, benzodiazepines are contraindicated in comatose patients. [CL: KN]

9. **(c)** During REM sleep, colorful dreams and nightmares take place. [CL: KN]

CHAPTER 25

1. **(c)** Most oral concentrations are well absorbed from the gastrointestinal tract. Metabolism and biodegradation of antipsychotic drugs are highly variable; therefore, therapeutic serum concentrations have not been established. [CL: KN]

2. **(a)** While antipsychotic agents are not curative, they have been shown to be effective in controlling symptoms. [CL: KN]

3. **(d)** Antipsychotic drugs are highly lipophilic and are stored in fatty tissues. After the drugs are discontinued, they are slowly released by the tissues and excreted. [CL: CO]

4. **(b)** Impaired memory is likely to be produced by blockage of cholinergic sites within the brain. [CL: KN]

5. **(b)** Tardive dyskinesia is thought to be linked to dopamine receptor blockage, which is the same mechanism responsible for the positive effects of neuroleptic agents. [CL: CO]

6. **(c)** A characteristic of pseudoparkinsonism is motor retardation. [CL: KN]

7. **(a)** Patients with Parkinson's disease may demonstrate worsened symptoms when they take haloperidol. [CL: KN]

8. **(d)** Chlorpromazine (Thorazine) is classified as an aliphatic, a subgroup of the phenothiazines. [CL: KN]

9. **(b)** Alcohol potentiates and prolongs the effects of antipsychotic medications. For this reason, patients taking neuroleptic agents should avoid alcohol. [CL: CO]

CHAPTER 26

1. **(c)** Although the action of antidepressants is not completely understood, they are thought to act by regulating the processes which inactivate norepinephrine and serotonin. This results in prolonging the presence of norepinephrine (and serotonin) within the nerve synapses. [CL: CO]

2. **(b)** Antidepressants are highly lipid-soluble and are extensively distributed throughout body tissue. [CL: KN]

3. **(c)** Anticholinergic symptoms associated with antidepressants include blurred vision, dry mouth, constipation, and urinary hesitancy. [CL: KN]

4. **(c)** Phenelzine sulfate is an example of a monoamine oxidase (MAO) inhibitor. [CL: KN]

5. **(c)** The effectiveness of tricyclic antidepressants is enhanced when given with sodium bicarbonate. [CL: CO]

6. **(a)** Signs/symptoms of severe lithium toxicity include hyperreflexia, stupor, or seizures. [CL: KN]

7. **(b)** A potentially life-threatening interaction exists between mepridine (Demerol) and MAO inhibitors; therefore, the drugs should not be administered together. [CL: KN]

8. **(d)** Tricyclic antidepressants may increase blood glucose levels. [CL: CO]

9. **(b)** Lithium is thought to act by reducing the release of norepinephrine and increasing its reuptake. This results in a dampened effect at the synaptic junction. [CL: KN]

CHAPTER 27

1. **(c)** The myocardium is the tissue layer in which the major blood vessels are located. [CL: KN]

2. **(a)** The tricuspid valve separates the right atrium from the right ventricle. [CL: CO]

3. **(c)** Phase 2 of the action potential curve is the point at which calcium enters the cell via slow channels. [CL: CO]

4. **(c)** Ventricular depolarization is represented by the QRS complex on the electrocardiogram. [CL: CO]

5. **(c)** The bundle of His or AV junction initiates a heart rate of 60 to 40 beats per minute. The AV node has no pacemaking cells. [CL: CO]

6. **(b)** Cardiac output is calculated by stroke volume times heart rate. [CL: KN]

7. **(b)** Contractility refers to the ability of the heart to generate enough force to eject blood volume at a particular fiber length. [CL: KN]

8. **(d)** The right coronary artery supplies the posterior leaflet of the mitral valve. [CL: KN]

9. **(b)** Capillary filtration increases when capillary hydrostatic pressure is normal and colloid pressure is low, resulting in fluid shifts into the interstitial spaces (edema). [CL: KN]

10. **(a)** Approximately 90 percent of coronary artery perfusion occurs during diastole. [CL: KN]

CHAPTER 28

1. **(d)** Cardiac glycosides are positive inotropic agents, increasing the force of contraction. [CL: KN]

2. **(c)** Cardiac glycosides increase cardiac output, resulting in a secondary decrease in preload and diastolic volume. [CL: CO]

3. **(a)** The primary site of action by the digitalis glycosides is the AV node. [CL: KN]

4. **(b)** By reducing heart rate, digitalis glycosides exert a negative chronotropic effect. [CL: KN]

5. **(a)** In patients with cardiomegaly due to increased workload, digitalis preparations decrease heart size. [CL: KN]

6. **(d)** Digitalis glycosides slow the conduction through the AV node and are useful for atrial tachycardias such as paroxysmal atrial tachycardia. [CL: KN]

7. **(c)** Enzyme-inducing agents such as phenobarbital can potentially reduce digitoxin levels. [CL: CO]

8. **(b)** The calcium antagonist nifedipine (Procardia) increases digoxin concentration when given concurrently. [CL: KN]

9. **(a)** The interaction of quinidine and digoxin produces a greater potential for ventricular dysrhythmias. [CL: CO]

CHAPTER 29

1. **(d)** Guanethidine exerts its action as an antihypertensive by neuroeffector blockade. [CL: CO]

2. **(c)** Clonidine hydrochloride is useful in the treatment of opiate withdrawal. [CL: KN]

3. **(d)** Diazide seems to inhibit insulin release from pancreatic islet cells and can cause hyperglycemia if used for several days. [CL: CO]

4. **(a)** Reserpine causes gastric and intestinal irritation, resulting in abdominal cramps and diarrhea. [CL: KN]

5. **(b)** Guanethidine has negative inotropic effects, resulting in reduced cardiac output and reduced venous return. [CL: CO]

6. **(a)** Minoxidil causes increased cardiac output and reflex tachycardia. [CL: KN]

7. **(c)** Mecamylamine hydrochloride is a ganglionic blocker which blocks transmission of the sympathetic and parasympathetic nerve impulses. [CL: KN]

8. **(b)** Studies have shown that verapamil potentiates the effects of methyldopa (Aldomet). [CL: CO]

9. **(b)** Prazosin (Minipress) relaxes smooth muscle by blocking alpha$_1$-adrenergic receptors, thereby reducing peripheral vascular resistance. [CL: KN]

10. **(b)** Atenolol (Tenormin) is an example of a beta-adrenergic blocking agent which competes with epinephrine for beta-receptor sites, inhibiting beta-adrenergic stimuli. [CL: CO]

CHAPTER 30

1. **(c)** Atrial dysrhythmias such as atrial fibrillation are not usually life-threatening, but require treatment whether or not they are symptomatic. [CL: KN]

2. **(a)** Group IV calcium-channel antagonists depress phase 4 of depolarization and prolong phases 1 and 2 of repolarization. [CL: KN]

3. **(c)** Disopyramide (Norpace) is a Group 1a antidysrhythmia agent. [CL: KN]

4. **(b)** Procainamide is contraindicated for use in patients with myasthenia gravis, due to its anticholinergic effects. [CL: KN]

5. **(a)** Verapamil is effective in treating supraventricular tachycardias, such as atrial fibrillation and atrial flutter. [CL: KN]

6. **(a)** Bretylium is an example of a Group III antidysrhythmia drug which interferes with norepinephrine, increasing the threshold for developing ventricular fibrillation. [CL: KN]

7. **(c)** Group II agents act by blocking sympathetic stimulation at the sinus node. These agents are use-

ful in controlling ventricular dysrhythmias caused by exercise or excessive catecholamines. [CL: KN]

8. **(d)** Lorcainide is an investigational Group I drug, which suppresses ventricular ectopic beats with minimal adverse side effects. [CL: KN]

9. **(c)** Torsade de Pointe is a type of ventricular tachycardia associated with the presence of a prolonged Q-T interval. It is treated with beta blockers, isoproterenol, atropine, or by a cardiac pacemaker. [CL: CO]

10. **(b)** Mexiletine hydrochloride is structurally similar to lidocaine in that it depresses automaticity. [CL: KN]

CHAPTER 31

1. **(b)** Nitrates produce pooling of blood in the peripheral veins by reducing systemic venous tone. [CL: CO]

2. **(b)** Nitrates at high doses cause reduced peripheral resistance and ventricular outflow resistance (afterload). [CL: KN]

3. **(d)** Nitroglycerin is metabolized extensively by the liver. This first-pass characteristic reduces the effectiveness of the oral route. [CL: KN]

4. **(c)** Agents such as histamine and norepinephrine act as a physiologic antagonist to nitrates. [CL: KN]

5. **(d)** At the onset of chest pain, 1 or 2 metered doses of nitroglycerin translingual are sprayed into the oral mucosa. [CL: AP]

6. **(b)** Beta-adrenergic blockers decrease the force of cardiac contraction, thereby reducing myocardial oxygen demand. [CL: KN]

7. **(d)** Verapamil has a pronounced effect on AV node conduction and is contraindicated in patients with sick sinus syndrome who do not have a pacemaker. [CL: KN]

8. **(d)** Nylidrin hydrochloride, a beta-adrenergic stimulant, acts on beta$_2$ receptor cells in skeletal muscle to produce arteriole dilation. [CL: KN]

9. **(d)** Papaverine is a direct-acting vasodilator which has been used for relief of cerebral and peripheral ischemia related to arterial spasm and senile dementia. [CL: KN]

CHAPTER 32

1. **(c)** The greater the ratio of lipids to protein, the lower the density. Very low-density lipoproteins (VLDL) have larger amounts of lipids. [CL: CO]

2. **(d)** Dietary iron, as well as oral preparations, are re-

moved from the body via the loss of iron-containing cells from the bowel, skin, and genitourinary tract. Normal loss is 0.5 to 1 mg/day. [CL: KN]

3. **(c)** Deferoxamine binds with ferric iron into a water-soluble chelate which is excreted by the kidneys. [CL: KN]

4. **(a)** Triglyceride is an example of a simple lipid which consists of fatty acid and glycerol. [CL: KN]

5. **(b)** Type III hyperlipidemia is treated with diet alterations and nicotinic acid. [CL: KN]

6. **(d)** Gemfibrozil decreases serum triglycerides by 40 to 55 percent and is used to treat patients with Type IV and V hyperlipidemia. [CL: CO]

7. **(a)** Patients taking high doses of clofibrate are at risk for development of cancer of the biliary tract. The therapeutic use of this agent is limited. [CL: KN]

8. **(c)** Pernicious anemia is a type of megaloblastic anemia which is characterized by large germ cells in the bone marrow and by large immature red cells in the plasma. [CL: KN]

9. **(c)** Clofibrate inhibits the synthesis of cholesterol. [CL: KN]

CHAPTER 33

1. **(d)** Stage II of the clotting process involves the conversion of prothrombin to thrombin by thromboplastin. [CL: KN]

2. **(a)** The intrinsic cascade of the clotting system is activated when the endothelium lining the blood vessels is damaged. [CL: KN]

3. **(c)** Anticoagulants do not dissolve existing clots; rather, they retard the clotting process at various stages. [CL: KN]

4. **(d)** Heparin can be extracted from many cells, but highest concentrations are found in the lungs and intestines. [CL: CO]

5. **(d)** Conditions such as precordial effusion may result in bleeding and represent a contraindication to oral anticoagulant therapy. [CL: KN]

6. **(a)** Dipyridamole blocks ADP-induced platelet aggregation and is classified as an antiplatelet agent. [CL: KN]

7. **(b)** A blood clotting factor which is dependent on vitamin K is prothrombin. Synthesis of prothrombin is promoted by vitamin K in the liver. [CL: CO]

8. **(d)** Heparin acts to inhibit the first stages of the clotting process by: preventing the formation of fibrin in stage III; reducing the amount of thromboplastin in stage I; and exerting an antiprothrombin action in stage II. [CL: KN]

Key to [Codes]: CL = Cognitive level; KN = Knowledge; CO = Comprehension; AP = Application; AN = Analysis

9. **(d)** Streptokinase is a thrombolytic agent which is contraindicated in patients with cerebrovascular accident due to the potential for intracerebral bleeding. [CL: KN]

CHAPTER 34

1. **(d)** The upper airway is composed of the nose, mouth, and throat. The purpose of these structures is to warm and filter the inhaled air. [CL: KN]

2. **(a)** The larynx contains structures which protect the lower airway by playing a vital role in the coughing mechanism. The larynx closes tightly when food or liquid enters the oropharynx. [CL: CO]

3. **(c)** The mucus secreted by the glands of the bronchial epithelium is sticky and traps most of the dust and bacteria which bypass the upper airway defense mechanisms. [CL: CO]

4. **(c)** Specialized neurons, known as chemoreceptors, are sensitive to changes in blood pH and carbon dioxide levels. [CL: KN]

5. **(d)** Humoral mediators released from mast cells and basophils overstimulate the parasympathetic nervous system, causing bronchial constriction. [CL: CO]

6. **(c)** The physiological work of breathing can be increased by any factor which weakens the muscles of respiration. [CL: KN]

7. **(a)** Infection is the most common cause of reduced lung compliance. Inflammatory exudate impedes lung expansion. [CL: KN]

8. **(b)** Excessive mucus production, a common feature of many lung diseases, partially obstructs the airway and results in increased airway resistance. [CL: CO]

9. **(d)** Beta$_2$ are specific receptors of the sympathetic branch of the autonomic nervous system and are found in bronchial smooth muscle. [CL: KN]

10. **(d)** Chemoreceptors in the medulla are highly sensitive to changes in arterial carbon dioxide levels. A rise in carbon dioxide levels causes an increase in ventilation, which continues until the level of carbon dioxide returns to normal. [CL: CO]

CHAPTER 35

1. **(c)** Catecholamine compounds are useful in controlling bronchospasm; however, their popularity has declined, due to short duration of action and cardiovascular side effects. [CL: KN]

2. **(b)** Beta-blocking agents act as antagonists to sympathomimetics. Concomitant use of beta-blockers reduces the effectiveness of both agents. [CL: CO]

3. **(d)** Xanthine agents such as theophylline have the ability to inhibit activity of the enzyme that inacti-

vates cAMP. The effect is an indirect relaxation of bronchial smooth muscle. [CL: KN]

4. **(a)** Cimetidine is an example of a drug which decreases the rate of metabolism of theophylline, resulting in greater risk of toxicity. [CL: KN]

5. **(d)** Corticosteroids are agents used to reduce bronchial inflammation, thereby reducing bronchial obstruction. They are thought to act by decreasing the release of inflammatory mediators from injured tissue. [CL: CO]

6. **(b)** Cromolyn sodium is an anti-inflammatory agent used to prevent asthma attacks. This drug is not a bronchodilator and can aggravate bronchospasm. [CL: CO]

7. **(b)** Major side effects of ephedrine involve cardiac irritability, such as premature atrial contractions. [CL: CO]

8. **(a)** Adverse side effects of isoproterenol involve the central nervous system and include nervousness, tremors, and restlessness. [CL: KN]

9. **(d)** The effect of parasympathetic stimulation is release of a cyclic nucleotide (cGMP) which constricts bronchial smooth muscle. Anticholinergic bronchodilators act by decreasing production of cGMP, allowing cAMP to have greater influence and resulting in bronchial relaxation. [CL: CO]

10. **(b)** In patients with severe bronchial obstruction, all breath sounds are greatly diminished due to the reduced volume of air passing into and out of the lungs. [CL: CO]

CHAPTER 36

1. **(b)** Theophylline is an example of a respiratory stimulant which is particularly useful in treating apnea. [CL: KN]

2. **(d)** Early signs of oxygen toxicity include cough, nasal congestion, sore throat, and increasing dyspnea. [CL: KN]

3. **(d)** Methadone has a rapid onset of action and long duration of effect. This agent has high addiction potential. [CL: KN]

4. **(a)** Carbon dioxide increases ventilation by stimulating the chemoreceptors which signal the respiratory center to increase rate and depth of ventilation. [CL: KN]

5. **(b)** This hormone increases responsiveness of the respiratory center to carbon dioxide and decreases the center's excitatory threshold. [CL: CO]

6. **(d)** Oxygen should be administered to premature infants at a sufficient level to prevent hypoxemia. These patients are best maintained below 80 mmHg. A range of 50 to 80 for the PaO$_2$ is generally acceptable. [CL: KN]

7. **(b)** Very precise oxygen concentrations, such as 35 percent, are delivered by Venturi mask devices. [CL: CO]

8. **(b)** Oxygen toxicity can occur if high oxygen concentrations are given over long periods of time. [CL: KN]

9. **(a)** Tidal volume is the amount of air that is inhaled and exhaled with each breath. [CL: KN]

CHAPTER 37

1. **(d)** The filtration of blood occurs in the glomerulus, forming glomerular filtrate. The proximal tubule then reabsorbs 70 to 80 percent of the filtrate and returns it to the systemic circulation. Fluid leaving the proximal tubule enters the loop of Henle and then moves into the collecting ducts, where the filtrate is either concentrated or diluted prior to excretion as urine. [CL: CO]

2. **(b)** The kidney maintains acid-base regulation by generation of HCO_3^- through H^+ excretion. [CL: KN]

3. **(c)** Parathyroid hormone (PTH) is secreted by the parathyroid glands when the plasma calcium is low. This hormone elevates plasma calcium by decreasing renal calcium excretion, increasing bone resorption, and increasing intestinal calcium absorption. [CL: KN]

4. **(a)** ADH acts on the cortical and medullary collecting ducts of the kidney to alter water permeability. [CL: KN]

5. **(b)** Aldosterone mediates the exchange of sodium for potassium in the distal convoluted tubule. [CL: KN]

6. **(d)** Vitamin D which is ingested through the diet is synthesized in the skin. [CL: KN]

7. **(b)** Erythropoietin, produced by the liver in response to hypoxia or other factors, stimulates erythrocyte production in the liver. [CL: KN]

8. **(b)** As much as 20 percent of insulin produced by the pancreas is degraded in the renal tubular cells. Therefore, diabetic patients with renal disease may require less insulin. [CL: KN]

9. **(d)** The distal convoluted tubule is impermeable to water and urea, but contains a sodium pumping mechanism which is the site of action for thiazide diuretics. [CL: CO]

10. **(a)** Ammonia (NH_3) diffuses into the lumen, combining with H^+ to form ammonium (NH_4) which is eliminated through the urine. This results in a reduction of H^+. [CL: CO]

CHAPTER 38

1. **(d)** Carbonic anyhydrase inhibitors block the formation of carbonic acid, resulting in excretion of Na^+ and HCO_3^- in the urine. This creates a state of systemic hyperchloremic acidosis. [CL: KN]

2. **(b)** These diuretic agents compete with aldosterone and prevent the reabsorption of sodium (in exchange for potassium) in the distal tubules. [CL: KN]

3. **(a)** Hydrostatic pressure is that which is created by the contraction of the heart. [CL: KN]

4. **(c)** Fluid accumulates within the interstitial space when there exists an alteration in capillary permeability, an increase in intravascular hydrostatic pressure, or a decrease in intravascular oncotic pressure. [CL: KN]

5. **(c)** Angiotensin I is converted to angiotensin II in the lungs. [CL: KN]

6. **(a)** Overdiuresis of patients with ascites results in depletion of intravascular volume. Peripheral edema fluid is mobilized faster than ascitic fluid. Patients without peripheral edema should not diurese over 900 ml/day. [CL: KN]

7. **(b)** Carbonic anyhydrase inhibitors should not be used in situations, such as pulmonary obstruction, in which the resulting acidotic state would increase the respiratory rate. [CL: KN]

8. **(d)** Urea (Ureaphil) is an osmotic diuretic which is used to reduce intracranial and intraocular pressure. [CL: KN]

9. **(d)** Triamterene is a potassium-sparing agent with mild diuretic action. Patients taking this drug should not be given potassium supplements. [CL: AP]

10. **(b)** Anasarca is a term referring to severe generalized edema. [CL: KN]

CHAPTER 39

1. **(d)** Vitamin D metabolism is suppressed in patients with chronic renal failure. This results in altered absorption of calcium from the gastrointestinal system. [CL: CO]

2. **(b)** In response to a decrease in arterial pH in metabolic acidosis, the body attempts to compensate by increasing the rate and depth of respirations, blowing off carbon dioxide. [CL: CO]

3. **(b)** Metabolic alkalosis is characterized by elevated plasma concentration of bicarbonate (HCO_3^-), causing elevated pH levels. [CL: KN]

Key to [Codes]: CL = Cognitive level; KN = Knowledge; CO = Comprehension; AP = Application; AN = Analysis

4. **(a)** Oliguria is defined as urine output which is less than 20 ml/hour or 500 ml/day. [CL: KN]

5. **(c)** Reduced calcium levels stimulate the production of parathormone from the parathyroid gland. As renal failure progresses, a condition of hyperparathyroidism develops. [CL: KN]

6. **(c)** For moderate potassium deficits (not below 2.5 mEq/L), the intravenous potassium concentrations should not exceed 30 mEq/L, and the flow rate should be ≤10 mEq/hour. [CL: AP]

7. **(c)** Proximal renal tubular acidosis is caused by altered bicarbonate reabsorption. This results in increased excretion of bicarbonate. [CL: CO]

8. **(b)** A creatinine clearance of 30 ml/minute is classified as moderate renal failure. [CL: KN]

9. **(d)** Pre-renal azotemia is said to exist in the oliguric patient when an elevation in the BUN is greater than the rise in the serum creatinine. [CL: KN]

CHAPTER 40

1. **(a)** The function of the thymus involves the immune system, particularly in the newborn. The pancreas, parathyroid, and pituitary are all part of the endocrine system. [CL: CO]

2. **(c)** The polypeptide hormones secreted by the anterior pituitary include growth hormone, prolactin, and corticotropin. [CL: KN]

3. **(c)** Regulation of hormonal activity is by negative feedback mechanisms. The endocrine gland will continue to excrete hormone until the target organ responds appropriately. When the target organ's response is strong, the hormonal activity is suppressed. [CL: CO]

4. **(b)** Calcitonin is secreted by the thyroid gland and functions to regulate calcium and phosphorus levels. [CL: KN]

5. **(a)** Somatostatin, a hormone secreted by the delta cells of the pancreas, depresses insulin and glucogon secretion. [CL: KN]

6. **(d)** Aldosterone is the major mineralocorticoid produced by the adrenal cortex. This hormone functions to stimulate reabsorption of sodium and chloride in the renal distal tubule. [CL: KN]

7. **(c)** Parathormone, released by the parathyroid gland, increases serum calcium levels. [CL: CO]

8. **(a)** Estrogens increase osteoblastic activity which is concerned with the formation of bone tissue. [CL: KN]

9. **(a)** By stimulating gluconeogenesis in the liver, cortisol maintains serum blood levels. [CL: KN]

10. **(c)** Testosterone is an example of a more insoluble hormone which requires a protein carrier. [CL: KN]

CHAPTER 41

1. **(a)** Somatotropin (growth hormone) stimulates a protein-building cycle, increasing the nitrogen balance. This hormone has no specific target organ; instead, generalized tissue growth occurs. [CL: CO]

2. **(c)** The lipolytic or ketogenic effect of growth hormone results in increased fat stores in the liver and leads to the conversion of fatty acids to ketone bodies. [CL: KN]

3. **(c)** Drugs such as nicotine and chlorpropamide (Diabinese) stimulate vasopressin release. [CL: KN]

4. **(d)** In larger doses, vasopressin stimulates smooth muscle contraction, which is particularly evident in small arterioles. [CL: KN]

5. **(b)** Desmopressin increases factor VIII levels and is used to maintain hemostasis during and after surgery in patients with von Willebrand's disease. [CL: KN]

6. **(c)** Vasopressin is produced in the hypothalamus and stored in the posterior pituitary, to be released as needed by the body. [CL: KN]

7. **(a)** Somatotropin therapy is quite expensive, costing around $5,000 to $25,000 per year. [CL: CO]

8. **(d)** Secretion of growth hormone is suppressed by glucocorticoid drugs. [CL: KN]

9. **(b)** Alcohol inhibits vasopressin release. Other agents which depress vasopressin release included phenytoin and chlorpromazide. [CL: KN]

CHAPTER 42

1. **(b)** Common signs of adrenal cortex hypofunction (as in Addison's disease) include fluid and electrolyte imbalances resulting in water and sodium loss and potassium retention. [CL: KN]

2. **(d)** Angiotensin stimulates the release of aldosterone from the adrenal cortex. [CL: KN]

3. **(a)** Desoxycorticosterone pivalate (Pivalate) is a mineralocorticoid used to provide maintenance therapy for patients with salt-losing adrenogenital syndrome and adrenocortical insufficiency. [CL: KN]

4. **(d)** Corticotropin (ACTH) secreted by the anterior pituitary gland controls the release of glucocorticoids from the adrenal cortex. [CL: KN]

5. **(b)** The effect of glucocorticoids on protein metabolism leads to muscle weakness in all extremities, especially the lower extremities. [CL: KN]

6. **(c)** In some cases, glucocorticoid drugs are adjusted to mimic the normal diurnal pattern of cortisol excretion. [CL: CO]

7. **(b)** Redistribution of fat stores is associated with glucocorticoid therapy, resulting in a cervicodorsal fat pad or buffalo hump. [CL: CO]

8. **(a)** Abrupt withdrawal of long-term glucocorticoid therapy may result in syncope, muscular weakness, nausea, anorexia, and hypotension. [CL: KN]

9. **(c)** The synthetic corticosteroids are more potent than cortisone and hydrocortisone, which are natural products. Additionally, the sodium-retaining potential is greatly decreased or eliminated in synthetic products. [CL: KN]

CHAPTER 43

1. **(c)** Testosterone, the male sex hormone, produces a positive nitrogen balance and an increase in musculature as a result of its anabolic activity. [CL: KN]

2. **(c)** Certain carcinomas (prostate and male breast) may be exacerbated by the use of male hormone therapy. [CL: KN]

3. **(a)** Ethylestrenol (Maxibolin) is an anabolic steroid which promotes weight gain and bodybuilding processes.

4. **(a)** Estrogen increases the effects of hydrocortisone by potentiating the anti-inflammatory effect. [CL: KN]

5. **(c)** Androgens decrease the effect of oral anticoagulants, which, in the case of coumadin therapy, would be seen in subtherapeutic prothrombin times. [CL: AP]

6. **(d)** Oral contraceptives are contraindicated in patients with thrombophlebitis. When signs of calf pain and tenderness are reported, these agents should be discontinued. [CL: KN]

7. **(b)** The triphasic pill provides greater protection at midcycle, reducing the occurrence of breakthrough bleeding. [CL: KN]

8. **(b)** Patients using spermicidal creams should not douche for 6 to 8 hours after use, in order to maintain protection against pregnancy. [CL: KN]

9. **(d)** One milligram of diethylstilbesterol equals 0.5 mg of estradiol, 5 mg of conjugated estrogen, and 0.8 mg of mestranol. [CL: KN]

CHAPTER 44

1. **(d)** The fragments of fatty acid metabolism, which occurs in the absence of insulin, are referred to as ketone bodies. The presence of excess ketone bodies is termed ketosis. [CL: KN]

2. **(a)** A reduction in insulin availability results in increased triglycerides and increased conversion of fatty acids into phospholipids and cholesterol. This results in a greater risk for the development of atherosclerosis. [CL: CO]

3. **(b)** An insulin compound with longer action can be made by adding zinc, protamine, or globin. [CL: KN]

4. **(a)** Humalin insulin is recommended for those individuals who will be on insulin therapy intermittently, such as the gestational diabetic or the nondiabetic receiving parenteral nutrition. [CL: CO]

5. **(d)** Long-acting insulins are usually given with a short-acting insulin. In low doses, they suppress gluconeolysis and gluconeogenesis, mimicking physiologic insulin release. [CL: CO]

6. **(c)** Generally, a single dose of intermediate-acting insulin does not maintain adequate glucose control 24 hours a day. This method of treatment is often limited to the Type II diabetic over 60 years old. Strict control is not as urgent in these patients. [CL: KN]

7. **(a)** Concerning the biotransformation of insulin, the plasma half-life of insulin injected intravenously is less than 9 minutes. Antibody formation may extend the half-life up to 13 hours. [CL: KN]

8. **(c)** Late symptoms of hypoglycemia include blurred vision and disorientation. [CL: KN]

9. **(b)** Epinephrine antagonizes the effect of insulin by mobilizing glycogen to increase the blood glucose. [CL: KN]

10. **(b)** The presence of food delays absorption of glipizide (Glucotrol); therefore, it must be taken on an empty stomach. [CL: KN]

CHAPTER 45

1. **(b)** The ratio of T_4 to T_3 is 4:1. Decreased serum levels of T_3 and T_4 stimulate the pituitary gland to secrete TSh, which controls the release of thyroid hormones. [CL: KN]

2. **(b)** T_3 and T_4 function as regulators of metabolic rate and cell growth. They accelerate chemical reactions, oxygen consumption, and heat production. [CL: KN]

3. **(a)** The normal T/S ratio is 20:1. Hyperactivity or hypoactivity is reflected by this ratio. [CL: KN]

4. **(c)** Thyrocalcitonin is released in response to high serum calcium. It acts to decrease calcium absorption in the gut and to prevent resorption of calcium in the bone. [CL: KN]

5. **(d)** Parathormone affects bone, causing calcium resorption. [CL: CO]

6. **(a)** Thyroid hormones strengthen the rate and force of cardiac contraction, thereby increasing cardiac output to the tissues. [CL: KN]

Key to [Codes]: CL = Cognitive level; KN = Knowledge; CO = Comprehension; AP = Application; AN = Analysis

7. **(c)** Iodides act as antithyroid drugs by inhibiting the release of hormones into circulation, increasing the quantity of bound (inactive) hormone and reducing the vascularity of the thyroid gland. [CL: CO]

8. **(c)** In addition to inhibition of the synthesis of thyroid hormones, propylthiouracil partially inhibits the peripheral conversion of T_4 to T_3. [CL: KN]

9. **(c)** Vitamin D agents elevate serum calcium levels by stimulation of calcium absorption in the intestine and mobilization of calcium from bones. [CL: KN]

10. **(b)** Pruritus and urticaria are the most common adverse effects of antithyroid medications. [CL: KN]

CHAPTER 46

1. **(d)** Areas of the body where various bacteria, fungi, and protozoa exist include the skin, intestine, oropharynx, conjunctiva, and lower genitourinary tract. [CL: CO]

2. **(c)** An important factor to be considered when selecting an antibiotic for therapy is the sensitivity of the organism to antibiotics. [CL: KN]

3. **(b)** Ampicillin is stable in gastric contents and is well absorbed following oral administration. [CL: CO]

4. **(b)** While most antibiotics must be reduced or the interval increased in patients with renal insufficiency, some agents require no reduction in dosage. An example is clindamycin. [CL: KN]

5. **(a)** The addition of clavulanic acid, which is a beta-lactamase inhibitor, broadens the penicillin activity to include penicillinase-producing organisms. [CL: CO]

6. **(c)** Aztreonam, a monocyclic antibiotic, has an antibiotic activity which is limited to aerobic gramnegative rods. [CL: KN]

7. **(b)** Cilastatin inhibits dehydropeptidase in the proximal tubules. This enzyme inactivates imipenem. Cilastatin has no antibacterial activity. [CL: KN]

8. **(a)** Sulfonamides compete for the enzyme which synthesizes folic acid in bacterial cells. The effect is suppression of purine and DNA synthesis, resulting in cell death. [CL: CO]

9. **(d)** Erythromycin inhibits the metabolism of theophylline and may precipitate signs of theophylline toxicity. [CL: KN]

10. **(c)** The most common side effect of clindamycin therapy is diarrhea. If significant diarrhea occurs, the antibiotic should be discontinued. [CL: KN]

CHAPTER 47

1. **(a)** The prostaglandins, produced and released under certain circumstances, have actions which include increased capillary permeability, vasodilaton, increased cardiac output, and inhibition of platelet aggregation. [CL: KN]

2. **(d)** The release of prostaglandins inhibits gastric acid secretion and stabilizes the gastric mucosa. [CL: KN]

3. **(a)** Misoprostol produces urterine contractions which may endanger pregnancy. [CL: CO]

4. **(c)** Anti-inflammatory medications developed for short-term use provide pain relief and should be administered for only one to four weeks. Severe side effects can develop as a result of short-term therapy. [CL: CO]

5. **(b)** Histamines encourage phagocytic cells in the bloodstream to migrate to the place of injury. The phagocytic cells then attempt to engulf foreign particles present, releasing proteases and hydrolases in the process. [CL: KN]

6. **(d)** Salicylates act to relive the pain associated with arthritis by inhibiting prostaglandin synthesis. [CL: KN]

7. **(a)** Nonsteroidal anti-inflammatory agents decrease glomerular filtration rate and decrease renal blood flow; therefore, they should be used cautiously in patients with renal disease. [CL: CO]

8. **(c)** Phenylbutazone (Butazolidin) has many adverse side effects and is used only for short-term therapy. [CL: KN]

9. **(b)** D-penicillamine (Cuprimine) is a nonsteroidal anti-inflammatory agent which is used to treat rheumatoid arthritis. It is thought to have immunosupressive activity. [CL: KN]

10. **(a)** Meclofenamate sodium, a salicylate-like medication, has been known to cause diarrhea which can be severe in some cases. [CL: KN]

CHAPTER 48

1. **(d)** Malignant tumors or neoplasms differ from benign tumors in that they have the ability to invade surrounding tissue and metastasize. [CL: CO]

2. **(b)** During the S phase, actual DNA synthesis occurs, taking from 10 to 20 hours to double the DNA complement. [CL: KN]

3. **(d)** According to the Stem Cell Theory, only a small cell population has the potential to reproduce the entire tissue from its genetic storehouse. [CL: KN]

4. **(a)** In 1919 it was discovered that nitrogen mustard had leukopenic activity. Administration of chemotherapy began around 50 years ago. [CL: KN]

5. **(b)** Adjuvant chemotherapy is the administration of chemotherapy for the purpose of destroying micrometastasis and preventing the development of secondary tumors following the removal of the primary tumor. [CL: KN]

6. **(c)** Cell cycle-specific chemotherapeutic agents are designed to affect the cell during a specific phase of the cell life cycle. [CL: KN]

7. **(a)** Cisplatin is an example of an alkylating or cell-nonspecific agent used to treat disseminated carcinomas of the breast, ovaries, testes, and lungs. [CL: KN]

8. **(c)** Historically, chemotherapy was not considered first-line treatment for malignant disease. The major use of these agents was for treatment of hematologic and metastatic tumors. [CL: KN]

9. **(c)** Mechlorethamine (Mustargen) was first administered to patients in 1942. [CL: KN]

10. **(d)** Chemotherapeutic agents are generally more effective against dividing cells than against resting cells. [CL: KN]

CHAPTER 49

1. **(a)** The most accurate means of calculating dosages for all antineoplastic drugs is by using body surface area. [CL: KN]

2. **(d)** When mixing chemotherapeutic agents, the preparer should wear a face mask and protective clothing to guard against airborne particles or aerosolization of the drug. [CL: KN]

3. **(b)** Alkylating agents are derived from sulfur mustard gases and form electrophilic bonds with the guanine in DNA, thereby inactivating the cell replication process. [CL: CO]

4. **(d)** Cyclophosphamide is not a tumor-specific antimetabolite and is capable of cross-linking DNA in many normal cells as well as abnormal cells. [CL: KN]

5. **(c)** As an alkylating nitrosourea, carmustine is useful against primary and metastatic brain tumors because it is lipid soluble and crosses the blood-brain barrier. [CL: CO]

6. **(a)** Antimetabolites interfere with the metabolic pathways of dividing cells by their similarity to vitamins, coenzymes, or normal cell intermediary products. [CL: CO]

7. **(c)** Methotrexate is a folic acid antagonist which affects normal as well as malignant cell growth. In order to reduce potentially fatal toxic effects, leucovorin is administered to "rescue" the normal cells. Leucovorin provides a form of folic acid which can only be used by normal cells. [CL: KN]

8. **(d)** The antimetabolite fluorouracil (5-FU) works by inhibiting pyrimidine synthesis and, thereby, altering DNA synthesis. [CL: KN]

9. **(b)** Thioguanine is a purine antagonist, resulting in increased purine and uric acid levels. Secondary gouty arthritis is associated with abnormally high uric acid levels. [CL: CO]

10. **(b)** The vinca alkaloids are derivatives of the periwinkle plant and are cell cycle-specific. [CL: KN]

CHAPTER 50

1. **(b)** T-cells assist the B-cells in the synthesis of antibodies. This is a "helper" role only as they do not produce antibodies or antibody-like proteins. [CL: KN]

2. **(d)** B-cells mature in bursa-equivalent areas located in Peyer's patches in the intestines. [CL: KN]

3. **(c)** The presence of blocking factors or antibodies by tumor cells can inhibit the ability of the host organism to recognize the tumor cells as foreign. [CL: CO]

4. **(a)** Passive nonspecific immunotherapy is the injection of serum from healthy individuals into cancer patients. [CL: CO]

5. **(b)** Patients with lymphocyte predominant breast tumors have a well-documented improved prognosis over patients without lymphocytic infiltration. [CL: CO]

6. **(c)** When T-cells are sensitized by foreign antigens, soluble factors called lymphokines are released. An example is migration inhibitory factor (MIF), which activates and draws tissue macrophages to the tumor cell site. [CL: CO]

7. **(c)** One of the basic goals in cancer immunotherapy is to promote and stimulate immunocompetence by active or passive methods. [CL: KN]

8. **(b)** Immunorestorative immunotherapy uses substances such as interferon to augment the patient's own immune system. [CL: KN]

9. **(b)** The vaccine BCG should be protected from light and kept in refrigeration to retain potency. [CL: KN]

10. **(a)** Commonly seen side effects of interferon therapy include flu-like symptoms, such as fever, chills, myalgia, fatigue, and/or headache. [CL: KN]

CHAPTER 51

1. **(a)** The pyloric glands produce mucus which protects the gastric mucosa. [CL: KN]

2. **(c)** Enterogastrone, a hormone produced in the small intestine, helps to regulate gastric emptying. [CL: KN]

3. **(c)** The large intestine is composed of the cecum, colon, and rectum and is about 1.5 meters long. [CL: KN]

Key to [Codes]: CL = Cognitive level; KN = Knowledge; CO = Comprehension; AP = Application; AN = Analysis

4. **(a)** Villikinin is a hormone secreted by the intestinal wall which allows the villi to absorb increased nutrients through active transport and passive diffusion. [CL: CO]

5. **(d)** The crypts of Lieberkuhn are small glands located along the surface of the small intestine. These glands secrete approximately 2000 ml of alkaline secretions daily. The secretions contain special enzymes which enable final digestion of food before absorption. [CL: KN]

6. **(d)** Bacterial action in the small intestine helps in splitting food by-products. [CL: KN]

7. **(b)** The effect of the sympathetic nervous system on the gastrointestinal system results in slowing or cessation of function. [CL: KN]

8. **(c)** The liver stores, rather than synthesizes, Vitamins A, D, and B$_{12}$. The liver performs more than 500 individual functions. [CL: CO]

9. **(c)** The pancreas produces insulin and glucagon as an endocrine function. Chymotrypsin is released as an exocrine function. [CL: KN]

10. **(b)** Cytochrome P-450 is a substance produced in the liver which plays a vital role in drug biotransformation. [CL: KN]

CHAPTER 52

1. **(d)** Antacids interact with gastric secretions, neutralizing some of the hydrochloric acid secretion and increasing the gastric pH. [CL: CO]

2. **(d)** Milk-alkali syndrome, caused by overuse of sodium bicarbonate and calcium carbonate, is characterized by hypercalcemia, alkalosis, and renal failure. [CL: KN]

3. **(a)** Anticholinergics are used as adjuncts in the management of peptic ulcers. They relieve pain by inhibiting motility and secretions. [CL: KN]

4. **(b)** Antacids decrease the absorption of tetracycline antibiotics by binding with them to form complexes which are difficult to absorb. [CL: KN]

5. **(c)** Anticholinergics suppress perspiration; therefore, patients should avoid excessive heat for they are at risk for heat strokes. [CL: KN]

6. **(b)** The belladonna alkaloids are readily absorbed from the gastrointestinal tract and readily cross the blood-brain barrier. [CL: KN]

7. **(b)** When aluminum antacids bind with phosphate in the bowel, they produce hypophosphatemia with prolonged use. Symptoms of this adverse effect include muscle weakness, anorexia, and malaise. [CL: KN]

8. **(c)** Aluminum antacids relax gastric smooth muscles and delay gastric emptying in addition to their neutralizing action. [CL: KN]

9. **(a)** The Acid Neutralizing Capacity (ANC) is expressed as the mEq of hydrochloride required to keep an antacid suspension at pH 3.0 for 2 hours in vitro. A high ANC denotes an effective antacid. [CL: KN]

CHAPTER 53

1. **(b)** Antiemetics act locally or centrally to relieve nausea and vomiting. They are used to prevent nausea and vomiting rather than to treat the cause. [CL: KN]

2. **(a)** Extrapyramidal symptoms seen with high doses of phenothiazines include acute dystonia, which is characterized by spasms of the tongue, face, neck, and back. [CL: CO]

3. **(d)** Scopolamine is an anticholinergic agent which is most effective in preventing motion sickness. Major side effects are blurred vision and dry mouth. [CL: KN]

4. **(d)** Antihistamines inhibit the transmission of impulses along the vestibular portion of the eighth cranial nerve. They also act on the vomiting center to reduce stimulation. [CL: KN]

5. **(c)** Antidopaminergics work by reducing sensitivity to dopamine stimulation in the chemoreceptor trigger zone in the vomiting center. An example of such an agent is promethazine (Phenergan). [CL: KN]

6. **(c)** Akathisia refers to motor restlessness and anxiety. Patients may pace back and forth or have continuous nonpurposeful movement of an extremity. [CL: KN]

7. **(d)** Patients using the Transderm-Scop system need to be cautioned about drowsiness, a common side effect. Patients using the patch should not operate heavy equipment. [CL: CO]

8. **(b)** Due to possible teratogenic effects, antiemetics are contraindicated during pregnancy. [CL: KN]

9. **(a)** Dronabinol (Marinol) is a cannabinoid which has the principal psychoactive substance found in *Cannabis sativa* (marijuana). This controlled substance is indicated for persons receiving chemotherapy who have not responded to other antiemetics.

CHAPTER 54

1. **(c)** Pancrelipase is used for symptomatic treatment of malabsorption syndromes, such as cystic fibrosis. [CL: KN]

2. **(a)** Absorbents have a tendency to bind with drugs given concurrently, thereby inhibiting their absorption. It is best to separate absorbents and routine medications by at least 2 hours. [CL: KN]

3. **(d)** Lomotil contains a small amount of atropine, which can cause side effects such as dry mouth, blurred vision, nausea, and vomiting. [CL: KN]

4. **(c)** Paregoric tincture contains 2 mg morphine per 5 ml and 45 percent alcohol. Morphine is very effective

in treating diarrhea, but is not commonly used. [CL: KN]

5. **(b)** Patients on antibiotic therapy often have diarrhea because the normal bacterial flora of the intestine are destroyed. Lactinex encourages the growth of normal intestinal flora and reduces gastrointestinal complications associated with antibiotic therapy. [CL: CO]

6. **(d)** Donnagel contains atropine and hyoscyamine sulfate. These medications are contraindicated in patients with narrow-angle glaucoma. [CL: KN]

7. **(b)** Castor oil is a contact/stimulant laxative which directly stimulates small intestine smooth muscle and inhibits water and electrolyte reabsorption from the intestinal lumen. [CL: KN]

8. **(d)** Patients taking cascara may notice a change in urine color. The drug may tint acid urine a yellow-brown or alkaline urine a reddish color. [CL: CO]

9. **(a)** Senna, an anthraquinone derivative, is converted to active aglycones in the colon. The aglycones stimulate Auerbach's plexus to induce peristalsis and bowel evacuation. [CL: KN]

CHAPTER 55

1. **(d)** Mucomyst provides glutathione to the liver cells, preventing cell damage from the buildup of acetaminophen metabolites. [CL: KN]

2. **(a)** In hepatic disease, ascites develops because of several factors, one of which is increased aldosterone production. Fluid retention is further increased due to decreased aldosterone metabolism in the liver. Spironolactone (Aldactone) is an aldosterone antagonist which produces a helpful diuresis. [CL: KN]

3. **(c)** The symptoms related to phase I of hepatic encephalopathy are personality changes, agitation, vacant stare, and difficulty performing calculations. [CL: KN]

4. **(a)** The most common adverse effect of Heptavax B is pain and soreness at the injection site. [CL: KN]

5. **(c)** Lactulose is effective in reducing ammonia levels in patients with encephalopathy and improving protein tolerance in patients with advanced cirrhosis. [CL: CO]

CHAPTER 56

1. **(c)** Anabolism is the synthesis of cellular elements for the process of cellular growth, maintenance, and tissue repair. When food intake exceeds metabolic demands, anabolism occurs and weight gain results. [CL: KN]

2. **(b)** Epinephrine acts to mobilize substrates to provide energy, resulting in catabolism. The action of epinephrine results in inhibition of protein and carbohydrate synthesis. [CL: KN]

3. **(b)** When nutrients are not supplied to the body in adequate amounts, as in starvation, the body begins to break down fats to fatty acids and ketone bodies for energy in order to spare protein. [CL: KN]

4. **(a)** Meal replacement formulas which are milk-based are nutritionally complete and used in patients with an intact digestive system. They are high in lactose and should not be used for patients who are lactose intolerant. [CL: CO]

5. **(c)** The fat content in most commercial formulas can be up to 47 percent of the total calories. Fats increase the calorie content without increasing osmolarity. [CL: KN]

6. **(d)** PFE administration is contraindicated for patients with disturbances in fat metabolism, such as patients with acute pancreatitis associated with hyperlipemia. [CL: KN]

7. **(b)** Adverse reactions to intravenous lipid emulsion can include allergic reactions, such as chills, fever, diaphoresis, chest pain, or back pain. Initial administration should begin at 1 ml/minute for the first 15 to 30 minutes. [CL: KN]

8. **(a)** Thirst is one of the first signs of impending dehydration from administration of hyperosmolar enteral formulas. [CL: KN]

9. **(c)** When tube feeding is administered too rapidly, the distended stomach may be pushed up against the diaphragm and interfere with adequate chest expansion. This may result in respiratory distress. [CL: CO]

10. **(a)** A TPN solution should be initiated slowly, usually at a rate of 40 to 50 ml/hour and increased over a 24-hour period to the desired rate. This allows for the body to adjust to utilization of the TPN products. [CL: KN]

CHAPTER 57

1. **(c)** Five minerals are considered to be essential for maintaining health and are needed by the body daily. These are calcium, magnesium, sodium, potassium, and phosphorus. [CL: KN]

2. **(d)** Minerals are naturally occurring nonorganic solid substances which are carried via the blood to target organs. [CL: KN]

3. **(c)** Four fat-soluble vitamins are utilized by the body. They include Vitamins, A, D, E, and K. [CL: KN]

4. **(b)** Toxic side effects of Vitamin A are numerous. Alopecia, skin changes, hepatic dysfunction, and diplopia have been reported. [CL: KN]

5. **(b)** Vitamin D increases the absorption of calcium in the gut and the reabsorption of phosphorus by the renal tubules. This vitamin is used in the treatment of hypocalcemia. [CL: KN]

6. **(a)** Vitamin E appears to retard the hemolysis of red blood cells and has been found to be therapeutic in the management of certain anemias. [CL: CO]

7. **(c)** Aquamephyton is a derivative identical to Vitamin K_1. It should be given slowly by intravenous administration, not to exceed 1 mg/minute. Severe reactions have been reported as the result of rapid IV infusion. [CL: KN]

8. **(d)** Alcoholics are most likely to develop thiamine deficiencies due to inadequate dietary intake during periods of heavy drinking. [CL: KN]

9. **(a)** Pyridoxine enhances the peripheral metabolism of levodopa when taken in doses of greater than 5 mg daily. When Vitamin B_6 and levodopa are taken concurrently, the dosage of levodopa may need to be increased. [CL: KN]

10. **(b)** Elevated copper levels may be produced by estrogen compounds, thyroid, or corticotropin. [CL: KN]

CHAPTER 58

1. **(b)** As the major cation in the extracellular fluid, sodium maintains osmotic pressure and serum osmolarity. [CL: KN]

2. **(b)** Potassium products should not be given concurrently with potassium-sparing diuretics, such as spironolactone. Hyperkalemia can result in 1 to 2 days. [CL: KN]

3. **(a)** Skeletal muscle weakness is a common symptom of hypokalemia. In addition, patients may exhibit decreased reflexes and ST depression on the ECG. [CL: KN]

4. **(c)** This suspension lowers potassium by exchanging it with sodium in the intestine. When administering agent rectally, the patient should retain the enema for 30 to 60 minutes for optimal action. [CL: KN]

5. **(d)** Signs/symptoms associated with hypocalcemia include drowsiness and lethargy due to neurological hypofunction. [CL: KN]

6. **(a)** Magnesium slows conduction in the heart; therefore, intravenous administration is contraindicated in patients with heart block. [CL: KN]

7. **(d)** In acidosis there is more ionized or free calcium, and serum calcium levels increase. [CL: CO]

8. **(c)** Calcium products bind with tetracycline and inhibit absorption. Patients should avoid taking calcium with tetracycline antibiotics. [CL: KN]

9. **(d)** Phosphate promotes white blood cells' phagocytic action as well as supplying essential metabolic processes, such as ATP production. [CL: KN]

10. **(a)** Hyperkalemia, potassium excess, can produce high peaked T waves on the ECG. [CL: CO]

CHAPTER 59

1. **(a)** The vascular middle layer of the eye is composed of the ciliary body, iris, and choroid. [CL: KN]

2. **(c)** The retina, inner layer of the eye, is composed of several layers of nerve cells which translate light waves into neural impulses which are then transmitted via the optic nerve to the brain. [CL: KN]

3. **(b)** The fovea centralis is composed of cone cells and is the portion of the retina where visual acuity is the greatest. [CL: KN]

4. **(c)** The image enters the eye through the cornea and aqueous humor. It is then transmitted through the lens and the vitreous humor to the retina. [CL: CO]

5. **(b)** Myopia is the inability to see distant objects. In this condition, the image focuses in front of the retina. [CL: KN]

6. **(d)** The accommodation reflex allows the pupil to become smaller when the gaze shifts from a distant to a close object. This allows us to see printed material as well as large or distant objects. [CL: KN]

7. **(d)** The vestibule is a portion of the inner ear that is involved with changes in posture and balance. [CL: KN]

8. **(b)** The cochlea is stimulated by sound vibrations and the cilia of the organ of Corti send impulses to the brain via the acoustic nerve. [CL: CO]

9. **(c)** The function of the inner ear, which is composed of the auricle and meatus, is to funnel sound through the auditory canal to the middle and inner ear. [CL: CO]

10. **(a)** Normally, intraocular pressure is maintained at 12 to 25 mmHg. In conditions such as glaucoma, the intraocular pressure rises to 60 mmHg or more. [CL: KN]

CHAPTER 60

1. **(b)** Fluorescein sodium, a nontoxic water-soluble dye, stains denuded areas of the epithelium of the eye. The preparation can be used to test lacrimal patency, demonstrated by the appearance of dye in nasal secretions. [CL: KN]

2. **(a)** Idoxuridine should be administered for 5 to 7 days after healing has occurred in order to prevent a recurrence of herpes. [CL: KN]

3. **(d)** Anti-inflammatory medications are used to treat some nonpyrogenic inflammatory conditions of the eye. Their action reduces inflammation and permanent scarring. [CL: KN]

4. **(d)** The direct-acting cholinergic miotics reduce intraocular pressure by constricting the pupil, causing spasms of the ciliary muscle and decreasing the resistance to outflow of aqueous humor. [CL: CO]

5. **(b)** Ocusert is an eye insert which releases pilocarpine slowly into the eye for a period of about 1 week. The insert should be rinsed gently with tap water prior to insertion to prevent a large initial release of pilocarpine. [CL: KN]

6. **(c)** Physostigmine is a cholinesterase inhibitor which inhibits cholinesterase and enhances the effect of endogenous acetylcholine on the eye. [CL: KN]

7. **(b)** Concurrent use of beta-blocker ophthalmic agents with digitalis products may have an addictive slowing effect on the cardiac conduction system. [CL: CO]

8. **(b)** Acetazolamide is a carbonic anhydrase inhibitor which interferes with production of carbonic acid. This leads to systemic acidosis and reduced aqueous humor formation. [CL: CO]

9. **(c)** Alpha-adrenergic agents contract the dilator muscle of the iris, causing dilation of the pupil. These agents have only a slight effect on the ciliary muscle. [CL: KN]

10. **(d)** Osmotic diuretics are used to treat glaucoma in patients resistant to the effects of miotics of carbonic anhydrase. Osmotic agents are given cautiously to patients with congestive heart failure because the heart may not be able to handle the larger fluid volume produced by the pulling of fluid from the tissues. [CL: KN]

CHAPTER 61

1. **(d)** The most frequently used irrigating solution for the ear is Burow's solution (aluminum acetate solution). [CL: KN]

2. **(b)** First line drugs which are effective in treating otitis media are amoxicillin (Amoxil) and ampicillin (Polycillin). [CL: KN]

3. **(a)** Antihistamine-decongestants are thought to improve eustachian tube patency and enhance drainage from the middle ear. [CL: KN]

4. **(c)** Aminoglycoside antibiotics may damage the eighth cranial nerve, causing irreversible hearing loss. [CL: KN]

5. **(c)** Penicillin G and penicillin V are not effective against *Hemophilus influenzae*. The agent of choice is ampicillin. [CL: KN]

CHAPTER 62

1. **(b)** Enzymes are proteins which are synthesized from plant and animal sources. Enzymes are catalysts for chemical reactions, but are not altered by the reaction. [CL: CO]

2. **(c)** Sutilains functions best at a pH range of 6.0 to 6.8. This proteolytic enzyme is inactive on viable tissue. Loose, wet dressings should be placed on wound after sutilains is applied. [CL: KN]

3. **(b)** The skin should be cleansed with water or isotonic saline prior to applying sutilains. The use of iodine, hexachlorophene, or detergents decreases the effectiveness of sutilains. [CL: KN]

4. **(d)** Elase is a proteolytic and fibrinolytic enzyme derived from bovine sources. Patients allergic to beef may exhibit allergic reactions to this enzyme. [CL: CO]

5. **(b)** When digestive enzymes are absorbed bucally, mild stinging may occur. This is usually relieved by removing the tablet. [CL: KN]

CHAPTER 63

1. **(a)** The second main layer of skin is the dermis, which contains collagen and elastin in addition to a network of nerves and capillaries. [CL: KN]

2. **(c)** Emollients have fixed oils, such as olive, flaxseed, or cottonseed, as a base and are used to treat dry, cracked skin. [CL: KN]

3. **(c)** Mild pain and transient burning are the major side effects of acyclovir. [CL: KN]

4. **(b)** Corticosteroids have vasoconstrictive actions when used topically. In addition, they are anti-inflammatory and antipruritic. [CL: KN]

5. **(d)** The area to be treated is cleansed well with soap and water. Any scales or crusts are removed before applying the medication. [CL: CO]

6. **(b)** Treatment of skin lesions may take considerable time. Some skin conditions are slow to heal and must be evaluated frequently, usually on a daily basis. [CL: KN]

Key to [Codes]: CL = Cognitive level; KN = Knowledge; CO = Comprehension; AP = Application; AN = Analysis

7. **(b)** Reactions to medications may occur up to a year after discontinuing; therefore, a complete medication history should be obtained. Generally, the patient is taken off all medications, if possible, to discover the problem. [CL: CO]

CHAPTER 64

1. **(b)** Passive immunity provides immediate protection, but does not last for an extended period of time. Its effectiveness in treating disease is limited. [CL: CO]

2. **(c)** Diphtheria is a toxoid vaccine in which detoxified but antigenically active poisons are administered. Toxoids provide an excellent immunity. [CL: KN]

3. **(a)** Children younger than 15 months have passive immunity acquired from the mother. If immunized earlier than 15 months, the maternal antibodies will destroy the attenuated virus before the child's active immunity is stimulated. [CL: CO]

4. **(d)** Neomycin is utilized in the production of the attenuated virus for the measles vaccine. Persons allergic to neomycin may react hypersensitively. [CL: KN]

5. **(c)** By changing the needle after the vaccine has been withdrawn from the vial, local tissue reaction to the injection can be reduced. [CL: KN]

6. **(b)** Varicella-zoster virus is the infective organism responsible for chickenpox. [CL: KN]

7. **(c)** Active immunity may take from 5 to 14 days to develop after primary immunization. [CL: KN]

8. **(a)** The child who is at high risk should be vaccinated for Hib if between the ages of 18 and 23 months. Otherwise, the initial vaccination should be given at 24 months. [CL: KN]

9. **(c)** If active TB treatment drugs are given along with BCG, they will cause the vaccine to be ineffective. [CL: KN]

CHAPTER 65

1. **(b)** The intravenous route for medication is preferable for the patient with heart failure. [CL: CO]

2. **(a)** If an IV access is not available, drugs such as epinephrine, atropine, and lidocaine can be administered endotracheally. [CL: KN]

3. **(a)** Beta-blockers block sympathetic response to increased fluid volume, worsening congestive heart failure. [CL: CO]

4. **(c)** Assessment findings related to pulmonary edema are severe dyspnea, pink, frothy sputum, rales, hypertension, and tachycardia. [CL: KN]

5. **(b)** Dobutamine (Dobutrex) is a positive inotropic agent which improves cardiac output and performance. [CL: KN]

6. **(a)** For the control of seizures in status epilepticus, diazepam (Valium) should be given slowly intravenously. [CL: KN]

7. **(c)** The patient is exhibiting signs and symptoms of thyroid storm. Propylthiouracil is a drug which can be used in this situation because it blocks the release of thyroid hormone. [CL: KN]

8. **(a)** A patent airway must be maintained and is a top priority for the nurse in an emergency situation. [CL: KN]

9. **(d)** Patients in acute adrenal insufficiency exhibit signs of dehydration, hypotension, weakness, and abdominal pain. [CL: KN]

10. **(c)** Atropine sulfate produces an anticholinergic response to block release of acetylcholine and improves the patient's condition. [CL: KN]

CHAPTER 66

1. **(d)** Dimercaprol is the antidote for arsenic, gold, and/or mercury toxicity by promoting urinary excretion. In order to protect the kidneys, the urine is kept alkaline. [CL: KN]

2. **(b)** Sotradecol and morrhuate can cause asthmatic symptoms as an adverse effect; therefore, they are contraindicated in patients with the disease. [CL: KN]

3. **(c)** In order to ensure even buccal absorption of nicotine, the gum should be chewed slowly and intermittently for 30 minutes. [CL: KN]

4. **(b)** Adverse effects of antihemophilic A factor include chest tightness, wheezing, and other signs of allergic response. The physician should be notified of these effects immediately. [CL: KN]

5. **(d)** Changes in blood pressure may occur in patients using minoxidil for male pattern baldness; therefore, monitoring blood pressure regularly is important. [CL: CO]

ANSWERS, RATIONALES, AND CODES FOR SITUATION QUESTIONS

SITUATION 1–1

1. **(c)** Hypothetical questions are useful in determining patient comprehension of previously learned material. [NP: AS, CL: AN]

2. **(a)** An allergic reaction may be manifested by a rash. The other symptoms are considered undesirable adverse drug effects. [NP: AS, CL: CO]

3. **(a)** Heavy smokers may require higher doses of theophylline in order for it to be effective. [NP: EV, CL: AN]

4. **(b)** Barbiturates may cause unexpected abnormal reactions, such as restlessness and excitability, in the elderly. [NP: EV, CL: AN]

5. **(d)** Alcohol may cause a rapid rise in blood pressure when taken with MAO inhibitors. [NP: IM, CL: AP]

6. **(c)** A drug interaction between Warfarin and aspirin may result in bleeding. [NP: EV, CL: AN]

SITUATION 2–1

1. **(c)** One of the nurse's major responsibilities is to provide education regarding drug effectiveness and adverse effects. [NP: IM, CL: CO]

2. **(a)** Hospital orders for Valium are valid for 7 days and require a physician's reorder for continuation. [NP: PL, CL: KN]

3. **(c)** Talwin is classified as a Schedule IV controlled drug, and a prescription must be rewritten after 6 months or 5 refills. [NP: IM, CL: KN]

4. **(d)** Even with FDA approval, medications may be discovered to be toxic or fatal once administered to a large group of individuals. [NP: PL, CL: CO]

5. **(a)** Narcotics which are drawn up and not used must be returned to the point of origin, usually the hospital pharmacy. The nurse cannot discard the entire dose. [NP: IM, CL: AP]

6. **(c)** In obtaining a verbal order for a Schedule II substance, such as Demerol, the physician must countersign the order within 48 hours. [NP: IM, CL: AP]

SITUATION 3–1

1. **(d)** Local medications produce effects that are confined to one area of the body; a caplet is an oral dosage form that is absorbed systemically. [NP: IM, CL: CO]

2. **(a)** Administration of water with guaifenesin will ensure entry into the stomach and enhance absorption. [NP: IM, CL: AP]

3. **(c)** Crushing a sustained-release drug will interfere with the timed-release property of the drug preparation. [NP: IM, CL: AP]

4. **(c)** IV administration places the drug directly into the vasculature, thus bypassing all barriers to drug absorption. [NP: IM, CL: KN]

5. **(b)** Suppositories are designed to melt at body temperature; thus, they are stored in a cool place. [NP: AN, CL: AP]

6. **(c)** Transdermal scopolamine disks are applied be-

Key to [Codes]; NP = Nursing process phase; AS = Assessment; AN = Analysis; PL = Planning; IM = Implementation; EV = Evaluation; CL = Cognitive level; KN = Knowledge; CO = Comprehension; AP = Application; AN = Analysis

hind the ear and are not affected by water. [NP: IM, CL: AP]

SITUATION 3–2

1. **(d)** Antibiotics are best given around the clock at regular intervals to maintain therapeutic blood levels. [NP: PL, CL: CO]

2. **(d)** The nurse is responsible for administering the correct dose of the ordered drug. The physician is responsible for changing the dosage if needed. [NP: IM, CL: CO]

3. **(d)** The implementation of IV therapy has no direct effect on social interaction. [NP: AN, CL: AP]

4. **(a)** Answers b, c, and d are all important for the nurse to assess prior to administering medications. A rapid pulse may not be a reason to withhold medication. [NP: IM, CL: CO]

5. **(c)** Effective handwashing will decrease the chance of infection. [NP: IM, CL: AP]

6. **(b)** A concentrated, or bolus, dose is given directly into the vein over a period of at least 1 to 2 minutes. [NP: IM, CO: KN)

SITUATION 4–1

1. **(c)** A prior occurrence of hives following penicillin administration indicates that the patient has developed an allergy to the drug and should not receive penicillin or related preparations again. [NP: IM, CL: AN]

2. **(d)** Food decreases the absorption rate of erythromycin. [NP: IM, CL: AP]

3. **(a)** Aspirin, an acidic drug, is better absorbed in the small intestine if administered with an antacid. [NP: IM, CL: AP]

4. **(a)** Penicillin G is able to cross the blood–brain barrier and provide effective treatment for central nervous system pathology. [NP: PL, CL: CO]

5. **(c)** Elderly patients may have decreased function of the liver enzyme systems needed for drug biotransformation, with resultant toxic drug complications. [NP: IM, CL: AN]

6. **(b)** Desensitization may occur with repeated use of beta-adrenergic bronchodilators, resulting in decreased response to treatment. [NP: AS, CL: AP]

SITUATION 5–1

1. **(b)** Quinidine is capable of displacing digoxin from its tissue binding sites. When these drugs are given together, digoxin dosage needs to be reduced. [NP: AN, CL: AN]

2. **(d)** Ototoxicity is the manifestation of a combined toxicity when an aminoglycoside antibiotic and furosemide are used together in therapy. [NP: EV, CL: AN]

3. **(d)** Calcium, a heavy metal found in milk, forms a complex with tetracycline, thus decreasing absorption of this antibiotic. [NP: EV, CL: CO]

4. **(b)** Drug absorption is affected by altering the intestinal mucosa as with antineoplastic therapy. [NP: PL, CL: AN]

5. **(a)** Biotransformation, which occurs in the liver, can affect drug concentration at the site of action. [NP: AN, CL: AN]

6. **(b)** Tagamet alters GI pH and thus may alter oral drug absorption. [NP: AS, CL: AN]

SITUATION 5–2

1. **(d)** An additive effect occurs when two drugs with the same effect, such as aspirin and codeine, are combined. The result is an enhanced effect. [NP: IM, CL: AP]

2. **(c)** The two drugs, working to lower the blood pressure by different mechanisms, produce an antihypertensive effect greater than either drug would by itself. This is an example of synergism. [NP: AN, CL: CO]

3. **(b)** Calcium binds with chocolate, thus reducing the absorption of the drug. [NP: IM, CL: AP]

4. **(c)** Licorice promotes potassium excretion, which is also a major adverse effect of diuretics such as Lasix. [NP: EV, CL: AP]

5. **(d)** Chinese food often contains large amounts of monosodium glutamate, which can enhance the effects of MAO inhibitors. [NP: EV, CL: AP]

6. **(a)** Tuna fish contains a high histamine content, which may interact with isoniazid to produce a histamine reaction. [NP: EV, CL: AP]

SITUATION 6–1

1. **(b)** Type II allergic reactions are often seen in patients receiving diphtheria and tetanus antitoxin. Symptoms include fever, rash, arthralgia, splenomegaly, and lymph node enlargement. [NP: AS, CL: AP]

2. **(d)** This patient presents signs and symptoms related to an anaphylactic reaction due to penicillin. Emergency treatment includes epinephrine, antihistamines, bronchodilators, and vasopressors. [NP: PL, CL: AN]

3. **(c)** One of the most common drugs which cause a delayed hypersensitivity reaction is benzene. If symptoms of contact dermatitis occur, the product should be completely washed from the skin and not used again. [NP: IM, CL: CO]

4. **(a)** An idiosyncratic reaction is one that occurs unexpectedly in a small portion of patients. An example of this type of reaction would be symptoms of systemic lupus erythematosus related to Pronestyl. The reaction is due to a deficiency of N-acetyltransferase. [NP: AN, CL: CO]

5. **(b)** Quinidine is a drug known to cause thrombocytopenia (reduced platelets). [NP: AS, CL: AP]

6. **(d)** The first action should be to take a set of vital signs as a baseline assessment. [NP: AS, CL: AP]

SITUATION 7–1

1. **(a)** Taking antihistamines at bedtime will reduce the effect of sedation. [NP: IM, CL: AP]

2. **(d)** In elderly patients, antihistamines may cause dizziness, confusion, and hypotension. Reduced rhinorrhea is a desired effect. [NP: IM, CL: CO]

3. **(c)** Calcium carbonate, a calcium-containing antacid, may cause increased gastric secretion and should be avoided when ulcer healing is indicated. [NP: AN, CL: AP]

4. **(a)** Antihistamines are contraindicated for patients with narrow-angle glaucoma. [NP: IM, CL: AP]

5. **(b)** Arrhythmias may occur when digitalis preparations are taken with decongestants. [NP: AN, CL: CO]

6. **(b)** Aluminum hydroxide is used to treat hyperphosphatemia, common in renal failure patients, because it prevents absorption of phosphate from the GI tract. [NP: PL, CL: AP]

SITUATION 8–1

1. **(a)** An individual will not learn until readiness to learn is displayed. [NP: AS, CL: CO]

2. **(c)** If printed material is not readable by the patient, the written information will not be understood. [NP: AN, CL: KN]

3. **(b)** Skinner's conditioning theory focuses on reinforcement as a motivator. [NP: PL, CL: KN]

4. **(b)** Personal involvement in the learning event is a component of experiential learning. [NP: AN, CL: CO]

5. **(d)** A recent diagnosis may increase the patient's stress and anxiety level, thus interfering with effective learning. [NP: AS, CL: AN]

6. **(a)** One of the major ways by which experiential learning becomes responsible learning is through self-evaluation. [NP: EV, CL: KN]

SITUATION 8–2

1. **(b)** The pre-teaching phase of Ausubel's theory is probably the most useful in assessing the patient's readiness to learn. [NP: AS, CL: CO]

2. **(d)** By posing questions, an individual displays motivation by desiring greater knowledge about practical health care. [NP: AS, CL: AN]

3. **(b)** Anxiety may occur when a lack of knowledge regarding a specific event is identified. [NP: AN, CL: AN]

4. **(a)** Teaching goals related to discharge are realized well in advance of discharge to avoid misunderstanding and noncompliance. [NP: PL, CL: CO]

5. **(d)** Medication teaching responsibilities for the nurse include the purpose of drug therapy as well as method and proper timing of medication administration. [NP: IM, CL: CO]

6. **(c)** Smiling is an example of a universal non-verbal positive reinforcer. [NP: IM, CL: AP]

SITUATION 9–1

1. **(d)** Barium is eliminated unchanged in the feces, requiring several days for evacuation. For this reason, the barium enema should be performed before the barium swallow. [NP: PL, CL: CO]

2. **(b)** Barium administration is contraindicated in patients with perforation of the gastrointestinal tract or intestinal obstruction. If signs of perforation or obstruction are observed, such as increased abdominal pain, rigidity, or nausea, the physician should be informed. [NP: IM, CL: AN]

3. **(a)** Nursing actions following barium enema include encouraging intake of oral fluids. [NP: PL, CL: CO]

4. **(d)** Administration of a barium enema may stimulate a vagal response resulting in bradycardia and hypotension. This occurs more frequently in the older adult. [NP: AS, CL: CO]

5. **(c)** Dehydration can occur when elderly patients are kept NPO and receive numerous enemas. [NP: AN, CL: AN]

6. **(d)** Determining the effect of the patient's past experiences with diagnostic testing is an aspect of nursing assessment. [NP: EV, CL: CO]

SITUATION 10–1

1. **(b)** Halothane is associated with myocardial and respiratory depressant effects. The drug can also cause hepatotoxicity. [NP: IM, CL: CO]

Key to [Codes]; NP = Nursing process phase; AS = Assessment; AN = Analysis; PL = Planning; IM = Implementation; EV = Evaluation; CL = Cognitive level; KN = Knowledge; CO = Comprehension; AP = Application; AN = Analysis

2. **(d)** Mental alertness is generally depressed for 2 to 3 hours following use of isoflurane. Postanesthesia nausea and excitation are rare. There is less of a tendency to develop dysrhythmias than with other agents. [NP: PL, CL: KN]

3. **(c)** About 12 percent of patients receiving Ketamine experience disturbing dreams. [NP: IM, CL: KN]

4. **(c)** Narcan is a narcotic antagonist; when administered, patients can experience intense pain. [NP: IM, CL: AP]

5. **(a)** When Pavulon, a nondepolarizing block, is no longer needed, it can be reversed by administration of an antidote mixture of neostigmine and atropine. [NP: PL, CL: CO]

6. **(b)** A possible reaction to general anesthesia related to Inderal taken preoperatively is hypotension. [NP: AS, CL: KN]

SITUATION 10–2

1. **(c)** Methohexital sodium (Brevital) is less likely to cause bronchospasm and may, therefore, be administered cautiously to patients with asthma. [NP: AS, CL: AP]

2. **(a)** Droperidol/fentanyl can cause bradycardia; therefore, it is essential that atropine be kept readily available. [NP: PL, CL: CO]

3. **(d)** After administration of succinylcholine, potassium is forced out of muscle cells and into circulation. Hyperkalemia is a relative contraindication to its use. [NP: AN, CL: CO]

4. **(c)** Severe hypertension may result if Xylocaine with epinephrine is given to patients taking MAO inhibitors or tricyclic antidepressant drugs. [NP: AN, CL: KN]

5. **(b)** Procaine hydrochloride is not irritating to soft tissues or nerves. [NP: PL, CL: CO]

6. **(a)** Alfenta should be used with caution in patients with impaired renal function as reflected by creatinine levels. [NP: AS, CL: AN]

SITUATION 11–1

1. **(a)** A clinical sign of dehydrating is poor skin turgor. [NP: AS, CL: AP]

2. **(c)** Baseline data, such as patient weights, electrolytes, and laboratory tests, are obtained prior to starting the IV. [NP: AS, CL: CO]

3. **(a)** When intake is less than output, dehydration occurs. This results in greater concentration of particles in the extracellular space. To compensate, fluid moves from the intracellular space to the extracellular space, and the cells become shrunken. [NP: AN, CL: AP]

4. **(c)** 2.5 percent dextrose + 0.45 percent sodium chloride is an example of a hydrating solution which is hypotonic in composition. [NP: AN, CL: AN]

5. **(d)** Hypotonic solutions should be given slowly because a sudden shift of fluid into the cells can occur. [NP: PL, CL: KN]

6. **(b)** With adequate hydration and renal function, urine output should exceed 30 cc per hour. [NP: EV, CL: AN]

SITUATION 11–2

1. **(d)** Respiratory alkalosis is caused by excessive loss of carbon dioxide. It is treated by eliminating the cause and helping the patient to breathe more deeply and slowly. A rebreather bag helps to retain carbon dioxide. [NP: IM, CL: AP]

2. **(a)** Edema results from increased hydrostatis pressure in addition to reduced oncotic pressure, increased capillary permeability, and/or reduced lymphatic drainage. [NP: AS, CL: KN]

3. **(b)** If metabolic alkalosis is related to gastrointestinal losses, chloride levels will be low. Potassium levels will also be low because potassium will move into the cells in exchange for hydrogen ions. [NP: AN, CL: AN]

4. **(b)** A moderate weight loss is 2 to 5 percent of total body weight. In this case, 5 percent of 154 lb is 7.7 lb. [NP: AS, CL: CO]

5. **(c)** Patients with metabolic acidosis are often severely dehydrated and need to have adequate volume restored. [NP: PL, CL: AP]

6. **(d)** In compensated states, the pH approaches normal, while significant changes may exist in the acid-base components. [NP: AN, CL: AN]

SITUATION 12–1

1. **(c)** Blood is usually started at 20 gtt per minute for the first 10 minutes. If no reaction is noted, the rate may be increased to 50 to 70 gtt per minute. [NP: IM, CL: AP]

2. **(c)** Patients are often premedicated with acetaminophen and antihistamines in order to decrease sensitivity reactions. [NP: PL, CL: CO]

3. **(a)** If problems develop, the infusion can be stopped and the normal saline solution turned on. When a reaction occurs, hospital policy should be followed. [NP: IM, CL: AP]

4. **(b)** Blood preservatives contain citric acid which binds with free calcium in the blood. Patients who receive multiple blood transfusions may require a calcium supplement. [NP: AN, CL: CO]

5. **(d)** Von Willebrand's disease is a congenital clotting disorder involving a deficiency of factor VIII. [NP: AN, CL: CO]

6. **(d)** In evaluating the effectiveness of blood transfusion, a unit of packed red cells should raise the hematocrit by about 3 grams. [NP: EV, CL: KN]

SITUATION 12–2

1. **(a)** Platelets are administered quickly within 10 minutes. [NP: IM, CL: AP]

2. **(c)** The administration of blood may be traumatic for the family. The nurse will inform the family of the reason for the transfusion and allay their fears. [NP: IM, CL: AN]

3. **(b)** After 10 to 15 transfusions with random donor platelets, patients become senitized and the life span of subsequent transfused platelets is reduced. The platelets will need to be matched for the human histocompatibility antigen. [NP: PL, CL: AP]

4. **(b)** If special platelet administration sets are not available, a filter with a pore size of at least 170 microns may be used. This prevents excess filtration of the platelets. [NP: IM, CL: KN]

5. **(d)** Urine flow greater than .5 ml/kg/hour is an appropriate finding indicating adequate volume expansion. [NP: EV, CL: CO]

6. **(a)** Patients receiving multiple blood transfusions need to have their acidbase balance checked due to the accumulation of citric acid. [NP: AN, CL: CO]

SITUATION 13–1

1. **(b)** Signs of intoxication from cocaine include cardiac arrhythmias. [NP: AS, CL: KN]

2. **(c)** Mixed addition is a condition in which the person is dependent on more than one substance, such as cocaine and alcohol. [NP: AN, CL: AP]

3. **(d)** The nurse should obtain information about drug use, but refrain from lengthy interpersonal interactions which might increase agitation. [NP: IM, CL: CO]

4. **(d)** Non-pharmacologic nursing interventions such as relaxation techniques promote sleep and rest. Administering strong sedatives may induce dependence. [NP: IM, CL: KN]

5. **(a)** During the acute phase of intoxication, the nurse is primarily concerned with deterring life-threatening effects. Education, however, is an important aspect of care and should be initiated whether or not the patient appears receptive. [NP: PL, CL: CO]

6. **(c)** This response reflects an understanding of the need to confront the problem rather than to deny it. [NP: EV, CL: AN]

SITUATION 13–2

1. **(b)** Signs of intoxication from depressant drugs include loss of superficial reflexes, diminished respiratory volume, and hypotension. [NP: AS, CL: KN]

2. **(a)** Signs of phencyclidine intoxication include severe anxiety, feelings of panic, and potential for aggressive/violent behavior. [NP: AN, CL: AP]

3. **(c)** The nurse will administer decreasing amounts of opioids, usually in the form of methadone, as indicated. [NP: PL, CL: KN]

4. **(b)** In patients with mixed alcoholbenzodiazepine (Valium, Librium) dependence, seizures may occur between days 7 and 14. [NP: AN, CL: KN]

5. **(a)** The use of antipsychotic medications should be avoided in treating patients for hallucinogen intoxication. [NP: PL, CL: AP]

6. **(d)** The goals associated with acute intoxication induced by depressants include provisions for a safe environment and a stable physiologic status. The patient may or may not verbalize a desire to abstain from further drug use. [NP: PL, CL: CO]

SITUATION 14–1

1. **(c)** While it is preferable to insert the scalp vein needle in the direction of venous flow, the needle may be placed in either direction, since scalp veins have no valves. [NP: PL, CL: KN]

2. **(c)** After a medication is given via the volume control chamber, a portion of the drug remains in the tubing. For the neonate receiving slow infusion rates, routine IV tubing changes should be performed before the medication is given. [NP: IM, CL: KN]

3. **(a)** The neonate has less albumin available for binding with drugs. Due to the larger proportion of unbound drug, there is greater likelihood of developing a toxic reaction. It may be necessary to decrease the drug and shorten the interval time between dosages. [NP: AN, CL: AP]

4. **(b)** Drugs such as salicylates have a stronger binding power for albumin than bilirubin. This would release free bilirubin to cross the blood-brain barrier, potentially causing brain damage. [NP: AS, CL: CO]

5. **(d)** The neonate's liver is immature at birth and less effective for drug metabolism. A prolonged therapeutic effect may be observed due to an increased half life. [NP: IM, CL: AP]

6. **(a)** Drugs such as digoxin are dependent on glomerular filtration rate (GFR). The GFR increases rapidly during the first weeks of life. [NP: EV, CL: CO]

Key to [Codes]; NP = Nursing process phase; AS = Assessment; AN = Analysis; PL = Planning; IM = Implementation; EV = Evaluation; CL = Cognitive level; KN = Knowledge; CO = Comprehension; AP = Application; AN = Analysis

SITUATION 14–2

1. **(d)** Conditions such as gastritis may cause gastric motility to increase suddenly. When this occurs, the opposite timing of the therapeutic effect may be seen. [NP: OL, CL: CO]

2. **(c)** The deltoid muscle in children less than 3 to 4 years old is not well developed and is usually avoided. The area is small, but has a rapid rate of absorption. [NP: IM, CL: CO]

3. **(a)** The rate of metabolism of theophylline can be increased in the child and necessitate a decrease in the dosage interval. [NP: AN, CL: AP]

4. **(a)** Young children may not want to identify themselves in order to avoid taking the medication. It is imperative to check the armband for identification prior to administering medications. [NP: IM, CL: KN]

5. **(c)** For some medications, such as theophylline, the best method to evaluate effectiveness of the medication is by measuring serum concentration. [NP: EV, CL: KN]

6. **(d)** This response indicates a desire to fit the medication schedule into the family's routine, thereby increasing compliance. [NP: EV, CL: AN]

SITUATION 15–1

1. **(a)** Proteinuria is one of the triad of symptoms which characterize pre-eclampsia. Edema and hypertension are the other classic symptoms. [NP: AS, CL: KN]

2. **(c)** For a continuous infusion, 32 mEq of magnesium sulfate is added to 250 cc 5 percent dextrose and given at a rate not to exceed 4 ml per minute. [NP: IM, CL: AP]

3. **(b)** The patient should be observed for diminished neuromuscular functioning, including hyporeflexia, which is associated with hypermagnesemia. [NP: AS, CL: CO]

4. **(d)** Calcium is the antidote for magnesium toxicity. [NP: PL, CL: KN]

5. **(c)** The patient with eclampsia should demonstrate an absence of seizure activity. [NP: EV, CL: AN]

6. **(d)** Following delivery, infants of mothers who received magnesium sulfate need to be observed closely for signs of neuromuscular depression during the first 24 to 48 hours. [NP: IM, CL: KN]

SITUATION 15–2

1. **(c)** Since Demerol prolongs the latent phase of labor, it should be administered after labor is well established. [NP: AS, CL: KN]

2. **(a)** Hypotension is a side effect of epidural anesthesia. By placing a noncompressible sandbag under the right hip, the uterus is displaced to the left. This position maintains vena caval blood return. [NP: IM, CL: AP]

3. **(d)** Systemic hypotension related to epidural anesthesia may be treated with the administration of oxygen, epinephrine, intravenous fluids, as well as left lateral positioning. Trendelenburg position further compounds the problem by reducing uteroplacental blood flow and vena caval blood return. [NP: PL, CL: CO]

4. **(c)** The action of Ergotrate is to stimulate smooth muscle, thereby controlling postpartal hemorrhage and uterine atony. [NP: AN, CL: KN]

5. **(d)** Rho(D)immune globulin (RhoGam) is administered intramuscularly to women who are Rh-negative and give birth to Rh-positive infants. [NP: IM, CL: CO]

6. **(c)** The patient needs to be aware of the side effects of bromocriptine, which include hypotension, dizziness, headache, and nausea. [NP: IM, CL: KN]

SITUATION 16–1

1. **(b)** Gentamycin is a nephrotoxic agent; therefore, creatinine levels should be checked as a reflection of renal function. [NP: IM, CL: AP]

2. **(c)** A fluid restriction would potentiate dehydration. Since gentamycin is a water-soluble drug, more would remain in circulation and lead to possible toxicity. [NP: IM, CL: AN]

3. **(d)** Drugs such as gentamycin can produce ototoxicity. [NP: IM, CL: CO]

4. **(a)** The reduced metabolism of barbiturates by the liver is partly responsible for the "hangover" effect seen in the elderly. [NP: AS, CL: AP]

5. **(d)** Orinase is an example of a medication which is bound to protein for distribution. Hypoproteinemia can cause an increase in the amount of unbound drug, resulting in an increased action. [NP: AS, CL: CO]

6. **(b)** Drugs such as procainamide are primarily excreted by the kidneys. Careful monitoring of renal function is important so that possible problems leading to drug toxicity can be identified. [NP: IM, CL: KN]

SITUATION 18–1

1. **(b)** Acetylcholine is given intraocularly during ophthalmic surgery to obtain complete miosis. [NP: AN, CL: KN]

2. **(c)** The onset of action of Miochol is immediate, with effects lasting 10 minutes. [NP: PL, CL: KN]

3. **(a)** Signs of muscarinic excess can occur if Urecholine is given intramuscularly or intravenously. The usual route is oral or subcutaneous. [NP: AN, CL: CO]

4. **(a)** Due to the cholinergic effect of increased gastric secretions, bethanechol is contraindicated in patients with peptic ulcer disease. [NP: AS, CL: CO]

5. **(d)** Atropine, an anticholinergic drug, is the agent of choice in the event that toxic effects of bethanechol occur. [NP: PL, CL: KN]

6. **(d)** Bethanechol should be kept in a light-resistent container. The patient should also be taught to report any adverse side effects immediately. [NP: EV, CL: AN]

SITUATION 18–2

1. **(b)** Cholinesterase inhibitors block the breakdown of acetylcholine and contribute to the stimulation of cholinergic receptors. This stimulation produces an increase in gastric secretions and is contraindicated in patients with peptic ulcer disease. [NP: AN, CL: CO]

2. **(d)** Adverse side effects of propantheline bromide include photophobia, tachycardia, headache, and urinary retention. [NP: IM, CL: CO]

3. **(c)** A very common side effect of propantheline is dryness of the mouth; therefore, alteration in oral mucous membrane is an appropriate nursing diagnosis. [NP: AN, CL: AP]

4. **(b)** Restriction of fluid intake would exacerbate dry mucous membranes. Increasing oral intake is indicated unless ordered otherwise. [NP: PL, CL: CO]

5. **(b)** Robinul is extremely potent in its ability to decrease pharyngeal, tracheal, and bronchial secretions. [NP: AN, CL: KN]

6. **(a)** Anticholinergic drugs, such as Robinul and propantheline, produce mydriasis. [NP: AS, CL: CO]

SITUATION 19–1

1. **(c)** More common side effects of ergotamine tartrate (Ergomar) are nausea and vomiting. [NP: PL, CL: CO]

2. **(b)** The sublingual tablets should be taken when a headache develops, and the dosage should not exceed three tablets in a 24-hour period. [NP: IM, CL: CO]

3. **(d)** Beta blockers are contraindicated in patients with congestive heart failure. [NP: AS, CL: KN]

4. **(b)** Antacids reduce the bioavailability of propranolol. [NP: EV, CL: AP]

5. **(c)** Fatigue is a common side effect of beta blockers and results from hemodynamic effects or peripheral metabolic effects. [NP: AN, CL: AN]

6. **(d)** Concurrent administration of cimetidine and furosemide can cause adverse effects. Patients who are diabetic and on insulin or oral hyperglycemic agents need to be assessed for potential for hyperglycemia. [NP: PL, CL: CO]

SITUATION 19–2

1. **(b)** At low doses, 1 μg/kg/min, dopamine dilates renal and mesenteric arteries, producing increased urine output and improved creatinine clearance. At the lower infusion rate, blood pressure is not expected to increase. [NP: EV, CL: AP]

2. **(d)** When administering vasopressor agents, such as dopamine, it is important to maintain adequate blood volume in order to ensure tissue perfusion. [NP: PL, CL: CO]

3. **(a)** In the event of extravasation of dopamine, an alpha-adrenergic blocker such as phentolamine hydrochloride is infiltrated into the same location. [NP: IM, CL: AP]

4. **(b)** At infusion rates of 10 to 20 μg/kg/min, dopamine stimulates alpha-adrenergic activity, resulting in increased blood pressure. [NP: EV, CL: KN]

5. **(d)** Nitroglycerin ointment may be used with catecholamine infusions to increase peripheral blood flow without affecting blood pressure. [NP: PL, CL: CO]

6. **(d)** In some cases, discontinuing dopamine may be difficult, due in part to the short half-life of the drug. The dosage should be tapered slowly and vital signs taken frequently. [NP: IM, CL: AP]

SITUATION 20–1

1. **(d)** Meperidine (Demerol) may cause biliary tract spasm. [NP: PL, CL: AP]

2. **(b)** The most common adverse reactions include nausea, euphoria, agitation, and constipation. [NP: AS, CL: CO]

3. **(a)** Epidural morphine is more water soluble than lipid soluble, and the onset of action is related to the slow diffusion through the lipid neural membrane. [NP: PL, CL: KN]

4. **(c)** Pruritis or rash is commonly associated with the administration of epidural opiates, which may be due in part to histamine release. [NP: IM, CL: KN]

5. **(d)** Signs and symptoms of paresthesia may be related to nerve tissue compression caused by catheter migration. Throbbing occipital headache may indicate dural puncture. Poor pain relief may be a sign

---

Key to [Codes]; NP = Nursing process phase; AS = Assessment; AN = Analysis; PL = Planning; IM = Implementation; EV = Evaluation; CL = Cognitive level; KN = Knowledge; CO = Comprehension; AP = Application; AN = Analysis

that the catheter is malfunctioning. Drowsiness is more likely related to a side effect of morphine rather than catheter malposition. [NP: PL, CL: CO]

6. **(b)** Constipation is a commonly reported adverse effect of codeine. [NP: IM, CL: AP]

SITUATION 20–2

1. **(d)** A sign of tolerance is the report that a drug is not as effective as it once was. [NP: AS, CL: AP]

2. **(a)** Chronic pain is usually burning or nagging and may become the pathology, altering the patient's lifestyle. [NP: AN, CL: AP]

3. **(d)** Dilaudid may exert an additive effect if given with general anesthetics. In addition, this drug is a semi-synthetic derivative of morphine which is ten times more potent. [NP: PL, CL: KN]

4. **(c)** Pain medication should be given promptly when needed. Nurses should not rely on their own perception of the pain experience. Pain medication will not be as effective if given after the patient is in severe pain. [NP: IM, CL: AP]

5. **(c)** Nausea and vomiting usually are related to adverse effects of the medication, but may indicate poor pain control. [NP: IM, CL: KN]

6. **(b)** Neostigmine reduces urinary spasms which may cause urinary retention. [NP: IM, CL: KN]

SITUATION 21–1

1. **(b)** The usual initial dosage for Ritalin, as the treatment for ADD, is 5 mg before breakfast. [NP: IM, CL: AP]

2. **(b)** Usually the drug is given only on school days. Drug holidays are planned to evaluate behavioral response to the agents. [NP: PL, CL: KN]

3. **(d)** Prenatal, perinatal, and postnatal information should be obtained in order to determine factors contributing to ADD. [NP: AS, CL: KN]

4. **(a)** Adverse effects of Ritalin use in children include retarded growth and development. [NP: AN, CL: AP]

5. **(c)** Drug therapy for children with attention deficit disorders is not a panacea, but usually does improve attention span and coordination and may enhance peer relationships. [NP: PL, CL: CO]

6. **(b)** Reducing caffeine-containing products may help in reducing hyperactivity and behavioral problems. [NP: IM, CL: KN]

SITUATION 21–2

1. **(a)** Amphetamine therapy is contraindicated for patients with glaucoma, due to mydriatic effects. [NP: AS, CL: CO]

2. **(c)** The dosage for Benzedrine as treatment for nar-

colepsy is 20 to 60 mg 1 day po. The dosage is age-specific and dependent on severity of the condition. [NP: AN, CL: KN]

3. **(a)** For the patient with narcolepsy, the nurse should perform a baseline neurological assessment. [NP: AS, CL: AP]

4. **(d)** Patients who are taking amphetamines report tachycardia and palpitations. Other effects include depression, headaches, and increased motor activity. [NP: IM, CL: CO]

5. **(c)** Anorexia is a frequently reported side effect of amphetamine therapy and represents a potential nutritional problem. [NP: AN, CL: AP]

6. **(c)** Patients should be taught to plan a varied and interesting daily schedule and to incorporate recreational activity. They should avoid monotony and routines at home which can be boring. Air travel can precipitate narcolepsy attacks. [NP: EV, CL: AN]

SITUATION 22–1

1. **(c)** Phenytoin should be given slowly at a rate of 50 mg/minute via the intravenous route. [NP: IM, CL: KN]

2. **(c)** Phenytoin can cause hypotension when given intravenously. [NP: IM, CL: KN]

3. **(a)** The therapeutic range for serum phenytoin (Dilantin) is 10 to 20 μg/ml; therefore, the nurse will anticipate continuing the dosage as ordered. [NP: EV, CL: AP]

4. **(d)** The standard drug of choice for status epilepticus is diazepam (Valium). [NP: PL, CL: CO]

5. **(c)** Due to the side effect of gingival hyperplasia related to Dilantin therapy, patients should be taught to perform good oral hygiene. [NP: IM, CL: KN]

6. **(b)** Glycosuria is a secondary endocrine effect of phenytoin, due to the inhibition of insulin secretion. [NP: AS, CL: KN]

SITUATION 22–2

1. **(a)** For therapeutic results, a serum concentration of 10 to 25 μg/ml is recommended. [NP: EV, CL: KN]

2. **(d)** The major side effects of phenobarbital relate to neurotoxicity. [NP: IM, CL: CO]

3. **(a)** Control of partial seizures is an example of an outcome or goal for patients on anticonvulsants. [NP: PL, CL: KN]

4. **(c)** Trough levels are obtained prior to administration to determine if the minimum effective serum concentration is present. [NP: IM, CL: CO]

5. **(a)** To reduce the risk of status epilepticus, the phenobarbital should be reduced gradually before discontinuing. [NP: PL, CL: AP]

6. **(b)** Tegretol affects the secretion of ADH, causing a decrease in serum osmolality and sodium levels. [NP: IM, CL: CO]

SITUATION 23–1

1. **(a)** The tremors and rigidity of Parkinson's disease relate to the excitatory effect of the cholinergic system. [NP: AS, CL: AP]

2. **(d)** The use of anticholinergics is contraindicated in patients with tachycardia. [NP: AS, CL: CO]

3. **(b)** Antihistamines give additive anticholinergic effects. [NP: IM, CL: KN]

4. **(b)** Long-term therapy with levodopa agents may produce adverse effects such as abnormal involuntary movements, akinetic spells, and behavioral disturbances. [NP: IM, CL: CO]

5. **(d)** Trihexyphenidyl delays gastric emptying, thereby delaying absorpiton of Sinemet. [NP: AN, CL: CO]

6. **(a)** Cardiac dysrhythmias are common cardiovascular effects of Sinemet therapy. [NP: PL, CL: KN]

SITUATION 23–2

1. **(b)** Myasthenia gravis is characterized by muscle weakness which becomes severe with activity and improves with rest. [NP: AS, CL: KN]

2. **(b)** The onset of action of edrophonium is 30 to 60 seconds. [NP: PL, CL: KN]

3. **(a)** When giving an anticholinesterase, the buildup of acetylcholine may cause bradycardia and decreased cardiac output. [NP: IM, CL: AP]

4. **(c)** Adverse effects of Mestinon include those due to stimulation of cholinergic receptors, such as diarrhea, nausea, and vomiting. [NP: IM, CL: KN]

5. **(b)** The oral dosage of medication for control of myasthenia should be divided into three or four intervals during the day. [NP: IM, CL: CO]

6. **(a)** With higher doses of corticosteroids, a period of "early worsening" of the signs and symptoms of myasthenia will occur. [NP: IM, CL: KN]

SITUATION 24–1

1. **(a)** During the assessment, it is important for the nurse to determine the physical as well as psychological symptoms that the patient is experiencing. The nurse should focus on the response to the anxiety as the core of the illness. [NP: AS, CL: AP]

2. **(b)** Alcohol enhances the effect of the anxiolytic agent and should not be used in combination. [NP: IM, CL: KN]

3. **(b)** A common adverse reaction associated with this agent is slurred speech. Other neurological effects include dizziness and confusion. [NP: IM, CL: CO]

4. **(d)** Patients taking anxiolytic agents may spend less time in REM sleep, resulting in continued altered sleep patterns and a sense of not sleeping well. [NP: AN, CL: AP]

5. **(c)** Cigarette smoking may decrease the effectiveness of the benzodiazepine by enhancing its metabolism. [NP: EV, CL: AP]

6. **(a)** Because alprazolam clears the system rapidly, abruptly stopping the drug may result in seizures. [NP: IM, CL: KN]

SITUATION 24–2

1. **(d)** Patients with severe levels of anxiety will demonstrate physiologic responses such as increased respirations, pulse, and blood pressure. [NP: AS, CL: AP]

2. **(b)** When diazepam is to be given intramuscularly, the deltoid muscle provides rapid and complete absorption. [NP: PL, CL: KN]

3. **(c)** In this situation, a measurable outcome of anxiolytic therapy is reduction of blood pressure, respirations, and pulse to preanxiety levels. [NP: EV, CL: AP]

4. **(d)** Unusual excitement may indicate a paradoxic reaction, which may occur with benzodiazepines, especially in elderly patients. [NP: PL, CL: CO]

5. **(a)** Due to the potential for dry mouth and constipation associated with diazepam therapy, patients should be encouraged to maintain adequate hydration. [NP: IM, CL: AN]

6. **(c)** Benzodiazepines may elevate bilirubin levels. Patient evaluation should include monitoring this laboratory result. [NP: EV, CL: KN]

SITUATION 25–1

1. **(c)** It may be difficult to question the patient about her history or her feelings at this time. It will be important for the nurse to list the symptoms which the patient is exhibiting to be used as a baseline for evaluation of drug therapy. [NP: AS, CL: AP]

2. **(b)** The intramuscular loading dose for Thorazine is 400 to 1500 mg/day. [NP: PL, CL: KN]

3. **(b)** The best approach with psychotically ill patients is to be kind, firm, and positive. It is best not to have the patient make any decisions at this time or carry on lengthy conversations. [NP: IM, CL: KN]

Key to [Codes]; NP = Nursing process phase; AS = Assessment; AN = Analysis; PL = Planning; IM = Implementation; EV = Evaluation; CL = Cognitive level; KN = Knowledge; CO = Comprehension; AP = Application; AN = Analysis

4. **(c)** The predicted onset of action for intramuscular Thorazine is 30 minutes. [NP: PL, CL: KN]

5. **(c)** In the early period of drug therapy, sedation is the predominant side effect. [NP: EV, CL: CO]

6. **(d)** After two days from the initial dose, the nurse can anticipate increased socialization. [NP: EV, CL: CO]

SITUATION 25–2

1. **(d)** Thiothixene is available only in intramuscular forms. [NP: PL, CL: KN]

2. **(c)** Antipsychotic agents are often incompatible with other injectable drugs and should be administered separately. [NP: PL, CL: KN]

3. **(b)** Patients need to understand that they must adhere to long-term therapeutic measures despite feelings of well-being. Most psychotic reactions will recur unless patients follow the treatment schedule. [NP: IM, CL: CO]

4. **(c)** Symptoms such as a sore throat may be related to problems of agranulocytosis and should be reported immediately. [NP: PL, CL: CO]

5. **(b)** Difficulty swallowing and chewing food may indicate extrapyramidal side effects related to neuroleptic therapy. [NP: EV, CL: AP]

6. **(c)** Symptoms described are related to cholestatic jaundice. The treatment for this condition includes discontinuing the neuroleptic drug, providing bedrest, and encouraging a high protein/carbohydrate diet. [NP: PL, CL: CO]

SITUATION 26–1

1. **(a)** Depressed patients are particularly prone to suicide. The nurse needs to be aware of cues, both verbal and nonverbal, which indicate suicidal tendencies. [NP: AS, CL: AP]

2. **(c)** Behavior which indicates major depression includes decreased energy and loss of interest in activities. [NP: AS, CL: KN]

3. **(b)** Nursing mothers should not take imipramine because it is excreted in the breast milk in low concentrations. [NP: AS, CL: CO]

4. **(a)** Tricyclic antidepressives should not be taken with substances containing ascorbic acid, which causes decreased effectiveness. [NP: IM, CL: AP]

5. **(d)** Side effects such as sedation and drowsiness are common; therefore, the patient should avoid driving or operating machinery. [NP: IM, CL: CO]

6. **(d)** Evidence of successful treatment of depression includes demonstration of interest in personal appearance. [NP: EV, CL: KN]

SITUATION 26–2

1. **(b)** Due to the potential for drug interactions, the patient should be maintained on a low monoamine diet for 1 to 2 weeks prior to isocarboxazid therapy. [NP: PL, CL: CO]

2. **(b)** A common adverse reaction to isocarboxazid therapy is orthostatic hypotension. This side effect is less pronounced as therapy continues. [NP: IM, CL: KN]

3. **(a)** Toxic symptoms related to overdose include neurological symptoms such as headache or confusion. [NP: EV, CL: CO]

4. **(b)** An increased effect of amoxapine may be seen with the addition of an MAO inhibitor. [NP: AN, CL: AP]

5. **(c)** A hypertensive crisis can arise after contraindicated food or medication is taken. Hypertension is the result of supranormal release of catecholamine stores. [NP: AN, CL: KN]

6. **(d)** The patient taking an MAO inhibitor needs to avoid foods high in tyramine, such as cheese, red wines, and smoked meats. [NP: IM, CL: KN]

SITUATION 28–1

1. **(b)** Electrolytes and acid-base imbalances are corrected in the case of digoxin toxicity. Potassium may or may not need to be supplemented. [NP: PL, CL: KN]

2. **(d)** Atrial dysrhythmias related to digoxin toxicity can be treated with phenytoin (Dilantin). [NP: PL, CL: CO]

3. **(d)** Hypomagnesemia tends to increase the sensitivity to digitalis preparations. [NP: AS, CL: KN]

4. **(a)** The therapeutic range for serum digoxin is 0.5 to 2.0 ng/ml. [NP: EV, CL: KN]

5. **(b)** It will be very important for the patient to monitor her pulse rate daily and to report a pulse rate <60 or >110 before taking the medicaton. [NP: IM, CL: AP]

6. **(b)** Patient education about digoxin administration is critical to preventing toxic manifestations of the drug and expensive hospital costs. The patient in this case demonstrates a lack of understanding concerning the potential for toxic effects. [NP: AN, CL: AN]

SITUATION 28–2

1. **(b)** The loading dose in adults is approximately .010 to .020 mg/kg, administered as three to four equally divided doses over 24 hours. [NP: AN, CL: KN]

2. **(d)** The usual route of digoxin administration is by intravenous injection if the patient is symptomatic. [NP: PL, CL: AP]

3. **(c)** Blood pressure may be increased in patients with limited cardiac reserve who are receiving digoxin by the intravenous route. [NP: IM, CL: CO]

4. **(a)** Because the primary elimination of digoxin is by renal mechanisms, the maintenance dose is based on creatinine clearance. [NP: AN, CL: CO]

5. **(b)** A rapid pulse may indicate that the patient needs to have the digoxin dosage increased or to have serum levels evaluated. [NP: IM, CL: CO]

6. **(b)** Patients should be taught not to try to "catch up" on missed dosages by taking two pills in one day. If a dosage is missed, then it should be eliminated. [NP: EV, CL: AN]

SITUATION 29–1

1. **(d)** Initial therapy with prazosin tends to produce orthostatic hypotension; therefore, the patient should be taught to rise slowly from a supine position. [NP: IM, CL: KN]

2. **(a)** Prazosin is metabolized by the liver. The drug half-life is prolonged in patients with hepatic disease. [NP: AS, CL: CO]

3. **(d)** Compliance can be improved by involving the patients in their own care, such as taking daily blood pressure. [NP: PL, CL: CO]

4. **(a)** Patients who are just being started on a new drug regime need close follow-up, preferably within five days of initial drug administration. [NP: EV, CL: AN]

5. **(c)** Patients with hypertension should avoid caffeine-containing products which may potentially increase blood pressure. [NP: IM, CL: CO]

6. **(d)** Patients should be taught not to discontinue the medication. If the patient has adverse side effects, then she should contact the nurse or physician. [NP: EV, CL: AN]

SITUATION 29–2

1. **(d)** The range of nitroprusside dosage is .5 to 10 mcg/kg/minute. Doses above 10 mcg/kg/minute should be administered only if necessary. [NP: OL, CL: KN]

2. **(b)** Nitroprusside solutions should be protected from light to prevent deterioration. [NP: IM, CL: KN]

3. **(a)** Thiocyanate is a metabolite of nitroprusside which can accumulate and cause adverse effects. Thiocyanate levels should be monitored in patients receiving intravenous nitroprusside longer than one to two days. [NP: PL, CL: KN]

4. **(a)** Because of the potential for rapid reduction in blood pressure with intravenous nitroprusside, resulting in cerebral hypoperfusion, the mean arterial blood pressure should not be reduced more than 20 to 30 percent in the first 24 hours. [NP: IM, CL: AP]

5. **(c)** Nitroprusside reduces both preload and afterload, increasing cardiac output and renal blood flow. The expected outcome would be increased urine output. [NP: EV, CL: CO]

6. **(c)** A reduction in diastolic pressure along with increased cardiac output can potentiate cardiac ischemia. [NP: IM, CL: KN]

SITUATION 30–1

1. **(c)** Quinidine action results in prolongation of the Q-T interval; therefore, basline data documenting the Q-T interval are important. [NP: AS, CL: AP]

2. **(c)** Quinidine reacts with digoxin to increase serum digoxin levels. [NP: AN, CL: CO]

3. **(a)** The most common side effects related to quinidine therapy are gastrointestinal complaints, such as diarrhea. [NP: IM, CL: KN]

4. **(b)** Taking quinidine with meals may reduce gastrointestinal side effects. [NP: IM, CL: KN]

5. **(d)** Patients on quinidine therapy may develop thrombocytopenia, which is due to quinidine-platelet complexes, resulting in destruction of platelets. [NP: IM, CL: AP]

6. **(b)** Evidence of increasing weight may indicate congestive heart failure and should be reported to the physician or nurse. [NP: EV, CL: AN]

SITUATION 30–2

1. **(a)** The standard IV bolus dose for lidocaine is 1mg/kg. [NP: PL, CL: KN]

2. **(d)** The standard dosage range for lidocaine infusion is 1 to 4 mg/minute. [NP: PL, CL: KN]

3. **(d)** Mixing lidocaine with other drugs may potentiate deterioration or precipitation. [NP: IM, CL: CO]

4. **(a)** Due to anesthetic properties and distribution into the central nervous system, side effects include disorientation, agitation, numbness, and more severe CNS effects. [NP: PL, CL: KN]

5. **(c)** The half-life of lidocaine in patients with ischemic heart disease is 4 to 5 hours after discontinuation of infusions of 24 hours' duration. [NP: AN, CL: KN]

6. **(a)** Thrombocytopenia can occur with tocainide therapy; therefore, the patient should be alert to signs of increased bruising. [NP: IM, CL: CO]

Key to [Codes]; NP = Nursing process phase; AS = Assessment; AN = Analysis; PL = Planning; IM = Implementation; EV = Evaluation; CL = Cognitive level; KN = Knowledge; CO = Comprehension; AP = Application; AN = Analysis

SITUATION 31–1

1. **(b)** If high dose therapy is to be used, the infusion is titrated by 20 to 50 mcg increments. It is also important to monitor the blood pressure and pulse frequently, particularly with initial intravenous therapy. [NP: IM, CL: KN]

2. **(d)** Nitrates can cause reflex tachycardia in patients with normal cardiac function. [NP: AS, CL: AP]

3. **(b)** A pounding headache represents an adverse side effect which is usually relieved by reducing the dosage or discontinuing the infusion. [NP: AN, CL: CO]

4. **(d)** Altering nitrate levels by allowing nitrate-free periods reduced the development of nitrate tolerance. [NP: AN, CL: AP]

5. **(c)** Transdermal nitroglycerin patches can be applied to any non-hairy part of the body. [NP: IM, CL: CO]

6. **(b)** Nitroglycerin tablets should be taken before any activity that is likely to induce angina, such as exercise or sexual activity. [NP: IM, CL: KN]

SITUATION 31–2

1. **(c)** Isosorbide dinitrate sustained-release tablets should not be chewed or crushed, as this would interfere with the sustained release action. [NP: IM, CL: KN]

2. **(a)** Nifedipine reduces peripheral vascular resistance and, along with concurrent use with nitrates, can cause hypotension with initial administration. [NP: IM, CL: AP]

3. **(a)** The presence of kidney dysfunction may increase nifedipine levels and is important to note with assessment data. [NP: AS, CL: KN]

4. **(b)** Nifedipine can cause a noncardiac dependent peripheral edema, which can be treated with diuretics. [NP: AN, CL: CO]

5. **(c)** The patient should avoid excessive strenuous exercise, but exercise activity which is tolerated without angina is acceptable. [NP: IM, CL: CO]

6. **(d)** Nitroglycerin tablets are not habit-forming and can be taken as needed. It should be stressed, however, that if chest pain becomes severe or is not relieved with nitroglycerin, the physician should be notified. [NP: EV, CL: AP]

SITUATION 32–1

1. **(b)** Lifestyle patterns are important to note in patients with hyperlipidemia, especially the amount of stress which they may encounter. [NP: AS, CL: AP]

2. **(a)** Cholestyramine, a bile sequestrant agent, may elevate triglyceride levels and should not be given to patients with triglyceride levels above 400 mg/dl. [NP: AS, CL: CO]

3. **(d)** Cholestyramine should be mixed with fluids or high-moisture-content foods to disguise the taste and to dissolve the medication. [NP: IM, CL: KN]

4. **(c)** Cholestyramine may interfere with the absorption of thiazide diuretics; therefore, the diuretic should be taken within 1 hour before or 4 to 6 hours after cholestyramine. [NP: IM, CL: CO]

5. **(a)** Adverse effects related to cholestyramine therapy include bleeding tendencies. Patients taking this agent should be assessed for the potential for bleeding. [NP: EV, CL: AP]

6. **(a)** A fall in LDL levels is apparent within 4 to 7 days of treatment with cholestyramine. [NP: EV, CL: KN]

SITUATION 32–2

1. **(c)** Red blood cells which appear hypochromic are characteristic of iron deficiency anemia. [NP: AS, CL: KN]

2. **(c)** Oral iron is contraindicated in patients with peptic ulcer disease. [NP: AS, CL: CO]

3. **(c)** Constipation is a local effect of orally administered iron products. [NP: PL, CL: AP]

4. **(b)** Eggs consumed with iron products can inhibit absorption. [NP: IM, CL: CO]

5. **(c)** Coffee and tea consumed with meals can reduce iron absorption. [NP: IM, CL: AP]

6. **(b)** As the hemoglobin level rises due to iron therapy, the patient notes less fatigue and increased feelings of well-being. [NP: EV, CL: KN]

SITUATION 33–1

1. **(b)** The adult intravenous bolus of heparin is approximately 100 units per kg of body weight. [NP: PL, CL: AP]

2. **(c)** When patients are receiving heparin infusions, they should not be given intramuscular injections because of the increased risk of bleeding. [NP: IM, CL: KN]

3. **(c)** Protamine is a heparin antagonist which acts by neutralizing heparin. [NP: PL, CL: CO]

4. **(c)** Partial thromboplastin time is monitored for evaluation of heparin therapy. [NP: EV, CL: KN]

5. **(a)** After subcutaneous injection, pressure is applied at the site. However, the site should not be massaged. [NP: IM, CL: KN]

6. **(b)** Due to increased potential for bleeding, the patient receiving heparin therapy should not take aspirin, ibuprofen, or indomethacin. Acetaminophen

would be the most appropriate choice in this case. [NP: AN, CL: CO]

SITUATION 33–2

1. **(c)** The peripheral intravenous dosage of streptokinase for occluded coronary arteries is 1.5 million units given over 1 hour. [NP: PL, CL: KN]

2. **(b)** Because streptokinase is a foreign protein, allergic reactions may be produced, as demonstrated by urticaria, warm flushed skin, or fever. [NP: IM, CL: CO]

3. **(a)** Initial coumadin therapy is based on daily prothrombin time. [NP: EV, CL: AP]

4. **(b)** Drinking alcoholic beverages (especially in excess) may increase the potential for bleeding by affecting hepatic metabolism. [NP: IM, CL: AP]

5. **(d)** Vitamin K is the antagonist of coumadin and is the drug of choice when signs of hemorrhage are observed with coumadin therapy. The coumadin dosage may also need to be held until bleeding subsides. [NP: PL, CL: CO]

6. **(b)** Using an electric razor reduces the potential for bleeding related to shaving. [NP: EV, CL: AP]

SITUATION 35–1

1. **(b)** The maintenance intravenous dose for aminophylline is 0.2 to 0.9 mg/kg/min, depending on serum levels. [NP: PL, CL: KN]

2. **(a)** The therapeutic range for serum aminophylline is 10 to 20 mcg/ml. [NP: EV, CL: AP]

3. **(c)** Theophylline increases gastric acid secretion, aggravating gastric mucosa. [NP: IM, CL: AP]

4. **(c)** Side effects of theophylline frequently include palpitations, nervousness, insomnia, and frequent urination. [NP: IM, CL: AP]

5. **(a)** Caffeine and caffeine-containing foods may accentuate some of the stimulating effects of theophylline. [NP: IM, CL: AP]

6. **(d)** The metabolism of theophylline is accelerated by tobacco smoking; therefore, the dosage may need to be increased if the patient smokes cigarettes. [NP: AN, CL: CO]

SITUATION 35–2

1. **(b)** Signs of bronchial obstruction include the use of accessory muscles, wheezing on auscultation, increased heart rate, and/or mental status changes. [NP: AS, CL: AP]

2. **(d)** Side effects of terbutaline therapy include tachy-

cardia, dysrhythmias, and other cardiac complications. Patients receiving this drug should be monitored closely for evidence of cardiovascular effects. [NP: IM, CL: CO]

3. **(b)** Terbutaline has been known to cause paradoxical bronchospasm and reduced Pao_2 levels. Arterial blood gases should be monitored closely. [NP: IM, CL: AP]

4. **(a)** Common side effects of inhaled steroid agents, such as beclomethasone, include hoarseness, sore throat, and sinusitis. These effects can be reduced by thoroughly rinsing the mouth after each dose. [NP: IM, CL: AP]

5. **(c)** Patients using aerosol medication delivery systems should hold their breath for several seconds after instillation to allow for maximum absorption of the medication. [NP: AS, CL: CO]

6. **(a)** The puff of medication must be delivered at the beginning of inhalation to ensure that the distal airways receive the dosage. The patient should begin a deep, slow inhalation through the mouth, while depressing the cartridge fully. [NP: EV, CL: AN]

SITUATION 36–1

1. **(b)** Patients with chronic obstructive disease are at risk for oxygen-induced hypoventilation. Oxygen should be delivered at the lowest rate possible, while at the same time reducing the threat of hypoxemia. [NP: PL, CL: AN]

2. **(c)** For patients with chronic obstructive pulmonary disease, a range of 60 to 70 mmHg is appropriate. [NP: EV, CL: AP]

3. **(a)** Patients with chronic obstructive pulmonary disease are at risk for oxygen-induced hypoventilation. Signs of this condition include lethargy and decreasing respiratory rate and depth. [NP: IM, CL: AP]

4. **(b)** Humidification reduces the drying effect of oxygen on mucous membrane. [NP: IM, CL: KN]

5. **(a)** To deliver 24 percent oxygen via nasal cannula, the flow meter should be set at one liter per minute. [NP: IM, CL: CO]

6. **(c)** Adventitious breath sounds such as wheezes or rales indicate pulmonary problems which may alter the exchange of oxygen at the capillary level. [NP: AS, CL: CO]

SITUATION 38–1

1. **(c)** Because of the patient's history of ETOH abuse and potential for hepatic dysfunction, albumin levels

should be noted. Patients with hypoalbuminemia may need protein replacement as well as diuretic therapy. [NP: AS, CL: AN]

2. **(d)** Ototoxicity has been associated with loop diuretics such as furosemide. This may occur, in particular, with patients receiving large doses by intravenous infusion. [NP: IM, CL: CO]

3. **(a)** Furosemide potentiates the excretion of sodium, causing hyponatremia. [NP: IM, CL: KN]

4. **(c)** Due to the diuretic effect, patients should weigh daily and report any rapid changes in weight. Rapid weight loss can cause dehydration and hypotension. [NP: IM, CL: KN]

5. **(c)** Due to potassium depletion with diuretics, patients should include foods high in potassium, such as dried fruits. [NP: IM, CL: CO]

6. **(a)** Patients on diuretic therapy should be observed for evidence of altered coagulation. [NP: EV, CL: AP]

SITUATION 38–2

1. **(d)** To reduce intracranial pressure, the usual dosage for a 15 to 25 percent solution is 1.5 to 2.0 gms per kg. [NP: PL, CL: KN]

2. **(c)** In general, a reduction in the ICP will be noted within 15 minutes of starting the infusion of mannitol. [NP: PL, CL: KN]

3. **(c)** Mannitol solutions frequently crystalize, but may be rewarmed gently to dissolve formed crystals. [NP: IM, CL: KN]

4. **(a)** Dry mucous membranes are a common adverse effect of mannitol therapy; therefore, Alteration in Oral Mucous Membranes is an appropriate nursing diagnostic category. [NP: AN, CL: AP]

5. **(d)** It is recommended that mannitol be infused with an inline IV filter to prevent infusion of microcrystals. [NP: PL, CL: KN]

6. **(a)** A therapeutic outcome of mannitol therapy for patients with increased intracranial pressure would be best demonstrated by improved neurological status. [NP: EV, CL: AN]

SITUATION 39–1

1. **(d)** Due to the potential for ototoxicity, the furosemide infusion rate should not exceed 4 mg/minute. [NP: PL, CL: KN]

2. **(a)** In diseases such as ATN, the kidneys lose the ability to concentrate urine. A specific gravity of greater than 1.010 reflects impaired renal concentration. [NP: IM, CL: CO]

3. **(c)** For stimulation of dopaminergic sites and dilation of renal and mesenteric arteries, the dopamine infusion should be between 2 and 5 mcg/kg/min for optimum glomerular filtration rate. [NP: IM, CL: KN]

4. **(a)** Restricting dietary sodium may be an important aspect of management of hypertension related to acute renal failure. [NP: PL, CL: AP]

5. **(d)** Sorbitol is an osmotic laxative which reduces the potential for constipation and prevents intestinal obstruction. [NP: AN, CL: KN]

6. **(a)** Maximal results from one Kayexalate enema may lower the serum potassium by .5 to 1.0 mEq/L. In this case, a reduction of the serum potassium from 7.0 to 5.5 mEq/L is an appropriate outcome. [NP: EV, CL: AP]

SITUATION 39–2

1. **(a)** Aluminum-containing antacids bind with phosphate, reducing absorption of phosphate in the gastrointestinal tract. [NP: AN, CL: CO]

2. **(b)** The phosphate binding effect is greater when Basagel is given with meals. [NP: PL, CL: KN]

3. **(b)** Patients with a secondary cardiac condition may demonstrate fluid volume excess related to Bicitra administration, which provides increased sodium in the form of $NaHCO_3$. [NP: AN, CL: CO]

4. **(d)** Allopurinol is a xanthine oxidase inhibitor which decreases the production of uric acid. Hyperuricemia (gout) is a common result of renal failure. [NP: EV, CL: AP]

5. **(c)** The dilutional phenomena of renal failure must be considered when assessing for anemia in patients with renal failure. [NP: AS, CL: KN]

6. **(d)** Recombinant human erythropoietin has been shown to increase the erythrocyte count in 7 to 14 days following intravenous injection. This polypeptide acts on the bone marrow to accelerate maturation of red blood cells. [NP: EV, CL: AP]

SITUATION 41–1

1. **(d)** Due to removal of pituitary tumor, this patient is at risk for development of hypothalamic diabetes insipidus. This condition exists due to the reduced release of anti-diuretic hormone. [NP: AS, CL: AP]

2. **(b)** Vasopressin tannate is given intramuscularly. It is not to be used intravenously. Vasopressin is destroyed by digestive enzymes and cannot be given orally. [NP: PL, CL: KN]

3. **(c)** Vasopressin tannate is an oil suspension which must be thoroughly mixed to ensure that all the particles are included in the suspension. [NP: IM, CL: KN]

4. **(b)** Adverse effects of vasopressin tannate include pounding in the head, pallor, and sweating. [NP: AN, CL: AP]

5. **(a)** Patients on antidiuretic therapy should have the

medication adjusted to maintain a urine output of 1.5 to 2 liters per day. [NP: PL, CL: CO]

6. **(d)** Signs of dehydration, such as thirst, should be reported promptly because they indicate a need for alteration of the dosage. [NP: IM, CL: KN]

SITUATION 42–1

1. **(c)** In patients with primary adrenal insufficiency, the second 24-hour urine after ACTH stimulation will reveal no increase in urinary steroid levels. In the normal individual, urinary steroid levels will increase threefold to fivefold after ACTH stimulation. [NP: AS, CL: KN]

2. **(d)** A major adverse effect of mineralocorticoids is sodium and water retention, increasing blood volume. This can lead to increased blood pressure in some cases. [NP: IM, CL: CO]

3. **(d)** Reduced potassium levels are associated with mineralocorticoid therapy, and patients should be encouraged to increase dietary intake of potassium-rich foods. [NP: IM, CL: KN]

4. **(d)** Due to the high potential for gastric irritation with adrenal cortical drugs, patients should avoid excessive intake of coffee and alcoholic beverages. [NP: IM, CL: CO]

5. **(a)** An outcome or goal which indicates appropriate therapy for Addison's disease would be increased energy, resulting in less fatigue. [NP: PL, CL: AP]

6. **(a)** Cholesterol and triglyceride levels increase as a result of steroid therapy. [NP: EV, CL: KN]

SITUATION 42–2

1. **(c)** Peptic ulcer disease represents a condition in which steroids should be given cautiously, due to exacerbation of the disease and gastrointestinal bleeding. [NP: AS, CL: KN]

2. **(b)** Intravenous infusions of Solu-Medrol should be given over 10 to 20 minutes. [NP: IM, CL: KN]

3. **(d)** Glucocorticoids increase blood sugar levels, particularly in those patients with diabetes mellitus who are taking hypoglycemic agents. [NP: AN, CL: AP]

4. **(b)** Prior to long-term therapy with glucocorticoids, patients should be tested for the presence of active or arrested tuberculosis. If this condition exists, careful monitoring is indicated, as well as prophylactic INH therapy. [NP: PL, CL: KN]

5. **(b)** Although there are fewer side effects with a steroidal inhaler (local application) than with the systemic route, overuse or abuse can lead to hypotha-

lamic-pituitary-adrenal (HPA) suppression. [NP: EV, CL: CO]

6. **(a)** For patients on glucocorticoids for anti-inflammatory purposes, maintenance on the smallest dose possible for the shortest period of time reduces the potential for serious side effects. [NP: PL, CL: CO]

SITUATION 43–1

1. **(a)** Assessment of the patient in his late teens with hypogonadism will reveal excessive growth of long bones, absence of male pattern hair growth, and small external genitalia. [NP: AS, CL: CO]

2. **(c)** Testosterone cypionate is an androgen which is administered intramuscularly on a regular schedule until sexual characteristics have developed. Oral agents are less effective initially, due to high first-pass effect. [NP: PL, CL: KN]

4. **(a)** A side effect related to testosterone therapy is sleeplessness. Other nervous system effects are excitation and changes in libido. [NP: IM, CL: KN]

5. **(d)** Common side effects of oral testosterone therapy are nausea, vomiting, and diarrhea. Taking the drug with meals will reduce these effects. [NP: IM, CL: KN]

6. **(c)** Hepatic function can be altered by testosterone therapy. Liver function should be monitored at regular intervals. [NP: EV, CL: CO]

SITUATION 43–2

1. **(d)** Conjugated estrogen optimally should be administered in a cyclic fashion, three weeks on and one week off. [NP: PL, CL: KN]

2. **(d)** Estrogen therapy is contraindicated in patients with liver dysfunction. Estrogens are metabolized extensively by the liver. [NP: AS, CL: CO]

3. **(b)** Sodium and water retention have been associated with estrogen therapy. Patients should be taught to weigh regularly and to report sudden weight gain. [NP: IM, CP: CO]

4. **(d)** Patients taking estrogen should be encouraged to reduce or eliminate cigarette smoking, due to the link with increased risk of vascular disease. [NP: AS, CL: KN]

5. **(c)** The side effect of nausea and vomiting may be reduced to taking estrogen agents on a full stomach. [NP: IM, CL: AP]

6. **(c)** Postmenopausal women should increase their dietary intake of calcium in order to prevent osteoporosis. [NP: IM, CL: AP]

Key to [Codes]; NP = Nursing process phase; AS = Assessment; AN = Analysis; PL = Planning; IM = Implementation; EV = Evaluation; CL = Cognitive level; KN = Knowledge; CO = Comprehension; AP = Application; AN = Analysis

SITUATION 44–1

1. **(b)** The onset of action of regular insulin is 15 minutes to 1 hour. Regular Humulin Insulin has an even more rapid onset. [NP: PL, CL: CO]

2. **(d)** The most likely time for an insulin reaction to occur in a patient who takes an intermediate-acting insulin in the morning is prior to supper. [NP: AN, CL: AP]

3. **(a)** Sweating is an early sign of hypoglycemia and is related to the release of epinephrine as a compensatory response. [NP: IM, CL: AP]

4. **(c)** Regular insulin should be drawn up first if mixed with an intermediate-acting insulin such as NPH. If NPH is drawn up first, it may contaminate the vial of regular insulin. [NP: IM, CL: KN]

5. **(a)** Children with diabetes mellitus are at risk for Altered Growth and Development related to the effects of impaired glucose regulation. [NP: AN, CL: AN]

6. **(d)** Periods of increased exercise may require a reduced insulin dosage because exercise increases glucose utilization. [NP: EV, CL: AN]

SITUATION 44–2

1. **(c)** Chlorpropamide is a long-acting first generation agent which is not recommended for the diabetic with renal failure (as evidenced by elevated creatinine) because hypoglycemia may last for several days. [NP: AS, CL: AP]

2. **(c)** Cross sensitivity may occur in patients taking chlorpropamide (a sulfonyl-urea) who are allergic to sulfa medications. [NP: AS, CL: CO]

3. **(a)** Patients taking chlorpropamide are prone to inappropriate antidiuretic hormone secretion. Symptoms related to this condition correspond to hyponatremia. The patient should report headache, lethargy, and signs of swelling promptly. [NP: IM, CL: AP]

4. **(d)** Salicylates may displace sulfonyl-urease from protein binding sites, resulting in enhanced hypoglycemic activity. [NP: IM, CL: CO]

5. **(d)** Oral hypoglycemia agents may enhance the metabolism of digoxin by microsomal enzyme induction. [NP: EV, CL: CO]

6. **(b)** Chlorpropamide is a long-acting agent which begins activity one hour after administration and peaks 12 hours later. [NP: PL, CL: AP]

SITUATION 45–1

1. **(d)** Patients with hyperthyroidism may exhibit exophthalmos, which is an abnormal protrusion of the eyeball. [NP: AS, CL: KN]

2. **(b)** Propylthiouracil is effectively absorbed via the gastrointestinal tract and is not available in parenteral forms. [NP: PL, CL: KN]

3. **(d)** Thyroid crisis can be fatal because of excessive cardiac stimulation. As a beta-blocker, propranolol can protect the heart from life-threatening tachycardia, a manifestation of catecholamine release. [NP: AN, CL: AP]

4. **(a)** Side effects of sodium iodide include those related to iodism: increased salivation, burning sensations in the mouth and throat, and gingivial soreness. [NP: AS, CL: AP]

5. **(a)** Patients on antithyroid medications should be taught to limit iodine-rich foods such as seafood. [NP: IM, CL: AP]

6. **(a)** Bleeding related to thrombocytopenia may occur with antithyroid therapy; therefore, prothrombin times and cell counts should be evaluated on a routine basis. [NP: EV, CL: KN]

SITUATION 46–1

1. **(c)** Neurological side effects are common with INH therapy. These include muscle twitching, peripheral neuritis, and paresthesias. [NP: IM, CL: AP]

2. **(a)** INH interferes with the normal action of pyridoxine, Vitamin B_6, which is an essential component in nerve conduction. Supplementing pyridoxine can help to alleviate neurotoxicities. [NP: IM, CL: CO]

3. **(d)** Rifampin may produce a reddish-orange discoloration of urine, sweat, or tears. [NP: AS, CL: KN]

4. **(a)** Food may delay absorption of rifampin; therefore, it should be taken on an empty stomach. [NP: PL, CL: CO]

5. **(c)** Liver damage may occur due to concomitant use of INH and rifampin. Liver enzymes should be monitored on a routine basis. [NP: EV, CL: AP]

6. **(b)** Mental status changes may occur in patients taking INH. The family should be aware of this and report signs of psychosis promptly. [NP: EV, CL: AN]

SITUATION 46–2

1. **(b)** Patients on aminoglycoside therapy should be monitored for the development of nephrotoxicity, which is indicated by an elevation in serum creatinine levels. [NP: AS, CL: AP]

2. **(a)** Peak serum concentrations of gentamycin should range between 4 and 10 μg/ml. [NP: EV, CL: AP]

3. **(c)** Patients on antibiotic therapy should be monitored for elevated or depressed WBC levels. Elevated WBCs indicate continuing infection, while very low levels may indicate depressed bone marrow function as a result of antibiotic therapy. [NP: IM, CL: CO]

4. **(b)** Timentin may inhibit platelet aggregation, resulting in a prolonged bleeding time and potential for injury due to coagulation abnormalities. [NP: AN, CL: AN]

5. **(d)** Penicillins may induce hypokalemia due to enhanced renal distal tubular secretion of potassium. [NP: PL, CL: CO]

6. **(b)** A common side effect of aminoglycoside therapy is ototoxicity; therefore, patients should be monitored closely for evidence of hearing disturbances. [NP: AS, CL: AP]

SITUATION 47-1

1. **(d)** A common effect of ibuprofen use is gastric irritation. If this should occur, the drug should be taken with food, milk, or an antacid. [NP: IM, CL: AP]

2. **(b)** Nonsteroidal anti-inflammatory agents such as ibuprofen impair platelet aggregation and prolong bleeding time. Patients need to be evaluated on a routine basis for evidence of bleeding disorders. [NP: EV, CL: KN]

3. **(d)** Contraindications of gold sodium therapy include patients with congestive heart disease, since gold deposits can worsen the condition. [NP: AS, CL: CO]

4. **(a)** The bottle of gold sodium thiomalate should be agitated by rolling the vial between hands to warm the solution and ensure uniform suspension. [NP: PL, CL: KN]

5. **(c)** The most common adverse side effects occur as a result of gold deposits in the skin causing rashes, puritis, and pigment changes. [NP: IM, CL: CO]

6. **(c)** Gold sodium thiomalate is slow acting and 6 to 8 weeks may be required before benefits will be noticed. [NP: EV, CL: AN]

SITUATION 49-1

1. **(c)** Because of side effects of bone marrow depression, patients receiving fluorouracil should be assessed prior to treatment for a WBC of $<3,500/mm^3$ or platelets below $100,000/mm^3$. [NP: AS, CL: AP]

2. **(b)** Stomatitis is a frequent effect of fluorouracil therapy; therefore, frequent oral care limits the occurrence and severity of this side effect. [NP: PL, CL: CO]

3. **(b)** Side effects of fluorouracil include gastro-intestinal ulcers. Patients should be taught to be aware of and report evidence of GI bleeding, such as dark, tarry stools. [NP: IM, CL: CO]

4. **(d)** Bladder toxicity is related to Cytoxan therapy, especially on long-term oral use. Drinking plenty of fluids reduces the risk of developing related complications. [NP: IM, CL: AP]

5. **(a)** Liver dysfunction may be noted in patients taking Cytoxan. Liver enzymes should be monitored closely. [NP: EV, CL: AP]

6. **(c)** Red urine is an indication of severe hematuria and should be reported immediately. This is a sign of hemorrhagic cystitis and is related to Cytoxan therapy. Sudden weight gain may indicate retention of water resulting from syndrome of inappropriate antidiuretic hormone (SIADH), also related to Cytoxan therapy. [NP: EV, CL: AN]

SITUATION 49-2

1. **(a)** Cardiac toxicity has been related to Adriamycin use. The ECG should be monitored for changes on a routine basis. [NP: AS, CL: AP]

2. **(d)** If extravasation of Adriamycin is suspected, the specific antidote is 3–5 ml of 7–8.5% sodium bicarbonate injected subcutaneously at the site. Ice packs may also be used intermittently for 18 to 24 hours. [NP: IM, CL: AP]

3. **(c)** Nausea and vomiting are acute toxic effects of BCNU and occur approximately 6 hours after beginning the infusion. Antiemetics should be given along with the chemotherapy. [NP: PL, CL: CO]

4. **(b)** Bone marrow depression related to BCNU therapy occurs approximately 3–6 weeks after administration. [NP: EV, CL: KN]

5. **(a)** A unique toxic effect of mithramycin is a hemorrhagic syndrome causing facial flushing, epistaxis, and/or hematemesis. [NP: IM, CL: AP]

6. **(b)** Mithramycin causes bone marrow depression (especially thrombocytopenia), and patients are at risk for bleeding. [NP: AN, CL: AN]

SITUATION 50-1

1. **(c)** Because of the short half-life of AZT, the drug must be taken every 4 hours around the clock in order to achieve therapeutic drug levels. [NP: PL, CL: KN]

2. **(d)** Common side effects of AZT therapy include nausea, anorexia, and severe headaches. [NP: IM, CL: CO]

3. **(a)** Severe bone marrow depression is an acute toxic effect of AZT therapy. The CBC should be evaluated

routinely and, if patient becomes severely anemic, therapy may need to be altered. [NP: EV, CL: CO]

4. **(b)** Drugs such as indomethacin and acetaminophen may increase toxic effects of AZT. Patients should be taught to contact the physician before using any medications. [NP: IM, CL: AP]

5. **(b)** AIDS patients on AZT are still able to transmit the virus to others; therefore, appropriate precautions need to be observed. [NP: PL, CL: AP]

6. **(c)** An intact integument is the best first line of defense against invading organisms, particularly in patients susceptible to infection. [NP: AS, CL: AP]

SITUATION 52–1

1. **(c)** During rapid intravenous infusion of cimetidine, patients may develop bradycardia and cardiac arrest. [NP: PL, CL: AP]

2. **(b)** Patients on cimetidine therapy may experience gastrointestinal side effects such as nausea, diarrhea, and/or abdominal pain. [NP: IM, CL: AP]

3. **(d)** Patients taking aluminum products commonly experience constipation due to the combination of aluminum and bile salts. [NP: PL, CL: CO]

4. **(a)** The stimulation of bowel mobility may be dangerous in the case of bowel obstruction, perforation, or hemorrhage. [NP: AN, CL: CO]

5. **(c)** There is a high incidence of central nervous system effects related to metoclopramide therapy. These include restlessness, drowsiness, and extrapyramidal and parkinsonism-like reactions. [NP: IM, CL: AP]

6. **(b)** Patients on drugs to prevent hyperacidity will be evaluated in terms of evidence of gastric bleeding or irritation. An outcome of successful treatment would be stool specimens negative for occult blood. [NP: EV, CL: AP]

SITUATION 53–1

1. **(b)** Due to potential for hypotension and orthostatic hypotension, the patient's blood pressure should be assessed prior to administration of phenothiazines. [NP: AS, CL: AP]

2. **(c)** An adverse side effect related to therapy with phenothiazines, such as prochlorperazine, is dry mouth. The nurse should provide frequent oral care to increase comfort. [NP: IM, CL: AP]

3. **(c)** Many of the side effects related to prochlorperazine therapy involve neurological effects such as blurred vision and sedation. [NP: IM, CL: CO]

4. **(a)** Auditory and visual hallucinations have been reported with the use of diphenidol. The patient should report these side effects to the physician. [NP: IM, CL: AP]

5. **(b)** Antiemetics may have an additive effect when taken with alcohol. Patients should be taught to avoid drinking alcohol when taking this medication. [NP: EV, CL: AN]

6. **(d)** Optimally patients on antiemetic therapy will not experience nausea or vomiting and will not demonstrate evidence of dehydration or acid-base imbalance. [NP: EV, CL: CO]

SITUATION 54–1

1. **(b)** Laxatives are contraindicated if there is evidence of abdominal obstruction or if the patient has a fecal impaction. [NP: AS, CL: AP]

2. **(a)** Bisacodyl is best taken with water. It should not be taken with an alkaline solution such as milk or an antacid because the enteric coating dissolves in the stomach, where the medications can cause severe cramping. [NP: IM, CL: KN]

3. **(a)** Metamucil should be administered in juice or fluid and followed with at least 8 ounces of fluid to prevent intestinal impaction or obstruction. [NP: IM, CL: AP]

4. **(d)** Metamucil contains sugar, which can affect the blood glucose level in patients with diabetes mellitus. [NP: IM, CL: AP]

5. **(b)** Bulk-producing agents may take from 1 to 3 days to be effective. [NP: PL, CL: KN]

6. **(d)** Because of a high concentration of sodium, magnesium hydroxide should be given cautiously to patients with renal disease. [NP: AS, CL: AP]

SITUATION 55–1

1. **(b)** Lactulose is a synthetic derivative of the sugar lactose and is a nonosmotic cathartic which induces evacuation of the bowel. [NP: PL, CL: CO]

2. **(c)** The action of lactulose in the bowel is the conversion of ammonia to ammonium for evacuation in the stool. The reduction in the ammonia level alleviates some of the symptoms associated with hepatic failure. [NP: EV, CL: AP]

3. **(d)** When treating hepatic encephalopathy, neomycin is given only orally or via the nasogastric tube. The agent acts directly in the colon to reduce the breakdown products of urea and protein. Only a small percentage of neomycin is absorbed systemically. [NP: PL, CL: CO]

4. **(b)** Patients with normal renal function excrete the small amount of neomycin which is absorbed systemically. If renal impairment is present, the drug may accumulate and cause further renal damage. [NP: AS, CL: AP]

5. **(a)** The therapeutic effect of cholestyramine is not usually noted until 1 to 3 weeks after initiation of therapy. [NP: PL, CL: KN]

6. **(a)** The breakdown of protein further increases the buildup of urea and ammonia during the acute stage of encephalopathy. Protein is slowly added to the diet as the patient recovers. [NP: PL, CL: CO]

SITUATION 60-1

1. **(d)** Adverse ophthalmic effects of pilocarpine which are most commonly reported are burning and itching. [NP: IM, CL: KN]

2. **(c)** Pilocarpine is a direct-acting cholinergic which will cause pupil constriction. [NP: AS, CL: CO]

3. **(b)** Patients using pilocarpine will experience reduced visual acuity in dim light as a result of the miotic action on pupils and cilliary muscles. [NP: IM, CL: KN]

4. **(c)** Timolol is a non-cardioselective beta 1 and beta 2 blocker. Therefore, patients with bronchial asthma or COPD should not receive this agent. [NP: AS, CL: AP]

5. **(d)** When necessary to switch from one antiglaucoma agent to timolol, discontinue the first agent (pilocarpine) on the second day of timolol therapy. [NP: PL, CL: CO]

6. **(a)** A side effect of timolol therapy is hypotension; therefore, the blood pressure should be monitored during initial therapy. [NP: IM, CL: CO]

SITUATION 62-1

1. **(b)** During the first 24 hours of collagenase treatment, a fever may occur due to the accumulation of leucocytes at the wound site. This can be reduced by frequent aspiration of wound exudate. [NP: AS, CL: CO]

2. **(d)** Itching and stinging often occur with initial therapy with topically administered enzymes. These symptoms should subside. If itching and stinging continue, the physician should be notified. [NP: EV, CL: KN]

3. **(b)** Hydrogen peroxide is compatible with collagenase and can be used to prepare and clean the wound prior to application. The hydrogen peroxide should be folowed by sterile normal saline. [NP: IM, CL: AP]

4. **(a)** The purpose of collagenase is to debride wounds for promotion of healing. Collagenase has no antibacterial properties. [NP: PL, CL: CO]

5. **(d)** Collagenase should be applied to injured tissue only, because it can cause erythema of healthy tissue. The surrounding tissue can be protected by an agent such as zinc oxide ointment. [NP: IM, CL: KN]

6. **(d)** Collagenase can induce bleeding and hemorrhage and should be used cautiously if evidence of hemorrhage exists. [NP: AN, CL: AP]

SITUATION 63-1

1. **(d)** Benzoyl peroxide is applied to the skin and left on for 15 minutes on the first evening. The length of time which benzoyl peroxide is left on the skin increases gradually until it can be left on overnight. [NP: IM, CL: KN]

2. **(b)** Side effects of acne products, such as extreme dryness of skin, are increased with overuse of these products. [NP: IM, CL: AP]

3. **(c)** After applying tretinoin to affected skin areas once a day, the hands should be washed thoroughly. Irritation will result if the agent is in contact with delicate mucous membranes. [NP: IM, CL: KN]

4. **(d)** Within 48 hours, the skin generally becomes red and begins to peel. Pigment changes may occur, but these are temporary. [NP: EV, CL: AP]

5. **(b)** Alcohol intake should be eliminated during therapy with isotretinoin because of potentiation of adverse effects. [NP: IM, CL: KN]

6. **(a)** Approximately one-fourth of patients on isotretinoin demonstrate elevated triglyceride levels with potential for increased cholesterol. [NP: EV, CL: CO]

SITUATION 64-1

1. **(a)** The Rho(D) Immune Globulin (RhoGAM) is used to suppress the immune response in nonsensitized Rh negative women who receive Rh positive blood, as in the case of delivery of an Rh positive baby. [NP: AN, CL: CO]

2. **(b)** Administration of RhoGAM should be within 72 hours of delivery. [NP: PL, CL: KN]

3. **(d)** The recommended schedule for childhood immunizations should begin at 2 months of age. [NP: IM, CL: KN]

4. **(c)** Evidence of an active infection, such as a high fever, is a contraindication to immunization. [NP: AS, CL: AP]

5. **(c)** Common adverse effects related to DPT vaccine include anorexia and fretfulness, in addition to redness and pain at the site of injection. [NP: IM, CL: AP]

6. **(c)** It is recommended that children at age 15 months receive DPT, poliovirus, and measles, mumps, and rubella (MMR) vaccines. [NP: PL, CL: KN]

Key to [Codes]; NP = Nursing process phase; AS = Assessment; AN = Analysis; PL = Planning; IM = Implementation;
EV = Evaluation; CL = Cognitive level; KN = Knowledge; CO = Comprehension; AP = Application; AN = Analysis

APPENDIX D DILUTION AND STORAGE TIME OF IV DRUGS

Drug	Type and Amount of Diluent to Use	Storage Time	
		Frozen or Refrigerated After Initial Reconstitution in Manufacturer's Vial	**Refrigerated After Dilution for IV Administration**
ACTH (corticotropin for injection) (Acthar)	D$_5$W or NSS At least 250 ml for whatever diagnostic dose doctor orders; dilution is often 500 ml (don't mix in Soluset)	Information not available	24 hours
Alteplase, recombinant (Activase)	Sterile water only 50 mg in 50 ml 100 mg dose; 60 mg in 1 hour, 20 mg in 2 hours, 20 mg in 30 hours	Use immediately	Use immediately
Amikacin sulfate (Amikin)	D$_5$W 5 mg/ml (500 mg in 200 ml of diluent)	Not applicable (packaged in liquid form)	72 hours
Aminocaproic acid (Amicar)	D$_5$W or NSS 1 g in 50 ml of diluent	Refrigerated: 24 hours	24 hours
Aminophylline (multi-source)	D$_5$W or NSS 250 ml or more (don't mix in a Soluset)	Not applicable (packaged in liquid form)	24 hours
Amphotericin B (Fungizone)	Reconstitute as follows: 1. With sterile needle and syringe, rapidly inject 10 ml sterile water for injection (without additives). 2. Shake vial well until clear. 3. Dilute with D$_5$W (with pH of above 4.2) 1 mg/10 ml. Don't use NSS (suspension will precipitate). Don't filter (filter may block passage of antibiotic dispersion). Wrap bottle in foil to protect from exposure to light.	Refrigerated: 7 days. Frozen: 30 days.	7 days
Ampicillin (Omnipen, Polycillin, others)	Sterile water or NSS 2–30 mg/ml over 10–15 minutes	Use immediately	Use immediately
Anistreplase (APSAC, Eminase)	Sterile water 5 ml to 30 U over 2–5 minutes Do not shake.	—	30 minutes
Aztreonam (Azactam)	Most solutions 1 g in 100 ml over 20–60 minutes 1 g in 6–10 ml bolus over 3–5 minutes	Refrigerated: 7 days Frozen: 3 months	24–72 hours
Calcium disodium versenate (Calcium disodium edetate)	D$_5$W or NSS 1 g in 250–500 ml	Not applicable (packaged in liquid form)	24 hours
Carbenicillin disodium (Geopen, Pyopen)	Most solutions 1 g in 10–20 ml	Refrigerated: 3–14 days depending on solution	3–14 days
Cefamandole naftate (Mandol)	D$_5$W or NSS 1 g in 10 ml (IV push) 1 or 2 g in 50 ml (infusion)	Refrigerated: 96 hours Frozen: 6 months	96 hours

CONTINUED ON THE FOLLOWING PAGE

APPENDIX D DILUTION AND STORAGE TIME OF IV DRUGS–*CONTINUED*

Drug	Type and Amount of Diluent to Use	Storage Time	
		Frozen or Refrigerated After Initial Reconstitution in Manufacturer's Vial	**Refrigerated After Dilution for IV Administration**
Cefotetan disodium (Cefotan)	D$_5$W or NSS 1–2 g in 10–20 ml over 3–5 minutes	Refrigerated: 96 hours Frozen: 1 week	24 hours
Cefoxitin sodium (Mefoxin)	D$_5$W, NSS, sterile water for injection, lactated Ringer's solution 1 to 2 g in 50 ml	Refrigerated: 48 hours Frozen: 26 weeks	48 hours
Ceftizoxime sodium (Cefizox)	D$_5$, D$_{10}$W, D/NS, invert sugar, or lactated Ringer's solution 1 g in 50–100 ml bolus over 2–3 minutes	Refrigerated: 96 hours	96 hours
Cephapirin sodium (Cefadyl)	D$_5$W or NSS 1 g in 50 ml; 2 g in 100 ml	Refrigerated: 10 days Frozen: 60 days	10 days
Cimetidine HCl (Tagamet)	D$_5$W 300 mg in 100 ml	Information not available	48 hours
Cortisol sodium succinate (Solu-Cortef, A-hydroCort)	D$_5$W or NSS At least 1 cc of diluent per mg	Refrigerated: 72 hours	48 hours
Dexamethasone phosphate (Decadron, Hexadrol)	D$_5$W, NSS, D$_5$NSS, or lactated Ringer's solution 1 mg–40 mg in 500 ml	Not applicable (packaged in liquid form)	48 hours
Erythromycin gluceptate (Ilotycin)	D$_5$W or 0.9% sodium chloride injection less than 500 mg in 100 ml 500 mg in 250 ml 1 g in 1000 ml (Reconstitute with sterile water—no preservatives. Add 2.5 ml sodium bicarbonate to 100 ml of IV solution and 5 ml sodium bicarbonate to 250 ml. Without sodium bicarbonate, solution remains stable for only 4 hours and is extremely irritating to the vein wall. Solution MUST run over 1 hour.)	Refrigerated: 7 days Freezing not recommended	24 hours (in buffered diluents)
Famotidine (Pepcid)	0.9% NSS, D$_5$W, or lactated Ringer's solution 2 ml in 100 ml infused over 15–30 minutes	Refrigerated: 30 days	48 hours
Heparin sodium (multisource)	Usually D$_5$W or NSS At least 250 ml and usually 500 ml or 1000 ml depending on physician's order. Heparin is given by IV push bolus or slow IV infusion. Don't mix in Soluset.	Not applicable (packaged in liquid form)	24 hours
Imipenem-cilastatin (Primaxin)	Most solutions 250 mg in 100 ml over 20–30 minutes 1 g over 40–60 minutes	Do not freeze.	24 hours

APPENDIX D DILUTION AND STORAGE TIME OF IV DRUGS–*CONTINUED*

Drug	Type and Amount of Diluent to Use	Storage Time Frozen or Refrigerated After Initial Reconstitution in Manufacturer's Vial	Refrigerated After Dilution for IV Administration
Iron dextran injection (Imferon, Chromagen D, Dextraron-50)	Administer undiluted (drug comes already reconstituted with NSS) by slow IV push bolus (1 minute per ml). Drug is sometimes mixed with at least 250 ml NSS and given by slow IV infusion (over 1–3 hours)—but this is not a manufacturer's recommendation. Physician should give initial test dose to check for adverse reactions.	Not applicable	Not approved for dilution
Methicillin sodium (Staphcillin, Celbenin)	D_5W, NSS, or sterile water for injection: 1 g in 50 ml 2 g in 100 ml	Refrigerated: 96 hours Frozen: 30 days	7 days (Celbenin: 14 days in concentrations of 10–60 mg/ml)
Methyldopate hydrochloride (Aldomet Ester)	D_5W 100 ml Usual dosage is 250–500 mg, but up to 1 g can be given in 100 ml. Solution usually runs over 30–60 minutes.	Information not available	24 hours
Methylprednisolone sodium succinate (Solu-Medrol, A-Methapred)	D_5W or NSS Less than 1 g in 50 ml 1 g or more in 100 ml For initial reconstitution of drug in manufactuer's vial, use *only* the diluent provided by the manufactuer.	Refrigerated: 48 hours	48 hours
Metronidazole hydrochloride (Flagyl IV)	D_5W, NSS, or lactated Ringer's solution 1. Reconstitute with 4.4 ml of diluent 2. Add to IV solution in concentration not to exceed 8 mg/ml 3. Neutralize with 5 mEq sodium bicarbonate for each 500 mg of metronidazole	96 hours at room temperature. DO NOT REFRIGERATE OR FREEZE	24 hours at room temperature. DO NOT REFRIGERATE
Mezlocillin sodium (Mezlin)	0.9% NSS 10–100 mg/ml Lactated Ringer's solution 10–100 mg/ml 0.9% NSS 250 mg/ml	Refrigerated: 7 days Frozen: 28 days Refrigerated: 7 days —	48 hours 72 hours 24 hours
Nafcillin sodium (Nafcil, Unipen, Nallpen)	Sterile water, NSS, Ringer's injection, D_5W 1 g in 15–30 ml bolus over 10–15 minutes	Refrigerated: 24 hours Frozen: 96 hours	— —
Oxacillin sodium (Prostaphlin)	NSS or sterile water 1 g in 10–20 ml bolus over 10 minutes	Refrigerated: 24 hours	6 hours
Oxytocin (Pitocin, Syntocinon)	D_5W or NSS 10 to 40 units in 1000 ml	Not applicable (packaged in liquid form)	7 days

CONTINUED ON THE FOLLOWING PAGE

APPENDIX D DILUTION AND STORAGE TIME OF IV DRUGS–*CONTINUED*

Drug	Type and Amount of Diluent to Use	Storage Time Frozen or Refrigerated After Initial Reconstitution in Manufacturer's Vial	Refrigerated After Dilution for IV Administration
Penicillin G sodium	D₅W or NSS 3 million units or less in 50 ml More than 3 million units in 100 ml	Refrigerated: 7 days	7 days
Piperacillin sodium (Pipracil)	Sterile water, NSS, D₅W 1 g in 50–100 ml over 30 minutes or as bolus over 3–5 minutes	Refrigerated: 1 week Frozen: 1 month	48 hours
Potassium chloride (multisource)	Any standard diluent (D5W, NSS, Ringer's lactate, etc.) as ordered by physician. Don't mix in Soluset (too great a concentration can cause cardiac irritability and phlebitis). Common concentrations are: 40 mEq in 500 ml; 80 mEq in 1000 ml	Not applicable (packaged in liquid form)	96 hours
Potassium phosphate (multisource)	Any standard diluent as ordered by physician. At least 500 cc. Use vials once only; don't store used vial (solution does not contain a bacteriostatic agent.) Don't mix in Soluset.	Not applicable (packaged in liquid form)	96 hours
Ranitidine (Zantac)	0.9% NSS, D₅W, D₁₀W, lactated Ringer's solution 50 mg in 20 ml injected over 5 minutes	Refrigerated: 10 days Frozen: 30 days	24 hours
Streptokinase (Streptase)	NSS, D₅W 5 ml to vial. Do not shake. Withdraw and dilute with additional 45 ml. 15 ml/hour over 30 minutes; 3 ml/hour maintenance dose.	Use immediately	Use immediately
Ticarcillin disodium (Ticar)	D₅W, NSS, or sterile water for injection 1.0 g to 5.0 g in 100 ml	Refrigerated: 14 days Frozen: 30 days	14 days
Tobramycin sulfate (Nebcin)	D₅W or NSS 40 mg or less in 50 ml; 41–100 mg in 100 ml; more than 100 mg: 1 mg/ml	Freezing and refrigeration not recommended	96 hours
Vancomycin HCl (Vancocin)	D₅W or NSS less than 500 mg in 100 ml 500 mg in 200 ml	Refrigerated: 96 hours	96 hours
Vitamins: (Folvite—5 mg; Betalin-5—100 mg; Berocca C—1 amp; Hexabetalin)	All common diluents in amounts ordered by physican Added to 500 ml or more of solution, usually a liter	Not applicable (packaged in liquid form only)	72 hours

Adapted and updated (1990) from Hickman, R: *When you have to reconstitute meds.* RN 41(5):40–43, 1981, with permission.

INDEX

See also the Drug and Agent Index, which follows this index, on pp. DA1 through DA25. An "f" following a page number indicates a figure. A "t" indicates a table.

DRUG AND AGENT INDEX

See also the general index, which precedes this index, on pp I1 through I23.
An ''f'' following a page number indicates a figure. A ''t'' indicates a table.

NURSING PROCESS TABLES ─────────────────

Nursing Process for the Patient With . . .